From the most trusted source:

the only CPT® codebook with official coding rules and guidelines!

D0580473

Your trusted source

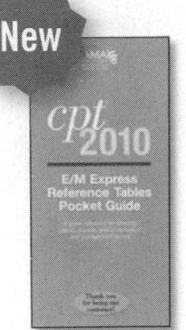

Loaded with new features to increase coding accuracy, the *CPT® 2010 Professional Edition* includes section specific table of contents for easier navigation and quicker code look-ups in a given section, relevant anatomical and procedural illustrations now incorporated within the code sections, and more!

New

Purchase direct from the AMA and receive a FREE E/M Express Reference Tables Pocket Guide*!

A quick reference guide that provides a side-by-side comparison of E/M codes in a CPT section. Easy to use, each table summarizes the requirements for reporting E/M services and helps the user select and validate proper E/M coding.

AMA
AMERICAN
MEDICAL
ASSOCIATION

Available October 2009, spiralbound, 8½" x 11", 700 pages

Order #: EP888810
Price: $107.95

ISBN: 978-1-60359-119-5
AMA member price: $75.95

Phone: (800) 621-8335   Order online: www.amabookstore.com

*Not available for wholesalers/resellers. Supplies are limited. The AMA reserves the right to determine order eligibility.

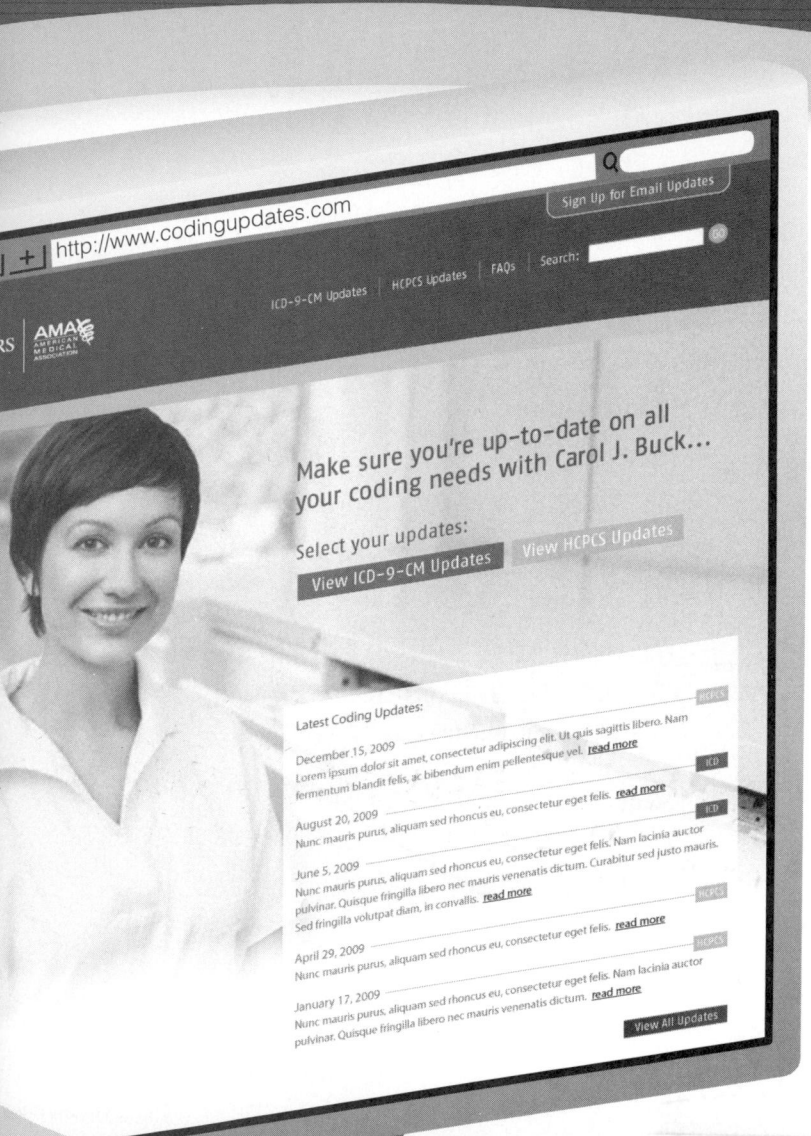

Stay up to Date!
Access the Latest ICD-9-CM and HCPCS Code Updates Throughout the Year

FREE! Access is included with your ICD-9-CM or HCPCS Manual from the AMA and Elsevier!

Trust *Carol J. Buck,* the *AMA* and *Elsevier* to give you quick access to the most up-to-date codes!

Access the mid-year code updates as soon as they are published by the government

Sign up now for email alerts that let you know when new codes are posted

SAUNDERS ELSEVIER

AMERICAN MEDICAL ASSOCIATION

http://codingupdates.com
gives you access to the latest mid-year code updates for ICD-9-CM and HCPCS!

GW10-02

STANDARD EDITION

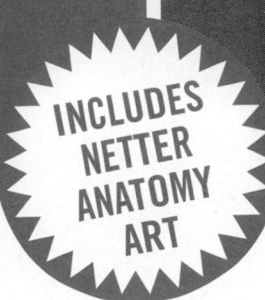

INCLUDES NETTER ANATOMY ART

2010
ICD-9-CM

VOLUMES 1, 2, & 3

FOR HOSPITALS

STANDARD EDITION

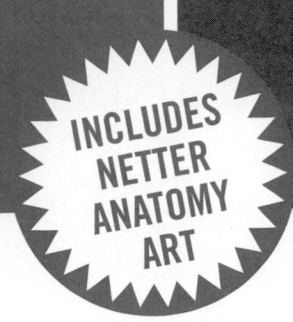

INCLUDES
NETTER
ANATOMY
ART

2010
ICD-9-CM

VOLUMES 1, 2, & 3

FOR HOSPITALS

Carol J. Buck

MS, CPC-I, CPC, CPC-H, CCS-P

Program Director, Retired
Medical Secretary Programs
Northwest Technical College
East Grand Forks, Minnesota

SAUNDERS
ELSEVIER

AMA
AMERICAN
MEDICAL
ASSOCIATION

SAUNDERS

ELSEVIER

3251 Riverport Lane
Maryland Heights, Missouri 63043

2010 ICD-9-CM FOR HOSPITALS, VOLUMES 1, 2, & 3, STANDARD EDITION   ISBN: 978-1-4377-0747-2

Copyright © 2010, 2009, 2008, 2007, 2006, 2005, 2004, 2003, 2002, 2001, 2000 by Saunders, an imprint of Elsevier Inc.

All rights reserved. No part of this publication may be reproduced or transmitted in any form or by any means, electronic or mechanical, including photocopying, recording, or any information storage and retrieval system, without permission in writing from the publisher. Permissions may be sought directly from Elsevier's Rights Department: phone: (+1) 215 239 3804 (US) or (+44) 1865 843830 (UK); fax: (+44) 1865 853333; e-mail: healthpermissions@elsevier.com. You may also complete your request on-line via the Elsevier website at http://www.elsevier.com/permissions.

Notice

Knowledge and best practice in this field are constantly changing. As new research and experience broaden our knowledge, changes in practice, treatment, and drug therapy may become necessary or appropriate. Readers are advised to check the most current information provided (i) on procedures featured or (ii) by the manufacturer of each product to be administered, to verify the recommended dose or formula, the method and duration of administration, and contraindications. It is the responsibility of the practitioner, relying on his or her own experience and knowledge of the patient, to make diagnoses, to determine dosages and the best treatment for each individual patient, and to take all appropriate safety precautions. To the fullest extent of the law, neither the Publisher nor the Author assumes any liability for any injury and/or damage to persons or property arising out of or related to any use of the material contained in this book.

The Publisher

Current Procedural Terminology (CPT) is copyright 2009 American Medical Association. All Rights Reserved. No fee schedules, basic units, relative values, or related listings are included in CPT. The AMA assumes no liability for the data contained herein. Applicable FARS/DFARS restrictions apply to government use.

ISBN: 978-1-4377-0747-2

Publisher: Michael S. Ledbetter
Developmental Editor: Jenna Johnson
Publishing Services Manager: Pat Joiner-Myers

Working together to grow
libraries in developing countries

www.elsevier.com | www.bookaid.org | www.sabre.org

ELSEVIER   BOOK AID International   Sabre Foundation

Printed in the United States of America

Last digit is the print number: 9 8 7 6 5 4 3 2 1

COLLABORATORS

Technical Collaborators:

Jacqueline Klitz Grass, MA, CPC
Coding Specialist
Grand Forks, North Dakota

Nancy Maguire, ACS, CRT, PCS, FCS, CPC, CPC-H, HCS-D, APC, AFC
Physician Consultant for Auditing and Education
Universal City, Texas

Technical Assistant:

Judith Neppel, RN, MS
Executive Director
Minnesota Rural Health Association
University of Minnesota, Crookston
Crookston, Minnesota

Hospital Reimbursement Specialist:

Lynn-Marie D. Wozniak, MS, RHIT
Product Manager
New York

Elsevier/MC Strategies Revenue Cycle, Coding and Compliance Staff

"Experts in providing e-learning on revenue cycle, coding and compliance."

Deborah Neville, RHIA, CCS-P
Director
Minnesota

Elizabeth Wheeler, RHIA, CCS-P
Product Manager
New York

Lynn-Marie D. Wozniak, MS, RHIT
Product Manager
New York

Therese M. Jorwic, MPH, RHIA, CCS, CCS-P, FAHIMA
Product Specialist
Illinois

Sandra L. Macica, MS, RHIA, CCS, ROCC
Product Specialist
New York

CONTENTS

Part IV   Procedures Volume 3   1231

Part V   2009 Inpatient Procedures   1475

Part VI   2010 MS-DRG, Version 27 (Proposed)   1481

GUIDE TO USING THE 2010 ICD-9-CM FOR HOSPITALS, VOLUMES 1, 2, & 3, STANDARD EDITION

Medical coding has long been a part of the health care profession. Through the years medical coding systems have become more complex and extensive. Today, medical coding is an intricate and immense process that is present in every health care setting. The increased use of electronic submissions for health care services only increases the need for coders who understand the coding process.

2010 ICD-9-CM for Hospitals, Volumes 1, 2, & 3, Standard Edition was developed to help meet the needs of students preparing for a career in medical coding by offering a comprehensive coding text at a reasonable price. This text combines the official coding guidelines and all three volumes of the ICD-9-CM in one book.

All material strictly adheres to the latest government versions available at the time of printing.

ILLUSTRATIONS AND ITEMS

The ICD-9-CM, Volume 1, Tabular List contains illustrations, pictures, and items to assist you in understanding difficult terminology, diseases/ conditions, or coding in a specific category. Items are always printed in ▆▆▆▆ ink so the added material is not mistaken for official notations or instructions. ▆▆▆▆ ink is also used for other annotations in the text. Your ideas on what other descriptions or illustrations should be in future editions of this text are always appreciated.

Annotated

Throughout the volumes, revisions, additions, and deleted codes or words are indicated by the following symbols:

◀▦ **Revised:** Revisions within the line or code from the previous edition are indicated by the arrow.

◀ **New:** Additions to the previous edition are indicated by the triangle.

~~deleted~~ **Deleted:** Deletions from previous edition are struck through.

ICD-9-CM, Volume 2, Index to Diseases Symbol

▆▆ **Omit code:** Identifies a term that is not reported. The words *omit code* are highlighted in ▆▆ for easier reference in Volume 1.

ICD-9-CM, Volume 1, Tabular List Symbols

● **Unacceptable Principal Diagnosis:** These codes have a black dot before them and give additional information or describe the circumstances affecting the health care encounter but are unacceptable as principal diagnosis in the Medicare code edits for inpatient admission.

❶ **First Listed:** The number 1 inside a circle appears before V codes that may be listed as the first code according to the V Code Table in the *ICD-9-CM Official Guidelines for Coding and Reporting*.

❶⁄₂ **First Listed or Additional:** The 1/2 inside a circle appears before V codes that may be listed as the first code and may also be listed as an additional V code according to the V Code Table in the *ICD-9-CM Official Guidelines for Coding and Reporting*.

❷ **Additional Only:** The number 2 inside a circle appears before V codes that may only be listed as an additional code. These codes may not be listed as a first code according to the V Code Table in the *ICD-9-CM Official Guidelines for Coding and Reporting*.

- **Use Additional Digit(s):** The colored dot cautions that the code requires additional digit(s) to ensure the greatest specificity.

OGCR **OGCR:** The Official Guidelines for Coding and Reporting symbol indicates the placement of a portion of a guideline as that guideline pertains to the code by which it is located. The complete OGCR are located in Part I.

Coding Clinic identifies the year, quarter, and page number that presents information about an ICD-9-CM code in the American Hospital Association's **Coding Clinic.**

Excludes: Terms following the word "Excludes" are to be coded elsewhere and are highlighted in ⬜ for easier reference.

Includes: This note appears immediately to further define or give examples of the content of codes and is highlighted in ▬ for easier reference.

Use additional: The words indicate an instructional note that another code may be needed, and are highlighted in ▬ for easier reference.

Code first: The words indicate an instructional note that directs the coder to sequence the underlying condition before the manifestation. "Code first" is highlighted in ▬ for easier reference.

Omit code: Identifies a term that is not reported. The words "omit code" are highlighted in ▬ for easier reference.

🅒🅒 Indicates 2009 complications and comorbidities and major complications and comorbidities according to the Inpatient Prospective Payment System (IPPS) rule published in the *Federal Register*. For the latest updates, reference http://www.cms.hhs.gov/AcuteInpatientPPS/FFD/list.asp#TopOfPage.

🅟 **Present on Admission:** These code categories represent circumstances regarding the health care encounter or factors influencing health status that do not represent a current disease or injury or are always present on admission according to Appendix I, Present on Admission Reporting Guidelines in the *ICD-9-CM Official Guidelines for Coding and Reporting*.

🅗 HAC is a Hospital-Acquired Condition that, when present as a secondary diagnosis in an inpatient setting, is a higher cost, higher volume, or both and results in a higher MS-DRG assignment according to the Inpatient Prospective Payment System (IPPS) rule published in the *Federal Register*.

At the time of publication, the final list of HAC codes for 2010 had not been released. Please check our website at http://codingupdates.com for updates or http://www.cms.hhs.gov/HospitalAcqCond/06 Hospital-Acquired Conditions.asp#T on the CMS website.

Age conflict: The Medicare Code Editor detects inconsistencies between a patient's age and diagnosis. For example, a 5-year-old patient with benign prostatic hypertrophy or a 78-year-old pregnant female.

The diagnosis is clinically and virtually impossible in a patient of the stated age. Therefore, either the diagnosis or the age is presumed to be incorrect. There are four age categories for diagnoses in the Medicare Code Editor:

N • **Newborn.** Age of 0 years; a subset of diagnoses intended only for newborns and neonates (e.g., fetal distress, perinatal jaundice).

P • **Pediatric.** Age range is 0–17 years (e.g., Reye's syndrome, routine child health exam).

M • **Maternity.** Age range is 12–55 years (e.g., diabetes in pregnancy, antepartum pulmonary complication).

A • **Adult.** Age range is 15–124 years (e.g., senile delirium, mature cataract).

♀ ♂ **Sex conflict:** Medicare Code Editor detects inconsistencies between a patient's sex and diagnosis. For example, a male patient with cervical cancer (diagnosis) or a female patient with a prostatectomy (procedure). In both instances, the indicated diagnosis or the procedure conflicts with the stated sex of the patient. Therefore, either the patient's diagnosis, procedure, or sex is presumed to be incorrect.

▶ **Manifestation Code:** The symbol indicates codes that report manifestations (symptoms) and should not be assigned as a principal (first-listed) diagnosis.

ICD-9-CM, Volume 3, Tabular List Symbols

● **Use Additional Digit(s):** The colored dot cautions that the code requires additional digit(s) to ensure the greatest specificity.

✱ **Valid O.R. Procedure:** The colored "x" is placed before a code that is a valid operating room (O.R.) procedure according to the MS-DRG grouper.

◆ **Non-O.R. Procedure:** Indicates updates based on the Medicare Code Edits (MCE) to those procedures that Medicare would not normally reimburse.

♀ ♂ **Sex conflict:** Medicare Code Editor detects inconsistencies between a patient's sex and procedure. For example, a male patient with cervical cancer (diagnosis) or a female patient with a prostatectomy (procedure). In both instances, the indicated diagnosis or the procedure conflicts with the stated sex of the patient. Therefore, the patient's diagnosis, procedure, or sex is presumed to be incorrect.

▭ **Excludes:** Terms following the word "Excludes" are to be coded elsewhere and are highlighted in ▭ for easier reference.

▬ **Includes:** This note appears immediately under a code to further define or give examples of the content of codes and is highlighted in ▬ for easier reference.

▬ **Use additional:** The words indicate an instructional note that another code may be needed, and they are highlighted in ▬ for easier reference.

▬ **Code also:** This identifies synchronous procedures, which require reporting of individual components of a procedure.

▬ **Omit code:** Identifies procedures that are included in another larger procedure. The words are highlighted in ▬ for easier reference.

Part VI 2010 MS-DRG, Version 27 (Proposed)

Included in Part VI are the MS-DRG Definitions Manual Appendixes A, B, C, D, and the Procedure Code Tables from Appendix E.

MS-DRG, Appendix A List of Medicare Severity Diagnosis Related Groups, Version 27 (Proposed) contains a list of each MS-DRG with a specification of the MDC and whether the MS-DRG is medical or surgical.

MS-DRG, Appendix B Diagnosis Code/MDC/MS-DRG Index lists each diagnosis code, as well as the MDC, and the MS-DRGs to which the diagnosis is assigned when used as the principal diagnosis.

MS-DRG, Appendix D MS-DRG Surgical Hierarchy by MDC and MS-DRG presents the surgical hierarchy for each MDC.

MS-DRG, Appendix E MS-DRG, Procedure Code/MS-DRG Tables contain the following reference tables:

Table 1 Pacemaker Lead/Device Reference Table

Table 2 Abdominal Aorta/Thoracic Vessel Resection Reference Table

Table 3 Cardioverter-Defibrillator Lead/Generator Reference Table

Table 4 Spinal Fusion Reference Table

Table 5 Kidney/Pancreas Transplant Reference Table

Table 6 Lead/Device Reference Table

SYMBOLS AND CONVENTIONS

ICD-9-CM, Volumes 1, 2, & 3
Symbols Used to Identify New, Revised, or Deleted Material

Volume 1, Tabular List

237.70   Neurofibromatosis, unspecified ◄

Indicates **new** information or a new code.

V01.1   Cholera ◄

Indicates a **revision** within the line or code.

~~244.3   Other iatrogenic hypothyroidism~~
~~Hypothyroidism resulting from:~~
~~P-aminosalicylic acid [PAS]~~
~~Phenylbutazone~~
~~Resorcinol~~
~~Iatrogenic hypothyroidism NOS~~
~~Use additional E code to identify drug~~

Indicates **deleted** words/codes in the current edition.

Volume 2, Alphabetic Index

Congestion, congestive ~~(chronic) (passive)~~ ◄

Indicates a **deleted** entry in the current edition.

Volume 3, Procedures, Index

Biopsy
    peritoneum
        closed 54.24 ◄

Lung ~~(complete)~~ (with mediastinal dissection) ~~32.5~~ 32.59 ◄

Indicates a **deleted** entry in the current edition.

Volume 3, Procedures, Tabular List

00.74   Hip ~~replacement~~ bearing surface, metal-on-polyethylene ◄

Indicates a **deleted** entry in the current edition.

Codes or index entries are for purposes of illustration only and may not be current.

Symbols for Volume 1, Tabular List

Use Additional Digit(s): The colored dot cautions you that the code requires additional digit(s) to ensure the greatest specificity.

Indicates **proposed** 2010 complications and comorbidities and major complications and comorbidities according to the Inpatient Prospective Payment System (IPPS) rule published in the *Federal Register*. For the latest updates, reference http://www.cms.hhs.gov/AcuteInpatientPPS/FFD/list.asp#TopOfPage.

● **237.7   Neurofibromatosis**
von Recklinghausen's disease

Unacceptable Principal Diagnosis: These codes have a black dot before them and give additional information or describe the circumstances affecting the health care encounter but are unacceptable as principal diagnosis in the Medicare Code Edits for inpatient admission.

● **284.2   Myelophthisis**

242.1   Toxic uninodular goiter
Thyroid nodule, toxic or with hyperthyroidism
Uninodular goiter, toxic or with hyperthyroidism

Present on Admission: Are exempt codes that do not represent a current disease or injury or are always present on admission.

OGCR Section I.C.3.a.2
If the type of diabetes mellitus is not documented in the medical record the default is type II.

First Listed: This symbol appears before V codes that are acceptable as first-listed codes according to the V Code Table in the *ICD-9-CM Official Guidelines for Coding and Reporting*.

❶ **V46.13   Encounter for weaning from respirator [ventilator]**

First Listed or Additional: This symbol appears before V codes that may be either first-listed or additional codes according to the V Code Table in the *ICD-9-CM Official Guidelines for Coding and Reporting*.

V46.14   Mechanical complication of respirator [ventilator]

Additional Only: This symbol appears before V codes that may be reported as additional codes, not as first-listed codes, according to the V Code Table in the *ICD-9-CM Official Guidelines for Coding and Reporting*.

❷ **V46.11   Dependence on respirator, status**

007.4   Cryptosporidiosis
Coding Clinic: 1997, Q4, P30-31

Indicates a Volume 1 reference in the American Hospital Association *Coding Clinic for ICD-9-CM*.

112.2   Of other urogenital sites

This symbol indicates a Hospital-Acquired Condition (HAC). The Deficit Reduction Act of 2005 (DRA) required an adjustment in Medicare Severity Diagnosis Related Group (MS-DRG) payment for certain hospital-acquired conditions.

Medicare Code Editor **Newborn** edit (age 0 years) indicating diagnoses intended only for newborns and neonates (e.g., fetal distress, perinatal jaundice).

747.83   Persistent fetal circulation   **N**

783.41   Failure to thrive   **P**

Medicare Code Editor **Pediatric** edit (age 0–17 years), e.g., Reye's syndrome, routine child health examination.

Medicare Code Editor **Maternity** edit (age 12–55 years), e.g., diabetes in pregnancy, antepartum pulmonary complications.

632   Missed abortion   **M**

256.31   Premature menopause   **A**

Medicare Code Editor **Adult** edit (age 15–124 years), e.g., senile delirium, mature cataract.

Codes or index entries are for purposes of illustration only and may not be current.

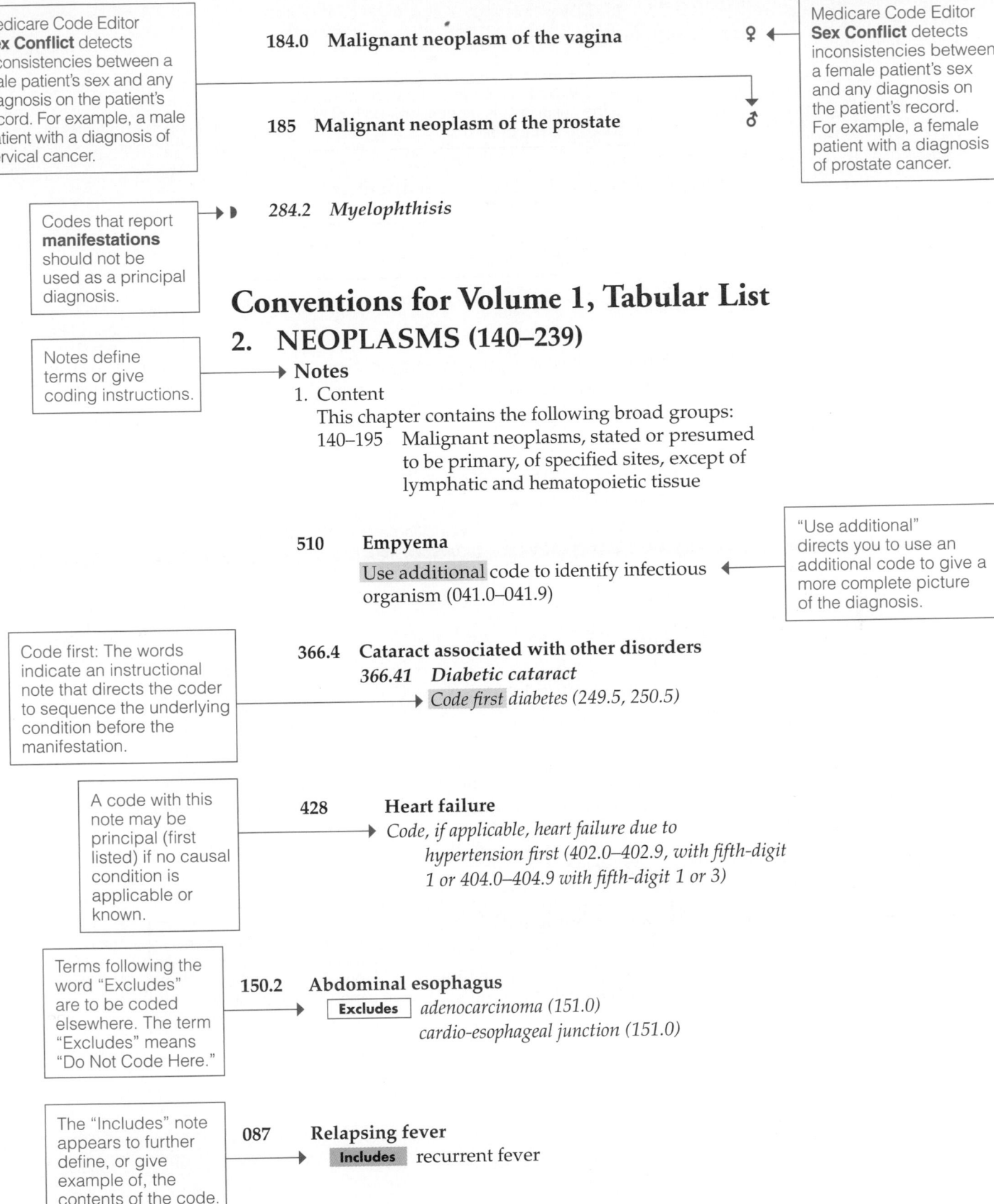

Medicare Code Editor **Sex Conflict** detects inconsistencies between a male patient's sex and any diagnosis on the patient's record. For example, a male patient with a diagnosis of cervical cancer.

184.0   Malignant neoplasm of the vagina   ♀

185   Malignant neoplasm of the prostate   ♂

Medicare Code Editor **Sex Conflict** detects inconsistencies between a female patient's sex and any diagnosis on the patient's record. For example, a female patient with a diagnosis of prostate cancer.

Codes that report **manifestations** should not be used as a principal diagnosis.

284.2   *Myelophthisis*

Conventions for Volume 1, Tabular List
2. NEOPLASMS (140–239)

Notes define terms or give coding instructions.

Notes
1. Content
   This chapter contains the following broad groups:
   140–195   Malignant neoplasms, stated or presumed to be primary, of specified sites, except of lymphatic and hematopoietic tissue

510   Empyema
Use additional code to identify infectious organism (041.0–041.9)

"Use additional" directs you to use an additional code to give a more complete picture of the diagnosis.

Code first: The words indicate an instructional note that directs the coder to sequence the underlying condition before the manifestation.

366.4   Cataract associated with other disorders
366.41   Diabetic cataract
Code first diabetes (249.5, 250.5)

A code with this note may be principal (first listed) if no causal condition is applicable or known.

428   Heart failure
Code, if applicable, heart failure due to hypertension first (402.0–402.9, with fifth-digit 1 or 404.0–404.9 with fifth-digit 1 or 3)

Terms following the word "Excludes" are to be coded elsewhere. The term "Excludes" means "Do Not Code Here."

150.2   Abdominal esophagus
Excludes   *adenocarcinoma (151.0)*
cardio-esophageal junction (151.0)

The "Includes" note appears to further define, or give example of, the contents of the code.

087   Relapsing fever
Includes   recurrent fever

Codes or index entries are for purposes of illustration only and may not be current.

474   **Chronic disease of tonsils and adenoids**

"and" indicates a code that can be assigned if either of the conditions is present or if both of the conditions are present.

366.4   **Cataract associated with other disorders**

"with" indicates a code that can be used only if both conditions are present.

NEC means Not Elsewhere Classifiable and is to be used only when the information at hand specifies a condition but there is no more specific code for that condition.

244.8   **Other specified acquired hypothyroidism**
          Secondary hypothyroidism NEC

Bold type is used for all codes and titles.

159.0   **Intestinal tract, part unspecified**
          Intestine NOS

NOS means Not Otherwise Specified and is the equivalent of "unspecified."

426.89   **Other**
          Dissociation:
                atrioventricular [AV]

Brackets are used to enclose synonyms, alternative wording, or explanatory phrases.

158.8   **Specified parts of peritoneum**
          Cul-de-sac (of Douglas)
          Mesentery

Parentheses are used to enclose supplementary words that may be present or absent in the statement of a disease without affecting the code.

628.4   **Of cervical or vaginal origin**
          Infertility associated with:
                anomaly of cervical mucus
                congenital structural anomaly

A colon is used after an incomplete term that needs one or more of the modifiers that follow in order to make it assignable to a given category.

Codes or index entries are for purposes of illustration only and may not be current.

Conventions for Volume 2, Alphabetic Index

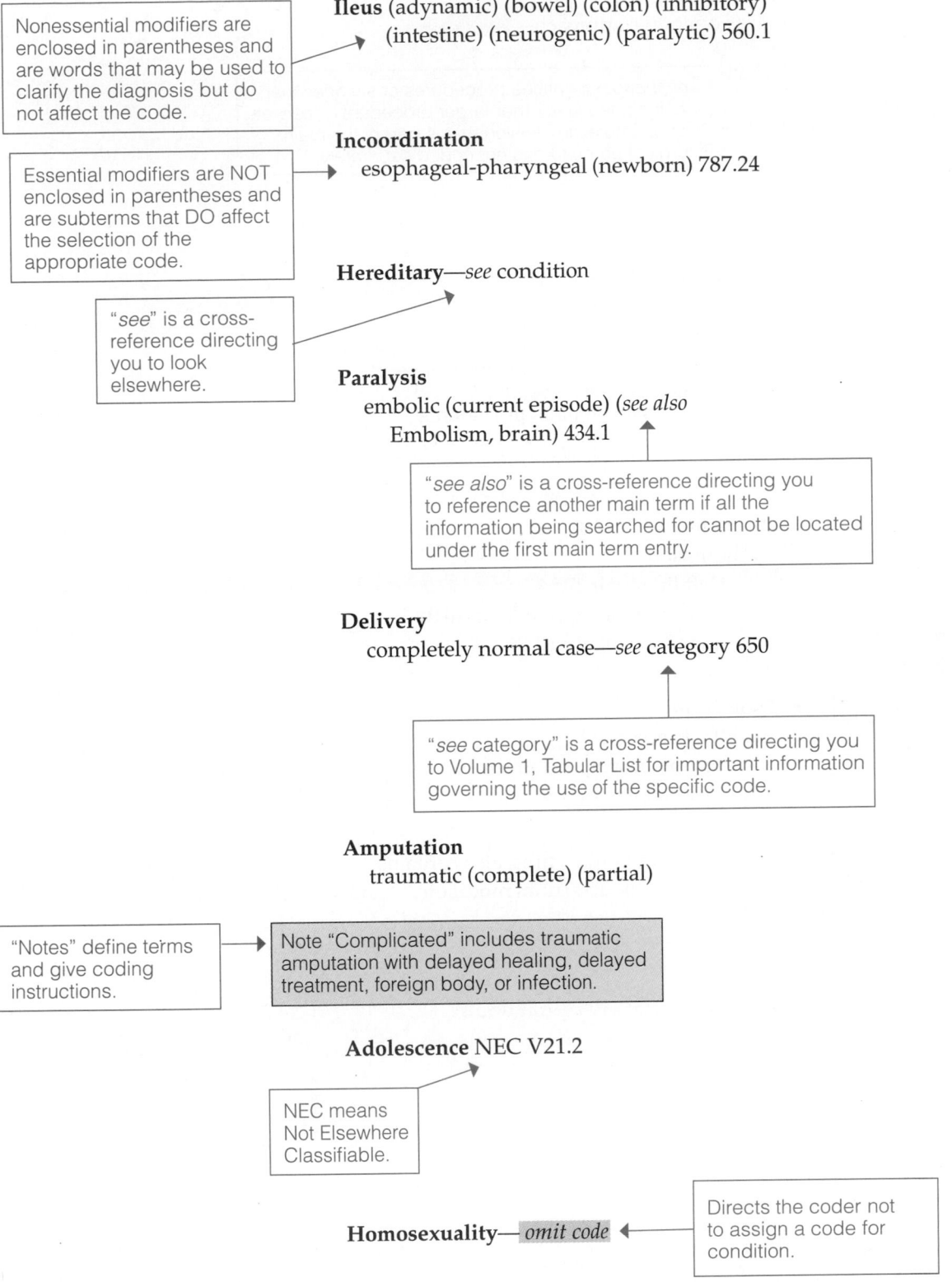

Ileus (adynamic) (bowel) (colon) (inhibitory) (intestine) (neurogenic) (paralytic) 560.1

Nonessential modifiers are enclosed in parentheses and are words that may be used to clarify the diagnosis but do not affect the code.

Incoordination
esophageal-pharyngeal (newborn) 787.24

Essential modifiers are NOT enclosed in parentheses and are subterms that DO affect the selection of the appropriate code.

Hereditary—*see* condition

"*see*" is a cross-reference directing you to look elsewhere.

Paralysis
embolic (current episode) (*see also* Embolism, brain) 434.1

"*see also*" is a cross-reference directing you to reference another main term if all the information being searched for cannot be located under the first main term entry.

Delivery
completely normal case—*see* category 650

"*see category*" is a cross-reference directing you to Volume 1, Tabular List for important information governing the use of the specific code.

Amputation
traumatic (complete) (partial)

"Notes" define terms and give coding instructions.

Note "Complicated" includes traumatic amputation with delayed healing, delayed treatment, foreign body, or infection.

Adolescence NEC V21.2

NEC means Not Elsewhere Classifiable.

Directs the coder not to assign a code for condition.

Homosexuality—*omit code*

Codes or index entries are for purposes of illustration only and may not be current.

Conventions for Volume 3, Procedures, Index

Arthrotomy 80.10

  as operative approach—*omit code*

> "*omit code*" identifies procedures or services that are included in another larger procedure or service. For example, an incision that is part of the main surgical procedure is not coded separately.

Ileal

  bladder

    closed 57.87 [*45.51*]

> For some operative procedures it is necessary to record the individual components of the procedure. These procedures are termed **"synchronous procedures"** and are listed together in the Index. The codes are sequenced in the same order as displayed in the Index.

Operation

  Thompson

    cleft lip repair 27.54

    correction of lymphedema 40.9

    quadricepsplasty 83.86

> Eponyms are operations named for people and are listed in the Index both under the eponym and under the term "Operation."

Thompson

  cleft lip repair 27.54

  correction of lymphedema 40.9

  quadricepsplasty 83.86

Volume 3, Index to Procedures, also contains "*see*," "*see also*," "*see* category," "essential modifiers," "nonessential modifiers," "notes," NEC, and NOS as in Volume 2, Alphabetic Index.

Codes or index entries are for purposes of illustration only and may not be current.

Symbols for Volume 3, Procedures, Tabular List

Use Additional Digit(s):
The colored dot cautions that the code requires additional digit(s) to ensure the greatest specificity.

● **31.9**   Other operations on larynx and trachea
✖ **31.91**   Division of laryngeal nerve

Valid O.R. Procedure:
The "x" is placed before a code that is a valid operating room (O.R.) procedure according to the MS-DRG grouper.

00.0   Theropeutic ultrasound
→ Coding Clinic: 2002, Q4, P90-91

Indicates a Volume 3 reference in the American Hospital Association *Coding Clinic for ICD-9-CM.*

65.01   Laparoscopic oophorotomy   ♀

Medicare Code Editor **Sex Conflict** detects inconsistencies between a female patient's sex and any procedure on the patient's record. For example, a female patient assigned a procedure code for a prostatectomy.

Medicare Code Editor **Sex Conflict** detects inconsistencies between a male patient's sex and any procedure on the patient's record. For example, a male patient assigned a procedure code for a hysterectomy.

60.0   Incision of prostate   ♂

✖ **00.10**   Implantation of chemotherapeutic agent
Brain wafer chemotherapy
Interstitial/intracavitary
    Excludes   *injection or infusion of cancer chemotherapeutic substance (99.25)*
Coding Clinic: 2020, Q4, P93
→ ♦ Non-OR Procedure with MDC 01, MS-DRG 023

Non-OR Procedure indicates updates based on the Medicare Code Edits (MCE) to those procedures that Medicare would not normally reimburse.

Conventions for Volume 3, Procedures, Tabular List

The "Includes" note appears to further define, or give example of, the contents of the code.

88.4   Arteriography using contrast material   ← **Bold** type is used for all codes and titles.
→ **Includes**   angiography of arteries
    arterial puncture for injection of contrast material
    radiography of arteries (by fluoroscopy)
    retrograde arteriography

The fifth-digit subclassification identifies the site to be viewed, not the site of injection

Terms following the word "Excludes" are to be coded elsewhere. The term means "Do Not Code Here."

→ **Excludes**   *arteriography using:
    radioisotopes or radionuclides (92.01–92.19)*

For some operative procedures it is necessary to record the individual components of the procedure. These procedures are termed "synchronous procedures."

45.5   Isolation of intestinal segment
→ **Code also** any synchronous:
    anastomosis other than end-to-end (45.90–45.94)
    enterostomy (46.10–46.39)

Codes or index entries are for purposes of illustration only and may not be current.

GUIDE TO THE 2010 ICD-9-CM UPDATES

VOLUME 1 CHANGES EFFECTIVE OCTOBER 1, 2009

1. INFECTIOUS AND PARASITIC DISEASES (001-139)

Revise   **Excludes** *influenza (487.0-487.8, <u>488.0-488.1</u>)*

008 Intestinal infections due to other organisms

    008.6 Enteritis due to specified virus

       008.63 Norwalk virus

Add   Norovirus

Revise   **008.65 <u>Calicivirus</u>**

035 Erysipelas

Revise   **Excludes** *postpartum or puerperal erysipelas (<u>670.8</u>)*

037 Tetanus

   Excludes *tetanus:*

Revise   *puerperal (<u>670.8</u>)*

041 Bacterial infection in conditions classified elsewhere and of unspecified site

Revise   **041.3** ~~Friedländer's bacillus~~ Klebsiella pneumoniae

Delete   ~~Infection by Klebsiella pneumoniae~~

     041.8 Other specified bacterial infections

Revise   **041.86 Helicobacter pylori** ~~(H. pylori)~~ [H. pylori]

046 Slow virus infections and prion diseases of central nervous system

     046.1 Jakob-Creutzfeldt disease

Add   Use additional code to identify dementia:

Add   with behavioral disturbance (294.11)

Add   without behavioral disturbance (294.10)

Revise   **VIRAL DISEASES GENERALLY ACCOMPANIED BY EXANTHEM (050-059)**

078 Other diseases due to viruses and Chlamydiae

     078.8 Other specified diseases due to viruses and Chlamydiae

       078.89 Other specified diseases due to viruses

Delete   ~~Tanapox~~

190 Malignant neoplasm of eye

Add   **Excludes** *dark area on retina and choroid (239.81)*

Add   *retinal freckle (239.81)*

196 Secondary and unspecified malignant neoplasm of lymph nodes

Add   **Excludes** *secondary neuroendocrine tumor of (distant) lymph nodes (209.71)*

197 Secondary malignant neoplasm of respiratory and digestive systems

Add   **Excludes** *secondary neuroendocrine tumor of liver (209.72)*

Add   *secondary neuroendocrine tumor of respiratory organs (209.79)*

198 Secondary malignant neoplasm of other specified sites

Add   **Excludes** *secondary neuroendocrine tumor of other specified sites (209.79)*

199 Malignant neoplasm without specification of site

Add   **Excludes** *malignant (poorly differentiated) neuroendocrine carcinoma, any site (209.30)*

Revise   *malignant (<u>poorly differentiated</u>) neuroendocrine tumor, any site (209.30)*

Revise   *neuroendocrine carcinoma (<u>high grade</u>), any site (209.30)*

     199.2 Malignant neoplasm associated with transplanted organ

Revise   Use additional code for specific malignancy ~~site~~

MALIGNANT NEOPLASM OF LYMPHATIC AND HEMATOPOIETIC TISSUE (200-208)

Add   **Excludes** *autoimmune lymphoproliferative syndrome (279.41)*

202 Other malignant neoplasms of lymphoid and histiocytic tissue

     202.0 Nodular lymphoma

       Lymphoma:

Revise   follicular (giant) (<u>large cell</u>)

     202.1 Mycosis fungoides

Add   **Excludes** *peripheral T-cell lymphoma (202.7)*

209 Neuroendocrine tumors

Add   **Excludes** *benign pancreatic islet cell tumors (211.7)*

Revise   *<u>malignant pancreatic islet cell tumors</u> (157.4)*

     209.3 Malignant poorly differentiated neuroendocrine tumors

       209.30 Malignant poorly differentiated neuroendocrine carcinoma, any site

Add   **Excludes** *Merkel cell carcinoma (209.31-209.36)*

New code   **209.31 Merkel cell carcinoma of the face**
         Merkel cell carcinoma of the ear
         Merkel cell carcinoma of the eyelid, including canthus
         Merkel cell carcinoma of the lip

New code   **209.32 Merkel cell carcinoma of the scalp and neck**

New code   **209.33 Merkel cell carcinoma of the upper limb**

New code   **209.34 Merkel cell carcinoma of the lower limb**

New code   **209.35 Merkel cell carcinoma of the trunk**

New code   **209.36 Merkel cell carcinoma of other sites**
Merkel cell carcinoma of the buttock
Merkel cell carcinoma of the genitals
Merkel cell carcinoma NOS

New sub   **209.7 Secondary neuroendocrine tumors**
Secondary carcinoid tumors

New code   **209.70 Secondary neuroendocrine tumor, unspecified site**

New code   **209.71 Secondary neuroendocrine tumor of distant lymph nodes**
Mesentery metastasis of neuroendocrine tumor

New code   **209.72 Secondary neuroendocrine tumor of liver**

New code   **209.73 Secondary neuroendocrine tumor of bone**

New code   **209.74 Secondary neuroendocrine tumor of peritoneum**

New code   **209.75 Secondary Merkel cell carcinoma**
Merkel cell carcinoma nodal presentation
Merkel cell carcinoma visceral metastatic presentation
Secondary Merkel cell carcinoma, any site

New code   **209.79 Secondary neuroendocrine tumor of other sites**

238 Neoplasm of uncertain behavior of other and unspecified sites and tissues

238.7 Other lymphatic and hematopoietic tissues

238.72 Low grade myelodysplastic syndrome lesions

Add   Refractory anemia with excess blasts-1 (RAEB-1)

238.73 High grade myelodysplastic syndrome lesions

Delete   ~~Refractory anemia with excess blasts-1 (RAEB-1)~~

239 Neoplasms of unspecified nature

239.8 Other specified sites

New code   **239.81 Retina and choroid**
Dark area on retina
Retinal freckle

New code   **239.89 Other specified sites**

251 Other disorders of pancreatic internal secretion

251.3 Postsurgical hypoinsulinemia

Add   Use additional code to identify (any associated):

Add   acquired absence of pancreas (V45.79)
Add   insulin use (V58.67)
Add   secondary diabetes mellitus (249.00-249.91)

Add   **Excludes** *transient hyperglycemia post procedure (790.29)*
transient hypoglycemia post procedure (251.2)

269 Other nutritional deficiencies

269.8 Other nutritional deficiency

Excludes *feeding problems (783.3)*
Revise   *newborn (779.31-779.34)*

270 Disorders of amino-acid transport and metabolism

Revise   **Excludes** *gout (274.00-274.9)*

272 Disorders of lipoid metabolism

272.2 Mixed hyperlipidemia

Add   Combined hyperlipidemia
Add   Elevated cholesterol with elevated triglycerides NEC

272.4 Other and unspecified hyperlipidemia

Delete   ~~Combined hyperlipidemia~~

274 Gout

274.0 Gouty arthropathy

New code   **274.00 Gouty arthropathy, unspecified**

New code   **274.01 Acute gouty arthropathy**
Acute gout
Gout attack
Gout flare
Podagra

New code   **274.02 Chronic gouty arthropathy without mention of tophus (tophi)**
Chronic gout

New code   **274.03 Chronic gouty arthropathy with tophus (tophi)**
Chronic tophaceous gout
Gout with tophi NOS

274.8 Gout with other specified manifestations

274.82 Gouty tophi of other sites

Add   **Excludes** *gout with tophi NOS (274.03)*
Add   *gouty arthropathy with tophi (274.03)*

277 Other and unspecified disorders of metabolism

277.2 Other disorders of purine and pyrimidine metabolism

Revise   **Excludes** *gout (274.00-274.9)*

277.8 Other specified disorders of metabolism

New code   **277.88 Tumor lysis syndrome**
Spontaneous tumor lysis syndrome
Tumor lysis syndrome following antineoplastic drug therapy
Use additional E code to identify cause, if drug-induced

279 Disorders involving the immune mechanism

279.4 Autoimmune disease, not elsewhere classified

Delete   ~~Autoimmune disease NOS~~

New code   **279.41 Autoimmune lymphoproliferative syndrome**
ALPS

New code   **279.49 Autoimmune disease, not elsewhere classified**
Autoimmune disease NOS

279.5 Graft-versus-host disease

Code first *underlying cause, such as:*
Revise   complication of blood transfusion (999.89)
Revise   complication of transplanted organ ~~(bone marrow)~~ (996.80-996.89)

285 Other and unspecified anemias

285.2 Anemia of chronic disease

Revise   Anemia in (due to) (with) chronic illness

285.22 Anemia in neoplastic disease

Add   **Excludes** *anemia due to antineoplastic chemotherapy (285.3)*

New code   **285.3 Antineoplastic chemotherapy induced anemia**

Anemia due to antineoplastic chemotherapy

Excludes *anemia due to drug NEC – code to type of anemia*
anemia in neoplastic disease (285.22)
aplastic anemia due to antineoplastic chemotherapy (284.89)

290 Dementias

290.0 Senile dementia, uncomplicated

Revise   **Excludes** *mild memory disturbances, not amounting to dementia, associated with senile brain disease (310.8)*

294 Persistent mental disorders due to conditions classified elsewhere

294.1 Dementia in conditions classified elsewhere

Code first any underlying physical condition as:
dementia in:
Jakob-Creutzfeldt disease

Revise   (046.11-046.19)

294.8 Other persistent mental disorders due to conditions classified elsewhere

Revise   **Excludes** *mild memory disturbances, not amounting to dementia (310.8)*

305 Nondependent abuse of drugs

305.1 Tobacco use disorder

Delete   [0-3]

307 Special symptoms or syndromes, not elsewhere classified

307.0 Stuttering

Revise   **Excludes** *dysphasia (784.59)*
Add   *stuttering (fluency disorder) due to late effect of cerebrovascular accident (438.14)*

310 Specific nonpsychotic mental disorders due to brain damage

310.1 Personality change due to conditions classified elsewhere

Delete   **Excludes** *memory loss of unknown cause (780.93)*

Add   *mild cognitive impairment (331.83)*
Add   *postconcussion syndrome (310.2)*
Add   *signs and symptoms involving emotional state (799.21-799.29)*

310.8 Other specified nonpsychotic mental disorders following organic brain damage

Add   **Excludes** *memory loss of unknown cause (780.93)*

331 Other cerebral degenerations

331.7 Cerebral degeneration in diseases classified elsewhere

Revise   **Excludes** *cerebral degeneration in: Jakob-Creutzfeldt disease (046.11-046.19)*

331.8 Other cerebral degeneration

331.83 Mild cognitive impairment, so stated

Add   **Excludes** *cognitive impairment due to skull fracture (800-801, 803-804)*

333 Other extrapyramidal disease and abnormal movement disorders

333.2 Myoclonus

Add   Palatal myoclonus
Delete   Progressive myoclonic epilepsy
Delete   Unverricht-Lundborg disease

Add   **Excludes** *progressive myoclonic epilepsy (345.1)*
Add   *Unverricht-Lundborg disease (345.1)*

345 Epilepsy and recurrent seizures

The following fifth-digit subclassification is for use with categories 345.0, .1, .4-.9:

1   with intractable epilepsy
Add   pharmacoresistant (pharmacologically resistant)
Add   poorly controlled
Add   refractory (medically)
Add   treatment resistant

Add   **Excludes** *hippocampal sclerosis (348.81)*
Add   *mesial temporal sclerosis (348.81)*
Add   *temporal sclerosis (348.81)*

345.1 Generalized convulsive epilepsy

Add   Progressive myoclonic epilepsy
Add   Unverricht-Lundborg disease

348 Other conditions of brain

348.8 Other conditions of brain

Delete   Cerebral:
Delete   calcification
Delete   fungus

New code   **348.81 Temporal sclerosis**
Hippocampal sclerosis
Mesial temporal sclerosis

New code   **348.89 Other conditions of brain**
Cerebral:
calcification
fungus

359 Muscular dystrophies and other myopathies

359.2 Myotonic disorders

359.22 Myotonia congenita

Add   Myotonia levior

359.29 Other specified myotonic disorder

Delete   Myotonia levior

New sub   **359.7 Inflammatory and immune myopathies, NEC**

New code   **359.71 Inclusion body myositis**
IBM

New code   **359.79 Other inflammatory and immune myopathies, NEC**
Inflammatory myopathy NOS

372 Disorders of conjunctiva

372.0 Acute conjunctivitis

New code | 372.06 Acute chemical conjunctivitis
Acute toxic conjunctivitis

> Use additional E code to identify the chemical or toxic agent
>
> Excludes *burn of eye and adnexa (940.0-940.9)*
> *chemical corrosion injury of eye (940.2-940.3)*

372.3 Other and unspecified conjunctivitis

372.34 Pingueculitis

Add |
> Excludes *pinguecula (372.51)*

372.5 Conjunctival degenerations and deposits

372.51 Pinguecula

Add |
> Excludes *pingueculitis (372.34)*

403 Hypertensive chronic kidney disease

Revise |
> Excludes *acute ~~renal~~ kidney failure (584.5-584.9)*

413 Angina pectoris

413.9 Other and unspecified angina pectoris
Angina:

Add | equivalent

Add |
> Use additional code(s) for symptoms associated with angina equivalent

415 Acute pulmonary heart disease

415.1 Pulmonary embolism and infarction

Add |
> Excludes *chronic pulmonary embolism (416.2)*

Add |
> *personal history of pulmonary embolism (V12.51)*

416 Chronic pulmonary heart disease

New code | 416.2 Chronic pulmonary embolism

> Use additional code, if applicable, for associated long-term (current) use of anticoagulants (V58.61)
>
> Excludes *personal history of pulmonary embolism (V12.51)*

438 Late effects of cerebrovascular disease

438.1 Speech and language deficits

New code | 438.13 Dysarthria

New code | 438.14 Fluency disorder
Stuttering

445 Atheroembolism

445.8 Of other sites

445.81 Kidney

Revise |
> Use additional code for any associated acute ~~renal~~ kidney failure or chronic kidney disease (584, 585)

453 Other venous embolism and thrombosis

Delete |
> Excludes *~~that with inflammation, phlebitis, and thrombophlebitis (451.0-451.9)~~*

Revise | 453.2 Of inferior vena cava

Revise | 453.4 Acute venous embolism and thrombosis of deep vessels of lower extremity

Revise | 453.40 Acute venous embolism and thrombosis of unspecified deep vessels of lower extremity

Revise | 453.41 Acute venous embolism and thrombosis of deep vessels of proximal lower extremity

Revise | 453.42 Acute venous embolism and thrombosis of deep vessels of distal lower extremity

New sub | 453.5 Chronic venous embolism and thrombosis of deep vessels of lower extremity

> Use additional code, if applicable, for associated long-term (current) use of anticoagulants (V58.61)
>
> Excludes *personal history of venous thrombosis and embolism (V12.51)*

New code | 453.50 Chronic venous embolism and thrombosis of unspecified deep vessels of lower extremity

New code | 453.51 Chronic venous embolism and thrombosis of deep vessels of proximal lower extremity

New code | 453.52 Chronic venous embolism and thrombosis of deep vessels of distal lower extremity

New code | 453.6 Venous embolism and thrombosis of superficial vessels of lower extremity
Saphenous vein (greater) (lesser)

New sub | 453.7 Chronic venous embolism and thrombosis of other specified vessels

> Use additional code, if applicable, for associated long-term (current) use of anticoagulants (V58.61)
>
> Excludes *personal history of venous thrombosis and embolism (V12.51)*

New code | 453.71 Chronic venous embolism and thrombosis of superficial veins of upper extremity
Antecubital vein
Basilic vein
Cephalic vein

New code | 453.72 Chronic venous embolism and thrombosis of deep veins of upper extremity
Brachial vein
Radial vein
Ulnar vein

New code | 453.73 Chronic venous embolism and thrombosis of upper extremity, unspecified

New code | 453.74 Chronic venous embolism and thrombosis of axillary veins

New code | 453.75 Chronic venous embolism and thrombosis of subclavian veins

New code | 453.76 Chronic venous embolism and thrombosis of internal jugular veins

New code | 453.77 Chronic venous embolism and thrombosis of other thoracic veins
Brachiocephalic (innominate)
Superior vena cava

New code | 453.79 Chronic venous embolism and thrombosis of other specified veins

Revise	**453.8**	<u>Acute venous embolism and thrombosis</u> of other specified veins
New code		**453.81 Acute venous embolism and thrombosis of superficial veins of upper extremity** Antecubital vein Basilic vein Cephalic vein
New code		**453.82 Acute venous embolism and thrombosis of deep veins of upper extremity** Brachial vein Radial vein Ulnar vein
New code		**453.83 Acute venous embolism and thrombosis of upper extremity, unspecified**
New code		**453.84 Acute venous embolism and thrombosis of axillary veins**
New code		**453.85 Acute venous embolism and thrombosis of subclavian veins**
New code		**453.86 Acute venous embolism and thrombosis of internal jugular veins**
New code		**453.87 Acute venous embolism and thrombosis of other thoracic veins** Brachiocephalic (innominate) Superior vena cava
New code		**453.89 Acute venous embolism and thrombosis of other specified veins**

487 Influenza

Add	Influenza caused by unspecified influenza virus

Excludes	*Hemophilus influenzae [H. influenzae]:*
Add	*influenza due to 2009 H1N1 [swine] influenza virus (488.1)*
Revise	*influenza due to identified avian influenza virus (<u>488.0</u>)*
Add	*influenza due to identified novel H1N1 influenza virus (488.1)*

Revise	**488 Influenza due to <u>certain</u> identified ~~avian~~ influenza <u>viruses</u>**
Delete	~~Note: Influenza caused by influenza viruses that normally infect only birds and, less commonly, other animals~~

Excludes	*influenza caused by ~~other~~ <u>unspecified</u> influenza viruses (487.0-487.8)*
Revise	

New code	**488.0 Influenza due to identified avian influenza virus** Avian influenza Bird flu Influenza A/H5N1
New code	**488.1 Influenza due to identified novel H1N1 influenza virus** 2009 H1N1 [swine] influenza virus Novel 2009 influenza H1N1 Novel H1N1 influenza Novel influenza A/H1N1 Swine flu

536 Disorders of function of stomach

    536.2 Persistent vomiting

Add	**Excludes** *bilious emesis (vomiting) (787.04)*
Add	*vomiting of fecal matter (569.87)*

567 Peritonitis and retroperitoneal infections

Excludes	*peritonitis:*
Revise	*puerperal (<u>670.8</u>)*

569 Other disorders of intestine

New sub	**569.7 Complications of intestinal pouch**
New code	**569.71 Pouchitis** Inflammation of internal ileoanal pouch
New code	**569.79 Other complications of intestinal pouch**
	569.8 Other specified disorders of intestine
New code	**569.87 Vomiting of fecal matter**

572 Liver abscess and sequelae of chronic liver disease

Revise	**572.2 Hepatic ~~coma~~ <u>encephalopathy</u>**
Delete	~~Hepatic encephalopathy~~
Add	Hepatic coma
Revise	**584 Acute ~~renal~~ <u>kidney</u> failure**
Add	**Includes** Acute renal failure
Revise	**584.5 <u>Acute kidney failure</u> ~~W~~<u>w</u>ith lesion of tubular necrosis**
Revise	**584.6 <u>Acute kidney failure</u> ~~W~~<u>w</u>ith lesion of renal cortical necrosis**
Revise	**584.7 <u>Acute kidney failure</u> ~~W~~<u>w</u>ith lesion of renal medullary [papillary] necrosis**
Revise	**584.8 <u>Acute kidney failure</u> ~~W~~<u>w</u>ith other specified pathological lesion in kidney**
Revise	**584.9 <u>Acute kidney failure</u> ~~Acute renal failure~~, unspecified**

587 Renal sclerosis, unspecified

Revise	**Includes** Atrophy of kidney
Delete	~~Atrophy of kidney~~

611 Other disorders of breast

    611.8 Other specified disorders of breast

        611.82 Hypoplasia of breast

Add	**Excludes** *congenital absence of breast (757.6)*

614 Inflammatory disease of ovary, fallopian tube, pelvic cellular tissue, and peritoneum

Revise	**Excludes** *major infection following delivery (<u>670.0-670.8</u>)*

615 Inflammatory diseases of uterus, except cervix

Revise	**Excludes** *following delivery (670.0-670.8)*
Revise	*hyperplastic endometritis (621.30-<u>621.35</u>)*

621 Disorders of uterus, not elsewhere classified

621.3 Endometrial hyperplasia

Delete
~~Hyperplasia (adenomatous) (cystic) (glandular) of endometrium~~
~~Hyperplastic endometritis~~

621.30 Endometrial hyperplasia, unspecified

Add
Hyperplasia (adenomatous) (cystic) (glandular) of endometrium

Add
Hyperplastic endometritis

621.31 Simple endometrial hyperplasia without atypia

Add
| **Excludes** | *benign endometrial hyperplasia (621.34)* |

621.32 Complex endometrial hyperplasia without atypia

Add
| **Excludes** | *benign endometrial hyperplasia (621.34)* |

621.33 Endometrial hyperplasia with atypia

Add
| **Excludes** | *endometrial intraepithelial neoplasia [EIN] (621.35)* |

New code
621.34 Benign endometrial hyperplasia

New code
621.35 Endometrial intraepithelial neoplasia [EIN]

| **Excludes** | *malignant neoplasm of endometrium with endometrial intraepithelial neoplasia [EIN] (182.0)* |

624 Noninflammatory disorders of vulva and perineum

Revise
| **Excludes** | *condyloma acuminatum (078.11)* |

639 Complications following abortion and ectopic and molar pregnancies

639.3 Kidney failure

Revise
Revise
Renal (kidney):

646 Other complications of pregnancy, not elsewhere classified

646.6 Infections of genitourinary tract in pregnancy

Revise
| **Excludes** | *major puerperal infection (670.0-670.8)* |

649 Other conditions or status of the mother complicating pregnancy, childbirth, or the puerperium

649.3 Coagulation defects complicating pregnancy, childbirth, or the puerperium

Revise
Conditions classifiable to 286, 287, 289

Revise
Use additional code to identify the specific coagulation defect (286.0-286.9, 287.0-287.9, 289.0-289.9)

669 Other complications of labor and delivery, not elsewhere classified

Revise
669.3 Acute ~~renal~~ kidney failure following labor and delivery

670 Major puerperal infection
[0,2,4]

Delete   ~~Use 0 as fourth digit for category 670~~
Delete   ~~Puerperal:~~
Delete   ~~endometritis~~
Delete   ~~fever (septic)~~
Delete   ~~pelvic:~~
Delete   ~~cellulitis~~
Delete   ~~sepsis~~
Delete   ~~peritonitis~~
Delete   ~~pyemia~~
Delete   ~~salpingitis~~
Delete   ~~septicemia~~

Revise sub
670.0 Major puerperal infection, unspecified
[0,2,4]

New sub
670.1 Puerperal endometritis
[0,2,4]

New sub
670.2 Puerperal sepsis
[0,2,4]   Puerperal pyemia

New sub
670.3 Puerperal septic thrombophlebitis
[0,2,4]

New sub
670.8 Other major puerperal infection
[0,2,4]   Puerperal:
pelvic cellulitis
peritonitis
salpingitis

671 Venous complications in pregnancy and the puerperium

Add
| **Excludes** | *personal history of venous complications prior to pregnancy, such as:* |

Add
thrombophlebitis (V12.52)

Add
thrombosis and embolism (V12.51)

671.2 Superficial thrombophlebitis

Add
Phlebitis NOS

Add
Thrombosis NOS

671.3 Deep phlebothrombosis, antepartum

Add
Use additional code to identify the deep vein thrombosis (453.40-453.42, 453.50-453.52, 453.72-453.79, 453.82-453.89)

Add
Use additional code for long term (current) use of anticoagulants, if applicable (V58.61)

671.4 Deep phlebothrombosis, postpartum

Add
Use additional code to identify the deep vein thrombosis (453.40-453.42, 453.50-453.52, 453.72-453.79, 453.82-453.89)

Add
Use additional code for long term (current) use of anticoagulants, if applicable (V58.61)

671.9 Unspecified venous complication

Delete   ~~Phlebitis NOS~~
Delete   ~~Thrombosis NOS~~

INFECTIONS OF SKIN AND SUBCUTANEOUS TISSUE (680-686)

| **Excludes** | *certain infections of skin classified under "Infectious and Parasitic Diseases," such as:* |

Revise
viral warts (078.10-078.19)

707 Chronic ulcer of skin

707.0 Pressure ulcer

707.03 Lower back

Add
Coccyx

712 Crystal arthropathies

Revise | **Excludes** *gouty arthropathy (274.00-274.03)*

713 Arthropathy associated with other disorders classified elsewhere

    713.0 Arthropathy associated with other endocrine and metabolic disorders

Revise | **Excludes** *arthropathy associated with:*
gouty arthropathy
(274.00-274.03)

727 Other disorders of synovium, tendon, and bursa

    727.01 Synovitis and tenosynovitis in diseases classified elsewhere

Revise | **Excludes** *gouty (274.00-274.03)*

733 Other disorders of bone and cartilage

    733.1 Pathologic fracture

Add | Chronic fracture

756 Other congenital musculoskeletal anomalies

    756.7 Anomalies of abdominal wall

New code | **756.72 Omphalocele**
      Exomphalos

New code | **756.73 Gastroschisis**

    756.79 Other congenital anomalies of abdominal wall

Delete | Exomphalos
Delete | Gastroschisis
Delete | Omphalocele

757 Congenital anomalies of the integument

Revise | **757.6 Specified congenital anomalies of breast**
Revise | Congenital aAbsent breast or nipple
Add | **Excludes** *micromastia (611.82)*

762 Fetus or newborn affected by complications of placenta, cord, and membranes

    762.3 Placental transfusion syndromes

Revise | Use additional code to indicate resultant condition in fetus or newborn:

768 Intrauterine hypoxia and birth asphyxia

    768.5 Severe birth asphyxia

Revise | **Excludes** *hypoxic-ischemic encephalopathy (HIE) (768.70-768.73)*

    768.6 Mild or moderate birth asphyxia

Revise | **Excludes** *hypoxic-ischemic encephalopathy (HIE) (768.70-768.73)*

    768.7 Hypoxic-ischemic encephalopathy (HIE)

New code | **768.70 Hypoxic-ischemic encephalopathy, unspecified**

New code | **768.71 Mild hypoxic-ischemic encephalopathy**

New code | **768.72 Moderate hypoxic-ischemic encephalopathy**

New code | **768.73 Severe hypoxic-ischemic encephalopathy**

772 Fetal and neonatal hemorrhage

Add | **Excludes** *fetal hematologic conditions complicating pregnancy (678.0)*

Revise | **772.0 Fetal blood loss affecting newborn**

776 Hematological disorders of newborn

Revise | **Includes** disorders specific to the fetus or newborn though possibly originating in utero

Revise | **776.9 Unspecified hematological disorder specific to fetus or newborn**

777 Perinatal disorders of digestive system

    777.5 Necrotizing enterocolitis in newborn

Delete | Pseudomembranous enterocolitis in newborn

    777.51 Stage I necrotizing enterocolitis in newborn

Add | Necrotizing enterocolitis without pneumatosis, without perforation

779 Other and ill-defined conditions originating in the perinatal period

Revise | **779.3 Disorder of stomach function and feeding problems in newborn**
Delete | Regurgitation of food in newborn
Delete | Slow feeding in newborn
Delete | Vomiting in newborn
New code | **779.31 Feeding problems in newborn**
    Slow feeding in newborn

    Excludes *feeding problem in child over 28 days old (783.3)*

New code | **779.32 Bilious vomiting in newborn**

    Excludes *bilious vomiting in child over 28 days old (787.04)*

New code | **779.33 Other vomiting in newborn**
    Regurgitation of food in newborn

    Excludes *vomiting in child over 28 days old (536.2, 787.01-787.03, 787.04)*

New code | **779.34 Failure to thrive in newborn**

    Excludes *failure to thrive in child over 28 days old (783.41)*

780 General symptoms

    780.0 Alteration of consciousness

Add | **Excludes** *alteration of consciousness due to:*
Add | *intracranial injuries (850.0-854.19)*
Add | *skull fractures (800.00-801.99, 803.00-804.99)*

    780.9 Other general symptoms

    780.93 Memory loss

Add | **Excludes** *memory loss due to:*
Add | *intracranial injuries (850.0-854.19)*
Add | *skull fractures (800.00-801.99, 803.00-804.99)*
Revise | *mild memory disturbance due to organic brain damage (310.8)*

783 Symptoms concerning nutrition, metabolism, and development

    783.3 Feeding difficulties and mismanagement

    Excludes *feeding disturbance or problems:*
Revise | *in newborn (779.31-779.34)*

    783.4 Lack of expected normal physiological development in childhood

    783.41 Failure to thrive

Add | **Excludes** *failure to thrive in newborn (779.34)*

784 Symptoms involving head and neck

Revise   784.4 Voice ~~disturbance~~ and resonance disorders

Revise   784.40 Voice ~~disturbance~~ and resonance disorder, unspecified

New code   784.42 Dysphonia
Hoarseness

New code   784.43 Hypernasality

New code   784.44 Hyponasality

Revise   784.49 Other voice and resonance disorders

Delete   ~~Dsyphonia~~
Delete   ~~Hoarseness~~
Delete   ~~Hypernasality~~
Delete   ~~Hyponasality~~

784.5 Other speech disturbance

Delete   ~~Dysarthria~~
Delete   ~~Dysphasia~~
Delete   ~~Slurred speech~~

Add | Excludes | *speech disorder due to late effect of cerebrovascular accident (438.10-438.19)*

New code   784.51 Dysarthria

| Excludes | *dysarthria due to late effect of cerebrovascular accident (438.13)*

New code   784.59 Other speech disturbance
Dysphasia
Slurred speech
Speech disturbance NOS

787 Symptoms involving digestive system

787.0 Nausea and vomiting

| Excludes | *vomiting*
Add   *fecal matter (569.87)*
Revise   *of newborn (779.32, 779.33)*
Add   *persistent (536.2)*

New code   787.04 Bilious emesis
Bilious vomiting

| Excludes | *bilious emesis (vomiting) in newborn (779.32)*

789 Other symptoms involving abdomen and pelvis

789.0 Abdominal pain
[0-7, 9]

Delete   ~~Colic:~~
~~NOS~~
~~infantile~~

Delete | Excludes | ~~renal colic (788.0)~~

New code   789.7 Colic
Colic NOS
Infantile colic

| Excludes | *colic in adult and child over 12 months old (789.0)*
renal colic (788.0)

790 Nonspecific findings on examination of blood

790.01 Precipitous drop in hematocrit
Drop in hemoglobin
Add

Revise   **793 Nonspecific (abnormal) findings on radiological and other examination of body structure**

793.8 Breast

New code   793.82 Inconclusive mammogram
Dense breasts NOS
Inconclusive mammogram NEC
Inconclusive mammography due to dense breasts
Inconclusive mammography NEC

Revise   793.89 Other (abnormal) findings on radiological examination of breast

793.9 Other

Revise   793.99 Other nonspecific (abnormal) findings on radiological and other examinations of body structure

795 Other and nonspecific abnormal cytological, histological, immunological and DNA test findings

795.0 Abnormal Papanicolaou smear of cervix and cervical HPV

Revise | Excludes | *carcinoma ~~in-situ~~ in situ of cervix (233.1)*

795.3 Nonspecific positive culture findings
795.39 Other nonspecific positive culture findings

Add | Excludes | *colonization status (V02.0-V02.9)*

796 Other nonspecific abnormal findings

796.7 Abnormal cytologic smear of anus and anal HPV

Revise | Excludes | *severe anal dysplasia (histologically confirmed) (230.5, 230.6)*

799 Other ill-defined and unknown causes of morbidity and mortality

Revise   799.2 ~~Nervousness~~ Signs and symptoms involving emotional state
Delete   ~~"Nerves"~~
Add | Excludes | *anxiety (293.84, 300.00-300.09)*
Add   *depression (311)*

New code   799.21 Nervousness
Nervous

New code   799.22 Irritability
Irritable

New code   799.23 Impulsiveness
Impulsive

| Excludes | *impulsive neurosis (300.3)*

New code   799.24 Emotional lability

New code   799.25 Demoralization and apathy
Apathetic

New code   799.29 Other signs and symptoms involving emotional state

799.8 Other ill-defined conditions

New code   799.82 Apparent life threatening event in infant
ALTE
Apparent life threatening event in newborn and infant

Use additional code(s) for associated signs and symptoms

| Excludes | *signs and symptoms associated with a confirmed diagnosis-code to confirmed diagnosis*

FRACTURE OF SKULL (800-804)

Add   **Includes** traumatic brain injury due to fracture of skull

813 Fracture of radius and ulna

    813.4 Lower end, closed

Revise   813.45 Torus fracture of radius (alone)

Add   **Excludes** *Torus fracture of radius and ulna (813.47)*

New code   813.46 Torus fracture of ulna (alone)

             Excludes *Torus fracture of radius and ulna (813.47)*

New code   813.47 Torus fracture of radius and ulna

832 Dislocation of elbow

Revise   The following fifth-digit subclassification is for use with ~~category 832~~ subcategories 832.0 and 832.1:

New code   **832.2 Nursemaid's elbow**
          Subluxation of radial head

INTRACRANIAL INJURY, EXCLUDING THOSE WITH SKULL FRACTURE (850-854)

Add   **Includes** traumatic brain injury without skull fracture

854 Intracranial injury of other and unspecified nature

Revise   **Includes** injury:
Revise   brain ~~injury~~ NOS
Revise   intracranial ~~injury~~
Add   traumatic brain NOS

OPEN WOUNDS (870-897)

Delete   ~~Use additional code to identify infection~~

945 Burn of lower limb(s)

    945.0 Unspecified degree
Revise   [0-6, 9]

    945.1 Erythema [first degree]
Revise   [0-6, 9]

    945.2 Blisters, epidermal loss [second degree]
Revise   [0-6, 9]

    945.3 Full-thickness skin loss [third degree NOS]
Revise   [0-6, 9]

    945.4 Deep necrosis of underlying tissues [deep third degree] without mention of loss of a body part
Revise   [0-6, 9]

    945.5 Deep necrosis of underlying tissues [deep third degree] with loss of a body part
Revise   [0-6, 9]

969 Poisoning by psychotropic agents

    969.0 Antidepressants
Delete   ~~Amitriptyline~~
Delete   ~~Imipramine~~
Delete   ~~Monoamine oxidase [MAO] inhibitors~~

New code   969.00 Antidepressant, unspecified

New code   969.01 Monoamine oxidase inhibitors
             MAOI

New code   969.02 Selective serotonin and norepinephrine reuptake inhibitors
             SSNRI antidepressants

New code   969.03 Selective serotonin reuptake inhibitors
             SSRI antidepressants

New code   969.04 Tetracyclic antidepressants
New code   969.05 Tricyclic antidepressants
New code   969.09 Other antidepressants

    969.7 Psychostimulants
Delete   ~~Amphetamine~~
Delete   ~~Caffeine~~

New code   969.70 Psychostimulant, unspecified
New code   969.71 Caffeine
New code   969.72 Amphetamines
             Methamphetamines
New code   969.73 Methylphenidate
New code   969.79 Other psychostimulants

974 Poisoning by water, mineral, and uric acid metabolism drugs

    974.1 Purine derivative diuretics
Revise   **Excludes** *caffeine (969.71)*

995 Certain adverse effects not elsewhere classified

    995.2 Other and unspecified adverse effect of drug, medicinal and biological substance (due) to correct medicinal substance properly administered

New code   **995.24 Failed moderate sedation during procedure**
          Failed conscious sedation during procedure

    995.9 Systemic inflammatory response syndrome (SIRS)

       995.92 Severe sepsis
          Use additional code to specify acute organ dysfunction, such as:
Revise   acute ~~renal~~ kidney failure (584.5-584.9)

       995.94 Systemic inflammatory response syndrome due to non-infectious process with acute organ dysfunction
          Use additional code to specify acute organ dysfunction, such as:
Revise   acute ~~renal~~ kidney failure (584.5-584.9)

996 Complications peculiar to certain specified procedures

    996.4 Mechanical complication of internal orthopedic device, implant, and graft

Revise   **996.43** ~~Prosthetic joint implant failure~~ Broken prosthetic joint implant

       996.47 Other mechanical complication of prosthetic joint implant
Add   Prosthetic joint implant failure NOS

    996.7 Other complications of internal (biological) (synthetic) prosthetic device, implant, and graft
       Use additional code to identify complication, such as:
Add   venous embolism and thrombosis (453.2-453.9)

997 Complications affecting specified body systems, not elsewhere classified

997.3 Respiratory complications

997.31 Ventilator associated pneumonia

Add
Ventilator associated pneumonitis

997.4 Digestive system complications

| Excludes | specified gastrointestinal complications classified elsewhere, such as: |

Add
complications of intestinal pouch (569.71-569.79)

Add
pouchitis (569.71)

997.5 Urinary complications

Revise
Renal (kidney):

999 Complications of medical care, not elsewhere classified

999.6 ABO incompatibility reaction

Add
| Excludes | minor blood group antigens reactions (Duffy) (E) (K(ell)) (Kidd) (Lewis) (M) (N) (P) (S) (999.89) |

V07 Need for isolation and other prophylactic measures

V07.5 Prophylactic use of agents affecting estrogen receptors and estrogen levels

V07.52 Prophylactic use of aromatase inhibitors
Prophylactic use of:

Revise
exemestane exemestar (Aromasin)

V10 Personal history of malignant neoplasm

Delete
Code first any continuing functional activity, such as:

Delete
carcinoid syndrome (259.2)

V10.0 Gastrointestinal tract

Add
| Excludes | personal history of malignant carcinoid tumor (V10.91) |

Add
personal history of malignant neuroendocrine tumor (V10.91)

V10.1 Trachea, bronchus, and lung

Add
| Excludes | personal history of malignant carcinoid tumor (V10.91) |

Add
personal history of malignant neuroendocrine tumor (V10.91)

V10.8 Personal history of malignant neoplasm of other sites

Add
| Excludes | personal history of malignant carcinoid tumor (V10.91) |

Add
personal history of malignant neuroendocrine tumor (V10.91)

Revise
V10.9 Other and Uunspecified personal history of malignant neoplasm

New code
V10.90 Personal history of unspecified malignant neoplasm

Add
Personal history of malignant neoplasm NOS

| Excludes | personal history of malignant carcinoid tumor (V10.91) |
personal history of malignant neuroendocrine tumor (V10.91)
personal history of Merkel cell carcinoma (V10.91)

New code
V10.91 Personal history of malignant neuroendocrine tumor
"Personal history of malignant carcinoid tumor NOS
Personal history of malignant neuroendocrine tumor NOS
Personal history of Merkel cell carcinoma NOS

Code first any continuing functional activity, such as:
carcinoid syndrome (259.2)

V12 Personal history of certain other diseases

V12.5 Diseases of circulatory system

V12.54 Transient ischemic attack (TIA), and cerebral infarction without residual deficits

Add
| Excludes | history of traumatic brain injury (V15.52) |

V15 Other personal history presenting hazards to health

V15.0 Allergy, other than to medicinal agents

Revise
V15.06 Allergy to insects and arachnids

V15.5 Injury

New code
V15.52 History of traumatic brain injury

| Excludes | personal history of cerebrovascular accident (cerebral infarction) without residual deficits (V12.54) |

	V15.8	**Other specified personal history presenting hazards to health**
New code	**V15.80**	**History of failed moderate sedation**
		History of failed conscious sedation
New code	**V15.83**	**Underimmunization status**
		Delinquent immunization status
		Lapsed immunization schedule status
Revise	**V15.84**	**Contact with and (suspected) exposure to ~~Exposure to~~ asbestos**
Revise	**V15.85**	**Contact with and (suspected) exposure to ~~Exposure to~~ potentially hazardous body fluids**
Revise	**V15.86**	**Contact with and (suspected) exposure to ~~Exposure to~~ lead**

V20 Health supervision of infant or child

	V20.2	**Routine infant or child health check**
Delete		~~Initial and subsequent routine newborn check~~
Add		Health check for child over 28 days old
Add		[Excludes] *health check for child under 29 days old (V20.31-V20.32)*
Add		*newborn health supervision (V20.31-V20.32)*
New sub	**V20.3**	**Newborn health supervision**
		Health check for child under 29 days old
		[Excludes] *health check for child over 28 days old (V20.2)*
New code	**V20.31**	**Health supervision for newborn under 8 days old**
		Health check for newborn under 8 days old
New code	**V20.32**	**Health supervision for newborn 8 to 28 days old**
		Health check for newborn 8 to 28 days old
		Newborn weight check

V23 Supervision of high-risk pregnancy

	V23.8	**Other high-risk pregnancy**
	V23.86	**Pregnancy with history of in utero procedure during previous pregnancy**
Revise		[Excludes] *management of pregnancy affected by in utero procedure during current pregnancy (679.0-679.1)*

	V26	**Procreative management**
	V26.4	**General counseling and advice**
New code	**V26.42**	**Encounter for fertility preservation counseling**
		Encounter for fertility preservation counseling prior to cancer therapy
		Encounter for fertility preservation counseling prior to surgical removal of gonads
	V26.8	**Other specified procreative management**
New code	**V26.82**	**Encounter for fertility preservation procedure**
		Encounter for fertility preservation procedure prior to cancer therapy
		Encounter for fertility preservation procedure prior to surgical removal of gonads

V45 Other postprocedural states

	V45.7	**Acquired absence of organ**
	V45.71	**Acquired absence of breast and nipple**
Add		[Excludes] *congenital absence of breast and nipple (757.6)*

V53 Fitting and adjustment of other device

Revise	**V53.5**	**Other gastrointestinal appliance and device**
New code	**V53.50**	**Fitting and adjustment of intestinal appliance and device**
New code	**V53.51**	**Fitting and adjustment of gastric lap band**
New code	**V53.59**	**Fitting and adjustment of other gastrointestinal appliance and device**

V54 Other orthopedic aftercare

	V54.1	**Aftercare for healing traumatic fracture**
Add		[Excludes] *aftercare following joint replacement (V54.81)*
	V54.2	**Aftercare for healing pathologic fracture**
Add		[Excludes] *aftercare following joint replacement (V54.81)*

V57 Care involving use of rehabilitation procedures

Revise	**V57.3**	**Speech-language therapy**

V60 Housing, household, and economic circumstances

	V60.8	**Other specified housing or economic circumstances**
New code	**V60.81**	**Foster care (status)**
New code	**V60.89**	**Other specified housing or economic circumstances**

V61 Other family circumstances

   V61.0 Family disruption

      V61.01 Family disruption due to family member on military deployment

Add
         Excludes *family disruption due to family member on non-military extended absence from home (V61.08)*

New code
      V61.07 Family disruption due to death of family member

         Excludes *bereavement (V62.82)*

New code
      V61.08 Family disruption due to other extended absence of family member

         Excludes *family disruption due to family member on military deployment (V61.01)*

   V61.2 Parent-child problems

New code
      V61.23 Counseling for parent-biological child problem

         Concern about behavior of biological child
         Parent-biological child conflict
         Parent-biological child relationship problem

New code
      V61.24 Counseling for parent-adopted child problem

         Concern about behavior of adopted child
         Parent-adopted child conflict
         Parent-adopted child relationship problem

New code
      V61.25 Counseling for parent (guardian)-foster child problem

         Concern about behavior of foster child
         Parent (guardian)-foster child conflict
         Parent (guardian)-foster child relationship problem

Revise
      V61.29 Other parent-child problems

Delete
         ~~Problem concerning adopted or foster child~~

   V61.4 Health problems within family

New code
      V61.42 Substance abuse in family

V62 Other psychosocial circumstances

   V62.8 Other psychological or physical stress, not elsewhere classified

      V62.82 Bereavement, uncomplicated

Add
         Excludes *family disruption due to death of family member (V61.07)*

V65 Other persons seeking consultation

   V65.1 Person consulting on behalf of another person

Revise
      V65.11 Pediatric pre-birth visit for expectant ~~mother~~ parent(s)

         Pre-adoption visit for adoptive parent(s)

Add
V70 General medical examination

   V70.0 Routine general medical examination at a health care facility

Revise
      Excludes *health checkup of infant or child over 28 days old (V20.2)*

Add
        health supervision of newborn 8 to 28 days old (V20.32)

Add
        health supervision of newborn under 8 days old (V20.31)

V72 Special investigations and examinations

Add
      Excludes *health supervision of newborn 8 to 28 days old (V20.32)*

Add
        health supervision of newborn under 8 days old (V20.31)

Revise
        routine examination of infant or child over 28 days old (V20.2)

   V72.5 Radiological examination, not elsewhere classified

Delete
      Excludes ~~examination for suspected tuberculosis (V71.2)~~

Add
        radiologic examinations as part of pre-procedural testing (V72.81-V72.84)

   V72.6 Laboratory examination

Add
      Encounters for blood and urine testing

Delete
      Excludes ~~that for suspected disorder (V71.0-V71.9)~~

New code
      V72.60 Laboratory examination, unspecified

New code
      V72.61 Antibody response examination

         Immunity status testing

         Excludes *encounter for allergy testing (V72.7)*

New code
      V72.62 Laboratory examination ordered as part of a routine general medical examination

         Blood tests for routine general physical examination

New code
      V72.63 Pre-procedural laboratory examination

         Blood tests prior to treatment or procedure
         Pre-operative laboratory examination

New code
      V72.69 Other laboratory examination

   V72.8 Other specified examinations

Add
      Excludes *pre-procedural laboratory examinations (V72.63)*

      V72.83 Other specified preoperative examination

Add
        Examination prior to chemotherapy

V80 Special screening for neurological, eye, and ear diseases

V80.0 Neurological conditions

New code V80.01 Traumatic brain injury

New code V80.09 Other neurological conditions

V87 Other specified personal exposures and history presenting hazards to health

V87.3 Contact with and (suspected) exposure to other potentially hazardous substances

New code V87.32 Contact with and (suspected) exposure to algae bloom

V87.4 Personal history of drug therapy

New code V87.43 Personal history of estrogen therapy

New code V87.44 Personal history of inhaled steroid therapy

New code V87.45 Personal history of systemic steroid therapy
Personal history of steroid therapy NOS

New code V87.46 Personal history of immunosuppression therapy

Excludes *personal history of steroid therapy (V87.44, V87.45)*

Revise **SUPPLEMENTARY CLASSIFICATION OF EXTERNAL CAUSES OF INJURY AND POISONING (E000-E999)**

Revise section: Machinery accidents [other than those connected with transport] are classifiable to category E919, in which the fourth digit allows a broad classification of the type of machinery involved. ~~If a more detailed classification of type of machinery is required, it is suggested that the "Classification of Industrial Accidents according to Agency," prepared by the International Labor Office, be used in addition; it is included in this publication.~~

Categories for "late effects" of accidents and other external causes are to be found at E929, E959, E969, E977, E989, and E999.

~~Definitions and examples related to transport accidents~~

New section **EXTERNAL CAUSE STATUS (E000)**

Add **Note:** A code from category E000 should be used in conjunction with the external cause code(s) assigned to a record to indicate the status of the person at the time the event occurred. A single code from category E000 should be assigned for an encounter.

New category E000 **External cause status**

New code E000.0 **Civilian activity done for income or pay**
Civilian activity done for financial or other compensation
Excludes *military activity (E000.1)*

New code E000.1 **Military activity**
Excludes *activity of off duty military personnel (E000.8)*

New code E000.8 **Other external cause status**
Activity NEC
Hobby not done for income
Leisure activity
Off-duty activity of military personnel
Recreation or sport not for income or while a student
Student activity
Volunteer activity
Excludes *civilian activity done for income or compensation (E000.0)*
military activity (E000.1)

New code E000.9 **Unspecified external cause status**

New section **ACTIVITY (E001-E030)**

Note: Categories E001 to E030 are provided for use to indicate the activity of the person seeking healthcare for an injury or health condition, such as a heart attack while shoveling snow, which resulted from, or was contributed to, by the activity. These codes are appropriate for use for both acute injuries, such as those from chapter 17, and conditions that are due to the long-term, cumulative effects of an activity, such as those from chapter 13. They are also appropriate for use with external cause codes for cause and intent if identifying the activity provides additional information on the event.

These codes should be used in conjunction with other external cause codes for external cause status (E000) and place of occurrence (E849).

This section contains the following broad activity categories:

E001 Activities involving walking and running

E002 Activities involving water and water craft

E003 Activities involving ice and snow

E004 Activities involving climbing, rappelling, and jumping off

E005 Activities involving dancing and other rhythmic movement

E006 Activities involving other sports and athletics played individually

E007 Activities involving other sports and athletics played as a team or group

E008 Activities involving other specified sports and athletics

E009 Activity involving other cardiorespiratory exercise

E010 Activity involving other muscle strengthening exercises

E011 Activities involving computer technology and electronic devices

E012 Activities involving arts and handcrafts

E013 Activities involving personal hygiene and household maintenance

E014 Activities involving person providing caregiving

E015 Activities involving food preparation, cooking and grilling

E016 Activities involving property and land maintenance, building and construction

E017 Activities involving roller coasters and other types of external motion

E018 Activities involving playing musical instrument

E019 Activities involving animal care

E029 Other activity

E030 Unspecified activity

E001 Activities involving walking and running

New category

| **Excludes** | walking an animal (E019.0) |
| | walking or running on a treadmill (E009.0) |

New code **E001.0 Walking, marching and hiking**
Walking, marching and hiking on level or elevated terrain

| **Excludes** | mountain climbing (E004.0) |

New code **E001.1 Running**

New category **E002 Activities involving water and water craft**

| **Excludes** | activities involving ice (E003.0-E003.9) |
| | boating and other watercraft transport accidents (E830-E838) |

New code **E002.0 Swimming**

New code **E002.1 Springboard and platform diving**

New code **E002.2 Water polo**

New code **E002.3 Water aerobics and water exercise**

New code **E002.4 Underwater diving and snorkeling**
SCUBA diving

New code **E002.5 Rowing, canoeing, kayaking, rafting and tubing**
Canoeing, kayaking, rafting and tubing in calm and turbulent water

New code **E002.6 Water skiing and wake boarding**

New code **E002.7 Surfing, windsurfing and boogie boarding**

New code **E002.8 Water sliding**

New code **E002.9 Other activity involving water and watercraft**
Activity involving water NOS
Parasailing
Water survival training and testing

New category **E003 Activities involving ice and snow**

| **Excludes** | shoveling ice and snow (E016.0) |

New code **E003.0 Ice skating**
Figure skating (singles) (pairs)
Ice dancing

| **Excludes** | ice hockey (E003.1) |

New code **E003.1 Ice hockey**

New code **E003.2 Snow (alpine) (downhill) skiing, snow boarding, sledding, tobogganing and snow tubing**

| **Excludes** | cross country skiing (E003.3) |

New code **E003.3 Cross country skiing**
Nordic skiing

New code **E003.9 Other activity involving ice and snow**
Activity involving ice and snow NOS

New category **E004 Activities involving climbing, rappelling and jumping off**

Excludes	hiking on level or elevated terrain (E001.0)
	jumping rope (E006.5)
	sky diving (E840-E844)
	trampoline jumping (E005.3)

New code **E004.0 Mountain climbing, rock climbing and wall climbing**

New code **E004.1 Rappelling**

New code **E004.2 BASE jumping**
Building, Antenna, Span, Earth jumping

New code **E004.3 Bungee jumping**

New code **E004.4 Hang gliding**

New code **E004.9 Other activity involving climbing, rappelling and jumping off**

New category **E005 Activities involving dancing and other rhythmic movement**

| **Excludes** | martial arts (E008.4) |

New code **E005.0 Dancing**

New code **E005.1 Yoga**

New code **E005.2 Gymnastics**
Rhythmic gymnastics

| **Excludes** | trampoline (E005.3) |

New code **E005.3 Trampoline**

New code **E005.4 Cheerleading**

New code **E005.9 Other activity involving dancing and other rhythmic movements**

New category **E006 Activities involving other sports and athletics played individually**

Excludes	dancing (E005.0)
	gymnastic (E005.2)
	trampoline (E005.3)
	yoga (E005.1)

New code **E006.0 Roller skating (inline) and skateboarding**

New code **E006.1 Horseback riding**

New code **E006.2 Golf**

New code **E006.3 Bowling**

New code **E006.4 Bike riding**

| **Excludes** | transport accident involving bike riding (E800-E829) |

New code **E006.5 Jumping rope**

New code **E006.6 Non-running track and field events**

| **Excludes** | running (any form) (E001.1) |

New code **E006.9 Other activity involving other sports and athletics played individually**

Excludes	activities involving climbing, rappelling, and jumping (E004.0-E004.9)
	activities involving ice and snow (E003.0-E003.9)
	activities involving walking and running (E001.0-E001.9)
	activities involving water and watercraft (E002.0-E002.9)

New category	**E007**	**Activities involving other sports and athletics played as a team or group**

> **Excludes** *ice hockey (E003.1)*
> *water polo (E002.2)*

New code **E007.0 American tackle football**
Football NOS

New code **E007.1 American flag or touch football**

New code **E007.2 Rugby**

New code **E007.3 Baseball**
Softball

New code **E007.4 Lacrosse and field hockey**

New code **E007.5 Soccer**

New code **E007.6 Basketball**

New code **E007.7 Volleyball (beach) (court)**

New code **E007.8 Physical games generally associated with school recess, summer camp and children**
Capture the flag
Dodge ball
Four square
Kickball

New code **E007.9 Other activity involving other sports and athletics played as a team or group**
Cricket

New category **E008 Activities involving other specified sports and athletics**

New code **E008.0 Boxing**

New code **E008.1 Wrestling**

New code **E008.2 Racquet and hand sports**
Handball
Racquetball
Squash
Tennis

New code **E008.3 Frisbee**
Ultimate frisbee

New code **E008.4 Martial arts**
Combatives

New code **E008.9 Other specified sports and athletics activity**

> **Excludes** *sports and athletics activities specified in categories E001-E007*

New category **E009 Activity involving other cardiorespiratory exercise**
Activity involving physical training

New code **E009.0 Exercise machines primarily for cardiorespiratory conditioning**
Elliptical and stepper machines
Stationary bike
Treadmill

New code **E009.1 Calisthenics**
Jumping jacks
Warm up and cool down

New code **E009.2 Aerobic and step exercise**

New code **E009.3 Circuit training**

New code **E009.4 Obstacle course**
Challenge course
Confidence course

New code **E009.5 Grass drills**
Guerilla drills

New code **E009.9 Other activity involving other cardiorespiratory exercise**

> **Excludes** *activities involving cardio-respiratory exercise specified in categories E001-E008*

New category **E010 Activity involving other muscle strengthening exercises**

New code **E010.0 Exercise machines primarily for muscle strengthening**

New code **E010.1 Push-ups, pull-ups, sit-ups**

New code **E010.2 Free weights**
Barbells
Dumbbells

New code **E010.3 Pilates**

New code **E010.9 Other activity involving other muscle strengthening exercises**

> **Excludes** *activities involving muscle strengthening specified in categories E001-E009*

New category **E011 Activities involving computer technology and electronic devices**

> **Excludes** *electronic musical keyboard or instruments (E018.0)*

New code **E011.0 Computer keyboarding**
Electronic game playing using keyboard or other stationary device

New code **E011.1 Hand held interactive electronic device**
Cellular telephone and communication device
Electronic game playing using interactive device

> **Excludes** *electronic game playing using keyboard or other stationary device (E011.0)*

New code **E011.9 Other activity involving computer technology and electronic devices**

New category **E012 Activities involving arts and handcrafts**

> **Excludes** *activities involving playing musical instrument (E018.0-E018.3)*

New code **E012.0 Knitting and crocheting**

New code **E012.1 Sewing**

New code **E012.2 Furniture building and finishing**
Furniture repair

New code **E012.9 Activity involving other arts and handcrafts**

New category **E013 Activities involving personal hygiene and household maintenance**

> **Excludes** *activities involving cooking and grilling (E015.0-E015.9)*
> *activities involving property and land maintenance, building and construction (E016.0-E016.9)*
> *activity involving persons providing caregiving (E014.0-E014.9)*
> *dishwashing (E015.0)*
> *food preparation (E015.0)*
> *gardening (E016.1)*

New code **E013.0 Personal bathing and showering**

New code **E013.1 Laundry**

New code	E013.2	Vacuuming
New code	E013.3	Ironing
New code	E013.4	Floor mopping and cleaning
New code	E013.5	Residential relocation
		Packing up and unpacking involved in moving to a new residence
New code	E013.8	Other personal hygiene activity
New code	E013.9	Other household maintenance
New category	E014	Activities involving person providing caregiving
New code	E014.0	Caregiving involving bathing
New code	E014.1	Caregiving involving lifting
New code	E014.9	Other activity involving person providing caregiving
New category	E015	Activities involving food preparation, cooking and grilling
New code	E015.0	Food preparation and clean up
		Dishwashing
New code	E015.1	Grilling and smoking food
New code	E015.2	Cooking and baking
		Use of stove, oven and microwave oven
New code	E015.9	Other activity involving cooking and grilling
New category	E016	Activities involving property and land maintenance, building and construction
New code	E016.0	Digging, shoveling and raking
		Dirt digging
		Raking leaves
		Snow shoveling
New code	E016.1	Gardening and landscaping
		Pruning, trimming shrubs, weeding
New code	E016.2	Building and construction
New code	E016.9	Other activity involving property and land maintenance, building and construction
New category	E017	Activities involving roller coasters and other types of external motion
New code	E017.0	Rollercoaster riding
New code	E017.9	Other activity involving external motion
New category	E018	Activities involving playing musical instrument
		Activity involving playing electric musical instrument
New code	E018.0	Piano playing
		Musical keyboard (electronic) playing
New code	E018.1	Drum and other percussion instrument playing
New code	E018.2	String instrument playing
New code	E018.3	Wind and brass instrument playing
New category	E019	Activities involving animal care
		Excludes _horseback riding (E006.1)_
New code	E019.0	Walking an animal
New code	E019.1	Milking an animal
New code	E019.2	Grooming and shearing an animal
New code	E019.9	Other activity involving animal care

New category	E029	Other activity
New code	E029.0	Refereeing a sports activity
New code	E029.1	Spectator at an event
New code	E029.2	Rough housing and horseplay
New code	E029.9	Other activity
New code	E030	Unspecified activity

New section

TRANSPORT ACCIDENTS (E800-E848)

Add   Definitions and examples related to transport accidents

(a) A transport accident (E800-E848) is any accident involving a device designed primarily for, or being used at the time primarily for, conveying persons or goods from one place to another.

WATER TRANSPORT ACCIDENTS (E830-E838)

The following fourth-digit subdivisions are for use with categories E830-E838 to identify the injured person:

New fourth-digit sub   .7 Occupant of military watercraft, any type

	E876	**Other and unspecified misadventures during medical care**
Revise	E876.5	Performance of ~~inappropriate~~ wrong operation (procedure) on correct patient
Add		Wrong device implanted into correct surgical site
Add		**Excludes** _correct operation (procedure) performed on wrong body part (E876.7)_
New code	E876.6	Performance of operation (procedure) on patient not scheduled for surgery
		Performance of operation (procedure) intended for another patient
		Performance of operation (procedure) on wrong patient
New code	E876.7	Performance of correct operation (procedure) on wrong side/body part
		Performance of correct operation (procedure) on wrong side
		Performance of correct operation (procedure) on wrong site
	E918	**Caught accidentally in or between objects**
Add		**Excludes** _injury caused by:_ _mechanism or component of firearm and air gun (E928.7)_
	E919	**Accidents caused by machinery**
Add		**Excludes** _injury caused by:_ _mechanism or component of firearm and air gun (E928.7)_
	E920	**Accidents caused by cutting and piercing instruments or objects**
Add		**Excludes** _injury caused by mechanism or component of firearm and air gun (E928.7)_
	E922	**Accident caused by firearm and air gun missile**
Add		**Excludes** _injury caused by mechanism or component of firearm and air gun (E928.7)_
	E923	**Accident caused by explosive material**
Add		**Excludes** _injury caused by mechanism or component of firearm and air gun (E928.7)_

	E927 Overexertion and strenuous and repetitive movements or loads
Add	Use additional code to identify activity (E001-E030)
	E928 Other and unspecified environmental and accidental causes
New code	**E928.7 Mechanism or component of firearm and air gun**

Injury due to:
   explosion of gun parts
   recoil
Pierced, cut, crushed, or pinched
   by slide trigger mechanism,
   scope or other gun part
Powder burn from firearm or air
   gun

   Excludes   accident caused by firearm
             and air gun missile
             (E922.0-E922.9)

DRUGS, MEDICINAL AND BIOLOGICAL SUBSTANCES CAUSING ADVERSE EFFECTS IN THERAPEUTIC USE (E930-E949)

| Revise | Excludes   administration with suicidal or homicidal intent or intent to harm, or in circumstances classifiable to ~~E980-E989~~ (E950.0-E950.5, E962.0, E980.0-E980.5) |

INJURY RESULTING FROM OPERATIONS OF WAR (E990-E999)

| Revise | Includes   injuries to military personnel and civilians caused by war and civil insurrections and occurring during the time of war and insurrection, and peacekeeping missions |

E990 Injury due to war operations by fires and conflagrations

	E990.0 From gasoline bomb
Add	Incendiary bomb
New code	**E990.1 From flamethrower**
New code	**E990.2 From incendiary bullet**
New code	**E990.3 From fire caused indirectly from conventional weapon**

   Excludes   fire aboard military aircraft
             (E994.3)

E991 Injury due to war operations by bullets and fragments

| Add | Excludes   injury due to bullets and fragments due to war operations, but occurring after cessation of hostilities (E998.0)
injury due to explosion of artillery shells and mortars (E993.2)
injury due to explosion of improvised explosive device [IED] (E993.3-E993.5)
injury due to sea-based artillery shell (E992.3) |

| New code | **E991.4 Fragments from munitions** |

Fragments from:
   artillery shell
   bombs, except antipersonnel
   detonation of unexploded
      ordnance [UXO]
   grenade
   guided missile
   land mine
   rockets
   shell

| New code | **E991.5 Fragments from person-borne improvised explosive device [IED]** |
| New code | **E991.6 Fragments from vehicle-borne improvised explosive device [IED]** |

IED borne by land, air, or water
   transport vehicle

| New code | **E991.7 Fragments from other improvised explosive device [IED]** |

Roadside IED

| New code | **E991.8 Fragments from weapons** |

Fragments from:
   artillery
   autocannons
   automatic grenade launchers
   missile launchers
   mortars
   small arms

E991.9 Other and unspecified fragments

| Delete | ~~Fragments from:~~
~~artillery shell~~
~~bombs, except antipersonnel~~
~~grenade~~
~~guided missile~~
~~land mine~~
~~rockets~~
~~shell~~ |
| Revise | Shrapnel NOS |

E992 Injury due to war operations by explosion of marine weapons

| Delete | ~~Depth charge~~
~~Marine mines~~
~~Mine NOS, at sea or in harbor~~
~~Sea-based artillery shell~~
~~Torpedo~~
~~Underwater blast~~ |
New code	**E992.0 Torpedo**
New code	**E992.1 Depth charge**
New code	**E992.2 Marine mines**

Marine mines at sea or in harbor

New code	**E992.3 Sea-based artillery shell**
New code	**E992.8 Other by other marine weapons**
New code	**E992.9 Unspecified marine weapon**

Underwater blast NOS

E993 Injury due to war operations by other explosion

| Delete | ~~Accidental explosion of munitions being used in war~~
~~Accidental explosion of own weapons~~
~~Air blast NOS~~
~~Blast NOS~~
~~Explosion NOS~~
~~Explosion of:~~
~~artillery shell~~
~~breech block~~
~~cannon block~~
~~mortar bomb~~
~~Injury by weapon burst~~ |
Add	Injuries due to direct or indirect pressure or air blast of an explosion occurring during war operations
Add	Excludes injury due to fragments resulting from an explosion (E991.0-E991.9)
Add	injury due to detonation of unexploded ordnance but occurring after cessation of hostilities (E998.0-E998.9)
Add	injury due to nuclear weapons (E996.0-E996.9)
New code	**E993.0 Aerial bomb**
New code	**E993.1 Guided missile**

New code	**E993.2**	**Mortar** Artillery shell
New code	**E993.3**	**Person-borne improvised explosive device [IED]**
New code	**E993.4**	**Vehicle-borne improvised explosive device [IED]** IED borne by land, air, or water transport vehicle
New code	**E993.5**	**Other improvised explosive device [IED]** Roadside IED
New code	**E993.6**	**Unintentional detonation of own munitions** Unintentional detonation of own ammunition (artillery) (mortars)
New code	**E993.7**	**Unintentional discharge of own munitions launch device** Unintentional explosion of own: Autocannons Automatic grenade launchers Missile launchers Small arms
New code	**E993.8**	**Other specified explosion** Bomb Grenade Land mine
New code	**E993.9**	**Unspecified explosion** Air blast NOS Blast NOS Blast wave NOS Blast wind NOS Explosion NOS
	E994	**Injury due to war operations by destruction of aircraft**
Delete		~~Airplane:~~ ~~burned~~ ~~exploded~~ ~~shot down~~ ~~Crushed by falling airplane~~
New code	**E994.0**	**Destruction of aircraft due to enemy fire or explosives** Air to air missile Explosive device placed on aircraft Rocket propelled grenade [RPG] Small arms fire Surface to air missile
New code	**E994.1**	**Unintentional destruction of aircraft due to own onboard explosives**
New code	**E994.2**	**Destruction of aircraft due to collision with other aircraft**
New code	**E994.3**	**Destruction of aircraft due to onboard fire**
New code	**E994.8**	**Other destruction of aircraft**
New code	**E994.9**	**Unspecified destruction of aircraft**

	E995	**Injury due to war operations by other and unspecified forms of conventional warfare**
Delete		~~Battle wounds~~ ~~Bayonet injury~~ ~~Drowned in war operations~~
New code	**E995.0**	**Unarmed hand-to-hand combat** **Excludes** *intentional restriction of airway (E995.3)*
New code	**E995.1**	**Struck by blunt object** Baton (nightstick) Stave
New code	**E995.2**	**Piercing object** Bayonet Knife Sword
New code	**E995.3**	**Intentional restriction of air and airway** Intentional submersion Strangulation Suffocation
New code	**E995.4**	**Unintentional drowning due to inability to surface or obtain air** Submersion
New code	**E995.8**	**Other forms of conventional warfare**
New code	**E995.9**	**Unspecified form of conventional warfare**
	E996	**Injury due to war operations by nuclear weapons**
Delete		~~Blast effects~~ ~~Exposure to ionizing radiation from nuclear weapons~~ ~~Fireball effects~~ ~~Heat~~ ~~Other direct and secondary effects of nuclear weapons~~
Add		Dirty bomb NOS
Add		**Excludes** *late effects of injury due to nuclear weapons (E999.1, E999.0)*
New code	**E996.0**	**Direct blast effect of nuclear weapon** Injury to bodily organs due to blast pressure
New code	**E996.1**	**Indirect blast effect of nuclear weapon** Injury due to being thrown by blast Injury due to being struck or crushed by blast debris
New code	**E996.2**	**Thermal radiation effect of nuclear weapon** Burns due to thermal radiation Fireball effects Flash burns Heat effects
New code	**E996.3**	**Nuclear radiation effects** Acute radiation exposure Beta burns Fallout exposure Radiation sickness Secondary effects of nuclear weapons
New code	**E996.8**	**Other effects of nuclear weapons**
New code	**E996.9**	**Unspecified effect of nuclear weapon**

	E997	Injury due to war operations by other forms of unconventional warfare
New code	E997.3	Weapon of mass destruction [WMD], unspecified
	E998	Injury due to war operations but occurring after cessation of hostilities
New code	E998.0	Explosion of mines
New code	E998.1	Explosion of bombs
New code	E998.8	Injury due to other war operations but occurring after cessation of hostilities
New code	E998.9	Injury due to unspecified war operations but occurring after cessation of hostilities

VOLUME 3 CHANGES EFFECTIVE OCTOBER 1, 2009

Tabular List

Add
inclusion
term

00.2 Intravascular imaging of blood vessels
Virtual histology intravascular
ultrasound [VH-IVUS]

Add
exclusion
note

Excludes *intravascular imaging of vessel(s) by OCT (38.24-38.25)*

Revise
code title

00.56 Insertion or replacement of implantable pressure sensor (lead) for intracardiac or great vessel hemodynamic monitoring

Revise
code title

00.57 Implantation or replacement of subcutaneous device for intracardiac or great vessel hemodynamic monitoring

01.59 Other excision or destruction of lesion or tissue of brain

Add
exclusion
term

Excludes *laser interstitial thermal therapy [LITT] of lesion or tissue of brain under guidance (17.61)*

06.31 Excision of lesion of thyroid

Add
exclusion
term

Excludes *laser interstitial thermal therapy [LITT] of lesion or tissue of neck under guidance (17.62)*

13.2 Extracapsular extraction of lens by linear extraction technique

Add code
also note

Code also any synchronous insertion of pseudophakos (13.71)

13.3 Extracapsular extraction of lens by simple aspiration (and irrigation) technique

Add code
also note

Code also any synchronous insertion of pseudophakos (13.71)

13.4 Extracapsular extraction of lens by fragmentation and aspiration technique

Add code
also note

Code also any synchronous insertion of pseudophakos (13.71)

New sub   **17. 5 Additional cardiovascular procedures**

New code   **17.51 Implantation of rechargeable cardiac contractility modulation [CCM], total system**

Note: Device testing during procedure – *omit code*
Implantation of CCM system includes formation of pocket, transvenous leads, including placement of leads, placement of catheter into left ventricle, intraoperative procedures for evaluation of lead signals, obtaining sensing threshold measurements, obtaining defibrillator threshold measurements.

Includes implantation of device with removal of existing device

Code also any concomitant:
coronary bypass (36.10– 6.19)
extracorporeal circulation (39.61)
insertion or replacement of automatic cardioverter/ defibrillator, total system [AICD] (37.94)

Excludes *implantation of CCM pulse generator only (17.52)*

New code   **17.52 Implantation or replacement of cardiac contractility modulation [CCM] rechargeable pulse generator only**

Note: Device testing during procedure – *omit code*
Implantation of CCM device with removal of any existing CCM device

Code also any concomitant:
revision of device pocket (37.79)
revision of lead [electrode] (37.75)

New sub   **17.6 Laser interstitial thermal therapy [LITT] under guidance**
Focused laser interstitial thermal therapy [f-LITT] under MRI guidance
MRI-guided LITT

New code   **17.61 Laser interstitial thermal therapy [LITT] of lesion or tissue of brain under guidance**
Focused laser interstitial thermal therapy [f-LITT] under MRI guidance
MRI-guided LITT of lesion or tissue of brain

Excludes *laser interstitial thermal therapy [LITT] of lesion or tissue of head under guidance (17.62)*

New code

17.62 Laser interstitial thermal therapy [LITT] of lesion or tissue of head and neck under guidance
Focused laser interstitial thermal therapy [f-LITT] under MRI guidance
MRI-guided LITT of lesion or tissue of head and neck

Excludes *laser interstitial thermal therapy [LITT] of lesion or tissue of brain under guidance (17.61)*

New code

17.63 Laser interstitial thermal therapy [LITT] of lesion or tissue of liver under guidance
Focused laser interstitial thermal therapy [f-LITT] under MRI guidance
MRI-guided LITT of lesion or tissue of liver

New code

17.69 Laser interstitial thermal therapy [LITT] of lesion or tissue of other and unspecified site under guidance
Focused laser interstitial thermal therapy [f-LITT] under MRI guidance
MRI-guided LITT of lesion or tissue of breast
MRI-guided LITT of lesion or tissue of lung
MRI-guided LITT of lesion or tissue of prostate

Excludes *laser interstitial thermal therapy [LITT] of lesion or tissue of brain under guidance (17.61)*
laser interstitial thermal therapy [LITT] of lesion or tissue of head and neck under guidance (17.62)
laser interstitial thermal therapy [LITT] of lesion or tissue of liver under guidance (17.63)

New sub

17.7 Other diagnostic and therapeutic procedures

New code

17.70 Intravenous infusion of clofarabine

Excludes *injection or infusion of cancer chemotherapeutic substance (99.25)*

Revise sub title

27.5 Plastic repair of lip and mouth

32.29 Other local excision or destruction of lesion or tissue of lung

Add exclusion term

Excludes *laser interstitial thermal therapy [LITT] of lesion or tissue of lung under guidance (17.69)*

Add inclusion term

33.24 Closed [endoscopic] biopsy of bronchus
Transbronchoscopic needle aspiration [TBNA]

Revise code title

33.71 Endoscopic insertion or replacement of bronchial valve(s), single lobe

Add exclusion term

Excludes *endoscopic insertion or replacement of bronchial valve(s), multiple lobes (33.73)*

New Code

33.73 Endoscopic insertion or replacement of bronchial valve(s), multiple lobes

Excludes *endoscopic insertion or replacement of bronchial valve(s), single lobe (33.71)*

34.1 Incision of mediastinum

Add code also note

Code also any biopsy, if performed

34.22 Mediastinoscopy

Revise code also note

Code also any ~~lymph node~~ biopsy, if performed ~~(40.11)~~

37.79 Revision or relocation of cardiac device pocket
Removal of implantable hemodynamic presssure sensor (lead) and monitor device

Revise inclusion term

37.94 Implantation or replacement of automatic cardioverter/ defibrillator, total system [AICD]

Revise code also note

Code also any concomitant procedure [e.g., coronary bypass] (36.010-36.19) or CCM, total system (17.51)]

38.23 Intravascular spectroscopy

Revise Includes term

Includes ~~imaging~~ spectroscopy of both coronary and peripheral vessels

Revise exclusion term

Excludes *intravascular imaging of: coronary vessels (00.24, 38.24) peripheral vessels (00.23, 38.25)*

New code

38.24 Intravascular imaging of coronary vessel(s) by optical coherence tomography [OCT]

New code

38.25 Intravascular imaging of non-coronary vessel(s) by optical coherence tomography [OCT]

Excludes *intravascular imaging of coronary vessel(s) by OCT (38.24)*

39.50 Angioplasty or atherectomy of other non-coronary vessel(s)

Add code also note

Code also any:
insertion of drug-eluting peripheral vessel stent (00.55)

Revise code also note

insertion of non- ~~coronary~~ drug-eluting peripheral vessel stent(s) or stent graft(s) (39.90)

Revise sub title	**39.7**	**Endovascular ~~repair~~ procedures <u>on</u> ~~of~~ vessel(s)**
Add inclusion term		<u>Embolization</u>
Add inclusion term		<u>Implantation</u>
Add inclusion term		<u>Occlusion</u>
Add inclusion term		<u>Removal</u>
Add inclusion term		<u>Repair</u>
Revise code title	**39.72**	**Endovascular ~~repair~~ <u>embolization or occlusion</u> of head and neck vessels**
Delete inclusion term		~~Coil embolization or occlusion~~

Excludes
Add exclusion term		*<u>embolization of head or neck vessels using bare coils (39.75)</u>*
Add exclusion term		*<u>embolization of head or neck vessels using bioactive coils (39.76)</u>*

39.74 Endovascular removal of obstruction from head and neck vessel(s)

Excludes
Revise exclusion term		*occlusive endovascular ~~repair~~ <u>embolization</u> of head or neck vessel(s) using bare coils ~~(39.72)~~ ~~(39.75)~~*
Add exclusion term		*<u>occlusive endovascular embolization of head or neck vessel(s) using bioactive coils (39.76)</u>*

New code	**39.75**	**Endovascular embolization or occlusion of vessel(s) of head or neck using bare coils**
		Bare metal coils
		Bare platinum coils [BPC]
		That for treatment of aneurysm, arteriovenous malformation [AVM] or fistula
New code	**39.76**	**Endovascular embolization or occlusion of vessel(s) of head or neck using bioactive coils**
		Biodegradable inner luminal polymer coils
		Coil embolization or occlusion utilizing bioactive coils
		Coils containing polyglycolic acid [PGA]
		That for treatment of aneurysm, arteriovenous malformation [AVM] or fistula

Revise code title	**39.79**	**Other endovascular ~~repair~~ procedures ~~(of aneurysm)~~ ~~of~~ <u>on</u> other vessels**
Revise inclusion term		<u>Other</u> ~~C~~<u>c</u>oil embolization or occlusion
Add inclusion term		<u>Repair of aneurysm</u>

Excludes
Add exclusion term		*<u>abdominal aortic aneurysm resection [AAA] (38.44)</u>*
Add exclusion term		*<u>endovascular implantation of graft in abdominal aorta (39.71)</u>*
Revise exclusion term		*endovascular ~~repair~~ <u>embolization or occlusion</u> of head and neck vessels, <u>bare metal coils</u> ~~(39.72)~~ <u>(39.75)</u>*
Add exclusion term		*<u>endovascular embolization or occlusion of head and neck vessels, bioactive coils (39.76)</u>*
Add exclusion term		*thoracic aortic aneurysm resection (38.45)*

Revise code title	**39.90**	**Insertion of non-drug-eluting peripheral <u>(non-coronary)</u> vessel stent(s)**
	46.85	**Dilation of intestine**
Add exclusion term		**Excludes** *<u>with insertion of colonic stent (46.86-46.87)</u>*
New code	**46.86**	**Endoscopic insertion of colonic stent(s)**
		Colonoscopy (flexible) (through stoma) with transendoscopic stent placement
		Combined with fluoroscopic-guided insertion
		Stent endoprosthesis of colon
		Through the scope [TTS] technique

Excludes *other non-endoscopic insertion of colonic stent (46.87)*

New code	**46.87**	**Other insertion of colonic stent(s)**

Includes that by:
fluoroscopic guidance only
rectal guiding tube
Non-endoscopic insertion

Code also any synchronous diagnostic procedure(s)

Excludes *endoscopic insertion of colonic stent (46.86)*

50.29 Other destruction of lesion of liver

Add exclusion term

| Excludes | *laser interstitial thermal therapy [LITT] of lesion or tissue of liver under guidance (17.63)* |

60.61 Local excision of lesion of prostate

Delete inclusion term

~~Excision of prostatic lesion by any approach~~

Add exclusion term

| Excludes | *laser interstitial thermal therapy [LITT] of lesion or tissue of prostate under guidance (17.69)* |

Revise code title

80.00 Arthrotomy for removal of prosthesis without replacement, unspecified site

Revise code title

80.01 Arthrotomy for removal of prosthesis without replacement, shoulder

Revise code title

80.02 Arthrotomy for removal of prosthesis without replacement, elbow

Revise code title

80.03 Arthrotomy for removal of prosthesis without replacement, wrist

Revise code title

80.04 Arthrotomy for removal of prosthesis without replacement, hand and finger

Revise code title

80.05 Arthrotomy for removal of prosthesis without replacement, hip

Revise code title

80.06 Arthrotomy for removal of prosthesis without replacement, knee

Revise code title

80.07 Arthrotomy for removal of prosthesis without replacement, ankle

Revise code title

80.08 Arthrotomy for removal of prosthesis without replacement, foot and toe

Revise code title

80.09 Arthrotomy for removal of prosthesis without replacement, other specified sites

81.5 Joint replacement of lower extremity

Add note

Note: Removal of prior prosthesis – omit code

81.54 Total knee replacement

Add inclusion term

Partial knee replacement

Add inclusion term

81.84 Total elbow replacement

Partial elbow replacement

85.20 Excision or destruction of breast tissue, not otherwise specified

Add exclusion term

| Excludes | *laser interstitial thermal therapy [LITT] of lesion or tissue of breast under guidance (17.69)* |

88.91 Magnetic resonance imaging of brain and brain stem

Add exclusion term

| Excludes | *laser interstitial thermal therapy [LITT] of lesion or tissue of brain under guidance (17.61)* |

88.92 Magnetic resonance imaging of chest and myocardium

Add exclusion term

| Excludes | *laser interstitial thermal therapy [LITT] of lesion or tissue of breast under guidance (17.69) laser interstitial thermal therapy [LITT] of lesion or tissue of lung under guidance (17.69)* |

88.95 Magnetic resonance imaging of pelvis, prostate, and bladder

Add exclusion term

| Excludes | *laser interstitial thermal therapy [LITT] of lesion or tissue of prostate under guidance (17.69)* |

88.97 Magnetic resonance imaging of other and unspecified sites

Add exclusion term

| Excludes | *laser interstitial thermal therapy [LITT] of lesion or tissue of other and unspecified site under guidance (17.69)* |

99.25 Injection or infusion of cancer chemotherapeutic substance

Add exclusion term

| Excludes | *intravenous infusion of clofarabine (17.70)* |

STANDARD EDITION

INCLUDES NETTER ANATOMY ART

2010

ICD-9-CM

VOLUMES 1, 2, & 3

FOR HOSPITALS

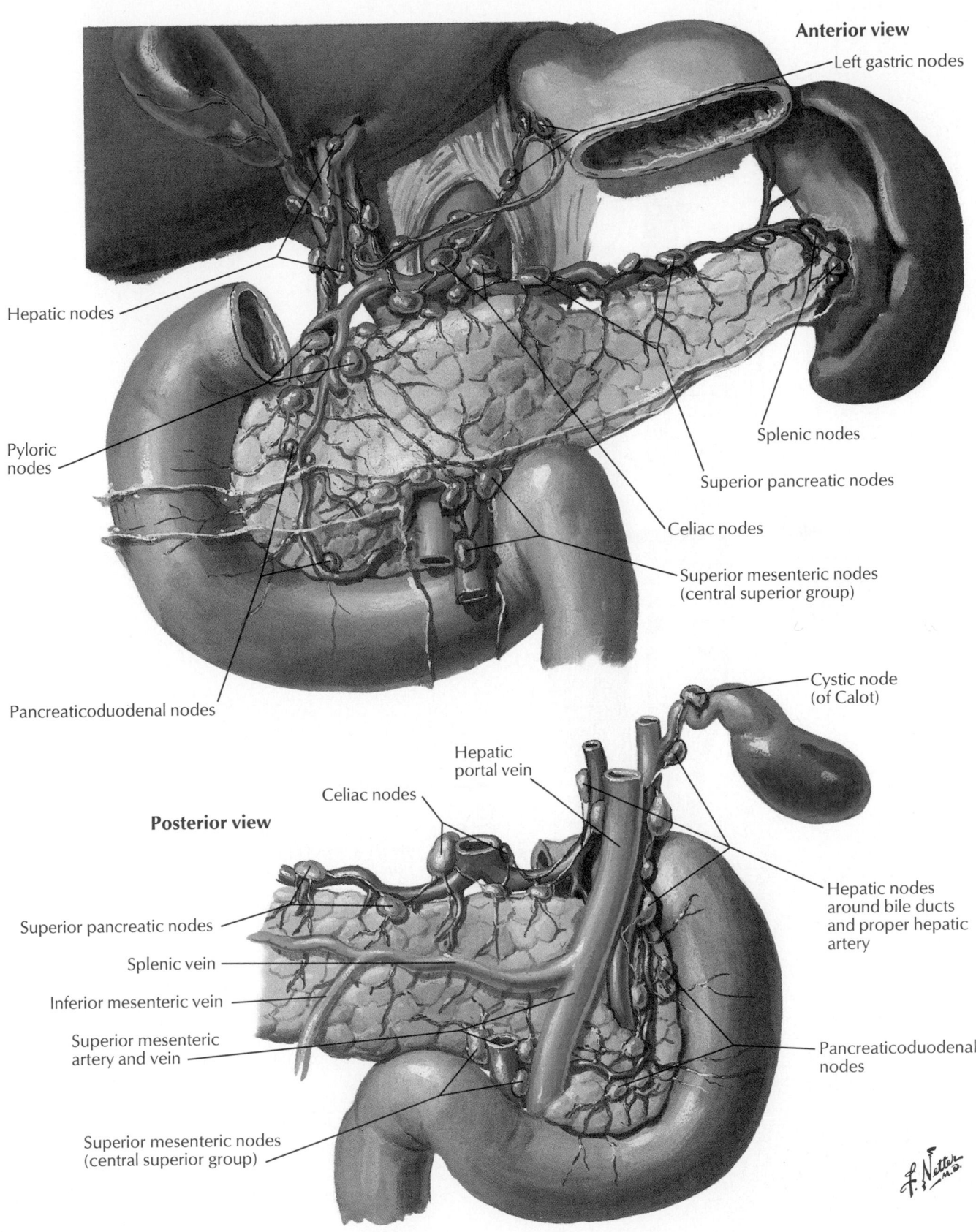

Anterior view

Left gastric nodes

Hepatic nodes

Pyloric nodes

Pancreaticoduodenal nodes

Splenic nodes

Superior pancreatic nodes

Celiac nodes

Superior mesenteric nodes (central superior group)

Cystic node (of Calot)

Hepatic portal vein

Celiac nodes

Posterior view

Superior pancreatic nodes

Splenic vein

Inferior mesenteric vein

Superior mesenteric artery and vein

Superior mesenteric nodes (central superior group)

Hepatic nodes around bile ducts and proper hepatic artery

Pancreaticoduodenal nodes

Plate 315 Lymph Vessels and Nodes of Pancreas. (Netter: Atlas of Human Anatomy, 4 ed, 2006, Saunders.)

Dermatome pattern

Levels of principal dermatomes

C5	Clavicles
C5, 6, 7	Lateral parts of upper limbs
C8; T1	Medial sides of upper limbs
C6	Thumb
C6, 7, 8	Hand
C8	Ring and little fingers
T4	Level of nipples
T10	Level of umbilicus
T12	Inguinal or groin regions
L1, 2, 3, 4	Anterior and inner surfaces of lower limbs
L4, 5; S1	Foot
L4	Medial side of great toe
L5; S1, 2	Outer and posterior sides of lower limbs
S1	Lateral margin of foot and little toe
S2, 3, 4	Perineum

Plate 164 Dermatomes. (Netter: Atlas of Human Anatomy, 4 ed, 2006, Saunders.)

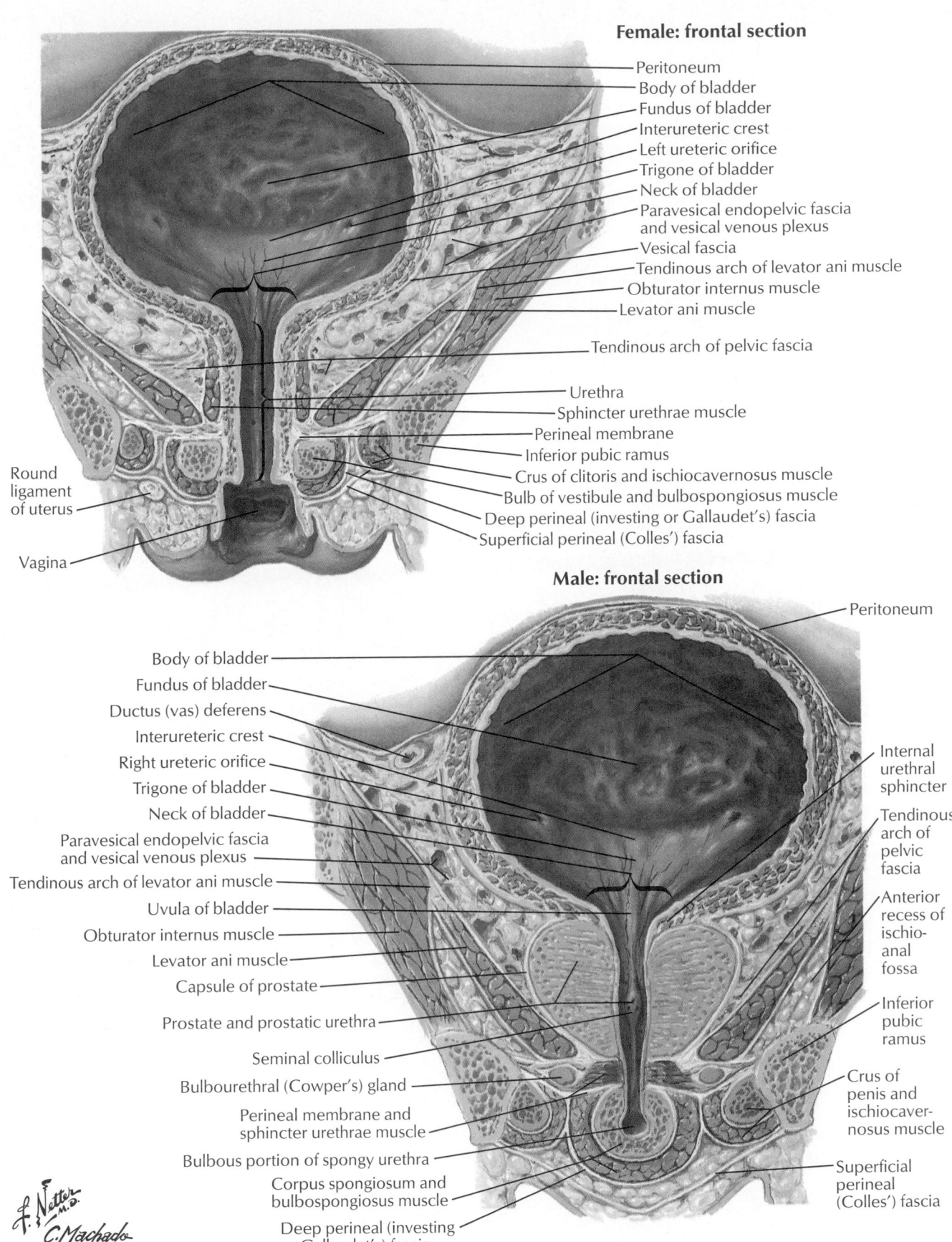

Female: frontal section

Peritoneum
Body of bladder
Fundus of bladder
Interureteric crest
Left ureteric orifice
Trigone of bladder
Neck of bladder
Paravesical endopelvic fascia and vesical venous plexus
Vesical fascia
Tendinous arch of levator ani muscle
Obturator internus muscle
Levator ani muscle

Tendinous arch of pelvic fascia

Urethra
Sphincter urethrae muscle
Perineal membrane
Inferior pubic ramus
Crus of clitoris and ischiocavernosus muscle
Bulb of vestibule and bulbospongiosus muscle
Deep perineal (investing or Gallaudet's) fascia
Superficial perineal (Colles') fascia

Round ligament of uterus

Vagina

Male: frontal section

Peritoneum

Body of bladder
Fundus of bladder
Ductus (vas) deferens
Interureteric crest
Right ureteric orifice
Trigone of bladder
Neck of bladder
Paravesical endopelvic fascia and vesical venous plexus
Tendinous arch of levator ani muscle
Uvula of bladder
Obturator internus muscle
Levator ani muscle
Capsule of prostate
Prostate and prostatic urethra
Seminal colliculus
Bulbourethral (Cowper's) gland
Perineal membrane and sphincter urethrae muscle
Bulbous portion of spongy urethra
Corpus spongiosum and bulbospongiosus muscle
Deep perineal (investing or Gallaudet's) fascia

Internal urethral sphincter
Tendinous arch of pelvic fascia
Anterior recess of ischio-anal fossa
Inferior pubic ramus
Crus of penis and ischiocavernosus muscle
Superficial perineal (Colles') fascia

Plate 366 Urinary Bladder: Female and Male. (Netter: Atlas of Human Anatomy, 4 ed, 2006, Saunders.)

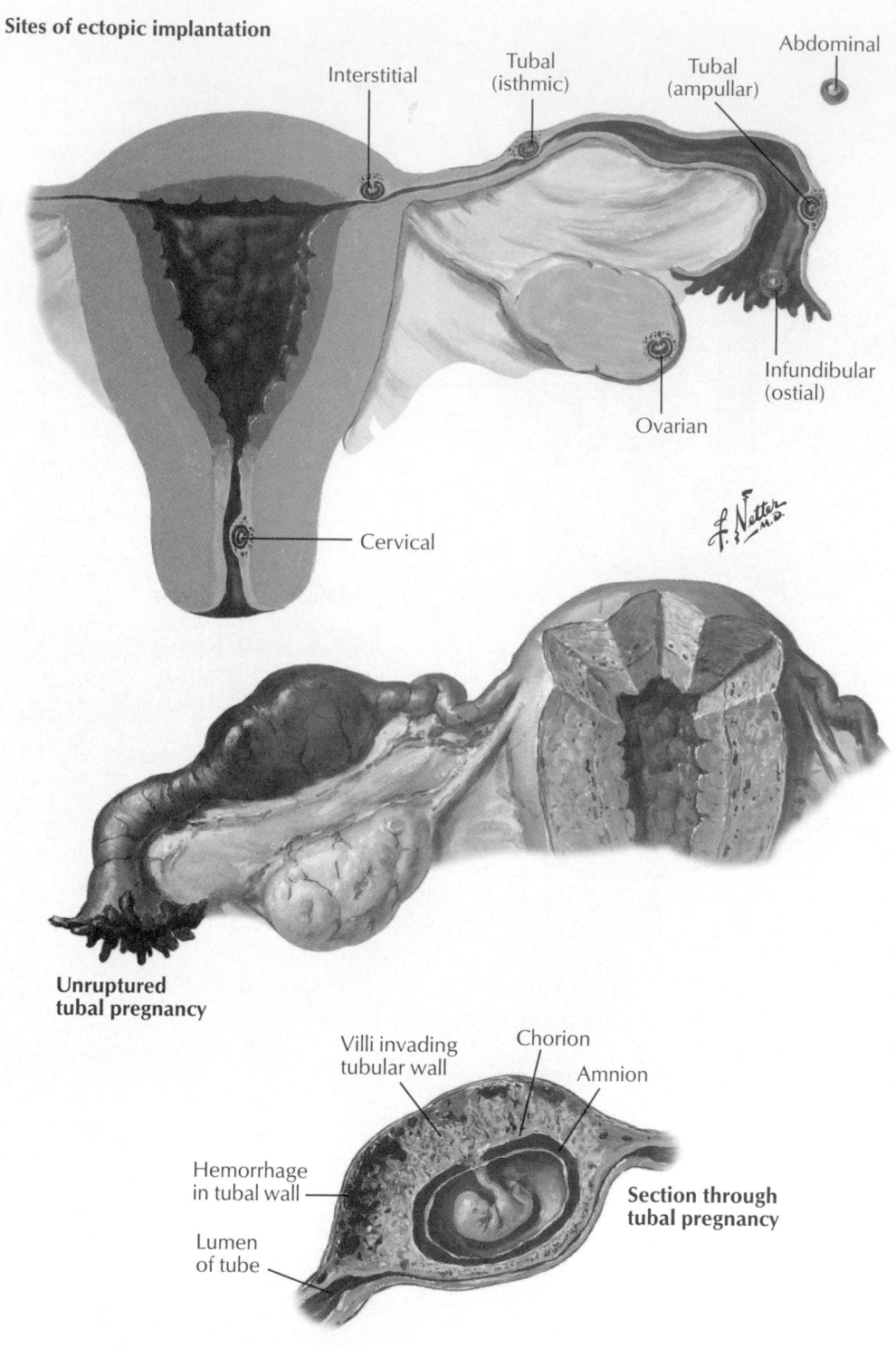

Sites of ectopic implantation

Interstitial

Tubal (isthmic)

Tubal (ampullar)

Abdominal

Infundibular (ostial)

Ovarian

Cervical

Unruptured tubal pregnancy

Villi invading tubular wall

Chorion

Amnion

Hemorrhage in tubal wall

Lumen of tube

Section through tubal pregnancy

Plate 375   Ectopic Pregnancy. (Netter: Atlas of Human Anatomy, 4 ed, 2006, Saunders.)

NAP-4

NETTER ANATOMY PLATE

Superficial inguinal ring

External spermatic fascia

Cremaster muscle and fascia

Septum of scrotum (formed by dartos fascia)

Superficial (dartos) fascia of scrotum

Skin of scrotum

Skin of penis

Superficial fascia of penis (Colles' fascia)

Deep (Buck's) fascia of penis

Testicular artery

Ductus deferens

Artery to ductus deferens

Genital branch of genitofemoral nerve

Pampiniform (venous) plexus

Epididymis

Appendix of epididymis

Appendix of testis

Testis (covered by visceral layer of tunica vaginalis)

Parietal layer of tunica vaginalis

Superficial (dartos) fascia of scrotum

External spermatic fascia

Cremaster muscle and fascia

Internal spermatic fascia

Parietal layer of tunica vaginalis

Epididymis

Testis (covered by visceral layer of tunica vaginalis)

Skin of scrotum

Plate 387   Scrotum and Contents. (Netter: Atlas of Human Anatomy, 4 ed, 2006, Saunders.)

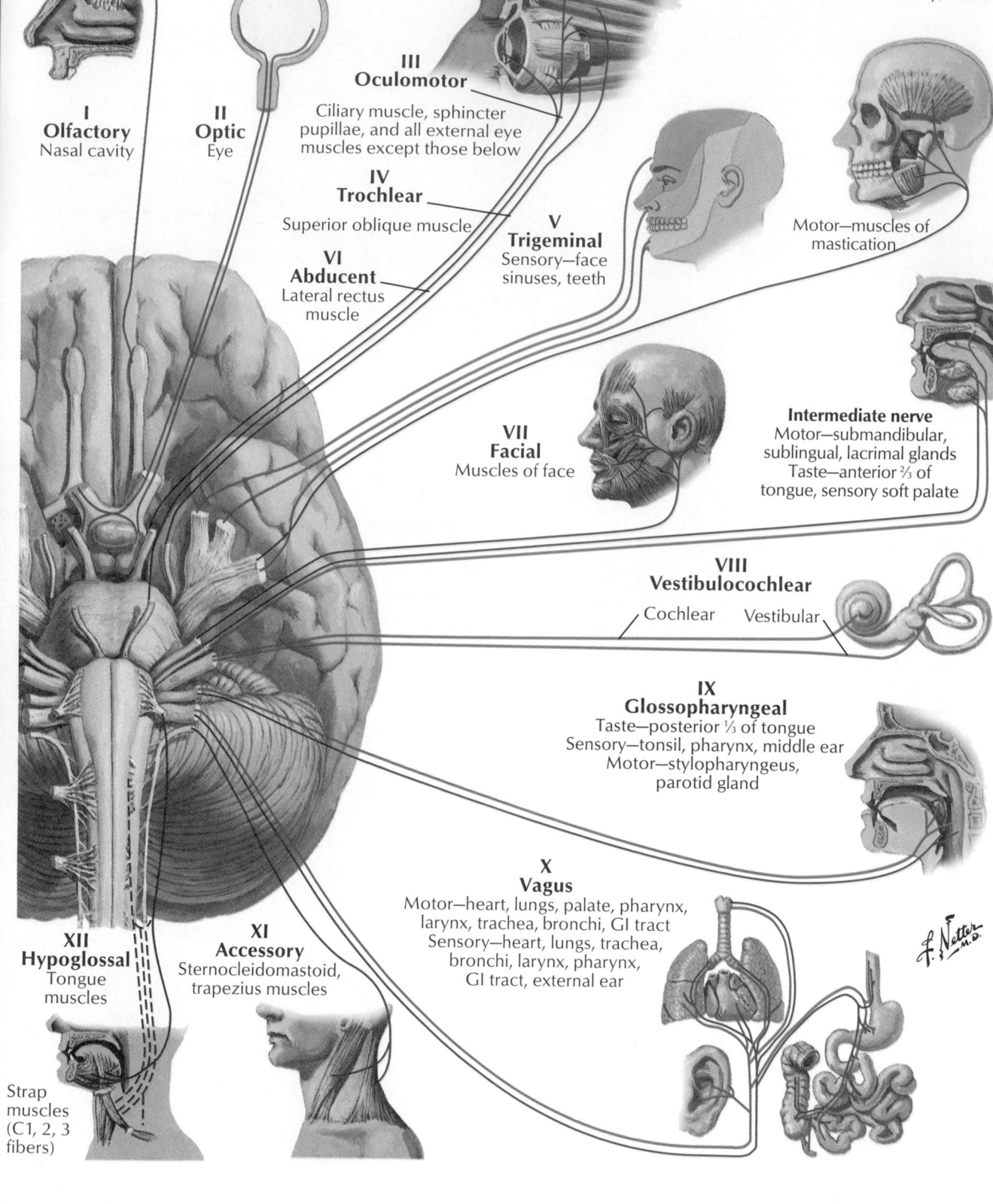

- - - - - - Spinal nerve fibers
———— Efferent (motor) fibers
———— Afferent (sensory) fibers

I
Olfactory
Nasal cavity

II
Optic
Eye

III
Oculomotor
Ciliary muscle, sphincter
pupillae, and all external eye
muscles except those below

IV
Trochlear
Superior oblique muscle

VI
Abducent
Lateral rectus
muscle

V
Trigeminal
Sensory—face
sinuses, teeth

Motor—muscles of
mastication

VII
Facial
Muscles of face

Intermediate nerve
Motor—submandibular,
sublingual, lacrimal glands
Taste—anterior ⅔ of
tongue, sensory soft palate

VIII
Vestibulocochlear
Cochlear   Vestibular

IX
Glossopharyngeal
Taste—posterior ⅓ of tongue
Sensory—tonsil, pharynx, middle ear
Motor—stylopharyngeus,
parotid gland

X
Vagus
Motor—heart, lungs, palate, pharynx,
larynx, trachea, bronchi, GI tract
Sensory—heart, lungs, trachea,
bronchi, larynx, pharynx,
GI tract, external ear

XII
Hypoglossal
Tongue
muscles

Strap
muscles
(C1, 2, 3
fibers)

XI
Accessory
Sternocleidomastoid,
trapezius muscles

f. Netter
m.d.

NETTER ANATOMY PLATE

Plate 118 Cranial Nerves (Motor and Sensory Distribution): Schema. (Netter: Atlas of Human Anatomy, 4 ed, 2006, Saunders.)

Superior view

Supratrochlear nerve

Medial rectus muscle

Superior oblique muscle

Infratrochlear nerve

Nasociliary nerve

Trochlear nerve (IV)

Common tendinous ring

Ophthalmic nerve (V₁)

Optic nerve (II)

Internal carotid artery and nerve plexus

Oculomotor nerve (III)

Trochlear nerve (IV)

Abducent nerve (VI)

Tentorium cerebelli

Medial branch } Supraorbital nerve
Lateral branch

Levator palpebrae superioris muscle

Superior rectus muscle

Lacrimal gland

Lacrimal nerve

Lateral rectus muscle

Frontal nerve

Maxillary nerve (V₂)

Meningeal branch of maxillary nerve

Mandibular nerve (V₃)

Lesser petrosal nerve

Meningeal branch of mandibular nerve

Greater petrosal nerve

Trigeminal (semilunar) ganglion

Tentorial (meningeal) branch of ophthalmic nerve

Superior view:
levator palpebrae superioris, superior rectus, and superior oblique muscles partially cut away

Supratrochlear nerve *(cut)*

Supraorbital nerve branches *(cut)*

Infratrochlear nerve

Anterior ethmoidal nerve

Optic nerve (II)

Posterior ethmoidal nerve

Superior branch of oculomotor nerve (III) *(cut)*

Nasociliary nerve

Internal carotid plexus

Trochlear nerve (IV) *(cut)*

Oculomotor nerve (III)

Abducent nerve (VI)

Long ciliary nerves

Short ciliary nerves

Lacrimal nerve

Ciliary ganglion

Parasympathetic root of ciliary ganglion (from inferior branch of oculomotor nerve)

Sympathetic root of ciliary ganglion (from internal carotid plexus)

Sensory root of ciliary ganglion (from nasociliary nerve)

Branches to inferior and medial rectus muscles

Abducent nerve (VI)

Inferior branch of oculomotor nerve (III)

Lacrimal nerve

Frontal nerve *(cut)*

Ophthalmic nerve (V₁)

Plate 86 Nerves of Orbit. (Netter: Atlas of Human Anatomy, 4 ed, 2006, Saunders.)

NETTER ANATOMY PLATE

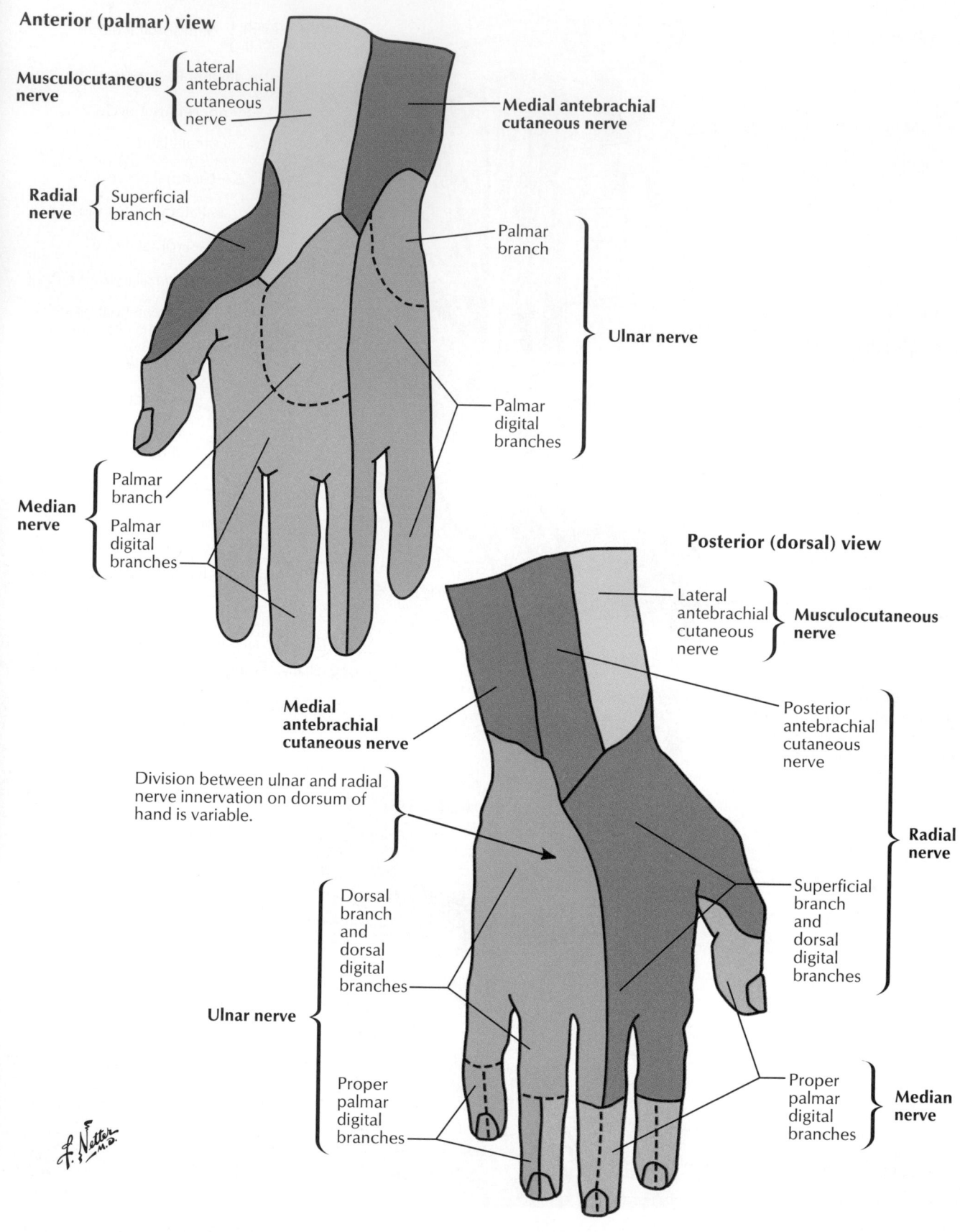

Anterior (palmar) view

Musculocutaneous nerve { Lateral antebrachial cutaneous nerve

Medial antebrachial cutaneous nerve

Radial nerve { Superficial branch

Palmar branch } Ulnar nerve

Palmar digital branches

Median nerve { Palmar branch / Palmar digital branches

Posterior (dorsal) view

Lateral antebrachial cutaneous nerve } **Musculocutaneous nerve**

Posterior antebrachial cutaneous nerve

Medial antebrachial cutaneous nerve

Division between ulnar and radial nerve innervation on dorsum of hand is variable.

Radial nerve

Superficial branch and dorsal digital branches

Dorsal branch and dorsal digital branches

Ulnar nerve

Proper palmar digital branches

Proper palmar digital branches } **Median nerve**

Plate 472 Cutaneous Innervation of Wrist and Hand. (Netter: Atlas of Human Anatomy, 4 ed, 2006, Saunders.)

NAP-8

Anterior view

Deltoid muscle

Coracobrachialis muscle

Biceps brachii muscle { Short head (*cut*)
Long head (*cut*)

Musculocutaneous nerve

Brachialis muscle

Biceps brachii muscle (*cut*) and tendon

Lateral antebrachial cutaneous nerve
(from musculocutaneous nerve)

Radial nerve { Deep branch
Superficial branch

Supinator muscle

Brachioradialis muscle

Radial artery

Pronator teres muscle (*partially cut*)

Median nerve

Flexor pollicis longus muscle

Flexor carpi radialis tendon (*cut*)

Flexor retinaculum (transverse carpal ligament)

Superficial branch of radial nerve

Recurrent (motor) branch of median nerve to thenar muscles

Common palmar digital branches of median nerve

Proper palmar digital branches of median nerve

Intercostobrachial nerve

Medial brachial cutaneous nerve

Radial nerve

Ulnar nerve

Medial antebrachial cutaneous nerve

Median nerve

Brachial artery

Bicipital aponeurosis

Humeral head (*cut*) } Pronator teres muscle
Ulnar head

Flexor carpi radialis muscle (*cut*)

Humeroulnar head } Flexor digitorum superficialis muscle (*cut*)
Radial head

Flexor digitorum profundus muscle

Flexor carpi ulnaris muscle

Ulnar artery and nerve

Dorsal branch of ulnar nerve

Flexor digitorum superficialis tendons (*cut*)

Deep palmar branch of ulnar artery and deep branch of ulnar nerve

Superficial branch of ulnar nerve

Superficial palmar arch (*cut*)

Common palmar digital branch of ulnar nerve

Communicating branch of median nerve with ulnar nerve

Proper palmar digital branches of ulnar nerve

Plate 473   Arteries and Nerves of Upper Limb. (Netter: Atlas of Human Anatomy, 4 ed, 2006, Saunders.)

Lateral cutaneous branch of subcostal nerve

Inguinal ligament (Poupart's)

Superficial circumflex iliac vein

Femoral branches of genitofemoral nerve

Lateral femoral cutaneous nerve

Saphenous opening (fossa ovalis)

Fascia lata

Anterior cutaneous branches of femoral nerve

Patellar nerve plexus

Branches of lateral sural cutaneous nerve (from common fibular [peroneal] nerve)

Deep fascia of leg (crural fascia)

Superficial fibular (peroneal) nerve
Medial dorsal cutaneous branch

Intermediate dorsal cutaneous branch

Small saphenous vein and lateral dorsal cutaneous nerve (from sural nerve)

Lateral dorsal digital nerve and vein of 5th toe

Dorsal metatarsal veins

Dorsal digital nerves and veins

Superficial epigastric vein

Ilioinguinal nerve (scrotal branch) (usually passes through superficial inguinal ring)

Genital branch of genitofemoral nerve

Femoral vein

Superficial external pudendal vein

Accessory saphenous vein

Great saphenous vein

Cutaneous branches of obturator nerve

Infrapatellar branch of saphenous nerve

Saphenous nerve (terminal branch of femoral nerve)

Great saphenous vein

Dorsal digital nerves

Dorsal venous arch

Dorsal digital nerve and vein of medial side of great toe

Dorsal digital branch of deep fibular (peroneal) nerve

Plate 544 Superficial Nerves and Veins of Lower Limb: Anterior View. (Netter: Atlas of Human Anatomy, 4 ed, 2006, Saunders.)

NAP-10

NETTER ANATOMY PLATE

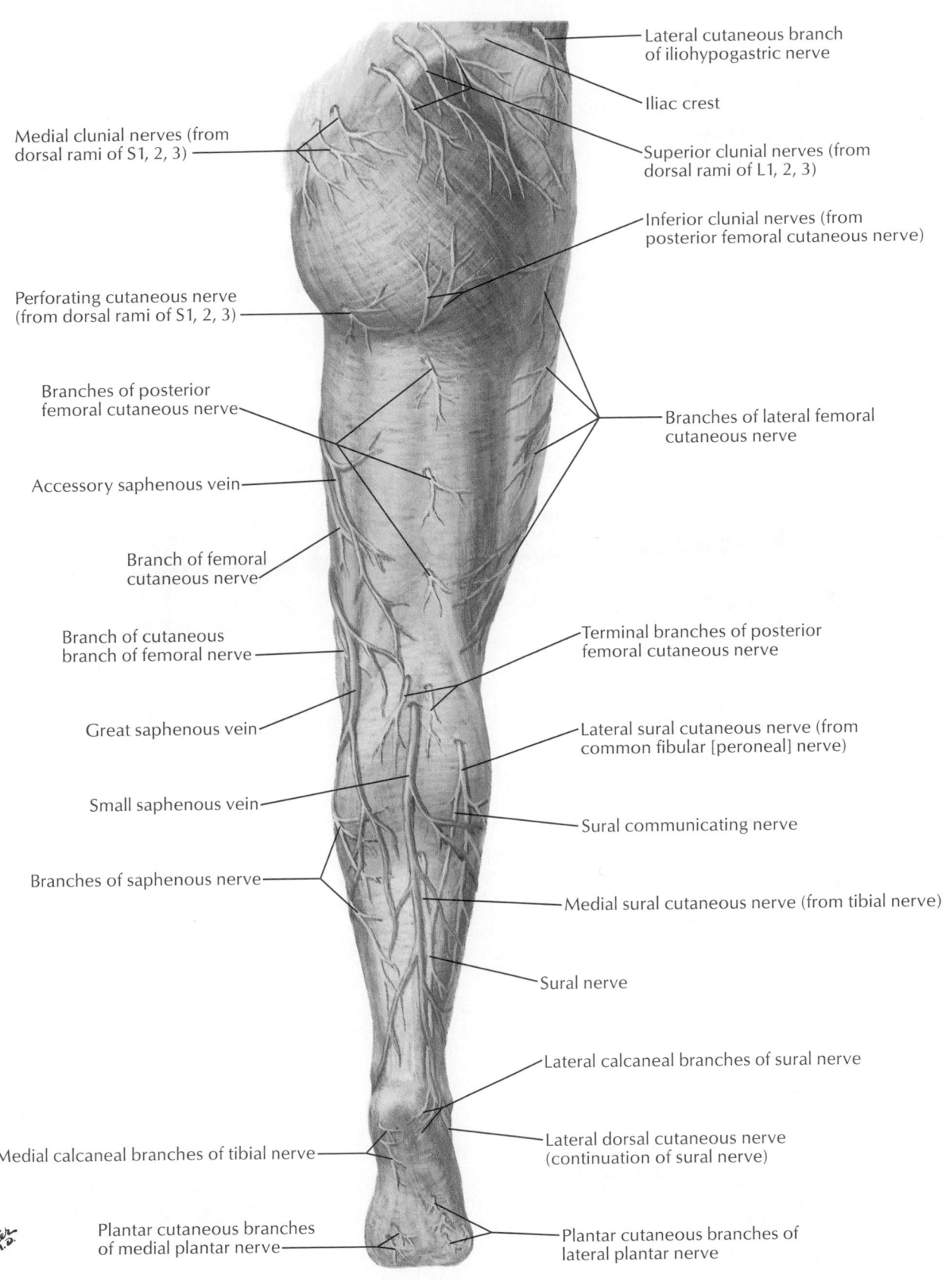

Lateral cutaneous branch of iliohypogastric nerve

Iliac crest

Superior clunial nerves (from dorsal rami of L1, 2, 3)

Inferior clunial nerves (from posterior femoral cutaneous nerve)

Medial clunial nerves (from dorsal rami of S1, 2, 3)

Perforating cutaneous nerve (from dorsal rami of S1, 2, 3)

Branches of posterior femoral cutaneous nerve

Branches of lateral femoral cutaneous nerve

Accessory saphenous vein

Branch of femoral cutaneous nerve

Branch of cutaneous branch of femoral nerve

Terminal branches of posterior femoral cutaneous nerve

Great saphenous vein

Lateral sural cutaneous nerve (from common fibular [peroneal] nerve)

Small saphenous vein

Sural communicating nerve

Branches of saphenous nerve

Medial sural cutaneous nerve (from tibial nerve)

Sural nerve

Lateral calcaneal branches of sural nerve

Medial calcaneal branches of tibial nerve

Lateral dorsal cutaneous nerve (continuation of sural nerve)

Plantar cutaneous branches of medial plantar nerve

Plantar cutaneous branches of lateral plantar nerve

Plate 545   Superficial Nerves and Veins of Lower Limb: Posterior View. (Netter: Atlas of Human Anatomy, 4 ed, 2006, Saunders.)

NETTER ANATOMY PLATE

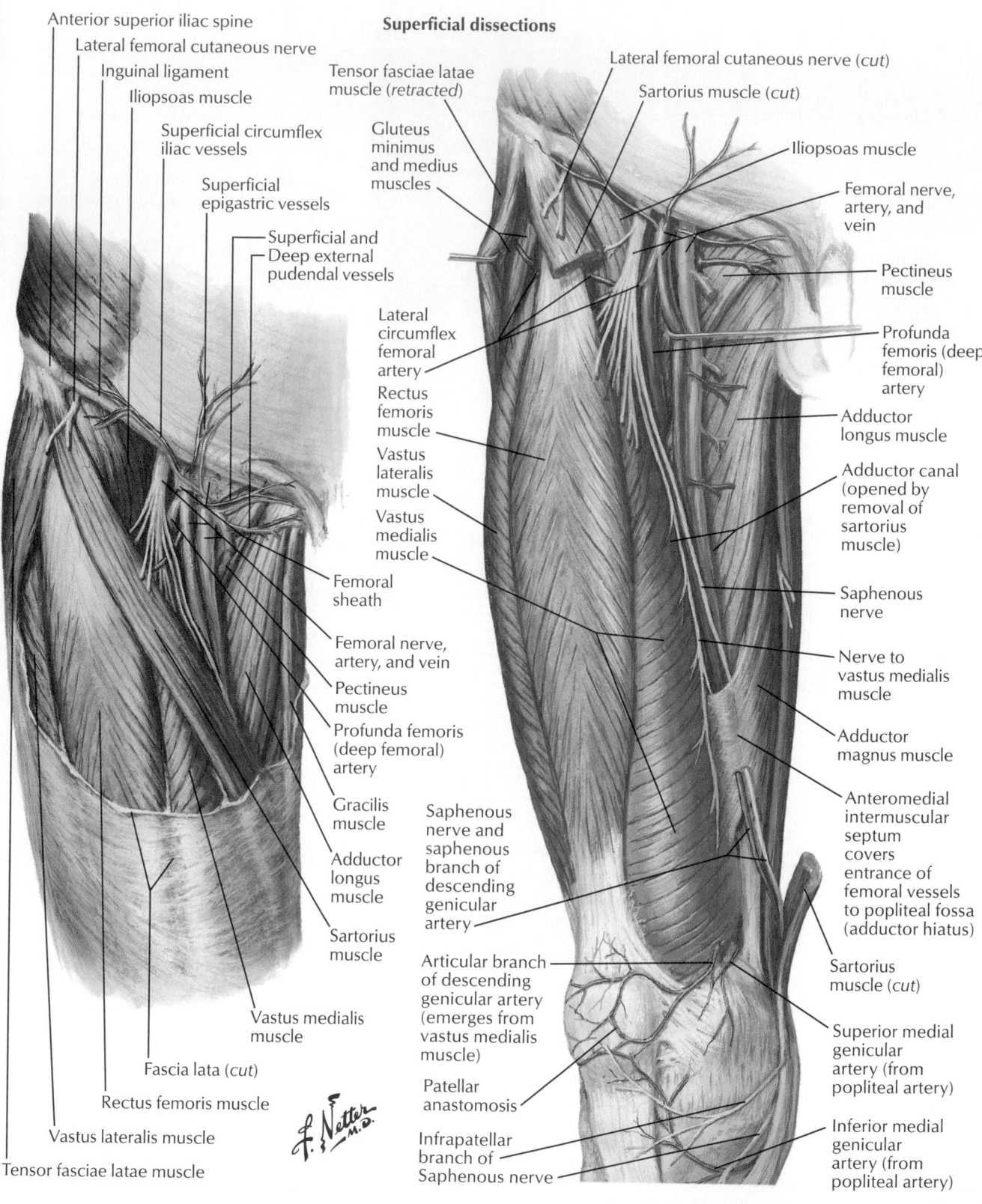

Superficial dissections

Anterior superior iliac spine
Lateral femoral cutaneous nerve
Inguinal ligament
Iliopsoas muscle
Superficial circumflex iliac vessels
Superficial epigastric vessels
Superficial and Deep external pudendal vessels

Tensor fasciae latae muscle (*retracted*)
Gluteus minimus and medius muscles
Lateral circumflex femoral artery
Rectus femoris muscle
Vastus lateralis muscle
Vastus medialis muscle
Femoral sheath
Femoral nerve, artery, and vein
Pectineus muscle
Profunda femoris (deep femoral) artery
Gracilis muscle
Adductor longus muscle
Sartorius muscle
Vastus medialis muscle
Fascia lata (*cut*)
Rectus femoris muscle
Vastus lateralis muscle
Tensor fasciae latae muscle

Lateral femoral cutaneous nerve (*cut*)
Sartorius muscle (*cut*)
Iliopsoas muscle
Femoral nerve, artery, and vein
Pectineus muscle
Profunda femoris (deep femoral) artery
Adductor longus muscle
Adductor canal (opened by removal of sartorius muscle)
Saphenous nerve
Nerve to vastus medialis muscle
Adductor magnus muscle
Anteromedial intermuscular septum covers entrance of femoral vessels to popliteal fossa (adductor hiatus)
Sartorius muscle (*cut*)
Superior medial genicular artery (from popliteal artery)
Inferior medial genicular artery (from popliteal artery)

Saphenous nerve and saphenous branch of descending genicular artery
Articular branch of descending genicular artery (emerges from vastus medialis muscle)
Patellar anastomosis
Infrapatellar branch of Saphenous nerve

F. Netter M.D.

Plate 500 Arteries and Nerves of Thigh: Anterior View. (Netter: Atlas of Human Anatomy, 4 ed, 2006, Saunders.)

Deep dissection

Deep circumflex iliac artery

Lateral femoral cutaneous nerve

Sartorius muscle (*cut*)

Iliopsoas muscle

Tensor fasciae latae muscle (*retracted*)

Gluteus medius and minimus muscles

Femoral nerve

Rectus femoris muscle (*cut*)

Ascending, transverse and descending branches of Lateral circumflex femoral artery

Medial circumflex femoral artery

Pectineus muscle (*cut*)

Profunda femoris (deep femoral) artery

Perforating branches

Adductor longus muscle (*cut*)

Vastus lateralis muscle

Vastus intermedius muscle

Rectus femoris muscle (*cut*)

Saphenous nerve

Anteromedial intermuscular septum (*opened*)

Vastus medialis muscle

Quadriceps femoris tendon

Patella and patellar anastomosis

Medial patellar retinaculum

Patellar ligament

External iliac artery and vein

Inguinal ligament (Poupart's)

Femoral artery and vein (*cut*)

Pectineus muscle (*cut*)

Obturator canal

Obturator externus muscle

Adductor longus muscle (*cut*)

Anterior branch and Posterior branch of obturator nerve

Quadratus femoris muscle

Adductor brevis muscle

Branches of posterior branch of obturator nerve

Adductor magnus muscle

Gracilis muscle

Cutaneous branch of obturator nerve

Femoral artery and vein (*cut*)

Descending genicular artery
Articular branch
Saphenous branch

Adductor hiatus

Sartorius muscle (*cut*)

Adductor magnus tendon

Adductor tubercle on medial epicondyle of femur

Superior medial genicular artery (from popliteal artery)

Infrapatellar branch of Saphenous nerve

Inferior medial genicular artery (from popliteal artery)

Plate 501   Arteries and Nerves of Thigh: Anterior View. (Netter: Atlas of Human Anatomy, 4 ed, 2006, Saunders.)

Deep dissection

Superior clunial nerves

Gluteus maximus muscle (*cut*)

Medial clunial nerves

Inferior gluteal artery and nerve

Pudendal nerve

Nerve to obturator internus (and superior gemellus)

Posterior femoral cutaneous nerve

Sacrotuberous ligament

Ischial tuberosity

Inferior clunial nerves (*cut*)

Adductor magnus muscle

Gracilis muscle

Sciatic nerve

Muscular branches of sciatic nerve

Semitendinosus muscle (*retracted*)

Semimembranosus muscle

Sciatic nerve

Articular branch

Adductor hiatus

Popliteal vein and artery

Superior medial genicular artery

Medial epicondyle of femur

Tibial nerve

Gastrocnemius muscle (medial head)

Medial sural cutaneous nerve

Small saphenous vein

Iliac crest

Gluteal aponeurosis and gluteus medius muscle (*cut*)

Superior gluteal artery and nerve

Gluteus minimus muscle

Tensor fasciae latae muscle

Piriformis muscle

Gluteus medius muscle (*cut*)

Superior gemellus muscle

Greater trochanter of femur

Obturator internus muscle

Inferior gemellus muscle

Gluteus maximus muscle (*cut*)

Quadratus femoris muscle

Medial circumflex femoral artery

Vastus lateralis muscle and iliotibial tract

Adductor minimus part of adductor magnus muscle

1st perforating artery (from profunda femoris artery)

Adductor magnus muscle

2nd and 3rd perforating arteries (from profunda femoris artery)

4th perforating artery (from profunda femoris artery)

Long head (*retracted*) ⎫ Biceps femoris
Short head ⎬ muscle

Superior lateral genicular artery

Common fibular (peroneal) nerve

Plantaris muscle

Gastrocnemius muscle (lateral head)

Lateral sural cutaneous nerve

Plate 502   Arteries and Nerves of Thigh: Posterior View. (Netter: Atlas of Human Anatomy, 4 ed, 2006, Saunders.)

Horizontal section

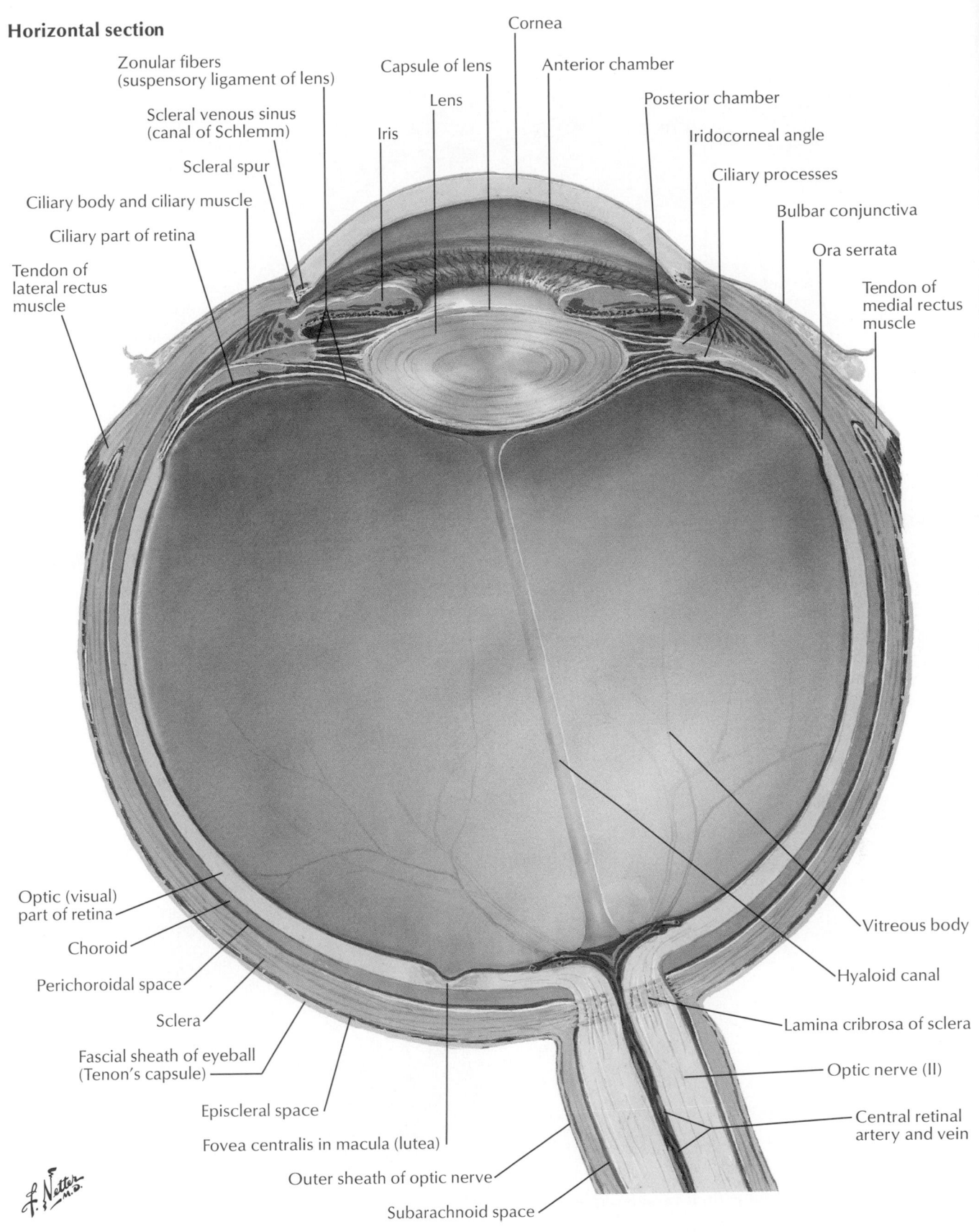

Zonular fibers (suspensory ligament of lens)

Scleral venous sinus (canal of Schlemm)

Scleral spur

Ciliary body and ciliary muscle

Ciliary part of retina

Tendon of lateral rectus muscle

Iris

Lens

Capsule of lens

Cornea

Anterior chamber

Posterior chamber

Iridocorneal angle

Ciliary processes

Bulbar conjunctiva

Ora serrata

Tendon of medial rectus muscle

Optic (visual) part of retina

Choroid

Perichoroidal space

Sclera

Fascial sheath of eyeball (Tenon's capsule)

Episcleral space

Fovea centralis in macula (lutea)

Outer sheath of optic nerve

Subarachnoid space

Vitreous body

Hyaloid canal

Lamina cribrosa of sclera

Optic nerve (II)

Central retinal artery and vein

Plate 87 Eyeball. (Netter: Atlas of Human Anatomy, 4 ed, 2006, Saunders.)

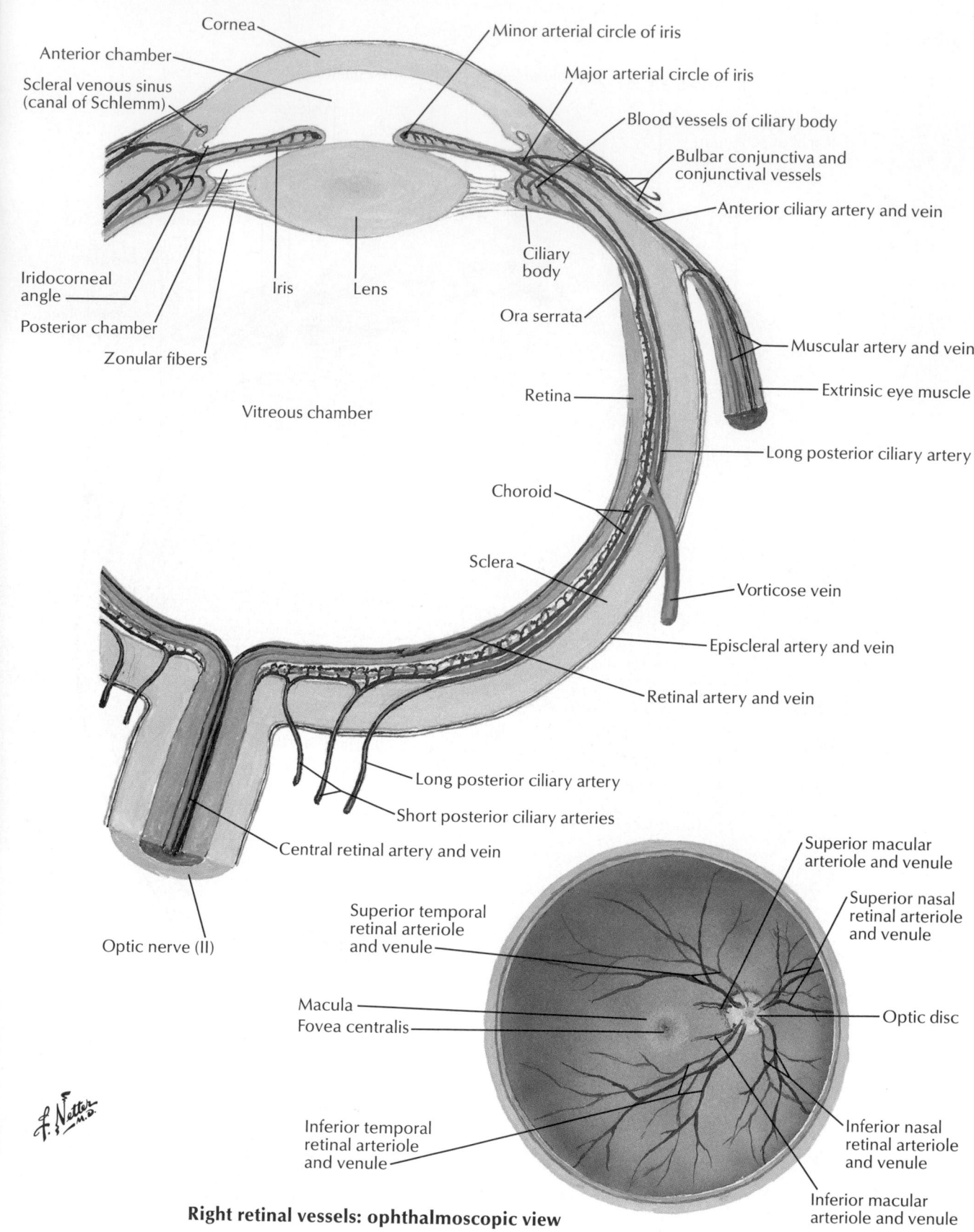

Cornea

Anterior chamber

Scleral venous sinus
(canal of Schlemm)

Minor arterial circle of iris

Major arterial circle of iris

Blood vessels of ciliary body

Bulbar conjunctiva and
conjunctival vessels

Anterior ciliary artery and vein

Ciliary
body

Ora serrata

Muscular artery and vein

Extrinsic eye muscle

Long posterior ciliary artery

Iridocorneal
angle

Iris

Lens

Posterior chamber

Zonular fibers

Vitreous chamber

Retina

Choroid

Sclera

Vorticose vein

Episcleral artery and vein

Retinal artery and vein

Long posterior ciliary artery

Short posterior ciliary arteries

Central retinal artery and vein

Optic nerve (II)

Superior temporal
retinal arteriole
and venule

Macula

Fovea centralis

Superior macular
arteriole and venule

Superior nasal
retinal arteriole
and venule

Optic disc

Inferior temporal
retinal arteriole
and venule

Inferior nasal
retinal arteriole
and venule

Inferior macular
arteriole and venule

Right retinal vessels: ophthalmoscopic view

Plate 90   Intrinsic Arteries and Veins of Eye. (Netter: Atlas of Human Anatomy, 4 ed, 2006, Saunders.)

NAP-16

NETTER ANATOMY PLATE

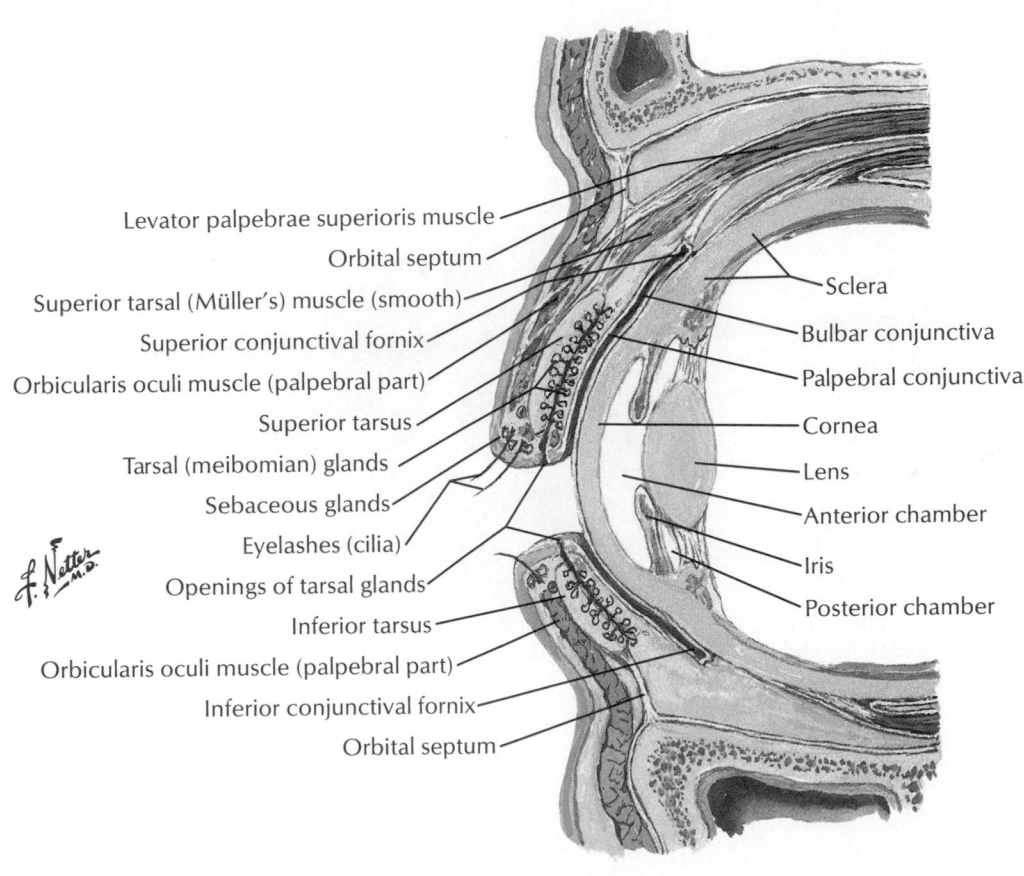

Levator palpebrae superioris muscle

Orbital septum

Superior tarsal (Müller's) muscle (smooth)

Superior conjunctival fornix

Orbicularis oculi muscle (palpebral part)

Superior tarsus

Tarsal (meibomian) glands

Sebaceous glands

Eyelashes (cilia)

Openings of tarsal glands

Inferior tarsus

Orbicularis oculi muscle (palpebral part)

Inferior conjunctival fornix

Orbital septum

Sclera

Bulbar conjunctiva

Palpebral conjunctiva

Cornea

Lens

Anterior chamber

Iris

Posterior chamber

Plate 81, Middle   Eyelid. (Netter: Atlas of Human Anatomy, 4 ed, 2006, Saunders.)

NAP-17

Superior palpebral conjunctiva:
tarsal (meibomian) glands
shining through

Seen through { Pupil
cornea { Iris

Corneoscleral junction
(corneal limbus)

Bulbar conjunctiva
over sclera

Inferior conjunctival fornix

Inferior palpebral conjunctiva:
tarsal glands shining through

Superior lacrimal papilla and
punctum

Plica semilunaris

Lacrimal caruncle in
lacrimal lake (lacus lacrimalis)

Inferior lacrimal papilla and
punctum

Plate 81, Upper   Eyelid. (Netter: Atlas of Human Anatomy, 4 ed, 2006, Saunders.)

Superior lacrimal papilla and punctum

Orbital part of lacrimal gland

Palpebral part of lacrimal gland

Excretory ducts of lacrimal gland

Plica semilunaris

Lacrimal caruncle

Inferior lacrimal papilla and punctum

Lacrimal canaliculi

Lacrimal sac

Nasolacrimal duct

Opening of nasolacrimal duct

Superior lacrimal papilla and punctum

Frontal bone (*cut away*)

Orbital part of lacrimal gland

Palpebral part of lacrimal gland

Excretory ducts of lacrimal gland

Plica semilunaris and lacrimal lake

Lacrimal caruncle

Inferior lacrimal papilla and punctum

Opening of nasolacrimal duct

Lacrimal canaliculi

Lacrimal sac

Nasolacrimal duct

Middle nasal concha

Nasal cavity

Inferior nasal concha (*cut*)

Inferior nasal meatus

Plate 82   Lacrimal Apparatus. (Netter: Atlas of Human Anatomy, 4 ed, 2006, Saunders.)

Frontal section

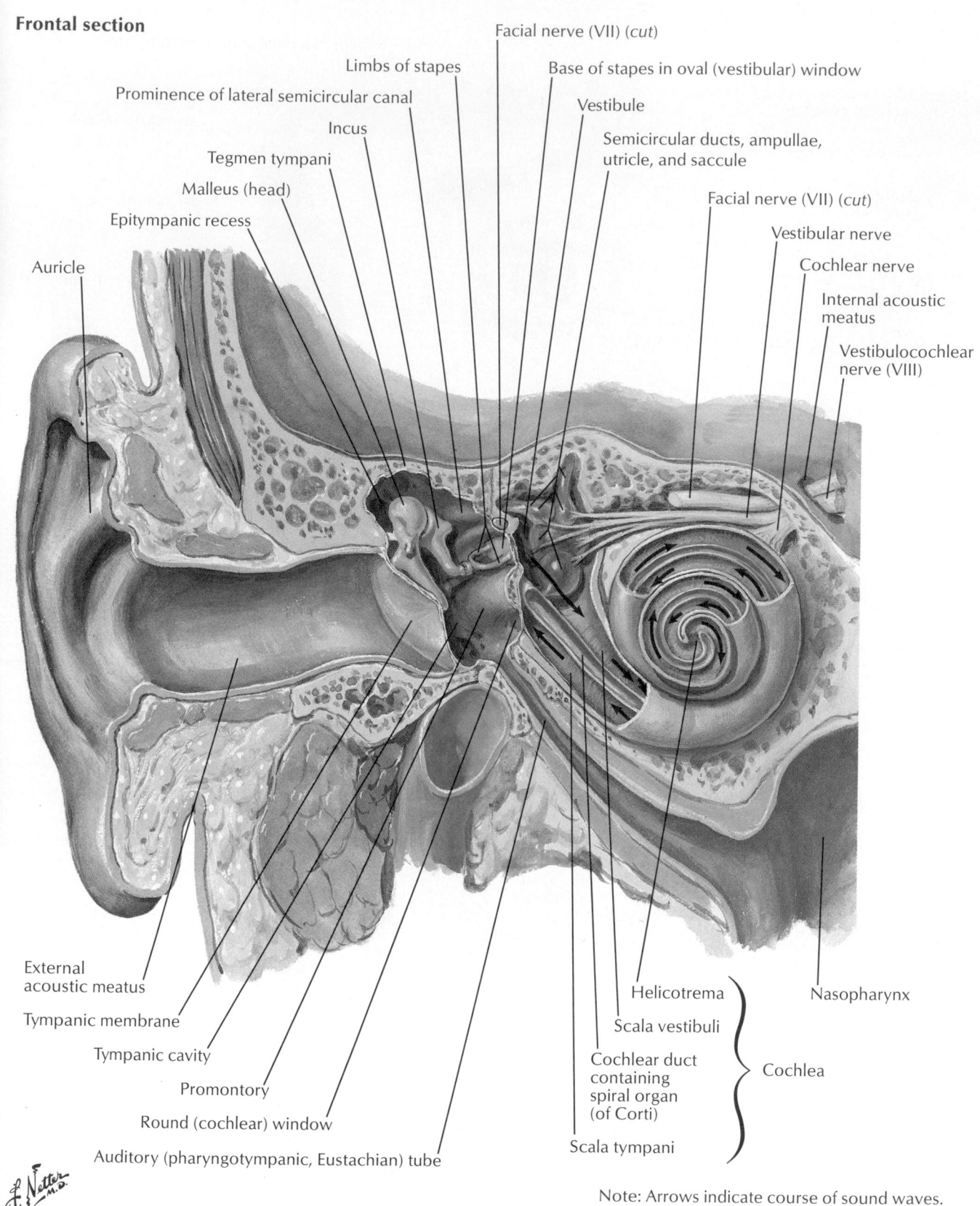

Plate 92 labels:
- Facial nerve (VII) (*cut*)
- Limbs of stapes
- Base of stapes in oval (vestibular) window
- Prominence of lateral semicircular canal
- Vestibule
- Incus
- Semicircular ducts, ampullae, utricle, and saccule
- Tegmen tympani
- Malleus (head)
- Facial nerve (VII) (*cut*)
- Epitympanic recess
- Vestibular nerve
- Cochlear nerve
- Auricle
- Internal acoustic meatus
- Vestibulocochlear nerve (VIII)
- External acoustic meatus
- Tympanic membrane
- Tympanic cavity
- Promontory
- Round (cochlear) window
- Auditory (pharyngotympanic, Eustachian) tube
- Helicotrema
- Scala vestibuli
- Cochlear duct containing spiral organ (of Corti)
- Scala tympani
- Cochlea
- Nasopharynx

Note: Arrows indicate course of sound waves.

Plate 92 Pathway of Sound Reception. (Netter: Atlas of Human Anatomy, 4 ed, 2006, Saunders.)

Medial wall of tympanic cavity: lateral view

Mastoid antrum

Prominence of lateral semicircular canal

Prominence of facial canal

Geniculum (geniculate ganglion) of facial nerve

Greater petrosal nerve

Base of stapes in fossa of oval (vestibular) window

Tensor tympani muscle (*tendon cut*)

Limbs of stapes

Auditory (pharyngotympanic, Eustachian) tube

Pyramidal eminence

Levator veli palatini muscle

Chorda tympani nerve (*cut*)

Mastoid cells

Tendon of stapedius muscle

Promontory with tympanic nerve (of Jacobson) and plexus under mucosa

Fossa of round (cochlear) window

Jugular fossa

Internal carotid artery

Facial nerve (VII) in stylomastoid foramen

Tympanic cells

Plate 94   Tympanic Cavity. (Netter: Atlas of Human Anatomy, 4 ed, 2006, Saunders.)

Otoscopic view of right tympanic membrane

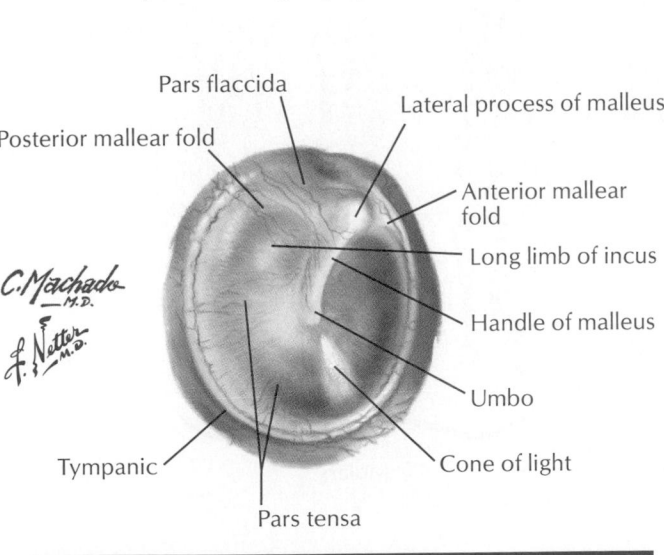

Pars flaccida

Posterior mallear fold

Lateral process of malleus

Anterior mallear fold

Long limb of incus

Handle of malleus

Umbo

Tympanic

Cone of light

Pars tensa

Plate 93   Tympanic Cavity. (Netter: Atlas of Human Anatomy, 4 ed, 2006, Saunders.)

Dissected right bony labyrinth (otic capsule): membranous labyrinth removed

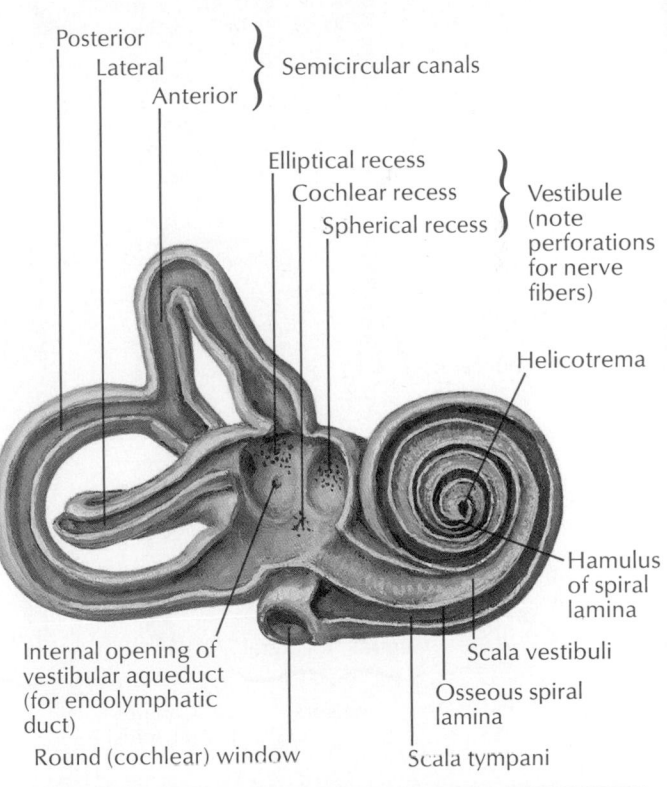

Posterior

Lateral

Anterior

Semicircular canals

Elliptical recess

Cochlear recess

Spherical recess

Vestibule (note perforations for nerve fibers)

Helicotrema

Hamulus of spiral lamina

Scala vestibuli

Osseous spiral lamina

Scala tympani

Internal opening of vestibular aqueduct (for endolymphatic duct)

Round (cochlear) window

Plate 95   Bony Membranous Labyrinth. (Netter: Atlas of Human Anatomy, 4 ed, 2006, Saunders.)

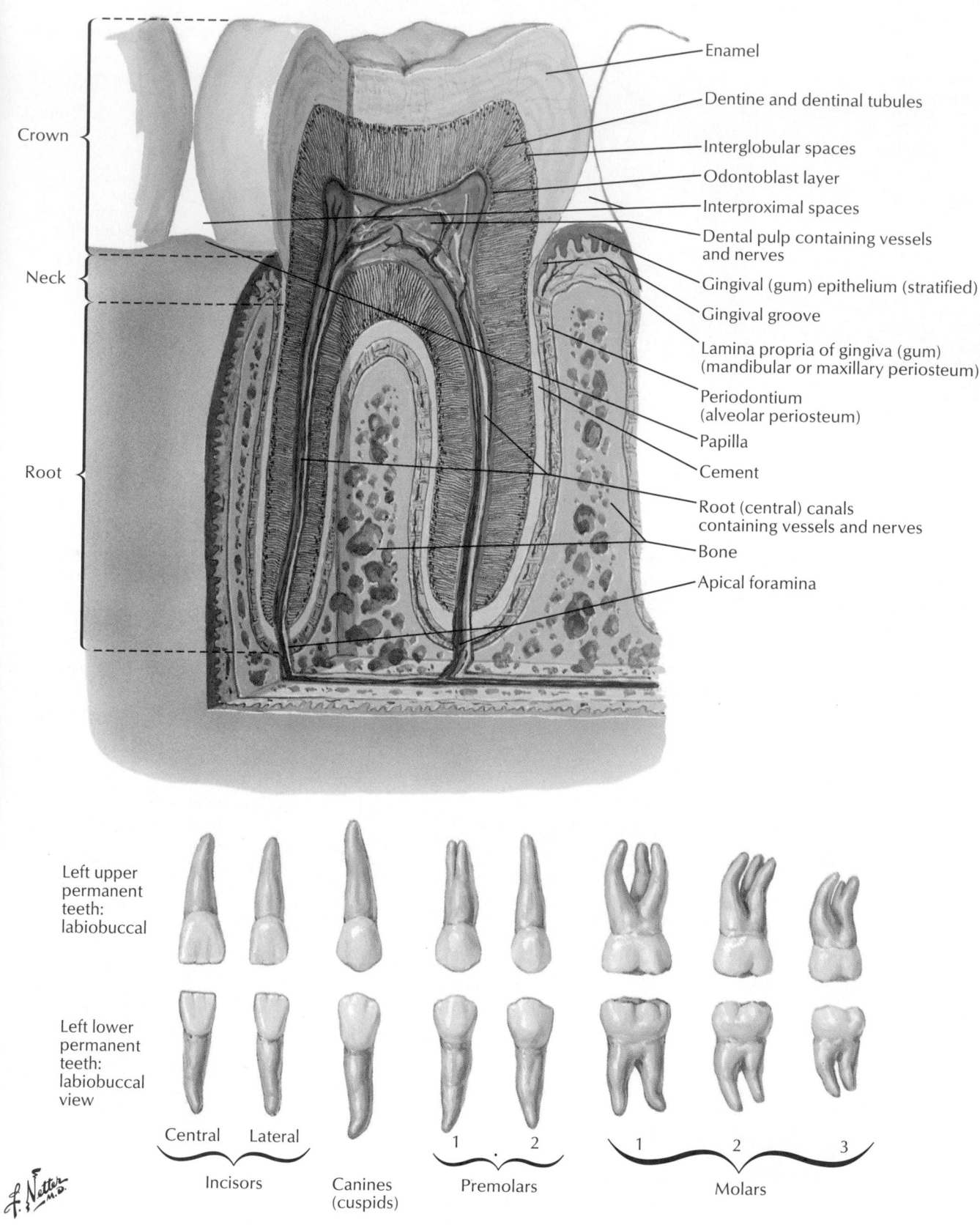

Crown

Neck

Root

Enamel

Dentine and dentinal tubules

Interglobular spaces

Odontoblast layer

Interproximal spaces

Dental pulp containing vessels and nerves

Gingival (gum) epithelium (stratified)

Gingival groove

Lamina propria of gingiva (gum) (mandibular or maxillary periosteum)

Periodontium (alveolar periosteum)

Papilla

Cement

Root (central) canals containing vessels and nerves

Bone

Apical foramina

Left upper permanent teeth: labiobuccal

Left lower permanent teeth: labiobuccal view

Central   Lateral

Incisors

Canines (cuspids)

1   2

Premolars

1   2   3

Molars

Plate 57   Teeth. (Netter: Atlas of Human Anatomy, 4 ed, 2006, Saunders.)

NAP-22

Tongue

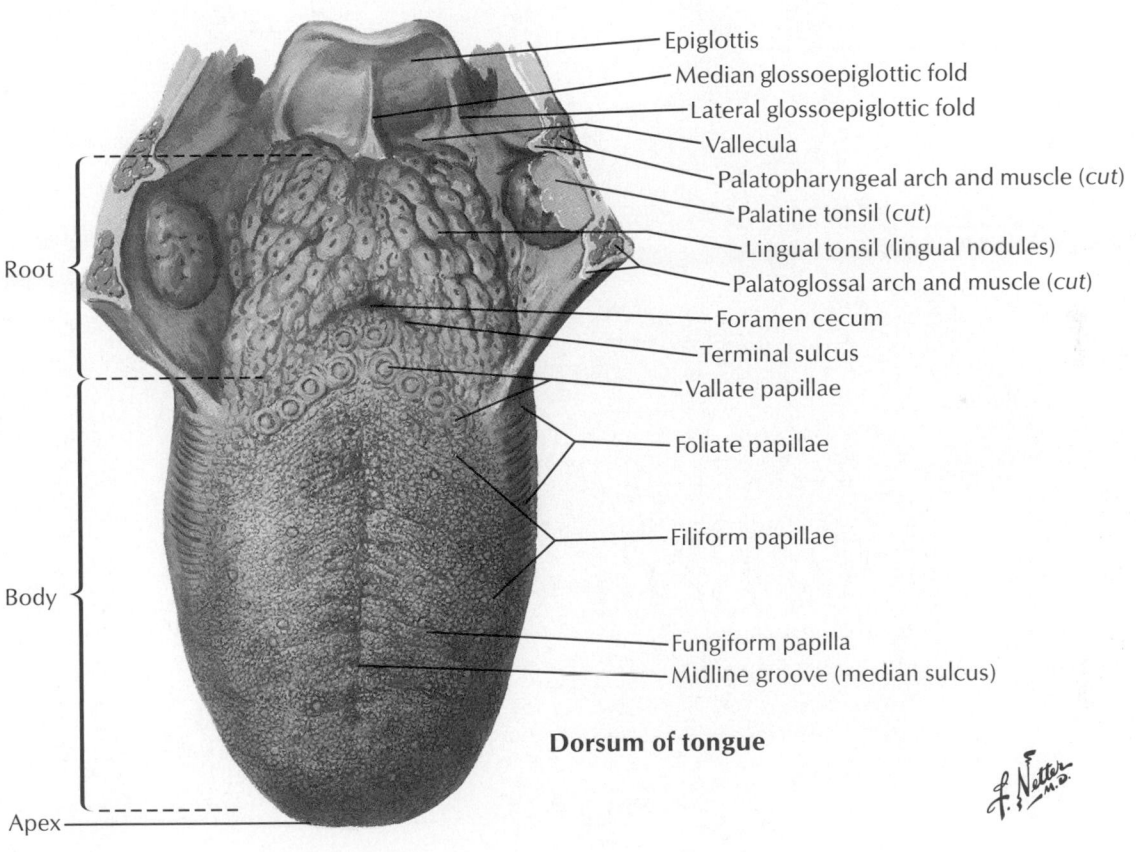

Epiglottis
Median glossoepiglottic fold
Lateral glossoepiglottic fold
Vallecula
Palatopharyngeal arch and muscle (*cut*)
Palatine tonsil (*cut*)
Lingual tonsil (lingual nodules)
Palatoglossal arch and muscle (*cut*)
Foramen cecum
Terminal sulcus
Vallate papillae
Foliate papillae
Filiform papillae
Fungiform papilla
Midline groove (median sulcus)

Root

Body

Apex

Dorsum of tongue

Plate 58   Tongue. (Netter: Atlas of Human Anatomy, 4 ed, 2006, Saunders.)

NAP-23

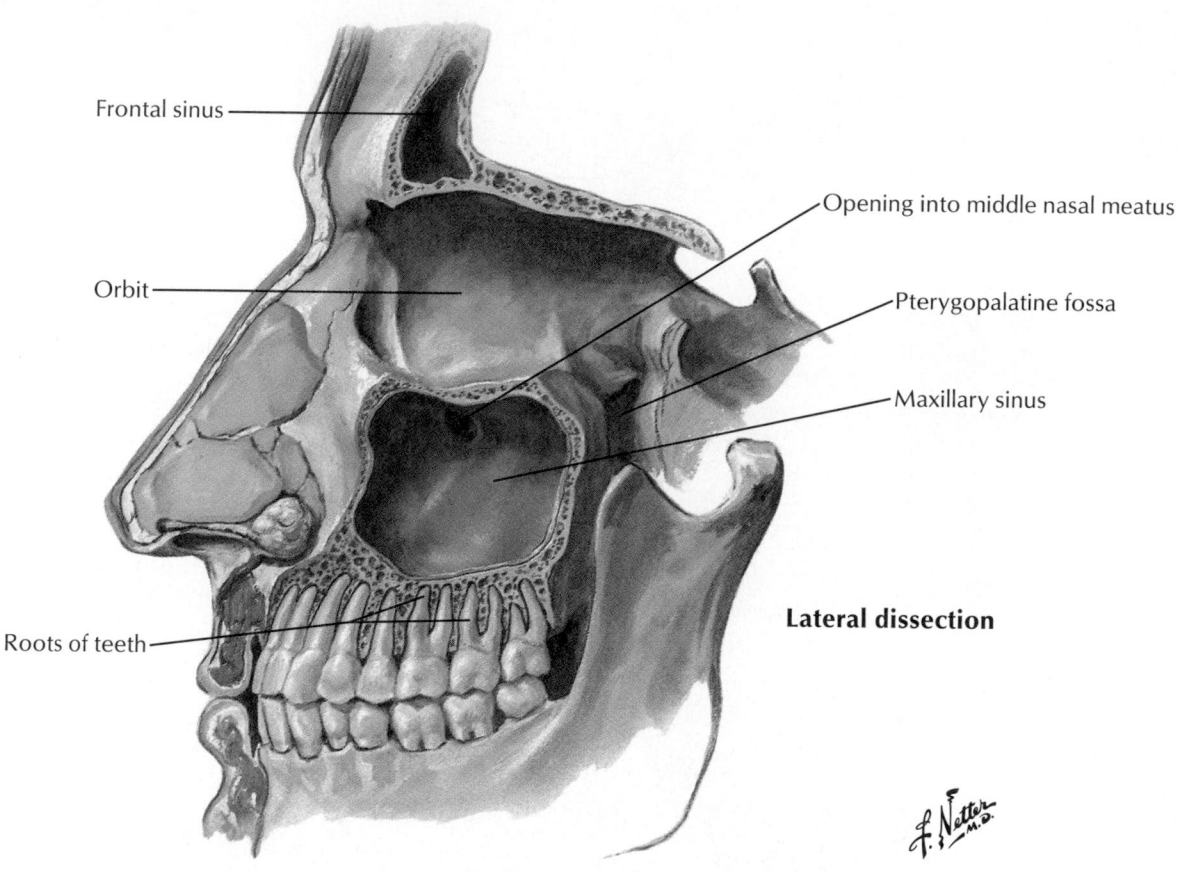

Frontal sinus

Opening into middle nasal meatus

Orbit

Pterygopalatine fossa

Maxillary sinus

Lateral dissection

Roots of teeth

Plate 49 Paranasal Sinuses. (Netter: Atlas of Human Anatomy, 4 ed, 2006, Saunders.)

Superficial temporal artery and vein and auriculotemporal nerve

Branches of facial nerve

Transverse facial artery

Accessory parotid gland

Parotid duct

Buccinator muscle (*cut*)

Masseter muscle

Lingual nerve

Submandibular ganglion

Tongue

Frenulum of tongue

Sublingual fold with openings of sublingual ducts

Sublingual caruncle with opening of submandibular duct

Sublingual gland

Submandibular duct

Sublingual artery and vein

Mylohyoid muscle (*cut*)

Digastric muscle (anterior belly)

Submandibular gland

Facial artery and vein

Hyoid bone

Parotid gland

Retromandibular vein (anterior and posterior branches)

Digastric muscle (posterior belly)

Stylohyoid muscle

External jugular vein

Sternocleidomastoid muscle

Common trunk receiving facial, anterior branch of retromandibular, and lingual veins (common facial vein)

Internal jugular vein

External carotid artery

Parotid gland: totally serous

Submandibular gland: mostly serous, partially mucous

Sublingual gland: almost completely mucous

Plate 61   Salivary Glands. (Netter: Atlas of Human Anatomy, 4 ed, 2006, Saunders.)

Right coronary artery: left anterior oblique view

Sinuatrial (SA) nodal branch

Right coronary artery

Atrioventricular (AV) nodal branch

Branches to back of left ventricle

Right marginal branch

Posterior interventricular branch (posterior descending artery)

Arteriogram

Right coronary artery: right anterior oblique view

Sinuatrial (SA) nodal branch

Conus (arteriosus) branch

Right coronary artery

Right marginal branch

Arteriogram

Atrioventricular (AV) nodal branch

Right posterolateral branches (to back of left ventricle)

Posterior interventricular branch (posterior descending artery)

Plate 218 Coronary Arteries: Arteriographic Views. (Netter: Atlas of Human Anatomy, 4 ed, 2006, Saunders.)

Left coronary artery: left anterior oblique view

Left coronary artery

Circumflex branch

Arteriogram

Anterior interventricular branch (left anterior descending)

Diagonal branches of anterior interventricular branch

Atrioventricular branch of circumflex branch

Left (obtuse) marginal branch

Posterolateral branches

(Perforating) interventricular septal branches

Left coronary artery: right anterior oblique view

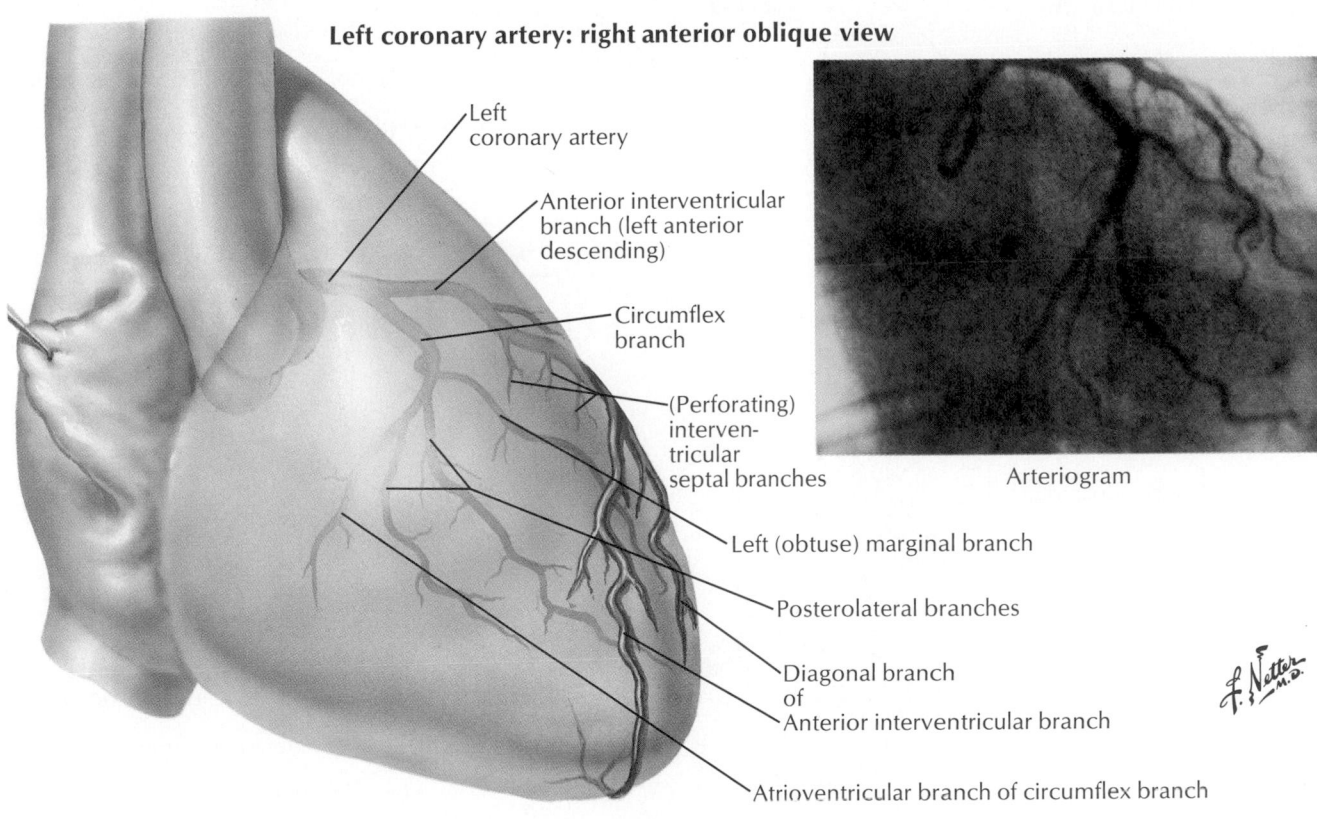

Left coronary artery

Anterior interventricular branch (left anterior descending)

Circumflex branch

(Perforating) interventricular septal branches

Arteriogram

Left (obtuse) marginal branch

Posterolateral branches

Diagonal branch of Anterior interventricular branch

Atrioventricular branch of circumflex branch

Plate 219   Coronary Arteries: Arteriographic Views. (Netter: Atlas of Human Anatomy, 4 ed, 2006, Saunders.)

Corpus callosum

Anterolateral central (lenticulostriate) arteries

Lateral frontobasal (orbitofrontal) artery

Prefrontal artery

Precentral (pre-Rolandic) and central (Rolandic) sulcal arteries

Anterior parietal (postcentral sulcal) artery

Posterior parietal artery

Branch to angular gyrus

Temporal branches (anterior, middle, and posterior)

Middle cerebral artery and branches (deep in lateral cerebral [Sylvian] sulcus)

Anterior communicating artery

Posterior communicating artery

Anterior inferior cerebellar artery (AICA)

Posterior spinal artery

Paracentral artery

Medial frontal branches

Pericallosal artery

Callosomarginal artery

Polar frontal artery

Anterior cerebral arteries

Medial frontobasal (orbitofrontal) artery

Distal medial striate artery (recurrent artery of Heubner)

Internal carotid artery

Anterior choroidal artery

Posterior cerebral artery

Superior cerebellar artery

Basilar and pontine arteries

Labyrinthine (internal acoustic) artery

Vertebral artery

Posterior inferior cerebellar artery (PICA)

Anterior spinal artery

Corpus striatum (caudate and lentiform nuclei)

Anterolateral central (lenticulostriate) arteries

Insula (island of Reil)

Limen of insula

Precentral (pre-Rolandic), central (Rolandic) sulcal, and parietal arteries

Lateral cerebral (Sylvian) sulcus

Temporal branches of middle cerebral artery

Temporal lobe

Middle cerebral artery

Internal carotid artery

Falx cerebri

Callosomarginal arteries and Pericallosal arteries (branches of anterior cerebral arteries)

Trunk of corpus callosum

Internal capsule

Septum pellucidum

Rostrum of corpus callosum

Anterior cerebral arteries

Distal medial striate artery (recurrent artery of Heubner)

Anterior communicating artery

Optic chiasm

Plate 141   Arteries of Brain: Frontal View and Section. (Netter: Atlas of Human Anatomy, 4 ed, 2006, Saunders.)

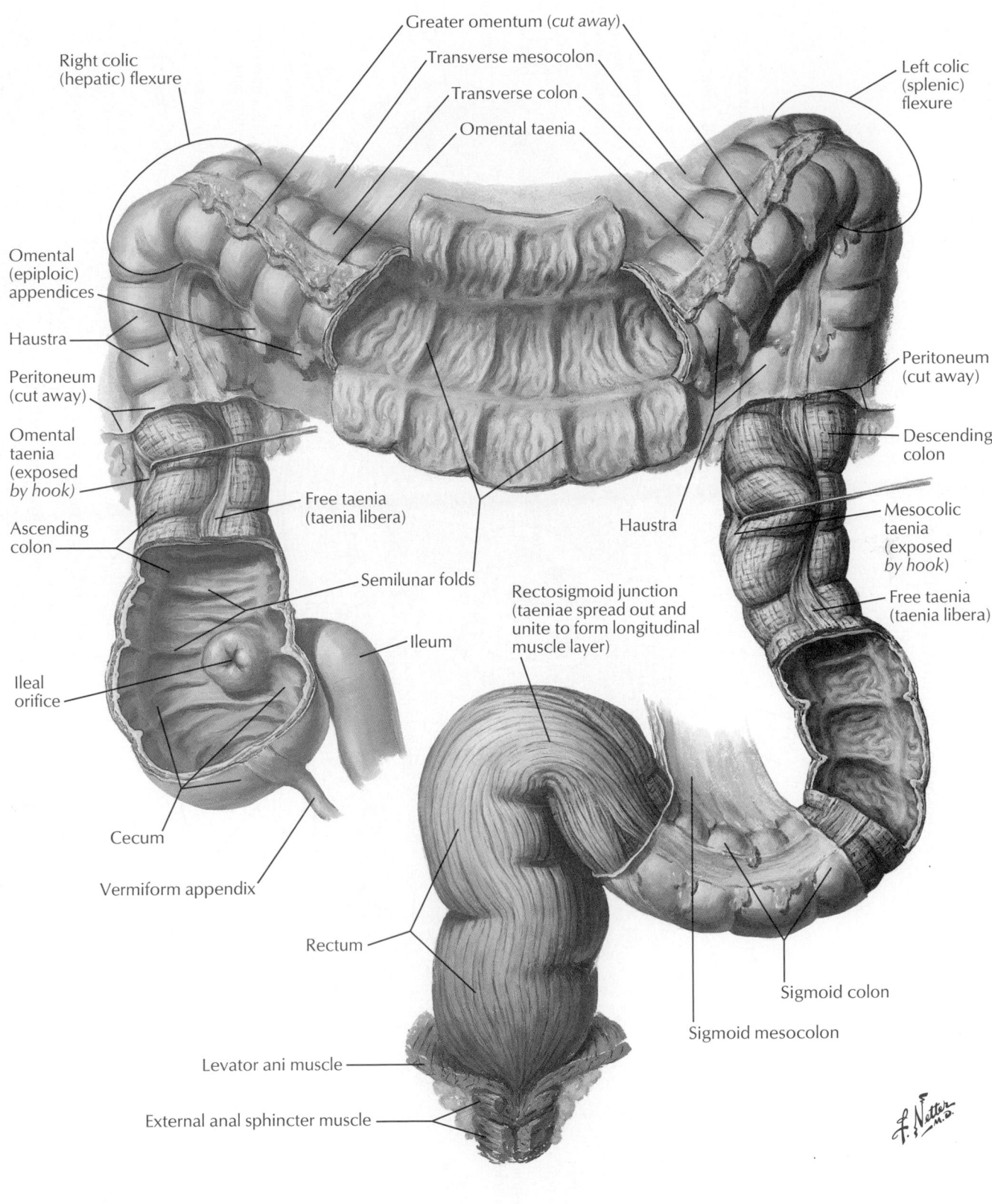

Right colic (hepatic) flexure

Greater omentum (*cut away*)

Transverse mesocolon

Transverse colon

Omental taenia

Left colic (splenic) flexure

Omental (epiploic) appendices

Haustra

Peritoneum (cut away)

Omental taenia (exposed *by hook*)

Ascending colon

Ileal orifice

Cecum

Vermiform appendix

Rectum

Levator ani muscle

External anal sphincter muscle

Free taenia (taenia libera)

Semilunar folds

Ileum

Rectosigmoid junction (taeniae spread out and unite to form longitudinal muscle layer)

Haustra

Peritoneum (cut away)

Descending colon

Mesocolic taenia (exposed *by hook*)

Free taenia (taenia libera)

Sigmoid colon

Sigmoid mesocolon

f. Netter m.d.

Plate 284   Mucosa and Musculature of Large Intestine. (Netter: Atlas of Human Anatomy, 4 ed, 2006, Saunders.)

Transverse Section: T3–4 Intervertebral Disc, Manubrium

T3–4

Plate 244

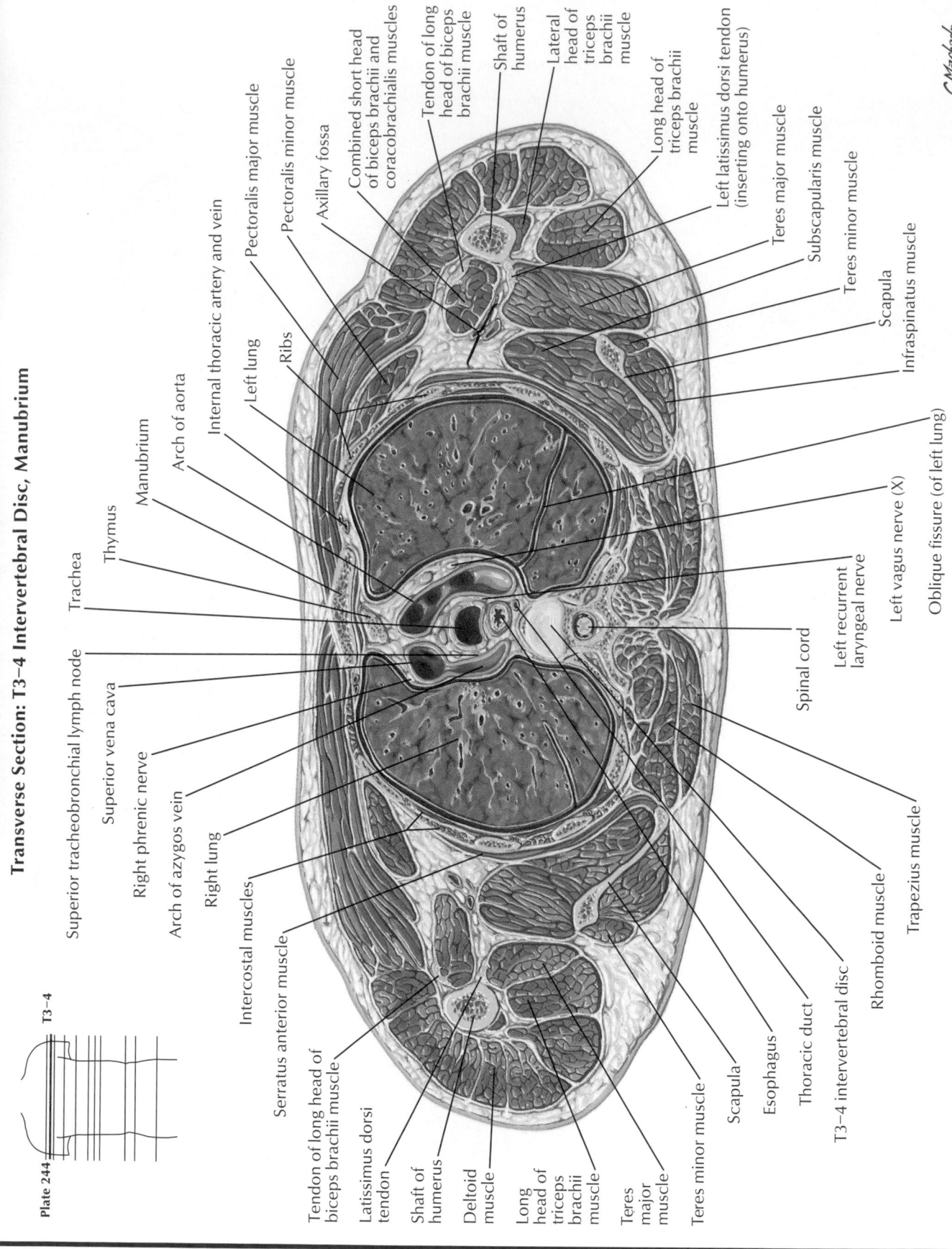

Superior tracheobronchial lymph node
Superior vena cava
Right phrenic nerve
Arch of azygos vein
Right lung
Intercostal muscles
Serratus anterior muscle
Tendon of long head of biceps brachii muscle
Latissimus dorsi tendon
Shaft of humerus
Deltoid muscle
Long head of triceps brachii muscle
Teres major muscle
Teres minor muscle
Scapula
Esophagus
Thoracic duct
T3–4 intervertebral disc
Rhomboid muscle
Trapezius muscle

Trachea
Thymus
Manubrium
Arch of aorta
Internal thoracic artery and vein
Left lung
Ribs
Axillary fossa
Combined short head of biceps brachii and coracobrachialis muscles
Tendon of long head of biceps brachii muscle
Shaft of humerus
Lateral head of triceps brachii muscle
Long head of triceps brachii muscle
Left latissimus dorsi tendon (inserting onto humerus)
Teres major muscle
Subscapularis muscle
Teres minor muscle
Scapula
Infraspinatus muscle

Pectoralis major muscle
Pectoralis minor muscle

Left vagus nerve (X)
Oblique fissure (of left lung)
Spinal cord
Left recurrent laryngeal nerve

Plate 244   Cross Section of Thorax at T3-4 Disc Level. (Netter: Atlas of Human Anatomy, 4 ed, 2006, Saunders.)

Right knee in extension: posterior view

Posterior cruciate ligament

Anterior cruciate ligament

Posterior meniscofemoral ligament

Lateral condyle of femur (articular surface)

Popliteus tendon

Fibular collateral ligament

Lateral meniscus

Head of fibula

Adductor tubercle on medial epicondyle of femur

Medial condyle of femur (articular surface)

Medial meniscus

Tibial collateral ligament

Medial condyle of tibia

Plate 509   Knee: Cruciate and Collateral Ligaments. (Netter: Atlas of Human Anatomy, 4 ed, 2006, Saunders.)

Paramedian (sagittal) dissection

Ureter

Uterine (fallopian) tube

Ovary

Ligament of ovary

Round ligament of uterus

Broad ligament (*cut*)

Superior pubic ramus (*cut*)

Inferior pubic ramus (*cut*)

Ischiocavernosus muscle

Body of clitoris

Labia minora

Labium majus

Rectouterine pouch (of Douglas)

Peritoneum (*cut edge*)

Vesicouterine pouch

Rectum

Ureter

Urinary bladder

Vagina

Pelvic diaphragm (levator ani muscle)

Deep transverse perineal muscle (*cut*)

External anal sphincter muscle

Median (sagittal) section

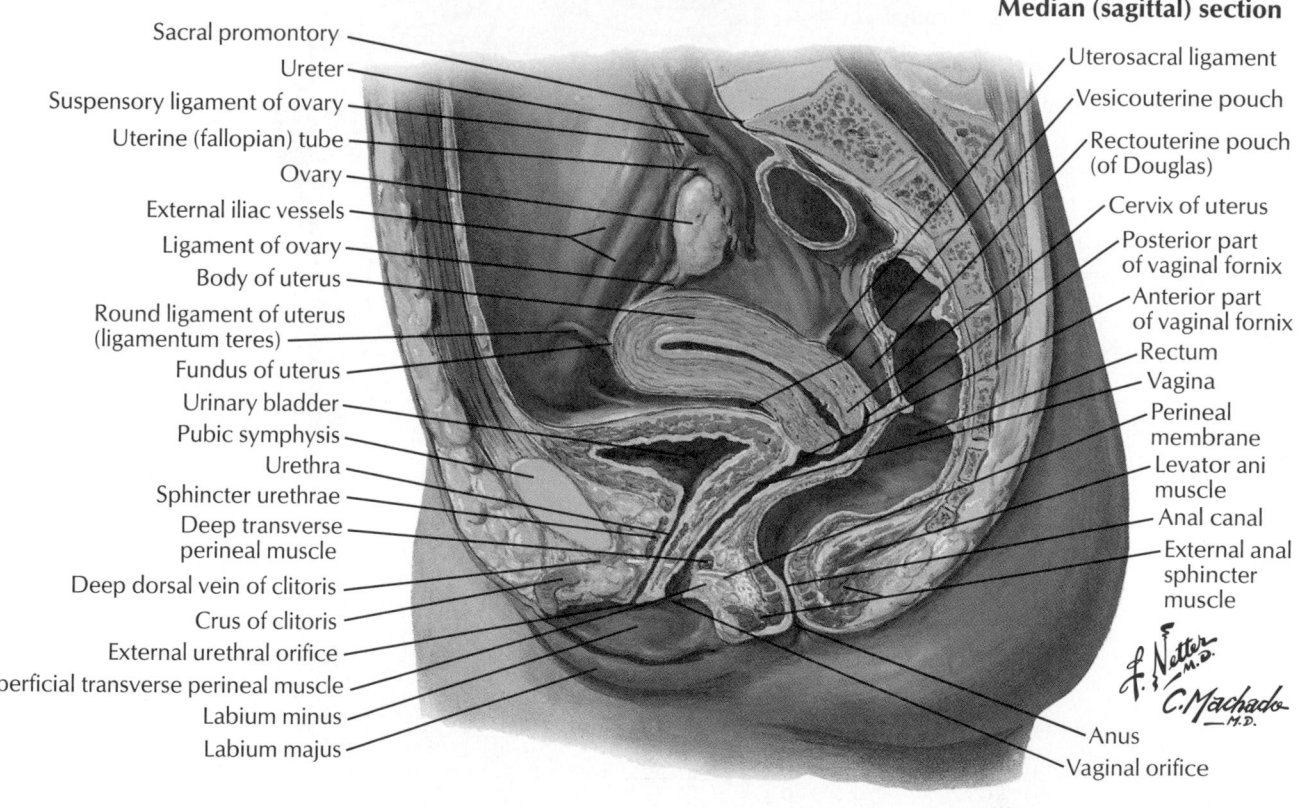

Sacral promontory

Ureter

Suspensory ligament of ovary

Uterine (fallopian) tube

Ovary

External iliac vessels

Ligament of ovary

Body of uterus

Round ligament of uterus (ligamentum teres)

Fundus of uterus

Urinary bladder

Pubic symphysis

Urethra

Sphincter urethrae

Deep transverse perineal muscle

Deep dorsal vein of clitoris

Crus of clitoris

External urethral orifice

Superficial transverse perineal muscle

Labium minus

Labium majus

Uterosacral ligament

Vesicouterine pouch

Rectouterine pouch (of Douglas)

Cervix of uterus

Posterior part of vaginal fornix

Anterior part of vaginal fornix

Rectum

Vagina

Perineal membrane

Levator ani muscle

Anal canal

External anal sphincter muscle

Anus

Vaginal orifice

f. Netter M.D.

C.Machado M.D.

Plate 360 Pelvic Viscera and Perineum: Female. (Netter: Atlas of Human Anatomy, 4 ed, 2006, Saunders.)

NETTER ANATOMY PLATE

Introduction

ICD-9-CM BACKGROUND

The International Classification of Diseases, 9th Revision, Clinical Modification (ICD-9-CM) is based on the official version of the World Health Organization's 9th Revision, International Classification of Diseases (ICD-9). ICD-9 is designed for the classification of morbidity and mortality information for statistical purposes, and for the indexing of hospital records by disease and operations, for data storage and retrieval. The historical background of the International Classification of Diseases may be found in the Introduction to ICD-9 (Manual of the International Classification of Diseases, Injuries, and Causes of Death, World Health Organization, Geneva, Switzerland, 1977).

ICD-9-CM is a clinical modification of the World Health Organization's International Classification of Diseases, 9th Revision (ICD-9). The term "clinical" is used to emphasize the modification's intent: to serve as a useful tool in the area of classification of morbidity data for indexing of medical records, medical care review, and ambulatory and other medical care programs, as well as for basic health statistics. To describe the clinical picture of the patient, the codes must be more precise than those needed only for statistical groupings and trend analysis.

COORDINATION AND MAINTENANCE COMMITTEE

Annual modifications are made to the ICD-9-CM through the ICD-9-CM Coordination and Maintenance Committee (C&M). The Committee is made up of representatives from two Federal Government agencies, the National Center for Health Statistics and the Health Care Financing Administration. The Committee holds meetings twice a year which are open to the public. Modification proposals submitted to the Committee for consideration are presented at the meetings for public discussion. Those modification proposals which are approved are incorporated into the official government version of the ICD-9-CM and become effective for use October 1 of the year following their presentation. The C&M also prepares updates for use April 1 of each year. To date, no April 1 updates have been released.

1

CHARACTERISTICS OF ICD-9-CM

ICD-9-CM far exceeds its predecessors in the number of codes provided. The disease classification has been expanded to include health-related conditions and to provide greater specificity at the fifth-digit level of detail. These fifth digits are not optional; they are intended for use in recording the information substantiated in the clinical record.

Volume I of ICD-9-CM contains five appendices:

Appendix A   Morphology of Neoplasms
Appendix B   Glossary of Mental Disorders (Deleted in 2004)
Appendix C   Classification of Drugs by American Hospital Formulary Service
              List Number and Their ICD-9-CM Equivalents
Appendix D   Classification of Industrial Accidents According to Agency
Appendix E   List of Three-Digit Categories

These appendices are included as a reference to the user in order to provide further information about the patient's clinical picture, to further define a diagnostic statement, to aid in classifying new drugs, or to reference three-digit categories.

Volume 2 of ICD-9-CM contains many diagnostic terms which do not appear in Volume 1 since the index includes most diagnostic terms currently in use.

The Disease Classification

ICD-9-CM is totally compatible with its parent system, ICD-9, thus meeting the need for comparability of morbidity and mortality statistics at the international level. A few fourth-digit codes were created in existing three-digit rubrics only when the necessary detail could not be accommodated by the use of a fifth-digit subclassification. To ensure that each rubric of ICD-9-CM collapses back to its ICD-9 counterpart, the following specifications governed the ICD-9-CM disease classification:

Specifications for the Tabular List

1. Three-digit rubrics and their contents are unchanged from ICD-9.
2. The sequence of three-digit rubrics is unchanged from ICD-9.
3. Unsubdivided three-digit rubrics are subdivided where necessary to:
   a) Add clinical detail
   b) Isolate terms for clinical accuracy
4. The modification in ICD-9-CM is accomplished by the addition of a fifth digit to existing ICD-9 rubrics.
5. The optional dual classification in ICD-9 is modified.
   a) Duplicate rubrics are deleted:
      1) Four-digit manifestation categories duplicating etiology entries.
      2) Manifestation inclusion terms duplicating etiology entries.
   b) Manifestations of diseases are identified, to the extent possible, by creating five-digit codes in the etiology rubrics.
   c) When the manifestation of a disease cannot be included in the etiology rubrics, provision for its identification is made by retaining the ICD-9 rubrics used for classifying manifestations of disease.
6. The format of ICD-9-CM is revised from that used in ICD-9.
   a) American spelling of medical terms is used.
   b) Inclusion terms are indented beneath the titles of codes.
   c) Codes not to be used for principal tabulation of disease are printed with the notation, "Code first underlying disease."

Specifications for the Alphabetic Index

1. Format of the Alphabetic Index follows the format of ICD-9.
2. When two codes are required to indicate etiology and manifestation, the manifestation code appears in brackets, e.g., diabetic cataract 250.5X [366.41]. The etiology code is always sequenced first followed by the manifestation code.

The following guidelines were the most current at the time of publication. Check the website at http://codingupdates.com for the latest updates to the Guidelines.

ICD-9-CM OFFICIAL GUIDELINES FOR CODING AND REPORTING

Effective October 1, 2008
Narrative changes appear in bold text
Items underlined have been moved within the guidelines since October 1, 2007
The guidelines include the updated V Code Table

The Centers for Medicare and Medicaid Services (CMS) and the National Center for Health Statistics (NCHS), two departments within the U.S. Federal Government's Department of Health and Human Services (DHHS) provide the following guidelines for coding and reporting using the International Classification of Diseases, 9th Revision, Clinical Modification (ICD-9-CM). These guidelines should be used as a companion document to the official version of the ICD-9-CM as published on CD-ROM by the U.S. Government Printing Office (GPO).

These guidelines have been approved by the four organizations that make up the Cooperating Parties for the ICD-9-CM: the American Hospital Association (AHA), the American Health Information Management Association (AHIMA), CMS, and NCHS. These guidelines are included on the official government version of the ICD-9-CM, and also appear in "Coding Clinic for ICD-9-CM" published by the AHA.

These guidelines are a set of rules that have been developed to accompany and complement the official conventions and instructions provided within the ICD-9-CM itself. These guidelines are based on the coding and sequencing instructions in Volumes I, II and III of ICD-9-CM, but provide additional instruction. Adherence to these guidelines when assigning ICD-9-CM diagnosis and procedure codes is required under the Health Insurance Portability and Accountability Act (HIPAA). The diagnosis codes (Volumes 1-2) have been adopted under HIPAA for all healthcare settings. Volume 3 procedure codes have been adopted for inpatient procedures reported by hospitals. A joint effort between the healthcare provider and the coder is essential to achieve complete and accurate documentation, code assignment, and reporting of diagnoses and procedures. These guidelines have been developed to assist both the healthcare provider and the coder in identifying those diagnoses and procedures that are to be reported. The importance of consistent, complete documentation in the medical record cannot be overemphasized. Without such documentation accurate coding cannot be achieved. The entire record should be reviewed to determine the specific reason for the encounter and the conditions treated.

The term encounter is used for all settings, including hospital admissions. In the context of these guidelines, the term provider is used throughout the guidelines to mean physician or any qualified health care practitioner who is legally accountable for establishing the patient's diagnosis. Only this set of guidelines, approved by the Cooperating Parties, is official.

The guidelines are organized into sections. Section I includes the structure and conventions of the classification and general guidelines that apply to the entire classification, and chapter-specific guidelines that correspond to the chapters as they are arranged in the classification. Section II includes guidelines for selection of principal diagnosis for non-outpatient settings. Section III includes guidelines for reporting additional diagnoses in non-outpatient settings. Section IV is for outpatient coding and reporting.

ICD-9-CM Official Guidelines for Coding and Reporting

Section I. Conventions, general coding guidelines and chapter specific guidelines

A. Conventions for the ICD-9-CM
  1. Format:
  2. Abbreviations
     a. Index abbreviations
     b. Tabular abbreviations
  3. Punctuation
  4. Includes and Excludes Notes and Inclusion terms
  5. Other and Unspecified codes
     a. "Other" codes
     b. "Unspecified" codes
  6. Etiology/manifestation convention ("code first", "use additional code" and "in diseases classified elsewhere" notes)
  7. "And"
  8. "With"
  9. "See" and "See Also"

B. General Coding Guidelines
  1. Use of Both Alphabetic Index and Tabular List
  2. Locate each term in the Alphabetic Index
  3. Level of Detail in Coding
  4. Code or codes from 001.0 through V89
  5. Selection of codes 001.0 through 999.9
  6. Signs and symptoms
  7. Conditions that are an integral part of a disease process
  8. Conditions that are not an integral part of a disease process
  9. Multiple coding for a single condition
  10. Acute and Chronic Conditions
  11. Combination Code
  12. Late Effects
  13. Impending or Threatened Condition
  14. **Reporting Same Diagnosis Code More than Once**
  15. **Admissions/Encounters for Rehabilitation**
  16. **Documentation for BMI and Pressure Ulcer Stages**

C. Chapter-Specific Coding Guidelines
  1. Chapter 1: Infectious and Parasitic Diseases (001-139)
     a. Human Immunodeficiency Virus (HIV) Infections
     b. Septicemia, Systemic Inflammatory Response Syndrome (SIRS), Sepsis, Severe Sepsis, and Septic Shock
     c. **Methicillin Resistant *Staphylococcus aureus* (MRSA) Conditions**

2. Chapter 2: Neoplasms (140-239)
   a. Treatment directed at the malignancy
   b. Treatment of secondary site
   c. Coding and sequencing of complications
   d. Primary malignancy previously excised
   e. Admissions/Encounters involving chemotherapy, immunotherapy and radiation therapy
   f. Admission/encounter to determine extent of malignancy
   g. Symptoms, signs, and ill-defined conditions listed in Chapter 16 associated with neoplasms
   h. Admission/encounter for pain control/management
   i. Malignant neoplasm associated with transplanted organ
3. Chapter 3: Endocrine, Nutritional, and Metabolic Diseases and Immunity Disorders (240-279)
   a. Diabetes mellitus
4. Chapter 4: Diseases of Blood and Blood Forming Organs (280-289)
   a. Anemia of chronic disease
5. Chapter 5: Mental Disorders (290-319)
   Reserved for future guideline expansion
6. Chapter 6: Diseases of Nervous System and Sense Organs (320-389)
   a. Pain - Category 338
7. Chapter 7: Diseases of Circulatory System (390-459)
   a. Hypertension
   b. Cerebral infarction/stroke/cerebrovascular accident (CVA)
   c. Postoperative cerebrovascular accident
   d. Late Effects of Cerebrovascular Disease
   e. Acute myocardial infarction (AMI)
8. Chapter 8: Diseases of Respiratory System (460-519)
   a. Chronic Obstructive Pulmonary Disease [COPD] and Asthma
   b. Chronic Obstructive Pulmonary Disease [COPD] and Bronchitis
   c. Acute Respiratory Failure
   d. Influenza due to identified avian influenza virus (avian influenza)
9. Chapter 9: Diseases of Digestive System (520-579)
   Reserved for future guideline expansion
10. Chapter 10: Diseases of Genitourinary System (580-629)
    a. Chronic kidney disease
11. Chapter 11: Complications of Pregnancy, Childbirth, and the Puerperium (630-679)
    a. General Rules for Obstetric Cases
    b. Selection of OB Principal or First-listed Diagnosis
    c. Fetal Conditions Affecting the Management of the Mother
    d. HIV Infection in Pregnancy, Childbirth and the Puerperium
    e. Current Conditions Complicating Pregnancy
    f. Diabetes mellitus in pregnancy
    g. Gestational diabetes
    h. Normal Delivery, Code 650
    i. The Postpartum and Peripartum Periods
    j. Code 677, Late effect of complication of pregnancy
    k. Abortions

Section II. Selection of Principal Diagnosis

A. Codes for symptoms, signs, and ill-defined conditions
B. Two or more interrelated conditions, each potentially meeting the definition for principal diagnosis
C. Two or more diagnoses that equally meet the definition for principal diagnosis
D. Two or more comparative or contrasting conditions
E. A symptom(s) followed by contrasting/comparative diagnoses
F. Original treatment plan not carried out
G. Complications of surgery and other medical care
H. Uncertain Diagnosis
 I. Admission from Observation Unit
    1. Admission Following Medical Observation
    2. Admission Following Post-Operative Observation
 J. Admission from Outpatient Surgery

Section III. Reporting Additional Diagnoses

A. Previous conditions
B. Abnormal findings
C. Uncertain Diagnosis

Section IV. Diagnostic Coding and Reporting Guidelines for Outpatient Services

A. Selection of first-listed condition
    1. Outpatient Surgery
    2. Observation Stay
B. Codes from 001.0 through **V89.09**
C. Accurate reporting of ICD-9-CM diagnosis codes
D. Selection of codes 001.0 through 999.9
E. Codes that describe symptoms and signs
F. Encounters for circumstances other than a disease or injury
G. Level of Detail in Coding
    1. ICD-9-CM codes with 3, 4, or 5 digits
    2. Use of full number of digits required for a code
H. ICD-9-CM code for the diagnosis, condition, problem, or other reason for encounter/visit
 I. Uncertain diagnosis
 J. Chronic diseases
K. Code all documented conditions that coexist
L. Patients receiving diagnostic services only
M. Patients receiving therapeutic services only
N. Patients receiving preoperative evaluations only
O. Ambulatory surgery
P. Routine outpatient prenatal visits

Appendix I: Present on Admission Reporting Guidelines

Section I. Conventions, general coding guidelines and chapter specific guidelines

The conventions, general guidelines and chapter-specific guidelines are applicable to all health care settings unless otherwise indicated.

A. Conventions for the ICD-9-CM

The conventions for the ICD-9-CM are the general rules for use of the classification independent of the guidelines. These conventions are incorporated within the index and tabular of the ICD-9-CM as instructional notes. The conventions are as follows:

1. Format:

The ICD-9-CM uses an indented format for ease in reference

2. Abbreviations

a. Index abbreviations

NEC "Not elsewhere classifiable"
This abbreviation in the index represents "other specified" when a specific code is not available for a condition the index directs the coder to the "other specified" code in the tabular.

b. Tabular abbreviations

NEC "Not elsewhere classifiable"
This abbreviation in the tabular represents "other specified". When a specific code is not available for a condition the tabular includes an NEC entry under a code to identify the code as the "other specified" code.
(See Section I.A.5.a. "Other" codes").

NOS "Not otherwise specified"
This abbreviation is the equivalent of unspecified.
(See Section I.A.5.b., "Unspecified" codes)

3. Punctuation

[ ] Brackets are used in the tabular list to enclose synonyms, alternative wording or explanatory phrases. Brackets are used in the index to identify manifestation codes.
(See Section I.A.6. "Etiology/manifestations")

( ) Parentheses are used in both the index and tabular to enclose supplementary words that may be present or absent in the statement of a disease or procedure without affecting the code number to which it is assigned. The terms within the parentheses are referred to as nonessential modifiers.

: Colons are used in the Tabular list after an incomplete term which needs one or more of the modifiers following the colon to make it assignable to a given category.

4. Includes and Excludes Notes and Inclusion terms

Includes: This note appears immediately under a three-digit code title to further define, or give examples of, the content of the category.

Excludes: An excludes note under a code indicates that the terms excluded from the code are to be coded elsewhere. In some cases the codes for the excluded terms should not be used in conjunction with the code from which it is excluded. An example of this is a congenital condition excluded from an acquired form of the same condition. The congenital and acquired codes should not be used together. In other cases, the excluded terms may be used together with an excluded code. An example of this is when fractures of different bones are coded to different codes. Both codes may be used together if both types of fractures are present.

Inclusion terms: List of terms is included under certain four and five digit codes. These terms are the conditions for which that code number is to be used. The terms may be synonyms of the code title, or, in the case of "other specified" codes, the terms are a list of the various conditions assigned to that code. The inclusion terms are not necessarily exhaustive. Additional terms found only in the index may also be assigned to a code.

5. **Other and Unspecified codes**

a. **"Other" codes**

Codes titled "other" or "other specified" (usually a code with a 4th digit 8 or fifth-digit 9 for diagnosis codes) are for use when the information in the medical record provides detail for which a specific code does not exist. Index entries with NEC in the line designate "other" codes in the tabular. These index entries represent specific disease entities for which no specific code exists so the term is included within an "other" code.

b. **"Unspecified" codes**

Codes (usually a code with a 4th digit 9 or 5th digit 0 for diagnosis codes) titled "unspecified" are for use when the information in the medical record is insufficient to assign a more specific code.

6. **Etiology/manifestation convention ("code first", "use additional code" and "in diseases classified elsewhere" notes)**

Certain conditions have both an underlying etiology and multiple body system manifestations due to the underlying etiology. For such conditions, the ICD-9-CM has a coding convention that requires the underlying condition be sequenced first followed by the manifestation. Wherever such a combination exists, there is a "use additional code" note at the etiology code, and a "code first" note at the manifestation code. These instructional notes indicate the proper sequencing order of the codes, etiology followed by manifestation.

In most cases the manifestation codes will have in the code title, "in diseases classified elsewhere." Codes with this title are a component of the etiology/ manifestation convention. The code title indicates that it is a manifestation code. "In diseases classified elsewhere" codes are never permitted to be used as first listed or principal diagnosis codes. They must be used in conjunction with an underlying condition code and they must be listed following the underlying condition.

There are manifestation codes that do not have "in diseases classified elsewhere" in the title. For such codes a "use additional code" note will still be present and the rules for sequencing apply.

In addition to the notes in the tabular, these conditions also have a specific index entry structure. In the index both conditions are listed together with the etiology code first followed by the manifestation codes in brackets. The code in brackets is always to be sequenced second.

The most commonly used etiology/manifestation combinations are the codes for Diabetes mellitus, category 250. For each code under category 250 there is a use additional code note for the manifestation that is specific for that particular diabetic manifestation. Should a patient have more than one manifestation of diabetes, more than one code from category 250 may be used with as many manifestation codes as are needed to fully describe the patient's complete diabetic condition. The category 250 diabetes codes should be sequenced first, followed by the manifestation codes.

"Code first" and "Use additional code" notes are also used as sequencing rules in the classification for certain codes that are not part of an etiology/ manifestation combination.

See - Section I.B.9. "Multiple coding for a single condition".

7. **"And"**

The word "and" should be interpreted to mean either "and" or "or" when it appears in a title.

8. **"With"**

The word "with" in the alphabetic index is sequenced immediately following the main term, not in alphabetical order.

9. **"See" and "See Also"**

The "see" instruction following a main term in the index indicates that another term should be referenced. It is necessary to go to the main term referenced with the "see" note to locate the correct code.

A "see also" instruction following a main term in the index instructs that there is another main term that may also be referenced that may provide additional index entries that may be useful. It is not necessary to follow the "see also" note when the original main term provides the necessary code.

B. **General Coding Guidelines**

1. **Use of Both Alphabetic Index and Tabular List**

Use both the Alphabetic Index and the Tabular List when locating and assigning a code. Reliance on only the Alphabetic Index or the Tabular List leads to errors in code assignments and less specificity in code selection.

2. **Locate each term in the Alphabetic Index**

Locate each term in the Alphabetic Index and verify the code selected in the Tabular List. Read and be guided by instructional notations that appear in both the Alphabetic Index and the Tabular List.

3. **Level of Detail in Coding**

Diagnosis and procedure codes are to be used at their highest number of digits available.

ICD-9-CM diagnosis codes are composed of codes with 3, 4, or 5 digits. Codes with three digits are included in ICD-9-CM as the heading of a category of codes that may be further subdivided by the use of fourth and/or fifth digits, which provide greater detail.

A three-digit code is to be used only if it is not further subdivided. Where fourth-digit subcategories and/or fifth-digit subclassifications are provided, they must be assigned. A code is invalid if it has not been coded to the full number of digits required for that code. For example, Acute myocardial infarction, code 410, has fourth digits that describe the location of the infarction (e.g., 410.2, Of inferolateral wall), and fifth digits that identify the episode of care. It would be incorrect to report a code in category 410 without a fourth and fifth digit.

ICD-9-CM Volume 3 procedure codes are composed of codes with either 3 or 4 digits. Codes with two digits are included in ICD-9-CM as the heading of a category of codes that may be further subdivided by the use of third and/or fourth digits, which provide greater detail.

4. **Code or codes from 001.0 through V89.09**

The appropriate code or codes from 001.0 through V89.09 must be used to identify diagnoses, symptoms, conditions, problems, complaints or other reason(s) for the encounter/visit.

5. **Selection of codes 001.0 through 999.9**

   The selection of codes 001.0 through 999.9 will frequently be used to describe the reason for the admission/encounter. These codes are from the section of ICD-9-CM for the classification of diseases and injuries (e.g., infectious and parasitic diseases; neoplasms; symptoms, signs, and ill-defined conditions, etc.).

6. **Signs and symptoms**

   Codes that describe symptoms and signs, as opposed to diagnoses, are acceptable for reporting purposes when a related definitive diagnosis has not been established (confirmed) by the provider. Chapter 16 of ICD-9-CM, Symptoms, Signs, and Ill-defined conditions (codes 780.0 - 799.9) contain many, but not all codes for symptoms.

7. **Conditions that are an integral part of a disease process**

   Signs and symptoms that are associated routinely with a disease process should not be assigned as additional codes, unless otherwise instructed by the classification.

8. **Conditions that are not an integral part of a disease process**

   Additional signs and symptoms that may not be associated routinely with a disease process should be coded when present.

9. **Multiple coding for a single condition**

   In addition to the etiology/manifestation convention that requires two codes to fully describe a single condition that affects multiple body systems, there are other single conditions that also require more than one code. "Use additional code" notes are found in the tabular at codes that are not part of an etiology/manifestation pair where a secondary code is useful to fully describe a condition. The sequencing rule is the same as the etiology/manifestation pair - , "use additional code" indicates that a secondary code should be added.

   For example, for infections that are not included in chapter 1, a secondary code from category 041, Bacterial infection in conditions classified elsewhere and of unspecified site, may be required to identify the bacterial organism causing the infection. A "use additional code" note will normally be found at the infectious disease code, indicating a need for the organism code to be added as a secondary code.

   "Code first" notes are also under certain codes that are not specifically manifestation codes but may be due to an underlying cause. When a "code first" note is present and an underlying condition is present the underlying condition should be sequenced first.

   "Code, if applicable, any causal condition first", notes indicate that this code may be assigned as a principal diagnosis when the causal condition is unknown or not applicable. If a causal condition is known, then the code for that condition should be sequenced as the principal or first-listed diagnosis.

   Multiple codes may be needed for late effects, complication codes and obstetric codes to more fully describe a condition. See the specific guidelines for these conditions for further instruction.

10. **Acute and Chronic Conditions**

    If the same condition is described as both acute (subacute) and chronic, and separate subentries exist in the Alphabetic Index at the same indentation level, code both and sequence the acute (subacute) code first.

11. Combination Code

A combination code is a single code used to classify:
Two diagnoses, or
A diagnosis with an associated secondary process (manifestation)
A diagnosis with an associated complication

Combination codes are identified by referring to subterm entries in the Alphabetic Index and by reading the inclusion and exclusion notes in the Tabular List.

Assign only the combination code when that code fully identifies the diagnostic conditions involved or when the Alphabetic Index so directs. Multiple coding should not be used when the classification provides a combination code that clearly identifies all of the elements documented in the diagnosis. When the combination code lacks necessary specificity in describing the manifestation or complication, an additional code should be used as a secondary code.

12. Late Effects

A late effect is the residual effect (condition produced) after the acute phase of an illness or injury has terminated. There is no time limit on when a late effect code can be used. The residual may be apparent early, such as in cerebrovascular accident cases, or it may occur months or years later, such as that due to a previous injury. Coding of late effects generally requires two codes sequenced in the following order: The condition or nature of the late effect is sequenced first. The late effect code is sequenced second.

An exception to the above guidelines are those instances where the code for late effect is followed by a manifestation code identified in the Tabular List and title, or the late effect code has been expanded (at the fourth and fifth-digit levels) to include the manifestation(s). The code for the acute phase of an illness or injury that led to the late effect is never used with a code for the late effect.

13. Impending or Threatened Condition

Code any condition described at the time of discharge as "impending" or "threatened" as follows:

If it did occur, code as confirmed diagnosis.

If it did not occur, reference the Alphabetic Index to determine if the condition has a subentry term for "impending" or "threatened" and also reference main term entries for "Impending" and for "Threatened."

If the subterms are listed, assign the given code.

If the subterms are not listed, code the existing underlying condition(s) and not the condition described as impending or threatened.

14. Reporting Same Diagnosis Code More than Once

Each unique ICD-9-CM diagnosis code may be reported only once for an encounter. This applies to bilateral conditions or two different conditions classified to the same ICD-9-CM diagnosis code.

15. Admissions/Encounters for Rehabilitation

When the purpose for the admission/encounter is rehabilitation, sequence the appropriate V code from category V57, Care involving use of rehabilitation procedures, as the principal/first-listed diagnosis. The code for the condition for which the service is being performed should be reported as an additional diagnosis.

Only one code from category V57 is required. Code V57.89, Other specified rehabilitation procedures, should be assigned if more than one type of rehabilitation is performed during a single encounter. A procedure code should be reported to identify each type of rehabilitation therapy actually performed.

16. **Documentation for BMI and Pressure Ulcer Stages**

For the Body Mass Index (BMI) and pressure ulcer stage codes, code assignment may be based on medical record documentation from clinicians who are not the patient's provider (i.e., physician or other qualified healthcare practitioner legally accountable for establishing the patient's diagnosis), since this information is typically documented by other clinicians involved in the care of the patient (e.g., a dietitian often documents the BMI and nurses often documents the pressure ulcer stages). However, the associated diagnosis (such as overweight, obesity, or pressure ulcer) must be documented by the patient's provider. If there is conflicting medical record documentation, either from the same clinician or different clinicians, the patient's attending provider should be queried for clarification.

The BMI and pressure ulcer stage codes should only be reported as secondary diagnoses. As with all other secondary diagnosis codes, the BMI and pressure ulcer stage codes should only be assigned when they meet the definition of a reportable additional diagnosis (see Section III, Reporting Additional Diagnoses).

C. **Chapter-Specific Coding Guidelines**

In addition to general coding guidelines, there are guidelines for specific diagnoses and/or conditions in the classification. Unless otherwise indicated, these guidelines apply to all health care settings. Please refer to Section II for guidelines on the selection of principal diagnosis.

1. **Chapter 1: Infectious and Parasitic Diseases (001-139)**

a. **Human Immunodeficiency Virus (HIV) Infections**

1) **Code only confirmed cases**

Code only confirmed cases of HIV infection/illness. This is an exception to the hospital inpatient guideline Section II, H.

In this context, "confirmation" does not require documentation of positive serology or culture for HIV; the provider's diagnostic statement that the patient is HIV positive, or has an HIV-related illness is sufficient.

2) **Selection and sequencing of HIV codes**

(a) **Patient admitted for HIV-related condition**

If a patient is admitted for an HIV-related condition, the principal diagnosis should be 042, followed by additional diagnosis codes for all reported HIV-related conditions.

(b) **Patient with HIV disease admitted for unrelated condition**

If a patient with HIV disease is admitted for an unrelated condition (such as a traumatic injury), the code for the unrelated condition (e.g., the nature of injury code) should be the principal diagnosis. Other diagnoses would be 042 followed by additional diagnosis codes for all reported HIV-related conditions.

(c) **Whether the patient is newly diagnosed**

Whether the patient is newly diagnosed or has had previous admissions/encounters for HIV conditions is irrelevant to the sequencing decision.

(d) **Asymptomatic human immunodeficiency virus**

V08 Asymptomatic human immunodeficiency virus [HIV] infection, is to be applied when the patient without any documentation of symptoms is listed as being "HIV positive," "known HIV," "HIV test positive," or similar terminology. Do not use this code if the term "AIDS" is used or if the patient is treated for any HIV-related illness or is described as having any condition(s) resulting from his/her HIV positive status; use 042 in these cases.

(e) Patients with inconclusive HIV serology

Patients with inconclusive HIV serology, but no definitive diagnosis or manifestations of the illness, may be assigned code 795.71, Inconclusive serologic test for Human Immunodeficiency Virus [HIV].

(f) Previously diagnosed HIV-related illness

Patients with any known prior diagnosis of an HIV-related illness should be coded to 042. Once a patient has developed an HIV-related illness, the patient should always be assigned code 042 on every subsequent admission/encounter. Patients previously diagnosed with any HIV illness (042) should never be assigned to 795.71 or V08.

(g) HIV Infection in Pregnancy, Childbirth and the Puerperium

During pregnancy, childbirth or the puerperium, a patient admitted (or presenting for a health care encounter) because of an HIV-related illness should receive a principal diagnosis code of 647.6X, Other specified infectious and parasitic diseases in the mother classifiable elsewhere, but complicating the pregnancy, childbirth or the puerperium, followed by 042 and the code(s) for the HIV-related illness(es). Codes from Chapter 15 always take sequencing priority.

Patients with asymptomatic HIV infection status admitted (or presenting for a health care encounter) during pregnancy, childbirth, or the puerperium should receive codes of 647.6X and V08.

(h) Encounters for testing for HIV

If a patient is being seen to determine his/her HIV status, use code V73.89, Screening for other specified viral disease. Use code V69.8, Other problems related to lifestyle, as a secondary code if an asymptomatic patient is in a known high risk group for HIV. Should a patient with signs or symptoms or illness, or a confirmed HIV related diagnosis be tested for HIV, code the signs and symptoms or the diagnosis. An additional counseling code V65.44 may be used if counseling is provided during the encounter for the test.

When a patient returns to be informed of his/her HIV test results use code V65.44, HIV counseling, if the results of the test are negative.

If the results are positive but the patient is asymptomatic use code V08, Asymptomatic HIV infection. If the results are positive and the patient is symptomatic use code 042, HIV infection, with codes for the HIV related symptoms or diagnosis. The HIV counseling code may also be used if counseling is provided for patients with positive test results.

b. **Septicemia, Systemic Inflammatory Response Syndrome (SIRS), Sepsis, Severe Sepsis, and Septic Shock**

1) **SIRS, Septicemia, and Sepsis**

(a) The terms *septicemia* and *sepsis* are often used interchangeably by providers, however they are not considered synonymous terms. The following descriptions are provided for reference but do not preclude querying the provider for clarification about terms used in the documentation:

(i) Septicemia generally refers to a systemic disease associated with the presence of pathological microorganisms or toxins in the blood, which can include bacteria, viruses, fungi or other organisms.

(ii) Systemic inflammatory response syndrome (SIRS) generally refers to the systemic response to infection, trauma/burns, or other insult (such as cancer) with symptoms including fever, tachycardia, tachypnea, and leukocytosis.

(iii) Sepsis generally refers to SIRS due to infection.

(iv) Severe sepsis generally refers to sepsis with associated acute organ dysfunction.

(b) **The Coding of SIRS, sepsis and severe sepsis**

The coding of SIRS, sepsis and severe sepsis requires a minimum of 2 codes: a code for the underlying cause (such as infection or trauma) and a code from subcategory 995.9 Systemic inflammatory response syndrome (SIRS).

(i) The code for the underlying cause (such as infection or trauma) must be sequenced before the code from subcategory 995.9 Systemic inflammatory response syndrome (SIRS).

(ii) Sepsis and severe sepsis require a code for the systemic infection (038.xx, 112.5, etc.) and either code 995.91, Sepsis, or 995.92, Severe sepsis. If the causal organism is not documented, assign code 038.9, Unspecified septicemia.

(iii) Severe sepsis requires additional code(s) for the associated acute organ dysfunction(s).

(iv) If a patient has sepsis with multiple organ dysfunctions, follow the instructions for coding severe sepsis.

(v) Either the term sepsis or SIRS must be documented to assign a code from subcategory 995.9.

(vi) *See Section I.C.17.g), Injury and poisoning, for information regarding systemic inflammatory response syndrome (SIRS) due to trauma/burns and other non-infectious processes.*

(c) Due to the complex nature of sepsis and severe sepsis, some cases may require querying the provider prior to assignment of the codes.

2) **Sequencing sepsis and severe sepsis**

   (a) **Sepsis and severe sepsis as principal diagnosis**

   If sepsis or severe sepsis is present on admission, and meets the definition of principal diagnosis, the systemic infection code (e.g., 038.xx, 112.5, etc) should be assigned as the principal diagnosis, followed by code 995.91, Sepsis, or 995.92, Severe sepsis, as required by the sequencing rules in the Tabular List. Codes from subcategory 995.9 can never be assigned as a principal diagnosis. A code should also be assigned for any localized infection, if present.

   If the sepsis or severe sepsis is due to a postprocedural infection, see Section I.C.1.b.10 for guidelines related to sepsis due to postprocedural infection.

   (b) **Sepsis and severe sepsis as secondary diagnoses**

   When sepsis or severe sepsis develops during the encounter (it was not present on admission), the systemic infection code and code 995.91 or 995.92 should be assigned as secondary diagnoses.

   (c) **Documentation unclear as to whether sepsis or severe sepsis is present on admission**

   Sepsis or severe sepsis may be present on admission but the diagnosis may not be confirmed until sometime after admission. If the documentation is not clear whether the sepsis or severe sepsis was present on admission, the provider should be queried.

3) **Sepsis/SIRS with Localized Infection**

   If the reason for admission is both sepsis, severe sepsis, or SIRS and a localized infection, such as pneumonia or cellulitis, a code for the systemic infection (038.xx, 112.5, etc) should be assigned first, then code 995.91 or 995.92, followed by the code for the localized infection. If the patient is admitted with a localized infection, such as pneumonia, and sepsis/SIRS doesn't develop until after admission, see guideline I.C.1.b.2.b).

   If the localized infection is postprocedural, *see Section I.C.1.b.10 for guidelines related to sepsis due to postprocedural infection.*

   Note: The term urosepsis is a nonspecific term. If that is the only term documented then only code 599.0 should be assigned based on the default for the term in the ICD-9-CM index, in addition to the code for the causal organism if known.

4) **Bacterial Sepsis and Septicemia**

   In most cases, it will be a code from category 038, Septicemia, that will be used in conjunction with a code from subcategory 995.9 such as the following:

   (a) **Streptococcal sepsis**

   If the documentation in the record states streptococcal sepsis, codes 038.0, Streptococcal septicemia, and code 995.91 should be used, in that sequence.

   (b) **Streptococcal septicemia**

   If the documentation states streptococcal septicemia, only code 038.0 should be assigned, however, the provider should be queried whether the patient has sepsis, an infection with SIRS.

5) **Acute organ dysfunction that is not clearly associated with the sepsis**

   If a patient has sepsis and an acute organ dysfunction, but the medical record documentation indicates that the acute organ dysfunction is related to a medical condition other than the sepsis, do not assign code 995.92, Severe sepsis. An acute organ dysfunction must be associated with the sepsis in order to assign the severe sepsis code. If the documentation is not clear as to whether an acute organ dysfunction is related to the sepsis or another medical condition, query the provider.

6) **Septic shock**

   (a) **Sequencing of septic shock**

   Septic shock generally refers to circulatory failure associated with severe sepsis, and, therefore, it represents a type of acute organ dysfunction.

   For all cases of septic shock, the code for the systemic infection should be sequenced first, followed by codes 995.92 and 785.52. Any additional codes for other acute organ dysfunctions should also be assigned. As noted in the sequencing instructions in the Tabular List, the code for septic shock cannot be assigned as a principal diagnosis.

   (b) **Septic Shock without documentation of severe sepsis**

   Septic shock indicates the presence of severe sepsis.

   Code 995.92, Severe sepsis, must be assigned with code 785.52, Septic shock, even if the term severe sepsis is not documented in the record. The "use additional code" note and the "code first" note in the tabular support this guideline.

7) **Sepsis and septic shock complicating abortion and pregnancy**

   Sepsis and septic shock complicating abortion, ectopic pregnancy, and molar pregnancy are classified to category codes in Chapter 11 (630-639).

   See section I.C.11.

8) **Negative or inconclusive blood cultures**

   Negative or inconclusive blood cultures do not preclude a diagnosis of septicemia or sepsis in patients with clinical evidence of the condition, however, the provider should be queried.

9) **Newborn sepsis**

   See Section I.C.15.j for information on the coding of newborn sepsis.

10) **Sepsis due to a Postprocedural Infection**

   (a) **Documentation of causal relationship**

   As with all postprocedural complications, code assignment is based on the provider's documentation of the relationship between the infection and the procedure.

   (b) **Sepsis due to postprocedural infection**

   In cases of postprocedural sepsis, the complication code, such as code 998.59, Other postoperative infection, or 674.3x, Other complications of obstetrical surgical wounds should be coded first followed by the appropriate sepsis codes (systemic infection code and either code 995.91or 995.92). An additional code(s) for any acute organ dysfunction should also be assigned for cases of severe sepsis.

11) **External cause of injury codes with SIRS**

   Refer to Section I.C.19.a.7 for instruction on the use of external cause of injury codes with codes for SIRS resulting from trauma.

12) **Sepsis and Severe Sepsis Associated with Non-infectious Process**

In some cases, a non-infectious process, such as trauma, may lead to an infection which can result in sepsis or severe sepsis. If sepsis or severe sepsis is documented as associated with a non-infectious condition, such as a burn or serious injury, and this condition meets the definition for principal diagnosis, the code for the non-infectious condition should be sequenced first, followed by the code for the systemic infection and either code 995.91, Sepsis, or 995.92, Severe sepsis. Additional codes for any associated acute organ dysfunction(s) should also be assigned for cases of severe sepsis. If the sepsis or severe sepsis meets the definition of principal diagnosis, the systemic infection and sepsis codes should be sequenced before the non-infectious condition. When both the associated non-infectious condition and the sepsis or severe sepsis meet the definition of principal diagnosis, either may be assigned as principal diagnosis.

See Section I.C.1.b.2)(a) for guidelines pertaining to sepsis or severe sepsis as the principal diagnosis.

Only one code from subcategory 995.9 should be assigned. Therefore, when a non-infectious condition leads to an infection resulting in sepsis or severe sepsis, assign either code 995.91 or 995.92. Do not additionally assign code 995.93, Systemic inflammatory response syndrome due to non-infectious process without acute organ dysfunction, or 995.94, Systemic inflammatory response syndrome with acute organ dysfunction.

See Section I.C.17.g for information on the coding of SIRS due to trauma/burns or other non-infectious disease processes.

c. **Methicillin Resistant *Staphylococcus aureus* (MRSA) Conditions**

1) **Selection and sequencing of MRSA codes**

(a) **Combination codes for MRSA infection**

When a patient is diagnosed with an infection that is due to methicillin resistant *Staphylococcus aureus* (MRSA), and that infection has a combination code that includes the causal organism (e.g., septicemia, pneumonia) assign the appropriate code for the condition (e.g., code 038.12, Methicillin resistant Staphylococcus aureus septicemia or code 482.42, Methicillin resistant pneumonia due to Staphylococcus aureus). Do not assign code 041.12, Methicillin resistant Staphylococcus aureus, as an additional code because the code includes the type of infection and the MRSA organism. Do not assign a code from subcategory V09.0, Infection with microorganisms resistant to penicillins, as an additional diagnosis.

See Section C.1.b.1 for instructions on coding and sequencing of septicemia.

(b) **Other codes for MRSA infection**

When there is documentation of a current infection (e.g., wound infection, stitch abscess, urinary tract infection) due to MRSA, and that infection does not have a combination code that includes the causal organism, select the appropriate code to identify the condition along with code 041.12, Methicillin resistant Staphylococcus aureus, for the MRSA infection. Do not assign a code from subcategory V09.0, Infection with microorganisms resistant to penicillins.

(c) **Methicillin susceptible Staphylococcus aureus (MSSA) and MRSA colonization**

The condition or state of being colonized or carrying MSSA or MRSA is called colonization or carriage, while an individual person is described as being colonized or being a carrier. Colonization means that MSSA or MSRA is present on or in the body without necessarily causing illness. A positive MRSA colonization test might be documented by the provider as "MRSA screen positive" or "MRSA nasal swab positive".

Assign code V02.54, Carrier or suspected carrier, Methicillin resistant Staphylococcus aureus, for patients documented as having MRSA colonization. Assign code V02.53, Carrier or suspected carrier, Methicillin susceptible Staphylococcus aureus, for patient documented as having MSSA colonization. Colonization is not necessarily indicative of a disease process or as the cause of a specific condition the patient may have unless documented as such by the provider.

Code V02.59, Other specified bacterial diseases, should be assigned for other types of staphylococcal colonization (e.g., S. *epidermidis*, S. *saprophyticus*). Code V02.59 should not be assigned for colonization with any type of *Staphylococcus aureus* (MRSA, MSSA).

(d) **MRSA colonization and infection**

If a patient is documented as having both MRSA colonization and infection during a hospital admission, code V02.54, Carrier or suspected carrier, Methicillin resistant *Staphylococcus aureus*, and a code for the MRSA infection may both be assigned.

2. **Chapter 2: Neoplasms (140-239)**

<u>General guidelines</u>

Chapter 2 of the ICD-9-CM contains the codes for most benign and all malignant neoplasms. Certain benign neoplasms, such as prostatic adenomas, may be found in the specific body system chapters. To properly code a neoplasm it is necessary to determine from the record if the neoplasm is benign, in-situ, malignant, or of uncertain histologic behavior. If malignant, any secondary (metastatic) sites should also be determined.

The neoplasm table in the Alphabetic Index should be referenced first. However, if the histological term is documented, that term should be referenced first, rather than going immediately to the Neoplasm Table, in order to determine which column in the Neoplasm Table is appropriate. For example, if the documentation indicates "adenoma," refer to the term in the Alphabetic Index to review the entries under this term and the instructional note to "see also neoplasm, by site, benign." The table provides the proper code based on the type of neoplasm and the site. It is important to select the proper column in the table that corresponds to the type of neoplasm. The tabular should then be referenced to verify that the correct code has been selected from the table and that a more specific site code does not exist.

See Section I. C. 18.d.4. for information regarding V codes for genetic susceptibility to cancer.

a. **Treatment directed at the malignancy**

If the treatment is directed at the malignancy, designate the malignancy as the principal diagnosis.

The only exception to this guideline is if a patient admission/encounter is solely for the administration of chemotherapy, immunotherapy or radiation therapy, assign the appropriate V58.x code as the first-listed or principal diagnosis, and the diagnosis or problem for which the service is being performed as a secondary diagnosis.

b. **Treatment of secondary site**

When a patient is admitted because of a primary neoplasm with metastasis and treatment is directed toward the secondary site only, the secondary neoplasm is designated as the principal diagnosis even though the primary malignancy is still present.

c. **Coding and sequencing of complications**

Coding and sequencing of complications associated with the malignancies or with the therapy thereof are subject to the following guidelines:

1) **Anemia associated with malignancy**

When admission/encounter is for management of an anemia associated with the malignancy, and the treatment is only for anemia, the appropriate anemia code (such as code 285.22, Anemia in neoplastic disease) is designated as the principal diagnosis and is followed by the appropriate code(s) for the malignancy.

Code 285.22 may also be used as a secondary code if the patient suffers from anemia and is being treated for the malignancy.

2) **Anemia associated with chemotherapy, immunotherapy and radiation therapy**

When the admission/encounter is for management of an anemia associated with chemotherapy, immunotherapy or radiotherapy and the only treatment is for the anemia, the anemia is sequenced first followed by code E933.1. The appropriate neoplasm code should be assigned as an additional code.

3) **Management of dehydration due to the malignancy**

When the admission/encounter is for management of dehydration due to the malignancy or the therapy, or a combination of both, and only the dehydration is being treated (intravenous rehydration), the dehydration is sequenced first, followed by the code(s) for the malignancy.

4) **Treatment of a complication resulting from a surgical procedure**

When the admission/encounter is for treatment of a complication resulting from a surgical procedure, designate the complication as the principal or first-listed diagnosis if treatment is directed at resolving the complication.

d. **Primary malignancy previously excised**

When a primary malignancy has been previously excised or eradicated from its site and there is no further treatment directed to that site and there is no evidence of any existing primary malignancy, a code from category V10, Personal history of malignant neoplasm, should be used to indicate the former site of the malignancy. Any mention of extension, invasion, or metastasis to another site is coded as a secondary malignant neoplasm to that site. The secondary site may be the principal or first-listed with the V10 code used as a secondary code.

e. **Admissions/Encounters involving chemotherapy, immunotherapy and radiation therapy**

1) **Episode of care involves surgical removal of neoplasm**

When an episode of care involves the surgical removal of a neoplasm, primary or secondary site, followed by adjunct chemotherapy or radiation treatment during the same episode of care, the neoplasm code should be assigned as principal or first-listed diagnosis, using codes in the 140-198 series or where appropriate in the 200-203 series.

2) **Patient admission/encounter solely for administration of chemotherapy, immunotherapy and radiation therapy**

If a patient admission/encounter is solely for the administration of chemotherapy, immunotherapy or radiation therapy assign code V58.0, Encounter for radiation therapy, or V58.11, Encounter for antineoplastic chemotherapy, or V58.12, Encounter for antineoplastic immunotherapy as the first-listed or principal diagnosis. If a patient receives more than one of these therapies during the same admission more than one of these codes may be assigned, in any sequence.

The malignancy for which the therapy is being administered should be assigned as a secondary diagnosis.

3) **Patient admitted for radiotherapy/chemotherapy and immunotherapy and develops complications**

When a patient is admitted for the purpose of radiotherapy, immunotherapy or chemotherapy and develops complications such as uncontrolled nausea and vomiting or dehydration, the principal or first-listed diagnosis is V58.0, Encounter for radiotherapy, or V58.11, Encounter for antineoplastic chemotherapy, or V58.12, Encounter for antineoplastic immunotherapy followed by any codes for the complications.

f. **Admission/encounter to determine extent of malignancy**

When the reason for admission/encounter is to determine the extent of the malignancy, or for a procedure such as paracentesis or thoracentesis, the primary malignancy or appropriate metastatic site is designated as the principal or first-listed diagnosis, even though chemotherapy or radiotherapy is administered.

g. **Symptoms, signs, and ill-defined conditions listed in Chapter 16 associated with neoplasms**

Symptoms, signs, and ill-defined conditions listed in Chapter 16 characteristic of, or associated with, an existing primary or secondary site malignancy cannot be used to replace the malignancy as principal or first-listed diagnosis, regardless of the number of admissions or encounters for treatment and care of the neoplasm.

See section I.C.18.d.14, Encounter for prophylactic organ removal.

h. **Admission/encounter for pain control/management**

See Section I.C.6.a.5 for information on coding admission/encounter for pain control/management.

i. **Malignant neoplasm associated with transplanted organ**

A malignant neoplasm of a transplanted organ should be coded as a transplant complication. Assign first the appropriate code from subcategory 996.8, Complications of transplanted organ, followed by code 199.2, Malignant neoplasm associated with transplanted organ. Use an additional code for the specific malignancy.

3. **Chapter 3: Endocrine, Nutritional, and Metabolic Diseases and Immunity Disorders (240-279)**

   a. **Diabetes mellitus**

   Codes under category 250, Diabetes mellitus, identify complications/ manifestations associated with diabetes mellitus. A fifth-digit is required for all category 250 codes to identify the type of diabetes mellitus and whether the diabetes is controlled or uncontrolled.

   See I.C.3.a.7 for secondary diabetes

   1) **Fifth-digits for category 250:**

      The following are the fifth-digits for the codes under category 250:

      0 type II or unspecified type, not stated as uncontrolled

      1 type I, [juvenile type], not stated as uncontrolled

      2 type II or unspecified type, uncontrolled

      3 type I, [juvenile type], uncontrolled

      The age of a patient is not the sole determining factor, though most type I diabetics develop the condition before reaching puberty. For this reason type I diabetes mellitus is also referred to as juvenile diabetes.

   2) **Type of diabetes mellitus not documented**

      If the type of diabetes mellitus is not documented in the medical record the default is type II.

   3) **Diabetes mellitus and the use of insulin**

      All type I diabetics must use insulin to replace what their bodies do not produce. However, the use of insulin does not mean that a patient is a type I diabetic. Some patients with type II diabetes mellitus are unable to control their blood sugar through diet and oral medication alone and do require insulin. If the documentation in a medical record does not indicate the type of diabetes but does indicate that the patient uses insulin, the appropriate fifth-digit for type II must be used. For type II patients who routinely use insulin, code V58.67, Long-term (current) use of insulin, should also be assigned to indicate that the patient uses insulin. Code V58.67 should not be assigned if insulin is given temporarily to bring a type II patient's blood sugar under control during an encounter.

   4) **Assigning and sequencing diabetes codes and associated conditions**

      When assigning codes for diabetes and its associated conditions, the code(s) from category 250 must be sequenced before the codes for the associated conditions. The diabetes codes and the secondary codes that correspond to them are paired codes that follow the etiology/manifestation convention of the classification *(See Section I.A.6., Etiology/manifestation convention)*. Assign as many codes from category 250 as needed to identify all of the associated conditions that the patient has. The corresponding secondary codes are listed under each of the diabetes codes.

      (a) **Diabetic retinopathy/diabetic macular edema**

         Diabetic macular edema, code 362.07, is only present with diabetic retinopathy. Another code from subcategory 362.0, Diabetic retinopathy, must be used with code 362.07. Codes under subcategory 362.0 are diabetes manifestation codes, so they must be used following the appropriate diabetes code.

5) **Diabetes mellitus in pregnancy and gestational diabetes**

   (a) For diabetes mellitus complicating pregnancy, see Section I.C.11.f., Diabetes mellitus in pregnancy.

   (b) For gestational diabetes, see Section I.C.11, g., Gestational diabetes.

6) **Insulin pump malfunction**

   (a) **Underdose of insulin due insulin pump failure**

   An underdose of insulin due to an insulin pump failure should be assigned 996.57, Mechanical complication due to insulin pump, as the principal or first listed code, followed by the appropriate diabetes mellitus code based on documentation.

   (b) **Overdose of insulin due to insulin pump failure**

   The principal or first listed code for an encounter due to an insulin pump malfunction resulting in an overdose of insulin, should also be 996.57, Mechanical complication due to insulin pump, followed by code 962.3, Poisoning by insulins and antidiabetic agents, and the appropriate diabetes mellitus code based on documentation.

7) **Secondary Diabetes Mellitus**

   Codes under category 249, Secondary diabetes mellitus, identify complications/manifestations associated with secondary diabetes mellitus. Secondary diabetes is always caused by another condition or event (e.g., cystic fibrosis, malignant neoplasm of pancreas, pancreatectomy, adverse effect of drug, or poisoning).

   (a) **Fifth-digits for category 249:**

   A fifth-digit is required for all category 249 codes to identify whether the diabetes is controlled or uncontrolled.

   (b) **Secondary diabetes mellitus and the use of insulin**

   For patients who routinely use insulin, code V58.67, Long-term (current) use of insulin, should also be assigned. Code V58.67 should not be assigned if insulin is given temporarily to bring a patient's blood sugar under control during an encounter.

   (c) **Assigning and sequencing secondary diabetes codes and associated conditions**

   When assigning codes for secondary diabetes and its associated conditions (e.g. renal manifestations), the code(s) from category 249 must be sequenced before the codes for the associated conditions. The secondary diabetes codes and the diabetic manifestation codes that correspond to them are paired codes that follow the etiology/manifestation convention of the classification. Assign as many codes from category 249 as needed to identify all of the associated conditions that the patient has. The corresponding codes for the associated conditions are listed under each of the secondary diabetes codes. For example, secondary diabetes with diabetic nephrosis is assigned to code 249.40, followed by 581.81.

(d) Assigning and sequencing secondary diabetes codes and its causes

The sequencing of the secondary diabetes codes in relationship to codes for the cause of the diabetes is based on the reason for the encounter, applicable ICD-9-CM sequencing conventions, and chapter-specific guidelines.

If a patient is seen for treatment of the secondary diabetes or one of its associated conditions, a code from category 249 is sequenced as the principal or first-listed diagnosis, with the cause of the secondary diabetes (e.g. cystic fibrosis) sequenced as an additional diagnosis.

If, however, the patient is seen for the treatment of the condition causing the secondary diabetes (e.g., malignant neoplasm of pancreas), the code for the cause of the secondary diabetes should be sequenced as the principal or first-listed diagnosis followed by a code from category 249.

(i) Secondary diabetes mellitus due to pancreatectomy

For postpancreatectomy diabetes mellitus (lack of insulin due to the surgical removal of all or part of the pancreas), assign code 251.3, Postsurgical hypoinsulinemia. A code from subcategory 249 should not be assigned for secondary diabetes mellitus due to pancreatectomy. Code also any diabetic manifestations (e.g. diabetic nephrosis 581.81).

(ii) Secondary diabetes due to drugs

Secondary diabetes may be caused by an adverse effect of correctly administered medications, poisoning or late effect of poisoning.

See section I.C.17.e for coding of adverse effects and poisoning, and section I.C.19 for E code reporting.

4. Chapter 4: Diseases of Blood and Blood Forming Organs (280-289)

a. Anemia of chronic disease

Subcategory 285.2, Anemia in chronic illness, has codes for anemia in chronic kidney disease, code 285.21; anemia in neoplastic disease, code 285.22; and anemia in other chronic illness, code 285.29. These codes can be used as the principal/first listed code if the reason for the encounter is to treat the anemia. They may also be used as secondary codes if treatment of the anemia is a component of an encounter, but not the primary reason for the encounter. When using a code from subcategory 285 it is also necessary to use the code for the chronic condition causing the anemia.

1) Anemia in chronic kidney disease

When assigning code 285.21, Anemia in chronic kidney disease, it is also necessary to assign a code from category 585, Chronic kidney disease, to indicate the stage of chronic kidney disease.

See I.C.10.a. Chronic kidney disease (CKD).

2) Anemia in neoplastic disease

When assigning code 285.22, Anemia in neoplastic disease, it is also necessary to assign the neoplasm code that is responsible for the anemia. Code 285.22 is for use for anemia that is due to the malignancy, not for anemia due to antineoplastic chemotherapy drugs, which is an adverse effect.

See I.C.2.c.1 Anemia associated with malignancy.

See I.C.2.c.2 Anemia associated with chemotherapy, immunotherapy and radiation therapy.

See I.C.17.e.1. Adverse effects.

5. **Chapter 5: Mental Disorders (290-319)**

   Reserved for future guideline expansion

6. **Chapter 6: Diseases of Nervous System and Sense Organs (320-389)**

   a. **Pain - Category 338**

      1) **General coding information**

         Codes in category 338 may be used in conjunction with codes from other categories and chapters to provide more detail about acute or chronic pain and neoplasm-related pain, unless otherwise indicated below.

         If the pain is not specified as acute or chronic, do not assign codes from category 338, except for post-thoracotomy pain, postoperative pain, neoplasm related pain, or central pain syndrome.

         A code from subcategories 338.1 and 338.2 should not be assigned if the underlying (definitive) diagnosis is known, unless the reason for the encounter is pain control/ management and not management of the underlying condition.

      (a) **Category 338 Codes as Principal or First-Listed Diagnosis**

         Category 338 codes are acceptable as principal diagnosis or the first-listed code:

         • When pain control or pain management is the reason for the admission/encounter (e.g., a patient with displaced intervertebral disc, nerve impingement and severe back pain presents for injection of steroid into the spinal canal). The underlying cause of the pain should be reported as an additional diagnosis, if known.

         • When an admission or encounter is for a procedure aimed at treating the underlying condition (e.g., spinal fusion, kyphoplasty), a code for the underlying condition (e.g., vertebral fracture, spinal stenosis) should be assigned as the principal diagnosis. No code from category 338 should be assigned.

         • When a patient is admitted for the insertion of a neurostimulator for pain control, assign the appropriate pain code as the principal or first listed diagnosis. When an admission or encounter is for a procedure aimed at treating the underlying condition and a neurostimulator is inserted for pain control during the same admission/encounter, a code for the underlying condition should be assigned as the principal diagnosis and the appropriate pain code should be assigned as a secondary diagnosis.

      (b) **Use of Category 338 Codes in Conjunction with Site Specific Pain Codes**

         (i) **Assigning Category 338 Codes and Site-Specific Pain Codes**

            Codes from category 338 may be used in conjunction with codes that identify the site of pain (including codes from chapter 16) if the category 338 code provides additional information. For example, if the code describes the site of the pain, but does not fully describe whether the pain is acute or chronic, then both codes should be assigned.

(ii) **Sequencing of Category 338 Codes with Site-Specific Pain Codes**

The sequencing of category 338 codes with site-specific pain codes (including chapter 16 codes), is dependent on the circumstances of the encounter/admission as follows:

- If the encounter is for pain control or pain management, assign the code from category 338 followed by the code identifying the specific site of pain (e.g., encounter for pain management for acute neck pain from trauma is assigned code 338.11, Acute pain due to trauma, followed by code 723.1, Cervicalgia, to identify the site of pain).

- If the encounter is for any other reason except pain control or pain management, and a related definitive diagnosis has not been established (confirmed) by the provider, assign the code for the specific site of pain first, followed by the appropriate code from category 338.

2) **Pain due to devices, implants and grafts**

Pain associated with devices, implants or grafts left in a surgical site (for example painful hip prosthesis) is assigned to the appropriate code(s) found in Chapter 17, Injury and Poisoning. Use additional code(s) from category 338 to identify acute or chronic pain due to presence of the device, implant or graft (338.18-338.19 or 338.28-338.29).

3) **Postoperative Pain**

Post-thoracotomy pain and other postoperative pain are classified to subcategories 338.1 and 338.2, depending on whether the pain is acute or chronic. The default for post-thoracotomy and other postoperative pain not specified as acute or chronic is the code for the acute form.

Routine or expected postoperative pain immediately after surgery should not be coded.

(a) **Postoperative pain not associated with specific postoperative complication**

Postoperative pain not associated with a specific postoperative complication is assigned to the appropriate postoperative pain code in category 338.

(b) **Postoperative pain associated with specific postoperative complication**

Postoperative pain associated with a specific postoperative complication (such as painful wire sutures) is assigned to the appropriate code(s) found in Chapter 17, Injury and Poisoning. If appropriate, use additional code(s) from category 338 to identify acute or chronic pain (338.18 or 338.28). If pain control/management is the reason for the encounter, a code from category 338 should be assigned as the principal or first-listed diagnosis in accordance with *Section I.C.6.a.1.a above*.

(c) **Postoperative pain as principal or first-listed diagnosis**

Postoperative pain may be reported as the principal or first-listed diagnosis when the stated reason for the admission/encounter is documented as postoperative pain control/management.

(d) Postoperative pain as secondary diagnosis

Postoperative pain may be reported as a secondary diagnosis code when a patient presents for outpatient surgery and develops an unusual or inordinate amount of postoperative pain.

The provider's documentation should be used to guide the coding of postoperative pain, as well as *Section III. Reporting Additional Diagnoses* and *Section IV. Diagnostic Coding and Reporting in the Outpatient Setting.*

See Section II.I.2 for information on sequencing of diagnoses for patients admitted to hospital inpatient care following post-operative observation.

See Section II.J for information on sequencing of diagnoses for patients admitted to hospital inpatient care from outpatient surgery.

See Section IV.A.2 for information on sequencing of diagnoses for patients admitted for observation.

4) Chronic pain

Chronic pain is classified to subcategory 338.2. There is no time frame defining when pain becomes chronic pain. The provider's documentation should be used to guide use of these codes.

5) Neoplasm Related Pain

Code 338.3 is assigned to pain documented as being related, associated or due to cancer, primary or secondary malignancy, or tumor. This code is assigned regardless of whether the pain is acute or chronic.

This code may be assigned as the principal or first-listed code when the stated reason for the admission/encounter is documented as pain control/pain management. The underlying neoplasm should be reported as an additional diagnosis.

When the reason for the admission/encounter is management of the neoplasm and the pain associated with the neoplasm is also documented, code 338.3 may be assigned as an additional diagnosis.

See Section I.C.2 for instructions on the sequencing of neoplasms for all other stated reasons for the admission/encounter (except for pain control/ pain management).

6) Chronic pain syndrome

This condition is different than the term "chronic pain," and therefore this code should only be used when the provider has specifically documented this condition.

7. Chapter 7: Diseases of Circulatory System (390-459)

a. Hypertension

Hypertension Table

The Hypertension Table, found under the main term, "Hypertension", in the Alphabetic Index, contains a complete listing of all conditions due to or associated with hypertension and classifies them according to malignant, benign, and unspecified.

1) Hypertension, Essential, or NOS

Assign hypertension (arterial) (essential) (primary) (systemic) (NOS) to category code 401 with the appropriate fourth digit to indicate malignant (.0), benign (.1), or unspecified (.9). Do not use either .0 malignant or .1 benign unless medical record documentation supports such a designation.

2) Hypertension with Heart Disease

Heart conditions (425.8, 429.0-429.3, 429.8, 429.9) are assigned to a code from category 402 when a causal relationship is stated (due to hypertension) or implied (hypertensive). Use an additional code from category 428 to identify the type of heart failure in those patients with heart failure. More than one code from category 428 may be assigned if the patient has systolic or diastolic failure and congestive heart failure.

The same heart conditions (425.8, 429.0-429.3, 429.8, 429.9) with hypertension, but without a stated causal relationship, are coded separately. Sequence according to the circumstances of the admission/encounter.

3) Hypertensive Chronic Kidney Disease

Assign codes from category 403, Hypertensive chronic kidney disease, when conditions classified to category 585 are present. Unlike hypertension with heart disease, ICD-9-CM presumes a cause-and-effect relationship and classifies chronic kidney disease (CKD) with hypertension as hypertensive chronic kidney disease.

Fifth digits for category 403 should be assigned as follows:

- 0 with CKD stage I through stage IV, or unspecified.
- 1 with CKD stage V or end stage renal disease.

The appropriate code from category 585, Chronic kidney disease, should be used as a secondary code with a code from category 403 to identify the stage of chronic kidney disease.

See Section I.C.10.a for information on the coding of chronic kidney disease.

4) Hypertensive Heart and Chronic Kidney Disease

Assign codes from combination category 404, Hypertensive heart and chronic kidney disease, when both hypertensive kidney disease and hypertensive heart disease are stated in the diagnosis. Assume a relationship between the hypertension and the chronic kidney disease, whether or not the condition is so designated. Assign an additional code from category 428, to identify the type of heart failure. More than one code from category 428 may be assigned if the patient has systolic or diastolic failure and congestive heart failure.

Fifth digits for category 404 should be assigned as follows:

- 0 without heart failure and with chronic kidney disease (CKD) stage I through stage IV, or unspecified
- 1 with heart failure and with CKD stage I through stage IV, or unspecified
- 2 without heart failure and with CKD stage V or end stage renal disease
- 3 with heart failure and with CKD stage V or end stage renal disease

The appropriate code from category 585, Chronic kidney disease, should be used as a secondary code with a code from category 404 to identify the stage of kidney disease.

See Section I.C.10.a for information on the coding of chronic kidney disease.

5) Hypertensive Cerebrovascular Disease

First assign codes from 430-438, Cerebrovascular disease, then the appropriate hypertension code from categories 401-405.

6) **Hypertensive Retinopathy**

Two codes are necessary to identify the condition. First assign the code from subcategory 362.11, Hypertensive retinopathy, then the appropriate code from categories 401-405 to indicate the type of hypertension.

7) **Hypertension, Secondary**

Two codes are required: one to identify the underlying etiology and one from category 405 to identify the hypertension. Sequencing of codes is determined by the reason for admission/ encounter.

8) **Hypertension, Transient**

Assign code 796.2, Elevated blood pressure reading without diagnosis of hypertension, unless patient has an established diagnosis of hypertension. Assign code 642.3x for transient hypertension of pregnancy.

9) **Hypertension, Controlled**

Assign appropriate code from categories 401-405. This diagnostic statement usually refers to an existing state of hypertension under control by therapy.

10) **Hypertension, Uncontrolled**

Uncontrolled hypertension may refer to untreated hypertension or hypertension not responding to current therapeutic regimen. In either case, assign the appropriate code from categories 401-405 to designate the stage and type of hypertension. Code to the type of hypertension.

11) **Elevated Blood Pressure**

For a statement of elevated blood pressure without further specificity, assign code 796.2, Elevated blood pressure reading without diagnosis of hypertension, rather than a code from category 401.

b. **Cerebral infarction/stroke/cerebrovascular accident (CVA)**

The terms stroke and CVA are often used interchangeably to refer to a cerebral infarction. The terms stroke, CVA, and cerebral infarction NOS are all indexed to the default code 434.91, Cerebral artery occlusion, unspecified, with infarction. Code 436, Acute, but ill-defined, cerebrovascular disease, should not be used when the documentation states stroke or CVA.

See Section I.C.18.d.3 for information on coding status post administration of tPA in a different facility within the last 24 hours.

c. **Postoperative cerebrovascular accident**

A cerebrovascular hemorrhage or infarction that occurs as a result of medical intervention is coded to 997.02, Iatrogenic cerebrovascular infarction or hemorrhage. Medical record documentation should clearly specify the cause- and-effect relationship between the medical intervention and the cerebrovascular accident in order to assign this code. A secondary code from the code range 430-432 or from a code from subcategories 433 or 434 with a fifth digit of "1" should also be used to identify the type of hemorrhage or infarct.

This guideline conforms to the use additional code note instruction at category 997. Code 436, Acute, but ill-defined, cerebrovascular disease, should not be used as a secondary code with code 997.02.

d. Late Effects of Cerebrovascular Disease

1) Category 438, Late Effects of Cerebrovascular disease

Category 438 is used to indicate conditions classifiable to categories 430-437 as the causes of late effects (neurologic deficits), themselves classified elsewhere. These "late effects" include neurologic deficits that persist after initial onset of conditions classifiable to 430-437. The neurologic deficits caused by cerebrovascular disease may be present from the onset or may arise at any time after the onset of the condition classifiable to 430-437.

2) Codes from category 438 with codes from 430-437

Codes from category 438 may be assigned on a health care record with codes from 430-437, if the patient has a current cerebrovascular accident (CVA) and deficits from an old CVA.

3) Code V12.54

Assign code V12.54, Transient ischemic attack (TIA), and cerebral infarction without residual deficits (and not a code from category 438) as an additional code for history of cerebrovascular disease when no neurologic deficits are present.

e. Acute myocardial infarction (AMI)

1) ST elevation myocardial infarction (STEMI) and non ST elevation myocardial infarction (NSTEMI)

The ICD-9-CM codes for acute myocardial infarction (AMI) identify the site, such as anterolateral wall or true posterior wall. Subcategories 410.0-410.6 and 410.8 are used for ST elevation myocardial infarction (STEMI). Subcategory 410.7, Subendocardial infarction, is used for non ST elevation myocardial infarction (NSTEMI) and nontransmural MIs.

2) Acute myocardial infarction, unspecified

Subcategory 410.9 is the default for the unspecified term acute myocardial infarction. If only STEMI or transmural MI without the site is documented, query the provider as to the site, or assign a code from subcategory 410.9.

3) AMI documented as nontransmural or subendocardial but site provided

If an AMI is documented as nontransmural or subendocardial, but the site is provided, it is still coded as a subendocardial AMI. If NSTEMI evolves to STEMI, assign the STEMI code. If STEMI converts to NSTEMI due to thrombolytic therapy, it is still coded as STEMI.

See Section I.C.18.d.3 for information on coding status post administration of tPA in a different facility within the last 24 hours.

8. Chapter 8: Diseases of Respiratory System (460-519)

See I.C.17.f. for ventilator-associated pneumonia.

a. Chronic Obstructive Pulmonary Disease [COPD] and Asthma

1) Conditions that comprise COPD and Asthma

The conditions that comprise COPD are obstructive chronic bronchitis, subcategory 491.2, and emphysema, category 492. All asthma codes are under category 493, Asthma. Code 496, Chronic airway obstruction, not elsewhere classified, is a nonspecific code that should only be used when the documentation in a medical record does not specify the type of COPD being treated.

2) **Acute exacerbation of chronic obstructive bronchitis and asthma**

The codes for chronic obstructive bronchitis and asthma distinguish between uncomplicated cases and those in acute exacerbation. An acute exacerbation is a worsening or a decompensation of a chronic condition. An acute exacerbation is not equivalent to an infection superimposed on a chronic condition, though an exacerbation may be triggered by an infection.

3) **Overlapping nature of the conditions that comprise COPD and asthma**

Due to the overlapping nature of the conditions that make up COPD and asthma, there are many variations in the way these conditions are documented. Code selection must be based on the terms as documented. When selecting the correct code for the documented type of COPD and asthma, it is essential to first review the index, and then verify the code in the tabular list. There are many instructional notes under the different COPD subcategories and codes. It is important that all such notes be reviewed to assure correct code assignment.

4) **Acute exacerbation of asthma and status asthmaticus**

An acute exacerbation of asthma is an increased severity of the asthma symptoms, such as wheezing and shortness of breath. Status asthmaticus refers to a patient's failure to respond to therapy administered during an asthmatic episode and is a life threatening complication that requires emergency care. If status asthmaticus is documented by the provider with any type of COPD or with acute bronchitis, the status asthmaticus should be sequenced first. It supersedes any type of COPD including that with acute exacerbation or acute bronchitis. It is inappropriate to assign an asthma code with 5th digit 2, with acute exacerbation, together with an asthma code with 5th digit 1, with status asthmatics. Only the 5th digit 1 should be assigned.

b. **Chronic Obstructive Pulmonary Disease [COPD] and Bronchitis**

1) **Acute bronchitis with COPD**

Acute bronchitis, code 466.0, is due to an infectious organism. When acute bronchitis is documented with COPD, code 491.22, Obstructive chronic bronchitis with acute bronchitis, should be assigned. It is not necessary to also assign code 466.0. If a medical record documents acute bronchitis with COPD with acute exacerbation, only code 491.22 should be assigned. The acute bronchitis included in code 491.22 supersedes the acute exacerbation. If a medical record documents COPD with acute exacerbation without mention of acute bronchitis, only code 491.21 should be assigned.

c. **Acute Respiratory Failure**

1) **Acute respiratory failure as principal diagnosis**

Code 518.81, Acute respiratory failure, may be assigned as a principal diagnosis when it is the condition established after study to be chiefly responsible for occasioning the admission to the hospital, and the selection is supported by the Alphabetic Index and Tabular List. However, chapter-specific coding guidelines (such as obstetrics, poisoning, HIV, newborn) that provide sequencing direction take precedence.

2) **Acute respiratory failure as secondary diagnosis**

Respiratory failure may be listed as a secondary diagnosis if it occurs after admission, or if it is present on admission, but does not meet the definition of principal diagnosis.

3) **Sequencing of acute respiratory failure and another acute condition**

When a patient is admitted with respiratory failure and another acute condition, (e.g., myocardial infarction, cerebrovascular accident, **aspiration pneumonia**), the principal diagnosis will not be the same in every situation. **This applies whether the other acute condition is a respiratory or nonrespiratory condition.** Selection of the principal diagnosis will be dependent on the circumstances of admission. If both the respiratory failure and the other acute condition are equally responsible for occasioning the admission to the hospital, and there are no chapter-specific sequencing rules, the guideline regarding two or more diagnoses that equally meet the definition for principal diagnosis *(Section II, C.)* may be applied in these situations.

If the documentation is not clear as to whether acute respiratory failure and another condition are equally responsible for occasioning the admission, query the provider for clarification.

d. **Influenza due to identified avian influenza virus (avian influenza)**

Code only confirmed cases of avian influenza. This is an exception to the hospital inpatient guideline Section II, H. (Uncertain Diagnosis).

In this context, "confirmation" does not require documentation of positive laboratory testing specific for avian influenza. However, coding should be based on the provider's diagnostic statement that the patient has avian influenza.

If the provider records "suspected or possible or probable avian influenza," the appropriate influenza code from category 487 should be assigned. Code 488, Influenza due to identified avian influenza virus, should not be assigned.

9. **Chapter 9: Diseases of Digestive System (520-579)**

Reserved for future guideline expansion

10. **Chapter 10: Diseases of Genitourinary System (580-629)**

a. **Chronic kidney disease**

1) **Stages of chronic kidney disease (CKD)**

The ICD-9-CM classifies CKD based on severity. The severity of CKD is designated by stages I-V. Stage II, code 585.2, equates to mild CKD; stage III, code 585.3, equates to moderate CKD; and stage IV, code 585.4, equates to severe CKD. Code 585.6, End stage renal disease (ESRD), is assigned when the provider has documented end-stage-renal disease (ESRD).

If both a stage of CKD and ESRD are documented, assign code 585.6 only.

2) **Chronic kidney disease and kidney transplant status**

Patients who have undergone kidney transplant may still have some form of CKD, because the kidney transplant may not fully restore kidney function. Therefore, the presence of CKD alone does not constitute a transplant complication. Assign the appropriate 585 code for the patient's stage of CKD and code V42.0. If a transplant complication such as failure or rejection is documented, see section I.C.17.f.2.b for information on coding complications of a kidney transplant. If the documentation is unclear as to whether the patient has a complication of the transplant, query the provider.

3) Chronic kidney disease with other conditions

Patients with CKD may also suffer from other serious conditions, most commonly diabetes mellitus and hypertension. The sequencing of the CKD code in relationship to codes for other contributing conditions is based on the conventions in the tabular list.

See I.C.3.a.4 for sequencing instructions for diabetes.

See I.C.4.a.1 for anemia in CKD.

See I.C.7.a.3 for hypertensive chronic kidney disease.

See I.C.17.f.2.b, Kidney transplant complications, for instructions on coding of documented rejection or failure.

11. **Chapter 11: Complications of Pregnancy, Childbirth, and the Puerperium (630-679)**

a. **General Rules for Obstetric Cases**

1) **Codes from chapter 11 and sequencing priority**

Obstetric cases require codes from chapter 11, codes in the range 630-679, Complications of Pregnancy, Childbirth, and the Puerperium. Chapter 11 codes have sequencing priority over codes from other chapters. Additional codes from other chapters may be used in conjunction with chapter 11 codes to further specify conditions. Should the provider document that the pregnancy is incidental to the encounter, then code V22.2 should be used in place of any chapter 11 codes. It is the provider's responsibility to state that the condition being treated is not affecting the pregnancy.

2) **Chapter 11 codes used only on the maternal record**

Chapter 11 codes are to be used only on the maternal record, never on the record of the newborn.

3) **Chapter 11 fifth-digits**

Categories 640-648, 651-676 have required fifth-digits, which indicate whether the encounter is antepartum, postpartum and whether a delivery has also occurred.

4) **Fifth-digits, appropriate for each code**

The fifth-digits, which are appropriate for each code number, are listed in brackets under each code. The fifth-digits on each code should all be consistent with each other. That is, should a delivery occur all of the fifth-digits should indicate the delivery.

b. **Selection of OB Principal or First-listed Diagnosis**

1) **Routine outpatient prenatal visits**

For routine outpatient prenatal visits when no complications are present codes V22.0, Supervision of normal first pregnancy, and V22.1, Supervision of other normal pregnancy, should be used as the first-listed diagnoses. These codes should not be used in conjunction with chapter 11 codes.

2) **Prenatal outpatient visits for high-risk patients**

For prenatal outpatient visits for patients with high-risk pregnancies, a code from category V23, Supervision of high-risk pregnancy, should be used as the first-listed diagnosis. Secondary chapter 11 codes may be used in conjunction with these codes if appropriate.

3) Episodes when no delivery occurs

In episodes when no delivery occurs, the principal diagnosis should correspond to the principal complication of the pregnancy, which necessitated the encounter. Should more than one complication exist, all of which are treated or monitored, any of the complications codes may be sequenced first.

4) When a delivery occurs

When a delivery occurs, the principal diagnosis should correspond to the main circumstances or complication of the delivery. In cases of cesarean delivery, the selection of the principal diagnosis should correspond to the reason the cesarean delivery was performed unless the reason for admission/encounter was unrelated to the condition resulting in the cesarean delivery.

5) Outcome of delivery

An outcome of delivery code, V27.0-V27.9, should be included on every maternal record when a delivery has occurred. These codes are not to be used on subsequent records or on the newborn record.

c. Fetal Conditions Affecting the Management of the Mother

1) Codes from category 655

Known or suspected fetal abnormality affecting management of the mother, and category 656, Other fetal and placental problems affecting the management of the mother, are assigned only when the fetal condition is actually responsible for modifying the management of the mother, i.e., by requiring diagnostic studies, additional observation, special care, or termination of pregnancy. The fact that the fetal condition exists does not justify assigning a code from this series to the mother's record.

See I.C.18.d. for suspected maternal and fetal conditions not found

2) In utero surgery

In cases when surgery is performed on the fetus, a diagnosis code from category 655, Known or suspected fetal abnormalities affecting management of the mother, should be assigned identifying the fetal condition. Procedure code 75.36, Correction of fetal defect, should be assigned on the hospital inpatient record.

No code from Chapter 15, the perinatal codes, should be used on the mother's record to identify fetal conditions. Surgery performed in utero on a fetus is still to be coded as an obstetric encounter.

d. HIV Infection in Pregnancy, Childbirth and the Puerperium

During pregnancy, childbirth or the puerperium, a patient admitted because of an HIV-related illness should receive a principal diagnosis of 647.6X, Other specified infectious and parasitic diseases in the mother classifiable elsewhere, but complicating the pregnancy, childbirth or the puerperium, followed by 042 and the code(s) for the HIV-related illness(es).

Patients with asymptomatic HIV infection status admitted during pregnancy, childbirth, or the puerperium should receive codes of 647.6X and V08.

e. Current Conditions Complicating Pregnancy

Assign a code from subcategory 648.x for patients that have current conditions when the condition affects the management of the pregnancy, childbirth, or the puerperium. Use additional secondary codes from other chapters to identify the conditions, as appropriate.

f. **Diabetes mellitus in pregnancy**

Diabetes mellitus is a significant complicating factor in pregnancy. Pregnant women who are diabetic should be assigned code 648.0x, Diabetes mellitus complicating pregnancy, and a secondary code from category 250, Diabetes mellitus, **or category 249, Secondary diabetes** to identify the type of diabetes.

Code V58.67, Long-term (current) use of insulin, should also be assigned if the diabetes mellitus is being treated with insulin.

g. **Gestational diabetes**

Gestational diabetes can occur during the second and third trimester of pregnancy in women who were not diabetic prior to pregnancy. Gestational diabetes can cause complications in the pregnancy similar to those of pre-existing diabetes mellitus. It also puts the woman at greater risk of developing diabetes after the pregnancy. Gestational diabetes is coded to 648.8x, Abnormal glucose tolerance. Codes 648.0x and 648.8x should never be used together on the same record.

Code V58.67, Long-term (current) use of insulin, should also be assigned if the gestational diabetes is being treated with insulin.

h. **Normal Delivery, Code 650**

1) **Normal delivery**

Code 650 is for use in cases when a woman is admitted for a full-term normal delivery and delivers a single, healthy infant without any complications antepartum, during the delivery, or postpartum during the delivery episode. Code 650 is always a principal diagnosis. It is not to be used if any other code from chapter 11 is needed to describe a current complication of the antenatal, delivery, or perinatal period. Additional codes from other chapters may be used with code 650 if they are not related to or are in any way complicating the pregnancy.

2) **Normal delivery with resolved antepartum complication**

Code 650 may be used if the patient had a complication at some point during her pregnancy, but the complication is not present at the time of the admission for delivery.

3) **V27.0, Single liveborn, outcome of delivery**

V27.0, Single liveborn, is the only outcome of delivery code appropriate for use with 650.

i. **The Postpartum and Peripartum Periods**

1) **Postpartum and peripartum periods**

The postpartum period begins immediately after delivery and continues for six weeks following delivery. The peripartum period is defined as the last month of pregnancy to five months postpartum.

2) **Postpartum complication**

A postpartum complication is any complication occurring within the six-week period.

3) **Pregnancy-related complications after 6 week period**

Chapter 11 codes may also be used to describe pregnancy-related complications after the six-week period should the provider document that a condition is pregnancy related.

4) **Postpartum complications occurring during the same admission as delivery**

Postpartum complications that occur during the same admission as the delivery are identified with a fifth digit of "2." Subsequent admissions/encounters for postpartum complications should be identified with a fifth digit of "4."

5) **Admission for routine postpartum care following delivery outside hospital**

When the mother delivers outside the hospital prior to admission and is admitted for routine postpartum care and no complications are noted, code V24.0, Postpartum care and examination immediately after delivery, should be assigned as the principal diagnosis.

6) **Admission following delivery outside hospital with postpartum conditions**

A delivery diagnosis code should not be used for a woman who has delivered prior to admission to the hospital. Any postpartum conditions and/or postpartum procedures should be coded.

j. **Code 677, Late effect of complication of pregnancy**

1) **Code 677**

Code 677, Late effect of complication of pregnancy, childbirth, and the puerperium is for use in those cases when an initial complication of a pregnancy develops a sequelae requiring care or treatment at a future date.

2) **After the initial postpartum period**

This code may be used at any time after the initial postpartum period.

3) **Sequencing of Code 677**

This code, like all late effect codes, is to be sequenced following the code describing the sequelae of the complication.

k. **Abortions**

1) **Fifth-digits required for abortion categories**

Fifth-digits are required for abortion categories 634-637. Fifth-digit 1, incomplete, indicates that all of the products of conception have not been expelled from the uterus. Fifth-digit 2, complete, indicates that all products of conception have been expelled from the uterus.

2) **Code from categories 640-648 and 651-659**

A code from categories 640-648 and 651-659 may be used as additional codes with an abortion code to indicate the complication leading to the abortion.

Fifth digit 3 is assigned with codes from these categories when used with an abortion code because the other fifth digits will not apply. Codes from the 660-669 series are not to be used for complications of abortion.

3) **Code 639 for complications**

Code 639 is to be used for all complications following abortion. Code 639 cannot be assigned with codes from categories 634-638.

4) **Abortion with Liveborn Fetus**

When an attempted termination of pregnancy results in a liveborn fetus assign code 644.21, Early onset of delivery, with an appropriate code from category V27, Outcome of Delivery. The procedure code for the attempted termination of pregnancy should also be assigned.

5) **Retained Products of Conception following an abortion**

Subsequent admissions for retained products of conception following a spontaneous or legally induced abortion are assigned the appropriate code from category 634, Spontaneous abortion, or 635 Legally induced abortion, with a fifth digit of "1" (incomplete). This advice is appropriate even when the patient was discharged previously with a discharge diagnosis of complete abortion.

12. **Chapter 12: Diseases Skin and Subcutaneous Tissue (680-709)**
    a. Pressure ulcer stage codes
       1) Pressure ulcer stages

          Two codes are needed to completely describe a pressure ulcer: A code from subcategory 707.0, Pressure ulcer, to identify the site of the pressure ulcer and a code from subcategory 707.2, Pressure ulcer stages.

          The codes in subcategory 707.2, Pressure ulcer stages, are to be used as an additional diagnosis with a code(s) from subcategory 707.0, Pressure Ulcer. Codes from 707.2, Pressure ulcer stages, may not be assigned as a principal or first-listed diagnosis. The pressure ulcer stage codes should only be used with pressure ulcers and not with other types of ulcers (e.g., stasis ulcer).

          The ICD-9-CM classifies pressure ulcer stages based on severity, which is designated by stages I-IV and unstageable.

       2) Unstageable pressure ulcers

          Assignment of code 707.25, Pressure ulcer, unstageable, should be based on the clinical documentation. Code 707.25 is used for pressure ulcers whose stage cannot be clinically determined (e.g., the ulcer is covered by eschar or has been treated with a skin or muscle graft) and pressure ulcers that are documented as deep tissue injury but not documented as due to trauma. This code should not be confused with code 707.20, Pressure ulcer, stage unspecified. Code 707.20 should be assigned when there is no documentation regarding the stage of the pressure ulcer.

       3) Documented pressure ulcer stage

          Assignment of the pressure ulcer stage code should be guided by clinical documentation of the stage or documentation of the terms found in the index. For clinical terms describing the stage that are not found in the index, and there is no documentation of the stage, the provider should be queried.

       4) Bilateral pressure ulcers with same stage

          When a patient has bilateral pressure ulcers (e.g., both buttocks) and both pressure ulcers are documented as being the same stage, only the code for the site and one code for the stage should be reported.

       5) Bilateral pressure ulcers with different stages

          When a patient has bilateral pressure ulcers at the same site (e.g., both buttocks) and each pressure ulcer is documented as being at a different stage, assign one code for the site and the appropriate codes for the pressure ulcer stage.

       6) Multiple pressure ulcers of different sites and stages

          When a patient has multiple pressure ulcers at different sites (e.g., buttock, heel, shoulder) and each pressure ulcer is documented as being at different stages (e.g., stage 3 and stage 4), assign the appropriate codes for each different site and a code for each different pressure ulcer stage.

       7) Patients admitted with pressure ulcers documented as healed

          No code is assigned if the documentation states that the pressure ulcer is completely healed.

8) **Patients admitted with pressure ulcers documented as healing**

Pressure ulcers described as healing should be assigned the appropriate pressure ulcer stage code based on the documentation in the medical record. If the documentation does not provide information about the stage of the healing pressure ulcer, assign code 707.20, Pressure ulcer stage, unspecified.

If the documentation is unclear as to whether the patient has a current (new) pressure ulcer or if the patient is being treated for a healing pressure ulcer, query the provider.

9) **Patient admitted with pressure ulcer evolving into another stage during the admission**

If a patient is admitted with a pressure ulcer at one stage and it progresses to a higher stage, assign the code for highest stage reported for that site.

13. **Chapter 13: Diseases of Musculoskeletal and Connective Tissue (710-739)**

a. **Coding of Pathologic Fractures**

1) **Acute Fractures vs. Aftercare**

Pathologic fractures are reported using subcategory 733.1, when the fracture is newly diagnosed. Subcategory 733.1 may be used while the patient is receiving active treatment for the fracture. Examples of active treatment are: surgical treatment, emergency department encounter, evaluation and treatment by a new physician.

Fractures are coded using the aftercare codes (subcategories V54.0, V54.2, V54.8 or V54.9) for encounters after the patient has completed active treatment of the fracture and is receiving routine care for the fracture during the healing or recovery phase. Examples of fracture aftercare are: cast change or removal, removal of external or internal fixation device, medication adjustment, and follow up visits following fracture treatment.

Care for complications of surgical treatment for fracture repairs during the healing or recovery phase should be coded with the appropriate complication codes.

Care of complications of fractures, such as malunion and nonunion, should be reported with the appropriate codes.

See Section I. C. 17.b for information on the coding of traumatic fractures.

14. **Chapter 14: Congenital Anomalies (740-759)**

a. **Codes in categories 740-759, Congenital Anomalies**

Assign an appropriate code(s) from categories 740-759, Congenital Anomalies, when an anomaly is documented. A congenital anomaly may be the principal/first listed diagnosis on a record or a secondary diagnosis.

When a congenital anomaly does not have a unique code assignment, assign additional code(s) for any manifestations that may be present.

When the code assignment specifically identifies the congenital anomaly, manifestations that are an inherent component of the anomaly should not be coded separately. Additional codes should be assigned for manifestations that are not an inherent component.

Codes from Chapter 14 may be used throughout the life of the patient. If a congenital anomaly has been corrected, a personal history code should be used to identify the history of the anomaly. Although present at birth, a congenital anomaly may not be identified until later in life. Whenever the condition is diagnosed by the physician, it is appropriate to assign a code from codes 740-759.

For the birth admission, the appropriate code from category V30, Liveborn infants, according to type of birth should be sequenced as the principal diagnosis, followed by any congenital anomaly codes, 740-759.

15. **Chapter 15: Newborn (Perinatal) Guidelines (760-779)**

For coding and reporting purposes the perinatal period is defined as before birth through the 28th day following birth. The following guidelines are provided for reporting purposes. Hospitals may record other diagnoses as needed for internal data use.

a. **General Perinatal Rules**

1) **Chapter 15 Codes**

They are <u>never</u> for use on the maternal record. Codes from Chapter 11, the obstetric chapter, are never permitted on the newborn record. Chapter 15 code may be used throughout the life of the patient if the condition is still present.

2) **Sequencing of perinatal codes**

Generally, codes from Chapter 15 should be sequenced as the principal/first-listed diagnosis on the newborn record, with the exception of the appropriate V30 code for the birth episode, followed by codes from any other chapter that provide additional detail. The "use additional code" note at the beginning of the chapter supports this guideline. If the index does not provide a specific code for a perinatal condition, assign code 779.89, Other specified conditions originating in the perinatal period, followed by the code from another chapter that specifies the condition. Codes for signs and symptoms may be assigned when a definitive diagnosis has not been established.

3) **Birth process or community acquired conditions**

If a newborn has a condition that may be either due to the birth process or community acquired and the documentation does not indicate which it is, the default is due to the birth process and the code from Chapter 15 should be used. If the condition is community-acquired, a code from Chapter 15 should not be assigned.

4) **Code all clinically significant conditions**

All clinically significant conditions noted on routine newborn examination should be coded. A condition is clinically significant if it requires:

- clinical evaluation; or
- therapeutic treatment; or
- diagnostic procedures; or
- extended length of hospital stay; or
- increased nursing care and/or monitoring; or
- has implications for future health care needs

Note: The perinatal guidelines listed above are the same as the general coding guidelines for "additional diagnoses", except for the final point regarding implications for future health care needs. Codes should be assigned for conditions that have been specified by the provider as having implications for future health care needs. Codes from the perinatal chapter should not be assigned unless the provider has established a definitive diagnosis.

b. **Use of codes V30-V39**

When coding the birth of an infant, assign a code from categories V30-V39, according to the type of birth. A code from this series is assigned as a principal diagnosis, and assigned only once to a newborn at the time of birth.

c. **Newborn transfers**

If the newborn is transferred to another institution, the V30 series is not used at the receiving hospital.

d. **Use of category V29**

1) **Assigning a code from category V29**

Assign a code from category V29, Observation and evaluation of newborns and infants for suspected conditions not found, to identify those instances when a healthy newborn is evaluated for a suspected condition that is determined after study not to be present. Do not use a code from category V29 when the patient has identified signs or symptoms of a suspected problem; in such cases, code the sign or symptom.

A code from category V29 may also be assigned as a principal code for readmissions or encounters when the V30 code no longer applies. Codes from category V29 are for use only for healthy newborns and infants for which no condition after study is found to be present.

2) **V29 code on a birth record**

A V29 code is to be used as a secondary code after the V30, Outcome of delivery, code.

e. **Use of other V codes on perinatal records**

V codes other than V30 and V29 may be assigned on a perinatal or newborn record code. The codes may be used as a principal or first-listed diagnosis for specific types of encounters or for readmissions or encounters when the V30 code no longer applies.

See Section I.C.18 for information regarding the assignment of V codes.

f. **Maternal Causes of Perinatal Morbidity**

Codes from categories 760-763, Maternal causes of perinatal morbidity and mortality, are assigned only when the maternal condition has actually affected the fetus or newborn. The fact that the mother has an associated medical condition or experiences some complication of pregnancy, labor or delivery does not justify the routine assignment of codes from these categories to the newborn record.

g. **Congenital Anomalies in Newborns**

For the birth admission, the appropriate code from category V30, Liveborn infants according to type of birth, should be used, followed by any congenital anomaly codes, categories 740-759. Use additional secondary codes from other chapters to specify conditions associated with the anomaly, if applicable.

Also, see Section I.C.14 for information on the coding of congenital anomalies.

h. **Coding Additional Perinatal Diagnoses**

1) **Assigning codes for conditions that require treatment**

Assign codes for conditions that require treatment or further investigation, prolong the length of stay, or require resource utilization.

2) **Codes for conditions specified as having implications for future health care needs**

Assign codes for conditions that have been specified by the provider as having implications for future health care needs.

Note: This guideline should not be used for adult patients.

3) **Codes for newborn conditions originating in the perinatal period**

Assign a code for newborn conditions originating in the perinatal period (categories 760-779), as well as complications arising during the current episode of care classified in other chapters, only if the diagnoses have been documented by the responsible provider at the time of transfer or discharge as having affected the fetus or newborn.

i. **Prematurity and Fetal Growth Retardation**

Providers utilize different criteria in determining prematurity. A code for prematurity should not be assigned unless it is documented. The 5th digit assignment for codes from category 764 and subcategories 765.0 and 765.1 should be based on the recorded birth weight and estimated gestational age.

A code from subcategory 765.2, Weeks of gestation, should be assigned as an additional code with category 764 and codes from 765.0 and 765.1 to specify weeks of gestation as documented by the provider in the record.

j. **Newborn sepsis**

Code 771.81, Septicemia [sepsis] of newborn, should be assigned with a secondary code from category 041, Bacterial infections in conditions classified elsewhere and of unspecified site, to identify the organism. A code from category 038, Septicemia, should not be used on a newborn record. **Do not assign code 995.91, Sepsis, as** code 771.81 describes the sepsis. **If applicable, use additional codes to identify severe sepsis (995.92) and any associated acute organ dysfunction.**

16. **Chapter 16: Signs, Symptoms and Ill-Defined Conditions (780-799)**

Reserved for future guideline expansion

17. **Chapter 17: Injury and Poisoning (800-999)**

a. **Coding of Injuries**

When coding injuries, assign separate codes for each injury unless a combination code is provided, in which case the combination code is assigned. Multiple injury codes are provided in ICD-9-CM, but should not be assigned unless information for a more specific code is not available. These codes are not to be used for normal, healing surgical wounds or to identify complications of surgical wounds.

The code for the most serious injury, as determined by the provider and the focus of treatment, is sequenced first.

1) **Superficial injuries**

Superficial injuries such as abrasions or contusions are not coded when associated with more severe injuries of the same site.

2) **Primary injury with damage to nerves/blood vessels**

When a primary injury results in minor damage to peripheral nerves or blood vessels, the primary injury is sequenced first with additional code(s) from categories 950-957, Injury to nerves and spinal cord, and/or 900-904, Injury to blood vessels. When the primary injury is to the blood vessels or nerves, that injury should be sequenced first.

b. Coding of Traumatic Fractures

The principles of multiple coding of injuries should be followed in coding fractures. Fractures of specified sites are coded individually by site in accordance with both the provisions within categories 800-829 and the level of detail furnished by medical record content. Combination categories for multiple fractures are provided for use when there is insufficient detail in the medical record (such as trauma cases transferred to another hospital), when the reporting form limits the number of codes that can be used in reporting pertinent clinical data, or when there is insufficient specificity at the fourth-digit or fifth-digit level. More specific guidelines are as follows:

1) Acute Fractures vs. Aftercare

Traumatic fractures are coded using the acute fracture codes (800-829) while the patient is receiving active treatment for the fracture. Examples of active treatment are: surgical treatment, emergency department encounter, and evaluation and treatment by a new physician.

Fractures are coded using the aftercare codes (subcategories V54.0, V54.1, V54.8, or V54.9) for encounters after the patient has completed active treatment of the fracture and is receiving routine care for the fracture during the healing or recovery phase. Examples of fracture aftercare are: cast change or removal, removal of external or internal fixation device, medication adjustment, and follow up visits following fracture treatment.

Care for complications of surgical treatment for fracture repairs during the healing or recovery phase should be coded with the appropriate complication codes.

Care of complications of fractures, such as malunion and nonunion, should be reported with the appropriate codes.

Pathologic fractures are not coded in the 800-829 range, but instead are assigned to subcategory 733.1. *See Section I.C.13.a for additional information.*

2) Multiple fractures of same limb

Multiple fractures of same limb classifiable to the same three-digit or four-digit category are coded to that category.

3) Multiple unilateral or bilateral fractures of same bone

Multiple unilateral or bilateral fractures of same bone(s) but classified to different fourth-digit subdivisions (bone part) within the same three-digit category are coded individually by site.

4) Multiple fracture categories 819 and 828

Multiple fracture categories 819 and 828 classify bilateral fractures of both upper limbs (819) and both lower limbs (828), but without any detail at the fourth-digit level other than open and closed type of fractures.

5) **Multiple fractures sequencing**

Multiple fractures are sequenced in accordance with the severity of the fracture. The provider should be asked to list the fracture diagnoses in the order of severity.

c. **Coding of Burns**

Current burns (940-948) are classified by depth, extent and by agent (E code). Burns are classified by depth as first degree (erythema), second degree (blistering), and third degree (full-thickness involvement).

1) **Sequencing of burn and related condition codes**

Sequence first the code that reflects the highest degree of burn when more than one burn is present.

   a. When the reason for the admission or encounter is for treatment of external multiple burns, sequence first the code that reflects the burn of the highest degree.

   b. When a patient has both internal and external burns, the circumstances of admission govern the selection of the principal diagnosis or first-listed diagnosis.

   c. When a patient is admitted for burn injuries and other related conditions such as smoke inhalation and/or respiratory failure, the circumstances of admission govern the selection of the principal or first-listed diagnosis.

2) **Burns of the same local site**

Classify burns of the same local site (three-digit category level, 940-947) but of different degrees to the subcategory identifying the highest degree recorded in the diagnosis.

3) **Non-healing burns**

Non-healing burns are coded as acute burns.

Necrosis of burned skin should be coded as a non-healed burn.

4) **Code 958.3, Posttraumatic wound infection**

Assign code 958.3, Posttraumatic wound infection, not elsewhere classified, as an additional code for any documented infected burn site.

5) **Assign separate codes for each burn site**

When coding burns, assign separate codes for each burn site. Category 946 Burns of Multiple specified sites, should only be used if the location of the burns are not documented. Category 949, Burn, unspecified, is extremely vague and should rarely be used.

6) **Assign codes from category 948, Burns**

Burns classified according to extent of body surface involved, when the site of the burn is not specified or when there is a need for additional data. It is advisable to use category 948 as additional coding when needed to provide data for evaluating burn mortality, such as that needed by burn units. It is also advisable to use category 948 as an additional code for reporting purposes when there is mention of a third-degree burn involving 20 percent or more of the body surface.

In assigning a code from category 948:

Fourth-digit codes are used to identify the percentage of total body surface involved in a burn (all degree).

Fifth-digits are assigned to identify the percentage of body surface involved in third-degree burn.

Fifth-digit zero (0) is assigned when less than 10 percent or when no body surface is involved in a third-degree burn.

Category 948 is based on the classic "rule of nines" in estimating body surface involved: head and neck are assigned nine percent, each arm nine percent, each leg 18 percent, the anterior trunk 18 percent, posterior trunk 18 percent, and genitalia one percent. Providers may change these percentage assignments where necessary to accommodate infants and children who have proportionately larger heads than adults and patients who have large buttocks, thighs, or abdomen that involve burns.

7) **Encounters for treatment of late effects of burns**

Encounters for the treatment of the late effects of burns (i.e., scars or joint contractures) should be coded to the residual condition (sequelae) followed by the appropriate late effect code (906.5-906.9). A late effect E code may also be used, if desired.

8) **Sequelae with a late effect code and current burn**

When appropriate, both a sequelae with a late effect code, and a current burn code may be assigned on the same record (when both a current burn and sequelae of an old burn exist).

d. **Coding of Debridement of Wound, Infection, or Burn**

Excisional debridement involves surgical removal or cutting away, as opposed to a mechanical (brushing, scrubbing, washing) debridement.

For coding purposes, excisional debridement is assigned to code 86.22.

Nonexcisional debridement is assigned to code 86.28.

e. **Adverse Effects, Poisoning and Toxic Effects**

The properties of certain drugs, medicinal and biological substances or combinations of such substances, may cause toxic reactions. The occurrence of drug toxicity is classified in ICD-9-CM as follows:

1) **Adverse Effect**

When the drug was correctly prescribed and properly administered, code the reaction plus the appropriate code from the E930-E949 series. Codes from the E930-E949 series must be used to identify the causative substance for an adverse effect of drug, medicinal and biological substances, correctly prescribed and properly administered. The effect, such as tachycardia, delirium, gastrointestinal hemorrhaging, vomiting, hypokalemia, hepatitis, renal failure, or respiratory failure, is coded and followed by the appropriate code from the E930-E949 series.

Adverse effects of therapeutic substances correctly prescribed and properly administered (toxicity, synergistic reaction, side effect, and idiosyncratic reaction) may be due to (1) differences among patients, such as age, sex, disease, and genetic factors, and (2) drug-related factors, such as type of drug, route of administration, duration of therapy, dosage, and bioavailability.

2) **Poisoning**

(a) **Error was made in drug prescription**

Errors made in drug prescription or in the administration of the drug by provider, nurse, patient, or other person, use the appropriate poisoning code from the 960-979 series.

(b) **Overdose of a drug intentionally taken**

If an overdose of a drug was intentionally taken or administered and resulted in drug toxicity, it would be coded as a poisoning (960-979 series).

(c) **Nonprescribed drug taken with correctly prescribed and properly administered drug**

If a nonprescribed drug or medicinal agent was taken in combination with a correctly prescribed and properly administered drug, any drug toxicity or other reaction resulting from the interaction of the two drugs would be classified as a poisoning.

(d) **Interaction of drug(s) and alcohol**

When a reaction results from the interaction of a drug(s) and alcohol, this would be classified as poisoning.

(e) <u>**Sequencing of poisoning**</u>

<u>When coding a poisoning or reaction to the improper use of a medication (e.g., wrong dose, wrong substance, wrong route of administration) the poisoning code is sequenced first, followed by a code for the manifestation. If there is also a diagnosis of drug abuse or dependence to the substance, the abuse or dependence is coded as an additional code.</u>

See Section I.C.3.a.6.b. if poisoning is the result of insulin pump malfunctions and Section I.C.19 for general use of E-codes.

3) **Toxic Effects**

(a) **Toxic effect codes**

When a harmful substance is ingested or comes in contact with a person, this is classified as a toxic effect. The toxic effect codes are in categories 980-989.

(b) **Sequencing toxic effect codes**

A toxic effect code should be sequenced first, followed by the code(s) that identify the result of the toxic effect.

(c) **External cause codes for toxic effects**

An external cause code from categories E860-E869 for accidental exposure, codes E950.6 or E950.7 for intentional self-harm, category E962 for assault, or categories E980-E982, for undetermined, should also be assigned to indicate intent.

f. **Complications of care**

1) **Complications of care**

(a) **Documentation of complications of care**

As with all procedural or postprocedural complications, code assignment is based on the provider's documentation of the relationship between the condition and the procedure.

2) Transplant complications

(a) Transplant complications other than kidney

Codes under subcategory 996.8, Complications of transplanted organ, are for use for both complications and rejection of transplanted organs. A transplant complication code is only assigned if the complication affects the function of the transplanted organ. Two codes are required to fully describe a transplant complication, the appropriate code from subcategory 996.8 and a secondary code that identifies the complication.

Pre-existing conditions or conditions that develop after the transplant are not coded as complications unless they affect the function of the transplanted organs.

See I.C.18.d.3) for transplant organ removal status

See I.C.2.i for malignant neoplasm associated with transplanted organ.

(b) Chronic kidney disease and kidney transplant complications

Patients who have undergone kidney transplant may still have some form of chronic kidney disease (CKD) because the kidney transplant may not fully restore kidney function. Code 996.81 should be assigned for documented complications of a kidney transplant, such as transplant failure or rejection **or other transplant complication.** Code 996.81 should not be assigned for post kidney transplant patients who have chronic kidney (CKD) unless a transplant complication such as transplant failure or rejection is documented. If the documentation is unclear as to whether the patient has a complication of the transplant, query the provider.

For patients with CKD following a kidney transplant, but who do not have a complication such as failure or rejection, *see section I.C.10.a.2, Chronic kidney disease and kidney transplant status.*

3) Ventilator associated pneumonia

(a) Documentation of Ventilator associated Pneumonia

As with all procedural or postprocedural complications, code assignment is based on the provider's documentation of the relationship between the condition and the procedure.

Code 997.31, Ventilator associated pneumonia, should be assigned only when the provider has documented ventilator associated pneumonia (VAP). An additional code to identify the organism (e.g., Pseudomonas aeruginosa, code 041.7) should also be assigned. Do not assign an additional code from categories 480-484 to identify the type of pneumonia.

Code 997.31 should not be assigned for cases where the patient has pneumonia and is on a mechanical ventilator but the provider has not specifically stated that the pneumonia is ventilator-associated pneumonia.

If the documentation is unclear as to whether the patient has a pneumonia that is a complication attributable to the mechanical ventilator, query the provider.

(b) Patient admitted with pneumonia and develops VAP

A patient may be admitted with one type of pneumonia (e.g., code 481, Pneumococcal pneumonia) and subsequently develop VAP. In this instance, the principal diagnosis would be the appropriate code from categories 480-484 for the pneumonia diagnosed at the time of admission. Code 997.31, Ventilator associated pneumonia, would be assigned as an additional diagnosis when the provider has also documented the presence of ventilator associated pneumonia.

g. **SIRS due to Non-infectious Process**

The systemic inflammatory response syndrome (SIRS) can develop as a result of certain non-infectious disease processes, such as trauma, malignant neoplasm, or pancreatitis. When SIRS is documented with a noninfectious condition, and no subsequent infection is documented, the code for the underlying condition, such as an injury, should be assigned, followed by code 995.93, Systemic inflammatory response syndrome due to noninfectious process without acute organ dysfunction, or 995.94, Systemic inflammatory response syndrome due to non-infectious process with acute organ dysfunction. If an acute organ dysfunction is documented, the appropriate code(s) for the associated acute organ dysfunction(s) should be assigned in addition to code 995.94. If acute organ dysfunction is documented, but it cannot be determined if the acute organ dysfunction is associated with SIRS or due to another condition (e.g., directly due to the trauma), the provider should be queried.

When the non-infectious condition has led to an infection that results in SIRS, *see Section I.C.1.b.12 for the guideline for sepsis and severe sepsis associated with a non-infectious process.*

18. **Classification of Factors Influencing Health Status and Contact with Health Service (Supplemental V01-V89)**

Note: The chapter specific guidelines provide additional information about the use of V codes for specified encounters.

a. **Introduction**

ICD-9-CM provides codes to deal with encounters for circumstances other than a disease or injury. The Supplementary Classification of Factors Influencing Health Status and Contact with Health Services (V01.0 - **V89.09**) is provided to deal with occasions when circumstances other than a disease or injury (codes 001-999) are recorded as a diagnosis or problem.

There are four primary circumstances for the use of V codes:

1) A person who is not currently sick encounters the health services for some specific reason, such as to act as an organ donor, to receive prophylactic care, such as inoculations or health screenings, or to receive counseling on health related issues.

2) A person with a resolving disease or injury, or a chronic, long-term condition requiring continuous care, encounters the health care system for specific aftercare of that disease or injury (e.g., dialysis for renal disease; chemotherapy for malignancy; cast change). A diagnosis/symptom code should be used whenever a current, acute, diagnosis is being treated or a sign or symptom is being studied.

3) Circumstances or problems influence a person's health status but are not in themselves a current illness or injury.

4) Newborns, to indicate birth status

b. **V codes use in any healthcare setting**

V codes are for use in any healthcare setting. V codes may be used as either a first listed (principal diagnosis code in the inpatient setting) or secondary code, depending on the circumstances of the encounter. Certain V codes may only be used as first listed, others only as secondary codes.

See Section I.C.18.e, V Code Table.

c. **V Codes indicate a reason for an encounter**

They are not procedure codes. A corresponding procedure code must accompany a V code to describe the procedure performed.

d. Categories of V Codes

1) Contact/Exposure

Category V01 indicates contact with or exposure to communicable diseases. These codes are for patients who do not show any sign or symptom of a disease but have been exposed to it by close personal contact with an infected individual or are in an area where a disease is epidemic. These codes may be used as a first listed code to explain an encounter for testing, or, more commonly, as a secondary code to identify a potential risk.

2) Inoculations and vaccinations

Categories V03-V06 are for encounters for inoculations and vaccinations. They indicate that a patient is being seen to receive a prophylactic inoculation against a disease. The injection itself must be represented by the appropriate procedure code. A code from V03-V06 may be used as a secondary code if the inoculation is given as a routine part of preventive health care, such as a well-baby visit.

3) Status

Status codes indicate that a patient is either a carrier of a disease or has the sequelae or residual of a past disease or condition. This includes such things as the presence of prosthetic or mechanical devices resulting from past treatment. A status code is informative, because the status may affect the course of treatment and its outcome. A status code is distinct from a history code. The history code indicates that the patient no longer has the condition.

A status code should not be used with a diagnosis code from one of the body system chapters, if the diagnosis code includes the information provided by the status code. For example, code V42.1, Heart transplant status, should not be used with code 996.83, Complications of transplanted heart. The status code does not provide additional information. The complication code indicates that the patient is a heart transplant patient.

The status V codes/categories are:

V02   Carrier or suspected carrier of infectious diseases

Carrier status indicates that a person harbors the specific organisms of a disease without manifest symptoms and is capable of transmitting the infection.

V07.5X   Prophylactic use of agents affecting estrogen receptors and estrogen level

This code indicates when a patient is receiving a drug that affects estrogen receptors and estrogen levels for prevention of cancer.

V08   Asymptomatic HIV infection status

This code indicates that a patient has tested positive for HIV but has manifested no signs or symptoms of the disease.

V09   Infection with drug-resistant microorganisms

This category indicates that a patient has an infection that is resistant to drug treatment. Sequence the infection code first.

| V21 | Constitutional states in development |
| V22.2 | Pregnant state, incidental |

This code is a secondary code only for use when the pregnancy is in no way complicating the reason for visit. Otherwise, a code from the obstetric chapter is required.

V26.5x	Sterilization status
V42	Organ or tissue replaced by transplant
V43	Organ or tissue replaced by other means
V44	Artificial opening status
V45	Other postsurgical states

Assign code V45.87, Transplant organ removal status, to indicate that a transplanted organ has been previously removed. This code should not be assigned for the encounter in which the transplanted organ is removed. The complication necessitating removal of the transplant organ should be assigned for that encounter.

See section I.C17.f.2. for information on the coding of organ transplant complications.

Assign code V45.88, Status post administration of tPA (rtPA) in a different facility within the last 24 hours prior to admission to the current facility, as a secondary diagnosis when a patient is received by transfer into a facility and documentation indicates they were administered tissue plasminogen activator (tPA) within the last 24 hours prior to admission to the current facility.

This guideline applies even if the patient is still receiving the tPA at the time they are received into the current facility.

The appropriate code for the condition for which the tPA was administered (such as cerebrovascular disease or myocardial infarction) should be assigned first.

Code V45.88 is only applicable to the receiving facility record and not to the transferring facility record.

V46	Other dependence on machines
V49.6	Upper limb amputation status
V49.7	Lower limb amputation status

Note: Categories V42-V46, and subcategories V49.6, V49.7 are for use only if there are no complications or malfunctions of the organ or tissue replaced, the amputation site or the equipment on which the patient is dependent.

V49.81	Postmenopausal status
V49.82	Dental sealant status
V49.83	Awaiting organ transplant status

V58.6x   Long-term (current) drug use

Codes from this subcategory indicate a patient's continuous use of a prescribed drug (including such things as aspirin therapy) for the long-term treatment of a condition or for prophylactic use. It is not for use for patients who have addictions to drugs. **This subcategory is not for use of medications for detoxification or maintenance programs to prevent withdrawal symptoms in patients with drug dependence (e.g., methadone maintenance for opiate dependence). Assign the appropriate code for the drug dependence instead.**

Assign a code from subcategory V58.6, Long-term (current) drug use, if the patient is receiving a medication for an extended period as a prophylactic measure (such as for the prevention of deep vein thrombosis) or as treatment of a chronic condition (such as arthritis) or a disease requiring a lengthy course of treatment (such as cancer). Do not assign a code from subcategory V58.6 for medication being administered for a brief period of time to treat an acute illness or injury (such as a course of antibiotics to treat acute bronchitis).

V83   Genetic carrier status

Genetic carrier status indicates that a person carries a gene, associated with a particular disease, which may be passed to offspring who may develop that disease. The person does not have the disease and is not at risk of developing the disease.

V84   Genetic susceptibility status

Genetic susceptibility indicates that a person has a gene that increases the risk of that person developing the disease.

Codes from category V84, Genetic susceptibility to disease, should not be used as principal or first-listed codes. If the patient has the condition to which he/she is susceptible, and that condition is the reason for the encounter, the code for the current condition should be sequenced first. If the patient is being seen for follow-up after completed treatment for this condition, and the condition no longer exists, a follow-up code should be sequenced first, followed by the appropriate personal history and genetic susceptibility codes. If the purpose of the encounter is genetic counseling associated with procreative management, a code from subcategory V26.3, Genetic counseling and testing, should be assigned as the first-listed code, followed by a code from category V84. Additional codes should be assigned for any applicable family or personal history.

See Section I.C. 18.d.14 for information on prophylactic organ removal due to a genetic susceptibility.

V86   Estrogen receptor status

V88   Acquired absence of other organs and tissue

4) **History (of)**

There are two types of history V codes, personal and family. Personal history codes explain a patient's past medical condition that no longer exists and is not receiving any treatment, but that has the potential for recurrence, and therefore may require continued monitoring. The exceptions to this general rule are category V14, Personal history of allergy to medicinal agents, and subcategory V15.0, Allergy, other than to medicinal agents.

A person who has had an allergic episode to a substance or food in the past should always be considered allergic to the substance.

Family history codes are for use when a patient has a family member(s) who has had a particular disease that causes the patient to be at higher risk of also contracting the disease.

Personal history codes may be used in conjunction with follow-up codes and family history codes may be used in conjunction with screening codes to explain the need for a test or procedure. History codes are also acceptable on any medical record regardless of the reason for visit. A history of an illness, even if no longer present, is important information that may alter the type of treatment ordered.

The history V code categories are:

V10	Personal history of malignant neoplasm
V12	Personal history of certain other diseases
V13	Personal history of other diseases
	Except: V13.4, Personal history of arthritis, and V13.6, Personal history of congenital malformations. These conditions are life-long so are not true history codes.
V14	Personal history of allergy to medicinal agents
V15	Other personal history presenting hazards to health
	Except: V15.7, Personal history of contraception.
V16	Family history of malignant neoplasm
V17	Family history of certain chronic disabling diseases
V18	Family history of certain other specific diseases
V19	Family history of other conditions
V87	**Other specified personal exposures and history presenting hazards to health**

5) **Screening**

Screening is the testing for disease or disease precursors in seemingly well individuals so that early detection and treatment can be provided for those who test positive for the disease. Screenings that are recommended for many subgroups in a population include: routine mammograms for women over 40, a fecal occult blood test for everyone over 50, an amniocentesis to rule out a fetal anomaly for pregnant women over 35, because the incidence of breast cancer and colon cancer in these subgroups is higher than in the general population, as is the incidence of Down's syndrome in older mothers.

The testing of a person to rule out or confirm a suspected diagnosis because the patient has some sign or symptom is a diagnostic examination, not a screening. In these cases, the sign or symptom is used to explain the reason for the test.

A screening code may be a first listed code if the reason for the visit is specifically the screening exam. It may also be used as an additional code if the screening is done during an office visit for other health problems. A screening code is not necessary if the screening is inherent to a routine examination, such as a pap smear done during a routine pelvic examination.

Should a condition be discovered during the screening then the code for the condition may be assigned as an additional diagnosis.

The V code indicates that a screening exam is planned. A procedure code is required to confirm that the screening was performed.

The screening V code categories:

V28	Antenatal screening
V73-V82	Special screening examinations

6) **Observation**

There are three observation V code categories. They are for use in very limited circumstances when a person is being observed for a suspected condition that is ruled out. The observation codes are not for use if an injury or illness or any signs or symptoms related to the suspected condition are present. In such cases the diagnosis/symptom code is used with the corresponding E code to identify any external cause.

The observation codes are to be used as principal diagnosis only. The only exception to this is when the principal diagnosis is required to be a code from the V30, Live born infant, category. Then the V29 observation code is sequenced after the V30 code. Additional codes may be used in addition to the observation code but only if they are unrelated to the suspected condition being observed.

Codes from subcategory V89.0, Suspected maternal and fetal conditions not found, may either be used as a first listed or as an additional code assignment depending on the case. They are for use in very limited circumstances on a maternal record when an encounter is for a suspected maternal or fetal condition that is ruled out during that encounter (for example, a maternal or fetal condition may be suspected due to an abnormal test result). These codes should not be used when the condition is confirmed. In those cases, the confirmed condition should be coded. In addition, these codes are not for use if an illness or any signs or symptoms related to the suspected condition or problem are present. In such cases the diagnosis/symptom code is used.

Additional codes may be used in addition to the code from subcategory V89.0, but only if they are unrelated to the suspected condition being evaluated.

Codes from subcategory V89.0 may not be used for encounters for antenatal screening of mother. *See Section I.C.18.d., Screening).*

For encounters for suspected fetal condition that are inconclusive following testing and evaluation, assign the appropriate code from category 655, 656, 657 or 658.

The observation V code categories:

V29   Observation and evaluation of newborns for suspected condition not found

For the birth encounter, a code from category V30 should be sequenced before the V29 code.

V71   Observation and evaluation for suspected condition not found

V89   Suspected maternal and fetal conditions not found

7) **Aftercare**

Aftercare visit codes cover situations when the initial treatment of a disease or injury has been performed and the patient requires continued care during the healing or recovery phase, or for the long-term consequences of the disease. The aftercare V code should not be used if treatment is directed at a current, acute disease or injury. The diagnosis code is to be used in these cases. Exceptions to this rule are codes V58.0, Radiotherapy, and codes from subcategory V58.1, Encounter for chemotherapy and immunotherapy for neoplastic conditions. These codes are to be first listed, followed by the diagnosis code when a patient's encounter is solely to receive radiation therapy or chemotherapy for the treatment of a neoplasm. Should a patient receive both chemotherapy and radiation therapy during the same encounter code V58.0 and V58.1 may be used together on a record with either one being sequenced first.

The aftercare codes are generally first listed to explain the specific reason for the encounter. An aftercare code may be used as an additional code when some type of aftercare is provided in addition to the reason for admission and no diagnosis code is applicable. An example of this would be the closure of a colostomy during an encounter for treatment of another condition.

Aftercare codes should be used in conjunction with any other aftercare codes or other diagnosis codes to provide better detail on the specifics of an aftercare encounter visit, unless otherwise directed by the classification. The sequencing of multiple aftercare codes is discretionary.

Certain aftercare V code categories need a secondary diagnosis code to describe the resolving condition or sequelae, for others, the condition is inherent in the code title.

Additional V code aftercare category terms include fitting and adjustment, and attention to artificial openings.

Status V codes may be used with aftercare V codes to indicate the nature of the aftercare. For example code V45.81, Aortocoronary bypass status, may be used with code V58.73, Aftercare following surgery of the circulatory system, NEC, to indicate the surgery for which the aftercare is being performed. Also, a transplant status code may be used following code V58.44, Aftercare following organ transplant, to identify the organ transplanted. A status code should not be used when the aftercare code indicates the type of status, such as using V55.0, Attention to tracheostomy with V44.0, Tracheostomy status.

See Section I. B.16 Admissions/Encounter for Rehabilitation

The aftercare V category/codes:

V51.0	**Encounter for breast reconstruction following mastectomy**
V52	Fitting and adjustment of prosthetic device and implant
V53	Fitting and adjustment of other device
V54	Other orthopedic aftercare
V55	Attention to artificial openings
V56	Encounter for dialysis and dialysis catheter care
V57	Care involving the use of rehabilitation procedures
V58.0	Radiotherapy
V58.11	Encounter for antineoplastic chemotherapy
V58.12	Encounter for antineoplastic immunotherapy
V58.3x	Attention to dressings and sutures
V58.41	Encounter for planned post-operative wound closure
V58.42	Aftercare, surgery, neoplasm
V58.43	Aftercare, surgery, trauma
V58.44	Aftercare involving organ transplant
V58.49	Other specified aftercare following surgery
V58.7x	Aftercare following surgery
V58.81	Fitting and adjustment of vascular catheter
V58.82	Fitting and adjustment of non-vascular catheter
V58.83	Monitoring therapeutic drug
V58.89	Other specified aftercare

8) Follow-up

The follow-up codes are used to explain continuing surveillance following completed treatment of a disease, condition, or injury. They imply that the condition has been fully treated and no longer exists. They should not be confused with aftercare codes that explain current treatment for a healing condition or its sequelae. Follow-up codes may be used in conjunction with history codes to provide the full picture of the healed condition and its treatment. The follow-up code is sequenced first, followed by the history code.

A follow-up code may be used to explain repeated visits. Should a condition be found to have recurred on the follow-up visit, then the diagnosis code should be used in place of the follow-up code.

The follow-up V code categories:

V24	Postpartum care and evaluation
V67	Follow-up examination

9) Donor

Category V59 is the donor codes. They are used for living individuals who are donating blood or other body tissue. These codes are only for individuals donating for others, not for self donations. They are not for use to identify cadaveric donations.

10) Counseling

Counseling V codes are used when a patient or family member receives assistance in the aftermath of an illness or injury, or when support is required in coping with family or social problems. They are not necessary for use in conjunction with a diagnosis code when the counseling component of care is considered integral to standard treatment.

The counseling V categories/codes:

V25.0	General counseling and advice for contraceptive management
V26.3	Genetic counseling
V26.4	General counseling and advice for procreative management
V61.**X**	Other family circumstances
V65.1	Person consulted on behalf of another person
V65.3	Dietary surveillance and counseling
V65.4	Other counseling, not elsewhere classified

11) Obstetrics and related conditions

See Section I.C.11., the Obstetrics guidelines for further instruction on the use of these codes.

V codes for pregnancy are for use in those circumstances when none of the problems or complications included in the codes from the Obstetrics chapter exist (a routine prenatal visit or postpartum care). Codes V22.0, Supervision of normal first pregnancy, and V22.1, Supervision of other normal pregnancy, are always first listed and are not to be used with any other code from the OB chapter.

The outcome of delivery, category V27, should be included on all maternal delivery records. It is always a secondary code.

V codes for family planning (contraceptive) or procreative management and counseling should be included on an obstetric record either during the pregnancy or the postpartum stage, if applicable.

Obstetrics and related conditions V code categories:

V22	Normal pregnancy
V23	Supervision of high-risk pregnancy

Except: V23.2, Pregnancy with history of abortion. Code 646.3, Habitual aborter, from the OB chapter is required to indicate a history of abortion during a pregnancy.

V24	Postpartum care and evaluation
V25	Encounter for contraceptive management

Except V25.0x

(See Section I.C.18.d.11, Counseling)

V26	Procreative management

Except V26.5x, Sterilization status, V26.3 and V26.4

(See Section I.C.18.d.11., Counseling)

V27	Outcome of delivery
V28	Antenatal screening

(See Section I.C.18.d.6., Screening)

12) Newborn, infant and child

See Section I.C.15, the Newborn guidelines for further instruction on the use of these codes.

Newborn V code categories:

V20	Health supervision of infant or child
V29	Observation and evaluation of newborns for suspected condition not found

(See Section I.C.18.d.7, Observation)

V30-V39 Liveborn infant according to type of birth

13) Routine and administrative examinations

The V codes allow for the description of encounters for routine examinations, such as, a general check-up, or, examinations for administrative purposes, such as, a pre-employment physical. The codes are not to be used if the examination is for diagnosis of a suspected condition or for treatment purposes. In such cases the diagnosis code is used. During a routine exam, should a diagnosis or condition be discovered, it should be coded as an additional code. Pre-existing and chronic conditions and history codes may also be included as additional codes as long as the examination is for administrative purposes and not focused on any particular condition.

Pre-operative examination V codes are for use only in those situations when a patient is being cleared for surgery and no treatment is given.

The V codes categories/code for routine and administrative examinations:

V20.2	Routine infant or child health check

Any injections given should have a corresponding procedure code.

V70	General medical examination
V72	Special investigations and examinations

Codes V72.5 and V72.6 may be used if the reason for the patient encounter is for routine laboratory/radiology testing in the absence of any signs, symptoms, or associated diagnosis. If routine testing is performed during the same encounter as a test to evaluate a sign, symptom, or diagnosis, it is appropriate to assign both the V code and the code describing the reason for the non-routine test.

14) **Miscellaneous V codes**

The miscellaneous V codes capture a number of other health care encounters that do not fall into one of the other categories. Certain of these codes identify the reason for the encounter, others are for use as additional codes that provide useful information on circumstances that may affect a patient's care and treatment.

Prophylactic Organ Removal

For encounters specifically for prophylactic removal of breasts, ovaries, or another organ due to a genetic susceptibility to cancer or a family history of cancer, the principal or first listed code should be a code from subcategory V50.4, Prophylactic organ removal, followed by the appropriate genetic susceptibility code and the appropriate family history code.

If the patient has a malignancy of one site and is having prophylactic removal at another site to prevent either a new primary malignancy or metastatic disease, a code for the malignancy should also be assigned in addition to a code from subcategory V50.4. A V50.4 code should not be assigned if the patient is having organ removal for treatment of a malignancy, such as the removal of the testes for the treatment of prostate cancer.

Miscellaneous V code categories/codes:

V07	Need for isolation and other prophylactic measures
	Except V07.5, Prophylactic use of agents affecting estrogen receptors and estrogen levels
V50	Elective surgery for purposes other than remedying health states
V58.5	Orthodontics
V60	Housing, household, and economic circumstances
V62	Other psychosocial circumstances
V63	Unavailability of other medical facilities for care
V64	Persons encountering health services for specific procedures, not carried out
V66	Convalescence and Palliative Care
V68	Encounters for administrative purposes
V69	Problems related to lifestyle
V85	Body Mass Index

15) Nonspecific V codes

Certain V codes are so non-specific, or potentially redundant with other codes in the classification, that there can be little justification for their use in the inpatient setting. Their use in the outpatient setting should be limited to those instances when there is no further documentation to permit more precise coding. Otherwise, any sign or symptom or any other reason for visit that is captured in another code should be used.

Nonspecific V code categories/codes:

V11	Personal history of mental disorder
	A code from the mental disorders chapter, with an in remission fifth-digit, should be used.
V13.4	Personal history of arthritis
V13.6	Personal history of congenital malformations
V15.7	Personal history of contraception
V23.2	Pregnancy with history of abortion
V40	Mental and behavioral problems
V41	Problems with special senses and other special functions
V47	Other problems with internal organs
V48	Problems with head, neck, and trunk
V49	Problems with limbs and other problems

Exceptions:

V49.6	Upper limb amputation status
V49.7	Lower limb amputation status
V49.81	Postmenopausal status
V49.82	Dental sealant status
V49.83	Awaiting organ transplant status

V51.8	**Other** aftercare involving the use of plastic surgery
V58.2	Blood transfusion, without reported diagnosis
V58.9	Unspecified aftercare

See Section IV.K. and Section IV.L. of the Outpatient guidelines.

V CODE TABLE
October 1, 2008 (FY2009)
Items in bold indicate a new entry or change from the October 2007 table
Items underlined have been moved within the table since October 2007

The V code table below contains columns for 1st listed, 1st or additional, additional only, and non-specific. Each code or category is listed in the left hand column, and the allowable sequencing of the code or codes within the category is noted under the appropriate column.

As indicated by the footnote in the "1st Dx Only" column, the V codes designated as first-listed only are generally intended to be limited for use as a first-listed only diagnosis, but may be reported as an additional diagnosis in those situations when the patient has more than one encounter on a single day and the codes for the multiple encounters are combined, or when there is more than one V code that meets the definition of principal diagnosis (e.g., a patient is admitted to home healthcare for both aftercare and rehabilitation and they equally meet the definition of principal diagnosis). The V codes designated as first-listed only should not be reported if they do not meet the definition of principal or first-listed diagnosis.

See Section II and Section IV.A for information on selection of principal and first-listed diagnosis.

See Section II.C for information on two or more diagnoses that equally meet the definition for principal diagnosis.

Code(s)	Description	1st Dx Only[1]	1st or Add'l Dx[2]	Add'l Dx Only[3]	Non-Specific Diagnosis[4]
V01.X	Contact with or exposure to communicable diseases		X		
V02.X	Carrier or suspected carrier of infectious diseases		X		
V03.X	Need for prophylactic vaccination and inoculation against bacterial diseases		X		
V04.X	Need for prophylactic vaccination and inoculation against certain diseases		X		
V05.X	Need for prophylactic vaccination and inoculation against single diseases		X		
V06.X	Need for prophylactic vaccination and inoculation against combinations of diseases		X		
V07.0	**Isolation**	**X**			
V07.1	**Desensitization to allergens**	**X**			
V07.2	**Prophylactic immunotherapy**	**X**			
V07.3X	**Other prophylactic chemotherapy**	**X**			
V07.4	**Hormone replacement therapy (postmenopausal)**			**X**	
V07.5X	**Prophylactic use of agents affecting estrogen receptors and estrogen levels**			**X**	
V07.8	**Other specified prophylactic measure**	**X**			
V07.9	**Unspecified prophylactic measure**				**X**
V08	Asymptomatic HIV infection status		X		
V09.X	Infection with drug resistant organisms			X	
V10.X	Personal history of malignant neoplasm		X		
V11.X	Personal history of mental disorder				X
V12.X	Personal history of certain other diseases		X		
V13.0X	Personal history of other disorders of urinary system		X		
V13.1	Personal history of trophoblastic disease		X		
V13.2X	Personal history of other genital system and obstetric disorders		X		
V13.3	Personal history of diseases of skin and subcutaneous tissue		X		
V13.4	Personal history of arthritis				X
V13.5**X**	Personal history of other musculoskeletal disorders		X		

[1]*Generally for use as first listed only but may be used as additional if patient has more than one encounter on one day or there is more than one reason for the encounter*
[2]*These codes may be used as first listed or additional codes*
[3]*These codes are only for use as additional codes*
[4]*These codes are primarily for use in the nonacute setting and should be limited to encounters for which no sign or symptom or reason for visit is documented in the record. Their use may be as either a first listed or additional code.*

Code(s)	Description	1st Dx Only[1]	1st or Add'l Dx[2]	Add'l Dx Only[3]	Non-Specific Diagnosis[4]
V13.61	Personal history of hypospadias			X	
V13.69	Personal history of congenital malformations				X
V13.7	Personal history of perinatal problems		X		
V13.8	Personal history of other specified diseases		X		
V13.9	Personal history of unspecified disease				X
V14.X	Personal history of allergy to medicinal agents			X	
V15.0X	Personal history of allergy, other than to medicinal agents			X	
V15.1	Personal history of surgery to heart and great vessels			X	
V15.2X	**Personal history of surgery to other organs**			X	
V15.3	Personal history of irradiation			X	
V15.4X	Personal history of psychological trauma			X	
V15.5X	Personal history of injury			X	
V15.6	Personal history of poisoning			X	
V15.7	Personal history of contraception				X
V15.81	Personal history of noncompliance with medical treatment			X	
V15.82	Personal history of tobacco use			X	
V15.84	Personal history of exposure to asbestos			X	
V15.85	Personal history of exposure to potentially hazardous body fluids			X	
V15.86	Personal history of exposure to lead			X	
V15.87	Personal history of extracorporeal membrane oxygenation [ECMO]			X	
V15.88	History of fall		X		
V15.89	Other specified personal history presenting hazards to health			X	
V16.X	Family history of malignant neoplasm		X		
V17.X	Family history of certain chronic disabling diseases		X		
V18.X	Family history of certain other specific conditions		X		
V19.X	Family history of other conditions		X		
V20.X	Health supervision of infant or child	X			
V21.X	Constitutional states in development			X	
V22.0	Supervision of normal first pregnancy	X			
V22.1	Supervision of other normal pregnancy	X			
V22.2	Pregnancy state, incidental			X	
V23.X	Supervision of high-risk pregnancy		X		
V24.X	Postpartum care and examination	X			
V25.X	Encounter for contraceptive management		X		
V26.0	Tuboplasty or vasoplasty after previous sterilization		X		
V26.1	Artificial insemination		X		
V26.2X	Procreative management investigation and testing		X		
V26.3X	Procreative management, genetic counseling and testing		X		
V26.4X	Procreative management, genetic counseling and advice		X		
V26.5X	Procreative management, sterilization status			X	
V26.81	Encounter for assisted reproductive fertility procedure cycle	X			
V26.89	Other specified procreative management		X		

[1]Generally for use as first listed only but may be used as additional if patient has more than one encounter on one day or there is more than one reason for the encounter
[2]These codes may be used as first listed or additional codes
[3]These codes are only for use as additional codes
[4]These codes are primarily for use in the nonacute setting and should be limited to encounters for which no sign or symptom or reason for visit is documented in the record. Their use may be as either a first listed or additional code.

GUIDELINES - V CODE TABLE

Code(s)	Description	1st Dx Only[1]	1st or Add'l Dx[2]	Add'l Dx Only[3]	Non-Specific Diagnosis[4]
V26.9	Unspecified procreative management		X		
V27.X	Outcome of delivery			X	
V28.X	Encounter for antenatal screening of mother		X		
V29.X	Observation and evaluation of newborns for suspected condition not found		X		
V30.X	Single liveborn	X			
V31.X	Twin, mate liveborn	X			
V32.X	Twin, mate stillborn	X			
V33.X	Twin, unspecified	X			
V34.X	Other multiple, mates all liveborn	X			
V35.X	Other multiple, mates all stillborn	X			
V36.X	Other multiple, mates live- and stillborn	X			
V37.X	Other multiple, unspecified	X			
V39.X	Unspecified	X			
V40.X	Mental and behavioral problems				X
V41.X	Problems with special senses and other special functions				X
V42.X	Organ or tissue replaced by transplant			X	
V43.0	Organ or tissue replaced by other means, eye globe			X	
V43.1	Organ or tissue replaced by other means, lens			X	
V43.21	Organ or tissue replaced by other means, heart assist device			X	
V43.22	Fully implantable artificial heart status		X		
V43.3	Organ or tissue replaced by other means, heart valve			X	
V43.4	Organ or tissue replaced by other means, blood vessel			X	
V43.5	Organ or tissue replaced by other means, bladder			X	
V43.6X	Organ or tissue replaced by other means, joint			X	
V43.7	Organ or tissue replaced by other means, limb			X	
V43.8X	Other organ or tissue replaced by other means			X	
V44.X	Artificial opening status			X	
V45.0X	Cardiac device in situ			X	
V45.1X	Renal dialysis status			X	
V45.2	Presence of cerebrospinal fluid drainage device			X	
V45.3	Intestinal bypass or anastomosis status			X	
V45.4	Arthrodesis status			X	
V45.5X	Presence of contraceptive device			X	
V45.6X	States following surgery of eye and adnexa			X	
V45.7X	Acquired absence of organ		X		
V45.8X	Other postprocedural status			X	
V46.0	Other dependence on machines, aspirator			X	
V46.11	Dependence on respiratory, status			X	.
V46.12	Encounter for respirator dependence during power failure	X			
V46.13	Encounter for weaning from respirator [ventilator]	X			
V46.14	Mechanical complication of respirator [ventilator]		X		
V46.2	Other dependence on machines, supplemental oxygen			X	

[1]Generally for use as first listed only but may be used as additional if patient has more than one encounter on one day or there is more than one reason for the encounter
[2]These codes may be used as first listed or additional codes
[3]These codes are only for use as additional codes
[4]These codes are primarily for use in the nonacute setting and should be limited to encounters for which no sign or symptom or reason for visit is documented in the record. Their use may be as either a first listed or additional code.

Code(s)	Description	1st Dx Only[1]	1st or Add'l Dx[2]	Add'l Dx Only[3]	Non-Specific Diagnosis[4]
V46.3	**Wheelchair dependence**			X	
V46.8	Other dependence on other enabling machines			X	
V46.9	Unspecified machine dependence				X
V47.X	Other problems with internal organs				X
V48.X	Problems with head, neck and trunk				X
V49.0	Deficiencies of limbs				X
V49.1	Mechanical problems with limbs				X
V49.2	Motor problems with limbs				X
V49.3	Sensory problems with limbs				X
V49.4	Disfigurements of limbs				X
V49.5	Other problems with limbs				X
V49.6X	Upper limb amputation status		X		
V49.7X	Lower limb amputation status		X		
V49.81	Asymptomatic postmenopausal status (age-related) (natural)		X		
V49.82	Dental sealant status			X	
V49.83	Awaiting organ transplant status			X	
V49.84	Bed confinement status		X		
V49.85	Dual sensory impairment			X	
V49.89	Other specified conditions influencing health status		X		
V49.9	Unspecified condition influencing health status				X
V50.X	Elective surgery for purposes other than remedying health states		X		
V51.0	**Encounter for breast reconstruction following mastectomy**	X			
V51.8	**Other aftercare involving the use of plastic surgery**				X
V52.X	Fitting and adjustment of prosthetic device and implant		X		
V53.X	Fitting and adjustment of other device		X		
V54.X	Other orthopedic aftercare		X		
V55.X	Attention to artificial openings		X		
V56.0	Extracorporeal dialysis	X			
V56.1	Encounter for fitting and adjustment of extracorporeal dialysis catheter		X		
V56.2	Encounter for fitting and adjustment of peritoneal dialysis catheter		X		
V56.3X	Encounter for adequacy testing for dialysis		X		
V56.8	Encounter for other dialysis and dialysis catheter care		X		
V57.X	Care involving use of rehabilitation procedures	X			
V58.0	Radiotherapy	X			
V58.11	Encounter for antineoplastic chemotherapy	X			
V58.12	Encounter for antineoplastic immunotherapy	X			
V58.2	Blood transfusion without reported diagnosis				X
V58.3X	Attention to dressings and sutures		X		
V58.4X	Other aftercare following surgery		X		
V58.5	Encounter for orthodontics				X
V58.6X	Long term (current) drug use			X	
V58.7X	Aftercare following surgery to specified body systems, not elsewhere classified		X		

[1]Generally for use as first listed only but may be used as additional if patient has more than one encounter on one day or there is more than one reason for the encounter
[2]These codes may be used as first listed or additional codes
[3]These codes are only for use as additional codes
[4]These codes are primarily for use in the nonacute setting and should be limited to encounters for which no sign or symptom or reason for visit is documented in the record. Their use may be as either a first listed or additional code.

GUIDELINES - V CODE TABLE

Code(s)	Description	1st Dx Only[1]	1st or Add'l Dx[2]	Add'l Dx Only[3]	Non-Specific Diagnosis[4]
V58.8X	Other specified procedures and aftercare		X		
V58.9	Unspecified aftercare				X
V59.X	Donors	X			
V60.X	Housing, household, and economic circumstances			X	
V61.X	Other family circumstances		X		
V62.X	Other psychosocial circumstances			X	
V63.X	Unavailability of other medical facilities for care		X		
V64.X	Persons encountering health services for specified procedure, not carried out			X	
V65.X	Other persons seeking consultation without complaint or sickness		X		
V66.0	Convalescence and palliative care following surgery	X			
V66.1	Convalescence and palliative care following radiotherapy	X			
V66.2	Convalescence and palliative care following chemotherapy	X			
V66.3	Convalescence and palliative care following psychotherapy and other treatment for mental disorder	X			
V66.4	Convalescence and palliative care following treatment of fracture	X			
V66.5	Convalescence and palliative care following other treatment	X			
V66.6	Convalescence and palliative care following combined treatment	X			
V66.7	Encounter for palliative care			X	
V66.9	Unspecified convalescence	X			
V67.X	Follow-up examination		X		
V68.X	Encounters for administrative purposes	X			
V69.X	Problems related to lifestyle		X		
V70.0	Routine general medical examination at a health care facility	X			
V70.1	General psychiatric examination, requested by the authority	X			
V70.2	General psychiatric examination, other and unspecified	X			
V70.3	Other medical examination for administrative purposes	X			
V70.4	Examination for medicolegal reasons	X			
V70.5	Health examination of defined subpopulations	X			
V70.6	Health examination in population surveys	X			
V70.7	Examination of participant in clinical trial		X		
V70.8	Other specified general medical examinations	X			
V70.9	Unspecified general medical examination	X			
V71.X	Observation and evaluation for suspected conditions not found	X			
V72.0	Examination of eyes and vision		X		
V72.1X	Examination of ears and hearing		X		
V72.2	Dental examination		X		
V72.3X	Gynecological examination		X		
V72.4X	Pregnancy examination or test		X		
V72.5	Radiological examination, NEC		X		
V72.6	Laboratory examination		X		
V72.7	Diagnostic skin and sensitization tests		X		
V72.81	Preoperative cardiovascular examination		X		

[1]Generally for use as first listed only but may be used as additional if patient has more than one encounter on one day or there is more than one reason for the encounter
[2]These codes may be used as first listed or additional codes
[3]These codes are only for use as additional codes
[4]These codes are primarily for use in the nonacute setting and should be limited to encounters for which no sign or symptom or reason for visit is documented in the record. Their use may be as either a first listed or additional code.

Code(s)	Description	1st Dx Only[1]	1st or Add'l Dx[2]	Add'l Dx Only[3]	Non-Specific Diagnosis[4]
V72.82	Preoperative respiratory examination		X		
V72.83	Other specified preoperative examination		X		
V72.84	Preoperative examination, unspecified		X		
V72.85	Other specified examination		X		
V72.86	Encounter for blood typing		X		
V72.9	Unspecified examination				X
V73.X	Special screening examination for viral and chlamydial diseases		X		
V74.X	Special screening examination for bacterial and spirochetal diseases		X		
V75.X	Special screening examination for other infectious diseases		X		
V76.X	Special screening examination for malignant neoplasms		X		
V77.X	Special screening examination for endocrine, nutritional, metabolic and immunity disorders		X		
V78.X	Special screening examination for disorders of blood and blood-forming organs		X		
V79.X	Special screening examination for mental disorders and developmental handicaps		X		
V80.X	Special screening examination for neurological, eye, and ear diseases		X		
V81.X	Special screening examination for cardiovascular, respiratory, and genitourinary diseases		X		
V82.X	Special screening examination for other conditions		X		
V83.X	Genetic carrier status		X		
V84.X	Genetic susceptibility to disease			X	
V85	Body mass index			X	
V86	Estrogen receptor status			X	
V87.0X	**Contact with and (suspected) exposure to hazardous metals**		X		
V87.1X	**Contact with and (suspected) exposure to hazardous aromatic compounds**		X		
V87.2	**Contact with and (suspected) exposure to other potentially hazardous chemicals**		X		
V87.3X	**Contact with and (suspected) exposure to other potentially hazardous substances**		X		
V87.4X	**Personal history of drug therapy**			X	
V88.0X	**Acquired absence of cervix and uterus**			X	
V89.0X	**Suspected maternal and fetal anomalies not found**		X		

[1]Generally for use as first listed only but may be used as additional if patient has more than one encounter on one day or there is more than one reason for the encounter
[2]These codes may be used as first listed or additional codes
[3]These codes are only for use as additional codes
[4]These codes are primarily for use in the nonacute setting and should be limited to encounters for which no sign or symptom or reason for visit is documented in the record. Their use may be as either a first listed or additional code.

19. **Supplemental Classification of External Causes of Injury and Poisoning (E-codes, E800-E999)**

Introduction: These guidelines are provided for those who are currently collecting E codes in order that there will be standardization in the process. If your institution plans to begin collecting E codes, these guidelines are to be applied. The use of E codes is supplemental to the application of ICD-9-CM diagnosis codes. E codes are never to be recorded as principal diagnoses (first-listed in non-inpatient setting) and are not required for reporting to CMS.

External causes of injury and poisoning codes (E codes) are intended to provide data for injury research and evaluation of injury prevention strategies. E codes capture how the injury or poisoning happened (cause), the intent (unintentional or accidental; or intentional, such as suicide or assault), and the place where the event occurred.

Some major categories of E codes include:

transport accidents

poisoning and adverse effects of drugs, medicinal substances and biologicals

accidental falls

accidents caused by fire and flames

accidents due to natural and environmental factors

late effects of accidents, assaults or self injury

assaults or purposely inflicted injury

suicide or self inflicted injury

These guidelines apply for the coding and collection of E codes from records in hospitals, outpatient clinics, emergency departments, other ambulatory care settings and provider offices, and nonacute care settings, except when other specific guidelines apply.

a. **General E Code Coding Guidelines**

1) **Used with any code in the range of 001-V89**

An E code may be used with any code in the range of 001-V89, which indicates an injury, poisoning, or adverse effect due to an external cause.

2) **Assign the appropriate E code for all initial treatments**

Assign the appropriate E code for the initial encounter of an injury, poisoning, or adverse effect of drugs, not for subsequent treatment.

External cause of injury codes (E-codes) may be assigned while the acute fracture codes are still applicable.

See Section I.C.17.b.1 for coding of acute fractures.

3) **Use the full range of E codes**

Use the full range of E codes to completely describe the cause, the intent and the place of occurrence, if applicable, for all injuries, poisonings, and adverse effects of drugs.

4) **Assign as many E codes as necessary**

Assign as many E codes as necessary to fully explain each cause. If only one E code can be recorded, assign the E code most related to the principal diagnosis.

5) **The selection of the appropriate E code**

The selection of the appropriate E code is guided by the Index to External Causes, which is located after the alphabetical index to diseases and by Inclusion and Exclusion notes in the Tabular List.

6) **E code can never be a principal diagnosis**

An E code can never be a principal (first listed) diagnosis.

7) **External cause code(s) with systemic inflammatory response syndrome (SIRS)**

An external cause code is not appropriate with a code from subcategory 995.9, unless the patient also has an injury, poisoning, or adverse effect of drugs.

b. **Place of Occurrence Guideline**

Use an additional code from category E849 to indicate the Place of Occurrence for injuries and poisonings. The Place of Occurrence describes the place where the event occurred and not the patient's activity at the time of the event.

Do not use E849.9 if the place of occurrence is not stated.

c. **Adverse Effects of Drugs, Medicinal and Biological Substances Guidelines**

1) **Do not code directly from the Table of Drugs**

Do not code directly from the Table of Drugs and Chemicals. Always refer back to the Tabular List.

2) **Use as many codes as necessary to describe**

Use as many codes as necessary to describe completely all drugs, medicinal or biological substances.

3) **If the same E code would describe the causative agent**

If the same E code would describe the causative agent for more than one adverse reaction, assign the code only once.

4) **If two or more drugs, medicinal or biological substances**

If two or more drugs, medicinal or biological substances are reported, code each individually unless the combination code is listed in the Table of Drugs and Chemicals. In that case, assign the E code for the combination.

5) **When a reaction results from the interaction of a drug(s)**

When a reaction results from the interaction of a drug(s) and alcohol, use poisoning codes and E codes for both.

6) **If the reporting format limits the number of E codes**

If the reporting format limits the number of E codes that can be used in reporting clinical data, code the one most related to the principal diagnosis. Include at least one from each category (cause, intent, place) if possible.

If there are different fourth digit codes in the same three digit category, use the code for "Other specified" of that category. If there is no "Other specified" code in that category, use the appropriate "Unspecified" code in that category.

If the codes are in different three digit categories, assign the appropriate E code for other multiple drugs and medicinal substances.

7) **Codes from the E930-E949 series**

Codes from the E930-E949 series must be used to identify the causative substance for an adverse effect of drug, medicinal and biological substances, correctly prescribed and properly administered. The effect, such as tachycardia, delirium, gastrointestinal hemorrhaging, vomiting, hypokalemia, hepatitis, renal failure, or respiratory failure, is coded and followed by the appropriate code from the E930-E949 series.

d. Multiple Cause E Code Coding Guidelines

If two or more events cause separate injuries, an E code should be assigned for each cause. The first listed E code will be selected in the following order:

E codes for child and adult abuse take priority over all other E codes.

See Section I.C.19.e., Child and Adult abuse guidelines.

E codes for terrorism events take priority over all other E codes except child and adult abuse

E codes for cataclysmic events take priority over all other E codes except child and adult abuse and terrorism.

E codes for transport accidents take priority over all other E codes except cataclysmic events and child and adult abuse and terrorism.

The first-listed E code should correspond to the cause of the most serious diagnosis due to an assault, accident, or self-harm, following the order of hierarchy listed above.

e. Child and Adult Abuse Guideline

1) Intentional injury

When the cause of an injury or neglect is intentional child or adult abuse, the first listed E code should be assigned from categories E960-E968, Homicide and injury purposely inflicted by other persons, (except category E967). An E code from category E967, Child and adult battering and other maltreatment, should be added as an additional code to identify the perpetrator, if known.

2) Accidental intent

In cases of neglect when the intent is determined to be accidental E code E904.0, Abandonment or neglect of infant and helpless person, should be the first listed E code.

f. Unknown or Suspected Intent Guideline

1) If the intent (accident, self-harm, assault) of the cause of an injury or poisoning is unknown

If the intent (accident, self-harm, assault) of the cause of an injury or poisoning is unknown or unspecified, code the intent as undetermined E980-E989.

2) If the intent (accident, self-harm, assault) of the cause of an injury or poisoning is questionable

If the intent (accident, self-harm, assault) of the cause of an injury or poisoning is questionable, probable or suspected, code the intent as undetermined E980-E989.

g. Undetermined Cause

When the intent of an injury or poisoning is known, but the cause is unknown, use codes: E928.9, Unspecified accident, E958.9, Suicide and self-inflicted injury by unspecified means, and E968.9, Assault by unspecified means.

These E codes should rarely be used, as the documentation in the medical record, in both the inpatient outpatient and other settings, should normally provide sufficient detail to determine the cause of the injury.

h. Late Effects of External Cause Guidelines

1) Late effect E codes

Late effect E codes exist for injuries and poisonings but not for adverse effects of drugs, misadventures and surgical complications.

2) Late effect E codes (E929, E959, E969, E977, E989, or E999.1)

A late effect E code (E929, E959, E969, E977, E989, or E999.1) should be used with any report of a late effect or sequela resulting from a previous injury or poisoning (905-909).

3) Late effect E code with a related current injury

A late effect E code should never be used with a related current nature of injury code.

4) Use of late effect E codes for subsequent visits

Use a late effect E code for subsequent visits when a late effect of the initial injury or poisoning is being treated. There is no late effect E code for adverse effects of drugs.

Do not use a late effect E code for subsequent visits for follow-up care (e.g., to assess healing, to receive rehabilitative therapy) of the injury or poisoning when no late effect of the injury has been documented.

i. Misadventures and Complications of Care Guidelines

1) Code range E870-E876

Assign a code in the range of E870-E876 if misadventures are stated by the provider.

2) Code range E878-E879

Assign a code in the range of E878-E879 if the provider attributes an abnormal reaction or later complication to a surgical or medical procedure, but does not mention misadventure at the time of the procedure as the cause of the reaction.

j. Terrorism Guidelines

1) Cause of injury identified by the Federal Government (FBI) as terrorism

When the cause of an injury is identified by the Federal Government (FBI) as terrorism, the first-listed E-code should be a code from category E979, Terrorism. The definition of terrorism employed by the FBI is found at the inclusion note at E979. The terrorism E-code is the only E-code that should be assigned. Additional E codes from the assault categories should not be assigned.

2) Cause of an injury is suspected to be the result of terrorism

When the cause of an injury is suspected to be the result of terrorism a code from category E979 should not be assigned. Assign a code in the range of E codes based circumstances on the documentation of intent and mechanism.

3) Code E979.9, Terrorism, secondary effects

Assign code E979.9, Terrorism, secondary effects, for conditions occurring subsequent to the terrorist event. This code should not be assigned for conditions that are due to the initial terrorist act.

4) Statistical tabulation of terrorism codes

For statistical purposes these codes will be tabulated within the category for assault, expanding the current category from E960-E969 to include E979 and E999.1.

Section II. Selection of Principal Diagnosis

The circumstances of inpatient admission always govern the selection of principal diagnosis. The principal diagnosis is defined in the Uniform Hospital Discharge Data Set (UHDDS) as "that condition established after study to be chiefly responsible for occasioning the admission of the patient to the hospital for care."

The UHDDS definitions are used by hospitals to report inpatient data elements in a standardized manner. These data elements and their definitions can be found in the July 31, 1985, Federal Register (Vol. 50, No, 147), pp. 31038-40.

Since that time the application of the UHDDS definitions has been expanded to include all non-outpatient settings (acute care, short term, long term care and psychiatric hospitals; home health agencies; rehab facilities; nursing homes, etc).

In determining principal diagnosis the coding conventions in the ICD-9-CM, Volumes I and II take precedence over these official coding guidelines.

(See Section I.A., Conventions for the ICD-9-CM)

The importance of consistent, complete documentation in the medical record cannot be overemphasized. Without such documentation the application of all coding guidelines is a difficult, if not impossible, task.

A. Codes for symptoms, signs, and ill-defined conditions

Codes for symptoms, signs, and ill-defined conditions from Chapter 16 are not to be used as principal diagnosis when a related definitive diagnosis has been established.

B. Two or more interrelated conditions, each potentially meeting the definition for principal diagnosis.

When there are two or more interrelated conditions (such as diseases in the same ICD-9-CM chapter or manifestations characteristically associated with a certain disease) potentially meeting the definition of principal diagnosis, either condition may be sequenced first, unless the circumstances of the admission, the therapy provided, the Tabular List, or the Alphabetic Index indicate otherwise.

C. Two or more diagnoses that equally meet the definition for principal diagnosis

In the unusual instance when two or more diagnoses equally meet the criteria for principal diagnosis as determined by the circumstances of admission, diagnostic workup and/or therapy provided, and the Alphabetic Index, Tabular List, or another coding guidelines does not provide sequencing direction, any one of the diagnoses may be sequenced first.

D. Two or more comparative or contrasting conditions.

In those rare instances when two or more contrasting or comparative diagnoses are documented as "either/or" (or similar terminology), they are coded as if the diagnoses were confirmed and the diagnoses are sequenced according to the circumstances of the admission. If no further determination can be made as to which diagnosis should be principal, either diagnosis may be sequenced first.

E. A symptom(s) followed by contrasting/comparative diagnoses

When a symptom(s) is followed by contrasting/comparative diagnoses, the symptom code is sequenced first. All the contrasting/comparative diagnoses should be coded as additional diagnoses.

F. **Original treatment plan not carried out**

Sequence as the principal diagnosis the condition, which after study occasioned the admission to the hospital, even though treatment may not have been carried out due to unforeseen circumstances.

G. **Complications of surgery and other medical care**

When the admission is for treatment of a complication resulting from surgery or other medical care, the complication code is sequenced as the principal diagnosis. If the complication is classified to the 996-999 series and the code lacks the necessary specificity in describing the complication, an additional code for the specific complication should be assigned.

H. **Uncertain Diagnosis**

If the diagnosis documented at the time of discharge is qualified as "probable", "suspected", "likely", "questionable", "possible", or "still to be ruled out", or other similar terms indicating uncertainty, code the condition as if it existed or was established. The bases for these guidelines are the diagnostic workup, arrangements for further workup or observation, and initial therapeutic approach that correspond most closely with the established diagnosis.

Note: This guideline is applicable only to inpatient admissions to short-term, acute, long-term care and psychiatric hospitals.

I. **Admission from Observation Unit**

1. **Admission Following Medical Observation**

   When a patient is admitted to an observation unit for a medical condition, which either worsens or does not improve, and is subsequently admitted as an inpatient of the same hospital for this same medical condition, the principal diagnosis would be the medical condition which led to the hospital admission.

2. **Admission Following Post-Operative Observation**

   When a patient is admitted to an observation unit to monitor a condition (or complication) that develops following outpatient surgery, and then is subsequently admitted as an inpatient of the same hospital, hospitals should apply the Uniform Hospital Discharge Data Set (UHDDS) definition of principal diagnosis as "that condition established after study to be chiefly responsible for occasioning the admission of the patient to the hospital for care."

J. **Admission from Outpatient Surgery**

When a patient receives surgery in the hospital's outpatient surgery department and is subsequently admitted for continuing inpatient care at the same hospital, the following guidelines should be followed in selecting the principal diagnosis for the inpatient admission:

- If the reason for the inpatient admission is a complication, assign the complication as the principal diagnosis.
- If no complication, or other condition, is documented as the reason for the inpatient admission, assign the reason for the outpatient surgery as the principal diagnosis.
- If the reason for the inpatient admission is another condition unrelated to the surgery, assign the unrelated condition as the principal diagnosis.

Section III. Reporting Additional Diagnoses

GENERAL RULES FOR OTHER (ADDITIONAL) DIAGNOSES

For reporting purposes the definition for "other diagnoses" is interpreted as additional conditions that affect patient care in terms of requiring:

> clinical evaluation; or
> therapeutic treatment; or
> diagnostic procedures; or
> extended length of hospital stay; or
> increased nursing care and/or monitoring.

The UHDDS item #11-b defines Other Diagnoses as "all conditions that coexist at the time of admission, that develop subsequently, or that affect the treatment received and/or the length of stay. Diagnoses that relate to an earlier episode which have no bearing on the current hospital stay are to be excluded." UHDDS definitions apply to inpatients in acute care, short-term, long term care and psychiatric hospital setting. The UHDDS definitions are used by acute care short-term hospitals to report inpatient data elements in a standardized manner. These data elements and their definitions can be found in the July 31, 1985, Federal Register (Vol. 50, No, 147), pp. 31038-40.

Since that time the application of the UHDDS definitions has been expanded to include all non-outpatient settings (acute care, short term, long term care and psychiatric hospitals; home health agencies; rehab facilities; nursing homes, etc).

The following guidelines are to be applied in designating "other diagnoses" when neither the Alphabetic Index nor the Tabular List in ICD-9-CM provide direction. The listing of the diagnoses in the patient record is the responsibility of the attending provider.

A. Previous conditions

If the provider has included a diagnosis in the final diagnostic statement, such as the discharge summary or the face sheet, it should ordinarily be coded. Some providers include in the diagnostic statement resolved conditions or diagnoses and status-post procedures from previous admission that have no bearing on the current stay. Such conditions are not to be reported and are coded only if required by hospital policy.

However, history codes (V10-V19) may be used as secondary codes if the historical condition or family history has an impact on current care or influences treatment.

B. Abnormal findings

Abnormal findings (laboratory, x-ray, pathologic, and other diagnostic results) are not coded and reported unless the provider indicates their clinical significance. If the findings are outside the normal range and the attending provider has ordered other tests to evaluate the condition or prescribed treatment, it is appropriate to ask the provider whether the abnormal finding should be added.

Please note: This differs from the coding practices in the outpatient setting for coding encounters for diagnostic tests that have been interpreted by a provider.

C. Uncertain Diagnosis

If the diagnosis documented at the time of discharge is qualified as "probable", "suspected", "likely", "questionable", "possible", or "still to be ruled out" or other similar terms indicating uncertainty, code the condition as if it existed or was established. The bases for these guidelines are the diagnostic workup, arrangements for further workup or observation, and initial therapeutic approach that correspond most closely with the established diagnosis.

Note: This guideline is applicable only to inpatient admissions to short-term, acute, long-term care and psychiatric hospitals.

Section IV. Diagnostic Coding and Reporting Guidelines for Outpatient Services

These coding guidelines for outpatient diagnoses have been approved for use by hospitals/ providers in coding and reporting hospital-based outpatient services and provider-based office visits.

Information about the use of certain abbreviations, punctuation, symbols, and other conventions used in the ICD-9-CM Tabular List (code numbers and titles), can be found in Section IA of these guidelines, under "Conventions Used in the Tabular List." Information about the correct sequence to use in finding a code is also described in Section I.

The terms encounter and visit are often used interchangeably in describing outpatient service contacts and, therefore, appear together in these guidelines without distinguishing one from the other.

Though the conventions and general guidelines apply to all settings, coding guidelines for outpatient and provider reporting of diagnoses will vary in a number of instances from those for inpatient diagnoses, recognizing that:

> The Uniform Hospital Discharge Data Set (UHDDS) definition of principal diagnosis applies only to inpatients in acute, short-term, long-term care and psychiatric hospitals.

> Coding guidelines for inconclusive diagnoses (probable, suspected, rule out, etc.) were developed for inpatient reporting and do not apply to outpatients.

A. Selection of first-listed condition

In the outpatient setting, the term first-listed diagnosis is used in lieu of principal diagnosis.

In determining the first-listed diagnosis the coding conventions of ICD-9-CM, as well as the general and disease specific guidelines take precedence over the outpatient guidelines.

Diagnoses often are not established at the time of the initial encounter/visit. It may take two or more visits before the diagnosis is confirmed.

The most critical rule involves beginning the search for the correct code assignment through the Alphabetic Index. Never begin searching initially in the Tabular List as this will lead to coding errors.

1. Outpatient Surgery

When a patient presents for outpatient surgery, code the reason for the surgery as the first-listed diagnosis (reason for the encounter), even if the surgery is not performed due to a contraindication.

2. Observation Stay

When a patient is admitted for observation for a medical condition, assign a code for the medical condition as the first-listed diagnosis.

When a patient presents for outpatient surgery and develops complications requiring admission to observation, code the reason for the surgery as the first reported diagnosis (reason for the encounter), followed by codes for the complications as secondary diagnoses.

B. Codes from 001.0 through V89

The appropriate code or codes from 001.0 through **V89** must be used to identify diagnoses, symptoms, conditions, problems, complaints, or other reason(s) for the encounter/visit.

C. Accurate reporting of ICD-9-CM diagnosis codes

For accurate reporting of ICD-9-CM diagnosis codes, the documentation should describe the patient's condition, using terminology which includes specific diagnoses as well as symptoms, problems, or reasons for the encounter. There are ICD-9-CM codes to describe all of these.

D. Selection of codes 001.0 through 999.9

The selection of codes 001.0 through 999.9 will frequently be used to describe the reason for the encounter. These codes are from the section of ICD-9-CM for the classification of diseases and injuries (e.g. infectious and parasitic diseases; neoplasms; symptoms, signs, and ill-defined conditions, etc.).

E. Codes that describe symptoms and signs

Codes that describe symptoms and signs, as opposed to diagnoses, are acceptable for reporting purposes when a diagnosis has not been established (confirmed) by the provider. Chapter 16 of ICD-9-CM, Symptoms, Signs, and Ill-defined conditions (codes 780.0 - 799.9) contain many, but not all codes for symptoms.

F. Encounters for circumstances other than a disease or injury

ICD-9-CM provides codes to deal with encounters for circumstances other than a disease or injury. The Supplementary Classification of factors Influencing Health Status and Contact with Health Services (V01.0- **V89**) is provided to deal with occasions when circumstances other than a disease or injury are recorded as diagnosis or problems. *See Section I.C. 18 for information on V-codes.*

G. Level of Detail in Coding

1. ICD-9-CM codes with 3, 4, or 5 digits

ICD-9-CM is composed of codes with either 3, 4, or 5 digits. Codes with three digits are included in ICD-9-CM as the heading of a category of codes that may be further subdivided by the use of fourth and/or fifth digits, which provide greater specificity.

2. Use of full number of digits required for a code

A three-digit code is to be used only if it is not further subdivided. Where fourth-digit subcategories and/or fifth-digit subclassifications are provided, they must be assigned. A code is invalid if it has not been coded to the full number of digits required for that code.

See also discussion under Section I.b.3., General Coding Guidelines, Level of Detail in Coding.

H. ICD-9-CM code for the diagnosis, condition, problem, or other reason for encounter/visit

List first the ICD-9-CM code for the diagnosis, condition, problem, or other reason for encounter/visit shown in the medical record to be chiefly responsible for the services provided. List additional codes that describe any coexisting conditions. In some cases the first-listed diagnosis may be a symptom when a diagnosis has not been established (confirmed) by the physician.

I. Uncertain diagnosis

Do not code diagnoses documented as "probable", "suspected," "questionable," "rule out," or "working diagnosis" or other similar terms indicating uncertainty. Rather, code the condition(s) to the highest degree of certainty for that encounter/visit, such as symptoms, signs, abnormal test results, or other reason for the visit.

Please note: This differs from the coding practices used by short-term, acute care, long-term care and psychiatric hospitals.

J. Chronic diseases

Chronic diseases treated on an ongoing basis may be coded and reported as many times as the patient receives treatment and care for the condition(s)

K. **Code all documented conditions that coexist**

Code all documented conditions that coexist at the time of the encounter/visit, and require or affect patient care treatment or management. Do not code conditions that were previously treated and no longer exist. However, history codes (V10-V19) may be used as secondary codes if the historical condition or family history has an impact on current care or influences treatment.

L. **Patients receiving diagnostic services only**

For patients receiving diagnostic services only during an encounter/visit, sequence first the diagnosis, condition, problem, or other reason for encounter/visit shown in the medical record to be chiefly responsible for the outpatient services provided during the encounter/visit. Codes for other diagnoses (e.g., chronic conditions) may be sequenced as additional diagnoses.

For encounters for routine laboratory/radiology testing in the absence of any signs, symptoms, or associated diagnosis, assign V72.5 and V72.6. If routine testing is performed during the same encounter as a test to evaluate a sign, symptom, or diagnosis, it is appropriate to assign both the V code and the code describing the reason for the non-routine test.

For outpatient encounters for diagnostic tests that have been interpreted by a physician, and the final report is available at the time of coding, code any confirmed or definitive diagnosis(es) documented in the interpretation. Do not code related signs and symptoms as additional diagnoses.

Please note: This differs from the coding practice in the hospital inpatient setting regarding abnormal findings on test results.

M. **Patients receiving therapeutic services only**

For patients receiving therapeutic services only during an encounter/visit, sequence first the diagnosis, condition, problem, or other reason for encounter/visit shown in the medical record to be chiefly responsible for the outpatient services provided during the encounter/visit. Codes for other diagnoses (e.g., chronic conditions) may be sequenced as additional diagnoses.

The only exception to this rule is that when the primary reason for the admission/encounter is chemotherapy, radiation therapy, or rehabilitation, the appropriate V code for the service is listed first, and the diagnosis or problem for which the service is being performed listed second.

N. **Patients receiving preoperative evaluations only**

For patients receiving preoperative evaluations only, sequence first a code from category V72.8, Other specified examinations, to describe the pre-op consultations. Assign a code for the condition to describe the reason for the surgery as an additional diagnosis. Code also any findings related to the pre-op evaluation.

O. **Ambulatory surgery**

For ambulatory surgery, code the diagnosis for which the surgery was performed. If the postoperative diagnosis is known to be different from the preoperative diagnosis at the time the diagnosis is confirmed, select the postoperative diagnosis for coding, since it is the most definitive.

P. **Routine outpatient prenatal visits**

For routine outpatient prenatal visits when no complications are present, codes V22.0, Supervision of normal first pregnancy, or V22.1, Supervision of other normal pregnancy, should be used as the principal diagnosis. These codes should not be used in conjunction with chapter 11 codes.

Appendix I
Present on Admission Reporting Guidelines

Introduction

These guidelines are to be used as a supplement to the *ICD-9-CM Official Guidelines for Coding and Reporting* to facilitate the assignment of the Present on Admission (POA) indicator for each diagnosis and external cause of injury code reported on claim forms (UB-04 and 837 Institutional).

These guidelines are not intended to replace any guidelines in the main body of the *ICD-9-CM Official Guidelines for Coding and Reporting*. The POA guidelines are not intended to provide guidance on when a condition should be coded, but rather, how to apply the POA indicator to the final set of diagnosis codes that have been assigned in accordance with Sections I, II, and III of the official coding guidelines. Subsequent to the assignment of the ICD-9-CM codes, the POA indicator should then be assigned to those conditions that have been coded.

As stated in the Introduction to the ICD-9-CM Official Guidelines for Coding and Reporting, a joint effort between the healthcare provider and the coder is essential to achieve complete and accurate documentation, code assignment, and reporting of diagnoses and procedures. The importance of consistent, complete documentation in the medical record cannot be overemphasized. Medical record documentation from any provider involved in the care and treatment of the patient may be used to support the determination of whether a condition was present on admission or not. In the context of the official coding guidelines, the term "provider" means a physician or any qualified healthcare practitioner who is legally accountable for establishing the patient's diagnosis.

These guidelines are not a substitute for the provider's clinical judgment as to the determination of whether a condition was/was not present on admission. The provider should be queried regarding issues related to the linking of signs/symptoms, timing of test results, and the timing of findings.

General Reporting Requirements

All claims involving inpatient admissions to general acute care hospitals or other facilities that are subject to a law or regulation mandating collection of present on admission information.

Present on admission is defined as present at the time the order for inpatient admission occurs — conditions that develop during an outpatient encounter, including emergency department, observation, or outpatient surgery, are considered as present on admission.

POA indicator is assigned to principal and secondary diagnoses (as defined in Section II of the Official Guidelines for Coding and Reporting) and the external cause of injury codes.

Issues related to inconsistent, missing, conflicting or unclear documentation must still be resolved by the provider.

If a condition would not be coded and reported based on UHDDS definitions and current official coding guidelines, then the POA indicator would not be reported.

Reporting Options

Y - Yes

N - No

U - Unknown

W – Clinically undetermined

Unreported/Not used **(or "1" for Medicare usage)** – (Exempt from POA reporting)

For more specific instructions on Medicare POA indicator reporting options, refer to http://www.cms.hhs.gov/HospitalAcqCond/02_Statute_Regulations _Program_Instructions.asp#TopOfPage

Reporting Definitions

Y = present at the time of inpatient admission

N = not present at the time of inpatient admission

U = documentation is insufficient to determine if condition is present on admission

W = provider is unable to clinically determine whether condition was present on admission or not

Timeframe for POA Identification and Documentation

There is no required timeframe as to when a provider (per the definition of "provider" used in these guidelines) must identify or document a condition to be present on admission. In some clinical situations, it may not be possible for a provider to make a definitive diagnosis (or a condition may not be recognized or reported by the patient) for a period of time after admission. In some cases it may be several days before the provider arrives at a definitive diagnosis. This does not mean that the condition was not present on admission. Determination of whether the condition was present on admission or not will be based on the applicable POA guideline as identified in this document, or on the provider's best clinical judgment.

If at the time of code assignment the documentation is unclear as to whether a condition was present on admission or not, it is appropriate to query the provider for clarification.

Assigning the POA Indicator

Condition is on the "Exempt from Reporting" list

Leave the "present on admission" field blank if the condition is on the list of ICD-9-CM codes for which this field is not applicable. This is the only circumstance in which the field may be left blank.

POA Explicitly Documented

Assign Y for any condition the provider explicitly documents as being present on admission.

Assign N for any condition the provider explicitly documents as not present at the time of admission.

Conditions diagnosed prior to inpatient admission

Assign "Y" for conditions that were diagnosed prior to admission (example: hypertension, diabetes mellitus, asthma)

Conditions diagnosed during the admission but clearly present before admission

Assign "Y" for conditions diagnosed during the admission that were clearly present but not diagnosed until after admission occurred.

Diagnoses subsequently confirmed after admission are considered present on admission if at the time of admission they are documented as suspected, possible, rule out, differential diagnosis, or constitute an underlying cause of a symptom that is present at the time of admission.

Condition develops during outpatient encounter prior to inpatient admission

Assign Y for any condition that develops during an outpatient encounter prior to a written order for inpatient admission.

Documentation does not indicate whether condition was present on admission

Assign "U" when the medical record documentation is unclear as to whether the condition was present on admission. "U" should not be routinely assigned and used only in very limited circumstances. Coders are encouraged to query the providers when the documentation is unclear.

Documentation states that it cannot be determined whether the condition was or was not present on admission

Assign "W" when the medical record documentation indicates that it cannot be clinically determined whether or not the condition was present on admission.

Chronic condition with acute exacerbation during the admission

If the code is a combination code that identifies both the chronic condition and the acute exacerbation, see POA guidelines pertaining to combination codes.

If the combination code only identifies the chronic condition and not the acute exacerbation (e.g., acute exacerbation of CHF), assign "Y."

Conditions documented as possible, probable, suspected, or rule out at the time of discharge

If the final diagnosis contains a possible, probable, suspected, or rule out diagnosis, and this diagnosis was suspected at the time of inpatient admission, assign "Y."

If the final diagnosis contains a possible, probable, suspected, or rule out diagnosis, and this diagnosis was based on symptoms or clinical findings that were not present on admission, assign "N".

Conditions documented as impending or threatened at the time of discharge

If the final diagnosis contains an impending or threatened diagnosis, and this diagnosis is based on symptoms or clinical findings that were present on admission, assign "Y".

If the final diagnosis contains an impending or threatened diagnosis, and this diagnosis is based on symptoms or clinical findings that were not present on admission, assign "N".

Acute and Chronic Conditions

Assign "Y" for acute conditions that are present at time of admission and N for acute conditions that are not present at time of admission.

Assign "Y" for chronic conditions, even though the condition may not be diagnosed until after admission.

If a single code identifies both an acute and chronic condition, see the POA guidelines for combination codes.

Combination Codes

Assign "N" if any part of the combination code was not present on admission (e.g., obstructive chronic bronchitis with acute exacerbation and the exacerbation was not present on admission; gastric ulcer that does not start bleeding until after admission; asthma patient develops status asthmaticus after admission)

Assign "Y" if all parts of the combination code were present on admission (e.g., patient with diabetic nephropathy is admitted with uncontrolled diabetes)

If the final diagnosis includes comparative or contrasting diagnoses, and both were present, or suspected, at the time of admission, assign "Y".

For infection codes that include the causal organism, assign "Y" if the infection (or signs of the infection) was present on admission, even though the culture results may not be known until after admission (e.g., patient is admitted with pneumonia and the provider documents pseudomonas as the causal organism a few days later).

Same Diagnosis Code for Two or More Conditions

When the same ICD-9-CM diagnosis code applies to two or more conditions during the same encounter (e.g. bilateral condition, or two separate conditions classified to the same ICD-9-CM diagnosis code):

Assign "Y" if all conditions represented by the single ICD-9-CM code were present on admission (e.g. bilateral fracture of the same bone, same site, and both fractures were present on admission)

Assign "N" if any of the conditions represented by the single ICD-9-CM code was not present on admission (e.g. dehydration with hyponatremia is assigned to code 276.1, but only one of these conditions was present on admission).

Obstetrical conditions

Whether or not the patient delivers during the current hospitalization does not affect assignment of the POA indicator. The determining factor for POA assignment is whether the pregnancy complication or obstetrical condition described by the code was present at the time of admission or not.

If the pregnancy complication or obstetrical condition was present on admission (e.g., patient admitted in preterm labor), assign "Y".

If the pregnancy complication or obstetrical condition was not present on admission (e.g., 2nd degree laceration during delivery, postpartum hemorrhage that occurred during current hospitalization, fetal distress develops after admission), assign "N".

If the obstetrical code includes more than one diagnosis and any of the diagnoses identified by the code were not present on admission assign "N".

(e.g., Code 642.7, Pre-eclampsia or eclampsia superimposed on pre-existing hypertension).

If the obstetrical code includes information that is not a diagnosis, do not consider that information in the POA determination.

(e.g. Code 652.1x, Breech or other malpresentation successfully converted to cephalic presentation should be reported as present on admission if the fetus was breech on admission but was converted to cephalic presentation after admission (since the conversion to cephalic presentation does not represent a diagnosis, the fact that the conversion occurred after admission has no bearing on the POA determination).

Perinatal conditions

Newborns are not considered to be admitted until after birth. Therefore, any condition present at birth or that developed in utero is considered present at admission and should be assigned "Y". This includes conditions that occur during delivery (e.g., injury during delivery, meconium aspiration, exposure to streptococcus B in the vaginal canal).

Congenital conditions and anomalies

Assign "Y" for congenital conditions and anomalies. Congenital conditions are always considered present on admission.

External cause of injury codes

Assign "Y" for any E code representing an external cause of injury or poisoning that occurred prior to inpatient admission (e.g., patient fell out of bed at home, patient fell out of bed in emergency room prior to admission)

Assign "N" for any E code representing an external cause of injury or poisoning that occurred during inpatient hospitalization (e.g., patient fell out of hospital bed during hospital stay, patient experienced an adverse reaction to a medication administered after inpatient admission)

Categories and Codes Exempt from Diagnosis Present on Admission Requirement
Effective Date: October 1, 2008

Note: "Diagnosis present on admission" for these code categories are exempt because they represent circumstances regarding the healthcare encounter or factors influencing health status that do not represent a current disease or injury or are always present on admission

137-139, Late effects of infectious and parasitic diseases

268.1, Rickets, late effect

326, Late effects of intracranial abscess or pyogenic infection

412, Old myocardial infarction

438, Late effects of cerebrovascular disease

650, Normal delivery

660.7, Failed forceps or vacuum extractor, unspecified

677, Late effect of complication of pregnancy, childbirth, and the puerperium

905-909, Late effects of injuries, poisonings, toxic effects, and other external causes

V02, Carrier or suspected carrier of infectious diseases

V03, Need for prophylactic vaccination and inoculation against bacterial diseases

V04, Need for prophylactic vaccination and inoculation against certain viral diseases

V05, Need for other prophylactic vaccination and inoculation against single diseases

V06, Need for prophylactic vaccination and inoculation against combinations of diseases

V07, Need for isolation and other prophylactic measures

V10, Personal history of malignant neoplasm

V11, Personal history of mental disorder

V12, Personal history of certain other diseases

V13, Personal history of other diseases

V14, Personal history of allergy to medicinal agents

V15.01-V15.09, Other personal history, Allergy, other than to medicinal agents

V15.1, Other personal history, Surgery to heart and great vessels

V15.2, Other personal history, Surgery to other major organs

V15.3, Other personal history, Irradiation

V15.4, Other personal history, Psychological trauma

V15.5, Other personal history, Injury

V15.6, Other personal history, Poisoning

V15.7, Other personal history, Contraception

V15.81, Other personal history, Noncompliance with medical treatment

V15.82, Other personal history, History of tobacco use

V15.88, Other personal history, History of fall

V15.89, Other personal history, Other

V15.9 Unspecified personal history presenting hazards to health

V16, Family history of malignant neoplasm

V17, Family history of certain chronic disabling diseases

V18, Family history of certain other specific conditions

V19, Family history of other conditions

V20, Health supervision of infant or child

V21, Constitutional states in development

V22, Normal pregnancy

V23, Supervision of high-risk pregnancy

V24, Postpartum care and examination

V25, Encounter for contraceptive management

V26, Procreative management

V27, Outcome of delivery

V28, Antenatal screening

V29, Observation and evaluation of newborns for suspected condition not found

V30-V39, Liveborn infants according to type of birth

V42, Organ or tissue replaced by transplant

V43, Organ or tissue replaced by other means

V44, Artificial opening status

V45, Other postprocedural states

V46, Other dependence on machines

V49.60-V49.77, Upper and lower limb amputation status

V49.81-V49.84, Other specified conditions influencing health status

V50, Elective surgery for purposes other than remedying health states

V51, Aftercare involving the use of plastic surgery

V52, Fitting and adjustment of prosthetic device and implant

V53, Fitting and adjustment of other device

V54, Other orthopedic aftercare

V55, Attention to artificial openings

V56, Encounter for dialysis and dialysis catheter care

V57, Care involving use of rehabilitation procedures

V58, Encounter for other and unspecified procedures and aftercare

V59, Donors

V60, Housing, household, and economic circumstances

V61, Other family circumstances

V62, Other psychosocial circumstances

V64, Persons encountering health services for specific procedures, not carried out

V65, Other persons seeking consultation

V66, Convalescence and palliative care

V67, Follow-up examination

V68, Encounters for administrative purposes

V69, Problems related to lifestyle

V70, General medical examination

V71, Observation and evaluation for suspected condition not found

V72, Special investigations and examinations

V73, Special screening examination for viral and chlamydial diseases

V74, Special screening examination for bacterial and spirochetal diseases

V75, Special screening examination for other infectious diseases

V76, Special screening for malignant neoplasms

V77, Special screening for endocrine, nutritional, metabolic, and immunity disorders

V78, Special screening for disorders of blood and blood-forming organs

V79, Special screening for mental disorders and developmental handicaps

V80, Special screening for neurological, eye, and ear diseases

V81, Special screening for cardiovascular, respiratory, and genitourinary diseases

V82, Special screening for other conditions

V83, Genetic carrier status

V84, Genetic susceptibility to disease

V85, Body Mass Index

V86, Estrogen receptor status

V87.4, Personal history of drug therapy

V88, Acquired absence of cervix and uterus

V89, Suspected maternal and fetal conditions not found

E800-E807, Railway accidents

E810-E819, Motor vehicle traffic accidents

E820-E825, Motor vehicle nontraffic accidents

E826-E829, Other road vehicle accidents

E830-E838, Water transport accidents

E840-E845, Air and space transport accidents

E846-E848, Vehicle accidents not elsewhere classifiable

E849.0-E849.6, Place of occurrence

E849.8-E849.9, Place of occurrence

E883.1, Accidental fall into well

E883.2, Accidental fall into storm drain or manhole

E884.0, Fall from playground equipment

E884.1, Fall from cliff

E885.0, Fall from (nonmotorized) scooter

E885.1, Fall from roller skates

E885.2, Fall from skateboard

E885.3, Fall from skis

E885.4, Fall from snowboard

E886.0, Fall on same level from collision, pushing, or shoving, by or with other person, In sports

E890.0-E890.9, Conflagration in private dwelling

E893.0, Accident caused by ignition of clothing, from controlled fire in private dwelling

E893.2, Accident caused by ignition of clothing, from controlled fire not in building or structure

E894, Ignition of highly inflammable material

E895, Accident caused by controlled fire in private dwelling

E897, Accident caused by controlled fire not in building or structure

E898.0-E898.1, Accident caused by other specified fire and flames

E917.0, Striking against or struck accidentally by objects or persons, in sports without subsequent fall

E917.1, Striking against or struck accidentally by objects or persons, caused by a crowd, by collective fear or panic without subsequent fall

E917.2, Striking against or struck accidentally by objects or persons, in running water without subsequent fall

E917.5, Striking against or struck accidentally by objects or persons, object in sports with subsequent fall

E917.6, Striking against or struck accidentally by objects or persons, caused by a crowd, by collective fear or panic with subsequent fall

E919.0-E919.1, Accidents caused by machinery

E919.3-E919.9, Accidents caused by machinery

E921.0-E921.9, Accident caused by explosion of pressure vessel

E922.0-E922.9, Accident caused by firearm and air gun missile

E924.1, Caustic and corrosive substances

E926.2, Visible and ultraviolet light sources

E928.0-E928.8, Other and unspecified environmental and accidental causes

E929.0-E929.9, Late effects of accidental injury

E959, Late effects of self-inflicted injury

E970-E978, Legal intervention

E979, Terrorism

E981.0-E981.8, Poisoning by gases in domestic use, undetermined whether accidentally or purposely inflicted

E982.0-E982.9, Poisoning by other gases, undetermined whether accidentally or purposely inflicted

E985.0-E985.7, Injury by firearms, air guns and explosives, undetermined whether accidentally or purposely inflicted

E987.0, Falling from high place, undetermined whether accidentally or purposely inflicted, residential premises

E987.2, Falling from high place, undetermined whether accidentally or purposely inflicted, natural sites

E989, Late effects of injury, undetermined whether accidentally or purposely inflicted

E990-E999, Injury resulting from operations of war

POA Examples

General Medical Surgical

1. Patient is admitted for diagnostic work-up for cachexia. The final diagnosis is malignant neoplasm of lung with metastasis.

   Assign "Y" on the POA field for the malignant neoplasm. The malignant neoplasm was clearly present on admission, although it was not diagnosed until after the admission occurred.

2. A patient undergoes outpatient surgery. During the recovery period, the patient develops atrial fibrillation and the patient is subsequently admitted to the hospital as an inpatient.

   Assign "Y" on the POA field for the atrial fibrillation since it developed prior to a written order for inpatient admission.

3. A patient is treated in observation and while in Observation, the patient falls out of bed and breaks a hip. The patient is subsequently admitted as an inpatient to treat the hip fracture.

   Assign "Y" on the POA field for the hip fracture since it developed prior to a written order for inpatient admission.

4. A patient with known congestive heart failure is admitted to the hospital after he develops decompensated congestive heart failure.

   Assign "Y" on the POA field for the congestive heart failure. The ICD-9-CM code identifies the chronic condition and does not specify the acute exacerbation.

5. A patient undergoes inpatient surgery. After surgery, the patient develops fever and is treated aggressively. The physician's final diagnosis documents "possible postoperative infection following surgery."

   Assign "N" on the POA field for the postoperative infection since final diagnoses that contain the terms "possible", "probable", "suspected" or "rule out" and that are based on symptoms or clinical findings that were not present on admission should be reported as "N".

6. A patient with severe cough and difficulty breathing was diagnosed during his hospitalization to have lung cancer.

   Assign "Y" on the POA field for the lung cancer. Even though the cancer was not diagnosed until after admission, it is a chronic condition that was clearly present before the patient's admission.

7. A patient is admitted to the hospital for a coronary artery bypass surgery. Postoperatively he developed a pulmonary embolism.

   Assign "N" on the POA field for the pulmonary embolism. This is an acute condition that was not present on admission.

8. A patient is admitted with a known history of coronary atherosclerosis, status post myocardial infarction five years ago is now admitted for treatment of impending myocardial infarction. The final diagnosis is documented as "impending myocardial infarction."

   Assign "Y" to the impending myocardial infarction because the condition is present on admission.

9. A patient with diabetes mellitus developed uncontrolled diabetes on day 3 of the hospitalization.

   Assign "N" to the diabetes code because the "uncontrolled" component of the code was not present on admission.

10. A patient is admitted with high fever and pneumonia. The patient rapidly deteriorates and becomes septic. The discharge diagnosis lists sepsis and pneumonia. The documentation is unclear as to whether the sepsis was present on admission or developed shortly after admission.

    Query the physician as to whether the sepsis was present on admission, developed shortly after admission, or it cannot be clinically determined as to whether it was present on admission or not.

11. A patient is admitted for repair of an abdominal aneurysm. However, the aneurysm ruptures after hospital admission.

    Assign "N" for the ruptured abdominal aneurysm. Although the aneurysm was present on admission, the "ruptured" component of the code description did not occur until after admission.

12. A patient with viral hepatitis B progresses to hepatic coma after admission.

    Assign "N" for the viral hepatitis B with hepatic coma because part of the code description did not develop until after admission.

13. A patient with a history of varicose veins and ulceration of the left lower extremity strikes the area against the side of his hospital bed during an inpatient hospitalization. It bleeds profusely. The final diagnosis lists varicose veins with ulcer and hemorrhage.

    Assign "Y" for the varicose veins with ulcer. Although the hemorrhage occurred after admission, the code description for varicose veins with ulcer does not mention hemorrhage.

14. The nursing initial assessment upon admission documents the presence of a decubitus ulcer. There is no mention of the decubitus ulcer in the physician documentation until several days after admission.

    Query the physician as to whether the decubitus ulcer was present on admission, or developed after admission. Both diagnosis code assignment and determination of whether a condition was present on admission must be based on provider documentation in the medical record (per the definition of "provider" found at the beginning of these POA guidelines and in the introductory section of the ICD-9-CM Official Guidelines for Coding and Reporting). If it cannot be determined from the provider documentation whether or not a condition was present on admission, the provider should be queried.

15. **A urine culture is obtained on admission. The provider documents urinary tract infection when the culture results become available a few days later.**

    Assign "Y" to the urinary tract infection since the diagnosis is based on test results from a specimen obtained on admission. It may not be possible for a provider to make a definitive diagnosis for a period of time after admission. There is no required timeframe as to when a provider must identify or document a condition to be present on admission.

16. **A patient tested positive for Methicillin resistant Staphylococcus (MRSA) on routine nasal culture on admission to the hospital. During the hospitalization, he underwent insertion of a central venous catheter and later developed an infection and was diagnosed with MRSA sepsis due to central venous catheter infection.**

    Assign "Y" to the positive MRSA colonization. Assign "N" for the MRSA sepsis due to central venous catheter infection since the patient did not have a MRSA infection at the time of admission.

Obstetrics

1. A female patient was admitted to the hospital and underwent a normal delivery.

    Leave the "present on admission" (POA) field blank. Code 650, Normal delivery, is on the "exempt from reporting" list.

2. Patient admitted in late pregnancy due to excessive vomiting and dehydration. During admission patient goes into premature labor

    Assign "Y" for the excessive vomiting and the dehydration.

    Assign "N" for the premature labor

3. Patient admitted in active labor. During the stay, a breast abscess is noted when mother attempted to breast feed. Provider is unable to determine whether the abscess was present on admission

    Assign "W" for the breast abscess.

4. Patient admitted in active labor. After 12 hours of labor it is noted that the infant is in fetal distress and a Cesarean section is performed

   Assign "N" for the fetal distress.

5. **Pregnant female was admitted in labor and fetal nuchal cord entanglement was diagnosed. Physician is queried, but is unable to determine whether the cord entanglement was present on admission or not.**

   Assign "W" for the fetal nuchal cord entanglement.

Newborn

1. A single liveborn infant was delivered in the hospital via Cesarean section. The physician documented fetal bradycardia during labor in the final diagnosis in the newborn record.

   Assign " Y" because the bradycardia developed prior to the newborn admission (birth).

2. A newborn developed diarrhea which was believed to be due to the hospital baby formula.

   Assign " N" because the diarrhea developed after admission.

3. **A newborn born in the hospital, birth complicated by nuchal cord entanglement.**

   Assign "Y" for the nuchal cord entanglement on the baby's record. Any condition that is present at birth or that developed in utero is considered present at admission, including conditions that occur during delivery.

A

AAT (alpha-1 antitrypsin) deficiency 273.4
AAV (disease) (illness) (infection) - *see* Human immunodeficiency virus (disease) (illness) (infection)
Abactio - *see* Abortion, induced
Abactus venter - *see* Abortion, induced
Abarognosis 781.99
Abasia (-astasia) 307.9
  atactica 781.3
  choreic 781.3
  hysterical 300.11
  paroxysmal trepidant 781.3
  spastic 781.3
  trembling 781.3
  trepidans 781.3
Abderhalden-Kaufmann-Lignac syndrome (cystinosis) 270.0
Abdomen, abdominal - *see also* condition
  accordion 306.4
  acute 789.0●
  angina 557.1
  burst 868.00
  convulsive equivalent (*see also* Epilepsy) 345.5●
  heart 746.87
  muscle deficiency syndrome 756.79
  obstipum 756.79
Abdominalgia 789.0●
  periodic 277.31
Abduction contracture, hip or other joint - *see* Contraction, joint
Abercrombie's syndrome (amyloid degeneration) 277.39
Aberrant (congenital) - *see also* Malposition, congenital
  adrenal gland 759.1
  blood vessel NEC 747.60
    arteriovenous NEC 747.60
    cerebrovascular 747.81
    gastrointestinal 747.61
    lower limb 747.64
    renal 747.62
    spinal 747.82
    upper limb 747.63
  breast 757.6
  endocrine gland NEC 759.2
  gastrointestinal vessel (peripheral) 747.61
  hepatic duct 751.69
  lower limb vessel (peripheral) 747.64
  pancreas 751.7
  parathyroid gland 759.2
  peripheral vascular vessel NEC 747.60
  pituitary gland (pharyngeal) 759.2
  renal blood vessel 747.62
  sebaceous glands, mucous membrane, mouth 750.26
  spinal vessel 747.82
  spleen 759.0
  testis (descent) 752.51
  thymus gland 759.2
  thyroid gland 759.2
  upper limb vessel (peripheral) 747.63
Aberratio
  lactis 757.6
  testis 752.51
Aberration - *see also* Anomaly
  chromosome - *see* Anomaly, chromosome(s)
  distantial 368.9
  mental (*see also* Disorder, mental, nonpsychotic) 300.9

Abetalipoproteinemia 272.5
Abionarce 780.79
Abiotrophy 799.89
Ablatio
  placentae - *see* Placenta, ablatio
  retinae (*see also* Detachment, retina) 361.9
Ablation
  pituitary (gland) (with hypofunction) 253.7
  placenta - *see* Placenta, ablatio
  uterus 621.8
Ablepharia, ablepharon, ablephary 743.62
Ablepsia - *see* Blindness
Ablepsy - *see* Blindness
Ablutomania 300.3
Abnormal, abnormality, abnormalities - *see also* Anomaly
  acid-base balance 276.4
    fetus or newborn - *see* Distress, fetal
  adaptation curve, dark 368.63
  alveolar ridge 525.9
  amnion 658.9●
    affecting fetus or newborn 762.9
  anatomical relationship NEC 759.9
  apertures, congenital, diaphragm 756.6
  auditory perception NEC 388.40
  autosomes NEC 758.5
    13 758.1
    18 758.2
    21 or 22 758.0
    D_1 758.1
    E_3 758.2
    G 758.0
  ballistocardiogram 794.39
  basal metabolic rate (BMR) 794.7
  biosynthesis, testicular androgen 257.2
  blood level (of)
    cobalt 790.6
    copper 790.6
    iron 790.6
    lead 790.6
    lithium 790.6
    magnesium 790.6
    mineral 790.6
    zinc 790.6
  blood pressure
    elevated (without diagnosis of hypertension) 796.2
    low (*see also* Hypotension) 458.9
      reading (incidental) (isolated) (nonspecific) 796.3
  blood sugar 790.29
  bowel sounds 787.5
  breathing behavior - *see* Respiration
  caloric test 794.19
  cervix (acquired) NEC 622.9
    congenital 752.40
    in pregnancy or childbirth 654.6●
      causing obstructed labor 660.2●
        affecting fetus or newborn 763.1
  chemistry, blood NEC 790.6
  chest sounds 786.7
  chorion 658.9●
    affecting fetus or newborn 762.9
  chromosomal NEC 758.89
    analysis, nonspecific result 795.2
    autosomes (*see also* Abnormal, autosomes NEC) 758.5

Abnormal, abnormality, abnormalities (*Continued*)
  chromosomal NEC (*Continued*)
    fetal, (suspected) affecting management of pregnancy 655.1●
    sex 758.81
  clinical findings NEC 796.4
  communication - *see* Fistula
  configuration of pupils 379.49
  coronary
    artery 746.85
    vein 746.9
  cortisol-binding globulin 255.8
  course, Eustachian tube 744.24
  creatinine clearance 794.4
  dentofacial NEC 524.9
    functional 524.50
    specified type NEC 524.89
  development, developmental NEC 759.9
    bone 756.9
    central nervous system 742.9
  direction, teeth 524.30
  dynia (*see also* Defect, coagulation) 286.9
  Ebstein 746.2
  echocardiogram 793.2
  echoencephalogram 794.01
  echogram NEC - *see* Findings, abnormal, structure
  electrocardiogram (ECG) (EKG) 794.31
  electroencephalogram (EEG) 794.02
  electromyogram (EMG) 794.17
    ocular 794.14
  electro-oculogram (EOG) 794.12
  electroretinogram (ERG) 794.11
  erythrocytes 289.9
    congenital, with perinatal jaundice 282.9 [774.0]
  eustachian valve 746.9
  excitability under minor stress 301.9
  fat distribution 782.9
  feces 787.7
  fetal heart rate - *see* Distress, fetal
  fetus NEC
    affecting management of pregnancy - *see* Pregnancy, management affected by, fetal
    causing disproportion 653.7●
      affecting fetus or newborn 763.1
      causing obstructed labor 660.1●
        affecting fetus or newborn 763.1
  findings without manifest disease - *see* Findings, abnormal
  fluid
    amniotic 792.3
    cerebrospinal 792.0
    peritoneal 792.9
    pleural 792.9
    synovial 792.9
    vaginal 792.9
  forces of labor NEC 661.9●
    affecting fetus or newborn 763.7
  form, teeth 520.2
  function studies
    auditory 794.15
    bladder 794.9
    brain 794.00
    cardiovascular 794.30
    endocrine NEC 794.6
    kidney 794.4

◀ New   ◀▥ Revised   deleted Deleted   ● Use Additional Digit(s)   ▥ Omit code

Abnormal, abnormality, abnormalities
(Continued)
function studies (Continued)
liver 794.8
nervous system
central 794.00
peripheral 794.19
oculomotor 794.14
pancreas 794.9
placenta 794.9
pulmonary 794.2
retina 794.11
special senses 794.19
spleen 794.9
thyroid 794.5
vestibular 794.16
gait 781.2
hysterical 300.11
gastrin secretion 251.5
globulin
cortisol-binding 255.8
thyroid-binding 246.8
glucagon secretion 251.4
glucose 790.29
in pregnancy, childbirth, or
puerperium 648.8 ●
fetus or newborn 775.0
non-fasting 790.29
gravitational (G) forces or states 994.9
hair NEC 704.2
hard tissue formation in pulp 522.3
head movement 781.0
heart
rate
fetus, affecting liveborn infant
before the onset of labor 763.81
during labor 763.82
unspecified as to time of onset
763.83
intrauterine
before the onset of labor 763.81
during labor 763.82
unspecified as to time of onset
763.83
newborn
before the onset of labor 763.81
during labor 763.82
unspecified as to time of onset
763.83
shadow 793.2
sounds NEC 785.3
hemoglobin (see also Disease,
hemoglobin) 282.7
trait - see Trait, hemoglobin,
abnormal
hemorrhage, uterus - see Hemorrhage,
uterus
histology NEC 795.4
increase in
appetite 783.6
development 783.9
involuntary movement 781.0
jaw closure 524.51
karyotype 795.2
knee jerk 796.1
labor NEC 661.9 ●
affecting fetus or newborn 763.7
laboratory findings - see Findings,
abnormal
length, organ or site, congenital - see
Distortion
liver function test 790.6
loss of height 781.91
loss of weight 783.21

Abnormal, abnormality, abnormalities
(Continued)
lung shadow 793.1
mammogram 793.80
calcification 793.89
calculus 793.89
microcalcification 793.81
Mantoux test 795.5
membranes (fetal)
affecting fetus or newborn 762.9
complicating pregnancy 658.8 ●
menstruation - see Menstruation
metabolism (see also condition) 783.9
movement 781.0
disorder NEC 333.90
sleep related, unspecified 780.58
specified NEC 333.99
head 781.0
involuntary 781.0
specified type NEC 333.99
muscle contraction, localized 728.85
myoglobin (Aberdeen) (Annapolis)
289.9
narrowness, eyelid 743.62
optokinetic response 379.57
organs or tissues of pelvis NEC
in pregnancy or childbirth 654.9 ●
affecting fetus or newborn
763.89
causing obstructed labor 660.2 ●
affecting fetus or newborn
763.1
origin - see Malposition, congenital
palmar creases 757.2
Papanicolaou (smear)
anus 796.70
with
atypical squamous cells
cannot exclude high grade
squamous
intraepithelial lesion
(ASC-H) 796.72
of undetermined
significance (ASC-US)
796.71
cytologic evidence of
malignancy 796.76
high grade squamous
intraepithelial lesion
(HGSIL) 796.74
low grade squamous
intraepithelial lesion
(LGSIL) 796.73
glandular 796.70
specified finding NEC 796.79
cervix 795.00
with
atypical squamous cells
cannot exclude high grade
squamous
intraepithelial lesion
(ASC-H) 795.02
of undetermined
significance (ASC-US)
795.01
cytologic evidence of
malignancy 795.06
high grade squamous
intraepithelial lesion
(HGSIL) 795.04
low grade squamous
intraepithelial lesion
(LGSIL) 795.03
nonspecific finding NEC 795.09

Abnormal, abnormality, abnormalities
(Continued)
Papanicolaou (smear) (Continued)
other site 796.9
vagina 795.10
with
atypical squamous cells
cannot exclude high grade
squamous
intraepithelial lesion
(ASC-H) 795.12
of undetermined
significance (ASC-US)
795.11
cytologic evidence of
malignancy 795.16
high grade squamous
intraepithelial lesion
(HGSIL)795.14
low grade squamous
intraepithelial lesion
(LGSIL) 795.13
glandular 795.10
specified finding NEC 795.19
parturition
affecting fetus or newborn 763.9
mother - see Delivery, complicated
pelvis (bony) - see Deformity, pelvis
percussion, chest 786.7
periods (grossly) (see also
Menstruation) 626.9
phonocardiogram 794.39
placenta - see Placenta, abnormal
plantar reflex 796.1
plasma protein - see Deficiency, plasma,
protein
pleural folds 748.8
position - see also Malposition
gravid uterus 654.4 ●
causing obstructed labor 660.2 ●
affecting fetus or newborn
763.1
posture NEC 781.92
presentation (fetus) - see Presentation,
fetus, abnormal
product of conception NEC 631
puberty - see Puberty
pulmonary
artery 747.3
function, newborn 770.89
test results 794.2
ventilation, newborn 770.89
hyperventilation 786.01
pulsations in neck 785.1
pupil reflexes 379.40
quality of milk 676.8 ●
radiological examination 793.99
abdomen NEC 793.6
biliary tract 793.3
breast 793.89
mammogram NOS 793.80
mammographic
calcification 793.89
calculus 793.89
microcalcification 793.81
gastrointestinal tract 793.4
genitourinary organs 793.5
head 793.0
image test inconclusive due to
excess body fat 793.91
intrathoracic organ NEC 793.2
lung (field) 793.1
musculoskeletal system 793.7
retroperitoneum 793.6

Abnormal, abnormality, abnormalities
(*Continued*)
  radiological examination (*Continued*)
    skin and subcutaneous tissue 793.99
    skull 793.0
  red blood cells 790.09
    morphology 790.09
    volume 790.09
  reflex NEC 796.1
  renal function test 794.4
  respiration signs - *see* Respiration
  response to nerve stimulation 794.10
  retinal correspondence 368.34
  rhythm, heart - *see also* Arrhythmia
    fetus - *see* Distress, fetal
  saliva 792.4
  scan
    brain 794.09
    kidney 794.4
    liver 794.8
    lung 794.2
    thyroid 794.5
  secretion
    gastrin 251.5
    glucagon 251.4
  semen 792.2
  serum level (of)
    acid phosphatase 790.5
    alkaline phosphatase 790.5
    amylase 790.5
    enzymes NEC 790.5
    lipase 790.5
  shape
    cornea 743.41
    gallbladder 751.69
    gravid uterus 654.4●
      affecting fetus or newborn
        763.89
      causing obstructed labor 660.2●
        affecting fetus or newborn
          763.1
    head (*see also* Anomaly, skull) 756.0
    organ or site, congenital NEC - *see*
      Distortion
  sinus venosus 747.40
  size
    fetus, complicating delivery 653.5●
      causing obstructed labor 660.1●
    gallbladder 751.69
    head (*see also* Anomaly, skull) 756.0
    organ or site, congenital NEC - *see*
      Distortion
    teeth 520.2
  skin and appendages, congenital NEC
    757.9
  soft parts of pelvis - *see* Abnormal,
    organs or tissues of pelvis
  spermatozoa 792.2
  sputum (amount) (color) (excessive)
    (odor) (purulent) 786.4
  stool NEC 787.7
    bloody 578.1
      occult 792.1
    bulky 787.7
    color (dark) (light) 792.1
    content (fat) (mucus) (pus) 792.1
    occult blood 792.1
  synchondrosis 756.9
  test results without manifest disease -
    see Findings, abnormal
  thebesian valve 746.9
  thermography - *see* Findings, abnormal,
    structure
  threshold, cones or rods (eye) 368.63

Abnormal, abnormality, abnormalities
(*Continued*)
  thyroid-binding globulin 246.8
  thyroid product 246.8
  toxicology (findings) NEC 796.0
  tracheal cartilage (congenital) 748.3
  transport protein 273.8
  ultrasound results - *see* Findings,
    abnormal, structure
  umbilical cord
    affecting fetus or newborn 762.6
    complicating delivery 663.9●
    specified NEC 663.8●
  union
    cricoid cartilage and thyroid
      cartilage 748.3
    larynx and trachea 748.3
    thyroid cartilage and hyoid bone
      748.3
  urination NEC 788.69
    psychogenic 306.53
    stream
      intermittent 788.61
      slowing 788.62
      splitting 788.61
      weak 788.62
    urgency 788.63
  urine (constituents) NEC 791.9
  uterine hemorrhage (*see also*
    Hemorrhage, uterus) 626.9
    climacteric 627.0
    postmenopausal 627.1
  vagina (acquired) (congenital)
    in pregnancy or childbirth 654.7●
      affecting fetus or newborn
        763.89
      causing obstructed labor 660.2●
        affecting fetus or newborn
          763.1
  vascular sounds 785.9
  vectorcardiogram 794.39
  visually evoked potential (VEP)
    794.13
  vulva (acquired) (congenital)
    in pregnancy or childbirth 654.8●
      affecting fetus or newborn
        763.89
      causing obstructed labor 660.2●
        affecting fetus or newborn
          763.1
  weight
    gain 783.1
      of pregnancy 646.1●
        with hypertension - *see*
          Toxemia, of pregnancy
    loss 783.21
  x-ray examination - *see* Abnormal,
    radiological examination
Abnormally formed uterus - *see* Anomaly,
  uterus
Abnormity (any organ or part) - *see*
  Anomaly
ABO
  hemolytic disease 773.1
  incompatibility reaction 999.6
Abocclusion 524.20
Abolition, language 784.69
Aborter, habitual or recurrent NEC
  without current pregnancy 629.81
  current abortion (*see also* Abortion,
    spontaneous) 634.9●
    affecting fetus or newborn 761.8
  observation in current pregnancy
    646.3●

Abortion (complete) (incomplete)
  (inevitable) (with retained products
  of conception) 637.9●

Note 01   Use the following fifth-digit subclassification with categories 634-637:
0   unspecified
1   incomplete
2   complete

  with
    complication(s) (any) following
      previous abortion - *see*
      category 639
    damage to pelvic organ (laceration)
      (rupture) (tear) 637.2●
    embolism (air) (amniotic fluid)
      (blood clot) (pulmonary)
      (pyemic) (septic) (soap) 637.6●
    genital tract and pelvic infection
      637.0●
    hemorrhage, delayed or excessive
      637.1●
    metabolic disorder 637.4●
    renal failure (acute) 637.3●
    sepsis (genital tract) (pelvic organ)
      637.0●
      urinary tract 637.7●
    shock (postoperative) (septic)
      637.5●
    specified complication NEC 637.7●
    toxemia 637.3●
    unspecified complication(s) 637.8●
    urinary tract infection 637.7●
  accidental - *see* Abortion, spontaneous
  artificial - *see* Abortion, induced
  attempted (failed) - *see* Abortion, failed
  criminal - *see* Abortion, illegal
  early - *see* Abortion, spontaneous
  elective - *see* Abortion, legal
  failed (legal) 638.9
    with
      damage to pelvic organ
        (laceration) (rupture) (tear)
        638.2
      embolism (air) (amniotic fluid)
        (blood clot) (pulmonary)
        (pyemic) (septic) (soap)
        638.6
      genital tract and pelvic infection
        638.0
      hemorrhage, delayed or excessive
        638.1
      metabolic disorder 638.4
      renal failure (acute) 638.3
      sepsis (genital tract) (pelvic
        organ) 638.0
        urinary tract 638.7
      shock (postoperative) (septic)
        638.5
      specified complication NEC 638.7
      toxemia 638.3
      unspecified complication(s) 638.8
      urinary tract infection 638.7
  fetal indication - *see* Abortion, legal
  fetus 779.6
  following threatened abortion - *see*
    Abortion, by type
  habitual or recurrent (care during
    pregnancy) 646.3●
    with current abortion (*see also*
      Abortion, spontaneous) 634.9●
      affecting fetus or newborn 761.8
    without current pregnancy 629.81

◀ New   ◀▥ Revised   ~~deleted~~ Deleted   ● Use Additional Digit(s)   ▨ Omit code

Abortion (*Continued*)
homicidal - *see* Abortion, illegal
illegal 636.9 ●
with
damage to pelvic organ
(laceration) (rupture) (tear)
636.2 ●
embolism (air) (amniotic fluid)
(blood clot) (pulmonary)
(pyemic) (septic) (soap)
636.6 ●
genital tract and pelvic infection
636.0 ●
hemorrhage, delayed or excessive
636.1 ●
metabolic disorder 636.4 ●
renal failure 636.3 ●
sepsis (genital tract) (pelvic
organ) 636.0 ●
urinary tract 636.7 ●
shock (postoperative) (septic)
636.5 ●
specified complication NEC
636.7 ●
toxemia 636.3 ●
unspecified complication(s)
636.8 ●
urinary tract infection 636.7 ●
fetus 779.6
induced 637.9 ●
illegal - *see* Abortion, illegal
legal indications - *see* Abortion, legal
medical indications - *see* Abortion,
legal
therapeutic - *see* Abortion, legal
late - *see* Abortion, spontaneous
legal (legal indication) (medical
indication) (under medical
supervision) 635.9 ●
with
damage to pelvic organ
(laceration) (rupture) (tear)
635.2 ●
embolism (air) (amniotic fluid)
(blood clot) (pulmonary)
(pyemic) (septic) (soap)
635.6 ●
genital tract and pelvic infection
635.0 ●
hemorrhage, delayed or excessive
635.1 ●
metabolic disorder 635.4 ●
renal failure (acute) 635.3 ●
sepsis (genital tract) (pelvic
organ) 635.0 ●
urinary tract 635.7 ●
shock (postoperative) (septic)
635.5 ●
specified complication NEC
635.7 ●
toxemia 635.3 ●
unspecified complication(s)
635.8 ●
urinary tract infection 635.7 ●
fetus 779.6
medical indication - *see* Abortion,
legal
mental hygiene problem - *see* Abortion,
legal
missed 632
operative - *see* Abortion, legal
psychiatric indication - *see* Abortion,
legal
recurrent - *see* Abortion, spontaneous

Abortion (*Continued*)
self-induced - *see* Abortion, illegal
septic - *see* Abortion, by type, with
sepsis
spontaneous 634.9 ●
with
damage to pelvic organ
(laceration) (rupture) (tear)
634.2 ●
embolism (air) (amniotic fluid)
(blood clot) (pulmonary)
(pyemic) (septic) (soap)
634.6 ●
genital tract and pelvic infection
634.0 ●
hemorrhage, delayed or excessive
634.1 ●
metabolic disorder 634.4 ●
renal failure 634.3 ●
sepsis (genital tract) (pelvic
organ) 634.0 ●
urinary tract 634.7 ●
shock (postoperative) (septic)
634.5 ●
specified complication NEC
634.7 ●
toxemia 634.3 ●
unspecified complication(s)
634.8 ●
urinary tract infection 634.7 ●
fetus 761.8
threatened 640.0 ●
affecting fetus or newborn
762.1
surgical - *see* Abortion, legal
therapeutic - *see* Abortion, legal
threatened 640.0 ●
affecting fetus or newborn 762.1
tubal - *see* Pregnancy, tubal
voluntary - *see* Abortion, legal
Abortus fever 023.9
Aboulomania 301.6
Abrachia 755.20
Abrachiatism 755.20
Abrachiocephalia 759.89
Abrachiocephalus 759.89
Abrami's disease (acquired hemolytic
jaundice) 283.9
Abramov-Fiedler myocarditis (acute
isolated myocarditis) 422.91
Abrasion - *see also* Injury, superficial, by
site
cornea 918.1
dental 521.20
extending into
dentine 521.22
pulp 521.23
generalized 521.25
limited to enamel 521.21
localized 521.24
teeth, tooth (dentifrice) (habitual)
(hard tissues) (occupational)
(ritual) (traditional) (wedge
defect) (*see also* Abrasion, dental)
521.20
Abrikossov's tumor (M9580/0) - *see also*
Neoplasm, connective tissue, benign
malignant (M9580/3) - *see* Neoplasm,
connective tissue, malignant
Abrism 988.8
Abruption, placenta - *see* Placenta,
abruptio
Abruptio placentae - *see* Placenta,
abruptio

Abscess (acute) (chronic) (infectional)
(lymphangitic) (metastatic)
(multiple) (pyogenic) (septic) (with
lymphangitis) (*see also* Cellulitis)
682.9
abdomen, abdominal
cavity 567.22
wall 682.2
abdominopelvic 567.22
accessory sinus (chronic) (*see also*
Sinusitis) 473.9
adrenal (capsule) (gland) 255.8
alveolar 522.5
with sinus 522.7
ambic 006.3
bladder 006.8
brain (with liver or lung abscess)
006.5
liver (without mention of brain or
lung abscess) 006.3
with
brain abscess (and lung
abscess) 006.5
lung abscess 006.4
lung (with liver abscess) 006.4
with brain abscess 006.5
seminal vesicle 006.8
specified site NEC 006.8
spleen 006.8
anaerobic 040.0
ankle 682.6
anorectal 566
antecubital space 682.3
antrum (chronic) (Highmore) (*see also*
Sinusitis, maxillary) 473.0
anus 566
apical (tooth) 522.5
with sinus (alveolar) 522.7
appendix 540.1
areola (acute) (chronic) (nonpuerperal)
611.0
puerperal, postpartum 675.1 ●
arm (any part, above wrist) 682.3
artery (wall) 447.2
atheromatous 447.2
auditory canal (external) 380.10
auricle (ear) (staphylococcal)
(streptococcal) 380.10
axilla, axillary (region) 682.3
lymph gland or node 683
back (any part) 682.2
Bartholin's gland 616.3
with
abortion - *see* Abortion, by type,
with sepsis
ectopic pregnancy (*see also*
categories 633.0-633.9)
639.0
molar pregnancy (*see also*
categories 630-632)
639.0
complicating pregnancy or
puerperium 646.6 ●
following
abortion 639.0
ectopic or molar pregnancy
639.0
bartholinian 616.3
Bezold's 383.01
bile, biliary, duct or tract (*see also*
Cholecystitis) 576.8
bilharziasis 120.1
bladder (wall) 595.89
amebic 006.8

Abscess *(Continued)*
  bone (subperiosteal) *(see also*
    Osteomyelitis)* 730.0●
    accessory sinus (chronic) *(see also*
      Sinusitis)* 473.9
    acute 730.0●
    chronic or old 730.1●
    jaw (lower) (upper) 526.4
    mastoid - *see* Mastoiditis, acute
    petrous *(see also* Petrositis)
      383.20
    spinal (tuberculous) *(see also*
      Tuberculosis)* 015.0●
      [730.88]
      nontuberculous 730.08
  bowel 569.5
  brain (any part) 324.0
    amebic (with liver or lung abscess)
      006.5
    cystic 324.0
    late effect - *see* category 326
    otogenic 324.0
    tuberculous *(see also* Tuberculosis)
      013.3●
  breast (acute) (chronic) (nonpuerperal)
    611.0
    newborn 771.5
    puerperal, postpartum 675.1●
    tuberculous *(see also* Tuberculosis)
      017.9●
  broad ligament (chronic) *(see also*
    Disease, pelvis, inflammatory)*
    614.4
    acute 614.3
  Brodie's (chronic) (localized) *(see also*
    Osteomyelitis)* 730.1●
  bronchus 519.19
  buccal cavity 528.3
  bulbourethral gland 597.0
  bursa 727.89
    pharyngeal 478.29
  buttock 682.5
  canaliculus, breast 611.0
  canthus 372.20
  cartilage 733.99
  cecum 569.5
    with appendicitis 540.1
  cerebellum, cerebellar 324.0
    late effect - *see* category 326
  cerebral (embolic) 324.0
    late effect - *see* category 326
  cervical (neck region) 682.1
    lymph gland or node 683
    stump *(see also* Cervicitis) 616.0
  cervix (stump) (uteri) *(see also*
    Cervicitis)* 616.0
  cheek, external 682.0
    inner 528.3
  chest 510.9
    with fistula 510.0
    wall 682.2
  chin 682.0
  choroid 363.00
  ciliary body 364.3
  circumtonsillar 475
  cold (tuberculous) - *see also*
    Tuberculosis, abscess
    articular - *see* Tuberculosis, joint
  colon (wall) 569.5
  colostomy or enterostomy 569.61
  conjunctiva 372.00
  connective tissue NEC 682.9
  cornea 370.55
    with ulcer 370.00

Abscess *(Continued)*
  corpus
    cavernosum 607.2
    luteum *(see also* Salpingo-oophoritis)
      614.2
  Cowper's gland 597.0
  cranium 324.0
  cul-de-sac (Douglas') (posterior) *(see*
    also* Disease, pelvis,
    inflammatory) 614.4
    acute 614.3
  dental 522.5
    with sinus (alveolar) 522.7
  dentoalveolar 522.5
    with sinus (alveolar) 522.7
  diaphragm, diaphragmatic 567.22
  digit NEC 681.9
  Douglas' cul-de-sac or pouch *(see also*
    Disease, pelvis, inflammatory)*
    614.4
    acute 614.3
  Dubois' 090.5
  ductless gland 259.8
  ear
    acute 382.00
    external 380.10
    inner 386.30
    middle - *see* Otitis media
  elbow 682.3
  endamebic - *see* Abscess, amebic
  entamebic - *see* Abscess, amebic
  enterostomy 569.61
  epididymis 604.0
  epidural 324.9
    brain 324.0
    late effect - *see* category 326
    spinal cord 324.1
  epiglottis 478.79
  epiploon, epiploic 567.22
  erysipelatous *(see also* Erysipelas) 035
  esophagostomy 530.86
  esophagus 530.19
  ethmoid (bone) (chronic) (sinus) *(see*
    also* Sinusitis, ethmoidal) 473.2
  external auditory canal 380.10
  extradural 324.9
    brain 324.0
    late effect - *see* category 326
    spinal cord 324.1
  extraperitoneal - *see* Abscess,
    peritoneum
  eye 360.00
  eyelid 373.13
  face (any part, except eye) 682.0
  fallopian tube *(see also* Salpingo-
    oophoritis) 614.2
  fascia 728.89
  fauces 478.29
  fecal 569.5
  femoral (region) 682.6
  filaria, filarial *(see also* Infestation,
    filarial) 125.9
  finger (any) (intrathecal) (periosteal)
    (subcutaneous) (subcuticular)
    681.00
  fistulous NEC 682.9
  flank 682.2
  foot (except toe) 682.7
  forearm 682.3
  forehead 682.0
  frontal (sinus) (chronic) *(see also*
    Sinusitis, frontal) 473.1
  gallbladder *(see also* Cholecystitis,
    acute) 575.0

Abscess *(Continued)*
  gastric 535.0●
  genital organ or tract NEC
    female 616.9
      with
        abortion - *see* Abortion, by
          type, with sepsis
        ectopic pregnancy *(see also*
          categories 633.0-633.9)
          639.0
        molar pregnancy *(see also*
          categories 630-632)
          639.0
      following
        abortion 639.0
        ectopic or molar pregnancy
          639.0
      puerperal, postpartum, childbirth
        670.8●   ◀▥
    male 608.4
  genitourinary system, tuberculous *(see*
    also* Tuberculosis) 016.9●
  gingival 523.30
  gland, glandular (lymph) (acute) NEC
    683
  glottis 478.79
  gluteal (region) 682.5
  gonorrheal NEC *(see also* Gonococcus)
    098.0
  groin 682.2
  gum 523.30
  hand (except finger or thumb) 682.4
  head (except face) 682.8
  heart 429.89
  heel 682.7
  helminthic *(see also* Infestation, by
    specific parasite) 128.9
  hepatic 572.0
    amebic *(see also* Abscess, liver,
      amebic) 006.3
    duct 576.8
  hip 682.6
    tuberculous (active) *(see also*
      Tuberculosis) 015.1●
  ileocecal 540.1
  ileostomy (bud) 569.61
  iliac (region) 682.2
    fossa 540.1
  iliopsoas 567.31
    tuberculous *(see also* Tuberculosis)
      015.0● [730.88]
  infraclavicular (fossa) 682.3
  inguinal (region) 682.2
    lymph gland or node 683
  intersphincteric (anus) 566
  intestine, intestinal 569.5
    rectal 566
  intra-abdominal *(see also* Abscess,
    peritoneum) 567.22
    postoperative 998.59
  intracranial 324.0
    late effect - *see* category 326
  intramammary - *see* Abscess, breast
  intramastoid *(see also* Mastoiditis,
    acute) 383.00
  intraorbital 376.01
  intraperitoneal 567.22
  intraspinal 324.1
    late effect - *see* category 326
  intratonsillar 475
  iris 364.3
  ischiorectal 566
  jaw (bone) (lower) (upper) 526.4
    skin 682.0

Abscess *(Continued)*
  joint *(see also* Arthritis, pyogenic)
      711.0●
    vertebral (tuberculous) *(see also*
        Tuberculosis) 015.0● *[730.88]*
      nontuberculous 724.8
  kidney 590.2
    with
      abortion - *see* Abortion, by type,
          with urinary tract infection
      calculus 592.0
      ectopic pregnancy *(see also*
          categories 633.0-633.9)
          639.8
      molar pregnancy *(see also*
          categories 630-632) 639.8
      complicating pregnancy or
          puerperium 646.6●
        affecting fetus or newborn
          760.1
      following
        abortion 639.8
        ectopic or molar pregnancy
          639.8
  knee 682.6
    joint 711.06
    tuberculous (active) *(see also*
        Tuberculosis) 015.2●
  labium (majus) (minus) 616.4
    complicating pregnancy, childbirth,
        or puerperium 646.6●
  lacrimal (passages) (sac) *(see also*
      Dacryocystitis) 375.30
    caruncle 375.30
    gland *(see also* Dacryoadenitis)
        375.00
  lacunar 597.0
  larynx 478.79
  lateral (alveolar) 522.5
    with sinus 522.7
  leg, except foot 682.6
  lens 360.00
  lid 373.13
  lingual 529.0
    tonsil 475
  lip 528.5
  Littre's gland 597.0
  liver 572.0
    amebic 006.3
      with
        brain abscess (and lung
            abscess) 006.5
        lung abscess 006.4
      due to Entamoeba histolytica 006.3
    dysenteric *(see also* Abscess, liver,
        amebic) 006.3
    pyogenic 572.0
    tropical *(see also* Abscess, liver,
        amebic) 006.3
  loin (region) 682.2
  lumbar (tuberculous) *(see also*
      Tuberculosis) 015.0● *[730.88]*
    nontuberculous 682.2
  lung (miliary) (putrid) 513.0
    amebic (with liver abscess) 006.4
      with brain abscess 006.5
  lymph, lymphatic, gland or node
      (acute) 683
    any site, except mesenteric 683
    mesentery 289.2
  lymphangitic, acute - *see* Cellulitis
  malar 526.4
  mammary gland - *see* Abscess, breast
  marginal (anus) 566

Abscess *(Continued)*
  mastoid (process) *(see also* Mastoiditis,
      acute) 383.00
    subperiosteal 383.01
  maxilla, maxillary 526.4
    molar (tooth) 522.5
      with sinus 522.7
    premolar 522.5
    sinus (chronic) *(see also* Sinusitis,
        maxillary) 473.0
  mediastinum 513.1
  meibomian gland 373.12
  meninges *(see also* Meningitis) 320.9
  mesentery, mesenteric 567.22
  mesosalpinx *(see also* Salpingo-
      oophoritis) 614.2
  milk 675.1●
  Monro's (psoriasis) 696.1
  mons pubis 682.2
  mouth (floor) 528.3
  multiple sites NEC 682.9
  mural 682.2
  muscle 728.89
    psoas 567.31
  myocardium 422.92
  nabothian (follicle) *(see also* Cervicitis)
      616.0
  nail (chronic) (with lymphangitis) 681.9
    finger 681.02
    toe 681.11
  nasal (fossa) (septum) 478.19
    sinus (chronic) *(see also* Sinusitis)
        473.9
  nasopharyngeal 478.29
  nates 682.5
  navel 682.2
    newborn NEC 771.4
  neck (region) 682.1
    lymph gland or node 683
  nephritic *(see also* Abscess, kidney)
      590.2
  nipple 611.0
    puerperal, postpartum 675.0●
  nose (septum) 478.19
    external 682.0
  omentum 567.22
  operative wound 998.59
  orbit, orbital 376.01
  ossifluent - *see* Abscess, bone
  ovary, ovarian (corpus luteum) *(see also*
      Salpingo-oophoritis) 614.2
  oviduct *(see also* Salpingo-oophoritis)
      614.2
  palate (soft) 528.3
    hard 526.4
  palmar (space) 682.4
  pancreas (duct) 577.0
  paradontal 523.30
  parafrenal 607.2
  parametric, parametrium (chronic) *(see
      also* Disease, pelvis,
      inflammatory) 614.4
    acute 614.3
  paranephric 590.2
  parapancreatic 577.0
  parapharyngeal 478.22
  pararectal 566
  parasinus *(see also* Sinusitis) 473.9
  parauterine *(see also* Disease, pelvis,
      inflammatory) 614.4
    acute 614.3
  paravaginal *(see also* Vaginitis) 616.10
  parietal region 682.8
  parodontal 523.30

Abscess *(Continued)*
  parotid (duct) (gland) 527.3
    region 528.3
  parumbilical 682.2
    newborn 771.4
  pectoral (region) 682.2
  pelvirectal 567.22
  pelvis, pelvic
    female (chronic) *(see also* Disease,
        pelvis, inflammatory) 614.4
      acute 614.3
    male, peritoneal (cellular tissue) - *see*
        Abscess, peritoneum
    tuberculous *(see also* Tuberculosis)
        016.9●
  penis 607.2
    gonococcal (acute) 098.0
      chronic or duration of 2 months
          or over 098.2
  perianal 566
  periapical 522.5
    with sinus (alveolar) 522.7
  periappendiceal 540.1
  pericardial 420.99
  pericecal 540.1
  pericemental 523.30
  pericholecystic *(see also* Cholecystitis,
      acute) 575.0
  pericoronal 523.30
  peridental 523.30
  perigastric 535.0●
  perimetric *(see also* Disease, pelvis,
      inflammatory) 614.4
    acute 614.3
  perinephric, perinephritic *(see also*
      Abscess, kidney) 590.2
  perineum, perineal (superficial) 682.2
    deep (with urethral involvement)
        597.0
    urethra 597.0
  periodontal (parietal) 523.31
    apical 522.5
  periosteum, periosteal *(see also*
      Periostitis) 730.3●
    with osteomyelitis *(see also*
        Osteomyelitis) 730.2●
      acute or subacute 730.0●
      chronic or old 730.1●
  peripleuritic 510.9
    with fistula 510.0
  periproctic 566
  periprostatic 601.2
  perirectal (staphylococcal) 566
  perirenal (tissue) *(see also* Abscess,
      kidney) 590.2
  perisinuous (nose) *(see also* Sinusitis)
      473.9
  peritoneum, peritoneal (perforated)
      (ruptured) 567.22
    with
      abortion - *see* Abortion, by type,
          with sepsis
      appendicitis 540.1
      ectopic pregnancy *(see also*
          categories 633.0-633.9)
          639.0
      molar pregnancy *(see also*
          categories 630-632) 639.0
    following
      abortion 639.0
      ectopic or molar pregnancy 639.0
    pelvic, female *(see also* Disease,
        pelvis, inflammatory) 614.4
      acute 614.3

◄ New   ◄▦ Revised   ~~deleted~~ Deleted   ● Use Additional Digit(s)   ▦ Omit code

Abscess *(Continued)*
  peritoneum, peritoneal *(Continued)*
    postoperative 998.59
    puerperal, postpartum, childbirth
      670.8●   ◀▥
    tuberculous *(see also* Tuberculosis)
      014.0●
  peritonsillar 475
  perityphlic 540.1
  periureteral 593.89
  periurethral 597.0
    gonococcal (acute) 098.0
      chronic or duration of 2 months
        or over 098.2
  periuterine *(see also* Disease, pelvis,
    inflammatory) 614.4
    acute 614.3
  perivesical 595.89
  pernicious NEC 682.9
  petrous bone - *see* Petrositis
  phagedenic NEC 682.9
    chancroid 099.0
  pharynx, pharyngeal (lateral)
    478.29
  phlegmonous NEC 682.9
  pilonidal 685.0
  pituitary (gland) 253.8
  pleura 510.9
    with fistula 510.0
  popliteal 682.6
  postanal 566
  postcecal 540.1
  postlaryngeal 478.79
  postnasal 478.19
  postpharyngeal 478.24
  posttonsillar 475
  posttyphoid 002.0
  Pott's *(see also* Tuberculosis) 015.0●
    [730.88]
  pouch of Douglas (chronic) *(see also*
    Disease, pelvis, inflammatory)
    614.4
  premammary - *see* Abscess, breast
  prepatellar 682.6
  prostate *(see also* Prostatitis) 601.2
    gonococcal (acute) 098.12
      chronic or duration of 2 months
        or over 098.32
  psoas 567.31
    tuberculous *(see also* Tuberculosis)
      015.0● *[730.88]*
  pterygopalatine fossa 682.8
  pubis 682.2
  puerperal - *see* Puerperal, abscess, by
    site
  pulmonary - *see* Abscess, lung
  pulp, pulpal (dental) 522.0
    finger 681.01
    toe 681.10
  pyemic - *see* Septicemia
  pyloric valve 535.0●
  rectovaginal septum 569.5
  rectovesical 595.89
  rectum 566
  regional NEC 682.9
  renal *(see also* Abscess, kidney) 590.2
  retina 363.00
  retrobulbar 376.01
  retrocecal 567.22
  retrolaryngeal 478.79
  retromammary - *see* Abscess, breast
  retroperineal 682.2
  retroperitoneal 567.38
    postprocedural 998.59

Abscess *(Continued)*
  retropharyngeal 478.24
    tuberculous *(see also* Tuberculosis)
      012.8●
  retrorectal 566
  retrouterine *(see also* Disease, pelvis,
    inflammatory) 614.4
    acute 614.3
  retrovesical 595.89
  root, tooth 522.5
    with sinus (alveolar) 522.7
  round ligament *(see also* Disease, pelvis,
    inflammatory) 614.4
    acute 614.3
  rupture (spontaneous) NEC 682.9
  sacrum (tuberculous) *(see also*
    Tuberculosis) 015.0● *[730.88]*
    nontuberculous 730.08
  salivary duct or gland 527.3
  scalp (any part) 682.8
  scapular 730.01
  sclera 379.09
  scrofulous *(see also* Tuberculosis)
    017.2●
  scrotum 608.4
  seminal vesicle 608.0
    amebic 006.8
  septal, dental 522.5
    with sinus (alveolar) 522.7
  septum (nasal) 478.19
  serous *(see also* Periostitis) 730.3●
  shoulder 682.3
  side 682.2
  sigmoid 569.5
  sinus (accessory) (chronic) (nasal) *(see*
    also Sinusitis) 473.9
    intracranial venous (any) 324.0
    late effect - *see* category 326
  Skene's duct or gland 597.0
  skin NEC 682.9
    tuberculous (primary) *(see also*
      Tuberculosis) 017.0●
  sloughing NEC 682.9
  specified site NEC 682.8
    amebic 006.8
  spermatic cord 608.4
  sphenoidal (sinus) *(see also* Sinusitis,
    sphenoidal) 473.3
  spinal
    cord (any part) (staphylococcal)
      324.1
      tuberculous *(see also* Tuberculosis)
        013.5●
    epidural 324.1
  spine (column) (tuberculous) *(see also*
    Tuberculosis) 015.0● *[730.88]*
    nontuberculous 730.08
  spleen 289.59
    amebic 006.8
  staphylococcal NEC 682.9
  stitch 998.59
  stomach (wall) 535.0●
  strumous (tuberculous) *(see also*
    Tuberculosis) 017.2●
  subarachnoid 324.9
    brain 324.0
    cerebral 324.0
    late effect - *see* category 326
    spinal cord 324.1
  subareolar - *see also* Abscess, breast
    puerperal, postpartum 675.1●
  subcecal 540.1
  subcutaneous NEC 682.9
  subdiaphragmatic 567.22

Abscess *(Continued)*
  subdorsal 682.2
  subdural 324.9
    brain 324.0
    late effect - *see* category 326
    spinal cord 324.1
  subgaleal 682.8
  subhepatic 567.22
  sublingual 528.3
    gland 527.3
  submammary - *see* Abscess, breast
  submandibular (region) (space)
    (triangle) 682.0
    gland 527.3
  submaxillary (region) 682.0
    gland 527.3
  submental (pyogenic) 682.0
    gland 527.3
  subpectoral 682.2
  subperiosteal - *see* Abscess, bone
  subperitoneal 567.22
  subphrenic - *see also* Abscess,
    peritoneum 567.22
    postoperative 998.59
  subscapular 682.2
  subungual 681.9
  suburethral 597.0
  sudoriparous 705.89
  suppurative NEC 682.9
  supraclavicular (fossa) 682.3
  suprahepatic 567.22
  suprapelvic *(see also* Disease, pelvis,
    inflammatory) 614.4
    acute 614.3
  suprapubic 682.2
  suprarenal (capsule) (gland) 255.8
  sweat gland 705.89
  syphilitic 095.8
  teeth, tooth (root) 522.5
    with sinus (alveolar) 522.7
    supporting structures NEC 523.30
  temple 682.0
  temporal region 682.0
  temporosphenoidal 324.0
    late effect - *see* category 326
  tendon (sheath) 727.89
  testicle - *see* Orchitis
  thecal 728.89
  thigh (acquired) 682.6
  thorax 510.9
    with fistula 510.0
  throat 478.29
  thumb (intrathecal) (periosteal)
    (subcutaneous) (subcuticular)
    681.00
  thymus (gland) 254.1
  thyroid (gland) 245.0
  toe (any) (intrathecal) (periosteal)
    (subcutaneous) (subcuticular)
    681.10
  tongue (staphylococcal) 529.0
  tonsil(s) (lingual) 475
  tonsillopharyngeal 475
  tooth, teeth (root) 522.5
    with sinus (alveolar) 522.7
    supporting structure NEC 523.30
  trachea 478.9
  trunk 682.2
  tubal *(see also* Salpingo-oophoritis)
    614.2
  tuberculous - *see* Tuberculosis, abscess
  tubo-ovarian *(see also* Salpingo-
    oophoritis) 614.2
  tunica vaginalis 608.4

◀ New   ◀▥ Revised   ~~deleted~~ Deleted   ● Use Additional Digit(s)   ▥ Omit code

Abscess *(Continued)*
umbilicus NEC 682.2
   newborn 771.4
upper arm 682.3
upper respiratory 478.9
urachus 682.2
urethra (gland) 597.0
urinary 597.0
uterus, uterine (wall) *(see also*
   Endometritis) 615.9
   ligament *(see also* Disease, pelvis,
      inflammatory) 614.4
      acute 614.3
   neck *(see also* Cervicitis) 616.0
uvula 528.3
vagina (wall) *(see also* Vaginitis) 616.10
vaginorectal *(see also* Vaginitis) 616.10
vas deferens 608.4
vermiform appendix 540.1
vertebra (column) (tuberculous) *(see
   also* Tuberculosis) 015.0● *[730.88]*
   nontuberculous 730.0●
vesical 595.89
vesicouterine pouch *(see also* Disease,
   pelvis, inflammatory) 614.4
vitreous (humor) (pneumococcal)
   360.04
vocal cord 478.5
von Bezold's 383.01
vulva 616.4
   complicating pregnancy, childbirth,
      or puerperium 646.6●
vulvovaginal gland *(see also* Vaginitis)
   616.3
web-space 682.4
wrist 682.4

Absence (organ or part) (complete or
   partial)
acoustic nerve 742.8
adrenal (gland) (congenital) 759.1
   acquired V45.79
albumin (blood) 273.8
alimentary tract (complete) (congenital)
   (partial) 751.8
   lower 751.5
   upper 750.8
alpha-fucosidase 271.8
alveolar process (acquired) 525.8
   congenital 750.26
anus, anal (canal) (congenital) 751.2
aorta (congenital) 747.22
aortic valve (congenital) 746.89
appendix, congenital 751.2
arm (acquired) V49.60
   above elbow V49.66
   below elbow V49.65
   congenital *(see also* Deformity,
      reduction, upper limb) 755.20
      lower - *see* Absence, forearm,
         congenital
      upper (complete) (partial) (with
         absence of distal elements,
         incomplete) 755.24
         with
            complete absence of distal
               elements 755.21
            forearm (incomplete)
               755.23
artery (congenital) (peripheral) NEC
   (see also Anomaly, peripheral
   vascular system) 747.60
   brain 747.81
   cerebral 747.81
   coronary 746.85

Absence *(Continued)*
artery NEC *(Continued)*
   pulmonary 747.3
   umbilical 747.5
atrial septum 745.69
auditory canal (congenital) (external)
   744.01
auricle (ear) (with stenosis or atresia of
   auditory canal), congenital 744.01
bile, biliary duct (common) or passage
   (congenital) 751.61
bladder (acquired) V45.74
   congenital 753.8
bone (congenital) NEC 756.9
   marrow 284.9
      acquired (secondary) 284.89
      congenital 284.09
      hereditary 284.09
      idiopathic 284.9
   skull 756.0
bowel sounds 787.5
brain 740.0
   specified part 742.2
breast(s) (acquired) V45.71
   congenital 757.6
broad ligament (congenital) 752.19
bronchus (congenital) 748.3
calvarium, calvaria (skull) 756.0
canaliculus lacrimalis, congenital
   743.65
carpal(s) (congenital) (complete)
   (partial) (with absence of distal
   elements, incomplete) *(see also*
   Deformity, reduction, upper limb)
   755.28
   with complete absence of distal
      elements 755.21
cartilage 756.9
caudal spine 756.13
cecum (acquired) (postoperative)
   (posttraumatic) V45.72
   congenital 751.2
cementum 520.4
cerebellum (congenital) (vermis)
   742.2
cervix (acquired) (uteri) V88.01
   with remaining uterus V88.03
   and uterus V88.01
   congenital 752.49
chin, congenital 744.89
cilia (congenital) 743.63
   acquired 374.89
circulatory system, part NEC 747.89
clavicle 755.51
clitoris (congenital) 752.49
coccyx, congenital 756.13
cold sense *(see also* Disturbance,
   sensation) 782.0
colon (acquired) (postoperative) V45.72
   congenital 751.2
congenital
   lumen - *see* Atresia
   organ or site NEC - *see* Agenesis
   septum - *see* Imperfect, closure
corpus callosum (congenital) 742.2
cricoid cartilage 748.3
diaphragm (congenital) (with hernia)
   756.6
   with obstruction 756.6
digestive organ(s) or tract, congenital
   (complete) (partial) 751.8
   acquired V45.79
   lower 751.5
   upper 750.8

Absence *(Continued)*
ductus arteriosus 747.89
duodenum (acquired) (postoperative)
   V45.72
   congenital 751.1
ear, congenital 744.09
   acquired V45.79
   auricle 744.01
   external 744.01
   inner 744.05
   lobe, lobule 744.21
   middle, except ossicles 744.03
      ossicles 744.04
   ossicles 744.04
ejaculatory duct (congenital) 752.89
endocrine gland NEC (congenital)
   759.2
epididymis (congenital) 752.89
   acquired V45.77
epiglottis, congenital 748.3
epileptic (atonic) (typical) *(see also*
   Epilepsy) 345.0●
erythrocyte 284.9
erythropoiesis 284.9
   congenital 284.01
esophagus (congenital) 750.3
eustachian tube (congenital) 744.24
extremity (acquired)
   congenital *(see also* Deformity,
      reduction) 755.4
   lower V49.70
   upper V49.60
extrinsic muscle, eye 743.69
eye (acquired) V45.78
   adnexa (congenital) 743.69
   congenital 743.00
   muscle (congenital) 743.69
eyelid (fold), congenital 743.62
   acquired 374.89
face
   bones NEC 756.0
   specified part NEC 744.89
fallopian tube(s) (acquired)
   V45.77
   congenital 752.19
femur, congenital (complete)
   (partial) (with absence of
   distal elements, incomplete)
   (see also Deformity, reduction,
   lower limb) 755.34
   with
      complete absence of distal
         elements 755.31
      tibia and fibula (incomplete)
         755.33
fibrin 790.92
fibrinogen (congenital) 286.3
   acquired 286.6
fibula, congenital (complete)
   (partial) (with absence of
   distal elements, incomplete)
   (see also Deformity, reduction,
   lower limb) 755.37
   with
      complete absence of distal
         elements 755.31
      tibia 755.35
      with
         complete absence of distal
            elements 755.31
         femur (incomplete) 755.33
            with complete absence
               of distal elements
               755.31

Absence (Continued)
  finger (acquired) V49.62
    congenital (complete) (partial) (see
      also Deformity, reduction,
      upper limb) 755.29
      meaning all fingers (complete)
        (partial) 755.21
      transverse 755.21
  fissures of lungs (congenital) 748.5
  foot (acquired) V49.73
    congenital (complete) 755.31
  forearm (acquired) V49.65
    congenital (complete) (partial)
      (with absence of distal
      elements, incomplete) (see also
      Deformity, reduction, upper
      limb) 755.25
      with
        complete absence of distal
          elements (hand and
          fingers) 755.21
        humerus (incomplete) 755.23
  fovea centralis 743.55
  fucosidase 271.8
  gallbladder (acquired) V45.79
    congenital 751.69
  gamma globulin (blood) 279.00
  genital organs
    acquired V45.77
    congenital
      female 752.89
        external 752.49
        internal NEC 752.89
      male 752.89
        penis 752.69
  genitourinary organs, congenital NEC
    752.89
  glottis 748.3
  gonadal, congenital NEC 758.6
  hair (congenital) 757.4
    acquired - see Alopecia
  hand (acquired) V49.63
    congenital (complete) (see also
      Deformity, reduction, upper
      limb) 755.21
  heart (congenital) 759.89
    acquired - see Status, organ
      replacement
  heat sense (see also Disturbance,
    sensation) 782.0
  humerus, congenital (complete)
    (partial) (with absence of distal
    elements, incomplete) (see also
    Deformity, reduction, upper
    limb) 755.24
    with
      complete absence of distal
        elements 755.21
      radius and ulna (incomplete)
        755.23
  hymen (congenital) 752.49
  ileum (acquired) (postoperative)
    (posttraumatic) V45.72
    congenital 751.1
  immunoglobulin, isolated NEC 279.03
    IgA 279.01
    IgG 279.03
    IgM 279.02
  incus (acquired) 385.24
    congenital 744.04
  internal ear (congenital) 744.05
  intestine (acquired) (small) V45.72
    congenital 751.1
      large 751.2

Absence (Continued)
  intestine (Continued)
    large V45.72
      congenital 751.2
  iris (congenital) 743.45
  jaw - see Absence, mandible
  jejunum (acquired) V45.72
    congenital 751.1
  joint, congenital NEC 755.8
  kidney(s) (acquired) V45.73
    congenital 753.0
  labium (congenital) (majus) (minus)
    752.49
  labyrinth, membranous 744.05
  lacrimal apparatus (congenital) 743.65
  larynx (congenital) 748.3
  leg (acquired) V49.70
    above knee V49.76
    below knee V49.75
    congenital (partial) (unilateral) (see
      also Deformity, reduction,
      lower limb) 755.31
      lower (complete) (partial) (with
        absence of distal elements,
        incomplete) 755.35
        with
          complete absence of distal
            elements (foot and
            toes) 755.31
          thigh (incomplete) 755.33
            with complete absence of
              distal elements
              755.31
      upper - see Absence, femur
  lens (congenital) 743.35
    acquired 379.31
  ligament, broad (congenital) 752.19
  limb (acquired)
    congenital (complete) (partial) (see
      also Deformity, reduction)
      755.4
      lower 755.30
        complete 755.31
        incomplete 755.32
        longitudinal - see Deficiency,
          lower limb, longitudinal
        transverse 755.31
      upper 755.20
        complete 755.21
        incomplete 755.22
        longitudinal - see Deficiency,
          upper limb, longitudinal
        transverse 755.21
    lower NEC V49.70
    upper NEC V49.60
  lip 750.26
  liver (congenital) (lobe) 751.69
  lumbar (congenital) (vertebra)
    756.13
    isthmus 756.11
    pars articularis 756.11
  lumen - see Atresia
  lung (bilateral) (congenital) (fissure)
    (lobe) (unilateral) 748.5
    acquired (any part) V45.76
  mandible (congenital) 524.09
  maxilla (congenital) 524.09
  menstruation 626.0
  metacarpal(s), congenital (complete)
    (partial) (with absence of distal
    elements, incomplete) (see also
    Deformity, reduction, upper limb)
    755.28
    with all fingers, complete 755.21

Absence (Continued)
  metatarsal(s), congenital (complete)
    (partial) (with absence of distal
    elements, incomplete) (see also
    Deformity, reduction, lower limb)
    755.38
    with complete absence of distal
      elements 755.31
  muscle (congenital) (pectoral)
    756.81
    ocular 743.69
  musculoskeletal system (congenital)
    NEC 756.9
  nail(s) (congenital) 757.5
  neck, part 744.89
  nerve 742.8
  nervous system, part NEC 742.8
  neutrophil 288.00
  nipple (congenital) 757.6
    acquired V45.71
  nose (congenital) 748.1
    acquired 738.0
  nuclear 742.8
  ocular muscle (congenital) 743.69
  organ
    of Corti (congenital) 744.05
    or site
      acquired V45.79
      congenital NEC 759.89
  osseous meatus (ear) 744.03
  ovary (acquired) V45.77
    congenital 752.0
  oviduct (acquired) V45.77
    congenital 752.19
  pancreas (congenital) 751.7
    acquired (postoperative)
      (posttraumatic) V45.79
  parathyroid gland (congenital)
    759.2
  parotid gland(s) (congenital)
    750.21
  patella, congenital 755.64
  pelvic girdle (congenital) 755.69
  penis (congenital) 752.69
    acquired V45.77
  pericardium (congenital) 746.89
  perineal body (congenital) 756.81
  phalange(s), congenital 755.4
    lower limb (complete) (intercalary)
      (partial) (terminal) (see also
      Deformity, reduction, lower
      limb) 755.39
      meaning all toes (complete)
        (partial) 755.31
      transverse 755.31
    upper limb (complete) (intercalary)
      (partial) (terminal) (see also
      Deformity, reduction, upper
      limb) 755.29
      meaning all digits (complete)
        (partial) 755.21
      transverse 755.21
  pituitary gland (congenital) 759.2
  postoperative - see Absence, by site,
    acquired
  prostate (congenital) 752.89
    acquired V45.77
  pulmonary
    artery 747.3
    trunk 747.3
    valve (congenital) 746.01
    vein 747.49
  punctum lacrimale (congenital)
    743.65

◀ New   ◀╫║ Revised   ~~deleted~~ Deleted   ● Use Additional Digit(s)   ▓▓ Omit code

Absence *(Continued)*
  radius, congenital (complete) (partial)
        (with absence of distal elements,
        incomplete) 755.26
     with
        complete absence of distal
              elements 755.21
        ulna 755.25
           with
              complete absence of distal
                    elements 755.21
              humerus (incomplete) 755.23
  ray, congenital 755.4
     lower limb (complete) (partial) *(see
           also* Deformity, reduction,
           lower limb) 755.38
        meaning all rays 755.31
        transverse 755.31
     upper limb (complete) (partial) *(see
           also* Deformity, reduction,
           upper limb) 755.28
        meaning all rays 755.21
        transverse 755.21
  rectum (congenital) 751.2
     acquired V45.79
  red cell 284.9
     acquired (secondary) 284.81
     congenital 284.01
     hereditary 284.01
     idiopathic 284.9
  respiratory organ (congenital) NEC
        748.9
  rib (acquired) 738.3
     congenital 756.3
  roof of orbit (congenital) 742.0
  round ligament (congenital) 752.89
  sacrum, congenital 756.13
  salivary gland(s) (congenital) 750.21
  scapula 755.59
  scrotum, congenital 752.89
  seminal tract or duct (congenital)
        752.89
     acquired V45.77
  septum (congenital) - *see also* Imperfect,
        closure, septum
     atrial 745.69
        and ventricular 745.7
     between aorta and pulmonary
           artery 745.0
     ventricular 745.3
        and atrial 745.7
  sex chromosomes 758.81
  shoulder girdle, congenital (complete)
        (partial) 755.59
  skin (congenital) 757.39
  skull bone 756.0
     with
        anencephalus 740.0
        encephalocele 742.0
        hydrocephalus 742.3
           with spina bifida *(see also*
                 Spina bifida) 741.0●
        microcephalus 742.1
  spermatic cord (congenital) 752.89
  spinal cord 742.59
  spine, congenital 756.13
  spleen (congenital) 759.0
     acquired V45.79
  sternum, congenital 756.3
  stomach (acquired) (partial)
        (postoperative) V45.75
     with postgastric surgery syndrome
           564.2
     congenital 750.7

Absence *(Continued)*
  submaxillary gland(s) (congenital)
        750.21
  superior vena cava (congenital)
        747.49
  tarsal(s), congenital (complete)
        (partial) (with absence of distal
        elements, incomplete) *(see also*
        Deformity, reduction, lower
        limb) 755.38
  teeth, tooth (congenital) 520.0
     with abnormal spacing 524.30
     acquired 525.10
        with malocclusion 524.30
        due to
           caries 525.13
           extraction 525.10
           periodontal disease 525.12
           trauma 525.11
  tendon (congenital) 756.81
  testis (congenital) 752.89
     acquired V45.77
  thigh (acquired) 736.89
  thumb (acquired) V49.61
     congenital 755.29
  thymus gland (congenital) 759.2
  thyroid (gland) (surgical) 246.8
     with hypothyroidism 244.0
     cartilage, congenital 748.3
     congenital 243
  tibia, congenital (complete) (partial)
        (with absence of distal elements,
        incomplete) *(see also* Deformity,
        reduction, lower limb) 755.36
     with
        complete absence of distal
              elements 755.31
        fibula 755.35
           with
              complete absence of distal
                    elements 755.31
              femur (incomplete)
                    755.33
                 with complete absence
                       of distal elements
                       755.31
  toe (acquired) V49.72
     congenital (complete) (partial)
           755.39
        meaning all toes 755.31
        transverse 755.31
     great V49.71
  tongue (congenital) 750.11
  tooth, teeth (congenital) 520.0
     with abnormal spacing 524.30
     acquired 525.10
        with malocclusion 524.30
        due to
           caries 525.13
           extraction 525.10
           periodontal disease 525.12
           trauma 525.11
  trachea (cartilage) (congenital) (rings)
        748.3
  transverse aortic arch (congenital)
        747.21
  tricuspid valve 746.1
  ulna, congenital (complete) (partial)
        (with absence of distal elements,
        incomplete) *(see also* Deformity,
        reduction, upper limb) 755.27
     with
        complete absence of distal
              elements 755.21

Absence *(Continued)*
  ulna, congenital *(Continued)*
     with *(Continued)*
        radius 755.25
           with
              complete absence of distal
                    elements 755.21
              humerus (incomplete)
                    755.23
  umbilical artery (congenital) 747.5
  ureter (congenital) 753.4
     acquired V45.74
  urethra, congenital 753.8
     acquired V45.74
  urinary system, part NEC, congenital
        753.8
     acquired V45.74
  uterus (acquired) V88.01
     with remaining cervical stump
           V88.02
     and cervix V88.01
     congenital 752.3
  uvula (congenital) 750.26
  vagina, congenital 752.49
     acquired V45.77
  vas deferens (congenital) 752.89
     acquired V45.77
  vein (congenital) (peripheral) NEC *(see
        also* Anomaly, peripheral vascular
        system) 747.60
     brain 747.81
     great 747.49
     portal 747.49
     pulmonary 747.49
  vena cava (congenital) (inferior)
        (superior) 747.49
  ventral horn cell 742.59
  ventricular septum 745.3
  vermis of cerebellum 742.2
  vertebra, congenital 756.13
  vulva, congenital 752.49
Absentia epileptica *(see also* Epilepsy)
     345.0●
Absinthemia *(see also* Dependence)
     304.6●
Absinthism *(see also* Dependence)
     304.6●
Absorbent system disease 459.89
Absorption
  alcohol, through placenta or breast
        milk 760.71
  antibiotics, through placenta or breast
        milk 760.74
  anticonvulsants, through placenta or
        breast milk 760.77
  antifungals, through placenta or breast
        milk 760.74
  anti-infective, through placenta or
        breast milk 760.74
  antimetabolics, through placenta or
        breast milk 760.78
  chemical NEC 989.9
     specified chemical or substance - *see*
           Table of Drugs and Chemicals
     through placenta or breast milk
           (fetus or newborn) 760.70
        alcohol 760.71
        anticonvulsants 760.77
        antifungals 760.74
        anti-infective agents 760.74
        antimetabolics 760.78
        cocaine 760.75
        "crack" 760.75
        diethylstilbestrol [DES] 760.76

Absorption (Continued)
  chemical NEC (Continued)
    through placenta or breast milk (Continued)
      hallucinogenic agents 760.73
      medicinal agents NEC 760.79
      narcotics 760.72
      obstetric anesthetic or analgesic drug 763.5
      specified agent NEC 760.79
      suspected, affecting management of pregnancy 655.5●
  cocaine, through placenta or breast milk 760.75
  drug NEC (see also Reaction, drug)
    through placenta or breast milk (fetus or newborn) 760.70
      alcohol 760.71
      anticonvulsants 760.77
      antifungals 760.74
      anti-infective agents 760.74
      antimetabolics 760.78
      cocaine 760.75
      "crack" 760.75
      diethylstilbestrol (DES) 760.76
      hallucinogenic agents 760.73
      medicinal agents NEC 760.79
      narcotics 760.72
      obstetric anesthetic or analgesic drug 763.5
      specified agent NEC 760.79
      suspected, affecting management of pregnancy 655.5●
  fat, disturbance 579.8
  hallucinogenic agents, through placenta or breast milk 760.73
  immune sera, through placenta or breast milk 760.79
  lactose defect 271.3
  medicinal agents NEC, through placenta or breast milk 760.79
  narcotics, through placenta or breast milk 760.72
  noxious substance - see Absorption, chemical
  protein, disturbance 579.8
  pus or septic, general - see Septicemia
  quinine, through placenta or breast milk 760.74
  toxic substance - see Absorption, chemical
  uremic - see Uremia
Abstinence symptoms or syndrome
  alcohol 291.81
  drug 292.0
  neonatal 779.5 ◄
Abt-Letterer-Siwe syndrome (acute histiocytosis X) (M9722/3) 202.5●
Abulia 799.89
Abulomania 301.6
Abuse
  adult 995.80
    emotional 995.82
    multiple forms 995.85
    neglect (nutritional) 995.84
    physical 995.81
    psychological 995.82
    sexual 995.83
  alcohol (see also Alcoholism) 305.0●
    dependent 303.9●
    nondependent 305.0●

Abuse (Continued)
  child 995.50
    counseling
      perpetrator
        non-parent V62.83
        parent V61.22
      victim V61.21
    emotional 995.51
    multiple forms 995.59
    neglect (nutritional) 995.52
    physical 995.54
      shaken infant syndrome 995.55
    psychological 995.51
    sexual 995.53
  drugs, nondependent 305.9●

┌───┐
│ Note 02   Use the following fifth-digit   │
│ subclassification with the following   │
│ codes: 305.0, 305.2-305.9:   │
│   │
│ 0   unspecified   │
│ 1   continuous   │
│ 2   episodic   │
│ 3   in remission   │
└───┘

      amphetamine type 305.7●
      antidepressants 305.8●
      anxiolytic 305.4●
      barbiturates 305.4●
      caffeine 305.9●
      cannabis 305.2●
      cocaine type 305.6●
      hallucinogens 305.3●
      hashish 305.2●
      hypnotic 305.4●
      inhalant 305.9●
      LSD 305.3●
      marijuana 305.2●
      mixed 305.9●
      morphine type 305.5●
      opioid type 305.5●
      phencyclidine (PCP) 305.9●
      sedative 305.4●
      specified NEC 305.9●
      tranquilizers 305.4●
    spouse 995.80
    tobacco 305.1
Acalcerosis 275.40
Acalcicosis 275.40
Acalculia 784.69
  developmental 315.1
Acanthocheilonemiasis 125.4
Acanthocytosis 272.5
Acanthokeratodermia 701.1
Acantholysis 701.8
  bullosa 757.39
Acanthoma (benign) (M8070/0) - see also Neoplasm, by site, benign
  malignant (M8070/3) - see Neoplasm, by site, malignant
Acanthosis (acquired) (nigricans) 701.2
  adult 701.2
  benign (congenital) 757.39
  congenital 757.39
  glycogenic
    esophagus 530.89
  juvenile 701.2
  tongue 529.8
Acanthrocytosis 272.5
Acapnia 276.3
Acarbia 276.2
Acardia 759.89
Acardiacus amorphus 759.89
Acardiotrophia 429.1
Acardius 759.89

Acariasis 133.9
  sarcoptic 133.0
Acaridiasis 133.9
Acarinosis 133.9
Acariosis 133.9
Acarodermatitis 133.9
  urticarioides 133.9
Acarophobia 300.29
Acatalasemia 277.89
Acatalasia 277.89
Acatamathesia 784.69
Acataphasia 784.59   ◄▥
Acathisia 781.0
  due to drugs 333.99
Acceleration, accelerated
  atrioventricular conduction 426.7
  idioventricular rhythm 427.89
Accessory (congenital)
  adrenal gland 759.1
  anus 751.5
  appendix 751.5
  atrioventricular conduction 426.7
  auditory ossicles 744.04
  auricle (ear) 744.1
  autosome(s) NEC 758.5
    21 or 22 758.0
  biliary duct or passage 751.69
  bladder 753.8
  blood vessels (peripheral) (congenital) NEC (see also Anomaly, peripheral vascular system) 747.60
    cerebral 747.81
    coronary 746.85
  bone NEC 756.9
    foot 755.67
  breast tissue, axilla 757.6
  carpal bones 755.56
  cecum 751.5
  cervix 752.49
  chromosome(s) NEC 758.5
    13-15 758.1
    16-18 758.2
    21 or 22 758.0
    autosome(s) NEC 758.5
    D₁ 758.1
    E₃ 758.2
    G 758.0
    sex 758.81
  coronary artery 746.85
  cusp(s), heart valve NEC 746.89
    pulmonary 746.09
  cystic duct 751.69
  digits 755.00
  ear (auricle) (lobe) 744.1
  endocrine gland NEC 759.2
  external os 752.49
  eyelid 743.62
  eye muscle 743.69
  face bone(s) 756.0
  fallopian tube (fimbria) (ostium) 752.19
  fingers 755.01
  foreskin 605
  frontonasal process 756.0
  gallbladder 751.69
  genital organ(s)
    female 752.89
      external 752.49
      internal NEC 752.89
    male NEC 752.89
      penis 752.69
  genitourinary organs NEC 752.89

◄ New   ◄▥ Revised   ~~deleted~~ Deleted   ● Use Additional Digit(s)   � Omit code

Accessory (Continued)
heart 746.89
valve NEC 746.89
pulmonary 746.09
hepatic ducts 751.69
hymen 752.49
intestine (large) (small) 751.5
kidney 753.3
lacrimal canal 743.65
leaflet, heart valve NEC 746.89
pulmonary 746.09
ligament, broad 752.19
liver (duct) 751.69
lobule (ear) 744.1
lung (lobe) 748.69
muscle 756.82
navicular of carpus 755.56
nervous system, part NEC 742.8
nipple 757.6
nose 748.1
organ or site NEC - see Anomaly,
specified type NEC
ovary 752.0
oviduct 752.19
pancreas 751.7
parathyroid gland 759.2
parotid gland (and duct) 750.22
pituitary gland 759.2
placental lobe - see Placenta, abnormal
preauricular appendage 744.1
prepuce 605
renal arteries (multiple) 747.62
rib 756.3
cervical 756.2
roots (teeth) 520.2
salivary gland 750.22
sesamoids 755.8
sinus - see Condition
skin tags 757.39
spleen 759.0
sternum 756.3
submaxillary gland 750.22
tarsal bones 755.67
teeth, tooth 520.1
causing crowding 524.31
tendon 756.89
thumb 755.01
thymus gland 759.2
thyroid gland 759.2
toes 755.02
tongue 750.13
tragus 744.1
ureter 753.4
urethra 753.8
urinary organ or tract NEC 753.8
uterus 752.2
vagina 752.49
valve, heart NEC 746.89
pulmonary 746.09
vertebra 756.19
vocal cords 748.3
vulva 752.49
Accident, accidental - see also condition
birth NEC 767.9
cardiovascular (see also Disease,
cardiovascular) 429.2
cerebral (see also Disease,
cerebrovascular, acute) 434.91
cerebrovascular (current) (CVA) (see
also Disease, cerebrovascular,
acute) 434.91
aborted 434.91
embolic 434.11
healed or old V12.54

Accident, accidental (Continued)
cerebrovascular (Continued)
hemorrhagic - see Hemorrhage,
brain
impending 435.9
ischemic 434.91
late effect - see Late effect(s) (of)
cerebrovascular disease
postoperative 997.02
thrombotic 434.01
coronary (see also Infarct, myocardium)
410.9●
craniovascular (see also Disease,
cerebrovascular, acute) 436
during pregnancy, to mother, affecting
fetus or newborn 760.5
heart, cardiac (see also Infarct,
myocardium) 410.9●
intrauterine 779.89
vascular - see Disease, cerebrovascular,
acute
Accommodation
disorder of 367.51
drug-induced 367.89
toxic 367.89
insufficiency of 367.4
paralysis of 367.51
hysterical 300.11
spasm of 367.53
Accouchement - see Delivery
Accreta placenta (without hemorrhage)
667.0●
with hemorrhage 666.0●
Accretio cordis (nonrheumatic) 423.1
Accretions on teeth 523.6
Accumulation secretion, prostate 602.8
Acephalia, acephalism, acephaly 740.0
Acephalic 740.0
Acephalobrachia 759.89
Acephalocardia 759.89
Acephalocardius 759.89
Acephalochiria 759.89
Acephalochirus 759.89
Acephalogaster 759.89
Acephalostomus 759.89
Acephalothorax 759.89
Acephalus 740.0
Acetonemia 790.6
diabetic 250.1●
due to secondary diabetes 249.1●
Acetonglycosuria 982.8
Acetonuria 791.6
Achalasia 530.0
cardia 530.0
digestive organs congenital NEC 751.8
esophagus 530.0
pelvirectal 751.3
psychogenic 306.4
pylorus 750.5
sphincteral NEC 564.89
Achard-Thiers syndrome (adrenogenital)
255.2
Ache(s) - see Pain
Acheilia 750.26
Acheiria 755.21
Achillobursitis 726.71
Achillodynia 726.71
Achlorhydria, achlorhydric 536.0
anemia 280.9
diarrhea 536.0
neurogenic 536.0
postvagotomy 564.2
psychogenic 306.4
secondary to vagotomy 564.2

Achloroblepsia 368.52
Achloropsia 368.52
Acholia 575.8
Acholuric jaundice (familial)
(splenomegalic) (see also
Spherocytosis) 282.0
acquired 283.9
Achondroplasia 756.4
Achrestic anemia 281.8
Achroacytosis, lacrimal gland 375.00
tuberculous (see also Tuberculosis)
017.3●
Achroma, cutis 709.00
Achromate (congenital) 368.54
Achromatopia 368.54
Achromatopsia (congenital) 368.54
Achromia
congenital 270.2
parasitica 111.0
unguium 703.8
Achylia
gastrica 536.8
neurogenic 536.3
psychogenic 306.4
pancreatica 577.1
Achylosis 536.8
Acid
burn - see also Burn, by site
from swallowing acid - see Burn,
internal organs
deficiency
amide nicotinic 265.2
amino 270.9
ascorbic 267
folic 266.2
nicotinic (amide) 265.2
pantothenic 266.2
intoxication 276.2
peptic disease 536.8
stomach 536.8
psychogenic 306.4
Acidemia 276.2
arginosuccinic 270.6
fetal
affecting management of pregnancy
656.3●
before onset of labor, in liveborn
infant 768.2
during labor and delivery, in
liveborn infant 768.3
intrauterine 656.3●
unspecified as to time of onset, in
liveborn infant 768.4
newborn 775.81
pipecolic 270.7
Acidity, gastric (high) (low) 536.8
psychogenic 306.4
Acidocytopenia 288.59
Acidocytosis 288.3
Acidopenia 288.59
Acidosis 276.2
diabetic 250.1●
due to secondary diabetes
249.1●
fetal, affecting management of
pregnancy 656.8●
fetal, affecting newborn 775.81
kidney tubular 588.89
lactic 276.2
metabolic NEC 276.2
with respiratory acidosis 276.4
of newborn 775.81
late, of newborn 775.7
newborn 775.81

Acidosis (Continued)
  renal
    hyperchloremic 588.89
    tubular (distal) (proximal) 588.89
  respiratory 276.2
    complicated by
      metabolic acidosis 276.4
        of newborn 775.81
      metabolic alkalosis 276.4
Aciduria 791.9
  arginosuccinic 270.6
  beta-aminoisobutyric (BAIB) 277.2
  glutaric
    type I 270.7
    type II (type IIA, IIB, IIC) 277.85
    type III 277.86
  glycolic 271.8
  methylmalonic 270.3
    with glycinemia 270.7
  organic 270.9
  orotic (congenital) (hereditary)
    (pyrimidine deficiency) 281.4
Acladiosis 111.8
  skin 111.8
Aclasis
  diaphyseal 756.4
  tarsoepiphyseal 756.59
Acleistocardia 745.5
Aclusion 524.4
Acmesthesia 782.0
Acne (pustular) (vulgaris) 706.1
  agminata (see also Tuberculosis) 017.0●
  artificialis 706.1
  atrophica 706.0
  cachecticorum (Hebra) 706.1
  conglobata 706.1
  conjunctiva 706.1
  cystic 706.1
  decalvans 704.09
  erythematosa 695.3
  eyelid 706.1
  frontalis 706.0
  indurata 706.1
  keloid 706.1
  lupoid 706.0
  necrotic, necrotica 706.0
    miliaris 704.8
  neonatal 706.1
  nodular 706.1
  occupational 706.1
  papulosa 706.1
  rodens 706.0
  rosacea 695.3
  scorbutica 267
  scrofulosorum (Bazin) (see also
    Tuberculosis) 017.0●
  summer 692.72
  tropical 706.1
  varioliformis 706.0
Acneiform drug eruptions 692.3
Acnitis (primary) (see also Tuberculosis)
    017.0●
Acomia 704.00
Acontractile bladder 344.61
Aconuresis (see also Incontinence) 788.30
Acosta's disease 993.2
Acousma 780.1
Acoustic - see condition
Acousticophobia 300.29
Acquired - see condition
Acquired immune deficiency
    syndrome - see Human
      immunodeficiency virus (disease)
      (illness) (infection)

Acquired immunodeficiency
    syndrome - see Human
      immunodeficiency virus (disease)
      (illness) (infection)
Acragnosis 781.99
Acrania 740.0
Acroagnosis 781.99
Acroasphyxia, chronic 443.89
Acrobrachycephaly 756.0
Acrobystiolith 608.89
Acrobystitis 607.2
Acrocephalopolysyndactyly 755.55
Acrocephalosyndactyly 755.55
Acrocephaly 756.0
Acrochondrohyperplasia 759.82
Acrocyanosis 443.89
  newborn 770.83
    meaning transient blue hands and
      feet - omit code
Acrodermatitis 686.8
  atrophicans (chronica) 701.8
  continua (Hallopeau) 696.1
  enteropathica 686.8
  Hallopeau's 696.1
  perstans 696.1
  pustulosa continua 696.1
  recalcitrant pustular 696.1
Acrodynia 985.0
Acrodysplasia 755.55
Acrohyperhidrosis (see also
    Hyperhidrosis) 780.8
Acrokeratosis verruciformis 757.39
Acromastitis 611.0
Acromegaly, acromegalia (skin) 253.0
Acromelalgia 443.82
Acromicria, acromikria 756.59
Acronyx 703.0
Acropachy, thyroid (see also
    Thyrotoxicosis) 242.9●
Acropachyderma 757.39
Acroparesthesia 443.89
  simple (Schultz's type) 443.89
  vasomotor (Nothnagel's type) 443.89
Acropathy thyroid (see also
    Thyrotoxicosis) 242.9●
Acrophobia 300.29
Acroposthitis 607.2
Acroscleriasis (see also Scleroderma) 710.1
Acroscleroderma (see also Scleroderma)
    710.1
Acrosclerosis (see also Scleroderma)
    710.1
Acrosphacelus 785.4
Acrosphenosyndactylia 755.55
Acrospiroma, eccrine (M8402/0) - see
    Neoplasm, skin, benign
Acrostealgia 732.9
Acrosyndactyly (see also Syndactylism)
    755.10
Acrotrophodynia 991.4
Actinic - see also condition
  cheilitis (due to sun) 692.72
    chronic NEC 692.74
    due to radiation, except from sun
      692.82
  conjunctivitis 370.24
  dermatitis (due to sun) (see also
    Dermatitis, actinic) 692.70
  due to
    roentgen rays or radioactive
      substance 692.82
    ultraviolet radiation, except from
      sun 692.82
    sun NEC 692.70

Actinic (Continued)
  elastosis solare 692.74
  granuloma 692.73
  keratitis 370.24
  ophthalmia 370.24
  reticuloid 692.73
Actinobacillosis, general 027.8
Actinobacillus
  lignieresii 027.8
  mallei 024
  muris 026.1
Actinocutitis NEC (see also Dermatitis,
    actinic) 692.70
Actinodermatitis NEC (see also
    Dermatitis, actinic) 692.70
Actinomyces
  israelii (infection) - see
    Actinomycosis
  muris-ratti (infection) 026.1
Actinomycosis, actinomycotic 039.9
  with
    pneumonia 039.1
  abdominal 039.2
  cervicofacial 039.3
  cutaneous 039.0
  pulmonary 039.1
  specified site NEC 039.8
  thoracic 039.1
Actinoneuritis 357.89
Action, heart
  disorder 427.9
    postoperative 997.1
  irregular 427.9
    postoperative 997.1
    psychogenic 306.2
Active - see condition
Activity decrease, functional 780.99
Acute - see also condition
  abdomen NEC 789.0●
  gallbladder (see also Cholecystitis,
    acute) 575.0
Acyanoblepsia 368.53
Acyanopsia 368.53
Acystia 753.8
Acystinervia - see Neurogenic, bladder
Acystineuria - see Neurogenic, bladder
Adactylia, adactyly (congenital) 755.4
  lower limb (complete) (intercalary)
    (partial) (terminal) (see also
      Deformity, reduction, lower limb)
    755.39
    meaning all digits (complete)
      (partial) 755.31
    transverse (complete) (partial)
      755.31
  upper limb (complete) (intercalary)
    (partial) (terminal) (see also
      Deformity, reduction, upper limb)
    755.29
    meaning all digits (complete)
      (partial) 755.21
    transverse (complete) (partial)
      755.21
Adair-Dighton syndrome (brittle bones
    and blue sclera, deafness) 756.51
Adamantinoblastoma (M9310/0) - see
    Ameloblastoma
Adamantinoma (M9310/0) - see
    Ameloblastoma
Adamantoblastoma (M9310/0) - see
    Ameloblastoma
Adams-Stokes (-Morgagni) disease or
    syndrome (syncope with heart
    block) 426.9

◀ New   ◀▬ Revised   deleted Deleted   ● Use Additional Digit(s)   ▨ Omit code

Adaptation reaction (see also Reaction, adjustment) 309.9
ADEM (acute disseminated encephalomy-elitis)(postinfectious) 136.9 [323.61]
  infectious 136.9 [323.61]
  noninfectious 323.81
Addiction - see also Dependence
  absinthe 304.6 ●
  alcoholic (ethyl) (methyl) (wood) 303.9 ●
    complicating pregnancy, childbirth, or puerperium 648.4 ●
      affecting fetus or newborn 760.71
    suspected damage to fetus affecting management of pregnancy 655.4 ●
  drug (see also Dependence) 304.9 ●
  ethyl alcohol 303.9 ●
  heroin 304.0 ●
  hospital 301.51
  methyl alcohol 303.9 ●
  methylated spirit 303.9 ●
  morphine (-like substances) 304.0 ●
  nicotine 305.1
  opium 304.0 ●
  tobacco 305.1
  wine 303.9 ●
Addison's
  anemia (pernicious) 281.0
  disease (bronze) (primary adrenal insufficiency) 255.41
    tuberculous (see also Tuberculosis) 017.6 ●
  keloid (morphea) 701.0
  melanoderma (adrenal cortical hypofunction) 255.41
Addison-Biermer anemia (pernicious) 281.0
Addison-Gull disease - see Xanthoma
Addisonian crisis or melanosis (acute adrenocortical insufficiency) 255.41
Additional - see also Accessory
  chromosome(s) 758.5
    13-15 758.1
    16-18 758.2
    21 758.0
    autosome(s) NEC 758.5
    sex 758.81
Adduction contracture, hip or other joint - see Contraction, joint
Adenasthenia gastrica 536.0
Aden fever 061
Adenitis (see also Lymphadenitis) 289.3
  acute, unspecified site 683
    epidemic infectious 075
  axillary 289.3
    acute 683
    chronic or subacute 289.1
  Bartholin's gland 616.89
  bulbourethral gland (see also Urethritis) 597.89
  cervical 289.3
    acute 683
    chronic or subacute 289.1
  chancroid (Ducrey's bacillus) 099.0
  chronic (any lymph node, except mesenteric) 289.1
    mesenteric 289.2
  Cowper's gland (see also Urethritis) 597.89
  epidemic, acute 075
  gangrenous 683
  gonorrheal NEC 098.89

Adenitis (Continued)
  groin 289.3
    acute 683
    chronic or subacute 289.1
  infectious 075
  inguinal (region) 289.3
    acute 683
    chronic or subacute 289.1
  lymph gland or node, except mesenteric 289.3
    acute 683
    chronic or subacute 289.1
    mesenteric (acute) (chronic) (nonspecific) (subacute) 289.2
  mesenteric (acute) (chronic) (nonspecific) (subacute) 289.2
    due to Pasteurella multocida (P. septica) 027.2
  parotid gland (suppurative) 527.2
  phlegmonous 683
  salivary duct or gland (any) (recurring) (suppurative) 527.2
  scrofulous (see also Tuberculosis) 017.2 ●
  septic 289.3
  Skene's duct or gland (see also Urethritis) 597.89
  strumous, tuberculous (see also Tuberculosis) 017.2 ●
  subacute, unspecified site 289.1
  sublingual gland (suppurative) 527.2
  submandibular gland (suppurative) 527.2
  submaxillary gland (suppurative) 527.2
  suppurative 683
  tuberculous - see Tuberculosis, lymph gland
  urethral gland (see also Urethritis) 597.89
  venereal NEC 099.8
  Wharton's duct (suppurative) 527.2
Adenoacanthoma (M8570/3) - see Neoplasm, by site, malignant
Adenoameloblastoma (M9300/0) 213.1
  upper jaw (bone) 213.0
Adenocarcinoma (M8140/3) - see also Neoplasm, by site, malignant

> Note 03   The list of adjectival modifiers below is not exhaustive. A description of adenocarcinoma that does not appear in this list should be coded in the same manner as carcinoma with that description. Thus, "mixed acidophil-basophil adenocarcinoma," should be coded in the same manner as "mixed acidophil-basophil carcinoma," which appears in the list under "Carcinoma."
>
> Except where otherwise indicated, the morphological varieties of adenocarcinoma in the list below should be coded by site as for "Neoplasm, malignant."

  with
    apocrine metaplasia (M8573/3)
    cartilaginous (and osseous) metaplasia (M8571/3)
    osseous (and cartilaginous) metaplasia (M8571/3)
    spindle cell metaplasia (M8572/3)
    squamous metaplasia (M8570/3)

Adenocarcinoma (Continued)
  acidophil (M8280/3)
    specified site - see Neoplasm, by site, malignant
    unspecified site 194.3
  acinar (M8550/3)
  acinic cell (M8550/3)
  adrenal cortical (M8370/3) 194.0
  alveolar (M8251/3)
    and
      epidermoid carcinoma, mixed (M8560/3)
      squamous cell carcinoma, mixed (M8560/3)
  apocrine (M8401/3)
    breast - see Neoplasm, breast, malignant
    specified site NEC - see Neoplasm, skin, malignant
    unspecified site 173.9
  basophil (M8300/3)
    specified site - see Neoplasm, by site, malignant
    unspecified site 194.3
  bile duct type (M8160/3)
    liver 155.1
    specified site NEC - see Neoplasm, by site, malignant
    unspecified site 155.1
  bronchiolar (M8250/3) - see Neoplasm, lung, malignant
  ceruminous (M8420/3) 173.2
  chromophobe (M8270/3)
    specified site - see Neoplasm, by site, malignant
    unspecified site 194.3
  clear cell (mesonephroid type) (M8310/3)
  colloid (M8480/3)
  cylindroid type (M8200/3)
  diffuse type (M8145/3)
    specified site - see Neoplasm, by site, malignant
    unspecified site 151.9
  duct (infiltrating) (M8500/3)
    with Paget's disease (M8541/3) - see Neoplasm, breast, malignant
    specified site - see Neoplasm, by site, malignant
    unspecified site 174.9
  embryonal (M9070/3)
  endometrioid (M8380/3) - see Neoplasm, by site, malignant
  eosinophil (M8280/3)
    specified site - see Neoplasm, by site, malignant
    unspecified site 194.3
  follicular (M8330/3)
    and papillary (M8340/3) 193
    moderately differentiated type (M8332/3) 193
    pure follicle type (M8331/3) 193
    specified site - see Neoplasm, by site, malignant
    trabecular type (M8332/3) 193
    unspecified type 193
    well differentiated type (M8331/3) 193
  gelatinous (M8480/3)
  granular cell (M8320/3)
  Hürthle cell (M8290/3) 193
  in
    adenomatous
      polyp (M8210/3)
      polyposis coli (M8220/3) 153.9

Adenocarcinoma (Continued)
in (Continued)
polypoid adenoma (M8210/3)
tubular adenoma (M8210/3)
villous adenoma (M8261/3)
infiltrating duct (M8500/3)
with Paget's disease (M8541/3) -
see Neoplasm, breast,
malignant
specified site - see Neoplasm, by site,
malignant
unspecified site 174.9
inflammatory (M8530/3)
specified site - see Neoplasm, by site,
malignant
unspecified site 174.9
in situ (M8140/2) - see Neoplasm, by
site, in situ
intestinal type (M8144/3)
specified site - see Neoplasm, by site,
malignant
unspecified site 151.9
intraductal (noninfiltrating)
(M8500/2)
papillary (M8503/2)
specified site - see Neoplasm, by
site, in situ
unspecified site 233.0
specified site - see Neoplasm, by site,
in situ
unspecified site 233.0
islet cell (M8150/3)
and exocrine, mixed (M8154/3)
specified site - see Neoplasm, by
site, malignant
unspecified site 157.9
pancreas 157.4
specified site NEC - see Neoplasm,
by site, malignant
unspecified site 157.4
lobular (M8520/3)
specified site - see Neoplasm, by site,
malignant
unspecified site 174.9
medullary (M8510/3)
mesonephric (M9110/3)
mixed cell (M8323/3)
mucinous (M8480/3)
mucin-producing (M8481/3)
mucoid (M8480/3) - see also Neoplasm,
by site, malignant
cell (M8300/3)
specified site - see Neoplasm, by
site, malignant
unspecified site 194.3
nonencapsulated sclerosing (M8350/3)
193
oncocytic (M8290/3)
oxyphilic (M8290/3)
papillary (M8260/3)
and follicular (M8340/3) 193
intraductal (noninfiltrating)
(M8503/2)
specified site - see Neoplasm, by
site, in situ
unspecified site 233.0
serous (M8460/3)
specified site - see Neoplasm, by
site, malignant
unspecified site 183.0
papillocystic (M8450/3)
specified site - see Neoplasm, by site,
malignant
unspecified site 183.0

Adenocarcinoma (Continued)
pseudomucinous (M8470/3)
specified site - see Neoplasm, by site,
malignant
unspecified site 183.0
renal cell (M8312/3) 189.0
sebaceous (M8410/3)
serous (M8441/3) - see also Neoplasm,
by site, malignant
papillary
specified site - see Neoplasm, by
site, malignant
unspecified site 183.0
signet ring cell (M8490/3)
superficial spreading (M8143/3)
sweat gland (M8400/3) - see Neoplasm,
skin, malignant
trabecular (M8190/3)
tubular (M8211/3)
villous (M8262/3)
water-clear cell (M8322/3) 194.1
Adenofibroma (M9013/0)
clear cell (M8313/0) - see Neoplasm, by
site, benign
endometrioid (M8381/0) 220
borderline malignancy (M8381/1)
236.2
malignant (M8381/3) 183.0
mucinous (M9015/0)
specified site - see Neoplasm, by site,
benign
unspecified site 220
prostate 600.20
with
other lower urinary tract
symptoms (LUTS) 600.21
urinary
obstruction 600.21
retention 600.21
serous (M9014/0)
specified site - see Neoplasm, by site,
benign
unspecified site 220
specified site - see Neoplasm, by site,
benign
unspecified site 220
Adenofibrosis
breast 610.2
endometrioid 617.0
Adenoiditis 474.01
acute 463
chronic 474.01
with chronic tonsillitis 474.02
Adenoids (congenital) (of nasal fossa) 474.9
hypertrophy 474.12
vegetations 474.2
Adenolipomatosis (symmetrical) 272.8
Adenolymphoma (M8561/0)
specified site - see Neoplasm, by site,
benign
unspecified 210.2
Adenoma (sessile) (M8140/0) - see also
Neoplasm, by site, benign

Note 04   Except where otherwise
indicated, the morphological varieties
of adenoma in the list below should
be coded by site as for "Neoplasm,
benign."

acidophil (M8280/0)
specified site - see Neoplasm, by site,
benign
unspecified site 227.3

Adenoma (Continued)
acinar (cell) (M8550/0)
acinic cell (M8550/0)
adrenal (cortex) (cortical) (functioning)
(M8370/0) 227.0
clear cell type (M8373/0) 227.0
compact cell type (M8371/0) 227.0
glomerulosa cell type (M8374/0)
227.0
heavily pigmented variant
(M8372/0) 227.0
mixed cell type (M8375/0) 227.0
alpha cell (M8152/0)
pancreas 211.7
specified site NEC - see Neoplasm,
by site, benign
unspecified site 211.7
alveolar (M8251/0)
apocrine (M8401/0)
breast 217
specified site NEC - see Neoplasm,
skin, benign
unspecified site 216.9
basal cell (M8147/0)
basophil (M8300/0)
specified site - see Neoplasm, by site,
benign
unspecified site 227.3
beta cell (M8151/0)
pancreas 211.7
specified site NEC - see Neoplasm,
by site, benign
unspecified site 211.7
bile duct (M8160/0) 211.5
black (M8372/0) 227.0
bronchial (M8140/1) 235.7
carcinoid type (M8240/3) - see
Neoplasm, lung, malignant
cylindroid type (M8200/3) - see
Neoplasm, lung, malignant
ceruminous (M8420/0) 216.2
chief cell (M8321/0) 227.1
chromophobe (M8270/0)
specified site - see Neoplasm, by site,
benign
unspecified site 227.3
clear cell (M8310/0)
colloid (M8334/0)
specified site - see Neoplasm, by site,
benign
unspecified site 226
cylindroid type, bronchus (M8200/3) -
see Neoplasm, lung, malignant
duct (M8503/0)
embryonal (M8191/0)
endocrine, multiple (M8360/1)
single specified site - see Neoplasm,
by site, uncertain behavior
two or more specified sites 237.4
unspecified site 237.4
endometrioid (M8380/0) - see also
Neoplasm, by site, benign
borderline malignancy (M8380/1) -
see Neoplasm, by site,
uncertain behavior
eosinophil (M8280/0)
specified site - see Neoplasm, by site,
benign
unspecified site 227.3
fetal (M8333/0)
specified site - see Neoplasm, by site,
benign
unspecified site 226

◀ New   ◀▥ Revised   deleted Deleted   ● Use Additional Digit(s)   ▬ Omit code

Adenoma *(Continued)*
  follicular (M8330/0)
    specified site - *see* Neoplasm, by site, benign
    unspecified site 226
  hepatocellular (M8170/0) 211.5
  Hürthle cell (M8290/0) 226
  intracystic papillary (M8504/0)
  islet cell (functioning) (M8150/0)
    pancreas 211.7
    specified site NEC - *see* Neoplasm, by site, benign
    unspecified site 211.7
  liver cell (M8170/0) 211.5
  macrofollicular (M8334/0)
    specified site NEC - *see* Neoplasm, by site, benign
    unspecified site 226
  malignant, malignum (M8140/3) - *see* Neoplasm, by site, malignant
  mesonephric (M9110/0)
  microfollicular (M8333/0)
    specified site - *see* Neoplasm, by site, benign
    unspecified site 226
  mixed cell (M8323/0)
  monomorphic (M8146/0)
  mucinous (M8480/0)
  mucoid cell (M8300/0)
    specified site - *see* Neoplasm, by site, benign
    unspecified site 227.3
  multiple endocrine (M8360/1)
    single specified site - *see* Neoplasm, by site, uncertain behavior
    two or more specified sites 237.4
    unspecified site 237.4
  nipple (M8506/0) 217
  oncocytic (M8290/0)
  oxyphilic (M8290/0)
  papillary (M8260/0) - *see also* Neoplasm, by site, benign
    intracystic (M8504/0)
  papillotubular (M8263/0)
  Pick's tubular (M8640/0)
    specified site - *see* Neoplasm, by site, benign
    unspecified site
      female 220
      male 222.0
  pleomorphic (M8940/0)
  polypoid (M8210/0)
  prostate (benign) 600.20
    with
      other lower urinary tract symptoms (LUTS) 600.21
      urinary
        obstruction 600.21
        retention 600.21
  rete cell 222.0
  sebaceous, sebaceum (gland) (senile) (M8410/0) - *see also* Neoplasm, skin, benign
    disseminata 759.5
  Sertoli cell (M8640/0)
    specified site - *see* Neoplasm, by site, benign
    unspecified site
      female 220
      male 222.0
  skin appendage (M8390/0) - *see* Neoplasm, skin, benign
  sudoriferous gland (M8400/0) - *see* Neoplasm, skin, benign

Adenoma *(Continued)*
  sweat gland or duct (M8400/0) - *see* Neoplasm, skin, benign
  testicular (M8640/0)
    specified site - *see* Neoplasm, by site, benign
    unspecified site
      female 220
      male 222.0
  thyroid 226
  trabecular (M8190/0)
  tubular (M8211/0) - *see also* Neoplasm, by site, benign
    papillary (M8460/3)
    Pick's (M8640/0)
      specified site - *see* Neoplasm, by site, benign
      unspecified site
        female 220
        male 222.0
  tubulovillous (M8263/0)
  villoglandular (M8263/0)
  villous (M8261/1) - *see* Neoplasm, by site, uncertain behavior
  water-clear cell (M8322/0) 227.1
  wolffian duct (M9110/0)
Adenomatosis (M8220/0)
  endocrine (multiple) (M8360/1)
    single specified site - *see* Neoplasm, by site, uncertain behavior
    two or more specified sites 237.4
    unspecified site 237.4
  erosive of nipple (M8506/0) 217
  pluriendocrine - *see* Adenomatosis, endocrine
  pulmonary (M8250/1) 235.7
    malignant (M8250/3) - *see* Neoplasm, lung, malignant
  specified site - *see* Neoplasm, by site, benign
  unspecified site 211.3
Adenomatous
  cyst, thyroid (gland) - *see* Goiter, nodular
  goiter (nontoxic) (*see also* Goiter, nodular) 241.9
    toxic or with hyperthyroidism 242.3●
Adenomyoma (M8932/0) - *see also* Neoplasm, by site, benign
  prostate 600.20
    with
      other lower urinary tract symptoms (LUTS) 600.21
      urinary
        obstruction 600.21
        retention 600.21
Adenomyometritis 617.0
Adenomyosis (uterus) (internal) 617.0
Adenopathy (lymph gland) 785.6
  inguinal 785.6
  mediastinal 785.6
  mesentery 785.6
  syphilitic (secondary) 091.4
  tracheobronchial 785.6
    tuberculous (*see also* Tuberculosis) 012.1●
      primary, progressive 010.8●
  tuberculous (*see also* Tuberculosis, lymph gland) 017.2●
    tracheobronchial 012.1●
      primary, progressive 010.8●
Adenopharyngitis 462
Adenophlegmon 683

Adenosalpingitis 614.1
Adenosarcoma (M8960/3) 189.0
Adenosclerosis 289.3
Adenosis
  breast (sclerosing) 610.2
  vagina, congenital 752.49
Adentia (complete) (partial) (*see also* Absence, teeth) 520.0
Adherent
  labium (minus) 624.4
  pericardium (nonrheumatic) 423.1
    rheumatic 393
  placenta 667.0●
    with hemorrhage 666.0●
  prepuce 605
  scar (skin) NEC 709.2
  tendon in scar 709.2
Adhesion(s), adhesive (postinfectional) (postoperative)
  abdominal (wall) (*see also* Adhesions, peritoneum) 568.0
  amnion to fetus 658.8●
    affecting fetus or newborn 762.8
  appendix 543.9
  arachnoiditis - *see* Meningitis
  auditory tube (Eustachian) 381.89
  bands - *see also* Adhesions, peritoneum
    cervix 622.3
    uterus 621.5
  bile duct (any) 576.8
  bladder (sphincter) 596.8
  bowel (*see also* Adhesions, peritoneum) 568.0
  cardiac 423.1
    rheumatic 398.99
  cecum (*see also* Adhesions, peritoneum) 568.0
  cervicovaginal 622.3
    congenital 752.49
    postpartal 674.8●
    old 622.3
  cervix 622.3
  clitoris 624.4
  colon (*see also* Adhesions, peritoneum) 568.0
  common duct 576.8
  congenital - *see also* Anomaly, specified type NEC
    fingers (*see also* Syndactylism, fingers) 755.11
    labium (majus) (minus) 752.49
    omental, anomalous 751.4
    ovary 752.0
    peritoneal 751.4
    toes (*see also* Syndactylism, toes) 755.13
    tongue (to gum or roof of mouth) 750.12
  conjunctiva (acquired) (localized) 372.62
    congenital 743.63
    extensive 372.63
  cornea - *see* Opacity, cornea
  cystic duct 575.8
  diaphragm (*see also* Adhesions, peritoneum) 568.0
  due to foreign body - *see* Foreign body
  duodenum (*see also* Adhesions, peritoneum) 568.0
    with obstruction 537.3
  ear, middle - *see* Adhesions, middle ear
  epididymis 608.89
  epidural - *see* Adhesions, meninges

Adhesion(s) *(Continued)*
  epiglottis 478.79
  Eustachian tube 381.89
  eyelid 374.46
    postoperative 997.99
      surgically created V45.69
  gallbladder *(see also* Disease,
    gallbladder) 575.8
  globe 360.89
  heart 423.1
    rheumatic 398.99
  ileocecal (coil) *(see also* Adhesions,
    peritoneum) 568.0
  ileum *(see also* Adhesions, peritoneum)
    568.0
  intestine (postoperative) *(see also*
    Adhesions, peritoneum) 568.0
    with obstruction 560.81
      with hernia - *see also* Hernia, by
        site, with obstruction
          gangrenous - *see* Hernia, by
            site, with gangrene
  intra-abdominal *(see also* Adhesions,
    peritoneum) 568.0
  iris 364.70
    to corneal graft 996.79
  joint *(see also* Ankylosis) 718.5●
  kidney 593.89
  labium (majus) (minus), congenital
    752.49
  liver 572.8
  lung 511.0
  mediastinum 519.3
  meninges 349.2
    cerebral (any) 349.2
      congenital 742.4
    congenital 742.8
    spinal (any) 349.2
      congenital 742.59
    tuberculous (cerebral) (spinal) *(see
      also* Tuberculosis, meninges)
        013.0●
  mesenteric *(see also* Adhesions,
    peritoneum) 568.0
  middle ear (fibrous) 385.10
    drum head 385.19
      to
        incus 385.11
        promontorium 385.13
        stapes 385.12
      specified NEC 385.19
  nasal (septum) (to turbinates)
    478.19
  nerve NEC 355.9
    spinal 355.9
      root 724.9
        cervical NEC 723.4
        lumbar NEC 724.4
        lumbosacral 724.4
        thoracic 724.4
  ocular muscle 378.60
  omentum *(see also* Adhesions,
    peritoneum) 568.0
  organ or site, congenital NEC -
    see Anomaly, specified type
      NEC
  ovary 614.6
    congenital (to cecum, kidney, or
      omentum) 752.0
  parauterine 614.6
  parovarian 614.6
  pelvic (peritoneal)
    female (postoperative)
      (postinfection) 614.6

Adhesion(s) *(Continued)*
  pelvic *(Continued)*
    male (postoperative) (postinfection)
      (see also Adhesions,
        peritoneum) 568.0
    postpartal (old) 614.6
    tuberculous *(see also* Tuberculosis)
      016.9●
  penis to scrotum (congenital) 752.69
  periappendiceal *(see also* Adhesions,
    peritoneum) 568.0
  pericardium (nonrheumatic) 423.1
    rheumatic 393
    tuberculous *(see also* Tuberculosis)
      017.9● [420.0]
  pericholecystic 575.8
  perigastric *(see also* Adhesions,
    peritoneum) 568.0
  periovarian 614.6
  periprostatic 602.8
  perirectal *(see also* Adhesions,
    peritoneum) 568.0
  perirenal 593.89
  peritoneum, peritoneal (fibrous)
    (postoperative) 568.0
    with obstruction (intestinal) 560.81
      with hernia - *see also* Hernia, by
        site, with obstruction
          gangrenous - *see* Hernia, by
            site, with gangrene
    duodenum 537.3
    congenital 751.4
    female (postoperative)
      (postinfective) 614.6
    pelvic, female 614.6
    pelvic, male 568.0
    postpartal, pelvic 614.6
    to uterus 614.6
  peritubal 614.6
  periureteral 593.89
  periuterine 621.5
  perivesical 596.8
  perivesicular (seminal vesicle) 608.89
  pleura, pleuritic 511.0
    tuberculous *(see also* Tuberculosis,
      pleura) 012.0●
  pleuropericardial 511.0
  postoperative (gastrointestinal tract)
    (see also Adhesions, peritoneum)
    eyelid 997.99
      surgically created V45.69
    pelvic, female 614.9
    pelvic, male 568.0
    urethra 598.2
  postpartal, old 624.4
  preputial, prepuce 605
  pulmonary 511.0
  pylorus *(see also* Adhesions,
    peritoneum) 568.0
  Rosenmüller's fossa 478.29
  sciatic nerve 355.0
  seminal vesicle 608.89
  shoulder (joint) 726.0
  sigmoid flexure *(see also* Adhesions,
    peritoneum) 568.0
  spermatic cord (acquired) 608.89
    congenital 752.89
  spinal canal 349.2
    nerve 355.9
      root 724.9
        cervical NEC 723.4
        lumbar NEC 724.4
        lumbosacral 724.4
        thoracic 724.4

Adhesion(s) *(Continued)*
  stomach *(see also* Adhesions,
    peritoneum) 568.0
  subscapular 726.2
  tendonitis 726.90
    shoulder 726.0
  testicle 608.89
  tongue (congenital) (to gum or roof of
    mouth) 750.12
    acquired 529.8
  trachea 519.19
  tubo-ovarian 614.6
  tunica vaginalis 608.89
  ureter 593.89
  uterus 621.5
    to abdominal wall 614.6
      in pregnancy or childbirth 654.4●
        affecting fetus or newborn
          763.89
  vagina (chronic) (postoperative)
    (postradiation) 623.2
  vaginitis (congenital) 752.49
  vesical 596.8
  vitreous 379.29
Adie (-Holmes) syndrome (tonic pupillary
  reaction) 379.46
Adiponecrosis neonatorum 778.1
Adiposa dolorosa 272.8
Adiposalgia 272.8
Adiposis 278.0●
  cerebralis 253.8
  dolorosa 272.8
  tuberosa simplex 272.8
Adiposity 278.02
  heart *(see also* Degeneration,
    myocardial) 429.1
  localized 278.1
Adiposogenital dystrophy 253.8
Adjustment
  prosthesis or other device - *see* Fitting
    of
  reaction - *see* Reaction, adjustment
Administration, prophylactic
  antibiotics V07.39
  antitoxin, any V07.2
  antivenin V07.2
  chemotherapeutic agent NEC V07.39
  chemotherapy NEC V07.39
  diphtheria antitoxin V07.2
  fluoride V07.31
  gamma globulin V07.2
  immune sera (gamma globulin) V07.2
  passive immunization agent V07.2
  RhoGAM V07.2
Admission (encounter)
  as organ donor - *see* Donor
  by mistake V68.9
  for
    adequacy testing (for)
      hemodialysis V56.31
      peritoneal dialysis V56.32
    adjustment (of)
      artificial
        arm (complete) (partial)
          V52.0
        eye V52.2
        leg (complete) (partial) V52.1
      brain neuropacemaker V53.02
      breast
        implant V52.4
          exchange (different
            material) (different
              size) V52.4
        prosthesis V52.4

◄ New   ◄▥ Revised   ~~deleted~~ Deleted   ● Use Additional Digit(s)   ▨ Omit code

Admission *(Continued)*
  for *(Continued)*
    adjustment (of) *(Continued)*
      cardiac device V53.39
        defibrillator, automatic
          implantable V53.32
        pacemaker V53.31
          carotid sinus V53.39
      catheter
        non-vascular V58.82
        vascular V58.81
      cerebral ventricle
        (communicating)
        shunt V53.01
      colostomy belt V55.3
      contact lenses V53.1
      cystostomy device V53.6
      dental prosthesis V52.3
      device, unspecified type V53.90
        abdominal V53.59 ◀▥
        cardiac V53.39
          defibrillator, automatic
            implantable V53.32
          pacemaker V53.31
          carotid sinus V53.39
        cerebral ventricle
          (communicating)
          shunt V53.01
        gastrointestinal NEC V53.59 ◀
        insulin pump V53.91
        intestinal V53.50 ◀
        intrauterine contraceptive V25.1
        nervous system V53.09
        orthodontic V53.4
        other device V53.99
        prosthetic V52.9
          breast V52.4
          dental V52.3
          eye V52.2
          specified type NEC V52.8
        special senses V53.09
        substitution
          auditory V53.09
          nervous system V53.09
          visual V53.09
        urinary V53.6
      dialysis catheter
        extracorporeal V56.1
        peritoneal V56.2
      diaphragm (contraceptive) V25.02
      gastric lap band V53.51 ◀
      gastrointestinal appliance and
        device NEC V53.59 ◀
      growth rod V54.02
      hearing aid V53.2
      ileostomy device V55.2
      intestinal appliance and ~~or~~ device
        ~~NEC~~ V53.50 ◀▥
      intrauterine contraceptive device
        V25.1
      neuropacemaker (brain)
        (peripheral nerve) (spinal
        cord) V53.02
      orthodontic device V53.4
      orthopedic (device) V53.7
        brace V53.7
        cast V53.7
        shoes V53.7
      pacemaker
        brain V53.02
        cardiac V53.31
        carotid sinus V53.39
        peripheral nerve V53.02
        spinal cord V53.02

Admission *(Continued)*
  for *(Continued)*
    adjustment (of) *(Continued)*
      prosthesis V52.9
        arm (complete) (partial) V52.0
        breast V52.4
        dental V52.3
        eye V52.2
        leg (complete) (partial) V52.1
        specified type NEC V52.8
      spectacles V53.1
      wheelchair V53.8
    adoption referral or proceedings
      V68.89
    aftercare *(see also* Aftercare) V58.9
      cardiac pacemaker V53.31
      chemotherapy (oral) (intravenous)
        V58.11 ◀▥
      dialysis
        extracorporeal (renal) V56.0
        peritoneal V56.8
        renal V56.0
      fracture *(see also* Aftercare,
        fracture) V54.9
      medical NEC V58.89
      organ transplant V58.44
      orthopedic V54.9
        specified care NEC V54.89
      pacemaker device
        brain V53.02
        cardiac V53.31
        carotid sinus V53.39
        nervous system V53.02
        spinal cord V53.02
      postoperative NEC V58.49
        wound closure, planned V58.41
      postpartum
        immediately after delivery
          V24.0
        routine follow-up V24.2
      postradiation V58.0
      radiation therapy V58.0
      removal of
        non-vascular catheter V58.82
        vascular catheter V58.81
      specified NEC V58.89
      surgical NEC V58.49
        wound closure, planned V58.41
    antineoplastic
      chemotherapy (oral) (intravenous)
        V58.11 ◀▥
      immunotherapy V58.12
    artificial insemination V26.1
    assisted reproductive fertility
      procedure cycle V26.81
    attention to artificial opening (of)
      V55.9
      artificial vagina V55.7
      colostomy V55.3
      cystostomy V55.5
      enterostomy V55.4
      gastrostomy V55.1
      ileostomy V55.2
      jejunostomy V55.4
      nephrostomy V55.6
      specified site NEC V55.8
        intestinal tract V55.4
        urinary tract V55.6
      tracheostomy V55.0
      ureterostomy V55.6
      urethrostomy V55.6
    battery replacement
      cardiac pacemaker V53.31
    blood typing V72.86
      Rh typing V72.86

Admission *(Continued)*
  for *(Continued)*
    boarding V65.0
    breast
      augmentation or reduction V50.1
      implant exchange (different
        material) (different size)
        V52.4
      reconstruction following
        mastectomy V51.0
      removal
        prophylactic V50.41
        tissue expander without
          synchronous insertion of
          permanent implant V52.4
    change of
      cardiac pacemaker (battery) 53.31
      carotid sinus pacemaker V53.39
      catheter in artificial opening - *see*
        Attention to, artificial,
        opening
      drains V58.49
      dressing
        wound V58.30
          nonsurgical V58.30
          surgical V58.31
      fixation device
        external V54.89
        internal V54.01
      Kirschner wire V54.89
      neuropacemaker device (brain)
        (peripheral nerve) (spinal
        cord) V53.02
      nonsurgical wound dressing
        V58.30
      pacemaker device
        brain V53.02
        cardiac V53.31
        carotid sinus V53.39
        nervous system V53.02
      plaster cast V54.89
      splint, external V54.89
      Steinmann pin V54.89
      surgical wound dressing V58.31
      traction device V54.89
      wound packing V58.30
        nonsurgical V58.30
        surgical V58.31
    checkup only V70.0
    chemotherapy, (oral) (intravenous)
      antineoplastic V58.11 ◀▥
    circumcision, ritual or routine (in
      absence of medical indication)
      V50.2
    clinical research investigation
      (control) (normal comparison)
      (participant) V70.7
    closure of artificial opening - *see*
      Attention to, artificial, opening
    contraceptive
      counseling V25.09
        emergency V25.03
        postcoital V25.03
      management V25.9
        specified type NEC V25.8
    convalescence following V66.9
      chemotherapy V66.2
      psychotherapy V66.3
      radiotherapy V66.1
      surgery V66.0
      treatment (for) V66.5
        combined V66.6
        fracture V66.4
        mental disorder NEC V66.3
        specified condition NEC V66.5

Admission (*Continued*)
  for (*Continued*)
    cosmetic surgery NEC V50.1
      breast reconstruction following mastectomy V51.0
      following healed injury or operation V51.8
    counseling (*see also* Counseling) V65.40
      without complaint or sickness V65.49
    contraceptive management V25.09
      emergency V25.03
      postcoital V25.03
    dietary V65.3
    exercise V65.41
    fertility preservation (prior to cancer therapy) (prior to surgical removal of gonads) V26.42
    for
      nonattending third party V65.19
      pediatric pre-birth visit for expectant mother V65.11
        pre-adoption visit for adoptive parent(s) V65.11
        pre-birth visit for expectant parent(s) V65.11
      victim of abuse
        child V61.21
        partner or spouse V61.11
    genetic V26.33
    gonorrhea V65.45
    HIV V65.44
    human immunodeficiency virus V65.44
    injury prevention V65.43
    insulin pump training V65.46
    natural family planning
      procreative V26.41
      to avoid pregnancy V25.04
    procreative management V26.49
      using natural family planning V26.41
    sexually transmitted disease NEC V65.45
      HIV V65.44
    specified reason NEC V65.49
    substance use and abuse V65.42
    syphilis V65.45
    victim of abuse
      child V61.21
      partner or spouse V61.11
  desensitization to allergens V07.1
  dialysis V56.0
    catheter
      fitting and adjustment
        extracorporeal V56.1
        peritoneal V56.2
      removal or replacement
        extracorporeal V56.1
        peritoneal V56.2
    extracorporeal (renal) V56.0
    peritoneal V56.8
    renal V56.0
  dietary surveillance and counseling V65.3
  drug monitoring, therapeutic V58.83
  ear piercing V50.3

Admission (*Continued*)
  for (*Continued*)
    elective surgery
      breast
        augmentation or reduction V50.1
        reconstruction following mastectomy V51.0
        removal, prophylactic V50.41
      circumcision, ritual or routine (in absence of medical indication) V50.2
      cosmetic NEC V50.1
        breast reconstruction following mastectomy V51.0
        following healed injury or operation V51.8
      ear piercing V50.3
      face-lift V50.1
      hair transplant V50.0
      plastic
        breast reconstruction following mastectomy V51.0
        cosmetic NEC V50.1
        following healed injury or operation V51.8
      prophylactic organ removal V50.49
        breast V50.41
        ovary V50.42
      repair of scarred tissue (following healed injury or operation) V51.8
      specified type NEC V50.8
    end-of-life care V66.7
    examination (*see also* Examination) V70.9
      administrative purpose NEC V70.3
      adoption V70.3
      allergy V72.7
      antibody response V72.61
      at health care facility V70.0
      athletic team V70.3
      camp V70.3
      cardiovascular, preoperative V72.81
      clinical research investigation (control) (participant) V70.7
      dental V72.2
      developmental testing (child) (infant) V20.2
      donor (potential) V70.8
      driver's license V70.3
      ear V72.19
      employment V70.5
      eye V72.0
      follow-up (routine) - *see* Examination, follow-up
      for admission to
        old age home V70.3
        school V70.3
      general V70.9
        specified reason NEC V70.8
      gynecological V72.31
      health supervision (child) (infant) V20.2
        child (over 28 days old) V20.2
        infant (over 28 days old) V20.2
        newborn
          8 to 28 days old V20.32
          under 8 days old V20.31
      hearing V72.19
        following failed hearing screening V72.11

Admission (*Continued*)
  for (*Continued*)
    examination(*Continued*)
      immigration V70.3
      infant, routine V20.2
        8 to 28 days old V20.32
        over 28 days old, routine V20.2
        under 8 days old V20.31
      insurance certification V70.3
      laboratory V72.60
        ordered as part of a routine general medical examination V72.62
        pre-operative V72.63
        pre-procedural V72.63
        specified NEC V72.69
      marriage license V70.3
      medical (general) (*see also* Examination, medical) V70.9
      medicolegal reasons V70.4
      naturalization V70.3
      pelvic (annual) (periodic) V72.31
      postpartum checkup V24.2
      pregnancy (possible) (unconfirmed) V72.40
        negative result V72.41
        positive result V72.42
      preoperative V72.84
        cardiovascular V72.81
        respiratory V72.82
        specified NEC V72.83
      preprocedural V72.84
        cardiovascular V72.81
        general physical V72.83
        respiratory V72.82
        specified NEC V72.83
      prior to chemotherapy V72.83
      prison V70.3
      psychiatric (general) V70.2
        requested by authority V70.1
      radiological NEC V72.5
      respiratory, preoperative V72.82
      school V70.3
      screening - *see* Screening
      skin hypersensitivity V72.7
      specified type NEC V72.85
      sport competition V70.3
      vision V72.0
      well baby and child care V20.2
    exercise therapy V57.1
    face-lift, cosmetic reason V50.1
    fertility preservation (prior to cancer therapy) (prior to surgical removal of gonads) V26.82
    fitting (of)
      artificial
        arm (complete) (partial) V52.0
        eye V52.2
        leg (complete) (partial) V52.1
      biliary drainage tube V58.82
      brain neuropacemaker V53.02
      breast V52.4
        implant V52.4
        prosthesis V52.4
      cardiac pacemaker V53.31
      catheter
        non-vascular V58.82
        vascular V58.81
      cerebral ventricle (communicating) shunt V53.01
      chest tube V58.82
      colostomy belt V55.2
      contact lenses V53.1
      cystostomy device V53.6
      dental prosthesis V52.3

◀ New   ◀▥ Revised   ~~deleted~~ Deleted   ● Use Additional Digit(s)   ▨ Omit code

Admission (*Continued*)
  for (*Continued*)
    fitting (*Continued*)
      device, unspecified type V53.90
        abdominal V53.59 ◀▥
        cerebral ventricle
          (communicating) shunt
          V53.01
        gastrointestinal NEC V53.59 ◀
        insulin pump V53.91
        intestinal V53.50 ◀
        intrauterine contraceptive
          V25.1
        nervous system V53.09
        orthodontic V53.4
        other device V53.99
        prosthetic V52.9
          breast V52.4
          dental V52.3
          eye V52.2
        special senses V53.09
        substitution
          auditory V53.09
          nervous system V53.09
          visual V53.09
      diaphragm (contraceptive)
        V25.02
      fistula (sinus tract) drainage tube
        V58.82
      gastric lap band V53.51 ◀
      gastrointestinal appliance and
        device NEC V53.59 ◀
      growth rod V54.02
      hearing aid V53.2
      ileostomy device V55.2
      intestinal appliance and ~~or~~ device
        ~~NEC~~ V53.50 ◀▥
      intrauterine contraceptive device
        V25.1
      neuropacemaker (brain)
        (peripheral nerve) (spinal
        cord) V53.02
      orthodontic device V53.4
      orthopedic (device) V53.7
        brace V53.7
        cast V53.7
        shoes V53.7
      pacemaker
        brain V53.02
        cardiac V53.31
        carotid sinus V53.39
        spinal cord V53.02
      pleural drainage tube V58.82
      portacath V58.81
      prosthesis V52.9
        arm (complete) (partial) V52.0
        breast V52.4
        dental V52.3
        eye V52.2
        leg (complete) (partial) V52.1
        specified type NEC V52.8
      spectacles V53.1
      wheelchair V53.8
    follow-up examination (routine)
      (following) V67.9
      cancer chemotherapy V67.2
      chemotherapy V67.2
      high-risk medication NEC V67.51
      injury NEC V67.59
      psychiatric V67.3
      psychotherapy V67.3
      radiotherapy V67.1
      specified surgery NEC V67.09
      surgery V67.00
        vaginal pap smear V67.01

Admission (*Continued*)
  for (*Continued*)
    follow-up examination (*Continued*)
      treatment (for) V67.9
        combined V67.6
        fracture V67.4
        involving high-risk medication
          NEC V67.51
        mental disorder V67.3
        specified NEC V67.59
    hair transplant, for cosmetic reason
      V50.0
    health advice, education, or
      instruction V65.4
    hearing conservation and treatment
      V72.12
    hormone replacement therapy
      (postmenopausal) V07.4
    hospice care V66.7
    immunizations (childhood)
      appropriate for age V20.2 ◀
    immunotherapy, antineoplastic
      V58.12
    insertion (of)
      subdermal implantable
        contraceptive V25.5
    insulin pump titration V53.91
    insulin pump training V65.46
    intrauterine device
      insertion V25.1
      management V25.42
    investigation to determine further
      disposition V63.8
    in vitro fertilization cycle V26.81
    isolation V07.0
    issue of
      disability examination certificate
        V68.01
      medical certificate NEC V68.09
      repeat prescription NEC V68.1
        contraceptive device NEC
          V25.49
    kidney dialysis V56.0
    lengthening of growth rod V54.02
    mental health evaluation V70.2
      requested by authority V70.1
    natural family planning counseling
      and advice
      procreative V26.41
      to avoid pregnancy V25.04
    nonmedical reason NEC V68.89
    nursing care evaluation V63.8
    observation (without need for
      further medical care) (*see also*
      Observation) V71.9
      accident V71.4
      alleged rape or seduction V71.5
      criminal assault V71.6
      following accident V71.4
        at work V71.3
      foreign body ingestion V71.89
      growth and development
        variations, childhood
        V21.0
      inflicted injury NEC V71.6
      ingestion of deleterious agent or
        foreign body V71.89
      injury V71.6
      malignant neoplasm V71.1
      mental disorder V71.09
      newborn - *see* Observation,
        suspected, condition,
        newborn
      rape V71.5
      specified NEC V71.89

Admission (*Continued*)
  for (*Continued*)
    observation (*Continued*)
      suspected
        disorder V71.9
          abuse V71.81
          accident V71.4
            at work V71.3
          benign neoplasm V71.89
          cardiovascular V71.7
          exposure
            anthrax V71.82
            biological agent NEC
              V71.83
            SARS V71.83
          heart V71.7
          inflicted injury NEC V71.6
          malignant neoplasm V71.1
          mental NEC V71.09
          neglect V71.81
          specified condition NEC
            V71.89
          tuberculosis V71.2
        maternal and fetal problem not
          found
          amniotic cavity and
            membrane V89.01
          cervical shortening V89.05
          fetal anomaly V89.03
          fetal growth V89.04
          oligohydramnios V89.01
          other specified NEC V89.09
          placenta V89.02
          polyhydramnios V89.01
      tuberculosis V71.2
    occupational therapy V57.21
    organ transplant, donor - *see* Donor
    ovary, ovarian removal, prophylactic
      V50.42
    palliative care V66.7
    Papanicolaou smear
      cervix V76.2
        for suspected malignant
          neoplasm V76.2
        no disease found V71.1
        routine, as part of
          gynecological
          examination V72.31
        to confirm findings of recent
          normal smear following
          initial abnormal smear
          V72.32
      vaginal V76.47
        following hysterectomy for
          malignant condition
          V67.01
    passage of sounds or bougie in
      artificial opening - *see*
      Attention to, artificial, opening
    paternity testing V70.4
    peritoneal dialysis V56.32
    physical therapy NEC V57.1
    plastic surgery
      breast reconstruction following
        mastectomy V51.0
      cosmetic NEC V50.1
      following healed injury or
        operation V51.8
    postmenopausal hormone
      replacement therapy V07.4
    postpartum observation
      immediately after delivery
      V24.0
      routine follow-up V24.2
    poststerilization (for restoration)
      V26.0

◀ New   ◀▥ Revised   ~~deleted~~ Deleted   ● Use Additional Digit(s)   ▨ Omit code

Admission *(Continued)*
  for *(Continued)*
    procreative management V26.9
      assisted reproductive fertility
        procedure cycle V26.81
      in vitro fertilization cycle V26.81
      specified type NEC V26.89
    prophylactic
      administration of
        antibiotics V07.39
        antitoxin, any V07.2
        antivenin V07.2
        chemotherapeutic agent NEC
          V07.39
        chemotherapy NEC V07.39
        diphtheria antitoxin V07.2
        fluoride V07.31
        gamma globulin V07.2
        immune sera (gamma
          globulin) V07.2
        RhoGAM V07.2
        tetanus antitoxin V07.2
      breathing exercises V57.0
      chemotherapy NEC V07.39
        fluoride V07.31
      measure V07.9
        specified type NEC V07.8
      organ removal V50.49
        breast V50.41
        ovary V50.42
    psychiatric examination (general)
      V70.2
    requested by authority V70.1
    radiation management V58.0
    radiotherapy V58.0
    reconstruction following
      mastectomy V51.0
    reforming of artificial opening -
      see Attention to, artificial,
        opening
    rehabilitation V57.9
      multiple types V57.89
      occupational V57.21
      orthoptic V57.4
      orthotic V57.81
      physical NEC V57.1
      specified type NEC V57.89
      speech(-language) V57.3   ◄▥
      vocational V57.22
    removal of
      breast tissue expander without
        synchronous insertion of
        permanent implant V52.4
      cardiac pacemaker V53.31
      cast (plaster) V54.89
      catheter from artificial opening -
        see Attention to, artificial,
          opening
      cerebral ventricle
        (communicating) shunt
          V53.01
      cystostomy catheter V55.5
      device
        cerebral ventricle
          (communicating)
          shunt V53.01
        fixation
          external V54.89
          internal V54.01
        intrauterine contraceptive
          V25.42
        traction, external V54.89
      drains V58.49
      dressing
        wound V58.30
          nonsurgical V58.30
          surgical V58.31

Admission *(Continued)*
  for *(Continued)*
    removal of *(Continued)*
      fixation device
        external V54.89
        internal V54.01
      intrauterine contraceptive device
        V25.42
      Kirschner wire V54.89
      neuropacemaker (brain)
        (peripheral nerve) (spinal
          cord) V53.02
      nonsurgical wound dressing
        V58.30
      orthopedic fixation device
        external V54.89
        internal V54.01
      pacemaker device
        brain V53.02
        cardiac V53.31
        carotid sinus V53.39
        nervous system V53.02
      plaster cast V54.89
      plate (fracture) V54.01
      rod V54.01
      screw (fracture) V54.01
      splint, traction V54.89
      staples V58.32
      Steinmann pin V54.89
      subdermal implantable
        contraceptive V25.43
      surgical wound dressing V58.31
      sutures V58.32
      traction device, external V54.89
      ureteral stent V53.6
      wound packing V58.30
        nonsurgical V58.30
        surgical V58.31
    repair of scarred tissue (following
      healed injury or operation)
        V51.8
    reprogramming of cardiac
      pacemaker V53.31
    respirator [ventilator] dependence
      during
        mechanical failure V46.14
        power failure V46.12
      for weaning V46.13
    restoration of organ continuity
      (poststerilization) (tuboplasty)
      (vasoplasty) V26.0
    Rh typing V72.86
    routine infant and child vision and
      hearing testing V20.2   ◄
    sensitivity test - *see also* Test, skin
      allergy NEC V72.7
      bacterial disease NEC V74.9
      Dick V74.8
      Kveim V82.89
      Mantoux V74.1
      mycotic infection NEC V75.4
      parasitic disease NEC V75.8
      Schick V74.3
      Schultz-Charlton V74.8
    social service (agency) referral or
      evaluation V63.8
    speech(-language) therapy V57.3 ◄▥
    sterilization V25.2
    suspected disorder (ruled out)
      (without need for further
      care) - *see* Observation
    terminal care V66.7
    tests only - *see* Test
    therapeutic drug monitoring V58.83
    therapy
      blood transfusion, without
        reported diagnosis V58.2

Admission *(Continued)*
  for *(Continued)*
    therapy *(Continued)*
      breathing exercises V57.0
      chemotherapy, antineoplastic
        V58.11
        prophylactic NEC V07.39
        fluoride V07.31
      dialysis (intermittent) (treatment)
        extracorporeal V56.0
        peritoneal V56.8
        renal V56.0
        specified type NEC V56.8
      exercise (remedial) NEC V57.1
        breathing V57.0
      immunotherapy, antineoplastic
        V58.12
      long-term (current) drug use
        NEC V58.69
        antibiotics V58.62
        anticoagulants V58.61
        anti-inflammatories, non-
          steroidal (NSAID) V58.64
        antiplatelets V58.63
        antithrombotics V58.63
        aspirin V58.66
        high-risk medications NEC
          V58.69
        insulin V58.67
        methadone V58.69
        opiate analgesic V58.69
        steroids V58.65
      occupational V57.21
      orthoptic V57.4
      physical NEC V57.1
      radiation V58.0
      speech(-language) V57.3   ◄▥
      vocational V57.22
    toilet or cleaning
      of artificial opening - *see*
        Attention to, artificial,
          opening
      of non-vascular catheter V58.82
      of vascular catheter V58.81
    tubal ligation V25.2
    tuboplasty for previous sterilization
      V26.0
    ultrasound, routine fetal V28.3
    vaccination, prophylactic (against)
      arthropod-borne virus, viral NEC
        V05.1
        disease NEC V05.1
        encephalitis V05.0
      Bacille Calmette Guérin (BCG)
        V03.2
      BCG V03.2
      chickenpox V05.4
      cholera alone V03.0
        with typhoid-paratyphoid
          (cholera + TAB) V06.0
      common cold V04.7
      dengue V05.1
      diphtheria alone V03.5
      diphtheria-tetanus-pertussis
        (DTP) (DTaP) V06.1
        with
          poliomyelitis (DTP polio)
            V06.3
          typhoid-paratyphoid
            (DTP + TAB) V06.2
      diphtheria-tetanus [Td] [DT]
        without pertussis V06.5
      disease (single) NEC V05.9
        bacterial NEC V03.9
          specified type NEC V03.89
        combinations NEC V06.9
          specified type NEC V06.8

◄ New   ◄▥ Revised   ~~deleted~~ Deleted   ● Use Additional Digit(s)   ▬ Omit code

Admission *(Continued)*
  for *(Continued)*
    vaccination, prophylactic *(Continued)*
      disease *(Continued)*
        specified type NEC V05.8
        viral NEC V04.89
      encephalitis, viral, arthropod-
          borne V05.0
      Hemophilus influenzae, type B
          [Hib] V03.81
      hepatitis, viral V05.3
      human papillomavirus (HPV)
          V04.89
      immune sera (gamma globulin)
          V07.2
      influenza V04.81
        with
          Streptococcus pneumoniae
              [pneumococcus] V06.6
      Leishmaniasis V05.2
      measles alone V04.2
      measles-mumps-rubella (MMR)
          V06.4
      mumps alone V04.6
        with measles and rubella
            (MMR) V06.4
      not done because of
          contraindication V64.09
      pertussis alone V03.6
      plague V03.3
      pneumonia V03.82
      poliomyelitis V04.0
        with diphtheria-tetanus-
            pertussis (DTP polio)
            V06.3
      rabies V04.5
      respiratory syncytial virus (RSV)
          V04.82
      rubella alone V04.3
        with measles and mumps
            (MMR) V06.4
      smallpox V04.1
      specified type NEC V05.8
      Streptococcus pneumoniae
          [pneumococcus] V03.82
        with
          influenza V06.6
      tetanus toxoid alone V03.7
        with diphtheria [Td] [DT] V06.5
            and pertussis (DTP) (DTaP)
            V06.1
      tuberculosis (BCG) V03.2
      tularemia V03.4
      typhoid alone V03.1
        with diphtheria-tetanus-
            pertussis (TAB + DTP)
            V06.2
      typhoid-paratyphoid alone (TAB)
          V03.1
      typhus V05.8
      varicella (chicken pox) V05.4
      viral encephalitis, arthropod-
          borne V05.0
      viral hepatitis V05.3
      yellow fever V04.4
    vasectomy V25.2
    vasoplasty for previous sterilization
        V26.0
    vision examination V72.0
    vocational therapy V57.22
    waiting period for admission to
        other facility V63.2
      undergoing social agency
          investigation V63.8
    well baby and child care V20.2
    x-ray of chest
      for suspected tuberculosis V71.2
      routine V72.5

Adnexitis (suppurative) *(see also* Salpingo-
    oophoritis) 614.2
Adolescence NEC V21.2
Adoption
  agency referral V68.89
  examination V70.3
  held for V68.89
Adrenal gland - *see* condition
Adrenalism 255.9
  tuberculous *(see also* Tuberculosis)
      017.6●
Adrenalitis, adrenitis 255.8
  meningococcal hemorrhagic 036.3
Adrenarche, precocious 259.1
Adrenocortical syndrome 255.2
Adrenogenital syndrome (acquired)
    (congenital) 255.2
  iatrogenic, fetus or newborn 760.79
Adrenoleukodystrophy 277.86
  neonatal 277.86
  x-linked 277.86
Adrenomyeloneuropathy 277.86
Adventitious bursa - *see* Bursitis
Adynamia (episodica) (hereditary)
    (periodic) 359.3
Adynamic
  ileus or intestine *(see also* Ileus) 560.1
  ureter 753.22
Aeration lung, imperfect, newborn 770.5
Aerobullosis 993.3
Aerocele - *see* Embolism, air
Aerodermectasia
  subcutaneous (traumatic) 958.7
    surgical 998.81
  surgical 998.81
Aerodontalgia 993.2
Aeroembolism 993.3
Aerogenes capsulatus infection *(see also*
    Gangrene, gas) 040.0
Aero-otitis media 993.0
Aerophagy, aerophagia 306.4
  psychogenic 306.4
Aerosinusitis 993.1
Aerotitis 993.0
Affection, affections - *see also* Disease
  sacroiliac (joint), old 724.6
  shoulder region NEC 726.2
Afibrinogenemia 286.3
  acquired 286.6
  congenital 286.3
  postpartum 666.3●
African
  sleeping sickness 086.5
  tick fever 087.1
  trypanosomiasis 086.5
    Gambian 086.3
    Rhodesian 086.4
Aftercare V58.9
  amputation stump V54.89
  artificial openings - *see* Attention to,
      artificial, opening
  blood transfusion without reported
      diagnosis V58.2
  breathing exercise V57.0
  cardiac device V53.39
    defibrillator, automatic implantable
        V53.32
    pacemaker V53.31
      carotid sinus V53.39
  carotid sinus pacemaker V53.39
  cerebral ventricle (communicating)
      shunt V53.01
  chemotherapy (oral) (intravenous)
      session (adjunctive)
      (maintenance) V58.11   ◀▥
  defibrillator, automatic implantable
      cardiac V53.32

Aftercare *(Continued)*
  exercise (remedial) (therapeutic) V57.1
    breathing V57.0
  extracorporeal dialysis (intermittent)
      (treatment) V56.0
  following surgery NEC V58.49
    for
      injury V58.43
      neoplasm V58.42
      organ transplant V58.44
      trauma V58.43
    joint replacement V54.81
    of
      circulatory system V58.73
      digestive system V58.75
      genital organs V58.76
      genitourinary system V58.76
      musculoskeletal system V58.78
      nervous system V58.72
      oral cavity V58.75
      respiratory system V58.74
      sense organs V58.71
      skin V58.77
      subcutaneous tissue V58.77
      teeth V58.75
      urinary system V58.76
    spinal - *see* Aftercare, following
        surgery, of, specified body
        system
    wound closure, planned V58.41
  fracture V54.9
    healing V54.89
      pathologic
        ankle V54.29
        arm V54.20
          lower V54.22
          upper V54.21
        finger V54.29
        foot V54.29
        hand V54.29
        hip V54.23
        leg V54.24
          lower V54.26
          upper V54.25
        pelvis V54.29
        specified site NEC V54.29
        toe(s) V54.29
        vertebrae V54.27
        wrist V54.29
      traumatic
        ankle V54.19
        arm V54.10
          lower V54.12
          upper V54.11
        finger V54.19
        foot V54.19
        hand V54.19
        hip V54.13
        leg V54.14
          lower V54.16
          upper V54.15
        pelvis V54.19
        specified site NEC V54.19
        toe(s) V54.19
        vertebrae V54.17
        wrist V54.19
    removal of
      external fixation device V54.89
      internal fixation device V54.01
    specified care NEC V54.89
  gait training V57.1
    for use of artificial limb(s) V57.81
  internal fixation device V54.09
  involving
    dialysis (intermittent) (treatment)
      extracorporeal V56.0
      peritoneal V56.8
      renal V56.0

Aftercare (Continued)
  involving (Continued)
    gait training V57.1
      for use of artificial limb(s) V57.81
    growth rod
      adjustment V54.02
      lengthening V54.02
    internal fixation device V54.09
    orthoptic training V57.4
    orthotic training V57.81
    radiotherapy session V58.0
    removal of
      drains V58.49
      dressings
        wound V58.30
          nonsurgical V58.30
          surgical V58.31
      fixation device
        external V54.89
        internal V54.01
      fracture plate V54.01
      nonsurgical wound dressing
        V58.30
      pins V54.01
      plaster cast V54.89
      rods V54.01
      screws V54.01
      staples V58.32
      surgical wound dressings V58.31
      sutures V58.32
      traction device, external V54.89
      wound packing V58.30
        nonsurgical V58.30
        surgical V58.31
  neuropacemaker (brain) (peripheral
    nerve) (spinal cord) V53.02
  occupational therapy V57.21
  orthodontic V58.5
  orthopedic V54.9
    change of external fixation or
      traction device V54.89
    following joint replacement V54.81
    internal fixation device V54.09
    removal of fixation device
      external V54.89
      internal V54.01
    specified care NEC V54.89
  orthoptic training V57.4
  orthotic training V57.81
  pacemaker
    brain V53.02
    cardiac V53.31
    carotid sinus V53.39
    peripheral nerve V53.02
    spinal cord V53.02
  peritoneal dialysis (intermittent)
    (treatment) V56.8
  physical therapy NEC V57.1
    breathing exercises V57.0
  radiotherapy session V58.0
  rehabilitation procedure V57.9
    breathing exercises V57.0
    multiple types V57.89
    occupational V57.21
    orthoptic V57.4
    orthotic V57.81
    physical therapy NEC V57.1
    remedial exercises V57.1
    specified type NEC V57.89
    speech(-language) V57.3   ◄▦
    therapeutic exercises V57.1
    vocational V57.22
  renal dialysis (intermittent) (treatment)
    V56.0

Aftercare (Continued)
  specified type NEC V58.89
    removal of non-vascular cathether
      V58.82
    removal of vascular catheter V58.81
  speech(-language) therapy V57.3   ◄▦
  stump, amputation V54.89
  vocational rehabilitation V57.22
After-cataract 366.50
  obscuring vision 366.53
  specified type, not obscuring vision
    366.52
Agalactia 676.4●
Agammaglobulinemia 279.00
  with lymphopenia 279.2
  acquired (primary) (secondary) 279.06
  Bruton's X-linked 279.04
  infantile sex-linked (Bruton's)
    (congenital) 279.04
  Swiss-type 279.2
Aganglionosis (bowel) (colon) 751.3
Age (old) (see also Senile) 797
Agenesis - see also Absence, by site,
    congenital
  acoustic nerve 742.8
  adrenal (gland) 759.1
  alimentary tract (complete) (partial)
    NEC 751.8
    lower 751.2
    upper 750.8
  anus, anal (canal) 751.2
  aorta 747.22
  appendix 751.2
  arm (complete) (partial) (see also
    Deformity, reduction, upper limb)
    755.20
  artery (peripheral) NEC (see also
    Anomaly, peripheral vascular
    system) 747.60
    brain 747.81
    coronary 746.85
    pulmonary 747.3
    umbilical 747.5
  auditory (canal) (external) 744.01
  auricle (ear) 744.01
  bile, biliary duct or passage 751.61
  bone NEC 756.9
  brain 740.0
    specified part 742.2
  breast 757.6
  bronchus 748.3
  canaliculus lacrimalis 743.65
  carpus NEC (see also Deformity,
    reduction, upper limb) 755.28
  cartilage 756.9
  cecum 751.2
  cerebellum 742.2
  cervix 752.49
  chin 744.89
  cilia 743.63
  circulatory system, part NEC 747.89
  clavicle 755.51
  clitoris 752.49
  coccyx 756.13
  colon 751.2
  corpus callosum 742.2
  cricoid cartilage 748.3
  diaphragm (with hernia) 756.6
  digestive organ(s) or tract (complete)
    (partial) NEC 751.8
    lower 751.2
    upper 750.8
  ductus arteriosus 747.89
  duodenum 751.1

Agenesis (Continued)
  ear NEC 744.09
    auricle 744.01
    lobe 744.21
  ejaculatory duct 752.89
  endocrine (gland) NEC 759.2
  epiglottis 748.3
  esophagus 750.3
  Eustachian tube 744.24
  extrinsic muscle, eye 743.69
  eye 743.00
    adnexa 743.69
  eyelid (fold) 743.62
  face
    bones NEC 756.0
    specified part NEC 744.89
  fallopian tube 752.19
  femur NEC (see also Absence, femur,
    congenital) 755.34
  fibula NEC (see also Absence, fibula,
    congenital) 755.37
  finger NEC (see also Absence, finger,
    congenital) 755.29
  foot (complete) (see also Deformity,
    reduction, lower limb) 755.31
  gallbladder 751.69
  gastric 750.8
  genitalia, genital (organ)
    female 752.89
      external 752.49
      internal NEC 752.89
    male 752.89
      penis 752.69
  glottis 748.3
  gonadal 758.6
  hair 757.4
  hand (complete) (see also Deformity,
    reduction, upper limb) 755.21
  heart 746.89
    valve NEC 746.89
      aortic 746.89
      mitral 746.89
      pulmonary 746.01
  hepatic 751.69
  humerus NEC (see also Absence,
    humerus, congenital) 755.24
  hymen 752.49
  ileum 751.1
  incus 744.04
  intestine (small) 751.1
    large 751.2
  iris (dilator fibers) 743.45
  jaw 524.09
  jejunum 751.1
  kidney(s) (partial) (unilateral) 753.0
  labium (majus) (minus) 752.49
  labyrinth, membranous 744.05
  lacrimal apparatus (congenital) 743.65
  larynx 748.3
  leg NEC (see also Deformity, reduction,
    lower limb) 755.30
  lens 743.35
  limb (complete) (partial) (see also
    Deformity, reduction) 755.4
    lower NEC 755.30
    upper 755.20
  lip 750.26
  liver 751.69
  lung (bilateral) (fissures) (lobe)
    (unilateral) 748.5
  mandible 524.09
  maxilla 524.09
  metacarpus NEC 755.28
  metatarsus NEC 755.38

Agenesis (Continued)
muscle (any) 756.81
musculoskeletal system NEC 756.9
nail(s) 757.5
neck, part 744.89
nerve 742.8
nervous system, part NEC 742.8
nipple 757.6
nose 748.1
nuclear 742.8
organ
of Corti 744.05
or site not listed - see Anomaly,
specified type NEC
osseous meatus (ear) 744.03
ovary 752.0
oviduct 752.19
pancreas 751.7
parathyroid (gland) 759.2
patella 755.64
pelvic girdle (complete) (partial) 755.69
penis 752.69
pericardium 746.89
perineal body 756.81
pituitary (gland) 759.2
prostate 752.89
pulmonary
artery 747.3
trunk 747.3
vein 747.49
punctum lacrimale 743.65
radioulnar NEC (see also Absence,
forearm, congenital) 755.25
radius NEC (see also Absence, radius,
congenital) 755.26
rectum 751.2
renal 753.0
respiratory organ NEC 748.9
rib 756.3
roof of orbit 742.0
round ligament 752.89
sacrum 756.13
salivary gland 750.21
scapula 755.59
scrotum 752.89
seminal duct or tract 752.89
septum
atrial 745.69
between aorta and pulmonary
artery 745.0
ventricular 745.3
shoulder girdle (complete) (partial)
755.59
skull (bone) 756.0
with
anencephalus 740.0
encephalocele 742.0
hydrocephalus 742.3
with spina bifida (see also
Spina bifida) 741.0●
microcephalus 742.1
spermatic cord 752.89
spinal cord 742.59
spine 756.13
lumbar 756.13
isthmus 756.11
pars articularis 756.11
spleen 759.0
sternum 756.3
stomach 750.7
tarsus NEC 755.38
tendon 756.81
testicular 752.89
testis 752.89

Agenesis (Continued)
thymus (gland) 759.2
thyroid (gland) 243
cartilage 748.3
tibia NEC (see also Absence, tibia,
congenital) 755.36
tibiofibular NEC 755.35
toe (complete) (partial) (see also
Absence, toe, congenital) 755.39
tongue 750.11
trachea (cartilage) 748.3
ulna NEC (see also Absence, ulna,
congenital) 755.27
ureter 753.4
urethra 753.8
urinary tract NEC 753.8
uterus 752.3
uvula 750.26
vagina 752.49
vas deferens 752.89
vein(s) (peripheral) NEC (see also
Anomaly, peripheral vascular
system) 747.60
brain 747.81
great 747.49
portal 747.49
pulmonary 747.49
vena cava (inferior) (superior) 747.49
vermis of cerebellum 742.2
vertebra 756.13
lumbar 756.13
isthmus 756.11
pars articularis 756.11
vulva 752.49
Ageusia (see also Disturbance, sensation)
781.1
Aggressiveness 301.3
Aggressive outburst (see also Disturbance,
conduct) 312.0●
in children or adolescents 313.9
Aging skin 701.8
Agitated - see condition
Agitation 307.9
catatonic (see also Schizophrenia) 295.2●
Aglossia (congenital) 750.11
Aglycogenosis 271.0
Agnail (finger) (with lymphangitis) 681.02
Agnosia (body image) (tactile) 784.69
verbal 784.69
auditory 784.69
secondary to organic lesion 784.69
developmental 315.8
secondary to organic lesion 784.69
visual 368.16
object 368.16
suspected
Agoraphobia 300.22
with panic disorder 300.21
Agrammatism 784.69
Agranulocytopenia (see also
Agranulocytosis) 288.09
Agranulocytosis (angina) (see also
Neutropenia) 288.09 ◀▬
chronic 288.09
cyclical 288.02
due to infection 288.04 ◀
genetic 288.01
infantile 288.01
periodic 288.02
pernicious 288.09
Agraphia (absolute) 784.69
with alexia 784.61
developmental 315.39
Agrypnia (see also Insomnia) 780.52

Ague (see also Malaria) 084.6
brass-founders' 985.8
dumb 084.6
tertian 084.1
Agyria 742.2
Ahumada-del Castillo syndrome
(nonpuerperal galactorrhea and
amenorrhea) 253.1
AIDS 042
AIDS-associated retrovirus (disease)
(illness) 042
infection - see Human
immunodeficiency virus,
infection
AIDS-associated virus (disease) (illness)
042
infection - see Human
immunodeficiency virus,
infection
AIDS-like disease (illness) (syndrome)
042
AIDS-related complex 042
AIDS-related conditions 042
AIDS-related virus (disease) (illness) 042
infection - see Human
immunodeficiency virus,
infection
AIDS virus (disease) (illness) 042
infection - see Human
immunodeficiency virus,
infection
Ailment, heart - see Disease, heart
Ailurophobia 300.29
AIN I [anal intraepithelial neoplasia I]
(histologically confirmed) 569.44
AIN II [anal intraepithelial neoplasia II]
(histologically confirmed) 569.44
AIN III [anal intraepithelial neoplasia III]
230.6
anal canal 230.5
Ainhum (disease) 136.0
Air
anterior mediastinum 518.1
compressed, disease 993.3
embolism (any site) (artery) (cerebral)
958.0
with
abortion - see Abortion, by type,
with embolism
ectopic pregnancy (see also
categories 633.0-633.9) 639.6
molar pregnancy (see also
categories 630-632) 639.6
due to implanted device - see
Complications, due to
(presence of) any device,
implant, or graft classified to
996.0-996.5 NEC
following
abortion 639.6
ectopic or molar pregnancy 639.6
infusion, perfusion, or
transfusion 999.1
in pregnancy, childbirth, or
puerperium 673.0●
traumatic 958.0
hunger 786.09
psychogenic 306.1
leak (lung) (pulmonary) (thorax) 512.8
iatrogenic 512.1
postoperative 512.1
rarefied, effects of - see Effect, adverse,
high altitude
sickness 994.6

Airplane sickness 994.6
Akathisia, acathisia 781.0
  due to drugs 333.99
    neuroleptic-induced acute 333.99
Akinesia algeria 352.6
Akiyami 100.89
Akureyri disease (epidemic
    neuromyasthenia) 049.8
Alacrima (congenital) 743.65
Alactasia (hereditary) 271.3
Alagille syndrome 759.89
Alalia 784.3
  developmental 315.31
    receptive-expressive 315.32
  secondary to organic lesion 784.3
Alaninemia 270.8
Alastrim 050.1
Albarrán's disease (colibacilluria) 791.9
Albers-Schönberg's disease (marble
    bones) 756.52
Albert's disease 726.71
Albinism, albino (choroid) (cutaneous)
    (eye) (generalized) (isolated)
    (ocular) (oculocutaneous) (partial)
    270.2
Albinismus 270.2
Albright (-Martin) (-Bantam) disease
    (pseudohypoparathyroidism)
    275.49
Albright (-McCune) (-Sternberg)
    syndrome (osteitis fibrosa
    disseminata) 756.59
Albuminous - see Condition
Albuminuria, albuminuric (acute)
    (chronic) (subacute) 791.0
  Bence-Jones 791.0
  cardiac 785.9
  complicating pregnancy, childbirth, or
    puerperium 646.2●
    with hypertension - see Toxemia, of
      pregnancy
    affecting fetus or newborn 760.1
  cyclic 593.6
  gestational 646.2●
  gravidarum 646.2●
    with hypertension - see Toxemia, of
      pregnancy
    affecting fetus or newborn 760.1
  heart 785.9
  idiopathic 593.6
  orthostatic 593.6
  postural 593.6
  pre-eclamptic (mild) 642.4●
    affecting fetus or newborn 760.0
    severe 642.5●
      affecting fetus or newborn 760.0
  recurrent physiologic 593.6
  scarlatinal 034.1
Albumosuria 791.0
  Bence-Jones 791.0
  myelopathic (M9730/3) 203.0●
Alcaptonuria 270.2
Alcohol, alcoholic
  abstinence 291.81
  acute intoxication 305.0●
    with dependence 303.0●
  addiction (see also Alcoholism) 303.9●
    maternal
      with suspected fetal damage
        affecting management of
        pregnancy 655.4●
      affecting fetus or newborn 760.71
  amnestic disorder, persisting 291.1
  anxiety 291.89

Alcohol, alcoholic (Continued)
  brain syndrome, chronic 291.2
  cardiopathy 425.5
  chronic (see also Alcoholism) 303.9●
  cirrhosis (liver) 571.2
  delirium 291.0
    acute 291.0
    chronic 291.1
    tremens 291.0
    withdrawal 291.0
  dementia NEC 291.2
  deterioration 291.2
  drunkenness (simple) 305.0●
  hallucinosis (acute) 291.3
  induced
    circadian rhythm sleep disorder
      291.82
    hypersomnia 291.82
    insomnia 291.82
    mental disorder 291.9
      anxiety 291.89
      mood 291.89
      sexual 291.89
      sleep 291.82
      specified type 291.89
    parasomnia 291.82
    persisting
      amnestic disorder 291.1
      dementia 291.2
    psychotic disorder
      with
        delusions 291.5
        hallucinations 291.3
    sleep disorder 291.82
  insanity 291.9
  intoxication (acute) 305.0●
    with dependence 303.0●
    pathological 291.4
  jealousy 291.5
  Korsakoff's, Korsakov's, Korsakow's
    291.1
  liver NEC 571.3
    acute 571.1
    chronic 571.2
  mania (acute) (chronic) 291.9
  mood 291.89
  paranoia 291.5
  paranoid (type) psychosis 291.5
  pellagra 265.2
  poisoning, accidental (acute) NEC 980.9
    specified type of alcohol - see Table
      of Drugs and Chemicals
  psychosis (see also Psychosis, alcoholic)
    291.9
    Korsakoff's, Korsakov's, Korsakow's
      291.1
    polyneuritic 291.1
    with
      delusions 291.5
      hallucinations 291.3
  related disorder 291.9
  withdrawal symptoms, syndrome NEC
    291.81
    delirium 291.0
    hallucinosis 291.3
Alcoholism 303.9●

> Note 05   Use the following fifth-digit
> subclassification with category 303:
>
> 0   unspecified
> 1   continuous
> 2   episodic
> 3   in remission

Alcoholism (Continued)
  with psychosis (see also Psychosis,
    alcoholic) 291.9
  acute 303.0●
  chronic 303.9●
    with psychosis 291.9
  complicating pregnancy, childbirth, or
    puerperium 648.4●
    affecting fetus or newborn 760.71
  history V11.3
  Korsakoff's, Korsakov's, Korsakow's
    291.1
  suspected damage to fetus affecting
    management of pregnancy
    655.4●
Alder's anomaly or syndrome (leukocyte
    granulation anomaly) 288.2
Alder-Reilly anomaly (leukocyte
    granulation) 288.2
Aldosteronism (primary) 255.10
  congenital 255.10
  familial type I 255.11
  glucocorticoid-remediable 255.11
  secondary 255.14
Aldosteronoma (M8370/1) 237.2
Aldrich (-Wiskott) syndrome (eczema-
    thrombocytopenia) 279.12
Aleppo boil 085.1
Aleukemic - see condition
Aleukia
  congenital 288.09
  hemorrhagica 284.9
    acquired (secondary) 284.89
    congenital 284.09
    idiopathic 284.9
  splenica 289.4
Alexia (congenital) (developmental)
    315.01
  secondary to organic lesion 784.61
Algoneurodystrophy 733.7
Algophobia 300.29
Alibert's disease (mycosis fungoides)
    (M9700/3) 202.1●
Alibert-Bazin disease (M9700/3) 202.1●
Alice in Wonderland syndrome 293.89
Alienation, mental (see also Psychosis)
    298.9
Alkalemia 276.3
Alkalosis 276.3
  metabolic 276.3
    with respiratory acidosis 276.4
  respiratory 276.3
Alkaptonuria 270.2
Allen-Masters syndrome 620.6
Allergic bronchopulmonary aspergillosis
    518.6
Allergy, allergic (reaction) 995.3
  air-borne substance (see also Fever, hay)
    477.9
    specified allergen NEC 477.8
  alveolitis (extrinsic) 495.9
    due to
      Aspergillus clavatus 495.4
      cryptostroma corticale 495.6
      organisms (fungal, thermophilic
        actinomycete, other)
        growing in ventilation
        (air conditioning systems)
        495.7
    specified type NEC 495.8
  anaphylactic shock 999.4
    due to food - see Anaphylactic shock,
      due to, food
  angioneurotic edema 995.1

◀ New   ◀▥ Revised   ~~deleted~~ Deleted   ● Use Additional Digit(s)   ▨ Omit code

A

Allergy, allergic (Continued)
  animal (cat) (dog) (epidermal) 477.8
    dander 477.2
    hair 477.2
  arthritis (see also Arthritis, allergic)
      716.2●
  asthma - see Asthma
  bee sting (anaphylactic shock) 989.5
  biological - see Allergy, drug
  bronchial asthma - see Asthma
  conjunctivitis (eczematous) 372.14
  dander, animal (cat) (dog) 477.2
  dandruff 477.8
  dermatitis (venenata) - see Dermatitis
  diathesis V15.09
  drug, medicinal substance, and
      biological (any) (correct medicinal
      substance properly administered)
      (external) (internal) 995.27
    wrong substance given or taken
      NEC 977.9
    specified drug or substance - see
      Table of Drugs and
      Chemicals
  dust (house) (stock) 477.8
  eczema - see Eczema
  endophthalmitis 360.19
  epidermal (animal) 477.8
  existing dental restorative material
      525.66
  feathers 477.8
  food (any) (ingested) 693.1
    atopic 691.8
    in contact with skin 692.5
  gastritis 535.4●
  gastroenteritis 558.3
  gastrointestinal 558.3
  grain 477.0
  grass (pollen) 477.0
    asthma (see also Asthma) 493.0●
    hay fever 477.0
  hair, animal (cat) (dog) 477.2
  hay fever (grass) (pollen) (ragweed)
      (tree) (see also Fever, hay) 477.9
  history (of) V15.09
    to
      arachnid bite V15.06
      eggs V15.03
      food additives V15.05
      insect bite V15.06
      latex V15.07
      milk products V15.02
      nuts V15.05
        peanuts V15.01
      radiographic dye V15.08
      seafood V15.04
      specified food NEC V15.05
      spider bite V15.06
  horse serum - see Allergy, serum
  inhalant 477.9
    dust 477.8
    pollen 477.0
    specified allergen other than pollen
      477.8
  kapok 477.8
  medicine - see Allergy, drug
  migraine 339.00
  milk protein 558.3
  pannus 370.62
  pneumonia 518.3
  pollen (any) (hay fever) 477.0
    asthma (see also Asthma) 493.0●
  primrose 477.0
  primula 477.0
  purpura 287.0

Allergy, allergic (Continued)
  ragweed (pollen) (Senecio jacobae)
      477.0
    asthma (see also Asthma) 493.0●
    hay fever 477.0
  respiratory (see also Allergy, inhalant)
      477.9
    due to
      drug - see Allergy, drug
      food - see Allergy, food
  rhinitis (see also Fever, hay) 477.9
    due to food 477.1
  rose 477.0
  Senecio jacobae 477.0
  serum (prophylactic) (therapeutic)
      999.5
    anaphylactic shock 999.4
  shock (anaphylactic) (due to adverse
      effect of correct medicinal
      substance properly administered)
      995.0
    food - see Anaphylactic shock, due
      to, food
    from serum or immunization 999.5
      anaphylactic 999.4
  sinusitis (see also Fever, hay) 477.9
  skin reaction 692.9
    specified substance - see Dermatitis,
      due to
  tree (any) (hay fever) (pollen) 477.0
    asthma (see also Asthma) 493.0●
  upper respiratory (see also Fever, hay)
      477.9
  urethritis 597.89
  urticaria 708.0
  vaccine - see Allergy, serum
Allescheriosis 117.6
Alligator skin disease (ichthyosis
    congenita) 757.1
  acquired 701.1
Allocheiria, allochiria (see also
    Disturbance, sensation) 782.0
Almeida's disease (Brazilian
    blastomycosis) 116.1
Alopecia (atrophicans) (pregnancy)
    (premature) (senile) 704.00
  adnata 757.4
  areata 704.01
  celsi 704.01
  cicatrisata 704.09
  circumscripta 704.01
  congenital, congenitalis 757.4
  disseminata 704.01
  effluvium (telogen) 704.02
  febrile 704.09
  generalisata 704.09
  hereditaria 704.09
  marginalis 704.01
  mucinosa 704.09
  postinfectional 704.09
  seborrheica 704.09
  specific 091.82
  syphilitic (secondary) 091.82
  telogen effluvium 704.02
  totalis 704.09
  toxica 704.09
  universalis 704.09
  x-ray 704.09
Alpers' disease 330.8
Alpha-lipoproteinemia 272.4
Alpha thalassemia 282.49
Alphos 696.1
Alpine sickness 993.2
Alport's syndrome (hereditary hematuria-
    nephropathy-deafness) 759.89

ALPS (autoimmune lymphoproliferative
    syndrome) 279.41 ◄
ALTE (apparent life threatening event) in
    newborn and infant 799.82 ◄
Alteration (of), altered
  awareness 780.09
    transient 780.02
  consciousness 780.09
    persistent vegetative state 780.03
    transient 780.02
  mental status 780.97
    amnesia (retrograde) 780.93
    memory loss 780.93
Alternaria (infection) 118
Alternating - see condition
Altitude, high (effects) - see Effect,
    adverse, high altitude
Aluminosis (of lung) 503
Alvarez syndrome (transient cerebral
    ischemia) 435.9
Alveolar capillary block syndrome 516.3
Alveolitis
  allergic (extrinsic) 495.9
    due to organisms (fungal,
      thermophilic actinomycete,
      other) growing in ventilation
      (air conditioning systems) 495.7
    specified type NEC 495.8
  due to
    Aspergillus clavatus 495.4
    Cryptostroma corticale 495.6
  fibrosing (chronic) (cryptogenic) (lung)
      516.3
    idiopathic 516.3
    rheumatoid 714.81
  jaw 526.5
  sicca dolorosa 526.5
Alveolus, alveolar - see condition
Alymphocytosis (pure) 279.2
Alymphoplasia, thymic 279.2
Alzheimer's
  dementia (senile)
    with behavioral disturbance 331.0
      [294.11]
    without behavioral disturbance
      331.0 [294.10]
  disease or sclerosis 331.0
    with dementia - see Alzheimer's,
      dementia
Amastia (see also Absence, breast) 611.89
Amaurosis (acquired) (congenital) (see
    also Blindness) 369.00
  fugax 362.34
  hysterical 300.11
  Leber's (congenital) 362.76
  tobacco 377.34
  uremic - see Uremia
Amaurotic familial idiocy (infantile)
    (juvenile) (late) 330.1
Ambisexual 752.7
Amblyopia (acquired) (congenital)
    (partial) 368.00
  color 368.59
    acquired 368.55
  deprivation 368.02
  ex anopsia 368.00
  hysterical 300.11
  nocturnal 368.60
    vitamin A deficiency 264.5
  refractive 368.03
  strabismic 368.01
  suppression 368.01
  tobacco 377.34
  toxic NEC 377.34
  uremic - see Uremia

Ameba, amebic (histolytica) - *see also*
　Amebiasis
　abscess 006.3
　　bladder 006.8
　　brain (with liver and lung abscess)
　　　006.5
　　liver 006.3
　　　with
　　　　brain abscess (and lung
　　　　　abscess) 006.5
　　　　lung abscess 006.4
　　lung (with liver abscess) 006.4
　　　with brain abscess 006.5
　　seminal vesicle 006.8
　　spleen 006.8
　carrier (suspected of) V02.2
　meningoencephalitis
　　due to Naegleria (gruberi) 136.29
　　primary 136.29
Amebiasis NEC 006.9
　with
　　brain abscess (with liver or lung
　　　abscess) 006.5
　　liver abscess (without mention of
　　　brain or lung abscess) 006.3
　　lung abscess (with liver abscess)
　　　006.4
　　　with brain abscess 006.5
　acute 006.0
　bladder 006.8
　chronic 006.1
　cutaneous 006.6
　cutis 006.6
　due to organism other than Entamoeba
　　histolytica 007.8
　hepatic (*see also* Abscess, liver, amebic)
　　006.3
　nondysenteric 006.2
　seminal vesicle 006.8
　specified
　　organism NEC 007.8
　　site NEC 006.8
Ameboma 006.8
Amelia 755.4
　lower limb 755.31
　upper limb 755.21
Ameloblastoma (M9310/0) 213.1
　jaw (bone) (lower) 213.1
　　upper 213.0
　long bones (M9261/3) - *see* Neoplasm,
　　bone, malignant
　malignant (M9310/3) 170.1
　　jaw (bone) (lower) 170.1
　　　upper 170.0
　mandible 213.1
　tibial (M9261/3) 170.7
Amelogenesis imperfecta 520.5
　nonhereditaria (segmentalis) 520.4
Amenorrhea (primary) (secondary) 626.0
　due to ovarian dysfunction 256.8
　hyperhormonal 256.8
Amentia (*see also* Retardation, mental) 319
　Meynert's (nonalcoholic) 294.0
　　alcoholic 291.1
　nevoid 759.6
American
　leishmaniasis 085.5
　mountain tick fever 066.1
　trypanosomiasis - *see* Trypanosomiasis,
　　American
Ametropia (*see also* Disorder,
　accommodation) 367.9
Amianthosis 501
Amimia 784.69

Amino acid
　deficiency 270.9
　　anemia 281.4
　metabolic disorder (*see also* Disorder,
　　amino acid) 270.9
Aminoaciduria 270.9
　imidazole 270.5
Amnesia (retrograde) 780.93
　auditory 784.69
　　developmental 315.31
　　secondary to organic lesion 784.69
　dissociative 300.12
　hysterical or dissociative type 300.12
　psychogenic 300.12
　transient global 437.7
Amnestic (confabulatory) syndrome 294.0
　alcohol-induced persisting 291.1
　drug-induced persisting 292.83
　posttraumatic 294.0
Amniocentesis screening (for) V28.2
　alphafetoprotein level, raised V28.1
　chromosomal anomalies V28.0
Amnion, amniotic - *see also* condition
　nodosum 658.8●
Amnionitis (complicating pregnancy)
　658.4●
　affecting fetus or newborn 762.7
Amoral trends 301.7
Amotio retinae (*see also* Detachment,
　retina) 361.9
Ampulla
　lower esophagus 530.89
　phrenic 530.89
Amputation
　any part of fetus, to facilitate delivery
　　763.89
　cervix (supravaginal) (uteri) 622.8
　　in pregnancy or childbirth 654.6●
　　　affecting fetus or newborn
　　　　763.89
　clitoris - *see* Wound, open, clitoris
　congenital
　　lower limb 755.31
　　upper limb 755.21
　neuroma (traumatic) - *see also* Injury,
　　nerve, by site
　　surgical complication (late) 997.61
　penis - *see* Amputation, traumatic,
　　penis
　status (without complication) - *see*
　　Absence, by site, acquired
　stump (surgical) (posttraumatic)
　　abnormal, painful, or with
　　　complication (late) 997.60
　　healed or old NEC - *see also* Absence,
　　　by site, acquired
　　　lower V49.70
　　　upper V49.60
　traumatic (complete) (partial)

Note 06　"Complicated" includes
traumatic amputation with delayed
healing, delayed treatment, foreign
body, or infection.

　　arm 887.4
　　　at or above elbow 887.2
　　　　complicated 887.3
　　　below elbow 887.0
　　　　complicated 887.1
　　　both (bilateral) (any level(s))
　　　　887.6
　　　　complicated 887.7
　　　complicated 887.5

Amputation (*Continued*)
　traumatic (*Continued*)
　　finger(s) (one or both hands) 886.0
　　　with thumb(s) 885.0
　　　　complicated 885.1
　　　complicated 886.1
　　foot (except toe(s) only) 896.0
　　　and other leg 897.6
　　　　complicated 897.7
　　　both (bilateral) 896.2
　　　　complicated 896.3
　　　complicated 896.1
　　toe(s) only (one or both feet) 895.0
　　　complicated 895.1
　　genital organ(s) (external) NEC
　　　878.8
　　　complicated 878.9
　　hand (except finger(s) only) 887.0
　　　and other arm 887.6
　　　　complicated 887.7
　　　both (bilateral) 887.6
　　　　complicated 887.7
　　　complicated 887.1
　　finger(s) (one or both hands)
　　　886.0
　　　with thumb(s) 885.0
　　　　complicated 885.1
　　　complicated 886.1
　　thumb(s) (with fingers of either
　　　hand) 885.0
　　　complicated 885.1
　　head 874.9
　　late effect - *see* Late, effects (of),
　　　amputation
　　leg 897.4
　　　and other foot 897.6
　　　　complicated 897.7
　　　at or above knee 897.2
　　　　complicated 897.3
　　　below knee 897.0
　　　　complicated 897.1
　　　both (bilateral) 897.6
　　　　complicated 897.7
　　　complicated 897.5
　　lower limb(s) except toe(s) - *see*
　　　Amputation, traumatic, leg
　　nose - *see* Wound, open, nose
　　penis 878.0
　　　complicated 878.1
　　sites other than limbs - *see* Wound,
　　　open, by site
　　thumb(s) (with finger(s) of either
　　　hand) 885.0
　　　complicated 885.1
　　toe(s) (one or both feet) 895.0
　　　complicated 895.1
　　upper limb(s) - *see* Amputation,
　　　traumatic, arm
Amputee (bilateral) (old) - *see also*
　Absence, by site, acquired V49.70
Amusia 784.69
　developmental 315.39
　secondary to organic lesion 784.69
Amyelencephalus 740.0
Amyelia 742.59
Amygdalitis - *see* Tonsillitis
Amygdalolith 474.8
Amyloid disease or degeneration 277.30
　heart 277.39 *[425.7]*
Amyloidosis (familial) (general)
　(generalized) (genetic) (primary)
　277.30
　with lung involvement 277.39 *[517.8]*
　cardiac, hereditary 277.39

◀ New　　◀▥ Revised　　~~deleted~~ Deleted　　● Use Additional Digit(s)　　▦ Omit code

Amyloidosis (Continued)
  heart 277.39 [425.7]
  nephropathic 277.39 [583.81]
  neuropathic (Portuguese) (Swiss)
    277.39 [357.4]
  pulmonary 277.39 [517.8]
  secondary 277.39
  systemic, inherited 277.39
Amylopectinosis (brancher enzyme
  deficiency) 271.0
Amylophagia 307.52
Amyoplasia, congenita 756.89
Amyotonia 728.2
  congenita 358.8
Amyotrophia, amyotrophy, amyotrophic
  728.2
  congenita 756.89
  diabetic 250.6● [353.5]
    due to secondary diabetes 249.6●
      [353.5]
  lateral sclerosis (syndrome)
    335.20
  neuralgic 353.5
  sclerosis (lateral) 335.20
  spinal progressive 335.21
Anacidity, gastric 536.0
  psychogenic 306.4
Anaerosis of newborn 770.88
Analbuminemia 273.8
Analgesia (see also Anesthesia) 782.0
Analphalipoproteinemia 272.5
Anaphylactic shock or reaction (correct
  substance properly administered)
  995.0
  due to
    food 995.60
      additives 995.66
      crustaceans 995.62
      eggs 995.68
      fish 995.65
      fruits 995.63
      milk products 995.67
      nuts (tree) 995.64
      peanuts 995.61
      seeds 995.64
      specified NEC 995.69
      tree nuts 995.64
      vegetables 995.63
    immunization 999.4
    overdose or wrong substance given
      or taken 977.9
      specified drug - see Table of
        Drugs and Chemicals
    serum 999.4
  following sting(s) 989.5
  purpura 287.0
  serum 999.4
Anaphylactoid shock or reaction - see
  Anaphylactic shock
Anaphylaxis - see Anaphylactic shock
Anaplasia, cervix 622.10
Anarthria 784.51 ◀━━
Anarthritic rheumatoid disease
  446.5
Anasarca 782.3
  cardiac (see also Failure, heart)
    428.0
  fetus or newborn 778.0
  lung 514
  nutritional 262
  pulmonary 514
  renal (see also Nephrosis) 581.9
Anaspadias 752.62

Anastomosis
  aneurysmal - see Aneurysm
  arteriovenous, congenital NEC (see also
    Anomaly, arteriovenous) 747.60
    ruptured, of brain (see also
      Hemorrhage, subarachnoid)
      430
  intestinal 569.89
    complicated NEC 997.4
      involving urinary tract 997.5
  retinal and choroidal vessels 743.58
    acquired 362.17
Anatomical narrow angle (glaucoma)
  365.02
Ancylostoma (infection) (infestation)
  126.9
  americanus 126.1
  braziliense 126.2
  caninum 126.8
  ceylanicum 126.3
  duodenale 126.0
  Necator americanus 126.1
Ancylostomiasis (intestinal) 126.9
  ancylostoma
    americanus 126.1
    caninum 126.8
    ceylanicum 126.3
    duodenale 126.0
  braziliense 126.2
  Necator americanus 126.1
Anders' disease or syndrome (adiposis
  tuberosa simplex) 272.8
Andersen's glycogen storage disease
  271.0
Anderson's disease 272.7
Andes disease 993.2
Andrews' disease (bacterid) 686.8
Androblastoma (M8630/1)
  benign (M8630/0)
    specified site - see Neoplasm, by site,
      benign
    unspecified site
      female 220
      male 222.0
  malignant (M8630/3)
    specified site - see Neoplasm, by site,
      malignant
    unspecified site
      female 183.0
      male 186.9
  specified site - see Neoplasm, by site,
    uncertain behavior
  tubular (M8640/0)
    with lipid storage (M8641/0)
      specified site - see Neoplasm, by
        site, benign
      unspecified site
        female 220
        male 222.0
    specified site - see Neoplasm, by site,
      benign
    unspecified site
      female 220
      male 222.0
  unspecified site
    female 236.2
    male 236.4
Android pelvis 755.69
  with disproportion (fetopelvic) 653.3●
    affecting fetus or newborn 763.1
    causing obstructed labor 660.1●
      affecting fetus or newborn 763.1
Anectasis, pulmonary (newborn or fetus)
  770.5

Anemia 285.9
  with
    disorder of
      anaerobic glycolysis 282.3
      pentose phosphate pathway 282.2
    koilonychia 280.9
  6-phosphogluconic dehydrogenase
    deficiency 282.2
  achlorhydric 280.9
  achrestic 281.8
  Addison's (pernicious) 281.0
  Addison-Biermer (pernicious) 281.0
  agranulocytic 288.09
  amino acid deficiency 281.4
  antineoplastic chemotherapy induced
    285.3 ◀
  aplastic 284.9
    acquired (secondary) 284.89
    congenital 284.01
    constitutional 284.01
    due to
      antineoplastic chemotherapy
        284.89
      chronic systemic disease 284.89
      drugs 284.89
      infection 284.89
      radiation 284.89
    idiopathic 284.9
    myxedema 244.9
    of or complicating pregnancy 648.2●
    red cell (acquired) (adult) (with
      thymoma) 284.81
      congenital 284.01
      pure 284.01
    specified type NEC 284.89
    toxic (paralytic) 284.89
  aregenerative 284.9
    congenital 284.01
  asiderotic 280.9
  atypical (primary) 285.9
  autohemolysis of Selwyn and Dacie
    (type I) 282.2
  autoimmune hemolytic 283.0
  Baghdad Spring 282.2
  Balantidium coli 007.0
  Biermer's (pernicious) 281.0
  blood loss (chronic) 280.0
    acute 285.1
  bothriocephalus 123.4
  brickmakers' (see also Ancylostomiasis)
    126.9
  cerebral 437.8
  childhood 282.9
  chlorotic 280.9
  chronica congenita aregenerativa
    284.01
  chronic simple 281.9
  combined system disease NEC 281.0
    [336.2]
    due to dietary deficiency 281.1 [336.2]
  complicating pregnancy or childbirth
    648.2●
  congenital (following fetal blood loss)
    776.5
    aplastic 284.01
    due to isoimmunization NEC 773.2
    Heinz-body 282.7
    hereditary hemolytic NEC 282.9
    nonspherocytic
      type I 282.2
      type II 282.3
    pernicious 281.0
    spherocytic (see also Spherocytosis)
      282.0

Anemia (*Continued*)
  Cooley's (erythroblastic) 282.49
  crescent - *see* Disease, sickle-cell
  cytogenic 281.0
  Dacie's (nonspherocytic)
    type I 282.2
    type II 282.3
  Davidson's (refractory) 284.9
  deficiency 281.9
    2, 3 diphosphoglycurate mutase 282.3
    2, 3 PG 282.3
    6-PGD 282.2
    6-phosphogluronic dehydrogenase 282.2
    amino acid 281.4
    combined B_{12} and folate 281.3
    enzyme, drug-induced (hemolytic) 282.2
    erythrocytic glutathione 282.2
    folate 281.2
      dietary 281.2
      drug-induced 281.2
    folic acid 281.2
      dietary 281.2
      drug-induced 281.2
    G-6-PD 282.2
    GGS-R 282.2
    glucose-6-phosphate dehydrogenase (G-6-PD) 282.2
    glucose-phosphate isomerase 282.3
    glutathione peroxidase 282.2
    glutathione reductase 282.2
    glyceraldehyde phosphate dehydrogenase 282.3
    GPI 282.3
    G SH 282.2
    hexokinase 282.3
    iron (Fe) 280.9
      specified NEC 280.8
    nutritional 281.9
      with
        poor iron absorption 280.9
        specified deficiency NEC 281.8
      due to inadequate dietary iron intake 280.1
      specified type NEC 281.8
    of or complicating pregnancy 648.2●
    pentose phosphate pathway 282.2
    PFK 282.3
    phosphofructo-aldolase 282.3
    phosphofructokinase 282.3
    phosphoglycerate kinase 282.3
    PK 282.3
    protein 281.4
    pyruvate kinase (PK) 282.3
    TPI 282.3
    triosephosphate isomerase 282.3
    vitamin B_{12} NEC 281.1
      dietary 281.1
      pernicious 281.0
  Diamond-Blackfan (congenital hypoplastic) 284.01
  dibothriocephalus 123.4
  dimorphic 281.9
  diphasic 281.8
  diphtheritic 032.89
  Diphyllobothrium 123.4
  drepanocytic (*see also* Disease, sickle-cell) 282.60
  due to
    antineoplastic chemotherapy 285.3 ◀
    blood loss (chronic) 280.0
      acute 285.1

Anemia (*Continued*)
  due to (*Continued*)
    chemotherapy, antineoplastic 285.3 ◀
    defect of Embden-Meyerhof pathway glycolysis 282.3
    disorder of glutathione metabolism 282.2
    drug - *see* Anemia, by type (*see also* Table of Drugs and Chemicals)
    chemotherapy, antineoplastic 285.3 ◀
    fetal blood loss 776.5
    fish tapeworm (D. latum) infestation 123.4
    glutathione metabolism disorder 282.2
    hemorrhage (chronic) 280.0
      acute 285.1
    hexose monophosphate (HMP) shunt deficiency 282.2
    impaired absorption 280.9
    loss of blood (chronic) 280.0
      acute 285.1
    myxedema 244.9
    Necator americanus 126.1
    prematurity 776.6
    selective vitamin B_{12} malabsorption with proteinuria 281.1
  Dyke-Young type (secondary) (symptomatic) 283.9
  dyserythropoietic (congenital) (types I, II, III) 285.8
  dyshemopoietic (congenital) 285.8
  Egypt (*see also* Ancylostomiasis) 126.9
  elliptocytosis (*see also* Elliptocytosis) 282.1
  enzyme deficiency, drug-induced 282.2
  epidemic (*see also* Ancylostomiasis) 126.9
  EPO resistant 285.21
  erythroblastic
    familial 282.49
    fetus or newborn (*see also* Disease, hemolytic) 773.2
      late 773.5
  erythrocytic glutathione deficiency 282.2
  erythropoietin-resistant (EPO resistant anemia) 285.21
  essential 285.9
  Faber's (achlorhydric anemia) 280.9
  factitious (self-induced bloodletting) 280.0
  familial erythroblastic (microcytic) 282.49
  Fanconi's (congenital pancytopenia) 284.09
  favism 282.2
  fetal 678.0●
    following blood loss, affecting newborn 776.5
  fetus or newborn
    due to
      ABO
        antibodies 773.1
        incompatibility, maternal/fetal 773.1
        isoimmunization 773.1
      Rh
        antibodies 773.0
        incompatibility, maternal/fetal 773.0
        isoimmunization 773.0
    following fetal blood loss 776.5
  fish tapeworm (D. latum) infestation 123.4

Anemia (*Continued*)
  folate (folic acid) deficiency 281.2
    dietary 281.2
    drug-induced 281.2
  folate malabsorption, congenital 281.2
  folic acid deficiency 281.2
    dietary 281.2
    drug-induced 281.2
  G-6-PD 282.2
  general 285.9
  glucose-6-phosphate dehydrogenase deficiency 282.2
  glutathione-reductase deficiency 282.2
  goat's milk 281.2
  granulocytic 288.09
  Heinz-body, congenital 282.7
  hemoglobin deficiency 285.9
  hemolytic 283.9
    acquired 283.9
      with hemoglobinuria NEC 283.2
      autoimmune (cold type) (idiopathic) (primary) (secondary) (symptomatic) (warm type) 283.0
      due to
        cold reactive antibodies 283.0
        drug exposure 283.0
        warm reactive antibodies 283.0
      fragmentation 283.19
      idiopathic (chronic) 283.9
      infectious 283.19
        autoimmune 283.0
        non-autoimmune 283.10
      toxic 283.19
      traumatic cardiac 283.19
    acute 283.9
      due to enzyme deficiency NEC 282.3
      fetus or newborn (*see also* Disease, hemolytic) 773.2
        late 773.5
      Lederer's (acquired infectious hemolytic anemia) 283.19
    autoimmune (acquired) 283.0
    chronic 282.9
      idiopathic 283.9
    cold type (secondary) (symptomatic) 283.0
    congenital (spherocytic) (*see also* Spherocytosis) 282.0
      nonspherocytic - *see* Anemia, hemolytic, nonspherocytic, congenital
    drug-induced 283.0
      enzyme deficiency 282.2
    due to
      cardiac conditions 283.19
      drugs 283.0
      enzyme deficiency NEC 282.3
        drug-induced 282.2
      presence of shunt or other internal prosthetic device 283.19
      thrombotic thrombocytopenic purpura 446.6
    elliptocytotic (*see also* Elliptocytosis) 282.1
    familial 282.9
    hereditary 282.9
      due to enzyme deficiency NEC 282.3
      specified NEC 282.8
    idiopathic (chronic) 283.9
    infectious (acquired) 283.19

◀ New   ◀▦ Revised   ~~deleted~~ Deleted   ● Use Additional Digit(s)   ▦ Omit code

Anemia *(Continued)*
  hemolytic *(Continued)*
    mechanical 283.19
    microangiopathic 283.19
    nonautoimmune 283.10
    nonspherocytic
      congenital or hereditary NEC
        282.3
        glucose-6-phosphate
          dehydrogenase
          deficiency 282.2
        pyruvate kinase (PK)
          deficiency 282.3
        type I 282.2
        type II 282.3
        type I 282.2
        type II 282.3
      of or complicating pregnancy
        648.2●
    resulting from presence of shunt or
      other internal prosthetic
      device 283.19
    secondary 283.19
      autoimmune 283.0
    sickle-cell - *see* Disease, sickle-cell
    Stransky-Regala type (Hb-E) *(see also*
      Disease, hemoglobin) 282.7
    symptomatic 283.19
      autoimmune 283.0
    toxic (acquired) 283.19
    uremic (adult) (child) 283.11
    warm type (secondary)
      (symptomatic) 283.0
  hemorrhagic (chronic) 280.0
    acute 285.1
  HEMPAS 285.8
  hereditary erythroblast
    multinuclearity-positive acidified
    serum test 285.8
  Herrick's (hemoglobin S disease)
    282.61
  hexokinase deficiency 282.3
  high A₂ 282.49
  hookworm *(see also* Ancylostomiasis)
    126.9
  hypochromic (idiopathic) (microcytic)
    (normoblastic) 280.9
    with iron loading 285.0
    due to blood loss (chronic) 280.0
      acute 285.1
    familial sex linked 285.0
    pyridoxine-responsive 285.0
  hypoplasia, red blood cells 284.81
    congenital or familial 284.01
  hypoplastic (idiopathic) 284.9
    congenital 284.01
    familial 284.01
    of childhood 284.09
  idiopathic 285.9
    hemolytic, chronic 283.9
  in (due to) (with)   ◄▥
    chronic illness NEC 285.29
    chronic kidney disease 285.21
    end-stage renal disease 285.21
    neoplastic disease 285.22
  infantile 285.9
  infective, infectional 285.9
  intertropical *(see also* Ancylostomiasis)
    126.9
  iron (Fe) deficiency 280.9
    due to blood loss (chronic) 280.0
      acute 285.1
    of or complicating pregnancy 648.2●
    specified NEC 280.8

Anemia *(Continued)*
  Jaksch's (pseudoleukemia infantum)
    285.8
  Joseph-Diamond-Blackfan (congenital
    hypoplastic) 284.01
  labyrinth 386.50
  Lederer's (acquired infectious
    hemolytic anemia) 283.19
  leptocytosis (hereditary) 282.49
  leukoerythroblastic 284.2
  macrocytic 281.9
    nutritional 281.2
    of or complicating pregnancy 648.2●
    tropical 281.2
  malabsorption (familial), selective B₁₂
    with proteinuria 281.1
  malarial *(see also* Malaria) 084.6
  malignant (progressive) 281.0
  malnutrition 281.9
  marsh *(see also* Malaria) 084.6
  Mediterranean (with
    hemoglobinopathy) 282.49
  megaloblastic 281.9
    combined B₁₂ and folate deficiency
      281.3
    nutritional (of infancy) 281.2
    of infancy 281.2
    of or complicating pregnancy 648.2●
    refractory 281.3
    specified NEC 281.3
  megalocytic 281.9
  microangiopathic hemolytic 283.19
  microcytic (hypochromic) 280.9
    due to blood loss (chronic) 280.0
      acute 285.1
    familial 282.49
    hypochromic 280.9
  microdrepanocytosis 282.49
  miners' *(see also* Ancylostomiasis) 126.9
  myelopathic 285.8
  myelophthisic (normocytic) 284.2
  newborn *(see also* Disease, hemolytic)
    773.2
    due to isoimmunization *(see also*
      Disease, hemolytic) 773.2
    late, due to isoimmunization 773.5
    posthemorrhagic 776.5
  nonregenerative 284.9
  nonspherocytic hemolytic - *see* Anemia,
    hemolytic, nonspherocytic
  normocytic (infectional) (not due to
    blood loss) 285.9
    due to blood loss (chronic) 280.0
      acute 285.1
    myelophthisic 284.2
  nutritional (deficiency) 281.9
    with
      poor iron absorption 280.9
      specified deficiency NEC 281.8
    due to inadequate dietary iron
      intake 280.1
    megaloblastic (of infancy) 281.2
  of childhood 282.9
  of chronic
    disease NEC 285.29
    illness NEC 285.29
  of or complicating pregnancy 648.2●
    affecting fetus or newborn 760.8
  of prematurity 776.6
  orotic aciduric (congenital) (hereditary)
    281.4
  osteosclerotic 289.89
  ovalocytosis (hereditary) *(see also*
    Elliptocytosis) 282.1

Anemia *(Continued)*
  paludal *(see also* Malaria) 084.6
  pentose phosphate pathway deficiency
    282.2
  pernicious (combined system
    disease) (congenital)
    (dorsolateral spinal
    degeneration) (juvenile)
    (myelopathy) (neuropathy)
    (posterior sclerosis) (primary)
    (progressive) (spleen) 281.0
    of or complicating pregnancy
      648.2●
  pleochromic 285.9
    of sprue 281.8
  portal 285.8
  posthemorrhagic (chronic) 280.0
    acute 285.1
    newborn 776.5
  postoperative
    due to (acute) blood loss 285.1
      chronic blood loss 280.0
    other 285.9
  postpartum 648.2●
  pressure 285.9
  primary 285.9
  profound 285.9
  progressive 285.9
    malignant 281.0
    pernicious 281.0
  protein-deficiency 281.4
  pseudoleukemica infantum 285.8
  puerperal 648.2●
  pure red cell 284.81
    congenital 284.01
  pyridoxine-responsive (hypochromic)
    285.0
  pyruvate kinase (PK) deficiency
    282.3
  refractoria sideroblastica 238.72
  refractory (primary) 238.72
    with
      excess
        blasts-1 (RAEB-1) 238.72   ◄▥
        blasts-2 (RAEB-2) 238.73
      hemochromatosis 238.72
      ringed sideroblasts (RARS)
        238.72
    due to
      drug 285.0
      myelodysplastic syndrome
        238.72
      toxin 285.0
    hereditary 285.0
    idiopathic 238.72
    megaloblastic 281.3
    sideroblastic 238.72
      hereditary 285.0
    sideropenic 280.9
  Rietti-Greppi-Micheli (thalassemia
    minor) 282.49
  scorbutic 281.8
  secondary (to) 285.9
    blood loss (chronic) 280.0
      acute 285.1
    hemorrhage 280.0
      acute 285.1
    inadequate dietary iron intake
      280.1
  semiplastic 284.9
  septic 285.9
  sickle-cell *(see also* Disease, sickle-cell)
    282.60
  sideroachrestic 285.0

Anemia *(Continued)*
  sideroblastic (acquired) (any type)
      (congenital) (drug-induced) (due
      to disease) (hereditary) (primary)
      (secondary) (sex-linked
      hypochromic) (vitamin B$_6$
      responsive) 285.0
    refractory 238.72
      congenital 285.0
      drug-induced 285.0
      hereditary 285.0
      sex-linked hypochromic 285.0
      vitamin B$_6$-responsive 285.0
  sideropenic 280.9
    due to blood loss (chronic) 280.0
      acute 285.1
  simple chronic 281.9
  specified type NEC 285.8
  spherocytic (hereditary) *(see also*
      Spherocytosis) 282.0
  splenic 285.8
    familial (Gaucher's) 272.7
  splenomegalic 285.8
  stomatocytosis 282.8
  syphilitic 095.8
  target cell (oval) 282.49
  thalassemia 282.49
  thrombocytopenic *(see also*
      Thrombocytopenia) 287.5
  toxic 284.89
  triosephosphate isomerase deficiency
      282.3
  tropical, macrocytic 281.2
  tuberculous *(see also* Tuberculosis)
      017.9●
  Vegan's 281.1
  vitamin
    B$_6$-responsive 285.0
    B$_{12}$ deficiency (dietary) 281.1
      pernicious 281.0
  von Jaksch's (pseudoleukemia
      infantum) 285.8
  Witts' (achlorhydric anemia) 280.9
  Zuelzer (-Ogden) (nutritional
      megaloblastic anemia) 281.2
Anencephalus, anencephaly 740.0
  fetal, affecting management of
      pregnancy 655.0●
Anergasia *(see also* Psychosis, organic)
      294.9
  senile 290.0
Anesthesia, anesthetic 782.0
  complication or reaction NEC 995.22
    due to
      correct substance properly
          administered 995.22
      overdose or wrong substance
          given 968.4
      specified anesthetic - *see* Table
          of Drugs and Chemicals
  cornea 371.81
  death from
    correct substance properly
        administered 995.4
    during delivery 668.9●
    overdose or wrong substance given
        968.4
    specified anesthetic - *see* Table of
        Drugs and Chemicals
  eye 371.81
  functional 300.11
  hyperesthetic, thalamic 338.0
  hysterical 300.11
  local skin lesion 782.0

Anesthesia, anesthetic *(Continued)*
  olfactory 781.1
  sexual (psychogenic) 302.72
  shock
    due to
      correct substance properly
          administered 995.4
      overdose or wrong substance
          given 968.4
      specified anesthetic - *see* Table
          of Drugs and Chemicals
  skin 782.0
  tactile 782.0
  testicular 608.9
  thermal 782.0
Anetoderma (maculosum) 701.3
Aneuploidy NEC 758.5
Aneurin deficiency 265.1
Aneurysm (anastomotic) (artery)
      (cirsoid) (diffuse) (false) (fusiform)
      (multiple) (ruptured) (saccular)
      (varicose) 442.9
  abdominal (aorta) 441.4
    ruptured 441.3
    syphilitic 093.0
  aorta, aortic (nonsyphilitic) 441.9
    abdominal 441.4
      dissecting 441.02
      ruptured 441.3
      syphilitic 093.0
    arch 441.2
      ruptured 441.1
    arteriosclerotic NEC 441.9
      ruptured 441.5
    ascending 441.2
      ruptured 441.1
    congenital 747.29
    descending 441.9
      abdominal 441.4
        ruptured 441.3
      ruptured 441.5
      thoracic 441.2
        ruptured 441.1
    dissecting 441.00
      abdominal 441.02
      thoracic 441.01
      thoracoabdominal 441.03
    due to coarctation (aorta) 747.10
    ruptured 441.5
    sinus, right 747.29
    syphilitic 093.0
    thoracoabdominal 441.7
      ruptured 441.6
    thorax, thoracic (arch)
        (nonsyphilitic) 441.2
      dissecting 441.01
      ruptured 441.1
      syphilitic 093.0
    transverse 441.2
      ruptured 441.1
    valve (heart) *(see also* Endocarditis,
        aortic) 424.1
  arteriosclerotic NEC 442.9
    cerebral 437.3
      ruptured *(see also* Hemorrhage,
          subarachnoid) 430
  arteriovenous (congenital)
      (peripheral) NEC *(see also*
      Anomaly, arteriovenous) 747.60
    acquired NEC 447.0
    brain 437.3
      ruptured *(see also* Hemorrhage,
          subarachnoid) 430

Aneurysm *(Continued)*
  arteriovenous *(Continued)*
    acquired NEC *(Continued)*
      coronary 414.11
      pulmonary 417.0
    brain (cerebral) 747.81
      ruptured *(see also* Hemorrhage,
          subarachnoid) 430
    coronary 746.85
    pulmonary 747.3
    retina 743.58
    specified site NEC 747.89
      acquired 447.0
    traumatic *(see also* Injury, blood
        vessel, by site) 904.9
  basal - *see* Aneurysm, brain
  berry (congenital) (ruptured)
      (see also Hemorrhage,
      subarachnoid) 430
  brain 437.3
    arteriosclerotic 437.3
      ruptured *(see also* Hemorrhage,
          subarachnoid) 430
    arteriovenous 747.81
      acquired 437.3
        ruptured *(see also* Hemorrhage,
            subarachnoid) 430
      ruptured *(see also* Hemorrhage,
          subarachnoid) 430
    berry (congenital) (ruptured) *(see
        also* Hemorrhage,
        subarachnoid) 430
    congenital 747.81
      ruptured *(see also* Hemorrhage,
          subarachnoid) 430
    meninges 437.3
      ruptured *(see also* Hemorrhage,
          subarachnoid) 430
    miliary (congenital) (ruptured) *(see
        also* Hemorrhage,
        subarachnoid) 430
    mycotic 421.0
      ruptured *(see also* Hemorrhage,
          subarachnoid) 430
    nonruptured 437.3
    ruptured *(see also* Hemorrhage,
        subarachnoid) 430
    syphilitic 094.87
  syphilitic (hemorrhage) 094.87
  traumatic - *see* Injury, intracranial
  cardiac (false) *(see also* Aneurysm,
      heart) 414.10
  carotid artery (common) (external)
      442.81
    internal (intracranial portion) 437.3
      extracranial portion 442.81
      ruptured into brain *(see also*
          Hemorrhage, subarachnoid)
          430
    syphilitic 093.89
      intracranial 094.87
  cavernous sinus *(see also* Aneurysm,
      brain) 437.3
    arteriovenous 747.81
      ruptured *(see also* Hemorrhage,
          subarachnoid) 430
    congenital 747.81
      ruptured *(see also* Hemorrhage,
          subarachnoid) 430
  celiac 442.84
  central nervous system, syphilitic
      094.89
  cerebral - *see* Aneurysm, brain
  chest - *see* Aneurysm, thorax

◄ New   ◄▥ Revised   ~~deleted~~ Deleted   ● Use Additional Digit(s)   ▨ Omit code

Aneurysm *(Continued)*
  circle of Willis *(see also* Aneurysm,
    brain) 437.3
    congenital 747.81
      ruptured *(see also* Hemorrhage,
        subarachnoid) 430
    ruptured *(see also* Hemorrhage,
      subarachnoid) 430
  common iliac artery 442.2
  congenital (peripheral) NEC 747.60
    brain 747.81
      ruptured *(see also* Hemorrhage,
        subarachnoid) 430
    cerebral - *see* Aneurysm, brain,
      congenital
    coronary 746.85
    gastrointestinal 747.61
    lower limb 747.64
    pulmonary 747.3
    renal 747.62
    retina 743.58
    specified site NEC 747.89
    spinal 747.82
    upper limb 747.63
  conjunctiva 372.74
  conus arteriosus *(see also* Aneurysm,
    heart) 414.10
  coronary (arteriosclerotic) (artery)
    (vein) *(see also* Aneurysm, heart)
    414.11
    arteriovenous 746.85
    congenital 746.85
    syphilitic 093.89
  cylindrical 441.9
    ruptured 441.5
    syphilitic 093.9
  dissecting 442.9
    aorta 441.00
      abdominal 441.02
      thoracic 441.01
      thoracoabdominal 441.03
    syphilitic 093.9
  ductus arteriosus 747.0
  embolic - *see* Embolism, artery
  endocardial, infective (any valve)
    421.0
  femoral 442.3
  gastroduodenal 442.84
  gastroepiploic 442.84
  heart (chronic or with a stated duration
    of over 8 weeks) (infectional)
    (wall) 414.10
    acute or with a stated duration of 8
      weeks or less *(see also* Infarct,
      myocardium) 410.9●
    congenital 746.89
    valve - *see* Endocarditis
  hepatic 442.84
  iliac (common) 442.2
  infective (any valve) 421.0
  innominate (nonsyphilitic) 442.89
    syphilitic 093.89
  interauricular septum *(see also*
    Aneurysm, heart) 414.10
  interventricular septum *(see also*
    Aneurysm, heart) 414.10
  intracranial - *see* Aneurysm, brain
  intrathoracic (nonsyphilitic) 441.2
    ruptured 441.1
    syphilitic 093.0
  jugular vein 453.89 ◀▥
  lower extremity 442.3
  lung (pulmonary artery) 417.1
  malignant 093.9

Aneurysm *(Continued)*
  mediastinal (nonsyphilitic) 442.89
    syphilitic 093.89
  miliary (congenital) (ruptured) *(see also*
    Hemorrhage, subarachnoid) 430
  mitral (heart) (valve) 424.0
  mural (arteriovenous) (heart) *(see also*
    Aneurysm, heart) 414.10
  mycotic, any site 421.0
    without endocarditis - *see*
      Aneurysm, by site
    ruptured, brain *(see also*
      Hemorrhage, subarachnoid)
      430
  myocardium *(see also* Aneurysm, heart)
    414.10
  neck 442.81
  pancreaticoduodenal 442.84
  patent ductus arteriosus 747.0
  peripheral NEC 442.89
    congenital NEC *(see also* Aneurysm,
      congenital) 747.60
  popliteal 442.3
  pulmonary 417.1
    arteriovenous 747.3
      acquired 417.0
    syphilitic 093.89
    valve (heart) *(see also* Endocarditis,
      pulmonary) 424.3
  racemose 442.9
    congenital (peripheral) NEC 747.60
  radial 442.0
  Rasmussen's *(see also* Tuberculosis)
    011.2●
  renal 442.1
  retinal (acquired) 362.17
    congenital 743.58
    diabetic 250.5● *[362.01]*
      due to secondary diabetes 249.5●
        [362.01]
  sinus, aortic (of Valsalva) 747.29
  specified site NEC 442.89
  spinal (cord) 442.89
    congenital 747.82
    syphilitic (hemorrhage) 094.89
  spleen, splenic 442.83
  subclavian 442.82
    syphilitic 093.89
  superior mesenteric 442.84
  syphilitic 093.9
    aorta 093.0
    central nervous system 094.89
    congenital 090.5
    spine, spinal 094.89
  thoracoabdominal 441.7
    ruptured 441.6
  thorax, thoracic (arch) (nonsyphilitic)
    441.2
    dissecting 441.0●
    ruptured 441.1
    syphilitic 093.0
  traumatic (complication) (early) - *see*
    Injury, blood vessel, by site
  tricuspid (heart) (valve) - *see*
    Endocarditis, tricuspid
  ulnar 442.0
  upper extremity 442.0
  valve, valvular - *see* Endocarditis
  venous 456.8
    congenital NEC *(see also* Aneurysm,
      congenital) 747.60
  ventricle (arteriovenous) *(see also*
    Aneurysm, heart) 414.10
  visceral artery NEC 442.84

Angiectasis 459.89
Angiectopia 459.9
Angiitis 447.6
  allergic granulomatous 446.4
  hypersensitivity 446.20
    Goodpasture's syndrome 446.21
    specified NEC 446.29
  necrotizing 446.0
  Wegener's (necrotizing respiratory
    granulomatosis) 446.4
Angina (attack) (cardiac) (chest) (effort)
  (heart) (pectoris) (syndrome)
  (vasomotor) 413.9
  abdominal 557.1
  accelerated 411.1
  agranulocytic 288.03
  aphthous 074.0
  catarrhal 462
  crescendo 411.1
  croupous 464.4
  cruris 443.9
    due to atherosclerosis NEC *(see also*
      Arteriosclerosis, extremities)
      440.20
  decubitus 413.0
  diphtheritic (membranous) 032.0 ◀
  equivalent 413.9
  erysipelatous 034.0
  erythematous 462
  exudative, chronic 476.0
  faucium 478.29
  gangrenous 462
    diphtheritic 032.0
  infectious 462
  initial 411.1
  intestinal 557.1
  ludovici 528.3
  Ludwig's 528.3
  malignant 462
    diphtheritic 032.0
  membranous 464.4
    diphtheritic 032.0
  mesenteric 557.1
  monocytic 075
  nocturnal 413.0
  phlegmonous 475
    diphtheritic 032.0
  preinfarctional 411.1
  Prinzmetal's 413.1
  progressive 411.1
  pseudomembranous 101
  psychogenic 306.2
  pultaceous, diphtheritic 032.0
  scarlatinal 034.1
  septic 034.0
  simple 462
  stable NEC 413.9
  staphylococcal 462
  streptococcal 034.0
  stridulous, diphtheritic 032.3
  syphilitic 093.9
    congenital 090.5
  tonsil 475
  trachealis 464.4
  unstable 411.1
  variant 413.1
  Vincent's 101
Angioblastoma (M9161/1) - *see*
  Neoplasm, connective tissue,
  uncertain behavior
Angiocholecystitis *(see also* Cholecystitis,
  acute) 575.0
Angiocholitis *(see also* Cholecystitis,
  acute) 576.1

Angiodysgensis spinalis 336.1
Angiodysplasia (intestinalis) (intestine) 569.84
  with hemorrhage 569.85
  duodenum 537.82
    with hemorrhage 537.83
  stomach 537.82
    with hemorrhage 537.83
Angioedema (allergic) (any site) (with urticaria) 995.1
  hereditary 277.6
Angioendothelioma (M9130/1) - see also Neoplasm, by site, uncertain behavior
  benign (M9130/0) (see also Hemangioma, by site) 228.00
  bone (M9260/3) - see Neoplasm, bone, malignant
  Ewing's (M9260/3) - see Neoplasm, bone, malignant
  nervous system (M9130/0) 228.09
Angiofibroma (M9160/0) - see also Neoplasm, by site, benign
  juvenile (M9160/0) 210.7
    specified site - see Neoplasm, by site, benign
    unspecified site 210.7
Angiohemophilia (A) (B) 286.4
Angioid streaks (choroid) (retina) 363.43
Angiokeratoma (M9141/0) - see also Neoplasm, skin, benign
  corporis diffusum 272.7
Angiokeratosis
  diffuse 272.7
Angioleiomyoma (M8894/0) - see Neoplasm, connective tissue, benign
Angioleucitis 683
Angiolipoma (M8861/0) (see also Lipoma, by site) 214.9
  infiltrating (M8861/1) - see Neoplasm, connective tissue, uncertain behavior
Angioma (M9120/0) (see also Hemangioma, by site) 228.00
  capillary 448.1
  hemorrhagicum hereditaria 448.0
  malignant (M9120/3) - see Neoplasm, connective tissue, malignant
  pigmentosum et atrophicum 757.33
  placenta - see Placenta, abnormal
  plexiform (M9131/0) - see Hemangioma, by site
  senile 448.1
  serpiginosum 709.1
  spider 448.1
  stellate 448.1
Angiomatosis 757.32
  bacillary 083.8
  corporis diffusum universale 272.7
  cutaneocerebral 759.6
  encephalocutaneous 759.6
  encephalofacial 759.6
  encephalotrigeminal 759.6
  hemorrhagic familial 448.0
  hereditary familial 448.0
  heredofamilial 448.0
  meningo-oculofacial 759.6
  multiple sites 228.09
  neuro-oculocutaneous 759.6
  retina (Hippel's disease) 759.6
  retinocerebellosa 759.6
  retinocerebral 759.6
  systemic 228.09

Angiomyolipoma (M8860/0)
  specified site - see Neoplasm, connective tissue, benign
  unspecified site 223.0
Angiomyoliposarcoma (M8860/3) - see Neoplasm, connective tissue, malignant
Angiomyoma (M8894/0) - see Neoplasm, connective tissue, benign
Angiomyosarcoma (M8894/3) - see Neoplasm, connective tissue, malignant
Angioneurosis 306.2
Angioneurotic edema (allergic) (any site) (with urticaria) 995.1
  hereditary 277.6
Angiopathia, angiopathy 459.9
  diabetic (peripheral) 250.7● [443.81]
    due to secondary diabetes 249.7● [443.81]
  peripheral 443.9
    diabetic 250.7● [443.81]
      due to secondary diabetes 249.7● [443.81]
    specified type NEC 443.89
  retinae syphilitica 093.89
  retinalis (juvenilis) 362.18
    background 362.10
    diabetic 250.5● [362.01]
      due to secondary diabetes 249.5● [362.01]
    proliferative 362.29
  tuberculous (see also Tuberculosis) 017.3● [362.18]
Angiosarcoma (M9120/3) - see Neoplasm, connective tissue, malignant
Angiosclerosis - see Arteriosclerosis
Angioscotoma, enlarged 368.42
Angiospasm 443.9
  brachial plexus 353.0
  cerebral 435.9
  cervical plexus 353.2
  nerve
    arm 354.9
      axillary 353.0
      median 354.1
      ulnar 354.2
    autonomic (see also Neuropathy, peripheral, autonomic) 337.9
    axillary 353.0
    leg 355.8
      plantar 355.6
    lower extremity - see Angiospasm, nerve, leg
    median 354.1
    peripheral NEC 355.9
    spinal NEC 355.9
    sympathetic (see also Neuropathy, peripheral, autonomic) 337.9
    ulnar 354.2
    upper extremity - see Angiospasm, nerve, arm
  peripheral NEC 443.9
  traumatic 443.9
    foot 443.9
    leg 443.9
  vessel 443.9
Angiospastic disease or edema 443.9
Angle's
  class I 524.21
  class II 524.22
  class III 524.23
Anguillulosis 127.2

Angulation
  cecum (see also Obstruction, intestine) 560.9
  coccyx (acquired) 738.6
    congenital 756.19
  femur (acquired) 736.39
    congenital 755.69
  intestine (large) (small) (see also Obstruction, intestine) 560.9
  sacrum (acquired) 738.5
    congenital 756.19
  sigmoid (flexure) (see also Obstruction, intestine) 560.9
  spine (see also Curvature, spine) 737.9
  tibia (acquired) 736.89
    congenital 755.69
  ureter 593.3
  wrist (acquired) 736.09
    congenital 755.59
Angulus infectiosus 686.8
Anhedonia 780.99
Anhidrosis (lid) (neurogenic) (thermogenic) 705.0
Anhydration 276.51
  with
    hypernatremia 276.0
    hyponatremia 276.1
Anhydremia 276.52
  with
    hypernatremia 276.0
    hyponatremia 276.1
Anidrosis 705.0
Aniridia (congenital) 743.45
Anisakiasis (infection) (infestation) 127.1
Anisakis larva infestation 127.1
Aniseikonia 367.32
Anisocoria (pupil) 379.41
  congenital 743.46
Anisocytosis 790.09
Anisometropia (congenital) 367.31
Ankle - see condition
Ankyloblepharon (acquired) (eyelid) 374.46
  filiforme (adnatum) (congenital) 743.62
  total 743.62
Ankylodactly (see also Syndactylism) 755.10
Ankyloglossia 750.0
Ankylosis (fibrous) (osseous) 718.50
  ankle 718.57
  any joint, produced by surgical fusion V45.4
  cricoarytenoid (cartilage) (joint) (larynx) 478.79
  dental 521.6
  ear ossicle NEC 385.22
    malleus 385.21
  elbow 718.52
  finger 718.54
  hip 718.55
  incostapedial joint (infectional) 385.22
  joint, produced by surgical fusion NEC V45.4
  knee 718.56
  lumbosacral (joint) 724.6
  malleus 385.21
  multiple sites 718.59
  postoperative (status) V45.4
  sacroiliac (joint) 724.6
  shoulder 718.51
  specified site NEC 718.58
  spine NEC 724.9
  surgical V45.4
  teeth, tooth (hard tissues) 521.6

◀ New　◀▥ Revised　deleted Deleted　● Use Additional Digit(s)　▨ Omit code

Ankylosis *(Continued)*
  temporomandibular joint 524.61
  wrist 718.53
Ankylostoma - *see* Ancylostoma
Ankylostomiasis (intestinal) - *see*
  Ancylostomiasis
Ankylurethria (*see also* Stricture, urethra)
  598.9
Annular - *see also* condition
  detachment, cervix 622.8
  organ or site, congenital NEC - *see*
    Distortion
  pancreas (congenital) 751.7
Anodontia (complete) (partial) (vera) 520.0
  with abnormal spacing 524.30
  acquired 525.10
    causing malocclusion 524.30
    due to
      caries 525.13
      extraction 525.10
      periodontal disease 525.12
      trauma 525.11
Anomaly, anomalous (congenital)
  (unspecified type) 759.9
  abdomen 759.9
  abdominal wall 756.70
  acoustic nerve 742.9
  adrenal (gland) 759.1
  Alder (-Reilly) (leukocyte granulation)
    288.2
  alimentary tract 751.9
    lower 751.5
      specified type NEC 751.8
    upper (any part, except tongue)
      750.9
      tongue 750.10
        specified type NEC 750.19
  alveolar 524.70
    ridge (process) 525.8
      specified NEC 524.79
  ankle (joint) 755.69
  anus, anal (canal) 751.5
  aorta, aortic 747.20
    arch 747.21
    coarctation (postductal) (preductal)
      747.10
    cusp or valve NEC 746.9
    septum 745.0
    specified type NEC 747.29
  aorticopulmonary septum 745.0
  apertures, diaphragm 756.6
  appendix 751.5
  aqueduct of Sylvius 742.3
    with spina bifida (*see also* Spina
      bifida) 741.0●
  arm 755.50
    reduction (*see also* Deformity,
      reduction, upper limb) 755.20
  arteriovenous (congenital) (peripheral)
    NEC 747.60
    brain 747.81
    cerebral 747.81
    coronary 746.85
    gastrointestinal 747.61
      acquired - *see* Angiodysplasia
    lower limb 747.64
    renal 747.62
    specified site NEC 747.69
    spinal 747.82
    upper limb 747.63
  artery (*see also* Anomaly, peripheral
    vascular system) NEC 747.60
    brain 747.81
    cerebral 747.81

Anomaly, anomalous *(Continued)*
  artery NEC *(Continued)*
    coronary 746.85
    eye 743.9
    pulmonary 747.3
    renal 747.62
    retina 743.9
    umbilical 747.5
  arytenoepiglottic folds 748.3
  atrial
    bands 746.9
    folds 746.9
    septa 745.5
  atrioventricular
    canal 745.69
    common 745.69
    conduction 426.7
    excitation 426.7
    septum 745.4
  atrium - *see* Anomaly, atrial
  auditory canal 744.3
    specified type NEC 744.29
      with hearing impairment 744.02
  auricle
    ear 744.3
      causing impairment of hearing
        744.02
    heart 746.9
      septum 745.5
  autosomes, autosomal NEC 758.5
  Axenfeld's 743.44
  back 759.9
  band
    atrial 746.9
    heart 746.9
    ventricular 746.9
  Bartholin's duct 750.9
  biliary duct or passage 751.60
    atresia 751.61
  bladder (neck) (sphincter) (trigone) 753.9
    specified type NEC 753.8
  blood vessel 747.9
    artery - *see* Anomaly, artery
    peripheral vascular - *see* Anomaly,
      peripheral vascular system
    vein - *see* Anomaly, vein
  bone NEC 756.9
    ankle 755.69
    arm 755.50
    chest 756.3
    cranium 756.0
    face 756.0
    finger 755.50
    foot 755.67
    forearm 755.50
    frontal 756.0
    head 756.0
    hip 755.63
    leg 755.60
    lumbosacral 756.10
    nose 748.1
    pelvic girdle 755.60
    rachitic 756.4
    rib 756.3
    shoulder girdle 755.50
    skull 756.0
      with
        anencephalus 740.0
        encephalocele 742.0
        hydrocephalus 742.3
          with spina bifida (*see also*
            Spina bifida) 741.0●
        microcephalus 742.1
    toe 755.66

Anomaly, anomalous *(Continued)*
  brain 742.9
    multiple 742.4
    reduction 742.2
    specified type NEC 742.4
    vessel 747.81
  branchial cleft NEC 744.49
    cyst 744.42
    fistula 744.41
    persistent 744.41
    sinus (external) (internal) 744.41 ◀▥
  breast 757.6
  broad ligament 752.10
    specified type NEC 752.19
  bronchus 748.3
  bulbar septum 745.0
  bulbus cordis 745.9
    persistent (in left ventricle) 745.8
  bursa 756.9
  canal of Nuck 752.9
  canthus 743.9
  capillary NEC (*see also* Anomaly,
    peripheral vascular system)
    747.60
  cardiac 746.9
    septal closure 745.9
      acquired 429.71
    valve NEC 746.9
      pulmonary 746.00
      specified type NEC 746.89
  cardiovascular system 746.9
    complicating pregnancy, childbirth,
      or puerperium 648.5 ●
  carpus 755.50
  cartilage, trachea 748.3
  cartilaginous 756.9
  caruncle, lacrimal, lachrymal 743.9
  cascade stomach 750.7
  cauda equina 742.59
  cecum 751.5
  cerebral - *see also* Anomaly, brain
    vessels 747.81
  cerebrovascular system 747.81
  cervix (uterus) 752.40
    with doubling of vagina and uterus
      752.2
    in pregnancy or childbirth 654.6 ●
      affecting fetus or newborn 763.89
      causing obstructed labor 660.2 ●
        affecting fetus or newborn
          763.1
  Chédiak-Higashi (-Steinbrinck)
    (congenital gigantism of
    peroxidase granules) 288.2
  cheek 744.9
  chest (wall) 756.3
  chin 744.9
    specified type NEC 744.89
  chordae tendineae 746.9
  choroid 743.9
    plexus 742.9
  chromosomes, chromosomal 758.9
    13 (13-15) 758.1
    18 (16-18) 758.2
    21 or 22 758.0
    autosomes NEC (*see also* Abnormal,
      autosomes) 758.5
      deletion 758.39
    Christchurch 758.39
    D_1 758.1
    E_3 758.2
    G 758.0
    mitochondrial 758.9

Anomaly, anomalous (*Continued*)
  chromosomes, chromosomal
    (*Continued*)
    mosaics 758.89
    sex 758.81
      complement, XO 758.6
      complement, XXX 758.81
      complement, XXY 758.7
      complement, XYY 758.81
      gonadal dysgenesis 758.6
      Klinefelter's 758.7
      Turner's 758.6
    trisomy 21 758.0
  cilia 743.9
  circulatory system 747.9
    specified type NEC 747.89
  clavicle 755.51
  clitoris 752.40
  coccyx 756.10
  colon 751.5
  common duct 751.60
  communication
    coronary artery 746.85
    left ventricle with right atrium
      745.4
  concha (ear) 744.3
  connection
    renal vessels with kidney 747.62
    total pulmonary venous 747.41
  connective tissue 756.9
    specified type NEC 756.89
  cornea 743.9
    shape 743.41
    size 743.41
    specified type NEC 743.49
  coronary
    artery 746.85
    vein 746.89
  cranium - *see* Anomaly, skull
  cricoid cartilage 748.3
  cushion, endocardial 745.60
    specified type NEC 745.69
  cystic duct 751.60
  dental arch 524.20
    specified NEC 524.29
  dental arch relationship 524.20
    angle's class I 524.21
    angle's class II 524.22
    angle's class III 524.23
    articulation
      anterior 524.27
      posterior 524.27
      reverse 524.27
    disto-occlusion 524.22
      division I 524.22
      division II 524.22
    excessive horizontal overlap 524.26
    interarch distance (excessive)
      (inadequate) 524.28
    mesio-occlusion 524.23
    neutro-occlusion 524.21
    open
      anterior occlusal relationship
        524.24
      posterior occlusal relationship
        524.25
    specified NEC 524.29
  dentition 520.6
  dentofacial NEC 524.9
    functional 524.50
    specified type NEC 524.89
  dermatoglyphic 757.2
  Descemet's membrane 743.9
    specified type NEC 743.49

Anomaly, anomalous (*Continued*)
  development
    cervix 752.40
    vagina 752.40
    vulva 752.40
  diaphragm, diaphragmatic (apertures)
    NEC 756.6
  digestive organ(s) or system 751.9
    lower 751.5
    specified type NEC 751.8
    upper 750.9
  distribution, coronary artery 746.85
  ductus
    arteriosus 747.0
    Botalli 747.0
  duodenum 751.5
  dura 742.9
    brain 742.4
    spinal cord 742.59
  ear 744.3
    causing impairment of hearing
      744.00
      specified type NEC 744.09
    external 744.3
      causing impairment of hearing
        744.02
      specified type NEC 744.29
    inner (causing impairment of
      hearing) 744.05
    middle, except ossicles (causing
      impairment of hearing) 744.03
      ossicles 744.04
    ossicles 744.04
    prominent auricle 744.29
    specified type NEC 744.29
      with hearing impairment 744.09
  Ebstein's (heart) 746.2
    tricuspid valve 746.2
  ectodermal 757.9
  Eisenmenger's (ventricular septal
    defect) 745.4
  ejaculatory duct 752.9
    specified type NEC 752.89
  elbow (joint) 755.50
  endocardial cushion 745.60
    specified type NEC 745.69
  endocrine gland NEC 759.2
  epididymis 752.9
  epiglottis 748.3
  esophagus 750.9
    specified type NEC 750.4
  Eustachian tube 744.3
    specified type NEC 744.24
  eye (any part) 743.9
    adnexa 743.9
      specified type NEC 743.69
    anophthalmos 743.00
    anterior
      chamber and related structures
        743.9
      angle 743.9
        specified type NEC 743.44
      specified type NEC 743.44
      segment 743.9
        combined 743.48
        multiple 743.48
        specified type NEC 743.49
    cataract (*see also* Cataract) 743.30
    glaucoma (*see also* Buphthalmia)
      743.20
    lid 743.9
      specified type NEC 743.63
    microphthalmos (*see also*
      Microphthalmos) 743.10

Anomaly, anomalous (*Continued*)
  eye (*Continued*)
    posterior segment 743.9
      specified type NEC 743.59
      vascular 743.58
      vitreous 743.9
        specified type NEC 743.51
    ptosis (eyelid) 743.61
    retina 743.9
      specified type NEC 743.59
    sclera 743.9
      specified type NEC 743.47
    specified type NEC 743.8
  eyebrow 744.89
  eyelid 743.9
    specified type NEC 743.63
  face (any part) 744.9
    bone(s) 756.0
    specified type NEC 744.89
  fallopian tube 752.10
    specified type NEC 752.19
  fascia 756.9
    specified type NEC 756.89
  femur 755.60
  fibula 755.60
  finger 755.50
    supernumerary 755.01
    webbed (*see also* Syndactylism,
      fingers) 755.11
  fixation, intestine 751.4
  flexion (joint) 755.9
    hip or thigh (*see also* Dislocation,
      hip, congenital) 754.30
  folds, heart 746.9
  foot 755.67
  foramen
    Botalli 745.5
    ovale 745.5
  forearm 755.50
  forehead (*see also* Anomaly, skull)
    756.0
  form, teeth 520.2
  fovea centralis 743.9
  frontal bone (*see also* Anomaly, skull)
    756.0
  gallbladder 751.60
  Gartner's duct 752.41
  gastrointestinal tract 751.9
    specified type NEC 751.8
    vessel 747.61
  genitalia, genital organ(s) or system
    female 752.9
      external 752.40
        specified type NEC 752.49
      internal NEC 752.9
    male (external and internal) 752.9
      epispadias 752.62
      hidden penis 752.65
      hydrocele, congenital 778.6
      hypospadias 752.61
      micropenis 752.64
      testis, undescended 752.51
        retractile 752.52
      specified type NEC 752.89
  genitourinary NEC 752.9
  Gerbode 745.4
  globe (eye) 743.9
  glottis 748.3
  granulation or granulocyte, genetic
    288.2
    constitutional 288.2
    leukocyte 288.2
  gum 750.9
  gyri 742.9

◀ New   ◀▥ Revised   ~~deleted~~ Deleted   ● Use Additional Digit(s)   ▨ Omit code

Anomaly, anomalous (*Continued*)
  hair 757.9
    specified type NEC 757.4
  hand 755.50
  hard tissue formation in pulp 522.3
  head (*see also* Anomaly, skull) 756.0
  heart 746.9
    auricle 746.9
    bands 746.9
    fibroelastosis cordis 425.3
    folds 746.9
    malposition 746.87
    maternal, affecting fetus or newborn
        760.3
    obstructive NEC 746.84
    patent ductus arteriosus (Botalli)
        747.0
    septum 745.9
      acquired 429.71
      aortic 745.0
      aorticopulmonary 745.0
      atrial 745.5
      auricular 745.5
      between aorta and pulmonary
          artery 745.0
      endocardial cushion type 745.60
        specified type NEC 745.69
      interatrial 745.5
      interventricular 745.4
        with pulmonary stenosis or
            atresia, dextraposition of
            aorta, and hypertrophy of
            right ventricle 745.2
        acquired 429.71
      specified type NEC 745.8
      ventricular 745.4
        with pulmonary stenosis or
            atresia, dextraposition of
            aorta, and hypertrophy
            of right ventricle 745.2
        acquired 429.71
    specified type NEC 746.89
    tetralogy of Fallot 745.2
    valve NEC 746.9
      aortic 746.9
        atresia 746.89
        bicuspid valve 746.4
        insufficiency 746.4
        specified type NEC 746.89
        stenosis 746.3
          subaortic 746.81
          supravalvular 747.22
      mitral 746.9
        atresia 746.89
        insufficiency 746.6
        specified type NEC 746.89
        stenosis 746.5
      pulmonary 746.00
        atresia 746.01
        insufficiency 746.09
        stenosis 746.02
          infundibular 746.83
          subvalvular 746.83
      tricuspid 746.9
        atresia 746.1
        stenosis 746.1
    ventricle 746.9
  heel 755.67
  Hegglin's 288.2
  hemianencephaly 740.0
  hemicephaly 740.0
  hemicrania 740.0
  hepatic duct 751.60
  hip (joint) 755.63

Anomaly, anomalous (*Continued*)
  hourglass
    bladder 753.8
    gallbladder 751.69
    stomach 750.7
  humerus 755.50
  hymen 752.40
  hypersegmentation of neutrophils,
      hereditary 288.2
  hypophyseal 759.2
  ileocecal (coil) (valve) 751.5
  ileum (intestine) 751.5
  ilium 755.60
  integument 757.9
    specified type NEC 757.8
  interarch distance (excessive)
      (inadequate) 524.28
  intervertebral cartilage or disc 756.10
  intestine (large) (small) 751.5
    fixational type 751.4
  iris 743.9
    specified type NEC 743.46
  ischium 755.60
  jaw NEC 524.9
    closure 524.51
    size (major) NEC 524.00
    specified type NEC 524.89
  jaw-cranial base relationship 524.10
    specified NEC 524.19
  jejunum 751.5
  joint 755.9
    hip
      dislocation (*see also* Dislocation,
          hip, congenital) 754.30
      predislocation (*see also*
          Subluxation, congenital,
          hip) 754.32
      preluxation (*see also* Subluxation,
          congenital, hip) 754.32
      subluxation (*see also* Subluxation,
          congenital, hip) 754.32
    lumbosacral 756.10
      spondylolisthesis 756.12
      spondylosis 756.11
    multiple arthrogryposis 754.89
    sacroiliac 755.69
  Jordan's 288.2
  kidney(s) (calyx) (pelvis) 753.9
    vessel 747.62
  Klippel-Feil (brevicollis) 756.16
  knee (joint) 755.64
  labium (majus) (minus) 752.40
  labyrinth, membranous (causing
      impairment of hearing) 744.05
  lacrimal
    apparatus, duct or passage 743.9
      specified type NEC 743.65
    gland 743.9
      specified type NEC 743.64
  Langdon Down (mongolism) 758.0
  larynx, laryngeal (muscle) 748.3
    web, webbed 748.2
  leg (lower) (upper) 755.60
    reduction NEC (*see also* Deformity,
        reduction, lower limb) 755.30
  lens 743.9
    shape 743.36
    specified type NEC 743.39
  leukocytes, genetic 288.2
    granulation (constitutional) 288.2
  lid (fold) 743.9
  ligament 756.9
    broad 752.10
    round 752.9

Anomaly, anomalous (*Continued*)
  limb, except reduction deformity 755.8
    lower 755.60
      reduction deformity (*see also*
          Deformity, reduction, lower
          limb) 755.30
      specified type NEC 755.69
    upper 755.50
      reduction deformity (*see also*
          Deformity, reduction, upper
          limb) 755.20
      specified type NEC 755.59
  lip 750.9
    harelip (*see also* Cleft, lip) 749.10
    specified type NEC 750.26
  liver (duct) 751.60
    atresia 751.69
  lower extremity 755.60
    vessel 747.64
  lumbosacral (joint) (region) 756.10
  lung (fissure) (lobe) NEC 748.60
    agenesis 748.5
    specified type NEC 748.69
  lymphatic system 759.9
  Madelung's (radius) 755.54
  mandible 524.9
    size NEC 524.00
  maxilla 524.90
    size NEC 524.00
  May (-Hegglin) 288.2
  meatus urinarius 753.9
    specified type NEC 753.8
  meningeal bands or folds, constriction
      of 742.8
  meninges 742.9
    brain 742.4
    spinal 742.59
  meningocele (*see also* Spina bifida)
      741.9 ●
    acquired 349.2
  mesentery 751.9
  metacarpus 755.50
  metatarsus 755.67
  middle ear, except ossicles (causing
      impairment of hearing) 744.03
    ossicles 744.04
  mitral (leaflets) (valve) 746.9
    atresia 746.89
    insufficiency 746.6
    specified type NEC 746.89
    stenosis 746.5
  mouth 750.9
    specified type NEC 750.26
  multiple NEC 759.7
    specified type NEC 759.89
  muscle 756.9
    eye 743.9
      specified type NEC 743.69
    specified type NEC 756.89
  musculoskeletal system, except limbs
      756.9
    specified type NEC 756.9
  nail 757.9
    specified type NEC 757.5
  narrowness, eyelid 743.62
  nasal sinus or septum 748.1
  neck (any part) 744.9
    specified type NEC 744.89
  nerve 742.9
    acoustic 742.9
      specified type NEC 742.8
    optic 742.9
      specified type NEC 742.8
    specified type NEC 742.8

Anomaly, anomalous (*Continued*)
  nervous system NEC 742.9
    brain 742.9
      specified type NEC 742.4
    specified type NEC 742.8
  neurological 742.9
  nipple 757.6
  nonteratogenic NEC 754.89
  nose, nasal (bone) (cartilage) (septum)
    (sinus) 748.1
  ocular muscle 743.9
  omphalomesenteric duct 751.0
  opening, pulmonary veins 747.49
  optic
    disc 743.9
      specified type NEC 743.57
    nerve 742.9
  opticociliary vessels 743.9
  orbit (eye) 743.9
    specified type NEC 743.66
  organ
    of Corti (causing impairment of
      hearing) 744.05
    or site 759.9
      specified type NEC 759.89
  origin
    both great arteries from same
      ventricle 745.11
    coronary artery 746.85
    innominate artery 747.69
    left coronary artery from pulmonary
      artery 746.85
    pulmonary artery 747.3
    renal vessels 747.62
    subclavian artery (left) (right) 747.21
  osseous meatus (ear) 744.03
  ovary 752.0
  oviduct 752.10
  palate (hard) (soft) 750.9
    cleft (*see also* Cleft, palate) 749.00
  pancreas (duct) 751.7
  papillary muscles 746.9
  parathyroid gland 759.2
  paraurethral ducts 753.9
  parotid (gland) 750.9
  patella 755.64
  Pelger-Huët (hereditary
    hyposegmentation) 288.2
  pelvic girdle 755.60
    specified type NEC 755.69
  pelvis (bony) 755.60
    complicating delivery 653.0●
    rachitic 268.1
      fetal 756.4
  penis (glans) 752.69
  pericardium 746.89
  peripheral vascular system NEC
    747.60
    gastrointestinal 747.61
    lower limb 747.64
    renal 747.62
    specified site NEC 747.69
    spinal 747.82
    upper limb 747.63
  Peter's 743.44
  pharynx 750.9
    branchial cleft 744.41
    specified type NEC 750.29
  Pierre Robin 756.0
  pigmentation 709.00
    congenital 757.33
    specified NEC 709.09
  pituitary (gland) 759.2
  pleural folds 748.8

Anomaly, anomalous (*Continued*)
  portal vein 747.40
  position tooth, teeth 524.30
    crowding 524.31
    displacement 524.30
      horizontal 524.33
      vertical 524.34
    distance
      interocclusal
        excessive 524.37
        insufficient 524.36
    excessive spacing 524.32
    rotation 524.35
    specified NEC 524.39
  preauricular sinus 744.46
  prepuce 752.9
  prostate 752.9
  pulmonary 748.60
    artery 747.3
    circulation 747.3
    specified type NEC 748.69
    valve 746.00
      atresia 746.01
      insufficiency 746.09
      specified type NEC 746.09
      stenosis 746.02
        infundibular 746.83
        subvalvular 746.83
    vein 747.40
    venous
      connection 747.49
        partial 747.42
        total 747.41
      return 747.49
        partial 747.42
        total (TAPVR) (complete)
          (subdiaphragmatic)
          (supradiaphragmatic)
          747.41
  pupil 743.9
  pylorus 750.9
    hypertrophy 750.5
    stenosis 750.5
  rachitic, fetal 756.4
  radius 755.50
  rectovaginal (septum) 752.40
  rectum 751.5
  refraction 367.9
  renal 753.9
    vessel 747.62
  respiratory system 748.9
    specified type NEC 748.8
  rib 756.3
    cervical 756.2
  Rieger's 743.44
  rings, trachea 748.3
  rotation - *see also* Malrotation
    hip or thigh (*see also* Subluxation,
      congenital, hip) 754.32
  round ligament 752.9
  sacroiliac (joint) 755.69
  sacrum 756.10
  saddle
    back 754.2
    nose 754.0
      syphilitic 090.5
  salivary gland or duct 750.9
    specified type NEC 750.26
  scapula 755.50
  sclera 743.9
    specified type NEC 743.47
  scrotum 752.9
  sebaceous gland 757.9

Anomaly, anomalous (*Continued*)
  seminal duct or tract 752.9
  sense organs 742.9
    specified type NEC 742.8
  septum
    heart - *see* Anomaly, heart, septum
    nasal 748.1
  sex chromosomes NEC (*see also*
    Anomaly, chromosomes)
    758.81
  shoulder (girdle) (joint) 755.50
    specified type NEC 755.59
  sigmoid (flexure) 751.5
  sinus of Valsalva 747.29
  site NEC 759.9
  skeleton generalized NEC 756.50
  skin (appendage) 757.9
    specified type NEC 757.39
  skull (bone) 756.0
    with
      anencephalus 740.0
      encephalocele 742.0
      hydrocephalus 742.3
        with spina bifida (*see also*
          Spina bifida) 741.0●
      microcephalus 742.1
  specified type NEC
    adrenal (gland) 759.1
    alimentary tract (complete) (partial)
      751.8
      lower 751.5
      upper 750.8
    ankle 755.69
    anus, anal (canal) 751.5
    aorta, aortic 747.29
      arch 747.21
    appendix 751.5
    arm 755.59
    artery (peripheral) NEC (*see also*
      Anomaly, peripheral vascular
      system) 747.60
      brain 747.81
      coronary 746.85
      eye 743.58
      pulmonary 747.3
      retinal 743.58
      umbilical 747.5
    auditory canal 744.29
      causing impairment of hearing
        744.02
    bile duct or passage 751.69
    bladder 753.8
      neck 753.8
    bone(s) 756.9
      arm 755.59
      face 756.0
      leg 755.69
      pelvic girdle 755.69
      shoulder girdle 755.59
      skull 756.0
        with
          anencephalus 740.0
          encephalocele 742.0
          hydrocephalus 742.3
            with spina bifida (*see
              also* Spina bifida)
              741.0●
          microcephalus 742.1
    brain 742.4
    breast 757.6
    broad ligament 752.19
    bronchus 748.3
    canal of Nuck 752.89

◄ New   ◄||| Revised   ~~deleted~~ Deleted   ● Use Additional Digit(s)   ▨ Omit code

Anomaly, anomalous *(Continued)*
  specified type NEC *(Continued)*
    cardiac septal closure 745.8
    carpus 755.59
    cartilaginous 756.9
    cecum 751.5
    cervix 752.49
    chest (wall) 756.3
    chin 744.89
    ciliary body 743.46
    circulatory system 747.89
    clavicle 755.51
    clitoris 752.49
    coccyx 756.19
    colon 751.5
    common duct 751.69
    connective tissue 756.89
    cricoid cartilage 748.3
    cystic duct 751.69
    diaphragm 756.6
    digestive organ(s) or tract 751.8
      lower 751.5
      upper 750.8
    duodenum 751.5
    ear 744.29
      auricle 744.29
        causing impairment of
            hearing 744.02
      causing impairment of hearing
          744.09
      inner (causing impairment of
          hearing) 744.05
      middle, except ossicles 744.03
        ossicles 744.04
    ejaculatory duct 752.89
    endocrine 759.2
    epiglottis 748.3
    esophagus 750.4
    eustachian tube 744.24
    eye 743.8
      lid 743.63
      muscle 743.69
    face 744.89
      bone(s) 756.0
    fallopian tube 752.19
    fascia 756.89
    femur 755.69
    fibula 755.69
    finger 755.59
    foot 755.67
    fovea centralis 743.55
    gallbladder 751.69
    Gartner's duct 752.89
    gastrointestinal tract 751.8
    genitalia, genital organ(s)
      female 752.89
        external 752.49
        internal NEC 752.89
      male 752.89
        penis 752.69
        scrotal transposition
            752.81
    genitourinary tract NEC 752.89
    glottis 748.3
    hair 757.4
    hand 755.59
    heart 746.89
      valve NEC 746.89
        pulmonary 746.09
    hepatic duct 751.69
    hydatid of Morgagni 752.89
    hymen 752.49
    integument 757.8

Anomaly, anomalous *(Continued)*
  specified type NEC *(Continued)*
    intestine (large) (small) 751.5
      fixational type 751.4
    iris 743.46
    jejunum 751.5
    joint 755.8
    kidney 753.3
    knee 755.64
    labium (majus) (minus) 752.49
    labyrinth, membranous 744.05
    larynx 748.3
    leg 755.69
    lens 743.39
    limb, except reduction deformity
        755.8
      lower 755.69
        reduction deformity *(see also*
            Deformity, reduction,
            lower limb) 755.30
      upper 755.59
        reduction deformity *(see also*
            Deformity, reduction,
            upper limb) 755.20
    lip 750.26
    liver 751.69
    lung (fissure) (lobe) 748.69
    meatus urinarius 753.8
    metacarpus 755.59
    mouth 750.26
    muscle 756.89
      eye 743.69
    musculoskeletal system, except
        limbs 756.9
    nail 757.5
    neck 744.89
    nerve 742.8
      acoustic 742.8
      optic 742.8
    nervous system 742.8
    nipple 757.6
    nose 748.1
    organ NEC 759.89
      of Corti 744.05
    osseous meatus (ear) 744.03
    ovary 752.0
    oviduct 752.19
    pancreas 751.7
    parathyroid 759.2
    patella 755.64
    pelvic girdle 755.69
    penis 752.69
    pericardium 746.89
    peripheral vascular system NEC
        (see also Anomaly, peripheral
        vascular system) 747.60
    pharynx 750.29
    pituitary 759.2
    prostate 752.89
    radius 755.59
    rectum 751.5
    respiratory system 748.8
    rib 756.3
    round ligament 752.89
    sacrum 756.19
    salivary duct or gland 750.26
    scapula 755.59
    sclera 743.47
    scrotum 752.89
      transposition 752.81
    seminal duct or tract 752.89
    shoulder girdle 755.59
    site NEC 759.89

Anomaly, anomalous *(Continued)*
  specified type NEC *(Continued)*
    skin 757.39
    skull (bone(s)) 756.0
      with
        anencephalus 740.0
        encephalocele 742.0
        hydrocephalus 742.3
          with spina bifida *(see also*
              Spina bifida) 741.0●
        microcephalus 742.1
    specified organ or site NEC 759.89
    spermatic cord 752.89
    spinal cord 742.59
    spine 756.19
    spleen 759.0
    sternum 756.3
    stomach 750.7
    tarsus 755.67
    tendon 756.89
    testis 752.89
    thorax (wall) 756.3
    thymus 759.2
    thyroid (gland) 759.2
      cartilage 748.3
    tibia 755.69
    toe 755.66
    tongue 750.19
    trachea (cartilage) 748.3
    ulna 755.59
    urachus 753.7
    ureter 753.4
      obstructive 753.29
    urethra 753.8
      obstructive 753.6
    urinary tract 753.8
    uterus 752.3
    uvula 750.26
    vagina 752.49
    vascular NEC *(see also* Anomaly,
        peripheral vascular system)
        747.60
      brain 747.81
    vas deferens 752.89
    vein(s) (peripheral) NEC *(see also*
        Anomaly, peripheral vascular
        system) 747.60
      brain 747.81
      great 747.49
      portal 747.49
      pulmonary 747.49
    vena cava (inferior) (superior) 747.49
    vertebra 756.19
    vulva 752.49
  spermatic cord 752.9
  spine, spinal 756.10
    column 756.10
    cord 742.9
      meningocele *(see also* Spina
          bifida) 741.9●
      specified type NEC 742.59
      spina bifida *(see also* Spina bifida)
          741.9●
      vessel 747.82
    meninges 742.59
    nerve root 742.9
  spleen 759.0
  Sprengel's 755.52
  sternum 756.3
  stomach 750.9
    specified type NEC 750.7
  submaxillary gland 750.9
  superior vena cava 747.40
  talipes - *see* Talipes

Anomaly, anomalous *(Continued)*
  tarsus 755.67
    with complete absence of distal
      elements 755.31
  teeth, tooth NEC 520.9
    position 524.30
      crowding 524.31
      displacement 524.30
        horizontal 524.33
        vertical 524.34
      distance
        interocclusal
          excessive 524.37
          insufficient 524.36
      excessive spacing 524.32
      rotation 524.35
      specified NEC 524.39
    spacing 524.30
  tendon 756.9
    specified type NEC 756.89
  termination
    coronary artery 746.85
  testis 752.9
  thebesian valve 746.9
  thigh 755.60
    flexion *(see also* Subluxation,
      congenital, hip) 754.32
  thorax (wall) 756.3
  throat 750.9
  thumb 755.50
    supernumerary 755.01
  thymus gland 759.2
  thyroid (gland) 759.2
    cartilage 748.3
  tibia 755.60
    saber 090.5
  toe 755.66
    supernumerary 755.02
    webbed *(see also* Syndactylism,
      toes) 755.13
  tongue 750.10
    specified type NEC 750.19
  trachea, tracheal 748.3
    cartilage 748.3
    rings 748.3
  tragus 744.3
  transverse aortic arch 747.21
  trichromata 368.59
  trichromatopsia 368.59
  tricuspid (leaflet) (valve) 746.9
    atresia 746.1
    Ebstein's 746.2
    specified type NEC 746.89
    stenosis 746.1
  trunk 759.9
  Uhl's (hypoplasia of myocardium,
    right ventricle) 746.84
  ulna 755.50
  umbilicus 759.9
    artery 747.5
  union, trachea with larynx 748.3
  unspecified site 759.9
  upper extremity 755.50
    vessel 747.63
  urachus 753.7
    specified type NEC 753.7
  ureter 753.9
    obstructive 753.20
    specified type NEC 753.4
      obstructive 753.29
  urethra (valve) 753.9
    obstructive 753.6
    specified type NEC 753.8

Anomaly, anomalous *(Continued)*
  urinary tract or system (any part,
    except urachus) 753.9
    specified type NEC 753.8
    urachus 753.7
  uterus 752.3
    with only one functioning horn
      752.3
    in pregnancy or childbirth 654.0●
      affecting fetus or newborn 763.89
      causing obstructed labor 660.2●
        affecting fetus or newborn
          763.1
  uvula 750.9
  vagina 752.40
  valleculae 748.3
  valve (heart) NEC 746.9
    formation, ureter 753.29
    pulmonary 746.00
    specified type NEC 746.89
  vascular NEC *(see also* Anomaly,
    peripheral vascular system)
    747.60
    ring 747.21
  vas deferens 752.9
  vein(s) (peripheral) NEC *(see also*
    Anomaly, peripheral vascular
    system) 747.60
    brain 747.81
    cerebral 747.81
    coronary 746.89
    great 747.40
      specified type NEC 747.49
    portal 747.40
    pulmonary 747.40
    retina 743.9
  vena cava (inferior) (superior) 747.40
  venous - *see* Anomaly, vein
  venous return (pulmonary) 747.49
    partial 747.42
    total 747.41
  ventricle, ventricular (heart) 746.9
    bands 746.9
    folds 746.9
    septa 745.4
  vertebra 756.10
  vesicourethral orifice 753.9
  vessels NEC *(see also* Anomaly,
    peripheral vascular system)
    747.60
    optic papilla 743.9
  vitelline duct 751.0
  vitreous humor 743.9
    specified type NEC 743.51
  vulva 752.40
  wrist (joint) 755.50
Anomia 784.69
Anonychia 757.5
  acquired 703.8
Anophthalmos, anophthalmus (clinical)
  (congenital) (globe) 743.00
  acquired V45.78
Anopsia (altitudinal) (quadrant) 368.46
Anorchia 752.89
Anorchism, anorchidism 752.89
Anorexia 783.0
  hysterical 300.11
  nervosa 307.1
Anosmia *(see also* Disturbance, sensation)
  781.1
  hysterical 300.11
  postinfectional 478.9
  psychogenic 306.7
  traumatic 951.8

Anosognosia 780.99
Anosphrasia 781.1
Anosteoplasia 756.50
Anotia 744.09
Anovulatory cycle 628.0
Anoxemia 799.02
  newborn 770.88
Anoxia 799.02
  altitude 993.2
  cerebral 348.1
    with
      abortion - *see* Abortion, by type,
        with specified complication
        NEC
      ectopic pregnancy *(see also*
        categories 633.0-633.9) 639.8
      molar pregnancy *(see also*
        categories 630-632) 639.8
    complicating
      delivery (cesarean) (instrumental)
        669.4●
      ectopic or molar pregnancy 639.8
      obstetric anesthesia or sedation
        668.2●
    during or resulting from a
      procedure 997.01
    following
      abortion 639.8
      ectopic or molar pregnancy
        639.8
    newborn *(see also* Distress, fetal,
      liveborn infant) 770.88
  due to drowning 994.1
  fetal, affecting newborn 770.88
  heart - *see* Insufficiency, coronary
  high altitude 993.2
  intrauterine
    fetal death (before onset of labor)
      768.0
      during labor 768.1
    liveborn infant - *see* Distress, fetal,
      liveborn infant
  myocardial - *see* Insufficiency, coronary
  newborn 768.9
    mild or moderate 768.6
    severe 768.5
  pathological 799.02
Anteflexion - *see* Anteversion
Antenatal
  care, normal pregnancy V22.1
    first V22.0
  sampling
    chorionic villus V28.89
  screening of mother (for) V28.9
    based on amniocentesis NEC V28.2
      chromosomal anomalies V28.0
      raised alphafetoprotein levels
        V28.1
    chromosomal anomalies V28.0
    fetal growth retardation using
      ultrasonics V28.4
    genomic V28.89
    isoimmunization V28.5
    malformations using ultrasonics
      V28.3
    proteomic V28.89
    raised alphafetoprotein levels in
      amniotic fluid V28.1
    risk
      pre-term labor V28.82
    specified condition NEC V28.89
    Streptococcus B V28.6
  survey
    fetal anatomic V28.81

◀ New   ◀▥ Revised   ~~deleted~~ Deleted   ● Use Additional Digit(s)   ▨ Omit code

Antenatal (Continued)
  testing
    nuchal translucency V28.89
Antepartum - see condition
Anterior - see also condition
  spinal artery compression syndrome
    721.1
Antero-occlusion 524.24
Anteversion
  cervix - see Anteversion, uterus
  femur (neck), congenital 755.63
  uterus, uterine (cervix) (postinfectional)
    (postpartal, old) 621.6
    congenital 752.3
    in pregnancy or childbirth 654.4●
      affecting fetus or newborn 763.89
      causing obstructed labor 660.2●
        affecting fetus or newborn
          763.1
Anthracosilicosis (occupational) 500
Anthracosis (lung) (occupational) 500
  lingua 529.3
Anthrax 022.9
  with pneumonia 022.1 [484.5]
  colitis 022.2
  cutaneous 022.0
  gastrointestinal 022.2
  intestinal 022.2
  pulmonary 022.1
  respiratory 022.1
  septicemia 022.3
  specified manifestation NEC 022.8
Anthropoid pelvis 755.69
  with disproportion (fetopelvic) 653.2●
    affecting fetus or newborn 763.1
    causing obstructed labor 660.1●
      affecting fetus or newborn 763.1
Anthropophobia 300.29
Antibioma, breast 611.0
Antibodies
  maternal (blood group) (see also
    Incompatibility) 656.2●
    anti-D, cord blood 656.1●
      fetus or newborn 773.0
Antibody deficiency syndrome
  agammaglobulinemic 279.00
  congenital 279.04
  hypogammaglobulinemic 279.00
Anticoagulant, intrinsic, circulating,
    causing hemorrhagic disorder
    (see also Circulating anticoagulants)
    286.5   ◀▥
Antimongolism syndrome 758.39
Antimonial cholera 985.4
Antisocial personality 301.7
Antithrombinemia (see also Circulating
    anticoagulants) 286.5
Antithromboplastinemia (see also
    Circulating anticoagulants) 286.5
Antithromboplastinogenemia (see also
    Circulating anticoagulants) 286.5
Antitoxin complication or reaction - see
    Complications, vaccination
Anton (-Babinski) syndrome
    (hemiasomatognosia) 307.9
Antritis (chronic) 473.0
  maxilla 473.0
    acute 461.0
  stomach 535.4●
Antrum, antral - see condition
Anuria 788.5
  with
    abortion - see Abortion, by type,
      with renal failure

Anuria (Continued)
  with (Continued)
    ectopic pregnancy (see also
      categories 633.0-633.9) 639.3
    molar pregnancy (see also categories
      630-632) 639.3
  calculus (impacted) (recurrent) 592.9
    kidney 592.0
    ureter 592.1
  congenital 753.3
  due to a procedure 997.5
  following
    abortion 639.3
    ectopic or molar pregnancy 639.3
  newborn 753.3
  postrenal 593.4
  puerperal, postpartum, childbirth
    669.3●
  specified as due to a procedure 997.5
  sulfonamide
    correct substance properly
      administered 788.5
    overdose or wrong substance given
      or taken 961.0
  traumatic (following crushing) 958.5
Anus, anal - see also condition
  high risk human papillomavirus (HPV)
    DNA test positive 796.75
  low risk human papillomavirus (HPV)
    DNA test positive 796.79
Anusitis 569.49
Anxiety (neurosis) (reaction) (state) 300.00
  alcohol-induced 291.89
  depression 300.4
  drug-induced 292.89
  due to or associated with physical
    condition 293.84
  generalized 300.02
  hysteria 300.20
  in
    acute stress reaction 308.0
    transient adjustment reaction 309.24
  panic type 300.01
  separation, abnormal 309.21
  syndrome (organic) (transient) 293.84
Aorta, aortic - see condition
Aortectasia 441.9
Aortitis (nonsyphilitic) 447.6
  arteriosclerotic 440.0
  calcific 447.6
  Döhle-Heller 093.1
  luetic 093.1
  rheumatic (see also Endocarditis, acute,
    rheumatic) 391.1
  rheumatoid - see Arthritis, rheumatoid
  specific 093.1
  syphilitic 093.1
    congenital 090.5
Apathetic ~~thyroid storm~~ (~~see also~~
    ~~Thyrotoxicosis~~) ~~242.9~~ 799.25   ◀▥
  thyroid storm (see also Thyrotoxicosis)
    242.9●   ◀
Apathy 799.25   ◀
Apepsia 536.8
  achlorhydric 536.0
  psychogenic 306.4
Aperistalsis, esophagus 530.0
Apert's syndrome
    (acrocephalosyndactyly) 755.55
Apert-Gallais syndrome (adrenogenital)
    255.2
Apertognathia 524.20
Aphagia 787.20
  psychogenic 307.1

Aphakia (acquired) (bilateral)
    (postoperative) (unilateral) 379.31
  congenital 743.35
Aphalangia (congenital) 755.4
  lower limb (complete) (intercalary)
    (partial) (terminal) 755.39
    meaning all digits (complete)
      (partial) 755.31
    transverse 755.31
  upper limb (complete) (intercalary)
    (partial) (terminal) 755.29
    meaning all digits (complete)
      (partial) 755.21
    transverse 755.21
Aphasia (amnestic) (ataxic) (auditory)
    (Broca's) (choreatic) (classic)
    (expressive) (global) (ideational)
    (ideokinetic) (ideomotor) (jargon)
    (motor) (nominal) (receptive)
    (semantic) (sensory) (syntactic)
    (verbal) (visual) (Wernicke's) 784.3
  developmental 315.31
  syphilis, tertiary 094.89
  uremic - see Uremia
Aphemia 784.3
  uremic - see Uremia
Aphonia 784.41
  clericorum 784.49
  hysterical 300.11
  organic 784.41
  psychogenic 306.1
Aphthae, aphthous - see also condition
  Bednar's 528.2
  cachectic 529.0
  epizootic 078.4
  fever 078.4
  oral 528.2
  stomatitis 528.2
  thrush 112.0
  ulcer (oral) (recurrent) 528.2
    genital organ(s) NEC
      female 616.50
      male 608.89
    larynx 478.79
Apical - see condition
Apical ballooning syndrome 429.83
Aplasia - see also Agenesis
  alveolar process (acquired) 525.8
    congenital 750.26
  aorta (congenital) 747.22
  aortic valve (congenital) 746.89
  axialis extracorticalis (congenital) 330.0
  bone marrow (myeloid) 284.9
    acquired (secondary) 284.89
    congenital 284.01
    idiopathic 284.9
  brain 740.0
    specified part 742.2
  breast 757.6
  bronchus 748.3
  cementum 520.4
  cerebellar 742.2
  congenital (pure) red cell 284.01
  corpus callosum 742.2
  erythrocyte 284.81
    congenital 284.01
  extracortical axial 330.0
  eye (congenital) 743.00
  fovea centralis (congenital) 743.55
  germinal (cell) 606.0
  iris 743.45
  labyrinth, membranous 744.05
  limb (congenital) 755.4
    lower NEC 755.30
    upper NEC 755.20

Aplasia (Continued)
  lung (bilateral) (congenital) (unilateral)
      748.5
  nervous system NEC 742.8
  nuclear 742.8
  ovary 752.0
  Pelizaeus-Merzbacher 330.0
  prostate (congenital) 752.89
  red cell (with thymoma) (adult) 284.81
      acquired (secondary) 284.81
      congenital 284.01
      hereditary 284.01
      of infants 284.01
      primary 284.01
      pure 284.01
  round ligament (congenital) 752.89
  salivary gland 750.21
  skin (congenital) 757.39
  spinal cord 742.59
  spleen 759.0
  testis (congenital) 752.89
  thymic, with immunodeficiency 279.2
  thyroid 243
  uterus 752.3
  ventral horn cell 742.59
Apleuria 756.3
Apnea, apneic (spells) 786.03
  newborn, neonatorum 770.81
      essential 770.81
      obstructive 770.82
      primary 770.81
      sleep 770.81
      specified NEC 770.82
  psychogenic 306.1
  sleep 780.57
      with
          hypersomnia, unspecified 780.53
          hyposomnia, unspecified 780.51
          insomnia, unspecified 780.51
          sleep disturbance 780.57
      central, in conditions classified
          elsewhere 327.27
      obstructive (adult) (pediatric)
          327.23
      organic 327.20
          other 327.29
      primary central 327.21
Apneumatosis newborn 770.4
Apodia 755.31
Apophysitis (bone) (see also
      Osteochondrosis) 732.9
  calcaneus 732.5
  juvenile 732.6
Apoplectiform convulsions (see also
      Disease, cerebrovascular, acute) 436
Apoplexia, apoplexy, apoplectic (see also
      Disease, cerebrovascular, acute) 436
  abdominal 569.89
  adrenal 036.3
  attack 436
  basilar (see also Disease,
      cerebrovascular, acute) 436
  brain (see also Disease, cerebrovascular,
      acute) 436
  bulbar (see also Disease,
      cerebrovascular, acute) 436
  capillary (see also Disease,
      cerebrovascular, acute) 436
  cardiac (see also Infarct, myocardium)
      410.9●
  cerebral (see also Disease,
      cerebrovascular, acute) 436
  chorea (see also Disease,
      cerebrovascular, acute) 436

Apoplexia, apoplexy, apoplectic
      (Continued)
  congestive (see also Disease,
      cerebrovascular, acute) 436
      newborn 767.4
  embolic (see also Embolism, brain)
      434.1●
  fetus 767.0
  fit (see also Disease, cerebrovascular,
      acute) 436
  healed or old V12.54
  heart (auricle) (ventricle) (see also
      Infarct, myocardium) 410.9●
  heat 992.0
  hemiplegia (see also Disease,
      cerebrovascular, acute) 436
  hemorrhagic (stroke) (see also
      Hemorrhage, brain) 432.9
  ingravescent (see also Disease,
      cerebrovascular, acute) 436
  late effect - see Late effect(s) (of)
      cerebrovascular disease
  lung - see Embolism, pulmonary
  meninges, hemorrhagic (see also
      Hemorrhage, subarachnoid) 430
  neonatorum 767.0
  newborn 767.0
  pancreatitis 577.0
  placenta 641.2●
  progressive (see also Disease,
      cerebrovascular, acute) 436
  pulmonary (artery) (vein) - see
      Embolism, pulmonary
  sanguineous (see also Disease,
      cerebrovascular, acute) 436
  seizure (see also Disease,
      cerebrovascular, acute) 436
  serous (see also Disease,
      cerebrovascular, acute) 436
  spleen 289.59
  stroke (see also Disease, cerebrovascular,
      acute) 436
  thrombotic (see also Thrombosis, brain)
      434.0●
  uremic - see Uremia
  uteroplacental 641.2●
Appendage
  fallopian tube (cyst of Morgagni) 752.11
  intestine (epiploic) 751.5
  preauricular 744.1
  testicular (organ of Morgagni) 752.89
Appendicitis 541
  with
      perforation, peritonitis
          (generalized), or rupture 540.0
      with peritoneal abscess 540.1
      peritoneal abscess 540.1
  acute (catarrhal) (fulminating)
      (gangrenous) (inflammatory)
      (obstructive) (retrocecal)
      (suppurative) 540.9
      with
          perforation, peritonitis, or
              rupture 540.0
          with peritoneal abscess 540.1
          peritoneal abscess 540.1
  amebic 006.8
  chronic (recurrent) 542
  exacerbation - see Appendicitis, acute
  fulminating - see Appendicitis, acute
  gangrenous - see Appendicitis, acute
  healed (obliterative) 542
  interval 542
  neurogenic 542

Appendicitis (Continued)
  obstructive 542
  pneumococcal 541
  recurrent 542
  relapsing 542
  retrocecal 541
  subacute (adhesive) 542
  subsiding 542
  suppurative - see Appendicitis, acute
  tuberculous (see also Tuberculosis)
      014.8●
Appendiclausis 543.9
Appendicolithiasis 543.9
Appendicopathia oxyurica 127.4
Appendix, appendicular - see also
      condition
  Morgagni (male) 752.89
      fallopian tube 752.11
Appetite
  depraved 307.52
  excessive 783.6
      psychogenic 307.51
  lack or loss (see also Anorexia) 783.0
      nonorganic origin 307.59
  perverted 307.52
      hysterical 300.11
Apprehension, apprehensiveness
      (abnormal) (state) 300.00
  specified type NEC 300.09
Approximal wear 521.10
Apraxia (classic) (ideational) (ideokinetic)
      (ideomotor) (motor) 784.69
  oculomotor, congenital 379.51
  verbal 784.69
Aptyalism 527.7
Aqueous misdirection 365.83
Arabicum elephantiasis (see also
      Infestation, filarial) 125.9
Arachnidism 989.5
Arachnitis - see Meningitis
Arachnodactyly 759.82
Arachnoidism 989.5
Arachnoiditis (acute) (adhesive) (basic)
      (brain) (cerebrospinal) (chiasmal)
      (chronic) (spinal) (see also
      Meningitis) 322.9
  meningococcal (chronic) 036.0
  syphilitic 094.2
  tuberculous (see also Tuberculosis,
      meninges) 013.0●
Araneism 989.5
Arboencephalitis, Australian 062.4
Arborization block (heart) 426.6
Arbor virus, arbovirus (infection) NEC
      066.9
ARC 042
Arches - see condition
Arcuatus uterus 752.3
Arcus (cornea)
  juvenilis 743.43
      interfering with vision 743.42
  senilis 371.41
Arc-welders' lung 503
Arc-welders' syndrome (photokeratitis)
      370.24
Areflexia 796.1
Areola - see condition
Argentaffinoma (M8241/1) - see also
      Neoplasm, by site, uncertain
      behavior
  benign (M8241/0) - see Neoplasm, by
      site, benign
  malignant (M8241/3) - see Neoplasm,
      by site, malignant
  syndrome 259.2

◄ New   ◄▥ Revised   ~~deleted~~ Deleted   ● Use Additional Digit(s)   ▨ Omit code

Argentinian hemorrhagic fever 078.7
Arginosuccinicaciduria 270.6
Argonz-Del Castillo syndrome
  (nonpuerperal galactorrhea and
  amenorrhea) 253.1
Argyll-Robertson phenomenon, pupil, or
  syndrome (syphilitic) 094.89
  atypical 379.45
  nonluetic 379.45
  nonsyphilitic 379.45
  reversed 379.45
Argyria, argyriasis NEC 985.8
  conjunctiva 372.55
  cornea 371.16
  from drug or medicinal agent
    correct substance properly
      administered 709.09
    overdose or wrong substance given
      or taken 961.2
Arhinencephaly 742.2
Arias-Stella phenomenon 621.30
Ariboflavinosis 266.0
Arizona enteritis 008.1
Arm - see condition
Armenian disease 277.31
Arnold-Chiari obstruction or syndrome
  (see also Spina bifida) 741.0●
  type I 348.4
  type II (see also Spina bifida) 741.0●
  type III 742.0
  type IV 742.2
Arousals
  confusional 327.41
Arrest, arrested
  active phase of labor 661.1●
    affecting fetus or newborn 763.7
  any plane in pelvis
    complicating delivery 660.1●
      affecting fetus or newborn 763.1
  bone marrow (see also Anemia, aplastic)
    284.9
  cardiac 427.5
    with
      abortion - see Abortion, by type,
        with specified complication
        NEC
      ectopic pregnancy (see also
        categories 633.0-633.9) 639.8
      molar pregnancy (see also
        categories 630-632) 639.8
    complicating
      anesthesia
        correct substance properly
          administered 427.5
        obstetric 668.1●
        overdose or wrong substance
          given 968.4
        specified anesthetic - see
          Table of Drugs and
          Chemicals
      delivery (cesarean) (instrumental)
        669.4●
      ectopic or molar pregnancy 639.8
      surgery (nontherapeutic)
        (therapeutic) 997.1
    fetus or newborn 779.85
    following
      abortion 639.8
      ectopic or molar pregnancy 639.8
    personal history, successfully
      rescucitated V12.53
    postoperative (immediate) 997.1
      long-term effect of cardiac
        surgery 429.4

Arrest, arrested (Continued)
  cardiorespiratory (see also Arrest,
    cardiac) 427.5
  deep transverse 660.3●
    affecting fetus or newborn 763.1
  development or growth
    bone 733.91
    child 783.40
    fetus 764.9●
      affecting management of
        pregnancy 656.5●
    tracheal rings 748.3
  epiphyseal 733.91
  granulopoiesis 288.09
  heart - see Arrest, cardiac
  respiratory 799.1
    newborn 770.87
  sinus 426.6
  transverse (deep) 660.3●
    affecting fetus or newborn 763.1
Arrhenoblastoma (M8630/1)
  benign (M8630/0)
    specified site - see Neoplasm, by site,
      benign
    unspecified site
      female 220
      male 222.0
  malignant (M8630/3)
    specified site - see Neoplasm, by site,
      malignant
    unspecified site
      female 183.0
      male 186.9
  specified site - see Neoplasm, by site,
    uncertain behavior
  unspecified site
    female 236.2
    male 236.4
Arrhinencephaly 742.2
  due to
    trisomy 13 (13-15) 758.1
    trisomy 18 (16-18) 758.2
Arrhythmia (auricle) (cardiac) (cordis)
  (gallop rhythm) (juvenile) (nodal)
  (reflex) (sinus) (supraventricular)
  (transitory) (ventricle) 427.9
  bigeminal rhythm 427.89
  block 426.9
  bradycardia 427.89
  contractions, premature 427.60
  coronary sinus 427.89
  ectopic 427.89
  extrasystolic 427.60
  postoperative 997.1
  psychogenic 306.2
  vagal 780.2
Arrillaga-Ayerza syndrome (pulmonary
  artery sclerosis with pulmonary
  hypertension) 416.0
Arsenical
  dermatitis 692.4
  keratosis 692.4
  pigmentation 985.1
    from drug or medicinal agent
      correct substance properly
        administered 709.09
      overdose or wrong substance
        given or taken 961.1
Arsenism 985.1
  from drug or medicinal agent
    correct substance properly
      administered 692.4
    overdose or wrong substance given
      or taken 961.1

Arterial - see condition
Arteriectasis 447.8
Arteriofibrosis - see Arteriosclerosis
Arteriolar sclerosis - see Arteriosclerosis
Arteriolith - see Arteriosclerosis
Arteriolitis 447.6
  necrotizing, kidney 447.5
  renal - see Hypertension, kidney
Arteriolosclerosis - see Arteriosclerosis
Arterionephrosclerosis (see also
  Hypertension, kidney) 403.90
Arteriopathy 447.9
Arteriosclerosis, arteriosclerotic (artery)
  (deformans) (diffuse) (disease)
  (endarteritis) (general) (obliterans)
  (obliterative) (occlusive) (senile)
  (with calcification) 440.9
  with
    gangrene 440.24
    psychosis (see also Psychosis,
      arteriosclerotic) 290.40
    ulceration 440.23
  aorta 440.0
  arteries of extremities - see
    Arteriosclerosis, extremities
  basilar (artery) (see also Occlusion,
    artery, basilar) 433.0●
  brain 437.0
  bypass graft
    coronary artery 414.05
      autologous artery
        (gastroepiploic) (internal
        mammary) 414.04
      autologous vein 414.02
      nonautologous biological 414.03
      of transplanted heart 414.07
    extremity 440.30
      autologous vein 440.31
      nonautologous biological 440.32
  cardiac - see Arteriosclerosis, coronary
  cardiopathy - see Arteriosclerosis,
    coronary
  cardiorenal (see also Hypertension,
    cardiorenal) 404.90
  cardiovascular (see also Disease,
    cardiovascular) 429.2
  carotid (artery) (common) (internal)
    (see also Occlusion, artery, carotid)
    433.1●
  central nervous system 437.0
  cerebral 437.0
    late effect - see Late effect(s) (of)
      cerebrovascular disease
  cerebrospinal 437.0
  cerebrovascular 437.0
  coronary (artery) 414.00
    due to lipid rich plaque 414.3
    graft - see Arteriosclerosis, bypass
      graft
    native artery 414.01
      of transplanted heart 414.06
  extremities (native artery) NEC 440.20
    bypass graft 440.30
      autologous vein 440.31
      nonautologous biological 440.32
    claudication (intermittent) 440.21
      and
        gangrene 440.24
        rest pain 440.22
          and
            gangrene 440.24
            ulceration 440.23
              and gangrene 440.24
        ulceration 440.23
          and gangrene 440.24

Arteriosclerosis, arteriosclerotic
(Continued)
  extremities NEC (Continued)
    gangrene 440.24
    rest pain 440.22
    and
      gangrene 440.24
      ulceration 440.23
        and gangrene 440.24
    specified site NEC 440.29
    ulceration 440.23
      and gangrene 440.24
  heart (disease) - see also
    Arteriosclerosis, coronary
    valve 424.99
      aortic 424.1
      mitral 424.0
      pulmonary 424.3
      tricuspid 424.2
  kidney (see also Hypertension, kidney)
    403.90
  labyrinth, labyrinthine 388.00
  medial NEC (see also Arteriosclerosis,
    extremities) 440.20
  mesentery (artery) 557.1
  Mönckeberg's (see also Arteriosclerosis,
    extremities) 440.20
  myocarditis 429.0
  nephrosclerosis (see also Hypertension,
    kidney) 403.90
  peripheral (of extremities) - see
    Arteriosclerosis, extremities
  precerebral 433.9●
    specified artery NEC 433.8●
  pulmonary (idiopathic) 416.0
  renal (see also Hypertension, kidney)
    403.90
    arterioles (see also Hypertension,
      kidney) 403.90
    artery 440.1
  retinal (vascular) 440.8 [362.13]
  specified artery NEC 440.8
    with gangrene 440.8 [785.4]
  spinal (cord) 437.0
  vertebral (artery) (see also Occlusion,
    artery, vertebral) 433.2●
Arteriospasm 443.9
Arteriovenous - see condition
Arteritis 447.6
  allergic (see also Angiitis,
    hypersensitivity) 446.20
  aorta (nonsyphilitic) 447.6
    syphilitic 093.1
  aortic arch 446.7
  brachiocephalica 446.7
  brain 437.4
    syphilitic 094.89
  branchial 446.7
  cerebral 437.4
    late effect - see Late effect(s) (of)
      cerebrovascular disease
    syphilitic 094.89
  coronary (artery) - see also
    Arteriosclerosis, coronary
    rheumatic 391.9
      chronic 398.99
    syphilitic 093.89
  cranial (left) (right) 446.5
  deformans - see Arteriosclerosis
  giant cell 446.5
  necrosing or necrotizing 446.0
  nodosa 446.0
  obliterans - see also Arteriosclerosis
    subclaviocarotica 446.7

Arteritis (Continued)
  pulmonary 417.8
  retina 362.18
  rheumatic - see Fever, rheumatic
  senile - see Arteriosclerosis
  suppurative 447.2
  syphilitic (general) 093.89
    brain 094.89
    coronary 093.89
    spinal 094.89
  temporal 446.5
  young female, syndrome 446.7
Artery, arterial - see condition
Arthralgia (see also Pain, joint) 719.4●
  allergic (see also Pain, joint) 719.4●
  in caisson disease 993.3
  psychogenic 307.89
  rubella 056.71
  Salmonella 003.23
  temporomandibular joint 524.62
Arthritis, arthritic (acute) (chronic)
    (subacute) 716.9●
  meaning Osteoarthritis - see
    Osteoarthrosis

> Note 08　Use the following fifth-digit
> subclassification with categories
> 711-712, 715-716:
>
> 0　　site unspecified
> 1　　shoulder region
> 2　　upper arm
> 3　　forearm
> 4　　hand
> 5　　pelvic region and thigh
> 6　　lower leg
> 7　　ankle and foot
> 8　　other specified sites
> 9　　multiple sites

  allergic 716.2●
  ankylosing (crippling) (spine) 720.0
    [713.2]
    sites other than spine 716.9●
  atrophic 714.0
    spine 720.9
  back (see also Arthritis, spine) 721.90
  Bechterew's (ankylosing spondylitis)
    720.0
  blennorrhagic 098.50 [711.6]●
  cervical, cervicodorsal (see also
    Spondylosis, cervical) 721.0
  Charcôt's 094.0 [713.5]
    diabetic 250.6● [713.5]
      due to secondary diabetes 249.6●
        [713.5]
    syringomyelic 336.0 [713.5]
    tabetic 094.0 [713.5]
  chylous (see also Filariasis) 125.9
    [711.7]●
  climacteric NEC 716.3●
  coccyx 721.8
  cricoarytenoid 478.79
  crystal (-induced) - see Arthritis, due to
    crystals
  deformans (see also Osteoarthrosis)
    715.9●
    spine 721.90
      with myelopathy 721.91
  degenerative (see also Osteoarthrosis)
    715.9●
    idiopathic 715.09
    polyarticular 715.09
    spine 721.90
      with myelopathy 721.91

Arthritis, arthritic (Continued)
  dermatoarthritis, lipoid 272.8 [713.0]
  due to or associated with
    acromegaly 253.0 [713.0]
    actinomycosis 039.8 [711.4]●
    amyloidosis 277.39 [713.7]
    bacterial disease NEC 040.89
      [711.4]●
    Behçet's syndrome 136.1 [711.2]●
    blastomycosis 116.0 [711.6]●
    brucellosis (see also Brucellosis) 023.9
      [711.4]●
    caisson disease 993.3
    coccidioidomycosis 114.3 [711.6]●
    coliform (Escherichia coli) 711.0●
    colitis, ulcerative - (see also Colitis,
      ulcerative) 556.9 [713.1]
    cowpox 051.01 [711.5]●
    crystals -(see also Gout)
      dicalcium phosphate 275.49
        [712.1]●
      pyrophosphate 275.49 [712.2]●
      specified NEC 275.49 [712.8]●
    dermatoarthritis, lipoid 272.8 [713.0]
    dermatological disorder NEC 709.9
      [713.3]
    diabetes 250.6● [713.5]
      due to secondary diabetes 249.6●
        [713.5]
    diphtheria 032.89 [711.4]●
    dracontiasis 125.7 [711.7]●
    dysentery 009.0 [711.3]●
    endocrine disorder NEC 259.9
      [713.0]
    enteritis NEC 009.1 [711.3]●
      infectious (see also Enteritis,
        infectious) 009.0 [711.3]●
        specified organism NEC 008.8
          [711.3]●
      regional (see also Enteritis,
        regional) 555.9 [713.1]
        specified organism NEC 008.8
          [711.3]●
    epiphyseal slip, nontraumatic (old)
      716.8●
    erysipelas 035 [711.4]●
    erythema
      epidemic 026.1
      multiforme 695.10 [713.3]
      nodosum 695.2 [713.3]
    Escherichia coli 711.0●
    filariasis NEC 125.9 [711.7]●
    gastrointestinal condition NEC 569.9
      [713.1]
    glanders 024 [711.4]●
    Gonococcus 098.50
    gout 274.00　　　　　　　◀▥▥
    H. influenzae 711.0●
    helminthiasis NEC 128.9 [711.7]●
    hematological disorder NEC 289.9
      [713.2]
    hemochromatosis 275.0 [713.0]
    hemoglobinopathy NEC (see also
      Disease, hemoglobin) 282.7
      [713.2]
    hemophilia (see also Hemophilia)
      286.0 [713.2]
    Hemophilus influenzae (H.
      influenzae) 711.0●
    Henoch (-Schönlein) purpura 287.0
      [713.6]
    histoplasmosis NEC (see also
      Histoplasmosis) 115.99
      [711.6]●

◀ New　　◀▥▥ Revised　　deleted Deleted　　● Use Additional Digit(s)　　▥▥ Omit code

Arthritis, arthritic (*Continued*)
  due to or associated with (*Continued*)
    human parvovirus 079.83
      [711.5]●
    hyperparathyroidism 252.00
      [713.0]
    hypersensitivity reaction NEC
      995.3 [713.6]
    hypogammaglobulinemia (*see also*
      Hypogammaglobulinemia)
      279.00 [713.0]
    hypothyroidism NEC 244.9
      [713.0]
    infection (*see also* Arthritis,
      infectious) 711.9●
    infectious disease NEC 136.9
      [711.8]●
    leprosy (*see also* Leprosy) 030.9
      [711.4]●
    leukemia NEC (M9800/3) 208.9●
      [713.2]
    lipoid dermatoarthritis 272.8
      [713.0]
    Lyme disease 088.81 [711.8]●
    Mediterranean fever, familial 277.31
      [713.7]
    meningococcal infection 036.82
    metabolic disorder NEC 277.9
      [713.0]
    multiple myelomatosis (M9730/3)
      203.0● [713.2]
    mumps 072.79 [711.5]●
    mycobacteria 031.8 [711.4]●
    mycosis NEC 117.9 [711.6]●
    neurological disorder NEC 349.9
      [713.5]
    ochronosis 270.2 [713.0]
    O'Nyong Nyong 066.3 [711.5]●
    parasitic disease NEC 136.9
      [711.8]●
    paratyphoid fever (*see also* Fever,
      paratyphoid) 002.9 [711.3]●
    parvovirus B19 079.83 [711.5]●
    Pneumococcus 711.0●
    poliomyelitis (*see also* Poliomyelitis)
      045.9● [711.5]●
    Pseudomonas 711.0●
    psoriasis 696.0
    pyogenic organism (E. coli) (H.
      influenzae) (Pseudomonas)
      (Streptococcus) 711.0●
    rat-bite fever 026.1 [711.4]●
    regional enteritis (*see also* Enteritis,
      regional) 555.9 [713.1]
    Reiter's disease 099.3 [711.1]●
    respiratory disorder NEC 519.9
      [713.4]
    reticulosis, malignant (M9720/3)
      202.3● [713.2]
    rubella 056.71
    salmonellosis 003.23
    sarcoidosis 135 [713.7]
    serum sickness 999.5 [713.6]
    Staphylococcus 711.0●
    Streptococcus 711.0●
    syphilis (*see also* Syphilis) 094.0
      [711.4]●
    syringomyelia 336.0 [713.5]
    thalassemia 282.49 [713.2]
    tuberculosis (*see also* Tuberculosis,
      arthritis) 015.9● [711.4]●
    typhoid fever 002.0 [711.3]●
    ulcerative colitis - (*see also* Colitis,
      ulcerative) 556.9 [713.1]

Arthritis, arthritic (*Continued*)
  due to or associated with (*Continued*)
    urethritis
      nongonococcal (*see also* Urethritis,
        nongonococcal) 099.40
        [711.1]●
      nonspecific (*see also* Urethritis,
        nongonococcal) 099.40
        [711.1]●
      Reiter's 099.3 [711.1]●
    viral disease NEC 079.99 [711.5]●
  erythema epidemic 026.1
  gonococcal 098.50
  gouty (acute) 274.00   ◀🞀
    acute 274.01   ◀
  hypertrophic (*see also* Osteoarthrosis)
    715.9●
    spine 721.90
      with myelopathy 721.91
  idiopathic, blennorrheal 099.3
  in caisson disease 993.3 [713.8]
  infectious or infective (acute) (chronic)
    (subacute) NEC 711.9●
    nonpyogenic 711.9●
    spine 720.9
  inflammatory NEC 714.9
  juvenile rheumatoid (chronic)
    (polyarticular) 714.30
    acute 714.31
    monoarticular 714.33
    pauciarticular 714.32
  lumbar (*see also* Spondylosis, lumbar)
    721.3
  meningococcal 036.82
  menopausal NEC 716.3●
  migratory - *see* Fever, rheumatic
  neuropathic (Charcôt's) 094.0 [713.5]
    diabetic 250.6● [713.5]
      due to secondary diabetes 249.6●
        [713.5]
    nonsyphilitic NEC 349.9 [713.5]
    syringomyelic 336.0 [713.5]
    tabetic 094.0 [713.5]
  nodosa (*see also* Osteoarthrosis) 715.9●
    spine 721.90
      with myelopathy 721.91
  nonpyogenic NEC 716.9●
    spine 721.90
      with myelopathy 721.91
  ochronotic 270.2 [713.0]
  palindromic (*see also* Rheumatism,
    palindromic) 719.3●
  pneumococcal 711.0●
  postdysenteric 009.0 [711.3]●
  postrheumatic, chronic (Jaccoud's)
    714.4
  primary progressive 714.0
    spine 720.9
  proliferative 714.0
    spine 720.0
  psoriatic 696.0
  purulent 711.0●
  pyogenic or pyemic 711.0●
  rheumatic 714.0
    acute or subacute - *see* Fever,
      rheumatic
    chronic 714.0
    spine 720.9
  rheumatoid (nodular) 714.0
    with
      splenoadenomegaly and
        leukopenia 714.1
      visceral or systemic involvement
        714.2

Arthritis, arthritic (*Continued*)
  rheumatoid (*Continued*)
    aortitis 714.89
    carditis 714.2
    heart disease 714.2
    juvenile (chronic) (polyarticular)
      714.30
      acute 714.31
      monoarticular 714.33
      pauciarticular 714.32
    spine 720.0
    rubella 056.71
    sacral, sacroiliac, sacrococcygeal (*see
      also* Spondylosis, sacral) 721.3
    scorbutic 267
    senile or senescent (*see also*
      Osteoarthrosis) 715.9●
      spine 721.90
        with myelopathy 721.91
    septic 711.0●
    serum (nontherapeutic) (therapeutic)
      999.5 [713.6]
    specified form NEC 716.8●
    spine 721.90
      with myelopathy 721.91
      atrophic 720.9
      degenerative 721.90
        with myelopathy 721.91
      hypertrophic (with deformity) 721.90
        with myelopathy 721.91
      infectious or infective NEC 720.9
      Marie-Strümpell 720.0
      nonpyogenic 721.90
        with myelopathy 721.91
      pyogenic 720.9
      rheumatoid 720.0
      traumatic (old) 721.7
      tuberculous (*see also* Tuberculosis)
        015.0● [720.81]
    staphylococcal 711.0●
    streptococcal 711.0●
    suppurative 711.0●
    syphilitic 094.0 [713.5]
      congenital 090.49 [713.5]
    syphilitica deformans (Charcôt) 094.0
      [713.5]
    temporomandibular joint 524.69
    thoracic (*see also* Spondylosis, thoracic)
      721.2
    toxic of menopause 716.3●
    transient 716.4●
    traumatic (chronic) (old) (post) 716.1●
      current injury - *see* nature of injury
    tuberculous (*see also* Tuberculosis,
      arthritis) 015.9● [711.4]●
    urethritica 099.3 [711.1]●
    urica, uratic 274.00   🞀
    venereal 099.3 [711.1]●
    vertebral (*see also* Arthritis, spine)
      721.90
    villous 716.8●
    von Bechterew's 720.0
Arthrocele (*see also* Effusion, joint) 719.0●
Arthrochondritis - *see* Arthritis
Arthrodesis status V45.4
Arthrodynia (*see also* Pain, joint) 719.4●
  psychogenic 307.89
Arthrodysplasia 755.9
Arthrofibrosis, joint (*see also* Ankylosis)
  718.5●
Arthrogryposis 728.3
  multiplex, congenita 754.89
Arthrokatadysis 715.35
Arthrolithiasis 274.00   🞀

Arthro-onychodysplasia 756.89
Arthro-osteo-onychodysplasia 756.89
Arthropathy (see also Arthritis) 716.9●

Note 09   Use the following fifth-digit
subclassification with categories 711-
712, 716:

0   site unspecified
1   shoulder region
2   upper arm
3   forearm
4   hand
5   pelvic region and thigh
6   lower leg
7   ankle and foot
8   other specified sites
9   multiple sites

Behçet's 136.1 [711.2]●
Charcôt's 094.0 [713.5]
    diabetic 250.6● [713.5]
        due to secondary diabetes 249.6●
            [713.5]
    syringomyelic 336.0 [713.5]
    tabetic 094.0 [713.5]
crystal (-induced) - see Arthritis, due to
    crystals
gouty 274.00   ◄▥
    acute 274.01   ◄
    chronic (without mention of tophus
        (tophi)) 274.02   ◄
    with tophus (tophi) 274.03   ◄
neurogenic, neuropathic (Charcôt's)
    (tabetic) 094.0 [713.5]
    diabetic 250.6● [713.5]
        due to secondary diabetes 249.6●
            [713.5]
    nonsyphilitic NEC 349.9 [713.5]
    syringomyelic 336.0 [713.5]
postdysenteric NEC 009.0 [711.3]●
postrheumatic, chronic (Jaccoud's) 714.4
psoriatic 696.0
pulmonary 731.2
specified NEC 716.8●
syringomyelia 336.0 [713.5]
tabes dorsalis 094.0 [713.5]
tabetic 094.0 [713.5]
transient 716.4●
traumatic 716.1●
uric acid 274.00   ◄▥
Arthrophyte (see also Loose, body, joint)
    718.1●
Arthrophytis 719.80
    ankle 719.87
    elbow 719.82
    foot 719.87
    hand 719.84
    hip 719.85
    knee 719.86
    multiple sites 719.89
    pelvic region 719.85
    shoulder (region) 719.81
    specified site NEC 719.88
    wrist 719.83
Arthropyosis (see also Arthritis, pyogenic)
    711.0●
Arthroscopic surgical procedure
    converted to open procedure V64.43
Arthrosis (deformans) (degenerative)
    (see also Osteoarthrosis) 715.9●
    Charcôt's 094.0 [713.5]
    polyarticular 715.09
    spine (see also Spondylosis) 721.90

Arthus phenomenon 995.21
    due to
        correct substance properly
            administered 995.21
        overdose or wrong substance given
            or taken 977.9
            specified drug - see Table of
                Drugs and Chemicals
        serum 999.5
Articular - see also condition
    disc disorder (reducing or non-
        reducing) 524.63
    spondylolisthesis 756.12
Articulation
    anterior 524.27
    posterior 524.27
    reverse 524.27
Artificial
    device (prosthetic) - see Fitting, device
    insemination V26.1
    menopause (states) (symptoms)
        (syndrome) 627.4
    opening status (functioning) (without
        complication) V44.9
        anus (colostomy) V44.3
        colostomy V44.3
        cystostomy V44.50
            appendico-vesicostomy V44.52
            cutaneous-vesicostomy V44.51
            specified type NEC V44.59
        enterostomy V44.4
        gastrostomy V44.1
        ileostomy V44.2
        intestinal tract NEC V44.4
        jejunostomy V44.4
        nephrostomy V44.6
        specified site NEC V44.8
    tracheostomy V44.0
    ureterostomy V44.6
    urethrostomy V44.6
    urinary tract NEC V44.6
    vagina V44.7
    vagina status V44.7
ARV (disease) (illness) (infection) - see
    Human immunodeficiency virus
    (disease) (illness) (infection)
Arytenoid - see condition
Asbestosis (occupational) 501
Asboe-Hansen's disease (incontinentia
    pigmenti) 757.33
Ascariasis (intestinal) (lung) 127.0
Ascaridiasis 127.0
Ascaridosis 127.0
Ascaris 127.0
    lumbricoides (infestation) 127.0
    pneumonia 127.0
Ascending - see condition
Aschoff's bodies (see also Myocarditis,
    rheumatic) 398.0
Ascites 789.59
    abdominal NEC 789.59
    cancerous (M8000/6) 789.51
    cardiac 428.0
    chylous (nonfilarial) 457.8
        filarial (see also Infestation, filarial)
            125.9
    congenital 778.0
    due to S. japonicum 120.2
    fetal, causing fetopelvic disproportion
        653.7●
    heart 428.0
    joint (see also Effusion, joint) 719.0●
    malignant (M8000/6) 789.51
    pseudochylous 789.59

Ascites (Continued)
    syphilitic 095.2
    tuberculous (see also Tuberculosis)
        014.0●
Ascorbic acid (vitamin C) deficiency
    (scurvy) 267
ASC-H (atypical squamous cells cannot
    exclude high grade squamous
    intraepithelial lesion)
    anus 796.72
    cervix 795.02
    vagina 795.12
ASC-US (atypical squamous cells of
    undetermined significance)
    anus 796.71
    cervix 795.01
    vagina 795.11
ASCVD (arteriosclerotic cardiovascular
    disease) 429.2
Aseptic - see condition
Asherman's syndrome 621.5
Asialia 527.7
Asiatic cholera (see also Cholera) 001.9
Asocial personality or trends 301.7
Asomatognosia 781.8
Aspergillosis 117.3
    with pneumonia 117.3 [484.6]
    allergic bronchopulmonary 518.6
    nonsyphilitic NEC 117.3
Aspergillus (flavus) (fumigatus)
    (infection) (terreus) 117.3
Aspermatogenesis 606.0
Aspermia (testis) 606.0
Asphyxia, asphyxiation (by) 799.01
    antenatal - see Distress, fetal
    bedclothes 994.7
    birth (see also Asphyxia, newborn)
        768.9
    bunny bag 994.7
    carbon monoxide 986
    caul (see also Asphyxia, newborn)
        768.9
    cave-in 994.7
        crushing - see Injury, internal,
            intrathoracic organs
    constriction 994.7
    crushing - see Injury, internal,
        intrathoracic organs
    drowning 994.1
    fetal, affecting newborn 768.9
    food or foreign body (in larynx) 933.1
        bronchioles 934.8
        bronchus (main) 934.1
        lung 934.8
        nasopharynx 933.0
        nose, nasal passages 932
        pharynx 933.0
        respiratory tract 934.9
            specified part NEC 934.8
        throat 933.0
        trachea 934.0
    gas, fumes, or vapor NEC 987.9
        specified - see Table of Drugs and
            Chemicals
    gravitational changes 994.7
    hanging 994.7
    inhalation - see Inhalation
    intrauterine
        fetal death (before onset of labor)
            768.0
            during labor 768.1
        liveborn infant - see Distress, fetal,
            liveborn infant
    local 443.0

◄ New   ◄▥ Revised   ~~deleted~~ Deleted   ● Use Additional Digit(s)   ▬ Omit code

Asphyxia, asphyxiation (*Continued*)
mechanical 994.7
during birth (*see also* Distress, fetal)
768.9
mucus 933.1
bronchus (main) 934.1
larynx 933.1
lung 934.8
nasal passages 932
newborn 770.18
pharynx 933.0
respiratory tract 934.9
specified part NEC 934.8
throat 933.0
trachea 934.0
vaginal (fetus or newborn) 770.18
newborn 768.9
with neurologic involvement 768.5
blue 768.6
livida 768.6
mild or moderate 768.6
pallida 768.5
severe 768.5
white 768.5
pathological 799.01
plastic bag 994.7
postnatal (*see also* Asphyxia, newborn)
768.9
mechanical 994.7
pressure 994.7
reticularis 782.61
strangulation 994.7
submersion 994.1
traumatic NEC - *see* Injury, internal,
intrathoracic organs
vomiting, vomitus - *see* Asphyxia, food
or foreign body
Aspiration
acid pulmonary (syndrome) 997.39
obstetric 668.0 ●
amniotic fluid 770.13
with respiratory symptoms 770.14
bronchitis 507.0
clear amniotic fluid 770.13
with
pneumonia 770.14
pneumonitis 770.14
respiratory symptoms 770.14
contents of birth canal 770.17
with respiratory symptoms 770.18
fetal 770.10
blood 770.15
with
pneumonia 770.16
pneumonitis 770.16
pneumonitis 770.18
food, foreign body, or gasoline (with
asphyxiation) - *see* Asphyxia,
food or foreign body
meconium 770.11
with
pneumonia 770.12
pneumonitis 770.12
respiratory symptoms 770.12
below vocal cords 770.11
with respiratory symptoms
770.12
mucus 933.1
into
bronchus (main) 934.1
lung 934.8
respiratory tract 934.9
specified part NEC 934.8
trachea 934.0

Aspiration (*Continued*)
mucus (*Continued*)
newborn 770.17
vaginal (fetus or newborn) 770.17
newborn 770.10
with respiratory symptoms 770.18
blood 770.15
with
pneumonia 770.16
pneumonitis 770.16
respiratory symptoms
770.16
pneumonia 507.0
fetus or newborn 770.18
meconium 770.12
pneumonitis 507.0
fetus or newborn 770.18
meconium 770.12
obstetric 668.0 ●
postnatal stomach contents 770.85
with
pneumonia 770.86
pneumonitis 770.86
respiratory symptoms 770.86
syndrome of newborn (massive)
770.18
meconium 770.12
vernix caseosa 770.17
Asplenia 759.0
with mesocardia 746.87
Assam fever 085.0
Assimilation, pelvis
with disproportion 653.2 ●
affecting fetus or newborn 763.1
causing obstructed labor 660.1 ●
affecting fetus or newborn
763.1
Assmann's focus (*see also* Tuberculosis)
011.0 ●
Astasia (-abasia) 307.9
hysterical 300.11
Asteatosis 706.8
cutis 706.8
Astereognosis 780.99
Asterixis 781.3
in liver disease 572.8
Asteroid hyalitis 379.22
Asthenia, asthenic 780.79
cardiac (*see also* Failure, heart) 428.9
psychogenic 306.2
cardiovascular (*see also* Failure, heart)
428.9
psychogenic 306.2
heart (*see also* Failure, heart) 428.9
psychogenic 306.2
hysterical 300.11
myocardial (*see also* Failure, heart)
428.9
psychogenic 306.2
nervous 300.5
neurocirculatory 306.2
neurotic 300.5
psychogenic 300.5
psychoneurotic 300.5
psychophysiologic 300.5
reaction, psychoneurotic 300.5
senile 797
Stiller's 780.79
tropical anhidrotic 705.1
Asthenopia 368.13
accommodative 367.4
hysterical (muscular) 300.11
psychogenic 306.7
Asthenospermia 792.2

Asthma, asthmatic (bronchial) (catarrh)
(spasmodic) 493.9 ●

> Note 10   The following fifth digit
> subclassification is for use with codes
> 493.0-493.2, 493.9:
>
> 0   unspecified
> 1   with status asthmaticus
> 2   with (acute) exacerbation

with
chronic obstructive pulmonary
disease (COPD) 493.2 ●
hay fever 493.0 ●
rhinitis, allergic 493.0 ●
allergic 493.9 ●
stated cause (external allergen)
493.0 ●
atopic 493.0 ●
cardiac (*see also* Failure, ventricular,
left) 428.1
cardiobronchial (*see also* Failure,
ventricular, left) 428.1
cardiorenal (*see also* Hypertension,
cardiorenal) 404.90
childhood 493.0 ●
Colliers' 500
cough variant 493.82
croup 493.9 ●
detergent 507.8
due to
detergent 507.8
inhalation of fumes 506.3
internal immunological process
493.0 ●
endogenous (intrinsic) 493.1 ●
eosinophilic 518.3
exercise induced bronchospasm 493.81
exogenous (cosmetics) (dander or dust)
(drugs) (dust) (feathers) (food)
(hay) (platinum) (pollen) 493.0 ●
extrinsic 493.0 ●
grinders' 502
hay 493.0 ●
heart (*see also* Failure, ventricular, left)
428.1
IgE 493.0 ●
infective 493.1 ●
intrinsic 493.1 ●
Kopp's 254.8
late-onset 493.1 ●
meat-wrappers' 506.9
Millar's (laryngismus stridulus) 478.75
millstone makers' 502
miners' 500
Monday morning 504
New Orleans (epidemic) 493.0 ●
platinum 493.0 ●
pneumoconiotic (occupational) NEC 505
potters' 502
psychogenic 316 [493.9] ●
pulmonary eosinophilic 518.3
red cedar 495.8
Rostan's (*see also* Failure, ventricular,
left) 428.1
sandblasters' 502
sequoiosis 495.8
stonemasons' 502
thymic 254.8
tuberculous (*see also* Tuberculosis,
pulmonary) 011.9 ●
Wichmann's (laryngismus stridulus)
478.75
wood 495.8

Astigmatism (compound) (congenital) 367.20
  irregular 367.22
  regular 367.21
Astroblastoma (M9430/3)
  nose 748.1
  specified site - see Neoplasm, by site, malignant
  unspecified site 191.9
Astrocytoma (cystic) (M9400/3)
  anaplastic type (M9401/3)
    specified site - see Neoplasm, by site, malignant
    unspecified site 191.9
  fibrillary (M9420/3)
    specified site - see Neoplasm, by site, malignant
    unspecified site 191.9
  fibrous (M9420/3)
    specified site - see Neoplasm, by site, malignant
    unspecified site 191.9
  gemistocytic (M9411/3)
    specified site - see Neoplasm, by site, malignant
    unspecified site 191.9
  juvenile (M9421/3)
    specified site - see Neoplasm, by site, malignant
    unspecified site 191.9
  nose 748.1
  pilocytic (M9421/3)
    specified site - see Neoplasm, by site, malignant
    unspecified site 191.9
  piloid (M9421/3)
    specified site - see Neoplasm, by site, malignant
    unspecified site 191.9
  protoplasmic (M9410/3)
    specified site - see Neoplasm, by site, malignant
    unspecified site 191.9
  specified site - see Neoplasm, by site, malignant
  subependymal (M9383/1) 237.5
    giant cell (M9384/1) 237.5
  unspecified site 191.9
Astroglioma (M9400/3)
  nose 748.1
  specified site - see Neoplasm, by site, malignant
  unspecified site 191.9
Asymbolia 784.60
Asymmetrical breathing 786.09
Asymmetry - see also Distortion
  breast, between native and reconstructed 612.1
  chest 786.9
  face 754.0
  jaw NEC 524.12
    maxillary 524.11
  pelvis with disproportion 653.0●
    affecting fetus or newborn 763.1
    causing obstructed labor 660.1●
      affecting fetus or newborn 763.1
Asynergia 781.3
Asynergy 781.3
  ventricular 429.89
Asystole (heart) (see also Arrest, cardiac) 427.5
At risk for falling V15.88

Ataxia, ataxy, ataxic 781.3
  acute 781.3
  brain 331.89
  cerebellar 334.3
    hereditary (Marie's) 334.2
    in
      alcoholism 303.9● [334.4]
      myxedema (see also Myxedema) 244.9 [334.4]
      neoplastic disease NEC 239.9 [334.4]
  cerebral 331.89
  family, familial 334.2
    cerebral (Marie's) 334.2
    spinal (Friedreich's) 334.0
  Friedreich's (heredofamilial) (spinal) 334.0
  frontal lobe 781.3
  gait 781.2
    hysterical 300.11
  general 781.3
  hereditary NEC 334.2
    cerebellar 334.2
    spastic 334.1
    spinal 334.0
  heredofamilial (Marie's) 334.2
  hysterical 300.11
  locomotor (progressive) 094.0
    diabetic 250.6● [337.1]
      due to secondary diabetes 249.6● [337.1]
  Marie's (cerebellar) (heredofamilial) 334.2
  nonorganic origin 307.9
  partial 094.0
  postchickenpox 052.7
  progressive locomotor 094.0
  psychogenic 307.9
  Sanger-Brown's 334.2
  spastic 094.0
    hereditary 334.1
    syphilitic 094.0
  spinal
    hereditary 334.0
    progressive locomotor 094.0
  telangiectasia 334.8
Ataxia-telangiectasia 334.8
Atelectasis (absorption collapse) (complete) (compression) (massive) (partial) (postinfective) (pressure collapse) (pulmonary) (relaxation) 518.0
  newborn (congenital) (partial) 770.5
    primary 770.4
  primary 770.4
  tuberculous (see also Tuberculosis, pulmonary) 011.9●
Ateleiosis, ateliosis 253.3
Atelia - see Distortion
Ateliosis 253.3
Atelocardia 746.9
Atelomyelia 742.59
Athelia 757.6
Atheroembolism
  extremity
    lower 445.02
    upper 445.01
  kidney 445.81
  specified site NEC 445.89
Atheroma, atheromatous (see also Arteriosclerosis) 440.9
  aorta, aortic 440.0
    valve (see also Endocarditis, aortic) 424.1

Atheroma, atheromatous (Continued)
  artery - see Arteriosclerosis
  basilar (artery) (see also Occlusion, artery, basilar) 433.0●
  carotid (artery) (common) (internal) (see also Occlusion, artery, carotid) 433.1●
  cerebral (arteries) 437.0
  coronary (artery) - see Arteriosclerosis, coronary
  degeneration - see Arteriosclerosis
  heart, cardiac - see Arteriosclerosis, coronary
  mitral (valve) 424.0
  myocardium, myocardial - see Arteriosclerosis, coronary
  pulmonary valve (heart) (see also Endocarditis, pulmonary) 424.3
  skin 706.2
  tricuspid (heart) (valve) 424.2
  valve, valvular - see Endocarditis
  vertebral (artery) (see also Occlusion, artery, vertebral) 433.2●
Atheromatosis - see also Arteriosclerosis
  arterial, congenital 272.8
Atherosclerosis - see Arteriosclerosis
Athetosis (acquired) 781.0
  bilateral 333.79
  congenital (bilateral) 333.6
  double 333.71
  unilateral 781.0
Athlete's
  foot 110.4
  heart 429.3
Athletic team examination V70.3
Athrepsia 261
Athyrea (acquired) (see also Hypothyroidism) 244.9
  congenital 243
Athyreosis (congenital) 243
  acquired - see Hypothyroidism
Athyroidism (acquired) (see also Hypothyroidism) 244.9
  congenital 243
Atmospheric pyrexia 992.0
Atonia, atony, atonic
  abdominal wall 728.2
  bladder (sphincter) 596.4
    neurogenic NEC 596.54
      with cauda equina syndrome 344.61
  capillary 448.9
  cecum 564.89
    psychogenic 306.4
  colon 564.89
    psychogenic 306.4
  congenital 779.89
  dyspepsia 536.3
    psychogenic 306.4
  intestine 564.89
    psychogenic 306.4
  stomach 536.3
    neurotic or psychogenic 306.4
    psychogenic 306.4
  uterus 661.2●
    with hemorrhage (postpartum) 666.1●
      affecting fetus or newborn 763.7
    without hemorrhage
      intrapartum 661.2●
      postpartum 669.8●
  vesical 596.4
Atopy NEC V15.09
Atransferrinemia, congenital 273.8

◀ New   ◀▦ Revised   deleted Deleted   ● Use Additional Digit(s)   ▦ Omit code

Atresia, atretic (congenital) 759.89
  alimentary organ or tract NEC
      751.8
    lower 751.2
    upper 750.8
  ani, anus, anal (canal) 751.2
  aorta 747.22
    with hypoplasia of ascending aorta
        and defective development of
        left ventricle (with mitral valve
        atresia) 746.7
    arch 747.11
    ring 747.21
  aortic (orifice) (valve) 746.89
    arch 747.11
  aqueduct of Sylvius 742.3
    with spina bifida (see also Spina
        bifida) 741.0●
  artery NEC (see also Atresia, blood
      vessel) 747.60
    cerebral 747.81
    coronary 746.85
    eye 743.58
    pulmonary 747.3
    umbilical 747.5
  auditory canal (external) 744.02
  bile, biliary duct (common) or passage
      751.61
    acquired (see also Obstruction,
        biliary) 576.2
  bladder (neck) 753.6
  blood vessel (peripheral) NEC
      747.60
    cerebral 747.81
    gastrointestinal 747.61
    lower limb 747.64
    pulmonary artery 747.3
    renal 747.62
    spinal 747.82
    upper limb 747.63
  bronchus 748.3
  canal, ear 744.02
  cardiac
    valve 746.89
      aortic 746.89
      mitral 746.89
      pulmonary 746.01
      tricuspid 746.1
  cecum 751.2
  cervix (acquired) 622.4
    congenital 752.49
    in pregnancy or childbirth 654.6●
      affecting fetus or newborn
          763.89
      causing obstructed labor 660.2●
        affecting fetus or newborn
            763.1
  choana 748.0
  colon 751.2
  cystic duct 751.61
    acquired 575.8
      with obstruction (see also
          Obstruction, gallbladder)
          575.2
  digestive organs NEC 751.8
  duodenum 751.1
  ear canal 744.02
  ejaculatory duct 752.89
  epiglottis 748.3
  esophagus 750.3
  Eustachian tube 744.24
  fallopian tube (acquired) 628.2
    congenital 752.19
  follicular cyst 620.0

Atresia, atretic (Continued)
  foramen of
    Luschka 742.3
      with spina bifida (see also Spina
          bifida) 741.0●
    Magendie 742.3
      with spina bifida (see also Spina
          bifida) 741.0●
  gallbladder 751.69
  genital organ
    external
      female 752.49
      male NEC 752.89
        penis 752.69
    internal
      female 752.89
      male 752.89
  glottis 748.3
  gullet 750.3
  heart
    valve NEC 746.89
      aortic 746.89
      mitral 746.89
      pulmonary 746.01
      tricuspid 746.1
  hymen 752.42
    acquired 623.3
    postinfective 623.3
  ileum 751.1
  intestine (small) 751.1
    large 751.2
  iris, filtration angle (see also
      Buphthalmia) 743.20
  jejunum 751.1
  kidney 753.3
  lacrimal, apparatus 743.65
    acquired - see Stenosis, lacrimal
  larynx 748.3
  ligament, broad 752.19
  lung 748.5
  meatus urinarius 753.6
  mitral valve 746.89
    with atresia or hypoplasia of aortic
        orifice or valve, with
        hypoplasia of ascending aorta
        and defective development of
        left ventricle 746.7
  nares (anterior) (posterior) 748.0
  nasolacrimal duct 743.65
  nasopharynx 748.8
  nose, nostril 748.0
    acquired 738.0
  organ or site NEC - see Anomaly,
      specified type NEC
  osseous meatus (ear) 744.03
  oviduct (acquired) 628.2
    congenital 752.19
  parotid duct 750.23
    acquired 527.8
  pulmonary (artery) 747.3
    valve 746.01
    vein 747.49
  pulmonic 746.01
  pupil 743.46
  rectum 751.2
  salivary duct or gland 750.23
    acquired 527.8
  sublingual duct 750.23
    acquired 527.8
  submaxillary duct or gland 750.23
    acquired 527.8
  trachea 748.3
  tricuspid valve 746.1
  ureter 753.29

Atresia, atretic (Continued)
  ureteropelvic junction 753.21
  ureterovesical orifice 753.22
  urethra (valvular) 753.6
  urinary tract NEC 753.29
  uterus 752.3
    acquired 621.8
  vagina (acquired) 623.2
    congenital 752.49
    postgonococcal (old) 098.2
    postinfectional 623.2
    senile 623.2
  vascular NEC (see also Atresia, blood
      vessel) 747.60
    cerebral 747.81
  vas deferens 752.89
  vein NEC (see also Atresia, blood
      vessel) 747.60
    cardiac 746.89
    great 747.49
    portal 747.49
    pulmonary 747.49
  vena cava (inferior) (superior) 747.49
  vesicourethral orifice 753.6
  vulva 752.49
    acquired 624.8
Atrichia, atrichosis 704.00
  congenital (universal) 757.4
Atrioventricularis commune 745.69
Atrophia - see also Atrophy
  alba 709.09
  cutis 701.8
    idiopathica progressiva 701.8
    senilis 701.8
  dermatological, diffuse (idiopathic)
      701.8
  flava hepatis (acuta) (subacuta) (see also
      Necrosis, liver) 570
  gyrata of choroid and retina (central)
      363.54
    generalized 363.57
  senilis 797
    dermatological 701.8
  unguium 703.8
    congenita 757.5
Atrophoderma, atrophodermia 701.9
  diffusum (idiopathic) 701.8
  maculatum 701.3
    et striatum 701.3
      due to syphilis 095.8
    syphilitic 091.3
  neuriticum 701.8
  pigmentosum 757.33
  reticulatum symmetricum faciei 701.8
  senile 701.8
  symmetrical 701.8
  vermiculata 701.8
Atrophy, atrophic
  adrenal (autoimmune) (capsule)
      (cortex) (gland) 255.41
    with hypofunction 255.41
  alveolar process or ridge (edentulous)
      525.20
    mandible 525.20
      minimal 525.21
      moderate 525.22
      severe 525.23
    maxilla 525.20
      minimal 525.24
      moderate 525.25
      severe 525.26
  appendix 543.9
  Aran-Duchenne muscular 335.21
  arm 728.2

Atrophy, atrophic *(Continued)*
  arteriosclerotic - *see* Arteriosclerosis
  arthritis 714.0
    spine 720.9
  bile duct (any) 576.8
  bladder 596.8
  blanche (of Milian) 701.3
  bone (senile) 733.99
    due to
      disuse 733.7
      infection 733.99
      tabes dorsalis (neurogenic)
        094.0
    posttraumatic 733.99
  brain (cortex) (progressive) 331.9
    with dementia 290.10
    Alzheimer's 331.0
      with dementia - *see* Alzheimer's,
        dementia
    circumscribed (Pick's) 331.11
      with dementia
        with behavioral disturbance
          331.11 *[294.11]*
        without behavioral
          disturbance 331.11
          [294.10]
    congenital 742.4
    hereditary 331.9
    senile 331.2
  breast 611.4
    puerperal, postpartum 676.3●
  buccal cavity 528.9
  cardiac (brown) (senile) *(see also*
      Degeneration, myocardial)
      429.1
  cartilage (infectional) (joint) 733.99
  cast, plaster of Paris 728.2
  cerebellar - *see* Atrophy, brain
  cerebral - *see* Atrophy, brain
  cervix (endometrium) (mucosa)
      (myometrium) (senile) (uteri)
      622.8
    menopausal 627.8
  Charcôt-Marie-Tooth 356.1
  choroid 363.40
    diffuse secondary 363.42
    hereditary *(see also* Dystrophy,
        choroid) 363.50
      gyrate
        central 363.54
        diffuse 363.57
        generalized 363.57
    senile 363.41
  ciliary body 364.57
  colloid, degenerative 701.3
  conjunctiva (senile) 372.89
  corpus cavernosum 607.89
  cortical *(see also* Atrophy, brain) 331.9
  Cruveilhier's 335.21
  cystic duct 576.8
  dacryosialadenopathy 710.2
  degenerative
    colloid 701.3
    senile 701.3
  Déjérine-Thomas 333.0
  diffuse idiopathic, dermatological
      701.8
  disuse
    bone 733.7
    muscle 728.2
    pelvic muscles and anal sphincter
      618.83
  Duchenne-Aran 335.21
  ear 388.9

Atrophy, atrophic *(Continued)*
  edentulous alveolar ridge 525.20
    mandible 525.20
      minimal 525.21
      moderate 525.22
      severe 525.23
    maxilla 525.20
      minimal 525.24
      moderate 525.25
      severe 525.26
  emphysema, lung 492.8
  endometrium (senile) 621.8
    cervix 622.8
  enteric 569.89
  epididymis 608.3
  eyeball, cause unknown 360.41
  eyelid (senile) 374.50
  facial (skin) 701.9
  facioscapulohumeral (Landouzy-
      Déjérine) 359.1
  fallopian tube (senile), acquired 620.3
  fatty, thymus (gland) 254.8
  gallbladder 575.8
  gastric 537.89
  gastritis (chronic) 535.1●
  gastrointestinal 569.89
  genital organ, male 608.89
  glandular 289.3
  globe (phthisis bulbi) 360.41
  gum *(see also* Recession, gingival)
      523.20
  hair 704.2
  heart (brown) (senile) *(see also*
      Degeneration, myocardial) 429.1
  hemifacial 754.0
    Romberg 349.89
  hydronephrosis 591
  infantile 261
    paralysis, acute *(see also*
        Poliomyelitis, with paralysis)
        045.1●
  intestine 569.89
  iris (generalized) (postinfectional)
      (sector shaped) 364.59
    essential 364.51
    progressive 364.51
    sphincter 364.54
  kidney (senile) *(see also* Sclerosis, renal)
      587
    with hypertension *(see also*
        Hypertension, kidney) 403.90
    congenital 753.0
    hydronephrotic 591
    infantile 753.0
  lacrimal apparatus (primary) 375.13
    secondary 375.14
  Landouzy-Déjérine 359.1
  laryngitis, infection 476.0
  larynx 478.79
  Leber's optic 377.16
  lip 528.5
  liver (acute) (subacute) *(see also*
      Necrosis, liver) 570
    chronic (yellow) 571.8
    yellow (congenital) 570
      with
        abortion - *see* Abortion, by
          type, with specified
          complication NEC
        ectopic pregnancy *(see also*
          categories 633.0-633.9)
          639.8
        molar pregnancy *(see also*
          categories 630-632) 639.8

Atrophy, atrophic *(Continued)*
  liver *(Continued)*
    yellow *(Continued)*
      chronic 571.8
      complicating pregnancy 646.7●
      following
        abortion 639.8
        ectopic or molar pregnancy
          639.8
      from injection, inoculation or
        transfusion (onset within 8
        months after
        administration) - *see*
        Hepatitis, viral
      healed 571.5
      obstetric 646.7●
      postabortal 639.8
      postimmunization - *see* Hepatitis,
        viral
      posttransfusion - *see* Hepatitis,
        viral
      puerperal, postpartum 674.8●
  lung (senile) 518.89
    congenital 748.69
  macular (dermatological) 701.3
    syphilitic, skin 091.3
      striated 095.8
  muscle, muscular 728.2
    disuse 728.2
    Duchenne-Aran 335.21
    extremity (lower) (upper) 728.2
    familial spinal 335.11
    general 728.2
    idiopathic 728.2
    infantile spinal 335.0
    myelopathic (progressive) 335.10
    myotonic 359.21
    neuritic 356.1
    neuropathic (peroneal) (progressive)
      356.1
    peroneal 356.1
    primary (idiopathic) 728.2
    progressive (familial) (hereditary)
      (pure) 335.21
      adult (spinal) 335.19
      infantile (spinal) 335.0
      juvenile (spinal) 335.11
      spinal 335.10
        adult 335.19
        hereditary or familial
          335.11
        infantile 335.0
    pseudohypertrophic 359.1
    spinal (progressive) 335.10
      adult 335.19
      Aran-Duchenne 335.21
      familial 335.11
      hereditary 335.11
      infantile 335.0
      juvenile 335.11
    syphilitic 095.6
  myocardium *(see also* Degeneration,
      myocardial) 429.1
  myometrium (senile) 621.8
    cervix 622.8
  myotatic 728.2
  myotonia 359.21
  nail 703.8
    congenital 757.5
  nasopharynx 472.2
  nerve - *see also* Disorder, nerve
    abducens 378.54
    accessory 352.4
    acoustic or auditory 388.5

◀ New   ◀▥ Revised   ~~deleted~~ Deleted   ● Use Additional Digit(s)   ▨ Omit code

Atrophy, atrophic (Continued)
nerve (Continued)
cranial 352.9
first (olfactory) 352.0
second (optic) (see also Atrophy,
optic nerve) 377.10
third (oculomotor) (partial)
378.51
total 378.52
fourth (trochlear) 378.53
fifth (trigeminal) 350.8
sixth (abducens) 378.54
seventh (facial) 351.8
eighth (auditory) 388.5
ninth (glossopharyngeal) 352.2
tenth (pneumogastric) (vagus)
352.3
eleventh (accessory) 352.4
twelfth (hypoglossal) 352.5
facial 351.8
glossopharyngeal 352.2
hypoglossal 352.5
oculomotor (partial) 378.51
total 378.52
olfactory 352.0
peripheral 355.9
pneumogastric 352.3
trigeminal 350.8
trochlear 378.53
vagus (pneumogastric) 352.3
nervous system, congenital 742.8
neuritic (see also Disorder, nerve) 355.9
neurogenic NEC 355.9
bone
tabetic 094.0
nutritional 261
old age 797
olivopontocerebellar 333.0
optic nerve (ascending) (descending)
(infectional) (nonfamilial)
(papillomacular bundle)
(postretinal) (secondary NEC)
(simple) 377.10
associated with retinal dystrophy
377.13
dominant hereditary 377.16
glaucomatous 377.14
hereditary (dominant) (Leber's)
377.16
Leber's (hereditary) 377.16
partial 377.15
postinflammatory 377.12
primary 377.11
syphilitic 094.84
congenital 090.49
tabes dorsalis 094.0
orbit 376.45
ovary (senile), acquired 620.3
oviduct (senile), acquired 620.3
palsy, diffuse 335.20
pancreas (duct) (senile) 577.8
papillary muscle 429.81
paralysis 355.9
parotid gland 527.0
patches skin 701.3
senile 701.8
penis 607.89
pharyngitis 472.1
pharynx 478.29
pluriglandular 258.8
polyarthritis 714.0
prostate 602.2
pseudohypertrophic 359.1
renal (see also Sclerosis, renal) 587

Atrophy, atrophic (Continued)
reticulata 701.8
retina (see also Degeneration, retina)
362.60
hereditary (see also Dystrophy,
retina) 362.70
rhinitis 472.0
salivary duct or gland 527.0
scar NEC 709.2
sclerosis, lobar (of brain) 331.0
with dementia
with behavioral disturbance 331.0
[294.11]
without behavioral disturbance
331.0 [294.10]
scrotum 608.89
seminal vesicle 608.89
senile 797
degenerative, of skin 701.3
skin (patches) (senile) 701.8
spermatic cord 608.89
spinal (cord) 336.8
acute 336.8
muscular (chronic) 335.10
adult 335.19
familial 335.11
juvenile 335.10
paralysis 335.10
acute (see also Poliomyelitis, with
paralysis) 045.1●
spine (column) 733.99
spleen (senile) 289.59
spots (skin) 701.3
senile 701.8
stomach 537.89
striate and macular 701.3
syphilitic 095.8
subcutaneous 701.9
due to injection 999.9
sublingual gland 527.0
submaxillary gland 527.0
Sudeck's 733.7
suprarenal (autoimmune) (capsule)
(gland) 255.41
with hypofunction 255.41
tarso-orbital fascia, congenital 743.66
testis 608.3
thenar, partial 354.0
throat 478.29
thymus (fat) 254.8
thyroid (gland) 246.8
with
cretinism 243
myxedema 244.9
congenital 243
tongue (senile) 529.8
papillae 529.4
smooth 529.4
trachea 519.19
tunica vaginalis 608.89
turbinate 733.99
tympanic membrane (nonflaccid)
384.82
flaccid 384.81
ulcer (see also Ulcer, skin) 707.9
upper respiratory tract 478.29
uterus, uterine (acquired) (senile) 621.8
cervix 622.8
due to radiation (intended effect) 621.8
vagina (senile) 627.3
vascular 459.89
vas deferens 608.89
vertebra (senile) 733.99
vulva (primary) (senile) 624.1

Atrophy, atrophic (Continued)
Werdnig-Hoffmann 335.0
yellow (acute) (congenital) (liver)
(subacute) (see also Necrosis,
liver) 570
chronic 571.8
resulting from administration of
blood, plasma, serum, or other
biological substance (within 8
months of administration) - see
Hepatitis, viral
Attack
akinetic (see also Epilepsy) 345.0●
angina - see Angina
apoplectic (see also Disease,
cerebrovascular, acute) 436
benign shuddering 333.93
bilious - see Vomiting
cataleptic 300.11
cerebral (see also Disease,
cerebrovascular, acute) 436
coronary (see also Infarct, myocardium)
410.9●
cyanotic, newborn 770.83
epileptic (see also Epilepsy) 345.9●
epileptiform 780.39
heart (see also Infarct, myocardium)
410.9●
hemiplegia (see also Disease,
cerebrovascular, acute) 436
hysterical 300.11
jacksonian (see also Epilepsy) 345.5●
myocardium, myocardial (see also
Infarct, myocardium) 410.9●
myoclonic (see also Epilepsy) 345.1●
panic 300.01
paralysis (see also Disease,
cerebrovascular, acute) 436
paroxysmal 780.39
psychomotor (see also Epilepsy) 345.4●
salaam (see also Epilepsy) 345.6●
schizophreniform (see also
Schizophrenia) 295.4●
sensory and motor 780.39
syncope 780.2
toxic, cerebral 780.39
transient ischemic (TIA) 435.9
unconsciousness 780.2
hysterical 300.11
vasomotor 780.2
vasovagal (idiopathic) (paroxysmal)
780.2
Attention to
artificial
opening (of) V55.9
digestive tract NEC V55.4
specified site NEC V55.8
urinary tract NEC V55.6
vagina V55.7
colostomy V55.3
cystostomy V55.5
dressing
wound V58.30
nonsurgical V58.30
surgical V58.31
gastrostomy V55.1
ileostomy V55.2
jejunostomy V55.4
nephrostomy V55.6
surgical dressings V58.31
sutures V58.32
tracheostomy V55.0
ureterostomy V55.6
urethrostomy V55.6

Attrition
    gum (*see also* Recession, gingival)
        523.20
    teeth (hard tissues) 521.10
        excessive 521.10
            extending into
                dentine 521.12
                pulp 521.13
            generalized 521.15
            limited to enamel 521.11
            localized 521.14
Atypical - *see also* condition
    cells
        endocervical 795.00
        endometrial 795.00
        glandular
            anus 796.70
            cervical 795.00
            vaginal 795.10
    distribution, vessel (congenital)
        (peripheral) NEC 747.60
    endometrium 621.9
    kidney 593.89
Atypism, cervix 622.10
Audible tinnitus (*see also* Tinnitus) 388.30
Auditory - *see* condition
Audry's syndrome (acropachyderma) 757.39
Aujeszky's disease 078.89
Aura
    jacksonian (*see also* Epilepsy) 345.5●
    persistent migraine 346.5●
        with cerebral infarction 346.6●
        without cerebral infarction 346.5●
Aurantiasis, cutis 278.3
Auricle, auricular - *see* condition
Auriculotemporal syndrome 350.8
Australian
    Q fever 083.0
    X disease 062.4
Autism, autistic (child) (infantile) 299.0●
Autodigestion 799.89
Autoerythrocyte sensitization 287.2
Autographism 708.3
Autoimmune
    cold sensitivity 283.0
    disease NEC 279.49   ◄▦▦
    hemolytic anemia 283.0
    lymphoproliferative syndrome (ALPS)
        279.41   ◄
    thyroiditis 245.2
Autoinfection, septic - *see* Septicemia
Autointoxication 799.89
Automatism 348.89   ◄▦▦
    epileptic (*see also* Epilepsy) 345.4●
    paroxysmal, idiopathic (*see also*
        Epilepsy) 345.4●

Autonomic, autonomous
    bladder 596.54
        neurogenic 596.54
            with cauda equina 344.61
    dysreflexia 337.3
    faciocephalalgia (*see also* Neuropathy,
        peripheral, autonomic) 337.9
    hysterical seizure 300.11
    imbalance (*see also* Neuropathy,
        peripheral, autonomic 337.9
Autophony 388.40
Autosensitivity, erythrocyte 287.2
Autotopagnosia 780.99
Autotoxemia 799.89
Autumn - *see* condition
Avellis' syndrome 344.89
Aviators
    disease or sickness (*see also* Effect,
        adverse, high altitude) 993.2
    ear 993.0
    effort syndrome 306.2
Avitaminosis (multiple NEC) (*see also*
        Deficiency, vitamin) 269.2
    A 264.9
    B 266.9
        with
            beriberi 265.0
            pellagra 265.2
    B_1 265.1
    B_2 266.0
    B_6 266.1
    B_{12} 266.2
    C (with scurvy) 267
    D 268.9
        with
            osteomalacia 268.2
            rickets 268.0
    E 269.1
    G 266.0
    H 269.1
    K 269.0
    multiple 269.2
    nicotinic acid 265.2
    P 269.1
Avulsion (traumatic) 879.8
    blood vessel - *see* Injury, blood vessel,
        by site
    cartilage - *see also* Dislocation, by site
        knee, current (*see also* Tear,
            meniscus) 836.2
        symphyseal (inner), complicating
            delivery 665.6●
    complicated 879.9
    diaphragm - *see* Injury, internal,
        diaphragm

Avulsion (*Continued*)
    ear - *see* Wound, open, ear
    epiphysis of bone - *see* Fracture, by site
    external site other than limb - *see*
        Wound, open, by site
    eye 871.3
    fingernail - *see* Wound, open, finger
    fracture - *see* Fracture, by site
    genital organs, external - *see* Wound,
        open, genital organs
    head (intracranial) NEC - *see also* Injury,
        intracranial, with open
        intracranial wound
        complete 874.9
        external site NEC 873.8
        complicated 873.9
    internal organ or site - *see* Injury,
        internal, by site
    joint - *see also* Dislocation, by site
        capsule - *see* Sprain, by site
    ligament - *see* Sprain, by site
    limb - *see also* Amputation, traumatic,
        by site
        skin and subcutaneous tissue - *see*
            Wound, open, by site
    muscle - *see* Sprain, by site
    nerve (root) - *see* Injury, nerve, by site
    scalp - *see* Wound, open, scalp
    skin and subcutaneous tissue - *see*
        Wound, open, by site
    symphyseal cartilage (inner),
        complicating delivery 665.6●
    tendon - *see also* Sprain, by site
        with open wound - *see* Wound,
            open, by site
    toenail - *see* Wound, open, toe(s)
    tooth 873.63
        complicated 873.73
Awaiting organ transplant status V49.83
Awareness of heart beat 785.1
Axe grinders' disease 502
Axenfeld's anomaly or syndrome 743.44
Axilla, axillary - *see also* condition
    breast 757.6
Axonotmesis - *see* Injury, nerve, by site
Ayala's disease 756.89
Ayerza's disease or syndrome
        (pulmonary artery sclerosis with
        pulmonary hypertension) 416.0
Azoospermia 606.0
Azorean disease (of the nervous system)
        334.8
Azotemia 790.6
    meaning uremia (*see also* Uremia) 586
Aztec ear 744.29
Azygos lobe, lung (fissure) 748.69

◄ New   ◄▦▦ Revised   ~~deleted~~ Deleted   ● Use Additional Digit(s)   ▦▦ Omit code

B

Baader's syndrome (erythema multiforme exudativum) 695.19
Baastrup's syndrome 721.5
Babesiasis 088.82
Babesiosis 088.82
Babington's disease (familial hemorrhagic telangiectasia) 448.0
Babinski's syndrome (cardiovascular syphilis) 093.89
Babinski-Fröhlich syndrome (adiposogenital dystrophy) 253.8
Babinski-Nageotte syndrome 344.89
Bacillary - see condition
Bacilluria 791.9
  asymptomatic, in pregnancy or puerperium 646.5●
  tuberculous (see also Tuberculosis) 016.9●
Bacillus - see also Infection, bacillus
  abortus infection 023.1
  anthracis infection 022.9
  coli
    infection 041.4
      generalized 038.42
      intestinal 008.00
    pyemia 038.42
    septicemia 038.42
  Flexner's 004.1
  fusiformis infestation 101
  mallei infection 024
  Shiga's 004.0
  suipestifer infection (see also Infection, Salmonella) 003.9
Back - see condition
Backache (postural) 724.5
  psychogenic 307.89
  sacroiliac 724.6
Backflow (pyelovenous) (see also Disease, renal) 593.9
Backknee (see also Genu, recurvatum) 736.5
Bacteremia 790.7
  newborn 771.83
Bacteria
  in blood (see also Bacteremia) 790.7
  in urine (see also Bacteriuria) 791.9
Bacterial - see condition
Bactericholia (see also Cholecystitis, acute) 575.0
Bacterid, bacteride (Andrews' pustular) 686.8
Bacteriuria, bacteruria 791.9
  with
    urinary tract infection 599.0
  asymptomatic 791.9
    in pregnancy or puerperium 646.5●
      affecting fetus or newborn 760.1
Bad
  breath 784.99
  heart - see Disease, heart
  trip (see also Abuse, drugs, nondependent) 305.3●
Baehr-Schiffrin disease (thrombotic thrombocytopenic purpura) 446.6
Baelz's disease (cheilitis glandularis apostematosa) 528.5
Baerensprung's disease (eczema marginatum) 110.3
Bagassosis (occupational) 495.1
Baghdad boil 085.1
Bagratuni's syndrome (temporal arteritis) 446.5

Baker's
  cyst (knee) 727.51
    tuberculous (see also Tuberculosis) 015.2●
  itch 692.89
Bakwin-Krida syndrome (craniometaphyseal dysplasia) 756.89
Balanitis (circinata) (gangraenosa) (infectious) (vulgaris) 607.1
  amebic 006.8
  candidal 112.2
  chlamydial 099.53
  due to Ducrey's bacillus 099.0
  erosiva circinata et gangraenosa 607.1
  gangrenous 607.1
  gonococcal (acute) 098.0
    chronic or duration of 2 months or over 098.2
  nongonococcal 607.1
  phagedenic 607.1
  venereal NEC 099.8
  xerotica obliterans 607.81
Balanoposthitis 607.1
  chlamydial 099.53
  gonococcal (acute) 098.0
    chronic or duration of 2 months or over 098.2
  ulcerative NEC 099.8
Balanorrhagia - see Balanitis
Balantidiasis 007.0
Balantidiosis 007.0
Balbuties, balbutio 307.0
Bald
  patches on scalp 704.00
  tongue 529.4
Baldness (see also Alopecia) 704.00
Balfour's disease (chloroma) 205.3●
Balint's syndrome (psychic paralysis of visual fixation) 368.16
Balkan grippe 083.0
Ball
  food 938
  hair 938
Ballantyne (-Runge) syndrome (postmaturity) 766.22
Balloon disease (see also Effect, adverse, high altitude) 993.2
Ballooning posterior leaflet syndrome 424.0
Baló's disease or concentric sclerosis 341.1
Bamberger's disease (hypertrophic pulmonary osteoarthropathy) 731.2
Bamberger-Marie disease (hypertrophic pulmonary osteoarthropathy) 731.2
Bamboo spine 720.0
Bancroft's filariasis 125.0
Band(s)
  adhesive (see also Adhesions, peritoneum) 568.0
  amniotic 658.8●
    affecting fetus or newborn 762.8
  anomalous or congenital - see also Anomaly, specified type NEC
    atrial 746.9
    heart 746.9
    intestine 751.4
    omentum 751.4
    ventricular 746.9
  cervix 622.3
  gallbladder (congenital) 751.69
  intestinal (adhesive) (see also Adhesions, peritoneum) 568.0
    congenital 751.4

Band(s) (Continued)
  obstructive (see also Obstruction, intestine) 560.81
  periappendiceal (congenital) 751.4
  peritoneal (adhesive) (see also Adhesions, peritoneum) 568.0
    with intestinal obstruction 560.81
    congenital 751.4
  uterus 621.5
  vagina 623.2
Bandemia (without diagnosis of specific infection) 288.66
Bandl's ring (contraction)
  complicating delivery 661.4●
    affecting fetus or newborn 763.7
Bang's disease (Brucella abortus) 023.1
Bangkok hemorrhagic fever 065.4
Bannister's disease 995.1
Bantam-Albright-Martin disease (pseudohypoparathyroidism) 275.49
Banti's disease or syndrome (with cirrhosis) (with portal hypertension) - see Cirrhosis, liver
Bar
  calcaneocuboid 755.67
  calcaneonavicular 755.67
  cubonavicular 755.67
  prostate 600.90
    with
      other lower urinary tract symptoms (LUTS) 600.91
      urinary
        obstruction 600.91
        retention 600.91
  talocalcaneal 755.67
Baragnosis 780.99
Barasheh, barashek 266.2
Barcoo disease or rot (see also Ulcer, skin) 707.9
Bard-Pic syndrome (carcinoma, head of pancreas) 157.0
Bärensprung's disease (eczema marginatum) 110.3
Baritosis 503
Barium lung disease 503
Barlow's syndrome (meaning mitral valve prolapse) 424.0
Barlow (-Möller) disease or syndrome (meaning infantile scurvy) 267
Barodontalgia 993.2
Baron Münchausen syndrome 301.51
Barosinusitis 993.1
Barotitis 993.0
Barotrauma 993.2
  odontalgia 993.2
  otitic 993.0
  sinus 993.1
Barraquer's disease or syndrome (progressive lipodystrophy) 272.6
Barré-Guillain syndrome 357.0
Barré-Liéou syndrome (posterior cervical sympathetic) 723.2
Barrel chest 738.3
Barrett's esophagus 530.85
Barrett's syndrome or ulcer (chronic peptic ulcer of esophagus) 530.85
Bársony-Polgár syndrome (corkscrew esophagus) 530.5
Bársony-Teschendorf syndrome (corkscrew esophagus) 530.5
Barth syndrome 759.89
Bartholin's
  adenitis (see also Bartholinitis) 616.89
  gland - see condition

Bartholinitis (suppurating) 616.89
  gonococcal (acute) 098.0
    chronic or duration of 2 months or
      over 098.2
Bartonellosis 088.0
Bartter's syndrome (secondary
  hyperaldosteronism with
  juxtaglomerular hyperplasia)
  255.13
Basal - see condition
Basan's (hidrotic) ectodermal dysplasia
  757.31
Baseball finger 842.13
Basedow's disease or syndrome
  (exophthalmic goiter) 242.0●
Basic - see condition
Basilar - see condition
Bason's (hidrotic) ectodermal dysplasia
  757.31
Basopenia 288.59
Basophilia 288.65
Basophilism (corticoadrenal) (Cushing's)
  (pituitary) (thymic) 255.0
Bassen-Kornzweig syndrome
  (abetalipoproteinemia) 272.5
Bat ear 744.29
Bateman's
  disease 078.0
  purpura (senile) 287.2
Bathing cramp 994.1
Bathophobia 300.23
Batten's disease, retina 330.1 [362.71]
Batten-Mayou disease 330.1 [362.71]
Batten-Steinert syndrome 359.21
Battered
  adult (syndrome) 995.81
  baby or child (syndrome) 995.54
  spouse (syndrome) 995.81
Battey mycobacterium infection 031.0
Battledore placenta - see Placenta,
  abnormal
Battle exhaustion (see also Reaction,
  stress, acute) 308.9
Baumgarten-Cruveilhier (cirrhosis)
  disease, or syndrome 571.5
Bauxite
  fibrosis (of lung) 503
  workers' disease 503
Bayle's disease (dementia paralytica)
  094.1
Bazin's disease (primary) (see also
  Tuberculosis) 017.1●
Beach ear 380.12
Beaded hair (congenital) 757.4
Beals syndrome 759.82
Beard's disease (neurasthenia) 300.5
Bearn-Kunkel (-Slater) syndrome (lupoid
  hepatitis) 571.49
Beat
  elbow 727.2
  hand 727.2
  knee 727.2
Beats
  ectopic 427.60
  escaped, heart 427.60
    postoperative 997.1
  premature (nodal) 427.60
    atrial 427.61
    auricular 427.61
    postoperative 997.1
    specified type NEC 427.69
    supraventricular 427.61
    ventricular 427.69

Beau's
  disease or syndrome (see also
    Degeneration, myocardial) 429.1
  lines (transverse furrows on
    fingernails) 703.8
Bechterew's disease (ankylosing
  spondylitis) 720.0
Bechterew-Strümpell-Marie syndrome
  (ankylosing spondylitis) 720.0
Beck's syndrome (anterior spinal artery
  occlusion) 433.8●
Becker's
  disease
    idiopathic mural endomyocardial
      disease 425.2
    myotonia congenita, recessive form
      359.22
  dystrophy 359.22
Beckwith (-Wiedemann) syndrome
  759.89
Bedbugs bite(s) - see Injury, superficial,
  by site
Bedclothes, asphyxiation or suffocation
  by 994.7
Bed confinement status V49.84
Bednar's aphthae 528.2
Bedsore (see also Ulcer, pressure)
  707.00
  with gangrene 707.00 [785.4]
Bedwetting (see also Enuresis) 788.36
Beer-drinkers' heart (disease) 425.5
Bee sting (with allergic or anaphylactic
  shock) 989.5
Begbie's disease (exophthalmic goiter)
  242.0●
Behavior disorder, disturbance - see also
  Disturbance, conduct
  antisocial, without manifest psychiatric
    disorder
    adolescent V71.02
    adult V71.01
    child V71.02
  dyssocial, without manifest psychiatric
    disorder
    adolescent V71.02
    adult V71.01
    child V71.02
  high-risk- see problem
Behçet's syndrome 136.1
Behr's disease 362.50
Beigel's disease or morbus (white piedra)
  111.2
Bejel 104.0
Bekhterev's disease (ankylosing
  spondylitis) 720.0
Bekhterev-Strümpell-Marie syndrome
  (ankylosing spondylitis) 720.0
Belching (see also Eructation) 787.3
Bell's
  disease (see also Psychosis, affective)
    296.0●
  mania (see also Psychosis, affective)
    296.0●
  palsy, paralysis 351.0
    infant 767.5
    newborn 767.5
    syphilitic 094.89
  spasm 351.0
Bence-Jones albuminuria,
  albuminosuria, or proteinuria
  791.0
Bends 993.3
Benedikt's syndrome (paralysis)
  344.89

Benign - see also condition
  cellular changes, cervix 795.09
  prostate
    hyperplasia 600.20
      with
        other lower urinary tract
          symptoms (LUTS)
          600.21
        urinary
          obstruction 600.21
          retention 600.21
  neoplasm 222.2
Bennett's
  disease (leukemia) 208.9●
  fracture (closed) 815.01
    open 815.11
Benson's disease 379.22
Bent
  back (hysterical) 300.11
  nose 738.0
    congenital 754.0
Bereavement V62.82
  as adjustment reaction 309.0
Berger's paresthesia (lower limb)
  782.0
Bergeron's disease (hysteroepilepsy)
  300.11
Beriberi (acute) (atrophic) (chronic)
  (dry) (subacute) (wet) 265.0
  with polyneuropathy 265.0 [357.4]
  heart (disease) 265.0 [425.7]
  leprosy 030.1
  neuritis 265.0 [357.4]
Berlin's disease or edema (traumatic)
  921.3
Berloque dermatitis 692.72
Bernard-Horner syndrome (see also
  Neuropathy, peripheral, autonomic)
  337.9
Bernard-Sergent syndrome (acute
  adrenocortical insufficiency)
  255.41
Bernard-Soulier disease or
  thrombopathy 287.1
Bernhardt's disease or paresthesia
  355.1
Bernhardt-Roth disease or syndrome
  (parasthesia) 355.1
Bernheim's syndrome (see also Failure,
  heart) 428.0
Bertielliasis 123.8
Bertolotti's syndrome (sacralization of
  fifth lumbar vertebra) 756.15
Berylliosis (acute) (chronic) (lung)
  (occupational) 503
Besnier's
  lupus pernio 135
  prurigo (atopic dermatitis) (infantile
    eczema) 691.8
Besnier-Boeck disease or sarcoid
  135
Besnier-Boeck-Schaumann disease
  (sarcoidosis) 135
Best's disease 362.76
Bestiality 302.1
Beta-adrenergic hyperdynamic
  circulatory state 429.82
Beta-aminoisobutyric aciduria 277.2
Beta-mercaptolactate-cysteine
  disulfiduria 270.0
Beta thalassemia (major) (minor) (mixed)
  282.49
Beurmann's disease (sporotrichosis)
  117.1

◀ New　◀ Revised　~~deleted~~ Deleted　● Use Additional Digit(s)　▨ Omit code

Bezoar 938
  intestine 936
  stomach 935.2
Bezold's abscess (see also Mastoiditis)
  383.01
Bianchi's syndrome (aphasia-apraxia-
  alexia) 784.69
Bicornuate or bicornis uterus 752.3
  in pregnancy or childbirth 654.0●
    with obstructed labor 660.2●
      affecting fetus or newborn 763.1
    affecting fetus or newborn 763.89
Bicuspid aortic valve 746.4
Biedl-Bardet syndrome 759.89
Bielschowsky's disease 330.1
Bielschowsky-Jansky
  amaurotic familial idiocy 330.1
  disease 330.1
Biemond's syndrome (obesity, polydactyly,
  and mental retardation) 759.89
Biermer's anemia or disease (pernicious
  anemia) 281.0
Biett's disease 695.4
Bifid (congenital) - see also Imperfect,
  closure
  apex, heart 746.89
  clitoris 752.49
  epiglottis 748.3
  kidney 753.3
  nose 748.1
  patella 755.64
  scrotum 752.89
  toe 755.66
  tongue 750.13
  ureter 753.4
  uterus 752.3
  uvula 749.02
    with cleft lip (see also Cleft, palate,
      with cleft lip) 749.20
Biforis uterus (suprasimplex) 752.3
Bifurcation (congenital) - see also
  Imperfect, closure
  gallbladder 751.69
  kidney pelvis 753.3
  renal pelvis 753.3
  rib 756.3
  tongue 750.13
  trachea 748.3
  ureter 753.4
  urethra 753.8
  uvula 749.02
    with cleft lip (see also Cleft, palate,
      with cleft lip) 749.20
  vertebra 756.19
Bigeminal pulse 427.89
Bigeminy 427.89
Big spleen syndrome 289.4
Bilateral - see condition
Bile duct - see condition
Bile pigments in urine 791.4
Bilharziasis (see also Schistosomiasis)
  120.9
  chyluria 120.0
  cutaneous 120.3
  galacturia 120.0
  hematochyluria 120.0
  intestinal 120.1
  lipemia 120.9
  lipuria 120.0
  Oriental 120.2
  piarhemia 120.9
  pulmonary 120.2
  tropical hematuria 120.0
  vesical 120.0

Biliary - see condition
Bilious (attack) - see also Vomiting
  fever, hemoglobinuric 084.8
Bilirubinuria 791.4
Biliuria 791.4
Billroth's disease
  meningocele (see also Spina bifida)
    741.9●
Bilobate placenta - see Placenta, abnormal
Bilocular
  heart 745.7
  stomach 536.8
Bing-Horton syndrome (histamine
  cephalgia) 339.00
Binswanger's disease or dementia
  290.12
Biörck (-Thorson) syndrome (malignant
  carcinoid) 259.2
Biparta, bipartite - see also Imperfect,
  closure
  carpal scaphoid 755.59
  patella 755.64
  placenta - see Placenta, abnormal
  vagina 752.49
Bird
  face 756.0
  fanciers' lung or disease 495.2
  flu 488.0   ◀
Bird's disease (oxaluria) 271.8
Birth
  abnormal fetus or newborn 763.9
  accident, fetus or newborn - see Birth,
    injury
  complications in mother - see Delivery,
    complicated
  compression during NEC 767.9
  defect - see Anomaly
  delayed, fetus 763.9
  difficult NEC, affecting fetus or
    newborn 763.9
  dry, affecting fetus or newborn 761.1
  forced, NEC, affecting fetus or
    newborn 763.89
  forceps, affecting fetus or newborn
    763.2
  hematoma of sternomastoid 767.8
  immature 765.1●
    extremely 765.0●
  inattention, after or at 995.52
  induced, affecting fetus or newborn
    763.89
  infant - see Newborn
  injury NEC 767.9
    adrenal gland 767.8
    basal ganglia 767.0
    brachial plexus (paralysis) 767.6
    brain (compression) (pressure)
      767.0
    cerebellum 767.0
    cerebral hemorrhage 767.0
    conjunctiva 767.8
    eye 767.8
    fracture
      bone, any except clavicle or spine
        767.3
      clavicle 767.2
      femur 767.3
      humerus 767.3
      long bone 767.3
      radius and ulna 767.3
      skeleton NEC 767.3
      skull 767.3
      spine 767.4
      tibia and fibula 767.3

Birth (Continued)
  injury NEC (Continued)
    hematoma 767.8
      liver (subcapsular) 767.8
      mastoid 767.8
      skull 767.19
      sternomastoid 767.8
      testes 767.8
      vulva 767.8
    intracranial (edema) 767.0
    laceration
      brain 767.0
      by scalpel 767.8
      peripheral nerve 767.7
    liver 767.8
    meninges
      brain 767.0
      spinal cord 767.4
    nerves (cranial, peripheral) 767.7
      brachial plexus 767.6
      facial 767.5
    paralysis 767.7
      brachial plexus 767.6
      Erb (-Duchenne) 767.6
      facial nerve 767.5
      Klumpke (-Déjérine) 767.6
      radial nerve 767.6
      spinal (cord) (hemorrhage)
        (laceration) (rupture) 767.4
    rupture
      intracranial 767.0
      liver 767.8
      spinal cord 767.4
      spleen 767.8
      viscera 767.8
    scalp 767.19
    scalpel wound 767.8
    skeleton NEC 767.3
    specified NEC 767.8
    spinal cord 767.4
    spleen 767.8
    subdural hemorrhage 767.0
    tentorial, tear 767.0
    testes 767.8
    vulva 767.8
  instrumental, NEC, affecting fetus or
    newborn 763.2
  lack of care, after or at 995.52
  multiple
    affected by maternal complications
      of pregnancy 761.5
    healthy liveborn - see Newborn,
      multiple
  neglect, after or at 995.52
  newborn - see Newborn
  palsy or paralysis NEC 767.7
  precipitate, fetus or newborn 763.6
  premature (infant) 765.1●
  prolonged, affecting fetus or newborn
    763.9
  retarded, fetus or newborn 763.9
  shock, newborn 779.89
  strangulation or suffocation
    due to aspiration of clear amniotic
      fluid 770.13
      with respiratory symptoms
        770.14
    mechanical 767.8
  trauma NEC 767.9
  triplet
    affected by maternal complications
      of pregnancy 761.5
    healthy liveborn - see Newborn,
      multiple

Birth (Continued)
twin
affected by maternal complications
of pregnancy 761.5
healthy liveborn - see Newborn, twin
ventouse, affecting fetus or newborn
763.3
Birthmark 757.32
Birt-Hogg-Dube syndrome 759.89
Bisalbuminemia 273.8
Biskra button 085.1
Bite(s)
with intact skin surface - see Contusion
animal - see Wound, open, by site
intact skin surface - see Contusion
bedbug - see Injury, superficial, by site
centipede 989.5
chigger 133.8
fire ant 989.5
flea - see Injury, superficial, by site
human (open wound) - see also Wound,
open, by site
intact skin surface - see Contusion
insect
nonvenomous - see Injury,
superficial, by site
venomous 989.5
mad dog (death from) 071
open
anterior 524.24
posterior 524.25
poisonous 989.5
red bug 133.8
reptile 989.5
nonvenomous - see Wound, open, by
site
snake 989.5
nonvenomous - see Wound, open, by
site
spider (venomous) 989.5
nonvenomous - see Injury,
superficial, by site
venomous 989.5
Biting
cheek or lip 528.9
nail 307.9
Black
death 020.9
eye NEC 921.0
hairy tongue 529.3
heel 924.20
lung disease 500
palm 923.20
Blackfan-Diamond anemia or syndrome
(congenital hypoplastic anemia)
284.01
Blackhead 706.1
Blackout 780.2
Blackwater fever 084.8
Bladder - see condition
Blast
blindness 921.3
concussion - see Blast, injury
injury 869.0
with open wound into cavity 869.1
abdomen or thorax - see Injury,
internal, by site
brain (see also Concussion, brain)
850.9
with skull fracture - see Fracture,
skull
ear (acoustic nerve trauma) 951.5
with perforation, tympanic
membrane - see Wound,
open, ear, drum

Blast (Continued)
injury (Continued)
lung (see also Injury, internal, lung)
861.20
otitic (explosive) 388.11
Blastomycosis, blastomycotic (chronic)
(cutaneous) (disseminated) (lung)
(pulmonary) (systemic) 116.0
Brazilian 116.1
European 117.5
keloidal 116.2
North American 116.0
primary pulmonary 116.0
South American 116.1
Bleb(s) 709.8
emphysematous (bullous) (diffuse)
(lung) (ruptured) (solitary) 492.0
filtering, eye (postglaucoma) (status)
V45.69
with complication 997.99
postcataract extraction
(complication) 997.99
lung (ruptured) 492.0
congenital 770.5
subpleural (emphysematous) 492.0
Bleeder (familial) (hereditary) (see also
Defect, coagulation) 286.9
nonfamilial 286.9
Bleeding (see also Hemorrhage) 459.0
anal 569.3
anovulatory 628.0
atonic, following delivery 666.1●
capillary 448.9
due to subinvolution 621.1
puerperal 666.2●
ear 388.69
excessive, associated with menopausal
onset 627.0
familial (see also Defect, coagulation)
286.9
following intercourse 626.7
gastrointestinal 578.9
gums 523.8
hemorrhoids - see Hemorrhoids,
bleeding
intermenstrual
irregular 626.6
regular 626.5
intraoperative 998.11
irregular NEC 626.4
menopausal 627.0
mouth 528.9
nipple 611.79
nose 784.7
ovulation 626.5
postclimacteric 627.1
postcoital 626.7
postmenopausal 627.1
following induced menopause 627.4
postoperative 998.11
preclimacteric 627.0
puberty 626.3
excessive, with onset of menstrual
periods 626.3
rectum, rectal 569.3
tendencies (see also Defect, coagulation)
286.9
throat 784.8
umbilical stump 772.3
umbilicus 789.9
unrelated to menstrual cycle 626.6
uterus, uterine 626.9
climacteric 627.0
dysfunctional 626.8

Bleeding (Continued)
uterus, uterine (Continued)
functional 626.8
unrelated to menstrual cycle
626.6
vagina, vaginal 623.8
functional 626.8
vicarious 625.8
Blennorrhagia, blennorrhagic - see
Blennorrhea
Blennorrhea (acute) 098.0
adultorum 098.40
alveolaris 523.40
chronic or duration of 2 months or over
098.2
gonococcal (neonatorum) 098.40
inclusion (neonatal) (newborn) 771.6
neonatorum 098.40
Blepharelosis (see also Entropion) 374.00
Blepharitis (eyelid) 373.00
angularis 373.01
ciliaris 373.00
with ulcer 373.01
marginal 373.00
with ulcer 373.01
scrofulous (see also Tuberculosis)
017.3● [373.00]
squamous 373.02
ulcerative 373.01
Blepharochalasis 374.34
congenital 743.62
Blepharoclonus 333.81
Blepharoconjunctivitis (see also
Conjunctivitis) 372.20
angular 372.21
contact 372.22
Blepharophimosis (eyelid) 374.46
congenital 743.62
Blepharoplegia 374.89
Blepharoptosis 374.30
congenital 743.61
Blepharopyorrhea 098.49
Blepharospasm 333.81
due to drugs 333.85
Blessig's cyst 362.62
Blighted ovum 631
Blind
bronchus (congenital) 748.3
eye - see also Blindness
hypertensive 360.42
hypotensive 360.41
loop syndrome (postoperative) 579.2
sac, fallopian tube (congenital) 752.19
spot, enlarged 368.42
tract or tube (congenital) NEC - see
Atresia
Blindness (acquired) (congenital) (both
eyes) 369.00
with deafness V49.85
blast 921.3
with nerve injury - see Injury, nerve,
optic
Bright's - see Uremia
color (congenital) 368.59
acquired 368.55
blue 368.53
green 368.52
red 368.51
total 368.54
concussion 950.9
cortical 377.75
day 368.10
acquired 368.10
congenital 368.10

◀ New ◀▥ Revised ~~deleted~~ Deleted ● Use Additional Digit(s) ▨ Omit code

B

Blindness *(Continued)*
  day *(Continued)*
    hereditary 368.10
    specified type NEC 368.10
  due to
    injury NEC 950.9
    refractive error - *see* Error, refractive
  eclipse (total) 363.31
  emotional 300.11
  face 368.16
  hysterical 300.11
  legal (both eyes) (USA definition) 369.4
    with impairment of better (less
      impaired) eye
    near-total 369.02
      with
        lesser eye impairment 369.02
          near-total 369.04
          total 369.03
    profound 369.05
      with
        lesser eye impairment
          369.05
          near-total 369.07
          profound 369.08
          total 369.06
    severe 369.21
      with
        lesser eye impairment
          369.21
          blind 369.11
          near-total 369.13
          profound 369.14
          severe 369.22
          total 369.12
    total
      with lesser eye impairment
        total 369.01
  mind 784.69
  moderate
    both eyes 369.25
      with impairment of lesser eye
        (specified as)
        blind, not further specified
          369.15
        low vision, not further
          specified 369.23
        near-total 369.17
        profound 369.18
        severe 369.24
        total 369.16
    one eye 369.74
      with vision of other eye (specified
        as)
        near-normal 369.75
        normal 369.76
  near-total
    both eyes 369.04
      with impairment of lesser eye
        (specified as)
        blind, not further specified
          369.02
        total 369.03
    one eye 369.64
      with vision of other eye (specified
        as)
        near-normal 369.65
        normal 369.66
  night 368.60
    acquired 368.62
    congenital (Japanese) 368.61
    hereditary 368.61
    specified type NEC 368.69
    vitamin A deficiency 264.5

Blindness *(Continued)*
  nocturnal - *see* Blindness, night
  one eye 369.60
    with low vision of other eye 369.10
  profound
    both eyes 369.08
      with impairment of lesser eye
        (specified as)
        blind, not further specified
          369.05
        near-total 369.07
        total 369.06
    one eye 369.67
      with vision of other eye (specified
        as)
        near-normal 369.68
        normal 369.69
  psychic 784.69
  severe
    both eyes 369.22
      with impairment of lesser eye
        (specified as)
        blind, not further specified
          369.11
        low vision, not further
          specified 369.21
        near-total 369.13
        profound 369.14
        total 369.12
    one eye 369.71
      with vision of other eye (specified
        as)
        near-normal 369.72
        normal 369.73
  snow 370.24
  sun 363.31
  temporary 368.12
  total
    both eyes 369.01
    one eye 369.61
      with vision of other eye (specified
        as)
        near-normal 369.62
        normal 369.63
  transient 368.12
  traumatic NEC 950.9
  word (developmental) 315.01
    acquired 784.61
    secondary to organic lesion 784.61
Blister - *see also* Injury, superficial,
  by site
  beetle dermatitis 692.89
  due to burn - *see* Burn, by site, second
    degree
  fever 054.9
  multiple, skin, nontraumatic 709.8
Bloating 787.3
Bloch-Siemens syndrome (incontinentia
  pigmenti) 757.33
Bloch-Stauffer dyshormonal dermatosis
  757.33
Bloch-Sulzberger disease or syndrome
  (incontinentia pigmenti)
  (melanoblastosis) 757.33
Block
  alveolar capillary 516.3
  arborization (heart) 426.6
  arrhythmic 426.9
  atrioventricular (AV) (incomplete)
    (partial) 426.10
    with
      2:1 atrioventricular response
        block 426.13
      atrioventricular dissociation 426.0

Block *(Continued)*
  atrioventricular *(Continued)*
    first degree (incomplete) 426.11
    second degree (Mobitz type I)
      426.13
      Mobitz (type II) 426.12
    third degree 426.0
    complete 426.0
      congenital 746.86
    congenital 746.86
    Mobitz (incomplete)
      type I (Wenckebach's) 426.13
      type II 426.12
    partial 426.13
  auriculoventricular (*see also* Block,
    atrioventricular) 426.10
    complete 426.0
      congenital 746.86
    congenital 746.86
  bifascicular (cardiac) 426.53
  bundle branch (complete) (false)
    (incomplete) 426.50
    bilateral 426.53
    left (complete) (main stem) 426.3
      with right bundle branch block
        426.53
      anterior fascicular 426.2
        with
          posterior fascicular block
            426.3
          right bundle branch block
            426.52
      hemiblock 426.2
      incomplete 426.2
        with right bundle branch block
          426.53
      posterior fascicular 426.2
        with
          anterior fascicular block
            426.3
          right bundle branch block
            426.51
    right 426.4
      with
        left bundle branch block
          (incomplete) (main stem)
          426.53
        left fascicular block 426.53
          anterior 426.52
          posterior 426.51
    Wilson's type 426.4
  cardiac 426.9
  conduction 426.9
    complete 426.0
  Eustachian tube (*see also* Obstruction,
    Eustachian tube) 381.60
  fascicular (left anterior) (left posterior)
    426.2
  foramen Magendie (acquired) 331.3
    congenital 742.3
      with spina bifida (*see also* Spina
        bifida) 741.0●
  heart 426.9
    first degree (atrioventricular) 426.11
    second degree (atrioventricular)
      426.13
    third degree (atrioventricular) 426.0
    bundle branch (complete) (false)
      (incomplete) 426.50
      bilateral 426.53
      left (*see also* Block, bundle branch,
        left) 426.3
      right (*see also* Block, bundle
        branch, right) 426.4

Block *(Continued)*
  heart *(Continued)*
    complete (atrioventricular) 426.0
    congenital 746.86
    incomplete 426.13
    intra-atrial 426.6
    intraventricular NEC 426.6
    sinoatrial 426.6
    specified type NEC 426.6
  hepatic vein 453.0
  intraventricular (diffuse) (myofibrillar)
      426.6
    bundle branch (complete) (false)
        (incomplete) 426.50
      bilateral 426.53
      left *(see also* Block, bundle branch,
          left) 426.3
      right *(see also* Block, bundle
          branch, right) 426.4
  kidney *(see also* Disease, renal) 593.9
    postcystoscopic 997.5
  myocardial *(see also* Block, heart) 426.9
  nodal 426.10
  optic nerve 377.49
  organ or site (congenital) NEC - *see*
      Atresia
  parietal 426.6
  peri-infarction 426.6
  portal (vein) 452
  sinoatrial 426.6
  sinoauricular 426.6
  spinal cord 336.9
  trifascicular 426.54
  tubal 628.2
  vein NEC 453.9
Blocq's disease or syndrome (astasia-
    abasia) 307.9
Blood
  constituents, abnormal NEC 790.6
  disease 289.9
    specified NEC 289.89
  donor V59.01
    other blood components V59.09
    stem cells V59.02
    whole blood V59.01
  dyscrasia 289.9
    with
      abortion - *see* Abortion, by type,
          with hemorrhage, delayed
          or excessive
      ectopic pregnancy *(see also*
          categories 633.0–633.9) 639.1
      molar pregnancy *(see also*
          categories 630–632) 639.1
      ~~fetus or newborn NEC 776.9~~
    following
      abortion 639.1
      ectopic or molar pregnancy 639.1
    newborn NEC 776.9 ◄
    puerperal, postpartum 666.3●
  flukes NEC *(see also* Infestation,
      Schistosoma) 120.9
  in
    feces *(see also* Melena) 578.1
      occult 792.1
    urine *(see also* Hematuria) 599.70
  mole 631
  occult 792.1
  poisoning *(see also* Septicemia) 038.9
  pressure
    decreased, due to shock following
        injury 958.4
    fluctuating 796.4

Blood *(Continued)*
  pressure *(Continued)*
    high *(see also* Hypertension) 401.9
      incidental reading (isolated)
          (nonspecific), without
          diagnosis of hypertension
          796.2
    low *(see also* Hypotension) 458.9
      incidental reading (isolated)
          (nonspecific), without
          diagnosis of hypotension
          796.3
  spitting *(see also* Hemoptysis) 786.3
  staining cornea 371.12
  transfusion
    without reported diagnosis V58.2
    donor V59.01
      stem cells V59.02
    reaction or complication - *see*
        Complications, transfusion
  tumor - *see* Hematoma
  vessel rupture - *see* Hemorrhage
  vomiting *(see also* Hematemesis)
      578.0
Blood-forming organ disease 289.9
Bloodgood's disease 610.1
Bloodshot eye 379.93
Bloom (-Machacek) (-Torre) syndrome
    757.39
Blotch, palpebral 372.55
Blount's disease (tibia vara) 732.4
Blount-Barber syndrome (tibia vara)
    732.4
Blue
  baby 746.9
  bloater 491.20
    with
      acute bronchitis 491.22
      exacerbation (acute) 491.21
  diaper syndrome 270.0
  disease 746.9
  dome cyst 610.0
  drum syndrome 381.02
  sclera 743.47
    with fragility of bone and deafness
        756.51
  toe syndrome 445.02
Blueness *(see also* Cyanosis) 782.5
Blurring, visual 368.8
Blushing (abnormal) (excessive) 782.62
BMI (body mass index)
  adult
    25.0–25.9 V85.21
    26.0–26.9 V85.22
    27.0–27.9 V85.23
    28.0–28.9 V85.24
    29.0–29.9 V85.25
    30.0–30.9 V85.30
    31.0–31.9 V85.31
    32.0–32.9 V85.32
    33.0–33.9 V85.33
    34.0–34.9 V85.34
    35.0–35.9 V85.35
    36.0–36.9 V85.36
    37.0–37.9 V85.37
    38.0–38.9 V85.38
    39.0–39.9 V85.39
    40 and over V85.4
    between 19–24 V85.1
    less than 19 V85.0
  pediatric
    5th percentile to less than 85th
        percentile for age V85.52

BMI *(Continued)*
  pediatric *(Continued)*
    85th percentile to less than 95th
        percentile for age V85.53
    greater than or equal to 95th
        percentile for age V85.54
    less than 5th percentile for age
        V85.51
Boarder, hospital V65.0
  infant V65.0
Bockhart's impetigo (superficial
    folliculitis) 704.8
Bodechtel-Guttmann disease (subacute
    sclerosing panencephalitis) 046.2
Boder-Sedgwick syndrome (ataxia-
    telangiectasia) 334.8
Body, bodies
  Aschoff *(see also* Myocarditis,
      rheumatic) 398.0
  asteroid, vitreous 379.22
  choroid, colloid (degenerative) 362.57
    hereditary 362.77
  cytoid (retina) 362.82
  drusen (retina) *(see also* Drusen) 362.57
    optic disc 377.21
  fibrin, pleura 511.0
  foreign - *see* Foreign body
  Hassall-Henle 371.41
  loose
    joint *(see also* Loose, body, joint)
        718.1●
      knee 717.6
    knee 717.6
    sheath, tendon 727.82
  Mallory's 034.1
  mass index (BMI)
    adult
      25.0–25.9 V85.21
      26.0–26.9 V85.22
      27.0–27.9 V85.23
      28.0–28.9 V85.24
      29.0–29.9 V85.25
      30.0–30.9 V85.30
      31.0–31.9 V85.31
      32.0–32.9 V85.32
      33.0–33.9 V85.33
      34.0–34.9 V85.34
      35.0–35.9 V85.35
      36.0–36.9 V85.36
      37.0–37.9 V85.37
      38.0–38.9 V85.38
      39.0–39.9 V85.39
      40 and over V85.4
      between 19–24 V85.1
      less than 19 V85.0
    pediatric
      5th percentile to less than 85th
          percentile for age V85.52
      85th percentile to less than 95th
          percentile for age V85.53
      greater than or equal to 95th
          percentile for age V85.54
      less than 5th percentile for age
          V85.51
  Mooser 081.0
  Negri 071
  rice (joint) *(see also* Loose, body, joint)
      718.1●
    knee 717.6
  rocking 307.3
Boeck's
  disease (sarcoidosis) 135
  lupoid (miliary) 135
  sarcoid 135

◄ New   ◄▥ Revised   ~~deleted~~ Deleted   ● Use Additional Digit(s)   ▨ Omit code

Boerhaave's syndrome (spontaneous esophageal rupture) 530.4
Boggy
  cervix 622.8
  uterus 621.8
Boil (see also Carbuncle) 680.9
  abdominal wall 680.2
  Aleppo 085.1
  ankle 680.6
  anus 680.5
  arm (any part, above wrist) 680.3
  auditory canal, external 680.0
  axilla 680.3
  back (any part) 680.2
  Baghdad 085.1
  breast 680.2
  buttock 680.5
  chest wall 680.2
  corpus cavernosum 607.2
  Delhi 085.1
  ear (any part) 680.0
  eyelid 373.13
  face (any part, except eye) 680.0
  finger (any) 680.4
  flank 680.2
  foot (any part) 680.7
  forearm 680.3
  Gafsa 085.1
  genital organ, male 608.4
  gluteal (region) 680.5
  groin 680.2
  hand (any part) 680.4
  head (any part, except face) 680.8
  heel 680.7
  hip 680.6
  knee 680.6
  labia 616.4
  lacrimal (see also Dacryocystitis) 375.30
    gland (see also Dacryoadenitis) 375.00
    passages (duct) (sac) (see also Dacryocystitis) 375.30
  leg, any part, except foot 680.6
  multiple sites 680.9
  natal 085.1
  neck 680.1
  nose (external) (septum) 680.0
  orbit, orbital 376.01
  partes posteriores 680.5
  pectoral region 680.2
  penis 607.2
  perineum 680.2
  pinna 680.0
  scalp (any part) 680.8
  scrotum 608.4
  seminal vesicle 608.0
  shoulder 680.3
  skin NEC 680.9
  specified site NEC 680.8
  spermatic cord 608.4
  temple (region) 680.0
  testis 608.4
  thigh 680.6
  thumb 680.4
  toe (any) 680.7
  tropical 085.1
  trunk 680.2
  tunica vaginalis 608.4
  umbilicus 680.2
  upper arm 680.3
  vas deferens 608.4
  vulva 616.4
  wrist 680.4

Bold hives (see also Urticaria) 708.9
Bolivian hemorrhagic fever 078.7
Bombé, iris 364.74
Bomford-Rhoads anemia (refractory) 238.72
Bone - see condition
Bonnevie-Ullrich syndrome 758.6
Bonnier's syndrome 386.19
Bonvale Dam fever 780.79
Bony block of joint 718.80
  ankle 718.87
  elbow 718.82
  foot 718.87
  hand 718.84
  hip 718.85
  knee 718.86
  multiple sites 718.89
  pelvic region 718.85
  shoulder (region) 718.81
  specified site NEC 718.88
  wrist 718.83
BOOP (bronchiolitis obliterans organized pneumonia) 516.8
Borderline
  intellectual functioning V62.89
  osteopenia 733.90
  pelvis 653.1●
    with obstruction during labor 660.1●
      affecting fetus or newborn 763.1
  psychosis (see also Schizophrenia) 295.5●
    of childhood (see also Psychosis, childhood) 299.8●
  schizophrenia (see also Schizophrenia) 295.5●
Borna disease 062.9
Bornholm disease (epidemic pleurodynia) 074.1
Borrelia vincentii (mouth) (pharynx) (tonsils) 101
Bostock's catarrh (see also Fever, hay) 477.9
Boston exanthem 048
Botalli, ductus (patent) (persistent) 747.0
Bothriocephalus latus infestation 123.4
Botulism 005.1
  food poisoning 005.1
  infant 040.41
  non-foodborne 040.42
  wound 040.42
Bouba (see also Yaws) 102.9
Bouffée délirante 298.3
Bouillaud's disease or syndrome (rheumatic heart disease) 391.9
Bourneville's disease (tuberous sclerosis) 759.5
Boutonneuse fever 082.1
Boutonniere
  deformity (finger) 736.21
  hand (intrinsic) 736.21
Bouveret (-Hoffmann) disease or syndrome (paroxysmal tachycardia) 427.2
Bovine heart - see Hypertrophy, cardiac
Bowel - see condition
Bowen's
  dermatosis (precancerous) (M8081/2) - see Neoplasm, skin, in situ
  disease (M8081/2) - see Neoplasm, skin, in situ
  epithelioma (M8081/2) - see Neoplasm, skin, in situ

Bowen's (Continued)
  type
    epidermoid carcinoma in situ (M8081/2) - see Neoplasm, skin, in situ
    intraepidermal squamous cell carcinoma (M8081/2) - see Neoplasm, skin, in situ
Bowing
  femur 736.89
    congenital 754.42
  fibula 736.89
    congenital 754.43
  forearm 736.09
    away from midline (cubitus valgus) 736.01
    toward midline (cubitus varus) 736.02
  leg(s), long bones, congenital 754.44
  radius 736.09
    away from midline (cubitus valgus) 736.01
    toward midline (cubitus varus) 736.02
  tibia 736.89
    congenital 754.43
Bowleg(s) 736.42
  congenital 754.44
  rachitic 268.1
Boyd's dysentery 004.2
Brachial - see condition
Brachman-de Lange syndrome (Amsterdam dwarf, mental retardation, and brachycephaly) 759.89
Brachycardia 427.89
Brachycephaly 756.0
Brachymorphism and ectopia lentis 759.89
Bradley's disease (epidemic vomiting) 078.82
Bradycardia 427.89
  chronic (sinus) 427.81
  newborn 779.81
  nodal 427.89
  postoperative 997.1
  reflex 337.09
  sinoatrial 427.89
    with paroxysmal tachyarrhythmia or tachycardia 427.81
    chronic 427.81
  sinus 427.89
    with paroxysmal tachyarrhythmia or tachycardia 427.81
    chronic 427.81
    persistent 427.81
    severe 427.81
  tachycardia syndrome 427.81
  vagal 427.89
Bradykinesia 781.0 ◀
Bradypnea 786.09
Brailsford's disease 732.3
  radial head 732.3
  tarsal scaphoid 732.5
Brailsford-Morquio disease or syndrome (mucopolysaccharidosis IV) 277.5
Brain - see also condition
  death 348.89 ◀▥
  syndrome (acute) (chronic) (nonpsychotic) (organic) (with neurotic reaction) (with behavioral reaction) (see also Syndrome, brain) 310.9
  with
    presenile brain disease 290.10
    psychosis, psychotic reaction (see also Psychosis, organic) 294.9

Brain (*Continued*)
  syndrome (*Continued*)
    congenital (*see also* Retardation, mental) 319
Branched-chain amino-acid disease 270.3
Branchial - *see* condition
Brandt's syndrome (acrodermatitis enteropathica) 686.8
Brash (water) 787.1
Brass-founders' ague 985.8
Bravais-Jacksonian epilepsy (*see also* Epilepsy) 345.5●
Braxton Hicks contractions 644.1●
Braziers' disease 985.8
Brazilian
  blastomycosis 116.1
  leishmaniasis 085.5
BRBPR (bright red blood per rectum) 569.3
Break
  cardiorenal - *see* Hypertension, cardiorenal
  retina (*see also* Defect, retina) 361.30
Breakbone fever 061
Breakdown
  device, implant, or graft - *see* Complications, mechanical
  nervous (*see also* Disorder, mental, nonpsychotic) 300.9
    perineum 674.2●
Breast - *see also* condition
  buds 259.1
    in newborn 779.89
  dense 793.82
  nodule 793.89
Breast feeding difficulties 676.8●
Breath
  foul 784.99
  holder, child 312.81
  holding spells 786.9
  shortness 786.05
Breathing
  asymmetrical 786.09
  bronchial 786.09
  exercises V57.0
  labored 786.09
  mouth 784.99
    causing malocclusion 524.59
  periodic 786.09
    high altitude 327.22
  tic 307.20
Breathlessness 786.09
Breda's disease (*see also* Yaws) 102.9
Breech
  delivery, affecting fetus or newborn 763.0
  extraction, affecting fetus or newborn 763.0
  presentation (buttocks) (complete) (frank) 652.2●
    with successful version 652.1●
    before labor, affecting fetus or newborn 761.7
    during labor, affecting fetus or newborn 763.0
Breisky's disease (kraurosis vulvae) 624.09
Brennemann's syndrome (acute mesenteric lymphadenitis) 289.2
Brenner's
  tumor (benign) (M9000/0) 220
    borderline malignancy (M9000/1) 236.2
    malignant (M9000/3) 183.0
    proliferating (M9000/1) 236.2

Bretonneau's disease (diphtheritic malignant angina) 032.0
Breus' mole 631
Brevicollis 756.16
Bricklayers' itch 692.89
Brickmakers' anemia 126.9
Bridge
  myocardial 746.85
Bright red blood per rectum (BRBPR) 569.3
Bright's
  blindness - *see* Uremia
  disease (*see also* Nephritis) 583.9
    arteriosclerotic (*see also* Hypertension, kidney) 403.90
Brill's disease (recrudescent typhus) 081.1
  flea-borne 081.0
  louse-borne 081.1
Brill-Symmers disease (follicular lymphoma) (M9690/3) 202.0●
Brill-Zinsser disease (recrudescent typhus) 081.1
Brinton's disease (linitis plastica) (M8142/3) 151.9
Brion-Kayser disease (*see also* Fever, paratyphoid) 002.9
Briquet's disorder or syndrome 300.81
Brissaud's
  infantilism (infantile myxedema) 244.9
  motor-verbal tic 307.23
Brissaud-Meige syndrome (infantile myxedema) 244.9
Brittle
  bones (congenital) 756.51
  nails 703.8
    congenital 757.5
Broad - *see also* condition
  beta disease 272.2
  ligament laceration syndrome 620.6
Brock's syndrome (atelectasis due to enlarged lymph nodes) 518.0
Brocq's disease 691.8
  atopic (diffuse) neurodermatitis 691.8
  lichen simplex chronicus 698.3
  parakeratosis psoriasiformis 696.2
  parapsoriasis 696.2
Brocq-Duhring disease (dermatitis herpetiformis) 694.0
Brodie's
  abscess (localized) (chronic) (*see also* Osteomyelitis) 730.1●
  disease (joint) (*see also* Osteomyelitis) 730.1●
Broken
  arches 734
    congenital 755.67
  back - *see* Fracture, vertebra, by site
  bone - *see* Fracture, by site
  compensation - *see* Disease, heart
  heart syndrome 429.83
  implant or internal device - *see* listing under Complications, mechanical
  neck - *see* Fracture, vertebra, cervical
  nose 802.0
    open 802.1
  tooth, teeth 873.63
    complicated 873.73
Bromhidrosis 705.89
Bromidism, bromism
  acute 967.3
    correct substance properly administered 349.82
    overdose or wrong substance given or taken 967.3
  chronic (*see also* Dependence) 304.1●

Bromidrosiphobia 300.23
Bromidrosis 705.89
Bronchi, bronchial - *see* condition
Bronchiectasis (cylindrical) (diffuse) (fusiform) (localized) (moniliform) (postinfectious) (recurrent) (saccular) 494.0
  with acute exacerbation 494.1
  congenital 748.61
  tuberculosis (*see also* Tuberculosis) 011.5●
Bronchiolectasis - *see* Bronchiectasis
Bronchiolitis (acute) (infectious) (subacute) 466.19
  with
    bronchospasm or obstruction 466.19
    influenza, flu, or grippe 487.1
  catarrhal (acute) (subacute) 466.19
  chemical 506.0
    chronic 506.4
  chronic (obliterative) 491.8
  due to external agent - *see* Bronchitis, acute, due to
  fibrosa obliterans 491.8
  influenzal 487.1
  obliterans 491.8
    with organizing pneumonia (BOOP) 516.8
    status post lung transplant 996.84
  obliterative (chronic) (diffuse) (subacute) 491.8
    due to fumes or vapors 506.4
  respiratory syncytial virus 466.11
  vesicular - *see* Pneumonia, broncho-
Bronchitis (diffuse) (hypostatic) (infectious) (inflammatory) (simple) 490
  with
    emphysema - *see* Emphysema
    influenza, flue, or grippe 487.1
    obstruction airway, chronic 491.20
      with
        acute bronchitis 491.22
        exacerbation (acute) 491.21
    tracheitis 490
      acute or subacute 466.0
        with bronchospasm or obstruction 466.0
      chronic 491.8
  acute or subacute 466.0
    with
      bronchiectasis 494.1
      bronchospasm 466.0
      obstruction 466.0
      tracheitis 466.0
    chemical (due to fumes or vapors) 506.0
    due to
      fumes or vapors 506.0
      radiation 508.8
  allergic (acute) (*see also* Asthma) 493.9●
  arachidic 934.1
  aspiration 507.0
    due to fumes or vapors 506.0
  asthmatic (acute) 493.90
    with
      acute exacerbation 493.92
      status asthmaticus 493.91
    chronic 493.2●
  capillary 466.19
    with bronchospasm or obstruction 466.19
    chronic 491.8
  caseous (*see also* Tuberculosis) 011.3●

◄ New   ⬅ Revised   ~~deleted~~ Deleted   ● Use Additional Digit(s)   ▓ Omit code

Bronchitis *(Continued)*
Castellani's 104.8
catarrhal 490
  acute - *see* Bronchitis, acute
  chronic 491.0
chemical (acute) (subacute) 506.0
  chronic 506.4
  due to fumes or vapors (acute)
    (subacute) 506.0
    chronic 506.4
chronic 491.9
  with
    tracheitis (chronic) 491.8
  asthmatic 493.2●
  catarrhal 491.0
  chemical (due to fumes and vapors)
    506.4
  due to
    fumes or vapors (chemical)
      (inhalation) 506.4
    radiation 508.8
    tobacco smoking 491.0
  mucopurulent 491.1
  obstructive 491.20
    with
      acute bronchitis 491.22
      exacerbation (acute) 491.21
  purulent 491.1
  simple 491.0
  specified type NEC 491.8
croupous 466.0
  with bronchospasm or obstruction
    466.0
  due to fumes or vapors 506.0
emphysematous 491.20
  with
    acute bronchitis 491.22
    exacerbation (acute) 491.21
exudative 466.0
fetid (chronic) (recurrent) 491.1
fibrinous, acute or subacute 466.0
  with bronchospasm or obstruction
    466.0
grippal 487.1
influenzal 487.1
membranous, acute or subacute 466.0
  with bronchospasm or obstruction
    466.0
moulders' 502
mucopurulent (chronic) (recurrent)
  491.1
  acute or subacute 466.0
obliterans 491.8
obstructive (chronic) 491.20
  with
    acute bronchitis 491.22
    exacerbation (acute) 491.21
pituitous 491.1
plastic (inflammatory) 466.0
pneumococcal, acute or subacute 466.0
  with bronchospasm or obstruction
    466.0
pseudomembranous 466.0
purulent (chronic) (recurrent) 491.1
  acute or subacute 466.0
    with bronchospasm or
      obstruction 466.0
putrid 491.1
scrofulous (*see also* Tuberculosis)
  011.3●
senile 491.9
septic, acute or subacute 466.0
  with bronchospasm or obstruction
    466.0

Bronchitis *(Continued)*
smokers' 491.0
spirochetal 104.8
suffocative, acute or subacute 466.0
summer (*see also* Asthma) 493.9●
suppurative (chronic) 491.1
  acute or subacute 466.0
tuberculous (*see also* Tuberculosis)
  011.3●
ulcerative 491.8
  Vincent's 101
Vincent's 101
viral, acute or subacute 466.0
Bronchoalveolitis 485
Bronchoaspergillosis 117.3
Bronchocele
  meaning
    dilatation of bronchus 519.19
    goiter 240.9
Bronchogenic carcinoma 162.9
Bronchohemisporosis 117.9
Broncholithiasis 518.89
  tuberculous (*see also* Tuberculosis)
    011.3●
Bronchomalacia 748.3
Bronchomoniliasis 112.89
Bronchomycosis 112.89
Bronchonocardiosis 039.1
Bronchopleuropneumonia - *see*
  Pneumonia, broncho-
Bronchopneumonia - *see* Pneumonia,
  broncho-
Bronchopneumonitis - *see* Pneumonia,
  broncho-
Bronchopulmonary - *see* condition
Bronchopulmonitis - *see* Pneumonia,
  broncho-
Bronchorrhagia 786.3
  newborn 770.3
  tuberculous (*see also* Tuberculosis)
    011.3●
Bronchorrhea (chronic) (purulent)
  491.0
  acute 466.0
Bronchospasm 519.11
  with
    asthma - *see* Asthma
    bronchiolitis, acute 466.19
      due to respiratory syncytial
        virus 466.11
    bronchitis - *see* Bronchitis
    chronic obstructive pulmonary
      disease (COPD) 496
    emphysema - *see* Emphysema
    due to external agent - *see*
      Condition, respiratory,
      acute, due to
    acute 519.11
    exercise induced 493.81
Bronchospirochetosis 104.8
Bronchostenosis 519.19
Bronchus - *see* condition
Bronze, bronzed
  diabetes 275.0
  disease (Addison's) (skin) 255.41
    tuberculous (*see also* Tuberculosis)
      017.6●
Brooke's disease or tumor (M8100/0) -
  see Neoplasm, skin, benign
Brown's tendon sheath syndrome
  378.61
Brown enamel of teeth (hereditary)
  520.5

Brown-Séquard's paralysis (syndrome)
  344.89
Brow presentation complicating delivery
  652.4●
Brucella, brucellosis (infection) 023.9
  abortus 023.1
  canis 023.3
  dermatitis, skin 023.9
  melitensis 023.0
  mixed 023.8
  suis 023.2
Bruck's disease 733.99
Bruck-de Lange disease or syndrome
  (Amsterdam dwarf, mental
  retardation, and brachycephaly)
  759.89
Brugada syndrome 746.89
Brug's filariasis 125.1
Brugsch's syndrome (acropachyderma)
  757.39
Bruhl's disease (splenic anemia with
  fever) 285.8
Bruise (skin surface intact) - *see also*
  Contusion
  with
    fracture - *see* Fracture, by site
    open wound - *see* Wound, open, by
      site
    internal organ (abdomen, chest, or
      pelvis) - *see* Injury, internal, by
      site
    umbilical cord 663.6●
      affecting fetus or newborn 762.6
Bruit 785.9
  arterial (abdominal) (carotid) 785.9
  supraclavicular 785.9
Brushburn - *see* Injury, superficial, by
  site
Bruton's X-linked agammaglobulinemia
  279.04
Bruxism 306.8
  sleep related 327.53
Bubbly lung syndrome 770.7
Bubo 289.3
  blennorrhagic 098.89
  chancroidal 099.0
  climatic 099.1
  due to Hemophilus ducreyi 099.0
  gonococcal 098.89
  indolent NEC 099.8
  inguinal NEC 099.8
    chancroidal 099.0
    climatic 099.1
    due to H. ducreyi 099.0
  scrofulous (*see also* Tuberculosis)
    017.2●
  soft chancre 099.0
  suppurating 683
  syphilitic 091.0
    congenital 090.0
  tropical 099.1
  venereal NEC 099.8
  virulent 099.0
Bubonic plague 020.0
Bubonocele - *see* Hernia, inguinal
Buccal - *see* condition
Buchanan's disease (juvenile
  osteochondrosis of iliac crest)
  732.1
Buchem's syndrome (hyperostosis
  corticalis) 733.3
Buchman's disease (osteochondrosis,
  juvenile) 732.1

◀ New   ◀ⅢⅡ Revised   ~~deleted~~ Deleted   ● Use Additional Digit(s)   ▨ Omit code

Bucket handle fracture (semilunar cartilage) (*see also* Tear, meniscus) 836.2
Budd-Chiari syndrome (hepatic vein thrombosis) 453.0
Budgerigar-fanciers' disease or lung 495.2
Büdinger-Ludloff-Läwen disease 717.89
Buds
  breast 259.1
  in newborn 779.89
Buerger's disease (thromboangiitis obliterans) 443.1
Bulbar - *see* condition
Bulbus cordis 745.9
  persistent (in left ventricle) 745.8
Bulging fontanels (congenital) 756.0
Bulimia 783.6
  nervosa 307.51
  nonorganic origin 307.51
Bulky uterus 621.2
Bulla(e) 709.8
  lung (emphysematous) (solitary) 492.0
Bullet wound - *see also* Wound, open, by site
  fracture - *see* Fracture, by site, open
  internal organ (abdomen, chest, or pelvis) - *see* Injury, internal, by site, with open wound
  intracranial - *see* Laceration, brain, with open wound
Bullis fever 082.8
Bullying (*see also* Disturbance, conduct) 312.0●
Bundle
  branch block (complete) (false) (incomplete) 426.50
    bilateral 426.53
    left (*see also* Block, bundle branch, left) 426.3
      hemiblock 426.2
    right (*see also* Block, bundle branch, right) 426.4
  of His - *see* condition
  of Kent syndrome (anomalous atrioventricular excitation) 426.7
Bungpagga 040.81
Bunion 727.1
Bunionette 727.1
Bunyamwera fever 066.3
Buphthalmia, buphthalmos (congenital) 743.20
  associated with
    keratoglobus, congenital 743.22
    megalocornea 743.22
    ocular anomalies NEC 743.22
  isolated 743.21
  simple 743.21
Bürger-Grütz disease or syndrome (essential familial hyperlipemia) 272.3
Buried roots 525.3
Burke's syndrome 577.8
Burkitt's
  tumor (M9750/3) 200.2●
  type malignant, lymphoma, lymphoblastic, or undifferentiated (M9750/3) 200.2●

Burn (acid) (cathode ray) (caustic) (chemical) (electric heating appliance) (electricity) (fire) (flame) (hot liquid or object) (irradiation) (lime) (radiation) (steam) (thermal) (x-ray) 949.0

Note 11	Use the following fifth-digit subclassification with category 948 to indicate the percent of body surface with third degree burn:
0	less than 10 percent or unspecified
1	10–19 percent
2	20–29 percent
3	30–39 percent
4	40–49 percent
5	50–59 percent
6	60–69 percent
7	70–79 percent
8	80–89 percent
9	90 percent or more of body surface

with
  blisters - *see* Burn, by site, second degree
  erythema - *see* Burn, by site, first degree
  skin loss (epidermal) - *see also* Burn, by site, second degree
  full thickness - *see also* Burn, by site, third degree
    with necrosis of underlying tissues - *see* Burn, by site, third degree, deep
first degree - *see* Burn, by site, first degree
second degree - *see* Burn, by site, second degree
third degree - *see also* Burn, by site, third degree
  deep - *see* Burn, by site, third degree, deep
abdomen, abdominal (muscle) (wall) 942.03
  with
    trunk - *see* Burn, trunk, multiple sites
  first degree 942.13
  second degree 942.23
  third degree 942.33
    deep 942.43
      with loss of body part 942.53
ankle 945.03
  with
    lower limb(s) - *see* Burn, leg, multiple sites
  first degree 945.13
  second degree 945.23
  third degree 945.33
    deep 945.43
      with loss of body part 945.53
anus - *see* Burn, trunk, specified site NEC
arm(s) 943.00
  first degree 943.10
  second degree 943.20
  third degree 943.30
    deep 943.40
      with loss of body part 943.50
  lower - *see* Burn, forearm(s)

Burn (*Continued*)
  arm(s) (*Continued*)
    multiple sites, except hand(s) or wrist(s) 943.09
    first degree 943.19
    second degree 943.29
    third degree 943.39
      deep 943.49
        with loss of body part 943.59
    upper 943.03
    first degree 943.13
    second degree 943.23
    third degree 943.33
      deep 943.43
        with loss of body part 943.53
  auditory canal (external) - *see* Burn, ear
  auricle (ear) - *see* Burn, ear
  axilla 943.04
    with
      upper limb(s), except hand(s) or wrist(s) - *see* Burn, arm(s), multiple sites
    first degree 943.14
    second degree 943.24
    third degree 943.34
      deep 943.44
        with loss of body part 943.54
  back 942.04
    with
      trunk - *see* Burn, trunk, multiple sites
    first degree 942.14
    second degree 942.24
    third degree 942.34
      deep 942.44
        with loss of body part 942.54
  biceps
    brachii - *see* Burn, arm(s), upper
    femoris - *see* Burn, thigh
  breast(s) 942.01
    with
      trunk - *see* Burn, trunk, multiple sites
    first degree 942.11
    second degree 942.21
    third degree 942.31
      deep 942.41
        with loss of body part 942.51
  brow - *see* Burn, forehead
  buttock(s) - *see* Burn, back
  canthus (eye) 940.1
    chemical 940.0
  cervix (uteri) 947.4
  cheek (cutaneous) 941.07
    with
      face or head - *see* Burn, head, multiple sites
    first degree 941.17
    second degree 941.27
    third degree 941.37
      deep 941.47
        with loss of body part 941.57
  chest wall (anterior) 942.02
    with
      trunk - *see* Burn, trunk, multiple sites
    first degree 942.12
    second degree 942.22
    third degree 942.32
      deep 942.42
        with loss of body part 942.52

◀ New   ◀▥ Revised   ~~deleted~~ Deleted   ● Use Additional Digit(s)   ▨ Omit code

Burn *(Continued)*
  chin 941.04
    with
      face or head - *see* Burn, head,
        multiple sites
    first degree 941.14
    second degree 941.24
    third degree 941.34
      deep 941.44
        with loss of body part 941.54
  clitoris - *see* Burn, genitourinary
    organs, external
  colon 947.3
  conjunctiva (and cornea) 940.4
    chemical
      acid 940.3
      alkaline 940.2
  cornea (and conjunctiva) 940.4
    chemical
      acid 940.3
      alkaline 940.2
  costal region - *see* Burn, chest wall
  due to ingested chemical agent - *see*
    Burn, internal organs
  ear (auricle) (canal) (drum) (external)
    941.01
    with
      face or head - *see* Burn, head,
        multiple sites
    first degree 941.11
    second degree 941.21
    third degree 941.31
      deep 941.41
        with loss of a body part 941.51
  elbow 943.02
    with
      hand(s) and wrist(s) - *see* Burn,
        multiple specified sites
      upper limb(s), except hand(s) or
        wrist(s) - *see also* Burn,
        arm(s), multiple sites
    first degree 943.12
    second degree 943.22
    third degree 943.32
      deep 943.42
        with loss of body part 943.52
  electricity, electric current - *see* Burn, by
    site
  entire body - *see* Burn, multiple,
    specified sites
  epididymis - *see* Burn, genitourinary
    organs, external
  epigastric region - *see* Burn, abdomen
  epiglottis 947.1
  esophagus 947.2
  extent (percent of body surface)
    less than 10 percent 948.0●
    10–19 percent 948.1●
    20–29 percent 948.2●
    30–39 percent 948.3●
    40–49 percent 948.4●
    50–59 percent 948.5●
    60–69 percent 948.6●
    70–79 percent 948.7●
    80–89 percent 948.8●
    90 percent or more 948.9●
  extremity
    lower - *see* Burn, leg
    upper - *see* Burn, arm(s)
  eye(s) (and adnexa) (only) 940.9
    with
      face, head, or neck 941.02
        first degree 941.12
        second degree 941.22

Burn *(Continued)*
  eye(s) *(Continued)*
    with *(Continued)*
      face, head, or neck *(Continued)*
        third degree 941.32
          deep 941.42
            with loss of body part
              941.52
      other sites (classifiable to more
        than one category in 940–
        945) - *see* Burn, multiple,
        specified sites
      resulting rupture and destruction
        of eyeball 940.5
    specified part - *see* Burn, by site
  eyeball - *see also* Burn, eye
    with resulting rupture and
      destruction of eyeball 940.5
  eyelid(s) 940.1
    chemical 940.0
  face - *see* Burn, head
  finger (nail) (subungual) 944.01
    with
      hand(s) - *see* Burn, hand(s),
        multiple sites
      other sites - *see* Burn, multiple,
        specified sites
      thumb 944.04
        first degree 944.14
        second degree 944.24
        third degree 944.34
          deep 944.44
            with loss of body part
              944.54
    first degree 944.11
    second degree 944.21
    third degree 944.31
      deep 944.41
        with loss of body part 944.51
    multiple (digits) 944.03
      with thumb - *see* Burn, finger,
        with thumb
      first degree 944.13
      second degree 944.23
      third degree 944.33
        deep 944.43
          with loss of body part
            944.53
  flank - *see* Burn, abdomen
  foot 945.02
    with
      lower limb(s) - *see* Burn, leg,
        multiple sites
    first degree 945.12
    second degree 945.22
    third degree 945.32
      deep 945.42
        with loss of body part 945.52
  forearm(s) 943.01
    with
      upper limb(s), except hand(s) or
        wrist(s) - *see* Burn, arm(s),
        multiple sites
    first degree 943.11
    second degree 943.21
    third degree 943.31
      deep 943.41
        with loss of body part 943.51
  forehead 941.07
    with
      face or head - *see* Burn, head,
        multiple sites
    first degree 941.17
    second degree 941.27

Burn *(Continued)*
  forehead *(Continued)*
    third degree 941.37
      deep 941.47
        with loss of body part 941.57
  fourth degree - *see* Burn, by site, third
    degree, deep
  friction - *see* Injury, superficial, by site
  from swallowing caustic or corrosive
    substance NEC - *see* Burn,
    internal organs
  full thickness - *see* Burn, by site, third
    degree
  gastrointestinal tract 947.3
  genitourinary organs
    external 942.05
      with
        trunk - *see* Burn, trunk,
          multiple sites
      first degree 942.15
      second degree 942.25
      third degree 942.35
        deep 942.45
          with loss of body part
            942.55
    internal 947.8
  globe (eye) - *see* Burn, eyeball
  groin - *see* Burn, abdomen
  gum 947.0
  hand(s) (phalanges) (and wrist) 944.00
    first degree 944.10
    second degree 944.20
    third degree 944.30
      deep 944.40
        with loss of body part 944.50
    back (dorsal surface) 944.06
      first degree 944.16
      second degree 944.26
      third degree 944.36
        deep 944.46
          with loss of body part
            944.56
    multiple sites 944.08
      first degree 944.18
      second degree 944.28
      third degree 944.38
        deep 944.48
          with loss of body part
            944.58
  head (and face) 941.00
    eye(s) only 940.9
      specified part - *see* Burn, by site
    first degree 941.10
    second degree 941.20
    third degree 941.30
      deep 941.40
        with loss of body part 941.50
    multiple sites 941.09
      with eyes - *see* Burn, eyes, with
        face, head, or neck
      first degree 941.19
      second degree 941.29
      third degree 941.39
        deep 941.49
          with loss of body part
            941.59
  heel - *see* Burn, foot
  hip - *see* Burn, trunk, specified site
    NEC
  iliac region - *see* Burn, trunk, specified
    site NEC
  infected 958.3
  inhalation (*see also* Burn, internal
    organs) 947.9

Burn (Continued)

internal organs 947.9
    from caustic or corrosive substance (swallowing) NEC 947.9
    specified NEC (see also Burn, by site) 947.8
interscapular region - see Burn, back
intestine (large) (small) 947.3
iris - see Burn, eyeball
knee 945.05
    with
        lower limb(s) - see Burn, leg, multiple sites
    first degree 945.15
    second degree 945.25
    third degree 945.35
        deep 945.45
            with loss of body part 945.55
labium (majus) (minus) - see Burn, genitourinary organs, external
lacrimal apparatus, duct, gland, or sac 940.1
    chemical 940.0
larynx 947.1
late effect - see Late, effects (of), burn
leg 945.00
    first degree 945.10
    second degree 945.20
    third degree 945.30
        deep 945.40
            with loss of body part 945.50
    lower 945.04
        with other part(s) of lower limb(s) - see Burn, leg, multiple sites
        first degree 945.14
        second degree 945.24
        third degree 945.34
            deep 945.44
                with loss of body part 945.54
    multiple sites 945.09
        first degree 945.19
        second degree 945.29
        third degree 945.39
            deep 945.49
                with loss of body part 945.59
    upper - see Burn, thigh
lightning - see Burn, by site
limb(s)
    lower (including foot or toe(s)) - see Burn, leg
    upper (except wrist and hand) - see Burn, arm(s)
lip(s) 941.03
    with
        face or head - see Burn, head, multiple sites
    first degree 941.13
    second degree 941.23
    third degree 941.33
        deep 941.43
            with loss of body part 941.53
lumbar region - see Burn, back
lung 947.1
malar region - see Burn, cheek
mastoid region - see Burn, scalp
membrane, tympanic - see Burn, ear
midthoracic region - see Burn, chest wall
mouth 947.0

Burn (Continued)

multiple (see also Burn, unspecified) 949.0
    specified sites classifiable to more than one category in 940–945 946.0
    first degree 946.1
    second degree 946.2
    third degree 946.3
        deep 946.4
            with loss of body part 946.5
muscle, abdominal - see Burn, abdomen
nasal (septum) - see Burn, nose
neck 941.08
    with
        face or head - see Burn, head, multiple sites
    first degree 941.18
    second degree 941.28
    third degree 941.38
        deep 941.48
            with loss of body part 941.58
nose (septum) 941.05
    with
        face or head - see Burn, head, multiple sites
    first degree 941.15
    second degree 941.25
    third degree 941.35
        deep 941.45
            with loss of body part 941.55
occipital region - see Burn, scalp
orbit region 940.1
    chemical 940.0
oronasopharynx 947.0
palate 947.0
palm(s) 944.05
    with
        hand(s) and wrist(s) - see Burn, hand(s), multiple sites
    first degree 944.15
    second degree 944.25
    third degree 944.35
        deep 944.45
            with loss of a body part 944.55
parietal region - see Burn, scalp
penis - see Burn, genitourinary organs, external
perineum - see Burn, genitourinary organs, external
periocular area 940.1
    chemical 940.0
pharynx 947.0
pleura 947.1
popliteal space - see Burn, knee
prepuce - see Burn, genitourinary organs, external
pubic region - see Burn, genitourinary organs, external
pudenda - see Burn, genitourinary organs, external
rectum 947.3
sac, lacrimal 940.1
    chemical 940.0
sacral region - see Burn, back
salivary (ducts) (glands) 947.0
scalp 941.06
    with
        face or neck - see Burn, head, multiple sites
    first degree 941.16
    second degree 941.26

Burn (Continued)

scalp (Continued)
    third degree 941.36
        deep 941.46
            with loss of body part 941.56
scapular region 943.06
    with
        upper limb(s), except hand(s) or wrist(s) - see Burn, arm(s), multiple sites
    first degree 943.16
    second degree 943.26
    third degree 943.36
        deep 943.46
            with loss of body part 943.56
sclera - see Burn, eyeball
scrotum - see Burn, genitourinary organs, external
septum, nasal - see Burn, nose
shoulder(s) 943.05
    with
        hand(s) and wrist(s) - see Burn, multiple, specified sites
        upper limb(s), except hand(s) or wrist(s) - see Burn, arm(s), multiple sites
    first degree 943.15
    second degree 943.25
    third degree 943.35
        deep 943.45
            with loss of body part 943.55
skin NEC (see also Burn, unspecified) 949.0
skull - see Burn, head
small intestine 947.3
sternal region - see Burn, chest wall
stomach 947.3
subconjunctival - see Burn, conjunctiva
subcutaneous - see Burn, by site, third degree
submaxillary region - see Burn, head
submental region - see Burn, chin
sun - see Sunburn
supraclavicular fossa - see Burn, neck
supraorbital - see Burn, forehead
temple - see Burn, scalp
temporal region - see Burn, scalp
testicle - see Burn, genitourinary organs, external
testis - see Burn, genitourinary organs, external
thigh 945.06
    with
        lower limb(s) - see Burn, leg, multiple sites
    first degree 945.16
    second degree 945.26
    third degree 945.36
        deep 945.46
            with loss of body part 945.56
thorax (external) - see Burn, chest wall
throat 947.0
thumb(s) (nail) (subungual) 944.02
    with
        finger(s) - see Burn, finger, with other sites, thumb
        hand(s) and wrist(s) - see Burn, hand(s), multiple sites
    first degree 944.12
    second degree 944.22
    third degree 944.32
        deep 944.42
            with loss of body part 944.52

◄ New   ◄≡ Revised   ~~deleted~~ Deleted   ● Use Additional Digit(s)   ▬ Omit code

Burn (*Continued*)
  toe (nail) (subungual) 945.01
    with
      lower limb(s) - *see* Burn, leg,
        multiple sites
    first degree 945.11
    second degree 945.21
    third degree 945.31
      deep 945.41
        with loss of body part 945.51
  tongue 947.0
  tonsil 947.0
  trachea 947.1
  trunk 942.00
    first degree 942.10
    second degree 942.20
    third degree 942.30
      deep 942.40
        with loss of body part 942.50
    multiple sites 942.09
      first degree 942.19
      second degree 942.29
      third degree 942.39
        deep 942.49
          with loss of body part
            942.59
    specified site NEC 942.09
      first degree 942.19
      second degree 942.29
      third degree 942.39
        deep 942.49
          with loss of body part
            942.59
  tunica vaginalis - *see* Burn,
    genitourinary organs, external
  tympanic membrane - *see* Burn, ear
  tympanum - *see* Burn, ear
  ultraviolet 692.82
  unspecified site (multiple) 949.0
    with extent of body surface involved
      specified
      less than 10 percent 948.0●
      10–19 percent 948.1●
      20–29 percent 948.2●
      30–39 percent 948.3●
      40–49 percent 948.4●
      50–59 percent 948.5●
      60–69 percent 948.6●
      70–79 percent 948.7●
      80–89 percent 948.8●
      90 percent or more 948.9●

Burn (*Continued*)
  unspecified site (*Continued*)
    first degree 949.1
    second degree 949.2
    third degree 949.3
      deep 949.4
        with loss of body part 949.5
  uterus 947.4
  uvula 947.0
  vagina 947.4
  vulva - *see* Burn, genitourinary organs,
    external
  wrist(s) 944.07
    with
      hand(s) - *see* Burn, hand(s),
        multiple sites
    first degree 944.17
    second degree 944.27
    third degree 944.37
      deep 944.47
        with loss of body part
          944.57
Burnett's syndrome (milk-alkali)
  275.42
Burnier's syndrome (hypophyseal
  dwarfism) 253.3
Burning
  feet syndrome 266.2
  sensation (*see also* Disturbance,
    sensation) 782.0
  tongue 529.6
Burns' disease (osteochondrosis, lower
  ulna) 732.3
Bursa - *see also* condition
  pharynx 478.29
Bursitis NEC 727.3
  Achilles tendon 726.71
  adhesive 726.90
    shoulder 726.0
  ankle 726.79
  buttock 726.5
  calcaneal 726.79
  collateral ligament
    fibular 726.63
    tibial 726.62
  Duplay's 726.2
  elbow 726.33
  finger 726.8
  foot 726.79
  gonococcal 098.52
  hand 726.4

Bursitis NEC (*Continued*)
  hip 726.5
  infrapatellar 726.69
  ischiogluteal 726.5
  knee 726.60
  occupational NEC 727.2
  olecranon 726.33
  pes anserinus 726.61
  pharyngeal 478.29
  popliteal 727.51
  prepatellar 726.65
  radiohumeral 727.3
  scapulohumeral 726.19
    adhesive 726.0
  shoulder 726.10
    adhesive 726.0
  subacromial 726.19
    adhesive 726.0
  subcoracoid 726.19
  subdeltoid 726.19
    adhesive 726.0
  subpatellar 726.69
  syphilitic 095.7
  Thornwaldt's, Tornwaldt's
    (pharyngeal) 478.29
  toe 726.79
  trochanteric area 726.5
  wrist 726.4
Burst stitches or sutures (complication of
  surgery) (external) (*see also*
  Dehiscence) 998.32
  internal 998.31
Buruli ulcer 031.1
Bury's disease (erythema elevatum
  diutinum) 695.89
Buschke's disease or scleredema
  (adultorum) 710.1
Busquet's disease (osteoperiostitis) (*see
  also* Osteomyelitis) 730.1●
Busse-Buschke disease (cryptococcosis)
  117.5
Buttock - *see* condition
Button
  Biskra 085.1
  Delhi 085.1
  oriental 085.1
Buttonhole hand (intrinsic) 736.21
Bwamba fever (encephalitis) 066.3
Byssinosis (occupational) 504
Bywaters' syndrome 958.5

C

Cacergasia 300.9
Cachexia 799.4
  cancerous - *see also* Neoplasm, by site,
    malignant 799.4
  cardiac - *see* Disease, heart
  dehydration 276.51
    with
      hypernatremia 276.0
      hyponatremia 276.1
    due to malnutrition 799.4
  exophthalmic 242.0●
  heart - *see* Disease, heart
  hypophyseal 253.2
  hypopituitary 253.2
  lead 984.9
    specified type of lead - *see* Table of
      Drugs and Chemicals
  malaria 084.9
  malignant *see also* Neoplasm, by site,
    malignant 799.4
  marsh 084.9
  nervous 300.5
  old age 797
  pachydermic - *see* Hypothyroidism
  paludal 084.9
  pituitary (postpartum) 253.2
  renal (*see also* Disease, renal) 593.9
  saturnine 984.9
    specified type of lead - *see* Table of
      Drugs and Chemicals
  senile 797
  Simmonds' (pituitary cachexia) 253.2
  splenica 289.59
  strumipriva (*see also* Hypothyroidism)
    244.9
  tuberculous NEC (*see also* Tuberculosis)
    011.9●
Café au lait spots 709.09
Caffey's disease or syndrome (infantile
  cortical hyperostosis) 756.59
Caisson disease 993.3
Caked breast (puerperal, postpartum)
  676.2●
Cake kidney 753.3
Calabar swelling 125.2
Calcaneal spur 726.73
Calcaneoapophysitis 732.5
Calcaneonavicular bar 755.67
Calcareous - *see* condition
Calcicosis (occupational) 502
Calciferol (vitamin D) deficiency 268.9
  with
    osteomalacia 268.2
    rickets (*see also* Rickets) 268.0
Calcification
  adrenal (capsule) (gland) 255.41
    tuberculous (*see also* Tuberculosis)
      017.6●
  aorta 440.0
  artery (annular) - *see* Arteriosclerosis
  auricle (ear) 380.89
  bladder 596.8
    due to S. hematobium 120.0
  brain (cortex) - *see* Calcification,
    cerebral
  bronchus 519.19
  bursa 727.82
  cardiac (*see also* Degeneration,
    myocardial) 429.1
  cartilage (postinfectional) 733.99
  cerebral (cortex) 348.89 ◀═
    artery 437.0

Calcification (*Continued*)
  cervix (uteri) 622.8
  choroid plexus 349.2
  conjunctiva 372.54
  corpora cavernosa (penis) 607.89
  cortex (brain) - *see* Calcification,
    cerebral
  dental pulp (nodular) 522.2
  dentinal papilla 520.4
  disc, intervertebral 722.90
    cervical, cervicothoracic 722.91
    lumbar, lumbosacral 722.93
    thoracic, thoracolumbar 722.92
  fallopian tube 620.8
  falx cerebri - *see* Calcification, cerebral
  fascia 728.89
  gallbladder 575.8
  general 275.40
  heart (*see also* Degeneration,
    myocardial) 429.1
    valve - *see* Endocarditis
  intervertebral cartilage or disc
    (postinfectional) 722.90
    cervical, cervicothoracic 722.91
    lumbar, lumbosacral 722.93
    thoracic, thoracolumbar 722.92
  intracranial - *see* Calcification, cerebral
  intraspinal ligament 728.89
  joint 719.80
    ankle 719.87
    elbow 719.82
    foot 719.87
    hand 719.84
    hip 719.85
    knee 719.86
    multiple sites 719.89
    pelvic region 719.85
    shoulder (region) 719.81
    specified site NEC 719.88
    wrist 719.83
  kidney 593.89
    tuberculous (*see also* Tuberculosis)
      016.0●
  larynx (senile) 478.79
  lens 366.8
  ligament 728.89
    intraspinal 728.89
    knee (medial collateral) 717.89
  lung 518.89
    active 518.89
    postinfectional 518.89
    tuberculous (*see also* Tuberculosis,
      pulmonary) 011.9●
  lymph gland or node (postinfectional)
    289.3
    tuberculous (*see also* Tuberculosis,
      lymph gland) 017.2●
  mammographic 793.89
  massive (paraplegic) 728.10
  medial (*see also* Arteriosclerosis,
    extremities) 440.20
  meninges (cerebral) 349.2
  metastatic 275.40
  Mönckeberg's - *see* Arteriosclerosis
  muscle 728.10
    heterotopic, postoperative 728.13
  myocardium, myocardial (*see also*
    Degeneration, myocardial) 429.1
  ovary 620.8
  pancreas 577.8
  penis 607.89
  periarticular 728.89
  pericardium (*see also* Pericarditis) 423.8
  pineal gland 259.8

Calcification (*Continued*)
  pleura 511.0
    postinfectional 518.89
    tuberculous (*see also* Tuberculosis,
      pleura) 012.0●
  pulp (dental) (nodular) 522.2
  renal 593.89
  Rider's bone 733.99
  sclera 379.16
  semilunar cartilage 717.89
  spleen 289.59
  subcutaneous 709.3
  suprarenal (capsule) (gland) 255.41
  tendon (sheath) 727.82
    with bursitis, synovitis or
      tenosynovitis 727.82
  trachea 519.19
  ureter 593.89
  uterus 621.8
  vitreous 379.29
Calcified - *see also* Calcification
  hematoma NEC 959.9
Calcinosis (generalized) (interstitial)
  (tumoral) (universalis) 275.49
  circumscripta 709.3
  cutis 709.3
  intervertebralis 275.49 [722.90]
  Raynaud's phenomenon
    sclerodactylytelangiectasis
    (CRST) 710.1
Calciphylaxis (*see also* Calcification, by
  site) 275.49
Calcium
  blood
    high (*see also* Hypercalcemia) 275.42
    low (*see also* Hypocalcemia) 275.41
  deposits - *see also* Calcification, by site
    in bursa 727.82
    in tendon (sheath) 727.82
      with bursitis, synovitis or
        tenosynovitis 727.82
  salts or soaps in vitreous 379.22
Calciuria 791.9
Calculi - *see* Calculus
Calculosis, intrahepatic - *see*
  Choledocholithiasis
Calculus, calculi, calculous 592.9
  ampulla of Vater - *see*
    Choledocholithiasis
  anuria (impacted) (recurrent) 592.0
  appendix 543.9
  bile duct (any) - *see* Choledocholithiasis
  biliary - *see* Cholelithiasis
  bilirubin, multiple - *see* Cholelithiasis
  bladder (encysted) (impacted)
    (urinary) 594.1
    diverticulum 594.0
  bronchus 518.89
  calyx (kidney) (renal) 592.0
    congenital 753.3
  cholesterol (pure) (solitary) - *see*
    Cholelithiasis
  common duct (bile) - *see*
    Choledocholithiasis
  conjunctiva 372.54
  cystic 594.1
    duct - *see* Cholelithiasis
  dental 523.6
    subgingival 523.6
    supragingival 523.6
  epididymis 608.89
  gallbladder - *see also* Cholelithiasis
    congenital 751.69
  hepatic (duct) - *see* Choledocholithiasis

◀ New   ◀═ Revised   ~~deleted~~ Deleted   ● Use Additional Digit(s)   ▨ Omit code

Calculus, calculi, calculous *(Continued)*
  intestine (impaction) (obstruction) 560.39
  kidney (impacted) (multiple) (pelvis)
      (recurrent) (staghorn) 592.0
    congenital 753.3
  lacrimal (passages) 375.57
  liver (impacted) - *see* Choledocholithiasis
  lung 518.89
  mammographic 793.89
  nephritic (impacted) (recurrent) 592.0
  nose 478.19
  pancreas (duct) 577.8
  parotid gland 527.5
  pelvis, encysted 592.0
  prostate 602.0
  pulmonary 518.89
  renal (impacted) (recurrent) 592.0
    congenital 753.3
  salivary (duct) (gland) 527.5
  seminal vesicle 608.89
  staghorn 592.0
  Stensen's duct 527.5
  sublingual duct or gland 527.5
    congenital 750.26
  submaxillary duct, gland, or region 527.5
  suburethral 594.8
  tonsil 474.8
  tooth, teeth 523.6
  tunica vaginalis 608.89
  ureter (impacted) (recurrent) 592.1
  urethra (impacted) 594.2
  urinary (duct) (impacted) (passage)
      (tract) 592.9
    lower tract NEC 594.9
      specified site 594.8
  vagina 623.8
  vesical (impacted) 594.1
  Wharton's duct 527.5
Caliectasis 593.89
California
  disease 114.0
  encephalitis 062.5
Caligo cornea 371.03
Callositas, callosity (infected) 700
Callus (infected) 700
  bone 726.91
  excessive, following fracture - *see also*
      Late, effect (of), fracture
Calvé (-Perthes) disease (osteochondrosis,
      femoral capital) 732.1
Calvities (*see also* Alopecia) 704.00
Cameroon fever (*see also* Malaria) 084.6
Camptocormia 300.11
Camptodactyly (congenital) 755.59
Camurati-Engelmann disease
      (diaphyseal sclerosis) 756.59
Canal - *see* condition
Canaliculitis (lacrimal) (acute) 375.31
  Actinomyces 039.8
  chronic 375.41
Canavan's disease 330.0
Cancer (M8000/3) - *see also* Neoplasm, by
      site, malignant

Note 12   The term "cancer" when
modified by an adjective or adjectival
phrase indicating a morphological type
should be coded in the same manner
as "carcinoma" with that adjective or
phrase. Thus, "squamous-cell cancer"
should be coded in the same manner as
"squamous-cell carcinoma," which appears in the list under "Carcinoma."

Cancer *(Continued)*
  bile duct type (M8160/3), liver 155.1
  hepatocellular (M8170/3) 155.0
Cancerous (M8000/3) - *see* Neoplasm, by
      site, malignant
Cancerphobia 300.29
Cancrum oris 528.1
Candidiasis, candidal 112.9
  with pneumonia 112.4
  balanitis 112.2
  congenital 771.7
  disseminated 112.5
  endocarditis 112.81
  esophagus 112.84
  intertrigo 112.3
  intestine 112.85
  lung 112.4
  meningitis 112.83
  mouth 112.0
  nails 112.3
  neonatal 771.7
  onychia 112.3
  otitis externa 112.82
  otomycosis 112.82
  paronychia 112.3
  perionyxis 112.3
  pneumonia 112.4
  pneumonitis 112.4
  skin 112.3
  specified site NEC 112.89
  systemic 112.5
  urogenital site NEC 112.2
  vagina 112.1
  vulva 112.1
  vulvovaginitis 112.1
Candidiosis - *see* Candidiasis
Candiru infection or infestation 136.8
Canities (premature) 704.3
  congenital 757.4
Canker (mouth) (sore) 528.2
  rash 034.1
Cannabinosis 504
Canton fever 081.9
Cap
  cradle 690.11
Capillariasis 127.5
Capillary - *see* condition
Caplan's syndrome 714.81
Caplan-Colinet syndrome 714.81
Capsule - *see* condition
Capsulitis (joint) 726.90
  adhesive (shoulder) 726.0
  hip 726.5
  knee 726.60
  labyrinthine 387.8
  thyroid 245.9
  wrist 726.4
Caput
  crepitus 756.0
  medusae 456.8
  succedaneum 767.19
Carapata disease 087.1
Carate - *see* Pinta
Carbohydrate-deficient glycoprotein
      syndrome (CDGS) 271.8
Carboxyhemoglobinemia 986
Carbuncle 680.9
  abdominal wall 680.2
  ankle 680.6
  anus 680.5
  arm (any part, above wrist) 680.3
  auditory canal, external 680.0
  axilla 680.3
  back (any part) 680.2

Carbuncle *(Continued)*
  breast 680.2
  buttock 680.5
  chest wall 680.2
  corpus cavernosum 607.2
  ear (any part) (external) 680.0
  eyelid 373.13
  face (any part, except eye) 680.0
  finger (any) 680.4
  flank 680.2
  foot (any part) 680.7
  forearm 680.3
  genital organ (male) 608.4
  gluteal (region) 680.5
  groin 680.2
  hand (any part) 680.4
  head (any part, except face) 680.8
  heel 680.7
  hip 680.6
  kidney (*see also* Abscess, kidney)
      590.2
  knee 680.6
  labia 616.4
  lacrimal
    gland (*see also* Dacryoadenitis)
        375.00
    passages (duct) (sac) (*see also*
        Dacryocystitis) 375.30
  leg, any part except foot 680.6
  lower extremity, any part except foot
      680.6
  malignant 022.0
  multiple sites 680.9
  neck 680.1
  nose (external) (septum) 680.0
  orbit, orbital 376.01
  partes posteriores 680.5
  pectoral region 680.2
  penis 607.2
  perineum 680.2
  pinna 680.0
  scalp (any part) 680.8
  scrotum 608.4
  seminal vesicle 608.0
  shoulder 680.3
  skin NEC 680.9
  specified site NEC 680.8
  spermatic cord 608.4
  temple (region) 680.0
  testis 608.4
  thigh 680.6
  thumb 680.4
  toe (any) 680.7
  trunk 680.2
  tunica vaginalis 608.4
  umbilicus 680.2
  upper arm 680.3
  urethra 597.0
  vas deferens 608.4
  vulva 616.4
  wrist 680.4
Carbunculus (*see also* Carbuncle) 680.9
Carcinoid (tumor) (M8240/1) - *see* Tumor,
      carcinoid
  and struma ovarii (M9091/1) 236.2
  argentaffin (M8241/1) - *see* Neoplasm,
      by site, uncertain behavior
    malignant (M8241/3) - *see*
        Neoplasm, by site, malignant
  benign (M9091/0) 220
  composite (M8244/3) - *see* Neoplasm,
      by site, malignant
  goblet cell (M8243/3) - *see* Neoplasm,
      by site, malignant

Carcinoid (Continued)
  malignant (M8240/3) - see Neoplasm,
      by site, malignant
  nonargentaffin (M8242/1) - see also
      Neoplasm, by site, uncertain
      behavior
    malignant (M8242/3) - see
        Neoplasm, by site, malignant
  strumal (M9091/1) 236.2
  syndrome (intestinal) (metastatic)
      259.2
  type bronchial adenoma (M8240/3) -
      see Neoplasm, lung, malignant
Carcinoidosis 259.2
Carcinoma (M8010/3) - see also Neoplasm,
    by site, malignant

Note 13   Except where otherwise
indicated, the morphological varieties
of carcinoma in the list below should
be coded by site as for "Neoplasm,
malignant."

  with
    apocrine metaplasia (M8573/3)
    cartilaginous (and osseous)
        metaplasia (M8571/3)
    osseous (and cartilaginous)
        metaplasia (M8571/3)
    productive fibrosis (M8141/3)
    spindle cell metaplasia (M8572/3)
    squamous metaplasia (M8570/3)
  acidophil (M8280/3)
    specified site - see Neoplasm, by site,
        malignant
    unspecified site 194.3
  acidophil-basophil, mixed (M8281/3)
    specified site - see Neoplasm, by site,
        malignant
    unspecified site 194.3
  acinar (cell) (M8550/3)
  acinic cell (M8550/3)
  adenocystic (M8200/3)
  adenoid
    cystic (M8200/3)
    squamous cell (M8075/3)
  adenosquamous (M8560/3)
  adnexal (skin) (M8390/3) - see
      Neoplasm, skin, malignant
  adrenal cortical (M8370/3) 194.0
  alveolar (M8251/3)
    cell (M8250/3) - see Neoplasm, lung,
        malignant
  anaplastic type (M8021/3)
  apocrine (M8401/3)
    breast - see Neoplasm, breast,
        malignant
    specified site NEC - see Neoplasm,
        skin, malignant
    unspecified site 173.9
  basal cell (pigmented) (M8090/3) -
      see also Neoplasm, skin,
      malignant
    fibro-epithelial type (M8093/3) -
        see Neoplasm, skin,
        malignant
    morphea type (M8092/3) - see
        Neoplasm, skin, malignant
    multicentric (M8091/3) - see
        Neoplasm, skin, malignant
  basaloid (M8123/3)
  basal-squamous cell, mixed
      (M8094/3) - see Neoplasm, skin,
      malignant

Carcinoma (Continued)
  basophil (M8300/3)
    specified site - see Neoplasm, by site,
        malignant
    unspecified site 194.3
  basophil-acidophil, mixed (M8281/3)
    specified site - see Neoplasm, by site,
        malignant
    unspecified site 194.3
  basosquamous (M8094/3) - see
      Neoplasm, skin, malignant
  bile duct type (M8160/3)
    and hepatocellular, mixed
        (M8180/3) 155.0
    liver 155.1
    specified site NEC - see Neoplasm,
        by site, malignant
    unspecified site 155.1
  branchial or branchiogenic 146.8
  bronchial or bronchogenic - see
      Neoplasm, lung, malignant
  bronchiolar (terminal) (M8250/3) -
      see Neoplasm, lung,
      malignant
  bronchiolo-alveolar (M8250/3) -
      see Neoplasm, lung,
      malignant
  bronchogenic (epidermoid) 162.9
  C cell (M8510/3)
    specified site - see Neoplasm, by site,
        malignant
    unspecified site 193
  ceruminous (M8420/3) 173.2
  chorionic (M9100/3)
    specified site - see Neoplasm, by site,
        malignant
    unspecified site
      female 181
      male 186.9
  chromophobe (M8270/3)
    specified site - see Neoplasm, by site,
        malignant
    unspecified site 194.3
  clear cell (mesonephroid type)
      (M8310/3)
  cloacogenic (M8124/3)
    specified site - see Neoplasm, by site,
        malignant
    unspecified site 154.8
  colloid (M8480/3)
  cribriform (M8201/3)
  cylindroid type (M8200/3)
  diffuse type (M8145/3)
    specified site - see Neoplasm, by site,
        malignant
    unspecified site 151.9
  duct (cell) (M8500/3)
    with Paget's disease (M8541/3) -
        see Neoplasm, breast,
        malignant
    infiltrating (M8500/3)
      specified site - see Neoplasm, by
          site, malignant
      unspecified site 174.9
  ductal (M8500/3)
  ductular, infiltrating (M8521/3)
  embryonal (M9070/3)
    and teratoma, mixed (M9081/3)
    combined with choriocarcinoma
        (M9101/3) - see Neoplasm, by
        site, malignant
    infantile type (M9071/3)
    liver 155.0
    polyembryonal type (M9072/3)

Carcinoma (Continued)
  endometrioid (M8380/3)
  eosinophil (M8280/3)
    specified site - see Neoplasm, by site,
        malignant
    unspecified site 194.3
  epidermoid (M8070/3) - see also
      Carcinoma, squamous cell
    and adenocarcinoma, mixed
        (M8560/3)
    in situ, Bowen's type (M8081/2) - see
        Neoplasm, skin, in situ
    intradermal - see Neoplasm, skin, in
        situ
  fibroepithelial type basal cell
      (M8093/3) - see Neoplasm, skin,
      malignant
  follicular (M8330/3)
    and papillary (mixed) (M8340/3) 193
    moderately differentiated type
        (M8332/3) 193
    pure follicle type (M8331/3) 193
    specified site - see Neoplasm, by site,
        malignant
    trabecular type (M8332/3) 193
    unspecified site 193
    well differentiated type (M8331/3)
        193
  gelatinous (M8480/3)
  giant cell (M8031/3)
    and spindle cell (M8030/3)
  granular cell (M8320/3)
  granulosa cell (M8620/3) 183.0
  hepatic cell (M8170/3) 155.0
  hepatocellular (M8170/3) 155.0
    and bile duct, mixed (M8180/3) 155.0
  hepatocholangiolitic (M8180/3) 155.0
  Hürthle cell (thyroid) 193
  hypernephroid (M8311/3)
  in
    adenomatous
      polyp (M8210/3)
      polyposis coli (M8220/3) 153.9
    pleomorphic adenoma (M8940/3)
    polypoid adenoma (M8210/3)
    situ (M8010/3) - see Carcinoma, in
        situ
    tubular adenoma (M8210/3)
    villous adenoma (M8261/3)
  infiltrating duct (M8500/3)
    with Paget's disease (M8541/3) - see
        Neoplasm, breast, malignant
    specified site - see Neoplasm, by site,
        malignant
    unspecified site 174.9
  inflammatory (M8530/3)
    specified site - see Neoplasm, by site,
        malignant
    unspecified site 174.9
  in situ (M8010/2) - see also Neoplasm,
      by site, in situ
    epidermoid (M8070/2) - see also
        Neoplasm, by site, in situ
      with questionable stromal
          invasion (M8076/2)
        specified site - see Neoplasm,
            by site, in situ
        unspecified site 233.1
      Bowen's type (M8081/2) - see
          Neoplasm, skin, in situ
    intraductal (M8500/2)
      specified site - see Neoplasm, by
          site, in situ
      unspecified site 233.0

◀ New   ◀▥ Revised   ~~deleted~~ Deleted   ● Use Additional Digit(s)   ▬ Omit code

Carcinoma (Continued)
  in situ (Continued)
    lobular (M8520/2)
      specified site - see Neoplasm, by
        site, in situ
      unspecified site 233.0
    papillary (M8050/2) - see Neoplasm,
      by site, in situ
    squamous cell (M8070/2) - see also
      Neoplasm, by site, in situ
      with questionable stromal
        invasion (M8076/2)
      specified site - see Neoplasm,
        by site, in situ
      unspecified site 233.1
    transitional cell (M8120/2) - see
      Neoplasm, by site, in situ
  intestinal type (M8144/3)
    specified site - see Neoplasm, by site,
      malignant
    unspecified site 151.9
  intraductal (noninfiltrating)
    (M8500/2)
    papillary (M8503/2)
      specified site - see Neoplasm, by
        site, in situ
      unspecified site 233.0
    specified site - see Neoplasm, by site,
      in situ
    unspecified site 233.0
  intraepidermal (M8070/2) - see also
    Neoplasm, skin, in situ
    squamous cell, Bowen's type
      (M8081/2) - see Neoplasm,
      skin, in situ
  intraepithelial (M8010/2) - see also
    Neoplasm, by site, in situ
    squamous cell (M8072/2) - see
      Neoplasm, by site, in situ
  intraosseous (M9270/3) 170.1
    upper jaw (bone) 170.0
  islet cell (M8150/3)
    and exocrine, mixed (M8154/3)
      specified site - see Neoplasm, by
        site, malignant
      unspecified site 157.9
    pancreas 157.4
    specified site NEC - see Neoplasm,
      by site, malignant
    unspecified site 157.4
  juvenile, breast (M8502/3) - see
    Neoplasm, breast, malignant
  Kulchitsky's cell (carcinoid tumor of
    intestine) 259.2
  large cell (M8012/3)
    squamous cell, non-keratinizing
      type (M8072/3)
  Leydig cell (testis) (M8650/3)
    specified site - see Neoplasm, by site,
      malignant
    unspecified site 186.9
      female 183.0
      male 186.9
  liver cell (M8170/3) 155.0
  lobular (infiltrating) (M8520/3)
    noninfiltrating (M8520/3)
      specified site - see Neoplasm, by
        site, in situ
      unspecified site 233.0
    specified site - see Neoplasm, by site,
      malignant
    unspecified site 174.9
  lymphoepithelial (M8082/3)

Carcinoma (Continued)
  medullary (M8510/3)
    with
      amyloid stroma (M8511/3)
        specified site - see Neoplasm,
          by site, malignant
        unspecified site 193
      lymphoid stroma (M8512/3)
        specified site - see Neoplasm,
          by site, malignant
        unspecified site 174.9
  Merkel cell 209.36 ◀
    buttock 209.36 ◀
    ear 209.31 ◀
    eyelid, including canthus 209.31 ◀
    face 209.31 ◀
    genitals 209.36 ◀
    lip 209.31 ◀
    lower limb 209.34 ◀
    neck 209.32 ◀
    nodal presentation 209.75 ◀
    scalp 209.32 ◀
    secondary (any site) 209.75 ◀
    specified site NEC 209.36 ◀
    trunk 209.35 ◀
    unknown primary site 209.75 ◀
    upper limb 209.33 ◀
    visceral metastatic presentation
      209.75 ◀
  mesometanephric (M9110/3)
  mesonephric (M9110/3)
  metastatic (M8010/6) - see Metastasis,
    cancer
  metatypical (M8095/3) - see Neoplasm,
    skin, malignant
  morphea type basal cell (M8092/3) - see
    Neoplasm, skin, malignant
  mucinous (M8480/3)
  mucin-producing (M8481/3)
  mucin-secreting (M8481/3)
  mucoepidermoid (M8430/3)
  mucoid (M8480/3)
    cell (M8300/3)
      specified site - see Neoplasm, by
        site, malignant
      unspecified site 194.3
  mucous (M8480/3)
  neuroendocrine
    high grade (M8240/3) 209.30
    malignant poorly differentiated
      (M8240/3) 209.30
  nonencapsulated sclerosing (M8350/3)
    193
  noninfiltrating
    intracystic (M8504/2) - see
      Neoplasm, by site, in situ
    intraductal (M8500/2)
      papillary (M8503/2)
        specified site - see Neoplasm,
          by site, in situ
        unspecified site 233.0
      specified site - see Neoplasm, by
        site, in situ
      unspecified site 233.0
    lobular (M8520/2)
      specified site - see Neoplasm, by
        site, in situ
      unspecified site 233.0
  oat cell (M8042/3)
    specified site - see Neoplasm, by site,
      malignant
    unspecified site 162.9
  odontogenic (M9270/3) 170.1
    upper jaw (bone) 170.0
  onocytic (M8290/3)

Carcinoma (Continued)
  oxyphilic (M8290/3)
  papillary (M8050/3)
    and follicular (mixed) (M8340/3) 193
    epidermoid (M8052/3)
    intraductal (noninfiltrating)
      (M8503/2)
      specified site - see Neoplasm, by
        site, in situ
      unspecified site 233.0
    serous (M8460/3)
      specified site - see Neoplasm, by
        site, malignant
      surface (M8461/3)
        specified site - see Neoplasm,
          by site, malignant
        unspecified site 183.0
      unspecified site 183.0
    squamous cell (M8052/3)
    transitional cell (M8130/3)
  papillocystic (M8450/3)
    specified site - see Neoplasm, by site,
      malignant
    unspecified site 183.0
  parafollicular cell (M8510/3)
    specified site - see Neoplasm, by site,
      malignant
    unspecified site 193
  pleomorphic (M8022/3)
  polygonal cell (M8034/3)
  prickle cell (M8070/3)
  pseudoglandular, squamous cell
    (M8075/3)
  pseudomucinous (M8470/3)
    specified site - see Neoplasm, by site,
      malignant
    unspecified site 183.0
  pseudosarcomatous (M8033/3)
  regaud type (M8082/3) - see
    Neoplasm, nasopharynx,
    malignant
  renal cell (M8312/3) 189.0
  reserve cell (M8041/3)
  round cell (M8041/3)
  Schmincke (M8082/3) - see
    Neoplasm, nasopharynx,
    malignant
  Schneiderian (M8121/3)
    specified site - see Neoplasm, by site,
      malignant
    unspecified site 160.0
  scirrhous (M8141/3)
  sebaceous (M8410/3) - see Neoplasm,
    skin, malignant
  secondary (M8010/6) - see Neoplasm,
    by site, malignant, secondary
  secretory, breast (M8502/3) - see
    Neoplasm, breast, malignant
  serous (M8441/3)
    papillary (M8460/3)
      specified site - see Neoplasm, by
        site, malignant
      unspecified site 183.0
    surface, papillary (M8461/3)
      specified site - see Neoplasm, by
        site, malignant
      unspecified site 183.0
  Sertoli cell (M8640/3)
    specified site - see Neoplasm, by site,
      malignant
    unspecified site 186.9
  signet ring cell (M8490/3)
    metastatic (M8490/6) - see
      Neoplasm, by site, secondary
  simplex (M8231/3)

Carcinoma (*Continued*)
  skin appendage (M8390/3) - *see*
    Neoplasm, skin, malignant
  small cell (M8041/3)
    fusiform cell type (M8043/3)
    squamous cell, nonkeratinizing type
      (M8073/3)
  solid (M8230/3)
    with amyloid stroma (M8511/3)
      specified site - *see* Neoplasm, by
        site, malignant
      unspecified site 193
  spheroidal cell (M8035/3)
  spindle cell (M8032/3)
    and giant cell (M8030/3)
  spinous cell (M8070/3)
  squamous (cell) (M8070/3)
    adenoid type (M8075/3)
    and adenocarcinoma, mixed
      (M8560/3)
    intraepidermal, Bowen's type - *see*
      Neoplasm, skin, in situ
    keratinizing type (large cell)
      (M8071/3)
    large cell, nonkeratinizing type
      (M8072/3)
    microinvasive (M8076/3)
      specified site - *see* Neoplasm, by
        site, malignant
      unspecified site 180.9
    nonkeratinizing type (M8072/3)
    papillary (M8052/3)
    pseudoglandular (M8075/3)
    small cell, nonkeratinizing type
      (M8073/3)
    spindle cell type (M8074/3)
    verrucous (M8051/3)
  superficial spreading (M8143/3)
  sweat gland (M8400/3) - *see* Neoplasm,
    skin, malignant
  theca cell (M8600/3) 183.0
  thymic (M8580/3) 164.0
  trabecular (M8190/3)
  transitional (cell) (M8120/3)
    papillary (M8130/3)
    spindle cell type (M8122/3)
  tubular (M8211/3)
  undifferentiated type (M8020/3)
  urothelial (M8120/3)
  ventriculi 151.9
  verrucous (epidermoid) (squamous
    cell) (M8051/3)
  villous (M8262/3)
  water-clear cell (M8322/3) 194.1
  wolffian duct (M9110/3)
Carcinomaphobia 300.29
Carcinomatosis
  peritonei (M8010/6) 197.6
  specified site NEC (M8010/3) - *see*
    Neoplasm, by site, malignant
  unspecified site (M8010/6) 199.0
Carcinosarcoma (M8980/3) - *see also*
  Neoplasm, by site, malignant
  embryonal type (M8981/3) - *see*
    Neoplasm, by site, malignant
Cardia, cardial - *see* condition
Cardiac - *see also* condition
  death - *see* Disease, heart
  device
    defibrillator, automatic implantable
      V45.02
    in situ NEC V45.00
    pacemaker
      cardiac
        fitting or adjustment
          V53.31
        in situ V45.01

Cardiac (*Continued*)
  device (*Continued*)
    carotid sinus
      fitting or adjustment V53.39
      in situ V45.09
    pacemaker - *see* Cardiac, device,
      pacemaker
    tamponade 423.3
Cardialgia (*see also* Pain, precordial)
  786.51
Cardiectasis - *see* Hypertrophy, cardiac
Cardiochalasia 530.81
Cardiomalacia (*see also* Degeneration,
  myocardial) 429.1
Cardiomegalia glycogenica diffusa 271.0
Cardiomegaly (*see also* Hypertrophy,
  cardiac) 429.3
  congenital 746.89
  glycogen 271.0
  hypertensive (*see also* Hypertension,
    heart) 402.90
  idiopathic 425.4
Cardiomyoliposis (*see also* Degeneration,
  myocardial) 429.1
Cardiomyopathy (congestive) (constrictive)
  (familial) (infiltrative) (obstructive)
  (restrictive) (sporadic) 425.4
  alcoholic 425.5
  amyloid 277.39 [425.7]
  beriberi 265.0 [425.7]
  cobalt-beer 425.5
  congenital 425.3
  due to
    amyloidosis 277.39 [425.7]
    beriberi 265.0 [425.7]
    cardiac glycogenosis 271.0 [425.7]
    Chagas' disease 086.0
    Friedreich's ataxia 334.0 [425.8]
    hypertension - *see* Hypertension,
      with, heart involvement
    mucopolysaccharidosis 277.5 [425.7]
    myotonia atrophica 359.21 [425.8]
    progressive muscular dystrophy
      359.1 [425.8]
    sarcoidosis 135 [425.8]
  glycogen storage 271.0 [425.7]
  hypertensive - *see* Hypertension, with,
    heart involvement
  hypertrophic
    nonobstructive 425.4
    obstructive 425.1
      congenital 746.84
  idiopathic (concentric) 425.4
  in
    Chagas' disease 086.0
    sarcoidosis 135 [425.8]
  ischemic 414.8
  metabolic NEC 277.9 [425.7]
    amyloid 277.39 [425.7]
    thyrotoxic (*see also* Thyrotoxicosis)
      242.9● [425.7]
    thyrotoxicosis (*see also*
      Thyrotoxicosis) 242.9● [425.7]
  newborn 425.4
    congenital 425.3
  nutritional 269.9 [425.7]
    beriberi 265.0 [425.7]
  obscure of Africa 425.2
  peripartum 674.5●
  postpartum 674.5●
  primary 425.4
  secondary 425.9
  stress induced 429.83
  takotsubo 429.83
  thyrotoxic (*see also* Thyrotoxicosis)
    242.9● [425.7]

Cardiomyopathy (*Continued*)
  toxic NEC 425.9
  tuberculous (*see also* Tuberculosis)
    017.9● [425.8]
Cardionephritis - *see* Hypertension,
  cardiorenal
Cardionephropathy - *see* Hypertension,
  cardiorenal
Cardionephrosis - *see* Hypertension,
  cardiorenal
Cardioneurosis 306.2
Cardiopathia nigra 416.0
Cardiopathy (*see also* Disease, heart)
  429.9
  hypertensive (*see also* Hypertension,
    heart) 402.90
  idiopathic 425.4
  mucopolysaccharidosis 277.5 [425.7]
Cardiopericarditis (*see also* Pericarditis)
  423.9
Cardiophobia 300.29
Cardioptosis 746.87
Cardiorenal - *see* condition
Cardiorrhexis (*see also* Infarct,
  myocardium) 410.9●
Cardiosclerosis - *see* Arteriosclerosis,
  coronary
Cardiosis - *see* Disease, heart
Cardiospasm (esophagus) (reflex)
  (stomach) 530.0
  congenital 750.7
Cardiostenosis - *see* Disease, heart
Cardiosymphysis 423.1
Cardiothyrotoxicosis - *see*
  Hyperthyroidism
Cardiovascular - *see* condition
Carditis (acute) (bacterial) (chronic)
  (subacute) 429.89
  Coxsackie 074.20
  hypertensive (*see also* Hypertension,
    heart) 402.90
  meningococcal 036.40
  rheumatic - *see* Disease, heart,
    rheumatic
  rheumatoid 714.2
Care (of)
  child (routine) V20.1
  convalescent following V66.9
    chemotherapy V66.2
    medical NEC V66.5
    psychotherapy V66.3
    radiotherapy V66.1
    surgery V66.0
    surgical NEC V66.0
    treatment (for) V66.5
      combined V66.6
      fracture V66.4
      mental disorder NEC V66.3
      specified type NEC V66.5
  end-of-life V66.7
  family member (handicapped) (sick)
    creating problem for family V61.49
    provided away from home for
      holiday relief V60.5
    unavailable, due to
      absence (person rendering care)
        (sufferer) V60.4
      inability (any reason) of person
        rendering care V60.4
  holiday relief V60.5
  hospice V66.7
  lack of (at or after birth) (infant) (child)
    995.52
    adult 995.84
  lactation of mother V24.1
  palliative V66.7

◀ New   ◀▥ Revised   ~~deleted~~ Deleted   ● Use Additional Digit(s)   ▨ Omit code

Care (*Continued*)
  postpartum
    immediately after delivery V24.0
    routine follow-up V24.2
  prenatal V22.1
    first pregnancy V22.0
    high-risk pregnancy V23.9
      specified problem NEC V23.89
  terminal V66.7
  unavailable, due to
    absence of person rendering care
      V60.4
    inability (any reason) of person
      rendering care V60.4
  well baby V20.1
Caries (bone) (*see also* Tuberculosis, bone)
  015.9● [*730.8*]●
  arrested 521.04
  cementum 521.03
  cerebrospinal (tuberculous) 015.0●
    [*730.88*]
  dental (acute) (chronic) (incipient)
    (infected) 521.00
    with pulp exposure 521.03
    extending to
      dentine 521.02
      pulp 521.03
    other specified NEC 521.09
    pit and fissure 521.06
    primary
      pit and fissure origin 521.06
      root surface 521.08
      smooth surface origin 521.07
    root surface 521.08
    smooth surface 521.07
  dentin (acute) (chronic) 521.02
  enamel (acute) (chronic) (incipient)
    521.01
  external meatus 380.89
  hip (*see also* Tuberculosis) 015.1● [*730.85*]
  initial 521.01
  knee 015.2● [*730.86*]
  labyrinth 386.8
  limb NEC 015.7● [*730.88*]
  mastoid (chronic) (process) 383.1
  middle ear 385.89
  nose 015.7● [*730.88*]
  orbit 015.7● [*730.88*]
  ossicle 385.24
  petrous bone 383.20
  sacrum (tuberculous) 015.0● [*730.88*]
  spine, spinal (column) (tuberculous)
    015.0● [*730.88*]
  syphilitic 095.5
    congenital 090.0 [*730.8*]●
  teeth (internal) 521.00
    initial 521.01
  vertebra (column) (tuberculous) 015.0●
    [*730.88*]
Carini's syndrome (ichthyosis congenita)
  757.1
Carious teeth 521.00
Carneous mole 631
Carnosinemia 270.5
Carotid body or sinus syndrome 337.01
Carotidynia 337.01
Carotinemia (dietary) 278.3
Carotinosis (cutis) (skin) 278.3
Carpal tunnel syndrome 354.0
Carpenter's syndrome 759.89
Carpopedal spasm (*see also* Tetany) 781.7
Carpoptosis 736.05
Carrier (suspected) of
  amebiasis V02.2
  bacterial disease (meningococcal,
    staphylococcal) NEC V02.59

Carrier (*Continued*)
  cholera V02.0
  cystic fibrosis gene V83.81
  defective gene V83.89
  diphtheria V02.4
  dysentery (bacillary) V02.3
    amebic V02.2
  Endamoeba histolytica V02.2
  gastrointestinal pathogens NEC V02.3
  genetic defect V83.89
  gonorrhea V02.7
  group B streptococcus V02.51
  HAA (hepatitis Australian-antigen)
    V02.61
  hemophilia A (asymptomatic) V83.01
    symptomatic V83.02
  hepatitis V02.60
    Australian-antigen (HAA) V02.61
    B V02.61
    C V02.62
    specified type NEC V02.69
    serum V02.61
    viral V02.60
  infective organism NEC V02.9
  malaria V02.9
  paratyphoid V02.3
  Salmonella V02.3
    typhosa V02.1
  serum hepatitis V02.61
  Shigella V02.3
  Staphylococcus NEC V02.59
    methicillin
      resistant Staphylococcus aureus
        V02.54
      susceptible Staphylococcus
        aureus V02.53
  Streptococcus NEC V02.52
    group B V02.51
  typhoid V02.1
  venereal disease NEC V02.8
Carrión's disease (Bartonellosis) 088.0
Car sickness 994.6
Carter's
  relapsing fever (Asiatic) 087.0
Cartilage - *see* condition
Caruncle (inflamed)
  abscess, lacrimal (*see also*
    Dacryocystitis) 375.30
  conjunctiva 372.00
    acute 372.00
  eyelid 373.00
  labium (majus) (minus) 616.89
  lacrimal 375.30
  urethra (benign) 599.3
  vagina (wall) 616.89
Cascade stomach 537.6
Caseation lymphatic gland (*see also*
  Tuberculosis) 017.2●
Caseous
  bronchitis - *see* Tuberculosis,
    pulmonary
  meningitis 013.0●
  pneumonia - *see* Tuberculosis,
    pulmonary
Cassidy (-Scholte) syndrome (malignant
  carcinoid) 259.2
Castellani's bronchitis 104.8
Castleman's tumor or lymphoma
  (mediastinal lymph node
  hyperplasia) 785.6
Castration, traumatic 878.2
  complicated 878.3
Casts in urine 791.7
Cat's ear 744.29
Catalepsy 300.11
  catatonic (acute) (*see also*
    Schizophrenia) 295.2●

Catalepsy (*Continued*)
  hysterical 300.11
  schizophrenic (*see also* Schizophrenia)
    295.2●
Cataphasia 307.0
Cataplexy (idiopathic) *see also*
  Narcolepsy
Cataract (anterior cortical) (anterior polar)
  (black) (capsular) (central) (cortical)
  (hypermature) (immature)
  (incipient) (mature) 366.9
  anterior
    and posterior axial embryonal
      743.33
    pyramidal 743.31
    subcapsular polar
      infantile, juvenile, or presenile
        366.01
      senile 366.13
  associated with
    calcinosis 275.40 [*366.42*]
    craniofacial dysostosis 756.0 [*366.44*]
    galactosemia 271.1 [*366.44*]
    hypoparathyroidism 252.1 [*366.42*]
    myotonic disorders 359.21 [*366.43*]
    neovascularization 366.33
  blue dot 743.39
  cerulean 743.39
  complicated NEC 366.30
  congenital 743.30
    capsular or subcapsular 743.31
    cortical 743.32
    nuclear 743.33
    specified type NEC 743.39
    total or subtotal 743.34
    zonular 743.32
  coronary (congenital) 743.39
    acquired 366.12
  cupuliform 366.14
  diabetic 250.5● [*366.41*]
    due to secondary diabetes 249.5●
      [*366.41*]
  drug-induced 366.45
  due to
    chalcosis 360.24 [*366.34*]
    chronic choroiditis (*see also*
      Choroiditis) 363.20 [*366.32*]
    degenerative myopia 360.21 [*366.34*]
    glaucoma (*see also* Glaucoma) 365.9
      [*366.31*]
    infection, intraocular NEC 366.32
    inflammatory ocular disorder NEC
      366.32
    iridocyclitis, chronic 364.10 [*366.33*]
    pigmentary retinal dystrophy 362.74
      [*366.34*]
    radiation 366.46
  electric 366.46
  glassblowers' 366.46
  heat ray 366.46
  heterochromic 366.33
  in eye disease NEC 366.30
  infantile (*see also* Cataract, juvenile)
    366.00
  intumescent 366.12
  irradiational 366.46
  juvenile 366.00
    anterior subcapsular polar 366.01
    combined forms 366.09
    cortical 366.03
    lamellar 366.03
    nuclear 366.04
    posterior subcapsular polar 366.02
    specified NEC 366.09
    zonular 366.03

Cataract *(Continued)*
  lamellar 743.32
    infantile juvenile, or presenile 366.03
  morgagnian 366.18
  myotonic 359.21 *[366.43]*
  myxedema 244.9 *[366.44]*
    nuclear 366.16
  posterior, polar (capsular) 743.31
    infantile, juvenile, or presenile 366.02
    senile 366.14
  presenile *(see also* Cataract, juvenile) 366.00
  punctate
    acquired 366.12
    congenital 743.39
  secondary (membrane) 366.50
    obscuring vision 366.53
    specified type, not obscuring vision 366.52
  senile 366.10
    anterior subcapsular polar 366.13
    combined forms 366.19
    cortical 366.15
    hypermature 366.18
    immature 366.12
    incipient 366.12
    mature 366.17
    nuclear 366.16
    posterior subcapsular polar 366.14
    specified NEC 366.19
    total or subtotal 366.17
  snowflake 250.5● *[366.41]*
    due to secondary diabetes 249.5● *[366.41]*
  specified NEC 366.8
  subtotal (senile) 366.17
    congenital 743.34
  sunflower 360.24 *[366.34]*
  tetanic NEC 252.1 *[366.42]*
  total (mature) (senile) 366.17
    congenital 743.34
    localized 366.21
    traumatic 366.22
  toxic 366.45
  traumatic 366.20
    partially resolved 366.23
    total 366.22
  zonular (perinuclear) 743.32
    infantile, juvenile, or presenile 366.03
Cataracta 366.10
  brunescens 366.16
  cerulea 743.39
  complicata 366.30
  congenita 743.30
  coralliformis 743.39
  coronaria (congenital) 743.39
    acquired 366.12
  diabetic 250.5● *[366.41]*
    due to secondary diabetes 249.5● *[366.41]*
  floriformis 360.24 *[366.34]*
  membranacea
    accreta 366.50
    congenita 743.39
  nigra 366.16
Catarrh, catarrhal (inflammation) *(see also* condition) 460
  acute 460
  asthma, asthmatic *(see also* Asthma) 493.9●
  Bostock's *(see also* Fever, hay) 477.9
  bowel - *see* Enteritis

Catarrh, catarrhal *(Continued)*
  bronchial 490
    acute 466.0
    chronic 491.0
    subacute 466.0
  cervix, cervical (canal) (uteri) - *see* Cervicitis
  chest *(see also* Bronchitis) 490
  chronic 472.0
  congestion 472.0
  conjunctivitis 372.03
  due to syphilis 095.9
    congenital 090.0
  enteric - *see* Enteritis
  epidemic 487.1
  Eustachian 381.50
  eye (acute) (vernal) 372.03
  fauces *(see also* Pharyngitis) 462
  febrile 460
  fibrinous acute 466.0
  gastroenteric - *see* Enteritis
  gastrointestinal - *see* Enteritis
  gingivitis 523.00
  hay *(see also* Fever, hay) 477.9
  infectious 460
  intestinal - *see* Enteritis
  larynx *(see also* Laryngitis, chronic) 476.0
  liver 070.1
    with hepatic coma 070.0
  lung *(see also* Bronchitis) 490
    acute 466.0
    chronic 491.0
  middle ear (chronic) - *see* Otitis media, chronic
  mouth 528.00
  nasal (chronic) *(see also* Rhinitis) 472.0
    acute 460
  nasobronchial 472.2
  nasopharyngeal (chronic) 472.2
    acute 460
  nose - *see* Catarrh, nasal
  ophthalmia 372.03
  pneumococcal, acute 466.0
  pulmonary *(see also* Bronchitis) 490
    acute 466.0
    chronic 491.0
  spring (eye) 372.13
  suffocating *(see also* Asthma) 493.9●
  summer (hay) *(see also* Fever, hay) 477.9
  throat 472.1
  tracheitis 464.10
    with obstruction 464.11
  tubotympanal 381.4
    acute *(see also* Otitis media, acute, nonsuppurative) 381.00
    chronic 381.10
  vasomotor *(see also* Fever, hay) 477.9
  vesical (bladder) - *see* Cystitis
Catarrhus aestivus *(see also* Fever, hay) 477.9
Catastrophe, cerebral *(see also* Disease, cerebrovascular, acute) 436
Catatonia, catatonic (acute) 781.99
  with
    affective psychosis - *see* Psychosis, affective
  agitation 295.2●
  dementia (praecox) 295.2●
  due to or associated with physical condition 293.89
  excitation 295.2●

Catatonia, catatonic *(Continued)*
  excited type 295.2●
  in conditions classified elsewhere 293.89
  schizophrenia 295.2●
  stupor 295.2●
Cat-scratch - *see also* Injury, superficial
  disease or fever 078.3
Cauda equina - *see also* condition
  syndrome 344.60
Cauliflower ear 738.7
Caul over face 768.9
Causalgia 355.9
  lower limb 355.71
  upper limb 354.4
Cause
  external, general effects NEC 994.9
  not stated 799.9
  unknown 799.9
Caustic burn - *see also* Burn, by site
  from swallowing caustic or corrosive substance - *see* Burn, internal organs
Cavare's disease (familial periodic paralysis) 359.3
Cave-in, injury
  crushing (severe) *(see also* Crush, by site) 869.1
  suffocation 994.7
Cavernitis (penis) 607.2
  lymph vessel - *see* Lymphangioma
Cavernositis 607.2
Cavernous - *see* condition
Cavitation of lung *(see also* Tuberculosis) 011.2●
  nontuberculous 518.89
  primary, progressive 010.8●
Cavity
  lung - *see* Cavitation of lung
  optic papilla 743.57
  pulmonary - *see* Cavitation of lung
  teeth 521.00
  vitreous (humor) 379.21
Cavovarus foot, congenital 754.59
Cavus foot (congenital) 754.71
  acquired 736.73
Cazenave's
  disease (pemphigus) NEC 694.4
  lupus (erythematosus) 695.4
CDGS (carbohydrate-deficient glycoprotein syndrome) 271.8
Cecitis - *see* Appendicitis
Cecocele - *see* Hernia
Cecum - *see* condition
Celiac
  artery compression syndrome 447.4
  disease 579.0
  infantilism 579.0
Cell, cellular - *see also* condition
  anterior chamber (eye) (positive aqueous ray) 364.04
Cellulitis (diffuse) (with lymphangitis) *(see also* Abscess) 682.9
  abdominal wall 682.2
  anaerobic *(see also* Gas gangrene) 040.0
  ankle 682.6
  anus 566
  areola 611.0
  arm (any part, above wrist) 682.3
  auditory canal (external) 380.10
  axilla 682.3
  back (any part) 682.2
  breast 611.0
    postpartum 675.1●

◀ New   ◀▥ Revised   ~~deleted~~ Deleted   ● Use Additional Digit(s)   ▨ Omit code

Cellulitis (Continued)
  broad ligament (see also Disease, pelvis,
      inflammatory) 614.4
    acute 614.3
  buttock 682.5
  cervical (neck region) 682.1
  cervix (uteri) (see also Cervicitis) 616.0
  cheek, external 682.0
    internal 528.3
  chest wall 682.2
  chronic NEC 682.9
  colostomy 569.61
  corpus cavernosum 607.2
  digit 681.9
  Douglas' cul-de-sac or pouch (chronic)
      (see also Disease, pelvis,
      inflammatory) 614.4
    acute 614.3
  drainage site (following operation)
      998.59
  ear, external 380.10
  enterostomy 569.61
  erysipelar (see also Erysipelas) 035
  esophagostomy 530.86
  eyelid 373.13
  face (any part, except eye) 682.0
  finger (intrathecal) (periosteal)
      (subcutaneous) (subcuticular)
      681.00
  flank 682.2
  foot (except toe) 682.7
  forearm 682.3
  gangrenous (see also Gangrene) 785.4
  genital organ NEC
    female - see Abscess, genital organ,
        female
    male 608.4
  glottis 478.71
  gluteal (region) 682.5
  gonococcal NEC 098.0
  groin 682.2
  hand (except finger or thumb) 682.4
  head (except face) NEC 682.8
  heel 682.7
  hip 682.6
  jaw (region) 682.0
  knee 682.6
  labium (majus) (minus) (see also
      Vulvitis) 616.10
  larynx 478.71
  leg, except foot 682.6
  lip 528.5
  mammary gland 611.0
  mouth (floor) 528.3
  multiple sites NEC 682.9
  nasopharynx 478.21
  navel 682.2
    newborn NEC 771.4
  neck (region) 682.1
  nipple 611.0
  nose 478.19
    external 682.0
  orbit, orbital 376.01
  palate (soft) 528.3
  pectoral (region) 682.2
  pelvis, pelvic
    with
      abortion - see Abortion, by type,
          with sepsis
      ectopic pregnancy (see also
          categories 633.0–633.9)
          639.0
      molar pregnancy (see also
          categories 630–632) 639.0

Cellulitis (Continued)
  pelvis, pelvic (Continued)
    female (see also Disease, pelvis,
        inflammatory) 614.4
      acute 614.3
      following
        abortion 639.0
        ectopic or molar pregnancy 639.0
    male 567.21
    puerperal, postpartum, childbirth
        670.8 ◀▥
  penis 607.2
  perineal, perineum 682.2
  perirectal 566
  peritonsillar 475
  periurethral 597.0
  periuterine (see also Disease, pelvis,
      inflammatory) 614.4
    acute 614.3
  pharynx 478.21
  phlegmonous NEC 682.9
  rectum 566
  retromammary 611.0
  retroperitoneal (see also Peritonitis)
      567.38
  round ligament (see also Disease, pelvis,
      inflammatory) 614.4
    acute 614.3
  scalp (any part) 682.8
    dissecting 704.8
  scrotum 608.4
  seminal vesicle 608.0
  septic NEC 682.9
  shoulder 682.3
  specified sites NEC 682.8
  spermatic cord 608.4
  submandibular (region) (space)
      (triangle) 682.0
    gland 527.3
  submaxillary 528.3
    gland 527.3
  submental (pyogenic) 682.0
    gland 527.3
  suppurative NEC 682.9
  testis 608.4
  thigh 682.6
  thumb (intrathecal) (periosteal) (sub-
      cutaneous) (subcuticular) 681.00
  toe (intrathecal) (periosteal)
      (subcutaneous) (subcuticular)
      681.10
  tonsil 475
  trunk 682.2
  tuberculous (primary) (see also
      Tuberculosis) 017.0●
  tunica vaginalis 608.4
  umbilical 682.2
    newborn NEC 771.4
  vaccinal 999.39
  vagina - see Vaginitis
  vas deferens 608.4
  vocal cords 478.5
  vulva (see also Vulvitis) 616.10
  wrist 682.4
Cementoblastoma, benign (M9273/0)
    213.1
  upper jaw (bone) 213.0
Cementoma (M9273/0) 213.1
  gigantiform (M9276/0) 213.1
    upper jaw (bone) 213.0
  upper jaw (bone) 213.0
Cementoperiostitis 523.40
  acute 523.33
  apical 523.40

Cephalgia, cephalagia (see also Headache)
    784.0
  histamine 339.00
  nonorganic origin 307.81
  other trigeminal autonomic (TACS)
      339.09
  psychogenic 307.81
  tension 307.81
Cephalhematocele, cephalematocele
  due to birth injury 767.19
  fetus or newborn 767.19
  traumatic (see also Contusion, head) 920
Cephalhematoma, cephalematoma
    (calcified)
  due to birth injury 767.19
  fetus or newborn 767.19
  traumatic (see also Contusion, head) 920
Cephalic - see condition
Cephalitis - see Encephalitis
Cephalocele 742.0
Cephaloma - see Neoplasm, by site,
    malignant
Cephalomenia 625.8
Cephalopelvic - see condition
Cercomoniasis 007.3
Cerebellitis - see Encephalitis
Cerebellum (cerebellar) - see condition
Cerebral - see condition
Cerebritis - see Encephalitis
Cerebrohepatorenal syndrome 759.89
Cerebromacular degeneration 330.1
Cerebromalacia (see also Softening, brain)
    434.9●
Cerebrosidosis 272.7
Cerebrospasticity - see Palsy, cerebral
Cerebrospinal - see condition
Cerebrum - see condition
Ceroid storage disease 272.7
Cerumen (accumulation) (impacted)
    380.4
Cervical - see also condition
  auricle 744.43
  high risk human papillomavirus (HPV)
      DNA test positive 795.05
  intraepithelial glandular neoplasia
      233.1
  low risk human papillomavirus (HPV)
      DNA test positive 795.09
  rib 756.2
  shortening - see Short, cervical
Cervicalgia 723.1
Cervicitis (acute) (chronic) (nonvenereal)
    (subacute) (with erosion or
    ectropion) 616.0
  with
    abortion - see Abortion, by type,
        with sepsis
    ectopic pregnancy (see also
        categories 633.0-633.9) 639.0
    molar pregnancy (see also categories
        630-632) 639.0
    ulceration 616.0
  chlamydial 099.53
  complicating pregnancy or puerperium
      646.6●
    affecting fetus or newborn 760.8
  following
    abortion 639.0
    ectopic or molar pregnancy 639.0
  gonococcal (acute) 098.15
    chronic or duration of 2 months or
        more 098.35
  senile (atrophic) 616.0
  syphilitic 095.8

Cervicitis (*Continued*)
  trichomonal 131.09
  tuberculous (*see also* Tuberculosis)
    016.7●
Cervicoaural fistula 744.49
Cervicocolpitis (emphysematosa) (*see also*
  Cervicitis) 616.0
Cervix - *see* condition
Cesarean delivery, operation or section
  NEC 669.7●
  affecting fetus or newborn 763.4
  post mortem, affecting fetus or
    newborn 761.6
  previous, affecting management of
    pregnancy 654.2●
Céstan's syndrome 344.89
Céstan-Chenais paralysis 344.89
Céstan-Raymond syndrome 433.8●
Cestode infestation NEC 123.9
  specified type NEC 123.8
Cestodiasis 123.9
CGF (congenital generalized fibromatosis)
  759.89
Chabert's disease 022.9
Chacaleh 266.2
Chafing 709.8
Chagas' disease (*see also* Trypanosomiasis,
  American) 086.2
  with heart involvement 086.0
Chagres fever 084.0
Chalasia (cardiac sphincter) 530.81
Chalazion 373.2
Chalazoderma 757.39
Chalcosis 360.24
  cornea 371.15
  crystalline lens 360.24 [366.34]
  retina 360.24
Chalicosis (occupational) (pulmonum) 502
Chancre (any genital site) (hard)
  (indurated) (infecting) (primary)
  (recurrent) 091.0
  congenital 090.0
  conjunctiva 091.2
  Ducrey's 099.0
  extragenital 091.2
  eyelid 091.2
  Hunterian 091.0
  lip (syphilis) 091.2
  mixed 099.8
  nipple 091.2
  Nisbet's 099.0
  of
    carate 103.0
    pinta 103.0
    yaws 102.0
  palate, soft 091.2
  phagedenic 099.0
  Ricord's 091.0
  Rollet's (syphilitic) 091.0
  seronegative 091.0
  seropositive 091.0
  simple 099.0
  soft 099.0
    bubo 099.0
  urethra 091.0
  yaws 102.0
Chancriform syndrome 114.1
Chancroid 099.0
  anus 099.0
  penis (Ducrey's bacillus) 099.0
  perineum 099.0
  rectum 099.0
  scrotum 099.0
  urethra 099.0
  vulva 099.0

Chandipura fever 066.8
Chandler's disease (osteochondritis
  dissecans, hip) 732.7
Change(s) (of) - *see also* Removal of
  arteriosclerotic - *see* Arteriosclerosis
  battery
    cardiac pacemaker V53.31
  bone 733.90
    diabetic 250.8● [731.8]
      due to secondary diabetes 249.8●
      [731.8]
    in disease, unknown cause 733.90
  bowel habits 787.99
  cardiorenal (vascular) (*see also*
    Hypertension, cardiorenal) 404.90
  cardiovascular - *see* Disease,
    cardiovascular
  circulatory 459.9
  cognitive or personality change of
    other type, nonpsychotic 310.1
  color, teeth, tooth
    during formation 520.8
    extrinsic 523.6
    intrinsic posteruptive 521.7
  contraceptive device V25.42
  cornea, corneal
    degenerative NEC 371.40
    membrane NEC 371.30
    senile 371.41
  coronary (*see also* Ischemia, heart) 414.9
  degenerative
    chamber angle (anterior) (iris) 364.56
    ciliary body 364.57
    spine or vertebra (*see also*
      Spondylosis) 721.90
  dental pulp, regressive 522.2
  drains V58.49
  dressing
    wound V58.30
      nonsurgical V58.30
      surgical V58.31
  fixation device V54.89
    external V54.89
    internal V54.01
  heart - *see also* Disease, heart
  hip joint 718.95
  hyperplastic larynx 478.79
  hypertrophic
    nasal sinus (*see also* Sinusitis) 473.9
    turbinate, nasal 478.0
    upper respiratory tract 478.9
  inflammatory - *see* Inflammation
  joint (*see also* Derangement, joint) 718.90
    sacroiliac 724.6
  Kirschner wire V54.89
  knee 717.9
  macular, congenital 743.55
  malignant (M----/3) - *see also*
    Neoplasm, by site, malignant

> Note 14   For malignant change occur-
> ring in a neoplasm, use the appropriate
> M code with behavior digit/3 e.g.,
> malignant change in uterine fibroid-
> M8890/3. For malignant change occur-
> ring in a nonneoplastic condition (e.g.,
> gastric ulcer) use the M code M8000/3.

  mental (status) NEC 780.97
    due to or associated with physical
      condition - *see* Syndrome, brain
  myocardium, myocardial - *see*
    Degeneration, myocardial
  of life (*see also* Menopause) 627.2
  pacemaker battery (cardiac) V53.31

Change(s) (*Continued*)
  peripheral nerve 355.9
  personality (nonpsychotic) NEC 310.1
  plaster cast V54.89
  refractive, transient 367.81
  regressive, dental pulp 522.2
  retina 362.9
    myopic (degenerative) (malignant)
      360.21
    vascular appearance 362.13
  sacroiliac joint 724.6
  scleral 379.19
    degenerative 379.16
  senile (*see also* Senility) 797
  sensory (*see also* Disturbance,
    sensation) 782.0
  skin texture 782.8
  spinal cord 336.9
  splint, external V54.89
  subdermal implantable contraceptive
    V25.5
  suture V58.32
  traction device V54.89
  trophic 355.9
    arm NEC 354.9
    leg NEC 355.8
    lower extremity NEC 355.8
    upper extremity NEC 354.9
  vascular 459.9
  vasomotor 443.9
  voice 784.49
    psychogenic 306.1
  wound packing V58.30
    nonsurgical V58.30
    surgical V58.31
Changing sleep-work schedule, affecting
  sleep 327.36
Changuinola fever 066.0
Chapping skin 709.8
Character
  depressive 301.12
Charcôt's
  arthropathy 094.0 [713.5]
  cirrhosis - *see* Cirrhosis, biliary
  disease 094.0
    spinal cord 094.0
  fever (biliary) (hepatic) (intermittent) -
    see Choledocholithiasis
  joint (disease) 094.0 [713.5]
    diabetic 250.6● [713.5]
      due to secondary diabetes 249.6●
      [713.5]
    syringomyelic 336.0 [713.5]
  syndrome (intermittent claudication)
    443.9
    due to atherosclerosis 440.21
Charcôt-Marie-Tooth disease, paralysis,
  or syndrome 356.1
CHARGE association (syndrome) 759.89
Charleyhorse (quadriceps) 843.8
  muscle, except quadriceps - *see* Sprain,
    by site
Charlouis' disease (*see also* Yaws) 102.9
Chauffeur's fracture - *see* Fracture, ulna,
  lower end
Cheadle (-Möller) (-Barlow) disease or
  syndrome (infantile scurvy) 267
Checking (of)
  contraceptive device (intrauterine)
    V25.42
  device
    fixation V54.89
      external V54.89
      internal V54.09
    traction V54.89

◄ New   ◄|||| Revised   ~~deleted~~ Deleted   ● Use Additional Digit(s)   ▨ Omit code

Checking (Continued)
  Kirschner wire V54.89
  plaster cast V54.89
  splint, external V54.89
Checkup
  following treatment - see Examination
  health V70.0
  infant (over 28 days old) (not sick)
      V20.2 ◄▥
  newborn, routine
      initial V20.2
      subsequent V20.2
      8 to 28 days old V20.32 ◄
      over 28 days old, routine V20.2 ◄
      under 8 days old V20.31 ◄
      weight V20.32 ◄
  pregnancy (normal) V22.1
      first V22.0
      high-risk pregnancy V23.9
          specified problem NEC V23.89
Chédiak-Higashi (-Steinbrinck) anomaly,
      disease, or syndrome (congenital
      gigantism of peroxidase granules)
      288.2
Cheek - see also condition
  biting 528.9
Cheese itch 133.8
Cheese washers' lung 495.8
Cheilitis 528.5
  actinic (due to sun) 692.72
      chronic NEC 692.74
          due to radiation, except from sun
              692.82
          due to radiation, except from sun
              692.82
  acute 528.5
  angular 528.5
  catarrhal 528.5
  chronic 528.5
  exfoliative 528.5
  gangrenous 528.5
  glandularis apostematosa 528.5
  granulomatosa 351.8
  infectional 528.5
  membranous 528.5
  Miescher's 351.8
  suppurative 528.5
  ulcerative 528.5
  vesicular 528.5
Cheilodynia 528.5
Cheilopalatoschisis (see also Cleft, palate,
      with cleft lip) 749.20
Cheilophagia 528.9
Cheiloschisis (see also Cleft, lip) 749.10
Cheilosis 528.5
  with pellagra 265.2
  angular 528.5
  due to
      dietary deficiency 266.0
      vitamin deficiency 266.0
Cheiromegaly 729.89
Cheiropompholyx 705.81
Cheloid (see also Keloid) 701.4
Chemical burn - see also Burn, by site
  from swallowing chemical - see Burn,
      internal organs
Chemodectoma (M8693/1) - see
      Paraganglioma, nonchromaffin
Chemoprophylaxis NEC V07.39
Chemosis, conjunctiva 372.73
Chemotherapy
  convalescence V66.2
  encounter (for) (oral) (intravenous)
      V58.11 ◄▥
  maintenance (oral) (intravenous)
      V58.11 ◄▥

Chemotherapy (Continued)
  prophylactic NEC V07.39
      fluoride V07.31
Cherubism 526.89
Chest - see condition
Cheyne-Stokes respiration (periodic)
      786.04
Chiari's
  disease or syndrome (hepatic vein
      thrombosis) 453.0
  malformation
      type I 348.4
      type II (see also Spina bifida) 741.0●
      type III 742.0
      type IV 742.2
  network 746.89
Chiari-Frommel syndrome 676.6●
Chicago disease (North American
      blastomycosis) 116.0
Chickenpox (see also Varicella) 052.9
  exposure to V01.71
  vaccination and inoculation
      (prophylactic) V05.4
Chiclero ulcer 085.4
Chiggers 133.8
Chignon 111.2
  fetus or newborn (from vacuum
      extraction) 767.19
Chigoe disease 134.1
Chikungunya fever 066.3
Chilaiditi's syndrome (subphrenic
      displacement, colon) 751.4
Chilblains 991.5
  lupus 991.5
Child
  behavior causing concern V61.20
      adopted child V61.24 ◄
      biological child V61.23 ◄
      foster child V61.25 ◄
Childbed fever 670.8 ◄▥
Childbirth - see also Delivery
  puerperal complications - see Puerperal
Childhood, period of rapid growth V21.0
Chill(s) 780.64
  with fever 780.60
  without fever 780.64
  congestive 780.99
      in malarial regions 084.6
  septic - see Septicemia
  urethral 599.84
Chilomastigiasis 007.8
Chin - see condition
Chinese dysentery 004.9
Chiropractic dislocation (see also Lesion,
      nonallopathic, by site) 739.9
Chitral fever 066.0
Chlamydia, chlamydial - see condition
Chloasma 709.09
  cachecticorum 709.09
  eyelid 374.52
      congenital 757.33
      hyperthyroid 242.0●
  gravidarum 646.8●
  idiopathic 709.09
  skin 709.09
  symptomatic 709.09
Chloroma (M9930/3) 205.3●
Chlorosis 280.9
  Egyptian (see also Ancylostomiasis) 126.9
  miners' (see also Ancylostomiasis) 126.9
Chlorotic anemia 280.9
Chocolate cyst (ovary) 617.1
Choked
  disk or disc - see Papilledema
  on food, phlegm, or vomitus NEC (see
      also Asphyxia, food) 933.1

Choked (Continued)
  phlegm 933.1
  while vomiting NEC (see also Asphyxia,
      food) 933.1
Chokes (resulting from bends) 993.3
Choking sensation 784.99
Cholangiectasis (see also Disease,
      gallbladder) 575.8
Cholangiocarcinoma (M8160/3)
  and hepatocellular carcinoma,
      combined (M8180/3) 155.0
  liver 155.1
  specified site NEC - see Neoplasm, by
      site, malignant
  unspecified site 155.1
Cholangiohepatitis 575.8
  due to fluke infestation 121.1
Cholangiohepatoma (M8180/3) 155.0
Cholangiolitis (acute) (chronic)
      (extrahepatic) (gangrenous) 576.1
  intrahepatic 575.8
  paratyphoidal (see also Fever,
      paratyphoid) 002.9
  typhoidal 002.0
Cholangioma (M8160/0) 211.5
  malignant - see Cholangiocarcinoma
Cholangitis (acute) (ascending)
      (catarrhal) (chronic) (infective)
      (malignant) (primary) (recurrent)
      (sclerosing) (secondary) (stenosing)
      (suppurative) 576.1
  chronic nonsuppurative destructive
      571.6
  nonsuppurative destructive (chronic)
      571.6
Cholecystdocholithiasis - see
      Choledocholithiasis
Cholecystitis 575.10
  with
      calculus, stones in
          bile duct (common) (hepatic) -
              see Choledocholithiasis
          gallbladder - see Cholelithiasis
  acute 575.0
  acute and chronic 575.12
  chronic 575.11
  emphysematous (acute) (see also
      Cholecystitis, acute) 575.0
  gangrenous (see also Cholecystitis,
      acute) 575.0
  paratyphoidal, current (see also Fever,
      paratyphoid) 002.9
  suppurative (see also Cholecystitis,
      acute) 575.0
  typhoidal 002.0
Choledochitis (suppurative) 576.1
Choledocholith - see Choledocholithiasis
Choledocholithiasis 574.5●

Note 15   Use the following fifth-digit
subclassification with category 574:

0   without mention of obstruction
1   with obstruction

  with
      cholecystitis 574.4●
          acute 574.3●
          chronic 574.4●
      cholelithiasis 574.9●
          with
              cholecystitis 574.7●
                  acute 574.6●
                      and chronic 574.8●
                  chronic 574.7●

◄ New   ◄▥ Revised   deleted Deleted   ● Use Additional Digit(s)   ▨ Omit code   **159**

Cholelithiasis (impacted) (multiple) 574.2●

Note 16   Use the following fifth-digit subclassification with category 574:

0   without mention of obstruction
1   with obstruction

with
cholecystitis 574.1●
acute 574.0●
chronic 574.1●
choledocholithiasis 574.9●
with
cholecystitis 574.7●
acute 574.6●
and chronic 574.8●
chronic cholecystitis 574.7●
Cholemia (see also Jaundice) 782.4
familial 277.4
Gilbert's (familial nonhemolytic) 277.4
Cholemic gallstone - see Cholelithiasis
Choleperitoneum, choleperitonitis (see also Disease, gallbladder) 567.81
Cholera (algid) (Asiatic) (asphyctic) (epidemic) (gravis) (Indian) (malignant) (morbus) (pestilential) (spasmodic) 001.9
antimonial 985.4
carrier (suspected) of V02.0
classical 001.0
contact V01.0
due to
Vibrio
cholerae (Inaba, Ogawa, Hikojima serotypes) 001.0
el Tor 001.1
el Tor 001.1
exposure to V01.0
vaccination, prophylactic (against) V03.0
Cholerine (see also Cholera) 001.9
Cholestasis 576.8
due to total parenteral nutrition (TPN) 573.8
Cholesteatoma (ear) 385.30
attic (primary) 385.31
diffuse 385.35
external ear (canal) 380.21
marginal (middle ear) 385.32
with involvement of mastoid cavity 385.33
secondary (with middle ear involvement) 385.33
mastoid cavity 385.30
middle ear (secondary) 385.32
with involvement of mastoid cavity 385.33
postmastoidectomy cavity (recurrent) 383.32
primary 385.31
recurrent, postmastoidectomy cavity 383.32
secondary (middle ear) 385.32
with involvement of mastoid cavity 385.33
Cholesteatosis (middle ear) (see also Cholesteatoma) 385.30
diffuse 385.35
Cholesteremia 272.0
Cholesterin
granuloma, middle ear 385.82
in vitreous 379.22

Cholesterol
deposit
retina 362.82
vitreous 379.22
elevated (high) 272.0
with elevated (high) triglycerides 272.2
imbibition of gallbladder (see also Disease, gallbladder) 575.6
Cholesterolemia 272.0
essential 272.0
familial 272.0
hereditary 272.0
Cholesterosis, cholesterolosis (gallbladder) 575.6
with
cholecystitis - see Cholecystitis
cholelithiasis - see Cholelithiasis
middle ear (see also Cholesteatoma) 385.30
Cholocolic fistula (see also Fistula, gallbladder) 575.5
Choluria 791.4
Chondritis (purulent) 733.99
auricle 380.03
costal 733.6
Tietze's 733.6
patella, posttraumatic 717.7
pinna 380.03
posttraumatica patellae 717.7
tuberculous (active) (see also Tuberculosis) 015.9●
intervertebral 015.0● [730.88]
Chondroangiopathia calcarea seu punctate 756.59
Chondroblastoma (M9230/0) - see also Neoplasm, bone, benign
malignant (M9230/3) - see Neoplasm, bone, malignant
Chondrocalcinosis (articular) (crystal deposition) (dihydrate) (see also Arthritis, due to, crystals) 275.49 [712.3]●
due to
calcium pyrophosphate 275.49 [712.2]●
dicalcium phosphate crystals 275.49 [712.1]●
pyrophosphate crystals 275.49 [712.2]●
Chondrodermatitis nodularis helicis 380.00
Chondrodysplasia 756.4
angiomatose 756.4
calcificans congenita 756.59
epiphysialis punctata 756.59
hereditary deforming 756.4
rhizomelic punctata 277.86
Chondrodystrophia (fetalis) 756.4
calcarea 756.4
calcificans congenita 756.59
fetalis hypoplastica 756.59
hypoplastica calcinosa 756.59
punctata 756.59
tarda 277.5
Chondrodystrophy (familial) (hypoplastic) 756.4
myotonic (congenital) 359.23
Chondroectodermal dysplasia 756.55
Chondrolysis 733.99
Chondroma (M9220/0) - see also Neoplasm, cartilage, benign
juxtacortical (M9221/0) - see Neoplasm, bone, benign

Chondroma (Continued)
periosteal (M9221/0) - see Neoplasm, bone, benign
Chondromalacia 733.92
epiglottis (congenital) 748.3
generalized 733.92
knee 717.7
larynx (congenital) 748.3
localized, except patella 733.92
patella, patellae 717.7
systemic 733.92
tibial plateau 733.92
trachea (congenital) 748.3
Chondromatosis (M9220/1) - see Neoplasm, cartilage, uncertain behavior
Chondromyxosarcoma (M9220/3) - see Neoplasm, cartilage, malignant
Chondro-osteodysplasia (Morquio-Brailsford type) 277.5
Chondro-osteodystrophy 277.5
Chondro-osteoma (M9210/0) - see Neoplasm, bone, benign
Chondropathia tuberosa 733.6
Chondrosarcoma (M9220/3) - see also Neoplasm, cartilage, malignant
juxtacortical (M9221/3) - see Neoplasm, bone, malignant
mesenchymal (M9240/3) - see Neoplasm, connective tissue, malignant
Chordae tendineae rupture (chronic) 429.5
Chordee (nonvenereal) 607.89
congenital 752.63
gonococcal 098.2
Chorditis (fibrinous) (nodosa) (tuberosa) 478.5
Chordoma (M9370/3) - see Neoplasm, by site, malignant
Chorea (gravis) (minor) (spasmodic) 333.5
with
heart involvement - see Chorea with rheumatic heart disease
rheumatic heart disease (chronic, inactive, or quiescent) (conditions classifiable to 393–398) - see- rheumatic heart condition involved,
active or acute (conditions classifiable to 391) 392.0
acute - see Chorea, Sydenham's
apoplectic (see also Disease, cerebrovascular, acute) 436
chronic 333.4
electric 049.8
gravidarum - see Eclampsia, pregnancy
habit 307.22
hereditary 333.4
Huntington's 333.4
posthemiplegic 344.89
pregnancy - see Eclampsia, pregnancy
progressive 333.4
chronic 333.4
hereditary 333.4
rheumatic (chronic) 392.9
with heart disease or involvement - see Chorea, with rheumatic heart disease
senile 333.5
Sydenham's 392.9
with heart involvement - see Chorea, with rheumatic heart disease
nonrheumatic 333.5
variabilis 307.23

Choreoathetosis (paroxysmal) 333.5
Chorioadenoma (destruens) (M9100/1)
236.1
Chorioamnionitis 658.4●
affecting fetus or newborn 762.7
Chorioangioma (M9120/0) 219.8
Choriocarcinoma (M9100/3)
combined with
embryonal carcinoma (M9101/3) -
see Neoplasm, by site,
malignant
teratoma (M9101/3) - see Neoplasm,
by site, malignant
specified site - see Neoplasm, by site,
malignant
unspecified site
female 181
male 186.9
Chorioencephalitis, lymphocytic (acute)
(serous) 049.0
Chorioepithelioma (M9100/3) - see
Choriocarcinoma
Choriomeningitis (acute) (benign)
(lymphocytic) (serous) 049.0
Chorionepithelioma (M9100/3) - see
Choriocarcinoma
Chorionitis (see also Scleroderma)
710.1
Chorioretinitis 363.20
disseminated 363.10
generalized 363.13
in
neurosyphilis 094.83
secondary syphilis 091.51
peripheral 363.12
posterior pole 363.11
tuberculous (see also Tuberculosis)
017.3● [363.13]
due to
histoplasmosis (see also
Histoplasmosis) 115.92
toxoplasmosis (acquired) 130.2
congenital (active) 771.2
focal 363.00
juxtapapillary 363.01
peripheral 363.04
posterior pole NEC 363.03
juxtapapillaris, juxtapapillary 363.01
progressive myopia (degeneration)
360.21
syphilitic (secondary) 091.51
congenital (early) 090.0 [363.13]
late 090.5 [363.13]
late 095.8 [363.13]
tuberculous (see also Tuberculosis)
017.3● [363.13]
Choristoma - see Neoplasm, by site,
benign
Choroid - see condition
Choroideremia, choroidermia (initial
stage) (late stage) (partial or total
atrophy) 363.55
Choroiditis (see also Chorioretinitis)
363.20
leprous 030.9 [363.13]
senile guttate 363.41
sympathetic 360.11
syphilitic (secondary) 091.51
congenital (early) 090.0 [363.13]
late 090.5 [363.13]
late 095.8 [363.13]
Tay's 363.41
tuberculous (see also Tuberculosis)
017.3● [363.13]

Choroidopathy NEC 363.9
degenerative (see also Degeneration,
choroid) 363.40
hereditary (see also Dystrophy, choroid)
363.50
specified type NEC 363.8
Choroidoretinitis - see Chorioretinitis
Choroidosis, central serous 362.41
Choroidretinopathy, serous 362.41
Christian's syndrome (chronic
histiocytosis X) 277.89
Christian-Weber disease (nodular
nonsuppurative panniculitis) 729.30
Christmas disease 286.1
Chromaffinoma (M8700/0) - see also
Neoplasm, by site, benign
malignant (M8700/3) - see Neoplasm,
by site, malignant
Chromatopsia 368.59
Chromhidrosis, chromidrosis 705.89
Chromoblastomycosis 117.2
Chromomycosis 117.2
Chromophytosis 111.0
Chromotrichomycosis 111.8
Chronic - see condition
Churg-Strauss syndrome 446.4
Chyle cyst, mesentery 457.8
Chylocele (nonfilarial) 457.8
filarial (see also Infestation, filarial)
125.9
tunica vaginalis (nonfilarial) 608.84
filarial (see also Infestation, filarial)
125.9
Chylomicronemia (fasting) (with
hyperprebetalipoproteinemia)
272.3
Chylopericardium (acute) 420.90
Chylothorax (nonfilarial) 457.8
filarial (see also Infestation, filarial)
125.9
Chylous
ascites 457.8
cyst of peritoneum 457.8
hydrocele 603.9
hydrothorax (nonfilarial) 457.8
filarial (see also Infestation, filarial)
125.9
Chyluria 791.1
bilharziasis 120.0
due to
Brugia (malayi) 125.1
Wuchereria (bancrofti) 125.0
malayi 125.1
filarial (see also Infestation, filarial)
125.9
filariasis (see also Infestation, filarial)
125.9
nonfilarial 791.1
Cicatricial (deformity) - see Cicatrix
Cicatrix (adherent) (contracted) (painful)
(vicious) 709.2
adenoid 474.8
alveolar process 525.8
anus 569.49
auricle 380.89
bile duct (see also Disease, biliary)
576.8
bladder 596.8
bone 733.99
brain 348.89 ◀▥
cervix (postoperative) (postpartal)
622.3
in pregnancy or childbirth 654.6●
causing obstructed labor 660.2●

Cicatrix (Continued)
chorioretinal 363.30
disseminated 363.35
macular 363.32
peripheral 363.34
posterior pole NEC 363.33
choroid - see Cicatrix, chorioretinal
common duct (see also Disease, biliary)
576.8
congenital 757.39
conjunctiva 372.64
cornea 371.00
tuberculous (see also Tuberculosis)
017.3● [371.05]
duodenum (bulb) 537.3
esophagus 530.3
eyelid 374.46
with
ectropion - see Ectropion
entropion - see Entropion
hypopharynx 478.29
knee, semilunar cartilage 717.5
lacrimal
canaliculi 375.53
duct
acquired 375.56
neonatal 375.55
punctum 375.52
sac 375.54
larynx 478.79
limbus (cystoid) 372.64
lung 518.89
macular 363.32
disseminated 363.35
peripheral 363.34
middle ear 385.89
mouth 528.9
muscle 728.89
nasolacrimal duct
acquired 375.56
neonatal 375.55
nasopharynx 478.29
palate (soft) 528.9
penis 607.89
prostate 602.8
rectum 569.49
retina 363.30
disseminated 363.35
macular 363.32
peripheral 363.34
posterior pole NEC 363.33
semilunar cartilage - see Derangement,
meniscus
seminal vesicle 608.89
skin 709.2
infected 686.8
postinfectional 709.2
tuberculous (see also Tuberculosis)
017.0●
specified site NEC 709.2
throat 478.29
tongue 529.8
tonsil (and adenoid) 474.8
trachea 478.9
tuberculous NEC (see also Tuberculosis)
011.9●
ureter 593.89
urethra 599.84
uterus 621.8
vagina 623.4
in pregnancy or childbirth 654.7●
causing obstructed labor 660.2●
vocal cord 478.5
wrist, constricting (annular) 709.2

CIDP (chronic inflammatory demyelinating polyneuropathy) 357.81
CIN I [cervical intraepithelial neoplasia I] 622.11
CIN II [cervical intraepithelial neoplasia II] 622.12
CIN III [cervical intraepithelial neoplasia III] 233.1
Cinchonism
  correct substance properly administered 386.9
  overdose or wrong substance given or taken 961.4
Circine herpes 110.5
Circle of Willis - *see* condition
Circular - *see also* condition
  hymen 752.49
Circulating, intrinsic anticoagulants causing hemorrhagic disorder 286.5 ◀▥
  following childbirth 666.3●
  postpartum 666.3●
Circulation
  collateral (venous), any site 459.89
  defective 459.9
    congenital 747.9
    lower extremity 459.89
  embryonic 747.9
  failure 799.89
    fetus or newborn 779.89
    peripheral 785.59
  fetal, persistent 747.83
  heart, incomplete 747.9
Circulatory system - *see* condition
Circulus senilis 371.41
Circumcision
  in absence of medical indication V50.2
  ritual V50.2
  routine V50.2
Circumscribed - *see* condition
Circumvallata placenta - *see* Placenta, abnormal
Cirrhosis, cirrhotic 571.5
  with alcoholism 571.2
  alcoholic (liver) 571.2
  atrophic (of liver) - *see* Cirrhosis, portal
  Baumgarten-Cruveilhier 571.5
  biliary (cholangiolitic) (cholangitic) (cholestatic) (extrahepatic) (hypertrophic) (intrahepatic) (nonobstructive) (obstructive) (pericholangiolitic) (posthepatic) (primary) (secondary) (xanthomatous) 571.6
    due to
      clonorchiasis 121.1
      flukes 121.3
  brain 331.9
  capsular - *see* Cirrhosis, portal
  cardiac 571.5
    alcoholic 571.2
  central (liver) - *see* Cirrhosis, liver
  Charcôt's 571.6
  cholangiolitic - *see* Cirrhosis, biliary
  cholangitic - *see* Cirrhosis, biliary
  cholestatic - *see* Cirrhosis, biliary
  clitoris (hypertrophic) 624.2
  coarsely nodular 571.5
  congestive (liver) - *see* Cirrhosis, cardiac
  Cruveilhier-Baumgarten 571.5
  cryptogenic (of liver) 571.5
    alcoholic 571.2
  dietary (*see also* Cirrhosis, portal) 571.5

Cirrhosis, cirrhotic (*Continued*)
  due to
    bronzed diabetes 275.0
    congestive hepatomegaly - *see* Cirrhosis, cardiac
    cystic fibrosis 277.00
    hemochromatosis 275.0
    hepatolenticular degeneration 275.1
    passive congestion (chronic) - *see* Cirrhosis, cardiac
    Wilson's disease 275.1
    xanthomatosis 272.2
  extrahepatic (obstructive) - *see* Cirrhosis, biliary
  fatty 571.8
    alcoholic 571.0
  florid 571.2
  Glisson's - *see* Cirrhosis, portal
  Hanot's (hypertrophic) - *see* Cirrhosis, biliary
  hepatic - *see* Cirrhosis, liver
  hepatolienal - *see* Cirrhosis, liver
  hobnail - *see* Cirrhosis, portal
  hypertrophic - *see also* Cirrhosis, liver
    biliary - *see* Cirrhosis, biliary
    Hanot's - *see* Cirrhosis, biliary
  infectious NEC - *see* Cirrhosis, portal
  insular - *see* Cirrhosis, portal
  intrahepatic (obstructive) (primary) (secondary) - *see* Cirrhosis, biliary
  juvenile (*see also* Cirrhosis, portal) 571.5
  kidney (*see also* Sclerosis, renal) 587
  Laennec's (of liver) 571.2
    nonalcoholic 571.5
  liver (chronic) (hepatolienal) (hypertrophic) (nodular) (splenomegalic) (unilobar) 571.5
    with alcoholism 571.2
    alcoholic 571.2
    congenital (due to failure of obliteration of umbilical vein) 777.8
    cryptogenic 571.5
      alcoholic 571.2
    fatty 571.8
      alcoholic 571.0
    macronodular 571.5
      alcoholic 571.2
    micronodular 571.5
      alcoholic 571.2
    nodular, diffuse 571.5
      alcoholic 571.2
    pigmentary 275.0
    portal 571.5
      alcoholic 571.2
    postnecrotic 571.5
      alcoholic 571.2
    syphilitic 095.3
  lung (chronic) (*see also* Fibrosis, lung) 515
  macronodular (of liver) 571.5
    alcoholic 571.2
  malarial 084.9
  metabolic NEC 571.5
  micronodular (of liver) 571.5
    alcoholic 571.2
  monolobular - *see* Cirrhosis, portal
  multilobular - *see* Cirrhosis, portal
  nephritis (*see also* Sclerosis, renal) 587
  nodular - *see* Cirrhosis, liver
  nutritional (fatty) 571.5
  obstructive (biliary) (extrahepatic) (intrahepatic) - *see* Cirrhosis, biliary

Cirrhosis, cirrhotic (*Continued*)
  ovarian 620.8
  paludal 084.9
  pancreas (duct) 577.8
  pericholangiolitic - *see* Cirrhosis, biliary
  periportal - *see* Cirrhosis, portal
  pigment, pigmentary (of liver) 275.0
  portal (of liver) 571.5
    alcoholic 571.2
  posthepatitic (*see also* Cirrhosis, postnecrotic) 571.5
  postnecrotic (of liver) 571.5
    alcoholic 571.2
  primary (intrahepatic) - *see* Cirrhosis, biliary
  pulmonary (*see also* Fibrosis, lung) 515
  renal (*see also* Sclerosis, renal) 587
  septal (*see also* Cirrhosis, postnecrotic) 571.5
  spleen 289.51
  splenomegalic (of liver) - *see* Cirrhosis, liver
  stasis (liver) - *see* Cirrhosis, liver
  stomach 535.4●
  Todd's (*see also* Cirrhosis, biliary) 571.6
  toxic (nodular) - *see* Cirrhosis, postnecrotic
  trabecular - *see* Cirrhosis, postnecrotic
  unilobar - *see* Cirrhosis, liver
  vascular (of liver) - *see* Cirrhosis, liver
  xanthomatous (biliary) (*see also* Cirrhosis, biliary) 571.6
    due to xanthomatosis (familial) (metabolic) (primary) 272.2
Cistern, subarachnoid 793.0
Citrullinemia 270.6
Citrullinuria 270.6
Ciuffini-Pancoast tumor (M8010/3) (carcinoma, pulmonary apex) 162.3
Civatte's disease or poikiloderma 709.09
CJD (Creutzfeldt-Jakob disease) 046.19
  variant (vCJD) 046.11
Clam diggers' itch 120.3
Clap - *see* Gonorrhea
Clark's paralysis 343.9
Clarke-Hadfield syndrome (pancreatic infantilism) 577.8
Clastothrix 704.2
Claude's syndrome 352.6
Claude Bernard-Horner syndrome (*see also* Neuropathy, peripheral, autonomic) 337.9
Claudication, intermittent 443.9
  cerebral (artery) (*see also* Ischemia, cerebral, transient) 435.9
  due to atherosclerosis 440.21
  spinal cord (arteriosclerotic) 435.1
    syphilitic 094.89
  spinalis 435.1
  venous (axillary) 453.89 ◀▥
Claudicatio venosa intermittens 453.89 ◀▥
Claustrophobia 300.29
Clavus (infected) 700
Clawfoot (congenital) 754.71
  acquired 736.74
Clawhand (acquired) 736.06
  congenital 755.59
Clawtoe (congenital) 754.71
  acquired 735.5
Clay eating 307.52
Clay shovelers' fracture - *see* Fracture, vertebra, cervical
Cleansing of artificial opening (*see also* Attention to artificial opening) V55.9

◀ New   ◀▥ Revised   ~~deleted~~ Deleted   ● Use Additional Digit(s)   ▨ Omit code

Cleft (congenital) - *see also* Imperfect, closure
  alveolar process 525.8
  branchial (persistent) 744.41
    cyst 744.42
  clitoris 752.49
  cricoid cartilage, posterior 748.3
  facial (*see also* Cleft, lip) 749.10
  lip 749.10
    with cleft palate 749.20
      bilateral (lip and palate) 749.24
        with unilateral lip or palate 749.25
        complete 749.23
        incomplete 749.24
      unilateral (lip and palate) 749.22
        with bilateral lip or palate 749.25
        complete 749.21
        incomplete 749.22
    bilateral 749.14
      with cleft palate, unilateral 749.25
      complete 749.13
      incomplete 749.14
    unilateral 749.12
      with cleft palate, bilateral 749.25
      complete 749.11
      incomplete 749.12
  nose 748.1
  palate 749.00
    with cleft lip 749.20
      bilateral (lip and palate) 749.24
        with unilateral lip or palate 749.25
        complete 749.23
        incomplete 749.24
      unilateral (lip and palate) 749.22
        with bilateral lip or palate 749.25
        complete 749.21
        incomplete 749.22
    bilateral 749.04
      with cleft lip, unilateral 749.25
      complete 749.03
      incomplete 749.04
    unilateral 749.02
      with cleft lip, bilateral 749.25
      complete 749.01
      incomplete 749.02
  penis 752.69
  posterior, cricoid cartilage 748.3
  scrotum 752.89
  sternum (congenital) 756.3
  thyroid cartilage (congenital) 748.3
  tongue 750.13
  uvula 749.02
    with cleft lip (*see also* Cleft, lip, with cleft palate) 749.20
  water 366.12
Cleft hand (congenital) 755.58
Cleidocranial dysostosis 755.59
Cleidotomy, fetal 763.89
Cleptomania 312.32
Clérambault's syndrome 297.8
  erotomania 302.89
Clergyman's sore throat 784.49
Click, clicking
  systolic syndrome 785.2
Clifford's syndrome (postmaturity) 766.22
Climacteric (*see also* Menopause) 627.2
  arthritis NEC (*see also* Arthritis, climacteric) 716.3●

Climacteric (*Continued*)
  depression (*see also* Psychosis, affective) 296.2●
  disease 627.2
    recurrent episode 296.3●
    single episode 296.2●
  female (symptoms) 627.2
  male (symptoms) (syndrome) 608.89
  melancholia (*see also* Psychosis, affective) 296.2●
    recurrent episode 296.3●
    single episode 296.2●
  paranoid state 297.2
  paraphrenia 297.2
  polyarthritis NEC 716.39
    male 608.89
  symptoms (female) 627.2
Clinical research investigation (control) (participant) V70.7
Clinodactyly 755.59
Clitoris - *see* condition
Cloaca, persistent 751.5
Clonorchiasis 121.1
Clonorchiosis 121.1
Clonorchis infection, liver 121.1
Clonus 781.0
Closed bite 524.20
Closed surgical procedure converted to open procedure
  arthroscopic V64.43
  laparoscopic V64.41
  thoracoscopic V64.42
Closure
  artificial opening (*see also* Attention to artificial opening) V55.9
  congenital, nose 748.0
  cranial sutures, premature 756.0
  defective or imperfect NEC - *see* Imperfect, closure
  fistula, delayed - *see* Fistula
  fontanelle, delayed 756.0
  foramen ovale, imperfect 745.5
  hymen 623.3
  interauricular septum, defective 745.5
  interventricular septum, defective 745.4
  lacrimal duct 375.56
    congenital 743.65
    neonatal 375.55
  nose (congenital) 748.0
    acquired 738.0
  vagina 623.2
  valve - *see* Endocarditis
  vulva 624.8
Clot (blood)
  artery (obstruction) (occlusion) (*see also* Embolism) 444.9
  atrial appendage 429.89
  bladder 596.7
  brain (extradural or intradural) (*see also* Thrombosis, brain) 434.0●
    late effect - *see* Late effect(s) (of) cerebrovascular disease
  circulation 444.9
  heart (*see also* Infarct, myocardium) 410.9●
    without myocardial infarction 429.89
  vein (*see also* Thrombosis) 453.9
Clotting defect NEC (*see also* Defect, coagulation) 286.9
Clouded state 780.09
  epileptic (*see also* Epilepsy) 345.9●
  paroxysmal (idiopathic) (*see also* Epilepsy) 345.9●

Clouding
  corneal graft 996.51
Cloudy
  antrum, antra 473.0
  dialysis effluent 792.5
Clouston's (hidrotic) ectodermal dysplasia 757.31
Clubbing of fingers 781.5
Clubfinger 736.29
  acquired 736.29
  congenital 754.89
Clubfoot (congenital) 754.70
  acquired 736.71
  equinovarus 754.51
  paralytic 736.71
Club hand (congenital) 754.89
  acquired 736.07
Clubnail (acquired) 703.8
  congenital 757.5
Clump kidney 753.3
Clumsiness 781.3
  syndrome 315.4
Cluttering 307.0
Clutton's joints 090.5
Coagulation, intravascular (diffuse) (disseminated) (*see also* Fibrinolysis) 286.6
  newborn 776.2
Coagulopathy (*see also* Defect, coagulation) 286.9
  consumption 286.6
  intravascular (disseminated) NEC 286.6
    newborn 776.2
Coalition
  calcaneoscaphoid 755.67
  calcaneus 755.67
  tarsal 755.67
Coal miners'
  elbow 727.2
  lung 500
Coal workers' lung or pneumoconiosis 500
Coarctation
  aorta (postductal) (preductal) 747.10
  pulmonary artery 747.3
Coated tongue 529.3
Coats' disease 362.12
Cocainism (*see also* Dependence) 304.2●
Coccidioidal granuloma 114.3
Coccidioidomycosis 114.9
  with pneumonia 114.0
  cutaneous (primary) 114.1
  disseminated 114.3
  extrapulmonary (primary) 114.1
  lung 114.5
    acute 114.0
    chronic 114.4
    primary 114.0
  meninges 114.2
  primary (pulmonary) 114.0
    acute 114.0
  prostate 114.3
  pulmonary 114.5
    acute 114.0
    chronic 114.4
    primary 114.0
  specified site NEC 114.3
Coccidioidosis 114.9
  lung 114.5
    acute 114.0
    chronic 114.4
    primary 114.0
  meninges 114.2

Coccidiosis (colitis) (diarrhea) (dysentery) 007.2
Cocciuria 791.9
Coccus in urine 791.9
Coccydynia 724.79
Coccygodynia 724.79
Coccyx - *see* condition
Cochin-China
   diarrhea 579.1
      anguilluliasis 127.2
   ulcer 085.1
Cock's peculiar tumor 706.2
Cockayne's disease or syndrome
      (microcephaly and dwarfism) 759.89
Cockayne-Weber syndrome
      (epidermolysis bullosa) 757.39
Cocked-up toe 735.2
Codman's tumor (benign
      chondroblastoma) (M9230/0) - *see*
      Neoplasm, bone, benign
Coenurosis 123.8
Coffee workers' lung 495.8
Cogan's syndrome 370.52
   congenital oculomotor apraxia 379.51
   nonsyphilitic interstitial keratitis 370.52
Coiling, umbilical cord - *see*
      Complications, umbilical cord
Coitus, painful (female) 625.0
   male 608.89
   psychogenic 302.76
Cold 460
   with influenza, flu, or grippe 487.1
   abscess - *see also* Tuberculosis, abscess
      articular - *see* Tuberculosis, joint
   agglutinin
      disease (chronic) or syndrome 283.0
      hemoglobinuria 283.0
         paroxysmal (cold) (nocturnal)
            283.2
   allergic (*see also* Fever, hay) 477.9
   bronchus or chest - *see* Bronchitis
      with grippe or influenza 487.1
   common (head) 460
      vaccination, prophylactic (against)
         V04.7
   deep 464.10
   effects of 991.9
      specified effect NEC 991.8
   excessive 991.9
      specified effect NEC 991.8
   exhaustion from 991.8
   exposure to 991.9
      specified effect NEC 991.8
   grippy 487.1
   head 460
   injury syndrome (newborn) 778.2
   intolerance 780.99
   on lung - *see* Bronchitis
   rose 477.0
   sensitivity, autoimmune 283.0
   virus 460
Coldsore (*see also* Herpes, simplex) 054.9
Colibacillosis 041.4
   generalized 038.42
Colibacilluria 791.9
Colic (recurrent) 789.7 ◀▥
   abdomen 789.7 ◀▥
      psychogenic 307.89
   appendicular 543.9
   appendix 543.9
   bile duct - *see* Choledocholithiasis
   biliary - *see* Cholelithiasis
   bilious - *see* Cholelithiasis
   common duct - *see* Choledocholithiasis

Colic (*Continued*)
   Devonshire NEC 984.9
      specified type of lead - *see* Table of
         Drugs and Chemicals
   flatulent 787.3
   gallbladder or gallstone - *see*
      Cholelithiasis
   gastric 536.8
   hepatic (duct) - *see* Choledocholithiasis
   hysterical 300.11
   in ◀
      adult 789.0 ◀
      child over 12 months old 789.0 ◀
      infant 789.7 ◀
   infantile 789.7 ◀▥
   intestinal 789.7 ◀▥
   kidney 788.0
   lead NEC 984.9
      specified type of lead - *see* Table of
         Drugs and Chemicals
   liver (duct) - *see* Choledocholithiasis
   mucous 564.9
      psychogenic 316 *[564.9]*
   nephritic 788.0
   Painter's NEC 984.9
   pancreas 577.8
   psychogenic 306.4
   renal 788.0
   saturnine NEC 984.9
      specified type of lead - *see* Table of
         Drugs and Chemicals
   spasmodic 789.7 ◀▥
   ureter 788.0
   urethral 599.84
      due to calculus 594.2
   uterus 625.8
      menstrual 625.3
   vermicular 543.9
   virus 460
   worm NEC 128.9
Colicystitis (*see also* Cystitis) 595.9
Colitis (acute) (catarrhal) (croupous)
      (cystica superficialis) (exudative)
      (hemorrhagic) (noninfectious)
      (phlegmonous) (presumed
      noninfectious) 558.9
   adaptive 564.9
   allergic 558.3
   amebic (*see also* Amebiasis) 006.9
      nondysenteric 006.2
   anthrax 022.2
   bacillary (*see also* Infection, Shigella)
      004.9
   balantidial 007.0
   chronic 558.9
      ulcerative (*see also* Colitis, ulcerative)
         556.9
   coccidial 007.2
   dietetic 558.9
   due to radiation 558.1
   eosinophilic 558.42 ◀▥
   functional 558.9
   gangrenous 009.0
   giardial 007.1
   granulomatous 555.1
   gravis (*see also* Colitis, ulcerative) 556.9
   infectious (*see also* Enteritis, due to,
      specific organism) 009.0
      presumed 009.1
   ischemic 557.9
      acute 557.0
      chronic 557.1
      due to mesenteric artery
         insufficiency 557.1

Colitis (*Continued*)
   membranous 564.9
      psychogenic 316 *[564.9]*
   mucous 564.9
      psychogenic 316 *[564.9]*
   necrotic 009.0
   polyposa (*see also* Colitis, ulcerative)
      556.9
   protozoal NEC 007.9
   pseudomembranous 008.45
   pseudomucinous 564.9
   regional 555.1
   segmental 555.1
   septic (*see also* Enteritis, due to, specific
      organism) 009.0
   spastic 564.9
      psychogenic 316 *[564.9]*
   Staphylococcus 008.41
      food 005.0
   thromboulcerative 557.0
   toxic 558.2
   transmural 555.1
   trichomonal 007.3
   tuberculous (ulcerative) 014.8●
   ulcerative (chronic) (idiopathic)
      (nonspecific) 556.9
      entero- 556.0
      fulminant 557.0
      ileo- 556.1
      left-sided 556.5
      procto- 556.2
      proctosigmoid 556.3
      psychogenic 316 *[556]*
      specified NEC 556.8
      universal 556.6
Collagen disease NEC 710.9
   nonvascular 710.9
   vascular (allergic) (*see also* Angiitis,
      hypersensitivity) 446.20
Collagenosis (*see also* Collagen disease)
   710.9
   cardiovascular 425.4
   mediastinal 519.3
Collapse 780.2
   adrenal 255.8
   cardiorenal (*see also* Hypertension,
      cardiorenal) 404.90
   cardiorespiratory 785.51
      fetus or newborn 779.85
   cardiovascular (*see also* Disease, heart)
      785.51
      fetus or newborn 779.85
   circulatory (peripheral) 785.59
      with
         abortion - *see* Abortion, by type,
            with shock
         ectopic pregnancy (*see also*
            categories 633.0–633.9) 639.5
         molar pregnancy (*see also*
            categories 630–632) 639.5
      during or after labor and delivery
         669.1●
      fetus or newborn 779.85
      following
         abortion 639.5
         ectopic or molar pregnancy 639.5
      during or after labor and delivery
         669.1●
      fetus or newborn 779.89
   external ear canal 380.50
      secondary to
         inflammation 380.53
         surgery 380.52
         trauma 380.51
   general 780.2

◀ New   ◀▥ Revised   ~~deleted~~ Deleted   ● Use Additional Digit(s)   ▨ Omit code

C

Collapse (Continued)
- heart - see Disease, heart
- heat 992.1
- hysterical 300.11
- labyrinth, membranous (congenital) 744.05
- lung (massive) (see also Atelectasis) 518.0
  - pressure, during labor 668.0●
- myocardial - see Disease, heart
- nervous (see also Disorder, mental, nonpsychotic) 300.9
- neurocirculatory 306.2
- nose 738.0
- postoperative (cardiovascular) 998.0
- pulmonary (see also Atelectasis) 518.0
  - fetus or newborn 770.5
    - partial 770.5
    - primary 770.4
- thorax 512.8
  - iatrogenic 512.1
  - postoperative 512.1
- trachea 519.19
- valvular - see Endocarditis
- vascular (peripheral) 785.59
  - with
    - abortion - see Abortion, by type, with shock
    - ectopic pregnancy (see also categories 633.0–633.9) 639.5
    - molar pregnancy (see also categories 630–632) 639.5
  - cerebral (see also Disease, cerebrovascular, acute) 436
  - during or after labor and delivery 669.1●
  - fetus or newborn 779.89
  - following
    - abortion 639.5
    - ectopic or molar pregnancy 639.5
- vasomotor 785.59
- vertebra 733.13

Collateral - see also condition
- circulation (venous) 459.89
- dilation, veins 459.89

Colles' fracture (closed) (reversed) (separation) 813.41
- open 813.51

Collet's syndrome 352.6

Collet-Sicard syndrome 352.6

Colliculitis urethralis (see also Urethritis) 597.89

Colliers'
- asthma 500
- lung 500
- phthisis (see also Tuberculosis) 011.4●

Collodion baby (ichthyosis congenita) 757.1

Colloid milium 709.3

Coloboma NEC 743.49
- choroid 743.59
- fundus 743.52
- iris 743.46
- lens 743.36
- lids 743.62
- optic disc (congenital) 743.57
  - acquired 377.23
- retina 743.56
- sclera 743.47

Coloenteritis - see Enteritis

Colon - see condition

Colonization
- MRSA (methicillin resistant Staphylococcus aureus) V02.54
- MSSA (methicillin susceptible Staphylococcus aureus) V02.53

Coloptosis 569.89

Color
- amblyopia NEC 368.59
  - acquired 368.55
- blindness NEC (congenital) 368.59
  - acquired 368.55

Colostomy
- attention to V55.3
- fitting or adjustment V55.3
- malfunctioning 569.62
- status V44.3

Colpitis (see also Vaginitis) 616.10

Colpocele 618.6

Colpocystitis (see also Vaginitis) 616.10

Colporrhexis 665.4●

Colpospasm 625.1

Column, spinal, vertebral - see condition

Coma 780.01
- apoplectic (see also Disease, cerebrovascular, acute) 436
- diabetic (with ketoacidosis) 250.3●
  - due to secondary diabetes 249.3●
  - hyperosmolar 250.2●
    - due to secondary diabetes 249.2●
- eclamptic (see also Eclampsia) 780.39
- epileptic 345.3
- hepatic 572.2
- hyperglycemic 250.2●
  - due to secondary diabetes 249.2●
- hyperosmolar (diabetic) (nonketotic) 250.2●
  - due to secondary diabetes 249.2●
- hypoglycemic 251.0
  - diabetic 250.3●
    - due to secondary diabetes 249.3●
- insulin 250.3●
  - due to secondary diabetes 249.3●
  - hyperosmolar 250.2●
    - due to secondary diabetes 249.2●
  - nondiabetic 251.0
  - organic hyperinsulinism 251.0
- Kussmaul's (diabetic) 250.3●
  - due to secondary diabetes 249.3●
- liver 572.2
- newborn 779.2
- prediabetic 250.2●
  - due to secondary diabetes 249.2●
- uremic - see Uremia

Combat fatigue (see also Reaction, stress, acute) 308.9

Combined - see condition

Comedo 706.1

Comedocarcinoma (M8501/3) - see also Neoplasm, breast, malignant
- noninfiltrating (M8501/2)
  - specified site - see Neoplasm, by site, in situ
  - unspecified site 233.0

Comedomastitis 610.4

Comedones 706.1
- lanugo 757.4

Comma bacillus, carrier (suspected) of V02.3

Comminuted fracture - see Fracture, by site

Common
- aortopulmonary trunk 745.0
- atrioventricular canal (defect) 745.69
- atrium 745.69
- cold (head) 460
  - vaccination, prophylactic (against) V04.7

Common (Continued)
- truncus (arteriosus) 745.0
- ventricle 745.3

Commotio (current)
- cerebri (see also Concussion, brain) 850.9
  - with skull fracture - see Fracture, skull, by site
- retinae 921.3
- spinalis - see Injury, spinal, by site

Commotion (current)
- brain (without skull fracture) (see also Concussion, brain) 850.9
  - with skull fracture - see Fracture, skull, by site
- spinal cord - see Injury, spinal, by site

Communication
- abnormal - see also Fistula
  - between
    - base of aorta and pulmonary artery 745.0
    - left ventricle and right atrium 745.4
    - pericardial sac and pleural sac 748.8
    - pulmonary artery and pulmonary vein 747.3
  - congenital, between uterus and anterior abdominal wall 752.3
    - bladder 752.3
    - intestine 752.3
    - rectum 752.3
  - left ventricular-right atrial 745.4
  - pulmonary artery-pulmonary vein 747.3

Compartment syndrome - see Syndrome, compartment

Compensation
- broken - see Failure, heart
- failure - see Failure, heart
- neurosis, psychoneurosis 300.11

Complaint - see also Disease
- bowel, functional 564.9
  - psychogenic 306.4
- intestine, functional 564.9
  - psychogenic 306.4
- kidney (see also Disease, renal) 593.9
- liver 573.9
- miners' 500

Complete - see condition

Complex
- cardiorenal (see also Hypertension, cardiorenal) 404.90
- castration 300.9
- Costen's 524.60
- ego-dystonic homosexuality 302.0
- Eisenmenger's (ventricular septal defect) 745.4
- homosexual, ego-dystonic 302.0
- hypersexual 302.89
- inferiority 301.9
- jumped process
  - spine - see Dislocation, vertebra
- primary, tuberculosis (see also Tuberculosis) 010.0●
- regional pain syndrome 355.9
  - type I 337.20
    - lower limb 337.22
    - specified site NEC 337.29
    - upper limb 337.21
  - type II
    - lower limb 355.71
    - upper limb 354.4
- Taussig-Bing (transposition, aorta and overriding pulmonary artery) 745.11

◄ New   ◄ Revised   ~~deleted~~ Deleted   ● Use Additional Digit(s)   ▨ Omit code

Complications

abortion NEC - *see* categories 634–639
accidental puncture or laceration
    during a procedure 998.2
amniocentesis, fetal 679.1●
amputation stump (late) (surgical)
    997.60
    traumatic - *see* Amputation,
      traumatic
anastomosis (and bypass) - *see also*
    Complications, due to (presence
    of) any device, implant, or graft
    classified to 996.0–996.5 NEC
    hemorrhage NEC 998.11
    intestinal (internal) NEC 997.4
      involving urinary tract 997.5
    mechanical - *see* Complications,
      mechanical, graft
    urinary tract (involving intestinal
      tract) 997.5
anesthesia, anesthetic NEC (*see also*
    Anesthesia, complication)
    995.22
    in labor and delivery 668.9●
      affecting fetus or newborn 763.5
      cardiac 668.1●
      central nervous system 668.2●
      pulmonary 668.0●
      specified type NEC 668.8●
aortocoronary (bypass) graft 996.03
    atherosclerosis - *see* Arteriosclerosis,
      coronary
    embolism 996.72
    occlusion NEC 996.72
    thrombus 996.72
arthroplasty (*see also* Complications,
    prosthetic joint) 996.49
artificial opening
    cecostomy 569.60
    colostomy 569.60
    cystostomy 997.5
    enterostomy 569.60
    esophagostomy 530.87
      infection 530.86
      mechanical 530.87
    gastrostomy 536.40
    ileostomy 569.60
    jejunostomy 569.60
    nephrostomy 997.5
    tracheostomy 519.00
    ureterostomy 997.5
    urethrostomy 997.5
bariatric surgery 997.4
bile duct implant (prosthetic) NEC
    996.79
    infection or inflammation 996.69
    mechanical 996.59
bleeding (intraoperative)
    (postoperative) 998.11
blood vessel graft 996.1
    aortocoronary 996.03
      atherosclerosis - *see*
        Arteriosclerosis, coronary
      embolism 996.72
      occlusion NEC 996.72
      thrombus 996.72
    atherosclerosis - *see* Arteriosclerosis,
      extremities
    embolism 996.74
    occlusion NEC 996.74
    thrombus 996.74
bone growth stimulator NEC 996.78
    infection or inflammation 996.67
bone marrow transplant 996.85

Complications (*Continued*)

breast implant (prosthetic) NEC
    996.79
    infection or inflammation 996.69
    mechanical 996.54
bypass - *see also* Complications,
    anastomosis
    aortocoronary 996.03
      atherosclerosis - *see*
        Arteriosclerosis, coronary
      embolism 996.72
      occlusion NEC 996.72
      thrombus 996.72
    carotid artery 996.1
      atherosclerosis - *see*
        Arteriosclerosis, coronary
      embolism 996.74
      occlusion NEC 996.74
      thrombus 996.74
cardiac (*see also* Disease, heart) 429.9
    device, implant, or graft NEC 996.72
      infection or inflammation 996.61
      long-term effect 429.4
      mechanical (*see also*
        Complications, mechanical,
        by type) 996.00
      valve prosthesis 996.71
        infection or inflammation
          996.61
    postoperative NEC 997.1
      long-term effect 429.4
cardiorenal (*see also* Hypertension,
    cardiorenal) 404.90
carotid artery bypass graft 996.1
    atherosclerosis - *see* Arteriosclerosis,
      coronary
    embolism 996.74
    occlusion NEC 996.74
    thrombus 996.74
cataract fragments in eye 998.82
catheter device NEC - *see also*
    Complications, due to (presence
    of) any device, implant, or graft
    classified to 996.0-996.5 NEC
    mechanical - *see* Complications,
      mechanical, catheter
cecostomy 569.60
cesarean section wound 674.3●
chemotherapy (antineoplastic) 995.29
chin implant (prosthetic) NEC 996.79
    infection or inflammation 996.69
    mechanical 996.59
colostomy (enterostomy) 569.60
    specified type NEC 569.69
contraceptive device, intrauterine NEC
    996.76
    infection 996.65
    inflammation 996.65
    mechanical 996.32
cord (umbilical) - *see* Complications,
    umbilical cord
cornea
    due to
      contact lens 371.82
coronary (artery) bypass (graft) NEC
    996.03
    atherosclerosis - *see* Arteriosclerosis,
      coronary
    embolism 996.72
    infection or inflammation 996.61
    mechanical 996.03
    occlusion NEC 996.72
    specified type NEC 996.72
    thrombus 996.72

Complications (*Continued*)

cystostomy 997.5
delivery 669.9●
    procedure (instrumental) (manual)
      (surgical) 669.4●
    specified type NEC 669.8●
dialysis (hemodialysis) (peritoneal)
    (renal) NEC 999.9
    catheter NEC - *see also*
      Complications, due to
      (presence of) any device,
      implant, or graft classified to
      996.0–996.5 NEC
      infection or inflammation 996.62
        peritoneal 996.68
      mechanical 996.1
        peritoneal 996.56
drug NEC 995.29
due to (presence of) any device,
    implant, or graft classified to
    996.0–996.5 NEC 996.70
    with infection or inflammation - *see*
      Complications, infection or
      inflammation, due to (presence
      of) any device, implant, or
      graft classified to 996.0–996.5
      NEC
    arterial NEC 996.74
      coronary NEC 996.03
        atherosclerosis - *see*
          Arteriosclerosis,
          coronary
        embolism 996.72
        occlusion NEC 996.72
        specified type NEC 996.72
        thrombus 996.72
      renal dialysis 996.73
    arteriovenous fistula or shunt NEC
      996.74
    bone growth stimulator 996.78
    breast NEC 996.79
    cardiac NEC 996.72
      defibrillator 996.72
      pacemaker 996.72
      valve prosthesis 996.71
    catheter NEC 996.79
      spinal 996.75
      urinary, indwelling 996.76
      vascular NEC 996.74
        renal dialysis 996.73
      ventricular shunt 996.75
    coronary (artery) bypass (graft) NEC
      996.03
      atherosclerosis - *see*
        Arteriosclerosis, coronary
      embolism 996.72
      occlusion NEC 996.72
      thrombus 996.72
    electrodes
      brain 996.75
      heart 996.72
    esophagostomy 530.87
    gastrointestinal NEC 996.79
    genitourinary NEC 996.76
    heart valve prosthesis NEC
      996.71
    infusion pump 996.74
    insulin pump 996.57
    internal
      joint prosthesis 996.77
      orthopedic NEC 996.78
      specified type NEC 996.79
    intrauterine contraceptive device
      NEC 996.76

◀ New   ◀■ Revised   ~~deleted~~ Deleted   ● Use Additional Digit(s)   ▨ Omit code

Complications (Continued)
due to any device, implant, or graft
classified to 996.0–996.5 NEC
(Continued)
joint prosthesis, internal NEC 996.77
mechanical - see Complications,
mechanical
nervous system NEC 996.75
ocular lens NEC 996.79
orbital NEC 996.79
orthopedic NEC 996.78
joint, internal 996.77
renal dialysis 996.73
specified type NEC 996.79
urinary catheter, indwelling 996.76
vascular NEC 996.74
ventricular shunt 996.75
during dialysis NEC 999.9
ectopic or molar pregnancy NEC 639.9
electroshock therapy NEC 999.9
enterostomy 569.60
specified type NEC 569.69
esophagostomy 530.87
infection 530.86
mechanical 530.87
external (fixation) device with internal
component(s) NEC 996.78
infection or inflammation 996.67
mechanical 996.49
extracorporeal circulation NEC 999.9
eye implant (prosthetic) NEC 996.79
infection or inflammation 996.69
mechanical
ocular lens 996.53
orbital globe 996.59
fetal, from amniocentesis 679.1●
gastrointestinal, postoperative NEC
(see also Complications, surgical
procedures) 997.4
gastrostomy 536.40
specified type NEC 536.49
genitourinary device, implant or graft
NEC 996.76
infection or inflammation 996.65
urinary catheter, indwelling 996.64
mechanical (see also Complications,
mechanical, by type) 996.30
specified NEC 996.39
graft (bypass) (patch) - see also
Complications, due to (presence
of) any device, implant, or graft
classified to 996.0–996.5 NEC
bone marrow 996.85
corneal NEC 996.79
infection or inflammation 996.69
rejection or reaction 996.51
mechanical - see Complications,
mechanical, graft
organ (immune or nonimmune
cause) (partial) (total) 996.80
bone marrow 996.85
heart 996.83
intestines 996.87
kidney 996.81
liver 996.82
lung 996.84
pancreas 996.86
specified NEC 996.89
skin NEC 996.79
infection or inflammation 996.69
rejection 996.52
artificial 996.55
decellularized allodermis
996.55

Complications (Continued)
heart - see also Disease, heart transplant
(immune or nonimmune cause)
996.83
hematoma (intraoperative)
(postoperative) 998.12
hemorrhage (intraoperative)
(postoperative) 998.11
hyperalimentation therapy NEC 999.9
immunization (procedure) - see
Complications, vaccination
implant - see also Complications, due to
(presence of) any device, implant,
or graft classified to 996.0–996.5
NEC
dental placement, hemorrhagic
525.71
mechanical, - see Complications,
mechanical, implant
infection and inflammation
due to (presence of) any device,
implant or graft classified to
996.0–996.5 NEC 996.60
arterial NEC 996.62
coronary 996.61
renal dialysis 996.62
arteriovenous fistula or shunt
996.62
artificial heart 996.61
bone growth stimulator 996.67
breast 996.69
cardiac 996.61
catheter NEC 996.69
central venous 999.31
Hickman 999.31
peripherally inserted central
(PICC) 999.31
peritoneal 996.68
portacath (port-a-cath) 999.31
spinal 996.63
triple lumen 999.31
umbilical venous 999.31
urinary, indwelling 996.64
vascular (arterial) (dialysis)
(peripheral venous) NEC
996.62
ventricular shunt 996.63
central venous catheter 999.31
coronary artery bypass 996.61
electrodes
brain 996.63
heart 996.61
gastrointestinal NEC 996.69
genitourinary NEC 996.65
indwelling urinary catheter
996.64
heart assist device 996.61
heart valve 996.61
Hickman catheter 999.31
infusion pump 996.62
insulin pump 996.69
intrauterine contraceptive device
996.65
joint prosthesis, internal 996.66
ocular lens 996.69
orbital (implant) 996.69
orthopedic NEC 996.67
joint, internal 996.66
peripherally inserted central
catheter (PICC) 999.31
portacath (port-a-cath) 999.31
specified type NEC 996.69
triple lumen catheter 999.31
umbilical venous catheter 999.31

Complications (Continued)
infection and inflammation (Continued)
due to any device (Continued)
urinary catheter, indwelling 996.64
ventricular shunt 996.63
infusion (procedure) 999.88
blood - see Complications,
transfusion
infection NEC 999.39
sepsis NEC 999.39
inhalation therapy NEC 999.9
injection (procedure) 999.9
drug reaction (see also Reaction,
drug) 995.27
infection NEC 999.39
sepsis NEC 999.39
serum (prophylactic) (therapeutic) -
see Complications, vaccination
vaccine (any) - see Complications,
vaccination
inoculation (any) - see Complications,
vaccination
insulin pump 996.57
internal device (catheter) (electronic)
(fixation) (prosthetic) - see also
Complications, due to (presence
of) any device, implant, or graft
classified to 996.0–996.5 NEC
mechanical - see Complications,
mechanical
intestinal pouch, specified NEC
569.79   ◀
intestinal transplant (immune or
nonimmune cause) 996.87
intraoperative bleeding or hemorrhage
998.11
intrauterine contraceptive device (see
also Complications, contraceptive
device) 996.76
with fetal damage affecting
management of pregnancy
655.8●
infection or inflammation 996.65
in utero procedure
fetal 679.1●
maternal 679.0●
jejunostomy 569.60
kidney transplant (immune or
nonimmune cause) 996.81
labor 669.9●
specified condition NEC 669.8●
liver transplant (immune or
nonimmune cause) 996.82
lumbar puncture 349.0
mechanical
anastomosis - see Complications,
mechanical, graft
artificial heart 996.09
bypass - see Complications,
mechanical, graft
catheter NEC 996.59
cardiac 996.09
cystostomy 996.39
dialysis (hemodialysis) 996.1
peritoneal 996.56
during a procedure 998.2
urethral, indwelling 996.31
colostomy 569.62
device NEC 996.59
balloon (counterpulsation),
intra-aortic 996.1
cardiac 996.00
automatic implantable
defibrillator 996.04
long-term effect 429.4
specified NEC 996.09

Complications *(Continued)*
  mechanical *(Continued)*
    device NEC *(Continued)*
      contraceptive, intrauterine 996.32
      counterpulsation, intra-aortic
        996.1
      fixation, external, with internal
        components 996.49
      fixation, internal (nail, rod, plate)
        996.40
      genitourinary 996.30
        specified NEC 996.39
      insulin pump 996.57
      nervous system 996.2
      orthopedic, internal 996.40
        prosthetic joint *(see also*
          Complications,
          mechanical, device,
          orthopedic, prosthetic,
          joint) 996.47
      prosthetic NEC 996.59
        joint *(see also Complications,*
          prosthetic joint) 996.47 ◀▥
          articular bearing surface
            wear 996.46
          aseptic loosening 996.41
          breakage 996.43
          dislocation 996.42
          failure 996.47   ◀▥
          fracture 996.43
            around prosthetic 996.44
            peri-prosthetic 996.44
          instability 996.42
          loosening 996.41
          peri-prosthetic osteolysis
            996.45
          subluxation 996.42
          wear 996.46
      umbrella, vena cava 996.1
      vascular 996.1
    dorsal column stimulator 996.2
    electrode NEC 996.59
      brain 996.2
      cardiac 996.01
      spinal column 996.2
    enterostomy 569.62
    esophagostomy 530.87
    fistula, arteriovenous, surgically
      created 996.1
    gastrostomy 536.42
    graft NEC 996.52
      aortic (bifurcation) 996.1
      aortocoronary bypass 996.03
      blood vessel NEC 996.1
      bone 996.49
      cardiac 996.00
      carotid artery bypass 996.1
      cartilage 996.49
      corneal 996.51
      coronary bypass 996.03
      decellularized allodermis 996.55
      genitourinary 996.30
        specified NEC 996.39
      muscle 996.49
      nervous system 996.2
      organ (immune or nonimmune
        cause) 996.80
        heart 996.83
        intestines 996.87
        kidney 996.81
        liver 996.82
        lung 996.84
        pancreas 996.86
        specified NEC 996.89

Complications *(Continued)*
  mechanical *(Continued)*
    graft NEC *(Continued)*
      orthopedic, internal 996.49
      peripheral nerve 996.2
      prosthetic NEC 996.59
      skin 996.52
        artificial 996.55
      specified NEC 996.59
      tendon 996.49
      tissue NEC 996.52
      tooth 996.59
      ureter, without mention of
        resection 996.39
      vascular 996.1
    heart valve prosthesis 996.02
      long-term effect 429.4
    implant NEC 996.59
      cardiac 996.00
        automatic implantable defibril-
          lator 996.04
        long-term effect 429.4
        specified NEC 996.09
      electrode NEC 996.59
        brain 996.2
        cardiac 996.01
        spinal column 996.2
      genitourinary 996.30
      nervous system 996.2
      orthopedic, internal 996.49
      prosthetic NEC 996.59
        in
          bile duct 996.59
          breast 996.54
          chin 996.59
          eye
            ocular lens 996.53
            orbital globe 996.59
      vascular 996.1
    insulin pump 996.57
    nonabsorbable surgical material
      996.59
    pacemaker NEC 996.59
      brain 996.2
      cardiac 996.01
      nerve (phrenic) 996.2
    patch - *see* Complications,
      mechanical, graft
    prosthesis NEC 996.59
      bile duct 996.59
      breast 996.54
      chin 996.59
      ocular lens 996.53
      reconstruction, vas deferens
        996.39
    reimplant NEC 996.59
      extremity *(see also* Complications,
        reattached, extremity)
        996.90
      organ *(see also* Complications,
        transplant, organ, by site)
        996.80
    repair - *see* Complications,
      mechanical, graft
    respirator [ventilator] V46.14
    shunt NEC 996.59
      arteriovenous, surgically created
        996.1
      ventricular (communicating)
        996.2
    stent NEC 996.59
    tracheostomy 519.02
    vas deferens reconstruction 996.39
    ventilator [respirator] V46.14

Complications *(Continued)*
  medical care NEC 999.9
    cardiac NEC 997.1
    gastrointestinal NEC 997.4
    nervous system NEC 997.00
    peripheral vascular NEC 997.2
    respiratory NEC 997.39
    urinary NEC 997.5
    vascular
      mesenteric artery 997.71
      other vessels 997.79
      peripheral vessels 997.2
      renal artery 997.72
  nephrostomy 997.5
  nervous system
    device, implant, or graft NEC 349.1
      mechanical 996.2
    postoperative NEC 997.00
  obstetric 669.9●
    procedure (instrumental) (manual)
      (surgical) 669.4●
    specified NEC 669.8●
    surgical wound 674.3●
  ocular lens implant NEC 996.79
    infection or inflammation 996.69
    mechanical 996.53
  organ transplant - *see* Complications,
    transplant, organ, by site
  orthopedic device, implant, or graft
    internal (fixation) (nail) (plate) (rod)
      NEC 996.78
      infection or inflammation 996.67
      joint prosthesis 996.77
        infection or inflammation
          996.66
      mechanical 996.40
  pacemaker (cardiac) 996.72
    infection or inflammation 996.61
    mechanical 996.01
  pancreas transplant (immune or
    nonimmune cause) 996.86
  perfusion NEC 999.9
  perineal repair (obstetrical) 674.3●
    disruption 674.2●
  pessary (uterus) (vagina) - *see*
    Complications, contraceptive
    device
  phototherapy 990
  postcystoscopic 997.5
  postmastoidectomy NEC 383.30
  postoperative - *see* Complications,
    surgical procedures
  pregnancy NEC 646.9●
    affecting fetus or newborn 761.9
  prosthetic device, internal - *see also*
    Complications, due to (presence
    of) any device, implant or graft
    classified to 996.0–996.5 NEC
    mechanical NEC *(see also*
      Complications, mechanical)
      996.59
  puerperium NEC *(see also* Puerperal)
    674.9●
  puncture, spinal 349.0
  pyelogram 997.5
  radiation 990
  radiotherapy 990
  reattached
    body part, except extremity 996.99
    extremity (infection) (rejection)
      996.90
      arm(s) 996.94
      digit(s) (hand) 996.93
        foot 996.95

◀ New   ◀▥ Revised   ~~deleted~~ Deleted   ● Use Additional Digit(s)   ▬ Omit code

Complications *(Continued)*
 reattached *(Continued)*
 extremity *(Continued)*
 finger(s) 996.93
 foot 996.95
 forearm 996.91
 hand 996.92
 leg 996.96
 lower NEC 996.96
 toe(s) 996.95
 upper NEC 996.94
 reimplant NEC - *see also* Complications,
 due to (presence of) any device,
 implant, or graft classified to
 996.0–996.5 NEC
 bone marrow 996.85
 extremity *(see also* Complications,
 reattached, extremity) 996.90
 due to infection 996.90
 mechanical - *see* Complications,
 mechanical, reimplant
 organ (immune or nonimmune
 cause) (partial) (total) *(see also*
 Complications, transplant,
 organ, by site) 996.80
 renal allograft 996.81
 renal dialysis - *see* Complications,
 dialysis
 respirator [ventilator], mechanical
 V46.14
 respiratory 519.9
 device, implant or graft NEC
 996.79
 infection or inflammation 996.69
 mechanical 996.59
 distress syndrome, adult, following
 trauma or surgery 518.5
 insufficiency, acute, postoperative
 518.5
 postoperative NEC 997.39
 therapy NEC 999.9
 sedation during labor and delivery
 668.9●
 affecting fetus or newborn 763.5
 cardiac 668.1●
 central nervous system 668.2●
 pulmonary 668.0●
 specified type NEC 668.8●
 seroma (intraoperative) (postoperative)
 (noninfected) 998.13
 infected 998.51
 shunt - *see also* Complications, due to
 (presence of) any device, implant,
 or graft classified to 996.0–996.5
 NEC
 mechanical - *see* Complications,
 mechanical, shunt
 specified body system NEC
 device, implant, or graft - *see*
 Complications, due to
 (presence of) any device,
 implant, or graft classified to
 996.0–996.5 NEC
 postoperative NEC 997.99
 spinal puncture or tap 349.0
 stoma, external
 gastrointestinal tract
 colostomy 569.60
 enterostomy 569.60
 esophagostomy 530.87
 infection 530.86
 mechanical 530.87
 gastrostomy 536.40
 urinary tract 997.5

Complications *(Continued)*
 stomach banding 997.4
 stomach stapling 997.4
 surgical procedures 998.9
 accidental puncture or laceration
 998.2
 amputation stump (late) 997.60
 anastomosis - *see* Complications,
 anastomosis
 burst stitches or sutures (external)
 (see also Dehiscence) 998.32
 internal 998.31
 cardiac 997.1
 long-term effect following cardiac
 surgery 429.4
 catheter device - *see* Complications,
 catheter device
 cataract fragments in eye 998.82
 cecostomy malfunction 569.62
 colostomy malfunction 569.62
 cystostomy malfunction 997.5
 dehiscence (of incision) (external)
 (see also Dehiscence) 998.32
 internal 998.31
 dialysis NEC *(see also* Complications,
 dialysis) 999.9
 disruption *(see also* Dehiscence)
 anastomosis (internal) - *see*
 Complications, mechanical,
 graft
 internal suture (line) 998.31
 wound (external) 998.32
 internal 998.31
 dumping syndrome
 (postgastrectomy) 564.2
 elephantiasis or lymphedema 997.99
 postmastectomy 457.0
 emphysema (surgical) 998.81
 enterostomy malfunction 569.62
 esophagostomy malfunction 530.87
 evisceration 998.32
 fistula (persistent postoperative)
 998.6
 foreign body inadvertently left in
 wound (sponge) (suture)
 (swab) 998.4
 from nonabsorbable surgical
 material (Dacron) (mesh)
 (permanent suture)
 (reinforcing) (Teflon) - *see*
 Complications due to
 (presence of) any device,
 implant, or graft classified to
 996.0–996.5 NEC
 gastrointestinal NEC 997.4
 gastrostomy malfunction 536.42
 hematoma 998.12
 hemorrhage 998.11
 ileostomy malfunction 569.62
 internal prosthetic device NEC *(see
 also* Complications, internal
 device) 996.70
 hemolytic anemia 283.19
 infection or inflammation 996.60
 malfunction - *see* Complications,
 mechanical
 mechanical complication - *see*
 Complications, mechanical
 thrombus 996.70
 jejunostomy malfunction 569.62
 nervous system NEC 997.00
 obstruction, internal anastomosis -
 see Complications, mechanical,
 graft

Complications *(Continued)*
 surgical procedures *(Continued)*
 other body system NEC 997.99
 peripheral vascular NEC 997.2
 postcardiotomy syndrome 429.4
 postcholecystectomy syndrome 576.0
 postcommissurotomy syndrome
 429.4
 postgastrectomy dumping
 syndrome 564.2
 postmastectomy lymphedema
 syndrome 457.0
 postmastoidectomy 383.30
 cholesteatoma, recurrent 383.32
 cyst, mucosal 383.31
 granulation 383.33
 inflammation, chronic 383.33
 postvagotomy syndrome 564.2
 postvalvulotomy syndrome 429.4
 reattached extremity (infection)
 (rejection) *(see also*
 Complications, reattached,
 extremity) 996.90
 respiratory NEC 997.39
 seroma 998.13
 shock (endotoxic) (hypovolemic)
 (septic) 998.0
 shunt, prosthetic (thrombus) - *see
 also* Complications, due to
 (presence of) any device,
 implant, or graft classified to
 996.0–996.5 NEC
 hemolytic anemia 283.19
 specified complication NEC 998.89
 stitch abscess 998.59
 transplant - *see* Complications, graft
 ureterostomy malfunction 997.5
 urethrostomy malfunction 997.5
 urinary NEC 997.5
 vascular
 mesenteric artery 997.71
 other vessels 997.79
 peripheral vessels 997.2
 renal artery 997.72
 wound infection 998.59
 therapeutic misadventure NEC 999.9
 surgical treatment 998.9
 tracheostomy 519.00
 transfusion (blood) (lymphocytes)
 (plasma) NEC 999.89
 acute lung injury (TRALI) 518.7
 atrophy, liver, yellow, subacute
 (within 8 months of
 administration) - *see* Hepatitis,
 viral
 bone marrow 996.85
 embolism
 air 999.1
 thrombus 999.2
 hemolysis NEC 999.89
 bone marrow 996.85
 hepatitis (serum) (type B) (within 8
 months after administration) -
 see Hepatitis, viral
 incompatibility reaction ~~(ABO)~~
 ~~(blood group) 999.6~~ ◀▥
 ABO 999.6 ◀
 minor blood group 999.89 ◀
 Rh (factor) 999.7
 infection 999.39
 jaundice (serum) (within 8 months
 after administration) - *see*
 Hepatitis, viral
 sepsis 999.39

Complications (*Continued*)
  transfusion NEC (*Continued*)
    shock or reaction NEC 999.89
      bone marrow 996.85
    subacute yellow atrophy of liver
      (within 8 months after
      administration) - *see* Hepatitis,
      viral
    thromboembolism 999.2
  transplant NEC - *see also*
    Complications, due to (presence
    of) any device, implant, or graft
    classified to 996.0–996.5 NEC
    bone marrow 996.85
    organ (immune or nonimmune
      cause) (partial) (total) 996.80
      bone marrow 996.85
      heart 996.83
      intestines 996.87
      kidney 996.81
      liver 996.82
      lung 996.84
      pancreas 996.86
      specified NEC 996.89
  trauma NEC (early) 958.8
  ultrasound therapy NEC 999.9
  umbilical cord
    affecting fetus or newborn 762.6
    complicating delivery 663.9●
      affecting fetus or newborn 762.6
      specified type NEC 663.8●
  urethral catheter NEC 996.76
    infection or inflammation 996.64
    mechanical 996.31
  urinary, postoperative NEC 997.5
  vaccination 999.9
    anaphylaxis NEC 999.4
    cellulitis 999.39
    encephalitis or encephalomyelitis
      323.51
    hepatitis (serum) (type B) (within 8
      months after administration) -
      see Hepatitis, viral
    infection (general) (local) NEC
      999.39
    jaundice (serum) (within 8 months
      after administration) - *see*
      Hepatitis, viral
    meningitis 997.09 [321.8]
    myelitis 323.52
    protein sickness 999.5
    reaction (allergic) 999.5
      Herxheimer's 995.0
      serum 999.5
    sepsis 999.39
    serum intoxication, sickness, rash, or
      other serum reaction NEC
      999.5
    shock (allergic) (anaphylactic) 999.4
    subacute yellow atrophy of liver
      (within 8 months after
      administration) - *see* Hepatitis,
      viral
    vaccinia (generalized) 999.0
      localized 999.39
  vascular
    device, implant, or graft NEC 996.74
      infection or inflammation 996.62
      mechanical NEC 996.1
        cardiac (*see also* Complications,
        mechanical, by type)
        996.00
    following infusion, perfusion, or
      transfusion 999.2

Complications (*Continued*)
  vascular (*Continued*)
    postoperative NEC 997.2
      mesenteric artery 997.71
      other vessels 997.79
      peripheral vessels 997.2
      renal artery 997.72
  ventilation therapy NEC 999.9
  ventilator [respirator], mechanical
    V46.14
Compound presentation, complicating
  delivery 652.8●
  causing obstructed labor 660.0●
Compressed air disease 993.3
Compression
  with injury - *see* specific injury
  arm NEC 354.9
  artery 447.1
    celiac, syndrome 447.4
  brachial plexus 353.0
  brain (stem) 348.4
    due to
      contusion, brain - *see* Contusion,
        brain
      injury NEC - *see also* Hemorrhage,
        brain, traumatic
        birth - *see* Birth, injury, brain
      laceration, brain - *see* Laceration,
        brain
    osteopathic 739.0
  bronchus 519.19
  by cicatrix - *see* Cicatrix
  cardiac 423.9
  cauda equina 344.60
    with neurogenic bladder 344.61
  celiac (artery) (axis) 447.4
  cerebral - *see* Compression, brain
  cervical plexus 353.2
  cord (umbilical) - *see* Compression,
    umbilical cord
  cranial nerve 352.9
    second 377.49
    third (partial) 378.51
      total 378.52
    fourth 378.53
    fifth 350.8
    sixth 378.54
    seventh 351.8
  divers' squeeze 993.3
  duodenum (external) (*see also*
    Obstruction, duodenum) 537.3
  during birth 767.9
  esophagus 530.3
    congenital, external 750.3
  Eustachian tube 381.63
  facies (congenital) 754.0
  fracture - *see* Fracture, by site
  heart - *see* Disease, heart
  intestine (*see also* Obstruction, intestine)
    560.9
    with hernia - *see* Hernia, by site,
      with obstruction
  laryngeal nerve, recurrent 478.79
  leg NEC 355.8
  lower extremity NEC 355.8
  lumbosacral plexus 353.1
  lung 518.89
  lymphatic vessel 457.1
  medulla - *see* Compression, brain
  nerve NEC - *see also* Disorder, nerve
    arm NEC 354.9
    autonomic nervous system (*see also*
      Neuropathy, peripheral,
      autonomic) 337.9

Compression (*Continued*)
  nerve NEC (*Continued*)
    axillary 353.0
    cranial NEC 352.9
    due to displacement of
      intervertebral disc 722.2
      with myelopathy 722.70
      cervical 722.0
        with myelopathy 722.71
      lumbar, lumbosacral 722.10
        with myelopathy 722.73
      thoracic, thoracolumbar 722.11
        with myelopathy 722.72
    iliohypogastric 355.79
    ilioinguinal 355.79
    leg NEC 355.8
    lower extremity NEC 355.8
    median (in carpal tunnel) 354.0
    obturator 355.79
    optic 377.49
    plantar 355.6
    posterior tibial (in tarsal tunnel)
      355.5
    root (by scar tissue) NEC 724.9
      cervical NEC 723.4
      lumbar NEC 724.4
      lumbosacral 724.4
      thoracic 724.4
    saphenous 355.79
    sciatic (acute) 355.0
    sympathetic 337.9
    traumatic - *see* Injury, nerve
    ulnar 354.2
    upper extremity NEC 354.9
  peripheral - *see* Compression, nerve
  spinal (cord) (old or nontraumatic)
    336.9
    by displacement of intervertebral
      disc - *see* Displacement,
      intervertebral disc
    nerve
      root NEC 724.9
        postoperative 722.80
          cervical region 722.81
          lumbar region 722.83
          thoracic region 722.82
        traumatic - *see* Injury, nerve,
          spinal
      traumatic - *see* Injury, nerve,
        spinal
    spondylogenic 721.91
      cervical 721.1
      lumbar, lumbosacral 721.42
      thoracic 721.41
    traumatic - *see also* Injury, spinal, by
      site
      with fracture, vertebra - *see*
        Fracture, vertebra, by site,
        with spinal cord injury
  spondylogenic - *see* Compression,
    spinal cord, spondylogenic
  subcostal nerve (syndrome) 354.8
  sympathetic nerve NEC 337.9
  syndrome 958.5
  thorax 512.8
    iatrogenic 512.1
    postoperative 512.1
  trachea 519.19
    congenital 748.3
  ulnar nerve (by scar tissue) 354.2
  umbilical cord
    affecting fetus or newborn
      762.5
      cord prolapsed 762.4

◀ New   ◀▥ Revised   ~~deleted~~ Deleted   ● Use Additional Digit(s)   ▨ Omit code

Compression (Continued)
umbilical cord (Continued)
complicating delivery 663.2●
cord around neck 663.1●
cord prolapsed 663.0●
upper extremity NEC 354.9
ureter 593.3
urethra - see Stricture, urethra
vein 459.2
vena cava (inferior) (superior) 459.2
vertebral NEC - see Compression,
spinal (cord)
Compulsion, compulsive
eating 307.51
neurosis (obsessive) 300.3
personality 301.4
states (mixed) 300.3
swearing 300.3
in Gilles de la Tourette's syndrome
307.23
tics and spasms 307.22
water drinking NEC (syndrome) 307.9
Concato's disease (pericardial
polyserositis) 423.2
peritoneal 568.82
pleural - see Pleurisy
Concavity, chest wall 738.3
Concealed
hemorrhage NEC 459.0
penis 752.65
Concentric fading 368.12
Concern (normal) about sick person in
family V61.49
Concrescence (teeth) 520.2
Concretio cordis 423.1
rheumatic 393
Concretion - see also Calculus
appendicular 543.9
canaliculus 375.57
clitoris 624.8
conjunctiva 372.54
eyelid 374.56
intestine (impaction) (obstruction)
560.39
lacrimal (passages) 375.57
prepuce (male) 605
female (clitoris) 624.8
salivary gland (any) 527.5
seminal vesicle 608.89
stomach 537.89
tonsil 474.8
Concussion (current) 850.9
with
loss of consciousness 850.5
brief (less than one hour)
30 minutes or less 850.11
31–59 minutes 850.12
moderate (1–24 hours) 850.2
prolonged (more than 24 hours)
(with complete recovery)
(with return to pre-existing
conscious level) 850.3
without return to pre-existing
conscious level 850.4
mental confusion or disorientation
(without loss of consciousness)
850.0
with loss of consciousness - see
Concussion, with, loss of
consciousness
without loss of consciousness 850.0
blast (air) (hydraulic) (immersion)
(underwater) 869.0
with open wound into cavity 869.1

Concussion (Continued)
blast (Continued)
abdomen or thorax - see Injury,
internal, by site
brain - see Concussion, brain
ear (acoustic nerve trauma) 951.5
with perforation, tympanic
membrane - see Wound,
open, ear drum
thorax - see Injury, internal,
intrathoracic organs NEC
brain or cerebral (without skull
fracture) 850.9
with
loss of consciousness 850.5
brief (less than one hour)
30 minutes or less 850.11
31–59 minutes 850.12
moderate (1–24 hours) 850.2
prolonged (more than 24
hours) (with complete
recovery) (with return to
pre-existing conscious
level) 850.3
without return to pre-
existing conscious
level 850.4
mental confusion or
disorientation (without loss
of consciousness) 850.0
with loss of consciousness - see
Concussion, brain, with,
loss of consciousness
skull fracture - see Fracture, skull,
by site
without loss of consciousness 850.0
cauda equina 952.4
cerebral - see Concussion, brain
conus medullaris (spine) 952.4
hydraulic - see Concussion, blast
internal organs - see Injury, internal, by
site
labyrinth - see Injury, intracranial
ocular 921.3
osseous labyrinth - see Injury,
intracranial
spinal (cord) - see also Injury, spinal, by
site
due to
broken
back - see Fracture, vertebra,
by site, with spinal cord
injury
neck - see Fracture, vertebra,
cervical, with spinal cord
injury
fracture, fracture dislocation, or
compression fracture of
spine or vertebra - see
Fracture, vertebra, by site,
with spinal cord injury
syndrome 310.2
underwater blast - see Concussion, blast
Condition - see also Disease
fetal hematologic 678.0●
psychiatric 298.9
respiratory NEC 519.9
acute or subacute NEC 519.9
due to
external agent 508.9
specified type NEC 508.8
fumes or vapors (chemical)
(inhalation) 506.3
radiation 508.0

Condition (Continued)
respiratory NEC (Continued)
chronic NEC 519.9
due to
external agent 508.9
specified type NEC 508.8
fumes or vapors (chemical)
(inhalation) 506.4
radiation 508.1
due to
external agent 508.9
specified type NEC 508.8
fumes or vapors (chemical)
inhalation 506.9
Conduct disturbance (see also
Disturbance, conduct) 312.9
adjustment reaction 309.3
hyperkinetic 314.2
Condyloma NEC 078.11
acuminatum 078.11
gonorrheal 098.0
latum 091.3
syphilitic 091.3
congenital 090.0
venereal, syphilitic 091.3
Confinement - see Delivery
Conflagration - see also Burn, by site
asphyxia (by inhalation of smoke,
gases, fumes, or vapors) 987.9
specified agent - see Table of Drugs
and Chemicals
Conflict
family V61.9
specified circumstance NEC V61.8
interpersonal NEC V62.81
marital V61.10
involving
divorce V61.03
estrangement V61.09
parent (guardian)-child V61.20   ◄▥
adopted child V61.24   ◄
biological child V61.23   ◄
foster child V61.25   ◄
partner V61.10
Confluent - see condition
Confusion, confused (mental) (state) (see
also State, confusional) 298.9
acute 293.0
epileptic 293.0
postoperative 293.9
psychogenic 298.2
reactive (from emotional stress,
psychological trauma) 298.2
subacute 293.1
Confusional arousals 327.41
Congelation 991.9
Congenital - see also condition
aortic septum 747.29
generalized fibromatosis (CGF) 759.89
intrinsic factor deficiency 281.0
malformation - see Anomaly
Congestion, congestive
asphyxia, newborn 768.9
bladder 596.8
bowel 569.89
brain (see also Disease, cerebrovascular
NEC) 437.8
malarial 084.9
breast 611.79
bronchi 519.19
bronchial tube 519.19
catarrhal 472.0
cerebral - see Congestion, brain
cerebrospinal - see Congestion, brain
chest 786.9

Congestion, congestive (*Continued*)
  chill 780.99
    malarial (*see also* Malaria) 084.6
  circulatory NEC 459.9
  conjunctiva 372.71
  due to disturbance of circulation 459.9
  duodenum 537.3
  enteritis - *see* Enteritis
  eye 372.71
  fibrosis syndrome (pelvic) 625.5
  gastroenteritis - *see* Enteritis
  general 799.89
  glottis 476.0
  heart (*see also* Failure, heart) 428.0
  hepatic 573.0
  hypostatic (lung) 514
  intestine 569.89
  intracranial - *see* Congestion, brain
  kidney 593.89
  labyrinth 386.50
  larynx 476.0
  liver 573.0
  lung 786.9
    active or acute (*see also* Pneumonia) 486
      congenital 770.0
    chronic 514
    hypostatic 514
    idiopathic, acute 518.5
    passive 514
  malaria, malarial (brain) (fever) (*see also* Malaria) 084.6
  medulla - *see* Congestion, brain
  nasal 478.19
  nose 478.19
  orbit, orbital 376.33
    inflammatory (chronic) 376.10
      acute 376.00
  ovary 620.8
  pancreas 577.8
  pelvic, female 625.5
  pleural 511.0
  prostate (active) 602.1
  pulmonary - *see* Congestion, lung
  renal 593.89
  retina 362.89
  seminal vesicle 608.89
  spinal cord 336.1
  spleen 289.51
    chronic 289.51
  stomach 537.89
  trachea 464.11
  urethra 599.84
  uterus 625.5
    with subinvolution 621.1
  viscera 799.89
Congestive - *see* Congestion
Conical
  cervix 622.6
  cornea 371.60
  teeth 520.2
Conjoined twins 759.4
  causing disproportion (fetopelvic) 678.1●
  fetal 678.1●
Conjugal maladjustment V61.10
  involving
    divorce V61.03
    estrangement V61.09
Conjunctiva - *see* condition
Conjunctivitis (exposure) (infectious) (nondiphtheritic) (pneumococcal) (pustular) (staphylococcal) (streptococcal) NEC 372.30
  actinic 370.24

Conjunctivitis (*Continued*)
  acute 372.00
    atopic 372.05
    chemical 372.06　◄
    contagious 372.03
    follicular 372.02
    hemorrhagic (viral) 077.4
    toxic 372.06　◄
  adenoviral (acute) 077.3
  allergic (chronic) 372.14
    with hay fever 372.05
  anaphylactic 372.05
  angular 372.03
  Apollo (viral) 077.4
  atopic 372.05
  blennorrhagic (neonatorum) 098.40
  catarrhal 372.03
  chemical 372.06　◄▥
    allergic 372.05
    meaning corrosion - *see* Burn, conjunctiva
  chlamydial 077.98
    due to
      Chlamydia trachomatis - *see* Trachoma
      paratrachoma 077.0
  chronic 372.10
    allergic 372.14
    follicular 372.12
    simple 372.11
    specified type NEC 372.14
    vernal 372.13
  diphtheritic 032.81
  due to
    dust 372.05
    enterovirus type 70 077.4
    erythema multiforme 695.10 [372.33]
    filariasis (*see also* Filariasis) 125.9 [372.15]
    mucocutaneous
      disease NEC 372.33
      leishmaniasis 085.5 [372.15]
    Reiter's disease 099.3 [372.33]
    syphilis 095.8 [372.10]
    toxoplasmosis (acquired) 130.1
      congenital (active) 771.2
    trachoma - *see* Trachoma
  dust 372.05
  eczematous 370.31
  epidemic 077.1
    hemorrhagic 077.4
  follicular (acute) 372.02
    adenoviral (acute) 077.3
    chronic 372.12
  glare 370.24
  gonococcal (neonatorum) 098.40
  granular (trachomatous) 076.1
    late effect 139.1
  hemorrhagic (acute) (epidemic) 077.4
  herpetic (simplex) 054.43
    zoster 053.21
  inclusion 077.0
  infantile 771.6
  influenzal 372.03
  Koch-Weeks 372.03
  light 372.05
  medicamentosa 372.05
  membranous 372.04
  meningococcic 036.89
  Morax-Axenfeld 372.02
  mucopurulent NEC 372.03
  neonatal 771.6
    gonococcal 098.40
  Newcastle's 077.8

Conjunctivitis (*Continued*)
  nodosa 360.14
  of Beal 077.3
  parasitic 372.15
    filariasis (*see also* Filariasis) 125.9 [372.15]
    mucocutaneous leishmaniasis 085.5 [372.15]
  Parinaud's 372.02
  petrificans 372.39
  phlyctenular 370.31
  pseudomembranous 372.04
    diphtheritic 032.81
  purulent 372.03
  Reiter's 099.3 [372.33]
  rosacea 695.3 [372.31]
  serous 372.01
    viral 077.99
  simple chronic 372.11
  specified NEC 372.39
  sunlamp 372.04
  swimming pool 077.0
  toxic 372.06　◄
  trachomatous (follicular) 076.1
    acute 076.0
    late effect 139.1
  traumatic NEC 372.39
  tuberculous (*see also* Tuberculosis) 017.3● [370.31]
  tularemic 021.3
  tularensis 021.3
  vernal 372.13
    limbar 372.13 [370.32]
  viral 077.99
    acute hemorrhagic 077.4
    specified NEC 077.8
Conjunctivochalasis 372.81
Conjunctoblepharitis - *see* Conjunctivitis
Conn (-Louis) syndrome (primary aldosteronism) 255.12
Connective tissue - *see* condition
Conradi (-Hünermann) syndrome or disease (chondrodysplasia calcificans congenita) 756.59
Consanguinity V19.7
Consecutive - *see* condition
Consolidated lung (base) - *see* Pneumonia, lobar
Constipation 564.00
  atonic 564.09
  drug induced
    correct substance properly administered 564.09
    overdose or wrong substance given or taken 977.9
    specified drug - *see* Table of Drugs and Chemicals
  neurogenic 564.09
  other specified NEC 564.09
  outlet dysfunction 564.02
  psychogenic 306.4
  simple 564.00
  slow transit 564.01
  spastic 564.09
Constitutional - *see also* condition
  arterial hypotension (*see also* Hypotension) 458.9
  obesity 278.00
    morbid 278.01
  psychopathic state 301.9
  short stature in childhood 783.43
  state, developmental V21.9
    specified development NEC V21.8
  substandard 301.6

◄ New　◄▥ Revised　~~deleted~~ Deleted　● Use Additional Digit(s)　▢ Omit code

Constitutionally substandard 301.6
Constriction
 anomalous, meningeal bands or folds
  742.8
 aortic arch (congenital) 747.10
 asphyxiation or suffocation by 994.7
 bronchus 519.19
 canal, ear (*see also* Stricture, ear canal,
  acquired) 380.50
 duodenum 537.3
 gallbladder (*see also* Obstruction,
  gallbladder) 575.2
  congenital 751.69
 intestine (*see also* Obstruction, intestine)
  560.9
 larynx 478.74
  congenital 748.3
 meningeal bands or folds, anomalous
  742.8
 organ or site, congenital NEC - *see*
  Atresia
 prepuce (congenital) 605
 pylorus 537.0
  adult hypertrophic 537.0
  congenital or infantile 750.5
  newborn 750.5
 ring (uterus) 661.4●
  affecting fetus or newborn 763.7
 spastic - *see also* Spasm
  ureter 593.3
  urethra - *see* Stricture, urethra
 stomach 537.89
 ureter 593.3
 urethra - *see* Stricture, urethra
 visual field (functional) (peripheral)
  368.45
Constrictive - *see* condition
Consultation V65.9
 medical - *see also* Counseling, medical
 specified reason NEC V65.8
 without complaint or sickness V65.9
  feared complaint unfounded V65.5
  specified reason NEC V65.8
Consumption - *see* Tuberculosis
Contact
 with
  AIDS virus V01.79
  anthrax V01.81
  asbestos V15.84 ◀
  cholera V01.0
  communicable disease V01.9
   specified type NEC V01.89
   viral NEC V01.79
  Escherichia coli (E. coli) V01.83
  German measles V01.4
  gonorrhea V01.6
  HIV V01.79
  human immunodeficiency virus
   V01.79
  lead V15.86 ◀
  meningococcus V01.84
  parasitic disease NEC V01.89
  poliomyelitis V01.2
  potentially hazardous body fluids
   V15.85 ◀
  rabies V01.5
  rubella V01.4
  SARS-associated coronavirus V01.82
  smallpox V01.3
  syphilis V01.6
  tuberculosis V01.1
  varicella V01.71
  venereal disease V01.6
  viral disease NEC V01.79
 dermatitis - *see* Dermatitis

Contamination, food (*see also* Poisoning,
 food) 005.9
Contraception, contraceptive
 advice NEC V25.09
  family planning V25.09
  fitting of diaphragm V25.02
  prescribing or use of
   oral contraceptive agent V25.01
   specified agent NEC V25.02
 counseling NEC V25.09
  emergency V25.03
  family planning V25.09
  fitting of diaphragm V25.02
  prescribing or use of
   oral contraceptive agent V25.01
    emergency V25.03
    postcoital V25.03
   specified agent NEC V25.02
 device (in situ) V45.59
  causing menorrhagia 996.76
  checking V25.42
  complications 996.32
  insertion V25.1
  intrauterine V45.51
  reinsertion V25.42
  removal V25.42
  subdermal V45.52
 fitting of diaphragm V25.02
 insertion
  intrauterine contraceptive device
   V25.1
  subdermal implantable V25.5
 maintenance V25.40
  examination V25.40
   intrauterine device V25.42
   oral contraceptive V25.41
   specified method NEC V25.49
   subdermal implantable V25.43
  intrauterine device V25.42
  oral contraceptive V25.41
  specified method NEC V25.49
  subdermal implantable V25.43
 management NEC V25.49
 prescription
  oral contraceptive agent V25.01
   emergency V25.03
   postcoital V25.03
   repeat V25.41
  specified agent NEC V25.02
   repeat V25.49
 sterilization V25.2
 surveillance V25.40
  intrauterine device V25.42
  oral contraceptive agent V25.41
  specified method NEC V25.49
  subdermal implantable V25.43
Contraction, contracture, contracted
 Achilles tendon (*see also* Short, tendon,
  Achilles) 727.81
 anus 564.89
 axilla 729.90
 bile duct (*see also* Disease, biliary) 576.8
 bladder 596.8
  neck or sphincter 596.0
 bowel (*see also* Obstruction, intestine)
  560.9
 Braxton Hicks 644.1●
 breast implant, capsular 611.83
 bronchus 519.19
 burn (old) - *see* Cicatrix
 capsular, of breast implant 611.83
 cecum (*see also* Obstruction, intestine)
  560.9
 cervix (*see also* Stricture, cervix) 622.4
  congenital 752.49

Contraction, contracture, contracted
 (*Continued*)
 cicatricial - *see* Cicatrix
 colon (*see also* Obstruction, intestine)
  560.9
 conjunctiva, trachomatous, active
  076.1
  late effect 139.1
 Dupuytren's 728.6
 eyelid 374.41
 eye socket (after enucleation) 372.64
 face 729.90
 fascia (lata) (postural) 728.89
  Dupuytren's 728.6
  palmar 728.6
  plantar 728.71
 finger NEC 736.29
  congenital 755.59
  joint (*see also* Contraction, joint)
   718.44
 flaccid, paralytic
  joint (*see also* Contraction, joint)
   718.4●
  muscle 728.85
   ocular 378.50
 gallbladder (*see also* Obstruction,
  gallbladder) 575.2
 hamstring 728.89
  tendon 727.81
 heart valve - *see* Endocarditis
 Hicks' 644.1●
 hip (*see also* Contraction, joint) 718.4●
 hourglass
  bladder 596.8
   congenital 753.8
  gallbladder (*see also* Obstruction,
   gallbladder) 575.2
   congenital 751.69
  stomach 536.8
   congenital 750.7
   psychogenic 306.4
  uterus 661.4●
   affecting fetus or newborn 763.7
 hysterical 300.11
 infantile (*see also* Epilepsy) 345.6●
 internal os (*see also* Stricture, cervix)
  622.4
 intestine (*see also* Obstruction, intestine)
  560.9
 joint (abduction) (acquired)
  (adduction) (flexion) (rotation)
  718.40
  ankle 718.47
  congenital NEC 755.8
   generalized or multiple 754.89
    lower limb joints 754.89
   hip (*see also* Subluxation,
    congenital, hip) 754.32
   lower limb (including pelvic
    girdle) not involving hip
    754.89
   upper limb (including shoulder
    girdle) 755.59
  elbow 718.42
  foot 718.47
  hand 718.44
  hip 718.45
  hysterical 300.11
  knee 718.46
  multiple sites 718.49
  pelvic region 718.45
  shoulder (region) 718.41
  specified site NEC 718.48
  wrist 718.43

Contraction, contracture, contracted
(*Continued*)
kidney (granular) (secondary) (*see also*
Sclerosis, renal) 587
congenital 753.3
hydronephritic 591
pyelonephritic (*see also* Pyelitis,
chronic) 590.00
tuberculous (*see also* Tuberculosis)
016.0●
ligament 728.89
congenital 756.89
liver - *see* Cirrhosis, liver
muscle (postinfectional) (postural)
NEC 728.85
congenital 756.89
sternocleidomastoid 754.1
extraocular 378.60
eye (extrinsic) (*see also* Strabismus)
378.9
paralytic (*see also* Strabismus,
paralytic) 378.50
flaccid 728.85
hysterical 300.11
ischemic (Volkmann's) 958.6
paralytic 728.85
posttraumatic 958.6
psychogenic 306.0
specified as conversion reaction
300.11
myotonic 728.85
neck (*see also* Torticollis) 723.5
congenital 754.1
psychogenic 306.0
ocular muscle (*see also* Strabismus)
378.9
paralytic (*see also* Strabismus,
paralytic) 378.50
organ or site, congenital NEC - *see*
Atresia
outlet (pelvis) - *see* Contraction, pelvis
palmar fascia 728.6
paralytic
joint (*see also* Contraction, joint)
718.4●
muscle 728.85
ocular (*see also* Strabismus,
paralytic) 378.50
pelvis (acquired) (general) 738.6
affecting fetus or newborn 763.1
complicating delivery 653.1●
causing obstructed labor
660.1●
generally contracted 653.1●
causing obstructed labor
660.1●
inlet 653.2●
causing obstructed labor
660.1●
midpelvic 653.8●
causing obstructed labor
660.1●
midplane 653.8●
causing obstructed labor
660.1●
outlet 653.3●
causing obstructed labor
660.1●
plantar fascia 728.71
premature
atrial 427.61
auricular 427.61
auriculoventricular 427.61
heart (junctional) (nodal) 427.60

Contraction, contracture, contracted
(*Continued*)
premature (*Continued*)
supraventricular 427.61
ventricular 427.69
prostate 602.8
pylorus (*see also* Pylorospasm) 537.81
rectosigmoid (*see also* Obstruction,
intestine) 560.9
rectum, rectal (sphincter) 564.89
psychogenic 306.4
ring (Bandl's) 661.4●
affecting fetus or newborn 763.7
scar - *see* Cicatrix
sigmoid (*see also* Obstruction, intestine)
560.9
socket, eye 372.64
spine (*see also* Curvature, spine) 737.9
stomach 536.8
hourglass 536.8
congenital 750.7
psychogenic 306.4
psychogenic 306.4
tendon (sheath) (*see also* Short, tendon)
727.81
toe 735.8
ureterovesical orifice (postinfectional)
593.3
urethra 599.84
uterus 621.8
abnormal 661.9●
affecting fetus or newborn 763.7
clonic, hourglass or tetanic 661.4●
affecting fetus or newborn 763.7
dyscoordinate 661.4●
affecting fetus or newborn 763.7
hourglass 661.4●
affecting fetus or newborn 763.7
hypotonic NEC 661.2●
affecting fetus or newborn 763.7
incoordinate 661.4●
affecting fetus or newborn 763.7
inefficient or poor 661.2●
affecting fetus or newborn 763.7
irregular 661.2●
affecting fetus or newborn 763.7
tetanic 661.4●
affecting fetus or newborn 763.7
vagina (outlet) 623.2
vesical 596.8
neck or urethral orifice 596.0
visual field, generalized 368.45
Volkmann's (ischemic) 958.6
Contusion (skin surface intact) 924.9
with
crush injury - *see* Crush
dislocation - *see* Dislocation, by site
fracture - *see* Fracture, by site
internal injury - *see also* Injury,
internal, by site
heart - *see* Contusion, cardiac
kidney - *see* Contusion, kidney
liver - *see* Contusion, liver
lung - *see* Contusion, lung
spleen - *see* Contusion, spleen
intracranial injury - *see* Injury,
intracranial
nerve injury - *see* Injury, nerve
open wound - *see* Wound, open, by
site
abdomen, abdominal (muscle) (wall)
922.2
organ(s) NEC 868.00
adnexa, eye NEC 921.9

Contusion (*Continued*)
ankle 924.21
with other parts of foot 924.20
arm 923.9
lower (with elbow) 923.10
upper 923.03
with shoulder or axillary region
923.09
auditory canal (external) (meatus) (and
other part(s) of neck, scalp, or
face, except eye) 920
auricle, ear (and other part(s) of neck,
scalp, or face except eye) 920
axilla 923.02
with shoulder or upper arm 923.09
back 922.31
bone NEC 924.9
brain (cerebral) (membrane) (with
hemorrhage) 851.8●

Note 17 Use the following fifth-
digit subclassification with categories
851–854:

0 unspecified state of consciousness
1 with no loss of consciousness
2 with brief [less than one hour]
loss of consciousness
3 with moderate [1-24 hours] loss
of consciousness
4 with prolonged [more than
24 hours] loss of
consciousness and return to
pre-existing conscious level
5 with prolonged [more than
24 hours] loss of
consciousness, without
return to pre-existing
conscious level

Use fifth-digit 5 to designate when a
patient is unconscious and dies before
regaining consciousness, regardless of
the duration of the loss of consciousness

6 with loss of consciousness of
unspecified duration
9 with concussion, unspecified

---

with
open intracranial wound 851.9●
skull fracture - *see* Fracture, skull,
by site
cerebellum 851.4●
with open intracranial wound
851.5●
cortex 851.0●
with open intracranial wound
851.1●
occipital lobe 851.4●
with open intracranial wound
851.5●
stem 851.4●
with open intracranial wound
851.5●
breast 922.0
brow (and other part(s) of neck, scalp,
or face, except eye) 920
buttock 922.32
canthus 921.1
cardiac 861.01
with open wound into thorax 861.11
cauda equina (spine) 952.4
cerebellum - *see* Contusion, brain,
cerebellum

◀ New   ◀|||| Revised   ~~deleted~~ Deleted   ● Use Additional Digit(s)   ▨ Omit code

Contusion (*Continued*)

cerebral - *see* Contusion, brain
cheek(s) (and other part(s) of neck,
    scalp, or face, except eye) 920
chest (wall) 922.1
chin (and other part(s) of neck, scalp,
    or face, except eye) 920
clitoris 922.4
conjunctiva 921.1
conus medullaris (spine) 952.4
cornea 921.3
corpus cavernosum 922.4
cortex (brain) (cerebral) - *see* Contusion,
    brain, cortex
costal region 922.1
ear (and other part(s) of neck, scalp, or
    face except eye) 920
elbow 923.11
    with forearm 923.10
epididymis 922.4
epigastric region 922.2
eye NEC 921.9
eyeball 921.3
eyelid(s) (and periocular area) 921.1
face (and neck, or scalp, any part,
    except eye) 920
femoral triangle 922.2
fetus or newborn 772.6
finger(s) (nail) (subungual) 923.3
flank 922.2
foot (with ankle) (excluding toe(s))
    924.20
forearm (and elbow) 923.10
forehead (and other part(s) of neck,
    scalp, or face, except eye) 920
genital organs, external 922.4
globe (eye) 921.3
groin 922.2
gum(s) (and other part(s) of neck,
    scalp, or face, except eye) 920
hand(s) (except fingers alone)
    923.20
head (any part, except eye) (and
    face) (and neck) 920
heart - *see* Contusion, cardiac
heel 924.20
hip 924.01
    with thigh 924.00
iliac region 922.2
inguinal region 922.2
internal organs (abdomen, chest, or
    pelvis) NEC - *see* Injury, internal,
    by site
interscapular region 922.33
iris (eye) 921.3
kidney 866.01
    with open wound into cavity
      866.11
knee 924.11
    with lower leg 924.10
labium (majus) (minus) 922.4
lacrimal apparatus, gland, or sac
    921.1
larynx (and other part(s) of neck,
    scalp, or face, except eye) 920
late effect - *see* Late, effects (of),
    contusion
leg 924.5
    lower (with knee) 924.10
lens 921.3
lingual (and other part(s) of neck,
    scalp, or face, except eye) 920
lip(s) (and other part(s) of neck, scalp,
    or face, except eye) 920

Contusion (*Continued*)

liver 864.01
    with
      laceration - *see* Laceration, liver
      open wound into cavity 864.11
lower extremity 924.5
    multiple sites 924.4
lumbar region 922.31
lung 861.21
    with open wound into thorax 861.31
malar region (and other part(s) of neck,
    scalp, or face, except eye) 920
mandibular joint (and other part(s) of
    neck, scalp, or face, except eye)
    920
mastoid region (and other part(s) of
    neck, scalp, or face, except eye)
    920
membrane, brain - *see* Contusion, brain
midthoracic region 922.1
mouth (and other part(s) of neck, scalp,
    or face, except eye) 920
multiple sites (not classifiable to same
    three-digit category) 924.8
    lower limb 924.4
    trunk 922.8
    upper limb 923.8
muscle NEC 924.9
myocardium - *see* Contusion, cardiac
nasal (septum) (and other part(s) of
    neck, scalp, or face, except eye)
    920
neck (and scalp, or face, any part,
    except eye) 920
nerve - *see* Injury, nerve, by site
nose (and other part(s) of neck, scalp,
    or face, except eye) 920
occipital region (scalp) (and neck or
    face, except eye) 920
    lobe - *see* Contusion, brain, occipital
      lobe
orbit (region) (tissues) 921.2
palate (soft) (and other part(s) of neck,
    scalp, or face, except eye) 920
parietal region (scalp) (and neck, or
    face, except eye) 920
    lobe - *see* Contusion, brain
penis 922.4
pericardium - *see* Contusion, cardiac
perineum 922.4
periocular area 921.1
pharynx (and other part(s) of neck,
    scalp, or face, except eye) 920
popliteal space (*see also* Contusion,
    knee) 924.11
prepuce 922.4
pubic region 922.4
pudenda 922.4
pulmonary - *see* Contusion, lung
quadriceps femoralis 924.00
rib cage 922.1
sacral region 922.32
salivary ducts or glands (and other
    part(s) of neck, scalp, or face,
    except eye) 920
scalp (and neck, or face, any part,
    except eye) 920
scapular region 923.01
    with shoulder or upper arm 923.09
sclera (eye) 921.3
scrotum 922.4
shoulder 923.00
    with upper arm or axillar regions
      923.09

Contusion (*Continued*)

skin NEC 924.9
skull 920
spermatic cord 922.4
spinal cord - *see also* Injury, spinal, by
    site
    cauda equina 952.4
    conus medullaris 952.4
spleen 865.01
    with open wound into cavity
      865.11
sternal region 922.1
stomach - *see* Injury, internal, stomach
subconjunctival 921.1
subcutaneous NEC 924.9
submaxillary region (and other part(s)
    of neck, scalp, or face, except eye)
    920
submental region (and other part(s) of
    neck, scalp, or face, except eye)
    920
subperiosteal NEC 924.9
supraclavicular fossa (and other part(s)
    of neck, scalp, or face, except eye)
    920
supraorbital (and other part(s) of
    neck, scalp, or face, except eye)
    920
temple (region) (and other part(s) of
    neck, scalp, or face, except eye)
    920
testis 922.4
thigh (and hip) 924.00
thorax 922.1
    organ - *see* Injury, internal,
      intrathoracic
throat (and other part(s) of neck, scalp,
    or face, except eye) 920
thumb(s) (nail) (subungual) 923.3
toe(s) (nail) (subungual) 924.3
tongue (and other part(s) of neck,
    scalp, or face, except eye) 920
trunk 922.9
    multiple sites 922.8
    specified site - *see* Contusion, by site
tunica vaginalis 922.4
tympanum (membrane) (and other
    part(s) of neck, scalp, or face,
    except eye) 920
upper extremity 923.9
    multiple sites 923.8
uvula (and other part(s) of neck, scalp,
    or face, except eye) 920
vagina 922.4
vocal cord(s) (and other part(s) of neck,
    scalp, or face, except eye) 920
vulva 922.4
wrist 923.21
    with hand(s), except finger(s) alone
      923.20
Conus (any type) (congenital) 743.57
acquired 371.60
medullaris syndrome 336.8
Convalescence (following) V66.9
chemotherapy V66.2
medical NEC V66.5
psychotherapy V66.3
radiotherapy V66.1
surgery NEC V66.0
treatment (for) NEC V66.5
    combined V66.6
    fracture V66.4
    mental disorder NEC V66.3
    specified disorder NEC V66.5

◀ New   ◀▥ Revised   ~~deleted~~ Deleted   ● Use Additional Digit(s)   ▨ Omit code

Conversion
  closed surgical procedure to open procedure
    arthroscopic V64.43
    laparoscopic V64.41
    thoracoscopic V64.42
  hysteria, hysterical, any type 300.11
  neurosis, any 300.11
  reaction, any 300.11
Converter, tuberculosis (test reaction) 795.5
Convulsions (idiopathic) 780.39
  apoplectiform (*see also* Disease, cerebrovascular, acute) 436
  brain 780.39
  cerebral 780.39
  cerebrospinal 780.39
  due to trauma NEC - *see* Injury, intracranial
  eclamptic (*see also* Eclampsia) 780.39
  epileptic (*see also* Epilepsy) 345.9●
  epileptiform (*see also* Seizure, epileptiform) 780.39
  epileptoid (*see also* Seizure, epileptiform) 780.39
  ether
    anesthetic
      correct substance properly administered 780.39
      overdose or wrong substance given 968.2
    other specified type - *see* Table of Drugs and Chemicals
  febrile (simple) 780.31
    complex 780.32
  generalized 780.39
  hysterical 300.11
  infantile 780.39
    epilepsy - *see* Epilepsy
  internal 780.39
  jacksonian (*see also* Epilepsy) 345.5●
  myoclonic 333.2
  newborn 779.0
  paretic 094.1
  pregnancy (nephritic) (uremic) - *see* Eclampsia, pregnancy
  psychomotor (*see also* Epilepsy) 345.4●
  puerperal, postpartum - *see* Eclampsia, pregnancy
  recurrent 780.39
    epileptic - *see* Epilepsy
  reflex 781.0
  repetitive 780.39
    epileptic - *see* Epilepsy
  salaam (*see also* Epilepsy) 345.6●
  scarlatinal 034.1
  spasmodic 780.39
  tetanus, tetanic (*see also* Tetanus) 037
  thymic 254.8
  uncinate 780.39
  uremic 586
Convulsive - *see also* Convulsions
  disorder or state 780.39
    epileptic - *see* Epilepsy
  equivalent, abdominal (*see also* Epilepsy) 345.5●
Cooke-Apert-Gallais syndrome (adrenogenital) 255.2
Cooley's anemia (erythroblastic) 282.49
Coolie itch 126.9
Cooper's
  disease 610.1
  hernia - *see* Hernia, Cooper's

Coordination disturbance 781.3
Copper wire arteries, retina 362.13
Copra itch 133.8
Coprolith 560.39
Coprophilia 302.89
Coproporphyria, hereditary 277.1
Coprostasis 560.39
  with hernia - *see also* Hernia, by site, with obstruction
    gangrenous - *see* Hernia, by site, with gangrene
Cor
  biloculare 745.7
  bovinum - *see* Hypertrophy, cardiac
  bovis - *see also* Hypertrophy, cardiac
  pulmonale (chronic) 416.9
    acute 415.0
  triatriatum, triatrium 746.82
  triloculare 745.8
    biatriatum 745.3
    biventriculare 745.69
Corbus' disease 607.1
Cord - *see also* condition
  around neck (tightly) (with compression)
    affecting fetus or newborn 762.5
    complicating delivery 663.1●
      without compression 663.3●
        affecting fetus or newborn 762.6
  bladder NEC 344.61
    tabetic 094.0
  prolapse
    affecting fetus or newborn 762.4
    complicating delivery 663.0●
Cord's angiopathy (*see also* Tuberculosis) 017.3● [362.18]
Cordis ectopia 746.87
Corditis (spermatic) 608.4
Corectopia 743.46
Cori type glycogen storage disease - *see* Disease, glycogen storage
Cork-handlers' disease or lung 495.3
Corkscrew esophagus 530.5
Corlett's pyosis (impetigo) 684
Corn (infected) 700
Cornea - *see also* condition
  donor V59.5
  guttata (dystrophy) 371.57
  plana 743.41
Cornelia de Lange's syndrome (Amsterdam dwarf, mental retardation, and brachycephaly) 759.89
Cornual gestation or pregnancy - *see* Pregnancy, cornual
Cornu cutaneum 702.8
Coronary (artery) - *see also* condition
  arising from aorta or pulmonary trunk 746.85
Corpora - *see also* condition
  amylacea (prostate) 602.8
  cavernosa - *see* condition
Corpulence (*see also* Obesity)
Corpus - *see* condition
Corrigan's disease - *see* Insufficiency, aortic
Corrosive burn - *see* Burn, by site
Corsican fever (*see also* Malaria) 084.6
Cortical - *see also* condition
  blindness 377.75
  necrosis, kidney (bilateral) 583.6
Corticoadrenal - *see* condition
Corticosexual syndrome 255.2

Coryza (acute) 460
  with grippe or influenza 487.1
  syphilitic 095.8
    congenital (chronic) 090.0
Costen's syndrome or complex 524.60
Costiveness (*see also* Constipation) 564.00
Costochondritis 733.6
Cotard's syndrome (paranoia) 297.1
Cot death 798.0
Cotia virus 059.8
Cotungo's disease 724.3
Cough 786.2
  with hemorrhage (*see also* Hemoptysis) 786.3
  affected 786.2
  bronchial 786.2
    with grippe or influenza 487.1
  chronic 786.2
  epidemic 786.2
  functional 306.1
  hemorrhagic 786.3
  hysterical 300.11
  laryngeal, spasmodic 786.2
  nervous 786.2
  psychogenic 306.1
  smokers' 491.0
  tea tasters' 112.89
Counseling NEC V65.40
  without complaint or sickness V65.49
  abuse victim NEC V62.89
    child V61.21
    partner V61.11
    spouse V61.11
  child abuse, maltreatment, or neglect V61.21
  contraceptive NEC V25.09
    device (intrauterine) V25.02
    maintenance V25.40
      intrauterine contraceptive device V25.42
      oral contraceptive (pill) V25.41
      specified type NEC V25.49
      subdermal implantable V25.43
    management NEC V25.9
    oral contraceptive (pill) V25.01
      emergency V25.03
      postcoital V25.03
    prescription NEC V25.02
      oral contraceptive (pill) V25.01
        emergency V25.03
        postcoital V25.03
        repeat prescription V25.41
      repeat prescription V25.40
    subdermal implantable V25.43
    surveillance NEC V25.40
  dietary V65.3
  exercise V65.41
  expectant parent(s), ~~pediatric pre-birth visit V65.11~~
    pediatric pre-adoption visit V65.11 ◀
    pediatric pre-birth visit V65.11 ◀
  explanation of
    investigation finding NEC V65.49
    medication NEC V65.49
  family planning V25.09
    natural
      procreative V26.41
      to avoid pregnancy V25.04
  for nonattending third party V65.19
  genetic V26.33
  gonorrhea V65.45
  health (advice) (education) (instruction) NEC V65.49
  HIV V65.44
  human immunodeficiency virus V65.44

◀ New   ◀||| Revised   ~~deleted~~ Deleted   ● Use Additional Digit(s)   ▨ Omit code

Counseling NEC *(Continued)*
  injury prevention V65.43
  insulin pump training V65.46
  marital V61.10
  medical (for) V65.9
    boarding school resident V60.6
    condition not demonstrated V65.5
    feared complaint and no disease
        found V65.5
    institutional resident V60.6
    on behalf of another V65.19
    person living alone V60.3
  natural family planning
    procreative V26.41
    to avoid pregnancy V25.04
  parent (guardian)-child conflict
      V61.20 ◀▥
    adopted child V61.24 ◀
    biological child V61.23 ◀
    foster child V61.25 ◀
    specified problem NEC V61.29
  partner abuse
    perpetrator V61.12
    victim V61.11
  pediatric pre-birth visit for expectant
      mother V65.11 ◀▥
    pre-adoption visit for adoptive
        parent(s) V65.11 ◀
    pre-birth visit for expectant parents
        V65.11 ◀
  perpetrator of
    child abuse V62.83
      parental V61.22
    partner abuse V61.12
    spouse abuse V61.12
  procreative V65.49
  sex NEC V65.49
    transmitted disease NEC V65.45
      HIV V65.44
  specified reason NEC V65.49
  spousal abuse
    perpetrator V61.12
    victim V61.11
  substance use and abuse V65.42
  syphilis V65.45
  victim (of)
    abuse NEC V62.89
    child abuse V61.21
    partner abuse V61.11
    spousal abuse V61.11
Coupled rhythm 427.89
Couvelaire uterus (complicating
    delivery) - *see* Placenta, separation
Cowper's gland - *see* condition
Cowperitis (*see also* Urethritis) 597.89
  gonorrheal (acute) 098.0
    chronic or duration of 2 months or
        over 098.2
Cowpox (abortive) 051.01
  due to vaccination 999.0
  eyelid 051.01 *[373.5]*
    postvaccination 999.0 *[373.5]*
Coxa
  plana 732.1
  valga (acquired) 736.31
    congenital 755.61
    late effect of rickets 268.1
  vara (acquired) 736.32
    congenital 755.62
    late effect of rickets 268.1
Coxae malum senilis 715.25
Coxalgia (nontuberculous) 719.45
  tuberculous (*see also* Tuberculosis)
      015.1● *[730.85]*
Coxalgic pelvis 736.30

Coxitis 716.65
Coxsackie (infection) (virus) 079.2
  central nervous system NEC 048
  endocarditis 074.22
  enteritis 008.67
  meningitis (aseptic) 047.0
  myocarditis 074.23
  pericarditis 074.21
  pharyngitis 074.0
  pleurodynia 074.1
  specific disease NEC 074.8
Crabs, meaning pubic lice 132.2
Crack baby 760.75
Cracked
  nipple 611.2
    puerperal, postpartum 676.1●
  tooth 521.81
Cradle cap 690.11
Craft neurosis 300.89
Craigiasis 007.8
Cramp(s) 729.82
  abdominal 789.0●
  bathing 994.1
  colic 789.7● ◀▥
    infantle 789.7 ◀
    psychogenic 306.4
  due to immersion 994.1
  extremity (lower) (upper) NEC
      729.82
  fireman 992.2
  heat 992.2
  hysterical 300.11
  immersion 994.1
  intestinal 789.0●
    psychogenic 306.4
  linotypist's 300.89
    organic 333.84
  muscle (extremity) (general) 729.82
    due to immersion 994.1
    hysterical 300.11
  occupational (hand) 300.89
    organic 333.84
  psychogenic 307.89
  salt depletion 276.1
  sleep related leg 327.52
  stoker 992.2
  stomach 789.0●
  telegraphers' 300.89
    organic 333.84
  typists' 300.89
    organic 333.84
  uterus 625.8
    menstrual 625.3
  writers' 333.84
    organic 333.84
    psychogenic 300.89
Cranial - *see* condition
Cranioclasis, fetal 763.89
Craniocleidodysostosis 755.59
Craniofenestria (skull) 756.0
Craniolacunia (skull) 756.0
Craniopagus 759.4
Craniopathy, metabolic 733.3
Craniopharyngeal - *see* condition
Craniopharyngioma (M9350/1) 237.0
Craniorachischisis (totalis) 740.1
Cranioschisis 756.0
Craniostenosis 756.0
Craniosynostosis 756.0
Craniotabes (cause unknown) 733.3
  rachitic 268.1
  syphilitic 090.5
Craniotomy, fetal 763.89
Cranium - *see* condition
Craw-craw 125.3

CRBSI (catheter-related bloodstream
    infection) 999.31
Creaking joint 719.60
  ankle 719.67
  elbow 719.62
  foot 719.67
  hand 719.64
  hip 719.65
  knee 719.66
  multiple sites 719.69
  pelvic region 719.65
  shoulder (region) 719.61
  specified site NEC 719.68
  wrist 719.63
Creeping
  eruption 126.9
  palsy 335.21
  paralysis 335.21
Crenated tongue 529.8
Creotoxism 005.9
Crepitus
  caput 756.0
  joint 719.60
    ankle 719.67
    elbow 719.62
    foot 719.67
    hand 719.64
    hip 719.65
    knee 719.66
    multiple sites 719.69
    pelvic region 719.65
    shoulder (region) 719.61
    specified site NEC 719.68
    wrist 719.63
Crescent or conus choroid, congenital
    743.57
Cretin, cretinism (athyrotic) (congenital)
    (endemic) (metabolic) (nongoitrous)
    (sporadic) 243
  goitrous (sporadic) 246.1
  pelvis (dwarf type) (male type) 243
    with disproportion (fetopelvic)
        653.1●
      affecting fetus or newborn
          763.1
      causing obstructed labor 660.1●
        affecting fetus or newborn
            763.1
  pituitary 253.3
Cretinoid degeneration 243
Creutzfeldt-Jakob disease (CJD)
    (syndrome) 046.19
  with dementia
    with behavioral disturbance 046.19
        [294.11]
    without behavioral disturbance
        046.19 *[294.10]*
  familial 046.19
  iatrogenic 046.19
  specified NEC 046.19
  sporadic 046.19
  variant (vCJD) 046.11
    with dementia
      with behavioral disturbance
          046.11 *[294.11]*
      without behavioral disturbance
          046.11 *[294.10]*
Crib death 798.0
Cribriform hymen 752.49
Cri-du-chat syndrome 758.31
Crigler-Najjar disease or syndrome
    (congenital hyperbilirubinemia)
    277.4
Crimean hemorrhagic fever 065.0
Criminalism 301.7

Crisis
- abdomen 789.0●
- addisonian (acute adrenocortical insufficiency) 255.41
- adrenal (cortical) 255.41
- asthmatic - *see* Asthma
- brain, cerebral (*see also* Disease, cerebrovascular, acute) 436
- celiac 579.0
- Dietl's 593.4
- emotional NEC 309.29
    - acute reaction to stress 308.0
    - adjustment reaction 309.9
    - specific to childhood or adolescence 313.9
- gastric (tabetic) 094.0
- glaucomatocyclitic 364.22
- heart (*see also* Failure, heart) 428.9
- hypertensive - *see* Hypertension
- nitritoid
    - correct substance properly administered 458.29
    - overdose or wrong substance given or taken 961.1
- oculogyric 378.87
    - psychogenic 306.7
- Pel's 094.0
- psychosexual identity 302.6
- rectum 094.0
- renal 593.81
- sickle cell 282.62
- stomach (tabetic) 094.0
- tabetic 094.0
- thyroid (*see also* Thyrotoxicosis) 242.9●
- thyrotoxic (*see also* Thyrotoxicosis) 242.9●
- vascular - *see* Disease, cerebrovascular, acute

Crocq's disease (acrocyanosis) 443.89
Crohn's disease (*see also* Enteritis, regional) 555.9
Cronkhite-Canada syndrome 211.3
Crooked septum, nasal 470
Cross
- birth (of fetus) complicating delivery 652.3●
    - with successful version 652.1●
    - causing obstructed labor 660.0●
- bite, anterior or posterior 524.27
- eye (*see also* Esotropia) 378.00

Crossed ectopia of kidney 753.3
Crossfoot 754.50
Croup, croupous (acute) (angina) (catarrhal) (infective) (inflammatory) (laryngeal) (membranous) (nondiphtheritic) (pseudomembranous) 464.4
- asthmatic (*see also* Asthma) 493.9●
- bronchial 466.0
- diphtheritic (membranous) 032.3
- false 478.75
- spasmodic 478.75
    - diphtheritic 032.3
- stridulous 478.75
    - diphtheritic 032.3

Crouzon's disease (craniofacial dysostosis) 756.0
Crowding, teeth 524.31
CRST syndrome (cutaneous systemic sclerosis) 710.1
Cruchet's disease (encephalitis lethargica) 049.8
Cruelty in children (*see also* Disturbance, conduct) 312.9

Crural ulcer (*see also* Ulcer, lower extremity) 707.10
Crush, crushed, crushing (injury) 929.9
- abdomen 926.19
    - internal - *see* Injury, internal, abdomen
- ankle 928.21
    - with other parts of foot 928.20
- arm 927.9
    - lower (and elbow) 927.10
    - upper 927.03
        - with shoulder or axillary region 927.09
- axilla 927.02
    - with shoulder or upper arm 927.09
- back 926.11
- breast 926.19
- buttock 926.12
- cheek 925.1
- chest - *see* Injury, internal, chest
- ear 925.1
- elbow 927.11
    - with forearm 927.10
- face 925.1
- finger(s) 927.3
    - with hand(s) 927.20
        - and wrist(s) 927.21
- flank 926.19
- foot, excluding toe(s) alone (with ankle) 928.20
- forearm (and elbow) 927.10
- genitalia, external (female) (male) 926.0
    - internal - *see* Injury, internal, genital organ NEC
- hand, except finger(s) alone (and wrist) 927.20
- head - *see* Fracture, skull, by site
- heel 928.20
- hip 928.01
    - with thigh 928.00
- internal organ (abdomen, chest, or pelvis) - *see* Injury, internal, by site
- knee 928.11
    - with leg, lower 928.10
- labium (majus) (minus) 926.0
- larynx 925.2
- late effect - *see* Late, effects (of), crushing
- leg 928.9
    - lower 928.10
        - and knee 928.11
    - upper 928.00
- limb
    - lower 928.9
        - multiple sites 928.8
    - upper 927.9
        - multiple sites 927.8
- multiple sites NEC 929.0
- neck 925.2
- nerve - *see* Injury, nerve, by site
- nose 802.0
    - open 802.1
- penis 926.0
- pharynx 925.2
- scalp 925.1
- scapular region 927.01
    - with shoulder or upper arm 927.09
- scrotum 926.0
- shoulder 927.00
    - with upper arm or axillary region 927.09
- skull or cranium - *see* Fracture, skull, by site
- spinal cord - *see* Injury, spinal, by site

Crush, crushed, crushing (*Continued*)
- syndrome (complication of trauma) 958.5
- testis 926.0
- thigh (with hip) 928.00
- throat 925.2
- thumb(s) (and fingers) 927.3
- toe(s) 928.3
    - with foot 928.20
        - and ankle 928.21
- tonsil 925.2
- trunk 926.9
    - chest - *see* Injury, internal, intrathoracic organs NEC
    - internal organ - *see* Injury, internal, by site
    - multiple sites 926.8
    - specified site NEC 926.19
- vulva 926.0
- wrist 927.21
    - with hand(s), except fingers alone 927.20

Crusta lactea 690.11
Crusts 782.8
Crutch paralysis 953.4
Cruveilhier's disease 335.21
Cruveilhier-Baumgarten cirrhosis, disease, or syndrome 571.5
Cruz-Chagas disease (*see also* Trypanosomiasis) 086.2
Crying
- constant, continuous
    - adolescent 780.95
    - adult 780.95
    - baby 780.92
    - child 780.95
    - infant 780.92
    - newborn 780.92
- excessive
    - adolescent 780.95
    - adult 780.95
    - baby 780.92
    - child 780.95
    - infant 780.92
    - newborn 780.92

Cryofibrinogenemia 273.2
Cryoglobulinemia (mixed) 273.2
Crypt (anal) (rectal) 569.49
Cryptitis (anal) (rectal) 569.49
Cryptococcosis (European) (pulmonary) (systemic) 117.5
Cryptococcus 117.5
- epidermicus 117.5
- neoformans, infection by 117.5
Cryptopapillitis (anus) 569.49
Cryptophthalmos (eyelid) 743.06
Cryptorchid, cryptorchism, cryptorchidism 752.51
Cryptosporidiosis 007.4
- hepatobiliary 136.8 ◄
- respiratory 136.8 ◄
Cryptotia 744.29
Crystallopathy
- calcium pyrophosphate (*see also* Arthritis) 275.49 [712.2]●
- dicalcium phosphate (*see also* Arthritis) 275.49 [712.1]●
- gouty 274.00 ◄ɪɪ
- pyrophosphate NEC (*see also* Arthritis) 275.49 [712.2]●
- uric acid 274.00 ◄ɪɪ
Crystalluria 791.9
Csillag's disease (lichen sclerosus et atrophicus) 701.0
Cuban itch 050.1

◄ New   ◄ɪɪ Revised   ~~deleted~~ Deleted   ● Use Additional Digit(s)   ▭ Omit code

Cubitus
  valgus (acquired) 736.01
    congenital 755.59
    late effect of rickets 268.1
  varus (acquired) 736.02
    congenital 755.59
    late effect of rickets 268.1
Cultural deprivation V62.4
Cupping of optic disc 377.14
Curling's ulcer - see Ulcer, duodenum
Curling esophagus 530.5
Curschmann (-Batten) (-Steinert) disease
    or syndrome 359.21
Curvature
  organ or site, congenital NEC - see
      Distortion
  penis (lateral) 752.69
  Pott's (spinal) (see also Tuberculosis)
      015.0● [737.43]
  radius, idiopathic, progressive
      (congenital) 755.54
  spine (acquired) (angular) (idiopathic)
      (incorrect) (postural) 737.9
    congenital 754.2
    due to or associated with
        Charcôt-Marie-Tooth disease
            356.1 [737.40]
        mucopolysaccharidosis 277.5
            [737.40]
        neurofibromatosis 237.71 [737.40]
        osteitis
            deformans 731.0 [737.40]
            fibrosa cystica 252.01 [737.40]
        osteoporosis (see also
            Osteoporosis) 733.00
            [737.40]
        poliomyelitis (see also
            Poliomyelitis) 138 [737.40]
        tuberculosis (Pott's curvature) (see
            also Tuberculosis) 015.0●
            [737.43]
    kyphoscoliotic (see also
        Kyphoscoliosis) 737.30
    kyphotic (see also Kyphosis) 737.10
    late effect of rickets 268.1 [737.40]
    Pott's 015.0● [737.40]
    scoliotic (see also Scoliosis) 737.30
    specified NEC 737.8
    tuberculous 015.0● [737.40]
Cushing's
  basophilism, disease, or syndrome
      (iatrogenic) (idiopathic) (pituitary
      basophilism) (pituitary
      dependent) 255.0
  ulcer - see Ulcer, peptic
Cushingoid due to steroid therapy
  correct substance properly
      administered 255.0
  overdose or wrong substance given or
      taken 962.0
Cut (external) - see Wound, open, by site
Cutaneous - see also condition
  hemorrhage 782.7
  horn (cheek) (eyelid) (mouth) 702.8
  larva migrans 126.9
Cutis - see also condition
  hyperelastic 756.83
    acquired 701.8
  laxa 756.83
    senilis 701.8
  marmorata 782.61
  osteosis 709.3
  pendula 756.83
    acquired 701.8

Cutis (Continued)
  rhomboidalis nuchae 701.8
  verticis gyrata 757.39
    acquired 701.8
Cyanopathy, newborn 770.83
Cyanosis 782.5
  autotoxic 289.7
  common atrioventricular canal
      745.69
  congenital 770.83
  conjunctiva 372.71
  due to
    endocardial cushion defect
        745.60
    nonclosure, foramen botalli 745.5
    patent foramen botalli 745.5
    persistent foramen ovale 745.5
  enterogenous 289.7
  fetus or newborn 770.83
  ostium primum defect 745.61
  paroxysmal digital 443.0
  retina, retinal 362.10
Cycle
  anovulatory 628.0
  menstrual, irregular 626.4
Cyclencephaly 759.89
Cyclical vomiting 536.2
  associated with migraine 346.2●
  psychogenic 306.4
Cyclitic membrane 364.74
Cyclitis (see also Iridocyclitis) 364.3
  acute 364.00
    primary 364.01
    recurrent 364.02
  chronic 364.10
    in
        sarcoidosis 135 [364.11]
        tuberculosis (see also Tuberculosis)
            017.3● [364.11]
  Fuchs' heterochromic 364.21
  granulomatous 364.10
  lens induced 364.23
  nongranulomatous 364.00
  posterior 363.21
  primary 364.01
  recurrent 364.02
  secondary (noninfectious) 364.04
    infectious 364.03
  subacute 364.00
    primary 364.01
    recurrent 364.02
Cyclokeratitis - see Keratitis
Cyclophoria 378.44
Cyclopia, cyclops 759.89
Cycloplegia 367.51
Cyclospasm 367.53
Cyclosporiasis 007.5
Cyclothymia 301.13
Cyclothymic personality 301.13
Cyclotropia 378.33
Cyesis - see Pregnancy
Cylindroma (M8200/3) - see also
    Neoplasm, by site, malignant
  eccrine dermal (M8200/0) - see
      Neoplasm, skin, benign
  skin (M8200/0) - see Neoplasm, skin,
      benign
Cylindruria 791.7
Cyllosoma 759.89
Cynanche
  diphtheritic 032.3
  tonsillaris 475
Cynorexia 783.6
Cyphosis - see Kyphosis

Cyprus fever (see also Brucellosis) 023.9
Cyriax's syndrome (slipping rib) 733.99
Cyst (mucus) (retention) (serous) (simple)

> Note 18   In general, cysts are not
> neoplastic and are classified to the
> appropriate category for disease of
> the specified anatomical site. This
> generalization does not apply to certain
> types of cysts which are neoplastic in
> nature, for example, dermoid, nor does
> it apply to cysts of certain structures,
> for example, branchial cleft, which are
> classified as developmental anomalies.
>
> The following listing includes some
> of the most frequently reported sites
> of cysts as well as qualifiers which
> indicate the type of cyst. The latter
> qualifiers usually are not repeated
> under the anatomical sites. Since the
> code assignment for a given site may
> vary depending upon the type of cyst,
> the coder should refer to the listings
> under the specified type of cyst before
> consideration is given to the site.

  accessory, fallopian tube 752.11
  adenoid (infected) 474.8
  adrenal gland 255.8
    congenital 759.1
  air, lung 518.89
  allantoic 753.7
  alveolar process (jaw bone) 526.2
  amnion, amniotic 658.8●
  anterior chamber (eye) 364.60
    exudative 364.62
    implantation (surgical) (traumatic)
        364.61
    parasitic 360.13
  anterior nasopalatine 526.1
  antrum 478.19
  anus 569.49
  apical (periodontal) (tooth) 522.8
  appendix 543.9
  arachnoid, brain 348.0
  arytenoid 478.79
  auricle 706.2
  Baker's (knee) 727.51
    tuberculous (see also Tuberculosis)
        015.2●
  Bartholin's gland or duct 616.2
  bile duct (see also Disease, biliary)
      576.8
  bladder (multiple) (trigone) 596.8
  Blessig's 362.62
  blood, endocardial (see also
      Endocarditis) 424.90
  blue dome 610.0
  bone (local) 733.20
    aneurysmal 733.22
    jaw 526.2
        developmental (odontogenic)
            526.0
        fissural 526.1
        latent 526.89
    solitary 733.21
    unicameral 733.21
  brain 348.0
    congenital 742.4
    hydatid (see also Echinococcus)
        122.9
    third ventricle (colloid) 742.4
  branchial (cleft) 744.42
  branchiogenic 744.42

Cyst *(Continued)*
  breast (benign) (blue dome)
      (pedunculated) (solitary)
      (traumatic) 610.0
    involution 610.4
    sebaceous 610.8
  broad ligament (benign) 620.8
    embryonic 752.11
  bronchogenic (mediastinal)
      (sequestration) 518.89
    congenital 748.4
  buccal 528.4
  bulbourethral gland (Cowper's) 599.89
  bursa, bursal 727.49
    pharyngeal 478.26
  calcifying odontogenic (M9301/0) 213.1
    upper jaw (bone) 213.0
  canal of Nuck (acquired) (serous) 629.1
    congenital 752.41
  canthus 372.75
  carcinomatous (M8010/3) - *see*
      Neoplasm, by site, malignant
  cartilage (joint) - *see* Derangement, joint
  cauda equina 336.8
  cavum septi pellucidi NEC 348.0
  celomic (pericardium) 746.89
  cerebellopontine (angle) - *see* Cyst,
      brain
  cerebellum - *see* Cyst, brain
  cerebral - *see* Cyst, brain
  cervical lateral 744.42
  cervix 622.8
    embryonal 752.41
    nabothian (gland) 616.0
  chamber, anterior (eye) 364.60
    exudative 364.62
    implantation (surgical) (traumatic)
        364.61
    parasitic 360.13
  chiasmal, optic NEC (*see also* Lesion,
      chiasmal) 377.54
  chocolate (ovary) 617.1
  choledochal (congenital) 751.69
    acquired 576.8
  choledochus 751.69
  chorion 658.8 ●
  choroid plexus 348.0
  chyle, mesentery 457.8
  ciliary body 364.60
    exudative 364.64
    implantation 364.61
    primary 364.63
  clitoris 624.8
  coccyx (*see also* Cyst, bone) 733.20
  colloid
    third ventricle (brain) 742.4
    thyroid gland - *see* Goiter
  colon 569.89
  common (bile) duct (*see also* Disease,
      biliary) 576.8
  congenital NEC 759.89
    adrenal glands 759.1
    epiglottis 748.3
    esophagus 750.4
    fallopian tube 752.11
    kidney 753.10
      multiple 753.19
      single 753.11
    larynx 748.3
    liver 751.62
    lung 748.4
    mediastinum 748.8
    ovary 752.0
    oviduct 752.11

Cyst *(Continued)*
  congenital NEC *(Continued)*
    pancreas 751.7
    periurethral (tissue) 753.8
    prepuce NEC 752.69
      penis 752.69
    sublingual 750.26
    submaxillary gland 750.26
    thymus (gland) 759.2
    tongue 750.19
    ureterovesical orifice 753.4
    vulva 752.41
  conjunctiva 372.75
  cornea 371.23
  corpora quadrigemina 348.0
  corpus
    albicans (ovary) 620.2
    luteum (ruptured) 620.1
  Cowper's gland (benign) (infected)
      599.89
  cranial meninges 348.0
  craniobuccal pouch 253.8
  craniopharyngeal pouch 253.8
  cystic duct (*see also* Disease,
      gallbladder) 575.8
  Cysticercus (any site) 123.1
  Dandy-Walker 742.3
    with spina bifida (*see also* Spina
        bifida) 741.0 ●
  dental 522.8
    developmental 526.0
    eruption 526.0
    lateral periodontal 526.0
    primordial (keratocyst) 526.0
    root 522.8
  dentigerous 526.0
    mandible 526.0
    maxilla 526.0
  dermoid (M9084/0) - *see also*
      Neoplasm, by site, benign
    with malignant transformation
        (M9084/3) 183.0
    implantation
      external area or site (skin) NEC
          709.8
      iris 364.61
      skin 709.8
      vagina 623.8
      vulva 624.8
    mouth 528.4
    oral soft tissue 528.4
    sacrococcygeal 685.1
      with abscess 685.0
  developmental of ovary, ovarian
      752.0
  dura (cerebral) 348.0
    spinal 349.2
  ear (external) 706.2
  echinococcal (*see also* Echinococcus)
      122.9
  embryonal
    cervix uteri 752.41
    genitalia, female external 752.41
    uterus 752.3
    vagina 752.41
  endometrial 621.8
    ectopic 617.9
  endometrium (uterus) 621.8
    ectopic - *see* Endometriosis
  enteric 751.5
  enterogenous 751.5
  epidermal (inclusion) (*see also* Cyst,
      skin) 706.2

Cyst *(Continued)*
  epidermoid (inclusion) (*see also* Cyst,
      skin) 706.2
    mouth 528.4
    not of skin - *see* Cyst, by site
    oral soft tissue 528.4
  epididymis 608.89
  epiglottis 478.79
  epiphysis cerebri 259.8
  epithelial (inclusion) (*see also* Cyst,
      skin) 706.2
  epoophoron 752.11
  eruption 526.0
  esophagus 530.89
  ethmoid sinus 478.19
  eye (retention) 379.8
    congenital 743.03
    posterior segment, congenital 743.54
  eyebrow 706.2
  eyelid (sebaceous) 374.84
    infected 373.13
    sweat glands or ducts 374.84
  falciform ligament (inflammatory)
      573.8
  fallopian tube 620.8
    congenital 752.11
  female genital organs NEC 629.89
  fimbrial (congenital) 752.11
  fissural (oral region) 526.1
  follicle (atretic) (graafian) (ovarian)
      620.0
    nabothian (gland) 616.0
  follicular (atretic) (ovarian) 620.0
    dentigerous 526.0
  frontal sinus 478.19
  gallbladder or duct 575.8
  ganglion 727.43
  Gartner's duct 752.41
  gas, of mesentery 568.89
  gingiva 523.8
  gland of moll 374.84
  globulomaxillary 526.1
  graafian follicle 620.0
  granulosal lutein 620.2
  hemangiomatous (M9121/0) (*see also*
      Hemangioma) 228.00
  hydatid (*see also* Echinococcus) 122.9
    fallopian tube (Morgagni) 752.11
    liver NEC 122.8
    lung NEC 122.9
    Morgagni 752.89
      fallopian tube 752.11
    specified site NEC 122.9
  hymen 623.8
    embryonal 752.41
  hypopharynx 478.26
  hypophysis, hypophyseal (duct)
      (recurrent) 253.8
    cerebri 253.8
  implantation (dermoid)
    anterior chamber (eye) 364.61
    external area or site (skin) NEC
        709.8
    iris 364.61
    vagina 623.8
    vulva 624.8
  incisor, incisive canal 526.1
  inclusion (epidermal) (epithelial)
      (epidermoid) (mucous)
      (squamous) (*see also* Cyst, skin)
      706.2
    not of skin - *see* Neoplasm, by site,
        benign
  intestine (large) (small) 569.89

◀ New   ◀▥ Revised   ~~deleted~~ Deleted   ● Use Additional Digit(s)   ▬ Omit code

Cyst *(Continued)*
  intracranial - *see* Cyst, brain
  intraligamentous 728.89
    knee 717.89
  intrasellar 253.8
  iris (idiopathic) 364.60
    exudative 364.62
    implantation (surgical) (traumatic)
      364.61
    miotic pupillary 364.55
    parasitic 360.13
  Iwanoff's 362.62
  jaw (bone) (aneurysmal)
    (extravasation) (hemorrhagic)
    (traumatic) 526.2
    developmental (odontogenic) 526.0
    fissural 526.1
  keratin 706.2
  kidney (congenital) 753.10
    acquired 593.2
    calyceal (*see also* Hydronephrosis)
      591
    multiple 753.19
    pyelogenic (*see also* Hydronephrosis)
      591
    simple 593.2
    single 753.11
    solitary (not congenital) 593.2
  labium (majus) (minus) 624.8
    sebaceous 624.8
  lacrimal
    apparatus 375.43
    gland or sac 375.12
  larynx 478.79
  lens 379.39
    congenital 743.39
  lip (gland) 528.5
  liver 573.8
    congenital 751.62
    hydatid (*see also* Echinococcus) 122.8
      granulosis 122.0
      multilocularis 122.5
  lung 518.89
    congenital 748.4
    giant bullous 492.0
  lutein 620.1
  lymphangiomatous (M9173/0) 228.1
  lymphoepithelial
    mouth 528.4
    oral soft tissue 528.4
  macula 362.54
  malignant (M8000/3) - *see* Neoplasm,
    by site, malignant
  mammary gland (sweat gland) (*see also*
    Cyst, breast) 610.0
  mandible 526.2
    dentigerous 526.0
    radicular 522.8
  maxilla 526.2
    dentigerous 526.0
    radicular 522.8
  median
    anterior maxillary 526.1
    palatal 526.1
  mediastinum (congenital) 748.8
  meibomian (gland) (retention) 373.2
    infected 373.12
  membrane, brain 348.0
  meninges (cerebral) 348.0
    spinal 349.2
  meniscus knee 717.5
  mesentery, mesenteric (gas) 568.89
    chyle 457.8
    gas 568.89

Cyst *(Continued)*
  mesonephric duct 752.89
  mesothelial
    peritoneum 568.89
    pleura (peritoneal) 568.89
  milk 611.5
  miotic pupillary (iris) 364.55
  Morgagni (hydatid) 752.89
    fallopian tube 752.11
  mouth 528.4
  Müllerian duct 752.89
    appendix testis 608.89
    cervix (embryonal) 752.41
    fallopian tube 752.11
    prostatic utricle 599.89
    vagina (embryonal) 752.41
  multilocular (ovary) (M8000/1)
    239.5
  myometrium 621.8
  nabothian (follicle) (ruptured) 616.0
  nasal sinus 478.19
  nasoalveolar 528.4
  nasolabial 528.4
  nasopalatine (duct) 526.1
    anterior 526.1
  nasopharynx 478.26
  neoplastic (M8000/1) - *see also*
    Neoplasm, by site, unspecified
    nature
    benign (M8000/0) - *see* Neoplasm,
      by site, benign
    uterus 621.8
  nervous system - *see* Cyst, brain
  neuroenteric 742.59
  neuroepithelial ventricle 348.0
  nipple 610.0
  nose 478.19
    skin of 706.2
  odontogenic, developmental 526.0
  omentum (lesser) 568.89
    congenital 751.8
  oral soft tissue (dermoid) (epidermoid)
    (lymphoepithelial) 528.4
  ora serrata 361.19
  orbit 376.81
  ovary, ovarian (twisted) 620.2
    adherent 620.2
    chocolate 617.1
    corpus
      albicans 620.2
      luteum 620.1
    dermoid (M9084/0) 220
    developmental 752.0
    due to failure of involution NEC
      620.2
    endometrial 617.1
    follicular (atretic) (graafian)
      (hemorrhagic) 620.0
    hemorrhagic 620.2
    in pregnancy or childbirth 654.4●
      affecting fetus or newborn 763.89
      causing obstructed labor 660.2●
      affecting fetus or newborn
        763.1
    multilocular (M8000/1) 239.5
    pseudomucinous (M8470/0) 220
    retention 620.2
    serous 620.2
    theca lutein 620.2
    tuberculous (*see also* Tuberculosis)
      016.6●
    unspecified 620.2
  oviduct 620.8
  palatal papilla (jaw) 526.1

Cyst *(Continued)*
  palate 526.1
    fissural 526.1
    median (fissural) 526.1
  palatine, of papilla 526.1
  pancreas, pancreatic 577.2
    congenital 751.7
    false 577.2
    hemorrhagic 577.2
    true 577.2
  paralabral
    hip 718.85
    shoulder 840.7
  paramesonephric duct - *see* Cyst,
    Müllerian duct
  paranephric 593.2
  paraovarian 752.11
  paraphysis, cerebri 742.4
  parasitic NEC 136.9
  parathyroid (gland) 252.8
  paratubal (fallopian) 620.8
  paraurethral duct 599.89
  paroophoron 752.11
  parotid gland 527.6
    mucous extravasation or retention
      527.6
  parovarian 752.11
  pars planus 364.60
    exudative 364.64
    primary 364.63
  pelvis, female
    in pregnancy or childbirth 654.4●
      affecting fetus or newborn 763.89
      causing obstructed labor 660.2●
      affecting fetus or newborn
        763.1
  penis (sebaceous) 607.89
  periapical 522.8
  pericardial (congenital) 746.89
    acquired (secondary) 423.8
  pericoronal 526.0
  perineural (Tarlov's) 355.9
  periodontal 522.8
    lateral 526.0
  peripancreatic 577.2
  peripelvic (lymphatic) 593.2
  peritoneum 568.89
    chylous 457.8
  pharynx (wall) 478.26
  pilonidal (infected) (rectum) 685.1
    with abscess 685.0
    malignant (M9084/3) 173.5
  pituitary (duct) (gland) 253.8
  placenta (amniotic) - *see* Placenta,
    abnormal
  pleura 519.8
  popliteal 727.51
  porencephalic 742.4
    acquired 348.0
  postanal (infected) 685.1
    with abscess 685.0
  posterior segment of eye, congenital
    743.54
  postmastoidectomy cavity 383.31
  preauricular 744.47
  prepuce 607.89
    congenital 752.69
  primordial (jaw) 526.0
  prostate 600.3
  pseudomucinous (ovary) (M8470/0) 220
  pudenda (sweat glands) 624.8
  pupillary, miotic 364.55
    sebaceous 624.8
  radicular (residual) 522.8

Cyst (*Continued*)
  radiculodental 522.8
  ranular 527.6
  Rathke's pouch 253.8
  rectum (epithelium) (mucous) 569.49
  renal - *see* Cyst, kidney
  residual (radicular) 522.8
  retention (ovary) 620.2
  retina 361.19
    macular 362.54
    parasitic 360.13
    primary 361.13
    secondary 361.14
  retroperitoneal 568.89
  sacrococcygeal (dermoid) 685.1
    with abscess 685.0
  salivary gland or duct 527.6
    mucous extravasation or retention 527.6
  Sampson's 617.1
  sclera 379.19
  scrotum (sebaceous) 706.2
    sweat glands 706.2
  sebaceous (duct) (gland) 706.2
    breast 610.8
    eyelid 374.84
    genital organ NEC
      female 629.89
      male 608.89
    scrotum 706.2
  semilunar cartilage (knee) (multiple) 717.5
  seminal vesicle 608.89
  serous (ovary) 620.2
  sinus (antral) (ethmoidal) (frontal) (maxillary) (nasal) (sphenoidal) 478.19
  Skene's gland 599.89
  skin (epidermal) (epidermoid, inclusion) (epithelial) (inclusion) (retention) (sebaceous) 706.2
    breast 610.8
    eyelid 374.84
    genital organ NEC
      female 629.89
      male 608.89
    neoplastic 216.3
    scrotum 706.2
    sweat gland or duct 705.89
  solitary
    bone 733.21
    kidney 593.2
  spermatic cord 608.89
  sphenoid sinus 478.19
  spinal meninges 349.2
  spine (*see also* Cyst, bone) 733.20
  spleen NEC 289.59
    congenital 759.0
    hydatid (*see also* Echinococcus) 122.9
  spring water (pericardium) 746.89
  subarachnoid 348.0
    intrasellar 793.0
  subdural (cerebral) 348.0
    spinal cord 349.2
  sublingual gland 527.6
    mucous extravasation or retention 527.6
  submaxillary gland 527.6
    mucous extravasation or retention 527.6
  suburethral 599.89
  suprarenal gland 255.8
  suprasellar - *see* Cyst, brain
  sweat gland or duct 705.89

Cyst (*Continued*)
  sympathetic nervous system 337.9
  synovial 727.40
    popliteal space 727.51
  Tarlov's 355.9
  tarsal 373.2
  tendon (sheath) 727.42
  testis 608.89
  theca-lutein (ovary) 620.2
  Thornwaldt's, Tornwaldt's 478.26
  thymus (gland) 254.8
  thyroglossal (duct) (infected) (persistent) 759.2
  thyroid (gland) 246.2
    adenomatous - *see* Goiter, nodular
    colloid (*see also* Goiter) 240.9
  thyrolingual duct (infected) (persistent) 759.2
  tongue (mucous) 529.8
  tonsil 474.8
  tooth (dental root) 522.8
  tubo-ovarian 620.8
    inflammatory 614.1
  tunica vaginalis 608.89
  turbinate (nose) (*see also* Cyst, bone) 733.20
  Tyson's gland (benign) (infected) 607.89
  umbilicus 759.89
  urachus 753.7
  ureter 593.89
  ureterovesical orifice 593.89
    congenital 753.4
  urethra 599.84
  urethral gland (Cowper's) 599.89
  uterine
    ligament 620.8
      embryonic 752.11
    tube 620.8
  uterus (body) (corpus) (recurrent) 621.8
    embryonal 752.3
  utricle (ear) 386.8
    prostatic 599.89
  utriculus masculinus 599.89
  vagina, vaginal (squamous cell) (wall) 623.8
    embryonal 752.41
    implantation 623.8
    inclusion 623.8
  vallecula, vallecular 478.79
  ventricle, neuroepithelial 348.0
  verumontanum 599.89
  vesical (orifice) 596.8
  vitreous humor 379.29
  vulva (sweat glands) 624.8
    congenital 752.41
    implantation 624.8
    inclusion 624.8
    sebaceous gland 624.8
  vulvovaginal gland 624.8
  wolffian 752.89

Cystadenocarcinoma (M8440/3) - *see also* Neoplasm, by site, malignant
  bile duct type (M8161/3) 155.1
  endometrioid (M8380/3) - *see* Neoplasm, by site, malignant
  mucinous (M8470/3)
    papillary (M8471/3)
      specified site - *see* Neoplasm, by site, malignant
      unspecified site 183.0
    specified site - *see* Neoplasm, by site, malignant
    unspecified site 183.0

Cystadenocarcinoma (*Continued*)
  papillary (M8450/3)
    mucinous (M8471/3)
      specified site - *see* Neoplasm, by site, malignant
      unspecified site 183.0
    pseudomucinous (M8471/3)
      specified site - *see* Neoplasm, by site, malignant
      unspecified site 183.0
    serous (M8460/3)
      specified site - *see* Neoplasm, by site, malignant
      unspecified site 183.0
    specified site - *see* Neoplasm, by site, malignant
    unspecified 183.0
  pseudomucinous (M8470/3)
    papillary (M8471/3)
      specified site - *see* Neoplasm, by site, malignant
      unspecified site 183.0
    specified site - *see* Neoplasm, by site, malignant
    unspecified site 183.0
  serous (M8441/3)
    papillary (M8460/3)
      specified site - *see* Neoplasm, by site, malignant
      unspecified site 183.0
    specified site - *see* Neoplasm, by site, malignant
    unspecified site 183.0
Cystadenofibroma (M9013/0)
  clear cell (M8313/0) - *see* Neoplasm, by site, benign
  endometrioid (M8381/0) 220
    borderline malignancy (M8381/1) 236.2
    malignant (M8381/3) 183.0
  mucinous (M9015/0)
    specified site - *see* Neoplasm, by site, benign
    unspecified site 220
  serous (M9014/0)
    specified site - *see* Neoplasm, by site, benign
    unspecified site 220
  specified site - *see* Neoplasm, by site, benign
  unspecified site 220
Cystadenoma (M8440/0) - *see also* Neoplasm, by site, benign
  bile duct (M8161/0) 211.5
  endometrioid (M8380/0) - *see also* Neoplasm, by site, benign
    borderline malignancy (M8380/1) - *see* Neoplasm, by site, uncertain behavior
  malignant (M8440/3) - *see* Neoplasm, by site, malignant
  mucinous (M8470/0)
    borderline malignancy (M8470/1)
      specified site - *see* Neoplasm, uncertain behavior
      unspecified site 236.2
    papillary (M8471/0)
      borderline malignancy (M8471/1)
        specified site - *see* Neoplasm, by site, uncertain behavior
      unspecified site 236.2

◀ New ◀▥ Revised ~~deleted~~ Deleted ● Use Additional Digit(s) ▨ Omit code

Cystadenoma *(Continued)*
  mucinous *(Continued)*
    papillary *(Continued)*
      specified site - *see* Neoplasm, by
        site, benign
      unspecified site 220
    specified site - *see* Neoplasm, by site,
      benign
    unspecified site 220
  papillary (M8450/0)
    borderline malignancy (M8450/1)
      specified site - *see* Neoplasm, by
        site, uncertain behavior
      unspecified site 236.2
    lymphomatosum (M8561/0) 210.2
    mucinous (M8471/0)
      borderline malignancy (M8471/1)
        specified site - *see* Neoplasm, by
          site, uncertain behavior
        unspecified site 236.2
      specified site - *see* Neoplasm, by
        site, benign
      unspecified site 220
    pseudomucinous (M8471/0)
      borderline malignancy (M8471/1)
        specified site - *see* Neoplasm,
          by site uncertain
          behavior
        unspecified site 236.2
      specified site - *see* Neoplasm, by
        site, benign
      unspecified site 220
    serous (M8460/0)
      borderline malignancy (M8460/1)
        specified site - *see* Neoplasm,
          by site, uncertain
          behavior
        unspecified site 236.2
      specified site - *see* Neoplasm, by
        site, benign
      unspecified site 220
    specified site - *see* Neoplasm, by site,
      benign
    unspecified site 220
  pseudomucinous (M8470/0)
    borderline malignancy (M8470/1)
      specified site - *see* Neoplasm, by
        site uncertain behavior
      unspecified site 236.2
    papillary (M8471/0)
      borderline malignancy (M8471/1)
        specified site - *see* Neoplasm,
          by site uncertain
          behavior
        unspecified site 236.2
      specified site - *see* Neoplasm, by
        site, benign
      unspecified site 220
    specified site - *see* Neoplasm, by site,
      benign
    unspecified site 220
  serous (M8441/0)
    borderline malignancy (M8441/1)
      specified site - *see* Neoplasm, by
        site, uncertain behavior
      unspecified site 236.2
    papillary (M8460/0)
      borderline malignancy (M8460/1)
        specified site - *see* Neoplasm,
          by site, uncertain
          behavior
        unspecified site 236.2
      specified site - *see* Neoplasm, by
        site, benign
      unspecified site 220

Cystadenoma *(Continued)*
  serous *(Continued)*
    specified site - *see* Neoplasm, by site,
      benign
    unspecified site 220
  thyroid 226
Cystathioninemia 270.4
Cystathioninuria 270.4
Cystic - *see also* condition
  breast, chronic 610.1
  corpora lutea 620.1
  degeneration, congenital
    brain 742.4
    kidney (*see also* Cystic, disease,
      kidney) 753.10
  disease
    breast, chronic 610.1
    kidney, congenital 753.10
      medullary 753.16
      multiple 753.19
      polycystic - *see* Polycystic, kidney
      single 753.11
      specified NEC 753.19
    liver, congenital 751.62
    lung 518.89
      congenital 748.4
    pancreas, congenital 751.7
    semilunar cartilage 717.5
  duct - *see* condition
  eyeball, congenital 743.03
  fibrosis (pancreas) 277.00
    with
      manifestations
        gastrointestinal 277.03
        pulmonary 277.02
        specified NEC 277.09
      meconium ileus 277.01
      pulmonary exacerbation 277.02
  hygroma (M9173/0) 228.1
  kidney, congenital 753.10
    medullary 753.16
    multiple 753.19
    polycystic - *see* Polycystic, kidney
    single 753.11
    specified NEC 753.19
  liver, congenital 751.62
  lung 518.89
    congenital 748.4
  mass - *see* Cyst
  mastitis, chronic 610.1
  ovary 620.2
  pancreas, congenital 751.7
Cysticerciasis 123.1
Cysticercosis (mammary) (subretinal)
  123.1
Cysticercus 123.1
  cellulosae infestation 123.1
Cystinosis (malignant) 270.0
Cystinuria 270.0
Cystitis (bacillary) (colli) (diffuse)
      (exudative) (hemorrhagic)
      (purulent) (recurrent) (septic)
      (suppurative) (ulcerative) 595.9
  with
    abortion - *see* Abortion, by type,
      with urinary tract infection
    ectopic pregnancy (*see also*
      categories 633.0–633.9) 639.8
    fibrosis 595.1
    leukoplakia 595.1
    malakoplakia 595.1
    metaplasia 595.1
    molar pregnancy (*see also* categories
      630–632) 639.8

Cystitis *(Continued)*
  actinomycotic 039.8 *[595.4]*
  acute 595.0
    of trigone 595.3
  allergic 595.89
  amebic 006.8 *[595.4]*
  bilharzial 120.9 *[595.4]*
  blennorrhagic (acute) 098.11
    chronic or duration of 2 months or
      more 098.31
  bullous 595.89
  calculous 594.1
  chlamydial 099.53
  chronic 595.2
    interstitial 595.1
    of trigone 595.3
  complicating pregnancy, childbirth, or
    puerperium 646.6 ●
    affecting fetus or newborn 760.1
  cystic(a) 595.81
  diphtheritic 032.84
  echinococcal
    glanulosus 122.3 *[595.4]*
    multilocularis 122.6 *[595.4]*
  emphysematous 595.89
  encysted 595.81
  follicular 595.3
  following
    abortion 639.8
    ectopic or molar pregnancy 639.8
  gangrenous 595.89
  glandularis 595.89
  gonococcal (acute) 098.11
    chronic or duration of 2 months or
      more 098.31
  incrusted 595.89
  interstitial 595.1
  irradiation 595.82
  irritation 595.89
  malignant 595.89
  monilial 112.2
  of trigone 595.3
  panmural 595.1
  polyposa 595.89
  prostatic 601.3
  radiation 595.82
  Reiter's (abacterial) 099.3
  specified NEC 595.89
  subacute 595.2
  submucous 595.1
  syphilitic 095.8
  trichomoniasis 131.09
  tuberculous (*see also* Tuberculosis)
    016.1 ●
  ulcerative 595.1
Cystocele
  female (without uterine prolapse)
    618.01
    with uterine prolapse 618.4
      complete 618.3
      incomplete 618.2
    lateral 618.02
    midline 618.01
    paravaginal 618.02
  in pregnancy or childbirth 654.4 ●
    affecting fetus or newborn 763.89
    causing obstructed labor 660.2 ●
      affecting fetus or newborn 763.1
  male 596.8
Cystoid
  cicatrix limbus 372.64
  degeneration macula 362.53
Cystolithiasis 594.1

Cystoma (M8440/0) - *see also* Neoplasm,
　　by site, benign
　endometrial, ovary 617.1
　mucinous (M8470/0)
　　specified site - *see* Neoplasm, by site,
　　　benign
　　unspecified site 220
　serous (M8441/0)
　　specified site - *see* Neoplasm, by site,
　　　benign
　　unspecified site 220
　simple (ovary) 620.2
Cystoplegia 596.53
Cystoptosis 596.8
Cystopyelitis (*see also* Pyelitis) 590.80
Cystorrhagia 596.8

Cystosarcoma phyllodes (M9020/1) 238.3
　benign (M9020/0) 217
　malignant (M9020/3) - *see* Neoplasm,
　　breast, malignant
Cystostomy status V44.50
　with complication 997.5
　appendico-vesicostomy V44.52
　cutaneous-vesicostomy V44.51
　specified type NEC V44.59
Cystourethritis (*see also* Urethritis) 597.89
Cystourethrocele (*see also* Cystocele)
　female (without uterine prolapse) 618.09
　　with uterine prolapse 618.4
　　　complete 618.3
　　　incomplete 618.2
　male 596.8

Cytomegalic inclusion disease 078.5
　congenital 771.1
Cytomycosis, reticuloendothelial (*see also*
　　Histoplasmosis, American) 115.00
Cytopenia 289.9
　refractory
　　with
　　　multilineage dysplasia (RCMD)
　　　　238.72
　　　and ringed sideroblasts
　　　　(RCMD-RS) 238.72

◀ New ◀ Revised ~~deleted~~ Deleted ● Use Additional Digit(s) Omit code

D

Daae (-Finsen) disease (epidemic pleurodynia) 074.1
Dabney's grip 074.1
Da Costa's syndrome (neurocirculatory asthenia) 306.2
Dacryoadenitis, dacryadenitis 375.00
  acute 375.01
  chronic 375.02
Dacryocystitis 375.30
  acute 375.32
  chronic 375.42
  neonatal 771.6
  phlegmonous 375.33
  syphilitic 095.8
    congenital 090.0
  trachomatous, active 076.1
    late effect 139.1
  tuberculous (see also Tuberculosis) 017.3 ●
Dacryocystoblenorrhea 375.42
Dacryocystocele 375.43
Dacryolith, dacryolithiasis 375.57
Dacryoma 375.43
Dacryopericystitis (acute) (subacute) 375.32
  chronic 375.42
Dacryops 375.11
Dacryosialadenopathy, atrophic 710.2
Dacryostenosis 375.56
  congenital 743.65
Dactylitis
  bone (see also Osteomyelitis) 730.2 ●
  sickle-cell 282.62
    Hb-C 282.64
    Hb-SS 282.62
    specified NEC 282.69
  syphilitic 095.5
  tuberculous (see also Tuberculosis) 015.5 ●
Dactylolysis spontanea 136.0
Dactylosymphysis (see also Syndactylism) 755.10
Damage
  arteriosclerotic - see Arteriosclerosis
  brain 348.9
    anoxic, hypoxic 348.1
      during or resulting from a procedure 997.01
      ischemic, in newborn 768.70 ◀⊪⊪
        mild 768.71 ◀
        moderate 768.72 ◀
        severe 768.73 ◀
    child NEC 343.9
    due to birth injury 767.0
    minimal (child) (see also Hyperkinesia) 314.9
    newborn 767.0
  cardiac - see also Disease, heart
  cardiorenal (vascular) (see also Hypertension, cardiorenal) 404.90
  central nervous system - see Damage, brain
  cerebral NEC - see Damage, brain
  coccyx, complicating delivery 665.6 ●
  coronary (see also Ischemia, heart) 414.9
  eye, birth injury 767.8
  heart - see also Disease, heart
    valve - see Endocarditis
  hypothalamus NEC 348.9
  liver 571.9
    alcoholic 571.3
  medication 995.20
  myocardium (see also Degeneration, myocardial) 429.1
  pelvic

Damage (Continued)
  pelvic (Continued)
    joint or ligament, during delivery 665.6 ●
    organ NEC
      with
        abortion - see Abortion, by type, with damage to pelvic organs
        ectopic pregnancy (see also categories 633.0–633.9) 639.2
        molar pregnancy (see also categories 630–632) 639.2
      during delivery 665.5 ●
      following
        abortion 639.2
        ectopic or molar pregnancy 639.2
  renal (see also Disease, renal) 593.9
  skin, solar 692.79
    acute 692.72
    chronic 692.74
  subendocardium, subendocardial (see also Degeneration, myocardial) 429.1
  vascular 459.9
Dameshek's syndrome (erythroblastic anemia) 282.49
Dana-Putnam syndrome (subacute combined sclerosis with pernicious anemia) 281.0 [336.2]
Danbolt (-Closs) syndrome (acrodermatitis enteropathica) 686.8
Dandruff 690.18
Dandy fever 061
Dandy-Walker deformity or syndrome (atresia, foramen of Magendie) 742.3
  with spina bifida (see also Spina bifida) 741.0 ●
Dangle foot 736.79
Danielssen's disease (anesthetic leprosy) 030.1
Danlos' syndrome 756.83
Darier's disease (congenital) (keratosis follicularis) 757.39
  due to vitamin A deficiency 264.8
  meaning erythema annulare centrifugum 695.0
Darier-Roussy sarcoid 135
Dark area on retina 239.81 ◀
Darling's
  disease (see also Histoplasmosis, American) 115.00
  histoplasmosis (see also Histoplasmosis, American) 115.00
Dartre 054.9
Darwin's tubercle 744.29
Davidson's anemia (refractory) 284.9
Davies' disease 425.0
Davies-Colley syndrome (slipping rib) 733.99
Dawson's encephalitis 046.2
Day blindness (see also Blindness, day) 368.60
Dead
  fetus
    retained (in utero) 656.4 ●
      early pregnancy (death before 22 completed weeks' gestation) 632
      late (death after 22 completed weeks' gestation) 656.4 ●
    syndrome 641.3 ●

Dead (Continued)
  labyrinth 386.50
  ovum, retained 631
Deaf and dumb NEC 389.7
Deaf mutism (acquired) (congenital) NEC 389.7
  endemic 243
  hysterical 300.11
  syphilitic, congenital 090.0
Deafness (acquired) (complete) (congenital) (hereditary) (middle ear) (partial) 389.9
  with
    blindness V49.85
    blue sclera and fragility of bone 756.51
  auditory fatigue 389.9
  aviation 993.0
    nerve injury 951.5
  boilermakers' 951.5
  central 389.14
    with conductive hearing loss 389.20
      bilateral 389.22
      unilateral 389.21
  conductive (air) 389.00
    with sensorineural hearing loss 389.20
      bilateral 389.22
      unilateral 389.21
    bilateral 389.06
    combined types 389.08
    external ear 389.01
    inner ear 389.04
    middle ear 389.03
    multiple types 389.08
    tympanic membrane 389.02
    unilateral 389.05
  emotional (complete) 300.11
  functional (complete) 300.11
  high frequency 389.8
  hysterical (complete) 300.11
  injury 951.5
  low frequency 389.8
  mental 784.69
  mixed conductive and sensorineural 389.20
    bilateral 389.22
    unilateral 389.21
  nerve
    with conductive hearing loss 389.20
      bilateral 389.22
      unilateral 389.21
    bilateral 389.12
    unilateral 389.13
  neural
    with conductive hearing loss 389.20
      bilateral 389.22
      unilateral 389.21
    bilateral 389.12
    unilateral 389.13
  noise-induced 388.12
    nerve injury 951.5
  nonspeaking 389.7
  perceptive 389.10
    with conductive hearing loss 389.20
      bilateral 389.22
      unilateral 389.21
    central 389.14
    neural
      bilateral 389.12
      unilateral 389.13

Deafness *(Continued)*
    perceptive *(Continued)*
        sensorineural 389.10
            asymmetrical 389.16
            bilateral 389.18
            unilateral 389.15
        sensory
            bilateral 389.11
            unilateral 389.17
    psychogenic (complete) 306.7
    sensorineural *(see also* Deafness,
        perceptive) 389.10
        asymmetrical 389.16
        bilateral 389.18
        unilateral 389.15
    sensory
        with conductive hearing loss 389.20
            bilateral 389.22
            unilateral 389.21
        bilateral 389.11
        unilateral 389.17
    specified type NEC 389.8
    sudden NEC 388.2
    syphilitic 094.89
    transient ischemic 388.02
    transmission - *see* Deafness, conductive
    traumatic 951.5
    word (secondary to organic lesion)
        784.69
        developmental 315.31
Death
    after delivery (cause not stated)
        (sudden) 674.9●
    anesthetic
        due to
            correct substance properly
                administered 995.4
            overdose or wrong substance
                given 968.4
            specified anesthetic - *see* Table
                of Drugs and Chemicals
        during delivery 668.9●
    brain 348.89   ◀▥
    cardiac (sudden) (SCD) - *code to*
        underlying condition
        family history of V17.41
        personal history of, successfully
            resuscitated V12.53
    cause unknown 798.2
    cot (infant) 798.0
    crib (infant) 798.0
    fetus, fetal (cause not stated)
        (intrauterine) 779.9
        early, with retention (before 22
            completed weeks' gestation)
            632
        from asphyxia or anoxia (before
            labor) 768.0
            during labor 768.1
        late, affecting management of
            pregnancy (after 22 completed
            weeks' gestation) 656.4●
    from pregnancy NEC 646.9●
    instantaneous 798.1
    intrauterine *(see also* Death, fetus)
        779.9
        complicating pregnancy 656.4●
    maternal, affecting fetus or newborn
        761.6
    neonatal NEC 779.9
    sudden (cause unknown) 798.1
        cardiac (SCD)
            family history of V17.41
            personal history of, successfully
                resuscitated V12.53

Death *(Continued)*
    sudden *(Continued)*
        during delivery 669.9●
            under anesthesia NEC 668.9●
        infant, syndrome (SIDS) 798.0
        puerperal, during puerperium
            674.9●
    unattended (cause unknown) 798.9
    under anesthesia NEC
        due to
            correct substance properly
                administered 995.4
            overdose or wrong substance
                given 968.4
            specified anesthetic - *see*
                Table of Drugs and
                Chemicals
        during delivery 668.9●
    violent 798.1
de Beurmann-Gougerot disease
    (sporotrichosis) 117.1
Debility (general) (infantile)
    (postinfectional) 799.3
    with nutritional difficulty 269.9
    congenital or neonatal NEC 779.9
    nervous 300.5
    old age 797
    senile 797
Débove's disease (splenomegaly) 789.2
Decalcification
    bone *(see also* Osteoporosis) 733.00
    teeth 521.89
Decapitation 874.9
    fetal (to facilitate delivery) 763.89
Decapsulation, kidney 593.89
Decay
    dental 521.00
    senile 797
    tooth, teeth 521.00
Decensus, uterus - *see* Prolapse, uterus
Deciduitis (acute)
    with
        abortion - *see* Abortion, by type,
            with sepsis
        ectopic pregnancy *(see also*
            categories 633.0–633.9)
            639.0
        molar pregnancy *(see also* categories
            630–632) 639.0
    affecting fetus or newborn 760.8
    following
        abortion 639.0
        ectopic or molar pregnancy 639.0
    in pregnancy 646.6●
    puerperal, postpartum 670.1   ◀▥
Deciduoma malignum (M9100/3) 181
Deciduous tooth (retained) 520.6
Decline (general) *(see also* Debility)
    799.3
Decompensation
    cardiac (acute) (chronic) *(see also*
        Disease, heart) 429.9
        failure - *see* Failure, heart
    cardiorenal *(see also* Hypertension,
        cardiorenal) 404.90
    cardiovascular *(see also* Disease,
        cardiovascular) 429.2
    heart *(see also* Disease, heart) 429.9
        failure - *see* Failure, heart
    hepatic 572.2
    myocardial (acute) (chronic) *(see also*
        Disease, heart) 429.9
        failure - *see* Failure, heart
    respiratory 519.9
Decompression sickness 993.3

Decrease, decreased
    blood
        platelets *(see also* Thrombocytopenia)
            287.5
        pressure 796.3
            due to shock following
                injury 958.4
                operation 998.0
        white cell count 288.50
            specified NEC 288.59
    cardiac reserve - *see* Disease, heart
    estrogen 256.39
        postablative 256.2
    fetal movements 655.7●
    fragility of erythrocytes 289.89
    function
        adrenal (cortex) 255.41
            medulla 255.5
        ovary in hypopituitarism 253.4
        parenchyma of pancreas 577.8
        pituitary (gland) (lobe) (anterior)
            253.2
            posterior (lobe) 253.8
    functional activity 780.99
    glucose 790.29
    haptoglobin (serum) NEC 273.8
    leukocytes 288.50
    libido 799.81
    lymphocytes 288.51
    platelets *(see also* Thrombocytopenia)
        287.5
    pulse pressure 785.9
    respiration due to shock following
        injury 958.4
    sexual desire 799.81
    tear secretion NEC 375.15
    tolerance
        fat 579.8
        salt and water 276.9
    vision NEC 369.9
    white blood cell count 288.50
Decubital gangrene *(see also* Ulcer,
    pressure) 707.00 *[785.4]*
Decubiti *(see also* Ulcer, pressure)
    707.00
Decubitus (ulcer) *(see also* Ulcer, pressure)
    707.00
    with gangrene 707.00 *[785.4]*
    ankle 707.06
    back
        lower 707.03
        upper 707.02
    buttock 707.05
    coccyx 707.03   ◀▥
    elbow 707.01
    head 707.09
    heel 707.07
    hip 707.04
    other site 707.09
    sacrum 707.03
    shoulder blades 707.02
Deepening acetabulum 718.85
Defect, defective 759.9
    3-beta-hydroxysteroid dehydrogenase
        255.2
    11-hydroxylase 255.2
    21-hydroxylase 255.2
    abdominal wall, congenital 756.70
    aorticopulmonary septum 745.0
    aortic septal 745.0
    atrial septal (ostium secundum type)
        745.5
        acquired 429.71
        ostium primum type 745.61
        sinus venosus 745.8

◀ New   ◀▥ Revised   ~~deleted~~ Deleted   ● Use Additional Digit(s)   ▥ Omit code

Defect, defective (Continued)
 atrioventricular
  canal 745.69
  septum 745.4
   acquired 429.71
 atrium secundum 745.5
  acquired 429.71
 auricular septal 745.5
  acquired 429.71
 bilirubin excretion 277.4
 biosynthesis, testicular androgen
   257.2
 bridge 525.60
 bulbar septum 745.0
 butanol-insoluble iodide 246.1
 chromosome - see Anomaly,
   chromosome
 circulation (acquired) 459.9
  congenital 747.9
  newborn 747.9
 clotting NEC (see also Defect,
   coagulation) 286.9
 coagulation (factor) (see also
   Deficiency, coagulation factor)
   286.9
  with
   abortion - see Abortion, by type,
    with hemorrhage
   ectopic pregnancy (see also
    categories 634–638)
    639.1
   molar pregnancy (see also
    categories 630–632)
    639.1
  acquired (any) 286.7
  antepartum or intrapartum
    641.3●
   affecting fetus or newborn
    762.1
  causing hemorrhage of pregnancy
    or delivery 641.3●
  complicating pregnancy,
    childbirth, or puerperium
    649.3●
  due to
   liver disease 286.7
   vitamin K deficiency 286.7
  newborn, transient 776.3
  postpartum 666.3●
  specified type NEC 286.9
 conduction (heart) 426.9
  bone (see also Deafness, conductive)
    389.00
 congenital, organ or site NEC - see also
   Anomaly
  circulation 747.9
  Descemet's membrane 743.9
   specified type NEC 743.49
  diaphragm 756.6
  ectodermal 757.9
  esophagus 750.9
  pulmonic cusps - see Anomaly, heart
    valve
  respiratory system 748.9
   specified type NEC 748.8
 crown 525.60
 cushion endocardial 745.60
 dental restoration 525.60
 dentin (hereditary) 520.5
 Descemet's membrane (congenital)
   743.9
  acquired 371.30
  specific type NEC 743.49
 deutan 368.52

Defect, defective (Continued)
 developmental - see also Anomaly, by
   site
  cauda equina 742.59
  left ventricle 746.9
   with atresia or hypoplasia of
    aortic orifice or valve, with
    hypoplasia of ascending
    aorta 746.7
   in hypoplastic left heart
    syndrome 746.7
  testis 752.9
  vessel 747.9
 diaphragm
  with elevation, eventration, or
    hernia - see Hernia, diaphragm
  congenital 756.6
   with elevation, eventration, or
    hernia 756.6
   gross (with elevation,
    eventration, or hernia) 756.6
 ectodermal, congenital 757.9
 Eisenmenger's (ventricular septal
   defect) 745.4
 endocardial cushion 745.60
  specified type NEC 745.69
 esophagus, congenital 750.9
 extensor retinaculum 728.9
 fibrin polymerization (see also Defect,
   coagulation) 286.3
 filling
  biliary tract 793.3
  bladder 793.5
  dental 525.60
  gallbladder 793.3
  kidney 793.5
  stomach 793.4
  ureter 793.5
 fossa ovalis 745.5
 gene, carrier (suspected) of V83.89
 Gerbode 745.4
 glaucomatous, without elevated
   tension 365.89
 Hageman (factor) (see also Defect,
   coagulation) 286.3
 hearing (see also Deafness) 389.9
 high grade 317
 homogentisic acid 270.2
 interatrial septal 745.5
  acquired 429.71
 interauricular septal 745.5
  acquired 429.71
 interventricular septal 745.4
  with pulmonary stenosis or atresia,
    dextraposition of aorta, and
    hypertrophy of right ventricle
    745.2
  acquired 429.71
  in tetralogy of Fallot 745.2
 iodide trapping 246.1
 iodotyrosine dehalogenase 246.1
 kynureninase 270.2
 learning, specific 315.2
 major osseous 731.3
 mental (see also Retardation, mental)
   319
 osseous, major 731.3
 osteochondral NEC 738.8
 ostium
  primum 745.61
  secundum 745.5
 pericardium 746.89
 peroxidase-binding 246.1
 placental blood supply - see Placenta,
   insufficiency
 platelet (qualitative) 287.1
  constitutional 286.4

Defect, defective (Continued)
 postural, spine 737.9
 protan 368.51
 pulmonic cusps, congenital 746.00
 renal pelvis 753.9
  obstructive 753.29
  specified type NEC 753.3
 respiratory system, congenital 748.9
  specified type NEC 748.8
 retina, retinal 361.30
  with detachment (see also
    Detachment, retina, with retinal
    defect) 361.00
  multiple 361.33
   with detachment 361.02
  nerve fiber bundle 362.85
  single 361.30
   with detachment 361.01
 septal (closure) (heart) NEC 745.9
  acquired 429.71
  atrial 745.5
  specified type NEC 745.8
 speech NEC 784.59   ◄▥
  developmental 315.39
  late effect of cerebrovascular disease
    - see Late effect(s) (of)
    cerebrovascular disease,
    speech and language
    deficit   ◄
  secondary to organic lesion 784.59   ◄▥
  Taussig-Bing (transposition, aorta
    and overriding pulmonary
    artery) 745.11
 teeth, wedge 521.20
 thyroid hormone synthesis 246.1
 tritan 368.53
 ureter 753.9
  obstructive 753.29
 vascular (acquired) (local) 459.9
  congenital (peripheral) NEC 747.60
   gastrointestinal 747.61
   lower limb 747.64
   renal 747.62
   specified NEC 747.69
   spinal 747.82
   upper limb 747.63
 ventricular septal 745.4
  with pulmonary stenosis or atresia,
    dextraposition of aorta, and
    hypertrophy of right ventricle
    745.2
  acquired 429.71
  atrioventricular canal type 745.69
  between infundibulum and anterior
    portion 745.4
  in tetralogy of Fallot 745.2
  isolated anterior 745.4
 vision NEC 369.9
 visual field 368.40
  arcuate 368.43
  heteronymous, bilateral 368.47
  homonymous, bilateral 368.46
  localized NEC 368.44
  nasal step 368.44
  peripheral 368.44
  sector 368.43
 voice and resonance 784.40   ◄▥
 wedge, teeth (abrasion) 521.20
Defeminization syndrome 255.2
Deferentitis 608.4
 gonorrheal (acute) 098.14
  chronic or duration of 2 months or
    over 098.34
Defibrination syndrome (see also
   Fibrinolysis) 286.6

Deficiency, deficient
  3-beta-hydroxysteroid dehydrogenase
    255.2
  6-phosphogluconic dehydrogenase
    (anemia) 282.2
  11-beta-hydroxylase 255.2
  17-alpha-hydroxylase 255.2
  18-hydroxysteroid dehydrogenase
    255.2
  20-alpha-hydroxylase 255.2
  21-hydroxylase 255.2
  AAT (alpha-1 antitrypsin) 273.4
  abdominal muscle syndrome 756.79
  accelerator globulin (Ac G) (blood) (*see
    also* Defect, coagulation) 286.3
  AC globulin (congenital) (*see also*
    Defect, coagulation) 286.3
    acquired 286.7
  activating factor (blood) (*see also* Defect,
    coagulation) 286.3
  adenohypophyseal 253.2
  adenosine deaminase 277.2
  aldolase (hereditary) 271.2
  alpha-1-antitrypsin 273.4
  alpha-1-trypsin inhibitor 273.4
  alpha-fucosidase 271.8
  alpha-lipoprotein 272.5
  alpha-mannosidase 271.8
  amino acid 270.9
  anemia - *see* Anemia, deficiency
  aneurin 265.1
    with beriberi 265.0
  antibody NEC 279.00
  antidiuretic hormone 253.5
  antihemophilic
    factor (A) 286.0
      B 286.1
      C 286.2
    globulin (AHG) NEC 286.0
  antithrombin III 289.81
  antitrypsin 273.4
  argininosuccinate synthetase or lyase
    270.6
  ascorbic acid (with scurvy) 267
  autoprothrombin
    I (*see also* Defect, coagulation) 286.3
    II 286.1
    C (*see also* Defect, coagulation)
      286.3
  bile salt 579.8
  biotin 266.2
  biotinidase 277.6
  bradykinase-1 277.6
  brancher enzyme (amylopectinosis)
    271.0
  calciferol 268.9
    with
      osteomalacia 268.2
      rickets (*see also* Rickets) 268.0
  calcium 275.40
    dietary 269.3
  calorie, severe 261
  carbamyl phosphate synthetase 270.6
  cardiac (*see also* Insufficiency,
    myocardial) 428.0
  carnitine 277.81
    due to
      hemodialysis 277.83
      inborn errors of metabolism
        277.82
      valproic acid therapy 277.83
    iatrogenic 277.83
    palmitoyltransferase (CPT1, CPT2)
      277.85

Deficiency, deficient (*Continued*)
  carnitine (*Continued*)
    palmityl transferase (CPT1, CPT2)
      277.85
    primary 277.81
    secondary 277.84
  carotene 264.9
  Carr factor (*see also* Defect, coagulation)
    286.9
  central nervous system 349.9
  ceruloplasmin 275.1
  cevitamic acid (with scurvy) 267
  choline 266.2
  Christmas factor 286.1
  chromium 269.3
  citrin 269.1
  clotting (blood) (*see also* Defect,
    coagulation) 286.9
  coagulation factor NEC 286.9
    with
      abortion - *see* Abortion, by type,
        with hemorrhage
      ectopic pregnancy (*see also*
        categories 634–638) 639.1
      molar pregnancy (*see also*
        categories 630–632) 639.1
    acquired (any) 286.7
    antepartum or intrapartum 641.3●
      affecting fetus or newborn
        762.1
    complicating pregnancy,
      childbirth, or puerperium
      649.3●
    due to
      liver disease 286.7
      vitamin K deficiency 286.7
    newborn, transient 776.3
    postpartum 666.3●
    specified type NEC 286.3
  color vision (congenital) 368.59
    acquired 368.55
  combined glucocorticoid and
    mineralocorticoid 255.41
  combined, two or more coagulation
    factors (*see also* Defect,
    coagulation) 286.9
  complement factor NEC 279.8
  contact factor (*see also* Defect,
    coagulation) 286.3
  copper NEC 275.1
  corticoadrenal 255.41
  craniofacial axis 756.0
  cyanocobalamin (vitamin B$_{12}$) 266.2
  debrancher enzyme (limit dextrinosis)
    271.0
  desmolase 255.2
  diet 269.9
  dihydrofolate reductase 281.2
  dihydropteridine reductase 270.1
  disaccharidase (intestinal) 271.3
  disease NEC 269.9
  ear(s) V48.8
  edema 262
  endocrine 259.9
  enzymes, circulating NEC (*see also*
    Deficiency, by specific enzyme)
    277.6
  ergosterol 268.9
    with
      osteomalacia 268.2
      rickets (*see also* Rickets) 268.0
  erythrocytic glutathione (anemia)
    282.2
  eyelid(s) V48.8

Deficiency, deficient (*Continued*)
  factor (*see also* Defect, coagulation)
    286.9
    I (congenital) (fibrinogen) 286.3
      antepartum or intrapartum
        641.3●
      affecting fetus or newborn
        762.1
      newborn, transient 776.3
      postpartum 666.3●
    II (congenital) (prothrombin) 286.3
    V (congenital) (labile) 286.3
    VII (congenital) (stable) 286.3
    VIII (congenital) (functional) 286.0
      with
        functional defect 286.0
        vascular defect 286.4
    IX (Christmas) (congenital)
      (functional) 286.1
    X (congenital) (Stuart-Prower) 286.3
    XI (congenital) (plasma
      thromboplastin antecedent)
      286.2
    XII (congenital) (Hageman) 286.3
    XIII (congenital) (fibrin stabilizing)
      286.3
    Hageman 286.3
    multiple (congenital) 286.9
      acquired 286.7
  fibrinase (*see also* Defect, coagulation)
    286.3
  fibrinogen (congenital) (*see also* Defect,
    coagulation) 286.3
    acquired 286.6
  fibrin-stabilizing factor (congenital) (*see
    also* Defect, coagulation) 286.3
    acquired 286.7
  finger - *see* Absence, finger
  fletcher factor (*see also* Defect,
    coagulation) 286.9
  fluorine 269.3
  folate, anemia 281.2
  folic acid (vitamin B$_c$) 266.2
    anemia 281.2
  follicle-stimulating hormone (FSH)
    253.4
  fructokinase 271.2
  fructose-1, 6-diphosphate 271.2
  fructose-1-phosphate aldolase 271.2
  FSH (follicle-stimulating hormone)
    253.4
  fucosidase 271.8
  galactokinase 271.1
  galactose-1-phosphate uridyl
    transferase 271.1
  gamma globulin in blood 279.00
  glass factor (*see also* Defect,
    coagulation) 286.3
  glucocorticoid 255.41
  glucose-6-phosphatase 271.0
  glucose-6-phosphate dehydrogenase
    anemia 282.2
  glucuronyl transferase 277.4
  glutathione-reductase (anemia) 282.2
  glycogen synthetase 271.0
  growth hormone 253.3
  Hageman factor (congenital) (*see also*
    Defect, coagulation) 286.3
  head V48.0
  hemoglobin (*see also* Anemia) 285.9
  hepatophosphorylase 271.0
  hexose monophosphate (HMP) shunt
    282.2
  HGH (human growth hormone) 253.3

◄ New   ◄ Revised   ~~deleted~~ Deleted   ● Use Additional Digit(s)   ▓ Omit code

Deficiency, deficient (*Continued*)
 HG-PRT 277.2
 homogentisic acid oxidase 270.2
 hormone - *see also* Deficiency, by
   specific hormone
   anterior pituitary (isolated) (partial)
     NEC 253.4
     growth (human) 253.3
   follicle-stimulating 253.4
   growth (human) (isolated) 253.3
   human growth 253.3
   interstitial cell-stimulating 253.4
   luteinizing 253.4
   melanocyte-stimulating 253.4
   testicular 257.2
 human growth hormone 253.3
 humoral 279.00
   with
     hyper-IgM 279.05
       autosomal recessive 279.05
       X-linked 279.05
     increased IgM 279.05
     congenital hypogammaglobulinemia
       279.04
     non-sex-linked 279.06
     selective immunoglobulin NEC
       279.03
       IgA 279.01
       IgG 279.03
       IgM 279.02
         increased 279.05
   specified NEC 279.09
 hydroxylase 255.2
 hypoxanthine-guanine
   phosphoribosyltransferase
   (HG-PRT) 277.2
 ICSH (interstitial cell-stimulating
   hormone) 253.4
 immunity NEC 279.3
   cell-mediated 279.10
     with
       hyperimmunoglobulinemia
         279.2
       thrombocytopenia and eczema
         279.12
     specified NEC 279.19
   combined (severe) 279.2
     syndrome 279.2
   common variable 279.06
   humoral NEC 279.00
     IgA (secretory) 279.01
     IgG 279.03
     IgM 279.02
 immunoglobulin, selective NEC 279.03
   IgA 279.01
   IgG 279.03
   IgM 279.02
 inositol (B complex) 266.2
 interferon 279.49   ◄▥
 internal organ V47.0
 interstitial cell-stimulating hormone
   (ICSH) 253.4
 intrinsic factor (Castle's) (congenital)
   281.0
 intrinsic (urethral) sphincter (ISD)
   599.82
 invertase 271.3
 iodine 269.3
 iron, anemia 280.9
 labile factor (congenital) (*see also*
   Defect, coagulation) 286.3
   acquired 286.7
 lacrimal fluid (acquired) 375.15
   congenital 743.64

Deficiency, deficient (*Continued*)
 lactase 271.3
 Laki-Lorand factor (*see also* Defect,
   coagulation) 286.3
 lecithin-cholesterol acyltranferase
   272.5
 LH (luteinizing hormone) 253.4
 limb V49.0
   lower V49.0
     congenital (*see also* Deficiency,
       lower limb, congenital)
       755.30
   upper V49.0
     congenital (*see also* Deficiency,
       upper limb, congenital)
       755.20
 lipocaic 577.8
 lipoid (high-density) 272.5
 lipoprotein (familial) (high-density)
   272.5
 liver phosphorylase 271.0
 long chain 3-hydroxyacyl CoA
   dehydrogenase (LCHAD) 277.85
 long chain/very long chain acyl CoA
   dehydrogenase (LCAD, VLCAD)
   277.85
 lower limb V49.0
   congenital 755.30
     with complete absence of distal
       elements 755.31
     longitudinal (complete) (partial)
       (with distal deficiencies,
       incomplete) 755.32
       with complete absence of
         distal elements 755.31
       combined femoral, tibial,
         fibular (incomplete)
         755.33
       femoral 755.34
       fibular 755.37
       metatarsal(s) 755.38
       phalange(s) 755.39
         meaning all digits 755.31
       tarsal(s) 755.38
       tibia 755.36
       tibiofibular 755.35
     transverse 755.31
 luteinizing hormone (LH) 253.4
 lysosomal alpha-1, 4 glucosidase
   271.0
 magnesium 275.2
 mannosidase 271.8
 medium chain acyl CoA
   dehydrogenase (MCAD) 277.85
 melanocyte-stimulating hormone
   (MSH) 253.4
 menadione (vitamin K) 269.0
   newborn 776.0
 mental (familial) (hereditary) (*see also*
   Retardation, mental) 319
 methylenetetrahydrofolate reductase
   (MTHFR) 270.4
 mineral NEC 269.3
 mineralocorticoid 255.42
 molybdenum 269.3
 moral 301.7
 multiple, syndrome 260
 myocardial (*see also* Insufficiency,
   myocardial) 428.0
 myophosphorylase 271.0
 NADH (DPNH)-methemoglobin-
   reductase (congenital) 289.7
 NADH diaphorase or reductase
   (congenital) 289.7

Deficiency, deficient (*Continued*)
 neck V48.1
 niacin (amide) (-tryptophan) 265.2
 nicotinamide 265.2
 nicotinic acid (amide) 265.2
 nose V48.8
 number of teeth (*see also* Anodontia)
   520.0
 nutrition, nutritional 269.9
   specified NEC 269.8
 ornithine transcarbamylase 270.6
 ovarian 256.39
 oxygen (*see also* Anoxia) 799.02
 pantothenic acid 266.2
 parathyroid (gland) 252.1
 phenylalanine hydroxylase 270.1
 phosphoenolpyruvate carboxykinase
   271.8
 phosphofructokinase 271.2
 phosphoglucomutase 271.0
 phosphohexosisomerase 271.0
 phosphomannomutase 271.8
 phosphomannose isomerase 271.8
 phosphomannosyl mutase 271.8
 phosphorylase kinase, liver 271.0
 pituitary (anterior) 253.2
   posterior 253.5
 placenta - *see* Placenta, insufficiency
 plasma
   cell 279.00
     protein (paraproteinemia)
       (pyroglobulinemia) 273.8
     gamma globulin 279.00
   thromboplastin
     antecedent (PTA) 286.2
     component (PTC) 286.1
 platelet NEC 287.1
   constitutional 286.4
 polyglandular 258.9
 potassium (K) 276.8
 proaccelerin (congenital) (*see also*
   Defect, congenital) 286.3
   acquired 286.7
 proconvertin factor (congenital) (*see
   also* Defect, coagulation) 286.3
   acquired 286.7
 prolactin 253.4
 protein 260
   anemia 281.4
   C 289.81
   plasma - *see* Deficiency, plasma,
     protein
   S 289.81
 prothrombin (congenital) (*see also*
   Defect, coagulation) 286.3
   acquired 286.7
 Prower factor (*see also* Defect,
   coagulation) 286.3
 PRT 277.2
 pseudocholinesterase 289.89
 psychobiological 301.6
 PTA 286.2
 PTC 286.1
 purine nucleoside phosphorylase 277.2
 pyracin (alpha) (beta) 266.1
 pyridoxal 266.1
 pyridoxamine 266.1
 pyridoxine (derivatives) 266.1
 pyruvate carboxylase 271.8
 pyruvate dehydrogenase 271.8
 pyruvate kinase (PK) 282.3
 riboflavin (vitamin B_2) 266.0
 saccadic eye movements 379.57
 salivation 527.7

Deficiency, deficient (Continued)
salt 276.1
secretion
ovary 256.39
salivary gland (any) 527.7
urine 788.5
selenium 269.3
serum
antitrypsin, familial 273.4
protein (congenital) 273.8
short chain acyl CoA dehydrogenase (SCAD) 277.85
short stature homeobox gene (SHOX)
with
dyschondrosteosis 756.89
short stature (idiopathic) 783.43
Turner's syndrome 758.6
smooth pursuit movements (eye) 379.58
sodium (Na) 276.1
SPCA (see also Defect, coagulation) 286.3
specified NEC 269.8
stable factor (congenital) (see also Defect, coagulation) 286.3
acquired 286.7
Stuart (-Prower) factor (see also Defect, coagulation) 286.3
sucrase 271.3
sucrase-isomaltase 271.3
sulfite oxidase 270.0
syndrome, multiple 260
thiamine, thiaminic (chloride) 265.1
thrombokinase (see also Defect, coagulation) 286.3
newborn 776.0
thrombopoieten 287.39
thymolymphatic 279.2
thyroid (gland) 244.9
tocopherol 269.1
toe - see Absence, toe
tooth bud (see also Anodontia) 520.0
trunk V48.1
UDPG-glycogen transferase 271.0
upper limb V49.0
congenital 755.20
with complete absence of distal elements 755.21
longitudinal (complete) (partial) (with distal deficiencies, incomplete) 755.22
carpal(s) 755.28
combined humeral, radial, ulnar (incomplete) 755.23
humeral 755.24
metacarpal(s) 755.28
phalange(s) 755.29
meaning all digits 755.21
radial 755.26
radioulnar 755.25
ulnar 755.27
transverse (complete) (partial) 755.21
vascular 459.9
vasopressin 253.5
viosterol (see also Deficiency, calciferol) 268.9
vitamin (multiple) NEC 269.2
A 264.9
with
Bitôt's spot 264.1
corneal 264.2
with corneal ulceration 264.3

Deficiency, deficient (Continued)
vitamin (Continued)
A (Continued)
with (Continued)
keratomalacia 264.4
keratosis, follicular 264.8
night blindness 264.5
scar of cornea, xerophthalmic 264.6
specified manifestation NEC 264.8
ocular 264.7
xeroderma 264.8
xerophthalmia 264.7
xerosis
conjunctival 264.0
with Bitôt's spot 264.1
corneal 264.2
with corneal ulceration 264.3
B (complex) NEC 266.9
with
beriberi 265.0
pellagra 265.2
specified type NEC 266.2
B_1 NEC 265.1
beriberi 265.0
B_2 266.0
B_6 266.1
B_{12} 266.2
B_C (folic acid) 266.2
C (ascorbic acid) (with scurvy) 267
D (calciferol) (ergosterol) 268.9
with
osteomalacia 268.2
rickets (see also Rickets) 268.0
E 269.1
folic acid 266.2
G 266.0
H 266.2
K 269.0
of newborn 776.0
nicotinic acid 265.2
P 269.1
PP 265.2
specified NEC 269.1
zinc 269.3
Deficient - see also Deficiency
blink reflex 374.45
craniofacial axis 756.0
number of teeth (see also Anodontia) 520.0
secretion of urine 788.5
Deficit
neurologic NEC 781.99
due to
cerebrovascular lesion (see also Disease, cerebrovascular, acute) 436
late effect - see Late effect(s) (of) cerebrovascular disease
transient ischemic attack 435.9
ischemic
reversible (RIND) 434.91
history of (personal) V12.54
prolonged (PRIND) 434.91
history of (personal) V12.54
oxygen 799.02
Deflection
radius 736.09
septum (acquired) (nasal) (nose) 470
spine - see Curvature, spine
turbinate (nose) 470

Defluvium
capillorum (see also Alopecia) 704.00
ciliorum 374.55
unguium 703.8
Deformity 738.9
abdomen, congenital 759.9
abdominal wall
acquired 738.8
congenital 756.70
muscle deficiency syndrome 756.79
acquired (unspecified site) 738.9
specified site NEC 738.8
adrenal gland (congenital) 759.1
alimentary tract, congenital 751.9
lower 751.5
specified type NEC 751.8
upper (any part, except tongue) 750.9
specified type NEC 750.8
tongue 750.10
specified type NEC 750.19
ankle (joint) (acquired) 736.70
abduction 718.47
congenital 755.69
contraction 718.47
specified NEC 736.79
anus (congenital) 751.5
acquired 569.49
aorta (congenital) 747.20
acquired 447.8
arch 747.21
acquired 447.8
coarctation 747.10
aortic
arch 747.21
acquired 447.8
cusp or valve (congenital) 746.9
acquired (see also Endocarditis, aortic) 424.1
ring 747.21
appendix 751.5
arm (acquired) 736.89
congenital 755.50
arteriovenous (congenital) (peripheral) NEC 747.60
gastrointestinal 747.61
lower limb 747.64
renal 747.62
specified NEC 747.69
spinal 747.82
upper limb 747.63
artery (congenital) (peripheral) NEC (see also Deformity, vascular) 747.60
acquired 447.8
cerebral 747.81
coronary (congenital) 746.85
acquired (see also Ischemia, heart) 414.9
retinal 743.9
umbilical 747.5
atrial septal (congenital) (heart) 745.5
auditory canal (congenital) (external) (see also Deformity, ear) 744.3
acquired 380.50
auricle
ear (congenital) (see also Deformity, ear) 744.3
acquired 380.32
heart (congenital) 746.9
back (acquired) - see Deformity, spine
Bartholin's duct (congenital) 750.9

◀ New　◀▥ Revised　~~deleted~~ Deleted　● Use Additional Digit(s)　▨ Omit code

Deformity (Continued)
  bile duct (congenital) 751.60
    acquired 576.8
      with calculus, choledocholithiasis,
        or stones - see
        Choledocholithiasis
  biliary duct or passage (congenital)
    751.60
    acquired 576.8
      with calculus, choledocholithiasis,
        or stones - see
        Choledocholithiasis
  bladder (neck) (sphincter) (trigone)
    (acquired) 596.8
    congenital 753.9
  bone (acquired) NEC 738.9
    congenital 756.9
    turbinate 738.0
  boutonniere (finger) 736.21
  brain (congenital) 742.9
    acquired 348.89   ◄▦
      multiple 742.4
      reduction 742.2
      vessel (congenital) 747.81
  breast (acquired) 611.89
    congenital 757.6   ◄▦
    reconstructed 612.0
  bronchus (congenital) 748.3
    acquired 519.19
  bursa, congenital 756.9
  canal of Nuck 752.9
  canthus (congenital) 743.9
    acquired 374.89
  capillary (acquired) 448.9
    congenital NEC (see also Deformity,
      vascular) 747.60
  cardiac - see Deformity, heart
  cardiovascular system (congenital)
    746.9
  caruncle, lacrimal (congenital)
    743.9
    acquired 375.69
  cascade, stomach 537.6
  cecum (congenital) 751.5
    acquired 569.89
  cerebral (congenital) 742.9
    acquired 348.89   ◄▦
  cervix (acquired) (uterus) 622.8
    congenital 752.40
  cheek (acquired) 738.19
    congenital 744.9
  chest (wall) (acquired) 738.3
    congenital 754.89
    late effect of rickets 268.1
  chin (acquired) 738.19
    congenital 744.9
  choroid (congenital) 743.9
    acquired 363.8
    plexus (congenital) 742.9
      acquired 349.2
  cicatricial - see Cicatrix
  cilia (congenital) 743.9
    acquired 374.89
  circulatory system (congenital)
    747.9
  clavicle (acquired) 738.8
    congenital 755.51
  clitoris (congenital) 752.40
    acquired 624.8
  clubfoot - see Clubfoot
  coccyx (acquired) 738.6
    congenital 756.10
  colon (congenital) 751.5
    acquired 569.89

Deformity (Continued)
  concha (ear) (congenital) (see also
    Deformity, ear) 744.3
    acquired 380.32
  congenital, organ or site not listed (see
    also Anomaly) 759.9
  cornea (congenital) 743.9
    acquired 371.70
  coronary artery (congenital) 746.85
    acquired (see also Ischemia, heart)
      414.9
  cranium (acquired) 738.19
    congenital (see also Deformity, skull,
      congenital) 756.0
  cricoid cartilage (congenital) 748.3
    acquired 478.79
  cystic duct (congenital) 751.60
    acquired 575.8
  Dandy-Walker 742.3
    with spina bifida (see also Spina
      bifida) 741.0●
  diaphragm (congenital) 756.6
    acquired 738.8
  digestive organ(s) or system
    (congenital) NEC 751.9
    specified type NEC 751.8
  ductus arteriosus 747.0
  duodenal bulb 537.89
  duodenum (congenital) 751.5
    acquired 537.89
  dura (congenital) 742.9
    brain 742.4
      acquired 349.2
    spinal 742.59
      acquired 349.2
  ear (congenital) 744.3
    acquired 380.32
    auricle 744.3
      causing impairment of hearing
        744.02
      causing impairment of hearing
        744.00
    external 744.3
      causing impairment of hearing
        744.02
    internal 744.05
    lobule 744.3
    middle 744.03
      ossicles 744.04
    ossicles 744.04
  ectodermal (congenital) NEC 757.9
    specified type NEC 757.8
  ejaculatory duct (congenital) 752.9
    acquired 608.89
  elbow (joint) (acquired) 736.00
    congenital 755.50
    contraction 718.42
  endocrine gland NEC 759.2
  epididymis (congenital) 752.9
    acquired 608.89
    torsion 608.24
  epiglottis (congenital) 748.3
    acquired 478.79
  esophagus (congenital) 750.9
    acquired 530.89
  Eustachian tube (congenital) NEC
    744.3
    specified type NEC 744.24
  extremity (acquired) 736.9
    congenital, except reduction
      deformity 755.9
    lower 755.60
    upper 755.50
  reduction - see Deformity, reduction

Deformity (Continued)
  eye (congenital) 743.9
    acquired 379.8
    muscle 743.9
  eyebrow (congenital) 744.89
  eyelid (congenital) 743.9
    acquired 374.89
    specified type NEC 743.62
  face (acquired) 738.19
    congenital (any part) 744.9
      due to intrauterine malposition
        and pressure 754.0
  fallopian tube (congenital) 752.10
    acquired 620.8
  femur (acquired) 736.89
    congenital 755.60
  fetal
    with fetopelvic disproportion
      653.7●
        affecting fetus or newborn 763.1
      causing obstructed labor 660.1●
        affecting fetus or newborn 763.1
    known or suspected, affecting
      management of pregnancy
      655.9●
  finger (acquired) 736.20
    boutonniere type 736.21
    congenital 755.50
    flexion contracture 718.44
    swan neck 736.22
  flexion (joint) (acquired) 736.9
    congenital NEC 755.9
    hip or thigh (acquired) 736.39
      congenital (see also Subluxation,
        congenital, hip) 754.32
  foot (acquired) 736.70
    cavovarus 736.75
      congenital 754.59
    congenital NEC 754.70
      specified type NEC 754.79
    valgus (acquired) 736.79
      congenital 754.60
        specified type NEC 754.69
    varus (acquired) 736.79
      congenital 754.50
        specified type NEC 754.59
  forearm (acquired) 736.00
    congenital 755.50
  forehead (acquired) 738.19
    congenital (see also Deformity, skull,
      congenital) 756.0
  frontal bone (acquired) 738.19
    congenital (see also Deformity, skull,
      congenital) 756.0
  gallbladder (congenital) 751.60
    acquired 575.8
  gastrointestinal tract (congenital) NEC
    751.9
    acquired 569.89
    specified type NEC 751.8
  genitalia, genital organ(s) or system
    NEC
    congenital 752.9
    female (congenital) 752.9
      acquired 629.89
      external 752.40
      internal 752.9
    male (congenital) 752.9
      acquired 608.89
  globe (eye) (congenital) 743.9
    acquired 360.89
  gum (congenital) 750.9
    acquired 523.9
  gunstock 736.02

Deformity *(Continued)*
  hand (acquired) 736.00
    claw 736.06
    congenital 755.50
    minus (and plus) (intrinsic) 736.09
    pill roller (intrinsic) 736.09
    plus (and minus) (intrinsic) 736.09
    swan neck (intrinsic) 736.09
  head (acquired) 738.10
    congenital (*see also* Deformity, skull,
      congenital) 756.0
    specified NEC 738.19
  heart (congenital) 746.9
    auricle (congenital) 746.9
    septum 745.9
      auricular 745.5
      specified type NEC 745.8
      ventricular 745.4
    valve (congenital) NEC 746.9
      acquired - *see* Endocarditis
      pulmonary (congenital) 746.00
      specified type NEC 746.89
    ventricle (congenital) 746.9
  heel (acquired) 736.76
    congenital 755.67
  hepatic duct (congenital) 751.60
    acquired 576.8
      with calculus, choledocholithiasis,
        or stones - *see*
        Choledocholithiasis
  hip (joint) (acquired) 736.30
    congenital NEC 755.63
    flexion 718.45
      congenital (*see also* Subluxation,
        congenital, hip) 754.32
  hourglass - *see* Contraction, hourglass
  humerus (acquired) 736.89
    congenital 755.50
  hymen (congenital) 752.40
  hypophyseal (congenital) 759.2
  ileocecal (coil) (valve) (congenital)
    751.5
    acquired 569.89
  ileum (intestine) (congenital) 751.5
    acquired 569.89
  ilium (acquired) 738.6
    congenital 755.60
  integument (congenital) 757.9
  intervertebral cartilage or disc
    (acquired) - *see also* Displacement,
    intervertebral disc
    congenital 756.10
  intestine (large) (small) (congenital)
    751.5
    acquired 569.89
  iris (acquired) 364.75
    congenital 743.9
    prolapse 364.89
  ischium (acquired) 738.6
    congenital 755.60
  jaw (acquired) (congenital) NEC 524.9
    due to intrauterine malposition and
      pressure 754.0
  joint (acquired) NEC 738.8
    congenital 755.9
    contraction (abduction) (adduction)
      (extension) (flexion) - *see*
      Contraction, joint
  kidney(s) (calyx) (pelvis) (congenital)
    753.9
    acquired 593.89
    vessel 747.62
      acquired 459.9
  Klippel-Feil (brevicollis) 756.16

Deformity *(Continued)*
  knee (acquired) NEC 736.6
    congenital 755.64
  labium (majus) (minus) (congenital)
    752.40
    acquired 624.8
  lacrimal apparatus or duct (congenital)
    743.9
    acquired 375.69
  larynx (muscle) (congenital)
    748.3
    acquired 478.79
    web (glottic) (subglottic) 748.2
  leg (lower) (upper) (acquired) NEC
    736.89
    congenital 755.60
    reduction - *see* Deformity,
      reduction, lower limb
  lens (congenital) 743.9
    acquired 379.39
  lid (fold) (congenital) 743.9
    acquired 374.89
  ligament (acquired) 728.9
    congenital 756.9
  limb (acquired) 736.9
    congenital, except reduction
      deformity 755.9
      lower 755.60
        reduction (*see also*
          Deformity, reduction,
          lower limb) 755.30
      upper 755.50
        reduction (*see also*
          Deformity, reduction,
          lower limb) 755.20
    specified NEC 736.89
  lip (congenital) NEC 750.9
    acquired 528.5
    specified type NEC 750.26
  liver (congenital) 751.60
    acquired 573.8
    duct (congenital) 751.60
      acquired 576.8
        with calculus,
          choledocholithiasis,
          or stones - *see*
          Choledocholithiasis
  lower extremity - *see* Deformity, leg
  lumbosacral (joint) (region)
    (congenital) 756.10
    acquired 738.5
  lung (congenital) 748.60
    acquired 518.89
    specified type NEC 748.69
  lymphatic system, congenital
    759.9
  Madelung's (radius) 755.54
  maxilla (acquired) (congenital)
    524.9
  meninges or membrane (congenital)
    742.9
    brain 742.4
      acquired 349.2
    spinal (cord) 742.59
      acquired 349.2
  mesentery (congenital) 751.9
    acquired 568.89
  metacarpus (acquired) 736.00
    congenital 755.50
  metatarsus (acquired) 736.70
    congenital 754.70
  middle ear, except ossicles (congenital)
    744.03
    ossicles 744.04

Deformity *(Continued)*
  mitral (leaflets) (valve) (congenital)
    746.9
    acquired - *see* Endocarditis, mitral
    Ebstein's 746.89
    parachute 746.5
    specified type NEC 746.89
    stenosis, congenital 746.5
  mouth (acquired) 528.9
    congenital NEC 750.9
      specified type NEC 750.26
  multiple, congenital NEC 759.7
    specified type NEC 759.89
  muscle (acquired) 728.9
    congenital 756.9
      specified type NEC 756.89
      sternocleidomastoid (due to
        intrauterine malposition
        and pressure) 754.1
  musculoskeletal system, congenital
    NEC 756.9
    specified type NEC 756.9
  nail (acquired) 703.9
    congenital 757.9
  nasal - *see* Deformity, nose
  neck (acquired) NEC 738.2
    congenital (any part) 744.9
      sternocleidomastoid 754.1
  nervous system (congenital) 742.9
  nipple (congenital) 757.6
    acquired 611.89
  nose, nasal (cartilage) (acquired) 738.0
    bone (turbinate) 738.0
    congenital 748.1
      bent 754.0
      squashed 754.0
    saddle 738.0
      syphilitic 090.5
    septum 470
      congenital 748.1
    sinus (wall) (congenital) 748.1
      acquired 738.0
    syphilitic (congenital) 090.5
      late 095.8
  ocular muscle (congenital) 743.9
    acquired 378.60
  opticociliary vessels (congenital) 743.9
  orbit (congenital) (eye) 743.9
    acquired NEC 376.40
      associated with craniofacial
        deformities 376.44
      due to
        bone disease 376.43
        surgery 376.47
        trauma 376.47
  organ of Corti (congenital) 744.05
  ovary (congenital) 752.0
    acquired 620.8
  oviduct (congenital) 752.10
    acquired 620.8
  palate (congenital) 750.9
    acquired 526.89
    cleft (congenital) (*see also* Cleft,
      palate) 749.00
    hard, acquired 526.89
    soft, acquired 528.9
  pancreas (congenital) 751.7
    acquired 577.8
  parachute, mitral valve 746.5
  parathyroid (gland) 759.2
  parotid (gland) (congenital) 750.9
    acquired 527.8
  patella (acquired) 736.6
    congenital 755.64

◄ New   ⬅ Revised   ~~deleted~~ Deleted   ● Use Additional Digit(s)   ▨ Omit code

Deformity *(Continued)*
  pelvis, pelvic (acquired) (bony) 738.6
    with disproportion (fetopelvic)
      653.0 ●
      affecting fetus or newborn 763.1
      causing obstructed labor 660.1 ●
        affecting fetus or newborn
          763.1
    congenital 755.60
    rachitic (late effect) 268.1
  penis (glans) (congenital) 752.9
    acquired 607.89
  pericardium (congenital) 746.9
    acquired - *see* Pericarditis
  pharynx (congenital) 750.9
    acquired 478.29
  Pierre Robin (congenital) 756.0
  pinna (acquired) 380.32
    congenital 744.3
  pituitary (congenital) 759.2
  pleural folds (congenital) 748.8
  portal vein (congenital) 747.40
  posture - *see* Curvature, spine
  prepuce (congenital) 752.9
    acquired 607.89
  prostate (congenital) 752.9
    acquired 602.8
  pulmonary valve - *see* Endocarditis,
    pulmonary
  pupil (congenital) 743.9
    acquired 364.75
  pylorus (congenital) 750.9
    acquired 537.89
  rachitic (acquired), healed or old 268.1
  radius (acquired) 736.00
    congenital 755.50
      reduction - *see* Deformity,
        reduction, upper limb
  rectovaginal septum (congenital)
    752.40
    acquired 623.8
  rectum (congenital) 751.5
    acquired 569.49
  reduction (extremity) (limb) 755.4
    brain 742.2
    lower limb 755.30
      with complete absence of distal
        elements 755.31
      longitudinal (complete) (partial)
        (with distal deficiencies,
        incomplete) 755.32
        with complete absence of
          distal elements 755.31
        combined femoral, tibial,
          fibular (incomplete)
          755.33
        femoral 755.34
        fibular 755.37
        metatarsal(s) 755.38
        phalange(s) 755.39
          meaning all digits 755.31
        tarsal(s) 755.38
        tibia 755.36
        tibiofibular 755.35
        transverse 755.31
    upper limb 755.20
      with complete absence of distal
        elements 755.21
      longitudinal (complete) (partial)
        (with distal deficiencies,
        incomplete) 755.22
        with complete absence of
          distal elements 755.21
        carpal(s) 755.28

Deformity *(Continued)*
  reduction *(Continued)*
    upper limb *(Continued)*
      longitudinal *(Continued)*
        combined humeral, radial,
          ulnar (incomplete) 755.23
        humeral 755.24
        metacarpal(s) 755.28
        phalange(s) 755.29
          meaning all digits 755.21
        radial 755.26
        radioulnar 755.25
        ulnar 755.27
      transverse (complete) (partial)
        755.21
    renal - *see* Deformity, kidney
  respiratory system (congenital) 748.9 ●
    specified type NEC 748.8
  rib (acquired) 738.3
    congenital 756.3
    cervical 756.2
  rotation (joint) (acquired) 736.9
    congenital 755.9
    hip or thigh 736.39
      congenital (*see also* Subluxation,
        congenital, hip) 754.32
  sacroiliac joint (congenital) 755.69
    acquired 738.5
  sacrum (acquired) 738.5
    congenital 756.10
  saddle
    back 737.8
    nose 738.0
      syphilitic 090.5
  salivary gland or duct (congenital)
    750.9
    acquired 527.8
  scapula (acquired) 736.89
    congenital 755.50
  scrotum (congenital) 752.9
    acquired 608.89
  sebaceous gland, acquired 706.8
  seminal tract or duct (congenital)
    752.9
    acquired 608.89
  septum (nasal) (acquired) 470
    congenital 748.1
  shoulder (joint) (acquired) 736.89
    congenital 755.50
      specified type NEC 755.59
    contraction 718.41
  sigmoid (flexure) (congenital) 751.5
    acquired 569.89
  sinus of Valsalva 747.29
  skin (congenital) 757.9
    acquired NEC 709.8
  skull (acquired) 738.19
    congenital 756.0
      with
        anencephalus 740.0
        encephalocele 742.0
        hydrocephalus 742.3
          with spina bifida (*see also*
            Spina bifida) 741.0 ●
        microcephalus 742.1
      due to intrauterine malposition
        and pressure 754.0
  soft parts, organs or tissues (of pelvis)
    in pregnancy or childbirth NEC
      654.9 ●
      affecting fetus or newborn 763.89
      causing obstructed labor 660.2 ●
        affecting fetus or newborn
          763.1

Deformity *(Continued)*
  spermatic cord (congenital) 752.9
    acquired 608.89
      torsion 608.22
        extravaginal 608.21
        intravaginal 608.22
  spinal
    column - *see* Deformity, spine
    cord (congenital) 742.9
      acquired 336.8
      vessel (congenital) 747.82
    nerve root (congenital) 742.9
      acquired 724.9
  spine (acquired) NEC 738.5
    congenital 756.10
      due to intrauterine malposition
        and pressure 754.2
    kyphoscoliotic (*see also*
      Kyphoscoliosis) 737.30
    kyphotic (*see also* Kyphosis) 737.10
    lordotic (*see also* Lordosis) 737.20
    rachitic 268.1
    scoliotic (*see also* Scoliosis) 737.30
  spleen
    acquired 289.59
    congenital 759.0
  Sprengel's (congenital) 755.52
  sternum (acquired) 738.3
    congenital 756.3
  stomach (congenital) 750.9
    acquired 537.89
  submaxillary gland (congenital) 750.9
    acquired 527.8
  swan neck (acquired)
    finger 736.22
    hand 736.09
  talipes - *see* Talipes
  teeth, tooth NEC 520.9
  testis (congenital) 752.9
    acquired 608.89
      torsion 608.20
  thigh (acquired) 736.89
    congenital 755.60
  thorax (acquired) (wall) 738.3
    congenital 754.89
    late effect of rickets 268.1
  thumb (acquired) 736.20
    congenital 755.50
  thymus (tissue) (congenital) 759.2
  thyroid (gland) (congenital) 759.2
    cartilage 748.3
      acquired 478.79
  tibia (acquired) 736.89
    congenital 755.60
    saber 090.5
  toe (acquired) 735.9
    congenital 755.66
    specified NEC 735.8
  tongue (congenital) 750.10
    acquired 529.8
  tooth, teeth NEC 520.9
  trachea (rings) (congenital) 748.3
    acquired 519.19
  transverse aortic arch (congenital)
    747.21
  tricuspid (leaflets) (valve) (congenital)
    746.9
    acquired - *see* Endocarditis, tricuspid
    atresia or stenosis 746.1
    specified type NEC 746.89
  trunk (acquired) 738.3
    congenital 759.9
  ulna (acquired) 736.00
    congenital 755.50

Deformity (*Continued*)
　upper extremity - *see* Deformity, arm
　urachus (congenital) 753.7
　ureter (opening) (congenital) 753.9
　　acquired 593.89
　urethra (valve) (congenital) 753.9
　　acquired 599.84
　urinary tract or system (congenital) 753.9
　　urachus 753.7
　uterus (congenital) 752.3
　　acquired 621.8
　uvula (congenital) 750.9
　　acquired 528.9
　vagina (congenital) 752.40
　　acquired 623.8
　valve, valvular (heart) (congenital) 746.9
　　acquired - *see* Endocarditis
　　pulmonary 746.00
　　specified type NEC 746.89
　vascular (congenital) (peripheral) NEC 747.60
　　acquired 459.9
　　gastrointestinal 747.61
　　lower limb 747.64
　　renal 747.62
　　specified site NEC 747.69
　　spinal 747.82
　　upper limb 747.63
　vas deferens (congenital) 752.9
　　acquired 608.89
　vein (congenital) NEC (*see also* Deformity, vascular) 747.60
　　brain 747.81
　　coronary 746.9
　　great 747.40
　vena cava (inferior) (superior) (congenital) 747.40
　vertebra - *see* Deformity, spine
　vesicourethral orifice (acquired) 596.8
　　congenital NEC 753.9
　　　specified type NEC 753.8
　vessels of optic papilla (congenital) 743.9
　visual field (contraction) 368.45
　vitreous humor (congenital) 743.9
　　acquired 379.29
　vulva (congenital) 752.40
　　acquired 624.8
　wrist (joint) (acquired) 736.00
　　congenital 755.50
　　contraction 718.43
　　valgus 736.03
　　　congenital 755.59
　　varus 736.04
　　　congenital 755.59

Degeneration, degenerative
　adrenal (capsule) (gland) 255.8
　　with hypofunction 255.41
　　fatty 255.8
　　hyaline 255.8
　　infectional 255.8
　　lardaceous 277.39
　amyloid (any site) (general) 277.39
　anterior cornua, spinal cord 336.8
　anterior labral 840.8
　aorta, aortic 440.0
　　fatty 447.8
　　valve (heart) (*see also* Endocarditis, aortic) 424.1
　arteriovascular - *see* Arteriosclerosis

Degeneration, degenerative (*Continued*)
　artery, arterial (atheromatous) (calcareous) - *see also* Arteriosclerosis
　　amyloid 277.39
　　lardaceous 277.39
　　medial NEC (*see also* Arteriosclerosis, extremities) 440.20
　articular cartilage NEC (*see also* Disorder, cartilage, articular) 718.0●
　　elbow 718.02
　　knee 717.5
　　patella 717.7
　　shoulder 718.01
　　spine (*see also* Spondylosis) 721.90
　atheromatous - *see* Arteriosclerosis
　bacony (any site) 277.39
　basal nuclei or ganglia NEC 333.0
　bone 733.90
　brachial plexus 353.0
　brain (cortical) (progressive) 331.9
　　arteriosclerotic 437.0
　　childhood 330.9
　　　specified type NEC 330.8
　　congenital 742.4
　　cystic 348.0
　　　congenital 742.4
　　familial NEC 331.89
　　grey matter 330.8
　　heredofamilial NEC 331.89
　　in
　　　alcoholism 303.9● [331.7]
　　　beriberi 265.0 [331.7]
　　　cerebrovascular disease 437.9 [331.7]
　　　congenital hydrocephalus 742.3 [331.7]
　　　　with spina bifida (*see also* Spina bifida) 741.0● [331.7]
　　　Babry's disease 272.7 [330.2]
　　　Gaucher's disease 272.7 [330.2]
　　　Hunter's disease or syndrome 277.5 [330.3]
　　　lipidosis
　　　　cerebral 330.1
　　　　generalized 272.7 [330.2]
　　　mucopolysaccharidosis 277.5 [330.3]
　　　myxedema (*see also* Myxedema) 244.9 [331.7]
　　　neoplastic disease NEC (M8000/1) 239.9 [331.7]
　　　Niemann-Pick disease 272.7 [330.2]
　　　sphingolipidosis 272.7 [330.2]
　　　vitamin B$_{12}$ deficiency 266.2 [331.7]
　　motor centers 331.89
　　senile 331.2
　　specified type NEC 331.89
　breast - *see* Disease, breast
　Bruch's membrane 363.40
　bundle of His 426.50
　　left 426.3
　　right 426.4
　calcareous NEC 275.49
　capillaries 448.9
　　amyloid 277.39
　　fatty 448.9
　　lardaceous 277.39

Degeneration, degenerative (*Continued*)
　cardiac (brown) (calcareous) (fatty) (fibrous) (hyaline) (mural) (muscular) (pigmentary) (senile) (with arteriosclerosis) (*see also* Degeneration, myocardial) 429.1
　　valve, valvular - *see* Endocarditis
　cardiorenal (*see also* Hypertension, cardiorenal) 404.90
　cardiovascular (*see also* Disease, cardiovascular) 429.2
　　renal (*see also* Hypertension, cardiorenal) 404.90
　cartilage (joint) - *see* Derangement, joint
　cerebellar NEC 334.9
　　primary (hereditary) (sporadic) 334.2
　cerebral - *see* Degeneration, brain
　cerebromacular 330.1
　cerebrovascular 437.1
　　due to hypertension 437.2
　　late effect - *see* Late effect(s) (of) cerebrovascular disease
　cervical plexus 353.2
　cervix 622.8
　　due to radiation (intended effect) 622.8
　　　adverse effect or misadventure 622.8
　changes, spine or vertebra (*see also* Spondylosis) 721.90
　chitinous 277.39
　chorioretinal 363.40
　　congenital 743.53
　　hereditary 363.50
　choroid (colloid) (drusen) 363.40
　　hereditary 363.50
　　senile 363.41
　　　diffuse secondary 363.42
　cochlear 386.8
　collateral ligament (knee) (medial) 717.82
　　lateral 717.81
　combined (spinal cord) (subacute) 266.2 [336.2]
　　with anemia (pernicious) 281.0 [336.2]
　　　due to dietary deficiency 281.1 [336.2]
　　due to vitamin B$_{12}$ deficiency anemia (dietary) 281.1 [336.2]
　conjunctiva 372.50
　　amyloid 277.39 [372.50]
　cornea 371.40
　　calcerous 371.44
　　familial (hereditary) (*see also* Dystrophy, cornea) 371.50
　　　macular 371.55
　　　reticular 371.54
　　hyaline (of old scars) 371.41
　　marginal (Terrien's) 371.48
　　mosaic (shagreen) 371.41
　　nodular 371.46
　　peripheral 371.48
　　senile 371.41
　cortical (cerebellar) (parenchymatous) 334.2
　　alcoholic 303.9● [334.4]
　　diffuse, due to arteriopathy 437.0
　corticostriatal-spinal 334.8
　cretinoid 243
　cruciate ligament (knee) (posterior) 717.84
　　anterior 717.83

◀ New　◀||| Revised　~~deleted~~ Deleted　● Use Additional Digit(s)　▓ Omit code

Degeneration, degenerative *(Continued)*
cutis 709.3
   amyloid 277.39
dental pulp 522.2
disc disease - *see* Degeneration,
   intervertebral disc
dorsolateral (spinal cord) - *see*
   Degeneration, combined
endocardial 424.90
extrapyramidal NEC 333.90
eye NEC 360.40
   macular (*see also* Degeneration,
      macula) 362.50
      congenital 362.75
      hereditary 362.76
fatty (diffuse) (general) 272.8
   liver 571.8
      alcoholic 571.0
   localized site - *see* Degeneration, by
      site, fatty
   placenta - *see* Placenta, abnormal
globe (eye) NEC 360.40
   macular - *see* Degeneration,
      macula
grey matter 330.8
heart (brown) (calcareous) (fatty)
   (fibrous) (hyaline) (mural)
   (muscular) (pigmentary) (senile)
   (with arteriosclerosis) (*see also*
   Degeneration, myocardial)
   429.1
   amyloid 277.39 *[425.7]*
   atheromatous - *see* Arteriosclerosis,
      coronary
   gouty 274.82
   hypertensive (*see also* Hypertension,
      heart) 402.90
   ischemic 414.9
   valve, valvular - *see* Endocarditis
hepatolenticular (Wilson's) 275.1
hepatorenal 572.4
heredofamilial
   brain NEC 331.89
   spinal cord NEC 336.8
hyaline (diffuse) (generalized) 728.9
   localized - *see also* Degeneration, by
      site
      cornea 371.41
      keratitis 371.41
hypertensive vascular - *see*
   Hypertension
infrapatellar fat pad 729.31
internal semilunar cartilage 717.3
intervertebral disc 722.6
   with myelopathy 722.70
   cervical, cervicothoracic 722.4
      with myelopathy 722.71
   lumbar, lumbosacral 722.52
      with myelopathy 722.73
   thoracic, thoracolumbar 722.51
      with myelopathy 722.72
intestine 569.89
   amyloid 277.39
   lardaceous 277.39
iris (generalized) (*see also* Atrophy, iris)
   364.59
   pigmentary 364.53
   pupillary margin 364.54
ischemic - *see* Ischemia
joint disease (*see also* Osteoarthrosis)
   715.9●
   multiple sites 715.09
   spine (*see also* Spondylosis)
      721.90

Degeneration, degenerative *(Continued)*
kidney (*see also* Sclerosis, renal) 587
   amyloid 277.39 *[583.81]*
   cyst, cystic (multiple) (solitary) 593.2
      congenital (*see also* Cystic,
         disease, kidney) 753.10
   fatty 593.89
   fibrocystic (congenital) 753.19
   lardaceous 277.39 *[583.81]*
   polycystic (congenital) 753.12
      adult type (APKD) 753.13
      autosomal dominant 753.13
      autosomal recessive 753.14
      childhood type (CPKD) 753.14
      infantile type 753.14
   waxy 277.39 *[583.81]*
Kuhnt-Junius (retina) 362.52
labyrinth, osseous 386.8
lacrimal passages, cystic 375.12
lardaceous (any site) 277.39
lateral column (posterior), spinal cord
   (*see also* Degeneration, combined)
   266.2 *[336.2]*
lattice 362.63
lens 366.9
   infantile, juvenile, or presenile
      366.00
   senile 366.10
lenticular (familial) (progressive)
   (Wilson's) (with cirrhosis of liver)
   275.1
   striate artery 437.0
lethal ball, prosthetic heart valve 996.02
ligament
   collateral (knee) (medial) 717.82
      lateral 717.81
   cruciate (knee) (posterior) 717.84
      anterior 717.83
liver (diffuse) 572.8
   amyloid 277.39
   congenital (cystic) 751.62
   cystic 572.8
      congenital 751.62
   fatty 571.8
      alcoholic 571.0
   hypertrophic 572.8
   lardaceous 277.39
   parenchymatous, acute or subacute
      (*see also* Necrosis, liver) 570
   pigmentary 572.8
   toxic (acute) 573.8
   waxy 277.39
lung 518.89
lymph gland 289.3
   hyaline 289.3
   lardaceous 277.39
macula (acquired) (senile) 362.50
   atrophic 362.51
   Best's 362.76
   congenital 362.75
   cystic 362.54
   cystoid 362.53
   disciform 362.52
   dry 362.51
   exudative 362.52
   familial pseudoinflammatory
      362.77
   hereditary 362.76
   hole 362.54
   juvenile (Stargardt's) 362.75
   nonexudative 362.51
   pseudohole 362.54
   wet 362.52
medullary - *see* Degeneration, brain

Degeneration, degenerative *(Continued)*
membranous labyrinth, congenital
   (causing impairment of hearing)
   744.05
meniscus - *see* Derangement, joint
microcystoid 362.62
mitral - *see* Insufficiency, mitral
Mönckeberg's (*see also* Arteriosclerosis,
   extremities) 440.20
moral 301.7
motor centers, senile 331.2
mural (*see also* Degeneration,
   myocardial) 429.1
   heart, cardiac (*see also* Degeneration,
      myocardial) 429.1
   myocardium, myocardial (*see also*
      Degeneration, myocardial)
      429.1
muscle 728.9
   fatty 728.9
   fibrous 728.9
   heart (*see also* Degeneration,
      myocardial) 429.1
   hyaline 728.9
muscular progressive 728.2
myelin, central nervous system NEC
   341.9
myocardium, myocardial (brown)
   (calcareous) (fatty) (fibrous)
   (hyaline) (mural) (muscular)
   (pigmentary) (senile) (with
   arteriosclerosis) 429.1
   with rheumatic fever (conditions
      classifiable to 390) 398.0
      active, acute, or subacute 391.2
         with chorea 392.0
      inactive or quiescent (with
         chorea) 398.0
   amyloid 277.39 *[425.7]*
   congenital 746.89
   fetus or newborn 779.89
   gouty 274.82
   hypertensive (*see also* Hypertension,
      heart) 402.90
   ischemic 414.8
   rheumatic (*see also* Degeneration,
      myocardium, with rheumatic
      fever) 398.0
   syphilitic 093.82
nasal sinus (mucosa) (*see also* Sinusitis)
   473.9
   frontal 473.1
   maxillary 473.0
nerve - *see* Disorder, nerve
nervous system 349.89
   amyloid 277.39 *[357.4]*
   autonomic (*see also* Neuropathy,
      peripheral, autonomic) 337.9
   fatty 349.89
   peripheral autonomic NEC (*see also*
      Neuropathy, peripheral,
      autonomic) 337.9
nipple 611.9
nose 478.19
oculoacousticocerebral, congenital
   (progressive) 743.8
olivopontocerebellar (familial)
   (hereditary) 333.0
osseous labyrinth 386.8
ovary 620.8
   cystic 620.2
   microcystic 620.2
pallidal, pigmentary (progressive)
   333.0

Degeneration, degenerative (Continued)
pancreas 577.8
  tuberculous (see also Tuberculosis) 017.9●
papillary muscle 429.81
paving stone 362.61
penis 607.89
peritoneum 568.89
pigmentary (diffuse) (general)
  localized - see Degeneration, by site
  pallidal (progressive) 333.0
  secondary 362.65
pineal gland 259.8
pituitary (gland) 253.8
placenta (fatty) (fibrinoid) (fibroid) - see Placenta, abnormal
popliteal fat pad 729.31
posterolateral (spinal cord) (see also Degeneration, combined) 266.2 [336.2]
pulmonary valve (heart) (see also Endocarditis, pulmonary) 424.3
pulp (tooth) 522.2
pupillary margin 364.54
renal (see also Sclerosis, renal) 587
  fibrocystic 753.19
  polycystic 753.12
    adult type (APKD) 753.13
    autosomal dominant 753.13
    autosomal recessive 753.14
    childhood type (CPKD) 753.14
    infantile type 753.14
reticuloendothelial system 289.89
retina (peripheral) 362.60
  with retinal defect (see also Detachment, retina, with retinal defect) 361.00
  cystic (senile) 362.50
  cystoid 362.53
  hereditary (see also Dystrophy, retina) 362.70
    cerebroretinal 362.71
    congenital 362.75
    juvenile (Stargardt's) 362.75
    macula 362.76
  Kuhnt-Junius 362.52
  lattice 362.63
  macular (see also Degeneration, macula) 362.50
  microcystoid 362.62
  palisade 362.63
  paving stone 362.61
  pigmentary (primary) 362.74
    secondary 362.65
  posterior pole (see also Degeneration, macula) 362.50
  secondary 362.66
  senile 362.60
    cystic 362.53
    reticular 362.64
saccule, congenital (causing impairment of hearing) 744.05
sacculocochlear 386.8
senile 797
  brain 331.2
  cardiac, heart, or myocardium (see also Degeneration, myocardial) 429.1
  motor centers 331.2
  reticule 362.64
  retina, cystic 362.50
  vascular - see Arteriosclerosis
silicone rubber poppet (prosthetic valve) 996.02

Degeneration, degenerative (Continued)
sinus (cystic) (see also Sinusitis) 473.9
  polypoid 471.1
skin 709.3
  amyloid 277.39
  colloid 709.3
spinal (cord) 336.8
  amyloid 277.39
  column 733.90
  combined (subacute) (see also Degeneration, combined) 266.2 [336.2]
    with anemia (pernicious) 281.0 [336.2]
  dorsolateral (see also Degeneration, combined) 266.2 [336.2]
  familial NEC 336.8
  fatty 336.8
  funicular (see also Degeneration, combined) 266.2 [336.2]
  heredofamilial NEC 336.8
  posterolateral (see also Degeneration, combined) 266.2 [336.2]
  subacute combined - see Degeneration, combined
  tuberculous (see also Tuberculosis) 013.8
spine 733.90
spleen 289.59
  amyloid 277.39
  lardaceous 277.39
stomach 537.89
  lardaceous 277.39
strionigral 333.0
sudoriparous (cystic) 705.89
suprarenal (capsule) (gland) 255.8
  with hypofunction 255.41
sweat gland 705.89
synovial membrane (pulpy) 727.9
tapetoretinal 362.74
  adult or presenile form 362.50
testis (postinfectional) 608.89
thymus (gland) 254.8
  fatty 254.8
  lardaceous 277.39
thyroid (gland) 246.8
tricuspid (heart) (valve) - see Endocarditis, tricuspid
tuberculous NEC (see also Tuberculosis) 011.9●
turbinate 733.90
uterus 621.8
  cystic 621.8
vascular (senile) - see also Arteriosclerosis
  hypertensive - see Hypertension
vitreoretinal (primary) 362.73
  secondary 362.66
vitreous humor (with infiltration) 379.21
wallerian NEC - see Disorder, nerve
waxy (any site) 277.39
Wilson's hepatolenticular 275.1
Deglutition
paralysis 784.99
  hysterical 300.11
pneumonia 507.0
Degos' disease or syndrome 447.8
Degradation disorder, branched-chain amino-acid 270.3
Dehiscence
anastomosis - see Complications, anastomosis
cesarean wound 674.1●

Dehiscence (Continued)
closure of
  cornea 998.32
  fascia, superficial or muscular 998.31
  internal organ 998.31
  mucosa 998.32
  muscle or muscle flap 998.31
  ribs or rib cage 998.31
  skin 998.32
  skull or craniotomy 998.31
  sternum or sternotomy 998.31
  subcutaneous tissue 998.32
  tendon or ligament 998.31
  traumatic laceration (external) (internal) 998.33
episiotomy 674.2●
operation wound 998.32
  deep 998.31
  external 998.32
  internal 998.31
  superficial 998.32
perineal wound (postpartum) 674.2●
postoperative 998.32
  abdomen 998.32
    internal 998.31
  internal 998.31
traumatic injury wound repair 998.33
uterine wound 674.1●
Dehydration (cachexia) 276.51
with
  hypernatremia 276.0
  hyponatremia 276.1
  newborn 775.5
Deiters' nucleus syndrome 386.19
Déjérine's disease 356.0
Déjérine-Klumpke paralysis 767.6
Déjérine-Roussy syndrome 338.0
Déjérine-Sottas disease or neuropathy (hypertrophic) 356.0
Déjérine-Thomas atrophy or syndrome 333.0
de Lange's syndrome (Amsterdam dwarf, mental retardation, and brachycephaly) 759.89
Delay, delayed
adaptation, cones or rods 368.63
any plane in pelvis
  affecting fetus or newborn 763.1
  complicating delivery 660.1●
birth or delivery NEC 662.1●
  affecting fetus or newborn 763.9
  second twin, triplet, or multiple mate 662.3●
closure - see also Fistula
  cranial suture 756.0
  fontanel 756.0
coagulation NEC 790.92
conduction (cardiac) (ventricular) 426.9
delivery NEC 662.1●
  second twin, triplet, etc. 662.3●
    affecting fetus or newborn 763.89
development
  in childhood 783.40
    physiological 783.40
  intellectual NEC 315.9
  learning NEC 315.2
  reading 315.00
  sexual 259.0
  speech 315.39
    and language due to hearing loss 315.34
    associated with hyperkinesis 314.1
  spelling 315.09

◀ New   ◀ Revised   deleted Deleted   ● Use Additional Digit(s)   Omit code

Delay, delayed (Continued)
gastric emptying 536.8
menarche 256.39
due to pituitary hypofunction
253.4
menstruation (cause unknown)
626.8
milestone in childhood 783.42
motility - see Hypomotility
passage of meconium (newborn)
777.1
primary respiration 768.9
puberty 259.0
separation of umbilical cord 779.83
sexual maturation, female 259.0
vaccination V64.00
Del Castillo's syndrome (germinal
aplasia) 606.0
Deleage's disease 359.89
Deletion syndrome
5p 758.31
22q11.2 758.32
autosomal NEC 758.39
constitutional 5q deletion 758.39
Delhi (boil) (button) (sore) 085.1
Delinquency (juvenile) 312.9
group (see also Disturbance, conduct)
312.2●
neurotic 312.4
Delirium, delirious 780.09
acute (psychotic) 293.0
alcoholic 291.0
acute 291.0
chronic 291.1
alcoholicum 291.0
chronic (see also Psychosis) 293.89
due to or associated with physical
condition - see Psychosis,
organic
drug-induced 292.81
due to conditions classified elsewhere
293.0
eclamptic (see also Eclampsia)
780.39
exhaustion (see also Reaction, stress,
acute) 308.9
hysterical 300.11
in
presenile dementia 290.11
senile dementia 290.3
induced by drug 292.81
manic, maniacal (acute) (see also
Psychosis, affective) 296.0●
recurrent episode 296.1●
single episode 296.0●
puerperal 293.9
senile 290.3
subacute (psychotic) 293.1
thyroid (see also Thyrotoxicosis)
242.9●
traumatic - see also Injury,
intracranial
with
lesion, spinal cord - see Injury,
spinal, by site
shock, spinal - see Injury, spinal,
by site
tremens (impending) 291.0
uremic - see Uremia
withdrawal
alcoholic (acute) 291.0
chronic 291.1
drug 292.0

Delivery

Note 19   Use the following fifth-digit
subclassification with categories
640–649, 651–676:

0   unspecified as to episode of care
1   delivered, with or without
mention of antepartum
condition
2   delivered, with mention of
postpartum complication
3   antepartum condition or
complication
4   postpartum condition or
complication

breech (assisted) (buttocks) (complete)
(frank) (spontaneous) 652.2●
affecting fetus or newborn 763.0
extraction NEC 669.6●
cesarean (for) 669.7●
abnormal
cervix 654.6●
pelvic organs of tissues 654.9●
pelvis (bony) (major) NEC 653.0●
presentation or position 652.9●
in multiple gestation 652.6●
size, fetus 653.5●
soft parts (of pelvis) 654.9●
uterus, congenital 654.0●
vagina 654.7●
vulva 654.8●
abruptio placentae 641.2●
acromion presentation 652.8●
affecting fetus or newborn 763.4
anteversion, cervix or uterus 654.4●
atony, uterus 661.2●
with hemorrhage 666.1●
bicornis or bicornuate uterus 654.0●
breech presentation (buttocks)
(complete) (frank) 652.2●
brow presentation 652.4●
cephalopelvic disproportion
(normally formed fetus)
653.4●
chin presentation 652.4●
cicatrix of cervix 654.6●
contracted pelvis (general) 653.1●
inlet 653.2●
outlet 653.3●
cord presentation or prolapse 663.0●
cystocele 654.4●
deformity (acquired) (congenital)
pelvic organs or tissues NEC
654.9●
pelvis (bony) NEC 653.0●
displacement, uterus NEC 654.4●
disproportion NEC 653.9●
distress
fetal 656.8●
maternal 669.0●
eclampsia 642.6●
face presentation 652.4●
failed
forceps 660.7●
trial of labor NEC 660.6●
vacuum extraction 660.7●
ventouse 660.7●
fetal deformity 653.7●
fetal-maternal hemorrhage 656.0●
fetus, fetal
distress 656.8●
prematurity 656.8●
fibroid (tumor) (uterus) 654.1●

Delivery (Continued)
cesarean (Continued)
footling 652.8●
with successful version 652.1●
hemorrhage (antepartum)
(intrapartum) NEC 641.9●
hydrocephalic fetus 653.6●
incarceration of uterus 654.3●
incoordinate uterine action 661.4●
inertia, uterus 661.2●
primary 661.0●
secondary 661.1●
lateroversion, uterus or cervix
654.4●
mal lie 652.9●
malposition
fetus 652.9●
in multiple gestation 652.6●
pelvic organs or tissues NEC
654.9●
uterus NEC or cervix 654.4●
malpresentation NEC 652.9●
in multiple gestation 652.6●
maternal
diabetes mellitus (conditions
classifiable to 249 and 250)
648.0●
heart disease NEC 648.6●
meconium in liquor 656.8●
staining only 792.3
oblique presentation 652.3●
oversize fetus 653.5●
pelvic tumor NEC 654.9●
placental insufficiency 656.5●
placenta previa 641.0●
with hemorrhage 641.1●
poor dilation, cervix 661.0●
pre-eclampsia 642.4●
severe 642.5●
previous
cesarean delivery, section
654.2●
surgery (to)
cervix 654.6●
gynecological NEC 654.9●
rectum 654.8●
uterus NEC 654.9●
previous cesarean delivery,
section 654.2●
vagina 654.7●
prolapse
arm or hand 652.7●
uterus 654.4●
prolonged labor 662.1●
rectocele 654.4●
retroversion, uterus or cervix
654.3●
rigid
cervix 654.6●
pelvic floor 654.4●
perineum 654.8●
vagina 654.7●
vulva 654.8●
sacculation, pregnant uterus 654.4●
scar(s)
cervix 654.6●
cesarean delivery, section 654.2●
uterus NEC 654.9●
due to previous cesarean
delivery, section 654.2●
Shirodkar suture in situ 654.5●
shoulder presentation 652.8●
stenosis or stricture, cervix 654.6●
transverse presentation or lie 652.3●

Delivery *(Continued)*
　cesarean *(Continued)*
　　tumor, pelvic organs or tissues NEC
　　　654.4●
　　umbilical cord presentation or
　　　prolapse 663.0●
　completely normal case - *see* category
　　650
　complicated (by) NEC 669.9●
　　abdominal tumor, fetal 653.7●
　　　causing obstructed labor 660.1●
　　abnormal, abnormality of
　　　cervix 654.6●
　　　　causing obstructed labor
　　　　　660.2●
　　　forces of labor 661.9●
　　　formation of uterus 654.0●
　　　pelvic organs or tissues 654.9●
　　　　causing obstructed labor
　　　　　660.2●
　　　pelvis (bony) (major) NEC 653.0●
　　　　causing obstructed labor
　　　　　660.1●
　　　presentation or position NEC
　　　　652.9●
　　　　causing obstructed labor
　　　　　660.0●
　　　size, fetus 653.5●
　　　　causing obstructed labor
　　　　　660.1●
　　　soft parts (of pelvis) 654.9●
　　　　causing obstructed labor
　　　　　660.2●
　　　uterine contractions NEC 661.9●
　　　uterus (formation) 654.0●
　　　　causing obstructed labor
　　　　　660.2●
　　　vagina 654.7●
　　　　causing obstructed labor
　　　　　660.2●
　　abnormally formed uterus (any
　　　type) (congenital) 654.0●
　　　causing obstructed labor 660.2●
　　acromion presentation 652.8●
　　　causing obstructed labor 660.0●
　　adherent placenta 667.0●
　　　with hemorrhage 666.0●
　　adhesions, uterus (to abdominal
　　　wall) 654.4●
　　advanced maternal age NEC
　　　659.6●
　　　multigravida 659.6●
　　　primigravida 659.5●
　　air embolism 673.0●
　　amnionitis 658.4●
　　amniotic fluid embolism 673.1●
　　anesthetic death 668.9●
　　annular detachment, cervix 665.3●
　　antepartum hemorrhage - *see*
　　　Delivery, complicated,
　　　hemorrhage
　　anteversion, cervix or uterus 654.4●
　　　causing obstructed labor 660.2●
　　apoplexy 674.0●
　　　placenta 641.2●
　　arrested active phase 661.1●
　　asymmetrical pelvis bone 653.0●
　　　causing obstructed labor 660.1●
　　atony, uterus with hemorrhage
　　　(hypotonic) (inertia) 666.1●
　　　hypertonic 661.4●
　　Bandl's ring 661.4●
　　Battledore placenta - *see* Placenta,
　　　abnormal

Delivery *(Continued)*
　complicated (by) NEC *(Continued)*
　　bicornis or bicornuate uterus
　　　654.0●
　　　causing obstructed labor 660.2●
　　birth injury to mother NEC 665.9●
　　bleeding (*see also* Delivery,
　　　complicated, hemorrhage)
　　　641.9●
　　breech presentation (assisted)
　　　(buttocks) (complete) (frank)
　　　(spontaneous) 652.2●
　　　with successful version 652.1●
　　brow presentation 652.4●
　　cephalopelvic disproportion
　　　(normally formed fetus)
　　　653.4●
　　　causing obstructed labor 660.1●
　　cerebral hemorrhage 674.0●
　　cervical dystocia 661.2●
　　chin presentation 652.4●
　　　causing obstructed labor 660.0●
　　cicatrix
　　　cervix 654.6●
　　　　causing obstructed labor
　　　　　660.2●
　　　vagina 654.7●
　　　　causing obstructed labor
　　　　　660.2●
　　coagulation defect 649.3●
　　colporrhexis 665.4●
　　　with perineal laceration 664.0●
　　compound presentation 652.8●
　　　causing obstructed labor 660.0●
　　compression of cord (umbilical)
　　　663.2●
　　　around neck 663.1●
　　　cord prolapsed 663.0●
　　contraction, contracted pelvis
　　　653.1●
　　　causing obstructed labor 660.1●
　　　general 653.1●
　　　　causing obstructed labor
　　　　　660.1●
　　　inlet 653.2●
　　　　causing obstructed labor
　　　　　660.1●
　　　midpelvic 653.8●
　　　　causing obstructed labor
　　　　　660.1●
　　　midplane 653.8●
　　　　causing obstructed labor
　　　　　660.1●
　　　outlet 653.3●
　　　　causing obstructed labor
　　　　　660.1●
　　contraction ring 661.4●
　　cord (umbilical) 663.9●
　　　around neck, tightly or with
　　　　compression 663.1●
　　　　without compression 663.3●
　　　bruising 663.6●
　　　complication NEC 663.9●
　　　　specified type NEC 663.8●
　　　compression NEC 663.2●
　　　entanglement NEC 663.3●
　　　　with compression 663.2●
　　　forelying 663.0●
　　　hematoma 663.6●
　　　marginal attachment 663.8●
　　　presentation 663.0●
　　　prolapse (complete) (occult)
　　　　(partial) 663.0●
　　　short 663.4●

Delivery *(Continued)*
　complicated (by) NEC *(Continued)*
　　cord *(Continued)*
　　　specified complication NEC
　　　　663.8●
　　　thrombosis (vessels) 663.6●
　　　vascular lesion 663.6●
　　　velamentous insertion 663.8●
　　Couvelaire uterus 641.2●
　　cretin pelvis (dwarf type) (male
　　　type) 653.1●
　　　causing obstructed labor 660.1●
　　crossbirth 652.3●
　　　with successful version 652.1●
　　　causing obstructed labor 660.0●
　　cyst (Gartner's duct) 654.7●
　　cystocele 654.4●
　　　causing obstructed labor 660.2●
　　death of fetus (near term) 656.4●
　　　early (before 22 completed weeks'
　　　　gestation) 632
　　deformity (acquired) (congenital)
　　　fetus 653.7●
　　　　causing obstructed labor
　　　　　660.1●
　　　pelvic organs or tissues NEC
　　　　654.9●
　　　　causing obstructed labor
　　　　　660.2●
　　　pelvis (bony) NEC 653.0●
　　　　causing obstructed labor
　　　　　660.1●
　　delay, delayed
　　　delivery in multiple pregnancy
　　　　662.3●
　　　　due to locked mates 660.5●
　　　following rupture of membranes
　　　　(spontaneous) 658.2●
　　　　artificial 658.3●
　　depressed fetal heart tones 659.7●
　　diastasis recti 665.8●
　　dilatation
　　　bladder 654.4●
　　　　causing obstructed labor
　　　　　660.2●
　　　cervix, incomplete, poor or slow
　　　　661.0●
　　diseased placenta 656.7●
　　displacement uterus NEC 654.4●
　　　causing obstructed labor 660.2●
　　disproportion NEC 653.9●
　　　causing obstructed labor 660.1●
　　disruptio uteri - *see* Delivery,
　　　complicated, rupture, uterus
　　distress
　　　fetal 656.8●
　　　maternal 669.0●
　　double uterus (congenital) 654.0●
　　　causing obstructed labor
　　　　660.2●
　　dropsy amnion 657●
　　dysfunction, uterus 661.9●
　　　hypertonic 661.4●
　　　hypotonic 661.2●
　　　　primary 661.0●
　　　　secondary 661.1●
　　　incoordinate 661.4●
　　dystocia
　　　cervical 661.2●
　　　fetal - *see* Delivery, complicated,
　　　　abnormal, presentation
　　　maternal - *see* Delivery,
　　　　complicated, prolonged
　　　　labor

◄ New　◄▦ Revised　~~deleted~~ Deleted　● Use Additional Digit(s)　▓ Omit code

Delivery *(Continued)*
  complicated (by) NEC *(Continued)*
    dystocia *(Continued)*
      pelvic - *see* Delivery, complicated, contraction pelvis
      positional 652.8●
      shoulder girdle 660.4●
    eclampsia 642.6●
    ectopic kidney 654.4●
      causing obstructed labor 660.2●
    edema, cervix 654.6●
      causing obstructed labor 660.2●
    effusion, amniotic fluid 658.1●
    elderly multigravida 659.6●
    elderly primigravida 659.5●
    embolism (pulmonary) 673.2●
      air 673.0●
      amniotic fluid 673.1●
      blood-clot 673.2●
      cerebral 674.0●
      fat 673.8●
      pyemic 673.3●
      septic 673.3●
    entanglement, umbilical cord 663.3●
      with compression 663.2●
      around neck (with compression) 663.1●
    eversion, cervix or uterus 665.2●
    excessive
      fetal growth 653.5●
        causing obstructed labor 660.1●
      size of fetus 653.5●
        causing obstructed labor 660.1●
    face presentation 652.4●
      causing obstructed labor 660.0●
      to pubes 660.3●
    failure, fetal head to enter pelvic brim 652.5●
      causing obstructed labor 660.0●
    female genital mutilation 660.8●
    fetal
      acid-base balance 656.8●
      death (near term) NEC 656.4●
        early (before 22 completed weeks' gestation) 632
      deformity 653.7●
        causing obstructed labor 660.1●
      distress 656.8●
      heart rate or rhythm 659.7●
      reduction of multiple fetuses reduced to single fetus 651.7●
    fetopelvic disproportion 653.4●
      causing obstructed labor 660.1●
    fever during labor 659.2●
    fibroid (tumor) (uterus) 654.1●
      causing obstructed labor 660.2●
    fibromyomata 654.1●
      causing obstructed labor 660.2●
    forelying umbilical cord 663.0●
    fracture of coccyx 665.6●
    hematoma 664.5●
      broad ligament 665.7●
      ischial spine 665.7●
      pelvic 665.7●
      perineum 664.5●
      soft tissues 665.7●
      subdural 674.0●
      umbilical cord 663.6●
      vagina 665.7●
      vulva or perineum 664.5●

Delivery *(Continued)*
  complicated (by) NEC *(Continued)*
    hemorrhage (uterine) (antepartum) (intrapartum) (pregnancy) 641.9●
      accidental 641.2●
      associated with
        afibrinogenemia 641.3●
        coagulation defect 641.3●
          hyperfibrinolysis 641.3●
          hypofibrinogenemia 641.3●
      cerebral 674.0●
      due to
        low-lying placenta 641.1●
        placenta previa 641.1●
        premature separation of placenta (normally implanted) 641.2●
        retained placenta 666.0●
        trauma 641.8●
        uterine leiomyoma 641.8●
      marginal sinus rupture 641.2●
      placenta NEC 641.9●
      postpartum (atonic) (immediate) (within 24 hours) 666.1●
        with retained or trapped placenta 666.0●
        delayed 666.2●
        secondary 666.2●
        third stage 666.0●
    hourglass contraction, uterus 661.4●
    hydramnios 657●
    hydrocephalic fetus 653.6●
      causing obstructed labor 660.1●
    hydrops fetalis 653.7●
      causing obstructed labor 660.1●
    hypertension - *see* Hypertension, complicating pregnancy
    hypertonic uterine dysfunction 661.4●
    hypotonic uterine dysfunction 661.2●
    impacted shoulders 660.4●
    incarceration, uterus 654.3●
      causing obstructed labor 660.2●
    incomplete dilation (cervix) 661.0●
    incoordinate uterus 661.4●
    indication NEC 659.9●
      specified type NEC 659.8●
    inertia, uterus 661.2●
      hypertonic 661.4●
      hypotonic 661.2●
      primary 661.0●
      secondary 661.1●
    infantile
      genitalia 654.4●
        causing obstructed labor 660.2●
      uterus (os) 654.4●
        causing obstructed labor 660.2●
    injury (to mother) NEC 665.9●
    intrauterine fetal death (near term) NEC 656.4●
      early (before 22 completed weeks' gestation) 632
    inversion, uterus 665.2●
    kidney, ectopic 654.4●
      causing obstructed labor 660.2●
    knot (true), umbilical cord 663.2●
    labor, premature (before 37 completed weeks' gestation) 644.2●

Delivery *(Continued)*
  complicated (by) NEC *(Continued)*
    laceration 664.9●
      anus (sphincter) (healed) (old) 654.8●
        with mucosa 664.3●
        not associated with third-degree perineal laceration 664.6●
      bladder (urinary) 665.5●
      bowel 665.5●
      central 664.4●
      cervix (uteri) 665.3●
      fourchette 664.0●
      hymen 664.0●
      labia (majora) (minora) 664.0●
      pelvic
        floor 664.1●
        organ NEC 665.5●
      perineum, perineal 664.4●
        first degree 664.0●
        second degree 664.1●
        third degree 664.2●
        fourth degree 664.3●
        central 664.4●
        extensive NEC 664.4●
        muscles 664.1●
        skin 664.0●
        slight 664.0●
      peritoneum 665.5●
      periurethral tissue 664.8●
      rectovaginal (septum) (without perineal laceration) 665.4●
        with perineum 664.2●
          with anal or rectal mucosa 664.3●
      skin (perineum) 664.0●
      specified site or type NEC 664.8●
      sphincter ani (healed) (old) 654.8●
        with mucosa 664.3●
        not associated with third-degree perineal laceration 664.6●
      urethra 665.5●
      uterus 665.1●
        before labor 665.0●
      vagina, vaginal (deep) (high) (sulcus) (wall) (without perineal laceration) 665.4●
        with perineum 664.0●
        muscles, with perineum 664.1●
      vulva 664.0●
    lateroversion, uterus or cervix 654.4●
      causing obstructed labor 660.2●
    locked mates 660.5●
    low implantation of placenta - *see* Delivery, complicated, placenta, previa
    mal lie 652.9●
    malposition
      fetus NEC 652.9●
        causing obstructed labor 660.0●
      pelvic organs or tissues NEC 654.9●
        causing obstructed labor 660.2●
      placenta 641.1●
        without hemorrhage 641.0●

Delivery *(Continued)*
  complicated (by) NEC *(Continued)*
    malposition *(Continued)*
      uterus NEC or cervix 654.4●
        causing obstructed labor
          660.2●
    malpresentation 652.9●
      causing obstructed labor 660.0●
    marginal sinus (bleeding) (rupture)
      641.2●
    maternal hypotension syndrome
      669.2●
    meconium in liquor 656.8●
    membranes, retained - *see* Delivery,
      complicated, placenta,
      retained
    mentum presentation 652.4●
      causing obstructed labor 660.0●
    metrorrhagia (myopathia) - *see*
      Delivery, complicated,
      hemorrhage
    metrorrhexis - *see* Delivery,
      complicated, rupture, uterus
    multiparity (grand) 659.4●
    myelomeningocele, fetus 653.7●
      causing obstructed labor 660.1●
    Nägele's pelvis 653.0●
      causing obstructed labor 660.1●
    nonengagement, fetal head 652.5●
      causing obstructed labor 660.0●
    oblique presentation 652.3●
      causing obstructed labor
        660.0●
    obstetric
      shock 669.1●
      trauma NEC 665.9●
    obstructed labor 660.9●
      due to
        abnormality of pelvic organs
          or tissues (conditions
          classifiable to 654.0–
          654.9) 660.2●
        deep transverse arrest 660.3●
        impacted shoulders 660.4●
        locked twins 660.5●
        malposition and
          malpresentation of fetus
          (conditions classifiable to
          652.0–652.9) 660.0●
        persistent occipitoposterior
          660.3●
        shoulder dystocia 660.4●
    occult prolapse of umbilical cord
      663.0●
    oversize fetus 653.5●
      causing obstructed labor 660.1●
    pathological retraction ring, uterus
      661.4●
    pelvic
      arrest (deep) (high) (of fetal head)
        (transverse) 660.3●
      deformity (bone) - *see also*
        Deformity, pelvis, with
        disproportion
      soft tissue 654.9●
        causing obstructed labor
          660.2●
      tumor NEC 654.9●
        causing obstructed labor
          660.2●
    penetration, pregnant uterus by
      instrument 665.1●
    perforation - *see* Delivery,
      complicated, laceration

Delivery *(Continued)*
  complicated (by) NEC *(Continued)*
    persistent
      hymen 654.8●
        causing obstructed labor
          660.2●
      occipitoposterior 660.3●
    placenta, placental
      ablatio 641.2●
      abnormality 656.7●
        with hemorrhage 641.2●
      abruptio 641.2●
      accreta 667.0●
        with hemorrhage 666.0●
      adherent (without hemorrhage)
        667.0●
        with hemorrhage 666.0●
      apoplexy 641.2●
      Battledore - *see* Placenta,
        abnormal
      detachment (premature)
        641.2●
      disease 656.7●
      hemorrhage NEC 641.9●
      increta (without hemorrhage)
        667.0●
        with hemorrhage 666.0●
      low (implantation) 641.1●
        without hemorrhage 641.0●
      malformation 656.7●
        with hemorrhage 641.2●
      malposition 641.1●
        without hemorrhage 641.0●
      marginal sinus rupture 641.2●
      percreta 667.0●
        with hemorrhage 666.0●
      premature separation 641.2●
      previa (central) (lateral)
        (marginal) (partial) 641.1●
        without hemorrhage 641.0●
      retained (with hemorrhage)
        666.0●
        without hemorrhage 667.0●
      rupture of marginal sinus 641.2●
      separation (premature) 641.2●
      trapped 666.0●
        without hemorrhage 667.0●
      vicious insertion 641.1●
    polyhydramnios 657●
    polyp, cervix 654.6●
      causing obstructed labor 660.2●
    precipitate labor 661.3●
    premature
      labor (before 37 completed
        weeks' gestation) 644.2●
      rupture, membranes 658.1●
        delayed delivery following
          658.2●
    presenting umbilical cord 663.0●
    previous
      cesarean delivery, section 654.2●
      surgery
        cervix 654.6●
          causing obstructed labor
            660.2●
        gynecological NEC 654.9●
          causing obstructed labor
            660.2●
        perineum 654.8●
        rectum 654.8●
        uterus NEC 654.9●
          due to previous cesarean
            delivery, section
            654.2●

Delivery *(Continued)*
  complicated (by) NEC *(Continued)*
    previous *(Continued)*
      surgery *(Continued)*
        vagina 654.7●
          causing obstructed labor
            660.2●
        vulva 654.8●
    primary uterine inertia 661.0●
    primipara, elderly or old 659.5●
    prolapse
      arm or hand 652.7●
        causing obstructed labor
          660.0●
      cord (umbilical) 663.0●
      fetal extremity 652.8●
      foot or leg 652.8●
        causing obstructed labor
          660.0●
      umbilical cord (complete) (occult)
        (partial) 663.0●
      uterus 654.4●
        causing obstructed labor
          660.2●
    prolonged labor 662.1●
      first stage 662.0●
      second stage 662.2●
      active phase 661.2●
      due to
        cervical dystocia 661.2●
        contraction ring 661.4●
        tetanic uterus 661.4●
        uterine inertia 661.2●
          primary 661.0●
          secondary 661.1●
      latent phase 661.0●
    pyrexia during labor 659.2●
    rachitic pelvis 653.2●
      causing obstructed labor 660.1●
    rectocele 654.4●
      causing obstructed labor 660.2●
    retained membranes or portions of
      placenta 666.2●
      without hemorrhage 667.1●
    retarded (prolonged) birth 662.1●
    retention secundines (with
      hemorrhage) 666.2●
      without hemorrhage 667.1●
    retroversion, uterus or cervix
      654.3●
      causing obstructed labor 660.2●
    rigid
      cervix 654.6●
        causing obstructed labor
          660.2●
      pelvic floor 654.4●
        causing obstructed labor
          660.2●
      perineum or vulva 654.8●
        causing obstructed labor
          660.2●
      vagina 654.7●
        causing obstructed labor
          660.2●
    Robert's pelvis 653.0●
      causing obstructed labor
        660.1●
    rupture - *see also* Delivery,
      complicated, laceration
      bladder (urinary) 665.5●
      cervix 665.3●
      marginal sinus 641.2●
      membranes, premature 658.1●
      pelvic organ NEC 665.5●

◄ New   ◄▥ Revised   ~~deleted~~ Deleted   ● Use Additional Digit(s)   ▨ Omit code

Delivery (*Continued*)
  complicated (by) NEC (*Continued*)
    rupture (*Continued*)
      perineum (without mention of
        other laceration) - *see*
        Delivery, complicated,
        laceration, perineum
      peritoneum 665.5●
      urethra 665.5●
      uterus (during labor) 665.1●
        before labor 665.0●
    sacculation, pregnant uterus 654.4●
    sacral teratomas, fetal 653.7●
      causing obstructed labor 660.1●
    scar(s)
      cervix 654.6●
        causing obstructed labor
          660.2●
      cesarean delivery, section 654.2●
        causing obstructed labor
          660.2●
      perineum 654.8●
        causing obstructed labor
          660.2●
      uterus NEC 654.9●
        causing obstructed labor
          660.2●
        due to previous cesarean
          delivery, section 654.2●
      vagina 654.7●
        causing obstructed labor
          660.2●
      vulva 654.8●
        causing obstructed labor
          660.2●
    scoliotic pelvis 653.0●
      causing obstructed labor 660.1●
    secondary uterine inertia 661.1●
    secundines, retained - *see* Delivery,
      complicated, placenta,
      retained
    separation
      placenta (premature) 641.2●
      pubic bone 665.6●
      symphysis pubis 665.6●
    septate vagina 654.7●
      causing obstructed labor 660.2●
    shock (birth) (obstetric) (puerperal)
      669.1●
    short cord syndrome 663.4●
    shoulder
      girdle dystocia 660.4●
      presentation 652.8●
        causing obstructed labor
          660.0●
    Siamese twins 678.1●
      ~~causing obstructed labor 660.1~~
    slow slope active phase 661.2●
    spasm
      cervix 661.4●
      uterus 661.4●
    spondylolisthesis, pelvis 653.3●
      causing obstructed labor 660.1●
    spondylolysis (lumbosacral) 653.3●
      causing obstructed labor 660.1●
    spondylosis 653.0●
      causing obstructed labor 660.1●
    stenosis or stricture
      cervix 654.6●
        causing obstructed labor
          660.2●
      vagina 654.7●
        causing obstructed labor
          660.2●

Delivery (*Continued*)
  complicated (by) NEC (*Continued*)
    sudden death, unknown cause
      669.9●
    tear (pelvic organ) (*see also* Delivery,
      complicated, laceration)
      664.9●
      anal sphincter (healed) (old)
        654.8●
        not associated with third-
          degree perineal
          laceration 664.6●
    teratomas, sacral, fetal 653.7●
      causing obstructed labor 660.1●
    tetanic uterus 661.4●
    tipping pelvis 653.0●
      causing obstructed labor 660.1●
    transverse
      arrest (deep) 660.3●
      presentation or lie 652.3●
        with successful version
          652.1●
        causing obstructed labor
          660.0●
    trauma (obstetrical) NEC 665.9●
    tumor
      abdominal, fetal 653.7●
        causing obstructed labor
          660.1●
      pelvic organs or tissues NEC
        654.9●
        causing obstructed labor
          660.2●
    umbilical cord (*see also* Delivery,
      complicated, cord) 663.9●
      around neck tightly, or with
        compression 663.1●
      entanglement NEC 663.3●
        with compression 663.2●
      prolapse (complete) (occult)
        (partial) 663.0●
    unstable lie 652.0●
      causing obstructed labor
        660.0●
    uterine
      inertia (*see also* Delivery,
        complicated, inertia,
        uterus) 661.2●
        spasm 661.4●
    vasa previa 663.5●
    velamentous insertion of cord
      663.8●
    young maternal age 659.8●
  delayed NEC 662.1●
    following rupture of membranes
      (spontaneous) 658.2●
      artificial 658.3●
    second twin, triplet, etc. 662.3●
  difficult NEC 669.9●
    previous, affecting management of
      pregnancy or childbirth
      V23.49
    specified type NEC 669.8●
  early onset (spontaneous) 644.2●
  footling 652.8●
    with successful version 652.1●
  forceps NEC 669.5●
    affecting fetus or newborn 763.2
  missed (at or near term) 656.4●
  multiple gestation NEC 651.9●
    with fetal loss and retention of one
      or more fetus(es) 651.6●
    following (elective) fetal reduction
      651.7●

Delivery (*Continued*)
  multiple gestation NEC (*Continued*)
    specified type NEC 651.8●
      with fetal loss and retention of
        one or more fetus(es)
        651.6●
      following (elective) fetal
        reduction 651.7●
  nonviable infant 656.4●
  normal - *see* category 650
  precipitate 661.3●
    affecting fetus or newborn 763.6
  premature NEC (before 37 completed
    weeks' gestation) 644.2●
  previous, affecting management of
    pregnancy V23.41
  quadruplet NEC 651.2●
    with fetal loss and retention of one
      or more fetus(es) 651.5●
    following (elective) fetal reduction
      651.7●
  quintuplet NEC 651.8●
    with fetal loss and retention of one
      or more fetus(es) 651.6●
    following (elective) fetal reduction
      651.7●
  sextuplet NEC 651.8●
    with fetal loss and retention of one
      or more fetus(es) 651.6●
    following (elective) fetal reduction
      651.7●
  specified complication NEC
    669.8●
  stillbirth (near term) NEC 656.4●
    early (before 22 completed weeks'
      gestation) 632
  term pregnancy (live birth) NEC - *see*
    category 650
    stillbirth NEC 656.4●
  threatened premature 644.2●
  triplets NEC 651.1●
    with fetal loss and retention of one
      or more fetus(es) 651.4●
    delayed delivery (one or more
      mates) 662.3●
    following (elective) fetal reduction
      651.7●
    locked mates 660.5●
  twins NEC 651.0●
    with fetal loss and retention of one
      fetus 651.3●
    delayed delivery (one or more
      mates) 662.3●
    following (elective) fetal reduction
      651.7●
    locked mates 660.5●
  uncomplicated - *see* category 650
  vacuum extractor NEC 669.5●
    affecting fetus or newborn
      763.3
  ventouse NEC 669.5●
    affecting fetus or newborn
      763.3
Dellen, cornea 371.41
Delusions (paranoid) 297.9
  grandiose 297.1
  parasitosis 300.29
  systematized 297.1
Dementia 294.8
  alcohol-induced persisting (*see
    also* Psychosis, alcoholic)
    291.2
  Alzheimer's - *see* Alzheimer's,
    dementia

◀ New   ◀‖‖ Revised   ~~deleted~~ Deleted   ● Use Additional Digit(s)   ▨ Omit code

Dementia (*Continued*)
  arteriosclerotic (simple type)
    (uncomplicated) 290.40
    with
      acute confusional state 290.41
      delirium 290.41
      delusions 290.42
      depressed mood 290.43
      depressed type 290.43
      paranoid type 290.42
  Binswanger's 290.12
  catatonic (acute) (*see also*
    Schizophrenia) 295.2 ●
  congenital (*see also* Retardation, mental)
    319
  degenerative 290.9
    presenile-onset - *see* Dementia,
      presenile
    senile-onset - *see* Dementia, senile
  developmental (*see also* Schizophrenia)
    295.9 ●
  dialysis 294.8
    transient 293.9
  drug-induced persisting (*see also*
    Psychosis, drug) 292.82
  due to or associated with condition(s)
    classified elsewhere
    Alzheimer's
      with behavioral disturbance 331.0
        [294.11]
      without behavioral disturbance
        331.0 [294.10]
    cerebral lipidoses
      with behavioral disturbance 330.1
        [294.11]
      without behavioral disturbance
        330.1 [294.10]
    epilepsy
      with behavioral disturbance
        345.9 ● [294.11]
      without behavioral disturbance
        345.9 ● [294.10]
    hepatolenticular degeneration
      with behavioral disturbance 275.1
        [294.11]
      without behavioral disturbance
        275.1 [294.10]
    HIV
      with behavioral disturbance 042
        [294.11]
      without behavioral disturbance
        042 [294.10]
    Huntington's chorea
      with behavioral disturbance 333.4
        [294.11]
      without behavioral disturbance
        333.4 [294.10]
    Jakob-Creutzfeldt disease (CJD)
      with behavioral disturbance
        046.19 [294.11]
      without behavioral disturbance
        046.19 [294.10]
      variant (vCJD) 046.11
        with dementia
          with behavioral disturbance
            046.11 [294.11]
          without behavioral
            disturbance 046.11
            [294.10]
    Lewy bodies
      with behavioral disturbance
        331.82 [294.11]
      without behavioral disturbance
        331.82 [294.10]

Dementia (*Continued*)
  due to or associated with condition(s)
    classified elsewhere (*Continued*)
    multiple sclerosis
      with behavioral disturbance 340
        [294.11]
      without behavioral disturbance
        340 [294.10]
    neurosyphilis
      with behavioral disturbance 094.9
        [294.11]
      without behavioral disturbance
        094.9 [294.10]
    Parkinsonism
      with behavioral disturbance
        331.82 [294.11]
      without behavioral disturbance
        331.82 [294.10]
    Pelizaeus-Merzbacher disease
      with behavioral disturbance 333.0
        [294.11]
      without behavioral disturbance
        333.0 [294.10]
    Pick's disease
      with behavioral disturbance
        331.11 [294.11]
      without behavioral disturbance
        331.11 [294.10]
    polyarteritis nodosa
      with behavioral disturbance 446.0
        [294.11]
      without behavioral disturbance
        446.0 [294.10]
    syphilis
      with behavioral disturbance 094.1
        [294.11]
      without behavioral disturbance
        094.1 [294.10]
    Wilson's disease
      with behavioral disturbance 275.1
        [294.11]
      without behavioral disturbance
        275.1 [294.10]
  frontal 331.19
    with behavioral disturbance 331.19
      [294.11]
    without behavioral disturbance
      331.19 [294.10]
  frontotemporal 331.19
    with behavioral disturbance 331.19
      [294.11]
    without behavioral disturbance
      331.19 [294.10]
  hebephrenic (acute) 295.1 ●
  Heller's (infantile psychosis) (*see also*
    Psychosis, childhood) 299.1 ●
  idiopathic 290.9
    presenile-onset - *see* Dementia,
      presenile
    senile-onset - *see* Dementia, senile
  in
    arteriosclerotic brain disease 290.40
    senility 290.0
  induced by drug 292.82
  infantile, infantilia (*see also* Psychosis,
    childhood) 299.0 ●
  Lewy body 331.82
    with behavioral disturbance 331.82
      [294.11]
    without behavioral disturbance
      331.82 [294.10]
  multi-infarct (cerebrovascular) (*see also*
    Dementia, arteriosclerotic) 290.40
  old age 290.0

Dementia (*Continued*)
  paralytica, paralytic 094.1
    juvenilis 090.40
    syphilitic 094.1
      congenital 090.40
    tabetic form 094.1
  paranoid (*see also* Schizophrenia)
    295.3 ●
  paraphrenic (*see also* Schizophrenia)
    295.3 ●
  paretic 094.1
  praecox (*see also* Schizophrenia) 295.9 ●
  presenile 290.10
    with
      acute confusional state 290.11
      delirium 290.11
      delusional features 290.12
      depressive features 290.13
    depressed type 290.13
    paranoid type 290.12
    simple type 290.10
    uncomplicated 290.10
  primary (acute) (*see also* Schizophrenia)
    295.0 ●
  progressive, syphilitic 094.1
  puerperal - *see* Psychosis, puerperal
  schizophrenic (*see also* Schizophrenia)
    295.9 ●
  senile 290.0
    with
      acute confusional state 290.3
      delirium 290.3
      delusional features 290.20
      depressive features 290.21
    depressed type 290.21
    exhaustion 290.0
    paranoid type 290.20
  simple type (acute) (*see also*
    Schizophrenia) 295.0 ●
  simplex (acute) (*see also* Schizophrenia)
    295.0 ●
  syphilitic 094.1
  uremic - *see* Uremia
  vascular 290.40
    with
      delirium 290.41
      delusions 290.42
      depressed mood 290.43
Demerol dependence (*see also*
  Dependence) 304.0 ●
Demineralization, ankle (*see also*
  Osteoporosis) 733.00
Demodex folliculorum (infestation) 133.8
Demoralization 799.25 ◀
de Morgan's spots (senile angiomas) 448.1
Demyelinating
  polyneuritis, chronic inflammatory
    357.81
Demyelination, demyelinization
  central nervous system 341.9
    specified NEC 341.8
  corpus callosum (central) 341.8
  global 340
Dengue (fever) 061
  sandfly 061
  vaccination, prophylactic (against)
    V05.1
  virus hemorrhagic fever 065.4
Dens
  evaginatus 520.2
  in dente 520.2
  invaginatus 520.2
Dense
  breast(s) - *omit code*

◀ New   ◀▥ Revised   ~~deleted~~ Deleted   ● Use Additional Digit(s)   ▬ Omit code

Density
   increased, bone (disseminated)
      (generalized) (spotted) 733.99
   lung (nodular) 518.89
Dental - see also condition
   examination only V72.2
Dentia praecox 520.6
Denticles (in pulp) 522.2
Dentigerous cyst 526.0
Dentin
   irregular (in pulp) 522.3
   opalescent 520.5
   secondary (in pulp) 522.3
   sensitive 521.89
Dentinogenesis imperfecta 520.5
Dentinoma (M9271/0) 213.1
   upper jaw (bone) 213.0
Dentition 520.7
   abnormal 520.6
   anomaly 520.6
   delayed 520.6
   difficult 520.7
   disorder of 520.6
   precocious 520.6
   retarded 520.6
Denture sore (mouth) 528.9
Dependence

Note 20   Use the following fifth-digit subclassification with category 304:

0   unspecified
1   continuous
2   episodic
3   in remission

   with
      withdrawal symptoms
         alcohol 291.81
         drug 292.0
   14-hydroxy-dihydromorphinone
      304.0●
   absinthe 304.6●
   acemorphan 304.0●
   acetanilid(e) 304.6●
   acetophenetidin 304.6●
   acetorphine 304.0●
   acetyldihydrocodeine 304.0●
   acetyldihydrocodeinone 304.0●
   Adalin 304.1●
   Afghanistan black 304.3●
   agrypnal 304.1●
   alcohol, alcoholic (ethyl) (methyl)
      (wood) 303.9●
      maternal, with suspected fetal
         damage affecting management
         of pregnancy 655.4●
   allobarbitone 304.1●
   allonal 304.1●
   allylisopropylacetylurea 304.1●
   alphaprodine (hydrochloride) 304.0●
   Alurate 304.1●
   Alvodine 304.0●
   amethocaine 304.6●
   amidone 304.0●
   amidopyrine 304.6●
   aminopyrine 304.6●
   amobarbital 304.1●
   amphetamine(s) (type) (drugs
      classifiable to 969.7) 304.4●
   amylene hydrate 304.6●
   amylobarbitone 304.1●
   amylocaine 304.6●
   Amytal (sodium) 304.1●

Dependence (Continued)
   analgesic (drug) NEC 304.6●
      synthetic with morphine-like effect
         304.0●
   anesthetic (agent) (drug) (gas) (general)
      (local) NEC 304.6●
   Angel dust 304.6●
   anileridine 304.0●
   antipyrine 304.6●
   anxiolytic 304.1●
   aprobarbital 304.1●
   aprobarbitone 304.1●
   atropine 304.6●
   Avertin (bromide) 304.6●
   barbenyl 304.1●
   barbital(s) 304.1●
   barbitone 304.1●
   barbiturate(s) (compounds) (drugs
      classifiable to 967.0) 304.1●
   barbituric acid (and compounds)
      304.1●
   benzedrine 304.4●
   benzylmorphine 304.0●
   Beta-chlor 304.1●
   bhang 304.3●
   blue velvet 304.0●
   Brevital 304.1●
   bromal (hydrate) 304.1●
   bromide(s) NEC 304.1●
   bromine compounds NEC 304.1●
   bromisovalum 304.1●
   bromoform 304.1●
   Bromo-seltzer 304.1●
   bromural 304.1●
   butabarbital (sodium) 304.1●
   butabarpal 304.1●
   butallylonal 304.1●
   butethal 304.1●
   buthalitone (sodium) 304.1●
   Butisol 304.1●
   butobarbitone 304.1●
   butyl chloral (hydrate) 304.1●
   caffeine 304.4●
   cannabis (indica) (sativa) (resin)
      (derivatives) (type) 304.3●
   carbamazepine 304.6●
   Carbrital 304.1●
   carbromal 304.1●
   carisoprodol 304.6●
   Catha (edulis) 304.4●
   chloral (betaine) (hydrate) 304.1●
   chloralamide 304.1●
   chloralformamide 304.1●
   chloralose 304.1●
   chlordiazepoxide 304.1●
   Chloretone 304.1●
   chlorobutanol 304.1●
   chlorodyne 304.1●
   chloroform 304.6●
   Cliradon 304.0●
   coca (leaf) and derivatives 304.2●
   cocaine 304.2●
      hydrochloride 304.2●
      salt (any) 304.2●
   codeine 304.0●
   combination of drugs (excluding
      morphine or opioid type drug)
      NEC 304.8●
      morphine or opioid type drug with
         any other drug 304.7●
   croton-chloral 304.1●
   cyclobarbital 304.1●
   cyclobarbitone 304.1●
   dagga 304.3●

Dependence (Continued)
   Delvinal 304.1●
   Demerol 304.0●
   desocodeine 304.0●
   desomorphine 304.0●
   desoxyephedrine 304.4●
   DET 304.5●
   dexamphetamine 304.4●
   dexedrine 304.4●
   dextromethorphan 304.0●
   dextromoramide 304.0●
   dextronorpseudoephedrine 304.4●
   dextrorphan 304.0●
   diacetylmorphine 304.0●
   Dial 304.1●
   diallylbarbituric acid 304.1●
   diamorphine 304.0●
   diazepam 304.1●
   dibucaine 304.6●
   dichloroethane 304.6●
   diethyl barbituric acid 304.1●
   diethylsulfone-diethylmethane 304.1●
   difencloxazine 304.0●
   dihydrocodeine 304.0●
   dihydrocodeinone 304.0●
   dihydrohydroxycodeinone 304.0●
   dihydroisocodeine 304.0●
   dihydromorphine 304.0●
   dihydromorphinone 304.0●
   dihydroxcodeinone 304.0●
   Dilaudid 304.0●
   dimenhydrinate 304.6●
   dimethylmeperidine 304.0●
   dimethyltriptamine 304.5●
   Dionin 304.0●
   diphenoxylate 304.6●
   dipipanone 304.0●
   d-lysergic acid diethylamide 304.5●
   DMT 304.5●
   Dolophine 304.0●
   DOM 304.2●
   doriden 304.1●
   dormiral 304.1●
   Dormison 304.1●
   Dromoran 304.0●
   drug NEC 304.9●
      analgesic NEC 304.6●
      combination (excluding morphine
         or opioid type drug) NEC
         304.8●
      morphine or opioid type drug
         with any other drug 304.7●
      complicating pregnancy, childbirth,
         or puerperium 648.3●
         affecting fetus or newborn 779.5
      hallucinogenic 304.5●
      hypnotic NEC 304.1●
      narcotic NEC 304.9
      psychostimulant NEC 304.4●
      sedative 304.1●
      soporific NEC 304.1●
      specified type NEC 304.6●
      suspected damage to fetus affecting
         management of pregnancy
         655.5●
      synthetic, with morphine-like effect
         304.0●
      tranquilizing 304.1●
   duboisine 304.6●
   ectylurea 304.1●
   Endocaine 304.6●
   Equanil 304.1●
   Eskabarb 304.1●
   ethchlorvynol 304.1●

Dependence (*Continued*)
 ether (ethyl) (liquid) (vapor) (vinyl)
  304.6●
 ethidene 304.6●
 ethinamate 304.1●
 ethoheptazine 304.6●
 ethyl
  alcohol 303.9●
  bromide 304.6●
  carbamate 304.6●
  chloride 304.6●
  morphine 304.0●
 ethylene (gas) 304.6●
  dichloride 304.6●
 ethylidene chloride 304.6●
 etilfen 304.1●
 etorphine 304.0●
 etoval 304.1●
 eucodal 304.0●
 euneryl 304.1●
 Evipal 304.1●
 Evipan 304.1●
 fentanyl 304.0●
 ganja 304.3●
 gardenal 304.1●
 gardenpanyl 304.1●
 gelsemine 304.6●
 Gelsemium 304.6●
 Gemonil 304.1●
 glucochloral 304.1●
 glue (airplane) (sniffing) 304.6●
 glutethimide 304.1●
 hallucinogenics 304.5●
 hashish 304.3●
 headache powder NEC 304.6●
 Heavenly Blue 304.5●
 hedonal 304.1●
 hemp 304.3●
 heptabarbital 304.1●
 Heptalgin 304.0●
 heptobarbitone 304.1●
 heroin 304.0●
  salt (any) 304.0●
 hexethal (sodium) 304.1●
 hexobarbital 304.1●
 Hycodan 304.0●
 hydrocodone 304.0●
 hydromorphinol 304.0●
 hydromorphinone 304.0●
 hydromorphone 304.0●
 hydroxycodeine 304.0●
 hypnotic NEC 304.1●
 Indian hemp 304.3●
 inhalant 304.6●
 intranarcon 304.1●
 Kemithal 304.1●
 ketobemidone 304.0●
 khat 304.4●
 kif 304.3●
 Lactuca (virosa) extract 304.1●
 lactucarium 304.1●
 laudanum 304.0●
 Lebanese red 304.3●
 Leritine 304.0●
 lettuce opium 304.1●
 Levanil 304.1●
 Levo-Dromoran 304.0●
 levo-iso-methadone 304.0●
 levorphanol 304.0●
 Librium 304.1●
 Lomotil 304.6●
 Lotusate 304.1●
 LSD (-25) (and derivatives) 304.5●
 Luminal 304.1●

Dependence (*Continued*)
 lysergic acid 304.5●
  amide 304.5●
 maconha 304.3●
 magic mushroom 304.5●
 marihuana 304.3●
 MDA (methylene dioxyamphetamine)
  304.4●
 Mebaral 304.1●
 Medinal 304.1●
 Medomin 304.1●
 megahallucinogenics 304.5●
 meperidine 304.0●
 mephobarbital 304.1●
 meprobamate 304.1●
 mescaline 304.5●
 methadone 304.0●
 methamphetamine(s) 304.4●
 methaqualone 304.1●
 metharbital 304.1●
 methitural 304.1●
 methobarbitone 304.1●
 methohexital 304.1●
 methopholine 304.6●
 methyl●
  alcohol 303.9●
  bromide 304.6●
  morphine 304.0●
  sulfonal 304.1●
 methylated spirit 303.9●
 methylbutinol 304.6●
 methyldihydromorphinone 304.0●
 methylene●
  chloride 304.6●
  dichloride 304.6●
  dioxyamphetamine (MDA) 304.4●
 methylparafynol 304.1●
 methylphenidate 304.4●
 methyprylone 304.1●
 metopon 304.0●
 Miltown 304.1●
 morning glory seeds 304.5●
 morphinan(s) 304.0●
 morphine (sulfate) (sulfite) (type)
   (drugs classifiable to 965.00–
   965.09) 304.0●
 morphine or opioid type drug (drugs
   classifiable to 965.00–965.09) with
   any other drug 304.7●
 morphinol(s) 304.0●
 morphinon 304.0●
 morpholinylethylmorphine 304.0●
 mylomide 304.1●
 myristicin 304.5●
 narcotic (drug) NEC 304.9●
 nealbarbital 304.1●
 nealbarbitone 304.1●
 Nembutal 304.1●
 Neonal 304.1●
 Neraval 304.1●
 Neravan 304.1●
 neurobarb 304.1●
 nicotine 305.1
 Nisentil 304.0●
 nitrous oxide 304.6●
 Noctec 304.1●
 Noludar 304.1●
 nonbarbiturate sedatives and
   tranquilizers with similar effect
   304.1●
 noptil 304.1●
 normorphine 304.0●
 noscapine 304.0●
 Novocaine 304.6●
 Numorphan 304.0●

Dependence (*Continued*)
 nunol 304.1●
 Nupercaine 304.6●
 Oblivon 304.1●
 on
  aspirator V46.0
  hemodialysis V45.11
  hyperbaric chamber V46.8
  iron lung V46.11
  machine (enabling) V46.9
   specified type NEC V46.8
  peritoneal dialysis V45.11
  Possum (patient-operated-selector-
   mechanism) V46.8
  renal dialysis machine V45.11
  respirator [ventilator] V46.11
   encounter
    during
     power failure V46.12
     mechanical failure V46.14
    for weaning V46.13
  supplemental oxygen V46.2
  wheelchair V46.3
 opiate 304.0●
 opioids 304.0●
 opioid type drug 304.0●
  with any other drug 304.7●
 opium (alkaloids) (derivatives)
   (tincture) 304.0●
 ortal 304.1●
 oxazepam 304.1●
 oxycodone 304.0●
 oxymorphone 304.0●
 Palfium 304.0●
 Panadol 304.6●
 pantopium 304.0●
 pantopon 304.0●
 papaverine 304.0●
 paracetamol 304.6●
 paracodin 304.0●
 paraldehyde 304.1●
 paregoric 304.0●
 Parzone 304.0●
 PCP (phencyclidine) 304.6●
 Pearly Gates 304.5●
 pentazocine 304.0●
 pentobarbital 304.1●
 pentobarbitone (sodium) 304.1●
 Pentothal 304.1●
 Percaine 304.6●
 Percodan 304.0●
 Perichlor 304.1●
 Pernocton 304.1●
 Pernoston 304.1●
 peronine 304.0●
 pethidine (hydrochloride) 304.0●
 petrichloral 304.1●
 peyote 304.5●
 Phanodorn 304.1●
 phenacetin 304.6●
 phenadoxone 304.0●
 phenaglycodol 304.1●
 phenazocine 304.0●
 phencyclidine 304.6●
 phenmetrazine 304.4●
 phenobal 304.1●
 phenobarbital 304.1●
 phenobarbitone 304.1●
 phenomorphan 304.0●
 phenonyl 304.1●
 phenoperidine 304.0●
 pholcodine 304.0●
 piminodine 304.0●
 Pipadone 304.0●
 Pitkin's solution 304.6●

◀ New   ◀▥ Revised   ~~deleted~~ Deleted   ● Use Additional Digit(s)   ▬ Omit code

Dependence (Continued)
Placidyl 304.1●
polysubstance 304.8●
Pontocaine 304.6●
pot 304.3●
potassium bromide 304.1●
Preludin 304.4●
Prinadol 304.0●
probarbital 304.1●
procaine 304.6●
propanal 304.1●
propoxyphene 304.6●
psilocibin 304.5●
psilocin 304.5●
psilocybin 304.5●
psilocyline 304.5●
psilocyn 304.5●
psychedelic agents 304.5●
psychostimulant NEC 304.4●
psychotomimetic agents 304.5●
pyrahexyl 304.3●
Pyramidon 304.6●
quinalbarbitone 304.1●
racemoramide 304.0●
racemorphan 304.0●
Rela 304.6●
scopolamine 304.6●
secobarbital 304.1●
seconal 304.1●
sedative NEC 304.1●
    nonbarbiturate with barbiturate
        effect 304.1●
Sedormid 304.1●
sernyl 304.1●
sodium bromide 304.1●
Soma 304.6●
Somnal 304.1●
Somnos 304.1●
Soneryl 304.1●
soporific (drug) NEC 304.1●
specified drug NEC 304.6●
speed 304.4●
spinocaine 304.6●
stovaine 304.6●
STP 304.5●
stramonium 304.6●
Sulfonal 304.1●
sulfonethylmethane 304.1●
sulfonmethane 304.1●
Surital 304.1●
synthetic drug with morphine-like
    effect 304.0●
talbutal 304.1●
tetracaine 304.6●
tetrahydrocannabinol 304.3●
tetronal 304.1●
THC 304.3●
thebacon 304.0●
thebaine 304.0●
thiamil 304.1●
thiamylal 304.1●
thiopental 304.1●
tobacco 305.1
toluene, toluol 304.6●
tranquilizer NEC 304.1●
    nonbarbiturate with barbiturate
        effect 304.1●
tribromacetaldehyde 304.6●
tribromethanol 304.6●
tribromomethane 304.6●
trichloroethanol 304.6●
trichoroethyl phosphate 304.1●
triclofos 304.1●
Trional 304.1●
Tuinal 304.1●

Dependence (Continued)
Turkish green 304.3●
urethan(e) 304.6●
Valium 304.1●
Valmid 304.1●
veganin 304.0●
veramon 304.1●
Veronal 304.1●
versidyne 304.6●
vinbarbital 304.1●
vinbarbitone 304.1●
vinyl bitone 304.1●
vitamin B₆ 266.1
wine 303.9●
Zactane 304.6●
Dependency
passive 301.6
reactions 301.6
Depersonalization (episode, in neurotic
    state) (neurotic) (syndrome) 300.6
Depletion
carbohydrates 271.9
complement factor 279.8
extracellular fluid 276.52
plasma 276.52
potassium 276.8
    nephropathy 588.89
salt or sodium 276.1
    causing heat exhaustion or
        prostration 992.4
    nephropathy 593.9
volume 276.50
    extracellular fluid 276.52
    plasma 276.52
Deployment (military) ◀
personal history of V62.22 ◀
returned from V62.22 ◀
status V62.21 ◀
Deposit
argentous, cornea 371.16
bone, in Boeck's sarcoid 135
calcareous, calcium - see
    Calcification
cholesterol
    retina 362.82
    skin 709.3
    vitreous (humor) 379.22
conjunctival 372.56
cornea, corneal NEC 371.10
    argentous 371.16
    in
        cystinosis 270.0 [371.15]
        mucopolysaccharidosis 277.5
            [371.15]
crystalline, vitreous (humor) 379.22
hemosiderin, in old scars of cornea
    371.11
metallic, in lens 366.45
skin 709.3
teeth, tooth (betel) (black) (green)
    (materia alba) (orange) (soft)
    (tobacco) 523.6
urate, in kidney (see also Disease, renal)
    593.9
Depraved appetite 307.52
Depression 311
acute (see also Psychosis, affective)
    296.2●
    recurrent episode 296.3●
    single episode 296.2●
agitated (see also Psychosis, affective)
    296.2●
    recurrent episode 296.3●
    single episode 296.2●
anaclitic 309.21

Depression (Continued)
anxiety 300.4
arches 734
    congenital 754.61
autogenous (see also Psychosis,
    affective) 296.2●
    recurrent episode 296.3●
    single episode 296.2●
basal metabolic rate (BMR) 794.7
bone marrow 289.9
central nervous system 799.1
    newborn 779.2
cerebral 331.9
    newborn 779.2
cerebrovascular 437.8
    newborn 779.2
chest wall 738.3
endogenous (see also Psychosis,
    affective) 296.2●
    recurrent episode 296.3●
    single episode 296.2●
functional activity 780.99
hysterical 300.11
involutional, climacteric, or
    menopausal (see also Psychosis,
        affective) 296.2●
    recurrent episode 296.3●
    single episode 296.2●
manic (see also Psychosis, affective)
    296.80
medullary 348.89   ◀▥
    newborn 779.2
mental 300.4
metatarsal heads - see Depression,
    arches
metatarsus - see Depression, arches
monopolar (see also Psychosis,
    affective) 296.2●
    recurrent episode 296.3●
    single episode 296.2●
nervous 300.4
neurotic 300.4
nose 738.0
postpartum 648.4●
psychogenic 300.4
    reactive 298.0
psychoneurotic 300.4
psychotic (see also Psychosis, affective)
    296.2●
    reactive 298.0
    recurrent episode 296.3●
    single episode 296.2●
reactive 300.4
    neurotic 300.4
    psychogenic 298.0
    psychoneurotic 300.4
    psychotic 298.0
recurrent 296.3●
respiratory center 348.89   ◀▥
    newborn 770.89
scapula 736.89
senile 290.21
situational (acute) (brief) 309.0
    prolonged 309.1
skull 754.0
sternum 738.3
visual field 368.40
Depressive reaction - see also Reaction,
    depressive
acute (transient) 309.0
    with anxiety 309.28
prolonged 309.1
situational (acute) 309.0
    prolonged 309.1

Deprivation
- cultural V62.4
- emotional V62.89
  - affecting
    - adult 995.82
    - infant or child 995.51
- food 994.2
  - specific substance NEC 269.8
- protein (familial) (kwashiorkor) 260
- sleep V69.4
- social V62.4
  - affecting
    - adult 995.82
    - infant or child 995.51
- symptoms, syndrome
  - alcohol 291.81
  - drug 292.0
- vitamins (see also Deficiency, vitamin) 269.2
- water 994.3

de Quervain's
- disease (tendon sheath) 727.04
- syndrome 259.51
- thyroiditis (subacute granulomatous thyroiditis) 245.1

Derangement
- ankle (internal) 718.97
  - current injury (see also Dislocation, ankle) 837.0
  - recurrent 718.37
- cartilage (articular) NEC (see also Disorder, cartilage, articular) 718.0●
  - knee 717.9
    - recurrent 718.36
  - recurrent 718.3●
- collateral ligament (knee) (medial) (tibial) 717.82
  - current injury 844.1
    - lateral (fibular) 844.0
  - lateral (fibular) 717.81
    - current injury 844.0
- cruciate ligament (knee) (posterior) 717.84
  - anterior 717.83
    - current injury 844.2
  - current injury 844.2
- elbow (internal) 718.92
  - current injury (see also Dislocation, elbow) 832.00
  - recurrent 718.32
- gastrointestinal 536.9
- heart - see Disease, heart
- hip (joint) (internal) (old) 718.95
  - current injury (see also Dislocation, hip) 835.00
  - recurrent 718.35
- intervertebral disc - see Displacement, intervertebral disc
- joint (internal) 718.90
  - ankle 718.97
  - current injury - see also Dislocation, by site
    - knee, meniscus or cartilage (see also Tear, meniscus) 836.2
  - elbow 718.92
  - foot 718.97
  - hand 718.94
  - hip 718.95
  - knee 717.9
  - multiple sites 718.99
  - pelvic region 718.95

Derangement (Continued)
- joint (Continued)
  - recurrent 718.30
    - ankle 718.37
    - elbow 718.32
    - foot 718.37
    - hand 718.34
    - hip 718.35
    - knee 718.36
    - multiple sites 718.39
    - pelvic region 718.35
    - shoulder (region) 718.31
    - specified site NEC 718.38
    - temporomandibular (old) 524.69
    - wrist 718.33
  - shoulder (region) 718.91
  - specified site NEC 718.98
  - spine NEC 724.9
  - temporomandibular 524.69
  - wrist 718.93
- knee (cartilage) (internal) 717.9
  - current injury (see also Tear, meniscus) 836.2
  - ligament 717.89
    - capsular 717.85
    - collateral - see Derangement, collateral ligament
    - cruciate - see Derangement, cruciate ligament
    - specified NEC 717.85
  - recurrent 718.36
- low back NEC 724.9
- meniscus NEC (knee) 717.5
  - current injury (see also Tear, meniscus) 836.2
  - lateral 717.40
    - anterior horn 717.42
    - posterior horn 717.43
    - specified NEC 717.49
  - medial 717.3
    - anterior horn 717.1
    - posterior horn 717.2
  - recurrent 718.3●
  - site other than knee - see Disorder, cartilage, articular
- mental (see also Psychosis) 298.9
- rotator cuff (recurrent) (tear) 726.10
  - current 840.4
- sacroiliac (old) 724.6
  - current - see Dislocation, sacroiliac
- semilunar cartilage (knee) 717.5
  - current injury 836.2
    - lateral 836.1
    - medial 836.0
  - recurrent 718.3●
- shoulder (internal) 718.91
  - current injury (see also Dislocation, shoulder) 831.00
  - recurrent 718.31
- spine (recurrent) NEC 724.9
  - current - see Dislocation, spine
- temporomandibular (internal) (joint) (old) 524.69
  - current - see Dislocation, jaw

Dercum's disease or syndrome (adiposis dolorosa) 272.8

Derealization (neurotic) 300.6

Dermal - see condition

Dermaphytid - see Dermatophytosis

Dermatergosis - see Dermatitis

Dermatitis (allergic) (contact) (occupational) (venenata) 692.9
- ab igne 692.82
- acneiform 692.9

Dermatitis (Continued)
- actinic (due to sun) 692.70
  - acute 692.72
  - chronic NEC 692.74
  - other than from sun NEC 692.82
- ambustionis
  - due to
    - burn or scald - see Burn, by site
    - sunburn (see also Sunburn) 692.71
- amebic 006.6
- ammonia 691.0
- anaphylactoid NEC 692.9
- arsenical 692.4
- artefacta 698.4
  - psychogenic 316 [698.4]
- asthmatic 691.8
- atopic (allergic) (intrinsic) 691.8
  - psychogenic 316 [691.8]
- atrophicans 701.8
  - diffusa 701.8
  - maculosa 701.3
- autoimmune progesterone 279.49 ◄
- berlock, berloque 692.72
- blastomycetic 116.0
- blister beetle 692.89
- Brucella NEC 023.9
- bullosa 694.9
  - striata pratensis 692.6
- bullous 694.9
  - mucosynechial, atrophic 694.60
    - with ocular involvement 694.61
  - seasonal 694.8
- calorica
  - due to
    - burn or scald - see Burn, by site
    - cold 692.89
    - sunburn (see also Sunburn) 692.71
- caterpillar 692.89
- cercarial 120.3
- combustionis
  - due to
    - burn or scald - see Burn, by site
    - sunburn (see also Sunburn) 692.71
- congelationis 991.5
- contusiformis 695.2
- diabetic 250.8●
- diaper 691.0
- diphtheritica 032.85
- due to
  - acetone 692.2
  - acids 692.4
  - adhesive plaster 692.4
  - alcohol (skin contact) (substances classifiable to 980.0–980.9) 692.4
    - taken internally 693.8
  - alkalis 692.4
  - allergy NEC 692.9
  - ammonia (household) (liquid) 692.4
  - animal
    - dander (cat) (dog) 692.84
    - hair (cat) (dog) 692.84
  - arnica 692.3
  - arsenic 692.4
    - taken internally 693.8
  - blister beetle 692.89
  - cantharides 692.3
  - carbon disulphide 692.2
  - caterpillar 692.89
  - caustics 692.4

◄ New   ◄▪ Revised   ~~deleted~~ Deleted   ● Use Additional Digit(s)   ▨ Omit code

Dermatitis (Continued)
due to (Continued)
cereal (ingested) 693.1
contact with skin 692.5
chemical(s) NEC 692.4
internal 693.8
irritant NEC 692.4
taken internally 693.8
chlorocompounds 692.2
coffee (ingested) 693.1
contact with skin 692.5
cold weather 692.89
cosmetics 692.81
cyclohexanes 692.2
dander, animal (cat) (dog)
692.84
deodorant 692.81
detergents 692.0
dichromate 692.4
drugs and medicinals (correct
substance properly
administered) (internal use)
693.0
external (in contact with skin)
692.3
wrong substance given or
taken 976.9
specified substance - see
Table of Drugs and
Chemicals
wrong substance given or taken
977.9
specified substance - see
Table of Drugs and
Chemicals
dyes 692.89
hair 692.89
epidermophytosis - see
Dermatophytosis
esters 692.2
external irritant NEC 692.9
specified agent NEC 692.89
eye shadow 692.81
fish (ingested) 693.1
contact with skin 692.5
flour (ingested) 693.1
contact with skin 692.5
food (ingested) 693.1
in contact with skin 692.5
fruit (ingested) 693.1
contact with skin 692.5
fungicides 692.3
furs 692.84
glycols 692.2
greases NEC 692.1
hair, animal (cat) (dog) 692.84
hair dyes 692.89
hot
objects and materials - see Burn,
by site
weather or places 692.89
hydrocarbons 692.2
infrared rays, except from sun
692.82
solar NEC (see also Dermatitis,
due to, sun) 692.70
ingested substance 693.9
drugs and medicinals (see
also Dermatitis, due to,
drugs and medicinals)
693.0
food 693.1
specified substance NEC
693.8

Dermatitis (Continued)
due to (Continued)
ingestion or injection of
chemical 693.8
drug (correct substance properly
administered) 693.0
wrong substance given or
taken 977.9
specified substance - see
Table of Drugs and
Chemicals
insecticides 692.4
internal agent 693.9
drugs and medicinals (see also
Dermatitis, due to, drugs
and medicinals) 693.0
food (ingested) 693.1
in contact with skin 692.5
specified agent NEC 693.8
iodine 692.3
iodoform 692.3
irradiation 692.82
jewelry 692.83
keratolytics 692.3
ketones 692.2
lacquer tree (Rhus verniciflua)
692.6
light (sun) NEC (see also Dermatitis,
due to, sun) 692.70
other 692.82
low temperature 692.89
mascara 692.81
meat (ingested) 693.1
contact with skin 692.5
mercury, mercurials 692.3
metals 692.83
milk (ingested) 693.1
contact with skin 692.5
Neomycin 692.3
nylon 692.4
oils NEC 692.1
paint solvent 692.2
pediculocides 692.3
petroleum products (substances
classifiable to 981) 692.4
phenol 692.3
photosensitiveness, photosensitivity
(sun) 692.72
other light 692.82
plants NEC 692.6
plasters, medicated (any) 692.3
plastic 692.4
poison
ivy (Rhus toxicodendron) 692.6
oak (Rhus diversiloba) 692.6
plant or vine 692.6
sumac (Rhus venenata) 692.6
vine (Rhus radicans) 692.6
preservatives 692.89
primrose (primula) 692.6
primula 692.6
radiation 692.82
sun NEC (see also Dermatitis,
due to, sun) 692.70
tanning bed 692.82
radioactive substance 692.82
radium 692.82
ragweed (Senecio jacobae) 692.6
Rhus (diversiloba) (radicans)
(toxicodendron) (venenata)
(verniciflua) 692.6
rubber 692.4
scabicides 692.3
Senecio jacobae 692.6

Dermatitis (Continued)
due to (Continued)
solar radiation - see Dermatitis, due
to, sun
solvents (any) (substances
classifiable to 982.0–982.8)
692.2
chlorocompound group 692.2
cyclohexane group 692.2
ester group 692.2
glycol group 692.2
hydrocarbon group 692.2
ketone group 692.2
paint 692.2
specified agent NEC 692.89
sun 692.70
acute 692.72
chronic NEC 692.74
specified NEC 692.79
sunburn (see also Sunburn) 692.71
sunshine NEC (see also Dermatitis,
due to, sun) 692.70
tanning bed 692.82
tetrachlorethylene 692.2
toluene 692.2
topical medications 692.3
turpentine 692.2
ultraviolet rays, except from sun
692.82
sun NEC (see also Dermatitis, due
to, sun) 692.70
vaccine or vaccination (correct
substance properly
administered) 693.0
wrong substance given or taken
bacterial vaccine 978.8
specified - see Table
of Drugs and
Chemicals
other vaccines NEC 979.9
specified - see Table of
Drugs and
Chemicals
varicose veins (see also Varicose,
vein, inflamed or infected)
454.1
x-rays 692.82
dyshydrotic 705.81
dysmenorrheica 625.8
eczematoid NEC 692.9
infectious 690.8
eczematous NEC 692.9
epidemica 695.89
erysipelatosa 695.81
escharotica - see Burn, by site
exfoliativa, exfoliative 695.89
generalized 695.89
infantum 695.81
neonatorum 695.81
eyelid 373.31
allergic 373.32
contact 373.32
eczematous 373.31
herpes (zoster) 053.20
simplex 054.41
infective 373.5
due to
actinomycosis 039.3 [373.5]
herpes
simplex 054.41
zoster 053.20
impetigo 684 [373.5]
leprosy (see also Leprosy) 030.0
[373.4]

Dermatitis (Continued)
  eyelid (Continued)
    infective (Continued)
      due to (Continued)
        lupus vulgaris (tuberculous)
          (see also Tuberculosis)
          017.0 ● [373.4]
        mycotic dermatitis (see also
          Dermatomycosis) 111.9
          [373.5]
        vaccinia 051.02 [373.5]
          postvaccination 999.0
          [373.5]
        yaws (see also Yaws) 102.9 [373.4]
  facta, factitia 698.4
    psychogenic 316 [698.4]
  ficta 698.4
    psychogenic 316 [698.4]
  flexural 691.8
  follicularis 704.8
  friction 709.8
  fungus 111.9
    specified type NEC 111.8
  gangrenosa, gangrenous (infantum)
    (see also Gangrene) 785.4
  gestationis 646.8●
  gonococcal 098.89
  gouty 274.89
  harvest mite 133.8
  heat 692.89
  herpetiformis (bullous) (erythematous)
    (pustular) (vesicular) 694.0
    juvenile 694.2
    senile 694.5
  hiemalis 692.89
  hypostatic, hypostatica 454.1
    with ulcer 454.2
  impetiginous 684
  infantile (acute) (chronic)
    (intertriginous) (intrinsic)
    (seborrheic) 690.12
  infectiosa eczematoides 690.8
  infectious (staphylococcal)
    (streptococcal) 686.9
    eczematoid 690.8
  infective eczematoid 690.8
  Jacquet's (diaper dermatitis) 691.0
  leptus 133.8
  lichenified NEC 692.9
  lichenoid, chronic 701.0
  lichenoides purpurica pigmentosa
    709.1
  meadow 692.6
  medicamentosa (correct substance
    properly administered) (internal
    use) (see also Dermatitis, due to,
    drugs or medicinals) 693.0
    due to contact with skin 692.3
  mite 133.8
  multiformis 694.0
    juvenile 694.2
    senile 694.5
  napkin 691.0
  neuro 698.3
  neurotica 694.0
  nummular NEC 692.9
  osteatosis, osteatotic 706.8
  papillaris capillitii 706.1
  pellagrous 265.2
  perioral 695.3
  perstans 696.1
  photosensitivity (sun) 692.72
    other light 692.82
  pigmented purpuric lichenoid 709.1

Dermatitis (Continued)
  polymorpha dolorosa 694.0
  primary irritant 692.9
  pruriginosa 694.0
  pruritic NEC 692.9
  psoriasiform nodularis 696.2
  psychogenic 316
  purulent 686.00
  pustular contagious 051.2
  pyococcal 686.00
  pyocyaneus 686.09
  pyogenica 686.00
  radiation 692.82
  repens 696.1
  Ritter's (exfoliativa) 695.81
  Schamberg's (progressive pigmentary
    dermatosis) 709.09
  schistosome 120.3
  seasonal bullous 694.8
  seborrheic 690.10
    infantile 690.12
  sensitization NEC 692.9
  septic (see also Septicemia) 686.00
    gonococcal 098.89
  solar, solare NEC (see also Dermatitis,
    due to, sun) 692.70
  stasis 454.1
    due to
      postphlebitic syndrome 459.12
        with ulcer 459.13
      varicose veins - see Varicose
    ulcerated or with ulcer (varicose)
      454.2
  sunburn (see also Sunburn) 692.71
  suppurative 686.00
  traumatic NEC 709.8
  trophoneurotica 694.0
  ultraviolet, except from sun 692.82
    due to sun NEC (see also Dermatitis,
      due to, sun) 692.70
  varicose 454.1
    with ulcer 454.2
  vegetans 686.8
  verrucosa 117.2
  xerotic 706.8
Dermatoarthritis, lipoid 272.8 [713.0]
Dermatochalasia, dermatochalasis 374.87
Dermatofibroma (lenticulare) (M8832/0) -
  see also Neoplasm, skin, benign
  protuberans (M8832/1) - see Neoplasm,
    skin, uncertain behavior
Dermatofibrosarcoma (protuberans)
  (M8832/3) - see Neoplasm, skin,
  malignant
Dermatographia 708.3
Dermatolysis (congenital) (exfoliativa)
  757.39
  acquired 701.8
  eyelids 374.34
  palpebrarum 374.34
  senile 701.8
Dermatomegaly NEC 701.8
Dermatomucomyositis 710.3
Dermatomycosis 111.9
  furfuracea 111.0
  specified type NEC 111.8
Dermatomyositis (acute) (chronic) 710.3
Dermatoneuritis of children 985.0
Dermatophiliasis 134.1
Dermatophytide - see Dermatophytosis
Dermatophytosis (Epidermophyton)
  (infection) (microsporum) (tinea)
  (Trichophyton) 110.9
  beard 110.0

Dermatophytosis (Continued)
  body 110.5
  deep seated 110.6
  fingernails 110.1
  foot 110.4
  groin 110.3
  hand 110.2
  nail 110.1
  perianal (area) 110.3
  scalp 110.0
  scrotal 110.8
  specified site NEC 110.8
  toenails 110.1
  vulva 110.8
Dermatopolyneuritis 985.0
Dermatorrhexis 756.83
  acquired 701.8
Dermatosclerosis (see also Scleroderma)
  710.1
  localized 701.0
Dermatosis 709.9
  Andrews' 686.8
  atopic 691.8
  Bowen's (M8081/2) - see Neoplasm,
    skin, in situ
  bullous 694.9
    specified type NEC 694.8
  erythematosquamous 690.8
  exfoliativa 695.89
  factitial 698.4
  gonococcal 098.89
  herpetiformis 694.0
    juvenile 694.2
    senile 694.5
  hysterical 300.11
  linear IgA 694.8
  menstrual NEC 709.8
  neutrophilic, acute febrile 695.89
  occupational (see also Dermatitis)
    692.9
  papulosa nigra 709.8
  pigmentary NEC 709.00
    progressive 709.09
    Schamberg's 709.09
    Siemens-Bloch 757.33
  progressive pigmentary 709.09
  psychogenic 316
  pustular subcorneal 694.1
  Schamberg's (progressive pigmentary)
    709.09
  senile NEC 709.3
  specified NEC 702.8
  Unna's (seborrheic dermatitis) 690.10
Dermographia 708.3
Dermographism 708.3
Dermoid (cyst) (M9084/0) - see also
  Neoplasm, by site, benign
  with malignant transformation
    (M9084/3) 183.0
Dermopathy
  infiltrative, with thyrotoxicosis
    242.0●
  nephrogenic fibrosing 701.8
  senile NEC 709.3
Dermophytosis - see Dermatophytosis
Descemet's membrane - see condition
Descemetocele 371.72
Descending - see condition
Descensus uteri (complete) (incomplete)
  (partial) (without vaginal wall
  prolapse) 618.1
  with mention of vaginal wall prolapse -
    see Prolapse, uterovaginal
Desensitization to allergens V07.1

◄ New   ◄▥ Revised   ~~deleted~~ Deleted   ● Use Additional Digit(s)   ▨ Omit code

Desert
 rheumatism 114.0
 sore (see also Ulcer, skin) 707.9
Desertion (child) (newborn) 995.52
 adult 995.84
Desmoid (extra-abdominal) (tumor)
  (M8821/1) - see also Neoplasm,
  connective tissue, uncertain
  behavior
 abdominal (M8822/1) - see Neoplasm, ·
  connective tissue, uncertain
  behavior
Despondency 300.4
Desquamative dermatitis NEC 695.89
Destruction
 articular facet (see also Derangement,
  joint) 718.9●
  vertebra 724.9
 bone 733.90
  syphilitic 095.5
 joint (see also Derangement, joint)
  718.9●
  sacroiliac 724.6
 kidney 593.89
 live fetus to facilitate birth NEC 763.89
 ossicles (ear) 385.24
 rectal sphincter 569.49
 septum (nasal) 478.19
 tuberculous NEC (see also Tuberculosis)
  011.9●
 tympanic membrane 384.82
 tympanum 385.89
 vertebral disc - see Degeneration,
  intervertebral disc
Destructiveness (see also Disturbance,
  conduct) 312.9
 adjustment reaction 309.3
Detachment
 cartilage - see also Sprain, by site
  knee - see Tear, meniscus
 cervix, annular 622.8
  complicating delivery 665.3●
 choroid (old) (postinfectional)
  (simple) (spontaneous)
  363.70
  hemorrhagic 363.72
  serous 363.71
 knee, medial meniscus (old) 717.3
  current injury 836.0
 ligament - see Sprain, by site
 placenta (premature) - see Placenta,
  separation
 retina (recent) 361.9
  with retinal defect
   (rhegmatogenous) 361.00
   giant tear 361.03
   multiple 361.02
   partial
    with
     giant tear 361.03
     multiple defects 361.02
     retinal dialysis (juvenile)
      361.04
     single defect 361.01
    retinal dialysis (juvenile)
     361.04
    single 361.01
    subtotal 361.05
    total 361.05
  delimited (old) (partial) 361.06
  old
   delimited 361.06
   partial 361.06
   total or subtotal 361.07

Detachment (Continued)
 retina (Continued)
  pigment epithelium (RPE) (serous)
   362.42
   exudative 362.42
   hemorrhagic 362.43
  rhegmatogenous (see also
   Detachment, retina, with retinal
   defect) 361.00
  serous (without retinal defect)
   361.2
  specified type NEC 361.89
  traction (with vitreoretinal
   organization) 361.81
 vitreous humor 379.21
Detergent asthma 507.8
Deterioration
 epileptic
  with behavioral disturbance 345.9●
   [294.11]
  without behavioral disturbance
   345.9● [294.10]
 heart, cardiac (see also Degeneration,
  myocardial) 429.1
 mental (see also Psychosis) 298.9
 myocardium, myocardial (see also
  Degeneration, myocardial)
  429.1
 senile (simple) 797
  transplanted organ - see
   Complications, transplant,
   organ, by site
de Toni-Fanconi syndrome (cystinosis)
  270.0
Deuteranomaly 368.52
Deuteranopia (anomalous trichromat)
  (complete) (incomplete) 368.52
Deutschländer's disease - see Fracture,
  foot
Development
 abnormal, bone 756.9
 arrested 783.40
  bone 733.91
  child 783.40
  due to malnutrition (protein-calorie)
   263.2
  fetus or newborn 764.9●
  tracheal rings (congenital) 748.3
 defective, congenital - see also Anomaly
  cauda equina 742.59
  left ventricle 746.9
   with atresia or hypoplasia of
    aortic orifice or valve with
    hypoplasia of ascending
    aorta 746.7
   in hypoplastic left heart
    syndrome 746.7
 delayed (see also Delay, development)
  783.40
  arithmetical skills 315.1
  language (skills) 315.31
   and speech due to hearing loss
    315.34
   expressive 315.31
   mixed receptive-expressive
    315.32
  learning skill, specified NEC 315.2
  mixed skills 315.5
  motor coordination 315.4
  reading 315.00
  specified
   learning skill NEC 315.2
   type NEC, except learning
    315.8

Development (Continued)
 delayed (Continued)
  speech 315.39
   and language due to hearing loss
    315.34
   associated with hyperkinesia
    314.1
   phonological 315.39
   spelling 315.09
  written expression 315.2
 imperfect, congenital - see also Anomaly
  heart 746.9
  lungs 748.60
 improper (fetus or newborn) 764.9●
 incomplete (fetus or newborn) 764.9●
  affecting management of pregnancy
   656.5●
  bronchial tree 748.3
  organ or site not listed - see
   Hypoplasia
  respiratory system 748.9
 sexual, precocious NEC 259.1
 tardy, mental (see also Retardation,
  mental) 319
Developmental - see condition
Devergie's disease (pityriasis rubra
  pilaris) 696.4
Deviation
 conjugate (eye) 378.87
  palsy 378.81
  spasm, spastic 378.82
 esophagus 530.89
 eye, skew 378.87
 mandible, opening and closing 524.53
 midline (jaw) (teeth) 524.29
  specified site NEC - see Malposition
 occlusal plane 524.76
 organ or site, congenital NEC - see
  Malposition, congenital
 septum (acquired) (nasal) 470
  congenital 754.0
 sexual 302.9
  bestiality 302.1
  coprophilia 302.89
  ego-dystonic
   homosexuality 302.0
   lesbianism 302.0
  erotomania 302.89
   Clérambault's 297.8
  exhibitionism (sexual) 302.4
  fetishism 302.81
   transvestic 302.3
  frotteurism 302.89
  homosexuality, ego-dystonic 302.0
   pedophilic 302.2
  lesbianism, ego-dystonic 302.0
  masochism 302.83
  narcissism 302.89
  necrophilia 302.89
  nymphomania 302.89
  pederosis 302.2
  pedophilia 302.2
  sadism 302.84
  sadomasochism 302.84
  satyriasis 302.89
  specified type NEC 302.89
  transvestic fetishism 302.3
  transvestism 302.3
  voyeurism 302.82
  zoophilia (erotica) 302.1
 teeth, midline 524.29
 trachea 519.19
 ureter (congenital) 753.4
Devic's disease 341.0

Device
  cerebral ventricle (communicating) in situ V45.2
  contraceptive - *see* Contraceptive, device
  drainage, cerebrospinal fluid V45.2
Devil's
  grip 074.1
  pinches (purpura simplex) 287.2
Devitalized tooth 522.9
Devonshire colic 984.9
  specified type of lead - *see* Table of Drugs and Chemicals
Dextraposition, aorta 747.21
  with ventricular septal defect, pulmonary stenosis or atresia, and hypertrophy of right ventricle 745.2
  in tetralogy of Fallot 745.2
Dextratransposition, aorta 745.11
Dextrinosis, limit (debrancher enzyme deficiency) 271.0
Dextrocardia (corrected) (false) (isolated) (secondary) (true) 746.87
  with
    complete transposition of viscera 759.3
    situs inversus 759.3
Dextroversion, kidney (left) 753.3
Dhobie itch 110.3
Diabetes, diabetic (brittle) (congenital) (familial) (mellitus) (poorly-controlled) (severe) (slight) (without complication) 250.0● ◄▥

Note 21   Use the following fifth-digit subclassification with category 250:

0   type II or unspecified type, not stated as uncontrolled

    Fifth-digit 0 is for use for type II patients, even if the patient requires insulin

1   type I [juvenile type], not stated as uncontrolled

2   type II or unspecified type, uncontrolled

    Fifth-digit 2 is for use for type II patients, even if the patient requires insulin

3   type I [juvenile type], uncontrolled

---

  with
    coma (with ketoacidosis) 250.3●
      due to secondary diabetes 249.3●
    hyperosmolar (nonketotic) 250.2●
      due to secondary diabetes 249.2●
    complication NEC 250.9●
      due to secondary diabetes 249.9●
      specified NEC 250.8●
        due to secondary diabetes 249.8●
    gangrene 250.7● [785.4]
      due to secondary diabetes 249.7● [785.4]
    hyperglycemia - *code to* Diabetes, by type, with 5th digit for not stated as uncontrolled

Diabetes, diabetic (*Continued*)
  with (*Continued*)
    hyperosmolarity 250.2●
      due to secondary diabetes 249.2●
    ketosis, ketoacidosis 250.1●
      due to secondary diabetes 249.1●
    osteomyelitis 250.8● [731.8]
      due to secondary diabetes 249.8● [731.8]
    specified manifestations NEC 250.8●
      due to secondary diabetes 249.8●
  acetonemia 250.1●
    due to secondary diabetes 249.1●
  acidosis 250.1●
    due to secondary diabetes 249.1●
  amyotrophy 250.6● [353.5]
    due to secondary diabetes 249.6● [353.5]
  angiopathy, peripheral 250.7● [443.81]
    due to secondary diabetes 249.7● [443.81]
  asymptomatic 790.29
  autonomic neuropathy (peripheral) 250.6● [337.1]
    due to secondary diabetes 249.6● [337.1]
  bone change 250.8● [731.8]
    due to secondary diabetes 249.8● [731.8]
  bronze, bronzed 275.0
  cataract 250.5● [366.41]
    due to secondary diabetes 249.5● [366.41]
  chemical induced - *see* Diabetes, secondary
  complicating pregnancy, childbirth, or puerperium 648.0●
  coma (with ketoacidosis) 250.3●
    due to secondary diabetes 249.3●
    hyperglycemic 250.3●
      due to secondary diabetes 249.3●
    hyperosmolar (nonketotic) 250.2●
      due to secondary diabetes 249.2●
    hypoglycemic 250.3●
      due to secondary diabetes 249.3●
    insulin 250.3●
      due to secondary diabetes 249.3●
  complicating pregnancy, childbirth, or puerperium (maternal) (conditions classifiable to 249 and 250) 648.0●
    affecting fetus or newborn 775.0
  complication NEC 250.9●
    due to secondary diabetes 249.9●
    specified NEC 250.8●
      due to secondary diabetes 249.8●
  dorsal sclerosis 250.6● [340]
    due to secondary diabetes 249.6● [340]
  drug-induced - *see also* Diabetes, secondary
    overdose or wrong substance given or taken - *see* Table of Drugs and Chemicals
  due to
    cystic fibrosis - *see* Diabetes, secondary
    infection - *see* Diabetes, secondary
  dwarfism-obesity syndrome 258.1
  gangrene 250.7● [785.4]
    due to secondary diabetes 249.7● [785.4]
  gastroparesis 250.6● [536.3]
    due to secondary diabetes 249.6● [536.3]

Diabetes, diabetic (*Continued*)
  gestational 648.8●
    complicating pregnancy, childbirth, or puerperium 648.8●
  glaucoma 250.5● [365.44]
    due to secondary diabetes 249.5● [365.44]
  glomerulosclerosis (intercapillary) 250.4● [581.81]
    due to secondary diabetes 249.4● [581.81]
  glycogenosis, secondary 250.8● [259.8]
    due to secondary diabetes 249.8● [259.8]
  hemochromatosis 275.0
  hyperosmolar coma 250.2●
    due to secondary diabetes 249.2●
  hyperosmolarity 250.2●
    due to secondary diabetes 249.2●
  hypertension-nephrosis syndrome 250.4● [581.81]
    due to secondary diabetes 249.4● [581.81]
  hypoglycemia 250.8●
    due to secondary diabetes 249.8●
  hypoglycemic shock 250.8●
    due to secondary diabetes 249.8●
  inadequately controlled - *code to* Diabetes, by type, with 5th digit for not stated as uncontrolled
  insipidus 253.5
    nephrogenic 588.1
    pituitary 253.5
    vasopression-resistant 588.1
  intercapillary glomerulosclerosis 250.4● [581.81]
    due to secondary diabetes 249.4● [581.81]
  iritis 250.5● [364.42]
    due to secondary diabetes 249.5● [364.42]
  ketosis, ketoacidosis 250.1●
    due to secondary diabetes 249.1●
  Kimmelstiel (-Wilson) disease or syndrome (intercapillary glomerulosclerosis) 250.4● [581.81]
    due to secondary diabetes 249.4● [581.81]
  Lancereaux's (diabetes mellitus with marked emaciation) 250.8● [261]
    due to secondary diabetes 249.8● [261]
  latent (chemical) - *see* Diabetes, secondary
    complicating pregnancy, childbirth, or puerperium 648.0●
  lipoidosis 250.8● [272.7]
    due to secondary diabetes 249.8● [272.7]
  macular edema 250.5● [362.07]
    due to secondary diabetes 249.5● [362.07]
  maternal
    with manifest disease in the infant 775.1
    affecting fetus or newborn 775.0
  microaneurysms, retinal 250.5● [362.01]
    due to secondary diabetes 249.5● [362.01]
  mononeuropathy 250.6● [355.9]
    due to secondary diabetes 249.6● [355.9]
  neonatal, transient 775.1

◄ New   ◄▥ Revised   ~~deleted~~ Deleted   ● Use Additional Digit(s)   ▓ Omit code

Diabetes, diabetic (Continued)
- nephropathy 250.4● [583.81]
  - due to secondary diabetes 249.4● [583.81] ◀▥
- nephrosis (syndrome) 250.4● [581.81]
  - due to secondary diabetes 249.4● [583.81]
- neuralgia 250.6● [357.2]
  - due to secondary diabetes 249.6● [357.2]
- neuritis 250.6● [357.2]
  - due to secondary diabetes 249.6● [357.2]
- neurogenic arthropathy 250.6● [713.5]
  - due to secondary diabetes 249.6● [713.5]
- neuropathy 250.6● [357.2]
  - autonomic (peripheral) 250.6 [337.1] ◀
    - due to secondary diabetes 249.6 [337.1] ◀
  - due to secondary diabetes 249.6● [357.2]
- nonclinical 790.29
- osteomyelitis 250.8● [731.8]
  - due to secondary diabetes 249.8● [731.8]
- out of control - code to Diabetes, by type, with 5th digit for uncontrolled
- peripheral autonomic neuropathy 250.6● [337.1]
  - due to secondary diabetes 249.6● [337.1]
- phosphate 275.3
- polyneuropathy 250.6● [357.2]
  - due to secondary diabetes 249.6● [357.2]
- poorly controlled - code to Diabetes, by type, with 5th digit for not stated as uncontrolled
- renal (true) 271.4
- retinal
  - edema 250.5● [362.07]
    - due to secondary diabetes 249.5● [362.07]
  - hemorrhage 250.5● [362.01]
    - due to secondary diabetes 249.5● [362.01]
  - microaneurysms 250.5● [362.01]
    - due to secondary diabetes 249.5● [362.01]
  - retinitis 250.5● [362.01]
    - due to secondary diabetes 249.5● [362.01]
  - retinopathy 250.5● [362.01]
    - due to secondary diabetes 249.5● [362.01]
    - background 250.5● [362.01]
      - due to secondary diabetes 249.5● [362.01]
    - nonproliferative 250.5● [362.03]
      - due to secondary diabetes 249.5● [362.03]
      - mild 250.5● [362.04]
        - due to secondary diabetes 249.5● [362.04]
      - moderate 250.5● [362.05]
        - due to secondary diabetes 249.5● [362.05]
      - severe 250.5● [362.06]
        - due to secondary diabetes 249.5● [362.06]

Diabetes, diabetic (Continued)
- retinopathy (Continued)
  - proliferative 250.5● [362.02]
    - due to secondary diabetes 249.5● [362.02]
- secondary (chemical-induced) (due to chronic condition) (due to infection) (drug-induced) 249.0●
  - with
    - coma (with ketoacidosis) 249.3●
      - hyperosmolar (nonketotic) 249.2●
    - complication NEC 249.9●
      - specified NEC 249.8●
    - gangrene 249.7● [785.4]
    - hyperosmolarity 249.2●
    - ketosis, ketoacidosis 249.1●
    - osteomyelitis 249.8● [731.8]
    - specified manifestations NEC 249.8●
  - acetonemia 249.1●
  - acidosis 249.1●
  - amyotrophy 249.6● [353.5]
  - angiopathy, peripheral 249.7● [443.81]
  - autonomic neuropathy (peripheral) 249.6● [337.1]
  - bone change 249.8● [731.8]
  - cataract 249.5● [366.41]
  - coma (with ketoacidosis) 249.3●
    - hyperglycemic 249.3●
    - hyperosmolar (nonketotic) 249.2●
    - hypoglycemic 249.3●
    - insulin 249.3●
  - complicating pregnancy, childbirth, or puerperium (maternal) 648.0●
    - affecting fetus or newborn 775.0
  - complication NEC 249.9●
    - specified NEC 249.8●
  - dorsal sclerosis 249.6● [340]
  - due to overdose or wrong substance given or taken - see Table of Drugs and Chemicals
  - gangrene 249.7● [785.4]
  - gastroparesis 249.6● [536.3]
  - glaucoma 249.5● [365.44]
  - glomerulosclerosis (intercapillary) 249.4● [581.81]
  - glycogenosis, secondary 249.8● [259.8]
  - hyperosmolar coma 249.2●
  - hyperosmolarity 249.2●
  - hypertension-nephrosis syndrome 249.4● [581.81]
  - hypoglycemia 249.8●
  - hypoglycemic shock 249.8●
  - intercapillary glomerulosclerosis 249.4● [581.81]
  - iritis 249.5● [364.42]
  - ketosis, ketoacidosis 249.1●
  - Kimmelstiel (-Wilson) disease or syndrome (intercapillary glomerulosclerosis) 249.4● [581.81]
  - Lancereaux's (diabetes mellitus with marked emaciation) 249.8● [261]
  - lipoidosis 249.8● [272.7]
  - macular edema 249.5● [362.07]

Diabetes, diabetic (Continued)
- secondary (Continued)
  - maternal
    - with manifest disease in the infant 775.1
    - affecting fetus or newborn 775.0
  - microaneurysms, retinal 249.5● [362.01]
  - mononeuropathy 249.6● [355.9]
  - nephropathy 249.4● [583.81] ◀▥
  - nephrosis (syndrome) 249.4● [581.81]
  - neuralgia 249.6● [357.2]
  - neuritis 249.6● [357.2]
  - neurogenic arthropathy 249.6● [713.5]
  - neuropathy 249.6● [357.2]
    - autonomic (peripheral) 249.6 [337.1] ◀
  - osteomyelitis 249.8● [731.8]
  - peripheral autonomic neuropathy 249.6● [337.1]
  - polyneuropathy 249.6● [357.2]
  - retinal
    - edema 249.5● [362.07]
    - hemorrhage 249.5● [362.01]
    - microaneurysms 249.5● [362.01]
  - retinitis 249.5● [362.01]
  - retinopathy 249.5● [362.01]
    - background 249.5● [362.01]
    - nonproliferative 249.5● [362.03]
      - mild 249.5● [362.04]
      - moderate 249.5● [362.05]
      - severe 249.5● [362.06]
    - proliferative 249.5● [362.02]
  - ulcer (skin) 249.8● [707.9]
    - lower extremity 249.8● [707.10]
      - ankle 249.8● [707.13]
      - calf 249.8● [707.12]
      - foot 249.8● [707.15]
      - heel 249.8● [707.14]
      - knee 249.8● [707.19]
      - specified site NEC 249.8● [707.19]
      - thigh 249.8● [707.11]
      - toes 249.8● [707.15]
    - specified site NEC 249.8● [707.8]
  - xanthoma 249.8● [272.2]
- steroid induced - see also Diabetes, secondary
  - overdose or wrong substance given or taken 962.0
- stress 790.29
- subclinical 790.29
- subliminal 790.29
- sugar 250.0●
- ulcer (skin) 250.8● [707.9]
  - due to secondary diabetes 249.8● [707.9]
  - lower extremity 250.8● [707.10]
    - due to secondary diabetes 249.8● [707.10]
    - ankle 250.8● [707.13]
      - due to secondary diabetes 249.8● [707.13]
    - calf 250.8● [707.12]
      - due to secondary diabetes 249.8● [707.12]
    - foot 250.8● [707.15]
      - due to secondary diabetes 249.8● [707.15]
    - heel 250.8● [707.14]
      - due to secondary diabetes 249.8● [707.14]
    - knee 250.8● [707.19]
      - due to secondary diabetes 249.8● [707.19]

◀ New ◀▥ Revised deleted Deleted ● Use Additional Digit(s) ▧ Omit code

Diabetes, diabetic *(Continued)*
  ulcer *(Continued)*
    lower extremity *(Continued)*
      specified site NEC 250.8●
        [707.19]
        due to secondary diabetes
          249.8● [707.19]
      thigh 250.8● [707.11]
        due to secondary diabetes
          249.8● [707.11]
      toes 250.8● [707.15]
        due to secondary diabetes
          249.8● [707.15]
    specified site NEC 250.8● [707.8]
      due to secondary diabetes 249.8●
        [707.8]
    xanthoma 250.8● [272.2]
      due to secondary diabetes 249.8●
        [272.2]
Diacyclothrombopathia 287.1
Diagnosis deferred 799.9
Dialysis (intermittent) (treatment)
  anterior retinal (juvenile) (with
    detachment) 361.04
  extracorporeal V56.0
  hemodialysis V56.0
    status only V45.11
  peritoneal V56.8
    status only V45.11
  renal V56.0
    status only V45.11
  specified type NEC V56.8
Diamond-Blackfan anemia or syndrome
  (congenital hypoplastic anemia)
  284.01
Diamond-Gardener syndrome
  (autoerythrocyte sensitization)
  287.2
Diaper rash 691.0
Diaphoresis (excessive) NEC *(see also*
  Hyperhidrosis) 780.8
Diaphragm - *see* condition
Diaphragmalgia 786.52
Diaphragmitis 519.4
Diaphyseal aclasis 756.4
Diaphysitis 733.99
Diarrhea, diarrheal (acute) (autumn)
  (bilious) (bloody) (catarrhal)
  (choleraic) (chronic) (gravis) (green)
  (infantile) (lienteric) (noninfectious)
  (presumed noninfectious)
  (putrefactive) (secondary) (sporadic)
  (summer) (symptomatic) (thermic)
  787.91
  achlorhydric 536.0
  allergic 558.3
  amebic *(see also* Amebiasis) 006.9
    with abscess - *see* Abscess, amebic
    acute 006.0
    chronic 006.1
    nondysenteric 006.2
  bacillary - *see* Dysentery, bacillary
  bacterial NEC 008.5
  balantidial 007.0
  bile salt-induced 579.8
  cachectic NEC 787.91
  chilomastix 007.8
  choleriformis 001.1
  coccidial 007.2
  Cochin-China 579.1
    anguilluliasis 127.2
    psilosis 579.1
  Dientamoeba 007.8
  dietetic 787.91

Diarrhea, diarrheal *(Continued)*
  due to
    achylia gastrica 536.8
    Aerobacter aerogenes 008.2
    Bacillus coli - *see* Enteritis, E. coli
    bacteria NEC 008.5
    bile salts 579.8
    Capillaria
      hepatica 128.8
      philippinensis 127.5
    Clostridium perfringens (C) (F)
      008.46
    Enterobacter aerogenes 008.2
    enterococci 008.49
    Escherichia coli - *see* Enteritis, E. coli
    Giardia lamblia 007.1
    Heterophyes heterophyes 121.6
    irritating foods 787.91
    Metagonimus yokogawai 121.5
    Necator americanus 126.1
    Paracolobactrum arizonae 008.1
    Paracolon bacillus NEC 008.47
      Arizona 008.1
    Proteus (bacillus) (mirabilis)
      (Morganii) 008.3
    Pseudomonas aeruginosa 008.42
    S. japonicum 120.2
    specified organism NEC 008.8
      bacterial 008.49
      viral NEC 008.69
    Staphylococcus 008.41
    Streptococcus 008.49
      anaerobic 008.46
    Strongyloides stercoralis 127.2
    Trichuris trichiuria 127.3
    virus NEC *(see also* Enteritis, viral)
      008.69
  dysenteric 009.2
    due to specified organism NEC
      008.8
  dyspeptic 787.91
  endemic 009.3
    due to specified organism NEC
      008.8
  epidemic 009.2
    due to specified organism NEC
      008.8
  fermentative 787.91
  flagellate 007.9
  Flexner's (ulcerative) 004.1
  functional 564.5
    following gastrointestinal surgery
      564.4
    psychogenic 306.4
  giardial 007.1
  Giardia lamblia 007.1
  hill 579.1
  hyperperistalsis (nervous) 306.4
  infectious 009.2
    due to specified organism NEC
      008.8
    presumed 009.3
  inflammatory 787.91
    due to specified organism NEC
      008.8
  malarial *(see also* Malaria) 084.6
  mite 133.8
  mycotic 117.9
  nervous 306.4
  neurogenic 564.5
  parenteral NEC 009.2
  postgastrectomy 564.4
  postvagotomy 564.4
  prostaglandin induced 579.8

Diarrhea, diarrheal *(Continued)*
  protozoal NEC 007.9
  psychogenic 306.4
  septic 009.2
    due to specified organism NEC
      008.8
  specified organism NEC 008.8
    bacterial 008.49
    viral NEC 008.69
  Staphylococcus 008.41
  Streptococcus 008.49
    anaerobic 008.46
  toxic 558.2
  travelers' 009.2
    due to specified organism NEC
      008.8
  trichomonal 007.3
  tropical 579.1
  tuberculous 014.8●
  ulcerative (chronic) *(see also* Colitis,
    ulcerative) 556.9
  viral *(see also* Enteritis, viral) 008.8
  zymotic NEC 009.2
Diastasis
  cranial bones 733.99
    congenital 756.0
  joint (traumatic) - *see* Dislocation, by
    site
  muscle 728.84
    congenital 756.89
  recti (abdomen) 728.84
    complicating delivery 665.8●
    congenital 756.79
Diastema, teeth, tooth 524.30
Diastematomyelia 742.51
Diataxia, cerebral, infantile 343.0
Diathesis
  allergic V15.09
  bleeding (familial) 287.9
  cystine (familial) 270.0
  gouty 274.9
  hemorrhagic (familial) 287.9
    newborn NEC 776.0
  oxalic 271.8
  scrofulous *(see also* Tuberculosis)
    017.2●
  spasmophilic *(see also* Tetany) 781.7
  ulcer 536.9
  uric acid 274.9
Diaz's disease or osteochondrosis 732.5
Dibothriocephaliasis 123.4
  larval 123.5
Dibothriocephalus (infection)
  (infestation) (latus) 123.4
  larval 123.5
Dicephalus 759.4
Dichotomy, teeth 520.2
Dichromat, dichromata (congenital)
  368.59
Dichromatopsia (congenital) 368.59
Dichuchwa 104.0
Dicroceliasis 121.8
Didelphys, didelphic *(see also* Double
  uterus) 752.2
Didymitis *(see also* Epididymitis) 604.90
Died - *see also* Death
  without
    medical attention (cause unknown)
      798.9
    sign of disease 798.2
Dientamoeba diarrhea 007.8
Dietary
  inadequacy or deficiency 269.9
  surveillance and counseling V65.3

◀ New   ◀ Revised   ~~deleted~~ Deleted   ● Use Additional Digit(s)   ▨ Omit code

Dietl's crisis 593.4
Dieulafoy lesion (hemorrhagic)
of
    duodenum 537.84
    esophagus 530.82
    intestine 569.86
    stomach 537.84
Difficult
birth, affecting fetus or newborn
    763.9
delivery NEC 669.9●
Difficulty
feeding 783.3
    adult 783.3
    breast 676.8●
    child 783.3
    elderly 783.3
    infant 783.3
    newborn 779.31 ◀▥
    nonorganic (infant) NEC 307.59
mechanical, gastroduodenal stoma
    537.89
reading 315.00
specific, spelling 315.09
swallowing (*see also* Dysphagia)
    787.20
walking 719.7
Diffuse - *see* condition
Diffused ganglion 727.42
Di George's syndrome (thymic
    hypoplasia) 279.11
Digestive - *see* condition
Di Guglielmo's disease or syndrome
    (M9841/3) 207.0●
Diktyoma (M9051/3) - *see* Neoplasm, by
    site, malignant
Dilaceration, tooth 520.4
Dilatation
anus 564.89
    venule - *see* Hemorrhoids
aorta (focal) (general) (*see also*
    Aneurysm, aorta) 441.9
    congenital 747.29
    infectional 093.0
    ruptured 441.5
    syphilitic 093.0
appendix (cystic) 543.9
artery 447.8
bile duct (common) (cystic)
    (congenital) 751.69
    acquired 576.8
bladder (sphincter) 596.8
    congenital 753.8
    in pregnancy or childbirth
        654.4●
        causing obstructed labor
            660.2●
            affecting fetus or newborn
                763.1
blood vessel 459.89
bronchus, bronchi 494.0
    with acute exacerbation 494.1
calyx (due to obstruction) 593.89
capillaries 448.9
cardiac (acute) (chronic) (*see also*
    Hypertrophy, cardiac) 429.3
    congenital 746.89
    valve NEC 746.89
        pulmonary 746.09
    hypertensive (*see also* Hypertension,
        heart) 402.90
cavum septi pellucidi 742.4
cecum 564.89
    psychogenic 306.4

Dilatation (*Continued*)
cervix (uteri) - *see also* Incompetency,
    cervix
    incomplete, poor, slow
        affecting fetus or newborn 763.7
        complicating delivery 661.0●
            affecting fetus or newborn
                763.7
colon 564.7
    congenital 751.3
    due to mechanical obstruction
        560.89
    psychogenic 306.4
common bile duct (congenital) 751.69
    acquired 576.8
        with calculus,
            choledocholithiasis, or
            stones - *see*
            Choledocholithiasis
cystic duct 751.69
    acquired (any bile duct) 575.8
duct, mammary 610.4
duodenum 564.89
esophagus 530.89
    congenital 750.4
    due to
        achalasia 530.0
        cardiospasm 530.0
Eustachian tube, congenital 744.24
fontanel 756.0
gallbladder 575.8
    congenital 751.69
gastric 536.8
    acute 536.1
    psychogenic 306.4
heart (acute) (chronic) (*see also*
    Hypertrophy, cardiac) 429.3
    congenital 746.89
    hypertensive (*see also* Hypertension,
        heart) 402.90
    valve - *see also* Endocarditis
        congenital 746.89
ileum 564.89
    psychogenic 306.4
inguinal rings - *see* Hernia, inguinal
jejunum 564.89
    psychogenic 306.4
kidney (calyx) (collecting structures)
    (cystic) (parenchyma) (pelvis)
    593.89
lacrimal passages 375.69
lymphatic vessel 457.1
mammary duct 610.4
Meckel's diverticulum (congenital)
    751.0
meningeal vessels, congenital 742.8
myocardium (acute) (chronic) (*see also*
    Hypertrophy, cardiac) 429.3
organ or site, congenital NEC - *see*
    Distortion
pancreatic duct 577.8
pelvis, kidney 593.89
pericardium - *see* Pericarditis
pharynx 478.29
prostate 602.8
pulmonary
    artery (idiopathic) 417.8
        congenital 747.3
    valve, congenital 746.09
pupil 379.43
rectum 564.89
renal 593.89
saccule vestibularis, congenital 744.05
salivary gland (duct) 527.8

Dilatation (*Continued*)
sphincter ani 564.89
stomach 536.8
    acute 536.1
    psychogenic 306.4
submaxillary duct 527.8
trachea, congenital 748.3
ureter (idiopathic) 593.89
    congenital 753.20
    due to obstruction 593.5
urethra (acquired) 599.84
vasomotor 443.9
vein 459.89
ventricular, ventricle (acute) (chronic)
    (*see also* Hypertrophy, cardiac)
    429.3
    cerebral, congenital 742.4
    hypertensive (*see also* Hypertension,
        heart) 402.90
venule 459.89
    anus - *see* Hemorrhoids
vesical orifice 596.8
Dilated, dilation - *see* Dilatation
Diminished
hearing (acuity) (*see also* Deafness)
    389.9
pulse pressure 785.9
vision NEC 369.9
vital capacity 794.2
Diminuta taenia 123.6
Diminution, sense or sensation (cold)
    (heat) (tactile) (vibratory) (*see also*
    Disturbance, sensation) 782.0
Dimitri-Sturge-Weber disease
    (encephalocutaneous angiomatosis)
    759.6
Dimple
parasacral 685.1
    with abscess 685.0
pilonidal 685.1
    with abscess 685.0
postanal 685.1
    with abscess 685.0
Dioctophyma renale (infection)
    (infestation) 128.8
Dipetalonemiasis 125.4
Diphallus 752.69
Diphtheria, diphtheritic (gangrenous)
    (hemorrhagic) 032.9
carrier (suspected) of V02.4
cutaneous 032.85
cystitis 032.84
faucial 032.0
infection of wound 032.85
inoculation (anti) (not sick) V03.5
laryngeal 032.3
myocarditis 032.82
nasal anterior 032.2
nasopharyngeal 032.1
neurological complication 032.89
peritonitis 032.83
specified site NEC 032.89
Diphyllobothriasis (intestine) 123.4
larval 123.5
Diplacusis 388.41
Diplegia (upper limbs) 344.2
brain or cerebral 437.8
congenital 343.0
facial 351.0
    congenital 352.6
infantile or congenital (cerebral)
    (spastic) (spinal) 343.0
lower limbs 344.1
syphilitic, congenital 090.49

◀ New   ◀▥ Revised   ~~deleted~~ Deleted   ● Use Additional Digit(s)   ▭ Omit code

Diplococcus, diplococcal - *see* condition
Diplomyelia 742.59
Diplopia 368.2
  refractive 368.15
Dipsomania (*see also* Alcoholism) 303.9●
  with psychosis (*see also* Psychosis,
    alcoholic) 291.9
Dipylidiasis 123.8
  intestine 123.8
Direction, teeth, abnormal 524.30
Dirt-eating child 307.52
Disability
  heart - *see* Disease, heart
  learning NEC 315.2
  special spelling 315.09
Disarticulation (*see also* Derangement,
    joint) 718.9●
  meaning
    amputation
      status - *see* Absence, by site
      traumatic - *see* Amputation,
        traumatic
    dislocation, traumatic or congenital -
      see Dislocation
Disaster, cerebrovascular (*see also*
    Disease, cerebrovascular, acute) 436
Discharge
  anal NEC 787.99
  breast (female) (male) 611.79
  conjunctiva 372.89
  continued locomotor idiopathic (*see*
    also Epilepsy) 345.5●
  diencephalic autonomic idiopathic (*see*
    also Epilepsy) 345.5●
  ear 388.60
    blood 388.69
    cerebrospinal fluid 388.61
  excessive urine 788.42
  eye 379.93
  nasal 478.19
  nipple 611.79
  patterned motor idiopathic (*see also*
    Epilepsy) 345.5●
  penile 788.7
  postnasal - *see* Sinusitis
  sinus, from mediastinum 510.0
  umbilicus 789.9
  urethral 788.7
    bloody 599.84
  vaginal 623.5
Discitis 722.90
  cervical, cervicothoracic 722.91
  lumbar, lumbosacral 722.93
  thoracic, thoracolumbar 722.92
Discogenic syndrome - *see* Displacement,
    intervertebral disc
Discoid
  kidney 753.3
  meniscus, congenital 717.5
  semilunar cartilage 717.5
Discoloration
  mouth 528.9
  nails 703.8
  teeth 521.7
    due to
      drugs 521.7
      metals (copper) (silver) 521.7
      pulpal bleeding 521.7
    during formation 520.8
    extrinsic 523.6
    intrinsic posteruptive 521.7
Discomfort
  chest 786.59
  visual 368.13

Discomycosis - *see* Actinomycosis
Discontinuity, ossicles, ossicular chain
  385.23
Discrepancy
  centric occlusion
    maximum intercuspation 524.55
    of teeth 524.55
  leg length (acquired) 736.81
    congenital 755.30
  uterine size-date 649.6●
Discrimination
  political V62.4
  racial V62.4
  religious V62.4
  sex V62.4
Disease, diseased - *see also* Syndrome
  Abrami's (acquired hemolytic jaundice)
    283.9
  absorbent system 459.89
  accumulation - *see* Thesaurismosis
  acid-peptic 536.8
  Acosta's 993.2
  Adams-Stokes (-Morgagni) (syncope
    with heart block) 426.9
  Addison's (bronze) (primary adrenal
    insufficiency) 255.41
    anemia (pernicious) 281.0
    tuberculous (*see also* Tuberculosis)
      017.6●
  Addison-Gull - *see* Xanthoma
  adenoids (and tonsils) (chronic) 474.9
  adrenal (gland) (capsule) (cortex)
    255.9
    hyperfunction 255.3
    hypofunction 255.41
    specified type NEC 255.8
  ainhum (dactylolysis spontanea)
    136.0
  akamushi (scrub typhus) 081.2
  Akureyri (epidemic neuromyasthenia)
    049.8
  Albarrán's (colibacilluria) 791.9
  Albers-Schönberg's (marble bones)
    756.52
  Albert's 726.71
  Albright (-Martin) (-Bantam) 275.49
  Alibert's (mycosis fungoides)
    (M9700/3) 202.1●
  Alibert-Bazin (M9700/3) 202.1●
  alimentary canal 569.9
  alligator skin (ichthyosis congenita)
    757.1
    acquired 701.1
  Almeida's (Brazilian blastomycosis)
    116.1
  Alpers' 330.8
  alpine 993.2
  altitude 993.2
  alveoli, teeth 525.9
  Alzheimer's - *see* Alzheimer's
  amyloid (any site) 277.30
  anarthritic rheumatoid 446.5
  Anders' (adiposis tuberosa simplex)
    272.8
  Andersen's (glycogenosis IV) 271.0
  Anderson's (angiokeratoma corporis
    diffusum) 272.7
  Andes 993.2
  Andrews' (bacterid) 686.8
  angiopastic, angiospasmodic 443.9
    cerebral 435.9
      with transient neurologic deficit
        435.9
    vein 459.89

Disease, diseased (*Continued*)
  anterior
    chamber 364.9
    horn cell 335.9
      specified type NEC 335.8
  antral (chronic) 473.0
    acute 461.0
  anus NEC 569.49
  aorta (nonsyphilitic) 447.9
    syphilitic NEC 093.89
  aortic (heart) (valve) (*see also*
    Endocarditis, aortic) 424.1
  apollo 077.4
  aponeurosis 726.90
  appendix 543.9
  aqueous (chamber) 364.9
  arc-welders' lung 503
  Armenian 277.31
  Arnold-Chiari (*see also* Spina bifida)
    741.0●
  arterial 447.9
    occlusive (*see also* Occlusion, by site)
      444.22
      with embolus or thrombus - *see*
        Occlusion, by site
      due to stricture or stenosis 447.1
    specified type NEC 447.8
  arteriocardiorenal (*see also*
    Hypertension, cardiorenal) 404.90
  arteriolar (generalized) (obliterative)
    447.90
    specified type NEC 447.8
  arteriorenal - *see* Hypertension, kidney
  arteriosclerotic - *see also* Arteriosclerosis
    cardiovascular 429.2
    coronary - *see* Arteriosclerosis,
      coronary
    heart - *see* Arteriosclerosis, coronary
    vascular - *see* Arteriosclerosis
  artery 447.9
    cerebral 437.9
    coronary - *see* Arteriosclerosis,
      coronary
    specified type NEC 447.8
  arthropod-borne NEC 088.9
    specified type NEC 088.89
  Asboe-Hansen's (incontinentia
    pigmenti) 757.33
  atticoantral, chronic (with posterior or
    superior marginal perforation of
    ear drum) 382.2
  auditory canal, ear 380.9
  Aujeszky's 078.89
  auricle, ear NEC 380.30
  Australian X 062.4
  autoimmune NEC 279.49   ◀▥▥
    hemolytic (cold type) (warm type)
      283.0
    parathyroid 252.1
    thyroid 245.2
  aviators' (*see also* Effect, adverse, high
    altitude) 993.2
  ax(e)-grinders' 502
  Ayala's 756.89
  Ayerza's (pulmonary artery sclerosis
    with pulmonary hypertension)
    416.0
  Azorean (of the nervous system) 334.8
  Babington's (familial hemorrhagic
    telangiectasia) 448.0
  back bone NEC 733.90
  bacterial NEC 040.89
    zoonotic NEC 027.9
      specified type NEC 027.8

◀ New   ◀▥▥ Revised   ~~deleted~~ Deleted   ● Use Additional Digit(s)   ▥▥ Omit code

Disease, diseased *(Continued)*
  Baehr-Schiffrin (thrombotic
    thrombocytopenic purpura)
    446.6
  Baelz's (cheilitis glandularis
    apostematosa) 528.5
  Baerensprung's (eczema marginatum)
    110.3
  Balfour's (chloroma) 205.3 ●
  balloon *(see also* Effect, adverse, high
    altitude) 993.2
  Baló's 341.1
  Bamberger (-Marie) (hypertrophic
    pulmonary osteoarthropathy)
    731.2
  Bang's (Brucella abortus) 023.1
  Bannister's 995.1
  Banti's (with cirrhosis) (with portal
    hypertension) - *see* Cirrhosis, liver
  Barcoo *(see also* Ulcer, skin) 707.9
  barium lung 503
  Barlow (-Möller) (infantile scurvy) 267
  barometer makers' 985.0
  Barraquer (-Simons) (progressive
    lipodystrophy) 272.6
  basal ganglia 333.90
    degenerative NEC 333.0
    specified NEC 333.89
  Basedow's (exophthalmic goiter)
    242.0 ●
  basement membrane NEC 583.89
    with
      pulmonary hemorrhage
        (Goodpasture's syndrome)
        446.21 *[583.81]*
  Bateman's 078.0
    purpura (senile) 287.2
  Batten's 330.1 *[362.71]*
  Batten-Mayou (retina) 330.1 *[362.71]*
  Batten-Steinert 359.21
  Battey 031.0
  Baumgarten-Cruveilhier (cirrhosis of
    liver) 571.5
  bauxite-workers' 503
  Bayle's (dementia paralytica) 094.1
  Bazin's (primary) *(see also* Tuberculosis)
    017.1 ●
  Beard's (neurasthenia) 300.5
  Beau's *(see also* Degeneration,
    myocardial) 429.1
  Bechterew's (ankylosing spondylitis)
    720.0
  Becker's
    idiopathic mural endomyocardial
      disease 425.2
    myotonia congenita, recessive form
      359.22
  Begbie's (exophthalmic goiter) 242.0 ●
  Behr's 362.50
  Beigel's (white piedra) 111.2
  Bekhterev's (ankylosing spondylitis)
    720.0
  Bell's *(see also* Psychosis, affective)
    296.0 ●
  Bennett's (leukemia) 208.9 ●
  Benson's 379.22
  Bergeron's (hysteroepilepsy) 300.11
  Berlin's 921.3
  Bernard-Soulier (thrombopathy) 287.1
  Bernhardt (-Roth) 355.1
  beryllium 503
  Besnier-Boeck (-Schaumann)
    (sarcoidosis) 135
  Best's 362.76

Disease, diseased *(Continued)*
  Beurmann's (sporotrichosis) 117.1
  Bielschowsky (-Jansky) 330.1
  Biermer's (pernicious anemia) 281.0
  Biett's (discoid lupus erythematosus)
    695.4
  bile duct *(see also* Disease, biliary) 576.9
  biliary (duct) (tract) 576.9
    with calculus, choledocholithiasis,
      or stones - *see*
        Choledocholithiasis
  Billroth's (meningocele) *(see also* Spina
    bifida) 741.9 ●
  Binswanger's 290.12
  Bird's (oxaluria) 271.8
  bird fanciers' 495.2
  black lung 500
  bladder 596.9
    specified NEC 596.8
  bleeder's 286.0
  Bloch-Sulzberger (incontinentia
    pigmenti) 757.33
  Blocq's (astasia-abasia) 307.9
  blood (-forming organs) 289.9
    specified NEC 289.89
    vessel 459.9
  Bloodgood's 610.1
  Blount's (tibia vara) 732.4
  blue 746.9
  Bodechtel-Guttmann (subacute
    sclerosing panencephalitis) 046.2
  Boeck's (sarcoidosis) 135
  bone 733.90
    fibrocystic NEC 733.29
      jaw 526.2
    marrow 289.9
    Paget's (osteitis deformans) 731.0
    specified type NEC 733.99
    von Recklinghausen's (osteitis
      fibrosa cystica) 252.01
  Bonfils' - *see* Disease, Hodgkin's
  Borna 062.9
  Bornholm (epidemic pleurodynia)
    074.1
  Bostock's *(see also* Fever, hay) 477.9
  Bouchard's (myopathic dilatation of
    the stomach) 536.1
  Bouillaud's (rheumatic heart disease)
    391.9
  Bourneville (-Brissaud) (tuberous
    sclerosis) 759.5
  Bouveret (-Hoffmann) (paroxysmal
    tachycardia) 427.2
  bowel 569.9
    functional 564.9
      psychogenic 306.4
  Bowen's (M8081/2) - *see* Neoplasm,
    skin, in situ
  Bozzolo's (multiple myeloma)
    (M9730/3) 203.0 ●
  Bradley's (epidemic vomiting)
    078.82
  Brailsford's 732.3
    radius, head 732.3
    tarsal, scaphoid 732.5
  Brailsford-Morquio
    (mucopolysaccharidosis IV)
    277.5
  brain 348.9
    Alzheimer's 331.0
      · with dementia - *see* Alzheimer's,
        dementia
    arterial, artery 437.9
    arteriosclerotic 437.0

Disease, diseased *(Continued)*
  brain *(Continued)*
    congenital 742.9
    degenerative - *see* Degeneration,
      brain
    inflammatory - *see also* Encephalitis
      late effect - *see* category 326
    organic 348.9
      arteriosclerotic 437.0
    parasitic NEC 123.9
    Pick's 331.11
      with dementia
        with behavioral disturbance
          331.11 *[294.11]*
        without behavioral
          disturbance 331.11
          [294.10]
    senile 331.2
  braziers' 985.8
  breast 611.9
    cystic (chronic) 610.1
    fibrocystic 610.1
    inflammatory 611.0
    Paget's (M8540/3) 174.0
    puerperal, postpartum NEC 676.3 ●
    specified NEC 611.89
  Breda's *(see also* Yaws) 102.9
  Breisky's (kraurosis vulvae) 624.09
  Bretonneau's (diphtheritic malignant
    angina) 032.0
  Bright's *(see also* Nephritis) 583.9
    arteriosclerotic *(see also*
      Hypertension, kidney) 403.90
  Brill's (recrudescent typhus) 081.1
    flea-borne 081.0
    louse-borne 081.1
  Brill-Symmers (follicular lymphoma)
    (M9690/3) 202.0 ●
  Brill-Zinsser (recrudescent typhus)
    081.1
  Brinton's (leather bottle stomach)
    (M8142/3) 151.9
  Brion-Kayser *(see also* Fever,
    paratyphoid) 002.9
  broad
    beta 272.2
    ligament, noninflammatory 620.9
      specified NEC 620.8
  Brocq's 691.8
    meaning
      atopic (diffuse) neurodermatitis
        691.8
      dermatitis herpetiformis 694.0
      lichen simplex chronicus 698.3
      parapsoriasis 696.2
      prurigo 698.2
  Brocq-Duhring (dermatitis
    herpetiformis) 694.0
  Brodie's (joint) *(see also* Osteomyelitis)
    730.1 ●
  bronchi 519.19
  bronchopulmonary 519.19
  bronze (Addison's) 255.41
    tuberculous *(see also* Tuberculosis)
      017.6 ●
  Brown-Séquard 344.89
  Bruck's 733.99
  Bruck-de Lange (Amsterdam dwarf,
    mental retardation, and
    brachycephaly) 759.89
  Bruhl's (splenic anemia with fever)
    285.8
  Bruton's (X-linked
    agammaglobulinemia) 279.04

Disease, diseased (*Continued*)
buccal cavity 528.9
Buchanan's (juvenile osteochondrosis, iliac crest) 732.1
Buchman's (osteochondrosis juvenile) 732.1
Budgerigar-Fanciers' 495.2
Budinger-Ludloff-Läwen 717.89
Büerger's (thromboangiitis obliterans) 443.1
Burger-Grütz (essential familial hyperlipemia) 272.3
Burns' (lower ulna) 732.3
bursa 727.9
Bury's (erythema elevatum diutinum) 695.89
Buschke's 710.1
Busquet's (*see also* Osteomyelitis) 730.1●
Busse-Buschke (cryptococcosis) 117.5
C₂ (*see also* Alcoholism) 303.9●
Caffey's (infantile cortical hyperostosis) 756.59
caisson 993.3
calculous 592.9
California 114.0
Calvé (-Perthes) (osteochondrosis, femoral capital) 732.1
Camurati-Engelmann (diaphyseal sclerosis) 756.59
Canavan's 330.0
capillaries 448.9
Carapata 087.1
cardiac - *see* Disease, heart
cardiopulmonary, chronic 416.9
cardiorenal (arteriosclerotic) (hepatic) (hypertensive) (vascular) (*see also* Hypertension, cardiorenal) 404.90
cardiovascular (arteriosclerotic) 429.2
congenital 746.9
hypertensive (*see also* Hypertension, heart) 402.90
benign 402.10
malignant 402.00
renal (*see also* Hypertension, cardiorenal) 404.90
syphilitic (asymptomatic) 093.9
carotid gland 259.8
Carrión's (Bartonellosis) 088.0
cartilage NEC 733.90
specified NEC 733.99
Castellani's 104.8
cat-scratch 078.3
Cavare's (familial periodic paralysis) 359.3
Cazenave's (pemphigus) 694.4
cecum 569.9
celiac (adult) 579.0
infantile 579.0
cellular tissue NEC 709.9
central core 359.0
cerebellar, cerebellum - *see* Disease, brain
cerebral (*see also* Disease, brain) 348.9
arterial, artery 437.9
degenerative - *see* Degeneration, brain
cerebrospinal 349.9
cerebrovascular NEC 437.9
acute 436
embolic - *see* Embolism, brain
late effect - *see* Late effect(s) (of) cerebrovascular disease

Disease, diseased (*Continued*)
cerebrovascular NEC (*Continued*)
acute (*Continued*)
puerperal, postpartum, childbirth 674.0●
thrombotic - *see* Thrombosis, brain
arteriosclerotic 437.0
embolic - *see* Embolism, brain
ischemic, generalized NEC 437.1
late effect - *see* Late effect(s) (of) cerebrovascular disease
occlusive 437.1
puerperal, postpartum, childbirth 674.0●
specified type NEC 437.8
thrombotic - *see* Thrombosis, brain
ceroid storage 272.7
cervix (uteri)
inflammatory 616.0
noninflammatory 622.9
specified NEC 622.8
Chabert's 022.9
Chagas' (*see also* Trypanosomiasis, American) 086.2
Chandler's (osteochondritis dissecans, hip) 732.7
Charcôt's (joint) 094.0 [713.5]
spinal cord 094.0
Charcôt-Marie-Tooth 356.1
Charlouis' (*see also* Yaws) 102.9
Cheadle (-Möller) (-Barlow) (infantile scurvy) 267
Chédiak-Steinbrinck (-Higashi) (congenital gigantism of peroxidase granules) 288.2
cheek, inner 528.9
chest 519.9
Chiari's (hepatic vein thrombosis) 453.0
Chicago (North American blastomycosis) 116.0
chignon (white piedra) 111.2
chigoe, chigo (jigger) 134.1
childhood granulomatous 288.1
Chinese liver fluke 121.1
chlamydial NEC 078.88
cholecystic (*see also* Disease, gallbladder) 575.9
choroid 363.9
degenerative (*see also* Degeneration, choroid) 363.40
hereditary (*see also* Dystrophy, choroid) 363.50
specified type NEC 363.8
Christian's (chronic histiocytosis X) 277.89
Christian-Weber (nodular nonsuppurative panniculitis) 729.30
Christmas 286.1
ciliary body 364.9
specified NEC 364.89
circulatory (system) NEC 459.9
chronic, maternal, affecting fetus or newborn 760.3
specified NEC 459.89
syphilitic 093.9
congenital 090.5
Civatte's (poikiloderma) 709.09
climacteric 627.2
male 608.89
coagulation factor deficiency (congenital) (*see also* Defect, coagulation) 286.9

Disease, diseased (*Continued*)
Coats' 362.12
coccidioidal pulmonary 114.5
acute 114.0
chronic 114.4
primary 114.0
residual 114.4
Cockayne's (microcephaly and dwarfism) 759.89
Cogan's 370.52
cold
agglutinin 283.0
or hemoglobinuria 283.0
paroxysmal (cold) (nocturnal) 283.2
hemagglutinin (chronic) 283.0
collagen NEC 710.9
nonvascular 710.9
specified NEC 710.8
vascular (allergic) (*see also* Angiitis, hypersensitivity) 446.20
colon 569.9
functional 564.9
congenital 751.3
ischemic 557.0
combined system (of spinal cord) 266.2 [336.2]
with anemia (pernicious) 281.0 [336.2]
compressed air 993.3
Concato's (pericardial polyserositis) 423.2
peritoneal 568.82
pleural - *see* Pleurisy
congenital NEC 799.89
conjunctiva 372.9
chlamydial 077.98
specified NEC 077.8
specified type NEC 372.89
viral 077.99
specified NEC 077.8
connective tissue, diffuse (*see also* Disease, collagen) 710.9
Conor and Bruch's (boutonneuse fever) 082.1
Conradi (-Hünermann) 756.59
Cooley's (erythroblastic anemia) 282.49
Cooper's 610.1
Corbus' 607.1
cork-handlers' 495.3
cornea (*see also* Keratopathy) 371.9
coronary (*see also* Ischemia, heart) 414.9
congenital 746.85
ostial, syphilitic 093.20
aortic 093.22
mitral 093.21
pulmonary 093.24
tricuspid 093.23
Corrigan's - *see* Insufficiency, aortic
Cotugno's 724.3
Coxsackie (virus) NEC 074.8
cranial nerve NEC 352.9
Creutzfeldt-Jakob (CJD) 046.19
with dementia
with behavioral disturbance 046.19 [294.11]
without behavioral disturbance 046.19 [294.10]
familial 046.19
iatrogenic 046.19
specified NEC 046.19
sporadic 046.19

◀ New   ◀▥ Revised   ~~deleted~~ Deleted   ● Use Additional Digit(s)   ▭ Omit code

Disease, diseased *(Continued)*
  Creutzfeldt-Jakob *(Continued)*
    variant (vCJD) 046.11
      with dementia
        with behavioral disturbance
          046.11 *[294.11]*
        without behavioral
          disturbance 046.11
          [294.10]
  Crigler-Najjar (congenital
    hyperbilirubinemia) 277.4
  Crocq's (acrocyanosis) 443.89
  Crohn's (intestine) *(see also* Enteritis,
    regional) 555.9
  Crouzon's (craniofacial dysostosis)
    756.0
  Cruchet's (encephalitis lethargica)
    049.8
  Cruveilhier's 335.21
  Cruz-Chagas *(see also*
    Trypanosomiasis,
    American) 086.2
  crystal deposition *(see also* Arthritis,
    due to, crystals) 712.9 ●
  Csillag's (lichen sclerosus et
    atrophicus) 701.0
  Curschmann's 359.21
  Cushing's (pituitary basophilism)
    255.0
  cystic
    breast (chronic) 610.1
    kidney, congenital *(see also* Cystic,
      disease, kidney) 753.10
    liver, congenital 751.62
    lung 518.89
      congenital 748.4
    pancreas 577.2
      congenital 751.7
    renal, congenital *(see also* Cystic,
      disease, kidney) 753.10
    semilunar cartilage 717.5
  cysticercus 123.1
  cystine storage (with renal sclerosis)
    270.0
  cytomegalic inclusion (generalized)
    078.5
    with
      pneumonia 078.5 *[484.1]*
    congenital 771.1
  Daae (-Finsen) (epidemic pleurodynia)
    074.1
  dancing 297.8
  Danielssen's (anesthetic leprosy)
    030.1
  Darier's (congenital) (keratosis
    follicularis) 757.39
    erythema annulare centrifugum
      695.0
    vitamin A deficiency 264.8
  Darling's (histoplasmosis) *(see also*
    Histoplasmosis, American)
    115.00
  Davies' 425.0
  de Beurmann-Gougerot
    (sporotrichosis) 117.1
  Débove's (splenomegaly) 789.2
  deer fly *(see also* Tularemia) 021.9
  deficiency 269.9
  degenerative - *see also* Degeneration
    disc - *see* Degeneration,
      intervertebral disc
  Degos' 447.8
  Déjérine (-Sottas) 356.0
  Déleage's 359.89

Disease, diseased *(Continued)*
  demyelinating, demyelinizating (brain
    stem) (central nervous system)
    341.9
    multiple sclerosis 340
    specified NEC 341.8
  de Quervain's (tendon sheath) 727.04
    thyroid (subacute granulomatous
      thyroiditis) 245.1
  Dercum's (adiposis dolorosa) 272.8
  Deutschländer's - *see* Fracture, foot
  Devergie's (pityriasis rubra pilaris)
    696.4
  Devic's 341.0
  diaphorase deficiency 289.7
  diaphragm 519.4
  diarrheal, infectious 009.2
  diatomaceous earth 502
  Diaz's (osteochondrosis astragalus)
    732.5
  digestive system 569.9
  Di Guglielmo's (erythemic myelosis)
    (M9841/3) 207.0 ●
  Dimitri-Sturge-Weber
    (encephalocutaneous
    angiomatosis) 759.6
  disc, degenerative - *see* Degeneration,
    intervertebral disc
  discogenic *(see also* Disease,
    intervertebral disc) 722.90
  diverticular - *see* Diverticula
  Down's (mongolism) 758.0
  Dubini's (electric chorea) 049.8
  Dubois' (thymus gland) 090.5
  Duchenne's 094.0
    locomotor ataxia 094.0
    muscular dystrophy 359.1
    paralysis 335.22
    pseudohypertrophy, muscles 359.1
  Duchenne-Griesinger 359.1
  ductless glands 259.9
  Duhring's (dermatitis herpetiformis)
    694.0
  Dukes (-Filatov) 057.8
  duodenum NEC 537.9
    specified NEC 537.89
  Duplay's 726.2
  Dupré's (meningism) 781.6
  Dupuytren's (muscle contracture) 728.6
  Durand-Nicolas-Favre (climatic bubo)
    099.1
  Duroziez's (congenital mitral stenosis)
    746.5
  Dutton's (trypanosomiasis) 086.9
  Eales' 362.18
  ear (chronic) (inner) NEC 388.9
    middle 385.9
      adhesive *(see also* Adhesions,
        middle ear) 385.10
      specified NEC 385.89
  Eberth's (typhoid fever) 002.0
  Ebstein's
    heart 746.2
    meaning diabetes 250.4 ● *[581.81]*
      due to secondary diabetes 249.4 ●
        [581.81]
  Echinococcus *(see also* Echinococcus)
    122.9
  ECHO virus NEC 078.89
  Economo's (encephalitis lethargica)
    049.8
  Eddowes' (brittle bones and blue
    sclera) 756.51
  Edsall's 992.2

Disease, diseased *(Continued)*
  Eichstedt's (pityriasis versicolor) 111.0
  Ellis-van Creveld (chondroectodermal
    dysplasia) 756.55
  endocardium - *see* Endocarditis
  endocrine glands or system NEC 259.9
    specified NEC 259.8
  endomyocardial, idiopathic mural 425.2
  Engel-von Recklinghausen (osteitis
    fibrosa cystica) 252.01
  Engelmann's (diaphyseal sclerosis)
    756.59
  English (rickets) 268.0
  Engman's (infectious eczematoid
    dermatitis) 690.8
  enteroviral, enterovirus NEC 078.89
    central nervous system NEC 048
  epidemic NEC 136.9
  epididymis 608.9
  epigastric, functional 536.9
    psychogenic 306.4
  Erb (-Landouzy) 359.1
  Erb-Goldflam 358.00
  Erdheim-Chester (ECD) 277.89 ◀
  Erichsen's (railway spine) 300.16
  esophagus 530.9
    functional 530.5
    psychogenic 306.4
  Eulenburg's (congenital paramyotonia)
    359.29
  Eustachian tube 381.9
  Evans' (thrombocytopenic purpura)
    287.32
  external auditory canal 380.9
  extrapyramidal NEC 333.90
  eye 379.90
    anterior chamber 364.9
    inflammatory NEC 364.3
    muscle 378.9
  eyeball 360.9
  eyelid 374.9
  eyeworm of Africa 125.2
  Fabry's (angiokeratoma corporis
    diffusum) 272.7
  facial nerve (seventh) 351.9
    newborn 767.5
  Fahr-Volhard (malignant
    nephrosclerosis) 403.00
  fallopian tube, noninflammatory 620.9
    specified NEC 620.8
  familial periodic 277.31
    paralysis 359.3
  Fanconi's (congenital pancytopenia)
    284.09
  Farber's (disseminated
    lipogranulomatosis) 272.8
  fascia 728.9
    inflammatory 728.9
  Fauchard's (periodontitis) 523.40
  Favre-Durand-Nicolas (climatic bubo)
    099.1
  Favre-Racouchot (elastoidosis cutanea
    nodularis) 701.8
  Fede's 529.0
  Feer's 985.0
  Felix's (juvenile osteochondrosis, hip)
    732.1
  Fenwick's (gastric atrophy) 537.89
  Fernels' (aortic aneurysm) 441.9
  fibrocaseous, of lung *(see also*
    Tuberculosis, pulmonary) 011.9 ●
  fibrocystic - *see also* Fibrocystic, disease
    newborn 277.01
  Fiedler's (leptospiral jaundice) 100.0

Disease, diseased (Continued)
fifth 057.0
Filatoff's (infectious mononucleosis) 075
Filatov's (infectious mononucleosis) 075
file-cutters' 984.9
specified type of lead - see Table of Drugs and Chemicals
filterable virus NEC 078.89
fish skin 757.1
acquired 701.1
Flajani (-Basedow) (exophthalmic goiter) 242.0●
Flatau-Schilder 341.1
flax-dressers' 504
Fleischner's 732.3
flint 502
fluke - see Infestation, fluke
Følling's (phenylketonuria) 270.1
foot and mouth 078.4
foot process 581.3
Forbes' (glycogenosis III) 271.0
Fordyce's (ectopic sebaceous glands) (mouth) 750.26
Fordyce-Fox (apocrine miliaria) 705.82
Fothergill's
meaning scarlatina anginosa 034.1
neuralgia (see also Neuralgia, trigeminal) 350.1
Fournier's 608.83
fourth 057.8
Fox (-Fordyce) (apocrine miliaria) 705.82
Francis' (see also Tularemia) 021.9
Franklin's (heavy chain) 273.2
Frei's (climatic bubo) 099.1
Freiberg's (flattening metatarsal) 732.5
Friedländer's (endarteritis obliterans) - see Arteriosclerosis
Friedreich's
combined systemic or ataxia 334.0
facial hemihypertrophy 756.0
myoclonia 333.2
Fröhlich's (adiposogenital dystrophy) 253.8
Frommel's 676.6●
frontal sinus (chronic) 473.1
acute 461.1
Fuller's earth 502
fungus, fungous NEC 117.9
Gaisböck's (polycythemia hypertonica) 289.0
gallbladder 575.9
congenital 751.60
Gamna's (siderotic splenomegaly) 289.51
Gamstorp's (adynamia episodica hereditaria) 359.3
Gandy-Nanta (siderotic splenomegaly) 289.51
Gannister (occupational) 502
Garré's (see also Osteomyelitis) 730.1●
gastric (see also Disease, stomach) 537.9
gastroesophageal reflux (GERD) 530.81
gastrointestinal (tract) 569.9
amyloid 277.39
functional 536.9
psychogenic 306.4
Gaucher's (adult) (cerebroside lipidosis) (infantile) 272.7
Gayet's (superior hemorrhagic polioencephalitis) 265.1

Disease, diseased (Continued)
Gee (-Herter) (-Heubner) (-Thaysen) (nontropical sprue) 579.0
generalized neoplastic (M8000/6) 199.0
genital organs NEC
female 629.9
specified NEC 629.89
male 608.9
Gerhardt's (erythromelalgia) 443.82
Gerlier's (epidemic vertigo) 078.81
Gibert's (pityriasis rosea) 696.3
Gibney's (perispondylitis) 720.9
Gierke's (glycogenosis I) 271.0
Gilbert's (familial nonhemolytic jaundice) 277.4
Gilchrist's (North American blastomycosis) 116.0
Gilford (-Hutchinson) (progeria) 259.8
Gilles de la Tourette's (motor-verbal tic) 307.23
Giovannini's 117.9
gland (lymph) 289.9
Glanzmann's (hereditary hemorrhagic thrombasthenia) 287.1
glassblowers' 527.1
Glénard's (enteroptosis) 569.89
Glisson's (see also Rickets) 268.0
glomerular
membranous, idiopathic 581.1
minimal change 581.3
glycogen storage (Andersen's) (Cori types 1-7) (Forbes') (McArdle-Schmid-Pearson) (Pompe's) (types I-VII) 271.0
cardiac 271.0 [425.7]
generalized 271.0
glucose-6-phosphatase deficiency 271.0
heart 271.0 [425.7]
hepatorenal 271.0
liver and kidneys 271.0
myocardium 271.0 [425.7]
von Gierke's (glycogenosis I) 271.0
Goldflam-Erb 358.00
Goldscheider's (epidermolysis bullosa) 757.39
Goldstein's (familial hemorrhagic telangiectasia) 448.0
gonococcal NEC 098.0
Goodall's (epidemic vomiting) 078.82
Gordon's (exudative enteropathy) 579.8
Gougerot's (trisymptomatic) 709.1
Gougerot-Carteaud (confluent reticulate papillomatosis) 701.8
Gougerot-Hailey-Hailey (benign familial chronic pemphigus) 757.39
graft-versus-host 279.50
acute 279.51
on chronic 279.53
chronic 279.52
grain-handlers' 495.8
Grancher's (splenopneumonia) - see Pneumonia
granulomatous (childhood) (chronic) 288.1
graphite lung 503
Graves' (exophthalmic goiter) 242.0●
Greenfield's 330.0
green monkey 078.89
Griesinger's (see also Ancylostomiasis) 126.9

Disease, diseased (Continued)
grinders' 502
Grisel's 723.5
Gruby's (tinea tonsurans) 110.0
Guertin's (electric chorea) 049.8
Guillain-Barré 357.0
Guinon's (motor-verbal tic) 307.23
Gull's (thyroid atrophy with myxedema) 244.8
Gull and Sutton's - see Hypertension, kidney
gum NEC 523.9
Günther's (congenital erythropoietic porphyria) 277.1
gynecological 629.9
specified NEC 629.89
H 270.0
Haas' 732.3
Habermann's (acute parapsoriasis varioliformis) 696.2
Haff 985.1
Hageman (congenital factor XII deficiency) (see also Defect, congenital) 286.3
Haglund's (osteochondrosis os tibiale externum) 732.5
Hagner's (hypertrophic pulmonary osteoarthropathy) 731.2
Hailey-Hailey (benign familial chronic pemphigus) 757.39
hair (follicles) NEC 704.9
specified type NEC 704.8
Hallervorden-Spatz 333.0
Hallopeau's (lichen sclerosus et atrophicus) 701.0
Hamman's (spontaneous mediastinal emphysema) 518.1
hand, foot, and mouth 074.3
Hand-Schüller-Christian (chronic histiocytosis X) 277.89
Hanot's - see Cirrhosis, biliary
Hansen's (leprosy) 030.9
benign form 030.1
malignant form 030.0
Harada's 363.22
Harley's (intermittent hemoglobinuria) 283.2
Hart's (pellagra-cerebellar ataxia-renal aminoaciduria) 270.0
Hartnup (pellagra-cerebellar ataxia-renal aminoaciduria) 270.0
Hashimoto's (struma lymphomatosa) 245.2
Hb - see Disease, hemoglobin
heart (organic) 429.9
with
acute pulmonary edema (see also Failure, ventricular, left) 428.1
hypertensive 402.91
with renal failure 404.92
benign 402.11
with renal failure 404.12
malignant 402.01
with renal failure 404.02
kidney disease - see Hypertension, cardiorenal
rheumatic fever (conditions classifiable to 390)
active 391.9
with chorea 392.0
inactive or quiescent (with chorea) 398.90

◄ New   ◄▥ Revised   ~~deleted~~ Deleted   ● Use Additional Digit(s)   ▨ Omit code

Disease, diseased *(Continued)*
  heart *(Continued)*
    amyloid 277.39 *[425.7]*
    aortic (valve) *(see also* Endocarditis, aortic) 424.1
    arteriosclerotic or sclerotic (minimal) (senile) - *see* Arteriosclerosis, coronary
    artery, arterial - *see* Arteriosclerosis, coronary
    atherosclerotic - *see* Arteriosclerosis, coronary
    beer drinkers' 425.5
    beriberi 265.0 *[425.7]*
    black 416.0
    congenital NEC 746.9
      cyanotic 746.9
      maternal, affecting fetus or newborn 760.3
      specified type NEC 746.89
    congestive *(see also* Failure, heart) 428.0
    coronary 414.9
    cryptogenic 429.9
    due to
      amyloidosis 277.39 *[425.7]*
      beriberi 265.0 *[425.7]*
      cardiac glycogenosis 271.0 *[425.7]*
      Friedreich's ataxia 334.0 *[425.8]*
      gout 274.82
      mucopolysaccharidosis 277.5 *[425.7]*
      myotonia atrophica 359.21 *[425.8]*
      progressive muscular dystrophy 359.1 *[425.8]*
      sarcoidosis 135 *[425.8]*
    fetal 746.9
      inflammatory 746.89
    fibroid *(see also* Myocarditis) 429.0
    functional 427.9
      postoperative 997.1
      psychogenic 306.2
    glycogen storage 271.0 *[425.7]*
    gonococcal NEC 098.85
    gouty 274.82
    hypertensive *(see also* Hypertension, heart) 402.90
      benign 402.10
      malignant 402.00
    hyperthyroid *(see also* Hyperthyroidism) 242.9● *[425.7]*
    incompletely diagnosed - *see* Disease, heart
    ischemic (chronic) *(see also* Ischemia, heart) 414.9
      acute *(see also* Infarct, myocardium) 410.9●
        without myocardial infarction 411.89
          with coronary (artery) occlusion 411.81
      asymptomatic 412
      diagnosed on ECG or other special investigation but currently presenting no symptoms 412
    kyphoscoliotic 416.1
    mitral *(see also* Endocarditis, mitral) 394.9
    muscular *(see also* Degeneration, myocardial) 429.1
    postpartum 674.8●
    psychogenic (functional) 306.2

Disease, diseased *(Continued)*
  heart *(Continued)*
    pulmonary (chronic) 416.9
      acute 415.0
      specified NEC 416.8
    rheumatic (chronic) (inactive) (old) (quiescent) (with chorea) 398.90
      active or acute 391.9
        with chorea (active) (rheumatic) (Sydenham's) 392.0
        specified type NEC 391.8
      maternal, affecting fetus or newborn 760.3
    rheumatoid - *see* Arthritis, rheumatoid
    sclerotic - *see* Arteriosclerosis, coronary
    senile *(see also* Myocarditis) 429.0
    specified type NEC 429.89
    syphilitic 093.89
      aortic 093.1
        aneurysm 093.0
      asymptomatic 093.89
      congenital 090.5
    thyroid (gland) *(see also* Hyperthyroidism) 242.9● *[425.7]*
    thyrotoxic *(see also* Thyrotoxicosis) 242.9● *[425.7]*
    tuberculous *(see also* Tuberculosis) 017.9● *[425.8]*
    valve, valvular (obstructive) (regurgitant) - *see also* Endocarditis
      congenital NEC *(see also* Anomaly, heart, valve) 746.9
      pulmonary 746.00
      specified type NEC 746.89
    vascular - *see* Disease, cardiovascular
  heavy-chain (gamma G) 273.2
  Heberden's 715.04
  Hebra's
    dermatitis exfoliativa 695.89
    erythema multiforme exudativum 695.19
    pityriasis
      maculata et circinata 696.3
      rubra 695.89
        pilaris 696.4
    prurigo 698.2
  Heerfordt's (uveoparotitis) 135
  Heidenhain's 290.10
    with dementia 290.10
  Heilmeyer-Schöner (M9842/3) 207.1●
  Heine-Medin *(see also* Poliomyelitis) 045.9●
  Heller's *(see also* Psychosis, childhood) 299.1●
  Heller-Döhle (syphilitic aortitis) 093.1
  hematopoietic organs 289.9
  hemoglobin (Hb) 282.7
    with thalassemia 282.49
    abnormal (mixed) NEC 282.7
      with thalassemia 282.49
    AS genotype 282.5
    Bart's 282.49
    C (Hb-C) 282.7
      with other abnormal hemoglobin NEC 282.7
      elliptocytosis 282.7

Disease, diseased *(Continued)*
  hemoglobin (Hb) *(Continued)*
    C (Hb-C) *(Continued)*
      Hb-S (without crisis) 282.63
        with
          crisis 282.64
          vaso-occlusive pain 282.64
      sickle-cell (without crisis) 282.63
        with
          crisis 282.64
          vaso-occlusive pain 282.64
      thalassemia 282.49
    constant spring 282.7
    D (Hb-D) 282.7
      with other abnormal hemoglobin NEC 282.7
      Hb-S (without crisis) 282.68
        with crisis 282.69
      sickle-cell (without crisis) 282.68
        with crisis 282.69
      thalassemia 282.49
    E (Hb-E) 282.7
      with other abnormal hemoglobin NEC 282.7
      Hb-S (without crisis) 282.68
        with crisis 282.69
      sickle-cell (without crisis) 282.68
        with crisis 282.69
      thalassemia 282.49
    elliptocytosis 282.7
    F (Hb-F) 282.7
    G (Hb-G) 282.7
    H (Hb-H) 282.49
    hereditary persistence, fetal (HPFH) ("Swiss variety") 282.7
    high fetal gene 282.7
    I thalassemia 282.49
    M 289.7
    S - *see also* Disease, sickle-cell, Hb-S
      thalassemia (without crisis) 282.41
        with
          crisis 282.42
          vaso-occlusive pain 282.42
    spherocytosis 282.7
    unstable, hemolytic 282.7
    Zurich (Hb-Zurich) 282.7
  hemolytic (fetus) (newborn) 773.2
    autoimmune (cold type) (warm type) 283.0
    due to or with
      incompatibility
        ABO (blood group) 773.1
        blood (group) (Duffy) (Kell) (Kidd) (Lewis) (M) (S) NEC 773.2
        Rh (blood group) (factor) 773.0
        Rh negative mother 773.0
    unstable hemoglobin 282.7
  hemorrhagic 287.9
    newborn 776.0
  Henoch (-Schönlein) (purpura nervosa) 287.0
  hepatic - *see* Disease, liver
  hepatolenticular 275.1
  heredodegenerative NEC
    brain 331.89
    spinal cord 336.8
  Hers' (glycogenosis VI) 271.0
  Herter (-Gee) (-Heubner) (nontropical sprue) 579.0
  Herxheimer's (diffuse idiopathic cutaneous atrophy) 701.8
  Heubner's 094.89

Disease, diseased (*Continued*)
Heubner-Herter (nontropical sprue) 579.0
high fetal gene or hemoglobin thalassemia 282.49
Hildenbrand's (typhus) 081.9
hip (joint) NEC 719.95
  congenital 755.63
  suppurative 711.05
  tuberculous (*see also* Tuberculosis) 015.1● [*730.85*]
Hippel's (retinocerebral angiomatosis) 759.6
Hirschfeld's (acute diabetes mellitus) (*see also* Diabetes) 250.0●
  due to secondary diabetes 249.0●
Hirschsprung's (congenital megacolon) 751.3
His (-Werner) (trench fever) 083.1
HIV 042
Hodgkin's (M9650/3) 201.9●

> Note 22 Use the following fifth-digit subclassification with category 201:
>
> 0   unspecified site
> 1   lymph nodes of head, face, and neck
> 2   intrathoracic lymph nodes
> 3   intra-abdominal lymph nodes
> 4   lymph nodes of axilla and upper limb
> 5   lymph nodes of inguinal region and lower limb
> 6   intrapelvic lymph nodes
> 7   spleen
> 8   lymph nodes of multiple sites

  lymphocytic
    depletion (M9653/3) 201.7●
      diffuse fibrosis (M9654/3) 201.7●
      reticular type (M9655/3) 201.7●
    predominance (M9651/3) 201.4●
  lymphocytic-histiocytic predominance (M9651/3) 201.4●
  mixed cellularity (M9652/3) 201.6●
  nodular sclerosis (M9656/3) 201.5●
    cellular phase (M9657/3) 201.5●
Hodgson's 441.9
  ruptured 441.5
Hoffa (-Kastert) (liposynovitis prepatellaris) 272.8
Holla (*see also* Spherocytosis) 282.0
homozygous-Hb-S 282.61
hoof and mouth 078.4
hookworm (*see also* Ancylostomiasis) 126.9
Horton's (temporal arteritis) 446.5
host-versus-graft (immune or nonimmune cause) 279.50
HPFH (hereditary persistence of fetal hemoglobin) ("Swiss variety") 282.7
Huchard's (continued arterial hypertension) 401.9
Huguier's (uterine fibroma) 218.9

Disease, diseased (*Continued*)
human immunodeficiency (virus) 042
hunger 251.1
Hunt's
  dyssynergia cerebellaris myoclonica 334.2
  herpetic geniculate ganglionitis 053.11
Huntington's 333.4
Huppert's (multiple myeloma) (M9730/3) 203.0●
Hurler's (mucopolysaccharidosis I) 277.5
Hutchinson's, meaning
  angioma serpiginosum 709.1
  cheiropompholyx 705.81
  prurigo estivalis 692.72
Hutchinson-Boeck (sarcoidosis) 135
Hutchinson-Gilford (progeria) 259.8
hyaline (diffuse) (generalized) 728.9
  membrane (lung) (newborn) 769
hydatid (*see also* Echinococcus) 122.9
Hyde's (prurigo nodularis) 698.3
hyperkinetic (*see also* Hyperkinesia) 314.9
  heart 429.82
hypertensive (*see also* Hypertension) 401.9
hypophysis 253.9
  hyperfunction 253.1
  hypofunction 253.2
Iceland (epidemic neuromyasthenia) 049.8
I cell 272.7
ill-defined 799.89
immunologic NEC 279.9
immunoproliferative 203.8●
inclusion 078.5
  salivary gland 078.5
infancy, early NEC 779.9
infective NEC 136.9
inguinal gland 289.9
internal semilunar cartilage, cystic 717.5
intervertebral disc 722.90
  with myelopathy 722.70
  cervical, cervicothoracic 722.91
    with myelopathy 722.71
  lumbar, lumbosacral 722.93
    with myelopathy 722.73
  thoracic, thoracolumbar 722.92
    with myelopathy 722.72
intestine 569.9
  functional 564.9
    congenital 751.3
    psychogenic 306.4
  lardaceous 277.39
  organic 569.9
  protozoal NEC 007.9
iris 364.9
  specified NEC 364.89
iron
  metabolism 275.0
  storage 275.0
Isambert's (*see also* Tuberculosis, larynx) 012.3●
Iselin's (osteochondrosis, fifth metatarsal) 732.5
island (scrub typhus) 081.2
itai-itai 985.5
Jadassohn's (maculopapular erythroderma) 696.2
Jadassohn-Pellizari's (anetoderma) 701.3

Disease, diseased (*Continued*)
Jakob-Creutzfeldt (CJD) 046.19
  with dementia
    with behavioral disturbance 046.19 [*294.11*]
    without behavioral disturbance 046.19 [*294.10*]
  familial 046.19
  iatrogenic 046.19
  specified NEC 046.19
  sporadic 046.19
  variant (vCJD) 046.11
    with dementia
      with behavioral disturbance 046.11 [*294.11*]
      without behavioral disturbance 046.11 [*294.10*]
Jaksch (-Luzet) (pseudoleukemia infantum) 285.8
Janet's 300.89
Jansky-Bielschowsky 330.1
jaw NEC 526.9
  fibrocystic 526.2
Jensen's 363.05
Jeune's (asphyxiating thoracic dystrophy) 756.4
Jigger 134.1
Johnson-Stevens (erythema multiforme exudativum) 695.13
joint NEC 719.9●
  ankle 719.97
  Charcôt 094.0 [*713.5*]
  degenerative (*see also* Osteoarthrosis) 715.9●
    multiple 715.09
    spine (*see also* Spondylosis) 721.90
  elbow 719.92
  foot 719.97
  hand 719.94
  hip 719.95
  hypertrophic (chronic) (degenerative) (*see also* Osteoarthrosis) 715.9●
    spine (*see also* Spondylosis) 721.90
  knee 719.96
  Luschka 721.90
  multiple sites 719.99
  pelvic region 719.95
  sacroiliac 724.6
  shoulder (region) 719.91
  specified site NEC 719.98
  spine NEC 724.9
    pseudarthrosis following fusion 733.82
    sacroiliac 724.6
  wrist 719.93
Jourdain's (acute gingivitis) 523.00
Jüngling's (sarcoidosis) 135
Kahler (-Bozzolo) (multiple myeloma) (M9730/3) 203.0●
Kalischer's 759.6
Kaposi's 757.33
  lichen ruber 697.8
    acuminatus 696.4
    moniliformis 697.8
  xeroderma pigmentosum 757.33
Kaschin-Beck (endemic polyarthritis) 716.00
  ankle 716.07
  arm 716.02
    lower (and wrist) 716.03
    upper (and elbow) 716.02
  foot (and ankle) 716.07

◄ New   ◄▥ Revised   ~~deleted~~ Deleted   ● Use Additional Digit(s)   ▨ Omit code

Disease, diseased (*Continued*)
 Kaschin-Beck (*Continued*)
  forearm (and wrist) 716.03
  hand 716.04
  leg 716.06
   lower 716.06
   upper 716.05
  multiple sites 716.09
  pelvic region (hip) (thigh) 716.05
  shoulder region 716.01
  specified site NEC 716.08
 Katayama 120.2
 Kawasaki 446.1
 Kedani (scrub typhus) 081.2
 kidney (functional) (pelvis) (*see also*
   Disease, renal) 593.9
  chronic 585.9
   requiring chronic dialysis 585.6
   stage
    I 585.1
    II (mild) 585.2
    III (moderate) 585.3
    IV (severe) 585.4
    V 585.5
  cystic (congenital) 753.10
   multiple 753.19
   single 753.11
   specified NEC 753.19
  fibrocystic (congenital) 753.19
  in gout 274.10
  polycystic (congenital) 753.12
   adult type (APKD) 753.13
   autosomal dominant 753.13
   autosomal recessive 753.14
   childhood type (CPKD) 753.14
   infantile type 753.14
 Kienböck's (carpal lunate) (wrist) 732.3
 Kimmelstiel (-Wilson) (intercapillary
   glomerulosclerosis) 250.4●
   [581.81]
  due to secondary diabetes 249.4●
   [581.81]
 Kinnier Wilson's (hepatolenticular
   degeneration) 275.1
 kissing 075
 Kleb's (*see also* Nephritis) 583.9
 Klinger's 446.4
 Klippel's 723.8
 Klippel-Feil (brevicollis) 756.16
 Knight's 911.1
 Köbner's (epidermolysis bullosa)
   757.39
 Koenig-Wichmann (pemphigus) 694.4
 Köhler's
  first (osteoarthrosis juvenilis) 732.5
  second (Freiberg's infraction,
    metatarsal head) 732.5
  patellar 732.4
  tarsal navicular (bone)
    (osteoarthrosis juvenilis) 732.5
 Köhler-Freiberg (infraction, metatarsal
   head) 732.5
 Köhler-Mouchet (osteoarthrosis
   juvenilis) 732.5
 Köhler-Pellegrini-Stieda (calcification,
   knee joint) 726.62
 Kok 759.89
 König's (osteochondritis dissecans)
   732.7
 Korsakoff's (nonalcoholic) 294.0
  alcoholic 291.1
 Kostmann's (infantile genetic
   agranulocytosis) 288.01
 Krabbe's 330.0

Disease, diseased (*Continued*)
 Kraepelin-Morel (*see also*
   Schizophrenia) 295.9●
 Kraft-Weber-Dimitri 759.6
 Kufs' 330.1
 Kugelberg-Welander 335.11
 Kuhnt-Junius 362.52
 Kümmell's (-Verneuil) (spondylitis)
   721.7
 Kundrat's (lymphosarcoma) 200.1●
 kuru 046.0
 Kussmaul (-Meier) (polyarteritis
   nodosa) 446.0
 Kyasanur Forest 065.2
 Kyrle's (hyperkeratosis follicularis in
   cutem penetrans) 701.1
 labia
  inflammatory 616.10
  noninflammatory 624.9
   specified NEC 624.8
 labyrinth, ear 386.8
 lacrimal system (apparatus) (passages)
   375.9
  gland 375.00
  specified NEC 375.89
 Lafora's 333.2
 Lagleyze-von Hippel (retinocerebral
   angiomatosis) 759.6
 Lancereaux-Mathieu (leptospiral
   jaundice) 100.0
 Landry's 357.0
 Lane's 569.89
 lardaceous (any site) 277.39
 Larrey-Weil (leptospiral jaundice)
   100.0
 Larsen (-Johansson) (juvenile
   osteopathia patellae) 732.4
 larynx 478.70
 Lasègue (persecution mania) 297.9
 Leber's 377.16
 Lederer's (acquired infectious
   hemolytic anemia) 283.19
 Legg's (capital femoral
   osteochondrosis) 732.1
 Legg-Calvé-Perthes (capital femoral
   osteochondrosis) 732.1
 Legg-Calvé-Waldenström (femoral
   capital osteochondrosis) 732.1
 Legg-Perthes (femoral capital
   osteochrondosis) 732.1
 Legionnaires' 482.84
 Leigh's 330.8
 Leiner's (exfoliative dermatitis)
   695.89
 Leloir's (lupus erythematosus) 695.4
 Lenegre's 426.0
 lens (eye) 379.39
 Leriche's (osteoporosis, posttraumatic)
   733.7
 Letterer-Siwe (acute histiocytosis X)
   (M9722/3) 202.5●
 Lev's (acquired complete heart block)
   426.0
 Lewandowski's (*see also* Tuberculosis)
   017.0●
 Lewandowski-Lutz
   (epidermodysplasia
   verruciformis) 078.19
 Lewy body 331.82
  with dementia
   with behavioral disturbance
     331.82 [294.11]
   without behavioral disturbance
     331.82 [294.10]

Disease, diseased (*Continued*)
 Leyden's (periodic vomiting) 536.2
 Libman-Sacks (verrucous endocarditis)
   710.0 [424.91]
 Lichtheim's (subacute combined
   sclerosis with pernicious anemia)
   281.0 [336.2]
 ligament 728.9
 light chain 203.0●
 Lightwood's (renal tubular acidosis)
   588.89
 Lignac's (cystinosis) 270.0
 Lindau's (retinocerebral angiomatosis)
   759.6
 Lindau-von Hippel (angiomatosis
   retinocerebellosa) 759.6
 lip NEC 528.5
 lipidosis 272.7
 lipoid storage NEC 272.7
 Lipschütz's 616.50
 Little's - *see* Palsy, cerebral
 liver 573.9
  alcoholic 571.3
   acute 571.1
   chronic 571.3
  chronic 571.9
   alcoholic 571.3
  cystic, congenital 751.62
  drug-induced 573.3
  due to
   chemicals 573.3
   fluorinated agents 573.3
   hypersensitivity drugs 573.3
   isoniazids 573.3
  end stage NEC 572.8
   due to hepatitis - *see* Hepatitis
  fibrocystic (congenital) 751.62
  glycogen storage 271.0
  organic 573.9
  polycystic (congenital) 751.62
 Lobo's (keloid blastomycosis) 116.2
 Lobstein's (brittle bones and blue
   sclera) 756.51
 locomotor system 334.9
 Lorain's (pituitary dwarfism) 253.3
 Lou Gehrig's 335.20
 Lucas-Championnière (fibrinous
   bronchitis) 466.0
 Ludwig's (submaxillary cellulitis)
   528.3
 luetic - *see* Syphilis
 lumbosacral region 724.6
 lung NEC 518.89
  black 500
  congenital 748.60
  cystic 518.89
   congenital 748.4
  fibroid (chronic) (*see also* Fibrosis,
    lung) 515
  fluke 121.2
   oriental 121.2
  in
   amyloidosis 277.39 [517.8]
   polymyositis 710.4 [517.8]
   sarcoidosis 135 [517.8]
   Sjögren's syndrome 710.2
     [517.8]
   syphilis 095.1
   systemic lupus erythematosus
     710.0 [517.8]
   systemic sclerosis 710.1 [517.2]
  interstitial (chronic) 515
   acute 136.3
  nonspecific, chronic 496

Disease, diseased *(Continued)*
  lung NEC *(Continued)*
    obstructive (chronic) (COPD) 496
      with
        acute
          bronchitis 491.22
          exacerbation NEC 491.21
        alveolitis, allergic (*see also*
          Alveolitis, allergic) 495.9
        asthma (chronic) (obstructive)
          493.2●
        bronchiectasis 494.0
          with acute exacerbation
            494.1
        bronchitis (chronic) 491.20
          with
            acute bronchitis 491.22
            exacerbation (acute)
              491.21
        decompensated 491.21
          with exacerbation 491.21
        emphysema NEC 492.8
        diffuse (with fibrosis) 496
    polycystic 518.89
      asthma (chronic) (obstructive)
        493.2●
      congenital 748.4
    purulent (cavitary) 513.0
    restrictive 518.89
    rheumatoid 714.81
      diffuse interstitial 714.81
    specified NEC 518.89
  Lutembacher's (atrial septal defect
    with mitral stenosis) 745.5
  Lutz-Miescher (elastosis perforans
    serpiginosa) 701.1
  Lutz-Splendore-de Almeida (Brazilian
    blastomycosis) 116.1
  Lyell's (toxic epidermal necrolysis)
    695.15
    due to drug
      correct substance properly
        administered 695.15
      overdose or wrong substance
        given or taken 977.9
      specific drug - *see* Table of
        Drugs and Chemicals
  Lyme 088.81
  lymphatic (gland) (system) 289.9
    channel (noninfective) 457.9
    vessel (noninfective) 457.9
      specified NEC 457.8
  lymphoproliferative (chronic)
    (M9970/1) 238.79
  Machado-Joseph 334.8
  Madelung's (lipomatosis) 272.8
  Madura (actinomycotic) 039.9
    mycotic 117.4
  Magitot's 526.4
  Majocchi's (purpura annularis
    telangiectodes) 709.1
  malarial (*see also* Malaria) 084.6
  Malassez's (cystic) 608.89
  Malibu 919.8
    infected 919.9
  malignant (M8000/3) - *see also*
    Neoplasm, by site, malignant
    previous, affecting management of
      pregnancy V23.89
  Manson's 120.1
  maple bark 495.6
  maple syrup (urine) 270.3
  Marburg (virus) 078.89
  Marchiafava (-Bignami) 341.8

Disease, diseased *(Continued)*
  Marfan's 090.49
    congenital syphilis 090.49
    meaning Marfan's syndrome 759.82
  Marie-Bamberger (hypertrophic
    pulmonary osteoarthropathy)
    (secondary) 731.2
    primary or idiopathic
      (acropachyderma) 757.39
    pulmonary (hypertrophic
      osteoarthropathy) 731.2
  Marie-Strümpell (ankylosing
    spondylitis) 720.0
  Marion's (bladder neck obstruction)
    596.0
  Marsh's (exophthalmic goiter) 242.0●
  Martin's 715.27
  mast cell 757.33
    systemic (M9741/3) 202.6●
  mastoid (*see also* Mastoiditis) 383.9
    process 385.9
  maternal, unrelated to pregnancy NEC,
    affecting fetus or newborn 760.9
  Mathieu's (leptospiral jaundice) 100.0
  Mauclaire's 732.3
  Mauriac's (erythema nodosum
    syphiliticum) 091.3
  Maxcy's 081.0
  McArdle (-Schmid-Pearson)
    (glycogenosis V) 271.0
  mediastinum NEC 519.3
  Medin's (*see also* Poliomyelitis) 045.9●
  Mediterranean (with
    hemoglobinopathy) 282.49
  medullary center (idiopathic)
    (respiratory) 348.89 ◄▬
  Meige's (chronic hereditary edema)
    757.0
  Meleda 757.39
  Ménétrier's (hypertrophic gastritis)
    535.2●
  Ménière's (active) 386.00
    cochlear 386.02
    cochleovestibular 386.01
    inactive 386.04
    in remission 386.04
    vestibular 386.03
  meningeal - *see* Meningitis
  mental (*see also* Psychosis) 298.9
  Merzbacher-Pelizaeus 330.0
  mesenchymal 710.9
  mesenteric embolic 557.0
  metabolic NEC 277.9
  metal polishers' 502
  metastatic - *see* Metastasis
  Mibelli's 757.39
  microdrepanocytic 282.49
  microvascular - *code to* condition
  Miescher's 709.3
  Mikulicz's (dryness of mouth, absent
    or decreased lacrimation) 527.1
  Milkman (-Looser) (osteomalacia with
    pseudofractures) 268.2
  Miller's (osteomalacia) 268.2
  Mills' 335.29
  Milroy's (chronic hereditary edema)
    757.0
  Minamata 985.0
  Minor's 336.1
  Minot's (hemorrhagic disease,
    newborn) 776.0
  Minot-von Willebrand-Jürgens
    (angiohemophilia) 286.4
  Mitchell's (erythromelalgia) 443.82

Disease, diseased *(Continued)*
  mitral - *see* Endocarditis, mitral
  Mljet (mal de Meleda) 757.39
  Möbius', Moebius' 346.2●
  Möeller's 267
  Möller (-Barlow) (infantile scurvy)
    267
  Mönckeberg's (*see also* Arteriosclerosis,
    extremities) 440.20
  Mondor's (thrombophlebitis of breast)
    451.89
  Monge's 993.2
  Morel-Kraepelin (*see also*
    Schizophrenia) 295.9●
  Morgagni's (syndrome) (hyperostosis
    frontalis interna) 733.3
  Morgagni-Adams-Stokes (syncope
    with heart block) 426.9
  Morquio (-Brailsford) (-Ullrich)
    (mucopolysaccharidosis IV) 277.5
  Morton's (with metatarsalgia) 355.6
  Morvan's 336.0
  motor neuron (bulbar) (mixed type)
    335.20
  Mouchet's (juvenile osteochondrosis,
    foot) 732.5
  mouth 528.9
  Moyamoya 437.5
  Mucha's (acute parapsoriasis
    varioliformis) 696.2
  mu-chain 273.2
  mucolipidosis (I) (II) (III) 272.7
  Münchmeyer's (exostosis luxurians)
    728.11
  Murri's (intermittent hemoglobinuria)
    283.2
  muscle 359.9
    inflammatory 728.9
    ocular 378.9
  musculoskeletal system 729.90
  mushroom workers' 495.5
  Myà's (congenital dilation, colon) 751.3
  mycotic 117.9
  myeloproliferative (chronic) (M9960/1)
    238.79
  myocardium, myocardial (*see also*
    Degeneration, myocardial) 429.1
    hypertensive (*see also* Hypertension,
      heart) 402.90
    primary (idiopathic) 425.4
  myoneural 358.9
  Naegeli's 287.1
  nail 703.9
    specified type NEC 703.8
  Nairobi sheep 066.1
  nasal 478.19
    cavity NEC 478.19
    sinus (chronic) - *see* Sinusitis
  navel (newborn) NEC 779.89
    delayed separation of umbilical cord
      779.83
  nemaline body 359.0
  neoplastic, generalized (M8000/6)
    199.0
  nerve - *see* Disorder, nerve
  nervous system (central) 349.9
    autonomic, peripheral (*see also*
      Neuropathy, peripheral,
      autonomic) 337.9
    congenital 742.9
    inflammatory - *see* Encephalitis
    parasympathetic (*see also*
      Neuropathy, peripheral,
      autonomic) 337.9

◄ New   ◄▬ Revised   ~~deleted~~ Deleted   ● Use Additional Digit(s)   ▭ Omit code

Disease, diseased *(Continued)*
  nervous system *(Continued)*
    peripheral NEC 355.9
    prion NEC 046.79
    specified NEC 349.89
    sympathetic *(see also* Neuropathy,
        peripheral, autonomic) 337.9
    vegetative *(see also* Neuropathy,
        peripheral, autonomic) 337.9
  Nettleship's (urticaria pigmentosa)
      757.33
  Neumann's (pemphigus vegetans)
      694.4
  neurologic (central) NEC *(see also*
      Disease, nervous system) 349.9
    peripheral NEC 355.9
  neuromuscular system NEC 358.9
  Newcastle 077.8
  Nicolas (-Durand) -Favre (climatic
      bubo) 099.1
  Niemann-Pick (lipid histiocytosis)
      272.7
  nipple 611.9
    Paget's (M8540/3) 174.0
  Nishimoto (-Takeuchi) 437.5
  nonarthropod-borne NEC 078.89
    central nervous system NEC 049.9
    enterovirus NEC 078.89
  nonautoimmune hemolytic NEC 283.10
  Nonne-Milroy-Meige (chronic
      hereditary edema) 757.0
  Norrie's (congenital progressive
      oculoacousticocerebral
      degeneration) 743.8
  nose 478.19
  nucleus pulposus - *see* Disease,
      intervertebral disc
  nutritional 269.9
    maternal, affecting fetus or newborn
        760.4
  oasthouse, urine 270.2
  obliterative vascular 447.1
  Odelberg's (juvenile osteochondrosis)
      732.1
  Oguchi's (retina) 368.61
  Ohara's *(see also* Tularemia) 021.9
  Ollier's (chondrodysplasia) 756.4
  Opitz's (congestive splenomegaly)
      289.51
  Oppenheim's 358.8
  Oppenheim-Urbach (necrobiosis
      lipoidica diabeticorum) 250.8●
      [709.3]
    due to secondary diabetes 249.8●
        [709.3]
  optic nerve NEC 377.49
  orbit 376.9
    specified NEC 376.89
  Oriental liver fluke 121.1
  Oriental lung fluke 121.2
  Ormond's 593.4
  Osgood's tibia (tubercle) 732.4
  Osgood-Schlatter 732.4
  Osler (-Vaquez) (polycythemia vera)
      (M9950/1) 238.4
  Osler-Rendu (familial hemorrhagic
      telangiectasia) 448.0
  osteofibrocystic 252.01
  Otto's 715.35
  outer ear 380.9
  ovary (noninflammatory) NEC 620.9
    cystic 620.2
    polycystic 256.4
    specified NEC 620.8

Disease, diseased *(Continued)*
  Owren's (congenital) *(see also* Defect,
      coagulation) 286.3
  Paas' 756.59
  Paget's (osteitis deformans) 731.0
    with infiltrating duct carcinoma of
        the breast (M8541/3) - *see*
        Neoplasm, breast, malignant
    bone 731.0
      osteosarcoma in (M9184/3) - *see*
          Neoplasm, bone, malignant
    breast (M8540/3) 174.0
    extramammary (M8542/3) - *see also*
        Neoplasm, skin, malignant
      anus 154.3
      skin 173.5
    malignant (M8540/3)
      breast 174.0
      specified site NEC (M8542/3) -
          see Neoplasm, skin,
          malignant
      unspecified site 174.0
    mammary (M8540/3) 174.0
    nipple (M8540/3) 174.0
  palate (soft) 528.9
  Paltauf-Sternberg 201.9●
  pancreas 577.9
    cystic 577.2
      congenital 751.7
    fibrocystic 277.00
  Panner's 732.3
    capitellum humeri 732.3
    head of humerus 732.3
    tarsal navicular (bone)
        (osteochondrosis) 732.5
  panvalvular - *see* Endocarditis, mitral
  parametrium 629.9
  parasitic NEC 136.9
    cerebral NEC 123.9
    intestinal NEC 129
    mouth 112.0
    skin NEC 134.9
    specified type - *see* Infestation
    tongue 112.0
  parathyroid (gland) 252.9
    specified NEC 252.8
  Parkinson's 332.0
  parodontal 523.9
  Parrot's (syphilitic osteochondritis)
      090.0
  Parry's (exophthalmic goiter) 242.0●
  Parson's (exophthalmic goiter)
      242.0●
  Pavy's 593.6
  Paxton's (white piedra) 111.2
  Payr's (splenic flexure syndrome)
      569.89
  pearl-workers' (chronic osteomyelitis)
      (see also Osteomyelitis) 730.1●
  Pel-Ebstein - *see* Disease, Hodgkin's
  Pelizaeus-Merzbacher 330.0
    with dementia
      with behavioral disturbance 330.0
          [294.11]
      without behavioral disturbance
          330.0 *[294.10]*
  Pellegrini-Stieda (calcification, knee
      joint) 726.62
  pelvis, pelvic
    female NEC 629.9
      specified NEC 629.89
    gonococcal (acute) 098.19
      chronic or duration of 2 months
          or over 098.39

Disease, diseased *(Continued)*
  pelvis, pelvic *(Continued)*
    infection *(see also* Disease, pelvis,
        inflammatory) 614.9
    inflammatory (female) (PID) 614.9
      with
        abortion - *see* Abortion, by
            type, with sepsis
        ectopic pregnancy *(see also*
            categories 633.0–633.9)
            639.0
        molar pregnancy *(see also*
            categories 630–632) 639.0
      acute 614.3
      chronic 614.4
      complicating pregnancy 646.6●
        affecting fetus or newborn
            760.8
      following
        abortion 639.0
        ectopic or molar pregnancy
            639.0
      peritonitis (acute) 614.5
        chronic NEC 614.7
      puerperal, postpartum, childbirth
          670.8   ◀▦
      specified NEC 614.8
    organ, female NEC 629.9
      specified NEC 629.89
    peritoneum, female NEC 629.9
      specified NEC 629.89
  penis 607.9
    inflammatory 607.2
  peptic NEC 536.9
    acid 536.8
  periapical tissues NEC 522.9
  pericardium 423.9
    specified type NEC 423.8
  perineum
    female
      inflammatory 616.9
        specified NEC 616.89
      noninflammatory 624.9
        specified NEC 624.8
    male (inflammatory) 682.2
  periodic (familial) (Reimann's) NEC
      277.31
    paralysis 359.3
  periodontal NEC 523.9
    specified NEC 523.8
  periosteum 733.90
  peripheral
    arterial 443.9
    autonomic nervous system *(see also*
        Neuropathy, autonomic) 337.9
    nerve NEC *(see also* Neuropathy)
        356.9
      multiple - *see* Polyneuropathy
    vascular 443.9
      specified type NEC 443.89
  peritoneum 568.9
    pelvic, female 629.9
      specified NEC 629.89
  Perrin-Ferraton (snapping hip) 719.65
  persistent mucosal (middle ear) (with
      posterior or superior marginal
      perforation of ear drum) 382.2
  Perthes' (capital femoral
      osteochondrosis) 732.1
  Petit's *(see also* Hernia, lumbar) 553.8
  Peutz-Jeghers 759.6
  Peyronie's 607.85
  Pfeiffer's (infectious mononucleosis)
      075

Disease, diseased (*Continued*)
pharynx 478.20
Phocas' 610.1
photochromogenic (acid-fast bacilli)
    (pulmonary) 031.0
    nonpulmonary 031.9
Pick's
    brain 331.11
       with dementia
          with behavioral disturbance
            331.11 *[294.11]*
          without behavioral
            disturbance 331.11
            [294.10]
    cerebral atrophy 331.11
       with dementia
          with behavioral disturbance
            331.11 *[294.11]*
          without behavioral
            disturbance 331.11
            [294.10]
    lipid histiocytosis 272.7
    liver (pericardial pseudocirrhosis of
       liver) 423.2
    pericardium (pericardial
       pseudocirrhosis of liver) 423.2
    polyserositis (pericardial
       pseudocirrhosis of liver)
       423.2
Pierson's (osteochondrosis) 732.1
pigeon fanciers' or breeders' 495.2
pineal gland 259.8
pink 985.0
Pinkus' (lichen nitidus) 697.1
pinworm 127.4
pituitary (gland) 253.9
    hyperfunction 253.1
    hypofunction 253.2
pituitary snuff-takers' 495.8
placenta
    affecting fetus or newborn 762.2
    complicating pregnancy or
       childbirth 656.7●
pleura (cavity) (*see also* Pleurisy)
    511.0
Plummer's (toxic nodular goiter)
    242.3●
pneumatic
    drill 994.9
    hammer 994.9
policeman's 729.2
Pollitzer's (hidradenitis suppurativa)
    705.83
polycystic (congenital) 759.89
    kidney or renal 753.12
       adult type (APKD) 753.13
       autosomal dominant 753.13
       autosomal recessive 753.14
       childhood type (CPKD) 753.14
       infantile type 753.14
    liver or hepatic 751.62
    lung or pulmonary 518.89
       congenital 748.4
    ovary, ovaries 256.4
    spleen 759.0
Pompe's (glycogenosis II) 271.0
Poncet's (tuberculous rheumatism) (*see
    also* Tuberculosis) 015.9●
Posada-Wernicke 114.9
Potain's (pulmonary edema) 514
Pott's (*see also* Tuberculosis) 015.0 ●
    [730.88]
    osteomyelitis 015.0● *[730.88]*
    paraplegia 015.0 ● *[730.88]*

Disease, diseased (*Continued*)
Pott's (*Continued*)
    spinal curvature 015.0● *[737.43]*
    spondylitis 015.0● *[720.81]*
Potter's 753.0
Poulet's 714.2
pregnancy NEC (*see also* Pregnancy)
    646.9●
Preiser's (osteoporosis) 733.09
Pringle's (tuberous sclerosis) 759.5
Profichet's 729.90
prostate 602.9
    specified type NEC 602.8
protozoal NEC 136.8
    intestine, intestinal NEC 007.9
pseudo-Hurler's (mucolipidosis III)
    272.7
psychiatric (*see also* Psychosis) 298.9
psychotic (*see also* Psychosis) 298.9
Puente's (simple glandular cheilitis)
    528.5
puerperal NEC (*see also* Puerperal)
    674.9●
pulmonary - *see also* Disease, lung
    amyloid 277.39 *[517.8]*
    artery 417.9
    circulation, circulatory 417.9
       specified NEC 417.8
    diffuse obstructive (chronic) 496
       with
          acute bronchitis 491.22
          asthma (chronic) (obstructive)
            493.2●
          exacerbation NEC (acute)
            491.21
    heart (chronic) 416.9
       specified NEC 416.8
    hypertensive (vascular) 416.0
       cardiovascular 416.0
    obstructive diffuse (chronic) 496
       with
          acute bronchitis 491.22
          asthma (chronic) (obstructive)
            493.2●
          bronchitis (chronic) 491.20
            with
               exacerbation (acute)
                 491.21
               acute 491.22
          exacerbation NEC (acute)
            491.21
       decompensated 491.21
          with exacerbation 491.21
    valve (*see also* Endocarditis,
       pulmonary) 424.3
pulp (dental) NEC 522.9
pulseless 446.7
Putnam's (subacute combined sclerosis
    with pernicious anemia) 281.0
    [336.2]
Pyle (-Cohn) (craniometaphyseal
    dysplasia) 756.89
pyramidal tract 333.90
Quervain's
    tendon sheath 727.04
    thyroid (subacute granulomatous
       thyroiditis) 245.1
Quincke's - *see* Edema,
    angioneurotic
Quinquaud (acne decalvans)
    704.09
rag sorters' 022.1
Raynaud's (paroxysmal digital
    cyanosis) 443.0

Disease, diseased (*Continued*)
reactive airway - *see* Asthma
Recklinghausen's (M9540/1) 237.71
    bone (osteitis fibrosa cystica) 252.01
Recklinghausen-Applebaum
    (hemochromatosis) 275.0
Reclus' (cystic) 610.1
rectum NEC 569.49
Refsum's (heredopathia atactica
    polyneuritiformis) 356.3
Reichmann's (gastrosuccorrhea) 536.8
Reimann's (periodic) 277.31
Reiter's 099.3
renal (functional) (pelvis) (*see also*
    Disease, kidney) 593.9
    with
       edema (*see also* Nephrosis) 581.9
       exudative nephritis 583.89
       lesion of interstitial nephritis
          583.89
       stated generalized cause - *see*
          Nephritis
    acute 593.9
    basement membrane NEC 583.89
       with
          pulmonary hemorrhage
            (Goodpasture's
            syndrome) 446.21
            [583.81]
    chronic (*see also* Disease, kidney,
       chronic) 585.9
    complicating pregnancy or
       puerperium NEC 646.2●
       with hypertension - *see* Toxemia,
          of pregnancy
       affecting fetus or newborn 760.1
    cystic, congenital (*see also* Cystic,
       disease, kidney) 753.10
    diabetic 250.4● *[583.81]*
       due to secondary diabetes 249.4●
          [581.81]
    due to
       amyloidosis 277.39 *[583.81]*
       diabetes mellitus 250.4 ●
          [583.81]
          due to secondary diabetes
            249.4 ● *[581.81]*
       systemic lupus erythematosis
          710.0 *[583.81]*
    end-stage 585.6
    exudative 583.89
    fibrocystic (congenital) 753.19
    gonococcal 098.19 *[583.81]*
    gouty 274.10
    hypertensive (*see also* Hypertension,
       kidney) 403.90
    immune complex NEC 583.89
    interstitial (diffuse) (focal) 583.89
    lupus 710.0 *[583.81]*
    maternal, affecting fetus or newborn
       760.1
       hypertensive 760.0
    phosphate-losing (tubular) 588.0
    polycystic (congenital) 753.12
       adult type (APKD) 753.13
       autosomal dominant 753.13
       autosomal recessive 753.14
       childhood type (CPKD) 753.14
       infantile type 753.14
    specified lesion or cause NEC (*see
       also* Glomerulonephritis)
       583.89
    subacute 581.9
    syphilitic 095.4

◄ New   ◄▥ Revised   ~~deleted~~ Deleted   ● Use Additional Digit(s)   ▩ Omit code

Disease, diseased (*Continued*)
 renal (*Continued*)
  tuberculous (*see also* Tuberculosis)
   016.0● [*583.81*]
  tubular (*see also* Nephrosis, tubular)
   584.5
 Rendu-Osler-Weber (familial
   hemorrhagic telangiectasia) 448.0
 renovascular (arteriosclerotic) (*see also*
   Hypertension, kidney) 403.90
 respiratory (tract) 519.9
  acute or subacute (upper) NEC
    465.9
   due to fumes or vapors 506.3
   multiple sites NEC 465.8
   noninfectious 478.9
   streptococcal 034.0
  chronic 519.9
   arising in the perinatal period
     770.7
   due to fumes or vapors 506.4
  due to
   aspiration of liquids or solids
     508.9
   external agents NEC 508.9
    specified NEC 508.8
   fumes or vapors 506.9
    acute or subacute NEC 506.3
    chronic 506.4
  fetus or newborn NEC 770.9
  obstructive 496
  specified type NEC 519.8
  upper (acute) (infectious) NEC
    465.9
   multiple sites NEC 465.8
   noninfectious NEC 478.9
   streptococcal 034.0
 retina, retinal NEC 362.9
  Batten's or Batten-Mayou 330.1
    [*362.71*]
  degeneration 362.89
  vascular lesion 362.17
 rheumatic (*see also* Arthritis) 716.8●
  heart - *see* Disease, heart, rheumatic
 rheumatoid (heart) - *see* Arthritis,
   rheumatoid
 rickettsial NEC 083.9
  specified type NEC 083.8
 Riedel's (ligneous thyroiditis) 245.3
 Riga (-Fede) (cachectic aphthae) 529.0
 Riggs' (compound periodontitis)
   523.40
 Ritter's 695.81
 Rivalta's (cervicofacial actinomycosis)
   039.3
 Robles' (onchocerciasis) 125.3 [*360.13*]
 Roger's (congenital interventricular
   septal defect) 745.4
 Rokitansky's (*see also* Necrosis, liver)
   570
 Romberg's 349.89
 Rosenthal's (factor XI deficiency) 286.2
 Rossbach's (hyperchlorhydria) 536.8
  psychogenic 306.4
 Roth (-Bernhardt) 355.1
 Runeberg's (progressive pernicious
   anemia) 281.0
 Rust's (tuberculous spondylitis) (*see
   also* Tuberculosis) 015.0 ● [*720.81*]
 Rustitskii's (multiple myeloma)
   (M9730/3) 203.0●
 Ruysch's (Hirschsprung's disease) 751.3
 Sachs (-Tay) 330.1
 sacroiliac NEC 724.6

Disease, diseased (*Continued*)
 salivary gland or duct NEC 527.9
  inclusion 078.5
   streptococcal 034.0
  virus 078.5
 Sander's (paranoia) 297.1
 Sandhoff's 330.1
 sandworm 126.9
 Savill's (epidemic exfoliative
   dermatitis) 695.89
 Schamberg's (progressive pigmentary
   dermatosis) 709.09
 Schaumann's (sarcoidosis) 135
 Schenck's (sporotrichosis) 117.1
 Scheuermann's (osteochondrosis) 732.0
 Schilder (-Flatau) 341.1
 Schimmelbusch's 610.1
 Schlatter's tibia (tubercle) 732.4
 Schlatter-Osgood 732.4
 Schmorl's 722.30
  cervical 722.39
  lumbar, lumbosacral 722.32
  specified region NEC 722.39
  thoracic, thoracolumbar 722.31
 Scholz's 330.0
 Schönlein (-Henoch) (purpura
   rheumatica) 287.0
 Schottmüller's (*see also* Fever,
   paratyphoid) 002.9
 Schüller-Christian (chronic
   histiocytosis X) 277.89
 Schultz's (agranulocytosis) 288.09
 Schwalbe-Ziehen-Oppenheimer 333.6
 Schwartz-Jampel 359.23
 Schweninger-Buzzi (macular atrophy)
   701.3
 sclera 379.19
 scrofulous (*see also* Tuberculosis)
   017.2●
 scrotum 608.9
 sebaceous glands NEC 706.9
 Secretan's (posttraumatic edema) 782.3
 semilunar cartilage, cystic 717.5
 seminal vesicle 608.9
 Senear-Usher (pemphigus
   erythematosus) 694.4
 serum NEC 999.5
 Sever's (osteochondrosis calcaneum)
   732.5
 sexually transmitted - *see* Disease,
   venereal
 Sézary's (reticulosis) (M9701/3)
   202.2●
 Shaver's (bauxite pneumoconiosis)
   503
 Sheehan's (postpartum pituitary
   necrosis) 253.2
 shimamushi (scrub typhus) 081.2
 shipyard 077.1
 sickle-cell 282.60
  with
   crisis 282.62
   Hb-S disease 282.61
   other abnormal hemoglobin
     (Hb-D) (Hb-E) (Hb-G)
     (Hb-J) (Hb-K) (Hb-O)
     (Hb-P) (high fetal gene)
     (without crisis) 282.68
    with crisis 282.69
  elliptocytosis 282.60
  Hb-C (without crisis) 282.63
   with
    crisis 282.64
    vaso-occlusive pain 282.64

Disease, diseased (*Continued*)
 sickle-cell (*Continued*)
  Hb-S 282.61
   with
    crisis 282.62
    Hb-C (without crisis) 282.63
     with
      crisis 282.64
      vaso-occlusive pain
        282.64
    other abnormal hemoglobin
      (Hb-D) (Hb-E) (Hb-G)
      (Hb-J) (Hb-K) (Hb-O)
      (Hb-P) (high fetal gene)
      (without crisis) 282.68
     with crisis 282.69
  spherocytosis 282.60
  thalassemia (without crisis) 282.41
   with
    crisis 282.42
    vaso-occlusive pain 282.42
 Siegal-Cattan-Mamou (periodic) 277.31
 silo fillers' 506.9
 Simian B 054.3
 Simmonds' (pituitary cachexia) 253.2
 Simons' (progressive lipodystrophy)
   272.6
 Sinding-Larsen (juvenile osteopathia
   patellae) 732.4
 sinus - *see also* Sinusitis
  brain 437.9
  specified NEC 478.19
 Sirkari's 085.0
 sixth (*see also* Exanthem subitum)
   058.10
 Sjögren (-Gougerot) 710.2
  with lung involvement 710.2 [*517.8*]
 Skevas-Zerfus 989.5
 skin NEC 709.9
  due to metabolic disorder 277.9
  specified type NEC 709.8
 sleeping (*see also* Narcolepsy) 347.00
  meaning sleeping sickness (*see also*
    Trypanosomiasis) 086.5
 small vessel 443.9
 Smith-Strang (oasthouse urine) 270.2
 Sneddon-Wilkinson (subcorneal
   pustular dermatosis) 694.1
 South African creeping 133.8
 Spencer's (epidemic vomiting) 078.82
 Spielmeyer-Stock 330.1
 Spielmeyer-Vogt 330.1
 spine, spinal 733.90
  combined system (*see also*
    Degeneration, combined) 266.2
    [*336.2*]
   with pernicious anemia 281.0
     [*336.2*]
  cord NEC 336.9
   congenital 742.9
  demyelinating NEC 341.8
  joint (*see also* Disease, joint, spine)
    724.9
  tuberculous 015.0● [*730.8*]●
 spinocerebellar 334.9
  specified NEC 334.8
 spleen (organic) (postinfectional)
   289.50
  amyloid 277.39
  lardaceous 277.39
  polycystic 759.0
  specified NEC 289.59
 sponge divers' 989.5
 Stanton's (melioidosis) 025

Disease, diseased (Continued)
   Stargardt's 362.75
   Startle 759.89
   Steinert's 359.21
   Sternberg's - see Disease, Hodgkin's
   Stevens-Johnson (erythema multiforme
      exudativum) 695.13
   Sticker's (erythema infectiosum) 057.0
   Stieda's (calcification, knee joint) 726.62
   Still's (juvenile rheumatoid arthritis)
      714.30
     adult onset 714.2
   Stiller's (asthenia) 780.79
   Stokes' (exophthalmic goiter) 242.0●
   Stokes-Adams (syncope with heart
      block) 426.9
   Stokvis (-Talma) (enterogenous
      cyanosis) 289.7
   stomach NEC (organic) 537.9
     functional 536.9
       psychogenic 306.4
     lardaceous 277.39
   stonemasons' 502
   storage
     glycogen (see also Disease, glycogen
       storage) 271.0
     lipid 272.7
     mucopolysaccharide 277.5
   striatopallidal system 333.90
     specified NEC 333.89
   Strümpell-Marie (ankylosing
      spondylitis) 720.0
   Stuart's (congenital factor X deficiency)
      (see also Defect, coagulation) 286.3
   Stuart-Prower (congenital factor X
      deficiency) (see also Defect,
      coagulation) 286.3
   Sturge (-Weber) (-Dimitri)
      (encephalocutaneous
      angiomatosis) 759.6
   Stuttgart 100.89
   Sudeck's 733.7
   supporting structures of teeth NEC
      525.9
   suprarenal (gland) (capsule) 255.9
     hyperfunction 255.3
     hypofunction 255.41
   Sutton's 709.09
   Sutton and Gull's - see Hypertension,
      kidney
   sweat glands NEC 705.9
     specified type NEC 705.89
   sweating 078.2
   Sweeley-Klionsky 272.4
   Swift (-Feer) 985.0
   swimming pool (bacillus) 031.1
   swineherd's 100.89
   Sylvest's (epidemic pleurodynia) 074.1
   Symmers (follicular lymphoma)
      (M9690/3) 202.0●
   sympathetic nervous system (see also
      Neuropathy, peripheral,
      autonomic) 337.9
   synovium 727.9
   syphilitic - see Syphilis
   systemic tissue mast cell (M9741/3)
      202.6●
   Taenzer's 757.4
   Takayasu's (pulseless) 446.7
   Talma's 728.85
   Tangier (familial high-density
      lipoprotein deficiency) 272.5
   Tarral-Besnier (pityriasis rubra pilaris)
      696.4

Disease, diseased (Continued)
   Tay-Sachs 330.1
   Taylor's 701.8
   tear duct 375.69
   teeth, tooth 525.9
     hard tissues 521.9
       specified NEC 521.89
     pulp NEC 522.9
   tendon 727.9
     inflammatory NEC 727.9
   terminal vessel 443.9
   testis 608.9
   Thaysen-Gee (nontropical sprue) 579.0
   Thomsen's 359.22
   Thomson's (congenital poikiloderma)
      757.33
   Thornwaldt's, Tornwaldt's (pharyngeal
      bursitis) 478.29
   throat 478.20
     septic 034.0
   thromboembolic (see also Embolism)
      444.9
   thymus (gland) 254.9
     specified NEC 254.8
   thyroid (gland) NEC 246.9
     heart (see also Hyperthyroidism)
      242.9● [425.7]
     lardaceous 277.39
     specified NEC 246.8
   Tietze's 733.6
   Tommaselli's
     correct substance properly
      administered 599.70
     overdose or wrong substance given
      or taken 961.4
   tongue 529.9
   tonsils, tonsillar (and adenoids)
      (chronic) 474.9
     specified NEC 474.8
   tooth, teeth 525.9
     hard tissues 521.9
       specified NEC 521.89
     pulp NEC 522.9
   Tornwaldt's (pharyngeal bursitis)
      478.29
   Tourette's 307.23
   trachea 519.19
   tricuspid - see Endocarditis, tricuspid
   triglyceride-storage, type I, II, III
      272.7
   triple vessel - see Arteriosclerosis,
      coronary
   trisymptomatic, Gougerot's 709.1
   trophoblastic (see also Hydatidiform
      mole) 630
     previous, affecting management of
      pregnancy V23.1
   tsutsugamushi (scrub typhus) 081.2
   tube (fallopian), noninflammatory
      620.9
     specified NEC 620.8
   tuberculous NEC (see also Tuberculosis)
      011.9●
   tubo-ovarian
     inflammatory (see also Salpingo-
      oophoritis) 614.2
     noninflammatory 620.9
      specified NEC 620.8
   tubotympanic, chronic (with anterior
      perforation of ear drum) 382.1
   tympanum 385.9
   Uhl's 746.84
   umbilicus (newborn) NEC 779.89
     delayed separation 779.83

Disease, diseased (Continued)
   Underwood's (sclerema neonatorum)
      778.1
   undiagnosed 799.9
   Unna's (seborrheic dermatitis) 690.18
   unstable hemoglobin hemolytic
      282.7
   Unverricht (-Lundborg) 345.1   ◄▥
   Urbach-Oppenheim (necrobiosis
      lipoidica diabeticorum) 250.8●
      [709.3]
     due to secondary diabetes 249.8●
      [709.3]
   Urbach-Wiethe (lipoid proteinosis)
      272.8
   ureter 593.9
   urethra 599.9
     specified type NEC 599.84
   urinary (tract) 599.9
     bladder 596.9
      specified NEC 596.8
     maternal, affecting fetus or newborn
      760.1
   Usher-Senear (pemphigus
      erythematosus) 694.4
   uterus (organic) 621.9
     infective (see also Endometritis) 615.9
     inflammatory (see also Endometritis)
      615.9
     noninflammatory 621.9
      specified type NEC 621.8
   uveal tract
     anterior 364.9
     posterior 363.9
   vagabonds' 132.1
   vagina, vaginal
     inflammatory 616.10
     noninflammatory 623.9
      specified NEC 623.8
   Valsuani's (progressive pernicious
      anemia, puerperal) 648.2●
     complicating pregnancy or
      puerperium 648.2●
   valve, valvular - see also Endocarditis
     congenital NEC (see also Anomaly,
      heart, valve) 746.9
     pulmonary 746.00
     specified type NEC 746.89
   van Bogaert-Nijssen (-Peiffer) 330.0
   van Creveld-von Gierke (glycogenosis
      I) 271.0
   van den Bergh's (enterogenous
      cyanosis) 289.7
   van Neck's (juvenile osteochondrosis)
      732.1
   Vaquez (-Osler) (polycythemia vera)
      (M9950/1) 238.4
   vascular 459.9
     arteriosclerotic - see Arteriosclerosis
     hypertensive - see Hypertension
     obliterative 447.1
      peripheral 443.9
     occlusive 459.9
     peripheral (occlusive) 443.9
      in (due to) (with) diabetes
       mellitus 250.7● [443.81] ◄▥
      in (due to) (with) secondary
       diabetes 249.7●
       [443.81] ◄▥
     specified type NEC 443.89
   vas deferens 608.9
   vasomotor 443.9
   vasospastic 443.9
   vein 459.9

◄ New   ◄▥ Revised   ~~deleted~~ Deleted   ● Use Additional Digit(s)   ▥ Omit code

Disease, diseased (Continued)
venereal 099.9
  chlamydial NEC 099.50
    anus 099.52
    bladder 099.53
    cervix 099.53
    epididymis 099.54
    genitourinary NEC 099.55
      lower 099.53
      specified NEC 099.54
    pelvic inflammatory disease 099.54
    perihepatic 099.56
    peritoneum 099.56
    pharynx 099.51
    rectum 099.52
    specified site NEC 099.59
    testis 099.54
    vagina 099.53
    vulva 099.53
  fifth 099.1
  sixth 099.1
  complicating pregnancy, childbirth, or puerperium 647.2●
  specified nature or type NEC 099.8
    chlamydial - see Disease, venereal, chlamydial
Verneuil's (syphilitic bursitis) 095.7
Verse's (calcinosis intervertebralis) 275.49 [722.90]
vertebra, vertebral NEC 733.90
  disc - see Disease, Intervertebral disc
vibration NEC 994.9
Vidal's (lichen simplex chronicus) 698.3
Vincent's (trench mouth) 101
Virchow's 733.99
virus (filterable) NEC 078.89
  arbovirus NEC 066.9
  arthropod-borne NEC 066.9
  central nervous system NEC 049.9
    specified type NEC 049.8
  complicating pregnancy, childbirth, or puerperium 647.6●
  contact (with) V01.79
    varicella V01.71
  exposure to V01.79
    varicella V01.71
  Marburg 078.89
  maternal
    with fetal damage affecting management of pregnancy 655.3●
  nonarthropod-borne NEC 078.89
    central nervous system NEC 049.9
      specified NEC 049.8
  vaccination, prophylactic (against) V04.89
vitreous 379.29
vocal cords NEC 478.5
Vogt's (Cecile) 333.71
Vogt-Spielmeyer 330.1
Volhard-Fahr (malignant nephrosclerosis) 403.00
Volkmann's
  acquired 958.6
von Bechterew's (ankylosing spondylitis) 720.0
von Economo's (encephalitis lethargica) 049.8
von Eulenburg's (congenital paramyotonia) 359.29

Disease, diseased (Continued)
von Gierke's (glycogenosis I) 271.0
von Graefe's 378.72
von Hippel's (retinocerebral angiomatosis) 759.6
von Hippel-Lindau (angiomatosis retinocerebellosa) 759.6
von Jaksch's (pseudoleukemia infantum) 285.8
von Recklinghausen's (M9540/1) 237.71
  bone (osteitis fibrosa cystica) 252.01
von Recklinghausen-Applebaum (hemochromatosis) 275.0
von Willebrand (-Jürgens) (angiohemophilia) 286.4
von Zambusch's (lichen sclerosus et atrophicus) 701.0
Voorhoeve's (dyschondroplasia) 756.4
Vrolik's (osteogenesis imperfecta) 756.51
vulva
  inflammatory 616.10
  noninflammatory 624.9
    specified NEC 624.8
Wagner's (colloid milium) 709.3
Waldenström's (osteochondrosis capital femoral) 732.1
Wallgren's (obstruction of splenic vein with collateral circulation) 459.89
Wardrop's (with lymphangitis) 681.9
  finger 681.02
  toe 681.11
Wassilieff's (leptospiral jaundice) 100.0
wasting NEC 799.4
  due to malnutrition 261
  paralysis 335.21
Waterhouse-Friderichsen 036.3
waxy (any site) 277.39
Weber-Christian (nodular nonsuppurative panniculitis) 729.30
Wegner's (syphilitic osteochondritis) 090.0
Weil's (leptospiral jaundice) 100.0
  of lung 100.0
Weir Mitchell's (erythromelalgia) 443.82
Werdnig-Hoffmann 335.0
Werlhof's (see also Purpura, thrombocytopenic) 287.39
Wermer's 258.01
Werner's (progeria adultorum) 259.8
Werner-His (trench fever) 083.1
Werner-Schultz (agranulocytosis) 288.09
Wernicke's (superior hemorrhagic polioencephalitis) 265.1
Wernicke-Posadas 114.9
Whipple's (intestinal lipodystrophy) 040.2
whipworm 127.3
white
  blood cell 288.9
    specified NEC 288.8
  spot 701.0
White's (congenital) (keratosis follicularis) 757.39
Whitmore's (melioidosis) 025
Widal-Abrami (acquired hemolytic jaundice) 283.9
Wilkie's 557.1
Wilkinson-Sneddon (subcorneal pustular dermatosis) 694.1

Disease, diseased (Continued)
Willis' (diabetes mellitus) (see also Diabetes) 250.0●
  due to secondary diabetes 249.0●
Wilson's (hepatolenticular degeneration) 275.1
Wilson-Brocq (dermatitis exfoliativa) 695.89
winter vomiting 078.82
Wise's 696.2
Wohlfart-Kugelberg-Welander 335.11
Woillez's (acute idiopathic pulmonary congestion) 518.5
Wolman's (primary familial xanthomatosis) 272.7
wool-sorters' 022.1
Zagari's (xerostomia) 527.7
Zahorsky's (exanthem subitum) 058.10
Ziehen-Oppenheim 333.6
zoonotic, bacterial NEC 027.9
  specified type NEC 027.8
Disfigurement (due to scar) 709.2
  head V48.6
  limb V49.4
  neck V48.7
  trunk V48.7
Disgerminoma - see Dysgerminoma
Disinsertion, retina 361.04
Disintegration, complete, of the body 799.89
  traumatic 869.1
Disk kidney 753.3
Dislocatable hip, congenital (see also Dislocation, hip, congenital) 754.30
Dislocation (articulation) (closed) (displacement) (simple) (subluxation) 839.8

Note 23

"Closed" includes simple, complete, partial, uncomplicated, and unspecified dislocation.

"Open" includes dislocation specified as infected or compound and dislocation with foreign body.

"Chronic," "habitual," "old," or "recurrent" dislocations should be coded as indicated under the entry "Dislocation, recurrent"; and "pathological" as indicated under the entry "Dislocation, pathological."

For late effect of dislocation see Late, effect, dislocation.

---

  with fracture - see Fracture, by site
acromioclavicular (joint) (closed) 831.04
  open 831.14
anatomical site (closed)
  specified NEC 839.69
    open 839.79
  unspecified or ill-defined 839.8
    open 839.9
ankle (scaphoid bone) (closed) 837.0
  open 837.1
arm (closed) 839.8
  open 839.9
astragalus (closed) 837.0
  open 837.1
atlanto-axial (closed) 839.01
  open 839.11

Dislocation *(Continued)*
  atlas (closed) 839.01
    open 839.11
  axis (closed) 839.02
    open 839.12
  back (closed) 839.8
    open 839.9
  Bell-Daly 723.8
  breast bone (closed) 839.61
    open 839.71
  capsule, joint - *see* Dislocation, by site
  carpal (bone) - *see* Dislocation, wrist
  carpometacarpal (joint) (closed) 833.04
    open 833.14
  cartilage (joint) - *see also* Dislocation, by site
    knee - *see* Tear, meniscus
  cervical, cervicodorsal, or cervicothoracic (spine) (vertebra) - *see* Dislocation, vertebra, cervical
  chiropractic (*see also* Lesion, nonallopathic) 739.9
  chondrocostal - *see* Dislocation, costochondral
  chronic - *see* Dislocation, recurrent
  clavicle (closed) 831.04
    open 831.14
  coccyx (closed) 839.41
    open 839.51
  collar bone (closed) 831.04
    open 831.14
  compound (open) NEC 839.9
  congenital NEC 755.8
    hip (*see also* Dislocation, hip, congenital) 754.30
    lens 743.37
    rib 756.3
    sacroiliac 755.69
    spine NEC 756.19
    vertebra 756.19
  coracoid (closed) 831.09
    open 831.19
  costal cartilage (closed) 839.69
    open 839.79
  costochondral (closed) 839.69
    open 839.79
  cricoarytenoid articulation (closed) 839.69
    open 839.79
  cricothyroid (cartilage) articulation (closed) 839.69
    open 839.79
  dorsal vertebrae (closed) 839.21
    open 839.31
  ear ossicle 385.23
  elbow (closed) 832.00
    anterior (closed) 832.01
      open 832.11
    congenital 754.89
    divergent (closed) 832.09
      open 832.19
    lateral (closed) 832.04
      open 832.14
    medial (closed) 832.03
      open 832.13
    open 832.10
    posterior (closed) 832.02
      open 832.12
    recurrent 718.32
    specified type NEC 832.09
      open 832.19
  eye 360.81
    lateral 376.36

Dislocation *(Continued)*
  eyeball 360.81
    lateral 376.36
  femur
    distal end (closed) 836.50
      anterior 836.52
        open 836.62
      lateral 836.54 ◀▥
        open 836.64 ◀▥
      medial 836.53 ◀▥
        open 836.63 ◀▥
      open 836.60
      posterior 836.51
        open 836.61
    proximal end (closed) 835.00
      anterior (pubic) 835.03
        open 835.13
      obturator 835.02
        open 835.12
      open 835.10
      posterior 835.01
        open 835.11
  fibula
    distal end (closed) 837.0
      open 837.1
    proximal end (closed) 836.59
      open 836.69
  finger(s) (phalanx) (thumb) (closed) 834.00
    interphalangeal (joint) 834.02
      open 834.12
    metacarpal (bone), distal end 834.01
      open 834.11
    metacarpophalangeal (joint) 834.01
      open 834.11
    open 834.10
    recurrent 718.34
  foot (closed) 838.00
    open 838.10
    recurrent 718.37
  forearm (closed) 839.8
    open 839.9
  fracture - *see* Fracture, by site
  glenoid (closed) 831.09
    open 831.19
  habitual - *see* Dislocation, recurrent
  hand (closed) 839.8
    open 839.9
  hip (closed) 835.00
    anterior 835.03
      obturator 835.02
        open 835.12
      open 835.13
    congenital (unilateral) 754.30
      with subluxation of other hip 754.35
      bilateral 754.31
    developmental 718.75
    open 835.10
    posterior 835.01
      open 835.11
    recurrent 718.35
  humerus (closed) 831.00
    distal end (*see also* Dislocation, elbow) 832.00
    open 831.10
    proximal end (closed) 831.00
      anterior (subclavicular) (subcoracoid) (subglenoid) (closed) 831.01
        open 831.11
      inferior (closed) 831.03
        open 831.13

Dislocation *(Continued)*
  humerus *(Continued)*
    proximal end *(Continued)*
      open 831.10
      posterior (closed) 831.02
        open 831.12
  implant - *see* Complications, mechanical
  incus 385.23
  infracoracoid (closed) 831.01
    open 831.11
  innominate (pubic junction) (sacral junction) (closed) 839.69
    acetabulum (*see also* Dislocation, hip) 835.00
    open 839.79
  interphalangeal (joint)
    finger or hand (closed) 834.02
      open 834.12
    foot or toe (closed) 838.06
      open 838.16
  jaw (cartilage) (meniscus) (closed) 830.0
    open 830.1
    recurrent 524.69
  joint NEC (closed) 839.8
    developmental 718.7●
    open 839.9
    pathological - *see* Dislocation, pathological
    recurrent - *see* Dislocation, recurrent
  knee (closed) 836.50
    anterior 836.51
      open 836.61
    congenital (with genu recurvatum) 754.41
    habitual 718.36
    lateral 836.54
      open 836.64
    medial 836.53
      open 836.63
    old 718.36
    open 836.60
    posterior 836.52
      open 836.62
    recurrent 718.36
    rotatory 836.59
      open 836.69
  lacrimal gland 375.16
  leg (closed) 839.8
    open 839.9
  lens (crystalline) (complete) (partial) 379.32
    anterior 379.33
    congenital 743.37
    ocular implant 996.53
    posterior 379.34
    traumatic 921.3
  ligament - *see* Dislocation, by site
  lumbar (vertebrae) (closed) 839.20
    open 839.30
  lumbosacral (vertebrae) (closed) 839.20
    congenital 756.19
    open 839.30
  mandible (closed) 830.0
    open 830.1
  maxilla (inferior) (closed) 830.0
    open 830.1
  meniscus (knee) - *see also* Tear, meniscus
    other sites - *see* Dislocation, by site

◀ New   ◀▥ Revised   ~~deleted~~ Deleted   ● Use Additional Digit(s)   ▨ Omit code

Dislocation (*Continued*)
  metacarpal (bone)
    distal end (closed) 834.01
      open 834.11
    proximal end (closed) 833.05
      open 833.15
  metacarpophalangeal (joint) (closed)
    834.01
    open 834.11
  metatarsal (bone) (closed) 838.04
    open 838.14
  metatarsophalangeal (joint) (closed)
    838.05
    open 838.15
  midcarpal (joint) (closed) 833.03
    open 833.13
  midtarsal (joint) (closed) 838.02
    open 838.12
  Monteggia's - *see* Dislocation, hip
  multiple locations (except fingers only
    or toes only) (closed) 839.8
    open 839.9
  navicular (bone) foot (closed) 837.0
    open 837.1
  neck (*see also* Dislocation, vertebra,
    cervical) 839.00
  Nélaton's - *see* Dislocation, ankle
  nontraumatic (joint) - *see* Dislocation,
    pathological
  nose (closed) 839.69
    open 839.79
  not recurrent, not current injury - *see*
    Dislocation, pathological
  occiput from atlas (closed) 839.01
    open 839.11
  old - *see* Dislocation, recurrent
  open (compound) NEC 839.9
  ossicle, ear 385.23
  paralytic (flaccid) (spastic) - *see*
    Dislocation, pathological
  patella (closed) 836.3
    congenital 755.64
    open 836.4
  pathological NEC 718.20
    ankle 718.27
    elbow 718.22
    foot 718.27
    hand 718.24
    hip 718.25
    knee 718.26
    lumbosacral joint 724.6
    multiple sites 718.29
    pelvic region 718.25
    sacroiliac 724.6
    shoulder (region) 718.21
    specified site NEC 718.28
    spine 724.8
      sacroiliac 724.6
    wrist 718.23
  pelvis (closed) 839.69
    acetabulum (*see also* Dislocation,
      hip) 835.00
    open 839.79
  phalanx
    foot or toe (closed) 838.09
      open 838.19
    hand or finger (*see also* Dislocation,
      finger) 834.00
  postpoliomyelitic - *see* Dislocation,
    pathological
  prosthesis, internal - *see* Complications,
    mechanical
  radiocarpal (joint) (closed) 833.02
    open 833.12

Dislocation (*Continued*)
  radioulnar (joint)
    distal end (closed) 833.01
      open 833.11
    proximal end (*see also* Dislocation,
      elbow) 832.00
  radius
    distal end (closed) 833.00
      open 833.10
    proximal end (closed) 832.01
      open 832.11
  recurrent (*see also* Derangement, joint,
    recurrent) 718.3●
    elbow 718.32
    hip 718.35
    joint NEC 718.38
    knee 718.36
    lumbosacral (joint) 724.6
    patella 718.36
    sacroiliac 724.6
    shoulder 718.31
    temporomandibular 524.69
  rib (cartilage) (closed) 839.69
    congenital 756.3
    open 839.79
  sacrococcygeal (closed) 839.42
    open 839.52
  sacroiliac (joint) (ligament) (closed)
    839.42
    congenital 755.69
    open 839.52
    recurrent 724.6
  sacrum (closed) 839.42
    open 839.52
  scaphoid (bone)
    ankle or foot (closed) 837.0
      open 837.1
    wrist (closed) (*see also* Dislocation,
      wrist) 833.00
      open 833.10
  scapula (closed) 831.09
    open 831.19
  semilunar cartilage, knee - *see* Tear,
    meniscus
  septal cartilage (nose) (closed) 839.69
    open 839.79
  septum (nasal) (old) 470
  sesamoid bone - *see* Dislocation, by site
  shoulder (blade) (ligament) (closed)
    831.00
    anterior (subclavicular) (subcoracoid)
      (subglenoid) (closed) 831.01
      open 831.11
    chronic 718.31
    inferior 831.03
      open 831.13
    open 831.10
    posterior (closed) 831.02
      open 831.12
    recurrent 718.31
  skull - *see* Injury, intracranial
  Smith's - *see* Dislocation, foot
  spine (articular process) (*see also*
    Dislocation, vertebra) (closed)
    839.40
    atlanto-axial (closed) 839.01
      open 839.11
      recurrent 723.8
    cervical, cervicodorsal,
      cervicothoracic (closed) (*see
      also* Dislocation, vertebrae,
      cervical) 839.00
      open 839.10
      recurrent 723.8

Dislocation (*Continued*)
  spine (*Continued*)
    coccyx 839.41
      open 839.51
    congenital 756.19
    due to birth trauma 767.4
    open 839.50
    recurrent 724.9
    sacroiliac 839.42
      recurrent 724.6
    sacrum (sacrococcygeal) (sacroiliac)
      839.42
      open 839.52
  spontaneous - *see* Dislocation,
    pathological
  sternoclavicular (joint) (closed)
    839.61
    open 839.71
  sternum (closed) 839.61
    open 839.71
  subastragalar - *see* Dislocation, foot
  subglenoid (closed) 831.01
    open 831.11
  symphysis
    jaw (closed) 830.0
      open 830.1
    mandibular (closed) 830.0
      open 830.1
    pubis (closed) 839.69
      open 839.79
  tarsal (bone) (joint) 838.01
    open 838.11
  tarsometatarsal (joint) 838.03
    open 838.13
  temporomandibular (joint) (closed)
    830.0
    open 830.1
    recurrent 524.69
  thigh
    distal end (*see also* Dislocation,
      femur, distal end) 836.50
    proximal end (*see also* Dislocation,
      hip) 835.00
  thoracic (vertebrae) (closed) 839.21
    open 839.31
  thumb(s) (*see also* Dislocation, finger)
    834.00
  thyroid cartilage (closed) 839.69
    open 839.79
  tibia
    distal end (closed) 837.0
      open 837.1
    proximal end (closed) 836.50
      anterior 836.51
        open 836.61
      lateral 836.54
        open 836.64
      medial 836.53
        open 836.63
      open 836.60
      posterior 836.52
        open 836.62
      rotatory 836.59
        open 836.69
  tibiofibular
    distal (closed) 837.0
      open 837.1
    superior (closed) 836.59
      open 836.69
  toe(s) (closed) 838.09
    open 838.19
  trachea (closed) 839.69
    open 839.79

Dislocation (*Continued*)
  ulna
    distal end (closed) 833.09
      open 833.19
    proximal end - *see* Dislocation,
        elbow
  vertebra (articular process) (body)
      (closed) (traumatic) 839.40
    cervical, cervicodorsal or
        cervicothoracic (closed) 839.00
      first (atlas) 839.01
        open 839.11
      second (axis) 839.02
        open 839.12
      third 839.03
        open 839.13
      fourth 839.04
        open 839.14
      fifth 839.05
        open 839.15
      sixth 839.06
        open 839.16
      seventh 839.07
        open 839.17
      congenital 756.19
      multiple sites 839.08
        open 839.18
      open 839.10
    congenital 756.19
    dorsal 839.21
      open 839.31
      recurrent 724.9
    lumbar, lumbosacral 839.20
      open 839.30
    non-traumatic - *see* Displacement,
        intervertebral disc
    open NEC 839.50
    recurrent 724.9
    specified region NEC 839.49
      open 839.59
    thoracic 839.21
      open 839.31
  wrist (carpal bone) (scaphoid)
      (semilunar) (closed) 833.00
    carpometacarpal (joint) 833.04
      open 833.14
    metacarpal bone, proximal end
        833.05
      open 833.15
    midcarpal (joint) 833.03
      open 833.13
    open 833.10
    radiocarpal (joint) 833.02
      open 833.12
    radioulnar (joint) 833.01
      open 833.11
    recurrent 718.33
    specified site NEC 833.09
      open 833.19
  xiphoid cartilage (closed) 839.61
    open 839.71
Dislodgement
  artificial skin graft 996.55
  decellularized allodermis graft
      996.55
Disobedience, hostile (covert) (overt)
    (*see also* Disturbance, conduct)
    312.0●
Disorder - *see also* Disease
  academic underachievement,
      childhood and adolescence 313.83
  accommodation 367.51
    drug-induced 367.89
    toxic 367.89

Disorder (*Continued*)
  adjustment (*see also* Reaction,
      adjustment) 309.9
    with
      anxiety 309.24
      anxiety and depressed mood
          309.28
      depressed mood 309.0
      disturbance of conduct 309.3
      disturbance of emotions and
          conduct 309.4
  adrenal (capsule) (cortex) (gland) 255.9
    specified type NEC 255.8
  adrenogenital 255.2
  affective (*see also* Psychosis, affective)
      296.90
    atypical 296.81
  aggressive, unsocialized (*see also*
      Disturbance, conduct) 312.0●
  alcohol, alcoholic (*see also* Alcohol)
      291.9
  allergic - *see* Allergy
  amino acid (metabolic) (*see also*
      Disturbance, metabolism, amino
      acid) 270.9
    albinism 270.2
    alkaptonuria 270.2
    argininosuccinicaciduria 270.6
    beta-amino-isobutyricaciduria 277.2
    cystathioninuria 270.4
    cystinosis 270.0
    cystinuria 270.0
    glycinuria 270.0
    homocystinuria 270.4
    imidazole 270.5
    maple syrup (urine) disease 270.3
    neonatal, transitory 775.89
    oasthouse urine disease 270.2
    ochronosis 270.2
    phenylketonuria 270.1
    phenylpyruvic oligophrenia 270.1
    purine NEC 277.2
    pyrimidine NEC 277.2
    renal transport NEC 270.0
    specified type NEC 270.8
    transport NEC 270.0
      renal 270.0
    xanthinuria 277.2
  amnestic (*see also* Amnestic syndrome)
      294.8
    alcohol-induced persisting 291.1
    drug-induced persisting 292.83
    in conditions classified elsewhere
        294.0
  anaerobic glycolysis with anemia 282.3
  anxiety (*see also* Anxiety) 300.00
    due to or associated with physical
        condition 293.84
  arteriole 447.9
    specified type NEC 447.8
  artery 447.9
    specified type NEC 447.8
  articulation - *see* Disorder, joint
  Asperger's 299.8●
  attachment of infancy or early
      childhood 313.89
  attention deficit 314.00
    with hyperactivity 314.01
    predominantly
    combined hyperactive/inattentive
        314.01
      hyperactive/impulsive 314.01
      inattentive 314.00
    residual type 314.8

Disorder (*Continued*)
  auditory processing disorder 388.45
    acquired 388.45
    developmental 315.32
  autistic 299.0●
  autoimmune NEC 279.49   ◀▦
    hemolytic (cold type) (warm type)
        283.0
    parathyroid 252.1
    thyroid 245.2
  avoidant, childhood or adolescence
      313.21
  balance
    acid-base 276.9
      mixed (with hypercapnia)
          276.4
    electrolyte 276.9
    fluid 276.9
  behavior NEC (*see also* Disturbance,
      conduct) 312.9
    disruptive 312.9
  bilirubin excretion 277.4
  bipolar (affective) (alternating)
      296.80

> Note 63   Use the following fifth-
> digit subclassification with categories
> 296.0–296.6:
>
> 0   unspecified
> 1   mild
> 2   moderate
> 3   severe, without mention of
>   psychotic behavior
> 4   severe, specified as with
>   psychotic behavior
> 5   in partial or unspecified
>   remission
> 6   in full remission

    atypical 296.7
    specified type NEC 296.89
    type I 296.7
      most recent episode (or current)
        depressed 296.5●
        hypomanic 296.4●
        manic 296.4●
        mixed 296.6●
        unspecified 296.7
      single manic episode 296.0●
    type II (recurrent major depressive
        episodes with hypomania)
        296.89
  bladder 596.9
    functional NEC 596.59
    specified NEC 596.8
  bleeding 286.9
  bone NEC 733.90
    specified NEC 733.99
  brachial plexus 353.0
  branched-chain amino-acid
      degradation 270.3
  breast 611.9
    puerperal, postpartum 676.3●
    specified NEC 611.89
  Briquet's 300.81
  bursa 727.9
    shoulder region 726.10
  carbohydrate metabolism, congenital
      271.9
  cardiac, functional 427.9
    postoperative 997.1
    psychogenic 306.2
  cardiovascular, psychogenic 306.2

◀ New   ◀▦ Revised   ~~deleted~~ Deleted   ● Use Additional Digit(s)   ▦ Omit code

Disorder *(Continued)*
cartilage NEC 733.90
  articular 718.00
    ankle 718.07
    elbow 718.02
    foot 718.07
    hand 718.04
    hip 718.05
    knee 717.9
    multiple sites 718.09
    pelvic region 718.05
    shoulder region 718.01
    specified
      site NEC 718.08
      type NEC 733.99
    wrist 718.03
catatonic - *see* Catatonia
central auditory processing 315.32
  acquired 388.45
  developmental 315.32
cervical region NEC 723.9
cervical root (nerve) NEC 353.2
character NEC (*see also* Disorder,
  personality) 301.9
ciliary body 364.9
  specified NEC 364.89
coagulation (factor) (*see also* Defect,
  coagulation) 286.9
  factor VIII (congenital) (functional)
    286.0
  factor IX (congenital) (functional)
    286.1
  neonatal, transitory 776.3
coccyx 724.70
  specified NEC 724.79
cognitive 294.9
colon 569.9
  functional 564.9
    congenital 751.3
communication 307.9
conduct (*see also* Disturbance, conduct)
  312.9
  adjustment reaction 309.3
  adolescent onset type 312.82
  childhood onset type 312.81
  compulsive 312.30
    specified type NEC 312.39
  hyperkinetic 314.2
  onset unspecified 312.89
  socialized (type) 312.20
    aggressive 312.23
    unaggressive 312.21
  specified NEC 312.89
conduction, heart 426.9
  specified NEC 426.89
conflict
  sexual orientation 302.0
congenital
  glycosylation (CDG) 271.8
  convulsive (secondary) (*see also*
    Convulsions) 780.39
    due to injury at birth 767.0
    idiopathic 780.39
  coordination 781.3
cornea NEC 371.89
  due to contact lens 371.82
corticosteroid metabolism NEC
  255.2
cranial nerve - *see* Disorder, nerve,
  cranial
cyclothymic 301.13
degradation, branched-chain amino
  acid 270.3
delusional 297.1

Disorder *(Continued)*
dentition 520.6
depersonalization 300.6
depressive NEC 311
  atypical 296.82
  major (*see also* Psychosis, affective)
    296.2●
    recurrent episode 296.3●
    single episode 296.2●
development, specific 315.9
  associated with hyperkinesia
    314.1
  coordination 315.4
  language 315.31
    and speech due to hearing loss
      315.34
  learning 315.2
    arithmetical 315.1
    reading 315.00
  mixed 315.5
  motor coordination 315.4
  specified type NEC 315.8
  speech 315.39
    and language due to hearing loss
      315.34
diaphragm 519.4
digestive 536.9
  fetus or newborn 777.9
    specified NEC 777.8
  psychogenic 306.4
disintegrative childhood 299.1●
dissociative 300.15
  identity 300.14
  nocturnal 307.47
drug-related 292.9
dysmorphic body 300.7
dysthymic 300.4
ear 388.9
  degenerative NEC 388.00
  external 380.9
    specified 380.89
  pinna 380.30
  specified type NEC 388.8
  vascular NEC 388.00
eating NEC 307.50
electrolyte NEC 276.9
  with
    abortion - *see* Abortion, by type,
      with metabolic disorder
    ectopic pregnancy (*see also*
      categories 633.0–633.9)
      639.4
    molar pregnancy (*see also*
      categories 630–632) 639.4
  acidosis 276.2
    metabolic 276.2
    respiratory 276.2
  alkalosis 276.3
    metabolic 276.3
    respiratory 276.3
  following
    abortion 639.4
    ectopic or molar pregnancy
      639.4
  neonatal, transitory NEC 775.5
emancipation as adjustment reaction
  309.22
emotional (*see also* Disorder, mental,
  nonpsychotic) V40.9
endocrine 259.9
  specified type NEC 259.8
esophagus 530.9
  functional 530.5
  psychogenic 306.4

Disorder *(Continued)*
explosive
  intermittent 312.34
  isolated 312.35
expressive language 315.31
eye 379.90
  globe - *see* Disorder, globe
  ill-defined NEC 379.99
  limited duction NEC 378.63
  specified NEC 379.8
eyelid 374.9
  degenerative 374.50
  sensory 374.44
  specified type NEC 374.89
  vascular 374.85
factitious (with combined
    psychological and physical
    signs and symptoms) (with
    predominantly physical signs
    and symptoms) 300.19
  with predominantly psychological
    signs and symptoms 300.16
factor, coagulation (*see also* Defect,
  coagulation) 286.9
  VIII (congenital) (functional)
    286.0
  IX (congenital) (functional) 286.1
fascia 728.9
fatty acid oxidation 277.85
feeding - *see* Feeding
female sexual arousal 302.72
fluid NEC 276.9
gastric (functional) 536.9
  motility 536.8
  psychogenic 306.4
  secretion 536.8
gastrointestinal (functional) NEC
  536.9
  newborn (neonatal) 777.9
    specified NEC 777.8
  psychogenic 306.4
gender (child) 302.6
  adult 302.85
gender identity (childhood) 302.6
  adolescents 302.85
  adults (-life) 302.85
genitourinary system, psychogenic
  306.50
globe 360.9
  degenerative 360.20
    specified NEC 360.29
  specified type NEC 360.89
hearing - *see also* Deafness
  conductive type (air) (*see also*
    Deafness, conductive)
    389.00
  mixed conductive and
    sensorineural 389.20
    bilateral 389.22
    unilateral 389.21
  nerve
    bilateral 389.12
    unilateral 389.13
  perceptive (*see also* Deafness,
    perceptive) 389.10
  sensorineural type NEC (*see also*
    Deafness, sensorineural)
    389.10
heart action 427.9
  postoperative 997.1
hematological, transient neonatal
  776.9
  specified type NEC 776.8
hematopoietic organs 289.9

Disorder *(Continued)*
  hemorrhagic NEC 287.9
    due to intrinsic circulating
        anticoagulants 286.5
    specified type NEC 287.8
  hemostasis *(see also* Defect, coagulation)
        286.9
  homosexual conflict 302.0
  hypomanic (chronic) 301.11
  identity
    childhood and adolescence 313.82
      gender 302.6
  immune mechanism (immunity) 279.9
    single complement (C_1–C_9) 279.8
    specified type NEC 279.8
  impulse control *(see also* Disturbance,
        conduct, compulsive) 312.30
  infant sialic acid storage 271.8
  integument, fetus or newborn 778.9
    specified type NEC 778.8
  interactional psychotic (childhood) *(see
        also* Psychosis, childhood)
        299.1●
  intermittent explosive 312.34
  intervertebral disc 722.90
    cervical, cervicothoracic 722.91
    lumbar, lumbosacral 722.93
    thoracic, thoracolumbar 722.92
  intestinal 569.9
    functional NEC 564.9
      congenital 751.3
      postoperative 564.4
    psychogenic 306.4
  introverted, of childhood and
        adolescence 313.22
  involuntary emotional expression
        (IEED) 310.8
  iris 364.9
    specified NEC 364.89
  iron, metabolism 275.0
  isolated explosive 312.35
  joint NEC 719.90
    ankle 719.97
    elbow 719.92
    foot 719.97
    hand 719.94
    hip 719.95
    knee 719.96
    multiple sites 719.99
    pelvic region 719.95
    psychogenic 306.0
    shoulder (region) 719.91
    specified site NEC 719.98
    temporomandibular 524.60
      sounds on opening or closing
          524.64
      specified NEC 524.69
    wrist 719.93
  kidney 593.9
    functional 588.9
      specified NEC 588.89
  labyrinth, labyrinthine 386.9
    specified type NEC 386.8
  lactation 676.9●
  language (developmental) (expressive)
        315.31
    mixed receptive-expressive 315.32
  learning 315.9
  ligament 728.9
  ligamentous attachments, peripheral -
        see also Enthesopathy
    spine 720.1
  limb NEC 729.90
    psychogenic 306.0

Disorder *(Continued)*
  lipid
    metabolism, congenital 272.9
    storage 272.7
  lipoprotein deficiency (familial) 272.5
  low back NEC 724.9
    psychogenic 306.0
  lumbosacral
    plexus 353.1
    root (nerve) NEC 353.4
  lymphoproliferative (chronic) NEC
        (M9970/1) 238.79
    post-transplant (PTLD) 238.77
  major depressive *(see also* Psychosis,
        affective) 296.2●
    recurrent episode 296.3●
    single episode 296.2●
  male erectile 607.84
    nonorganic origin 302.72
  manic *(see also* Psychosis, affective)
        296.0●
    atypical 296.81
  mathematics 315.1
  meniscus NEC *(see also* Disorder,
        cartilage, articular) 718.0●
  menopausal 627.9
    specified NEC 627.8
  menstrual 626.9
    psychogenic 306.52
    specified NEC 626.8
  mental (nonpsychotic) 300.9
    affecting management of pregnancy,
        childbirth, or puerperium
        648.4●
    drug-induced 292.9
      hallucinogen persisting
          perception 292.89
      specified type NEC 292.89
    due to or associated with
        alcoholism 291.9
        drug consumption NEC 292.9
          specified type NEC 292.89
        physical condition NEC 293.9
    induced by drug 292.9
      specified type NEC 292.89
    neurotic *(see also* Neurosis) 300.9
    of infancy, childhood or adolescence
        313.9
    persistent
      other
        due to conditions classified
            elsewhere 294.8
      unspecified
        due to conditions classified
            elsewhere 294.9
    presenile 310.1
      psychotic NEC 290.10
    previous, affecting management of
        pregnancy V23.89
    psychoneurotic *(see also* Neurosis)
        300.9
    psychotic *(see also* Psychosis) 298.9
      brief 298.8
      senile 290.20
    specific, following organic brain
        damage 310.9
      cognitive or personality change
          of other type 310.1
      frontal lobe syndrome 310.0
      postconcussional syndrome 310.2
      specified type NEC 310.8
    transient
      in conditions classified elsewhere
          293.9

Disorder *(Continued)*
  metabolism NEC 277.9
    with
      abortion - *see* Abortion, by type,
          with metabolic disorder
      ectopic pregnancy *(see also*
          categories 633.0–633.9)
          639.4
      molar pregnancy *(see also*
          categories 630–632) 639.4
    alkaptonuria 270.2
    amino acid *(see also* Disorder, amino
          acid) 270.9
      specified type NEC 270.8
    ammonia 270.6
    arginine 270.6
    argininosuccinic acid 270.6
    basal 794.7
    bilirubin 277.4
    calcium 275.40
    carbohydrate 271.9
      specified type NEC 271.8
    cholesterol 272.9
    citrulline 270.6
    copper 275.1
    corticosteroid 255.2
    cystine storage 270.0
    cystinuria 270.0
    fat 272.9
      fatty acid oxidation 277.85
    following
      abortion 639.4
      ectopic or molar pregnancy
          639.4
    fructosemia 271.2
    fructosuria 271.2
    fucosidosis 271.8
    galactose-1-phosphate uridyl
          transferase 271.1
    glutamine 270.7
    glycine 270.7
    glycogen storage NEC 271.0
      hepatorenal 271.0
    hemochromatosis 275.0
    in labor and delivery 669.0●
    iron 275.0
    lactose 271.3
    lipid 272.9
      specified type NEC 272.8
      storage 272.7
    lipoprotein - *see also* Hyperlipemia
      deficiency (familial) 272.5
    lysine 270.7
    magnesium 275.2
    mannosidosis 271.8
    mineral 275.9
      specified type NEC 275.8
      mitochondrial 277.87
    mucopolysaccharide 277.5
    nitrogen 270.9
    ornithine 270.6
    oxalosis 271.8
    pentosuria 271.8
    phenylketonuria 270.1
    phosphate 275.3
    phosphorus 275.3
    plasma protein 273.9
      specified type NEC 273.8
    porphyrin 277.1
    purine 277.2
    pyrimidine 277.2
    serine 270.7
    sodium 276.9
    specified type NEC 277.89

◀ New   ◀▐▐ Revised   ~~deleted~~ Deleted   ● Use Additional Digit(s)   ▩ Omit code

Disorder (Continued)
  metabolism NEC (Continued)
    steroid 255.2
    threonine 270.7
    urea cycle 270.6
    xylose 271.8
  micturition NEC 788.69
    psychogenic 306.53
  misery and unhappiness, of childhood
    and adolescence 313.1
  mitochondrial metabolism 277.87
  mitral valve 424.0
  mood (see also Disorder, bipolar) 296.90
    episodic 296.90
      specified NEC 296.99
    in conditions classified elsewhere
      293.83
  motor tic 307.20
    chronic 307.22
    transient (childhood) 307.21
  movement NEC 333.90
    hysterical 300.11
    medication-induced 333.90
    periodic limb 327.51
    sleep related unspecified 780.58
      other organic 327.59
    specified type NEC 333.99
    stereotypic 307.3
  mucopolysaccharide 277.5
  muscle 728.9
    psychogenic 306.0
    specified type NEC 728.3
  muscular attachments, peripheral - see
      also Enthesopathy
    spine 720.1
  musculoskeletal system NEC 729.90
    psychogenic 306.0
  myeloproliferative (chronic) NEC
      (M9960/1) 238.79
  myoneural 358.9
    due to lead 358.2
    specified type NEC 358.8
    toxic 358.2
  myotonic 359.29
  neck region NEC 723.9
  nerve 349.9
    abducens NEC 378.54
    accessory 352.4
    acoustic 388.5
    auditory 388.5
    auriculotemporal 350.8
    axillary 353.0
    cerebral - see Disorder, nerve, cranial
    cranial 352.9
      first 352.0
      second 377.49
      third
        partial 378.51
        total 378.52
      fourth 378.53
      fifth 350.9
      sixth 378.54
      seventh NEC 351.9
      eighth 388.5
      ninth 352.2
      tenth 352.3
      eleventh 352.4
      twelfth 352.5
      multiple 352.6
    entrapment - see Neuropathy,
        entrapment
    facial 351.9
      specified NEC 351.8
    femoral 355.2

Disorder (Continued)
  nerve (Continued)
    glossopharyngeal NEC 352.2
    hypoglossal 352.5
    iliohypogastric 355.79
    ilioinguinal 355.79
    intercostal 353.8
    lateral
      cutaneous of thigh 355.1
      popliteal 355.3
    lower limb NEC 355.8
    medial, popliteal 355.4
    median NEC 354.1
    obturator 355.79
    oculomotor
      partial 378.51
      total 378.52
    olfactory 352.0
    optic 377.49
      hypoplasia 377.43
      ischemic 377.41
      nutritional 377.33
      toxic 377.34
    peroneal 355.3
    phrenic 354.8
    plantar 355.6
    pneumogastric 352.3
    posterior tibial 355.5
    radial 354.3
    recurrent laryngeal 352.3
    root 353.9
      specified NEC 353.8
    saphenous 355.79
    sciatic NEC 355.0
    specified NEC 355.9
      lower limb 355.79
      upper limb 354.8
    spinal 355.9
    sympathetic NEC 337.9
    trigeminal 350.9
      specified NEC 350.8
    trochlear 378.53
    ulnar 354.2
    upper limb NEC 354.9
    vagus 352.3
  nervous system NEC 349.9
    autonomic (peripheral) (see also
        Neuropathy, peripheral,
        autonomic) 337.9
    cranial 352.9
    parasympathetic (see also
        Neuropathy, peripheral,
        autonomic) 337.9
    specified type NEC 349.89
    sympathetic (see also Neuropathy,
        peripheral, autonomic) 337.9
    vegetative (see also Neuropathy,
        peripheral, autonomic) 337.9
  neurohypophysis NEC 253.6
  neurological NEC 781.99
    peripheral NEC 355.9
  neuromuscular NEC 358.9
    hereditary NEC 359.1
    specified NEC 358.8
    toxic 358.2
  neurotic 300.9
    specified type NEC 300.89
  neutrophil, polymorphonuclear
      (functional) 288.1
  nightmare 307.47
  night terror 307.46
  obsessive-compulsive 300.3
  oppositional defiant, childhood and
      adolescence 313.81

Disorder (Continued)
  optic
    chiasm 377.54
      associated with
        inflammatory disorders 377.54
        neoplasm NEC 377.52
          pituitary 377.51
        pituitary disorders 377.51
        vascular disorders 377.53
    nerve 377.49
    radiations 377.63
    tracts 377.63
  orbit 376.9
    specified NEC 376.89
  orgasmic
    female 302.73
    male 302.74
  overanxious, of childhood and
      adolescence 313.0
  oxidation, fatty acid 277.85
  pancreas, internal secretion (other than
      diabetes mellitus) 251.9
    specified type NEC 251.8
  panic 300.01
    with agoraphobia 300.21
  papillary muscle NEC 429.81
  paranoid 297.9
    induced 297.3
    shared 297.3
  parathyroid 252.9
    specified type NEC 252.8
  paroxysmal, mixed 780.39
  pentose phosphate pathway with
      anemia 282.2
  periodic limb movement 327.51
  peroxisomal 277.86
  personality 301.9
    affective 301.10
    aggressive 301.3
    amoral 301.7
    anancastic, anankastic 301.4
    antisocial 301.7
    asocial 301.7
    asthenic 301.6
    avoidant 301.82
    borderline 301.83
    compulsive 301.4
    cyclothymic 301.13
    dependent-passive 301.6
    dyssocial 301.7
    emotional instability 301.59
    epileptoid 301.3
    explosive 301.3
    following organic brain damage
        310.1
    histrionic 301.50
    hyperthymic 301.11
    hypomanic (chronic) 301.11
    hypothymic 301.12
    hysterical 301.50
    immature 301.89
    inadequate 301.6
    introverted 301.21
    labile 301.59
    moral deficiency 301.7
    narcissistic 301.81
    obsessional 301.4
    obsessive-compulsive 301.4
    overconscientious 301.4
    paranoid 301.0
    passive (-dependent) 301.6
    passive-aggressive 301.84
    pathological NEC 301.9
    pseudosocial 301.7

Disorder (Continued)
  personality (Continued)
    psychopathic 301.9
    schizoid 301.20
      introverted 301.21
      schizotypal 301.22
    schizotypal 301.22
    seductive 301.59
    type A 301.4
    unstable 301.59
  pervasive developmental 299.9●
    childhood-onset 299.8●
    specified NEC 299.8●
  phonological 315.39
  pigmentation, choroid (congenital)
    743.53
  pinna 380.30
    specified type NEC 380.39
  pituitary, thalamic 253.9
    anterior NEC 253.4
    iatrogenic 253.7
    postablative 253.7
    specified NEC 253.8
  pityriasis-like NEC 696.8
  platelets (blood) 287.1
  polymorphonuclear neutrophils
    (functional) 288.1
  porphyrin metabolism 277.1
  postmenopausal 627.9
    specified type NEC 627.8
  post-transplant lymphoproliferative
    (PTLD) 238.77
  post-traumatic stress (PTSD) 309.81
  posttraumatic stress 309.81
    acute 309.81
    brief 309.81
    chronic 309.81
  premenstrual dysphoric (PMDD)
    625.4
  psoriatic-like NEC 696.8
  psychic, with diseases classified
    elsewhere 316
  psychogenic NEC (see also condition)
    300.9
    allergic NEC
      respiratory 306.1
    anxiety 300.00
      atypical 300.00
      generalized 300.02
    appetite 307.59
    articulation, joint 306.0
    asthenic 300.5
    blood 306.8
    cardiovascular (system) 306.2
    compulsive 300.3
    cutaneous 306.3
    depressive 300.4
    digestive (system) 306.4
    dysmenorrheic 306.52
    dyspneic 306.1
    eczematous 306.3
    endocrine (system) 306.6
    eye 306.7
    feeding 307.59
    functional NEC 306.9
    gastric 306.4
    gastrointestinal (system) 306.4
    genitourinary (system) 306.50
    heart (function) (rhythm) 306.2
    hemic 306.8
    hyperventilatory 306.1
    hypochondriacal 300.7
    hysterical 300.10
    intestinal 306.4

Disorder (Continued)
  psychogenic NEC (Continued)
    joint 306.0
    learning 315.2
    limb 306.0
    lymphatic (system) 306.8
    menstrual 306.52
    micturition 306.53
    monoplegic NEC 306.0
    motor 307.9
    muscle 306.0
    musculoskeletal 306.0
    neurocirculatory 306.2
    obsessive 300.3
    occupational 300.89
    organ or part of body NEC 306.9
    organs of special sense 306.7
    paralytic NEC 306.0
    phobic 300.20
    physical NEC 306.9
    pruritic 306.3
    rectal 306.4
    respiratory (system) 306.1
    rheumatic 306.0
    sexual (function) 302.70
      specified type NEC 302.79
    sexual orientation conflict 302.0
    skin (allergic) (eczematous)
      (pruritic) 306.3
    sleep 307.40
      initiation or maintenance 307.41
        persistent 307.42
        transient 307.41
      movement 780.58
      sleep terror 307.46
      specified type NEC 307.49
    specified part of body NEC 306.8
    stomach 306.4
  psychomotor NEC 307.9
    hysterical 300.11
  psychoneurotic (see also Neurosis) 300.9
    mixed NEC 300.89
  psychophysiologic (see also Disorder,
    psychosomatic) 306.9
  psychosexual identity (childhood)
    302.6
    adult-life 302.85
  psychosomatic NEC 306.9
    allergic NEC
      respiratory 306.1
    articulation, joint 306.0
    cardiovascular (system) 306.2
    cutaneous 306.3
    digestive (system) 306.4
    dysmenorrheic 306.52
    dyspneic 306.1
    endocrine (system) 306.6
    eye 306.7
    gastric 306.4
    gastrointestinal (system) 306.4
    genitourinary (system) 306.50
    heart (functional) (rhythm) 306.2
    hyperventilatory 306.1
    intestinal 306.4
    joint 306.0
    limb 306.0
    lymphatic (system) 306.8
    menstrual 306.52
    micturition 306.53
    monoplegic NEC 306.0
    muscle 306.0
    musculoskeletal 306.0
    neurocirculatory 306.2
    organs of special sense 306.7

Disorder (Continued)
  psychosomatic NEC (Continued)
    paralytic NEC 306.0
    pruritic 306.3
    rectal 306.4
    respiratory (system) 306.1
    rheumatic 306.0
    sexual (function) 302.70
      specified type NEC 302.79
    skin 306.3
    specified part of body NEC 306.8
    stomach 306.4
  psychotic (see also Psychosis) 298.9
    brief 298.8
  purine metabolism NEC 277.2
  pyrimidine metabolism NEC 277.2
  reactive attachment of infancy or early
    childhood 313.89
  reading, developmental 315.00
  reflex 796.1
  REM sleep behavior 327.42
  renal function, impaired 588.9
    specified type NEC 588.89
  renal transport NEC 588.89
  respiration, respiratory NEC 519.9
    due to
      aspiration of liquids or solids
        508.9
      inhalation of fumes or vapors
        506.9
    psychogenic 306.1
  retina 362.9
    specified type NEC 362.89
  rumination 307.53
  sacroiliac joint NEC 724.6
  sacrum 724.6
  schizo-affective (see also Schizophrenia)
    295.7●
  schizoid, childhood or adolescence
    313.22
  schizophreniform 295.4●
  schizotypal personality 301.22
  secretion, thyrocalcitonin 246.0
  seizure 345.9●
    recurrent 345.9●
    epileptic - see Epilepsy
  semantic pragmatic 315.39
    with autism 299.0●
  sense of smell 781.1
    psychogenic 306.7
  separation anxiety 309.21
  sexual (see also Deviation, sexual) 302.9
    aversion 302.79
    desire, hypoactive 302.71
    function, psychogenic 302.70
  shyness, of childhood and adolescence
    313.21
  single complement (C_1–C_9) 279.8
  skin NEC 709.9
    fetus or newborn 778.9
      specified type 778.8
    psychogenic (allergic) (eczematous)
      (pruritic) 306.3
    specified type NEC 709.8
    vascular 709.1
  sleep 780.50
    with apnea - see Apnea, sleep
    alcohol induced 291.82
    arousal 307.46
      confusional 327.41
    circadian rhythm 327.30
      advanced sleep phase type 327.32
      alcohol induced 291.82
      delayed sleep phase type 327.31

◀ New   ◀━ Revised   ~~deleted~~ Deleted   ● Use Additional Digit(s)   ▨ Omit code

Disorder (Continued)
  sleep (Continued)
    circadian rhythm (Continued)
      drug induced 292.85
      free running type 327.34
      in conditions classified elsewhere 327.37
      irregular sleep-wake type 327.33
      jet lag type 327.35
      other 327.39
      shift work type 327.36
    drug induced 292.85
    initiation or maintenance (see also Insomnia) 780.52
    nonorganic origin (transient) 307.41
      persistent 307.42
    nonorganic origin 307.40
      specified type NEC 307.49
    organic specified type NEC 327.8
    periodic limb movement 327.51
    specified NEC 780.59
    wake
      cycle - see Disorder, sleep, circadian rhythm
      schedule - see Disorder, sleep, circadian rhythm
  social, of childhood and adolescence 313.22
  soft tissue 729.90
    specified type NEC 729.99
  somatization 300.81
  somatoform (atypical) (undifferentiated) 300.82
    severe 300.81
    specified type NEC 300.89
  speech NEC 784.59 ◀▥
    nonorganic origin 307.9
  spine NEC 724.9
    ligamentous or muscular attachments, peripheral 720.1
  steroid metabolism NEC 255.2
  stomach (functional) (see also Disorder, gastric) 536.9
    psychogenic 306.4
  storage, iron 275.0
  stress (see also Reaction, stress, acute) 308.3
    posttraumatic
      acute 309.81
      brief 309.81
      chronic (motor or vocal) 309.81
  substitution 300.11
  suspected - see Observation
  synovium 727.9
  temperature regulation, fetus or newborn 778.4
  temporomandibular joint NEC 524.60
    sounds on opening or closing 524.64
    specified NEC 524.69
  tendon 727.9
    shoulder region 726.10
  thoracic root (nerve) NEC 353.3
  thyrocalcitonin secretion 246.0
  thyroid (gland) NEC 246.9
    specified type NEC 246.8
  tic 307.20
    chronic (motor or vocal) 307.22
    motor-verbal 307.23
    organic origin 333.1
    transient (of childhood) 307.21

Disorder (Continued)
  tooth NEC 525.9
    development NEC 520.9
      specified type NEC 520.8
    eruption 520.6
    specified type NEC 525.8
  Tourette's 307.23
  transport, carbohydrate 271.9
    specified type NEC 271.8
  tubular, phosphate-losing 588.0
  tympanic membrane 384.9
  unaggressive, unsocialized (see also Disturbance, conduct) 312.1●
  undersocialized, unsocialized (see also Disturbance, conduct)
    aggressive (type) 312.0●
    unaggressive (type) 312.1●
  vision, visual NEC 368.9
    binocular NEC 368.30
    cortex 377.73
      associated with
        inflammatory disorders 377.73
        neoplasms 377.71
        vascular disorders 377.72
    pathway NEC 377.63
      associated with
        inflammatory disorders 377.63
        neoplasms 377.61
        vascular disorders 377.62
  vocal tic
    chronic 307.22
  wakefulness (see also Hypersomnia) 780.54
    nonorganic origin (transient) 307.43
    persistent 307.44
  written expression 315.2
Disorganized globe 360.29
Displacement, displaced

> **Note 24** For acquired displacement of bones, cartilage, joints, tendons, due to injury, see also Dislocation.
>
> Displacements at ages under one year should be considered congenital, provided there is no indication the condition was acquired after birth.

  acquired traumatic of bone, cartilage, joint, tendon NEC (without fracture) (see also Dislocation) 839.8
    with fracture - see Fracture, by site
  adrenal gland (congenital) 759.1
  alveolus and teeth, vertical 524.75
  appendix, retrocecal (congenital) 751.5
  auricle (congenital) 744.29
  bladder (acquired) 596.8
    congenital 753.8
  brachial plexus (congenital) 742.8
  brain stem, caudal 742.4
  canaliculus lacrimalis 743.65
  cardia, through esophageal hiatus 750.6
  cerebellum, caudal 742.4
  cervix - see Displacement, uterus
  colon (congenital) 751.4
  device, implant, or graft - see Complications, mechanical
  epithelium
    columnar of cervix 622.10
    cuboidal, beyond limits of external os (uterus) 752.49
  esophageal mucosa into cardia of stomach, congenital 750.4

Displacement, displaced (Continued)
  esophagus (acquired) 530.89
    congenital 750.4
  eyeball (acquired) (old) 376.36
    congenital 743.8
    current injury 871.3
    lateral 376.36
  fallopian tube (acquired) 620.4
    congenital 752.19
    opening (congenital) 752.19
  gallbladder (congenital) 751.69
  gastric mucosa 750.7
    into
      duodenum 750.7
      esophagus 750.7
      Meckel's diverticulum, congenital 750.7
  globe (acquired) (lateral) (old) 376.36
    current injury 871.3
  graft
    artificial skin graft 996.55
    decellularized allodermis graft 996.55
  heart (congenital) 746.87
    acquired 429.89
  hymen (congenital) (upward) 752.49
  internal prosthesis NEC - see Complications, mechanical
  intervertebral disc (with neuritis, radiculitis, sciatica, or other pain) 722.2
    with myelopathy 722.70
    cervical, cervicodorsal, cervicothoracic 722.0
      with myelopathy 722.71
      due to major trauma - see Dislocation, vertebra, cervical
    due to trauma - see Dislocation, vertebra
    lumbar, lumbosacral 722.10
      with myelopathy 722.73
      due to major trauma - see Dislocation, vertebra, lumbar
    thoracic, thoracolumbar 722.11
      with myelopathy 722.72
      due to major trauma - see Dislocation, vertebra, thoracic
  intrauterine device 996.32
  kidney (acquired) 593.0
    congenital 753.3
  lacrimal apparatus or duct (congenital) 743.65
  macula (congenital) 743.55
  Meckel's diverticulum (congenital) 751.0
  nail (congenital) 757.5
    acquired 703.8
  opening of Wharton's duct in mouth 750.26
  organ or site, congenital NEC - see Malposition, congenital
  ovary (acquired) 620.4
    congenital 752.0
    free in peritoneal cavity (congenital) 752.0
    into hernial sac 620.4
  oviduct (acquired) 620.4
    congenital 752.19
  parathyroid (gland) 252.8
  parotid gland (congenital) 750.26
  punctum lacrimale (congenital) 743.65

Displacement, displaced *(Continued)*
  sacroiliac (congenital) (joint) 755.69
    current injury - *see* Dislocation,
      sacroiliac
    old 724.6
  spine (congenital) 756.19
  spleen, congenital 759.0
  stomach (congenital) 750.7
    acquired 537.89
  subglenoid (closed) 831.01
  sublingual duct (congenital) 750.26
  teeth, tooth 524.30
    horizontal 524.33
    vertical 524.34
  tongue (congenital) (downward)
    750.19
  trachea (congenital) 748.3
  ureter or ureteric opening or orifice
    (congenital) 753.4
  uterine opening of oviducts or
    fallopian tubes 752.19
  uterus, uterine (*see also* Malposition,
    uterus) 621.6
    congenital 752.3
  ventricular septum 746.89
    with rudimentary ventricle 746.89
  xyphoid bone (process) 738.3
Disproportion 653.9●
  affecting fetus or newborn 763.1
  breast, reconstructed 612.1
    between native and reconstructed
      612.1
  caused by
    conjoined twins 678.1●
    contraction, pelvis (general) 653.1●
      inlet 653.2●
      midpelvic 653.8●
      midplane 653.8●
      outlet 653.3●
    fetal
      ascites 653.7●
      hydrocephalus 653.6●
      hydrops 653.7●
      meningomyelocele 653.7●
      sacral teratoma 653.7●
      tumor 653.7●
    hydrocephalic fetus 653.6●
    pelvis, pelvic, abnormality (bony)
      NEC 653.0●
    unusually large fetus 653.5●
  causing obstructed labor 660.1●
  cephalopelvic, normally formed fetus
    653.4●
    causing obstructed labor 660.1●
  fetal NEC 653.5●
    causing obstructed labor 660.1●
  fetopelvic, normally formed fetus
    653.4●
    causing obstructed labor 660.1●
  mixed maternal and fetal origin,
    normally, formed fetus 653.4●
  pelvis, pelvic (bony) NEC 653.1●
    causing obstructed labor 660.1●
  specified type NEC 653.8●
Disruption
  cesarean wound 674.1●
  family V61.09
    due to
      child in
        care of non-parental family
          member V61.06
        foster care V61.06
        welfare custody V61.05
      death of family member V61.07 ◀
      divorce V61.03

Disruption *(Continued)*
  family *(Continued)*
    due to *(Continued)*
      estrangement V61.09
        parent-child V61.04
      extended absence of family
        member NEC V61.08 ◀
      family member
        on military deployment V61.01
        return from military
          deployment V61.02
      legal separation V61.03
  gastrointestinal anastomosis 997.4
  ligament(s) - *see also* Sprain
    knee
      current injury - *see* Dislocation,
        knee
      old 717.89
        capsular 717.85
        collateral (medial) 717.82
          lateral 717.81
        cruciate (posterior) 717.84
          anterior 717.83
        specified site NEC 717.85
  marital V61.10
    involving
      divorce V61.03
      estrangement V61.09
  operation wound (external) (*see also*
    Dehiscence) 998.32
    internal 998.31
  organ transplant, anastomosis site - *see*
    Complications, transplant, organ,
    by site
  ossicles, ossicular chain 385.23
    traumatic - *see* Fracture, skull, base
  parenchyma
    liver (hepatic) - *see* Laceration, liver,
      major
    spleen - *see* Laceration, spleen,
      parenchyma, massive
  phase-shift, of 24 hour sleep-wake
    cycle, unspecified 780.55
    nonorganic origin 307.45
  sleep-wake cycle (24 hour), unspecified
    780.55
    circadian rhythm 327.33
    nonorganic origin 307.45
  suture line (external) (*see also*
    Dehiscence) 998.32
    internal 998.31
  wound 998.30
    cesarean operation 674.1●
    episiotomy 674.2●
    operation (surgical) 998.32
      cesarean 674.1●
      internal 998.31
    perineal (obstetric) 674.2●
    uterine 674.1●
Disruptio uteri - *see also* Rupture, uterus
  complicating delivery - *see* Delivery,
    complicated, rupture, uterus
Dissatisfaction with
  employment V62.29
  school environment V62.3
Dissecting - *see* condition
Dissection
  aorta 441.00
    abdominal 441.02
    thoracic 441.01
    thoracoabdominal 441.03
  artery, arterial
    carotid 443.21
    coronary 414.12
    iliac 443.22

Dissection *(Continued)*
  artery, arterial *(Continued)*
    renal 443.23
    specified NEC 443.29
    vertebral 443.24
  vascular 459.9
  wound - *see* Wound, open, by site
Disseminated - *see* condition
Dissociated personality NEC 300.15
Dissociation
  auriculoventricular or atrioventricular
    (any degree) (AV) 426.89
    with heart block 426.0
  interference 426.89
  isorhythmic 426.89
  rhythm
    atrioventricular (AV) 426.89
    interference 426.89
Dissociative
  identity disorder 300.14
  reaction NEC 300.15
Dissolution, vertebra (*see also*
  Osteoporosis) 733.00
Distention
  abdomen (gaseous) 787.3
  bladder 596.8
  cecum 569.89
  colon 569.89
  gallbladder 575.8
  gaseous (abdomen) 787.3
  intestine 569.89
  kidney 593.89
  liver 573.9
  seminal vesicle 608.89
  stomach 536.8
    acute 536.1
    psychogenic 306.4
  ureter 593.5
  uterus 621.8
Distichia, distichiasis (eyelid) 743.63
Distoma hepaticum infestation 121.3
Distomiasis 121.9
  bile passages 121.3
    due to Clonorchis sinensis 121.1
  hemic 120.9
  hepatic (liver) 121.3
    due to Clonorchis sinensis
      (clonorchiasis) 121.1
  intestinal 121.4
  liver 121.3
    due to Clonorchis sinensis 121.1
  lung 121.2
  pulmonary 121.2
Distomolar (fourth molar) 520.1
  causing crowding 524.31
Disto-occlusion (division I) (division II)
  524.22
Distortion (congenital)
  adrenal (gland) 759.1
  ankle (joint) 755.69
  anus 751.5
  aorta 747.29
  appendix 751.5
  arm 755.59
  artery (peripheral) NEC (*see also*
    Distortion, peripheral vascular
    system) 747.60
    cerebral 747.81
    coronary 746.85
    pulmonary 747.3
    retinal 743.58
    umbilical 747.5
  auditory canal 744.29
    causing impairment of hearing
      744.02

◀ New   ◀▥ Revised   ~~deleted~~ Deleted   ● Use Additional Digit(s)   ▨ Omit code

Distortion (Continued)
  bile duct or passage 751.69
  bladder 753.8
  brain 742.4
  bronchus 748.3
  cecum 751.5
  cervix (uteri) 752.49
  chest (wall) 756.3
  clavicle 755.51
  clitoris 752.49
  coccyx 756.19
  colon 751.5
  common duct 751.69
  cornea 743.41
  cricoid cartilage 748.3
  cystic duct 751.69
  duodenum 751.5
  ear 744.29
    auricle 744.29
      causing impairment of hearing
          744.02
    causing impairment of hearing
        744.09
    external 744.29
      causing impairment of hearing
          744.02
    inner 744.05
    middle, except ossicles 744.03
      ossicles 744.04
    ossicles 744.04
  endocrine (gland) NEC 759.2
  epiglottis 748.3
  Eustachian tube 744.24
  eye 743.8
    adnexa 743.69
  face bone(s) 756.0
  fallopian tube 752.19
  femur 755.69
  fibula 755.69
  finger(s) 755.59
  foot 755.67
  gallbladder 751.69
  genitalia, genital organ(s)
    female 752.89
      external 752.49
      internal NEC 752.89
    male 752.89
      penis 752.69
  glottis 748.3
  gyri 742.4
  hand bone(s) 755.59
  heart (auricle) (ventricle) 746.89
    valve (cusp) 746.89
  hepatic duct 751.69
  humerus 755.59
  hymen 752.49
  ileum 751.5
  intestine (large) (small) 751.5
    with anomalous adhesions, fixation
        or malrotation 751.4
  jaw NEC 524.89
  jejunum 751.5
  kidney 753.3
  knee (joint) 755.64
  labium (majus) (minus) 752.49
  larynx 748.3
  leg 755.69
  lens 743.36
  liver 751.69
  lumbar spine 756.19
    with disproportion (fetopelvic)
        653.0●
      affecting fetus or newborn
          763.1
      causing obstructed labor 660.1●

Distortion (Continued)
  lumbosacral (joint) (region) 756.19
  lung (fissures) (lobe) 748.69
  nerve 742.8
  nose 748.1
  organ
    of Corti 744.05
    of site not listed - see Anomaly,
        specified type NEC
  ossicles, ear 744.04
  ovary 752.0
  oviduct 752.19
  pancreas 751.7
  parathyroid (gland) 759.2
  patella 755.64
  peripheral vascular system NEC
      747.60
    gastrointestinal 747.61
    lower limb 747.64
    renal 747.62
    spinal 747.82
    upper limb 747.63
  pituitary (gland) 759.2
  radius 755.59
  rectum 751.5
  rib 756.3
  sacroiliac joint 755.69
  sacrum 756.19
  scapula 755.59
  shoulder girdle 755.59
  site not listed - see Anomaly, specified
      type NEC
  skull bone(s) 756.0
    with
      anencephalus 740.0
      encephalocele 742.0
      hydrocephalus 742.3
        with spina bifida (see also
            Spina bifida) 741.0●
      microcephalus 742.1
  spinal cord 742.59
  spine 756.19
  spleen 759.0
  sternum 756.3
  thorax (wall) 756.3
  thymus (gland) 759.2
  thyroid (gland) 759.2
    cartilage 748.3
  tibia 755.69
  toe(s) 755.66
  tongue 750.19
  trachea (cartilage) 748.3
  ulna 755.59
  ureter 753.4
    causing obstruction 753.20
  urethra 753.8
    causing obstruction 753.6
  uterus 752.3
  vagina 752.49
  vein (peripheral) NEC (see also
      Distortion, peripheral vascular
      system) 747.60
    great 747.49
    portal 747.49
    pulmonary 747.49
  vena cava (inferior) (superior)
      747.49
  vertebra 756.19
  visual NEC 368.15
    shape or size 368.14
  vulva 752.49
  wrist (bones) (joint) 755.59
Distress
  abdomen 789.0●
  colon 564.9

Distress (Continued)
  emotional V40.9
  epigastric 789.0●
  fetal (syndrome) 768.4
    affecting management of
        pregnancy or childbirth
        656.8●
    liveborn infant 768.4
      first noted
        before onset of labor 768.2
        during labor and delivery
            768.3
    stillborn infant (death before onset
        of labor) 768.0
      death during labor 768.1
  gastrointestinal (functional) 536.9
    psychogenic 306.4
  intestinal (functional) NEC 564.9
    psychogenic 306.4
  intrauterine - see Distress, fetal
  leg 729.5
  maternal 669.0●
  mental V40.9
  respiratory 786.09
    acute (adult) 518.82
    adult syndrome (following
        shock, surgery, or trauma)
        518.5
      specified NEC 518.82
    fetus or newborn 770.89
    syndrome (idiopathic) (newborn)
        769
  stomach 536.9
    psychogenic 306.4
Distribution vessel, atypical NEC
    747.60
  coronary artery 746.85
  spinal 747.82
Districhiasis 704.2
Disturbance - see also Disease
  absorption NEC 579.9
    calcium 269.3
    carbohydrate 579.8
    fat 579.8
    protein 579.8
    specified type NEC 579.8
    vitamin (see also Deficiency,
        vitamin) 269.2
  acid-base equilibrium 276.9
  activity and attention, simple, with
      hyperkinesis 314.01
  amino acid (metabolic) (see also
      Disorder, amino acid) 270.9
    imidazole 270.5
    maple syrup (urine) disease
        270.3
    transport 270.0
  assimilation, food 579.9
  attention, simple 314.00
    with hyperactivity 314.01
  auditory, nerve, except deafness
      388.5
  behavior (see also Disturbance, conduct)
      312.9
  blood clotting (hypoproteinemia)
      (mechanism) (see also Defect,
      coagulation) 286.9
  central nervous system NEC
      349.9
  cerebral nerve NEC 352.9
  circulatory 459.9
  conduct 312.9
    adjustment reaction 309.3
    adolescent onset type 312.82

Disturbance (Continued)
  conduct (Continued)
    childhood onset type 312.81

> Note 25 Use the following fifth-digit subclassification with categories 312.0–312.2:
>
> 0   unspecified
> 1   mild
> 2   moderate
> 3   severe

    compulsive 312.30
      intermittent explosive disorder 312.34
      isolated explosive disorder 312.35
      kleptomania 312.32
      pathological gambling 312.31
      pyromania 312.33
    hyperkinetic 314.2
    intermittent explosive 312.34
    isolated explosive 312.35
    mixed with emotions 312.4
    socialized (type) 312.20
      aggressive 312.23
      unaggressive 312.21
    specified type NEC 312.89
    undersocialized, unsocialized
      aggressive (type) 312.0●
      unaggressive (type) 312.1●
  coordination 781.3
  cranial nerve NEC 352.9
  deep sensibility - see Disturbance, sensation
  digestive 536.9
    psychogenic 306.4
  electrolyte - see Imbalance, electrolyte
  emotions specific to childhood or adolescence 313.9
    with
      academic underachievement 313.83
      anxiety and fearfulness 313.0
      elective mutism 313.23
      identity disorder 313.82
      jealousy 313.3
      misery and unhappiness 313.1
      oppositional defiant disorder 313.81
      overanxiousness 313.0
      sensitivity 313.21
      shyness 313.21
      social withdrawal 313.22
      withdrawal reaction 313.22
    involving relationship problems 313.3
    mixed 313.89
    specified type NEC 313.89
  endocrine (gland) 259.9
    neonatal, transitory 775.9
      specified NEC 775.89
  equilibrium 780.4
  feeding (elderly) (infant) 783.3
    newborn 779.31
    nonorganic origin NEC 307.59
    psychogenic NEC 307.59
  fructose metabolism 271.2
  gait 781.2
    hysterical 300.11
  gastric (functional) 536.9
    motility 536.8
    psychogenic 306.4
    secretion 536.8

Disturbance (Continued)
  gastrointestinal (functional) 536.9
    psychogenic 306.4
  habit, child 307.9
  hearing, except deafness 388.40
  heart, functional (conditions classifiable to 426, 427, 428)
    due to presence of (cardiac) prosthesis 429.4
    postoperative (immediate) 997.1
      long-term effect of cardiac surgery 429.4
    psychogenic 306.2
  hormone 259.9
  innervation uterus, sympathetic, parasympathetic 621.8
  keratinization NEC
    gingiva 523.10
    lip 528.5
    oral (mucosa) (soft tissue) 528.79
      residual ridge mucosa
        excessive 528.72
        minimal 528.71
    tongue 528.79
  labyrinth, labyrinthine (vestibule) 386.9
  learning, specific NEC 315.2
  memory (see also Amnesia) 780.93
    mild, following organic brain damage 310.8
  mental (see also Disorder, mental) 300.9
    associated with diseases classified elsewhere 316
  metabolism (acquired) (congenital) (see also Disorder, metabolism) 277.9
    with
      abortion - see Abortion, by type, with metabolic disorder
      ectopic pregnancy (see also categories 633.0–633.9) 639.4
      molar pregnancy (see also categories 630–632) 639.4
    amino acid (see also Disorder, amino acid) 270.9
      aromatic NEC 270.2
      branched-chain 270.3
      specified type NEC 270.8
      straight-chain NEC 270.7
      sulfur-bearing 270.4
      transport 270.0
    ammonia 270.6
    arginine 270.6
    argininosuccinic acid 270.6
    carbohydrate NEC 271.9
    cholesterol 272.9
    citrulline 270.6
    cystathionine 270.4
    fat 272.9
    following
      abortion 639.4
      ectopic or molar pregnancy 639.4
    general 277.9
      carbohydrate 271.9
      iron 275.0
      phosphate 275.3
      sodium 276.9
    glutamine 270.7
    glycine 270.7
    histidine 270.5
    homocystine 270.4
    in labor or delivery 669.0●
    iron 275.0
    isoleucine 270.3

Disturbance (Continued)
  metabolism (Continued)
    leucine 270.3
    lipoid 272.9
      specified type NEC 272.8
    lysine 270.7
    methionine 270.4
    neonatal, transitory 775.9
      specified type NEC 775.89
    nitrogen 788.99
    ornithine 270.6
    phosphate 275.3
    phosphatides 272.7
    serine 270.7
    sodium NEC 276.9
    threonine 270.7
    tryptophan 270.2
    tyrosine 270.2
    urea cycle 270.6
    valine 270.3
  motor 796.1
  nervous functional 799.21
  neuromuscular mechanism (eye) due to syphilis 094.84
  nutritional 269.9
    nail 703.8
  ocular motion 378.87
    psychogenic 306.7
  oculogyric 378.87
    psychogenic 306.7
  oculomotor NEC 378.87
    psychogenic 306.7
  olfactory nerve 781.1
  optic nerve NEC 377.49
  oral epithelium, including tongue 528.79
    residual ridge mucosa
      excessive 528.72
      minimal 528.71
  personality (pattern) (trait) (see also Disorder, personality) 301.9
    following organic brain damage 310.1
  polyglandular 258.9
  psychomotor 307.9
  pupillary 379.49
  reflex 796.1
  rhythm, heart 427.9
    postoperative (immediate) 997.1
      long-term effect of cardiac surgery 429.4
    psychogenic 306.2
  salivary secretion 527.7
  sensation (cold) (heat) (localization) (tactile discrimination localization) (texture) (vibratory) NEC 782.0
    hysterical 300.11
    skin 782.0
    smell 781.1
    taste 781.1
  sensory (see also Disturbance, sensation) 782.0
    innervation 782.0
  situational (transient) (see also Reaction, adjustment) 309.9
    acute 308.3
  sleep 780.50
    with apnea - see Apnea, sleep
    initiation or maintenance (see also Insomnia) 780.52
      nonorganic origin 307.41
    nonorganic origin 307.40
      specified type NEC 307.49

Disturbance *(Continued)*
  sleep *(Continued)*
    specified NEC 780.59
      nonorganic origin 307.49
    wakefulness *(see also* Hypersomnia)
      780.54
      nonorganic origin 307.43
  sociopathic 301.7
  speech NEC 784.59 ◀▥
    developmental 315.39
      associated with hyperkinesis
        314.1
    secondary to organic lesion 784.59 ◀▥
  stomach (functional) *(see also*
    Disturbance, gastric) 536.9
  sympathetic (nerve) *(see also*
    Neuropathy, peripheral,
    autonomic) 337.9
  temperature sense 782.0
    hysterical 300.11
  tooth
    eruption 520.6
    formation 520.4
    structure, hereditary NEC 520.5
  touch *(see also* Disturbance, sensation)
    782.0
  vascular 459.9
    arteriosclerotic - *see* Arteriosclerosis
  vasomotor 443.9
  vasospastic 443.9
  vestibular labyrinth 386.9
  vision, visual NEC 368.9
    psychophysical 368.16
    specified NEC 368.8
    subjective 368.10
  voice and resonance 784.40 ◀▥
  wakefulness (initiation or
    maintenance) *(see also*
    Hypersomnia) 780.54
    nonorganic origin 307.43
Disulfiduria, beta-mercaptolactate-
  cysteine 270.0
Disuse atrophy, bone 733.7
Ditthomska syndrome 307.81
Diuresis 788.42
Divers'
  palsy or paralysis 993.3
  squeeze 993.3
Diverticula, diverticulosis, diverticulum
  (acute) (multiple) (perforated)
  (ruptured) 562.10
  with diverticulitis 562.11
  aorta (Kommerell's) 747.21
  appendix (noninflammatory) 543.9
  bladder (acquired) (sphincter) 596.3
    congenital 753.8
  broad ligament 620.8
  bronchus (congenital) 748.3
    acquired 494.0
      with acute exacerbation 494.1
  calyx, calyceal (kidney) 593.89
  cardia (stomach) 537.1
  cecum 562.10
    with
      diverticulitis 562.11
        with hemorrhage 562.13
      hemorrhage 562.12
    congenital 751.5
  colon (acquired) 562.10
    with
      diverticulitis 562.11
        with hemorrhage 562.13
      hemorrhage 562.12
    congenital 751.5

Diverticula, diverticulosis,
  diverticulum *(Continued)*
  duodenum 562.00
    with
      diverticulitis 562.01
        with hemorrhage 562.03
      hemorrhage 562.02
    congenital 751.5
  epiphrenic (esophagus) 530.6
  esophagus (congenital) 750.4
    acquired 530.6
    epiphrenic 530.6
    pulsion 530.6
    traction 530.6
    Zenker's 530.6
  Eustachian tube 381.89
  fallopian tube 620.8
  gallbladder (congenital) 751.69
  gastric 537.1
  heart (congenital) 746.89
  ileum 562.00
    with
      diverticulitis 562.01
        with hemorrhage 562.03
      hemorrhage 562.03
  intestine (large) 562.10
    with
      diverticulitis 562.11
        with hemorrhage 562.13
      hemorrhage 562.12
    congenital 751.5
    small 562.00
      with
        diverticulitis 562.01
          with hemorrhage 562.03
        hemorrhage 562.02
      congenital 751.5
  jejunum 562.00
    with
      diverticulitis 562.01
        with hemorrhage 562.03
      hemorrhage 562.02
  kidney (calyx) (pelvis) 593.89
    with calculus 592.0
  Kommerell's 747.21
  laryngeal ventricle (congenital)
    748.3
  Meckel's (displaced) (hypertrophic)
    751.0
  midthoracic 530.6
  organ or site, congenital NEC - *see*
    Distortion
  pericardium (congenital) (cyst)
    746.89
    acquired (true) 423.8
  pharyngoesophageal (pulsion)
    530.6
  pharynx (congenital) 750.27
  pulsion (esophagus) 530.6
  rectosigmoid 562.10
    with
      diverticulitis 562.11
        with hemorrhage 562.13
      hemorrhage 562.12
    congenital 751.5
  rectum 562.10
    with
      diverticulitis 562.11
        with hemorrhage 562.13
      hemorrhage 562.12
  renal (calyces) (pelvis) 593.89
    with calculus 592.0
  Rokitansky's 530.6
  seminal vesicle 608.0

Diverticula, diverticulosis,
  diverticulum *(Continued)*
  sigmoid 562.10
    with
      diverticulitis 562.11
        with hemorrhage 562.13
      hemorrhage 562.12
    congenital 751.5
  small intestine 562.00
    with
      diverticulitis 562.01
        with hemorrhage 562.03
      hemorrhage 562.02
  stomach (cardia) (juxtacardia)
    (juxtapyloric) (acquired) 537.1
    congenital 750.7
  subdiaphragmatic 530.6
  trachea (congenital) 748.3
    acquired 519.19
  traction (esophagus) 530.6
  ureter (acquired) 593.89
    congenital 753.4
  ureterovesical orifice 593.89
  urethra (acquired) 599.2
    congenital 753.8
  ventricle, left (congenital) 746.89
  vesical (urinary) 596.3
    congenital 753.8
  Zenker's (esophagus) 530.6
Diverticulitis (acute) *(see also* Diverticula)
  562.11
  with hemorrhage 562.13
  bladder (urinary) 596.3
  cecum (perforated) 562.11
    with hemorrhage 562.13
  colon (perforated) 562.11
    with hemorrhage 562.13
  duodenum 562.01
    with hemorrhage 562.03
  esophagus 530.6
  ileum (perforated) 562.01
    with hemorrhage 562.03
  intestine (large) (perforated) 562.11
    with hemorrhage 562.13
    small 562.01
      with hemorrhage 562.03
  jejunum (perforated) 562.01
    with hemorrhage 562.03
  Meckel's (perforated) 751.0
  pharyngoesophageal 530.6
  rectosigmoid (perforated) 562.11
    with hemorrhage 562.13
  rectum 562.11
    with hemorrhage 562.13
  sigmoid (old) (perforated) 562.11
    with hemorrhage 562.13
  small intestine (perforated) 562.01
    with hemorrhage 562.03
  vesical (urinary) 596.3
Diverticulosis - *see* Diverticula
Division
  cervix uteri 622.8
    external os into two openings by
      frenum 752.49
    external (cervical) into two openings
      by frenum 752.49
  glans penis 752.69
  hymen 752.49
  labia minora (congenital) 752.49
  ligament (partial or complete)
    (current) - *see also* Sprain, by
    site
    with open wound - *see* Wound,
      open, by site

Division (*Continued*)
  muscle (partial or complete) (current) - *see also* Sprain, by site
    with open wound - *see* Wound, open, by site
  nerve - *see* Injury, nerve, by site
  penis glans 752.69
  spinal cord - *see* Injury, spinal, by site
  vein 459.9
    traumatic - *see* Injury, vascular, by site
Divorce V61.03
Dix-Hallpike neurolabyrinthitis 386.12
Dizziness 780.4
  hysterical 300.11
  psychogenic 306.9
Doan-Wiseman syndrome (primary splenic neutropenia) 289.53
Dog bite - *see* Wound, open, by site
Döhle-Heller aortitis 093.1
Döhle body-panmyelopathic syndrome 288.2
Dolichocephaly, dolichocephalus 754.0
Dolichocolon 751.5
Dolichostenomelia 759.82
Donohue's syndrome (leprechaunism) 259.8
Donor
  blood V59.01
    other blood components V59.09
    stem cells V59.02
    whole blood V59.01
  bone V59.2
    marrow V59.3
  cornea V59.5
  egg (oocyte) (ovum) V59.70
    over age 35 V59.73
      anonymous recipient V59.73
      designated recipient V59.74
    under age 35 V59.71
      anonymous recipient V59.71
      designated recipient V59.72
  heart V59.8
  kidney V59.4
  liver V59.6
  lung V59.8
  lymphocyte V59.8
  organ V59.9
    specified NEC V59.8
  potential, examination of V70.8
  skin V59.1
  specified organ or tissue NEC V59.8
  sperm V59.8
  stem cells V59.02
  tissue V59.9
    specified type NEC V59.8
Donovanosis (granuloma venereum) 099.2
DOPS (diffuse obstructive pulmonary syndrome) 496
Double
  albumin 273.8
  aortic arch 747.21
  auditory canal 744.29
  auricle (heart) 746.82
  bladder 753.8
  external (cervical) os 752.49
  kidney with double pelvis (renal) 753.3
  larynx 748.3
  meatus urinarius 753.8
  organ or site NEC - *see* Accessory

Double (*Continued*)
  orifice
    heart valve NEC 746.89
      pulmonary 746.09
  outlet, right ventricle 745.11
  pelvis (renal) with double ureter 753.4
  penis 752.69
  tongue 750.13
  ureter (one or both sides) 753.4
    with double pelvis (renal) 753.4
  urethra 753.8
  urinary meatus 753.8
  uterus (any degree) 752.2
    with doubling of cervix and vagina 752.2
    in pregnancy or childbirth 654.0●
      affecting fetus or newborn 763.89
  vagina 752.49
    with doubling of cervix and uterus 752.2
  vision 368.2
  vocal cords 748.3
  vulva 752.49
  whammy (syndrome) 360.81
Douglas' pouch, cul-de-sac - *see* condition
Down's disease or syndrome (mongolism) 758.0
Down-growth, epithelial (anterior chamber) 364.61
Dracontiasis 125.7
Dracunculiasis 125.7
Dracunculosis 125.7
Drainage
  abscess (spontaneous) - *see* Abscess
  anomalous pulmonary veins to hepatic veins or right atrium 747.41
  stump (amputation) (surgical) 997.62
  suprapubic, bladder 596.8
Dream state, hysterical 300.13
Drepanocytic anemia (*see also* Disease, sickle cell) 282.60
Dresbach's syndrome (elliptocytosis) 282.1
Dreschlera (infection) 118
  hawaiiensis 117.8
Dressler's syndrome (postmyocardial infarction) 411.0
Dribbling (post-void) 788.35
Drift, ulnar 736.09
Drinking (alcohol) - *see also* Alcoholism
  excessive, to excess NEC (*see also* Abuse, drugs, nondependent) 305.0●
    bouts, periodic 305.0●
    continual 303.9●
    episodic 305.0●
    habitual 303.9●
    periodic 305.0●
Drip, postnasal (chronic) 784.91
  due to:
    allergic rhinitis - *see* Rhinitis, allergic
    common cold 460
    gastroesophageal reflux - *see* Reflux, gastroesophageal
    nasopharyngitis - *see* Nasopharyngitis
    other known condition - *code to* condition
    sinusitis - *see* Sinusitis
Drivers' license examination V70.3
Droop
  Cooper's 611.81
  facial 781.94

Drop
  finger 736.29
  foot 736.79
  hematocrit (precipitous) 790.01
  hemoglobin 790.01 ◄
  toe 735.8
  wrist 736.05
Dropped
  dead 798.1
  heart beats 426.6
Dropsy, dropsical (*see also* Edema) 782.3
  abdomen 789.59
  amnion (*see also* Hydramnios) 657●
  brain - *see* Hydrocephalus
  cardiac (*see also* Failure, heart) 428.0
  cardiorenal (*see also* Hypertension, cardiorenal) 404.90
  chest 511.9
  fetus or newborn 778.0
    due to isoimmunization 773.3
  gangrenous (*see also* Gangrene) 785.4
  heart (*see also* Failure, heart) 428.0
  hepatic - *see* Cirrhosis, liver
  infantile - *see* Hydrops, fetalis
  kidney (*see also* Nephrosis) 581.9
  liver - *see* Cirrhosis, liver
  lung 514
  malarial (*see also* Malaria) 084.9
  neonatorum - *see* Hydrops, fetalis
  nephritic 581.9
  newborn - *see* Hydrops, fetalis
  nutritional 269.9
  ovary 620.8
  pericardium (*see also* Pericarditis) 423.9
  renal (*see also* Nephrosis) 581.9
  uremic - *see* Uremia
Drowned, drowning (near) 994.1
  lung 518.5
Drowsiness 780.09
Drug - *see also* condition
  addiction (*see also* Dependence) 304.9●
  adverse effect NEC, correct substance properly administered 995.20
  allergy 995.27
  dependence (*see also* Dependence) 304.9●
  habit (*see also* Dependence) 304.9●
  hypersensitivity 995.27
  induced
    circadian rhythm sleep disorder 292.85
    hypersomnia 292.85
    insomnia 292.85
    mental disorder 292.9
      anxiety 292.89
      mood 292.84
      sexual 292.89
      sleep 292.85
      specified type 292.89
    parasomnia 292.85
    persisting
      amnestic disorder 292.83
      dementia 292.82
    psychotic disorder
      with
        delusions 292.11
        hallucinations 292.12
    sleep disorder 292.85
  intoxication 292.89
  overdose - *see* Table of Drugs and Chemicals
  poisoning - *see* Table of Drugs and Chemicals

◄ New   ◄ Revised   ~~deleted~~ Deleted   ● Use Additional Digit(s)   ▭ Omit code

Drug (Continued)
  therapy (maintenance) status NEC
    chemotherapy, antineoplastic
      V58.11
    immunotherapy, antineoplastic
      V58.12
    long-term (current) use V58.69
      antibiotics V58.62
      anticoagulants V58.61
      anti-inflammatories, non-
        steroidal (NSAID) V58.64
      antiplatelets V58.63
      antithrombotics V58.63
      aspirin V58.66
      high-risk medications NEC
        V58.69
      insulin V58.67
      methadone V58.69
      opiate analgesic V58.69
      steroids V58.65
  wrong substance given or taken in
    error - see Table of Drugs and
    Chemicals
Drunkenness (see also Abuse, drugs,
  nondependent) 305.0●
  acute in alcoholism (see also
    Alcoholism) 303.0●
  chronic (see also Alcoholism) 303.9●
  pathologic 291.4
  simple (acute) 305.0●
    in alcoholism 303.0●
  sleep 307.47
Drusen
  optic disc or papilla 377.21
  retina (colloid) (hyaloid degeneration)
    362.57
    hereditary 362.77
Drusenfieber 075
Dry, dryness - see also condition
  eye 375.15
    syndrome 375.15
  larynx 478.79
  mouth 527.7
  nose 478.19
  skin syndrome 701.1
  socket (teeth) 526.5
  throat 478.29
DSAP (disseminated superficial actinic
  porokeratosis) 692.75
Duane's retraction syndrome 378.71
Duane-Stilling-Türk syndrome (ocular
  retraction syndrome) 378.71
Dubin-Johnson disease or syndrome
  277.4
Dubini's disease (electric chorea) 049.8
Dubois' abscess or disease 090.5
Duchenne's
  disease 094.0
    locomotor ataxia 094.0
    muscular dystrophy 359.1
    pseudohypertrophy, muscles
      359.1
  paralysis 335.22
  syndrome 335.22
Duchenne-Aran myelopathic, muscular
  atrophy (nonprogressive)
  (progressive) 335.21
Duchenne-Griesinger disease 359.1
Ducrey's
  bacillus 099.0
  chancre 099.0
  disease (chancroid) 099.0
Duct, ductus - see condition
Duengero 061

Duhring's disease (dermatitis
  herpetiformis) 694.0
Dukes (-Filatov) disease 057.8
Dullness
  cardiac (decreased) (increased) 785.3
Dumb ague (see also Malaria) 084.6
Dumbness (see also Aphasia) 784.3
Dumdum fever 085.0
Dumping syndrome (postgastrectomy)
  564.2
  nonsurgical 536.8
Duodenitis (nonspecific) (peptic)
  535.60
  with hemorrhage 535.61
  due to
    strongyloides stercoralis 127.2
Duodenocholangitis 575.8
Duodenum, duodenal - see condition
Duplay's disease, periarthritis, or
  syndrome 726.2
Duplex - see also Accessory
  kidney 753.3
  placenta - see Placenta, abnormal
  uterus 752.2
Duplication - see also Accessory
  anus 751.5
  aortic arch 747.21
  appendix 751.5
  biliary duct (any) 751.69
  bladder 753.8
  cecum 751.5
    and appendix 751.5
  clitoris 752.49
  cystic duct 751.69
  digestive organs 751.8
  duodenum 751.5
  esophagus 750.4
  fallopian tube 752.19
  frontonasal process 756.0
  gallbladder 751.69
  ileum 751.5
  intestine (large) (small) 751.5
  jejunum 751.5
  kidney 753.3
  liver 751.69
  nose 748.1
  pancreas 751.7
  penis 752.69
  respiratory organs NEC 748.9
  salivary duct 750.22
  spinal cord (incomplete) 742.51
  stomach 750.7
  ureter 753.4
  vagina 752.49
  vas deferens 752.89
  vocal cords 748.3
Dupré's disease or syndrome
  (meningism) 781.6
Dupuytren's
  contraction 728.6
  disease (muscle contracture) 728.6
  fracture (closed) 824.4
    ankle (closed) 824.4
      open 824.5
    fibula (closed) 824.4
      open 824.5
    open 824.5
    radius (closed) 813.42
      open 813.52
  muscle contracture 728.6
Durand-Nicolas-Favre disease (climatic
  bubo) 099.1
Durotomy, incidental (inadvertent) (see
  also Tear, dural) 349.31

Duroziez's disease (congenital mitral
  stenosis) 746.5
Dust
  conjunctivitis 372.05
  reticulation (occupational) 504
Dutton's
  disease (trypanosomiasis) 086.9
  relapsing fever (West African) 087.1
Dwarf, dwarfism 259.4
  with infantilism (hypophyseal) 253.3
  achondroplastic 756.4
  Amsterdam 759.89
  bird-headed 759.89
  congenital 259.4
  constitutional 259.4
  hypophyseal 253.3
  infantile 259.4
  Levi type 253.3
  Lorain-Levi (pituitary) 253.3
  Lorain type (pituitary) 253.3
  metatropic 756.4
  nephrotic-glycosuric, with
    hypophosphatemic rickets
    270.0
  nutritional 263.2
  ovarian 758.6
  pancreatic 577.8
  pituitary 253.3
  polydystrophic 277.5
  primordial 253.3
  psychosocial 259.4
  renal 588.0
    with hypertension - see
      Hypertension, kidney
  Russell's (uterine dwarfism and
    craniofacial dysostosis) 759.89
Dyke-Young anemia or syndrome
  (acquired macrocytic hemolytic
  anemia) (secondary) (symptomatic)
  283.9
Dynia abnormality (see also Defect,
  coagulation) 286.9
Dysacousis 388.40
Dysadrenocortism 255.9
  hyperfunction 255.3
  hypofunction 255.41
Dysarthria 784.51 ◄▥
  due to late effect of cerebrovascular
    disease (see also Late effect(s) (of)
    cerebrovascular disease) 438.13 ◄
Dysautonomia (see also Neuropathy,
  peripheral, autonomic) 337.9
  familial 742.8
Dysbarism 993.3
Dysbasia 719.7
  angiosclerotica intermittens 443.9
    due to atherosclerosis 440.21
  hysterical 300.11
  lordotica (progressiva) 333.6
  nonorganic origin 307.9
  psychogenic 307.9
Dysbetalipoproteinemia (familial)
  272.2
Dyscalculia 315.1
Dyschezia (see also Constipation) 564.00
Dyschondroplasia (with hemangiomata)
  756.4
  Voorhoeve's 756.4
Dyschondrosteosis 756.59
Dyschromia 709.00
Dyscollagenosis 710.9
Dyscoria 743.41
Dyscraniopyophalangy 759.89

Dyscrasia
  blood 289.9
    with antepartum hemorrhage 641.3●
    fetus or newborn NEC 76.9
    hemorrhage, subungual 287.8
    puerperal, postpartum 666.3●
  ovary 256.8
  plasma cell 273.9
  pluriglandular 258.9
  polyglandular 258.9
Dysdiadochokinesia 781.3
Dysectasia, vesical neck 596.8
Dysendocrinism 259.9
Dysentery, dysenteric (bilious)
    (catarrhal) (diarrhea) (epidemic)
    (gangrenous) (hemorrhagic)
    (infectious) (sporadic) (tropical)
    (ulcerative) 009.0
  abscess, liver (*see also* Abscess, amebic)
    006.3
  amebic (*see also* Amebiasis) 006.9
    with abscess - *see* Abscess, amebic
    acute 006.0
    carrier (suspected) of V02.2
    chronic 006.1
  arthritis (*see also* Arthritis, due to,
      dysentery) 009.0 [711.3]●
    bacillary 004.9 [711.3]●
  asylum 004.9
  bacillary 004.9
    arthritis 004.9 [711.3]●
    Boyd 004.2
    Flexner 004.1
    Schmitz (-Stutzer) 004.0
    Shiga 004.0
    Shigella 004.9
      group A 004.0
      group B 004.1
      group C 004.2
      group D 004.3
      specified type NEC 004.8
    Sonne 004.3
    specified type NEC 004.8
  bacterium 004.9
  balantidial 007.0
  Balantidium coli 007.0
  Boyd's 004.2
  Chilomastix 007.8
  Chinese 004.9
  choleriform 001.1
  coccidial 007.2
  Dientamoeba fragilis 007.8
  due to specified organism NEC - *see*
      Enteritis, due to, by organism
  Embadomonas 007.8
  Endolimax nana - *see* Dysentery,
      amebic
  Entamoba, entamebic - *see* Dysentery,
      amebic
  Flexner's 004.1
  Flexner-Boyd 004.2
  giardial 007.1
  Giardia lamblia 007.1
  Hiss-Russell 004.1
  lamblia 007.1
  leishmanial 085.0
  malarial (*see also* Malaria) 084.6
  metazoal 127.9
  Monilia 112.89
  protozoal NEC 007.9
  Russell's 004.8
  salmonella 003.0
  schistosomal 120.1
  Schmitz (-Stutzer) 004.0

Dysentery, dysenteric (*Continued*)
  Shiga 004.0
  Shigella NEC (*see also* Dysentery,
      bacillary) 004.9
    boydii 004.2
    dysenteriae 004.0
      Schmitz 004.0
      Shiga 004.0
    flexneri 004.1
    group A 004.0
    group B 004.1
    group C 004.2
    group D 004.3
    Schmitz 004.0
    Shiga 004.0
    Sonnei 004.3
  Sonne 004.3
  strongyloidiasis 127.2
  trichomonal 007.3
  tuberculous (*see also* Tuberculosis)
      014.8●
  viral (*see also* Enteritis, viral) 008.8
Dysequilibrium 780.4
Dysesthesia 782.0
  hysterical 300.11
Dysfibrinogenemia (congenital) (*see also*
    Defect, coagulation) 286.3
Dysfunction
  adrenal (cortical) 255.9
    hyperfunction 255.3
    hypofunction 255.41
  associated with sleep stages or arousal
      from sleep 780.56
    nonorganic origin 307.47
  bladder NEC 596.59
  bleeding, uterus 626.8
  brain, minimal (*see also* Hyperkinesia)
      314.9
  cerebral 348.30
  colon 564.9
    psychogenic 306.4
  colostomy or enterostomy 569.62
  cystic duct 575.8
  diastolic 429.9
    with heart failure - *see* Failure, heart
    due to
      cardiomyopathy - *see*
          Cardiomyopathy
      hypertension - *see* Hypertension,
          heart
  endocrine NEC 259.9
  endometrium 621.8
  enteric stoma 569.62
  enterostomy 569.62
  erectile 607.84
    nonorganic origin 302.72
  esophagostomy 530.87
  Eustachian tube 381.81
  gallbladder 575.8
  gastrointestinal 536.9
  gland, glandular NEC 259.9
  heart 427.9
    postoperative (immediate) 997.1
      long-term effect of cardiac
          surgery 429.4
  hemoglobin 289.89
  hepatic 573.9
  hepatocellular NEC 573.9
  hypophysis 253.9
    hyperfunction 253.1
    hypofunction 253.2
    posterior lobe 253.6
      hypofunction 253.5
  kidney (*see also* Disease, renal) 593.9

Dysfunction (*Continued*)
  labyrinthine 386.50
    specified NEC 386.58
  liver 573.9
    constitutional 277.4
  minimal brain (child) (*see also*
      Hyperkinesia) 314.9
  ovary, ovarian 256.9
    hyperfunction 256.1
      estrogen 256.0
    hypofunction 256.39
      postablative 256.2
    postablative 256.2
    specified NEC 256.8
  papillary muscle 429.81
    with myocardial infarction 410.8●
  parathyroid 252.8
    hyperfunction 252.00
    hypofunction 252.1
  pineal gland 259.8
  pituitary (gland) 253.9
    hyperfunction 253.1
    hypofunction 253.2
    posterior 253.6
      hypofunction 253.5
  placental - *see* Placenta, insufficiency
  platelets (blood) 287.1
  polyglandular 258.9
    specified NEC 258.8
  psychosexual 302.70
    with
      dyspareunia (functional)
          (psychogenic) 302.76
      frigidity 302.72
      impotence 302.72
      inhibition
        orgasm
          female 302.73
          male 302.74
        sexual
          desire 302.71
          excitement 302.72
      premature ejaculation 302.75
      sexual aversion 302.79
      specified disorder NEC 302.79
      vaginismus 306.51
  pylorus 537.9
  rectum 564.9
    psychogenic 306.4
  segmental (*see also* Dysfunction,
      somatic) 739.9
  senile 797
  sexual 302.70
  sinoatrial node 427.81
  somatic 739.9
    abdomen 739.9
    acromioclavicular 739.7
    cervical 739.1
    cervicothoracic 739.1
    costochondral 739.8
    costovertebral 739.8
    extremities
      lower 739.6
      upper 739.7
    head 739.0
    hip 739.5
    lumbar, lumbosacral 739.3
    occipitocervical 739.0
    pelvic 739.5
    pubic 739.5
    rib cage 739.8
    sacral 739.4
    sacrococcygeal 739.4
    sacroiliac 739.4

◀ New   ◀▥ Revised   ~~deleted~~ Deleted   ● Use Additional Digit(s)   ▨ Omit code

Dysfunction (Continued)
  somatic (Continued)
    specified site NEC 739.9
    sternochondral 739.8
    sternoclavicular 739.7
    temporomandibular 739.0
    thoracic, thoracolumbar 739.2
  stomach 536.9
    psychogenic 306.4
  suprarenal 255.9
    hyperfunction 255.3
    hypofunction 255.41
  symbolic NEC 784.60
    specified type NEC 784.69
  systolic 429.9
    with heart failure - see Failure, heart
  temporomandibular (joint) (joint-pain-syndrome) NEC 524.60
    sounds on opening or closing 524.64
    specified NEC 524.69
  testicular 257.9
    hyperfunction 257.0
    hypofunction 257.2
    specified type NEC 257.8
  thymus 254.9
  thyroid 246.9
    complicating pregnancy, childbirth, or puerperium 648.1●
    hyperfunction - see Hyperthyroidism
    hypofunction - see Hypothyroidism
  uterus, complicating delivery 661.9●
    affecting fetus or newborn 763.7
    hypertonic 661.4●
    hypotonic 661.2●
      primary 661.0●
      secondary 661.1●
  velopharyngeal (acquired) 528.9
    congenital 750.29
  ventricular 429.9
    with congestive heart failure (see also Failure, heart) 428.0
    due to
      cardiomyopathy - see Cardiomyopathy
      hypertension - see Hypertension, heart
    left, reversible following sudden emotional stress 429.83
  vesicourethral NEC 596.59
  vestibular 386.50
    specified type NEC 386.58
Dysgammaglobulinemia 279.06
Dysgenesis
  gonadal (due to chromosomal anomaly) 758.6
    pure 752.7
  kidney(s) 753.0
  ovarian 758.6
  renal 753.0
  reticular 279.2
  seminiferous tubules 758.6
  tidal platelet 287.31
Dysgerminoma (M9060/3)
  specified site - see Neoplasm, by site, malignant
  unspecified site
    female 183.0
    male 186.9
Dysgeusia 781.1
Dysgraphia 781.3
Dyshidrosis 705.81
Dysidrosis 705.81

Dysinsulinism 251.8
Dyskaryotic cervical smear 795.09
Dyskeratosis (see also Keratosis) 701.1
  bullosa hereditaria 757.39
  cervix 622.10
  congenital 757.39
  follicularis 757.39
    vitamin A deficiency 264.8
  gingiva 523.8
  oral soft tissue NEC 528.79
  tongue 528.79
  uterus NEC 621.8
Dyskinesia 781.3
  biliary 575.8
  esophagus 530.5
  hysterical 300.11
  intestinal 564.89
  neuroleptic-induced tardive 333.85
  nonorganic origin 307.9
  orofacial 333.82
    due to drugs 333.85
  psychogenic 307.9
  subacute, due to drugs 333.85
  tardive (oral) 333.85
Dyslalia 784.59 ◄▥
  developmental 315.39
Dyslexia 784.61
  developmental 315.02
  secondary to organic lesion 784.61
Dyslipidemia 272.4
Dysmaturity (see also Immaturity) 765.1●
  lung 770.4
  pulmonary 770.4
Dysmenorrhea (essential) (exfoliative) (functional) (intrinsic) (membranous) (primary) (secondary) 625.3
  psychogenic 306.52
Dysmetabolic syndrome X 277.7
Dysmetria 781.3
Dysmorodystrophia mesodermalis congenita 759.82
Dysnomia 784.3
Dysorexia 783.0
  hysterical 300.11
Dysostosis
  cleidocranial, cleidocranialis 755.59
  craniofacial 756.0
  Fairbank's (idiopathic familial generalized osteophytosis) 756.50
  mandibularis 756.0
  mandibulofacial, incomplete 756.0
  multiplex 277.5
  orodigitofacial 759.89
Dyspareunia (female) 625.0
  male 608.89
  psychogenic 302.76
Dyspepsia (allergic) (congenital) (fermentative) (flatulent) (functional) (gastric) (gastrointestinal) (neurogenic) (occupational) (reflex) 536.8
  acid 536.8
  atonic 536.3
    psychogenic 306.4
  diarrhea 787.91
    psychogenic 306.4
  intestinal 564.89
    psychogenic 306.4
  nervous 306.4
  neurotic 306.4
  psychogenic 306.4

Dysphagia 787.20
  cervical 787.29
  functional 300.11
  hysterical 300.11
  nervous 300.11
  neurogenic 787.29
  oral phase 787.21
  oropharyngeal phase 787.22
  pharyngeal phase 787.23
  pharyngoesophageal phase 787.24
  psychogenic 306.4
  sideropenic 280.8
  spastica 530.5
  specified NEC 787.29
Dysphagocytosis, congenital 288.1 ◄▥
Dysphasia 784.59 ◄▥
Dysphonia 784.42 ◄▥
  clericorum 784.49
  functional 300.11
  hysterical 300.11
  psychogenic 306.1
  spastica 478.79
Dyspigmentation - see also Pigmentation
  eyelid (acquired) 374.52
Dyspituitarism 253.9
  hyperfunction 253.1
  hypofunction 253.2
  posterior lobe 253.6
Dysplasia - see also Anomaly
  anus 569.44
    intraepithelial neoplasia I [AIN I] (histologically confirmed) 569.44
    intraepithelial neoplasia II [AIN II] (histologically confirmed) 569.44
    intraepithelial neoplasia III [AIN III] 230.6
      anal canal 230.5
    mild (histologically confirmed) 569.44
    moderate (histologically confirmed) 569.44
    severe 230.6
      anal canal 230.5
  artery
    fibromuscular NEC 447.8
      carotid 447.8
      renal 447.3
  bladder 596.8
  bone (fibrous) NEC 733.29
    diaphyseal, progressive 756.59
    jaw 526.89
    monostotic 733.29
    polyostotic 756.54
    solitary 733.29
  brain 742.9
  bronchopulmonary, fetus or newborn 770.7
  cervix (uteri) 622.10
    cervical intraepithelial neoplasia I [CIN I] 622.11
    cervical intraepithelial neoplasia II [CIN II] 622.12
    cervical intraepithelial neoplasia III [CIN III] 233.1
    CIN I 622.11
    CIN II 622.12
    CIN III 233.1
    mild 622.11
    moderate 622.12
    severe 233.1
  chondroectodermal 756.55
  chondromatose 756.4

Dysplasia (Continued)
  colon 211.3
  craniocarpotarsal 759.89
  craniometaphyseal 756.89
  dentinal 520.5
  diaphyseal, progressive 756.59
  ectodermal (anhidrotic) (Bason)
      (Clouston's) (congenital)
      (Feinmesser) (hereditary)
      (hidrotic) (Marshall)
      (Robinson's) 757.31
  epiphysealis 756.9
    multiplex 756.56
    punctata 756.59
  epiphysis 756.9
    multiple 756.56
  epithelial
    epiglottis 478.79
    uterine cervix 622.10
  erythroid NEC 289.89
  eye (see also Microphthalmos)
      743.10
  familial metaphyseal 756.89
  fibromuscular, artery NEC 447.8
    carotid 447.8
    renal 447.3
  fibrous
    bone NEC 733.29
    diaphyseal, progressive 756.59
    jaw 526.89
    monostotic 733.29
    polyostotic 756.54
    solitary 733.29
  high grade, focal - see Neoplasm, by
      site, benign
  hip (congenital) 755.63
    with dislocation (see also Dislocation,
        hip, congenital) 754.30
  hypohidrotic ectodermal 757.31
  joint 755.8
  kidney 753.15
  leg 755.69
  linguofacialis 759.89
  lung 748.5
  macular 743.55
  mammary (benign) (gland) 610.9
    cystic 610.1
    specified type NEC 610.8
  metaphyseal 756.9
    familial 756.89
  monostotic fibrous 733.29
  muscle 756.89
  myeloid NEC 289.89
  nervous system (general) 742.9
  neuroectodermal 759.6
  oculoauriculovertebral 756.0
  oculodentodigital 759.89
  olfactogenital 253.4
  osteo-onycho-arthro (hereditary) 756.89
  periosteum 733.99
  polyostotic fibrous 756.54
  progressive diaphyseal 756.59
  prostate 602.3
    intraepithelial neoplasia I
        [PIN I] 602.3
    intraepithelial neoplasia II
        [PIN II] 602.3
    intraepithelial neoplasia III
        [PIN III] 233.4
  renal 753.15
  renofacialis 753.0
  retinal NEC 743.56
  retrolental (see also Retinopathy of
      prematurity) 362.21

Dysplasia (Continued)
  skin 709.8
  spinal cord 742.9
  thymic, with immunodeficiency
      279.2
  vagina 623.0
    mild 623.0
    moderate 623.0
    severe 233.31
  vocal cord 478.5
  vulva 624.8
    intraepithelial neoplasia I [VIN I]
        624.01
    intraepithelial neoplasia II [VIN II]
        624.02
    intraepithelial neoplasia III [VIN III]
        233.32
    mild 624.01
    moderate 624.02
    severe 233.32
    VIN I 624.01
    VIN II 624.02
    VIN III 233.32
Dyspnea (nocturnal) (paroxysmal) 786.09
  asthmatic (bronchial) (see also Asthma)
      493.9●
    with bronchitis (see also Asthma)
        493.9●
    chronic 493.2●
  cardiac (see also Failure, ventricular,
      left) 428.1
  cardiac (see also Failure, ventricular,
      left) 428.1
  functional 300.11
  hyperventilation 786.01
  hysterical 300.11
  Monday morning 504
  newborn 770.89
  psychogenic 306.1
  uremic - see Uremia
Dyspraxia 781.3
  syndrome 315.4
Dysproteinemia 273.8
  transient with copper deficiency
      281.4
Dysprothrombinemia (constitutional)
    (see also Defect, coagulation) 286.3
Dysreflexia, autonomic 337.3
Dysrhythmia
  cardiac 427.9
    postoperative (immediate) 997.1
      long-term effect of cardiac
          surgery 429.4
    specified type NEC 427.89
  cerebral or cortical 348.30
Dyssecretosis, mucoserous 710.2
Dyssocial reaction, without manifest
    psychiatric disorder
  adolescent V71.02
  adult V71.01
  child V71.02
Dyssomnia NEC 780.56
  nonorganic origin 307.47
Dyssplenism 289.4
Dyssynergia
  biliary (see also Disease, biliary)
      576.8
  cerebellaris myoclonica 334.2
  detrusor sphincter (bladder) 596.55
  ventricular 429.89
Dystasia, hereditary areflexic 334.3
Dysthymia 300.4
Dysthymic disorder 300.4
Dysthyroidism 246.9

Dystocia 660.9●
  affecting fetus or newborn 763.1
  cervical 661.2●
    affecting fetus or newborn 763.7
  contraction ring 661.4●
    affecting fetus or newborn 763.7
  fetal 660.9●
    abnormal size 653.5●
    affecting fetus or newborn 763.1
    deformity 653.7●
  maternal 660.9●
    affecting fetus or newborn 763.1
  positional 660.0●
    affecting fetus or newborn 763.1
  shoulder (girdle) 660.4●
    affecting fetus or newborn 763.1
  uterine NEC 661.4●
    affecting fetus or newborn 763.7
Dystonia
  acute
    due to drugs 333.72
    neuroleptic-induced acute 333.72
  deformans progressiva 333.6
  lenticularis 333.6
  musculorum deformans 333.6
  torsion (idiopathic) 333.6
    acquired 333.79
    fragments (of) 333.89
    genetic 333.6
    symptomatic 333.79
Dystonic
  movements 781.0
Dystopia kidney 753.3
Dystrophy, dystrophia 783.9
  adiposogenital 253.8
  asphyxiating thoracic 756.4
  Becker's type 359.22
  brevicollis 756.16
  Bruch's membrane 362.77
  cervical (sympathetic) NEC 337.09
  chondro-osseus with punctate
      epiphyseal dysplasia 756.59
  choroid (hereditary) 363.50
    central (areolar) (partial) 363.53
      total (gyrate) 363.54
    circinate 363.53
    circumpapillary (partial) 363.51
      total 363.52
    diffuse
      partial 363.56
      total 363.57
    generalized
      partial 363.56
      total 363.57
    gyrate
      central 363.54
      generalized 363.57
    helicoid 363.52
    peripapillary - see Dystrophy,
        choroid, circumpapillary
    serpiginous 363.54
  cornea (hereditary) 371.50
    anterior NEC 371.52
    Cogan's 371.52
    combined 371.57
    crystalline 371.56
    endothelial (Fuchs') 371.57
    epithelial 371.50
      juvenile 371.51
      microscopic cystic 371.52
    granular 371.53
    lattice 371.54
    macular 371.55
    marginal (Terrien's) 371.48

◄ New   ◄Ⅲ Revised   ~~deleted~~ Deleted   ● Use Additional Digit(s)   ▦ Omit code

Dystrophy, dystrophia *(Continued)*
  cornea *(Continued)*
    Meesman's 371.51
    microscopic cystic (epithelial)
      371.52
    nodular, Salzmann's 371.46
    polymorphous 371.58
    posterior NEC 371.58
    ring-like 371.52
    Salzmann's nodular 371.46
    stromal NEC 371.56
  dermatochondrocorneal 371.50
  Duchenne's 359.1
  due to malnutrition 263.9
  Erb's 359.1
  familial
    hyperplastic periosteal 756.59
    osseous 277.5
  foveal 362.77
  Fuchs', cornea 371.57
  Gowers' muscular 359.1
  hair 704.2
  hereditary, progressive muscular
    359.1
  hypogenital, with diabetic tendency
    759.81
  Landouzy-Déjérine 359.1
  Leyden-Möbius 359.1
  mesodermalis congenita 759.82
  muscular 359.1
    congenital (hereditary) 359.0
      myotonic 359.22
    distal 359.1
    Duchenne's 359.1
    Erb's 359.1
    fascioscapulohumeral 359.1
    Gowers' 359.1
    hereditary (progressive) 359.1

Dystrophy, dystrophia *(Continued)*
  muscular *(Continued)*
    Landouzy-Déjérine 359.1
    limb-girdle 359.1
    myotonic 359.21
    progressive (hereditary) 359.1
      Charcôt-Marie-Tooth 356.1
    pseudohypertrophic (infantile)
      359.1
  myocardium, myocardial *(see also*
    Degeneration, myocardial)*
    429.1
  myotonic 359.21
  myotonica 359.21
  nail 703.8
    congenital 757.5
  neurovascular (traumatic) *(see also*
    Neuropathy, peripheral,
    autonomic)* 337.9
  nutritional 263.9
  ocular 359.1
  oculocerebrorenal 270.8
  oculopharyngeal 359.1
  ovarian 620.8
  papillary (and pigmentary) 701.1
  pelvicrural atrophic 359.1
  pigmentary *(see also* Acanthosis)
    701.2
  pituitary (gland) 253.8
  polyglandular 258.8
  posttraumatic sympathetic - *see*
    Dystrophy, symphatic
  progressive ophthalmoplegic 359.1
  reflex neuromuscular - *see* Dystrophy,
    sympathetic
  retina, retinal (hereditary) 362.70
    albipunctate 362.74
    Bruch's membrane 362.77

Dystrophy, dystrophia *(Continued)*
  retina, retinal *(Continued)*
    cone, progressive 362.75
    hyaline 362.77
    in
      Bassen-Kornzweig syndrome
        272.5 *[362.72]*
      cerebroretinal lipidosis 330.1
        [362.71]
      Refsum's disease 356.3 *[362.72]*
      systemic lipidosis 272.7 *[362.71]*
    juvenile (Stargardt's) 362.75
    pigmentary 362.74
    pigment epithelium 362.76
    progressive cone (-rod) 362.75
    pseudoinflammatory foveal
      362.77
    rod, progressive 362.75
    sensory 362.75
    vitelliform 362.76
  Salzmann's nodular 371.46
  scapuloperoneal 359.1
  skin NEC 709.9
  sympathetic (posttraumatic) (reflex)
    337.20
    lower limb 337.22
    specified site NEC 337.29
    upper limb 337.21
  tapetoretinal NEC 362.74
  thoracic asphyxiating 756.4
  unguium 703.8
    congenital 757.5
  vitreoretinal (primary) 362.73
    secondary 362.66
  vulva 624.09
Dysuria 788.1
  psychogenic 306.53

E

Eagle-Barrett syndrome 756.71
Eales' disease (syndrome) 362.18
Ear - *see also* condition
  ache 388.70
    otogenic 388.71
    referred 388.72
  lop 744.29
  piercing V50.3
  swimmers' acute 380.12
  tank 380.12
  tropical 111.8 *[380.15]*
  wax 380.4
Earache 388.70
  otogenic 388.71
  referred 388.72
Early satiety 780.94
Eaton-Lambert syndrome (*see also*
  Neoplasm, by site, malignant)
  199.1 *[358.1]*
Eberth's disease (typhoid fever) 002.0
Ebstein's
  anomaly or syndrome (downward
    displacement, tricuspid valve
    into right ventricle) 746.2
  disease (diabetes) 250.4● *[581.81]*
    due to secondary diabetes 249.4●
      [581.81]
Eccentro-osteochondrodysplasia
  277.5
Ecchondroma (M9210/0) - *see* Neoplasm,
  bone, benign
Ecchondrosis (M9210/1) 238.0
Ecchordosis physaliphora 756.0
Ecchymosis (multiple) 459.89
  conjunctiva 372.72
  eye (traumatic) 921.0
  eyelids (traumatic) 921.1
  newborn 772.6
  spontaneous 782.7
  traumatic - *see* Contusion
ECD (Erdheim-Chester disease) 277.89 ◄
Echinococciasis - *see* Echinococcus
Echinococcosis - *see* Echinococcus
Echinococcus (infection) 122.9
  granulosus 122.4
    liver 122.0
    lung 122.1
    orbit 122.3 *[376.13]*
    specified site NEC 122.3
    thyroid 122.2
  liver NEC 122.8
    granulosus 122.0
    multilocularis 122.5
  lung NEC 122.9
    granulosus 122.1
    multilocularis 122.6
  multilocularis 122.7
    liver 122.5
    specified site NEC 122.6
  orbit 122.9 *[376.13]*
    granulosus 122.3 *[376.13]*
    multilocularis 122.6 *[376.13]*
  specified site NEC 122.9
    granulosus 122.3
    multilocularis 122.6 *[376.13]*
  thyroid NEC 122.9
    granulosus 122.2
    multilocularis 122.6
Echinorhynchiasis 127.7
Echinostomiasis 121.8
Echolalia 784.69
ECHO virus infection NEC 079.1

Eclampsia, eclamptic (coma)
  (convulsions) (delirium) 780.39
  female, child-bearing age NEC - *see*
    Eclampsia, pregnancy
  gravidarum - *see* Eclampsia, pregnancy
  male 780.39
  not associated with pregnancy or
    childbirth 780.39
  pregnancy, childbirth, or puerperium
    642.6●
    with pre-existing hypertension
      642.7●
    affecting fetus or newborn 760.0
  uremic 586
Eclipse blindness (total) 363.31
Economic circumstance affecting care
  V60.9
  specified type NEC V60.89   ◄▥
Economo's disease (encephalitis
  lethargica) 049.8
Ectasia, ectasis
  aorta (*see also* Aneurysm, aorta) 441.9
    ruptured 441.5
  breast 610.4
  capillary 448.9
  cornea (marginal) (postinfectional)
    371.71
  duct (mammary) 610.4
  gastric antral vascular (GAVE) 537.82
    with hemorrhage 537.83
    without hemorrhage 537.82
  kidney 593.89
  mammary duct (gland) 610.4
  papillary 448.9
  renal 593.89
  salivary gland (duct) 527.8
  scar, cornea 371.71
  sclera 379.11
Ecthyma 686.8
  contagiosum 051.2
  gangrenosum 686.09
  infectiosum 051.2
Ectocardia 746.87
Ectodermal dysplasia, congenital 757.31
Ectodermosis erosiva pluriorificialis
  695.19
Ectopic, ectopia (congenital) 759.89
  abdominal viscera 751.8
    due to defect in anterior abdominal
      wall 756.79
  ACTH syndrome 255.0
  adrenal gland 759.1
  anus 751.5
  auricular beats 427.61
  beats 427.60
  bladder 753.5
  bone and cartilage in lung 748.69
  brain 742.4
  breast tissue 757.6
  cardiac 746.87
  cerebral 742.4
  cordis 746.87
  endometrium 617.9
  gallbladder 751.69
  gastric mucosa 750.7
  gestation - *see* Pregnancy, ectopic
  heart 746.87
  hormone secretion NEC 259.3
  hyperparathyroidism 259.3
  kidney (crossed) (intrathoracic) (pelvis)
    753.3
    in pregnancy or childbirth 654.4●
      causing obstructed labor 660.2●
  lens 743.37

Ectopic, ectopia (*Continued*)
  lentis 743.37
  mole - *see* Pregnancy, ectopic
  organ or site NEC - *see* Malposition,
    congenital
  ovary 752.0
  pancreas, pancreatic tissue 751.7
  pregnancy - *see* Pregnancy, ectopic
  pupil 364.75
  renal 753.3
  sebaceous glands of mouth 750.26
  secretion
    ACTH 255.0
    adrenal hormone 259.3
    adrenalin 259.3
    adrenocorticotropin 255.0
    antidiuretic hormone (ADH) 259.3
    epinephrine 259.3
    hormone NEC 259.3
    norepinephrine 259.3
    pituitary (posterior) 259.3
  spleen 759.0
  testis 752.51
  thyroid 759.2
  ureter 753.4
  ventricular beats 427.69
  vesicae 753.5
Ectrodactyly 755.4
  finger (*see also* Absence, finger,
    congenital) 755.29
  toe (*see also* Absence, toe, congenital)
    755.39
Ectromelia 755.4
  lower limb 755.30
  upper limb 755.20
Ectropion 374.10
  anus 569.49
  cervix 622.0
    with mention of cervicitis 616.0
  cicatricial 374.14
  congenital 743.62
  eyelid 374.10
    cicatricial 374.14
    congenital 743.62
    mechanical 374.12
    paralytic 374.12
    senile 374.11
    spastic 374.13
  iris (pigment epithelium) 364.54
  lip (congenital) 750.26
    acquired 528.5
  mechanical 374.12
  paralytic 374.12
  rectum 569.49
  senile 374.11
  spastic 374.13
  urethra 599.84
  uvea 364.54
Eczema (acute) (allergic) (chronic)
  (erythematous) (fissum)
  (occupational) (rubrum) (squamous)
  692.9
  asteatotic 706.8
  atopic 691.8
  contact NEC 692.9
  dermatitis NEC 692.9
  due to specified cause - *see* Dermatitis,
    due to
  dyshidrotic 705.81
  external ear 380.22
  flexural 691.8
  gouty 274.89
  herpeticum 054.0
  hypertrophicum 701.8

◄ New   ◄▥ Revised   ~~deleted~~ Deleted   ● Use Additional Digit(s)   ▥ Omit code

Eczema *(Continued)*
  hypostatic - *see* Varicose, vein
  impetiginous 684
  infantile (acute) (chronic) (due to any
      substance) (intertriginous)
      (seborrheic) 690.12
  intertriginous NEC 692.9
    infantile 690.12
  intrinsic 691.8
  lichenified NEC 692.9
  marginatum 110.3
  nummular 692.9
  pustular 686.8
  seborrheic 690.18
    infantile 690.12
  solare 692.72
  stasis (lower extremity) 454.1
    ulcerated 454.2
  vaccination, vaccinatum 999.0
  varicose (lower extremity) - *see*
      Varicose, vein
  verrucosum callosum 698.3
Eczematoid, exudative 691.8
Eddowes' syndrome (brittle bones and
    blue sclera) 756.51
Edema, edematous 782.3
  with nephritis (*see also* Nephrosis)
      581.9
  allergic 995.1
  angioneurotic (allergic) (any site)
      (with urticaria) 995.1
    hereditary 277.6
  angiospastic 443.9
  Berlin's (traumatic) 921.3
  brain 348.5
    due to birth injury 767.8
    fetus or newborn 767.8
  cardiac (*see also* Failure, heart) 428.0
  cardiovascular (*see also* Failure, heart)
      428.0
  cerebral - *see* Edema, brain
  cerebrospinal vessel - *see* Edema,
      brain
  cervix (acute) (uteri) 622.8
    puerperal, postpartum 674.8 ●
  chronic hereditary 757.0
  circumscribed, acute 995.1
    hereditary 277.6
  complicating pregnancy (gestational)
      646.1 ●
    with hypertension - *see* Toxemia, of
        pregnancy
  conjunctiva 372.73
  connective tissue 782.3
  cornea 371.20
    due to contact lenses 371.24
    idiopathic 371.21
    secondary 371.22
  cystoid macular 362.53
  due to
    lymphatic obstruction - *see* Edema,
        lymphatic
    salt retention 276.0
  epiglottis - *see* Edema, glottis
  essential, acute 995.1
    hereditary 277.6
  extremities, lower - *see* Edema, legs
  eyelid NEC 374.82
  familial, hereditary (legs) 757.0
  famine 262
  fetus or newborn 778.5
  genital organs
    female 629.89
    male 608.86

Edema, edematous *(Continued)*
  gestational 646.1 ●
    with hypertension - *see* Toxemia, of
        pregnancy
  glottis, glottic, glottides (obstructive)
      (passive) 478.6
    allergic 995.1
      hereditary 277.6
    due to external agent - *see*
        Condition, respiratory, acute,
        due to specified agent
  heart (*see also* Failure, heart) 428.0
    newborn 779.89
  heat 992.7
  hereditary (legs) 757.0
  inanition 262
  infectious 782.3
  intracranial 348.5
    due to injury at birth 767.8
  iris 364.89
  joint (*see also* Effusion, joint) 719.0 ●
  larynx (*see also* Edema, glottis) 478.6
  legs 782.3
    due to venous obstruction 459.2
    hereditary 757.0
  localized 782.3
    due to venous obstruction 459.2
      lower extremity 459.2
  lower extremities - *see* Edema, legs
  lung 514
    acute 518.4
      with heart disease or failure (*see
          also* Failure, ventricular, left)
          428.1
        congestive 428.0
      chemical (due to fumes or
          vapors) 506.1
      due to
        external agent(s) NEC 508.9
          specified NEC 508.8
        fumes and vapors (chemical)
            (inhalation) 506.1
        radiation 508.0
    chemical (acute) 506.1
      chronic 506.4
    chronic 514
      chemical (due to fumes or
          vapors) 506.4
      due to
        external agent(s) NEC 508.9
          specified NEC 508.8
        fumes or vapors (chemical)
            (inhalation) 506.4
        radiation 508.1
    due to
      external agent 508.9
        specified NEC 508.8
      high altitude 993.2
      near drowning 994.1
    postoperative 518.4
    terminal 514
  lymphatic 457.1
    due to mastectomy operation
        457.0
  macula 362.83
    cystoid 362.53
    diabetic 250.5 ● [362.07]
      due to secondary diabetes 249.5 ●
          [362.07]
  malignant (*see also* Gangrene, gas)
      040.0
  Milroy's 757.0
  nasopharynx 478.25
  neonatorum 778.5

Edema, edematous *(Continued)*
  nutritional (newborn) 262
    with dyspigmentation, skin and hair
        260
  optic disc or nerve - *see* Papilledema
  orbit 376.33
    circulatory 459.89
  palate (soft) (hard) 528.9
  pancreas 577.8
  penis 607.83
  periodic 995.1
    hereditary 277.6
  pharynx 478.25
  pitting 782.3
  pulmonary - *see* Edema, lung
  Quincke's 995.1
    hereditary 277.6
  renal (*see also* Nephrosis) 581.9
  retina (localized) (macular) (peripheral)
      362.83
    cystoid 362.53
    diabetic 250.5 ● [362.07]
      due to secondary diabetes 249.5 ●
          [362.07]
  salt 276.0
  scrotum 608.86
  seminal vesicle 608.86
  spermatic cord 608.86
  spinal cord 336.1
  starvation 262
  stasis - *see also* Hypertension, venous
      459.30
  subconjunctival 372.73
  subglottic (*see also* Edema, glottis) 478.6
  supraglottic (*see also* Edema, glottis)
      478.6
  testis 608.86
  toxic NEC 782.3
  traumatic NEC 782.3
  tunica vaginalis 608.86
  vas deferens 608.86
  vocal cord - *see* Edema, glottis
  vulva (acute) 624.8
Edentia (complete) (partial) (*see also*
    Absence, tooth) 520.0
  acquired (*see also* Edentulism) 525.40
    due to
      caries 525.13
      extraction 525.10
      periodontal disease 525.12
      specified NEC 525.19
      trauma 525.11
  causing malocclusion 524.30
  congenital (deficiency of tooth buds)
      520.0
Edentulism 525.40
  complete 525.40
    class I 525.41
    class II 525.42
    class III 525.43
    class IV 525.44
  partial 525.50
    class I 525.51
    class II 525.52
    class III 525.53
    class IV 525.54
Edsall's disease 992.2
Educational handicap V62.3
Edwards' syndrome 758.2
Effect, adverse NEC
  abnormal gravitational (G) forces or
      states 994.9
  air pressure - *see* Effect, adverse,
      atmospheric pressure

Effect, adverse NEC (*Continued*)
altitude (high) - *see* Effect, adverse,
    high altitude
anesthetic
    in labor and delivery NEC 668.9●
      affecting fetus or newborn 763.5
antitoxin - *see* Complications,
    vaccination
atmospheric pressure 993.9
    due to explosion 993.4
    high 993.3
    low - *see* Effect, adverse, high
      altitude
    specified effect NEC 993.8
biological, correct substance properly
    administered (*see also* Effect,
    adverse, drug) 995.20
blood (derivatives) (serum)
    (transfusion) - *see* Complications,
    transfusion
chemical substance NEC 989.9
    specified - *see* Table of Drugs and
    Chemicals
cobalt, radioactive (*see also* Effect,
    adverse, radioactive substance)
    990
cold (temperature) (weather) 991.9
    chilblains 991.5
    frostbite - *see* Frostbite
    specified effect NEC 991.8
drugs and medicinals 995.20
    correct substance properly
      administered 995.20
    overdose or wrong substance given
      or taken 977.9
    specified drug - *see* Table of
      Drugs and Chemicals
electric current (shock) 994.8
    burn - *see* Burn, by site
electricity (electrocution) (shock) 994.8
    burn - *see* Burn, by site
exertion (excessive) 994.5
exposure 994.9
    exhaustion 994.4
external cause NEC 994.9
fallout (radioactive) NEC 990
fluoroscopy NEC 990
foodstuffs
    allergic reaction (*see also* Allergy,
    food) 693.1
    anaphylactic shock due to food
      NEC 995.60
    noxious 988.9
    specified type NEC (*see also*
      Poisoning, by name of
      noxious foodstuff) 988.8
gases, fumes, or vapors - *see* Table of
    Drugs and Chemicals
glue (airplane) sniffing 304.6●
heat - *see* Heat
high altitude NEC 993.2
    anoxia 993.2
    on
      ears 993.0
      sinuses 993.1
    polycythemia 289.0
hot weather - *see* Heat
hunger 994.2
immersion, foot 991.4
immunization - *see* Complications,
    vaccination
immunological agents - *see*
    Complications, vaccination
implantation (removable) of isotope or
    radium NEC 990

Effect, adverse NEC (*Continued*)
infrared (radiation) (rays) NEC 990
    burn - *see* Burn, by site
    dermatitis or eczema 692.82
infusion - *see* Complications, infusion
ingestion or injection of isotope
    (therapeutic) NEC 990
irradiation NEC (*see also* Effect,
    adverse, radiation) 990
isotope (radioactive) NEC 990
lack of care (child) (infant) (newborn)
    995.52
    adult 995.84
lightning 994.0
    burn - *see* Burn, by site
Lirugin - *see* Complications,
    vaccination
medicinal substance, correct, properly
    administered (*see also* Effect,
    adverse, drugs) 995.20
mesothorium NEC 990
motion 994.6
noise, inner ear 388.10
other drug, medicinal and biological
    substance 995.29
overheated places - *see* Heat
polonium NEC 990
psychosocial, of work environment
    V62.1
radiation (diagnostic) (fallout)
    (infrared) (natural source)
    (therapeutic) (tracer) (ultraviolet)
    (x-ray) NEC 990
    with pulmonary manifestations
      acute 508.0
      chronic 508.1
    dermatitis or eczema 692.82
      due to sun NEC (*see also*
        Dermatitis, due to, sun)
        692.70
    fibrosis of lungs 508.1
    maternal with suspected damage to
      fetus affecting management of
      pregnancy 655.6●
    pneumonitis 508.0
radioactive substance NEC 990
    dermatitis or eczema 692.82
radioactivity NEC 990
radiotherapy NEC 990
    dermatitis or eczema 692.82
radium NEC 990
reduced temperature 991.9
    frostbite - *see* Frostbite
    immersion, foot (hand) 991.4
    specified effect NEC 991.8
roentgenography NEC 990
roentgenoscopy NEC 990
roentgen rays NEC 990
serum (prophylactic) (therapeutic)
    NEC 999.5
specified NEC 995.89
    external cause NEC 994.9
strangulation 994.7
submersion 994.1
teletherapy NEC 990
thirst 994.3
transfusion - *see* Complications,
    transfusion
ultraviolet (radiation) (rays) NEC 990
    burn - *see also* Burn, by site
      from sun (*see also* Sunburn) 692.71
    dermatitis or eczema 692.82
      due to sun NEC (*see also*
        Dermatitis, due to, sun)
        692.70

Effect, adverse NEC (*Continued*)
uranium NEC 990
vaccine (any) - *see* Complications,
    vaccination
weightlessness 994.9
whole blood - *see also* Complications,
    transfusion
    overdose or wrong substance given
      (*see also* Table of Drugs and
      Chemicals) 964.7
working environment V62.1
x-rays NEC 990
    dermatitis or eczema 692.82
Effect, remote
of cancer - *see* condition
Effects, late - *see* Late, effect (of)
Effluvium, telogen 704.02
Effort
intolerance 306.2
syndrome (aviators) (psychogenic)
    306.2
Effusion
amniotic fluid (*see also* Rupture,
    membranes, premature) 658.1●
brain (serous) 348.5
bronchial (*see also* Bronchitis) 490
cerebral 348.5
cerebrospinal (*see also* Meningitis) 322.9
    vessel 348.5
chest - *see* Effusion, pleura
intracranial 348.5
joint 719.00
    ankle 719.07
    elbow 719.02
    foot 719.07
    hand 719.04
    hip 719.05
    knee 719.06
    multiple sites 719.09
    pelvic region 719.05
    shoulder (region) 719.01
    specified site NEC 719.08
    wrist 719.03
meninges (*see also* Meningitis) 322.9
pericardium, pericardial (*see also*
    Pericarditis) 423.9
    acute 420.90
peritoneal (chronic) 568.82
pleura, pleurisy, pleuritic,
    pleuropericardial 511.9
    bacterial, nontuberculous 511.1
    fetus or newborn 511.9
    malignant 511.81
    nontuberculous 511.9
      bacterial 511.1
    pneumococcal 511.1
    staphylococcal 511.1
    streptococcal 511.1
    traumatic 862.29
      with open wound 862.39
    tuberculous (*see also* Tuberculosis,
      pleura) 012.0●
      primary progressive 010.1●
pulmonary - *see* Effusion, pleura
spinal (*see also* Meningitis) 322.9
thorax, thoracic - *see* Effusion, pleura
Egg (oocyte) (ovum)
donor V59.70
    over age 35 V59.73
      anonymous recipient V59.73
      designated recipient V59.74
    under age 35 V59.71
      anonymous recipient V59.71
      designated recipient V59.72
Eggshell nails 703.8
congenital 757.5

Ego-dystonic
    homosexuality 302.0
    lesbianism 302.0
    sexual orientation 302.0
Egyptian splenomegaly 120.1
Ehlers-Danlos syndrome 756.83
Ehrlichiosis 082.40
    chaffeensis 082.41
    specified type NEC 082.49
Eichstedt's disease (pityriasis versicolor)
    111.0
EIN (endometrial intraepithelial
    neoplasia) 621.35 ◄
Eisenmenger's complex or syndrome
    (ventricular septal defect) 745.4
Ejaculation, semen
    painful 608.89
        psychogenic 306.59
    premature 302.75
    retrograde 608.87
Ekbom syndrome (restless legs) 333.94
Ekman's syndrome (brittle bones and
    blue sclera) 756.51
Elastic skin 756.83
    acquired 701.8
Elastofibroma (M8820/0) - see Neoplasm,
    connective tissue, benign
Elastoidosis
    cutanea nodularis 701.8
    cutis cystica et comedonica 701.8
Elastoma 757.39
    juvenile 757.39
    Miescher's (elastosis perforans
        serpiginosa) 701.1
Elastomyofibrosis 425.3
Elastosis 701.8
    atrophicans 701.8
    perforans serpiginosa 701.1
    reactive perforating 701.1
    senilis 701.8
    solar (actinic) 692.74
Elbow - see condition
Electric
    current, electricity, effects (concussion)
        (fatal) (nonfatal) (shock) 994.8
        burn - see Burn, by site
    feet (foot) syndrome 266.2
    shock from electroshock gun (taser)
        994.8
Electrocution 994.8
Electrolyte imbalance 276.9
    with
        abortion - see Abortion, by type,
            with metabolic disorder
        ectopic pregnancy (see also
            categories 633.0–633.9) 639.4
        hyperemesis gravidarum (before 22
            completed weeks' gestation)
            643.1 ●
        molar pregnancy (see also categories
            630–632) 639.4
    following
        abortion 639.4
        ectopic or molar pregnancy 639.4
Elephant man syndrome 237.71
Elephantiasis (nonfilarial) 457.1
    arabicum (see also Infestation, filarial)
        125.9
    congenita hereditaria 757.0
    congenital (any site) 757.0
    due to
        Brugia (malayi) 125.1
        mastectomy operation 457.0
        Wuchereria (bancrofti) 125.0
            malayi 125.1

Elephantiasis (Continued)
    eyelid 374.83
    filarial (see also Infestation, filarial)
        125.9
    filariensis (see also Infestation, filarial)
        125.9
    gingival 523.8
    glandular 457.1
    graecorum 030.9
    lymphangiectatic 457.1
    lymphatic vessel 457.1
        due to mastectomy operation 457.0
    neuromatosa 237.71
    postmastectomy 457.0
    scrotum 457.1
    streptococcal 457.1
    surgical 997.99
        postmastectomy 457.0
    telangiectodes 457.1
    vulva (nonfilarial) 624.8
Elevated - see Elevation
    findings on laboratory examination -
        see Findings, abnormal, without
        diagnosis (examination)
        (laboratory test) ◄
    GFR (glomerular filtration rate) -
        see Findings, abnormal, without
        diagnosis (examination)
        (laboratory test) ◄
Elevation
    17-ketosteroids 791.9
    acid phosphatase 790.5
    alkaline phosphatase 790.5
    amylase 790.5
    antibody titers 795.79
    basal metabolic rate (BMR) 794.7
    blood pressure (see also Hypertension)
        401.9
        reading (incidental) (isolated)
            (nonspecific), no diagnosis of
            hypertension 796.2
    blood sugar 790.29
    body temperature (of unknown origin)
        (see also Pyrexia) 780.60
    cancer antigen 125 [CA 125] 795.82
    carcinoembryonic antigen [CEA]
        795.81
    cholesterol 272.0
        with high triglycerides 272.2
    conjugate, eye 378.81
    C-reactive protein (CRP) 790.95
    CRP (C-reactive protein) 790.95
    diaphragm, congenital 756.6
    GFR (glomerular filtration rate) - see
        Findings, abnormal, without
        diagnosis (examination)
        (laboratory test) ◄
    glucose
        fasting 790.21
        tolerance test 790.22
    immunoglobulin level 795.79
    indolacetic acid 791.9
    lactic acid dehydrogenase (LDH) level
        790.4
    leukocytes 288.60
    lipase 790.5
    lipoprotein a level 272.8
    liver function test (LFT) 790.6
        alkaline phosphatase 790.5
        aminotransferase 790.4
        bilirubin 782.4
        hepatic enzyme NEC 790.5
        lactate dehydrogenase 790.4
    lymphocytes 288.61
    prostate specific antigen (PSA)
        790.93

Elevation (Continued)
    renin 790.99
        in hypertension (see also
            Hypertension, renovascular)
            405.91
    Rh titer 999.7
    scapula, congenital 755.52
    sedimentation rate 790.1
    SGOT 790.4
    SGPT 790.4
    transaminase 790.4
    triglycerides 272.1
        with high cholesterol 272.2
    vanillylmandelic acid 791.9
    venous pressure 459.89
    VMA 791.9
    white blood cell count 288.60
        specified NEC 288.69
Elliptocytosis (congenital) (hereditary)
    282.1
    Hb-C (disease) 282.7
    hemoglobin disease 282.7
    sickle-cell (disease) 282.60
        trait 282.5
Ellis-van Creveld disease or syndrome
    (chondroectodermal dysplasia)
    756.55
Ellison-Zollinger syndrome
    (gastric hypersecretion with pancreatic
    islet cell tumor) 251.5
Elongation, elongated (congenital) - see
    also Distortion
    bone 756.9
    cervix (uteri) 752.49
        acquired 622.6
        hypertrophic 622.6
    colon 751.5
    common bile duct 751.69
    cystic duct 751.69
    frenulum, penis 752.69
    labia minora, acquired 624.8
    ligamentum patellae 756.89
    petiolus (epiglottidis) 748.3
    styloid bone (process) 733.99
    tooth, teeth 520.2
    uvula 750.26
        acquired 528.9
Elschnig bodies or pearls 366.51
El Tor cholera 001.1
Emaciation (due to malnutrition) 261
Emancipation disorder 309.22
Embadomoniasis 007.8
Embarrassment heart, cardiac - see
    Disease, heart
Embedded tooth, teeth 520.6
    root only 525.3
Embolic - see condition
Embolism 444.9
    with
        abortion - see Abortion, by type,
            with embolism
        ectopic pregnancy (see also
            categories 633.0–633.9) 639.6
        molar pregnancy (see also categories
            630–632) 639.6
    air (any site) 958.0
        with
            abortion - see Abortion, by type,
                with embolism
            ectopic pregnancy (see also
                categories 633.0–633.9)
                639.6
            molar pregnancy (see also
                categories 630–632)
                639.6

Embolism (Continued)
  air (Continued)
    due to implanted device - see
      Complications, due to
      (presence of) any device,
      implant, or graft classified to
      996.0–996.5 NEC
    following
      abortion 639.6
      ectopic or molar pregnancy 639.6
      infusion, perfusion, or
        transfusion 999.1
    in pregnancy, childbirth, or
      puerperium 673.0●
    traumatic 958.0
  amniotic fluid (pulmonary) 673.1●
    with
      abortion - see Abortion, by type,
        with embolism
      ectopic pregnancy (see also
        categories 633.0–633.9) 639.6
      molar pregnancy (see also
        categories 630–632) 639.6
    following
      abortion 639.6
      ectopic or molar pregnancy 639.6
  aorta, aortic 444.1
    abdominal 444.0
    bifurcation 444.0
    saddle 444.0
    thoracic 444.1
  artery 444.9
    auditory, internal 433.8●
    basilar (see also Occlusion, artery,
      basilar) 433.0●
    bladder 444.89
    carotid (common) (internal) (see also
      Occlusion, artery, carotid)
      433.1●
    cerebellar (anterior inferior)
      (posterior inferior) (superior)
      433.8●
    cerebral (see also Embolism, brain)
      434.1●
    choroidal (anterior) 433.8●
    communicating posterior 433.8●
    coronary (see also Infarct,
      myocardium) 410.9●
      without myocardial infarction
        411.81
    extremity 444.22
      lower 444.22
      upper 444.21
    hypophyseal 433.8●
    mesenteric (with gangrene)
      557.0
    ophthalmic (see also Occlusion,
      retina) 362.30
    peripheral 444.22
    pontine 433.8●
    precerebral NEC - see Occlusion,
      artery, precerebral
    pulmonary - see Embolism,
      pulmonary
    pyemic 449
      pulmonary 415.12
    renal 593.81
    retinal (see also Occlusion, retina)
      362.30
    septic 449
      pulmonary 415.12
    specified site NEC 444.89
    vertebral (see also Occlusion, artery,
      vertebral) 433.2●
  auditory, internal 433.8●
  basilar (artery) (see also Occlusion,
    artery, basilar) 433.0●

Embolism (Continued)
  birth, mother - see Embolism,
    obstetrical
  blood-clot
    with
      abortion - see Abortion, by type,
        with embolism
      ectopic pregnancy (see also
        categories 633.0–633.9) 639.6
      molar pregnancy (see also
        categories 630–632) 639.6
    following
      abortion 639.6
      ectopic or molar pregnancy 639.6
    in pregnancy, childbirth, or
      puerperium 673.2●
  brain 434.1●
    with
      abortion - see Abortion, by type,
        with embolism
      ectopic pregnancy (see also
        categories 633.0–633.9)
        639.6
      molar pregnancy (see also
        categories 630–632) 639.6
    following
      abortion 639.6
      ectopic or molar pregnancy 639.6
    late effect - see Late effect(s) (of)
      cerebrovascular disease
    puerperal, postpartum, childbirth
      674.0●
  capillary 448.9
  cardiac (see also Infarct, myocardium)
    410.9●
  carotid (artery) (common) (internal)
    (see also Occlusion, artery, carotid)
    433.1●
  cavernous sinus (venous) - see
    Embolism, intracranial venous
    sinus
  cerebral (see also Embolism, brain)
    434.1●
  cholesterol - see Atheroembolism
  choroidal (anterior) (artery) 433.8●
  coronary (artery or vein) (systemic) (see
    also Infarct, myocardium) 410.9●
    without myocardial infarction 411.81
  due to (presence of) any device,
    implant, or graft classifiable to
    996.0–996.5 - see Complications,
    due to (presence of) any device,
    implant, or graft classified to
    996.0–996.5 NEC
  encephalomalacia (see also Embolism,
    brain) 434.1●
  extremities 444.22
    lower 444.22
    upper 444.21
  eye 362.30
  fat (cerebral) (pulmonary) (systemic)
    958.1
    with
      abortion - see Abortion, by type,
        with embolism
      ectopic pregnancy (see also
        categories 633.0–633.9) 639.6
      molar pregnancy (see also
        categories 630–632) 639.6
    complicating delivery or
      puerperium 673.8●
    following
      abortion 639.6
      ectopic or molar pregnancy
        639.6
    in pregnancy, childbirth, or the
      puerperium 673.8●

Embolism (Continued)
  femoral (artery) 444.22
    vein 453.6
      deep 453.41
    following
      abortion 639.6
      ectopic or molar pregnancy
        639.6
      infusion, perfusion, or transfusion
        air 999.1
        thrombus 999.2
  heart (fatty) (see also Infarct,
    myocardium) 410.9●
  hepatic (vein) 453.0
  iliac (artery) 444.81
  iliofemoral 444.81
  in pregnancy, childbirth, or
    puerperium (pulmonary) - see
    Embolism, obstetrical
  intestine (artery) (vein) (with gangrene)
    557.0
  intracranial (see also Embolism, brain)
    434.1●
    venous sinus (any) 325
      late effect - see category 326
      nonpyogenic 437.6
        in pregnancy or puerperium
          671.5●
  kidney (artery) 593.81
  lateral sinus (venous) - see
    Embolism, intracranial venous
    sinus
  longitudinal sinus (venous) - see
    Embolism, intracranial venous
    sinus
  lower extremity 444.22
  lung (massive) - see Embolism,
    pulmonary
  meninges (see also Embolism, brain)
    434.1●
  mesenteric (artery) (with gangrene)
    557.0
  multiple NEC 444.9
  obstetrical (pulmonary) 673.2●
    air 673.0●
    amniotic fluid (pulmonary) 673.1●
    blood-clot 673.2●
    cardiac 674.8●
    fat 673.8●
    heart 674.8●
    pyemic 673.3●
    septic 673.3●
    specified NEC 674.8●
  ophthalmic (see also Occlusion, retina)
    362.30
  paradoxical NEC 444.9
  penis 607.82
  peripheral arteries NEC 444.22
    lower 444.22
    upper 444.21
  pituitary 253.8
  popliteal (artery) 444.22
  portal (vein) 452
  postoperative NEC 997.2
    cerebral 997.02
    mesenteric artery 997.71
    other vessels 997.79
    peripheral vascular 997.2
    pulmonary 415.11
      septic 415.11
    renal artery 997.72
  precerebral artery (see also
    Occlusion, artery, precerebral)
    433.9●
  puerperal - see Embolism,
    obstetrical

◀ New   ◀▥ Revised   ~~deleted~~ Deleted   ● Use Additional Digit(s)   ▨ Omit code

Embolism (Continued)
pulmonary (acute) (artery) (vein)
415.19 ◀
with
abortion - see Abortion, by type,
with embolism
ectopic pregnancy (see also
categories 633.0–633.9) 639.6
molar pregnancy (see also
categories 630–632) 639.6
chronic 416.2 ◀
following
abortion 639.6
ectopic or molar pregnancy 639.6
healed or old V12.51 ◀
iatrogenic 415.11
in pregnancy, childbirth, or
puerperium - see Embolism,
obstetrical
personal history of V12.51 ◀
postoperative 415.11
septic 415.12
pyemic (multiple) (see also Septicemia)
415.12
with
abortion - see Abortion, by type,
with embolism
ectopic pregnancy (see also
categories 633.0–633.9) 639.6
molar pregnancy (see also
categories 630–632) 639.6
Aerobacter aerogenes 415.12
enteric gram-negative bacilli 415.12

Enterobacter aerogenes 415.12
Escherichia coli 415.12
following
abortion 639.6
ectopic or molar pregnancy 639.6
Hemophilus influenzae 415.12
pneumococcal 415.12
Proteus vulgaris 415.12
Pseudomonas (aeruginosa) 415.12
puerperal, postpartum, childbirth
(any organism) 673.3●
Serratia 415.12
specified organism NEC 415.12
staphylococcal 415.12
aureus 415.12
specified organism NEC 415.12
streptococcal 415.12
renal (artery) 593.81
vein 453.3
retina, retinal (see also Occlusion, retina)
362.30
saddle (aorta) 444.0
septic 415.12
arterial 449
septicemic - see Embolism, pyemic
sinus - see Embolism, intracranial
venous sinus
soap
with
abortion - see Abortion, by type,
with embolism
ectopic pregnancy (see also
categories 633.0–633.9) 639.6
molar pregnancy (see also
categories 630–632) 639.6
following
abortion 639.6
ectopic or molar pregnancy 639.6
spinal cord (nonpyogenic) 336.1
in pregnancy or puerperium 671.5●
pyogenic origin 324.1
late effect - see category 326
spleen, splenic (artery) 444.89

Embolism (Continued)
thrombus (thromboembolism)
following infusion, perfusion, or
transfusion 999.2
upper extremity 444.21
vein 453.9
with inflammation or phlebitis - see
Thrombophlebitis
antecubital ◀
acute 453.81
chronic 453.71 ◀
axillary
acute 453.84 ◀
chronic 453.74 ◀
basilic
acute 453.81 ◀
chronic 453.71 ◀
brachial
acute 453.82 ◀
chronic 453.72 ◀
brachiocephalic (innominate)
acute 453.87 ◀
chronic 453.77 ◀
cephalic
acute 453.81 ◀
chronic 453.71 ◀
cerebral (see also Embolism, brain)
434.1●
coronary (see also Infarct,
myocardium) 410.9●
without myocardial infarction
411.81
hepatic 453.0
internal jugular ◀
acute 453.86 ◀
chronic 453.76 ◀
lower extremity (superficial)
453.6 ◀
deep 453.40
acute 453.40 ◀
calf 453.42 ◀
distal (lower leg) 453.42 ◀
femoral 453.41 ◀
iliac 453.41 ◀
lower leg 453.42 ◀
peroneal 453.42 ◀
popliteal 453.41 ◀
proximal (upper leg)
453.41 ◀
thigh 453.41 ◀
tibial 453.42 ◀
calf 453.42
chronic 453.50 ◀
calf 453.52 ◀
distal (lower leg) 453.52 ◀
femoral 453.51 ◀
iliac 453.51 ◀
lower leg 453.52 ◀
peroneal 453.52 ◀
popliteal 453.51 ◀
proximal (upper leg)
453.51 ◀
thigh 453.51 ◀
tibial 453.52 ◀
distal (lower leg) 453.42
femoral 453.41
iliac 453.41
lower leg 453.42
peroneal 453.42
popliteal 453.41
proximal (upper leg) 453.41
thigh 453.41
tibial 453.42
saphenous (greater) (lesser)
453.6 ◀
superficial 453.6 ◀

Embolism (Continued)
vein (Continued)
mesenteric (with gangrene) 557.0
portal 452
pulmonary - see Embolism, pulmonary
radial
acute 453.82 ◀
chronic 453.72 ◀
renal 453.3
saphenous (greater) (lesser) 453.6 ◀
specified NEC (acute) 453.89 ◀
chronic 453.79
with inflammation or phlebitis -
see Thrombophlebitis
subclavian ◀
acute 453.85 ◀
chronic 453.75 ◀
superior vena cava
acute 453.87 ◀
chronic 453.77 ◀
thoracic
acute 453.87 ◀
chronic 453.77 ◀
ulnar
acute 453.82 ◀
chronic 453.72 ◀
upper extremity 453.83 ◀
acute 453.83 ◀
deep 453.82 ◀
superficial 453.81 ◀
chronic 453.73 ◀
deep 453.72 ◀
superficial 453.71 ◀
vena cava (inferior) (superior) 453.2 ◀
inferior 453.2 ◀
superior
acute 453.87 ◀
chronic 453.77 ◀
vessels of brain (see also Embolism,
brain) 434.1●
Embolization - see Embolism
Embolus - see Embolism
Embryoma (M9080/1) - see also
Neoplasm, by site, uncertain
behavior
benign (M9080/0) - see Neoplasm, by
site, benign
kidney (M8960/3) 189.0
liver (M8970/3) 155.0
malignant (M9080/3) - see also
Neoplasm, by site, malignant
kidney (M8960/3) 189.0
liver (M8970/3) 155.0
testis (M9070/3) 186.9
undescended 186.0
testis (M9070/3) 186.9
undescended 186.0
Embryonic
circulation 747.9
heart 747.9
vas deferens 752.89
Embryopathia NEC 759.9
Embryotomy, fetal 763.89
Embryotoxon 743.43
interfering with vision 743.42
Emesis - see also Vomiting
bilious 787.04 ◀
gravidarum - see Hyperemesis,
gravidarum
Emissions, nocturnal (semen) 608.89
Emotional
crisis - see Crisis, emotional
disorder (see also Disorder, mental) 300.9
instability (excessive) 301.3
lability 799.24 ◀
overlay - see Reaction, adjustment
upset 300.9

Emotionality, pathological 301.3
Emotogenic disease (see also Disorder, psychogenic) 306.9
Emphysema (atrophic) (centriacinar) (centrilobular) (chronic) (diffuse) (essential) (hypertrophic) (interlobular) (lung) (obstructive) (panlobular) (paracicatricial) (paracinar) (postural) (pulmonary) (senile) (subpleural) (traction) (unilateral) (unilobular) (vesicular) 492.8
  with bronchitis
    chronic 491.20
      with
        acute bronchitis 491.22
        exacerbation (acute) 491.21
  bullous (giant) 492.0
  cellular tissue 958.7
    surgical 998.81
  compensatory 518.2
  congenital 770.2
  conjunctiva 372.89
  connective tissue 958.7
    surgical 998.81
  due to fumes or vapors 506.4
  eye 376.89
  eyelid 374.85
    surgical 998.81
    traumatic 958.7
  fetus or newborn (interstitial) (mediastinal) (unilobular) 770.2
  heart 416.9
  interstitial 518.1
    congenital 770.2
    fetus or newborn 770.2
  laminated tissue 958.7
    surgical 998.81
  mediastinal 518.1
    fetus or newborn 770.2
  newborn (interstitial) (mediastinal) (unilobular) 770.2
  obstructive diffuse with fibrosis 492.8
  orbit 376.89
  subcutaneous 958.7
    due to trauma 958.7
    nontraumatic 518.1
    surgical 998.81
  surgical 998.81
  thymus (gland) (congenital)254.8
  traumatic 958.7
  tuberculous (see also Tuberculosis, pulmonary) 011.9●
Employment examination (certification) V70.5
Empty sella (turcica) syndrome 253.8
Empyema (chest) (diaphragmatic) (double) (encapsulated) (general) (interlobar) (lung) (medial) (necessitatis) (perforating chest wall) (pleura) (pneumococcal) (residual) (sacculated) (streptococcal) (supradiaphragmatic) 510.9
  with fistula 510.0
  accessory sinus (chronic) (see also Sinusitis) 473.9
  acute 510.9
    with fistula 510.0
  antrum (chronic) (see also Sinusitis, maxillary) 473.0
  brain (any part) (see also Abscess, brain) 324.0
  ethmoidal (sinus) (chronic) (see also Sinusitis, ethmoidal) 473.2
  extradural (see also Abscess, extradural) 324.9

Empyema (Continued)
  frontal (sinus) (chronic) (see also Sinusitis, frontal) 473.1
  gallbladder (see also Cholecystitis, acute) 575.0
  mastoid (process) (acute) (see also Mastoiditis, acute) 383.00
  maxilla, maxillary 526.4
    sinus (chronic) (see also Sinusitis, maxillary) 473.0
  nasal sinus (chronic) (see also Sinusitis) 473.9
    sinus (accessory) (nasal) (see also Sinusitis) 473.9
  sphenoidal (chronic) (sinus) (see also Sinusitis, sphenoidal) 473.3
  subarachnoid (see also Abscess, extradural) 324.9
  subdural (see also Abscess, extradural) 324.9
  tuberculous (see also Tuberculosis, pleura) 012.0●
  ureter (see also Ureteritis) 593.89
  ventricular (see also Abscess, brain) 324.0
Enameloma 520.2
Encephalitis (bacterial) (chronic) (hemorrhagic) (idiopathic) (nonepidemic) (spurious) (subacute) 323.9
  acute - see also Encephalitis, viral
    disseminated (postinfectious) NEC 136.9 [323.61]
      postimmunization or postvaccination 323.51
    inclusional 049.8
    inclusion body 049.8
    necrotizing 049.8
  arboviral, arbovirus NEC 064
  arthropod-borne (see also Encephalitis, viral, arthropod-borne) 064
  Australian X 062.4
  Bwamba fever 066.3
  California (virus) 062.5
  Central European 063.2
  Czechoslovakian 063.2
  Dawson's (inclusion body) 046.2
  diffuse sclerosing 046.2
  due to
    actinomycosis 039.8 [323.41]
    cat-scratch disease 078.3 [323.01]
    human herpesvirus 6 058.21
    human herpesvirus 7 058.29
    human herpesvirus NEC 058.29
    infection classified elsewhere 136.9 [323.41]
    infectious mononucleosis 075 [323.01]
    malaria (see also Malaria) 084.6 [323.2]
    Negishi virus 064
    ornithosis 073.7 [323.01]
    prophylactic inoculation against smallpox 323.51
    rickettsiosis (see also Rickettsiosis) 083.9 [323.1]
    rubella 056.01
    toxoplasmosis (acquired) 130.0
      congenital (active) 771.2 [323.41]
    typhus (fever) (see also Typhus) 081.9 [323.1]
    vaccination (smallpox) 323.51
  Eastern equine 062.2
  endemic 049.8
  epidemic 049.8
  equine (acute) (infectious) (viral) 062.9
    eastern 062.2
    Venezuelan 066.2
    western 062.1

Encephalitis (Continued)
  Far Eastern 063.0
  following vaccination or other immunization procedure 323.51
  herpes 054.3
  human herpesvirus 6 058.21
  human herpesvirus 7 058.29
  human herpesvirus NEC 058.29
  Ilheus (virus) 062.8
  inclusion body 046.2
  infectious (acute) (virus) NEC 049.8
  influenzal 487.8 [323.41]
    lethargic 049.8
  Japanese (B type) 062.0
  La Crosse 062.5
  Langat 063.8
  late effect - see Late, effect, encephalitis
  lead 984.9 [323.71]
  lethargic (acute) (infectious) (influenzal) 049.8
  lethargica 049.8
  louping ill 063.1
  lupus 710.0 [323.81]
  lymphatica 049.0
  Mengo 049.8
  meningococcal 036.1
  mumps 072.2
  Murray Valley 062.4
  myoclonic 049.8
  Negishi virus 064
  otitic NEC 382.4 [323.41]
  parasitic NEC 123.9 [323.41]
  periaxialis (concentrica) (diffusa) 341.1
  postchickenpox 052.0
  postexanthematous NEC 057.9 [323.62]
  postimmunization 323.51
  postinfectious NEC 136.9 [323.62]
  postmeasles 055.0
  posttraumatic 323.81
  postvaccinal (smallpox) 323.51
  postvaricella 052.0
  postviral NEC 079.99 [323.62]
    postexanthematous 057.9 [323.62]
    specified NEC 057.8 [323.62]
  Powassan 063.8
  progressive subcortical (Binswanger's) 290.12
  Rasmussen 323.81
  Rio Bravo 049.8
  rubella 056.01
  Russian
    autumnal 062.0
    spring-summer type (taiga) 063.0
  saturnine 984.9 [323.71]
  Semliki Forest 062.8
  serous 048
  slow-acting virus NEC 046.8
  specified cause NEC 323.81
  St. Louis type 062.3
  subacute sclerosing 046.2
  subcorticalis chronica 290.12
  summer 062.0
  suppurative 324.0
  syphilitic 094.81
    congenital 090.41
  tick-borne 063.9
  torula, torular 117.5 [323.41]
  toxic NEC 989.9 [323.71]
  toxoplasmic (acquired) 130.0
    congenital (active) 771.2 [323.41]
  trichinosis 124 [323.41]
  Trypanosomiasis (see also Trypanosomiasis) 086.9 [323.2]
  tuberculous (see also Tuberculosis) 013.6●
  type B (Japanese) 062.0

◀ New   ◀▥ Revised   deleted Deleted   ● Use Additional Digit(s)   ▬ Omit code

Encephalitis (Continued)
  type C 062.3
  van Bogaert's 046.2
  Venezuelan 066.2
  Vienna type 049.8
  viral, virus 049.9
    arthropod-borne NEC 064
      mosquito-borne 062.9
        Australian X disease 062.4
        California virus 062.5
        Eastern equine 062.2
        Ilheus virus 062.8
        Japanese (B type) 062.0
        Murray Valley 062.4
        specified type NEC 062.8
        St. Louis 062.3
        type B 062.0
        type C 062.3
        Western equine 062.1
      tick-borne 063.9
        biundulant 063.2
        Central European 063.2
        Czechoslovakian 063.2
        diphasic meningoencephalitis
          063.2
        Far Eastern 063.0
        Langat 063.8
        louping ill 063.1
        Powassan 063.8
        Russian spring-summer (taiga)
          063.0
        specified type NEC 063.8
        vector unknown 064
      slow acting NEC 046.8
      specified type NEC 049.8
  vaccination, prophylactic (against)
    V05.0
  von Economo's 049.8
  Western equine 062.1
  West Nile type 066.41
Encephalocele 742.0
  orbit 376.81
Encephalocystocele 742.0
Encephalomalacia (brain) (cerebellar)
    (cerebral) (cerebrospinal) (see also
    Softening, brain) 434.9●
  due to
    hemorrhage (see also Hemorrhage,
      brain) 431
    recurrent spasm of artery 435.9
  embolic (cerebral) (see also Embolism,
    brain) 434.1●
  subcorticalis chronicus arteriosclerotica
    290.12
  thrombotic (see also Thrombosis, brain)
    434.0●
Encephalomeningitis - see
    Meningoencephalitis
Encephalomeningocele 742.0
Encephalomeningomyelitis - see
    Meningoencephalitis
Encephalomeningopathy (see also
    Meningoencephalitis) 349.9
Encephalomyelitis (chronic)
    (granulomatous) (myalgic, benign)
    (see also Encephalitis) 323.9
  abortive disseminated 049.8
  acute disseminated (ADEM)
    (postinfectious) 136.9
    [323.61]
    infectious 136.9 [323.61]
    noninfectious 323.81
    postimmunization 323.51
  due to
    cat-scratch disease 078.3 [323.01]
    infectious mononucleosis 075
      [323.01]

Encephalitis (Continued)
  due to (Continued)
    ornithosis 073.7 [323.01]
    vaccination (any) 323.51
  equine (acute) (infectious) 062.9
    eastern 062.2
    Venezuelan 066.2
    western 062.1
  funicularis infectiosa 049.8
  late effect - see Late, effect, encephalitis
  Munch-Peterson's 049.8
  postchickenpox 052.0
  postimmunization 323.51
  postmeasles 055.0
  postvaccinal (smallpox) 323.51
  rubella 056.01
  specified cause NEC 323.81
  syphilitic 094.81
  West Nile 066.41
Encephalomyelocele 742.0
Encephalomyelomeningitis - see
    Meningoencephalitis
Encephalomyeloneuropathy 349.9
Encephalomyelopathy 349.9
  subacute necrotizing (infantile) 330.8
Encephalomyeloradiculitis (acute) 357.0
Encephalomyeloradiculoneuritis (acute)
    357.0
Encephalomyeloradiculopathy 349.9
Encephalomyocarditis 074.23
Encephalopathia hyperbilirubinemica,
    newborn 774.7
  due to isoimmunization (conditions
    classifiable to 773.0–773.2) 773.4
Encephalopathy (acute) 348.30
  alcoholic 291.2
  anoxic - see Damage, brain, anoxic
  arteriosclerotic 437.0
    late effect - see Late effect(s) (of)
      cerebrovascular disease
  bilirubin, newborn 774.7
    due to isoimmunization 773.4
  congenital 742.9
  demyelinating (callosal) 341.8
  due to
    birth injury (intracranial) 767.8
    dialysis 294.8
      transient 293.9
    drugs - (see also Table of Drugs and
      Chemicals) 348.39
    hyperinsulinism - see
      Hyperinsulinism
    influenza (virus) 487.8
    lack of vitamin (see also Deficiency,
      vitamin) 269.2
    nicotinic acid deficiency 291.2
    serum (nontherapeutic)
      (therapeutic) 999.5
    syphilis 094.81
    trauma (postconcussional) 310.2
      current (see also Concussion,
        brain) 850.9
        with skull fracture - see
          Fracture, skull, by site,
          with intracranial injury
    vaccination 323.51
  hepatic 572.2
  hyperbilirubinemic, newborn 774.7
    due to isoimmunization (conditions
      classifiable to 773.0–773.2) 773.4
  hypertensive 437.2
  hypoglycemic 251.2
  hypoxic - see also Damage, brain, anoxic
    ischemic (HIE) 768.70 ◀▥
      mild 768.71 ◀
      moderate 768.72 ◀
      severe 768.73 ◀

Encephalopathy (Continued)
  infantile cystic necrotizing (congenital)
    341.8
  lead 984.9 [323.71]
  leukopolio 330.0
  metabolic (see also Delirium) 348.31
    toxic 349.82
  necrotizing
    hemorrhagic (acute) 323.61
    subacute 330.8
  other specified type NEC 348.39
  pellagrous 265.2
  portal-systemic 572.2
  postcontusional 310.2
  posttraumatic 310.2
  saturnine 984.9 [323.71]
  septic 348.31
  spongioform, subacute (viral) 046.19
  subacute
    necrotizing 330.8
    spongioform 046.19
    viral, spongioform 046.19
  subcortical progressive (Schilder) 341.1
    chronic (Binswanger's) 290.12
  toxic 349.82
    metabolic 349.82
  traumatic (postconcussional) 310.2
    current (see also Concussion, brain)
      850.9
        with skull fracture - see Fracture,
          skull, by site, with
          intracranial injury
  vitamin B deficiency NEC 266.9
  Wernicke's (superior hemorrhagic
    polioencephalitis) 265.1
Encephalorrhagia (see also Hemorrhage,
    brain) 432.9
  healed or old V12.54
  late effect - see Late effect(s) (of)
    cerebrovascular disease
Encephalosis, posttraumatic 310.2
Enchondroma (M9220/0) - see also
    Neoplasm, bone, benign
  multiple, congenital 756.4
Enchondromatosis (cartilaginous)
    (congenital) (multiple) 756.4
Enchondroses, multiple (cartilaginous)
    (congenital) 756.4
Encopresis (see also Incontinence, feces) 787.6
  nonorganic origin 307.7
Encounter for - see also Admission for
  administrative purpose only V68.9
    referral of patient without exami-
      nation or treatment V68.81
    specified purpose NEC V68.89
  chemotherapy, (oral) (intravenous),
    antineoplastic V58.11 ◀▥
  dialysis
    extracorporeal (renal) V56.0
    peritoneal V56.8
  disability examination V68.01
  end-of-life care V66.7
  hospice care V66.7
  immunizations (childhood)
    appropriate for age V20.2 ◀
  immunotherapy, antineoplastic V58.12
  palliative care V66.7
  paternity testing V70.4
  radiotherapy V58.0
  respirator [ventilator] dependence
    during
      mechanical failure V46.14
      power failure V46.12
    for weaning V46.13
  routine infant and child vision and
    hearing testing V20.2 ◀
  school examination V70.3 ◀
    following surgery V67.09 ◀

◀ New   ◀▥ Revised   ~~deleted~~ Deleted   ● Use Additional Digit(s)   ▥ Omit code

Encounter for *(Continued)*
  screening mammogram NEC V76.12
    for high-risk patient V76.11
  terminal care V66.7
  weaning from respirator [ventilator]
    V46.13
Encystment - *see* Cyst
End-of-life care V66.7
Endamebiasis - *see* Amebiasis
Endamoeba - *see* Amebiasis
Endarteritis (bacterial, subacute)
  (infective) (septic) 447.6
  brain, cerebral or cerebrospinal 437.4
    late effect - *see* Late effect(s) (of)
      cerebrovascular disease
  coronary (artery) - *see* Arteriosclerosis,
    coronary
  deformans - *see* Arteriosclerosis
  embolic (*see also* Embolism) 444.9
  obliterans - *see also* Arteriosclerosis
    pulmonary 417.8
  pulmonary 417.8
  retina 362.18
  senile - *see* Arteriosclerosis
  syphilitic 093.89
    brain or cerebral 094.89
    congenital 090.5
    spinal 094.89
  tuberculous (*see also* Tuberculosis)
    017.9●
Endemic - *see* condition
Endocarditis (chronic) (indeterminate)
  (interstitial) (marantic) (nonbacterial
  thrombotic) (residual) (sclerotic)
  (sclerous) (senile) (valvular) 424.90
  with
    rheumatic fever (conditions
      classifiable to 390)
      active - *see* Endocarditis, acute,
        rheumatic
      inactive or quiescent (with
        chorea) 397.9
  acute or subacute 421.9
    rheumatic (aortic) (mitral)
      (pulmonary) (tricuspid) 391.1
      with chorea (acute) (rheumatic)
        (Sydenham's) 392.0
  aortic (heart) (nonrheumatic) (valve)
    424.1
    with
      mitral (valve) disease 396.9
        active or acute 391.1
          with chorea (acute)
            (rheumatic)
            (Sydenham's) 392.0
        bacterial 421.0
      rheumatic fever (conditions
        classifiable to 390)
        active - *see* Endocarditis, acute,
          rheumatic
        inactive or quiescent (with
          chorea) 395.9
          with mitral disease 396.9
    acute or subacute 421.9
    arteriosclerotic 424.1
    congenital 746.89
    hypertensive 424.1
    rheumatic (chronic) (inactive) 395.9
      with mitral (valve) disease 396.9
        active or acute 391.1
          with chorea (acute)
            (rheumatic)
            (Sydenham's) 392.0
      active or acute 391.1
        with chorea (acute)
          (rheumatic)
          (Sydenham's) 392.0

Endocarditis *(Continued)*
  aortic *(Continued)*
    specified cause, except rheumatic
      424.1
    syphilitic 093.22
  arteriosclerotic or due to
    arteriosclerosis 424.99
  atypical verrucous (Libman-Sacks)
    710.0 *[424.91]*
  bacterial (acute) (any valve) (chronic)
    (subacute) 421.0
  blastomycotic 116.0 *[421.1]*
  candidal 112.81
  congenital 425.3
  constrictive 421.0
  Coxsackie 074.22
  due to
    blastomycosis 116.0 *[421.1]*
    candidiasis 112.81
    Coxsackie (virus) 074.22
    disseminated lupus erythematosus
      710.0 *[424.91]*
    histoplasmosis (*see also*
      Histoplasmosis) 115.94
    hypertension (benign) 424.99
    moniliasis 112.81
    prosthetic cardiac valve 996.61
    Q fever 083.0 *[421.1]*
    serratia marcescens 421.0
    typhoid (fever) 002.0 *[421.1]*
  fetal 425.3
  gonococcal 098.84
  hypertensive 424.99
  infectious or infective (acute) (any
    valve) (chronic) (subacute)
    421.0
  lenta (acute) (any valve) (chronic)
    (subacute) 421.0
  Libman-Sacks 710.0 *[424.91]*
  Loeffler's (parietal fibroplastic)
    421.0
  malignant (acute) (any valve) (chronic)
    (subacute) 421.0
  meningococcal 036.42
  mitral (chronic) (double) (fibroid)
    (heart) (inactive) (valve) (with
    chorea) 394.9
    with
      aortic (valve) disease 396.9
        active or acute 391.1
          with chorea (acute)
            (rheumatic)
            (Sydenham's) 392.0
      rheumatic fever (conditions
        classifiable to 390)
        active - *see* Endocarditis,
          acute, rheumatic
        inactive or quiescent (with
          chorea) 394.9
          with aortic valve disease
            396.9
    active or acute 391.1
      with chorea (acute) (rheumatic)
        (Sydenham's) 392.0
      bacterial 421.0
    arteriosclerotic 424.0
    congenital 746.89
    hypertensive 424.0
    nonrheumatic 424.0
      acute or subacute 421.9
    syphilitic 093.21
  monilial 112.81
  mycotic (acute) (any valve) (chronic)
    (subacute) 421.0
  pneumococcic (acute) (any valve)
    (chronic) (subacute)
    421.0

Endocarditis *(Continued)*
  pulmonary (chronic) (heart) (valve) 424.3
    with
      rheumatic fever (conditions
        classifiable to 390)
        active - *see* Endocarditis, acute,
          rheumatic
        inactive or quiescent (with
          chorea) 397.1
    acute or subacute 421.9
      rheumatic 391.1
        with chorea (acute)
          (rheumatic)
          (Sydenham's) 392.0
    arteriosclerotic or due to
      arteriosclerosis 424.3
    congenital 746.09
    hypertensive or due to hypertension
      (benign) 424.3
    rheumatic (chronic) (inactive) (with
      chorea) 397.1
      active or acute 391.1
        with chorea (acute)
          (rheumatic)
          (Sydenham's) 392.0
    syphilitic 093.24
  purulent (acute) (any valve) (chronic)
    (subacute) 421.0
  rheumatic (chronic) (inactive) (with
    chorea) 397.9
    active or acute (aortic) (mitral)
      (pulmonary) (tricuspid) 391.1
      with chorea (acute) (rheumatic)
        (Sydenham's) 392.0
  septic (acute) (any valve) (chronic)
    (subacute) 421.0
  specified cause, except rheumatic
    424.99
  streptococcal (acute) (any valve)
    (chronic) (subacute) 421.0
  subacute - *see* Endocarditis, acute
  suppurative (any valve) (acute)
    (chronic) (subacute) 421.0
  syphilitic NEC 093.20
  toxic (*see also* Endocarditis, acute) 421.9
  tricuspid (chronic) (heart) (inactive)
    (rheumatic) (valve) (with chorea)
    397.0
    with
      rheumatic fever (conditions
        classifiable to 390)
        active - *see* Endocarditis, acute,
          rheumatic
        inactive or quiescent (with
          chorea) 397.0
    active or acute 391.1
      with chorea (acute) (rheumatic)
        (Sydenham's) 392.0
    arteriosclerotic 424.2
    congenital 746.89
    hypertensive 424.2
    nonrheumatic 424.2
      acute or subacute 421.9
    specified cause, except rheumatic
      424.2
    syphilitic 093.23
  tuberculous (*see also* Tuberculosis)
    017.9● *[424.91]*
  typhoid 002.0 *[421.1]*
  ulcerative (acute) (any valve) (chronic)
    (subacute) 421.0
  vegetative (acute) (any valve) (chronic)
    (subacute) 421.0
  verrucous (acute) (any valve) (chronic)
    (subacute) NEC 710.0 *[424.91]*
    nonbacterial 710.0 *[424.91]*
    nonrheumatic 710.0 *[424.91]*

◄ New   ◄▌ Revised   ~~deleted~~ Deleted   ● Use Additional Digit(s)   ▬ Omit code

Endocardium, endocardial - *see also* condition
  cushion defect 745.60
    specified type NEC 745.69
Endocervicitis (*see also* Cervicitis) 616.0
  due to
    intrauterine (contraceptive) device 996.65
  gonorrheal (acute) 098.15
    chronic or duration of 2 months or over 098.35
  hyperplastic 616.0
  syphilitic 095.8
  trichomonal 131.09
  tuberculous (*see also* Tuberculosis) 016.7●
Endocrine - *see* condition
Endocrinopathy, pluriglandular 258.9
Endodontitis 522.0
Endomastoiditis (*see also* Mastoiditis) 383.9
Endometrioma 617.9
Endometriosis 617.9
  appendix 617.5
  bladder 617.8
  bowel 617.5
  broad ligament 617.3
  cervix 617.0
  colon 617.5
  cul-de-sac (Douglas') 617.3
  exocervix 617.0
  fallopian tube 617.2
  female genital organ NEC 617.8
  gallbladder 617.8
  in scar of skin 617.6
  internal 617.0
  intestine 617.5
  lung 617.8
  myometrium 617.0
  ovary 617.1
  parametrium 617.3
  pelvic peritoneum 617.3
  peritoneal (pelvic) 617.3
  rectovaginal septum 617.4
  rectum 617.5
  round ligament 617.3
  skin 617.6
  specified site NEC 617.8
  stromal (M8931/1) 236.0
  umbilicus 617.8
  uterus 617.0
    internal 617.0
  vagina 617.4
  vulva 617.8
Endometritis (nonspecific) (purulent) (septic) (suppurative) 615.9
  with
    abortion - *see* Abortion, by type, with sepsis
    ectopic pregnancy (*see also* categories 633.0-633.9) 639.0
    molar pregnancy (*see also* categories 630-632) 639.0
  acute 615.0
  blennorrhagic 098.16
    acute 098.16
    chronic or duration of 2 months or over 098.36
  cervix, cervical (*see also* Cervicitis) 616.0
    hyperplastic 616.0
  chronic 615.1
  complicating pregnancy 670.1   ◀▥
    affecting fetus or newborn 760.8
    septic 670.2   ◀
  decidual 615.9
  following
    abortion 639.0
    ectopic or molar pregnancy 639.0

Endometritis (*Continued*)
  gonorrheal (acute) 098.16
    chronic or duration of 2 months or over 098.36
  hyperplastic (*see also* Hyperplasia, endometrium) 621.30
    cervix 616.0
  polypoid - *see* Endometritis, hyperplastic
  puerperal, postpartum, childbirth 670.1   ◀▥
    septic 670.2   ◀
  senile (atrophic) 615.9
  subacute 615.0
  tuberculous (*see also* Tuberculosis) 016.7●
Endometrium - *see* condition
Endomyocardiopathy, South African 425.2
Endomyocarditis - *see* Endocarditis
Endomyofibrosis 425.0
Endomyometritis (*see also* Endometritis) 615.9
Endopericarditis - *see* Endocarditis
Endoperineuritis - *see* Disorder, nerve
Endophlebitis (*see also* Phlebitis) 451.9
  leg 451.2
    deep (vessels) 451.19
    superficial (vessels) 451.0
  portal (vein) 572.1
  retina 362.18
  specified site NEC 451.89
  syphilitic 093.89
Endophthalmia (*see also* Endophthalmitis) 360.00
  gonorrheal 098.42
Endophthalmitis (globe) (infective) (metastatic) (purulent) (subacute) 360.00
  acute 360.01
  bleb associated 379.63
  chronic 360.03
  parasitic 360.13
  phacoanaphylactic 360.19
  specified type NEC 360.19
  sympathetic 360.11
Endosalpingioma (M9111/1) 236.2
Endosalpingiosis 629.89
Endosteitis - *see* Osteomyelitis
Endothelioma, bone (M9260/3) - *see* Neoplasm, bone, malignant
Endotheliosis 287.8
  hemorrhagic infectional 287.8
Endotoxemia - *code to* condition
Endotoxic shock 785.52
Endotrachelitis (*see also* Cervicitis) 616.0
Enema rash 692.89
Engel-von Recklinghausen disease or syndrome (osteitis fibrosa cystica) 252.01
Engelmann's disease (diaphyseal sclerosis) 756.59
English disease (*see also* Rickets) 268.0
Engman's disease (infectious eczematoid dermatitis) 690.8
Engorgement
  breast 611.79
    newborn 778.7
    puerperal, postpartum 676.2●
  liver 573.9
  lung 514
  pulmonary 514
  retina, venous 362.37
  stomach 536.8
  venous, retina 362.37
Enlargement, enlarged - *see also* Hypertrophy

Enlargement, enlarged (*Continued*)
  abdomen 789.3●
  adenoids 474.12
    and tonsils 474.10
  alveolar process or ridge 525.8
  apertures of diaphragm (congenital) 756.6
  blind spot, visual field 368.42
  gingival 523.8
  heart, cardiac (*see also* Hypertrophy, cardiac) 429.3
  lacrimal gland, chronic 375.03
  liver (*see also* Hypertrophy, liver) 789.1
  lymph gland or node 785.6
  orbit 376.46
  organ or site, congenital NEC - *see* Anomaly, specified type NEC
  parathyroid (gland) 252.01
  pituitary fossa 793.0
  prostate (simple) (soft) 600.00
    with
      other lower urinary tract symptoms (LUTS) 600.01
      urinary
        obstruction 600.01
        retention 600.01
  sella turcica 793.0
  spleen (*see also* Splenomegaly) 789.2
    congenital 759.0
  thymus (congenital) (gland) 254.0
  thyroid (gland) (*see also* Goiter) 240.9
  tongue 529.8
  tonsils 474.11
    and adenoids 474.10
  uterus 621.2
Enophthalmos 376.50
  due to
    atrophy of orbital tissue 376.51
    surgery 376.52
    trauma 376.52
Enostosis 526.89
Entamebiasis - *see* Amebiasis
Entamebic - *see* Amebiasis
Entanglement, umbilical cord(s) 663.3●
  with compression 663.2●
  affecting fetus or newborn 762.5
  around neck with compression 663.1●
  twins in monoamniotic sac 663.2●
Enteralgia 789.0●
Enteric - *see* condition
Enteritis (acute) (catarrhal) (choleraic) (chronic) (congestive) (diarrheal) (exudative) (follicular) (hemorrhagic) (infantile) (lienteric) (noninfectious) (perforative) (phlegmonous) (presumed noninfectious) (pseudomembranous) 558.9
  adaptive 564.9
  aertrycke infection 003.0
  allergic 558.3
  amebic (*see also* Amebiasis) 006.9
    with abscess - *see* Abscess, amebic
    acute 006.0
      with abscess - *see* Abscess, amebic nondysenteric 006.2
    chronic 006.1
      with abscess - *see* Abscess, amebic nondysenteric 006.2
    nondysenteric 006.2
  anaerobic (cocci) (gram-negative) (gram-positive) (mixed) NEC 008.46
  bacillary NEC 004.9
  bacterial NEC 008.5
    specified NEC 008.49

Enteritis *(Continued)*
 Bacteroides (fragilis)
   (melaninogeniscus) (oralis) 008.46
 Butyrivibrio (fibriosolvens) 008.46
 Campylobacter 008.43
 Candida 112.85
 Chilomastix 007.8
 choleriformis 001.1
 chronic 558.9
   ulcerative *(see also* Colitis, ulcerative)
     556.9
 cicatrizing (chronic) 555.0
 Clostridium
   botulinum 005.1
   difficile 008.45
   haemolyticum 008.46
   novyi 008.46
   perfringens (C) (F) 008.46
   specified type NEC 008.46
 coccidial 007.2
 dietetic 558.9
 due to
   achylia gastrica 536.8
   adenovirus 008.62
   Aerobacter aerogenes 008.2
   anaerobes *(see also* Enteritis,
     anaerobic) 008.46
   Arizona (bacillus) 008.1
   astrovirus 008.66
   Bacillus coli - *see* Enteritis, E. coli
   bacteria NEC 008.5
     specified NEC 008.49
   Bacteroides *(see also* Enteritis,
     Bacteroides) 008.46
   Butyrivibrio (fibriosolvens)
     008.46
   calicivirus 008.65   ◄▥
   Campylobacter 008.43
   Clostridium - *see* Enteritis,
     Clostridium
   Cockle agent 008.64
   Coxsackie (virus) 008.67
   Ditchling agent 008.64
   ECHO virus 008.67
   Enterobacter aerogenes 008.2
   enterococci 008.49
   enterovirus NEC 008.67
   Escherichia coli - *see* Enteritis, E. coli
   Eubacterium 008.46
   Fusobacterium (nucleatum) 008.46
   gram-negative bacteria NEC 008.47
     anaerobic NEC 008.46
   Hawaii agent 008.63
   irritating foods 558.9
   Klebsiella aerogenes 008.47
   Marin County agent 008.66
   Montgomery County agent 008.63
   noroviris 008.63   ◄
   Norwalk-like agent 008.63
   Norwalk virus 008.63
   Otofuke agent 008.63
   Paracolobactrum arizonae 008.1
   paracolon bacillus NEC 008.47
     Arizona 008.1
   Paramatta agent 008.64
   Peptococcus 008.46
   Peptostreptococcus 008.46
   Proprionibacterium 008.46
   Proteus (bacillus) (mirabilis)
     (morganii) 008.3
   Pseudomonas aeruginosa 008.42
   Rotavirus 008.61
   Sapporo agent 008.63
   small round virus (SRV) NEC
     008.64
     featureless NEC 008.63
     structured NEC 008.63

Enteritis *(Continued)*
 due to *(Continued)*
   Snow Mountain (SM) agent 008.63
   specified
     bacteria NEC 008.49
     organism, nonbacterial NEC 008.8
     virus NEC 008.69
   Staphylococcus 008.41
   Streptococcus 008.49
     anaerobic 008.46
   Taunton agent 008.63
   Torovirus 008.69
   Treponema 008.46
   Veillonella 008.46
   virus 008.8
     specified type NEC 008.69
   Wollan (W) agent 008.64
   Yersinia enterocolitica 008.44
 dysentery - *see* Dysentery
 E. coli 008.00
   enterohemorrhagic 008.04
   enteroinvasive 008.03
   enteropathogenic 008.01
   enterotoxigenic 008.02
   specified type NEC 008.09
 El Tor 001.1
 embadomonial 007.8
 eosinophilic 558.41
 epidemic 009.0
 Eubacterium 008.46
 fermentative 558.9
 fulminant 557.0
 Fusobacterium (nucleatum) 008.46
 gangrenous *(see also* Enteritis, due to,
   by organism) 009.0
 giardial 007.1
 gram-negative bacteria NEC 008.47
   anaerobic NEC 008.46
 infectious NEC *(see also* Enteritis, due
   to, by organism) 009.0
   presumed 009.1
 influenzal 487.8
 ischemic 557.9
   acute 557.0
   chronic 557.1
   due to mesenteric artery
     insufficiency 557.1
 membranous 564.9
 mucous 564.9
 myxomembranous 564.9
 necrotic *(see also* Enteritis, due to, by
   organism) 009.0
 necroticans 005.2
 necrotizing of fetus or newborn *(see also*
   Enterocolitis, necrotizing,
   newborn) 777.50
 neurogenic 564.9
 newborn 777.8
   necrotizing *(see also* Enterocolitis,
     necrotizing, newborn)
     777.50
 parasitic NEC 129
 paratyphoid (fever) *(see also* Fever,
   paratyphoid) 002.9
 Peptococcus 008.46
 Peptostreptococcus 008.46
 Proprionibacterium 008.46
 protozoal NEC 007.9
 radiation 558.1
 regional (of) 555.9
   intestine
     large (bowel, colon, or rectum)
       555.1
       with small intestine 555.2
     small (duodenum, ileum, or
       jejunum) 555.0
       with large intestine 555.2

Enteritis *(Continued)*
 Salmonella infection 003.0
 salmonellosis 003.0
 segmental *(see also* Enteritis, regional)
   555.9
 septic *(see also* Enteritis, due to, by
   organism) 009.0
 Shigella 004.9
 simple 558.9
 spasmodic 564.9
 spastic 564.9
 staphylococcal 008.41
   due to food 005.0
 streptococcal 008.49
   anaerobic 008.46
 toxic 558.2
 Treponema (denticola) (macrodentium)
   008.46
 trichomonal 007.3
 tuberculous *(see also* Tuberculosis) 014.8●
 typhosa 002.0
 ulcerative (chronic) *(see also* Colitis,
   ulcerative) 556.9
 Veillonella 008.46
 viral 008.8
   adenovirus 008.62
   enterovirus 008.67
   specified virus NEC 008.69
 Yersinia enterocolitica 008.44
 zymotic 009.0
Enteroarticular syndrome 099.3
Enterobiasis 127.4
Enterobius vermicularis 127.4
Enterocele *(see also* Hernia) 553.9
 pelvis, pelvic (acquired) (congenital)
   618.6
 vagina, vaginal (acquired) (congenital)
   618.6
Enterocolitis - *see also* Enteritis
 fetus or newborn *(see also* Enterocolitis,
   necrotizing, newborn) 777.8
   necrotizing 777.50
 fulminant 557.0
 granulomatous 555.2
 hemorrhagic (acute) 557.0
   chronic 557.1
 necrotizing (acute) (membranous) 557.0
   newborn 777.50
     with
       perforation 777.53
       pneumatosis without
         perforation 777.52
       pneumatosis and perforation
         777.53
     without pneumatosis, without
       perforation 777.51   ◄
     stage I 777.51
     stage II 777.52
     stage III 777.53
 primary necrotizing *(see also*
   Enterocolitis, necrotizing,
   newborn) 777.50
 pseudomembranous 008.45
   newborn 008.45   ◄
 radiation 558.1
   newborn *(see also* Enterocolitis,
     necrotizing, newborn) 777.50
 ulcerative 556.0
Enterocystoma 751.5
Enterogastritis - *see* Enteritis
Enterogenous cyanosis 289.7
Enterolith, enterolithiasis (impaction)
 560.39
 with hernia - *see also* Hernia, by site,
   with obstruction
   gangrenous - *see* Hernia, by site,
     with gangrene

Enteropathy 569.9
  exudative (of Gordon) 579.8
  gluten 579.0
  hemorrhagic, terminal 557.0
  protein-losing 579.8
Enteroperitonitis (see also Peritonitis)
  567.9
Enteroptosis 569.89
Enterorrhagia 578.9
Enterospasm 564.9
  psychogenic 306.4
Enterostenosis (see also Obstruction,
  intestine) 560.9
Enterostomy status V44.4
  with complication 569.60
Enthesopathy 726.90
  ankle and tarsus 726.70
  elbow region 726.30
    specified NEC 726.39
  hip 726.5
  knee 726.60
  peripheral NEC 726.8
  shoulder region 726.10
    adhesive 726.0
  spinal 720.1
  wrist and carpus 726.4
Entrance, air into vein - see Embolism,
  air
Entrapment, nerve - see Neuropathy,
  entrapment
Entropion (eyelid) 374.00
  cicatricial 374.04
  congenital 743.62
  late effect of trachoma (healed)
    139.1
  mechanical 374.02
  paralytic 374.02
  senile 374.01
  spastic 374.03
Enucleation of eye (current) (traumatic)
  871.3
Enuresis 788.30
  habit disturbance 307.6
  nocturnal 788.36
    psychogenic 307.6
  nonorganic origin 307.6
  psychogenic 307.6
Enzymopathy 277.9
Eosinopenia 288.59
Eosinophilia 288.3
  allergic 288.3
  hereditary 288.3
  idiopathic 288.3
  infiltrative 518.3
  Loeffler's 518.3
  myalgia syndrome 710.5
  pulmonary (tropical) 518.3
  secondary 288.3
  tropical 518.3
Eosinophilic - see also condition
  fasciitis 728.89
  granuloma (bone) 277.89
  infiltration lung 518.3
Ependymitis (acute) (cerebral) (chronic)
  (granular) (see also Meningitis)
  322.9
Ependymoblastoma (M9392/3)
  specified site - see Neoplasm, by site,
    malignant
  unspecified site 191.9
Ependymoma (epithelial) (malignant)
  (M9391/3)
  anaplastic type (M9392/3)
    specified site - see Neoplasm, by site,
      malignant
    unspecified site 191.9

Ependymoma (Continued)
  benign (M9391/0)
    specified site - see Neoplasm, by site,
      benign
    unspecified site 225.0
  myxopapillary (M9394/1) 237.5
  papillary (M9393/1) 237.5
  specified site - see Neoplasm, by site,
    malignant
  unspecified site 191.9
Ependymopathy 349.2
  spinal cord 349.2
Ephelides, ephelis 709.09
Ephemeral fever (see also Pyrexia)
  780.60
Epiblepharon (congenital) 743.62
Epicanthus, epicanthic fold (congenital)
  (eyelid) 743.63
Epicondylitis (elbow) (lateral) 726.32
  medial 726.31
Epicystitis (see also Cystitis) 595.9
Epidemic - see condition
Epidermidalization, cervix - see condition
Epidermidization, cervix - see condition
Epidermis, epidermal - see condition
Epidermization, cervix - see condition
Epidermodysplasia verruciformis
  078.19
Epidermoid
  cholesteatoma - see Cholesteatoma
  inclusion (see also Cyst, skin) 706.2
Epidermolysis
  acuta (combustiformis) (toxica)
    695.15
  bullosa 757.39
  necroticans combustiformis 695.15
    due to drug
      correct substance properly
        administered 695.15
      overdose or wrong substance
        given or taken 977.9
      specified drug - see Table of
        Drugs and Chemicals
Epidermophytid - see Dermatophytosis
Epidermophytosis (infected) - see
  Dermatophytosis
Epidermosis, ear (middle) (see also
  Cholesteatoma) 385.30
Epididymis - see condition
Epididymitis (nonvenereal) 604.90
  with abscess 604.0
  acute 604.99
  blennorrhagic (acute) 098.0
    chronic or duration of 2 months or
      over 098.2
  caseous (see also Tuberculosis) 016.4 ●
  chlamydial 099.54
  diphtheritic 032.89 [604.91]
  filarial 125.9 [604.91]
  gonococcal (acute) 098.0
    chronic or duration of 2 months or
      over 098.2
  recurrent 604.99
  residual 604.99
  syphilitic 095.8 [604.91]
  tuberculous (see also Tuberculosis)
    016.4 ●
Epididymo-orchitis (see also Epididymitis)
  604.90
  with abscess 604.0
  chlamydial 099.54
  gonococcal (acute) 098.13
    chronic or duration of 2 months or
      over 098.33
Epidural - see condition
Epigastritis (see also Gastritis) 535.5 ●
Epigastrium, epigastric - see condition

Epigastrocele (see also Hernia, epigastric)
  553.29
Epiglottiditis (acute) 464.30
  with obstruction 464.31
  chronic 476.1
  viral 464.30
    with obstruction 464.31
Epiglottis - see condition
Epiglottitis (acute) 464.30
  with obstruction 464.31
  chronic 476.1
  viral 464.30
    with obstruction 464.31
Epignathus 759.4
Epilepsia
  partialis continua (see also Epilepsy)
    345.7 ●
  procursiva (see also Epilepsy)
    345.8 ●
Epilepsy, epileptic (idiopathic)
  345.9 ●

Note 26   use the following fifth-digit
subclassifications with categories 345.0,
345.1, 345.4–345.9

0   without mention of intractable
        epilepsy
1   with intractable epilepsy
        pharmacoresistant
          (pharmacologically
            resistant)   ◄
        poorly controlled   ◄
        refractory (medically) ◄
        treatment resistant   ◄

  abdominal 345.5 ●
  absence (attack) 345.0 ●
  akinetic 345.0 ●
    psychomotor 345.4 ●
  automatism 345.4 ●
  autonomic diencephalic 345.5 ●
  brain 345.9 ●
  Bravais-Jacksonian 345.5 ●
  cerebral 345.9 ●
  climacteric 345.9 ●
  clonic 345.1 ●
  clouded state 345.9 ●
  coma 345.3 ●
  communicating 345.4 ●
  complicating pregnancy, childbirth, or
    the puerperium 649.4 ●
  congenital 345.9 ●
  convulsions 345.9 ●
  cortical (focal) (motor) 345.5 ●
  cursive (running) 345.8 ●
  cysticercosis 123.1
  deterioration
    with behavioral disturbance 345.9 ●
      [294.11]
    without behavioral disturbance
      345.9 ● [294.10]
  due to syphilis 094.89
  equivalent 345.5 ●
  fit 345.9 ●
  focal (motor) 345.5 ●
  gelastic 345.8 ●
  generalized 345.9 ●
    convulsive 345.1 ●
    flexion 345.1 ●
    nonconvulsive 345.0 ●
  grand mal (idiopathic) 345.1 ●
  Jacksonian (motor) (sensory)
    345.5 ●
  Kojevnikoff's, Kojevnikov's,
    Kojewnikoff's 345.7 ●
  laryngeal 786.2
  limbic system 345.4 ●

Epilepsy, epileptic *(Continued)*
  localization related (focal) (partial) and
      epileptic syndromes
    with
        complex partial seizures 345.4●
        simple partial seizures 345.5●
    major (motor) 345.1●
    minor 345.0●
    mixed (type) 345.9●
    motor partial 345.5●
    musicogenic 345.1●
    myoclonus, myoclonic 345.1●
        progressive (familial) 345.1   ◀▥
    nonconvulsive, generalized
        345.0●
    parasitic NEC 123.9
    partial (focalized) 345.5●
    with
        impairment of consciousness
            345.4●
        memory and ideational
            disturbances 345.4●
        without impairment of
            consciousness 345.5●
        abdominal type 345.5●
        motor type 345.5●
        psychomotor type 345.4●
        psychosensory type 345.4●
        secondarily generalized
            345.4●
        sensory type 345.5●
        somatomotor type 345.5●
        somatosensory type 345.5●
        temporal lobe type 345.4●
        visceral type 345.5●
        visual type 345.5●
    peripheral 345.9●
    petit mal 345.0●
    photokinetic 345.8●
    progressive myoclonic (familial)
        345.1   ◀▥
    psychic equivalent 345.5●
    psychomotor 345.4●
    psychosensory 345.4●
    reflex 345.1●
    seizure 345.9●
    senile 345.9●
    sensory-induced 345.5●
    sleep *(see also* Narcolepsy) 347.00
    somatomotor type 345.5●
    somatosensory 345.5●
    specified type NEC 345.8●
    status (grand mal) 345.3
        focal motor 345.7●
        petit mal 345.2●
        psychomotor 345.7●
        temporal lobe 345.7●
    symptomatic 345.9●
    temporal lobe 345.4●
    tonic (-clonic) 345.1●
    traumatic (injury unspecified)
        907.0
        injury specified - *see* Late, effect (of)
            specified injury
    twilight 293.0
    uncinate (gyrus) 345.4●
    Unverricht (-Lundborg) (familial
        myoclonic) 345.1   ◀▥
    visceral 345.5●
    visual 345.5●
Epileptiform
    convulsions 780.39
    seizure 780.39
Epiloia 759.5
Epimenorrhea 626.2
Epipharyngitis *(see also* Nasopharyngitis)
    460

Epiphora 375.20
    due to
        excess lacrimation 375.21
        insufficient drainage 375.22
Epiphyseal arrest 733.91
    femoral head 732.2
Epiphyseolysis, epiphysiolysis *(see also*
    Osteochondrosis) 732.9
Epiphysitis *(see also* Osteochondrosis)
    732.9
    juvenile 732.6
    marginal (Scheuermann's) 732.0
    os calcis 732.5
    syphilitic (congenital) 090.0
    vertebral (Scheuermann's) 732.0
Epiplocele *(see also* Hernia)553.9
Epiploitis *(see also* Peritonitis) 567.9
Epiplosarcomphalocele *(see also* Hernia,
    umbilicus) 553.1
Episcleritis 379.00
    gouty 274.89 *[379.09]*
    nodular 379.02
    periodica fugax 379.01
        angioneurotic - *see* Edema,
            angioneurotic
    specified NEC 379.09
    staphylococcal 379.00
    suppurative 379.00
    syphilitic 095.0
    tuberculous *(see also* Tuberculosis)
        017.3● *[379.09]*
Episode
    brain *(see also* Disease, cerebrovascular,
        acute) 436
    cerebral *(see also* Disease,
        cerebrovascular, acute) 436
    depersonalization (in neurotic
        state) 300.6
    hyporesponsive 780.09
    psychotic *(see also* Psychosis) 298.9
        organic, transient 293.9
    schizophrenic (acute) NEC *(see also*
        Schizophrenia) 295.4●
Epispadias
    female 753.8
    male 752.62
Episplenitis 289.59
Epistaxis (multiple) 784.7
    hereditary 448.0
    vicarious menstruation 625.8
Epithelioma (malignant) (M8011/3) - *see*
    also Neoplasm, by site, malignant
    adenoides cysticum (M8100/0) - *see*
        Neoplasm, skin, benign
    basal cell (M8090/3) - *see* Neoplasm,
        skin, malignant
    benign (M8011/0) - *see* Neoplasm, by
        site, benign
    Bowen's (M8081/2) - *see* Neoplasm,
        skin, in situ
    calcifying (benign) (Malherbe's)
        (M8110/0) - *see* Neoplasm, skin,
        benign
    external site - *see* Neoplasm, skin,
        malignant
    intraepidermal, Jadassohn (M8096/0) -
        see Neoplasm, skin, benign
    squamous cell (M8070/3) - *see*
        Neoplasm, by site, malignant
Epitheliopathy
    pigment, retina 363.15
    posterior multifocal placoid (acute)
        363.15
Epithelium, epithelial - *see* condition
Epituberculosis (allergic) (with
    atelectasis) *(see also* Tuberculosis)
    010.8●

Eponychia 757.5
Epstein's
    nephrosis or syndrome *(see also*
        Nephrosis) 581.9
    pearl (mouth) 528.4
Epstein-Barr infection (viral) 075
    chronic 780.79 *[139.8]*
Epulis (giant cell) (gingiva) 523.8
Equinia 024
Equinovarus (congenital) 754.51
    acquired 736.71
Equivalent
    angina 413.9   ◀
    convulsive (abdominal) *(see also*
        Epilepsy) 345.5●
    epileptic (psychic) *(see also* Epilepsy)
        345.5●
Erb's
    disease 359.1
    palsy, paralysis (birth) (brachial)
        (newborn) 767.6
        spinal (spastic) syphilitic 094.89
    pseudohypertrophic muscular
        dystrophy 359.1
Erb (-Duchenne) paralysis (birth injury)
    (newborn) 767.6
Erb-Goldflam disease or syndrome
    358.00
Erdheim-Chester disease (ECD) 277.89   ◀
Erdheim's syndrome (acromegalic
    macrospondylitis) 253.0
Erection, painful (persistent) 607.3
Ergosterol deficiency (vitamin D) 268.9
    with
        osteomalacia 268.2
        rickets *(see also* Rickets) 268.0
Ergotism (ergotized grain) 988.2
    from ergot used as drug (migraine
        therapy)
        correct substance properly
            administered 349.82
        overdose or wrong substance given
            or taken 975.0
Erichsen's disease (railway spine) 300.16
Erlacher-Blount syndrome (tibia vara)
    732.4
Erosio interdigitalis blastomycetica 112.3
Erosion
    arteriosclerotic plaque - *see*
        Arteriosclerosis, by site
    artery NEC 447.2
        without rupture 447.8
    bone 733.99
    bronchus 519.19
    cartilage (joint) 733.99
    cervix (uteri) (acquired) (chronic)
        (congenital) 622.0
        with mention of cervicitis 616.0
    cornea (recurrent) *(see also* Keratitis)
        371.42
        traumatic 918.1
    dental (idiopathic) (occupational)
        521.30
        extending into
            dentine 521.32
            pulp 521.33
        generalized 521.35
        limited to enamel 521.31
        localized 521.34
    duodenum, postpyloric - *see* Ulcer,
        duodenum
    esophagus 530.89
    gastric 535.4●
    intestine 569.89
    lymphatic vessel 457.8
    pylorus, pyloric (ulcer) 535.4●
    sclera 379.16

◀ New   ◀▥ Revised   ~~deleted~~ Deleted   ● Use Additional Digit(s)   ▦ Omit code

Erosion (Continued)
spine, aneurysmal 094.89
spleen 289.59
stomach 535.4●
teeth (idiopathic) (occupational) (see
     also Erosion, dental) 521.30
  due to
     medicine 521.30
     persistent vomiting 521.30
urethra 599.84
uterus 621.8
vertebra 733.99
Erotomania 302.89
Clerambault's 297.8
Error
in diet 269.9
refractive 367.9
  astigmatism (see also Astigmatism)
       367.20
  drug-induced 367.89
  hypermetropia 367.0
  hyperopia 367.0
  myopia 367.1
  presbyopia 367.4
  toxic 367.89
Eructation 787.3
nervous 306.4
psychogenic 306.4
Eruption
creeping 126.9
drug - see Dermatitis, due to, drug
Hutchinson, summer 692.72
Kaposi's varicelliform 054.0
napkin (psoriasiform) 691.0
polymorphous
  light (sun) 692.72
     other source 692.82
psoriasiform, napkin 691.0
recalcitrant pustular 694.8
ringed 695.89
skin (see also Dermatitis) 782.1
  creeping (meaning hookworm) 126.9
  due to
     chemical(s) NEC 692.4
       internal use 693.8
     drug - see Dermatitis, due to, drug
     prophylactic inoculation or
          vaccination against
          disease - see Dermatitis, due
          to, vaccine
     smallpox vaccination NEC - see
          Dermatitis, due to, vaccine
  erysipeloid 027.1
  feigned 698.4
  Hutchinson, summer 692.72
  Kaposi's, varicelliform 054.0
     vaccinia 999.0
  lichenoid, axilla 698.3
  polymorphous, due to light 692.72
  toxic NEC 695.0
  vesicular 709.8
teeth, tooth
  accelerated 520.6
  delayed 520.6
  difficult 520.6
  disturbance of 520.6
  in abnormal sequence 520.6
  incomplete 520.6
  late 520.6
  natal 520.6
  neonatal 520.6
  obstructed 520.6
  partial 520.6
  persistent primary 520.6
  premature 520.6
  prenatal 520.6
vesicular 709.8

Erysipelas (gangrenous) (infantile)
     (newborn) (phlegmonous)
     (suppurative) 035
external ear 035 [380.13]
puerperal, postpartum, childbirth
     670.8 ◀━
Erysipelatoid (Rosenbach's) 027.1
Erysipeloid (Rosenbach's) 027.1
Erythema, erythematous (generalized)
     695.9
ab igne - see Burn, by site, first degree
annulare (centrifugum) (rheumaticum)
     695.0
arthriticum epidemicum 026.1
brucellum (see also Brucellosis) 023.9
bullosum 695.19
caloricum - see Burn, by site, first
     degree
chronicum migrans 088.81
circinatum 695.19
diaper 691.0
due to
  chemical (contact) NEC 692.4
     internal 693.8
  drug (internal use) 693.0
     contact 692.3
elevatum diutinum 695.89
endemic 265.2
epidemic, arthritic 026.1
figuratum perstans 695.0
gluteal 691.0
gyratum (perstans) (repens)
     695.19
heat - see Burn, by site, first degree
ichthyosiforme congenitum 757.1
induratum (primary) (scrofulosorum)
     (see also Tuberculosis) 017.1●
  nontuberculous 695.2
infantum febrile 057.8
infectional NEC 695.9
infectiosum 057.0
inflammation NEC 695.9
intertrigo 695.89
iris 695.10
lupus (discoid) (localized) (see also
     Lupus, erythematosus) 695.4
marginatum 695.0
  rheumaticum - see Fever, rheumatic
medicamentosum - see Dermatitis, due
     to, drug
migrans 529.1
  chronicum 088.81
multiforme 695.10
  bullosum 695.19
  conjunctiva 695.19
  exudativum (Hebra) 695.19
  major 695.12
  minor 695.11
  pemphigoides 694.5
napkin 691.0
neonatorum 778.8
nodosum 695.2
  tuberculous (see also Tuberculosis)
       017.1●
nummular, nummulare 695.19
palmar 695.0
palmaris hereditarium 695.0
pernio 991.5
perstans solare 692.72
rash, newborn 778.8
scarlatiniform (exfoliative) (recurrent)
     695.0
simplex marginatum 057.8
solare (see also Sunburn) 692.71
streptogenes 696.5
toxic, toxicum NEC 695.0
  newborn 778.8

Erythema, erythematous (Continued)
tuberculous (primary) (see also
     Tuberculosis) 017.0●
venenatum 695.0
Erythematosus - see condition
Erythematous - see condition
Erythermalgia (primary) 443.82
Erythralgia 443.82
Erythrasma 039.0
Erythredema 985.0
polyneuritica 985.0
polyneuropathy 985.0
Erythremia (acute) (M9841/3) 207.0●
chronic (M9842/3) 207.1●
secondary 289.0
Erythroblastopenia (acquired) 284.89
congenital 284.01
Erythroblastophthisis 284.01
Erythroblastosis (fetalis) (newborn) 773.2
due to
  ABO
     antibodies 773.1
     incompatibility, maternal/fetal
          773.1
     isoimmunization 773.1
  Rh
     antibodies 773.0
     incompatibility, maternal/fetal
          773.0
     isoimmunization 773.0
Erythrocyanosis (crurum) 443.89
Erythrocythemia - see Erythremia
Erythrocytopenia 285.9
Erythrocytosis (megalosplenic)
familial 289.6
oval, hereditary (see also Elliptocytosis)
     282.1
secondary 289.0
stress 289.0
Erythroderma (see also Erythema) 695.9
desquamativa (in infants) 695.89
exfoliative 695.89
ichthyosiform, congenital 757.1
infantum 695.89
maculopapular 696.2
neonatorum 778.8
psoriaticum 696.1
secondary 695.9
Erythrodysesthesia, palmar plantar (PPE)
     693.0
Erythrogenesis imperfecta 284.09
Erythroleukemia (M9840/3) 207.0●
Erythromelalgia 443.82
Erythromelia 701.8
Erythropenia 285.9
Erythrophagocytosis 289.9
Erythrophobia 300.23
Erythroplakia
oral mucosa 528.79
tongue 528.79
Erythroplasia (Queyrat) (M8080/2)
specified site - see Neoplasm, skin, in
     situ
unspecified site 233.5
Erythropoiesis, idiopathic ineffective
     285.0
Escaped beats, heart 427.60
postoperative 997.1
Esoenteritis - see Enteritis
Esophagalgia 530.89
Esophagectasis 530.89
due to cardiospasm 530.0
Esophagismus 530.5
Esophagitis (alkaline) (chemical)
     (chronic) (infectional) (necrotic)
     (peptic) (postoperative)
     (regurgitant) 530.10

Esophagitis *(Continued)*
  acute 530.12
  candidal 112.84
  eosinophilic 530.13
  reflux 530.11
  specified NEC 530.19
  tuberculous *(see also* Tuberculosis)
    017.8●
  ulcerative 530.19
Esophagocele 530.6
Esophagodynia 530.89
Esophagomalacia 530.89
Esophagoptosis 530.89
Esophagospasm 530.5
Esophagostenosis 530.3
Esophagostomiasis 127.7
Esophagostomy
  complication 530.87
    infection 530.86
    malfunctioning 530.87
    mechanical 530.87
Esophagotracheal - *see* condition
Esophagus - *see* condition
Esophoria 378.41
  convergence, excess 378.84
  divergence, insufficiency 378.85
Esotropia (nonaccommodative) 378.00
  accommodative 378.35
  alternating 378.05
    with
      A pattern 378.06
      specified noncomitancy NEC
        378.08
      V pattern 378.07
      X pattern 378.08
      Y pattern 378.08
    intermittent 378.22
  intermittent 378.20
    alternating 378.22
    monocular 378.21
  monocular 378.01
    with
      A pattern 378.02
      specified noncomitancy NEC
        378.04
      V pattern 378.03
      X pattern 378.04
      Y pattern 378.04
    intermittent 378.21
Espundia 085.5
Essential - *see* condition
Esterapenia 289.89
Esthesioneuroblastoma (M9522/3) 160.0
Esthesioneurocytoma (M9521/3) 160.0
Esthesioneuroepithelioma (M9523/3)
  160.0
Esthiomene 099.1
Estivo-autumnal
  fever 084.0
  malaria 084.0
Estrangement V61.09
Estriasis 134.0
Ethanolaminuria 270.8
Ethanolism *(see also* Alcoholism) 303.9●
Ether dependence, dependency *(see also*
    Dependence) 304.6●
Etherism *(see also* Dependence) 304.6●
Ethmoid, ethmoidal - *see* condition
Ethmoiditis (chronic) (nonpurulent)
    (purulent) *(see also* Sinusitis,
    ethmoidal) 473.2
  influenzal 487.1
  Woakes' 471.1
Ethylism *(see also* Alcoholism) 303.9●

Eulenburg's disease (congenital
    paramyotonia) 359.29
Eunuchism 257.2
Eunuchoidism 257.2
  hypogonadotropic 257.2
European blastomycosis 117.5
Eustachian - *see* condition
Euthyroid sick syndrome 790.94
Euthyroidism 244.9
Evaluation
  fetal lung maturity 659.8●
  for suspected condition *(see also*
      Observation) V71.9
    abuse V71.81
    exposure
      anthrax V71.82
      biologic agent NEC V71.83
      SARS V71.83
    neglect V71.81
    newborn - *see* Observation,
        suspected, condition, newborn
    specified condition NEC V71.89
  mental health V70.2
    requested by authority V70.1
  nursing care V63.8
  social service V63.8
Evans' syndrome (thrombocytopenic
    purpura) 287.32
Event, apparent life threatening in
    newborn and infant (ALTE) 799.82 ◄
Eventration
  colon into chest - *see* Hernia,
      diaphragm
  diaphragm (congenital) 756.6
Eversion
  bladder 596.8
  cervix (uteri) 622.0
    with mention of cervicitis 616.0
  foot NEC 736.79
    congenital 755.67
  lacrimal punctum 375.51
  punctum lacrimale (postinfectional)
      (senile) 375.51
  ureter (meatus) 593.89
  urethra (meatus) 599.84
  uterus 618.1
    complicating delivery 665.2●
      affecting fetus or newborn 763.89
    puerperal, postpartum 674.8●
Evidence
  of malignancy
    cytologic
      without histologic confirmation
        anus 796.76
        cervix 795.06
        vagina 795.16
Evisceration
  birth injury 767.8
  bowel (congenital) - *see* Hernia, ventral
  congenital *(see also* Hernia, ventral)
      553.29
  operative wound 998.32
  traumatic NEC 869.1
    eye 871.3
Evulsion - *see* Avulsion
Ewing's
  angioendothelioma (M9260/3) - *see*
      Neoplasm, bone, malignant
  sarcoma (M9260/3) - *see* Neoplasm,
      bone, malignant
  tumor (M9260/3) - *see* Neoplasm, bone,
      malignant
Exaggerated lumbosacral angle (with
    impinging spine) 756.12

Examination (general) (routine) (of) (for)
    V70.9
  allergy V72.7
  annual V70.0
  cardiovascular preoperative V72.81
  cervical Papanicolaou smear V76.2
    as a part of routine gynecological
        examination V72.31
    to confirm findings of recent normal
        smear following initial
        abnormal smear V72.32
  child care (routine) V20.2
  clinical research investigation (normal
      control patient) (participant)
      V70.7
  dental V72.2
  developmental testing (child) (infant)
      V20.2
  donor (potential) V70.8
  ear V72.19
  eye V72.0
  following
    accident (motor vehicle) V71.4
    alleged rape or seduction (victim or
        culprit) V71.5
    inflicted injury (victim or culprit)
        NEC V71.6
    rape or seduction, alleged (victim or
        culprit) V71.5
    treatment (for) V67.9
      combined V67.6
      fracture V67.4
      involving high-risk medication
          NEC V67.51
      mental disorder V67.3
      specified condition NEC V67.59
  follow-up (routine) (following) V67.9
    cancer chemotherapy V67.2
    chemotherapy V67.2
    disease NEC V67.59
    high-risk medication NEC V67.51
    injury NEC V67.59
    population survey V70.6
    postpartum V24.2
    psychiatric V67.3
    psychotherapy V67.3
    radiotherapy V67.1
    specified surgery NEC V67.09
    surgery V67.00
      vaginal pap smear V67.01
  gynecological V72.31
    for contraceptive maintenance V25.40
      intrauterine device V25.42
      pill V25.41
      specified method NEC V25.49
  health (of)
    armed forces personnel V70.5
    checkup V70.0
    child, routine V20.2
    defined subpopulation NEC V70.5
    inhabitants of institutions V70.5
    occupational V70.5
    pre-employment screening V70.5
    preschool children V70.5
      for admission to school V70.3
    prisoners V70.5
      for entrance into prison V70.3
    prostitutes V70.5
    refugees V70.5
    school children V70.5
    students V70.5
  hearing V72.19
    following failed hearing screening
        V72.11

◄ New   ◄▥ Revised   ~~deleted~~ Deleted   ● Use Additional Digit(s)   ▨ Omit code

Examination (*Continued*)
  infant ~~V20.2~~ ◀◀◀
    8 to 28 days old V20.32 ◀
    over 28 days old, routine V20.2 ◀
    under 8 days old V20.31 ◀
  laboratory V72.60 ◀◀◀
    ordered as part of a routine general
      medical examination V72.62 ◀
    pre-operative V72.63 ◀
    pre-procedural V72.63 ◀
    specified NEC V72.69 ◀
  lactating mother V24.1
  medical (for) (of) V70.9
    administrative purpose NEC
      V70.3
    admission to
      old age home V70.3
      prison V70.3
      school V70.3
    adoption V70.3
    armed forces personnel V70.5
    at health care facility V70.0
    camp V70.3
    child, routine V20.2
    clinical research (control) (normal
      comparison) (participant)
      V70.7
    defined subpopulation NEC V70.5
    donor (potential) V70.8
    driving license V70.3
    general V70.9
      routine V70.0
      specified reason NEC V70.8
    immigration V70.3
    inhabitants of institutions V70.5
    insurance certification V70.3
    marriage V70.3
    medicolegal reasons V70.4
    naturalization V70.3
    occupational V70.5
    population survey V70.6
    pre-employment V70.5
    preschool children V70.5
      for admission to school V70.3
    prison V70.3
    prisoners V70.5
      for entrance into prison V70.3
    prostitutes V70.5
    refugees V70.5
    school children V70.5
    specified reason NEC V70.8
    sport competition V70.3
    students V70.5
  medicolegal reason V70.4
  pelvic (annual) (periodic) V72.31
  periodic (annual) (routine) V70.0
  postpartum
    immediately after delivery V24.0
    routine follow-up V24.2
  pregnancy (unconfirmed) (possible)
    V72.40
    negative result V72.41
    positive result V72.42
  prenatal V22.1
    first pregnancy V22.0
    high-risk pregnancy V23.9
      specified problem NEC V23.89
  preoperative V72.84
    cardiovascular V72.81
    respiratory V72.82
    specified NEC V72.83
  preprocedural V72.84
    cardiovascular V72.81
    general physical V72.83
    respiratory V72.82
    specified NEC V72.83

Examination (*Continued*)
  prior to chemotherapy V72.83 ◀
  psychiatric V70.2
    follow-up not needing further care
      V67.3
    requested by authority V70.1
  radiological NEC V72.5
  respiratory preoperative V72.82
  screening - *see* Screening
  sensitization V72.7
  skin V72.7
    hypersensitivity V72.7
  special V72.9
  specified type or reason NEC V72.85
    preoperative V72.83
      specified NEC V72.83
  teeth V72.2
  vaginal Papanicolaou smear V76.47
    following hysterectomy for
      malignant condition V67.01
  victim or culprit following
    alleged rape or seduction V71.5
    inflicted injury NEC V71.6
  vision V72.0
  well baby V20.2
Exanthem, exanthema (*see also* Rash) 782.1
  Boston 048
  epidemic, with meningitis 048
  lichenoid psoriasiform 696.2
  subitum 058.10
    due to
      human herpesvirus 6 058.11
      human herpesvirus 7 058.12
  viral, virus NEC 057.9
    specified type NEC 057.8
Excess, excessive, excessively
  alcohol level in blood 790.3
  carbohydrate tissue, localized 278.1
  carotene (dietary) 278.3
  cold 991.9
    specified effect NEC 991.8
  convergence 378.84
  crying 780.95
    of
      adolescent 780.95
      adult 780.95
      baby 780.92
      child 780.95
      infant (baby) 780.92
      newborn 780.92
  development, breast 611.1
  diaphoresis (*see also* Hyperhidrosis)
    780.8
  distance, interarch 524.28
  divergence 378.85
  drinking (alcohol) NEC (*see also*
    Abuse, drugs, nondependent)
    305.0●
    continual (*see also* Alcoholism)
      303.9●
    habitual (*see also* Alcoholism) 303.9●
  eating 783.6
  eyelid fold (congenital) 743.62
  fat 278.02
    in heart (*see also* Degeneration,
      myocardial) 429.1
    tissue, localized 278.1
  foreskin 605
  gas 787.3
  gastrin 251.5
  glucagon 251.4
  heat (*see also* Heat) 992.9
  horizontal
    overjet 524.26
    overlap 524.26
  interarch distance 524.28

Excess, excessive, excessively (*Continued*)
  intermaxillary vertical dimension
    524.37
  interocclusal distance of teeth 524.37
  large
    colon 564.7
      congenital 751.3
    fetus or infant 766.0
      with obstructed labor 660.1●
      affecting management of
        pregnancy 656.6●
      causing disproportion 653.5●
    newborn (weight of 4500 grams or
      more) 766.0
    organ or site, congenital NEC - *see*
      Anomaly, specified type NEC
  lid fold (congenital) 743.62
  long
    colon 751.5
    organ or site, congenital NEC - *see*
      Anomaly, specified type NEC
    umbilical cord (entangled)
      affecting fetus or newborn 762.5
      in pregnancy or childbirth 663.3●
        with compression 663.2●
  menstruation 626.2
  number of teeth 520.1
    causing crowding 524.31
  nutrients (dietary) NEC 783.6
  potassium (K) 276.7
  salivation (*see also* Ptyalism) 527.7
  secretion - *see also* Hypersecretion
    milk 676.6●
    sputum 786.4
    sweat (*see also* Hyperhidrosis)
      780.8
  short
    organ or site, congenital NEC - *see*
      Anomaly, specified type NEC
    umbilical cord
      affecting fetus or newborn 762.6
      in pregnancy or childbirth
        663.4●
  skin NEC 701.9
    eyelid 743.62
      acquired 374.30
  sodium (Na) 276.0
  spacing of teeth 524.32
  sputum 786.4
  sweating (*see also* Hyperhidrosis)
    780.8
  tearing (ducts) (eye) (*see also* Epiphora)
    375.20
  thirst 783.5
    due to deprivation of water 994.3
  tissue in reconstructed breast 612.0
  tuberosity 524.07
  vitamin
    A (dietary) 278.2
      administered as drug (chronic)
        (prolonged excessive
        intake) 278.2
      reaction to sudden overdose
        963.5
    D (dietary) 278.4
      administered as drug (chronic)
        (prolonged excessive
        intake) 278.4
      reaction to sudden overdose
        963.5
  weight 278.02
    gain 783.1
      of pregnancy 646.1●
    loss 783.21
Excitability, abnormal, under minor
  stress 309.29

Excitation
  catatonic (see also Schizophrenia)
      295.2●
  psychogenic 298.1
  reactive (from emotional stress,
      psychological trauma) 298.1
Excitement
  manic (see also Psychosis, affective)
      296.0●
    recurrent episode 296.1●
    single episode 296.0●
  mental, reactive (from emotional stress,
      psychological trauma) 298.1
  state, reactive (from emotional stress,
      psychological trauma) 298.1
Excluded pupils 364.76
Excoriation (traumatic) (see also Injury,
    superficial, by site) 919.8
  neurotic 698.4
Excyclophoria 378.44
Excyclotropia 378.33
Exencephalus, exencephaly 742.0
Exercise
  breathing V57.0
  remedial NEC V57.1
  therapeutic NEC V57.1
Exfoliation
  skin
    due to erythematous condition
        695.50
      involving (percent of body
          surface)
        less than 10 percent 695.50
        10-19 percent 695.51
        20-29 percent 695.52
        30-39 percent 695.53
        40-49 percent 695.54
        50-59 percent 695.55
        60-69 percent 695.56
        70-79 percent 695.57
        80-89 percent 695.58
        90 percent or more 695.59
  teeth
    due to systemic causes 525.0
Exfoliative - see also condition
  dermatitis 695.89
Exhaustion, exhaustive (physical NEC)
    780.79
  battle (see also Reaction, stress, acute)
      308.9
  cardiac (see also Failure, heart) 428.9
  delirium (see also Reaction, stress,
      acute) 308.9
  due to
    cold 991.8
    excessive exertion 994.5
    exposure 994.4
    overexertion 994.5
  fetus or newborn 779.89
  heart (see also Failure, heart) 428.9
  heat 992.5
    due to
      salt depletion 992.4
      water depletion 992.3
  manic (see also Psychosis, affective)
      296.0●
    recurrent episode 296.1●
    single episode 296.0●
  maternal, complicating delivery 669.8●
    affecting fetus or newborn 763.89
  mental 300.5
  myocardium, myocardial (see also
      Failure, heart) 428.9
  nervous 300.5

Exhaustion, exhaustive (Continued)
  old age 797
  postinfectional NEC 780.79
  psychogenic 300.5
  psychosis (see also Reaction, stress,
      acute) 308.9
  senile 797
    dementia 290.0
Exhibitionism (sexual) 302.4
Exomphalos 756.72
Exophoria 378.42
  convergence, insufficiency 378.83
  divergence, excess 378.85
Exophthalmic
  cachexia 242.0●
  goiter 242.0●
  ophthalmoplegia 242.0● [376.22]
Exophthalmos 376.30
  congenital 743.66
  constant 376.31
  endocrine NEC 259.9 [376.22]
  hyperthyroidism 242.0● [376.21]
  intermittent NEC 376.34
  malignant 242.0● [376.21]
  pulsating 376.35
    endocrine NEC 259.9 [376.22]
  thyrotoxic 242.0● [376.21]
Exostosis 726.91
  cartilaginous (M9210/0) - see
      Neoplasm, bone, benign
  congenital 756.4
  ear canal, external 380.81
  gonococcal 098.89
  hip 726.5
  intracranial 733.3
  jaw (bone) 526.81
  luxurians 728.11
  multiple (cancellous) (congenital)
      (hereditary) 756.4
  nasal bones 726.91
  orbit, orbital 376.42
  osteocartilaginous (M9210/0) - see
      Neoplasm, bone, benign
  spine 721.8
    with spondylosis - see
        Spondylosis
  syphilitic 095.5
  wrist 726.4
Exotropia 378.10
  alternating 378.15
    with
      A pattern 378.16
      specified noncomitancy NEC
          378.18
      V pattern 378.17
      X pattern 378.18
      Y pattern 378.18
    intermittent 378.24
  intermittent 378.20
    alternating 378.24
    monocular 378.23
  monocular 378.11
    with
      A pattern 378.12
      specified noncomitancy NEC
          378.14
      V pattern 378.13
      X pattern 378.14
      Y pattern 378.14
    intermittent 378.23
Explanation of
  investigation finding V65.4
  medication V65.4

Exposure (suspected) 994.9
  algae bloom V87.32
  cold 991.9
    specified effect NEC 991.8
  effects of 994.9
  exhaustion due to 994.4
  to
    AIDS virus V01.79
    anthrax V01.81
    aromatic
      amines V87.11
      dyes V87.19
    arsenic V87.01
    asbestos V15.84
    benzene V87.12
    body fluids (hazardous) V15.85
    cholera V01.0
    chromium compounds V87.09
    communicable disease V01.9
      specified type NEC V01.89
    dyes V87.2
      aromatic V87.19
    Escherichia coli (E. coli) V01.83
    German measles V01.4
    gonorrhea V01.6
    hazardous
      aromatic compounds NEC
          V87.19
      body fluids V15.85
      chemicals NEC V87.2
      metals V87.09
      substances V87.39
    HIV V01.79
    human immunodeficiency virus
        V01.79
    lead V15.86
    meningococcus V01.84
    mold V87.31
    nickel dust V87.09
    parasitic disease V01.89
    poliomyelitis V01.2
    polycyclic aromatic hydrocarbons
        V87.19
    potentially hazardous body fluids
        V15.85
    rabies V01.5
    rubella V01.4
    SARS-associated coronavirus V01.82
    smallpox V01.3
    syphilis V01.6
    tuberculosis V01.1
    varicella V01.71
    venereal disease V01.6
    viral disease NEC V01.79
      varicella V01.71
Exsanguination, fetal 772.0
Exstrophy
  abdominal content 751.8
  bladder (urinary) 753.5
Extensive - see condition
Extra - see also Accessory
  rib 756.3
    cervical 756.2
Extraction
  with hook 763.89
  breech NEC 669.6●
    affecting fetus or newborn 763.0
  cataract postsurgical V45.61
  manual NEC 669.8●
    affecting fetus or newborn 763.89
Extrasystole 427.60
  atrial 427.61
  postoperative 997.1
  ventricular 427.69

◀ New   ◀║║ Revised   deleted Deleted   ● Use Additional Digit(s)   Omit code

Extrauterine gestation or pregnancy - *see*
    Pregnancy, ectopic
Extravasation
    blood 459.0
        lower extremity 459.0
    chemotherapy, vesicant 999.81 ◀▥
    chyle into mesentery 457.8
    pelvicalyceal 593.4
    pyelosinus 593.4
    urine 788.8
        from ureter 788.8
    vesicant
        agent NEC 999.82 ◀▥
        chemotherapy 999.81 ◀▥
Extremity - *see* condition

Extrophy - *see* Exstrophy
Extroversion
    bladder 753.5
    uterus 618.1
        complicating delivery 665.2●
            affecting fetus or newborn
                763.89
        postpartal (old) 618.1
Extruded tooth 524.34
Extrusion
    alveolus and teeth 524.75
    breast implant (prosthetic) 996.54
    device, implant, or graft - *see*
        Complications, mechanical
    eye implant (ball) (globe) 996.59

Extrusion *(Continued)*
    intervertebral disc - *see* Displacement,
        intervertebral disc
    lacrimal gland 375.43
    mesh (reinforcing) 996.59
    ocular lens implant 996.53
    prosthetic device NEC - *see*
        Complications, mechanical
    vitreous 379.26
Exudate, pleura - *see* Effusion, pleura
Exudates, retina 362.82
Exudative - *see* condition
Eye, eyeball, eyelid - *see* condition
Eyestrain 368.13
Eyeworm disease of Africa 125.2

F

Faber's anemia or syndrome
(achlorhydric anemia) 280.9
Fabry's disease (angiokeratoma corporis
diffusum) 272.7
Face, facial - *see* condition
Facet of cornea 371.44
Faciocephalalgia, autonomic (*see also*
Neuropathy, peripheral, autonomic)
337.9
Facioscapulohumeral myopathy 359.1
Factitious disorder, illness - *see* Illness,
factitious
Factor
deficiency - *see* Deficiency, factor
psychic, associated with diseases
classified elsewhere 316
risk-see problem
Fahr-Volhard disease (malignant
nephrosclerosis) 403.00
Failure, failed
adenohypophyseal 253.2
attempted abortion (legal) (*see also*
Abortion, failed) 638.9
bone marrow (anemia) 284.9
acquired (secondary) 284.89
congenital 284.09
idiopathic 284.9
cardiac (*see also* Failure, heart) 428.9
newborn 779.89
cardiorenal (chronic) 428.9
hypertensive (*see also* Hypertension,
cardiorenal) 404.93
cardiorespiratory 799.1
specified during or due to a
procedure 997.1
long-term effect of cardiac
surgery 429.4
cardiovascular (chronic) 428.9
cerebrovascular 437.8
cervical dilatation in labor 661.0 ●
affecting fetus or newborn 763.7
circulation, circulatory 799.89
fetus or newborn 779.89
peripheral 785.50
compensation - *see* Disease, heart
congestive (*see also* Failure, heart) 428.0
conscious sedation, during
procedure 995.24   ◀
coronary (*see also* Insufficiency,
coronary) 411.89
dental implant 525.79
due to
infection 525.71
lack of attached gingiva
525.72
occlusal trauma (caused by poor
prosthetic design) 525.72
parafunctional habits 525.72
periodontal infection
(periimplantitis) 525.72
poor oral hygiene 525.72
unintentional loading 525.71
endosseous NEC 525.79
mechanical 525.73
osseointegration 525.71
due to
complications of systemic
disease 525.71
poor bone quality 525.71
premature loading 525.71
~~following intentional prosthetic~~
~~loading 525.72~~
iatrogenic 525.71
prior to intentional prosthetic
loading 525.71

Failure, failed (*Continued*)
dental implant (*Continued*)
post-osseointegration
biological 525.72
iatrogenic 525.72
due to complications of systemic
disease 525.72
mechanical 525.73
pre-integration 525.71
pre-osseointegration 525.71
dental prosthesis causing loss of dental
implant 525.73
dental restoration
marginal integrity 525.61
periodontal anatomical integrity
525.65
descent of head (at term) 652.5 ●
affecting fetus or newborn 763.1
in labor 660.0 ●
affecting fetus or newborn
763.1
device, implant, or graft - *see*
Complications, mechanical
engagement of head NEC 652.5 ●
in labor 660.0 ●
extrarenal 788.99
fetal head to enter pelvic brim
652.5 ●
affecting fetus or newborn 763.1
in labor 660.0 ●
affecting fetus or newborn 763.1
forceps NEC 660.7 ●
affecting fetus or newborn 763.1
fusion (joint) (spinal) 996.49
growth in childhood 783.43
heart (acute) (sudden) 428.9
with
abortion - *see* Abortion, by type,
with specified complication
NEC
acute pulmonary edema (*see also*
Failure, ventricular, left)
428.1
with congestion (*see also*
Failure, heart) 428.0
decompensation (*see also* Failure,
heart) 428.0
dilation - *see* Disease, heart
ectopic pregnancy (*see also*
categories 633.0–633.9)
639.8
molar pregnancy (*see also*
categories 630–632) 639.8
arteriosclerotic 440.9
combined left-right sided 428.0
combined systolic and diastolic
428.40
acute 428.41
acute on chronic 428.43
chronic 428.42
compensated (*see also* Failure, heart)
428.0
complicating
abortion - *see* Abortion, by type,
with specified complication
NEC
delivery (cesarean) (instrumental)
669.4 ●
ectopic pregnancy (*see also*
categories 633.0–633.9) 639.8
molar pregnancy (*see also*
categories 630–632) 639.8
obstetric anesthesia or sedation
668.1 ●
surgery 997.1

Failure, failed (*Continued*)
heart (*Continued*)
congestive (compensated)
(decompensated) (*see also*
Failure, heart) 428.0
with rheumatic fever (conditions
classifiable to 390)
active 391.8
inactive or quiescent (with
chorea) 398.91
fetus or newborn 779.89
hypertensive (*see also*
Hypertension, heart)
402.91
with renal disease (*see also*
Hypertension,
cardiorenal) 404.91
with renal failure 404.93
benign 402.11
malignant 402.01
rheumatic (chronic) (inactive)
(with chorea) 398.91
active or acute 391.8
with chorea (Sydenham's)
392.0
decompensated (*see also* Failure,
heart) 428.0
degenerative (*see also* Degeneration,
myocardial) 429.1
diastolic 428.30
acute 428.31
acute on chronic 428.33
chronic 428.32
due to presence of (cardiac)
prosthesis 429.4
fetus or newborn 779.89
following
abortion 639.8
cardiac surgery 429.4
ectopic or molar pregnancy
639.8
high output NEC 428.9
hypertensive (*see also* Hypertension,
heart) 402.91
with renal disease (*see also*
Hypertension, cardiorenal)
404.91
with renal failure 404.93
benign 402.11
malignant 402.01
left (ventricular) (*see also* Failure,
ventricular, left) 428.1
with right-sided failure (*see also*
Failure, heart) 428.0
low output (syndrome) NEC
428.9
organic - *see* Disease, heart
postoperative (immediate) 997.1
long term effect of cardiac
surgery 429.4
rheumatic (chronic) (congestive)
(inactive) 398.91
right (secondary to left heart failure,
conditions classifiable to 428.1)
(ventricular) (*see also* Failure,
heart) 428.0
senile 797
specified during or due to a
procedure 997.1
long-term effect of cardiac
surgery 429.4
systolic 428.20
acute 428.21
acute on chronic 428.23
chronic 428.22

◀ New   ◀▥ Revised   ~~deleted~~ Deleted   ● Use Additional Digit(s)   ▨ Omit code

Failure, failed (Continued)
  heart (Continued)
    thyrotoxic (see also Thyrotoxicosis)
        242.9● [425.7]
    valvular - see Endocarditis
  hepatic 572.8
    acute 570
    due to a procedure 997.4
  hepatorenal 572.4
  hypertensive heart (see also
      Hypertension, heart) 402.91
    benign 402.11
    malignant 402.01
  induction (of labor) 659.1●
    abortion (legal) (see also Abortion,
        failed) 638.9
    affecting fetus or newborn 763.89
    by oxytocic drugs 659.1●
    instrumental 659.0●
    mechanical 659.0●
    medical 659.1●
    surgical 659.0●
  initial alveolar expansion, newborn
      770.4
  involution, thymus (gland) 254.8
  kidney - see Failure, renal
  lactation 676.4●
  Leydig's cell, adult 257.2
  liver 572.8
    acute 570
  medullary 799.89
  mitral - see Endocarditis, mitral
  moderate sedation, during
      procedure 995.24   ◀
  myocardium, myocardial (see also
      Failure, heart) 428.9
    chronic (see also Failure, heart)
        428.0
    congestive (see also Failure, heart)
        428.0
  ovarian (primary) 256.39
    iatrogenic 256.2
    postablative 256.2
    postirradiation 256.2
    postsurgical 256.2
  ovulation 628.0
  prerenal 788.99
  renal (kidney) 586   ◀▥
    with
      abortion - see Abortion, by type,
          with renal failure
      ectopic pregnancy (see also
          categories 633.0–633.9) 639.3
      edema (see also Nephrosis) 581.9
      hypertension (see also
          Hypertension, kidney)
          403.91
      hypertensive heart disease
          (conditions classifiable to
          402) 404.92
        with heart failure 404.93
        benign 404.12
          with heart failure 404.13
        malignant 404.02
          with heart failure 404.03
      molar pregnancy (see also
          categories 630–632) 639.3
      tubular necrosis (acute) 584.5
    acute 584.9
      with lesion of
        necrosis
          cortical (renal) 584.6
          medullary (renal)
              (papillary) 584.7
          tubular 584.5
        specified pathology NEC
            584.8

Failure, failed (Continued)
  renal (Continued)
    chronic 585.9
      hypertensive or with
          hypertension (see also
          Hypertension, kidney)
          403.91
    due to a procedure 997.5
    following
      abortion 639.3
      crushing 958.5
      ectopic or molar pregnancy
          639.3
      labor and delivery (acute)
          669.3●
    hypertensive (see also Hypertension,
        kidney) 403.91
    puerperal, postpartum 669.3●
  respiration, respiratory 518.81
    acute 518.81
    acute and chronic 518.84
    center 348.89   ◀▥
      newborn 770.84
    chronic 518.83
    due to trauma, surgery or shock
        518.5
    newborn 770.84
  rotation
    cecum 751.4
    colon 751.4
    intestine 751.4
    kidney 753.3
  sedation, during procedure   ◀
    conscious 995.24   ◀
    moderate 995.24   ◀
  segmentation - see also Fusion
    fingers (see also Syndactylism,
        fingers) 755.11
    toes (see also Syndactylism, toes)
        755.13
  seminiferous tubule, adult 257.2
  senile (general) 797
    with psychosis 290.20
  testis, primary (seminal) 257.2
  to progress 661.2●
  to thrive
    adult 783.7
    child 783.41
    newborn 779.34   ◀
  transplant 996.80
    bone marrow 996.85
    organ (immune or nonimmune
        cause) 996.80
      bone marrow 996.85
      heart 996.83
      intestines 996.87
      kidney 996.81
      liver 996.82
      lung 996.84
      pancreas 996.86
      specified NEC 996.89
    skin 996.52
      artificial 996.55
      decellularized allodermis
          996.55
      temporary allograft or pigskin
          graft - omit code
  trial of labor NEC 660.6●
    affecting fetus or newborn 763.1
  tubal ligation 998.89
  urinary 586
  vacuum extraction
    abortion - see Abortion, failed
    delivery NEC 660.7●
      affecting fetus or newborn
          763.1
  vasectomy 998.89

Failure, failed (Continued)
  ventouse NEC 660.7●
    affecting fetus or newborn 763.1
  ventricular (see also Failure, heart) 428.9
    left 428.1
      with rheumatic fever (conditions
          classifiable to 390)
        active 391.8
          with chorea 392.0
        inactive or quiescent (with
            chorea) 398.91
      hypertensive (see also
          Hypertension, heart)
          402.91
        benign 402.11
        malignant 402.01
      rheumatic (chronic) (inactive)
          (with chorea) 398.91
        active or acute 391.8
          with chorea 392.0
    right (see also Failure, heart) 428.0
  vital centers, fetus or newborn
      779.89
  weight gain in childhood 783.41
Fainting (fit) (spell) 780.2
Falciform hymen 752.49
Fall, maternal, affecting fetus or
    newborn 760.5
Fallen arches 734
Falling, any organ or part - see Prolapse
Fallopian
  insufflation
    fertility testing V26.21
    following sterilization reversal
        V26.22
  tube - see condition
Fallot's
  pentalogy 745.2
  tetrad or tetralogy 745.2
  triad or trilogy 746.09
Fallout, radioactive (adverse effect) NEC
    990
False - see also condition
  bundle branch block 426.50
  bursa 727.89
  croup 478.75
  joint 733.82
  labor (pains) 644.1●
  opening, urinary, male 752.69
  passage, urethra (prostatic) 599.4
  positive
    serological test for syphilis 795.6
    Wassermann reaction 795.6
  pregnancy 300.11
Family, familial - see also condition
  affected by
    family member
      currently on deployment
          (military) V61.01
      returned from deployment
          (military) (current or past
          conflict) V61.02
  disruption (see also Disruption, family)
      V61.09
  estrangement V61.09
  hemophagocytic
    lymphohistiocytosis 288.4
    reticulosis 288.4
  Li-Fraumeni (syndrome) V84.01
  planning advice V25.09
    natural
      procreative V26.41
      to avoid pregnancy V25.04
  problem V61.9
    specified circumstance NEC
        V61.8
  retinoblastoma (syndrome) 190.5

Famine 994.2
edema 262
Fanconi's anemia (congenital
pancytopenia) 284.09
Fanconi (-de Toni) (-Debré) syndrome
(cystinosis) 270.0
Farber (-Uzman) syndrome or disease
(disseminated lipogranulomatosis)
272.8
Farcin 024
Farcy 024
Farmers'
lung 495.0
skin 692.74
Farsightedness 367.0
Fascia - see condition
Fasciculation 781.0
Fasciculitis optica 377.32
Fasciitis 729.4
eosinophilic 728.89
necrotizing 728.86
nodular 728.79
perirenal 593.4
plantar 728.71
pseudosarcomatous 728.79
traumatic (old) NEC 728.79
current - see Sprain, by site
Fasciola hepatica infestation 121.3
Fascioliasis 121.3
Fasciolopsiasis (small intestine) 121.4
Fasciolopsis (small intestine) 121.4
Fast pulse 785.0
Fat
embolism (cerebral) (pulmonary)
(systemic) 958.1
with
abortion - see Abortion, by type,
with embolism
ectopic pregnancy (see also
categories 633.0–633.9) 639.6
molar pregnancy (see also
categories 630–632) 639.6
complicating delivery or
puerperium 673.8●
following
abortion 639.6
ectopic or molar pregnancy
639.6
in pregnancy, childbirth, or the
puerperium 673.8●
excessive 278.02
in heart (see also Degeneration,
myocardial) 429.1
general 278.02
hernia, herniation 729.30
eyelid 374.34
knee 729.31
orbit 374.34
retro-orbital 374.34
retropatellar 729.31
specified site NEC 729.39
indigestion 579.8
in stool 792.1
localized (pad) 278.1
heart (see also Degeneration,
myocardial) 429.1
knee 729.31
retropatellar 729.31
necrosis - see also Fatty, degeneration
breast (aseptic) (segmental) 611.3
mesentery 567.82
omentum 567.82
peritoneum 567.82
pad 278.1

Fatal familial insomnia (FFI) 046.72
Fatal syncope 798.1
Fatigue 780.79
auditory deafness (see also Deafness)
389.9
chronic, syndrome 780.71
combat (see also Reaction, stress, acute)
308.9
during pregnancy 646.8●
general 780.79
psychogenic 300.5
heat (transient) 992.6
muscle 729.89
myocardium (see also Failure, heart)
428.9
nervous 300.5
neurosis 300.5
operational 300.89
postural 729.89
posture 729.89
psychogenic (general) 300.5
senile 797
syndrome NEC 300.5
chronic 780.71
undue 780.79
voice 784.49
Fatness 278.02
Fatty - see also condition
apron 278.1
degeneration (diffuse) (general) NEC
272.8
localized - see Degeneration, by site,
fatty
placenta - see Placenta, abnormal
heart (enlarged) (see also Degeneration,
myocardial) 429.1
infiltration (diffuse) (general) (see also
Degeneration, by site, fatty) 272.8
heart (enlarged) (see also
Degeneration, myocardial)
429.1
liver 571.8
alcoholic 571.0
necrosis - see Degeneration, fatty
phanerosis 272.8
Fauces - see condition
Fauchard's disease (periodontitis) 523.40
Faucitis 478.29
Faulty - see also condition
position of teeth 524.30
Favism (anemia) 282.2
Favre-Racouchot disease (elastoidosis
cutanea nodularis) 701.8
Favus 110.9
beard 110.0
capitis 110.0
corporis 110.5
eyelid 110.8
foot 110.4
hand 110.2
scalp 110.0
specified site NEC 110.8
Fear, fearfulness (complex) (reaction)
300.20
child 313.0
of
animals 300.29
closed spaces 300.29
crowds 300.29
eating in public 300.23
heights 300.29
open spaces 300.22
with panic attacks 300.21
public speaking 300.23

Fear, fearfulness (Continued)
of (Continued)
streets 300.22
with panic attacks 300.21
travel 300.22
with panic attacks 300.21
washing in public 300.23
transient 308.0
Feared complaint unfounded V65.5
Febricula (continued) (simple) (see also
Pyrexia) 780.60
Febrile (see also Pyrexia) 780.60
convulsion (simple) 780.31
complex 780.32
seizure (simple) 780.31
atypical 780.32
complex 780.32
complicated 780.32
Febris (see also Fever) 780.60
aestiva (see also Fever, hay) 477.9
flava (see also Fever, yellow) 060.9
melitensis 023.0
pestis (see also Plague) 020.9
puerperalis 672●
recurrens (see also Fever, relapsing)
087.9
pediculo vestimenti 087.0
rubra 034.1
typhoidea 002.0
typhosa 002.0
Fecal - see condition
Fecalith (impaction) 560.39
with hernia - see also Hernia, by site,
with obstruction
gangrenous - see Hernia, by site,
with gangrene
appendix 543.9
congenital 777.1
Fede's disease 529.0
Feeble-minded 317
Feeble rapid pulse due to shock
following injury 958.4
Feeding
faulty (elderly) (infant) 783.3
newborn 779.31   ◀▥
formula check V20.2
improper (elderly) (infant) 783.3
newborn 779.31   ◀▥
problem (elderly) (infant) 783.3
newborn 779.31   ◀▥
nonorganic origin 307.59
Feeling of foreign body in throat
784.99
Feer's disease 985.0
Feet - see condition
Feigned illness V65.2
Feil-Klippel syndrome (brevicollis) 756.16
Feinmesser's (hidrotic) ectodermal
dysplasia 757.31
Felix's disease (juvenile osteochondrosis,
hip) 732.1
Felon (any digit) (with lymphangitis)
681.01
herpetic 054.6
Felty's syndrome (rheumatoid arthritis
with splenomegaly and leukopenia)
714.1
Feminism in boys 302.6
Feminization, testicular 259.51
with pseudohermaphroditism, male
259.51
Femoral hernia - see Hernia, femoral
Femora vara 736.32
Femur, femoral - see condition

◀ New   ◀▥ Revised   ~~deleted~~ Deleted   ● Use Additional Digit(s)   ▓ Omit code

Fenestrata placenta - *see* Placenta, abnormal
Fenestration, fenestrated - *see also*
    Imperfect, closure
  aorta-pulmonary 745.0
  aorticopulmonary 745.0
  aortopulmonary 745.0
  cusps, heart valve NEC 746.89
    pulmonary 746.09
  hymen 752.49
  pulmonic cusps 746.09
Fenwick's disease 537.89
Fermentation (gastric) (gastrointestinal)
    (stomach) 536.8
  intestine 564.89
    psychogenic 306.4
  psychogenic 306.4
Fernell's disease (aortic aneurysm) 441.9
Fertile eunuch syndrome 257.2
Fertility, meaning multiparity - *see*
    Multiparity
Fetal
  alcohol syndrome 760.71
  anemia 678.0●
  thrombocytopenia 678.0●
  twin to twin transfusion 678.0●
Fetalis uterus 752.3
Fetid
  breath 784.99
  sweat 705.89
Fetishism 302.81
  transvestic 302.3
Fetomaternal hemorrhage
  affecting management of pregnancy
    656.0●
  fetus or newborn 772.0
Fetus, fetal - *see also* condition
  papyraceous 779.89
  type lung tissue 770.4
Fever 780.60
  with chills 780.60
    in malarial regions (*see also* Malaria)
      084.6
  abortus NEC 023.9
  aden 061
  African tick-borne 087.1
  American
    mountain tick 066.1
    spotted 082.0
  and ague (*see also* Malaria) 084.6
  aphthous 078.4
  arbovirus hemorrhagic 065.9
  Assam 085.0
  Australian A or Q 083.0
  Bangkok hemorrhagic 065.4
  biliary, Charcôt's intermittent - *see*
    Choledocholithiasis
  bilious, hemoglobinuric 084.8
  blackwater 084.8
  blister 054.9
  Bonvale Dam 780.79
  boutonneuse 082.1
  brain 323.9
    late effect - *see* category 326
  breakbone 061
  Bullis 082.8
  Bunyamwera 066.3
  Burdwan 085.0
  Bwamba (encephalitis) 066.3
  Cameroon (*see also* Malaria) 084.6
  Canton 081.9
  catarrhal (acute) 460
    chronic 472.0
  cat-scratch 078.3
  cerebral 323.9
    late effect - *see* category 326

Fever (*Continued*)
  cerebrospinal (meningococcal) (*see also*
    Meningitis, cerebrospinal) 036.0
  Chagres 084.0
  Chandipura 066.8
  changuinola 066.0
  Charcôt's (biliary) (hepatic)
    (intermittent) *see*
    Choledocholithiasis
  Chikungunya (viral) 066.3
    hemorrhagic 065.4
  childbed 670.8 ◀▦
  Chitral 066.0
  Colombo (*see also* Fever, paratyphoid)
    002.9
  Colorado tick (virus) 066.1
  congestive
    malarial (*see also* Malaria) 084.6
    remittent (*see also* Malaria) 084.6
  Congo virus 065.0
  continued 780.60
    malarial 084.0
  Corsican (*see also* Malaria) 084.6
  Crimean hemorrhagic 065.0
  Cyprus (*see also* Brucellosis) 023.9
  dandy 061
  deer fly (*see also* Tularemia) 021.9
  dehydration, newborn 778.4
  dengue (virus) 061
    hemorrhagic 065.4
  desert 114.0
  due to heat 992.0
  Dumdum 085.0
  enteric 002.0
  ephemeral (of unknown origin) (*see also*
    Pyrexia) 780.60
  epidemic, hemorrhagic of the Far East
    065.0
  erysipelatous (*see also* Erysipelas) 035
  estivo-autumnal (malarial) 084.0
  etiocholanolone 277.31
  famine - *see also* Fever, relapsing
    meaning typhus - *see* Typhus
  Far Eastern hemorrhagic 065.0
  five day 083.1
  Fort Bragg 100.89
  gastroenteric 002.0
  gastromalarial (*see also* Malaria) 084.6
  Gibraltar (*see also* Brucellosis) 023.9
  glandular 075
  Guama (viral) 066.3
  Haverhill 026.1
  hay (allergic) (with rhinitis) 477.9
    with
      asthma (bronchial) (*see also*
        Asthma) 493.0●
    due to
      dander, animal (cat) (dog) 477.2
      dust 477.8
      fowl 477.8
      hair, animal (cat) (dog) 477.2
      pollen, any plant or tree 477.0
      specified allergen other than
        pollen 477.8
  heat (effects) 992.0
  hematuric, bilious 084.8
  hemoglobinuric (malarial) 084.8
    bilious 084.8
  hemorrhagic (arthropod-borne) NEC
    065.9
    with renal syndrome 078.6
    arenaviral 078.7
    Argentine 078.7
    Bangkok 065.4

Fever (*Continued*)
  hemorrhagic NEC (*Continued*)
    Bolivian 078.7
    Central Asian 065.0
    chikungunya 065.4
    Crimean 065.0
    dengue (virus) 065.4
    Ebola 065.8
    epidemic 078.6
      of Far East 065.0
    Far Eastern 065.0
    Junin virus 078.7
    Korean 078.6
    Kyasanur forest 065.2
    Machupo virus 078.7
    mite-borne NEC 065.8
    mosquito-borne 065.4
    Omsk 065.1
    Philippine 065.4
    Russian (Yaroslav) 078.6
    Singapore 065.4
    Southeast Asia 065.4
    Thailand 065.4
    tick-borne NEC 065.3
  hepatic (*see also* Cholecystitis) 575.8
    intermittent (Charcôt's) - *see*
      Choledocholithiasis
  herpetic (*see also* Herpes) 054.9
  hyalomma tick 065.0
  icterohemorrhagic 100.0
  inanition 780.60
    newborn 778.4
  in conditions classified elsewhere
    780.61
  infective NEC 136.9
  intermittent (bilious) (*see also* Malaria)
    084.6
    hepatic (Charcôt) - *see*
      Choledocholithiasis
    of unknown origin (*see also* Pyrexia)
      780.60
    pernicious 084.0
  iodide
    correct substance properly
      administered 780.60
    overdose or wrong substance given
      or taken 975.5
  Japanese river 081.2
  jungle yellow 060.0
  Junin virus, hemorrhagic 078.7
  Katayama 120.2
  Kedani 081.2
  Kenya 082.1
  Korean hemorrhagic 078.6
  Lassa 078.89
  Lone Star 082.8
  lung - *see* Pneumonia
  Machupo virus, hemorrhagic 078.7
  malaria, malarial (*see also* Malaria)
    084.6
  Malta (*see also* Brucellosis) 023.9
  Marseilles 082.1
  marsh (*see also* Malaria) 084.6
  Mayaro (viral) 066.3
  Mediterranean (*see also* Brucellosis)
    023.9
    familial 277.31
    tick 082.1
  meningeal - *see* Meningitis
  metal fumes NEC 985.8
  Meuse 083.1
  Mexican - *see* Typhus, Mexican
  Mianeh 087.1
  miasmatic (*see also* Malaria) 084.6

Fever *(Continued)*
 miliary 078.2
 milk, female 672●
 mill 504
 mite-borne hemorrhagic 065.8
 Monday 504
 mosquito-borne NEC 066.3
  hemorrhagic NEC 065.4
 mountain 066.1
  meaning
   Rocky Mountain spotted 082.0
   undulant fever *(see also*
    Brucellosis) 023.9
  tick (American) 066.1
 Mucambo (viral) 066.3
 mud 100.89
 Neapolitan *(see also* Brucellosis) 023.9
 neutropenic 288.00
 newborn (environmentally-induced)
  778.4
 nine-mile 083.0
 nonexanthematous tick 066.1
 North Asian tick-borne typhus 082.2
 Omsk hemorrhagic 065.1
 O'nyong nyong (viral) 066.3
 Oropouche (viral) 066.3
 Oroya 088.0
 paludal *(see also* Malaria) 084.6
 Panama 084.0
 pappataci 066.0
 paratyphoid 002.9
  A 002.1
  B (Schottmüller's) 002.2
  C (Hirschfeld) 002.3
 parrot 073.9
 periodic 277.31
 pernicious, acute 084.0
 persistent (of unknown origin) *(see also*
  Pyrexia) 780.60
 petechial 036.0
 pharyngoconjunctival 077.2
  adenoviral type 3 077.2
 Philippine hemorrhagic 065.4
 phlebotomus 066.0
 Piry 066.8
 Pixuna (viral) 066.3
 Plasmodium ovale 084.3
 pleural *(see also* Pleurisy) 511.0
 pneumonic - *see* Pneumonia
 polymer fume 987.8
 postimmunization 780.63
 postoperative 780.62
  due to infection 998.59
 postvaccination 780.63
 pretibial 100.89
 puerperal, postpartum 672●
 putrid - *see* Septicemia
 pyemic - *see* Septicemia
 Q 083.0
  with pneumonia 083.0 *[484.8]*
 quadrilateral 083.0
 quartan (malaria) 084.2
 Queensland (coastal) 083.0
  seven-day 100.89
 Quintan (A) 083.1
 quotidian 084.0
 rabbit *(see also* Tularemia) 021.9
 rat-bite 026.9
  due to
   Spirillum minor or minus 026.0
   Spirochaeta morsus muris 026.0
   Streptobacillus moniliformis
    026.1
 recurrent - *see* Fever, relapsing

Fever *(Continued)*
 relapsing 087.9
  Carter's (Asiatic) 087.0
  Dutton's (West African) 087.1
  Koch's 087.9
  louse-borne (epidemic) 087.0
  Novy's (American) 087.1
  Obermeyer's (European) 087.0
  spirillum NEC 087.9
  tick-borne (endemic) 087.1
 remittent (bilious) (congestive) (gastric)
  (see also Malaria) 084.6
 rheumatic (active) (acute) (chronic)
  (subacute) 390
  with heart involvement 391.9
   carditis 391.9
   endocarditis (aortic) (mitral)
    (pulmonary) (tricuspid)
    391.1
   multiple sites 391.8
   myocarditis 391.2
   pancarditis, acute 391.8
   pericarditis 391.0
   specified type NEC 391.8
   valvulitis 391.1
  inactive or quiescent with
   cardiac hypertrophy 398.99
   carditis 398.90
   endocarditis 397.9
    aortic (valve) 395.9
     with mitral (valve) disease
      396.9
    mitral (valve) 394.9
     with aortic (valve) disease
      396.9
    pulmonary (valve) 397.1
    tricuspid (valve) 397.0
   heart conditions (classifiable to
    429.3, 429.6, 429.9) 398.99
    failure (congestive) (conditions
     classifiable to 428.0,
     428.9) 398.91
   left ventricular failure
    (conditions classifiable
    to 428.1) 398.91
   myocardial degeneration
    (conditions classifiable to
    429.1) 398.0
   myocarditis (conditions
    classifiable to 429.0) 398.0
   pancarditis 398.99
   pericarditis 393
 Rift Valley (viral) 066.3
 Rocky Mountain spotted 082.0
 rose 477.0
 Ross river (viral) 066.3
 Russian hemorrhagic 078.6
 sandfly 066.0
 San Joaquin (valley) 114.0
 Sao Paulo 082.0
 scarlet 034.1
 septic - *see* Septicemia
 seven-day 061
  Japan 100.89
  Queensland 100.89
 shin bone 083.1
 Singapore hemorrhagic 065.4
 solar 061
 sore 054.9
 South African tick-bite 087.1
 Southeast Asia hemorrhagic 065.4
 spinal - *see* Meningitis
 spirillary 026.0
 splenic *(see also* Anthrax) 022.9

Fever *(Continued)*
 spotted (Rocky Mountain) 082.0
  American 082.0
  Brazilian 082.0
  Colombian 082.0
  meaning
   cerebrospinal meningitis 036.0
   typhus 082.9
 spring 309.23
 steroid
  correct substance properly
   administered 780.60
  overdose or wrong substance given
   or taken 962.0
 streptobacillary 026.1
 subtertian 084.0
 Sumatran mite 081.2
 sun 061
 swamp 100.89
 sweating 078.2
 swine 003.8
 sylvatic yellow 060.0
 Tahyna 062.5
 tertian - *see* Malaria, tertian
 Thailand hemorrhagic 065.4
 thermic 992.0
 three day 066.0
  with Coxsackie exanthem 074.8
 tick
  American mountain 066.1
  Colorado 066.1
  Kemerovo 066.1
  Mediterranean 082.1
  mountain 066.1
  nonexanthematous 066.1
  Quaranfil 066.1
 tick-bite NEC 066.1
 tick-borne NEC 066.1
  hemorrhagic NEC 065.3
 transitory of newborn 778.4
 trench 083.1
 tsutsugamushi 081.2
 typhogastric 002.0
 typhoid (abortive) (ambulant) (any
  site) (hemorrhagic) (infection)
  (intermittent) (malignant)
  (rheumatic) 002.0
 typhomalarial *(see also* Malaria) 084.6
 typhus - *see* Typhus
 undulant *(see also* Brucellosis) 023.9
 unknown origin *(see also* Pyrexia)
  780.60
 uremic - *see* Uremia
 uveoparotid 135
 valley (Coccidioidomycosis) 114.0
 Venezuelan equine 066.2
 Volhynian 083.1
 Wesselsbron (viral) 066.3
 West
  African 084.8
  Nile (viral) 066.40
   with
    cranial nerve disorders
     066.42
    encephalitis 066.41
    optic neuritis 066.42
    other complications 066.49
    other neurologic manifestations
     066.42
    polyradiculitis 066.42
 Whitmore's 025
 Wolhynian 083.1
 worm 128.9
 Yaroslav hemorrhagic 078.6

◄ New   ◄▬ Revised   ~~deleted~~ Deleted   ● Use Additional Digit(s)   ▬ Omit code

Fever (Continued)
  yellow 060.9
    jungle 060.0
    sylvatic 060.0
    urban 060.1
    vaccination, prophylactic (against)
      V04.4
  Zika (viral) 066.3
Fibrillation
  atrial (established) (paroxysmal) 427.31
  auricular (atrial) (established) 427.31
  cardiac (ventricular) 427.41
  coronary (see also Infarct, myocardium)
    410.9●
  heart (ventricular) 427.41
  muscular 728.9
  postoperative 997.1
  ventricular 427.41
Fibrin
  ball or bodies, pleural (sac) 511.0
  chamber, anterior (eye) (gelatinous
    exudate) 364.04
Fibrinogenolysis (hemorrhagic) - see
  Fibrinolysis
Fibrinogenopenia (congenital) (hereditary)
  (see also Defect, coagulation) 286.3
  acquired 286.6
Fibrinolysis (acquired) (hemorrhagic)
  (pathologic) 286.6
  with
    abortion - see Abortion, by type, with
      hemorrhage, delayed or
      excessive
    ectopic pregnancy (see also
      categories 633.0–633.9) 639.1
    molar pregnancy (see also categories
      630–632) 639.1
  antepartum or intrapartum 641.3●
    affecting fetus or newborn 762.1
  following
    abortion 639.1
    ectopic or molar pregnancy 639.1
  newborn, transient 776.2
  postpartum 666.3●
Fibrinopenia (hereditary) (see also Defect,
  coagulation) 286.3
  acquired 286.6
Fibrinopurulent - see condition
Fibrinous - see condition
Fibroadenoma (M9010/0)
  cellular intracanalicular (M9020/0) 217
  giant (intracanalicular) (M9020/0) 217
  intracanalicular (M9011/0)
    cellular (M9020/0) 217
    giant (M9020/0) 217
    specified site - see Neoplasm, by site,
      benign
    unspecified site 217
  juvenile (M9030/0) 217
  pericanicular (M9012/0)
    specified site - see Neoplasm, by site,
      benign
    unspecified site 217
  phyllodes (M9020/0) 217
  prostate 600.20
    with
      other lower urinary tract
        symptoms (LUTS) 600.21
      urinary
        obstruction 600.21
        retention 600.21
  specified site - see Neoplasm, by site,
    benign
  unspecified site 217

Fibroadenosis, breast (chronic) (cystic)
  (diffuse) (periodic) (segmental) 610.2
Fibroangioma (M9160/0) - see also
  Neoplasm, by site, benign
  juvenile (M9160/0)
    specified site - see Neoplasm, by site,
      benign
    unspecified site 210.7
Fibrocellulitis progressiva ossificans
  728.11
Fibrochondrosarcoma (M9220/3) - see
  Neoplasm, cartilage, malignant
Fibrocystic
  disease 277.00
    bone NEC 733.29
    breast 610.1
    jaw 526.2
    kidney (congenital) 753.19
    liver 751.62
    lung 518.89
      congenital 748.4
    pancreas 277.00
  kidney (congenital) 753.19
Fibrodysplasia ossificans multiplex
  (progressiva) 728.11
Fibroelastosis (cordis) (endocardial)
  (endomyocardial) 425.3
Fibroid (tumor) (M8890/0) - see also
  Neoplasm, connective tissue, benign
  disease, lung (chronic) (see also Fibrosis,
    lung) 515
  heart (disease) (see also Myocarditis)
    429.0
  induration, lung (chronic) (see also
    Fibrosis, lung) 515
  in pregnancy or childbirth 654.1●
    affecting fetus or newborn 763.89
    causing obstructed labor 660.2●
      affecting fetus or newborn
        763.1
  liver - see Cirrhosis, liver
  lung (see also Fibrosis, lung) 515
  pneumonia (chronic) (see also Fibrosis,
    lung) 515
  uterus (M8890/0) (see also Leiomyoma,
    uterus) 218.9
Fibrolipoma (M8851/0) (see also Lipoma,
  by site) 214.9
Fibroliposarcoma (M8850/3) - see
  Neoplasm, connective tissue,
  malignant
Fibroma (M8810/0) - see also Neoplasm,
  connective tissue, benign
  ameloblastic (M9330/0) 213.1
    upper jaw (bone) 213.0
  bone (nonossifying) 733.99
    ossifying (M9262/0) - see Neoplasm,
      bone, benign
  cementifying (M9274/0) - see
    Neoplasm, bone, benign
  chondromyxoid (M9241/0) - see
    Neoplasm, bone, benign
  desmoplastic (M8823/1) - see
    Neoplasm, connective tissue,
    uncertain behavior
  facial (M8813/0) - see Neoplasm,
    connective tissue, benign
  invasive (M8821/1) - see Neoplasm,
    connective tissue, uncertain
    behavior
  molle (M8851/0) (see also Lipoma, by
    site) 214.9
  myxoid (M8811/0) - see Neoplasm,
    connective tissue, benign

Fibroma (Continued)
  nasopharynx, nasopharyngeal
    (juvenile) (M9160/0) 210.7
  nonosteogenic (nonossifying) - see
    Dysplasia, fibrous
  odontogenic (M9321/0) 213.1
    upper jaw (bone) 213.0
  ossifying (M9262/0) - see Neoplasm,
    bone, benign
  periosteal (M8812/0) - see Neoplasm,
    bone, benign
  prostate 600.20
    with
      other lower urinary tract
        symptoms (LUTS) 600.21
      urinary
        obstruction 600.21
        retention 600.21
  soft (M8851/0) (see also Lipoma, by
    site) 214.9
Fibromatosis 728.79
  abdominal (M8822/1) - see Neoplasm,
    connective tissue, uncertain
    behavior
  aggressive (M8821/1) - see Neoplasm,
    connective tissue, uncertain
    behavior
  congenital generalized (CGF) 759.89
  Dupuytren's 728.6
  gingival 523.8
  plantar fascia 728.71
  proliferative 728.79
  pseudosarcomatous (proliferative)
    (subcutaneous) 728.79
  subcutaneous pseudosarcomatous
    (proliferative) 728.79
Fibromyalgia 729.1
Fibromyoma (M8890/0) - see also
  Neoplasm, connective tissue, benign
  uterus (corpus) (see also Leiomyoma,
    uterus) 218.9
  in pregnancy or childbirth 654.1●
    affecting fetus or newborn 763.89
    causing obstructed labor 660.2●
      affecting fetus or newborn
        763.1
Fibromyositis (see also Myositis) 729.1
  scapulohumeral 726.2
Fibromyxolipoma (M8852/0) (see also
  Lipoma, by site) 214.9
Fibromyxoma (M8811/0) - see Neoplasm,
  connective tissue, benign
Fibromyxosarcoma (M8811/3) - see
  Neoplasm, connective tissue,
  malignant
Fibro-odontoma, ameloblastic (M9290/0)
  213.1
  upper jaw (bone) 213.0
Fibro-osteoma (M9262/0) - see Neoplasm,
  bone, benign
Fibroplasia, retrolental (see also
  Retinopathy of prematurity) 362.21
Fibropurulent - see condition
Fibrosarcoma (M8810/3) - see also
  Neoplasm, connective tissue,
  malignant
  ameloblastic (M9330/3) 170.1
    upper jaw (bone) 170.0
  congenital (M8814/3) - see Neoplasm,
    connective tissue, malignant
  fascial (M8813/3) - see Neoplasm,
    connective tissue, malignant
  infantile (M8814/3) - see Neoplasm,
    connective tissue, malignant

Fibrosarcoma *(Continued)*
  odontogenic (M9330/3) 170.1
    upper jaw (bone) 170.0
  periosteal (M8812/3) - *see* Neoplasm,
    bone, malignant
Fibrosclerosis
  breast 610.3
  corpora cavernosa (penis) 607.89
  familial multifocal NEC 710.8
  multifocal (idiopathic) NEC 710.8
  penis (corpora cavernosa) 607.89
Fibrosis, fibrotic
  adrenal (gland) 255.8
  alveolar (diffuse) 516.3
  amnion 658.8●
  anal papillae 569.49
  anus 569.49
  appendix, appendiceal,
    noninflammatory 543.9
  arteriocapillary - *see* Arteriosclerosis
  bauxite (of lung) 503
  biliary 576.8
    due to Clonorchis sinensis 121.1
  bladder 596.8
    interstitial 595.1
    localized submucosal 595.1
    panmural 595.1
  bone, diffuse 756.59
  breast 610.3
  capillary - *see also* Arteriosclerosis
    lung (chronic) (*see also* Fibrosis,
      lung) 515
  cardiac (*see also* Myocarditis) 429.0
  cervix 622.8
  chorion 658.8●
  corpus cavernosum 607.89
  cystic (of pancreas) 277.00
    with
      manifestations
        gastrointestinal 277.03
        pulmonary 277.02
        specified NEC 277.09
      meconium ileus 277.01
      pulmonary exacerbation 277.02
  due to (presence of) any device,
    implant, or graft - *see*
    Complications, due to
    (presence of) any device, implant,
    or graft classified to 996.0–996.5
    NEC
  ejaculatory duct 608.89
  endocardium (*see also* Endocarditis)
    424.90
  endomyocardial (African) 425.0
  epididymis 608.89
  eye muscle 378.62
  graphite (of lung) 503
  heart (*see also* Myocarditis) 429.0
  hepatic - *see also* Cirrhosis, liver
    due to Clonorchis sinensis 121.1
  hepatolienal - *see* Cirrhosis, liver
  hepatosplenic - *see* Cirrhosis, liver
  infrapatellar fat pad 729.31
  interstitial pulmonary, newborn
    770.7
  intrascrotal 608.89
  kidney (*see also* Sclerosis, renal) 587
  liver - *see* Cirrhosis, liver
  lung (atrophic) (capillary) (chronic)
    (confluent) (massive)
    (perialveolar) (peribronchial)
    515
    with
      anthracosilicosis (occupational)
        500

Fibrosis, fibrotic *(Continued)*
  lung *(Continued)*
    with *(Continued)*
      anthracosis (occupational) 500
      asbestosis (occupational) 501
      bagassosis (occupational) 495.1
      bauxite 503
      berylliosis (occupational) 503
      byssinosis (occupational) 504
      calcicosis (occupational) 502
      chalicosis (occupational) 502
      dust reticulation (occupational)
        504
      farmers' lung 495.0
      gannister disease (occupational)
        502
      graphite 503
      pneumonoconiosis (occupational)
        505
      pneumosiderosis (occupational)
        503
      siderosis (occupational) 503
      silicosis (occupational) 502
      tuberculosis (*see also* Tuberculosis)
        011.4●
    diffuse (idiopathic) (interstitial)
      516.3
    due to
      bauxite 503
      fumes or vapors (chemical)
        (inhalation) 506.4
      graphite 503
    following radiation 508.1
    postinflammatory 515
    silicotic (massive) (occupational)
      502
    tuberculous (*see also* Tuberculosis)
      011.4●
  lymphatic gland 289.3
  median bar 600.90
    with
      other lower urinary tract
        symptoms (LUTS) 600.91
      urinary
        obstruction 600.91
        retention 600.91
  mediastinum (idiopathic) 519.3
  meninges 349.2
  muscle NEC 728.2
    iatrogenic (from injection) 999.9
  myocardium, myocardial (*see also*
    Myocarditis) 429.0
  oral submucous 528.8
  ovary 620.8
  oviduct 620.8
  pancreas 577.8
    cystic 277.00
      with
        manifestations
          gastrointestinal 277.03
          pulmonary 277.02
          specified NEC 277.09
        meconium ileus 277.01
        pulmonary exacerbation
          277.02
  penis 607.89
  periappendiceal 543.9
  periarticular (*see also* Ankylosis)
    718.5●
  pericardium 423.1
  perineum, in pregnancy or childbirth
    654.8●
    affecting fetus or newborn 763.89
    causing obstructed labor 660.2●
      affecting fetus or newborn 763.1

Fibrosis, fibrotic *(Continued)*
  perineural NEC 355.9
    foot 355.6
  periureteral 593.89
  placenta - *see* Placenta, abnormal
  pleura 511.0
  popliteal fat pad 729.31
  preretinal 362.56
  prostate (chronic) 600.90
    with
      other lower urinary tract
        symptoms (LUTS) 600.91
      urinary
        obstruction 600.91
        retention 600.91
  pulmonary (chronic) (*see also* Fibrosis,
    lung) 515
    alveolar capillary block 516.3
    interstitial
      diffuse (idiopathic) 516.3
      newborn 770.7
  radiation - *see* Effect, adverse, radiation
  rectal sphincter 569.49
  retroperitoneal, idiopathic 593.4
  sclerosing mesenteric (idiopathic)
    567.82
  scrotum 608.89
  seminal vesicle 608.89
  senile 797
  skin NEC 709.2
  spermatic cord 608.89
  spleen 289.59
    bilharzial (*see also* Schistosomiasis)
      120.9
  subepidermal nodular (M8832/0) - *see*
    Neoplasm, skin, benign
  submucous NEC 709.2
    oral 528.8
    tongue 528.8
  syncytium - *see* Placenta, abnormal
  testis 608.89
    chronic, due to syphilis 095.8
  thymus (gland) 254.8
  tunica vaginalis 608.89
  ureter 593.89
  urethra 599.84
  uterus (nonneoplastic) 621.8
    bilharzial (*see also* Schistosomiasis)
      120.9
    neoplastic (*see also* Leiomyoma,
      uterus) 218.9
  vagina 623.8
  valve, heart (*see also* Endocarditis)
    424.90
  vas deferens 608.89
  vein 459.89
    lower extremities 459.89
  vesical 595.1
Fibrositis (periarticular) (rheumatoid)
  729.0
  humeroscapular region 726.2
  nodular, chronic
    Jaccoud's 714.4
    rheumatoid 714.4
  ossificans 728.11
  scapulohumeral 726.2
Fibrothorax 511.0
Fibrotic - *see* Fibrosis
Fibrous - *see* condition
Fibroxanthoma (M8831/0) - *see also*
  Neoplasm, connective tissue,
  benign
  atypical (M8831/1) - *see* Neoplasm,
    connective tissue, uncertain
    behavior

◀ New   ◀▥ Revised   ~~deleted~~ Deleted   ● Use Additional Digit(s)   ▨ Omit code

Fibroxanthoma (*Continued*)
  malignant (M8831/3) - *see* Neoplasm,
    connective tissue, malignant
Fibroxanthosarcoma (M8831/3) - *see*
  Neoplasm, connective tissue,
  malignant
Fiedler's
  disease (leptospiral jaundice) 100.0
  myocarditis or syndrome (acute
    isolated myocarditis) 422.91
Fiessinger-Leroy (-Reiter) syndrome 099.3
Fiessinger-Rendu syndrome (erythema
  muliforme exudativum) 695.19
Fifth disease (eruptive) 057.0
  venereal 099.1
Filaria, filarial - *see* Infestation, filarial
Filariasis (*see also* Infestation, filarial) 125.9
  bancroftian 125.0
  Brug's 125.1
  due to
    bancrofti 125.0
    Brugia (Wuchereria) (malayi) 125.1
    Loa loa 125.2
    malayi 125.1
    organism NEC 125.6
    Wuchereria (bancrofti) 125.0
      malayi 125.1
  Malayan 125.1
  ozzardi 125.5
  specified type NEC 125.6
Filatoff's, Filatov's, Filatow's disease
  (infectious mononucleosis) 075
File-cutters' disease 984.9
  specified type of lead - *see* Table of
    Drugs and Chemicals
Filling defect
  biliary tract 793.3
  bladder 793.5
  duodenum 793.4
  gallbladder 793.3
  gastrointestinal tract 793.4
  intestine 793.4
  kidney 793.5
  stomach 793.4
  ureter 793.5
Filtering bleb, eye (postglaucoma)
  (status) V45.69
  with complication or rupture 997.99
  postcataract extraction (complication)
    997.99
Fimbrial cyst (congenital) 752.11
Fimbriated hymen 752.49
Financial problem affecting care V60.2
Findings, (abnormal), without diagnosis
  (examination) (laboratory
  test) 796.4 ◄▥
  17-ketosteroids, elevated 791.9
  acetonuria 791.6
  acid phosphatase 790.5
  albumin-globulin ratio 790.99
  albuminuria 791.0
  alcohol in blood 790.3
  alkaline phosphatase 790.5
  amniotic fluid 792.3
  amylase 790.5
  antenatal screening 796.5
  anisocytosis 790.09
  anthrax, positive 795.31
  antibody titers, elevated 795.79
  anticardiolipin antibody 795.79
  antigen-antibody reaction 795.79
  antiphospholipid antibody 795.79
  bacteriuria 791.9
  ballistocardiogram 794.39
  bicarbonate 276.9
  bile in urine 791.4
  bilirubin 277.4

Findings, abnormal, without diagnosis
  (*Continued*)
  bleeding time (prolonged) 790.92
  blood culture, positive 790.7
  blood gas level (arterial) 790.91
  blood sugar level 790.29
    high 790.29
      fasting glucose 790.21
      glucose tolerance test 790.22
    low 251.2
  C-reactive protein (CRP) 790.95
  calcium 275.40
  cancer antigen 125 [CA 125] 795.82
  carbonate 276.9
  carcinoembryonic antigen [CEA] 795.81
  casts, urine 791.7
  catecholamines 791.9
  cells, urine 791.7
  cerebrospinal fluid (color) (content)
    (pressure) 792.0
  cervical
    high risk human papillomavirus
      (HPV) DNA test positive
      795.05
    low risk human papillomavirus
      (HPV) DNA test positive
      795.09
  chloride 276.9
  cholesterol 272.9
    high 272.0
      with high triglycerides 272.2
  chromosome analysis 795.2
  chyluria 791.1
  circulation time 794.39
  cloudy dialysis effluent 792.5
  cloudy urine 791.9
  coagulation study 790.92
  cobalt, blood 790.6
  color of urine (unusual) NEC 791.9
  copper, blood 790.6
  creatinine clearance 794.4
  crystals, urine 791.9
  culture, positive NEC 795.39
    blood 790.7
    HIV V08
    human immunodeficiency virus
      V08
    nose 795.39
      Staphylococcus - *see* Carrier
        (suspected) of,
        Staphylococcus
    skin lesion NEC 795.39
    spinal fluid 792.0
    sputum 795.39
    stool 792.1
    throat 795.39
    urine 791.9
    viral
      human immunodeficiency V08
    wound 795.39
  cytology specified site NEC 796.9 ◄
  echocardiogram 793.2
  echoencephalogram 794.01
  echogram NEC - *see* Findings,
    abnormal, structure
  electrocardiogram (ECG) (EKG)
    794.31
  electroencephalogram (EEG) 794.02
  electrolyte level, urinary 791.9
  electromyogram (EMG) 794.17
    ocular 794.14
  electro-oculogram (EOG) 794.12
  electroretinogram (ERG) 794.11
  enzymes, serum NEC 790.5
  fibrinogen titer coagulation study
    790.92
  filling defect - *see* Filling defect

Findings, abnormal, without diagnosis
  (*Continued*)
  function study NEC 794.9
    auditory 794.15
    bladder 794.9
    brain 794.00
    cardiac 794.30
    endocrine NEC 794.6
      thyroid 794.5
    kidney 794.4
    liver 794.8
    nervous system
      central 794.00
      peripheral 794.19
    oculomotor 794.14
    pancreas 794.9
    placenta 794.9
    pulmonary 794.2
    retina 794.11
    special senses 794.19
    spleen 794.9
    vestibular 794.16
  gallbladder, nonvisualization 793.3
  glucose 790.29
    elevated
      fasting 790.21
      tolerance test 790.22
  glycosuria 791.5
  heart
    shadow 793.2
    sounds 785.3
  hematinuria 791.2
  hematocrit
    drop (precipitous) 790.01
    elevated 282.7
    low 285.9
  hematologic NEC 790.99
  hematuria 599.70
  hemoglobin ◄
    drop 790.01
    elevated 282.7
    low 285.9
  hemoglobinuria 791.2
  histological NEC 795.4
  hormones 259.9
  immunoglobulins, elevated 795.79
  indolacetic acid, elevated 791.9
  iron 790.6
  karyotype 795.2
  ketonuria 791.6
  lactic acid dehydrogenase
    (LDH) 790.4
  lead 790.6
  lipase 790.5
  lipids NEC 272.9
  lithium, blood 790.6
  liver function test 790.6
  lung field (coin lesion) (shadow)
    793.1
  magnesium, blood 790.6
  mammogram 793.80
    calcification 793.89
    calculus 793.89
    dense breasts 793.82 ◄
    inconclusive 793.82 ◄
      due to dense breasts 793.82 ◄
    microcalcification 793.81
  mediastinal shift 793.2
  melanin, urine 791.9
  microbiologic NEC 795.39
  mineral, blood NEC 790.6
  myoglobinuria 791.3
  nasal swab, anthrax 795.31
  neonatal screening 796.6
  nitrogen derivatives, blood 790.6
  nonvisualization of gallbladder 793.3
  nose culture, positive 795.39

Findings, abnormal, without diagnosis
(Continued)
odor of urine (unusual) NEC 791.9
oxygen saturation 790.91
Papanicolaou (smear) 796.9
  anus 796.70
    with
      atypical squamous cells
        cannot exclude high
          grade squamous
          intraepithelial
          lesion (ASC-H)
          796.72
        of undetermined
          significance
          (ASC-US) 796.71
      cytologic evidence of
        malignancy 796.76
      high grade squamous
        intraepithelial lesion
        (HGSIL) 796.74
      low grade squamous
        intraepithelial lesion
        (LGSIL) 796.73
    glandular 796.70
    specified finding NEC 796.79
  cervix 795.00
    with
      atypical squamous cells
        cannot exclude high grade
          squamous
          intraepithelial lesion
          (ASC-H) 795.02
        of undetermined
          significance
          (ASC-US) 795.01
      cytologic evidence of
        malignancy 795.06
      high grade squamous
        intraepithelial lesion
        (HGSIL) 795.04
      low grade squamous
        intraepithelial lesion
        (LGSIL) 795.03
    dyskaryotic 795.09
    nonspecific finding NEC
      795.09
  other site 796.9
  vagina 795.10
    with
      atypical squamous cells
        cannot exclude high grade
          squamous
          intraepithelial lesion
          (ASC-H) 795.12
        of undetermined
          significance
          (ASC-US) 795.11
      cytologic evidence of
        malignancy 795.16
      high grade squamous
        intraepithelial lesion
        (HGSIL) 795.14
      low grade squamous
        intraepithelial lesion
        (LGSIL) 795.13
    glandular 795.10
    specified NEC 795.19
peritoneal fluid 792.9
phonocardiogram 794.39
phosphorus 275.3
pleural fluid 792.9
pneumoencephalogram 793.0
PO₂-oxygen ratio 790.91
poikilocytosis 790.09

Findings, abnormal, without diagnosis
(Continued)
potassium
  deficiency 276.8
  excess 276.7
PPD 795.5
prostate specific antigen (PSA)
  790.93
protein, serum NEC 790.99
proteinuria 791.0
prothrombin time (prolonged) (partial)
  (PT) (PTT) 790.92
pyuria 791.9
radiologic (x-ray) 793.99
  abdomen 793.6
  biliary tract 793.3
  breast 793.89
    abnormal mammogram NOS
      793.80
    mammographic
      calcification 793.89
      calculus 793.89
      microcalcification 793.81
  gastrointestinal tract 793.4
  genitourinary organs 793.5
  head 793.0
  image test inconclusive due to
    excess body fat 793.91
  intrathoracic organs NEC 793.2
  lung 793.1
  musculoskeletal 793.7
  placenta 793.99
  retroperitoneum 793.6
  skin 793.99
  skull 793.0
  subcutaneous tissue 793.99
red blood cell 790.09
  count 790.09
  morphology 790.09
  sickling 790.09
  volume 790.09
saliva 792.4
scan NEC 794.9
  bladder 794.9
  bone 794.9
  brain 794.09
  kidney 794.4
  liver 794.8
  lung 794.2
  pancreas 794.9
  placental 794.9
  spleen 794.9
  thyroid 794.5
sedimentation rate, elevated 790.1
semen 792.2
serological (for)
  human immunodeficiency virus
    (HIV)
      inconclusive 795.71
      positive V08
  syphilis - *see* Findings, serology for
    syphilis
serology for syphilis
  false positive 795.6
  positive 097.1
    false 795.6
    follow-up of latent syphilis - *see*
      Syphilis, latent
    only finding - *see* Syphilis, latent
serum 790.99
  blood NEC 790.99
  enzymes NEC 790.5
  proteins 790.99
SGOT 790.4
SGPT 790.4

Findings, abnormal, without diagnosis
(Continued)
sickling of red blood cells 790.09
skin test, positive 795.79
  tuberculin (without active
    tuberculosis) 795.5
sodium 790.6
  deficiency 276.1
  excess 276.0
specified NEC 796.9 ◄
spermatozoa 792.2
spinal fluid 792.0
  culture, positive 792.0
sputum culture, positive 795.39
  for acid-fast bacilli 795.39
stool NEC 792.1
  bloody 578.1
    occult 792.1
  color 792.1
  culture, positive 792.1
  occult blood 792.1
stress test 794.39
structure, body (echogram)
  (thermogram) (ultrasound) (x-ray)
  NEC 793.99
  abdomen 793.6
  breast 793.89
    abnormal mammogram 793.80
    mammographic
      calcification 793.89
      calculus 793.89
      microcalcification 793.81
  gastrointestinal tract 793.4
  genitourinary organs 793.5
  head 793.0
    echogram (ultrasound) 794.01
  intrathoracic organs NEC 793.2
  lung 793.1
  musculoskeletal 793.7
  placenta 793.99
  retroperitoneum 793.6
  skin 793.99
  subcutaneous tissue NEC 793.99
synovial fluid 792.9
thermogram - *see* Findings, abnormal,
  structure
throat culture, positive 795.39
thyroid (function) 794.5
  metabolism (rate) 794.5
  scan 794.5
  uptake 794.5
total proteins 790.99
toxicology (drugs) (heavy metals) 796.0
transaminase (level) 790.4
triglycerides 272.9
  high 272.1
    with high cholesterol 272.2
tuberculin skin test (without active
    tuberculosis) 795.5
tumor markers NEC 795.89
ultrasound - *see also* Findings,
    abnormal, structure
  cardiogram 793.2
uric acid, blood 790.6
urine, urinary constituents 791.9
  acetone 791.6
  albumin 791.0
  bacteria 791.9
  bile 791.4
  blood 599.70
  casts or cells 791.7
  chyle 791.1
  culture, positive 791.9
  glucose 791.5
  hemoglobin 791.2

◄ New   ◄▥ Revised   ~~deleted~~ Deleted   ● Use Additional Digit(s)   ▦ Omit code

Findings, abnormal, without diagnosis
(Continued)
  urine, urinary constituents (Continued)
    ketone 791.6
    protein 791.0
    pus 791.9
    sugar 791.5
  vaginal
    fluid 792.9
    high risk human papillomavirus
      (HPV) DNA test positive
      795.15
    low risk human papillomavirus
      (HPV) DNA test positive
      795.19
  vanillylmandelic acid, elevated 791.9
  vectorcardiogram (VCG) 794.39
  ventriculogram (cerebral) 793.0
  VMA, elevated 791.9
  Wassermann reaction
    false positive 795.6
    positive 097.1
      follow-up of latent syphilis - see
        Syphilis, latent
      only finding - see Syphilis, latent
  white blood cell 288.9
    count 288.9
      elevated 288.60
      low 288.50
    differential 288.9
    morphology 288.9
  wound culture 795.39
  xerography 793.89
  zinc, blood 790.6
Finger - see condition
Finnish type nephrosis (congenital)
  759.89
Fire, St. Anthony's (see also Erysipelas) 035
Fish
  hook stomach 537.89
  meal workers' lung 495.8
Fisher's syndrome 357.0
Fissure, fissured
  abdominal wall (congenital) 756.79
  anus, anal 565.0
    congenital 751.5
  buccal cavity 528.9
  clitoris (congenital) 752.49
  ear, lobule (congenital) 744.29
  epiglottis (congenital) 748.3
  larynx 478.79
    congenital 748.3
  lip 528.5
    congenital (see also Cleft, lip) 749.10
  nipple 611.2
    puerperal, postpartum 676.1●
  palate (congenital) (see also Cleft,
    palate) 749.00
  postanal 565.0
  rectum 565.0
  skin 709.8
    streptococcal 686.9
  spine (congenital) (see also Spina bifida)
    741.9●
  sternum (congenital) 756.3
  tongue (acquired) 529.5
    congenital 750.13
Fistula (sinus) 686.9
  abdomen (wall) 569.81
    bladder 596.2
    intestine 569.81
    ureter 593.82
    uterus 619.2
  abdominorectal 569.81
  abdominosigmoidal 569.81

Fistula (Continued)
  abdominothoracic 510.0
  abdominouterine 619.2
    congenital 752.3
  abdominovesical 596.2
  accessory sinuses (see also Sinusitis)
    473.9
  actinomycotic - see Actinomycosis
  alveolar
    antrum (see also Sinusitis, maxillary)
      473.0
    process 522.7
  anorectal 565.1
  antrobuccal (see also Sinusitis,
    maxillary) 473.0
  antrum (see also Sinusitis, maxillary)
    473.0
  anus, anal (infectional) (recurrent)
    565.1
    congenital 751.5
    tuberculous (see also Tuberculosis)
      014.8●
  aortic sinus 747.29
  aortoduodenal 447.2
  appendix, appendicular 543.9
  arteriovenous (acquired) 447.0
    brain 437.3
      congenital 747.81
        ruptured (see also
          Hemorrhage,
          subarachnoid) 430
      ruptured (see also Hemorrhage,
        subarachnoid) 430
    cerebral 437.3
      congenital 747.81
    congenital (peripheral) 747.60
      brain - see Fistula,
        arteriovenous,
        brain, congenital
      coronary 746.85
      gastrointestinal 747.61
      lower limb 747.64
      pulmonary 747.3
      renal 747.62
      specified site NEC 747.69
      upper limb 747.63
    coronary 414.19
      congenital 746.85
    heart 414.19
    pulmonary (vessels) 417.0
      congenital 747.3
    surgically created (for dialysis)
      V45.11
      complication NEC 996.73
        atherosclerosis - see
          Arteriosclerosis,
          extremities
        embolism 996.74
        infection or inflammation
          996.62
        mechanical 996.1
        occlusion NEC 996.74
        thrombus 996.74
    traumatic - see Injury, blood vessel,
      by site
  artery 447.2
  aural 383.81
    congenital 744.49
  auricle 383.81
    congenital 744.49
  Bartholin's gland 619.8
  bile duct (see also Fistula, biliary)
    576.4
  biliary (duct) (tract) 576.4
    congenital 751.69

Fistula (Continued)
  bladder (neck) (sphincter) 596.2
    into seminal vesicle 596.2
  bone 733.99
  brain 348.89 ◀▥
    arteriovenous - see Fistula,
      arteriovenous, brain
  branchial (cleft) 744.41
  branchiogenous 744.41
  breast 611.0
    puerperal, postpartum 675.1●
  bronchial 510.0
  bronchocutaneous,
    bronchomediastinal,
    bronchopleural,
    bronchopleuromediastinal
    (infective) 510.0
    tuberculous (see also Tuberculosis)
      011.3●
  bronchoesophageal 530.84
    congenital 750.3
  buccal cavity (infective) 528.3
  canal, ear 380.89
  carotid-cavernous
    congenital 747.81
      with hemorrhage 430
    traumatic 900.82
      with hemorrhage (see also
        Hemorrhage, brain,
        traumatic) 853.0●
    late effect 908.3
  cecosigmoidal 569.81
  cecum 569.81
  cerebrospinal (fluid) 349.81
  cervical, lateral (congenital)
    744.41
  cervicoaural (congenital) 744.49
  cervicosigmoidal 619.1
  cervicovesical 619.0
  cervix 619.8
  chest (wall) 510.0
  cholecystocolic (see also Fistula,
    gallbladder) 575.5
  cholecystocolonic (see also Fistula,
    gallbladder) 575.5
  cholecystoduodenal (see also Fistula,
    gallbladder) 575.5
  cholecystoenteric (see also Fistula,
    gallbladder) 575.5
  cholecystogastric (see also Fistula,
    gallbladder) 575.5
  cholecystointestinal (see also Fistula,
    gallbladder) 575.5
  choledochoduodenal 576.4
  cholocolic (see also Fistula, gallbladder)
    575.5
  coccyx 685.1
    with abscess 685.0
  colon 569.81
  colostomy 569.69
  colovaginal (acquired) 619.1
  common duct (bile duct) 576.4
  congenital, NEC - see Anomaly,
    specified type NEC
  cornea, causing hypotony
    360.32
  coronary, arteriovenous 414.19
    congenital 746.85
  costal region 510.0
  cul-de-sac, Douglas' 619.8
  cutaneous 686.9
  cystic duct (see also Fistula, gallbladder)
    575.5
    congenital 751.69
  dental 522.7

Fistula (*Continued*)
diaphragm 510.0
  bronchovisceral 510.0
  pleuroperitoneal 510.0
  pulmonoperitoneal 510.0
duodenum 537.4
ear (canal) (external) 380.89
enterocolic 569.81
enterocutaneous 569.81
enteroenteric 569.81
entero-uterine 619.1
  congenital 752.3
enterovaginal 619.1
  congenital 752.49
enterovesical 596.1
epididymis 608.89
  tuberculous (*see also* Tuberculosis)
    016.4●
esophagobronchial 530.89
  congenital 750.3
esophagocutaneous 530.89
esophagopleurocutaneous 530.89
esophagotracheal 530.84
  congenital 750.3
esophagus 530.89
  congenital 750.4
ethmoid (*see also* Sinusitis, ethmoidal)
  473.2
eyeball (cornea) (sclera) 360.32
eyelid 373.11
fallopian tube (external) 619.2
fecal 569.81
  congenital 751.5
from periapical lesion 522.7
frontal sinus (*see also* Sinusitis, frontal)
  473.1
gallbladder 575.5
  with calculus, cholelithiasis, stones
    (*see also* Cholelithiasis) 574.2●
  congenital 751.69
gastric 537.4
gastrocolic 537.4
  congenital 750.7
  tuberculous (*see also* Tuberculosis)
    014.8●
gastroenterocolic 537.4
gastroesophageal 537.4
gastrojejunal 537.4
gastrojejunocolic 537.4
genital
  organs
    female 619.9
      specified site NEC 619.8
    male 608.89
  tract-skin (female) 619.2
hepatopleural 510.0
hepatopulmonary 510.0
horseshoe 565.1
ileorectal 569.81
ileosigmoidal 569.81
ileostomy 569.69
ileovesical 596.1
ileum 569.81
in ano 565.1
  tuberculous (*see also* Tuberculosis)
    014.8●
inner ear (*see also* Fistula, labyrinth)
  386.40
intestine 569.81
intestinocolonic (abdominal) 569.81
intestinoureteral 593.82
intestinouterine 619.1
intestinovaginal 619.1
  congenital 752.49

Fistula (*Continued*)
intestinovesical 596.1
involving female genital tract 619.9
  digestive-genital 619.1
  genital tract-skin 619.2
  specified site NEC 619.8
  urinary-genital 619.0
ischiorectal (fossa) 566
jejunostomy 569.69
jejunum 569.81
joint 719.80
  ankle 719.87
  elbow 719.82
  foot 719.87
  hand 719.84
  hip 719.85
  knee 719.86
  multiple sites 719.89
  pelvic region 719.85
  shoulder (region) 719.81
  specified site NEC 719.88
  tuberculous - *see* Tuberculosis, joint
  wrist 719.83
kidney 593.89
labium (majus) (minus) 619.8
labyrinth, labyrinthine NEC 386.40
  combined sites 386.48
  multiple sites 386.48
  oval window 386.42
  round window 386.41
  semicircular canal 386.43
lacrimal, lachrymal (duct) (gland) (sac)
  375.61
lacrimonasal duct 375.61
laryngotracheal 748.3
larynx 478.79
lip 528.5
  congenital 750.25
lumbar, tuberculous (*see also*
  Tuberculosis) 015.0● [730.8]●
lung 510.0
lymphatic (node) (vessel) 457.8
mamillary 611.0
mammary (gland) 611.0
  puerperal, postpartum 675.1●
mastoid (process) (region) 383.1
maxillary (*see also* Sinusitis, maxillary)
  473.0
mediastinal 510.0
mediastinobronchial 510.0
mediastinocutaneous 510.0
middle ear 385.89
mouth 528.3
nasal 478.19
  sinus (*see also* Sinusitis) 473.9
nasopharynx 478.29
nipple - *see* Fistula, breast
nose 478.19
oral (cutaneous) 528.3
  maxillary (*see also* Sinusitis,
    maxillary) 473.0
  nasal (with cleft palate) (*see also*
    Cleft, palate) 749.00
orbit, orbital 376.10
oro-antral (*see also* Sinusitis, maxillary)
  473.0
oval window (internal ear) 386.42
oviduct (external) 619.2
palate (hard) 526.89
  soft 528.9
pancreatic 577.8
pancreaticoduodenal 577.8
parotid (gland) 527.4
  region 528.3

Fistula (*Continued*)
pelvoabdominointestinal 569.81
penis 607.89
perianal 565.1
pericardium (pleura) (sac) (*see also*
  Pericarditis) 423.8
pericecal 569.81
perineal - *see* Fistula, perineum
perineorectal 569.81
perineosigmoidal 569.81
perineo-urethroscrotal 608.89
perineum, perineal (with urethral
  involvement) NEC 599.1
  tuberculous (*see also* Tuberculosis)
    017.9●
  ureter 593.82
perirectal 565.1
  tuberculous (*see also* Tuberculosis)
    014.8●
peritoneum (*see also* Peritonitis) 567.22
periurethral 599.1
pharyngo-esophageal 478.29
pharynx 478.29
  branchial cleft (congenital) 744.41
pilonidal (infected) (rectum) 685.1
  with abscess 685.0
pleura, pleural, pleurocutaneous,
  pleuroperitoneal 510.0
  stomach 510.0
  tuberculous (*see also* Tuberculosis)
    012.0●
pleuropericardial 423.8
postauricular 383.81
postoperative, persistent 998.6
preauricular (congenital) 744.46
prostate 602.8
pulmonary 510.0
  arteriovenous 417.0
    congenital 747.3
  tuberculous (*see also* Tuberculosis,
    pulmonary) 011.9●
pulmonoperitoneal 510.0
rectolabial 619.1
rectosigmoid (intercommunicating)
  569.81
rectoureteral 593.82
rectourethral 599.1
  congenital 753.8
rectouterine 619.1
  congenital 752.3
rectovaginal 619.1
  congenital 752.49
  old, postpartal 619.1
  tuberculous (*see also* Tuberculosis)
    014.8●
rectovesical 596.1
  congenital 753.8
rectovesicovaginal 619.1
rectovulvar 619.1
  congenital 752.49
rectum (to skin) 565.1
  tuberculous (*see also* Tuberculosis)
    014.8●
renal 593.89
retroauricular 383.81
round window (internal ear) 386.41
salivary duct or gland 527.4
  congenital 750.24
sclera 360.32
scrotum (urinary) 608.89
  tuberculous (*see also* Tuberculosis)
    016.5●
semicircular canals (internal ear)
  386.43

◀ New   ◀▥ Revised   ~~deleted~~ Deleted   ● Use Additional Digit(s)   ▦ Omit code

Fistula *(Continued)*
  sigmoid 569.81
    vesicoabdominal 596.1
  sigmoidovaginal 619.1
    congenital 752.49
  skin 686.9
    ureter 593.82
    vagina 619.2
  sphenoidal sinus *(see also* Sinusitis,
    sphenoidal) 473.3
  splenocolic 289.59
  stercoral 569.81
  stomach 537.4
  sublingual gland 527.4
    congenital 750.24
  submaxillary
    gland 527.4
      congenital 750.24
    region 528.3
  thoracic 510.0
    duct 457.8
  thoracicoabdominal 510.0
  thoracicogastric 510.0
  thoracicointestinal 510.0
  thoracoabdominal 510.0
  thoracogastric 510.0
  thorax 510.0
  thyroglossal duct 759.2
  thyroid 246.8
  trachea (congenital) (external)
    (internal) 748.3
  tracheoesophageal 530.84
    congenital 750.3
    following tracheostomy 519.09
  traumatic
    arteriovenous *(see also* Injury, blood
      vessel, by site) 904.9
      brain - *see* Injury, intracranial
  tuberculous - *see* Tuberculosis, by site
  typhoid 002.0
  umbilical 759.89
  umbilico-urinary 753.8
  urachal, urachus 753.7
  ureter (persistent) 593.82
  ureteroabdominal 593.82
  ureterocervical 593.82
  ureterorectal 593.82
  ureterosigmoido-abdominal 593.82
  ureterovaginal 619.0
  ureterovesical 596.2
  urethra 599.1
    congenital 753.8
    tuberculous *(see also* Tuberculosis)
      016.3●
  urethroperineal 599.1
  urethroperineovesical 596.2
  urethrorectal 599.1
    congenital 753.8
  urethroscrotal 608.89
  urethrovaginal 619.0
  urethrovesical 596.2
  urethrovesicovaginal 619.0
  urinary (persistent) (recurrent) 599.1
  uteroabdominal (anterior wall)
    619.2
    congenital 752.3
  uteroenteric 619.1
  uterofecal 619.1
  uterointestinal 619.1
    congenital 752.3
  uterorectal 619.1
    congenital 752.3
  uteroureteric 619.0
  uterovaginal 619.8

Fistula *(Continued)*
  uterovesical 619.0
    congenital 752.3
  uterus 619.8
  vagina (wall) 619.8
    postpartal, old 619.8
  vaginocutaneous (postpartal) 619.2
  vaginoileal (acquired) 619.1
  vaginoperineal 619.2
  vesical NEC 596.2
  vesicoabdominal 596.2
  vesicocervicovaginal 619.0
  vesicocolic 596.1
  vesicocutaneous 596.2
  vesicoenteric 596.1
  vesicointestinal 596.1
  vesicometrorectal 619.1
  vesicoperineal 596.2
  vesicorectal 596.1
    congenital 753.8
  vesicosigmoidal 596.1
  vesicosigmoidovaginal 619.1
  vesicoureteral 596.2
  vesicoureterovaginal 619.0
  vesicourethral 596.2
  vesicourethrorectal 596.1
  vesicouterine 619.0
    congenital 752.3
  vesicovaginal 619.0
  vulvorectal 619.1
    congenital 752.49
Fit 780.39
  apoplectic *(see also* Disease,
    cerebrovascular, acute) 436
    late effect - *see* Late effect(s) (of)
      cerebrovascular disease
  epileptic *(see also* Epilepsy) 345.9●
  fainting 780.2
  hysterical 300.11
  newborn 779.0
Fitting (of)
  artificial
    arm (complete) (partial) V52.0
    breast V52.4
      implant exchange (different
        material) (different size)
        V52.4
    eye(s) V52.2
    leg(s) (complete) (partial) V52.1
  brain neuropacemaker V53.02
  cardiac pacemaker V53.31
  carotid sinus pacemaker V53.39
  cerebral ventricle (communicating)
    shunt V53.01
  colostomy belt V55.3
  contact lenses V53.1
  cystostomy device V53.6
  defibrillator, automatic implantable
    cardiac V53.32
  dentures V52.3
  device, unspecified type V53.90
    abdominal V53.59   ◀▥
    cardiac
      defibrillator, automatic
        implantable V53.32
      pacemaker V53.31
      specified NEC V53.39
    cerebral ventricle (communicating)
      shunt V53.01
    gastrointestinal NEC V53.59 ◀
    insulin pump V53.91 ◀
    intestinal V53.50 ◀
    intrauterine contraceptive V25.1
    nervous system V53.09

Fitting *(Continued)*
  device, unspecified type *(Continued)*
    orthodontic V53.4
    orthoptic V53.1
    other device V53.99
    prosthetic V52.9
      breast V52.4
      dental V52.3
      eye V52.2
      specified type NEC V52.8
    special senses V53.09
    substitution
      auditory V53.09
      nervous system V53.09
      visual V53.09
    urinary V53.6
  diaphragm (contraceptive) V25.02
  gastric lap band V53.51 ◀
  gastrointestinal appliance and device
    NEC V53.59 ◀
  glasses (reading) V53.1
  growth rod V54.02
  hearing aid V53.2
  ileostomy device V55.2
  intestinal appliance and ~~or~~ device ~~NEC~~
    V53.50 ◀▥
  intrauterine contraceptive device V25.1
  neuropacemaker (brain) (peripheral
    nerve) (spinal cord) V53.02
  orthodontic device V53.4
  orthopedic (device) V53.7
    brace V53.7
    cast V53.7
    corset V53.7
    shoes V53.7
  pacemaker (cardiac) V53.31
    brain V53.02
    carotid sinus V53.39
    peripheral nerve V53.02
    spinal cord V53.02
  prosthesis V52.9
    arm (complete) (partial) V52.0
    breast V52.4
      implant exchange (different
        material) (different size)
        V52.4
    dental V52.3
    eye V52.2
    leg (complete) (partial) V52.1
    specified type NEC V52.8
  spectacles V53.1
  wheelchair V53.8
Fitz's syndrome (acute hemorrhagic
  pancreatitis) 577.0
Fitz-Hugh and **Curtis syndrome** 098.86
  due to
    Chlamydia trachomatis 099.56
    Neisseria gonorrhoeae (gonococcal
      peritonitis) 098.86
Fixation
  joint - *see* Ankylosis
  larynx 478.79
  pupil 364.76
  stapes 385.22
    deafness *(see also* Deafness,
      conductive) 389.04
  uterus (acquired) - *see* Malposition,
    uterus
  vocal cord 478.5
Flaccid - *see also* condition
  foot 736.79
  forearm 736.09
  palate, congenital 750.26
Flail
  chest 807.4
    newborn 767.3

Flail *(Continued)*
  joint (paralytic) 718.80
    ankle 718.87
    elbow 718.82
    foot 718.87
    hand 718.84
    hip 718.85
    knee 718.86
    multiple sites 718.89
    pelvic region 718.85
    shoulder (region) 718.81
    specified site NEC 718.88
    wrist 718.83
Flajani (-Basedow) syndrome or disease
    (exophthalmic goiter) 242.0●
Flap, liver 572.8
Flare, anterior chamber (aqueous) (eye)
    364.04
Flashback phenomena (drug)
    (hallucinogenic) 292.89
Flat
  chamber (anterior) (eye) 360.34
  chest, congenital 754.89
  electroencephalogram (EEG) 348.89 ◀▥
  foot (acquired) (fixed type) (painful)
    (postural) (spastic) 734
    congenital 754.61
      rocker bottom 754.61
      vertical talus 754.61
    rachitic 268.1
    rocker bottom (congenital) 754.61
    vertical talus, congenital 754.61
  organ or site, congenital NEC - *see*
    Anomaly, specified type NEC
  pelvis 738.6
    with disproportion (fetopelvic)
      653.2●
      affecting fetus or newborn 763.1
      causing obstructed labor 660.1●
        affecting fetus or newborn
        763.1
    congenital 755.69
Flatau-Schilder disease 341.1
Flattening
  head, femur 736.39
  hip 736.39
  lip (congenital) 744.89
  nose (congenital) 754.0
    acquired 738.0
Flatulence 787.3
Flatus 787.3
  vaginalis 629.89
Flax dressers' disease 504
Flea bite - *see* Injury, superficial, by site
Fleischer (-Kayser) ring (corneal
    pigmentation) 275.1 *[371.14]*
Fleischner's disease 732.3
Fleshy mole 631
Flexibilitas cerea (*see also* Catalepsy) 300.11
Flexion
  cervix - *see* Flexion, uterus
  contracture, joint (*see also* Contraction,
    joint) 718.4●
  deformity, joint (*see also* Contraction,
    joint) 736.9
    hip, congenital (*see also* Subluxation,
      congenital, hip) 754.32
  uterus (*see also* Malposition, uterus)
    621.6
Flexner's
  bacillus 004.1
  diarrhea (ulcerative) 004.1
  dysentery 004.1
Flexner-Boyd dysentery 004.2

Flexure - *see* condition
Floater, vitreous 379.24
Floating
  cartilage (joint) (*see also* Disorder,
    cartilage, articular) 718.0●
    knee 717.6
  gallbladder (congenital) 751.69
  kidney 593.0
    congenital 753.3
  liver (congenital) 751.69
  rib 756.3
  spleen 289.59
Flooding 626.2
Floor - *see* condition
Floppy
  infant NEC 781.99
  iris syndrome 364.81
  valve syndrome (mitral) 424.0
Flu - *see also* Influenza
  bird 488.0   ◀
  gastric NEC 008.8
  swine 488.1   ◀
Fluctuating blood pressure 796.4
Fluid
  abdomen 789.59
  chest (*see also* Pleurisy, with effusion)
    511.9
  heart (*see also* Failure, heart) 428.0
  joint (*see also* Effusion, joint) 719.0●
  loss (acute) 276.50
    with
      hypernatremia 276.0
      hyponatremia 276.1
  lung - *see also* Edema, lung
    encysted 511.89
  peritoneal cavity 789.59
    malignant 789.51
  pleural cavity (*see also* Pleurisy, with
    effusion) 511.9
  retention 276.6
Flukes NEC (*see also* Infestation, fluke)
    121.9
  blood NEC (*see also* Infestation,
    Schistosoma) 120.9
  liver 121.3
Fluor (albus) (vaginalis) 623.5
  trichomonal (Trichomonas vaginalis)
    131.00
Fluorosis (dental) (chronic) 520.3
Flushing 782.62
  menopausal 627.2
Flush syndrome 259.2
Flutter
  atrial or auricular 427.32
  heart (ventricular) 427.42
    atrial 427.32
  impure 427.32
  postoperative 997.1
  ventricular 427.42
Flux (bloody) (serosanguineous) 009.0
Focal - *see* condition
Fochier's abscess - *see* Abscess, by site
Focus, Assmann's (*see also* Tuberculosis)
    011.0●
Fogo selvagem 694.4
Foix-Alajouanine syndrome 336.1
Folds, anomalous - *see also* Anomaly,
    specified type NEC
  Bowman's membrane 371.31
  Descemet's membrane 371.32
  epicanthic 743.63
  heart 746.89
  posterior segment of eye, congenital
    743.54

Folie a deux 297.3
Follicle
  cervix (nabothian) (ruptured) 616.0
  graafian, ruptured, with hemorrhage
    620.0
  nabothian 616.0
Folliclis (primary) (*see also* Tuberculosis)
    017.0●
Follicular - *see also* condition
  cyst (atretic) 620.0
Folliculitis 704.8
  abscedens et suffodiens 704.8
  decalvans 704.09
  gonorrheal (acute) 098.0
    chronic or duration of 2 months or
      more 098.2
  keloid, keloidalis 706.1
  pustular 704.8
  ulerythematosa reticulata 701.8
Folliculosis, conjunctival 372.02
Følling's disease (phenylketonuria) 270.1
Follow-up (examination) (routine)
    (following) V67.9
  cancer chemotherapy V67.2
  chemotherapy V67.2
  fracture V67.4
  high-risk medication V67.51
  injury NEC V67.59
  postpartum
    immediately after delivery V24.0
    routine V24.2
  psychiatric V67.3
  psychotherapy V67.3
  radiotherapy V67.1
  specified condition NEC V67.59
  specified surgery NEC V67.09
  surgery V67.00
    vaginal pap smear V67.01
  treatment V67.9
    combined NEC V67.6
    fracture V67.4
    involving high-risk medication NEC
      V67.51
    mental disorder V67.3
    specified NEC V67.59
Fong's syndrome (hereditary
    osteoonychodysplasia) 756.89
Food
  allergy 693.1
  anaphylactic shock - *see* Anaphylactic
    shock, due to food
  asphyxia (from aspiration or
    inhalation) (*see also* Asphyxia,
    food) 933.1
  choked on (*see also* Asphyxia, food) 933.1
  deprivation 994.2
    specified kind of food NEC 269.8
  intoxication (*see also* Poisoning, food)
    005.9
  lack of 994.2
  poisoning (*see also* Poisoning, food)
    005.9
  refusal or rejection NEC 307.59
  strangulation or suffocation (*see also*
    Asphyxia, food) 933.1
  toxemia (*see also* Poisoning, food) 005.9
Foot - *see also* condition
  and mouth disease 078.4
  process disease 581.3
Foramen ovale (nonclosure) (patent)
    (persistent) 745.5
Forbes' (glycogen storage) disease 271.0
Forbes-Albright syndrome (nonpuerperal
    amenorrhea and lactation associated
    with pituitary tumor) 253.1

◀ New   ◀▥ Revised   ~~deleted~~ Deleted   ● Use Additional Digit(s)   ▬ Omit code

Forced birth or delivery NEC 669.8●
    affecting fetus or newborn NEC 763.89
Forceps
    delivery NEC 669.5●
        affecting fetus or newborn 763.2
Fordyce's disease (ectopic sebaceous
        glands) (mouth) 750.26
Fordyce-Fox disease (apocrine miliaria)
        705.82
Forearm - *see* condition
Foreign body

> **Note 27** For foreign body with open
> wound or other injury, see Wound,
> open, or the type of injury specified.

    accidentally left during a procedure
        998.4
    anterior chamber (eye) 871.6
        magnetic 871.5
            retained or old 360.51
        retained or old 360.61
    ciliary body (eye) 871.6
        magnetic 871.5
            retained or old 360.52
        retained or old 360.62
    entering through orifice (current) (old)
        accessory sinus 932
        air passage (upper) 933.0
            lower 934.8
        alimentary canal 938
        alveolar process 935.0
        antrum (Highmore) 932
        anus 937
        appendix 936
        asphyxia due to (*see also* Asphyxia,
            food) 933.1
        auditory canal 931
        auricle 931
        bladder 939.0
        bronchioles 934.8
        bronchus (main) 934.1
        buccal cavity 935.0
        canthus (inner) 930.1
        cecum 936
        cervix (canal) uterine 939.1
        coil, ileocecal 936
        colon 936
        conjunctiva 930.1
        conjunctival sac 930.1
        cornea 930.0
        digestive organ or tract NEC 938
        duodenum 936
        ear (external) 931
        esophagus 935.1
        eye (external) 930.9
            combined sites 930.8
            intraocular - *see* Foreign body, by
                site
            specified site NEC 930.8
        eyeball 930.8
            intraocular - *see* Foreign body,
                intraocular
        eyelid 930.1
            retained or old 374.86
        frontal sinus 932
        gastrointestinal tract 938
        genitourinary tract 939.9
        globe 930.8
            penetrating 871.6
                magnetic 871.5
                    retained or old 360.50
                retained or old 360.60
        gum 935.0

Foreign body (*Continued*)
    entering through orifice (*Continued*)
        Highmore's antrum 932
        hypopharynx 933.0
        ileocecal coil 936
        ileum 936
        inspiration (of) 933.1
        intestine (large) (small) 936
        lacrimal apparatus, duct, gland, or
            sac 930.2
        larynx 933.1
        lung 934.8
        maxillary sinus 932
        mouth 935.0
        nasal sinus 932
        nasopharynx 933.0
        nose (passage) 932
        nostril 932
        oral cavity 935.0
        palate 935.0
        penis 939.3
        pharynx 933.0
        pyriform sinus 933.0
        rectosigmoid 937
            junction 937
        rectum 937
        respiratory tract 934.9
            specified part NEC 934.8
        sclera 930.1
        sinus 932
            accessory 932
            frontal 932
            maxillary 932
            nasal 932
            pyriform 933.0
        small intestine 936
        stomach (hairball) 935.2
        suffocation by (*see also* Asphyxia,
            food) 933.1
        swallowed 938
            tongue 933.0
        tear ducts or glands 930.2
        throat 933.0
        tongue 935.0
            swallowed 933.0
        tonsil, tonsillar 933.0
            fossa 933.0
        trachea 934.0
        ureter 939.0
        urethra 939.0
        uterus (any part) 939.1
        vagina 939.2
        vulva 939.2
        wind pipe 934.0
    feeling of, in throat 784.99
    granuloma (old) 728.82
        bone 733.99
        in operative wound (inadvertently
            left) 998.4
            due to surgical material
                intentionally left - *see*
                Complications, due to
                (presence of) any device,
                implant, or graft classified
                to 996.0–996.5 NEC
        muscle 728.82
        skin 709.4
        soft tissue NEC 709.4
        subcutaneous tissue 709.4
    in
        bone (residual) 733.99
        open wound - *see* Wound, open, by
            site complicated
        soft tissue (residual) 729.6

Foreign body (*Continued*)
    inadvertently left in operation
        wound (causing adhesions,
        obstruction, or perforation)
        998.4
    ingestion, ingested NEC 938
    inhalation or inspiration (*see also*
        Asphyxia, food) 933.1
    internal organ, not entering
        through an orifice - *see* Injury,
        internal, by site, with open
        wound
    intraocular (nonmagnetic) 871.6
        combined sites 871.6
            magnetic 871.5
                retained or old 360.59
            retained or old 360.69
        magnetic 871.5
            retained or old 360.50
        retained or old 360.60
        specified site NEC 871.6
            magnetic 871.5
                retained or old 360.59
            retained or old 360.69
    iris (nonmagnetic) 871.6
        magnetic 871.5
            retained or old 360.52
        retained or old 360.62
    lens (nonmagnetic) 871.6
        magnetic 871.5
            retained or old 360.53
        retained or old 360.63
    lid, eye 930.1
    ocular muscle 870.4
        retained or old 376.6
    old or residual
        bone 733.99
        eyelid 374.86
        middle ear 385.83
        muscle 729.6
            ocular 376.6
        retrobulbar 376.6
        skin 729.6
            with granuloma 709.4
        soft tissue 729.6
            with granuloma 709.4
        subcutaneous tissue 729.6
            with granuloma 709.4
    operation wound, left accidentally
        998.4
    orbit 870.4
        retained or old 376.6
    posterior wall, eye 871.6
        magnetic 871.5
            retained or old 360.55
        retained or old 360.65
    respiratory tree 934.9
        specified site NEC 934.8
    retained (old) (nonmagnetic) (in)
        anterior chamber (eye) 360.61
            magnetic 360.51
        ciliary body 360.62
            magnetic 360.52
        eyelid 374.86
        globe 360.60
            magnetic 360.50
        intraocular 360.60
            magnetic 360.50
            specified site NEC 360.69
                magnetic 360.59
        iris 360.62
            magnetic 360.52
        lens 360.63
            magnetic 360.53

Foreign body (Continued)
retained (Continued)
muscle 729.6
orbit 376.6
posterior wall of globe 360.65
magnetic 360.55
retina 360.65
magnetic 360.55
retrobulbar 376.6
skin 729.6
with granuloma 709.4
soft tissue 729.6
with granuloma 709.4
subcutaneous tissue 729.6
with granuloma 709.4
vitreous 360.64
magnetic 360.54
retina 871.6
magnetic 871.5
retained or old 360.55
retained or old 360.65
superficial, without major open wound
(see also Injury, superficial, by site)
919.6
swallowed NEC 938
throat, feeling of 784.99
vitreous (humor) 871.6
magnetic 871.5
retained or old 360.54
retained or old 360.64
Forking, aqueduct of Sylvius
742.3
with spina bifida (see also
Spina bifida) 741.0●
Formation
bone in scar tissue (skin) 709.3
connective tissue in vitreous
379.25
Elschnig pearls (postcataract
extraction) 366.51
hyaline in cornea 371.49
sequestrum in bone (due to infection)
(see also Osteomyelitis)
730.1●
valve
colon, congenital 751.5
ureter (congenital) 753.29
Formication 782.0
Fort Bragg fever 100.89
Fossa - see also condition
pyriform - see condition
Foster care (status) V60.81 ◄
Foster-Kennedy syndrome 377.04
Fothergill's
disease, meaning scarlatina anginosa
034.1
neuralgia (see also Neuralgia,
trigeminal) 350.1
Foul breath 784.99
Found dead (cause unknown)
798.9
Foundling V20.0
Fournier's disease (idiopathic gangrene)
608.83
Fourth
cranial nerve - see condition
disease 057.8
molar 520.1
Foville's syndrome 344.89
Fox's
disease (apocrine miliaria) 705.82
impetigo (contagiosa) 684
Fox-Fordyce disease (apocrine miliaria)
705.82

Fracture (abduction) (adduction)
(avulsion) (compression) (crush)
(dislocation) (oblique) (separation)
(closed) 829.0

Note 28   For fracture of any of the
following sites with fracture of other
bones - see Fracture, multiple.

"Closed" includes the following descriptions of fractures, with or without
delayed healing, unless they are specified as open or compound:

comminuted
depressed
elevated
fissured
greenstick
impacted
linear
simple
slipped epiphysis
spiral
unspecified

"Open" includes the following descriptions of fractures, with or without
delayed healing:

compound
infected
missile
puncture
with foreign body

For late effect of fracture, see Late, effect, fracture, by site.

with
internal injuries in same region
(conditions classifiable to
860–869) - see also Injury,
internal, by site
pelvic region - see Fracture,
pelvis
acetabulum (with visceral injury)
(closed) 808.0
open 808.1
acromion (process) (closed) 811.01
open 811.11
alveolus (closed) 802.8
open 802.9
ankle (malleolus) (closed) 824.8
bimalleolar (Dupuytren's) (Pott's)
824.4
open 824.5
bone 825.21
open 825.31
lateral malleolus only (fibular)
824.2
open 824.3
medial malleolus only (tibial) 824.0
open 824.1
open 824.9
pathologic 733.16
talus 825.21
open 825.31
trimalleolar 824.6
open 824.7
antrum - see Fracture, skull, base
arm (closed) 818.0
and leg(s) (any bones) 828.0
open 828.1
both (any bones) (with rib(s)) (with
sternum) 819.0
open 819.1

Fracture (Continued)
arm (Continued)
lower 813.80
open 813.90
open 818.1
upper - see Fracture, humerus
astragalus (closed) 825.21
open 825.31
atlas - see Fracture, vertebra, cervical,
first
axis - see Fracture, vertebra, cervical,
second
back - see Fracture, vertebra, by site
Barton's - see Fracture, radius, lower end
basal (skull) - see Fracture, skull, base
Bennett's (closed) 815.01
open 815.11
bimalleolar (closed) 824.4
open 824.5
bone (closed) NEC 829.0
birth injury NEC 767.3
open 829.1
pathological NEC (see also Fracture,
pathologic) 733.10
stress NEC (see also Fracture, stress)
733.95
boot top - see Fracture, fibula
boxers' - see Fracture, metacarpal
bone(s)
breast bone - see Fracture, sternum
buckle - see Fracture, torus ◄
bucket handle (semilunar cartilage) -
see Tear, meniscus
burst - see Fracture, traumatic, by site
bursting - see Fracture, phalanx, hand,
distal
calcaneus (closed) 825.0
open 825.1
capitate (bone) (closed) 814.07
open 814.17
capitellum (humerus) (closed) 812.49
open 812.59
carpal bone(s) (wrist NEC) (closed)
814.00
open 814.10
specified site NEC 814.09
open 814.19
cartilage, knee (semilunar) - see Tear,
meniscus
cervical - see Fracture, vertebra, cervical
chauffeur's - see Fracture, ulna, lower
end
chisel - see Fracture, radius, upper end
chronic - see Fracture, pathologic ◄
clavicle (interligamentous part)
(closed) 810.00
acromial end 810.03
open 810.13
due to birth trauma 767.2
open 810.10
shaft (middle third) 810.02
open 810.12
sternal end 810.01
open 810.11
clayshovelers' - see Fracture, vertebra,
cervical
coccyx - see also Fracture, vertebra,
coccyx
complicating delivery 665.6●
collar bone - see Fracture, clavicle
Colles' (reversed) (closed) 813.41
open 813.51
comminuted - see Fracture, by site
compression - see also Fracture, by site
nontraumatic - see Fracture,
pathologic

◄ New   ◄▥ Revised   ~~deleted~~ Deleted   ● Use Additional Digit(s)   ▨ Omit code

Fracture *(Continued)*
 congenital 756.9
 coracoid process (closed) 811.02
  open 811.12
 coronoid process (ulna) (closed)
  813.02
  mandible (closed) 802.23
   open 802.33
  open 813.12
 corpus cavernosum penis 959.13
 costochondral junction - *see* Fracture,
  rib
 costosternal junction - *see* Fracture, rib
 cranium - *see* Fracture, skull, by site
 cricoid cartilage (closed) 807.5
  open 807.6
 cuboid (ankle) (closed) 825.23
  open 825.33
 cuneiform
  foot (closed) 825.24
   open 825.34
  wrist (closed) 814.03
   open 814.13
 dental implant 525.73
 dental restorative material
  with loss of material 525.64
  without loss of material 525.63
 due to
  birth injury - *see* Birth injury, fracture
  gunshot - *see* Fracture, by site, open
  neoplasm - *see* Fracture, pathologic
  osteoporosis - *see* Fracture,
   pathologic
 Dupuytren's (ankle) (fibula) (closed)
  824.4
  open 824.5
  radius 813.42
   open 813.52
 Duverney's - *see* Fracture, ilium
 elbow - *see also* Fracture, humerus,
  lower end
  olecranon (process) (closed) 813.01
   open 813.11
  supracondylar (closed) 812.41
   open 812.51
 ethmoid (bone) (sinus) - *see* Fracture,
  skull, base
 face bone(s) (closed) NEC 802.8
  with
   other bone(s) - *see* Fracture,
    multiple, skull
   skull - *see also* Fracture, skull
    involving other bones - *see*
     Fracture, multiple, skull
  open 802.9
 fatigue - *see* Fracture, march
 femur, femoral (closed) 821.00
  cervicotrochanteric 820.03
   open 820.13
  condyles, epicondyles 821.21
   open 821.31
  distal end - *see* Fracture, femur,
   lower end
  epiphysis (separation)
   capital 820.01
    open 820.11
   head 820.01
    open 820.11
   lower 821.22
    open 821.32
   trochanteric 820.01
    open 820.11
   upper 820.01
    open 820.11

Fracture *(Continued)*
 femur, femoral *(Continued)*
  head 820.09
   open 820.19
  lower end or extremity (distal end)
   (closed) 821.20
   condyles, epicondyles 821.21
    open 821.31
   epiphysis (separation) 821.22
    open 821.32
   multiple sites 821.29
    open 821.39
   open 821.30
   specified site NEC 821.29
    open 821.39
   supracondylar 821.23
    open 821.33
   T-shaped 821.21
    open 821.31
  neck (closed) 820.8
   base (cervicotrochanteric)
    820.03
    open 820.13
   extracapsular 820.20
    open 820.30
   intertrochanteric (section)
    820.21
    open 820.31
   intracapsular 820.00
    open 820.10
   intratrochanteric 820.21
    open 820.31
   midcervical 820.02
    open 820.12
   open 820.9
   pathologic 733.14
    specified part NEC 733.15
   specified site NEC 820.09
    open 820.19
   transcervical 820.02
    open 820.12
   transtrochanteric 820.20
    open 820.30
  open 821.10
  pathologic 733.14
   specified part NEC 733.15
  peritrochanteric (section) 820.20
   open 820.30
  shaft (lower third) (middle third)
   (upper third) 821.01
   open 821.11
  subcapital 820.09
   open 820.19
  subtrochanteric (region) (section)
   820.22
   open 820.32
  supracondylar 821.23
   open 821.33
  transepiphyseal 820.01
   open 820.11
  trochanter (greater) (lesser) (*see also*
   Fracture, femur, neck, by site)
   820.20
   open 820.30
  T-shaped, into knee joint
   821.21
   open 821.31
  upper end 820.8
   open 820.9
 fibula (closed) 823.81
  with tibia 823.82
   open 823.92
  distal end 824.8
   open 824.9

Fracture *(Continued)*
 fibula *(Continued)*
  epiphysis
   lower 824.8
    open 824.9
   upper - *see* Fracture, fibula, upper
    end
  head - *see* Fracture, fibula, upper end
  involving ankle 824.2
   open 824.3
  lower end or extremity 824.8
   open 824.9
  malleolus (external) (lateral) 824.2
   open 824.3
  open NEC 823.91
  pathologic 733.16
  proximal end - *see* Fracture, fibula,
   upper end
  shaft 823.21
   with tibia 823.22
    open 823.32
   open 823.31
  stress 733.93
  torus 823.41
   with tibia 823.42
  upper end or extremity (epiphysis)
   (head) (proximal end) (styloid)
   823.01
   with tibia 823.02
    open 823.12
   open 823.11
 finger(s), of one hand (closed) (*see also*
  Fracture, phalanx, hand) 816.00
  with
   metacarpal bone(s), of same hand
    817.0
    open 817.1
   thumb of same hand 816.03
    open 816.13
  open 816.10
 foot, except toe(s) alone (closed) 825.20
  open 825.30
 forearm (closed) NEC 813.80
  lower end (distal end) (lower
   epiphysis) 813.40
   open 813.50
  open 813.90
  shaft 813.20
   open 813.30
  upper end (proximal end) (upper
   epiphysis) 813.00
   open 813.10
 fossa, anterior, middle, or posterior -
  see Fracture, skull, base
 frontal (bone) - *see also* Fracture, skull,
  vault
  sinus - *see* Fracture, skull, base
 Galeazzi's - *see* Fracture, radius, lower
  end
 glenoid (cavity) (fossa) (scapula)
  (closed) 811.03
  open 811.13
 Gosselin's - *see* Fracture, ankle
 greenstick - *see* Fracture, by site
 grenade-throwers' - *see* Fracture,
  humerus, shaft
 gutter - *see* Fracture, skull, vault
 hamate (closed) 814.08
  open 814.18
 hand, one (closed) 815.00
  carpals 814.00
   open 814.10
   specified site NEC 814.09
    open 814.19

Fracture (Continued)
  hand, one (Continued)
    metacarpals 815.00
      open 815.10
    multiple, bones of one hand
      817.0
      open 817.1
    open 815.10
    phalanges (see also Fracture,
      phalanx, hand) 816.00
      open 816.10
  healing
    aftercare (see also Aftercare, fracture)
      V54.89
    change of cast V54.89
    complications - see condition
    convalescence V66.4
    removal of
      cast V54.89
      fixation device
        external V54.89
        internal V54.01
  heel bone (closed) 825.0
    open 825.1
  Hill-Sachs 812.09
  hip (closed) (see also Fracture, femur,
    neck) 820.8
    open 820.9
    pathologic 733.14
  humerus (closed) 812.20
    anatomical neck 812.02
      open 812.12
    articular process (see also Fracture
      humerus, condyle(s)) 812.44
      open 812.54
    capitellum 812.49
      open 812.59
    condyle(s) 812.44
      lateral (external) 812.42
        open 812.52
      medial (internal epicondyle)
        812.43
        open 812.53
      open 812.54
    distal end - see Fracture, humerus,
      lower end
    epiphysis
      lower (see also Fracture, humerus,
        condyle(s)) 812.44
        open 812.54
      upper 812.09
        open 812.19
    external condyle 812.42
      open 812.52
    great tuberosity 812.03
      open 812.13
    head 812.09
      open 812.19
    internal epicondyle 812.43
      open 812.53
    lesser tuberosity 812.09
      open 812.19
    lower end or extremity (distal end)
      (see also Fracture, humerus, by
      site) 812.40
      multiple sites NEC 812.49
        open 812.59
      open 812.50
      specified site NEC 812.49
        open 812.59
    neck 812.01
      open 812.11
    open 812.30
    pathologic 733.11

Fracture (Continued)
  humerus (Continued)
    proximal end - see Fracture,
      humerus, upper end
    shaft 812.21
      open 812.31
    supracondylar 812.41
      open 812.51
    surgical neck 812.01
      open 812.11
    trochlea 812.49
      open 812.59
    T-shaped 812.44
      open 812.54
    tuberosity - see Fracture, humerus,
      upper end
    upper end or extremity (proximal
      end) (see also Fracture,
      humerus, by site) 812.00
      open 812.10
      specified site NEC 812.09
        open 812.19
  hyoid bone (closed) 807.5
    open 807.6
  hyperextension - see Fracture, radius,
    lower end
  ilium (with visceral injury) (closed)
    808.41
    open 808.51
  impaction, impacted - see Fracture, by
    site
  incus - see Fracture, skull, base
  innominate bone (with visceral injury)
    (closed) 808.49
    open 808.59
  instep, of one foot (closed) 825.20
    with toe(s) of same foot 827.0
      open 827.1
    open 825.30
  insufficiency - see Fracture, pathologic,
    by site
  internal
    ear - see Fracture, skull, base
    semilunar cartilage, knee - see Tear,
      meniscus, medial
  intertrochanteric - see Fracture, femur,
    neck, intertrochanteric
  ischium (with visceral injury) (closed)
    808.42
    open 808.52
  jaw (bone) (lower) (closed) (see also
    Fracture, mandible) 802.20
    angle 802.25
      open 802.35
    open 802.30
    upper - see Fracture, maxilla
  knee
    cap (closed) 822.0
      open 822.1
    cartilage (semilunar) - see Tear,
      meniscus
  labyrinth (osseous) - see Fracture, skull,
    base
  larynx (closed) 807.5
    open 807.6
  late effect - see Late, effects (of),
    fracture
  Le Fort's - see Fracture, maxilla
  leg (closed) 827.0
    with rib(s) or sternum 828.0
      open 828.1
    both (any bones) 828.0
      open 828.1
    lower - see Fracture, tibia

Fracture (Continued)
  leg (Continued)
    open 827.1
    upper - see Fracture, femur
  limb
    lower (multiple) (closed) NEC
      827.0
      open 827.1
    upper (multiple) (closed) NEC
      818.0
      open 818.1
  long bones, due to birth trauma - see
    Birth injury, fracture
  lumbar - see Fracture, vertebra,
    lumbar
  lunate bone (closed) 814.02
    open 814.12
  malar bone (closed) 802.4
    open 802.5
  Malgaigne's (closed) 808.43
    open 808.53
  malleolus (closed) 824.8
    bimalleolar 824.4
      open 824.5
    lateral 824.2
      and medial - see also Fracture,
        malleolus, bimalleolar
        with lip of tibia - see
          Fracture, malleolus,
          trimalleolar
      open 824.3
    medial (closed) 824.0
      and lateral - see also Fracture,
        malleolus, bimalleolar
        with lip of tibia - see
          Fracture, malleolus,
          trimalleolar
      open 824.1
    open 824.9
    trimalleolar (closed) 824.6
      open 824.7
  malleus - see Fracture, skull, base
  malunion 733.81
  mandible (closed) 802.20
    angle 802.25
      open 802.35
    body 802.28
      alveolar border 802.27
        open 802.37
      open 802.38
      symphysis 802.26
        open 802.36
    condylar process 802.21
      open 802.31
    coronoid process 802.23
      open 802.33
    multiple sites 802.29
      open 802.39
    open 802.30
    ramus NEC 802.24
      open 802.34
    subcondylar 802.22
      open 802.32
  manubrium - see Fracture, sternum
  march 733.95
    fibula 733.93
    metatarsals 733.94
    tibia 733.93
  maxilla, maxillary (superior) (upper
    jaw) (closed) 802.4
    inferior - see Fracture, mandible
    open 802.5
  meniscus, knee - see Tear, meniscus

◄ New   ◄▥ Revised   deleted Deleted   ● Use Additional Digit(s)   Omit code

Fracture *(Continued)*
  metacarpus, metacarpal (bone(s)), of
      one hand (closed) 815.00
    with phalanx, phalanges, hand
        (finger(s)) (thumb) of same
        hand 817.0
      open 817.1
    base 815.02
      first metacarpal 815.01
        open 815.11
        open 815.12
      thumb 815.01
        open 815.11
    multiple sites 815.09
      open 815.19
    neck 815.04
      open 815.14
    open 815.10
    shaft 815.03
      open 815.13
  metatarsus, metatarsal (bone(s)), of one
      foot (closed) 825.25
    with tarsal bone(s) 825.29
      open 825.39
    open 825.35
  Monteggia's (closed) 813.03
    open 813.13
  Moore's - *see* Fracture, radius, lower
      end
  multangular bone (closed)
    larger 814.05
      open 814.15
    smaller 814.06
      open 814.16
  multiple (closed) 829.0

Note 29 Multiple fractures of sites
classifiable to the same three- or
four-digit category are coded to that
category, except for sites classifiable
to 810–818 or 820–827 in different
limbs.

Multiple fractures of sites classifiable
to different fourth-digit subdivisions
within the same three-digit category
should be dealt with according to
coding rules.

Multiple fractures of sites classifiable
to different three-digit categories
(identifiable from the listing under
"Fracture"), and of sites classifiable to
810–818 or 820–827 in different limbs
should be coded according to the
following list, which should be referred
to in the following priority order:
skull or face bones, pelvis or vertebral
column, legs, arms.

---

    arm (multiple bones in same arm
        except in hand alone) (sites
        classifiable to 810–817 with
        sites classifiable to a different
        three-digit category in
        810–817 in same arm) (closed)
        818.0
      open 818.1
    arms, both or arm(s) with rib(s) or
        sternum (sites classifiable to
        810–818 with sites classifiable
        to same range of categories in
        other limb or to 807) (closed)
        819.0
      open 819.1

Fracture *(Continued)*
  multiple *(Continued)*
    bones of trunk NEC (closed) 809.0
      open 809.1
    hand, metacarpal bone(s) with
        phalanx or phalanges of same
        hand (sites classifiable to 815
        with sites classifiable to 816 in
        same hand) (closed) 817.0
      open 817.1
    leg (multiple bones in same leg)
        (sites classifiable to 820–826
        with sites classifiable to a
        different three-digit category
        in that range in same leg)
        (closed) 827.0
      open 827.1
    legs, both or leg(s) with arm(s),
        rib(s), or sternum (sites
        classifiable to 820–827 with
        sites classifiable to same range
        of categories in other leg or to
        807 or 810–819) (closed) 828.0
      open 828.1
    open 829.1
    pelvis with other bones except skull
        or face bones (sites classifiable
        to 808 with sites classifiable to
        805–807 or 810–829) (closed)
        809.0
      open 809.1
    skull, specified or unspecified bones,
        or face bone(s) with any other
        bone(s) (sites classifiable to
        800–803 with sites classifiable
        to 805–829) (closed) 804.0 ●

Note 30 Use the following fifth-digit
subclassification with categories 800,
801, 803, and 804:

0	unspecified state of consciousness
1	with no loss of consciousness
2	with brief [less than one hour] loss of consciousness
3	with moderate [1–24 hours] loss of consciousness
4	with prolonged [more than 24 hours] loss of consciousness and return to pre-existing conscious level
5	with prolonged [more than 24 hours] loss of consciousness, without return to pre-existing conscious level

Use fifth-digit 5 to designate when a
patient is unconscious and dies before
regaining consciousness, regardless of
the duration of the loss of consciousness

6	with loss of consciousness of unspecified duration
9	with concussion, unspecified

---

    with
      contusion, cerebral 804.1 ●
      epidural hemorrhage 804.2 ●
      extradural hemorrhage 804.2 ●
      hemorrhage (intracranial) NEC
          804.3 ●
      intracranial injury NEC 804.4 ●
      laceration, cerebral 804.1 ●

Fracture *(Continued)*
  multiple *(Continued)*
    with *(Continued)*
        subarachnoid hemorrhage 804.2 ●
        subdural hemorrhage 804.2 ●
      open 804.5 ●
        with
            contusion, cerebral 804.6 ●
            epidural hemorrhage 804.7 ●
            extradural hemorrhage 804.7 ●
            hemorrhage (intracranial)
                NEC 804.8 ●
            intracranial injury NEC 804.9 ●
            laceration, cerebral 804.6 ●
            subarachnoid hemorrhage
                804.7 ●
            subdural hemorrhage 804.7 ●
    vertebral column with other bones,
        except skull or face bones (sites
        classifiable to 805 or 806 with
        sites classifiable to 807–808 or
        810–829) (closed) 809.0
      open 809.1
  nasal (bone(s)) (closed) 802.0
    open 802.1
    sinus - *see* Fracture, skull, base
  navicular
    carpal (wrist) (closed) 814.01
      open 814.11
    tarsal (ankle) (closed) 825.22
      open 825.32
  neck - *see* Fracture, vertebra, cervical
  neural arch - *see* Fracture, vertebra, by
      site
  nonunion 733.82
  nose, nasal, (bone) (septum) (closed)
      802.0
    open 802.1
  occiput - *see* Fracture, skull, base
  odontoid process - *see* Fracture,
      vertebra, cervical
  olecranon (process) (ulna) (closed)
      813.01
    open 813.11
  open 829.1
  orbit, orbital (bone) (region) (closed)
      802.8
    floor (blow-out) 802.6
      open 802.7
    open 802.9
    roof - *see* Fracture, skull, base
    specified part NEC 802.8
      open 802.9
  os
    calcis (closed) 825.0
      open 825.1
    magnum (closed) 814.07
      open 814.17
    pubis (with visceral injury) (closed)
        808.2
      open 808.3
    triquetrum (closed) 814.03
      open 814.13
  osseous
    auditory meatus - *see* Fracture, skull,
        base
    labyrinth - *see* Fracture, skull, base
  ossicles, auditory (incus) (malleus)
      (stapes) - *see* Fracture, skull, base
  osteoporotic - *see* Fracture, pathologic
  palate (closed) 802.8
    open 802.9
  paratrooper - *see* Fracture, tibia, lower
      end

Fracture *(Continued)*
  parietal bone - *see* Fracture, skull, vault
  parry - *see* Fracture, Monteggia's
  patella (closed) 822.0
    open 822.1
  pathologic (cause unknown)
      733.10
    ankle 733.16
    femur (neck) 733.14
      specified NEC 733.15
    fibula 733.16
    hip 733.14
    humerus 733.11
    radius (distal) 733.12
    specified site NEC 733.19
    tibia 733.16
    ulna 733.12
    vertebrae (collapse) 733.13
    wrist 733.12
  pedicle (of vertebral arch) - *see*
      Fracture, vertebra, by site
  pelvis, pelvic (bone(s)) (with visceral
      injury) (closed) 808.8
    multiple (with disruption of pelvic
        circle) 808.43
      open 808.53
    open 808.9
    rim (closed) 808.49
      open 808.59
  peritrochanteric (closed) 820.20
    open 820.30
  phalanx, phalanges, of one
    foot (closed) 826.0
      with bone(s) of same lower limb
          827.0
        open 827.1
      open 826.1
    hand (closed) 816.00
      with metacarpal bone(s) of same
          hand 817.0
        open 817.1
      distal 816.02
        open 816.12
      middle 816.01
        open 816.11
      multiple sites NEC 816.03
        open 816.13
      open 816.10
      proximal 816.01
        open 816.11
  pisiform (closed) 814.04
    open 814.14
  pond - *see* Fracture, skull, vault
  Pott's (closed) 824.4
    open 824.5
  prosthetic device, internal - *see*
      Complications, mechanical
  pubis (with visceral injury) (closed)
      808.2
    open 808.3
  Quervain's (closed) 814.01
    open 814.11
  radius (alone) (closed) 813.81
    with ulna NEC 813.83
      open 813.93
    distal end - *see* Fracture, radius,
        lower end
    epiphysis
      lower - *see* Fracture, radius, lower
          end
      upper - *see* Fracture, radius,
          upper end
    head - *see* Fracture, radius, upper
        end

Fracture *(Continued)*
  radius *(Continued)*
    lower end or extremity (distal end)
        (lower epiphysis) 813.42
      with ulna (lower end) 813.44
        open 813.54
      open 813.52
      torus 813.45
        with ulna 813.47 ◄
    neck - *see* Fracture, radius, upper
        end
    open NEC 813.91
    pathologic 733.12
    proximal end - *see* Fracture, radius,
        upper end
    shaft (closed) 813.21
      with ulna (shaft) 813.23
        open 813.33
      open 813.31
    upper end 813.07
      with ulna (upper end) 813.08
        open 813.18
      epiphysis 813.05
        open 813.15
      head 813.05
        open 813.15
      multiple sites 813.07
        open 813.17
      neck 813.06
        open 813.16
        open 813.17
      specified site NEC 813.07
        open 813.17
  ramus
    inferior or superior (with visceral
        injury) (closed) 808.2
      open 808.3
    ischium - *see* Fracture, ischium
    mandible 802.24
      open 802.34
  rib(s) (closed) 807.0●

Note 31   Use the following fifth-digit
subclassification with categories
807.0–807.1:

0   rib(s), unspecified
1   one rib
2   two ribs
3   three ribs
4   four ribs
5   five ribs
6   six ribs
7   seven ribs
8   eight or more ribs
9   multiple ribs, unspecified

    with flail chest (open) 807.4
      open 807.1●
  root, tooth 873.63
    complicated 873.73
  sacrum - *see* Fracture, vertebra, sacrum
  scaphoid
    ankle (closed) 825.22
      open 825.32
    wrist (closed) 814.01
      open 814.11
  scapula (closed) 811.00
    acromial, acromion (process) 811.01
      open 811.11
    body 811.09
      open 811.19
    coracoid process 811.02
      open 811.12

Fracture *(Continued)*
  scapula *(Continued)*
    glenoid (cavity) (fossa) 811.03
      open 811.13
    neck 811.03
      open 811.13
    open 811.10
  semilunar
    bone, wrist (closed) 814.02
      open 814.12
    cartilage (interior) (knee) - *see* Tear,
        meniscus
  sesamoid bone - *see* Fracture, by site
  Shepherd's (closed) 825.21
    open 825.31
  shoulder - *see also* Fracture, humerus,
      upper end
    blade - *see* Fracture, scapula
  silverfork - *see* Fracture, radius, lower
      end
  sinus (ethmoid) (frontal) (maxillary)
      (nasal) (sphenoidal) - *see* Fracture,
      skull, base
  Skillern's - *see* Fracture, radius, shaft
  skull (multiple NEC) (with face bones)
      (closed) 803.0●

Note 32   Use the following fifth-digit
subclassification with categories 800,
801, 803, and 804:

0   unspecified state of
        consciousness
1   with no loss of consciousness
2   with brief [less than one hour]
        loss of consciousness
3   with moderate [1-24 hours] loss
        of consciousness
4   with prolonged [more than
        24 hours] loss of
        consciousness and return to
        pre-existing conscious level
5   with prolonged [more than
        24 hours] loss of
        consciousness, without
        return to pre-existing
        conscious level

Use fifth-digit 5 to designate when a
patient is unconscious and dies before
regaining consciousness, regardless of
the duration of the loss of consciousness

6   with loss of consciousness of
        unspecified duration
9   with concussion, unspecified

    with
      contusion, cerebral 803.1●
      epidural hemorrhage 803.2●
      extradural hemorrhage 803.2●
      hemorrhage (intracranial) NEC
          803.3●
      intracranial injury NEC 803.4●
      laceration, cerebral 803.1●
      other bones - *see* Fracture,
          multiple, skull
      subarachnoid hemorrhage 803.2●
      subdural hemorrhage 803.2●
    base (antrum) (ethmoid bone) (fossa)
        (internal ear) (nasal sinus)
        (occiput) (sphenoid) (temporal
        bone) (closed) 801.0●
      with
        contusion, cerebral 801.1●
        epidural hemorrhage 801.2●

Fracture *(Continued)*
  skull *(Continued)*
    base *(Continued)*
      with *(Continued)*
        extradural hemorrhage 801.2●
        hemorrhage (intracranial)
          NEC 801.3●
        intracranial injury NEC 801.4●
        laceration, cerebral 801.1●
        subarachnoid hemorrhage
          801.2●
        subdural hemorrhage 801.2●
      open 801.5●
        with
          contusion, cerebral 801.6●
          epidural hemorrhage
            801.7●
          extradural hemorrhage
            801.7●
          hemorrhage (intracranial)
            NEC 801.8●
          intracranial injury NEC
            801.9●
          laceration, cerebral 801.6●
          subarachnoid hemorrhage
            801.7●
          subdural hemorrhage
            801.7●
    birth injury 767.3
    face bones - *see* Fracture, face bones
    open 803.5●
      with
        contusion, cerebral 803.6●
        epidural hemorrhage 803.7●
        extradural hemorrhage 803.7●
        hemorrhage (intracranial)
          NEC 803.8●
        intracranial injury NEC 803.9●
        laceration, cerebral 803.6●
        subarachnoid hemorrhage
          803.7●
        subdural hemorrhage 803.7●
    vault (frontal bone) (parietal bone)
      (vertex) (closed) 800.0●
      with
        contusion, cerebral 800.1●
        epidural hemorrhage 800.2●
        extradural hemorrhage 800.2●
        hemorrhage (intracranial)
          NEC 800.3●
        intracranial injury NEC
          800.4●
        laceration, cerebral 800.1●
        subarachnoid hemorrhage
          800.2●
        subdural hemorrhage
          800.2●
      open 800.5●
        with
          contusion, cerebral
            800.6●
          epidural hemorrhage
            800.7●
          extradural hemorrhage
            800.7●
          hemorrhage (intracranial)
            NEC 800.8●
          intracranial injury NEC
            800.9●
          laceration, cerebral 800.6●
          subarachnoid hemorrhage
            800.7●
          subdural hemorrhage
            800.7●

Fracture *(Continued)*
  Smith's 813.41
    open 813.51
  sphenoid (bone) (sinus) - *see* Fracture,
    skull, base
  spine - *see also* Fracture, vertebra,
    by site due to birth trauma
    767.4
  spinous process - *see* Fracture,
    vertebra, by site
  spontaneous - *see* Fracture, pathologic
  sprinters' - *see* Fracture, ilium
  stapes - *see* Fracture, skull, base
  stave - *see also* Fracture, metacarpus,
    metacarpal bone(s)
    spine - *see* Fracture, tibia, upper
      end
  sternum (closed) 807.2
    with flail chest (open) 807.4
    open 807.3
  Stieda's - *see* Fracture, femur, lower
    end
  stress 733.95
    fibula 733.93
    metatarsals 733.94
    specified site NEC 733.95
    tibia 733.93
  styloid process
    metacarpal (closed) 815.02
      open 815.12
    radius - *see* Fracture, radius, lower
      end
    temporal bone - *see* Fracture, skull,
      base
    ulna - *see* Fracture, ulna, lower
      end
  supracondylar, elbow 812.41
    open 812.51
  symphysis pubis (with visceral injury)
    (closed) 808.2
    open 808.3
  talus (ankle bone) (closed) 825.21
    open 825.31
  tarsus, tarsal bone(s) (with
    metatarsus) of one foot
    (closed) NEC 825.29
    open 825.39
  temporal bone (styloid) - *see* Fracture,
    skull, base
  tendon - *see* Sprain, by site
  thigh - *see* Fracture, femur, shaft
  thumb (and finger(s)) of one hand
    (closed) (*see also* Fracture,
    phalanx, hand) 816.00
    with metacarpal bone(s) of same
      hand 817.0
      open 817.1
    metacarpal(s) - *see* Fracture,
      metacarpus
    open 816.10
  thyroid cartilage (closed) 807.5
    open 807.6
  tibia (closed) 823.80
    with fibula 823.82
      open 823.92
    condyles - *see* Fracture, tibia, upper
      end
    distal end 824.8
      open 824.9
    epiphysis
      lower 824.8
        open 824.9
      upper - *see* Fracture, tibia, upper
        end

Fracture *(Continued)*
  tibia *(Continued)*
    head (involving knee joint) - *see*
      Fracture, tibia, upper end
    intercondyloid eminence - *see*
      Fracture, tibia, upper end
    involving ankle 824.0
      open 824.1
    lower end or extremity (anterior
      lip) (posterior lip) 824.8
      open 824.9
    malleolus (internal) (medial) 824.0
      open 824.1
    open NEC 823.90
    pathologic 733.16
    proximal end - *see* Fracture, tibia,
      upper end
    shaft 823.20
      with fibula 823.22
        open 823.32
      open 823.30
    spine - *see* Fracture, tibia, upper end
    stress 733.93
    torus 823.40
      with fibula 823.42
    tuberosity - *see* Fracture, tibia, upper
      end
    upper end or extremity (condyle)
      (epiphysis) (head) (spine)
      (proximal end) (tuberosity)
      823.00
      with fibula 823.02
        open 823.12
      open 823.10
  toe(s), of one foot (closed) 826.0
    with bone(s) of same lower limb
      827.0
      open 827.1
    open 826.1
  tooth (root) 873.63
    complicated 873.73
  torus
    fibula 823.41
      with tibia 823.42
    humerus 812.49   ◄
    radius (alone) 813.45   ◄▥
      with ulna 813.47   ◄
    tibia 823.40
      with fibula 823.42
    ulna (alone) 813.46   ◄
      with radius 813.47   ◄
  trachea (closed) 807.5
    open 807.6
  transverse process - *see* Fracture,
    vertebra, by site
  trapezium (closed) 814.05
    open 814.15
  trapezoid bone (closed) 814.06
    open 814.16
  trimalleolar (closed) 824.6
    open 824.7
  triquetral (bone) (closed) 814.03
    open 814.13
  trochanter (greater) (lesser) (closed)
    (*see also* Fracture, femur, neck,
    by site) 820.20
    open 820.30
  trunk (bones) (closed) 809.0
    open 809.1
  tuberosity (external) - *see* Fracture,
    by site
  ulna (alone) (closed) 813.82
    with radius NEC 813.83
      open 813.93

Fracture *(Continued)*
ulna *(Continued)*
coronoid process (closed) 813.02
open 813.12
distal end - *see* Fracture, ulna, lower end
epiphysis
lower - *see* Fracture, ulna, lower end
upper - *see* Fracture, ulna, upper, end
head - *see* Fracture, ulna, lower end
lower end (distal end) (head) (lower epiphysis) (styloid process) 813.43
with radius (lower end) 813.44
open 813.54
open 813.53
olecranon process (closed) 813.01
open 813.11
open NEC 813.92
pathologic 733.12
proximal end - *see* Fracture, ulna, upper end
shaft 813.22
with radius (shaft) 813.23
open 813.33
open 813.32
styloid process - *see* Fracture, ulna, lower end
torus 813.46 ◀
with radius 813.47 ◀
transverse - *see* Fracture, ulna, by site
upper end (epiphysis) 813.04
with radius (upper end) 813.08
open 813.18
multiple sites 813.04
open 813.14
open 813.14
specified site NEC 813.04
open 813.14
unciform (closed) 814.08
open 814.18
vertebra, vertebral (back) (body) (column) (neural arch) (pedicle) (spine) (spinous process) (transverse process) (closed) 805.8
with
hematomyelia - *see* Fracture, vertebra, by site, with spinal cord injury
injury to
cauda equina - *see* Fracture, vertebra, sacrum, with spinal cord injury
nerve - *see* Fracture, vertebra, by site, with spinal cord injury
paralysis - *see* Fracture, vertebra, by site, with spinal cord injury
paraplegia - *see* Fracture, vertebra, by site, with spinal cord injury
quadriplegia - *see* Fracture, vertebra, by site, with spinal cord injury
spinal concussion - *see* Fracture, vertebra, by site, with spinal cord injury

Fracture *(Continued)*
vertebra, vertebral *(Continued)*
with *(Continued)*
spinal cord injury (closed) NEC 806.8

Note 33   Use the following fifth-digit subclassification with categories 806.0–806.3:

C_1–C_4 or unspecified level and D_1–D_6 (T_1–T_6) or unspecified level with:

0   unspecified spinal cord injury
1   complete lesion of cord
2   anterior cord syndrome
3   central cord syndrome
4   specified injury NEC

level and D_1–D_{12} level with:

5   unspecified spinal cord injury
6   complete lesion of cord
7   anterior cord syndrome
8   central cord syndrome
9   specified injury NEC

cervical 806.0●
open 806.1●
chronic 733.13
dorsal, dorsolumbar 806.2●
open 806.3●
open 806.9
thoracic, thoracolumbar 806.2●
open 806.3●
atlanto-axial - *see* Fracture, vertebra, cervical
cervical (hangman) (teardrop) (closed) 805.00
with spinal cord injury - *see* Fracture, vertebra, with spinal cord injury, cervical
first (atlas) 805.01
open 805.11
second (axis) 805.02
open 805.12
third 805.03
open 805.13
fourth 805.04
open 805.14
fifth 805.05
open 805.15
sixth 805.06
open 805.16
seventh 805.07
open 805.17
multiple sites 805.08
open 805.18
open 805.10
coccyx (closed) 805.6
with spinal cord injury (closed) 806.60
cauda equina injury 806.62
complete lesion 806.61
open 806.71
open 806.72
open 806.70
specified type NEC 806.69
open 806.79
open 805.7
collapsed 733.13
compression, not due to trauma 733.13

Fracture *(Continued)*
dorsal (closed) 805.2
with spinal cord injury - *see* Fracture, vertebra, with spinal cord injury, dorsal
open 805.3
dorsolumbar (closed) 805.2
with spinal cord injury - *see* Fracture, vertebra, with spinal cord injury, dorsal
open 805.3
due to osteoporosis 733.13
fetus or newborn 767.4
lumbar (closed) 805.4
with spinal cord injury (closed) 806.4
open 806.5
open 805.5
nontraumatic 733.13
open NEC 805.9
pathologic (any site) 733.13
sacrum (closed) 805.6
with spinal cord injury 806.60
cauda equina injury 806.62
complete lesion 806.61
open 806.71
open 806.72
open 806.70
specified type NEC 806.69
open 806.79
open 805.7
site unspecified (closed) 805.8
with spinal cord injury (closed) 806.8
open 806.9
open 805.9
stress (any site) 733.95
thoracic (closed) 805.2
with spinal cord injury - *see* Fracture, vertebra, with spinal cord injury, thoracic
open 805.3
vertex - *see* Fracture, skull, vault
vomer (bone) 802.0
open 802.1
Wagstaffe's - *see* Fracture, ankle
wrist (closed) 814.00
open 814.10
pathologic 733.12
xiphoid (process) - *see* Fracture, sternum
zygoma (zygomatic arch) (closed) 802.4
open 802.5
Fragile X syndrome 759.83
Fragilitas
crinium 704.2
hair 704.2
ossium 756.51
with blue sclera 756.51
unguium 703.8
congenital 757.5
Fragility
bone 756.51
with deafness and blue sclera 756.51
capillary (hereditary) 287.8
hair 704.2
nails 703.8
Fragmentation - *see* Fracture, by site
Frailty 797
Frambesia, frambesial (tropica) (*see also* Yaws) 102.9
initial lesion or ulcer 102.0
primary 102.0

◀ New   ⬅ Revised   ~~deleted~~ Deleted   ● Use Additional Digit(s)   ▬ Omit code

Frambeside
gummatous 102.4
of early yaws 102.2
Frambesioma 102.1
Franceschetti's syndrome
(mandibulofacial dysostosis)
756.0
Francis' disease (*see also* Tularemia)
021.9
Frank's essential thrombocytopenia (*see
also* Purpura, thrombocytopenic)
287.39
Franklin's disease (heavy chain) 273.2
Fraser's syndrome 759.89
Freckle 709.09
malignant melanoma in (M8742/3) - *see*
Melanoma
melanotic (of Hutchinson) (M8742/2) -
see Neoplasm, skin, in situ
retinal 239.81 ◀
Freeman-Sheldon syndrome 759.89
Freezing 991.9
specified effect NEC 991.8
Frei's disease (climatic bubo) 099.1
Freiberg's
disease (osteochondrosis, second
metatarsal) 732.5
infraction of metatarsal head 732.5
osteochondrosis 732.5
Fremitus, friction, cardiac 785.3
Frenulum linguae 750.0
Frenum
external os 752.49
tongue 750.0
Frequency (urinary) NEC 788.41
micturition 788.41
nocturnal 788.43
polyuria 788.42
psychogenic 306.53
Frey's syndrome (auriculotemporal
syndrome) 705.22
Friction
burn (*see also* Injury, superficial, by site)
919.0
fremitus, cardiac 785.3
precordial 785.3
sounds, chest 786.7
Friderichsen-Waterhouse syndrome or
disease 036.3
Friedländer's
B (bacillus) NEC (*see also* condition)
041.3
sepsis or septicemia 038.49
disease (endarteritis obliterans) - *see*
Arteriosclerosis
Friedreich's
ataxia 334.0
combined systemic disease 334.0
disease 333.2
combined systemic 334.0
myoclonia 333.2
sclerosis (spinal cord) 334.0
Friedrich-Erb-Arnold syndrome
(acropachyderma) 757.39
Frigidity 302.72
psychic or psychogenic 302.72
Fröhlich's disease or syndrome
(adiposogenital dystrophy) 253.8
Froin's syndrome 336.8
Frommel's disease 676.6●
Frommel-Chiari syndrome 676.6●
Frontal - *see also* condition
lobe syndrome 310.0

Frostbite 991.3
face 991.0
foot 991.2
hand 991.1
specified site NEC 991.3
Frotteurism 302.89
Frozen 991.9
pelvis 620.8
shoulder 726.0
Fructosemia 271.2
Fructosuria (benign) (essential) 271.2
Fuchs'
black spot (myopic) 360.21
corneal dystrophy (endothelial)
371.57
heterochromic cyclitis 364.21
Fucosidosis 271.8
Fugue 780.99
dissociative 300.13
hysterical (dissociative) 300.13
reaction to exceptional stress (transient)
308.1
Fukuhara syndrome 277.87
Fuller Albright's syndrome (osteitis
fibrosa disseminata) 756.59
Fuller's earth disease 502
Fulminant, fulminating - *see* condition
Functional - *see* condition
Functioning
borderline intellectual V62.89
Fundus - *see also* condition
flavimaculatus 362.76
Fungemia 117.9
Fungus, fungous
cerebral 348.89 ◀⃫
disease NEC 117.9
infection - *see* Infection, fungus
testis (*see also* Tuberculosis) 016.5●
[608.81]
Funiculitis (acute) 608.4
chronic 608.4
endemic 608.4
gonococcal (acute) 098.14
chronic or duration of 2 months or
over 098.34
tuberculous (*see also* Tuberculosis)
016.5●
FUO (*see also* Pyrexia) 780.60
Funnel
breast (acquired) 738.3
congenital 754.81
late effect of rickets 268.1
chest (acquired) 738.3
congenital 754.81
late effect of rickets 268.1
pelvis (acquired) 738.6
with disproportion (fetopelvic)
653.3●
affecting fetus or newborn
763.1
causing obstructed labor
660.1●
affecting fetus or newborn
763.1
congenital 755.69
tuberculous (*see also* Tuberculosis)
016.9●
Furfur 690.18
microsporon 111.0
Furor, paroxysmal (idiopathic) (*see also*
Epilepsy) 345.8●
Furriers' lung 495.8
Furrowed tongue 529.5
congenital 750.13

Furrowing nail(s) (transverse) 703.8
congenital 757.5
Furuncle 680.9
abdominal wall 680.2
ankle 680.6
anus 680.5
arm (any part, above wrist) 680.3
auditory canal, external 680.0
axilla 680.3
back (any part) 680.2
breast 680.2
buttock 680.5
chest wall 680.2
corpus cavernosum 607.2
ear (any part) 680.0
eyelid 373.13
face (any part, except eye) 680.0
finger (any) 680.4
flank 680.2
foot (any part) 680.7
forearm 680.3
gluteal (region) 680.5
groin 680.2
hand (any part) 680.4
head (any part, except face) 680.8
heel 680.7
hip 680.6
kidney (*see also* Abscess, kidney) 590.2
knee 680.6
labium (majus) (minus) 616.4
lacrimal
gland (*see also* Dacryoadenitis)
375.00
passages (duct) (sac) (*see also*
Dacryocystitis) 375.30
leg, any part except foot 680.6
malignant 022.0
multiple sites 680.9
neck 680.1
nose (external) (septum) 680.0
orbit 376.01
partes posteriores 680.5
pectoral region 680.2
penis 607.2
perineum 680.2
pinna 680.0
scalp (any part) 680.8
scrotum 608.4
seminal vesicle 608.0
shoulder 680.3
skin NEC 680.9
specified site NEC 680.8
spermatic cord 608.4
temple (region) 680.0
testis 604.90
thigh 680.6
thumb 680.4
toe (any) 680.7
trunk 680.2
tunica vaginalis 608.4
umbilicus 680.2
upper arm 680.3
vas deferens 608.4
vulva 616.4
wrist 680.4
Furunculosis (*see also* Furuncle) 680.9
external auditory meatus 680.0 [380.13]
Fusarium (infection) 118
Fusion, fused (congenital)
anal (with urogenital canal) 751.5
aorta and pulmonary artery 745.0
astragaloscaphoid 755.67
atria 745.5
atrium and ventricle 745.69

Fusion, fused *(Continued)*
  auditory canal 744.02
  auricles, heart 745.5
  binocular, with defective stereopsis
      368.33
  bone 756.9
  cervical spine - *see* Fusion, spine
  choanal 748.0
  commissure, mitral valve 746.5
  cranial sutures, premature 756.0
  cusps, heart valve NEC 746.89
    mitral 746.5
    tricuspid 746.89
  ear ossicles 744.04
  fingers *(see also* Syndactylism, fingers)
     755.11
  hymen 752.42
  hymeno-urethral 599.89
    causing obstructed labor 660.1●
      affecting fetus or newborn
        763.1
  joint (acquired) - *see also* Ankylosis
    congenital 755.8
  kidneys (incomplete) 753.3

Fusion, fused *(Continued)*
  labium (majus) (minus) 752.49
  larynx and trachea 748.3
  limb 755.8
    lower 755.69
    upper 755.59
  lobe, lung 748.5
  lumbosacral (acquired) 724.6
    congenital 756.15
    surgical V45.4
  nares (anterior) (posterior) 748.0
  nose, nasal 748.0
  nostril(s) 748.0
  organ or site NEC - *see* Anomaly,
    specified type NEC
  ossicles 756.9
    auditory 744.04
  pulmonary valve segment 746.02
  pulmonic cusps 746.02
  ribs 756.3
  sacroiliac (acquired) (joint) 724.6
    congenital 755.69
    surgical V45.4
  skull, imperfect 756.0

Fusion, fused *(Continued)*
  spine (acquired) 724.9
    arthrodesis status V45.4
    congenital (vertebra) 756.15
    postoperative status V45.4
  sublingual duct with submaxillary duct
    at opening in mouth 750.26
  talonavicular (bar) 755.67
  teeth, tooth 520.2
  testes 752.89
  toes *(see also* Syndactylism, toes) 755.13
  trachea and esophagus 750.3
  twins 759.4
  urethral-hymenal 599.89
  vagina 752.49
  valve cusps - *see* Fusion, cusps, heart
    valve
  ventricles, heart 745.4
  vertebra (arch) - *see* Fusion, spine
  vulva 752.49
Fusospirillosis (mouth) (tongue) (tonsil)
  101
Fussy infant (baby) 780.91

◀ New   ◀▥ Revised   ~~deleted~~ Deleted   ● Use Additional Digit(s)   ▨ Omit code

G

Gafsa boil 085.1
Gain, weight (abnormal) (excessive) (*see also* Weight, gain) 783.1
Gaisböck's disease or syndrome (polycythemia hypertonica) 289.0
Gait
  abnormality 781.2
    hysterical 300.11
  ataxic 781.2
    hysterical 300.11
  disturbance 781.2
    hysterical 300.11
  paralytic 781.2
  scissor 781.2
  spastic 781.2
  staggering 781.2
    hysterical 300.11
Galactocele (breast) (infected) 611.5
  puerperal, postpartum 676.8●
Galactophoritis 611.0
  puerperal, postpartum 675.2●
Galactorrhea 676.6●
  not associated with childbirth 611.6
Galactosemia (classic) (congenital) 271.1
Galactosuria 271.1
Galacturia 791.1
  bilharziasis 120.0
Galen's vein - *see* condition
Gallbladder - *see also* condition
  acute (*see also* Disease, gallbladder) 575.0
Gall duct - *see* condition
Gallop rhythm 427.89
Gallstone (cholemic) (colic) (impacted) - *see also* Cholelithiasis
  causing intestinal obstruction 560.31
Gambling, pathological 312.31
Gammaloidosis 277.39
Gammopathy 273.9
  macroglobulinemia 273.3
  monoclonal (benign) (essential) (idiopathic) (with lymphoplasmacytic dyscrasia) 273.1
Gamna's disease (siderotic splenomegaly) 289.51
Gampsodactylia (congenital) 754.71
Gamstorp's disease (adynamia episodica hereditaria) 359.3
Gandy-Nanta disease (siderotic splenomegaly) 289.51
Gang activity, without manifest psychiatric disorder V71.09
  adolescent V71.02
  adult V71.01
  child V71.02
Gangliocytoma (M9490/0) - *see* Neoplasm, connective tissue, benign
Ganglioglioma (M9505/1) - *see* Neoplasm, by site, uncertain behavior
Ganglion 727.43
  joint 727.41
  of yaws (early) (late) 102.6
  periosteal (*see also* Periostitis) 730.3●
  tendon sheath (compound) (diffuse) 727.42
  tuberculous (*see also* Tuberculosis) 015.9●
Ganglioneuroblastoma (M9490/3) - *see* Neoplasm, connective tissue, malignant

Ganglioneuroma (M9490/0) - *see also* Neoplasm, connective tissue, benign
  malignant (M9490/3) - *see* Neoplasm, connective tissue, malignant
Ganglioneuromatosis (M9491/0) - *see* Neoplasm, connective tissue, benign
Ganglionitis
  fifth nerve (*see also* Neuralgia, trigeminal) 350.1
  gasserian 350.1
  geniculate 351.1
    herpetic 053.11
    newborn 767.5
  herpes zoster 053.11
  herpetic geniculate (Hunt's syndrome) 053.11
Gangliosidosis 330.1
Gangosa 102.5
Gangrene, gangrenous (anemia) (artery) (cellulitis) (dermatitis) (dry) (infective) (moist) (pemphigus) (septic) (skin) (stasis) (ulcer) 785.4
  with
    arteriosclerosis (native artery) 440.24
      bypass graft 440.30
        autologous vein 440.31
        nonautologous biological 440.32
    diabetes (mellitus) 250.7● [785.4]
      due to secondary diabetes 249.7● [785.4]
  abdomen (wall) 785.4
  adenitis 683
  alveolar 526.5
  angina 462
    diphtheritic 032.0
  anus 569.49
  appendices epiploicae - *see* Gangrene, mesentery
  appendix - *see* Appendicitis, acute
  arteriosclerotic - *see* Arteriosclerosis, with, gangrene
  auricle 785.4
  Bacillus welchii (*see also* Gangrene, gas) 040.0
  bile duct (*see also* Cholangitis) 576.8
  bladder 595.89
  bowel - *see* Gangrene, intestine
  cecum - *see* Gangrene, intestine
  Clostridium perfringens or welchii (*see also* Gangrene, gas) 040.0
  colon - *see* Gangrene, intestine
  connective tissue 785.4
  cornea 371.40
  corpora cavernosa (infective) 607.2
    noninfective 607.89
  cutaneous, spreading 785.4
  decubital (*see also* Ulcer, pressure) 707.00 [785.4]
  diabetic (any site) 250.7● [785.4]
    due to secondary diabetes 249.7● [785.4]
  dropsical 785.4
  emphysematous (*see also* Gangrene, gas) 040.0
  epidemic (ergotized grain) 988.2
  epididymis (infectional) (*see also* Epididymitis) 604.99
  erysipelas (*see also* Erysipelas) 035
  extremity (lower) (upper) 785.4
  gallbladder or duct (*see also* Cholecystitis, acute) 575.0

Gangrene, gangrenous (*Continued*)
  gas (bacillus) 040.0
    with
      abortion - *see* Abortion, by type, with sepsis
      ectopic pregnancy (*see also* categories 633.0–633.9) 639.0
      molar pregnancy (*see also* categories 630–632) 639.0
    following
      abortion 639.0
      ectopic or molar pregnancy 639.0
    puerperal, postpartum, childbirth 670.8 ◀▦
  glossitis 529.0
  gum 523.8
  hernia - *see* Hernia, by site, with gangrene
  hospital noma 528.1
  intestine, intestinal (acute) (hemorrhagic) (massive) 557.0
    with
      hernia - *see* Hernia, by site, with gangrene
      mesenteric embolism or infarction 557.0
      obstruction (*see also* Obstruction, intestine) 560.9
  laryngitis 464.00
    with obstruction 464.01
  liver 573.8
  lung 513.0
    spirochetal 104.8
  lymphangitis 457.2
  Meleney's (cutaneous) 686.09
  mesentery 557.0
    with
      embolism or infarction 557.0
      intestinal obstruction (*see also* Obstruction, intestine) 560.9
  mouth 528.1
  noma 528.1
  orchitis 604.90
  ovary (*see also* Salpingo-oophoritis) 614.2
  pancreas 577.0
  penis (infectional) 607.2
    noninfective 607.89
  perineum 785.4
  pharynx 462
    septic 034.0
  pneumonia 513.0
  Pott's 440.24
  presenile 443.1
  pulmonary 513.0
  pulp, tooth 522.1
  quinsy 475
  Raynaud's (symmetric gangrene) 443.0 [785.4]
  rectum 569.49
  retropharyngeal 478.24
  rupture - *see* Hernia, by site, with gangrene
  scrotum 608.4
    noninfective 608.83
  senile 440.24
  sore throat 462
  spermatic cord 608.4
    noninfective 608.89
  spine 785.4
  spirochetal NEC 104.8
  spreading cutaneous 785.4
  stomach 537.89
  stomatitis 528.1

Gangrene, gangrenous (Continued)
symmetrical 443.0 [785.4]
testis (infectional) (see also Orchitis)
604.99
noninfective 608.89
throat 462
diphtheritic 032.0
thyroid (gland) 246.8
tonsillitis (acute) 463
tooth (pulp) 522.1
tuberculous NEC (see also Tuberculosis)
011.9●
tunica vaginalis 608.4
noninfective 608.89
umbilicus 785.4
uterus (see also Endometritis) 615.9
uvulitis 528.3
vas deferens 608.4
noninfective 608.89
vulva (see also Vulvitis) 616.10
Gannister disease (occupational) 502
with tuberculosis - see Tuberculosis,
pulmonary
Ganser's syndrome, hysterical 300.16
Gardner-Diamond syndrome
(autoerythrocyte sensitization) 287.2
Gargoylism 277.5
Garré's
disease (see also Osteomyelitis) 730.1●
osteitis (sclerosing) (see also
Osteomyelitis) 730.1●
osteomyelitis (see also Osteomyelitis)
730.1●
Garrod's pads, knuckle 728.79
Gartner's duct
cyst 752.41
persistent 752.41
Gas 787.3
asphyxia, asphyxiation, inhalation,
poisoning, suffocation NEC 987.9
specified gas - see Table of Drugs
and Chemicals
bacillus gangrene or infection - see Gas,
gangrene
cyst, mesentery 568.89
excessive 787.3
gangrene 040.0
with
abortion - see Abortion, by type,
with sepsis
ectopic pregnancy (see also
categories 633.0–633.9) 639.0
molar pregnancy (see also
categories 630–632) 639.0
following
abortion 639.0
ectopic or molar pregnancy
639.0
puerperal, postpartum,
childbirth 670.8   ◄▥
on stomach 787.3
pains 787.3
Gastradenitis 535.0●
Gastralgia 536.8
psychogenic 307.89
Gastrectasis, gastrectasia 536.1
psychogenic 306.4
Gastric - see condition
Gastrinoma (M8153/1)
malignant (M8153/3)
pancreas 157.4
specified site NEC - see Neoplasm,
by site, malignant
unspecified site 157.4

Gastrinoma (Continued)
specified site - see Neoplasm, by site,
uncertain behavior
unspecified site 235.5
Gastritis 535.5●

Note 34   Use the following fifth-digit subclassification for category 535:
0   without mention of hemorrhage
1   with hemorrhage

acute 535.0●
alcoholic 535.3●
allergic 535.4●
antral 535.4●
atrophic 535.1●
atrophic-hyperplastic 535.1●
bile-induced 535.4●
catarrhal 535.0●
chronic (atrophic) 535.1●
cirrhotic 535.4●
corrosive (acute) 535.4●
dietetic 535.4●
due to diet deficiency 269.9 [535.4]●
eosinophilic 535.7●
erosive 535.4●
follicular 535.4●
chronic 535.1●
giant hypertrophic 535.2●
glandular 535.4●
chronic 535.1●
hypertrophic (mucosa) 535.2●
chronic giant 211.1
irritant 535.4●
nervous 306.4
phlegmonous 535.0●
psychogenic 306.4
sclerotic 535.4●
spastic 536.8
subacute 535.0●
superficial 535.4●
suppurative 535.0●
toxic 535.4●
tuberculous (see also Tuberculosis)
017.9●
Gastrocarcinoma (M8010/3) 151.9
Gastrocolic - see condition
Gastrocolitis - see Enteritis
Gastrodisciasis 121.8
Gastroduodenitis (see also Gastritis)
535.5●
catarrhal 535.0●
infectional 535.0●
virus, viral 008.8
specified type NEC 008.69
Gastrodynia 536.8
Gastroenteritis (acute) (catarrhal)
(congestive) (hemorrhagic)
(noninfectious) (see also Enteritis)
558.9
aertrycke infection 003.0
allergic 558.3
chronic 558.9
ulcerative (see also Colitis, ulcerative)
556.9
dietetic 558.9
due to
antineoplastic chemotherapy 558.9
food poisoning (see also Poisoning,
food) 005.9
radiation 558.1
eosinophilic 558.41
epidemic 009.0

Gastroenteritis (Continued)
functional 558.9
infectious (see also Enteritis, due to, by
organism) 009.0
presumed 009.1
salmonella 003.0
septic (see also Enteritis, due to, by
organism) 009.0
toxic 558.2
tuberculous (see also Tuberculosis)
014.8●
ulcerative (see also Colitis, ulcerative)
556.9
viral NEC 008.8
specified type NEC 008.69
zymotic 009.0
Gastroenterocolitis - see Enteritis
Gastroenteropathy, protein-losing 579.8
Gastroenteroptosis 569.89
Gastroesophageal laceration-hemorrhage
syndrome 530.7
Gastroesophagitis 530.19
Gastrohepatitis (see also Gastritis) 535.5●
Gastrointestinal - see condition
Gastrojejunal - see condition
Gastrojejunitis (see also Gastritis) 535.5●
Gastrojejunocolic - see condition
Gastroliths 537.89
Gastromalacia 537.89
Gastroparalysis 536.3
diabetic 250.6● [536.3]
due to secondary diabetes 249.6●
[536.3]
Gastroparesis 536.3
diabetic 250.6● [536.3]
due to secondary diabetes 249.6●
[536.3]
Gastropathy 537.9
congestive portal 537.89
erythematous 535.5●
exudative 579.8
portal hypertensive 537.89
Gastroptosis 537.5
Gastrorrhagia 578.0
Gastrorrhea 536.8
psychogenic 306.4
Gastroschisis (congenital) 756.73   ◄▥
acquired 569.89
Gastrospasm (neurogenic) (reflex) 536.8
neurotic 306.4
psychogenic 306.4
Gastrostaxis 578.0
Gastrostenosis 537.89
Gastrostomy
attention to V55.1
complication 536.40
specified type 536.49
infection 536.41
malfunctioning 536.42
status V44.1
Gastrosuccorrhea (continuous)
(intermittent) 536.8
neurotic 306.4
psychogenic 306.4
Gaucher's
disease (adult) (cerebroside lipidosis)
(infantile) 272.7
hepatomegaly 272.7
splenomegaly (cerebroside lipidosis)
272.7
GAVE (gastric antral vascular ectasia)
537.82
with hemorrhage 537.83
without hemorrhage 537.82

◄ New   ◄▥ Revised   ~~deleted~~ Deleted   ● Use Additional Digit(s)   ▨ Omit code

Gayet's disease (superior hemorrhagic polioencephalitis) 265.1
Gayet-Wernicke's syndrome (superior hemorrhagic polioencephalitis) 265.1
Gee (-Herter) (-Heubner) (-Thaysen) disease or syndrome (nontropical sprue) 579.0
Gélineau's syndrome (see also Narcolepsy) 347.00
Gemination, teeth 520.2
Gemistocytoma (M9411/3)
    specified site - see Neoplasm, by site, malignant
    unspecified site 191.9
General, generalized - see condition
Genetic
    susceptibility to
        MEN (multiple endocrine neoplasia) V84.81
        neoplasia
            multiple endocrine [MEN] V84.81
        neoplasm
            malignant, of
                breast V84.01
                endometrium V84.04
                other V84.09
                ovary V84.02
                prostate V84.03
            specified disease NEC V84.89
Genital - see condition
    warts 078.11
Genito-anorectal syndrome 099.1
Genitourinary system - see condition
Genu
    congenital 755.64
    extrorsum (acquired) 736.42
        congenital 755.64
        late effects of rickets 268.1
    introrsum (acquired) 736.41
        congenital 755.64
        late effects of rickets 268.1
    rachitic (old) 268.1
    recurvatum (acquired) 736.5
        congenital 754.40
            with dislocation of knee 754.41
        late effects of rickets 268.1
    valgum (acquired) (knock-knee) 736.41
        congenital 755.64
        late effects of rickets 268.1
    varum (acquired) (bowleg) 736.42
        congenital 755.64
        late effect of rickets 268.1
Geographic tongue 529.1
Geophagia 307.52
Geotrichosis 117.9
    intestine 117.9
    lung 117.9
    mouth 117.9
Gephyrophobia 300.29
Gerbode defect 745.4
GERD (gastroesophageal reflux disease) 530.81
Gerhardt's
    disease (erythromelalgia) 443.82
    syndrome (vocal cord paralysis) 478.30
Gerlier's disease (epidemic vertigo) 078.81
German measles 056.9
    exposure to V01.4
Germinoblastoma (diffuse) (M9614/3) 202.8●
    follicular (M9692/3) 202.0●
Germinoma (M9064/3) - see Neoplasm, by site, malignant

Gerontoxon 371.41
Gerstmann-Sträussler-Scheinker syndrome (GSS) 046.71
Gerstmann's syndrome (finger agnosia) 784.69
Gestation (period) - see also Pregnancy
    ectopic NEC (see also Pregnancy, ectopic) 633.90
        with intrauterine pregnancy 633.91
Gestational proteinuria 646.2●
    with hypertension - see Toxemia, of pregnancy
Ghon tubercle primary infection (see also Tuberculosis) 010.0●
Ghost
    teeth 520.4
    vessels, cornea 370.64
Ghoul hand 102.3
Gianotti Crosti syndrome 057.8
    due to known virus - see Infection, virus
    due to unknown virus 057.8
Giant
    cell
        epulis 523.8
        peripheral (gingiva) 523.8
        tumor, tendon sheath 727.02
    colon (congenital) 751.3
    esophagus (congenital) 750.4
    kidney 753.3
    urticaria 995.1
        hereditary 277.6
Giardia lamblia infestation 007.1
Giardiasis 007.1
Gibert's disease (pityriasis rosea) 696.3
Gibraltar fever - see Brucellosis
Giddiness 780.4
    hysterical 300.11
    psychogenic 306.9
Gierke's disease (glycogenosis I) 271.0
Gigantism (cerebral) (hypophyseal) (pituitary) 253.0
Gilbert's disease or cholemia (familial nonhemolytic jaundice) 277.4
Gilchrist's disease (North American blastomycosis) 116.0
Gilford (-Hutchinson) disease or syndrome (progeria) 259.8
Gilles de la Tourette's disease (motor-verbal tic) 307.23
Gillespie's syndrome (dysplasia oculodentodigitalis) 759.89
Gingivitis 523.10
    acute 523.00
        necrotizing 101
        non-plaque induced 523.01
        plaque induced 523.00
    catarrhal 523.00
    chronic 523.10
        non-plaque induced 523.11
    desquamative 523.10
    expulsiva 523.40
    hyperplastic 523.10
    marginal, simple 523.10
    necrotizing, acute 101
    non-plaque induced 523.11
    pellagrous 265.2
    plaque induced 523.10
    ulcerative 523.10
        acute necrotizing 101
    Vincent's 101
Gingivoglossitis 529.0
Gingivopericementitis 523.40
Gingivosis 523.10

Gingivostomatitis 523.10
    herpetic 054.2
Giovannini's disease 117.9
GISA (glycopeptide intermediate staphylococcus aureus) V09.8
Gland, glandular - see condition
Glanders 024
Glanzmann (-Naegeli) disease or thrombasthenia 287.1
Glassblowers' disease 527.1
Glaucoma (capsular) (inflammatory) (noninflammatory) (primary) 365.9
    with increased episcleral venous pressure 365.82
    absolute 360.42
    acute 365.22
        narrow angle 365.22
        secondary 365.60
    angle closure 365.20
        acute 365.22
        chronic 365.23
        intermittent 365.21
        interval 365.21
        residual stage 365.24
        subacute 365.21
    borderline 365.00
    chronic 365.11
        noncongestive 365.11
        open angle 365.11
        simple 365.11
    closed angle - see Glaucoma, angle closure
    congenital 743.20
        associated with other eye anomalies 743.22
        simple 743.21
    congestive - see Glaucoma, narrow angle
    corticosteroid-induced (glaucomatous stage) 365.31
        residual stage 365.32
    hemorrhagic 365.60
    hypersecretion 365.81
    in or with
        aniridia 365.42
        Axenfeld's anomaly 365.41
        congenital syndromes NEC 759.89 [365.44]
        disorder of lens NEC 365.59
        inflammation, ocular 365.62   ◄
        iris
            anomalies NEC 365.42
            atrophy, essential 365.42
            bombé 365.61
        microcornea 365.43
        neurofibromatosis 237.71 [365.44]
        ocular
            cysts NEC 365.64
            disorders NEC 365.60
            trauma 365.65
            tumors NEC 365.64
        pupillary block or seclusion 365.61
        Rieger's anomaly or syndrome 365.41
        seclusion of pupil 365.61
        Sturge-Weber (-Dimitri) syndrome 759.6 [365.44]
        systemic syndrome NEC 365.44
        tumor of globe 365.64
        vascular disorders NEC 365.63
    infantile 365.14
        congenital 743.20
            associated with other eye anomalies 743.22
            simple 743.21

Glaucoma *(Continued)*
   juvenile 365.14
   low tension 365.12
   malignant 365.83
   narrow angle (primary) 365.20
      acute 365.22
      chronic 365.23
      intermittent 365.21
      interval 365.21
      residual stage 365.24
      subacute 365.21
   newborn 743.20
      associated with other eye anomalies 743.22
      simple 743.21
   noncongestive (chronic) 365.11
   nonobstructive (chronic) 365.11
   obstructive 365.60
      due to lens changes 365.59
   open angle 365.10
      with
         borderline intraocular pressure 365.01
         cupping of optic discs 365.01
         primary 365.11
         residual stage 365.15
   phacolytic 365.51
   pigmentary 365.13
   postinfectious 365.60
   pseudoexfoliation 365.52
   secondary NEC 365.60
   simple (chronic) 365.11
   simplex 365.11
   steroid responders 365.03
   suspect 365.00
   syphilitic 095.8
   traumatic NEC 365.65
      newborn 767.8
   wide angle (*see also* Glaucoma, open angle) 365.10
Glaucomatous flecks (subcapsular) 366.31
Glazed tongue 529.4
Gleet 098.2
Glénard's disease or syndrome (enteroptosis) 569.89
Glinski-Simmonds syndrome (pituitary cachexia) 253.2
Glioblastoma (multiforme) (M9440/3)
   with sarcomatous component (M9442/3)
      specified site - *see* Neoplasm, by site, malignant
      unspecified site 191.9
   giant cell (M9441/3)
      specified site - *see* Neoplasm, by site, malignant
      unspecified site 191.9
   specified site - *see* Neoplasm, by site, malignant
   unspecified site 191.9
Glioma (malignant) (M9380/3)
   astrocytic (M9400/3)
      specified site - *see* Neoplasm, by site, malignant
      unspecified site 191.9
   mixed (M9382/3)
      specified site - *see* Neoplasm, by site, malignant
      unspecified site 191.9
   nose 748.1
   specified site NEC - *see* Neoplasm, by site, malignant
   subependymal (M9383/1) 237.5
   unspecified site 191.9

Gliomatosis cerebri (M9381/3) 191.0
Glioneuroma (M9505/1) - *see* Neoplasm, by site, uncertain behavior
Gliosarcoma (M9380/3)
   specified site - *see* Neoplasm, by site, malignant
   unspecified site 191.9
Gliosis (cerebral) 349.89
   spinal 336.0
Glisson's
   cirrhosis - *see* Cirrhosis, portal
   disease (*see also* Rickets) 268.0
Glissonitis 573.3
Globinuria 791.2
Globus 306.4
   hystericus 300.11
Glomangioma (M8712/0) (*see also* Hemangioma) 228.00
Glomangiosarcoma (M8710/3) - *see* Neoplasm, connective tissue, malignant
Glomerular nephritis (*see also* Nephritis) 583.9
Glomerulitis (*see also* Nephritis) 583.9
Glomerulonephritis (*see also* Nephritis) 583.9
   with
      edema (*see also* Nephrosis) 581.9
      lesion of
         exudative nephritis 583.89
         interstitial nephritis (diffuse) (focal) 583.89
         necrotizing glomerulitis 583.4
            acute 580.4
            chronic 582.4
         renal necrosis 583.9
            cortical 583.6
            medullary 583.7
         specified pathology NEC 583.89
            acute 580.89
            chronic 582.89
      necrosis, renal 583.9
         cortical 583.6
         medullary (papillary) 583.7
      specified pathology or lesion NEC 583.89
   acute 580.9
      with
         exudative nephritis 580.89
         interstitial nephritis (diffuse) (focal) 580.89
         necrotizing glomerulitis 580.4
      extracapillary with epithelial crescents 580.4
      poststreptococcal 580.0
      proliferative (diffuse) 580.0
      rapidly progressive 580.4
      specified pathology NEC 580.89
   arteriolar (*see also* Hypertension, kidney) 403.90
   arteriosclerotic (*see also* Hypertension, kidney) 403.90
   ascending (*see also* Pyelitis) 590.80
   basement membrane NEC 583.89
      with
         pulmonary hemorrhage (Goodpasture's syndrome) 446.21 [583.81]
   chronic 582.9
      with
         exudative nephritis 582.89
         interstitial nephritis (diffuse) (focal) 582.89
         necrotizing glomerulitis 582.4

Glomerulonephritis *(Continued)*
   chronic *(Continued)*
      with *(Continued)*
         specified pathology or lesion NEC 582.89
      endothelial 582.2
      extracapillary with epithelial crescents 582.4
      hypocomplementemic persistent 582.2
      lobular 582.2
      membranoproliferative 582.2
      membranous 582.1
         and proliferative (mixed) 582.2
         sclerosing 582.1
      mesangiocapillary 582.2
      mixed membranous and proliferative 582.2
      proliferative (diffuse) 582.0
      rapidly progressive 582.4
      sclerosing 582.1
   cirrhotic - *see* Sclerosis, renal
   desquamative - *see* Nephrosis
   due to or associated with
      amyloidosis 277.39 [583.81]
         with nephrotic syndrome 277.39 [581.81]
         chronic 277.39 [582.81]
      diabetes mellitus 250.4● [583.81]
         due to secondary diabetes 249.4● [581.81]
         with nephrotic syndrome 250.4● [581.81]
            due to secondary diabetes 249.4● [581.81]
      diphtheria 032.89 [580.81]
      gonococcal infection (acute) 098.19 [583.81]
         chronic or duration of 2 months or over 098.39 [583.81]
      infectious hepatitis 070.9 [580.81]
      malaria (with nephrotic syndrome) 084.9 [581.81]
      mumps 072.79 [580.81]
      polyarteritis (nodosa) (with nephrotic syndrome) 446.0 [581.81]
      specified pathology NEC 583.89
         acute 580.89
         chronic 582.89
      streptotrichosis 039.8 [583.81]
      subacute bacterial endocarditis 421.0 [580.81]
      syphilis (late) 095.4
         congenital 090.5 [583.81]
         early 091.69 [583.81]
      systemic lupus erythematosus 710.0 [583.81]
         with nephrotic syndrome 710.0 [581.81]
         chronic 710.0 [582.81]
      tuberculosis (*see also* Tuberculosis) 016.0● [583.81]
      typhoid fever 002.0 [580.81]
   extracapillary with epithelial crescents 583.4
      acute 580.4
      chronic 582.4
   exudative 583.89
      acute 580.89
      chronic 582.89
   focal (*see also* Nephritis) 583.9
      embolic 580.4
   granular 582.89

◀ New   ◀▥ Revised   ~~deleted~~ Deleted   ● Use Additional Digit(s)   ▨ Omit code

Glomerulonephritis (Continued)
  granulomatous 582.89
  hydremic (see also Nephrosis) 581.9
  hypocomplementemic persistent 583.2
    with nephrotic syndrome 581.2
    chronic 582.2
  immune complex NEC 583.89
  infective (see also Pyelitis) 590.80
  interstitial (diffuse) (focal) 583.89
    with nephrotic syndrome 581.89
    acute 580.89
    chronic 582.89
  latent or quiescent 582.9
  lobular 583.2
    with nephrotic syndrome 581.2
    chronic 582.2
  membranoproliferative 583.2
    with nephrotic syndrome 581.2
    chronic 582.2
  membranous 583.1
    with nephrotic syndrome 581.1
    and proliferative (mixed) 583.2
      with nephrotic syndrome 581.2
      chronic 582.2
    chronic 582.1
    sclerosing 582.1
      with nephrotic syndrome 581.1
  mesangiocapillary 583.2
    with nephrotic syndrome 581.2
    chronic 582.2
  minimal change 581.3
  mixed membranous and proliferative
      583.2
    with nephrotic syndrome 581.2
    chronic 582.2
  necrotizing 583.4
    acute 580.4
    chronic 582.4
  nephrotic (see also Nephrosis) 581.9
  old - see Glomerulonephritis, chronic
  parenchymatous 581.89
  poststreptococcal 580.0
  proliferative (diffuse) 583.0
    with nephrotic syndrome 581.0
    acute 580.0
    chronic 582.0
  purulent (see also Pyelitis) 590.80
  quiescent - see Nephritis, chronic
  rapidly progressive 583.4
    acute 580.4
    chronic 582.4
  sclerosing membranous (chronic)
      582.1
    with nephrotic syndrome 581.1
  septic (see also Pyelitis) 590.80
  specified pathology or lesion NEC
      583.89
    with nephrotic syndrome 581.89
    acute 580.89
    chronic 582.89
  suppurative (acute) (disseminated) (see
      also Pyelitis) 590.80
  toxic - see Nephritis, acute
  tubal, tubular - see Nephrosis, tubular
  type II (Ellis) - see Nephrosis
  vascular - see Hypertension, kidney
Glomerulosclerosis (see also Sclerosis,
    renal) 587
  focal 582.1
    with nephrotic syndrome 581.1
  intercapillary (nodular) (with diabetes)
      250.4● [581.81]
    due to secondary diabetes 249.4●
      [581.81]

Glossagra 529.6
Glossalgia 529.6
Glossitis 529.0
  areata exfoliativa 529.1
  atrophic 529.4
  benign migratory 529.1
  gangrenous 529.0
  Hunter's 529.4
  median rhomboid 529.2
  Moeller's 529.4
  pellagrous 265.2
Glossocele 529.8
Glossodynia 529.6
  exfoliativa 529.4
Glossoncus 529.8
Glossophytia 529.3
Glossoplegia 529.8
Glossoptosis 529.8
Glossopyrosis 529.6
Glossotrichia 529.3
Glossy skin 701.9
Glottis - see condition
Glottitis - see Glossitis
Glucagonoma (M8152/0)
  malignant (M8152/3)
    pancreas 157.4
    specified site NEC - see Neoplasm,
      by site, malignant
    unspecified site 157.4
  pancreas 211.7
  specified site NEC - see Neoplasm, by
    site, benign
  unspecified site 211.7
Glucoglycinuria 270.7
Glue ear syndrome 381.20
Glue sniffing (airplane glue) (see also
    Dependence) 304.6●
Glycinemia (with methylmalonic
    acidemia) 270.7
Glycinuria (renal) (with ketosis) 270.0
Glycogen
  infiltration (see also Disease, glycogen
    storage) 271.0
  storage disease (see also Disease,
    glycogen storage) 271.0
Glycogenosis (see also Disease, glycogen
    storage) 271.0
  cardiac 271.0 [425.7]
  Cori, types I-VII 271.0
  diabetic, secondary 250.8● [259.8]
    due to secondary diabetes 249.8●
      [259.8]
  diffuse (with hepatic cirrhosis) 271.0
  generalized 271.0
  glucose-6-phosphatase deficiency
      271.0
  hepatophosphorylase deficiency
      271.0
  hepatorenal 271.0
  myophosphorylase deficiency 271.0
Glycopenia 251.2
Glycopeptide
  intermediate staphylococcus aureus
    (GISA) V09.8
  resistant
    enterococcus V09.8
    staphylococcus aureus (GRSA)
      V09.8
Glycoprolinuria 270.8
Glycosuria 791.5
  renal 271.4
Gnathostoma (spinigerum) (infection)
    (infestation) 128.1
  wandering swellings from 128.1

Gnathostomiasis 128.1
Goiter (adolescent) (colloid) (diffuse)
    (dipping) (due to iodine deficiency)
    (endemic) (euthyroid) (heart)
    (hyperplastic) (internal)
    (intrathoracic) (juvenile) (mixed
    type) (nonendemic)
    (parenchymatous) (plunging)
    (sporadic) (subclavicular)
    (substernal) 240.9
  with
    hyperthyroidism (recurrent) (see also
      Goiter, toxic) 242.0●
    thyrotoxicosis (see also Goiter, toxic)
      242.0●
  adenomatous (see also Goiter, nodular)
      241.9
  cancerous (M8000/3) 193
  complicating pregnancy, childbirth, or
      puerperium 648.1●
  congenital 246.1
  cystic (see also Goiter, nodular) 241.9
  due to enzyme defect in synthesis of
      thyroid hormone (butane-
      insoluble iodine) (coupling)
      (deiodinase) (iodide trapping or
      organification) (iodotyrosine
      dehalogenase) (peroxidase) 246.1
  dyshormonogenic 246.1
  exophthalmic (see also Goiter, toxic)
      242.0●
  familial (with deaf-mutism) 243
  fibrous 245.3
  lingual 759.2
  lymphadenoid 245.2
  malignant (M8000/3) 193
  multinodular (nontoxic) 241.1
    toxic or with hyperthyroidism (see
      also Goiter, toxic) 242.2●
  nodular (nontoxic) 241.9
    with
      hyperthyroidism (see also Goiter,
        toxic) 242.3●
      thyrotoxicosis (see also Goiter,
        toxic) 242.3●
    endemic 241.9
    exophthalmic (diffuse) (see also
      Goiter, toxic) 242.0●
    multinodular (nontoxic) 241.1
    sporadic 241.9
    toxic (see also Goiter, toxic) 242.3●
    uninodular (nontoxic) 241.0
  nontoxic (nodular) 241.9
    multinodular 241.1
    uninodular 241.0
  pulsating (see also Goiter, toxic) 242.0●
  simple 240.0
  toxic 242.0●

Note 35   Use the following fifth-digit
subclassification with category 242:

0   without mention of thyrotoxic
          crisis or storm
1   with mention of thyrotoxic crisis
          or storm

---

    adenomatous 242.3●
      multinodular 242.2●
      uninodular 242.1●
    multinodular 242.2●
    nodular 242.3●
      multinodular 242.2●
      uninodular 242.1●
    uninodular 242.1●

Goiter (Continued)
  uninodular (nontoxic) 241.0
    toxic or with hyperthyroidism (see
      also Goiter, toxic) 242.1●
Goldberg (-Maxwell) (-Morris) syndrome
  (testicular feminization) 259.51
Goldblatt's
  hypertension 440.1
  kidney 440.1
Goldenhar's syndrome
  (oculoauriculovertebral dysplasia)
  756.0
Goldflam-Erb disease or syndrome
  358.00
Goldscheider's disease (epidermolysis
  bullosa) 757.39
Goldstein's disease (familial hemorrhagic
  telangiectasia) 448.0
Golfer's elbow 726.32
Goltz-Gorlin syndrome (dermal
  hypoplasia) 757.39
Gonadoblastoma (M9073/1)
  specified site - see Neoplasm, by site
    uncertain behavior
  unspecified site
    female 236.2
    male 236.4
Gonecystitis (see also Vesiculitis) 608.0
Gongylonemiasis 125.6
  mouth 125.6
Goniosynechiae 364.73
Gonococcemia 098.89
Gonococcus, gonococcal (disease)
  (infection) (see also condition)
  098.0
  anus 098.7
  bursa 098.52
  chronic NEC 098.2
  complicating pregnancy, childbirth, or
    puerperium 647.1●
    affecting fetus or newborn 760.2
  conjunctiva, conjunctivitis
    (neonatorum) 098.40
  dermatosis 098.89
  endocardium 098.84
  epididymo-orchitis 098.13
    chronic or duration of 2 months or
      over 098.33
  eye (newborn) 098.40
  fallopian tube (chronic) 098.37
    acute 098.17
  genitourinary (acute) (organ) (system)
    (tract) (see also Gonorrhea) 098.0
    lower 098.0
      chronic 098.2
    upper 098.10
      chronic 098.30
  heart NEC 098.85
  joint 098.50
  keratoderma 098.81
  keratosis (blennorrhagica) 098.81
  lymphatic (gland) (node) 098.89
  meninges 098.82
  orchitis (acute) 098.13
    chronic or duration of 2 months or
      over 098.33
  pelvis (acute) 098.19
    chronic or duration of 2 months or
      over 098.39
  pericarditis 098.83
  peritonitis 098.86
  pharyngitis 098.6
  pharynx 098.6
  proctitis 098.7

Gonococcus, gonococcal (Continued)
  pyosalpinx (chronic) 098.37
    acute 098.17
  rectum 098.7
  septicemia 098.89
  skin 098.89
  specified site NEC 098.89
  synovitis 098.51
  tendon sheath 098.51
  throat 098.6
  urethra (acute) 098.0
    chronic or duration of 2 months or
      over 098.2
  vulva (acute) 098.0
    chronic or duration of 2 months or
      over 098.2
Gonocytoma (M9073/1)
  specified site - see Neoplasm, by site,
    uncertain behavior
  unspecified site
    female 236.2
    male 236.4
Gonorrhea 098.0
  acute 098.0
  Bartholin's gland (acute) 098.0
    chronic or duration of 2 months or
      over 098.2
  bladder (acute) 098.11
    chronic or duration of 2 months or
      over 098.31
  carrier (suspected of) V02.7
  cervix (acute) 098.15
    chronic or duration of 2 months or
      over 098.35
  chronic 098.2
  complicating pregnancy, childbirth, or
    puerperium 647.1●
    affecting fetus or newborn 760.2
  conjunctiva, conjunctivitis
    (neonatorum) 098.40
  contact V01.6
  Cowper's gland (acute) 098.0
    chronic or duration of 2 months or
      over 098.2
  duration of 2 months or over 098.2
  exposure to V01.6
  fallopian tube (chronic) 098.37
    acute 098.17
  genitourinary (acute) (organ) (system)
    (tract) 098.0
    chronic 098.2
    duration of 2 months or over 098.2
  kidney (acute) 098.19
    chronic or duration of 2 months or
      over 098.39
  ovary (acute) 098.19
    chronic or duration of 2 months or
      over 098.39
  pelvis (acute) 098.19
    chronic or duration of 2 months or
      over 098.39
  penis (acute) 098.0
    chronic or duration of 2 months or
      over 098.2
  prostate (acute) 098.12
    chronic or duration of 2 months or
      over 098.32
  seminal vesicle (acute) 098.14
    chronic or duration of 2 months or
      over 098.34
  specified site NEC - see Gonococcus
  spermatic cord (acute) 098.14
    chronic or duration of 2 months or
      over 098.34

Gonorrhea (Continued)
  urethra (acute) 098.0
    chronic or duration of 2 months or
      over 098.2
  vagina (acute) 098.0
    chronic or duration of 2 months or
      over 098.2
  vas deferens (acute) 098.14
    chronic or duration of 2 months or
      over 098.34
  vulva (acute) 098.0
    chronic or duration of 2 months or
      over 098.2
Goodpasture's syndrome (pneumorenal)
  446.21
Good's syndrome 279.06
Gopalan's syndrome (burning feet) 266.2
Gordon's disease (exudative enteropathy)
  579.8
Gorlin-Chaudhry-Moss syndrome
  759.89
Gougerot's syndrome (trisymptomatic)
  709.1
Gougerot-Blum syndrome (pigmented
  purpuric lichenoid dermatitis) 709.1
Gougerot-Carteaud disease or syndrome
  (confluent reticulate papillomatosis)
  701.8
Gougerot-Hailey-Hailey disease (benign
  familial chronic pemphigus)
  757.39
Gougerot (-Houwer)-Sjögren syndrome
  (keratoconjunctivitis sicca) 710.2
Gouley's syndrome (constrictive
  pericarditis) 423.2
Goundou 102.6
Gout, gouty 274.9
  with specified manifestations NEC
    274.89   ◄▥
    specified manifestations NEC
      274.89   ◄
    tophi (tophus) 274.03   ◄
  acute 274.01   ◄
  arthritis (acute) 274.00   ◄▥
    acute 274.01   ◄
  arthropathy 274.00   ◄▥
    acute 274.01   ◄
    chronic (without mention of tophus
      (tophi)) 274.02   ◄
      with tophus (tophi) 274.03   ◄
  attack 274.01   ◄
  chronic 274.02   ◄
    tophaceous 274.03   ◄
  degeneration, heart 274.82
  diathesis 274.9
  eczema 274.89
  episcleritis 274.89 [379.09]
  external ear (tophus) 274.81
  flare 274.01   ◄
  glomerulonephritis 274.10
  iritis 274.89 [364.11]
  joint 274.00   ◄▥
  kidney 274.10
  lead 984.9
    specified type of lead - see Table of
      Drugs and Chemicals
  nephritis 274.10
  neuritis 274.89 [357.4]
  phlebitis 274.89 [451.9]
  rheumatic 714.0
  saturnine 984.9
    specified type of lead - see Table of
      Drugs and Chemicals
  spondylitis 274.00   ◄▥

◄ New   ◄▥ Revised   deleted Deleted   ● Use Additional Digit(s)   ▥ Omit code

Gout, gouty (*Continued*)
  synovitis 274.00 ◀▥
  syphilitic 095.8
  tophi 274.03 ◀▥
    ear 274.81
    heart 274.82
    specified site NEC 274.82
Gowers'
  muscular dystrophy 359.1
  syndrome (vasovagal attack) 780.2
Gowers-Paton-Kennedy syndrome
  377.04
Gradenigo's syndrome 383.02
Graft-versus-host disease 279.50
  ~~bone marrow 996.85~~
  due to organ transplant NEC - *see*
    Complications, transplant, organ
Graham Steell's murmur (pulmonic
  regurgitation) (*see also* Endocarditis,
  pulmonary) 424.3
Grain-handlers' disease or lung 495.8
Grain mite (itch) 133.8
Grand
  mal (idiopathic) (*see also* Epilepsy)
    345.1●
    hysteria of Charcôt 300.11
    nonrecurrent or isolated 780.39
  multipara
    affecting management of labor and
      delivery 659.4●
    status only (not pregnant) V61.5
Granite workers' lung 502
Granular - *see also* condition
  inflammation, pharynx 472.1
  kidney (contracting) (*see also* Sclerosis,
    renal) 587
  liver - *see* Cirrhosis, liver
  nephritis - *see* Nephritis
Granulation tissue, abnormal - *see also*
  Granuloma
  abnormal or excessive 701.5
  postmastoidectomy cavity 383.33
  postoperative 701.5
  skin 701.5
Granulocytopenia, granulocytopenic
  (primary) 288.00
  malignant 288.09
Granuloma NEC 686.1
  abdomen (wall) 568.89
    skin (pyogenicum) 686.1
      from residual foreign body 709.4
  annulare 695.89
  anus 569.49
  apical 522.6
  appendix 543.9
  aural 380.23
  beryllium (skin) 709.4
    lung 503
  bone (*see also* Osteomyelitis) 730.1●
    eosinophilic 277.89
    from residual foreign body
      733.99
  canaliculus lacrimalis 375.81
  cerebral 348.89 ◀▥
  cholesterin, middle ear 385.82
  coccidioidal (progressive) 114.3
    lung 114.4
    meninges 114.2
    primary (lung) 114.0
  colon 569.89
  conjunctiva 372.61
  dental 522.6
  ear, middle (cholesterin) 385.82
    with otitis media - *see* Otitis media

Granuloma NEC (*Continued*)
  eosinophilic 277.89
    bone 277.89
    lung 277.89
    oral mucosa 528.9
  exuberant 701.5
  eyelid 374.89
  facial
    lethal midline 446.3
    malignant 446.3
  faciale 701.8
  fissuratum (gum) 523.8
  foot NEC 686.1
  foreign body (in soft tissue) NEC
    728.82
    bone 733.99
    in operative wound 998.4
    muscle 728.82
    skin 709.4
    subcutaneous tissue 709.4
  fungoides 202.1●
  gangraenescens 446.3
  giant cell (central) (jaw) (reparative)
    526.3
    gingiva 523.8
    peripheral (gingiva) 523.8
  gland (lymph) 289.3
  Hodgkin's (M9661/3) 201.1●
  ileum 569.89
  infectious NEC 136.9
  inguinale (Donovan) 099.2
    venereal 099.2
  intestine 569.89
  iridocyclitis 364.10
  jaw (bone) 526.3
    reparative giant cell 526.3
  kidney (*see also* Infection, kidney) 590.9
  lacrimal sac 375.81
  larynx 478.79
  lethal midline 446.3
  lipid 277.89
  lipoid 277.89
  liver 572.8
  lung (infectious) (*see also* Fibrosis, lung)
    515
    coccidioidal 114.4
    eosinophilic 277.89
  lymph gland 289.3
  Majocchi's 110.6
  malignant, face 446.3
  mandible 526.3
  mediastinum 519.3
  midline 446.3
  monilial 112.3
  muscle 728.82
    from residual foreign body 728.82
  nasal sinus (*see also* Sinusitis) 473.9
  operation wound 998.59
    foreign body 998.4
    stitch (external) 998.89
      internal wound 998.89
    talc 998.7
  oral mucosa, eosinophilic or pyogenic
    528.9
  orbit, orbital 376.11
  paracoccidioidal 116.1
  penis, venereal 099.2
  periapical 522.6
  peritoneum 568.89
    due to ova of helminths NEC (*see*
      also Helminthiasis) 128.9
  postmastoidectomy cavity 383.33
  postoperative - *see* Granuloma,
    operation wound

Granuloma NEC (*Continued*)
  prostate 601.8
  pudendi (ulcerating) 099.2
  pudendorum (ulcerative) 099.2
  pulp, internal (tooth) 521.49
  pyogenic, pyogenicum (skin) 686.1
    maxillary alveolar ridge 522.6
    oral mucosa 528.9
  rectum 569.49
  reticulohistiocytic 277.89
  rubrum nasi 705.89
  sarcoid 135
  Schistosoma 120.9
  septic (skin) 686.1
  silica (skin) 709.4
  sinus (accessory) (infectional) (nasal)
    (*see also* Sinusitis) 473.9
  skin (pyogenicum) 686.1
    from foreign body or material 709.4
  sperm 608.89
  spine
    syphilitic (epidural) 094.89
    tuberculous (*see also* Tuberculosis)
      015.0● [730.88]
  stitch (postoperative) 998.89
    internal wound 998.89
  suppurative (skin) 686.1
  suture (postoperative) 998.89
    internal wound 998.89
  swimming pool 031.1
  talc 728.82
    in operation wound 998.7
  telangiectaticum (skin) 686.1
  tracheostomy 519.09
  trichophyticum 110.6
  tropicum 102.4
  umbilicus 686.1
    newborn 771.4
  urethra 599.84
  uveitis 364.10
  vagina 099.2
  venereum 099.2
  vocal cords 478.5
  Wegener's (necrotizing respiratory
    granulomatosis) 446.4
Granulomatosis NEC 686.1
  disciformis chronica et progressiva 709.3
  infantiseptica 771.2
  lipoid 277.89
  lipophagic, intestinal 040.2
  miliary 027.0
  necrotizing, respiratory 446.4
  progressive, septic 288.1
  Wegener's (necrotizing respiratory)
    446.4
Granulomatous tissue - *see* Granuloma
Granulosis rubra nasi 705.89
Graphite fibrosis (of lung) 503
Graphospasm 300.89
  organic 333.84
Grating scapula 733.99
Gravel (urinary) (*see also* Calculus) 592.9
Graves' disease (exophthalmic goiter) (*see*
  also Goiter, toxic) 242.0●
Gravis - *see* condition
Grawitz's tumor (hypernephroma)
  (M8312/3) 189.0
Grayness, hair (premature) 704.3
  congenital 757.4
Gray or grey syndrome
  (chloramphenicol) (newborn)
  779.4
Greenfield's disease 330.0
Green sickness 280.9

Greenstick fracture - *see* Fracture, by site
Greig's syndrome (hypertelorism) 756.0
Grief 309.0
Griesinger's disease (*see also* Ancylostomiasis) 126.9
Grinders'
  asthma 502
  lung 502
  phthisis (*see also* Tuberculosis) 011.4●
Grinding, teeth 306.8
Grip
  Dabney's 074.1
  devil's 074.1
Grippe, grippal - *see also* Influenza
  Balkan 083.0
  intestinal 487.8
  summer 074.8
Grippy cold 487.1
Grisel's disease 723.5
Groin - *see* condition
Grooved
  nails (transverse) 703.8
  tongue 529.5
    congenital 750.13
Ground itch 126.9
Growing pains, children 781.99
Growth (fungoid) (neoplastic) (new) (M8000/1) - *see also* Neoplasm, by site, unspecified nature
  adenoid (vegetative) 474.12
  benign (M8000/0) - *see* Neoplasm, by site, benign
  fetal, poor 764.9●
    affecting management of pregnancy 656.5●
  malignant (M8000/3) - *see* Neoplasm, by site, malignant
  rapid, childhood V21.0
  secondary (M8000/6) - *see* Neoplasm, by site, malignant, secondary
GRSA (glycopeptide resistant staphylococcus aureus) V09.8
Gruber's hernia - *see* Hernia, Gruber's
Gruby's disease (tinea tonsurans) 110.0
GSS (Gerstmann-Sträussler-Scheinker syndrome) 046.71

G-trisomy 758.0
Guama fever 066.3
Gubler (-Millard) paralysis or syndrome 344.89
Guérin-Stern syndrome (arthrogryposis multiplex congenita) 754.89
Guertin's disease (electric chorea) 049.8
Guillain-Barré disease or syndrome 357.0
Guinea worms (infection) (infestation) 125.7
Guinon's disease (motor-verbal tic) 307.23
Gull's disease (thyroid atrophy with myxedema) 244.8
Gull and Sutton's disease - *see* Hypertension, kidney
Gum - *see* condition
Gumboil 522.7
Gumma (syphilitic) 095.9
  artery 093.89
    cerebral or spinal 094.89
  bone 095.5
    of yaws (late) 102.6
  brain 094.89
  cauda equina 094.89
  central nervous system NEC 094.9
  ciliary body 095.8 [364.11]
  congenital 090.5
    testis 090.5
  eyelid 095.8 [373.5]
  heart 093.89
  intracranial 094.89
  iris 095.8 [364.11]
  kidney 095.4
  larynx 095.8
  leptomeninges 094.2
  liver 095.3
  meninges 094.2
  myocardium 093.82
  nasopharynx 095.8
  neurosyphilitic 094.9
  nose 095.8
  orbit 095.8
  palate (soft) 095.8
  penis 095.8
  pericardium 093.81
  pharynx 095.8

Gumma(*Continued*)
  pituitary 095.8
  scrofulous (*see also* Tuberculosis) 017.0●
Gumma (*Continued*)
  skin 095.8
  specified site NEC 095.8
  spinal cord 094.89
  tongue 095.8
  tonsil 095.8
  trachea 095.8
  tuberculous (*see also* Tuberculosis) 017.0●
  ulcerative due to yaws 102.4
  ureter 095.8
  yaws 102.4
    bone 102.6
Gunn's syndrome (jaw-winking syndrome) 742.8
Gunshot wound - *see also* Wound, open, by site
  fracture - *see* Fracture, by site, open
  internal organs (abdomen, chest, or pelvis) - *see* Injury, internal, by site, with open wound
  intracranial - *see* Laceration, brain, with open intracranial wound
Günther's disease or syndrome (congenital erythropoietic porphyria) 277.1
Gustatory hallucination 780.1
Gynandrism 752.7
Gynandroblastoma (M8632/1)
  specified site - *see* Neoplasm, by site, uncertain behavior
  unspecified site
    female 236.2
    male 236.4
Gynandromorphism 752.7
Gynatresia (congenital) 752.49
Gynecoid pelvis, male 738.6
Gynecological examination V72.31
  for contraceptive maintenance V25.40
Gynecomastia 611.1
Gynephobia 300.29
Gyrate scalp 757.39

◀ New   ◀▥ Revised   ~~deleted~~ Deleted   ● Use Additional Digit(s)   ▨ Omit code

H

Haas' disease (osteochondrosis head of humerus) 732.3
Habermann's disease (acute parapsoriasis varioliformis) 696.2
Habit, habituation
  chorea 307.22
  disturbance, child 307.9
  drug (see also Dependence) 304.9●
  laxative (see also Abuse, drugs, nondependent) 305.9●
  spasm 307.20
    chronic 307.22
    transient (of childhood) 307.21
  tic 307.20
    chronic 307.22
    transient (of childhood) 307.21
  use of
    nonprescribed drugs (see also Abuse, drugs, nondependent) 305.9●
    patent medicines (see also Abuse, drugs, nondependent) 305.9●
  vomiting 536.2
Hadfield-Clarke syndrome (pancreatic infantilism) 577.8
Haff disease 985.1
Hag teeth, tooth 524.39
Hageman factor defect, deficiency, or disease (see also Defect, coagulation) 286.3
Haglund's disease (osteochondrosis os tibiale externum) 732.5
Haglund-Läwen-Fründ syndrome 717.89
Hagner's disease (hypertrophic pulmonary osteoarthropathy) 731.2
Hailey-Hailey disease (benign familial chronic pemphigus) 757.39
Hair - see also condition
  plucking 307.9
Hairball in stomach 935.2
Hairy black tongue 529.3
Half vertebra 756.14
Halitosis 784.99
Hallermann-Streiff syndrome 756.0
Hallervorden-Spatz disease or syndrome 333.0
Hallopeau's
  acrodermatitis (continua) 696.1
  disease (lichen sclerosis et atrophicus) 701.0
Hallucination (auditory) (gustatory) (olfactory) (tactile) 780.1
  alcohol-induced 291.3
  drug-induced 292.12
  visual 368.16
Hallucinosis 298.9
  alcohol-induced (acute) 291.3
  drug-induced 292.12
Hallus - see Hallux
Hallux 735.9
  limitus 735.8
  malleus (acquired) 735.3
  rigidus (acquired) 735.2
    congenital 755.66
    late effects of rickets 268.1
  valgus (acquired) 735.0
    congenital 755.66
  varus (acquired) 735.1
    congenital 755.66
Halo, visual 368.15
Hamartoblastoma 759.6

Hamartoma 759.6
  epithelial (gingival), odontogenic, central, or peripheral (M9321/0) 213.1
    upper jaw (bone) 213.0
  vascular 757.32
Hamartosis, hamartoses NEC 759.6
Hamman's disease or syndrome (spontaneous mediastinal emphysema) 518.1
Hamman-Rich syndrome (diffuse interstitial pulmonary fibrosis) 516.3
Hammer toe (acquired) 735.4
  congenital 755.66
  late effects of rickets 268.1
Hand - see condition
Hand-Schüller-Christian disease or syndrome (chronic histiocytosis x) 277.89
Hand-foot syndrome 693.0
Hanging (asphyxia) (strangulation) (suffocation) 994.7
Hangnail (finger) (with lymphangitis) 681.02
Hangover (alcohol) (see also Abuse, drugs, nondependent) 305.0●
Hanot's cirrhosis or disease - see Cirrhosis, biliary
Hanot-Chauffard (-Troisier) syndrome (bronze diabetes) 275.0
Hansen's disease (leprosy) 030.9
  benign form 030.1
  malignant form 030.0
Harada's disease or syndrome 363.22
Hard chancre 091.0
Hard firm prostate 600.10
  with
    urinary
      obstruction 600.11
      retention 600.11
Hardening
  artery - see Arteriosclerosis
  brain 348.89 ◀▥
  liver 571.8
Hare's syndrome (M8010/3) (carcinoma, pulmonary apex) 162.3
Harelip (see also Cleft, lip) 749.10
Harkavy's syndrome 446.0
Harlequin (fetus) 757.1
  color change syndrome 779.89
Harley's disease (intermittent hemoglobinuria) 283.2
Harris'
  lines 733.91
  syndrome (organic hyperinsulinism) 251.1
Hart's disease or syndrome (pellagra-cerebellar ataxia-renal aminoaciduria) 270.0
Hartmann's pouch (abnormal sacculation of gallbladder neck) 575.8
  of intestine V44.3
    attention to V55.3
Hartnup disease (pellagra-cerebellar ataxia-renal aminoaciduria) 270.0
Harvester lung 495.0
Hashimoto's disease or struma (struma lymphomatosa) 245.2
Hassall-Henle bodies (corneal warts) 371.41
Haut mal (see also Epilepsy) 345.1●
Haverhill fever 026.1
Hawaiian wood rose dependence 304.5●
Hawkins' keloid 701.4

Hay
  asthma (see also Asthma) 493.0●
  fever (allergic) (with rhinitis) 477.9
    with asthma (bronchial) (see also Asthma) 493.0●
    allergic, due to grass, pollen, ragweed, or tree 477.0
    conjunctivitis 372.05
    due to
      dander, animal (cat) (dog) 477.2
      dust 477.8
      fowl 477.8
      hair, animal (cat) (dog) 477.2
      pollen 477.0
      specified allergen other than pollen 477.8
Hayem-Faber syndrome (achlorhydric anemia) 280.9
Hayem-Widal syndrome (acquired hemolytic jaundice) 283.9
Haygarth's nodosities 715.04
Hazard-Crile tumor (M8350/3) 193
Hb (abnormal)
  disease - see Disease, hemoglobin
  trait - see Trait
H disease 270.0
Head - see also condition
  banging 307.3
Headache 784.0
  allergic 339.00
  associated with sexual activity 339.82
  cluster 339.00
    chronic 339.02
    episodic 339.01
  daily
    chronic 784.0
    new persistent (NPDH) 339.42
  drug induced 339.3
  due to
    loss, spinal fluid 349.0
    lumbar puncture 349.0
    saddle block 349.0
  emotional 307.81
  histamine 339.00
  hypnic 339.81
  lumbar puncture 349.0
  medication overuse 339.3
  menopausal 627.2
  menstrual 346.4●
  migraine 346.9●
  nasal septum 784.0
  nonorganic origin 307.81
  orgasmic 339.82
  postspinal 349.0
  post-traumatic 339.20
    acute 339.21
    chronic 339.22
  premenstrual 346.4●
  preorgasmic 339.82
  primary
    cough 339.83
    exertional 339.84
    stabbing 339.85
    thunderclap 339.43
  psychogenic 307.81
  psychophysiologic 307.81
  rebound 339.3
  short lasting unilateral neuralgiform with conjunctival injection and tearing (SUNCT) 339.05
  sick 346.9●

Headache (Continued)
  spinal 349.0
    complicating labor and delivery
        668.8●
      postpartum 668.8●
  spinal fluid loss 349.0
  syndrome
    cluster 339.00
    complicated NEC 339.44
    periodic in child or adolescent
        346.2●
    specified NEC 339.89
  tension 307.81
    type 339.10
      chronic 339.12
      episodic 339.11
  vascular 784.0
    migraine type 346.9●
  vasomotor 346.9●
Health
  advice V65.4
  audit V70.0
  checkup V70.0
  education V65.4
  hazard (see also History of) V15.9
    falling V15.88
    specified cause NEC V15.89
  instruction V65.4
  services provided because (of)
    boarding school residence V60.6
    holiday relief for person providing
        home care V60.5
    inadequate
      housing V60.1
      resources V60.2
    lack of housing V60.0
    no care available in home V60.4
    person living alone V60.3
    poverty V60.3
    residence in institution V60.6
    specified cause NEC V60.89   ◄▥
    vacation relief for person providing
        home care V60.5
Healthy
  donor (see also Donor) V59.9
  infant or child
    accompanying sick mother V65.0
    receiving care V20.1
  person
    accompanying sick relative V65.0
    admitted for sterilization V25.2
    receiving prophylactic inoculation
        or vaccination (see also
        Vaccination, prophylactic)
        V05.9
Hearing
  conservation and treatment V72.12
  examination V72.19
    following failed hearing screening
        V72.11
Heart - see condition
Heartburn 787.1
  psychogenic 306.4
Heat (effects) 992.9
  apoplexy 992.0
  burn - see also Burn, by site
    from sun (see also Sunburn) 692.71
  collapse 992.1
  cramps 992.2
  dermatitis or eczema 692.89
  edema 992.7
  erythema - see Burn, by site
  excessive 992.9
    specified effect NEC 992.8

Heat (Continued)
  exhaustion 992.5
    anhydrotic 992.3
    due to
      salt (and water) depletion
          992.4
      water depletion 992.3
  fatigue (transient) 992.6
  fever 992.0
  hyperpyrexia 992.0
  prickly 705.1
  prostration - see Heat, exhaustion
  pyrexia 992.0
  rash 705.1
  specified effect NEC 992.8
  stroke 992.0
  sunburn (see also Sunburn) 692.71
  syncope 992.1
Heavy-chain disease 273.2
Heavy-for-dates (fetus or infant) 766.1
  4500 grams or more 766.0
  exceptionally 766.0
Hebephrenia, hebephrenic (acute) (see
      also Schizophrenia) 295.1●
  dementia (praecox) (see also
      Schizophrenia) 295.1●
  schizophrenia (see also Schizophrenia)
      295.1●
Heberden's
  disease or nodes 715.04
  syndrome (angina pectoris) 413.9
Hebra's disease
  dermatitis exfoliativa 695.89
  erythema multiforme exudativum
      695.19
  pityriasis 695.89
    maculata et circinata 696.3
    rubra 695.89
      pilaris 696.4
  prurigo 698.2
Hebra, nose 040.1
Hedinger's syndrome (malignant
      carcinoid) 259.2
Heel - see condition
Heerfordt's disease or syndrome
      (uveoparotitis) 135
Hegglin's anomaly or syndrome 288.2
Heidenhain's disease 290.10
  with dementia 290.10
Heilmeyer-Schoner disease (M9842/3)
      207.1●
Heine-Medin disease (see also
      Poliomyelitis) 045.9●
Heinz-body anemia, congenital 282.7
Heller's disease or syndrome (infantile
      psychosis) (see also Psychosis,
      childhood) 299.1●
H.E.L.L.P. 642.5●
Helminthiasis (see also Infestation, by
      specific parasite) 128.9
  Ancylostoma (see also Ancylostoma)
      126.9
  intestinal 127.9
    mixed types (types classifiable to
        more than one of the
        categories 120.0–127.7) 127.8
    specified type 127.7
  mixed types (intestinal) (types
      classifiable to more than one
      of the categories 120.0–127.7)
      127.8
  Necator americanus 126.1
  specified type NEC 128.8
  Trichinella 124

Heloma 700
Hemangioblastoma (M9161/1) - see also
      Neoplasm, connective tissue,
      uncertain behavior
  malignant (M9161/3) - see Neoplasm,
      connective tissue, malignant
Hemangioblastomatosis, cerebelloretinal
      759.6
Hemangioendothelioma (M9130/1) - see
      also Neoplasm, by site, uncertain
      behavior
  benign (M9130/0) 228.00
  bone (diffuse) (M9130/3) - see
      Neoplasm, bone, malignant
  malignant (M9130/3) - see Neoplasm,
      connective tissue, malignant
  nervous system (M9130/0) 228.09
Hemangioendotheliosarcoma
      (M9130/3) - see Neoplasm,
      connective tissue, malignant
Hemangiofibroma (M9160/0) - see
      Neoplasm, by site, benign
Hemangiolipoma (M8861/0) - see
      Lipoma
Hemangioma (M9120/0) 228.00
  arteriovenous (M9123/0) - see
      Hemangioma, by site
  brain 228.02
  capillary (M9131/0) - see Hemangioma,
      by site
  cavernous (M9121/0) - see
      Hemangioma, by site
  central nervous system NEC
      228.09
  choroid 228.09
  heart 228.09
  infantile (M9131/0) - see Hemangioma,
      by site
  intra-abdominal structures 228.04
  intracranial structures 228.02
  intramuscular (M9132/0) - see
      Hemangioma, by site
  iris 228.09
  juvenile (M9131/0) - see Hemangioma,
      by site
  malignant (M9120/3) - see
      Neoplasm, connective
      tissue, malignant
  meninges 228.09
    brain 228.02
    spinal cord 228.09
  peritoneum 228.04
  placenta - see Placenta, abnormal
  plexiform (M9131/0) - see
      Hemangioma, by site
  racemose (M9123/0) - see
      Hemangioma, by site
  retina 228.03
  retroperitoneal tissue 228.04
  sclerosing (M8832/0) - see Neoplasm,
      skin, benign
  simplex (M9131/0) - see
      Hemangioma, by site
  skin and subcutaneous tissue
      228.01
  specified site NEC 228.09
  spinal cord 228.09
  venous (M9122/0) - see Hemangioma,
      by site
  verrucous keratotic (M9142/0) - see
      Hemangioma, by site
Hemangiomatosis (systemic) 757.32
  involving single site - see
      Hemangioma

◄ New   ◄▥ Revised   ~~deleted~~ Deleted   ● Use Additional Digit(s)   ▨ Omit code

Hemangiopericytoma (M9150/1) - *see also*
   Neoplasm, connective tissue,
   uncertain behavior
   benign (M9150/0) - *see* Neoplasm,
      connective tissue, benign
   malignant (M9150/3) - *see* Neoplasm,
      connective tissue, malignant
Hemangiosarcoma (M9120/3) - *see*
   Neoplasm, connective tissue,
   malignant
Hemarthrosis (nontraumatic) 719.10
   ankle 719.17
   elbow 719.12
   foot 719.17
   hand 719.14
   hip 719.15
   knee 719.16
   multiple sites 719.19
   pelvic region 719.15
   shoulder (region) 719.11
   specified site NEC 719.18
   traumatic - *see* Sprain, by site
   wrist 719.13
Hematemesis 578.0
   with ulcer - *see* Ulcer, by site, with
      hemorrhage
   due to S. japonicum 120.2
   Goldstein's (familial hemorrhagic
      telangiectasia) 448.0
   newborn 772.4
      due to swallowed maternal blood
         777.3
Hematidrosis 705.89
Hematinuria (*see also* Hemoglobinuria)
   791.2
   malarial 084.8
   paroxysmal 283.2
Hematite miners' lung 503
Hematobilia 576.8
Hematocele (congenital) (diffuse)
      (idiopathic) 608.83
   broad ligament 620.7
   canal of Nuck 629.0
   cord, male 608.83
   fallopian tube 620.8
   female NEC 629.0
   ischiorectal 569.89
   male NEC 608.83
   ovary 629.0
   pelvis, pelvic
      female 629.0
         with ectopic pregnancy (*see also*
            Pregnancy, ectopic) 633.90
            with intrauterine pregnancy
               633.91
      male 608.83
   periuterine 629.0
   retrouterine 629.0
   scrotum 608.83
   spermatic cord (diffuse) 608.83
   testis 608.84
   traumatic - *see* Injury, internal, pelvis
   tunica vaginalis 608.83
   uterine ligament 629.0
   uterus 621.4
   vagina 623.6
   vulva 624.5
Hematocephalus 742.4
Hematochezia (*see also* Melena) 578.1
Hematochyluria (*see also* Infestation,
   filarial) 125.9
Hematocolpos 626.8
Hematocornea 371.12
Hematogenous - *see* condition

Hematoma (skin surface intact)
   (traumatic) - *see also* Contusion

Note 36   Hematomas are coded according to origin and the nature and site of the hematoma or the accompanying injury. Hematomas of unspecified origin are coded as injuries of the sites involved, except:

(a)   hematomas of genital organs which are coded as diseases of the organ involved unless they complicate pregnancy or delivery
(b)   hematomas of the eye which are coded as diseases of the eye.

For late effect of hematoma classifiable to 920–924 *see* Late, effect, contusion.

---

   with
      crush injury - *see* Crush
      fracture - *see* Fracture, by site
      injury of internal organs - *see also*
         Injury, internal, by site
         kidney - *see* Hematoma, kidney,
            traumatic
         liver - *see* Hematoma, liver,
            traumatic
         spleen - *see* Hematoma, spleen
      nerve injury - *see* Injury, nerve
      open wound - *see* Wound, open, by
         site
      skin surface intact - *see* Contusion
   abdomen (wall) - *see* Contusion,
      abdomen
   amnion 658.8●
   aorta, dissecting 441.00
      abdominal 441.02
      thoracic 441.01
      thoracoabdominal 441.03
   arterial (complicating trauma) 904.9
      specified site - *see* Injury, blood
         vessel, by site
   auricle (ear) 380.31
   birth injury 767.8
      skull 767.19
   brain (traumatic) 853.0●

Note 37   Use the following fifth-digit subclassification with categories 851–854:

0   unspecified state of consciousness
1   with no loss of consciousness
2   with brief [less than one hour] loss of consciousness
3   with moderate [1–24 hours] loss of consciousness
4   with prolonged [more than 24 hours] loss of consciousness and return to pre-existing conscious level
5   with prolonged [more than 24 hours] loss of consciousness, without return to pre-existing conscious level

Use fifth-digit 5 to designate when a patient is unconscious and dies before regaining consciousness, regardless of the duration of the loss of consciousness

6   with loss of consciousness of unspecified duration
9   with concussion, unspecified

Hematoma (*Continued*)
   brain (*Continued*)
      with
         cerebral
            contusion - *see* Contusion,
               brain
            laceration - *see* Laceration,
               brain
            open intracranial wound
               853.1●
            skull fracture - *see* Fracture,
               skull, by site
      extradural or epidural 852.4●
         with open intracranial wound
            852.5●
         fetus or newborn 767.0
         nontraumatic 432.0
      fetus or newborn NEC 767.0
      nontraumatic (*see also* Hemorrhage,
         brain) 431
         epidural or extradural 432.0
         newborn NEC 772.8
         subarachnoid, arachnoid, or
            meningeal (*see also*
            Hemorrhage, subarachnoid)
            430
         subdural (*see also* Hemorrhage,
            subdural) 432.1
      subarachnoid, arachnoid, or
         meningeal 852.0●
         with open intracranial wound
            852.1●
         fetus or newborn 772.2
         nontraumatic (*see also*
            Hemorrhage,
            subarachnoid) 430
      subdural 852.2●
         with open intracranial wound
            852.3●
         fetus or newborn (localized)
            767.0
         nontraumatic (*see also*
            Hemorrhage, subdural)
            432.1
   breast (nontraumatic) 611.89
   broad ligament (nontraumatic)
      620.7
      complicating delivery 665.7●
      traumatic - *see* Injury, internal,
         broad ligament
   calcified NEC 959.9
   capitis 920
      due to birth injury 767.19
      newborn 767.19
   cerebral - *see* Hematoma, brain
   cesarean section wound 674.3●
   chorion - *see* Placenta, abnormal
   complicating delivery (perineum)
      (vulva) 664.5●
      pelvic 665.7●
      vagina 665.7●
   corpus
      cavernosum (nontraumatic)
         607.82
      luteum (nontraumatic) (ruptured)
         620.1
   dura (mater) - *see* Hematoma, brain,
      subdural
   epididymis (nontraumatic) 608.83
   epidural (traumatic) - *see also*
      Hematoma, brain, extradural
      spinal - *see* Injury, spinal, by site
   episiotomy 674.3●
   external ear 380.31

Hematoma (*Continued*)
extradural - *see also* Hematoma, brain,
extradural
fetus or newborn 767.0
nontraumatic 432.0
fetus or newborn 767.0
fallopian tube 620.8
genital organ (nontraumatic)
female NEC 629.89
male NEC 608.83
traumatic (external site) 922.4
internal - *see* Injury, internal,
genital organ
graafian follicle (ruptured) 620.0
internal organs (abdomen, chest, or
pelvis) - *see also* Injury, internal,
by site
kidney - *see* Hematoma, kidney,
traumatic
liver - *see* Hematoma, liver,
traumatic
spleen - *see* Hematoma, spleen
intracranial - *see* Hematoma, brain
kidney, cystic 593.81
traumatic 866.01
with open wound into cavity
866.11
labia (nontraumatic) 624.5
lingual (and other parts of neck, scalp,
or face, except eye) 920
liver (subcapsular) 573.8
birth injury 767.8
fetus or newborn 767.8
traumatic NEC 864.01
with
laceration - *see* Laceration,
liver
open wound into cavity 864.11
mediastinum - *see* Injury, internal,
mediastinum
meninges, meningeal (brain) - *see also*
Hematoma, brain, subarachnoid
spinal - *see* Injury, spinal, by site
mesosalpinx (nontraumatic) 620.8
traumatic - *see* Injury, internal, pelvis
muscle (traumatic) - *see* Contusion, by
site
nontraumatic 729.92
nasal (septum) (and other part(s) of
neck, scalp, or face, except eye)
920
obstetrical surgical wound 674.3 ●
orbit, orbital (nontraumatic) 376.32
traumatic 921.2
ovary (corpus luteum) (nontraumatic)
620.1
traumatic - *see* Injury, internal, ovary
pelvis (female) (nontraumatic)
629.89
complicating delivery 665.7 ●
male 608.83
traumatic - *see also* Injury, internal,
pelvis
specified organ NEC (*see also*
Injury, internal, pelvis)
867.6
penis (nontraumatic) 607.82
pericranial (and neck, or face any part,
except eye) 920
due to injury at birth 767.19
perineal wound (obstetrical) 674.3 ●
complicating delivery 664.5 ●
perirenal, cystic 593.81
pinna 380.31

Hematoma (*Continued*)
placenta - *see* Placenta, abnormal
postoperative 998.12
retroperitoneal (nontraumatic) 568.81
traumatic - *see* Injury, internal,
retroperitoneum
retropubic, male 568.81
scalp (and neck, or face any part,
except eye) 920
fetus or newborn 767.19
scrotum (nontraumatic) 608.83
traumatic 922.4
seminal vesicle (nontraumatic) 608.83
traumatic - *see* Injury, internal,
seminal, vesicle
soft tissue, nontraumatic 729.92
spermatic cord - *see also* Injury, internal,
spermatic cord
nontraumatic 608.83
spinal (cord) (meninges) - *see also*
Injury, spinal, by site
fetus or newborn 767.4
nontraumatic 336.1
spleen 865.01
with
laceration - *see* Laceration, spleen
open wound into cavity 865.11
sternocleidomastoid, birth injury 767.8
sternomastoid, birth injury 767.8
subarachnoid - *see also* Hematoma,
brain, subarachnoid
fetus or newborn 772.2
nontraumatic (*see also* Hemorrhage,
subarachnoid) 430
newborn 772.2
subdural - *see also* Hematoma, brain,
subdural
fetus or newborn (localized) 767.0
nontraumatic (*see also* Hemorrhage,
subdural) 432.1
subperiosteal (syndrome) 267
traumatic - *see* Hematoma, by site
superficial, fetus or newborn 772.6
syncytium - *see* Placenta, abnormal
testis (nontraumatic) 608.83
birth injury 767.8
traumatic 922.4
tunica vaginalis (nontraumatic) 608.83
umbilical cord 663.6 ●
affecting fetus or newborn 762.6
uterine ligament (nontraumatic) 620.7
traumatic - *see* Injury, internal, pelvis
uterus 621.4
traumatic - *see* Injury, internal, pelvis
vagina (nontraumatic) (ruptured) 623.6
complicating delivery 665.7 ●
traumatic 922.4
vas deferens (nontraumatic) 608.83
traumatic - *see* Injury, internal, vas
deferens
vitreous 379.23
vocal cord 920
vulva (nontraumatic) 624.5
complicating delivery 664.5 ●
fetus or newborn 767.8
traumatic 922.4
Hematometra 621.4
Hematomyelia 336.1
with fracture of vertebra (*see also*
Fracture, vertebra, by site, with
spinal cord injury) 806.8
fetus or newborn 767.4
Hematomyelitis 323.9
late effect - *see* category 326

Hematoperitoneum (*see also*
Hemoperitoneum) 568.81
Hematopneumothorax (*see also*
Hemothorax) 511.89
Hematopoiesis, cyclic 288.02
Hematoporphyria (acquired) (congenital)
277.1
Hematoporphyrinuria (acquired)
(congenital) 277.1
Hematorachis, hematorrhachis 336.1
fetus or newborn 767.4
Hematosalpinx 620.8
with
ectopic pregnancy (*see also*
categories 633.0–633.9) 639.2
molar pregnancy (*see also* categories
630–632) 639.2
infectional (*see also* Salpingo-
oophoritis) 614.2
Hematospermia 608.82
Hematothorax (*see also* Hemothorax) 511.89
Hematotympanum 381.03
Hematuria (benign) (essential)
(idiopathic) 599.70
due to S. hematobium 120.0
endemic 120.0
gross 599.71
intermittent 599.70
malarial 084.8
microscopic 599.72
paroxysmal 599.70
sulfonamide
correct substance properly
administered 599.70
overdose or wrong substance given
or taken 961.0
tropical (bilharziasis) 120.0
tuberculous (*see also* Tuberculosis)
016.9 ●
Hematuric bilious fever 084.8
Hemeralopia 368.10
Hemiabiotrophy 799.89
Hemi-akinesia 781.8
Hemianalgesia (*see also* Disturbance,
sensation) 782.0
Hemianencephaly 740.0
Hemianesthesia (*see also* Disturbance,
sensation) 782.0
Hemianopia, hemianopsia (altitudinal)
(homonymous) 368.46
binasal 368.47
bitemporal 368.47
heteronymous 368.47
syphilitic 095.8
Hemiasomatognosia 307.9
Hemiathetosis 781.0
Hemiatrophy 799.89
cerebellar 334.8
face 349.89
progressive 349.89
fascia 728.9
leg 728.2
tongue 529.8
Hemiballism (us) 333.5
Hemiblock (cardiac) (heart) (left) 426.2
Hemicardia 746.89
Hemicephalus, hemicephaly 740.0
Hemichorea 333.5
Hemicrania 346.9 ●
congenital malformation 740.0
continua 339.41
paroxysmal 339.03
chronic 339.04
episodic 339.03

◀ New   ◀▥ Revised   ~~deleted~~ Deleted   ● Use Additional Digit(s)   ▨ Omit code

Hemidystrophy - *see* Hemiatrophy
Hemiectromelia 755.4
Hemihypalgesia (*see also* Disturbance, sensation) 782.0
Hemihypertrophy (congenital) 759.89
   cranial 756.0
Hemihypesthesia (*see also* Disturbance, sensation) 782.0
Hemi-inattention 781.8
Hemimelia 755.4
   lower limb 755.30
      paraxial (complete) (incomplete) (intercalary) (terminal) 755.32
         fibula 755.37
         tibia 755.36
      transverse (complete) (partial) 755.31
   upper limb 755.20
      paraxial (complete) (incomplete) (intercalary) (terminal) 755.22
         radial 755.26
         ulnar 755.27
      transverse (complete) (partial) 755.21
Hemiparalysis (*see also* Hemiplegia) 342.9 ●
Hemiparesis (*see also* Hemiplegia) 342.9 ●
Hemiparesthesia (*see also* Disturbance, sensation) 782.0
Hemiplegia 342.9 ●
   acute (*see also* Disease, cerebrovascular, acute) 436
   alternans facialis 344.89
   apoplectic (*see also* Disease, cerebrovascular, acute) 436
      late effect or residual
         affecting
            dominant side 438.21
            nondominant side 438.22
            unspecified side 438.20
   arteriosclerotic 437.0
      late effect or residual
         affecting
            dominant side 438.21
            nondominant side 438.22
            unspecified side 438.20
   ascending (spinal) NEC 344.89
   attack (*see also* Disease, cerebrovascular, acute) 436
   brain, cerebral (current episode) 437.8
      congenital 343.1
   cerebral - *see* Hemiplegia, brain
   congenital (cerebral) (spastic) (spinal) 343.1
   conversion neurosis (hysterical) 300.11
   cortical - *see* Hemiplegia, brain
   due to
      arteriosclerosis 437.0
         late effect or residual
            affecting
               dominant side 438.21
               nondominant side 438.22
               unspecified side 438.20
      cerebrovascular lesion (*see also* Disease, cerebrovascular, acute) 436
         late effect
            affecting
               dominant side 438.21
               nondominant side 438.22
               unspecified side 438.20

Hemiplegia (*Continued*)
   embolic (current) (*see also* Embolism, brain) 434.1 ●
      late effect
         affecting
            dominant side 438.21
            nondominant side 438.22
            unspecified side 438.20
   flaccid 342.0 ●
   hypertensive (current episode) 437.8
   infantile (postnatal) 343.4
   late effect
      birth injury, intracranial or spinal 343.4
      cerebrovascular lesion - *see* Late effect(s) (of) cerebrovascular disease
      viral encephalitis 139.0
   middle alternating NEC 344.89
   newborn NEC 767.0
   seizure (current episode) (*see also* Disease, cerebrovascular, acute) 436
   spastic 342.1 ●
      congenital or infantile 343.1
   specified NEC 342.8 ●
   thrombotic (current) (*see also* Thrombosis, brain) 434.0 ●
   late effect - *see* Late effect(s) (of) cerebrovascular disease
Hemisection, spinal cord - *see* Fracture, vertebra, by site, with spinal cord injury
Hemispasm 781.0
   facial 781.0
Hemispatial neglect 781.8
Hemisporosis 117.9
Hemitremor 781.0
Hemivertebra 756.14
Hemobilia 576.8
Hemocholecyst 575.8
Hemochromatosis (acquired) (diabetic) (hereditary) (liver) (myocardium) (primary idiopathic) (secondary) 275.0
   with refractory anemia 238.72
Hemodialysis V56.0
Hemoglobin - *see also* condition
   abnormal (disease) - *see* Disease, hemoglobin
   AS genotype 282.5
   fetal, hereditary persistence 282.7
   high-oxygen-affinity 289.0
   low NEC 285.9
   S (Hb-S), heterozygous 282.5
Hemoglobinemia 283.2
   due to blood transfusion NEC 999.89
      bone marrow 996.85
   paroxysmal 283.2
Hemoglobinopathy (mixed) (*see also* Disease, hemoglobin) 282.7
   with thalassemia 282.49
   sickle-cell 282.60
      with thalassemia (without crisis) 282.41
         with
            crisis 282.42
            vaso-occlusive pain 282.42
Hemoglobinuria, hemoglobinuric 791.2
   with anemia, hemolytic, acquired (chronic) NEC 283.2
   cold (agglutinin) (paroxysmal) (with Raynaud's syndrome) 283.2

Hemoglobinuria, hemoglobinuric (*Continued*)
   due to
      exertion 283.2
      hemolysis (from external causes) NEC 283.2
   exercise 283.2
   fever (malaria) 084.8
   infantile 791.2
   intermittent 283.2
   malarial 084.8
   march 283.2
   nocturnal (paroxysmal) 283.2
   paroxysmal (cold) (nocturnal) 283.2
Hemolymphangioma (M9175/0) 228.1
Hemolysis
   fetal - *see* Jaundice, fetus or newborn
   intravascular (disseminated) NEC 286.6
      with
         abortion - *see* Abortion, by type, with hemorrhage, delayed or excessive
         ectopic pregnancy (*see also* categories 633.0–633.9) 639.1
         hemorrhage of pregnancy 641.3 ●
            affecting fetus or newborn 762.1
         molar pregnancy (*see also* categories 630–632) 639.1
      acute 283.2
      following
         abortion 639.1
         ectopic or molar pregnancy 639.1
   neonatal - *see* Jaundice, fetus or newborn
   transfusion NEC 999.89
      bone marrow 996.85
Hemolytic - *see also* condition
   anemia - *see* Anemia, hemolytic
   uremic syndrome 283.11
Hemometra 621.4
Hemopericardium (with effusion) 423.0
   newborn 772.8
   traumatic (*see also* Hemothorax, traumatic) 860.2
      with open wound into thorax 860.3
Hemoperitoneum 568.81
   infectional (*see also* Peritonitis) 567.29
   traumatic - *see* Injury, internal, peritoneum
Hemophagocytic syndrome 288.4
   infection-associated 288.4
Hemophilia (familial) (hereditary) 286.0
   A 286.0
      carrier (asymptomatic) V83.01
         symptomatic V83.02
   acquired 286.5
   B (Leyden) 286.1
   C 286.2
   calcipriva (*see also* Fibrinolysis) 286.7
   classical 286.0
   nonfamilial 286.7
   secondary 286.5
   vascular 286.4
Hemophilus influenzae NEC 041.5
   arachnoiditis (basic) (brain) (spinal) 320.0
      late effect - *see* category 326
   bronchopneumonia 482.2
   cerebral ventriculitis 320.0
      late effect - *see* category 326
   cerebrospinal inflammation 320.0
      late effect - *see* category 326

Hemophilus influenzae NEC (*Continued*)
infection NEC 041.5
leptomeningitis 320.0
late effect - *see* category 326
meningitis (cerebral) (cerebrospinal)
(spinal) 320.0
late effect - *see* category 326
meningomyelitis 320.0
late effect - *see* category 326
pachymeningitis (adhesive) (fibrous)
(hemorrhagic) (hypertrophic)
(spinal) 320.0
late effect - *see* category 326
pneumonia (broncho-) 482.2
Hemophthalmos 360.43
Hemopneumothorax (*see also*
Hemothorax) 511.89
traumatic 860.4
with open wound into thorax
860.5
Hemoptysis 786.3
due to Paragonimus (westermani)
121.2
newborn 770.3
tuberculous (*see also* Tuberculosis,
pulmonary) 011.9●
Hemorrhage, hemorrhagic
(nontraumatic) 459.0
abdomen 459.0
accidental (antepartum) 641.2●
affecting fetus or newborn 762.1
adenoid 474.8
adrenal (capsule) (gland) (medulla)
255.41
newborn 772.5
after labor - *see* Hemorrhage,
postpartum
alveolar
lung, newborn 770.3
process 525.8
alveolus 525.8
amputation stump (surgical) 998.11
secondary, delayed 997.69
anemia (chronic) 280.0
acute 285.1
antepartum - *see* Hemorrhage,
pregnancy
anus (sphincter) 569.3
apoplexy (stroke) 432.9
arachnoid - *see* Hemorrhage,
subarachnoid
artery NEC 459.0
brain (*see also* Hemorrhage, brain)
431
middle meningeal - *see* Hemorrhage,
subarachnoid
basilar (ganglion) (*see also* Hemorrhage,
brain) 431
bladder 596.8
blood dyscrasia 289.9
bowel 578.9
newborn 772.4
brain (miliary) (nontraumatic) 431
with
birth injury 767.0
arachnoid - *see* Hemorrhage,
subarachnoid
due to
birth injury 767.0
rupture of aneurysm (congenital)
(*see also* Hemorrhage,
subarachnoid) 430
mycotic 431
syphilis 094.89

Hemorrhage, hemorrhagic (*Continued*)
brain (*Continued*)
epidural or extradural - *see*
Hemorrhage, extradural
fetus or newborn (anoxic) (hypoxic)
(due to birth trauma)
(nontraumatic) 767.0
intraventricular 772.10
grade I 772.11
grade II 772.12
grade III 772.13
grade IV 772.14
iatrogenic 997.02
postoperative 997.02
puerperal, postpartum, childbirth
674.0●
stem 431
subarachnoid, arachnoid, or
meningeal - *see* Hemorrhage,
subarachnoid
subdural - *see* Hemorrhage, subdural
traumatic NEC 853.0●

Note 38   Use the following fifth-digit
subclassification with categories 851–854:

0   unspecified state of
consciousness
1   with no loss of consciousness
2   with brief [less than one hour]
loss of consciousness
3   with moderate [1–24 hours] loss
of consciousness
4   with prolonged [more than
24 hours] loss of
consciousness and return
to pre-existing conscious
level
5   with prolonged [more than
24 hours] loss of
consciousness, without
return to pre-existing
conscious level

Use fifth-digit 5 to designate when a
patient is unconscious and dies before
regaining consciousness, regardless of
the duration of the loss of consciousness

6   with loss of consciousness of
unspecified duration
9   with concussion, unspecified

---

with
cerebral
contusion - *see* Contusion,
brain
laceration - *see* Laceration,
brain
open intracranial wound
853.1●
skull fracture - *see* Fracture,
skull, by site
extradural or epidural 852.4●
with open intracranial wound
852.5●
subarachnoid 852.0●
with open intracranial wound
852.1●
subdural 852.2●
with open intracranial wound
852.3●
breast 611.79
bronchial tube - *see* Hemorrhage, lung
bronchopulmonary - *see* Hemorrhage,
lung

Hemorrhage, hemorrhagic (*Continued*)
bronchus (cause unknown) (*see also*
Hemorrhage, lung) 786.3
bulbar (*see also* Hemorrhage, brain) 431
bursa 727.89
capillary 448.9
primary 287.8
capsular - *see* Hemorrhage, brain
cardiovascular 429.89
cecum 578.9
cephalic (*see also* Hemorrhage, brain)
431
cerebellar (*see also* Hemorrhage, brain)
431
cerebellum (*see also* Hemorrhage, brain)
431
cerebral (*see also* Hemorrhage, brain)
431
fetus or newborn (anoxic)
(traumatic) 767.0
cerebromeningeal (*see also*
Hemorrhage, brain) 431
cerebrospinal (*see also* Hemorrhage,
brain) 431
cerebrovascular accident - *see*
Hemorrhage, brain
cerebrum (*see also* Hemorrhage, brain)
431
cervix (stump) (uteri) 622.8
cesarean section wound 674.3●
chamber, anterior (eye) 364.41
childbirth - *see* Hemorrhage,
complicating, delivery
choroid 363.61
expulsive 363.62
ciliary body 364.41
cochlea 386.8
colon - *see* Hemorrhage, intestine
complicating
delivery 641.9●
affecting fetus or newborn 762.1
associated with
afibrinogenemia 641.3●
affecting fetus or newborn
763.89
coagulation defect 641.3●
affecting fetus or newborn
763.89
hyperfibrinolysis 641.3●
affecting fetus or newborn
763.89
hypofibrinogenemia 641.3●
affecting fetus or newborn
763.89
due to
low-lying placenta 641.1●
affecting fetus or newborn
762.0
placenta previa 641.1●
affecting fetus or newborn
762.0
premature separation of
placenta 641.2●
affecting fetus or newborn
762.1
retained
placenta 666.0●
secundines 666.2●
trauma 641.8●
affecting fetus or newborn
763.89
uterine leiomyoma 641.8●
affecting fetus or newborn
763.89

◀ New   ◀▥ Revised   ~~deleted~~ Deleted   ● Use Additional Digit(s)   ▧ Omit code

Hemorrhage, hemorrhagic *(Continued)*
  complication(s)
    of dental implant placement 525.71
    surgical procedure 998.11
  concealed NEC 459.0
  congenital 772.9
  conjunctiva 372.72
    newborn 772.8
  cord, newborn 772.0
    slipped ligature 772.3
    stump 772.3
  corpus luteum (ruptured) 620.1
  cortical *(see also* Hemorrhage, brain)
    431
  cranial 432.9
  cutaneous 782.7
    newborn 772.6
  cyst, pancreas 577.2
  cystitis - *see* Cystitis
  delayed
    with
      abortion - *see* Abortion, by type,
        with hemorrhage, delayed
        or excessive
      ectopic pregnancy *(see also*
        categories 633.0–633.9) 639.1
      molar pregnancy *(see also*
        categories 630–632) 639.1
    following
      abortion 639.1
      ectopic or molar pregnancy
        639.1
    postpartum 666.2●
  diathesis (familial) 287.9
    newborn 776.0
  disease 287.9
    newborn 776.0
    specified type NEC 287.8
  disorder 287.9
    due to intrinsic circulating
      anticoagulants 286.5
    specified type NEC 287.8
  due to
    any device, implant, or graft
      (presence of) classifiable to
      996.0–996.5 - *see*
      Complications, due to
      (presence of) any device,
      implant, or graft classified to
      996.0–996.5 NEC
    intrinsic circulating anticoagulant
      286.5
  duodenum, duodenal 537.89
    ulcer - *see* Ulcer, duodenum, with
      hemorrhage
  dura mater - *see* Hemorrhage, subdural
  endotracheal - *see* Hemorrhage, lung
  epicranial subaponeurotic (massive)
    767.11
  epidural - *see* Hemorrhage, extradural
  episiotomy 674.3●
  esophagus 530.82
    varix *(see also* Varix, esophagus,
      bleeding) 456.0
  excessive
    with
      abortion - *see* Abortion, by type,
        with hemorrhage, delayed
        or excessive
      ectopic pregnancy *(see also*
        categories 633.0–633.9)
        639.1
      molar pregnancy *(see also*
        categories 630–632) 639.1

Hemorrhage, hemorrhagic *(Continued)*
  excessive *(Continued)*
    following
      abortion 639.1
      ectopic or molar pregnancy 639.1
  external 459.0
  extradural (traumatic) - *see also*
    Hemorrhage, brain, traumatic,
    extradural
    birth injury 767.0
    fetus or newborn (anoxic)
      (traumatic) 767.0
    nontraumatic 432.0
  eye 360.43
    chamber (anterior) (aqueous) 364.41
    fundus 362.81
  eyelid 374.81
  fallopian tube 620.8
  fetomaternal 772.0
    affecting management of pregnancy
      or puerperium 656.0●
  fetus, fetal, affecting newborn 772.0 ◀▥
    from
      cut end of co-twin's cord 772.0
      placenta 772.0
      ruptured cord 772.0
      vasa previa 772.0
    into
      co-twin 772.0
      mother's circulation 772.0
        affecting management of
          pregnancy or
          puerperium 656.0●
  fever *(see also* Fever, hemorrhagic) 065.9
    with renal syndrome 078.6
    arthropod-borne NEC 065.9
    Bangkok 065.4
    Crimean 065.0
    dengue virus 065.4
    epidemic 078.6
    Junin virus 078.7
    Korean 078.6
    Machupo virus 078.7
    mite-borne 065.8
    mosquito-borne 065.4
    Philippine 065.4
    Russian (Yaroslav) 078.6
    Singapore 065.4
    Southeast Asia 065.4
    Thailand 065.4
    tick-borne NEC 065.3
  fibrinogenolysis *(see also* Fibrinolysis)
    286.6
  fibrinolytic (acquired) *(see also*
    Fibrinolysis) 286.6
  fontanel 767.19
  from tracheostomy stoma 519.09
  fundus, eye 362.81
  funis
    affecting fetus or newborn 772.0
    complicating delivery 663.8●
  gastric *(see also* Hemorrhage, stomach)
    578.9
  gastroenteric 578.9
    newborn 772.4
  gastrointestinal (tract) 578.9
    newborn 772.4
  genitourinary (tract) NEC 599.89
  gingiva 523.8
  globe 360.43
  gravidarum - *see* Hemorrhage,
    pregnancy
  gum 523.8
  heart 429.89

Hemorrhage, hemorrhagic *(Continued)*
  hypopharyngeal (throat) 784.8
  intermenstrual 626.6
    irregular 626.6
    regular 626.5
  internal (organs) 459.0
    capsule *(see also* Hemorrhage brain)
      431
    ear 386.8
    newborn 772.8
  intestine 578.9
    congenital 772.4
    newborn 772.4
  into
    bladder wall 596.7
    bursa 727.89
    corpus luysii *(see also* Hemorrhage,
      brain) 431
  intra-abdominal 459.0
    during or following surgery 998.11
  intra-alveolar, newborn (lung) 770.3
  intracerebral *(see also* Hemorrhage,
    brain) 431
  intracranial NEC 432.9
    puerperal, postpartum, childbirth
      674.0●
    traumatic - *see* Hemorrhage, brain,
      traumatic
  intramedullary NEC 336.1
  intraocular 360.43
  intraoperative 998.11
  intrapartum - *see* Hemorrhage,
    complicating, delivery
  intrapelvic
    female 629.89
    male 459.0
  intraperitoneal 459.0
  intrapontine *(see also* Hemorrhage,
    brain) 431
  intrauterine 621.4
    complicating delivery - *see*
      Hemorrhage, complicating,
      delivery
    in pregnancy or childbirth - *see*
      Hemorrhage, pregnancy
    postpartum *(see also* Hemorrhage,
      postpartum) 666.1●
  intraventricular *(see also* Hemorrhage,
    brain) 431
    fetus or newborn (anoxic)
      (traumatic) 772.10
    grade I 772.11
    grade II 772.12
    grade III 772.13
    grade IV 772.14
  intravesical 596.7
  iris (postinfectional)
    (postinflammatory) (toxic) 364.41
  joint (nontraumatic) 719.10
    ankle 719.17
    elbow 719.12
    foot 719.17
    forearm 719.13
    hand 719.14
    hip 719.15
    knee 719.16
    lower leg 719.16
    multiple sites 719.19
    pelvic region 719.15
    shoulder (region) 719.11
    specified site NEC 719.18
    thigh 719.15
    upper arm 719.12
    wrist 719.13

Hemorrhage, hemorrhagic *(Continued)*
- kidney 593.81
- knee (joint) 719.16
- labyrinth 386.8
- leg NEC 459.0
- lenticular striate artery (*see also* Hemorrhage, brain) 431
- ligature, vessel 998.11
- liver 573.8
- lower extremity NEC 459.0
- lung 786.3
  - newborn 770.3
    - tuberculous (*see also* Tuberculosis, pulmonary) 011.9●
- malaria 084.8
- marginal sinus 641.2●
- massive subaponeurotic, birth injury 767.11
- maternal, affecting fetus or newborn 762.1
- mediastinum 786.3
- medulla (*see also* Hemorrhage, brain) 431
- membrane (brain) (*see also* Hemorrhage, subarachnoid) 430
  - spinal cord - *see* Hemorrhage, spinal cord
- meninges, meningeal (brain) (middle) (*see also* Hemorrhage, subarachnoid) 430
  - spinal cord - *see* Hemorrhage, spinal cord
- mesentery 568.81
- metritis 626.8
- midbrain (*see also* Hemorrhage, brain) 431
- mole 631
- mouth 528.9
- mucous membrane NEC 459.0
  - newborn 772.8
- muscle 728.89
- nail (subungual) 703.8
- nasal turbinate 784.7
  - newborn 772.8
- nasopharynx 478.29
- navel, newborn 772.3
- newborn 772.9
  - adrenal 772.5
  - alveolar (lung) 770.3
  - brain (anoxic) (hypoxic) (due to birth trauma) 767.0
  - cerebral (anoxic) (hypoxic) (due to birth trauma) 767.0
  - conjunctiva 772.8
  - cutaneous 772.6
  - diathesis 776.0
  - due to vitamin K deficiency 776.0
  - epicranial subaponeurotic (massive) 767.11
  - gastrointestinal 772.4
  - internal (organs) 772.8
  - intestines 772.4
  - intra-alveolar (lung) 770.3
  - intracranial (from any perinatal cause) 767.0
  - intraventricular (from any perinatal cause) 772.10
    - grade I 772.11
    - grade II 772.12
    - grade III 772.13
    - grade IV 772.14
  - lung 770.3

Hemorrhage, hemorrhagic *(Continued)*
- newborn *(Continued)*
  - pulmonary (massive) 770.3
  - spinal cord, traumatic 767.4
  - stomach 772.4
  - subaponeurotic (massive) 767.11
  - subarachnoid (from any perinatal cause) 772.2
  - subconjunctival 772.8
  - subgaleal 767.11
  - umbilicus 772.0
    - slipped ligature 772.3
    - vasa previa 772.0
- nipple 611.79
- nose 784.7
  - newborn 772.8
- obstetrical surgical wound 674.3●
- omentum 568.89
  - newborn 772.4
- optic nerve (sheath) 377.42
- orbit 376.32
- ovary 620.1
- oviduct 620.8
- pancreas 577.8
- parathyroid (gland) (spontaneous) 252.8
- parturition - *see* Hemorrhage, complicating, delivery
- penis 607.82
- pericardium, pericarditis 423.0
- perineal wound (obstetrical) 674.3●
- peritoneum, peritoneal 459.0
- peritonsillar tissue 474.8
  - after operation on tonsils 998.11
  - due to infection 475
- petechial 782.7
- pituitary (gland) 253.8
- placenta NEC 641.9●
  - affecting fetus or newborn 762.1
  - from surgical or instrumental damage 641.8●
    - affecting fetus or newborn 762.1
  - previa 641.1●
    - affecting fetus or newborn 762.0
- pleura - *see* Hemorrhage, lung
- polioencephalitis, superior 265.1
- polymyositis - *see* Polymyositis
- pons (*see also* Hemorrhage, brain) 431
- pontine (*see also* Hemorrhage, brain) 431
- popliteal 459.0
- postcoital 626.7
- postextraction (dental) 998.11
- postmenopausal 627.1
- postnasal 784.7
- postoperative 998.11
- postpartum (atonic) (following delivery of placenta) 666.1●
  - delayed or secondary (after 24 hours) 666.2●
  - retained placenta 666.0●
  - third stage 666.0●
- pregnancy (concealed) 641.9●
  - accidental 641.2●
    - affecting fetus or newborn 762.1
  - affecting fetus or newborn 762.1
  - before 22 completed weeks' gestation 640.9●
    - affecting fetus or newborn 762.1

Hemorrhage, hemorrhagic *(Continued)*
- pregnancy *(Continued)*
  - due to
    - abruptio placenta 641.2●
      - affecting fetus or newborn 762.1
    - afibrinogenemia or other coagulation defect (conditions classifiable to 286.0–286.9) 641.3●
      - affecting fetus or newborn 762.1
    - coagulation defect 641.3●
      - affecting fetus or newborn 762.1
    - hyperfibrinolysis 641.3●
      - affecting fetus or newborn 762.1
    - hypofibrinogenemia 641.3●
      - affecting fetus or newborn 762.1
    - leiomyoma, uterus 641.8●
      - affecting fetus or newborn 762.1
    - low-lying placenta 641.1●
      - affecting fetus or newborn 762.1
    - marginal sinus (rupture) 641.2●
      - affecting fetus or newborn 762.1
    - placenta previa 641.1●
      - affecting fetus or newborn 762.0
    - premature separation of placenta (normally implanted) 641.2●
      - affecting fetus or newborn 762.1
    - threatened abortion 640.0●
      - affecting fetus or newborn 762.1
    - trauma 641.8●
      - affecting fetus or newborn 762.1
  - early (before 22 completed weeks' gestation) 640.9●
    - affecting fetus or newborn 762.1
  - previous, affecting management of pregnancy or childbirth V23.49
  - unavoidable - *see* Hemorrhage, pregnancy, due to placenta previa
- prepartum (mother) - *see* Hemorrhage, pregnancy
- preretinal, cause unspecified 362.81
- prostate 602.1
- puerperal (*see also* Hemorrhage, postpartum) 666.1●
- pulmonary - *see also* Hemorrhage, lung
  - newborn (massive) 770.3
  - renal syndrome 446.21
- purpura (primary) (*see also* Purpura, thrombocytopenic) 287.39
- rectum (sphincter) 569.3
- recurring, following initial hemorrhage at time of injury 958.2
- renal 593.81
  - pulmonary syndrome 446.21
- respiratory tract (*see also* Hemorrhage, lung) 786.3

◄ New ◄▥ Revised ~~deleted~~ Deleted ● Use Additional Digit(s) ▨ Omit code

Hemorrhage, hemorrhagic *(Continued)*
retina, retinal (deep) (superficial)
(vessels) 362.81
diabetic 250.5● *[362.01]*
due to secondary diabetes 249.5●
[362.01]
due to birth injury 772.8
retrobulbar 376.89
retroperitoneal 459.0
retroplacental *(see also* Placenta,
separation) 641.2●
scalp 459.0
due to injury at birth 767.19
scrotum 608.83
secondary (nontraumatic) 459.0
following initial hemorrhage at time
of injury 958.2
seminal vesicle 608.83
skin 782.7
newborn 772.6
spermatic cord 608.83
spinal (cord) 336.1
aneurysm (ruptured) 336.1
syphilitic 094.89
due to birth injury 767.4
fetus or newborn 767.4
spleen 289.59
spontaneous NEC 459.0
petechial 782.7
stomach 578.9
newborn 772.4
ulcer - *see* Ulcer, stomach, with
hemorrhage
subaponeurotic, newborn 767.11
massive (birth injury) 767.11
subarachnoid (nontraumatic) 430
fetus or newborn (anoxic)
(traumatic) 772.2
puerperal, postpartum, childbirth
674.0●
traumatic - *see* Hemorrhage, brain,
traumatic, subarachnoid
subconjunctival 372.72
due to birth injury 772.8
newborn 772.8
subcortical *(see also* Hemorrhage, brain)
431
subcutaneous 782.7
subdiaphragmatic 459.0
subdural (nontraumatic) 432.1
due to birth injury 767.0
fetus or newborn (anoxic) (hypoxic)
(due to birth trauma) 767.0
puerperal, postpartum, childbirth
674.0●
spinal 336.1
traumatic - *see* Hemorrhage, brain,
traumatic, subdural
subgaleal 767.11
subhyaloid 362.81
subperiosteal 733.99
subretinal 362.81
subtentorial *(see also* Hemorrhage,
subdural) 432.1
subungual 703.8
due to blood dyscrasia 287.8
suprarenal (capsule) (gland) 255.41
fetus or newborn 772.5
tentorium (traumatic) - *see also*
Hemorrhage, brain, traumatic
fetus or newborn 767.0
nontraumatic - *see* Hemorrhage,
subdural
testis 608.83

Hemorrhage, hemorrhagic *(Continued)*
thigh 459.0
third stage 666.0●
thorax - *see* Hemorrhage, lung
throat 784.8
thrombocythemia 238.71
thymus (gland) 254.8
thyroid (gland) 246.3
cyst 246.3
tongue 529.8
tonsil 474.8
postoperative 998.11
tooth socket (postextraction) 998.11
trachea - *see* Hemorrhage, lung
traumatic - *see also* nature of injury
brain - *see* Hemorrhage, brain,
traumatic
recurring or secondary (following
initial hemorrhage at time of
injury) 958.2
tuberculous NEC *(see also* Tuberculosis,
pulmonary) 011.9●
tunica vaginalis 608.83
ulcer - *see* Ulcer, by site, with
hemorrhage
umbilicus, umbilical cord 772.0
after birth, newborn 772.3
complicating delivery 663.8●
affecting fetus or newborn
772.0
slipped ligature 772.3
stump 772.3
unavoidable (due to placenta previa)
641.1●
affecting fetus or newborn
762.0
upper extremity 459.0
urethra (idiopathic) 599.84
uterus, uterine (abnormal) 626.9
climacteric 627.0
complicating delivery - *see*
Hemorrhage, complicating,
delivery
due to
intrauterine contraceptive device
996.76
perforating uterus 996.32
functional or dysfunctional
626.8
in pregnancy - *see* Hemorrhage,
pregnancy
intermenstrual 626.6
irregular 626.6
regular 626.5
postmenopausal 627.1
postpartum *(see also* Hemorrhage,
postpartum) 666.1●
prepubertal 626.8
pubertal 626.3
puerperal (immediate) 666.1●
vagina 623.8
vasa previa 663.5●
affecting fetus or newborn
772.0
vas deferens 608.83
ventricular *(see also* Hemorrhage,
brain) 431
vesical 596.8
viscera 459.0
newborn 772.8
vitreous (humor) (intraocular)
379.23
vocal cord 478.5
vulva 624.8

Hemorrhoids (anus) (rectum) (without
complication) 455.6
bleeding, prolapsed, strangulated, or
ulcerated NEC 455.8
external 455.5
internal 455.2
complicated NEC 455.8
complicating pregnancy and
puerperium 671.8●
external 455.3
with complication NEC 455.5
bleeding, prolapsed, strangulated,
or ulcerated 455.5
thrombosed 455.4
internal 455.0
with complication NEC 455.2
bleeding, prolapsed, strangulated,
or ulcerated 455.2
thrombosed 455.1
residual skin tag 455.9
sentinel pile 455.9
thrombosed NEC 455.7
external 455.4
internal 455.1
Hemosalpinx 620.8
Hemosiderosis 275.0
dietary 275.0
pulmonary (idiopathic) 275.0 *[516.1]*
transfusion NEC 999.89
bone marrow 996.85
Hemospermia 608.82
Hemothorax 511.89
bacterial, nontuberculous 511.1
newborn 772.8
nontuberculous 511.89
bacterial 511.1
pneumococcal 511.1
postoperative 998.11
staphylococcal 511.1
streptococcal 511.1
traumatic 860.2
with
open wound into thorax 860.3
pneumothorax 860.4
with open wound into thorax
860.5
tuberculous *(see also* Tuberculosis,
pleura) 012.0●
Hemotympanum 385.89
Hench-Rosenberg syndrome
(palindromic arthritis) *(see also*
Rheumatism, palindromic)
719.3●
Henle's warts 371.41
Henoch (-Schönlein)
disease or syndrome (allergic purpura)
287.0
purpura (allergic) 287.0
Henpue, henpuye 102.6
Heparin-induced thrombocytopenia
(HIT) 289.84
Heparitinuria 277.5
Hepar lobatum 095.3
Hepatalgia 573.8
Hepatic - *see also* condition
flexure syndrome 569.89
Hepatitis 573.3
acute *(see also* Necrosis, liver) 570
alcoholic 571.1
infective 070.1
with hepatic coma 070.0
alcoholic 571.1
amebic - *see* Abscess, liver, amebic
anicteric (acute) - *see* Hepatitis, viral

Hepatitis *(Continued)*
    antigen-associated (HAA) - *see*
        Hepatitis, viral, type B
    Australian antigen (positive) - *see*
        Hepatitis, viral, type B
    autoimmune 571.42
    catarrhal (acute) 070.1
        with hepatic coma 070.0
        chronic 571.40
        newborn 070.1
            with hepatic coma 070.0
    chemical 573.3
    cholangiolitic 573.8
    cholestatic 573.8
    chronic 571.40
        active 571.49
            viral - *see* Hepatitis, viral
        aggressive 571.49
        persistent 571.41
        viral - *see* Hepatitis, viral
    cytomegalic inclusion virus 078.5 *[573.1]*
    diffuse 573.3
    "dirty needle" - *see* Hepatitis, viral
    drug-induced 573.3
    due to
        Coxsackie 074.8 *[573.1]*
        cytomegalic inclusion virus 078.5
            [573.1]
        infectious mononucleosis 075 *[573.1]*
        malaria 084.9 *[573.2]*
        mumps 072.71
        secondary syphilis 091.62
        toxoplasmosis (acquired) 130.5
            congenital (active) 771.2
    epidemic - *see* Hepatitis, viral, type A
    fetus or newborn 774.4
    fibrous (chronic) 571.49
        acute 570
    from injection, inoculation, or
        transfusion (blood) (other
        substance) (plasma) (serum)
        (onset within 8 months after
        administration) - *see* Hepatitis,
        viral
    fulminant (viral) *(see also* Hepatitis,
        viral) 070.9
        with hepatic coma 070.6
        type A 070.1
            with hepatic coma 070.0
        type B - *see* Hepatitis, viral, type B
    giant cell (neonatal) 774.4
    hemorrhagic 573.8
    history of
        B V12.09
        C V12.09
    homologous serum - *see* Hepatitis, viral
    hypertrophic (chronic) 571.49
        acute 570
    infectious, infective (acute) (chronic)
        (subacute) 070.1
        with hepatic coma 070.0
    inoculation - *see* Hepatitis, viral
    interstitial (chronic) 571.49
        acute 570
    lupoid 571.49
    malarial 084.9 *[573.2]*
    malignant *(see also* Necrosis, liver) 570
    neonatal (toxic) 774.4
    newborn 774.4
    parenchymatous (acute) *(see also*
        Necrosis, liver) 570
    peliosis 573.3
    persistent, chronic 571.41
    plasma cell 571.49

Hepatitis *(Continued)*
    postimmunization - *see* Hepatitis, viral
    postnecrotic 571.49
    posttransfusion - *see* Hepatitis, viral
    recurrent 571.49
    septic 573.3
    serum - *see* Hepatitis, viral
        carrier (suspected of) V02.61
    subacute *(see also* Necrosis, liver) 570
    suppurative (diffuse) 572.0
    syphilitic (late) 095.3
        congenital (early) 090.0 *[573.2]*
            late 090.5 *[573.2]*
        secondary 091.62
    toxic (noninfectious) 573.3
        fetus or newborn 774.4
    tuberculous *(see also* Tuberculosis)
        017.9●
    viral (acute) (anicteric) (cholangiolitic)
        (cholestatic) (chronic) (subacute)
        070.9
        with hepatic coma 070.6
        AU-SH type virus - *see* Hepatitis,
            viral, type B
        Australian antigen - *see* Hepatitis,
            viral, type B
        B-antigen - *see* Hepatitis, viral, type B
        Coxsackie 074.8 *[573.1]*
        cytomegalic inclusion 078.5 *[573.1]*
        IH (virus) - *see* Hepatitis, viral, type A
        infectious hepatitis virus - *see*
            Hepatitis, viral, type A
        serum hepatitis virus - *see* Hepatitis,
            viral, type B
        SH - *see* Hepatitis, viral, type B
        specified type NEC 070.59
            with hepatic coma 070.49
        type A 070.1
            with hepatic coma 070.0
        type B (acute) 070.30
            with
                hepatic coma 070.20
            carrier status V02.61
            chronic 070.32
                with
                    hepatic coma 070.22
                        with hepatitis delta
                            070.23
                    hepatitis delta 070.33
                        with hepatic coma 070.23
                        with hepatitis delta 070.21
                hepatitis delta 070.31
                    with hepatic coma 070.21
        type C
            acute 070.51
                with hepatic coma 070.41
            carrier status V02.62
            chronic 070.54
                with hepatic coma 070.44
            in remission 070.54
            unspecified 070.70
                with hepatic coma 070.71
        type delta (with hepatitis B carrier
            state) 070.52
            with
                active hepatitis B disease - *see*
                    Hepatitis, viral, type B
                hepatic coma 070.42
        type E 070.53
            with hepatic coma 070.43
        vaccination and inoculation
            (prophylactic) V05.3
    Waldenström's (lupoid hepatitis)
        571.49

Hepatization, lung (acute) - *see also*
        Pneumonia, lobar
    chronic *(see also* Fibrosis, lung) 515
Hepatoblastoma (M8970/3) 155.0
Hepatocarcinoma (M8170/3) 155.0
Hepatocholangiocarcinoma (M8180/3)
        155.0
Hepatocholangioma, benign (M8180/0)
        211.5
Hepatocholangitis 573.8
Hepatocystitis *(see also* Cholecystitis)
        575.10
Hepatodystrophy 570
Hepatolenticular degeneration 275.1
Hepatolithiasis - *see* Choledocholithiasis
Hepatoma (malignant) (M8170/3) 155.0
    benign (M8170/0) 211.5
    congenital (M8970/3) 155.0
    embryonal (M8970/3) 155.0
Hepatomegalia glycogenica diffusa 271.0
Hepatomegaly *(see also* Hypertrophy,
        liver) 789.1
    congenital 751.69
        syphilitic 090.0
    due to Clonorchis sinensis 121.1
    Gaucher's 272.7
    syphilitic (congenital) 090.0
Hepatoptosis 573.8
Hepatorrhexis 573.8
Hepatosis, toxic 573.8
Hepatosplenomegaly 571.8
    due to S. japonicum 120.2
    hyperlipemic (Bürger-Grutz type)
        272.3
Herald patch 696.3
Hereditary - *see* condition
Heredodegeneration 330.9
    macular 362.70
Heredopathia atactica polyneuritiformis
        356.3
Heredosyphilis *(see also* Syphilis,
        congenital) 090.9
Hermaphroditism (true) 752.7
    with specified chromosomal anomaly -
        see Anomaly, chromosomes, sex
Hernia, hernial (acquired) (recurrent)
        553.9
    with
        gangrene (obstructed) NEC 551.9
        obstruction NEC 552.9
            and gangrene 551.9
    abdomen (wall) - *see* Hernia, ventral
    abdominal, specified site NEC 553.8
        with
            gangrene (obstructed) 551.8
            obstruction 552.8
                and gangrene 551.8
    appendix 553.8
        with
            gangrene (obstructed) 551.8
            obstruction 552.8
                and gangrene 551.8
    bilateral (inguinal) - *see* Hernia,
        inguinal
    bladder (sphincter)
        congenital (female) (male) 756.71
        female *(see also* Cystocele, female)
            618.01
        male 596.8
    brain 348.4
        congenital 742.0
    broad ligament 553.8
    cartilage, vertebral - *see* Displacement,
        intervertebral disc

◀ New   ◀▥ Revised   ~~deleted~~ Deleted   ● Use Additional Digit(s)   ▥ Omit code

Hernia, hernial *(Continued)*
cerebral 348.4
  congenital 742.0
  endaural 742.0
ciliary body 364.89
  traumatic 871.1
colic 553.9
  with
    gangrene (obstructed) 551.9
    obstruction 552.9
      and gangrene 551.9
colon 553.9
  with
    gangrene (obstructed) 551.9
    obstruction 552.9
      and gangrene 551.9
colostomy (stoma) 569.69
Cooper's (retroperitoneal) 553.8
  with
    gangrene (obstructed) 551.8
    obstruction 552.8
      and gangrene 551.8
crural - *see* Hernia, femoral
diaphragm, diaphragmatic 553.3
  with
    gangrene (obstructed) 551.3
    obstruction 552.3
      and gangrene 551.3
  congenital 756.6
  due to gross defect of diaphragm
    756.6
  traumatic 862.0
    with open wound into cavity
      862.1
direct (inguinal) - *see* Hernia, inguinal
disc, intervertebral - *see* Displacement,
  intervertebral disc
diverticulum, intestine 553.9
  with
    gangrene (obstructed) 551.9
    obstruction 552.9
      and gangrene 551.9
double (inguinal) - *see* Hernia,
  inguinal
due to adhesion with obstruction
  560.81
duodenojejunal 553.8
  with
    gangrene (obstructed) 551.8
    obstruction 552.8
      and gangrene 551.8
en glissade - *see* Hernia, inguinal
enterostomy (stoma) 569.69
epigastric 553.29
  with
    gangrene (obstruction) 551.29
    obstruction 552.29
      and gangrene 551.29
  recurrent 553.21
    with
      gangrene (obstructed)
        551.21
      obstruction 552.21
        and gangrene 551.21
esophageal hiatus (sliding) 553.3
  with
    gangrene (obstructed) 551.3
    obstruction 552.3
      and gangrene 551.3
  congenital 750.6
external (inguinal) - *see* Hernia,
  inguinal
fallopian tube 620.4
fascia 728.89

Hernia, hernial *(Continued)*
fat 729.30
  eyelid 374.34
  orbital 374.34
  pad 729.30
    eye, eyelid 374.34
    knee 729.31
    orbit 374.34
    popliteal (space) 729.31
    specified site NEC 729.39
femoral (unilateral) 553.00
  with
    gangrene (obstructed) 551.00
    obstruction 552.00
      with gangrene 551.00
  bilateral 553.02
    gangrenous (obstructed)
      551.02
    obstructed 552.02
      with gangrene 551.02
    recurrent 553.03
      gangrenous (obstructed)
        551.03
      obstructed 552.03
        with gangrene 551.03
  recurrent (unilateral) 553.01
    bilateral 553.03
      gangrenous (obstructed)
        551.03
      obstructed 552.03
        with gangrene 551.03
    gangrenous (obstructed)
      551.01
    obstructed 552.01
      with gangrene 551.01
foramen
  Bochdalek 553.3
    with
      gangrene (obstructed) 551.3
      obstruction 552.3
        and gangrene 551.3
    congenital 756.6
  magnum 348.4
  Morgagni, Morgagnian 553.3
    with
      gangrene 551.3
      obstruction 552.3
        and gangrene 551.3
    congenital 756.6
funicular (umbilical) 553.1
  with
    gangrene (obstructed) 551.1
    obstruction 552.1
      and gangrene 551.1
  spermatic cord - *see* Hernia, inguinal
gangrenous - *see* Hernia, by site, with
  gangrene
gastrointestinal tract 553.9
  with
    gangrene (obstructed) 551.9
    obstruction 552.9
      and gangrene 551.9
gluteal - *see* Hernia, femoral
Gruber's (internal mesogastric)
  553.8
  with
    gangrene (obstructed) 551.8
    obstruction 552.8
      and gangrene 551.8
Hesselbach's 553.8
  with
    gangrene (obstructed) 551.8
    obstruction 552.8
      and gangrene 551.8

Hernia, hernial *(Continued)*
hiatal (esophageal) (sliding) 553.3
  with
    gangrene (obstructed) 551.3
    obstruction 552.3
      and gangrene 551.3
  congenital 750.6
incarcerated (*see also* Hernia, by site,
  with obstruction) 552.9
  gangrenous (*see also* Hernia, by site,
    with gangrene) 551.9
incisional 553.21
  with
    gangrene (obstructed) 551.21
    obstruction 552.21
      and gangrene 551.21
  lumbar - *see* Hernia, lumbar
  recurrent 553.21
    with
      gangrene (obstructed) 551.21
      obstruction 552.21
        and gangrene 551.21
indirect (inguinal) - *see* Hernia, inguinal
infantile - *see* Hernia, inguinal
infrapatellar fat pad 729.31
inguinal (direct) (double) (encysted)
  (external) (funicular) (indirect)
  (infantile) (internal) (interstitial)
  (oblique) (scrotal) (sliding)
  550.9●

> Note 41 Use the following fifth-digit
> subclassification with category 550:
>
> 0   unilateral or unspecified (not
>   specified as recurrent)
> 1   unilateral or unspecified,
>   recurrent
> 2   bilateral (not specified as
>   recurrent)
> 3   bilateral, recurrent

  with
    gangrene (obstructed) 550.0●
    obstruction 550.1●
      and gangrene 550.0●
internal 553.8
  with
    gangrene (obstructed) 551.8
    obstruction 552.8
      and gangrene 551.8
  inguinal - *see* Hernia, inguinal
interstitial 553.9
  with
    gangrene (obstructed) 551.9
    obstruction 552.9
      and gangrene 551.9
  inguinal - *see* Hernia, inguinal
intervertebral cartilage or disc - *see*
  Displacement, intervertebral disc
intestine, intestinal 553.9
  with
    gangrene (obstructed) 551.9
    obstruction 552.9
      and gangrene 551.9
intra-abdominal 553.9
  with
    gangrene (obstructed) 551.9
    obstruction 552.9
      and gangrene 551.9
intraparietal 553.9
  with
    gangrene (obstructed) 551.9
    obstruction 552.9
      and gangrene 551.9

Hernia, hernial *(Continued)*
    iris 364.89
        traumatic 871.1
    irreducible *(see also* Hernia, by site,
            with obstruction) 552.9
        gangrenous (with obstruction) *(see
            also* Hernia, by site, with
            gangrene) 551.9
    ischiatic 553.8
        with
            gangrene (obstructed) 551.8
            obstruction 552.8
                and gangrene 551.8
    ischiorectal 553.8
        with
            gangrene (obstructed) 551.8
            obstruction 552.8
                and gangrene 551.8
    lens 379.32
        traumatic 871.1
    linea
        alba - *see* Hernia, epigastric
        semilunaris - *see* Hernia,
            spigelian
    Littre's (diverticular) 553.9
        with
            gangrene (obstructed) 551.9
            obstruction 552.9
                and gangrene 551.9
    lumbar 553.8
        with
            gangrene (obstructed) 551.8
            obstruction 552.8
                and gangrene 551.8
        intervertebral disc 722.10
    lung (subcutaneous) 518.89
        congenital 748.69
    mediastinum 519.3
    mesenteric (internal) 553.8
        with
            gangrene (obstructed) 551.8
            obstruction 552.8
                and gangrene 551.8
    mesocolon 553.8
        with
            gangrene (obstructed) 551.8
            obstruction 552.8
                and gangrene 551.8
    muscle (sheath) 728.89
    nucleus pulposus - *see* Displacement,
        intervertebral disc
    oblique (inguinal) - *see* Hernia,
        inguinal
    obstructive *(see also* Hernia, by site,
            with obstruction) 552.9
        gangrenous (with obstruction)
            (see also Hernia, by site,
            with gangrene) 551.9
    obturator 553.8
        with
            gangrene (obstructed)
                551.8
            obstruction 552.8
                and gangrene 551.8
    omental 553.8
        with
            gangrene (obstructed)
                551.8
            obstruction 552.8
                and gangrene 551.8
    orbital fat (pad) 374.34
    ovary 620.4
    oviduct 620.4
    paracolostomy (stoma) 569.69

Hernia, hernial *(Continued)*
    paraduodenal 553.8
        with
            gangrene (obstructed) 551.8
            obstruction 552.8
                and gangrene 551.8
    paraesophageal 553.3
        with
            gangrene (obstructed) 551.3
            obstruction 552.3
                and gangrene 551.3
        congenital 750.6
    parahiatal 553.3
        with
            gangrene (obstructed) 551.3
            obstruction 552.3
                and gangrene 551.3
    paraumbilical 553.1
        with
            gangrene (obstructed) 551.1
            obstruction 552.1
                and gangrene 551.1
    parietal 553.9
        with
            gangrene (obstructed) 551.9
            obstruction 552.9
                and gangrene 551.9
    perineal 553.8
        with
            gangrene (obstructed) 551.8
            obstruction 552.8
                and gangrene 551.8
    peritoneal sac, lesser 553.8
        with
            gangrene (obstructed) 551.8
            obstruction 552.8
                and gangrene 551.8
    popliteal fat pad 729.31
    postoperative 553.21
        with
            gangrene (obstructed) 551.21
            obstruction 552.21
                and gangrene 551.21
    pregnant uterus 654.4●
    prevesical 596.8
    properitoneal 553.8
        with
            gangrene (obstructed) 551.8
            obstruction 552.8
                and gangrene 551.8
    pudendal 553.8
        with
            gangrene (obstructed) 551.8
            obstruction 552.8
                and gangrene 551.8
    rectovaginal 618.6
    retroperitoneal 553.8
        with
            gangrene (obstructed)
                551.8
            obstruction 552.8
                and gangrene 551.8
    Richter's (parietal) 553.9
        with
            gangrene (obstructed)
                551.9
            obstruction 552.9
                and gangrene 551.9
    Rieux's, Riex's (retrocecal) 553.8
        with
            gangrene (obstructed)
                551.8
            obstruction 552.8
                and gangrene 551.8

Hernia, hernial *(Continued)*
    sciatic 553.8
        with
            gangrene (obstructed) 551.8
            obstruction 552.8
                and gangrene 551.8
    scrotum, scrotal - *see* Hernia, inguinal
    sliding (inguinal) - *see also* Hernia,
        inguinal
    hiatus - *see* Hernia, hiatal
    spigelian 553.29
        with
            gangrene (obstructed) 551.29
            obstruction 552.29
                and gangrene 551.29
    spinal *(see also* Spina bifida) 741.9●
        with hydrocephalus 741.0●
    strangulated *(see also* Hernia, by site,
            with obstruction) 552.9
        gangrenous (with obstruction) *(see
            also* Hernia, by site, with
            gangrene) 551.9
    supraumbilicus (linea alba) - *see*
        Hernia, epigastric
    tendon 727.9
    testis (nontraumatic) 550.9●
        meaning
            scrotal hernia 550.9●
            symptomatic late syphilis 095.8
    Treitz's (fossa) 553.8
        with
            gangrene (obstructed) 551.8
            obstruction 552.8
                and gangrene 551.8
    tunica
        albuginea 608.89
        vaginalis 752.89
    umbilicus, umbilical 553.1
        with
            gangrene (obstructed) 551.1
            obstruction 552.1
                and gangrene 551.1
    ureter 593.89
        with obstruction 593.4
    uterus 621.8
        pregnant 654.4●
    vaginal (posterior) 618.6
    Velpeau's (femoral) *(see also* Hernia,
        femoral) 553.00
    ventral 553.20
        with
            gangrene (obstructed) 551.20
            obstruction 552.20
                and gangrene 551.20
        incisional 553.21
        recurrent 553.21
            with
                gangrene (obstructed) 551.21
                obstruction 552.21
                    and gangrene 551.21
    vesical
        congenital (female) (male) 756.71
        female *(see also* Cystocele, female)
            618.01
        male 596.8
    vitreous (into anterior chamber)
        379.21
        traumatic 871.1
Herniation - *see also* Hernia
    brain (stem) 348.4
    cerebral 348.4
    gastric mucosa (into duodenal bulb)
        537.89
    mediastinum 519.3

◄ New   ◄▥ Revised   ~~deleted~~ Deleted   ● Use Additional Digit(s)   ▨ Omit code

Herniation (Continued)
  nucleus pulposus - see Displacement,
    intervertebral disc
Herpangina 074.0
Herpes, herpetic 054.9
  auricularis (zoster) 053.71
    simplex 054.73
  blepharitis (zoster) 053.20
    simplex 054.41
  circinate 110.5
  circinatus 110.5
    bullous 694.5
  conjunctiva (simplex) 054.43
    zoster 053.21
  cornea (simplex) 054.43
    disciform (simplex) 054.43
    zoster 053.21
  encephalitis 054.3
  eye (zoster) 053.29
    simplex 054.40
  eyelid (zoster) 053.20
    simplex 054.41
  febrilis 054.9
  fever 054.9
  geniculate ganglionitis 053.11
  genital, genitalis 054.10
    specified site NEC 054.19
  gestationis 646.8●
  gingivostomatitis 054.2
  iridocyclitis (simplex) 054.44
    zoster 053.22
  iris (any site) 695.10
  iritis (simplex) 054.44
  keratitis (simplex) 054.43
    dendritic 054.42
    disciform 054.43
    interstitial 054.43
      zoster 053.21
  keratoconjunctivitis (simplex) 054.43
    zoster 053.21
  labialis 054.9
    meningococcal 036.89
  lip 054.9
  meningitis (simplex) 054.72
    zoster 053.0
  ophthalmicus (zoster) 053.20
    simplex 054.40
  otitis externa (zoster) 053.71
    simplex 054.73
  penis 054.13
  perianal 054.10
  pharyngitis 054.79
  progenitalis 054.10
  scrotum 054.19
  septicemia 054.5
  simplex 054.9
    complicated 054.8
      ophthalmic 054.40
        specified NEC 054.49
      specified NEC 054.79
    congenital 771.2
    external ear 054.73
    keratitis 054.43
      dendritic 054.42
    meningitis 054.72
    myelitis 054.74
    neuritis 054.79
    specified complication NEC 054.79
      ophthalmic 054.49
    visceral 054.71
  stomatitis 054.2
  tonsurans 110.0
    maculosus (of Hebra) 696.3
  visceral 054.71
  vulva 054.12

Herpes, herpetic (Continued)
  vulvovaginitis 054.11
  whitlow 054.6
  zoster 053.9
    auricularis 053.71
    complicated 053.8
      specified NEC 053.79
    conjunctiva 053.21
    cornea 053.21
    ear 053.71
    eye 053.29
    geniculate 053.11
    keratitis 053.21
      interstitial 053.21
    myelitis 053.14
    neuritis 053.10
    ophthalmicus(a) 053.20
    oticus 053.71
    otitis externa 053.71
    specified complication NEC 053.79
    specified site NEC 053.9
  zosteriform, intermediate type 053.9
Herrick's
  anemia (hemoglobin S disease) 282.61
  syndrome (hemoglobin S disease)
    282.61
Hers' disease (glycogenosis VI) 271.0
Herter's infantilism (nontropical sprue)
  579.0
Herter (-Gee) disease or syndrome
  (nontropical sprue) 579.0
Herxheimer's disease (diffuse idiopathic
  cutaneous atrophy) 701.8
Herxheimer's reaction 995.0
Hesitancy, urinary 788.64
Hesselbach's hernia - see Hernia,
  Hesselbach's
Heterochromia (congenital) 743.46
  acquired 364.53
  cataract 366.33
  cyclitis 364.21
  hair 704.3
  iritis 364.21
  retained metallic foreign body 360.62
    magnetic 360.52
  uveitis 364.21
Heterophoria 378.40
  alternating 378.45
  vertical 378.43
Heterophyes, small intestine 121.6
Heterophyiasis 121.6
Heteropsia 368.8
Heterotopia, heterotopic - see also
  Malposition, congenital
  cerebralis 742.4
  pancreas, pancreatic 751.7
  spinalis 742.59
Heterotropia 378.30
  intermittent 378.20
    vertical 378.31
  vertical (constant) (intermittent) 378.31
Heubner's disease 094.89
Heubner-Herter disease or syndrome
  (nontropical sprue) 579.0
Hexadactylism 755.00
Heyd's syndrome (hepatorenal) 572.4
HGSIL (high grade squamous
  intraepithelial lesion) (cytologic
  finding) (Pap smear finding)
  anus 796.74
  cervix 795.04
    biopsy finding - code to CIN II or
      CIN III
  vagina 795.14
Hibernoma (M8880/0) - see Lipoma

Hiccough 786.8
  epidemic 078.89
  psychogenic 306.1
Hiccup (see also Hiccough) 786.8
Hicks (-Braxton) contractures 644.1●
Hidden penis 752.65
Hidradenitis (axillaris) (suppurative)
  705.83
Hidradenoma (nodular) (M8400/0) -
  see also Neoplasm, skin, benign
  clear cell (M8402/0) - see Neoplasm,
    skin, benign
  papillary (M8405/0) - see Neoplasm,
    skin, benign
Hidrocystoma (M8404/0) - see Neoplasm,
  skin, benign
HIE (hypoxic-ischemic encephalopathy)
  768.70 ◄▥
  mild 768.71 ◄
  moderate 768.72 ◄
  severe 768.73 ◄
High
  A₂ anemia 282.49
  altitude effects 993.2
    anoxia 993.2
    on
      ears 993.0
      sinuses 993.1
    polycythemia 289.0
  arch
    foot 755.67
    palate 750.26
  artery (arterial) tension (see also
    Hypertension) 401.9
    without diagnosis of hypertension
      796.2
  basal metabolic rate (BMR) 794.7
  blood pressure (see also Hypertension)
    401.9
    incidental reading (isolated)
      (nonspecific), no diagnosis of
      hypertension 796.2
  cholesterol 272.0
    with high triglycerides 272.2
  compliance bladder 596.4
  diaphragm (congenital) 756.6
  frequency deafness (congenital)
    (regional) 389.8
  head at term 652.5●
    affecting fetus or newborn 763.1
  output failure (cardiac) (see also Failure,
    heart) 428.9
  oxygen-affinity hemoglobin 289.0
  palate 750.26
  risk
    behavior -see problem
    family situation V61.9
      specified circumstance NEC V61.8
    human papillomavirus (HPV) DNA
      test positive
      anal 796.75
      cervical 795.05
      vaginal 795.15
    individual NEC V62.89
    infant NEC V20.1
    patient taking drugs (prescribed)
      V67.51
      nonprescribed (see also Abuse,
        drugs, nondependent)
        305.9●
    pregnancy V23.9
      inadequate prenatal care V23.7
      specified problem NEC V23.89
  temperature (of unknown origin) (see
    also Pyrexia) 780.60

High (*Continued*)
 thoracic rib 756.3
 triglycerides 272.1
  with high cholesterol 272.2
Hildenbrand's disease (typhus) 081.9
Hilger's syndrome 337.09
Hill diarrhea 579.1
Hilliard's lupus (*see also* Tuberculosis)
  017.0●
Hilum - *see* condition
Hip - *see* condition
Hippel's disease (retinocerebral
  angiomatosis) 759.6
Hippus 379.49
Hirschfeld's disease (acute diabetes
  mellitus) (*see also* Diabetes) 250.0●
 due to secondary diabetes 249.0●
Hirschsprung's disease or megacolon
  (congenital) 751.3
Hirsuties (*see also* Hypertrichosis)
  704.1
Hirsutism (*see also* Hypertrichosis)
  704.1
Hirudiniasis (external) (internal)
  134.2
His-Werner disease (trench fever)
  083.1
Hiss-Russell dysentery 004.1
Histamine cephalgia 339.00
Histidinemia 270.5
Histidinuria 270.5
Histiocytic syndromes 288.4
Histiocytoma (M8832/0) - *see also*
  Neoplasm, skin, benign
 fibrous (M8830/0) - *see also* Neoplasm,
  skin, benign
  atypical (M8830/1) - *see* Neoplasm,
   connective tissue, uncertain
   behavior
  malignant (M8830/3) - *see*
   Neoplasm, connective tissue,
   malignant
Histiocytosis (acute) (chronic) (subacute)
  277.89
 acute differentiated progressive
  (M9722/3) 202.5●
 cholesterol 277.89
 essential 277.89
 lipid, lipoid (essential) 272.7
 lipochrome (familial) 288.1
 malignant (M9720/3) 202.3●
 non-Langerhans cell 277.89 ◄
 polyostotic sclerosing 277.89 ◄
 X (chronic) 277.89
  acute (progressive) (M9722/3)
   202.5●
Histoplasmosis 115.90
 with
  endocarditis 115.94
  meningitis 115.91
  pericarditis 115.93
  pneumonia 115.95
  retinitis 115.92
  specified manifestation NEC
   115.99
 African (due to Histoplasma duboisii)
  115.10
  with
   endocarditis 115.14
   meningitis 115.11
   pericarditis 115.13
   pneumonia 115.15
   retinitis 115.12
   specified manifestation NEC
    115.19

Histoplasmosis (*Continued*)
 American (due to Histoplasma
  capsulatum) 115.00
  with
   endocarditis 115.04
   meningitis 115.01
   pericarditis 115.03
   pneumonia 115.05
   retinitis 115.02
   specified manifestation NEC
    115.09
 Darling's - *see* Histoplasmosis,
  American
 large form (*see also* Histoplasmosis,
  African) 115.10
 lung 115.05
 small form (*see also* Histoplasmosis,
  American) 115.00
History (personal) of
 abuse
  emotional V15.42
  neglect V15.42
  physical V15.41
  sexual V15.41
 affective psychosis V11.1
 alcoholism V11.3
  specified as drinking problem (*see
   also* Abuse, drugs,
   nondependent) 305.0●
 allergy to
  analgesic agent NEC V14.6
  anesthetic NEC V14.4
  antibiotic agent NEC V14.1
   penicillin V14.0
  anti-infective agent NEC V14.3
  arachnid bite V15.06   ◄
  diathesis V15.09
  drug V14.9
   specified type NEC V14.8
  eggs V15.03
  food additives V15.05
  insect bite V15.06
  latex V15.07
  medicinal agents V14.9
   specified type NEC V14.8
  milk products V15.02
  narcotic agent NEC V14.5
  nuts V15.05
   peanuts V15.01
  penicillin V14.0
  radiographic dye V15.08
  seafood V15.04
  serum V14.7
  specified food NEC V15.05
  specified nonmedicinal agents NEC
   V15.09
  spider bite V15.06
  sulfa V14.2
  sulfonamides V14.2
  therapeutic agent NEC V15.09
  vaccine V14.7
 anemia V12.3
 arrest, sudden cardiac V12.53
 arthritis V13.4
 attack, transient ischemic (TIA)
  V12.54
 benign neoplasm of brain V12.41
 blood disease V12.3
 calculi, urinary V13.01
 cardiovascular disease V12.50
  myocardial infarction 412
 chemotherapy, antineoplastic
  V87.41
 child abuse V15.41
 cigarette smoking V15.82

History (personal) (*Continued*)
 circulatory system disease
  V12.50
  myocardial infarction 412
 congenital malformation
  V13.69
 contraception V15.7
 death, sudden, successfully
  resuscitated V12.53
 deficit
  prolonged reversible ischemic
   neurologic (PRIND)
   V12.54
  reversible ischemic neurologic
   (RIND) V12.54
 diathesis, allergic V15.09
 digestive system disease V12.70
  peptic ulcer V12.71
  polyps, colonic V12.72
  specified NEC V12.79
 disease (of) V13.9
  blood V12.3
  blood-forming organs V12.3
  cardiovascular system V12.50
  circulatory system V12.50
   specified NEC V12.59
  digestive system V12.70
   peptic ulcer V12.71
   polyps, colonic V12.72
   specified NEC V12.79
  infectious V12.00
   malaria V12.03
   methicillin resistant
    Staphylococcus aureus
    (MRSA) V12.04
   MRSA (methicillin resistant
    Staphylococcus aureus)
    V12.04
   poliomyelitis V12.02
   specified NEC V12.09
   tuberculosis V12.01
  parasitic V12.00
   specified NEC V12.09
  respiratory system V12.60
   pneumonia V12.61
   specified NEC V12.69
  skin V13.3
  specified site NEC V13.8
  subcutaneous tissue V13.3
  trophoblastic V13.1
   affecting management of
    pregnancy V23.1
 disorder (of) V13.9
  endocrine V12.2
  genital system V13.29
  hematological V12.3
  immunity V12.2
  mental V11.9
   affective type V11.1
   manic-depressive V11.1
   neurosis V11.2
   schizophrenia V11.0
   specified type NEC V11.8
  metabolic V12.2
  musculoskeletal NEC V13.59
  nervous system V12.40
   specified type NEC V12.49
  obstetric V13.29
   affecting management of current
    pregnancy V23.49
    pre-term labor V23.41
   pre-term labor V13.21
  sense organs V12.40
   specified type NEC V12.49
  specified site NEC V13.8

◄ New   ◄▥ Revised   ~~deleted~~ Deleted   ● Use Additional Digit(s)   ▨ Omit code

History (personal) *(Continued)*
  disorder *(Continued)*
    urinary system V13.00
      calculi V13.01
      infection V13.02
      nephrotic syndrome V13.03
      specified NEC V13.09
  drug use
    nonprescribed (*see also* Abuse,
      drugs, nondependent) 305.9●
    patent (*see also* Abuse, drugs,
      nondependent) 305.9●
  dysplasia
    cervical (conditions classifiable to
      622.10–622.12) V13.22
  effect NEC of external cause V15.89
  embolism (pulmonary) V12.51
  emotional abuse V15.42
  encephalitis V12.42
  endocrine disorder V12.2
  estrogen therapy V87.43 ◄
  extracorporeal membrane oxygenation
    (ECMO) V15.87
  failed ◄
    conscious sedation V15.80 ◄
    moderate sedation V15.80 ◄
  falling V15.88
  family
    allergy V19.6
    anemia V18.2
    arteriosclerosis V17.49
    arthritis V17.7
    asthma V17.5
    blindness V19.0
    blood disorder NEC V18.3
    cardiovascular disease V17.49
    carrier, genetic disease V18.9
    cerebrovascular disease V17.1
    chronic respiratory condition NEC
      V17.6
    colonic polyps V18.51
    congenital anomalies V19.5
    consanguinity V19.7
    coronary artery disease V17.3
    cystic fibrosis V18.19
    deafness V19.2
    diabetes mellitus V18.0
    digestive disorders V18.59
    disease or disorder (of)
      allergic V19.6
      blood NEC V18.3
      cardiovascular NEC V17.49
      cerebrovascular V17.1
      colonic polyps V18.51
      coronary artery V17.3
      death, sudden cardiac (SCD)
        V17.41
      digestive V18.59
      ear NEC V19.3
      endocrine V18.19
        multiple neoplasia [MEN]
          syndrome V18.11
      eye NEC V19.1
      genitourinary NEC V18.7
      hypertensive V17.49
      infectious V18.8
      ischemic heart V17.3
      kidney V18.69
        polycystic V18.61
      mental V17.0
      metabolic V18.19
      musculoskeletal NEC V17.89
        osteoporosis V17.81
      neurological NEC V17.2
      parasitic V18.8
      psychiatric condition V17.0
      skin condition V19.4

History *(Continued)*
  family *(Continued)*
    ear disorder NEC V19.3
    endocrine disease V18.19
      multiple neoplasia [MEN]
        syndrome V18.11
    epilepsy V17.2
    eye disorder NEC V19.1
    genetic disease carrier V18.9
    genitourinary disease NEC V18.7
    glomerulonephritis V18.69
    gout V18.19
    hay fever V17.6
    hearing loss V19.2
    hematopoietic neoplasia V16.7
    Hodgkin's disease V16.7
    Huntington's chorea V17.2
    hydrocephalus V19.5
    hypertension V17.49
    infarction, myocardial V17.3
    infectious disease V18.8
    ischemic heart disease V17.3
    kidney disease V18.69
      polycystic V18.61
    leukemia V16.6
    lymphatic malignant neoplasia
      NEC V16.7
    malignant neoplasm (of) NEC
      V16.9
     anorectal V16.0
     anus V16.0
     appendix V16.0
     bladder V16.52
     bone V16.8
     brain V16.8
     breast V16.3
      male V16.8
     bronchus V16.1
     cecum V16.0
     cervix V16.49
     colon V16.0
     duodenum V16.0
     esophagus V16.0
     eye V16.8
     gallbladder V16.0
     gastrointestinal tract V16.0
     genital organs V16.40
     hemopoietic NEC V16.7
     ileum V16.0
     ilium V16.8
     intestine V16.0
     intrathoracic organs NEC V16.2
     kidney V16.51
     larynx V16.2
     liver V16.0
     lung V16.1
     lymphatic NEC V16.7
     ovary V16.41
     oviduct V16.41
     pancreas V16.0
     penis V16.49
     prostate V16.42
     rectum V16.0
     respiratory organs NEC V16.2
     skin V16.8
     specified site NEC V16.8
     stomach V16.0
     testis V16.43
     trachea V16.1
     ureter V16.59
     urethra V16.59
     urinary organs V16.59
     uterus V16.49
     vagina V16.49
     vulva V16.49

History *(Continued)*
  family *(Continued)*
    MEN (multiple endocrine neoplasia
      syndrome) V18.11
    mental retardation V18.4
    metabolic disease NEC V18.19
    mongolism V19.5
    ~~monoclonal drug therapy V87.42~~
    multiple
      endocrine neoplasia [MEN]
        syndrome V18.11
      myeloma V16.7
    musculoskeletal disease NEC
      V17.89
      osteoporosis V17.81
    myocardial infarction V17.3
    nephritis V18.69
    nephrosis V18.69
      osteoporosis V17.81
    parasitic disease V18.8
    polycystic kidney disease V18.61
    psychiatric disorder V17.0
    psychosis V17.0
    retardation, mental V18.4
    retinitis pigmentosa V19.1
    schizophrenia V17.0
    skin conditions V19.4
    specified condition NEC V19.8
    stroke (cerebrovascular) V17.1
    sudden cardiac death (SCD)
      V17.41
    visual loss V19.0
  fracture, healed
    pathologic V13.51
    stress V13.52
    traumatic V15.51
  genital system disorder V13.29
    pre-term labor V13.21
  health hazard V15.9
    falling V15.88
    specified cause NEC V15.89
  hepatitis
    B V12.09
    C V12.09
  Hodgkin's disease V10.72
  hypospadias V13.61
  immunity disorder V12.2
  immunosuppression therapy V87.46 ◄
  infarction, cerebral, without residual
    deficits V12.54
  infection
    central nervous system V12.42
    urinary (tract) V13.02
  infectious disease V12.00
    malaria V12.03
    methicillin resistant Staphylococcus
      aureus (MRSA) V12.04
    MRSA (methicillin resistant
      Staphylococcus aureus)
      V12.04 poliomyelitis
      V12.02
    specified NEC V12.09
    tuberculosis V12.01
  injury NEC V15.59 ◄
    traumatic brain V15.52
  insufficient prenatal care V23.7
  in utero procedure
    during pregnancy V15.21
    while a fetus V15.22
  irradiation V15.3
  leukemia V10.60
    lymphoid V10.61
    monocytic V10.63
    myeloid V10.62
    specified type NEC V10.69

History (personal) (Continued)
little or no prenatal care V23.7
low birth weight (see also Status, low birth weight) V21.30
lymphosarcoma V10.71
malaria V12.03
malignant carcinoid tumor V10.91 ◄
malignant neoplasm (of) V10.90 ◄▥
    accessory sinus V10.22
    adrenal V10.88
    anus V10.06
    bile duct V10.09
    bladder V10.51
    bone V10.81
    brain V10.85
    breast V10.3
    bronchus V10.11
    cervix uteri V10.41
    colon V10.05
    connective tissue NEC V10.89
    corpus uteri V10.42
    digestive system V10.00
        specified part NEC V10.09
    duodenum V10.09
    endocrine gland NEC V10.88
    epididymis V10.48
    esophagus V10.03
    eye V10.84
    fallopian tube V10.44
    female genital organ V10.40
        specified site NEC V10.44
    gallbladder V10.09
    gastrointestinal tract V10.00
    gum V10.02
    hematopoietic NEC V10.79
    hypopharynx V10.02
    ileum V10.09
    intrathoracic organs NEC V10.20
    jejunum V10.09
    kidney V10.52
    large intestine V10.05
    larynx V10.21
    lip V10.02
    liver V10.07
    lung V10.11
    lymphatic NEC V10.79
    lymph glands or nodes NEC V10.79
    male genital organ V10.45
        specified site NEC V10.49
    mediastinum V10.29
    melanoma (of skin) V10.82
    middle ear V10.22
    mouth V10.02
        specified part NEC V10.02
    nasal cavities V10.22
    nasopharynx V10.02
    nervous system NEC V10.86
    nose V10.22
    oropharynx V10.02
    ovary V10.43
    pancreas V10.09
    parathyroid V10.88
    penis V10.49
    pharynx V10.02
    pineal V10.88
    pituitary V10.88
    placenta V10.44
    pleura V10.29
    prostate V10.46
    rectosigmoid junction V10.06
    rectum V10.06
    renal pelvis V10.53

History (personal) (Continued)
malignant neoplasm (Continued)
    respiratory organs NEC V10.20
    salivary gland V10.02
    skin V10.83
        melanoma V10.82
    small intestine NEC V10.09
    soft tissue NEC V10.89
    specified site NEC V10.89
    stomach V10.04
    testis V10.47
    thymus V10.29
    thyroid V10.87
    tongue V10.01
    trachea V10.12
    ureter V10.59
    urethra V10.59
    urinary organ V10.50
    uterine adnexa V10.44
    uterus V10.42
    vagina V10.44
    vulva V10.44
malignant neuroendocrine tumor V10.91 ◄
manic-depressive psychosis V11.1
meningitis V12.42
mental disorder V11.9
    affective type V11.1
    manic-depressive V11.1
    neurosis V11.2
    schizophrenia V11.0
    specified type NEC V11.8
Merkel cell carcinoma V10.91 ◄
metabolic disorder V12.2
methicillin resistant Staphylococcus aureus (MRSA) V12.04
MRSA (methicillin resistant Staphylococcus aureus) V12.04
musculoskeletal disorder NEC V13.59
myocardial infarction 412
neglect (emotional) V15.42
nephrotic syndrome V13.03
nervous system disorder V12.40
    specified type NEC V12.49
neurosis V11.2
noncompliance with medical treatment V15.81
nutritional deficiency V12.1
obstetric disorder V13.29
    affecting management of current pregnancy V23.49
        pre-term labor V23.41
    pre-term labor V13.21
parasitic disease V12.00
    specified NEC V12.09
perinatal problems V13.7
    low birth weight (see also Status, low birth weight) V21.30
physical abuse V15.41
poisoning V15.6
poliomyelitis V12.02
polyps, colonic V12.72
poor obstetric V13.29
    affecting management of current pregnancy V23.49
        pre-term labor V23.41
    pre-term labor V13.21
prolonged reversible ischemic neurologic deficit (PRIND) V12.54
psychiatric disorder V11.9
    affective type V11.1
    manic-depressive V11.1
    neurosis V11.2

History (personal) (Continued)
psychiatric disorder (Continued)
    schizophrenia V11.0
    specified type NEC V11.8
psychological trauma V15.49
    emotional abuse V15.42
    neglect V15.42
    physical abuse V15.41
    rape V15.41
psychoneurosis V11.2
radiation therapy V15.3
rape V15.41
respiratory system disease V12.60
    pneumonia V12.61
    specified NEC V12.69
reticulosarcoma V10.71
return from military deployment V62.22
reversible ischemic neurologic deficit (RIND) V12.54
schizophrenia V11.0
skin disease V13.3
smoking (tobacco) V15.82
steroid therapy V87.45 ◄
    inhaled V87.44 ◄
    systemic V87.45 ◄
stroke without residual deficits V12.54
subcutaneous tissue disease V13.3
sudden
    cardiac
        arrest V12.53
        death (successfully resuscitated) V12.53
surgery to
    great vessels V15.1
    heart V15.1
    in utero
        during pregnancy V15.21
        while a fetus V15.22
    organs NEC V15.29
syndrome, nephrotic V13.03
therapy
    antineoplastic drug V87.41
    drug NEC V87.49
    estrogen V87.43 ◄
    immunosuppression V87.46 ◄
    monoclonal drug V87.42
    steroid V87.45 ◄
        inhaled V87.44 ◄
        systemic V87.45 ◄
thrombophlebitis V12.52
thrombosis V12.51
tobacco use V15.82
trophoblastic disease V13.1
    affecting management of pregnancy V23.1
tuberculosis V12.01
ulcer, peptic V12.71
urinary system disorder V13.00
    calculi V13.01
    infection V13.02
    nephrotic syndrome V13.03
    specified NEC V13.09
HIT (heparin-induced thrombocytopenia) 289.84
HIV infection (disease) (illness) - see Human immunodeficiency virus (disease) (illness) (infection)
Hives (bold) (see also Urticaria) 708.9
Hoarseness 784.42 ◄▥
Hobnail liver - see Cirrhosis, portal
Hobo, hoboism V60.0

◄ New   ◄▥ Revised   ~~deleted~~ Deleted   ● Use Additional Digit(s)   ▥ Omit code

Hodgkin's
  disease (M9650/3) 201.9 ●
    lymphocytic
      depletion (M9653/3) 201.7 ●
        diffuse fibrosis (M9654/3)
          201.7 ●
        reticular type (M9655/3)
          201.7 ●
      predominance (M9651/3) 201.4 ●
    lymphocytic-histiocytic
      predominance (M9651/3)
        201.4 ●
Hodgkin's (Continued)
  disease (Continued)
    mixed cellularity (M9652/3) 201.6 ●
    nodular sclerosis (M9656/3) 201.5 ●
      cellular phase (M9657/3) 201.5 ●
    granuloma (M9661/3) 201.1 ●
    lymphogranulomatosis (M9650/3)
      201.9 ●
    lymphoma (M9650/3) 201.9 ●
    lymphosarcoma (M9650/3) 201.9 ●
    paragranuloma (M9660/3) 201.0 ●
    sarcoma (M9662/3) 201.2 ●
Hodgson's disease (aneurysmal dilatation
    of aorta) 441.9
  ruptured 441.5
Hodi-potsy 111.0
Hoffa (-Kastert) disease or syndrome
    (liposynovitis prepatellaris) 272.8
Hoffmann's syndrome 244.9 [359.5]
Hoffmann-Bouveret syndrome
    (paroxysmal tachycardia) 427.2
Hole
  macula 362.54
  optic disc, crater-like 377.22
  retina (macula) 362.54
    round 361.31
      with detachment 361.01
Holla disease (see also Spherocytosis) 282.0
Holländer-Simons syndrome
    (progressive lipodystrophy) 272.6
Hollow foot (congenital) 754.71
  acquired 736.73
Holmes' syndrome (visual disorientation)
    368.16
Holoprosencephaly 742.2
  due to
    trisomy 13 758.1
    trisomy 18 758.2
Holthouse's hernia - see Hernia,
    inguinal
Homesickness 309.89
Homocystinemia 270.4
Homocystinuria 270.4
Homologous serum jaundice
    (prophylactic) (therapeutic) - see
    Hepatitis, viral
Homosexuality - omit code
  ego-dystonic 302.0
  pedophilic 302.2
  problems with 302.0
Homozygous Hb-S disease 282.61
Honeycomb lung 518.89
  congenital 748.4
Hong Kong ear 117.3
HOOD (hereditary osteo-
    onychodysplasia) 756.89
Hooded
  clitoris 752.49
  penis 752.69
Hookworm (anemia) (disease)
    (infestation) - see Ancylostomiasis
Hoppe-Goldflam syndrome 358.00

Hordeolum (external) (eyelid) 373.11
  internal 373.12
Horn
  cutaneous 702.8
    cheek 702.8
    eyelid 702.8
    penis 702.8
    iliac 756.89
    nail 703.8
      congenital 757.5
    papillary 700
Horner's
  syndrome (see also Neuropathy,
      peripheral, autonomic) 337.9
    traumatic 954.0
  teeth 520.4
Horseshoe kidney (congenital) 753.3
Horton's
  disease (temporal arteritis) 446.5
  headache or neuralgia 339.00
Hospice care V66.7
Hospitalism (in children) NEC 309.83
Hourglass contraction, contracture
  bladder 596.8
  gallbladder 575.2
    congenital 751.69
  stomach 536.8
    congenital 750.7
    psychogenic 306.4
  uterus 661.4 ●
    affecting fetus or newborn 763.7
Household circumstance affecting care
    V60.9
  specified type NEC V60.89   ◀▥
Housemaid's knee 727.2
Housing circumstance affecting care V60.9
  specified type NEC V60.89   ◀▥
Huchard's disease (continued arterial
    hypertension) 401.9
Hudson-Stähli lines 371.11
Huguier's disease (uterine fibroma) 218.9
Hum, venous - omit code
Human bite (open wound) - (see also
    Wound, open, by site)
  intact skin surface - see Contusion
Human immunodeficiency virus
    (disease) (illness) 042
  infection V08
    with symptoms, symptomatic 042
Human immunodeficiency virus-2
    infection 079.53
Human immunovirus (disease) (illness)
    (infection) - see Human
    immunodeficiency virus (disease)
    (illness) (infection)
Human papillomavirus 079.4
  high risk, DNA test positive
    anal 796.75
    cervical 795.05
    vaginal 795.15
  low risk, DNA test positive
    anal 796.79
    cervical 795.09
    vaginal 795.19
Human parvovirus 079.83
Human T-cell lymphotrophic virus I
    infection 079.51
Human T-cell lymphotrophic virus II
    infection 079.52
Human T-cell lymphotropic virus-III
    (disease) (illness) (infection) - see
    Human immunodeficiency virus
    (disease) (illness) (infection)
HTLV-I infection 079.51

HTLV-II infection 079.52
HTLV-III (disease) (illness) (infection) -
    see Human immunodeficiency
    virus (disease) (illness)
    (infection)
HTLV-III/LAV (disease) (illness)
    (infection) - see Human
    immunodeficiency virus (disease)
    (illness) (infection)
Humpback (acquired) 737.9
  congenital 756.19
Hunchback (acquired) 737.9
  congenital 756.19
Hunger 994.2
  air, psychogenic 306.1
  disease 251.1
Hungry bone syndrome 275.5
Hunner's ulcer (see also Cystitis) 595.1
Hunt's
  neuralgia 053.11
  syndrome (herpetic geniculate
      ganglionitis) 053.11
    dyssynergia cerebellaris myoclonica
      334.2
Hunter's glossitis 529.4
Hunter (-Hurler) syndrome
    (mucopolysaccharidosis II) 277.5
Hunterian chancre 091.0
Huntington's
  chorea 333.4
  disease 333.4
Huppert's disease (multiple myeloma)
    (M9730/3) 203.0 ●
Hurler (-Hunter) disease or syndrome
    (mucopolysaccharidosis II) 277.5
Hürthle cell
  adenocarcinoma (M8290/3) 193
  adenoma (M8290/0) 226
  carcinoma (M8290/3) 193
  tumor (M8290/0) 226
Hutchinson's
  disease meaning
    angioma serpiginosum 709.1
    cheiropompholyx 705.81
    prurigo estivalis 692.72
    summer eruption, or summer
      prurigo 692.72
  incisors 090.5
  melanotic freckle (M8742/2) - see also
      Neoplasm, skin, in situ
    malignant melanoma in (M8742/3) -
      see Melanoma
  teeth or incisors (congenital syphilis)
    090.5
Hutchinson-Boeck disease or syndrome
    (sarcoidosis) 135
Hutchinson-Gilford disease or syndrome
    (progeria) 259.8
Hyaline
  degeneration (diffuse) (generalized)
    728.9
    localized - see Degeneration, by site
  membrane (disease) (lung) (newborn)
    769
Hyalinosis cutis et mucosae 272.8
Hyalin plaque, sclera, senile 379.16
Hyalitis (asteroid) 379.22
  syphilitic 095.8
Hydatid
  cyst or tumor - see also Echinococcus
    fallopian tube 752.11
  mole - see Hydatidiform mole
  Morgagni (congenital) 752.89
    fallopian tube 752.11

Hydatidiform mole (benign) (complicating pregnancy) (delivered) (undelivered) 630
  invasive (M9100/1) 236.1
  malignant (M9100/1) 236.1
  previous, affecting management of pregnancy V23.1
Hydatidosis - see Echinococcus
Hyde's disease (prurigo nodularis) 698.3
Hydradenitis 705.83
Hydradenoma (M8400/0) - see Hidradenoma
Hydralazine lupus or syndrome
  correct substance properly administered 695.4
  overdose or wrong substance given or taken 972.6
Hydramnios 657●
  affecting fetus or newborn 761.3
Hydrancephaly 742.3
  with spina bifida (see also Spina bifida) 741.0●
Hydranencephaly 742.3
  with spina bifida (see also Spina bifida) 741.0●
Hydrargyrism NEC 985.0
Hydrarthrosis (see also Effusion, joint) 719.0●
  gonococcal 098.50
  intermittent (see also Rheumatism, palindromic) 719.3●
  of yaws (early) (late) 102.6
  syphilitic 095.8
    congenital 090.5
Hydremia 285.9
Hydrencephalocele (congenital) 742.0
Hydrencephalomeningocele (congenital) 742.0
Hydroa 694.0
  aestivale 692.72
  gestationis 646.8●
  herpetiformis 694.0
  pruriginosa 694.0
  vacciniforme 692.72
Hydroadenitis 705.83
Hydrocalycosis (see also Hydronephrosis) 591
  congenital 753.29
Hydrocalyx (see also Hydronephrosis) 591
Hydrocele (calcified) (chylous) (idiopathic) (infantile) (inguinal canal) (recurrent) (senile) (spermatic cord) (testis) (tunica vaginalis) 603.9
  canal of Nuck (female) 629.1
    male 603.9
  congenital 778.6
  encysted 603.0
    congenital 778.6
  female NEC 629.89
  infected 603.1
  round ligament 629.89
  specified type NEC 603.8
    congenital 778.6
  spinalis (see also Spina bifida) 741.9●
  vulva 624.8
Hydrocephalic fetus
  affecting management or pregnancy 655.0●
  causing disproportion 653.6●
    with obstructed labor 660.1●
      affecting fetus or newborn 763.1

Hydrocephalus (acquired) (external) (internal) (malignant) (noncommunicating) (obstructive) (recurrent) 331.4
  aqueduct of Sylvius stricture 742.3
    with spina bifida (see also Spina bifida) 741.0●
  chronic 742.3
    with spina bifida (see also Spina bifida) 741.0●
Hydrocephalus (Continued)
  communicating 331.3
  congenital (external) (internal) 742.3
    with spina bifida (see also Spina bifida) 741.0●
  due to
    stricture of aqueduct of Sylvius 742.3
      with spina bifida (see also Spina bifida) 741.0●
    toxoplasmosis (congenital) 771.2
  fetal affecting management of pregnancy 655.0●
  foramen Magendie block (acquired) 331.3
    congenital 742.3
      with spina bifida (see also Spina bifida) 741.0●
  newborn 742.3
    with spina bifida (see also Spina bifida) 741.0●
  normal pressure 331.5
    idiopathic (INPH) 331.5
    secondary 331.3
  otitic 348.2
  syphilitic, congenital 090.49
  tuberculous (see also Tuberculosis) 013.8●
Hydrocolpos (congenital) 623.8
Hydrocystoma (M8404/0) - see Neoplasm, skin, benign
Hydroencephalocele (congenital) 742.0
Hydroencephalomeningocele (congenital) 742.0
Hydrohematopneumothorax (see also Hemothorax) 511.89
Hydromeningitis - see Meningitis
Hydromeningocele (spinal) (see also Spina bifida) 741.9●
  cranial 742.0
Hydrometra 621.8
Hydrometrocolpos 623.8
Hydromicrocephaly 742.1
Hydromphalus (congenital) (since birth) 757.39
Hydromyelia 742.53
Hydromyelocele (see also Spina bifida) 741.9●
Hydronephrosis 591
  atrophic 591
  congenital 753.29
  due to S. hematobium 120.0
  early 591
  functionless (infected) 591
  infected 591
  intermittent 591
  primary 591
  secondary 591
  tuberculous (see also Tuberculosis) 016.0●
Hydropericarditis (see also Pericarditis) 423.9
Hydropericardium (see also Pericarditis) 423.9
Hydroperitoneum 789.59
Hydrophobia 071

Hydrophthalmos (see also Buphthalmia) 743.20
Hydropneumohemothorax (see also Hemothorax) 511.89
Hydropneumopericarditis (see also Pericarditis) 423.9
Hydropneumopericardium (see also Pericarditis) 423.9
Hydropneumothorax 511.89
  nontuberculous 511.89
    bacterial 511.1
    pneumococcal 511.1
    staphylococcal 511.1
    streptococcal 511.1
  traumatic 860.0
    with open wound into thorax 860.1
  tuberculous (see also Tuberculosis, pleura) 012.0●
Hydrops 782.3
  abdominis 789.59
  amnii (complicating pregnancy) (see also Hydramnios) 657●
  articulorum intermittens (see also Rheumatism, palindromic) 719.3●
  cardiac (see also Failure, heart) 428.0
  congenital - see Hydrops, fetalis
  endolymphatic (see also Disease, Ménière's) 386.00
  fetal(is) or newborn 778.0
    due to isoimmunization 773.3
    not due to isoimmunization 778.0
  gallbladder 575.3
  idiopathic (fetus or newborn) 778.0
  joint (see also Effusion, joint) 719.0●
  labyrinth (see also Disease, Ménière's) 386.00
  meningeal NEC 331.4
  nutritional 262
  pericardium - see Pericarditis
  pleura (see also Hydrothorax) 511.89
  renal (see also Nephrosis) 581.9
  spermatic cord (see also Hydrocele) 603.9
Hydropyonephrosis (see also Pyelitis) 590.80
  chronic 590.00
Hydrorachis 742.53
Hydrorrhea (nasal) 478.19
  gravidarum 658.1●
  pregnancy 658.1●
Hydrosadenitis 705.83
Hydrosalpinx (fallopian tube) (follicularis) 614.1
Hydrothorax (double) (pleural) 511.89
  chylous (nonfilarial) 457.8
    filaria (see also Infestation, filarial) 125.9
  nontuberculous 511.89
    bacterial 511.1
    pneumococcal 511.1
    staphylococcal 511.1
    streptococcal 511.1
  traumatic 862.29
    with open wound into thorax 862.39
  tuberculous (see also Tuberculosis, pleura) 012.0●
Hydroureter 593.5
  congenital 753.22
Hydroureteronephrosis (see also Hydronephrosis) 591
Hydrourethra 599.84
Hydroxykynureninuria 270.2
Hydroxyprolinemia 270.8
Hydroxyprolinuria 270.8

◀ New ◀▥ Revised ~~deleted~~ Deleted ● Use Additional Digit(s) ▨ Omit code

Hygroma (congenital) (cystic) (M9173/0) 228.1
　prepatellar 727.3
　subdural - *see* Hematoma, subdural
Hymen - *see* condition
Hymenolepiasis (diminuta) (infection) (infestation) (nana) 123.6
Hymenolepsis (diminuta) (infection) (infestation) (nana) 123.6
Hypalgesia (*see also* Disturbance, sensation) 782.0
Hyperabduction syndrome 447.8
Hyperacidity, gastric 536.8
　psychogenic 306.4
Hyperactive, hyperactivity 314.01
　basal cell, uterine cervix 622.10
　bladder 596.51
　bowel (syndrome) 564.9
　　sounds 787.5
　cervix epithelial (basal) 622.10
　child 314.01
　colon 564.9
　gastrointestinal 536.8
　　psychogenic 306.4
　intestine 564.9
　labyrinth (unilateral) 386.51
　　with loss of labyrinthine reactivity 386.58
　　bilateral 386.52
　nasal mucous membrane 478.19
　stomach 536.8
　thyroid (gland) (*see also* Thyrotoxicosis) 242.9 ●
Hyperacusis 388.42
Hyperadrenalism (cortical) 255.3
　medullary 255.6
Hyperadrenocorticism 255.3
　congenital 255.2
　iatrogenic
　　correct substance properly administered 255.3
　　overdose or wrong substance given or taken 962.0
Hyperaffectivity 301.11
Hyperaldosteronism (atypical) (hyperplastic) (normoaldosteronal) (nor-motensive) (primary) 255.10
　secondary 255.14
Hyperalgesia (*see also* Disturbance, sensation) 782.0
Hyperalimentation 783.6
　carotene 278.3
　specified NEC 278.8
　vitamin A 278.2
　vitamin D 278.4
Hyperaminoaciduria 270.9
　arginine 270.6
　citrulline 270.6
　cystine 270.0
　glycine 270.0
　lysine 270.7
　ornithine 270.6
　renal (types I, II, III) 270.0
Hyperammonemia (congenital) 270.6
Hyperamnesia 780.99
Hyperamylasemia 790.5
Hyperaphia 782.0
Hyperazotemia 791.9
Hyperbetalipoproteinemia (acquired) (essential) (familial) (hereditary) (primary) (secondary) 272.0
　with prebetalipoproteinemia 272.2
Hyperbilirubinemia 782.4
　congenital 277.4
　constitutional 277.4
　neonatal (transient) (*see also* Jaundice, fetus or newborn) 774.6
　　of prematurity 774.2

Hyperbilirubinemica encephalopathia, newborn 774.7
　due to isoimmunization 773.4
Hypercalcemia, hypercalcemic (idiopathic) 275.42
　nephropathy 588.89
Hypercalcinuria 275.40
Hypercapnia 786.09
　with mixed acid-based disorder 276.4
　fetal, affecting newborn 770.89
Hypercarotinemia 278.3
Hypercementosis 521.5
Hyperchloremia 276.9
Hyperchlorhydria 536.8
　neurotic 306.4
　psychogenic 306.4
Hypercholesterinemia - *see* Hypercholesterolemia
Hypercholesterolemia 272.0
　with hyperglyceridemia, endogenous 272.2
　essential 272.0
　familial 272.0
　hereditary 272.0
　primary 272.0
　pure 272.0
Hypercholesterolosis 272.0
Hyperchylia gastrica 536.8
　psychogenic 306.4
Hyperchylomicronemia (familial) (with hyperbetalipoproteinemia) 272.3
Hypercoagulation syndrome (primary) 289.81
　secondary 289.82
Hypercorticosteronism
　correct substance properly administered 255.3
　overdose or wrong substance given or taken 962.0
Hypercortisonism
　correct substance properly administered 255.3
　overdose or wrong substance given or taken 962.0
Hyperdynamic beta-adrenergic state or syndrome (circulatory) 429.82
Hyperekplexia 759.89
Hyperelectrolytemia 276.9
Hyperemesis 536.2
　arising during pregnancy - *see* Hyperemesis, gravidarum
　gravidarum (mild) (before 22 completed weeks' gestation) 643.0 ●
　　with
　　　carbohydrate depletion 643.1 ●
　　　dehydration 643.1 ●
　　　electrolyte imbalance 643.1 ●
　　　metabolic disturbance 643.1 ●
　　affecting fetus or newborn 761.8
　　severe (with metabolic disturbance) 643.1 ●
　psychogenic 306.4
Hyperemia (acute) 780.99
　anal mucosa 569.49
　bladder 596.7
　cerebral 437.8
　conjunctiva 372.71
　ear, internal, acute 386.30
　enteric 564.89
　eye 372.71
　eyelid (active) (passive) 374.82
　intestine 564.89
　iris 364.41
　kidney 593.81

Hyperemia (*Continued*)
　labyrinth 386.30
　liver (active) (passive) 573.8
　lung 514
　ovary 620.8
　passive 780.99
　pulmonary 514
　renal 593.81
　retina 362.89
　spleen 289.59
　stomach 537.89
Hyperesthesia (body surface) (*see also* Disturbance, sensation) 782.0
　larynx (reflex) 478.79
　　hysterical 300.11
　pharynx (reflex) 478.29
Hyperestrinism 256.0
Hyperestrogenism 256.0
Hyperestrogenosis 256.0
Hyperexplexia 759.89
Hyperextension, joint 718.80
　ankle 718.87
　elbow 718.82
　foot 718.87
　hand 718.84
　hip 718.85
　knee 718.86
　multiple sites 718.89
　pelvic region 718.85
　shoulder (region) 718.81
　specified site NEC 718.88
　wrist 718.83
Hyperfibrinolysis - *see* Fibrinolysis
Hyperfolliculinism 256.0
Hyperfructosemia 271.2
Hyperfunction
　adrenal (cortex) 255.3
　　androgenic, acquired benign 255.3
　　medulla 255.6
　　virilism 255.2
　corticoadrenal NEC 255.3
　labyrinth - *see* Hyperactive, labyrinth
　medulloadrenal 255.6
　ovary 256.1
　　estrogen 256.0
　pancreas 577.8
　parathyroid (gland) 252.00
　pituitary (anterior) (gland) (lobe) 253.1
　testicular 257.0
Hypergammaglobulinemia 289.89
　monoclonal, benign (BMH) 273.1
　polyclonal 273.0
　Waldenström's 273.0
Hyperglobulinemia 273.8
Hyperglycemia 790.29
　maternal
　　affecting fetus or newborn 775.0
　　manifest diabetes in infant 775.1
　postpancreatectomy (complete) (partial) 251.3
Hyperglyceridemia 272.1
　endogenous 272.1
　essential 272.1
　familial 272.1
　hereditary 272.1
　mixed 272.3
　pure 272.1
Hyperglycinemia 270.7
Hypergonadism
　ovarian 256.1
　testicular (infantile) (primary) 257.0
Hyperheparinemia (*see also* Circulating anticoagulants) 286.5
Hyperhidrosis, hyperidrosis 705.21
　axilla 705.21
　face 705.21

Hyperhidrosis, hyperidrosis (*Continued*)
  focal (localized) 705.21
    primary 705.21
      axilla 705.21
      face 705.21
      palms 705.21
      soles 705.21
    secondary 705.22
      axilla 705.22
      face 705.22
      palms 705.22
      soles 705.22
  generalized 780.8
  palms 705.21
  psychogenic 306.3
  secondary 780.8
  soles 705.21
Hyperhistidinemia 270.5
Hyperinsulinism (ectopic) (functional)
    (organic) NEC 251.1
  iatrogenic 251.0
  reactive 251.2
  spontaneous 251.2
  therapeutic misadventure (from
      administration of insulin) 962.3
Hyperiodemia 276.9
Hyperirritability (cerebral), in newborn
    779.1
Hyperkalemia 276.7
Hyperkeratosis (*see also* Keratosis) 701.1
  cervix 622.2
  congenital 757.39
  cornea 371.89
  due to yaws (early) (late) (palmar or
      plantar) 102.3
  eccentrica 757.39
  figurata centrifuga atrophica 757.39
  follicularis 757.39
    in cutem penetrans 701.1
  limbic (cornea) 371.89
  palmoplantaris climacterica 701.1
  pinta (carate) 103.1
  senile (with pruritus) 702.0
  tongue 528.79
  universalis congenita 757.1
  vagina 623.1
  vocal cord 478.5
  vulva 624.09
Hyperkinesia, hyperkinetic (disease)
    (reaction) (syndrome) 314.9
  with
    attention deficit - *see* Disorder,
        attention deficit
    conduct disorder 314.2
    developmental delay 314.1
    simple disturbance of activity and
        attention 314.01
    specified manifestation NEC 314.8
  heart (disease) 429.82
  of childhood or adolescence NEC 314.9
Hyperlacrimation (*see also* Epiphora)
    375.20
Hyperlipemia (*see also* Hyperlipidemia)
    272.4
Hyperlipidemia 272.4
  carbohydrate-induced 272.1
  combined 272.2 ◄▥
  endogenous 272.1
  exogenous 272.3
  fat-induced 272.3
  group
    A 272.0
    B 272.1
    C 272.2
    D 272.3
  mixed 272.2
  specified type NEC 272.4

Hyperlipidosis 272.7
  hereditary 272.7
Hyperlipoproteinemia (acquired)
    (essential) (familial) (hereditary)
    (primary) (secondary) 272.4
  Fredrickson type
    I 272.3
    IIA 272.0
    IIB 272.2
    III 272.2
    IV 272.1
    V 272.3
  low-density-lipoid-type (LDL) 272.0
  very-low-density-lipoid-type [VLDL]
      272.1
Hyperlucent lung, unilateral 492.8
Hyperluteinization 256.1
Hyperlysinemia 270.7
Hypermagnesemia 275.2
  neonatal 775.5
Hypermaturity (fetus or newborn)
  post-term infant 766.21
  prolonged gestation infant 766.22
Hypermenorrhea 626.2
Hypermetabolism 794.7
Hypermethioninemia 270.4
Hypermetropia (congenital) 367.0
Hypermobility
  cecum 564.9
  coccyx 724.71
  colon 564.9
    psychogenic 306.4
  ileum 564.89
  joint (acquired) 718.80
    ankle 718.87
    elbow 718.82
    foot 718.87
    hand 718.84
    hip 718.85
    knee 718.86
    multiple sites 718.89
    pelvic region 718.85
    shoulder (region) 718.81
    specified site NEC 718.88
    wrist 718.83
  kidney, congenital 753.3
  meniscus (knee) 717.5
  scapula 718.81
  stomach 536.8
    psychogenic 306.4
  syndrome 728.5
  testis, congenital 752.52
  urethral 599.81
Hypermotility
  gastrointestinal 536.8
  intestine 564.9
    psychogenic 306.4
  stomach 536.8
Hypernasality 784.43 ◄▥
Hypernatremia 276.0
  with water depletion 276.0
Hypernephroma (M8312/3) 189.0
Hyperopia 367.0
Hyperorexia 783.6
Hyperornithinemia 270.6
Hyperosmia (*see also* Disturbance,
    sensation) 781.1
Hyperosmolality 276.0
Hyperosteogenesis 733.99
Hyperostosis 733.99
  calvarial 733.3
  cortical 733.3
    infantile 756.59
  frontal, internal of skull 733.3

Hyperostosis (*Continued*)
  interna frontalis 733.3
  monomelic 733.99
  skull 733.3
    congenital 756.0
  vertebral 721.8
    with spondylosis - *see* Spondylosis
    ankylosing 721.6
Hyperovarianism 256.1
Hyperovarism, hyperovaria 256.1
Hyperoxaluria (primary) 271.8
Hyperoxia 987.8
Hyperparathyroidism 252.00
  ectopic 259.3
  other 252.08
  primary 252.01
  secondary (of renal origin) 588.81
    non-renal 252.02
  tertiary 252.08
Hyperpathia (*see also* Disturbance,
    sensation) 782.0
  psychogenic 307.80
Hyperperistalsis 787.4
  psychogenic 306.4
Hyperpermeability, capillary 448.9
Hyperphagia 783.6
Hyperphenylalaninemia 270.1
Hyperphoria 378.40
  alternating 378.45
Hyperphosphatemia 275.3
Hyperpiesia (*see also* Hypertension) 401.9
Hyperpiesis (*see also* Hypertension) 401.9
Hyperpigmentation - *see* Pigmentation
Hyperpinealism 259.8
Hyperpipecolatemia 270.7
Hyperpituitarism 253.1
Hyperplasia, hyperplastic
  adenoids (lymphoid tissue) 474.12
    and tonsils 474.10
  adrenal (capsule) (cortex) (gland) 255.8
    with
      sexual precocity (male) 255.2
      virilism, adrenal 255.2
      virilization (female) 255.2
    congenital 255.2
    due to excess ACTH (ectopic)
        (pituitary) 255.0
    medulla 255.8
  alpha cells (pancreatic)
    with
      gastrin excess 251.5
      glucagon excess 251.4
  appendix (lymphoid) 543.0
  artery, fibromuscular NEC 447.8
    carotid 447.8
    renal 447.3
  bone 733.99
    marrow 289.9
  breast (*see also* Hypertrophy, breast)
      611.1
    ductal 610.8 ◄
      atypical 610.8 ◄
  carotid artery 447.8
  cementation, cementum (teeth) (tooth)
      521.5
  cervical gland 785.6
  cervix (uteri) 622.10
    basal cell 622.10
    congenital 752.49
    endometrium 622.10
    polypoid 622.10
  chin 524.05
  clitoris, congenital 752.49
  dentin 521.5
  endocervicitis 616.0

◄ New   ◄▥ Revised   ~~deleted~~ Deleted   ● Use Additional Digit(s)   ▥ Omit code

Hyperplasia, hyperplastic (Continued)
  endometrium, endometrial
    (adenomatous) (atypical) (cystic)
    (glandular) (polypoid) (uterus)
    621.30
    with atypia 621.33
    without atypia
      complex 621.32
      simple 621.31
    benign 621.34 ◄
    cervix 622.10
  epithelial 709.8
    focal, oral, including tongue 528.79
    mouth (focal) 528.79
    nipple 611.89
    skin 709.8
    tongue (focal) 528.79
    vaginal wall 623.0
  erythroid 289.9
  fascialis ossificans (progressiva) 728.11
  fibromuscular, artery NEC 447.8
    carotid 447.8
    renal 447.3
  genital
    female 629.89
    male 608.89
  gingiva 523.8
  glandularis
    cystica uteri 621.30
    endometrium (uterus) 621.30
    interstitialis uteri 621.30
  granulocytic 288.69
  gum 523.8
  hymen, congenital 752.49
  islands of Langerhans 251.1
  islet cell (pancreatic) 251.9
    alpha cells
      with excess
        gastrin 251.5
        glucagon 251.4
    beta cells 251.1
  juxtaglomerular (complex) (kidney)
    593.89
  kidney (congenital) 753.3
  liver (congenital) 751.69
  lymph node (gland) 785.6
  lymphoid (diffuse) (nodular) 785.6
    appendix 543.0
    intestine 569.89
  mandibular 524.02
    alveolar 524.72
    unilateral condylar 526.89
  Marchand multiple nodular (liver) -
    see Cirrhosis, postnecrotic
  maxillary 524.01
    alveolar 524.71
  medulla, adrenal 255.8
  myometrium, myometrial 621.2
  nose (lymphoid) (polypoid) 478.19
  oral soft tissue (inflammatory)
    (irritative) (mucosa) NEC 528.9
    gingiva 523.8
    tongue 529.8
  organ or site, congenital NEC - see
    Anomaly, specified type NEC
  ovary 620.8
  palate, papillary 528.9
  pancreatic islet cells 251.9
    alpha
      with excess
        gastrin 251.5
        glucagon 251.4
    beta 251.1
  parathyroid (gland) 252.01
  persistent, vitreous (primary) 743.51

Hyperplasia, hyperplastic (Continued)
  pharynx (lymphoid) 478.29
  prostate 600.90
    with
      other lower urinary tract
        symptoms (LUTS) 600.91
      urinary
        obstruction 600.91
        retention 600.91
    adenofibromatous 600.20
      with
        other lower urinary tract
          symptoms (LUTS)
          600.21
        urinary
          obstruction 600.21
          retention 600.21
    nodular 600.10
      with
        urinary
          obstruction 600.11
          retention 600.11
  renal artery (fibromuscular) 447.3
  reticuloendothelial (cell) 289.9
  salivary gland (any) 527.1
  Schimmelbusch's 610.1
  suprarenal (capsule) (gland) 255.8
  thymus (gland) (persistent) 254.0
  thyroid (see also Goiter) 240.9
    primary 242.0●
    secondary 242.2●
  tonsil (lymphoid tissue) 474.11
    and adenoids 474.10
  urethrovaginal 599.89
  uterus, uterine (myometrium) 621.2
    endometrium (see also Hyperplasia,
      endometrium) 621.30
  vitreous (humor), primary persistent
    743.51
  vulva 624.3
  zygoma 738.11
Hyperpnea (see also Hyperventilation)
  786.01
Hyperpotassemia 276.7
Hyperprebetalipoproteinemia 272.1
  with chylomicronemia 272.3
  familial 272.1
Hyperprolactinemia 253.1
Hyperprolinemia 270.8
Hyperproteinemia 273.8
Hyperprothrombinemia 289.89
Hyperpselaphesia 782.0
Hyperpyrexia 780.60
  heat (effects of) 992.0
  malarial (see also Malaria) 084.6
  malignant, due to anesthetic 995.86
  rheumatic - see Fever, rheumatic
  unknown origin (see also Pyrexia)
    780.60
Hyperreactor, vascular 780.2
Hyperreflexia 796.1
  bladder, autonomic 596.54
    with cauda equina 344.61
  detrusor 344.61
Hypersalivation (see also Ptyalism)
  527.7
Hypersarcosinemia 270.8
Hypersecretion
  ACTH 255.3
  androgens (ovarian) 256.1
  calcitonin 246.0
  corticoadrenal 255.3
  cortisol 255.0
  estrogen 256.0
  gastric 536.8
    psychogenic 306.4

Hypersecretion (Continued)
  gastrin 251.5
  glucagon 251.4
  hormone
    ACTH 255.3
    anterior pituitary 253.1
    growth NEC 253.0
    ovarian androgen 256.1
    testicular 257.0
    thyroid stimulating 242.8●
  insulin - see Hyperinsulinism
  lacrimal glands (see also Epiphora) 375.20
  medulloadrenal 255.6
  milk 676.6●
  ovarian androgens 256.1
  pituitary (anterior) 253.1
  salivary gland (any) 527.7
  testicular hormones 257.0
  thyrocalcitonin 246.0
  upper respiratory 478.9
Hypersegmentation, hereditary 288.2
  eosinophils 288.2
  neutrophil nuclei 288.2
Hypersensitive, hypersensitiveness,
  hypersensitivity - see also Allergy
  angiitis 446.20
    specified NEC 446.29
  carotid sinus 337.01
  colon 564.9
    psychogenic 306.4
  DNA (deoxyribonucleic acid)
    NEC 287.2
  drug (see also Allergy, drug) 995.27
  esophagus 530.89
  insect bites - see Injury, superficial, by
    site
  labyrinth 386.58
  pain (see also Disturbance, sensation)
    782.0
  pneumonitis NEC 495.9
  reaction (see also Allergy) 995.3
    upper respiratory tract NEC 478.8
  stomach (allergic) (nonallergic) 536.8
    psychogenic 306.4
Hypersomatotropism (classic) 253.0
Hypersomnia, unspecified 780.54
  with sleep apnea, unspecified 780.53
  alcohol induced 291.82
  drug induced 292.85
  due to
    medical condition classified
      elsewhere 327.14
    mental disorder 327.15
  idiopathic
    with long sleep time 327.11
    without long sleep time 327.12
  menstrual related 327.13
  nonorganic origin 307.43
    persistent (primary) 307.44
    transient 307.43
  organic 327.10
    other 327.19
  primary 307.44
  recurrent 327.13
Hypersplenia 289.4
Hypersplenism 289.4
Hypersteatosis 706.3
Hyperstimulation, ovarian 256.1
Hypersuprarenalism 255.3
Hypersusceptibility - see Allergy
Hyper-TBG-nemia 246.8
Hypertelorism 756.0
  orbit, orbital 376.41
Hypertension, hypertensive - see table
  on pg. 316–319

OGCR Section I.C.7.a.1

Assign hypertension (arterial) (essential) (systemic) (NOS) to category code 401 with appropriate fourth digit to indicate malignant (.0), benign (.1), or unspecified (.9). Do not use either .0 malignant or .1 benign unless medical record documentation supports such a designation.

	Malignant	Benign	Unspecified
Hypertension, hypertensive (arterial) (arteriolar) (crisis) (degeneration) (disease) (essential) (fluctuating) (idiopathic) (intermittent) (labile) (low renin) (orthostatic) (paroxysmal) (primary) (systemic) (uncontrolled) (vascular)	401.0	401.1	401.9
with			
chronic kidney disease	—	—	—
stage I through stage IV, or unspecified	403.00	403.10	403.90
stage V or end stage renal disease	403.01	403.11	403.91
heart involvement (conditions classifiable to 429.0–429.3, 429.8, 429.9 due to hypertension) (*see also* Hypertension, heart)	402.00	402.10	402.90
with kidney involvement - *see* Hypertension, cardiorenal			
renal (kidney) involvement (only conditions classifiable to 585, 586, 587) (excludes conditions classifiable to 584) (*see also* Hypertension, kidney)	403.00	403.10	403.90
with heart involvement - *see* Hypertension, cardiorenal failure (and sclerosis) (*see also* Hypertension, kidney)	403.01	403.11	403.91
sclerosis without failure (*see also* Hypertension, kidney)	403.00	403.10	403.90
accelerated (*see also* Hypertension, by type, malignant)	401.0	—	—
antepartum - *see* Hypertension, complicating pregnancy, childbirth, or the puerperium			
cardiorenal (disease)	404.00	404.10	404.90
with			
chronic kidney disease	—	—	—
stage I through stage IV, or unspecified	404.00	404.10	404.90
and heart failure	404.01	404.11	404.91
stage V or end stage renal disease	404.02	404.12	404.92
and heart failure	404.03	404.13	404.93
heart failure	404.01	404.11	404.91
and chronic kidney disease	404.01	404.11	404.91
stage I through stage IV or unspecified	404.01	404.11	404.91
stage V or end stage renal disease	404.03	404.13	404.93
cardiovascular disease (arteriosclerotic) (sclerotic)	402.00	402.10	402.90
with			
heart failure	402.01	402.11	402.91
renal involvement (conditions classifiable to 403) (*see also* Hypertension, cardiorenal)	404.00	404.10	404.90
cardiovascular renal (disease) (sclerosis) (*see also* Hypertension, cardiorenal)	404.00	404.10	404.90
cerebrovascular disease NEC	437.2	437.2	437.2
complicating pregnancy, childbirth, or the puerperium	642.2●	642.0●	642.9●
with			
albuminuria (and edema) (mild)	—	—	642.4●
severe	—	—	642.5●
chronic kidney disease	642.2●	642.2●	642.2●
and heart disease	642.2●	642.2●	642.2●
edema (mild)	—	—	642.4●
severe	—	—	642.5●
heart disease	642.2●	642.2●	642.2●
and chronic kidney disease	642.2●	642.2●	642.2●
renal disease	642.2●	642.2●	642.2●
and heart disease	642.2●	642.2●	642.2●

◀ New   ◀▥ Revised   ~~deleted~~ Deleted   ● Use Additional Digit(s)   ▨ Omit code

	Malignant	Benign	Unspecified
Hypertension, hypertensive *(Continued)*			
complicating pregnancy, childbirth, or the puerperium *(Continued)*			
chronic	642.2●	642.0●	642.0●
with pre-eclampsia or eclampsia	642.7●	642.7●	642.7●
fetus or newborn	760.0	760.0	760.0
essential	—	642.0●	642.0●
with pre-eclampsia or eclampsia	—	642.7●	642.7●
fetus or newborn	760.0	760.0	760.0
fetus or newborn	760.0	760.0	760.0
gestational	—	—	642.3●
pre-existing	642.2●	642.0●	642.0●
with pre-eclampsia or eclampsia	642.7●	642.7●	642.7●
fetus or newborn	760.0	760.0	760.0
secondary to renal disease	642.1●	642.1●	642.1●
with pre-eclampsia or eclampsia	642.7●	642.7●	642.7●
fetus or newborn	760.0	760.0	760.0
transient	—	—	642.3●
due to			
aldosteronism, primary	405.09	405.19	405.99
brain tumor	405.09	405.19	405.99
bulbar poliomyelitis	405.09	405.19	405.99
calculus			
kidney	405.09	405.19	405.99
ureter	405.09	405.19	405.99
coarctation, aorta	405.09	405.19	405.99
Cushing's disease	405.09	405.19	405.99
glomerulosclerosis (*see also* Hypertension, kidney)	403.00	403.10	403.90
periarteritis nodosa	405.09	405.19	405.99
pheochromocytoma	405.09	405.19	405.99
polycystic kidney(s)	405.09	405.19	405.99
polycythemia	405.09	405.19	405.99
porphyria	405.09	405.19	405.99
pyelonephritis	405.09	405.19	405.99
renal (artery)			
aneurysm	405.01	405.11	405.91
anomaly	405.01	405.11	405.91
embolism	405.01	405.11	405.91
fibromuscular hyperplasia	405.01	405.11	405.91
occlusion	405.01	405.11	405.91
stenosis	405.01	405.11	405.91
thrombosis	405.01	405.11	405.91
encephalopathy	437.2	437.2	437.2
gestational (transient) NEC	—	—	642.3●
Goldblatt's	440.1	440.1	440.1

◀ New   ◀▥ Revised   ~~deleted~~ Deleted   ● Use Additional Digit(s)   ▨ Omit code

	Malignant	Benign	Unspecified
Hypertension, hypertensive *(Continued)*			
heart (disease) (conditions classifiable to 429.0–429.3, 429.8, 429.9 due to hypertension)	402.00	402.10	402.90
with			
heart failure	402.01	402.11	402.91
hypertensive kidney disease (conditions classifiable to 403) (*see also* Hypertension, cardiorenal)	404.00	404.10	404.90
renal sclerosis (*see also* Hypertension, cardiorenal)	404.00	404.10	404.90
intracranial, benign	—	348.2	—
intraocular	—	—	365.04
kidney	403.00	403.10	403.90
with			
chronic kidney disease	—	—	—
stage I through stage IV, or unspecified	403.00	403.10	403.90
stage V or end stage renal disease	403.01	403.11	403.91
heart involvement (conditions classifiable to 429.0–429.3, 429.8, 429.9 due to hypertension) (*see also* Hypertension, cardiorenal)	404.00	404.10	404.90
hypertensive heart (disease) (conditions classifiable to 402) (*see also* Hypertension, cardiorenal)	404.00	404.10	404.90
lesser circulation	—	—	416.0
necrotizing	401.0	—	—
pancreatic duct - *code to* underlying condition			
with			
chronic pancreatitis	—	—	577.11
ocular			365.04
portal (due to chronic liver disease)	—	—	572.3
postoperative			997.91
psychogenic	—	—	306.2
puerperal, postpartum - *see* Hypertension, complicating pregnancy, childbirth, or the puerperium			
pulmonary (artery)	—	—	416.8
with cor pulmonale (chronic)	—	—	416.8
acute	—	—	415.0
idiopathic	—	—	416.0
primary	—	—	416.0
of newborn	—	—	747.83
secondary	—	—	416.8
renal (disease) (*see also* Hypertension, kidney)	403.00	403.10	403.90
renovascular NEC	405.01	405.11	405.91

◄ New   ⬅ Revised   ~~deleted~~ Deleted   ● Use Additional Digit(s)   ▨ Omit code

	Malignant	Benign	Unspecified
Hypertension, hypertensive *(Continued)*			
secondary NEC	405.09	405.19	405.99
due to			
aldosteronism, primary	405.09	405.19	405.99
brain tumor	405.09	405.19	405.99
bulbar poliomyelitis	405.09	405.19	405.99
calculus			
kidney	405.09	405.19	405.99
ureter	405.09	405.19	405.99
coarctation, aorta	405.09	405.19	405.99
Cushing's disease	405.09	405.19	405.99
glomerulosclerosis (*see also* Hypertension, kidney)	403.00	403.10	403.90
periarteritis nodosa	405.09	405.19	405.99
pheochromocytoma	405.09	405.19	405.99
polycystic kidney(s)	405.09	405.19	405.99
polycythemia	405.09	405.19	405.99
porphyria	405.09	405.19	405.99
pyelonephritis	405.09	405.19	405.99
renal (artery)			
aneurysm	405.01	405.11	405.91
anomaly	405.01	405.11	405.91
embolism	405.01	405.11	405.91
fibromuscular hyperplasia	405.01	405.11	405.91
occlusion	405.01	405.11	405.91
stenosis	405.01	405.11	405.91
thrombosis	405.01	405.11	405.91
transient	—	—	796.2
of pregnancy	—	—	642.3●
venous, chronic (asymptomatic) (idiopathic)	—	—	459.30
with			
complication, NEC	—	—	459.39
inflammation	—	—	459.32
with ulcer	—	—	459.33
ulcer	—	—	459.31
with inflammation	—	—	459.33
due to			
deep vein thrombosis (*see also* Syndrome, postphlebitic)	—	—	459.10

◄ New   ◀▥ Revised   ~~deleted~~ Deleted   ● Use Additional Digit(s)   ▨ Omit code

Hyperthecosis, ovary 256.8
Hyperthermia (of unknown origin) (*see also* Pyrexia) 780.60
  malignant (due to anesthesia) 995.86
  newborn 778.4
Hyperthymergasia (*see also* Psychosis, affective) 296.0●
  reactive (from emotional stress, psychological trauma) 298.1
  recurrent episode 296.1●
  single episode 296.0●
Hyperthymism 254.8
Hyperthyroid (recurrent) - *see* Hyperthyroidism
Hyperthyroidism (latent) (preadult) (recurrent) (without goiter) 242.9●

> Note 43   Use the following fifth-digit subclassification with category 242:
>
> 0   without mention of thyrotoxic crisis or storm
> 1   with mention of thyrotoxic crisis or storm

  with
      goiter (diffuse) 242.0●
        adenomatous 242.3●
          multinodular 242.2●
          uninodular 242.1●
        nodular 242.3●
          multinodular 242.2●
          uninodular 242.1●
        thyroid nodule 242.1●
  complicating pregnancy, childbirth, or puerperium 648.1●
  neonatal (transient) 775.3
Hypertonia - *see* Hypertonicity
Hypertonicity
  bladder 596.51
  fetus or newborn 779.89
  gastrointestinal (tract) 536.8
  infancy 779.89
    due to electrolyte imbalance 779.89
  muscle 728.85
  stomach 536.8
    psychogenic 306.4
  uterus, uterine (contractions) 661.4●
    affecting fetus or newborn 763.7
Hypertony - *see* Hypertonicity
Hypertransaminemia 790.4
Hypertrichosis 704.1
  congenital 757.4
  eyelid 374.54
  lanuginosa 757.4
    acquired 704.1
Hypertriglyceridemia, essential 272.1
Hypertrophy, hypertrophic
  adenoids (infectional) 474.12
    and tonsils (faucial) (infective) (lingual) (lymphoid) 474.10
  adrenal 255.8
  alveolar process or ridge 525.8
  anal papillae 569.49
  apocrine gland 705.82
  artery NEC 447.8
    carotid 447.8
    congenital (peripheral) NEC 747.60
      gastrointestinal 747.61
      lower limb 747.64
      renal 747.62
      specified NEC 747.69
      spinal 747.82
      upper limb 747.63
    renal 447.3

Hypertrophy, hypertrophic (*Continued*)
  arthritis (chronic) (*see also* Osteoarthrosis) 715.9●
    spine (*see also* Spondylosis) 721.90
  arytenoid 478.79
  asymmetrical (heart) 429.9
  auricular - *see* Hypertrophy, cardiac
  Bartholin's gland 624.8
  bile duct 576.8
  bladder (sphincter) (trigone) 596.8
  blind spot, visual field 368.42
  bone 733.99
  brain 348.89   ◄▥
  breast 611.1
    cystic 610.1
    fetus or newborn 778.7
    fibrocystic 610.1
    massive pubertal 611.1
    puerperal, postpartum 676.3●
    senile (parenchymatous) 611.1
  cardiac (chronic) (idiopathic) 429.3
    with
        rheumatic fever (conditions classifiable to 390)
          active 391.8
            with chorea 392.0
          inactive or quiescent (with chorea) 398.99
    congenital NEC 746.89
    fatty (*see also* Degeneration, myocardial) 429.1
    hypertensive (*see also* Hypertension, heart) 402.90
    rheumatic (with chorea) 398.99
      active or acute 391.8
        with chorea 392.0
    valve (*see also* Endocarditis) 424.90
      congenital NEC 746.89
  cartilage 733.99
  cecum 569.89
  cervix (uteri) 622.6
    congenital 752.49
    elongation 622.6
  clitoris (cirrhotic) 624.2
    congenital 752.49
  colon 569.89
    congenital 751.3
  conjunctiva, lymphoid 372.73
  cornea 371.89
  corpora cavernosa 607.89
  duodenum 537.89
  endometrium (uterus) (*see also* Hyperplasia, endometrium) 621.30
    cervix 622.6
  epididymis 608.89
  esophageal hiatus (congenital) 756.6
    with hernia - *see* Hernia, diaphragm
  eyelid 374.30
  falx, skull 733.99
  fat pad 729.30
    infrapatellar 729.31
    knee 729.31
    orbital 374.34
    popliteal 729.31
    prepatellar 729.31
    retropatellar 729.31
    specified site NEC 729.39
  foot (congenital) 755.67
  frenum, frenulum (tongue) 529.8
    linguae 529.8
    lip 528.5
  gallbladder or cystic duct 575.8

Hypertrophy, hypertrophic (*Continued*)
  gastric mucosa 535.2●
  gingiva 523.8
  gland, glandular (general) NEC 785.6
  gum (mucous membrane) 523.8
  heart (idiopathic) - *see also* Hypertrophy, cardiac
    valve - *see also* Endocarditis
      congenital NEC 746.89
  hemifacial 754.0
  hepatic - *see* Hypertrophy, liver
  hiatus (esophageal) 756.6
  hilus gland 785.6
  hymen, congenital 752.49
  ileum 569.89
  infrapatellar fat pad 729.31
  intestine 569.89
  jejunum 569.89
  kidney (compensatory) 593.1
    congenital 753.3
  labial frenulum 528.5
  labium (majus) (minus) 624.3
  lacrimal gland, chronic 375.03
  ligament 728.9
    spinal 724.8
  linguae frenulum 529.8
  lingual tonsil (infectional) 474.11
  lip (frenum) 528.5
    congenital 744.81
  liver 789.1
    acute 573.8
    cirrhotic - *see* Cirrhosis, liver
    congenital 751.69
    fatty - *see* Fatty, liver
  lymph gland 785.6
    tuberculous - *see* Tuberculosis, lymph gland
  mammary gland - *see* Hypertrophy, breast
  maxillary frenulum 528.5
  Meckel's diverticulum (congenital) 751.0
  medial meniscus, acquired 717.3
  median bar 600.90
    with
        other lower urinary tract symptoms (LUTS) 600.91
        urinary
          obstruction 600.91
          retention 600.91
  mediastinum 519.3
  meibomian gland 373.2
  meniscus, knee, congenital 755.64
  metatarsal head 733.99
  metatarsus 733.99
  mouth 528.9
  mucous membrane
    alveolar process 523.8
    nose 478.19
    turbinate (nasal) 478.0
  muscle 728.9
  muscular coat, artery NEC 447.8
    carotid 447.8
    renal 447.3
  myocardium (*see also* Hypertrophy, cardiac) 429.3
    idiopathic 425.4
  myometrium 621.2
  nail 703.8
    congenital 757.5
  nasal 478.19
    alae 478.19
    bone 738.0
    cartilage 478.19

◄ New   ◄▥ Revised   ~~deleted~~ Deleted   ● Use Additional Digit(s)   ▨ Omit code

Hypertrophy, hypertrophic (*Continued*)
  nasal (*Continued*)
    mucous membrane (septum)
        478.19
    sinus (*see also* Sinusitis) 473.9
    turbinate 478.0
  nasopharynx, lymphoid (infectional)
        (tissue) (wall) 478.29
  neck, uterus 622.6
  nipple 611.1
  normal aperture diaphragm
        (congenital) 756.6
  nose (*see also* Hypertrophy, nasal)
        478.19
  orbit 376.46
  organ or site, congenital NEC - *see*
        Anomaly, specified type NEC
  osteoarthropathy (pulmonary) 731.2
  ovary 620.8
  palate (hard) 526.89
    soft 528.9
  pancreas (congenital) 751.7
  papillae
    anal 569.49
    tongue 529.3
  parathyroid (gland) 252.01
  parotid gland 527.1
  penis 607.89
  phallus 607.89
    female (clitoris) 624.2
  pharyngeal tonsil 474.12
  pharyngitis 472.1
  pharynx 478.29
    lymphoid (infectional) (tissue) (wall)
        478.29
  pituitary (fossa) (gland) 253.8
  popliteal fat pad 729.31
  preauricular (lymph) gland
        (Hampstead) 785.6
  prepuce (congenital) 605
    female 624.2
  prostate (asymptomatic) (early)
        (recurrent) 600.90
    with
        other lower urinary tract
            symptoms (LUTS) 600.91
        urinary
            obstruction 600.91
            retention 600.91
    adenofibromatous 600.20
        with
            other lower urinary tract
                symptoms (LUTS)
                    600.21
            urinary
                obstruction 600.21
                retention 600.21
    benign 600.00
        with
            other lower urinary tract
                symptoms (LUTS)
                    600.01
            urinary
                obstruction 600.01
                retention 600.01
    congenital 752.89
  pseudoedematous hypodermal 757.0
  pseudomuscular 359.1
  pylorus (muscle) (sphincter) 537.0
    congenital 750.5
    infantile 750.5
  rectal sphincter 569.49
  rectum 569.49
  renal 593.1

Hypertrophy, hypertrophic (*Continued*)
  rhinitis (turbinate) 472.0
  salivary duct or gland 527.1
    congenital 750.26
  scaphoid (tarsal) 733.99
  scar 701.4
  scrotum 608.89
  sella turcica 253.8
  seminal vesicle 608.89
  sigmoid 569.89
  skin condition NEC 701.9
  spermatic cord 608.89
  spinal ligament 724.8
  spleen - *see* Splenomegaly
  spondylitis (spine) (*see also*
        Spondylosis) 721.90
  stomach 537.89
  subaortic stenosis (idiopathic) 425.1
  sublingual gland 527.1
    congenital 750.26
  submaxillary gland 527.1
  suprarenal (gland) 255.8
  tendon 727.9
  testis 608.89
    congenital 752.89
  thymic, thymus (congenital) (gland)
        254.0
  thyroid (gland) (*see also* Goiter) 240.9
    primary 242.0●
    secondary 242.2●
  toe (congenital) 755.65
    acquired 735.8
  tongue 529.8
    congenital 750.15
    frenum 529.8
    papillae (foliate) 529.3
  tonsil (faucial) (infective) (lingual)
        (lymphoid) 474.11
    with
        adenoiditis 474.01
        tonsillitis 474.00
            and adenoiditis 474.02
        and adenoids 474.10
  tunica vaginalis 608.89
  turbinate (mucous membrane) 478.0
  ureter 593.89
  urethra 599.84
  uterus 621.2
    puerperal, postpartum 674.8●
  uvula 528.9
  vagina 623.8
  vas deferens 608.89
  vein 459.89
  ventricle, ventricular (heart) (left)
        (right) - *see also* Hypertrophy,
        cardiac
    congenital 746.89
    due to hypertension (left) (right) (*see
        also* Hypertension, heart)
        402.90
        benign 402.10
        malignant 402.00
    right with ventricular septal defect,
        pulmonary stenosis or atresia,
        and dextraposition of aorta
        745.2
  verumontanum 599.89
  vesical 596.8
  vocal cord 478.5
  vulva 624.3
    stasis (nonfilarial) 624.3
Hypertropia (intermittent) (periodic)
        378.31
Hypertyrosinemia 270.2

Hyperuricemia 790.6
Hypervalinemia 270.3
Hyperventilation (tetany) 786.01
  hysterical 300.11
  psychogenic 306.1
  syndrome 306.1
Hyperviscidosis 277.00
Hyperviscosity (of serum) (syndrome)
        NEC 273.3
  polycythemic 289.0
  sclerocythemic 282.8
Hypervitaminosis (dietary) NEC 278.8
  A (dietary) 278.2
  D (dietary) 278.4
  from excessive administration or use of
        vitamin preparations (chronic)
        278.8
    reaction to sudden overdose 963.5
  vitamin A 278.2
    reaction to sudden overdose 963.5
  vitamin D 278.4
    reaction to sudden overdose 963.5
  vitamin K
    correct substance properly
        administered 278.8
    overdose or wrong substance
        given or taken 964.3
Hypervolemia 276.6
Hypesthesia (*see also* Disturbance,
        sensation) 782.0
  cornea 371.81
Hyphema (anterior chamber) (ciliary
        body) (iris) 364.41
  traumatic 921.3
Hyphemia - *see* Hyphema
Hypoacidity, gastric 536.8
  psychogenic 306.4
Hypoactive labyrinth (function) - *see*
        Hypofunction, labyrinth
Hypoadrenalism 255.41
  tuberculous (*see also* Tuberculosis)
        017.6●
Hypoadrenocorticism 255.41
  pituitary 253.4
Hypoalbuminemia 273.8
Hypoaldosteronism 255.42
Hypoalphalipoproteinemia 272.5
Hypobarism 993.2
Hypobaropathy 993.2
Hypobetalipoproteinemia (familial) 272.5
Hypocalcemia 275.41
  cow's milk 775.4
  dietary 269.3
  neonatal 775.4
  phosphate-loading 775.4
Hypocalcification, teeth 520.4
Hypochloremia 276.9
Hypochlorhydria 536.8
  neurotic 306.4
  psychogenic 306.4
Hypocholesteremia 272.5
Hypochondria (reaction) 300.7
Hypochondriac 300.7
Hypochondriasis 300.7
Hypochromasia blood cells 280.9
Hypochromic anemia 280.9
  due to blood loss (chronic) 280.0
    acute 285.1
  microcytic 280.9
Hypocoagulability (*see also* Defect,
        coagulation) 286.9
Hypocomplementemia 279.8
Hypocythemia (progressive) 284.9
Hypodontia (*see also* Anodontia) 520.0

◄ New   ◄▥ Revised   ~~deleted~~ Deleted   ● Use Additional Digit(s)   ▨ Omit code   **321**

Hypoeosinophilia 288.59
Hypoesthesia (*see also* Disturbance, sensation) 782.0
  cornea 371.81
  tactile 782.0
Hypoestrinism 256.39
Hypoestrogenism 256.39
Hypoferremia 280.9
  due to blood loss (chronic) 280.0
Hypofertility
  female 628.9
  male 606.1
Hypofibrinogenemia 286.3
  acquired 286.6
  congenital 286.3
Hypofunction
  adrenal (gland) 255.41
    cortex 255.41
    medulla 255.5
    specified NEC 255.5
  cerebral 331.9
  corticoadrenal NEC 255.41
  intestinal 564.89
  labyrinth (unilateral) 386.53
    with loss of labyrinthine reactivity 386.55
    bilateral 386.54
      with loss of labyrinthine reactivity 386.56
  Leydig cell 257.2
  ovary 256.39
    postablative 256.2
  pituitary (anterior) (gland) (lobe) 253.2
    posterior 253.5
  testicular 257.2
    iatrogenic 257.1
    postablative 257.1
    postirradiation 257.1
    postsurgical 257.1
Hypogammaglobulinemia 279.00
  acquired primary 279.06
  non-sex-linked, congenital 279.06
  sporadic 279.06
  transient of infancy 279.09
Hypogenitalism (congenital) (female) (male) 752.89
  penis 752.69
Hypoglycemia (spontaneous) 251.2
  coma 251.0
    diabetic 250.3●
      due to secondary diabetes 249.3●
    diabetic 250.8●
      due to secondary diabetes 249.8●
    due to insulin 251.0
      therapeutic misadventure 962.3
  familial (idiopathic) 251.2
  following gastrointestinal surgery 579.3
  infantile (idiopathic) 251.2
  in infant of diabetic mother 775.0
  leucine-induced 270.3
  neonatal 775.6
  reactive 251.2
  specified NEC 251.1
Hypoglycemic shock 251.0
  diabetic 250.8●
    due to secondary diabetes 249.8●
  due to insulin 251.0
  functional (syndrome) 251.1

Hypogonadism
  female 256.39
  gonadotrophic (isolated) 253.4
  hypogonadotropic (isolated) (with anosmia) 253.4
  isolated 253.4
  male 257.2
    hereditary familial (Reifenstein's syndrome) 259.52
  ovarian (primary) 256.39
  pituitary (secondary) 253.4
  testicular (primary) (secondary) 257.2
Hypohidrosis 705.0
Hypohidrotic ectodermal dysplasia 757.31
Hypoidrosis 705.0
Hypoinsulinemia, postsurgical 251.3
  postpancreatectomy (complete) (partial) 251.3
Hypokalemia 276.8
Hypokinesia 780.99
Hypoleukia splenica 289.4
Hypoleukocytosis 288.50
Hypolipidemia 272.5
Hypolipoproteinemia 272.5
Hypomagnesemia 275.2
  neonatal 775.4
Hypomania, hypomanic reaction (*see also* Psychosis, affective) 296.0●
  recurrent episode 296.1●
  single episode 296.0●
Hypomastia (congenital) 611.82
Hypomenorrhea 626.1
Hypometabolism 783.9
Hypomotility
  gastrointestinal tract 536.8
    psychogenic 306.4
  intestine 564.89
    psychogenic 306.4
  stomach 536.8
    psychogenic 306.4
Hyponasality 784.44 ◀▥
Hyponatremia 276.1
Hypo-ovarianism 256.39
Hypo-ovarism 256.39
Hypoparathyroidism (idiopathic) (surgically induced) 252.1
  neonatal 775.4
Hypopharyngitis 462
Hypophoria 378.40
Hypophosphatasia 275.3
Hypophosphatemia (acquired) (congenital) (familial) 275.3
  renal 275.3
Hypophyseal, hypophysis - *see also* condition
  dwarfism 253.3
  gigantism 253.0
  syndrome 253.8
Hypophyseothalamic syndrome 253.8
Hypopiesis - *see* Hypotension
Hypopigmentation 709.00
  eyelid 374.53
Hypopinealism 259.8
Hypopituitarism (juvenile) (syndrome) 253.2
  due to
    hormone therapy 253.7
    hypophysectomy 253.7
    radiotherapy 253.7
  postablative 253.7
  postpartum hemorrhage 253.2

Hypoplasia, hypoplasis 759.89
  adrenal (gland) 759.1
  alimentary tract 751.8
    lower 751.2
    upper 750.8
  anus, anal (canal) 751.2
  aorta 747.22
  aortic
    arch (tubular) 747.10
    orifice or valve with hypoplasia of ascending aorta and defective development of left ventricle (with mitral valve atresia) 746.7
  appendix 751.2
  areola 757.6
  arm (*see also* Absence, arm, congenital) 755.20
  artery (congenital) (peripheral) 747.60
    brain 747.81
    cerebral 747.81
    coronary 746.85
    gastrointestinal 747.61
    lower limb 747.64
    pulmonary 747.3
    renal 747.62
    retinal 743.58
    specified NEC 747.69
    spinal 747.82
    umbilical 747.5
    upper limb 747.63
  auditory canal 744.29
    causing impairment of hearing 744.02
  biliary duct (common) or passage 751.61
  bladder 753.8
  bone NEC 756.9
    face 756.0
    malar 756.0
    mandible 524.04
      alveolar 524.74
    marrow 284.9
      acquired (secondary) 284.89
      congenital 284.09
      idiopathic 284.9
    maxilla 524.03
      alveolar 524.73
    skull (*see also* Hypoplasia, skull) 756.0
  brain 742.1
    gyri 742.2
    specified part 742.2
  breast (areola) 611.82
  bronchus (tree) 748.3
  cardiac 746.89
    valve - *see* Hypoplasia, heart, valve
    vein 746.89
  carpus (*see also* Absence, carpal, congenital) 755.28
  cartilaginous 756.9
  cecum 751.2
  cementum 520.4
    hereditary 520.5
  cephalic 742.1
  cerebellum 742.2
  cervix (uteri) 752.49
  chin 524.06
  clavicle 755.51
  coccyx 756.19
  colon 751.2
  corpus callosum 742.2
  cricoid cartilage 748.3
  dermal, focal (Goltz) 757.39

◀ New   ◀▥ Revised   ~~deleted~~ Deleted   ● Use Additional Digit(s)   ▥ Omit code

Hypoplasia, hypoplasis (*Continued*)
digestive organ(s) or tract NEC 751.8
  lower 751.2
  upper 750.8
ear 744.29
  auricle 744.23
  lobe 744.29
  middle, except ossicles 744.03
    ossicles 744.04
  ossicles 744.04
enamel of teeth (neonatal) (postnatal)
    (prenatal) 520.4
  hereditary 520.5
endocrine (gland) NEC 759.2
endometrium 621.8
epididymis 752.89
epiglottis 748.3
erythroid, congenital 284.01
erythropoietic, chronic acquired 284.81
esophagus 750.3
Eustachian tube 744.24
eye (*see also* Microphthalmos) 743.10
  lid 743.62
face 744.89
  bone(s) 756.0
fallopian tube 752.19
femur (*see also* Absence, femur,
    congenital) 755.34
fibula (*see also* Absence, fibula,
    congenital) 755.37
finger (*see also* Absence, finger,
    congenital) 755.29
focal dermal 757.39
foot 755.31
gallbladder 751.69
genitalia, genital organ(s)
  female 752.89
    external 752.49
    internal NEC 752.89
  in adiposogenital dystrophy 253.8
  male 752.89
    penis 752.69
glottis 748.3
hair 757.4
hand 755.21
heart 746.89
  left (complex) (syndrome) 746.7
  valve NEC 746.89
    pulmonary 746.01
humerus (*see also* Absence, humerus,
    congenital) 755.24
hymen 752.49
intestine (small) 751.1
  large 751.2
iris 743.46
jaw 524.09
kidney(s) 753.0
labium (majus) (minus) 752.49
labyrinth, membranous 744.05
lacrimal duct (apparatus) 743.65
larynx 748.3
leg (*see also* Absence, limb, congenital,
    lower) 755.30
limb 755.4
  lower (*see also* Absence, limb,
    congenital, lower) 755.30
  upper (*see also* Absence, limb,
    congenital, upper) 755.20
liver 751.69
lung (lobe) 748.5
mammary (areolar) 611.82
mandibular 524.04
  alveolar 524.74
  unilateral condylar 526.89

Hypoplasia, hypoplasis (*Continued*)
maxillary 524.03
  alveolar 524.73
medullary 284.9
megakaryocytic 287.30
metacarpus (*see also* Absence,
    metacarpal, congenital) 755.28
metatarsus (*see also* Absence,
    metatarsal, congenital) 755.38
muscle 756.89
  eye 743.69
myocardium (congenital) (Uhl's
    anomaly) 746.84
nail(s) 757.5
nasolacrimal duct 743.65
nervous system NEC 742.8
neural 742.8
nose, nasal 748.1
ophthalmic (*see also* Microphthalmos)
    743.10
optic nerve 377.43
organ
  of Corti 744.05
  or site NEC - *see* Anomaly, by site
osseous meatus (ear) 744.03
ovary 752.0
oviduct 752.19
pancreas 751.7
parathyroid (gland) 759.2
parotid gland 750.26
patella 755.64
pelvis, pelvic girdle 755.69
penis 752.69
peripheral vascular system (congenital)
    NEC 747.60
  gastrointestinal 747.61
  lower limb 747.64
  renal 747.62
  specified NEC 747.69
  spinal 747.82
  upper limb 747.63
pituitary (gland) 759.2
pulmonary 748.5
  arteriovenous 747.3
  artery 747.3
  valve 746.01
punctum lacrimale 743.65
radioulnar (*see also* Absence, radius,
    congenital, with ulna) 755.25
radius (*see also* Absence, radius,
    congenital) 755.26
rectum 751.2
respiratory system NEC 748.9
rib 756.3
sacrum 756.19
scapula 755.59
shoulder girdle 755.59
skin 757.39
skull (bone) 756.0
  with
    anencephalus 740.0
    encephalocele 742.0
    hydrocephalus 742.3
      with spina bifida (*see also*
        Spina bifida) 741.0●
    microcephalus 742.1
spinal (cord) (ventral horn cell) 742.59
  vessel 747.82
spine 756.19
spleen 759.0
sternum 756.3
tarsus (*see also* Absence, tarsal,
    congenital) 755.38
testis, testicle 752.89

Hypoplasia, hypoplasis (*Continued*)
thymus (gland) 279.11
thyroid (gland) 243
  cartilage 748.3
tibiofibular (*see also* Absence, tibia,
    congenital, with fibula) 755.35
toe (*see also* Absence, toe, congenital)
    755.39
tongue 750.16
trachea (cartilage) (rings) 748.3
Turner's (tooth) 520.4
ulna (*see also* Absence, ulna, congenital)
    755.27
umbilical artery 747.5
ureter 753.29
uterus 752.3
vagina 752.49
vascular (peripheral) NEC (*see also*
    Hypoplasia, peripheral vascular
    system) 747.60
  brain 747.81
vein(s) (peripheral) NEC (*see also*
    Hypoplasia, peripheral vascular
    system) 747.60
  brain 747.81
  cardiac 746.89
  great 747.49
  portal 747.49
  pulmonary 747.49
  vena cava (inferior) (superior) 747.49
vertebra 756.19
vulva 752.49
zonule (ciliary) 743.39
zygoma 738.12
Hypopotassemia 276.8
Hypoproaccelerinemia (*see also* Defect,
    coagulation) 286.3
Hypoproconvertinemia (congenital) (*see
    also* Defect, coagulation) 286.3
Hypoproteinemia (essential)
    (hypermetabolic) (idiopathic) 273.8
Hypoproteinosis 260
Hypoprothrombinemia (congenital)
    (hereditary) (idiopathic) (*see also*
    Defect, coagulation) 286.3
  acquired 286.7
  newborn 776.3
Hypopselaphesia 782.0
Hypopyon (anterior chamber) (eye)
    364.05
  iritis 364.05
  ulcer (cornea) 370.04
Hypopyrexia 780.99
Hyporeflex 796.1
Hyporeninemia, extreme 790.99
  in primary aldosteronism 255.10
Hyporesponsive episode 780.09
Hyposecretion
  ACTH 253.4
  ovary 256.39
    postablative 256.2
  salivary gland (any) 527.7
Hyposegmentation of neutrophils,
    hereditary 288.2
Hyposiderinemia 280.9
Hyposmolality 276.1
  syndrome 276.1
Hyposomatotropism 253.3
Hyposomnia, unspecified (*see also*
    Insomnia) 780.52
  with sleep apnea, unspecified 780.51
Hypospadias (male) 752.61
  female 753.8
Hypospermatogenesis 606.1

◀ New   ◀▥ Revised   ~~deleted~~ Deleted   ● Use Additional Digit(s)   ▨ Omit code   **323**

◀ New   ◀▥ Revised   ~~deleted~~ Deleted   ● Use Additional Digit(s)   ▨ Omit code

I

Iatrogenic syndrome of excess cortisol 255.0
IBM (inclusion body myositis) 359.71 ◄
Iceland disease (epidemic neuromyasthenia) 049.8
Ichthyosis (congenita) 757.1
    acquired 701.1
    fetalis gravior 757.1
    follicularis 757.1
    hystrix 757.39
    lamellar 757.1
    lingual 528.6
    palmaris and plantaris 757.39
    simplex 757.1
    vera 757.1
    vulgaris 757.1
Ichthyotoxism 988.0
    bacterial (see also Poisoning, food) 005.9
Icteroanemia, hemolytic (acquired) 283.9
    congenital (see also Spherocytosis) 282.0
Icterus (see also Jaundice) 782.4
    catarrhal - see Icterus, infectious
    conjunctiva 782.4
        newborn 774.6
    epidemic - see Icterus, infectious
    febrilis - see Icterus, infectious
    fetus or newborn - see Jaundice, fetus or newborn
    gravis (see also Necrosis, liver) 570
        complicating pregnancy 646.7●
            affecting fetus or newborn 760.8
        fetus or newborn NEC 773.0
        obstetrical 646.7●
            affecting fetus or newborn 760.8
    hematogenous (acquired) 283.9
    hemolytic (acquired) 283.9
        congenital (see also Spherocytosis) 282.0
    hemorrhagic (acute) 100.0
        leptospiral 100.0
        newborn 776.0
        spirochetal 100.0
    infectious 070.1
        with hepatic coma 070.0
        leptospiral 100.0
        spirochetal 100.0
    intermittens juvenilis 277.4
    malignant (see also Necrosis, liver) 570
    neonatorum (see also Jaundice, fetus or newborn) 774.6
    pernicious (see also Necrosis, liver) 570
    spirochetal 100.0
Ictus solaris, solis 992.0
Id reaction (due to bacteria) 692.89
Ideation
    suicidal V62.84
Identity disorder 313.82
    dissociative 300.14
    gender role (child) 302.6
        adult 302.85
    psychosexual (child) 302.6
        adult 302.85
Idioglossia 307.9
Idiopathic - see condition
Idiosyncrasy (see also Allergy) 995.3
    drug, medicinal substance, and biological - see Allergy, drug
Idiot, idiocy (congenital) 318.2
    amaurotic (Bielschowsky) (-Jansky) (family) (infantile (late)) (juvenile (late)) (Vogt-Spielmeyer) 330.1
    microcephalic 742.1
    Mongolian 758.0
    oxycephalic 756.0

IEED (involuntary emotional expression disorder) 310.8
IFIS (intraoperative floppy iris syndrome) 364.81
IgE asthma 493.0●
Ileitis (chronic) (see also Enteritis) 558.9
    infectious 009.0
    noninfectious 558.9
    regional (ulcerative) 555.0
        with large intestine 555.2
    segmental 555.0
        with large intestine 555.2
    terminal (ulcerative) 555.0
        with large intestine 555.2
Ileocolitis (see also Enteritis) 558.9
    infectious 009.0
    regional 555.2
    ulcerative 556.1
Ileostomy status V44.2
    with complication 569.60
Ileotyphus 002.0
Ileum - see condition
Ileus (adynamic) (bowel) (colon) (inhibitory) (intestine) (neurogenic) (paralytic) 560.1
    arteriomesenteric duodenal 537.2
    due to gallstone (in intestine) 560.31
    duodenal, chronic 537.2
    following gastrointestinal surgery 997.4
    gallstone 560.31
    mechanical (see also Obstruction, intestine) 560.9
    meconium 777.1
        due to cystic fibrosis 277.01
    myxedema 564.89
    postoperative 997.4
    transitory, newborn 777.4
Iliac - see condition
Iliotibial band friction syndrome 728.89
Ill, louping 063.1
Illegitimacy V61.6
Illness - see also Disease
    factitious 300.19
        with
            combined psychological and physical signs and symptoms 300.19
            physical symptoms 300.19
            predominantly
                physical signs and symptoms 300.19
                psychological symptoms 300.16
        chronic (with physical symptoms) 301.51
    heart - see Disease, heart
    manic-depressive (see also Psychosis, affective) 296.80
    mental (see also Disorder, mental) 300.9
Imbalance 781.2
    autonomic (see also Neuropathy, peripheral, autonomic) 337.9
    electrolyte 276.9
        with
            abortion - see Abortion, by type, with metabolic disorder
            ectopic pregnancy (see also categories 633.0–633.9) 639.4
            hyperemesis gravidarum (before 22 completed weeks' gestation) 643.1●
            molar pregnancy (see also categories 630–632) 639.4

Imbalance (Continued)
    electrolyte (Continued)
        following
            abortion 639.4
            ectopic or molar pregnancy 639.4
        neonatal, transitory NEC 775.5
    endocrine 259.9
    eye muscle NEC 378.9
        heterophoria - see Heterophoria
    glomerulotubular NEC 593.89
    hormone 259.9
    hysterical (see also Hysteria) 300.10
    labyrinth NEC 386.50
    posture 729.90
    sympathetic (see also Neuropathy, peripheral, autonomic) 337.9
Imbecile, imbecility 318.0
    moral 301.7
    old age 290.9
    senile 290.9
    specified IQ - see IQ
    unspecified IQ 318.0
Imbedding, intrauterine device 996.32
Imbibition, cholesterol (gallbladder) 575.6
Imerslund (-Gräsbeck) syndrome (anemia due to familial selective vitamin B_{12} malabsorption) 281.1
Iminoacidopathy 270.8
Iminoglycinuria, familial 270.8
Immature - see also Immaturity
    personality 301.89
Immaturity 765.1●
    extreme 765.0●
    fetus or infant light-for-dates - see Light-for-dates
    lung, fetus or newborn 770.4
    organ or site NEC - see Hypoplasia
    pulmonary, fetus or newborn 770.4
    reaction 301.89
    sexual (female) (male) 259.0
Immersion 994.1
    foot 991.4
    hand 991.4
Immobile, immobility
    complete
        due to severe physical disability or frality 780.72
    intestine 564.89
    joint - see Ankylosis
    syndrome (paraplegic) 728.3
Immunization
    ABO
        affecting management of pregnancy 656.2●
            fetus or newborn 773.1
    complication - see Complications, vaccination
    Rh factor
        affecting management of pregnancy 656.1●
            fetus or newborn 773.0
        from transfusion 999.7
Immunodeficiency 279.3
    with
        adenosine-deaminase deficiency 279.2
        defect, predominant
            B-cell 279.00
            T-cell 279.10
        hyperimmunoglobulinemia 279.2
        lymphopenia, hereditary 279.2
        thrombocytopenia and eczema 279.12

Immunodeficiency (Continued)
 with (Continued)
  thymic
   aplasia 279.2
   dysplasia 279.2
  autosomal recessive, Swiss-type
    279.2
  common variable 279.06
  severe combined (SCID) 279.2
  to Rh factor
   affecting management of pregnancy
     656.1●
    fetus or newborn 773.0
  X-linked, with increased IgM 279.05
Immunotherapy, prophylactic V07.2
 antineoplastic V58.12
Impaction, impacted
 bowel, colon, rectum 560.30
  with hernia - see also Hernia, by site,
    with, obstruction
   gangrenous - see Hernia, by site,
     with gangrene
  by
    calculus 560.39
    gallstone 560.31
   fecal 560.39
   specified type NEC 560.39
 calculus - see Calculus
 cerumen (ear) (external) 380.4
 cuspid 520.6
 dental 520.6
 fecal, feces 560.39
  with hernia - see also Hernia, by site,
    with obstruction
   gangrenous - see Hernia, by site,
     with gangrene
 fracture - see Fracture, by site
 gallbladder - see Cholelithiasis
 gallstone(s) - see Cholelithiasis
   in intestine (any part) 560.31
 intestine(s) 560.30
  with hernia - see also Hernia, by site,
    with obstruction
   gangrenous - see Hernia, by site,
     with gangrene
  by
    calculus 560.39
    gallstone 560.31
   fecal 560.39
   specified type NEC 560.39
 intrauterine device (IUD) 996.32
 molar 520.6
 shoulder 660.4●
   affecting fetus or newborn 763.1
 tooth, teeth 520.6
 turbinate 733.99
Impaired, impairment (function)
 arm V49.1
  movement, involving
    musculoskeletal system V49.1
    nervous system V49.2
 auditory discrimination 388.43
 back V48.3
 body (entire) V49.89
 cognitive, mild, so stated 331.83
 combined visual hearing V49.85
 dual sensory V49.85
 glucose
  fasting 790.21
  tolerance test (oral) 790.22
 hearing (see also Deafness) 389.9
  combined with visual impairment
    V49.85
 heart - see Disease, heart

Impaired, impairment (Continued)
 kidney (see also Disease, renal)
   593.9
  disorder resulting from 588.9
   specified NEC 588.89
 leg V49.1
  movement, involving
    musculoskeletal system
     V49.1
    nervous system V49.2
 limb V49.1
  movement, involving
    musculoskeletal system
     V49.1
    nervous system V49.2
 liver 573.8
 mastication 524.9
 mild cognitive, so stated 331.83
 mobility
   ear ossicles NEC 385.22
   incostapedial joint 385.22
   malleus 385.21
 myocardium, myocardial (see also
    Insufficiency, myocardial)
    428.0
 neuromusculoskeletal NEC V49.89
   back V48.3
   head V48.2
   limb V49.2
   neck V48.3
   spine V48.3
   trunk V48.3
 rectal sphincter 787.99
 renal (see also Disease, renal) 593.9
  disorder resulting from 588.9
   specified NEC 588.89
 spine V48.3
 vision NEC 369.9
  both eyes NEC 369.3
  combined with hearing impairment
    V49.85
  moderate 369.74
   both eyes 369.25
    with impairment of lesser eye
      (specified as)
     blind, not further specified
       369.15
     low vision, not further
       specified 369.23
     near-total 369.17
     profound 369.18
     severe 369.24
     total 369.16
   one eye 369.74
    with vision of other eye
      (specified as)
     near-normal 369.75
     normal 369.76
  near-total 369.64
   both eyes 369.04
    with impairment of lesser eye
      (specified as)
     blind, not further specified
       369.02
     total 369.03
   one eye 369.64
    with vision of other eye
      (specified as)
     near-normal 369.65
     normal 369.66
   one eye 369.60
    with low vision of other eye
      369.10

Impaired, impairment (Continued)
 vision NEC (Continued)
  profound 369.67
   both eyes 369.08
    with impairment of lesser eye
      (specified as)
     blind, not further specified
       369.05
     near-total 369.07
     total 369.06
   one eye 369.67
    with vision of other eye
      (specified as)
     near-normal 369.68
     normal 369.69
  severe 369.71
   both eyes 369.22
    with impairment of lesser eye
      (specified as)
     blind, not further specified
       369.11
     low vision, not further
       specified 369.21
     near-total 369.13
     profound 369.14
     total 369.12
   one eye 369.71
    with vision of other eye
      (specified as)
     near-normal 369.72
     normal 369.73
  total
   both eyes 369.01
   one eye 369.61
    with vision of other eye
      (specified as)
     near-normal 369.62
     normal 369.63
Impaludism - see Malaria
Impediment, speech NEC 784.59 ◀|||
 psychogenic 307.9
 secondary to organic lesion 784.59 ◀|||
Impending
 cerebrovascular accident or attack 435.9
 coronary syndrome 411.1
 delirium tremens 291.0
 myocardial infarction 411.1
Imperception, auditory (acquired)
   (congenital) 389.9
Imperfect
 aeration, lung (newborn) 770.5
 closure (congenital)
  alimentary tract NEC 751.8
   lower 751.5
   upper 750.8
  atrioventricular ostium 745.69
  atrium (secundum) 745.5
   primum 745.61
  branchial cleft or sinus 744.41
  choroid 743.59
  cricoid cartilage 748.3
  cusps, heart valve NEC 746.89
   pulmonary 746.09
  ductus
   arteriosus 747.0
   Botalli 747.0
  ear drum 744.29
   causing impairment of hearing
     744.03
  endocardial cushion 745.60
  epiglottis 748.3
  esophagus with communication to
    bronchus or trachea 750.3
  Eustachian valve 746.89

◀ New   ◀||| Revised   ~~deleted~~ Deleted   ● Use Additional Digit(s)   ▨ Omit code

Imperfect (*Continued*)
 closure (*Continued*)
  eyelid 743.62
  face, facial (*see also* Cleft, lip) 749.10
  foramen
   Botalli 745.5
   ovale 745.5
  genitalia, genital organ(s) or system
   female 752.89
    external 752.49
    internal NEC 752.89
    uterus 752.3
   male 752.89
    penis 752.69
  glottis 748.3
  heart valve (cusps) NEC 746.89
  interatrial ostium or septum 745.5
  interauricular ostium or septum
   745.5
  interventricular ostium or septum
   745.4
  iris 743.46
  kidney 753.3
  larynx 748.3
  lens 743.36
  lip (*see also* Cleft, lip) 749.10
  nasal septum or sinus 748.1
  nose 748.1
  omphalomesenteric duct 751.0
  optic nerve entry 743.57
  organ or site NEC - *see* Anomaly,
   specified type, by site
  ostium
   interatrial 745.5
   interauricular 745.5
   interventricular 745.4
  palate (*see also* Cleft, palate) 749.00
  preauricular sinus 744.46
  retina 743.56
  roof of orbit 742.0
  sclera 743.47
  septum
   aortic 745.0
   aorticopulmonary 745.0
   atrial (secundum) 745.5
    primum 745.61
   between aorta and pulmonary
    artery 745.0
   heart 745.9
   interatrial (secundum) 745.5
    primum 745.61
   interauricular (secundum) 745.5
    primum 745.61
   interventricular 745.4
    with pulmonary stenosis or
     atresia, dextraposition of
     aorta, and hypertrophy
     of right ventricle 745.2
    in tetralogy of Fallot 745.2
   nasal 748.1
   ventricular 745.4
    with pulmonary stenosis or
     atresia, dextraposition of
     aorta, and hypertrophy
     of right ventricle 745.2
    in tetralogy of Fallot 745.2
  skull 756.0
   with
    anencephalus 740.0
    encephalocele 742.0
    hydrocephalus 742.3
     with spina bifida (*see also*
      Spina bifida) 741.0●
    microcephalus 742.1

Imperfect (*Continued*)
 closure (*Continued*)
  spine (with meningocele) (*see also*
   Spina bifida) 741.90
  thyroid cartilage 748.3
  trachea 748.3
  tympanic membrane 744.29
   causing impairment of hearing
    744.03
  uterus (with communication to
   bladder, intestine, or rectum)
   752.3
  uvula 749.02
   with cleft lip (*see also* Cleft,
    palate, with cleft lip)
    749.20
  vitelline duct 751.0
 development - *see* Anomaly, by site
 erection 607.84
 fusion - *see* Imperfect, closure
 inflation lung (newborn) 770.5
 intestinal canal 751.5
 poise 729.90
 rotation - *see* Malrotation
 septum, ventricular 745.4
Imperfectly descended testis 752.51
Imperforate (congenital) - *see also* Atresia
 anus 751.2
 bile duct 751.61
 cervix (uteri) 752.49
 esophagus 750.3
 hymen 752.42
 intestine (small) 751.1
  large 751.2
 jejunum 751.1
 pharynx 750.29
 rectum 751.2
 salivary duct 750.23
 urethra 753.6
 urinary meatus 753.6
 vagina 752.49
Impervious (congenital) - *see also* Atresia
 anus 751.2
 bile duct 751.61
 esophagus 750.3
 intestine (small) 751.1
  large 751.5
 rectum 751.2
 urethra 753.6
Impetiginization of other dermatoses
 684
Impetigo (any organism) (any site)
 (bullous) (circinate) (contagiosa)
 (neonatorum) (simplex) 684
 Bockhart's (superficial folliculitis)
  704.8
 external ear 684 *[380.13]*
 eyelid 684 *[373.5]*
 Fox's (contagiosa) 684
 furfuracea 696.5
 herpetiformis 694.3
  nonobstetrical 694.3
 staphylococcal infection 684
 ulcerative 686.8
 vulgaris 684
Impingement, soft tissue between teeth
 524.89
 anterior 524.81
 posterior 524.82
Implant, endometrial 617.9
Implantation
 anomalous - *see also* Anomaly, specified
  type, by site
  ureter 753.4

Implantation (*Continued*)
 cyst
  external area or site (skin) NEC
   709.8
  iris 364.61
  vagina 623.8
  vulva 624.8
 dermoid (cyst)
  external area or site (skin) NEC
   709.8
  iris 364.61
  vagina 623.8
  vulva 624.8
 placenta, low or marginal - *see* Placenta
  previa
Impotence (sexual) 607.84
 organic origin NEC 607.84
 psychogenic 302.72
Impoverished blood 285.9
Impression, basilar 756.0
Imprisonment V62.5
Improper
 development, infant 764.9●
Improperly tied umbilical cord (causing
 hemorrhage) 772.3
Impulses, obsessional 300.3
Impulsive ~~neurosis 300.3~~ 799.23   ◄▥
 neurosis 300.3   ◄
Impulsiveness 799.23   ◄
Inaction, kidney (*see also* Disease, renal)
 593.9
Inactive - *see* condition
Inadequate, inadequacy
 aesthetics of dental restoration
  525.67
 biologic 301.6
 cardiac and renal - *see* Hypertension,
  cardiorenal
 constitutional 301.6
 development
  child 783.40
  fetus 764.9●
   affecting management of
    pregnancy 656.5●
  genitalia
   after puberty NEC 259.0
   congenital - *see* Hypoplasia,
    genitalia
  lungs 748.5
  organ or site NEC - *see* Hypoplasia,
   by site
 dietary 269.9
 distance, interarch 524.28
 education V62.3
 environment
  economic problem V60.2
  household condition NEC V60.1
  poverty V60.2
  unemployment V62.0
 functional 301.6
 household care, due to
  family member
   handicapped or ill V60.4
   temporarily away from home
    V60.4
    on vacation V60.5
  technical defects in home V60.1
  temporary absence from home of
   person rendering care V60.4
 housing (heating) (space) V60.1
 interarch distance 524.28
 material resources V60.2
 mental (*see also* Retardation,
  mental) 319
 nervous system 799.29   ◄▥
 personality 301.6

Inadequate, inadequacy (Continued)
  prenatal care in current pregnancy
      V23.7
  pulmonary
      function 786.09
          newborn 770.89
      ventilation, newborn 770.89
  respiration 786.09
      newborn 770.89
  sample
      cytology
          anal 796.78
          cervical 795.08
          vaginal 795.18
  social 301.6
Inanition 263.9
  with edema 262
  due to
      deprivation of food 994.2
      malnutrition 263.9
  fever 780.60
Inappropriate secretion
  ACTH 255.0
  antidiuretic hormone (ADH)
      (excessive) 253.6
      deficiency 253.5
  ectopic hormone NEC 259.3
  pituitary (posterior) 253.6
Inattention after or at birth 995.52
Inborn errors of metabolism - see
      Disorder, metabolism
Incarceration, incarcerated
  bubonocele - see also Hernia, inguinal,
      with obstruction
      gangrenous - see Hernia, inguinal,
          with gangrene
  colon (by hernia) - see also Hernia, by
      site with obstruction
      gangrenous - see Hernia, by site,
          with gangrene
  enterocele 552.9
      gangrenous 551.9
  epigastrocele 552.29
      gangrenous 551.29
  epiplocele 552.9
      gangrenous 551.9
  exomphalos 552.1
      gangrenous 551.1
  fallopian tube 620.8
  hernia - see also Hernia, by site, with
      obstruction
      gangrenous - see Hernia, by site,
          with gangrene
  iris, in wound 871.1
  lens, in wound 871.1
  merocele (see also Hernia, femoral, with
      obstruction) 552.00
  omentum (by hernia) - see also Hernia,
      by site, with obstruction
      gangrenous - see Hernia, by site,
          with gangrene
  omphalocele 756.72   ◄▦
  rupture (meaning hernia) (see also
      Hernia, by site, with obstruction)
      552.9
      gangrenous (see also Hernia, by site,
          with gangrene) 551.9
  sarcoepiplocele 552.9
      gangrenous 551.9
  sarcoepiplomphalocele 552.1
      with gangrene 551.1
  uterus 621.8
      gravid 654.3●
          causing obstructed labor 660.2●
              affecting fetus or newborn
                  763.1

Incident, cerebrovascular (see also
      Disease, cerebrovascular, acute) 436
Incineration (entire body) (from fire,
      conflagration, electricity, or
      lightning) - see Burn, multiple,
      specified sites
Incised wound
  external - see Wound, open, by site
  internal organs (abdomen, chest, or
      pelvis) - see Injury, internal, by
      site, with open wound
Incision, incisional
  hernia - see Hernia, incisional
  surgical, complication - see
      Complications, surgical
      procedures
  traumatic
      external - see Wound, open, by site
      internal organs (abdomen, chest, or
          pelvis) - see Injury, internal, by
          site, with open wound
Inclusion
  azurophilic leukocytic 288.2
  blennorrhea (neonatal) (newborn)
      771.6
  cyst - see Cyst, skin
  gallbladder in liver (congenital) 751.69
Incompatibility
  ABO
      affecting management of pregnancy
          656.2●
      fetus or newborn 773.1
      infusion or transfusion reaction
          999.6
  blood (group) (Duffy) (E) (K(ell))
      (Kidd) (Lewis) (M) (N) (P) (S)
      NEC
      affecting management of pregnancy
          656.2●
      fetus or newborn 773.2
      infusion or transfusion reaction
          999.89   ◄▦
  contour of existing restoration of
      tooth
      with oral health 525.65
  marital V61.10
      involving
          divorce V61.03
          estrangement V61.09
  Rh (blood group) (factor)
      affecting management of pregnancy
          656.1●
      fetus or newborn 773.0
      infusion or transfusion reaction
          999.7
  Rhesus - see Incompatibility, Rh
Incompetency, incompetence,
      incompetent
  annular
      aortic (valve) (see also Insufficiency,
          aortic) 424.1
      mitral (valve) - (see also Insufficiency,
          mitral) 424.0
      pulmonary valve (heart) (see also
          Endocarditis, pulmonary)
          424.3
  aortic (valve) (see also Insufficiency,
      aortic) 424.1
      syphilitic 093.22
  cardiac (orifice) 530.0
  valve - see Endocarditis
  cervix, cervical (os) 622.5
      in pregnancy 654.5●
          affecting fetus or newborn
              761.0

Incompetency, incompetence, incompetent
      (Continued)
  chronotropic 426.89
      with
          autonomic dysfunction 337.9
          ischemic heart disease 414.9
          left ventricular dysfunction
              429.89   ◄▦
          sinus node dysfunction 427.81
  esophagogastric (junction) (sphincter)
      530.0
  heart valve, congenital 746.89
  mitral (valve) - see Insufficiency, mitral
  papillary muscle (heart) 429.81
  pelvic fundus
      pubocervical tissue 618.81
      rectovaginal tissue 618.82
  pulmonary valve (heart) (see also
      Endocarditis, pulmonary) 424.3
      congenital 746.09
  tricuspid (annular) (rheumatic) (valve)
      (see also Endocarditis, tricuspid)
      397.0
  valvular - see Endocarditis
  vein, venous (saphenous) (varicose)
      (see also Varicose, vein) 454.9
  velopharyngeal (closure)
      acquired 528.9
      congenital 750.29
Incomplete - see also condition
  bladder emptying 788.21
  expansion lungs (newborn) 770.5
  gestation (liveborn) - see Immaturity
  rotation - see Malrotation
Inconclusive   ◄
  image test due to excess body fat
      793.91   ◄
  mammogram, mammography 793.82 ◄
      due to dense breasts 793.82   ◄
Incontinence 788.30
  without sensory awareness 788.34
  anal sphincter 787.6
  continuous leakage 788.37
  feces 787.6
      due to hysteria 300.11
      nonorganic origin 307.7
  hysterical 300.11
  mixed (male) (female) (urge and stress)
      788.33
  overflow 788.38
  paradoxical 788.39
  rectal 787.6
  specified NEC 788.39
  stress (female) 625.6
      male NEC 788.32
  urethral sphincter 599.84
  urge 788.31
      and stress (male) (female) 788.33
  urine 788.30
      active 788.30
      due to
          cognitive impairment 788.91
          severe physical disability 788.91
          immobility 788.91
      functional 788.91
      male 788.30
          stress 788.32
              and urge 788.33
      neurogenic 788.39
      nonorganic origin 307.6
      stress (female) 625.6
          male NEC 788.32
      urge 788.31
          and stress 788.33
Incontinentia pigmenti 757.33

◄ New   ◄▦ Revised   ~~deleted~~ Deleted   ● Use Additional Digit(s)   ▓ Omit code

Incoordinate
uterus (action) (contractions) 661.4●
affecting fetus or newborn 763.7
Incoordination
esophageal-pharyngeal (newborn) 787.24
muscular 781.3
papillary muscle 429.81
Increase, increased
abnormal, in development 783.9
androgens (ovarian) 256.1
anticoagulants (antithrombin) (anti-VIIIa) (anti-IXa) (anti-Xa) (anti-XIa) 286.5
postpartum 666.3●
cold sense (see also Disturbance, sensation) 782.0
estrogen 256.0
function
adrenal (cortex) 255.3
medulla 255.6
pituitary (anterior) (gland) (lobe) 253.1
posterior 253.6
heat sense (see also Disturbance, sensation) 782.0
intracranial pressure 781.99
injury at birth 767.8
light reflex of retina 362.13
permeability, capillary 448.9
pressure
intracranial 781.99
injury at birth 767.8
intraocular 365.00
pulsations 785.9
pulse pressure 785.9
sphericity, lens 743.36
splenic activity 289.4
venous pressure 459.89
portal 572.3
Incrustation, cornea, lead, or zinc 930.0
Incyclophoria 378.44
Incyclotropia 378.33
Indeterminate sex 752.7
India rubber skin 756.83
Indicanuria 270.2
Indigestion (bilious) (functional) 536.8
acid 536.8
catarrhal 536.8
due to decomposed food NEC 005.9
fat 579.8
nervous 306.4
psychogenic 306.4
Indirect - see condition
Indolent bubo NEC 099.8
Induced
abortion - see Abortion, induced
birth, affecting fetus or newborn 763.89
delivery - see Delivery
labor - see Delivery
Induration, indurated
brain 348.89
breast (fibrous) 611.79
puerperal, postpartum 676.3●
broad ligament 620.8
chancre 091.0
anus 091.1
congenital 090.0
extragenital NEC 091.2
corpora cavernosa (penis) (plastic) 607.89
liver (chronic) 573.8
acute 573.8

Induration, indurated (Continued)
lung (black) (brown) (chronic) (fibroid) (see also Fibrosis, lung) 515
essential brown 275.0 [516.1]
penile 607.89
phlebitic - see Phlebitis
skin 782.8
stomach 537.89
Induratio penis plastica 607.89
Industrial - see condition
Inebriety (see also Abuse, drugs, nondependent) 305.0●
Inefficiency
kidney (see also Disease, renal) 593.9
thyroid (acquired) (gland) 244.9
Inelasticity, skin 782.8
Inequality, leg (acquired) (length) 736.81
congenital 755.30
Inertia
bladder 596.4
neurogenic 596.54
with cauda equina syndrome 344.61
stomach 536.8
psychogenic 306.4
uterus, uterine 661.2●
affecting fetus or newborn 763.7
primary 661.0●
secondary 661.1●
vesical 596.4
neurogenic 596.54
with cauda equina 344.61
Infant - see also condition
excessive crying of 780.92
fussy (baby) 780.91
held for adoption V68.89
newborn - see Newborn
post-term (gestation period over 40 completed weeks to 42 completed weeks) 766.21
prolonged gestation of (period over 42 completed weeks) 766.22
syndrome of diabetic mother 775.0
"Infant Hercules" syndrome 255.2
Infantile - see also condition
genitalia, genitals 259.0
in pregnancy or childbirth NEC 654.4●
affecting fetus or newborn 763.89
causing obstructed labor 660.2●
affecting fetus or newborn 763.1
heart 746.9
kidney 753.3
lack of care 995.52
macula degeneration 362.75
melanodontia 521.05
os, uterus (see also Infantile, genitalia) 259.0
pelvis 738.6
with disproportion (fetopelvic) 653.1●
affecting fetus or newborn 763.1
causing obstructed labor 660.1●
affecting fetus or newborn 763.1
penis 259.0
testis 257.2
uterus (see also Infantile, genitalia) 259.0
vulva 752.49
Infantilism 259.9
with dwarfism (hypophyseal) 253.3
Brissaud's (infantile myxedema) 244.9
celiac 579.0

Infantilism (Continued)
Herter's (nontropical sprue) 579.0
hypophyseal 253.3
hypothalamic (with obesity) 253.8
idiopathic 259.9
intestinal 579.0
pancreatic 577.8
pituitary 253.3
renal 588.0
sexual (with obesity) 259.0
Infants, healthy liveborn - see Newborn
Infarct, infarction
adrenal (capsule) (gland) 255.41
amnion 658.8●
anterior (with contiguous portion of intraventricular septum) NEC (see also Infarct, myocardium) 410.1●
appendices epiploicae 557.0
bowel 557.0
brain (stem) 434.91
embolic (see also Embolism, brain) 434.11
healed or old without residuals V12.54
iatrogenic 997.02
lacunar 434.91
late effect - see Late effect(s) (of) cerebrovascular disease
postoperative 997.02
puerperal, postpartum, childbirth 674.0●
thrombotic (see also Thrombosis, brain) 434.01
breast 611.89
Brewer's (kidney) 593.81
cardiac (see also Infarct, myocardium) 410.9●
cerebellar (see also Infarct, brain) 434.91
embolic (see also Embolism, brain) 434.11
cerebral (see also Infarct, brain) 434.91
aborted 434.91
embolic (see also Embolism, brain) 434.11
thrombotic (see also Infarct, brain) 434.01
chorion 658.8●
colon (acute) (agnogenic) (embolic) (hemorrhagic) (nonocclusive) (nonthrombotic) (occlusive) (segmental) (thrombotic) (with gangrene) 557.0
coronary artery (see also Infarct, myocardium) 410.9●
cortical 434.91
embolic (see also Embolism) 444.9
fallopian tube 620.8
gallbladder 575.8
heart (see also Infarct, myocardium) 410.9●
hepatic 573.4
impending (myocardium) 411.1
intestine (acute) (agnogenic) (embolic) (hemorrhagic) (nonocclusive) (nonthrombotic) (occlusive) (thrombotic) (with gangrene) 557.0
kidney 593.81
lacunar 434.91
liver 573.4

Infarct, infarction (Continued)
  lung (embolic) (thrombotic) 415.19
    with
      abortion - see Abortion, by type,
          with, embolism
      ectopic pregnancy (see also
          categories 633.0–633.9) 639.6
      molar pregnancy (see also
          categories 630–632) 639.6
    following
      abortion 639.6
      ectopic or molar pregnancy 639.6
    iatrogenic 415.11
    in pregnancy, childbirth, or
        puerperium - see Embolism,
        obstetrical
    postoperative 415.11
    septic 415.12
  lymph node or vessel 457.8
  medullary (brain) - see Infarct, brain
  meibomian gland (eyelid) 374.85
  mesentery, mesenteric (embolic)
      (thrombotic) (with gangrene)
      557.0
  midbrain - see Infarct, brain
  myocardium, myocardial (acute or
      with a stated duration of 8 weeks
      or less) (with hypertension)
      410.9●

Note 44   Use the following fifth-digit
subclassification with category 410:

0   episode unspecified
1   initial episode
2   subsequent episode without
          recurrence

---
    with symptoms after 8 weeks from
        date of infarction 414.8
    anterior (wall) (with contiguous
        portion of intraventricular
        septum) NEC 410.1●
    anteroapical (with contiguous
        portion of intraventricular
        septum) 410.1●
    anterolateral (wall) 410.0●
    anteroseptal (with contiguous
        portion of intraventricular
        septum) 410.1●
    apical-lateral 410.5●
    atrial 410.8●
    basal-lateral 410.5●
    chronic (with symptoms after 8
        weeks from date of infarction)
        414.8
    diagnosed on ECG, but presenting
        no symptoms 412
    diaphragmatic wall (with
        contiguous portion of
        intraventricular septum)
        410.4●
    healed or old, currently presenting
        no symptoms 412
    high lateral 410.5●
    impending 411.1
    inferior (wall) (with contiguous
        portion of intraventricular
        septum) 410.4●
    inferolateral (wall) 410.2●
    inferoposterior wall 410.3●
    intraoperative 997.1
    lateral wall 410.5●
    non-Q wave 410.7●

Infarct, infarction (Continued)
  myocardium, myocardial (Continued)
    non-ST elevation (NSTEMI) 410.7●
    nontransmural 410.7●
    papillary muscle 410.8●
    past (diagnosed on ECG or other
        special investigation, but
        currently presenting no
        symptoms) 412
      with symptoms NEC 414.8
    posterior (strictly) (true) (wall)
        410.6●
    posterobasal 410.6●
    posteroinferior 410.3●
    posterolateral 410.5●
    postprocedural 997.1
    previous, currently presenting no
        symptoms 412
    Q wave (see also Infarct,
        myocardium, by site) 410.9●
    septal 410.8●
    specified site NEC 410.8●
    ST elevation (STEMI) 410.9●
      anterior (wall) 410.1●
      anterolateral (wall) 410.0●
      inferior (wall) 410.4●
      inferolateral (wall) 410.2●
      inferoposterior wall 410.3●
      lateral wall 410.5●
      posterior (strictly) (true) (wall)
          410.6●
      specified site NEC 410.8●
    subendocardial 410.7●
    syphilitic 093.82
  non-ST elevation myocardial infarction
      (NSTEMI) 410.7●
  nontransmural 410.7●
  omentum 557.0
  ovary 620.8
  pancreas 577.8
  papillary muscle (see also Infarct,
      myocardium) 410.8●
  parathyroid gland 252.8
  pituitary (gland) 253.8
  placenta (complicating pregnancy)
      656.7●
    affecting fetus or newborn 762.2
  pontine - see Infarct, brain
  posterior NEC (see also Infarct,
      myocardium) 410.6●
  prostate 602.8
  pulmonary (artery) (hemorrhagic)
      (vein) 415.19
    with
      abortion - see Abortion, by type,
          with embolism
      ectopic pregnancy (see also
          categories 633.0–633.9)
          639.6
      molar pregnancy (see also
          categories 630–632) 639.6
    following
      abortion 639.6
      ectopic or molar pregnancy 639.6
    iatrogenic 415.11
    in pregnancy, childbirth, or
        puerperium - see Embolism,
        obstetrical
    postoperative 415.11
    septic 415.12
  renal 593.81
    embolic or thrombotic 593.81
  retina, retinal 362.84
    with occlusion - see Occlusion, retina

Infarct, infarction (Continued)
  spinal (acute) (cord) (embolic)
      (nonembolic) 336.1
  spleen 289.59
    embolic or thrombotic 444.89
  subchorionic - see Infarct, placenta
  subendocardial (see also Infarct,
      myocardium) 410.7●
  suprarenal (capsule) (gland) 255.41
  syncytium - see Infarct, placenta
  testis 608.83
  thrombotic (see also Thrombosis)
      453.9
    artery, arterial - see Embolism
  thyroid (gland) 246.3
  ventricle (heart) (see also Infarct,
      myocardium) 410.9●
Infecting - see condition
Infection, infected, infective
    (opportunistic) 136.9
  with lymphangitis - see Lymphangitis
  abortion - see Abortion, by type, with,
      sepsis
  abscess (skin) - see Abscess, by site
  Absidia 117.7
  acanthamoeba 136.21
  Acanthocheilonema (perstans) 125.4
    streptocerca 125.6
  accessory sinus (chronic) (see also
      Sinusitis) 473.9
  Achorion - see Dermatophytosis
  Acremonium falciforme 117.4
  acromioclavicular (joint) 711.91
  Actinobacillus
    lignieresii 027.8
    mallei 024
    muris 026.1
  Actinomadura - see Actinomycosis
  Actinomyces (israelii) - see also
      Actinomycosis
    muris-ratti 026.1
  Actinomycetales (Actinomadura)
      (Actinomyces) (Nocardia)
      (Streptomyces) - see
      Actinomycosis
  actinomycotic NEC (see also
      Actinomycosis) 039.9
  adenoid (chronic) 474.01
    acute 463
    and tonsil (chronic) 474.02
      acute or subacute 463
  adenovirus NEC 079.0
    in diseases classified elsewhere - see
        category 079
    unspecified nature or site 079.0
  Aerobacter aerogenes NEC 041.85
    enteritis 008.2
  Aerogenes capsulatus (see also
      Gangrene, gas) 040.0
  aertrycke (see also Infection,
      Salmonella) 003.9
  Ajellomyces dermatitidis 116.0
  alimentary canal NEC (see also
      Enteritis, due to, by organism)
      009.0
  Allescheria boydii 117.6
  Alternaria 118
  alveolus, alveolar (process) (pulpal
      origin) 522.4
  ameba, amebic (histolytica) (see also
      Amebiasis) 006.9
    acute 006.0
    chronic 006.1
    free-living 136.29

◀ New   ◀▥ Revised   ~~deleted~~ Deleted   ● Use Additional Digit(s)   ▨ Omit code

Infection, infected, infective (Continued)
  ameba, amebic (Continued)
    hartmanni 007.8
    specified
      site NEC 006.8
      type NEC 007.8
  amniotic fluid or cavity 658.4●
    affecting fetus or newborn 762.7
  anaerobes (cocci) (gram-negative)
    (gram-positive) (mixed) NEC
    041.84
  anal canal 569.49
  Ancylostoma braziliense 126.2
  Angiostrongylus cantonensis 128.8
  anisakiasis 127.1
  Anisakis larva 127.1
  anthrax (see also Anthrax) 022.9
  antrum (chronic) (see also Sinusitis,
    maxillary) 473.0
  anus (papillae) (sphincter) 569.49
  arbor virus NEC 066.9
  arbovirus NEC 066.9
  argentophil-rod 027.0
  Ascaris lumbricoides 127.0
  ascomycetes 117.4
  Aspergillus (flavus) (fumigatus)
    (terreus) 117.3
  atypical
    acid-fast (bacilli) (see also
      Mycobacterium, atypical)
      031.9
    mycobacteria (see also
      Mycobacterium, atypical)
      031.9
  auditory meatus (circumscribed)
    (diffuse) (external) (see also Otitis,
    externa) 380.10
  auricle (ear) (see also Otitis, externa)
    380.10
  axillary gland 683
  Babesiasis 088.82
  Babesiosis 088.82
  Bacillus NEC 041.89
    abortus 023.1
    anthracis (see also Anthrax) 022.9
    cereus (food poisoning) 005.89
    coli - see Infection, Escherichia coli
    coliform NEC 041.85
    Ducrey's (any location) 099.0
    Flexner's 004.1
    Friedländer's NEC 041.3
    fusiformis 101
    gas (gangrene) (see also Gangrene,
      gas) 040.0
    mallei 024
    melitensis 023.0
    paratyphoid, paratyphosus 002.9
      A 002.1
      B 002.2
      C 002.3
    Schmorl's 040.3
    Shiga 004.0
    suipestifer (see also Infection,
      Salmonella) 003.9
    swimming pool 031.1
    typhosa 002.0
    welchii (see also Gangrene, gas)
      040.0
    Whitmore's 025
  bacterial NEC 041.9
    specified NEC 041.89
      anaerobic NEC 041.84
      gram-negative NEC 041.85
        anaerobic NEC 041.84

Infection, infected, infective (Continued)
  Bacterium
    paratyphosum 002.9
      A 002.1
      B 002.2
      C 002.3
    typhosum 002.9
  Bacteroides (fragilis) (melaninogenicus)
    (oralis) NEC 041.82
  Balantidium coli 007.0
  Bartholin's gland 616.89
  Basidiobolus 117.7
  Bedsonia 079.98
    specified NEC 079.88
  bile duct 576.1
  bladder (see also Cystitis) 595.9
  Blastomyces, blastomycotic 116.0
    brasiliensis 116.1
    dermatitidis 116.0
    European 117.5
    loboi 116.2
    North American 116.0
    South American 116.1
  bleb
    postprocedural 379.60
      stage 1 379.61
      stage 2 379.62
      stage 3 379.63
  blood stream - see also Septicemia
    catheter-related (CRBSI) 999.31
  bone 730.9●
    specified - see Osteomyelitis
  Bordetella 033.9
    bronchiseptica 033.8
    parapertussis 033.1
    pertussis 033.0
  Borrelia
    bergdorfi 088.81
    vincentii (mouth) (pharynx) (tonsil)
      101
  bovine stomatitis 059.11
  brain (see also Encephalitis) 323.9
    late effect - see category 326
    membranes - (see also Meningitis)
      322.9
    septic 324.0
      late effect - see category 326
      meninges (see also Meningitis)
        320.9
  branchial cyst 744.42
  breast 611.0
    puerperal, postpartum 675.2●
      with nipple 675.9●
        specified type NEC 675.8●
      nonpurulent 675.2●
      purulent 675.1●
  bronchus (see also Bronchitis) 490
    fungus NEC 117.9
  Brucella 023.9
    abortus 023.1
    canis 023.3
    melitensis 023.0
    mixed 023.8
    suis 023.2
  Brugia (Wuchereria) malayi 125.1
  bursa - see Bursitis
  buttocks (skin) 686.9
  Candida (albicans) (tropicalis) (see also
    Candidiasis) 112.9
    congenital 771.7
  Candiru 136.8
  Capillaria
    hepatica 128.8
    philippinensis 127.5

Infection, infected, infective (Continued)
  cartilage 733.99
  cat liver fluke 121.0
  catheter-related bloodstream (CRBSI)
    999.31
  cellulitis - see Cellulitis, by site
  Cephalosporum falciforme 117.4
  Cercomonas hominis (intestinal) 007.3
  cerebrospinal (see also Meningitis) 322.9
    late effect - see category 326
  cervical gland 683
  cervix (see also Cervicitis) 616.0
  cesarean section wound 674.3●
  Chilomastix (intestinal) 007.8
  Chlamydia 079.98
    specified NEC 079.88
  Cholera (see also Cholera) 001.9
  chorionic plate 658.8●
  Cladosporium
    bantianum 117.8
    carrionii 117.2
    mansoni 111.1
    trichoides 117.8
    wernecki 111.1
  Clonorchis (sinensis) (liver) 121.1
  Clostridium (haemolyticum) (novyi)
    NEC 041.84
    botulinum 005.1
    histolyticum (see also Gangrene, gas)
      040.0
    oedematiens (see also Gangrene, gas)
      040.0
    perfringens 041.83
      due to food 005.2
    septicum (see also Gangrene, gas)
      040.0
    sordellii (see also Gangrene, gas)
      040.0
    welchii (see also Gangrene, gas)
      040.0
      due to food 005.2
  Coccidioides (immitis) (see also
    Coccidioidomycosis) 114.9
  coccus NEC 041.89
  colon (see also Enteritis, due to, by
    organism) 009.0
    bacillus - see Infection, Escherichia
      coli
  colostomy or enterostomy 569.61
  common duct 576.1
  complicating pregnancy, childbirth, or
    puerperium NEC 647.9●
    affecting fetus or newborn 760.2
  Condiobolus 117.7
  congenital NEC 771.89
    Candida albicans 771.7
    chronic 771.2
    Cytomegalovirus 771.1
    hepatitis, viral 771.2
    herpes simplex 771.2
    listeriosis 771.2
    malaria 771.2
    poliomyelitis 771.2
    rubella 771.0
    toxoplasmosis 771.2
    tuberculosis 771.2
    urinary (tract) 771.82
    vaccinia 771.2
  coronavirus 079.89
    SARS-associated 079.82
  corpus luteum (see also Salpingo-
    oophoritis) 614.2
  Corynebacterium diphtheriae - see
    Diphtheria

Infection, infected, infective (*Continued*)
cotia virus 059.8
Coxsackie (*see also* Coxsackie) 079.2
  endocardium 074.22
  heart NEC 074.20
  in diseases classified elsewhere - *see*
    category 079
  meninges 047.0
  myocardium 074.23
  pericardium 074.21
  pharynx 074.0
  specified disease NEC 074.8
  unspecified nature or site 079.2
Cryptococcus neoformans 117.5
Cryptosporidia 007.4
Cunninghamella 117.7
cyst - *see* Cyst
Cysticercus cellulosae 123.1
cytomegalovirus 078.5
  congenital 771.1
dental (pulpal origin) 522.4
deuteromycetes 117.4
Dicrocoelium dendriticum 121.8
Dipetalonema (perstans) 125.4
  streptocerca 125.6
diphtherial - *see* Diphtheria
Diphyllobothrium (adult) (latum)
  (pacificum) 123.4
  larval 123.5
Diplogonoporus (grandis) 123.8
Dipylidium (caninum) 123.8
Dirofilaria 125.6
dog tapeworm 123.8
Dracunculus medinensis 125.7
Dreschlera 118
  hawaiiensis 117.8
Ducrey's bacillus (any site) 099.0
due to or resulting from
  central venous catheter 999.31
  device, implant, or graft (any)
    (presence of) - *see*
    Complications, infection and
    inflammation, due to (presence
    of) any device, implant, or
    graft classified to 996.0–996.5
    NEC
  injection, inoculation, infusion,
    transfusion, or vaccination
    (prophylactic) (therapeutic)
    999.39
  injury NEC - *see* Wound, open, by
    site, complicated
  surgery 998.59
duodenum 535.6●
ear - *see also* Otitis
  external (*see also* Otitis, externa)
    380.10
  inner (*see also* Labyrinthitis) 386.30
  middle - *see* Otitis, media
Eaton's agent NEC 041.81
Eberthella typhosa 002.0
Ebola 078.89
echinococcosis 122.9
Echinococcus (*see also* Echinococcus)
  122.9
Echinostoma 121.8
ECHO virus 079.1
  in diseases classified elsewhere - *see*
    category 079
  unspecified nature or site 079.1
Ehrlichiosis 082.40
  chaffeensis 082.41
  specified type NEC 082.49
Endamoeba - *see* Infection, ameba

Infection, infected, infective (*Continued*)
endocardium (*see also* Endocarditis)
  421.0
endocervix (*see also* Cervicitis) 616.0
Entamoeba - *see* Infection, ameba
enteric (*see also* Enteritis, due to, by
  organism) 009.0
Enterobacter aerogenes NEC 041.85
Enterobacter sakazakii 041.85
Enterobius vermicularis 127.4
enterococcus NEC 041.04
enterovirus NEC 079.89
  central nervous system NEC 048
  enteritis 008.67
  meningitis 047.9
Entomophthora 117.7
Epidermophyton - *see* Dermatophytosis
epidermophytosis - *see*
  Dermatophytosis
episiotomy 674.3●
Epstein-Barr virus 075
  chronic 780.79 [139.8]
erysipeloid 027.1
Erysipelothrix (insidiosa)
  (rhusiopathiae) 027.1
erythema infectiosum 057.0
Escherichia coli NEC 041.4
  enteritis - *see* Enteritis, E. coli
  generalized 038.42
  intestinal - *see* Enteritis, E. coli
esophagostomy 530.86
ethmoidal (chronic) (sinus) (*see also*
  Sinusitis, ethmoidal) 473.2
Eubacterium 041.84
Eustachian tube (ear) 381.50
  acute 381.51
  chronic 381.52
exanthema subitum (*see also* Exanthem
  subitum) 058.10
external auditory canal (meatus) (*see*
  also Otitis, externa) 380.10
eye NEC 360.00
eyelid 373.9
  specified NEC 373.8
fallopian tube (*see also* Salpingo-
  oophoritis) 614.2
fascia 728.89
Fasciola
  gigantica 121.3
  hepatica 121.3
Fasciolopsis (buski) 121.4
fetus (intra-amniotic) - *see* Infection,
  congenital
filarial - *see* Infestation, filarial
finger (skin) 686.9
  abscess (with lymphangitis) 681.00
    pulp 681.01
  cellulitis (with lymphangitis)
    681.00
  distal closed space (with
    lymphangitis) 681.00
  nail 681.02
    fungus 110.1
fish tapeworm 123.4
  larval 123.5
flagellate, intestinal 007.9
fluke - *see* Infestation, fluke
focal
  teeth (pulpal origin) 522.4
  tonsils 474.00
    and adenoids 474.02
Fonsecaea
  compactum 117.2
  pedrosoi 117.2

Infection, infected, infective (*Continued*)
food (*see also* Poisoning, food) 005.9
foot (skin) 686.9
  fungus 110.4
Francisella tularensis (*see also*
  Tularemia) 021.9
frontal sinus (chronic) (*see also* Sinusitis,
  frontal) 473.1
fungus NEC 117.9
  beard 110.0
  body 110.5
  dermatiacious NEC 117.8
  foot 110.4
  groin 110.3
  hand 110.2
  nail 110.1
  pathogenic to compromised host
    only 118
  perianal (area) 110.3
  scalp 110.0
  scrotum 110.8
  skin 111.9
    foot 110.4
    hand 110.2
  toenails 110.1
  trachea 117.9
Fusarium 118
Fusobacterium 041.84
gallbladder (*see also* Cholecystitis,
  acute) 575.0
Gardnerella vaginalis 041.89
gas bacillus (*see also* Gas, gangrene)
  040.0
gastric (*see also* Gastritis) 535.5●
Gastrodiscoides hominis 121.8
gastroenteric (*see also* Enteritis, due to,
  by organism) 009.0
gastrointestinal (*see also* Enteritis, due
  to, by organism) 009.0
gastrostomy 536.41
generalized NEC (*see also* Septicemia)
  038.9
genital organ or tract NEC
  female 614.9
    with
      abortion - *see* Abortion, by
        type, with sepsis
      ectopic pregnancy (*see also*
        categories 633.0–633.9)
        639.0
      molar pregnancy (*see also*
        categories 630–632)
        639.0
    complicating pregnancy 646.6●
      affecting fetus or newborn
        760.8
    following
      abortion 639.0
      ectopic or molar pregnancy
        639.0
    puerperal, postpartum, childbirth
      670.8 ◀▦
      minor or localized 646.6●
        affecting fetus or newborn
        760.8
  male 608.4
genitourinary tract NEC 599.0
Ghon tubercle, primary (*see also*
  Tuberculosis) 010.0●
Giardia lamblia 007.1
gingival (chronic) 523.10
  acute 523.00
  Vincent's 101
glanders 024

◀ New   ◀▦ Revised   ~~deleted~~ Deleted   ● Use Additional Digit(s)   ▦ Omit code

Infection, infected, infective (*Continued*)
Glenosporopsis amazonica 116.2
Gnathostoma spinigerum 128.1
Gongylonema 125.6
gonococcal NEC (*see also* Gonococcus)
098.0
gram-negative bacilli NEC 041.85
anaerobic 041.84
guinea worm 125.7
gum (*see also* Infection, gingival) 523.10
Hantavirus 079.81
heart 429.89
Helicobacter pylori [H. pylori]
041.86 ◀▥
helminths NEC 128.9
intestinal 127.9
mixed (types classifiable to more
than one category in 120.0–
127.7) 127.8
specified type NEC 127.7
specified type NEC 128.8
Hemophilus influenzae NEC 041.5
generalized 038.41
Herpes (simplex) (*see also* Herpes,
simplex) 054.9
congenital 771.2
zoster (*see also* Herpes, zoster) 053.9
eye NEC 053.29
Heterophyes heterophyes 121.6
Histoplasma (*see also* Histoplasmosis)
115.90
capsulatum (*see also* Histoplasmosis,
American) 115.00
duboisii (*see also* Histoplasmosis,
African) 115.10
HIV V08
with symptoms, symptomatic 042
hookworm (*see also* Ancylostomiasis)
126.9
human herpesvirus 6 058.81
human herpesvirus 7 058.82
human herpesvirus 8 058.89
human herpesvirus NEC 058.89
human immunodeficiency virus V08
with symptoms, symptomatic 042
human papillomavirus 079.4
hydrocele 603.1
hydronephrosis 591
Hymenolepis 123.6
hypopharynx 478.29
inguinal glands 683
due to soft chancre 099.0
intestine, intestinal (*see also* Enteritis,
due to, by organism) 009.0
intrauterine (*see also* Endometritis)
615.9
complicating delivery 646.6●
isospora belli or hominis 007.2
Japanese B encephalitis 062.0
jaw (bone) (acute) (chronic) (lower)
(subacute) (upper) 526.4
joint - *see* Arthritis, infectious or
infective
Kaposi's sarcoma-associated
herpesvirus 058.89
kidney (cortex) (hematogenous) 590.9
with
abortion - *see* Abortion, by type,
with urinary tract infection
calculus 592.0
ectopic pregnancy (*see also*
categories 633.0–633.9) 639.8
molar pregnancy (*see also*
categories 630–632) 639.8

Infection, infected, infective (*Continued*)
kidney (*Continued*)
complicating pregnancy or
puerperium 646.6●
affecting fetus or newborn 760.1
following
abortion 639.8
ectopic or molar pregnancy 639.8
pelvis and ureter 590.3
Klebsiella pneumoniae NEC 041.3
knee (skin) NEC 686.9
joint - *see* Arthritis, infectious
Koch's (*see also* Tuberculosis,
pulmonary) 011.9●
labia (majora) (minora) (*see also*
Vulvitis) 616.10
lacrimal
gland (*see also* Dacryoadenitis)
375.00
passages (duct) (sac) (*see also*
Dacryocystitis) 375.30
larynx NEC 478.79
leg (skin) NEC 686.9
Leishmania (*see also* Leishmaniasis)
085.9
braziliensis 085.5
donovani 085.0
Ethiopica 085.3
furunculosa 085.1
infantum 085.0
Mexicana 085.4
tropica (minor) 085.1
major 085.2
Leptosphaeria senegalensis 117.4
Leptospira (*see also* Leptospirosis)
100.9
australis 100.89
bataviae 100.89
pyrogenes 100.89
specified type NEC 100.89
leptospirochetal NEC (*see also*
Leptospirosis) 100.9
Leptothrix - *see* Actinomycosis
Listeria monocytogenes (listeriosis)
027.0
congenital 771.2
liver fluke - *see* Infestation, fluke,
liver
Loa loa 125.2
eyelid 125.2 [373.6]
Loboa loboi 116.2
local, skin (staphylococcal)
(streptococcal) NEC 686.9
abscess - *see* Abscess, by site
cellulitis - *see* Cellulitis, by site
ulcer (*see also* Ulcer, skin) 707.9
Loefflerella
mallei 024
whitmori 025
lung 518.89
atypical Mycobacterium 031.0
tuberculous (*see also*
Tuberculosis,
pulmonary) 011.9●
basilar 518.89
chronic 518.89
fungus NEC 117.9
spirochetal 104.8
virus - *see* Pneumonia, virus
lymph gland (axillary) (cervical)
(inguinal) 683
mesenteric 289.2
lymphoid tissue, base of tongue or
posterior pharynx, NEC 474.00

Infection, infected, infective (*Continued*)
Madurella
grisea 117.4
mycetomii 117.4
major
with
abortion - *see* Abortion, by type,
with sepsis
ectopic pregnancy (*see also*
categories 633.0–633.9) 639.0
molar pregnancy (*see also*
categories 630–632) 639.0
following
abortion 639.0
ectopic or molar pregnancy
639.0
puerperal, postpartum,
childbirth 670.0 ◀▥
malarial - *see* Malaria
Malassezia furfur 111.0
Malleomyces
mallei 024
pseudomallei 025
mammary gland 611.0
puerperal, postpartum 675.2●
Mansonella (ozzardi) 125.5
mastoid (suppurative) - *see*
Mastoiditis
maxilla, maxillary 526.4
sinus (chronic) (*see also* Sinusitis,
maxillary) 473.0
mediastinum 519.2
medina 125.7
meibomian
cyst 373.12
gland 373.12
melioidosis 025
meninges (*see also* Meningitis) 320.9
meningococcal (*see also* condition)
036.9
brain 036.1
cerebrospinal 036.0
endocardium 036.42
generalized 036.2
meninges 036.0
meningococcemia 036.2
specified site NEC 036.89
mesenteric lymph nodes or glands
NEC 289.2
Metagonimus 121.5
metatarsophalangeal 711.97
methicillin
resistant Staphylococcus aureus
(MRSA) 041.12
susceptible Staphylococcus aureus
(MSSA) 041.11
microorganism resistant to drugs - *see*
Resistance (to), drugs by
microorganisms
Microsporidia 136.8
microsporum, microsporic - *see*
Dermatophytosis
mima polymorpha NEC 041.85
mixed flora NEC 041.89
Monilia (*see also* Candidiasis) 112.9
neonatal 771.7
monkeypox 059.01
Monosporium apiospermum 117.6
mouth (focus) NEC 528.9
parasitic 136.9
MRSA (methicillin resistant
Staphylococcus aureus) 041.12
MSSA (methicillin susceptible
Staphylococcus aureus) 041.11

◀ New   ◀▥ Revised   ~~deleted~~ Deleted   ● Use Additional Digit(s)   ▦ Omit code

Infection, infected, infective (*Continued*)
Mucor 117.7
muscle NEC 728.89
mycelium NEC 117.9
mycetoma
actinomycotic NEC (*see also*
Actinomycosis) 039.9
mycotic NEC 117.4
Mycobacterium, mycobacterial (*see also*
Mycobacterium) 031.9
Mycoplasma NEC 041.81
mycotic NEC 117.9
pathogenic to compromised host
only 118
skin NEC 111.9
systemic 117.9
myocardium NEC 422.90
nail (chronic) (with lymphangitis)
681.9
finger 681.02
fungus 110.1
ingrowing 703.0
toe 681.11
fungus 110.1
nasal sinus (chronic (*see also* Sinusitis)
473.9
nasopharynx (chronic) 478.29
acute 460
navel 686.9
newborn 771.4
Neisserian - *see* Gonococcus
Neotestudina rosatii 117.4
newborn, generalized 771.89
nipple 611.0
puerperal, postpartum 675.0●
with breast 675.9●
specified type NEC 675.8●
Nocardia - *see* Actinomycosis
nose 478.19
nostril 478.19
obstetrical surgical wound 674.3●
Oesophagostomum (apiostomum)
127.7
Oestrus ovis 134.0
Oidium albicans (*see also* Candidiasis)
112.9
Onchocerca (volvulus) 125.3
eye 125.3 [360.13]
eyelid 125.3 [373.6]
operation wound 998.59
Opisthorchis (felineus) (tenuicollis)
(viverrini) 121.0
orbit 376.00
chronic 376.10
orthopoxvirus 059.00
specified NEC 059.09
ovary (*see also* Salpingo-oophoritis)
614.2
Oxyuris vermicularis 127.4
pancreas 577.0
Paracoccidioides brasiliensis 116.1
Paragonimus (westermani) 121.2
parainfluenza virus 079.89
parameningococcus NEC 036.9
with meningitis 036.0
parapoxvirus 059.10
specified NEC 059.19
parasitic NEC 136.9
paratyphoid 002.9
type A 002.1
type B 002.2
type C 002.3
paraurethral ducts 597.89
parotid gland 527.2

Infection, infected, infective (*Continued*)
Pasteurella NEC 027.2
multocida (cat-bite) (dog-bite)
027.2
pestis (*see also* Plague) 020.9
pseudotuberculosis 027.2
septica (cat-bite) (dog-bite) 027.2
tularensis (*see also* Tularemia) 021.9
pelvic, female (*see also* Disease, pelvis,
inflammatory) 614.9
penis (glans) (retention) NEC 607.2
herpetic 054.13
Peptococcus 041.84
Peptostreptococcus 041.84
periapical (pulpal origin) 522.4
peridental 523.30
perineal wound (obstetrical) 674.3●
periodontal 523.31
periorbital 376.00
chronic 376.10
perirectal 569.49
perirenal (*see also* Infection, kidney)
590.9
peritoneal (*see also* Peritonitis) 567.9
periureteral 593.89
periurethral 597.89
Petriellidium boydii 117.6
pharynx 478.29
Coxsackie virus 074.0
phlegmonous 462
posterior, lymphoid 474.00
Phialophora
gougerotii 117.8
jeanselmei 117.8
verrucosa 117.2
Piedraia hortai 111.3
pinna, acute 380.11
pinta 103.9
intermediate 103.1
late 103.2
mixed 103.3
primary 103.0
pinworm 127.4
pityrosporum furfur 111.0
pleuropneumonia-like organisms NEC
(PPLO) 041.81
pneumococcal NEC 041.2
generalized (purulent) 038.2
Pneumococcus NEC 041.2
postoperative wound 998.59
posttraumatic NEC 958.3
postvaccinal 999.39
poxvirus 059.9
specified NEC 059.8
prepuce NEC 607.1
Proprionibacterium 041.84
prostate (capsule) (*see also* Prostatitis)
601.9
Proteus (mirabilis) (morganii)
(vulgaris) NEC 041.6
enteritis 008.3
protozoal NEC 136.8
intestinal NEC 007.9
Pseudomonas NEC 041.7
mallei 024
pneumonia 482.1
pseudomallei 025
psittacosis 073.9
puerperal, postpartum (major) 670.0 ◀▥
minor 646.6●
pulmonary - *see* Infection, lung
purulent - *see* Abscess
putrid, generalized - *see* Septicemia
pyemic - *see* Septicemia

Infection, infected, infective (*Continued*)
Pyrenochaeta romeroi 117.4
Q fever 083.0
rabies 071
rectum (sphincter) 569.49
renal (*see also* Infection, kidney) 590.9
pelvis and ureter 590.3
resistant to drugs - *see* Resistance (to),
drugs by microorganisms
respiratory 519.8
chronic 519.8
influenzal (acute) (upper) 487.1
lung 518.89
rhinovirus 460
syncytial virus 079.6
upper (acute) (infectious) NEC
465.9
with flu, grippe, or influenza
487.1
influenzal 487.1
multiple sites NEC 465.8
streptococcal 034.0
viral NEC 465.9
respiratory syncytial virus (RSV)
079.6
resulting from presence of shunt or
other internal prosthetic device -
see Complications, infection and
inflammation, due to (presence
of) any device, implant, or graft
classified to 996.0–996.5 NEC
retroperitoneal 567.39
retrovirus 079.50
human immunodeficiency virus
type 2 [HIV 2] 079.53
human T-cell lymphotrophic virus
type I [HTLV-I] 079.51
human T-cell lymphotrophic virus
type II [HTLV-II] 079.52
specified NEC 079.59
Rhinocladium 117.1
Rhinosporidium (seeberi) 117.0
rhinovirus
in diseases classified elsewhere - *see*
category 079
unspecified nature or site 079.3
Rhizopus 117.7
rickettsial 083.9
rickettsialpox 083.2
rubella (*see also* Rubella) 056.9
congenital 771.0
Saccharomyces (*see also* Candidiasis)
112.9
Saksenaea 117.7
salivary duct or gland (any) 527.2
Salmonella (aertrycke) (callinarum)
(choleraesuis) (enteritidis)
(suipestifer) (typhimurium)
003.9
with
arthritis 003.23
gastroenteritis 003.0
localized infection 003.20
specified type NEC 003.29
meningitis 003.21
osteomyelitis 003.24
pneumonia 003.22
septicemia 003.1
specified manifestation NEC
003.8
due to food (poisoning) (any
serotype) (*see also* Poisoning,
food, due to, Salmonella)
hirschfeldii 002.3

◀ New   ◀▥ Revised   ~~deleted~~ Deleted   ● Use Additional Digit(s)   ▨ Omit code

Infection, infected, infective (Continued)
  Salmonella (Continued)
    localized 003.20
      specified type NEC 003.29
    paratyphi 002.9
      A 002.1
      B 002.2
      C 002.3
    schottmuelleri 002.2
    specified type NEC 003.8
    typhi 002.0
    typhosa 002.0
  saprophytic 136.8
  Sarcocystis, lindemanni 136.5
  SARS-associated coronavirus 079.82
  scabies 133.0
  Schistosoma - see Infestation,
    Schistosoma
  Schmorl's bacillus 040.3
  scratch or other superficial injury - see
    Injury, superficial, by site
  scrotum (acute) NEC 608.4
  sealpox 059.12
  secondary, burn or open wound
    (dislocation) (fracture) 958.3
  seminal vesicle (see also Vesiculitis)
    608.0
  septic
    generalized - see Septicemia
    localized, skin (see also Abscess)
      682.9
  septicemic - see Septicemia
  seroma 998.51
  Serratia (marcescens) 041.85
    generalized 038.44
  sheep liver fluke 121.3
  Shigella 004.9
    boydii 004.2
    dysenteriae 004.0
    Flexneri 004.1
    group
      A 004.0
      B 004.1
      C 004.2
      D 004.3
    Schmitz (-Stutzer) 004.0
    Schmitzii 004.0
    Shiga 004.0
    Sonnei 004.3
    specified type NEC 004.8
  Sin Nombre virus 079.81
  sinus (see also Sinusitis) 473.9
    pilonidal 685.1
      with abscess 685.0
    skin NEC 686.9
  Skene's duct or gland (see also
    Urethritis) 597.89
  skin (local) (staphylococcal)
    (streptococcal) NEC 686.9
    abscess - see Abscess, by site
    cellulitis - see Cellulitis, by site
    due to fungus 111.9
      specified type NEC 111.8
    mycotic 111.9
      specified type NEC 111.8
    ulcer (see also Ulcer, skin) 707.9
  slow virus 046.9
    specified condition NEC 046.8
  Sparganum (mansoni) (proliferum)
    123.5
  spermatic cord NEC 608.4
  sphenoidal (chronic) (sinus) (see also
    Sinusitis, sphenoidal) 473.3
  Spherophorus necrophorus 040.3

Infection, infected, infective (Continued)
  spinal cord NEC (see also Encephalitis)
    323.9
    abscess 324.1
      late effect - see category 326
    late effect - see category 326
    meninges - see Meningitis
    streptococcal 320.2
  Spirillum
    minus or minor 026.0
    morsus muris 026.0
    obermeieri 087.0
  spirochetal NEC 104.9
    lung 104.8
    specified nature or site NEC
      104.8
  spleen 289.59
  Sporothrix schenckii 117.1
  Sporotrichum (schenckii) 117.1
  Sporozoa 136.8
  staphylococcal NEC 041.10
    aureus 041.11
      methicillin
        resistant (MRSA) 041.12
        susceptible MSSA) 041.11
    food poisoning 005.0
    generalized (purulent) 038.10
      aureus 038.11
        methicillin
          resistant 038.12
          susceptible 038.11
      specified organism NEC 038.19
    pneumonia 482.40
      aureus 482.41
        methicillin
          resistant (MRSA) 482.42
          susceptible (MSSA)
            482.41
      MRSA (methicillin resistant
        staphylococcus aureus)
        482.42
      MSSA (methicillin susceptible
        staphylococcus aureus)
        482.41
      specified type NEC 482.49
    septicemia 038.10
      aureus 038.11
        methicillin
          resistant (MRSA) 038.12
          susceptible (MSSA) 038.11
      MRSA (methicillin resistant
        staphylococcus aureus)
        038.12
      MSSA (methicillin susceptible
        staphylococcus aureus)
        038.11
      specified organism NEC 038.19
    specified NEC 041.19
  steatoma 706.2
  Stellantchasmus falcatus 121.6
  Streptobacillus moniliformis 026.1
  streptococcal NEC 041.00
    generalized (purulent) 038.0
    group
      A 041.01
      B 041.02
      C 041.03
      D [enterococcus] 041.04
      G 041.05
    pneumonia - see Pneumonia,
      streptococcal
    septicemia 038.0
    sore throat 034.0
    specified NEC 041.09

Infection, infected, infective (Continued)
  Streptomyces - see Actinomycosis
  streptotrichosis - see Actinomycosis
  Strongyloides (stercoralis) 127.2
  stump (amputation) (posttraumatic)
    (surgical) 997.62
    traumatic - see Amputation,
      traumatic, by site, complicated
  subcutaneous tissue, local NEC 686.9
  submaxillary region 528.9
  suipestifer (see also Infection,
    Salmonella) 003.9
  swimming pool bacillus 031.1
  syphilitic - see Syphilis
  systemic - see Septicemia
  Taenia - see Infestation, Taenia
  Taeniarhynchus saginatus 123.2
  tanapox 059.21
  tapeworm - see Infestation, tapeworm
  tendon (sheath) 727.89
  Ternidens diminutus 127.7
  testis (see also Orchitis) 604.90
  thigh (skin) 686.9
  threadworm 127.4
  throat 478.29
    pneumococcal 462
    staphylococcal 462
    streptococcal 034.0
    viral NEC (see also Pharyngitis) 462
  thumb (skin) 686.9
    abscess (with lymphangitis)
      681.00
      pulp 681.01
    cellulitis (with lymphangitis)
      681.00
    nail 681.02
  thyroglossal duct 529.8
  toe (skin) 686.9
    abscess (with lymphangitis)
      681.10
    cellulitis (with lymphangitis)
      681.10
    nail 681.11
      fungus 110.1
  tongue NEC 529.0
    parasitic 112.0
  tonsil (faucial) (lingual) (pharyngeal)
    474.00
    acute or subacute 463
    and adenoid 474.02
    tag 474.00
  tooth, teeth 522.4
    periapical (pulpal origin) 522.4
    peridental 523.30
    periodontal 523.31
    pulp 522.0
    socket 526.5
  TORCH - see Infection, congenital
    NEC
    without active infection 760.2
  Torula histolytica 117.5
  Toxocara (cani) (cati) (felis) 128.0
  Toxoplasma gondii (see also
    Toxoplasmosis) 130.9
  trachea, chronic 491.8
    fungus 117.9
  traumatic NEC 958.3
  trematode NEC 121.9
  trench fever 083.1
  Treponema
    denticola 041.84
    macrodenticum 041.84
    pallidum (see also Syphilis) 097.9
  Trichinella (spiralis) 124

Infection, infected, infective (*Continued*)
 Trichomonas 131.9
  bladder 131.09
  cervix 131.09
  hominis 007.3
  intestine 007.3
  prostate 131.03
  specified site NEC 131.8
  urethra 131.02
  urogenitalis 131.00
  vagina 131.01
  vulva 131.01
 Trichophyton, trichophytid - *see* Dermatophytosis
 Trichosporon (beigelii) cutaneum 111.2
 Trichostrongylus 127.6
 Trichuris (trichiuria) 127.3
 Trombicula (irritans) 133.8
 Trypanosoma (*see also* Trypanosomiasis) 086.9
  cruzi 086.2
 tubal (*see also* Salpingo-oophoritis) 614.2
 tuberculous NEC (*see also* Tuberculosis) 011.9●
 tubo-ovarian (*see also* Salpingo-oophoritis) 614.2
 tunica vaginalis 608.4
 tympanic membrane - *see* Myringitis
 typhoid (abortive) (ambulant) (bacillus) 002.0
 typhus 081.9
  flea-borne (endemic) 081.0
  louse-borne (epidemic) 080
  mite-borne 081.2
  recrudescent 081.1
  tick-borne 082.9
   African 082.1
   North Asian 082.2
 umbilicus (septic) 686.9
  newborn NEC 771.4
 ureter 593.89
 urethra (*see also* Urethritis) 597.80
 urinary (tract) NEC 599.0
  with
   abortion - *see* Abortion, by type, with urinary tract infection
   ectopic pregnancy (*see also* categories 633.0–633.9) 639.8
   molar pregnancy (*see also* categories 630–632) 639.8
  candidal 112.2
  complicating pregnancy, childbirth, or puerperium 646.6●
   affecting fetus or newborn 760.1
   asymptomatic 646.5●
    affecting fetus or newborn 760.1
  diplococcal (acute) 098.0
   chronic 098.2
  due to Trichomonas (vaginalis) 131.00
  following
   abortion 639.8
   ectopic or molar pregnancy 639.8
  gonococcal (acute) 098.0
   chronic or duration of 2 months or over 098.2
  newborn 771.82
  trichomonal 131.00
  tuberculous (*see also* Tuberculosis) 016.3●
 uterus, uterine (*see also* Endometritis) 615.9

Infection, infected, infective (*Continued*)
 utriculus masculinus NEC 597.89
 vaccination 999.39
 vagina (granulation tissue) (wall) (*see also* Vaginitis) 616.10
 varicella 052.9
 varicose veins - *see* Varicose, veins
 variola 050.9
  major 050.0
  minor 050.1
 vas deferens NEC 608.4
 Veillonella 041.84
 verumontanum 597.89
 vesical (*see also* Cystitis) 595.9
 Vibrio
  cholerae 001.0
   El Tor 001.1
  parahaemolyticus (food poisoning) 005.4
  vulnificus 041.85
 Vincent's (gums) (mouth) (tonsil) 101
 virus, viral 079.99
  adenovirus
   in diseases classified elsewhere - *see* category 079
   unspecified nature or site 079.0
  central nervous system NEC 049.9
   enterovirus 048
    meningitis 047.9
     specified type NEC 047.8
    slow virus 046.9
     specified condition NEC 046.8
  chest 519.8
  conjunctivitis 077.99
   specified type NEC 077.89
  coronavirus 079.89
   SARS-associated 079.82
  Coxsackie (*see also* Infection, Coxsackie) 079.2
  Ebola 065.8
  ECHO
   in diseases classified elsewhere - *see* category 079
   unspecified nature or site 079.1
  encephalitis 049.9
   arthropod-borne NEC 064
   tick-borne 063.9
    specified type NEC 063.8
  enteritis NEC (*see also* Enteritis, viral) 008.8
  exanthem NEC 057.9
  Hantavirus 079.81
  human papilloma 079.4
  in diseases classified elsewhere - *see* category 079
  intestine (*see also* Enteritis, viral) 008.8
  lung - *see* Pneumonia, viral
  respiratory syncytial (RSV) 079.6
  Retrovirus 079.50
  rhinovirus
   in diseases classified elsewhere - *see* category 079
   unspecified nature or site 079.3
  salivary gland disease 078.5
  slow 046.9
   specified condition NEC 046.8
  specified type NEC 079.89
   in diseases classified elsewhere - *see* category 079
  unspecified nature or site 079.99
  warts 078.10
   specified NEC 078.19
  yaba monkey tumor 059.22

Infection, infected, infective (*Continued*)
 vulva (*see also* Vulvitis) 616.10
 whipworm 127.3
 Whitmore's bacillus 025
 wound (local) (posttraumatic) NEC 958.3
  with
   dislocation - *see* Dislocation, by site, open
   fracture - *see* Fracture, by site, open
   open wound - *see* Wound, open, by site, complicated
  postoperative 998.59
  surgical 998.59
 Wuchereria 125.0
  bancrofti 125.0
  malayi 125.1
 yaba monkey tumor virus 059.22
 yatapoxvirus 059.20
 yaws - *see* Yaws
 yeast (*see also* Candidiasis) 112.9
 yellow fever (*see also* Fever, yellow) 060.9
 Yersinia pestis (*see also* Plague) 020.9
 Zeis' gland 373.12
 zoonotic bacterial NEC 027.9
 Zopfia senegalensis 117.4
Infective, infectious - *see* condition
Inferiority complex 301.9
 constitutional psychopathic 301.9
Infertility
 female 628.9
  age related 628.8
  associated with
   adhesions, peritubal 614.6 [628.2]
   anomaly
    cervical mucus 628.4
    congenital
     cervix 628.4
     fallopian tube 628.2
     uterus 628.3
     vagina 628.4
   anovulation 628.0
   dysmucorrhea 628.4
   endometritis, tuberculous (*see also* Tuberculosis) 016.7● [628.3]
   Stein-Leventhal syndrome 256.4 [628.0]
  due to
   adiposogenital dystrophy 253.8 [628.1]
   anterior pituitary disorder NEC 253.4 [628.1]
    hyperfunction 253.1 [628.1]
   cervical anomaly 628.4
   fallopian tube anomaly 628.2
   ovarian failure 256.39 [628.0]
   Stein-Leventhal syndrome 256.4 [628.0]
   uterine anomaly 628.3
   vaginal anomaly 628.4
  nonimplantation 628.3
  origin
   cervical 628.4
   pituitary-hypothalamus NEC 253.8 [628.1]
    anterior pituitary NEC 253.4 [628.1]
     hyperfunction NEC 253.1 [628.1]
    dwarfism 253.3 [628.1]
    panhypopituitarism 253.2 [628.1]

◀ New   ◀▥ Revised   ~~deleted~~ Deleted   ● Use Additional Digit(s)   ▨ Omit code

Infertility (Continued)
  female (Continued)
    origin (Continued)
      specified NEC 628.8
      tubal (block) (occlusion)
          (stenosis) 628.2
        adhesions 614.6 [628.2]
      uterine 628.3
      vaginal 628.4
    previous, requiring supervision of
        pregnancy V23.0
  male 606.9
    absolute 606.0
    due to
      azoospermia 606.0
      drug therapy 606.8
      extratesticular cause NEC
          606.8
      germinal cell
        aplasia 606.0
        desquamation 606.1
      hypospermatogenesis 606.1
      infection 606.8
      obstruction, afferent ducts 606.8
      oligospermia 606.1
      radiation 606.8
      spermatogenic arrest (complete)
          606.0
        incomplete 606.1
      systemic disease 606.8
Infestation 134.9
  Acanthocheilonema (perstans)
      125.4
    streptocerca 125.6
  Acariasis 133.9
    demodex folliculorum 133.8
    sarcoptes scabiei 133.0
    trombiculae 133.8
  Agamofilaria streptocerca 125.6
  Ancylostoma, Ankylostoma 126.9
    americanum 126.1
    braziliense 126.2
    canium 126.8
    ceylanicum 126.3
    duodenale 126.0
    new world 126.1
    old world 126.0
  Angiostrongylus cantonensis 128.8
  anisakiasis 127.1
  Anisakis larva 127.1
  arthropod NEC 134.1
  Ascaris lumbricoides 127.0
  Bacillus fusiformis 101
  Balantidium coli 007.0
  beef tapeworm 123.2
  Bothriocephalus (latus) 123.4
    larval 123.5
  broad tapeworm 123.4
    larval 123.5
  Brugia malayi 125.1
  Candiru 136.8
  Capillaria
    hepatica 128.8
    philippinensis 127.5
  cat liver fluke 121.0
  Cercomonas hominis (intestinal)
      007.3
  cestodes 123.9
    specified type NEC 123.8
  chigger 133.8
  chigoe 134.1
  Chilomastix 007.8
  Clonorchis (sinensis) (liver) 121.1
  coccidia 007.2

Infestation (Continued)
  complicating pregnancy, childbirth, or
      puerperium 647.9●
    affecting fetus or newborn 760.8
  Cysticercus cellulosae 123.1
  Demodex folliculorum 133.8
  Dermatobia (hominis) 134.0
  Dibothriocephalus (latus) 123.4
    larval 123.5
  Dicrocoelium dendriticum 121.8
  Diphyllobothrium (adult) (intestinal)
      (latum) (pacificum) 123.4
    larval 123.5
  Diplogonoporus (grandis) 123.8
  Dipylidium (caninum) 123.8
  Distoma hepaticum 121.3
  dog tapeworm 123.8
  Dracunculus medinensis 125.7
  dragon worm 125.7
  dwarf tapeworm 123.6
  Echinococcus (see also Echinococcus)
      122.9
  Echinostoma ilocanum 121.8
  Embadomonas 007.8
  Endamoeba (histolytica) - see Infection,
      ameba
  Entamoeba (histolytica) - see Infection,
      ameba
  Enterobius vermicularis 127.4
  Epidermophyton - see
      Dermatophytosis
  eyeworm 125.2
  Fasciola
    gigantica 121.3
    hepatica 121.3
  Fasciolopsis (buski) (small intestine)
      121.4
  filarial 125.9
    due to
      acanthocheilonema (perstans)
          125.4
        streptocerca 125.6
      Brugia (Wuchereria) malayi
          125.1
      Dracunculus medinensis 125.7
      guinea worms 125.7
      Mansonella (ozzardi) 125.5
      Onchocerca volvulus 125.3
        eye 125.3 [360.13]
        eyelid 125.3 [373.6]
      Wuchereria (bancrofti) 125.0
        malayi 125.1
    specified type NEC 125.6
  fish tapeworm 123.4
    larval 123.5
  fluke 121.9
    blood NEC (see also Schistosomiasis)
        120.9
    cat liver 121.0
    intestinal (giant) 121.4
    liver (sheep) 121.3
      cat 121.0
      Chinese 121.1
      clonorchiasis 121.1
      fascioliasis 121.3
      Oriental 121.1
    lung (oriental) 121.2
    sheep liver 121.3
  fly larva 134.0
  Gasterophilus (intestinalis) 134.0
  Gastrodiscoides hominis 121.8
  Giardia lamblia 007.1
  Gnathostoma (spinigerum) 128.1
  Gongylonema 125.6

Infestation (Continued)
  guinea worm 125.7
  helminth NEC 128.9
    intestinal 127.9
      mixed (types classifiable to more
          than one category in 120.0–
          127.7) 127.8
      specified type NEC 127.7
    specified type NEC 128.8
  Heterophyes heterophyes (small
      intestine) 121.6
  hookworm (see also Infestation,
      ancylostoma) 126.9
  Hymenolepis (diminuta) (nana) 123.6
  intestinal NEC 129
  leeches (aquatic) (land) 134.2
  Leishmania - see Leishmaniasis
  lice (see also Infestation, pediculus)
      132.9
  Linguatulidae, linguatula (pentastoma)
      (serrata) 134.1
  Loa loa 125.2
    eyelid 125.2 [373.6]
  louse (see also Infestation, pediculus)
      132.9
    body 132.1
    head 132.0
    pubic 132.2
  maggots 134.0
  Mansonella (ozzardi) 125.5
  medina 125.7
  Metagonimus yokogawai (small
      intestine) 121.5
  Microfilaria streptocerca 125.3
    eye 125.3 [360.13]
    eyelid 125.3 [373.6]
  Microsporon furfur 111.0
  microsporum - see Dermatophytosis
  mites 133.9
    scabic 133.0
    specified type NEC 133.8
  Monilia (albicans) (see also Candidiasis)
      112.9
    vagina 112.1
    vulva 112.1
  mouth 112.0
  Necator americanus 126.1
  nematode (intestinal) 127.9
    Ancylostoma (see also Ancylostoma)
        126.9
    Ascaris lumbricoides 127.0
    conjunctiva NEC 128.9
    Dioctophyma 128.8
    Enterobius vermicularis 127.4
    Gnathostoma spinigerum 128.1
    Oesophagostomum (apiostomum)
        127.7
    Physaloptera 127.4
    specified type NEC 127.7
    Strongyloides stercoralis 127.2
    Ternidens diminutus 127.7
    Trichinella spiralis 124
    Trichostrongylus 127.6
    Trichuris (trichiuria) 127.3
  Oesophagostomum (apiostomum)
      127.7
  Oestrus ovis 134.0
  Onchocerca (volvulus) 125.3
    eye 125.3 [360.13]
    eyelid 125.3 [373.6]
  Opisthorchis (felineus) (tenuicollis)
      (viverrini) 121.0
  Oxyuris vermicularis 127.4
  Paragonimus (westermani) 121.2

Infestation (*Continued*)
parasite, parasitic NEC 136.9
  eyelid 134.9 *[373.6]*
  intestinal 129
  mouth 112.0
  orbit 376.13
  skin 134.9
  tongue 112.0
pediculus 132.9
  capitis (humanus) (any site) 132.0
  corporis (humanus) (any site) 132.1
  eyelid 132.0 *[373.6]*
  mixed (classifiable to more than
    one category in 132.0–132.2)
    132.3
  pubis (any site) 132.2
phthirus (pubis) (any site) 132.2
  with any infestation classifiable to
    132.0 and 132.1 132.3
pinworm 127.4
pork tapeworm (adult) 123.0
protozoal NEC 136.8
pubic louse 132.2
rat tapeworm 123.6
red bug 133.8
roundworm (large) NEC 127.0
sand flea 134.1
saprophytic NEC 136.8
Sarcoptes scabiei 133.0
scabies 133.0
Schistosoma 120.9
  bovis 120.8
  cercariae 120.3
  hematobium 120.0
  intercalatum 120.8
  japonicum 120.2
  mansoni 120.1
  mattheii 120.8
  specified
    site - *see* Schistosomiasis
    type NEC 120.8
  spindale 120.8
screw worms 134.0
skin NEC 134.9
Sparganum (mansoni) (proliferum)
  123.5
  larval 123.5
specified type NEC 134.8
Spirometra larvae 123.5
Sporozoa NEC 136.8
Stellantchasmus falcatus 121.6
Strongyloides 127.2
Strongylus (gibsoni) 127.7
Taenia 123.3
  diminuta 123.6
  Echinococcus (*see also* Echinococcus)
    122.9
  mediocanellata 123.2
  nana 123.6
  saginata (mediocanellata) 123.2
  solium (intestinal form) 123.0
    larval form 123.1
Taeniarhynchus saginatus 123.2
tapeworm 123.9
  beef 123.2
  broad 123.4
    larval 123.5
  dog 123.8
  dwarf 123.6
  fish 123.4
    larval 123.5
  pork 123.0
  rat 123.6
Ternidens diminutus 127.7

Infestation (*Continued*)
Tetranychus molestissimus 133.8
threadworm 127.4
tongue 112.0
Toxocara (cani) (cati) (felis) 128.0
trematode(s) NEC 121.9
Trichina spiralis 124
Trichinella spiralis 124
Trichocephalus 127.3
Trichomonas 131.9
  bladder 131.09
  cervix 131.09
  intestine 007.3
  prostate 131.03
  specified site NEC 131.8
  urethra (female) (male) 131.02
  urogenital 131.00
  vagina 131.01
  vulva 131.01
Trichophyton - *see* Dermatophytosis
Trichostrongylus instabilis 127.6
Trichuris (trichiuria) 127.3
Trombicula (irritans) 133.8
Trypanosoma - *see* Trypanosomiasis
Tunga penetrans 134.1
Uncinaria americana 126.1
whipworm 127.3
worms NEC 128.9
  intestinal 127.9
Wuchereria 125.0
  bancrofti 125.0
  malayi 125.1

Infiltrate, infiltration
with an iron compound 275.0
amyloid (any site) (generalized)
  277.39
calcareous (muscle) NEC 275.49
  localized - *see* Degeneration, by
    site
calcium salt (muscle) 275.49
chemotherapy, vesicant 999.81 ◀▥
corneal (*see also* Edema, cornea)
  371.20
eyelid 373.9
fatty (diffuse) (generalized) 272.8
  localized - *see* Degeneration, by site,
    fatty
glycogen, glycogenic (*see also* Disease,
  glycogen storage) 271.0
heart, cardiac
  fatty (*see also* Degeneration,
    myocardial) 429.1
  glycogenic 271.0 *[425.7]*
inflammatory in vitreous 379.29
kidney (*see also* Disease, renal) 593.9
leukemic (M9800/3) - *see* Leukemia
liver 573.8
  fatty - *see* Fatty, liver
  glycogen (*see also* Disease, glycogen
    storage) 271.0
lung (*see also* Infiltrate, pulmonary)
  518.3
  eosinophilic 518.3
  x-ray finding only 793.1
lymphatic (*see also* Leukemia,
  lymphatic) 204.9●
  gland, pigmentary 289.3
muscle, fatty 728.9
myelogenous (*see also* Leukemia,
  myeloid) 205.9●
myocardium, myocardial
  fatty (*see also* Degeneration,
    myocardial) 429.1
  glycogenic 271.0 *[425.7]*

Infiltrate, infiltration (*Continued*)
pulmonary 518.3
  with
    eosinophilia 518.3
    pneumonia - *see* Pneumonia, by
      type
  x-ray finding only 793.1
Ranke's primary (*see also* Tuberculosis)
  010.0●
skin, lymphocytic (benign) 709.8
thymus (gland) (fatty) 254.8
urine 788.8
vesicant
  agent NEC 999.82 ◀▥
  chemotherapy 999.81 ◀▥
vitreous humor 379.29

Infirmity 799.89
senile 797

Inflammation, inflamed, inflammatory
(with exudation)
abducens (nerve) 378.54
accessory sinus (chronic) (*see also*
  Sinusitis) 473.9
adrenal (gland) 255.8
alimentary canal - *see* Enteritis
alveoli (teeth) 526.5
  scorbutic 267
amnion - *see* Amnionitis
anal canal 569.49
antrum (chronic) (*see also* Sinusitis,
  maxillary) 473.0
anus 569.49
appendix (*see also* Appendicitis) 541
arachnoid - *see* Meningitis
areola 611.0
  puerperal, postpartum 675.0●
areolar tissue NEC 686.9
artery - *see* Arteritis
auditory meatus (external) (*see also*
  Otitis, externa) 380.10
Bartholin's gland 616.89
bile duct or passage 576.1
bladder (*see also* Cystitis) 595.9
bleb
  postprocedural 379.60
    stage 1 379.61
    stage 2 379.62
    stage 3 379.63
bone - *see* Osteomyelitis
bowel (*see also* Enteritis) 558.9
brain (*see also* Encephalitis) 323.9
  late effect - *see* category 326
  membrane - *see* Meningitis
breast 611.0
  puerperal, postpartum 675.2●
broad ligament (*see also* Disease, pelvis,
  inflammatory) 614.4
  acute 614.3
bronchus - *see* Bronchitis
bursa - *see* Bursitis
capsule
  liver 573.3
  spleen 289.59
catarrhal (*see also* Catarrh) 460
  vagina 616.10
cecum (*see also* Appendicitis) 541
cerebral (*see also* Encephalitis) 323.9
  late effect - *see* category 326
  membrane - *see* Meningitis
cerebrospinal (*see also* Meningitis) 322.9
  late effect - *see* category 326
  meningococcal 036.0
  tuberculous (*see also* Tuberculosis)
    013.6●

◀ New   ◀▥ Revised   ~~deleted~~ Deleted   ● Use Additional Digit(s)   ▨ Omit code

Inflammation, inflamed, inflammatory
(Continued)
cervix (uteri) *(see also* Cervicitis) 616.0
chest 519.9
choroid NEC *(see also* Choroiditis)
363.20
cicatrix (tissue) - *see* Cicatrix
colon *(see also* Enteritis) 558.9
granulomatous 555.1
newborn 558.9
connective tissue (diffuse) NEC 728.9
cornea *(see also* Keratitis) 370.9
with ulcer *(see also* Ulcer, cornea)
370.00
corpora cavernosa (penis) 607.2
cranial nerve - *see* Disorder, nerve,
cranial
diarrhea - *see* Diarrhea
disc (intervertebral) (space) 722.90
cervical, cervicothoracic 722.91
lumbar, lumbosacral 722.93
thoracic, thoracolumbar 722.92
Douglas' cul-de-sac or pouch (chronic)
(see also Disease, pelvis,
inflammatory) 614.4
acute 614.3
due to (presence of) any device,
implant, or graft classifiable to
996.0–996.5 - *see* Complications,
infection and inflammation, due
to (presence of) any device,
implant, or graft classified to
996.0–996.5 NEC
duodenum 535.6●
dura mater - *see* Meningitis
ear - *see also* Otitis
external *(see also* Otitis, externa)
380.10
inner *(see also* Labyrinthitis) 386.30
middle - *see* Otitis media
esophagus 530.10
ethmoidal (chronic) (sinus) *(see also*
Sinusitis, ethmoidal) 473.2
Eustachian tube (catarrhal) 381.50
acute 381.51
chronic 381.52
extrarectal 569.49
eye 379.99
eyelid 373.9
specified NEC 373.8
fallopian tube *(see also* Salpingo-
oophoritis) 614.2
fascia 728.9
fetal membranes (acute) 658.4●
affecting fetus or newborn 762.7
follicular, pharynx 472.1
frontal (chronic) (sinus) *(see also*
Sinusitis, frontal) 473.1
gallbladder *(see also* Cholecystitis,
acute) 575.0
gall duct *(see also* Cholecystitis) 575.10
gastrointestinal *(see also* Enteritis)
558.9
genital organ (diffuse) (internal)
female 614.9
with
abortion - *see* Abortion, by
type, with sepsis
ectopic pregnancy *(see also*
categories 633.0–633.9)
639.0
molar pregnancy *(see also*
categories 630–632)
639.0

Inflammation, inflamed, inflammatory
(Continued)
genital organ *(Continued)*
female *(Continued)*
complicating pregnancy,
childbirth, or puerperium
646.6●
affecting fetus or newborn
760.8
following
abortion 639.0
ectopic or molar pregnancy
639.0
male 608.4
gland (lymph) *(see also* Lymphadenitis)
289.3
glottis *(see also* Laryngitis) 464.00
with obstruction 464.01
granular, pharynx 472.1
gum 523.10
heart *(see also* Carditis) 429.89
hepatic duct 576.8
hernial sac - *see* Hernia, by site
ileum *(see also* Enteritis) 558.9
terminal or regional 555.0
with large intestine 555.2
intervertebral disc 722.90
cervical, cervicothoracic 722.91
lumbar, lumbosacral 722.93
thoracic, thoracolumbar 722.92
intestine *(see also* Enteritis) 558.9
jaw (acute) (bone) (chronic) (lower)
(suppurative) (upper) 526.4
jejunum - *see* Enteritis
joint NEC *(see also* Arthritis) 716.9●
sacroiliac 720.2
kidney *(see also* Nephritis) 583.9
knee (joint) 716.66
tuberculous (active) *(see also*
Tuberculosis) 015.2●
labium (majus) (minus) *(see also*
Vulvitis) 616.10
lacrimal
gland *(see also* Dacryoadenitis)
375.00
passages (duct) (sac) *(see also*
Dacryocystitis) 375.30
larynx *(see also* Laryngitis) 464.00
with obstruction 464.01
diphtheritic 032.3
leg NEC 686.9
lip 528.5
liver (capsule) *(see also* Hepatitis) 573.3
acute 570
chronic 571.40
suppurative 572.0
lung (acute) *(see also* Pneumonia) 486
chronic (interstitial) 518.89
lymphatic vessel *(see also*
Lymphangitis) 457.2
lymph node or gland *(see also*
Lymphadenitis) 289.3
mammary gland 611.0
puerperal, postpartum 675.2●
maxilla, maxillary 526.4
sinus (chronic) *(see also* Sinusitis,
maxillary) 473.0
membranes of brain or spinal cord - *see*
Meningitis
meninges - *see* Meningitis
mouth 528.00
muscle 728.9
myocardium *(see also* Myocarditis)
429.0

Inflammation, inflamed, inflammatory
(Continued)
nasal sinus (chronic) *(see also* Sinusitis)
473.9
nasopharynx - *see* Nasopharyngitis
navel 686.9
newborn NEC 771.4
nerve NEC 729.2
nipple 611.0
puerperal, postpartum 675.0●
nose 478.19
suppurative 472.0
oculomotor nerve 378.51
optic nerve 377.30
orbit (chronic) 376.10
acute 376.00
chronic 376.10
ovary *(see also* Salpingo-oophoritis)
614.2
oviduct *(see also* Salpingo-oophoritis)
614.2
pancreas - *see* Pancreatitis
parametrium (chronic) *(see also* Disease,
pelvis, inflammatory) 614.4
acute 614.3
parotid region 686.9
gland 527.2
pelvis, female *(see also* Disease, pelvis,
inflammatory) 614.9
penis (corpora cavernosa) 607.2
perianal 569.49
pericardium *(see also* Pericarditis) 423.9
perineum (female) (male) 686.9
perirectal 569.49
peritoneum *(see also* Peritonitis) 567.9
periuterine *(see also* Disease, pelvis,
inflammatory) 614.9
perivesical *(see also* Cystitis) 595.9
petrous bone *(see also* Petrositis) 383.20
pharynx *(see also* Pharyngitis) 462
follicular 472.1
granular 472.1
pia mater - *see* Meningitis
pleura - *see* Pleurisy
postmastoidectomy cavity 383.30
chronic 383.33
pouch, internal ileoanal 569.71 ◄
prostate *(see also* Prostatitis) 601.9
rectosigmoid - *see* Rectosigmoiditis
rectum *(see also* Proctitis) 569.49
respiratory, upper *(see also* Infection,
respiratory, upper) 465.9
chronic, due to external agent - *see*
Condition, respiratory, chronic,
due to, external agent
due to
fumes or vapors (chemical)
(inhalation) 506.2
radiation 508.1
retina *(see also* Retinitis) 363.20
retrocecal *(see also* Appendicitis) 541
retroperitoneal *(see also* Peritonitis) 567.9
salivary duct or gland (any)
(suppurative) 527.2
scorbutic, alveoli, teeth 267
scrotum 608.4
sigmoid - *see* Enteritis
sinus *(see also* Sinusitis) 473.9
Skene's duct or gland *(see also*
Urethritis) 597.89
skin 686.9
spermatic cord 608.4
sphenoidal (sinus) *(see also* Sinusitis,
sphenoidal) 473.3

Inflammation, inflamed, inflammatory
(*Continued*)
spinal
  cord (*see also* Encephalitis) 323.9
    late effect - *see* category 326
  membrane - *see* Meningitis
  nerve - *see* Disorder, nerve
spine (*see also* Spondylitis) 720.9
spleen (capsule) 289.59
stomach - *see* Gastritis
stricture, rectum 569.49
subcutaneous tissue NEC 686.9
suprarenal (gland) 255.8
synovial (fringe) (membrane) - *see*
  Bursitis
tendon (sheath) NEC 726.90
testis (*see also* Orchitis) 604.90
thigh 686.9
throat (*see also* Sore throat) 462
thymus (gland) 254.8
thyroid (gland) (*see also* Thyroiditis)
  245.9
tongue 529.0
tonsil - *see* Tonsillitis
trachea - *see* Tracheitis
trochlear nerve 378.53
tubal (*see also* Salpingo-oophoritis)
  614.2
tuberculous NEC (*see also* Tuberculosis)
  011.9●
tubo-ovarian (*see also* Salpingo-
  oophoritis) 614.2
tunica vaginalis 608.4
tympanic membrane - *see* Myringitis
umbilicus, umbilical 686.9
  newborn NEC 771.4
uterine ligament (*see also* Disease,
  pelvis, inflammatory) 614.4
  acute 614.3
uterus (catarrhal) (*see also* Endometritis)
  615.9
uveal tract (anterior) (*see also*
  Iridocyclitis) 364.3
  posterior - *see* Chorioretinitis
  sympathetic 360.11
vagina (*see also* Vaginitis) 616.10
vas deferens 608.4
vein (*see also* Phlebitis) 451.9
  thrombotic 451.9
    cerebral (*see also* Thrombosis,
      brain) 434.0●
    leg 451.2
      deep (vessels) NEC 451.19
      superficial (vessels) 451.0
    lower extremity 451.2
      deep (vessels) NEC 451.19
      superficial (vessels) 451.0
vocal cord 478.5
vulva (*see also* Vulvitis) 616.10
Inflation, lung imperfect (newborn)
  770.5
Influenza, influenzal 487.1
with
  bronchitis 487.1
  bronchopneumonia 487.0
  cold (any type) 487.1
  digestive manifestations 487.8
  hemoptysis 487.1
  involvement of
    gastrointestinal tract 487.8
    nervous system 487.8
  laryngitis 487.1
  manifestations NEC 487.8
    respiratory 487.1
      pneumonia 487.0

Influenza, influenzal (*Continued*)
with (*Continued*)
  pharyngitis 487.1
  pneumonia (any form classifiable to
    480–483, 485–486) 487.0
  respiratory manifestations NEC
    487.1
  sinusitis 487.1
  sore throat 487.1
  tonsillitis 487.1
  tracheitis 487.1
  upper respiratory infection (acute)
    487.1
A/H5N1 488.0 ◀
abdominal 487.8
Asian 487.1
avian 488.0 ◀
bronchial 487.1
bronchopneumonia 487.0
catarrhal 487.1
due to identified ~~avian influenza~~
  ~~virus 488~~ ◀▥
  avian influenza virus 488.0 ◀
  novel H1N1 influenza virus 488.1 ◀
epidemic 487.1
gastric 487.8
intestinal 487.8
laryngitis 487.1
maternal affecting fetus or newborn
  760.2
  manifest influenza in infant 771.2
  novel (2009) H1N1 488.1 ◀
novel A/H1N1 488.1 ◀
pharyngitis 487.1
pneumonia (any form) 487.0
respiratory (upper) 487.1
specified NEC 487.1 ◀
stomach 487.8
vaccination, prophylactic (against)
  V04.81
Influenza-like disease 487.1
Infraction, Freiberg's (metatarsal head)
  732.5
Infraeruption, teeth 524.34
**Infusion complication, misadventure, or
  reaction** - *see* Complication, infusion
Ingestion
chemical - *see* Table of Drugs and
  Chemicals
drug or medicinal substance
  overdose or wrong substance given
    or taken 977.9
    specified drug - *see* Table of
      Drugs and Chemicals
foreign body NEC (*see also* Foreign
  body) 938
Ingrowing
hair 704.8
nail (finger) (toe) (infected) 703.0
Inguinal - *see also* condition
testis 752.51
Inhalation
carbon monoxide 986
flame
  mouth 947.0
  lung 947.1
food or foreign body (*see also* Asphyxia,
  food or foreign body) 933.1
gas, fumes, or vapor (noxious) 987.9
  specified agent - *see* Table of Drugs
    and Chemicals
liquid or vomitus (*see also* Asphyxia,
  food or foreign body) 933.1
  lower respiratory tract NEC
    934.9

Inhalation (*Continued*)
meconium (fetus or newborn) 770.11
  with respiratory symptoms 770.12
mucus (*see also* Asphyxia, mucus)
  933.1
oil (causing suffocation) (*see also*
  Asphyxia, food or foreign body)
  933.1
pneumonia - *see* Pneumonia, aspiration
smoke 987.9
steam 987.9
stomach contents or secretions (*see also*
  Asphyxia, food or foreign body)
  933.1
  in labor and delivery 668.0●
Inhibition, inhibited
academic as adjustment reaction
  309.23
orgasm
  female 302.73
  male 302.74
sexual
  desire 302.71
  excitement 302.72
work as adjustment reaction 309.23
Inhibitor, systemic lupus erythematosus
  (presence of) 286.5
Iniencephalus, iniencephaly 740.2
Injected eye 372.74
Injury 959.9

Note 45   For abrasion, insect bite
(nonvenomous), blister, or scratch, *see*
Injury, superficial.

For laceration, traumatic rupture, tear,
or penetrating wound of internal organs, such as heart, lung, liver, kidney,
pelvic organs, whether or not accompanied by open wound in the same
region, *see* Injury, internal.

For nerve injury, *see* Injury, nerve.

For late effect of injuries classifiable to
850–854, 860–869, 900–919, 950–959, *see*
Late, effect, injury, by type.

---

abdomen, abdominal (viscera) - *see also*
  Injury, internal, abdomen
  muscle or wall 959.12
acoustic, resulting in deafness 951.5
adenoid 959.09
adrenal (gland) - *see* Injury, internal,
  adrenal
alveolar (process) 959.09
ankle (and foot) (and knee) (and leg,
  except thigh) 959.7
anterior chamber, eye 921.3
anus 959.19
aorta (thoracic) 901.0
  abdominal 902.0
appendix - *see* Injury, internal,
  appendix
arm, upper (and shoulder) 959.2
artery (complicating trauma) (*see also*
  Injury, blood vessel, by site)
  904.9
  cerebral or meningeal (*see also*
    Hemorrhage, brain, traumatic,
    subarachnoid) 852.0●
auditory canal (external) (meatus)
  959.09
auricle, auris, ear 959.09
axilla 959.2
back 959.19

◀ New   ◀▥ Revised   ~~deleted~~ Deleted   ● Use Additional Digit(s)   ▦ Omit code

Injury (*Continued*)
bile duct - *see* Injury, internal, bile duct
birth - *see also* Birth, injury
  canal NEC, complicating delivery
    665.9 ●
bladder (sphincter) - *see* Injury, internal,
  bladder
blast (air) (hydraulic) (immersion)
  (underwater) NEC 869.0
  with open wound into cavity NEC
    869.1
  abdomen or thorax - *see* Injury,
    internal, by site
  brain - *see* Concussion, brain
  ear (acoustic nerve trauma) 951.5
    with perforation of tympanic
      membrane - *see* Wound,
      open, ear, drum
blood vessel NEC 904.9
  abdomen 902.9
    multiple 902.87
    specified NEC 902.89
  aorta (thoracic) 901.0
    abdominal 902.0
  arm NEC 903.9
  axillary 903.00
    artery 903.1
    vein 903.02
  azygos vein 901.89
  basilic vein 903.1
  brachial (artery) (vein) 903.1
  bronchial 901.89
  carotid artery 900.00
    common 900.01
    external 900.02
    internal 900.03
  celiac artery 902.20
    specified branch NEC 902.24
  cephalic vein (arm) 903.1
  colica dextra 902.26
  cystic
    artery 902.24
    vein 902.39
  deep plantar 904.6
  digital (artery) (vein) 903.5
  due to accidental puncture or
    laceration during procedure
    998.2
  extremity
    lower 904.8
      multiple 904.7
      specified NEC 904.7
    upper 903.9
      multiple 903.8
      specified NEC 903.8
  femoral
    artery (superficial) 904.1
      above profunda origin 904.0
      common 904.0
    vein 904.2
  gastric
    artery 902.21
    vein 902.39
  head 900.9
    intracranial - *see* Injury,
      intracranial
    multiple 900.82
    specified NEC 900.89
  hemiazygos vein 901.89
  hepatic
    artery 902.22
    vein 902.11
  hypogastric 902.59
    artery 902.51
    vein 902.52

Injury (*Continued*)
blood vessel (*Continued*)
  ileocolic
    artery 902.26
    vein 902.31
  iliac 902.50
    artery 902.53
    specified branch NEC 902.59
    vein 902.54
  innominate
    artery 901.1
    vein 901.3
  intercostal (artery) (vein) 901.81
  jugular vein (external) 900.81
    internal 900.1
  leg NEC 904.8
  mammary (artery) (vein) 901.82
  mesenteric
    artery 902.20
      inferior 902.27
      specified branch NEC 902.29
      superior (trunk) 902.25
        branches, primary 902.26
    vein 902.39
      inferior 902.32
      superior (and primary
        subdivisions) 902.31
  neck 900.9
    multiple 900.82
    specified NEC 900.89
  ovarian 902.89
    artery 902.81
    vein 902.82
  palmar artery 903.4
  pelvis 902.9
    multiple 902.87
    specified NEC 902.89
  plantar (deep) (artery) (vein)
    904.6
  popliteal 904.40
    artery 904.41
    vein 904.42
  portal 902.33
  pulmonary 901.40
    artery 901.41
    vein 901.42
  radial (artery) (vein) 903.2
  renal 902.40
    artery 902.41
    specified NEC 902.49
    vein 902.42
  saphenous
    artery 904.7
    vein (greater) (lesser) 904.3
  splenic
    artery 902.23
    vein 902.34
  subclavian
    artery 901.1
    vein 901.3
  suprarenal 902.49
  thoracic 901.9
    multiple 901.83
    specified NEC 901.89
  tibial 904.50
    artery 904.50
      anterior 904.51
      posterior 904.53
    vein 904.50
      anterior 904.52
      posterior 904.54
  ulnar (artery) (vein) 903.3
  uterine 902.59
    artery 902.55
    vein 902.56

Injury (*Continued*)
blood vessel (*Continued*)
  vena cava
    inferior 902.10
      specified branches NEC 902.19
    superior 901.2
brachial plexus 953.4
  newborn 767.6
brain (traumatic) NEC (*see also* Injury,
  intracranial) 854.0 ●   ⫸
  due to fracture of skull -
    see Fracture, skull, by site ◀
breast 959.19
broad ligament - *see* Injury, internal,
  broad ligament
bronchus, bronchi - *see* Injury, internal,
  bronchus
brow 959.09
buttock 959.19
canthus, eye 921.1
cathode ray 990
cauda equina 952.4
  with fracture, vertebra - *see* Fracture,
    vertebra, sacrum
cavernous sinus (*see also* Injury,
  intracranial) 854.0 ●
cecum - *see* Injury, internal, cecum
celiac ganglion or plexus 954.1
cerebellum (*see also* Injury, intracranial)
  854.0 ●
cervix (uteri) - *see* Injury, internal,
  cervix
cheek 959.09
chest - *see* Injury, internal, chest
  wall 959.11
childbirth - *see also* Birth, injury
  maternal NEC 665.9 ●
chin 959.09
choroid (eye) 921.3
clitoris 959.14
coccyx 959.19
  complicating delivery 665.6 ●
colon - *see* Injury, internal, colon
common duct - *see* Injury, internal,
  common duct
conjunctiva 921.1
  superficial 918.2
cord
  spermatic - *see* Injury, internal,
    spermatic cord
  spinal - *see* Injury, spinal, by site
cornea 921.3
  abrasion 918.1
  due to contact lens 371.82
  penetrating - *see* Injury, eyeball,
    penetrating
  superficial 918.1
    due to contact lens 371.82
cortex (cerebral) (*see also* Injury,
  intracranial) 854.0 ●
  visual 950.3
costal region 959.11
costochondral 959.11
cranial
  bones - *see* Fracture, skull, by site
  cavity (*see also* Injury, intracranial)
    854.0 ●
  nerve - *see* Injury, nerve, cranial
crushing - *see* Crush
cutaneous sensory nerve
  lower limb 956.4
  upper limb 955.5
deep tissue - *see* Contusion, by site
  meaning pressure ulcer 707.25
delivery - *see also* Birth, injury
  maternal NEC 665.9 ●

Injury (Continued)
Descemet's membrane - see Injury, eyeball, penetrating
diaphragm - see Injury, internal, diaphragm
diffuse axonal - see Injury, intracranial
duodenum - see Injury, internal, duodenum
ear (auricle) (canal) (drum) (external) 959.09
elbow (and forearm) (and wrist) 959.3
epididymis 959.14
epigastric region 959.12
epiglottis 959.09
epiphyseal, current - see Fracture, by site
esophagus - see Injury, internal, esophagus
Eustachian tube 959.09
extremity (lower) (upper) NEC 959.8
eye 921.9
    penetrating eyeball - see Injury, eyeball, penetrating
    superficial 918.9
eyeball 921.3
    penetrating 871.7
        with
            partial loss (of intraocular tissue) 871.2
            prolapse or exposure (of intraocular tissue) 871.1
            without prolapse 871.0
            foreign body (nonmagnetic) 871.6
                magnetic 871.5
    superficial 918.9
eyebrow 959.09
eyelid(s) 921.1
    laceration - see Laceration, eyelid
    superficial 918.0
face (and neck) 959.09
fallopian tube - see Injury, internal, fallopian tube
fingers(s) (nail) 959.5
flank 959.19
foot (and ankle) (and knee) (and leg, except thigh) 959.7
forceps NEC 767.9
    scalp 767.19
forearm (and elbow) (and wrist) 959.3
forehead 959.09
gallbladder - see Injury, internal, gallbladder
gasserian ganglion 951.2
gastrointestinal tract - see Injury, internal, gastrointestinal tract
genital organ(s)
    with
        abortion - see Abortion, by type, with, damage to pelvic organs
        ectopic pregnancy (see also categories 633.0–633.9) 639.2
        molar pregnancy (see also categories 630–632) 639.2
    external 959.14
    fracture of corpus cavernosum penis 959.13
    following
        abortion 639.2
        ectopic or molar pregnancy 639.2

Injury (Continued)
genital organ(s) (Continued)
    internal - see Injury, internal, genital organs
        obstetrical trauma NEC 665.9●
            affecting fetus or newborn 763.89
gland
    lacrimal 921.1
        laceration 870.8
    parathyroid 959.09
    salivary 959.09
    thyroid 959.09
globe (eye) (see also Injury, eyeball) 921.3
grease gun - see Wound, open, by site, complicated
groin 959.19   •
gum 959.09
hand(s) (except fingers) 959.4
head NEC 959.01
    with
        loss of consciousness 850.5
        skull fracture - see Fracture, skull, by site
heart - see Injury, internal, heart
heel 959.7
hip (and thigh) 959.6
hymen 959.14
hyperextension (cervical) (vertebra) 847.0
ileum - see Injury, internal, ileum
iliac region 959.19
infrared rays NEC 990
instrumental (during surgery) 998.2
    birth injury - see Birth, injury
    nonsurgical (see also Injury, by site) 959.9
    obstetrical 665.9●
        affecting fetus or newborn 763.89
        bladder 665.5●
        cervix 665.3●
        high vaginal 665.4●
        perineal NEC 664.9●
        urethra 665.5●
        uterus 665.5●
internal 869.0

Note 46   For injury of internal organ(s) by foreign body entering through a natural orifice (e.g., inhaled, ingested, or swallowed)-see Foreign body, entering through orifice.

For internal injury of any of the following sites with internal injury of any other of the sites-see Injury, internal, multiple.

    with
        fracture
            pelvis - see Fracture, pelvis
            specified site, except pelvis - see Injury, internal, by site
        open wound into cavity 869.1
    abdomen, abdominal (viscera) NEC 868.00
        with
            fracture, pelvis - see Fracture, pelvis
            open wound into cavity 868.10
        specified site NEC 868.09
            with open wound into cavity 868.19

Injury (Continued)
internal (Continued)
    adrenal (gland) 868.01
        with open wound into cavity 868.11
    aorta (thoracic) 901.0
        abdominal 902.0
    appendix 863.85
        with open wound into cavity 863.95
    bile duct 868.02
        with open wound into cavity 868.12
    bladder (sphincter) 867.0
        with
            abortion - see Abortion, by type, with, damage to pelvic organs
            ectopic pregnancy (see also categories 633.0–633.9) 639.2
            molar pregnancy (see also categories 630–632) 639.2
            open wound into cavity 867.1
        following
            abortion 639.2
            ectopic or molar pregnancy 639.2
        obstetrical trauma 665.5●
            affecting fetus or newborn 763.89
    blood vessel - see Injury, blood vessel, by site
    broad ligament 867.6
        with open wound into cavity 867.7
    bronchus, bronchi 862.21
        with open wound into cavity 862.31
    cecum 863.89
        with open wound into cavity 863.99
    cervix (uteri) 867.4
        with
            abortion - see Abortion, by type, with damage to pelvic organs
            ectopic pregnancy (see also categories 633.0–633.9) 639.2
            molar pregnancy (see also categories 630–632) 639.2
            open wound into cavity 867.5
        following
            abortion 639.2
            ectopic or molar pregnancy 639.2
        obstetrical trauma 665.3●
            affecting fetus or newborn 763.89
    chest (see also Injury, internal, intrathoracic organs) 862.8
        with open wound into cavity 862.9
    colon 863.40
        with
            open wound into cavity 863.50
            rectum 863.46
                with open wound into cavity 863.56
        ascending (right) 863.41
            with open wound into cavity 863.51

◄ New   ◀▥ Revised   ~~deleted~~ Deleted   ● Use Additional Digit(s)   ▨ Omit code

Injury *(Continued)*
  internal *(Continued)*
    colon *(Continued)*
      descending (left) 863.43
        with open wound into cavity
          863.53
      multiple sites 863.46
        with open wound into cavity
          863.56
      sigmoid 863.44
        with open wound into cavity
          863.54
      specified site NEC 863.49
        with open wound into cavity
          863.59
      transverse 863.42
        with open wound into cavity
          863.52
    common duct 868.02
      with open wound into cavity
        868.12
    complicating delivery 665.9 ●
      affecting fetus or newborn 763.89
    diaphragm 862.0
      with open wound into cavity
        862.1
    duodenum 863.21
      with open wound into cavity
        863.31
    esophagus (intrathoracic) 862.22
      with open wound into cavity
        862.32
      cervical region 874.4
        complicated 874.5
    fallopian tube 867.6
      with open wound into cavity
        867.7
    gallbladder 868.02
      with open wound into cavity
        868.12
    gastrointestinal tract NEC 863.80
      with open wound into cavity
        863.90
    genital organ NEC 867.6
      with open wound into cavity
        867.7
    heart 861.00
      with open wound into thorax
        861.10
    ileum 863.29
      with open wound into cavity
        863.39
    intestine NEC 863.89
      with open wound into cavity
        863.99
      large NEC 863.40
        with open wound into cavity
          863.50
      small NEC 863.20
        with open wound into cavity
          863.30
    intra-abdominal (organ) 868.00
      with open wound into cavity
        868.10
      multiple sites 868.09
        with open wound into cavity
          868.19
      specified site NEC 868.09
        with open wound into cavity
          868.19
    intrathoracic organs (multiple)
      862.8
      with open wound into cavity
        862.9

Injury *(Continued)*
  internal *(Continued)*
    intrathoracic organs *(Continued)*
      diaphragm (only) - *see* Injury,
        internal, diaphragm
      heart (only) - *see* Injury, internal,
        heart
      lung (only) - *see* Injury, internal,
        lung
      specified site NEC 862.29
        with open wound into cavity
          862.39
    intrauterine (*see also* Injury, internal,
      uterus) 867.4
      with open wound into cavity
        867.5
    jejunum 863.29
      with open wound into cavity
        863.39
    kidney (subcapsular) 866.00
      with
        disruption of parenchyma
          (complete) 866.03
          with open wound into
            cavity 866.13
        hematoma (without rupture of
          capsule) 866.01
          with open wound into
            cavity 866.11
        laceration 866.02
          with open wound into
            cavity 866.12
        open wound into cavity
          866.10
    liver 864.00
      with
        contusion 864.01
          with open wound into
            cavity 864.11
        hematoma 864.01
          with open wound into
            cavity 864.11
        laceration 864.05
          with open wound into
            cavity 864.15
          major (disruption of hepatic
            parenchyma) 864.04
            with open wound into
              cavity 864.14
          minor (capsule only)
            864.02
            with open wound into
              cavity 864.12
          moderate (involving
            parenchyma) 864.03
            with open wound into
              cavity 864.13
            multiple 864.04
          stellate 864.04
           with open wound into
            cavity 864.14
        open wound into cavity
          864.10
    lung 861.20
      with open wound into thorax
        861.30
      hemopneumothorax - *see*
        Hemopneumothorax,
        traumatic
      hemothorax - *see* Hemothorax,
        traumatic
      pneumohemothorax - *see*
        Pneumohemothorax,
        traumatic

Injury *(Continued)*
  internal *(Continued)*
    lung *(Continued)*
      pneumothorax - *see*
        Pneumothorax,
        traumatic
      transfusion related, acute
        (TRALI) 518.7
    mediastinum 862.29
      with open wound into cavity
        862.39
    mesentery 863.89
      with open wound into cavity
        863.99
    mesosalpinx 867.6
      with open wound into cavity
        867.7
    multiple 869.0

> **Note 47** Multiple internal injuries of
> sites classifiable to the same three- or
> four-digit category should be classified
> to that category.
>
> Multiple injuries classifiable to dif-
> ferent fourth-digit subdivisions of
> 861.-(heart and lung injuries) should be
> dealt with according to coding rules.

      internal 869.0
        with open wound into cavity
          869.1
      intra-abdominal organ (sites
        classifiable to 863–868)
        with
          intrathoracic organ(s) (sites
            classifiable to 861–862)
            869.0
            with open wound into
              cavity 869.1
          other intra-abdominal
            organ(s) (sites
            classifiable to
            863–868, except
            where classifiable
            to the same three-
            digit category)
            868.09
            with open wound into
              cavity 868.19
      intrathoracic organ (sites
        classifiable to 861–862)
        with
          intra-abdominal organ(s)
            (sites classifiable to
            863–868) 869.0
            with open wound into
              cavity 869.1
          other intrathoracic organs(s)
            (sites classifiable to
            861–862, except where
            classifiable to the same
            three-digit category)
            862.8
        with open wound into cavity
          862.9
    myocardium - *see* Injury, internal,
      heart
    ovary 867.6
      with open wound into cavity
        867.7
    pancreas (multiple sites) 863.84
      with open wound into cavity
        863.94

Injury *(Continued)*
  internal *(Continued)*
    pancreas *(Continued)*
      body 863.82
        with open wound into cavity
          863.92
      head 863.81
        with open wound into cavity
          863.91
      tail 863.83
        with open wound into cavity
          863.93
    pelvis, pelvic (organs) (viscera) 867.8
      with
        fracture, pelvis - *see* Fracture,
          pelvis
        open wound into cavity 867.9
      specified site NEC 867.6
        with open wound into cavity
          867.7
    peritoneum 868.03
      with open wound into cavity
        868.13
    pleura 862.29
      with open wound into cavity
        862.39
    prostate 867.6
      with open wound into cavity
        867.7
    rectum 863.45
      with
        colon 863.46
          with open wound into
            cavity 863.56
        open wound into cavity
          863.55
    retroperitoneum 868.04
      with open wound into cavity
        868.14
    round ligament 867.6
      with open wound into cavity
        867.7
    seminal vesicle 867.6
      with open wound into cavity
        867.7
    spermatic cord 867.6
      with open wound into cavity
        867.7
      scrotal - *see* Wound, open,
        spermatic cord
    spleen 865.00
      with
        disruption of parenchyma
          (massive) 865.04
          with open wound into
            cavity 865.14
        hematoma (without rupture of
          capsule) 865.01
          with open wound into
            cavity 865.11
        open wound into cavity 865.10
        tear, capsular 865.02
          with open wound into
            cavity 865.12
          extending into parenchyma
            865.03
            with open wound into
              cavity 865.13
    stomach 863.0
      with open wound into cavity
        863.1
    suprarenal gland (multiple) 868.01
      with open wound into cavity
        868.11

Injury *(Continued)*
  internal *(Continued)*
    thorax, thoracic (cavity) (organs)
      (multiple) *(see also* Injury,
      internal, intrathoracic organs)
      862.8
      with open wound into cavity
        862.9
    thymus (gland) 862.29
      with open wound into cavity
        862.39
    trachea (intrathoracic) 862.29
      with open wound into cavity
        862.39
      cervical region *(see also* Wound,
        open, trachea) 874.02
    ureter 867.2
      with open wound into cavity
        867.3
    urethra (sphincter) 867.0
      with
        abortion - *see* Abortion, by
          type, with, damage to
          pelvic organs
        ectopic pregnancy *(see also*
          categories 633.0–633.9)
          639.2
        molar pregnancy *(see also*
          categories 630–632)
          639.2
        open wound into cavity 867.1
      following
        abortion 639.2
        ectopic or molar pregnancy
          639.2
      obstetrical trauma 665.5●
        affecting fetus or newborn
          763.89
    uterus 867.4
      with
        abortion - *see* Abortion, by
          type, with, damage to
          pelvic organs
        ectopic pregnancy *(see also*
          categories 633.0–633.9)
          639.2
        molar pregnancy *(see also*
          categories 630–632)
          639.2
        open wound into cavity 867.5
      following
        abortion 639.2
        ectopic or molar pregnancy
          639.2
      obstetrical trauma NEC 665.5●
        affecting fetus or newborn
          763.89
    vas deferens 867.6
      with open wound into cavity
        867.7
    vesical (sphincter) 867.0
      with open wound into cavity
        867.1
    viscera (abdominal) *(see also* Injury,
      internal, multiple) 868.00
      with
        fracture, pelvis - *see* Fracture,
          pelvis
        open wound into cavity 868.10
      thoracic NEC *(see also* Injury,
        internal, intrathoracic
        organs) 862.8
      with open wound into cavity
        862.9

Injury *(Continued)*
  interscapular region 959.19
  intervertebral disc 959.19
  intestine - *see* Injury, internal, intestine
  intra-abdominal (organs) NEC - *see*
    Injury, internal, intra-abdominal
  intracranial (traumatic) 854.0   ◄▥

Note 48   Use the following fifth-
digit subclassification with categories
851–854:

0	unspecified state of consciousness
1	with no loss of consciousness
2	with brief [less than one hour] loss of consciousness
3	with moderate [1–24 hours] loss of consciousness
4	with prolonged [more than 24 hours] loss of consciousness and return to pre-existing conscious level
5	with prolonged [more than 24 hours] loss of consciousness, without return to pre-existing conscious level

Use fifth-digit 5 to designate when a
patient is unconscious and dies before
regaining consciousness, regardless of
the duration of the loss of consciousness

| 6 | with loss of consciousness of unspecified duration |
| 9 | with concussion, unspecified |

    with
      open intracranial wound
        854.1●
      skull fracture - *see* Fracture,
        skull, by site
    contusion 851.8●
      with open intracranial wound
        851.9●
      brain stem 851.4●
        with open intracranial wound
          851.5●
      cerebellum 851.4●
        with open intracranial wound
          851.5●
      cortex (cerebral) 851.0●
        with open intracranial wound
          851.2●
    hematoma - *see* Injury,
      intracranial, hemorrhage
    hemorrhage 853.0●
      with
        laceration - *see* Injury,
          intracranial,
          laceration
        open intracranial wound
          853.1●
      extradural 852.4●
        with open intracranial
          wound 852.5●
      subarachnoid 852.0●
        with open intracranial
          wound 852.1●
      subdural 852.2●
        with open intracranial
          wound 852.3●
    laceration 851.8●
      with open intracranial wound
        851.9●

◄ New   ◀▥ Revised   ~~deleted~~ Deleted   ● Use Additional Digit(s)   ▥ Omit code

Injury (Continued)
  intracranial (Continued)
    contusion (Continued)
      laceration (Continued)
        brain stem 851.6 ●
          with open intracranial
            wound 851.7 ●
        cerebellum 851.6 ●
          with open intracranial
            wound 851.7 ●
        cortex (cerebral) 851.2 ●
          with open intracranial
            wound 851.3 ●
  intraocular - see Injury, eyeball,
    penetrating
  intrathoracic organs (multiple) - see
    Injury, internal, intrathoracic
    organs
  intrauterine - see Injury, internal,
    intrauterine
  iris 921.3
    penetrating - see Injury, eyeball,
      penetrating
  jaw 959.09
  jejunum - see Injury, internal, jejunum
  joint NEC 959.9
    old or residual 718.80
      ankle 718.87
      elbow 718.82
      foot 718.87
      hand 718.84
      hip 718.85
      knee 718.86
      multiple sites 718.89
      pelvic region 718.85
      shoulder (region) 718.81
      specified site NEC 718.88
      wrist 718.83
  kidney - see Injury, internal, kidney
    acute (nontraumatic) 584.9
  knee (and ankle) (and foot) (and leg,
    except thigh) 959.7
  labium (majus) (minus) 959.14
  labyrinth, ear 959.09
  lacrimal apparatus, gland, or sac 921.1
    laceration 870.8
  larynx 959.09
  late effect - see Late, effects (of), injury
  leg, except thigh (and ankle) (and foot)
    (and knee) 959.7
    upper or thigh 959.6
  lens, eye 921.3
    penetrating - see Injury, eyeball,
      penetrating
  lid, eye - see Injury, eyelid
  lip 959.09
  liver - see Injury, internal, liver
  lobe, parietal - see Injury, intracranial
  lumbar (region) 959.19
    plexus 953.5
  lumbosacral (region) 959.19
    plexus 953.5
  lung - see Injury, internal, lung
  malar region 959.09
  mastoid region 959.09
  maternal, during pregnancy, affecting
    fetus or newborn 760.5
  maxilla 959.09
  mediastinum - see Injury, internal,
    mediastinum
  membrane
    brain (see also Injury, intracranial)
      854.0 ●
    tympanic 959.09

Injury (Continued)
  meningeal artery - see Hemorrhage,
    brain, traumatic, subarachnoid
  meninges (cerebral) - see Injury,
    intracranial
  mesenteric
    artery - see Injury, blood vessel,
      mesenteric, artery
    plexus, inferior 954.1
    vein - see Injury, blood vessel,
      mesenteric, vein
  mesentery - see Injury, internal,
    mesentery
  mesosalpinx - see Injury, internal,
    mesosalpinx
  middle ear 959.09
  midthoracic region 959.11
  mouth 959.09
  multiple (sites not classifiable to the
    same four-digit category in 959.0–
    959.7) 959.8
    internal 869.0
      with open wound into cavity
        869.1
  musculocutaneous nerve 955.4
  nail
    finger 959.5
    toe 959.7
  nasal (septum) (sinus) 959.09
  nasopharynx 959.09
  neck (and face) 959.09
  nerve 957.9
    abducens 951.3
    abducent 951.3
    accessory 951.6
    acoustic 951.5
    ankle and foot 956.9
    anterior crural, femoral 956.1
    arm (see also Injury, nerve, upper
      limb) 955.9
    auditory 951.5
    axillary 955.0
    brachial plexus 953.4
    cervical sympathetic 954.0
    cranial 951.9
      first or olfactory 951.8
      second or optic 950.0
      third or oculomotor 951.0
      fourth or trochlear 951.1
      fifth or trigeminal 951.2
      sixth or abducens 951.3
      seventh or facial 951.4
      eighth, acoustic, or auditory
        951.5
      ninth or glossopharyngeal 951.8
      tenth, pneumogastric, or vagus
        951.8
      eleventh or accessory 951.6
      twelfth or hypoglossal 951.7
      newborn 767.7
    cutaneous sensory
      lower limb 956.4
      upper limb 955.5
    digital (finger) 955.6
      toe 956.5
    facial 951.4
      newborn 767.5
    femoral 956.1
    finger 955.9
    foot and ankle 956.9
    forearm 955.9
    glossopharyngeal 951.8
    hand and wrist 955.9
    head and neck, superficial 957.0

Injury (Continued)
  nerve (Continued)
    hypoglossal 951.7
    involving several parts of body
      957.8
    leg (see also Injury, nerve, lower
      limb) 956.9
    lower limb 956.9
      multiple 956.8
      specified site NEC 956.5
    lumbar plexus 953.5
    lumbosacral plexus 953.5
    median 955.1
      forearm 955.1
      wrist and hand 955.1
    multiple (in several parts of body)
      (sites not classifiable to the
      same three-digit category)
      957.8
    musculocutaneous 955.4
    musculospiral 955.3
      upper arm 955.3
    oculomotor 951.0
    olfactory 951.8
    optic 950.0
    pelvic girdle 956.9
      multiple sites 956.8
      specified site NEC 956.5
    peripheral 957.9
      multiple (in several regions)
        (sites not classifiable to the
        same three-digit category)
        957.8
      specified site NEC 957.1
    peroneal 956.3
      ankle and foot 956.3
      lower leg 956.3
    plantar 956.5
    plexus 957.9
      celiac 954.1
      mesenteric, inferior 954.1
      spinal 953.9
        brachial 953.4
        lumbosacral 953.5
        multiple sites 953.8
      sympathetic NEC 954.1
    pneumogastric 951.8
    radial 955.3
      wrist and hand 955.3
    sacral plexus 953.5
    sciatic 956.0
      thigh 956.0
    shoulder girdle 955.9
      multiple 955.8
      specified site NEC 955.7
    specified site NEC 957.1
    spinal 953.9
      plexus - see Injury, nerve, plexus,
        spinal
      root 953.9
        cervical 953.0
        dorsal 953.1
        lumbar 953.2
        multiple sites 953.8
        sacral 953.3
    splanchnic 954.1
    sympathetic NEC 954.1
      cervical 954.0
    thigh 956.9
    tibial 956.5
      ankle and foot 956.2
      lower leg 956.5
      posterior 956.2
    toe 956.9

Injury (Continued)
  nerve (Continued)
    trigeminal 951.2
    trochlear 951.1
    trunk, excluding shoulder and
      pelvic girdles 954.9
      specified site NEC 954.8
      sympathetic NEC 954.1
    ulnar 955.2
      forearm 955.2
      wrist (and hand) 955.2
    upper limb 955.9
      multiple 955.8
      specified site NEC 955.7
    vagus 951.8
    wrist and hand 955.9
  nervous system, diffuse 957.8
  nose (septum) 959.09
  obstetrical NEC 665.9●
    affecting fetus or newborn 763.89
  occipital (region) (scalp) 959.09
    lobe (see also Injury, intracranial)
      854.0●
  optic 950.9
    chiasm 950.1
    cortex 950.3
    nerve 950.0
    pathways 950.2
  orbit, orbital (region) 921.2
    penetrating 870.3
      with foreign body 870.4
  ovary - see Injury, internal, ovary
  paint-gun - see Wound, open, by site,
    complicated
  palate (soft) 959.09
  pancreas - see Injury, internal, pancreas
  parathyroid (gland) 959.09
  parietal (region) (scalp) 959.09
    lobe - see Injury, intracranial
  pelvic
    floor 959.19
      complicating delivery 664.1●
        affecting fetus or newborn
          763.89
    joint or ligament, complicating
      delivery 665.6●
      affecting fetus or newborn
        763.89
    organs - see also Injury, internal,
      pelvis
      with
        abortion - see Abortion, by
          type, with damage to
          pelvic organs
        ectopic pregnancy (see also
          categories 633.0–633.9)
          639.2
        molar pregnancy (see also
          categories 633.0–633.9)
          639.2
        following
          abortion 639.2
          ectopic or molar pregnancy
            639.2
        obstetrical trauma 665.5●
          affecting fetus or newborn
            763.89
  pelvis 959.19
  penis 959.14
    fracture of corpus cavernosum
      959.13
  perineum 959.14
  peritoneum - see Injury, internal,
    peritoneum

Injury (Continued)
  periurethral tissue
    with
      abortion - see Abortion, by type,
        with damage to pelvic
        organs
      ectopic pregnancy (see also
        categories 633.0–633.9) 639.2
      molar pregnancy (see also
        categories 630–632) 639.2
    complicating delivery 665.5●
      affecting fetus or newborn 763.89
    following
      abortion 639.2
      ectopic or molar pregnancy
        639.2
  phalanges
    foot 959.7
    hand 959.5
  pharynx 959.09
  pleura - see Injury, internal, pleura
  popliteal space 959.7
  post-cardiac surgery (syndrome)
    429.4
  prepuce 959.14
  prostate - see Injury, internal, prostate
  pubic region 959.19
  pudenda 959.14
  radiation NEC 990
  radioactive substance or radium NEC
    990
  rectovaginal septum 959.14
  rectum - see Injury, internal, rectum
  retina 921.3
    penetrating - see Injury, eyeball,
      penetrating
  retroperitoneal - see Injury, internal,
    retroperitoneum
  roentgen rays NEC 990
  round ligament - see Injury, internal,
    round ligament
  sacral (region) 959.19
    plexus 953.5
  sacroiliac ligament NEC 959.19
  sacrum 959.19
  salivary ducts or glands 959.09
  scalp 959.09
    due to birth trauma 767.19
    fetus or newborn 767.19
  scapular region 959.2
  sclera 921.3
    penetrating - see Injury, eyeball,
      penetrating
    superficial 918.2
  scrotum 959.14
  seminal vesicle - see Injury, internal,
    seminal vesicle
  shoulder (and upper arm) 959.2
  sinus
    cavernous (see also Injury,
      intracranial) 854.0●
    nasal 959.09
  skeleton NEC, birth injury 767.3
  skin NEC 959.9
  skull - see Fracture, skull, by site
  soft tissue (of external sites) (severe) -
    see Wound, open, by site
  specified site NEC 959.8
  spermatic cord - see Injury, internal,
    spermatic cord
  spinal (cord) 952.9
    with fracture, vertebra - see Fracture,
      vertebra, by site, with spinal
      cord injury

Injury (Continued)
  spinal (Continued)
    cervical (C_1–C_4) 952.00
      with
        anterior cord syndrome 952.02
        central cord syndrome 952.03
        complete lesion of cord 952.01
        incomplete lesion NEC 952.04
        posterior cord syndrome
          952.04
      C_5–C_7 level 952.05
        with
          anterior cord syndrome
            952.07
          central cord syndrome
            952.08
          complete lesion of cord
            952.06
          incomplete lesion NEC
            952.09
          posterior cord syndrome
            952.09
        specified type NEC 952.09
      specified type NEC 952.04
    dorsal (D_1–D_6) (T_1–T_6) (thoracic)
      952.10
      with
        anterior cord syndrome
          952.12
        central cord syndrome
          952.13
        complete lesion of cord
          952.11
        incomplete lesion NEC
          952.14
        posterior cord syndrome
          952.14
      D_7–D_{12} level (T_7–T_{12}) 952.15
        with
          anterior cord syndrome
            952.17
          central cord syndrome
            952.18
          complete lesion of cord
            952.16
          incomplete lesion NEC
            952.19
          posterior cord syndrome
            952.19
        specified type NEC 952.19
      specified type NEC 952.14
    lumbar 952.2
    multiple sites 952.8
    nerve (root) NEC - see Injury, nerve,
      spinal, root
    plexus 953.9
      brachial 953.4
      lumbosacral 953.5
      multiple sites 953.8
    sacral 952.3
    thoracic (see also Injury, spinal,
      dorsal) 952.10
  spleen - see Injury, internal, spleen
  stellate ganglion 954.1
  sternal region 959.11
  stomach - see Injury, internal, stomach
  subconjunctival 921.1
  subcutaneous 959.9
  subdural - see Injury, intracranial
  submaxillary region 959.09
  submental region 959.09
  subungual
    fingers 959.5
    toes 959.7

◄ New   ◄▥ Revised   ~~deleted~~ Deleted   ● Use Additional Digit(s)   ▥ Omit code

Injury *(Continued)*
  superficial 919

> **Note 49** Use the following fourth-digit subdivisions with categories 910–919:
>
> .0 abrasion or friction burn without mention of infection
> .1 abrasion or friction burn, infected
> .2 blister without mention of infection
> .3 blister, infected
> .4 insect bite, nonvenomous, without mention of infection
> .5 insect bite, nonvenomous, infected
> .6 superficial foreign body (splinter) without major open wound and without mention of infection
> .7 superficial foreign body (splinter) without major open wound, infected
> .8 other and unspecified superficial injury without mention of infection
> .9 other and unspecified superficial injury, infected
>
> For late effects of superficial injury, *see* category 906.2.

    abdomen, abdominal (muscle) (wall) (and other part(s) of trunk) 911
    ankle (and hip, knee, leg, or thigh) 916
    anus (and other part(s) of trunk) 911
    arm 913
      upper (and shoulder) 912
    auditory canal (external) (meatus) (and other part(s) of face, neck, or scalp, except eye) 910
    axilla (and upper arm) 912
    back (and other part(s) of trunk) 911
    breast (and other part(s) of trunk) 911
    brow (and other part(s) of face, neck, or scalp, except eye) 910
    buttock (and other part(s) of trunk) 911
    canthus, eye 918.0
    cheek(s) (and other part(s) of face, neck, or scalp, except eye) 910
    chest wall (and other part(s) of trunk) 911
    chin (and other part(s) of face, neck, or scalp, except eye) 910
    clitoris (and other part(s) of trunk) 911
    conjunctiva 918.2
    cornea 918.1
      due to contact lens 371.82
    costal region (and other part(s) of trunk) 911
    ear(s) (auricle) (canal) (drum) (external) (and other part(s) of face, neck, or scalp, except eye) 910
    elbow (and forearm) (and wrist) 913

Injury *(Continued)*
  superficial *(Continued)*
    epididymis (and other part(s) of trunk) 911
    epigastric region (and other part(s) of trunk) 911
    epiglottis (and other part(s) of face, neck, or scalp, except eye) 910
    eye(s) (and adnexa) NEC 918.9
    eyelid(s) (and periocular area) 918.0
    face (any part(s), except eye) (and neck or scalp) 910
    finger(s) (nail) (any) 915
    flank (and other part(s) of trunk) 911
    foot (phalanges) (and toe(s)) 917
    forearm (and elbow) (and wrist) 913
    forehead (and other part(s) of face, neck, or scalp, except eye) 910
    globe (eye) 918.9
    groin (and other part(s) of trunk) 911
    gum(s) (and other part(s) of face, neck, or scalp, except eye) 910
    hand(s) (except fingers alone) 914
    head (and other part(s) of face, neck, or scalp, except eye) 910
    heel (and foot or toe) 917
    hip (and ankle, knee, leg, or thigh) 916
    iliac region (and other part(s) of trunk) 911
    interscapular region (and other part(s) of trunk) 911
    iris 918.9
    knee (and ankle, hip, leg, or thigh) 916
    labium (majus) (minus) (and other part(s) of trunk) 911
    lacrimal (apparatus) (gland) (sac) 918.0
    leg (lower) (upper) (and ankle, hip, knee, or thigh) 916
    lip(s) (and other part(s) of face, neck, or scalp, except eye) 910
    lower extremity (except foot) 916
    lumbar region (and other part(s) of trunk) 911
    malar region (and other part(s) of face, neck, or scalp, except eye) 910
    mastoid region (and other part(s) of face, neck, or scalp, except eye) 910
    midthoracic region (and other part(s) of trunk) 911
    mouth (and other part(s) of face, neck, or scalp, except eye) 910
    multiple sites (not classifiable to the same three-digit category) 919
    nasal (septum) (and other part(s) of face, neck, or scalp, except eye) 910
    neck (and face or scalp, any part(s), except eye) 910
    nose (septum) (and other part(s) of face, neck, or scalp, except eye) 910
    occipital region (and other part(s) of face, neck, or scalp, except eye) 910
    orbital region 918.0
    palate (soft) (and other part(s) of face, neck, or scalp, except eye) 910

Injury *(Continued)*
  superficial *(Continued)*
    parietal region (and other part(s) of face, neck, or scalp, except eye) 910
    penis (and other part(s) of trunk) 911
    perineum (and other part(s) of trunk) 911
    periocular area 918.0
    pharynx (and other part(s) of face, neck, or scalp, except eye) 910
    popliteal space (and ankle, hip, leg, or thigh) 916
    prepuce (and other part(s) of trunk) 911
    pubic region (and other part(s) of trunk) 911
    pudenda (and other part(s) of trunk) 911
    sacral region (and other part(s) of trunk) 911
    salivary (ducts) (glands) (and other part(s) of face, neck, or scalp, except eye) 910
    scalp (and other part(s) of face or neck, except eye) 910
    scapular region (and upper arm) 912
    sclera 918.2
    scrotum (and other part(s) of trunk) 911
    shoulder (and upper arm) 912
    skin NEC 919
    specified site(s) NEC 919
    sternal region (and other part(s) of trunk) 911
    subconjunctival 918.2
    subcutaneous NEC 919
    submaxillary region (and other part(s) of face, neck, or scalp, except eye) 910
    submental region (and other part(s) of face, neck, or scalp, except eye) 910
    supraclavicular fossa (and other part(s) of face, neck, or scalp, except eye) 910
    supraorbital 918.0
    temple (and other part(s) of face, neck, or scalp, except eye) 910
    temporal region (and other part(s) of face, neck, or scalp, except eye) 910
    testis (and other part(s) of trunk) 911
    thigh (and ankle, hip, knee, or leg) 916
    thorax, thoracic (external) (and other part(s) of trunk) 911
    throat (and other part(s) of face, neck, or scalp, except eye) 910
    thumb(s) (nail) 915
    toe(s) (nail) (subungual) (and foot) 917
    tongue (and other part(s) of face, neck, or scalp, except eye) 910
    tooth, teeth (*see also* Abrasion, dental) 521.20
    trunk (any part(s)) 911
    tunica vaginalis (and other part(s) of trunk) 911
    tympanum, tympanic membrane (and other part(s) of face, neck, or scalp, except eye) 910
    upper extremity NEC 913

Injury (Continued)
superficial (Continued)
uvula (and other part(s) of face, neck, or scalp, except eye) 910
vagina (and other part(s) of trunk) 911
vulva (and other part(s) of trunk) 911
wrist (and elbow) (and forearm) 913
supraclavicular fossa 959.19
supraorbital 959.09
surgical complication (external or internal site) 998.2
symphysis pubis 959.19
complicating delivery 665.6●
affecting fetus or newborn 763.89
temple 959.09
temporal region 959.09
testis 959.14
thigh (and hip) 959.6
thorax, thoracic (external) 959.11
cavity - see Injury, internal, thorax
internal - see Injury, internal, intrathoracic organs
throat 959.09
thumb(s) (nail) 959.5
thymus - see Injury, internal, thymus
thyroid (gland) 959.09
toe (nail) (any) 959.7
tongue 959.09
tonsil 959.09
tooth NEC 873.63
complicated 873.73
trachea - see Injury, internal, trachea
trunk 959.19
tunica vaginalis 959.14
tympanum, tympanic membrane 959.09
ultraviolet rays NEC 990
ureter - see Injury, internal, ureter
urethra (sphincter) - see Injury, internal, urethra
uterus - see Injury, internal, uterus
uvula 959.09
vagina 959.14
vascular - see Injury, blood vessel
vas deferens - see Injury, internal, vas deferens
vein (see also Injury, blood vessel, by site) 904.9
vena cava
inferior 902.10
superior 901.2
vesical (sphincter) - see Injury, internal, vesical
viscera (abdominal) - see Injury, internal, viscera
with fracture, pelvis - see Fracture, pelvis
visual 950.9
cortex 950.3
vitreous (humor) 871.2
vulva 959.14
whiplash (cervical spine) 847.0
wringer - see Crush, by site
wrist (and elbow) (and forearm) 959.3
x-ray NEC 990
Inoculation - see also Vaccination
complication or reaction - see Complication, vaccination
INPH (idiopathic normal pressure hydrocephalus) 331.5

Insanity, insane (see also Psychosis) 298.9
adolescent (see also Schizophrenia) 295.9●
alternating (see also Psychosis, affective, circular) 296.7
confusional 298.9
acute 293.0
subacute 293.1
delusional 298.9
paralysis, general 094.1
progressive 094.1
paresis, general 094.1
senile 290.20
Insect
bite - see Injury, superficial, by site
venomous, poisoning by 989.5
Insemination, artificial V26.1
Insensitivity
adrenocorticotropin hormone (ACTH) 255.41
androgen 259.50
complete 259.51
partial 259.52
Insertion
cord (umbilical) lateral or velamentous 663.8●
affecting fetus or newborn 762.6
intrauterine contraceptive device V25.1
placenta, vicious - see Placenta, previa
subdermal implantable contraceptive V25.5
velamentous, umbilical cord 663.8●
affecting fetus or newborn 762.6
Insolation 992.0
meaning sunstroke 992.0
Insomnia, unspecified 780.52
with sleep apnea, unspecified 780.51
adjustment 307.41
alcohol induced 291.82
behavioral, of childhood V69.5
drug induced 292.85
due to
medical condition classified elsewhere 327.01
mental disorder 327.02
fatal familial (FFI) 046.72
idiopathic 307.42
nonorganic origin 307.41
persistent (primary) 307.42
transient 307.41
organic 327.00
other 327.09
paradoxical 307.42
primary 307.42
psychophysiological 307.42
subjective complaint 307.49
Inspiration
food or foreign body (see also Asphyxia, food or foreign body) 933.1
mucus (see also Asphyxia, mucus) 933.1
Inspissated bile syndrome, newborn 774.4
Instability
detrusor 596.59
emotional (excessive) 301.3
joint (posttraumatic) 718.80
ankle 718.87
elbow 718.82
foot 718.87
hand 718.84
hip 718.85
knee 718.86
lumbosacral 724.6
multiple sites 718.89
pelvic region 718.85

Instability (Continued)
joint (Continued)
sacroiliac 724.6
shoulder (region) 718.81
specified site NEC 718.88
wrist 718.83
lumbosacral 724.6
nervous 301.89
personality (emotional) 301.59
thyroid, paroxysmal 242.9●
urethral 599.83
vasomotor 780.2
Insufficiency, insufficient
accommodation 367.4
adrenal (gland) (acute) (chronic) 255.41
medulla 255.5
primary 255.41
specified site NEC 255.5
adrenocortical 255.41
anterior (occlusal) guidance 524.54
anus 569.49
aortic (valve) 424.1
with
mitral (valve) disease 396.1
insufficiency, incompetence, or regurgitation 396.3
stenosis or obstruction 396.1
stenosis or obstruction 424.1
with mitral (valve) disease 396.8
congenital 746.4
rheumatic 395.1
with
mitral (valve) disease 396.1
insufficiency, incompetence, or regurgitation 396.3
stenosis or obstruction 396.1
stenosis or obstruction 395.2
with mitral (valve) disease 396.8
specified cause NEC 424.1
syphilitic 093.22
arterial 447.1
basilar artery 435.0
carotid artery 435.8
cerebral 437.1
coronary (acute or subacute) 411.89
mesenteric 557.1
peripheral 443.9
precerebral 435.9
vertebral artery 435.1
vertebrobasilar 435.3
arteriovenous 459.9
basilar artery 435.0
biliary 575.8
cardiac (see also Insufficiency, myocardial) 428.0
complicating surgery 997.1
due to presence of (cardiac) prosthesis 429.4
postoperative 997.1
long-term effect of cardiac surgery 429.4
specified during or due to a procedure 997.1
long-term effect of cardiac surgery 429.4
cardiorenal (see also Hypertension, cardiorenal) 404.90
cardiovascular (see also Disease, cardiovascular) 429.2
renal (see also Hypertension, cardiorenal) 404.90
carotid artery 435.8

◀ New   ⫶▪ Revised   ~~deleted~~ Deleted   ● Use Additional Digit(s)   ▬ Omit code

Insufficiency, insufficient (*Continued*)
 cerebral (vascular) 437.9
 cerebrovascular 437.9
  with transient focal neurological
    signs and symptoms 435.9
  acute 437.1
   with transient focal neurological
     signs and symptoms 435.9
 circulatory NEC 459.9
  fetus or newborn 779.89
 convergence 378.83
 coronary (acute or subacute) 411.89
  chronic or with a stated duration of
    over 8 weeks 414.8
 corticoadrenal 255.41
 dietary 269.9
 divergence 378.85
 food 994.2
 gastroesophageal 530.89
 gonadal
  ovary 256.39
  testis 257.2
 gonadotropic hormone secretion 253.4
 heart - *see also* Insufficiency, myocardial
  fetus or newborn 779.89
  valve (*see also* Endocarditis) 424.90
   congenital NEC 746.89
 hepatic 573.8
 idiopathic autonomic 333.0
 interocclusal distance of teeth (ridge)
   524.36
 kidney
  acute 593.9
  chronic 585.9
 labyrinth, labyrinthine (function)
   386.53
  bilateral 386.54
  unilateral 386.53
 lacrimal 375.15
 liver 573.8
 lung (acute) (*see also* Insufficiency,
   pulmonary) 518.82
  following trauma, surgery, or shock
    518.5
  newborn 770.89
 mental (congenital) (*see also*
   Retardation, mental) 319
 mesenteric 557.1
 mitral (valve) 424.0
  with
   aortic (valve) disease 396.3
    insufficiency, incompetence, or
      regurgitation 396.3
    stenosis or obstruction 396.2
   obstruction or stenosis 394.2
    with aortic valve disease 396.8
  congenital 746.6
  rheumatic 394.1
   with
    aortic (valve) disease 396.3
     insufficiency, incompetence,
       or regurgitation 396.3
     stenosis or obstruction 396.2
    obstruction or stenosis 394.2
     with aortic valve disease
       396.8
   active or acute 391.1
    with chorea, rheumatic
      (Sydenham's) 392.0
  specified cause, except rheumatic
    424.0
 muscle
  heart - *see* Insufficiency, myocardial
  ocular (*see also* Strabismus) 378.9

Insufficiency, insufficient (*Continued*)
 myocardial, myocardium (with
   arteriosclerosis) 428.0
  with rheumatic fever (conditions
    classifiable to 390)
   active, acute, or subacute 391.2
    with chorea 392.0
   inactive or quiescent (with
     chorea) 398.0
  congenital 746.89
  due to presence of (cardiac)
    prosthesis 429.4
  fetus or newborn 779.89
  following cardiac surgery 429.4
  hypertensive (*see also* Hypertension,
    heart) 402.91
   benign 402.11
   malignant 402.01
  postoperative 997.1
   long-term effect of cardiac
     surgery 429.4
  rheumatic 398.0
   active, acute, or subacute 391.2
    with chorea (Sydenham's)
      392.0
  syphilitic 093.82
 nourishment 994.2
 organic 799.89
 ovary 256.39
  postablative 256.2
 pancreatic 577.8
 parathyroid (gland) 252.1
 peripheral vascular (arterial) 443.9
 pituitary (anterior) 253.2
  posterior 253.5
 placental - *see* Placenta, insufficiency
 platelets 287.5
 prenatal care in current pregnancy
   V23.7
 progressive pluriglandular 258.9
 pseudocholinesterase 289.89
 pulmonary (acute) 518.82
  following
   shock 518.5
   surgery 518.5
   trauma 518.5
  newborn 770.89
  valve (*see also* Endocarditis,
    pulmonary) 424.3
   congenital 746.09
 pyloric 537.0
 renal 593.9
  acute 593.9
  chronic 585.9
  due to a procedure 997.5
 respiratory 786.09
  acute 518.82
   following shock, surgery, or
     trauma 518.5
  newborn 770.89
 rotation - *see* Malrotation
 suprarenal 255.41
  medulla 255.5
 tarso-orbital fascia, congenital 743.66
 tear film 375.15
 testis 257.2
 thyroid (gland) (acquired) - *see also*
   Hypothyroidism
  congenital 243
 tricuspid (*see also* Endocarditis,
   tricuspid) 397.0
  congenital 746.89
  syphilitic 093.23
 urethral sphincter 599.84

Insufficiency, insufficient (*Continued*)
 valve, valvular (heart) (*see also*
   Endocarditis) 424.90
 vascular 459.9
  intestine NEC 557.9
  mesenteric 557.1
  peripheral 443.9
  renal (*see also* Hypertension, kidney)
    403.90
 velopharyngeal
  acquired 528.9
  congenital 750.29
 venous (peripheral) 459.81
 ventricular - *see* Insufficiency,
   myocardial
 vertebral artery 435.1
 vertebrobasilar artery 435.3
 weight gain during pregnancy
   646.8●
 zinc 269.3
Insufflation
 fallopian
  fertility testing V26.21
  following sterilization reversal
    V26.22
 meconium 770.11
  with respiratory symptoms 770.12
Insular - *see* condition
Insulinoma (M8151/0)
 malignant (M8151/3)
  pancreas 157.4
  specified site - *see* Neoplasm, by site,
    malignant
  unspecified site 157.4
 pancreas 211.7
 specified site - *see* Neoplasm, by site,
   benign
 unspecified site 211.7
Insuloma - *see* Insulinoma
Insult
 brain 437.9
  acute 436
 cerebral 437.9
  acute 436
 cerebrovascular 437.9
  acute 436
 vascular NEC 437.9
  acute 436
Insurance examination (certification)
  V70.3
Intemperance (*see also* Alcoholism)
  303.9●
Interception of pregnancy (menstrual
  extraction) V25.3
Interference
 balancing side 524.56
 non-working side 524.56
Intermenstrual
 bleeding 626.6
  irregular 626.6
  regular 626.5
 hemorrhage 626.6
  irregular 626.6
  regular 626.5
 pain(s) 625.2
Intermittent - *see* condition
Internal - *see* condition
Interproximal wear 521.10
Interruption
 aortic arch 747.11
 bundle of His 426.50
 fallopian tube (for sterilization) V25.2
 phase-shift, sleep cycle 307.45
 repeated REM-sleep 307.48

Interruption (*Continued*)
sleep
due to perceived environmental
disturbances 307.48
phase-shift, of 24-hour sleep-wake
cycle 307.45
repeated REM-sleep type 307.48
vas deferens (for sterilization) V25.2
Intersexuality 752.7
Interstitial - *see* condition
Intertrigo 695.89
labialis 528.5
Intervertebral disc - *see* condition
Intestine, intestinal - *see also* condition
flu 487.8
Intolerance
carbohydrate NEC 579.8
cardiovascular exercise, with pain (at
rest) (with less than ordinary
activity) (with ordinary activity)
V47.2
cold 780.99
dissacharide (hereditary) 271.3
drug
correct substance properly
administered 995.27
wrong substance given or taken in
error 977.9
specified drug - *see* Table of
Drugs and Chemicals
effort 306.2
fat NEC 579.8
foods NEC 579.8
fructose (hereditary) 271.2
glucose (-galactose) (congenital) 271.3
gluten 579.0
lactose (hereditary) (infantile) 271.3
lysine (congenital) 270.7
milk NEC 579.8
protein (familial) 270.7
starch NEC 579.8
sucrose (-isomaltose) (congenital) 271.3
Intoxicated NEC (*see also* Alcoholism)
305.0●
Intoxication
acid 276.2
acute
alcoholic 305.0●
with alcoholism 303.0●
hangover effects 305.0●
caffeine 305.9●
hallucinogenic (*see also* Abuse,
drugs, nondependent) 305.3●
alcohol (acute) 305.0●
with alcoholism 303.0●
hangover effects 305.0●
idiosyncratic 291.4
pathological 291.4
alimentary canal 558.2
ammonia (hepatic) 572.2
caffeine 305.9●
chemical - *see also* Table of Drugs and
Chemicals
via placenta or breast milk 760.70
alcohol 760.71
anticonvulsants 760.77
antifungals 760.74
anti-infective agents 760.74
antimetabolics 760.78
cocaine 760.75
"crack" 760.75
hallucinogenic agents NEC 760.73
medicinal agents NEC 760.79
narcotics 760.72

Intoxication (*Continued*)
chemical (*Continued*)
via placenta or breast milk
(*Continued*)
obstetric anesthetic or analgesic
drug 763.5
specified agent NEC 760.79
suspected, affecting
management of
pregnancy 655.5●
cocaine, through placenta or breast
milk 760.75
delirium
alcohol 291.0
drug 292.81
drug 292.89
with delirium 292.81
correct substance properly
administered (*see also* Allergy,
drug) 995.27
newborn 779.4
obstetric anesthetic or sedation
668.9●
affecting fetus or newborn 763.5
overdose or wrong substance given
or taken - *see* Table of Drugs
and Chemicals
pathologic 292.2
specific to newborn 779.4
via placenta or breast milk 760.70
alcohol 760.71
anticonvulsants 760.77
antifungals 760.74
anti-infective agents 760.74
antimetabolics 760.78
cocaine 760.75
"crack" 760.75
hallucinogenic agents 760.73
medicinal agents NEC 760.79
narcotics 760.72
obstetric anesthetic or analgesic
drug 763.5
specified agent NEC 760.79
suspected, affecting
management of
pregnancy 655.5●
enteric - *see* Intoxication, intestinal
fetus or newborn, via placenta or breast
milk 760.70
alcohol 760.71
anticonvulsants 760.77
antifungals 760.74
anti-infective agents 760.74
antimetabolics 760.78
cocaine 760.75
"crack" 760.75
hallucinogenic agents 760.73
medicinal agents NEC 760.79
narcotics 760.72
obstetric anesthetic or analgesic
drug 763.5
specified agent NEC 760.79
suspected, affecting management of
pregnancy 655.5●
food - *see* Poisoning, food
gastrointestinal 558.2
hallucinogenic (acute) 305.3●
hepatocerebral 572.2
idiosyncratic alcohol 291.4
intestinal 569.89
due to putrefaction of food 005.9
methyl alcohol (*see also* Alcoholism)
305.0●
with alcoholism 303.0●

Intoxication (*Continued*)
non-foodborne due to toxins of
Clostridium botulinum [C.
botulinum] - *see* Botulism
pathologic 291.4
drug 292.2
potassium (K) 276.7
septic
with
abortion - *see* Abortion, by type,
with sepsis
ectopic pregnancy (*see also*
categories 633.0–633.9) 639.0
molar pregnancy (*see also*
categories 630–632) 639.0
during labor 659.3●
following
abortion 639.0
ectopic or molar pregnancy 639.0
generalized - *see* Septicemia
puerperal, postpartum,
childbirth 670.2   ◀▥
serum (prophylactic) (therapeutic)
999.5
uremic - *see* Uremia
water 276.6
Intracranial - *see* condition
Intrahepatic gallbladder 751.69
Intraligamentous - *see also* condition
pregnancy - *see* Pregnancy, cornual
Intraocular - *see also* condition
sepsis 360.00
Intrathoracic - *see also* condition
kidney 753.3
stomach - *see* Hernia, diaphragm
Intrauterine contraceptive device
checking V25.42
insertion V25.1
in situ V45.51
management V25.42
prescription V25.02
repeat V25.42
reinsertion V25.42
removal V25.42
Intraventricular - *see* condition
Intrinsic deformity - *see* Deformity
Intruded tooth 524.34
Intrusion, repetitive, of sleep (due to
environmental disturbances) (with
atypical polysomnographic features)
307.48
Intumescent, lens (eye) NEC 366.9
senile 366.12
Intussusception (colon) (enteric)
(intestine) (rectum) 560.0
appendix 543.9
congenital 751.5
fallopian tube 620.8
ileocecal 560.0
ileocolic 560.0
ureter (obstruction) 593.4
Invagination
basilar 756.0
colon or intestine 560.0
Invalid (since birth) 799.89
Invalidism (chronic) 799.89
Inversion
albumin-globulin (A-G) ratio 273.8
bladder 596.8
cecum (*see also* Intussusception) 560.0
cervix 622.8
nipple 611.79
congenital 757.6
puerperal, postpartum 676.3●

Inversion *(Continued)*
  optic papilla 743.57
  organ or site, congenital NEC - *see*
    Anomaly, specified type NEC
  sleep rhythm 327.39
    nonorganic origin 307.45
  testis (congenital) 752.51
  uterus (postinfectional) (postpartal,
    old) 621.7
    chronic 621.7
    complicating delivery 665.2●
      affecting fetus or newborn 763.89
  vagina - *see* Prolapse, vagina
Investigation
  allergens V72.7
  clinical research (control) (normal
    comparison) (participant) V70.7
Inviability - *see* Immaturity
Involuntary movement, abnormal 781.0
Involution, involutional - *see also*
    condition
  breast, cystic or fibrocystic 610.1
  depression (*see also* Psychosis, affective)
    296.2●
    recurrent episode 296.3●
    single episode 296.2●
  melancholia (*see also* Psychosis,
    affective) 296.2●
    recurrent episode 296.3●
    single episode 296.2●
  ovary, senile 620.3
  paranoid state (reaction) 297.2
  paraphrenia (climacteric) (menopause)
    297.2
  psychosis 298.8
  thymus failure 254.8
IQ
  under 20 318.2
  20–34 318.1
  35–49 318.0
  50–70 317
IRDS 769
Irideremia 743.45
Iridis rubeosis 364.42
  diabetic 250.5● *[364.42]*
    due to secondary diabetes 249.5●
      [364.42]
Iridochoroiditis (panuveitis) 360.12
Iridocyclitis NEC 364.3
  acute 364.00
    primary 364.01
    recurrent 364.02
  chronic 364.10
    in
      lepromatous leprosy 030.0
        [364.11]
      sarcoidosis 135 *[364.11]*
      tuberculosis (*see also* Tuberculosis)
        017.3● *[364.11]*
  due to allergy 364.04
  endogenous 364.01
  gonococcal 098.41
  granulomatous 364.10
  herpetic (simplex) 054.44
    zoster 053.22
  hypopyon 364.05
  lens induced 364.23
  nongranulomatous 364.00
  primary 364.01
  recurrent 364.02
  rheumatic 364.10
  secondary 364.04
    infectious 364.03
    noninfectious 364.04

Iridocyclitis NEC *(Continued)*
  subacute 364.00
    primary 364.01
    recurrent 364.02
  sympathetic 360.11
  syphilitic (secondary) 091.52
  tuberculous (chronic) (*see also*
    Tuberculosis) 017.3● *[364.11]*
Iridocyclochoroiditis (panuveitis)
  360.12
Iridodialysis 364.76
Iridodonesis 364.89
Iridoplegia (complete) (partial) (reflex)
  379.49
Iridoschisis 364.52
Iris - *see* condition
Iritis 364.3
  acute 364.00
    primary 364.01
    recurrent 364.02
  chronic 364.10
    in
      sarcoidosis 135 *[364.11]*
      tuberculosis (*see also*
        Tuberculosis) 017.3●
        [364.11]
  diabetic 250.5● *[364.42]*
    due to secondary diabetes 249.5●
      [364.42]
  due to
    allergy 364.04
    herpes simplex 054.44
    leprosy 030.0 *[364.11]*
  endogenous 364.01
  gonococcal 098.41
  gouty 274.89 *[364.11]*
  granulomatous 364.10
  hypopyon 364.05
  lens induced 364.23
  nongranulomatous 364.00
  papulosa 095.8 *[364.11]*
  primary 364.01
  recurrent 364.02
  rheumatic 364.10
  secondary 364.04
    infectious 364.03
    noninfectious 364.04
  subacute 364.00
    primary 364.01
    recurrent 364.02
  sympathetic 360.11
  syphilitic (secondary) 091.52
    congenital 090.0 *[364.11]*
    late 095.8 *[364.11]*
  tuberculous (*see also* Tuberculosis)
    017.3● *[364.11]*
  uratic 274.89 *[364.11]*
Iron
  deficiency anemia 280.9
  metabolism disease 275.0
  storage disease 275.0
Iron-miners' lung 503
Irradiated enamel (tooth, teeth) 521.89
Irradiation
  burn - *see* Burn, by site
  effects, adverse 990
Irreducible, irreducibility - *see*
    condition
Irregular, irregularity
  action, heart 427.9
  alveolar process 525.8
  bleeding NEC 626.4
  breathing 786.09
  colon 569.89

Irregular, irregularity *(Continued)*
  contour
    of cornea 743.41
      acquired 371.70
    reconstructed breast 612.0
  dentin in pulp 522.3
  eye movements NEC 379.59
  menstruation (cause unknown) 626.4
  periods 626.4
  prostate 602.9
  pupil 364.75
  respiratory 786.09
  septum (nasal) 470
  shape, organ or site, congenital NEC -
    see Distortion
  sleep-wake rhythm (non-24-hour)
    327.39
    nonorganic origin 307.45
  vertebra 733.99
Irritability ~~(nervous)~~ 799.22 ◀▥
  bladder 596.8
    neurogenic 596.54
      with cauda equina syndrome
        344.61
  bowel (syndrome) 564.1
  bronchial (*see also* Bronchitis) 490
  cerebral, newborn 779.1
  colon 564.1
    psychogenic 306.4
  duodenum 564.89
  heart (psychogenic) 306.2
  ileum 564.89
  jejunum 564.89
  myocardium 306.2
  nervousness 799.21 ◀
  rectum 564.89
  stomach 536.9
    psychogenic 306.4
  sympathetic (nervous system) (*see also*
    Neuropathy, peripheral,
    autonomic) 337.9
  urethra 599.84
  ventricular (heart) (psychogenic) 306.2
Irritable (*see also* Irritability) 799.22 ◀▥
Irritation
  anus 569.49
  axillary nerve 353.0
  bladder 596.8
  brachial plexus 353.0
  brain (traumatic) (*see also* Injury,
    intracranial) 854.0●
    nontraumatic - *see* Encephalitis
  bronchial (*see also* Bronchitis) 490
  cerebral (traumatic) (*see also* Injury,
    intracranial) 854.0●
    nontraumatic - *see* Encephalitis
  cervical plexus 353.2
  cervix (*see also* Cervicitis) 616.0
  choroid, sympathetic 360.11
  cranial nerve - *see* Disorder, nerve,
    cranial
  digestive tract 536.9
    psychogenic 306.4
  gastric 536.9
    psychogenic 306.4
  gastrointestinal (tract) 536.9
    functional 536.9
    psychogenic 306.4
  globe, sympathetic 360.11
  intestinal (bowel) 564.9
  labyrinth 386.50
  lumbosacral plexus 353.1
  meninges (traumatic) (*see also* Injury,
    intracranial) 854.0●
    nontraumatic - *see* Meningitis

Irritation (*Continued*)
  myocardium 306.2
  nerve - *see* Disorder, nerve
  nervous 799.21 ◄━
  nose 478.19
  penis 607.89
  perineum 709.9
  peripheral
    autonomic nervous system (*see also*
      Neuropathy, peripheral,
      autonomic) 337.9
    nerve - *see* Disorder, nerve
  peritoneum (*see also* Peritonitis) 567.9
  pharynx 478.29
  plantar nerve 355.6
  spinal (cord) (traumatic) - *see also*
      Injury, spinal, by site
    nerve - *see also* Disorder, nerve
      root NEC 724.9
        traumatic - *see* Injury, nerve,
          spinal
    nontraumatic - *see* Myelitis
  stomach 536.9
    psychogenic 306.4
  sympathetic nerve NEC (*see also*
    Neuropathy, peripheral,
    autonomic) 337.9
  ulnar nerve 354.2
  vagina 623.9
Isambert's disease 012.3●
Ischemia, ischemic 459.9
  basilar artery (with transient
    neurologic deficit) 435.0
  bone NEC 733.40
  bowel (transient) 557.9
    acute 557.0
    chronic 557.1
    due to mesenteric artery
      insufficiency 557.1
  brain - *see also* Ischemia, cerebral
    recurrent focal 435.9
  cardiac (*see also* Ischemia, heart) 414.9
  cardiomyopathy 414.8
  carotid artery (with transient
    neurologic deficit) 435.8
  cerebral (chronic) (generalized) 437.1
    arteriosclerotic 437.0
    intermittent (with transient
      neurologic deficit) 435.9
    newborn 779.2
    puerperal, postpartum, childbirth
      674.0●
    recurrent focal (with transient
      neurologic deficit) 435.9
    transient (with transient neurologic
      deficit) 435.9
  colon 557.9
    acute 557.0
    chronic 557.1
    due to mesenteric artery
      insufficiency 557.1
  coronary (chronic) (*see also* Ischemia,
    heart) 414.9

Ischemia, ischemic (*Continued*)
  heart (chronic or with a stated duration
      of over 8 weeks) 414.9
    acute or with a stated duration
      of 8 weeks or less (*see also*
      Infarct, myocardium)
      410.9●
      without myocardial infarction
        411.89
        with coronary (artery)
          occlusion 411.81
    subacute 411.89
  intestine (transient) 557.9
    acute 557.0
    chronic 557.1
    due to mesenteric artery
      insufficiency 557.1
  kidney 593.81
  labyrinth 386.50
  muscles, leg 728.89
  myocardium, myocardial (chronic or
      with a stated duration of over 8
      weeks) 414.8
    acute (*see also* Infarct, myocardium)
      410.9●
      without myocardial infarction
        411.89
        with coronary (artery)
          occlusion 411.81
  renal 593.81
  retina, retinal 362.84
  small bowel 557.9
    acute 557.0
    chronic 557.1
    due to mesenteric artery
      insufficiency 557.1
  spinal cord 336.1
  subendocardial (*see also* Insufficiency,
    coronary) 411.89
  vertebral artery (with transient
    neurologic deficit) 435.1
Ischialgia (*see also* Sciatica) 724.3
Ischiopagus 759.4
Ischium, ischial - *see* condition
Ischomenia 626.8
Ischuria 788.5
Iselin's disease or osteochondrosis
  732.5
Islands of
  parotid tissue in
    lymph nodes 750.26
    neck structures 750.26
  submaxillary glands in
    fascia 750.26
    lymph nodes 750.26
    neck muscles 750.26
Islet cell tumor, pancreas (M8150/0) 211.7
Isoimmunization NEC (*see also*
  Incompatibility) 656.2●
  anti-E 656.2●
  fetus or newborn 773.2
    ABO blood groups 773.1
    Rhesus (Rh) factor 773.0

Isolation V07.0
  social V62.4
Isosporosis 007.2
Issue
  medical certificate NEC V68.09
    cause of death V68.09
    disability examination V68.01
    fitness V68.09
    incapacity V68.09
  repeat prescription NEC V68.1
    appliance V68.1
    contraceptive V25.40
      device NEC V25.49
        intrauterine V25.42
        specified type NEC V25.49
      pill V25.41
    glasses V68.1
    medicinal substance V68.1
Itch (*see also* Pruritus) 698.9
  bakers' 692.89
  barbers' 110.0
  bricklayers' 692.89
  cheese 133.8
  clam diggers' 120.3
  coolie 126.9
  copra 133.8
  Cuban 050.1
  dew 126.9
  dhobie 110.3
  eye 379.99
  filarial (*see also* Infestation, filarial)
    125.9
  grain 133.8
  grocers' 133.8
  ground 126.9
  harvest 133.8
  jock 110.3
  Malabar 110.9
    beard 110.0
    foot 110.4
    scalp 110.0
  meaning scabies 133.0
  Norwegian 133.0
  perianal 698.0
  poultrymen's 133.8
  sarcoptic 133.0
  scrub 134..1
  seven year V61.10
    meaning scabies 133.0
  straw 133.8
  swimmers' 120.3
  washerwoman's 692.4
  water 120.3
  winter 698.8
Itsenko-Cushing syndrome (pituitary
  basophilism) 255.0
Ivemark's syndrome (asplenia with
  congenital heart disease) 759.0
Ivory bones 756.52
Ixodes 134.8
Ixodiasis 134.8

◄ New ◄━ Revised ~~deleted~~ Deleted ● Use Additional Digit(s) ▨ Omit code

J

Jaccoud's nodular fibrosis, chronic
(Jaccoud's syndrome) 714.4
Jackson's
membrane 751.4
paralysis or syndrome 344.89
veil 751.4
Jacksonian
epilepsy (*see also* Epilepsy) 345.5●
seizures (focal) (*see also* Epilepsy) 345.5●
Jacob's ulcer (M8090/3) - *see* Neoplasm,
skin, malignant, by site
Jacquet's dermatitis (diaper dermatitis)
691.0
Jadassohn's
blue nevus (M8780/0) - *see* Neoplasm,
skin, benign
disease (maculopapular erythroderma)
696.2
intraepidermal epithelioma
(M8096/0) - *see* Neoplasm, skin,
benign
Jadassohn-Lewandowski syndrome
(pachyonychia congenita) 757.5
Jadassohn-Pellizari's disease
(anetoderma) 701.3
Jadassohn-Tièche nevus (M8780/0) - *see*
Neoplasm, skin, benign
Jaffe-Lichtenstein (-Uehlinger) syndrome
252.01
Jahnke's syndrome (encephalocutaneous
angiomatosis) 759.6
Jakob-Creutzfeldt disease (CJD)
(syndrome) 046.19
with dementia
with behavioral disturba nce 046.19
[294.11]
without behavioral disturbance
046.19 [294.10]
familial 046.19
iatrogenic 046.19
specified NEC 046.19
sporadic 046.19
variant (vCJD) 046.11
with dementia
with behavioral disturbance
046.11 [294.11]
without behavioral disturbance
046.11 [294.10]
Jaksch (-Luzet) disease or syndrome
(pseudoleukemia infantum) 285.8
Jamaican
neuropathy 349.82
paraplegic tropical ataxic-spastic
syndrome 349.82
Janet's disease (psychasthenia) 300.89
Janiceps 759.4
Jansky-Bielschowsky amaurotic familial
idiocy 330.1
Japanese
B-type encephalitis 062.0
river fever 081.2
seven-day fever 100.89
Jaundice (yellow) 782.4
acholuric (familial) (splenomegalic) (*see*
also Spherocytosis) 282.0
acquired 283.9
breast milk 774.39
catarrhal (acute) 070.1
with hepatic coma 070.0
chronic 571.9
epidemic - *see* Jaundice, epidemic
cholestatic (benign) 782.4
chronic idiopathic 277.4

Jaundice (*Continued*)
epidemic (catarrhal) 070.1
with hepatic coma 070.0
leptospiral 100.0
spirochetal 100.0
febrile (acute) 070.1
with hepatic coma 070.0
leptospiral 100.0
spirochetal 100.0
fetus or newborn 774.6
due to or associated with
ABO
antibodies 773.1
incompatibility, maternal/fetal
773.1
isoimmunization 773.1
absence or deficiency of enzyme
system for bilirubin
conjugation (congenital)
774.39
blood group incompatibility NEC
773.2
breast milk inhibitors to
conjugation 774.39
associated with preterm
delivery 774.2
bruising 774.1
Crigler-Najjar syndrome 277.4
[774.31]
delayed conjugation 774.30
associated with preterm
delivery 774.2
development 774.39
drugs or toxins transmitted from
mother 774.1
G-6-PD deficiency 282.2 [774.0]
galactosemia 271.1 [774.5]
Gilbert's syndrome 277.4 [774.31]
hepatocellular damage 774.4
hereditary hemolytic anemia (*see
also* Anemia, hemolytic)
282.9 [774.0]
hypothyroidism, congenital 243
[774.31]
incompatibility, maternal/fetal
NEC 773.2
infection 774.1
inspissated bile syndrome 774.4
isoimmunization NEC 773.2
mucoviscidosis 277.01 [774.5]
obliteration of bile duct,
congenital 751.61 [774.5]
polycythemia 774.1
preterm delivery 774.2
red cell defect 282.9 [774.0]
Rh
antibodies 773.0
incompatibility, maternal/fetal
773.0
isoimmunization 773.0
spherocytosis (congenital) 282.0
[774.0]
swallowed maternal blood 774.1
physiological NEC 774.6
from injection, inoculation, infusion, or
transfusion (blood) (plasma)
(serum) (other substance) (onset
within 8 months after
administration) - *see* Hepatitis,
viral
Gilbert's (familial nonhemolytic) 277.4
hematogenous 283.9
hemolytic (acquired) 283.9
congenital (*see also* Spherocytosis)
282.0

Jaundice (*Continued*)
hemorrhagic (acute) 100.0
leptospiral 100.0
newborn 776.0
spirochetal 100.0
hepatocellular 573.8
homologous (serum) - *see* Hepatitis, viral
idiopathic, chronic 277.4
infectious (acute) (subacute) 070.1
with hepatic coma 070.0
leptospiral 100.0
spirochetal 100.0
leptospiral 100.0
malignant (*see also* Necrosis, liver) 570
newborn (physiological) (*see also*
Jaundice, fetus or newborn) 774.6
nonhemolytic, congenital familial
(Gilbert's) 277.4
nuclear, newborn (*see also* Kernicterus
of newborn) 774.7
obstructive NEC (*see also* Obstruction,
biliary) 576.8
postimmunization - *see* Hepatitis, viral
posttransfusion - *see* Hepatitis, viral
regurgitation (*see also* Obstruction,
biliary) 576.8
serum (homologous) (prophylactic)
(therapeutic) - *see* Hepatitis, viral
spirochetal (hemorrhagic) 100.0
symptomatic 782.4
newborn 774.6
Jaw - *see* condition
Jaw-blinking 374.43
congenital 742.8
Jaw-winking phenomenon or syndrome
742.8
Jealousy
alcoholic 291.5
childhood 313.3
sibling 313.3
Jejunitis (*see also* Enteritis) 558.9
Jejunostomy status V44.4
Jejunum, jejunal - *see* condition
Jensen's disease 363.05
Jericho boil 085.1
Jerks, myoclonic 333.2
Jervell-Lange-Nielsen syndrome 426.82
Jeune's disease or syndrome (asphyxiating
thoracic dystrophy) 756.4
Jigger disease 134.1
Job's syndrome (chronic granulomatous
disease) 288.1
Jod-Basedow phenomenon 242.8●
Johnson-Stevens disease (erythema
multiforme exudativum) 695.13
Joint - *see also* condition
Charcôt's 094.0 [713.5]
false 733.82
flail - *see* Flail, joint
mice - *see* Loose, body, joint, by site
sinus to bone 730.9●
von Gies' 095.8
Jordan's anomaly or syndrome 288.2
Josephs-Diamond-Blackfan anemia
(congenital hypoplastic) 284.01
Joubert syndrome 759.89
Jumpers' knee 727.2
Jungle yellow fever 060.0
Jungling's disease (sarcoidosis) 135
Junin virus hemorrhagic fever 078.7
Juvenile - *see also* condition
delinquent 312.9
group (*see also* Disturbance, conduct)
312.2●
neurotic 312.4

K

Kabuki syndrome 759.89
Kahler (-Bozzolo) disease (multiple myeloma) (M9730/3) 203.0●
Kakergasia 300.9
Kakke 265.0
Kala-azar (Indian) (infantile) (Mediterranean) (Sudanese) 085.0
Kalischer's syndrome (encephalocutaneous angiomatosis) 759.6
Kallmann's syndrome (hypogonadotropic hypogonadism with anosmia) 253.4
Kanner's syndrome (autism) (see also Psychosis, childhood) 299.0●
Kaolinosis 502
Kaposi's
    disease 757.33
        lichen ruber 696.4
            acuminatus 696.4
            moniliformis 697.8
        xeroderma pigmentosum 757.33
    sarcoma (M9140/3) 176.9
        adipose tissue 176.1
        aponeurosis 176.1
        artery 176.1
        associated herpesvirus infection 058.89
        blood vessel 176.1
        bursa 176.1
        connective tissue 176.1
        external genitalia 176.8
        fascia 176.1
        fatty tissue 176.1
        fibrous tissue 176.1
        gastrointestinal tract NEC 176.3
        ligament 176.1
        lung 176.4
        lymph
            gland(s) 176.5
            node(s) 176.5
        lymphatic(s) NEC 176.1
        muscle (skeletal) 176.1
        oral cavity NEC 176.8
        palate 176.2
        scrotum 176.8
        skin 176.0
        soft tissue 176.1
        specified site NEC 176.8
        subcutaneous tissue 176.1
        synovia 176.1
        tendon (sheath) 176.1
        vein 176.1
        vessel 176.1
        viscera NEC 176.9
        vulva 176.8
    varicelliform eruption 054.0
        vaccinia 999.0
Kartagener's syndrome or triad (sinusitis, bronchiectasis, situs inversus) 759.3
Kasabach-Merritt syndrome (capillary hemangioma associated with thrombocytopenic purpura) 287.39
Kaschin-Beck disease (endemic polyarthritis) - see Disease, Kaschin-Beck
Kast's syndrome (dyschondroplasia with hemangiomas) 756.4
Katatonia- see Catatonia
Katayama disease or fever 120.2
Kathisophobia 781.0
Kawasaki disease 446.1

Kayser-Fleischer ring (cornea) (pseudosclerosis) 275.1 [371.14]
Kaznelson's syndrome (congenital hypoplastic anemia) 284.01
Kearns-Sayre syndrome 277.87
Kedani fever 081.2
Kelis 701.4
Kelly (-Patterson) syndrome (sideropenic dysphagia) 280.8
Keloid, cheloid 701.4
    Addison's (morphea) 701.0
    cornea 371.00
    Hawkins' 701.4
    scar 701.4
Keloma 701.4
Kenya fever 082.1
Keratectasia 371.71
    congenital 743.41
Keratinization NEC
    alveolar ridge mucosa
        excessive 528.72
        minimal 528.71
Keratitis (nodular) (nonulcerative) (simple) (zonular) NEC 370.9
    with ulceration (see also Ulcer, cornea) 370.00
    actinic 370.24
    arborescens 054.42
    areolar 370.22
    bullosa 370.8
    deep - see Keratitis, interstitial
    dendritic(a) 054.42
    desiccation 370.34
    diffuse interstitial 370.52
    disciform(is) 054.43
        varicella 052.7 [370.44]
    epithelialis vernalis 372.13 [370.32]
    exposure 370.34
    filamentary 370.23
    gonococcal (congenital) (prenatal) 098.43
    herpes, herpetic (simplex) NEC 054.43
        zoster 053.21
    hypopyon 370.04
    in
        chickenpox 052.7 [370.44]
        exanthema (see also Exanthem) 057.9 [370.44]
        paravaccinia (see also Paravaccinia) 051.9 [370.44]
        smallpox (see also Smallpox) 050.9 [370.44]
        vernal conjunctivitis 372.13 [370.32]
    interstitial (nonsyphilitic) 370.50
        with ulcer (see also Ulcer, cornea) 370.00
        diffuse 370.52
        herpes, herpetic (simplex) 054.43
            zoster 053.21
        syphilitic (congenital) (hereditary) 090.3
        tuberculous (see also Tuberculosis) 017.3● [370.59]
    lagophthalmic 370.34
    macular 370.22
    neuroparalytic 370.35
    neurotrophic 370.35
    nummular 370.22
    oyster-shuckers' 370.8
    parenchymatous - see Keratitis, interstitial
    petrificans 370.8
    phlyctenular 370.31
    postmeasles 055.71

Keratitis (Continued)
    punctata, punctate 370.21
        leprosa 030.0 [370.21]
        profunda 090.3
        superficial (Thygeson's) 370.21
    purulent 370.8
    pustuliformis profunda 090.3
    rosacea 695.3 [370.49]
    sclerosing 370.54
    specified type NEC 370.8
    stellate 370.22
    striate 370.22
    superficial 370.20
        with conjunctivitis (see also Keratoconjunctivitis) 370.40
        punctate (Thygeson's) 370.21
    suppurative 370.8
    syphilitic (congenital) (prenatal) 090.3
    trachomatous 076.1
        late effect 139.1
    tuberculous (phlyctenular) (see also Tuberculosis) 017.3● [370.31]
    ulcerated (see also Ulcer, cornea) 370.00
    vesicular 370.8
    welders' 370.24
    xerotic (see also Keratomalacia) 371.45
        vitamin A deficiency 264.4
Keratoacanthoma 238.2
Keratocele 371.72
Keratoconjunctivitis (see also Keratitis) 370.40
    adenovirus type 8 077.1
    epidemic 077.1
    exposure 370.34
    gonococcal 098.43
    herpetic (simplex) 054.43
        zoster 053.21
    in
        chickenpox 052.7 [370.44]
        exanthema (see also Exanthem) 057.9 [370.44]
        paravaccinia (see also Paravaccinia) 051.9 [370.44]
        smallpox (see also Smallpox) 050.9 [370.44]
    infectious 077.1
    neurotrophic 370.35
    phlyctenular 370.31
    postmeasles 055.71
    shipyard 077.1
    sicca (Sjögren's syndrome) 710.2
        not in Sjögren's syndrome 370.33
    specified type NEC 370.49
    tuberculous (phlyctenular) (see also Tuberculosis) 017.3● [370.31]
Keratoconus 371.60
    acute hydrops 371.62
    congenital 743.41
    stable 371.61
Keratocyst (dental) 526.0
Keratoderma, keratodermia (congenital) (palmaris et plantaris) (symmetrical) 757.39
    acquired 701.1
    blennorrhagica 701.1
        gonococcal 098.81
    climacterium 701.1
    eccentrica 757.39
    gonorrheal 098.81
    punctata 701.1
    tylodes, progressive 701.1

◀ New   ◀▦ Revised   ~~deleted~~ Deleted   ● Use Additional Digit(s)   ▦ Omit code

Keratodermatocele 371.72
Keratoglobus 371.70
  congenital 743.41
    associated with buphthalmos
      743.22
Keratohemia 371.12
Keratoiritis (see also Iridocyclitis) 364.3
  syphilitic 090.3
  tuberculous (see also Tuberculosis)
    017.3● [364.11]
Keratolysis exfoliativa (congenital) 757.39
  acquired 695.89
  neonatorum 757.39
Keratoma 701.1
  congenital 757.39
  malignum congenitale 757.1
  palmaris et plantaris hereditarium
    757.39
  senile 702.0
Keratomalacia 371.45
  vitamin A deficiency 264.4
Keratomegaly 743.41
Keratomycosis 111.1
  nigricans (palmaris) 111.1
Keratopathy 371.40
  band (see also Keratitis) 371.43
  bullous (see also Keratitis) 371.23
  degenerative (see also Degeneration,
    cornea) 371.40
    hereditary (see also Dystrophy,
      cornea) 371.50
  discrete colliquative 371.49
Keratoscleritis, tuberculous (see also
  Tuberculosis) 017.3● [370.31]
Keratosis 701.1
  actinic 702.0
  arsenical 692.4
  blennorrhagica 701.1
    gonococcal 098.81
  congenital (any type) 757.39
  ear (middle) (see also Cholesteatoma)
    385.30
  female genital (external) 629.89
  follicular, vitamin A deficiency 264.8
  follicularis 757.39
    acquired 701.1
    congenital (acneiformis) (Siemens')
      757.39
    spinulosa (decalvans) 757.39
    vitamin A deficiency 264.8
  gonococcal 098.81
  larynx, laryngeal 478.79
  male genital (external) 608.89
  middle ear (see also Cholesteatoma)
    385.30
  nigricans 701.2
    congenital 757.39
  obturans 380.21
  oral epithelium
    residual ridge mucosa
      excessive 528.72
      minimal 528.71
  palmaris et plantaris (symmetrical)
    757.39
  penile 607.89
  pharyngeus 478.29
  pilaris 757.39
    acquired 701.1
  punctata (palmaris et plantaris) 701.1
  scrotal 608.89
  seborrheic 702.19
    inflamed 702.11
  senilis 702.0
  solar 702.0

Keratosis (Continued)
  suprafollicularis 757.39
  tonsillaris 478.29
  vagina 623.1
  vegetans 757.39
  vitamin A deficiency 264.8
Kerato-uveitis (see also Iridocyclitis) 364.3
Keraunoparalysis 994.0
Kerion (celsi) 110.0
Kernicterus of newborn (not due to
  isoimmunization) 774.7
  due to isoimmunization (conditions
    classifiable to 773.0–773.2) 773.4
Ketoacidosis 276.2
  diabetic 250.1●
    due to secondary diabetes 249.1●
Ketonuria 791.6
  branched-chain, intermittent 270.3
Ketosis 276.2
  diabetic 250.1●
    due to secondary diabetes 249.1●
Kidney - see condition
Kienböck's
  disease 732.3
    adult 732.8
  osteochondrosis 732.3
Kimmelstiel (-Wilson) disease or
  syndrome (intercapillary
  glomerulosclerosis) 250.4●
  [581.81]
  due to secondary diabetes 249.4●
  [581.81]
Kink, kinking
  appendix 543.9
  artery 447.1
  cystic duct, congenital 751.61
  hair (acquired) 704.2
  ileum or intestine (see also Obstruction,
    intestine) 560.9
  Lane's (see also Obstruction, intestine)
    560.9
  organ or site, congenital NEC - see
    Anomaly, specified type NEC, by
    site
  ureter (pelvic junction) 593.3
    congenital 753.20
  vein(s) 459.2
    caval 459.2
    peripheral 459.2
Kinnier Wilson's disease
  (hepatolenticular degeneration)
  275.1
Kissing
  osteophytes 721.5
  spine 721.5
  vertebra 721.5
Klauder's syndrome (erythema
  multiforme exudativum) 695.19
Klebs' disease (see also Nephritis)
  583.9
Klein-Waardenburg syndrome (ptosis-
  epicanthus) 270.2
Kleine-Levin syndrome 327.13
Kleptomania 312.32
Klinefelter's syndrome 758.7
Klinger's disease 446.4
Klippel's disease 723.8
Klippel-Feil disease or syndrome
  (brevicollis) 756.16
Klippel-Trenaunay syndrome 759.89
Klumpke (-Déjérine) palsy, paralysis
  (birth) (newborn) 767.6
Klüver-Bucy (-Terzian) syndrome 310.0
Knee - see condition

Knifegrinders' rot (see also Tuberculosis)
  011.4●
Knock-knee (acquired) 736.41
  congenital 755.64
Knot
  intestinal, syndrome (volvulus)
    560.2
  umbilical cord (true) 663.2●
    affecting fetus or newborn 762.5
Knots, surfer 919.8
  infected 919.9
Knotting (of)
  hair 704.2
  intestine 560.2
Knuckle pads (Garrod's) 728.79
Köbner's disease (epidermolysis bullosa)
  757.39
Koch's
  infection (see also Tuberculosis,
    pulmonary) 011.9●
  relapsing fever 087.9
Koch-Weeks conjunctivitis 372.03
Koenig-Wichman disease (pemphigus)
  694.4
Köhler's disease (osteochondrosis)
  732.5
  first (osteochondrosis juvenilis) 732.5
  second (Freiburg's infarction,
    metatarsal head) 732.5
  patellar 732.4
  tarsal navicular (bone) (osteoarthrosis
    juvenilis) 732.5
Köhler-Mouchet disease (osteoarthrosis
  juvenilis) 732.5
Köhler-Pellegrini-Stieda disease or
  syndrome (calcification, knee joint)
  726.62
Koilonychia 703.8
  congenital 757.5
Kojevnikov's, Kojewnikoff's epilepsy
  (see also Epilepsy) 345.7●
König's
  disease (osteochondritis dissecans)
    732.7
  syndrome 564.89
Koniophthisis (see also Tuberculosis)
  011.4●
Koplik's spots 055.9
Kopp's asthma 254.8
Korean hemorrhagic fever 078.6
Korsakoff (-Wernicke) disease, psychosis,
  or syndrome (nonalcoholic) 294.0
  alcoholic 291.1
Korsakov's disease - see Korsakoff's
  disease
Korsakow's disease - see Korsakoff's
  disease
Kostmann's disease or syndrome
  (infantile genetic agranulocytosis)
  288.01
Krabbe's
  disease (leukodystrophy) 330.0
  syndrome
    congenital muscle hypoplasia 756.89
    cutaneocerebral angioma 759.6
Kraepelin-Morel disease (see also
  Schizophrenia) 295.9●
Kraft-Weber-Dimitri disease 759.6
Kraurosis
  ani 569.49
  penis 607.0
  vagina 623.8
  vulva 624.09
Kreotoxism 005.9

Krukenberg's
  spindle 371.13
  tumor (M8490/6) 198.6
Kufs' disease 330.1
Kugelberg-Welander disease 335.11
Kuhnt-Junius degeneration or disease
  362.52
Kulchitsky's cell carcinoma (carcinoid
  tumor of intestine) 259.2
Kümmell's disease or spondylitis 721.7
Kundrat's disease (lymphosarcoma)
  200.1●
Kunekune - *see* Dermatophytosis
Kunkel syndrome (lupoid hepatitis)
  571.49
Kupffer cell sarcoma (M9124/3) 155.0
Kuru 046.0
Kussmaul's
  coma (diabetic) 250.3●
    due to secondary diabetes
      249.3●
  disease (polyarteritis nodosa) 446.0
  respiration (air hunger) 786.09
Kwashiorkor (marasmus type) 260
Kyasanur Forest disease 065.2

Kyphoscoliosis, kyphoscoliotic
  (acquired) (*see also* Scoliosis)
    737.30
  congenital 756.19
  due to radiation 737.33
  heart (disease) 416.1
  idiopathic 737.30
    infantile
      progressive 737.32
      resolving 737.31
  late effect of rickets 268.1 *[737.43]*
  specified NEC 737.39
  thoracogenic 737.34
  tuberculous (*see also* Tuberculosis)
    015.0● *[737.43]*
Kyphosis, kyphotic (acquired) (postural)
    737.10
  adolescent postural 737.0
  congenital 756.19
  dorsalis juvenilis 732.0
  due to or associated with
    Charcôt-Marie-Tooth disease 356.1
      [737.41]
    mucopolysaccharidosis 277.5
      [737.41]

Kyphosis, kyphotic (*Continued*)
  due to or associated with (*Continued*)
    neurofibromatosis 237.71 *[737.41]*
    osteitis
      deformans 731.0 *[737.41]*
      fibrosa cystica 252.01 *[737.41]*
    osteoporosis (*see also* Osteoporosis)
      733.0 *[737.41]*
    poliomyelitis (*see also* Poliomyelitis)
      138 *[737.41]*
    radiation 737.11
    tuberculosis (*see also* Tuberculosis)
      015.0● *[737.41]*
  Kümmell's 721.7
  late effect of rickets 268.1 *[737.41]*
  Morquio-Brailsford type (spinal) 277.5
    [737.41]
  pelvis 738.6
  postlaminectomy 737.12
  specified cause NEC 737.19
  syphilitic, congenital 090.5 *[737.41]*
  tuberculous (*see also* Tuberculosis)
    015.0● *[737.41]*
Kyrle's disease (hyperkeratosis
  follicularis in cutem penetrans) 701.1

◀ New   ◀◀ Revised   ~~deleted~~ Deleted   ● Use Additional Digit(s)   ▬ Omit code

L

Labia, labium - *see* condition
Labiated hymen 752.49
Labile
  blood pressure 796.2
  emotions, emotionality 301.3
  vasomotor system 443.9
Lability, emotional 799.24
Labioglossal paralysis 335.22
Labium leporinum (*see also* Cleft, lip)
  749.10
Labor (*see also* Delivery)
  with complications - *see* Delivery,
    complicated
  abnormal NEC 661.9●
    affecting fetus or newborn 763.7
  arrested active phase 661.1●
    affecting fetus or newborn 763.7
  desultory 661.2●
    affecting fetus or newborn 763.7
  dyscoordinate 661.4●
    affecting fetus or newborn 763.7
  early onset (22–36 weeks gestation)
    644.2●
  failed
    induction 659.1●
      mechanical 659.0●
      medical 659.1●
      surgical 659.0●
    trial (vaginal delivery) 660.6●
  false 644.1●
  forced or induced, affecting fetus or
    newborn 763.89
  hypertonic 661.4●
    affecting fetus or newborn 763.7
  hypotonic 661.2●
    affecting fetus or newborn 763.7
    primary 661.0●
      affecting fetus or newborn 763.7
    secondary 661.1●
      affecting fetus or newborn 763.7
  incoordinate 661.4●
    affecting fetus or newborn 763.7
  irregular 661.2●
    affecting fetus or newborn 763.7
  long - *see* Labor, prolonged
  missed (at or near term) 656.4●
  obstructed NEC 660.9●
    affecting fetus or newborn 763.1
    due to female genital mutilation
      660.8●
    specified cause NEC 660.8●
      affecting fetus or newborn 763.1
  pains, spurious 644.1●
  precipitate 661.3●
    affecting fetus or newborn 763.6
  premature 644.2●
    threatened 644.0●
  prolonged or protracted 662.1●
    affecting fetus or newborn 763.89
    first stage 662.0●
      affecting fetus or newborn 763.89
    second stage 662.2●
      affecting fetus or newborn 763.89
  threatened NEC 644.1●
  undelivered 644.1●
Labored breathing (*see also*
  Hyperventilation) 786.09
Labyrinthitis (inner ear) (destructive)
  (latent) 386.30
  circumscribed 386.32
  diffuse 386.31
  focal 386.32
  purulent 386.33

Labyrinthitis (*Continued*)
  serous 386.31
  suppurative 386.33
  syphilitic 095.8
  toxic 386.34
  viral 386.35
Laceration - *see also* Wound, open, by site
  accidental, complicating surgery
    998.2
  Achilles tendon 845.09
    with open wound 892.2
  anus (sphincter) 879.6
    with
      abortion - *see* Abortion, by type,
        with damage to pelvic
        organs
      ectopic pregnancy (*see also*
        categories 633.0–633.9) 639.2
      molar pregnancy (*see also*
        categories 630–632) 639.2
    complicated 879.7
    complicating delivery (healed) (old)
      654.8●
      with laceration of anal or rectal
        mucosa 664.3●
      not associated with third-degree
        perineal laceration 664.6●
    following
      abortion 639.2
      ectopic or molar pregnancy 639.2
    nontraumatic, nonpuerperal
      (healed) (old) 569.43
  bladder (urinary)
    with
      abortion - *see* Abortion, by type,
        with damage to pelvic
        organs
      ectopic pregnancy (*see also*
        categories 633.0–633.9) 639.2
      molar pregnancy (*see also*
        categories 630–632) 639.2
    following
      abortion 639.2
      ectopic or molar pregnancy 639.2
    obstetrical trauma 665.5●
  blood vessel - *see* Injury, blood vessel,
    by site
  bowel
    with
      abortion - *see* Abortion, by type,
        with damage to pelvic
        organs
      ectopic pregnancy (*see also*
        categories 633.0–633.9) 639.2
      molar pregnancy (*see also*
        categories 630–632) 639.2
    following
      abortion 639.2
      ectopic or molar pregnancy 639.2
    obstetrical trauma 665.5●
  brain (cerebral) (membrane) (with
    hemorrhage) 851.8●

Note 50 Use the following fifth-digit
subclassification with categories
851–854:

  0   unspecified state of
       consciousness
  1   with no loss of consciousness
  2   with brief [less than one hour]
       loss of consciousness
  3   with moderate [1–24 hours] loss
       of consciousness

Laceration (*Continued*)
  brain (*Continued*)

  4   with prolonged [more than
       24 hours] loss of
       consciousness and return to
       pre-existing conscious level
  5   with prolonged [more than
       24 hours] loss of
       consciousness, without
       return to pre-existing
       conscious level

Use fifth-digit 5 to designate when a
patient is unconscious and dies before
regaining consciousness, regardless of
the duration of the loss of
consciousness

  6   with loss of consciousness of
       unspecified duration
  9   with concussion, unspecified

    with
      open intracranial wound 851.9●
      skull fracture - *see* Fracture, skull,
        by site
    cerebellum 851.6●
      with open intracranial wound
        851.7●
    cortex 851.2●
      with open intracranial wound
        851.3●
    during birth 767.0
    stem 851.6●
      with open intracranial wound
        851.7●
  broad ligament
    with
      abortion - *see* Abortion, by type,
        with damage to pelvic
        organs
      ectopic pregnancy (*see also*
        categories 633.0–633.9)
        639.2
      molar pregnancy (*see also*
        categories 630–632) 639.2
    following
      abortion 639.2
      ectopic or molar pregnancy
        639.2
    nontraumatic 620.6
    obstetrical trauma 665.6●
    syndrome (nontraumatic) 620.6
  capsule, joint - *see* Sprain, by site
  cardiac - *see* Laceration, heart
  causing eversion of cervix uteri (old)
    622.0
  central, complicating delivery 664.4●
  cerebellum - *see* Laceration, brain,
    cerebellum
  cerebral - *see also* Laceration, brain
    during birth 767.0
  cervix (uteri)
    with
      abortion - *see* Abortion, by type,
        with damage to pelvic
        organs
      ectopic pregnancy (*see also*
        categories 633.0–633.9)
        639.2
      molar pregnancy (*see also*
        categories 630–632) 639.2
    following
      abortion 639.2
      ectopic or molar pregnancy 639.2

Laceration (*Continued*)
  cervix (*Continued*)
    nonpuerperal, nontraumatic 622.3
    obstetrical trauma (current) 665.3●
    old (postpartal) 622.3
    traumatic - *see* Injury, internal, cervix
  chordae heart 429.5
  complicated 879.9
  cornea - *see* Laceration, eyeball
    superficial 918.1
  cortex (cerebral) - *see* Laceration, brain,
    cortex
  esophagus 530.89
  eye(s) - *see* Laceration, ocular
  eyeball NEC 871.4
    with prolapse or exposure of
      intraocular tissue 871.1
    penetrating - *see* Penetrating wound,
      eyeball
    specified as without prolapse of
      intraocular tissue 871.0
  eyelid NEC 870.8
    full thickness 870.1
      involving lacrimal passages 870.2
    skin (and periocular area) 870.0
      penetrating - *see* Penetrating
        wound, orbit
  fourchette
    with
      abortion - *see* Abortion, by type,
        with damage to pelvic
        organs
      ectopic pregnancy (*see also*
        categories 633.0–633.9) 639.2
      molar pregnancy (*see also*
        categories 630–632) 639.2
    complicating delivery 664.0●
    following
      abortion 639.2
      ectopic or molar pregnancy 639.2
  heart (without penetration of heart
    chambers) 861.02
    with
      open wound into thorax 861.12
      penetration of heart chambers
        861.03
        with open wound into thorax
          861.13
  hernial sac - *see* Hernia, by site
  internal organ (abdomen) (chest)
    (pelvis) NEC - *see* Injury, internal,
    by site
  kidney (parenchyma) 866.02
    with
      complete disruption of
        parenchyma (rupture)
        866.03
        with open wound into cavity
          866.13
      open wound into cavity 866.12
  labia
    complicating delivery 664.0●
  ligament - *see also* Sprain, by site
    with open wound - *see* Wound,
      open, by site
  liver 864.05
    with open wound into cavity 864.15
    major (disruption of hepatic
      parenchyma) 864.04
      with open wound into cavity
        864.14
    minor (capsule only) 864.02
      with open wound into cavity
        864.12

Laceration (*Continued*)
  liver (*Continued*)
    moderate (involving parenchyma
      without major disruption)
      864.03
      with open wound into cavity
        864.13
      multiple 864.04
        with open wound into cavity
          864.14
    stellate 864.04
      with open wound into cavity
        864.14
  lung 861.22
    with open wound into thorax
      861.32
  meninges - *see* Laceration, brain
  meniscus (knee) (*see also* Tear,
    meniscus) 836.2
    old 717.5
    site other than knee - *see also* Sprain,
      by site
      old NEC (*see also* Disorder,
        cartilage, articular) 718.0●
  muscle - *see also* Sprain, by site
    with open wound - *see* Wound,
      open, by site
  myocardium - *see* Laceration, heart
  nerve - *see* Injury, nerve, by site
  ocular NEC (*see also* Laceration,
    eyeball) 871.4
    adnexa NEC 870.8
      penetrating 870.3
        with foreign body 870.4
  orbit (eye) 870.8
    penetrating 870.3
      with foreign body 870.4
  pelvic
    floor (muscles)
      with
        abortion - *see* Abortion, by type,
          with damage to pelvic
          organs
        ectopic pregnancy (*see also*
          categories 633.0–633.9)
          639.2
        molar pregnancy (*see also*
          categories 630–632)
          639.2
      complicating delivery 664.1●
      following
        abortion 639.2
        ectopic or molar pregnancy
          639.2
      nonpuerperal 618.7
      old (postpartal) 618.7
  organ NEC
    with
      abortion - *see* Abortion, by type,
        with damage to pelvic
        organs
      ectopic pregnancy (*see also*
        categories 633.0–633.9)
        639.2
      molar pregnancy (*see also*
        categories 630–632) 639.2
    complicating delivery 665.5●
      affecting fetus or newborn
        763.89
    following
      abortion 639.2
      ectopic or molar pregnancy
        639.2
    obstetrical trauma 665.5●

Laceration (*Continued*)
  perineum, perineal (old) (postpartal)
    618.7
    with
      abortion - *see* Abortion, by type,
        with damage to pelvic floor
      ectopic pregnancy (*see also*
        categories 633.0–633.9) 639.2
      molar pregnancy (*see also*
        categories 630–632) 639.2
    complicating delivery 664.4●
      first degree 664.0●
      second degree 664.1●
      third degree 664.2●
      fourth degree 664.3●
      central 664.4●
      involving
        anal sphincter (healed) (old)
          654.8●
          fourchette 664.0●
          hymen 664.0●
          labia 664.0●
          not associated with third-
            degree perineal
            laceration 664.6●
        pelvic floor 664.1●
        perineal muscles 664.1●
        rectovaginal with septum
          664.2●
          with anal mucosa 664.3●
        skin 664.0●
        sphincter (anal) (healed) (old)
          654.8●
          with anal mucosa 664.3●
          not associated with third-
            degree perineal
            laceration 664.6●
        vagina 664.0●
        vaginal muscles 664.1●
        vulva 664.0●
      secondary 674.2●
    following
      abortion 639.2
      ectopic or molar pregnancy 639.2
    male 879.6
      complicated 879.7
    muscles, complicating delivery
      664.1●
    nonpuerperal, current injury 879.6
      complicated 879.7
    secondary (postpartal) 674.2●
  peritoneum
    with
      abortion - *see* Abortion, by type,
        with damage to pelvic
        organs
      ectopic pregnancy (*see also*
        categories 633.0–633.9)
        639.2
      molar pregnancy (*see also*
        categories 630–632) 639.2
    following
      abortion 639.2
      ectopic or molar pregnancy 639.2
    obstetrical trauma 665.5●
  periurethral tissue
    with
      abortion - *see* Abortion, by type,
        with damage to pelvic
        organs
      ectopic pregnancy (*see also*
        categories 633.0–633.9) 639.2
      molar pregnancy (*see also*
        categories 630–632) 639.2

◀ New   ◀▥ Revised   ~~deleted~~ Deleted   ● Use Additional Digit(s)   ▥ Omit code

Laceration (Continued)
  periurethral tissue (Continued)
    following
      abortion 639.2
      ectopic or molar pregnancy 639.2
    obstetrical trauma 665.5●
  rectovaginal (septum)
    with
      abortion - see Abortion, by type,
        with damage to pelvic
        organs
      ectopic pregnancy (see also
        categories 633.0–633.9) 639.2
      molar pregnancy (see also
        categories 630–632) 639.2
    complicating delivery 665.4●
      with perineum 664.2●
        involving anal or rectal
          mucosa 664.3●
    following
      abortion 639.2
      ectopic or molar pregnancy
        639.2
    nonpuerperal 623.4
    old (postpartal) 623.4
  spinal cord (meninges) - see also Injury,
    spinal, by site
    due to injury at birth 767.4
    fetus or newborn 767.4
  spleen 865.09
    with
      disruption of parenchyma
        (massive) 865.04
        with open wound into cavity
          865.14
      open wound into cavity 865.19
    capsule (without disruption of
      parenchyma) 865.02
      with open wound into cavity
        865.12
    parenchyma 865.03
      with open wound into cavity
        865.13
      massive disruption (rupture)
        865.04
        with open wound into cavity
          865.14
  tendon 848.9
    with open wound - see Wound,
      open, by site
    Achilles 845.09
      with open wound 892.2
    lower limb NEC 844.9
      with open wound NEC 894.2
    upper limb NEC 840.9
      with open wound NEC 884.2
  tentorium cerebelli - see Laceration,
    brain, cerebellum
  tongue 873.64
    complicated 873.74
  urethra
    with
      abortion - see Abortion, by type,
        with damage to pelvic
        organs
      ectopic pregnancy (see also
        categories 633.0–633.9) 639.2
      molar pregnancy (see also
        categories 630–632) 639.2
    following
      abortion 639.2
      ectopic or molar pregnancy 639.2
    nonpuerperal, nontraumatic 599.84
    obstetrical trauma 665.5●

Laceration (Continued)
  uterus
    with
      abortion - see Abortion, by type,
        with damage to pelvic
        organs
      ectopic pregnancy (see also
        categories 633.0–633.9) 639.2
      molar pregnancy (see also
        categories 630–632) 639.2
    following
      abortion 639.2
      ectopic or molar pregnancy 639.2
    nonpuerperal, nontraumatic 621.8
    obstetrical trauma NEC 665.5●
    old (postpartal) 621.8
  vagina
    with
      abortion - see Abortion, by type,
        with damage to pelvic
        organs
      ectopic pregnancy (see also
        categories 633.0–633.9) 639.2
      molar pregnancy (see also
        categories 630–632) 639.2
      perineal involvement,
        complicating delivery
        664.0●
    complicating delivery 665.4●
      first degree 664.0●
      second degree 664.1●
      third degree 664.2●
      fourth degree 664.3●
      high 665.4●
      muscles 664.1●
      sulcus 665.4●
      wall 665.4●
    following
      abortion 639.2
      ectopic or molar pregnancy 639.2
    nonpuerperal, nontraumatic 623.4
    old (postpartal) 623.4
  valve, heart - see Endocarditis
  vulva
    with
      abortion - see Abortion, by type,
        with damage to pelvic
        organs
      ectopic pregnancy (see also
        categories 633.0–633.9) 639.2
      molar pregnancy (see also
        categories 630–632) 639.2
    complicating delivery 664.0●
    following
      abortion 639.2
      ectopic or molar pregnancy 639.2
    nonpuerperal, nontraumatic 624.4
    old (postpartal) 624.4
Lachrymal - see condition
Lachrymonasal duct - see condition
Lack of
  adequate intermaxillary vertical
    dimension 524.36
  appetite (see also Anorexia) 783.0
  care
    in home V60.4
    of adult 995.84
    of infant (at or after birth) 995.52
  coordination 781.3
  development - see also Hypoplasia
    physiological in childhood 783.40
  education V62.3
  energy 780.79
  financial resources V60.2

Lack of (Continued)
  food 994.2
    in environment V60.89 ◄▥
  growth in childhood 783.43
  heating V60.1
  housing (permanent) (temporary)
    V60.0
    adequate V60.1
  material resources V60.2
  medical attention 799.89
  memory (see also Amnesia) 780.93
    mild, following organic brain
      damage 310.8 ◄▥
  ovulation 628.0
  person able to render necessary care
    V60.4
  physical exercise V69.0
  physiologic development in childhood
    783.40
  posterior occlusal support 524.57
  prenatal care in current pregnancy
    V23.7
  shelter V60.0
  sleep V69.4
  water 994.3
Lacrimal - see condition
Lacrimation, abnormal (see also Epiphora)
  375.20
Lacrimonasal duct - see condition
Lactation, lactating (breast) (puerperal)
  (postpartum)
  defective 676.4●
  disorder 676.9●
    specified type NEC 676.8●
  excessive 676.6●
  failed 676.4●
  mastitis NEC 675.2●
  mother (care and/or examination)
    V24.1
  nonpuerperal 611.6
  suppressed 676.5●
Lacticemia 271.3
  excessive 276.2
Lactosuria 271.3
Lacunar skull 756.0
Laennec's cirrhosis (alcoholic) 571.2
  nonalcoholic 571.5
Lafora's disease 333.2
Lag, lid (nervous) 374.41
Lagleyze-von Hippel disease
  (retinocerebral angiomatosis) 759.6
Lagophthalmos (eyelid) (nervous)
  374.20
  cicatricial 374.23
  keratitis (see also Keratitis) 370.34
  mechanical 374.22
  paralytic 374.21
La grippe - see Influenza
Lahore sore 085.1
Lakes, venous (cerebral) 437.8
Laki-Lorand factor deficiency (see also
  Defect, coagulation) 286.3
Lalling 307.9
Lambliasis 007.1
Lame back 724.5
Lancereaux's diabetes (diabetes mellitus
  with marked emaciation) 250.8●
  [261]
  due to secondary diabetes 249.8●
    [261]
Landau-Kleffner syndrome 345.8●
Landouzy-Déjérine dystrophy
  (fascioscapulohumeral atrophy)
  359.1

Landry's disease or paralysis 357.0
Landry-Guillain-Barré syndrome 357.0
Lane's
  band 751.4
  disease 569.89
  kink (see also Obstruction, intestine)
    560.9
Langdon Down's syndrome (mongolism)
  758.0
Language abolition 784.69
Lanugo (persistent) 757.4
Laparoscopic surgical procedure
    converted to open procedure V64.41
Lardaceous
  degeneration (any site) 277.39
  disease 277.39
  kidney 277.39 [583.81]
  liver 277.39
Large
  baby (regardless of gestational age)
    766.1
    exceptionally (weight of 4500 grams
      or more) 766.0
    of diabetic mother 775.0
  ear 744.22
  fetus - see also Oversize, fetus
    causing disproportion 653.5●
      with obstructed labor 660.1●
  for dates
    fetus or newborn (regardless of
      gestational age) 766.1
      affecting management of
        pregnancy 656.6●
      exceptionally (weight of 4500
        grams or more) 766.0
  physiological cup 743.57
  stature 783.9
  waxy liver 277.39
  white kidney - see Nephrosis
Larsen's syndrome (flattened facies and
    multiple congenital dislocations)
    755.8
Larsen-Johansson disease (juvenile
    osteopathia patellae) 732.4
Larva migrans
  cutaneous NEC 126.9
    ancylostoma 126.9
  of Diptera in vitreous 128.0
  visceral NEC 128.0
Laryngeal - see also condition
  syncope 786.2
Laryngismus (acute) (infectious)
    (stridulous) 478.75
  congenital 748.3
  diphtheritic 032.3
Laryngitis (acute) (edematous) (fibrinous)
    (gangrenous) (infective) (infiltrative)
    (malignant) (membranous)
    (phlegmonous) (pneumococcal)
    (pseudomembranous) (septic)
    (subglottic) (suppurative) (ulcerative)
    (viral) 464.00
  with
    influenza, flu, or grippe 487.1
    obstruction 464.01
    tracheitis (see also Laryngotracheitis)
      464.20
      with obstruction 464.21
      acute 464.20
        with obstruction 464.21
      chronic 476.1
  atrophic 476.0
  Borrelia vincentii 101
  catarrhal 476.0

Laryngitis (Continued)
  chronic 476.0
    with tracheitis (chronic) 476.1
    due to external agent - see
        Condition, respiratory, chronic,
        due to
  diphtheritic (membranous) 032.3
  due to external agent - see
      Inflammation, respiratory, upper,
      due to
  H. influenzae 464.00
    with obstruction 464.01
  Hemophilus influenzae 464.00
    with obstruction 464.01
  hypertrophic 476.0
  influenzal 487.1
  pachydermic 478.79
  sicca 476.0
  spasmodic 478.75
    acute 464.00
      with obstruction 464.01
  streptococcal 034.0
  stridulous 478.75
  syphilitic 095.8
    congenital 090.5
  tuberculous (see also Tuberculosis,
    larynx) 012.3●
  Vincent's 101
Laryngocele (congenital) (ventricular)
  748.3
Laryngofissure 478.79
  congenital 748.3
Laryngomalacia (congenital) 748.3
Laryngopharyngitis (acute) 465.0
  chronic 478.9
    due to external agent - see
        Condition, respiratory, chronic,
        due to
  due to external agent - see
      Inflammation, respiratory, upper,
      due to
  septic 034.0
Laryngoplegia (see also Paralysis, vocal
  cord) 478.30
Laryngoptosis 478.79
Laryngospasm 478.75
  due to external agent - see Condition,
    respiratory, acute, due to
Laryngostenosis 478.74
  congenital 748.3
Laryngotracheitis (acute) (infectional)
    (viral) (see also Laryngitis) 464.20
  with obstruction 464.21
  atrophic 476.1
  Borrelia vincentii 101
  catarrhal 476.1
  chronic 476.1
    due to external agent - see
        Condition, respiratory, chronic,
        due to
  diphtheritic (membranous) 032.3
  due to external agent - see
      Inflammation, respiratory, upper,
      due to
  H. influenzae 464.20
    with obstruction 464.21
  hypertrophic 476.1
  influenzal 487.1
  pachydermic 478.75
  sicca 476.1
  spasmodic 478.75
    acute 464.20
      with obstruction 464.21
  streptococcal 034.0

Laryngotracheitis (Continued)
  stridulous 478.75
  syphilitic 095.8
    congenital 090.5
  tuberculous (see also Tuberculosis,
    larynx) 012.3●
  Vincent's 101
Laryngotracheobronchitis (see also
    Bronchitis) 490
  acute 466.0
  chronic 491.8
  viral 466.0
Laryngotracheobronchopneumonitis - see
    Pneumonia, broncho-
Larynx, laryngeal - see condition
Lasègue's disease (persecution mania)
  297.9
Lassa fever 078.89
Lassitude (see also Weakness) 780.79
Late - see also condition
  effect(s) (of) - see also condition
    abscess
      intracranial or intraspinal
          (conditions classifiable to
          324) - see category 326
    adverse effect of drug, medicinal or
        biological substance 909.5
    allergic reaction 909.9
    amputation
      postoperative (late) 997.60
      traumatic (injury classifiable to
          885–887 and 895–897)
          905.9
    burn (injury classifiable to 948–949)
        906.9
      extremities NEC (injury
          classifiable to 943 or 945)
          906.7
      hand or wrist (injury
          classifiable to 944) 906.6
      eye (injury classifiable to 940)
          906.5
      face, head, and neck (injury
          classifiable to 941) 906.5
      specified site NEC (injury
          classifiable to 942 and
          946–947) 906.8
    cerebrovascular disease (conditions
        classifiable to 430–437) 438.9
      with
        alterations of sensations
            438.6
        aphasia 438.11
        apraxia 438.81
        ataxia 438.84
        cognitive deficits 438.0
        disturbances of vision 438.7
        dysarthria 438.13   ◀
        dysphagia 438.82
        dysphasia 438.12
        facial droop 438.83
        facial weakness 438.83
        fluency disorder 438.14   ◀
        hemiplegia/hemiparesis
          affecting
            dominant side 438.21
            nondominant side 438.22
            unspecified side 438.20
        monoplegia of lower limb
          affecting
            dominant side 438.41
            nondominant side
                438.42
            unspecified side 438.40

◀ New   ◀▥ Revised   ~~deleted~~ Deleted   ● Use Additional Digit(s)   ▨ Omit code

Late *(Continued)*
 effect(s) (of) *(Continued)*
  cerebrovascular disease *(Continued)*
   with *(Continued)*
    monoplegia of upper limb
     affecting
      dominant side 438.31
      nondominant side 438.32
      unspecified side 438.30
    paralytic syndrome NEC
     affecting
      bilateral 438.53
      dominant side 438.51
      nondominant side
       438.52
      unspecified side 438.50
    speech and language deficit
     438.10
    specified type NEC
     438.19
    stuttering 438.14 ◄
    vertigo 438.85
   specified type NEC 438.89
  childbirth complication(s) 677
  complication(s) of
   childbirth 677
   delivery 677
   pregnancy 677
   puerperium 677
   surgical and medical care
    (conditions classifiable to
    996–999) 909.3
   trauma (conditions classifiable to
    958) 908.6
  contusion (injury classifiable to
   920–924) 906.3
  crushing (injury classifiable to
   925–929) 906.4
  delivery complication(s) 677
  dislocation (injury classifiable to
   830–839) 905.6
  encephalitis or encephalomyelitis
   (conditions classifiable to
   323) - *see* category 326
   in infectious diseases 139.8
    viral (conditions classifiable to
     049.8, 049.9, 062–064)
     139.0
  external cause NEC (conditions
   classifiable to 995) 909.9
   certain conditions classifiable to
    categories 991–994 909.4
  foreign body in orifice (injury
   classifiable to 930–939) 908.5
  fracture (multiple) (injury
   classifiable to 828–829) 905.5
   extremity
    lower (injury classifiable to
     821–827) 905.4
     neck of femur (injury
      classifiable to 820)
      905.3
    upper (injury classifiable to
     810–819) 905.2
   face and skull (injury classifiable
    to 800–804) 905.0
   skull and face (injury classifiable
    to 800–804) 905.0
   spine and trunk (injury
    classifiable to 805 and
    807–809) 905.1
    with spinal cord lesion (injury
     classifiable to 806)
     907.2

Late *(Continued)*
 effect(s) (of) *(Continued)*
  infection
   pyogenic, intracranial - *see*
    category 326
  infectious diseases (conditions
   classifiable to 001–136) NEC
   139.8
  injury (injury classifiable to 959)
   908.9
   blood vessel 908.3
    abdomen and pelvis (injury
     classifiable to 902) 908.4
    extremity (injury classifiable to
     903–904) 908.3
    head and neck (injury
     classifiable to 900) 908.3
    intracranial (injury
     classifiable to 850–854)
     907.0
     with skull fracture 905.0
    thorax (injury classifiable to
     901) 908.4
   internal organ NEC (injury
    classifiable to 867 and 869)
    908.2
    abdomen (injury classifiable to
     863–866 and 868) 908.1
    thorax (injury classifiable to
     860–862) 908.0
   intracranial (injury classifiable to
    850–854) 907.0
    with skull fracture (injury
     classifiable to 800–801
     and 803–804) 905.0
   nerve NEC (injury classifiable to
    957) 907.9
    cranial (injury classifiable to
     950–951) 907.1
    peripheral NEC (injury
     classifiable to 957)
     907.9
     lower limb and pelvic
      girdle (injury
      classifiable to 956)
      907.5
     upper limb and shoulder
      girdle (injury
      classifiable to 955)
      907.4
    roots and plexus(es), spinal
     (injury classifiable to 953)
     907.3
    trunk (injury classifiable to
     954) 907.3
   spinal
    cord (injury classifiable to 806
     and 952) 907.2
    nerve root(s) and plexus(es)
     (injury classifiable to 953)
     907.3
   superficial (injury classifiable to
    910–919) 906.2
   tendon (tendon injury classifiable
    to 840–848, 880–884 with .2,
    and 890–894 with .2) 905.8
  meningitis
   bacterial (conditions classifiable
    to 320) - *see* category 326
   unspecified cause (conditions
    classifiable to 322) - *see*
    category 326
  myelitis (*see also* Late, effect(s) (of),
   encephalitis) - *see* category 326

Late *(Continued)*
 effect(s) (of) *(Continued)*
  parasitic diseases (conditions
   classifiable to 001–136 NEC)
   139.8
  phlebitis or thrombophlebitis of
   intracranial venous sinuses
   (conditions classifiable to
   325) - *see* category 326
  poisoning due to drug, medicinal or
   biological substance
   (conditions classifiable to
   960–979) 909.0
  poliomyelitis, acute (conditions
   classifiable to 045) 138
  pregnancy complication(s) 677
  puerperal complication(s) 677
  radiation (conditions classifiable to
   990) 909.2
  rickets 268.1
  sprain and strain without mention
   of tendon injury (injury
   classifiable to 840–848, except
   tendon injury) 905.7
   tendon involvement 905.8
  toxic effect of
   drug, medicinal or biological
    substance (conditions
    classifiable to 960–979)
    909.0
   nonmedical substance
    (conditions classifiable
    to 980–989) 909.1
  trachoma (conditions classifiable
   to 076) 139.1
  tuberculosis 137.0
   bones and joints (conditions
    classifiable to 015) 137.3
   central nervous system
    (conditions classifiable to
    013) 137.1
   genitourinary (conditions
    classifiable to 016) 137.2
   pulmonary (conditions
    classifiable to 010–012)
    137.0
   specified organs NEC (conditions
    classifiable to 014, 017–018)
    137.4
  viral encephalitis (conditions
   classifiable to 049.8, 049.9,
   062–064) 139.0
  wound, open
   extremity (injury classifiable to
    880–884 and 890–894,
    except .2) 906.1
    tendon (injury classifiable to
     880–884 with .2 and
     890–894 with .2) 905.8
   head, neck, and trunk (injury
    classifiable to 870–879)
    906.0
 infant
  post-term (gestation period
   over 40 completed weeks
   to 42 completed weeks)
   766.21
  prolonged gestation (period
   over 42 completed weeks)
   766.22
Latent - *see* condition
Lateral - *see* condition
Laterocession - *see* Lateroversion
Lateroflexion - *see* Lateroversion

Lateroversion
  cervix - *see* Lateroversion, uterus
  uterus, uterine (cervix) (postinfectional)
      (postpartal, old) 621.6
    congenital 752.3
    in pregnancy or childbirth 654.4●
      affecting fetus or newborn 763.89
Lathyrism 988.2
Launois' syndrome (pituitary gigantism)
    253.0
Launois-Bensaude's lipomatosis 272.8
Launois-Cleret syndrome (adiposogenital
    dystrophy) 253.8
Laurence-Moon-Biedl syndrome (obesity,
    polydactyly, and mental retardation)
    759.89
LAV (disease) (illness) (infection) - *see*
    Human immunodeficiency virus
    (disease) (illness) (infection)
LAV/HTLV-III (disease) (illness)
    (infection) - *see* Human
    immunodeficiency virus (disease)
    (illness) (infection)
Lawford's syndrome
    (encephalocutaneous angiomatosis)
    759.6
Lax, laxity - *see also* Relaxation
  ligament 728.4
  skin (acquired) 701.8
    congenital 756.83
Laxative habit (*see also* Abuse, drugs,
    nondependent) 305.9●
Lazy leukocyte syndrome 288.09
LCAD (long chain/very long chain acyl
    CoA dehydrogenase deficiency,
    VLCAD) 277.85
LCHAD (long chain 3-hydroxyacyl CoA
    dehydrogenase deficiency) 277.85
Lead - *see also* condition
  exposure (suspected) to V15.86 ◄▥▥
  incrustation of cornea 371.15
  poisoning 984.9
    specified type of lead - *see* Table of
        Drugs and Chemicals
Lead miners' lung 503
Leakage
  amniotic fluid 658.1●
    with delayed delivery 658.2●
      affecting fetus or newborn 761.1
  bile from drainage tube (T tube) 997.4
  blood (microscopic), fetal, into
      maternal circulation 656.0●
    affecting management of pregnancy
        or puerperium 656.0●
  device, implant, or graft - *see*
      Complications, mechanical
  spinal fluid at lumbar puncture site
      997.09
  urine, continuous 788.37
Leaky heart - *see* Endocarditis
Learning defect, specific NEC
    (strephosymbolia) 315.2
Leather bottle stomach (M8142/3) 151.9
Leber's
  congenital amaurosis 362.76
  optic atrophy (hereditary) 377.16
Lederer's anemia or disease (acquired
    infectious hemolytic anemia) 283.19
Lederer-Brill syndrome (acquired
    infectious hemolytic anemia) 283.19
Leeches (aquatic) (land) 134.2
Left-sided neglect 781.8
Leg - *see* condition
Legal investigation V62.5

Legg (-Calvé)-Perthes disease or
    syndrome (osteochondrosis, femoral
    capital) 732.1
Legionnaires' disease 482.84
Leigh's disease 330.8
Leiner's disease (exfoliative dermatitis)
    695.89
Leiofibromyoma (M8890/0) - *see also*
    Leiomyoma
  uterus (cervix) (corpus) (*see also*
      Leiomyoma, uterus) 218.9
Leiomyoblastoma (M8891/1) - *see*
    Neoplasm, connective tissue,
    uncertain behavior
Leiomyofibroma (M8890/0) - *see also*
    Neoplasm, connective tissue, benign
  uterus (cervix) (corpus) (*see also*
      Leiomyoma, uterus) 218.9
Leiomyoma (M8890/0) - *see also*
    Neoplasm, connective tissue, benign
  bizarre (M8893/0) - *see* Neoplasm,
      connective tissue, benign
  cellular (M8892/1) - *see* Neoplasm,
      connective tissue, uncertain
      behavior
  epithelioid (M8891/1) - *see* Neoplasm,
      connective tissue, uncertain
      behavior
  prostate (polypoid) 600.20
    with
      other lower urinary tract
          symptoms (LUTS) 600.21
      urinary
        obstruction 600.21
        retention 600.21
  uterus (cervix) (corpus) 218.9
    interstitial 218.1
    intramural 218.1
    submucous 218.0
    subperitoneal 218.2
    subserous 218.2
  vascular (M8894/0) - *see* Neoplasm,
      connective tissue, benign
Leiomyomatosis (intravascular)
    (M8890/1) - *see* Neoplasm,
    connective tissue, uncertain
    behavior
Leiomyosarcoma (M8890/3) - *see also*
    Neoplasm, connective tissue,
    malignant
  epithelioid (M8891/3) - *see* Neoplasm,
      connective tissue, malignant
Leishmaniasis 085.9
  American 085.5
    cutaneous 085.4
    mucocutaneous 085.5
  Asian desert 085.2
  Brazilian 085.5
  cutaneous 085.9
    acute necrotizing 085.2
    American 085.4
    Asian desert 085.2
    diffuse 085.3
    dry form 085.1
    Ethiopian 085.3
    eyelid 085.5 [373.6]
    late 085.1
    lepromatous 085.3
    recurrent 085.1
    rural 085.2
    ulcerating 085.1
    urban 085.1
    wet form 085.2
    zoonotic form 085.2

Leishmaniasis (*Continued*)
  dermal - *see also* Leishmaniasis,
      cutaneous
    post kala-azar 085.0
  eyelid 085.5 [373.6]
  infantile 085.0
  Mediterranean 085.0
  mucocutaneous (American) 085.5
  naso-oral 085.5
  nasopharyngeal 085.5
  Old World 085.1
  tegumentaria diffusa 085.4
  vaccination, prophylactic (against)
      V05.2
  visceral (Indian) 085.0
Leishmanoid, dermal - *see also*
    Leishmaniasis, cutaneous
  post kala-azar 085.0
Leloir's disease 695.4
Lemiere syndrome 451.89
Lenegre's disease 426.0
Lengthening, leg 736.81
Lennox-Gastaut syndrome 345.0●
  with tonic seizures 345.1●
Lennox's syndrome (*see also* Epilepsy)
    345.0●
Lens - *see* condition
Lenticonus (anterior) (posterior)
    (congenital) 743.36
Lenticular degeneration, progressive
    275.1
Lentiglobus (posterior) (congenital) 743.36
Lentigo (congenital) 709.09
  juvenile 709.09
  Maligna (M8742/2) - *see also* Neoplasm,
      skin, in situ
    melanoma (M8742/3) - *see*
        Melanoma
  senile 709.09
Leonine leprosy 030.0
Leontiasis
  ossium 733.3
  syphilitic 095.8
    congenital 090.5
Léopold-Lévi's syndrome (paroxysmal
    thyroid instability) 242.9●
Lepore hemoglobin syndrome 282.49
Lepothrix 039.0
Lepra 030.9
  Willan's 696.1
Leprechaunism 259.8
Lepromatous leprosy 030.0
Leprosy 030.9
  anesthetic 030.1
  beriberi 030.1
  borderline (group B) (infiltrated)
      (neuritic) 030.3
  cornea (*see also* Leprosy, by type) 030.9
      [371.89]
  dimorphous (group B) (infiltrated)
      (lepromatous) (neuritic)
      (tuberculoid) 030.3
  eyelid 030.0 [373.4]
  indeterminate (group I) (macular)
      (neuritic) (uncharacteristic) 030.2
  leonine 030.0
  lepromatous (diffuse) (infiltrated)
      (macular) (neuritic) (nodular)
      (type L) 030.0
  macular (early) (neuritic) (simple) 030.2
  maculoanesthetic 030.1
  mixed 030.0
  neuro 030.1
  nodular 030.0

◄ New   ◄▥▥ Revised   ~~deleted~~ Deleted   ● Use Additional Digit(s)   ▥▥ Omit code

Leprosy (Continued)
  primary neuritic 030.3
  specified type or group NEC 030.8
  tubercular 030.1
  tuberculoid (macular)
    (maculoanesthetic) (major)
    (minor) (neuritic) (type T)
    030.1
Leptocytosis, hereditary 282.49
Leptomeningitis (chronic)
  (circumscribed) (hemorrhagic)
  (nonsuppurative) (see also
  Meningitis) 322.9
  aseptic 047.9
    adenovirus 049.1
    Coxsackie virus 047.0
    ECHO virus 047.1
    enterovirus 047.9
    lymphocytic choriomeningitis
      049.0
  epidemic 036.0
  late effect - see category 326
  meningococcal 036.0
  pneumococcal 320.1
  syphilitic 094.2
  tuberculous (see also Tuberculosis,
    meninges) 013.0●
Leptomeningopathy (see also Meningitis)
  322.9
Leptospiral - see condition
Leptospirochetal - see condition
Leptospirosis 100.9
  autumnalis 100.89
  canicula 100.89
  grippotyphosa 100.89
  hebdomadis 100.89
  icterohemorrhagica 100.0
  nanukayami 100.89
  pomona 100.89
  Weil's disease 100.0
Leptothricosis - see Actinomycosis
Leptothrix infestation - see
  Actinomycosis
Leptotricosis - see Actinomycosis
Leptus dermatitis 133.8
Léris pleonosteosis 756.89
Léri-Weill syndrome 756.59
Leriche's syndrome (aortic bifurcation
  occlusion) 444.0
Lermoyez's syndrome (see also Disease,
  Ménière's) 386.00
Lesbianism - omit code
  ego-dystonic 302.0
  problems with 302.0
Lesch-Nyhan syndrome (hypoxanthine-
  guanine-phosphoribosyltransferase
  deficiency) 277.2
Lesion(s)
  abducens nerve 378.54
  alveolar process 525.8
  anorectal 569.49
  aortic (valve) - see Endocarditis, aortic
  auditory nerve 388.5
  basal ganglion 333.90
  bile duct (see also Disease, biliary)
    576.8
  bladder 596.9
  bone 733.90
  brachial plexus 353.0
  brain 348.89 ◄▥
    congenital 742.9
    vascular (see also Lesion,
      cerebrovascular) 437.9
      degenerative 437.1

Lesion(s) (Continued)
  brain (Continued)
    vascular (Continued)
      healed or old without residuals
        V12.54
      hypertensive 437.2
      late effect - see Late effect(s) (of)
        cerebrovascular disease
  buccal 528.9
  calcified - see Calcification
  canthus 373.9
  carate - see Pinta, lesions
  cardia 537.89
  cardiac - see also Disease, heart
    congenital 746.9
    valvular - see Endocarditis
  cauda equina 344.60
    with neurogenic bladder 344.61
  cecum 569.89
  cerebral - see Lesion, brain
  cerebrovascular (see also Disease,
    cerebrovascular NEC) 437.9
    degenerative 437.1
    healed or old without residuals
      V12.54
    hypertensive 437.2
    specified type NEC 437.8
  cervical root (nerve) NEC 353.2
  chiasmal 377.54
    associated with
      inflammatory disorders
        377.54
      neoplasm NEC 377.52
        pituitary 377.51
      pituitary disorders 377.51
      vascular disorders 377.53
  chorda tympani 351.8
  coin, lung 793.1
  colon 569.89
  congenital - see Anomaly
  conjunctiva 372.9
  coronary artery (see also Ischemia,
    heart) 414.9
  cranial nerve 352.9
    first 352.0
    second 377.49
    third
      partial 378.51
      total 378.52
    fourth 378.53
    fifth 350.9
    sixth 378.54
    seventh 351.9
    eighth 388.5
    ninth 352.2
    tenth 352.3
    eleventh 352.4
    twelfth 352.5
  cystic - see Cyst
  degenerative - see Degeneration
  dermal (skin) 709.9
  Dieulafoy (hemorrhagic)
    of
      duodenum 537.84
      intestine 569.86
      stomach 537.84
  duodenum 537.89
    with obstruction 537.3
  eyelid 373.9
  gasserian ganglion 350.8
  gastric 537.89
  gastroduodenal 537.89
  gastrointestinal 569.89
  glossopharyngeal nerve 352.2

Lesion(s) (Continued)
  heart (organic) - see also Disease, heart
    vascular - see Disease,
      cardiovascular
  helix (ear) 709.9
  high grade myelodysplastic syndrome
    238.73
  hyperchromic, due to pinta (carate)
    103.1
  hyperkeratotic (see also Hyperkeratosis)
    701.1
  hypoglossal nerve 352.5
  hypopharynx 478.29
  hypothalamic 253.9
  ileocecal coil 569.89
  ileum 569.89
  iliohypogastric nerve 355.79
  ilioinguinal nerve 355.79
  in continuity - see Injury, nerve, by site
  inflammatory - see Inflammation
  intestine 569.89
  intracerebral - see Lesion, brain
  intrachiasmal (optic) (see also Lesion,
    chiasmal) 377.54
  intracranial, space-occupying NEC 784.2
  joint 719.90
    ankle 719.97
    elbow 719.92
    foot 719.97
    hand 719.94
    hip 719.95
    knee 719.96
    multiple sites 719.99
    pelvic region 719.95
    sacroiliac (old) 724.6
    shoulder (region) 719.91
    specified site NEC 719.98
    wrist 719.93
  keratotic (see also Keratosis) 701.1
  kidney (see also Disease, renal) 593.9
  laryngeal nerve (recurrent) 352.3
  leonine 030.0
  lip 528.5
  liver 573.8
  low grade myelodysplastic syndrome
    238.72
  lumbosacral
    plexus 353.1
    root (nerve) NEC 353.4
  lung 518.89
    coin 793.1
  maxillary sinus 473.0
  mitral - see Endocarditis, mitral
  Morel Lavallée - see Hematoma,
    by site ◄
  motor cortex 348.89 ◄▥
  nerve (see also Disorder, nerve) 355.9
  nervous system 349.9
    congenital 742.9
  nonallopathic NEC 739.9
    in region (of)
      abdomen 739.9
      acromioclavicular 739.7
      cervical, cervicothoracic 739.1
      costochondral 739.8
      costovertebral 739.8
      extremity
        lower 739.6
        upper 739.7
      head 739.0
      hip 739.5
      lower extremity 739.6
      lumbar, lumbosacral 739.3
      occipitocervical 739.0

Lesion(s) (Continued)
  nonallopathic NEC (Continued)
    in region (of) (Continued)
      pelvic 739.5
      pubic 739.5
      rib cage 739.8
      sacral, sacrococcygeal, sacroiliac
        739.4
      sternochondral 739.8
      sternoclavicular 739.7
      thoracic, thoracolumbar 739.2
      upper extremity 739.7
  nose (internal) 478.19
  obstructive - see Obstruction
  obturator nerve 355.79
  occlusive
    artery - see Embolism, artery
  organ or site NEC - see Disease, by
    site
  osteolytic 733.90
  paramacular, of retina 363.32
  peptic 537.89
  periodontal, due to traumatic occlusion
    523.8
  perirectal 569.49
  peritoneum (granulomatous)
    568.89
  pigmented (skin) 709.00
  pinta - see Pinta, lesions
  polypoid - see Polyp
  prechiasmal (optic) (see also Lesion,
    chiasmal) 377.54
  primary - see also Syphilis, primary
    carate 103.0
    pinta 103.0
    yaws 102.0
  pulmonary 518.89
    valve (see also Endocarditis,
      pulmonary) 424.3
  pylorus 537.89
  radiation NEC 990
  radium NEC 990
  rectosigmoid 569.89
  retina, retinal - see also Retinopathy
    vascular 362.17
  retroperitoneal 568.89
  romanus 720.1
  sacroiliac (joint) 724.6
  salivary gland 527.8
    benign lymphoepithelial 527.8
  saphenous nerve 355.79
  secondary - see Syphilis, secondary
  sigmoid 569.89
  sinus (accessory) (nasal) (see also
    Sinusitis) 473.9
  skin 709.9
    suppurative 686.00
  SLAP (superior glenoid labrum)
    840.7
  space-occupying, intracranial NEC
    784.2
  spinal cord 336.9
    congenital 742.9
    traumatic (complete) (incomplete)
      (transverse) - see also Injury,
      spinal, by site
      with
        broken
          back - see Fracture, vertebra,
            by site, with spinal
            cord injury
          neck - see Fracture, vertebra,
            cervical, with spinal
            cord injury

Lesion(s) (Continued)
  spinal cord (Continued)
    traumatic (Continued)
      with (Continued)
        fracture, vertebra - see
          Fracture, vertebra, by
          site, with spinal cord
          injury
  spleen 289.50
  stomach 537.89
  superior glenoid labrum (SLAP)
    840.7
  syphilitic - see Syphilis
  tertiary - see Syphilis, tertiary
  thoracic root (nerve) 353.3
  tonsillar fossa 474.9
  tooth, teeth 525.8
    white spot 521.01
  traumatic NEC (see also nature and site
    of injury) 959.9
  tricuspid (valve) - see Endocarditis,
    tricuspid
  trigeminal nerve 350.9
  ulcerated or ulcerative - see Ulcer
  uterus NEC 621.9
  vagina 623.8
  vagus nerve 352.3
  valvular - see Endocarditis
  vascular 459.9
    affecting central nervous system (see
      also Lesion, cerebrovascular)
      437.9
    following trauma (see also Injury,
      blood vessel, by site) 904.9
    retina 362.17
    traumatic - see Injury, blood vessel,
      by site
    umbilical cord 663.6●
      affecting fetus or newborn
        762.6
  visual
    cortex NEC (see also Disorder, visual,
      cortex) 377.73
    pathway NEC (see also Disorder,
      visual, pathway) 377.63
  warty - see Verruca
  white spot, on teeth 521.01
  x-ray NEC 990
Lethargic - see condition
Lethargy 780.79
Letterer-Siwe disease (acute histiocytosis
  X) (M9722/3) 202.5●
Leucinosis 270.3
Leucocoria 360.44
Leucosarcoma (M9850/3) 207.8●
Leukasmus 270.2
Leukemia, leukemic (congenital)
  (M9800/3) 208.9●

> Note 51 Use the following fifth-digit
> subclassification for categories 203–208:
>
> 0   without mention of having
>   achieved remission
>   failed remission
> 1   with remission
> 2   in relapse

  acute NEC (M9801/3) 208.0●
  aleukemic NEC (M9804/3) 208.8●
    granulocytic (M9864/3) 205.8●
  basophilic (M9870/3) 205.1●
  blast (cell) (M9801/3) 208.0●
  blastic (M9801/3) 208.0●
    granulocytic (M9861/3)
      205.0●

Leukemia, leukemic (Continued)
  chronic NEC (M9803/3) 208.1●
  compound (M9810/3) 207.8●
  eosinophilic (M9880/3) 205.1●
  giant cell (M9910/3) 207.2●
  granulocytic (M9860/3) 205.9●
    acute (M9861/3) 205.0●
    aleukemic (M9864/3) 205.8●
    blastic (M9861/3) 205.0●
    chronic (M9863/3) 205.1●
    subacute (M9862/3) 205.2●
    subleukemic (M9864/3) 205.8●
  hairy cell (M9940/3) 202.4●
  hemoblastic (M9801/3) 208.0●
  histiocytic (M9890/3) 206.9●
  lymphatic (M9820/3) 204.9●
    acute (M9821/3) 204.0●
    aleukemic (M9824/3) 204.8●
    chronic (M9823/3) 204.1●
    subacute (M9822/3) 204.2●
    subleukemic (M9824/3) 204.8●
  lymphoblastic (M9821/3) 204.0●
  lymphocytic (M9820/3) 204.9●
    acute (M9821/3) 204.0●
    aleukemic (M9824/3) 204.8●
    chronic (M9823/3) 204.1●
    granular ◄
      large T-cell 204.8● ◄
    subacute (M9822/3) 204.2●
    subleukemic (M9824/3) 204.8●
  lymphogenous (M9820/3) - see
    Leukemia, lymphoid
  lymphoid (M9820/3) 204.9●
    acute (M9821/3) 204.0●
    aleukemic (M9824/3) 204.8●
    blastic (M9821/3) 204.0●
    chronic (M9823/3) 204.1●
    subacute (M9822/3) 204.2●
    subleukemic (M9824/3) 204.8●
  lymphosarcoma cell (M9850/3)
    207.8●
  mast cell (M9900/3) 207.8●
  megakaryocytic (M9910/3) 207.2●
  megakaryocytoid (M9910/3) 207.2●
  mixed (cell) (M9810/3) 207.8●
  monoblastic (M9891/3) 206.0●
  monocytic (Schilling-type) (M9890/3)
    206.9●
    acute (M9891/3) 206.0●
    aleukemic (M9894/3) 206.8●
    chronic (M9893/3) 206.1●
    Naegeli-type (M9863/3) 205.1●
    subacute (M9892/3) 206.2●
    subleukemic (M9894/3) 206.8●
  monocytoid (M9890/3) 206.9●
    acute (M9891/3) 206.0●
    aleukemic (M9894/3) 206.8●
    chronic (M9893/3) 206.1●
    myelogenous (M9863/3) 205.1●
    subacute (M9892/3) 206.2●
    subleukemic (M9894/3) 206.8●
  monomyelocytic (M9860/3) - see
    Leukemia, myelomonocytic
  myeloblastic (M9861/3) 205.0●
  myelocytic (M9863/3) 205.1●
    acute (M9861/3) 205.0●
  myelogenous (M9860/3) 205.9●
    acute (M9861/3) 205.0●
    aleukemic (M9864/3) 205.8●
    chronic (M9863/3) 205.1●
    monocytoid (M9863/3) 205.1●
    subacute (M9862/3) 205.2●
    subleukemic (M9864) 205.8●
  myeloid (M9860/3) 205.9●
    acute (M9861/3) 205.0●

  ◄ New ◀▥ Revised ~~deleted~~ Deleted ● Use Additional Digit(s) ▨ Omit code

Leukemia, leukemic (Continued)
  myeloid (Continued)
    aleukemic (M9864/3) 205.8●
    chronic (M9863/3) 205.1●
    subacute (M9862/3) 205.2●
    subleukemic (M9864/3) 205.8●
  myelomonocytic (M9860/3) 205.9●
    acute (M9861/3) 205.0●
    chronic (M9863/3) 205.1●
  Naegeli-type monocytic (M9863/3)
    205.1●
  neutrophilic (M9865/3) 205.1●
  plasma cell (M9830/3) 203.1●
  plasmacytic (M9830/3) 203.1●
  prolymphocytic (M9825/3) - see
    Leukemia, lymphoid
  promyelocytic, acute (M9866/3)
    205.0●
  Schilling-type monocytic (M9890/3) -
    see Leukemia, monocytic
  stem cell (M9801/3) 208.0●
  subacute NEC (M9802/3) 208.2●
  subleukemic NEC (M9804/3) 208.8●
  thrombocytic (M9910/3) 207.2●
  undifferentiated (M9801/3) 208.0●
Leukemoid reaction (basophilic)
    (lymphocytic) (monocytic)
    (myelocytic) (neutrophilic) 288.62
Leukoaraiosis (hypertensive) 437.1 ◀
Leukoariosis - see Leukoaraiosis ◀
Leukoclastic vasculitis 446.29
Leukocoria 360.44
Leukocythemia - see Leukemia
Leukocytopenia 288.50
Leukocytosis 288.60
  basophilic 288.8
  eosinophilic 288.3
  lymphocytic 288.8
  monocytic 288.8
  neutrophilic 288.8
Leukoderma 709.09
  syphilitic 091.3
    late 095.8
Leukodermia (see also Leukoderma)
    709.09
Leukodystrophy (cerebral) (globoid cell)
    (metachromatic) (progressive)
    (sudanophilic) 330.0
Leukoedema, mouth or tongue 528.79
Leukoencephalitis
  acute hemorrhagic (postinfectious)
    NEC 136.9 [323.61]
    postimmunization or postvaccinal
      323.51
  subacute sclerosing 046.2
    van Bogaert's 046.2
    van Bogaert's (sclerosing) 046.2
Leukoencephalopathy (see also
    Encephalitis) 323.9
  acute necrotizing hemorrhagic
    (postinfectious) 136.9 [323.61]
    postimmunization or postvaccinal
      323.51
  Binswanger's 290.12 ◀
  metachromatic 330.0
  multifocal (progressive) 046.3
  progressive multifocal 046.3
  reversible, posterior 348.5
Leukoerythroblastosis 289.9
Leukoerythrosis 289.0
Leukokeratosis (see also Leukoplakia)
    702.8
  mouth 528.6
  nicotina palati 528.79
  tongue 528.6

Leukokoria 360.44
Leukokraurosis vulva, vulvae 624.09
Leukolymphosarcoma (M9850/3)
    207.8●
Leukoma (cornea) (interfering with
    central vision) 371.03
  adherent 371.04
Leukomalacia, periventricular 779.7
Leukomelanopathy, hereditary 288.2
Leukonychia (punctata) (striata) 703.8
  congenital 757.5
Leukopathia
  unguium 703.8
    congenital 757.5
Leukopenia 288.50
  basophilic 288.59
  cyclic 288.02
  eosinophilic 288.59
  familial 288.59
  malignant (see also Agranulocytosis)
    288.09
  periodic 288.02
  transitory neonatal 776.7
Leukopenic - see condition
Leukoplakia 702.8
  anus 569.49
  bladder (postinfectional) 596.8
  buccal 528.6
  cervix (uteri) 622.2
  esophagus 530.83
  gingiva 528.6
  kidney (pelvis) 593.89
  larynx 478.79
  lip 528.6
  mouth 528.6
  oral soft tissue (including tongue)
    (mucosa) 528.6
  palate 528.6
  pelvis (kidney) 593.89
  penis (infectional) 607.0
  rectum 569.49
  syphilitic 095.8
  tongue 528.6
  tonsil 478.29
  ureter (postinfectional) 593.89
  urethra (postinfectional) 599.84
  uterus 621.8
  vagina 623.1
  vesical 596.8
  vocal cords 478.5
  vulva 624.09
Leukopolioencephalopathy 330.0
Leukorrhea (vagina) 623.5
  due to Trichomonas (vaginalis)
    131.00
  trichomonal (Trichomonas vaginalis)
    131.00
Leukosarcoma (M9850/3) 207.8●
Leukosis (M9800/3) - see Leukemia
Lev's disease or syndrome (acquired
    complete heart block) 426.0
Levi's syndrome (pituitary dwarfism)
    253.3
Levocardia (isolated) 746.87
  with situs inversus 759.3
Levulosuria 271.2
Lewandowski's disease (primary) (see
    also Tuberculosis) 017.0●
Lewandowski-Lutz disease
    (epidermodysplasia verruciformis)
    078.19
Lewy body dementia 331.82
Lewy body disease 331.82
Leyden's disease (periodic vomiting)
    536.2

Leyden-Möbius dystrophy 359.1
Leydig cell
  carcinoma (M8650/3)
    specified site - see Neoplasm, by site,
      malignant
    unspecified site
      female 183.0
      male 186.9
  tumor (M8650/1)
    benign (M8650/0)
      specified site - see Neoplasm, by
        site, benign
      unspecified site
        female 220
        male 222.0
    malignant (M8650/3)
      specified site - see Neoplasm, by
        site, malignant
      unspecified site
        female 183.0
        male 186.9
    specified site - see Neoplasm, by site,
      uncertain behavior
    unspecified site
      female 236.2
      male 236.4
Leydig-Sertoli cell tumor (M8631/0)
  specified site - see Neoplasm, by site,
    benign
  unspecified site
    female 220
    male 222.0
LGSIL (low grade squamous
    intraepithelial lesion)
  anus 796.73
  cervix 795.03
  vagina 795.13
Liar, pathologic 301.7
Libman-Sacks disease or syndrome
    710.0 [424.91]
Lice (infestation) 132.9
  body (pediculus corporis) 132.1
  crab 132.2
  head (pediculus capitis) 132.0
  mixed (classifiable to more than one
    of the categories 132.0–132.2)
    132.3
  pubic (pediculus pubis) 132.2
Lichen 697.9
  albus 701.0
  annularis 695.89
  atrophicus 701.0
  corneus obtusus 698.3
  myxedematous 701.8
  nitidus 697.1
  pilaris 757.39
    acquired 701.1
  planopilaris 697.0
  planus (acute) (chronicus)
    (hypertrophic) (verrucous)
    697.0
    morphoeicus 701.0
    sclerosus (et atrophicus) 701.0
  ruber 696.4
    acuminatus 696.4
    moniliformis 697.8
    obtusus corneus 698.3
    of Wilson 697.0
    planus 697.0
  sclerosus (et atrophicus) 701.0
  scrofulosus (primary) (see also
    Tuberculosis) 017.0●
  simplex (Vidal's) 698.3
    chronicus 698.3
    circumscriptus 698.3

Lichen (Continued)
  spinulosus 757.39
    mycotic 117.9
  striata 697.8
  urticatus 698.2
Lichenification 698.3
  nodular 698.3
Lichenoides tuberculosis (primary) (see also Tuberculosis) 017.0
Lichtheim's disease or syndrome (subacute combined sclerosis with pernicious anemia) 281.0 [336.2]
Lien migrans 289.59
Lientery (see also Diarrhea) 787.91
  infectious 009.2
Life circumstance problem NEC V62.89
Li-Fraumeni cancer syndrome V84.01
Ligament - see condition
Light-for-dates (infant) 764.0●
  with signs of fetal malnutrition 764.1●
  affecting management of pregnancy 656.5●
Light-headedness 780.4
Lightning (effects) (shock) (stroke) (struck by) 994.0
  burn - see Burn, by site
  foot 266.2
Lightwood's disease or syndrome (renal tubular acidosis) 588.89
Lignac's disease (cystinosis) 270.0
Lignac (-de Toni) (-Fanconi) (-Debré) syndrome (cystinosis) 270.0
Lignac (-Fanconi) syndrome (cystinosis) 270.0
Ligneous thyroiditis 245.3
Likoff's syndrome (angina in menopausal women) 413.9
Limb - see condition
Limitation of joint motion (see also Stiffness, joint) 719.5●
  sacroiliac 724.6
Limit dextrinosis 271.0
Limited
  cardiac reserve - see Disease, heart
  duction, eye NEC 378.63
  mandibular range of motion 524.52
Lindau's disease (retinocerebral angiomatosis) 759.6
Lindau (-von Hippel) disease (angiomatosis retinocerebellosa) 759.6
Linea corneae senilis 371.41
Lines
  Beau's (transverse furrows on fingernails) 703.8
  Harris' 733.91
  Hudson-Stähli 371.11
  Stähli's 371.11
Lingua
  geographical 529.1
  nigra (villosa) 529.3
  plicata 529.5
    congenital 750.13
  tylosis 528.6
Lingual (tongue) - see also condition
  thyroid 759.2
Linitis (gastric) 535.4●
  plastica (M8142/3) 151.9
Lioderma essentialis (cum melanosis et telangiectasia) 757.33
Lip - see also condition
  biting 528.9
Lipalgia 272.8
Lipedema - see Edema

Lipemia (see also Hyperlipidemia) 272.4
  retina, retinalis 272.3
Lipidosis 272.7
  cephalin 272.7
  cerebral (infantile) (juvenile) (late) 330.1
  cerebroretinal 330.1 [362.71]
  cerebroside 272.7
  cerebrospinal 272.7
  chemically-induced 272.7
  cholesterol 272.7
  diabetic 250.8● [272.7]
    due to secondary diabetes 249.8● [272.7]
  dystopic (hereditary) 272.7
  glycolipid 272.7
  hepatosplenomegalic 272.3
  hereditary, dystopic 272.7
  sulfatide 330.0
Lipoadenoma (M8324/0 - see Neoplasm, by site, benign
Lipoblastoma (M8881/0) - see Lipoma, by site
Lipoblastomatosis (M8881/0) - see Lipoma, by site
Lipochondrodystrophy 277.5
Lipochrome histiocytosis (familial) 288.1
Lipodystrophia progressiva 272.6
Lipodystrophy (progressive) 272.6
  insulin 272.6
  intestinal 040.2
  mesenteric 567.82
Lipofibroma (M8851/0) - see Lipoma, by site
Lipoglycoproteinosis 272.8
Lipogranuloma, sclerosing 709.8
Lipogranulomatosis (disseminated) 272.8
  kidney 272.8
Lipoid - see also condition
  histiocytosis 272.7
    essential 272.7
  nephrosis (see also Nephrosis) 581.3
  proteinosis of Urbach 272.8
Lipoidemia (see also Hyperlipidemia) 272.4
Lipoidosis (see also Lipidosis) 272.7
Lipoma (M8850/0) 214.9
  breast (skin) 214.1
  face 214.0
  fetal (M8881/0) - see also Lipoma, by site
    fat cell (M8880/0) - see Lipoma, by site
  infiltrating (M8856/0) - see Lipoma, by site
  intra-abdominal 214.3
  intramuscular (M8856/0) - see Lipoma, by site
  intrathoracic 214.2
  kidney 214.3
  mediastinum 214.2
  muscle 214.8
  peritoneum 214.3
  retroperitoneum 214.3
  skin 214.1
    face 214.0
  spermatic cord 214.4
  spindle cell (M8857/0) - see Lipoma, by site
  stomach 214.3
  subcutaneous tissue 214.1
    face 214.0
  thymus 214.2
  thyroid gland 214.2

Lipomatosis (dolorosa) 272.8
  epidural 214.8
  fetal (M8881/0) - see Lipoma, by site
  Launois-Bensaude's 272.8
Lipomyohemangioma (M8860/0)
  specified site - see Neoplasm, connective tissue, benign
  unspecified site 223.0
Lipomyoma (M8860/0)
  specified site - see Neoplasm, connective tissue, benign
  unspecified site 223.0
Lipomyxoma (M8852/0) - see Lipoma, by site
Lipomyxosarcoma (M8852/3) - see Neoplasm, connective tissue, malignant
Lipophagocytosis 289.89
Lipoproteinemia (alpha) 272.4
  broad-beta 272.2
  floating-beta 272.2
  hyper-pre-beta 272.1
Lipoproteinosis (Rossle-Urbach-Wiethe) 272.8
Liposarcoma (M8850/3) - see also Neoplasm, connective tissue, malignant
  differentiated type (M8851/3) - see Neoplasm, connective tissue, malignant
  embryonal (M8852/3) - see Neoplasm, connective tissue, malignant
  mixed type (M8855/3) - see Neoplasm, connective tissue, malignant
  myxoid (M8852/3) - see Neoplasm, connective tissue, malignant
  pleomorphic (M8854/3) - see Neoplasm, connective tissue, malignant
  round cell (M8853/3) - see Neoplasm, connective tissue, malignant
  well differentiated type (M8851/3) - see Neoplasm, connective tissue, malignant
Liposynovitis prepatellaris 272.8
Lipping
  cervix 622.0
  spine (see also Spondylosis) 721.90
  vertebra (see also Spondylosis) 721.90
Lip pits (mucus), congenital 750.25
Lipschütz disease or ulcer 616.50
Lipuria 791.1
  bilharziasis 120.0
Liquefaction, vitreous humor 379.21
Lisping 307.9
Lissauer's paralysis 094.1
Lissencephalia, lissencephaly 742.2
Listerellose 027.0
Listeriose 027.0
Listeriosis 027.0
  congenital 771.2
  fetal 771.2
  suspected fetal damage affecting management of pregnancy 655.4●
Listlessness 780.79
Lithemia 790.6
Lithiasis - see also Calculus
  hepatic (duct) - see Choledocholithiasis
  urinary 592.9
Lithopedion 779.9
  affecting management of pregnancy 656.8●

◀ New   ◀┅ Revised   ~~deleted~~ Deleted   ● Use Additional Digit(s)   ▓▓ Omit code

Lithosis (occupational) 502
  with tuberculosis - *see* Tuberculosis,
    pulmonary
Lithuria 791.9
Litigation V62.5
Little
  league elbow 718.82
  stroke syndrome 435.9
Little's disease - *see* Palsy, cerebral
Littre's
  gland - *see* condition
  hernia - *see* Hernia, Littre's
Littritis (*see also* Urethritis) 597.89
Livedo 782.61
  annularis 782.61
  racemose 782.61
  reticularis 782.61
Live flesh 781.0
Liver - *see also* condition
  donor V59.6
Livida, asphyxia
  newborn 768.6
Living
  alone V60.3
    with handicapped person V60.4
Lloyd's syndrome 258.1
Loa loa 125.2
Loasis 125.2
Lobe, lobar - *see* condition
Lobo's disease or blastomycosis
  116.2
Lobomycosis 116.2
Lobotomy syndrome 310.0
Lobstein's disease (brittle bones and
  blue sclera) 756.51
Lobster-claw hand 755.58
Lobulation (congenital) - *see also*
    Anomaly, specified type NEC, by
    site
  kidney, fetal 753.3
  liver, abnormal 751.69
  spleen 759.0
Lobule, lobular - *see* condition
Local, localized - *see* condition
Locked bowel or intestine (*see also*
    Obstruction, intestine) 560.9
Locked-in state 344.81
Locked twins 660.5●
  affecting fetus or newborn 763.1
Locking
  joint (*see also* Derangement, joint)
    718.90
  knee 717.9
Lockjaw (*see also* Tetanus) 037
Locomotor ataxia (progressive) 094.0
Löffler's
  endocarditis 421.0
  eosinophilia or syndrome 518.3
  pneumonia 518.3
  syndrome (eosinophilic
    pneumonitis) 518.3
Löfgren's syndrome (sarcoidosis)
  135
Loiasis 125.2
  eyelid 125.2 *[373.6]*
Loneliness V62.89
Lone Star fever 082.8
Long labor 662.1●
  affecting fetus or newborn 763.89
  first stage 662.0●
  second stage 662.2●
Longitudinal stripes or grooves, nails
  703.8
  congenital 757.5

Long-term (current) drug use V58.69
  antibiotics V58.62
  anticoagulants V58.61
  anti-inflammatories, non-steroidal
    (NSAID) V58.64
  antiplatelets/antithrombotics
    V58.63
  aspirin V58.66
  high-risk medications NEC V58.69
  insulin V58.67
  methadone V58.69
  opiate analgesic V58.69
  pain killers V58.69
    anti-inflammatories, non-steroidal
      (NSAID) V58.64
    aspirin V58.66
  steroids V58.65
  tamoxifen V07.51   ◀▥▥
Loop
  intestine (*see also* Volvulus) 560.2
  intrascleral nerve 379.29
  vascular on papilla (optic) 743.57
Loose - *see also* condition
  body
    in tendon sheath 727.82
    joint 718.10
      ankle 718.17
      elbow 718.12
      foot 718.17
      hand 718.14
      hip 718.15
      knee 717.6
      multiple sites 718.19
      pelvic region 718.15
      prosthetic implant - *see*
        Complications, mechanical
      shoulder (region) 718.11
      specified site NEC 718.18
      wrist 718.13
    cartilage (joint) (*see also* Loose, body,
      joint) 718.1●
      knee 717.6
    facet (vertebral) 724.9
    prosthetic implant - *see* Complications,
      mechanical
    sesamoid, joint (*see also* Loose, body,
      joint) 718.1●
    tooth, teeth 525.8
Loosening epiphysis 732.9
Looser (-Debray)-Milkman syndrome
    (osteomalacia with
    pseudofractures) 268.2
Lop ear (deformity) 744.29
Lorain's disease or syndrome (pituitary
    dwarfism) 253.3
Lorain-Levi syndrome (pituitary
    dwarfism) 253.3
Lordosis (acquired) (postural) 737.20
  congenital 754.2
  due to or associated with
    Charcôt-Marie-Tooth disease 356.1
      [737.42]
    mucopolysaccharidosis 277.5
      [737.42]
    neurofibromatosis 237.71 *[737.42]*
    osteitis
      deformans 731.0 *[737.42]*
      fibrosa cystica 252.01 *[737.42]*
    osteoporosis (*see also* Osteoporosis)
      733.00 *[737.42]*
    poliomyelitis (*see also* Poliomyelitis)
      138 *[737.42]*
    tuberculosis (*see also* Tuberculosis)
      015.0● *[737.42]*

Lordosis (*Continued*)
  late effect of rickets 268.1 *[737.42]*
  postlaminectomy 737.21
  postsurgical NEC 737.22
  rachitic 268.1 *[737.42]*
  specified NEC 737.29
  tuberculous (*see also* Tuberculosis)
    015.0● *[737.42]*
Loss
  appetite 783.0
    hysterical 300.11
    nonorganic origin 307.59
    psychogenic 307.59
  blood - *see* Hemorrhage
  central vision 368.41
  consciousness 780.09
    transient 780.2
  control, sphincter, rectum 787.6
    nonorganic origin 307.7
  ear ossicle, partial 385.24
  elasticity, skin 782.8
  extremity or member, traumatic,
    current - *see* Amputation,
    traumatic
  fluid (acute) 276.50
    with
      hypernatremia 276.0
      hyponatremia 276.1
    fetus or newborn 775.5
  hair 704.00
  hearing - *see also* Deafness
    central 389.14
    conductive (air) 389.00
      with sensorineural hearing loss
        389.20
        bilateral 389.22
        unilateral 389.21
      bilateral 389.06
      combined types 389.08
      external ear 389.01
      inner ear 389.04
      middle ear 389.03
      multiple types 389.08
      tympanic membrane 389.02
      unilateral 389.05
    mixed conductive and sensorineural
      389.20
      bilateral 389.22
      unilateral 389.21
    mixed type 389.20
      bilateral 389.22
      unilateral 389.21
    nerve
      bilateral 389.12
      unilateral 389.13
    neural
      bilateral 389.12
      unilateral 389.13
    noise-induced 388.12
    perceptive NEC (*see also* Loss,
      hearing, sensorineural)
      389.10
    sensorineural 389.10
      with conductive hearing loss
        389.20
        bilateral 389.22
        unilateral 389.21
      asymmetrical 389.16
      bilateral 389.18
      central 389.14
      neural
        bilateral 389.12
        unilateral 389.13

Loss (*Continued*)
  hearing (*Continued*)
    sensorineural (*Continued*)
      sensory
        bilateral 389.11
          unilateral 389.17
        unilateral 389.15
      sensory
        bilateral 389.11
        unilateral 389.17
      specified type NEC 389.8
      sudden NEC 388.2
  height 781.91
  labyrinthine reactivity (unilateral) 386.55
    bilateral 386.56
  memory (*see also* Amnesia) 780.93
    mild, following organic brain damage 310.8 ◀▦
  mind (*see also* Psychosis) 298.9
  occusal vertical dimension 524.37
  organ or part - *see* Absence, by site, acquired
  sensation 782.0
  sense of
    smell (*see also* Disturbance, sensation) 781.1
    taste (*see also* Disturbance, sensation) 781.1
    touch (*see also* Disturbance, sensation) 781.1
  sight (acquired) (complete) (congenital) - *see* Blindness
  spinal fluid
    headache 349.0
  substance of
    bone (*see also* Osteoporosis) 733.00
    cartilage 733.99
      ear 380.32
    vitreous (humor) 379.26
  tooth, teeth
    acquired 525.10
      due to
        caries 525.13
        extraction 525.10
        periodontal disease 525.12
        specified NEC 525.19
        trauma 525.11
  vision, visual (*see also* Blindness) 369.9
    both eyes (*see also* Blindness, both eyes) 369.3
    complete (*see also* Blindness, both eyes) 369.00
    one eye 369.8
    sudden 368.11
    transient 368.12
  vitreous 379.26
  voice (*see also* Aphonia) 784.41
  weight (cause unknown) 783.21
Lou Gehrig's disease 335.20
Louis-Bar syndrome (ataxia-telangiectasia) 334.8
Louping ill 063.1
Lousiness - *see* Lice
Low
  back syndrome 724.2
  basal metabolic rate (BMR) 794.7
  birthweight 765.1●
    extreme (less than 1000 grams) 765.0●
    for gestational age 764.0●
    status (*see also* Status, low birth weight) V21.30
  bladder compliance 596.52

Low (*Continued*)
  blood pressure (*see also* Hypotension) 458.9
    reading (incidental) (isolated) (nonspecific) 796.3
  cardiac reserve - *see* Disease, heart
  compliance bladder 596.52
  frequency deafness - *see* Disorder, hearing
  function - *see also* Hypofunction
    kidney (*see also* Disease, renal) 593.9
    liver 573.9
  hemoglobin 285.9
  implantation, placenta - *see* Placenta, previa
  insertion, placenta - *see* Placenta, previa
  lying
    kidney 593.0
    organ or site, congenital - *see* Malposition, congenital
    placenta - *see* Placenta, previa
  output syndrome (cardiac) (*see also* Failure, heart) 428.9
  platelets (blood) (*see also* Thrombocytopenia) 287.5
  reserve, kidney (*see also* Disease, renal) 593.9
  risk
    human papillomavirus (HPV) DNA test positive
      anal 796.79
      cervical 795.09
      vaginal 795.19
  salt syndrome 593.9
  tension glaucoma 365.12
  vision 369.9
    both eyes 369.20
    one eye 369.70
Lowe (-Terrey-MacLachlan) **syndrome** (oculocerebrorenal dystrophy) 270.8
Lower extremity - *see* condition
Lown (-Ganong)-Levine **syndrome** (short P-R interval, normal QRS complex, and paroxysmal supraventricular tachycardia) 426.81
LSD reaction (*see also* Abuse, drugs, nondependent) 305.3●
L-shaped kidney 753.3
Lucas-Championnière disease (fibrinous bronchitis) 466.0
Lucey-Driscoll syndrome (jaundice due to delayed conjugation) 774.30
Ludwig's
  angina 528.3
  disease (submaxillary cellulitis) 528.3
Lues (venerea), luetic - *see* Syphilis
Luetscher's syndrome (dehydration) 276.51
Lumbago 724.2
  due to displacement, intervertebral disc 722.10
Lumbalgia 724.2
  due to displacement, intervertebral disc 722.10
Lumbar - *see* condition
Lumbarization, vertebra 756.15
Lumbermen's itch 133.8
Lump - *see also* Mass
  abdominal 789.3●
  breast 611.72
  chest 786.6
  epigastric 789.3●

Lump (*Continued*)
  head 784.2
  kidney 753.3
  liver 789.1
  lung 786.6
  mediastinal 786.6
  neck 784.2
  nose or sinus 784.2
  pelvic 789.3●
  skin 782.2
  substernal 786.6
  throat 784.2
  umbilicus 789.3●
Lunacy (*see also* Psychosis) 298.9
Lunatomalacia 732.3
Lung - *see also* condition
  donor V59.8
  drug addict's 417.8
  mainliners' 417.8
  vanishing 492.0
Lupoid (miliary) of Boeck 135
Lupus 710.0
  anticoagulant 289.81
  Cazenave's (erythematosus) 695.4
  discoid (local) 695.4
  disseminated 710.0
  erythematodes (discoid) (local) 695.4
  erythematosus (discoid) (local) 695.4
    disseminated 710.0
    eyelid 373.34
    systemic 710.0
      with
        encephalitis 710.0 *[323.81]*
        lung involvement 710.0 *[517.8]*
      inhibitor (presence of) 286.5
  exedens 017.0●
  eyelid (*see also* Tuberculosis) 017.0● *[373.4]*
  Hilliard's 017.0●
  hydralazine
    correct substance properly administered 695.4
    overdose or wrong substance given or taken 972.6
  miliaris disseminatus faciei 017.0●
  nephritis 710.0 *[583.81]*
    acute 710.0 *[580.81]*
    chronic 710.0 *[582.81]*
  nontuberculous, not disseminated 695.4
  pernio (Besnier) 135
  tuberculous (*see also* Tuberculosis) 017.0●
    eyelid (*see also* Tuberculosis) 017.0● *[373.4]*
  vulgaris 017.0●
Luschka's joint disease 721.90
Luteinoma (M8610/0) 220
Lutembacher's disease or syndrome (atrial septal defect with mitral stenosis) 745.5
Luteoma (M8610/0) 220
Lutz-Miescher disease (elastosis perforans serpiginosa) 701.1
Lutz-Splendore-de Almeida disease (Brazilian blastomycosis) 116.1
Luxatio
  bulbi due to birth injury 767.8
  coxae congenita (*see also* Dislocation, hip, congenital) 754.30
  erecta - *see* Dislocation, shoulder
  imperfecta - *see* Sprain, by site
  perinealis - *see* Dislocation, hip

◀ New   ◀▦ Revised   ~~deleted~~ Deleted   ● Use Additional Digit(s)   ▦ Omit code

Luxation - *see also* Dislocation, by site
  eyeball 360.81
    due to birth injury 767.8
    lateral 376.36
  genital organs (external) NEC - *see*
    Wound, open, genital organs
  globe (eye) 360.81
    lateral 376.36
  lacrimal gland (postinfectional) 375.16
  lens (old) (partial) 379.32
    congenital 743.37
      syphilitic 090.49 [379.32]
    Marfan's disease 090.49
    spontaneous 379.32
  penis - *see* Wound, open, penis
  scrotum - *see* Wound, open, scrotum
  testis - *see* Wound, open, testis
L-xyloketosuria 271.8
Lycanthropy (*see also* Psychosis) 298.9
Lyell's disease or syndrome (toxic
  epidermal necrolysis) 695.15
  due to drug
    correct substance properly
      administered 695.15
    overdose or wrong substance given
      or taken 977.9
      specified drug - *see* Table of
        Drugs and Chemicals
Lyme disease 088.81
Lymph
  gland or node - *see* condition
  scrotum (*see also* Infestation, filarial)
    125.9
Lymphadenitis 289.3
  with
    abortion - *see* Abortion, by type,
      with sepsis
    ectopic pregnancy (*see also*
      categories 633.0–633.9)
      639.0
    molar pregnancy (*see also* categories
      630–632) 639.0
  acute 683
    mesenteric 289.2
  any site, except mesenteric 289.3
    acute 683
    chronic 289.1
    mesenteric (acute) (chronic)
      (nonspecific) (subacute)
      289.2
    subacute 289.1
      mesenteric 289.2
  breast, puerperal, postpartum
    675.2●
  chancroidal (congenital) 099.0
  chronic 289.1
    mesenteric 289.2
  dermatopathic 695.89
  due to
    anthracosis (occupational) 500
    Brugia (Wuchereria) malayi
      125.1
    diphtheria (toxin) 032.89
    lymphogranuloma venereum
      099.1
    Wuchereria bancrofti 125.0
  following
    abortion 639.0
    ectopic or molar pregnancy
      639.0
  generalized 289.3
  gonorrheal 098.89
  granulomatous 289.1
  infectional 683

Lymphadenitis (*Continued*)
  mesenteric (acute) (chronic)
    (nonspecific) (subacute) 289.2
    due to Bacillus typhi 002.0
    tuberculous (*see also* Tuberculosis)
      014.8●
  mycobacterial 031.8
  purulent 683
  pyogenic 683
  regional 078.3
  septic 683
  streptococcal 683
  subacute, unspecified site 289.1
  suppurative 683
  syphilitic (early) (secondary) 091.4
    late 095.8
  tuberculous - *see* Tuberculosis, lymph
    gland
  venereal 099.1
Lymphadenoid goiter 245.2
Lymphadenopathy (general) 785.6
  due to toxoplasmosis (acquired)
    130.7
  congenital (active) 771.2
Lymphadenopathy-associated virus
  (disease) (illness) (infection) - *see*
    Human immunodeficiency virus
    (disease) (illness) (infection)
Lymphadenosis 785.6
  acute 075
Lymphangiectasis 457.1
  conjunctiva 372.89
  postinfectional 457.1
  scrotum 457.1
Lymphangiectatic elephantiasis,
  nonfilarial 457.1
Lymphangioendothelioma (M9170/0)
  228.1
  malignant (M9170/3) - *see* Neoplasm,
    connective tissue, malignant
Lymphangioma (M9170/0) 228.1
  capillary (M9171/0) 228.1
  cavernous (M9172/0) 228.1
  cystic (M9173/0) 228.1
  malignant (M9170/3) - *see* Neoplasm,
    connective tissue, malignant
Lymphangiomyoma (M9174/0) 228.1
Lymphangiomyomatosis (M9174/1) - *see*
  Neoplasm, connective tissue,
  uncertain behavior
Lymphangiosarcoma (M9170/3) - *see*
  Neoplasm, connective tissue,
  malig-nant
Lymphangitis 457.2
  with
    abortion - *see* Abortion, by type,
      with sepsis
    abscess - *see* Abscess, by site
    cellulitis - *see* Abscess, by site
    ectopic pregnancy (*see also*
      categories 633.0–633.9)
      639.0
    molar pregnancy (*see also* categories
      630–632) 639.0
  acute (with abscess or cellulitis)
    682.9
    specified site - *see* Abscess, by site
  breast, puerperal, postpartum
    675.2●
  chancroidal 099.0
  chronic (any site) 457.2
  due to
    Brugia (Wuchereria) malayi 125.1
    Wuchereria bancrofti 125.0

Lymphangitis (*Continued*)
  following
    abortion 639.0
    ectopic or molar pregnancy
      639.0
  gangrenous 457.2
  penis
    acute 607.2
    gonococcal (acute) 098.0
      chronic or duration of 2 months
        or more 098.2
  puerperal, postpartum,
    childbirth 670.8   ◀▥
  strumous, tuberculous (*see also*
    Tuberculosis) 017.2●
  subacute (any site) 457.2
  tuberculous - *see* Tuberculosis, lymph
    gland
Lymphatic (vessel) - *see* condition
Lymphatism 254.8
  scrofulous (*see also* Tuberculosis)
    017.2●
Lymphectasia 457.1
Lymphedema (*see also* Elephantiasis)
  457.1
  acquired (chronic) 457.1
  chronic hereditary 757.0
  congenital 757.0
  idiopathic hereditary 757.0
  praecox 457.1
  secondary 457.1
  surgical NEC 997.99
    postmastectomy (syndrome) 457.0
Lymph-hemangioma (M9120/0) - *see*
  Hemangioma, by site
Lymphoblastic - *see* condition
Lymphoblastoma (diffuse) (M9630/3)
  200.1●
  giant follicular (M9690/3) 202.0●
  macrofollicular (M9690/3) 202.0●
Lymphoblastosis, acute benign 075
Lymphocele 457.8
Lymphocythemia 288.51
Lymphocytic - *see also* condition
  chorioencephalitis (acute) (serous)
    049.0
  choriomeningitis (acute) (serous)
    049.0
Lymphocytoma (diffuse) (malignant)
  (M9620/3) 200.1●
Lymphocytomatosis (M9620/3) 200.1●
Lymphocytopenia 288.51
Lymphocytosis (symptomatic) 288.61
  infectious (acute) 078.89
Lymphoepithelioma (M8082/3) - *see*
  Neoplasm, by site, malignant
Lymphogranuloma (malignant)
  (M9650/3) 201.9●
  inguinale 099.1
  venereal (any site) 099.1
    with stricture of rectum 099.1
  venereum 099.1
Lymphogranulomatosis (malignant)
  (M9650/3) 201.9●
  benign (Boeck's sarcoid) (Schaumann's)
    135
  Hodgkin's (M9650/3) 201.9●
Lymphohistiocytosis, familial
  hemophagocytic 288.4
Lymphoid - *see* condition
Lympholeukoblastoma (M9850/3)
  207.8●
Lympholeukosarcoma (M9850/3)
  207.8●

Lymphoma (malignant) (M9590/3)
202.8●

Note 52   Use the following fifth-digit subclassification with categories 200–202:

0   unspecified site, extranodal and solid organ sites
1   lymph nodes of head, face, and neck
2   intrathoracic lymph nodes
3   intra-abdominal lymph nodes
4   lymph nodes of axilla and upper limb
5   lymph nodes of inguinal region and lower limb
6   intrapelvic lymph nodes
7   spleen
8   lymph nodes of multiple sites

benign (M9590/0) - *see* Neoplasm, by site, benign
Burkitt's type (lymphoblastic) (undifferentiated) (M9750/3) 200.2●
Castleman's (mediastinal lymph node hyperplasia) 785.6
centroblastic-centrocytic
    diffuse (M9614/3) 202.8●
    follicular (M9692/3) 202.0●
centroblastic type (diffuse) (M9632/3) 202.8●
    follicular (M9697/3) 202.0●
centrocytic (M9622/3) 202.8●
compound (M9613/3) 200.8●
convoluted cell type (lymphoblastic) (M9602/3) 202.8●
diffuse NEC (M9590/3) 202.8●
    large B cell 202.8●
follicular (giant) (M9690/3) 202.0●
    center cell (diffuse) (M9615/3) 202.8●
        cleaved (diffuse) (M9623/3) 202.8●
            follicular (M9695/3) 202.0●
        non-cleaved (diffuse) (M9633/3) 202.8●
            follicular (M9698/3) 202.0●
    centroblastic-centrocytic (M9692/3) 202.0●
    centroblastic type (M9697/3) 202.0●
    large cell 202.0●   ◄
    lymphocytic
        intermediate differentiation (M9694/3) 202.0●
        poorly differentiated (M9696/3) 202.0●
    mixed (cell type) (lymphocytic-histiocytic) (small cell and large cell) (M9691/3) 202.0●
germinocytic (M9622/3) 202.8●
giant, follicular or follicle (M9690/3) 202.0●

Lymphoma (*Continued*)
histiocytic (diffuse) (M9640/3) 200.0●
    nodular (M9642/3) 200.0●
    pleomorphic cell type (M9641/3) 200.0●
Hodgkin's (M9650/3) (*see also* Disease, Hodgkin's) 201.9●
immunoblastic (type) (M9612/3) 200.8●
large cell (M9640/3) 200.7●
    anaplastic 200.6●
    nodular (M9642/3) 202.0●   ◄▥
    pleomorphic cell type (M9641/3) 200.0●
lymphoblastic (diffuse) (M9630/3) 200.1●
    Burkitt's type (M9750/3) 200.2●
    convoluted cell type (M9602/3) 202.8●
lymphocytic (cell type) (diffuse) (M9620/3) 200.1●
    with plasmacytoid differentiation, diffuse (M9611/3) 200.8●
    intermediate differentiation (diffuse) (M9621/3) 200.1●
        follicular (M9694/3) 202.0●
        nodular (M9694/3) 202.0●
    nodular (M9690/3) 202.0●
    poorly differentiated (diffuse) (M9630/3) 200.1●
        follicular (M9696/3) 202.0●
        nodular (M9696/3) 202.0●
    well differentiated (diffuse) (M9620/3) 200.1●
        follicular (M9693/3) 202.0●
        nodular (M9693/3) 202.0●
lymphocytic-histiocytic, mixed (diffuse) (M9613/3) 200.8●
    follicular (M9691/3) 202.0●
    nodular (M9691/3) 202.0●
lymphoplasmacytoid type (M9611/3) 200.8●
lymphosarcoma type (M9610/3) 200.1●
macrofollicular (M9690/3) 202.0●
mantle cell 200.4●
marginal zone 200.3●
    extranodal B-cell 200.3●
    nodal B-cell 200.3●
    splenic B-cell 200.3●
mixed cell type (diffuse) (M9613/3) 200.8●
    follicular (M9691/3) 202.0●
    nodular (M9691/3) 202.0●
nodular (M9690/3) 202.0●
    histiocytic (M9642/3) 200.0●
    lymphocytic (M9690/3) 202.0●
        intermediate differentiation (M9694/3) 202.0●
        poorly differentiated (M9696/3) 202.0●
    mixed (cell type) (lymphocytic-histiocytic) (small cell and large cell) (M9691/3) 202.0●
non-Hodgkin's type NEC (M9591/3) 202.8●

Lymphoma (*Continued*)
peripheral T-cell 202.7●
primary central nervous system 200.5●
reticulum cell (type) (M9640/3) 200.0●
small cell and large cell, mixed (diffuse) (M9613/3) 200.8●
    follicular (M9691/3) 202.0●
    nodular (9691/3) 202.0●
stem cell (type) (M9601/3) 202.8●
T-cell 202.1●
    peripheral 202.7●
undifferentiated (cell type) (non-Burkitt's) (M9600/3) 202.8●
    Burkitt's type (M9750/3) 200.2●
Lymphomatosis (M9590/3) - *see also* Lymphoma
granulomatous 099.1
Lymphopathia
venereum 099.1
veneris 099.1
Lymphopenia 288.51
familial 279.2
Lymphoreticulosis, benign (of inoculation) 078.3
Lymphorrhea 457.8
Lymphosarcoma (M9610/3) 200.1●
diffuse (M9610/3) 200.1●
    with plasmacytoid differentiation (M9611/3) 200.8●
    lymphoplasmacytic (M9611/3) 200.8●
follicular (giant) (M9690/3) 202.0●
    lymphoblastic (M9696/3) 202.0●
    lymphocytic, intermediate differentiation (M9694/3) 202.0●
    mixed cell type (M9691/3) 202.0●
giant follicular (M9690/3) 202.0●
Hodgkin's (M9650/3) 201.9●
immunoblastic (M9612/3) 200.8●
lymphoblastic (diffuse) (M9630/3) 200.1●
    follicular (M9696/3) 202.0●
    nodular (M9696/3) 202.0●
lymphocytic (diffuse) (M9620/3) 200.1
    intermediate differentiation (diffuse) (M9621/3) 200.1●
        follicular (M9694/3) 202.0●
        nodular (M9694/3) 202.0●
    mixed cell type (diffuse) (M9613/3) 200.8●
        follicular (M9691/3) 202.0●
        nodular (M9691/3) 202.0●
nodular (M9690/3) 202.0●
    lymphoblastic (M9696/3) 202.0●
    lymphocytic, intermediate differentiation (M9694/3) 202.0●
    mixed cell type (M9691/3) 202.0●
prolymphocytic (M9631/3) 200.1●
reticulum cell (M9640/3) 200.0●
Lymphostasis 457.8
Lypemania (*see also* Melancholia) 296.2●
Lyssa 071

◄ New   ◄▥ Revised   ~~deleted~~ Deleted   ● Use Additional Digit(s)   ▥ Omit code

M

Macacus ear 744.29
Maceration
  fetus (cause not stated) 779.9
  wet feet, tropical (syndrome) 991.4
Machado-Joseph disease 334.8
Machupo virus hemorrhagic fever 078.7
Macleod's syndrome (abnormal
    transradiancy, one lung) 492.8
Macrocephalia, macrocephaly 756.0
Macrocheilia (congenital) 744.81
Macrochilia (congenital) 744.81
Macrocolon (congenital) 751.3
Macrocornea 743.41
  associated with buphthalmos 743.22
Macrocytic - *see* condition
Macrocytosis 289.89
Macrodactylia, macrodactylism (fingers)
    (thumbs) 755.57
  toes 755.65
Macrodontia 520.2
Macroencephaly 742.4
Macrogenia 524.05
Macrogenitosomia (female) (male)
    (praecox) 255.2
Macrogingivae 523.8
Macroglobulinemia (essential)
    (idiopathic) (monoclonal) (primary)
    (syndrome) (Waldenström's) 273.3
Macroglossia (congenital) 750.15
  acquired 529.8
Macrognathia, macrognathism
    (congenital) 524.00
  mandibular 524.02
    alveolar 524.72
  maxillary 524.01
    alveolar 524.71
Macrogyria (congenital) 742.4
Macrohydrocephalus (*see also*
    Hydrocephalus) 331.4
Macromastia (*see also* Hypertrophy,
    breast) 611.1
Macrophage activation syndrome 288.4
Macropsia 368.14
Macrosigmoid 564.7
  congenital 751.3
Macrospondylitis, acromegalic 253.0
Macrostomia (congenital) 744.83
Macrotia (external ear) (congenital)
    744.22
Macula
  cornea, corneal
    congenital 743.43
      interfering with vision 743.42
      interfering with central vision 371.03
      not interfering with central vision
        371.02
  degeneration (*see also* Degeneration,
    macula) 362.50
  hereditary (*see also* Dystrophy,
    retina) 362.70
  edema, cystoid 362.53
Maculae ceruleae 132.1
Macules and papules 709.8
Maculopathy, toxic 362.55
Madarosis 374.55
Madelung's
  deformity (radius) 755.54
  disease (lipomatosis) 272.8
  lipomatosis 272.8
Madness (*see also* Psychosis) 298.9
  myxedema (acute) 293.0
    subacute 293.1

Madura
  disease (actinomycotic) 039.9
    mycotic 117.4
  foot (actinomycotic) 039.4
    mycotic 117.4
Maduromycosis (actinomycotic) 039.9
  mycotic 117.4
Maffucci's syndrome (dyschondroplasia
    with hemangiomas) 756.4
Magenblase syndrome 306.4
Main en griffe (acquired) 736.06
  congenital 755.59
Maintenance
  chemotherapy regimen or treatment
    V58.11
  dialysis regimen or treatment
    extracorporeal (renal) V56.0
    peritoneal V56.8
    renal V56.0
  drug therapy or regimen
    chemotherapy, antineoplastic
      V58.11
    immunotherapy, antineoplastic
      V58.12
  external fixation NEC V54.89
  radiotherapy V58.0
  traction NEC V54.89
Majocchi's
  disease (purpura annularis
    telangiectodes) 709.1
  granuloma 110.6
Major - *see* condition
Mal
  cerebral (idiopathic) (*see also* Epilepsy)
    345.9●
  comital (*see also* Epilepsy) 345.9●
  de los pintos (*see also* Pinta) 103.9
  de Meleda 757.39
  de mer 994.6
  lie - *see* Presentation, fetal
  perforant (*see also* Ulcer, lower
    extremity) 707.15
Malabar itch 110.9
  beard 110.0
  foot 110.4
  scalp 110.0
Malabsorption 579.9
  calcium 579.8
  carbohydrate 579.8
  disaccharide 271.3
  drug-induced 579.8
  due to bacterial overgrowth 579.8
  fat 579.8
  folate, congenital 281.2
  galactose 271.1
  glucose-galactose (congenital) 271.3
  intestinal 579.9
  isomaltose 271.3
  lactose (hereditary) 271.3
  methionine 270.4
  monosaccharide 271.8
  postgastrectomy 579.3
  postsurgical 579.3
  protein 579.8
  sucrose (-isomaltose) (congenital)
    271.3
  syndrome 579.9
    postgastrectomy 579.3
    postsurgical 579.3
Malacia, bone 268.2
  juvenile (*see also* Rickets) 268.0
  Kienböck's (juvenile) (lunate) (wrist)
    732.3
  adult 732.8

Malacoplakia
  bladder 596.8
  colon 569.89
  pelvis (kidney) 593.89
  ureter 593.89
  urethra 599.84
Malacosteon 268.2
  juvenile (*see also* Rickets) 268.0
Maladaptation - *see* Maladjustment
Maladie de Roger 745.4
Maladjustment
  conjugal V61.10
    involving
      divorce V61.03
      estrangement V61.09
  educational V62.3
  family V61.9
    specified circumstance NEC
      V61.8
  marital V61.10
    involving
      divorce V61.03
      estrangement V61.09
  occupational V62.29
    current military deployment status
      V62.21
  simple, adult (*see also* Reaction,
    adjustment) 309.9
  situational acute (*see also* Reaction,
    adjustment) 309.9
  social V62.4
Malaise 780.79
Malakoplakia - *see* Malacoplakia
Malaria, malarial (fever) 084.6
  algid 084.9
  any type, with
    algid malaria 084.9
    blackwater fever 084.8
    fever
      blackwater 084.8
      hemoglobinuric (bilious)
        084.8
    hemoglobinuria, malarial 084.8
    hepatitis 084.9 [573.2]
    nephrosis 084.9 [581.81]
    pernicious complication NEC
      084.9
      cardiac 084.9
      cerebral 084.9
  cardiac 084.9
  carrier (suspected) of V02.9
  cerebral 084.9
  complicating pregnancy, childbirth,
    or puerperium 647.4●
  congenital 771.2
  congestion, congestive 084.6
    brain 084.9
  continued 084.0
  estivo-autumnal 084.0
  falciparum (malignant tertian)
    084.0
  hematinuria 084.8
  hematuria 084.8
  hemoglobinuria 084.8
  hemorrhagic 084.6
  induced (therapeutically) 084.7
    accidental - *see* Malaria, by type
  liver 084.9 [573.2]
  malariae (quartan) 084.2
  malignant (tertian) 084.0
  mixed infections 084.5
  monkey 084.4
  ovale 084.3
  pernicious, acute 084.0

Malaria, malarial (Continued)
  Plasmodium, P.
    falciparum 084.0
    malariae 084.2
    ovale 084.3
    vivax 084.1
  quartan 084.2
  quotidian 084.0
  recurrent 084.6
    induced (therapeutically) 084.7
      accidental - see Malaria, by type
  remittent 084.6
  specified types NEC 084.4
  spleen 084.6
  subtertian 084.0
  tertian (benign) 084.1
    malignant 084.0
  tropical 084.0
  typhoid 084.6
  vivax (benign tertian) 084.1
Malassez's disease (testicular cyst)
    608.89
Malassimilation 579.9
Maldescent, testis 752.51
Maldevelopment - see also Anomaly, by
    site
  brain 742.9
  colon 751.5
  hip (joint) 755.63
    congenital dislocation (see also
        Dislocation, hip, congenital)
        754.30
  mastoid process 756.0
  middle ear, except ossicles 744.03
    ossicles 744.04
  newborn (not malformation) 764.9●
  ossicles, ear 744.04
  spine 756.10
  toe 755.66
Male type pelvis 755.69
  with disproportion (fetopelvic) 653.2●
    affecting fetus or newborn 763.1
    causing obstructed labor 660.1●
      affecting fetus or newborn
        763.1
Malformation (congenital) - see also
    Anomaly
  bone 756.9
  bursa 756.9
  Chiari
    type I 348.4
    type II (see also Spina bifida)
        741.0●
    type III 742.0
    type IV 742.2
  circulatory system NEC 747.9
    specified type NEC 747.89
  cochlea 744.05
  digestive system NEC 751.9
    lower 751.5
    specified type NEC 751.8
    upper 750.9
  eye 743.9
  gum 750.9
  heart NEC 746.9
    specified type NEC 746.89
    valve 746.9
  internal ear 744.05
  joint NEC 755.9
    specified type NEC 755.8
  Mondini's (congenital) (malformation,
        cochlea) 744.05
  muscle 756.9
  nervous system (central) 742.9

Malformation (Continued)
  pelvic organs or tissues
    in pregnancy or childbirth 654.9●
      affecting fetus or newborn
        763.89
      causing obstructed labor 660.2●
        affecting fetus or newborn
          763.1
  placenta (see also Placenta, abnormal)
      656.7●
  respiratory organs 748.9
    specified type NEC 748.8
  Rieger's 743.44
  sense organs NEC 742.9
    specified type NEC 742.8
  skin 757.9
    specified type NEC 757.8
  spinal cord 742.9
  teeth, tooth NEC 520.9
  tendon 756.9
  throat 750.9
  umbilical cord (complicating delivery)
      663.9●
    affecting fetus or newborn 762.6
  umbilicus 759.9
  urinary system NEC 753.9
    specified type NEC 753.8
  venous - see Anomaly, vein
Malfunction - see also Dysfunction
  arterial graft 996.1
  cardiac pacemaker 996.01
  catheter device - see Complications,
      mechanical, catheter
  colostomy 569.62
    valve 569.62
  cystostomy 997.5
  device, implant, or graft NEC - see
      Complications, mechanical
  enteric stoma 569.62
  enterostomy 569.62
  esophagostomy 530.87
  gastroenteric 536.8
  gastrostomy 536.42
  ileostomy
    valve 569.62
  nephrostomy 997.5
  pacemaker - see Complications,
      mechanical, pacemaker
  prosthetic device, internal - see
      Complications, mechanical
  tracheostomy 519.02
  valve
    colostomy 569.62
    ileostomy 569.62
  vascular graft or shunt 996.1
Malgaigne's fracture (closed) 808.43
  open 808.53
Malherbe's
  calcifying epithelioma (M8110/0) - see
      Neoplasm, skin, benign
  tumor (M8110/0) - see Neoplasm, skin,
      benign
Malibu disease 919.8
  infected 919.9
Malignancy (M8000/3) - see Neoplasm,
    by site, malignant
Malignant - see condition
Malingerer, malingering V65.2
Mallet, finger (acquired) 736.1
  congenital 755.59
  late effect of rickets 268.1
Malleus 024
Mallory's bodies 034.1
Mallory-Weiss syndrome 530.7

Malnutrition (calorie) 263.9
  complicating pregnancy 648.9●
  degree
    first 263.1
    second 263.0
    third 262
    mild 263.1
    moderate 263.0
    severe 261
      protein-calorie 262
  fetus 764.2●
  "light-for-dates" 764.1●
  following gastrointestinal surgery 579.3
  intrauterine or fetal 764.2●
    fetus or infant "light-for-dates"
        764.1●
  lack of care, or neglect (child) (infant)
      995.52
    adult 995.84
  malignant 260
  mild 263.1
  moderate 263.0
  protein 260
  protein-calorie 263.9
    severe 262
    specified type NEC 263.8
  severe 261
    protein-calorie NEC 262
Malocclusion (teeth) 524.4
  angle's class I 524.21
  angle's class II 524.22
  angle's class III 524.23
  due to
    abnormal swallowing 524.59
    accessory teeth (causing crowding)
        524.31
    dentofacial abnormality NEC 524.89
    impacted teeth (causing crowding)
        520.6
    missing teeth 524.30
    mouth breathing 524.59
    sleep postures 524.59
    supernumerary teeth (causing
        crowding) 524.31
    thumb sucking 524.59
    tongue, lip, or finger habits 524.59
  temporomandibular (joint) 524.69
Malposition
  cardiac apex (congenital) 746.87
  cervix - see Malposition, uterus
  congenital
    adrenal (gland) 759.1
    alimentary tract 751.8
      lower 751.5
      upper 750.8
    aorta 747.21
    appendix 751.5
    arterial trunk 747.29
    artery (peripheral) NEC (see also
        Malposition, congenital,
        peripheral vascular system)
        747.60
      coronary 746.85
      pulmonary 747.3
    auditory canal 744.29
      causing impairment of hearing
          744.02
    auricle (ear) 744.29
      causing impairment of hearing
          744.02
    cervical 744.43
    biliary duct or passage 751.69
    bladder (mucosa) 753.8
      exteriorized or extroverted 753.5

◄ New   ◄ Revised   deleted Deleted   ● Use Additional Digit(s)   Omit code

Malposition *(Continued)*
  congenital *(Continued)*
    brachial plexus 742.8
    brain tissue 742.4
    breast 757.6
    bronchus 748.3
    cardiac apex 746.87
    cecum 751.5
    clavicle 755.51
    colon 751.5
    digestive organ or tract NEC 751.8
      lower 751.5
      upper 750.8
    ear (auricle) (external) 744.29
      ossicles 744.04
    endocrine (gland) NEC 759.2
    epiglottis 748.3
    Eustachian tube 744.24
    eye 743.8
    facial features 744.89
    fallopian tube 752.19
    finger(s) 755.59
      supernumerary 755.01
    foot 755.67
    gallbladder 751.69
    gastrointestinal tract 751.8
    genitalia, genital organ(s) or tract
      female 752.89
        external 752.49
        internal NEC 752.89
      male 752.89
        penis 752.69
        scrotal transposition 752.81
    glottis 748.3
    hand 755.59
    heart 746.87
      dextrocardia 746.87
        with complete transposition of
          viscera 759.3
    hepatic duct 751.69
    hip (joint) *(see also* Dislocation, hip,
      congenital) 754.30
    intestine (large) (small) 751.5
      with anomalous adhesions,
        fixation, or malrotation
        751.4
    joint NEC 755.8
    kidney 753.3
    larynx 748.3
    limb 755.8
      lower 755.69
      upper 755.59
    liver 751.69
    lung (lobe) 748.69
    nail(s) 757.5
    nerve 742.8
    nervous system NEC 742.8
    nose, nasal (septum) 748.1
    organ or site NEC - *see* Anomaly,
      specified type NEC, by site
    ovary 752.0
    pancreas 751.7
    parathyroid (gland) 759.2
    patella 755.64
    peripheral vascular system 747.60
      gastrointestinal 747.61
      lower limb 747.64
      renal 747.62
      specified NEC 747.69
      spinal 747.82
      upper limb 747.63
    pituitary (gland) 759.2
    respiratory organ or system NEC
      748.9

Malposition *(Continued)*
  congenital *(Continued)*
    rib (cage) 756.3
      supernumerary in cervical region
        756.2
    scapula 755.59
    shoulder 755.59
    spinal cord 742.59
    spine 756.19
    spleen 759.0
    sternum 756.3
    stomach 750.7
    symphysis pubis 755.69
    testis (undescended) 752.51
    thymus (gland) 759.2
    thyroid (gland) (tissue) 759.2
      cartilage 748.3
    toe(s) 755.66
      supernumerary 755.02
    tongue 750.19
    trachea 748.3
    uterus 752.3
    vein(s) (peripheral) NEC *(see also*
      Malposition, congenital,
      peripheral vascular system)
      747.60
      great 747.49
      portal 747.49
      pulmonary 747.49
      vena cava (inferior) (superior)
        747.49
  device, implant, or graft - *see*
    Complications, mechanical
  fetus NEC *(see also* Presentation, fetal)
    652.9●
    with successful version 652.1●
    affecting fetus or newborn 763.1
    before labor, affecting fetus or
      newborn 761.7
    causing obstructed labor 660.0●
    in multiple gestation (one fetus or
      more) 652.6●
      with locking 660.5●
      causing obstructed labor 660.0●
  gallbladder *(see also* Disease,
    gallbladder) 575.8
  gastrointestinal tract 569.89
    congenital 751.8
  heart *(see also* Malposition, congenital,
    heart) 746.87
  intestine 569.89
    congenital 751.5
  pelvic organs or tissues
    in pregnancy or childbirth 654.4●
      affecting fetus or newborn
        763.89
      causing obstructed labor 660.2●
        affecting fetus or newborn
          763.1
  placenta - *see* Placenta, previa
  stomach 537.89
    congenital 750.7
  tooth, teeth 524.30
    with impaction 520.6
  uterus (acquired) (acute) (adherent)
    (any degree) (asymptomatic)
    (postinfectional) (postpartal, old)
    621.6
    anteflexion or anteversion *(see also*
      Anteversion, uterus) 621.6
    congenital 752.3
    flexion 621.6
      lateral *(see also* Lateroversion,
        uterus) 621.6

Malposition *(Continued)*
  uterus *(Continued)*
    in pregnancy or childbirth 654.4●
      affecting fetus or newborn
        763.89
      causing obstructed labor 660.2●
        affecting fetus or newborn
          763.1
    inversion 621.6
    lateral (flexion) (version) *(see also*
      Lateroversion, uterus) 621.6
    lateroflexion *(see also* Lateroversion,
      uterus) 621.6
    lateroversion *(see also* Lateroversion,
      uterus) 621.6
    retroflexion or retroversion *(see also*
      Retroversion, uterus) 621.6
Malposture 729.90
Malpresentation, fetus *(see also*
  Presentation, fetal) 652.9●
Malrotation
  cecum 751.4
  colon 751.4
  intestine 751.4
  kidney 753.3
MALT (mucosa associated lymphoid
  tissue) 200.3●
Malt workers' lung 495.4
Malta fever *(see also* Brucellosis) 023.9
Maltosuria 271.3
Maltreatment (of)
  adult 995.80
    emotional 995.82
    multiple forms 995.85
    neglect (nutritional) 995.84
    physical 995.81
    psychological 995.82
    sexual 995.83
  child 995.50
    emotional 995.51
    multiple forms 995.59
    neglect (nutritional) 995.52
    physical 995.54
    shaken infant syndrome 995.55
    psychological 995.51
    sexual 995.53
  spouse *(see also* Maltreatment, adult)
    995.80
Malum coxae senilis 715.25
Malunion, fracture 733.81
Mammillitis *(see also* Mastitis) 611.0
  puerperal, postpartum 675.2●
Mammitis *(see also* Mastitis) 611.0
  puerperal, postpartum 675.2●
Mammographic
  calcification 793.89
  calculus 793.89
  microcalcification 793.81
Mammoplasia 611.1
Management
  contraceptive V25.9
    specified type NEC V25.8
  procreative V26.9
    specified type NEC V26.89
Mangled NEC *(see also* nature and site of
  injury) 959.9
Mania (monopolar) *(see also* Psychosis,
  affective) 296.0●
  alcoholic (acute) (chronic) 291.9
  Bell's - *see* Mania, chronic
  chronic 296.0●
    recurrent episode 296.1●
    single episode 296.0●
  compulsive 300.3

Mania (Continued)
  delirious (acute) 296.0●
    recurrent episode 296.1●
    single episode 296.0●
  epileptic (see also Epilepsy) 345.4●
  hysterical 300.10
  inhibited 296.89
  puerperal (after delivery) 296.0●
    recurrent episode 296.1●
    single episode 296.0●
  recurrent episode 296.1●
  senile 290.8
  single episode 296.0●
  stupor 296.89
  stuporous 296.89
  unproductive 296.89
Manic-depressive insanity, psychosis,
  reaction, or syndrome (see also
  Psychosis, affective) 296.80
  circular (alternating) 296.7
    currently
      depressed 296.5●
      episode unspecified 296.7
      hypomanic, previously depressed
        296.4●
      manic 296.4●
      mixed 296.6●
  depressed (type), depressive 296.2●
    atypical 296.82
    recurrent episode 296.3●
    single episode 296.2●
  hypomanic 296.0●
    recurrent episode 296.1●
    single episode 296.0●
  manic 296.0●
    atypical 296.81
    recurrent episode 296.1●
    single episode 296.0●
  mixed NEC 296.89
  perplexed 296.89
  stuporous 296.89
Manifestations, rheumatoid
  lungs 714.81
  pannus - see Arthritis, rheumatoid
  subcutaneous nodules - see Arthritis,
    rheumatoid
Mankowsky's syndrome (familial
  dysplastic osteopathy) 731.2
Mannoheptulosuria 271.8
Mannosidosis 271.8
Manson's
  disease (schistosomiasis) 120.1
  pyosis (pemphigus contagiosus) 684
  schistosomiasis 120.1
Mansonellosis 125.5
Manual - see condition
Maple bark disease 495.6
Maple bark-strippers' lung 495.6
Maple syrup (urine) disease or syndrome
  270.3
Marable's syndrome (celiac artery
  compression) 447.4
Marasmus 261
  brain 331.9
  due to malnutrition 261
  intestinal 569.89
  nutritional 261
  senile 797
  tuberculous NEC (see also Tuberculosis)
    011.9●
Marble
  bones 756.52
  skin 782.61
Marburg disease (virus) 078.89

March
  foot 733.94
  hemoglobinuria 283.2
Marchand multiple nodular hyperplasia
  (liver) 571.5
Marchesani (-Weill) syndrome
  (brachymorphism and ectopia
  lentis) 759.89
Marchiafava (-Bignami) disease or
  syndrome 341.8
Marchiafava-Micheli syndrome
  (paroxysmal nocturnal
  hemoglobinuria) 283.2
Marcus Gunn's syndrome (jaw-winking
  syndrome) 742.8
Marfan's
  congenital syphilis 090.49
  disease 090.49
  syndrome (arachnodactyly) 759.82
    meaning congenital syphilis
      090.49
      with luxation of lens 090.49
        [379.32]
Marginal
  implantation, placenta - see Placenta,
    previa
  placenta - see Placenta, previa
  sinus (hemorrhage) (rupture) 641.2●
    affecting fetus or newborn 762.1
Marie's
  cerebellar ataxia 334.2
  syndrome (acromegaly) 253.0
Marie-Bamberger disease or syndrome
  (hypertrophic) (pulmonary)
  (secondary) 731.2
  idiopathic (acropachyderma) 757.39
  primary (acropachyderma) 757.39
Marie-Charcôt-Tooth neuropathic
  atrophy, muscle 356.1
Marie-Strümpell arthritis or disease
  (ankylosing spondylitis) 720.0
Marihuana, marijuana
  abuse (see also Abuse, drugs,
    nondependent) 305.2●
  dependence (see also Dependence)
    304.3●
Marion's disease (bladder neck
  obstruction) 596.0
Marital conflict V61.10
Mark
  port wine 757.32
  raspberry 757.32
  strawberry 757.32
  stretch 701.3
  tattoo 709.09
Maroteaux-Lamy syndrome
  (mucopolysaccharidosis VI) 277.5
Marriage license examination V70.3
Marrow (bone)
  arrest 284.9
  megakaryocytic 287.30
  poor function 289.9
Marseilles fever 082.1
Marsh's disease (exophthalmic goiter)
  242.0●
Marshall's (hidrotic) ectodermal
  dysplasia 757.31
Marsh fever (see also Malaria) 084.6
Martin's disease 715.27
Martin-Albright syndrome
  (pseudohypoparathyroidism)
  275.49
Martorell-Fabre syndrome (pulseless
  disease) 446.7

Masculinization, female, with adrenal
  hyperplasia 255.2
Masculinovoblastoma (M8670/0)
  220
Masochism 302.83
Masons' lung 502
Mass
  abdominal 789.3●
  anus 787.99
  bone 733.90
  breast 611.72
  cheek 784.2
  chest 786.6
  cystic - see Cyst
  ear 388.8
  epigastric 789.3●
  eye 379.92
  female genital organ 625.8
  gum 784.2
  head 784.2
  intracranial 784.2
  joint 719.60
    ankle 719.67
    elbow 719.62
    foot 719.67
    hand 719.64
    hip 719.65
    knee 719.66
    multiple sites 719.69
    pelvic region 719.65
    shoulder (region) 719.61
    specified site NEC 719.68
    wrist 719.63
  kidney (see also Disease, kidney)
    593.9
  lung 786.6
  lymph node 785.6
  malignant (M8000/3) - see Neoplasm,
    by site, malignant
  mediastinal 786.6
  mouth 784.2
  muscle (limb) 729.89
  neck 784.2
  nose or sinus 784.2
  palate 784.2
  pelvis, pelvic 789.3●
  penis 607.89
  perineum 625.8
  rectum 787.99
  scrotum 608.89
  skin 782.2
  specified organ NEC - see Disease of
    specified organ or site
  splenic 789.2
  substernal 786.6
    thyroid (see also Goiter) 240.9
  superficial (localized) 782.2
  testes 608.89
  throat 784.2
  tongue 784.2
  umbilicus 789.3●
  uterus 625.8
  vagina 625.8
  vulva 625.8
Massive - see condition
Mastalgia 611.71
  psychogenic 307.89
Mast cell
  disease 757.33
    systemic (M9741/3) 202.6●
  leukemia (M9900/3) 207.8●
  sarcoma (M9742/3) 202.6●
  tumor (M9740/1) 238.5
    malignant (M9740/3) 202.6●

◀ New   ◀▥ Revised   ~~deleted~~ Deleted   ● Use Additional Digit(s)   ▨ Omit code

Masters-Allen syndrome 620.6
Mastitis (acute) (adolescent)
    (diffuse) (interstitial) (lobular)
    (nonpuerperal) (nonsuppurative)
    (parenchymatous) (phlegmonous)
    (simple) (subacute) (suppurative)
    611.0
  chronic (cystic) (fibrocystic) 610.1
  cystic 610.1
    Schimmelbusch's type 610.1
  fibrocystic 610.1
  infective 611.0
  lactational 675.2●
  lymphangitis 611.0
  neonatal (noninfective) 778.7
    infective 771.5
  periductal 610.4
  plasma cell 610.4
  puerperal, postpartum, (interstitial)
      (nonpurulent) (parenchymatous)
      675.2●
    purulent 675.1●
    stagnation 676.2●
  puerperalis 675.2●
  retromammary 611.0
    puerperal, postpartum 675.1●
  submammary 611.0
    puerperal, postpartum 675.1●
Mastocytoma (M9740/1) 238.5
  malignant (M9740/3) 202.6●
Mastocytosis 757.33
  malignant (M9741/3) 202.6●
  systemic (M9741/3) 202.6●
Mastodynia 611.71
  psychogenic 307.89
Mastoid - see condition
Mastoidalgia (see also Otalgia) 388.70
Mastoiditis (coalescent) (hemorrhagic)
    (pneumococcal) (streptococcal)
    (suppurative) 383.9
  acute or subacute 383.00
    with
      Gradenigo's syndrome 383.02
      petrositis 383.02
      specified complication NEC
        383.02
      subperiosteal abscess 383.01
  chronic (necrotic) (recurrent) 383.1
  tuberculous (see also Tuberculosis)
    015.6●
Mastopathy, mastopathia 611.9
  chronica cystica 610.1
  diffuse cystic 610.1
  estrogenic 611.89
  ovarian origin 611.89
Mastoplasia 611.1
Masturbation 307.9
Maternal condition, affecting fetus or
    newborn
  acute yellow atrophy of liver 760.8
  albuminuria 760.1
  anesthesia or analgesia 763.5
  blood loss 762.1
  chorioamnionitis 762.7
  circulatory disease, chronic
      (conditions classifiable
      to 390–459, 745–747) 760.3
  congenital heart disease (conditions
      classifiable to 745–746) 760.3
  cortical necrosis of kidney 760.1
  death 761.6
  diabetes mellitus 775.0
    manifest diabetes in the infant
      775.1

Maternal condition, affecting fetus or
    newborn (Continued)
  disease NEC 760.9
    circulatory system, chronic
        (conditions classifiable to
        390–459, 745–747) 760.3
    genitourinary system (conditions
        classifiable to 580–599)
        760.1
    respiratory (conditions classifiable
        to 490–519, 748) 760.3
  eclampsia 760.0
  hemorrhage NEC 762.1
  hepatitis acute, malignant, or subacute
      760.8
  hyperemesis (gravidarum) 761.8
  hypertension (arising during
      pregnancy) (conditions
      classifiable to 642) 760.0
  infection
    disease classifiable to 001–136
        760.2
    genital tract NEC 760.8
    urinary tract 760.1
  influenza 760.2
    manifest influenza in the infant
        771.2
  injury (conditions classifiable to
      800–996) 760.5
  malaria 760.2
    manifest malaria in infant or fetus
        771.2
  malnutrition 760.4
  necrosis of liver 760.8
  nephritis (conditions classifiable to
      580–583) 760.1
  nephrosis (conditions classifiable to
      581) 760.1
  noxious substance transmitted via
      breast milk or placenta 760.70
    alcohol 760.71
    anticonvulsants 760.77
    antifungals 760.74
    anti-infective agents 760.74
    antimetabolics 760.78
    cocaine 760.75
    "crack" 760.75
    diethylstilbestrol [DES] 760.76
    hallucinogenic agents 760.73
    medicinal agents NEC 760.79
    narcotics 760.72
    obstetric anesthetic or analgesic
        drug 760.72
    specified agent NEC 760.79
  nutritional disorder (conditions
      classifiable to 260–269) 760.4
  operation unrelated to current delivery
      (see also Newborn, affected by)
      760.64
  pre-eclampsia 760.0
  pyelitis or pyelonephritis, arising
      during pregnancy (conditions
      classifiable to 590) 760.1
  renal disease or failure 760.1
  respiratory disease, chronic
      (conditions classifiable to
      490–519, 748) 760.3
  rheumatic heart disease (chronic)
      (conditions classifiable to 393–
      398) 760.3
  rubella (conditions classifiable to 056)
      760.2
    manifest rubella in the infant or
        fetus 771.0

Maternal condition, affecting fetus or
    newborn (Continued)
  surgery unrelated to current delivery
      (see also Newborn, affected by)
      760.64
    to uterus or pelvic organs 760.64
  syphilis (conditions classifiable to 090–
      097) 760.2
    manifest syphilis in the infant or
        fetus 090.0
  thrombophlebitis 760.3
  toxemia (of pregnancy) 760.0
    pre-eclamptic 760.0
  toxoplasmosis (conditions classifiable
      to 130) 760.2
    manifest toxoplasmosis in the infant
        or fetus 771.2
  transmission of chemical substance
      through the placenta 760.70
    alcohol 760.71
    anticonvulsants 760.77
    antifungals 760.74
    anti-infective 760.74
    antimetabolics 760.78
    cocaine 760.75
    "crack" 760.75
    diethylstilbestrol [DES] 760.76
    hallucinogenic agents 760.73
    narcotics 760.72
    specified substance NEC 760.79
  uremia 760.1
  urinary tract conditions (conditions
      classifiable to 580–599) 760.1
  vomiting (pernicious) (persistent)
      (vicious) 761.8
Maternity - see Delivery
Matheiu's disease (leptospiral jaundice)
    100.0
Mauclaire's disease or osteochondrosis
    732.3
Maxcy's disease 081.0
Maxilla, maxillary - see condition
May (-Hegglin) anomaly or syndrome 288.2
Mayaro fever 066.3
Mazoplasia 610.8
MBD (minimal brain dysfunction), child
    (see also Hyperkinesia) 314.9
MCAD (medium chain acyl CoA
    dehydrogenase deficiency) 277.85
McArdle (-Schmid-Pearson) disease or
    syndrome (glycogenosis V) 271.0
McCune-Albright syndrome (osteitis
    fibrosa disseminata) 756.59
MCLS (mucocutaneous lymph node
    syndrome) 446.1
McQuarrie's syndrome (idiopathic
    familial hypoglycemia) 251.2
Measles (black) (hemorrhagic)
    (suppressed) 055.9
  with
    encephalitis 055.0
    keratitis 055.71
    keratoconjunctivitis 055.71
    otitis media 055.2
    pneumonia 055.1
  complication 055.8
    specified type NEC 055.79
  encephalitis 055.0
  French 056.9
  German 056.9
  keratitis 055.71
  keratoconjunctivitis 055.71
  liberty 056.9
  otitis media 055.2

Measles (*Continued*)
  pneumonia 055.1
  specified complications NEC 055.79
  vaccination, prophylactic (against)
    V04.2
Meatitis, urethral (*see also* Urethritis)
  597.89
Meat poisoning - *see* Poisoning, food
Meatus, meatal - *see* condition
Meat-wrappers' asthma 506.9
Meckel's
  diverticulitis 751.0
  diverticulum (displaced)
    (hypertrophic) 751.0
Meconium
  aspiration 770.11
    with
      pneumonia 770.12
      pneumonitis 770.12
      respiratory symptoms 770.12
      below vocal cords 770.11
        with respiratory symptoms
          770.12
      syndrome 770.12
  delayed passage in newborn 777.1
  ileus 777.1
    due to cystic fibrosis 277.01
  in liquor 792.3
    noted during delivery - 656.8●
  insufflation 770.11
    with respiratory symptoms 770.12
  obstruction
    fetus or newborn 777.1
      in mucoviscidosis 277.01
  passage of 792.3
    noted during delivery 763.84
  peritonitis 777.6
  plug syndrome (newborn) NEC
    777.1
  staining 779.84
Median - *see also* condition
  arcuate ligament syndrome 447.4
  bar (prostate) 600.90
    with
      other lower urinary tract
        symptoms (LUTS)
        600.91
      urinary
        obstruction 600.91
        retention 600.91
  rhomboid glossitis 529.2
  vesical orifice 600.90
    with
      other lower urinary tract
        symptoms (LUTS)
        600.91
      urinary
        obstruction 600.91
        retention 600.91
Mediastinal shift 793.2
Mediastinitis (acute) (chronic) 519.2
  actinomycotic 039.8
  syphilitic 095.8
  tuberculous (*see also* Tuberculosis)
    012.8●
Mediastinopericarditis (*see also*
  Pericarditis) 423.9
  acute 420.90
  chronic 423.8
    rheumatic 393
  rheumatic, chronic 393
Mediastinum, mediastinal - *see* condition
Medical services provided for - *see* Health,
  services provided because (of)

Medicine poisoning (by overdose)
  (wrong substance given or taken in
    error) 977.9
  specified drug or substance - *see* Table
    of Drugs and Chemicals
Medin's disease (poliomyelitis) 045.9●
Mediterranean
  anemia (with other hemoglobinopathy)
    282.49
  disease or syndrome (hemipathic)
    282.49
  fever (*see also* Brucellosis) 023.9
    familial 277.31
  kala-azar 085.0
  leishmaniasis 085.0
  tick fever 082.1
Medulla - *see* condition
Medullary
  cystic kidney 753.16
  sponge kidney 753.17
Medullated fibers
  optic (nerve) 743.57
  retina 362.85
Medulloblastoma (M9470/3)
  desmoplastic (M9471/3) 191.6
  specified site - *see* Neoplasm, by site,
    malignant
  unspecified site 191.6
Medulloepithelioma (M9501/3) - *see also*
  Neoplasm, by site, malignant
  teratoid (M9502/3) - *see* Neoplasm, by
    site, malignant
Medullomyoblastoma (M9472/3)
  specified site - *see* Neoplasm, by site,
    malignant
  unspecified site 191.6
Meekeren-Ehlers-Danlos syndrome
  756.83
Megacaryocytic - *see* condition
Megacolon (acquired) (functional) (not
  Hirschsprung's disease) 564.7
  aganglionic 751.3
  congenital, congenitum 751.3
  Hirschsprung's (disease) 751.3
  psychogenic 306.4
  toxic (*see also* Colitis, ulcerative) 556.9
Megaduodenum 537.3
Megaesophagus (functional) 530.0
  congenital 750.4
Megakaryocytic - *see* condition
Megalencephaly 742.4
Megalerythema (epidermicum)
  (infectiosum) 057.0
Megalia, cutis et ossium 757.39
Megaloappendix 751.5
Megalocephalus, megalocephaly NEC
  756.0
Megalocornea 743.41
  associated with buphthalmos 743.22
Megalocytic anemia 281.9
Megalodactylia (fingers) (thumbs) 755.57
  toes 755.65
Megaloduodenum 751.5
Megaloesophagus (functional) 530.0
  congenital 750.4
Megalogastria (congenital) 750.7
Megalomania 307.9
Megalophthalmos 743.8
Megalopsia 368.14
Megalosplenia (*see also* Splenomegaly)
  789.2
Megaloureter 593.89
  congenital 753.22
Megarectum 569.49

Megasigmoid 564.7
  congenital 751.3
Megaureter 593.89
  congenital 753.22
Megrim 346.9●
Meibomian
  cyst 373.2
    infected 373.12
  gland - *see* condition
  infarct (eyelid) 374.85
  stye 373.11
Meibomitis 373.12
Meige
  -Milroy disease (chronic hereditary
    edema) 757.0
  syndrome (blepharospasm-
    oromandibular dystonia) 333.82
Melalgia, nutritional 266.2
Melancholia (*see also* Psychosis, affective)
  296.90
  climacteric 296.2●
    recurrent episode 296.3●
    single episode 296.2●
  hypochondriac 300.7
  intermittent 296.2●
    recurrent episode 296.3●
    single episode 296.2●
  involutional 296.2●
    recurrent episode 296.3●
    single episode 296.2●
  menopausal 296.2●
    recurrent episode 296.3●
    single episode 296.2●
  puerperal 296.2●
  reactive (from emotional stress,
    psychological trauma) 298.0
  recurrent 296.3●
  senile 290.21
  stuporous 296.2●
    recurrent episode 296.3●
    single episode 296.2●
Melanemia 275.0
Melanoameloblastoma (M9363/0) - *see*
  Neoplasm, bone, benign
Melanoblastoma (M8720/3) - *see*
  Melanoma
Melanoblastosis
  Block-Sulzberger 757.33
  cutis linearis sive systematisata 757.33
Melanocarcinoma (M8720/3) - *see*
  Melanoma
Melanocytoma, eyeball (M8726/0) 224.0
Melanoderma, melanodermia 709.09
  Addison's (primary adrenal
    insufficiency) 255.41
Melanodontia, infantile 521.05
Melanodontoclasia 521.05
Melanoepithelioma (M8720/3) - *see*
  Melanoma
Melanoma (malignant) (M8720/3) 172.9

> **Note 53**   Except where otherwise
> indicated, the morphological varieties
> of melanoma in the list below should
> be coded by site as for "Melanoma
> (malignant)." Internal sites should be
> coded to malignant neoplasm of those
> sites.

  abdominal wall 172.5
  ala nasi 172.3
  amelanotic (M8730/3) - *see* Melanoma,
    by site

◄ New   ◄|||| Revised   ~~deleted~~ Deleted   ● Use Additional Digit(s)   ▨ Omit code

Melanoma (Continued)
  ankle 172.7
  anus, anal 154.3
    canal 154.2
  arm 172.6
  auditory canal (external) 172.2
  auricle (ear) 172.2
  auricular canal (external) 172.2
  axilla 172.5
  axillary fold 172.5
  back 172.5
  balloon cell (M8722/3) - see Melanoma,
    by site
  benign (M8720/0) - see Neoplasm, skin,
    benign
  breast (female) (male) 172.5
  brow 172.3
  buttock 172.5
  canthus (eye) 172.1
  cheek (external) 172.3
  chest wall 172.5
  chin 172.3
  choroid 190.6
  conjunctiva 190.3
  ear (external) 172.2
  epithelioid cell (M8771/3) - see also
    Melanoma, by site
    and spindle cell, mixed (M8775/3) -
      see Melanoma, by site
  external meatus (ear) 172.2
  eye 190.9
  eyebrow 172.3
  eyelid (lower) (upper) 172.1
  face NEC 172.3
  female genital organ (external) NEC
    184.4
  finger 172.6
  flank 172.5
  foot 172.7
  forearm 172.6
  forehead 172.3
  foreskin 187.1
  gluteal region 172.5
  groin 172.5
  hand 172.6
  heel 172.7
  helix 172.2
  hip 172.7
  in
    giant pigmented nevus (M8761/3) -
      see Melanoma, by site
    Hutchinson's melanotic freckle
      (M8742/3) - see Melanoma, by
      site
    junctional nevus (M8740/3) - see
      Melanoma, by site
    precancerous melanosis (M8741/3) -
      see Melanoma, by site
  in situ - see Melanoma, by site
    skin 172.9
  interscapular region 172.5
  iris 190.0
  jaw 172.3
  juvenile (M8770/0) - see Neoplasm,
    skin, benign
  knee 172.7
  labium
    majus 184.1
    minus 184.2
  lacrimal gland 190.2
  leg 172.7
  lip (lower) (upper) 172.0
  liver 197.7
  lower limb NEC 172.7

Melanoma (Continued)
  male genital organ (external) NEC
    187.9
  meatus, acoustic (external) 172.2
  meibomian gland 172.1
  metastatic
    of or from specified site - see
      Melanoma, by site
    site not of skin - see Neoplasm, by
      site, malignant, secondary
    to specified site - see Neoplasm, by
      site, malignant, secondary
    unspecified site 172.9
  nail 172.9
    finger 172.6
    toe 172.7
  neck 172.4
  nodular (M8721/3) - see Melanoma, by
    site
  nose, external 172.3
  orbit 190.1
  penis 187.4
  perianal skin 172.5
  perineum 172.5
  pinna 172.2
  popliteal (fossa) (space) 172.7
  prepuce 187.1
  pubes 172.5
  pudendum 184.4
  retina 190.5
  scalp 172.4
  scrotum 187.7
  septum nasal (skin) 172.3
  shoulder 172.6
  skin NEC 172.8
    in situ 172.9
  spindle cell (M8772/3) - see also
    Melanoma, by site
    type A (M8773/3) 190.0
    type B (M8774/3) 190.0
  submammary fold 172.5
  superficial spreading (M8743/3) - see
    Melanoma, by site
  temple 172.3
  thigh 172.7
  toe 172.7
  trunk NEC 172.5
  umbilicus 172.5
  upper limb NEC 172.6
  vagina vault 184.0
  vulva 184.4
Melanoplakia 528.9
Melanosarcoma (M8720/3) - see also
    Melanoma
  epithelioid cell (M8771/3) - see
    Melanoma
Melanosis 709.09
  addisonian (primary adrenal
    insufficiency) 255.41
    tuberculous (see also Tuberculosis)
      017.6●
  adrenal 255.41
  colon 569.89
  conjunctiva 372.55
    congenital 743.49
  corii degenerativa 757.33
  cornea (presenile) (senile) 371.12
    congenital 743.43
      interfering with vision 743.42
    prenatal 743.43
      interfering with vision 743.42
  eye 372.55
    congenital 743.49
  jute spinners' 709.09

Melanosis (Continued)
  lenticularis progressiva 757.33
  liver 573.8
  precancerous (M8741/2) - see also
    Neoplasm, skin, in situ
    malignant melanoma in (M8741/3) -
      see Melanoma
  Riehl's 709.09
  sclera 379.19
    congenital 743.47
  suprarenal 255.41
  tar 709.09
  toxic 709.09
Melanuria 791.9
MELAS syndrome (mitochondrial
    encephalopathy, lactic acidosis and
    stroke-like episodes) 277.87
Melasma 709.09
  adrenal (gland) 255.41
  suprarenal (gland) 255.41
Melena 578.1
  due to
    swallowed maternal blood 777.3
    ulcer - see Ulcer, by site, with
      hemorrhage
  newborn 772.4
    due to swallowed maternal blood
      777.3
Meleney's
  gangrene (cutaneous) 686.09
  ulcer (chronic undermining) 686.09
Melioidosis 025
Melitensis, febris 023.0
Melitococcosis 023.0
Melkersson (-Rosenthal) syndrome
    351.8
Mellitus, diabetes - see Diabetes
Melorheostosis (bone) (leri) 733.99
Meloschisis 744.83
Melotia 744.29
Membrana
  capsularis lentis posterior 743.39
  epipapillaris 743.57
Membranacea placenta - see Placenta,
    abnormal
Membranaceous uterus 621.8
Membrane, membranous - see also
    condition
  folds, congenital - see Web
  Jackson's 751.4
  over face (causing asphyxia), fetus or
    newborn 768.9
  premature rupture - see Rupture,
    membranes, premature
  pupillary 364.74
    persistent 743.46
  retained (complicating delivery)
    (with hemorrhage) 666.2●
    without hemorrhage 667.1●
  secondary (eye) 366.50
  unruptured (causing asphyxia)
    768.9
  vitreous humor 379.25
Membranitis, fetal 658.4
  affecting fetus or newborn 762.7
Memory disturbance, loss or lack (see also
    Amnesia) 780.93
  mild, following organic brain damage
    310.8   ◀▭
MEN (multiple endocrine neoplasia)
    syndromes
  type I 258.01
  type IIA 258.02
  type IIB 258.03

Menadione (vitamin K) deficiency 269.0
Menarche, precocious 259.1
Mendacity, pathologic 301.7
Mende's syndrome (ptosis-epicanthus) 270.2
Mendelson's syndrome (resulting from a procedure) 997.39
  obstetric 668.0●
Ménétrier's disease or syndrome (hypertrophic gastritis) 535.2●
Ménière's disease, syndrome, or vertigo 386.00
  cochlear 386.02
  cochleovestibular 386.01
  inactive 386.04
  in remission 386.04
  vestibular 386.03
Meninges, meningeal - see condition
Meningioma (M9530/0) - see also Neoplasm, meninges, benign
  angioblastic (M9535/0) - see Neoplasm, meninges, benign
  angiomatous (M9534/0) - see Neoplasm, meninges, benign
  endotheliomatous (M9531/0) - see Neoplasm, meninges, benign
  fibroblastic (M9532/0) - see Neoplasm, meninges, benign
  fibrous (M9532/0) - see Neoplasm, meninges, benign
  hemangioblastic (M9535/0) - see Neoplasm, meninges, benign
  hemangiopericytic (M9536/0) - see Neoplasm, meninges, benign
  malignant (M9530/3) - see Neoplasm, meninges, malignant
  meningiothelial (M9531/0) - see Neoplasm, meninges, benign
  meningotheliomatous (M9531/0) - see Neoplasm, meninges, benign
  mixed (M9537/0) - see Neoplasm, meninges, benign
  multiple (M9530/1) 237.6
  papillary (M9538/1) 237.6
  psammomatous (M9533/0) - see Neoplasm, meninges, benign
  syncytial (M9531/0) - see Neoplasm, meninges, benign
  transitional (M9537/0) - see Neoplasm, meninges, benign
Meningiomatosis (diffuse) (M9530/1) 237.6
Meningism (see also Meningismus) 781.6
Meningismus (infectional) (pneumococcal) 781.6
  due to serum or vaccine 997.09 [321.8]
  influenzal NEC 487.8
Meningitis (basal) (basic) (basilar) (brain) (cerebral) (cervical) (congestive) (diffuse) (hemorrhagic) (infantile) (membranous) (metastatic) (nonspecific) (pontine) (progressive) (simple) (spinal) (subacute) (sympathetica) (toxic) 322.9
  abacterial NEC (see also Meningitis, aseptic) 047.9
  actinomycotic 039.8 [320.7]
  adenoviral 049.1
  aerobacter aerogenes 320.82
  anaerobes (cocci) (gram-negative) (gram-positive) (mixed) (NEC) 320.81
  arbovirus NEC 066.9 [321.2]
    specified type NEC 066.8 [321.2]

Meningitis (Continued)
  aseptic (acute) NEC 047.9
    adenovirus 049.1
    Coxsackie virus 047.0
    due to
      adenovirus 049.1
      Coxsackie virus 047.0
      ECHO virus 047.1
      enterovirus 047.9
      mumps 072.1
      poliovirus (see also Poliomyelitis) 045.2● [321.2]
    ECHO virus 047.1
    herpes (simplex) virus 054.72
    zoster 053.0
    leptospiral 100.81
    lymphocytic choriomeningitis 049.0
    noninfective 322.0
  Bacillus pyocyaneus 320.89
  bacterial NEC 320.9
    anaerobic 320.81
    gram-negative 320.82
      anaerobic 320.81
  Bacteroides (fragilis) (oralis) (melaninogenicus) 320.81
  cancerous (M8000/6) 198.4
  candidal 112.83
  carcinomatous (M8010/6) 198.4
  caseous (see also Tuberculosis, meninges) 013.0●
  cerebrospinal (acute) (chronic) (diplococcal) (endemic) (epidemic) (fulminant) (infectious) (malignant) (meningococcal) (sporadic) 036.0
    carrier (suspected) of V02.59
  chronic NEC 322.2
  clear cerebrospinal fluid NEC 322.0
  Clostridium (haemolyticum) (novyi) NEC 320.81
  coccidioidomycosis 114.2
  Coxsackie virus 047.0
  cryptococcal 117.5 [321.0]
  diplococcal 036.0
    gram-negative 036.0
    gram-positive 320.1
  Diplococcus pneumoniae 320.1
  due to
    actinomycosis 039.8 [320.7]
    adenovirus 049.1
    coccidiomycosis 114.2
    enterovirus 047.9
      specified NEC 047.8
    histoplasmosis (see also Histoplasmosis) 115.91
    Listerosis 027.0 [320.7]
    Lyme disease 088.81 [320.7]
    moniliasis 112.83
    mumps 072.1
    neurosyphilis 094.2
    nonbacterial organisms NEC 321.8
    oidiomycosis 112.83
    poliovirus (see also Poliomyelitis) 045.2● [321.2]
    preventive immunization, inoculation, or vaccination 997.09 [321.8]
    sarcoidosis 135 [321.4]
    sporotrichosis 117.1 [321.1]
    syphilis 094.2
      acute 091.81
      congenital 090.42
      secondary 091.81

Meningitis (Continued)
  due to (Continued)
    trypanosomiasis (see also Trypanosomiasis) 086.9 [321.3]
    whooping cough 033.9 [320.7]
  E. coli 320.82
  ECHO virus 047.1
  endothelial-leukocytic, benign, recurrent 047.9
  Enterobacter aerogenes 320.82
  enteroviral 047.9
    specified type NEC 047.8
  enterovirus 047.9
    specified NEC 047.8
  eosinophilic 322.1
  epidemic NEC 036.0
  Escherichia coli (E. coli) 320.82
  Eubacterium 320.81
  fibrinopurulent NEC 320.9
    specified type NEC 320.89
  Friedländer (bacillus) 320.82
  fungal NEC 117.9 [321.1]
  Fusobacterium 320.81
  gonococcal 098.82
  gram-negative bacteria NEC 320.82
    anaerobic 320.81
    cocci 036.0
      specified NEC 320.82
  gram-negative cocci NEC 036.0
    specified NEC 320.82
  gram-positive cocci NEC 320.9
  H. influenzae 320.0
  herpes (simplex) virus 054.72
    zoster 053.0
  infectious NEC 320.9
  influenzal 320.0
  Klebsiella pneumoniae 320.82
  late effect - see Late, effect, meningitis
  leptospiral (aseptic) 100.81
  Listerella (monocytogenes) 027.0 [320.7]
  Listeria monocytogenes 027.0 [320.7]
  lymphocytic (acute) (benign) (serous) 049.0
    choriomeningitis virus 049.0
  meningococcal (chronic) 036.0
  Mima polymorpha 320.82
  Mollaret's 047.9
  monilial 112.83
  mumps (virus) 072.1
  mycotic NEC 117.9 [321.1]
  Neisseria 036.0
  neurosyphilis 094.2
  nonbacterial NEC (see also Meningitis, aseptic) 047.9
  nonpyogenic NEC 322.0
  oidiomycosis 112.83
  ossificans 349.2
  Peptococcus 320.81
  PeptoStreptococcus 320.81
  pneumococcal 320.1
  poliovirus (see also Poliomyelitis) 045.2● [321.2]
  Proprionibacterium 320.81
  Proteus morganii 320.82
  Pseudomonas (aeruginosa) (pyocyaneus) 320.82
  purulent NEC 320.9
    specified organism NEC 320.89
  pyogenic NEC 320.9
    specified organism NEC 320.89
  Salmonella 003.21
  septic NEC 320.9
    specified organism NEC 320.89

◄ New   ◄█║ Revised   ~~deleted~~ Deleted   ● Use Additional Digit(s)   ▒▒▒ Omit code

Meningitis (Continued)
  serosa circumscripta NEC 322.0
  serous NEC (see also Meningitis,
      aseptic) 047.9
    lymphocytic 049.0
    syndrome 348.2
  Serratia (marcescens) 320.82
  specified organism NEC 320.89
  sporadic cerebrospinal 036.0
  sporotrichosis 117.1 [321.1]
  staphylococcal 320.3
  sterile 997.09
  streptococcal (acute) 320.2
  suppurative 320.9
    specified organism NEC 320.89
  syphilitic 094.2
    acute 091.81
    congenital 090.42
    secondary 091.81
  torula 117.5 [321.0]
  traumatic (complication of injury)
      958.8
  Treponema (denticola)
      (macrodenticum) 320.81
  trypanosomiasis 086.1 [321.3]
  tuberculous (see also Tuberculosis,
      meninges) 013.0●
  typhoid 002.0 [320.7]
  Veillonella 320.81
  Vibrio vulnificus 320.82
  viral, virus NEC (see also Meningitis,
      aseptic) 047.9
  Wallgren's (see also Meningitis, aseptic)
      047.9
Meningocele (congenital) (spinal) (see also
    Spina bifida) 741.9●
  acquired (traumatic) 349.2
  cerebral 742.0
  cranial 742.0
Meningocerebritis - see
    Meningoencephalitis
Meningococcemia (acute) (chronic)
    036.2
Meningococcus, meningococcal (see also
    condition) 036.9
  adrenalitis, hemorrhagic 036.3
  carditis 036.40
  carrier (suspected) of V02.59
  cerebrospinal fever 036.0
  encephalitis 036.1
  endocarditis 036.42
  exposure to V01.84
  infection NEC 036.9
  meningitis (cerebrospinal) 036.0
  myocarditis 036.43
  optic neuritis 036.81
  pericarditis 036.41
  septicemia (chronic) 036.2
Meningoencephalitis (see also
    Encephalitis) 323.9
  acute NEC 048
  bacterial, purulent, pyogenic, or
      septic - see Meningitis
  chronic NEC 094.1
  diffuse NEC 094.1
  diphasic 063.2
  due to
    actinomycosis 039.8 [320.7]
    blastomycosis NEC (see also
        Blastomycosis) 116.0 [323.41]
    free-living amebae 136.29
    Listeria monocytogenes 027.0 [320.7]
    Lyme disease 088.81 [320.7]
    mumps 072.2

Meningoencephalitis (Continued)
  due to (Continued)
    Naegleria (amebae) (gruberi)
        (organisms) 136.29
    rubella 056.01
    sporotrichosis 117.1 [321.1]
    toxoplasmosis (acquired) 130.0
      congenital (active) 771.2
          [323.41]
    Trypanosoma 086.1 [323.2]
  epidemic 036.0
  herpes 054.3
  herpetic 054.3
  H. influenzae 320.0
  infectious (acute) 048
  influenzal 320.0
  late effect - see category 326
  Listeria monocytogenes 027.0 [320.7]
  lymphocytic (serous) 049.0
  mumps 072.2
  parasitic NEC 123.9 [323.41]
  pneumococcal 320.1
  primary amebic 136.29
  rubella 056.01
  serous 048
    lymphocytic 049.0
  specific 094.2
  staphylococcal 320.3
  streptococcal 320.2
  syphilitic 094.2
  toxic NEC 989.9 [323.71]
    due to
      carbon tetrachloride (vapor)
          987.8 [323.71]
      hydroxyquinoline derivatives
          poisoning 961.3 [323.71]
      lead 984.9 [323.71]
      mercury 985.0 [323.71]
      thallium 985.8 [323.71]
  toxoplasmosis (acquired) 130.0
  trypanosomic 086.1 [323.2]
  tuberculous (see also Tuberculosis,
      meninges) 013.0●
  virus NEC 048
Meningoencephalocele 742.0
  syphilitic 094.89
    congenital 090.49
Meningoencephalomyelitis (see also
    Meningoencephalitis) 323.9
  acute NEC 048
    disseminated (postinfectious) 136.9
        [323.61]
      postimmunization or
          postvaccination 323.51
  due to
    actinomycosis 039.8 [320.7]
    torula 117.5 [323.41]
    toxoplasma or toxoplasmosis
        (acquired) 130.0
      congenital (active) 771.2
          [323.41]
  late effect - see category 326
Meningoencephalomyelopathy (see also
    Meningoencephalomyelitis) 349.9
Meningoencephalopathy (see also
    Meningoencephalitis) 348.39
Meningoencephalopoliomyelitis (see also
    Poliomyelitis, bulbar) 045.0●
  late effect 138
Meningomyelitis (see also
    Meningoencephalitis) 323.9
  blastomycotic NEC (see also
      Blastomycosis) 116.0
          [323.41]

Meningomyelitis (Continued)
  due to
    actinomycosis 039.8 [320.7]
    blastomycosis (see also
        Blastomycosis) 116.0 [323.41]
    Meningococcus 036.0
    sporotrichosis 117.1 [323.41]
    torula 117.5 [323.41]
  late effect - see category 326
  lethargic 049.8
  meningococcal 036.0
  syphilitic 094.2
  tuberculous (see also Tuberculosis,
      meninges) 013.0●
Meningomyelocele (see also Spina bifida)
    741.9●
  syphilitic 094.89
Meningomyeloneuritis - see
    Meningoencephalitis
Meningoradiculitis - see Meningitis
Meningovascular - see condition
Meniscocytosis 282.60
Menkes' syndrome - see Syndrome,
    Menkes'
Menolipsis 626.0
Menometrorrhagia 626.2
Menopause, menopausal (symptoms)
    (syndrome) 627.2
  arthritis (any site) NEC 716.3●
  artificial 627.4
  bleeding 627.0
  crisis 627.2
  depression (see also Psychosis, affective)
      296.2●
    agitated 296.2●
      recurrent episode 296.3●
      single episode 296.2●
    psychotic 296.2●
      recurrent episode 296.3●
      single episode 296.2●
    recurrent episode 296.3●
    single episode 296.2●
  melancholia (see also Psychosis,
      affective) 296.2●
    recurrent episode 296.3●
    single episode 296.2●
  paranoid state 297.2
  paraphrenia 297.2
  postsurgical 627.4
  premature 256.31
    postirradiation 256.2
    postsurgical 256.2
  psychoneurosis 627.2
  psychosis NEC 298.8
  surgical 627.4
  toxic polyarthritis NEC 716.39
Menorrhagia (primary) 626.2
  climacteric 627.0
  menopausal 627.0
  postclimacteric 627.1
  postmenopausal 627.1
  preclimacteric 627.0
  premenopausal 627.0
  puberty (menses retained) 626.3
Menorrhalgia 625.3
Menoschesis 626.8
Menostaxis 626.2
Menses, retention 626.8
Menstrual - see also Menstruation
  cycle, irregular 626.4
  disorders NEC 626.9
  extraction V25.3
  fluid, retained 626.8
  molimen 625.4

Menstrual (*Continued*)
 period, normal V65.5
 regulation V25.3
Menstruation
 absent 626.0
 anovulatory 628.0
 delayed 626.8
 difficult 625.3
 disorder 626.9
  psychogenic 306.52
  specified NEC 626.8
 during pregnancy 640.8●
 excessive 626.2
 frequent 626.2
 infrequent 626.1
 irregular 626.4
 latent 626.8
 membranous 626.8
 painful (primary) (secondary) 625.3
  psychogenic 306.52
 passage of clots 626.2
 precocious 626.8
 protracted 626.8
 retained 626.8
 retrograde 626.8
 scanty 626.1
 suppression 626.8
 vicarious (nasal) 625.8
Mentagra (*see also* Sycosis) 704.8
Mental - *see also* condition
 deficiency (*see also* Retardation, mental)
  319
 deterioration (*see also* Psychosis) 298.9
 disorder (*see also* Disorder, mental)
  300.9
 exhaustion 300.5
 insufficiency (congenital) (*see also*
  Retardation, mental) 319
 observation without need for further
  medical care NEC V71.09
 retardation (*see also* Retardation,
  mental) 319
 subnormality (*see also* Retardation,
  mental) 319
  mild 317
  moderate 318.0
  profound 318.2
  severe 318.1
 upset (*see also* Disorder, mental) 300.9
Meralgia paresthetica 355.1
Mercurial - *see* condition
Mercurialism NEC 985.0
Merergasia 300.9
Merkel cell tumor - *see* ~~Neoplasm,~~
 ~~by site, malignant~~ Carcinoma,
  Merkel cell ◀▥
Merocele (*see also* Hernia, femoral) 553.00
Meromelia 755.4
 lower limb 755.30
  intercalary 755.32
   femur 755.34
    tibiofibular (complete)
     (incomplete) 755.33
   fibula 755.37
   metatarsal(s) 755.38
   tarsal(s) 755.38
   tibia 755.36
   tibiofibular 755.35
  terminal (complete) (partial)
   (transverse) 755.31
  longitudinal 755.32
   metatarsal(s) 755.38
   phalange(s) 755.39
   tarsal(s) 755.38
  transverse 755.31

Meromelia (*Continued*)
 upper limb 755.20
  intercalary 755.22
   carpal(s) 755.28
   humeral 755.24
    radioulnar (complete)
     (incomplete) 755.23
   metacarpal(s) 755.28
   phalange(s) 755.29
   radial 755.26
   radioulnar 755.25
   ulnar 755.27
  terminal (complete) (partial)
   (transverse) 755.21
  longitudinal 755.22
   carpal(s) 755.28
   metacarpal(s) 755.28
   phalange(s) 755.29
  transverse 755.21
Merosmia 781.1
MERRF syndrome (myoclonus with
  epilepsy and with ragged red fibers)
  277.87
Merycism - *see also* Vomiting
 psychogenic 307.53
Merzbacher-Pelizaeus disease 330.0
Mesaortitis - *see* Aortitis
Mesarteritis - *see* Arteritis
Mesencephalitis (*see also* Encephalitis)
  323.9
 late effect - *see* category 326
Mesenchymoma (M8990/1) - *see also*
  Neoplasm, connective tissue,
  uncertain behavior
 benign (M8990/0) - *see* Neoplasm,
  connective tissue, benign
 malignant (M8990/3) - *see* Neoplasm,
  connective tissue, malignant
Mesenteritis
 retractile 567.82
 sclerosing 567.82
Mesentery, mesenteric - *see* condition
Mesiodens, mesiodentes 520.1
 causing crowding 524.31
Mesio-occlusion 524.23
Mesocardia (with asplenia) 746.87
Mesocolon - *see* condition
Mesonephroma (malignant) (M9110/3) -
  see also Neoplasm, by site,
  malignant
 benign (M9110/0) - *see* Neoplasm, by
  site, benign
Mesophlebitis - *see* Phlebitis
Mesostromal dysgenesis 743.51
Mesothelioma (malignant) (M9050/3) -
  see also Neoplasm, by site,
  malignant
 benign (M9050/0) - *see* Neoplasm, by
  site, benign
 biphasic type (M9053/3) - *see also*
  Neoplasm, by site, malignant
 benign (M9053/0) - *see* Neoplasm,
  by site, benign
 epithelioid (M9052/3) - *see also*
  Neoplasm, by site, malignant
 benign (M9052/0) - *see* Neoplasm,
  by site, benign
 fibrous (M9051/3) - *see also* Neoplasm,
  by site, malignant
 benign (M9051/0) - *see* Neoplasm,
  by site, benign
Metabolic syndrome 277.7
Metabolism disorder 277.9
 specified type NEC 277.89
Metagonimiasis 121.5

Metagonimus infestation (small
  intestine) 121.5
Metal
 pigmentation (skin) 709.00
 polishers' disease 502
Metalliferous miners' lung 503
Metamorphopsia 368.14
Metaplasia
 bone, in skin 709.3
 breast 611.89
 cervix - *omit code*
 endometrium (squamous) 621.8
 esophagus 530.85
 intestinal, of gastric mucosa 537.89
 kidney (pelvis) (squamous) (*see also*
  Disease, renal) 593.89
 myelogenous 289.89
 myeloid 289.89
  agnogenic 238.76
  megakaryocytic 238.76
 spleen 289.59
 squamous cell
  amnion 658.8●
  bladder 596.8
  cervix - *see* condition
  trachea 519.19
  tracheobronchial tree 519.19
  uterus 621.8
  cervix - *see* condition
Metastasis, metastatic
 abscess - *see* Abscess
 calcification 275.40
 cancer, neoplasm, or disease
  from specified site (M8000/3) - *see*
   Neoplasm, by site, malignant
  to specified site (M8000/6) - *see*
   Neoplasm, by site, secondary
 deposits (in) (M8000/6) - *see* Neoplasm,
  by site, secondary
 mesentery, of neuroendocrine tumor
  209.71 ◀
 pneumonia 038.8 [484.8]
 spread (to) (M8000/6) - *see* Neoplasm,
  by site, secondary
Metatarsalgia 726.70
 anterior 355.6
 due to Freiberg's disease 732.5
 Morton's 355.6
Metatarsus, metatarsal - *see also*
  condition
 abductus valgus (congenital) 754.60
 adductus varus (congenital) 754.53
 primus varus 754.52
 valgus (adductus) (congenital) 754.60
 varus (abductus) (congenital) 754.53
 primus 754.52
Methadone use 304.00
Methemoglobinemia 289.7
 acquired (with sulfhemoglobinemia)
  289.7
 congenital 289.7
 enzymatic 289.7
 Hb-M disease 289.7
 hereditary 239.7
 toxic 289.7
Methemoglobinuria (*see also*
  Hemoglobinuria) 791.2
Methicillin
 resistant staphylococcus aureus
  (MRSA) 041.12
  colonization V02.54
  personal history of V12.04
 susceptible staphylococcus aureus
  (MSSA) 041.11
  colonization V02.53

Methioninemia 270.4
Metritis (catarrhal) (septic) (suppurative) (*see also* Endometritis) 615.9
  blennorrhagic 098.16
    chronic or duration of 2 months or over 098.36
  cervical (*see also* Cervicitis) 616.0
  gonococcal 098.16
    chronic or duration of 2 months or over 098.36
  hemorrhagic 626.8
  puerperal, postpartum, childbirth 670.1 ◄▦
  septic 670.2 ◄
  tuberculous (*see also* Tuberculosis) 016.7●
Metropathia hemorrhagica 626.8
Metroperitonitis (*see also* Peritonitis, pelvic, female) 614.5
Metrorrhagia 626.6
  arising during pregnancy - *see* Hemorrhage, pregnancy
  postpartum NEC 666.2●
  primary 626.6
  psychogenic 306.59
  puerperal 666.2●
Metrorrhexis - *see* Rupture, uterus
Metrosalpingitis (*see also* Salpingo-oophoritis) 614.2
Metrostaxis 626.6
Metrovaginitis (*see also* Endometritis) 615.9
  gonococcal (acute) 098.16
    chronic or duration of 2 months or over 098.36
Mexican fever - *see* Typhus, Mexican
Meyenburg-Altherr-Uehlinger syndrome 733.99
Meyer-Schwickerath and Weyers syndrome (dysplasia oculodentodigitalis) 759.89
Meynert's amentia (nonalcoholic) 294.0
  alcoholic 291.1
Mibelli's disease 757.39
Mice, joint (*see also* Loose, body, joint) 718.1●
  knee 717.6
Micheli-Rietti syndrome (thalassemia minor) 282.49
Michotte's syndrome 721.5
Micrencephalon, micrencephaly 742.1
Microalbuminuria 791.0
Microaneurysm, retina 362.14
  diabetic 250.5● [362.01]
    due to secondary diabetes 249.5● [362.01]
Microangiopathy 443.9
  diabetic (peripheral) 250.7● [443.81]
    due to secondary diabetes 249.7● [443.81]
    retinal 250.5● [362.01]
      due to secondary diabetes 249.5● [362.01]
  peripheral 443.9
    diabetic 250.7● [443.81]
      due to secondary diabetes 249.7● [443.81]
    retinal 362.18
      diabetic 250.5● [362.01]
        due to secondary diabetes 249.5● [362.01]
  thrombotic 446.6
    Moschcowitz's (thrombotic thrombocytopenic purpura) 446.6

Microcalcification, mammographic 793.81
Microcephalus, microcephalic, microcephaly 742.1
  due to toxoplasmosis (congenital) 771.2
Microcheilia 744.82
Microcolon (congenital) 751.5
Microcornea (congenital) 743.41
Microcytic - *see* condition
Microdeletions NEC 758.33
Microdontia 520.2
Microdrepanocytosis (thalassemia-Hb-S disease) 282.49
Microembolism
  atherothrombotic - *see* Atheroembolism
  retina 362.33
Microencephalon 742.1
Microfilaria streptocerca infestation 125.3
Microgastria (congenital) 750.7
Microgenia 524.06
Microgenitalia (congenital) 752.89
  penis 752.64
Microglioma (M9710/3)
  specified site - *see* Neoplasm, by site, malignant
  unspecified site 191.9
Microglossia (congenital) 750.16
Micrognathia, micrognathism (congenital) 524.00
  mandibular 524.04
    alveolar 524.74
  maxillary 524.03
    alveolar 524.73
Microgyria (congenital) 742.2
Microinfarct, heart (*see also* Insufficiency, coronary) 411.89
Microlithiasis, alveolar, pulmonary 516.2
Micromastia 611.82
Micromyelia (congenital) 742.59
Micropenis 752.64
Microphakia (congenital) 743.36
Microphthalmia (congenital) (*see also* Microphthalmos) 743.10
Microphthalmos (congenital) 743.10
  associated with eye and adnexal anomalies NEC 743.12
  due to toxoplasmosis (congenital) 771.2
  isolated 743.11
  simple 743.11
  syndrome 759.89
Micropsia 368.14
Microsporidiosis 136.8
Microsporosis (*see also* Dermatophytosis) 110.9
  nigra 111.1
Microsporum furfur infestation 111.0
Microstomia (congenital) 744.84
Microthelia 757.6
Microthromboembolism - *see* Embolism
Microtia (congenital) (external ear) 744.23
Microtropia 378.34
Micturition
  disorder NEC 788.69
    psychogenic 306.53
  frequency 788.41
    psychogenic 306.53
  nocturnal 788.43
  painful 788.1
    psychogenic 306.53

Middle
  ear - *see* condition
  lobe (right) syndrome 518.0
Midplane - *see* condition
Miescher's disease 709.3
  cheilitis 351.8
  granulomatosis disciformis 709.3
Miescher-Leder syndrome or granulomatosis 709.3
Mieten's syndrome 759.89
Migraine (idiopathic) 346.9●

> Note The following fifth digit subclassification is for use with category 346:
>
> 0   without mention of intractable migraine without mention of status migrainosus
> 1   with intractable migraine, so stated, without mention of status migrainosus
> 2   without mention of intractable migraine with status migrainosus
> 3   with intractable migraine, so stated, with status migrainosus

  with aura (acute-onset) (without headache) (prolonged) (typical) 346.0●
  without aura 346.1●
    chronic 346.7●
    transformed 346.7●
  abdominal (syndrome) 346.2●
  allergic (histamine) 346.2●
  atypical 346.8●
  basilar 346.0●
  chronic without aura 346.7●
  classic(al) 346.0●
  common 346.1●
  hemiplegic 346.3●
    familial 346.3●
    sporadic 346.3●
  lower-half 339.00
  menstrual 346.4●
  menstrually related 346.4●
  ophthalmic 346.8●
  ophthalmoplegic 346.2●
  premenstrual 346.4●
  pure menstrual 346.4●
  retinal 346.0●
  specified form NEC 346.8●
  transformed without aura 346.7●
  variant 346.2●
Migrant, social V60.0
Migratory, migrating - *see also* condition
  person V60.0
  testis, congenital 752.52
Mikulicz's disease or syndrome (dryness of mouth, absent or decreased lacrimation) 527.1
Milian atrophia blanche 701.3
Miliaria (crystallina) (rubra) (tropicalis) 705.1
  apocrine 705.82
Miliary - *see* condition
Milium (*see also* Cyst, sebaceous) 706.2
  colloid 709.3
  eyelid 374.84
Milk
  crust 690.11
  excess secretion 676.6●

Milk *(Continued)*
  fever, female 672●
  poisoning 988.8
  retention 676.2●
  sickness 988.8
  spots 423.1
Milkers' nodes 051.1
Milk-leg (deep vessels) 671.4●
  complicating pregnancy 671.3●
  nonpuerperal 451.19
  puerperal, postpartum, childbirth
    671.4●
Milkman (-Looser) disease or syndrome
    (osteomalacia with pseudofractures)
    268.2
Milky urine *(see also* Chyluria) 791.1
Millar's asthma (laryngismus stridulus)
    478.75
Millard-Gubler paralysis or syndrome
    344.89
Millard-Gubler-Foville paralysis 344.89
Miller-Dieker syndrome 758.33
Miller's disease (osteomalacia) 268.2
Miller Fisher's syndrome 357.0
Milles' syndrome (encephalocutaneous
    angiomatosis) 759.6
Mills' disease 335.29
Millstone makers' asthma or lung 502
Milroy's disease (chronic hereditary
    edema) 757.0
Miners' - *see also* condition
  asthma 500
  elbow 727.2
  knee 727.2
  lung 500
  nystagmus 300.89
  phthisis *(see also* Tuberculosis) 011.4●
  tuberculosis *(see also* Tuberculosis)
    011.4●
Minkowski-Chauffard syndrome *(see also*
    Spherocytosis) 282.0
Minor - *see* condition
Minor's disease 336.1
Minot's disease (hemorrhagic disease,
    newborn) 776.0
Minot-von Willebrand (-Jürgens) disease
    or syndrome (angiohemophilia)
    286.4
Minus (and plus) hand (intrinsic) 736.09
Miosis (persistent) (pupil) 379.42
Mirizzi's syndrome (hepatic duct
    stenosis) *(see also* Obstruction,
    biliary) 576.2
  with calculus, cholelithiasis, or stones -
    see Choledocholithiasis
Mirror writing 315.09
  secondary to organic lesion 784.69
Misadventure (prophylactic) (therapeutic)
    (see also Complications) 999.9
  administration of insulin 962.3
  infusion - *see* Complications, infusion
  local applications (of fomentations,
    plasters, etc.) 999.9
    burn or scald - *see* Burn, by site
  medical care (early) (late) NEC 999.9
    adverse effect of drugs or
      chemicals - *see* Table of Drugs
      and Chemicals
    burn or scald - *see* Burn, by site
  radiation NEC 990
  radiotherapy NEC 990
  surgical procedure (early) (late) - *see*
    Complications, surgical
    procedure

Misadventure *(Continued)*
  transfusion - *see* Complications,
    transfusion
  vaccination or other immunological
    procedure - *see* Complications,
    vaccination
Misanthropy 301.7
Miscarriage - *see* Abortion, spontaneous
Mischief, malicious, child *(see also*
    Disturbance, conduct) 312.0●
Misdirection
  aqueous 365.83
Mismanagement, feeding 783.3
Misplaced, misplacement
  kidney *(see also* Disease, renal)
    593.0
    congenital 753.3
  organ or site, congenital NEC - *see*
    Malposition, congenital
Missed
  abortion 632
  delivery (at or near term) 656.4●
  labor (at or near term) 656.4●
Misshapen reconstructed breast 612.0
Missing - *see also* Absence
  teeth (acquired) 525.10
    congenital *(see also* Anodontia)
      520.0
    due to
      caries 525.13
      extraction 525.10
      periodontal disease 525.12
      specified NEC 525.19
      trauma 525.11
  vertebrae (congenital) 756.13
Misuse of drugs NEC *(see also* Abuse,
    drug, nondependent) 305.9●
Mitchell's disease (erythromelalgia)
    443.82
Mite(s)
  diarrhea 133.8
  grain (itch) 133.8
  hair follicle (itch) 133.8
  in sputum 133.8
**Mitochondrial encephalopathy, lactic
    acidosis and stroke-like episodes**
    (MELAS syndrome) 277.87
**Mitochondrial neurogastrointestinal
    encephalopathy syndrome**
    (MNGIE) 277.87
Mitral - *see* condition
Mittelschmerz 625.2
Mixed - *see* condition
Mljet disease (mal de Meleda) 757.39
Mobile, mobility
  cecum 751.4
  coccyx 733.99
  excessive - *see* Hypermobility
  gallbladder 751.69
  kidney 593.0
    congenital 753.3
  organ or site, congenital NEC - *see*
    Malposition, congenital
  spleen 289.59
Mobitz heart block (atrioventricular)
    426.10
  type I (Wenckebach's) 426.13
  type II 426.12
Möbius'
  disease 346.2●
  syndrome
    congenital oculofacial paralysis
      352.6
    ophthalmoplegic migraine 346.2●

Moeller (-Barlow) disease (infantile
    scurvy) 267
  glossitis 529.4
Mohr's syndrome (types I and II) 759.89
Mola destruens (M9100/1) 236.1
Molarization, premolars 520.2
Molar pregnancy 631
  hydatidiform (delivered) (undelivered)
    630
Mold(s) in vitreous 117.9
Molding, head (during birth) - *omit code*
Mole (pigmented) (M8720/0) - *see also*
    Neoplasm, skin, benign
  blood 631
  Breus' 631
  cancerous (M8720/3) - *see* Melanoma
  carneous 631
  destructive (M9100/1) 236.1
  ectopic - *see* Pregnancy, ectopic
  fleshy 631
  hemorrhagic 631
  hydatid, hydatidiform (benign)
    (complicating pregnancy)
    (delivered) (undelivered) *(see also*
    Hydatidiform mole) 630
    invasive (M9100/1) 236.1
    malignant (M9100/1) 236.1
    previous, affecting management of
      pregnancy V23.1
  invasive (hydatidiform) (M9100/1)
    236.1
  malignant
    meaning
      malignant hydatidiform mole
        (9100/1) 236.1
      melanoma (M8720/3) - *see*
        Melanoma
  nonpigmented (M8730/0) - *see*
    Neoplasm, skin, benign
  pregnancy NEC 631
  skin (M8720/0) - *see* Neoplasm, skin,
    benign
  tubal - *see* Pregnancy, tubal
  vesicular *(see also* Hydatidiform mole)
    630
Molimen, molimina (menstrual) 625.4
Mollaret's meningitis 047.9
Mollities (cerebellar) (cerebral) 437.8
  ossium 268.2
Molluscum
  contagiosum 078.0
  epitheliale 078.0
  fibrosum (M8851/0) - *see* Lipoma, by
    site
  pendulum (M8851/0) - *see* Lipoma, by
    site
**Mönckeberg's arteriosclerosis,
    degeneration, disease, or sclerosis**
    (see also Arteriosclerosis, extremities)
    440.20
Monday fever 504
Monday morning dyspnea or asthma
    504
Mondini's malformation (cochlea) 744.05
Mondor's disease (thrombophlebitis of
    breast) 451.89
**Mongolian, mongolianism, mongolism,
    mongoloid** 758.0
  spot 757.33
Monilethrix (congenital) 757.4
Monilia infestation - *see* Candidiasis
Moniliasis - *see also* Candidiasis
  neonatal 771.7
  vulvovaginitis 112.1

Monkeypox 059.01
Monoarthritis 716.60
  ankle 716.67
  arm 716.62
    lower (and wrist) 716.63
    upper (and elbow) 716.62
  foot (and ankle) 716.67
  forearm (and wrist) 716.63
  hand 716.64
  leg 716.66
    lower 716.66
    upper 716.65
  pelvic region (hip) (thigh) 716.65
  shoulder (region) 716.61
  specified site NEC 716.68
Monoblastic - see condition
Monochromatism (cone) (rod)
    368.54
Monocytic - see condition
Monocytopenia 288.59
Monocytosis (symptomatic) 288.63
Monofixation syndrome 378.34
Monomania (see also Psychosis) 298.9
Mononeuritis 355.9
  cranial nerve - see Disorder, nerve,
    cranial
  femoral nerve 355.2
  lateral
    cutaneous nerve of thigh 355.1
    popliteal nerve 355.3
  lower limb 355.8
    specified nerve NEC 355.79
  medial popliteal nerve 355.4
  median nerve 354.1
  multiplex 354.5
  plantar nerve 355.6
  posterior tibial nerve 355.5
  radial nerve 354.3
  sciatic nerve 355.0
  ulnar nerve 354.2
  upper limb 354.9
    specified nerve NEC 354.8
  vestibular 388.5
Mononeuropathy (see also Mononeuritis)
    355.9
  diabetic NEC 250.6● [355.9]
    due to secondary diabetes 249.6●
      [355.9]
    lower limb 250.6● [355.8]
      due to secondary diabetes 249.6●
        [355.8]
    upper limb 250.6● [354.9]
      due to secondary diabetes 249.6●
        [354.9]
  iliohypogastric nerve 355.79
  ilioinguinal nerve 355.79
  obturator nerve 355.79
  saphenous nerve 355.79
Mononucleosis, infectious 075
  with hepatitis 075 [573.1]
Monoplegia 344.5
  brain (current episode) (see also
    Paralysis, brain) 437.8
    fetus or newborn 767.8
  cerebral (current episode) (see also
    Paralysis, brain) 437.8
  congenital or infantile (cerebral)
    (spastic) (spinal) 343.3
  embolic (current) (see also Embolism,
    brain) 434.1●
    late effect - see Late effect(s) (of)
      cerebrovascular disease
  infantile (cerebral) (spastic) (spinal)
    343.3

Monoplegia (Continued)
  lower limb 344.30
    affecting
      dominant side 344.31
      nondominant side 344.32
    due to late effect of cerebrovascular
      accident - see Late effect(s) (of)
        cerebrovascular accident
    newborn 767.8
    psychogenic 306.0
      specified as conversion reaction
        300.11
    thrombotic (current) (see also
      Thrombosis, brain) 434.0●
    late effect - see Late effect(s) (of)
      cerebrovascular disease
    transient 781.4
  upper limb 344.40
    affecting
      dominant side 344.41
      nondominant side 344.42
    due to late effect of cerebrovascular
      accident - see Late effect(s) (of)
        cerebrovascular accident
Monorchism, monorchidism 752.89
Monteggia's fracture (closed) 813.03
  open 813.13
Mood swings
  brief compensatory 296.99
  rebound 296.99
Moore's syndrome (see also Epilepsy)
    345.5●
Mooren's ulcer (cornea) 370.07
Mooser-Neill reaction 081.0
Mooser bodies 081.0
Moral
  deficiency 301.7
  imbecility 301.7
Morax-Axenfeld conjunctivitis 372.03
Morbilli (see also Measles) 055.9
Morbus
  anglicus, anglorum 268.0
  Beigel 111.2
  caducus (see also Epilepsy) 345.9●
  caeruleus 746.89
  celiacus 579.0
  comitialis (see also Epilepsy) 345.9●
  cordis - see also Disease, heart
    valvulorum - see Endocarditis
  coxae 719.95
    tuberculous (see also Tuberculosis)
      015.1●
  hemorrhagicus neonatorum 776.0
  maculosus neonatorum 772.6
  renum 593.0
  senilis (see also Osteoarthrosis) 715.9●
Morel-Kraepelin disease (see also
    Schizophrenia) 295.9●
Morel-Moore syndrome (hyperostosis
    frontalis interna) 733.3
Morel-Morgagni syndrome (hyperostosis
    frontalis interna) 733.3
Morgagni
  cyst, organ, hydatid, or appendage
    752.89
    fallopian tube 752.11
  disease or syndrome (hyperostosis
    frontalis interna) 733.3
Morgagni-Adams-Stokes syndrome
    (syncope with heart block) 426.9
Morgagni-Stewart-Morel syndrome
    (hyperostosis frontalis interna) 733.3
Moria (see also Psychosis) 298.9
Morning sickness 643.0●

Moron 317
Morphea (guttate) (linear) 701.0
Morphine dependence (see also
    Dependence) 304.0●
Morphinism (see also Dependence)
    304.0●
Morphinomania (see also Dependence)
    304.0●
Morphoea 701.0
Morquio (-Brailsford) (-Ullrich) disease or
    syndrome (mucopolysaccharidosis
    IV) 277.5
  kyphosis 277.5
Morris syndrome (testicular feminization)
    259.51
Morsus humanus (open wound) - see also
    Wound, open, by site
  skin surface intact - see Contusion
Mortification (dry) (moist) (see also
    Gangrene) 785.4
Morton's
  disease 355.6
  foot 355.6
  metatarsalgia (syndrome) 355.6
  neuralgia 355.6
  neuroma 355.6
  syndrome (metatarsalgia) (neuralgia)
    355.6
  toe 355.6
Morvan's disease 336.0
Mosaicism, mosaic (chromosomal) 758.9
  autosomal 758.5
  sex 758.81
Moschcowitz's syndrome (thrombotic
    thrombocytopenic purpura) 446.6
Mother yaw 102.0
Motion sickness (from travel, any
    vehicle) (from roundabouts or
    swings) 994.6
Mottled teeth (enamel) (endemic)
    (nonendemic) 520.3
Mottling enamel (endemic) (nonendemic)
    (teeth) 520.3
Mouchet's disease 732.5
Mould(s) (in vitreous) 117.9
Moulders'
  bronchitis 502
  tuberculosis (see also Tuberculosis)
    011.4●
Mounier-Kuhn syndrome 748.3
  with
    acute exacerbation 494.1
    bronchiectasis 494.0
      with (acute) exacerbation 494.1
  acquired 519.19
    with bronchiectasis 494.0
      with (acute) exacerbation 494.1
Mountain
  fever - see Fever, mountain
  sickness 993.2
    with polycythemia, acquired 289.0
    acute 289.0
  tick fever 066.1
Mouse, joint (see also Loose, body, joint)
    718.1●
  knee 717.6
Mouth - see condition
Movable
  coccyx 724.71
  kidney (see also Disease, renal) 593.0
    congenital 753.3
  organ or site, congenital NEC - see
    Malposition, congenital
  spleen 289.59

Movement
  abnormal (dystonic) (involuntary) 781.0
  decreased fetal 655.7●
  paradoxical facial 374.43
Moya Moya disease 437.5
Mozart's ear 744.29
MRSA (methicillin resistant staphylococcus aureus) 041.12
  colonization V02.54
  personal history of V12.04
MSSA (methicillin susceptible staphylococcus aureus) 041.11
  colonization V02.53
Mucha's disease (acute parapsoriasis varioliformis) 696.2
Mucha-Haberman syndrome (acute parapsoriasis varioliformis) 696.2
Mu-chain disease 273.2
Mucinosis (cutaneous) (papular) 701.8
Mucocele
  appendix 543.9
  buccal cavity 528.9
  gallbladder (see also Disease, gallbladder) 575.3
  lacrimal sac 375.43
  orbit (eye) 376.81
  salivary gland (any) 527.6
  sinus (accessory) (nasal) 478.19
  turbinate (bone) (middle) (nasal) 478.19
  uterus 621.8
Mucocutaneous lymph node syndrome (acute) (febrile) (infantile) 446.1
Mucoenteritis 564.9
Mucolipidosis I, II, III 272.7
Mucopolysaccharidosis (types 1–6) 277.5
  cardiopathy 277.5 [425.7]
Mucormycosis (lung) 117.7
Mucosa associated lymphoid tissue (MALT) 200.3●
Mucositis - see also Inflammation, by site 528.00
  cervix (ulcerative) 616.81
  due to
    antineoplastic therapy (ulcerative) 528.01
    other drugs (ulcerative) 528.02
    specified NEC 528.09
  gastrointestinal (ulcerative) 538
  nasal (ulcerative) 478.11
  necroticans agranulocytica (see also Agranulocytosis) 288.09
  ulcerative 528.00
  vagina (ulcerative) 616.81
  vulva (ulcerative) 616.81
Mucous - see also condition
  patches (syphilitic) 091.3
    congenital 090.0
Mucoviscidosis 277.00
  with meconium obstruction 277.01
Mucus
  asphyxia or suffocation (see also Asphyxia, mucus) 933.1
    newborn 770.18
  in stool 792.1
  plug (see also Asphyxia, mucus) 933.1
    aspiration, of newborn 770.17
    tracheobronchial 519.19
      newborn 770.18
Muguet 112.0
Mulberry molars 090.5
Müllerian mixed tumor (M8950/3) - see Neoplasm, by site, malignant

Multicystic kidney 753.19
Multilobed placenta - see Placenta, abnormal
Multinodular prostate 600.10
  with
    urinary
      obstruction 600.11
      retention 600.11
Multiparity V61.5
  affecting
    fetus or newborn 763.89
    management of
      labor and delivery 659.4●
      pregnancy V23.3
  requiring contraceptive management (see also Contraception) V25.9
Multipartita placenta - see Placenta, abnormal
Multiple, multiplex - see also condition
  birth
    affecting fetus or newborn 761.5
    healthy liveborn - see Newborn, multiple
  digits (congenital) 755.00
    fingers 755.01
    toes 755.02
  organ or site NEC - see Accessory
  personality 300.14
  renal arteries 747.62
Mumps 072.9
  with complication 072.8
    specified type NEC 072.79
  encephalitis 072.2
  hepatitis 072.71
  meningitis (aseptic) 072.1
  meningoencephalitis 072.2
  oophoritis 072.79
  orchitis 072.0
  pancreatitis 072.3
  polyneuropathy 072.72
  vaccination, prophylactic (against) V04.6
Mumu (see also Infestation, filarial) 125.9
Münchausen syndrome 301.51
Münchmeyer's disease or syndrome (exostosis luxurians) 728.11
Mural - see condition
Murmur (cardiac) (heart) (nonorganic) (organic) 785.2
  abdominal 787.5
  aortic (valve) (see also Endocarditis, aortic) 424.1
  benign - omit code
  cardiorespiratory 785.2
  diastolic - see condition
  Flint (see also Endocarditis, aortic) 424.1
  functional - omit code
  Graham Steell (pulmonic regurgitation) (see also Endocarditis, pulmonary) 424.3
  innocent - omit code
  insignificant - omit code
  midsystolic 785.2
  mitral (valve) - see Stenosis
  physiologic - see condition
  presystolic, mitral - see Insufficiency, mitral
  pulmonic (valve) (see also Endocarditis, pulmonary) 424.3
  Still's (vibratory) - omit code
  systolic (valvular) - see condition
  tricuspid (valve) - see Endocarditis, tricuspid

Murmur (Continued)
  undiagnosed 785.2
  valvular - see condition
  vibratory - omit code
Murri's disease (intermittent hemoglobinuria) 283.2
Muscae volitantes 379.24
Muscle, muscular - see condition
Musculoneuralgia 729.1
Mushrooming hip 718.95
Mushroom workers' (pickers') lung 495.5
Mutation
  factor V leiden 289.81
  prothrombin gene 289.81
Mutism (see also Aphasia) 784.3
  akinetic 784.3
  deaf (acquired) (congenital) 389.7
  hysterical 300.11
  selective (elective) 313.23
    adjustment reaction 309.83
Myà's disease (congenital dilation, colon) 751.3
Myalgia (intercostal) 729.1
  eosinophilia syndrome 710.5
  epidemic 074.1
    cervical 078.89
  psychogenic 307.89
  traumatic NEC 959.9
Myasthenia 358.00
  cordis - see Failure, heart
  gravis 358.00
    with exacerbation (acute) 358.01
    in crisis 358.01
    neonatal 775.2
    pseudoparalytica 358.00
  stomach 536.8
    psychogenic 306.4
  syndrome
    in
      botulism 005.1 [358.1]
      diabetes mellitus 250.6● [358.1]
        due to secondary diabetes 249.6● [358.1]
      hypothyroidism (see also Hypothyroidism) 244.9 [358.1]
      malignant neoplasm NEC 199.1 [358.1]
      pernicious anemia 281.0 [358.1]
      thyrotoxicosis (see also Thyrotoxicosis) 242.9● [358.1]
Myasthenic 728.87
Mycelium infection NEC 117.9
Mycetismus 988.1
Mycetoma (actinomycotic) 039.9
  bone 039.8
    mycotic 117.4
  foot 039.4
    mycotic 117.4
  madurae 039.9
    mycotic 117.4
  maduromycotic 039.9
    mycotic 117.4
  mycotic 117.4
  nocardial 039.9
Mycobacteriosis - see Mycobacterium
Mycobacterium, mycobacterial (infection) 031.9
  acid-fast (bacilli) 031.9
  anonymous (see also Mycobacterium, atypical) 031.9

◀ New   ◀█ Revised   ~~deleted~~ Deleted   ● Use Additional Digit(s)   ▒ Omit code

Mycobacterium, mycobacterial
  (Continued)
  atypical (acid-fast bacilli) 031.9
    cutaneous 031.1
    pulmonary 031.0
      tuberculous (*see also* Tuberculosis,
        pulmonary) 011.9●
    specified site NEC 031.8
  avium 031.0
    intracellulare complex bacteremia
      (MAC) 031.2
  balnei 031.1
  Battey 031.0
  cutaneous 031.1
  disseminated 031.2
    avium-intracellulare complex
      (DMAC) 031.2
  fortuitum 031.0
  intracellulare (battey bacillus) 031.0
  kakerifu 031.8
  kansasii 031.0
  kasongo 031.8
  leprae - *see* Leprosy
  luciflavum 031.0
  marinum 031.1
  pulmonary 031.0
    tuberculous (*see also* Tuberculosis,
      pulmonary) 011.9●
  scrofulaceum 031.1
  tuberculosis (human, bovine) - *see also*
    Tuberculosis
    avian type 031.0
  ulcerans 031.1
  xenopi 031.0
Mycosis, mycotic 117.9
  cutaneous NEC 111.9
  ear 111.8 *[380.15]*
  fungoides (M9700/3) 202.1●
  mouth 112.0
  pharynx 117.9
  skin NEC 111.9
  stomatitis 112.0
  systemic NEC 117.9
  tonsil 117.9
  vagina, vaginitis 112.1
Mydriasis (persistent) (pupil)
  379.43
Myelatelia 742.59
Myelinoclasis, perivascular, acute
  (postinfectious) NEC 136.9
  [323.61]
  postimmunization or postvaccinal
    323.51
Myelinosis, central pontine 341.8
Myelitis (ascending) (cerebellar)
  (childhood) (chronic) (descending)
  (diffuse) (disseminated) (pressure)
  (progressive) (spinal cord)
  (subacute) (*see also* Encephalitis)
  323.9
  acute (transverse) 341.20
    idiopathic 341.22
    in conditions classified elsewhere
      341.21
  due to
    infection classified elsewhere 136.9
      [323.42]
    specified cause NEC 323.82
    vaccination (any) 323.52
    viral diseases classified elsewhere
      323.02
  herpes simplex 054.74
  herpes zoster 053.14
  late effect - *see* category 326

Myelitis *(Continued)*
  optic neuritis in 341.0
  postchickenpox 052.2
  postimmunization 323.52
  postinfectious 136.9 *[323.63]*
  postvaccinal 323.52
  postvaricella 052.2
  syphilitic (transverse) 094.89
  toxic 989.9 *[323.72]*
  transverse 323.82
    acute 341.20
      idiopathic 341.22
      in conditions classified elsewhere
        341.21
    idiopathic 341.22
  tuberculous (*see also* Tuberculosis)
    013.6●
  virus 049.9
Myeloblastic - *see* condition
Myelocele (*see also* Spina bifida) 741.9●
  with hydrocephalus 741.0●
Myelocystocele (*see also* Spina bifida)
  741.9●
Myelocytic - *see* condition
Myelocytoma 205.1●
Myelodysplasia (spinal cord) 742.59
  meaning myelodysplastic syndrome -
    see Syndrome, myelodysplastic
Myeloencephalitis - *see* Encephalitis
Myelofibrosis 289.83
  with myeloid metaplasia 238.76
  idiopathic (chronic) 238.76
  megakaryocytic 238.79
  primary 238.76
  secondary 289.83
Myelogenous - *see* condition
Myeloid - *see* condition
Myelokathexis 288.09
Myeloleukodystrophy 330.0
Myelolipoma (M8870/0) - *see* Neoplasm,
  by site, benign
Myeloma (multiple) (plasma cell)
  (plasmacytic) (M9730/3) 203.0●
  monostotic (M9731/1) 238.6
  solitary (M9731/1) 238.6
Myelomalacia 336.8
Myelomata, multiple (M9730/3) 203.0●
Myelomatosis (M9730/3) 203.0●
Myelomeningitis - *see*
  Meningoencephalitis
Myelomeningocele (spinal cord) (*see also*
  Spina bifida) 741.9●
  fetal, causing fetopelvic disproportion
    653.7●
Myelo-osteo-musculodysplasia
  hereditaria 756.89
Myelopathic - *see* condition
Myelopathy (spinal cord) 336.9
  cervical 721.1
  diabetic 250.6● *[336.3]*
    due to secondary diabetes 249.6●
      [336.3]
  drug-induced 336.8
  due to or with
    carbon tetrachloride 987.8
      [323.72]
    degeneration or displacement,
      intervertebral disc 722.70
      cervical, cervicothoracic 722.71
      lumbar, lumbosacral 722.73
      thoracic, thoracolumbar 722.72
    hydroxyquinoline derivatives 961.3
      [323.72]
    infection - *see* Encephalitis

Myelopathy *(Continued)*
  due to or with *(Continued)*
    intervertebral disc disorder
      722.70
      cervical, cervicothoracic
        722.71
      lumbar, lumbosacral 722.73
      thoracic, thoracolumbar
        722.72
    lead 984.9 *[323.72]*
    mercury 985.0 *[323.72]*
    neoplastic disease (*see also*
      Neoplasm, by site) 239.9
      [336.3]
    pernicious anemia 281.0 *[336.3]*
    spondylosis 721.91
      cervical 721.1
      lumbar, lumbosacral 721.42
      thoracic 721.41
    thallium 985.8 *[323.72]*
  lumbar, lumbosacral 721.42
  necrotic (subacute) 336.1
  radiation-induced 336.8
  spondylogenic NEC 721.91
    cervical 721.1
    lumbar, lumbosacral 721.42
    thoracic 721.41
  thoracic 721.41
  toxic NEC 989.9 *[323.72]*
  transverse (*see also* Myelitis) 323.82
  vascular 336.1
Myelophthisis 284.2
Myeloproliferative disease (M9960/1)
  238.79
Myeloradiculitis (*see also*
  Polyneuropathy) 357.0
Myeloradiculodysplasia (spinal)
  742.59
Myelosarcoma (M9930/3) 205.3●
Myelosclerosis 289.89
  with myeloid metaplasia (M9961/1)
    238.76
  disseminated, of nervous system
    340
  megakaryocytic (M9961/1) 238.79
Myelosis (M9860/3) (*see also* Leukemia,
  myeloid) 205.9●
  acute (M9861/3) 205.0●
  aleukemic (M9864/3) 205.8●
  chronic (M9863/3) 205.1●
  erythremic (M9840/3) 207.0●
    acute (M9841/3) 207.0●
  megakaryocytic (M9920/3) 207.2●
  nonleukemic (chronic) 288.8
  subacute (M9862/3) 205.2●
Myesthenia - *see* Myasthenia
Myiasis (cavernous) 134.0
  orbit 134.0 *[376.13]*
Myoadenoma, prostate 600.20
  with
    other lower urinary tract symptoms
      (LUTS) 600.21
    urinary
      obstruction 600.21
      retention 600.21
Myoblastoma
  granular cell (M9580/0) - *see also*
    Neoplasm, connective tissue,
    benign
    malignant (M9580/3) - *see*
      Neoplasm, connective tissue,
      malignant
  tongue (M9580/0) 210.1
Myocardial - *see* condition

Myocardiopathy (congestive)
    (constrictive) (familial)
    (hypertrophic nonobstructive)
    (idiopathic) (infiltrative)
    (obstructive) (primary) (restrictive)
    (sporadic) 425.4
  alcoholic 425.5
  amyloid 277.39 [425.7]
  beriberi 265.0 [425.7]
  cobalt-beer 425.5
  due to
    amyloidosis 277.39 [425.7]
    beriberi 265.0 [425.7]
    cardiac glycogenosis 271.0 [425.7]
    Chagas' disease 086.0
    Friedreich's ataxia 334.0 [425.8]
    influenza 487.8 [425.8]
    mucopolysaccharidosis 277.5 [425.7]
    myotonia atrophica 359.21 [425.8]
    progressive muscular dystrophy
      359.1 [425.8]
    sarcoidosis 135 [425.8]
  glycogen storage 271.0 [425.7]
  hypertrophic obstructive 425.1
  metabolic NEC 277.9 [425.7]
  nutritional 269.9 [425.7]
  obscure (African) 425.2
  peripartum 674.5●
  postpartum 674.5●
  secondary 425.9
  thyrotoxic (see also Thyrotoxicosis)
    242.9 ● [425.7]
  toxic NEC 425.9
Myocarditis (fibroid) (interstitial) (old)
  (progressive) (senile) (with
  arteriosclerosis) 429.0
  with
    rheumatic fever (conditions
      classifiable to 390) 398.0
      active (see also Myocarditis, acute,
        rheumatic) 391.2
      inactive or quiescent (with
        chorea) 398.0
  active (nonrheumatic) 422.90
    rheumatic 391.2
      with chorea (acute) (rheumatic)
        (Sydenham's) 392.0
  acute or subacute (interstitial) 422.90
    due to Streptococcus (beta-
      hemolytic) 391.2
    idiopathic 422.91
    rheumatic 391.2
      with chorea (acute) (rheumatic)
        (Sydenham's) 392.0
    specified type NEC 422.99
  aseptic of newborn 074.23
  bacterial (acute) 422.92
  chagasic 086.0
  chronic (interstitial) 429.0
  congenital 746.89
  constrictive 425.4
  Coxsackie (virus) 074.23
  diphtheritic 032.82
  due to or in
    Coxsackie (virus) 074.23
    diphtheria 032.82
    epidemic louse-borne typhus 080
      [422.0]
    influenza 487.8 [422.0]
    Lyme disease 088.81 [422.0]
    scarlet fever 034.1 [422.0]
    toxoplasmosis (acquired) 130.3
    tuberculosis (see also Tuberculosis)
      017.9● [422.0]

Myocarditis (Continued)
  due to or in (Continued)
    typhoid 002.0 [422.0]
    typhus NEC 081.9 [422.0]
  eosinophilic 422.91
  epidemic of newborn 074.23
  Fiedler's (acute) (isolated) (subacute)
    422.91
  giant cell (acute) (subacute) 422.91
  gonococcal 098.85
  granulomatous (idiopathic) (isolated)
    (nonspecific) 422.91
  hypertensive (see also Hypertension,
    heart) 402.90
  idiopathic 422.91
    granulomatous 422.91
  infective 422.92
  influenzal 487.8 [422.0]
  isolated (diffuse) (granulomatous)
    422.91
  malignant 422.99
  meningococcal 036.43
  nonrheumatic, active 422.90
  parenchymatous 422.90
  pneumococcal (acute) (subacute) 422.92
  rheumatic (chronic) (inactive) (with
    chorea) 398.0
    active or acute 391.2
      with chorea (acute) (rheumatic)
        (Sydenham's) 392.0
  septic 422.92
  specific (giant cell) (productive)
    422.91
  staphylococcal (acute) (subacute)
    422.92
  suppurative 422.92
  syphilitic (chronic) 093.82
  toxic 422.93
    rheumatic (see also Myocarditis,
      acute rheumatic) 391.2
  tuberculous (see also Tuberculosis)
    017.9● [422.0]
  typhoid 002.0 [422.0]
  valvular - see Endocarditis
  viral, except Coxsackie 422.91
    Coxsackie 074.23
    of newborn (Coxsackie) 074.23
Myocardium, myocardial - see condition
Myocardosis (see also Cardiomyopathy)
  425.4
Myoclonia (essential) 333.2
  epileptica 345.1 ◀▥
  Friedrich's 333.2
  massive 333.2
Myoclonic
  epilepsy, familial (progressive) 345.1 ◀▥
  jerks 333.2
Myoclonus (familial essential)
  (multifocal) (simplex) 333.2
  with epilepsy and with ragged red
    fibers (MERRF syndrome)
    277.87
  facial 351.8
  massive (infantile) 333.2
  palatal 333.2 ◀
  pharyngeal 333.2 ◀▥
Myocytolysis 429.1 ◀
Myodiastasis 728.84
Myoendocarditis - see also Endocarditis
  acute or subacute 421.9
Myoepithelioma (M8982/0) - see
  Neoplasm, by site, benign
Myofascitis (acute) 729.1
  low back 724.2

Myofibroma (M8890/0) - see also
  Neoplasm, connective tissue, benign
  uterus (cervix) (corpus) (see also
    Leiomyoma) 218.9
Myofibromatosis
  infantile 759.89
Myofibrosis 728.2
  heart (see also Myocarditis) 429.0
  humeroscapular region 726.2
  scapulohumeral 726.2
Myofibrositis (see also Myositis) 729.1
  scapulohumeral 726.2
Myogelosis (occupational) 728.89
Myoglobinuria 791.3
Myoglobulinuria, primary 791.3
Myokymia - see also Myoclonus
  facial 351.8
Myolipoma (M8860/0)
  specified site - see Neoplasm,
    connective tissue, benign
  unspecified site 223.0
Myoma (M8895/0) - see also Neoplasm,
  connective tissue, benign
  cervix (stump) (uterus) (see also
    Leiomyoma) 218.9
  malignant (M8895/3) - see Neoplasm,
    connective tissue, malignant
  prostate 600.20
    with
      other lower urinary tract
        symptoms (LUTS) 600.21
      urinary
        obstruction 600.21
        retention 600.21
  uterus (cervix) (corpus) (see also
    Leiomyoma) 218.9
    in pregnancy or childbirth 654.1●
      affecting fetus or newborn 763.89
      causing obstructed labor 660.2●
        affecting fetus or newborn
          763.1
Myomalacia 728.9
  cordis, heart (see also Degeneration,
    myocardial) 429.1
Myometritis (see also Endometritis)
  615.9
Myometrium - see condition
Myonecrosis, clostridial 040.0
Myopathy 359.9
  alcoholic 359.4
  amyloid 277.39 [359.6]
  benign, congenital 359.0
  central core 359.0
  centronuclear 359.0
  congenital (benign) 359.0
  critical illness 359.81
  distal 359.1
  due to drugs 359.4
  endocrine 259.9 [359.5]
    specified type NEC 259.8 [359.5]
  extraocular muscles 376.82
  facioscapulohumeral 359.1
  in
    Addison's disease 255.41 [359.5]
    amyloidosis 277.39 [359.6]
    cretinism 243 [359.5]
    Cushing's syndrome 255.0 [359.5]
    disseminated lupus erythematosus
      710.0 [359.6]
    giant cell arteritis 446.5 [359.6]
    hyperadrenocorticism NEC 255.3
      [359.5]
    hyperparathyroidism 252.01 [359.5]
    hypopituitarism 253.2 [359.5]

◀ New   ◀▥ Revised   ~~deleted~~ Deleted   ● Use Additional Digit(s)   ▨ Omit code

Myopathy *(Continued)*
  in *(Continued)*
    hypothyroidism *(see also*
      Hypothyroidism) 244.9 *[359.5]*
    malignant neoplasm NEC
      (M8000/3) 199.1 *[359.6]*
    myxedema *(see also* Myxedema)
      244.9 *[359.5]*
    polyarteritis nodosa 446.0 *[359.6]*
    rheumatoid arthritis 714.0 *[359.6]*
    sarcoidosis 135 *[359.6]*
    scleroderma 710.1 *[359.6]*
    Sjögren's disease 710.2 *[359.6]*
    thyrotoxicosis *(see also*
      Thyrotoxicosis) 242.9● *[359.5]*
  inflammatory 359.79 ◀▥
    immune NEC 359.79 ◀
    specified NEC 359.79 ◀
  intensive care (ICU) 359.81
  limb-girdle 359.1
  myotubular 359.0
  necrotizing, acute 359.81
  nemaline 359.0
  ocular 359.1
  oculopharyngeal 359.1
  of critical illness 359.81
  primary 359.89
  progressive NEC 359.89
  proximal myotonic (PROMM) 359.21
  quadriplegic, acute 359.81
  rod body 359.0
  scapulohumeral 359.1
  specified type NEC 359.89
  toxic 359.4
Myopericarditis *(see also* Pericarditis)
  423.9
Myopia (axial) (congenital) (increased
  curvature or refraction, nucleus of
  lens) 367.1
  degenerative, malignant 360.21
  malignant 360.21
  progressive high (degenerative) 360.21
Myosarcoma (M8895/3) - *see* Neoplasm,
  connective tissue, malignant

Myosis (persistent) 379.42
  stromal (endolymphatic) (M8931/1)
    236.0
Myositis 729.1
  clostridial 040.0
  due to posture 729.1
  epidemic 074.1
  fibrosa or fibrous (chronic) 728.2
    Volkmann's (complicating trauma)
      958.6
  inclusion body (IBM) 359.71   ◀
  infective 728.0
  interstitial 728.81
  multiple - *see* Polymyositis
  occupational 729.1
  orbital, chronic 376.12
  ossificans 728.12
    circumscribed 728.12
    progressive 728.11
    traumatic 728.12
  progressive fibrosing 728.11
  purulent 728.0
  rheumatic 729.1
  rheumatoid 729.1
  suppurative 728.0
  syphilitic 095.6
  traumatic (old) 729.1
Myospasia impulsiva 307.23
Myotonia (acquisita) (intermittens) 728.85
  atrophica 359.21
  congenita 359.22
    acetazolamide responsive 359.22
    dominant form 359.22
    recessive form 359.22
  drug-induced 359.24
  dystrophica 359.21
  fluctuans 359.29
  levior 359.22   ◀▥
  permanens 359.29
Myotonic pupil 379.46
Myriapodiasis 134.1
Myringitis
  with otitis media - *see* Otitis media
  acute 384.00
    specified type NEC 384.09

Myringitis *(Continued)*
  bullosa hemorrhagica 384.01
  bullous 384.01
  chronic 384.1
Mysophobia 300.29
Mytilotoxism 988.0
Myxadenitis labialis 528.5
Myxedema (adult) (idiocy) (infantile)
  (juvenile) (thyroid gland) *(see also*
  Hypothyroidism) 244.9
  circumscribed 242.9●
  congenital 243
  cutis 701.8
  localized (pretibial) 242.9●
  madness (acute) 293.0
    subacute 293.1
  papular 701.8
  pituitary 244.8
  postpartum 674.8●
  pretibial 242.9●
  primary 244.9
Myxochondrosarcoma (M9220/3) -
  see Neoplasm, cartilage,
  malignant
Myxofibroma (M8811/0) - *see also*
  Neoplasm, connective tissue,
  benign
  odontogenic (M9320/0) 213.1
  upper jaw (bone) 213.0
Myxofibrosarcoma (M8811/3) - *see*
  Neoplasm, connective tissue,
  malignant
Myxolipoma (M8852/0) *(see also* Lipoma,
  by site) 214.9
Myxoliposarcoma (M8852/3) - *see*
  Neoplasm, connective tissue,
  malignant
Myxoma (M8840/0) - *see also* Neoplasm,
  connective tissue, benign
  odontogenic (M9320/0) 213.1
  upper jaw (bone) 213.0
Myxosarcoma (M8840/3) - *see* Neoplasm,
  connective tissue, malignant

N

Naegeli's
  disease (hereditary hemorrhagic thrombasthenia) 287.1
  leukemia, monocytic (M9863/3) 205.1●
  syndrome (incontinentia pigmenti) 757.33
Naffziger's syndrome 353.0
Naga sore (*see* also Ulcer, skin) 707.9
Nägele's pelvis 738.6
  with disproportion (fetopelvic) 653.0●
    affecting fetus or newborn 763.1
    causing obstructed labor 660.1●
      affecting fetus or newborn 763.1
Nager-de Reynier syndrome (dysostosis mandibularis) 756.0
Nail - *see* also condition
  biting 307.9
  patella syndrome (hereditary osteoonychodysplasia) 756.89
Nanism, nanosomia (*see* also Dwarfism) 259.4
  hypophyseal 253.3
  pituitary 253.3
  renis, renalis 588.0
Nanukayami 100.89
Napkin rash 691.0
Narcissism 301.81
Narcolepsy 347.00
  with cataplexy 347.01
  in conditions classified elsewhere 347.10
    with cataplexy 347.11
Narcosis
  carbon dioxide (respiratory) 786.09
  due to drug
    correct substance properly administered 780.09
    overdose or wrong substance given or taken 977.9
    specified drug - *see* Table of Drugs and Chemicals
Narcotism (chronic) (*see* also Dependence) 304.9●
  acute
    correct substance properly administered 349.82
    overdose or wrong substance given or taken 967.8
    specified drug - *see* Table of Drugs and Chemicals
NARP (ataxia and retinitis pigmentosa syndrome) 277.87
Narrow
  anterior chamber angle 365.02
  pelvis (inlet) (outlet) - *see* Contraction, pelvis
Narrowing
  artery NEC 447.1
    auditory, internal 433.8●
    basilar 433.0●
      with other precerebral artery 433.3●
        bilateral 433.3●
    carotid 433.1●
      with other precerebral artery 433.3●
        bilateral 433.3●
    cerebellar 433.8●
    choroidal 433.8●
    communicating posterior 433.8●

Narrowing *(Continued)*
  artery NEC *(Continued)*
    coronary - *see* also Arteriosclerosis, coronary
      congenital 746.85
        due to syphilis 090.5
    hypophyseal 433.8●
    pontine 433.8●
    precerebral NEC 433.9●
      multiple or bilateral 433.3●
      specified NEC 433.8●
    vertebral 433.2●
      with other precerebral artery 433.3●
      bilateral 433.3●
  auditory canal (external) (*see* also Stricture, ear canal, acquired) 380.50
  cerebral arteries 437.0
  cicatricial - *see* Cicatrix
  congenital - *see* Anomaly, congenital
  coronary artery - *see* Narrowing, artery, coronary
  ear, middle 385.22
  Eustachian tube (*see* also Obstruction, Eustachian tube) 381.60
  eyelid 374.46
    congenital 743.62
  intervertebral disc or space NEC - *see* Degeneration, intervertebral disc
  joint space, hip 719.85
  larynx 478.74
  lids 374.46
    congenital 743.62
  mesenteric artery (with gangrene) 557.0
  palate 524.89
  palpebral fissure 374.46
  retinal artery 362.13
  ureter 593.3
  urethra (*see* also Stricture, urethra) 598.9
Narrowness, abnormal, eyelid 743.62
Nasal - *see* condition
Nasolacrimal - *see* condition
Nasopharyngeal - *see* also condition
  bursa 478.29
  pituitary gland 759.2
  torticollis 723.5
Nasopharyngitis (acute) (infective) (subacute) 460
  chronic 472.2
    due to external agent - *see* Condition, respiratory, chronic, due to
  due to external agent - *see* Condition, respiratory, due to
  septic 034.0
  streptococcal 034.0
  suppurative (chronic) 472.2
  ulcerative (chronic) 472.2
Nasopharynx, nasopharyngeal - *see* condition
Natal tooth, teeth 520.6
Nausea (*see* also Vomiting) 787.02
  with vomiting 787.01
  epidemic 078.82
  gravidarum - *see* Hyperemesis, gravidarum
  marina 994.6
Naval - *see* condition
Neapolitan fever (*see* also Brucellosis) 023.9
Near drowning 994.1
Nearsightedness 367.1
Near-syncope 780.2

Nebécourt's syndrome 253.3
Nebula, cornea (eye) 371.01
  congenital 743.43
    interfering with vision 743.42
Necator americanus infestation 126.1
Necatoriasis 126.1
Neck - *see* condition
Necrencephalus (*see* also Softening, brain) 437.8
Necrobacillosis 040.3
Necrobiosis 799.89
  brain or cerebral (*see* also Softening, brain) 437.8
  lipoidica 709.3
    diabeticorum 250.8● [709.3]
      due to secondary diabetes 249.8● [709.3]
Necrodermolysis 695.15
Necrolysis, toxic epidermal 695.15
  due to drug
    correct substance properly administered 695.15
    overdose or wrong substance given or taken 977.9
    specified drug - *see* Table of Drugs and Chemicals
  Stevens-Johnson syndrome overlap (SJS-TEN overlap syndrome) 695.14
Necrophilia 302.89
Necrosis, necrotic
  adrenal (capsule) (gland) 255.8
  antrum, nasal sinus 478.19
  aorta (hyaline) (*see* also Aneurysm, aorta) 441.9
    cystic medial 441.00
      abdominal 441.02
      thoracic 441.01
      thoracoabdominal 441.03
    ruptured 441.5
  arteritis 446.0
  artery 447.5
  aseptic, bone 733.40
    femur (head) (neck) 733.42
      medial condyle 733.43
    humoral head 733.41
    jaw 733.45
    medial femoral condyle 733.43
    specific site NEC 733.49
    talus 733.44
  avascular, bone NEC (*see* also Necrosis, aseptic, bone) 733.40
  bladder (aseptic) (sphincter) 596.8
  bone (*see* also Osteomyelitis) 730.1●
    acute 730.0●
    aseptic or avascular 733.40
      femur (head) (neck) 733.42
        medial condyle 733.43
      humoral head 733.41
      jaw 733.45
      medial femoral condyle 733.43
      specified site NEC 733.49
      talus 733.44
    ethmoid 478.19
    ischemic 733.40
    jaw 526.4
      aseptic 733.45
    marrow 289.89
    Paget's (osteitis deformans) 731.0
    tuberculous - *see* Tuberculosis, bone
  brain (softening) (*see* also Softening, brain) 437.8
  breast (aseptic) (fat) (segmental) 611.3

◀ New   ◀▥ Revised   ~~deleted~~ Deleted   ● Use Additional Digit(s)   ▨ Omit code

Necrosis, necrotic (Continued)
bronchus, bronchi 519.19
central nervous system NEC (see also
Softening, brain) 437.8
cerebellar (see also Softening, brain) 437.8
cerebral (softening) (see also Softening,
brain) 437.8
cerebrospinal (softening) (see also
Softening, brain) 437.8
colon 557.0
cornea (see also Keratitis) 371.40
cortical, kidney 583.6
cystic medial (aorta) 441.00
abdominal 441.02
thoracic 441.01
thoracoabdominal 441.03
dental 521.09
pulp 522.1
due to swallowing corrosive
substance - see Burn, by site
ear (ossicle) 385.24
esophagus 530.89
ethmoid (bone) 478.19
eyelid 374.50
fat, fatty (generalized) (see also
Degeneration, fatty) 272.8
abdominal wall 567.82
breast (aseptic) (segmental) 611.3
intestine 569.89
localized - see Degeneration, by site,
fatty
mesentery 567.82
omentum 567.82
pancreas 577.8
peritoneum 567.82
skin (subcutaneous) 709.3
newborn 778.1
femur (aseptic) (avascular) 733.42
head 733.42
medial condyle 733.43
neck 733.42
gallbladder (see also Cholecystitis,
acute) 575.0
gangrenous 785.4
gastric 537.89
glottis 478.79
heart (myocardium) - see Infarct,
myocardium
hepatic (see also Necrosis, liver) 570
hip (aseptic) (avascular) 733.42
intestine (acute) (hemorrhagic)
(massive) 557.0
ischemic 785.4
jaw 526.4
aseptic 733.45
kidney (bilateral) 583.9
acute 584.9
cortical 583.6
acute 584.6
with
abortion - see Abortion, by
type, with renal
failure
ectopic pregnancy (see also
categories 633.0–633.9)
639.3
molar pregnancy (see also
categories 630–632)
639.3
complicating pregnancy 646.2●
affecting fetus or newborn
760.1
following labor and delivery
669.3●

Necrosis, necrotic (Continued)
kidney (Continued)
medullary (papillary) (see also
Pyelitis) 590.80
in
acute renal failure 584.7
nephritis, nephropathy 583.7
papillary (see also Pyelitis) 590.80
in
acute renal failure 584.7
nephritis, nephropathy 583.7
tubular 584.5
with
abortion - see Abortion, by
type, with renal failure
ectopic pregnancy (see also
categories 633.0–633.9)
639.3
molar pregnancy (see also
categories 630–632)
639.3
complicating
abortion 639.3
ectopic or molar pregnancy
639.3
pregnancy 646.2●
affecting fetus or newborn
760.1
following labor and delivery
669.3●
traumatic 958.5
larynx 478.79
liver (acute) (congenital) (diffuse)
(massive) (subacute) 570
with
abortion - see Abortion, by type,
with specified complication
NEC
ectopic pregnancy (see also
categories 633.0–633.9)
639.8
molar pregnancy (see also
categories 630–632) 639.8
complicating pregnancy 646.7●
affecting fetus or newborn
760.8
following
abortion 639.8
ectopic or molar pregnancy
639.8
obstetrical 646.7●
postabortal 639.8
puerperal, postpartum 674.8●
toxic 573.3
lung 513.0
lymphatic gland 683
mammary gland 611.3
mastoid (chronic) 383.1
mesentery 557.0
fat 567.82
mitral valve - see Insufficiency, mitral
myocardium, myocardial - see Infarct,
myocardium
nose (septum) 478.19
omentum 557.0
with mesenteric infarction 557.0
fat 567.82
orbit, orbital 376.10
ossicles, ear (aseptic) 385.24
ovary (see also Salpingo-oophoritis)
614.2
pancreas (aseptic) (duct) (fat) 577.8
acute 577.0
infective 577.0

Necrosis, necrotic (Continued)
papillary, kidney (see also Pyelitis)
590.80
perineum 624.8
peritoneum 557.0
with mesenteric infarction 557.0
fat 567.82
pharynx 462
in granulocytopenia 288.09
phosphorus 983.9
pituitary (gland) (postpartum)
(Sheehan) 253.2
placenta (see also Placenta, abnormal)
656.7●
pneumonia 513.0
pulmonary 513.0
pulp (dental) 522.1
pylorus 537.89
radiation - see Necrosis, by site
radium - see Necrosis, by site
renal - see Necrosis, kidney
sclera 379.19
scrotum 608.89
skin or subcutaneous tissue 709.8
due to burn - see Burn, by site
gangrenous 785.4
spine, spinal (column) 730.18
acute 730.18
cord 336.1
spleen 289.59
stomach 537.89
stomatitis 528.1
subcutaneous fat 709.3
fetus or newborn 778.1
subendocardial - see Infarct, myocardium
suprarenal (capsule) (gland) 255.8
teeth, tooth 521.09
testis 608.89
thymus (gland) 254.8
tonsil 474.8
trachea 519.19
tuberculous NEC - see Tuberculosis
tubular (acute) (anoxic) (toxic) 584.5
due to a procedure 997.5
umbilical cord, affecting fetus or
newborn 762.6
vagina 623.8
vertebra (lumbar) 730.18
acute 730.18
tuberculous (see also Tuberculosis)
015.0● [730.8]
vesical (aseptic) (bladder) 596.8
vulva 624.8
x-ray - see Necrosis, by site
Necrospermia 606.0
Necrotizing angiitis 446.0
Negativism 301.7
Neglect (child) (newborn) NEC 995.52
adult 995.84
after or at birth 995.52
hemispatial 781.8
left-sided 781.8
sensory 781.8
visuospatial 781.8
Negri bodies 071
Neill-Dingwall syndrome
(microcephaly and dwarfism)
759.89
Neisserian infection NEC - see
Gonococcus
Nematodiasis NEC (see also Infestation,
Nematode) 127.9
ancylostoma (see also Ancylostomiasis)
126.9

Neoformans cryptococcus infection
117.5
Neonatal - *see also* condition
abstinence syndrome 779.5 ◄
adrenoleukodystrophy
277.86
teeth, tooth 520.6
Neonatorum - *see* condition
Neoplasia
anal intraepithelial I [AIN I]
(histologically confirmed)
569.44

Neoplasia (*Continued*)
anal intraepithelial II [AIN II]
(histologically confirmed)
569.44
anal intraepithelial III [AIN III] 230.6
anal canal 230.5
endometrial intraepithelial
[EIN] 621.35 ◄
multiple endocrine [MEN]
type I 258.01
type IIA 258.02
type IIB 258.03

Neoplasia (*Continued*)
vaginal intraepithelial I [VAIN I]
623.0
vaginal intraepithelial II [VAIN II]
623.0
vaginal intraepithelial III [VAIN III]
233.31
vulvar intraepithelial I [VIN I] 624.01
vulvar intraepithelial II [VIN II] 624.02
vulvar intraepithelial III [VIN III]
233.32
Neoplasm, neoplastic see page 391–435

◄ New   ◄▪ Revised   ~~deleted~~ Deleted   ● Use Additional Digit(s)   ▨▨▨ Omit code

	Malignant					
	Primary	Secondary	Ca in situ	Benign	Uncertain Behavior	Unspecified
Neoplasm, neoplastic	199.1	199.1	234.9	229.9	238.9	239.9

Notes — 1. The list below gives the code numbers for neoplasms by anatomical site. For each site there are six possible code numbers according to whether the neoplasm in question is malignant, benign, in situ, of uncertain behavior, or of unspecified nature. The description of the neoplasm will often indicate which of the six columns is appropriate; e.g., malignant melanoma of skin, benign fibroadenoma of breast, carcinoma in situ of cervix uteri.

Where such descriptors are not present, the remainder of the Index should be consulted where guidance is given to the appropriate column for each morphological (histological) variety listed; e.g., Mesonephroma — see Neoplasm, malignant; Embryoma — see also Neoplasm, uncertain behavior; Disease, Bowen's — see Neoplasm, skin, in situ. However, the guidance in the Index can be overridden if one of the descriptors mentioned above is present; e.g., malignant adenoma of colon is coded to 153.9 and not to 211.3 as the adjective "malignant" overrides the Index entry "Adenoma - see also Neoplasm, benign."

*2. Sites marked with the sign * (e.g., face NEC*) should be classified to malignant neoplasm of skin of these sites if the variety of neoplasm is a squamous cell carcinoma or an epidermoid carcinoma and to benign neoplasm of skin of these sites if the variety of neoplasm is a papilloma (any type).*

	Primary	Secondary	Ca in situ	Benign	Uncertain Behavior	Unspecified
abdomen, abdominal	195.2	198.89	234.8	229.8	238.8	239.89 ◀️
cavity	195.2	198.89	234.8	229.8	238.8	239.89 ◀️
organ	195.2	198.89	234.8	229.8	238.8	239.89 ◀️
viscera	195.2	198.89	234.8	229.8	238.8	239.89 ◀️
wall	173.5	198.2	232.5	216.5	238.2	239.2
connective tissue	171.5	198.89	—	215.5	238.1	239.2
abdominopelvic	195.8	198.89	234.8	229.8	238.8	239.89 ◀️
accessory sinus - *see* Neoplasm, sinus						
acoustic nerve	192.0	198.4	—	225.1	237.9	239.7
acromion (process)	170.4	198.5	—	213.4	238.0	239.2
adenoid (pharynx) (tissue)	147.1	198.89	230.0	210.7	235.1	239.0
adipose tissue (*see also* Neoplasm, connective tissue)	171.9	198.89	—	215.9	238.1	239.2
adnexa (uterine)	183.9	198.82	233.39	221.8	236.3	239.5
adrenal (cortex) (gland) (medulla)	194.0	198.7	234.8	227.0	237.2	239.7
ala nasi (external)	173.3	198.2	232.3	216.3	238.2	239.2
alimentary canal or tract NEC	159.9	197.8	230.9	211.9	235.5	239.0
alveolar	143.9	198.89	230.0	210.4	235.1	239.0
mucosa	143.9	198.89	230.0	210.4	235.1	239.0
lower	143.1	198.89	230.0	210.4	235.1	239.0
upper	143.0	198.89	230.0	210.4	235.1	239.0
ridge or process	170.1	198.5	—	213.1	238.0	239.2
carcinoma	143.9	—	—	—	—	—
lower	143.1	—	—	—	—	—
upper	143.0	—	—	—	—	—
lower	170.1	198.5	—	213.1	238.0	239.2
mucosa	143.9	198.89	230.0	210.4	235.1	239.0
lower	143.1	198.89	230.0	210.4	235.1	239.0
upper	143.0	198.89	230.0	210.4	235.1	239.0
upper	170.0	198.5	—	213.0	238.0	239.2
sulcus	145.1	198.89	230.0	210.4	235.1	239.0

Neoplasm *(Continued)*	Malignant			Benign	Uncertain Behavior	Unspecified
	Primary	Secondary	Ca in situ			
alveolus	143.9	198.89	230.0	210.4	235.1	239.0
lower	143.1	198.89	230.0	210.4	235.1	239.0
upper	143.0	198.89	230.0	210.4	235.1	239.0
ampulla of Vater	156.2	197.8	230.8	211.5	235.3	239.0
ankle NEC*	195.5	198.89	232.7	229.8	238.8	239.89 ◀
anorectum, anorectal (junction)	154.8	197.5	230.7	211.4	235.2	239.0
antecubital fossa or space*	195.4	198.89	232.6	229.8	238.8	239.89 ◀
antrum (Highmore) (maxillary)	160.2	197.3	231.8	212.0	235.9	239.1
pyloric	151.2	197.8	230.2	211.1	235.2	239.0
tympanicum	160.1	197.3	231.8	212.0	235.9	239.1
anus, anal	154.3	197.5	230.6	211.4	235.5	239.0
canal	154.2	197.5	230.5	211.4	235.5	239.0
contiguous sites with rectosigmoid junction or rectum	154.8	—	—	—	—	—
margin	173.5	198.2	232.5	216.5	238.2	239.2
skin	173.5	198.2	232.5	216.5	238.2	239.2
sphincter	154.2	197.5	230.5	211.4	235.5	239.0
aorta (thoracic)	171.4	198.89	—	215.4	238.1	239.2
abdominal	171.5	198.89	—	215.5	238.1	239.2
aortic body	194.6	198.89	—	227.6	237.3	239.7
aponeurosis	171.9	198.89	—	215.9	238.1	239.2
palmar	171.2	198.89	—	215.2	238.1	239.2
plantar	171.3	198.89	—	215.3	238.1	239.2
appendix	153.5	197.5	230.3	211.3	235.2	239.0
arachnoid (cerebral)	192.1	198.4	—	225.2	237.6	239.7
spinal	192.3	198.4	—	225.4	237.6	239.7
areola (female)	174.0	198.81	233.0	217	238.3	239.3
male	175.0	198.81	233.0	217	238.3	239.3
arm NEC*	195.4	198.89	232.6	229.8	238.8	239.89 ◀
artery - *see* Neoplasm, connective tissue						
aryepiglottic fold	148.2	198.89	230.0	210.8	235.1	239.0
hypopharyngeal aspect	148.2	198.89	230.0	210.8	235.1	239.0
laryngeal aspect	161.1	197.3	231.0	212.1	235.6	239.1
marginal zone	148.2	198.89	230.0	210.8	235.1	239.0
arytenoid (cartilage)	161.3	197.3	231.0	212.1	235.6	239.1
fold - *see* Neoplasm, aryepiglottic						
associated with transplated organ	199.2	—	—	—	—	—
atlas	170.2	198.5	—	213.2	238.0	239.2
atrium, cardiac	164.1	198.89	—	212.7	238.8	239.89 ◀
auditory						
canal (external) (skin)	173.2	198.2	232.2	216.2	238.2	239.2
internal	160.1	197.3	231.8	212.0	235.9	239.1

◀ New   ◀ Revised   deleted Deleted   ● Use Additional Digit(s)   ▨ Omit code

| | Malignant | | | | | |
	Primary	Secondary	Ca in situ	Benign	Uncertain Behavior	Unspecified
Neoplasm *(Continued)*						
auditory *(Continued)*						
nerve	192.0	198.4	—	225.1	237.9	239.7
tube	160.1	197.3	231.8	212.0	235.9	239.1
opening	147.2	198.89	230.0	210.7	235.1	239.0
auricle, ear	173.2	198.2	232.2	216.2	238.2	239.2
cartilage	171.0	198.89	—	215.0	238.1	239.2
auricular canal (external)	173.2	198.2	232.2	216.2	238.2	239.2
internal	160.1	197.3	231.8	212.0	235.9	239.1
autonomic nerve or nervous system NEC	171.9	198.89	—	215.9	238.1	239.2
axilla, axillary	195.1	198.89	234.8	229.8	238.8	239.89◀▥
fold	173.5	198.2	232.5	216.5	238.2	239.2
back NEC*	195.8	198.89	232.5	229.8	238.8	239.89◀▥
Bartholin's gland	184.1	198.82	233.39	221.2	236.3	239.5
basal ganglia	191.0	198.3	—	225.0	237.5	239.6
basis pedunculi	191.7	198.3	—	225.0	237.5	239.6
bile or biliary (tract)	156.9	197.8	230.8	211.5	235.3	239.0
canaliculi (biliferi) (intrahepatic)	155.1	197.8	230.8	211.5	235.3	239.0
canals, interlobular	155.1	197.8	230.8	211.5	235.3	239.0
contiguous sites	156.8	—	—	—	—	—
duct or passage (common) (cystic) (extrahepatic)	156.1	197.8	230.8	211.5	235.3	239.0
contiguous sites						
with gallbladder	156.8	—	—	—	—	—
interlobular	155.1	197.8	230.8	211.5	235.3	239.0
intrahepatic	155.1	197.8	230.8	211.5	235.3	239.0
and extrahepatic	156.9	197.8	230.8	211.5	235.3	239.0
bladder (urinary)	188.9	198.1	233.7	223.3	236.7	239.4
contiguous sites	188.8	—	—	—	—	—
dome	188.1	198.1	233.7	223.3	236.7	239.4
neck	188.5	198.1	233.7	223.3	236.7	239.4
orifice	188.9	198.1	233.7	223.3	236.7	239.4
ureteric	188.6	198.1	233.7	223.3	236.7	239.4
urethral	188.5	198.1	233.7	223.3	236.7	239.4
sphincter	188.8	198.1	233.7	223.3	236.7	239.4
trigone	188.0	198.1	233.7	223.3	236.7	239.4
urachus	188.7	—	233.7	223.3	236.7	239.4
wall	188.9	198.1	233.7	223.3	236.7	239.4
anterior	188.3	198.1	233.7	223.3	236.7	239.4
lateral	188.2	198.1	233.7	223.3	236.7	239.4
posterior	188.4	198.1	233.7	223.3	236.7	239.4
blood vessel - *see* Neoplasm, connective tissue						

	Malignant					
	Primary	Secondary	Ca in situ	Benign	Uncertain Behavior	Unspecified
Neoplasm *(Continued)*						
bone (periosteum)	170.9	198.5	—	213.9	238.0	239.2

Note — Carcinomas and adenocarcinomas, of any type other than intraosseous or odontogenic, of the sites listed under "Neoplasm, bone" should be considered as constituting metastatic spread from an unspecified primary site and coded to 198.5 for morbidity coding.

acetabulum	170.6	198.5	—	213.6	238.0	239.2
acromion (process)	170.4	198.5	—	213.4	238.0	239.2
ankle	170.8	198.5	—	213.8	238.0	239.2
arm NEC	170.4	198.5	—	213.4	238.0	239.2
astragalus	170.8	198.5	—	213.8	238.0	239.2
atlas	170.2	198.5	—	213.2	238.0	239.2
axis	170.2	198.5	—	213.2	238.0	239.2
back NEC	170.2	198.5	—	213.2	238.0	239.2
calcaneus	170.8	198.5	—	213.8	238.0	239.2
calvarium	170.0	198.5	—	213.0	238.0	239.2
carpus (any)	170.5	198.5	—	213.5	238.0	239.2
cartilage NEC	170.9	198.5	—	213.9	238.0	239.2
clavicle	170.3	198.5	—	213.3	238.0	239.2
clivus	170.0	198.5	—	213.0	238.0	239.2
coccygeal vertebra	170.6	198.5	—	213.6	238.0	239.2
coccyx	170.6	198.5	—	213.6	238.0	239.2
costal cartilage	170.3	198.5	—	213.3	238.0	239.2
costovertebral joint	170.3	198.5	—	213.3	238.0	239.2
cranial	170.0	198.5	—	213.0	238.0	239.2
cuboid	170.8	198.5	—	213.8	238.0	239.2
cuneiform	170.9	198.5	—	213.9	238.0	239.2
ankle	170.8	198.5	—	213.8	238.0	239.2
wrist	170.5	198.5	—	213.5	238.0	239.2
digital	170.9	198.5	—	213.9	238.0	239.2
finger	170.5	198.5	—	213.5	238.0	239.2
toe	170.8	198.5	—	213.8	238.0	239.2
elbow	170.4	198.5	—	213.4	238.0	239.2
ethmoid (labyrinth)	170.0	198.5	—	213.0	238.0	239.2
face	170.0	198.5	—	213.0	238.0	239.2
lower jaw	170.1	198.5	—	213.1	238.0	239.2
femur (any part)	170.7	198.5	—	213.7	238.0	239.2
fibula (any part)	170.7	198.5	—	213.7	238.0	239.2
finger (any)	170.5	198.5	—	213.5	238.0	239.2
foot	170.8	198.5	—	213.8	238.0	239.2
forearm	170.4	198.5	—	213.4	238.0	239.2
frontal	170.0	198.5	—	213.0	238.0	239.2
hand	170.5	198.5	—	213.5	238.0	239.2

◀ New   ◀▥ Revised   ~~deleted~~ Deleted   ● Use Additional Digit(s)   ▨ Omit code

| | Malignant | | | | | |
	Primary	Secondary	Ca in situ	Benign	Uncertain Behavior	Unspecified
Neoplasm *(Continued)*						
bone *(Continued)*						
heel	170.8	198.5	—	213.8	238.0	239.2
hip	170.6	198.5	—	213.6	238.0	239.2
humerus (any part)	170.4	198.5	—	213.4	238.0	239.2
hyoid	170.0	198.5	—	213.0	238.0	239.2
ilium	170.6	198.5	—	213.6	238.0	239.2
innominate	170.6	198.5	—	213.6	238.0	239.2
intervertebral cartilage or disc	170.2	198.5	—	213.2	238.0	239.2
ischium	170.6	198.5	—	213.6	238.0	239.2
jaw (lower)	170.1	198.5	—	213.1	238.0	239.2
upper	170.0	198.5	—	213.0	238.0	239.2
knee	170.7	198.5	—	213.7	238.0	239.2
leg NEC	170.7	198.5	—	213.7	238.0	239.2
limb NEC	170.9	198.5	—	213.9	238.0	239.2
lower (long bones)	170.7	198.5	—	213.7	238.0	239.2
short bones	170.8	198.5	—	213.8	238.0	239.2
upper (long bones)	170.4	198.5	—	213.4	238.0	239.2
short bones	170.5	198.5	—	213.5	238.0	239.2
long	170.9	198.5	—	213.9	238.0	239.2
lower limbs NEC	170.7	198.5	—	213.7	238.0	239.2
upper limbs NEC	170.4	198.5	—	213.4	238.0	239.2
malar	170.0	198.5	—	213.0	238.0	239.2
mandible	170.1	198.5	—	213.1	238.0	239.2
marrow NEC	202.9●	198.5	—	—	—	238.79
mastoid	170.0	198.5	—	213.0	238.0	239.2
maxilla, maxillary (superior)	170.0	198.5	—	213.0	238.0	239.2
inferior	170.1	198.5	—	213.1	238.0	239.2
metacarpus (any)	170.5	198.5	—	213.5	238.0	239.2
metatarsus (any)	170.8	198.5	—	213.8	238.0	239.2
navicular (ankle)	170.8	198.5	—	213.8	238.0	239.2
hand	170.5	198.5	—	213.5	238.0	239.2
nose, nasal	170.0	198.5	—	213.0	238.0	239.2
occipital	170.0	198.5	—	213.0	238.0	239.2
orbit	170.0	198.5	—	213.0	238.0	239.2
parietal	170.0	198.5	—	213.0	238.0	239.2
patella	170.8	198.5	—	213.8	238.0	239.2
pelvic	170.6	198.5	—	213.6	238.0	239.2
phalanges	170.9	198.5	—	213.9	238.0	239.2
foot	170.8	198.5	—	213.8	238.0	239.2
hand	170.5	198.5	—	213.5	238.0	239.2

◀ New   ◀▥ Revised   ~~deleted~~ Deleted   ● Use Additional Digit(s)   ▨ Omit code

| | Malignant | | | | | |
	Primary	Secondary	Ca in situ	Benign	Uncertain Behavior	Unspecified
Neoplasm *(Continued)*						
bone *(Continued)*						
pubic	170.6	198.5	—	213.6	238.0	239.2
radius (any part)	170.4	198.5	—	213.4	238.0	239.2
rib	170.3	198.5	—	213.3	238.0	239.2
sacral vertebra	170.6	198.5	—	213.6	238.0	239.2
sacrum	170.6	198.5	—	213.6	238.0	239.2
scaphoid (of hand)	170.5	198.5	—	213.5	238.0	239.2
of ankle	170.8	198.5	—	213.8	238.0	239.2
scapula (any part)	170.4	198.5	—	213.4	238.0	239.2
sella turcica	170.0	198.5	—	213.0	238.0	239.2
short	170.9	198.5	—	213.9	238.0	239.2
lower limb	170.8	198.5	—	213.8	238.0	239.2
upper limb	170.5	198.5	—	213.5	238.0	239.2
shoulder	170.4	198.5	—	213.4	238.0	239.2
skeleton, skeletal NEC	170.9	198.5	—	213.9	238.0	239.2
skull	170.0	198.5	—	213.0	238.0	239.2
sphenoid	170.0	198.5	—	213.0	238.0	239.2
spine, spinal (column)	170.2	198.5	—	213.2	238.0	239.2
coccyx	170.6	198.5	—	213.6	238.0	239.2
sacrum	170.6	198.5	—	213.6	238.0	239.2
sternum	170.3	198.5	—	213.3	238.0	239.2
tarsus (any)	170.8	198.5	—	213.8	238.0	239.2
temporal	170.0	198.5	—	213.0	238.0	239.2
thumb	170.5	198.5	—	213.5	238.0	239.2
tibia (any part)	170.7	198.5	—	213.7	238.0	239.2
toe (any)	170.8	198.5	—	213.8	238.0	239.2
trapezium	170.5	198.5	—	213.5	238.0	239.2
trapezoid	170.5	198.5	—	213.5	238.0	239.2
turbinate	170.0	198.5	—	213.0	238.0	239.2
ulna (any part)	170.4	198.5	—	213.4	238.0	239.2
unciform	170.5	198.5	—	213.5	238.0	239.2
vertebra (column)	170.2	198.5	—	213.2	238.0	239.2
coccyx	170.6	198.5	—	213.6	238.0	239.2
sacrum	170.6	198.5	—	213.6	238.0	239.2
vomer	170.0	198.5	—	213.0	238.0	239.2
wrist	170.5	198.5	—	213.5	238.0	239.2
xiphoid process	170.3	198.5	—	213.3	238.0	239.2
zygomatic	170.0	198.5	—	213.0	238.0	239.2
book-leaf (mouth)	145.8	198.89	230.0	210.4	235.1	239.0
bowel - *see* Neoplasm, intestine						

◀ New   ◀▥ Revised   deleted Deleted   ● Use Additional Digit(s)   ▨ Omit code

	Malignant					
	Primary	Secondary	Ca in situ	Benign	Uncertain Behavior	Unspecified
Neoplasm *(Continued)*						
brachial plexus	171.2	198.89	—	215.2	238.1	239.2
brain NEC	191.9	198.3	—	225.0	237.5	239.6
basal ganglia	191.0	198.3	—	225.0	237.5	239.6
cerebellopontine angle	191.6	198.3	—	225.0	237.5	239.6
cerebellum NOS	191.6	198.3	—	225.0	237.5	239.6
cerebrum	191.0	198.3	—	225.0	237.5	239.6
choroid plexus	191.5	198.3	—	225.0	237.5	239.6
contiguous sites	191.8	—	—	—	—	—
corpus callosum	191.8	198.3	—	225.0	237.5	239.6
corpus striatum	191.0	198.3	—	225.0	237.5	239.6
cortex (cerebral)	191.0	198.3	—	225.0	237.5	239.6
frontal lobe	191.1	198.3	—	225.0	237.5	239.6
globus pallidus	191.0	198.3	—	225.0	237.5	239.6
hippocampus	191.2	198.3	—	225.0	237.5	239.6
hypothalamus	191.0	198.3	—	225.0	237.5	239.6
internal capsule	191.0	198.3	—	225.0	237.5	239.6
medulla oblongata	191.7	198.3	—	225.0	237.5	239.6
meninges	192.1	198.4	—	225.2	237.6	239.7
midbrain	191.7	198.3	—	225.0	237.5	239.6
occipital lobe	191.4	198.3	—	225.0	237.5	239.6
parietal lobe	191.3	198.3	—	225.0	237.5	239.6
peduncle	191.7	198.3	—	225.0	237.5	239.6
pons	191.7	198.3	—	225.0	237.5	239.6
stem	191.7	198.3	—	225.0	237.5	239.6
tapetum	191.8	198.3	—	225.0	237.5	239.6
temporal lobe	191.2	198.3	—	225.0	237.5	239.6
thalamus	191.0	198.3	—	225.0	237.5	239.6
uncus	191.2	198.3	—	225.0	237.5	239.6
ventricle (floor)	191.5	198.3	—	225.0	237.5	239.6
branchial (cleft) (vestiges)	146.8	198.89	230.0	210.6	235.1	239.0
breast (connective tissue) (female) (glandular tissue) (soft parts)	174.9	198.81	233.0	217	238.3	239.3
areola	174.0	198.81	233.0	217	238.3	239.3
male	175.0	198.81	233.0	217	238.3	239.3
axillary tail	174.6	198.81	233.0	217	238.3	239.3
central portion	174.1	198.81	233.0	217	238.3	239.3
contiguous sites	174.8	—	—	—	—	—
ectopic sites	174.8	198.81	233.0	217	238.3	239.3
inner	174.8	198.81	233.0	217	238.3	239.3
lower	174.8	198.81	233.0	217	238.3	239.3
lower-inner quadrant	174.3	198.81	233.0	217	238.3	239.3

◄ New   ◄▬ Revised   ~~deleted~~ Deleted   ● Use Additional Digit(s)   ▨ Omit code

	Malignant					
	Primary	Secondary	Ca in situ	Benign	Uncertain Behavior	Unspecified
Neoplasm *(Continued)*						
breast *(Continued)*						
lower-outer quadrant	174.5	198.81	233.0	217	238.3	239.3
male	175.9	198.81	233.0	217	238.3	239.3
areola	175.0	198.81	233.0	217	238.3	239.3
ectopic tissue	175.9	198.81	233.0	217	238.3	239.3
nipple	175.0	198.81	233.0	217	238.3	239.3
mastectomy site (skin)	173.5	198.2	—	—	—	—
specified as breast tissue	174.8	198.81	—	—	—	—
midline	174.8	198.81	233.0	217	238.3	239.3
nipple	174.0	198.81	233.0	217	238.3	239.3
male	175.0	198.81	233.0	217	238.3	239.3
outer	174.8	198.81	233.0	217	238.3	239.3
skin	173.5	198.2	232.5	216.5	238.2	239.2
tail (axillary)	174.6	198.81	233.0	217	238.3	239.3
upper	174.8	198.81	233.0	217	238.3	239.3
upper-inner quadrant	174.2	198.81	233.0	217	238.3	239.3
upper-outer quadrant	174.4	198.81	233.0	217	238.3	239.3
broad ligament	183.3	198.82	233.39	221.0	236.3	239.5
bronchiogenic, bronchogenic (lung)	162.9	197.0	231.2	212.3	235.7	239.1
bronchiole	162.9	197.0	231.2	212.3	235.7	239.1
bronchus	162.9	197.0	231.2	212.3	235.7	239.1
carina	162.2	197.0	231.2	212.3	235.7	239.1
contiguous sites with lung or trachea	162.8	—	—	—	—	—
lower lobe of lung	162.5	197.0	231.2	212.3	235.7	239.1
main	162.2	197.0	231.2	212.3	235.7	239.1
middle lobe of lung	162.4	197.0	231.2	212.3	235.7	239.1
upper lobe of lung	162.3	197.0	231.2	212.3	235.7	239.1
brow	173.3	198.2	232.3	216.3	238.2	239.2
buccal (cavity)	145.9	198.89	230.0	210.4	235.1	239.0
commissure	145.0	198.89	230.0	210.4	235.1	239.0
groove (lower) (upper)	145.1	198.89	230.0	210.4	235.1	239.0
mucosa	145.0	198.89	230.0	210.4	235.1	239.0
sulcus (lower) (upper)	145.1	198.89	230.0	210.4	235.1	239.0
bulbourethral gland	189.3	198.1	233.9	223.81	236.99	239.5
bursa - *see* Neoplasm, connective tissue						
buttock NEC*	195.3	198.89	232.5	229.8	238.8	239.89◄
calf*	195.5	198.89	232.7	229.8	238.8	239.89◄
calvarium	170.0	198.5	—	213.0	238.0	239.2
calyx, renal	189.1	198.0	233.9	223.1	236.91	239.5

◄ New   ◄▥ Revised   ~~deleted~~ Deleted   ● Use Additional Digit(s)   �Omit code

	Malignant					
	Primary	Secondary	Ca in situ	Benign	Uncertain Behavior	Unspecified
Neoplasm *(Continued)*						
canal						
anal	154.2	197.5	230.5	211.4	235.5	239.0
auditory (external)	173.2	198.2	232.2	216.2	238.2	239.2
auricular (external)	173.2	198.2	232.2	216.2	238.2	239.2
canaliculi, biliary (biliferi) (intrahepatic)	155.1	197.8	230.8	211.5	235.3	239.0
canthus (eye) (inner) (outer)	173.1	198.2	232.1	216.1	238.2	239.2
capillary - *see* Neoplasm, connective tissue						
caput coli	153.4	197.5	230.3	211.3	235.2	239.0
cardia (gastric)	151.0	197.8	230.2	211.1	235.2	239.0
cardiac orifice (stomach)	151.0	197.8	230.2	211.1	235.2	239.0
cardio-esophageal junction	151.0	197.8	230.2	211.1	235.2	239.0
cardio-esophagus	151.0	197.8	230.2	211.1	235.2	239.0
carina (bronchus) (trachea)	162.2	197.0	231.2	212.3	235.7	239.1
carotid (artery)	171.0	198.89	—	215.0	238.1	239.2
body	194.5	198.89	—	227.5	237.3	239.7
carpus (any bone)	170.5	198.5	—	213.5	238.0	239.2
cartilage (articular) (joint) NEC - *see also* Neoplasm, bone	170.9	198.5	—	213.9	238.0	239.2
arytenoid	161.3	197.3	231.0	212.1	235.6	239.1
auricular	171.0	198.89	—	215.0	238.1	239.2
bronchi	162.2	197.3	—	212.3	235.7	239.1
connective tissue - *see* Neoplasm, connective tissue						
costal	170.3	198.5	—	213.3	238.0	239.2
cricoid	161.3	197.3	231.0	212.1	235.6	239.1
cuneiform	161.3	197.3	231.0	212.1	235.6	239.1
ear (external)	171.0	198.89	—	215.0	238.1	239.2
ensiform	170.3	198.5	—	213.3	238.0	239.2
epiglottis	161.1	197.3	231.0	212.1	235.6	239.1
anterior surface	146.4	198.89	230.0	210.6	235.1	239.0
eyelid	171.0	198.89	—	215.0	238.1	239.2
intervertebral	170.2	198.5	—	213.2	238.0	239.2
larynx, laryngeal	161.3	197.3	231.0	212.1	235.6	239.1
nose, nasal	160.0	197.3	231.8	212.0	235.9	239.1
pinna	171.0	198.89	—	215.0	238.1	239.2
rib	170.3	198.5	—	213.3	238.0	239.2
semilunar (knee)	170.7	198.5	—	213.7	238.0	239.2
thyroid	161.3	197.3	231.0	212.1	235.6	239.1
trachea	162.0	197.3	231.1	212.2	235.7	239.1
cauda equina	192.2	198.3	—	225.3	237.5	239.7

	Malignant			Benign	Uncertain Behavior	Unspecified
	Primary	Secondary	Ca in situ	Benign	Uncertain Behavior	Unspecified
Neoplasm *(Continued)*						
cavity						
buccal	145.9	198.89	230.0	210.4	235.1	239.0
nasal	160.0	197.3	231.8	212.0	235.9	239.1
oral	145.9	198.89	230.0	210.4	235.1	239.0
peritoneal	158.9	197.6	—	211.8	235.4	239.0
tympanic	160.1	197.3	231.8	212.0	235.9	239.1
cecum	153.4	197.5	230.3	211.3	235.2	239.0
central						
nervous system - *see* Neoplasm, nervous system						
white matter	191.0	198.3	—	225.0	237.5	239.6
cerebellopontine (angle)	191.6	198.3	—	225.0	237.5	239.6
cerebellum, cerebellar	191.6	198.3	—	225.0	237.5	239.6
cerebrum, cerebral (cortex) (hemisphere) (white matter)	191.0	198.3	—	225.0	237.5	239.6
meninges	192.1	198.4	—	225.2	237.6	239.7
peduncle	191.7	198.3	—	225.0	237.5	239.6
ventricle (any)	191.5	198.3	—	225.0	237.5	239.6
cervical region	195.0	198.89	234.8	229.8	238.8	239.89◄
cervix (cervical) (uteri) (uterus)	180.9	198.82	233.1	219.0	236.0	239.5
canal	180.0	198.82	233.1	219.0	236.0	239.5
contiguous sites	180.8	—	—	—	—	—
endocervix (canal) (gland)	180.0	198.82	233.1	219.0	236.0	239.5
exocervix	180.1	198.82	233.1	219.0	236.0	239.5
external os	180.1	198.82	233.1	219.0	236.0	239.5
nabothian gland	180.0	198.82	233.1	219.0	236.0	239.5
squamocolumnar junction	180.8	198.82	233.1	219.0	236.0	239.5
stump	180.8	198.82	233.1	219.0	236.0	239.5
cheek	195.0	198.89	234.8	229.8	238.8	239.89◄
external	173.3	198.2	232.3	216.3	238.2	239.2
inner aspect	145.0	198.89	230.0	210.4	235.1	239.0
internal	145.0	198.89	230.0	210.4	235.1	239.0
mucosa	145.0	198.89	230.0	210.4	235.1	239.0
chest (wall) NEC	195.1	198.89	234.8	229.8	238.8	239.89◄
chiasma opticum	192.0	198.4	—	225.1	237.9	239.7
chin	173.3	198.2	232.3	216.3	238.2	239.2
choana	147.3	198.89	230.0	210.7	235.1	239.0
cholangiole	155.1	197.8	230.8	211.5	235.3	239.0
choledochal duct	156.1	197.8	230.8	211.5	235.3	239.0
choroid	190.6	198.4	234.0	224.6	238.8	239.81◄
plexus	191.5	198.3	—	225.0	237.5	239.6
ciliary body	190.0	198.4	234.0	224.0	238.8	239.89◄

◄ New   ◄▥ Revised   ~~deleted~~ Deleted   ● Use Additional Digit(s)   ▥ Omit code

	Malignant					
	Primary	Secondary	Ca in situ	Benign	Uncertain Behavior	Unspecified
Neoplasm *(Continued)*						
clavicle	170.3	198.5	—	213.3	238.0	239.2
clitoris	184.3	198.82	233.32	221.2	236.3	239.5
clivus	170.0	198.5	—	213.0	238.0	239.2
cloacogenic zone	154.8	197.5	230.7	211.4	235.5	239.0
coccygeal						
body or glomus	194.6	198.89	—	227.6	237.3	239.7
vertebra	170.6	198.5	—	213.6	238.0	239.2
coccyx	170.6	198.5	—	213.6	238.0	239.2
colon - *see also* Neoplasm, intestine, large and rectum	154.0	197.5	230.4	211.4	235.2	239.0
column, spinal - *see* Neoplasm, spine						
columnella	173.3	198.2	232.3	216.3	238.2	239.2
commissure						
labial, lip	140.6	198.89	230.0	210.4	235.1	239.0
laryngeal	161.0	197.3	231.0	212.1	235.6	239.1
common (bile) duct	156.1	197.8	230.8	211.5	235.3	239.0
concha	173.2	198.2	232.2	216.2	238.2	239.2
nose	160.0	197.3	231.8	212.0	235.9	239.1
conjunctiva	190.3	198.4	234.0	224.3	238.8	239.89 ◀
connective tissue NEC	171.9	198.89	—	215.9	238.1	239.2

Note — *For neoplasms of connective tissue (blood vessel, bursa, fascia, ligament, muscle, peripheral nerves, sympathetic and parasympathetic nerves and ganglia, synovia, tendon, etc.)*
or of morphological types that indicate connective tissue, code according to the list under "Neoplasm, connective tissue;" for sites that do not appear in this list, code to neoplasm of that
site; e.g.,

> *liposarcoma, shoulder 171.2*
>
> *leiomyosarcoma, stomach 151.9*
>
> *neurofibroma, chest wall 215.4*

Morphological types that indicate connective tissue appear in their proper place in the alphabetic index with the instruction "see Neoplasm, connective tissue ...."

	Primary	Secondary	Ca in situ	Benign	Uncertain Behavior	Unspecified
abdomen	171.5	198.89	—	215.5	238.1	239.2
abdominal wall	171.5	198.89	—	215.5	238.1	239.2
ankle	171.3	198.89	—	215.3	238.1	239.2
antecubital fossa or space	171.2	198.89	—	215.2	238.1	239.2
arm	171.2	198.89	—	215.2	238.1	239.2
auricle (ear)	171.0	198.89	—	215.0	238.1	239.2
axilla	171.4	198.89	—	215.4	238.1	239.2
back	171.7	198.89	—	215.7	238.1	239.2
breast (female) (*see also* Neoplasm, breast)	174.9	198.81	233.0	217	238.3	239.3
male	175.9	198.81	233.0	217	238.3	239.3
buttock	171.6	198.89	—	215.6	238.1	239.2
calf	171.3	198.89	—	215.3	238.1	239.2
cervical region	171.0	198.89	—	215.0	238.1	239.2
cheek	171.0	198.89	—	215.0	238.1	239.2

◀ New   ◀▥ Revised   ~~deleted~~ Deleted   ● Use Additional Digit(s)   ▬ Omit code

	Malignant			Benign	Uncertain Behavior	Unspecified
	Primary	Secondary	Ca in situ			
Neoplasm (Continued)						
connective tissue NEC (Continued)						
chest (wall)	171.4	198.89	—	215.4	238.1	239.2
chin	171.0	198.89	—	215.0	238.1	239.2
contiguous sites	171.8	—	—	—	—	—
diaphragm	171.4	198.89	—	215.4	238.1	239.2
ear (external)	171.0	198.89	—	215.0	238.1	239.2
elbow	171.2	198.89	—	215.2	238.1	239.2
extrarectal	171.6	198.89	—	215.6	238.1	239.2
extremity	171.8	198.89	—	215.8	238.1	239.2
lower	171.3	198.89	—	215.3	238.1	239.2
upper	171.2	198.89	—	215.2	238.1	239.2
eyelid	171.0	198.89	—	215.0	238.1	239.2
face	171.0	198.89	—	215.0	238.1	239.2
finger	171.2	198.89	—	215.2	238.1	239.2
flank	171.7	198.89	—	215.7	238.1	239.2
foot	171.3	198.89	—	215.3	238.1	239.2
forearm	171.2	198.89	—	215.2	238.1	239.2
forehead	171.0	198.89	—	215.0	238.1	239.2
gastric	171.5	198.89	—	215.5	238.1	—
gastrointestinal	171.5	198.89	—	215.5	238.1	—
gluteal region	171.6	198.89	—	215.6	238.1	239.2
great vessels NEC	171.4	198.89	—	215.4	238.1	239.2
groin	171.6	198.89	—	215.6	238.1	239.2
hand	171.2	198.89	—	215.2	238.1	239.2
head	171.0	198.89	—	215.0	238.1	239.2
heel	171.3	198.89	—	215.3	238.1	239.2
hip	171.3	198.89	—	215.3	238.1	239.2
hypochondrium	171.5	198.89	—	215.5	238.1	239.2
iliopsoas muscle	171.6	198.89	—	215.5	238.1	239.2
infraclavicular region	171.4	198.89	—	215.4	238.1	239.2
inguinal (canal) (region)	171.6	198.89	—	215.6	238.1	239.2
intestine	171.5	198.89	—	215.5	238.1	—
intrathoracic	171.4	198.89	—	215.4	238.1	239.2
ischorectal fossa	171.6	198.89	—	215.6	238.1	239.2
jaw	143.9	198.89	230.0	210.4	235.1	239.0
knee	171.3	198.89	—	215.3	238.1	239.2
leg	171.3	198.89	—	215.3	238.1	239.2
limb NEC	171.9	198.89	—	215.8	238.1	239.2
lower	171.3	198.89	—	215.3	238.1	239.2
upper	171.2	198.89	—	215.2	238.1	239.2

◀ New ◀▥ Revised ~~deleted~~ Deleted ● Use Additional Digit(s) ▭ Omit code

	Malignant					
	Primary	Secondary	Ca in situ	Benign	Uncertain Behavior	Unspecified
Neoplasm *(Continued)*						
connective tissue NEC *(Continued)*						
nates	171.6	198.89	—	215.6	238.1	239.2
neck	171.0	198.89	—	215.0	238.1	239.2
orbit	190.1	198.4	234.0	224.1	238.8	239.89 ◀
pararectal	171.6	198.89	—	215.6	238.1	239.2
para-urethral	171.6	198.89	—	215.6	238.1	239.2
paravaginal	171.6	198.89	—	215.6	238.1	239.2
pelvis (floor)	171.6	198.89	—	215.6	238.1	239.2
pelvo-abdominal	171.8	198.89	—	215.8	238.1	239.2
perineum	171.6	198.89	—	215.6	238.1	239.2
perirectal (tissue)	171.6	198.89	—	215.6	238.1	239.2
periurethral (tissue)	171.6	198.89	—	215.6	238.1	239.2
popliteal fossa or space	171.3	198.89	—	215.3	238.1	239.2
presacral	171.6	198.89	—	215.6	238.1	239.2
psoas muscle	171.5	198.89	—	215.5	238.1	239.2
pterygoid fossa	171.0	198.89	—	215.0	238.1	239.2
rectovaginal septum or wall	171.6	198.89	—	215.6	238.1	239.2
rectovesical	171.6	198.89	—	215.6	238.1	239.2
retroperitoneum	158.0	197.6	—	211.8	235.4	239.0
sacrococcygeal region	171.6	198.89	—	215.6	238.1	239.2
scalp	171.0	198.89	—	215.0	238.1	239.2
scapular region	171.4	198.89	—	215.4	238.1	239.2
shoulder	171.2	198.89	—	215.2	238.1	239.2
skin (dermis) NEC	173.9	198.2	232.9	216.9	238.2	239.2
stomach	171.5	198.89	—	215.5	238.1	—
submental	171.0	198.89	—	215.0	238.1	239.2
supraclavicular region	171.0	198.89	—	215.0	238.1	239.2
temple	171.0	198.89	—	215.0	238.1	239.2
temporal region	171.0	198.89	—	215.0	238.1	239.2
thigh	171.3	198.89	—	215.3	238.1	239.2
thoracic (duct) (wall)	171.4	198.89	—	215.4	238.1	239.2
thorax	171.4	198.89	—	215.4	238.1	239.2
thumb	171.2	198.89	—	215.2	238.1	239.2
toe	171.3	198.89	—	215.3	238.1	239.2
trunk	171.7	198.89	—	215.7	238.1	239.2
umbilicus	171.5	198.89	—	215.5	238.1	239.2
vesicorectal	171.6	198.89	—	215.6	238.1	239.2
wrist	171.2	198.89	—	215.2	238.1	239.2
conus medullaris	192.2	198.3	—	225.3	237.5	239.7

	Malignant					
	Primary	Secondary	Ca in situ	Benign	Uncertain Behavior	Unspecified
Neoplasm (Continued)						
cord (true) (vocal)	161.0	197.3	231.0	212.1	235.6	239.1
false	161.1	197.3	231.0	212.1	235.6	239.1
spermatic	187.6	198.82	233.6	222.8	236.6	239.5
spinal (cervical) (lumbar) (thoracic)	192.2	198.3	—	225.3	237.5	239.7
cornea (limbus)	190.4	198.4	234.0	224.4	238.8	239.89 ◄
corpus						
albicans	183.0	198.6	233.39	220	236.2	239.5
callosum, brain	191.8	198.3	—	225.0	237.5	239.6
cavernosum	187.3	198.82	233.5	222.1	236.6	239.5
gastric	151.4	197.8	230.2	211.1	235.2	239.0
penis	187.3	198.82	233.5	222.1	236.6	239.5
striatum, cerebrum	191.0	198.3	—	225.0	237.5	239.6
uteri	182.0	198.82	233.2	219.1	236.0	239.5
isthmus	182.1	198.82	233.2	219.1	236.0	239.5
cortex						
adrenal	194.0	198.7	234.8	227.0	237.2	239.7
cerebral	191.0	198.3	—	225.0	237.5	239.6
costal cartilage	170.3	198.5	—	213.3	238.0	239.2
costovertebral joint	170.3	198.5	—	213.3	238.0	239.2
Cowper's gland	189.3	198.1	233.9	223.81	236.99	239.5
cranial (fossa, any)	191.9	198.3	—	225.0	237.5	239.6
meninges	192.1	198.4	—	225.2	237.6	239.7
nerve (any)	192.0	198.4	—	225.1	237.9	239.7
craniobuccal pouch	194.3	198.89	234.8	227.3	237.0	239.7
craniopharyngeal (duct) (pouch)	194.3	198.89	234.8	227.3	237.0	239.7
cricoid	148.0	198.89	230.0	210.8	235.1	239.0
cartilage	161.3	197.3	231.0	212.1	235.6	239.1
cricopharynx	148.0	198.89	230.0	210.8	235.1	239.0
crypt of Morgagni	154.8	197.5	230.7	211.4	235.2	239.0
crystalline lens	190.0	198.4	234.0	224.0	238.8	239.89 ◄
cul-de-sac (Douglas')	158.8	197.6	—	211.8	235.4	239.0
cuneiform cartilage	161.3	197.3	231.0	212.1	235.6	239.1
cutaneous - see Neoplasm, skin						
cutis - see Neoplasm, skin						
cystic (bile) duct (common)	156.1	197.8	230.8	211.5	235.3	239.0
dermis - see Neoplasm, skin						
diaphragm	171.4	198.89	—	215.4	238.1	239.2
digestive organs, system, tube, or tract NEC	159.9	197.8	230.9	211.9	235.5	239.0
contiguous sites with peritoneum	159.8	—	—	—	—	—
disc, intervertebral	170.2	198.5	—	213.2	238.0	239.2

◄ New   ◄▦ Revised   ~~deleted~~ Deleted   ● Use Additional Digit(s)   ▦ Omit code

	Malignant					
	Primary	Secondary	Ca in situ	Benign	Uncertain Behavior	Unspecified
Neoplasm *(Continued)*						
disease, generalized	199.0	199.0	234.9	229.9	238.9	199.0
disseminated	199.0	199.0	234.9	229.9	238.9	199.0
Douglas' cul-de-sac or pouch	158.8	197.6	—	211.8	235.4	239.0
duodenojejunal junction	152.8	197.4	230.7	211.2	235.2	239.0
duodenum	152.0	197.4	230.7	211.2	235.2	239.0
dura (cranial) (mater)	192.1	198.4	—	225.2	237.6	239.7
cerebral	192.1	198.4	—	225.2	237.6	239.7
spinal	192.3	198.4	—	225.4	237.6	239.7
ear (external)	173.2	198.2	232.2	216.2	238.2	239.2
auricle or auris	173.2	198.2	232.2	216.2	238.2	239.2
canal, external	173.2	198.2	232.2	216.2	238.2	239.2
cartilage	171.0	198.89	—	215.0	238.1	239.2
external meatus	173.2	198.2	232.2	216.2	238.2	239.2
inner	160.1	197.3	231.8	212.0	235.9	239.89 ◄
lobule	173.2	198.2	232.2	216.2	238.2	239.2
middle	160.1	197.3	231.8	212.0	235.9	239.89 ◄
contiguous sites with accessory sinuses or nasal cavities	160.8	—	—	—	—	—
skin	173.2	198.2	232.2	216.2	238.2	239.2
earlobe	173.2	198.2	232.2	216.2	238.2	239.2
ejaculatory duct	187.8	198.82	233.6	222.8	236.6	239.5
elbow NEC*	195.4	198.89	232.6	229.8	238.8	239.89 ◄
endocardium	164.1	198.89	—	212.7	238.8	239.89 ◄
endocervix (canal) (gland)	180.0	198.82	233.1	219.0	236.0	239.5
endocrine gland NEC	194.9	198.89	—	227.9	237.4	239.7
pluriglandular NEC	194.8	198.89	234.8	227.8	237.4	239.7
endometrium (gland) (stroma)	182.0	198.82	233.2	219.1	236.0	239.5
ensiform cartilage	170.3	198.5	—	213.3	238.0	239.2
enteric - *see* Neoplasm, intestine						
ependyma (brain)	191.5	198.3	—	225.0	237.5	239.6
epicardium	164.1	198.89	—	212.7	238.8	239.89 ◄
epididymis	187.5	198.82	233.6	222.3	236.6	239.5
epidural	192.9	198.4	—	225.9	237.9	239.7
epiglottis	161.1	197.3	231.0	212.1	235.6	239.1
anterior aspect or surface	146.4	198.89	230.0	210.6	235.1	239.0
cartilage	161.3	197.3	231.0	212.1	235.6	239.1
free border (margin)	146.4	198.89	230.0	210.6	235.1	239.0
junctional region	146.5	198.89	230.0	210.6	235.1	239.0
posterior (laryngeal) surface	161.1	197.3	231.0	212.1	235.6	239.1
suprahyoid portion	161.1	197.3	231.0	212.1	235.6	239.1
esophagogastric junction	151.0	197.8	230.2	211.1	235.2	239.0

	Malignant			Benign	Uncertain Behavior	Unspecified
	Primary	Secondary	Ca in situ	Benign	Uncertain Behavior	Unspecified
Neoplasm (Continued)						
esophagus	150.9	197.8	230.1	211.0	235.5	239.0
abdominal	150.2	197.8	230.1	211.0	235.5	239.0
cervical	150.0	197.8	230.1	211.0	235.5	239.0
contiguous sites	150.8	—	—	—	—	—
distal (third)	150.5	197.8	230.1	211.0	235.5	239.0
lower (third)	150.5	197.8	230.1	211.0	235.5	239.0
middle (third)	150.4	197.8	230.1	211.0	235.5	239.0
proximal (third)	150.3	197.8	230.1	211.0	235.5	239.0
specified part NEC	150.8	197.8	230.1	211.0	235.5	239.0
thoracic	150.1	197.8	230.1	211.0	235.5	239.0
upper (third)	150.3	197.8	230.1	211.0	235.5	239.0
ethmoid (sinus)	160.3	197.3	231.8	212.0	235.9	239.1
bone or labyrinth	170.0	198.5	—	213.0	238.0	239.2
Eustachian tube	160.1	197.3	231.8	212.0	235.9	239.1
exocervix	180.1	198.82	233.1	219.0	236.0	239.5
external						
meatus (ear)	173.2	198.2	232.2	216.2	238.2	239.2
os, cervix uteri	180.1	198.82	233.1	219.0	236.0	239.5
extradural	192.9	198.4	—	225.9	237.9	239.7
extrahepatic (bile) duct	156.1	197.8	230.8	211.5	235.3	239.0
contiguous sites with gallbladder	156.8	—	—	—	—	—
extraocular muscle	190.1	198.4	234.0	224.1	238.8	239.89 ◀
extrarectal	195.3	198.89	234.8	229.8	238.8	239.89 ◀
extremity*	195.8	198.89	232.8	229.8	238.8	239.89 ◀
lower*	195.5	198.89	232.7	229.8	238.8	239.89 ◀
upper*	195.4	198.89	232.6	229.8	238.8	239.89 ◀
eye NEC	190.9	198.4	234.0	224.9	238.8	239.89 ◀
contiguous sites	190.8	—	—	—	—	—
specified sites NEC	190.8	198.4	234.0	224.8	238.8	239.89 ◀
eyeball	190.0	198.4	234.0	224.0	238.8	239.89 ◀
eyebrow	173.3	198.2	232.3	216.3	238.2	239.2
eyelid (lower) (skin) (upper)	173.1	198.2	232.1	216.1	238.2	239.2
cartilage	171.0	198.89	—	215.0	238.1	239.2
face NEC*	195.0	198.89	232.3	229.8	238.8	239.89 ◀
Fallopian tube (accessory)	183.2	198.82	233.39	221.0	236.3	239.5
falx (cerebella) (cerebri)	192.1	198.4	—	225.2	237.6	239.7
fascia - see also Neoplasm, connective tissue						
palmar	171.2	198.89	—	215.2	238.1	239.2
plantar	171.3	198.89	—	215.3	238.1	239.2
fatty tissue - see Neoplasm, connective tissue						

◀ New   ◀▥ Revised   ~~deleted~~ Deleted   ● Use Additional Digit(s)   ▬ Omit code

	Malignant			Benign	Uncertain Behavior	Unspecified
	Primary	Secondary	Ca in situ			
Neoplasm (*Continued*)						
fauces, faucial NEC	146.9	198.89	230.0	210.6	235.1	239.0
pillars	146.2	198.89	230.0	210.6	235.1	239.0
tonsil	146.0	198.89	230.0	210.5	235.1	239.0
femur (any part)	170.7	198.5	—	213.7	238.0	239.2
fetal membrane	181	198.82	233.2	219.8	236.1	239.5
fibrous tissue - *see* Neoplasm, connective tissue						
fibula (any part)	170.7	198.5	—	213.7	238.0	239.2
filum terminale	192.2	198.3	—	225.3	237.5	239.7
finger NEC*	195.4	198.89	232.6	229.8	238.8	239.89◄
flank NEC*	195.8	198.89	232.5	229.8	238.8	239.89◄
follicle, nabothian	180.0	198.82	233.1	219.0	236.0	239.5
foot NEC*	195.5	198.89	232.7	229.8	238.8	239.89◄
forearm NEC*	195.4	198.89	232.6	229.8	238.8	239.89◄
forehead (skin)	173.3	198.2	232.3	216.3	238.2	239.2
foreskin	187.1	198.82	233.5	222.1	236.6	239.5
fornix						
pharyngeal	147.3	198.89	230.0	210.7	235.1	239.0
vagina	184.0	198.82	233.31	221.1	236.3	239.5
fossa (of)						
anterior (cranial)	191.9	198.3	—	225.0	237.5	239.6
cranial	191.9	198.3	—	225.0	237.5	239.6
ischiorectal	195.3	198.89	234.8	229.8	238.8	239.89◄
middle (cranial)	191.9	198.3	—	225.0	237.5	239.6
pituitary	194.3	198.89	234.8	227.3	237.0	239.7
posterior (cranial)	191.9	198.3	—	225.0	237.5	239.6
pterygoid	171.0	198.89	—	215.0	238.1	239.2
pyriform	148.1	198.89	230.0	210.8	235.1	239.0
Rosenmüller	147.2	198.89	230.0	210.7	235.1	239.0
tonsillar	146.1	198.89	230.0	210.6	235.1	239.0
fourchette	184.4	198.82	233.32	221.2	236.3	239.5
frenulum						
labii - *see* Neoplasm, lip, internal						
linguae	141.3	198.89	230.0	210.1	235.1	239.0
frontal						
bone	170.0	198.5	—	213.0	238.0	239.2
lobe, brain	191.1	198.3	—	225.0	237.5	239.6
meninges	192.1	198.4	—	225.2	237.6	239.7
pole	191.1	198.3	—	225.0	237.5	239.6
sinus	160.4	197.3	231.8	212.0	235.9	239.1

	Malignant					
	Primary	Secondary	Ca in situ	Benign	Uncertain Behavior	Unspecified
Neoplasm (*Continued*)						
fundus						
stomach	151.3	197.8	230.2	211.1	235.2	239.0
uterus	182.0	198.82	233.2	219.1	236.0	239.5
gall duct (extrahepatic)	156.1	197.8	230.8	211.5	235.3	239.0
intrahepatic	155.1	197.8	230.8	211.5	235.3	239.0
gallbladder	156.0	197.8	230.8	211.5	235.3	239.0
contiguous sites with extrahepatic bile ducts	156.8	—	—	—	—	—
ganglia (*see also* Neoplasm, connective tissue)	171.9	198.89	—	215.9	238.1	239.2
basal	191.0	198.3	—	225.0	237.5	239.6
ganglion (*see also* Neoplasm, connective tissue)	171.9	198.89	—	215.9	238.1	239.2
cranial nerve	192.0	198.4	—	225.1	237.9	239.7
Gartner's duct	184.0	198.82	233.31	221.1	236.3	239.5
gastric - *see* Neoplasm, stomach						
gastrocolic	159.8	197.8	230.9	211.9	235.5	239.0
gastroesophageal junction	151.0	197.8	230.2	211.1	235.2	239.0
gastrointestinal (tract) NEC	159.9	197.8	230.9	211.9	235.5	239.0
generalized	199.0	199.0	234.9	229.9	238.9	199.0
genital organ or tract						
female NEC	184.9	198.82	233.39	221.9	236.3	239.5
contiguous sites	184.8					
specified site NEC	184.8	198.82	233.39	221.8	236.3	239.5
male NEC	187.9	198.82	233.6	222.9	236.6	239.5
contiguous sites	187.8	—	—	—	—	—
specified site NEC	187.8	198.82	233.6	222.8	236.6	239.5
genitourinary tract						
female	184.9	198.82	233.39	221.9	236.3	239.5
male	187.9	198.82	233.6	222.9	236.6	239.5
gingiva (alveolar) (marginal)	143.9	198.89	230.0	210.4	235.1	239.0
lower	143.1	198.89	230.0	210.4	235.1	239.0
mandibular	143.1	198.89	230.0	210.4	235.1	239.0
maxillary	143.0	198.89	230.0	210.4	235.1	239.0
upper	143.0	198.89	230.0	210.4	235.1	239.0
gland, glandular (lymphatic) (system) - *see also* Neoplasm, lymph gland						
endocrine NEC	194.9	198.89	—	227.9	237.4	239.7
salivary - *see* Neoplasm, salivary, gland						
glans penis	187.2	198.82	233.5	222.1	236.6	239.5
globus pallidus	191.0	198.3	—	225.0	237.5	239.6
glomus						
coccygeal	194.6	198.89	—	227.6	237.3	239.7
jugularis	194.6	198.89	—	227.6	237.3	239.7

◄ New   ◄ᴵᴵᴵᴵ Revised   deleted Deleted   ● Use Additional Digit(s)   ▬ Omit code

	Malignant					
	Primary	Secondary	Ca in situ	Benign	Uncertain Behavior	Unspecified
Neoplasm *(Continued)*						
glosso-epiglottic fold(s)	146.4	198.89	230.0	210.6	235.1	239.0
glossopalatine fold	146.2	198.89	230.0	210.6	235.1	239.0
glossopharyngeal sulcus	146.1	198.89	230.0	210.6	235.1	239.0
glottis	161.0	197.3	231.0	212.1	235.6	239.1
gluteal region*	195.3	198.89	232.5	229.8	238.8	239.89 ◄
great vessels NEC	171.4	198.89	—	215.4	238.1	239.2
groin NEC	195.3	198.89	232.5	229.8	238.8	239.89 ◄
gum	143.9	198.89	230.0	210.4	235.1	239.0
contiguous sites	143.8	—	—	—	—	—
lower	143.1	198.89	230.0	210.4	235.1	239.0
upper	143.0	198.89	230.0	210.4	235.1	239.0
hand NEC*	195.4	198.89	232.6	229.8	238.8	239.89 ◄
head NEC*	195.0	198.89	232.4	229.8	238.8	239.89 ◄
heart	164.1	198.89	—	212.7	238.8	239.89 ◄
contiguous sites with mediastinum or thymus	164.8	—	—	—	—	—
heel NEC*	195.5	198.89	232.7	229.8	238.8	239.89 ◄
helix	173.2	198.2	232.2	216.2	238.2	239.2
hematopoietic, hemopoietic tissue NEC	202.8 ●	198.89	—	—	—	238.79
hemisphere, cerebral	191.0	198.3	—	225.0	237.5	239.6
hemorrhoidal zone	154.2	197.5	230.5	211.4	235.5	239.0
hepatic	155.2	197.7	230.8	211.5	235.3	239.0
duct (bile)	156.1	197.8	230.8	211.5	235.3	239.0
flexure (colon)	153.0	197.5	230.3	211.3	235.2	239.0
primary	155.0	—	—	—	—	—
hilus of lung	162.2	197.0	231.2	212.3	235.7	239.1
hip NEC*	195.5	198.89	232.7	229.8	238.8	239.89 ◄
hippocampus, brain	191.2	198.3	—	225.0	237.5	239.6
humerus (any part)	170.4	198.5	—	213.4	238.0	239.2
hymen	184.0	198.82	233.31	221.1	236.3	239.5
hypopharynx, hypopharyngeal NEC	148.9	198.89	230.0	210.8	235.1	239.0
contiguous sites	148.8	—	—	—	—	—
postcricoid region	148.0	198.89	230.0	210.8	235.1	239.0
posterior wall	148.3	198.89	230.0	210.8	235.1	239.0
pyriform fossa (sinus)	148.1	198.89	230.0	210.8	235.1	239.0
specified site NEC	148.8	198.89	230.0	210.8	235.1	239.0
wall	148.9	198.89	230.0	210.8	235.1	239.0
posterior	148.3	198.89	230.0	210.8	235.1	239.0
hypophysis	194.3	198.89	234.8	227.3	237.0	239.7
hypothalamus	191.0	198.3	—	225.0	237.5	239.6
ileocecum, ileocecal (coil) (junction) (valve)	153.4	197.5	230.3	211.3	235.2	239.0

◄ New   ◄ Revised   deleted Deleted   ● Use Additional Digit(s)   ▓ Omit code

	Malignant					
	Primary	Secondary	Ca in situ	Benign	Uncertain Behavior	Unspecified
Neoplasm *(Continued)*						
ileum	152.2	197.4	230.7	211.2	235.2	239.0
ilium	170.6	198.5	—	213.6	238.0	239.2
immunoproliferative NEC	203.8●	—	—	—	—	—
infraclavicular (region)*	195.1	198.89	232.5	229.8	238.8	239.89◀▥
inguinal (region)*	195.3	198.89	232.5	229.8	238.8	239.89◀▥
insula	191.0	198.3	—	225.0	237.5	239.6
insular tissue (pancreas)	157.4	197.8	230.9	211.7	235.5	239.0
brain	191.0	198.3	—	225.0	237.5	239.6
interarytenoid fold	148.2	198.89	230.0	210.8	235.1	239.0
hypopharyngeal aspect	148.2	198.89	230.0	210.8	235.1	239.0
laryngeal aspect	161.1	197.3	231.0	212.1	235.6	239.1
marginal zone	148.2	198.89	230.0	210.8	235.1	239.0
interdental papillae	143.9	198.89	230.0	210.4	235.1	239.0
lower	143.1	198.89	230.0	210.4	235.1	239.0
upper	143.0	198.89	230.0	210.4	235.1	239.0
internal						
capsule	191.0	198.3	—	225.0	237.5	239.6
os (cervix)	180.0	198.82	233.1	219.0	236.0	239.5
intervertebral cartilage or disc	170.2	198.5	—	213.2	238.0	239.2
intestine, intestinal	159.0	197.8	230.7	211.9	235.2	239.0
large	153.9	197.5	230.3	211.3	235.2	239.0
appendix	153.5	197.5	230.3	211.3	235.2	239.0
caput coli	153.4	197.5	230.3	211.3	235.2	239.0
cecum	153.4	197.5	230.3	211.3	235.2	239.0
colon	153.9	197.5	230.3	211.3	235.2	239.0
and rectum	154.0	197.5	230.4	211.4	235.2	239.0
ascending	153.6	197.5	230.3	211.3	235.2	239.0
caput	153.4	197.5	230.3	211.3	235.2	239.0
contiguous sites	153.8	—	—	—	—	—
descending	153.2	197.5	230.3	211.3	235.2	239.0
distal	153.2	197.5	230.3	211.3	235.2	239.0
left	153.2	197.5	230.3	211.3	235.2	239.0
pelvic	153.3	197.5	230.3	211.3	235.2	239.0
right	153.6	197.5	230.3	211.3	235.2	239.0
sigmoid (flexure)	153.3	197.5	230.3	211.3	235.2	239.0
transverse	153.1	197.5	230.3	211.3	235.2	239.0
contiguous sites	153.8	—	—	—	—	—
hepatic flexure	153.0	197.5	230.3	211.3	235.2	239.0
ileocecum, ileocecal (coil) (valve)	153.4	197.5	230.3	211.3	235.2	239.0
sigmoid flexure (lower) (upper)	153.3	197.5	230.3	211.3	235.2	239.0
splenic flexure	153.7	197.5	230.3	211.3	235.2	239.0

◀ New   ◀▥ Revised   ~~deleted~~ Deleted   ● Use Additional Digit(s)   ▥ Omit code

	Malignant					
	Primary	Secondary	Ca in situ	Benign	Uncertain Behavior	Unspecified
Neoplasm *(Continued)*						
intestine, intestinal *(Continued)*						
small	152.9	197.4	230.7	211.2	235.2	239.0
contiguous sites	152.8	—	—	—	—	—
duodenum	152.0	197.4	230.7	211.2	235.2	239.0
ileum	152.2	197.4	230.7	211.2	235.2	239.0
jejunum	152.1	197.4	230.7	211.2	235.2	239.0
tract NEC	159.0	197.8	230.7	211.9	235.2	239.0
intra-abdominal	195.2	198.89	234.8	229.8	238.8	239.89◄||||
intracranial NEC	191.9	198.3	—	225.0	237.5	239.6
intrahepatic (bile) duct	155.1	197.8	230.8	211.5	235.3	239.0
intraocular	190.0	198.4	234.0	224.0	238.8	239.89◄||||
intraorbital	190.1	198.4	234.0	224.1	238.8	239.89◄||||
intrasellar	194.3	198.89	234.8	227.3	237.0	239.7
intrathoracic (cavity) (organs NEC)	195.1	198.89	234.8	229.8	238.8	239.89◄||||
contiguous sites with respiratory organs	165.8	—	—	—	—	—
iris	190.0	198.4	234.0	224.0	238.8	239.89◄||||
ischiorectal (fossa)	195.3	198.89	234.8	229.8	238.8	239.89◄||||
ischium	170.6	198.5	—	213.6	238.0	239.2
island of Reil	191.0	198.3	—	225.0	237.5	239.6
islands or islets of Langerhans	157.4	197.8	230.9	211.7	235.5	239.0
isthmus uteri	182.1	198.82	233.2	219.1	236.0	239.5
jaw	195.0	198.89	234.8	229.8	238.8	239.89◄||||
bone	170.1	198.5	—	213.1	238.0	239.2
carcinoma	143.9	—	—	—	—	—
lower	143.1	—	—	—	—	—
upper	143.0	—	—	—	—	—
lower	170.1	198.5	—	213.1	238.0	239.2
upper	170.0	198.5	—	213.0	238.0	239.2
carcinoma (any type) (lower) (upper)	195.0	—	—	—	—	—
skin	173.3	198.2	232.3	216.3	238.2	239.2
soft tissues	143.9	198.89	230.0	210.4	235.1	239.0
lower	143.1	198.89	230.0	210.4	235.1	239.0
upper	143.0	198.89	230.0	210.4	235.1	239.0
jejunum	152.1	197.4	230.7	211.2	235.2	239.0
joint NEC (*see also* Neoplasm, bone)	170.9	198.5	—	213.9	238.0	239.2
acromioclavicular	170.4	198.5	—	213.4	238.0	239.2
bursa or synovial membrane - *see* Neoplasm, connective tissue						
costovertebral	170.3	198.5	—	213.3	238.0	239.2
sternocostal	170.3	198.5	—	213.3	238.0	239.2
temporomandibular	170.1	198.5	—	213.1	238.0	239.2

	Malignant			Benign	Uncertain Behavior	Unspecified
	Primary	Secondary	Ca in situ	Benign	Uncertain Behavior	Unspecified
Neoplasm *(Continued)*						
junction						
anorectal	154.8	197.5	230.7	211.4	235.5	239.0
cardioesophageal	151.0	197.8	230.2	211.1	235.2	239.0
esophagogastric	151.0	197.8	230.2	211.1	235.2	239.0
gastroesophageal	151.0	197.8	230.2	211.1	235.2	239.0
hard and soft palate	145.5	198.89	230.0	210.4	235.1	239.0
ileocecal	153.4	197.5	230.3	211.3	235.2	239.0
pelvirectal	154.0	197.5	230.4	211.4	235.2	239.0
pelviureteric	189.1	198.0	233.9	223.1	236.91	239.5
rectosigmoid	154.0	197.5	230.4	211.4	235.2	239.0
squamocolumnar, of cervix	180.8	198.82	233.1	219.0	236.0	239.5
kidney (parenchymal)	189.0	198.0	233.9	223.0	236.91	239.5
calyx	189.1	198.0	233.9	223.1	236.91	239.5
hilus	189.1	198.0	233.9	223.1	236.91	239.5
pelvis	189.1	198.0	233.9	223.1	236.91	239.5
knee NEC*	195.5	198.89	232.7	229.8	238.8	239.89◄▦
labia (skin)	184.4	198.82	233.32	221.2	236.3	239.5
majora	184.1	198.82	233.32	221.2	236.3	239.5
minora	184.2	198.82	233.32	221.2	236.3	239.5
labial - *see also* Neoplasm, lip sulcus (lower) (upper)	145.1	198.89	230.0	210.4	235.1	239.0
labium (skin)	184.4	198.82	233.32	221.2	236.3	239.5
majus	184.1	198.82	233.32	221.2	236.3	239.5
minus	184.2	198.82	233.32	221.2	236.3	239.5
lacrimal						
canaliculi	190.7	198.4	234.0	224.7	238.8	239.89◄▦
duct (nasal)	190.7	198.4	234.0	224.7	238.8	239.89◄▦
gland	190.2	198.4	234.0	224.2	238.8	239.89◄▦
punctum	190.7	198.4	234.0	224.7	238.8	239.89◄▦
sac	190.7	198.4	234.0	224.7	238.8	239.89◄▦
Langerhans, islands or islets	157.4	197.8	230.9	211.7	235.5	239.0
laryngopharynx	148.9	198.89	230.0	210.8	235.1	239.0
larynx, laryngeal NEC	161.9	197.3	231.0	212.1	235.6	239.1
aryepiglottic fold	161.1	197.3	231.0	212.1	235.6	239.1
cartilage (arytenoid) (cricoid) (cuneiform) (thyroid)	161.3	197.3	231.0	212.1	235.6	239.1
commissure (anterior) (posterior)	161.0	197.3	231.0	212.1	235.6	239.1
contiguous sites	161.8	—	—	—	—	—
extrinsic NEC	161.1	197.3	231.0	212.1	235.6	239.1
meaning hypopharynx	148.9	198.89	230.0	210.8	235.1	239.0
interarytenoid fold	161.1	197.3	231.0	212.1	235.6	239.1
intrinsic	161.0	197.3	231.0	212.1	235.6	239.1

◄ New   ◄▦ Revised   ~~deleted~~ Deleted   ● Use Additional Digit(s)   ▦ Omit code

	Malignant			Benign	Uncertain Behavior	Unspecified
	Primary	Secondary	Ca in situ			
Neoplasm *(Continued)*						
larynx, laryngeal NEC *(Continued)*						
ventricular band	161.1	197.3	231.0	212.1	235.6	239.1
leg NEC*	195.5	198.89	232.7	229.8	238.8	239.89 ◀
lens, crystalline	190.0	198.4	234.0	224.0	238.8	239.89 ◀
lid (lower) (upper)	173.1	198.2	232.1	216.1	238.2	239.2
ligament - *see also* Neoplasm, connective tissue						
broad	183.3	198.82	233.39	221.0	236.3	239.5
Mackenrodt's	183.8	198.82	233.39	221.8	236.3	239.5
non-uterine - *see* Neoplasm, connective tissue						
round	183.5	198.82	—	221.0	236.3	239.5
sacro-uterine	183.4	198.82	—	221.0	236.3	239.5
uterine	183.4	198.82	—	221.0	236.3	239.5
utero-ovarian	183.8	198.82	233.39	221.8	236.3	239.5
uterosacral	183.4	198.82	—	221.0	236.3	239.5
limb*	195.8	198.89	232.8	229.8	238.8	239.89 ◀
lower*	195.5	198.89	232.7	229.8	238.8	239.89 ◀
upper*	195.4	198.89	232.6	229.8	238.8	239.89 ◀
limbus of cornea	190.4	198.4	234.0	224.4	238.8	239.89 ◀
lingual NEC (*see also* Neoplasm, tongue)	141.9	198.89	230.0	210.1	235.1	239.0
lingula, lung	162.3	197.0	231.2	212.3	235.7	239.1
lip (external) (lipstick area) (vermillion border)	140.9	198.89	230.0	210.0	235.1	239.0
buccal aspect - *see* Neoplasm, lip, internal						
commissure	140.6	198.89	230.0	210.4	235.1	239.0
contiguous sites	140.8	—	—	—	—	---
with oral cavity or pharynx	149.8	—	—	—	—	—
frenulum - *see* Neoplasm, lip, internal						
inner aspect - *see* Neoplasm, lip, internal						
internal (buccal) (frenulum) (mucosa) (oral)	140.5	198.89	230.0	210.0	235.1	239.0
lower	140.4	198.89	230.0	210.0	235.1	239.0
upper	140.3	198.89	230.0	210.0	235.1	239.0
lower	140.1	198.89	230.0	210.0	235.1	239.0
internal (buccal) (frenulum) (mucosa) (oral)	140.4	198.89	230.0	210.0	235.1	239.0
mucosa - *see* Neoplasm, lip, internal						
oral aspect - *see* Neoplasm, lip, internal						
skin (commissure) (lower) (upper)	173.0	198.2	232.0	216.0	238.2	239.2
upper	140.0	198.89	230.0	210.0	235.1	239.0
internal (buccal) (frenulum) (mucosa) (oral)	140.3	198.89	230.0	210.0	235.1	239.0
liver	155.2	197.7	230.8	211.5	235.3	239.0
primary	155.0	—	—	—	—	---

◀ New   ◀▥ Revised   ~~deleted~~ Deleted   ● Use Additional Digit(s)   ▨ Omit code

	Malignant			Benign	Uncertain Behavior	Unspecified
	Primary	Secondary	Ca in situ			
Neoplasm *(Continued)*						
lobe						
azygos	162.3	197.0	231.2	212.3	235.7	239.1
frontal	191.1	198.3	—	225.0	237.5	239.6
lower	162.5	197.0	231.2	212.3	235.7	239.1
middle	162.4	197.0	231.2	212.3	235.7	239.1
occipital	191.4	198.3	—	225.0	237.5	239.6
parietal	191.3	198.3	—	225.0	237.5	239.6
temporal	191.2	198.3	—	225.0	237.5	239.6
upper	162.3	197.0	231.2	212.3	235.7	239.1
lumbosacral plexus	171.6	198.4	—	215.6	238.1	239.2
lung	162.9	197.0	231.2	212.3	235.7	239.1
azygos lobe	162.3	197.0	231.2	212.3	235.7	239.1
carina	162.2	197.0	231.2	212.3	235.7	239.1
contiguous sites with bronchus or trachea	162.8	—	—	—	—	—
hilus	162.2	197.0	231.2	212.3	235.7	239.1
lingula	162.3	197.0	231.2	212.3	235.7	239.1
lobe NEC	162.9	197.0	231.2	212.3	235.7	239.1
lower lobe	162.5	197.0	231.2	212.3	235.7	239.1
main bronchus	162.2	197.0	231.2	212.3	235.7	239.1
middle lobe	162.4	197.0	231.2	212.3	235.7	239.1
upper lobe	162.3	197.0	231.2	212.3	235.7	239.1
lymph, lymphatic						
channel NEC (*see also* Neoplasm, connective tissue)	171.9	198.89	—	215.9	238.1	239.2
gland (secondary)	—	196.9	—	229.0	238.8	239.89 ◄
abdominal	—	196.2	—	229.0	238.8	239.89 ◄
aortic	—	196.2	—	229.0	238.8	239.89 ◄
arm	—	196.3	—	229.0	238.8	239.89 ◄
auricular (anterior) (posterior)	—	196.0	—	229.0	238.8	239.89 ◄
axilla, axillary	—	196.3	—	229.0	238.8	239.89 ◄
brachial	—	196.3	—	229.0	238.8	239.89 ◄
bronchial	—	196.1	—	229.0	238.8	239.89 ◄
bronchopulmonary	—	196.1	—	229.0	238.8	239.89 ◄
celiac	—	196.2	—	229.0	238.8	239.89 ◄
cervical	—	196.0	—	229.0	238.8	239.89 ◄
cervicofacial	—	196.0	—	229.0	238.8	239.89 ◄
Cloquet	—	196.5	—	229.0	238.8	239.89 ◄
colic	—	196.2	—	229.0	238.8	239.89 ◄
common duct	—	196.2	—	229.0	238.8	239.89 ◄
cubital	—	196.3	—	229.0	238.8	239.89 ◄
diaphragmatic	—	196.1	—	229.0	238.8	239.89 ◄

◄ New　◄■■ Revised　deleted Deleted　● Use Additional Digit(s)　▨ Omit code

	Malignant					
	Primary	Secondary	Ca in situ	Benign	Uncertain Behavior	Unspecified
Neoplasm *(Continued)*						
lymph, lymphatic *(Continued)*						
gland *(Continued)*						
epigastric, inferior	—	196.6	—	229.0	238.8	239.89 ◀
epitrochlear	—	196.3	—	229.0	238.8	239.89 ◀
esophageal	—	196.1	—	229.0	238.8	239.89 ◀
face	—	196.0	—	229.0	238.8	239.89 ◀
femoral	—	196.5	—	229.0	238.8	239.89 ◀
gastric	—	196.2	—	229.0	238.8	239.89 ◀
groin	—	196.5	—	229.0	238.8	239.89 ◀
head	—	196.0	—	229.0	238.8	239.89 ◀
hepatic	—	196.2	—	229.0	238.8	239.89 ◀
hilar (pulmonary)	—	196.1	—	229.0	238.8	239.89 ◀
splenic	—	196.2	—	229.0	238.8	239.89 ◀
hypogastric	—	196.6	—	229.0	238.8	239.89 ◀
ileocolic	—	196.2	—	229.0	238.8	239.89 ◀
iliac	—	196.6	—	229.0	238.8	239.89 ◀
infraclavicular	—	196.3	—	229.0	238.8	239.89 ◀
inguina, inguinal	—	196.5	—	229.0	238.8	239.89 ◀
innominate	—	196.1	—	229.0	238.8	239.89 ◀
intercostal	—	196.1	—	229.0	238.8	239.89 ◀
intestinal	—	196.2	—	229.0	238.8	239.89 ◀
intrabdominal	—	196.2	—	229.0	238.8	239.89 ◀
intrapelvic	—	196.6	—	229.0	238.8	239.89 ◀
intrathoracic	—	196.1	—	229.0	238.8	239.9
jugular	—	196.0	—	229.0	238.8	239.89 ◀
leg	—	196.5	—	229.0	238.8	239.89 ◀
limb						
lower	—	196.5	—	229.0	238.8	239.89 ◀
upper	—	196.3	—	229.0	238.8	239.89 ◀
lower limb	—	196.5	—	229.0	238.8	238.9
lumbar	—	196.2	—	229.0	238.8	239.89 ◀
mandibular	—	196.0	—	229.0	238.8	239.89 ◀
mediastinal	—	196.1	—	229.0	238.8	239.89 ◀
mesenteric (inferior) (superior)	—	196.2	—	229.0	238.8	239.89 ◀
midcolic	—	196.2	—	229.0	238.8	239.89 ◀
multiple sites in categories 196.0–196.6	—	196.8	—	229.0	238.8	239.89 ◀
neck	—	196.0	—	229.0	238.8	239.89 ◀
obturator	—	196.6	—	229.0	238.8	239.89 ◀
occipital	—	196.0	—	229.0	238.8	239.89 ◀
pancreatic	—	196.2	—	229.0	238.8	239.89 ◀

◀ New   ◀▥ Revised   ~~deleted~~ Deleted   ● Use Additional Digit(s)   ▥ Omit code

	Malignant			Benign	Uncertain Behavior	Unspecified
	Primary	Secondary	Ca in situ			
Neoplasm *(Continued)*						
lymph, lymphatic *(Continued)*						
gland *(Continued)*						
para-aortic	—	196.2	—	229.0	238.8	239.89
paracervical	—	196.6	—	229.0	238.8	239.89
parametrial	—	196.6	—	229.0	238.8	239.89
parasternal	—	196.1	—	229.0	238.8	239.89
parotid	—	196.0	—	229.0	238.8	239.89
pectoral	—	196.3	—	229.0	238.8	239.89
pelvic	—	196.6	—	229.0	238.8	239.89
peri-aortic	—	196.2	—	229.0	238.8	239.89
peripancreatic	—	196.2	—	229.0	238.8	239.89
popliteal	—	196.5	—	229.0	238.8	239.89
porta hepatis	—	196.2	—	229.0	238.8	239.89
portal	—	196.2	—	229.0	238.8	239.89
preauricular	—	196.0	—	229.0	238.8	239.89
prelaryngeal	—	196.0	—	229.0	238.8	239.89
presymphysial	—	196.6	—	229.0	238.8	239.89
pretracheal	—	196.0	—	229.0	238.8	239.89
primary (any site) NEC	202.9●	—	—	—	—	—
pulmonary (hiler)	—	196.1	—	229.0	238.8	239.89
pyloric	—	196.2	—	229.0	238.8	239.89
retroperitoneal	—	196.2	—	229.0	238.8	239.89
retropharyngeal	—	196.0	—	229.0	238.8	239.89
Rosenmüller's	—	196.5	—	229.0	238.8	239.89
sacral	—	196.6	—	229.0	238.8	239.89
scalene	—	196.0	—	229.0	238.8	239.89
site NEC	—	196.9	—	229.0	238.8	239.89
splenic (hilar)	—	196.2	—	229.0	238.8	239.89
subclavicular	—	196.3	—	229.0	238.8	239.89
subinguinal	—	196.5	—	229.0	238.8	239.89
sublingual	—	196.0	—	229.0	238.8	239.89
submandibular	—	196.0	—	229.0	238.8	239.89
submaxillary	—	196.0	—	229.0	238.8	239.89
submental	—	196.0	—	229.0	238.8	239.89
subscapular	—	196.3	—	229.0	238.8	239.89
supraclavicular	—	196.0	—	229.0	238.8	239.89
thoracic	—	196.1	—	229.0	238.8	239.89
tibial	—	196.5	—	229.0	238.8	239.89
tracheal		196.1	—	229.0	238.8	239.89
tracheobronchial	—	196.1	—	229.0	238.8	239.89

◀ New   ◀◀ Revised   ~~deleted~~ Deleted   ● Use Additional Digit(s)   ▨ Omit code

	Malignant					
	Primary	Secondary	Ca in situ	Benign	Uncertain Behavior	Unspecified
Neoplasm *(Continued)*						
lymph, lymphatic *(Continued)*						
gland *(Continued)*						
upper limb	—	196.3	—	229.0	238.8	239.89 ◀
Virchow's	—	196.0	—	229.0	238.8	239.89 ◀
node - *see also* Neoplasm, lymph gland	202.9●	—	—	—	—	—
primary NEC						
vessel (*see also* Neoplasm, connective tissue)	171.9	198.89	—	215.9	238.1	239.2
Mackenrodt's ligament	183.8	198.82	233.39	221.8	236.3	239.5
malar region - *see* Neoplasm, cheek	170.0	198.5	—	213.0	238.0	239.2
mammary gland - *see* Neoplasm, breast						
mandible	170.1	198.5	—	213.1	238.0	239.2
alveolar						
mucosa	143.1	198.89	230.0	210.4	235.1	239.0
ridge or process	170.1	198.5	—	213.1	238.0	239.2
carcinoma	143.1	—	—	—	—	—
carcinoma	143.1	—	—	—	—	—
marrow (bone) NEC	202.9●	198.5	—	—	—	238.79
mastectomy site (skin)	173.5	198.2	—	—	—	—
specified as breast tissue	174.8	198.81	—	—	—	—
mastoid (air cells) (antrum) (cavity)	160.1	197.3	231.8	212.0	235.9	239.1
bone or process	170.0	198.5	—	213.0	238.0	239.2
maxilla, maxillary (superior)	170.0	198.5	—	213.0	238.0	239.2
alveolar						
mucosa	143.0	198.89	230.0	210.4	235.1	239.0
ridge or process	170.0	198.5	—	213.0	238.0	239.2
carcinoma	143.0	—	—	—	—	—
antrum	160.2	197.3	231.8	212.0	235.9	239.1
carcinoma	143.0	—	—	—	—	—
inferior - *see* Neoplasm, mandible						
sinus	160.2	197.3	231.8	212.0	235.9	239.1
meatus						
external (ear)	173.2	198.2	232.2	216.2	238.2	239.2
Meckel's diverticulum	152.3	197.4	230.7	211.2	235.2	239.0
mediastinum, mediastinal	164.9	197.1	—	212.5	235.8	239.89 ◀
anterior	164.2	197.1	—	212.5	235.8	239.89 ◀
contiguous sites with heart and thymus	164.8	—	—	—	—	—
posterior	164.3	197.1	—	212.5	235.8	239.89 ◀
medulla						
adrenal	194.0	198.7	234.8	227.0	237.2	239.7
oblongata	191.7	198.3	—	225.0	237.5	239.6

◀ New   ◀▥ Revised   ~~deleted~~ Deleted   ● Use Additional Digit(s)   ▨ Omit code

	Malignant					
	Primary	Secondary	Ca in situ	Benign	Uncertain Behavior	Unspecified
Neoplasm *(Continued)*						
meibomian gland	173.1	198.2	232.1	216.1	238.2	239.2
melanoma - *see* Melanoma						
meninges (brain) (cerebral) (cranial) (intracranial)	192.1	198.4	—	225.2	237.6	239.7
spinal (cord)	192.3	198.4	—	225.4	237.6	239.7
meniscus, knee joint (lateral) (medial)	170.7	198.5	—	213.7	238.0	239.2
mesentery, mesenteric	158.8	197.6	—	211.8	235.4	239.0
mesoappendix	158.8	197.6	—	211.8	235.4	239.0
mesocolon	158.8	197.6	—	211.8	235.4	239.0
mesopharynx - *see* Neoplasm, oropharynx						
mesosalpinx	183.3	198.82	233.39	221.0	236.3	239.5
mesovarium	183.3	198.82	233.39	221.0	236.3	239.5
metacarpus (any bone)	170.5	198.5	—	213.5	238.0	239.2
metastatic NEC - *see also* Neoplasm, by site, secondary	—	199.1	—	—	—	—
metatarsus (any bone)	170.8	198.5	—	213.8	238.0	239.2
midbrain	191.7	198.3	—	225.0	237.5	239.6
milk duct - *see* Neoplasm, breast						
mons						
pubis	184.4	198.82	233.32	221.2	236.3	239.5
veneris	184.4	198.82	233.32	221.2	236.3	239.5
motor tract	192.9	198.4	—	225.9	237.9	239.7
brain	191.9	198.3	—	225.0	237.5	239.6
spinal	192.2	198.3	—	225.3	237.5	239.7
mouth	145.9	198.89	230.0	210.4	235.1	239.0
contiguous sites	145.8	—	—	—	—	—
floor	144.9	198.89	230.0	210.3	235.1	239.0
anterior portion	144.0	198.89	230.0	210.3	235.1	239.0
contiguous sites	144.8	—	—	—	—	—
lateral portion	144.1	198.89	230.0	210.3	235.1	239.0
roof	145.5	198.89	230.0	210.4	235.1	239.0
specified part NEC	145.8	198.89	230.0	210.4	235.1	239.0
vestibule	145.1	198.89	230.0	210.4	235.1	239.0
mucosa						
alveolar (ridge or process)	143.9	198.89	230.0	210.4	235.1	239.0
lower	143.1	198.89	230.0	210.4	235.1	239.0
upper	143.0	198.89	230.0	210.4	235.1	239.0
buccal	145.0	198.89	230.0	210.4	235.1	239.0
cheek	145.0	198.89	230.0	210.4	235.1	239.0
lip - *see* Neoplasm, lip, internal						
nasal	160.0	197.3	231.8	212.0	235.9	239.1
oral	145.0	198.89	230.0	210.4	235.1	239.0

◀ New   ◀▥ Revised   deleted Deleted   ● Use Additional Digit(s)   ▨ Omit code

	Malignant					
	Primary	Secondary	Ca in situ	Benign	Uncertain Behavior	Unspecified
Neoplasm *(Continued)*						
Müllerian duct						
female	184.8	198.82	233.39	221.8	236.3	239.5
male	187.8	198.82	233.6	222.8	236.6	239.5
multiple sites NEC	199.0	199.0	234.9	229.9	238.9	199.0
muscle - *see also* Neoplasm, connective tissue extraocular	190.1	198.4	234.0	224.1	238.8	239.89◀▥
myocardium	164.1	198.89	—	212.7	238.8	239.89◀▥
myometrium	182.0	198.82	233.2	219.1	236.0	239.5
myopericardium	164.1	198.89	—	212.7	238.8	239.89◀▥
nabothian gland (follicle)	180.0	198.82	233.1	219.0	236.0	239.5
nail	173.9	198.2	232.9	216.9	238.2	239.2
finger	173.6	198.2	232.6	216.6	238.2	239.2
toe	173.7	198.2	232.7	216.7	238.2	239.2
nares, naris (anterior) (posterior)	160.0	197.3	231.8	212.0	235.9	239.1
nasal - *see* Neoplasm, nose						
nasolabial groove	173.3	198.2	232.3	216.3	238.2	239.2
nasolacrimal duct	190.7	198.4	234.0	224.7	238.8	239.89◀▥
nasopharynx, nasopharyngeal	147.9	198.89	230.0	210.7	235.1	239.0
contiguous sites	147.8	—	—	—	—	—
floor	147.3	198.89	230.0	210.7	235.1	239.0
roof	147.0	198.89	230.0	210.7	235.1	239.0
specified site NEC	147.8	198.89	230.0	210.7	235.1	239.0
wall	147.9	198.89	230.0	210.7	235.1	239.0
anterior	147.3	198.89	230.0	210.7	235.1	239.0
lateral	147.2	198.89	230.0	210.7	235.1	239.0
posterior	147.1	198.89	230.0	210.7	235.1	239.0
superior	147.0	198.89	230.0	210.7	235.1	239.0
nates	173.5	198.2	232.5	216.5	238.2	239.2
neck NEC*	195.0	198.89	234.8	229.8	238.8	239.89◀▥
nerve (autonomic) (ganglion) (parasympathetic) (peripheral) (sympathetic) - *see also* Neoplasm, connective tissue						
abducens	192.0	198.4	—	225.1	237.9	239.7
accessory (spinal)	192.0	198.4	—	225.1	237.9	239.7
acoustic	192.0	198.4	—	225.1	237.9	239.7
auditory	192.0	198.4	—	225.1	237.9	239.7
brachial	171.2	198.89	—	215.2	238.1	239.2
cranial (any)	192.0	198.4	—	225.1	237.9	239.7
facial	192.0	198.4	—	225.1	237.9	239.7
femoral	171.3	198.89	—	215.3	238.1	239.2
glossopharyngeal	192.0	198.4	—	225.1	237.9	239.7
hypoglossal	192.0	198.4	—	225.1	237.9	239.7

	Malignant					
	Primary	Secondary	Ca in situ	Benign	Uncertain Behavior	Unspecified
Neoplasm *(Continued)*						
nerve *(Continued)*						
intercostal	171.4	198.89	—	215.4	238.1	239.2
lumbar	171.7	198.89	—	215.7	238.1	239.2
median	171.2	198.89	—	215.2	238.1	239.2
obturator	171.3	198.89	—	215.3	238.1	239.2
oculomotor	192.0	198.4	—	225.1	237.9	239.7
olfactory	192.0	198.4	—	225.1	237.9	239.7
optic	192.0	198.4	—	225.1	237.9	239.7
peripheral NEC	171.9	198.89	—	215.9	238.1	239.2
radial	171.2	198.89	—	215.2	238.1	239.2
sacral	171.6	198.89	—	215.6	238.1	239.2
sciatic	171.3	198.89	—	215.3	238.1	239.2
spinal NEC	171.9	198.89	—	215.9	238.1	239.2
trigeminal	192.0	198.4	—	225.1	237.9	239.7
trochlear	192.0	198.4	—	225.1	237.9	239.7
ulnar	171.2	198.89	—	215.2	238.1	239.2
vagus	192.0	198.4	—	225.1	237.9	239.7
nervous system (central) NEC	192.9	198.4	—	225.9	237.9	239.7
autonomic NEC	171.9	198.89	—	215.9	238.1	239.2
brain - *see also* Neoplasm, brain membrane or meninges	192.1	198.4	—	225.2	237.6	239.7
contiguous sites	192.8	—	—	—	—	—
parasympathetic NEC	171.9	198.89	—	215.9	238.1	239.2
sympathetic NEC	171.9	198.89	—	215.9	238.1	239.2
nipple (female)	174.0	198.81	233.0	217	238.3	239.3
male	175.0	198.81	233.0	217	238.3	239.3
nose, nasal	195.0	198.89	234.8	229.8	238.8	239.89 ◀
ala (external)	173.3	198.2	232.3	216.3	238.2	239.2
bone	170.0	198.5	—	213.0	238.0	239.2
cartilage	160.0	197.3	231.8	212.0	235.9	239.1
cavity	160.0	197.3	231.8	212.0	235.9	239.1
contiguous sites with accessory sinuses or middle ear	160.8	—	—	—	—	—
choana	147.3	198.89	230.0	210.7	235.1	239.0
external (skin)	173.3	198.2	232.3	216.3	238.2	239.2
fossa	160.0	197.3	231.8	212.0	235.9	239.1
internal	160.0	197.3	231.8	212.0	235.9	239.1
mucosa	160.0	197.3	231.8	212.0	235.9	239.1
septum	160.0	197.3	231.8	212.0	235.9	239.1
posterior margin	147.3	198.89	230.0	210.7	235.1	239.0
sinus - *see* Neoplasm, sinus						
skin	173.3	198.2	232.3	216.3	238.2	239.2

◀ New　◀▥ Revised　deleted Deleted　● Use Additional Digit(s)　▨ Omit code

	Malignant					
	Primary	Secondary	Ca in situ	Benign	Uncertain Behavior	Unspecified
Neoplasm *(Continued)*						
nose, nasal *(Continued)*						
turbinate (mucosa)	160.0	197.3	231.8	212.0	235.9	239.1
bone	170.0	198.5	—	213.0	238.0	239.2
vestibule	160.0	197.3	231.8	212.0	235.9	239.1
nostril	160.0	197.3	231.8	212.0	235.9	239.1
nucleus pulposus	170.2	198.5	—	213.2	238.0	230.2
occipital						
bone	170.0	198.5	—	213.0	238.0	239.2
lobe or pole, brain	191.4	198.3	—	225.0	237.5	239.6
odontogenic - *see* Neoplasm, jaw bone						
oesophagus - *see* Neoplasm, esophagus						
olfactory nerve or bulb	192.0	198.4	—	225.1	237.9	239.7
olive (brain)	191.7	198.3	—	225.0	237.5	239.6
omentum	158.8	197.6	—	211.8	235.4	239.0
operculum (brain)	191.0	198.3	—	225.0	237.5	239.6
optic nerve, chiasm, or tract	192.0	198.4	—	225.1	237.9	239.7
oral (cavity)	145.9	198.89	230.0	210.4	235.1	239.0
contiguous sites with lip or pharynx	149.8	—	—	—	—	—
ill-defined	149.9	198.89	230.0	210.4	235.1	239.0
mucosa	145.9	198.89	230.0	210.4	235.1	239.0
orbit	190.1	198.4	234.0	224.1	238.8	239.89 ◀
bone	170.0	198.5	—	213.0	238.0	239.2
eye	190.1	198.4	234.0	224.1	238.8	239.89 ◀
soft parts	190.1	198.4	234.0	224.1	238.8	239.89 ◀
organ of Zuckerkandl	194.6	198.89	—	227.6	237.3	239.7
oropharynx	146.9	198.89	230.0	210.6	235.1	239.0
branchial cleft (vestige)	146.8	198.89	230.0	210.6	235.1	239.0
contiguous sites	146.8	—	—	—	—	—
junctional region	146.5	198.89	230.0	210.6	235.1	239.0
lateral wall	146.6	198.89	230.0	210.6	235.1	239.0
pillars of fauces	146.2	198.89	230.0	210.6	235.1	239.0
posterior wall	146.7	198.89	230.0	210.6	235.1	239.0
specified part NEC	146.8	198.89	230.0	210.6	235.1	239.0
vallecula	146.3	198.89	230.0	210.6	235.1	239.0
os						
external	180.1	198.82	233.1	219.0	236.0	239.5
internal	180.0	198.82	233.1	219.0	236.0	239.5
ovary	183.0	198.6	233.39	220	236.2	239.5
oviduct	183.2	198.82	233.39	221.0	236.3	239.5

	Malignant					
	Primary	Secondary	Ca in situ	Benign	Uncertain Behavior	Unspecified
Neoplasm *(Continued)*						
palate	145.5	198.89	230.0	210.4	235.1	239.0
hard	145.2	198.89	230.0	210.4	235.1	239.0
junction of hard and soft palate	145.5	198.89	230.0	210.4	235.1	239.0
soft	145.3	198.89	230.0	210.4	235.1	239.0
nasopharyngeal surface	147.3	198.89	230.0	210.7	235.1	239.0
posterior surface	147.3	198.89	230.0	210.7	235.1	239.0
superior surface	147.3	198.89	230.0	210.7	235.1	239.0
palatoglossal arch	146.2	198.89	230.0	210.6	235.1	239.0
palatopharyngeal arch	146.2	198.89	230.0	210.6	235.1	239.0
pallium	191.0	198.3	—	225.0	237.5	239.6
palpebra	173.1	198.2	232.1	216.1	238.2	239.2
pancreas	157.9	197.8	230.9	211.6	235.5	239.0
body	157.1	197.8	230.9	211.6	235.5	239.0
contiguous sites	157.8	—	—	—	—	—
duct (of Santorini) (of Wirsung)	157.3	197.8	230.9	211.6	235.5	239.0
ectopic tissue	157.8	197.8				
head	157.0	197.8	230.9	211.6	235.5	239.0
islet cells	157.4	197.8	230.9	211.7	235.5	239.0
neck	157.8	197.8	230.9	211.6	235.5	239.0
tail	157.2	197.8	230.9	211.6	235.5	239.0
para-aortic body	194.6	198.89	—	227.6	237.3	239.7
paraganglion NEC	194.6	198.89	—	227.6	237.3	239.7
parametrium	183.4	198.82	—	221.0	236.3	239.5
paranephric	158.0	197.6	—	211.8	235.4	239.0
pararectal	195.3	198.89	—	229.8	238.8	239.89◀▥
parasagittal (region)	195.0	198.89	234.8	229.8	238.8	239.89◀▥
parasellar	192.9	198.4	—	225.9	237.9	239.7
parathyroid (gland)	194.1	198.89	234.8	227.1	237.4	239.7
paraurethral	195.3	198.89	—	229.8	238.8	239.89◀▥
gland	189.4	198.1	233.9	223.89	236.99	239.5
paravaginal	195.3	198.89	—	229.8	238.8	239.89◀▥
parenchyma, kidney	189.0	198.0	233.9	223.0	236.91	239.5
parietal						
bone	170.0	198.5	—	213.0	238.0	239.2
lobe, brain	191.3	198.3	—	225.0	237.5	239.6
paroophoron	183.3	198.82	233.39	221.0	236.3	239.5
parotid (duct) (gland)	142.0	198.89	230.0	210.2	235.0	239.0
parovarium	183.3	198.82	233.39	221.0	236.3	239.5
patella	170.8	198.5	—	213.8	238.0	239.2
peduncle, cerebral	191.7	198.3	—	225.0	237.5	239.6

◀ New   ◀▥ Revised   ~~deleted~~ Deleted   ● Use Additional Digit(s)   ▬ Omit code

	Malignant					
	Primary	Secondary	Ca in situ	Benign	Uncertain Behavior	Unspecified
Neoplasm *(Continued)*						
pelvirectal junction	154.0	197.5	230.4	211.4	235.2	239.0
pelvis, pelvic	195.3	198.89	234.8	229.8	238.8	239.89◄
bone	170.6	198.5	—	213.6	238.0	239.2
floor	195.3	198.89	234.8	229.8	238.8	239.89◄
renal	189.1	198.0	233.9	223.1	236.91	239.5
viscera	195.3	198.89	234.8	229.8	238.8	239.89◄
wall	195.3	198.89	234.8	229.8	238.8	239.89◄
pelvo-abdominal	195.8	198.89	234.8	229.8	238.8	239.89◄
penis	187.4	198.82	233.5	222.1	236.6	239.5
body	187.3	198.82	233.5	222.1	236.6	239.5
corpus (cavernosum)	187.3	198.82	233.5	222.1	236.6	239.5
glans	187.2	198.82	233.5	222.1	236.6	239.5
skin NEC	187.4	198.82	233.5	222.1	236.6	239.5
periadrenal (tissue)	158.0	197.6	—	211.8	235.4	239.0
perianal (skin)	173.5	198.2	232.5	216.5	238.2	239.2
pericardium	164.1	198.89	—	212.7	238.8	239.89◄
perinephric	158.0	197.6	—	211.8	235.4	239.0
perineum	195.3	198.89	234.8	229.8	238.8	239.89◄
periodontal tissue NEC	143.9	198.89	230.0	210.4	235.1	239.0
periosteum - *see* Neoplasm, bone						
peripancreatic	158.0	197.6	—	211.8	235.4	239.0
peripheral nerve NEC	171.9	198.89	—	215.9	238.1	239.2
perirectal (tissue)	195.3	198.89	—	229.8	238.8	239.89◄
perirenal (tissue)	158.0	197.6	—	211.8	235.4	239.0
peritoneum, peritoneal (cavity)	158.9	197.6	—	211.8	235.4	239.0
contiguous sites	158.8	—	—	—	—	—
with digestive organs	159.8	—	—	—	—	—
parietal	158.8	197.6	—	211.8	235.4	239.0
pelvic	158.8	197.6	—	211.8	235.4	239.0
specified part NEC	158.8	197.6	—	211.8	235.4	239.0
peritonsillar (tissue)	195.0	198.89	234.8	229.8	238.8	239.89◄
periurethral tissue	195.3	198.89	—	229.8	238.8	239.89◄
phalanges	170.9	198.5	—	213.9	238.0	239.2
foot	170.8	198.5	—	213.8	238.0	239.2
hand	170.5	198.5	—	213.5	238.0	239.2
pharynx, pharyngeal	149.0	198.89	230.0	210.9	235.1	239.0
bursa	147.1	198.89	230.0	210.7	235.1	239.0
fornix	147.3	198.89	230.0	210.7	235.1	239.0
recess	147.2	198.89	230.0	210.7	235.1	239.0
region	149.0	198.89	230.0	210.9	235.1	239.0

◄ New   ◄▥ Revised   deleted Deleted   ● Use Additional Digit(s)   ▥ Omit code

	Malignant			Benign	Uncertain Behavior	Unspecified
	Primary	Secondary	Ca in situ	Benign	Uncertain Behavior	Unspecified
Neoplasm *(Continued)*						
pharynx, pharyngeal *(Continued)*						
tonsil	147.1	198.89	230.0	210.7	235.1	239.0
wall (lateral) (posterior)	149.0	198.89	230.0	210.9	235.1	239.0
pia mater (cerebral) (cranial)	192.1	198.4	—	225.2	237.6	239.7
spinal	192.3	198.4	—	225.4	237.6	239.7
pillars of fauces	146.2	198.89	230.0	210.6	235.1	239.0
pineal (body) (gland)	194.4	198.89	234.8	227.4	237.1	239.7
pinna (ear) NEC	173.2	198.2	232.2	216.2	238.2	239.2
cartilage	171.0	198.89	—	215.0	238.1	239.2
piriform fossa or sinus	148.1	198.89	230.0	210.8	235.1	239.0
pituitary (body) (fossa) (gland) (lobe)	194.3	198.89	234.8	227.3	237.0	239.7
placenta	181	198.82	233.2	219.8	236.1	239.5
pleura, pleural (cavity)	163.9	197.2	—	212.4	235.8	239.1
contiguous sites	163.8	—	—	—	—	—
parietal	163.0	197.2	—	212.4	235.8	239.1
visceral	163.1	197.2	—	212.4	235.8	239.1
plexus						
brachial	171.2	198.89	—	215.2	238.1	239.2
cervical	171.0	198.89	—	215.0	238.1	239.2
choroid	191.5	198.3	—	225.0	237.5	239.6
lumbosacral	171.6	198.89	—	215.6	238.1	239.2
sacral	171.6	198.89	—	215.6	238.1	239.2
pluri-endocrine	194.8	198.89	234.8	227.8	237.4	239.7
pole						
frontal	191.1	198.3	—	225.0	237.5	239.6
occipital	191.4	198.3	—	225.0	237.5	239.6
pons (varolii)	191.7	198.3	—	225.0	237.5	239.6
popliteal fossa or space*	195.5	198.89	234.8	229.8	238.8	239.89◄
postcricoid (region)	148.0	198.89	230.0	210.8	235.1	239.0
posterior fossa (cranial)	191.9	198.3	—	225.0	237.5	239.6
postnasal space	147.9	198.89	230.0	210.7	235.1	239.0
prepuce	187.1	198.82	233.5	222.1	236.6	239.5
prepylorus	151.1	197.8	230.2	211.1	235.2	239.0
presacral (region)	195.3	198.89	—	229.8	238.8	239.89◄
prostate (gland)	185	198.82	233.4	222.2	236.5	239.5
utricle	189.3	198.1	233.9	223.81	236.99	239.5
pterygoid fossa	171.0	198.89	—	215.0	238.1	239.2
pubic bone	170.6	198.5	—	213.6	238.0	239.2
pudenda, pudendum (female)	184.4	198.82	233.32	221.2	236.3	239.5
pulmonary	162.9	197.0	231.2	212.3	235.7	239.1

◄ New   ◄▦ Revised   ~~deleted~~ Deleted   ● Use Additional Digit(s)   ▓ Omit code

	Malignant					
	Primary	Secondary	Ca in situ	Benign	Uncertain Behavior	Unspecified
Neoplasm *(Continued)*						
putamen	191.0	198.3	—	225.0	237.5	239.6
pyloric						
antrum	151.2	197.8	230.2	211.1	235.2	239.0
canal	151.1	197.8	230.2	211.1	235.2	239.0
pylorus	151.1	197.8	230.2	211.1	235.2	239.0
pyramid (brain)	191.7	198.3	—	225.0	237.5	239.6
pyriform fossa or sinus	148.1	198.89	230.0	210.8	235.1	239.0
radius (any part)	170.4	198.5	—	213.4	238.0	239.2
Rathke's pouch	194.3	198.89	234.8	227.3	237.0	239.7
rectosigmoid (colon) (junction)	154.0	197.5	230.4	211.4	235.2	239.0
contiguous sites with anus or rectum	154.8	—	—	—	—	—
rectouterine pouch	158.8	197.6	—	211.8	235.4	239.0
rectovaginal septum or wall	195.3	198.89	234.8	229.8	238.8	239.89◄
rectovesical septum	195.3	198.89	234.8	229.8	238.8	239.89◄
rectum (ampulla)	154.1	197.5	230.4	211.4	235.2	239.0
and colon	154.0	197.5	230.4	211.4	235.2	239.0
contiguous sites with anus or rectosigmoid junction	154.8	—	—	—	—	—
renal	189.0	198.0	233.9	223.0	236.91	239.5
calyx	189.1	198.0	233.9	223.1	236.91	239.5
hilus	189.1	198.0	233.9	223.1	236.91	239.5
parenchyma	189.0	198.0	233.9	223.0	236.91	239.5
pelvis	189.1	198.0	233.9	223.1	236.91	239.5
respiratory						
organs or system NEC	165.9	197.3	231.9	212.9	235.9	239.1
contiguous sites with intrathoracic organs	165.8	—	—	—	—	—
specified sites NEC	165.8	197.3	231.8	212.8	235.9	239.1
tract NEC	165.9	197.3	231.9	212.9	235.9	239.1
upper	165.0	197.3	231.9	212.9	235.9	239.1
retina	190.5	198.4	234.0	224.5	238.8	239.81◄
retrobulbar	190.1	198.4	—	224.1	238.8	239.89◄
retrocecal	158.0	197.6	—	211.8	235.4	239.0
retromolar (area) (triangle) (trigone)	145.6	198.89	230.0	210.4	235.1	239.0
retro-orbital	195.0	198.89	234.8	229.8	238.8	239.89◄
retroperitoneal (space) (tissue)	158.0	197.6	—	211.8	235.4	239.0
contiguous sites	158.8	—	—	—	—	—
retroperitoneum	158.0	197.6	—	211.8	235.4	239.0
contiguous sites	158.8	—	—	—	—	—
retropharyngeal	149.0	198.89	230.0	210.9	235.1	239.0
retrovesical (septum)	195.3	198.89	234.8	229.8	238.8	239.89◄
rhinencephalon	191.0	198.3	—	225.0	237.5	239.6

	Malignant			Benign	Uncertain Behavior	Unspecified
	Primary	Secondary	Ca in situ			
Neoplasm (Continued)						
rib	170.3	198.5	—	213.3	238.0	239.2
Rosenmüller's fossa	147.2	198.89	230.0	210.7	235.1	239.0
round ligament	183.5	198.82	—	221.0	236.3	239.5
sacrococcyx, sacrococcygeal	170.6	198.5	—	213.6	238.0	239.2
region	195.3	198.89	234.8	229.8	238.8	239.89 ◄
sacrouterine ligament	183.4	198.82	—	221.0	236.3	239.5
sacrum, sacral (vertebra)	170.6	198.5	—	213.6	238.0	239.2
salivary gland or duct (major)	142.9	198.89	230.0	210.2	235.0	239.0
contiguous sites	142.8	—	—	—	—	—
minor NEC	145.9	198.89	230.0	210.4	235.1	239.0
parotid	142.0	198.89	230.0	210.2	235.0	239.0
pluriglandular	142.8	198.89	230.0	210.2	235.0	239.0
sublingual	142.2	198.89	230.0	210.2	235.0	239.0
submandibular	142.1	198.89	230.0	210.2	235.0	239.0
submaxillary	142.1	198.89	230.0	210.2	235.0	239.0
salpinx (uterine)	183.2	198.82	233.39	221.0	236.3	239.5
Santorini's duct	157.3	197.8	230.9	211.6	235.5	239.0
scalp	173.4	198.2	232.4	216.4	238.2	239.2
scapula (any part)	170.4	198.5	—	213.4	238.0	239.2
scapular region	195.1	198.89	234.8	229.8	238.8	239.89 ◄
scar NEC (*see also* Neoplasm, skin)	173.9	198.2	232.9	216.9	238.2	239.2
sciatic nerve	171.3	198.89	—	215.3	238.1	239.2
sclera	190.0	198.4	234.0	224.0	238.8	239.89 ◄
scrotum (skin)	187.7	198.82	233.6	222.4	236.6	239.5
sebaceous gland - *see* Neoplasm, skin						
sella turcica	194.3	198.89	234.8	227.3	237.0	239.7
bone	170.0	198.5	—	213.0	238.0	239.2
semilunar cartilage (knee)	170.7	198.5	—	213.7	238.0	239.2
seminal vesicle	187.8	198.82	233.6	222.8	236.6	239.5
septum						
nasal	160.0	197.3	231.8	212.0	235.9	239.1
posterior margin	147.3	198.89	230.0	210.7	235.1	239.0
rectovaginal	195.3	198.89	234.8	229.8	238.8	239.89 ◄
rectovesical	195.3	198.89	234.8	229.8	238.8	239.89 ◄
urethrovaginal	184.9	198.82	233.39	221.9	236.3	239.5
vesicovaginal	184.9	198.82	233.39	221.9	236.3	239.5
shoulder NEC*	195.4	198.89	232.6	229.8	238.8	239.89 ◄
sigmoid flexure (lower) (upper)	153.3	197.5	230.3	211.3	235.2	239.0
sinus (accessory)	160.9	197.3	231.8	212.0	235.9	239.1
bone (any)	170.0	198.5	—	213.0	238.0	239.2

◄ New   ◄▬ Revised   ~~deleted~~ Deleted   ● Use Additional Digit(s)   ▬ Omit code

	Malignant					
	Primary	Secondary	Ca in situ	Benign	Uncertain Behavior	Unspecified
Neoplasm *(Continued)*						
sinus *(Continued)*						
contiguous sites with middle ear or nasal cavities	160.8	—	—	—	—	—
ethmoidal	160.3	197.3	231.8	212.0	235.9	239.1
frontal	160.4	197.3	231.8	212.0	235.9	239.1
maxillary	160.2	197.3	231.8	212.0	235.9	239.1
nasal, paranasal NEC	160.9	197.3	231.8	212.0	235.9	239.1
pyriform	148.1	198.89	230.0	210.8	235.1	239.0
sphenoidal	160.5	197.3	231.8	212.0	235.9	239.1
skeleton, skeletal NEC	170.9	198.5	—	213.9	238.0	239.2
Skene's gland	189.4	198.1	233.9	223.89	236.99	239.5
skin NEC	173.9	198.2	232.9	216.9	238.2	239.2
abdominal wall	173.5	198.2	232.5	216.5	238.2	239.2
ala nasi	173.3	198.2	232.3	216.3	238.2	239.2
ankle	173.7	198.2	232.7	216.7	238.2	239.2
antecubital space	173.6	198.2	232.6	216.6	238.2	239.2
anus	173.5	198.2	232.5	216.5	238.2	239.2
arm	173.6	198.2	232.6	216.6	238.2	239.2
auditory canal (external)	173.2	198.2	232.2	216.2	238.2	239.2
auricle (ear)	173.2	198.2	232.2	216.2	238.2	239.2
auricular canal (external)	173.2	198.2	232.2	216.2	238.2	239.2
axilla, axillary fold	173.5	198.2	232.5	216.5	238.2	239.2
back	173.5	198.2	232.5	216.5	238.2	239.2
breast	173.5	198.2	232.5	216.5	238.2	239.2
brow	173.3	198.2	232.3	216.3	238.2	239.2
buttock	173.5	198.2	232.5	216.5	238.2	239.2
calf	173.7	198.2	232.7	216.7	238.2	239.2
canthus (eye) (inner) (outer)	173.1	198.2	232.1	216.1	238.2	239.2
cervical region	173.4	198.2	232.4	216.4	238.2	239.2
cheek (external)	173.3	198.2	232.3	216.3	238.2	239.2
chest (wall)	173.5	198.2	232.5	216.5	238.2	239.2
chin	173.3	198.2	232.3	216.3	238.2	239.2
clavicular area	173.5	198.2	232.5	216.5	238.2	239.2
clitoris	184.3	198.82	233.32	221.2	236.3	239.5
columnella	173.3	198.2	232.3	216.3	238.2	239.2
concha	173.2	198.2	232.2	216.2	238.2	239.2
contiguous sites	173.8	—	—	—	—	—
ear (external)	173.2	198.2	232.2	216.2	238.2	239.2
elbow	173.6	198.2	232.6	216.6	238.2	239.2
eyebrow	173.3	198.2	232.3	216.3	238.2	239.2
eyelid	173.1	198.2	232.1	216.1	238.2	239.2

◀ New   ◀ⅢⅢ Revised   deleted Deleted   ● Use Additional Digit(s)   ▨ Omit code

	Malignant					
	Primary	**Secondary**	**Ca in situ**	**Benign**	**Uncertain Behavior**	**Unspecified**
Neoplasm *(Continued)*						
skin NEC *(Continued)*						
face NEC	173.3	198.2	232.3	216.3	238.2	239.2
female genital organs (external)	184.4	198.82	233.30	221.2	236.3	239.5
clitoris	184.3	198.82	233.32	221.2	236.3	239.5
labium NEC	184.4	198.82	233.32	221.2	236.3	239.5
majus	184.1	198.82	233.32	221.2	236.3	239.5
minus	184.2	198.82	233.32	221.2	236.3	239.5
pudendum	184.4	198.82	233.32	221.2	236.3	239.5
vulva	184.4	198.82	233.32	221.2	236.3	239.5
finger	173.6	198.2	232.6	216.6	238.2	239.2
flank	173.5	198.2	232.5	216.5	238.2	239.2
foot	173.7	198.2	232.7	216.7	238.2	239.2
forearm	173.6	198.2	232.6	216.6	238.2	239.2
forehead	173.3	198.2	232.3	216.3	238.2	239.2
glabella	173.3	198.2	232.3	216.3	238.2	239.2
gluteal region	173.5	198.2	232.5	216.5	238.2	239.2
groin	173.5	198.2	232.5	216.5	238.2	239.2
hand	173.6	198.2	232.6	216.6	238.2	239.2
head NEC	173.4	198.2	232.4	216.4	238.2	239.2
heel	173.7	198.2	232.7	216.7	238.2	239.2
helix	173.2	198.2	232.2	216.2	238.2	239.2
hip	173.7	198.2	232.7	216.7	238.2	239.2
infraclavicular region	173.5	198.2	232.5	216.5	238.2	239.2
inguinal region	173.5	198.2	232.5	216.5	238.2	239.2
jaw	173.3	198.2	232.3	216.3	238.2	239.2
knee	173.7	198.2	232.7	216.7	238.2	239.2
labia						
majora	184.1	198.82	233.32	221.2	236.3	239.5
minora	184.2	198.82	233.32	221.2	236.3	239.5
leg	173.7	198.2	232.7	216.7	238.2	239.2
lid (lower) (upper)	173.1	198.2	232.1	216.1	238.2	239.2
limb NEC	173.9	198.2	232.9	216.9	238.2	239.5
lower	173.7	198.2	232.7	216.7	238.2	239.2
upper	173.6	198.2	232.6	216.6	238.2	239.2
lip (lower) (upper)	173.0	198.2	232.0	216.0	238.2	239.2
male genital organs	187.9	198.82	233.6	222.9	236.6	239.5
penis	187.4	198.82	233.5	222.1	236.6	239.5
prepuce	187.1	198.82	233.5	222.1	236.6	239.5
scrotum	187.7	198.82	233.6	222.4	236.6	239.5

◄ New   ◄||| Revised   ~~deleted~~ Deleted   ● Use Additional Digit(s)   ▨ Omit code

| | Malignant | | | | | |
	Primary	Secondary	Ca in situ	Benign	Uncertain Behavior	Unspecified
Neoplasm *(Continued)*						
skin NEC *(Continued)*						
mastectomy site	173.5	198.2	—	—	—	—
specified as breast tissue	174.8	198.81	—	—	—	—
meatus, acoustic (external)	173.2	198.2	232.2	216.2	238.2	239.2
nates	173.5	198.2	232.5	216.5	238.2	239.2
neck	173.4	198.2	232.4	216.4	238.2	239.2
nose (external)	173.3	198.2	232.3	216.3	238.2	239.2
palm	173.6	198.2	232.6	216.6	238.2	239.2
palpebra	173.1	198.2	232.1	216.1	238.2	239.2
penis NEC	187.4	198.82	233.5	222.1	236.6	239.5
perianal	173.5	198.2	232.5	216.5	238.2	239.2
perineum	173.5	198.2	232.5	216.5	238.2	239.2
pinna	173.2	198.2	232.2	216.2	238.2	239.2
plantar	173.7	198.2	232.7	216.7	238.2	239.2
popliteal fossa or space	173.7	198.2	232.7	216.7	238.2	239.2
prepuce	187.1	198.82	233.5	222.1	236.6	239.5
pubes	173.5	198.2	232.5	216.5	238.2	239.2
sacrococcygeal region	173.5	198.2	232.5	216.5	238.2	239.2
scalp	173.4	198.2	232.4	216.4	238.2	239.2
scapular region	173.5	198.2	232.5	216.5	238.2	239.2
scrotum	187.7	198.82	233.6	222.4	236.6	239.5
shoulder	173.6	198.2	232.6	216.6	238.2	239.2
sole (foot)	173.7	198.2	232.7	216.7	238.2	239.2
specified sites NEC	173.8	198.2	232.8	216.8	232.8	239.2
submammary fold	173.5	198.2	232.5	216.5	238.2	239.2
supraclavicular region	173.4	198.2	232.4	216.4	238.2	239.2
temple	173.3	198.2	232.3	216.3	238.2	239.2
thigh	173.7	198.2	232.7	216.7	238.2	239.2
thoracic wall	173.5	198.2	232.5	216.5	238.2	239.2
thumb	173.6	198.2	232.6	216.6	238.2	239.2
toe	173.7	198.2	232.7	216.7	238.2	239.2
tragus	173.2	198.2	232.2	216.2	238.2	239.2
trunk	173.5	198.2	232.5	216.5	238.2	239.2
umbilicus	173.5	198.2	232.5	216.5	238.2	239.2
vulva	184.4	198.82	233.32	221.2	236.3	239.5
wrist	173.6	198.2	232.6	216.6	238.2	239.2
skull	170.0	198.5	—	213.0	238.0	239.2
soft parts or tissues - *see* Neoplasm, connective tissue						
specified site NEC	195.8	198.89	234.8	229.8	238.8	239.89 ◀

	Malignant					
	Primary	Secondary	Ca in situ	Benign	Uncertain Behavior	Unspecified
Neoplasm *(Continued)*						
spermatic cord	187.6	198.82	233.6	222.8	236.6	239.5
sphenoid	160.5	197.3	231.8	212.0	235.9	239.1
bone	170.0	198.5	—	213.0	238.0	239.2
sinus	160.5	197.3	231.8	212.0	235.9	239.1
sphincter						
anal	154.2	197.5	230.5	211.4	235.5	239.0
of Oddi	156.1	197.8	230.8	211.5	235.3	239.0
spine, spinal (column)	170.2	198.5	—	213.2	238.0	239.2
bulb	191.7	198.3	—	225.0	237.5	239.6
coccyx	170.6	198.5	—	213.6	238.0	239.2
cord (cervical) (lumbar) (sacral) (thoracic)	192.2	198.3	—	225.3	237.5	239.7
dura mater	192.3	198.4	—	225.4	237.6	239.7
lumbosacral	170.2	198.5	—	213.2	238.0	239.2
membrane	192.3	198.4	—	225.4	237.6	239.7
meninges	192.3	198.4	—	225.4	237.6	239.7
nerve (root)	171.9	198.89	—	215.9	238.1	239.2
pia mater	192.3	198.4	—	225.4	237.6	239.7
root	171.9	198.89	—	215.9	238.1	239.2
sacrum	170.6	198.5	—	213.6	238.0	239.2
spleen, splenic NEC	159.1	197.8	230.9	211.9	235.5	239.0
flexure (colon)	153.7	197.5	230.3	211.3	235.2	239.0
stem, brain	191.7	198.3	—	225.0	237.5	239.6
Stensen's duct	142.0	198.89	230.0	210.2	235.0	239.0
sternum	170.3	198.5	—	213.3	238.0	239.2
stomach	151.9	197.8	230.2	211.1	235.2	239.0
antrum (pyloric)	151.2	197.8	230.2	211.1	235.2	239.0
body	151.4	197.8	230.2	211.1	235.2	239.0
cardia	151.0	197.8	230.2	211.1	235.2	239.0
cardiac orifice	151.0	197.8	230.2	211.1	235.2	239.0
contiguous sites	151.8	—	—	—	—	—
corpus	151.4	197.8	230.2	211.1	235.2	239.0
fundus	151.3	197.8	230.2	211.1	235.2	239.0
greater curvature NEC	151.6	197.8	230.2	211.1	235.2	239.0
lesser curvature NEC	151.5	197.8	230.2	211.1	235.2	239.0
prepylorus	151.1	197.8	230.2	211.1	235.2	239.0
pylorus	151.1	197.8	230.2	211.1	235.2	239.0
wall NEC	151.9	197.8	230.2	211.1	235.2	239.0
anterior NEC	151.8	197.8	230.2	211.1	235.2	239.0
posterior NEC	151.8	197.8	230.2	211.1	235.2	239.0
stroma, endometrial	182.0	198.82	233.2	219.1	236.0	239.5

◀ New   ◀▮▮ Revised   deleted Deleted   ● Use Additional Digit(s)   ▨▨ Omit code

| | Malignant | | | | | |
	Primary	Secondary	Ca in situ	Benign	Uncertain Behavior	Unspecified
Neoplasm *(Continued)*						
stump, cervical	180.8	198.82	233.1	219.0	236.0	239.5
subcutaneous (nodule) (tissue) NEC - *see* Neoplasm, connective tissue						
subdural	192.1	198.4	—	225.2	237.6	239.7
subglottis, subglottic	161.2	197.3	231.0	212.1	235.6	239.1
sublingual	144.9	198.89	230.0	210.3	235.1	239.0
gland or duct	142.2	198.89	230.0	210.2	235.0	239.0
submandibular gland	142.1	198.89	230.0	210.2	235.0	239.0
submaxillary gland or duct	142.1	198.89	230.0	210.2	235.0	239.0
submental	195.0	198.89	234.8	229.8	238.8	239.89◄
subpleural	162.9	197.0	—	212.3	235.7	239.1
substernal	164.2	197.1	—	212.5	235.8	239.89◄
sudoriferous, sudoriparous gland, site unspecified	173.9	198.2	232.9	216.9	238.2	239.2
specified site - *see* Neoplasm, skin						
supraclavicular region	195.0	198.89	234.8	229.8	238.8	239.89◄
supraglottis	161.1	197.3	231.0	212.1	235.6	239.1
suprarenal (capsule) (cortex) (gland) (medulla)	194.0	198.7	234.8	227.0	237.2	239.7
suprasellar (region)	191.9	198.3	—	225.0	237.5	239.6
sweat gland (apocrine) (eccrine), site unspecified	173.9	198.2	232.9	216.9	238.2	239.2
specified site - *see* Neoplasm, skin						
sympathetic nerve or nervous system NEC	171.9	198.89	—	215.9	238.1	239.2
symphysis pubis	170.6	198.5	—	213.6	238.0	239.2
synovial membrane - *see* Neoplasm, connective tissue						
tapetum, brain	191.8	198.3	—	225.0	237.5	239.6
tarsus (any bone)	170.8	198.5	—	213.8	238.0	239.2
temple (skin)	173.3	198.2	232.3	216.3	238.2	239.2
temporal						
bone	170.0	198.5	—	213.0	238.0	239.2
lobe or pole	191.2	198.3	—	225.0	237.5	239.6
region	195.0	198.89	234.8	229.8	238.8	239.89◄
skin	173.3	198.2	232.3	216.3	238.2	239.2
tendon (sheath) - *see* Neoplasm, connective tissue						
tentorium (cerebelli)	192.1	198.4	—	225.2	237.6	239.7
testis, testes (descended) (scrotal)	186.9	198.82	233.6	222.0	236.4	239.5
ectopic	186.0	198.82	233.6	222.0	236.4	239.5
retained	186.0	198.82	233.6	222.0	236.4	239.5
undescended	186.0	198.82	233.6	222.0	236.4	239.5
thalamus	191.0	198.3	—	225.0	237.5	239.6
thigh NEC*	195.5	198.89	234.8	229.8	238.8	239.89◄
thorax, thoracic (cavity) (organs NEC)	195.1	198.89	234.8	229.8	238.8	239.89◄
duct	171.4	198.89	—	215.4	238.1	239.2
wall NEC	195.1	198.89	234.8	229.8	238.8	239.89◄

	Malignant					
	Primary	Secondary	Ca in situ	Benign	Uncertain Behavior	Unspecified
Neoplasm *(Continued)*						
throat	149.0	198.89	230.0	210.9	235.1	239.0
thumb NEC*	195.4	198.89	232.6	229.8	238.8	239.89 ◄
thymus (gland)	164.0	198.89	—	212.6	235.8	239.89 ◄
contiguous sites with heart and mediastinum	164.8	—	—	—	—	—
thyroglossal duct	193	198.89	234.8	226	237.4	239.7
thyroid (gland)	193	198.89	234.8	226	237.4	239.7
cartilage	161.3	197.3	231.0	212.1	235.6	239.1
tibia (any part)	170.7	198.5	—	213.7	238.0	239.2
toe NEC*	195.5	198.89	232.7	229.8	238.8	239.89 ◄
tongue	141.9	198.89	230.0	210.1	235.1	239.0
anterior (two-thirds) NEC	141.4	198.89	230.0	210.1	235.1	239.0
dorsal surface	141.1	198.89	230.0	210.1	235.1	239.0
ventral surface	141.3	198.89	230.0	210.1	235.1	239.0
base (dorsal surface)	141.0	198.89	230.0	210.1	235.1	239.0
border (lateral)	141.2	198.89	230.0	210.1	235.1	239.0
contiguous sites	141.8	—	—	—	—	—
dorsal surface NEC	141.1	198.89	230.0	210.1	235.1	239.0
fixed part NEC	141.0	198.89	230.0	210.1	235.1	239.0
foramen cecum	141.1	198.89	230.0	210.1	235.1	239.0
frenulum linguae	141.3	198.89	230.0	210.1	235.1	239.0
junctional zone	141.5	198.89	230.0	210.1	235.1	239.0
margin (lateral)	141.2	198.89	230.0	210.1	235.1	239.0
midline NEC	141.1	198.89	230.0	210.1	235.1	239.0
mobile part NEC	141.4	198.89	230.0	210.1	235.1	239.0
posterior (third)	141.0	198.89	230.0	210.1	235.1	239.0
root	141.0	198.89	230.0	210.1	235.1	239.0
surface (dorsal)	141.1	198.89	230.0	210.1	235.1	239.0
base	141.0	198.89	230.0	210.1	235.1	239.0
ventral	141.3	198.89	230.0	210.1	235.1	239.0
tip	141.2	198.89	230.0	210.1	235.1	239.0
tonsil	141.6	198.89	230.0	210.1	235.1	239.0
tonsil	146.0	198.89	230.0	210.5	235.1	239.0
fauces, faucial	146.0	198.89	230.0	210.5	235.1	239.0
lingual	141.6	198.89	230.0	210.1	235.1	239.0
palatine	146.0	198.89	230.0	210.5	235.1	239.0
pharyngeal	147.1	198.89	230.0	210.7	235.1	239.0
pillar (anterior) (posterior)	146.2	198.89	230.0	210.6	235.1	239.0
tonsillar fossa	146.1	198.89	230.0	210.6	235.1	239.0
tooth socket NEC	143.9	198.89	230.0	210.4	235.1	239.0

◄ New   ◄▥ Revised   ~~deleted~~ Deleted   ● Use Additional Digit(s)   ▨ Omit code

	Malignant					
	Primary	Secondary	Ca in situ	Benign	Uncertain Behavior	Unspecified
Neoplasm *(Continued)*						
trachea (cartilage) (mucosa)	162.0	197.3	231.1	212.2	235.7	239.1
contiguous sites with bronchus or lung	162.8	—	—	—	—	—
tracheobronchial	162.8	197.3	231.1	212.2	235.7	239.1
contiguous sites with lung	162.8	—	—	—	—	—
tragus	173.2	198.2	232.2	216.2	238.2	239.2
trunk NEC*	195.8	198.89	232.5	229.8	238.8	239.89 ◀
tubo-ovarian	183.8	198.82	233.39	221.8	236.3	239.5
tunica vaginalis	187.8	198.82	233.6	222.8	236.6	239.5
turbinate (bone)	170.0	198.5	—	213.0	238.0	239.2
nasal	160.0	197.3	231.8	212.0	235.9	239.1
tympanic cavity	160.1	197.3	231.8	212.0	235.9	239.1
ulna (any part)	170.4	198.5	—	213.4	238.0	239.2
umbilicus, umbilical	173.5	198.2	232.5	216.5	238.2	239.2
uncus, brain	191.2	198.3	—	225.0	237.5	239.6
unknown site or unspecified	199.1	199.1	234.9	229.9	238.9	239.9
urachus	188.7	198.1	233.7	223.3	236.7	239.4
ureter, ureteral	189.2	198.1	233.9	223.2	236.91	239.5
orifice (bladder)	188.6	198.1	233.7	223.3	236.7	239.4
ureter-bladder (junction)	188.6	198.1	233.7	223.3	236.7	239.4
urethra, urethral (gland)	189.3	198.1	233.9	223.81	236.99	239.5
orifice, internal	188.5	198.1	233.7	223.3	236.7	239.4
urethrovaginal (septum)	184.9	198.82	233.39	221.9	236.3	239.5
urinary organ or system NEC	189.9	198.1	233.9	223.9	236.99	239.5
bladder - *see* Neoplasm, bladder						
contiguous sites	189.8	—	—	—	—	—
specified sites NEC	189.8	198.1	233.9	223.89	236.99	239.5
utero-ovarian	183.8	198.82	233.39	221.8	236.3	239.5
ligament	183.3	198.82	—	221.0	236.3	239.5
uterosacral ligament	183.4	198.82	—	221.0	236.3	239.5
uterus, uteri, uterine	179	198.82	233.2	219.9	236.0	239.5
adnexa NEC	183.9	198.82	233.39	221.8	236.3	239.5
contiguous sites	183.8	—	—	—	—	—
body	182.0	198.82	233.2	219.1	236.0	239.5
contiguous sites	182.8	—	—	—	—	—
cervix	180.9	198.82	233.1	219.0	236.0	239.5
cornu	182.0	198.82	233.2	219.1	236.0	239.5
corpus	182.0	198.82	233.2	219.1	236.0	239.5
endocervix (canal) (gland)	180.0	198.82	233.1	219.0	236.0	239.5
endometrium	182.0	198.82	233.2	219.1	236.0	239.5

	Malignant					
	Primary	Secondary	Ca in situ	Benign	Uncertain Behavior	Unspecified
Neoplasm *(Continued)*						
uterus, uteri, uterine *(Continued)*						
exocervix	180.1	198.82	233.1	219.0	236.0	239.5
external os	180.1	198.82	233.1	219.0	236.0	239.5
fundus	182.0	198.82	233.2	219.1	236.0	239.5
internal os	180.0	198.82	233.1	219.0	236.0	239.5
isthmus	182.1	198.82	233.2	219.1	236.0	239.5
ligament	183.4	198.82	—	221.0	236.3	239.5
broad	183.3	198.82	233.39	221.0	236.3	239.5
round	183.5	198.82	—	221.0	236.3	239.5
lower segment	182.1	198.82	233.2	219.1	236.0	239.5
myometrium	182.0	198.82	233.2	219.1	236.0	239.5
squamocolumnar junction	180.8	198.82	233.1	219.0	236.0	239.5
tube	183.2	198.82	233.39	221.0	236.3	239.5
utricle, prostatic	189.3	198.1	233.9	223.81	236.99	239.5
uveal tract	190.0	198.4	234.0	224.0	238.8	239.89 ◀
uvula	145.4	198.89	230.0	210.4	235.1	239.0
vagina, vaginal (fornix) (vault) (wall)	184.0	198.82	233.31	221.1	236.3	239.5
vaginovesical	184.9	198.82	233.39	221.9	236.3	239.5
septum	184.9	198.82	233.39	221.9	236.3	239.5
vallecula (epiglottis)	146.3	198.89	230.0	210.6	235.1	239.0
vascular - *see* Neoplasm, connective tissue						
vas deferens	187.6	198.82	233.6	222.8	236.6	239.5
Vater's ampulla	156.2	197.8	230.8	211.5	235.3	239.0
vein, venous - *see* Neoplasm, connective tissue						
vena cava (abdominal) (inferior)	171.5	198.89	—	215.5	238.1	239.2
superior	171.4	198.89	—	215.4	238.1	239.2
ventricle (cerebral) (floor) (fourth) (lateral) (third)	191.5	198.3	—	225.0	237.5	239.6
cardiac (left) (right)	164.1	198.89	—	212.7	238.8	239.89 ◀
ventricular band of larynx	161.1	197.3	231.0	212.1	235.6	239.1
ventriculus - *see* Neoplasm, stomach						
vermillion border - *see* Neoplasm, lip						
vermis, cerebellum	191.6	198.3	—	225.0	237.5	239.6
vertebra (column)	170.2	198.5	—	213.2	238.0	239.2
coccyx	170.6	198.5	—	213.6	238.0	239.2
sacrum	170.6	198.5	—	213.6	238.0	239.2
vesical - *see* Neoplasm, bladder						
vesicle, seminal	187.8	198.82	233.6	222.8	236.6	239.5
vesicocervical tissue	184.9	198.82	233.39	221.9	236.3	239.5
vesicorectal	195.3	198.89	234.8	229.8	238.8	239.89 ◀
vesicovaginal	184.9	198.82	233.39	221.9	236.3	239.5
septum	184.9	198.82	233.39	221.9	236.3	239.5

◀ New   ◀▥ Revised   ~~deleted~~ Deleted   ● Use Additional Digit(s)   ▨ Omit code

	Malignant					
	Primary	Secondary	Ca in situ	Benign	Uncertain Behavior	Unspecified
Neoplasm *(Continued)*						
vessel (blood) - *see* Neoplasm, connective tissue						
vestibular gland, greater	184.1	198.82	233.32	221.2	236.3	239.5
vestibule						
mouth	145.1	198.89	230.0	210.4	235.1	239.0
nose	160.0	197.3	231.8	212.0	235.9	239.1
Virchow's gland	—	196.0	—	229.0	238.8	239.89◀▥
viscera NEC	195.8	198.89	234.8	229.8	238.8	239.89◀▥
vocal cords (true)	161.0	197.3	231.0	212.1	235.6	239.1
false	161.1	197.3	231.0	212.1	235.6	239.1
vomer	170.0	198.5	—	213.0	238.0	239.2
vulva	184.4	198.82	233.32	221.2	236.3	239.5
vulvovaginal gland	184.4	198.82	233.32	221.2	236.3	239.5
Waldeyer's ring	149.1	198.89	230.0	210.9	235.1	239.0
Wharton's duct	142.1	198.89	230.0	210.2	235.0	239.0
white matter (central) (cerebral)	191.0	198.3	—	225.0	237.5	239.6
windpipe	162.0	197.3	231.1	212.2	235.7	239.1
Wirsung's duct	157.3	197.8	230.9	211.6	235.5	239.0
wolffian (body) (duct)						
female	184.8	198.82	233.39	221.8	236.3	239.5
male	187.8	198.82	233.6	222.8	236.6	239.5
womb - *see* Neoplasm, uterus						
wrist NEC*	195.4	198.89	232.6	229.8	238.8	239.89◀▥
xiphoid process	170.3	198.5	—	213.3	238.0	239.2
Zuckerkandl's organ	194.6	198.89	—	227.6	237.3	239.7

Neovascularization
  choroid 362.16
  ciliary body 364.42
  cornea 370.60
    deep 370.63
    localized 370.61
  iris 364.42
  retina 362.16
  subretinal 362.16
Nephralgia 788.0
Nephritis, nephritic (albuminuric)
    (azotemic) (congenital)
    (degenerative) (diffuse)
    (disseminated) (epithelial) (familial)
    (focal) (granulomatous)
    (hemorrhagic) (infantile)
    (nonsuppurative, excretory)
    (uremic) 583.9
  with
    edema - see Nephrosis
    lesion of
      glomerulonephritis
        hypocomplementemic
            persistent 583.2
          with nephrotic syndrome
              581.2
          chronic 582.2
        lobular 583.2
          with nephrotic syndrome
              581.2
          chronic 582.2
        membranoproliferative
            583.2
          with nephrotic syndrome
              581.2
          chronic 582.2
        membranous 583.1
          with nephrotic syndrome
              581.1
          chronic 582.1
        mesangiocapillary 583.2
          with nephrotic syndrome
              581.2
          chronic 582.2
        mixed membranous and
            proliferative 583.2
          with nephrotic syndrome
              581.2
          chronic 582.2
        proliferative (diffuse) 583.0
          with nephrotic syndrome
              581.0
          acute 580.0
          chronic 582.0
        rapidly progressive 583.4
          acute 580.4
          chronic 582.4
        interstitial nephritis (diffuse)
            (focal) 583.89
          with nephrotic syndrome
              581.89
          acute 580.89
          chronic 582.89
      necrotizing glomerulitis 583.4
        acute 580.4
        chronic 582.4
      renal necrosis 583.9
        cortical 583.6
        medullary 583.7
      specified pathology NEC 583.89
        with nephrotic syndrome
            581.89
        acute 580.89
        chronic 582.89

Nephritis, nephritic (Continued)
  with (Continued)
    necrosis, renal 583.9
      cortical 583.6
      medullary (papillary) 583.7
    nephrotic syndrome (see also
        Nephrosis) 581.9
    papillary necrosis 583.7
    specified pathology NEC 583.89
  acute 580.9
    extracapillary with epithelial
        crescents 580.4
    hypertensive (see also Hypertension,
        kidney) 403.90
    necrotizing 580.4
    poststreptococcal 580.0
    proliferative (diffuse) 580.0
    rapidly progressive 580.4
    specified pathology NEC 580.89
  amyloid 277.39 [583.81]
    chronic 277.39 [582.81]
  arteriolar (see also Hypertension,
      kidney) 403.90
  arteriosclerotic (see also Hypertension,
      kidney) 403.90
  ascending (see also Pyelitis) 590.80
  atrophic 582.9
  basement membrane NEC 583.89
    with pulmonary hemorrhage
        (Goodpasture's syndrome)
        446.21 [583.81]
  calculous, calculus 592.0
  cardiac (see also Hypertension, kidney)
      403.90
  cardiovascular (see also Hypertension,
      kidney) 403.90
  chronic 582.9
    arteriosclerotic (see also
        Hypertension, kidney) 403.90
    hypertensive (see also Hypertension,
        kidney) 403.90
  cirrhotic (see also Sclerosis, renal) 587
  complicating pregnancy, childbirth, or
      puerperium 646.2●
    with hypertension 642.1●
      affecting fetus or newborn 760.0
    affecting fetus or newborn 760.1
  croupous 580.9
  desquamative - see Nephrosis
  due to
    amyloidosis 277.39 [583.81]
      chronic 277.39 [582.81]
    arteriosclerosis (see also
        Hypertension, kidney) 403.90
    diabetes mellitus 250.4● [583.81]
      due to secondary diabetes 249.4●
          [583.81]   ◀▥
      with nephrotic syndrome 250.4●
          [581.81]
        due to secondary diabetes
            249.4● [581.81]
    diphtheria 032.89 [580.81]
    gonococcal infection (acute) 098.19
        [583.81]
      chronic or duration of 2 months
          or over 098.39 [583.81]
    gout 274.10
    infectious hepatitis 070.9 [580.81]
    mumps 072.79 [580.81]
    specified kidney pathology NEC
        583.89
      acute 580.89
      chronic 582.89
    streptotrichosis 039.8 [583.81]

Nephritis, nephritic (Continued)
  due to (Continued)
    subacute bacterial endocarditis 421.0
        [580.81]
    systemic lupus erythematosus 710.0
        [583.81]
      chronic 710.0 [582.81]
    typhoid fever 002.0 [580.81]
  endothelial 582.2
  end state (chronic) (terminal) NEC
      585.6
  epimembranous 581.1
  exudative 583.89
    with nephrotic syndrome 581.89
    acute 580.89
    chronic 582.89
  gonococcal (acute) 098.19 [583.81]
    chronic or duration of 2 months or
        over 098.39 [583.81]
  gouty 274.10
  hereditary (Alport's syndrome)
      759.89
  hydremic - see Nephrosis
  hypertensive (see also Hypertension,
      kidney) 403.90
  hypocomplementemic persistent
      583.2
    with nephrotic syndrome 581.2
    chronic 582.2
  immune complex NEC 583.89
  infective (see also Pyelitis) 590.80
  interstitial (diffuse) (focal) 583.89
    with nephrotic syndrome 581.89
    acute 580.89
    chronic 582.89
  latent or quiescent - see Nephritis,
      chronic
  lead 984.9
    specified type of lead - see Table of
        Drugs and Chemicals
  lobular 583.2
    with nephrotic syndrome
        581.2
    chronic 582.2
  lupus 710.0 [583.81]
    acute 710.0 [580.81]
    chronic 710.0 [582.81]
  membranoproliferative 583.2
    with nephrotic syndrome 581.2
    chronic 582.2
  membranous 583.1
    with nephrotic syndrome 581.1
    chronic 582.1
  mesangiocapillary 583.2
    with nephrotic syndrome 581.2
    chronic 582.2
  minimal change 581.3
  mixed membranous and proliferative
      583.2
    with nephrotic syndrome 581.2
    chronic 582.2
  necrotic, necrotizing 583.4
    acute 580.4
    chronic 582.4
  nephrotic - see Nephrosis
  old - see Nephritis, chronic
  parenchymatous 581.89
  polycystic 753.12
    adult type (APKD) 753.13
    autosomal dominant 753.13
    autosomal recessive 753.14
    childhood type (CPKD) 753.14
    infantile type 753.14
  poststreptococcal 580.0

◀ New   ◀▥ Revised   ~~deleted~~ Deleted   ● Use Additional Digit(s)   ▬ Omit code

Nephritis, nephritic (Continued)
  pregnancy - see Nephritis, complicating
    pregnancy
  proliferative 583.0
    with nephrotic syndrome 581.0
    acute 580.0
    chronic 582.0
  purulent (see also Pyelitis) 590.80
  rapidly progressive 583.4
    acute 580.4
    chronic 582.4
  salt-losing or salt-wasting (see also
    Disease, renal) 593.9
  saturnine 584.9
    specified type of lead - see Table of
      Drugs and Chemicals
  septic (see also Pyelitis) 590.80
  specified pathology NEC 583.89
    acute 580.89
    chronic 582.89
  staphylococcal (see also Pyelitis) 590.80
  streptotrichosis 039.8 [583.81]
  subacute (see also Nephrosis) 581.9
  suppurative (see also Pyelitis) 590.80
  syphilitic (late) 095.4
    congenital 090.5 [583.81]
    early 091.69 [583.81]
  terminal (chronic) (end-stage) NEC
    585.6
  toxic - see Nephritis, acute
  tubal, tubular - see Nephrosis, tubular
  tuberculous (see also Tuberculosis)
    016.0● [583.81]
  type II (Ellis) - see Nephrosis
  vascular - see also Hypertension, kidney
  war 580.9
Nephroblastoma (M8960/3) 189.0
  epithelial (M8961/3) 189.0
  mesenchymal (M8962/3) 189.0
Nephrocalcinosis 275.49
Nephrocystitis, pustular (see also Pyelitis)
  590.80
Nephrolithiasis (congenital) (pelvis)
  (recurrent) 592.0
  uric acid 274.11
Nephroma (M8960/3) 189.0
  mesoblastic (M8960/1) 236.9
Nephronephritis (see also Nephrosis)
  581.9
Nephronopthisis 753.16
Nephropathy (see also Nephritis) 583.9
  with
    exudative nephritis 583.89
    interstitial nephritis (diffuse) (focal)
      583.89
    medullary necrosis 583.7
    necrosis 583.9
      cortical 583.6
      medullary or papillary 583.7
    papillary necrosis 583.7
    specified lesion or cause NEC 583.89
  analgesic 583.89
    with medullary necrosis, acute 584.7
  arteriolar (see also Hypertension,
    kidney) 403.90
  arteriosclerotic (see also Hypertension,
    kidney) 403.90
  complicating pregnancy 646.2●
  diabetic 250.4● [583.81]
    due to secondary diabetes 249.4●
      [583.81] ◄▬
  gouty 274.10
    specified type NEC 274.19
  hereditary amyloid 277.31

Nephropathy (Continued)
  hypercalcemic 588.89
  hypertensive (see also Hypertension,
    kidney) 403.90
  hypokalemic (vacuolar) 588.89
  IgA 583.9
  obstructive 593.89
    congenital 753.20
  phenacetin 584.7
  phosphate-losing 588.0
  potassium depletion 588.89
  proliferative (see also Nephritis,
    proliferative) 583.0
  protein-losing 588.89
  salt-losing or salt-wasting (see also
    Disease, renal) 593.9
  sickle-cell (see also Disease, sickle-cell)
    282.60 [583.81]
  toxic 584.5
  vasomotor 584.5
  water-losing 588.89
Nephroptosis (see also Disease, renal)
  593.0
  congenital (displaced) 753.3
Nephropyosis (see also Abscess, kidney)
  590.2
Nephrorrhagia 593.81
Nephrosclerosis (arteriolar)
  (arteriosclerotic) (chronic) (hyaline)
  (see also Hypertension, kidney)
  403.90
  gouty 274.10
  hyperplastic (arteriolar) (see also
    Hypertension, kidney) 403.90
  senile (see also Sclerosis, renal) 587
Nephrosis, nephrotic (Epstein's)
  (syndrome) 581.9
  with
    lesion of
      focal glomerulosclerosis 581.1
      glomerulonephritis
        endothelial 581.2
        hypocomplementemic
          persistent 581.2
        lobular 581.2
        membranoproliferative 581.2
        membranous 581.1
        mesangiocapillary 581.2
        minimal change 581.3
        mixed membranous and
          proliferative 581.2
        proliferative 581.0
      segmental hyalinosis 581.1
      specified pathology NEC 581.89
  acute - see Nephrosis, tubular
  anoxic - see Nephrosis, tubular
  arteriosclerotic (see also Hypertension,
    kidney) 403.90
  chemical - see Nephrosis, tubular
  cholemic 572.4
  complicating pregnancy, childbirth, or
    puerperium - see Nephritis,
    complicating pregnancy
  diabetic 250.4● [581.81]
    due to secondary diabetes 249.4●
      [581.81]
  Finnish type (congenital) 759.89
  hemoglobinuric - see Nephrosis,
    tubular
  in
    amyloidosis 277.39 [581.81]
    diabetes mellitus 250.4● [581.81]
      due to secondary diabetes 249.4●
        [581.81]

Nephrosis, nephrotic (Continued)
  in (Continued)
    epidemic hemorrhagic fever
      078.6
    malaria 084.9 [581.81]
    polyarteritis 446.0 [581.81]
    systemic lupus erythematosus
      710.0 [581.81]
  ischemic - see Nephrosis, tubular
  lipoid 581.3
  lower nephron - see Nephrosis,
    tubular
  lupoid 710.0 [581.81]
  lupus 710.0 [581.81]
  malarial 084.9 [581.81]
  minimal change 581.3
  necrotizing - see Nephrosis, tubular
  osmotic (sucrose) 588.89
  polyarteritic 446.0 [581.81]
  radiation 581.9
  specified lesion or cause NEC
    581.89
  syphilitic 095.4
  toxic - see Nephrosis, tubular
  tubular (acute) 584.5
    due to a procedure 997.5
    radiation 581.9
Nephrosonephritis hemorrhagic
  (endemic) 078.6
Nephrostomy status V44.6
  with complication 997.5
Nerve - see condition
Nerves 799.21 ◄▬
Nervous (see also condition) 799.21 ◄▬
  breakdown 300.9
  heart 306.2
  stomach 306.4
  tension 799.21 ◄▬
Nervousness 799.21 ◄▬
Nesidioblastoma (M8150/0)
  pancreas 211.7
  specified site NEC - see Neoplasm, by
    site, benign
  unspecified site 211.7
Netherton's syndrome (ichthyosiform
  erythroderma) 757.1
Nettle rash 708.8
Nettleship's disease (urticaria
  pigmentosa) 757.33
Neumann's disease (pemphigus
  vegetans) 694.4
Neuralgia, neuralgic (acute) (see also
  Neuritis) 729.2
  accessory (nerve) 352.4
  acoustic (nerve) 388.5
  ankle 355.8
  anterior crural 355.8
  anus 787.99
  arm 723.4
  auditory (nerve) 388.5
  axilla 353.0
  bladder 788.1
  brachial 723.4
  brain - see Disorder, nerve, cranial
  broad ligament 625.9
  cerebral - see Disorder, nerve, cranial
  ciliary 339.00
  cranial nerve - see also Disorder, nerve,
    cranial
    fifth or trigeminal (see also
      Neuralgia, trigeminal)
      350.1
  ear 388.71
    middle 352.1

◄ New   ◄▬ Revised   ~~deleted~~ Deleted   ● Use Additional Digit(s)   ▓ Omit code

Neuralgia, neuralgic (*Continued*)
  facial 351.8
  finger 354.9
  flank 355.8
  foot 355.8
  forearm 354.9
  Fothergill's (*see also* Neuralgia,
      trigeminal) 350.1
    postherpetic 053.12
  glossopharyngeal (nerve) 352.1
  groin 355.8
  hand 354.9
  heel 355.8
  Horton's 339.00
  Hunt's 053.11
  hypoglossal (nerve) 352.5
  iliac region 355.8
  infraorbital (*see also* Neuralgia,
      trigeminal) 350.1
  inguinal 355.8
  intercostal (nerve) 353.8
    postherpetic 053.19
  jaw 352.1
  kidney 788.0
  knee 355.8
  loin 355.8
  malarial (*see also* Malaria) 084.6
  mastoid 385.89
  maxilla 352.1
  median thenar 354.1
  metatarsal 355.6
  middle ear 352.1
  migrainous 339.00
  Morton's 355.6
  nerve, cranial - *see* Disorder, nerve,
      cranial
  nose 352.0
  occipital 723.8
  olfactory (nerve) 352.0
  ophthalmic 377.30
    postherpetic 053.19
  optic (nerve) 377.30
  penis 607.9
  perineum 355.8
  pleura 511.0
  postherpetic NEC 053.19
    geniculate ganglion 053.11
    ophthalmic 053.19
    trifacial 053.12
    trigeminal 053.12
  pubic region 355.8
  radial (nerve) 723.4
  rectum 787.99
  sacroiliac joint 724.3
  sciatic (nerve) 724.3
  scrotum 608.9
  seminal vesicle 608.9
  shoulder 354.9
  sluder's 337.09
  specified nerve NEC - *see* Disorder,
      nerve
  spermatic cord 608.9
  sphenopalatine (ganglion)
      337.09
  subscapular (nerve) 723.4
  suprascapular (nerve) 723.4
  testis 608.89
  thenar (median) 354.1
  thigh 355.8
  tongue 352.5
  trifacial (nerve) (*see also* Neuralgia,
      trigeminal) 350.1
  trigeminal (nerve) 350.1
    postherpetic 053.12
  tympanic plexus 388.71

Neuralgia, neuralgic (*Continued*)
  ulnar (nerve) 723.4
  vagus (nerve) 352.3
  wrist 354.9
  writers' 300.89
    organic 333.84
Neurapraxia - *see* Injury, nerve, by site
Neurasthenia 300.5
  cardiac 306.2
  gastric 306.4
  heart 306.2
  postfebrile 780.79
  postviral 780.79
Neurilemmoma (M9560/0) - *see also*
    Neoplasm, connective tissue,
    benign
  acoustic (nerve) 225.1
  malignant (M9560/3) - *see also*
      Neoplasm, connective tissue,
      malignant
    acoustic (nerve) 192.0
Neurilemmosarcoma (M9560/3) - *see*
    Neoplasm, connective tissue,
    malignant
Neurilemoma - *see* Neurilemmoma
Neurinoma (M9560/0) - *see*
    Neurilemmoma
Neurinomatosis (M9560/1) - *see also*
    Neoplasm, connective tissue,
    uncertain behavior
  centralis 759.5
Neuritis (*see also* Neuralgia) 729.2
  abducens (nerve) 378.54
  accessory (nerve) 352.4
  acoustic (nerve) 388.5
    syphilitic 094.86
  alcoholic 357.5
    with psychosis 291.1
  amyloid, any site 277.39 [357.4]
  anterior crural 355.8
  arising during pregnancy 646.4 ●
  arm 723.4
  ascending 355.2
  auditory (nerve) 388.5
  brachial (nerve) NEC 723.4
    due to displacement, intervertebral
        disc 722.0
  cervical 723.4
  chest (wall) 353.8
  costal region 353.8
  cranial nerve - *see also* Disorder, nerve,
      cranial
    first or olfactory 352.0
    second or optic 377.30
    third or oculomotor 378.52
    fourth or trochlear 378.53
    fifth or trigeminal (*see also*
        Neuralgia, trigeminal)
        350.1
    sixth or abducens 378.54
    seventh or facial 351.8
      newborn 767.5
    eighth or acoustic 388.5
    ninth or glossopharyngeal
        352.1
    tenth or vagus 352.3
    eleventh or accessory 352.4
    twelfth or hypoglossal 352.5
  Déjérine-Sottas 356.0
  diabetic 250.6 ● [357.2]
    due to secondary diabetes
        249.6 ● [357.2]
  diphtheritic 032.89 [357.4]

Neuritis (*Continued*)
  due to
    beriberi 265.0 [357.4]
    displacement, prolapse, protrusion,
        or rupture of intervertebral
        disc 722.2
      cervical 722.0
      lumbar, lumbosacral 722.10
      thoracic, thoracolumbar 722.11
    herniation, nucleus pulposus 722.2
      cervical 722.0
      lumbar, lumbosacral 722.10
      thoracic, thoracolumbar 722.11
  endemic 265.0 [357.4]
  facial (nerve) 351.8
    newborn 767.5
  general - *see* Polyneuropathy
  geniculate ganglion 351.1
    due to herpes 053.11
  glossopharyngeal (nerve) 352.1
  gouty 274.89 [357.4]
  hypoglossal (nerve) 352.5
  ilioinguinal (nerve) 355.8
  in diseases classified elsewhere - *see*
      Polyneuropathy, in
  infectious (multiple) 357.0
  intercostal (nerve) 353.8
  interstitial hypertrophic progressive
      NEC 356.9
  leg 355.8
  lumbosacral NEC 724.4
  median (nerve) 354.1
    thenar 354.1
  multiple (acute) (infective) 356.9
    endemic 265.0 [357.4]
  multiplex endemica 265.0 [357.4]
  nerve root (*see also* Radiculitis) 729.2
  oculomotor (nerve) 378.52
  olfactory (nerve) 352.0
  optic (nerve) 377.30
    in myelitis 341.0
    meningococcal 036.81
  pelvic 355.8
  peripheral (nerve) - *see also*
      Neuropathy, peripheral
    complicating pregnancy or
        puerperium 646.4 ●
    specified nerve NEC - *see*
        Mononeuritis
  pneumogastric (nerve) 352.3
  postchickenpox 052.7
  postherpetic 053.19
  progressive hypertrophic interstitial
      NEC 356.9
  puerperal, postpartum 646.4 ●
  radial (nerve) 723.4
  retrobulbar 377.32
    syphilitic 094.85
  rheumatic (chronic) 729.2
  sacral region 355.8
  sciatic (nerve) 724.3
    due to displacement of
        intervertebral disc 722.10
  serum 999.5
  specified nerve NEC - *see* Disorder,
      nerve
  spinal (nerve) 355.9
    root (*see also* Radiculitis) 729.2
  subscapular (nerve) 723.4
  suprascapular (nerve) 723.4
  syphilitic 095.8
  thenar (median) 354.1
  thoracic NEC 724.4
  toxic NEC 357.7
  trochlear (nerve) 378.53

◀ New   ◀▥ Revised   ~~deleted~~ Deleted   ● Use Additional Digit(s)   ▨▨ Omit code

Neuritis *(Continued)*
    ulnar (nerve) 723.4
    vagus (nerve) 352.3
Neuroangiomatosis, encephalofacial 759.6
Neuroastrocytoma (M9505/1) - *see* Neoplasm, by site, uncertain behavior
Neuro-avitaminosis 269.2
Neuroblastoma (M9500/3)
    olfactory (M9522/3) 160.0
    specified site - *see* Neoplasm, by site, malignant
    unspecified site 194.0
Neurochorioretinitis *(see also* Chorioretinitis) 363.20
Neurocirculatory asthenia 306.2
Neurocytoma (M9506/0) - *see* Neoplasm, by site, benign
Neurodermatitis (circumscribed) (circumscripta) (local) 698.3
    atopic 691.8
    diffuse (Brocq) 691.8
    disseminated 691.8
    nodulosa 698.3
Neuroencephalomyelopathy, optic 341.0
Neuroendocrine tumor - *see* Tumor, neuroendocrine
Neuroepithelioma (M9503/3) - *see also* Neoplasm, by site, malignant
    olfactory (M9521/3) 160.0
Neurofibroma (M9540/0) - *see also* Neoplasm, connective tissue, benign
    melanotic (M9541/0) - *see* Neoplasm, connective tissue, benign
    multiple (M9540/1) 237.70
        type 1 237.71
        type 2 237.72
    plexiform (M9550/0) - *see* Neoplasm, connective tissue, benign
Neurofibromatosis (multiple) (M9540/1) 237.70
    acoustic 237.72
    malignant (M9540/3) - *see* Neoplasm, connective tissue, malignant
    type 1 237.71
    type 2 237.72
    von Recklinghausen's 237.71
Neurofibrosarcoma (M9540/3) - *see* Neoplasm, connective tissue, malignant
Neurogenic - *see also* condition
    bladder (atonic) (automatic) (autonomic) (flaccid) (hypertonic) (hypotonic) (inertia) (infranuclear) (irritable) (motor) (nonreflex) (nuclear) (paralysis) (reflex) (sensory) (spastic) (supranuclear) (uninhibited) 596.54
        with cauda equina syndrome 344.61
    bowel 564.81
    heart 306.2
Neuroglioma (M9505/1) - *see* Neoplasm, by site, uncertain behavior
Neurolabyrinthitis (of Dix and Hallpike) 386.12
Neurolathyrism 988.2
Neuroleprosy 030.1
Neuroleptic malignant syndrome 333.92
Neurolipomatosis 272.8
Neuroma (M9570/0) - *see also* Neoplasm, connective tissue, benign
    acoustic (nerve) (M9560/0) 225.1
    amputation (traumatic) - *see also* Injury, nerve, by site
        surgical complication (late) 997.61

Neuroma *(Continued)*
    appendix 211.3
    auditory nerve 225.1
    digital 355.6
        toe 355.6
    interdigital (toe) 355.6
    intermetatarsal 355.6
    Morton's 355.6
    multiple 237.70
        type 1 237.71
        type 2 237.72
    nonneoplastic 355.9
        arm NEC 354.9
        leg NEC 355.8
        lower extremity NEC 355.8
        specified site NEC - *see* Mononeuritis, by site
        upper extremity NEC 354.9
    optic (nerve) 225.1
    plantar 355.6
    plexiform (M9550/0) - *see* Neoplasm, connective tissue, benign
    surgical (nonneoplastic) 355.9
        arm NEC 354.9
        leg NEC 355.8
        lower extremity NEC 355.8
        upper extremity NEC 354.9
    traumatic - *see also* Injury, nerve, by site old - *see* Neuroma, nonneoplastic
Neuromyalgia 729.1
Neuromyasthenia (epidemic) 049.8
Neuromyelitis 341.8
    ascending 357.0
    optica 341.0
Neuromyopathy NEC 358.9
Neuromyositis 729.1
Neuronevus (M8725/0) - *see* Neoplasm, skin, benign
Neuronitis 357.0
    ascending (acute) 355.2
    vestibular 386.12
Neuroparalytic - *see* condition
Neuropathy, neuropathic *(see also* Disorder, nerve) 355.9
    acute motor 357.82
    alcoholic 357.5
        with psychosis 291.1
    arm NEC 354.9
    ataxia and retinitis pigmentosa (NARP syndrome) 277.87
    autonomic (peripheral) - *see* Neuropathy, peripheral, autonomic
    axillary nerve 353.0
    brachial plexus 353.0
    cervical plexus 353.2
    chronic
        progressive segmentally demyelinating 357.89
        relapsing demyelinating 357.89
    congenital sensory 356.2
    Déjérine-Sottas 356.0
    diabetic 250.6 ● [357.2]
        autonomic (peripheral) 250.6 [337.1] ◄
        due to secondary diabetes 249.6 ● [357.2]
        autonomic (peripheral) 249.6 [337.1] ◄
    entrapment 355.9
        iliohypogastric nerve 355.79
        ilioinguinal nerve 355.79

Neuropathy, neuropathic *(Continued)*
    entrapment *(Continued)*
        lateral cutaneous nerve of thigh 355.1
        median nerve 354.0
        obturator nerve 355.79
        peroneal nerve 355.3
        posterior tibial nerve 355.5
        saphenous nerve 355.79
        ulnar nerve 354.2
    facial nerve 351.9
    hereditary 356.9
        peripheral 356.0
        sensory (radicular) 356.2
    hypertrophic
        Charcôt-Marie-Tooth 356.1
        Déjérine-Sottas 356.0
        interstitial 356.9
        Refsum 356.3
    intercostal nerve 354.8
    ischemic - *see* Disorder, nerve
    Jamaican (ginger) 357.7
    leg NEC 355.8
    lower extremity NEC 355.8
    lumbar plexus 353.1
    median nerve 354.1
    motor
        acute 357.82
    multiple (acute) (chronic) *(see also* Polyneuropathy) 356.9
    optic 377.39
        ischemic 377.41
        nutritional 377.33
        toxic 377.34
    peripheral (nerve) *(see also* Polyneuropathy) 356.9
        arm NEC 354.9
        autonomic 337.9
            amyloid 277.39 [337.1]
            idiopathic 337.00
            in
                amyloidosis 277.39 [337.1]
                diabetes (mellitus) 250.6 ● [337.1]
                    due to secondary diabetes 249.6 ● [337.1]
                diseases classified elsewhere 337.1
                gout 274.89 [337.1]
                hyperthyroidism 242.9 ● [337.1]
        due to
            antitetanus serum 357.6
            arsenic 357.7
            drugs 357.6
            lead 357.7
            organophosphate compounds 357.7
            toxic agent NEC 357.7
        hereditary 356.0
        idiopathic 356.9
            progressive 356.4
            specified type NEC 356.8
        in diseases classified elsewhere - *see* Polyneuropathy, in
        leg NEC 355.8
        lower extremity NEC 355.8
        upper extremity NEC 354.9
        plantar nerves 355.6
        progressive ~~hypertrophic interstitial 356.9~~ ◄
            hypertrophic interstitial 356.9 ◄
            inflammatory 357.89 ◄
    radicular NEC 729.2
        brachial 723.4
        cervical NEC 723.4

Neuropathy, neuropathic *(Continued)*
    radicular NEC *(Continued)*
        hereditary sensory 356.2
        lumbar 724.4
        lumbosacral 724.4
        thoracic NEC 724.4
    sacral plexus 353.1
    sciatic 355.0
    spinal nerve NEC 355.9
        root *(see also* Radiculitis) 729.2
    toxic 357.7
    trigeminal sensory 350.8
    ulnar nerve 354.2
    upper extremity NEC 354.9
    uremic 585.9 *[357.4]*
    vitamin B$_{12}$ 266.2 *[357.4]*
        with anemia (pernicious) 281.0
            [357.4]
            due to dietary deficiency 281.1
                [357.4]
Neurophthisis - *see also* Disorder, nerve
    peripheral 356.9
    diabetic 250.6● *[357.2]*
        due to secondary diabetes 249.6●
            [357.2]
Neuropraxia - *see* Injury, nerve
Neuroretinitis 363.05
    syphilitic 094.85
Neurosarcoma (M9540/3) - *see* Neoplasm,
    connective tissue, malignant
Neurosclerosis - *see* Disorder, nerve
Neurosis, neurotic 300.9
    accident 300.16
    anancastic, anankastic 300.3
    anxiety (state) 300.00
        generalized 300.02
        panic type 300.01
    asthenic 300.5
    bladder 306.53
    cardiac (reflex) 306.2
    cardiovascular 306.2
    climacteric, unspecified type 627.2
    colon 306.4
    compensation 300.16
    compulsive, compulsion 300.3
    conversion 300.11
    craft 300.89
    cutaneous 306.3
    depersonalization 300.6
    depressive (reaction) (type) 300.4
    endocrine 306.6
    environmental 300.89
    fatigue 300.5
    functional *(see also* Disorder,
        psychosomatic) 306.9
    gastric 306.4
    gastrointestinal 306.4
    genitourinary 306.50
    heart 306.2
    hypochondriacal 300.7
    hysterical 300.10
        conversion type 300.11
        dissociative type 300.15
    impulsive 300.3
    incoordination 306.0
        larynx 306.1
        vocal cord 306.1
    intestine 306.4
    larynx 306.1
        hysterical 300.11
        sensory 306.1
    menopause, unspecified type
        627.2
    mixed NEC 300.89

Neurosis, neurotic *(Continued)*
    musculoskeletal 306.0
    obsessional 300.3
        phobia 300.3
    obsessive-compulsive 300.3
    occupational 300.89
    ocular 306.7
    oral 307.0
    organ *(see also* Disorder,
        psychosomatic) 306.9
    pharynx 306.1
    phobic 300.20
    posttraumatic (acute) (situational)
        309.81
        chronic 309.81
    psychasthenic (type) 300.89
    railroad 300.16
    rectum 306.4
    respiratory 306.1
    rumination 306.4
    senile 300.89
    sexual 302.70
    situational 300.89
    specified type NEC 300.89
    state 300.9
        with depersonalization episode
            300.6
    stomach 306.4
    vasomotor 306.2
    visceral 306.4
    war 300.16
Neurospongioblastosis diffusa 759.5
Neurosyphilis (arrested) (early)
        (inactive) (late) (latent) (recurrent)
        094.9
    with ataxia (cerebellar) (locomotor)
        (spastic) (spinal) 094.0
    acute meningitis 094.2
    aneurysm 094.89
    arachnoid (adhesive) 094.2
    arteritis (any artery) 094.89
    asymptomatic 094.3
    congenital 090.40
    dura (mater) 094.89
    general paresis 094.1
    gumma 094.9
    hemorrhagic 094.9
    juvenile (asymptomatic) (meningeal)
        090.40
    leptomeninges (aseptic) 094.2
    meningeal 094.2
    meninges (adhesive) 094.2
    meningovascular (diffuse) 094.2
    optic atrophy 094.84
    parenchymatous (degenerative) 094.1
    paresis *(see also* Paresis, general) 094.1
    paretic *(see also* Paresis, general) 094.1
    relapse 094.9
    remission in (sustained) 094.9
    serological 094.3
    specified nature or site NEC
        094.89
    tabes (dorsalis) 094.0
        juvenile 090.40
    tabetic 094.0
        juvenile 090.40
    taboparesis 094.1
        juvenile 090.40
    thrombosis 094.89
    vascular 094.89
Neurotic *(see also* Neurosis) 300.9
    excoriation 698.4
        psychogenic 306.3
Neurotmesis - *see* Injury, nerve, by site

Neurotoxemia - *see* Toxemia
Neutro-occlusion 524.21
Neutropenia, neutropenic (idiopathic)
        (pernicious) (primary) 288.00
    chronic 288.09
        hypoplastic 288.09
    congenital (nontransient) 288.01
    cyclic 288.02
    drug induced 288.03
    due to infection 288.04
    fever 288.00
    genetic 288.01
    immune 288.09
    infantile 288.01
    malignant 288.09
    neonatal, transitory (isoimmune)
        (maternal transfer) 776.7
    periodic 288.02
    splenic 289.53
    splenomegaly 289.53
    toxic 288.09
Neutrophilia, hereditary giant
    288.2
Nevocarcinoma (M8720/3) - *see*
    Melanoma
Nevus (M8720/0) - *see also* Neoplasm,
    skin, benign

Note 55   Except where otherwise
indicated, varieties of nevus in the list
below that are followed by a morphology code number (M----/0) should be
coded by site as for "Neoplasm, skin,
benign."

---

    acanthotic 702.8
    achromic (M8730/0)
    amelanotic (M8730/0)
    anemic, anemicus 709.09
    angiomatous (M9120/0) *(see also*
        Hemangioma) 228.00
    araneus 448.1
    avasculosus 709.09
    balloon cell (M8722/0)
    bathing trunk (M8761/1) 238.2
    blue (M8780/0)
        cellular (M8790/0)
        giant (M8790/0)
        Jadassohn's (M8780/0)
        malignant (M8780/3) - *see*
            Melanoma
    capillary (M9131/0) *(see also*
        Hemangioma) 228.00
    cavernous (M9121/0) *(see also*
        Hemangioma) 228.00
    cellular (M8720/0)
        blue (M8790/0)
    comedonicus 757.33
    compound (M8760/0)
    conjunctiva (M8720/0) 224.3
    dermal (8750/0)
        and epidermal (M8760/0)
    epithelioid cell (and spindle cell)
        (M8770/0)
    flammeus 757.32
        osteohypertrophic 759.89
    hairy (M8720/0)
    halo (M8723/0)
    hemangiomatous (M9120/0) *(see also*
        Hemangioma) 228.00
    intradermal (M8750/0)
    intraepidermal (M8740/0)
    involuting (M8724/0)
    Jadassohn's (blue) (M8780/0)

◀ New   ◀▥ Revised   ~~deleted~~ Deleted   ● Use Additional Digit(s)   ▨ Omit code

Nevus (Continued)
  junction, junctional (M8740/0)
    malignant melanoma in (M8740/3) -
      see Melanoma
  juvenile (M8770/0)
  lymphatic (M9170/0) 228.1
  magnocellular (M8726/0)
    specified site - *see* Neoplasm, by site,
      benign
    unspecified site 224.0
  malignant (M8720/3) - *see* Melanoma
  meaning hemangioma (M9120/0) (*see*
    also Hemangioma) 228.00
  melanotic (pigmented) (M8720/0)
  multiplex 759.5
  nonneoplastic 448.1
  nonpigmented (M8730/0)
  nonvascular (M8720/0)
  oral mucosa, white sponge 750.26
  osteohypertrophic, flammeus
    759.89
  papillaris (M8720/0)
  papillomatosus (M8720/0)
  pigmented (M8720/0)
    giant (M8761/1) - *see also* Neoplasm,
      skin, uncertain behavior
      malignant melanoma in
        (M8761/3) - *see* Melanoma
    systematicus 757.33
  pilosus (M8720/0)
  port wine 757.32
  sanguineous 757.32
  sebaceous (senile) 702.8
  senile 448.1
  spider 448.1
  spindle cell (and epithelioid cell)
    (M8770/0)
  stellar 448.1
  strawberry 757.32
  syringocystadenomatous papilliferous
    (M8406/0)
  unius lateris 757.33
  Unna's 757.32
  vascular 757.32
  verrucous 757.33
  white sponge (oral mucosa) 750.26
Newborn (infant) (liveborn) ◄
  abstinence syndrome 779.5
  affected by
    amniocentesis 760.61
    maternal abuse of drugs
      (gestational) (via placenta) (via
      breast milk) (*see also* Noxious,
      substances transmitted
      through placenta
      or breast milk (affecting fetus
      or newborn)) 760.70
      methamphetamine(s) 760.72
    procedure
      amniocentesis 760.61
      in utero NEC 760.62
      surgical on mother
        during pregnancy NEC
          760.63
        previous not associated with
          pregnancy 760.64
  apnea 770.81
    obstructive 770.82
    specified NEC 770.82
  breast buds 779.89
  cardiomyopathy 425.4
    congenital 425.3
  convulsion 779.0
  electrolyte imbalance NEC (transitory)
    775.5

Newborn (Continued)
  fever (environmentally-induced)
    778.4
  gestation
    24 completed weeks 765.22
    25–26 completed weeks 765.23
    27–28 completed weeks 765.24
    29–30 completed weeks 765.25
    31–32 completed weeks 765.26
    33–34 completed weeks 765.27
    35–36 completed weeks 765.28
    37 or more completed weeks 765.29
    less than 24 completed weeks
      765.21
    unspecified completed weeks
      765.20
  infection 771.89
    candida 771.7
    mastitis 771.5
    specified NEC 771.89
    urinary tract 771.82
  mastitis 771.5
  multiple NEC
    born in hospital (without mention of
      cesarean delivery or section)
      V37.00
      with cesarean delivery or section
        V37.01
    born outside hospital
      hospitalized V37.1●
      not hospitalized V37.2●
    mates all liveborn
      born in hospital (without
        mention of cesarean
        delivery or section)
        V34.00
        with cesarean delivery or
          section V34.01
      born outside hospital
        hospitalized V34.1●
        not hospitalized V34.2●
    mates all stillborn
      born in hospital (without
        mention of cesarean
        delivery or section)
        V35.00
        with cesarean delivery or
          section V35.01
      born outside hospital
        hospitalized V35.1●
        not hospitalized V35.2●
    mates liveborn and stillborn
      born in hospital (without
        mention of cesarean
        delivery or section)
        V36.00
        with cesarean delivery or
          section V36.01
      born outside hospital
        hospitalized V36.1●
        not hospitalized V36.2●
  omphalitis 771.4
  seizure 779.0
  sepsis 771.81
  single
    born in hospital (without mention of
      cesarean delivery or section)
      V30.00
      with cesarean delivery or section
        V30.01
    born outside hospital
      hospitalized V30.1●
      not hospitalized V30.2●
  specified condition NEC 779.89

Newborn (Continued)
  twin NEC
    born in hospital (without mention of
      cesarean delivery or section)
      V33.00
      with cesarean delivery or section
        V33.01
    born outside hospital
      hospitalized V33.1●
      not hospitalized V33.2●
    mate liveborn
      born in hospital V31.0●
      born outside hospital
        hospitalized V31.1●
        not hospitalized V31.2●
    mate stillborn
      born in hospital V32.0●
      born outside hospital
        hospitalized V32.1●
        not hospitalized V32.2●
  unspecified as to single or multiple
    birth
    born in hospital (without mention of
      cesarean delivery or section)
      V39.00
      with cesarean delivery or section
        V39.01
    born outside hospital
      hospitalized V39.1●
      not hospitalized V39.2●
  weight check V20.32 ◄
Newcastle's conjunctivitis or disease
  077.8
Nezelof's syndrome (pure
  alymphocytosis) 279.13
Niacin (amide) deficiency 265.2
Nicolas-Durand-Favre disease (climatic
  bubo) 099.1
Nicolas-Favre disease (climatic bubo)
  099.1
Nicotinic acid (amide) deficiency
  265.2
Niemann-Pick disease (lipid
  histiocytosis) (splenomegaly)
  272.7
Night
  blindness (*see also* Blindness, night)
    368.60
    congenital 368.61
    vitamin A deficiency 264.5
  cramps 729.82
  sweats 780.8
  terrors, child 307.46
Nightmare 307.47
  REM-sleep type 307.47
Nipple - *see* condition
Nisbet's chancre 099.0
Nishimoto (-Takeuchi) disease 437.5
Nitritoid crisis or reaction - *see* Crisis,
  nitritoid
Nitrogen retention, extrarenal 788.99
Nitrosohemoglobinemia 289.89
Njovera 104.0
No
  diagnosis 799.9
  disease (found) V71.9
  room at the inn V65.0
Nocardiasis - *see* Nocardiosis
Nocardiosis 039.9
  with pneumonia 039.1
  lung 039.1
  specified type NEC 039.8
Nocturia 788.43
  psychogenic 306.53

Nocturnal - *see also* condition
  dyspnea (paroxysmal) 786.09
  emissions 608.89
  enuresis 788.36
    psychogenic 307.6
  frequency (micturition) 788.43
    psychogenic 306.53
Nodal rhythm disorder 427.89
Nodding of head 781.0
Node(s) - *see also* Nodules
  Heberden's 715.04
  larynx 478.79
  lymph - *see* condition
  milkers' 051.1
  Osler's 421.0
  rheumatic 729.89
  Schmorl's 722.30
    lumbar, lumbosacral 722.32
    specified region NEC 722.39
    thoracic, thoracolumbar 722.31
  singers' 478.5
  skin NEC 782.2
  tuberculous - *see* Tuberculosis, lymph
    gland
  vocal cords 478.5
Nodosities, Haygarth's 715.04
Nodule(s), nodular
  actinomycotic (*see also* Actinomycosis)
    039.9
  arthritic - *see* Arthritis, nodosa
  breast 793.89
  cutaneous 782.2
  Haygarth's 715.04
  inflammatory - *see* Inflammation
  juxta-articular 102.7
    syphilitic 095.7
    yaws 102.7
  larynx 478.79
  lung, solitary 518.89
    emphysematous 492.8
  milkers' 051.1
  prostate 600.10
    with
      urinary
        obstruction 600.11
        retention 600.11
  retrocardiac 785.9
  rheumatic 729.89
  rheumatoid - *see* Arthritis rheumatoid
  scrotum (inflammatory) 608.4
  singers' 478.5
  skin NEC 782.2
  solitary, lung 518.89
    emphysematous 492.8
  subcutaneous 782.2
  thyroid (gland) (nontoxic) (uninodular)
    241.0
    with
      hyperthyroidism 242.1●
      thyrotoxicosis 242.1●
    toxic or with hyperthyroidism
      242.1●
  vocal cords 478.5
Noma (gangrenous) (hospital) (infective)
    528.1
  auricle (*see also* Gangrene) 785.4
  mouth 528.1
  pudendi (*see also* Vulvitis) 616.10
  vulvae (*see also* Vulvitis) 616.10
Nomadism V60.0
Non-adherence
  artificial skin graft 996.55
  decellularized allodermis graft
    996.55

Non-autoimmune hemolytic anemia
    NEC 283.10
Nonclosure - *see also* Imperfect, closure
  ductus
    arteriosus 747.0
    Botalli 747.0
  Eustachian valve 746.89
  foramen
    Botalli 745.5
    ovale 745.5
Noncompliance with medical treatment
    V15.81
  renal dialysis V45.12
Nondescent (congenital) - *see also*
    Malposition, congenital
  cecum 751.4
  colon 751.4
  testis 752.51
Nondevelopment
  brain 742.1
    specified part 742.2
  heart 746.89
  organ or site, congenital NEC - *see*
    Hypoplasia
Nonengagement
  head NEC 652.5●
    in labor 660.1●
      affecting fetus or newborn 763.1
Nonexanthematous tick fever 066.1
Nonexpansion, lung (newborn) NEC 770.4
Nonfunctioning
  cystic duct (*see also* Disease,
    gallbladder) 575.8
  gallbladder (*see also* Disease,
    gallbladder) 575.8
  kidney (*see also* Disease, renal) 593.9
  labyrinth 386.58
Nonhealing
  stump (surgical) 997.69
  wound, surgical 998.83
Nonimplantation of ovum, causing
    infertility 628.3
Noninsufflation, fallopian tube 628.2
Nonne-Milroy-Meige syndrome (chronic
    hereditary edema) 757.0
Nonovulation 628.0
Nonpatent fallopian tube 628.2
Nonpneumatization, lung NEC 770.4
Nonreflex bladder 596.54
  with cauda equina 344.61
Nonretention of food - *see* Vomiting
Nonrotation - *see* Malrotation
Nonsecretion, urine (*see also* Anuria)
    788.5
  newborn 753.3
Nonunion
  fracture 733.82
  organ or site, congenital NEC - *see*
    Imperfect, closure
  symphysis pubis, congenital 755.69
  top sacrum, congenital 756.19
Nonviability 765.0●
Nonvisualization, gallbladder 793.3
Nonvitalized tooth 522.9
Non-working side interference 524.56
Normal
  delivery - *see* category 650
  menses V65.5
  state (feared complaint unfounded)
    V65.5
Normoblastosis 289.89
Normocytic anemia (infectional) 285.9
  due to blood loss (chronic) 280.0
    acute 285.1

Norrie's disease (congenital) (progressive
    oculoacousticocerebral
    degeneration) 743.8
North American blastomycosis
    116.0
Norwegian itch 133.0
Nose, nasal - *see* condition
Nosebleed 784.7
Nosomania 298.9
Nosophobia 300.29
Nostalgia 309.89
Notch of iris 743.46
Notched lip, congenital (*see also* Cleft,
    lip) 749.10
Notching nose, congenital (tip) 748.1
Nothnagel's
  syndrome 378.52
  vasomotor acroparesthesia 443.89
Novy's relapsing fever (American)
    087.1
Noxious
  foodstuffs, poisoning by
    fish 988.0
    fungi 988.1
    mushrooms 988.1
    plants (food) 988.2
    shellfish 988.0
    specified type NEC 988.8
    toadstool 988.1
  substances transmitted through
    placenta or breast milk
    (affecting fetus or newborn)
    760.70
    acetretin 760.78
    alcohol 760.71
    aminopterin 760.78
    antiandrogens 760.79
    anticonvulsant 760.77
    antifungal 760.74
    anti-infective agents 760.74
    antimetabolic 760.78
    atorvastatin 760.78
    carbamazepine 760.77
    cocaine 760.75
    "crack" 760.75
    diethylstilbestrol (DES) 760.76
    divalproex sodium 760.77
    endocrine disrupting chemicals
      760.79
    estrogens 760.79
    etretinate 760.78
    fluconazole 760.74
    fluvastatin 760.78
    hallucinogenic agents NEC 760.73
    hormones 760.79
    lithium 760.79
    lovastatin 760.78
    medicinal agents NEC 760.79
    methotrexate 760.78
    misoprostil 760.79
    narcotics 760.72
    obstetric anesthetic or analgesic
      763.5
    phenobarbital 760.77
    phenytoin 760.77
    pravastatin 760.78
    progestins 760.79
    retinoic acid 760.78
    simvastatin 760.78
    solvents 760.79
    specified agent NEC 760.79
    statins 760.78
    suspected, affecting management of
      pregnancy 655.5●

◀ New   ◀▥ Revised   ~~deleted~~ Deleted   ● Use Additional Digit(s)   ▥ Omit code

Noxious *(Continued)*
  substances transmitted through placenta
      or breast milk *(Continued)*
    tetracycline 760.74
    thalidomide 760.79
    trimethadione 760.77
    valproate 760.77
    valproic acid 760.77
    vitamin A 760.78
NPDH (new persistent daily headache)
    339.42
Nuchal hitch (arm) 652.8●
Nucleus pulposus - *see* condition
Numbness 782.0
Nuns' knee 727.2
Nursemaid's
  elbow 832.2●   ◀▥ Revised
  shoulder 831.0●

Nutmeg liver 573.8
Nutrition, deficient or insufficient
      (particular kind of food)
    269.9
  due to
    insufficient food 994.2
    lack of
        care (child) (infant) 995.52
          adult 995.84
        food 994.2
Nyctalopia (*see also* Blindness, night)
    368.60
  vitamin A deficiency 264.5
Nycturia 788.43
  psychogenic 306.53
Nymphomania 302.89

Nystagmus 379.50
  associated with vestibular system
      disorders 379.54
  benign paroxysmal positional 386.11
  central positional 386.2
  congenital 379.51
  deprivation 379.53
  dissociated 379.55
  latent 379.52
  miners' 300.89
  positional
    benign paroxysmal 386.11
    central 386.2
  specified NEC 379.56
  vestibular 379.54
  visual deprivation 379.53

O

Oasthouse urine disease 270.2
Obermeyer's relapsing fever (European) 087.0
Obesity (constitutional) (exogenous) (familial) (nutritional) (simple) 278.00
  adrenal 255.8
  complicating pregnancy, childbirth, or puerperium 649.1●
  due to hyperalimentation 278.00
  endocrine NEC 259.9
  endogenous 259.9
  Fröhlich's (adiposogenital dystrophy) 253.8
  glandular NEC 259.9
  hypothyroid (see also Hypothyroidism) 244.9
  morbid 278.01
  of pregnancy 649.1●
  pituitary 253.8
  severe 278.01
  thyroid (see also Hypothyroidism) 244.9
Oblique - see also condition
  lie before labor, affecting fetus or newborn 761.7
Obliquity, pelvis 738.6
Obliteration
  abdominal aorta 446.7
  appendix (lumen) 543.9
  artery 447.1
  ascending aorta 446.7
  bile ducts 576.8
    with calculus, choledocholithiasis, or stones - see Choledocholithiasis
    congenital 751.61
      jaundice from 751.61 [774.5]
  common duct 576.8
    with calculus, choledocholithiasis, or stones - see Choledocholithiasis
    congenital 751.61
  cystic duct 575.8
    with calculus, choledocholithiasis, or stones - see Choledocholithiasis
  disease, arteriolar 447.1
  endometrium 621.8
  eye, anterior chamber 360.34
  fallopian tube 628.2
  lymphatic vessel 457.1
    postmastectomy 457.0
  organ or site, congenital NEC - see Atresia
  placental blood vessels - see Placenta, abnormal
  supra-aortic branches 446.7
  ureter 593.89
  urethra 599.84
  vein 459.9
  vestibule (oral) 525.8
Observation (for) V71.9
  without need for further medical care V71.9
  accident NEC V71.4
    at work V71.3
  criminal assault V71.6
  deleterious agent ingestion V71.89
  disease V71.9
    cardiovascular V71.7
    heart V71.7

Observation (Continued)
  disease (Continued)
    mental V71.09
    specified condition NEC V71.89
  foreign body ingestion V71.89
  growth and development variations V21.8
  injuries (accidental) V71.4
    inflicted NEC V71.6
      during alleged rape or seduction V71.5
  malignant neoplasm, suspected V71.1
  postpartum
    immediately after delivery V24.0
    routine follow-up V24.2
  pregnancy
    high-risk V23.9
      specified problem NEC V23.89
    normal (without complication) V22.1
      with nonobstetric complication V22.2
      first V22.0
  rape or seduction, alleged V71.5
    injury during V71.5
  suicide attempt, alleged V71.89
  suspected (undiagnosed) (unproven)
    abuse V71.81
    cardiovascular disease V71.7
    child or wife battering victim V71.6
    concussion (cerebral) V71.6
    condition NEC V71.89
      infant - see Observation, suspected, condition, newborn
      maternal and fetal
        amniotic cavity and membrane problem V89.01
        cervical shortening V89.05
        fetal anomaly V89.03
        fetal growth problem V89.04
        oligohydramnios V89.01
        other specified problem NEC V89.09
        placental problem V89.02
        polyhydramnios V89.01
      newborn V29.9
        cardiovascular disease V29.8
        congenital anomaly V29.8
        genetic V29.3
        infectious V29.0
        ingestion foreign object V29.8
        injury V29.8
        metabolic V29.3
        neoplasm V29.8
        neurological V29.1
        poison, poisoning V29.8
        respiratory V29.2
        specified NEC V29.8
    exposure
      anthrax V71.82
      biologic agent NEC V71.83
      SARS V71.83
    infectious disease not requiring isolation V71.89
    malignant neoplasm V71.1
    mental disorder V71.09
    neglect V71.81
    neoplasm
      benign V71.89
      malignant V71.1
    specified condition NEC V71.89
    tuberculosis V71.2
  tuberculosis, suspected V71.2

Obsession, obsessional 300.3
  ideas and mental images 300.3
  impulses 300.3
  neurosis 300.3
  phobia 300.3
  psychasthenia 300.3
  ruminations 300.3
  state 300.3
  syndrome 300.3
Obsessive-compulsive 300.3
  neurosis 300.3
  personality 301.4
  reaction 300.3
Obstetrical trauma NEC (complicating delivery) 665.9●
  with
    abortion - see Abortion, by type, with damage to pelvic organs
    ectopic pregnancy (see also categories 633.0-633.9) 639.2
    molar pregnancy (see also categories 630-632) 639.2
  affecting fetus or newborn 763.89
  following
    abortion 639.2
    ectopic or molar pregnancy 639.2
Obstipation (see also Constipation) 564.00
  psychogenic 306.4
Obstruction, obstructed, obstructive
  airway NEC 519.8
    with
      allergic alveolitis NEC 495.9
      asthma NEC (see also Asthma) 493.9●
      bronchiectasis 494.0
        with acute exacerbation 494.1
      bronchitis (see also Bronchitis, with, obstruction) 491.20
      emphysema NEC 492.8
    chronic 496
      with
        allergic alveolitis NEC 495.5
        asthma NEC (see also Asthma) 493.2●
        bronchiectasis 494.0
          with acute exacerbation 494.1
        bronchitis (chronic) (see also Bronchitis, chronic, obstructive) 491.20
        emphysema NEC 492.8
    due to
      bronchospasm 519.11
      foreign body 934.9
      inhalation of fumes or vapors 506.9
      laryngospasm 478.75
  alimentary canal (see also Obstruction, intestine) 560.9
  ampulla of Vater 576.2
    with calculus, cholelithiasis, or stones - see Choledocholithiasis
  aortic (heart) (valve) (see also Stenosis, aortic) 424.1
    rheumatic (see also Stenosis, aortic, rheumatic) 395.0
  aortoiliac 444.0
  aqueduct of Sylvius 331.4
    congenital 742.3
      with spina bifida (see also Spina bifida) 741.0●
  Arnold-Chiari (see also Spina bifida) 741.0●

◀ New　　◀◀ Revised　　deleted Deleted　　● Use Additional Digit(s)　　▮ Omit code

Obstruction, obstructed, obstructive
(Continued)
artery (see also Embolism, artery) 444.9
  basilar (complete) (partial) (see also
    Occlusion, artery, basilar)
    433.0●
  carotid (complete) (partial) (see also
    Occlusion, artery, carotid)
    433.1●
  precerebral - see Occlusion, artery,
    precerebral NEC
  retinal (central) (see also Occlusion,
    retina) 362.30
  vertebral (complete) (partial) (see
    also Occlusion, artery,
    vertebral) 433.2●
asthma (chronic) (with obstructive
  pulmonary disease) 493.2●
band (intestinal) 560.81
bile duct or passage (see also
  Obstruction, biliary) 576.2
  congenital 751.61
    jaundice from 751.61 [774.5]
biliary (duct) (tract) 576.2
  with calculus 574.51
    with cholecystitis (chronic) 574.41
      acute 574.31
  congenital 751.61
    jaundice from 751.61 [774.5]
  gallbladder 575.2
    with calculus 574.21
      with cholecystitis (chronic)
        574.11
        acute 574.01
bladder neck (acquired) 596.0
  congenital 753.6
bowel (see also Obstruction, intestine)
  560.9
bronchus 519.19
canal, ear (see also Stricture, ear canal,
  acquired) 380.50
cardia 537.89
caval veins (inferior) (superior) 459.2
cecum (see also Obstruction, intestine)
  560.9
circulatory 459.9
colon (see also Obstruction, intestine)
  560.9
  sympathicotonic 560.89
common duct (see also Obstruction,
  biliary) 576.2
  congenital 751.61
coronary (artery) (heart) - (see also
  Arteriosclerosis, coronary)
  acute (see also Infarct, myocardium)
    410.9●
    without myocardial infarction
      411.81
cystic duct (see also Obstruction,
  gallbladder) 575.2
  congenital 751.61
device, implant, or graft - see
  Complications, due to (presence
  of) any device, implant, or graft
  classified to 996.0–996.5 NEC
due to foreign body accidentally left in
  operation wound 998.4
duodenum 537.3
  congenital 751.1
  due to
    compression NEC 537.3
    cyst 537.3
    intrinsic lesion or disease NEC
      537.3

Obstruction, obstructed, obstructive
(Continued)
duodenum (Continued)
  due to (Continued)
    scarring 537.3
    torsion 537.3
    ulcer 532.91
    volvulus 537.3
ejaculatory duct 608.89
endocardium 424.90
  arteriosclerotic 424.99
  specified cause, except rheumatic
    424.99
esophagus 530.3
Eustachian tube (complete) (partial)
  381.60
  cartilaginous
    extrinsic 381.63
    intrinsic 381.62
  due to
    cholesteatoma 381.61
    osseous lesion NEC 381.61
    polyp 381.61
  osseous 381.61
fallopian tube (bilateral) 628.2
fecal 560.39
  with hernia - see also Hernia, by site,
    with obstruction
    gangrenous - see Hernia, by site,
      with gangrene
foramen of Monro (congenital)
  742.3
  with spina bifida (see also Spina
    bifida) 741.0●
foreign body - see Foreign body
gallbladder 575.2
  with calculus, cholelithiasis, or
    stones 574.21
    with cholecystitis (chronic)
      574.11
      acute 574.01
  congenital 751.69
    jaundice from 751.69 [774.5]
gastric outlet 537.0
gastrointestinal (see also Obstruction,
  intestine) 560.9
glottis 478.79
hepatic 573.8
  duct (see also Obstruction, biliary)
    576.2
  congenital 751.61
icterus (see also Obstruction, biliary)
  576.8
  congenital 751.61
ileocecal coil (see also Obstruction,
  intestine) 560.9
ileum (see also Obstruction, intestine)
  560.9
iliofemoral (artery) 444.81
internal anastomosis - see
  Complications, mechanical, graft
intestine (mechanical) (neurogenic)
  (paroxysmal) (postinfectional)
  (reflex) 560.9
  with
    adhesions (intestinal) (peritoneal)
      560.81
    hernia - see also Hernia, by site,
      with obstruction
      gangrenous - see Hernia, by
        site, with gangrene
  adynamic (see also Ileus)
    560.1
  by gallstone 560.31

Obstruction, obstructed, obstructive
(Continued)
intestine (Continued)
  congenital or infantile (small)
    751.1
    large 751.2
  due to
    Ascaris lumbricoides 127.0
    mural thickening 560.89
    procedure 997.4
      involving urinary tract
        997.5
  impaction 560.39
  infantile - see Obstruction, intestine,
    congenital
  newborn
    due to
      fecaliths 777.1
      inspissated milk 777.2
      meconium (plug) 777.1
        in mucoviscidosis
          277.01
      transitory 777.4
  specified cause NEC 560.89
  transitory, newborn 777.4
  volvulus 560.2
intracardiac ball valve prosthesis
  996.02
jaundice (see also Obstruction, biliary)
  576.8
  congenital 751.61
jejunum (see also Obstruction, intestine)
  560.9
kidney 593.89
labor 660.9●
  affecting fetus or newborn
    763.1
  by
    bony pelvis (conditions
      classifiable to 653.0–653.9)
      660.1●
    deep transverse arrest 660.3●
    impacted shoulder 660.4●
    locked twins 660.5●
    malposition (fetus) (conditions
      classifiable to 652.0–652.9)
      660.0●
      head during labor 660.3●
    persistent occipitoposterior
      position 660.3●
    soft tissue, pelvic (conditions
      classifiable to 654.0–654.9)
      660.2●
lacrimal
  canaliculi 375.53
  congenital 743.65
  punctum 375.52
  sac 375.54
lacrimonasal duct 375.56
  congenital 743.65
  neonatal 375.55
lacteal, with steatorrhea 579.2
laryngitis (see also Laryngitis) 464.01
larynx 478.79
  congenital 748.3
liver 573.8
  cirrhotic (see also Cirrhosis, liver)
    571.5
lung 518.89
  with
    asthma - see Asthma
    bronchitis (chronic) 491.20
    emphysema NEC 492.8
  airway, chronic 496

Obstruction, obstructed, obstructive
(Continued)
  lung *(Continued)*
    chronic NEC 496
      with
        asthma (chronic) (obstructive)
          493.2●
    disease, chronic 496
      with
        asthma (chronic) (obstructive)
          493.2●
    emphysematous 492.8
  lymphatic 457.1
  meconium
    fetus or newborn 777.1
      in mucoviscidosis 277.01
    newborn due to fecaliths 777.1
  mediastinum 519.3
  mitral (rheumatic) - *see* Stenosis,
    mitral
  nasal 478.19
    duct 375.56
      neonatal 375.55
    sinus - *see* Sinusitis
  nasolacrimal duct 375.56
    congenital 743.65
    neonatal 375.55
  nasopharynx 478.29
  nose 478.19
  organ or site, congenital NEC - *see*
    Atresia
  pancreatic duct 577.8
  parotid gland 527.8
  pelviureteral junction *(see also*
    Obstruction, ureter) 593.4
  pharynx 478.29
  portal (circulation) (vein) 452
  prostate 600.90
    with
      other lower urinary tract
        symptoms (LUTS) 600.91
      urinary
        obstruction 600.91
        retention 600.91
    valve (urinary) 596.0
  pulmonary
    valve (heart) *(see also* Endocarditis,
      pulmonary) 424.3
    vein, isolated 747.49
  pyemic - *see* Septicemia
  pylorus (acquired) 537.0
    congenital 750.5
    infantile 750.5
  rectosigmoid *(see also* Obstruction,
    intestine) 560.9
  rectum 569.49
  renal 593.89
  respiratory 519.8
    chronic 496
  retinal (artery) (vein) (central) *(see also*
    Occlusion, retina) 362.30
  salivary duct (any) 527.8
    with calculus 527.5
  sigmoid *(see also* Obstruction, intestine)
    560.9
  sinus (accessory) (nasal) *(see also*
    Sinusitis) 473.9
  Stensen's duct 527.8
  stomach 537.89
    acute 536.1
    congenital 750.7
  submaxillary gland 527.8
    with calculus 527.5
  thoracic duct 457.1
  thrombotic - *see* Thrombosis
  tooth eruption 520.6

Obstruction, obstructed, obstructive
(Continued)
  trachea 519.19
  tracheostomy airway 519.09
  tricuspid - *see* Endocarditis, tricuspid
  upper respiratory, congenital 748.8
  ureter (functional) 593.4
    congenital 753.20
    due to calculus 592.1
  ureteropelvic junction, congenital
    753.21
  ureterovesical junction, congenital
    753.22
  urethra 599.60
    congenital 753.6
  urinary (moderate) 599.60
    organ or tract (lower) 599.60
      due to
        benign prostatic hypertrophy
          (BPH) - *see* category
          600
      specified NEC 599.69
        due to
          benign prostatic
            hypertrophy (BPH) -
            see category 600
    prostatic valve 596.0
    specified NEC 599.69
      due to
        benign prostatic hypertrophy
          (BPH) - *see* category
          600
  uropathy 599.60
  uterus 621.8
  vagina 623.2
  valvular - *see* Endocarditis
  vascular graft or shunt 996.1
    atherosclerosis - *see* Arteriosclerosis,
      coronary
    embolism 996.74
    occlusion NEC 996.74
    thrombus 996.74
  vein, venous 459.2
    caval (inferior) (superior) 459.2
    thrombotic - *see* Thrombosis
  vena cava (inferior) (superior)
    459.2
  ventricular shunt 996.2
  vesical 596.0
  vesicourethral orifice 596.0
  vessel NEC 459.9
Obturator - *see* condition
Occlusal
  plane deviation 524.76
  wear, teeth 521.10
Occlusion
  anus 569.49
    congenital 751.2
    infantile 751.2
  aortoiliac (chronic) 444.0
  aqueduct of Sylvius 331.4
    congenital 742.3
      with spina bifida *(see also* Spina
        bifida) 741.0●
  arteries of extremities, lower 444.22
    without thrombus or embolus *(see
      also* Arteriosclerosis,
      extremities) 440.20
    due to stricture or stenosis 447.1
    upper 444.21
      without thrombus or embolus
        (see also Arteriosclerosis,
        extremities) 440.20
      due to stricture or stenosis
        447.1

Occlusion *(Continued)*
  artery NEC *(see also* Embolism, artery)
    444.9
    auditory, internal 433.8●
    basilar 433.0●
      with other precerebral artery
        433.3●
      bilateral 433.3●
    brain or cerebral *(see also* Infarct,
      brain) 434.9●
    carotid 433.1●
      with other precerebral artery
        433.3●
      bilateral 433.3●
    cerebellar (anterior inferior)
      (posterior inferior) (superior)
      433.8●
    cerebral *(see also* Infarct, brain)
      434.9●
    choroidal (anterior) 433.8●
    chronic total
      coronary 414.2
      extremity(ies) 440.4
    communicating posterior 433.8●
    complete
      coronary 414.2
      extremity(ies) 440.4
    coronary (thrombotic) *(see also*
      Infarct, myocardium)
      410.9●
      acute 410.9●
        without myocardial infarction
          411.81
      chronic total 414.2
      complete 414.2
      healed or old 412
      total 414.2
    extremity(ies)
      chronic total 440.4
      complete 440.4
      total 440.4
    hypophyseal 433.8●
    iliac 444.81
    mesenteric (embolic) (thrombotic)
      (with gangrene) 557.0
    pontine 433.8●
    precerebral NEC 433.9●
      late effect - *see* Late effect(s) (of)
        cerebrovascular disease
      multiple or bilateral 433.3●
      puerperal, postpartum, childbirth
        674.0●
      specified NEC 433.8●
    renal 593.81
    retinal - *see* Occlusion, retina, artery
    spinal 433.8●
    vertebral 433.2●
      with other precerebral artery
        433.3●
      bilateral 433.3●
  basilar (artery) - *see* Occlusion, artery,
    basilar
  bile duct (any) *(see also* Obstruction,
    biliary) 576.2
  bowel *(see also* Obstruction, intestine)
    560.9
  brain (artery) (vascular) *(see also* Infarct,
    brain) 434.9●
  breast (duct) 611.89
  carotid (artery) (common) (internal) -
    see Occlusion, artery, carotid
  cerebellar (anterior inferior) (artery)
    (posterior inferior) (superior)
    433.8●
  cerebral (artery) *(see also* Infarct, brain)
    434.9●

◀ New   ◀▥ Revised   ~~deleted~~ Deleted   ● Use Additional Digit(s)   ▨ Omit code

Occlusion (Continued)
  cerebrovascular (see also Infarct, brain) 434.9●
    diffuse 437.0
  cervical canal (see also Stricture, cervix) 622.4
    by falciparum malaria 084.0
  cervix (uteri) (see also Stricture, cervix) 622.4
  choanal 748.0
  choroidal (artery) 433.8●
  colon (see also Obstruction, intestine) 560.9
  communicating posterior artery 433.8●
  coronary (artery) (thrombotic) (see also Infarct, myocardium) 410.9●
    acute 410.9●
      without myocardial infarction 411.81
    healed or old 412
  cystic duct (see also Obstruction, gallbladder) 575.2
    congenital 751.69
  disto
    division I 524.22
    division II 524.22
  embolic - see Embolism
  fallopian tube 628.2
    congenital 752.19
  gallbladder (see also Obstruction, gallbladder) 575.2
    congenital 751.69
      jaundice from 751.69 [744.5]
  gingiva, traumatic 523.8
  hymen 623.3
    congenital 752.42
  hypophyseal (artery) 433.8●
  iliac (artery) 444.81
  intestine (see also Obstruction, intestine) 560.9
  kidney 593.89
  lacrimal apparatus - see Stenosis, lacrimal
  lung 518.89
  lymph or lymphatic channel 457.1
  mammary duct 611.89
  mesenteric artery (embolic) (thrombotic) (with gangrene) 557.0
  nose 478.19
    congenital 748.0
  organ or site, congenital NEC - see Atresia
  oviduct 628.2
    congenital 752.19
  periodontal, traumatic 523.8
  peripheral arteries (lower extremity) 444.22
    without thrombus or embolus (see also Arteriosclerosis, extremities) 440.20
    due to stricture or stenosis 447.1
    upper extremity 444.21
      without thrombus or embolus (see also Arteriosclerosis, extremities) 440.20
      due to stricture or stenosis 447.1
  pontine (artery) 433.8●
  posterior lingual, of mandibular teeth 524.29
  precerebral artery - see Occlusion, artery, precerebral NEC
  puncta lacrimalia 375.52
  pupil 364.74
  pylorus (see also Stricture, pylorus) 537.0

Occlusion (Continued)
  renal artery 593.81
  retina, retinal (vascular) 362.30
    artery, arterial 362.30
      branch 362.32
      central (total) 362.31
      partial 362.33
      transient 362.34
      tributary 362.32
    vein 362.30
      branch 362.36
      central (total) 362.35
      incipient 362.37
      partial 362.37
      tributary 362.36
  spinal artery 433.8●
  stent
    coronary 996.72
  teeth (mandibular) (posterior lingual) 524.29
  thoracic duct 457.1
  tubal 628.2
  ureter (complete) (partial) 593.4
    congenital 753.29
  urethra (see also Stricture, urethra) 598.9
    congenital 753.6
  uterus 621.8
  vagina 623.2
  vascular NEC 459.9
  vein - see Thrombosis
  vena cava ~~(inferior) (superior)~~ ~~453.2~~ ◀▥
    inferior 453.2 ◀
    superior 453.87 ◀
      acute 453.87 ◀
      chronic 453.77 ◀
  ventricle (brain) NEC 331.4
  vertebral (artery) - see Occlusion, artery, vertebral
  vessel (blood) NEC 459.9
  vulva 624.8
Occlusio pupillae 364.74
Occupational
  problems NEC V62.29
  therapy V57.21
Ochlophobia 300.29
Ochronosis (alkaptonuric) (congenital) (endogenous) 270.2
  with chloasma of eyelid 270.2
Ocular muscle - see also condition
  myopathy 359.1
  torticollis 781.93
Oculoauriculovertebral dysplasia 756.0
Oculogyric
  crisis or disturbance 378.87
    psychogenic 306.7
Oculomotor syndrome 378.81
Oddi's sphincter spasm 576.5
Odelberg's disease (juvenile osteochondrosis) 732.1
Odontalgia 525.9
Odontoameloblastoma (M9311/0) 213.1
  upper jaw (bone) 213.0
Odontoclasia 521.05
Odontoclasis 873.63
  complicated 873.73
Odontodysplasia, regional 520.4
Odontogenesis imperfecta 520.5
Odontoma (M9280/0) 213.1
  ameloblastic (M9311/0) 213.1
    upper jaw (bone) 213.0
  calcified (M9280/0) 213.1
    upper jaw (bone) 213.0
  complex (M9282/0) 213.1
    upper jaw (bone) 213.0

Odontoma (Continued)
  compound (M9281/0) 213.1
    upper jaw (bone) 213.0
  fibroameloblastic (M9290/0) 213.1
    upper jaw (bone) 213.0
  follicular 526.0
    upper jaw (bone) 213.0
Odontomyelitis (closed) (open) 522.0
Odontonecrosis 521.09
Odontorrhagia 525.8
Odontosarcoma, ameloblastic (M9290/3) 170.1
  upper jaw (bone) 170.0
Odynophagia 787.20
Oesophagostomiasis 127.7
Oesophagostomum infestation 127.7
Oestriasis 134.0
Ogilvie's syndrome (sympathicotonic colon obstruction) 560.89
Oguchi's disease (retina) 368.61
Ohara's disease (see also Tularemia) 021.9
Oidiomycosis (see also Candidiasis) 112.9
Oidiomycotic meningitis 112.83
Oidium albicans infection (see also Candidiasis) 112.9
Old age 797
  dementia (of) 290.0
Olfactory - see condition
Oligemia 285.9
Oligergasia (see also Retardation, mental) 319
Oligoamnios 658.0●
  affecting fetus or newborn 761.2
Oligoastrocytoma, mixed (M9382/3)
  specified site - see Neoplasm, by site, malignant
  unspecified site 191.9
Oligocythemia 285.9
Oligodendroblastoma (M9460/3)
  specified site - see Neoplasm, by site, malignant
  unspecified site 191.9
Oligodendroglioma (M9450/3)
  anaplastic type (M9451/3)
    specified site - see Neoplasm, by site, malignant
    unspecified site 191.9
  specified site - see Neoplasm, by site, malignant
  unspecified site 191.9
Oligodendroma - see Oligodendroglioma
Oligodontia (see also Anodontia) 520.0
Oligoencephalon 742.1
Oligohydramnios 658.0●
  affecting fetus or newborn 761.2
  due to premature rupture of membranes 658.1●
    affecting fetus or newborn 761.2
Oligohydrosis 705.0
Oligomenorrhea 626.1
Oligophrenia (see also Retardation, mental) 319
  phenylpyruvic 270.1
Oligospermia 606.1
Oligotrichia 704.09
  congenita 757.4
Oliguria 788.5
  with
    abortion - see Abortion, by type, with renal failure
    ectopic pregnancy (see also categories 633.0–633.9) 639.3
    molar pregnancy (see also categories 630–632) 639.3

Oliguria (Continued)
  complicating
    abortion 639.3
    ectopic or molar pregnancy 639.3
    pregnancy 646.2●
      with hypertension - see Toxemia,
        of pregnancy
  due to a procedure 997.5
  following labor and delivery 669.3●
  heart or cardiac - see Failure, heart
  puerperal, postpartum 669.3●
  specified due to a procedure 997.5
Ollier's disease (chondrodysplasia)
  756.4
Omentitis (see also Peritonitis) 567.9
Omentocele (see also Hernia, omental)
  553.8
Omentum, omental - see condition
Omphalitis (congenital) (newborn)
  771.4
  not of newborn 686.9
  tetanus 771.3
Omphalocele 756.72   ◀▥
Omphalomesenteric duct, persistent
  751.0
Omphalorrhagia, newborn 772.3
Omsk hemorrhagic fever 065.1
Onanism 307.9
Onchocerciasis 125.3
  eye 125.3 [360.13]
Onchocercosis 125.3
Oncocytoma (M8290/0) - see Neoplasm,
  by site, benign
Ondine's curse 348.89   ◀▥
Oneirophrenia (see also Schizophrenia)
  295.4●
Onychauxis 703.8
  congenital 757.5
Onychia (with lymphangitis) 681.9
  dermatophytic 110.1
  finger 681.02
  toe 681.11
Onychitis (with lymphangitis) 681.9
  finger 681.02
  toe 681.11
Onychocryptosis 703.0
Onychodystrophy 703.8
  congenital 757.5
Onychogryphosis 703.8
Onychogryposis 703.8
Onycholysis 703.8
Onychomadesis 703.8
Onychomalacia 703.8
Onychomycosis 110.1
  finger 110.1
  toe 110.1
Onycho-osteodysplasia 756.89
Onychophagy 307.9
Onychoptosis 703.8
Onychorrhexis 703.8
  congenital 757.5
Onychoschizia 703.8
Onychotrophia (see also Atrophy, nail)
  703.8
O'Nyong Nyong fever 066.3
Onyxis (finger) (toe) 703.0
Onyxitis (with lymphangitis) 681.9
  finger 681.02
  toe 681.11
Oocyte (egg) (ovum)
  donor V59.70
    over age 35 V59.73
      anonymous recipient V59.73
      designated recipient V59.74

Oocyte (Continued)
  donor (Continued)
    under age 35 V59.71
      anonymous recipient V59.71
      designated recipient V59.72
Oophoritis (cystic) (infectional)
  (interstitial) (see also Salpingo-
  oophoritis) 614.2
  complicating pregnancy 646.6●
  fetal (acute) 752.0
  gonococcal (acute) 098.19
    chronic or duration of 2 months or
      over 098.39
  tuberculous (see also Tuberculosis)
    016.6●
Opacity, opacities
  cornea 371.00
    central 371.03
    congenital 743.43
      interfering with vision 743.42
    degenerative (see also Degeneration,
      cornea) 371.40
    hereditary (see also Dystrophy,
      cornea) 371.50
    inflammatory (see also Keratitis)
      370.9
    late effect of trachoma (healed)
      139.1
    minor 371.01
    peripheral 371.02
  enamel (fluoride) (nonfluoride) (teeth)
    520.3
  lens (see also Cataract) 366.9
  snowball 379.22
  vitreous (humor) 379.24
    congenital 743.51
Opalescent dentin (hereditary) 520.5
Open, opening
  abnormal, organ or site, congenital - see
    Imperfect, closure
  angle with
    borderline intraocular pressure
      365.01
    cupping of discs 365.01
  bite
    anterior 524.24
    posterior 524.25
  false - see Imperfect, closure
  margin on tooth restoration 525.61
  restoration margins 525.61
  wound - see Wound, open, by site
Operation
  causing mutilation of fetus 763.89
  destructive, on live fetus, to facilitate
    birth 763.89
  for delivery, fetus or newborn 763.89
  maternal, unrelated to current delivery,
    affecting fetus or newborn (see
    also Newborn, affected by) 760.64
Operational fatigue 300.89
Operative - see condition
Operculitis (chronic) 523.40
  acute 523.30
Operculum, retina 361.32
  with detachment 361.01
Ophiasis 704.01
Ophthalmia (see also Conjunctivitis)
  372.30
  actinic rays 370.24
  allergic (acute) 372.05
    chronic 372.14
  blennorrhagic (neonatorum) 098.40
  catarrhal 372.03
  diphtheritic 032.81

Ophthalmia (Continued)
  Egyptian 076.1
  electric, electrica 370.24
  gonococcal (neonatorum) 098.40
  metastatic 360.11
  migraine 346.8●
  neonatorum, newborn 771.6
    gonococcal 098.40
  nodosa 360.14
  phlyctenular 370.31
    with ulcer (see also Ulcer, cornea)
      370.00
  sympathetic 360.11
Ophthalmitis - see Ophthalmia
Ophthalmocele (congenital) 743.66
Ophthalmoneuromyelitis 341.0
Ophthalmopathy, infiltrative with
  thyrotoxicosis 242.0●
Ophthalmoplegia (see also Strabismus)
  378.9
  anterior internuclear 378.86
  ataxia-areflexia syndrome 357.0
  bilateral 378.9
  diabetic 250.5● [378.86]
    due to secondary diabetes 249.5●
      [378.86]
  exophthalmic 242.0● [376.22]
  external 378.55
    progressive 378.72
    total 378.56
  internal (complete) (total) 367.52
  internuclear 378.86
  migraine 346.2●
  painful 378.55
  Parinaud's 378.81
  progressive external 378.72
  supranuclear, progressive 333.0
  total (external) 378.56
    internal 367.52
  unilateral 378.9
Opisthognathism 524.00
Opisthorchiasis (felineus) (tenuicollis)
  (viverrini) 121.0
Opisthotonos, opisthotonus 781.0
Opitz's disease (congestive
  splenomegaly) 289.51
Opiumism (see also Dependence) 304.0●
Oppenheim's disease 358.8
Oppenheim-Urbach disease or syndrome
  (necrobiosis lipoidica diabeticorum)
  250.8● [709.3]
  due to secondary diabetes 249.8● [709.3]
Opsoclonia 379.59
Optic nerve - see condition
Orbit - see condition
Orchioblastoma (M9071/3) 186.9
Orchitis (nonspecific) (septic) 604.90
  with abscess 604.0
  blennorrhagic (acute) 098.13
    chronic or duration of 2 months or
      over 098.33
  diphtheritic 032.89 [604.91]
  filarial 125.9 [604.91]
  gangrenous 604.99
  gonococcal (acute) 098.13
    chronic or duration of 2 months or
      over 098.33
  mumps 072.0
  parotidea 072.0
  suppurative 604.99
  syphilitic 095.8 [604.91]
  tuberculous (see also Tuberculosis)
    016.5● [608.81]
Orf 051.2

Organic - *see also* condition
  heart - *see* Disease, heart
  insufficiency 799.89
Oriental
  bilharziasis 120.2
  schistosomiasis 120.2
  sore 085.1
Orientation
  ego-dystonic sexual 302.0
Orifice - *see* condition
Origin, both great vessels from right
    ventricle 745.11
Ormond's disease or syndrome 593.4
Ornithosis 073.9
  with
    complication 073.8
      specified NEC 073.7
    pneumonia 073.0
    pneumonitis (lobular) 073.0
Orodigitofacial dysostosis 759.89
Oropouche fever 066.3
Orotaciduria, oroticaciduria (congenital)
    (hereditary) (pyrimidine deficiency)
    281.4
Oroya fever 088.0
Orthodontics V58.5
  adjustment V53.4
  aftercare V58.5
  fitting V53.4
Orthopnea 786.02
Os, uterus - *see* condition
Osgood-Schlatter
  disease 732.4
  osteochondrosis 732.4
Osler's
  disease (M9950/1) (polycythemia vera)
    238.4
  nodes 421.0
Osler-Rendu disease (familial
    hemorrhagic telangiectasia) 448.0
Osler-Vaquez disease (M9950/1)
    (polycythemia vera) 238.4
Osler-Weber-Rendu syndrome (familial
    hemorrhagic telangiectasia) 448.0
Osmidrosis 705.89
Osseous - *see* condition
Ossification
  artery - *see* Arteriosclerosis
  auricle (ear) 380.39
  bronchus 519.19
  cardiac (*see also* Degeneration,
    myocardial) 429.1
  cartilage (senile) 733.99
  coronary - *see* Arteriosclerosis, coronary
  diaphragm 728.10
  ear 380.39
    middle (*see also* Otosclerosis) 387.9
  falx cerebri 349.2
  fascia 728.10
  fontanel
    defective or delayed 756.0
    premature 756.0
  heart (*see also* Degeneration,
    myocardial) 429.1
    valve - *see* Endocarditis
  larynx 478.79
  ligament
    posterior longitudinal 724.8
      cervical 723.7
  meninges (cerebral) 349.2
    spinal 336.8
  multiple, eccentric centers 733.99
  muscle 728.10
    heterotopic, postoperative 728.13

Ossification (*Continued*)
  myocardium, myocardial (*see also*
    Degeneration, myocardial) 429.1
  penis 607.81
  periarticular 728.89
  sclera 379.16
  tendon 727.82
  trachea 519.19
  tympanic membrane (*see also*
    Tympanosclerosis) 385.00
  vitreous (humor) 360.44
Osteitis (*see also* Osteomyelitis) 730.2 ●
  acute 730.0 ●
  alveolar 526.5
  chronic 730.1 ●
  condensans (ilii) 733.5
  deformans (Paget's) 731.0
    due to or associated with malignant
      neoplasm (*see also* Neoplasm,
      bone, malignant) 170.9 *[731.1]*
  due to yaws 102.6
  fibrosa NEC 733.29
    cystica (generalisata) 252.01
    disseminata 756.59
    osteoplastica 252.01
  fragilitans 756.51
  Garré's (sclerosing) 730.1 ●
  infectious (acute) (subacute) 730.0 ●
    chronic or old 730.1 ●
  jaw (acute) (chronic) (lower) (neonatal)
    (suppurative) (upper) 526.4
  parathyroid 252.01
  petrous bone (*see also* Petrositis) 383.20
  pubis 733.5
  sclerotic, nonsuppurative 730.1 ●
  syphilitic 095.5
  tuberculosa
    cystica (of Jüngling) 135
    multiplex cystoides 135
Osteoarthritica spondylitis (spine) (*see
    also* Spondylosis) 721.90
Osteoarthritis (*see also* Osteoarthrosis)
    715.9 ●
  distal interphalangeal 715.9 ●
  hyperplastic 731.2
  interspinalis (*see also* Spondylosis)
    721.90
  spine, spinal NEC (*see also* Spondylosis)
    721.90
Osteoarthropathy (*see also* Osteoarthrosis)
    715.9 ●
  chronic idiopathic hypertrophic 757.39
  familial idiopathic 757.39
  hypertrophic pulmonary 731.2
    secondary 731.2
  idiopathic hypertrophic 757.39
  primary hypertrophic 731.2
  pulmonary hypertrophic 731.2
  secondary hypertrophic 731.2
Osteoarthrosis (degenerative)
    (hypertrophic) (rheumatoid) 715.9 ●

> Note 56 Use the following fifth-digit
> subclassification with category 715:
>
> 0 site unspecified
> 1 shoulder region
> 2 upper arm
> 3 forearm
> 4 hand
> 5 pelvic region and thigh
> 6 lower leg
> 7 ankle and foot
> 8 other specified sites except spine
> 9 multiple sites

Osteoarthrosis (*Continued*)
  Deformans alkaptonurica 270.2
  generalized 715.09
  juvenilis (Köhler's) 732.5
  localized 715.3 ●
    idiopathic 715.1 ●
    primary 715.1 ●
    secondary 715.2 ●
  multiple sites, not specified as
    generalized 715.89
  polyarticular 715.09
  spine (*see also* Spondylosis) 721.90
  temporomandibular joint 524.69
Osteoblastoma (M9200/0) - *see*
    Neoplasm, bone, benign
Osteochondritis (*see also*
    Osteochondrosis) 732.9
  dissecans 732.7
    hip 732.7
  ischiopubica 732.1
  multiple 756.59
  syphilitic (congenital) 090.0
Osteochondrodermodysplasia 756.59
Osteochondrodystrophy 277.5
  deformans 277.5
  familial 277.5
  fetalis 756.4
Osteochondrolysis 732.7
Osteochondroma (M9210/0) - *see also*
    Neoplasm, bone, benign
  multiple, congenital 756.4
Osteochondromatosis (M9210/1) 238.0
  synovial 727.82
Osteochondromyxosarcoma (M9180/3) -
    see Neoplasm, bone, malignant
Osteochondropathy NEC 732.9
Osteochondrosarcoma (M9180/3) - *see*
    Neoplasm, bone, malignant
Osteochondrosis 732.9
  acetabulum 732.1
  adult spine 732.8
  astragalus 732.5
  Blount's 732.4
  Buchanan's (juvenile osteochondrosis
    of iliac crest) 732.1
  Buchman's (juvenile osteochondrosis)
    732.1
  Burns' 732.3
  calcaneus 732.5
  capitular epiphysis (femur) 732.1
  carpal
    lunate (wrist) 732.3
    scaphoid 732.3
  coxae juvenilis 732.1
  deformans juvenilis (coxae) (hip)
    732.1
    Scheuermann's 732.0
    spine 732.0
    tibia 732.4
    vertebra 732.0
  Diaz's (astragalus) 732.5
  dissecans (knee) (shoulder) 732.7
  femoral capital epiphysis 732.1
  femur (head) (juvenile) 732.1
  foot (juvenile) 732.5
  Freiberg's (disease) (second metatarsal)
    732.5
  Haas' 732.3
  Haglund's (os tibiale externum)
    732.5
  hand (juvenile) 732.3
  head of
    femur 732.1
    humerus (juvenile) 732.3

Osteochondrosis (*Continued*)
hip (juvenile) 732.1
humerus (juvenile) 732.3
iliac crest (juvenile) 732.1
ilium (juvenile) 732.1
ischiopubic synchondrosis 732.1
Iselin's (osteochondrosis fifth
metatarsal) 732.5
juvenile, juvenilis 732.6
arm 732.3
capital femoral epiphysis 732.1
capitellum humeri 732.3
capitular epiphysis 732.1
carpal scaphoid 732.3
clavicle, sternal epiphysis 732.6
coxae 732.1
deformans 732.1
foot 732.5
hand 732.3
hip and pelvis 732.1
lower extremity, except foot 732.4
lunate, wrist 732.3
medial cuneiform bone 732.5
metatarsal (head) 732.5
metatarsophalangeal 732.5
navicular, ankle 732.5
patella 732.4
primary patellar center (of Köhler)
732.4
specified site NEC 732.6
spine 732.0
tarsal scaphoid 732.5
tibia (epiphysis) (tuberosity) 732.4
upper extremity 732.3
vertebra (body) (Calvé) 732.0
epiphyseal plates (of
Scheuermann) 732.0
Kienböck's (disease) 732.3
Köhler's (disease) (navicular, ankle)
732.5
patellar 732.4
tarsal navicular 732.5
Legg-Calvé-Perthes (disease) 732.1
lower extremity (juvenile) 732.4
lunate bone 732.3
Mauclaire's 732.3
metacarpal heads (of Mauclaire) 732.3
metatarsal (fifth) (head) (second) 732.5
navicular, ankle 732.5
os calcis 732.5
Osgood-Schlatter 732.4
os tibiale externum 732.5
Panner's 732.3
patella (juvenile) 732.4
patellar center
primary (of Köhler) 732.4
secondary (of Sinding-Larsen) 732.4
pelvis (juvenile) 732.1
Pierson's 732.1
radial head (juvenile) 732.3
Scheuermann's 732.0
Sever's (calcaneum) 732.5
Sinding-Larsen (secondary patellar
center) 732.4
spine (juvenile) 732.0
adult 732.8
symphysis pubis (of Pierson) (juvenile)
732.1
syphilitic (congenital) 090.0
tarsal (navicular) (scaphoid) 732.5
tibia (proximal) (tubercle) 732.4
tuberculous - *see* Tuberculosis, bone
ulna 732.3
upper extremity (juvenile) 732.3

Osteochondrosis (*Continued*)
van Neck's (juvenile osteochondrosis)
732.1
vertebral (juvenile) 732.0
adult 732.8
Osteoclastoma (M9250/1) 238.0
malignant (M9250/3) - *see* Neoplasm,
bone, malignant
Osteocopic pain 733.90
Osteodynia 733.90
Osteodystrophy
azotemic 588.0
chronica deformans hypertrophica
731.0
congenital 756.50
specified type NEC 756.59
deformans 731.0
fibrosa localisata 731.0
parathyroid 252.01
renal 588.0
Osteofibroma (M9262/0) - *see* Neoplasm,
bone, benign
Osteofibrosarcoma (M9182/3) - *see*
Neoplasm, bone, malignant
Osteogenesis imperfecta 756.51
Osteogenic - *see* condition
Osteoma (M9180/0) - *see also* Neoplasm,
bone, benign
osteoid (M9191/0) - *see also* Neoplasm,
bone, benign
giant (M9200/0) - *see* Neoplasm,
bone, benign
Osteomalacia 268.2
chronica deformans hypertrophica
731.0
due to vitamin D deficiency 268.2
infantile (*see also* Rickets) 268.0
juvenile (*see also* Rickets) 268.0
pelvis 268.2
vitamin D-resistant 275.3
Osteomalacic bone 268.2
Osteomalacosis 268.2
Osteomyelitis (general) (infective)
(localized) (neonatal) (purulent)
(pyogenic) (septic) (staphylococcal)
(streptococcal) (suppurative) (with
periostitis) 730.2●

> Note 57   Use the following fifth-digit
> subclassification with category 730:
>
> 0   site unspecified
> 1   shoulder region
> 2   upper arm
> 3   forearm
> 4   hand
> 5   pelvic region and thigh
> 6   lower leg
> 7   ankle and foot
> 8   other specified sites
> 9   multiple sites

acute or subacute 730.0●
chronic or old 730.1●
due to or associated with
diabetes mellitus 250.8● [731.8]
due to secondary diabetes 249.8●
[731.8]
tuberculosis (*see also* Tuberculosis,
bone) 015.9● [730.8]●
limb bones 015.5● [730.8]●
specified bones NEC 015.7●
[730.8]●
spine 015.0● [730.8]●
typhoid 002.0 [730.8]●

Osteomyelitis (*Continued*)
Garré's 730.1●
jaw (acute) (chronic) (lower) (neonatal)
(suppurative) (upper) 526.4
nonsuppurating 730.1●
orbital 376.03
petrous bone (*see also* Petrositis)
383.20
Salmonella 003.24
sclerosing, nonsuppurative 730.1●
sicca 730.1●
syphilitic 095.5
congenital 090.0 [730.8]●
tuberculous - *see* Tuberculosis, bone
typhoid 002.0 [730.8]●
Osteomyelofibrosis 289.89
Osteomyelosclerosis 289.89
Osteonecrosis 733.40
meaning osteomyelitis 730.1●
Osteo-onycho-arthro dysplasia 756.89
Osteo-onychodysplasia, hereditary
756.89
Osteopathia
condensans disseminata 756.53
hyperostotica multiplex infantilis
756.59
hypertrophica toxica 731.2
striata 756.4
Osteopathy resulting from poliomyelitis
(*see also* Poliomyelitis) 045.9●
[730.7]
familial dysplastic 731.2
Osteopecilia 756.53
Osteopenia 733.90
borderline 733.90
Osteoperiostitis (*see also* Osteomyelitis)
730.2●
ossificans toxica 731.2
toxica ossificans 731.2
Osteopetrosis (familial) 756.52
Osteophyte - *see* Exostosis
Osteophytosis - *see* Exostosis
Osteopoikilosis 756.53
Osteoporosis (generalized) 733.00
circumscripta 731.0
disuse 733.03
drug-induced 733.09
idiopathic 733.02
postmenopausal 733.01
posttraumatic 733.7
screening V82.81
senile 733.01
specified type NEC 733.09
Osteoporosis-osteomalacia syndrome
268.2
Osteopsathyrosis 756.51
Osteoradionecrosis, jaw 526.89
Osteosarcoma (M9180/3) - *see also*
Neoplasm, bone, malignant
chondroblastic (M9181/3) - *see*
Neoplasm, bone, malignant
fibroblastic (M9182/3) - *see* Neoplasm,
bone, malignant
in Paget's disease of bone (M9184/3) -
see Neoplasm, bone, malignant
juxtacortical (M9190/3) - *see* Neoplasm,
bone malignant
parosteal (M9190/3) - *see* Neoplasm,
bone, malignant
telangiectatic (M9183/3) - *see*
Neoplasm, bone, malignant
Osteosclerosis 756.52
fragilis (generalisata) 756.52
Osteosclerotic anemia 289.89

Osteosis
  acromegaloid 757.39
  cutis 709.3
  parathyroid 252.01
  renal fibrocystic 588.0
Österreicher-Turner syndrome 756.89
Ostium
  atrioventriculare commune 745.69
  primum (arteriosum) (defect)
      (persistent) 745.61
  secundum (arteriosum) (defect)
      (patent) (persistent) 745.5
Ostrum-Furst syndrome 756.59
Otalgia 388.70
  otogenic 388.71
  referred 388.72
Othematoma 380.31
Otitic hydrocephalus 348.2
Otitis 382.9
  with effusion 381.4
      purulent 382.4
      secretory 381.4
      serous 381.4
      suppurative 382.4
  acute 382.9
  adhesive (see also Adhesions, middle
      ear) 385.10
  chronic 382.9
      with effusion 381.3
      mucoid, mucous (simple) 381.20
      purulent 382.3
      secretory 381.3
      serous 381.10
      suppurative 382.3
  diffuse parasitic 136.8
  externa (acute) (diffuse) (hemorrhagica)
      380.10
      actinic 380.22
      candidal 112.82
      chemical 380.22
      chronic 380.23
          mycotic - see Otitis, externa,
              mycotic
          specified type NEC 380.23
      circumscribed 380.10
      contact 380.22
      due to
          erysipelas 035 [380.13]
          impetigo 684 [380.13]
          seborrheic dermatitis 690.10
              [380.13]
      eczematoid 380.22
      furuncular 680.0 [380.13]
      infective 380.10
          chronic 380.16
      malignant 380.14
      mycotic (chronic) 380.15
          due to
              aspergillosis 117.3 [380.15]
              moniliasis 112.82
              otomycosis 111.8 [380.15]
      reactive 380.22
      specified type NEC 380.22
      tropical 111.8 [380.15]
  insidiosa (see also Otosclerosis) 387.9
  interna (see also Labyrinthitis) 386.30
  media (hemorrhagic) (staphylococcal)
      (streptococcal) 382.9
      acute 382.9
          with effusion 381.00
          allergic 381.04
              mucoid 381.05
              sanguineous 381.06
              serous 381.04

Otitis (Continued)
  media (Continued)
      acute (Continued)
          catarrhal 381.00
          exudative 381.00
          mucoid 381.02
              allergic 381.05
          necrotizing 382.00
              with spontaneous rupture of
                  ear drum 382.01
              in
                  influenza 487.8 [382.02]
                  measles 055.2
                  scarlet fever 034.1 [382.02]
          nonsuppurative 381.00
          purulent 382.00
              with spontaneous rupture of
                  ear drum 382.01
          sanguineous 381.03
              allergic 381.06
          secretory 381.01
          seromucinous 381.02
          serous 381.01
              allergic 381.04
          suppurative 382.00
              with spontaneous rupture of
                  ear drum 382.01
              due to
                  influenza 487.8 [382.02]
                  scarlet fever 034.1 [382.02]
          transudative 381.00
      adhesive (see also Adhesions, middle
          ear) 385.10
      allergic 381.4
          acute 381.04
              mucoid 381.05
              sanguineous 381.06
              serous 381.04
          chronic 381.3
      catarrhal 381.4
          acute 381.00
          chronic (simple) 381.10
      chronic 382.9
          with effusion 381.3
          adhesive (see also Adhesions,
              middle ear) 385.10
          allergic 381.3
          atticoantral, suppurative (with
              posterior or superior
              marginal perforation of ear
              drum) 382.2
          benign suppurative (with
              anterior perforation of ear
              drum) 382.1
          catarrhal 381.10
          exudative 381.3
          mucinous 381.20
          mucoid, mucous (simple)
              381.20
          mucosanguineous 381.29
          nonsuppurative 381.3
          purulent 382.3
          secretory 381.3
          seromucinous 381.3
          serosanguineous 381.19
          serous (simple) 381.10
          suppurative 382.3
              atticoantral (with posterior or
                  superior marginal
                  perforation of ear drum)
                  382.2
              benign (with anterior
                  perforation of ear drum)
                  382.1

Otitis (Continued)
  media (Continued)
      chronic (Continued)
          suppurative (Continued)
              tuberculous (see also
                  Tuberculosis) 017.4●
              tubotympanic 382.1
              transudative 381.3
          exudative 381.4
              acute 381.00
              chronic 381.3
          fibrotic (see also Adhesions, middle
              ear) 385.10
          mucoid, mucous 381.4
              acute 381.02
              chronic (simple) 381.20
          mucosanguineous, chronic 381.29
          nonsuppurative 381.4
              acute 381.00
              chronic 381.3
          postmeasles 055.2
          purulent 382.4
              acute 382.00
                  with spontaneous rupture of
                      ear drum 382.01
              chronic 382.3
          sanguineous, acute 381.03
              allergic 381.06
          secretory 381.4
              acute or subacute 381.01
              chronic 381.3
          seromucinous 381.4
              acute or subacute 381.02
              chronic 381.3
          serosanguineous, chronic 381.19
          serous 381.4
              acute or subacute 381.01
              chronic (simple) 381.10
          subacute - see Otitis, media, acute
          suppurative 382.4
              acute 382.00
                  with spontaneous rupture of
                      ear drum 382.01
              chronic 382.3
                  atticoantral 382.2
                  benign 382.1
                  tuberculous (see also
                      Tuberculosis)
                      017.4●
                  tubotympanic 382.1
              transudative 381.4
                  acute 381.00
                  chronic 381.3
              tuberculous (see also Tuberculosis)
                  017.4●
          postmeasles 055.2
Otoconia 386.8
Otolith syndrome 386.19
Otomycosis 111.8 [380.15]
  in
      aspergillosis 117.3 [380.15]
      moniliasis 112.82
Otopathy 388.9
Otoporosis (see also Otosclerosis)
  387.9
Otorrhagia 388.69
  traumatic - see nature of injury
Otorrhea 388.60
  blood 388.69
  cerebrospinal (fluid) 388.61
Otosclerosis (general) 387.9
  cochlear (endosteal) 387.2
  involving
      otic capsule 387.2

Otosclerosis (*Continued*)
  involving (*Continued*)
    oval window
      nonobliterative 387.0
      obliterative 387.1
    round window 387.2
  nonobliterative 387.0
  obliterative 387.1
  specified type NEC 387.8
Otospongiosis (*see also* Otosclerosis) 387.9
Otto's disease or pelvis 715.35
Outburst, aggressive (*see also*
    Disturbance, conduct) 312.0●
  in children or adolescents 313.9
Outcome of delivery
  multiple birth NEC V27.9
    all liveborn V27.5
    all stillborn V27.7
    some liveborn V27.6
    unspecified V27.9
  single V27.9
    liveborn V27.0
    stillborn V27.1
  twins V27.9
    both liveborn V27.2
    both stillborn V27.4
    one liveborn, one stillborn V27.3
Outlet - *see also* condition
  syndrome (thoracic) 353.0
Outstanding ears (bilateral) 744.29
Ovalocytosis (congenital) (hereditary) (*see
    also* Elliptocytosis) 282.1
Ovarian - *see also* condition
  pregnancy - *see* Pregnancy, ovarian
  remnant syndrome 620.8
  vein syndrome 593.4
Ovaritis (cystic) (*see also* Salpingo-
    oophoritis) 614.2
Ovary, ovarian - *see* condition
Overactive - *see also* Hyperfunction
  bladder 596.51
  eye muscle (*see also* Strabismus) 378.9
  hypothalamus 253.8
  thyroid (*see also* Thyrotoxicosis) 242.9●
Overactivity, child 314.01
Overbite (deep) (excessive) (horizontal)
    (vertical) 524.29

Overbreathing (*see also* Hyperventilation)
    786.01
Overconscientious personality 301.4
Overdevelopment - *see also* Hypertrophy
  breast (female) (male) 611.1
  nasal bones 738.0
  prostate, congenital 752.89
Overdistention - *see* Distention
Overdose overdosage (drug) 977.9
  specified drug or substance - *see* Table
    of Drugs and Chemicals
Overeating 783.6
  nonorganic origin 307.51
Overexertion (effects) (exhaustion)
    994.5
Overexposure (effects) 994.9
  exhaustion 994.4
Overfeeding (*see also* Overeating)
    783.6
Overfill, endodontic 526.62
Overgrowth, bone NEC 733.99
Overhanging
  tooth restoration 525.62
  unrepairable, dental restorative
    materials 525.62
Overheated (effects) (places) - *see* Heat
Overinhibited child 313.0
Overjet 524.29
  excessive horizontal 524.26
Overlaid, overlying (suffocation)
    994.7
Overlap
  excessive horizontal 524.26
Overlapping toe (acquired) 735.8
  congenital (fifth toe) 755.66
Overload
  fluid 276.6
  potassium (K) 276.7
  sodium (Na) 276.0
Overnutrition (*see also*
    Hyperalimentation) 783.6
Overproduction - *see also* Hypersecretion
  ACTH 255.3
  cortisol 255.0
  growth hormone 253.0
  thyroid-stimulating hormone (TSH)
    242.8●

Overriding
  aorta 747.21
  finger (acquired) 736.29
    congenital 755.59
  toe (acquired) 735.8
    congenital 755.66
Oversize
  fetus (weight of 4500 grams or more)
    766.0
    affecting management of pregnancy
      656.6●
    causing disproportion 653.5●
      with obstructed labor 660.1●
    affecting fetus or newborn 763.1
Overstimulation, ovarian 256.1
Overstrained 780.79
  heart - *see* Hypertrophy, cardiac
Overweight (*see also* Obesity) 278.02
Overwork 780.79
Oviduct - *see* condition
Ovotestis 752.7
Ovulation (cycle)
  failure or lack of 628.0
  pain 625.2
Ovum
  blighted 631
  donor V59.70
    over age 35 V59.73
      anonymous recipient V59.73
      designated recipient V59.74
    under age 35 V59.71
      anonymous recipient V59.71
      designated recipient V59.72
  dropsical 631
  pathologic 631
Owren's disease or syndrome
    (parahemophilia) (*see also* Defect,
    coagulation) 286.3
Oxalosis 271.8
Oxaluria 271.8
Ox heart - *see* Hypertrophy, cardiac
OX syndrome 758.6
Oxycephaly, oxycephalic 756.0
  syphilitic, congenital 090.0
Oxyuriasis 127.4
Oxyuris vermicularis (infestation) 127.4
Ozena 472.0

◀ New   ◀▥ Revised   ~~deleted~~ Deleted   ● Use Additional Digit(s)   ▨ Omit code

P

Pacemaker syndrome 429.4
Pachyderma, pachydermia 701.8
　laryngis 478.5
　laryngitis 478.79
　larynx (verrucosa) 478.79
Pachydermatitis 701.8
Pachydermatocele (congenital) 757.39
　acquired 701.8
Pachydermatosis 701.8
Pachydermoperiostitis
　secondary 731.2
Pachydermoperiostosis
　primary idiopathic 757.39
　secondary 731.2
Pachymeningitis (adhesive) (basal)
　　(brain) (cerebral) (cervical) (chronic)
　　(circumscribed) (external) (fibrous)
　　(hemorrhagic) (hypertrophic)
　　(internal) (purulent) (spinal)
　　(suppurative) (see also Meningitis)
　　322.9
　gonococcal 098.82
Pachyonychia (congenital) 757.5
　acquired 703.8
Pachyperiosteodermia
　primary or idiopathic 757.39
　secondary 731.2
Pachyperiostosis
　primary or idiopathic 757.39
　secondary 731.2
Pacinian tumor (M9507/0) - see
　　Neoplasm, skin, benign
Pads, knuckle or Garrod's 728.79
Paget's disease (osteitis deformans)
　　731.0
　with infiltrating duct carcinoma of the
　　　breast (M8541/3) - see Neoplasm,
　　　breast, malignant
　bone 731.0
　　osteosarcoma in (M9184/3) - see
　　　　Neoplasm, bone, malignant
　breast (M8540/3) 174.0
　extramammary (M8542/3) - see also
　　　Neoplasm, skin, malignant
　　anus 154.3
　　skin 173.5
　malignant (M8540/3)
　　breast 174.0
　　specified site NEC (M8542/3) - see
　　　　Neoplasm, skin, malignant
　　unspecified site 174.0
　mammary (M8540/3) 174.0
　necrosis of bone 731.0
　nipple (M8540/3) 174.0
　osteitis deformans 731.0
Paget-Schroetter syndrome (intermittent
　　venous claudication) 453.89　◀▥
Pain(s) (see also Painful) 780.96
　abdominal 789.0●
　acute 338.19
　　due to trauma 338.11
　　postoperative 338.18
　　　post-thoracotomy 338.12
　adnexa (uteri) 625.9
　alimentary, due to vascular
　　　insufficiency 557.9
　anginoid (see also Pain, precordial)
　　　786.51
　anus 569.42
　arch 729.5
　arm 729.5
　axillary 729.5

Pain(s) (Continued)
　back (postural) 724.5
　　low 724.2
　　psychogenic 307.89
　bile duct 576.9
　bladder 788.99
　bone 733.90
　breast 611.71
　　psychogenic 307.89
　broad ligament 625.9
　cancer associated 338.3
　cartilage NEC 733.90
　cecum 789.0●
　cervicobrachial 723.3
　chest (central) 786.50
　　atypical 786.59
　　midsternal 786.51
　　musculoskeletal 786.59
　　noncardiac 786.59
　　substernal 786.51
　　wall (anterior) 786.52
　chronic 338.29
　　associated with significant
　　　　psychosocial dysfunction
　　　　338.4
　　due to trauma 338.21
　　postoperative 338.28
　　　post-thoracotomy 338.22
　　syndrome 338.4
　coccyx 724.79
　colon 789.0●
　common duct 576.9
　coronary - see Angina
　costochondral 786.52
　diaphragm 786.52
　due to (presence of) any device,
　　　implant, or graft classifiable to
　　　996.0–996.5 - see Complications,
　　　due to (presence of) any device,
　　　implant, or graft classified to
　　　996.0–996.5 NEC
　　malignancy (primary) (secondary)
　　　338.3
　ear (see also Otalgia) 388.70
　epigastric, epigastrium 789.06
　extremity (lower) (upper) 729.5
　eye 379.91
　face, facial 784.0
　　atypical 350.2
　　nerve 351.8
　false (labor) 644.1●
　female genital organ NEC 625.9
　　psychogenic 307.89
　finger 729.5
　flank 789.0●
　foot 729.5
　gallbladder 575.9
　gas (intestinal) 787.3
　gastric 536.8
　generalized 780.96
　genital organ
　　female 625.9
　　male 608.9
　　psychogenic 307.89
　groin 789.0●
　growing 781.99
　hand 729.5
　head (see also Headache) 784.0
　heart (see also Pain, precordial)
　　　786.51
　infraorbital (see also Neuralgia,
　　　trigeminal) 350.1
　intermenstrual 625.2
　jaw 526.9

Pain(s) (Continued)
　joint 719.40
　　ankle 719.47
　　elbow 719.42
　　foot 719.47
　　hand 719.44
　　hip 719.45
　　knee 719.46
　　multiple sites 719.49
　　pelvic region 719.45
　　psychogenic 307.89
　　shoulder (region) 719.41
　　specified site NEC 719.48
　　wrist 719.43
　kidney 788.0
　labor, false or spurious 644.1●
　laryngeal 784.1
　leg 729.5
　limb 729.5
　low back 724.2
　lumbar region 724.2
　mastoid (see also Otalgia) 388.70
　maxilla 526.9
　menstrual 625.3
　metacarpophalangeal (joint)
　　　719.44
　metatarsophalangeal (joint)
　　　719.47
　mouth 528.9
　muscle 729.1
　　intercostal 786.59
　musculoskeletal (see also Pain, by site)
　　　729.1
　nasal 478.19
　nasopharynx 478.29
　neck NEC 723.1
　　psychogenic 307.89
　neoplasm related (acute) (chronic)
　　　338.3
　nerve NEC 729.2
　neuromuscular 729.1
　nose 478.19
　ocular 379.91
　ophthalmic 379.91
　orbital region 379.91
　osteocopic 733.90
　ovary 625.9
　　psychogenic 307.89
　over heart (see also Pain, precordial)
　　　786.51
　ovulation 625.2
　pelvic (female) 625.9
　　male NEC 789.0●
　　　psychogenic 307.89
　　psychogenic 307.89
　penis 607.9
　　psychogenic 307.89
　pericardial (see also Pain, precordial)
　　　786.51
　perineum
　　female 625.9
　　male 608.9
　pharynx 478.29
　pleura, pleural, pleuritic 786.52
　postoperative 338.18
　　acute 338.18
　　chronic 338.28
　post-thoracotomy 338.12
　　acute 338.12
　　chronic 338.22
　preauricular 388.70
　precordial (region) 786.51
　　psychogenic 307.89
　premenstrual 625.4

Pain(s) *(Continued)*
  psychogenic 307.80
    cardiovascular system 307.89
    gastrointestinal system 307.89
    genitourinary system 307.89
    heart 307.89
    musculoskeletal system 307.89
    respiratory system 307.89
    skin 306.3
  radicular (spinal) *(see also* Radiculitis)
    729.2
  rectum 569.42
  respiration 786.52
  retrosternal 786.51
  rheumatic NEC 729.0
    muscular 729.1
  rib 786.50
  root (spinal) *(see also* Radiculitis)
    729.2
  round ligament (stretch) 625.9
  sacroiliac 724.6
  sciatic 724.3
  scrotum 608.9
    psychogenic 307.89
  seminal vesicle 608.9
  sinus 478.19
  skin 782.0
  spermatic cord 608.9
  spinal root *(see also* Radiculitis)
    729.2
  stomach 536.8
    psychogenic 307.89
  substernal 786.51
  temporomandibular (joint) 524.62
  temporomaxillary joint 524.62
  testis 608.9
    psychogenic 307.89
  thoracic spine 724.1
    with radicular and visceral pain
      724.4
  throat 784.1
  tibia 733.90
  toe 729.5
  tongue 529.6
  tooth 525.9
  trigeminal *(see also* Neuralgia,
    trigeminal) 350.1
  tumor associated 338.3
  umbilicus 789.05
  ureter 788.0
  urinary (organ) (system) 788.0
  uterus 625.9
    psychogenic 307.89
  vagina 625.9
  vertebrogenic (syndrome) 724.5
  vesical 788.99
  vulva 625.9
  xiphoid 733.90
Painful - *see also* Pain
  arc syndrome 726.19
  coitus
    female 625.0
    male 608.89
    psychogenic 302.76
  ejaculation (semen) 608.89
    psychogenic 302.79
  erection 607.3
  feet syndrome 266.2
  menstruation 625.3
    psychogenic 306.52
  micturition 788.1
  ophthalmoplegia 378.55
  respiration 786.52
  scar NEC 709.2

Painful *(Continued)*
  total hip replacement 996.77
  total knee replacement 996.77
  urination 788.1
  wire sutures 998.89
Painters' colic 984.9
  specified type of lead - *see* Table of
    Drugs and Chemicals
Palate - *see* condition
Palatoplegia 528.9
Palatoschisis *(see also* Cleft, palate) 749.00
Palilalia 784.69
Palindromic arthritis *(see also*
  Rheumatism, palindromic) 719.3●
Palliative care V66.7
Pallor 782.61
  temporal, optic disc 377.15
Palmar - *see also* condition
  fascia - *see* condition
Palpable
  cecum 569.89
  kidney 593.89
  liver 573.9
  lymph nodes 785.6
  ovary 620.8
  prostate 602.9
  spleen *(see also* Splenomegaly) 789.2
  uterus 625.8
Palpitation (heart) 785.1
  psychogenic 306.2
Palsy *(see also* Paralysis) 344.9
  atrophic diffuse 335.20
  Bell's 351.0
    newborn 767.5
  birth 767.7
  brachial plexus 353.0
    fetus or newborn 767.6
  brain - *see also* Palsy, cerebral
    noncongenital or noninfantile 344.89
      late effect - *see* Late effect(s) (of)
        cerebrovascular disease
    syphilitic 094.89
      congenital 090.49
  bulbar (chronic) (progressive) 335.22
    pseudo NEC 335.23
    supranuclear NEC 344.89
  cerebral (congenital) (infantile)
    (spastic) 343.9
    athetoid 333.71
    diplegic 343.0
      late effect - *see* Late effect(s) (of)
        cerebrovascular disease
    hemiplegic 343.1
    monoplegic 343.3
    noncongenital or noninfantile 437.8
      late effect - *see* Late effect(s) (of)
        cerebrovascular disease
    paraplegic 343.0
    quadriplegic 343.2
    spastic, not congenital or infantile
      344.89
    syphilitic 094.89
      congenital 090.49
    tetraplegic 343.2
  cranial nerve - *see also* Disorder, nerve,
    cranial
    multiple 352.6
  creeping 335.21
  divers' 993.3
  Erb's (birth injury) 767.6
  facial 351.0
    newborn 767.5
  glossopharyngeal 352.2
  Klumpke (-Déjérine) 767.6

Palsy *(Continued)*
  lead 984.9
    specified type of lead - *see* Table of
      Drugs and Chemicals
  median nerve (tardy) 354.0
  peroneal nerve (acute) (tardy) 355.3
  progressive supranuclear 333.0
  pseudobulbar NEC 335.23
  radial nerve (acute) 354.3
  seventh nerve 351.0
    newborn 767.5
  shaking *(see also* Parkinsonism)
    332.0
  spastic (cerebral) (spinal) 343.9
    hemiplegic 343.1
  specified nerve NEC - *see* Disorder,
    nerve
  supranuclear NEC 356.8
    progressive 333.0
  ulnar nerve (tardy) 354.2
  wasting 335.21
Paltauf-Sternberg disease 201.9●
Paludism - *see* Malaria
Panama fever 084.0
Panaris (with lymphangitis) 681.9
  finger 681.02
  toe 681.11
Panaritium (with lymphangitis) 681.9
  finger 681.02
  toe 681.11
Panarteritis (nodosa) 446.0
  brain or cerebral 437.4
Pancake heart 793.2
  with cor pulmonale (chronic) 416.9
Pancarditis (acute) (chronic) 429.89
  with
    rheumatic
      fever (active) (acute) (chronic)
        (subacute) 391.8
        inactive or quiescent 398.99
  rheumatic, acute 391.8
    chronic or inactive 398.99
Pancoast's syndrome or tumor
  (carcinoma, pulmonary apex)
  (M8010/3) 162.3
Pancoast-Tobias syndrome (M8010/3)
  (carcinoma, pulmonary apex)
  162.3
Pancolitis 556.6
Pancreas, pancreatic - *see* condition
Pancreatitis 577.0
  acute (edematous) (hemorrhagic)
    (recurrent) 577.0
  annular 577.0
  apoplectic 577.0
  calcereous 577.0
  chronic (infectious) 577.1
    recurrent 577.1
  cystic 577.2
  fibrous 577.8
  gangrenous 577.0
  hemorrhagic (acute) 577.0
  interstitial (chronic) 577.1
    acute 577.0
  malignant 577.0
  mumps 072.3
  painless 577.1
  recurrent 577.1
  relapsing 577.1
  subacute 577.0
  suppurative 577.0
  syphilitic 095.8
Pancreatolithiasis 577.8
Pancytolysis 289.9

◄ New   ⬤▬ Revised   ~~deleted~~ Deleted   ● Use Additional Digit(s)   ▬▬ Omit code

Pancytopenia (acquired) 284.1
  with malformations 284.09
  congenital 284.09
Panencephalitis - *see also* Encephalitis
  subacute, sclerosing 046.2
Panhematopenia 284.81
  congenital 284.09
  constitutional 284.09
  splenic, primary 289.4
Panhemocytopenia 284.81
  congenital 284.09
  constitutional 284.09
Panhypogonadism 257.2
Panhypopituitarism 253.2
  prepubertal 253.3
Panic (attack) (state) 300.01
  reaction to exceptional stress (transient)
    308.0
Panmyelopathy, familial constitutional
  284.09
Panmyelophthisis 284.2
  acquired (secondary) 284.81
  congenital 284.2
  idiopathic 284.9
Panmyelosis (acute) (M9951/1) 238.79
Panner's disease 732.3
  capitellum humeri 732.3
  head of humerus 732.3
  tarsal navicular (bone)
    (osteochondrosis) 732.5
Panneuritis endemica 265.0 [357.4]
Panniculitis 729.30
  back 724.8
  knee 729.31
  mesenteric 567.82
  neck 723.6
  nodular, nonsuppurative 729.30
  sacral 724.8
  specified site NEC 729.39
Panniculus adiposus (abdominal)
  278.1
Pannus (corneal) 370.62
  abdominal (symptomatic) 278.1
  allergic eczematous 370.62
  degenerativus 370.62
  keratic 370.62
  rheumatoid - *see* Arthritis, rheumatoid
  trachomatosus, trachomatous (active)
    076.1 [370.62]
  late effect 139.1
Panophthalmitis 360.02
Panotitis - *see* Otitis media
Pansinusitis (chronic) (hyperplastic)
  (nonpurulent) (purulent) 473.8
  acute 461.8
  due to fungus NEC 117.9
  tuberculous (*see also* Tuberculosis)
    012.8●
Panuveitis 360.12
  sympathetic 360.11
Panvalvular disease - *see* Endocarditis,
  mitral
Papageienkrankheit 073.9
Papanicolaou smear
  anus 796.70
    with
      atypical squamous cells
        cannot exclude high grade
          squamous intraepithelial
          lesion (ASC-H) 796.72
        of undetermined significance
          (ASC-US) 796.71
      cytologic evidence of malignancy
        796.76

Papanicolaou smear *(Continued)*
  anus *(Continued)*
    with *(Continued)*
      high grade squamous
        intraepithelial lesion
        (HGSIL) 796.74
      low grade squamous
        intraepithelial lesion
        (LGSIL) 796.73
    glandular 796.70
    specified finding NEC 796.79
    unsatisfactory cytology 796.78
  cervix (screening test) V76.2
    as part of gynecological examination
      V72.31
    for suspected malignant neoplasm
      V76.2
    no disease found V71.1
    inadequate cytology sample
      795.08
    nonspecific abnormal finding
      795.00
      with
        atypical squamous cells
          cannot exclude high grade
            squamous
            intraepithelial lesion
            (ASC-H) 795.02
          of undetermined
            significance (ASC-US)
            795.01
        cytologic evidence of
          malignancy 795.06
        high grade squamous
          intraepithelial lesion
          (HGSIL) 795.04
        low grade squamous
          intraepithelial lesion
          (LGSIL) 795.03
      nonspecific finding NEC 795.09
      to confirm findings of recent
        normal smear following
        initial abnormal smear
        V72.32
    satisfactory smear but lacking
      transformation zone 795.07
    unsatisfactory cervical cytology
      795.08
  other specified site - *see also* Screening,
    malignant neoplasm
    for suspected malignant neoplasm -
      see also Screening, malignant
      neoplasm
    no disease found V71.1
    nonspecific abnormal finding
      796.9
    vagina V76.47
      with
        atypical squamous cells
          cannot exclude high grade
            squamous
            intraepithelial lesion
            (ASC-H) 795.12
          of undetermined
            significance (ASC-US)
            795.11
        cytologic evidence of
          malignancy 795.16
        high grade squamous
          intraepithelial lesion
          (HGSIL) 795.14
        low grade squamous
          intraepithelial lesion
          (LGSIL) 795.13

Papanicolaou smear *(Continued)*
  other specified site *(Continued)*
    vagina *(Continued)*
      abnormal NEC 795.19
      following hysterectomy for
        malignant condition V67.01
      inadequate cytology sample
        795.18
      unsatisfactory cytology 795.18
Papilledema 377.00
  associated with
    decreased ocular pressure 377.02
    increased intracranial pressure
      377.01
    retinal disorder 377.03
  choked disc 377.00
  infectional 377.00
Papillitis 377.31
  anus 569.49
  chronic lingual 529.4
  necrotizing, kidney 584.7
  optic 377.31
  rectum 569.49
  renal, necrotizing 584.7
  tongue 529.0
Papilloma (M8050/0) - *see also* Neoplasm,
  by site, benign

Note 58   Except where otherwise
indicated, the morphological varieties
of papilloma in the list below should
be coded by site as for "Neoplasm,
benign".

---

  acuminatum (female) (male) 078.11
  bladder (urinary) (transitional cell)
    (M8120/1) 236.7
    benign (M8120/0) 223.3
  choroid plexus (M9390/0) 225.0
    anaplastic type (M9390/3) 191.5
    malignant (M9390/3) 191.5
  ductal (M8503/0)
  dyskeratotic (M8052/0)
  epidermoid (M8052/0)
  hyperkeratotic (M8052/0)
  intracystic (M8504/0)
  intraductal (M8503/0)
  inverted (M8053/0)
  keratotic (M8052/0)
  parakeratotic (M8052/0)
  pinta (primary) 103.0
  renal pelvis (transitional cell)
    (M8120/1) 236.99
    benign (M8120/0) 223.1
  Schneiderian (M8121/0)
    specified site - *see* Neoplasm, by site,
      benign
    unspecified site 212.0
  serous surface (M8461/0)
    borderline malignancy (M8461/1)
      specified site - *see* Neoplasm, by
        site, uncertain behavior
      unspecified site 236.2
    specified site - *see* Neoplasm, by site,
      benign
    unspecified site 220
  squamous (cell) (M8052/0)
  transitional (cell) (M8120/0)
    bladder (urinary) (M8120/1) 236.7
    inverted type (M8121/1) - *see*
      Neoplasm, by site, uncertain
      behavior
    renal pelvis (M8120/1) 236.91
    ureter (M8120/1) 236.91

Papilloma (*Continued*)
  ureter (transitional cell) (M8120/1) 236.91
    benign (M8120/0) 223.2
  urothelial (M8120/1) - *see* Neoplasm, by site, uncertain behavior
  verrucous (M8051/0)
  villous (M8261/1) - *see* Neoplasm, by site, uncertain behavior
  yaws, plantar or palmar 102.1
Papillomata, multiple, of yaws 102.1
Papillomatosis (M8060/0) - *see also* Neoplasm, by site, benign
  confluent and reticulate 701.8
  cutaneous 701.8
  ductal, breast 610.1
  Gougerot-Carteaud (confluent reticulate) 701.8
  intraductal (diffuse) (M8505/0) - *see* Neoplasm, by site, benign
  subareolar duct (M8506/0) 217
Papillon-Léage and Psaume syndrome (orodigitofacial dysostosis) 759.89
Papule 709.8
  carate (primary) 103.0
  fibrous, of nose (M8724/0) 216.3
  pinta (primary) 103.0
Papulosis, malignant 447.8
Papyraceous fetus 779.89
  complicating pregnancy 646.0 ●
Paracephalus 759.7
Parachute mitral valve 746.5
Paracoccidioidomycosis 116.1
  mucocutaneous-lymphangitic 116.1
  pulmonary 116.1
  visceral 116.1
Paracoccidiomycosis - *see* Paracoccidioidomycosis
Paracusis 388.40
Paradentosis 523.5
Paradoxical facial movements 374.43
Paraffinoma 999.9
Paraganglioma (M8680/1)
  adrenal (M8700/0) 227.0
    malignant (M8700/3) 194.0
  aortic body (M8691/1) 237.3
    malignant (M8691/3) 194.6
  carotid body (M8692/1) 237.3
    malignant (M8692/3) 194.5
  chromaffin (M8700/0) - *see also* Neoplasm, by site, benign
    malignant (M8700/3) - *see* Neoplasm, by site, malignant
  extra-adrenal (M8693/1)
    malignant (M8693/3)
      specified site - *see* Neoplasm, by site, malignant
      unspecified site 194.6
    specified site - *see* Neoplasm, by site, uncertain behavior
    unspecified site 237.3
  glomus jugulare (M8690/1) 237.3
    malignant (M8690/3) 194.6
  jugular (M8690/1) 237.3
  malignant (M8680/3)
    specified site - *see* Neoplasm, by site, malignant
    unspecified site 194.6
  nonchromaffin (M8693/1)
    malignant (M8693/3)
      specified site - *see* Neoplasm, by site, malignant
      unspecified site 194.6

Paraganglioma (*Continued*)
  nonchromaffin (*Continued*)
    specified site - *see* Neoplasm, by site, uncertain behavior
    unspecified site 237.3
  parasympathetic (M8682/1)
    specified site - *see* Neoplasm, by site, uncertain behavior
    unspecified site 237.3
  specified site - *see* Neoplasm, by site, uncertain behavior
  sympathetic (M8681/1)
    specified site - *see* Neoplasm, by site, uncertain behavior
    unspecified site 237.3
  unspecified site 237.3
Parageusia 781.1
  psychogenic 306.7
Paragonimiasis 121.2
Paragranuloma, Hodgkin's (M9660/3) 201.0 ●
Parahemophilia (*see also* Defect, coagulation) 286.3
Parakeratosis 690.8
  psoriasiformis 696.2
  variegata 696.2
Paralysis, paralytic (complete) (incomplete) 344.9
  with
    broken
      back - *see* Fracture, vertebra, by site, with spinal cord injury
      neck - *see* Fracture, vertebra, cervical, with spinal cord injury
    fracture, vertebra - *see* Fracture, vertebra, by site, with spinal cord injury
    syphilis 094.89
  abdomen and back muscles 355.9
  abdominal muscles 355.9
  abducens (nerve) 378.54
  abductor 355.9
    lower extremity 355.8
    upper extremity 354.9
  accessory nerve 352.4
  accommodation 367.51
    hysterical 300.11
  acoustic nerve 388.5
  agitans 332.0
    arteriosclerotic 332.0
  alternating 344.89
    oculomotor 344.89
  amyotrophic 335.20
  ankle 355.8
  anterior serratus 355.9
  anus (sphincter) 569.49
  apoplectic (current episode) (*see also* Disease, cerebrovascular, acute) 436
    late effect - *see* Late effect(s) (of) cerebrovascular disease
  arm 344.40
    affecting
      dominant side 344.41
      nondominant side 344.42
    both 344.2
    hysterical 300.11
    late effect - *see* Late effect(s) (of) cerebrovascular disease
    psychogenic 306.0
    transient 781.4
      traumatic NEC (*see also* Injury, nerve, upper limb) 955.9

Paralysis, paralytic (*Continued*)
  arteriosclerotic (current episode) 437.0
    late effect - *see* Late effect(s) (of) cerebrovascular disease
  ascending (spinal), acute 357.0
  associated, nuclear 344.89
  asthenic bulbar 358.00
  ataxic NEC 334.9
    general 094.1
  athetoid 333.71
  atrophic 356.9
    infantile, acute (*see also* Poliomyelitis, with paralysis) 045.1 ●
    muscle NEC 355.9
    progressive 335.21
    spinal (acute) (*see also* Poliomyelitis, with paralysis) 045.1 ●
  attack (*see also* Disease, cerebrovascular, acute) 436
  axillary 353.0
  Babinski-Nageotte's 344.89
  Bell's 351.0
    newborn 767.5
  Benedikt's 344.89
  birth (injury) 767.7
    brain 767.0
    intracranial 767.0
    spinal cord 767.4
  bladder (sphincter) 596.53
    neurogenic 596.54
      with cauda equina syndrome 344.61
    puerperal, postpartum, childbirth 665.5 ●
    sensory 596.54
      with cauda equina 344.61
    spastic 596.54
      with cauda equina 344.61
  bowel, colon, or intestine (*see also* Ileus) 560.1
  brachial plexus 353.0
    due to birth injury 767.6
    newborn 767.6
  brain
    congenital - *see* Palsy, cerebral
    current episode 437.8
    diplegia 344.2
      late effect - *see* Late effect(s) (of) cerebrovascular disease
    hemiplegia 342.9 ●
      late effect - *see* Late effect(s) (of) cerebrovascular disease
    infantile - *see* Palsy, cerebral
    monoplegia - *see also* Monoplegia
      late effect - *see* Late effect(s) (of) cerebrovascular disease
    paraplegia 344.1
    quadriplegia - *see* Quadriplegia
    syphilitic, congenital 090.49
    triplegia 344.89
  bronchi 519.19
  Brown-Séquard's 344.89
  bulbar (chronic) (progressive) 335.22
    infantile (*see also* Poliomyelitis, bulbar) 045.0 ●
    poliomyelitic (*see also* Poliomyelitis, bulbar) 045.0 ●
    pseudo 335.23
    supranuclear 344.89
  bulbospinal 358.00
  cardiac (*see also* Failure, heart) 428.9

◀ New   ◀꜒ Revised   ~~deleted~~ Deleted   ● Use Additional Digit(s)   ▨ Omit code

Paralysis, paralytic *(Continued)*
  cerebral
    current episode 437.8
    spastic, infantile - *see* Palsy, cerebral
  cerebrocerebellar 437.8
    diplegic infantile 343.0
  cervical
    plexus 353.2
    sympathetic NEC 337.09
  Céstan-Chenais 344.89
  Charcôt-Marie-Tooth type 356.1
  childhood - *see* Palsy, cerebral
  Clark's 343.9
  colon (*see also* Ileus) 560.1
  compressed air 993.3
  compression
    arm NEC 354.9
    cerebral - *see* Paralysis, brain
    leg NEC 355.8
    lower extremity NEC 355.8
    upper extremity NEC 354.9
  congenital (cerebral) (spastic) (spinal) -
      see Palsy, cerebral
  conjugate movement (of eye) 378.81
    cortical (nuclear) (supranuclear)
        378.81
  convergence 378.83
  cordis (*see also* Failure, heart) 428.9
  cortical (*see also* Paralysis, brain)
      437.8
  cranial or cerebral nerve (*see also*
      Disorder, nerve, cranial) 352.9
  creeping 335.21
  crossed leg 344.89
  crutch 953.4
  deglutition 784.99
    hysterical 300.11
  dementia 094.1
  descending (spinal) NEC 335.9
  diaphragm (flaccid) 519.4
    due to accidental section of phrenic
        nerve during procedure 998.2
  digestive organs NEC 564.89
  diplegic - *see* Diplegia
  divergence (nuclear) 378.85
  divers' 993.3
  Duchenne's 335.22
  due to intracranial or spinal birth
      injury - *see* Palsy, cerebral
  embolic (current episode) (*see also*
      Embolism, brain) 434.1●
    late effect - *see* Late effect(s) (of)
        cerebrovascular disease
  enteric (*see also* Ileus) 560.1
    with hernia - *see* Hernia, by site,
        with obstruction
  Erb's syphilitic spastic spinal 094.89
  Erb (-Duchenne) (birth) (newborn)
      767.6
  esophagus 530.89
  essential, infancy (*see also* Poliomyelitis)
      045.9●
  extremity
    lower - *see* Paralysis, leg
    spastic (hereditary) 343.3
      noncongenital or noninfantile
          344.1
    transient (cause unknown) 781.4
    upper - *see* Paralysis, arm
  eye muscle (extrinsic) 378.55
    intrinsic 367.51
  facial (nerve) 351.0
    birth injury 767.5
    congenital 767.5

Paralysis, paralytic *(Continued)*
  facial *(Continued)*
    following operation NEC 998.2
    newborn 767.5
  familial 359.3
    periodic 359.3
    spastic 334.1
  fauces 478.29
  finger NEC 354.9
  foot NEC 355.8
  gait 781.2
  gastric nerve 352.3
  gaze 378.81
  general 094.1
    ataxic 094.1
    insane 094.1
    juvenile 090.40
    progressive 094.1
    tabetic 094.1
  glossopharyngeal (nerve) 352.2
  glottis (*see also* Paralysis, vocal cord)
      478.30
  gluteal 353.4
  Gubler (-Millard) 344.89
  hand 354.9
    hysterical 300.11
    psychogenic 306.0
  heart (*see also* Failure, heart) 428.9
  hemifacial, progressive 349.89
  hemiplegic - *see* Hemiplegia
  hyperkalemic periodic (familial) 359.3
  hypertensive (current episode) 437.8
  hypoglossal (nerve) 352.5
  hypokalemic periodic 359.3
  Hyrtl's sphincter (rectum) 569.49
  hysterical 300.11
  ileus (*see also* Ileus) 560.1
  infantile (*see also* Poliomyelitis) 045.9●
    atrophic acute 045.1●
    bulbar 045.0●
    cerebral - *see* Palsy, cerebral
    paralytic 045.1●
    progressive acute 045.9●
    spastic - *see* Palsy, cerebral
    spinal 045.9●
  infective (*see also* Poliomyelitis) 045.9●
  inferior nuclear 344.9
  insane, general or progressive 094.1
  internuclear 378.86
  interosseous 355.9
  intestine (*see also* Ileus) 560.1
  intracranial (current episode) (*see also*
      Paralysis, brain) 437.8
    due to birth injury 767.0
  iris 379.49
    due to diphtheria (toxin) 032.81
        [379.49]
  ischemic, Volkmann's (complicating
      trauma) 958.6
  isolated sleep, recurrent 327.43
  Jackson's 344.89
  jake 357.7
  Jamaica ginger (jake) 357.7
  juvenile general 090.40
  Klumpke (-Déjérine) (birth) (newborn)
      767.6
  labioglossal (laryngeal) (pharyngeal)
      335.22
  Landry's 357.0
  laryngeal nerve (recurrent) (superior)
      (*see also* Paralysis, vocal cord)
      478.30
  larynx (*see also* Paralysis, vocal cord)
      478.30
    due to diphtheria (toxin) 032.3

Paralysis, paralytic *(Continued)*
  late effect
    due to
      birth injury, brain or spinal
          (cord) - *see* Palsy, cerebral
      edema, brain or cerebral - *see*
          Paralysis, brain
      lesion
        late effect - *see* Late effect(s)
            (of) cerebrovascular
            disease
      spinal (cord) - *see* Paralysis,
          spinal
  lateral 335.24
  lead 984.9
    specified type of lead - *see* Table of
        Drugs and Chemicals
  left side - *see* Hemiplegia
  leg 344.30
    affecting
      dominant side 344.31
      nondominant side 344.32
    both (*see also* Paraplegia) 344.1
    crossed 344.89
    hysterical 300.11
    psychogenic 306.0
    transient or transitory 781.4
      traumatic NEC (*see also*
          Injury, nerve, lower limb)
          956.9
  levator palpebrae superioris 374.31
  limb NEC 344.5
    all four - *see* Quadriplegia
    quadriplegia - *see* Quadriplegia
  lip 528.5
  Lissauer's 094.1
  local 355.9
  lower limb - *see also* Paralysis,
      leg
    both (*see also* Paraplegia) 344.1
  lung 518.89
    newborn 770.89
  median nerve 354.1
  medullary (tegmental) 344.89
  mesencephalic NEC 344.89
    tegmental 344.89
  middle alternating 344.89
  Millard-Gubler-Foville 344.89
  monoplegic - *see* Monoplegia
  motor NEC 344.9
    cerebral - *see* Paralysis, brain
    spinal - *see* Paralysis, spinal
  multiple
    cerebral - *see* Paralysis, brain
    spinal - *see* Paralysis, spinal
  muscle (flaccid) 359.9
    due to nerve lesion NEC 355.9
    eye (extrinsic) 378.55
      intrinsic 367.51
      oblique 378.51
    iris sphincter 364.89
    ischemic (complicating trauma)
        (Volkmann's) 958.6
    pseudohypertrophic 359.1
  muscular (atrophic) 359.9
    progressive 335.21
  musculocutaneous nerve 354.9
  musculospiral 354.9
  nerve - *see also* Disorder, nerve
    third or oculomotor (partial)
        378.51
      total 378.52
    fourth or trochlear 378.53
    sixth or abducens 378.54

Paralysis, paralytic *(Continued)*
  nerve *(Continued)*
    seventh or facial 351.0
      birth injury 767.5
      due to
        injection NEC 999.9
        operation NEC 997.09
      newborn 767.5
    accessory 352.4
    auditory 388.5
    birth injury 767.7
    cranial or cerebral *(see also* Disorder, nerve, cranial) 352.9
    facial 351.0
      birth injury 767.5
      newborn 767.5
    laryngeal *(see also* Paralysis, vocal cord) 478.30
    newborn 767.7
    phrenic 354.8
      newborn 767.7
    radial 354.3
      birth injury 767.6
      newborn 767.6
    syphilitic 094.89
    traumatic NEC *(see also* Injury, nerve, by site) 957.9
    trigeminal 350.9
    ulnar 354.2
  newborn NEC 767.0
  normokalemic periodic 359.3
  obstetrical, newborn 767.7
  ocular 378.9
  oculofacial, congenital 352.6
  oculomotor (nerve) (partial) 378.51
    alternating 344.89
    external bilateral 378.55
    total 378.52
  olfactory nerve 352.0
  palate 528.9
  palatopharyngolaryngeal 352.6
  paratrigeminal 350.9
  periodic (familial) (hyperkalemic) (hypokalemic) (normokalemic) (potassium sensitive) (secondary) 359.3
  peripheral
    autonomic nervous system - *see* Neuropathy, peripheral, autonomic
    nerve NEC 355.9
  peroneal (nerve) 355.3
  pharynx 478.29
  phrenic nerve 354.8
  plantar nerves 355.6
  pneumogastric nerve 352.3
  poliomyelitis (current) *(see also* Poliomyelitis, with paralysis) 045.1 ●
    bulbar 045.0 ●
  popliteal nerve 355.3
  pressure *(see also* Neuropathy, entrapment) 355.9
  progressive 335.21
    atrophic 335.21
    bulbar 335.22
    general 094.1
    hemifacial 349.89
    infantile, acute *(see also* Poliomyelitis) 045.9 ●
    multiple 335.20
  pseudobulbar 335.23
  pseudohypertrophic 359.1
    muscle 359.1

Paralysis, paralytic *(Continued)*
  psychogenic 306.0
  pupil, pupillary 379.49
  quadriceps 355.8
  quadriplegic *(see also* Quadriplegia) 344.0
  radial nerve 354.3
    birth injury 767.6
  rectum (sphincter) 569.49
  rectus muscle (eye) 378.55
  recurrent
    isolated sleep 327.43
    laryngeal nerve *(see also* Paralysis, vocal cord) 478.30
  respiratory (muscle) (system) (tract) 786.09
    center NEC 344.89
      fetus or newborn 770.87
    congenital 768.9
    newborn 768.9
  right side - *see* Hemiplegia
  Saturday night 354.3
  saturnine 984.9
    specified type of lead - *see* Table of Drugs and Chemicals
  sciatic nerve 355.0
  secondary - *see* Paralysis, late effect
  seizure (cerebral) (current episode) *(see also* Disease, cerebrovascular, acute) 436
    late effect - *see* Late effect(s) (of) cerebrovascular disease
  senile NEC 344.9
  serratus magnus 355.9
  shaking *(see also* Parkinsonism) 332.0
  shock *(see also* Disease, cerebrovascular, acute) 436
    late effect - *see* Late effect(s) (of) cerebrovascular disease
  shoulder 354.9
  soft palate 528.9
  spasmodic - *see* Paralysis, spastic
  spastic 344.9
    cerebral infantile - *see* Palsy, cerebral
    congenital (cerebral) - *see* Palsy, cerebral
    familial 334.1
    hereditary 334.1
    infantile 343.9
    noncongenital or noninfantile, cerebral 344.9
    syphilitic 094.0
      spinal 094.89
  sphincter, bladder *(see also* Paralysis, bladder) 596.53
  spinal (cord) NEC 344.1
    accessory nerve 352.4
    acute *(see also* Poliomyelitis) 045.9 ●
    ascending acute 357.0
    atrophic (acute) *(see also* Poliomyelitis, with paralysis) 045.1 ●
      spastic, syphilitic 094.89
    congenital NEC 343.9
    hemiplegic - *see* Hemiplegia
    hereditary 336.8
    infantile *(see also* Poliomyelitis) 045.9 ●
    late effect NEC 344.89
    monoplegic - *see* Monoplegia
    nerve 355.9
    progressive 335.10
    quadriplegic - *see* Quadriplegia

Paralysis, paralytic *(Continued)*
  spinal (cord) NEC *(Continued)*
    spastic NEC 343.9
    traumatic - *see* Injury, spinal, by site
  sternomastoid 352.4
  stomach 536.3
    diabetic 250.6 ● *[536.3]*
      due to secondary diabetes 249.6 ● *[536.3]*
    nerve (nondiabetic) 352.3
  stroke (current episode) - *see* Infarct, brain
    late effect - *see* Late effect(s) (of) cerebrovascular disease
  subscapularis 354.8
  superior nuclear NEC 334.9
  supranuclear 356.8
  sympathetic
    cervical NEC 337.09
    nerve NEC *(see also* Neuropathy, peripheral, autonomic) 337.9
    nervous system - *see* Neuropathy, peripheral, autonomic
  syndrome 344.9
    specified NEC 344.89
  syphilitic spastic spinal (Erb's) 094.89
  tabetic general 094.1
  thigh 355.8
  throat 478.29
    diphtheritic 032.0
    muscle 478.29
  thrombotic (current episode) *(see also* Thrombosis, brain) 434.0 ●
    late effect - *see* Late effect(s) (of) cerebrovascular disease
  thumb NEC 354.9
  tick (-bite) 989.5
  Todd's (postepileptic transitory paralysis) 344.89
  toe 355.6
  tongue 529.8
  transient
    arm or leg NEC 781.4
    traumatic NEC *(see also* Injury, nerve, by site) 957.9
  trapezius 352.4
  traumatic, transient NEC *(see also* Injury, nerve, by site) 957.9
  trembling *(see also* Parkinsonism) 332.0
  triceps brachii 354.9
  trigeminal nerve 350.9
  trochlear nerve 378.53
  ulnar nerve 354.2
  upper limb - *see also* Paralysis, arm
    both *(see also* Diplegia) 344.2
  uremic - *see* Uremia
  uveoparotitic 135
  uvula 528.9
    hysterical 300.11
    postdiphtheritic 032.0
  vagus nerve 352.3
  vasomotor NEC 337.9
  velum palati 528.9
  vesical *(see also* Paralysis, bladder) 596.53
  vestibular nerve 388.5
  visual field, psychic 368.16
  vocal cord 478.30
    bilateral (partial) 478.33
      complete 478.34
    complete (bilateral) 478.34
    unilateral (partial) 478.31
      complete 478.32

◀ New   ◀▥ Revised   ~~deleted~~ Deleted   ● Use Additional Digit(s)   ▨ Omit code

Paralysis, paralytic (Continued)
  Volkmann's (complicating trauma) 958.6
  wasting 335.21
  Weber's 344.89
  wrist NEC 354.9
Paramedial orifice, urethrovesical 753.8
Paramenia 626.9
Parametritis (chronic) (see also Disease, pelvis, inflammatory) 614.4
  acute 614.3
  puerperal, postpartum, childbirth 670.8 ◀▦
Parametrium, parametric - see condition
Paramnesia (see also Amnesia) 780.93
Paramolar 520.1
  causing crowding 524.31
Paramyloidosis 277.30
Paramyoclonus multiplex 333.2
Paramyotonia 359.29
  congenita (of von Eulenburg) 359.29
Paraneoplastic syndrome - see condition
Parangi (see also Yaws) 102.9
Paranoia 297.1
  alcoholic 291.5
  querulans 297.8
  senile 290.20
Paranoid
  dementia (see also Schizophrenia) 295.3●
    praecox (acute) 295.3●
    senile 290.20
  personality 301.0
  psychosis 297.9
    alcoholic 291.5
    climacteric 297.2
    drug-induced 292.11
    involutional 297.2
    menopausal 297.2
    protracted reactive 298.4
    psychogenic 298.4
      acute 298.3
    senile 290.20
  reaction (chronic) 297.9
    acute 298.3
  schizophrenia (acute) (see also Schizophrenia) 295.3●
  state 297.9
    alcohol-induced 291.5
    climacteric 297.2
    drug-induced 292.11
    due to or associated with
      arteriosclerosis (cerebrovascular) 290.42
      presenile brain disease 290.12
      senile brain disease 290.20
    involutional 297.2
    menopausal 297.2
    senile 290.20
    simple 297.0
    specified type NEC 297.8
  tendencies 301.0
  traits 301.0
  trends 301.0
  type, psychopathic personality 301.0
Paraparesis (see also Paraplegia) 344.1
Paraphasia 784.3
Paraphilia (see also Deviation, sexual) 302.9
Paraphimosis (congenital) 605
  chancroidal 099.0
Paraphrenia, paraphrenic (late) 297.2
  climacteric 297.2
  dementia (see also Schizophrenia) 295.3●

Paraphrenia, paraphrenic (Continued)
  involutional 297.2
  menopausal 297.2
  schizophrenia (acute) (see also Schizophrenia) 295.3●
Paraplegia 344.1
  with
    broken back - see Fracture, vertebra, by site, with spinal cord injury
    fracture, vertebra - see Fracture, vertebra, by site, with spinal cord injury
  ataxic - see Degeneration, combined, spinal cord
  brain (current episode) (see also Paralysis, brain) 437.8
  cerebral (current episode) (see also Paralysis, brain) 437.8
  congenital or infantile (cerebral) (spastic) (spinal) 343.0
  cortical - see Paralysis, brain
  familial spastic 334.1
  functional (hysterical) 300.11
  hysterical 300.11
  infantile 343.0
  late effect 344.1
  Pott's (see also Tuberculosis) 015.0● [730.88]
  psychogenic 306.0
  spastic
    Erb's spinal 094.89
    hereditary 334.1
    not infantile or congenital 344.1
  spinal (cord)
    traumatic NEC - see Injury, spinal, by site
  syphilitic (spastic) 094.89
  traumatic NEC - see Injury, spinal, by site
Paraproteinemia 273.2
  benign (familial) 273.1
  monoclonal 273.1
  secondary to malignant or inflammatory disease 273.1
Parapsoriasis 696.2
  en plaques 696.2
  guttata 696.2
  lichenoides chronica 696.2
  retiformis 696.2
  varioliformis (acuta) 696.2
Parascarlatina 057.8
Parasitic - see also condition
  disease NEC (see also Infestation, parasitic) 136.9
    contact V01.89
    exposure to V01.89
    intestinal NEC 129
    skin NEC 134.9
  stomatitis 112.0
  sycosis 110.0
    beard 110.0
    scalp 110.0
  twin 759.4
Parasitism NEC 136.9
  intestinal NEC 129
  skin NEC 134.9
  specified - see Infestation
Parasitophobia 300.29
Parasomnia 307.47
  alcohol induced 291.82
  drug induced 292.85
  nonorganic origin 307.47

Parasomnia (Continued)
  organic 327.40
    in conditions classified elsewhere 327.44
    other 327.49
Paraspadias 752.69
Paraspasm facialis 351.8
Parathyroid gland - see condition
Parathyroiditis (autoimmune) 252.1
Parathyroprival tetany 252.1
Paratrachoma 077.0
Paratyphilitis (see also Appendicitis) 541
Paratyphoid (fever) - see Fever, paratyphoid
Paratyphus - see Fever, paratyphoid
Paraurethral duct 753.8
Para-urethritis 597.89
  gonococcal (acute) 098.0
    chronic or duration of 2 months or over 098.2
Paravaccinia NEC 051.9
  milkers' node 051.1
Paravaginitis (see also Vaginitis) 616.10
Parencephalitis (see also Encephalitis) 323.9
  late effect - see category 326
Parergasia 298.9
Paresis (see also Paralysis) 344.9
  accommodation 367.51
  bladder (spastic) (sphincter) (see also Paralysis, bladder) 596.53
    tabetic 094.0
  bowel, colon, or intestine (see also Ileus) 560.1
  brain or cerebral - see Paralysis, brain
  extrinsic muscle, eye 378.55
  general 094.1
    arrested 094.1
    brain 094.1
    cerebral 094.1
    insane 094.1
    juvenile 090.40
      remission 090.49
    progressive 094.1
    remission (sustained) 094.1
    tabetic 094.1
  heart (see also Failure, heart) 428.9
  infantile (see also Poliomyelitis) 045.9●
  insane 094.1
  juvenile 090.40
  late effect - see Paralysis, late effect
  luetic (general) 094.1
  peripheral progressive 356.9
  pseudohypertrophic 359.1
  senile NEC 344.9
  stomach 536.3
    diabetic 250.6● [536.3]
      due to secondary diabetes 249.6● [536.3]
  syphilitic (general) 094.1
    congenital 090.40
  transient, limb 781.4
  vesical (sphincter) NEC 596.53
Paresthesia (see also Disturbance, sensation) 782.0
  Berger's (paresthesia of lower limb) 782.0
  Bernhardt 355.1
  Magnan's 782.0
Paretic - see condition
Parinaud's
  conjunctivitis 372.02
  oculoglandular syndrome 372.02
  ophthalmoplegia 378.81

Parinaud's *(Continued)*
  syndrome (paralysis of conjugate
    upward gaze) 378.81
Parkes Weber and Dimitri syndrome
  (encephalocutaneous angiomatosis)
  759.6
Parkinson's disease, syndrome, or
  tremor - *see* Parkinsonism
Parkinsonism (arteriosclerotic)
  (idiopathic) (primary) 332.0
  associated with orthostatic hypotension
    (idiopathic) (symptomatic) 333.0
  due to drugs 332.1
  neuroleptic-induced 332.1
  secondary 332.1
  syphilitic 094.82
Parodontitis 523.40
Parodontosis 523.5
Paronychia (with lymphangitis) 681.9
  candidal (chronic) 112.3
  chronic 681.9
    candidal 112.3
    finger 681.02
    toe 681.11
  finger 681.02
  toe 681.11
  tuberculous (primary) (*see also*
    Tuberculosis) 017.0●
Parorexia NEC 307.52
  hysterical 300.11
Parosmia 781.1
  psychogenic 306.7
Parotid gland - *see* condition
Parotiditis (*see also* Parotitis) 527.2
  epidemic 072.9
  infectious 072.9
Parotitis 527.2
  allergic 527.2
  chronic 527.2
  epidemic (*see also* Mumps) 072.9
  infectious (*see also* Mumps) 072.9
  noninfectious 527.2
  nonspecific toxic 527.2
  not mumps 527.2
  postoperative 527.2
  purulent 527.2
  septic 527.2
  suppurative (acute) 527.2
  surgical 527.2
  toxic 527.2
Paroxysmal - *see also* condition
  dyspnea (nocturnal) 786.09
Parrot's disease (syphilitic
  osteochondritis) 090.0
Parrot fever 073.9
Parry's disease or syndrome
  (exophthalmic goiter) 242.0●
Parry-Romberg syndrome 349.89
Parson's disease (exophthalmic goiter)
  242.0●
Parsonage-Aldren-Turner syndrome 353.5
Parsonage-Turner syndrome 353.5
Pars planitis 363.21
Particolored infant 757.39
Parturition - *see* Delivery
Parvovirus 079.83
  B19 079.83
  human 079.83
Passage
  false, urethra 599.4
  meconium noted during delivery
    763.84
  of sounds or bougies (*see also* Attention
    to artificial opening) V55.9

Passive - *see* condition
Pasteurella septica 027.2
Pasteurellosis (*see also* Infection,
  Pasteurella) 027.2
PAT (paroxysmal atrial tachycardia)
  427.0
Patau's syndrome (trisomy D1) 758.1
Patch
  herald 696.3
Patches
  mucous (syphilitic) 091.3
    congenital 090.0
  smokers' (mouth) 528.6
Patellar - *see* condition
Patellofemoral syndrome 719.46
Patent - *see also* Imperfect closure
  atrioventricular ostium 745.69
  canal of Nuck 752.41
  cervix 622.5
    complicating pregnancy 654.5●
      affecting fetus or newborn 761.0
  ductus arteriosus or Botalli 747.0
  Eustachian
    tube 381.7
    valve 746.89
  foramen
    Botalli 745.5
    ovale 745.5
  interauricular septum 745.5
  interventricular septum 745.4
  omphalomesenteric duct 751.0
  os (uteri) - *see* Patent, cervix
  ostium secundum 745.5
  urachus 753.7
  vitelline duct 751.0
Paternity testing V70.4
Paterson's syndrome (sideropenic
  dysphagia) 280.8
Paterson (-Brown) (-Kelly) syndrome
  (sideropenic dysphagia) 280.8
Paterson-Kelly syndrome or web
  (sideropenic dysphagia) 280.8
Pathologic, pathological - *see also*
  condition
  asphyxia 799.01
  drunkenness 291.4
  emotionality 301.3
  fracture - *see* Fracture, pathologic
  liar 301.7
  personality 301.9
  resorption, tooth 521.40
    external 521.42
    internal 521.41
    specified NEC 521.49
  sexuality (*see also* Deviation, sexual)
    302.9
Pathology (of) - *see also* Disease
  periradicular, associated with previous
    endodontic treatment 526.69
Patterned motor discharge, idiopathic
  (*see also* Epilepsy) 345.5●
Patulous - *see also* Patent
  anus 569.49
  Eustachian tube 381.7
Pause, sinoatrial 427.81
Pavor nocturnus 307.46
Pavy's disease 593.6
Paxton's disease (white piedra) 111.2
Payr's disease or syndrome (splenic
  flexure syndrome) 569.89
PBA (pseudobulbar affect) 310.8
Pearls
  Elschnig 366.51
  enamel 520.2

Pearl-workers' disease (chronic
  osteomyelitis) (*see also*
  Osteomyelitis) 730.1●
Pectenitis 569.49
Pectenosis 569.49
Pectoral - *see* condition
Pectus
  carinatum (congenital) 754.82
    acquired 738.3
    rachitic (*see also* Rickets) 268.0
  excavatum (congenital) 754.81
    acquired 738.3
    rachitic (*see also* Rickets) 268.0
  recurvatum (congenital) 754.81
    acquired 738.3
Pedatrophia 261
Pederosis 302.2
Pediculosis (infestation) 132.9
  capitis (head louse) (any site) 132.0
  corporis (body louse) (any site) 132.1
  eyelid 132.0 [373.6]
  mixed (classifiable to more than one
    category in 132.0–132.2) 132.3
  pubis (pubic louse) (any site) 132.2
  vestimenti 132.1
  vulvae 132.2
Pediculus (infestation) - *see* Pediculosis
Pedophilia 302.2
Peg-shaped teeth 520.2
Pel's crisis 094.0
Pel-Ebstein disease - *see* Disease,
  Hodgkin's
Pelade 704.01
Pelger-Huët anomaly or syndrome
  (hereditary hyposegmentation) 288.2
Peliosis (rheumatica) 287.0
Pelizaeus-Merzbacher
  disease 330.0
  sclerosis, diffuse cerebral 330.0
Pellagra (alcoholic or with alcoholism)
  265.2
  with polyneuropathy 265.2 [357.4]
Pellagra-cerebellar-ataxia-renal
  aminoaciduria syndrome 270.0
Pellegrini's disease (calcification, knee
  joint) 726.62
Pellegrini (-Stieda) disease or syndrome
  (calcification, knee joint) 726.62
Pellizzi's syndrome (pineal) 259.8
Pelvic - *see also* condition
  congestion-fibrosis syndrome 625.5
  kidney 753.3
Pelvioectasis 591
Pelviolithiasis 592.0
Pelviperitonitis
  female (*see also* Peritonitis, pelvic,
    female) 614.5
  male (*see also* Peritonitis) 567.21
Pelvis, pelvic - *see also* condition or type
  infantile 738.6
  Nägele's 738.6
  obliquity 738.6
  Robert's 755.69
Pemphigoid 694.5
  benign, mucous membrane 694.60
    with ocular involvement 694.61
  bullous 694.5
  cicatricial 694.60
    with ocular involvement 694.61
  juvenile 694.2
Pemphigus 694.4
  benign 694.5
    chronic familial 757.39
  Brazilian 694.4

◀ New   ◀▥ Revised   ~~deleted~~ Deleted   ● Use Additional Digit(s)   ▨ Omit code

Pemphigus (*Continued*)
  circinatus 694.0
  congenital, traumatic 757.39
  conjunctiva 694.61
  contagiosus 684
  erythematodes 694.4
  erythematosus 694.4
  foliaceus 694.4
  frambesiodes 694.4
  gangrenous (*see also* Gangrene) 785.4
  malignant 694.4
  neonatorum, newborn 684
  ocular 694.61
  papillaris 694.4
  seborrheic 694.4
  South American 694.4
  syphilitic (congenital) 090.0
  vegetans 694.4
  vulgaris 694.4
  wildfire 694.4
Pendred's syndrome (familial goiter with
    deaf-mutism) 243
Pendulous
  abdomen 701.9
    in pregnancy or childbirth 654.4●
      affecting fetus or newborn
        763.89
  breast 611.89
Penetrating wound - *see also* Wound,
    open, by site
  with internal injury - *see* Injury,
      internal, by site, with open
      wound
  eyeball 871.7
    with foreign body (nonmagnetic)
        871.6
      magnetic 871.5
  ocular (*see also* Penetrating wound,
      eyeball) 871.7
    adnexa 870.3
      with foreign body 870.4
    orbit 870.3
      with foreign body 870.4
**Penetration, pregnant uterus by
    instrument**
  with
    abortion - *see* Abortion, by type,
        with damage to pelvic organs
    ectopic pregnancy (*see also*
        categories 633.0–633.9) 639.2
    molar pregnancy (*see also* categories
        630–632) 639.2
  complication of delivery 665.1●
    affecting fetus or newborn 763.89
  following
    abortion 639.2
    ectopic or molar pregnancy 639.2
Penfield's syndrome (*see also* Epilepsy)
    345.5●
Penicilliosis of lung 117.3
Penis - *see* condition
Penitis 607.2
Penta X syndrome 758.81
Pentalogy (of Fallot) 745.2
Pentosuria (benign) (essential) 271.8
Peptic acid disease 536.8
Peregrinating patient V65.2
Perforated - *see* Perforation
Perforation, perforative (nontraumatic)
  antrum (*see also* Sinusitis, maxillary)
      473.0
  appendix 540.0
    with peritoneal abscess 540.1
  atrial septum, multiple 745.5

Perforation, perforative (*Continued*)
  attic, ear 384.22
    healed 384.81
  bile duct, except cystic (*see also* Disease,
      biliary) 576.3
    cystic 575.4
  bladder (urinary) 596.6
    with
      abortion - *see* Abortion, by type,
          with damage to pelvic
          organs
      ectopic pregnancy (*see also*
          categories 633.0–633.9) 639.2
      molar pregnancy (*see also*
          categories 630–632) 639.2
    following
      abortion 639.2
      ectopic or molar pregnancy 639.2
    obstetrical trauma 665.5●
  bowel 569.83
    with
      abortion - *see* Abortion, by type,
          with damage to pelvic
          organs
      ectopic pregnancy (*see also*
          categories 633.0–633.9) 639.2
      molar pregnancy (*see also*
          categories 630–632) 639.2
    fetus or newborn 777.6
    following
      abortion 639.2
      ectopic or molar pregnancy 639.2
    obstetrical trauma 665.5●
  broad ligament
    with
      abortion - *see* Abortion, by type,
          with damage to pelvic
          organs
      ectopic pregnancy (*see also*
          categories 633.0–633.9) 639.2
      molar pregnancy (*see also*
          categories 630–632) 639.2
    following
      abortion 639.2
      ectopic or molar pregnancy 639.2
    obstetrical trauma 665.6●
  by
    device, implant, or graft - *see*
        Complications, mechanical
    foreign body left accidentally in
        operation wound 998.4
    instrument (any) during a
        procedure, accidental 998.2
  cecum 540.0
    with peritoneal abscess 540.1
  cervix (uteri) - *see also* Injury, internal,
      cervix
    with
      abortion - *see* Abortion, by type,
          with damage to pelvic
          organs
      ectopic pregnancy (*see also*
          categories 633.0–633.9) 639.2
      molar pregnancy (*see also*
          categories 630–632) 639.2
    following
      abortion 639.2
      ectopic or molar pregnancy 639.2
    obstetrical trauma 665.3●
  colon 569.83
  common duct (bile) 576.3
  cornea (*see also* Ulcer, cornea) 370.00
    due to ulceration 370.06
  cystic duct 575.4

Perforation, perforative (*Continued*)
  diverticulum (*see also* Diverticula)
      562.10
    small intestine 562.00
  duodenum, duodenal (ulcer) - *see*
      Ulcer, duodenum, with
      perforation
  ear drum - *see* Perforation, tympanum
  enteritis - *see* Enteritis
  esophagus 530.4
  ethmoidal sinus (*see also* Sinusitis,
      ethmoidal) 473.2
  foreign body (external site) - *see also*
      Wound, open, by site,
      complicated
    internal site, by ingested object - *see*
        Foreign body
  frontal sinus (*see also* Sinusitis, frontal)
      473.1
  gallbladder or duct (*see also* Disease,
      gallbladder) 575.4
  gastric (ulcer) - *see* Ulcer, stomach, with
      perforation
  heart valve - *see* Endocarditis
  ileum (*see also* Perforation, intestine)
      569.83
  instrumental
    external - *see* Wound, open, by site
    pregnant uterus, complicating
        delivery 665.9●
    surgical (accidental) (blood vessel)
        (nerve) (organ) 998.2
  intestine 569.83
    with
      abortion - *see* Abortion, by type,
          with damage to pelvic
          organs
      ectopic pregnancy (*see also*
          categories 633.0–633.9) 639.2
      molar pregnancy (*see also*
          categories 630–632) 639.2
    fetus or newborn 777.6
    obstetrical trauma 665.5●
    ulcerative NEC 569.83
  jejunum, jejunal 569.83
    ulcer - *see* Ulcer, gastrojejunal, with
        perforation
  mastoid (antrum) (cell) 383.89
  maxillary sinus (*see also* Sinusitis,
      maxillary) 473.0
  membrana tympani - *see* Perforation,
      tympanum
  nasal
    septum 478.19
      congenital 748.1
      syphilitic 095.8
    sinus (*see also* Sinusitis) 473.9
      congenital 748.1
  palate (hard) 526.89
    soft 528.9
      syphilitic 095.8
    syphilitic 095.8
  palatine vault 526.89
    syphilitic 095.8
      congenital 090.5
  pelvic
    floor
      with
        abortion - *see* Abortion, by
            type, with damage to
            pelvic organs
        ectopic pregnancy (*see also*
            categories 633.0–633.9)
            639.2

Perforation, perforative *(Continued)*
  pelvic *(Continued)*
    floor *(Continued)*
      with *(Continued)*
        molar pregnancy *(see also categories 630–632)* 639.2
      obstetrical trauma 664.1●
    organ
      with
        abortion - *see* Abortion, by type, with damage to pelvic organs
        ectopic pregnancy *(see also categories 633.0–633.9)* 639.2
        molar pregnancy *(see also categories 630–632)* 639.2
      following
        abortion 639.2
        ectopic or molar pregnancy 639.2
      obstetrical trauma 665.5●
  perineum - *see* Laceration, perineum
  periurethral tissue
    with
      abortion - *see* Abortion, by type, with damage to pelvic organs
      ectopic pregnancy *(see also categories 630–632)* 639.2
      molar pregnancy *(see also categories 630–632)* 639.2
  pharynx 478.29
  pylorus, pyloric (ulcer) - *see* Ulcer, stomach, with perforation
  rectum 569.49
  root canal space 526.61
  sigmoid 569.83
  sinus (accessory) (chronic) (nasal) *(see also* Sinusitis) 473.9
  sphenoidal sinus *(see also* Sinusitis, sphenoidal) 473.3
  stomach (due to ulcer) - *see* Ulcer, stomach, with perforation
  surgical (accidental) (by instrument) (blood vessel) (nerve) (organ) 998.2
  traumatic
    external - *see* Wound, open, by site
    eye *(see also* Penetrating wound, ocular) 871.7
    internal organ - *see* Injury, internal, by site
  tympanum (membrane) (persistent posttraumatic) (postinflammatory) 384.20
    with
      otitis media - *see* Otitis media
    attic 384.22
    central 384.21
    healed 384.81
    marginal NEC 384.23
    multiple 384.24
    pars flaccida 384.22
    total 384.25
    traumatic - *see* Wound, open, ear, drum
  typhoid, gastrointestinal 002.0
  ulcer - *see* Ulcer, by site, with perforation
  ureter 593.89

Perforation, perforative *(Continued)*
  urethra
    with
      abortion - *see* Abortion, by type, with damage to pelvic organs
      ectopic pregnancy *(see also categories 633.0–633.9)* 639.2
      molar pregnancy *(see also categories 630–632)* 639.2
    following
      abortion 639.2
      ectopic or molar pregnancy 639.2
    obstetrical trauma 665.5●
  uterus - *see also* Injury, internal, uterus
    with
      abortion - *see* Abortion, by type, with damage to pelvic organs
      ectopic pregnancy *(see also categories 633.0–633.9)* 639.2
      molar pregnancy *(see also categories 630–632)* 639.2
    by intrauterine contraceptive device 996.32
    following
      abortion 639.2
      ectopic or molar pregnancy 639.2
    obstetrical trauma - *see* Injury, internal, uterus, obstetrical trauma
  uvula 528.9
    syphilitic 095.8
  vagina - *see* Laceration, vagina
  viscus NEC 799.89
    traumatic 868.00
      with open wound into cavity 868.10
Periadenitis mucosa necrotica recurrens 528.2
Periangiitis 446.0
Periantritis 535.4●
Periappendicitis (acute) *(see also* Appendicitis) 541
Periarteritis (disseminated) (infectious) (necrotizing) (nodosa) 446.0
Periarthritis (joint) 726.90
  Duplay's 726.2
  gonococcal 098.50
  humeroscapularis 726.2
  scapulohumeral 726.2
  shoulder 726.2
  wrist 726.4
Periarthrosis (angioneural) - *see* Periarthritis
Peribronchitis 491.9
  tuberculous *(see also* Tuberculosis) 011.3●
Pericapsulitis, adhesive (shoulder) 726.0
Pericarditis (granular) (with decompensation) (with effusion) 423.9
  with
    rheumatic fever (conditions classifiable to 390)
      active *(see also* Pericarditis, rheumatic) 391.0
      inactive or quiescent 393
  actinomycotic 039.8 *[420.0]*
  acute (nonrheumatic) 420.90
    with chorea (acute) (rheumatic) (Sydenham's) 392.0
    bacterial 420.99
    benign 420.91

Pericarditis *(Continued)*
  acute *(Continued)*
    hemorrhagic 420.90
    idiopathic 420.91
    infective 420.90
    nonspecific 420.91
    rheumatic 391.0
      with chorea (acute) (rheumatic) (Sydenham's) 392.0
    sicca 420.90
    viral 420.91
  adhesive or adherent (external) (internal) 423.1
    acute - *see* Pericarditis, acute
    rheumatic (external) (internal) 393
  amebic 006.8 *[420.0]*
  bacterial (acute) (subacute) (with serous or seropurulent effusion) 420.99
  calcareous 423.2
  cholesterol (chronic) 423.8
    acute 420.90
  chronic (nonrheumatic) 423.8
    rheumatic 393
  constrictive 423.2
  Coxsackie 074.21
  due to
    actinomycosis 039.8 *[420.0]*
    amebiasis 006.8 *[420.0]*
    Coxsackie (virus) 074.21
    histoplasmosis *(see also* Histoplasmosis) 115.93
    nocardiosis 039.8 *[420.0]*
    tuberculosis *(see also* Tuberculosis) 017.9● *[420.0]*
  fibrinocaseous *(see also* Tuberculosis) 017.9● *[420.0]*
  fibrinopurulent 420.99
  fibrinous - *see* Pericarditis, rheumatic
  fibropurulent 420.99
  fibrous 423.1
  gonococcal 098.83
  hemorrhagic 423.0
  idiopathic (acute) 420.91
  infective (acute) 420.90
  meningococcal 036.41
  neoplastic (chronic) 423.8
    acute 420.90
  nonspecific 420.91
  obliterans, obliterating 423.1
  plastic 423.1
  pneumococcal (acute) 420.99
  postinfarction 411.0
  purulent (acute) 420.99
  rheumatic (active) (acute) (with effusion) (with pneumonia) 391.0
    with chorea (acute) (rheumatic) (Sydenham's) 392.0
    chronic or inactive (with chorea) 393
  septic (acute) 420.99
  serofibrinous - *see* Pericarditis, rheumatic
  staphylococcal (acute) 420.99
  streptococcal (acute) 420.99
  suppurative (acute) 420.99
  syphilitic 093.81
  tuberculous (acute) (chronic) *(see also* Tuberculosis) 017.9● *[420.0]*
  uremic 585.9 *[420.0]*
  viral (acute) 420.91
Pericardium, pericardial - *see* condition
Pericellulitis *(see also* Cellulitis) 682.9

◀ New   ◀▥ Revised   ~~deleted~~ Deleted   ● Use Additional Digit(s)   ▨ Omit code

Pericementitis 523.40
　acute 523.30
　chronic (suppurative) 523.40
Pericholecystitis (*see also* Cholecystitis)
　　575.10
Perichondritis
　auricle 380.00
　　acute 380.01
　　chronic 380.02
　bronchus 491.9
　ear (external) 380.00
　　acute 380.01
　　chronic 380.02
　larynx 478.71
　　syphilitic 095.8
　　typhoid 002.0 [478.71]
　nose 478.19
　pinna 380.00
　　acute 380.01
　　chronic 380.02
　trachea 478.9
Periclasia 523.5
Pericolitis 569.89
Pericoronitis (chronic) 523.40
　acute 523.33
Pericystitis (*see also* Cystitis) 595.9
Pericytoma (M9150/1) - *see also*
　　Neoplasm, connective tissue,
　　uncertain behavior
　benign (M9150/0) - *see* Neoplasm,
　　connective tissue, benign
　malignant (M9150/3) - *see* Neoplasm,
　　connective tissue, malignant
Peridacryocystitis, acute 375.32
Peridiverticulitis (*see also* Diverticulitis)
　　562.11
Periduodenitis 535.6●
Periendocarditis (*see also* Endocarditis)
　　424.90
　acute or subacute 421.9
Periepididymitis (*see also* Epididymitis)
　　604.90
Perifolliculitis (abscedens) 704.8
　capitis, abscedens et suffodiens 704.8
　dissecting, scalp 704.8
　scalp 704.8
　superficial pustular 704.8
Perigastritis (acute) 535.0●
Perigastrojejunitis (acute) 535.0●
Perihepatitis (acute) 573.3
　chlamydial 099.56
　gonococcal 098.86
Peri-ileitis (subacute) 569.89
Perilabyrinthitis (acute) - *see* Labyrinthitis
Perimeningitis - *see* Meningitis
Perimetritis (*see also* Endometritis) 615.9
Perimetrosalpingitis (*see also* Salpingo-
　　oophoritis) 614.2
Perineocele 618.05
Perinephric - *see* condition
Perinephritic - *see* condition
Perinephritis (*see also* Infection, kidney)
　　590.9
　purulent (*see also* Abscess, kidney)
　　590.2
Perineum, perineal - *see* condition
Perineuritis NEC 729.2
Periodic - *see also* condition
　disease (familial) 277.31
　edema 995.1
　　hereditary 277.6
　fever 277.31
　headache syndromes in child or
　　adolescent 346.2●

Periodic (*Continued*)
　limb movement disorder 327.51
　paralysis (familial) 359.3
　peritonitis 277.31
　polyserositis 277.31
　somnolence (*see also* Narcolepsy) 347.00
Periodontal
　cyst 522.8
　pocket 523.8
Periodontitis (chronic) (complex)
　　(compound) (simplex) 523.40
　acute 523.33
　aggressive 523.30
　　generalized 523.32
　　localized 523.31
　apical 522.6
　　acute (pulpal origin) 522.4
　generalized 523.42
　localized 523.41
Periodontoclasia 523.5
Periodontosis 523.5
Periods - *see also* Menstruation
　heavy 626.2
　irregular 626.4
Perionychia (with lymphangitis) 681.9
　finger 681.02
　toe 681.11
Perioophoritis (*see also* Salpingo-
　　oophoritis) 614.2
Periorchitis (*see also* Orchitis) 604.90
Periosteum, periosteal - *see* condition
Periostitis (circumscribed) (diffuse)
　　(infective) 730.3●

> **Note 59** Use the following fifth-digit
> subclassification with category 730:
>
> 0　site unspecified
> 1　shoulder region
> 2　upper arm
> 3　forearm
> 4　hand
> 5　pelvic region and thigh
> 6　lower leg
> 7　ankle and foot
> 8　other specified sites
> 9　multiple sites

　with osteomyelitis (*see also*
　　Osteomyelitis) 730.2●
　　acute or subacute 730.0●
　　chronic or old 730.1●
　albuminosa, albuminosus 730.3●
　alveolar 526.5
　alveolodental 526.5
　dental 526.5
　gonorrheal 098.89
　hyperplastica, generalized 731.2
　jaw (lower) (upper) 526.4
　monomelic 733.99
　orbital 376.02
　syphilitic 095.5
　　congenital 090.0 [730.8]●
　　secondary 091.61
　tuberculous (*see also* Tuberculosis,
　　bone) 015.9● [730.8]●
　yaws (early) (hypertrophic) (late)
　　102.6
Periostosis (*see also* Periostitis) 730.3●
　with osteomyelitis (*see also*
　　Osteomyelitis) 730.2●
　　acute or subacute 730.0●
　　chronic or old 730.1●
　hyperplastic 756.59
Peripartum cardiomyopathy 674.5●

Periphlebitis (*see also* Phlebitis) 451.9
　lower extremity 451.2
　　deep (vessels) 451.19
　　superficial (vessels) 451.0
　portal 572.1
　retina 362.18
　superficial (vessels) 451.0
　tuberculous (*see also* Tuberculosis)
　　017.9●
　　retina 017.3● [362.18]
Peripneumonia - *see* Pneumonia
Periproctitis 569.49
Periprostatitis (*see also* Prostatitis) 601.9
Perirectal - *see* condition
Perirenal - *see* condition
Perisalpingitis (*see also* Salpingo-
　　oophoritis) 614.2
Perisigmoiditis 569.89
Perisplenitis (infectional) 289.59
Perispondylitis - *see* Spondylitis
Peristalsis reversed or visible 787.4
Peritendinitis (*see also* Tenosynovitis)
　　726.90
　adhesive (shoulder) 726.0
Perithelioma (M9150/1) - *see* Pericytoma
Peritoneum, peritoneal - *see also* condition
　equilibration test V56.32
Peritonitis (acute) (adhesive) (fibrinous)
　　(hemorrhagic) (idiopathic)
　　(localized) (perforative) (primary)
　　(with adhesions) (with effusion)
　　567.9
　with or following
　　abortion - *see* Abortion, by type,
　　　with sepsis
　　abscess 567.21
　　appendicitis 540.0
　　　with peritoneal abscess 540.1
　　ectopic pregnancy (*see also*
　　　categories 633.0–633.9) 639.0
　　molar pregnancy (*see also* categories
　　　630–632) 639.0
　aseptic 998.7
　bacterial 567.29
　　spontaneous 567.23
　bile, biliary 567.81
　chemical 998.7
　chlamydial 099.56
　chronic proliferative 567.89
　congenital NEC 777.6
　diaphragmatic 567.22
　diffuse NEC 567.29
　diphtheritic 032.83
　disseminated NEC 567.29
　due to
　　bile 567.81
　　foreign
　　　body or object accidentally left
　　　　during a procedure
　　　　(instrument) (sponge)
　　　　(swab) 998.4
　　　substance accidentally left during
　　　　a procedure (chemical)
　　　　(powder) (talc) 998.7
　　talc 998.7
　　urine 567.89
　fibrinopurulent 567.29
　fibrinous 567.29
　fibrocaseous (*see also* Tuberculosis)
　　014.0●
　fibropurulent 567.29
　general, generalized (acute) 567.21
　gonococcal 098.86
　in infective disease NEC 136.9 [567.0]

Peritonitis (*Continued*)
  meconium (newborn) 777.6
  pancreatic 577.8
  paroxysmal, benign 277.31
  pelvic
    female (acute) 614.5
      chronic NEC 614.7
        with adhesions 614.6
      puerperal, postpartum, childbirth 670.8 ◀▦
    male (acute) 567.21
  periodic (familial) 277.31
  phlegmonous 567.29
  pneumococcal 567.1
  postabortal 639.0
  proliferative, chronic 567.89
  puerperal, postpartum, childbirth 670.8 ◀▦
  purulent 567.29
  septic 567.29
  spontaneous bacterial 567.23
  staphylococcal 567.29
  streptococcal 567.29
  subdiaphragmatic 567.29
  subphrenic 567.29
  suppurative 567.29
  syphilitic 095.2
    congenital 090.0 [567.0]
  talc 998.7
  tuberculous (*see also* Tuberculosis) 014.0●
  urine 567.89
Peritonsillar - *see* condition
Peritonsillitis 475
Perityphlitis (*see also* Appendicitis) 541
Periureteritis 593.89
Periurethral - *see* condition
Periurethritis (gangrenous) 597.89
Periuterine - *see* condition
Perivaginitis (*see also* Vaginitis) 616.10
Perivasculitis, retinal 362.18
Perivasitis (chronic) 608.4
Periventricular leukomalacia 779.7
Perivesiculitis (seminal) (*see also* Vesiculitis) 608.0
Perlèche 686.8
  due to
    moniliasis 112.0
    riboflavin deficiency 266.0
Pernicious - *see* condition
Pernio, perniosis 991.5
Persecution
  delusion 297.9
  social V62.4
Perseveration (tonic) 784.69
Persistence, persistent (congenital) 759.89
  anal membrane 751.2
  arteria stapedia 744.04
  atrioventricular canal 745.69
  bloody ejaculate 792.2
  branchial cleft 744.41
  bulbus cordis in left ventricle 745.8
  canal of Cloquet 743.51
  capsule (opaque) 743.51
  cilioretinal artery or vein 743.51
  cloaca 751.5
  communication - *see* Fistula, congenital
  convolutions
    aortic arch 747.21
    fallopian tube 752.19
    oviduct 752.19
    uterine tube 752.19
  double aortic arch 747.21

Persistence, persistent (*Continued*)
  ductus
    arteriosus 747.0
    Botalli 747.0
  fetal
    circulation 747.83
    form of cervix (uteri) 752.49
    hemoglobin (hereditary) ("Swiss variety") 282.7
    pulmonary hypertension 747.83
  foramen
    Botalli 745.5
    ovale 745.5
  Gartner's duct 752.41
  hemoglobin, fetal (hereditary) (HPFH) 282.7
  hyaloid
    artery (generally incomplete) 743.51
    system 743.51
  hymen (tag)
    in pregnancy or childbirth 654.8●
      causing obstructed labor 660.2●
  lanugo 757.4
  left
    posterior cardinal vein 747.49
    root with right arch of aorta 747.21
    superior vena cava 747.49
  Meckel's diverticulum 751.0
  mesonephric duct 752.89
    fallopian tube 752.11
  mucosal disease (middle ear) (with posterior or superior marginal perforation of ear drum) 382.2
  nail(s), anomalous 757.5
  occiput, anterior or posterior 660.3●
    fetus or newborn 763.1
  omphalomesenteric duct 751.0
  organ or site NEC - *see* Anomaly, specified type NEC
  ostium
    atrioventriculare commune 745.69
    primum 745.61
    secundum 745.5
  ovarian rests in fallopian tube 752.19
  pancreatic tissue in intestinal tract 751.5
  primary (deciduous)
    teeth 520.6
    vitreous hyperplasia 743.51
  pulmonary hypertension 747.83
  pupillary membrane 743.46
    iris 743.46
    Rhesus (Rh) titer 999.7
  right aortic arch 747.21
  sinus
    urogenitalis 752.89
    venosus with imperfect incorporation in right auricle 747.49
  thymus (gland) 254.8
    hyperplasia 254.0
  thyroglossal duct 759.2
  thyrolingual duct 759.2
  truncus arteriosus or communis 745.0
  tunica vasculosa lentis 743.39
  umbilical sinus 753.7
  urachus 753.7
  vegetative state 780.03
  vitelline duct 751.0
  wolffian duct 752.89

Person (with)
  admitted for clinical research, as participant or control subject V70.7
  affected by
    family member
      currently on deployment (military) V61.01
      returned from deployment (military) (current or past conflict) V61.02
  awaiting admission to adequate facility elsewhere V63.2
  undergoing social agency investigation V63.8
  concern (normal) about sick person in family V61.49
  consulting on behalf of another V65.19
    pediatric pre-birth visit for expectant mother V65.11 ◀▦
      pre-adoption visit for adoptive parents V65.11 ◀
      pre-birth visit for expectant parents V65.11 ◀
  currently deployed in theater or in support of military war, peacekeeping and humanitarian operations V62.21
  feared
    complaint in whom no diagnosis was made V65.5
    condition not demonstrated V65.5
  feigning illness V65.2
  healthy, accompanying sick person V65.0
  history of military war, peacekeeping and humanitarian deployment (current or past conflict) V62.22
  living (in)
    alone V60.3
    boarding school V60.6
    residence remote from hospital or medical care facility V63.0
    residential institution V60.6
    without
      adequate
        financial resources V60.2
        housing (heating) (space) V60.1
        housing (permanent) (temporary) V60.0
        material resources V60.2
      person able to render necessary care V60.4
      shelter V60.0
  medical services in home not available V63.1
  on waiting list V63.2
    undergoing social agency investigation V63.8
  sick or handicapped in family V61.49
  "worried well" V65.5
Personality
  affective 301.10
  aggressive 301.3
  amoral 301.7
  anancastic, anankastic 301.4
  antisocial 301.7
  asocial 301.7
  asthenic 301.6
  avoidant 301.82
  borderline 301.83
  change 310.1
  compulsive 301.4

◀ New   ◀▦ Revised   ~~deleted~~ Deleted   ● Use Additional Digit(s)   ▦ Omit code

Personality *(Continued)*
cycloid 301.13
cyclothymic 301.13
dependent 301.6
depressive (chronic) 301.12
disorder, disturbance NEC 301.9
with
antisocial disturbance 301.7
pattern disturbance NEC 301.9
sociopathic disturbance 301.7
trait disturbance 301.9
dual 300.14
dyssocial 301.7
eccentric 301.89
"haltlose" type 301.89
emotionally unstable 301.59
epileptoid 301.3
explosive 301.3
fanatic 301.0
histrionic 301.50
hyperthymic 301.11
hypomanic 301.11
hypothymic 301.12
hysterical 301.50
immature 301.89
inadequate 301.6
labile 301.59
masochistic 301.89
morally defective 301.7
multiple 300.14
narcissistic 301.81
obsessional 301.4
obsessive-compulsive 301.4
overconscientious 301.4
paranoid 301.0
passive (-dependent) 301.6
passive-aggressive 301.84
pathologic NEC 301.9
pattern defect or disturbance 301.9
pseudosocial 301.7
psychoinfantile 301.59
psychoneurotic NEC 301.89
psychopathic 301.9
with
amoral trend 301.7
antisocial trend 301.7
asocial trend 301.7
pathologic sexuality (*see also*
Deviation, sexual) 302.9
mixed types 301.9
schizoid 301.20
introverted 301.21
schizotypal 301.22
type A 301.4
unstable (emotional) 301.59
Perthes' disease (capital femoral
osteochondrosis) 732.1
Pertussis (*see also* Whooping cough) 033.9
vaccination, prophylactic (against)
V03.6
Peruvian wart 088.0
Perversion, perverted
appetite 307.52
hysterical 300.11
function
pineal gland 259.8
pituitary gland 253.9
anterior lobe
deficient 253.2
excessive 253.1
posterior lobe 253.6
placenta - *see* Placenta, abnormal
sense of smell or taste 781.1
psychogenic 306.7
sexual (*see also* Deviation, sexual) 302.9

Pervious, congenital - *see also* Imperfect,
closure
ductus arteriosus 747.0
Pes (congenital) (*see also* Talipes) 754.70
abductus (congenital) 754.60
acquired 736.79
acquired NEC 736.79
planus 734
adductus (congenital) 754.79
acquired 736.79
cavus 754.71
acquired 736.73
planovalgus (congenital) 754.69
acquired 736.79
planus (acquired) (any degree) 734
congenital 754.61
rachitic 268.1
valgus (congenital) 754.61
acquired 736.79
varus (congenital) 754.50
acquired 736.79
Pest (*see also* Plague) 020.9
Pestis (*see also* Plague) 020.9
bubonica 020.0
fulminans 020.0
minor 020.8
pneumonica - *see* Plague, pneumonic
Petechia, petechiae 782.7
fetus or newborn 772.6
Petechial
fever 036.0
typhus 081.9
Petges-Cléjat or Petges-Clégat syndrome
(poikilodermatomyositis) 710.3
Petit's
disease (*see also* Hernia, lumbar) 553.8
Petit mal (idiopathic) (*see also* Epilepsy)
345.0●
status 345.2
Petrellidosis 117.6
Petrositis 383.20
acute 383.21
chronic 383.22
Peutz-Jeghers disease or syndrome 759.6
Peyronie's disease 607.85
Pfeiffer's disease 075
Phacentocele 379.32
traumatic 921.3
Phacoanaphylaxis 360.19
Phacocele (old) 379.32
traumatic 921.3
Phaehyphomycosis 117.8
Phagedena (dry) (moist) (*see also*
Gangrene) 785.4
arteriosclerotic 440.24
geometric 686.09
penis 607.89
senile 440.24
sloughing 785.4
tropical (*see also* Ulcer, skin) 707.9
vulva 616.50
Phagedenic - *see also* condition
abscess - *see also* Abscess
chancroid 099.0
bubo NEC 099.8
chancre 099.0
ulcer (tropical) (*see also* Ulcer, skin)
707.9
Phagomania 307.52
Phakoma 362.89
Phantom limb (syndrome) 353.6
Pharyngeal - *see also* condition
arch remnant 744.41
pouch syndrome 279.11

Pharyngitis (acute) (catarrhal)
(gangrenous) (infective)
(malignant) (membranous)
(phlegmonous) (pneumococcal)
(pseudomembranous) (simple)
(staphylococcal) (subacute)
(suppurative) (ulcerative) (viral)
462
with influenza, flu, or grippe 487.1
aphthous 074.0
atrophic 472.1
chlamydial 099.51
chronic 472.1
Coxsackie virus 074.0
diphtheritic (membranous) 032.0
follicular 472.1
fusospirochetal 101
gonococcal 098.6
granular (chronic) 472.1
herpetic 054.79
hypertrophic 472.1
infectional, chronic 472.1
influenzal 487.1
lymphonodular, acute 074.8
septic 034.0
streptococcal 034.0
tuberculous (*see also* Tuberculosis)
012.8●
vesicular 074.0
Pharyngoconjunctival fever 077.2
Pharyngoconjunctivitis, viral 077.2
Pharyngolaryngitis (acute) 465.0
chronic 478.9
septic 034.0
Pharyngoplegia 478.29
Pharyngotonsillitis 465.8
tuberculous 012.8●
Pharyngotracheitis (acute) 465.8
chronic 478.9
Pharynx, pharyngeal - *see* condition
Phase of life problem NEC V62.89
Phenomenon
Arthus 995.21
flashback (drug) 292.89
jaw-winking 742.8
Jod-Basedow 242.8●
L. E. cell 710.0
lupus erythematosus cell 710.0
Pelger-Huët (hereditary
hyposegmentation) 288.2
Raynaud's (paroxysmal digital
cyanosis) (secondary) 443.0
Reilly's (*see also* Neuropathy,
peripheral, autonomic)
337.9
vasomotor 780.2
vasospastic 443.9
vasovagal 780.2
Wenckebach's, heart block (second
degree) 426.13
Phenylketonuria (PKU) 270.1
Phenylpyruvicaciduria 270.1
Pheochromoblastoma (M8700/3)
specified site - *see* Neoplasm, by site,
malignant
unspecified site 194.0
Pheochromocytoma (M8700/0)
malignant (M8700/3)
specified site - *see* Neoplasm, by site,
malignant
unspecified site 194.0
specified site - *see* Neoplasm, by site,
benign
unspecified site 227.0

Phimosis (congenital) 605
  chancroidal 099.0
  due to infection 605
Phlebectasia (*see also* Varicose, vein)
    454.9
  congenital NEC 747.60
  esophagus (*see also* Varix, esophagus)
    456.1
    with hemorrhage (*see also* Varix,
      esophagus, bleeding) 456.0
Phlebitis (infective) (pyemic) (septic)
    (suppurative) 451.9
  antecubital vein 451.82
  arm NEC 451.84
    axillary vein 451.89
    basilic vein 451.82
    deep 451.83
    superficial 451.82
  axillary vein 451.89
  basilic vein 451.82
  blue 451.9
  brachial vein 451.83
  breast, superficial 451.89
  cavernous (venous) sinus - *see*
      Phlebitis, intracranial sinus
  cephalic vein 451.82
  cerebral (venous) sinus - *see* Phlebitis,
      intracranial sinus
  chest wall, superficial 451.89
  complicating pregnancy or puerperium
    671.2● ◀▥
    affecting fetus or newborn 760.3
  cranial (venous) sinus - *see* Phlebitis,
      intracranial sinus
  deep (vessels) 451.19
    femoral vein 451.11
    specified vessel NEC 451.19
  due to implanted device - *see*
      Complications, due to (presence
      of) any device, implant, or graft
      classified to 996.0–996.5 NEC
  during or resulting from a procedure
    997.2
  femoral vein (deep) (superficial)
    451.11
  femoropopliteal 451.19
  following infusion, perfusion, or
      transfusion 999.2
  gouty 274.89 [451.9]
  hepatic veins 451.89
  iliac vein 451.81
  iliofemoral 451.11
  intracranial sinus (any) (venous) 325
    late effect - *see* category 326
    nonpyogenic 437.6
      in pregnancy or puerperium
        671.5●
  jugular vein 451.89
  lateral (venous) sinus - *see* Phlebitis,
      intracranial sinus
  leg 451.2
    deep (vessels) 451.19
      specified vessel NEC 451.19
    superficial (vessels) 451.0
      femoral vein 451.11
  longitudinal sinus - *see* Phlebitis,
      intracranial sinus
  lower extremity 451.2
    deep (vessels) 451.19
      specified vessel NEC 451.19
    superficial (vessels) 451.0
      femoral vein 451.11
  migrans, migrating (superficial)
    453.1

Phlebitis (*Continued*)
  pelvic
    with
      abortion - *see* Abortion, by type,
        with sepsis
      ectopic pregnancy (*see also*
          categories 633.0–633.9)
        639.0
      molar pregnancy (*see also*
          categories 630–632)
        639.0
    following
      abortion 639.0
      ectopic or molar pregnancy
        639.0
    puerperal, postpartum 671.4●
  popliteal vein 451.19
  portal (vein) 572.1
  postoperative 997.2
  pregnancy 671.2● ◀▥
    deep 671.3●
    specified type NEC 671.5●
  superficial 671.2●
  puerperal, postpartum, childbirth
    671.2● ◀▥
    deep 671.4●
    lower extremities 671.2●
    pelvis 671.4●
    specified site NEC 671.5●
    superficial 671.2●
  radial vein 451.83
  retina 362.18
  saphenous (great) (long) 451.0
    accessory or small 451.0
  sinus (meninges) - *see* Phlebitis,
      intracranial sinus
  specified site NEC 451.89
  subclavian vein 451.89
  syphilitic 093.89
  tibial vein 451.19
  ulcer, ulcerative 451.9
    leg 451.2
      deep (vessels) 451.19
        specified vessel NEC 451.19
      superficial (vessels) 451.0
        femoral vein 451.11
    lower extremity 451.2
      deep (vessels) 451.19
        femoral vein 451.11
        specified vessel NEC
          451.19
      superficial (vessels) 451.0
  ulnar vein 451.83
  umbilicus 451.89
  upper extremity - *see* Phlebitis, arm
    deep (veins) 451.83
      brachial vein 451.83
      radial vein 451.83
      ulnar vein 451.83
    superficial (veins) 451.82
      antecubital vein 451.82
      basilic vein 451.82
      cephalic vein 451.82
  uterus (septic) (*see also* Endometritis)
    615.9
  varicose (leg) (lower extremity)
      (*see also* Varicose, vein)
    454.1
Phlebofibrosis 459.89
Phleboliths 459.89
Phlebosclerosis 459.89
Phlebothrombosis - *see* Thrombosis
Phlebotomus fever 066.0
Phlegm, choked on 933.1

Phlegmasia
  alba dolens (deep vessels) 451.19
    complicating pregnancy 671.3●
    nonpuerperal 451.19
    puerperal, postpartum, childbirth
      671.4●
  cerulea dolens 451.19
Phlegmon (*see also* Abscess) 682.9
  erysipelatous (*see also* Erysipelas) 035
  iliac 682.2
    fossa 540.1
  throat 478.29
Phlegmonous - *see* condition
Phlyctenulosis (allergic)
    (keratoconjunctivitis)
    (nontuberculous) 370.31
  cornea 370.31
    with ulcer (*see also* Ulcer, cornea)
      370.00
  tuberculous (*see also* Tuberculosis)
    017.3● [370.31]
Phobia, phobic (reaction) 300.20
  animal 300.29
  isolated NEC 300.29
  obsessional 300.3
  simple NEC 300.29
  social 300.23
  specified NEC 300.29
  state 300.20
Phocas' disease 610.1
Phocomelia 755.4
  lower limb 755.32
    complete 755.33
    distal 755.35
    proximal 755.34
  upper limb 755.22
    complete 755.23
    distal 755.25
    proximal 755.24
Phoria (*see also* Heterophoria) 378.40
Phosphate-losing tubular disorder 588.0
Phosphatemia 275.3
Phosphaturia 275.3
Photoallergic response 692.72
Photocoproporphyria 277.1
Photodermatitis (sun) 692.72
  light other than sun 692.82
Photokeratitis 370.24
Photo-ophthalmia 370.24
Photophobia 368.13
Photopsia 368.15
Photoretinitis 363.31
Photoretinopathy 363.31
Photosensitiveness (sun) 692.72
  light other than sun 692.82
Photosensitization skin (sun) 692.72
  light other than sun 692.82
Phototoxic response 692.72
Phrenitis 323.9
Phrynoderma 264.8
Phthiriasis (pubis) (any site) 132.2
  with any infestation classifiable to 132.0
    and 132.1 132.3
Phthirus infestation - *see* Phthiriasis
Phthisis (*see also* Tuberculosis) 011.9●
  bulbi (infectional) 360.41
  colliers' 011.4●
  cornea 371.05
  eyeball (due to infection) 360.41
  millstone makers' 011.4●
  miners' 011.4●
  potters' 011.4●
  sandblasters' 011.4●
  stonemasons' 011.4●

◀ New   ◀▥ Revised   ~~deleted~~ Deleted   ● Use Additional Digit(s)   � Omit code

Phycomycosis 117.7
Physalopteriasis 127.7
Physical therapy NEC V57.1
  breathing exercises V57.0
Physiological cup, optic papilla
  borderline, glaucoma suspect 365.00
  enlarged 377.14
  glaucomatous 377.14
Phytobezoar 938
  intestine 936
  stomach 935.2
Pian (see also Yaws) 102.9
Pianoma 102.1
Piarhemia, piarrhemia (see also
    Hyperlipemia) 272.4
  bilharziasis 120.9
Pica 307.52
  hysterical 300.11
Pick's
  cerebral atrophy 331.11
    with dementia
      with behavioral disturbance
        331.11 [294.11]
      without behavioral disturbance
        331.11 [294.10]
  disease
    brain 331.11
      dementia in
        with behavioral disturbance
          331.11 [294.11]
        without behavioral
          disturbance 331.11
          [294.10]
    lipid histiocytosis 272.7
    liver (pericardial pseudocirrhosis of
      liver) 423.2
    pericardium (pericardial
      pseudocirrhosis of liver)
      423.2
    polyserositis (pericardial
      pseudocirrhosis of liver) 423.2
  syndrome
    heart (pericardial pseudocirrhosis of
      liver) 423.2
    liver (pericardial pseudocirrhosis of
      liver) 423.2
  tubular adenoma (M8640/0)
    specified site - see Neoplasm, by site,
      benign
    unspecified site
      female 220
      male 222.0
Pick-Herxheimer syndrome (diffuse
    idiopathic cutaneous atrophy) 701.8
Pick-Niemann disease (lipid
    histiocytosis) 272.7
Pickwickian syndrome (cardiopulmonary
    obesity) 278.8
Piebaldism, classic 709.09
Piedra 111.2
  beard 111.2
    black 111.3
    white 111.2
  black 111.3
  scalp 111.3
    black 111.3
    white 111.2
  white 111.2
Pierre Marie's syndrome (pulmonary
    hypertrophic osteoarthropathy)
    731.2
Pierre Marie-Bamberger syndrome
    (hypertrophic pulmonary
    osteoarthropathy) 731.2

Pierre Mauriac's syndrome (diabetes-
    dwarfism-obesity) 258.1
Pierre Robin deformity or syndrome
    (congenital) 756.0
Pierson's disease or osteochondrosis 732.1
Pigeon
  breast or chest (acquired) 738.3
    congenital 754.82
    rachitic (see also Rickets) 268.0
  breeders' disease or lung 495.2
  fanciers' disease or lung 495.2
  toe 735.8
Pigmentation (abnormal) 709.00
  anomalies NEC 709.00
    congenital 757.33
    specified NEC 709.09
  conjunctiva 372.55
  cornea 371.10
    anterior 371.11
    posterior 371.13
    stromal 371.12
  lids (congenital) 757.33
    acquired 374.52
  limbus corneae 371.10
  metals 709.00
  optic papilla, congenital 743.57
  retina (congenital) (grouped) (nevoid)
    743.53
    acquired 362.74
  scrotum, congenital 757.33
Piles - see Hemorrhoids
Pili
  annulati or torti (congenital) 757.4
  incarnati 704.8
Pill roller hand (intrinsic) 736.09
Pilomatrixoma (M8110/0) - see Neoplasm,
    skin, benign
Pilonidal - see condition
Pimple 709.8
PIN I (prostatic intraepithelial
    neoplasia I) 602.3
PIN II (prostatic intraepithelial
    neoplasia II) 602.3
PIN III (prostatic intraepithelial
    neoplasia III) 233.4
Pinched nerve - see Neuropathy,
    entrapment
Pineal body or gland - see condition
Pinealoblastoma (M9362/3) 194.4
Pinealoma (M9360/1) 237.1
  malignant (M9360/3) 194.4
Pineoblastoma (M9362/3) 194.4
Pineocytoma (M9361/1) 237.1
Pinguecula 372.51
Pingueculitis 372.34
Pinhole meatus (see also Stricture, urethra)
    598.9
Pink
  disease 985.0
  eye 372.03
  puffer 492.8
Pinkus' disease (lichen nitidus) 697.1
Pinpoint
  meatus (see also Stricture, urethra)
    598.9
  os (uteri) (see also Stricture, cervix)
    622.4
Pinselhaare (congenital) 757.4
Pinta 103.9
  cardiovascular lesions 103.2
  chancre (primary) 103.0
  erythematous plaques 103.1
  hyperchromic lesions 103.1
  hyperkeratosis 103.1

Pinta (Continued)
  lesions 103.9
    cardiovascular 103.2
    hyperchromic 103.1
    intermediate 103.1
    late 103.2
    mixed 103.3
    primary 103.0
    skin (achromic) (cicatricial)
      (dyschromic) 103.2
      hyperchromic 103.1
      mixed (achromic and
        hyperchromic) 103.3
  papule (primary) 103.0
  skin lesions (achromic) (cicatricial)
    (dyschromic) 103.2
    hyperchromic 103.1
    mixed (achromic and hyperchromic)
      103.3
  vitiligo 103.2
Pintid 103.0
Pinworms (disease) (infection)
    (infestation) 127.4
Piry fever 066.8
Pistol wound - see Gunshot wound
Pit, lip (mucus), congenital 750.25
Pitchers' elbow 718.82
Pithecoid pelvis 755.69
  with disproportion (fetopelvic)
    653.2●
    affecting fetus or newborn 763.1
    causing obstructed labor 660.1●
Pithiatism 300.11
Pitted - see also Pitting
  teeth 520.4
Pitting (edema) (see also Edema) 782.3
  lip 782.3
  nail 703.8
    congenital 757.5
Pituitary gland - see condition
Pituitary snuff-takers' disease 495.8
Pityriasis 696.5
  alba 696.5
  capitis 690.11
  circinata (et maculata) 696.3
  Hebra's (exfoliative dermatitis) 695.89
  lichenoides et varioliformis 696.2
  maculata (et circinata) 696.3
  nigra 111.1
  pilaris 757.39
    acquired 701.1
    Hebra's 696.4
  rosea 696.3
  rotunda 696.3
  rubra (Hebra) 695.89
    pilaris 696.4
  sicca 690.18
  simplex 690.18
  specified type NEC 696.5
  streptogenes 696.5
  versicolor 111.0
    scrotal 111.0
Placenta, placental
  ablatio 641.2●
    affecting fetus or newborn 762.1
  abnormal, abnormality 656.7●
    with hemorrhage 641.8●
      affecting fetus or newborn 762.1
    affecting fetus or newborn 762.2
  abruptio 641.2●
    affecting fetus or newborn 762.1
  accessory lobe - see Placenta, abnormal
  accreta (without hemorrhage) 667.0●
    with hemorrhage 666.0●

Placenta, placental (*Continued*)
adherent (without hemorrhage) 667.0●
  with hemorrhage 666.0●
apoplexy - *see* Placenta, separation
battledore - *see* Placenta, abnormal
bilobate - *see* Placenta, abnormal
bipartita - *see* Placenta, abnormal
carneous mole 631
centralis - *see* Placenta, previa
circumvallata - *see* Placenta, abnormal
cyst (amniotic) - *see* Placenta, abnormal
deficiency - *see* Placenta, insufficiency
degeneration - *see* Placenta,
    insufficiency
detachment (partial) (premature) (with
    hemorrhage) 641.2●
  affecting fetus or newborn 762.1
dimidiata - *see* Placenta, abnormal
disease 656.7●
  affecting fetus or newborn 762.2
duplex - *see* Placenta, abnormal
dysfunction - *see* Placenta,
    insufficiency
fenestrata - *see* Placenta, abnormal
fibrosis - *see* Placenta, abnormal
fleshy mole 631
hematoma - *see* Placenta, abnormal
hemorrhage NEC - *see* Placenta,
    separation
hormone disturbance or malfunction -
    see Placenta, abnormal
hyperplasia - *see* Placenta, abnormal
increta (without hemorrhage) 667.0●
  with hemorrhage 666.0●
infarction 656.7●
  affecting fetus or newborn 762.2
insertion, vicious - *see* Placenta, previa
insufficiency
  affecting
      fetus or newborn 762.2
      management of pregnancy
        656.5●
lateral - *see* Placenta, previa
low implantation or insertion - *see*
    Placenta, previa
low-lying - *see* Placenta, previa
malformation - *see* Placenta, abnormal
malposition - *see* Placenta, previa
marginalis, marginata - *see* Placenta,
    previa
marginal sinus (hemorrhage) (rupture)
    641.2●
  affecting fetus or newborn 762.1
membranacea - *see* Placenta, abnormal
multilobed - *see* Placenta, abnormal
multipartita - *see* Placenta, abnormal
necrosis - *see* Placenta, abnormal
percreta (without hemorrhage) 667.0●
  with hemorrhage 666.0●
polyp 674.4●
previa (central) (centralis) (complete)
    (lateral) (marginal) (marginalis)
    (partial) (partialis) (total) (with
    hemorrhage) 641.1●
  affecting fetus or newborn 762.0
  noted
      before labor, without hemorrhage
        (with cesarean delivery)
        641.0●
      during pregnancy (without
        hemorrhage) 641.0●
  without hemorrhage (before labor
      and delivery) (during
      pregnancy) 641.0●

Placenta, placental (*Continued*)
retention (with hemorrhage) 666.0
  fragments, complicating
      puerperium (delayed
      hemorrhage) 666.2●
    without hemorrhage 667.1●
  postpartum, puerperal 666.2●
    without hemorrhage 667.0●
separation (normally implanted)
    (partial) (premature) (with
    hemorrhage) 641.2●
  affecting fetus or newborn 762.1
septuplex - *see* Placenta, abnormal
small - *see* Placenta, insufficiency
softening (premature) - *see* Placenta,
    abnormal
spuria - *see* Placenta, abnormal
succenturiata - *see* Placenta, abnormal
syphilitic 095.8
transfusion syndromes 762.3
transmission of chemical substance -
    see Absorption, chemical, through
    placenta
trapped (with hemorrhage) 666.0●
  without hemorrhage 667.0●
trilobate - *see* Placenta, abnormal
tripartita - *see* Placenta, abnormal
triplex - *see* Placenta, abnormal
varicose vessel - *see* Placenta, abnormal
vicious insertion - *see* Placenta, previa
Placentitis
affecting fetus or newborn 762.7
complicating pregnancy 658.4●
Plagiocephaly (skull) 754.0
Plague 020.9
abortive 020.8
ambulatory 020.8
bubonic 020.0
cellulocutaneous 020.1
lymphatic gland 020.0
pneumonic 020.5
  primary 020.3
  secondary 020.4
pulmonary - *see* Plague, pneumonic
pulmonic - *see* Plague, pneumonic
septicemic 020.2
tonsillar 020.9
  septicemic 020.2
vaccination, prophylactic (against)
    V03.3
Planning, family V25.09
contraception V25.9
natural
    procreative V26.41
    to avoid pregnancy V25.04
procreation V26.49
    natural V26.41
Plaque
artery, arterial - *see* Arteriosclerosis
calcareous - *see* Calcification
Hollenhorst's (retinal) 362.33
tongue 528.6
Plasma cell myeloma 203.0●
Plasmacytoma, plasmocytoma (solitary)
    (M9731/1) 238.6
benign (M9731/0) - *see* Neoplasm, by
    site, benign
malignant (M9731/3) 203.8●
Plasmacytopenia 288.59
Plasmacytosis 288.64
Plaster ulcer (*see also* Ulcer, pressure)
    707.00
Plateau iris syndrome 364.82
Platybasia 756.0

Platyonychia (congenital) 757.5
acquired 703.8
Platypelloid pelvis 738.6
with disproportion (fetopelvic) 653.2●
    affecting fetus or newborn 763.1
    causing obstructed labor 660.1●
      affecting fetus or newborn 763.1
congenital 755.69
Platyspondylia 756.19
Plethora 782.62
newborn 776.4
Pleura, pleural - *see* condition
Pleuralgia 786.52
Pleurisy (acute) (adhesive) (chronic)
    (costal) (diaphragmatic) (double)
    (dry) (fetid) (fibrinous) (fibrous)
    (interlobar) (latent) (lung) (old)
    (plastic) (primary) (residual) (sicca)
    (sterile) (subacute) (unresolved)
    (with adherent pleura) 511.0
with
  effusion (without mention of cause)
      511.9
    bacterial, nontuberculous 511.1
    nontuberculous NEC 511.9
      bacterial 511.1
    pneumococcal 511.1
    specified type NEC 511.89
    staphylococcal 511.1
    streptococcal 511.1
    tuberculous (*see also* Tuberculosis,
        pleura) 012.0●
      primary, progressive 010.1●
  influenza, flu, or grippe 487.1
  tuberculosis - *see* Pleurisy,
      tuberculous
encysted 511.89
exudative (*see also* Pleurisy, with
    effusion) 511.9
  bacterial, nontuberculous 511.1
fibrinopurulent 510.9
  with fistula 510.0
fibropurulent 510.9
  with fistula 510.0
hemorrhagic 511.89
influenzal 487.1
pneumococcal 511.0
  with effusion 511.1
purulent 510.9
  with fistula 510.0
septic 510.9
  with fistula 510.0
serofibrinous (*see also* Pleurisy, with
    effusion) 511.9
  bacterial, nontuberculous 511.1
seropurulent 510.9
  with fistula 510.0
serous (*see also* Pleurisy, with effusion)
    511.9
  bacterial, nontuberculous 511.1
staphylococcal 511.0
  with effusion 511.1
streptococcal 511.0
  with effusion 511.1
suppurative 510.9
  with fistula 510.0
traumatic (post) (current) 862.29
  with open wound into cavity 862.39
tuberculous (with effusion) (*see also*
    Tuberculosis, pleura) 012.0●
  primary, progressive 010.1●
Pleuritis sicca - *see* Pleurisy
Pleurobronchopneumonia (*see also*
    Pneumonia, broncho-) 485

◀ New   ◀▥ Revised   ~~deleted~~ Deleted   ● Use Additional Digit(s)   ▬ Omit code

Pleurodynia 786.52
 epidemic 074.1
 viral 074.1
Pleurohepatitis 573.8
Pleuropericarditis (see also Pericarditis)
  423.9
 acute 420.90
Pleuropneumonia (acute) (bilateral)
  (double) (septic) (see also
  Pneumonia) 486
 chronic (see also Fibrosis, lung) 515
Pleurorrhea (see also Hydrothorax) 511.89

Plexitis, brachial 353.0
Plica
 knee 727.83
 polonica 132.0
 tonsil 474.8
Plicae dysphonia ventricularis 784.49
Plicated tongue 529.5
 congenital 750.13
Plug
 bronchus NEC 519.19
 meconium (newborn) NEC 777.1
 mucus - see Mucus, plug
Plumbism 984.9
 specified type of lead - see Table of
  Drugs and Chemicals
Plummer's disease (toxic nodular goiter)
  242.3●
Plummer-Vinson syndrome (sideropenic
  dysphagia) 280.8
Pluricarential syndrome of infancy 260
Plurideficiency syndrome of infancy 260
Plus (and minus) hand (intrinsic) 736.09
PMDD (premenstrual dysphoric
  disorder) 625.4
PMS 625.4
Pneumathemia - see Air, embolism, by type
Pneumatic drill or hammer disease 994.9
Pneumatocele (lung) 518.89
 intracranial 348.89 ◀▥▥
 tension 492.0
Pneumatosis
 cystoides intestinalis 569.89
 peritonei 568.89
 pulmonum 492.8
Pneumaturia 599.84
Pneumoblastoma (M8981/3) - see
  Neoplasm, lung, malignant
Pneumocephalus 348.89 ◀▥▥
Pneumococcemia 038.2
Pneumococcus, pneumococcal - see
  condition
Pneumoconiosis (due to) (inhalation of)
  505
 aluminum 503
 asbestos 501
 bagasse 495.1
 bauxite 503
 beryllium 503
 carbon electrode makers' 503
 coal
  miners' (simple) 500
  workers' (simple) 500
 cotton dust 504
 diatomite fibrosis 502
 dust NEC 504
  inorganic 503
  lime 502
  marble 502
  organic NEC 504
 fumes or vapors (from silo) 506.9
 graphite 503

Pneumoconiosis (Continued)
 hard metal 503
 mica 502
 moldy hay 495.0
 rheumatoid 714.81
 silica NEC 502
  and carbon 500
 silicate NEC 502
 talc 502
Pneumocystis carinii pneumonia
  136.3
Pneumocystis jiroveci pneumonia
  136.3
Pneumocystosis 136.3
 with pneumonia 136.3
Pneumoenteritis 025
Pneumohemopericardium (see also
  Pericarditis) 423.9
Pneumohemothorax (see also
  Hemothorax) 511.89
 traumatic 860.4
  with open wound into thorax
   860.5
Pneumohydropericardium (see also
  Pericarditis) 423.9
Pneumohydrothorax (see also
  Hydrothorax) 511.89
Pneumomediastinum 518.1
 congenital 770.2
 fetus or newborn 770.2
Pneumomycosis 117.9
Pneumonia (acute) (Alpenstich) (benign)
  (bilateral) (brain) (cerebral)
  (circumscribed) (congestive)
  (creeping) (delayed resolution)
  (double) (epidemic) (fever) (flash)
  (fulminant) (fungoid)
  (granulomatous) (hemorrhagic)
  (incipient) (infantile) (infectious)
  (infiltration) (insular) (intermittent)
  (latent) (lobe) (migratory) (newborn)
  (organized) (overwhelming)
  (primary) (progressive)
  (pseudolobar) (purulent) (resolved)
  (secondary) (senile) (septic)
  (suppurative) (terminal) (true)
  (unresolved) (vesicular) 486
 with influenza, flu, or grippe 487.0
 adenoviral 480.0
 adynamic 514
 alba 090.0
 allergic 518.3
 alveolar - see Pneumonia, lobar
 anaerobes 482.81
 anthrax 022.1 [484.5]
 apex, apical - see Pneumonia, lobar
 ascaris 127.0 [484.8]
 aspiration 507.0
  due to
   aspiration of microorganisms
    bacterial 482.9
     specified type NEC
      482.89
    specified organism NEC
     483.8
      bacterial NEC 482.89
    viral 480.9
     specified type NEC 480.8
   food (regurgitated) 507.0
   gastric secretions 507.0
   milk 507.0
   oils, essences 507.1
   solids, liquids NEC 507.8
   vomitus 507.0

Pneumonia (Continued)
 aspiration (Continued)
  fetal 770.18
   due to
    blood 770.16
    clear amniotic fluid
     770.14
    meconium 770.12
    postnatal stomach contents
     770.86
  newborn 770.18
   due to
    blood 770.16
    clear amniotic fluid
     770.14
    meconium 770.12
    postnatal stomach contents
     770.86
 asthenic 514
 atypical (disseminated) (focal)
   (primary) 486
  with influenza 487.0
 bacillus 482.9
  specified type NEC 482.89
 bacterial 482.9
  specified type NEC 482.89
 Bacteroides (fragilis) (oralis)
   (melaninogenicus) 482.81
 basal, basic, basilar - see Pneumonia,
   lobar
 bronchiolitis obliterans organized
   (BOOP) 516.8
 broncho-, bronchial (confluent)
   (croupous) (diffuse)
   (disseminated) (hemorrhagic)
   (involving lobes) (lobar)
   (terminal) 485
  with influenza 487.0
  allergic 518.3
  aspiration (see also Pneumonia,
    aspiration) 507.0
  bacterial 482.9
   specified type NEC 482.89
  capillary 466.19
   with bronchospasm or
     obstruction 466.19
  chronic (see also Fibrosis, lung)
    515
  congenital (infective) 770.0
  diplococcal 481
  Eaton's agent 483.0
  Escherichia coli (E. coli) 482.82
  Friedländer's bacillus 482.0
  Hemophilus influenzae 482.2
  hiberno-vernal 083.0 [484.8]
  hypostatic 514
  influenzal 487.0
  inhalation (see also Pneumonia,
    aspiration) 507.0
   due to fumes or vapors
     (chemical) 506.0
  Klebsiella 482.0
  lipid 507.1
   endogenous 516.8
  Mycoplasma (pneumoniae)
    483.0
  ornithosis 073.0
  pleuropneumonia-like organisms
    (PPLO) 483.0
  pneumococcal 481
  Proteus 482.83
  Pseudomonas 482.1
  specified organism NEC 483.8
   bacterial NEC 482.89

Pneumonia *(Continued)*
  broncho-, bronchial *(Continued)*
    staphylococcal 482.40
      aureus 482.41
        methicillin
          resistant (MRSA) 482.42
          susceptible (MSSA) 482.41
      specified type NEC 482.49
    streptococcal - *see* Pneumonia,
      streptococcal
    typhoid 002.0 *[484.8]*
    viral, virus (*see also* Pneumonia,
      viral) 480.9
  Butyrivibrio (fibriosolvens) 482.81
  Candida 112.4
  capillary 466.19
    with bronchospasm or obstruction
      466.19
  caseous (*see also* Tuberculosis) 011.6●
  catarrhal - *see* Pneumonia, broncho-
  central - *see* Pneumonia, lobar
  Chlamydia, chlamydial 483.1
    pneumoniae 483.1
    psittaci 073.0
    specified type NEC 483.1
    trachomatis 483.1
  cholesterol 516.8
  chronic (*see also* Fibrosis, lung) 515
  cirrhotic (chronic) (*see also* Fibrosis,
    lung) 515
  Clostridium (haemolyticum) (novyi)
    NEC 482.81
  confluent - *see* Pneumonia, broncho-
  congenital (infective) 770.0
    aspiration 770.18
  croupous - *see* Pneumonia, lobar
  cytomegalic inclusion 078.5 *[484.1]*
  deglutition (*see also* Pneumonia,
    aspiration) 507.0
  desquamative interstitial 516.8
  diffuse - *see* Pneumonia, broncho-
  diplococcal, diplococcus (broncho-)
    (lobar) 481
  disseminated (focal) - *see* Pneumonia,
    broncho-
  due to
    adenovirus 480.0
    anaerobes 482.81
    Bacterium anitratum 482.83
    Chlamydia, chlamydial 483.1
      pneumoniae 483.1
      psittaci 073.0
      specified type NEC 483.1
      trachomatis 483.1
    coccidioidomycosis 114.0
    Diplococcus (pneumoniae) 481
    Eaton's agent 483.0
    Escherichia coli (E. coli) 482.82
    Friedländer's bacillus 482.0
    fumes or vapors (chemical)
      (inhalation) 506.0
    fungus NEC 117.9 *[484.7]*
      coccidioidomycosis 114.0
    Hemophilus influenzae (H.
      influenzae) 482.2
    Herellea 482.83
    influenza 487.0
    Klebsiella pneumoniae 482.0
    Mycoplasma (pneumoniae) 483.0
    parainfluenza virus 480.2
    pleuropneumonia-like organism
      (PPLO) 483.0
    Pneumococcus 481
    Pneumocystis carinii 136.3

Pneumonia *(Continued)*
  due to *(Continued)*
    Pneumocystis jiroveci 136.3
    Proteus 482.83
    Pseudomonas 482.1
    respiratory syncytial virus 480.1
    rickettsia 083.9 *[484.8]*
    SARS-associated coronavirus 480.3
    specified
      bacteria NEC 482.89
      organism NEC 483.8
      virus NEC 480.8
    Staphylococcus 482.40
      aureus 482.41
        methicillin
          resistant (MRSA) 482.42
          susceptible (MSSA) 482.41
      specified type NEC 482.49
    Streptococcus - *see also* Pneumonia,
      streptococcal
      pneumoniae 481
    virus (*see also* Pneumonia, viral)
      480.9
      SARS-associated coronavirus
        480.3
  Eaton's agent 483.0
  embolic, embolism (*see* Embolism,
    pulmonary) 415.1●
  eosinophilic 518.3
  Escherichia coli (E. coli) 482.82
  Eubacterium 482.81
  fibrinous - *see* Pneumonia, lobar
  fibroid (chronic) (*see also* Fibrosis, lung)
    515
  fibrous (*see also* Fibrosis, lung) 515
  Friedländer's bacillus 482.0
  fusobacterium (nucleatum) 482.81
  gangrenous 513.0
  giant cell (*see also* Pneumonia, viral)
    480.9
  gram-negative bacteria NEC 482.83
    anaerobic 482.81
  grippal 487.0
  Hemophilus influenzae (bronchial)
    (lobar) 482.2
  hypostatic (broncho-) (lobar) 514
  in
    actinomycosis 039.1
    anthrax 022.1 *[484.5]*
    aspergillosis 117.3 *[484.6]*
    candidiasis 112.4
    coccidioidomycosis 114.0
    cytomegalic inclusion disease 078.5
      [484.1]
    histoplasmosis (*see also*
      Histoplasmosis) 115.95
    infectious disease NEC 136.9 *[484.8]*
    measles 055.1
    mycosis, systemic NEC 117.9 *[484.7]*
    nocardiasis, nocardiosis 039.1
    ornithosis 073.0
    pneumocystosis 136.3
    psittacosis 073.0
    Q fever 083.0 *[484.8]*
    salmonellosis 003.22
    toxoplasmosis 130.4
    tularemia 021.2
    typhoid (fever) 002.0 *[484.8]*
    varicella 052.1
    whooping cough (*see also* Whooping
      cough) 033.9 *[484.3]*
  infective, acquired prenatally 770.0
  influenzal (broncho) (lobar) (virus)
    487.0

Pneumonia *(Continued)*
  inhalation (*see also* Pneumonia,
    aspiration) 507.0
    fumes or vapors (chemical) 506.0
  interstitial 516.8
    with influenzal 487.0
    acute 136.3
    chronic (*see also* Fibrosis, lung) 515
    desquamative 516.8
    hypostatic 514
    lipoid 507.1
    lymphoid 516.8
    plasma cell 136.3
    Pseudomonas 482.1
  intrauterine (infective) 770.0
    aspiration 770.18
    blood 770.16
    clear amniotic fluid 770.14
    meconium 770.12
    postnatal stomach contents 770.86
  Klebsiella pneumoniae 482.0
  Legionnaires' 482.84
  lipid, lipoid (exogenous) (interstitial)
    507.1
    endogenous 516.8
  lobar (diplococcal) (disseminated)
    (double) (interstitial)
    (pneumococcal, any type) 481
    with influenza 487.0
    bacterial 482.9
      specified type NEC 482.89
    chronic (*see also* Fibrosis, lung) 515
    Escherichia coli (E. coli) 482.82
    Friedländer's bacillus 482.0
    Hemophilus influenzae (H.
      influenzae) 482.2
    hypostatic 514
    influenzal 487.0
    Klebsiella 482.0
    ornithosis 073.0
    Proteus 482.83
    Pseudomonas 482.1
    psittacosis 073.0
    specified organism NEC 483.8
      bacterial NEC 482.89
    staphylococcal 482.40
      aureus 482.41
        methicillin
          resistant (MRSA) 482.42
          susceptible (MSSA) 482.41
      specified type NEC 482.49
    streptococcal - *see* Pneumonia,
      streptococcal
    viral, virus (*see also* Pneumonia,
      viral) 480.9
  lobular (confluent) - *see* Pneumonia,
    broncho-
  Löffler's 518.3
  massive - *see* Pneumonia, lobar
  meconium aspiration 770.12
  metastatic NEC 038.8 *[484.8]*
  methicillin resistant Staphylococcus
    aureus (MRSA) 482.42
  methicillin susceptible Staphylococcus
    aureus (MSSA) 482.41
  MRSA (methicillin resistant
    Staphylococcus aureus) 482.42
  MSSA (methicillin susceptible
    Staphylococcus aureus) 482.41
  Mycoplasma (pneumoniae) 483.0
  necrotic 513.0
  nitrogen dioxide 506.9
  orthostatic 514
  parainfluenza virus 480.2

◀ New   ◀▥ Revised   ~~deleted~~ Deleted   ● Use Additional Digit(s)   ▭ Omit code

Pneumonia (Continued)
  parenchymatous (see also Fibrosis, lung) 515
  passive 514
  patchy - see Pneumonia, broncho
  Peptococcus 482.81
  Peptostreptococcus 482.81
  plasma cell 136.3
  pleurolobar - see Pneumonia, lobar
  pleuropneumonia-like organism (PPLO) 483.0
  pneumococcal (broncho) (lobar) 481
  Pneumocystis (carinii) (jiroveci) 136.3
  postinfectional NEC 136.9 [484.8]
  postmeasles 055.1
  postoperative 997.39
  primary atypical 486
  Proprionibacterium 482.81
  Proteus 482.83
  Pseudomonas 482.1
  psittacosis 073.0
  radiation 508.0
  respiratory syncytial virus 480.1
  resulting from a procedure 997.39
  rheumatic 390 [517.1]
  Salmonella 003.22
  SARS-associated coronavirus 480.3
  segmented, segmental - see Pneumonia, broncho-
  Serratia (marcascens) 482.83
  specified
    bacteria NEC 482.89
    organism NEC 483.8
    virus NEC 480.8
  spirochetal 104.8 [484]
  staphylococcal (broncho) (lobar) 482.40
    aureus 482.41
      methicillin
        resistant (MRSA) 482.42
        susceptible (MSSA) 482.41
    specified type NEC 482.49
  static, stasis 514
  streptococcal (broncho) (lobar) NEC 482.30
    Group
      A 482.31
      B 482.32
      specified NEC 482.39
    pneumoniae 481
    specified type NEC 482.39
  Streptococcus pneumoniae 481
  traumatic (complication) (early) (secondary) 958.8
  tuberculous (any) (see also Tuberculosis) 011.6 ●
  tularemic 021.2
  TWAR agent 483.1
  varicella 052.1
  Veillonella 482.81
  ventilator associated 997.31
  viral, virus (broncho) (interstitial) (lobar) 480.9
    with influenza, flu, or grippe 487.0
    adenoviral 480.0
    parainfluenza 480.2
    respiratory syncytial 480.1
    SARS-associated coronavirus 480.3
    specified type NEC 480.8
  white (congenital) 090.0
Pneumonic - see condition

Pneumonitis (acute) (primary) (see also Pneumonia) 486
  allergic 495.9
    specified type NEC 495.8
  aspiration 507.0
    due to fumes or gases 506.0
    fetal 770.18
      due to
        blood 770.16
        clear amniotic fluid 770.14
        meconium 770.12
        postnatal stomach contents 770.86
    newborn 770.18
      due to
        blood 770.16
        clear amniotic fluid 770.14
        meconium 770.12
        postnatal stomach contents 770.86
    obstetric 668.0 ●
  chemical 506.0
    due to fumes or gases 506.0
  cholesterol 516.8
  chronic (see also Fibrosis, lung) 515
  congenital rubella 771.0
  crack 506.0
  due to
    crack (cocaine) 506.0
    fumes or vapors 506.0
    inhalation
      food (regurgitated), milk, vomitus 507.0
      oils, essences 507.1
      saliva 507.0
      solids, liquids NEC 507.8
    toxoplasmosis (acquired) 130.4
      congenital (active) 771.2 [484.8]
  eosinophilic 518.3
  fetal aspiration 770.18
    due to
      blood 770.16
      clear amniotic fluid 770.14
      meconium 770.12
      postnatal stomach contents 770.86
  hypersensitivity 495.9
  interstitial (chronic) (see also Fibrosis, lung) 515
    lymphoid 516.8
  lymphoid, interstitial 516.8
  meconium aspiration 770.12
  postanesthetic
    correct substance properly administered 507.0
    obstetric 668.0 ●
    overdose or wrong substance given 968.4
    specified anesthetic - see Table of Drugs and Chemicals
  postoperative 997.39
    obstetric 668.0 ●
  radiation 508.0
  rubella, congenital 771.0
  "ventilation" 495.7
  ventilator associated 997.31 ◄▦
  wood-dust 495.8
Pneumonoconiosis - see Pneumoconiosis
Pneumoparotid 527.8
Pneumopathy NEC 518.89
  alveolar 516.9
    specified NEC 516.8
  due to dust NEC 504
  parietoalveolar 516.9
    specified condition NEC 516.8

Pneumopericarditis (see also Pericarditis) 423.9
  acute 420.90
Pneumopericardium - see also Pericarditis
  congenital 770.2
  fetus or newborn 770.2
  traumatic (post) (see also Pneumothorax, traumatic) 860.0
    with open wound into thorax 860.1
Pneumoperitoneum 568.89
  fetus or newborn 770.2
Pneumophagia (psychogenic) 306.4
Pneumopleurisy, pneumopleuritis (see also Pneumonia) 486
Pneumopyopericardium 420.99
Pneumopyothorax (see also Pyopneumothorax) 510.9
  with fistula 510.0
Pneumorrhagia 786.3
  newborn 770.3
  tuberculous (see also Tuberculosis, pulmonary) 011.9 ●
Pneumosiderosis (occupational) 503
Pneumothorax (acute) (chronic) 512.8
  congenital 770.2
  due to operative injury of chest wall or lung 512.1
    accidental puncture or laceration 512.1
  fetus or newborn 770.2
  iatrogenic 512.1
  postoperative 512.1
  spontaneous 512.8
    fetus or newborn 770.2
    tension 512.0
  sucking 512.8
    iatrogenic 512.1
    postoperative 512.1
  tense valvular, infectional 512.0
  tension 512.0
    iatrogenic 512.1
    postoperative 512.1
    spontaneous 512.0
  traumatic 860.0
    with
      hemothorax 860.4
        with open wound into thorax 860.5
      open wound into thorax 860.1
  tuberculous (see also Tuberculosis) 011.7 ●
Pocket(s)
  endocardial (see also Endocarditis) 424.90
  periodontal 523.8
Podagra 274.01   ◄▦
Podencephalus 759.89
Poikilocytosis 790.09
Poikiloderma 709.09
  Civatte's 709.09
  congenital 757.33
  vasculare atrophicans 696.2
Poikilodermatomyositis 710.3
Pointed ear 744.29
Poise imperfect 729.90
Poisoned - see Poisoning
Poisoning (acute) - see also Table of Drugs and Chemicals
  Bacillus, B.
    aertrycke (see also Infection, Salmonella) 003.9
    botulinus 005.1
    cholerae (suis) (see also Infection, Salmonella) 003.9

Poisoning *(Continued)*
  Bacillus, B. *(Continued)*
    paratyphosus *(see also* Infection, Salmonella) 003.9
    suipestifer *(see also* Infection, Salmonella) 003.9
  bacterial toxins NEC 005.9
  berries, noxious 988.2
  blood (general) - *see* Septicemia
  botulism 005.1
  bread, moldy, mouldy - *see* Poisoning, food
  Ciguatera 988.0
  damaged meat - *see* Poisoning, food
  death-cap (Amanita phalloides) (Amanita verna) 988.1
  decomposed food - *see* Poisoning, food
  diseased food - *see* Poisoning, food
  drug - *see* Table of Drugs and Chemicals
  epidemic, fish, meat, or other food - *see* Poisoning, food
  fava bean 282.2
  fish (bacterial) - *see also* Poisoning, food
    noxious 988.0
  food (acute) (bacterial) (diseased) (infected) NEC 005.9
    due to
      bacillus
        aertrycke *(see also* Poisoning, food, due to Salmonella) 003.9
        botulinus 005.1
        cereus 005.89
        choleraesuis *(see also* Poisoning, food, due to Salmonella) 003.9
        paratyphosus *(see also* Poisoning, food, due to Salmonella) 003.9
        suipestifer *(see also* Poisoning, food, due to Salmonella) 003.9
      Clostridium 005.3
        botulinum 005.1
        perfringens 005.2
        welchii 005.2
      Salmonella (aertrycke) (callinarum) (choleraesuis) (enteritidis) (paratyphi) (suipestifer) 003.9
        with
          gastroenteritis 003.0
          localized infection(s) *(see also* Infection, Salmonella) 003.20
          septicemia 003.1
          specified manifestation NEC 003.8
      specified bacterium NEC 005.89
      Staphylococcus 005.0
      Streptococcus 005.89
      Vibrio parahaemolyticus 005.4
      Vibrio vulnificus 005.81
    noxious or naturally toxic 988.0
      berries 988.2
      fish 988.0
      mushroom 988.1
      plants NEC 988.2
  ice cream - *see* Poisoning, food
  ichthyotoxism (bacterial) 005.9
  kreotoxism, food 005.9
  malarial - *see* Malaria
  meat - *see* Poisoning, food

Poisoning *(Continued)*
  mushroom (noxious) 988.1
  mussel - *see also* Poisoning, food
    noxious 988.0
  noxious foodstuffs *(see also* Poisoning, food, noxious) 988.9
    specified type NEC 988.8
  plants, noxious 988.2
  pork - *see also* Poisoning, food
    specified NEC 988.8
    Trichinosis 124
  ptomaine - *see* Poisoning, food
  putrefaction, food - *see* Poisoning, food
  radiation 508.0
  Salmonella *(see also* Infection, Salmonella) 003.9
  sausage - *see also* Poisoning, food
    Trichinosis 124
  saxitoxin 988.0
  shellfish - *see also* Poisoning, food
    noxious (amnesic) (azaspiracid) (diarrheic) (neurotoxic) (paralytic) 988.0
  Staphylococcus, food 005.0
  toxic, from disease NEC 799.89
  truffles - *see* Poisoning, food
  uremic - *see* Uremia
  uric acid 274.9
  water 276.6
Poison ivy, oak, sumac or other plant dermatitis 692.6
Poker spine 720.0
Policeman's disease 729.2
Polioencephalitis (acute) (bulbar) *(see also* Poliomyelitis, bulbar) 045.0●
  inferior 335.22
  influenzal 487.8
  superior hemorrhagic (acute) (Wernicke's) 265.1
  Wernicke's (superior hemorrhagic) 265.1
Polioencephalomyelitis (acute) (anterior) (bulbar) *(see also* Polioencephalitis) 045.0●
Polioencephalopathy, superior hemorrhagic 265.1
  with
    beriberi 265.0
    pellagra 265.2
Poliomeningoencephalitis - *see* Meningoencephalitis
Poliomyelitis (acute) (anterior) (epidemic) 045.9●

> Note 60   Use the following fifth-digit subclassification with category 045:
>
> 0   poliovirus, unspecified type
> 1   poliovirus, type I
> 2   poliovirus, type II
> 3   poliovirus, type III

  with
    paralysis 045.1●
      bulbar 045.0●
  abortive 045.2●
  ascending 045.9●
    progressive 045.9●
  bulbar 045.0●
  cerebral 045.0●
  chronic 335.21
  congenital 771.2
  contact V01.2
  deformities 138
  exposure to V01.2

Poliomyelitis *(Continued)*
  late effect 138
  nonepidemic 045.9●
  nonparalytic 045.2●
  old with deformity 138
  posterior, acute 053.19
  residual 138
  sequelae 138
  spinal, acute 045.9●
  syphilitic (chronic) 094.89
  vaccination, prophylactic (against) V04.0
Poliosis (eyebrow) (eyelashes) 704.3
  circumscripta (congenital) 757.4
    acquired 704.3
  congenital 757.4
Pollakiuria 788.41
  psychogenic 306.53
Pollinosis 477.0
Pollitzer's disease (hidradenitis suppurativa) 705.83
Polyadenitis *(see also* Adenitis) 289.3
  malignant 020.0
Polyalgia 729.99
Polyangiitis (essential) 446.0
Polyarteritis (nodosa) (renal) 446.0
Polyarthralgia 719.49
  psychogenic 306.0
Polyarthritis, polyarthropathy NEC 716.59
  due to or associated with other specified conditions - *see* Arthritis, due to or associated with
  endemic *(see also* Disease, Kaschin-Beck) 716.0●
  inflammatory 714.9
    specified type NEC 714.89
  juvenile (chronic) 714.30
    acute 714.31
  migratory - *see* Fever, rheumatic
  rheumatic 714.0
    fever (acute) - *see* Fever, rheumatic
Polycarential syndrome of infancy 260
Polychondritis (atrophic) (chronic) (relapsing) 733.99
Polycoria 743.46
Polycystic (congenital) (disease) 759.89
  degeneration, kidney - *see* Polycystic, kidney
  kidney (congenital) 753.12
    adult type (APKD) 753.13
    autosomal dominant 753.13
    autosomal recessive 753.14
    childhood type (CPKD) 753.14
    infantile type 753.14
  liver 751.62
  lung 518.89
    congenital 748.4
  ovary, ovaries 256.4
  spleen 759.0
Polycythemia (primary) (rubra) (vera) (M9950/1) 238.4
  acquired 289.0
  benign 289.0
    familial 289.6
  due to
    donor twin 776.4
    fall in plasma volume 289.0
    high altitude 289.0
    maternal-fetal transfusion 776.4
    stress 289.0

Polycythemia *(Continued)*
  emotional 289.0
  erythropoietin 289.0
  familial (benign) 289.6
  Gaisböck's (hypertonica) 289.0
  high altitude 289.0
  hypertonica 289.0
  hypoxemic 289.0
  neonatorum 776.4
  nephrogenous 289.0
  relative 289.0
  secondary 289.0
  spurious 289.0
  stress 289.0
Polycytosis cryptogenica 289.0
Polydactylism, polydactyly 755.00
  fingers 755.01
  toes 755.02
Polydipsia 783.5
Polydystrophic oligophrenia 277.5
Polyembryoma (M9072/3) - *see*
    Neoplasm, by site, malignant
Polygalactia 676.6 ●
Polyglandular
  deficiency 258.9
  dyscrasia 258.9
  dysfunction 258.9
  syndrome 258.8
Polyhydramnios *(see also* Hydramnios)
    657 ●
Polymastia 757.6
Polymenorrhea 626.2
Polymicrogyria 742.2
Polymyalgia 725
  arteritica 446.5
  rheumatica 725
Polymyositis (acute) (chronic)
    (hemorrhagic) 710.4
  with involvement of
    lung 710.4 *[517.8]*
    skin 710.3
  ossificans (generalisata) (progressiva)
    728.19
  Wagner's (dermatomyositis) 710.3
Polyneuritis, polyneuritic *(see also*
    Polyneuropathy) 356.9
  alcoholic 357.5
    with psychosis 291.1
  cranialis 352.6
  demyelinating, chronic inflammatory
    (CIDP) 357.81
  diabetic 250.6 ● *[357.2]*
    due to secondary diabetes 249.6 ●
      [357.2]
  due to lack of vitamin NEC 269.2
      [357.4]
  endemic 265.0 *[357.4]*
  erythredema 985.0
  febrile 357.0
  hereditary ataxic 356.3
  idiopathic, acute 357.0
  infective (acute) 357.0
  nutritional 269.9 *[357.4]*
  postinfectious 357.0
Polyneuropathy (peripheral) 356.9
  alcoholic 357.5
  amyloid 277.39 *[357.4]*
  arsenical 357.7
  critical illness 357.82
  demyelinating, chronic inflammatory
    (CIDP) 357.81
  diabetic 250.6 ● *[357.2]*
    due to secondary diabetes 249.6 ●
      [357.2]

Polyneuropathy *(Continued)*
  due to
    antitetanus serum 357.6
    arsenic 357.7
    drug or medicinal substance 357.6
      correct substance properly
        administered 357.6
      overdose or wrong substance
        given or taken 977.9
      specified drug - *see* Table of
        Drugs and Chemicals
    lack of vitamin NEC 269.2 *[357.4]*
    lead 357.7
    organophosphate compounds 357.7
    pellagra 265.2 *[357.4]*
    porphyria 277.1 *[357.4]*
    serum 357.6
    toxic agent NEC 357.7
  hereditary 356.0
  idiopathic 356.9
    progressive 356.4
  in
    amyloidosis 277.39 *[357.4]*
    avitaminosis 269.2 *[357.4]*
      specified NEC 269.1 *[357.4]*
    beriberi 265.0 *[357.4]*
    collagen vascular disease NEC 710.9
      [357.1]
    deficiency
      B-complex NEC 266.2 *[357.4]*
      vitamin B 266.9 *[357.4]*
      vitamin B₆ 266.1 *[357.4]*
    diabetes 250.6 ● *[357.2]*
      due to secondary diabetes 249.6 ●
        [357.2]
    diphtheria *(see also* Diphtheria)
      032.89 *[357.4]*
    disseminated lupus erythematosus
      710.0 *[357.1]*
    herpes zoster 053.13
    hypoglycemia 251.2 *[357.4]*
    malignant neoplasm (M8000/3)
      NEC 199.1 *[357.3]*
    mumps 072.72
    pellagra 265.2 *[357.4]*
    polyarteritis nodosa 446.0 *[357.1]*
    porphyria 277.1 *[357.4]*
    rheumatoid arthritis 714.0 *[357.1]*
    sarcoidosis 135 *[357.4]*
    uremia 585.9 *[357.4]*
  lead 357.7
  nutritional 269.9 *[357.4]*
    specified NEC 269.8 *[357.4]*
  postherpetic 053.13
  progressive 356.4
  sensory (hereditary) 356.2
  specified NEC 356.8
Polyonychia 757.5
Polyopia 368.2
  refractive 368.15
Polyorchism, polyorchidism (three testes)
    752.89
Polyorrhymenitis (peritoneal) *(see also*
    Polyserositis) 568.82
  pericardial 423.2
Polyostotic fibrous dysplasia 756.54
Polyotia 744.1
Polyp, polypus

Note 61   Polyps of organs or sites that
do not appear in the list below should
be coded to the residual category for
diseases of the organ or site concerned.

Polyp, polypus *(Continued)*
  accessory sinus 471.8
  adenoid tissue 471.0
  adenomatous (M8210/0) - *see also*
      Neoplasm, by site, benign
    adenocarcinoma in (M8210/3) - *see*
        Neoplasm, by site, malignant
    carcinoma in (M8210/3) - *see*
        Neoplasm, by site, malignant
    multiple (M8221/0) - *see* Neoplasm,
        by site, benign
  antrum 471.8
  anus, anal (canal) (nonadenomatous)
      569.0
    adenomatous 211.4
  Bartholin's gland 624.6
  bladder (M8120/1) 236.7
  broad ligament 620.8
  cervix (uteri) 622.7
    adenomatous 219.0
    in pregnancy or childbirth 654.6 ●
      affecting fetus or newborn
          763.89
      causing obstructed labor 660.2 ●
    mucous 622.7
    nonneoplastic 622.7
  choanal 471.0
  cholesterol 575.6
  clitoris 624.6
  colon (M8210/0) *(see also* Polyp,
      adenomatous) 211.3
  corpus uteri 621.0
  dental 522.0
  ear (middle) 385.30
  endometrium 621.0
  ethmoidal (sinus) 471.8
  fallopian tube 620.8
  female genital organs NEC 624.8
  frontal (sinus) 471.8
  gallbladder 575.6
  gingiva 523.8
  gum 523.8
  labia 624.6
  larynx (mucous) 478.4
  malignant (M8000/3) - *see* Neoplasm,
      by site, malignant
  maxillary (sinus) 471.8
  middle ear 385.30
  myometrium 621.0
  nares
    anterior 471.9
    posterior 471.0
  nasal (mucous) 471.9
    cavity 471.0
    septum 471.9
  nasopharyngeal 471.0
  neoplastic (M8210/0) - *see* Neoplasm,
      by site, benign
  nose (mucous) 471.9
  oviduct 620.8
  paratubal 620.8
  pharynx 478.29
    congenital 750.29
  placenta, placental 674.4 ●
  prostate 600.20
    with
      other lower urinary tract
          symptoms (LUTS) 600.21
      urinary
        obstruction 600.21
        retention 600.21
  pudenda 624.6
  pulp (dental) 522.0
  rectosigmoid 211.4

Polyp, polypus (Continued)
  rectum (nonadenomatous) 569.0
    adenomatous 211.4
  septum (nasal) 471.9
  sinus (accessory) (ethmoidal) (frontal)
      (maxillary) (sphenoidal) 471.8
  sphenoidal (sinus) 471.8
  stomach (M8210/0) 211.1
  tube, fallopian 620.8
  turbinate, mucous membrane 471.8
  ureter 593.89
  urethra 599.3
  uterine
    ligament 620.8
    tube 620.8
  uterus (body) (corpus) (mucous) 621.0
    in pregnancy or childbirth 654.1●
      affecting fetus or newborn 763.89
      causing obstructed labor 660.2●
  vagina 623.7
  vocal cord (mucous) 478.4
  vulva 624.6
Polyphagia 783.6
Polypoid - see condition
Polyposis - see also Polyp
  coli (adenomatous) (M8220/0) 211.3
    adenocarcinoma in (M8220/3) 153.9
    carcinoma in (M8220/3) 153.9
  familial (M8220/0) 211.3
  intestinal (adenomatous) (M8220/0)
      211.3
  multiple (M8221/0) - see Neoplasm, by
      site, benign
Polyradiculitis (acute) 357.0
Polyradiculoneuropathy (acute)
    (segmentally demyelinating) 357.0
Polysarcia 278.00
Polyserositis (peritoneal) 568.82
  due to pericarditis 423.2
  paroxysmal (familial) 277.31
  pericardial 423.2
  periodic (familial) 277.31
  pleural - see Pleurisy
  recurrent 277.31
  tuberculous (see also Tuberculosis,
      polyserositis) 018.9●
Polysialia 527.7
Polysplenia syndrome 759.0
Polythelia 757.6
Polytrichia (see also Hypertrichosis)
    704.1
Polyunguia (congenital) 757.5
  acquired 703.8
Polyuria 788.42
Pompe's disease (glycogenosis II) 271.0
Pompholyx 705.81
Poncet's disease (tuberculous
    rheumatism) (see also Tuberculosis)
    015.9●
Pond fracture - see Fracture, skull, vault
Ponos 085.0
Pons, pontine - see condition
Poor
  aesthetics of existing restoration of
      tooth 525.67
  contractions, labor 661.2●
    affecting fetus or newborn 763.7
  fetal growth NEC 764.9●
    affecting management of pregnancy
        656.5●
  incorporation
    artificial skin graft 996.55
    decellularized allodermis graft
        996.55

Poor (Continued)
  obstetrical history V13.29
    affecting management of current
        pregnancy V23.49
      pre-term labor V23.41
    pre-term labor V13.21
  sucking reflex (newborn) 796.1
  vision NEC 369.9
Poradenitis, nostras 099.1
Porencephaly (congenital)
    (developmental) (true) 742.4
  acquired 348.0
  nondevelopmental 348.0
  traumatic (post) 310.2
Porocephaliasis 134.1
Porokeratosis 757.39
  disseminated superficial actinic (DSAP)
      692.75
Poroma, eccrine (M8402/0) - see
    Neoplasm, skin, benign
Porphyria (acute) (congenital)
    (constitutional) (erythropoietic)
    (familial) (hepatica) (idiopathic)
    (idiosyncratic) (intermittent) (latent)
    (mixed hepatic) (photosensitive)
    (South African genetic) (Swedish)
    277.1
  acquired 277.1
  cutaneatarda
    hereditaria 277.1
    symptomatica 277.1
  due to drugs
    correct substance properly
        administered 277.1
    overdose or wrong substance given
        or taken 977.9
      specified drug - see Table of
          Drugs and Chemicals
  secondary 277.1
  toxic NEC 277.1
  variegata 277.1
Porphyrinuria (acquired) (congenital)
    (secondary) 277.1
Porphyruria (acquired) (congenital) 277.1
Portal - see condition
Port wine nevus or mark 757.32
Posadas-Wernicke disease 114.9
Position
  fetus, abnormal (see also Presentation,
      fetal) 652.9●
  teeth, faulty (see also Anomaly, position
      tooth) 524.30
Positive
  culture (nonspecific) 795.39
    AIDS virus V08
    blood 790.7
    HIV V08
    human immunodeficiency virus V08
    nose 795.39
      Staphylococcus - see Carrier
          (suspected) of,
          Staphylococcus
    skin lesion NEC 795.39
    spinal fluid 792.0
    sputum 795.39
    stool 792.1
    throat 795.39
    urine 791.9
    wound 795.39
  findings, anthrax 795.31
  HIV V08
  human immunodeficiency virus (HIV)
      V08
  PPD 795.5

Positive (Continued)
  serology
    AIDS virus V08
      inconclusive 795.71
    HIV V08
      inconclusive 795.71
    human immunodeficiency virus V08
      inconclusive 795.71
    syphilis 097.1
      with signs or symptoms - see
          Syphilis, by site and stage
      false 795.6
    skin test 795.7
      tuberculin (without active
          tuberculosis) 795.5
    VDRL 097.1
      with signs or symptoms - see
          Syphilis, by site and stage
      false 795.6
    Wassermann reaction 097.1
      false 795.6
Postcardiotomy syndrome 429.4
Postcaval ureter 753.4
Postcholecystectomy syndrome
    576.0
Postclimacteric bleeding 627.1
Postcommissurotomy syndrome
    429.4
Postconcussional syndrome 310.2
Postcontusional syndrome 310.2
Postcricoid region - see condition
Post-dates (pregnancy) - see Pregnancy
Postencephalitic - see also condition
  syndrome 310.8
Posterior - see condition
Posterolateral sclerosis (spinal cord) - see
    Degeneration, combined
Postexanthematous - see condition
Postfebrile - see condition
Postgastrectomy dumping syndrome
    564.2
Posthemiplegic chorea 344.89
Posthemorrhagic anemia (chronic) 280.0
  acute 285.1
  newborn 776.5
Posthepatitis syndrome 780.79
Postherpetic neuralgia (intercostal)
    (syndrome) (zoster) 053.19
  geniculate ganglion 053.11
  ophthalmica 053.19
  trigeminal 053.12
Posthitis 607.1
**Postimmunization complication or
    reaction** - see Complications,
    vaccination
Postinfectious - see condition
Postinfluenzal syndrome 780.79
Postlaminectomy syndrome 722.80
  cervical, cervicothoracic 722.81
  kyphosis 737.12
  lumbar, lumbosacral 722.83
  thoracic, thoracolumbar 722.82
Postleukotomy syndrome 310.0
Postlobectomy syndrome 310.0
Postmastectomy lymphedema
    (syndrome) 457.0
Postmaturity, postmature (fetus or
    newborn) (gestation period
    over 42 completed weeks)
    766.22
  affecting management of pregnancy
    post-term pregnancy 645.1●
    prolonged pregnancy 645.2●
  syndrome 766.22

◀ New   ◀▥ Revised   ~~deleted~~ Deleted   ● Use Additional Digit(s)   ▬ Omit code

Postmeasles - *see also* condition
  complication 055.8
    specified NEC 055.79
Postmenopausal
  endometrium (atrophic) 627.8
    suppurative (*see also* Endometritis)
      615.9
  hormone replacement therapy
    V07.4
  status (age related) (natural)
    V49.81
Postnasal drip 784.91
Postnatal - *see* condition
Postoperative - *see also* condition
  confusion state 293.9
  psychosis 293.9
  status NEC (*see also* Status (post))
    V45.89
Postpancreatectomy hyperglycemia
  251.3
Postpartum - *see also* condition
  anemia 648.2●
    cardiomyopathy 674.5●
  observation
    immediately after delivery
      V24.0
    routine follow-up V24.2
Postperfusion syndrome NEC
  999.89
  bone marrow 996.85
Postpoliomyelitic - *see* condition
Postsurgery status NEC (*see also* Status
  (post)) V45.89
Post-term (pregnancy) 645.1●
  infant (gestation period over 40
    completed weeks to 42
    completed weeks) 766.21
Post-transplant lymphoproliferative
  disorder (PTLD) 238.77
Posttraumatic - *see* condition
Posttraumatic brain syndrome,
  nonpsychotic 310.2
Post-Traumatic Stress Disorder (PTSD)
  309.81
Post-typhoid abscess 002.0
Postures, hysterical 300.11
Postvaccinal reaction or complication -
  see Complications, vaccination
Postvagotomy syndrome 564.2
Postvalvulotomy syndrome 429.4
Postvasectomy sperm count V25.8
Potain's disease (pulmonary edema)
  514
Potain's syndrome (gastrectasis with
  dyspepsia) 536.1
Pott's
  curvature (spinal) (*see also*
    Tuberculosis) 015.0● [737.43]
  disease or paraplegia (*see also*
    Tuberculosis) 015.0● [730.88]
  fracture (closed) 824.4
    open 824.5
  gangrene 440.24
  osteomyelitis (*see also* Tuberculosis)
    015.0● [730.88]
  spinal curvature (*see also* Tuberculosis)
    015.0● [737.43]
  tumor, puffy (*see also* Osteomyelitis)
    730.2●
Potter's
  asthma 502
  disease 753.0
  facies 754.0
  lung 502

Potter's (*Continued*)
  syndrome (with renal agenesis)
    753.0
Pouch
  bronchus 748.3
  Douglas' - *see* condition
  esophagus, esophageal (congenital)
    750.4
    acquired 530.6
  gastric 537.1
  Hartmann's (abnormal sacculation of
    gallbladder neck) 575.8
    of intestine V44.3
      attention to V55.3
  pharynx, pharyngeal (congenital)
    750.27
Pouchitis 569.71 ◀
Poulet's disease 714.2
Poultrymen's itch 133.8
Poverty V60.2
PPE (palmar plantar erythrodysesthesia)
  693.0
Prader-Labhart-Willi-Fanconi syndrome
  (hypogenital dystrophy with
  diabetic tendency) 759.81
Prader-Willi syndrome (hypogenital
  dystrophy with diabetic tendency)
  759.81
Preachers' voice 784.49
Pre-AIDS - *see* Human
  immunodeficiency virus
  (disease) (illness) (infection)
Preauricular appendage 744.1
Prebetalipoproteinemia (acquired)
  (essential) (familial) (hereditary)
  (primary) (secondary) 272.1
  with chylomicronemia 272.3
Precipitate labor 661.3●
  affecting fetus or newborn 763.6
Preclimacteric bleeding 627.0
  menorrhagia 627.0
Precocious
  adrenarche 259.1
  menarche 259.1
  menstruation 626.8
  pubarche 259.1
  puberty NEC 259.1
  sexual development NEC 259.1
  thelarche 259.1
Precocity, sexual (constitutional)
  (cryptogenic) (female) (idiopathic)
  (male) NEC 259.1
  with adrenal hyperplasia 255.2
Precordial pain 786.51
  psychogenic 307.89
Predeciduous teeth 520.2
Prediabetes, prediabetic 790.29
  complicating pregnancy, childbirth, or
    puerperium 648.8●
  fetus or newborn 775.89
Predislocation status of hip, at birth (*see
  also* Subluxation, congenital, hip)
  754.32
Pre-eclampsia (mild) 642.4●
  with pre-existing hypertension642.7●
  affecting fetus or newborn 760.0
  severe 642.5●
  superimposed on pre-existing
    hypertensive disease 642.7●
Preeruptive color change, teeth, tooth
  520.8
Preexcitation 426.7
  atrioventricular conduction 426.7
  ventricular 426.7

Preglaucoma 365.00
Pregnancy (single) (uterine) (without
  sickness) V22.2

Note 62 Use the following fifth-digit
subclassification with categories
640–649, 651–679: ◀▪▪

  0 unspecified as to episode of care
  1 delivered, with or without
      mention of antepartum
      condition
  2 delivered, with mention of
      postpartum complication
  3 antepartum condition or
      complication
  4 postpartum condition or
      complication

  abdominal (ectopic) 633.00
    with intrauterine pregnancy 633.01
    affecting fetus or newborn 761.4
  abnormal NEC 646.9●
  ampullar - *see* Pregnancy, tubal
  broad ligament - *see* Pregnancy, cornual
  cervical - *see* Pregnancy, cornual
  chemical 631 ◀
  combined (extrauterine and
    intrauterine) - *see* Pregnancy,
    cornual
  complicated (by) 646.9●
    abnormal, abnormality NEC 646.9●
      cervix 654.6●
      cord (umbilical) 663.9●
      glucose tolerance (conditions
        classifiable to 790.21–790.29)
        648.8●
      pelvic organs or tissues NEC
        654.9●
      pelvis (bony) 653.0●
      perineum or vulva 654.8●
      placenta, placental (vessel) 656.7●
      position
        cervix 654.4●
        placenta 641.1●
          without hemorrhage 641.0●
        uterus 654.4●
      size, fetus 653.5●
      uterus (congenital) 654.0●
    abscess or cellulitis
      bladder 646.6●
      genitourinary tract (conditions
        classifiable to 590, 595,
        597, 599.0, 614.0–614.5,
        614.7–614.9, 615) 646.6●
      kidney 646.6●
      urinary tract NEC 646.6●
    adhesion, pelvic peritoneal 648.9●
    air embolism 673.0●
    albuminuria 646.2●
      with hypertension - *see* Toxemia,
      of pregnancy
    amnionitis 658.4●
    amniotic fluid embolism 673.1●
    anemia (conditions classifiable to
      280–285) 648.2●
    appendicitis 648.9●
    atrophy, yellow (acute) (liver)
      (subacute) 646.7●
    bacilluria, asymptomatic 646.5●
    bacteriuria, asymptomatic 646.5●
    bariatric surgery status 649.2●
    bicornis or bicornuate uterus
      654.0●
    biliary problems 646.8●

Pregnancy *(Continued)*
 complicated *(Continued)*
 bone and joint disorders
   (conditions classifiable to
   720–724 or conditions
   affecting lower limbs
   classifiable to 711–719,
   725–738) 648.7●
 breech presentation (buttocks)
   (complete) (frank) 652.2●
  with successful version 652.1
 cardiovascular disease (conditions
   classifiable to 390–398, 410–
   429) 648.6●
  congenital (conditions classifiable
    to 745–747) 648.5●
 cerebrovascular disorders
   (conditions classifiable to
   430–434, 436–437) 674.0●
 cervicitis (conditions classifiable to
   616.0) 646.6●
 chloasma (gravidarum) 646.8●
 cholelithiasis 646.8●
 chorea (gravidarum) - *see* Eclampsia,
   pregnancy
 coagulation defect 649.3●
 conjoined twins 678.1●
 contraction, pelvis (general)
   653.1●
  inlet 653.2●
  outlet 653.3●
 convulsions (eclamptic) (uremic)
   642.6●
  with pre-existing hypertension
    642.7●
 current disease or condition
   (nonobstetric)
  abnormal glucose tolerance
    648.8●
  anemia 648.2●
  bone and joint (lower limb)
    648.7●
  cardiovascular 648.6●
   congenital 648.5●
  cerebrovascular 674.0●
  diabetes (conditions
    classifiable to 249 and
    250) 648.0●
  drug dependence 648.3●
  female genital mutilation
    648.9●
  genital organ or tract 646.6●
  gonorrheal 647.1●
  hypertensive 642.2●
   chronic kidney 642.2●
   renal 642.1●
  infectious 647.9
   specified type NEC 647.8●
  liver 646.7●
  malarial 647.4●
  nutritional deficiency 648.9●
  parasitic NEC 647.8●
  periodontal disease 648.9●
  renal 646.2●
   hypertensive 642.1●
  rubella 647.5●
  specified condition NEC
    648.9●
  syphilitic 647.0●
  thyroid 648.1●
  tuberculous 647.3●
  urinary 646.6●
  venereal 647.2●
  viral NEC 647.6●
 cystitis 646.6●
 cystocele 654.4●

Pregnancy *(Continued)*
 complicated *(Continued)*
 death of fetus (near term) 656.4●
  early pregnancy (before 22
    completed weeks'
    gestation) 632
 deciduitis 646.6●
 decreased fetal movements 655.7●
 diabetes (mellitus) (conditions
   classifiable to 249 and 250)
   648.0●
 disorders of liver 646.7●
 displacement, uterus NEC 654.4●
 disproportion - *see* Disproportion
 double uterus 654.0●
 drug dependence (conditions
   classifiable to 304) 648.3●
 dysplasia, cervix 654.6●
 early onset of delivery
   (spontaneous) 644.2●
 eclampsia, eclamptic (coma)
   (convulsions) (delirium)
   (nephritis) (uremia) 642.6●
  with pre-existing hypertension
    642.7●
 edema 646.1●
  with hypertension - *see* Toxemia,
    of pregnancy
 effusion, amniotic fluid 658.1●
  delayed delivery following
    658.2●
 embolism
  air 673.0●
  amniotic fluid 673.1●
  blood-clot 673.2●
  cerebral 674.0●
  pulmonary NEC 673.2●
  pyemic 673.3●
  septic 673.3●
 emesis (gravidarum) - *see* Pregnancy,
   complicated, vomiting
 endometritis (conditions classifiable
   to 615.0–615.9) 670.1● ◄▥
 decidual 646.6●
 epilepsy 649.4●
 excessive weight gain NEC 646.1●
 face presentation 652.4●
 failure, fetal head to enter pelvic
   brim 652.5●
 false labor (pains) 644.1●
 fatigue 646.8●
 fatty metamorphosis of liver
   646.7●
 female genital mutilation 648.9●
 fetal
  anemia 678.0 ●   ◄
  complications from in utero
    procedure 679.1●   ◄
  conjoined twins 678.1●
  death (near term) 656.4●
   early (before 22 completed
     weeks' gestation) 632
  deformity 653.7●
  distress 656.8●
  hematologic conditions
    678.0●   ◄
  reduction of multiple fetuses
    reduced to single fetus
    651.7●
  thrombocytopenia 678.0● ◄
  twin to twin transfusion
    678.0●   ◄
 fibroid (tumor) (uterus) 654.1●
 footling presentation 652.8●
  with successful version 652.1●
 gallbladder disease 646.8●

Pregnancy *(Continued)*
 complicated *(Continued)*
 gastric banding status 649.2●
 gastric bypass status for obesity
   649.2●
 goiter 648.1●
 gonococcal infection (conditions
   classifiable to 098) 647.1●
 gonorrhea (conditions classifiable to
   098) 647.1●
 hemorrhage 641.9●
  accidental 641.2●
  before 22 completed weeks'
    gestation NEC 640.9●
  cerebrovascular 674.0●
  due to
   afibrinogenemia or other
     coagulation defect
     (conditions classifiable t
     o 286.0–286.9) 641.3●
   leiomyoma, uterine 641.8●
   marginal sinus (rupture)
     641.2●
   premature separation, placenta
     641.2●
   trauma 641.8●
  early (before 22 completed weeks'
    gestation) 640.9●
  threatened abortion 640.0●
  unavoidable 641.1●
 hepatitis (acute) (malignant)
   (subacute) 646.7●
  viral 647.6●
 herniation of uterus 654.4●
 high head at term 652.5●
 hydatidiform mole (delivered)
   (undelivered) 630
 hydramnios 657●
 hydrocephalic fetus 653.6●
 hydrops amnii 657●
 hydrorrhea 658.1●
 hyperemesis (gravidarum) - *see*
   Hyperemesis, gravidarum
 hypertension - *see* Hypertension,
   complicating pregnancy
 hypertensive
  chronic kidney disease
    642.2●
  heart and chronic kidney
    disease 642.2●
  heart and renal disease 642.2●
  heart disease 642.2●
  renal disease 642.2●
 hypertensive heart and chronic
   kidney disease 642.2●
 hyperthyroidism 648.1●
 hypothyroidism 648.1●
 hysteralgia 646.8●
 icterus gravis 646.7●
 incarceration, uterus 654.3●
 incompetent cervix (os)
   654.5●
 infection 647.9●
  amniotic fluid 658.4●
  bladder 646.6●
  genital organ (conditions
    classifiable to 614.0–
    614.5, 614.7–614.9, 615)
    646.6●
  kidney (conditions classifiable to
    590.0–590.9) 646.6●
  urinary (tract) 646.6●
   asymptomatic 646.5●
 infective and parasitic diseases NEC
   647.8●

◄ New   ◄▥ Revised   ~~deleted~~ Deleted   ● Use Additional Digit(s)   ▤ Omit code

Pregnancy (Continued)
  complicated (Continued)
    inflammation●
      bladder 646.6●
      genital organ (conditions
          classifiable to 614.0–614.5,
          614.7–614.9, 615) 646.6●
      urinary tract NEC 646.6
    injury 648.9●
      obstetrical NEC 665.9●
    insufficient weight gain 646.8●
    intrauterine fetal death (near term)
        NEC 656.4●
      early (before 22 completed weeks'
          gestation) 632
    malaria (conditions classifiable to
        084) 647.4●
    malformation, uterus (congenital)
        654.0●
    malnutrition (conditions classifiable
        to 260–269) 648.9●
    malposition
      fetus - see Pregnancy,
          complicated,
          malpresentation
      uterus or cervix 654.4●
    malpresentation 652.9●
      with successful version 652.1●
      in multiple gestation 652.6●
      specified type NEC 652.8●
    marginal sinus hemorrhage or
        rupture 641.2●
    maternal complications from in
        utero procedure 679.0● ◀
    maternal drug abuse 648.4●
    maternal obesity syndrome 646.1●
    menstruation 640.8●
    mental disorders (conditions
        classifiable to 290–303, 305.0,
        305.2–305.9, 306–316, 317–319)
        648.4●
    mentum presentation 652.4●
    missed
      abortion 632
      delivery (at or near term) 656.4●
      labor (at or near term) 656.4●
    necrosis
      genital organ or tract (conditions
          classifiable to 614.0–614.5,
          614.7–614.9, 615) 646.6●
      liver (conditions classifiable to
          570) 646.7●
      renal, cortical 646.2●
    nephritis or nephrosis (conditions
        classifiable to 580–589)
        646.2●
      with hypertension 642.1●
    nephropathy NEC 646.2●
    neuritis (peripheral) 646.4●
    nutritional deficiency (conditions
        classifiable to 260–269) 648.9●
    obesity 649.1●
      surgery status 649.2●
    oblique lie or presentation 652.3●
      with successful version 652.1●
    obstetrical trauma NEC 665.9●
    oligohydramnios NEC 658.0●
    onset of contractions before 37
        weeks 644.0●
    oversize fetus 653.5●
    papyraceous fetus 646.0●
    patent cervix 654.5●
    pelvic inflammatory disease
        (conditions classifiable to
        614.0–614.5, 614.7–614.9, 615)
        646.6●

Pregnancy (Continued)
  complicated (Continued)
    pelvic peritoneal adhesion 648.9●
    placenta, placental
      abnormality 656.7●
      abruptio or ablatio 641.2●
      detachment 641.2●
      disease 656.7●
      infarct 656.7●
      low implantation 641.1●
        without hemorrhage 641.0●
      malformation 656.7●
      malposition 641.1●
        without hemorrhage 641.0●
      marginal sinus hemorrhage
          641.2●
      previa 641.1●
        without hemorrhage 641.0●
      separation (premature)
          (undelivered) 641.2●
    placentitis 658.4●
    polyhydramnios 657●
    postmaturity●
      post-term 645.1●
      prolonged 645.2●
    prediabetes 648.8●
    pre-eclampsia (mild) 642.4●
      severe 642.5●
      superimposed on pre-existing
          hypertensive disease 642.7●
    premature rupture of membranes
        658.1●
      with delayed delivery 658.2●
    previous
      infertility V23.0
      in utero procedure during
          previous pregnancy
          V23.86
      nonobstetric condition V23.89
      poor obstetrical history V23.49
      premature delivery V23.41
      trophoblastic disease (conditions
          classifiable to 630) V23.1
    prolapse, uterus 654.4●
    proteinuria (gestational) 646.2●
      with hypertension - see Toxemia,
          of pregnancy
    pruritus (neurogenic) 646.8●
    psychosis or psychoneurosis 648.4●
    ptyalism 646.8●
    pyelitis (conditions classifiable to
        590.0–590.9) 646.6●
    renal disease or failure NEC 646.2●
      with secondary hypertension
          642.1●
      hypertensive 642.2●
    retention, retained dead
        ovum 631●
    retroversion, uterus 654.3●
    Rh immunization, incompatibility,
        or sensitization 656.1●
    rubella (conditions classifiable to
        056) 647.5●
    rupture
      amnion (premature) 658.1●
        with delayed delivery 658.2●
      marginal sinus (hemorrhage)
          641.2●
      membranes (premature) 658.1●
        with delayed delivery 658.2●
      uterus (before onset of labor)
          665.0●
    salivation (excessive) 646.8●
    salpingo-oophoritis (conditions
        classifiable to 614.0–614.2)
        646.6●

Pregnancy (Continued)
  complicated (Continued)
    septicemia (conditions classifiable to
        038.0–038.9) 647.8●
      postpartum 670.2● ◀▦
      puerperal 670.2● ◀▦
      smoking 649.0●
    spasms, uterus (abnormal) 646.8●
    specified condition NEC 646.8●
    spotting 649.5●
    spurious labor pains 644.1●
    status post
      bariatric surgery 649.2●
      gastric banding 649.2●
      gastric bypass for obesity
          649.2●
      obesity surgery 649.2●
    superfecundation 651.9●
    superfetation 651.9●
    syphilis (conditions classifiable to
        090–097) 647.0●
    threatened
      abortion 640.0●
      premature delivery 644.2●
      premature labor 644.0●
    thrombophlebitis (superficial)
        671.2●
      deep 671.3●
      septic 670.3● ◀
    thrombosis 671.2● ◀▦
      venous (superficial) 671.2●
        deep 671.3●
    thyroid dysfunction (conditions
        classifiable to 240–246) 648.1●
    thyroiditis 648.1●
    thyrotoxicosis 648.1●
    tobacco use disorder 649.0●
    torsion of uterus 654.4●
    toxemia - see Toxemia, of pregnancy
    transverse lie or presentation 652.3●
      with successful version 652.1●
    trauma 648.9●
      obstetrical 665.9●
    tuberculosis (conditions classifiable
        to 010–018) 647.3●
    tumor
      cervix 654.6●
      ovary 654.4●
      pelvic organs or tissue NEC
          654.4●
      uterus (body) 654.1●
        cervix 654.6●
      vagina 654.7●
      vulva 654.8●
    unstable lie 652.0●
    uremia - see Pregnancy, complicated,
        renal disease
    urethritis 646.6●
    vaginitis or vulvitis (conditions
        classifiable to 616.1) 646.6●
    varicose
      placental vessels 656.7●
      veins (legs) 671.0●
        perineum 671.1●
        vulva 671.1●
    varicosity, labia or vulva 671.1●
    venereal disease NEC (conditions
        classifiable to 099) 647.2●
    venous complication 671.9● ◀
    viral disease NEC (conditions
        classifiable to 042, 050–055,
        057–079, 795.05, 795.15, 796.75)
        647.6●
    vomiting (incoercible) (pernicious)
        (persistent) (uncontrollable)
        (vicious) 643.9●

Pregnancy *(Continued)*
  complicated *(Continued)*
    vomiting *(Continued)*
      due to organic disease or other
        cause 643.8 ●
      early - *see* Hyperemesis,
        gravidarum
      late (after 22 completed weeks
        gestation) 643.2 ●
    young maternal age 659.8 ●
  complications NEC 646.9 ●
  cornual 633.80
    with intrauterine pregnancy 633.81
    affecting fetus or newborn 761.4
  death, maternal NEC 646.9 ●
  delivered - *see* Delivery
  ectopic (ruptured) NEC 633.90
    with intrauterine pregnancy 633.91
    abdominal - *see* Pregnancy,
      abdominal
    affecting fetus or newborn 761.4
    combined (extrauterine and
      intrauterine) - *see* Pregnancy,
      cornual
    ovarian - *see* Pregnancy, ovarian
    specified type NEC 633.80
      with intrauterine pregnancy
        633.81
      affecting fetus or newborn 761.4
    tubal - *see* Pregnancy, tubal
  examination, pregnancy
    negative result V72.41
    not confirmed V72.40
    positive result V72.42
  extrauterine - *see* Pregnancy, ectopic
  fallopian - *see* Pregnancy, tubal
  false 300.11
    labor (pains) 644.1 ●
  fatigue 646.8 ●
  illegitimate V61.6
  incidental finding V22.2
  in double uterus 654.0 ●
  interstitial - *see* Pregnancy, cornual
  intraligamentous - *see* Pregnancy,
    cornual
  intramural - *see* Pregnancy, cornual
  intraperitoneal - *see* Pregnancy,
    abdominal
  isthmian - *see* Pregnancy, tubal
  management affected by
    abnormal, abnormality
      fetus (suspected) 655.9 ●
        specified NEC 655.8 ●
      placenta 656.7 ●
    advanced maternal age NEC 659.6 ●
      multigravida 659.6 ●
      primigravida 659.5 ●
    antibodies (maternal)
      anti-c 656.1 ●
      anti-d 656.1 ●
      anti-e 656.1 ●
      blood group (ABO) 656.2 ●
        Rh(esus) 656.1 ●
    appendicitis 648.9 ●
    bariatric surgery status 649.2 ●
    coagulation defect 649.3 ●
    elderly multigravida 659.6 ●
    elderly primigravida 659.5 ●
    epilepsy 649.4 ●
    fetal (suspected) ●
      abnormality 655.9 ●
        abdominal 655.8 ●
        acid-base balance 656.8 ●
        cardiovascular 655.8 ●
        facial 655.8 ●
        gastrointestinal 655.8 ●

Pregnancy *(Continued)*
  management affected by *(Continued)*
    fetal *(Continued)*
      abnormality *(Continued)*
        genitourinary 655.8 ●
        heart rate or rhythm 659.7 ●
        limb 655.8 ●
        specified NEC 655.8 ●
      acidemia 656.3 ●
      anencephaly 655.0 ●
      aneuploidy 655.1 ●
      bradycardia 659.7 ●
      central nervous system
        malformation 655.0 ●
      chromosomal abnormalities
        (conditions classifiable to
        758.0–758.9) 655.1 ●
      damage from
        drugs 655.5 ●
          obstetric, anesthetic, or
            sedative 655.5 ●
        environmental toxins 655.8
        intrauterine contraceptive
          device 655.8 ●
        maternal
          alcohol addiction 655.4 ●
          disease NEC 655.4 ●
          drug use 655.5 ●
          listeriosis 655.4 ●
          rubella 655.3 ●
          toxoplasmosis 655.4 ●
          viral infection 655.3 ●
        radiation 655.6 ●
      death (near term) 656.4 ●
        early (before 22 completed
          weeks' gestation) 632
      distress 656.8 ●
      excessive growth 656.6 ●
      growth retardation 656.5 ●
      hereditary disease 655.2 ●
      hydrocephalus 655.0 ●
      intrauterine death 656.4 ●
      poor growth 656.5 ●
      spina bifida (with
        myelomeningocele)
        655.0 ●
    fetal-maternal hemorrhage 656.0 ●
    gastric banding status 649.2 ●
    gastric bypass status for obesity
      649.2 ●
    hereditary disease in family
      (possibly) affecting fetus
      655.2 ●
    incompatibility, blood groups (ABO)
      656.2 ●
      Rh(esus) 656.1 ●
    insufficient prenatal care V23.7
    intrauterine death 656.4 ●
    isoimmunization (ABO) 656.2 ●
      Rh(esus) 656.1 ●
    large-for-dates fetus 656.6 ●
    light-for-dates fetus 656.5 ●
    meconium in liquor 656.8 ●
    mental disorder (conditions
      classifiable to 290–303, 305.0,
      305.2–305.9, 306–316, 317–319)
      648.4 ●
    multiparity (grand) 659.4 ●
    obesity 649.1 ●
      surgery status 649.2 ●
    poor obstetric history V23.49
      pre-term labor V23.41
    postmaturity
      post-term 645.1 ●
      prolonged 645.2 ●
    post-term pregnancy 645.1 ●

Pregnancy *(Continued)*
  management affected by *(Continued)*
    previous
      abortion V23.2
        habitual 646.3 ●
      cesarean delivery 654.2 ●
      difficult delivery V23.49
      forceps delivery V23.49
      habitual abortions 646.3 ●
      hemorrhage, antepartum or
        postpartum V23.49
      hydatidiform mole V23.1
      infertility V23.0
      in utero procedure during
        previous pregnancy V23.86
      malignancy NEC V23.89
      nonobstetrical conditions V23.89
      premature delivery V23.41
      trophoblastic disease (conditions
        in 630) V23.1
      vesicular mole V23.1
    prolonged pregnancy 645.2 ●
    small-for-dates fetus 656.5 ●
    smoking 649.0 ●
    spotting 649.5 ●
    suspected conditions not found
      amniotic cavity and membrane
        problem V89.01
      cervical shortening V89.05
      fetal anomaly V89.03
      fetal growth problem V89.04
      oligohydramnios V89.01
      other specified problem NEC
        V89.09
      placental problem V89.02
      polyhydramnios V89.01
    tobacco use disorder 649.0 ●
    venous complication 671.9 ● ◀
    young maternal age 659.8 ●
  maternal death NEC 646.9 ●
  mesometric (mural) - *see* Pregnancy,
    cornual
  molar 631
    hydatidiform (*see also* Hydatidiform
      mole) 630
      previous, affecting management
        of pregnancy V23.1
      previous, affecting management of
        pregnancy V23.49
  multiple NEC 651.9 ●
    with fetal loss and retention of one
      or more fetus(es) 651.6 ●
    affecting fetus or newborn 761.5
    following (elective) fetal reduction
      651.7 ●
    specified type NEC 651.8 ●
      with fetal loss and retention of one
        or more fetus(es) 651.6 ●
      following (elective) fetal
        reduction 651.7 ●
  mural - *see* Pregnancy, cornual
  observation NEC V22.1
    first pregnancy V22.0
    high-risk V23.9
      specified problem NEC V23.89
  ovarian 633.20
    with intrauterine pregnancy 633.21
    affecting fetus or newborn 761.4
  possible, not (yet) confirmed V72.40
  postmature
    post-term 645.1 ●
    prolonged 645.2 ●
  post-term 645.1 ●
  prenatal care only V22.1
    first pregnancy V22.0
    high-risk V23.9
      specified problem NEC V23.89

◀ New   ◀▥ Revised   ~~deleted~~ Deleted   ● Use Additional Digit(s)   ▨ Omit code

Pregnancy (*Continued*)
    prolonged 645.2●
    quadruplet NEC 651.2●
        with fetal loss and retention of one
            or more fetus(es) 651.5●
        affecting fetus or newborn 761.5
        following (elective) fetal reduction
            651.7●
    quintuplet NEC 651.8●
        with fetal loss and retention of one
            or more fetus(es) 651.6●
        affecting fetus or newborn 761.5
        following (elective) fetal reduction
            651.7●
    resulting from
        assisted reproductive technology
            V23.85
        in vitro fertilization V23.85
    sextuplet NEC 651.8●
        with fetal loss and retention of one
            or more fetus(es) 651.6●
        affecting fetus or newborn 761.5
        following (elective) fetal reduction
            651.7●
    spurious 300.11
    superfecundation NEC 651.9●
        with fetal loss and retention of one
            or more fetus(es) 651.6●
        following (elective) fetal reduction
            651.7●
    superfetation NEC 651.9●
        with fetal loss and retention of one
            or more fetus(es) 651.6●
        following (elective) fetal reduction
            651.7●
    supervision (of) (for) - *see also*
        Pregnancy, management
        affected by
        elderly
            multigravida V23.82
            primigravida V23.81
        high-risk V23.9
            insufficient prenatal care V23.7
            specified problem NEC
                V23.89
        multiparity V23.3
        normal NEC V22.1
            first V22.0
        poor
            obstetric history V23.49
                pre-term labor V23.41
            reproductive history V23.5
        previous
            abortion V23.2
            hydatidiform mole V23.1
            infertility V23.0
            neonatal death V23.5
            stillbirth V23.5
            trophoblastic disease V23.1
            vesicular mole V23.1
        specified problem NEC V23.89
        young
            multigravida V23.84
            primigravida V23.83
    triplet NEC 651.1●
        with fetal loss and retention of one
            or more fetus(es) 651.4●
        affecting fetus or newborn 761.5
        following (elective) fetal reduction
            651.7●
    tubal (with rupture) 633.10
        with intrauterine pregnancy
            633.11
        affecting fetus or newborn
            761.4

Pregnancy (*Continued*)
    twin NEC 651.0●
        with fetal loss and retention of one
            fetus 651.3●
        affecting fetus or newborn 761.5
        conjoined 678.1●
        following (elective) fetal reduction
            651.7●
    unconfirmed V72.40
    undelivered (no other diagnosis) V22.2
        with false labor 644.1●
        high-risk V23.9
            specified problem NEC V23.89
    unwanted NEC V61.7
Pregnant uterus - *see* condition
Preiser's disease (osteoporosis) 733.09
Prekwashiorkor 260
Preleukemia 238.75
Preluxation of hip, congenital (*see also*
        Subluxation, congenital, hip) 754.32
Premature - *see also* condition
    beats (nodal) 427.60
        atrial 427.61
        auricular 427.61
        postoperative 997.1
        specified type NEC 427.69
        supraventricular 427.61
        ventricular 427.69
    birth NEC 765.1●
    closure
        cranial suture 756.0
        fontanel 756.0
        foramen ovale 745.8
    contractions 427.60
        atrial 427.61
        auricular 427.61
        auriculoventricular 427.61
        heart (extrasystole) 427.60
        junctional 427.60
        nodal 427.60
        postoperative 997.1
        ventricular 427.69
    ejaculation 302.75
    infant NEC 765.1●
        excessive 765.0●
        light-for-dates - *see* Light-for-dates
    labor 644.2●
        threatened 644.0●
    lungs 770.4
    menopause 256.31
    puberty 259.1
    rupture of membranes or amnion
        658.1●
        affecting fetus or newborn 761.1
        delayed delivery following 658.2●
    senility (syndrome) 259.8
    separation, placenta (partial) - *see*
        Placenta, separation
    ventricular systole 427.69
Prematurity NEC 765.1●
    extreme 765.0●
Premenstrual syndrome 625.4
Premenstrual tension 625.4
Premolarization, cuspids 520.2
Premyeloma 273.1
Prenatal
    care, normal pregnancy V22.1
        first V22.0
    death, cause unknown - *see* Death,
        fetus
    screening - *see* Antenatal, screening
    teeth 520.6
Prepartum - *see* condition
Preponderance, left or right ventricular
        429.3

Prepuce - *see* condition
PRES (posterior reversible
        encephalopathy syndrome) 348.39
Presbycardia 797
    hypertensive (*see also* Hypertension,
        heart) 402.90
Presbycusis 388.01
Presbyesophagus 530.89
Presbyophrenia 310.1
Presbyopia 367.4
Prescription of contraceptives NEC
        V25.02
    diaphragm V25.02
    oral (pill) V25.01
        emergency V25.03
        postcoital V25.03
        repeat V25.41
    repeat V25.40
        oral (pill) V25.41
Presenile - *see also* condition
    aging 259.8
    dementia (*see also* Dementia, presenile)
        290.10
Presenility 259.8
Presentation, fetal
    abnormal 652.9●
        with successful version 652.1●
        before labor, affecting fetus or
            newborn 761.7
        causing obstructed labor 660.0●
            affecting fetus or newborn, any,
                except breech 763.1
        in multiple gestation (one or more)
            652.6●
        specified NEC 652.8●
    arm 652.7●
        causing obstructed labor 660.0●
    breech (buttocks) (complete) (frank)
        652.2●
        with successful version 652.1●
            before labor, affecting fetus or
                newborn 761.7
        before labor, affecting fetus or
            newborn 761.7
    brow 652.4●
        causing obstructed labor 660.0●
    buttocks 652.2●
    chin 652.4●
    complete 652.2●
    compound 652.8●
    cord 663.0●
    extended head 652.4●
    face 652.4●
        to pubes 652.8●
    footling 652.8●
    frank 652.2●
    hand, leg, or foot NEC 652.8●
    incomplete 652.8●
    mentum 652.4●
    multiple gestation (one fetus or more)
        652.6●
    oblique 652.3●
        with successful version 652.1●
    shoulder 652.8●
        affecting fetus or newborn 763.1
    transverse 652.3●
        with successful version 652.1●
    umbilical cord 663.0●
    unstable 652.0●
Prespondylolisthesis (congenital)
        (lumbosacral) 756.11
Pressure
    area, skin ulcer (*see also* Ulcer, pressure)
        707.00
    atrophy, spine 733.99

Pressure (*Continued*)
  birth, fetus or newborn NEC 767.9
  brachial plexus 353.0
  brain 348.4
    injury at birth 767.0
  cerebral - *see* Pressure, brain
  chest 786.59
  cone, tentorial 348.4
    injury at birth 767.0
  funis - *see* Compression, umbilical cord
  hyposystolic (*see also* Hypotension)
    458.9
  increased
    intracranial 781.99
      due to
        benign intracranial
            hypertension 348.2
        hydrocephalus - *see*
            hydrocephalus
        injury at birth 767.8
    intraocular 365.00
  lumbosacral plexus 353.1
  mediastinum 519.3
  necrosis (chronic) (skin) (*see also*
    Decubitus) 707.00
  nerve - *see* Compression, nerve
  paralysis (*see also* Neuropathy,
    entrapment) 355.9
  pre-ulcer skin changes limited to
    persistent focal erythema (*see also*
    Ulcer, pressure) 707.21
  sore (chronic) (*see also* Ulcer, pressure)
    707.00
  spinal cord 336.9
  ulcer (chronic) (*see also* Ulcer, pressure)
    707.00
  umbilical cord - *see* Compression,
    umbilical cord
  venous, increased 459.89
Pre-syncope 780.2
Preterm infant NEC 765.1●
  extreme 765.0●
Priapism (penis) 607.3
Prickling sensation (*see also* Disturbance,
    sensation) 782.0
Prickly heat 705.1
Primary - *see* condition
Primigravida, elderly
  affecting
    fetus or newborn 763.89
    management of pregnancy, labor,
        and delivery 659.5●
Primipara, old
  affecting
    fetus or newborn 763.89
    management of pregnancy, labor,
        and delivery 659.5●
Primula dermatitis 692.6
Primus varus (bilateral) (metatarsus) 754.52
PRIND (prolonged reversible ischemic
    neurologic deficit) 434.91
  history of (personal) V12.54
Pringle's disease (tuberous sclerosis) 759.5
Prinzmetal's angina 413.1
Prinzmetal-Massumi syndrome (anterior
    chest wall) 786.52
Prizefighter ear 738.7
Problem (with) V49.9
  academic V62.3
  acculturation V62.4
  adopted child V61.24   ◀▥
  aged
    in-law V61.3
    parent V61.3
    person NEC V61.8

Problem (*Continued*)
  alcoholism in family V61.41
  anger reaction (*see also* Disturbance,
        conduct) 312.0●
  behavior, child 312.9
  behavioral V40.9
    specified NEC V40.3
  betting V69.3
  biological child V61.23   ◀
  cardiorespiratory NEC V47.2
  care of sick or handicapped person in
        family or household V61.49
  career choice V62.29
  communication V40.1
  conscience regarding medical care
        V62.6
  delinquency (juvenile) 312.9
  diet, inappropriate V69.1
  digestive NEC V47.3
  ear NEC V41.3
  eating habits, inappropriate V69.1
  economic V60.2
    affecting care V60.9
      specified type NEC V60.89   ◀▥
  educational V62.3
  enuresis, child 307.6
  exercise, lack of V69.0
  eye NEC V41.1
  family V61.9 .
    specified circumstance NEC V61.8
  fear reaction, child 313.0
  feeding (elderly) (infant) 783.3
    newborn 779.31   ◀▥
    nonorganic 307.59
  fetal, affecting management of
        pregnancy 656.9●
    specified type NEC 656.8●
  financial V60.2
  foster child V61.25   ◀▥
  ~~specified NEC V41.8~~
  functional V41.9
    specified type NEC V41.8
  gambling V69.3
  genital NEC V47.5
  head V48.9
    deficiency V48.0
    disfigurement V48.6
    mechanical V48.2
    motor V48.2
    movement of V48.2
    sensory V48.4
    specified condition NEC V48.8
  hearing V41.2
  high-risk sexual behavior V69.2
  identity 313.82
  influencing health status
        NEC V49.89
  internal organ NEC V47.9
    deficiency V47.0
    mechanical or motor V47.1
  interpersonal NEC V62.81
  jealousy, child 313.3
  learning V40.0
  legal V62.5
  life circumstance NEC V62.89
  lifestyle V69.9
    specified NEC V69.8
  limb V49.9
    deficiency V49.0
    disfigurement V49.4
    mechanical V49.1
    motor V49.2
    movement, involving
      musculoskeletal system V49.1
      nervous system V49.2

Problem (*Continued*)
  limb, (*Continued*)
    sensory V49.3
    specified condition NEC V49.5
  litigation V62.5
  living alone V60.3
  loneliness NEC V62.89
  marital V61.10
    involving
      divorce V61.03
      estrangement V61.09
      psychosexual disorder 302.9
      sexual function V41.7
    relationship V61.10
  mastication V41.6
  medical care, within family V61.49
  mental V40.9
    specified NEC V40.2
  mental hygiene, adult V40.9
  multiparity V61.5
  nail biting, child 307.9
  neck V48.9
    deficiency V48.1
    disfigurement V48.7
    mechanical V48.3
    motor V48.3
    movement V48.3
    sensory V48.5
    specified condition NEC V48.8
  neurological NEC 781.99
  none (feared complaint unfounded)
        V65.5
  occupational V62.29
  parent-child V61.20
    adopted child V61.24   ◀
    biological child V61.23   ◀
    foster child V61.25   ◀
    relationship V61.20
  partner V61.10
    relationship V61.10
  personal NEC V62.89
    interpersonal conflict NEC
        V62.81
  personality (*see also* Disorder,
        personality) 301.9
  phase of life V62.89
  placenta, affecting management of
        pregnancy 656.9●
    specified type NEC 656.8●
  poverty V60.2
  presence of sick or handicapped
        person in family or household
        V61.49
  psychiatric 300.9
  psychosocial V62.9
    specified type NEC V62.89
  relational NEC V62.81
  relationship, childhood 313.3
  religious or spiritual belief
    other than medical care V62.89
    regarding medical care V62.6
  self-damaging behavior V69.8
  sexual
    behavior, high-risk V69.2
    function NEC V41.7
  sibling
    relational V61.8
    relationship V61.8
  sight V41.0
  sleep, lack of V69.4
  sleep disorder, child 307.40
  smell V41.5
  speech V40.1
  spite reaction, child (*see also*
        Disturbance, conduct) 312.0●

Problem (Continued)
  spoiled child reaction (see also
      Disturbance, conduct) 312.1●
  substance abuse in family V61.42 ◄
  swallowing V41.6
  tantrum, child (see also Disturbance,
      conduct) 312.1●
  taste V41.5
  thumb sucking, child 307.9
  tic (child) 307.21
  trunk V48.9
      deficiency V48.1
      disfigurement V48.7
      mechanical V48.3
      motor V48.3
      movement V48.3
      sensory V48.5
      specified condition NEC V48.8
  unemployment V62.0
  urinary NEC V47.4
  voice production V41.4
Procedure (surgical) not done NEC
    V64.3
  because of
      contraindication V64.1
      patient's decision V64.2
          for reasons of conscience or
              religion V62.6
      specified reason NEC V64.3
Procidentia
  anus (sphincter) 569.1
  rectum (sphincter) 569.1
  stomach 537.89
  uteri 618.1
Proctalgia 569.42
  fugax 564.6
  spasmodic 564.6
      psychogenic 307.89
Proctitis 569.49
  amebic 006.8
  chlamydial 099.52
  gonococcal 098.7
  granulomatous 555.1
  idiopathic 556.2
      with ulcerative sigmoiditis
          556.3
  tuberculous (see also Tuberculosis)
      014.8●
  ulcerative (chronic) (nonspecific)
      556.2
      with ulcerative sigmoiditis 556.3
Proctocele
  female (without uterine prolapse)
      618.04
      with uterine prolapse 618.4
          complete 618.3
          incomplete 618.2
  male 569.49
Proctocolitis, idiopathic 556.2
  with ulcerative sigmoiditis 556.3
Proctoptosis 569.1
Proctosigmoiditis 569.89
  ulcerative (chronic) 556.3
Proctospasm 564.6
  psychogenic 306.4
Prodromal-AIDS - see Human
    immunodeficiency virus (disease)
    (illness) (infection)
Profichet's disease or syndrome
    729.90
Progeria (adultorum) (syndrome) 259.8
Prognathism (mandibular) (maxillary)
    524.00
Progonoma (melanotic) (M9363/0) - see
    Neoplasm, by site, benign

Progressive - see condition
Prolapse, prolapsed
  anus, anal (canal) (sphincter) 569.1
  arm or hand, complicating delivery
      652.7●
      causing obstructed labor 660.0●
          affecting fetus or newborn
              763.1
      fetus or newborn 763.1
  bladder (acquired) (mucosa)
      (sphincter)
      congenital (female) (male) 756.71
      female (see also Cystocele, female)
          618.01
      male 596.8
  breast implant (prosthetic) 996.54
  cecostomy 569.69
  cecum 569.89
  cervix, cervical (hypertrophied) 618.1
      anterior lip, obstructing labor
          660.2●
          affecting fetus or newborn 763.1
      congenital 752.49
      postpartal (old) 618.1
      stump 618.84
  ciliary body 871.1
  colon (pedunculated) 569.89
  colostomy 569.69
  conjunctiva 372.73
  cord - see Prolapse, umbilical cord
  disc (intervertebral) - see Displacement,
      intervertebral disc
  duodenum 537.89
  eye implant (orbital) 996.59
      lens (ocular) 996.53
  fallopian tube 620.4
  fetal extremity, complicating delivery
      652.8●
      causing obstructed labor 660.0●
      fetus or newborn 763.1
  funis - see Prolapse, umbilical cord
  gastric (mucosa) 537.89
  genital, female 618.9
      specified NEC 618.89
  globe 360.81
  ileostomy bud 569.69
  intervertebral disc - see Displacement,
      intervertebral disc
  intestine (small) 569.89
  iris 364.89
      traumatic 871.1
  kidney (see also Disease, renal) 593.0
      congenital 753.3
  laryngeal muscles or ventricle
      478.79
  leg, complicating delivery 652.8●
      causing obstructed labor 660.0●
      fetus or newborn 763.1
  liver 573.8
  meatus urinarius 599.5
  mitral valve 424.0
  ocular lens implant 996.53
  organ or site, congenital NEC - see
      Malposition, congenital
  ovary 620.4
  pelvic (floor), female 618.89
  perineum, female 618.89
  pregnant uterus 654.4●
  rectum (mucosa) (sphincter) 569.1
      due to Trichuris trichiuria 127.3
  spleen 289.59
  stomach 537.89
  umbilical cord
      affecting fetus or newborn 762.4
      complicating delivery 663.0●

Prolapse, prolapsed (Continued)
  ureter 593.89
      with obstruction 593.4
  ureterovesical orifice 593.89
  urethra (acquired) (infected) (mucosa)
      599.5
      congenital 753.8
  uterovaginal 618.4
      complete 618.3
      incomplete 618.2
      specified NEC 618.89
  uterus (first degree) (second degree)
      (third degree) (complete)
      (without vaginal wall prolapse)
      618.1
      with mention of vaginal wall
          prolapse - see Prolapse,
          uterovaginal
      congenital 752.3
      in pregnancy or childbirth
          654.4●
          affecting fetus or newborn
              763.1
          causing obstructed labor
              660.2●
              affecting fetus or newborn
                  763.1
      postpartal (old) 618.1
  uveal 871.1
  vagina (anterior) (posterior) (vault)
      (wall) (without uterine prolapse)
      618.00
      with uterine prolapse 618.4
          complete 618.3
          incomplete 618.2
      paravaginal 618.02
      posthysterectomy 618.5
      specified NEC 618.09
  vitreous (humor) 379.26
      traumatic 871.1
  womb - see Prolapse, uterus
Prolapsus, female 618.9
Proliferative - see condition
Prolinemia 270.8
Prolinuria 270.8
Prolonged, prolongation
  bleeding time (see also Defect,
      coagulation) 790.92
  "idiopathic" (in von Willebrand's
      disease) 286.4
  coagulation time (see also Defect,
      coagulation) 790.92
  gestation syndrome 766.22
  labor 662.1●
      affecting fetus or newborn
          763.89
      first stage 662.0●
      second stage 662.2●
  PR interval 426.11
  pregnancy 645.2●
  prothrombin time (see also Defect,
      coagulation) 790.92
  QT interval 794.31
      syndrome 426.82
  rupture of membranes (24 hours or
      more prior to onset of labor)
      658.2●
  uterine contractions in labor
      661.4●
      affecting fetus or newborn
          763.7
Prominauris 744.29
Prominence
  auricle (ear) (congenital) 744.29
      acquired 380.32

Prominence (Continued)
ischial spine or sacral promontory
with disproportion (fetopelvic)
653.3●
affecting fetus or newborn
763.1
causing obstructed labor
660.1●
affecting fetus or newborn
763.1
nose (congenital) 748.1
acquired 738.0
PROMM (proximal myotonic myotonia)
359.21
Pronation
ankle 736.79
foot 736.79
congenital 755.67
Prophylactic
administration of
agents affecting estrogen receptors
and estrogen levels NEC
V07.59
anastrozole (Arimidex) V07.52
antibiotics V07.39
antitoxin, any V07.2
antivenin V07.2
aromatase inhibitors V07.52
chemotherapeutic agent NEC V07.39
fluoride V07.31
diphtheria antitoxin V07.2
drug V07.39
estrogen receptor downregulators
V07.59
exemestane (Aromasin) V07.52 ◀▥
fulvestrant (Faslodex) V07.59
gamma globulin V07.2
gonadotropin-releasing hormone
(GnRH) agonist V07.59
goserelin acetate (Zoladex) V07.59
immune sera (gamma globulin)
V07.2
letrozole (Femara) V07.52
leuprolide acetate (leuprorelin)
(Lupron) V07.59
megestrol acetate (Megace)
V07.59
raloxifene (Evista) V07.51
RhoGAM V07.2
selective estrogen receptor
modulators (SERMs)
V07.51
tamoxifen (Nolvadex) V07.51
tetanus antitoxin V07.2
toremifene (Fareston) V07.51
chemotherapy NEC V07.39
fluoride V07.31
hormone replacement
(postmenopausal) V07.4
immunotherapy V07.2
measure V07.9
specified type NEC V07.8
medication V07.39
postmenopausal hormone replacement
V07.4
sterilization V25.2
Proptosis (ocular) (see also Exophthalmos)
376.30
thyroid 242.0●
Propulsion
eyeball 360.81
Prosecution, anxiety concerning V62.5
Prosopagnosia 368.16
Prostate, prostatic - see condition

Prostatism 600.90
with
other lower urinary tract symptoms
(LUTS) 600.91
urinary
obstruction 600.91
retention 600.91
Prostatitis (congestive) (suppurative)
601.9
acute 601.0
cavitary 601.8
chlamydial 099.54
chronic 601.1
diverticular 601.8
due to Trichomonas (vaginalis) 131.03
fibrous 600.90
with
other lower urinary tract
symptoms (LUTS) 600.91
urinary
obstruction 600.91
retention 600.91
gonococcal (acute) 098.12
chronic or duration of 2 months or
over 098.32
granulomatous 601.8
hypertrophic 600.00
with
other lower urinary tract
symptoms (LUTS) 600.01
urinary
obstruction 600.01
retention 600.01
specified type NEC 601.8
subacute 601.1
trichomonal 131.03
tuberculous (see also Tuberculosis)
016.5● [601.4]
Prostatocystitis 601.3
Prostatorrhea 602.8
Prostatoseminovesiculitis, trichomonal
131.03
Prostration 780.79
heat 992.5
anhydrotic 992.3
due to
salt (and water) depletion
992.4
water depletion 992.3
nervous 300.5
newborn 779.89
senile 797
Protanomaly 368.51
Protanopia (anomalous trichromat)
(complete) (incomplete) 368.51
Protection (against) (from) - see
Prophylactic
Protein
deficiency 260
malnutrition 260
sickness (prophylactic) (therapeutic)
999.5
Proteinemia 790.99
Proteinosis
alveolar, lung or pulmonary 516.0
lipid 272.8
lipoid (of Urbach) 272.8
Proteinuria (see also Albuminuria) 791.0
Bence-Jones NEC 791.0
gestational 646.2●
with hypertension - see Toxemia, of
pregnancy
orthostatic 593.6
postural 593.6

Proteolysis, pathologic 286.6
Protocoproporphyria 277.1
Protoporphyria (erythrohepatic)
(erythropoietic) 277.1
Protrusio acetabuli 718.65
Protrusion
acetabulum (into pelvis) 718.65
device, implant, or graft - see
Complications, mechanical
ear, congenital 744.29
intervertebral disc - see Displacement,
intervertebral disc
nucleus pulposus - see Displacement,
intervertebral disc
Proud flesh 701.5
Prune belly (syndrome) 756.71
Prurigo (ferox) (gravis) (Hebra's) (hebrae)
(mitis) (simplex) 698.2
agria 698.3
asthma syndrome 691.8
Besnier's (atopic dermatitis) (infantile
eczema) 691.8
eczematodes allergicum 691.8
estivalis (Hutchinson's) 692.72
Hutchinson's 692.72
nodularis 698.3
psychogenic 306.3
Pruritus, pruritic 698.9
ani 698.0
psychogenic 306.3
conditions NEC 698.9
psychogenic 306.3
due to Onchocerca volvulus 125.3
ear 698.9
essential 698.9
genital organ(s) 698.1
psychogenic 306.3
gravidarum 646.8●
hiemalis 698.8
neurogenic (any site) 306.3
perianal 698.0
psychogenic (any site) 306.3
scrotum 698.1
psychogenic 306.3
senile, senilis 698.8
Trichomonas 131.9
vulva, vulvae 698.1
psychogenic 306.3
Psammocarcinoma (M8140/3) - see
Neoplasm, by site, malignant
Pseudarthrosis, pseudoarthrosis (bone)
733.82
joint following fusion V45.4
Pseudoacanthosis
nigricans 701.8
Pseudoaneurysm - see Aneurysm
Pseudoangina (pectoris) - see Angina
Pseudoangioma 452
Pseudo-Argyll-Robertson pupil
379.45
Pseudoarteriosus 747.89
Pseudoarthrosis - see Pseudarthrosis
Pseudoataxia 799.89
Pseudobulbar affect (PBA) 310.8
Pseudobursa 727.89
Pseudocholera 025
Pseudochromidrosis 705.89
Pseudocirrhosis, liver, pericardial
423.2
Pseudocoarctation 747.21
Pseudocowpox 051.1
Pseudocoxalgia 732.1
Pseudocroup 478.75
Pseudocyesis 300.11

◀ New   ◀▥ Revised   ~~deleted~~ Deleted   ● Use Additional Digit(s)   ▒ Omit code

Pseudocyst
  lung 518.89
  pancreas 577.2
  retina 361.19
Pseudodementia 300.16
Pseudoelephantiasis neuroarthritica
    757.0
Pseudoemphysema 518.89
Pseudoencephalitis
  superior (acute) hemorrhagic 265.1
Pseudoerosion cervix, congenital 752.49
Pseudoexfoliation, lens capsule 366.11
Pseudofracture (idiopathic) (multiple)
    (spontaneous) (symmetrical) 268.2
Pseudoglanders 025
Pseudoglioma 360.44
Pseudogout - see Chondrocalcinosis
Pseudohallucination 780.1
Pseudohemianesthesia 782.0
Pseudohemophilia (Bernuth's)
    (hereditary) (type B) 286.4
  type A 287.8
  vascular 287.8
Pseudohermaphroditism 752.7
  with chromosomal anomaly - see
      Anomaly, chromosomal
  adrenal 255.2
  female (without adrenocortical
      disorder) 752.7
    with adrenocortical disorder
        255.2
      adrenal 255.2
  male (without gonadal disorder)
      752.7
    with
      adrenocortical disorder 255.2
      cleft scrotum 752.7
      feminizing testis 259.51
      gonadal disorder 257.9
      adrenal 255.2
Pseudohole, macula 362.54
Pseudo-Hurler's disease (mucolipidosis
    III) 272.7
Pseudohydrocephalus 348.2
Pseudohypertrophic muscular dystrophy
    (Erb's) 359.1
Pseudohypertrophy, muscle 359.1
Pseudohypoparathyroidism 275.49
Pseudoinfluenza 487.1
Pseudoinsomnia 307.49
Pseudoleukemia 288.8
  infantile 285.8
Pseudomembranous - see condition
Pseudomeningocele (cerebral) (infective)
    349.2
  postprocedural 997.01
  spinal 349.2
Pseudomenstruation 626.8
Pseudomucinous
  cyst (ovary) (M8470/0) 220
  peritoneum 568.89
Pseudomyeloma 273.1
Pseudomyxoma peritonei (M8480/6)
    197.6
Pseudoneuritis optic (nerve) 377.24
  papilla 377.24
    congenital 743.57
Pseudoneuroma - see Injury, nerve, by site
Pseudo-obstruction
  intestine (chronic) (idiopathic)
      (intermittent secondary)
      (primary) 564.89
    acute 560.89
Pseudopapilledema 377.24

Pseudoparalysis
  arm or leg 781.4
  atonic, congenital 358.8
Pseudopelade 704.09
Pseudophakia V43.1
Pseudopolycythemia 289.0
Pseudopolyposis, colon 556.4
Pseudoporencephaly 348.0
Pseudopseudohypoparathyroidism 275.49
Pseudopsychosis 300.16
Pseudopterygium 372.52
Pseudoptosis (eyelid) 374.34
Pseudorabies 078.89
Pseudoretinitis, pigmentosa 362.65
Pseudorickets 588.0
  senile (Pozzi's) 731.0
Pseudorubella 057.8
Pseudoscarlatina 057.8
Pseudosclerema 778.1
Pseudosclerosis (brain)
  Jakob's 046.19
  of Westphal (-Strümpell)
      (hepatolenticular degeneration)
      275.1
  spastic 046.19
    with dementia
      with behavioral disturbance
          046.19 [294.11]
      without behavioral disturbance
          046.19 [294.10]
Pseudoseizure 780.39
  non-psychiatric 780.39
  psychiatric 300.11
Pseudotabes 799.89
  diabetic 250.6● [337.1]
    due to secondary diabetes 249.6●
        [337.1]
Pseudotetanus (see also Convulsions)
    780.39
Pseudotetany 781.7
  hysterical 300.11
Pseudothalassemia 285.0
Pseudotrichinosis 710.3
Pseudotruncus arteriosus 747.29
Pseudotuberculosis, pasteurella
    (infection) 027.2
Pseudotumor
  cerebri 348.2
  orbit (inflammatory) 376.11
Pseudo-Turner's syndrome 759.89
Pseudoxanthoma elasticum 757.39
Psilosis (sprue) (tropical) 579.1
  Monilia 112.89
  nontropical 579.0
  not sprue 704.00
Psittacosis 073.9
Psoitis 728.89
Psora NEC 696.1
Psoriasis 696.1
  any type, except arthropathic 696.1
  arthritic, arthropathic 696.0
  buccal 528.6
  flexural 696.1
  follicularis 696.1
  guttate 696.1
  inverse 696.1
  mouth 528.6
  nummularis 696.1
  psychogenic 316 [696.1]
  punctata 696.1
  pustular 696.1
  rupioides 696.1
  vulgaris 696.1
Psorospermiasis 136.4

Psorospermosis 136.4
  follicularis (vegetans) 757.39
Psychalgia 307.80
Psychasthenia 300.89
  compulsive 300.3
  mixed compulsive states 300.3
  obsession 300.3
Psychiatric disorder or problem NEC
    300.9
Psychogenic - see also condition
  factors associated with physical
      conditions 316
Psychoneurosis, psychoneurotic (see also
    Neurosis) 300.9
  anxiety (state) 300.00
  climacteric 627.2
  compensation 300.16
  compulsion 300.3
  conversion hysteria 300.11
  depersonalization 300.6
  depressive type 300.4
  dissociative hysteria 300.15
  hypochondriacal 300.7
  hysteria 300.10
    conversion type 300.11
    dissociative type 300.15
  mixed NEC 300.89
  neurasthenic 300.5
  obsessional 300.3
  obsessive-compulsive 300.3
  occupational 300.89
  personality NEC 301.89
  phobia 300.20
  senile NEC 300.89
Psychopathic - see also condition
  constitution, posttraumatic 310.2
    with psychosis 293.9
  personality 301.9
    amoral trends 301.7
    antisocial trends 301.7
    asocial trends 301.7
    mixed types 301.7
    state 301.9
Psychopathy, sexual (see also Deviation,
    sexual) 302.9
Psychophysiologic, psychophysiological
    condition - see Reaction,
    psychophysiologic
Psychose passionelle 297.8
Psychosexual identity disorder 302.6
  adult-life 302.85
  childhood 302.6
Psychosis 298.9
  acute hysterical 298.1
  affecting management of pregnancy,
      childbirth, or puerperium 648.4●
  affective (see also Disorder, mood) 296.90

┌───┐
│ Note 63   Use the following fifth-digit │
│ subclassification with categories   │
│ 296.0–296.6:   │
│   │
│   0   unspecified   │
│   1   mild   │
│   2   moderate   │
│   3   severe, without mention of   │
│   psychotic behavior   │
│   4   severe, specified as with   │
│   psychotic behavior   │
│   5   in partial or unspecified remission│
│   6   in full remission   │
└───┘

  drug-induced 292.84
  due to or associated with physical
      condition 293.9

Psychosis (*Continued*)
  affective (*Continued*)
    involutional 293.83
      recurrent episode 296.3●
      single episode 296.2●
    manic-depressive 296.80
      circular (alternating) 296.7
        currently depressed 296.5●
        currently manic 296.4●
      depressed type 296.2●
        atypical 296.82
        recurrent episode 296.3●
        single episode 296.2●
      manic 296.0●
        atypical 296.81
        recurrent episode 296.1●
        single episode 296.0●
      mixed type NEC 296.89
      specified type NEC 296.89
    senile 290.21
    specified type NEC 296.99
  alcoholic 291.9
    with
      anxiety 291.89
      delirium tremens 291.0
      delusions 291.5
      dementia 291.2
      hallucinosis 291.3
      jealousy 291.5
      mood disturbance 291.89
      paranoia 291.5
      persisting amnesia 291.1
      sexual dysfunction 291.89
      sleep disturbance 291.89
    amnestic confabulatory 291.1
    delirium tremens 291.0
    hallucinosis 291.3
    Korsakoff's, Korsakov's, Korsakow's 291.1
    paranoid type 291.5
    pathological intoxication 291.4
    polyneuritic 291.1
    specified type NEC 291.89
  alternating (*see also* Psychosis, manic-depressive, circular) 296.7
  anergastic (*see also* Psychosis, organic) 294.9
  arteriosclerotic 290.40
    with
      acute confusional state 290.41
      delirium 290.41
      delusions 290.42
      depressed mood 290.43
    depressed type 290.43
    paranoid type 290.42
    simple type 290.40
    uncomplicated 290.40
  atypical 298.9
    depressive 296.82
    manic 296.81
  borderline (schizophrenia) (*see also* Schizophrenia) 295.5●
  of childhood (*see also* Psychosis, childhood) 299.8●
    prepubertal 299.8●
  brief reactive 298.8
  childhood, with origin specific to 299.9●

> Note 64　Use the following fifth-digit subclassification with category 299:
>
> 0　current or active state
> 1　residual state

Psychosis (*Continued*)
  childhood, with origin specific to (*Continued*)
    atypical 299.8●
    specified type NEC 299.8●
  circular (*see also* Psychosis, manic-depressive, circular) 296.7
  climacteric (*see also* Psychosis, involutional) 298.8
  confusional 298.9
    acute 293.0
    reactive 298.2
    subacute 293.1
  depressive (*see also* Psychosis, affective) 296.2●
    atypical 296.82
    involutional 296.2●
      with hypomania (bipolar II) 296.89
      recurrent episode 296.3●
      single episode 296.2●
    psychogenic 298.0
    reactive (emotional stress) (psychological trauma) 298.0
    recurrent episode 296.3●
      with hypomania (bipolar II) 296.89
    single episode 296.2●
  disintegrative, childhood (*see also* Psychosis, childhood) 299.1●
  drug 292.9
    with
      affective syndrome 292.84
      amnestic syndrome 292.83
      anxiety 292.89
      delirium 292.81
        withdrawal 292.0
      delusions 292.11
      dementia 292.82
      depressive state 292.84
      hallucinations 292.12
      hallucinosis 292.12
      mood disorder 292.84
      mood disturbance 292.84
      organic personality syndrome NEC 292.89
      sexual dysfunction 292.89
      sleep disturbance 292.89
      withdrawal syndrome (and delirium) 292.0
    affective syndrome 292.84
    delusions 292.11
    hallucinatory state 292.12
    hallucinosis 292.12
    paranoid state 292.11
    specified type NEC 292.89
    withdrawal syndrome (and delirium) 292.0
  due to or associated with physical condition (*see also* Psychosis, organic) 294.9
  epileptic NEC 293.9
  excitation (psychogenic) (reactive) 298.1
  exhaustive (*see also* Reaction, stress, acute) 308.9
  hypomanic (*see also* Psychosis, affective) 296.0●
    recurrent episode 296.1●
    single episode 296.0●
  hysterical 298.8
    acute 298.1
  incipient 298.8
    schizophrenic (*see also* Schizophrenia) 295.5●

Psychosis (*Continued*)
  induced 297.3
  infantile (*see also* Psychosis, childhood) 299.0●
  infective 293.9
    acute 293.0
    subacute 293.1
  in
    conditions classified elsewhere
      with
        delusions 293.81
        hallucinations 293.82
    pregnancy, childbirth, or puerperium 648.4●
  interactional (childhood) (*see also* Psychosis, childhood) 299.1●
  involutional 298.8
    depressive (*see also* Psychosis, affective) 296.2●
      recurrent episode 296.3●
      single episode 296.2●
    melancholic 296.2●
      recurrent episode 296.3●
      single episode 296.2●
    paranoid state 297.2
    paraphrenia 297.2
  Korsakoff's, Korakov's, Korsakow's (nonalcoholic) 294.0
    alcoholic 291.1
  mania (phase) (*see also* Psychosis, affective) 296.0●
    recurrent episode 296.1●
    single episode 296.0●
  manic (*see also* Psychosis, affective) 296.0●
    atypical 296.81
    recurrent episode 296.1●
    single episode 296.0●
  manic-depressive 296.80
    circular 296.7
      currently
        depressed 296.5●
        manic 296.4●
      mixed 296.6●
    depressive 296.2●
      recurrent episode 296.3●
        with hypomania (bipolar II) 296.89
      single episode 296.2●
    hypomanic 296.0●
      recurrent episode 296.1●
      single episode 296.0●
    manic 296.0●
      atypical 296.81
      recurrent episode 296.1●
      single episode 296.0●
    mixed NEC 296.89
    perplexed 296.89
    stuporous 296.89
  menopausal (*see also* Psychosis, involutional) 298.8
  mixed schizophrenic and affective (*see also* Schizophrenia) 295.7●
  multi-infarct (cerebrovascular) (*see also* Psychosis, arteriosclerotic) 290.40
  organic NEC 294.9
    due to or associated with
      addiction
        alcohol (*see also* Psychosis, alcoholic) 291.9
        drug (*see also* Psychosis, drug) 292.9

◄ New　◄▥ Revised　~~deleted~~ Deleted　● Use Additional Digit(s)　▨ Omit code

Psychosis (Continued)
organic NEC (Continued)
due to or associated with (Continued)
alcohol intoxication, acute (see also Psychosis, alcoholic) 291.9
alcoholism (see also Psychosis, alcoholic) 291.9
arteriosclerosis (cerebral) (see also Psychosis, arteriosclerotic) 290.40
cerebrovascular disease
acute (psychosis) 293.0
arteriosclerotic (see also Psychosis, arteriosclerotic) 290.40
childbirth - see Psychosis, puerperal
dependence
alcohol (see also Psychosis, alcoholic) 291.9
drug 292.9
disease
alcoholic liver (see also Psychosis, alcoholic) 291.9
brain
arteriosclerotic (see also Psychosis, arteriosclerotic) 290.40
cerebrovascular
acute (psychosis) 293.0
arteriosclerotic (see also Psychosis, arteriosclerotic) 290.40
endocrine or metabolic 293.9
acute (psychosis) 293.0
subacute (psychosis) 293.1
Jakob-Creutzfeldt 046.19
with behavioral disturbance 046.19 [294.11]
without behavioral disturbance 046.19 [294.10]
familial 046.19
iatrogenic 046.19
specified NEC 046.19
sporadic 046.19
variant 046.11
with dementia
with behavioral disturbance 046.11 [294.11]
without behavioral disturbance 046.11 [294.10]
liver, alcoholic (see also Psychosis, alcoholic) 291.9
disorder
cerebrovascular
acute (psychosis) 293.0
endocrine or metabolic 293.9
acute (psychosis) 293.0
subacute (psychosis) 293.1
epilepsy
with behavioral disturbance 345.9 [294.11]●
without behavioral disturbance 345.9 [294.10]●
transient (acute) 293.0

Psychosis (Continued)
organic NEC (Continued)
due to or associated with (Continued)
Huntington's chorea
with behavioral disturbance 333.4 [294.11]
without behavioral disturbance 333.4 [294.10]
infection
brain 293.9
acute (psychosis) 293.0
chronic 294.8
subacute (psychosis) 293.1
intracranial NEC 293.9
acute (psychosis) 293.0
chronic 294.8
subacute (psychosis) 293.1
intoxication
alcoholic (acute) (see also Psychosis, alcoholic) 291.9
pathological 291.4
drug (see also Psychosis, drug) 292.9
ischemia
cerebrovascular (generalized) (see also Psychosis, arteriosclerotic) 290.40
Jakob-Creutzfeldt disease (syndrome) 046.19
with behavioral disturbance 046.19 [294.11]
without behavioral disturbance 046.19 [294.10]
variant 046.11
with dementia
with behavioral disturbance 046.11 [294.11]
without behavioral disturbance 046.11 [294.10]
multiple sclerosis
with behavioral disturbance 340 [294.11]
without behavioral disturbance 340 [294.10]
physical condition NEC 293.9
with
delusions 293.81
hallucinations 293.82
presenility 290.10
puerperium - see Psychosis, puerperal
sclerosis, multiple
with behavioral disturbance 340 [294.11]
without behavioral disturbance 340 [294.10]
senility 290.20
status epilepticus
with behavioral disturbance 345.3 [294.11]
without behavioral disturbance 345.3 [294.10]
trauma
brain (birth) (from electrical current) (surgical) 293.9
acute (psychosis) 293.0
chronic 294.8
subacute (psychosis) 293.1

Psychosis (Continued)
organic NEC (Continued)
due to or associated with (Continued)
unspecified physical condition 293.9
with
delusions 293.81
hallucinations 293.82
infective 293.9
acute (psychosis) 293.0
subacute 293.1
posttraumatic 293.9
acute 293.0
subacute 293.1
specified type NEC 294.8
transient 293.9
with
anxiety 293.84
delusions 293.81
depression 293.83
hallucinations 293.82
depressive type 293.83
hallucinatory type 293.82
paranoid type 293.81
specified type NEC 293.89
paranoic 297.1
paranoid (chronic) 297.9
alcoholic 291.5
chronic 297.1
climacteric 297.2
involutional 297.2
menopausal 297.2
protracted reactive 298.4
psychogenic 298.4
acute 298.3
schizophrenic (see also Schizophrenia) 295.3●
senile 290.20
paroxysmal 298.9
senile 290.20
polyneuritic, alcoholic 291.1
postoperative 293.9
postpartum - see Psychosis, puerperal
prepsychotic (see also Schizophrenia) 295.5●
presbyophrenic (type) 290.8
presenile (see also Dementia, presenile) 290.10
prison 300.16
psychogenic 298.8
depressive 298.0
paranoid 298.4
acute 298.3
puerperal
specified type - see categories 295–298
unspecified type 293.89
acute 293.0
chronic 293.89
subacute 293.1
reactive (emotional stress) (psychological trauma) 298.8
brief 298.8
confusion 298.2
depressive 298.0
excitation 298.1
schizo-affective (depressed) (excited) (see also Schizophrenia) 295.7●
schizophrenia, schizophrenic (see also Schizophrenia) 295.9●
borderline type 295.5●
of childhood (see also Psychosis, childhood) 299.8●

Psychosis (Continued)
  schizophrenia, schizophrenic
    (Continued)
    catatonic (excited) (withdrawn)
      295.2●
    childhood type (see also Psychosis,
      childhood) 299.9●
    hebephrenic 295.1●
    incipient 295.5●
    latent 295.5●
    paranoid 295.3●
    prepsychotic 295.5●
    prodromal 295.5●
    pseudoneurotic 295.5●
    pseudopsychopathic 295.5●
    schizophreniform 295.4●
    simple 295.0●
    undifferentiated type 295.9●
  schizophreniform 295.4●
  senile NEC 290.20
    with
      delusional features 290.20
      depressive features 290.21
    depressed type 290.21
    paranoid type 290.20
    simple deterioration 290.20
    specified type - see categories 295–298
  shared 297.3
  situational (reactive) 298.8
  symbiotic (childhood) (see also
    Psychosis, childhood) 299.1●
  toxic (acute) 293.9
Psychotic (see also condition) 298.9
  episode 298.9
    due to or associated with physical
      conditions (see also Psychosis,
      organic) 293.9
Pterygium (eye) 372.40
  central 372.43
  colli 744.5
  double 372.44
  peripheral (stationary) 372.41
    progressive 372.42
  recurrent 372.45
Ptilosis 374.55
PTLD (post-transplant
  lymphoproliferative disorder)
  238.77
Ptomaine (poisoning) (see also Poisoning,
  food) 005.9
Ptosis (adiposa) 374.30
  breast 611.81
  cecum 569.89
  colon 569.89
  congenital (eyelid) 743.61
    specified site NEC - see Anomaly,
      specified type NEC
  epicanthus syndrome 270.2
  eyelid 374.30
    congenital 743.61
    mechanical 374.33
    myogenic 374.32
    paralytic 374.31
  gastric 537.5
  intestine 569.89
  kidney (see also Disease, renal) 593.0
    congenital 753.3
  liver 573.8
  renal (see also Disease, renal) 593.0
    congenital 753.3
  splanchnic 569.89
  spleen 289.59
  stomach 537.5
  viscera 569.89

PTSD (Post-Traumatic Stress Disorder)
  309.81
Ptyalism 527.7
  hysterical 300.11
  periodic 527.2
  pregnancy 646.8●
  psychogenic 306.4
Ptyalolithiasis 527.5
Pubalgia 848.8
Pubarche, precocious 259.1
Pubertas praecox 259.1
Puberty V21.1
  abnormal 259.9
  bleeding 626.3
  delayed 259.0
  precocious (constitutional)
    (cryptogenic) (idiopathic) NEC
    259.1
    due to
      adrenal
        cortical hyperfunction 255.2
        hyperplasia 255.2
      cortical hyperfunction 255.2
      ovarian hyperfunction 256.1
        estrogen 256.0
      pineal tumor 259.8
      testicular hyperfunction 257.0
  premature 259.1
    due to
      adrenal cortical hyperfunction
      255.2
      pineal tumor 259.8
      pituitary (anterior) hyperfunction
      253.1
Puckering, macula 362.56
Pudenda, pudendum - see condition
Puente's disease (simple glandular
  cheilitis) 528.5
Puerperal
  abscess
    areola 675.1●
    Bartholin's gland 646.6●
    breast 675.1●
    cervix (uteri) 670.8 ◀━
    fallopian tube 670.8 ◀━
    genital organ 670.8 ◀━
    kidney 646.6●
    mammary 675.1●
    mesosalpinx 670.8 ◀━
    nabothian 646.6●
    nipple 675.0●
    ovary, ovarian 670.8 ◀━
    oviduct 670.8 ◀━
    parametric 670.8 ◀━
    para-uterine 670.8 ◀━
    pelvic 670.8 ◀━
    perimetric 670.8 ◀━
    periuterine 670.8 ◀━
    retro-uterine 670.8 ◀━
    subareolar 675.1●
    suprapelvic 670.8 ◀━
    tubal (ruptured) 670.8 ◀━
    tubo-ovarian 670.8 ◀━
    urinary tract NEC 646.6●
    uterine, uterus 670.8 ◀━
    vagina (wall) 646.6●
    vaginorectal 646.6●
    vulvovaginal gland 646.6●
  accident 674.9●
  adnexitis 670.8 ◀━
  afibrinogenemia, or other coagulation
    defect 666.3●
  albuminuria (acute) (subacute) 646.2●
    pre-eclamptic 642.4●

Puerperal (Continued)
  anemia (conditions classifiable to
    280–285) 648.2●
  anuria 669.3●
  apoplexy 674.0●
  asymptomatic bacteriuria 646.5●
  atrophy, breast 676.3●
  blood dyscrasia 666.3●
  caked breast 676.2●
  cardiomyopathy 674.5●
  cellulitis - see Puerperal, abscess
  cerebrovascular disorder (conditions
    classifiable to 430–434, 436–437)
    674.0●
  cervicitis (conditions classifiable to
    616.0) 646.6●
  coagulopathy (any) 666.3●
  complications 674.9●
    specified type NEC 674.8●
  convulsions (eclamptic) (uremic)
    642.6●
    with pre-existing hypertension
      642.7●
  cracked nipple 676.1●
  cystitis 646.6●
  cystopyelitis 646.6●
  deciduitis (acute) 670.8 ◀━
  delirium NEC 293.9
  diabetes (mellitus) (conditions
    classifiable to 249 and 250)
    648.0●
  disease 674.9●
    breast NEC 676.3●
    cerebrovascular (acute) 674.0●
    nonobstetric NEC (see also
      Pregnancy, complicated,
      current disease or condition)
      648.9●
    pelvis inflammatory 670.8 ◀━
    renal NEC 646.2●
    tubo-ovarian 670.8 ◀━
    Valsuani's (progressive pernicious
      anemia) 648.2●
  disorder
    lactation 676.9●
      specified type NEC 676.8●
    nonobstetric NEC (see also
      Pregnancy, complicated,
      current disease or condition)
      648.9●
  disruption
    cesarean wound 674.1●
    episiotomy wound 674.2●
    perineal laceration wound 674.2●
  drug dependence (conditions
    classifiable to 304) 648.3●
  eclampsia 642.6●
    with pre-existing hypertension
      642.7●
  embolism (pulmonary) 673.2●
    air 673.0●
    amniotic fluid 673.1●
    blood clot 673.2●
    brain or cerebral 674.0●
    cardiac 674.8●
    fat 673.8●
    intracranial sinus (venous) 671.5●
    pyemic 673.3●
    septic 673.3●
    spinal cord 671.5●
  endometritis (conditions classifiable to
    615.0–615.9) 670.1 ◀━
  endophlebitis - see Puerperal, phlebitis
  endotrachelitis 646.6●

◀ New   ◀━ Revised   ~~deleted~~ Deleted   ● Use Additional Digit(s)   ▨ Omit code

Puerperal (Continued)
engorgement, breasts 676.2●
erysipelas 670.8 ⬅
failure
  lactation 676.4●
  renal, acute 669.3●
fever 670.8 ⬅
  meaning pyrexia (of unknown
    origin) 672●
  meaning sepsis 670.2 ⬅
  fissure, nipple 676.1●
fistula
  breast 675.1●
  mammary gland 675.1●
  nipple 675.0●
galactophoritis 675.2●
galactorrhea 676.6●
gangrene
  gas 670.8 ⬅
    with sepsis 670.2 ◀
  uterus 670.8 ⬅
gonorrhea (conditions classifiable to
  098) 647.1●
hematoma, subdural 674.0●
hematosalpinx, infectional 670.8 ⬅
hemiplegia, cerebral 674.0●
hemorrhage 666.1●
  brain 674.0●
  bulbar 674.0●
  cerebellar 674.0●
  cerebral 674.0●
  cortical 674.0●
  delayed (after 24 hours) (uterine)
    666.2●
  extradural 674.0●
  internal capsule 674.0●
  intracranial 674.0●
  intrapontine 674.0●
  meningeal 674.0●
  pontine 674.0●
  subarachnoid 674.0●
  subcortical 674.0●
  subdural 674.0●
  uterine, delayed 666.2●
  ventricular 674.0●
hemorrhoids 671.8●
hepatorenal syndrome 674.8●
hypertrophy
  breast 676.3●
  mammary gland 676.3●
induration breast (fibrous) 676.3●
infarction
  lung - see Puerperal, embolism
  pulmonary - see Puerperal,
    embolism
infection
  Bartholin's gland 646.6●
  breast 675.2●
    with nipple 675.9●
      specified type NEC 675.8●
  cervix 646.6●
  endocervix 646.6●
  fallopian tube 670.8 ⬅
  generalized 670.0 ⬅
  genital tract (major) 670.0 ⬅
    minor or localized 646.6●
  kidney (bacillus coli) 646.6●
  mammary gland 675.2●
    with nipple 675.9●
      specified type NEC 675.8●
  nipple 675.0●
    with breast 675.9●
      specified type NEC 675.8●
  ovary 670.8 ⬅

Puerperal (Continued)
infection (Continued)
  pelvic 670.8 ⬅
  peritoneum 670.8 ⬅
  renal 646.6●
  tubo-ovarian 670.8 ⬅
  urinary (tract) NEC 646.6●
    asymptomatic 646.5●
  uterus, uterine 670.8 ⬅
  vagina 646.6●
inflammation - see also Puerperal,
  infection
  areola 675.1●
  Bartholin's gland 646.6●
  breast 675.2●
  broad ligament 670.8 ⬅
  cervix (uteri) 646.6●
  fallopian tube 670.8 ⬅
  genital organs 670.8 ⬅
    localized 646.6●
  mammary gland 675.2●
  nipple 675.0●
  ovary 670.8 ⬅
  oviduct 670.8 ⬅
  pelvis 670.8 ⬅
  periuterine 670.8 ⬅
  tubal 670.8 ⬅
  vagina 646.6●
  vein - see Puerperal, phlebitis●
inversion, nipple 676.3●
ischemia, cerebral 674.0●
lymphangitis 670.8 ⬅
  breast 675.2●
malaria (conditions classifiable to 084)
  647.4●
malnutrition 648.9●
mammillitis 675.0●
mammitis 675.2●
mania 296.0●
  recurrent episode 296.1●
  single episode 296.0●
mastitis 675.2●
  purulent 675.1●
  retromammary 675.1●
  submammary 675.1●
melancholia 296.2●
  recurrent episode 296.3●
  single episode 296.2●
mental disorder (conditions
  classifiable to 290–303, 305.0,
  305.2–305.9, 306–316, 317–319)
  648.4●
metritis (septic) (suppurative) 670.1 ⬅
  septic 670.2 ◀
metroperitonitis 670.8 ⬅
metrorrhagia 666.2●
metrosalpingitis 670.8 ⬅
metrovaginitis 670.8 ⬅
milk leg 671.4●
monoplegia, cerebral 674.0●
necrosis
  kidney, tubular 669.3●
  liver (acute) (subacute) (conditions
    classifiable to 570) 674.8●
  ovary 670.8 ⬅
  renal cortex 669.3●
nephritis or nephrosis (conditions
  classifiable to 580–589) 646.2●
  with hypertension 642.1●
nutritional deficiency (conditions
  classifiable to 260–269) 648.9●
occlusion, precerebral artery 674.0●
oliguria 669.3●
oophoritis 670.8 ⬅
ovaritis 670.8 ⬅

Puerperal (Continued)
paralysis●
  bladder (sphincter) 665.5●
  cerebral 674.0●
paralytic stroke 674.0●
parametritis 670.8 ⬅
paravaginitis 646.6●
pelviperitonitis 670.8 ⬅
perimetritis 670.8 ⬅
perimetrosalpingitis 670.8 ⬅
perinephritis 646.6●
perioophoritis 670.8 ⬅
periphlebitis - see Puerperal, phlebitis
perisalpingitis 670.8 ⬅
peritoneal infection 670.8 ⬅
peritonitis (pelvic) 670.8 ⬅
perivaginitis 646.6●
phlebitis 671.2 ⬅
  deep 671.4●
  intracranial sinus (venous) 671.5●
  pelvic 671.4●
  specified site NEC 671.5●
  superficial 671.2●
phlegmasia alba dolens 671.4●
placental polyp 674.4●
pneumonia, embolic - see Puerperal,
  embolism
prediabetes 648.8●
pre-eclampsia (mild) 642.4●
  with pre-existing hypertension
    642.7●
  severe 642.5●
psychosis, unspecified (see also
  Psychosis, puerperal) 293.89●
pyelitis 646.6●
pyelocystitis 646.6●
pyelohydronephrosis 646.6●
pyelonephritis 646.6●
pyelonephrosis 646.6●
pyemia 670.2 ⬅
pyocystitis 646.6●
pyohemia 670.2 ⬅
pyometra 670.8 ⬅
pyonephritis 646.6●
pyonephrosis 646.6●
pyo-oophoritis 670.8 ⬅
pyosalpingitis 670.8 ⬅
pyosalpinx 670.8 ⬅
pyrexia (of unknown origin) 672●
renal
  disease NEC 646.2●
  failure, acute 669.3●
retention
  decidua (fragments) (with delayed
    hemorrhage) 666.2●
    without hemorrhage 667.1●
  placenta (fragments) (with delayed
    hemorrhage) 666.2●
    without hemorrhage 667.1●
  secundines (fragments) (with
    delayed hemorrhage) 666.2●
    without hemorrhage 667.1●
retracted nipple 676.0●
rubella (conditions classifiable to 056)
  647.5●
salpingitis 670.8 ⬅
salpingo-oophoritis 670.8 ⬅
salpingo-ovaritis 670.8 ⬅
salpingoperitonitis 670.8 ⬅
sapremia 670.2
secondary perineal tear 674.2●
sepsis (pelvic) 670.2 ⬅
septicemia 670.2 ⬅
subinvolution (uterus) 674.8●

Puerperal (Continued)
   sudden death (cause unknown) 674.9●
   suppuration - see Puerperal, abscess
   syphilis (conditions classifiable to 090–097) 647.0●
   tetanus 670.8 ◀▥
   thelitis 675.0●
   thrombocytopenia 666.3●
   thrombophlebitis (superficial) 671.2●
     deep 671.4●
     pelvic 671.4●
     septic 670.3 ◀
     specified site NEC 671.5●
   thrombosis (venous) - see Thrombosis, puerperal
   thyroid dysfunction (conditions classifiable to 240–246) 648.1●
   toxemia (see also Toxemia, of pregnancy) 642.4●
     eclamptic 642.6●
       with pre-existing hypertension 642.7●
     pre-eclamptic (mild) 642.4●
       with
         convulsions 642.6●
         pre-existing hypertension 642.7●
       severe 642.5●
   tuberculosis (conditions classifiable to 010–018) 647.3●
   uremia 669.3●
   vaginitis (conditions classifiable to 616.1) 646.6●
   varicose veins (legs) 671.0●
     vulva or perineum 671.1●
   venous complication 671.9 ◀
   vulvitis (conditions classifiable to 616.1) 646.6●
   vulvovaginitis (conditions classifiable to 616.1) 646.6●
   white leg 671.4●
Pulled muscle - see Sprain, by site
Pulmolithiasis 518.89
Pulmonary - see condition
Pulmonitis (unknown etiology) 486
Pulpitis (acute) (anachoretic) (chronic) (hyperplastic) (putrescent) (suppurative) (ulcerative) 522.0
Pulpless tooth 522.9
Pulse
   alternating 427.89
     psychogenic 306.2
   bigeminal 427.89
   fast 785.0
   feeble, rapid, due to shock following injury 958.4
   rapid 785.0
   slow 427.89
   strong 785.9
   trigeminal 427.89
   water-hammer (see also Insufficiency, aortic) 424.1
   weak 785.9
Pulseless disease 446.7
Pulsus
   alternans or trigeminy 427.89
     psychogenic 306.2
Punch drunk 310.2
Puncta lacrimalia occlusion 375.52
Punctiform hymen 752.49
Puncture (traumatic) - see also Wound, open, by site
   accidental, complicating surgery 998.2
   bladder, nontraumatic 596.6

Puncture (Continued)
   by
     device, implant, or graft - see Complications, mechanical
     foreign body
       internal organs - see also Injury, internal, by site
       by ingested object - see Foreign body
     left accidentally in operation wound 998.4
     instrument (any) during a procedure, accidental 998.2
   internal organs, abdomen, chest, or pelvis - see Injury, internal, by site
   kidney, nontraumatic 593.89
Pupil - see condition
Pupillary membrane 364.74
   persistent 743.46
Pupillotonia 379.46
   pseudotabetic 379.46
Purpura 287.2
   abdominal 287.0
   allergic 287.0
   anaphylactoid 287.0
   annularis telangiectodes 709.1
   arthritic 287.0
   autoerythrocyte sensitization 287.2
   autoimmune 287.0
   bacterial 287.0
   Bateman's (senile) 287.2
   capillary fragility (hereditary) (idiopathic) 287.8
   cryoglobulinemic 273.2
   devil's pinches 287.2
   fibrinolytic (see also Fibrinolysis) 286.6
   fulminans, fulminous 286.6
   gangrenous 287.0
   hemorrhagic (see also Purpura, thrombocytopenic) 287.39
     nodular 272.7
     nonthrombocytopenic 287.0
     thrombocytopenic 287.39
   Henoch's (purpura nervosa) 287.0
   Henoch-Schönlein (allergic) 287.0
   hypergammaglobulinemic (benign primary) (Waldenström's) 273.0
   idiopathic 287.31
     nonthrombocytopenic 287.0
     thrombocytopenic 287.31
   immune thrombocytopenic 287.31
   infectious 287.0
   malignant 287.0
   neonatorum 772.6
   nervosa 287.0
   newborn NEC 772.6
   nonthrombocytopenic 287.2
     hemorrhagic 287.0
     idiopathic 287.0
   nonthrombopenic 287.2
   peliosis rheumatica 287.0
   pigmentaria, progressiva 709.09
   posttransfusion 287.4
   primary 287.0
   primitive 287.0
   red cell membrane sensitivity 287.2
   rheumatica 287.0
   Schönlein (-Henoch) (allergic) 287.0
   scorbutic 267
   senile 287.2
   simplex 287.2
   symptomatica 287.0
   telangiectasia annularis 709.1

Purpura (Continued)
   thrombocytopenic (see also Thrombocytopenia) 287.30
     congenital 287.33
     essential 287.30
     hereditary 287.31
     idiopathic 287.31
     immune 287.31
     neonatal, transitory (see also Thrombocytopenia, neonatal transitory) 776.1
     primary 287.30
     puerperal, postpartum 666.3●
     thrombotic 446.6
   thrombohemolytic (see also Fibrinolysis) 286.6
   thrombopenic (see also Thrombocytopenia) 287.30
     congenital 287.33
     essential 287.30
   thrombotic 446.6
     thrombocytic 446.6
     thrombocytopenic 446.6
   toxic 287.0
   variolosa 050.0
   vascular 287.0
   visceral symptoms 287.0
   Werlhof's (see also Purpura, thrombocytopenic) 287.39
Purpuric spots 782.7
Purulent - see condition
Pus
   absorption, general - see Septicemia
   in
     stool 792.1
     urine 791.9
   tube (rupture) (see also Salpingo-oophoritis) 614.2
Pustular rash 782.1
Pustule 686.9
   malignant 022.0
   nonmalignant 686.9
Putnam's disease (subacute combined sclerosis with pernicious anemia) 281.0 [336.2]
Putnam-Dana syndrome (subacute combined sclerosis with pernicious anemia) 281.0 [336.2]
Putrefaction, intestinal 569.89
Putrescent pulp (dental) 522.1
Pyarthritis - see Pyarthrosis
Pyarthrosis (see also Arthritis, pyogenic) 711.0●
   tuberculous - see Tuberculosis, joint
Pycnoepilepsy, pycnolepsy (idiopathic) (see also Epilepsy) 345.0●
Pyelectasia 593.89
Pyelectasis 593.89
Pyelitis (congenital) (uremic) 590.80
   with
     abortion - see Abortion, by type, with specified complication NEC
     contracted kidney 590.00
     ectopic pregnancy (see also categories 633.0–633.9) 639.8
     molar pregnancy (see also categories 630–632) 639.8
   acute 590.10
     with renal medullary necrosis 590.11
   chronic 590.00
     with
       renal medullary necrosis 590.01

◀ New   ◀▥ Revised   ~~deleted~~ Deleted   ● Use Additional Digit(s)   ▥ Omit code

Pyelitis (*Continued*)
  complicating pregnancy, childbirth, or
      puerperium 646.6●
    affecting fetus or newborn 760.1
  cystica 590.3
  following
    abortion 639.8
    ectopic or molar pregnancy 639.8
  gonococcal 098.19
    chronic or duration of 2 months or
      over 098.39
  tuberculous (*see also* Tuberculosis)
    016.0● [*590.81*]
Pyelocaliectasis 593.89
Pyelocystitis (*see also* Pyelitis) 590.80
Pyelohydronephrosis 591
Pyelonephritis (*see also* Pyelitis) 590.80
  acute 590.10
    with renal medullary necrosis 590.11
  chronic 590.00
  syphilitic (late) 095.4
  tuberculous (*see also* Tuberculosis)
    016.0● [*590.81*]
Pyelonephrosis (*see also* Pyelitis) 590.80
  chronic 590.00
Pyelophlebitis 451.89
Pyelo-ureteritis cystica 590.3
Pyemia, pyemic (purulent) (*see also*
    Septicemia) 038.9
  abscess - *see* Abscess
  arthritis (*see also* Arthritis, pyogenic)
    711.0●
  Bacillus coli 038.42
  embolism (*see also* Septicemia) 415.12
  fever 038.9
  infection 038.9
  joint (*see also* Arthritis, pyogenic)
    711.0●
  liver 572.1
  meningococcal 036.2
  newborn 771.81
  phlebitis - *see* Phlebitis
  pneumococcal 038.2
  portal 572.1
  postvaccinal 999.39
  puerperal 670.2 ◀
  specified organism NEC 038.8
  staphylococcal 038.10
    aureus 038.11
      methicillin
        resistant 038.12
          susceptible 038.11
    specified organism NEC 038.19

Pyemia, pyemic (*Continued*)
  streptococcal 038.0
  tuberculous - *see* Tuberculosis,
    miliary
Pygopagus 759.4
Pykno-epilepsy, pyknolepsy
    (idiopathic) (*see also* Epilepsy)
    345.0●
Pyle (-Cohn) disease (craniometaphyseal
    dysplasia) 756.89
Pylephlebitis (suppurative) 572.1
Pylethrombophlebitis 572.1
Pylethrombosis 572.1
Pyloritis (*see also* Gastritis) 535.5●
Pylorospasm (reflex) 537.81
  congenital or infantile 750.5
  neurotic 306.4
  newborn 750.5
  psychogenic 306.4
Pylorus, pyloric - *see* condition
Pyoarthrosis - *see* Pyarthrosis
Pyocele
  mastoid 383.00
  sinus (accessory) (nasal) (*see also*
    Sinusitis) 473.9
  turbinate (bone) 473.9
  urethra (*see also* Urethritis) 597.0
Pyococcal dermatitis 686.00
Pyococcide, skin 686.00
Pyocolpos (*see also* Vaginitis)
    616.10
Pyocyaneus dermatitis 686.09
Pyocystitis (*see also* Cystitis) 595.9
Pyoderma, pyodermia 686.00
  gangrenosum 686.01
  specified type NEC 686.09
  vegetans 686.8
Pyodermatitis 686.00
  vegetans 686.8
Pyogenic - *see* condition
Pyohemia - *see* Septicemia
Pyohydronephrosis (*see also* Pyelitis)
    590.80
Pyometra 615.9
Pyometritis (*see also* Endometritis)
    615.9
Pyometrium (*see also* Endometritis)
    615.9
Pyomyositis 728.0
  ossificans 728.19
  tropical (bungpagga) 040.81
Pyonephritis (*see also* Pyelitis) 590.80
  chronic 590.00

Pyonephrosis (congenital) (*see also*
    Pyelitis) 590.80
  acute 590.10
Pyo-oophoritis (*see also* Salpingo-
    oophoritis) 614.2
Pyo-ovarium (*see also* Salpingo-
    oophoritis) 614.2
Pyopericarditis 420.99
Pyopericardium 420.99
Pyophlebitis - *see* Phlebitis
Pyopneumopericardium 420.99
Pyopneumothorax (infectional) 510.9
  with fistula 510.0
  subdiaphragmatic (*see also* Peritonitis)
    567.29
  subphrenic (*see also* Peritonitis)
    567.29
  tuberculous (*see also* Tuberculosis,
    pleura) 012.0●
Pyorrhea (alveolar) (alveolaris) 523.40
  degenerative 523.5
Pyosalpingitis (*see also* Salpingo-
    oophoritis) 614.2
Pyosalpinx (*see also* Salpingo-oophoritis)
    614.2
Pyosepticemia - *see* Septicemia
Pyosis
  Corlett's (impetigo) 684
  Manson's (pemphigus contagiosus)
    684
Pyothorax 510.9
  with fistula 510.0
  tuberculous (*see also* Tuberculosis,
    pleura) 012.0●
Pyoureter 593.89
  tuberculous (*see also* Tuberculosis)
    016.2●
Pyramidopallidonigral syndrome 332.0
Pyrexia (of unknown origin) (P.U.O.)
    780.60
  atmospheric 992.0
  during labor 659.2●
  environmentally-induced newborn
    778.4
  heat 992.0
  newborn, environmentally-induced
    778.4
  puerperal 672●
Pyroglobulinemia 273.8
Pyromania 312.33
Pyrosis 787.1
Pyrroloporphyria 277.1
Pyuria (bacterial) 791.9

Q

Q fever 083.0
  with pneumonia 083.0 *[484.8]*
Quadricuspid aortic valve 746.89
Quadrilateral fever 083.0
Quadriparesis - *see* Quadriplegia
  meaning muscle weakness 728.87
Quadriplegia 344.00
  with fracture, vertebra (process) - *see*
      Fracture, vertebra, cervical, with
      spinal cord injury
  brain (current episode) 437.8
  C₁–C₄
    complete 344.01
    incomplete 344.02
  C₅–C₇
    complete 344.03
    incomplete 344.04
  cerebral (current episode) 437.8
  congenital or infantile (cerebral)
      (spastic) (spinal) 343.2
  cortical 437.8
  embolic (current episode) (*see also*
      Embolism, brain) 434.1●
  functional 780.72

Quadriplegia (*Continued*)
  infantile (cerebral) (spastic) (spinal)
      343.2
  newborn NEC 767.0
  specified NEC 344.09
  thrombotic (current episode) (*see also*
      Thrombosis, brain) 434.0●
  traumatic - *see* Injury, spinal, cervical
Quadruplet
  affected by maternal complications of
      pregnancy 761.5
  healthy liveborn - *see* Newborn,
      multiple
  pregnancy (complicating delivery)
      NEC 651.8●
    with fetal loss and retention
        of one or more fetus(es)
        651.5●
    following (elective) fetal reduction
        651.7●
Quarrelsomeness 301.3
Quartan
  fever 084.2
  malaria (fever) 084.2
Queensland fever 083.0
  coastal 083.0
  seven-day 100.89

Quervain's disease 727.04
  thyroid (subacute granulomatous
      thyroiditis) 245.1
Queyrat's erythroplasia (M8080/2)
  specified site - *see* Neoplasm, skin, in
      situ
  unspecified site 233.5
Quincke's disease or edema - *see* Edema,
    angioneurotic
Quinquaud's disease (acne decalvans)
    704.09
Quinsy (gangrenous) 475
Quintan fever 083.1
Quintuplet
  affected by maternal complications of
      pregnancy 761.5
  healthy liveborn - *see* Newborn,
      multiple
  pregnancy (complicating delivery)
      NEC 651.2●
    with fetal loss and retention of one
        or more fetus(es) 651.6●
    following (elective) fetal reduction
        651.7●
Quotidian
  fever 084.0
  malaria (fever) 084.0

◄ New   ◄ⅢⅢ Revised   ~~deleted~~ Deleted   ● Use Additional Digit(s)   Omit code

R

Rabbia 071
Rabbit fever (*see also* Tularemia) 021.9
Rabies 071
    contact V01.5
    exposure to V01.5
    inoculation V04.5
        reaction - *see* Complications,
            vaccination
    vaccination, prophylactic (against)
        V04.5
Rachischisis (*see also* Spina bifida) 741.9●
Rachitic - *see also* condition
    deformities of spine 268.1
    pelvis 268.1
        with disproportion (fetopelvic)
            653.2●
            affecting fetus or newborn 763.1
            causing obstructed labor 660.1●
                affecting fetus or newborn
                    763.1
Rachitis, rachitism - *see also* Rickets
    acute 268.0
    fetalis 756.4
    renalis 588.0
    tarda 268.0
Racket nail 757.5
Radial nerve - *see* condition
Radiation effects or sickness - *see also*
    Effect, adverse, radiation
    cataract 366.46
    dermatitis 692.82
        sunburn (*see also* Sunburn) 692.71
Radiculitis (pressure) (vertebrogenic)
    729.2
    accessory nerve 723.4
    anterior crural 724.4
    arm 723.4
    brachial 723.4
    cervical NEC 723.4
    due to displacement of intervertebral
        disc - *see* Neuritis, due to,
        displacement intervertebral disc
    leg 724.4
    lumbar NEC 724.4
    lumbosacral 724.4
    rheumatic 729.2
    syphilitic 094.89
    thoracic (with visceral pain) 724.4
Radiculomyelitis 357.0
    toxic, due to
        Clostridium tetani 037
        corynebacterium diphtheriae 032.89
Radiculopathy (*see also* Radiculitis) 729.2
Radioactive substances, adverse effect -
    see Effect, adverse, radioactive
    substance
Radiodermal burns (acute) (chronic)
    (occupational) - *see* Burn, by site
Radiodermatitis 692.82
Radionecrosis - *see* Effect, adverse,
    radiation
Radiotherapy session V58.0
Radium, adverse effect - *see* Effect,
    adverse, radioactive substance
Raeder-Harbitz syndrome (pulseless
    disease) 446.7
Rage (*see also* Disturbance, conduct)
    312.0●
    meaning rabies 071
Rag sorters' disease 022.1
Raillietiniasis 123.8
Railroad neurosis 300.16

Railway spine 300.16
Raised - *see* Elevation
Raiva 071
Rake teeth, tooth 524.39
Rales 786.7
Ramifying renal pelvis 753.3
Ramsay Hunt syndrome (herpetic
    geniculate ganglionitis) 053.11
    meaning dyssynergia cerebellaris
        myoclonica 334.2
Ranke's primary infiltration (*see also*
    Tuberculosis) 010.0●
Ranula 527.6
    congenital 750.26
Rape
    adult 995.83
    alleged, observation or examination
        V71.5
    child 995.53
Rapid
    feeble pulse, due to shock, following
        injury 958.4
    heart (beat) 785.0
        psychogenic 306.2
    respiration 786.06
        psychogenic 306.1
    second stage (delivery) 661.3●
        affecting fetus or newborn 763.6
    time-zone change syndrome 327.35
Rarefaction, bone 733.99
Rash 782.1
    canker 034.1
    diaper 691.0
    drug (internal use) 693.0
        contact 692.3
    ECHO 9 virus 078.89
    enema 692.89
    food (*see also* Allergy, food) 693.1
    heat 705.1
    napkin 691.0
    nettle 708.8
    pustular 782.1
    rose 782.1
        epidemic 056.9
        of infants 057.8
    scarlet 034.1
    serum (prophylactic) (therapeutic)
        999.5
    toxic 782.1
    wandering tongue 529.1
Rasmussen's aneurysm (*see also*
    Tuberculosis) 011.2●
Rat-bite fever 026.9
    due to Streptobacillus moniliformis
        026.1
    spirochetal (morsus muris) 026.0
Rathke's pouch tumor (M9350/1) 237.0
Raymond (-Céstan) syndrome 433.8●
Raynaud's
    disease or syndrome (paroxysmal
        digital cyanosis) 443.0
    gangrene (symmetric) 443.0 [785.4]
    phenomenon (paroxysmal digital
        cyanosis) (secondary) 443.0
RDS 769
Reaction
    acute situational maladjustment (*see*
        also Reaction, adjustment) 309.9
    adaptation (*see also* Reaction,
        adjustment) 309.9
    adjustment 309.9
        with
            anxious mood 309.24
                with depressed mood 309.28

Reaction (*Continued*)
    adjustment (*Continued*)
        with (*Continued*)
            conduct disturbance 309.3
                combined with disturbance of
                    emotions 309.4
            depressed mood 309.0
                brief 309.0
                    with anxious mood
                      309.28
                prolonged 309.1
            elective mutism 309.83
            mixed emotions and conduct
                309.4
            mutism, elective 309.83
            physical symptoms 309.82
            predominant disturbance (of)
                conduct 309.3
                emotions NEC 309.29
                  mixed 309.28
                mixed, emotions and conduct
                  309.4
            specified type NEC 309.89
            specific academic or work
                inhibition 309.23
            withdrawal 309.83
        depressive 309.0
            with conduct disturbance
                309.4
            brief 309.0
            prolonged 309.1
            specified type NEC 309.89
    adverse food NEC 995.7
    affective (*see also* Psychosis, affective)
        296.90
        specified type NEC 296.99
    aggressive 301.3
        unsocialized (*see also* Disturbance,
            conduct) 312.0●
    allergic (*see also* Allergy) 995.3
        drug, medicinal substance, and
            biological - *see* Allergy, drug
        food - *see* Allergy, food
        serum 999.5
    anaphylactic - *see* Shock, anaphylactic
    anesthesia - *see* Anesthesia,
        complication
    anger 312.0●
    antisocial 301.7
    antitoxin (prophylactic) (therapeutic) -
        see Complications, vaccination
    anxiety 300.00
    Arthus 995.21
    asthenic 300.5
    compulsive 300.3
    conversion (anesthetic) (autonomic)
        (hyperkinetic) (mixed paralytic)
        (paresthetic) 300.11
    deoxyribonuclease (DNA)
        (DNase) hypersensitivity
        NEC 287.2
    depressive 300.4
        acute 309.0
        affective (*see also* Psychosis,
            affective) 296.2●
            recurrent episode 296.3●
            single episode 296.2●
        brief 309.0
        manic (*see also* Psychosis, affective)
            296.80
        neurotic 300.4
        psychoneurotic 300.4
        psychotic 298.0
    dissociative 300.15

Reaction (Continued)
  drug NEC (see also Table of Drugs and
      Chemicals) 995.20
    allergic - see also Allergy, drug
        995.27
    correct substance properly
        administered 995.20
    obstetric anesthetic or analgesic
        NEC 668.9●
      affecting fetus or newborn 763.5
    specified drug - see Table of
        Drugs and Chemicals
    overdose or poisoning 977.9
      specified drug - see Table of
          Drugs and Chemicals
    specific to newborn 779.4
    transmitted via placenta or breast
        milk - see Absorption, drug,
        through placenta
    withdrawal NEC 292.0
      infant of dependent mother
          779.5
    wrong substance given or taken in
        error 977.9
      specified drug - see Table of
          Drugs and Chemicals
  dyssocial 301.7
  dystonic, acute, due to drugs 333.72
  erysipeloid 027.1
  fear 300.20
    child 313.0
  fluid loss, cerebrospinal 349.0
  food - see also Allergy, food
    adverse NEC 995.7
    anaphylactic shock - see
        Anaphylactic shock, due to,
        food
  foreign
    body NEC 728.82
      in operative wound
          (inadvertently left) 998.4
        due to surgical material
            intentionally left - see
            Complications, due to
            (presence of) any device,
            implant, or graft
            classified to 996.0-996.5
            NEC
      substance accidentally left during a
          procedure (chemical) (powder)
          (talc) 998.7
      body or object (instrument)
          (sponge) (swab) 998.4
  graft-versus-host (GVH) 279.50
  grief (acute) (brief) 309.0
    prolonged 309.1
  gross stress (see also Reaction, stress,
      acute) 308.9
  group delinquent (see also Disturbance,
      conduct) 312.2●
  Herxheimer's 995.0
  hyperkinetic (see also Hyperkinesia)
      314.9
  hypochondriacal 300.7
  hypoglycemic, due to insulin 251.0
    therapeutic misadventure 962.3
  hypomanic (see also Psychosis,
      affective) 296.0●
    recurrent episode 296.1●
    single episode 296.0●
  hysterical 300.10
    conversion type 300.11
    dissociative 300.15
  id (bacterial cause) 692.89

Reaction (Continued)
  immaturity NEC 301.89
    aggressive 301.3
    emotional instability 301.59
  immunization - see Complications,
      vaccination
  incompatibility
    blood group (ABO) (infusion)
        (transfusion) 999.6   ◀▥
      ABO 999.6   ◀
      minor blood group 999.89   ◀
      Rh (factor) (infusion) (transfusion)
          999.7
  inflammatory - see Infection
  infusion - see Complications, infusion
  inoculation (immune serum) - see
      Complications, vaccination
  insulin 995.23
  involutional
    paranoid 297.2
    psychotic (see also Psychosis,
        affective, depressive) 296.2●
  leukemoid (basophilic) (lymphocytic)
      (monocytic) (myelocytic)
      (neutrophilic) 288.62
  LSD (see also Abuse, drugs,
      nondependent) 305.3●
  lumbar puncture 349.0
  manic-depressive (see also Psychosis,
      affective) 296.80
    depressed 296.2●
      recurrent episode 296.3●
      single episode 296.2●
    hypomanic 296.0●
  neurasthenic 300.5
  neurogenic (see also Neurosis) 300.9
  neurotic NEC 300.9
  neurotic-depressive 300.4
  nitritoid - see Crisis, nitritoid
  obsessive-compulsive 300.3
  organic 293.9
    acute 293.0
    subacute 293.1
  overanxious, child or adolescent 313.0
  paranoid (chronic) 297.9
    acute 298.3
    climacteric 297.2
    involutional 297.2
    menopausal 297.2
    senile 290.20
    simple 297.0
  passive
    aggressive 301.84
    dependency 301.6
  personality (see also Disorder,
      personality) 301.9
  phobic 300.20
  postradiation - see Effect, adverse,
      radiation
  psychogenic NEC 300.9
  psychoneurotic (see also Neurosis) 300.9
    anxiety 300.00
    compulsive 300.3
    conversion 300.11
    depersonalization 300.6
    depressive 300.4
    dissociative 300.15
    hypochondriacal 300.7
    hysterical 300.10
      conversion type 300.11
      dissociative type 300.15
    neurasthenic 300.5
    obsessive 300.3
    obsessive-compulsive 300.3
    phobic 300.20
    tension state 300.9

Reaction (Continued)
  psychophysiologic NEC (see also
      Disorder, psychosomatic) 306.9
    cardiovascular 306.2
    digestive 306.4
    endocrine 306.6
    gastrointestinal 306.4
    genitourinary 306.50
    heart 306.2
    hemic 306.8
    intestinal (large) (small) 306.4
    laryngeal 306.1
    lymphatic 306.8
    musculoskeletal 306.0
    pharyngeal 306.1
    respiratory 306.1
    skin 306.3
    special sense organs 306.7
  psychosomatic (see also Disorder,
      psychosomatic) 306.9
  psychotic (see also Psychosis) 298.9
    depressive 298.0
    due to or associated with physical
        condition (see also Psychosis,
        organic) 293.9
    involutional (see also Psychosis,
        affective) 296.2●
      recurrent episode 296.3●
      single episode 296.2●
  pupillary (myotonic) (tonic) 379.46
  radiation - see Effect, adverse,
      radiation
  runaway - see also Disturbance,
      conduct
    socialized 312.2●
    undersocialized, unsocialized
        312.1●
  scarlet fever toxin - see Complications,
      vaccination
  schizophrenic (see also Schizophrenia)
      295.9●
    latent 295.5●
  serological for syphilis - see Serology
      for syphilis
  serum (prophylactic) (therapeutic)
      999.5
    immediate 999.4
  situational (see also Reaction,
      adjustment) 309.9
    acute, to stress 308.3
    adjustment (see also Reaction,
        adjustment) 309.9
  somatization (see also Disorder,
      psychosomatic) 306.9
  spinal puncture 349.0
  spite, child (see also Disturbance,
      conduct) 312.0●
  stress, acute 308.9
    with predominant disturbance (of)
      consciousness 308.1
      emotions 308.0
      mixed 308.4
      psychomotor 308.2
      specified type NEC 308.3
    bone or cartilage - see Fracture, stress
  surgical procedure - see Complications,
      surgical procedure
  tetanus antitoxin - see Complications,
      vaccination
  toxin-antitoxin - see Complications,
      vaccination
  transfusion (blood) (bone marrow)
      (lymphocytes) (allergic) - see
      Complications, transfusion

◀ New   ◀▥ Revised   ~~deleted~~ Deleted   ● Use Additional Digit(s)   ▓ Omit code

Reaction (*Continued*)
  tuberculin skin test, nonspecific
      (without active tuberculosis)
      795.5
    positive (without active
        tuberculosis) 795.5
  ultraviolet - *see* Effect, adverse,
      ultraviolet
  undersocialized, unsocialized - *see also*
      Disturbance, conduct
    aggressive (type) 312.0●
    unaggressive (type) 312.1●
  vaccination (any) - *see* Complications,
      vaccination
  white graft (skin) 996.52
  withdrawing, child or adolescent
      313.22
  x-ray - *see* Effect, adverse, x-rays
Reactive depression (*see also* Reaction,
    depressive) 300.4
  neurotic 300.4
  psychoneurotic 300.4
  psychotic 298.0
Rebound tenderness 789.6●
Recalcitrant patient V15.81
Recanalization, thrombus - *see*
    Thrombosis
Recession, receding
  chamber angle (eye) 364.77
  chin 524.06
  gingival (postinfective) (postoperative)
      523.20
    generalized 523.25
    localized 523.24
    minimal 523.21
    moderate 523.22
    severe 523.23
Recklinghausen's disease (M9540/1)
    237.71
  bones (osteitis fibrosa cystica) 252.01
Recklinghausen-Applebaum disease
    (hemochromatosis) 275.0
Reclus' disease (cystic) 610.1
Recrudescent typhus (fever) 081.1
Recruitment, auditory 388.44
Rectalgia 569.42
Rectitis 569.49
Rectocele
  female (without uterine prolapse)
      618.04
    with uterine prolapse 618.4
      complete 618.3
      incomplete 618.2
    in pregnancy or childbirth 654.4●
      causing obstructed labor 660.2●
        affecting fetus or newborn 763.1
  male 569.49
  vagina, vaginal (outlet) 618.04
Rectosigmoiditis 569.89
  ulcerative (chronic) 556.3
Rectosigmoid junction - *see* condition
Rectourethral - *see* condition
Rectovaginal - *see* condition
Rectovesical - *see* condition
Rectum, rectal - *see* condition
Recurrent - *see* condition
Red bugs 133.8
Red cedar asthma 495.8
Redness
  conjunctiva 379.93
  eye 379.93
  nose 478.19
Reduced ventilatory or vital capacity
    794.2

Reduction
  function
    kidney (*see also* Disease, renal)
        593.9
    liver 573.8
  ventilatory capacity 794.2
  vital capacity 794.2
Redundant, redundancy
  abdomen 701.9
  anus 751.5
  cardia 537.89
  clitoris 624.2
  colon (congenital) 751.5
  foreskin (congenital) 605
  intestine 751.5
  labia 624.3
  organ or site, congenital NEC - *see*
      Accessory
  panniculus (abdominal) 278.1
  prepuce (congenital) 605
  pylorus 537.89
  rectum 751.5
  scrotum 608.89
  sigmoid 751.5
  skin (of face) 701.9
    eyelids 374.30
  stomach 537.89
  uvula 528.9
  vagina 623.8
Reduplication - *see* Duplication
Referral
  adoption (agency) V68.89
  nursing care V63.8
  patient without examination or
      treatment V68.81
  social services V63.8
Reflex - *see also* condition
  blink, deficient 374.45
  hyperactive gag 478.29
  neurogenic bladder NEC 596.54
    atonic 596.54
      with cauda equina syndrome
          344.61
  vasoconstriction 443.9
  vasovagal 780.2
Reflux 530.81
  acid 530.81
  esophageal 530.81
    with esophagitis 530.11
  esophagitis 530.11
  gastroesophageal 530.81
  mitral - *see* Insufficiency, mitral
  ureteral - *see* Reflux, vesicoureteral
  vesicoureteral 593.70
    with
      reflux nephropathy 593.73
        bilateral 593.72
        unilateral 593.71
Reformed gallbladder 576.0
Reforming, artificial openings (*see also*
    Attention to, artificial, opening)
    V55.9
Refractive error (*see also* Error, refractive)
    367.9
Refsum's disease or syndrome
    (heredopathia atactica
    polyneuritiformis) 356.3
Refusal of
  food 307.59
    hysterical 300.11
  treatment because of, due to
    patient's decision NEC V64.2
    reason of conscience or religion
        V62.6

Regaud
  tumor (M8082/3) - *see* Neoplasm,
      nasopharynx, malignant
  type carcinoma (M8082/3) - *see*
      Neoplasm, nasopharynx,
      malignant
Regional - *see* condition
Regulation feeding (elderly)
    (infant) 783.3
  newborn 779.31 ◀▥
Regurgitated
  food, choked on 933.1
  stomach contents, choked on 933.1
Regurgitation 787.03
  aortic (valve) (*see also* Insufficiency,
      aortic) 424.1
    congenital 746.4
    syphilitic 093.22
  food - *see also* Vomiting
    with reswallowing - *see* Rumination
    newborn 779.33 ◀▥
  gastric contents - *see* Vomiting
  heart - *see* Endocarditis
  mitral (valve) - *see also* Insufficiency,
      mitral
    congenital 746.6
  myocardial - *see* Endocarditis
  pulmonary (heart) (valve) (*see also*
      Endocarditis, pulmonary) 424.3
  stomach - *see* Vomiting
  tricuspid - *see* Endocarditis, tricuspid
  valve, valvular - *see* Endocarditis
  vesicoureteral - *see* Reflux,
      vesicoureteral
Rehabilitation V57.9
  multiple types V57.89
  occupational V57.21
  specified type NEC V57.89
  speech (-language) V57.3 ◀▥
  vocational V57.22
Reichmann's disease or syndrome
    (gastrosuccorrhea) 536.8
Reifenstein's syndrome (hereditary
    familial hypogonadism, male)
    259.52
Reilly's syndrome or phenomenon (*see
    also* Neuropathy, peripheral,
    autonomic) 337.9
Reimann's periodic disease 277.31
Reinsertion, contraceptive device V25.42
Reiter's disease, syndrome, or urethritis
    099.3 *[711.1]*●
Rejection
  food, hysterical 300.11
  transplant 996.80
    bone marrow 996.85
    corneal 996.51
    organ (immune or nonimmune
        cause) 996.80
      bone marrow 996.85
      heart 996.83
      intestines 996.87
      kidney 996.81
      liver 996.82
      lung 996.84
      pancreas 996.86
      specified NEC 996.89
    skin 996.52
      artificial 996.55
      decellularized allodermis 996.55
Relapsing fever 087.9
  Carter's (Asiatic) 087.0
  Dutton's (West African) 087.1
  Koch's 087.9

Relapsing fever (*Continued*)
  louse-borne (epidemic) 087.0
  Novy's (American) 087.1
  Obermeyer's (European) 087.0
  Spirillum 087.9
  tick-borne (endemic) 087.1
Relaxation
  anus (sphincter) 569.49
    due to hysteria 300.11
  arch (foot) 734
    congenital 754.61
  back ligaments 728.4
  bladder (sphincter) 596.59
  cardio-esophageal 530.89
  cervix (*see also* Incompetency, cervix)
    622.5
  diaphragm 519.4
  inguinal rings - *see* Hernia, inguinal
  joint (capsule) (ligament) (paralytic)
    (*see also* Derangement, joint)
    718.90
    congenital 755.8
  lumbosacral joint 724.6
  pelvic floor 618.89
  pelvis 618.89
  perineum 618.89
  posture 729.90
  rectum (sphincter) 569.49
  sacroiliac (joint) 724.6
  scrotum 608.89
  urethra (sphincter) 599.84
  uterus (outlet) 618.89
  vagina (outlet) 618.89
  vesical 596.59
Remains
  canal of Cloquet 743.51
  capsule (opaque) 743.51
Remittent fever (malarial) 084.6
Remnant
  canal of Cloquet 743.51
  capsule (opaque) 743.51
  cervix, cervical stump (acquired)
    (postoperative) 622.8
  cystic duct, postcholecystectomy 576.0
  fingernail 703.8
    congenital 757.5
  meniscus, knee 717.5
  thyroglossal duct 759.2
  tonsil 474.8
    infected 474.00
  urachus 753.7
Remote effect of cancer - *see* condition
Removal (of)
  catheter (urinary) (indwelling) V53.6
    from artificial opening - *see*
      Attention to, artificial, opening
    non-vascular V58.82
    vascular V58.81
  cerebral ventricle (communicating)
    shunt V53.01
  device - *see also* Fitting (of)
    contraceptive V25.42
    fixation
      external V54.89
      internal V54.01
    traction V54.89
  drains V58.49
  dressing
    wound V58.30
      nonsurgical V58.30
      surgical V58.31
  ileostomy V55.2
  Kirschner wire V54.89
  non-vascular catheter V58.82

Removal (of) (*Continued*)
  pin V54.01
  plaster cast V54.89
  plate (fracture) V54.01
  rod V54.01
  screw V54.01
  splint, external V54.89
  staples V58.32
  subdermal implantable contraceptive
    V25.43
  sutures V58.32
  traction device, external V54.89
  vascular catheter V58.81
  wound packing V58.30
    nonsurgical V58.30
    surgical V58.31
Ren
  arcuatus 753.3
  mobile, mobilis (*see also* Disease, renal)
    593.0
    congenital 753.3
  unguliformis 753.3
Renal - *see also* condition
  glomerulohyalinosis-diabetic
    syndrome 250.4● [581.81]
    due to secondary diabetes 249.4●
      [581.81]
Rendu-Osler-Weber disease or syndrome
  (familial hemorrhagic telangiectasia)
  448.0
Reninoma (M8361/1) 236.91
Rénon-Delille syndrome 253.8
Repair
  pelvic floor, previous, in pregnancy or
    childbirth 654.4●
    affecting fetus or newborn 763.89
  scarred tissue V51.8
Replacement by artificial or mechanical
  device or prosthesis of (*see also*
  Fitting (of))
  artificial skin V43.83
  bladder V43.5
  blood vessel V43.4
  breast V43.82
  eye globe V43.0
  heart
    with
      assist device V43.21
      fully implantable artificial heart
        V43.22
    valve V43.3
  intestine V43.89
  joint V43.60
    ankle V43.66
    elbow V43.62
    finger V43.69
    hip (partial) (total) V43.64
    knee V43.65
    shoulder V43.61
    specified NEC V43.69
    wrist V43.63
  kidney V43.89
  larynx V43.81
  lens V43.1
  limb(s) V43.7
  liver V43.89
  lung V43.89
  organ NEC V43.89
  pancreas V43.89
  skin (artificial) V43.83
  tissue NEC V43.89
Reprogramming
  cardiac pacemaker V53.31
Request for expert evidence V68.2

Reserve, decreased or low
  cardiac - *see* Disease, heart
    kidney (*see also* Disease, renal) 593.9
Residual - *see also* condition
  bladder 596.8
  foreign body - *see* Retention, foreign
    body
  state, schizophrenic (*see also*
    Schizophrenia) 295.6●
  urine 788.69
Resistance, resistant (to)
  activated protein C 289.81

> Note 65 Use the following subclas-
> sification for categories V09.5, V09.7,
> V09.8, V09.9
>
> 0   without mention of resistance to
>   multiple drugs
> 1   with resistance to multiple drugs
> V09.5 quinolones and
>   fluoro-quinolones
> V09.7 antimycobacterial agents
> V09.8 specified drugs NEC
> V09.9 unspecified drugs

  drugs by microorganisms V09.90
    amikacin V09.4
    aminoglycosides V09.4
    amodiaquine V09.5●
    amoxicillin V09.0
    ampicillin V09.0
    antimycobacterial agents V09.7●
    azithromycin V09.2
    azlocillin V09.0
    aztreonam V09.1
    B-lactam antibiotics V09.1
    bacampicillin V09.0
    bacitracin V09.8●
    benznidazole V09.8●
    capreomycin V09.7●
    carbenicillin V09.0
    cefaclor V09.1
    cefadroxil V09.1
    cefamandole V09.1
    cefatetan V09.1
    cefazolin V09.1
    cefixime V09.1
    cefonicid V09.1
    cefoperazone V09.1
    ceforanide V09.1
    cefotaxime V09.1
    cefoxitin V09.1
    ceftazidine V09.1
    ceftizoxime V09.1
    ceftriaxone V09.1
    cefuroxime V09.1
    cephalexin V09.1
    cephaloglycin V09.1
    cephaloridine V09.1
    cephalosporins V09.1
    cephalothin V09.1
    cephapirin V09.1
    cephradine V09.1
    chloramphenicol V09.8●
    chloraquine V09.5●
    chlorguanide V09.8●
    chlorproguanil V09.8●
    chlortetracycline V09.3
    cinoxacin V09.5●
    ciprofloxacin V09.5●
    clarithromycin V09.2
    clindamycin V09.8●
    clioquinol V09.5●
    clofazimine V09.7●

◄ New   ◄▥ Revised   ~~deleted~~ Deleted   ● Use Additional Digit(s)   ▓ Omit code

Resistance, resistant (Continued)
  drugs by microorganisms (Continued)
    cloxacillin V09.0
    cyclacillin V09.0
    cycloserine V09.7●
    dapsone [Dz] V09.7●
    demeclocycline V09.3
    dicloxacillin V09.0
    doxycycline V09.3
    enoxacin V09.5●
    erythromycin V09.2
    ethambutol [EMB] V09.7●
    ethionamide [ETA] V09.7●
    fluoroquinolones NEC V09.5●
    gentamicin V09.4
    halofantrine V09.8●
    imipenem V09.1
    iodoquinol V09.5●
    isoniazid [INH] V09.7●
    kanamycin V09.4
    macrolides V09.2
    mafenide V09.6
    MDRO (multiple drug resistant organisms) NOS V09.91
    mefloquine V09.8●
    melarsoprol V09.8●
    methicillin - see Infection, Methicillin
    methacycline V09.3
    methenamine V09.8●
    metronidazole V09.8●
    mezlocillin V09.0
    minocycline V09.3
    multiple drug resistant organisms NOS V09.91
    nafcillin V09.0
    nalidixic acid V09.5●
    natamycin V09.2
    neomycin V09.4
    netilmicin V09.4
    nimorazole V09.8●
    nitrofurantoin V09.8●
    norfloxacin V09.5●
    nystatin V09.2
    ofloxacin V09.5●
    oleandomycin V09.2
    oxacillin V09.0
    oxytetracycline V09.3
    para-amino salicyclic acid [PAS] V09.7●
    paromomycin V09.4
    penicillin (G) (V) (Vk) V09.0
    penicillins V09.0
    pentamidine V09.8●
    piperacillin V09.0
    primaquine V09.5●
    proguanil V09.8●
    pyrazinamide [PZA] V09.7●
    pyrimethamine/sulfalene V09.8●
    pyrimethamine/sulfodoxine V09.8●
    quinacrine V09.5●
    quinidine V09.8●
    quinine V09.8●
    quinolones V09.5●
    rifabutin V09.7●
    rifampin [Rif] V09.7●
    rifamycin V09.7●
    rolitetracycline V09.3
    specified drugs NEC V09.8●
    spectinomycin V09.8●
    spiramycin V09.2
    streptomycin [Sm] V09.4
    sulfacetamide V09.6
    sulfacytine V09.6

Resistance, resistant (Continued)
  drugs by microorganisms (Continued)
    sulfadiazine V09.6
    sulfadoxine V09.6
    sulfamethoxazole V09.6
    sulfapyridine V09.6
    sulfasalizine V09.6
    sulfasoxazone V09.6
    sulfonamides V09.6
    sulfoxone V09.7●
    tetracycline V09.3
    tetracyclines V09.3
    thiamphenicol V09.8●
    ticarcillin V09.0
    tinidazole V09.8●
    tobramycin V09.4
    triamphenicol V09.8●
    trimethoprim V09.8●
    vancomycin V09.8●
  insulin 277.7
  thyroid hormone 246.8
Resorption
  biliary 576.8
    purulent or putrid (see also Cholecystitis) 576.8
  dental (roots) 521.40
    alveoli 525.8
    pathological
      external 521.42
      internal 521.41
      specified NEC 521.49
  septic - see Septicemia
  teeth (roots) 521.40
    pathological
      external 521.42
      internal 521.41
      specified NEC 521.49
Respiration
  asymmetrical 786.09
  bronchial 786.09
  Cheyne-Stokes (periodic respiration) 786.04
  decreased, due to shock following injury 958.4
  disorder of 786.00
    psychogenic 306.1
    specified NEC 786.09
  failure 518.81
    acute 518.81
    acute and chronic 518.84
    chronic 518.83
    newborn 770.84
  insufficiency 786.09
    acute 518.82
    newborn NEC 770.89
  Kussmaul (air hunger) 786.09
  painful 786.52
  periodic 786.09
  high altitude 327.22
  poor 786.09
    newborn NEC 770.89
  sighing 786.7
    psychogenic 306.1
  wheezing 786.07
Respiratory - see also condition
  distress 786.09
    acute 518.82
    fetus or newborn NEC 770.89
    syndrome (newborn) 769
      adult (following shock, surgery, or trauma) 518.5
      specified NEC 518.82

Respiratory (Continued)
  failure 518.81
    acute 518.81
    acute and chronic 518.84
    chronic 518.83
Respiratory syncytial virus (RSV) 079.6
  bronchiolitis 466.11
  pneumonia 480.1
  vaccination, prophylactic (against) V04.82
Response
  photoallergic 692.72
  phototoxic 692.72
Rest, rests
  mesonephric duct 752.89
    fallopian tube 752.11
  ovarian, in fallopian tubes 752.19
  wolffian duct 752.89
Restless legs syndrome (RLS) 333.94
Restlessness 799.29
Restoration of organ continuity from previous sterilization (tuboplasty) (vasoplasty) V26.0
Restriction of housing space V60.1
Restzustand, schizophrenic (see also Schizophrenia) 295.6●
Retained - see Retention
Retardation
  development, developmental, specific (see also Disorder, development, specific) 315.9
    learning, specific 315.2
      arithmetical 315.1
      language (skills) 315.31
        expressive 315.31
        mixed receptive-expressive 315.32
      mathematics 315.1
      reading 315.00
        phonological 315.39
      written expression 315.2
    motor 315.4
  endochondral bone growth 733.91
  growth (physical) in childhood 783.43
    due to malnutrition 263.2
    fetal (intrauterine) 764.9●
      affecting management of pregnancy 656.5●
  intrauterine growth 764.9●
    affecting management of pregnancy 656.5●
  mental 319
    borderline V62.89
    mild, IQ 50-70 317
    moderate, IQ 35-49 318.0
    profound, IQ under 20 318.2
    severe, IQ 20-34 318.1
  motor, specific 315.4
  physical 783.43
    child 783.43
    due to malnutrition 263.2
    fetus (intrauterine) 764.9●
      affecting management of pregnancy 656.5●
  psychomotor NEC 307.9
  reading 315.00
Retching - see Vomiting
Retention, retained
  bladder (see also Retention, urine) 788.20
    psychogenic 306.53
  carbon dioxide 276.2
  cholelithisis 997.4
  cyst - see Cyst

Retention, retained (*Continued*)
 dead
  fetus (after 22 completed weeks'
    gestation) 656.4●
   early fetal death (before 22
     completed weeks'
     gestation) 632
  ovum 631
 decidua (following delivery)
   (fragments) (with hemorrhage)
   666.2●
  without hemorrhage 667.1●
 deciduous tooth 520.6
 dental root 525.3
 fecal (*see also* Constipation) 564.00
 fluid 276.6
 foreign body - *see also* Foreign body,
   retained
  bone 733.99
  current trauma - *see* Foreign body,
    by site or type
  middle ear 385.83
  muscle 729.6
  soft tissue NEC 729.6
 gallstones 997.4
 gastric 536.8
 membranes (following delivery) (with
   hemorrhage) 666.2●
  with abortion - *see* Abortion, by type
  without hemorrhage 667.1●
 menses 626.8
 milk (puerperal) 676.2●
 nitrogen, extrarenal 788.99
 placenta (total) (with hemorrhage)
   666.0●
  with abortion - *see* Abortion, by type
  portions or fragments 666.2●
   without hemorrhage 667.1●
  without hemorrhage 667.0●
 products of conception
  early pregnancy (fetal death before
    22 completed weeks'
    gestation) 632
  following
    abortion - *see* Abortion, by type
    delivery 666.2●
     with hemorrhage 666.2●
     without hemorrhage 667.1●
 secundines (following delivery) (with
   hemorrhage) 666.2●
  with abortion - *see* Abortion, by type
  complicating puerperium (delayed
    hemorrhage) 666.2●
  without hemorrhage 667.1●
 smegma, clitoris 624.8
 urine NEC 788.20
  bladder, incomplete emptying
    788.21
   due to
    benign prostatic hypertrophy
      (BPH) - *see* category 600
  due to
    benign prostatic hypertrophy
      (BPH) - *see* category 600
  psychogenic 306.53
  specified NEC 788.29
 water (in tissue) (*see also* Edema) 782.3
Reticulation, dust (occupational) 504
Reticulocytosis NEC 790.99
Reticuloendotheliosis
 acute infantile (M9722/3) 202.5●
 leukemic (M9940/3) 202.4●
 malignant (M9720/3) 202.3●
 nonlipid (M9722/3) 202.5●

Reticulohistiocytoma (giant cell) 277.89
Reticulohistiocytosis, multicentric
 272.8
Reticulolymphosarcoma (diffuse)
 (M9613/3) 200.8●
 follicular (M9691/3) 202.0●
 nodular (M9691/3) 202.0●
Reticulosarcoma (M9640/3) 200.0●
 nodular (M9642/3) 200.0●
 pleomorphic cell type (M9641/3)
   200.0●
Reticulosis (skin)
 acute of infancy (M9722/3) 202.5●
 familial hemophagocytic 288.4
 histiocytic medullary (M9721/3)
   202.3●
 lipomelanotic 695.89
 malignant (M9720/3) 202.3●
 Sezary's (M9701/3) 202.2●
Retina, retinal - *see* condition
Retinitis (*see also* Chorioretinitis) 363.20
 albuminurica 585.9 [363.10]
 arteriosclerotic 440.8 [362.13]
 central angiospastic 362.41
 Coat's 362.12
 diabetic 250.5● [362.01]
  due to secondary diabetes 249.5●
    [362.01]
 disciformis 362.52
 disseminated 363.10
  metastatic 363.14
  neurosyphilitic 094.83
  pigment epitheliopathy 363.15
 exudative 362.12
 focal 363.00
  in histoplasmosis 115.92
   capsulatum 115.02
   duboisii 115.12
  juxtapapillary 363.05
  macular 363.06
  paramacular 363.06
  peripheral 363.08
  posterior pole NEC 363.07
 gravidarum 646.8●
 hemorrhagica externa 362.12
 juxtapapillary (Jensen's) 363.05
 luetic - *see* Retinitis, syphilitic
 metastatic 363.14
 pigmentosa 362.74
 proliferans 362.29
 proliferating 362.29
 punctata albescens 362.76
 renal 585.9 [363.13]
 syphilitic (secondary) 091.51
  congenital 090.0 [363.13]
  early 091.51
  late 095.8 [363.13]
 syphilitica, central, recurrent 095.8
   [363.13]
 tuberculous (*see also* Tuberculous)
   017.3● [363.13]
Retinoblastoma (M9510/3) 190.5
 differentiated type (M9511/3) 190.5
 undifferentiated type (M9512/3) 190.5
Retinochoroiditis (*see also* Chorioretinitis)
 363.20
 central angiospastic 362.41
 disseminated 363.10
  metastatic 363.14
  neurosyphilitic 094.83
  pigment epitheliopathy 363.15
  syphilitic 094.83
 due to toxoplasmosis (acquired) (focal)
   130.2

Retinochoroiditis (*Continued*)
 focal 363.00
  in histoplasmosis 115.92
   capsulatum 115.02
   duboisii 115.12
  juxtapapillary (Jensen's) 363.05
  macular 363.06
  paramacular 363.06
  peripheral 363.08
  posterior pole NEC 363.07
 juxtapapillaris 363.05
 syphilitic (disseminated) 094.83
Retinopathy (background) 362.10
 arteriosclerotic 440.8 [362.13]
 atherosclerotic 440.8 [362.13]
 central serous 362.41
 circinate 362.10
 Coat's 362.12
 diabetic 250.5● [362.01]
  due to secondary diabetes 249.5●
    [362.01]
  nonproliferative 250.5● [362.03]
   due to secondary diabetes
     249.5● [362.03]
   mild 250.5● [362.04]
    due to secondary diabetes
      249.5● [362.04]
   moderate 250.5● [362.05]
    due to secondary diabetes
      249.5● [362.05]
   severe 250.5● [362.06]
    due to secondary diabetes
      249.5● [362.06]
  proliferative 250.5● [362.02]
   due to secondary diabetes 249.5●
     [362.02]
 exudative 362.12
 hypertensive 362.11
 nonproliferative
  diabetic 250.5● [362.03]
   due to secondary diabetes 249.5●
     [362.03]
   mild 250.5● [362.04]
    due to secondary diabetes
      249.5● [362.04]
   moderate 250.5● [362.05]
    due to secondary diabetes
      249.5● [362.05]
   severe 250.5● [362.06]
    due to secondary diabetes
      249.5● [362.06]
 of prematurity 362.20
  cicatricial 362.21
  stage
   0 362.22
   1 362.23
   2 362.24
   3 362.25
   4 362.26
   5 362.27
 pigmentary, congenital 362.74
 proliferative 362.29
  diabetic 250.5● [362.02]
   due to secondary diabetes
     249.5● [362.02]
  sickle-cell 282.60 [362.29]
 solar 363.31
Retinoschisis 361.10
 bullous 361.12
 congenital 743.56
 flat 361.11
 juvenile 362.73
Retractile testis 752.52

◀ New   ◀|||| Revised   ~~deleted~~ Deleted   ● Use Additional Digit(s)   ▬ Omit code

Retraction
  cervix - *see* Retraction, uterus
  drum (membrane) 384.82
  eyelid 374.41
  finger 736.29
  head 781.0
  lid 374.41
  lung 518.89
  mediastinum 519.3
  nipple 611.79
    congenital 757.6
    puerperal, postpartum 676.0●
  palmar fascia 728.6
  pleura (*see also* Pleurisy) 511.0
  ring, uterus (Bandl's) (pathological)
      661.4●
    affecting fetus or newborn 763.7
  sternum (congenital) 756.3
    acquired 738.3
    during respiration 786.9
  substernal 738.3
  supraclavicular 738.8
  syndrome (Duane's) 378.71
  uterus 621.6
  valve (heart) - *see* Endocarditis
Retrobulbar - *see* condition
Retrocaval ureter 753.4
Retrocecal - *see also* condition
  appendix (congenital) 751.5
Retrocession - *see* Retroversion
Retrodisplacement - *see* Retroversion
Retroflection, retroflexion - *see*
      Retroversion
Retrognathia, retrognathism
      (mandibular) (maxillary) 524.10
Retrograde
  ejaculation 608.87
  menstruation 626.8
Retroiliac ureter 753.4
Retroperineal - *see* condition
Retroperitoneal - *see* condition
Retroperitonitis 567.39
Retropharyngeal - *see* condition
Retroplacental - *see* condition
Retroposition - *see* Retroversion
Retrosternal thyroid (congenital) 759.2
Retroversion, retroverted
  cervix - *see* Retroversion, uterus
  female NEC (*see also* Retroversion,
      uterus) 621.6
  iris 364.70
  testis (congenital) 752.51
  uterus, uterine (acquired) (acute)
      (adherent) (any degree)
      (asymptomatic) (cervix)
      (postinfectional) (postpartal, old)
      621.6
    congenital 752.3
    in pregnancy or childbirth
        654.3●
      affecting fetus or newborn
          763.89
      causing obstructed labor
          660.2●
        affecting fetus or newborn
            763.1
Retrusion, premaxilla (developmental)
      524.04
Rett's syndrome 330.8
Reverse, reversed
  peristalsis 787.4
Reye's syndrome 331.81
Reye-Sheehan syndrome (postpartum
      pituitary necrosis) 253.2

Rh (factor)
  hemolytic disease 773.0
  incompatibility, immunization, or
      sensitization
    affecting management of pregnancy
        656.1●
    fetus or newborn 773.0
    transfusion reaction 999.7
  negative mother, affecting fetus or
      newborn 773.0
  titer elevated 999.7
  transfusion reaction 999.7
Rhabdomyolysis (idiopathic) 728.88
Rhabdomyoma (M8900/0) - *see also*
      Neoplasm, connective tissue,
      benign
  adult (M8904/0) - *see* Neoplasm,
      connective tissue, benign
  fetal (M8903/0) - *see* Neoplasm,
      connective tissue, benign
  glycogenic (M8904/0) - *see* Neoplasm,
      connective tissue, benign
Rhabdomyosarcoma (M8900/3) - *see also*
      Neoplasm, connective tissue,
      malignant
  alveolar (M8920/3) - *see* Neoplasm,
      connective tissue, malignant
  embryonal (M8910/3) - *see* Neoplasm,
      connective tissue, malignant
  mixed type (M8902/3) - *see* Neoplasm,
      connective tissue, malignant
  pleomorphic (M8901/3) - *see*
      Neoplasm, connective tissue,
      malignant
Rhabdosarcoma (M8900/3) - *see*
      Rhabdomyosarcoma
Rhesus (factor) (Rh) incompatibility - *see*
      Rh, incompatibility
Rheumaticosis - *see* Rheumatism
Rheumatism, rheumatic (acute NEC)
      729.0
  adherent pericardium 393
  arthritis
    acute or subacute - *see* Fever,
        rheumatic
    chronic 714.0
      spine 720.0
  articular (chronic) NEC (*see also*
      Arthritis) 716.9●
    acute or subacute - *see* Fever,
        rheumatic
  back 724.9
  blennorrhagic 098.59
  carditis - *see* Disease, heart, rheumatic
  cerebral - *see* Fever, rheumatic
  chorea (acute) - *see* Chorea, rheumatic
  chronic NEC 729.0
  coronary arteritis 391.9
    chronic 398.99
  degeneration, myocardium (*see also*
      Degeneration, myocardium, with
      rheumatic fever) 398.0
  desert 114.0
  febrile - *see* Fever, rheumatic
  fever - *see* Fever, rheumatic
  gonococcal 098.59
  gout 274.00   ◀▥
  heart
    disease (*see also* Disease, heart,
        rheumatic) 398.90
    failure (chronic) (congestive)
        (inactive) 398.91
  hemopericardium - *see* Rheumatic,
      pericarditis

Rheumatism, rheumatic (*Continued*)
  hydropericardium - *see* Rheumatic,
      pericarditis
  inflammatory (acute) (chronic)
      (subacute) - *see* Fever, rheumatic
  intercostal 729.0
    meaning Tietze's disease 733.6
  joint (chronic) NEC (*see also* Arthritis)
      716.9●
    acute - *see* Fever, rheumatic
  mediastinopericarditis - *see* Rheumatic,
      pericarditis
  muscular 729.0
  myocardial degeneration (*see also*
      Degeneration, myocardium, with
      rheumatic fever) 398.0
  myocarditis (chronic) (inactive) (with
      chorea) 398.0
    active or acute 391.2
      with chorea (acute) (rheumatic)
          (Sydenham's) 392.0
  myositis 729.1
  neck 724.9
  neuralgic 729.0
  neuritis (acute) (chronic) 729.2
  neuromuscular 729.0
  nodose - *see* Arthritis, nodosa
  nonarticular 729.0
  palindromic 719.30
    ankle 719.37
    elbow 719.32
    foot 719.37
    hand 719.34
    hip 719.35
    knee 719.36
    multiple sites 719.39
    pelvic region 719.35
    shoulder (region) 719.31
    specified site NEC 719.38
    wrist 719.33
  pancarditis, acute 391.8
    with chorea (acute) (rheumatic)
        (Sydenham's) 392.0
    chronic or inactive 398.99
  pericarditis (active) (acute) (with
      effusion) (with pneumonia)
      391.0
    with chorea (acute) (rheumatic)
        (Sydenham's) 392.0
    chronic or inactive 393
  pericardium - *see* Rheumatic,
      pericarditis
  pleuropericarditis - *see* Rheumatic,
      pericarditis
  pneumonia 390 [517.1]
  pneumonitis 390 [517.1]
  pneumopericarditis - *see* Rheumatic,
      pericarditis
  polyarthritis
    acute or subacute - *see* Fever,
        rheumatic
    chronic 714.0
  polyarticular NEC (*see also* Arthritis)
      716.9●
  psychogenic 306.0
  radiculitis 729.2
  sciatic 724.3
  septic - *see* Fever, rheumatic
  spine 724.9
  subacute NEC 729.0
  torticollis 723.5
  tuberculous NEC (*see also* Tuberculosis)
      015.9●
  typhoid fever 002.0

Rheumatoid - *see also* condition
lungs 714.81
Rhinitis (atrophic) (catarrhal) (chronic)
(croupous) (fibrinous) (hyperplastic)
(hypertrophic) (membranous)
(purulent) (suppurative) (ulcerative)
472.0
with
hay fever (*see also* Fever, hay) 477.9
with asthma (bronchial) 493.0●
sore throat - *see* Nasopharyngitis
acute 460
allergic (nonseasonal) (seasonal) (*see
also* Fever, hay) 477.9
with asthma (*see also* Asthma)
493.0●
due to food 477.1
granulomatous 472.0
infective 460
obstructive 472.0
pneumococcal 460
syphilitic 095.8
congenital 090.0
tuberculous (*see also* Tuberculosis)
012.8●
vasomotor (*see also* Fever, hay) 477.9
Rhinoantritis (chronic) 473.0
acute 461.0
Rhinodacryolith 375.57
Rhinolalia (aperta) (clausa) (open)
784.43
Rhinolith 478.19
nasal sinus (*see also* Sinusitis) 473.9
Rhinomegaly 478.19
Rhinopharyngitis (acute) (subacute) (*see
also* Nasopharyngitis) 460
chronic 472.2
destructive ulcerating 102.5
mutilans 102.5
Rhinophyma 695.3
Rhinorrhea 478.19
cerebrospinal (fluid) 349.81
paroxysmal (*see also* Fever, hay) 477.9
spasmodic (*see also* Fever, hay) 477.9
Rhinosalpingitis 381.50
acute 381.51
chronic 381.52
Rhinoscleroma 040.1
Rhinosporidiosis 117.0
Rhinovirus infection 079.3
Rhizomelic chrondrodysplasia punctata
277.86
Rhizomelique, pseudopolyarthritic 446.5
Rhoads and Bomford anemia (refractory)
238.72
Rhus
diversiloba dermatitis 692.6
radicans dermatitis 692.6
toxicodendron dermatitis 692.6
venenata dermatitis 692.6
verniciflua dermatitis 692.6
Rhythm
atrioventricular nodal 427.89
disorder 427.9
coronary sinus 427.89
ectopic 427.89
nodal 427.89
escape 427.89
heart, abnormal 427.9
fetus or newborn - *see* Abnormal,
heart rate
idioventricular 426.89
accelerated 427.89
nodal 427.89

Rhythm (Continued)
sleep, inversion 327.39
nonorganic origin 307.45
Rhytidosis facialis 701.8
Rib - *see also* condition
cervical 756.2
Riboflavin deficiency 266.0
Rice bodies (*see also* Loose, body, joint)
718.1●
knee 717.6
Richter's hernia - *see* Hernia, Richter's
Ricinism 988.2
Rickets (active) (acute) (adolescent)
(adult) (chest wall) (congenital)
(current) (infantile) (intestinal) 268.0
celiac 579.0
fetal 756.4
hemorrhagic 267
hypophosphatemic with nephrotic-
glycosuric dwarfism 270.0
kidney 588.0
late effect 268.1
renal 588.0
scurvy 267
vitamin D-resistant 275.3
Rickettsial disease 083.9
specified type NEC 083.8
Rickettsialpox 083.2
Rickettsiosis NEC 083.9
specified type NEC 083.8
tick-borne 082.9
specified type NEC 082.8
vesicular 083.2
Ricord's chancre 091.0
Riddoch's syndrome (visual
disorientation) 368.16
Rider's
bone 733.99
chancre 091.0
Ridge, alveolus - *see also* condition
edentulous
atrophy 525.20
mandible 525.20
minimal 525.21
moderate 525.22
severe 525.23
maxilla 525.20
minimal 525.24
moderate 525.25
severe 525.26
flabby 525.20
Ridged ear 744.29
Riedel's
disease (ligneous thyroiditis) 245.3
lobe, liver 751.69
struma (ligneous thyroiditis) 245.3
thyroiditis (ligneous) 245.3
Rieger's anomaly or syndrome
(mesodermal dysgenesis, anterior
ocular segment) 743.44
Riehl's melanosis 709.09
Rietti-Greppi-Micheli anemia or
syndrome 282.49
Rieux's hernia - *see* Hernia, Rieux's
Rift Valley fever 066.3
Riga's disease (cachectic aphthae) 529.0
Riga-Fede disease (cachectic aphthae)
529.0
Riggs' disease (compound periodontitis)
523.40
Right middle lobe syndrome 518.0
Rigid, rigidity - *see also* condition
abdominal 789.4●
articular, multiple congenital 754.89

Rigid, rigidity (Continued)
back 724.8
cervix uteri
in pregnancy or childbirth 654.6●
affecting fetus or newborn 763.89
causing obstructed labor 660.2●
affecting fetus or newborn
763.1
hymen (acquired) (congenital) 623.3
nuchal 781.6
pelvic floor
in pregnancy or childbirth 654.4●
affecting fetus or newborn 763.89
causing obstructed labor 660.2●
affecting fetus or newborn
763.1
perineum or vulva
in pregnancy or childbirth 654.8●
affecting fetus or newborn 763.89
causing obstructed labor 660.2●
affecting fetus or newborn
763.1
spine 724.8
vagina
in pregnancy or childbirth 654.7●
affecting fetus or newborn 763.89
causing obstructed labor 660.2●
affecting fetus or newborn 763.1
Rigors 780.99
Riley-Day syndrome (familial
dysautonomia) 742.8
RIND (reversible ischemic neurological
deficit) 434.91
history of (personal) V12.54
Ring(s)
aorta 747.21
Bandl's, complicating delivery 661.4●
affecting fetus or newborn 763.7
contraction, complicating delivery
661.4●
affecting fetus or newborn 763.7
esophageal (congenital) 750.3
Fleischer (-Kayser) (cornea) 275.1
[371.14]
hymenal, tight (acquired) (congenital)
623.3
Kayser-Fleischer (cornea) 275.1 *[371.14]*
retraction, uterus, pathological 661.4●
affecting fetus or newborn 763.7
Schatzki's (esophagus) (congenital)
(lower) 750.3
acquired 530.3
Soemmering's 366.51
trachea, abnormal 748.3
vascular (congenital) 747.21
Vossius' 921.3
late effect 366.21
Ringed hair (congenital) 757.4
Ringing in the ear (*see also* Tinnitus)
388.30
Ringworm 110.9
beard 110.0
body 110.5
Burmese 110.9
corporeal 110.5
foot 110.4
groin 110.3
hand 110.2
honeycomb 110.0
nails 110.1
perianal (area) 110.3
scalp 110.0
specified site NEC 110.8
Tokelau 110.5

◄ New   ◄|||| Revised   ~~deleted~~ Deleted   ● Use Additional Digit(s)   ▬ Omit code

Rise, venous pressure 459.89
Risk
　factor - *see* Problem
　falling V15.88
　suicidal 300.9
Ritter's disease (dermatitis exfoliativa
　　neonatorum) 695.81
Rivalry, sibling 313.3
Rivalta's disease (cervicofacial
　　actinomycosis) 039.3
River blindness 125.3 *[360.13]*
Robert's pelvis 755.69
　with disproportion (fetopelvic)
　　653.0●
　　affecting fetus or newborn 763.1
　　causing obstructed labor 660.1●
　　　affecting fetus or newborn
　　　763.1
Robin's syndrome 756.0
Robinson's (hidrotic) ectodermal
　　dysplasia 757.31
Robles' disease (onchocerciasis) 125.3
　　[360.13]
Rochalimea - *see* Rickettsial disease
Rocky Mountain fever (spotted) 082.0
Rodent ulcer (M8090/3) - *see also*
　　Neoplasm, skin, malignant
　cornea 370.07
Roentgen ray, adverse effect - *see* Effect,
　　adverse, x-ray
Roetheln 056.9
Roger's disease (congenital
　　interventricular septal defect) 745.4
Rokitansky's
　disease (*see also* Necrosis, liver) 570
　tumor 620.2
Rokitansky-Aschoff sinuses (mucosal
　　outpouching of gallbladder) (*see also*
　　Disease, gallbladder) 575.8
Rokitansky-Kuster-Hauser syndrome
　　(congenital absence vagina)
　　752.49
Rollet's chancre (syphilitic) 091.0
Rolling of head 781.0
Romano-Ward syndrome (prolonged QT
　　interval syndrome) 426.82
Romanus lesion 720.1
Romberg's disease or syndrome
　　349.89
Roof, mouth - *see* condition
Rosacea 695.3
　acne 695.3
　keratitis 695.3 *[370.49]*
Rosary, rachitic 268.0
Rose
　cold 477.0
　fever 477.0
　rash 782.1
　　epidemic 056.9
　　of infants 057.8
Rosen-Castleman-Liebow syndrome
　　(pulmonary proteinosis) 516.0
Rosenbach's erysipelatoid or erysipeloid
　　027.1
Rosenthal's disease (factor XI deficiency)
　　286.2
Roseola 057.8
　infantum, infantilis (*see also* Exanthem
　　subitum) 058.10
Rossbach's disease (hyperchlorhydria)
　　536.8
　psychogenic 306.4
Rossle-Urbach-Wiethe lipoproteinosis
　　272.8

Ross river fever 066.3
Rostan's asthma (cardiac) (*see also* Failure,
　　ventricular, left) 428.1
Rot
　Barcoo (*see also* Ulcer, skin) 707.9
　knife-grinders' (*see also* Tuberculosis)
　　011.4●
Rot-Bernhardt disease 355.1
Rotation
　anomalous, incomplete or insufficient -
　　see Malrotation
　cecum (congenital) 751.4
　colon (congenital) 751.4
　manual, affecting fetus or newborn
　　763.89
　spine, incomplete or insufficient
　　737.8
　tooth, teeth 524.35
　vertebra, incomplete or insufficient
　　737.8
Röteln 056.9
Roth's disease or meralgia 355.1
Roth-Bernhardt disease or syndrome
　　355.1
Rothmund (-Thomson) syndrome 757.33
Rotor's disease or syndrome (idiopathic
　　hyperbilirubinemia) 277.4
Rotundum ulcus - *see* Ulcer, stomach
Round
　back (with wedging of vertebrae)
　　737.10
　　late effect of rickets 268.1
　hole, retina 361.31
　　with detachment 361.01
　ulcer (stomach) - *see* Ulcer, stomach
　worms (infestation) (large) NEC
　　127.0
Roussy-Lévy syndrome 334.3
Routine postpartum follow-up V24.2
Roy (-Jutras) syndrome (acropachyderma)
　　757.39
Rubella (German measles) 056.9
　complicating pregnancy, childbirth, or
　　puerperium 647.5●
　complication 056.8
　　neurological 056.00
　　　encephalomyelitis 056.01
　　　specified type NEC 056.09
　　specified type NEC 056.79
　congenital 771.0
　contact V01.4
　exposure to V01.4
　maternal
　　with suspected fetal damage
　　　affecting management of
　　　pregnancy 655.3●
　　affecting fetus or newborn 760.2
　　　manifest rubella in infant 771.0
　specified complications NEC 056.79
　vaccination, prophylactic (against)
　　V04.3
Rubeola (measles) (*see also* Measles) 055.9
　complicated 055.8
　meaning rubella (*see also* Rubella) 056.9
　scarlatinosis 057.8
Rubeosis iridis 364.42
　diabetica 250.5● *[364.42]*
　　due to secondary diabetes 249.5●
　　　[364.42]
Rubinstein-Taybi's syndrome
　　(brachydactylia, short stature and
　　mental retardation) 759.89
Rud's syndrome (mental deficiency,
　　epilepsy, and infantilism) 759.89

Rudimentary (congenital) - *see also*
　　Agenesis
　arm 755.22
　bone 756.9
　cervix uteri 752.49
　eye (*see also* Microphthalmos) 743.10
　fallopian tube 752.19
　leg 755.32
　lobule of ear 744.21
　patella 755.64
　respiratory organs in thoracopagus
　　759.4
　tracheal bronchus 748.3
　uterine horn 752.3
　uterus 752.3
　　in male 752.7
　　solid or with cavity 752.3
　vagina 752.49
Ruiter-Pompen (-Wyers) syndrome
　　(angiokeratoma corporis diffusum)
　　272.7
Ruled out condition (*see also* Observation,
　　suspected) V71.9
Rumination - *see also* Vomiting
　disorder 307.53
　neurotic 300.3
　obsessional 300.3
　psychogenic 307.53
Runaway reaction - *see also* Disturbance,
　　conduct
　socialized 312.2●
　undersocialized, unsocialized 312.1●
Runeberg's disease (progressive
　　pernicious anemia) 281.0
Runge's syndrome (postmaturity)
　　766.22
Runny nose 784.99
Rupia 091.3
　congenital 090.0
　tertiary 095.9
Rupture, ruptured 553.9
　abdominal viscera NEC 799.89
　　obstetrical trauma 665.5●
　abscess (spontaneous) - *see* Abscess, by
　　site
　amnion - *see* Rupture, membranes
　aneurysm - *see* Aneurysm
　anus (sphincter) - *see* Laceration, anus
　aorta, aortic 441.5
　　abdominal 441.3
　　arch 441.1
　　ascending 441.1
　　descending 441.5
　　　abdominal 441.3
　　　thoracic 441.1
　　syphilitic 093.0
　　thoracoabdominal 441.6
　　thorax, thoracic 441.1
　　transverse 441.1
　　traumatic (thoracic) 901.0
　　　abdominal 902.0
　　valve or cusp (*see also* Endocarditis,
　　　aortic) 424.1
　appendix (with peritonitis) 540.0
　　with peritoneal abscess 540.1
　　traumatic - *see* Injury, internal,
　　　gastrointestinal tract
　arteriovenous fistula, brain (congenital)
　　430
　artery 447.2
　　brain (*see also* Hemorrhage, brain)
　　　431
　　coronary (*see also* Infarct,
　　　myocardium) 410.9●

Rupture, ruptured (*Continued*)
  artery (*Continued*)
    heart (*see also* Infarct, myocardium) 410.9●
    pulmonary 417.8
    traumatic (complication) (*see also* Injury, blood vessel, by site) 904.9
  bile duct, except cystic (*see also* Disease, biliary) 576.3
  cystic 575.4
    traumatic - *see* Injury, internal, intra-abdominal
  bladder (sphincter) 596.6
    with
      abortion - *see* Abortion, by type, with damage to pelvic organs
      ectopic pregnancy (*see also* categories 633.0–633.9) 639.2
      molar pregnancy (*see also* categories 630–632) 639.2
    following
      abortion 639.2
      ectopic or molar pregnancy 639.2
    nontraumatic 596.6
    obstetrical trauma 665.5●
    spontaneous 596.6
    traumatic - *see* Injury, internal, bladder
  blood vessel (*see also* Hemorrhage) 459.0
    brain (*see also* Hemorrhage, brain) 431
    heart (*see also* Infarct, myocardium) 410.9●
    traumatic (complication) (*see also* Injury, blood vessel, by site) 904.9
  bone - *see* Fracture, by site
  bowel 569.89
    traumatic - *see* Injury, internal, intestine
  Bowman's membrane 371.31
  brain
    aneurysm (congenital) (*see also* Hemorrhage, subarachnoid) 430
      late effect - *see* Late effect(s) (of) cerebrovascular disease
      syphilitic 094.87
    hemorrhagic (*see also* Hemorrhage, brain) 431
    injury at birth 767.0
    syphilitic 094.89
  capillaries 448.9
  cardiac (*see also* Infarct, myocardium) 410.9●
  cartilage (articular) (current) - *see also* Sprain, by site
    knee - *see* Tear, meniscus
    semilunar - *see* Tear, meniscus
  cecum (with peritonitis) 540.0
    with peritoneal abscess 540.1
    traumatic 863.89
      with open wound into cavity 863.99
  cerebral aneurysm (congenital) (*see also* Hemorrhage, subarachnoid) 430
    late effect - *see* Late effect(s) (of) cerebrovascular disease

Rupture, ruptured (*Continued*)
  cervix (uteri)
    with
      abortion - *see* Abortion, by type, with damage to pelvic organs
      ectopic pregnancy (*see also* categories 633.0–633.9) 639.2
      molar pregnancy (*see also* categories 630–632) 639.2
    following
      abortion 639.2
      ectopic or molar pregnancy 639.2
    obstetrical trauma 665.3●
    traumatic - *see* Injury, internal, cervix
  chordae tendineae 429.5
  choroid (direct) (indirect) (traumatic) 363.63
  circle of Willis (*see also* Hemorrhage, subarachnoid) 430
    late effect - *see* Late effect(s) (of) cerebrovascular disease
  colon 569.89
    traumatic - *see* Injury, internal, colon
  cornea (traumatic) - *see also* Rupture, eye
    due to ulcer 370.00
  coronary (artery) (thrombotic) (*see also* Infarct, myocardium) 410.9●
  corpus luteum (infected) (ovary) 620.1
  cyst - *see* Cyst
  cystic duct (*see also* Disease, gallbladder) 575.4
  Descemet's membrane 371.33
    traumatic - *see* Rupture, eye
  diaphragm - *see also* Hernia, diaphragm
    traumatic - *see* Injury, internal, diaphragm
  diverticulum
    bladder 596.3
    intestine (large) (*see also* Diverticula) 562.10
      small 562.00
  duodenal stump 537.89
  duodenum (ulcer) - *see* Ulcer, duodenum, with perforation
  ear drum (*see also* Perforation, tympanum) 384.20
    with otitis media - *see* Otitis media
    traumatic - *see* Wound, open, ear
  esophagus 530.4
    traumatic 862.22
      with open wound into cavity 862.32
      cervical region - *see* Wound, open, esophagus
  eye (without prolapse of intraocular tissue) 871.0
    with
      exposure of intraocular tissue 871.1
      partial loss of intraocular tissue 871.2
      prolapse of intraocular tissue 871.1
    due to burn 940.5
  fallopian tube 620.8
    due to pregnancy - *see* Pregnancy, tubal
    traumatic - *see* Injury, internal, fallopian tube
  fontanel 767.3
  free wall (ventricle) (*see also* Infarct, myocardium) 410.9●

Rupture, ruptured (*Continued*)
  gallbladder or duct (*see also* Disease, gallbladder) 575.4
    traumatic - *see* Injury, internal, gallbladder
  gastric (*see also* Rupture, stomach) 537.89
    vessel 459.0
  globe (eye) (traumatic) - *see* Rupture, eye
  graafian follicle (hematoma) 620.0
  heart (auricle) (ventricle) (*see also* Infarct, myocardium) 410.9●
    infectional 422.90
    traumatic - *see* Rupture, myocardium, traumatic
  hymen 623.8
  internal
    organ, traumatic - *see also* Injury, internal, by site
      heart - *see* Rupture, myocardium, traumatic
      kidney - *see* Rupture, kidney
      liver - *see* Rupture, liver
      spleen - *see* Rupture, spleen, traumatic
      semilunar cartilage - *see* Tear, meniscus
    intervertebral disc - *see* Displacement, intervertebral disc
    traumatic (current) - *see* Dislocation, vertebra
  intestine 569.89
    traumatic - *see* Injury, internal, intestine
  intracranial, birth injury 767.0
  iris 364.76
    traumatic - *see* Rupture, eye
  joint capsule - *see* Sprain, by site
  kidney (traumatic) 866.03
    with open wound into cavity 866.13
    due to birth injury 767.8
    nontraumatic 593.89
  lacrimal apparatus (traumatic) 870.2
  lens (traumatic) 366.20
  ligament - *see also* Sprain, by site
    with open wound - *see* Wound, open, by site
    old (*see also* Disorder, cartilage, articular) 718.0●
  liver (traumatic) 864.04
    with open wound into cavity 864.14
    due to birth injury 767.8
    nontraumatic 573.8
  lymphatic (node) (vessel) 457.8
  marginal sinus (placental) (with hemorrhage) 641.2●
    affecting fetus or newborn 762.1
  meaning hernia - *see* Hernia
  membrana tympani (*see also* Perforation, tympanum) 384.20
    with otitis media - *see* Otitis media
    traumatic - *see* Wound, open, ear
  membranes (spontaneous)
    artificial
      delayed delivery following 658.3●
      affecting fetus or newborn 761.1
    fetus or newborn 761.1
    delayed delivery following 658.2●
      affecting fetus or newborn 761.1

◀ New   ◀‖‖ Revised   ~~deleted~~ Deleted   ● Use Additional Digit(s)   ▓ Omit code

Rupture, ruptured *(Continued)*
  membranes *(Continued)*
    premature (less than 24 hours prior to onset of labor) 658.1●
      affecting fetus or newborn 761.1
      delayed delivery following 658.2●
        affecting fetus or newborn 761.1
  meningeal artery *(see also* Hemorrhage, subarachnoid) 430
    late effect - *see* Late effect(s) (of) cerebrovascular disease
  meniscus (knee) - *see also* Tear, meniscus
    old *(see also* Derangement, meniscus) 717.5
    site other than knee - *see* Disorder, cartilage, articular
    site other than knee - *see* Sprain, by site
  mesentery 568.89
    traumatic - *see* Injury, internal, mesentery
  mitral - *see* Insufficiency, mitral
  muscle (traumatic) NEC - *see also* Sprain, by site
    with open wound - *see* Wound, open, by site
    nontraumatic 728.83
  musculotendinous cuff (nontraumatic) (shoulder) 840.4
  mycotic aneurysm, causing cerebral hemorrhage *(see also* Hemorrhage, subarachnoid) 430
    late effect - *see* Late effect(s) (of) cerebrovascular disease
  myocardium, myocardial *(see also* Infarct, myocardium) 410.9●
    traumatic 861.03
      with open wound into thorax 861.13
  nontraumatic (meaning hernia) *(see also* Hernia, by site) 553.9
    obstructed *(see also* Hernia, by site, with obstruction) 552.9
      gangrenous *(see also* Hernia, by site, with gangrene) 551.9
  operation wound *(see also* Dehiscence) 998.32
    internal 998.31
  ovary, ovarian 620.8
    corpus luteum 620.1
    follicle (graafian) 620.0
  oviduct 620.8
    due to pregnancy - *see* Pregnancy, tubal
  pancreas 577.8
    traumatic - *see* Injury, internal, pancreas
  papillary muscle (ventricular) 429.6
  pelvic
    floor, complicating delivery 664.1●
    organ NEC - *see* Injury, pelvic, organs
  penis (traumatic) - *see* Wound, open, penis
  perineum 624.8
    during delivery *(see also* Laceration, perineum, complicating delivery) 664.4●
  pharynx (nontraumatic) (spontaneous) 478.29

Rupture, ruptured *(Continued)*
  pregnant uterus (before onset of labor) 665.0●
  prostate (traumatic) - *see* Injury, internal, prostate
  pulmonary
    artery 417.8
    valve (heart) *(see also* Endocarditis, pulmonary) 424.3
    vein 417.8
    vessel 417.8
  pupil, sphincter 364.75
  pus tube *(see also* Salpingo-oophoritis) 614.2
  pyosalpinx *(see also* Salpingo-oophoritis) 614.2
  rectum 569.49
    traumatic - *see* Injury, internal, rectum
  retina, retinal (traumatic) (without detachment) 361.30
    with detachment *(see also* Detachment, retina, with retinal defect) 361.00
  rotator cuff (capsule) (traumatic) 840.4
    nontraumatic, complete 727.61
  sclera 871.0
  semilunar cartilage, knee *(see also* Tear, meniscus) 836.2
    old *(see also* Derangement, meniscus) 717.5
  septum (cardiac) 410.8●
  sigmoid 569.89
    traumatic - *see* Injury, internal, colon, sigmoid
  sinus of Valsalva 747.29
  spinal cord - *see also* Injury, spinal, by site
    due to injury at birth 767.4
    fetus or newborn 767.4
    syphilitic 094.89
    traumatic - *see also* Injury, spinal, by site
      with fracture - *see* Fracture, vertebra, by site, with spinal cord injury
  spleen 289.59
    congenital 767.8
    due to injury at birth 767.8
    malarial 084.9
    nontraumatic 289.59
    spontaneous 289.59
    traumatic 865.04
      with open wound into cavity 865.14
  splenic vein 459.0
  stomach 537.89
    due to injury at birth 767.8
    traumatic - *see* Injury, internal, stomach
    ulcer - *see* Ulcer, stomach, with perforation
  synovium 727.50
    specified site NEC 727.59
  tendon (traumatic) - *see also* Sprain, by site
    with open wound - *see* Wound, open, by site
    Achilles 845.09
      nontraumatic 727.67
    ankle 845.09
      nontraumatic 727.68
    biceps (long bead) 840.8
      nontraumatic 727.62

Rupture, ruptured *(Continued)*
  tendon *(Continued)*
    foot 845.10
      interphalangeal (joint) 845.13
      metatarsophalangeal (joint) 845.12
      nontraumatic 727.68
      specified site NEC 845.19
      tarsometatarsal (joint) 845.11
    hand 842.10
      carpometacarpal (joint) 842.11
      interphalangeal (joint) 842.13
      metacarpophalangeal (joint) 842.12
      nontraumatic 727.63
        extensors 727.63
        flexors 727.64
      specified site NEC 842.19
    nontraumatic 727.60
      specified site NEC 727.69
    patellar 844.8
      nontraumatic 727.66
    quadriceps 844.8
      nontraumatic 727.65
    rotator cuff (capsule) 840.4
      nontraumatic, complete 727.61
    wrist 842.00
      carpal (joint) 842.01
      nontraumatic 727.63
        extensors 727.63
        flexors 727.64
      radiocarpal (joint) (ligament) 842.02
      radioulnar (joint), distal 842.09
      specified site NEC 842.09
  testis (traumatic) 878.2
    complicated 878.3
    due to syphilis 095.8
  thoracic duct 457.8
  tonsil 474.8
  traumatic
    with open wound - *see* Wound, open, by site
    aorta - *see* Rupture, aorta, traumatic
    ear drum - *see* Wound, open, ear, drum
    external site - *see* Wound, open, by site
    eye 871.2
    globe (eye) - *see* Wound, open, eyeball
    internal organ (abdomen, chest, or pelvis) - *see also* Injury, internal, by site
      heart - *see* Rupture, myocardium, traumatic
      kidney - *see* Rupture, kidney
      liver - *see* Rupture, liver
      spleen - *see* Rupture, spleen, traumatic
    ligament, muscle, or tendon - *see also* Sprain, by site
      with open wound - *see* Wound, open, by site
    meaning hernia - *see* Hernia
  tricuspid (heart) (valve) - *see* Endocarditis, tricuspid
  tube, tubal 620.8
    abscess *(see also* Salpingo-oophoritis) 614.2
    due to pregnancy - *see* Pregnancy, tubal

Rupture, ruptured (Continued)
  tympanum, tympanic (membrane) (see also Perforation, tympanum) 384.20
    with otitis media - see Otitis media
    traumatic - see Wound, open, ear, drum
  umbilical cord 663.8●
    fetus or newborn 772.0
  ureter (traumatic) (see also Injury, internal, ureter) 867.2
    nontraumatic 593.89
  urethra 599.84
    with
      abortion - see Abortion, by type, with damage to pelvic organs
      ectopic pregnancy (see also categories 633.0–633.9) 639.2
      molar pregnancy (see also categories 630–632) 639.2
    following
      abortion 639.2
      ectopic or molar pregnancy 639.2

Rupture, ruptured (Continued)
  urethra (Continued)
    obstetrical trauma 665.5●
    traumatic - see Injury, internal urethra
  uterosacral ligament 620.8
  uterus (traumatic) - see also Injury, internal uterus
    affecting fetus or newborn 763.89
    during labor 665.1●
    nonpuerperal, nontraumatic 621.8
    nontraumatic 621.8
    pregnant (during labor) 665.1●
      before labor 665.0●
  vagina 878.6
    complicated 878.7
    complicating delivery - see Laceration, vagina, complicating delivery
  valve, valvular (heart) - see Endocarditis
  varicose vein - see Varicose, vein
  varix - see Varix
  vena cava 459.0
  ventricle (free wall) (left) (see also Infarct, myocardium) 410.9●

Rupture, ruptured (Continued)
  vesical (urinary) 596.6
    traumatic - see Injury, internal, bladder
  vessel (blood) 459.0
    pulmonary 417.8
  viscus 799.89
  vulva 878.4
    complicated 878.5
    complicating delivery 664.0●
Russell's dwarf (uterine dwarfism and craniofacial dysostosis) 759.89
Russell's dysentery 004.8
Russell (-Silver) syndrome (congenital hemihypertrophy and short stature) 759.89
Russian spring-summer type encephalitis 063.0
Rust's disease (tuberculous spondylitis) 015.0● [720.81]
Rustitskii's disease (multiple myeloma) (M9730/3) 203.0●
Ruysch's disease (Hirschsprung's disease) 751.3
Rytand-Lipsitch syndrome (complete atrioventricular block) 426.0

◀ New　◀▥ Revised　~~deleted~~ Deleted　● Use Additional Digit(s)　▨ Omit code

S

Saber
- shin 090.5
- tibia 090.5

Sac, lacrimal - *see* condition

Saccharomyces infection (*see also* Candidiasis) 112.9

Saccharopinuria 270.7

Saccular - *see* condition

Sacculation
- aorta (nonsyphilitic) (*see also* Aneurysm, aorta) 441.9
  - ruptured 441.5
  - syphilitic 093.0
- bladder 596.3
- colon 569.89
- intralaryngeal (congenital) (ventricular) 748.3
- larynx (congenital) (ventricular) 748.3
- organ or site, congenital - *see* Distortion
- pregnant uterus, complicating delivery 654.4 ●
  - affecting fetus or newborn 763.1
  - causing obstructed labor 660.2 ●
    - affecting fetus or newborn 763.1
- rectosigmoid 569.89
- sigmoid 569.89
- ureter 593.89
- urethra 599.2
- vesical 596.3

Sachs (-Tay) disease (amaurotic familial idiocy) 330.1

Sacks-Libman disease 710.0 [424.91]

Sacralgia 724.6

Sacralization
- fifth lumbar vertebra 756.15
- incomplete (vertebra) 756.15

Sacrodynia 724.6

Sacroiliac joint - *see* condition

Sacroiliitis NEC 720.2

Sacrum - *see* condition

Saddle
- back 737.8
- embolus, aorta 444.0
- nose 738.0
  - congenital 754.0
  - due to syphilis 090.5

Sadism (sexual) 302.84

Saemisch's ulcer 370.04

Saenger's syndrome 379.46

Sago spleen 277.39

Sailors' skin 692.74

Saint
- Anthony's fire (*see also* Erysipelas) 035
- Guy's dance - *see* Chorea
- Louis-type encephalitis 062.3
- triad (*see also* Hernia, diaphragm) 553.3
- Vitus' dance - *see* Chorea

Salicylism
- correct substance properly administered 535.4 ●
- overdose or wrong substance given or taken 965.1

Salivary duct or gland - *see also* condition
- virus disease 078.5

Salivation (excessive) (*see also* Ptyalism) 527.7

Salmonella (aertrycke) (choleraesuis) (enteritidis) (gallinarum) (suipestifer) (typhimurium) (*see also* Infection, Salmonella) 003.9
- arthritis 003.23
- carrier (suspected) of V02.3
- meningitis 003.21
- osteomyelitis 003.24
- pneumonia 003.22
- septicemia 003.1
- typhosa 002.0
  - carrier (suspected) of V02.1

Salmonellosis 003.0
- with pneumonia 003.22

Salpingitis (catarrhal) (fallopian tube) (nodular) (pseudofollicular) (purulent) (septic) (*see also* Salpingo-oophoritis) 614.2
- ear 381.50
  - acute 381.51
  - chronic 381.52
- Eustachian (tube) 381.50
  - acute 381.51
  - chronic 381.52
- follicularis 614.1
- gonococcal (chronic) 098.37
  - acute 098.17
- interstitial, chronic 614.1
- isthmica nodosa 614.1
- old - *see* Salpingo-oophoritis, chronic
- puerperal, postpartum, childbirth 670.8 ◄▥
- specific (chronic) 098.37
  - acute 098.17
- tuberculous (acute) (chronic) (*see also* Tuberculosis) 016.6 ●
- venereal (chronic) 098.37
  - acute 098.17

Salpingocele 620.4

Salpingo-oophoritis (catarrhal) (purulent) (ruptured) (septic) (suppurative) 614.2
- acute 614.0
  - with
    - abortion - *see* Abortion, by type, with sepsis
    - ectopic pregnancy (*see also* categories 633.0–633.9) 639.0
    - molar pregnancy (*see also* categories 630–632) 639.0
  - following
    - abortion 639.0
    - ectopic or molar pregnancy 639.0
  - gonococcal 098.17
  - puerperal, postpartum, childbirth 670.8 ◄▥
  - tuberculous (*see also* Tuberculosis) 016.6 ●
- chronic 614.1
  - gonococcal 098.37
  - tuberculous (*see also* Tuberculosis) 016.6 ●
- complicating pregnancy 646.6 ●
  - affecting fetus or newborn 760.8
- gonococcal (chronic) 098.37
  - acute 098.17
- old - *see* Salpingo-oophoritis, chronic
- puerperal 670.8 ◄▥
- specific - *see* Salpingo-oophoritis, gonococcal
- subacute (*see also* Salpingo-oophoritis, acute) 614.0

Salpingo-oophoritis (*Continued*)
- tuberculous (acute) (chronic) (*see also* Tuberculosis) 016.6 ●
- venereal - *see* Salpingo-oophoritis, gonococcal

Salpingo-ovaritis (*see also* Salpingo-oophoritis) 614.2

Salpingoperitonitis (*see also* Salpingo-oophoritis) 614.2

Salt-losing
- nephritis (*see also* Disease, renal) 593.9
- syndrome (*see also* Disease, renal) 593.9

Salt-rheum (*see also* Eczema) 692.9

Salzmann's nodular dystrophy 371.46

Sampling
- chorionic villus V28.89

Sampson's cyst or tumor 617.1

Sandblasters'
- asthma 502
- lung 502

Sander's disease (paranoia) 297.1

Sandfly fever 066.0

Sandhoff's disease 330.1

Sanfilippo's syndrome (mucopolysaccharidosis III) 277.5

Sanger-Brown's ataxia 334.2

San Joaquin Valley fever 114.0

Sao Paulo fever or typhus 082.0

Saponification, mesenteric 567.89

Sapremia - *see* Septicemia

Sarcocele (benign)
- syphilitic 095.8
  - congenital 090.5

Sarcoepiplocele (*see also* Hernia) 553.9

Sarcoepiplomphalocele (*see also* Hernia, umbilicus) 553.1

Sarcoid (any site) 135
- with lung involvement 135 [517.8]
- Boeck's 135
- Darier-Roussy 135
- Spiegler-Fendt 686.8

Sarcoidosis 135
- cardiac 135 [425.8]
- lung 135 [517.8]

Sarcoma (M8800/3) - *see also* Neoplasm, connective tissue, malignant
- alveolar soft part (M9581/3) - *see* Neoplasm, connective tissue, malignant
- ameloblastic (M9330/3) 170.1
  - upper jaw (bone) 170.0
- botryoid (M8910/3) - *see* Neoplasm, connective tissue, malignant
- botryoides (M8910/3) - *see* Neoplasm, connective tissue, malignant
- cerebellar (M9480/3) 191.6
  - circumscribed (arachnoidal) (M9471/3) 191.6
- circumscribed (arachnoidal) cerebellar (M9471/3) 191.6
- clear cell, of tendons and aponeuroses (M9044/3) - *see* Neoplasm, connective tissue, malignant
- embryonal (M8991/3) - *see* Neoplasm, connective tissue, malignant
- endometrial (stromal) (M8930/3) 182.0
  - isthmus 182.1
- endothelial (M9130/3) - *see also* Neoplasm, connective tissue, malignant
  - bone (M9260/3) - *see* Neoplasm, bone, malignant

Sarcoma (Continued)
  epithelioid cell (M8804/3) - see
    Neoplasm, connective tissue,
    malignant
  Ewing's (M9260/3) - see Neoplasm,
    bone, malignant
  follicular dendritic cell 202.9●
  germinoblastic (diffuse) (M9632/3)
    202.8●
    follicular (M9697/3) 202.0●
  giant cell (M8802/3) - see also
    Neoplasm, connective tissue,
    malignant
    bone (M9250/3) - see Neoplasm,
      bone, malignant
  glomoid (M8710/3) - see Neoplasm,
    connective tissue, malignant
  granulocytic (M9930/3) 205.3●
  hemangioendothelial (M9130/3) - see
    Neoplasm, connective tissue,
    malignant
  hemorrhagic, multiple (M9140/3) - see
    Kaposi's, sarcoma
  Hodgkin's (M9662/3) 201.2●
  immunoblastic (M9612/3) 200.8●
  interdigitating dendritic cell 202.9●
  Kaposi's (M9140/3) - see Kaposi's,
    sarcoma
  Kupffer cell (M9124/3) 155.0
  Langerhans cell 202.9●
  leptomeningeal (M9530/3) - see
    Neoplasm, meninges,
    malignant
  lymphangioendothelial (M9170/3) - see
    Neoplasm, connective tissue,
    malignant
  lymphoblastic (M9630/3) 200.1●
  lymphocytic (M9620/3) 200.1●
  mast cell (M9740/3) 202.6●
  melanotic (M8720/3) - see Melanoma
  meningeal (M9530/3) - see Neoplasm,
    meninges, malignant
  meningothelial (M9530/3) - see
    Neoplasm, meninges,
    malignant
  mesenchymal (M8800/3) - see also
    Neoplasm, connective tissue,
    malignant
    mixed (M8990/3) - see Neoplasm,
      connective tissue, malignant
  mesothelial (M9050/3) - see Neoplasm,
    by site, malignant
  monstrocellular (M9481/3)
    specified site - see Neoplasm, by site,
      malignant
    unspecified site 191.9
  myeloid (M9930/3) 205.3●
  neurogenic (M9540/3) - see Neoplasm,
    connective tissue, malignant
  odontogenic (M9270/3) 170.1
    upper jaw (bone) 170.0
  osteoblastic (M9180/3) - see Neoplasm,
    bone, malignant
  osteogenic (M9180/3) - see also
    Neoplasm, bone, malignant
    juxtacortical (M9190/3) - see
      Neoplasm, bone, malignant
    periosteal (M9190/3) - see
      Neoplasm, bone, malignant
  periosteal (M8812/3) - see also
    Neoplasm, bone, malignant
    osteogenic (M9190/3) - see
      Neoplasm, bone, malignant
  plasma cell (M9731/3) 203.8●

Sarcoma (Continued)
  pleomorphic cell (M8802/3) - see
    Neoplasm, connective tissue,
    malignant
  reticuloendothelial (M9720/3)
    202.3●
  reticulum cell (M9640/3) 200.0●
    nodular (M9642/3) 200.0●
    pleomorphic cell type (M9641/3)
      200.0●
  round cell (M8803/3) - see
    Neoplasm, connective
    tissue, malignant
  small cell (M8803/3) - see
    Neoplasm, connective
    tissue, malignant
  spindle cell (M8801/3) - see
    Neoplasm, connective
    tissue, malignant
  stromal (endometrial) (M8930/3)
    182.0
    isthmus 182.1
  synovial (M9040/3) - see also
    Neoplasm, connective tissue,
    malignant
    biphasic type (M9043/3) - see
      Neoplasm, connective tissue,
      malignant
    epithelioid cell type (M9042/3) - see
      Neoplasm, connective tissue,
      malignant
    spindle cell type (M9041/3) - see
      Neoplasm, connective tissue,
      malignant
Sarcomatosis
  meningeal (M9539/3) - see Neoplasm,
    meninges, malignant
  specified site NEC (M8800/3) - see
    Neoplasm, connective tissue,
    malignant
  unspecified site (M8800/6) 171.9
Sarcosinemia 270.8
Sarcosporidiosis 136.5
Satiety, early 780.94
Satisfactory smear but lacking
    transformation zone
  anal 796.77
  cervical 795.07
Saturnine - see condition
Saturnism 984.9
  specified type of lead - see Table of
    Drugs and Chemicals
Satyriasis 302.89
Sauriasis - see Ichthyosis
Sauriderma 757.39
Sauriosis - see Ichthyosis
Savill's disease (epidemic exfoliative
    dermatitis) 695.89
SBE (subacute bacterial endocarditis)
    421.0
Scabies (any site) 133.0
Scabs 782.8
Scaglietti-Dagnini syndrome
    (acromegalic macrospondylitis)
    253.0
Scald, scalded - see also Burn, by site
  skin syndrome 695.81
Scalenus anticus (anterior) syndrome
    353.0
Scales 782.8
Scalp - see condition
Scaphocephaly 756.0
Scaphoiditis, tarsal 732.5
Scapulalgia 733.90

Scapulohumeral myopathy 359.1
Scar, scarring (see also Cicatrix) 709.2
  adherent 709.2
  atrophic 709.2
  cervix
    in pregnancy or childbirth 654.6●
      affecting fetus or newborn
        763.89
      causing obstructed labor 660.2●
        affecting fetus or newborn
          763.1
  cheloid 701.4
  chorioretinal 363.30
    disseminated 363.35
    macular 363.32
    peripheral 363.34
    posterior pole NEC 363.33
  choroid (see also Scar, chorioretinal)
    363.30
  compression, pericardial 423.9
  congenital 757.39
  conjunctiva 372.64
  cornea 371.00
    xerophthalmic 264.6
  due to previous cesarean delivery,
    complicating pregnancy or
    childbirth 654.2●
    affecting fetus or newborn 763.89
  duodenal (bulb) (cap) 537.3
  hypertrophic 701.4
  keloid 701.4
  labia 624.4
  lung (base) 518.89
  macula 363.32
    disseminated 363.35
    peripheral 363.34
  muscle 728.89
  myocardium, myocardial 412
  painful 709.2
  papillary muscle 429.81
  posterior pole NEC 363.33
    macular - see Scar, macula
  postnecrotic (hepatic) (liver) 571.9
  psychic V15.49
  retina (see also Scar, chorioretinal)
    363.30
  trachea 478.9
  uterus 621.8
    in pregnancy or childbirth NEC
      654.9●
      affecting fetus or newborn
        763.89
      from previous cesarean delivery
        654.2●
  vulva 624.4
Scarabiasis 134.1
Scarlatina 034.1
  anginosa 034.1
  maligna 034.1
  myocarditis, acute 034.1 [422.0]
    old (see also Myocarditis) 429.0
  otitis media 034.1 [382.02]
  ulcerosa 034.1
Scarlatinella 057.8
Scarlet fever (albuminuria) (angina)
    (convulsions) (lesions of lid) (rash)
    034.1
Schamberg's disease, dermatitis, or
    dermatosis (progressive pigmentary
    dermatosis) 709.09
Schatzki's ring (esophagus) (lower)
    (congenital) 750.3
  acquired 530.3
Schaufenster krankheit 413.9

◀ New   ⬅ Revised   deleted Deleted   ● Use Additional Digit(s)   Omit code

Schaumann's
  benign lymphogranulomatosis 135
  disease (sarcoidosis) 135
  syndrome (sarcoidosis) 135
Scheie's syndrome
    (mucopolysaccharidosis IS) 277.5
Schenck's disease (sporotrichosis) 117.1
Scheuermann's disease or
    osteochondrosis 732.0
Scheuthauer-Marie-Sainton syndrome
    (cleidocranialis dysostosis) 755.59
Schilder (-Flatau) disease 341.1
Schilling-type monocytic leukemia
    (M9890/3) 206.9 ●
Schimmelbusch's disease, cystic mastitis,
    or hyperplasia 610.1
Schirmer's syndrome
    (encephalocutaneous angiomatosis)
    759.6
Schistocelia 756.79
Schistoglossia 750.13
Schistosoma infestation - see Infestation,
    Schistosoma
Schistosomiasis 120.9
  Asiatic 120.2
  bladder 120.0
  chestermani 120.8
  colon 120.1
  cutaneous 120.3
  due to
    S. hematobium 120.0
    S. japonicum 120.2
    S. mansoni 120.1
    S. mattheii 120.8
  eastern 120.2
  genitourinary tract 120.0
  intestinal 120.1
  lung 120.2
  Manson's (intestinal) 120.1
  Oriental 120.2
  pulmonary 120.2
  specified type NEC 120.8
  vesical 120.0
Schizencephaly 742.4
Schizo-affective psychosis (see also
    Schizophrenia) 295.7 ●
Schizodontia 520.2
Schizoid personality 301.20
  introverted 301.21
  schizotypal 301.22
Schizophrenia, schizophrenic (reaction)
    295.9 ●

Note 66   Use the following fifth-digit
subclassification with category 295:

  0   unspecified
  1   subchronic
  2   chronic
  3   subchronic with acute
          exacerbation
  4   chronic with acute exacerbation
  5   in remission

  acute (attack) NEC 295.8 ●
    episode 295.4 ●
  atypical form 295.8 ●
  borderline 295.5 ●
  catalepsy 295.2 ●
  catatonic (type) (acute) (excited)
      (withdrawn) 295.2 ●
  childhood (type) (see also Psychosis,
      childhood) 299.9 ●
  chronic NEC 295.6 ●
  coenesthesiopathic 295.8 ●

Schizophrenia, schizophrenic (Continued)
  cyclic (type) 295.7 ●
  disorganized (type) 295.1 ●
  flexibilitas cerea 295.2 ●
  hebephrenic (type) (acute) 295.1 ●
  incipient 295.5 ●
  latent 295.5 ●
  paranoid (type) (acute) 295.3 ●
  paraphrenic (acute) 295.3 ●
  prepsychotic 295.5 ●
  primary (acute) 295.0 ●
  prodromal 295.5 ●
  pseudoneurotic 295.5 ●
  pseudopsychopathic 295.5 ●
  reaction 295.9 ●
  residual type (state) 295.6 ●
  restzustand 295.6 ●
  schizo-affective (type) (depressed)
      (excited) 295.7 ●
  schizophreniform type 295.4 ●
  simple (type) (acute) 295.0 ●
  simplex (acute) 295.0 ●
  specified type NEC 295.8 ●
  syndrome of childhood NEC (see also
      Psychosis, childhood) 299.9 ●
  undifferentiated type 295.9 ●
    acute 295.8 ●
    chronic 295.6 ●
Schizothymia 301.20
  introverted 301.21
  schizotypal 301.22
Schlafkrankheit 086.5
Schlatter's tibia (osteochondrosis) 732.4
Schlatter-Osgood disease
    (osteochondrosis, tibial tubercle)
    732.4
Schloffer's tumor (see also Peritonitis) 567.29
Schmidt's syndrome
    sphallo-pharyngo-laryngeal
        hemiplegia 352.6
    thyroid-adrenocortical insufficiency
        258.1
    vagoaccessory 352.6
Schmincke
    carcinoma (M8082/3) - see Neoplasm,
        nasopharynx, malignant
    tumor (M8082/3) - see Neoplasm,
        nasopharynx, malignant
Schmitz (-Stutzer) dysentery 004.0
Schmorl's disease or nodes 722.30
    lumbar, lumbosacral 722.32
    specified region NEC 722.39
    thoracic, thoracolumbar 722.31
Schneider's syndrome 047.9
Schneiderian
    carcinoma (M8121/3)
      specified site - see Neoplasm, by site,
          malignant
      unspecified site 160.0
    papilloma (M8121/0)
      specified site - see Neoplasm, by site,
          benign
      unspecified site 212.0
Schnitzler syndrome 273.1
Schoffer's tumor (see also Peritonitis) 567.29
Scholte's syndrome (malignant carcinoid)
    259.2
Scholz's disease 330.0
Scholz (-Bielschowsky-Henneberg)
    syndrome 330.0
Schönlein (-Henoch) disease (primary)
    (purpura) (rheumatic) 287.0
School examination V70.3
    following surgery V67.09 ◄

Schottmüller's disease (see also Fever,
    paratyphoid) 002.9
Schroeder's syndrome (endocrine-
    hypertensive) 255.3
Schüller-Christian disease or syndrome
    (chronic histiocytosis X) 277.89
Schultz's disease or syndrome
    (agranulocytosis) 288.09
Schultze's acroparesthesia, simple 443.89
Schwalbe-Ziehen-Oppenheimer disease
    333.6
Schwannoma (M9560/0) - see also
    Neoplasm, connective tissues,
    benign
  malignant (M9560/3) - see Neoplasm,
      connective tissue, malignant
Schwartz (-Jampel) syndrome 359.23
Schwartz-Bartter syndrome
    (inappropriate secretion of
    antidiuretic hormone) 253.6
Schweninger-Buzzi disease (macular
    atrophy) 701.3
Sciatic - see condition
Sciatica (infectional) 724.3
  due to
    displacement of intervertebral disc
        722.10
    herniation, nucleus pulposus 722.10
  wallet 724.3
Scimitar syndrome (anomalous venous
    drainage, right lung to inferior vena
    cava) 747.49
Sclera - see condition
Sclerectasia 379.11
Scleredema
  adultorum 710.1
  Buschke's 710.1
  newborn 778.1
Sclerema
  adiposum (newborn) 778.1
  adultorum 710.1
  edematosum (newborn) 778.1
  neonatorum 778.1
  newborn 778.1
Scleriasis - see Scleroderma
Scleritis 379.00
  with corneal involvement 379.05
  anterior (annular) (localized) 379.03
  brawny 379.06
  granulomatous 379.09
  posterior 379.07
  specified NEC 379.09
  suppurative 379.09
  syphilitic 095.0
  tuberculous (nodular) (see also
      Tuberculosis) 017.3 ● [379.09]
Sclerochoroiditis (see also Scleritis)
    379.00
Scleroconjunctivitis (see also Scleritis)
    379.00
Sclerocystic ovary (syndrome) 256.4
Sclerodactylia 701.0
Scleroderma, sclerodermia (acrosclerotic)
    (diffuse) (generalized) (progressive)
    (pulmonary) 710.1
  circumscribed 701.0
  linear 701.0
  localized (linear) 701.0
  newborn 778.1
Sclerokeratitis 379.05
  meaning sclerosing keratitis 370.54
  tuberculous (see also Tuberculosis)
      017.3 ● [379.09]
Scleroma, trachea 040.1

Scleromalacia
  multiple 731.0
  perforans 379.04
Scleromyxedema 701.8
Scleroperikeratitis 379.05
Sclerose en plaques 340
Sclerosis, sclerotic
  adrenal (gland) 255.8
  Alzheimer's 331.0
    with dementia - *see* Alzheimer's,
      dementia
  amyotrophic (lateral) 335.20
  annularis fibrosi
    aortic 424.1
    mitral 424.0
  aorta, aortic 440.0
    valve (*see also* Endocarditis, aortic)
      424.1
  artery, arterial, arteriolar,
    arteriovascular - *see*
    Arteriosclerosis
  ascending multiple 340
  Balo's (concentric) 341.1
  basilar - *see* Sclerosis, brain
  bone (localized) NEC 733.99
  brain (general) (lobular) 348.89 ◀▥
    Alzheimer's - *see* Alzheimer's,
      dementia
    artery, arterial 437.0
    atrophic lobar 331.0
      with dementia
        with behavioral disturbance
          331.0 *[294.11]*
        without behavioral
          disturbance 331.0
          [294.10]
    diffuse 341.1
      familial (chronic) (infantile) 330.0
      infantile (chronic) (familial) 330.0
      Pelizaeus-Merzbacher type 330.0
    disseminated 340
    hereditary 334.2
    hippocampal 348.81 ◀
    infantile (degenerative) (diffuse) 330.0
    insular 340
    Krabbe's 330.0
    mesial temporal 348.81 ◀
    miliary 340
    multiple 340
    Pelizaeus-Merzbacher 330.0
    progressive familial 330.0
    senile 437.0
    temporal 348.81 ◀
      mesial 348.81 ◀
    tuberous 759.5
  bulbar, progressive 340
  bundle of His 426.50
    left 426.3
    right 426.4
  cardiac - *see* Arteriosclerosis, coronary
  cardiorenal (*see also* Hypertension,
    cardiorenal) 404.90
  cardiovascular (*see also* Disease,
    cardiovascular) 429.2
  renal (*see also* Hypertension,
    cardiorenal) 404.90
  centrolobar, familial 330.0
  cerebellar - *see* Sclerosis, brain
  cerebral - *see* Sclerosis, brain
  cerebrospinal 340
    disseminated 340
    multiple 340
  cerebrovascular 437.0
  choroid 363.40
    diffuse 363.56

Sclerosis, sclerotic (*Continued*)
  combined (spinal cord) - *see also*
    Degeneration, combined
    multiple 340
  concentric, Balo's 341.1
  cornea 370.54
  coronary (artery) - *see* Arteriosclerosis,
    coronary
  corpus cavernosum
    female 624.8
    male 607.89
  Dewitzky's
    aortic 424.1
    mitral 424.0
  diffuse NEC 341.1
  disease, heart - *see* Arteriosclerosis,
    coronary
  disseminated 340
  dorsal 340
  dorsolateral (spinal cord) - *see*
    Degeneration, combined
  endometrium 621.8
  extrapyramidal 333.90
  eye, nuclear (senile) 366.16
  Friedreich's (spinal cord) 334.0
  funicular (spermatic cord) 608.89
  gastritis 535.4●
  general (vascular) - *see* Arteriosclerosis
  gland (lymphatic) 457.8
  hepatic 571.9
  hereditary
    cerebellar 334.2
    spinal 334.0
  hippocampal 348.81 ◀
  idiopathic cortical (Garre's) (*see also*
    Osteomyelitis) 730.1●
  ilium, piriform 733.5
  insular 340
    pancreas 251.8
  Islands of Langerhans 251.8
  kidney - *see* Sclerosis, renal
  larynx 478.79
  lateral 335.24
    amyotrophic 335.20
    descending 335.24
    primary 335.24
    spinal 335.24
  liver 571.9
  lobar, atrophic (of brain) 331.0
    with dementia
      with behavioral disturbance 331.0
        [294.11]
      without behavioral disturbance
        331.0 *[294.10]*
  lung (*see also* Fibrosis, lung) 515
  mastoid 383.1
  mesial temporal 348.81 ◀
  mitral - *see* Endocarditis, mitral
  Mönckeberg's (medial) (*see also*
    Arteriosclerosis, extremities)
    440.20
  multiple (brain stem) (cerebral)
    (generalized) (spinal cord) 340
  myocardium, myocardial - *see*
    Arteriosclerosis, coronary
  nuclear (senile), eye 366.16
  ovary 620.8
  pancreas 577.8
  penis 607.89
  peripheral arteries (*see also*
    Arteriosclerosis, extremities)
    440.20
  plaques 340
  pluriglandular 258.8
  polyglandular 258.8

Sclerosis, sclerotic (*Continued*)
  posterior (spinal cord) (syphilitic) 094.0
  posterolateral (spinal cord) - *see*
    Degeneration, combined
  prepuce 607.89
  primary lateral 335.24
  progressive systemic 710.1
  pulmonary (*see also* Fibrosis, lung) 515
    artery 416.0
    valve (heart) (*see also* Endocarditis,
      pulmonary) 424.3
  renal 587
    with
      cystine storage disease 270.0
      hypertension (*see also*
        Hypertension, kidney)
        403.90
      hypertensive heart disease
        (conditions classifiable to
        402) (*see also* Hypertension,
        cardiorenal) 404.90
      arteriolar (hyaline) (*see also*
        Hypertension, kidney) 403.90
      hyperplastic (*see also*
        Hypertension, kidney)
        403.90
  retina (senile) (vascular) 362.17
  rheumatic
    aortic valve 395.9
    mitral valve 394.9
  Schilder's 341.1
  senile - *see* Arteriosclerosis
  spinal (cord) (general) (progressive)
    (transverse) 336.8
    ascending 357.0
    combined - *see also* Degeneration,
      combined
      multiple 340
      syphilitic 094.89
    disseminated 340
    dorsolateral - *see* Degeneration,
      combined
    hereditary (Friedreich's) (mixed
      form) 334.0
    lateral (amyotrophic) 335.24
    multiple 340
    posterior (syphilitic) 094.0
  stomach 537.89
  subendocardial, congenital 425.3
  systemic (progressive) 710.1
    with lung involvement 710.1 *[517.2]*
  temporal 348.81 ◀
    mesial 348.81 ◀
  tricuspid (heart) (valve) - *see*
    Endocarditis, tricuspid
  tuberous (brain) 759.5
  tympanic membrane (*see also*
    Tympanosclerosis) 385.00
  valve, valvular (heart) - *see*
    Endocarditis
  vascular - *see* Arteriosclerosis
  vein 459.89
Sclerotenonitis 379.07
Sclerotitis (*see also* Scleritis) 379.00
  syphilitic 095.0
  tuberculous (*see also* Tuberculosis) 017.3
    ● *[379.09]*
Scoliosis (acquired) (postural) 737.30
  congenital 754.2
  due to or associated with
    Charcôt-Marie-Tooth disease 356.1
      [737.43]
    mucopolysaccharidosis 277.5
      [737.43]
    neurofibromatosis 237.71 *[737.43]*

◀ New   ◀▥ Revised   ~~deleted~~ Deleted   ● Use Additional Digit(s)   ▥ Omit code

Scoliosis (Continued)
  due to or associated with (Continued)
    osteitis
      deformans 731.0 [737.43]
      fibrosa cystica 252.01 [737.43]
    osteoporosis (see also Osteoporosis)
      733.00 [737.43]
    poliomyelitis 138 [737.43]
    radiation 737.33
    tuberculosis (see also Tuberculosis)
      015.0● [737.43]
  idiopathic 737.30
    infantile
      progressive 737.32
      resolving 737.31
  paralytic 737.39
  rachitic 268.1
  sciatic 724.3
  specified NEC 737.39
  thoracogenic 737.34
  tuberculous (see also Tuberculosis)
    015.0● [737.43]
Scoliotic pelvis 738.6
  with disproportion (fetopelvic) 653.0●
    affecting fetus or newborn 763.1
    causing obstructed labor 660.1●
      affecting fetus or newborn 763.1
Scorbutus, scorbutic 267
  anemia 281.8
Scotoma (ring) 368.44
  arcuate 368.43
  Bjerrum 368.43
  blind spot area 368.42
  central 368.41
  centrocecal 368.41
  paracecal 368.42
  paracentral 368.41
  scintillating 368.12
  Seidel 368.43
Scratch - see Injury, superficial, by site
Scratchy throat 784.99
Screening (for) V82.9
  alcoholism V79.1
  anemia, deficiency NEC V78.1
    iron V78.0
  anomaly, congenital V82.89
  antenatal, of mother V28.9
    alphafetoprotein levels, raised V28.1
    based on amniocentesis V28.2
      chromosomal anomalies V28.0
      raised alphafetoprotein levels
        V28.1
    fetal growth retardation using
      ultrasonics V28.4
    genomic V28.89
    isoimmunization V28.5
    malformations using ultrasonics
      V28.3
    proteomic V28.89
    raised alphafetoprotein levels V28.1
    risk
      pre-term labor V28.82
    specified condition NEC V28.89
    Streptococcus B V28.6
  arterial hypertension V81.1
  arthropod-borne viral disease NEC
    V73.5
  asymptomatic bacteriuria V81.5
  bacterial
    and spirochetal sexually transmitted
      diseases V74.5
    conjunctivitis V74.4
    disease V74.9
      sexually transmitted V74.5
      specified condition NEC V74.8

Screening (Continued)
  bacteriuria, asymptomatic V81.5
  blood disorder NEC V78.9
    specified type NEC V78.8
  bronchitis, chronic V81.3
  brucellosis V74.8
  cancer - see Screening, malignant
    neoplasm
  cardiovascular disease NEC V81.2
  cataract V80.2
  Chagas' disease V75.3
  chemical poisoning V82.5
  cholera V74.0
  cholesterol level V77.91
  chromosomal
    anomalies
      by amniocentesis, antenatal V28.0
      maternal postnatal V82.4
    athletes V70.3
  condition
    cardiovascular NEC V81.2
    eye NEC V80.2
    genitourinary NEC V81.6
    neurological NEC V80.09   ◄▬
    respiratory NEC V81.4
    skin V82.0
    specified NEC V82.89
  congenital
    anomaly V82.89
      eye V80.2
    dislocation of hip V82.3
    eye condition or disease V80.2
  conjunctivitis, bacterial V74.4
  contamination NEC (see also Poisoning)
    V82.5
  coronary artery disease V81.0
  cystic fibrosis V77.6
  deficiency anemia NEC V78.1
    iron V78.0
  dengue fever V73.5
  depression V79.0
  developmental handicap V79.9
    in early childhood V79.3
    specified type NEC V79.8
  diabetes mellitus V77.1
  diphtheria V74.3
  disease or disorder V82.9
    bacterial V74.9
      specified NEC V74.8
    blood V78.9
      specified type NEC V78.8
    blood-forming organ V78.9
      specified type NEC V78.8
    cardiovascular NEC V81.2
      hypertensive V81.1
      ischemic V81.0
    Chagas' V75.3
    chlamydial V73.98
      specified NEC V73.88
    ear NEC V80.3
    endocrine NEC V77.99
    eye NEC V80.2
    genitourinary NEC V81.6
    heart NEC V81.2
      hypertensive V81.1
      ischemic V81.0
    HPV (human papillomavirus)
      V73.81
    human papillomavirus (HPV)
      V73.81
    immunity NEC V77.99
    infectious NEC V75.9
    lipoid NEC V77.91
    mental V79.9
      specified type NEC V79.8

Screening (Continued)
  disease or disorder (Continued)
    metabolic NEC V77.99
      inborn NEC V77.7
    neurological NEC V80.09   ◄▬
    nutritional NEC V77.99
    rheumatic NEC V82.2
    rickettsial V75.0
    sexually transmitted V74.5
      bacterial V74.5
      spirochetal V74.5
    sickle-cell V78.2
      trait V78.2
    specified type NEC V82.89
    thyroid V77.0
    vascular NEC V81.2
      ischemic V81.0
    venereal V74.5
    viral V73.99
      arthropod-borne NEC V73.5
      specified type NEC V73.89
  dislocation of hip, congenital V82.3
  drugs in athletes V70.3
  elevated titer V82.9
  emphysema (chronic) V81.3
  encephalitis, viral (mosquito or tick
    borne) V73.5
  endocrine disorder NEC V77.99
  eye disorder NEC V80.2
    congenital V80.2
  fever
    dengue V73.5
    hemorrhagic V73.5
    yellow V73.4
  filariasis V75.6
  galactosemia V77.4
  genetic V82.79
    disease carrier status V82.71
  genitourinary condition NEC V81.6
  glaucoma V80.1
  gonorrhea V74.5
  gout V77.5
  Hansen's disease V74.2
  heart disease NEC V81.2
    hypertensive V81.1
    ischemic V81.0
  heavy metal poisoning V82.5
  helminthiasis, intestinal V75.7
  hematopoietic malignancy V76.89
  hemoglobinopathies NEC V78.3
  hemorrhagic fever V73.5
  Hodgkin's disease V76.89
  hormones in athletes V70.3
  HPV (human papillomavirus) V73.81
  human papillomavirus (HPV) V73.81
  hypercholesterolemia V77.91
  hyperlipidemia V77.91
  hypertension V81.1
  immunity disorder NEC V77.99
  inborn errors of metabolism NEC
    V77.7
  infection
    bacterial V74.9
      specified type NEC V74.8
    mycotic V75.4
    parasitic NEC V75.8
  infectious disease V75.9
    specified type NEC V75.8
  ingestion of radioactive substance
    V82.5
  intestinal helminthiasis V75.7
  iron deficiency anemia V78.0
  ischemic heart disease V81.0
  lead poisoning V82.5
  leishmaniasis V75.2

Screening (*Continued*)
leprosy V74.2
leptospirosis V74.8
leukemia V76.89
lipoid disorder NEC V77.91
lymphoma V76.89
malaria V75.1
malignant neoplasm (of) V76.9
  bladder V76.3
  blood V76.89
  breast V76.10
    mammogram NEC V76.12
      for high-risk patient V76.11
    specified type NEC V76.19
  cervix V76.2
  colon V76.51
  colorectal V76.51
  hematopoietic system V76.89
  intestine V76.50
    colon V76.51
    small V76.52
  lung V76.0
  lymph (glands) V76.89
  nervous system V76.81
  oral cavity V76.42
  other specified neoplasm NEC V76.89
  ovary V76.46
  prostate V76.44
  rectum V76.41
  respiratory organs V76.0
  skin V76.43
  specified sites NEC V76.49
  testis V76.45
  vagina V76.47
    following hysterectomy for malignant condition V67.01
malnutrition V77.2
mammogram NEC V76.12
  for high-risk patient V76.11
maternal postnatal chromosomal anomalies V82.4
measles V73.2
mental
  disorder V79.9
    specified type NEC V79.8
  retardation V79.2
metabolic disorder NEC V77.99
metabolic errors, inborn V77.7
mucoviscidosis V77.6
multiphasic V82.6
mycosis V75.4
mycotic infection V75.4
nephropathy V81.5
neurological condition NEC V80.09 ◄▦
nutritional disorder NEC V77.99
obesity V77.8
osteoporosis V82.81
parasitic infection NEC V75.8
phenylketonuria V77.3
plague V74.8
poisoning
  chemical NEC V82.5
    contaminated water supply V82.5
  heavy metal V82.5
poliomyelitis V73.0
postnatal chromosomal anomalies, maternal V82.4
prenatal - *see* Screening, antenatal
pulmonary tuberculosis V74.1
radiation exposure V82.5
renal disease V81.5
respiratory condition NEC V81.4

Screening (*Continued*)
rheumatic disorder NEC V82.2
rheumatoid arthritis V82.1
rickettsial disease V75.0
rubella V73.3
schistosomiasis V75.5
senile macular lesions of eye V80.2
sexually transmitted diseases V74.5
  bacterial V74.5
  spirochetal V74.5
sickle-cell anemia, disease, or trait V78.2
skin condition V82.0
sleeping sickness V75.3
smallpox V73.1
special V82.9
  specified condition NEC V82.89
specified type NEC V82.89
spirochetal disease V74.9
  sexually transmitted V74.5
  specified type NEC V74.8
stimulants in athletes V70.3
syphilis V74.5
tetanus V74.8
thyroid disorder V77.0
trachoma V73.6
traumatic brain injury V80.01 ◄
trypanosomiasis V75.3
tuberculosis, pulmonary V74.1
venereal disease V74.5
viral encephalitis
  mosquito-borne V73.5
  tick-borne V73.5
whooping cough V74.8
worms, intestinal V75.7
yaws V74.6
yellow fever V73.4
Scrofula (*see also* Tuberculosis) 017.2●
Scrofulide (primary) (*see also* Tuberculosis) 017.0●
Scrofuloderma, scrofulodermia (any site) (primary) (*see also* Tuberculosis) 017.0●
Scrofulosis (universal) (*see also* Tuberculosis) 017.2●
Scrofulosis lichen (primary) (*see also* Tuberculosis) 017.0●
Scrofulous - *see* condition
Scrotal tongue 529.5
  congenital 750.13
Scrotum - *see* condition
Scurvy (gum) (infantile) (rickets) (scorbutic) 267
Sea-blue histiocyte syndrome 272.7
Seabright-Bantam syndrome (pseudohypoparathyroidism) 275.49
Sealpox 059.12
Seasickness 994.6
Seatworm 127.4
Sebaceous
cyst (*see also* Cyst, sebaceous) 706.2
gland disease NEC 706.9
Sebocystomatosis 706.2
Seborrhea, seborrheic 706.3
adiposa 706.3
capitis 690.11
congestiva 695.4
corporis 706.3
dermatitis 690.10
  infantile 690.12
diathesis in infants 695.89
eczema 690.18
  infantile 690.12

Seborrhea, seborrheic (*Continued*)
keratosis 702.19
  inflamed 702.11
nigricans 759.89
sicca 690.18
wart 702.19
  inflamed 702.11
Seckel's syndrome 759.89
Seclusion pupil 364.74
Seclusiveness, child 313.22
Secondary - *see also* condition
neoplasm - *see* Neoplasm, by site, malignant, secondary
Secretan's disease or syndrome (posttraumatic edema) 782.3
Secretion
antidiuretic hormone, inappropriate (syndrome) 253.6
catecholamine, by pheochromocytoma 255.6
hormone
  antidiuretic, inappropriate (syndrome) 253.6
  by
    carcinoid tumor 259.2
    pheochromocytoma 255.6
  ectopic NEC 259.3
urinary
  excessive 788.42
  suppression 788.5
Section
cesarean
  affecting fetus or newborn 763.4
  post mortem, affecting fetus or newborn 761.6
  previous, in pregnancy or childbirth 654.2●
    affecting fetus or newborn 763.89
nerve, traumatic - *see* Injury, nerve, by site
Seeligmann's syndrome (ichthyosis congenita) 757.1
Segmentation, incomplete (congenital) - *see also* Fusion
bone NEC 756.9
lumbosacral (joint) 756.15
vertebra 756.15
  lumbosacral 756.15
Seizure(s) 780.39
akinetic (idiopathic) (*see also* Epilepsy) 345.0●
  psychomotor 345.4●
apoplexy, apoplectic (*see also* Disease, cerebrovascular, acute) 436
atonic (*see also* Epilepsy) 345.0●
autonomic 300.11
brain or cerebral (*see also* Disease, cerebrovascular, acute) 436
convulsive (*see also* Convulsions) 780.39
cortical (focal) (motor) (*see also* Epilepsy) 345.5●
disorder (*see also* Epilepsy) 345.9 ◄
due to stroke 438.89
epilepsy, epileptic (cryptogenic) (*see also* Epilepsy) 345.9●
epileptiform, epileptoid 780.39
  focal (*see also* Epilepsy) 345.5●
febrile (simple) 780.31
  with status epilepticus 345.3
  atypical 780.32
  complex 780.32
  complicated 780.32
heart - *see* Disease, heart
hysterical 300.11

◄ New   ◄▦ Revised   ~~deleted~~ Deleted   ● Use Additional Digit(s)   ▦ Omit code

Seizure(s) (Continued)
 Jacksonian (focal) (see also Epilepsy)
   345.5●
     motor type 345.5●
     sensory type 345.5●
 migraine triggered 346.0●
 newborn 779.0
 paralysis (see also Disease,
   cerebrovascular, acute) 436
 recurrent 345.9●
   epileptic - see Epilepsy
 repetitive 780.39
   epileptic - see Epilepsy
 salaam (see also Epilepsy) 345.6●
 uncinate (see also Epilepsy) 345.4●
Self-mutilation 300.9
Semicoma 780.09
Semiconsciousness 780.09
Seminal
 vesicle - see condition
 vesiculitis (see also Vesiculitis) 608.0
Seminoma (M9061/3)
 anaplastic type (M9062/3)
   specified site - see Neoplasm, by site,
     malignant
   unspecified site 186.9
 specified site - see Neoplasm, by site,
   malignant
 spermatocytic (M9063/3)
   specified site - see Neoplasm, by site,
     malignant
   unspecified site 186.9
 unspecified site 186.9
Semliki Forest encephalitis 062.8
Senear-Usher disease or syndrome
 (pemphigus erythematosus)
   694.4
Senecio jacobae dermatitis 692.6
Senectus 797
Senescence 797
Senile (see also condition) 797
 cervix (atrophic) 622.8
 degenerative atrophy, skin 701.3
 endometrium (atrophic) 621.8
 fallopian tube (atrophic) 620.3
 heart (failure) 797
 lung 492.8
 ovary (atrophic) 620.3
 syndrome 259.8
 vagina, vaginitis (atrophic) 627.3
 wart 702.0
Senility 797
 with
   acute confusional state 290.3
   delirium 290.3
   mental changes 290.9
   psychosis NEC (see also Psychosis,
     senile) 290.20
 premature (syndrome) 259.8
Sensation
 burning (see also Disturbance,
   sensation) 782.0
   tongue 529.6
 choking 784.99
 loss of (see also Disturbance, sensation)
   782.0
 prickling (see also Disturbance,
   sensation) 782.0
 tingling (see also Disturbance,
   sensation) 782.0
Sense loss (touch) (see also Disturbance,
   sensation) 782.0
 smell 781.1
 taste 781.1

Sensibility disturbance NEC (cortical)
 (deep) (vibratory) (see also
   Disturbance, sensation) 782.0
Sensitive dentine 521.89
Sensitiver Beziehungswahn 297.8
Sensitivity, sensitization - see also
   Allergy
 autoerythrocyte 287.2
 carotid sinus 337.01
 child (excessive) 313.21
 cold, autoimmune 283.0
 methemoglobin 289.7
 suxamethonium 289.89
 tuberculin, without clinical or
   radiological symptoms 795.5
Sensory
 extinction 781.8
 neglect 781.8
Separation
 acromioclavicular - see Dislocation,
   acromioclavicular
 anxiety, abnormal 309.21
 apophysis, traumatic - see Fracture, by
   site
 choroid 363.70
   hemorrhagic 363.72
   serous 363.71
 costochondral (simple) (traumatic) - see
   Dislocation, costochondral
 delayed
   umbilical cord 779.83
 epiphysis, epiphyseal
   nontraumatic 732.9
     upper femoral 732.2
   traumatic - see Fracture, by site
 fracture - see Fracture, by site
 infundibulum cardiac from right
   ventricle by a partition 746.83
 joint (current) (traumatic) - see
   Dislocation, by site
 placenta (normally implanted) - see
   Placenta, separation
 pubic bone, obstetrical trauma
   665.6●
 retina, retinal (see also Detachment,
   retina) 361.9
   layers 362.40
     sensory (see also Retinoschisis)
       361.10
   pigment epithelium (exudative)
     362.42
     hemorrhagic 362.43
 sternoclavicular (traumatic) - see
   Dislocation, sternoclavicular
 symphysis pubis, obstetrical trauma
   665.6●
 tracheal ring, incomplete (congenital)
   748.3
Sepsis (generalized) 995.91
 with
   abortion - see Abortion, by type,
     with sepsis
   acute organ dysfunction 995.92
   ectopic pregnancy (see also
     categories 633.0–633.9) 639.0
   molar pregnancy (see also categories
     630–632) 639.0
   multiple organ dysfunction (MOD)
     995.92
 buccal 528.3
 complicating labor 659.3●
 dental (pulpal origin) 522.4
 female genital organ NEC 614.9
 fetus (intrauterine) 771.81

Sepsis (Continued)
 following
   abortion 639.0
   ectopic or molar pregnancy 639.0
   infusion, perfusion, or transfusion
     999.39
 Friedländer's 038.49
 intraocular 360.00
 localized
   in operation wound 998.59
   skin (see also Abscess) 682.9
 malleus 024
 nadir 038.9
 newborn (organism unspecified) NEC
   771.81
 oral 528.3
 puerperal, postpartum, childbirth
   (pelvic) 670.2 ◄▥
 resulting from infusion, injection,
   transfusion, or vaccination
   999.39
 severe 995.92
 skin, localized (see also Abscess) 682.9
 umbilical (newborn) (organism
   unspecified) 771.89
   tetanus 771.3
 urinary 599.0
   meaning sepsis 995.91
   meaning urinary tract infection
     599.0
Septate - see also Septum
Septic - see also condition
 adenoids 474.01
   and tonsils 474.02
 arm (with lymphangitis) 682.3
 embolus - see Embolism
 finger (with lymphangitis) 681.00
 foot (with lymphangitis) 682.7
 gallbladder (see also Cholecystitis)
   575.8
 hand (with lymphangitis) 682.4
 joint (see also Arthritis, septic) 711.0●
 kidney (see also Infection, kidney)
   590.9
 leg (with lymphangitis) 682.6
 mouth 528.3
 nail 681.9
   finger 681.02
   toe 681.11
 shock (endotoxic) 785.52
 sore (see also Abscess) 682.9
   throat 034.0
     milk-borne 034.0
     streptococcal 034.0
 spleen (acute) 289.59
 teeth (pulpal origin) 522.4
 throat 034.0
 thrombus - see Thrombosis
 toe (with lymphangitis) 681.10
 tonsils 474.00
   and adenoids 474.02
 umbilical cord (newborn) (organism
   unspecified) 771.89
 uterus (see also Endometritis) 615.9
Septicemia, septicemic (generalized)
   (suppurative) 038.9
 with
   abortion - see Abortion, by type,
     with sepsis
   ectopic pregnancy (see also
     categories 633.0–633.9) 639.0
   molar pregnancy (see also categories
     630–632) 639.0
 Aerobacter aerogenes 038.49

Septicemia, septicemic (Continued)
anaerobic 038.3
anthrax 022.3
Bacillus coli 038.42
Bacteroides 038.3
Clostridium 038.3
complicating labor 659.3●
cryptogenic 038.9
enteric gram-negative bacilli
038.40
Enterobacter aerogenes 038.49
Erysipelothrix (insidiosa)
(rhusiopathiae) 027.1
Escherichia coli 038.42
following
abortion 639.0
ectopic or molar pregnancy
639.0
infusion, injection, transfusion, or
vaccination 999.39
Friedländer's (bacillus) 038.49
gangrenous 038.9
gonococcal 098.89
gram-negative (organism)
038.40
anaerobic 038.3
Hemophilus influenzae 038.41
herpes (simplex) 054.5
herpetic 054.5
Listeria monocytogenes 027.0
meningeal - see Meningitis
meningococcal (chronic) (fulminating)
036.2
methicillin
resistant Staphylococcus aureus
(MRSA) 038.12
susceptible Staphylococcus aureus
(MSSA) 038.11
MRSA (methicillin resistant
Staphylococcus aureus)
038.12
MSSA (methicillin susceptible
Staphylococcus aureus) 038.11
navel, newborn (organism unspecified)
771.89
newborn (organism unspecified)
771.81
plague 020.2
pneumococcal 038.2
postabortal 639.0
postoperative 998.59
Proteus vulgaris 038.49
Pseudomonas (aeruginosa) 038.43
puerperal, postpartum 670.2   ⬅
Salmonella (aertrycke) (callinarum)
(choleraesuis) (enteritidis)
(suipestifer) 003.1
Serratia 038.44
Shigella (see also Dysentery, bacillary)
004.9
specified organism NEC 038.8
staphylococcal 038.10
aureus 038.11
methicillin
resistant (MRSA) 038.12
susceptible (MSSA) 038.11
specified organism NEC 038.19
streptococcal (anaerobic) 038.0
Streptococcus pneumoniae 038.2
suipestifer 003.1
umbilicus, newborn (organism
unspecified) 771.89
viral 079.99
Yersinia enterocolitica 038.49

Septum, septate (congenital) - see also
Anomaly, specified type NEC
anal 751.2
aqueduct of Sylvius 742.3
with spina bifida (see also Spina
bifida) 741.0●
hymen 752.49
uterus (see also Double, uterus)
752.2
vagina 752.49
in pregnancy or childbirth
654.7●
affecting fetus or newborn 763.89
causing obstructed labor
660.2●
affecting fetus or newborn
763.1
Sequestration
lung (congenital) (extralobar)
(intralobar) 748.5
orbit 376.10
pulmonary artery (congenital)
747.3
splenic 289.52
Sequestrum
bone (see also Osteomyelitis)
730.1●
jaw 526.4
dental 525.8
jaw bone 526.4
sinus (accessory) (nasal) (see also
Sinusitis) 473.9
maxillary 473.0
Sequoiosis asthma 495.8
Serology for syphilis
doubtful
with signs or symptoms - see
Syphilis, by site and stage
follow-up of latent syphilis - see
Syphilis, latent
false positive 795.6
negative, with signs or symptoms - see
Syphilis, by site and stage
positive 097.1
with signs or symptoms - see
Syphilis, by site and stage
false 795.6
follow-up of latent syphilis - see
Syphilis, latent
only finding - see Syphilis, latent
reactivated 097.1
Seroma - (postoperative) (non-infected)
998.13
infected 998.51
post-traumatic 729.91
Seropurulent - see condition
Serositis, multiple 569.89
pericardial 423.2
peritoneal 568.82
pleural - see Pleurisy
Serotonin syndrome 333.99
Serous - see condition
Sertoli cell
adenoma (M8640/0)
specified site - see Neoplasm, by site,
benign
unspecified site
female 220
male 222.0
carcinoma (M8640/3)
specified site - see Neoplasm, by site,
malignant
unspecified site 186.9
syndrome (germinal aplasia) 606.0

Sertoli cell (Continued)
tumor (M8640/0)
with lipid storage (M8641/0)
specified site - see Neoplasm, by
site, benign
unspecified site
female 220
male 222.0
specified site - see Neoplasm, by site,
benign
unspecified site
female 220
male 222.0
Sertoli-Leydig cell tumor (M8631/0)
specified site - see Neoplasm, by site,
benign
unspecified site
female 220
male 222.0
Serum
allergy, allergic reaction 999.5
shock 999.4
arthritis 999.5 [713.6]
complication or reaction NEC 999.5
disease NEC 999.5
hepatitis 070.3●
intoxication 999.5
jaundice (homologous) - see Hepatitis,
viral, type B
neuritis 999.5
poisoning NEC 999.5
rash NEC 999.5
reaction NEC 999.5
sickness NEC 999.5
Sesamoiditis 733.99
Seven-day fever 061
of
Japan 100.89
Queensland 100.89
Sever's disease or osteochondrosis
(calcaneum) 732.5
Sex chromosome mosaics 758.81
Sex reassignment surgery status (see also
Trans-sexualism) 302.50   ⬅
Sextuplet
affected by maternal complication of
pregnancy 761.5
healthy liveborn - see Newborn,
multiple
pregnancy (complicating delivery)
NEC 651.8●
with fetal loss and retention of one
or more fetus(es) 651.6●
following (elective) fetal reduction
651.7●
Sexual
anesthesia 302.72
deviation (see also Deviation, sexual)
302.9
disorder (see also Deviation, sexual)
302.9
frigidity (female) 302.72
function, disorder of (psychogenic)
302.70
specified type NEC 302.79
immaturity (female) (male) 259.0
impotence 607.84
organic origin NEC 607.84
psychogenic 302.72
precocity (constitutional) (cryptogenic)
(female) (idiopathic) (male) NEC
259.1
with adrenal hyperplasia 255.2
sadism 302.84

Sexuality, pathological (*see also* Deviation, sexual) 302.9

Sézary's disease, reticulosis, or syndrome (M9701/3) 202.2●

Shadow, lung 793.1

Shaken infant syndrome 995.55

Shaking
head (tremor) 781.0
palsy or paralysis (*see also* Parkinsonism) 332.0

Shallowness, acetabulum 736.39

Shaver's disease or syndrome (bauxite pneumoconiosis) 503

Shearing
artificial skin graft 996.55
decellularized allodermis graft 996.55

Sheath (tendon) - *see* condition

Shedding
nail 703.8
teeth, premature, primary (deciduous) 520.6

Sheehan's disease or syndrome (postpartum pituitary necrosis) 253.2

Shelf, rectal 569.49

Shell
shock (current) (*see also* Reaction, stress, acute) 308.9
lasting state 300.16
teeth 520.5

Shield kidney 753.3

Shift, mediastinal 793.2

Shifting
pacemaker 427.89
sleep-work schedule (affecting sleep) 327.36

Shiga's
bacillus 004.0
dysentery 004.0

Shigella (dysentery) (*see also* Dysentery, bacillary) 004.9
carrier (suspected) of V02.3

Shigellosis (*see also* Dysentery, bacillary) 004.9

Shingles (*see also* Herpes, zoster) 053.9
eye NEC 053.29

Shin splints 844.9

Shipyard eye or disease 077.1

Shirodkar suture, in pregnancy 654.5●

Shock 785.50
with
abortion - *see* Abortion, by type, with shock
ectopic pregnancy (*see also* categories 633.0–633.9) 639.5
molar pregnancy (*see also* categories 630–632) 639.5
allergic - *see* Shock, anaphylactic
anaclitic 309.21
anaphylactic 995.0
chemical - *see* Table of Drugs and Chemicals
correct medicinal substance properly administered 995.0
drug or medicinal substance
correct substance properly administered 995.0
overdose or wrong substance given or taken 977.9
specified drug - *see* Table of Drugs and Chemicals
following sting(s) 989.5

Shock (*Continued*)
anaphylactic (*Continued*)
food - *see* Anaphylactic shock, due to, food
immunization 999.4
serum 999.4
anaphylactoid - *see* Shock, anaphylactic
anesthetic
correct substance properly administered 995.4
overdose or wrong substance given 968.4
specified anesthetic - *see* Table of Drugs and Chemicals
birth, fetus or newborn NEC 779.89
cardiogenic 785.51
chemical substance - *see* Table of Drugs and Chemicals
circulatory 785.59
complicating
abortion - *see* Abortion, by type, with shock
ectopic pregnancy - (*see also* categories 633.0–633.9) 639.5
labor and delivery 669.1●
molar pregnancy (*see also* categories 630–632) 639.5
culture 309.29
due to
drug 995.0
correct substance properly administered 995.0
overdose or wrong substance given or taken 977.9
specified drug - *see* Table of Drugs and Chemicals
food - *see* Anaphylactic shock, due to, food
during labor and delivery 669.1●
electric 994.8
from electroshock gun (taser) 994.8
endotoxic 785.52
due to surgical procedure 998.0
following
abortion 639.5
ectopic or molar pregnancy 639.5
injury (immediate) (delayed) 958.4
labor and delivery 669.1●
gram-negative 785.52
hematogenic 785.59
hemorrhagic
due to
disease 785.59
surgery (intraoperative) (postoperative) 998.0
trauma 958.4
hypovolemic NEC 785.59
surgical 998.0
traumatic 958.4
insulin 251.0
therapeutic misadventure 962.3
kidney 584.5
traumatic (following crushing) 958.5
lightning 994.0
lung 518.5
nervous (*see also* Reaction, stress, acute) 308.9

Shock (*Continued*)
obstetric 669.1●
with
abortion - *see* Abortion, by type, with shock
ectopic pregnancy (*see also* categories 633.0–633.9) 639.5
molar pregnancy (*see also* categories 630–632) 639.5
following
abortion 639.5
ectopic or molar pregnancy 639.5
paralysis, paralytic (*see also* Disease, cerebrovascular, acute) 436
late effect - *see* Late effect(s) (of) cerebrovascular disease
pleural (surgical) 998.0
due to trauma 958.4
postoperative 998.0
with
abortion - *see* Abortion, by type, with shock
ectopic pregnancy (*see also* categories 633.0–633.9) 639.5
molar pregnancy (*see also* categories 630–632) 639.5
following
abortion 639.5
ectopic or molar pregnancy 639.5
psychic (*see also* Reaction, stress, acute) 308.9
past history (of) V15.49
psychogenic (*see also* Reaction, stress, acute) 308.9
septic 785.52
with
abortion - *see* Abortion, by type, with shock
ectopic pregnancy (*see also* categories 633.0–633.9) 639.5
molar pregnancy (*see also* categories 630–632) 639.5
due to
surgical procedure 998.0
transfusion NEC 999.89 ◄▥
bone marrow 996.85
following
abortion 639.5
ectopic or molar pregnancy 639.5
surgical procedure 998.0
transfusion NEC 999.89 ◄▥
bone marrow 996.85
spinal - *see also* Injury, spinal, by site
with spinal bone injury - *see* Fracture, vertebra, by site, with spinal cord injury
surgical 998.0
therapeutic misadventure NEC (*see also* Complications) 998.89
thyroxin 962.7
toxic 040.82
transfusion - *see* Complications, transfusion
traumatic (immediate) (delayed) 958.4

Shoemakers' chest 738.3

Short, shortening, shortness
Achilles tendon (acquired) 727.81
arm 736.89
congenital 755.20
back 737.9
bowel syndrome 579.3
breath 786.05

Short, shortening, shortness (*Continued*)
cervical, cervix 649.7●
  gravid uterus 649.7●
  non-gravid uterus 622.5
    acquired 622.5
    congenital 752.49
chain acyl CoA dehydrogenase
    deficiency (SCAD) 277.85
common bile duct, congenital 751.69
cord (umbilical) 663.4●
  affecting fetus or newborn 762.6
cystic duct, congenital 751.69
esophagus (congenital) 750.4
femur (acquired) 736.81
  congenital 755.34
frenulum linguae 750.0
frenum, lingual 750.0
hamstrings 727.81
hip (acquired) 736.39
  congenital 755.63
leg (acquired) 736.81
  congenital 755.30
metatarsus (congenital) 754.79
  acquired 736.79
organ or site, congenital NEC - *see*
    Distortion
palate (congenital) 750.26
P-R interval syndrome 426.81
radius (acquired) 736.09
  congenital 755.26
round ligament 629.89
sleeper 307.49
stature, constitutional (hereditary)
    (idiopathic) 783.43
tendon 727.81
  Achilles (acquired) 727.81
    congenital 754.79
  congenital 756.89
thigh (acquired) 736.81
  congenital 755.34
tibialis anticus 727.81
umbilical cord 663.4●
  affecting fetus or newborn 762.6
urethra 599.84
uvula (congenital) 750.26
vagina 623.8
Shortsightedness 367.1
Shoshin (acute fulminating beriberi) 265.0
Shoulder - *see* condition
Shovel-shaped incisors 520.2
Shower, thromboembolic - *see* Embolism
Shunt (status)
aortocoronary bypass V45.81
arterial-venous (dialysis) V45.11
arteriovenous, pulmonary (acquired)
    417.0
  congenital 747.3
  traumatic (complication) 901.40
cerebral ventricle (communicating) in
    situ V45.2
coronary artery bypass V45.81
surgical, prosthetic, with
    complications - *see*
    Complications, shunt
vascular NEC V45.89
Shutdown
renal 586
  with
    abortion - *see* Abortion, by type,
      with renal failure
    ectopic pregnancy (*see also*
      categories 633.0–633.9) 639.3
    molar pregnancy (*see also*
      categories 630–632) 639.3

Shutdown (*Continued*)
complicating
  abortion 639.3
  ectopic or molar pregnancy 639.3
  following labor and delivery 669.3●
Shwachman's syndrome 288.02
Shy-Drager syndrome (orthostatic
    hypotension with multisystem
    degeneration) 333.0
Sialadenitis (any gland) (chronic)
    (supportive) 527.2
  epidemic - *see* Mumps
Sialadenosis, periodic 527.2
Sialaporia 527.7
Sialectasia 527.8
Sialitis 527.2
Sialoadenitis (*see also* Sialadenitis) 527.2
Sialoangitis 527.2
Sialodochitis (fibrinosa) 527.2
Sialodocholithiasis 527.5
Sialolithiasis 527.5
Sialorrhea (*see also* Ptyalism) 527.7
  periodic 527.2
Sialosis 527.8
  rheumatic 710.2
Siamese twin 759.4
  complicating pregnancy 678.1●
Sicard's syndrome 352.6
Sicca syndrome (keratoconjunctivitis)
    710.2
Sick 799.9
  cilia syndrome 759.89
  or handicapped person in family
    V61.49
Sickle-cell
anemia (*see also* Disease, sickle-cell)
    282.60
disease (*see also* Disease, sickle-cell)
    282.60
hemoglobin
  C disease (without crisis) 282.63
    with
      crisis 282.64
        vaso-occlusive pain 282.64
  D disease (without crisis) 282.68
    with crisis 282.69
  E disease (without crisis) 282.68
    with crisis 282.69
  thalassemia (without crisis) 282.41
    with
      crisis 282.42
        vaso-occlusive pain 282.42
trait 282.5
Sicklemia (*see also* Disease, sickle-cell)
    282.60
  trait 282.5
Sickness
air (travel) 994.6
airplane 994.6
alpine 993.2
altitude 993.2
Andes 993.2
aviators' 993.2
balloon 993.2
car 994.6
compressed air 993.3
decompression 993.3
green 280.9
harvest 100.89
milk 988.8
morning 643.0●
motion 994.6
mountain 993.2
  acute 289.0

Sickness (*Continued*)
protein (*see also* Complications,
    vaccination) 999.5
radiation NEC 990
roundabout (motion) 994.6
sea 994.6
serum NEC 999.5
sleeping (African) 086.5
  by Trypanosoma 086.5
    gambiense 086.3
    rhodesiense 086.4
  Gambian 086.3
  late effect 139.8
  Rhodesian 086.4
sweating 078.2
swing (motion) 994.6
train (railway) (travel) 994.6
travel (any vehicle) 994.6
Sick sinus syndrome 427.81
Sideropenia (*see also* Anemia, iron
    deficiency) 280.9
Siderosis (lung) (occupational) 503
cornea 371.15
eye (bulbi) (vitreous) 360.23
lens 360.23
Siegal-Cattan-Mamou disease (periodic)
    277.31
Siemens' syndrome
ectodermal dysplasia 757.31
keratosis follicularis spinulosa
    (decalvans) 757.39
Sighing respiration 786.7
Sigmoid
flexure - *see* condition
kidney 753.3
Sigmoiditis - *see* Enteritis
Silfverskiöld's syndrome 756.50
Silicosis, silicotic (complicated)
    (occupational) (simple) 502
fibrosis, lung (confluent) (massive)
    (occupational) 502
non-nodular 503
pulmonum 502
Silicotuberculosis (*see also* Tuberculosis)
    011.4●
Silo fillers' disease 506.9
Silver's syndrome (congenital
    hemihypertrophy and short
    stature) 759.89
Silver wire arteries, retina 362.13
Silvestroni-Bianco syndrome
    (thalassemia minima) 282.49
Simian crease 757.2
Simmonds' cachexia or disease
    (pituitary cachexia) 253.2
Simons' disease or syndrome
    (progressive lipodystrophy)
    272.6
Simple, simplex - *see* condition
Sinding-Larsen disease (juvenile
    osteopathia patellae) 732.4
Singapore hemorrhagic fever 065.4
Singers' node or nodule 478.5
Single
atrium 745.69
coronary artery 746.85
umbilical artery 747.5
ventricle 745.3
Singultus 786.8
epidemicus 078.89
Sinus - *see also* Fistula
abdominal 569.81
arrest 426.6
arrhythmia 427.89

◀ New ◀▥ Revised ~~deleted~~ Deleted ● Use Additional Digit(s) ▭ Omit code

Sinus *(Continued)*
  bradycardia 427.89
    chronic 427.81
  branchial cleft (external) (internal)
      744.41
  coccygeal (infected) 685.1
    with abscess 685.0
  dental 522.7
  dermal (congenital) 685.1
    with abscess 685.0
  draining - *see* Fistula
  infected, skin NEC 686.9
  marginal, rupture or bleeding
      641.2●
    affecting fetus or newborn
        762.1
  pause 426.6
  pericranii 742.0
  pilonidal (infected) (rectum) 685.1
    with abscess 685.0
  preauricular 744.46
  rectovaginal 619.1
  sacrococcygeal (dermoid) (infected)
      685.1
    with abscess 685.0
  skin
    infected NEC 686.9
    noninfected- *see* Ulcer, skin
  tachycardia 427.89
  tarsi syndrome 726.79
  testis 608.89
  tract (postinfectional) - *see* Fistula
  urachus 753.7
Sinuses, Rokitansky-Aschoff *(see also*
    Disease, gallbladder) 575.8
Sinusitis (accessory) (chronic)
    (hyperplastic) (nasal)
    (nonpurulent) (purulent)
    473.9
  with influenza, flu, or grippe
      487.1
  acute 461.9
    ethmoidal 461.2
    frontal 461.1
    maxillary 461.0
    specified type NEC 461.8
    sphenoidal 461.3
  allergic *(see also* Fever, hay)
      477.9
  antrum - *see* Sinusitis, maxillary
  due to
    fungus, any sinus 117.9
    high altitude 993.1
  ethmoidal 473.2
    acute 461.2
  frontal 473.1
    acute 461.1
  influenzal 487.1
  maxillary 473.0
    acute 461.0
  specified site NEC 473.8
  sphenoidal 473.3
    acute 461.3
  syphilitic, any sinus 095.8
  tuberculous, any sinus *(see also*
      Tuberculosis) 012.8●
Sinusitis-bronchiectasis-situs inversus
    (syndrome) (triad) 759.3
Sipple's syndrome (medullary thyroid
    carcinoma-pheochromocytoma)
    258.02
Sirenomelia 759.89
Siriasis 992.0
Sirkari's disease 085.0

SIRS (systemic inflammatory response
    syndrome) 995.90
  due to
    infectious process 995.91
      with acute organ dysfunction
          995.92
    non-infectious process 995.93
      with acute organ dysfunction
          995.94
Siti 104.0
Sitophobia 300.29
Situation, psychiatric 300.9
Situational
  disturbance (transient) *(see also*
      Reaction, adjustment) 309.9
    acute 308.3
  maladjustment, acute *(see also* Reaction,
      adjustment) 309.9
  reaction *(see also* Reaction, adjustment)
      309.9
    acute 308.3
Situs inversus or transversus 759.3
  abdominalis 759.3
  thoracis 759.3
Sixth disease
  due to
    human herpesvirus 6 058.11
    human herpesvirus 7 058.12
Sjögren (-Gougerot) syndrome or disease
    (keratoconjunctivitis sicca) 710.2
  with lung involvement 710.2 *[517.8]*
Sjögren-Larsson syndrome (ichthyosis
    congenita) 757.1
SJS-TEN (Stevens-Johnson syndrome-
    toxic epidermal necrolysis overlap
    syndrome) 695.14
Skeletal - *see* condition
Skene's gland - *see* condition
Skenitis *(see also* Urethritis) 597.89
  gonorrheal (acute) 098.0
    chronic or duration of 2 months or
        over 098.2
Skerljevo 104.0
Skevas-Zerfus disease 989.5
Skin - *see also* condition
  donor V59.1
  hidebound 710.9
SLAP lesion (superior glenoid labrum)
    840.7
Slate-dressers' lung 502
Slate-miners' lung 502
Sleep
  deprivation V69.4
  disorder 780.50
    with apnea - *see* Apnea, sleep
    child 307.40
    movement, unspecified 780.58
    nonorganic origin 307.40
      specified type NEC 307.49
  disturbance 780.50
    with apnea - *see* Apnea, sleep
    nonorganic origin 307.40
      specified type NEC 307.49
  drunkenness 307.47
  movement disorder, unspecified
      780.58
  paroxysmal *(see also* Narcolepsy)
      347.00
  related movement disorder,
      unspecified 780.58
  rhythm inversion 327.39
    nonorganic origin 307.45
  walking 307.46
    hysterical 300.13

Sleeping sickness 086.5
  late effect 139.8
Sleeplessness *(see also* Insomnia) 780.52
  menopausal 627.2
  nonorganic origin 307.41
Slipped, slipping
  epiphysis (postinfectional) 732.9
    traumatic (old) 732.9
      current - *see* Fracture, by site
    upper femoral (nontraumatic)
        732.2
  intervertebral disc - *see* Displacement,
      intervertebral disc
  ligature, umbilical 772.3
  patella 717.89
  rib 733.99
  sacroiliac joint 724.6
  tendon 727.9
  ulnar nerve, nontraumatic 354.2
  vertebra NEC *(see also*
      Spondylolisthesis) 756.12
Slocumb's syndrome 255.3
Sloughing (multiple) (skin) 686.9
  abscess - *see* Abscess, by site
  appendix 543.9
  bladder 596.8
  fascia 728.9
  graft - *see* Complications, graft
  phagedena *(see also* Gangrene) 785.4
  reattached extremity *(see also*
      Complications, reattached
      extremity) 996.90
  rectum 569.49
  scrotum 608.89
  tendon 727.9
  transplanted organ *(see also* Rejection,
      transplant, organ, by site)
      996.80
  ulcer *(see also* Ulcer, skin) 707.9
Slow
  feeding newborn 779.31   ◀▥
  fetal, growth NEC 764.9●
    affecting management of pregnancy
        656.5●
Slowing
  heart 427.89
  urinary stream 788.62
Sluder's neuralgia or syndrome 337.09   ◀▥
Slurred, slurring, speech 784.59   ◀▥
Small, smallness
  cardia reserve - *see* Disease, heart
  for dates
    fetus or newborn 764.0●
      with malnutrition 764.1●
      affecting management of
          pregnancy 656.5●
    infant, term 764.0●
      with malnutrition 764.1●
      affecting management of pregnancy
          656.5●
  introitus, vagina 623.3
  kidney, unknown cause 589.9
    bilateral 589.1
    unilateral 589.0
  ovary 620.8
  pelvis
    with disproportion (fetopelvic)
        653.1●
      affecting fetus or newborn 763.1
      causing obstructed labor 660.1●
        affecting fetus or newborn 763.1
  placenta - *see* Placenta, insufficiency
  uterus 621.8
  white kidney 582.9

Small-for-dates (see also Light-for-dates)
764.0●
affecting management of pregnancy
656.5●
Smallpox 050.9
contact V01.3
exposure to V01.3
hemorrhagic (pustular) 050.0
malignant 050.0
modified 050.2
vaccination
complications - see Complications,
vaccination
prophylactic (against) V04.1
Smith's fracture (separation) (closed)
813.41
open 813.51
Smith-Lemli-Opitz syndrome
(cerebrohepatorenal syndrome)
759.89
Smith-Magenis syndrome 758.33
Smith-Strang disease (oasthouse urine)
270.2
Smokers'
bronchitis 491.0
cough 491.0
syndrome (see also Abuse, drugs,
nondependent) 305.1
throat 472.1
tongue 528.6
Smoking complicating pregnancy,
childbirth, or the puerperium
649.0●
Smothering spells 786.09
Snaggle teeth, tooth 524.39
Snapping
finger 727.05
hip 719.65
jaw 524.69
temporomandibular joint sounds on
opening or closing 524.64
knee 717.9
thumb 727.05
Sneddon-Wilkinson disease or
syndrome (subcorneal pustular
dermatosis) 694.1
Sneezing 784.99
intractable 478.19
Sniffing
cocaine (see also Dependence) 304.2●
either (see also Dependence) 304.6●
glue (airplane) (see also Dependence)
304.6●
Snoring 786.09
Snow blindness 370.24
Snuffles (nonsyphilitic) 460
syphilitic (infant) 090.0
Social migrant V60.0
Sodoku 026.0
Soemmering's ring 366.51
Soft - see also condition
enlarged prostate 600.00
with
other lower urinary tract
symptoms (LUTS) 600.01
urinary
obstruction 600.01
retention 600.01
nails 703.8
Softening
bone 268.2
brain (necrotic) (progressive) 434.9●
arteriosclerotic 437.0
congenital 742.4

Softening (Continued)
brain (Continued)
embolic (see also Embolism, brain)
434.1●
hemorrhagic (see also Hemorrhage,
brain) 431
occlusive 434.9●
thrombotic (see also Thrombosis,
brain) 434.0●
cartilage 733.92
cerebellar - see Softening, brain
cerebral - see Softening, brain
cerebrospinal - see Softening, brain
myocardial, heart (see also
Degeneration, myocardial) 429.1
nails 703.8
spinal cord 336.8
stomach 537.89
Solar fever 061
Soldier's
heart 306.2
patches 423.1
Solitary
cyst
bone 733.21
kidney 593.2
kidney (congenital) 753.0
tubercle, brain (see also Tuberculosis,
brain) 013.2●
ulcer, bladder 596.8
Somatization reaction, somatic reaction
(see also Disorder, psychosomatic)
306.9
disorder 300.81
Somatoform disorder 300.82
atypical 300.82
severe 300.81
undifferentiated 300.82
Somnambulism 307.46
hysterical 300.13
Somnolence 780.09
nonorganic origin 307.43
periodic 349.89
Sonne dysentery 004.3
Soor 112.0
Sore
Delhi 085.1
desert (see also Ulcer, skin) 707.9
eye 379.99
Lahore 085.1
mouth 528.9
canker 528.2
due to dentures 528.9
muscle 729.1
naga (see also Ulcer, skin) 707.9
oriental 085.1
pressure (see also Ulcer, pressure)
707.00
with gangrene (see also Ulcer,
pressure) 707.00 [785.4]
skin NEC 709.9
soft 099.0
throat 462
with influenza, flu, or grippe 487.1
acute 462
chronic 472.1
clergyman's 784.49
Coxsackie (virus) 074.0
diphtheritic 032.0
epidemic 034.0
gangrenous 462
herpetic 054.79
influenzal 487.1
malignant 462

Sore (Continued)
throat (Continued)
purulent 462
putrid 462
septic 034.0
streptococcal (ulcerative) 034.0
ulcerated 462
viral NEC 462
Coxsackie 074.0
tropical (see also Ulcer, skin) 707.9
veldt (see also Ulcer, skin) 707.9
Sotos' syndrome (cerebral gigantism)
253.0
Sounds
friction, pleural 786.7
succussion, chest 786.7
temporomandibular joint
on opening or closing 524.64
South African cardiomyopathy
syndrome 425.2
South American
blastomycosis 116.1
trypanosomiasis - see Trypanosomiasis
Southeast Asian hemorrhagic fever 065.4
Spacing, teeth, abnormal 524.30
excessive 524.32
Spade-like hand (congenital) 754.89
Spading nail 703.8
congenital 757.5
Spanemia 285.9
Spanish collar 605
Sparganosis 123.5
Spasm, spastic, spasticity (see also
condition) 781.0
accommodation 367.53
ampulla of Vater (see also Disease,
gallbladder) 576.8
anus, ani (sphincter) (reflex) 564.6
psychogenic 306.4
artery NEC 443.9
basilar 435.0
carotid 435.8
cerebral 435.9
specified artery NEC 435.8
retinal (see also Occlusion, retinal,
artery) 362.30
vertebral 435.1
vertebrobasilar 435.3
Bell's 351.0
bladder (sphincter, external or internal)
596.8
bowel 564.9
psychogenic 306.4
bronchus, bronchiole 519.11
cardia 530.0
cardiac - see Angina
carpopedal (see also Tetany) 781.7
cecum 564.9
psychogenic 306.4
cerebral (arteries) (vascular) 435.9
specified artery NEC 435.8
cerebrovascular 435.9
cervix, complicating delivery 661.4●
affecting fetus or newborn 763.7
ciliary body (of accommodation)
367.53
colon 564.1
psychogenic 306.4
common duct (see also Disease, biliary)
576.8
compulsive 307.22
conjugate 378.82
convergence 378.84
coronary (artery) - see Angina

◀ New ◀◀ Revised ~~deleted~~ Deleted ● Use Additional Digit(s) ▨ Omit code

Spasm, spastic, spasticity (Continued)
diaphragm (reflex) 786.8
psychogenic 306.1
duodenum, duodenal (bulb) 564.89
esophagus (diffuse) 530.5
psychogenic 306.4
facial 351.8
fallopian tube 620.8
gait 781.2
gastrointestinal (tract) 536.8
psychogenic 306.4
glottis 478.75
hysterical 300.11
psychogenic 306.1
specified as conversion reaction
300.11
reflex through recurrent laryngeal
nerve 478.75
habit 307.20
chronic 307.22
transient (of childhood) 307.21
heart - see Angina
hourglass - see Contraction, hourglass
hysterical 300.11
infantile (see also Epilepsy) 345.6●
internal oblique, eye 378.51
intestinal 564.9
psychogenic 306.4
larynx, laryngeal 478.75
hysterical 300.11
psychogenic 306.1
specified as conversion reaction
300.11
levator palpebrae superioris 333.81
lightning (see also Epilepsy) 345.6●
mobile 781.0
muscle 728.85
back 724.8
psychogenic 306.0
nerve, trigeminal 350.1
nervous 306.0
nodding 307.3
infantile (see also Epilepsy) 345.6●
occupational 300.89
oculogyric 378.87
ophthalmic artery 362.30
orbicularis 781.0
perineal 625.8
peroneo-extensor (see also Flat, foot)
734
pharynx (reflex) 478.29
hysterical 300.11
psychogenic 306.1
specified as conversion reaction
300.11
pregnant uterus, complicating delivery
661.4●
psychogenic 306.0
pylorus 537.81
adult hypertrophic 537.0
congenital or infantile 750.5
psychogenic 306.4
rectum (sphincter) 564.6
psychogenic 306.4
retinal artery NEC (see also Occlusion,
retina, artery) 362.30
sacroiliac 724.6
salaam (infantile) (see also Epilepsy)
345.6●
saltatory 781.0
sigmoid 564.9
psychogenic 306.4
sphincter of Oddi (see also Disease,
gallbladder) 576.5

Spasm, spastic, spasticity (Continued)
stomach 536.8
neurotic 306.4
throat 478.29
hysterical 300.11
psychogenic 306.1
specified as conversion reaction
300.11
tic 307.20
chronic 307.22
transient (of childhood) 307.21
tongue 529.8
torsion 333.6
trigeminal nerve 350.1
postherpetic 053.12
ureter 593.89
urethra (sphincter) 599.84
uterus 625.8
complicating labor 661.4●
affecting fetus or newborn
763.7
vagina 625.1
psychogenic 306.51
vascular NEC 443.9
vasomotor NEC 443.9
vein NEC 459.89
vesical (sphincter, external or internal)
596.8
viscera 789.0●
Spasmodic - see condition
Spasmophilia (see also Tetany) 781.7
Spasmus nutans 307.3
Spastic - see also Spasm
child 343.9
Spasticity - see also Spasm
cerebral, child 343.9
Speakers' throat 784.49
Specific, specified - see condition
Speech
defect, disorder, disturbance,
impediment NEC 784.59 ◀▥
psychogenic 307.9 ◀▥
(language) therapy V57.3 ◀▥
Spells 780.39
breath-holding 786.9
Spencer's disease (epidemic vomiting)
078.82
Spens' syndrome (syncope with heart
block) 426.9
Spermatic cord - see condition
Spermatocele 608.1
congenital 752.89
Spermatocystitis 608.4
Spermatocytoma (M9063/3)
specified site - see Neoplasm, by site,
malignant
unspecified site 186.9
Spermatorrhea 608.89
Sperm counts
fertility testing V26.21
following sterilization reversal V26.22
postvasectomy V25.8
Sphacelus (see also Gangrene) 785.4
Sphenoidal - see condition
Sphenoiditis (chronic) (see also Sinusitis,
sphenoidal) 473.3
Sphenopalatine ganglion neuralgia
337.09
Sphericity, increased, lens 743.36
Spherocytosis (congenital) (familial)
(hereditary) 282.0
hemoglobin disease 282.7
sickle-cell (disease) 282.60
Spherophakia 743.36

Sphincter - see condition
Sphincteritis, sphincter of Oddi (see also
Cholecystitis) 576.8
Sphingolipidosis 272.7
Sphingolipodystrophy 272.7
Sphingomyelinosis 272.7
Spicule tooth 520.2
Spider
finger 755.59
nevus 448.1
vascular 448.1
Spiegler-Fendt sarcoid 686.8
Spielmeyer-Stock disease 330.1
Spielmeyer-Vogt disease 330.1
Spina bifida (aperta) 741.9●

> Note 67   Use the following fifth-digit
> subclassification with category 741:
>
> 0   unspecified region
> 1   cervical region
> 2   dorsal [thoracic] region
> 3   lumbar region

with hydrocephalus 741.0●
fetal (suspected), affecting
management of pregnancy
655.0●
occulta 756.17
Spindle, Krukenberg's 371.13
Spine, spinal - see condition
Spiradenoma (eccrine) (M8403/0) - see
Neoplasm, skin, benign
Spirillosis NEC (see also Fever, relapsing)
087.9
Spirillum minus 026.0
Spirillum obermeieri infection 087.0
Spirochetal - see condition
Spirochetosis 104.9
arthritic, arthritica 104.9 [711.8]●
bronchopulmonary 104.8
icterohemorrhagica 100.0
lung 104.8
Spitting blood (see also Hemoptysis) 786.3
Splanchnomegaly 569.89
Splanchnoptosis 569.89
Spleen, splenic - see also condition
agenesis 759.0
flexure syndrome 569.89
neutropenia syndrome 289.53
sequestration syndrome 289.52
Splenectasis (see also Splenomegaly)
789.2
Splenitis (interstitial) (malignant)
(nonspecific) 289.59
malarial (see also Malaria) 084.6
tuberculous (see also Tuberculosis)
017.7●
Splenocele 289.59
Splenomegalia - see Splenomegaly
Splenomegalic - see condition
Splenomegaly 789.2
Bengal 789.2
cirrhotic 289.51
congenital 759.0
congestive, chronic 289.51
cryptogenic 789.2
Egyptian 120.1
Gaucher's (cerebroside lipidosis) 272.7
idiopathic 789.2
malarial (see also Malaria) 084.6
neutropenic 289.53
Niemann-Pick (lipid histiocytosis)
272.7
siderotic 289.51

Splenomegaly *(Continued)*
  syphilitic 095.8
    congenital 090.0
  tropical (Bengal) (idiopathic) 789.2
Splenopathy 289.50
Splenopneumonia - *see* Pneumonia
Splenoptosis 289.59
Splinter - *see* Injury, superficial, by site
Split, splitting
  heart sounds 427.89
  lip, congenital (*see also* Cleft, lip)
    749.10
  nails 703.8
  urinary stream 788.61
Spoiled child reaction (*see also*
    Disturbance, conduct) 312.1●
Spondylarthritis (*see also* Spondylosis)
    721.90
Spondylarthrosis (*see also* Spondylosis)
    721.90
Spondylitis 720.9
  ankylopoietica 720.0
  ankylosing (chronic) 720.0
  atrophic 720.9
    ligamentous 720.9
  chronic (traumatic) (*see also*
      Spondylosis) 721.90
  deformans (chronic) (*see also*
      Spondylosis) 721.90
  gonococcal 098.53
  gouty 274.00   ◀▥
  hypertrophic (*see also* Spondylosis)
    721.90
  infectious NEC 720.9
  juvenile (adolescent) 720.0
  Kummell's 721.7
  Marie-Strümpell (ankylosing) 720.0
  muscularis 720.9
  ossificans ligamentosa 721.6
  osteoarthritica (*see also* Spondylosis)
    721.90
  posttraumatic 721.7
  proliferative 720.0
  rheumatoid 720.0
  rhizomelica 720.0
  sacroiliac NEC 720.2
  senescent (*see also* Spondylosis)
    721.90
  senile (*see also* Spondylosis) 721.90
  static (*see also* Spondylosis) 721.90
  traumatic (chronic) (*see also*
      Spondylosis) 721.90
  tuberculous (*see also* Tuberculosis)
      015.0● [720.81]
  typhosa 002.0 [720.81]
Spondyloarthrosis (*see also* Spondylosis)
    721.90
Spondylolisthesis (congenital)
    (lumbosacral) 756.12
  with disproportion (fetopelvic)
      653.3●
    affecting fetus or newborn
        763.1
    causing obstructed labor
        660.1●
      affecting fetus or newborn
          763.1
  acquired 738.4
  degenerative 738.4
  traumatic 738.4
    acute (lumbar) - *see* Fracture,
        vertebra, lumbar
      site other than lumbosacral - *see*
          Fracture, vertebra, by site

Spondylolysis (congenital) 756.11
  acquired 738.4
  cervical 756.19
  lumbosacral region 756.11
    with disproportion (fetopelvic)
        653.3●
      affecting fetus or newborn
          763.1
      causing obstructed labor 660.1●
        affecting fetus or newborn
            763.1
Spondylopathy
  inflammatory 720.9
    specified type NEC 720.89
  traumatic 721.7
Spondylose rhizomelique 720.0
Spondylosis 721.90
  with
      disproportion 653.3●
        affecting fetus or newborn
            763.1
        causing obstructed labor 660.1●
          affecting fetus or newborn
              763.1
    myelopathy NEC 721.91
  cervical, cervicodorsal 721.0
    with myelopathy 721.1
  inflammatory 720.9
  lumbar, lumbosacral 721.3
    with myelopathy 721.42
  sacral 721.3
    with myelopathy 721.42
  thoracic 721.2
    with myelopathy 721.41
  traumatic 721.7
Sponge
  divers' disease 989.5
  inadvertently left in operation wound
      998.4
  kidney (medullary) 753.17
Spongioblastoma (M9422/3)
  multiforme (M9440/3)
    specified site - *see* Neoplasm, by site,
        malignant
    unspecified site 191.9
  polare (M9423/3)
    specified site - *see* Neoplasm, by site,
        malignant
    unspecified site 191.9
  primitive polar (M9443/3)
    specified site - *see* Neoplasm, by site,
        malignant
    unspecified site 191.9
  specified site - *see* Neoplasm, by site,
      malignant
  unspecified site 191.9
Spongiocytoma (M9400/3)
  specified site - *see* Neoplasm, by site,
      malignant
  unspecified site 191.9
Spongioneuroblastoma (M9504/3) - *see*
    Neoplasm, by site, malignant
Spontaneous - *see also* condition
  fracture - *see* Fracture, pathologic
Spoon nail 703.8
  congenital 757.5
Sporadic - *see* condition
Sporotrichosis (bones) (cutaneous)
    (disseminated) (epidermal)
    (lymphatic) (lymphocutaneous)
    (mucous membranes) (pulmonary)
    (skeletal) (visceral) 117.1
Sporotrichum schenckii infection
    117.1

Spots, spotting
  atrophic (skin) 701.3
  Bitôt's (in the young child) 264.1
  café au lait 709.09
  cayenne pepper 448.1
  complicating pregnancy 649.5●
  cotton wool (retina) 362.83
  de Morgan's (senile angiomas) 448.1
  Fúchs' black (myopic) 360.21
  intermenstrual
    irregular 626.6
    regular 626.5
  interpalpebral 372.53
  Koplik's 055.9
  liver 709.09
  Mongolian (pigmented) 757.33
  of pregnancy 649.5●
  purpuric 782.7
  ruby 448.1
Spotted fever - *see* Fever, spotted
Sprain, strain (joint) (ligament) (muscle)
    (tendon) 848.9
  abdominal wall (muscle) 848.8
  Achilles tendon 845.09
  acromioclavicular 840.0
  ankle 845.00
    and foot 845.00
  anterior longitudinal, cervical 847.0
  arm 840.9
    upper 840.9
      and shoulder 840.9
  astragalus 845.00
  atlanto-axial 847.0
  atlanto-occipital 847.0
  atlas 847.0
  axis 847.0
  back (*see also* Sprain, spine) 847.9
  breast bone 848.40
  broad ligaments - *see* Injury, internal,
      broad ligament
  calcaneofibular 845.02
  carpal 842.01
  carpometacarpal 842.11
  cartilage
    costal, without mention of injury to
        sternum 848.3
      involving sternum 848.42
    ear 848.8
    knee 844.9
      with current tear (*see also* Tear,
          meniscus) 836.2
    semilunar (knee) 844.8
      with current tear (*see also* Tear,
          meniscus) 836.2
    septal, nose 848.0
    thyroid region 848.2
    xiphoid 848.49
  cervical, cervicodorsal, cervicothoracic
      847.0
  chondrocostal, without mention of
      injury to sternum 848.3
    involving sternum 848.42
  chondrosternal 848.42
  chronic (joint) - *see* Derangement,
      joint
  clavicle 840.9
  coccyx 847.4
  collar bone 840.9
  collateral, knee (medial) (tibial)
      844.1
    lateral (fibular) 844.0
    recurrent or old 717.89
      lateral 717.81
      medial 717.82

◀ New   ◀▥ Revised   ~~deleted~~ Deleted   ● Use Additional Digit(s)   ▭ Omit code

Sprain, strain *(Continued)*
  coracoacromial 840.8
  coracoclavicular 840.1
  coracohumeral 840.2
  coracoid (process) 840.9
  coronary, knee 844.8
  costal cartilage, without mention of
    injury to sternum 848.3
     involving sternum 848.42
  cricoarytenoid articulation 848.2
  cricothyroid articulation 848.2
  cruciate
    knee 844.2
    old 717.89
     anterior 717.83
     posterior 717.84
  deltoid
    ankle 845.01
    shoulder 840.8
  dorsal (spine) 847.1
  ear cartilage 848.8
  elbow 841.9
    and forearm 841.9
    specified site NEC 841.8
  femur (proximal end) 843.9
    distal end 844.9
  fibula (proximal end) 844.9
    distal end 845.00
  fibulocalcaneal 845.02
  finger(s) 842.10
  foot 845.10
    and ankle 845.00
  forearm 841.9
    and elbow 841.9
    specified site NEC 841.8
  glenoid (shoulder) - *(see also* SLAP
    lesion) 840.8
  hand 842.10
  hip 843.9
    and thigh 843.9
  humerus (proximal end) 840.9
    distal end 841.9
  iliofemoral 843.0
  infraspinatus 840.3
  innominate
    acetabulum 843.9
    pubic junction 848.5
    sacral junction 846.1
  internal
    collateral, ankle 845.01
    semilunar cartilage 844.8
     with current tear *(see also* Tear,
      meniscus) 836.2
     old 717.5
  interphalangeal
    finger 842.13
    toe 845.13
  ischiocapsular 843.1
  jaw (cartilage) (meniscus) 848.1
    old 524.69
  knee 844.9
    and leg 844.9
    old 717.5
     collateral
      lateral 717.81
      medial 717.82
     cruciate
      anterior 717.83
      posterior 717.84
  late effect - *see* Late, effects (of), sprain
  lateral collateral, knee 844.0
    old 717.81
  leg 844.9
    and knee 844.9

Sprain, strain *(Continued)*
  ligamentum teres femoris 843.8
  low back 846.9
  lumbar (spine) 847.2
  lumbosacral 846.0
    chronic or old 724.6
  mandible 848.1
    old 524.69
  maxilla 848.1
  medial collateral, knee 844.1
    old 717.82
  meniscus
    jaw 848.1
     old 524.69
    knee 844.8
     with current tear *(see also* Tear,
      meniscus) 836.2
     old 717.5
    mandible 848.1
     old 524.69
    specified site NEC 848.8
  metacarpal 842.10
    distal 842.12
    proximal 842.11
  metacarpophalangeal 842.12
  metatarsal 845.10
  metatarsophalangeal 845.12
  midcarpal 842.19
  midtarsal 845.19
  multiple sites, except fingers alone or
    toes alone 848.8
  neck 847.0
  nose (septal cartilage) 848.0
  occiput from atlas 847.0
  old - *see* Derangement, joint
  orbicular, hip 843.8
  patella(r) 844.8
    old 717.89
  pelvis 848.5
  phalanx
    finger 842.10
    toe 845.10
  radiocarpal 842.02
  radiohumeral 841.2
  radioulnar 841.9
    distal 842.09
  radius, radial (proximal end) 841.9
    and ulna 841.9
     distal 842.09
    collateral 841.0
    distal end 842.00
  recurrent - *see* Sprain, by site
  rib (cage), without mention of injury to
    sternum 848.3
    involving sternum 848.42
  rotator cuff (capsule) 840.4
  round ligament - *see also* Injury,
    internal, round ligament
    femur 843.8
  sacral (spine) 847.3
  sacrococcygeal 847.3
  sacroiliac (region) 846.9
    chronic or old 724.6
    ligament 846.1
    specified site NEC 846.8
  sacrospinatus 846.2
  sacrospinous 846.2
  sacrotuberous 846.3
  scaphoid bone, ankle 845.00
  scapula(r) 840.9
  semilunar cartilage (knee) 844.8
    with current tear *(see also* Tear,
     meniscus) 836.2
    old 717.5

Sprain, strain *(Continued)*
  septal cartilage (nose) 848.0
  shoulder 840.9
    and arm, upper 840.9
    blade 840.9
  specified site NEC 848.8
  spine 847.9
    cervical 847.0
    coccyx 847.4
    dorsal 847.1
    lumbar 847.2
    lumbosacral 846.0
     chronic or old 724.6
    sacral 847.3
    sacroiliac *(see also* Sprain, sacroiliac)
     846.9
     chronic or old 724.6
    thoracic 847.1
  sternoclavicular 848.41
  sternum 848.40
  subglenoid - *(see also* SLAP lesion)
    840.8
  subscapularis 840.5
  supraspinatus 840.6
  symphysis
    jaw 848.1
     old 524.69
    mandibular 848.1
     old 524.69
    pubis 848.5
  talofibular 845.09
  tarsal 845.10
  tarsometatarsal 845.11
  temporomandibular 848.1
    old 524.69
  teres
    ligamentum femoris 843.8
    major or minor 840.8
  thigh (proximal end) 843.9
    and hip 843.9
    distal end 844.9
  thoracic (spine) 847.1
  thorax 848.8
  thumb 842.10
  thyroid cartilage or region 848.2
  tibia (proximal end) 844.9
    distal end 845.00
  tibiofibular
    distal 845.03
    superior 844.3
  toe(s) 845.10
  trachea 848.8
  trapezoid 840.8
  ulna, ulnar (proximal end) 841.9
    collateral 841.1
    distal end 842.00
  ulnohumeral 841.3
  vertebrae *(see also* Sprain, spine)
    847.9
    cervical, cervicodorsal,
     cervicothoracic 847.0
  wrist (cuneiform) (scaphoid)
    (semilunar) 842.00
  xiphoid cartilage 848.49
Sprengel's deformity (congenital)
  755.52
Spring fever 309.23
Sprue 579.1
  celiac 579.0
  idiopathic 579.0
  meaning thrush 112.0
  nontropical 579.0
  tropical 579.1

Spur - *see also* Exostosis
  bone 726.91
    calcaneal 726.73
  calcaneal 726.73
  iliac crest 726.5
  nose (septum) 478.19
    bone 726.91
  septal 478.19
Spuria placenta - *see* Placenta, abnormal
Spurway's syndrome (brittle bones and
  blue sclera) 756.51
Sputum, abnormal (amount) (color)
  (excessive) (odor) (purulent) 786.4
  bloody 786.3
Squamous - *see also* condition
  cell metaplasia
    bladder 596.8
    cervix - *see* condition
  epithelium in
    cervical canal (congenital) 752.49
    uterine mucosa (congenital) 752.3
  metaplasia
    bladder 596.8
    cervix - *see* condition
Squashed nose 738.0
  congenital 754.0
Squeeze, divers' 993.3
Squint (*see also* Strabismus) 378.9
  accommodative (*see also* Esotropia)
    378.00
  concomitant (*see also* Heterotropia)
    378.30
Stab - *see also* Wound, open, by site
  internal organs - *see* Injury, internal, by
    site, with open wound
Staggering gait 781.2
  hysterical 300.11
Staghorn calculus 592.0
Stähl's
  ear 744.29
  pigment line (cornea) 371.11
Stähli's pigment lines (cornea) 371.11
Stain, staining
  meconium 779.84
  port wine 757.32
  tooth, teeth (hard tissues) 521.7
    due to
      accretions 523.6
      deposits (betel) (black) (green)
        (materia alba) (orange)
        (tobacco) 523.6
      metals (copper) (silver) 521.7
      nicotine 523.6
      pulpal bleeding 521.7
      tobacco 523.6
Stammering 307.0
Standstill
  atrial 426.6
  auricular 426.6
  cardiac (*see also* Arrest, cardiac) 427.5
  sinoatrial 426.6
  sinus 426.6
  ventricular (*see also* Arrest, cardiac)
    427.5
Stannosis 503
Stanton's disease (melioidosis) 025
Staphylitis (acute) (catarrhal) (chronic)
  (gangrenous) (membranous)
  (suppurative) (ulcerative) 528.3
Staphylococcemia 038.10
  aureus 038.11
  specified organism NEC 038.19
Staphylococcus, staphylococcal - *see*
  condition

Staphyloderma (skin) 686.00
Staphyloma 379.11
  anterior, localized 379.14
  ciliary 379.11
  cornea 371.73
  equatorial 379.13
  posterior 379.12
  posticum 379.12
  ring 379.15
  sclera NEC 379.11
Starch eating 307.52
Stargardt's disease 362.75
Starvation (inanition) (due to lack of
  food) 994.2
  edema 262
  voluntary NEC 307.1
Stasis
  bile (duct) (*see also* Disease, biliary)
    576.8
  bronchus (*see also* Bronchitis) 490
  cardiac (*see also* Failure, heart)
    428.0
  cecum 564.89
  colon 564.89
  dermatitis (*see also* Varix, with stasis
    dermatitis) 454.1
  duodenal 536.8
  eczema (*see also* Varix, with stasis
    dermatitis) 454.1
  edema (*see also* Hypertension, venous)
    459.30
  foot 991.4
  gastric 536.3
  ileocecal coil 564.89
  ileum 564.89
  intestinal 564.89
  jejunum 564.89
  kidney 586
  liver 571.9
    cirrhotic - *see* Cirrhosis, liver
  lymphatic 457.8
  pneumonia 514
  portal 571.9
  pulmonary 514
  rectal 564.89
  renal 586
    tubular 584.5
  stomach 536.3
  ulcer
    with varicose veins 454.0
    without varicose veins 459.81
  urine NEC (*see also* Retention, urine)
    788.20
  venous 459.81
State
  affective and paranoid, mixed, organic
    psychotic 294.8
  agitated 307.9
    acute reaction to stress 308.2
  anxiety (neurotic) (*see also* Anxiety)
    300.00
    specified type NEC 300.09
  apprehension (*see also* Anxiety) 300.00
    specified type NEC 300.09
  climacteric, female 627.2
    following induced menopause
      627.4
  clouded
    epileptic (*see also* Epilepsy)
      345.9●
    paroxysmal (idiopathic) (*see also*
      Epilepsy) 345.9●
  compulsive (mixed) (with obsession)
    300.3

State (*Continued*)
  confusional 298.9
    acute 293.0
      with
        arteriosclerotic dementia
          290.41
        presenile brain disease 290.11
        senility 290.3
    alcoholic 291.0
    drug-induced 292.81
    epileptic 293.0
    postoperative 293.9
    reactive (emotional stress)
      (psychological trauma) 298.2
    subacute 293.1
  constitutional psychopathic 301.9
  convulsive (*see also* Convulsions) 780.39
  depressive NEC 311
    induced by drug 292.84
    neurotic 300.4
  dissociative 300.15
  hallucinatory 780.1
    induced by drug 292.12
  hypercoagulable (primary) 289.81
    secondary 289.82
  hyperdynamic beta-adrenergic
    circulatory 429.82
  locked-in 344.81
  menopausal 627.2
    artificial 627.4
    following induced menopause
      627.4
  neurotic NEC 300.9
    with depersonalization episode
      300.6
  obsessional 300.3
  oneiroid (*see also* Schizophrenia)
    295.4●
  panic 300.01
  paranoid 297.9
    alcohol-induced 291.5
    arteriosclerotic 290.42
    climacteric 297.2
    drug-induced 292.11
    in
      presenile brain disease 290.12
      senile brain disease 290.20
    involutional 297.2
    menopausal 297.2
    senile 290.20
    simple 297.0
  postleukotomy 310.0
  pregnant (*see also* Pregnancy) V22.2
  psychogenic, twilight 298.2
  psychotic, organic (*see also* Psychosis,
    organic) 294.9
    mixed paranoid and affective
      294.8
  senile or presenile NEC 290.9
  transient NEC 293.9
    with
      anxiety 293.84
      delusions 293.81
      depression 293.83
      hallucinations 293.82
  residual schizophrenic (*see also*
    Schizophrenia) 295.6●
  tension (*see also* Anxiety) 300.9
  transient organic psychotic 293.9
    anxiety type 293.84
    depressive type 293.83
    hallucinatory type 293.83
    paranoid type 293.81
    specified type NEC 293.89

◀ New   ◀|||| Revised   ~~deleted~~ Deleted   ● Use Additional Digit(s)   ▨ Omit code

State *(Continued)*
  twilight
    epileptic 293.0
    psychogenic 298.2
  vegetative (persistent) 780.03
Status (post)
  absence
    epileptic *(see also* Epilepsy) 345.2
    of organ, acquired (postsurgical) -
      see Absence, by site, acquired
  administration of tPA (rtPA) in a
    different institution within the
    last 24 hours prior to admission
    to facility V45.88
  anastomosis of intestine (for bypass)
    V45.3
  anginosus 413.9
  angioplasty, percutaneous
    transluminal coronary
    V45.82
  ankle prosthesis V43.66
  aortocoronary bypass or shunt
    V45.81
  arthrodesis V45.4
  artificially induced condition NEC
    V45.89
  artificial opening (of) V44.9
    gastrointestinal tract NEC
      V44.4
    specified site NEC V44.8
    urinary tract NEC V44.6
    vagina V44.7
  aspirator V46.0
  asthmaticus *(see also* Asthma)
    493.9●
  awaiting organ transplant V49.83
  bariatric surgery V45.86
    complicating pregnancy,
      childbirth, or the
      puerperium 649.2●
  bed confinement V49.84
  breast
    correction V43.82
    implant removal V45.83
    reconstruction V43.82
  cardiac
    device (in situ) V45.00
      carotid sinus V45.09
        fitting or adjustment V53.39
      defibrillator, automatic
        implantable V45.02
      pacemaker V45.01
        fitting or adjustment V53.31
  carotid sinus stimulator V45.09
  cataract extraction V45.61
  chemotherapy V66.2
    current V58.69
  circumcision, female 629.20
  clitorectomy (female genital mutilation
    type I) 629.21
    with excision of labia minora
      (female genital mutilation
      type II) 629.22
  colonization - *see* Carrier (suspected) of
  colostomy V44.3
  contraceptive device V45.59
    intrauterine V45.51
    subdermal V45.52
  convulsivus idiopathicus *(see also*
    Epilepsy) 345.3
  coronary artery bypass or shunt
    V45.81
  ~~current military deployment status~~
    ~~V62.21~~

Status *(Continued)*
  cutting
    female genital 629.20
      specified NEC 629.29
      type I 629.21
      type II 629.22
      type III 629.23
      type IV 629.29
  cystostomy V44.50
    appendico-vesicostomy V44.52
    cutaneous-vesicostomy V44.51
    specifed type NEC V44.59
  defibrillator, automatic implantable
    cardiac V45.02
  delinquent immunization V15.83 ◄
  dental crowns V45.84
  dental fillings V45.84
  dental restoration V45.84
  dental sealant V49.82
  dialysis (hemo) (peritoneal) V45.11
  donor V59.9
  drug therapy or regimen V67.59
    high-risk medication NEC V67.51
  elbow prosthesis V43.62
  enterostomy V44.4
  epileptic, epilepticus (absence) (grand
    mal) *(see also* Epilepsy) 345.3
    focal motor 345.7●
    partial 345.7●
    petit mal 345.2
    psychomotor 345.7●
    temporal lobe 345.7●
  estrogen receptor
    negative [ER-] V86.1
    positive [ER+] V86.0
  eye (adnexa) surgery V45.69
  female genital
    cutting 629.20
      specified NEC 629.29
      type I 629.21
      type II 629.22
      type III 629.23
      type IV 629.29
    mutilation 629.20
      type I 629.21
      type II 629.22
      type III 629.23
      type IV 629.29
  filtering bleb (eye) (postglaucoma)
    V45.69
    with rupture or complication
      997.99
    postcataract extraction
      (complication) 997.99
  finger joint prosthesis V43.69 ◄
  foster care V60.81
  gastric
    banding V45.86
      complicating pregnancy,
        childbirth, or the
        puerperium 649.2●
    bypass for obesity V45.86
      complicating pregnancy,
        childbirth, or the
        puerperium 649.2●
  gastrostomy V44.1
  grand mal 345.3
  heart valve prosthesis V43.3
  hemodialysis V45.11
  hip prosthesis (joint) (partial) (total)
    V43.64
  hysterectomy V88.01
    partial with remaining cervical
      stump V88.02
    total V88.01
  ileostomy V44.2

Status *(Continued)*
  infibulation (female genital mutilation
    type III) 629.23
  insulin pump V45.85
  intestinal bypass V45.3
  intrauterine contraceptive device
    V45.51
  jejunostomy V44.4
  knee joint prosthesis V43.65
  lacunaris 437.8
  lacunosis 437.8
  lapsed immunization schedule
    V15.83   ◄
  low birth weight V21.30
    less than 500 grams V21.31
    500–999 grams V21.32
    1000–1499 grams V21.33
    1500–1999 grams V21.34
    2000–2500 grams V21.35
  lymphaticus 254.8
  malignant neoplasm, ablated or
    excised - *see* History, malignant
    neoplasm
  marmoratus 333.79
  military deployment V62.22   ◄
  mutilation, female 629.20
    type I 629.21
    type II 629.22
    type III 629.23
    type IV 629.29
  nephrostomy V44.6
  neuropacemaker NEC V45.89
    brain V45.89
    carotid sinus V45.09
    neurologic NEC V45.89
  obesity surgery V45.86
    complicating pregnancy, childbirth,
      or the puerperium 649.2●
  organ replacement
    by artificial or mechanical device or
      prosthesis of
      artery V43.4
      artificial skin V43.83
      bladder V43.5
      blood vessel V43.4
      breast V43.82
      eye globe V43.0
      heart
        assist device V43.21
        fully implantable artificial
          heart V43.22
        valve V43.3
      intestine V43.89
      joint V43.60
        ankle V43.66
        elbow V43.62
        finger V43.69
        hip (partial) (total) V43.64
        knee V43.65
        shoulder V43.61
        specified NEC V43.69
        wrist V43.63
      kidney V43.89
      larynx V43.81
      lens V43.1
      limb(s) V43.7
      liver V43.89
      lung V43.89
      organ NEC V43.89
      pancreas V43.89
      skin (artificial) V43.83
      tissue NEC V43.89
      vein V43.4
    by organ transplant (heterologous)
      (homologous) - *see* Status,
      transplant

◄ New   ◄▮ Revised   ~~deleted~~ Deleted   ● Use Additional Digit(s)   ▨ Omit code

Status (*Continued*)
  pacemaker
    brain V45.89
    cardiac V45.01
    carotid sinus V45.09
    neurologic NEC V45.89
    specified site NEC V45.89
  percutaneous transluminal coronary
    angioplasty V45.82
  peritoneal dialysis V45.11
  petit mal 345.2
  postcommotio cerebri 310.2
  postmenopausal (age related) (natural)
    V49.81
  postoperative NEC V45.89
  postpartum NEC V24.2
    care immediately following delivery
      V24.0
    routine follow-up V24.2
  postsurgical NEC V45.89
  renal dialysis V45.11
    noncompliance V45.12
  respirator [ventilator] V46.11
    encounter
      during
        mechanical failure V46.14
        power failure V46.12
      for weaning V46.13
  reversed jejunal transposition (for
    bypass) V45.3
  sex reassignment surgery (*see also*
    Trans-sexualism) 302.50
  shoulder prosthesis V43.61
  shunt
    aortocoronary bypass V45.81
    arteriovenous (for dialysis) V45.11
    cerebrospinal fluid V45.2
    vascular NEC V45.89
      aortocoronary (bypass) V45.81
    ventricular (communicating) (for
      drainage) V45.2
  sterilization
    tubal ligation V26.51
    vasectomy V26.52
  subdermal contraceptive device
    V45.52
  thymicolymphaticus 254.8
  thymicus 254.8
  thymolymphaticus 254.8
  tooth extraction 525.10
  tracheostomy V44.0
  transplant
    blood vessel V42.89
    bone V42.4
      marrow V42.81
    cornea V42.5
    heart V42.1
      valve V42.2
    intestine V42.84
    kidney V42.0
    liver V42.7
    lung V42.6
    organ V42.9
      removal (due to complication,
        failure, rejection or
        infection) V45.87
      specified site NEC V42.89
    pancreas V42.83
    peripheral stem cells V42.82
    skin V42.3
    stem cells, peripheral V42.82
    tissue V42.9
      specified type NEC V42.89
    vessel, blood V42.89

Status (*Continued*)
  tubal ligation V26.51
  underimmunization V15.83 ◄
  ureterostomy V44.6
  urethrostomy V44.6
  vagina, artificial V44.7
  vascular shunt NEC V45.89
    aortocoronary (bypass) V45.81
  vasectomy V26.52
  ventilator [respirator] V46.11
    encounter
      during
        mechanical failure V46.14
        power failure V46.12
      for weaning V46.13
  wheelchair confinement V46.3
  wrist prosthesis V43.63
Stave fracture - *see* Fracture, metacarpus,
  metacarpal bone(s)
Steal
  subclavian artery 435.2
  vertebral artery 435.1
Stealing, solitary, child problem (*see also*
  Disturbance, conduct) 312.1 ●
Steam burn - *see* Burn, by site
Steatocystoma multiplex 706.2
Steatoma (infected) 706.2
  eyelid (cystic) 374.84
    infected 373.13
Steatorrhea (chronic) 579.8
  with lacteal obstruction 579.2
  idiopathic 579.0
    adult 579.0
    infantile 579.0
  pancreatic 579.4
  primary 579.0
  secondary 579.8
  specified cause NEC 579.8
  tropical 579.1
Steatosis 272.8
  heart (*see also* Degeneration,
    myocardial) 429.1
  kidney 593.89
  liver 571.8
Steele-Richardson (-Olszewski)
  syndrome 333.0
Stein's syndrome (polycystic ovary) 256.4
Stein-Leventhal syndrome (polycystic
  ovary) 256.4
Steinbrocker's syndrome (*see also*
  Neuropathy, peripheral, autonomic)
  337.9
Steinert's disease 359.21
STEMI (ST elevation myocardial
  infarction) (*see also* - Infarct,
  myocardium, ST elevation) 410.9 ●
Stenocardia (*see also* Angina) 413.9
Stenocephaly 756.0
Stenosis (cicatricial) - *see also* Stricture
  ampulla of Vater 576.2
    with calculus, cholelithiasis, or
      stones - *see* Choledocholithiasis
  anus, anal (canal) (sphincter) 569.2
    congenital 751.2
  aorta (ascending) 747.22
    arch 747.10
    arteriosclerotic 440.0
    calcified 440.0
  aortic (valve) 424.1
    with
      mitral (valve)
        insufficiency or incompetence
        396.2
        stenosis or obstruction 396.0

Stenosis (*Continued*)
  aortic (*Continued*)
    atypical 396.0
    congenital 746.3
    rheumatic 395.0
      with
        insufficiency, incompetency or
          regurgitation 395.2
          with mitral (valve) disease
            396.8
        mitral (valve)
          disease (stenosis) 396.0
          insufficiency or
            incompetence 396.2
          stenosis or obstruction 396.0
    specified cause, except rheumatic
      424.1
    syphilitic 093.22
  aqueduct of Sylvius (congenital) 742.3
    with spina bifida (*see also* Spina
      bifida) 741.0 ●
    acquired 331.4
  artery NEC (*see also* Arteriosclerosis)
    447.1
    basilar - *see* Narrowing, artery,
      basilar
    carotid (common) (internal) - *see*
      Narrowing, artery, carotid
    celiac 447.4
    cerebral 437.0
      due to
        embolism (*see also* Embolism,
          brain) 434.1 ●
        thrombus (*see also* Thrombosis,
          brain) 434.0 ●
    extremities 440.20
    precerebral - *see* Narrowing, artery,
      precerebral
    pulmonary (congenital) 747.3
      acquired 417.8
    renal 440.1
    vertebral - *see* Narrowing, artery,
      vertebral
  bile duct or biliary passage (*see also*
    Obstruction, biliary) 576.2
    congenital 751.61
  bladder neck (acquired) 596.0
    congenital 753.6
  brain 348.89 ◄
  bronchus 519.19
    syphilitic 095.8
  cardia (stomach) 537.89
    congenital 750.7
  cardiovascular (*see also* Disease,
    cardiovascular) 429.2
  carotid artery - *see* Narrowing, artery,
    carotid
  cervix, cervical (canal) 622.4
    congenital 752.49
    in pregnancy or childbirth 654.6 ●
      affecting fetus or newborn
        763.89
      causing obstructed labor 660.2 ●
        affecting fetus or newborn
          763.1
  colon (*see also* Obstruction, intestine)
    560.9
    congenital 751.2
  colostomy 569.62
  common bile duct (*see also* Obstruction,
    biliary) 576.2
    congenital 751.61
  coronary (artery) - *see* Arteriosclerosis,
    coronary

◄ New   ◄▌ Revised   ~~deleted~~ Deleted   ● Use Additional Digit(s)   ▨ Omit code

Stenosis (*Continued*)
cystic duct (*see also* Obstruction,
     gallbladder) 575.2
   congenital 751.61
   due to (presence of) any device, implant,
        or graft classifiable to 996.0–996.5 -
        see Complications, due to
        (presence of) any device, implant,
        or graft classified to 996.0–996.5
        NEC
duodenum 537.3
   congenital 751.1
ejaculatory duct NEC 608.89
endocervical os - *see* Stenosis, cervix
enterostomy 569.62
esophagostomy 530.87
esophagus 530.3
   congenital 750.3
   syphilitic 095.8
      congenital 090.5
external ear canal 380.50
   secondary to
      inflammation 380.53
      surgery 380.52
      trauma 380.51
gallbladder (*see also* Obstruction,
     gallbladder) 575.2
glottis 478.74
heart valve (acquired) - *see also*
     Endocarditis
   congenital NEC 746.89
      aortic 746.3
      mitral 746.5
      pulmonary 746.02
      tricuspid 746.1
hepatic duct (*see also* Obstruction,
     biliary) 576.2
hymen 623.3
hypertrophic subaortic (idiopathic)
     425.1
infundibulum cardiac 746.83
intestine (*see also* Obstruction, intestine)
     560.9
   congenital (small) 751.1
      large 751.2
lacrimal
   canaliculi 375.53
   duct 375.56
      congenital 743.65
   punctum 375.52
      congenital 743.65
   sac 375.54
      congenital 743.65
lacrimonasal duct 375.56
   congenital 743.65
   neonatal 375.55
larynx 478.74
   congenital 748.3
   syphilitic 095.8
      congenital 090.5
mitral (valve) (chronic) (inactive) 394.0
   with
      aortic (valve)
         disease (insufficiency) 396.1
         insufficiency or incompetence
            396.1
         stenosis or obstruction 396.0
      incompetency, insufficiency or
         regurgitation 394.2
         with aortic valve disease
            396.8
   active or acute 391.1
      with chorea (acute) (rheumatic)
         (Sydenham's) 392.0

Stenosis (*Continued*)
mitral (*Continued*)
   congenital 746.5
   specified cause, except rheumatic
      424.0
   syphilitic 093.21
myocardium, myocardial (*see also*
     Degeneration, myocardial)
     429.1
   hypertrophic subaortic (idiopathic)
      425.1
nares (anterior) (posterior) 478.19
   congenital 748.0
nasal duct 375.56
   congenital 743.65
nasolacrimal duct 375.56
   congenital 743.65
   neonatal 375.55
organ or site, congenital NEC - *see*
     Atresia
papilla of Vater 576.2
   with calculus, cholelithiasis, or
      stones - *see* Choledocholithiasis
pulmonary (artery) (congenital) 747.3
   with ventricular septal defect,
      dextraposition of aorta and
      hypertrophy of right ventricle
      745.2
   acquired 417.8
   infundibular 746.83
   in tetralogy of Fallot 745.2
   subvalvular 746.83
   valve (*see also* Endocarditis,
      pulmonary) 424.3
      congenital 746.02
   vein 747.49
      acquired 417.8
   vessel NEC 417.8
pulmonic (congenital) 746.02
   infundibular 746.83
   subvalvular 746.83
pylorus (hypertrophic) 537.0
   adult 537.0
   congenital 750.5
   infantile 750.5
rectum (sphincter) (*see also* Stricture,
     rectum) 569.2
renal artery 440.1
salivary duct (any) 527.8
sphincter of Oddi (*see also* Obstruction,
     biliary) 576.2
spinal 724.00
   cervical 723.0
   lumbar, lumbosacral 724.02
   nerve (root) NEC 724.9
   specified region NEC 724.09
   thoracic, thoracolumbar 724.01
stomach, hourglass 537.6
subaortic 746.81
   hypertrophic (idiopathic) 425.1
supra (valvular)-aortic 747.22
trachea 519.19
   congenital 748.3
   syphilitic 095.8
   tuberculous (*see also* Tuberculosis)
      012.8●
tracheostomy 519.02
tricuspid (valve) (*see also* Endocarditis,
     tricuspid) 397.0
   congenital 746.1
   nonrheumatic 424.2
tubal 628.2
ureter (*see also* Stricture, ureter) 593.3
   congenital 753.29

Stenosis (*Continued*)
urethra (*see also* Stricture, urethra)
     598.9
vagina 623.2
   congenital 752.49
   in pregnancy or childbirth 654.7●
      affecting fetus or newborn
         763.89
      causing obstructed labor
         660.2●
         affecting fetus or newborn
            763.1
valve (cardiac) (heart) (*see also*
     Endocarditis) 424.90
   congenital NEC 746.89
      aortic 746.3
      mitral 746.5
      pulmonary 746.02
      tricuspid 746.1
      urethra 753.6
valvular (*see also* Endocarditis) 424.90
   congenital NEC 746.89
      urethra 753.6
vascular graft or shunt 996.1
   atherosclerosis - *see* Arteriosclerosis,
      extremities
   embolism 996.74
   occlusion NEC 996.74
   thrombus 996.74
vena cava (inferior) (superior) 459.2
   congenital 747.49
ventricular shunt 996.2
vulva 624.8
Stercolith (*see also* Fecalith) 560.39
   appendix 543.9
Stercoraceous, stercoral ulcer 569.82
   anus or rectum 569.41
Stereopsis, defective
   with fusion 368.33
   without fusion 368.32
Stereotypies NEC 307.3
Sterility
   female - *see* Infertility, female
   male (*see also* Infertility, male) 606.9
Sterilization, admission for V25.2
   status
      tubal ligation V26.51
      vasectomy V26.52
Sternalgia (*see also* Angina) 413.9
Sternopagus 759.4
Sternum bifidum 756.3
Sternutation 784.99
Steroid
   effects (adverse) (iatrogenic)
      cushingoid
         correct substance properly
            administered 255.0
         overdose or wrong substance
            given or taken 962.0
      diabetes - *see* Diabetes, secondary
         correct substance properly
            administered 251.8
         overdose or wrong substance
            given or taken 962.0
      due to
         correct substance properly
            administered 255.8
         overdose or wrong substance
            given or taken 962.0
      fever
         correct substance properly
            administered 780.60
         overdose or wrong substance
            given or taken 962.0

Steroid (*Continued*)
  effects (*Continued*)
    withdrawal
      correct substance properly
        administered 255.41
      overdose or wrong substance
        given or taken 962.0
  responder 365.03
Stevens-Johnson disease or syndrome
    (erythema multiforme exudativum)
    695.13
  toxic epidermal necrolysis overlap
    (SJS-TEN overlap syndrome)
    695.14
Stewart-Morel syndrome (hyperostosis
    frontalis interna) 733.3
Sticker's disease (erythema infectiosum)
    057.0
Stickler syndrome 759.89
Sticky eye 372.03
Stieda's disease (calcification, knee joint)
    726.62
Stiff
  back 724.8
  neck (*see also* Torticollis) 723.5
Stiff-baby 759.89
Stiff-man syndrome 333.91
Stiffness, joint NEC 719.50
  ankle 719.57
  back 724.8
  elbow 719.52
  finger 719.54
  hip 719.55
  knee 719.56
  multiple sites 719.59
  sacroiliac 724.6
  shoulder 719.51
  specified site NEC 719.58
  spine 724.9
  surgical fusion V45.4
  wrist 719.53
Stigmata, congenital syphilis 090.5
Still's disease or syndrome 714.30
  adult onset 714.2
Still-Felty syndrome (rheumatoid
    arthritis with splenomegaly and
    leukopenia) 714.1
Stillbirth, stillborn NEC 779.9
Stiller's disease (asthenia) 780.79
Stilling-Türk-Duane syndrome (ocular
    retraction syndrome) 378.71
Stimulation, ovary 256.1
Sting (animal) (bee) (fish) (insect)
    (jellyfish) (Portuguese man-o-war)
    (wasp) (venomous) 989.5
  anaphylactic shock or reaction
    989.5
  plant 692.6
Stippled epiphyses 756.59
Stitch
  abscess 998.59
  burst (in external operation
    wound) (*see also* Dehiscence)
    998.32
    internal 998.31
  in back 724.5
Stojano's (subcostal) **syndrome** 098.86
Stokes' disease (exophthalmic goiter)
    242.0●
Stokes-Adams syndrome (syncope with
    heart block) 426.9
Stokvis' (-Talma) **disease** (enterogenous
    cyanosis) 289.7
Stomach - *see* condition

Stoma malfunction
  colostomy 569.62
  cystostomy 997.5
  enterostomy 569.62
  esophagostomy 530.87
  gastrostomy 536.42
  ileostomy 569.62
  nephrostomy 997.5
  tracheostomy 519.02
  ureterostomy 997.5
Stomatitis 528.00
  angular 528.5
    due to dietary or vitamin deficiency
      266.0
  aphthous 528.2
  bovine 059.11
  candidal 112.0
  catarrhal 528.00
  denture 528.9
  diphtheritic (membranous) 032.0
  due to
    dietary deficiency 266.0
    thrush 112.0
    vitamin deficiency 266.0
  epidemic 078.4
  epizootic 078.4
  follicular 528.00
  gangrenous 528.1
  herpetic 054.2
  herpetiformis 528.2
  malignant 528.00
  membranous acute 528.00
  monilial 112.0
  mycotic 112.0
  necrotic 528.1
    ulcerative 101
  necrotizing ulcerative 101
  parasitic 112.0
  septic 528.00
  specified NEC 528.09
  spirochetal 101
  suppurative (acute) 528.00
  ulcerative 528.00
    necrotizing 101
  ulceromembranous 101
  vesicular 528.00
    with exanthem 074.3
  Vincent's 101
Stomatocytosis 282.8
Stomatomycosis 112.0
Stomatorrhagia 528.9
Stone(s) - *see also* Calculus
  bladder 594.1
    diverticulum 594.0
  cystine 270.0
  heart syndrome (*see also* Failure,
    ventricular, left) 428.1
  kidney 592.0
  prostate 602.0
  pulp (dental) 522.2
  renal 592.0
  salivary duct or gland (any) 527.5
  ureter 592.1
  urethra (impacted) 594.2
  urinary (duct) (impacted) (passage)
    592.9
    bladder 594.1
      diverticulum 594.0
    lower tract NEC 594.9
    specified site 594.8
  xanthine 277.2
Stonecutters' lung 502
  tuberculous (*see also* Tuberculosis)
    011.4●

Stonemasons'
  asthma, disease, or lung 502
    tuberculous (*see also* Tuberculosis)
      011.4●
  phthisis (*see also* Tuberculosis) 011.4●
Stoppage
  bowel (*see also* Obstruction, intestine)
    560.9
  heart (*see also* Arrest, cardiac) 427.5
  intestine (*see also* Obstruction, intestine)
    560.9
  urine NEC (*see also* Retention, urine)
    788.20
Storm, thyroid (apathetic) (*see also*
    Thyrotoxicosis) 242.9●
Strabismus (alternating) (congenital)
    (nonparalytic) 378.9
  concomitant (*see also* Heterotropia)
    378.30
    convergent (*see also* Esotropia)
      378.00
    divergent (*see also* Exotropia)
      378.10
  convergent (*see also* Esotropia) 378.00
  divergent (*see also* Exotropia) 378.10
  due to adhesions, scars - *see*
    Strabismus, mechanical
  in neuromuscular disorder NEC
    378.73
    intermittent 378.20
      vertical 378.31
  latent 378.40
    convergent (esophoria) 378.41
    divergent (exophoria) 378.42
    vertical 378.43
  mechanical 378.60
    due to
      Brown's tendon sheath syndrome
        378.61
      specified musculofascial disorder
        NEC 378.62
  paralytic 378.50
    third or oculomotor nerve (partial)
      378.51
      total 378.52
    fourth or trochlear nerve 378.53
    sixth or abducens nerve 378.54
  specified type NEC 378.73
  vertical (hypertropia) 378.31
Strain - *see also* Sprain, by site
  eye NEC 368.13
  heart - *see* Disease, heart
  meaning gonorrhea - *see* Gonorrhea
  on urination 788.65
  physical NEC V62.89
  postural 729.90
  psychological NEC V62.89
Strands
  conjunctiva 372.62
  vitreous humor 379.25
Strangulation, strangulated 994.7
  appendix 543.9
  asphyxiation or suffocation by 994.7
  bladder neck 596.0
  bowel - *see* Strangulation, intestine
  colon - *see* Strangulation, intestine
  cord (umbilical) - *see* Compression,
    umbilical cord
  due to birth injury 767.8
  food or foreign body (*see also* Asphyxia,
    food) 933.1
  hemorrhoids 455.8
    external 455.5
    internal 455.2

◀ New   ◀▦ Revised   ~~deleted~~ Deleted   ● Use Additional Digit(s)   ▦ Omit code

Strangulation, strangulated (Continued)
  hernia - see also Hernia, by site, with
      obstruction
    gangrenous - see Hernia, by site,
        with gangrene
  intestine (large) (small) 560.2
    with hernia - see also Hernia, by site,
        with obstruction
      gangrenous - see Hernia, by site,
          with gangrene
    congenital (small) 751.1
      large 751.2
  mesentery 560.2
  mucus (see also Asphyxia, mucus)
      933.1
    newborn 770.18
  omentum 560.2
  organ or site, congenital NEC - see
      Atresia
  ovary 620.8
    due to hernia 620.4
  penis 607.89
    foreign body 939.3
  rupture (see also Hernia, by site, with
      obstruction) 552.9
    gangrenous (see also Hernia, by site,
        with gangrene) 551.9
  stomach, due to hernia (see also
      Hernia, by site, with obstruction)
      552.9
    with gangrene (see also Hernia, by
        site, with gangrene) 551.9
  umbilical cord - see Compression,
      umbilical cord
  vesicourethral orifice 596.0
Strangury 788.1
Strawberry
  gallbladder (see also Disease,
      gallbladder) 575.6
  mark 757.32
  tongue (red) (white) 529.3
Straw itch 133.8
Streak, ovarian 752.0
Strephosymbolia 315.01
  secondary to organic lesion 784.69
Streptobacillary fever 026.1
Streptobacillus moniliformis 026.1
Streptococcemia 038.0
Streptococcicosis - see Infection,
      streptococcal
Streptococcus, streptococcal - see
      condition
Streptoderma 686.00
Streptomycosis - see Actinomycosis
Streptothricosis - see Actinomycosis
Streptothrix - see Actinomycosis
Streptotrichosis - see Actinomycosis
Stress 308.9
  fracture - see Fracture, stress
  polycythemia 289.0
  reaction (gross) (see also Reaction,
      stress, acute) 308.9
Stretching, nerve - see Injury, nerve, by
      site
Striae (albicantes) (atrophicae) (cutis
      distensae) (distensae) 701.3
Striations of nails 703.8
Stricture (see also Stenosis) 799.89
  ampulla of Vater 576.2
    with calculus, cholelithiasis, or
        stones - see Choledocholithiasis
  anus (sphincter) 569.2
    congenital 751.2
    infantile 751.2

Stricture (Continued)
  aorta (ascending) 747.22
    arch 747.10
    arteriosclerotic 440.0
    calcified 440.0
  aortic (valve) (see also Stenosis, aortic)
      424.1
    congenital 746.3
  aqueduct of Sylvius (congenital)
      742.3
    with spina bifida (see also Spina
        bifida) 741.0●
    acquired 331.4
  artery 447.1
    basilar - see Narrowing, artery,
        basilar
    carotid (common) (internal) - see
        Narrowing, artery, carotid
    celiac 447.4
    cerebral 437.0
      congenital 747.81
      due to
        embolism (see also Embolism,
            brain) 434.1●
        thrombus (see also Thrombosis,
            brain) 434.0●
    congenital (peripheral) 747.60
      cerebral 747.81
      coronary 746.85
      gastrointestinal 747.61
      lower limb 747.64
      renal 747.62
      retinal 743.58
      specified NEC 747.69
      spinal 747.82
      umbilical 747.5
      upper limb 747.63
    coronary - see Arteriosclerosis,
        coronary
      congenital 746.85
    precerebral - see Narrowing, artery,
        precerebral NEC
    pulmonary (congenital) 747.3
      acquired 417.8
    renal 440.1
    vertebral - see Narrowing, artery,
        vertebral
  auditory canal (congenital) (external)
      744.02
    acquired (see also Stricture, ear canal,
        acquired) 380.50
  bile duct or passage (any)
      (postoperative) (see also
      Obstruction, biliary) 576.2
    congenital 751.61
  bladder 596.8
    congenital 753.6
    neck 596.0
      congenital 753.6
  bowel (see also Obstruction, intestine)
      560.9
  brain 348.89 ◄▥
  bronchus 519.19
    syphilitic 095.8
  cardia (stomach) 537.89
    congenital 750.7
  cardiac - see also Disease, heart orifice
      (stomach) 537.89
  cardiovascular (see also Disease,
      cardiovascular) 429.2
  carotid artery - see Narrowing, artery,
      carotid
  cecum (see also Obstruction, intestine)
      560.9

Stricture (Continued)
  cervix, cervical (canal) 622.4
    congenital 752.49
    in pregnancy or childbirth
        654.6●
      affecting fetus or newborn
          763.89
      causing obstructed labor
          660.2●
        affecting fetus or newborn
            763.1
  colon (see also Obstruction, intestine)
      560.9
    congenital 751.2
  colostomy 569.62
  common bile duct (see also Obstruction,
      biliary) 576.2
    congenital 751.61
  coronary (artery) - see Arteriosclerosis,
      coronary
    congenital 746.85
  cystic duct (see also Obstruction,
      gallbladder) 575.2
    congenital 751.61
  cystostomy 997.5
  digestive organs NEC, congenital
      751.8
  duodenum 537.3
    congenital 751.1
  ear canal (external) (congenital)
      744.02
    acquired 380.50
      secondary to
        inflammation 380.53
        surgery 380.52
        trauma 380.51
  ejaculatory duct 608.85
  enterostomy 569.62
  esophagostomy 530.87
  esophagus (corrosive) (peptic)
      530.3
    congenital 750.3
    syphilitic 095.8
      congenital 090.5
  Eustachian tube (see also Obstruction,
      Eustachian tube) 381.60
    congenital 744.24
  fallopian tube 628.2
    gonococcal (chronic) 098.37
      acute 098.17
    tuberculous (see also Tuberculosis)
        016.6●
  gallbladder (see also Obstruction,
      gallbladder) 575.2
    congenital 751.69
  glottis 478.74
  heart - see also Disease, heart
    congenital NEC 746.89
    valve - see also Endocarditis
      congenital NEC 746.89
        aortic 746.3
        mitral 746.5
        pulmonary 746.02
        tricuspid 746.1
  hepatic duct (see also Obstruction,
      biliary) 576.2
  hourglass, of stomach 537.6
  hymen 623.3
  hypopharynx 478.29
  intestine (see also Obstruction, intestine)
      560.9
    congenital (small) 751.1
      large 751.2
    ischemic 557.1

Stricture (Continued)

lacrimal
  canaliculi 375.53
    congenital 743.65
  punctum 375.52
    congenital 743.65
  sac 375.54
    congenital 743.65
lacrimonasal duct 375.56
  congenital 743.65
  neonatal 375.55
larynx 478.79
  congenital 748.3
  syphilitic 095.8
    congenital 090.5
lung 518.89
meatus
  ear (congenital) 744.02
    acquired (see also Stricture, ear
      canal, acquired) 380.50
  osseous (congenital) (ear) 744.03
    acquired (see also Stricture, ear
      canal, acquired) 380.50
  urinarius (see also Stricture, urethra)
    598.9
    congenital 753.6
mitral (valve) (see also Stenosis, mitral)
  394.0
  congenital 746.5
  specified cause, except rheumatic
    424.0
myocardium, myocardial (see also
  Degeneration, myocardial)
  429.1
  hypertrophic subaortic (idiopathic)
    425.1
nares (anterior) (posterior) 478.19
  congenital 748.0
nasal duct 375.56
  congenital 743.65
  neonatal 375.55
nasolacrimal duct 375.56
  congenital 743.65
  neonatal 375.55
nasopharynx 478.29
  syphilitic 095.8
nephrostomy 997.5
nose 478.19
  congenital 748.0
nostril (anterior) (posterior) 478.19
  congenital 748.0
organ or site, congenital NEC - see
  Atresia
osseous meatus (congenital) (ear)
  744.03
  acquired (see also Stricture, ear canal,
    acquired) 380.50
os uteri (see also Stricture, cervix)
  622.4
oviduct - see Stricture, fallopian tube
pelviureteric junction 593.3
pharynx (dilation) 478.29
prostate 602.8
pulmonary, pulmonic
  artery (congenital) 747.3
    acquired 417.8
    noncongenital 417.8
  infundibulum (congenital) 746.83
  valve (see also Endocarditis,
    pulmonary) 424.3
    congenital 746.02
  vein (congenital) 747.49
    acquired 417.8
  vessel NEC 417.8

Stricture (Continued)

punctum lacrimale 375.52
  congenital 743.65
pylorus (hypertrophic) 537.0
  adult 537.0
  congenital 750.5
  infantile 750.5
rectosigmoid 569.89
rectum (sphincter) 569.2
  congenital 751.2
  due to
    chemical burn 947.3
    irradiation 569.2
    lymphogranuloma venereum
      099.1
  gonococcal 098.7
  inflammatory 099.1
  syphilitic 095.8
  tuberculous (see also Tuberculosis)
    014.8●
renal artery 440.1
salivary duct or gland (any) 527.8
sigmoid (flexure) (see also Obstruction,
  intestine) 560.9
spermatic cord 608.85
stoma (following) (of)
  colostomy 569.62
  cystostomy 997.5
  enterostomy 569.62
  esophagostomy 530.87
  gastrostomy 536.42
  ileostomy 569.62
  nephrostomy 997.5
  tracheostomy 519.02
  ureterostomy 997.5
stomach 537.89
  congenital 750.7
  hourglass 537.6
subaortic 746.81
  hypertrophic (acquired) (idiopathic)
    425.1
subglottic 478.74
syphilitic NEC 095.8
tendon (sheath) 727.81
trachea 519.19
  congenital 748.3
  syphilitic 095.8
  tuberculous (see also Tuberculosis)
    012.8●
tracheostomy 519.02
tricuspid (valve) (see also Endocarditis,
  tricuspid) 397.0
  congenital 746.1
  nonrheumatic 424.2
tunica vaginalis 608.85
ureter (postoperative) 593.3
  congenital 753.29
  tuberculous (see also Tuberculosis)
    016.2●
ureteropelvic junction 593.3
  congenital 753.21
ureterovesical orifice 593.3
  congenital 753.22
urethra (anterior) (meatal) (organic)
  (posterior) (spasmodic) 598.9
  associated with schistosomiasis (see
    also Schistosomiasis) 120.9
    [598.01]
  congenital (valvular) 753.6
  due to
    infection 598.00
      syphilis 095.8 [598.01]
    trauma 598.1
  gonococcal 098.2 [598.01]

Stricture (Continued)

urethra (Continued)
  gonorrheal 098.2 [598.01]
  infective 598.00
  late effect of injury 598.1
  postcatheterization 598.2
  postobstetric 598.1
  postoperative 598.2
  specified cause NEC 598.8
  syphilitic 095.8 [598.01]
  traumatic 598.1
  valvular, congenital 753.6
urinary meatus (see also Stricture,
  urethra) 598.9
  congenital 753.6
uterus, uterine 621.5
  os (external) (internal) - see Stricture,
    cervix
vagina (outlet) 623.2
  congenital 752.49
valve (cardiac) (heart) (see also
  Endocarditis) 424.90
  congenital (cardiac) (heart) NEC
    746.89
    aortic 746.3
    mitral 746.5
    pulmonary 746.02
    tricuspid 746.1
    urethra 753.6
valvular (see also Endocarditis)
  424.90
vascular graft or shunt 996.1
  atherosclerosis - see Arteriosclerosis,
    extremities
  embolism 996.74
  occlusion NEC 996.74
  thrombus 996.74
vas deferens 608.85
  congenital 752.89
vein 459.2
vena cava (inferior) (superior) NEC
  459.2
  congenital 747.49
ventricular shunt 996.2
vesicourethral orifice 596.0
  congenital 753.6
vulva (acquired) 624.8
Stridor 786.1
  congenital (larynx) 748.3
Stridulous - see condition
Strippling of nails 703.8
Stroke 434.91
  apoplectic (see also Disease,
    cerebrovascular, acute) 436
  brain - see Infarct, brain
  embolic 434.11
  epileptic - see Epilepsy
  healed or old V12.54
  heart - see Disease, heart
  heat 992.0
  hemorrhagic - see Hemorrhage, brain
  iatrogenic 997.02
  in evolution 434.91
  ischemic 434.91
  late effect - see Late effect(s) (of)
    cerebrovascular disease
  lightning 994.0
  paralytic - see Infarct, brain
  postoperative 997.02
  progressive 435.9
  thrombotic 434.01
Stromatosis, endometrial (M8931/1)
  236.0
Strong pulse 785.9

◀ New   ◀▥ Revised   ~~deleted~~ Deleted   ● Use Additional Digit(s)   ▨ Omit code

Strongyloides stercoralis infestation 127.2
Strongyloidiasis 127.2
Strongyloidosis 127.2
Strongylus (gibsoni) infestation 127.7
Strophulus (newborn) 779.89
   pruriginosus 698.2
Struck by lighting 994.0
Struma (see also Goiter) 240.9
   fibrosa 245.3
   Hashimoto (struma lymphomatosa) 245.2
   lymphomatosa 245.2
   nodosa (simplex) 241.9
      endemic 241.9
      multinodular 241.1
      sporadic 241.9
      toxic or with hyperthyroidism 242.3●
         multinodular 242.2●
         uninodular 242.1●
      toxicosa 242.3●
         multinodular 242.2●
         uninodular 242.1●
      uninodular 241.0
   ovarii (M9090/0) 220
      and carcinoid (M9091/1) 236.2
      malignant (M9090/3) 183.0
   Riedel's (ligneous thyroiditis) 245.3
   scrofulous (see also Tuberculosis) 017.2●
   tuberculous (see also Tuberculosis) 017.2●
      abscess 017.2●
      adenitis 017.2●
      lymphangitis 017.2●
      ulcer 017.2●
Strumipriva cachexia (see also Hypothyroidism) 244.9
Strümpell-Marie disease or spine (ankylosing spondylitis) 720.0
Strümpell-Westphal pseudosclerosis (hepatolenticular degeneration) 275.1
Stuart's disease (congenital factor X deficiency) (see also Defect, coagulation) 286.3
Stuart-Prower factor deficiency (congenital factor X deficiency) (see also Defect, coagulation) 286.3
Students' elbow 727.2
Stuffy nose 478.19
Stump - see also Amputation
   cervix, cervical (healed) 622.8
Stupor 780.09
   catatonic (see also Schizophrenia) 295.2●
   circular (see also Psychosis, manic-depressive, circular) 296.7
   manic 296.89
   manic-depressive (see also Psychosis, affective) 296.89
   mental (anergic) (delusional) 298.9
   psychogenic 298.8
   reaction to exceptional stress (transient) 308.2
   traumatic NEC - see also Injury, intracranial
      with spinal (cord)
         lesion - see Injury, spinal, by site
         shock - see Injury, spinal, by site
Sturge (-Weber) (-Dimitri) disease or syndrome (encephalocutaneous angiomatosis) 759.6
Sturge-Kalischer-Weber syndrome (encephalocutaneous angiomatosis) 759.6

Stuttering 307.0
   due to late effect of cerebrovascular disease (see also Late effect(s) (of) cerebrovascular disease) 438.14 ◄
Sty, stye 373.11
   external 373.11
   internal 373.12
   meibomian 373.12
Subacidity, gastric 536.8
   psychogenic 306.4
Subacute - see condition
Subarachnoid - see condition
Subclavian steal syndrome 435.2
Subcortical - see condition
Subcostal syndrome 098.86
   nerve compression 354.8
Subcutaneous, subcuticular - see condition
Subdelirium 293.1
Subdural - see condition
Subendocardium - see condition
Subependymoma (M9383/1) 237.5
Suberosis 495.3
Subglossitis - see Glossitis
Subhemophilia 286.0
Subinvolution (uterus) 621.1
   breast (postlactational) (postpartum) 611.89
   chronic 621.1
   puerperal, postpartum 674.8●
Sublingual - see condition
Sublinguitis 527.2
Subluxation - see also Dislocation, by site
   congenital NEC - see also Malposition, congenital
      hip (unilateral) 754.32
         with dislocation of other hip 754.35
         bilateral 754.33
      joint
         lower limb 755.69
         shoulder 755.59
         upper limb 755.59
      lower limb (joint) 755.69
      shoulder (joint) 755.59
      upper limb (joint) 755.59
   lens 379.32
      anterior 379.33
      posterior 379.34
   radial head 832.2 ◄
   rotary, cervical region of spine - see Fracture, vertebra, cervical
Submaxillary - see condition
Submersion (fatal) (nonfatal) 994.1
Submissiveness (undue), in child 313.0
Submucous - see condition
Subnormal, subnormality
   accommodation (see also Disorder, accommodation) 367.9
   mental (see also Retardation, mental) 319
      mild 317
      moderate 318.0
      profound 318.2
      severe 318.1
   temperature (accidental) 991.6
      not associated with low environmental temperature 780.99
Subphrenic - see condition
Subscapular nerve - see condition
Subseptus uterus 752.3
Subsiding appendicitis 542

Substance abuse in family V61.42 ◄
Substernal thyroid (see also Goiter) 240.9
   congenital 759.2
Substitution disorder 300.11
Subtentorial - see condition
Subtertian
   fever 084.0
   malaria (fever) 084.0
Subthyroidism (acquired) (see also Hypothyroidism) 244.9
   congenital 243
Succenturiata placenta - see Placenta, abnormal
Succussion sounds, chest 786.7
Sucking thumb, child 307.9
Sudamen 705.1
Sudamina 705.1
Sudanese kala-azar 085.0
Sudden
   death, cause unknown (less than 24 hours) 798.1
      cardiac (SCD)
         family history of V17.41
         personal history of, successfully resuscitated V12.53
      during childbirth 669.9●
      infant 798.0
      puerperal, postpartum 674.9●
   hearing loss NEC 388.2
   heart failure (see also Failure, heart) 428.9
   infant death syndrome 798.0
Sudeck's atrophy, disease, or syndrome 733.7
SUDS (Sudden unexplained death) 798.2
Suffocation (see also Asphyxia) 799.01
   by
      bed clothes 994.7
      bunny bag 994.7
      cave-in 994.7
      constriction 994.7
      drowning 994.1
      inhalation
         food or foreign body (see also Asphyxia, food or foreign body) 933.1
         oil or gasoline (see also Asphyxia, food or foreign body) 933.1
      overlying 994.7
      plastic bag 994.7
      pressure 994.7
      strangulation 994.7
   during birth 768.1
   mechanical 994.7
Sugar
   blood
      high 790.29
      low 251.2
   in urine 791.5
Suicide, suicidal (attempted)
   by poisoning - see Table of Drugs and Chemicals
   ideation V62.84
   risk 300.9
   tendencies 300.9
   trauma NEC (see also nature and site of injury) 959.9
Suipestifer infection (see also Infection, Salmonella) 003.9
Sulfatidosis 330.0
Sulfhemoglobinemia, sulphemoglobinemia (acquired) (congenital) 289.7

Sumatran mite fever 081.2
Summer - *see* condition
Sunburn 692.71
  dermatitis 692.71
  due to
    other ultraviolet radiation
      692.82
    tanning bed 692.82
  first degree 692.71
  second degree 692.76
  third degree 692.77
SUNCT (short lasting unilateral
  neuralgiform headache with
  conjunctival injection and tearing)
  339.05
Sunken
  acetabulum 718.85
  fontanels 756.0
Sunstroke 992.0
Superfecundation 651.9●
  with fetal loss and retention of one or
    more fetus(es) 651.6●
  following (elective) fetal reduction
    651.7●
Superfetation 651.9●
  with fetal loss and retention of one or
    more fetus(es) 651.6●
  following (elective) fetal reduction
    651.7●
Superinvolution uterus 621.8
Supernumerary (congenital)
  aortic cusps 746.89
  auditory ossicles 744.04
  bone 756.9
  breast 757.6
  carpal bones 755.56
  cusps, heart valve NEC 746.89
    mitral 746.5
    pulmonary 746.09
  digit(s) 755.00
    finger 755.01
    toe 755.02
  ear (lobule) 744.1
  fallopian tube 752.19
  finger 755.01
  hymen 752.49
  kidney 753.3
  lacrimal glands 743.64
  lacrimonasal duct 743.65
  lobule (ear) 744.1
  mitral cusps 746.5
  muscle 756.82
  nipples 757.6
  organ or site NEC - *see* Accessory
  ossicles, auditory 744.04
  ovary 752.0
  oviduct 752.19
  pulmonic cusps 746.09
  rib 756.3
    cervical or first 756.2
      syndrome 756.2
  roots (of teeth) 520.2
  spinal vertebra 756.19
  spleen 759.0
  tarsal bones 755.67
  teeth 520.1
    causing crowding 524.31
  testis 752.89
  thumb 755.01
  toe 755.02
  uterus 752.2
  vagina 752.49
  vertebra 756.19

Supervision (of)
  contraceptive method previously
    prescribed V25.40
    intrauterine device V25.42
    oral contraceptive (pill) V25.41
    specified type NEC V25.49
    subdermal implantable
      contraceptive V25.43
  dietary (for) V65.3
    allergy (food) V65.3
    colitis V65.3
    diabetes mellitus V65.3
    food allergy intolerance V65.3
    gastritis V65.3
    hypercholesterolemia V65.3
    hypoglycemia V65.3
    intolerance (food) V65.3
    obesity V65.3
    specified NEC V65.3
  lactation V24.1
  newborn health ◄
    8 to 28 days old V20.32 ◄
    under 8 days old V20.31 ◄
  pregnancy - *see* Pregnancy,
    supervision of
Supplemental teeth 520.1
  causing crowding 524.31
Suppression
  binocular vision 368.31
  lactation 676.5●
  menstruation 626.8
  ovarian secretion 256.39
  renal 586
  urinary secretion 788.5
  urine 788.5
Suppuration, suppurative - *see also*
    condition
  accessory sinus (chronic) (*see also*
    Sinusitis) 473.9
  adrenal gland 255.8
  antrum (chronic) (*see also* Sinusitis,
    maxillary) 473.0
  bladder (*see also* Cystitis) 595.89
  bowel 569.89
  brain 324.0
    late effect 326
  breast 611.0
    puerperal, postpartum 675.1●
  dental periosteum 526.5
  diffuse (skin) 686.00
  ear (middle) (*see also* Otitis media)
    382.4
    external (*see also* Otitis, externa)
      380.10
    internal 386.33
  ethmoidal (sinus) (chronic) (*see also*
    Sinusitis, ethmoidal) 473.2
  fallopian tube (*see also* Salpingo-
    oophoritis) 614.2
  frontal (sinus) (chronic) (*see also*
    Sinusitis, frontal) 473.1
  gallbladder (*see also* Cholecystitis,
    acute) 575.0
  gum 523.30
  hernial sac - *see* Hernia, by site
  intestine 569.89
  joint (*see also* Arthritis, suppurative)
    711.0●
  labyrinthine 386.33
  lung 513.0
  mammary gland 611.0
    puerperal, postpartum 675.1●
  maxilla, maxillary 526.4
    sinus (chronic) (*see also* Sinusitis,
      maxillary) 473.0
  muscle 728.0

Suppuration, suppurative (*Continued*)
  nasal sinus (chronic) (*see also* Sinusitis)
    473.9
  pancreas 577.0
  parotid gland 527.2
  pelvis, pelvic
    female (*see also* Disease, pelvis,
      inflammatory) 614.4
    acute 614.3
    male (*see also* Peritonitis) 567.21
  pericranial (*see also* Osteomyelitis)
    730.2●
  salivary duct or gland (any) 527.2
  sinus (nasal) (*see also* Sinusitis) 473.9
  sphenoidal (sinus) (chronic) (*see also*
    Sinusitis, sphenoidal) 473.3
  thymus (gland) 254.1
  thyroid (gland) 245.0
  tonsil 474.8
  uterus (*see also* Endometritis) 615.9
  vagina 616.10
  wound - *see also* Wound, open, by site,
    complicated
    dislocation - *see* Dislocation, by site,
      compound
    fracture - *see* Fracture, by site, open
    scratch or other superficial injury -
      see Injury, superficial, by site
Supraeruption, teeth 524.34
Supraglottitis 464.50
  with obstruction 464.51
Suprapubic drainage 596.8
Suprarenal (gland) - *see* condition
Suprascapular nerve - *see* condition
Suprasellar - *see* condition
Supraspinatus syndrome 726.10
Surfer knots 919.8
  infected 919.9
Surgery
  cosmetic NEC V50.1
    breast reconstruction following
      mastectomy V51.0
    following healed injury or operation
      V51.8
    hair transplant V50.0
  elective V50.9
    breast
      augmentation or reduction
        V50.1
      reconstruction following
        mastectomy V51.0
    circumcision, ritual or routine (in
      absence of medical indication)
      V50.2
    cosmetic NEC V50.1
    ear piercing V50.3
    face-lift V50.1
    following healed injury or operation
      V51.8
    hair transplant V50.0
  not done because of
    contraindication V64.1
    patient's decision V64.2
    specified reason NEC V64.3
  plastic
    breast
      augmentation or reduction
        V50.1
      reconstruction following
        mastectomy V51.0
    cosmetic V50.1
    face-lift V50.1
    following healed injury or operation
      V51.8

◄ New   ◄▦ Revised   ~~deleted~~ Deleted   ● Use Additional Digit(s)   ▦ Omit code

Surgery (Continued)
  plastic (Continued)
    repair of scarred tissue (following
        healed injury or operation)
        V51.8
    specified type NEC V50.8
  previous, in pregnancy or childbirth
    cervix 654.6●
      affecting fetus or newborn (see
          also Newborn, affected by)
          760.63
      causing obstructed labor 660.2●
        affecting fetus or newborn
            763.1
    pelvic soft tissues NEC 654.9●
      affecting fetus or newborn (see
          also Newborn, affected by)
          760.63
      causing obstructed labor
          660.2●
        affecting fetus or newborn
            763.1
    perineum or vulva 654.8●
    uterus NEC 654.9●
      affecting fetus or newborn (see
          also Newborn, affected by)
          760.63
      causing obstructed labor
          660.2●
        affecting fetus or newborn
            763.1
      from previous cesarean delivery
          654.2●
    vagina 654.7●
Surgical
  abortion - see Abortion, legal
  emphysema 998.81
  kidney (see also Pyelitis) 590.80
  operation NEC 799.9
  procedures, complication or
      misadventure - see Complications,
      surgical procedure
  shock 998.0
Survey
  fetal anatomic V28.81
Susceptibility
  genetic
    to
      MEN (multiple endocrine
          neoplasia) V84.81
      neoplasia
        multiple endocrine [MEN]
            V84.81
      neoplasm
        malignant, of
          breast V84.01
          endometrium V84.04
          other V84.09
          ovary V84.02
          prostate V84.03
        specified disease NEC
            V84.89
Suspected condition, ruled out (see also
    Observation, suspected) V71.9
  specified condition NEC V71.89
**Suspended uterus, in pregnancy or
    childbirth** 654.4●
  affecting fetus or newborn 763.89
  causing obstructed labor 660.2●
    affecting fetus or newborn 763.1
Sutton's disease 709.09
Sutton and Gull's disease (arteriolar
    nephrosclerosis) (see also
    Hypertension, kidney) 403.90

Suture
  burst (in external operation wound)
      (see also Dehiscence) 998.32
    internal 998.31
  inadvertently left in operation wound
      998.4
  removal V58.32
  Shirodkar, in pregnancy (with or
      without cervical incompetence)
      654.5●
**Swab inadvertently left in operation
    wound** 998.4
Swallowed, swallowing
  difficulty (see also Dysphagia) 787.20
  foreign body NEC (see also Foreign
      body) 938
Swamp fever 100.89
Swan neck hand (intrinsic) 736.09
Sweat(s), sweating
  disease or sickness 078.2
  excessive (see also Hyperhidrosis)
      780.8
  fetid 705.89
  fever 078.2
  gland disease 705.9
    specified type NEC 705.89
  miliary 078.2
  night 780.8
Sweeley-Klionsky disease
    (angiokeratoma corporis diffusum)
    272.7
Sweet's syndrome (acute febrile
    neutrophilic dermatosis) 695.89
Swelling 782.3
  abdominal (not referable to specific
      organ) 789.3●
  adrenal gland, cloudy 255.8
  ankle 719.07
  anus 787.99
  arm 729.81
  breast 611.72
  Calabar 125.2
  cervical gland 785.6
  cheek 784.2
  chest 786.6
  ear 388.8
  epigastric 789.3●
  extremity (lower) (upper) 729.81
  eye 379.92
  female genital organ 625.8
  finger 729.81
  foot 729.81
  glands 785.6
  gum 784.2
  hand 729.81
  head 784.2
  inflammatory - see Inflammation
  joint (see also Effusion, joint) 719.0●
    tuberculous - see Tuberculosis, joint
  kidney, cloudy 593.89
  leg 729.81
  limb 729.81
  liver 573.8
  lung 786.6
  lymph nodes 785.6
  mediastinal 786.6
  mouth 784.2
  muscle (limb) 729.81
  neck 784.2
  nose or sinus 784.2
  palate 784.2
  pelvis 789.3●
  penis 607.83
  perineum 625.8

Swelling (Continued)
  rectum 787.99
  scrotum 608.86
  skin 782.2
  splenic (see also Splenomegaly) 789.2
  substernal 786.6
  superficial, localized (skin) 782.2
  testicle 608.86
  throat 784.2
  toe 729.81
  tongue 784.2
  tubular (see also Disease, renal) 593.9
  umbilicus 789.3●
  uterus 625.8
  vagina 625.8
  vulva 625.8
  wandering, due to Gnathostoma
      (spinigerum) 128.1
  white - see Tuberculosis, arthritis
Swift's disease 985.0
Swimmers'
  ear (acute) 380.12
  itch 120.3
Swimming in the head 780.4
Swollen - see also Swelling
  glands 785.6
Swyer-James syndrome (unilateral
    hyperlucent lung) 492.8
Swyer's syndrome (XY pure gonadal
    dysgenesis) 752.7
Sycosis 704.8
  barbae (not parasitic) 704.8
  contagiosa 110.0
  lupoid 704.8
  mycotic 110.0
  parasitic 110.0
  vulgaris 704.8
Sydenham's chorea - see Chorea,
    Sydenham's
Sylvatic yellow fever 060.0
Sylvest's disease (epidemic pleurodynia)
    074.1
Symblepharon 372.63
  congenital 743.62
Symonds' syndrome 348.2
Sympathetic - see condition
Sympatheticotonia (see also Neuropathy,
    peripheral, autonomic) 337.9
Sympathicoblastoma (M9500/3)
  specified site - see Neoplasm, by site,
      malignant
  unspecified site 194.0
Sympathicogonioma (M9500/3) - see
    Sympathicoblastoma
Sympathoblastoma (M9500/3) - see
    Sympathicoblastoma
Sympathogonioma (M9500/3) - see
    Sympathicoblastoma
Symphalangy (see also Syndactylism) 755.10
Symptoms, specified (general) NEC
    780.99
  abdomen NEC 789.9
  bone NEC 733.90
  breast NEC 611.79
  cardiac NEC 785.9
  cardiovascular NEC 785.9
  chest NEC 786.9
  development NEC 783.9
  digestive system NEC 787.99
  emotional state NEC 799.29
  eye NEC 379.99
  gastrointestinal tract NEC 787.99
  genital organs NEC
    female 625.9
    male 608.9

Symptoms, specified (*Continued*)
  head and neck NEC 784.99
  heart NEC 785.9
  joint NEC 719.60
    ankle 719.67
    elbow 719.62
    foot 719.67
    hand 719.64
    hip 719.65
    knee 719.66
    multiple sites 719.69
    pelvic region 719.65
    shoulder (region) 719.61
    specified site NEC 719.68
    wrist 719.63
  larynx NEC 784.99
  limbs NEC 729.89
  lymphatic system NEC 785.9
  menopausal 627.2
  metabolism NEC 783.9
  mouth NEC 528.9
  muscle NEC 728.9
  musculoskeletal NEC 781.99
    limbs NEC 729.89
  nervous system NEC 781.99
  neurotic NEC 300.9
  nutrition, metabolism, and
      development NEC 783.9
  pelvis NEC 789.9
    female 625.9
  peritoneum NEC 789.9
  respiratory system NEC 786.9
  skin and integument NEC 782.9
  subcutaneous tissue NEC 782.9
  throat NEC 784.99
  tonsil NEC 784.99
  urinary system NEC 788.99
  vascular NEC 785.9
Sympus 759.89
Synarthrosis 719.80
  ankle 719.87
  elbow 719.82
  foot 719.87
  hand 719.84
  hip 719.85
  knee 719.86
  multiple sites 719.89
  pelvic region 719.85
  shoulder (region) 719.81
  specified site NEC 719.88
  wrist 719.83
Syncephalus 759.4
Synchondrosis 756.9
  abnormal (congenital) 756.9
  ischiopubic (van Neck's) 732.1
Synchysis (senile) (vitreous humor)
    379.21
  scintillans 379.22
Syncope (near) (pre-) 780.2
  anginosa 413.9
  bradycardia 427.89
  cardiac 780.2
  carotid sinus 337.01
  complicating delivery 669.2●
  due to lumbar puncture 349.0
  fatal 798.1
  heart 780.2
  heat 992.1
  laryngeal 786.2
  tussive 786.2
  vasoconstriction 780.2
  vasodepressor 780.2
  vasomotor 780.2
  vasovagal 780.2

Syncytial infarct - *see* Placenta, abnormal
Syndactylism, syndactyly (multiple sites)
    755.10
  fingers (without fusion of bone) 755.11
    with fusion of bone 755.12
  toes (without fusion of bone) 755.13
    with fusion of bone 755.14
Syndrome - *see also* Disease
  5q minus 238.74
  abdominal
    acute 789.0●
    migraine 346.2●
    muscle deficiency 756.79
  Abercrombie's (amyloid degeneration)
      277.39
  abnormal innervation 374.43
  abstinence
    alcohol 291.81
    drug 292.0
    neonatal 779.5   ◀
  Abt-Letterer-Siwe (acute histiocytosis
      X) (M9722/3) 202.5●
  Achard-Thiers (adrenogenital) 255.2
  acid pulmonary aspiration 997.39
    obstetric (Mendelson's) 668.0●
  acquired immune deficiency 042
  acquired immunodeficiency 042
  acrocephalosyndactylism 755.55
  acute abdominal 789.0●
  acute chest 517.3
  acute coronary 411.1
  Adair-Dighton (brittle bones and blue
      sclera, deafness) 756.51
  Adams-Stokes (-Morgagni) (syncope
      with heart block) 426.9
  Addisonian 255.41
  Adie (-Holmes) (pupil) 379.46
  adiposogenital 253.8
  adrenal
    hemorrhage 036.3
    meningococcic 036.3
  adrenocortical 255.3
  adrenogenital (acquired) (congenital)
      255.2
    feminizing 255.2
    iatrogenic 760.79
    virilism (acquired) (congenital) 255.2
  affective organic NEC 293.89
    drug-induced 292.84
  afferent loop NEC 537.89
  African macroglobulinemia 273.3
  Ahumada-Del Castillo (nonpuerperal
      galactorrhea and amenorrhea)
      253.1
  air blast concussion - *see* Injury,
      internal, by site
  Alagille 759.89
  Albright (-Martin)
      (pseudohypoparathyroidism)
      275.49
  Albright-McCune-Sternberg (osteitis
      fibrosa disseminata) 756.59
  alcohol withdrawal 291.81
  Alder's (leukocyte granulation
      anomaly) 288.2
  Aldrich (-Wiskott) (eczema-
      thrombocytopenia) 279.12
  Alibert-Bazin (mycosis fungoides)
      (M9700/3) 202.1●
  Alice in Wonderland 293.89
  alien hand 781.8
  Allen-Masters 620.6
  Alligator baby (ichthyosis congenita)
      757.1

Syndrome (*Continued*)
  Alport's (hereditary hematuria-
      nephropathy-deafness) 759.89
  Alvarez (transient cerebral ischemia)
      435.9
  alveolar capillary block 516.3
  Alzheimer's 331.0
    with dementia - *see* Alzheimer's,
      dementia
  amnestic (confabulatory) 294.0
    alcohol-induced persisting 291.1
    drug-induced 292.83
    posttraumatic 294.0
  amotivational 292.89
  amyostatic 275.1
  amyotrophic lateral sclerosis 335.20
  androgen insensitivity 259.51
    partial 259.52
  Angelman 759.89
  angina (*see also* Angina) 413.9
  ankyloglossia superior 750.0
  anterior
    chest wall 786.52
    compartment (tibial) 958.8
    spinal artery 433.8●
      compression 721.1
    tibial (compartment) 958.8
  antibody deficiency 279.00
    agammaglobulinemic 279.00
    congenital 279.04
    hypogammaglobulinemic 279.00
  anticardiolipin antibody 289.81
  antimongolism 758.39
  antiphospholipid antibody 289.81
  Anton (-Babinski)
      (hemiasomatognosia) 307.9
  anxiety (*see also* Anxiety) 300.00
    organic 293.84
  aortic
    arch 446.7
    bifurcation (occlusion) 444.0
    ring 747.21
  Apert's (acrocephalosyndactyly)
      755.55
  Apert-Gallais (adrenogenital) 255.2
  aphasia-apraxia-alexia 784.69
  apical ballooning 429.83
  "approximate answers" 300.16
  arcuate ligament (-celiac axis) 447.4
  arcus aortae 446.7
  arc welders' 370.24
  argentaffin, argentaffinoma 259.2
  Argonz-Del Castillo (nonpuerperal
      galactorrhea and amenorrhea)
      253.1
  Argyll Robertson's (syphilitic) 094.89
    nonsyphilitic 379.45
  Armenian 277.31
  arm-shoulder (*see also* Neuropathy,
      peripheral, autonomic) 337.9
  Arnold-Chiari (*see also* Spina bifida)
      741.0●
    type I 348.4
    type II 741.0●
    type III 742.0
    type IV 742.2
  Arrillaga-Ayerza (pulmonary artery
      sclerosis with pulmonary
      hypertension) 416.0
  arteriomesenteric duodenum occlusion
      537.89
  arteriovenous steal 996.73
  arteritis, young female (obliterative
      brachiocephalic) 446.7

◀ New   ◀▥ Revised   ~~deleted~~ Deleted   ● Use Additional Digit(s)   ▨ Omit code

Syndrome (Continued)

aseptic meningitis - *see* Meningitis, aseptic

Asherman's 621.5

Asperger's 299.8●

asphyctic (*see also* Anxiety) 300.00

aspiration, of newborn (massive 770.18)

    meconium 770.12

ataxia-telangiectasia 334.8

Audry's (acropachyderma) 757.39

auriculotemporal 350.8

autoimmune lymphoproliferative (ALPS) 279.41 ◀

autosomal - *see also* Abnormal, autosomes NEC

    deletion 758.39

        5p 758.31

        22q11.2 758.32

Avellis' 344.89

Axenfeld's 743.44

Ayerza (-Arrillaga) (pulmonary artery sclerosis with pulmonary hypertension) 416.0

Baader's (erythema multiforme exudativum) 695.19

Baastrup's 721.5

Babinski (-Vaquez) (cardiovascular syphilis) 093.89

Babinski-Fröhlich (adiposogenital dystrophy) 253.8

Babinski-Nageotte 344.89

Bagratuni's (temporal arteritis) 446.5

Bakwin-Krida (craniometaphyseal dysplasia) 756.89

Balint's (psychic paralysis of visual disorientation) 368.16

Ballantyne (-Runge) (postmaturity) 766.22

ballooning posterior leaflet 424.0

Banti's - *see* Cirrhosis, liver

Bard-Pic's (carcinoma, head of pancreas) 157.0

Bardet-Biedl (obesity, polydactyly, and mental retardation) 759.89

Barlow's (mitral valve prolapse) 424.0

Barlow (-Möller) (infantile scurvy) 267

Baron Munchausen's 301.51

Barré-Guillain 357.0

Barré-Liéou (posterior cervical sympathetic) 723.2

Barrett's (chronic peptic ulcer of esophagus) 530.85

Bársony-Pólgar (corkscrew esophagus) 530.5

Bársony-Teschendorf (corkscrew esophagus) 530.5

Barth 759.89

Bartter's (secondary hyperaldosteronism with juxtaglomerular hyperplasia) 255.13 ◀

basal cell nevus 759.89

Basedow's (exophthalmic goiter) 242.0●

basilar artery 435.0

basofrontal 377.04

Bassen-Kornzweig (abetalipoproteinemia) 272.5

Batten-Steinert 359.21

battered

    adult 995.81

    baby or child 995.54

    spouse 995.81

Baumgarten-Cruveilhier (cirrhosis of liver) 571.5

Syndrome (Continued)

Beals 759.82

Bearn-Kunkel (-Slater) (lupoid hepatitis) 571.49

Beau's (*see also* Degeneration, myocardial) 429.1

Bechterew-Strümpell-Marie (ankylosing spondylitis) 720.0

Beck's (anterior spinal artery occlusion) 433.8●

Beckwith (-Wiedemann) 759.89

Behçet's 136.1

Bekhterev-Strümpell-Marie (ankylosing spondylitis) 720.0

Benedikt's 344.89

Béquez César (-Steinbrinck-Chédiak-Higashi) (congenital gigantism of peroxidase granules) 288.2

Bernard-Horner (*see also* Neuropathy, peripheral, autonomic) 337.9

Bernard-Sergent (acute adrenocortical insufficiency) 255.41

Bernhardt-Roth 355.1

Bernheim's (*see also* Failure, heart) 428.0

Bertolotti's (sacralization of fifth lumbar vertebra) 756.15

Besnier-Boeck-Schaumann (sarcoidosis) 135

Bianchi's (aphasia-apraxia-alexia syndrome) 784.69

Biedl-Bardet (obesity, polydactyly, and mental retardation) 759.89

Biemond's (obesity, polydactyly, and mental retardation) 759.89

big spleen 289.4

bilateral polycystic ovarian 256.4

Bing-Horton's 339.00

Biörck (-Thorson) (malignant carcinoid) 259.2

Birt-Hogg-Dube 759.89

Blackfan-Diamond (congenital hypoplastic anemia) 284.01

black lung 500

black widow spider bite 989.5

bladder neck (*see also* Incontinence, urine) 788.30

blast (concussion) - *see* Blast, injury

blind loop (postoperative) 579.2

Block-Siemens (incontinentia pigmenti) 757.33

Bloch-Sulzberger (incontinentia pigmenti) 757.33

Bloom (-Machacek) (-Torre) 757.39

Blount-Barber (tibia vara) 732.4

blue

    bloater 491.20

        with

            acute bronchitis 491.22

            exacerbation (acute) 491.21

    diaper 270.0

    drum 381.02

    sclera 756.51

    toe 445.02

Boder-Sedgwick (ataxia-telangiectasia) 334.8

Boerhaave's (spontaneous esophageal rupture) 530.4

Bonnevie-Ullrich 758.6

Bonnier's 386.19

Borjeson-Forssman-Lehmann 759.89

Bouillaud's (rheumatic heart disease) 391.9

Bourneville (-Pringle) (tuberous sclerosis) 759.5

Syndrome (Continued)

Bouveret (-Hoffmann) (paroxysmal tachycardia) 427.2

brachial plexus 353.0

Brachman-de Lange (Amsterdam dwarf, mental retardation, and brachycephaly) 759.89

bradycardia-tachycardia 427.81

Brailsford-Morquio (dystrophy) (mucopolysaccharidosis IV) 277.5

brain (acute) (chronic) (nonpsychotic) (organic) (with behavioral reaction) (with neurotic reaction) 310.9

    with

        presenile brain disease (*see also* Dementia, presenile) 290.10

        psychosis, psychotic reaction (*see also* Psychosis, organic) 294.9

    chronic alcoholic 291.2

    congenital (*see also* Retardation, mental) 319

    postcontusional 310.2

    posttraumatic

        nonpsychotic 310.2

        psychotic 293.9

            acute 293.0

            chronic (*see also* Psychosis, organic) 294.8

            subacute 293.1

    psycho-organic (*see also* Syndrome, psycho-organic) 310.9

    psychotic (*see also* Psychosis, organic) 294.9

    senile (*see also* Dementia, senile) 290.0

branchial arch 744.41

Brandt's (acrodermatitis enteropathica) 686.8

Brennemann's 289.2

Briquet's 300.81

Brissaud-Meige (infantile myxedema) 244.9

broad ligament laceration 620.6

Brock's (atelectasis due to enlarged lymph nodes) 518.0

broken heart 429.83

Brown's tendon sheath 378.61

Brown-Séquard 344.89

brown spot 756.59

Brugada 746.89

Brugsch's (acropachyderma) 757.39

bubbly lung 770.7

Buchem's (hyperostosis corticalis) 733.3

Budd-Chiari (hepatic vein thrombosis) 453.0

Büdinger-Ludloff-Läwen 717.89

bulbar 335.22

    lateral (*see also* Disease, cerebrovascular, acute) 436

Bullis fever 082.8

bundle of Kent (anomalous atrioventricular excitation) 426.7

Bürger-Grutz (essential familial hyperlipemia) 272.3

Burke's (pancreatic insufficiency and chronic neutropenia) 577.8

Burnett's (milk-alkali) 275.42

Burnier's (hypophyseal dwarfism) 253.3

burning feet 266.2

Bywaters' 958.5

Syndrome *(Continued)*
 Caffey's (infantile cortical hyperostosis) 756.59
 Calvé-Legg-Perthes (osteochrondrosis, femoral capital) 732.1
 Caplan (-Colinet) syndrome 714.81
 capsular thrombosis (*see also* Thrombosis, brain) 434.0●
 carbohydrate-deficient glycoprotein (CDGS) 271.8
 carcinogenic thrombophlebitis 453.1
 carcinoid 259.2
 cardiac asthma (*see also* Failure, ventricular, left) 428.1
 cardiacos negros 416.0
 cardiofaciocutaneous 759.89 ◄
 cardiopulmonary obesity 278.8
 cardiorenal (*see also* Hypertension, cardiorenal) 404.90
 cardiorespiratory distress (idiopathic), newborn 769
 cardiovascular renal (*see also* Hypertension, cardiorenal) 404.90
 cardiovasorenal 272.7
 Carini's (ichthyosis congenita) 757.1
 carotid
  artery (internal) 435.8
  body or sinus 337.01
 carpal tunnel 354.0
 Carpenter's 759.89
 Cassidy (-Scholte) (malignant carcinoid) 259.2
 cat-cry 758.31
 cauda equina 344.60
 causalgia 355.9
  lower limb 355.71
  upper limb 354.4
 cavernous sinus 437.6
 celiac 579.0
  artery compression 447.4
  axis 447.4
 central pain 338.0
 cerebellomedullary malformation (*see also* Spina bifida) 741.0●
 cerebral gigantism 253.0
 cerebrohepatorenal 759.89
 cervical (root) (spine) NEC 723.8
  disc 722.71
  posterior, sympathetic 723.2
  rib 353.0
  sympathetic paralysis 337.09
  traumatic (acute) NEC 847.0
 cervicobrachial (diffuse) 723.3
 cervicocranial 723.2
 cervicodorsal outlet 353.2
 Céstan's 344.89
 Céstan (-Raymond) 433.8●
 Céstan-Chenais 344.89
 chancriform 114.1
 Charcôt's (intermittent claudication) 443.9
  angina cruris 443.9
  due to atherosclerosis 440.21
 Charcôt-Marie-Tooth 356.1
 Charcôt-Weiss-Baker 337.01
 CHARGE association 759.89
 Cheadle (-Möller) (-Barlow) (infantile scurvy) 267
 Chédiak-Higashi (-Steinbrinck) (congenital gigantism of peroxidase granules) 288.2
 chest wall 786.52
 Chiari's (hepatic vein thrombosis) 453.0
 Chiari-Frommel 676.6●

Syndrome *(Continued)*
 chiasmatic 368.41
 Chilaiditi's (subphrenic displacement, colon) 751.4
 chondroectodermal dysplasia 756.55
 chorea-athetosis-agitans 275.1
 Christian's (chronic histiocytosis X) 277.89
 chromosome 4 short arm deletion 758.39
 chronic pain 338.4
 Churg-Strauss 446.4
 Clarke-Hadfield (pancreatic infantilism) 577.8
 Claude's 352.6
 Claude Bernard-Horner (*see also* Neuropathy, peripheral, autonomic) 337.9
 Clérambault's
  automatism 348.89 ◄▄▄
  erotomania 297.8
 Clifford's (postmaturity) 766.22
 climacteric 627.2
 Clouston's (hidrotic ectodermal dysplasia) 757.31
 clumsiness 315.4
 Cockayne's (microencephaly and dwarfism) 759.89
 Cockayne-Weber (epidermolysis bullosa) 757.39
 Coffin-Lowry 759.89
 Cogan's (nonsyphilitic interstitial keratitis) 370.52
 cold injury (newborn) 778.2
 Collet (-Sicard) 352.6
 combined immunity deficiency 279.2
 compartment(al) (anterior) (deep) (posterior) 958.8
  nontraumatic
   abdomen 729.73
   arm 729.71
   buttock 729.72
   fingers 729.71
   foot 729.72
   forearm 729.71
   hand 729.71
   hip 729.72
   leg 729.72
   lower extremity 729.72
   shoulder 729.71
   specified site NEC 729.79
   thigh 729.72
   toes 729.72
   upper extremity 729.71
   wrist 729.71
  post-surgical (*see also* Syndrome, compartment, non-traumatic) 998.89
  traumatic 958.90
   abdomen 958.93
   arm 958.91
   buttock 958.92
   fingers 958.91
   foot 958.92
   forearm 958.91
   hand 958.91
   hip 958.92
   leg 958.92
   lower extremity 958.92
   shoulder 958.91
   specified site NEC 958.99
   thigh 958.92
   tibial 958.92

Syndrome *(Continued)*
 compartment(al) *(Continued)*
  traumatic *(Continued)*
   toes 958.92
   upper extremity 958.91
   wrist 958.91
 complex regional pain - *see also* Dystrophy, sympathetic
  type I - *see* Dystrophy, sympathetic (posttraumatic) (reflex)
  type II - *see* Causalgia
 compression 958.5
  cauda equina 344.60
   with neurogenic bladder 344.61
 concussion 310.2
 congenital
  affecting more than one system 759.7
   specified type NEC 759.89
  congenital central alveolar hypoventilation 327.25
  facial diplegia 352.6
  muscular hypertrophy-cerebral 759.89
 congestion-fibrosis (pelvic) 625.5
 conjunctivourethrosynovial 099.3
 Conn (-Louis) (primary aldosteronism) 255.12
 Conradi (-Hünermann) (chondrodysplasia calcificans congenita) 756.59
 conus medullaris 336.8
 Cooke-Apert-Gallais (adrenogenital) 255.2
 Cornelia de Lange's (Amsterdam dwarf, mental retardation, and brachycephaly) 759.8
 coronary insufficiency or intermediate 411.1
 cor pulmonale 416.9
 corticosexual 255.2
 Costen's (complex) 524.60
 costochondral junction 733.6
 costoclavicular 353.0
 costovertebral 253.0
 Cotard's (paranoia) 297.1
 Cowden 759.6
 craniovertebral 723.2
 Creutzfeldt-Jakob 046.19
  with dementia
   with behavioral disturbance 046.19 *[294.11]*
   without behavioral disturbance 046.19 *[294.10]*
  variant 046.11
   with dementia
    with behavioral disturbance 046.11 *[294.11]*
    without behavioral disturbance 046.11 *[294.10]*
 crib death 798.0
 cricopharyngeal 787.20
 cri-du-chat 758.31
 Crigler-Najjar (congenital hyperbilirubinemia) 277.4
 crocodile tears 351.8
 Cronkhite-Canada 211.3
 croup 464.4
 CRST (cutaneous systemic sclerosis) 710.1
 crush 958.5
 crushed lung (*see also* Injury, internal, lung) 861.20

◄ New   ◄▄▄ Revised   ~~deleted~~ Deleted   ● Use Additional Digit(s)   ▨▨▨ Omit code

Syndrome (Continued)

Cruveilhier-Baumgarten (cirrhosis of liver) 571.5
cubital tunnel 354.2
Cuiffini-Pancoast (M8010/3) (carcinoma, pulmonary apex) 162.3
Curschmann (-Batten) (-Steinert) 359.21
Cushing's (iatrogenic) (idiopathic) (pituitary basophilism) (pituitary-dependent) 255.0
  overdose or wrong substance given or taken 962.0
Cyriax's (slipping rib) 733.99
cystic duct stump 576.0
Da Costa's (neurocirculatory asthenia) 306.2
Dameshek's (erythroblastic anemia) 282.49
Dana-Putnam (subacute combined sclerosis with pernicious anemia) 281.0 [336.2]
Danbolt (-Closs) (acrodermatitis enteropathica) 686.8
Dandy-Walker (atresia, foramen of Magendie) 742.3
  with spina bifida (see also Spina bifida) 741.0●
Danlos' 756.83
Davies-Colley (slipping rib) 733.99
dead fetus 641.3●
defeminization 255.2
defibrination (see also Fibrinolysis) 286.6
Degos' 447.8
Deiters' nucleus 386.19
Déjérine-Roussy 338.0
Déjérine-Thomas 333.0
de Lange's (Amsterdam dwarf, mental retardation, and brachycephaly) (Cornelia) 759.89
Del Castillo's (germinal aplasia) 606.0
deletion chromosomes 758.39
delusional
  induced by drug 292.11
dementia-aphonia, of childhood (see also Psychosis, childhood) 299.1●
demyelinating NEC 341.9
denial visual hallucination 307.9
depersonalization 300.6
de Quervain's 259.51
Dercum's (adiposis dolorosa) 272.8
de Toni-Fanconi (-Debre) (cystinosis) 270.0
diabetes-dwarfism-obesity (juvenile) 258.1
diabetes mellitus-hypertension-nephrosis 250.4● [581.81]
  due to secondary diabetes 249.4● [581.81]
diabetes mellitus in newborn infant 775.1
diabetes-nephrosis 250.4● [581.81]
  due to secondary diabetes 249.4● [581.81]
diabetic amyotrophy 250.6● [353.5]
  due to secondary diabetes 249.6● [353.5]
Diamond-Blackfan (congenital hypoplastic anemia) 284.01
Diamond-Gardner (autoerythrocyte sensitization) 287.2

Syndrome (Continued)

DIC (diffuse or disseminated intravascular coagulopathy) (see also Fibrinolysis) 286.6
diencephalohypophyseal NEC 253.8
diffuse cervicobrachial 723.3
diffuse obstructive pulmonary 496
DiGeorge's (thymic hypoplasia) 279.11
Dighton's 756.51
Di Guglielmo's (erythremic myelosis) (M9841/3) 207.0●
disequilibrium 276.9
disseminated platelet thrombosis 446.6
Ditthomska 307.81
Doan-Wiseman (primary splenic neutropenia) 289.53
Döhle body-panmyelopathic 288.2
Donohue's (leprechaunism) 259.8
dorsolateral medullary (see also Disease, cerebrovascular, acute) 436
double athetosis 333.71
double whammy 360.81
Down's (mongolism) 758.0
Dresbach's (elliptocytosis) 282.1
Dressler's (postmyocardial infarction) 411.0
  hemoglobinuria 283.2
  postcardiotomy 429.4
drug withdrawal, infant, of dependent mother 779.5
dry skin 701.1
  eye 375.15
DSAP (disseminated superficial actinic porokeratosis) 692.75
Duane's (retraction) 378.71
Duane-Stilling-Türk (ocular retraction syndrome) 378.71
Dubin-Johnson (constitutional hyperbilirubinemia) 277.4
Dubin-Sprinz (constitutional hyperbilirubinemia) 277.4
Duchenne's 335.22
due to abnormality
  autosomal NEC (see also Abnormal, autosomes NEC) 758.5
    13 758.1
    18 758.2
    21 or 22 758.0
    D₁ 758.1
    E₃ 758.2
    G 758.0
  chromosomal 758.89
    sex 758.81
dumping 564.2
  nonsurgical 536.8
Duplay's 726.2
Dupré's (meningism) 781.6
Dyke-Young (acquired macrocytic hemolytic anemia) 283.9
dyspraxia 315.4
dystocia, dystrophia 654.9●
Eagle-Barret 756.71
Eales' 362.18
Eaton-Lambert (see also Neoplasm, by site, malignant) 199.1 [358.1]
Ebstein's (downward displacement, tricuspid valve into right ventricle) 746.2
ectopic ACTH secretion 255.0
eczema-thrombocytopenia 279.12
Eddowes' (brittle bones and blue sclera) 756.51

Syndrome (Continued)

Edwards' 758.2
efferent loop 537.89
effort (aviators') (psychogenic) 306.2
Ehlers-Danlos 756.83
Eisenmenger's (ventricular septal defect) 745.4
Ekbom's (restless legs) 333.94
Ekman's (brittle bones and blue sclera) 756.51
electric feet 266.2
Elephant man 237.71
Ellison-Zollinger (gastric hypersecretion with pancreatic islet cell tumor) 251.5
Ellis-van Creveld (chondroectodermal dysplasia) 756.55
embryonic fixation 270.2
empty sella (turcica) 253.8
endocrine-hypertensive 255.3
Engel-von Recklinghausen (osteitis fibrosa cystica) 252.01
enteroarticular 099.3
entrapment - see Neuropathy, entrapment
eosinophilia myalgia 710.5
epidemic vomiting 078.82
Epstein's - see Nephrosis
Erb (-Oppenheim)-Goldflam 358.00 ◄
Erdheim-Chester 277.89
Erdheim's (acromegalic macrospondylitis) 253.0
Erlacher-Blount (tibia vara) 732.4
erythrocyte fragmentation 283.19
euthyroid sick 790.94
Evans' (thrombocytopenic purpura) 287.32
excess cortisol, iatrogenic 255.0
exhaustion 300.5
extrapyramidal 333.90
eyelid-malar-mandible 756.0
eye retraction 378.71
Faber's (achlorhydric anemia) 280.9
Fabry (-Anderson) (angiokeratoma corporis diffusum) 272.7
facet 724.8
Fallot's 745.2
falx (see also Hemorrhage, brain) 431
familial eczema-thrombocytopenia 279.12
Fanconi's (anemia) (congenital pancytopenia) 284.09
Fanconi (-de Toni) (-Debré) (cystinosis) 270.0
Farber (-Uzman) (disseminated lipogranulomatosis) 272.8
fatigue NEC 300.5
  chronic 780.71
faulty bowel habit (idiopathic megacolon) 564.7
FDH (focal dermal hypoplasia) 757.39
fecal reservoir 560.39
Feil-Klippel (brevicollis) 756.16
Felty's (rheumatoid arthritis with splenomegaly and leukopenia) 714.1
fertile eunuch 257.2
fetal alcohol 760.71
  late effect 760.71
fibrillation-flutter 427.32
fibrositis (periarticular) 729.0
Fiedler's (acute isolated myocarditis) 422.91
Fiessinger-Leroy (-Reiter) 099.3

Syndrome (*Continued*)
  Fiessinger-Rendu (erythema
    multiforme exudativum)
    695.19
  first arch 756.0
  Fisher's 357.0
  fish odor 270.8
  Fitz's (acute hemorrhagic pancreatitis)
    577.0
  Fitz-Hugh and Curtis 098.86
    due to
      Chlamydia trachomatis 099.56
      Neisseria gonorrhoeae
        (gonococcal peritonitis)
        098.86
  Flajani (-Basedow) (exophthalmic
    goiter) 242.0●
  flat back
    acquired 737.29
    postprocedural 738.5
  floppy
    infant 781.99
    iris 364.81
    valve (mitral) 424.0
  flush 259.2
  Foix-Alajouanine 336.1
  Fong's (hereditary osteo-
    onychodysplasia) 756.89
  foramen magnum 348.4
  Forbes-Albright (nonpuerperal
    amenorrhea and lactation
    associated with pituitary tumor)
    253.1
  Foster-Kennedy 377.04
  Foville's (peduncular) 344.89
  fragile X 759.83
  Franceschetti's (mandibulofacial
    dysostosis) 756.0
  Fraser's 759.89
  Freeman-Sheldon 759.89
  Frey's (auriculotemporal) 705.22
  Friderichsen-Waterhouse 036.3
  Friedrich-Erb-Arnold
    (acropachyderma) 757.39
  Fröhlich's (adiposogenital dystrophy)
    253.8
  Froin's 336.8
  Frommel-Chiari 676.6●
  frontal lobe 310.0
  Fukuhara 277.87
  Fuller Albright's (osteitis fibrosa
    disseminata) 756.59
  functional
    bowel 564.9
    prepubertal castrate 752.89
  Gaisböck's (polycythemia hypertonica)
    289.0
  ganglion (basal, brain) 333.90
    geniculi 351.1
  Ganser's, hysterical 300.16
  Gardner-Diamond (autoerythrocyte
    sensitization) 287.2
  gastroesophageal junction 530.0
  gastroesophageal laceration-
    hemorrhage 530.7
  gastrojejunal loop obstruction 537.89
  Gayet-Wernicke's (superior
    hemorrhagic polioencephalitis)
    265.1
  Gee-Herter-Heubner (nontropical
    sprue) 579.0
  Gélineau's (*see also* Narcolepsy)
    347.00
  genito-anorectal 099.1

Syndrome (*Continued*)
  Gerhardt's (vocal cord paralysis)
    478.30
  Gerstmann's (finger agnosia) 784.69
  Gerstmann-Sträussler-Scheinker (GSS)
    046.71
  Gianotti Crosti 057.8
    due to known virus - *see* Infection,
      virus
    due to unknown virus 057.8
  Gilbert's 277.4
  Gilford (-Hutchinson) (progeria) 259.8
  Gilles de la Tourette's 307.23
  Gillespie's (dysplasia
    oculodentodigitalis) 759.89
  Glénard's (enteroptosis) 569.89
  Glinski-Simmonds (pituitary cachexia)
    253.2
  glucuronyl transferase 277.4
  glue ear 381.20
  Goldberg (-Maxwell) (-Morris)
    (testicular feminization) 259.51
  Goldenhar's (oculoauriculovertebral
    dysplasia) 756.0
  Goldflam-Erb 358.00
  Goltz-Gorlin (dermal hypoplasia)
    757.39
  Goodpasture's (pneumorenal) 446.21
  Good's 279.06
  Gopalan's (burning feet) 266.2
  Gorlin-Chaudhry-Moss 759.89
  Gorlin's 759.89   ◄
  Gougerot (-Houwer)-Sjögren
    (keratoconjunctivitis sicca) 710.2
  Gougerot-Blum (pigmented purpuric
    lichenoid dermatitis) 709.1
  Gougerot-Carteaud (confluent
    reticulate papillomatosis) 701.8
  Gouley's (constrictive pericarditis)
    423.2
  Gowers' (vasovagal attack) 780.2
  Gowers-Paton-Kennedy 377.04
  Gradenigo's 383.02
  Gray or grey (chloramphenicol)
    (newborn) 779.4
  Greig's (hypertelorism) 756.0
  GSS (Gerstmann-Sträussler-Scheinker)
    046.71
  Gubler-Millard 344.89
  Guérin-Stern (arthrogryposis multiplex
    congenita) 754.89
  Guillain-Barré (-Strohl) 357.0
  Gunn's (jaw-winking syndrome)
    742.8
  Günther's (congenital erythropoietic
    porphyria) 277.1
  gustatory sweating 350.8
  H₃O 759.81
  Hadfield-Clarke (pancreatic
    infantilism) 577.8
  Haglund-Läwen-Fründ 717.89
  hair tourniquet - *see also* Injury,
    superficial, by site
    finger 915.8
      infected 915.9
    penis 911.8
      infected 911.9
    toe 917.8
      infected 917.9
  hairless women 257.8
  Hallermann-Strieff 756.0
  Hallervorden-Spatz 333.0
  Hamman's (spontaneous mediastinal
    emphysema) 518.1

Syndrome (*Continued*)
  Hamman-Rich (diffuse interstitial
    pulmonary fibrosis) 516.3
  Hand-Schüller-Christian (chronic
    histiocytosis X) 277.89
  hand-foot 693.0
  Hanot-Chauffard (-Troisier) (bronze
    diabetes) 275.0
  Harada's 363.22
  Hare's (M8010/3) (carcinoma,
    pulmonary apex) 162.3
  Harkavy's 446.0
  harlequin color change 779.89
  Harris' (organic hyperinsulinism)
    251.1
  Hart's (pellagra-cerebellar ataxia-renal
    aminoaciduria) 270.0
  Hayem-Faber (achlorhydric anemia)
    280.9
  Hayem-Widal (acquired hemolytic
    jaundice) 283.9
  headache - *see* Headache, syndrome
  Heberden's (angina pectoris) 413.9
  Hedinger's (malignant carcinoid)
    259.2
  Hegglin's 288.2
  Heller's (infantile psychosis) (*see also*
    Psychosis, childhood) 299.1●
  H.E.L.L.P. 642.5●
  hemolytic-uremic (adult) (child) 283.11
  hemophagocytic 288.4
    infection-associated 288.4
  Hench-Rosenberg (palindromic
    arthritis) (*see also* Rheumatism,
    palindromic) 719.3●
  Henoch-Schönlein (allergic purpura)
    287.0
  hepatic flexure 569.89
  hepatorenal 572.4
    due to a procedure 997.4
    following delivery 674.8●
  hepatourologic 572.4
  Herrick's (hemoglobin S disease)
    282.61
  Herter (-Gee) (nontropical sprue) 579.0
  Heubner-Herter (nontropical sprue)
    579.0
  Heyd's (hepatorenal) 572.4
  HHHO 759.81
  high grade myelodysplastic 238.73
    with 5q deletion 238.73
  Hilger's 337.09
  histiocytic 288.4
  Hoffa (-Kastert) (liposynovitis
    prepatellaris) 272.8
  Hoffmann's 244.9 [359.5]
  Hoffmann-Bouveret (paroxysmal
    tachycardia) 427.2
  Hoffmann-Werdnig 335.0
  Holländer-Simons (progressive
    lipodystrophy) 272.6
  Holmes' (visual disorientation) 368.16
  Holmes-Adie 379.46
  Hoppe-Goldflam 358.00
  Horner's (*see also* Neuropathy,
    peripheral, autonomic) 337.9
    traumatic - *see* Injury, nerve, cervical
      sympathetic
  hospital addiction 301.51
  hungry bone 275.5
  Hunt's (herpetic geniculate
    ganglionitis) 053.11
    dyssynergia cerebellaris myoclonica
    334.2

◄ New   ◄꜡ Revised   ~~deleted~~ Deleted   ● Use Additional Digit(s)   ▬ Omit code

Syndrome *(Continued)*
   Hunter (-Hurler)
      (mucopolysaccharidosis II) 277.5
   hunterian glossitis 529.4
   Hurler (-Hunter)
      (mucopolysaccharidosis II)
      277.5
   Hutchinson's incisors or teeth 090.5
   Hutchinson-Boeck (sarcoidosis) 135
   Hutchinson-Gilford (progeria) 259.8
   hydralazine
      correct substance properly
         administered 695.4
      overdose or wrong substance given
         or taken 972.6
   hydraulic concussion (abdomen) *(see*
      also Injury, internal, abdomen)
      868.00
   hyperabduction 447.8
   hyperactive bowel 564.9
   hyperaldosteronism with hypokalemic
      alkalosis (Bartter's) 255.13
   hypercalcemic 275.42
   hypercoagulation NEC 289.89
   hypereosinophilic (idiopathic) 288.3
   hyperkalemic 276.7
   hyperkinetic - *see also* Hyperkinesia,
      heart 429.82
   hyperlipemia-hemolytic anemia-icterus
      571.1
   hypermobility 728.5
   hypernatremia 276.0
   hyperosmolarity 276.0
   hyperperfusion 997.01
   hypersomnia-bulimia 349.89
   hypersplenic 289.4
   hypersympathetic *(see also* Neuropathy,
      peripheral, autonomic) 337.9
   hypertransfusion, newborn 776.4
   hyperventilation, psychogenic 306.1
   hyperviscosity (of serum) NEC 273.3
      polycythemic 289.0
      sclerothymic 282.8
   hypoglycemic (familial) (neonatal)
      251.2
      functional 251.1
   hypokalemic 276.8
   hypophyseal 253.8
   hypophyseothalamic 253.8
   hypopituitarism 253.2
   hypoplastic left heart 746.7
   hypopotassemia 276.8
   hyposmolality 276.1
   hypotension, maternal 669.2●
   hypothenar hammer 443.89
   hypotonia-hypomentia-hypogonadism-
      obesity 759.81
   ICF (intravascular coagulation-
      fibrinolysis) *(see also* Fibrinolysis)
      286.6
   idiopathic cardiorespiratory distress,
      newborn 769
   idiopathic nephrotic (infantile) 581.9
   iliotibial band 728.89
   Imerslund (-Gräsbeck) (anemia due to
      familial selective vitamin B_{12}
      malabsorption) 281.1
   immobility (paraplegic) 728.3
   immunity deficiency, combined
      279.2
   impending coronary 411.1
   impingement
      shoulder 726.2
      vertebral bodies 724.4

Syndrome *(Continued)*
   inappropriate secretion of antidiuretic
      hormone (ADH) 253.6
   incomplete
      mandibulofacial 756.0
   infant
      death, sudden (SIDS) 798.0
      Hercules 255.2
      of diabetic mother 775.0
      shaken 995.55
   infantilism 253.3
   inferior vena cava 459.2
   influenza-like 487.1
   inspissated bile, newborn 774.4
   insufficient sleep 307.44
   intermediate coronary (artery) 411.1
   internal carotid artery *(see also*
      Occlusion, artery, carotid)
      433.1●
   interspinous ligament 724.8
   intestinal
      carcinoid 259.2
      gas 787.3
      knot 560.2
   intraoperative floppy iris (IFIS)
      364.81
   intravascular
      coagulation-fibrinolysis (ICF) *(see*
         also Fibrinolysis) 286.6
      coagulopathy *(see also* Fibrinolysis)
         286.6
   inverted Marfan's 759.89
   IRDS (idiopathic respiratory distress,
      newborn) 769
   irritable
      bowel 564.1
      heart 306.2
      weakness 300.5
   ischemic bowel (transient) 557.9
      chronic 557.1
      due to mesenteric artery
         insufficiency 557.1
   Itsenko-Cushing (pituitary
      basophilism) 255.0
   IVC (intravascular coagulopathy) *(see*
      also Fibrinolysis) 286.6
   Ivemark's (asplenia with congenital
      heart disease) 759.0
   Jaccoud's 714.4
   Jackson's 344.89
   Jadassohn-Lewandowski (pachyonchia
      congenita) 757.5
   Jaffe-Lichtenstein (-Uehlinger) 252.01
   Jahnke's (encephalocutaneous
      angiomatosis) 759.6
   Jakob-Creutzfeldt 046.19
      with dementia
         with behavioral disturbance
            046.19 *[294.11]*
         without behavioral disturbance
            046.19 *[294.10]*
      variant 046.11
         with dementia
            with behavioral disturbance
               046.11 *[294.11]*
            without behavioral
               disturbance 046.11
               [294.10]
   Jaksch's (pseudoleukemia infantum)
      285.8
   Jaksch-Hayem (-Luzet)
      (pseudoleukemia infantum) 285.8
   jaw-winking 742.8
   jejunal 564.2

Syndrome *(Continued)*
   Jervell-Lange-Nielsen 426.82
   jet lag 327.35
   Jeune's (asphyxiating thoracic
      dystrophy of newborn) 756.4
   Job's (chronic granulomatous disease)
      288.1
   Jordan's 288.2
   Joseph-Diamond-Blackfan (congenital
      hypoplastic anemia) 284.01
   Joubert 759.89
   jugular foramen 352.6
   Kabuki 759.89
   Kahler's (multiple myeloma)
      (M9730/3) 203.0●
   Kalischer's (encephalocutaneous
      angiomatosis) 759.6
   Kallmann's (hypogonadotropic
      hypogonadism with anosmia)
      253.4
   Kanner's (autism) *(see also* Psychosis,
      childhood) 299.0●
   Kartagener's (sinusitis, bronchiectasis,
      situs inversus) 759.3
   Kasabach-Merritt (capillary
      hemangioma associated with
      thrombocytopenic purpura)
      287.39
   Kast's (dyschondroplasia with
      hemangiomas) 756.4
   Kaznelson's (congenital hypoplastic
      anemia) 284.01
   Kearns-Sayre 277.87
   Kelly's (sideropenic dysphagia) 280.8
   Kimmelstiel-Wilson (intercapillary
      glomerulosclerosis) 250.4●
      [581.81]
      due to secondary diabetes 249.4●
      [581.81]
   Klauder's (erythema multiforme
      exudativum) 695.19
   Klein-Waardenburg (ptosis-epicanthus)
      270.2
   Kleine-Levin 327.13
   Klinefelter's 758.7
   Klippel-Feil (brevicollis) 756.16
   Klippel-Trenaunay 759.89
   Klumpke (-Déjérine) (injury to brachial
      plexus at birth) 767.6
   Klüver-Bucy (-Terzian) 310.0
   Köhler-Pelligrini-Stieda (calcification,
      knee joint) 726.62
   König's 564.89
   Korsakoff's (nonalcoholic) 294.0
      alcoholic 291.1
   Korsakoff (-Wernicke) (nonalcoholic)
      294.0
      alcoholic 291.1
   Kostmann's (infantile genetic
      agranulocytosis) 288.01
   Krabbe's
      congenital muscle hypoplasia 756.89
      cutaneocerebral angioma 759.6
   Kunkel (lupoid hepatitis) 571.49
   labyrinthine 386.50
   laceration, broad ligament 620.6
   Landau-Kleffner 345.8●
   Langdon Down (mongolism) 758.0
   Larsen's (flattened facies and multiple
      congenital dislocations) 755.8
   lateral
      cutaneous nerve of thigh 355.1
      medullary *(see also* Disease,
         cerebrovascular, acute) 436

Syndrome *(Continued)*
  Launois' (pituitary gigantism) 253.0
  Launois-Cléret (adiposogenital
    dystrophy) 253.8
  Laurence-Moon (-Bardet)-Biedl
    (obesity, polydactyly, and mental
    retardation) 759.89
  Lawford's (encephalocutaneous
    angiomatosis) 759.6
  lazy
    leukocyte 288.09
    posture 728.3
  Lederer-Brill (acquired infectious
    hemolytic anemia) 283.19
  Legg-Calvé-Perthes (osteochondrosis
    capital femoral) 732.1
  Lemiere 451.89
  Lennox-Gastaut syndrome 345.0●
    with tonic seizures 345.1●
  Lennox's (*see also* Epilepsy) 345.0●
  lenticular 275.1
  Léopold-Lévi's (paroxysmal thyroid
    instability) 242.9●
  Lepore hemoglobin 282.49
  Léri-Weill 756.59
  Leriche's (aortic bifurcation occlusion)
    444.0
  Lermoyez's (*see also* Disease, Ménière's)
    386.00
  Lesch-Nyhan (hypoxanthine-guanine-
    phosphoribosyltransferase
    deficiency) 277.2
  leukoencephalopathy, reversible,
    posterior 348.5
  Lev's (acquired complete heart block)
    426.0
  Levi's (pituitary dwarfism) 253.3
  Lévy-Roussy 334.3
  Lichtheim's (subacute combined
    sclerosis with pernicious anemia)
    281.0 [336.2]
  Li-Fraumeni V84.01
  Lightwood's (renal tubular acidosis)
    588.89
  Lignac (-de Toni) (-Fanconi) (-Debré)
    (cystinosis) 270.0
  Likoff's (angina in menopausal
    women) 413.9
  liver-kidney 572.4
  Lloyd's 258.1
  lobotomy 310.0
  Löffler's (eosinophilic pneumonitis)
    518.3
  Löfgren's (sarcoidosis) 135
  long arm 18 or 21 deletion 758.39
  Looser (-Debray)-Milkman
    (osteomalacia with
    pseudofractures) 268.2
  Lorain-Levi (pituitary dwarfism)
    253.3
  Louis-Bar (ataxia-telangiectasia)
    334.8
  low
    atmospheric pressure 993.2
    back 724.2
      psychogenic 306.0
    output (cardiac) (*see also* Failure,
      heart) 428.9
  Lowe's (oculocerebrorenal dystrophy)
    270.8
  Lowe-Terrey-MacLachlan
    (oculocerebrorenal
    dystrophy) 270.8
  lower radicular, newborn 767.4

Syndrome *(Continued)*
  Lown (-Ganong)-Levine (short P-R
    internal, normal QRS complex,
    and supraventricular tachycardia)
    426.81
  Lucey-Driscoll (jaundice due to
    delayed conjugation) 774.30
  Luetscher's (dehydration) 276.51
  lumbar vertebral 724.4
  Lutembacher's (atrial septal defect
    with mitral stenosis) 745.5
  Lyell's (toxic epidermal necrolysis)
    695.15
    due to drug
      correct substance properly
        administered 695.15
      overdose or wrong substance
        given or taken 977.9
      specified drug - *see* Table of
        Drugs and Chemicals
  MacLeod's 492.8
  macrogenitosomia praecox 259.8
  macroglobulinemia 273.3
  macrophage activation 288.4
  Maffucci's (dyschondroplasia with
    hemangiomas) 756.4
  Magenblase 306.4
  magnesium-deficiency 781.7
  malabsorption 579.9
    postsurgical 579.3
    spinal fluid 331.3
  Mal de Debarquement 780.4
  malignant carcinoid 259.2
  Mallory-Weiss 530.7
  mandibulofacial dysostosis 756.0
  manic-depressive (*see also* Psychosis,
    affective) 296.80
  Mankowsky's (familial dysplastic
    osteopathy) 731.2
  maple syrup (urine) 270.3
  Marable's (celiac artery compression)
    447.4
  Marchesani (-Weill) (brachymorphism
    and ectopia lentis) 759.89
  Marchiafava-Bignami 341.8
  Marchiafava-Micheli (paroxysmal
    nocturnal hemoglobinuria)
    283.2
  Marcus Gunn's (jaw-winking
    syndrome) 742.8
  Marfan's (arachnodactyly) 759.82
    meaning congenital syphilis 090.49
      with luxation of lens 090.49
        [379.32]
  Marie's (acromegaly) 253.0
    primary or idiopathic
      (acropachyderma) 757.39
    secondary (hypertrophic pulmonary
      osteoarthropathy) 731.2
  Markus-Adie 379.46
  Martin's 715.27
  Martin-Albright
    (pseudohypoparathyroidism)
    275.49
  Martorell-Fabré (pulseless disease)
    446.7
  massive aspiration of newborn 770.18
  Masters-Allen 620.6
  mastocytosis 757.33
  maternal hypotension 669.2●
  maternal obesity 646.1●

Syndrome *(Continued)*
  May (-Hegglin) 288.2
  McArdle (-Schmid) (-Pearson)
    (glycogenosis V) 271.0
  McCune-Albright (osteitis fibrosa
    disseminata) 756.59
  McQuarrie's (idiopathic familial
    hypoglycemia) 251.2
  meconium
    aspiration 770.12
    plug (newborn) NEC 777.1
  median arcuate ligament 447.4
  mediastinal fibrosis 519.3
  Meekeren-Ehlers-Danlos 756.83
  Meige (blepharospasm-oromandibular
    dystonia) 333.82
    -Milroy (chronic hereditary edema)
      757.0
  MELAS (mitochondrial
    encephalopathy, lactic acidosis
    and stroke-like episodes)
    277.87
  Melkersson (-Rosenthal) 351.8
  MEN (multiple endocrine neoplasia)
    type I 258.01
    type IIA 258.02
    type IIB 258.03
  Mende's (ptosis-epicanthus) 270.2
  Mendelson's (resulting from a
    procedure) 997.39
    during labor 668.0●
    obstetric 668.0●
  Ménétrier's (hypertrophic gastritis)
    535.2●
  Ménière's (*see also* Disease, Ménière's)
    386.00
  meningo-eruptive 047.1
  Menkes' 759.89
    glutamic acid 759.89
    maple syrup (urine) disease 270.3
  menopause 627.2
    postartificial 627.4
  menstruation 625.4
  MERRF (myoclonus with epilepsy and
    with ragged red fibers) 277.87
  mesenteric
    artery, superior 557.1
    vascular insufficiency (with
      gangrene) 557.1
  metabolic 277.7
  metastatic carcinoid 259.2
  Meyenburg-Altherr-Uehlinger 733.99
  Meyer-Schwickerath and Weyers
    (dysplasia oculodentodigitalis)
    759.89
  Micheli-Rietti (thalassemia minor)
    282.49
  Michotte's 721.5
  micrognathia-glossoptosis 756.0
  microphthalmos (congenital) 759.89
  midbrain 348.89 ◀▥
  middle
    lobe (lung) (right) 518.0
    radicular 353.0
  Miescher's
    familial acanthosis nigricans 701.2
    granulomatosis disciformis 709.3
  Mieten's 759.89
  migraine 346.0●
  Mikity-Wilson (pulmonary
    dysmaturity) 770.7
  Mikulicz's (dryness of mouth, absent
    or decreased lacrimation) 527.1
  milk alkali (milk drinkers') 275.42

◀ New   ◀▥ Revised   ~~deleted~~ Deleted   ● Use Additional Digit(s)   ▮ Omit code

Syndrome (Continued)

Milkman (-Looser) (osteomalacia with pseudofractures) 268.2
Millard-Gubler 344.89
Miller-Dieker 758.33
Miller Fisher's 357.0
Milles' (encephalocutaneous angiomatosis) 759.6
Minkowski-Chauffard (see also Spherocytosis) 282.0
Mirizzi's (hepatic duct stenosis) 576.2
with calculus, cholelithiasis, or stones - see Choledocholithiasis
mitochondrial neurogastrointestinal encephalopathy (MNGIE) 277.87
mitral
click (-murmur) 785.2
valve prolapse 424.0
MNGIE (mitochondrial neurogastrointestinal encephalopathy) 277.87
Möbius'
congenital oculofacial paralysis 352.6
ophthalmoplegic migraine 346.2 ●
Mohr's (types I and II) 759.89
monofixation 378.34
Moore's (see also Epilepsy) 345.5 ●
Morel-Moore (hyperostosis frontalis interna) 733.3
Morel-Morgagni (hyperostosis frontalis interna) 733.3
Morgagni (-Stewart-Morel) (hyperostosis frontalis interna) 733.3
Morgagni-Adams-Stokes (syncope with heart block) 426.9
Morquio (-Brailsford) (-Ullrich) (mucopolysaccharidosis IV) 277.5
Morris (testicular feminization) 259.51
Morton's (foot) (metatarsalgia) (metatarsal neuralgia) (neuralgia) (neuroma) (toe) 355.6
Moschcowitz (-Singer-Symmers) (thrombotic thrombocytopenic purpura) 446.6
Mounier-Kuhn 748.3
with
acute exacerbation 494.1
bronchiectasis 494.0
with (acute) exacerbation 494.1
acquired 519.19
with bronchiectasis 494.0
with (acute) exacerbation 494.1
Mucha-Haberman (acute parapsoriasis varioliformis) 696.2
mucocutaneous lymph node (acute) (febrile) (infantile) (MCLS) 446.1
multiple
deficiency 260
endocrine neoplasia (MEN)
type I 258.01
type IIA 258.02
type IIB 258.03
operations 301.51
Munchausen's 301.51
Munchmeyer's (exostosis luxurians) 728.11
Murchison-Sanderson - see Disease, Hodgkin's
myasthenic - see Myasthenia, syndrome

Syndrome (Continued)

myelodysplastic 238.75
with 5q deletion 238.74
high grade with 5q deletion 238.73
therapy-related 289.83
myeloproliferative (chronic) (M9960/1) 238.79
myofascial pain NEC 729.1
Naffziger's 353.0
Nager-de Reynier (dysostosis mandibularis) 756.0
nail-patella (hereditary osteo-onychodysplasia) 756.89
NARP (neuropathy, ataxia and retinitis pigmentosa) 277.87
Nebécourt's 253.3
Neill Dingwall (microencephaly and dwarfism) 759.89
nephrotic (see also Nephrosis) 581.9
diabetic 250.4 ● [581.81]
due to secondary diabetes 249.4 ● [581.81]
Netherton's (ichthyosiform erythroderma) 757.1
neurocutaneous 759.6
neuroleptic malignant 333.92
Nezelof's (pure alymphocytosis) 279.13
Niemann-Pick (lipid histiocytosis) 272.7
Nonne-Milroy-Meige (chronic hereditary edema) 757.0
nonsense 300.16
Noonan's 759.89
Nothnagel's
ophthalmoplegia-cerebellar ataxia 378.52
vasomotor acroparesthesia 443.89
nucleus ambiguous-hypoglossal 352.6
OAV (oculoauriculovertebral dysplasia) 756.0
obsessional 300.3
oculocutaneous 364.24
oculomotor 378.81
oculourethroarticular 099.3
Ogilvie's (sympathicotonic colon obstruction) 560.89
ophthalmoplegia-cerebellar ataxia 378.52
Oppenheim-Urbach (necrobiosis lipoidica diabeticorum) 250.8 ● [709.3]
due to secondary diabetes 249.8 ● [709.3]
oral-facial-digital 759.89
organic
affective NEC 293.83
drug-induced 292.84
anxiety 293.84
delusional 293.81
alcohol-induced 291.5
drug-induced 292.11
due to or associated with arteriosclerosis 290.42
presenile brain disease 290.12
senility 290.20
depressive 293.83
drug-induced 292.84
due to or associated with arteriosclerosis 290.43
presenile brain disease 290.13
senile brain disease 290.21
hallucinosis 293.82
drug-induced 292.84

Syndrome (Continued)

organic affective 293.83
induced by drug 292.84
organic personality 310.1
induced by drug 292.89
Ormond's 593.4
orodigitofacial 759.89
orthostatic hypotensive-dysautonomic-dyskinetic 333.0
Osler-Weber-Rendu (familial hemmorrhagic telangiectasia) 448.0
osteodermopathic hyperostosis 757.39
osteoporosis-osteomalacia 268.2
Österreicher-Turner (hereditary osteo-onychodysplasia) 756.89
os trigonum 755.69
Ostrum-Furst 756.59
otolith 386.19
otopalatodigital 759.89
outlet (thoracic) 353.0
ovarian remnant 620.8
Owren's (see also Defect, coagulation) 286.3
OX 758.6
pacemaker 429.4
Paget-Schroetter (intermittent venous claudication) 453.89 ◀▥
pain - see also Pain
central 338.0
chronic 338.4
complex regional 355.9
type I 337.20
lower limb 337.22
specified site NEC 337.29
upper limb 337.21
type II
lower limb 355.71
upper limb 354.4
myelopathic 338.0
thalamic (hyperesthetic) 338.0
painful
apicocostal vertebral (M8010/3) 162.3
arc 726.19
bruising 287.2
feet 266.2
Pancoast's (carcinoma, pulmonary apex) (M8010/3) 162.3
panhypopituitary (postpartum) 253.2
papillary muscle 429.81
with myocardial infarction 410.8 ●
Papillon-Léage and Psaume (orodigitofacial dysostosis) 759.89
parabiotic (transfusion)
donor (twin) 772.0
recipient (twin) 776.4
paralysis agitans 332.0
paralytic 344.9
specified type NEC 344.89
paraneoplastic - see Condition
Parinaud's (paralysis of conjugate upward gaze) 378.81
oculoglandular 372.02
Parkes Weber and Dimitri (encephalocutaneous angiomatosis) 759.6
Parkinson's (see also Parkinsonism) 332.0
parkinsonian (see also Parkinsonism) 332.0
Parry's (exophthalmic goiter) 242.0 ●
Parry-Romberg 349.89

Syndrome *(Continued)*
Parsonage-Aldren-Turner 353.5
Parsonage-Turner 353.5
Patau's (trisomy D$_1$) 758.1
patella clunk 719.66
patellofemoral 719.46
Paterson (-Brown) (-Kelly) (sideropenic dysphagia) 280.8
Payr's (splenic flexure syndrome) 569.89
pectoral girdle 447.8
pectoralis minor 447.8
Pelger-Huët (hereditary hyposegmentation) 288.2
pellagra-cerebellar ataxia-renal aminoaciduria 270.0
Pellegrini-Stieda 726.62
pellagroid 265.2
Pellizzi's (pineal) 259.8
pelvic congestion (-fibrosis) 625.5
Pendred's (familial goiter with deaf-mutism) 243
Penfield's (*see also* Epilepsy) 345.5●
Penta X 758.81
peptic ulcer - *see* Ulcer, peptic 533.9
perabduction 447.8
periodic 277.31
periurethral fibrosis 593.4
persistent fetal circulation 747.83
Petges-Cléjat (poikilodermatomyositis) 710.3
Peutz-Jeghers 759.6
Pfeiffer (acrocephalosyndactyly) 755.55
phantom limb 353.6
pharyngeal pouch 279.11
Pick's (pericardial pseudocirrhosis of liver) 423.2
heart 423.2
liver 423.2
Pick-Herxheimer (diffuse idiopathic cutaneous atrophy) 701.8
Pickwickian (cardiopulmonary obesity) 278.8
PIE (pulmonary infiltration with eosinophilia) 518.3
Pierre Marie-Bamberger (hypertrophic pulmonary osteoarthropathy) 731.2
Pierre Mauriac's (diabetes-dwarfism-obesity) 258.1
Pierre Robin 756.0
pigment dispersion, iris 364.53
pineal 259.8
pink puffer 492.8
pituitary 253.0
placental
dysfunction 762.2
insufficiency 762.2
transfusion 762.3
plantar fascia 728.71
plateau iris 364.82
plica knee 727.83
Plummer-Vinson (sideropenic dysphagia) 280.8
pluricarential of infancy 260
plurideficiency of infancy 260
pluriglandular (compensatory) 258.8
polycarential of infancy 260
polyglandular 258.8
polysplenia 759.0
pontine 433.8●
popliteal
artery entrapment 447.8
web 756.89

Syndrome *(Continued)*
postartificial menopause 627.4
postcardiac injury
postcardiotomy 429.4
postmyocardial infarction 411.0
postcardiotomy 429.4
postcholecystectomy 576.0
postcommissurotomy 429.4
postconcussional 310.2
postcontusional 310.2
postencephalitic 310.8
posterior
cervical sympathetic 723.2
fossa compression 348.4
inferior cerebellar artery (*see also* Disease, cerebrovascular, acute) 436
reversible encephalopathy (PRES) 348.39
postgastrectomy (dumping) 564.2
post-gastric surgery 564.2
posthepatitis 780.79
posttherpetic (neuralgia) (zoster) 053.19
geniculate ganglion 053.11
ophthalmica 053.19
postimmunization - *see* Complications, vaccination
postinfarction 411.0
postinfluenza (asthenia) 780.79
postirradiation 990
postlaminectomy 722.80
cervical, cervicothoracic 722.81
lumbar, lumbosacral 722.83
thoracic, thoracolumbar 722.82
postleukotomy 310.0
postlobotomy 310.0
postmastectomy lymphedema 457.0
postmature (of newborn) 766.22
postmyocardial infarction 411.0
postoperative NEC 998.9
blind loop 579.2
postpartum panhypopituitary 253.2
postperfusion NEC 999.89
bone marrow 996.85
postpericardiotomy 429.4
postphlebitic (asymptomatic) 459.10
with
complications NEC 459.19
inflammation 459.12
and ulcer 459.13
stasis dermatitis 459.12
with ulcer 459.13
ulcer 459.11
with inflammation 459.13
postpolio (myelitis) 138
postvagotomy 564.2
postvalvulotomy 429.4
postviral (asthenia) NEC 780.79
Potain's (gastrectasis with dyspepsia) 536.1
potassium intoxication 276.7
Potter's 753.0
Prader (-Labhart)-Willi (-Fanconi) 759.81
preinfarction 411.1
preleukemic 238.75
premature senility 259.8
premenstrual 625.4
premenstrual tension 625.4
pre ulcer 536.9

Syndrome *(Continued)*
Prinzmetal-Massumi (anterior chest wall syndrome) 786.52
Profichet's 729.90
progeria 259.8
progressive pallidal degeneration 333.0
prolonged gestation 766.22
Proteus (dermal hypoplasia) 757.39
prune belly 756.71
prurigo-asthma 691.8
pseudocarpal tunnel (sublimis) 354.0
pseudohermaphroditism-virilismhirsutism 255.2
pseudoparalytica 358.00
pseudo-Turner's 759.89
psycho-organic 293.9
acute 293.0
anxiety type 293.84
depressive type 293.83
hallucinatory type 293.82
nonpsychotic severity 310.1
specified focal (partial) NEC 310.8
paranoid type 293.81
specified type NEC 293.89
subacute 293.1
pterygolymphangiectasia 758.6
ptosis-epicanthus 270.2
pulmonary
arteriosclerosis 416.0
hypoperfusion (idiopathic) 769
renal (hemorrhagic) 446.21
pulseless 446.7
Putnam-Dana (subacute combined sclerosis with pernicious anemia) 281.0 [336.2]
pyloroduodenal 537.89
pyramidopallidonigral 332.0
pyriformis 355.0
QT interval prolongation 426.82
radicular NEC 729.2
lower limbs 724.4
upper limbs 723.4
newborn 767.4
Raeder-Harbitz (pulseless disease) 446.7
Ramsay Hunt's
dyssynergia cerebellaris myoclonica 334.2
herpetic geniculate ganglionitis 053.11
rapid time-zone change 327.35
Raymond (-Céstan) 433.8●
Raynaud's (paroxysmal digital cyanosis) 443.0
RDS (respiratory distress syndrome, newborn) 769
Refsum's (heredopathia atactica polyneuritiformis) 356.3
Reichmann's (gastrosuccorrhea) 536.8
Reifenstein's (hereditary familial hypogonadism, male) 259.52
Reilly's (*see also* Neuropathy, peripheral, autonomic 337.9
Reiter's 099.3
renal glomerulohyalinosis-diabetic 250.4● [581.81]
due to secondary diabetes 249.4● [581.81]
Rendu-Osler-Weber (familial hemorrhagic telangiectasia) 448.0
renofacial (congenital biliary fibroangiomatosis) 753.0
Rénon-Delille 253.8

◀ New ◀▥ Revised ~~deleted~~ Deleted ● Use Additional Digit(s) ▦ Omit code

Syndrome *(Continued)*

respiratory distress (idiopathic)
(newborn) 769
adult (following shock, surgery, or
trauma) 518.5
specified NEC 518.82
type II 770.6
restless legs (RLS) 333.94
retinoblastoma (familial) 190.5
retraction (Duane's) 378.71
retroperitoneal fibrosis 593.4
retroviral seroconversion (acute) V08
Rett's 330.8
Reye's 331.81
Reye-Sheehan (postpartum pituitary
necrosis) 253.2
Riddoch's (visual disorientation) 368.16
Ridley's (*see also* Failure, ventricular,
left) 428.1
Rieger's (mesodermal dysgenesis,
anterior ocular segment) 743.44
Rietti-Greppi-Micheli (thalassemia
minor) 282.49
right ventricular obstruction - *see*
Failure, heart
Riley-Day (familial dysautonomia)
742.8
Robin's 756.0
Rokitansky-Kuster-Hauser (congenital
absence, vagina) 752.49
Romano-Ward (prolonged QT interval
syndrome) 426.82
Romberg's 349.89
Rosen-Castleman-Liebow (pulmonary
proteinosis) 516.0
rotator cuff, shoulder 726.10
Roth's 355.1
Rothmund's (congenital poikiloderma)
757.33
Rotor's (idiopathic hyperbilirubinemia)
277.4
Roussy-Lévy 334.3
Roy (-Jutras) (acropachyderma)
757.39
rubella (congenital) 771.0
Rubinstein-Taybi's (brachydactylia,
short stature, and mental
retardation) 759.89
Rud's (mental deficiency, epilepsy, and
infantilism) 759.89
Ruiter-Pompen (-Wyers)
(angiokeratoma corporis
diffusum) 272.7
Runge's (postmaturity) 766.22
Russell (-Silver) (congenital
hemihypertrophy and short
stature) 759.89
Rytand-Lipsitch (complete
atrioventricular block) 426.0
sacralization-scoliosis-sciatica 756.15
sacroiliac 724.6
Saenger's 379.46
salt
depletion (*see also* Disease, renal)
593.9
due to heat NEC 992.8
causing heat exhaustion or
prostration 992.4
low (*see also* Disease, renal) 593.9
salt-losing (*see also* Disease, renal) 593.9
Sanfilippo's (mucopolysaccharidosis
III) 277.5
Scaglietti-Dagnini (acromegalic
macrospondylitis) 253.0

Syndrome *(Continued)*

scalded skin 695.81
scalenus anticus (anterior) 353.0
scapulocostal 354.8
scapuloperoneal 359.1
scapulovertebral 723.4
Schaumann's (sarcoidosis) 135
Scheie's (mucopolysaccharidosis IS)
277.5
Scheuthauer-Marie-Sainton
(cleidocranialis dysostosis) 755.59
Schirmer's (encephalocutaneous
angiomatosis) 759.6
schizophrenic, of childhood NEC (*see
also* Psychosis, childhood) 299.9 ●
Schmidt's
sphallo-pharyngo-laryngeal
hemiplegia 352.6
thyroid-adrenocortical insufficiency
258.1
vagoaccessory 352.6
Schneider's 047.9
Schnitzler 273.1
Scholte's (malignant carcinoid) 259.2
Scholz (-Bielschowsky-Henneberg)
330.0
Schroeder's (endocrine-hypertensive)
255.3
Schüller-Christian (chronic
histiocytosis X) 277.89
Schultz's (agranulocytosis) 288.09
Schwachman's - *see* Syndrome,
Shwachman's
Schwartz (-Jampel) 359.23
Schwartz-Bartter (inappropriate
secretion of antidiuretic hormone)
253.6
Scimitar (anomalous venous drainage,
right lung to inferior vena cava)
747.49
sclerocystic ovary 256.4
sea-blue histiocyte 272.7
Seabright-Bantam
(pseudohypoparathyroidism)
275.49
Seckel's 759.89
Secretan's (posttraumatic edema) 782.3
secretoinhibitor (keratoconjunctivitis
sicca) 710.2
Seeligmann's (ichthyosis congenita)
757.1
Senear-Usher (pemphigus
erythematosus) 694.4
senilism 259.8
seroconversion, retroviral (acute) V08
serotonin 333.99
serous meningitis 348.2
Sertoli cell (germinal aplasia) 606.0
sex chromosome mosaic 758.81
Sézary's (reticulosis) (M9701/3) 202.2 ●
shaken infant 995.55
Shaver's (bauxite pneumoconiosis) 503
Sheehan's (postpartum pituitary
necrosis) 253.2
shock (traumatic) 958.4
kidney 584.5
following crush injury 958.5
lung 518.5
neurogenic 308.9
psychic 308.9
Shone's 746.84
short
bowel 579.3
P-R interval 426.81

Syndrome *(Continued)*

shoulder-arm (*see also* Neuropathy,
peripheral, autonomic) 337.9
shoulder-girdle 723.4
shoulder-hand (*see also* Neuropathy,
peripheral, autonomic) 337.9
Shwachman's 288.02
Shy-Drager (orthostatic hypotension
with multisystem degeneration)
333.0
Sicard's 352.6
sicca (keratoconjunctivitis) 710.2
sick
cell 276.1
cilia 759.89
sinus 427.81
sideropenic 280.8
Siemens'
ectodermal dysplasia 757.31
keratosis follicularis spinulosa
(decalvans) 757.39
Silfverskiöld's (osteochondrodystrophy,
extremities) 756.50
Silver's (congenital hemihypertrophy
and short stature) 759.89
Silvestroni-Bianco (thalassemia
minima) 282.49
Simons' (progressive lipodystrophy)
272.6
sinus tarsi 726.79
sinusitis-bronchiectasis-situs inversus
759.3
Sipple's (medullary thyroid carcinoma-
pheochromocytoma) 258.02
Sjögren (-Gougerot)
(keratoconjunctivitis sicca) 710.2
with lung involvement 710.2 [517.8]
Sjögren-Larsson (ichthyosis congenita)
757.1
SJS-TEN (Stevens-Johnson syndrome-
toxic epidermal necrolysis
overlap) 695.14
Slocumb's 255.3
Sluder's 337.09
Smith-Lemli-Opitz (cerebrohepatorenal
syndrome) 759.89
Smith-Magenis 758.33
smokers' 305.1
Sneddon-Wilkinson (subcorneal
pustular dermatosis) 694.1
Sotos' (cerebral gigantism) 253.0
South African cardiomyopathy 425.2
spasmodic
upward movement, eye(s) 378.82
winking 307.20
Spens' (syncope with heart block) 426.9
spherophakia-brachymorphia 759.89
spinal cord injury - *see also* Injury,
spinal, by site
with fracture, vertebra - *see* Fracture,
vertebra, by site, with spinal
cord injury
cervical - *see* Injury, spinal, cervical
fluid malabsorption (acquired)
331.3
splenic
agenesis 759.0
flexure 569.89
neutropenia 289.53
sequestration 289.52
Spurway's (brittle bones and blue
sclera) 756.51
staphylococcal scalded skin 695.81
Stein's (polycystic ovary) 256.4

Syndrome (Continued)

Stein-Leventhal (polycystic ovary) 256.4

Steinbrocker's (see also Neuropathy, peripheral, autonomic) 337.9

Stevens-Johnson (erythema multiforme exudativum) 695.13

toxic epidermal necrolysis overlap (SJS-TEN overlap syndrome) 695.14

Stewart-Morel (hyperostosis frontalis interna) 733.3

Stickler 759.89

stiff-baby 759.89

stiff-man 333.91

Still's (juvenile rheumatoid arthritis) 714.30

Still-Felty (rheumatoid arthritis with splenomegaly and leukopenia) 714.1

Stilling-Türk-Duane (ocular retraction syndrome) 378.71

Stojano's (subcostal) 098.86

Stokes (-Adams) (syncope with heart block) 426.9

Stokvis-Talma (enterogenous cyanosis) 289.7

stone heart (see also Failure, ventricular, left) 428.1

straight-back 756.19

stroke (see also Disease, cerebrovascular, acute) 436

little 435.9

Sturge-Kalischer-Weber (encephalotrigeminal angiomatosis) 759.6

Sturge-Weber (-Dimitri) (encephalocutaneous angiomatosis) 759.6

subclavian-carotid obstruction (chronic) 446.7

subclavian steal 435.2

subcoracoid-pectoralis minor 447.8

subcostal 098.86

nerve compression 354.8

subperiosteal hematoma 267

subphrenic interposition 751.4

sudden infant death (SIDS) 798.0

Sudeck's 733.7

Sudeck-Leriche 733.7

superior

cerebellar artery (see also Disease, cerebrovascular, acute) 436

mesenteric artery 557.1

pulmonary sulcus (tumor) (M8010/3) 162.3

vena cava 459.2

suprarenal cortical 255.3

supraspinatus 726.10

Susac 348.39

swallowed blood 777.3

sweat retention 705.1

Sweet's (acute febrile neutrophilic dermatosis) 695.89

Swyer-James (unilateral hyperlucent lung) 492.8

Swyer's (XY pure gonadal dysgenesis) 752.7

Symonds' 348.2

sympathetic

cervical paralysis 337.09

pelvic 625.5

syndactylic oxycephaly 755.55

syphilitic-cardiovascular 093.89

Syndrome (Continued)

systemic

fibrosclerosing 710.8

inflammatory response (SIRS) 995.90

due to

infectious process 995.91

with acute organ dysfunction 995.92

non-infectious process 995.93

with acute organ dysfunction 995.94

systolic click (-murmur) 785.2

Tabagism 305.1

tachycardia-bradycardia 427.81

Takayasu (-Onishi) (pulseless disease) 446.7

Takotsubo 429.83

Tapia's 352.6

tarsal tunnel 355.5

Taussig-Bing (transposition, aorta and overriding pulmonary artery) 745.11

Taybi's (otopalatodigital) 759.89

Taylor's 625.5

teething 520.7

tegmental 344.89

telangiectasis-pigmentation-cataract 757.33

temporal 383.02

lobectomy behavior 310.0

temporomandibular joint-pain-dysfunction [TMJ] NEC 524.60

specified NEC 524.69

Terry's (see also Retinopathy of prematurity) 362.21

testicular feminization 259.51

testis, nonvirilizing 257.8

tethered (spinal) cord 742.59

thalamic 338.0

Thibierge-Weissenbach (cutaneous systemic sclerosis) 710.1

Thiele 724.6

thoracic outlet (compression) 353.0

thoracogenous rheumatic (hypertrophic pulmonary osteoarthropathy) 731.2

Thorn's (see also Disease, renal) 593.9

Thorson-Biörck (malignant carcinoid) 259.2

thrombopenia-hemangioma 287.39

thyroid-adrenocortical insufficiency 258.1

Tietze's 733.6

time-zone (rapid) 327.35

Tobias' (carcinoma, pulmonary apex) (M8010/3) 162.3

toilet seat 926.0

Tolosa-Hunt 378.55

Toni-Fanconi (cystinosis) 270.0

Touraine's (hereditary osteo-onychodysplasia) 756.89

Touraine-Solente-Golé (acropachyderma) 757.39

toxic

oil 710.5

shock 040.82

transfusion

fetal-maternal 772.0

twin

donor (infant) 772.0

recipient (infant) 776.4

transient left ventricular apical ballooning 429.83

Syndrome (Continued)

Treacher Collins' (incomplete mandibulofacial dysostosis) 756.0

trigeminal plate 259.8

triplex X female 758.81

trisomy NEC 758.5

13 or D₁ 758.1

16–18 or E 758.2

18 or E₃ 758.2

20 758.5

21 or G (mongolism) 758.0

22 or G (mongolism) 758.0

G 758.0

Troisier-Hanot-Chauffard (bronze diabetes) 275.0

tropical wet feet 991.4

Trousseau's (thrombophlebitis migrans visceral cancer) 453.1

tumor lysis (following antineoplastic drug therapy) (spontaneous) 277.88 ◀

Türk's (ocular retraction syndrome) 378.71

Turner's 758.6

Turner-Varny 758.6

Twiddler's (due to)

automatic implantable defibrillator 996.04

pacemaker 996.01

twin-to-twin transfusion 762.3

recipient twin 776.4

Uehlinger's (acropachyderma) 757.39

Ullrich (-Bonnevie) (-Turner) 758.6

Ullrich-Feichtiger 759.89

underwater blast injury (abdominal) (see also Injury, internal, abdomen) 868.00

universal joint, cervix 620.6

Unverricht (-Lundborg) 345.1 ◀▥

Unverricht-Wagner (dermatomyositis) 710.3

upward gaze 378.81

Urbach-Oppenheim (necrobiosis lipoidica diabeticorum) 250.8● [709.3]

due to secondary diabetes 249.8● [709.3]

Urbach-Wiethe (lipoid proteinosis) 272.8

uremia, chronic 585.9

urethral 597.81

urethro-oculoarticular 099.3

urethro-oculosynovial 099.3

urohepatic 572.4

uveocutaneous 364.24

uveomeningeal, uveomeningitis 363.22

vagohypoglossal 352.6

vagovagal 780.2

van Buchem's (hyperostosis corticalis) 733.3

van der Hoeve's (brittle bones and blue sclera, deafness) 756.51

van der Hoeve-Halbertsma-Waardenburg (ptosis-epicanthus) 270.2

van der Hoeve-Waarderburg-Gualdi (ptosis-epicanthus) 270.2

vanishing twin 651.33

van Neck-Odelberg (juvenile osteochondrosis) 732.1

vascular splanchnic 557.0

vasomotor 443.9

vasovagal 780.2

◀ New   ◀▥ Revised   ~~deleted~~ Deleted   ● Use Additional Digit(s)   ▨ Omit code

Syndrome (*Continued*)
VATER 759.89
Velo-cardio-facial 758.32
vena cava (inferior) (superior)
    (obstruction) 459.2
Verbiest's (claudicatio intermittens
    spinalis) 435.1
Vernet's 352.6
vertebral
    artery 435.1
        compression 721.1
    lumbar 724.4
    steal 435.1
vertebrogenic (pain) 724.5
vertiginous NEC 386.9
video display tube 723.8
Villaret's 352.6
Vinson-Plummer (sideropenic
    dysphagia) 280.8
virilizing adrenocortical hyperplasia,
    congenital 255.2
virus, viral 079.99
visceral larval migrans 128.0
visual disorientation 368.16
vitamin B₆ deficiency 266.1
vitreous touch 997.99
Vogt's (corpus striatum) 333.71
Vogt-Koyanagi 364.24
Volkmann's 958.6
von Bechterew-Stumpell (ankylosing
    spondylitis) 720.0
von Graefe's 378.72
von Hippel-Lindau (angiomatosis
    retinocerebellosa) 759.6
von Schroetter's (intermittent venous
    claudication) 453.89 ◀▥
von Willebrand (-Jürgens)
    (angiohemophilia) 286.4
Waardenburg-Klein (ptosis epicanthus)
    270.2
Wagner (-Unverricht)
    (dermatomyositis) 710.3
Waldenström's (macroglobulinemia)
    273.3
Waldenström-Kjellberg (sideropenic
    dysphagia) 280.8
Wallenberg's (posterior inferior
    cerebellar artery) (*see also* Disease,
    cerebrovascular, acute) 436
Waterhouse (-Friderichsen) 036.3
water retention 276.6
Weber's 344.89
Weber-Christian (nodular
    nonsuppurative panniculitis)
    729.30
Weber-Cockayne (epidermolysis
    bullosa) 757.39
Weber-Dimitri (encephalocutaneous
    angiomatosis) 759.6
Weber-Gubler 344.89
Weber-Leyden 344.89
Weber-Osler (familial hemorrhagic
    telangiectasia) 448.0
Wegener's (necrotizing respiratory
    granulomatosis) 446.4
Weill-Marchesani (brachymorphism
    and ectopia lentis) 759.89
Weingarten's (tropical eosinophilia)
    518.3
Weiss-Baker (carotid sinus syncope)
    337.01
Weissenbach-Thibierge (cutaneous
    systemic sclerosis) 710.1
Werdnig-Hoffmann 335.0

Syndrome (*Continued*)
Werlhof-Wichmann (*see also* Purpura,
    thrombocytopenic) 287.39
Wermer's (polyendocrine
    adenomatosis) 258.01
Werner's (progeria adultorum) 259.8
Wernicke's (nonalcoholic) (superior
    hemorrhagic polioencephalitis)
    265.1
Wernicke-Korsakoff (nonalcoholic) 294.0
    alcoholic 291.1
Westphal-Strümpell (hepatolenticular
    degeneration) 275.1
wet
    brain (alcoholic) 303.9●
    feet (maceration) (tropical) 991.4
    lung
        adult 518.5
        newborn 770.6
whiplash 847.0
Whipple's (intestinal lipodystrophy)
    040.2
"whistling face" (craniocarpotarsal
    dystrophy) 759.89
Widal (-Abrami) (acquired hemolytic
    jaundice) 283.9
Wilkie's 557.1
Wilkinson-Sneddon (subcorneal
    pustular dermatosis) 694.1
Willan-Plumbe (psoriasis) 696.1
Willebrand (-Jürgens)
    (angiohemophilia) 286.4
Willi-Prader (hypogenital dystrophy
    with diabetic tendency) 759.81
Wilson's (hepatolenticular
    degeneration) 275.1
Wilson-Mikity 770.7
Wiskott-Aldrich (eczema-
    thrombocytopenia) 279.12
withdrawal
    alcohol 291.81
    drug 292.0
        infant of dependent mother
        779.5
Woakes' (ethmoiditis) 471.1
Wolff-Parkinson-White (anomalous
    atrioventricular excitation)
    426.7
Wright's (hyperabduction) 447.8
X
    cardiac 413.9
    dysmetabolic 277.7
xiphoidalgia 733.99
XO 758.6
XXX 758.81
XXXXY 758.81
XXY 758.7
yellow vernix (placental dysfunction)
    762.2
Zahorsky's 074.0
Zellweger 277.86
Zieve's (jaundice, hyperlipemia and
    hemolytic anemia) 571.1
Zollinger-Ellison (gastric
    hypersecretion with pancreatic
    islet cell tumor) 251.5
Zuelzer-Ogden (nutritional
    megaloblastic anemia) 281.2
Synechia (iris) (pupil) 364.70
    anterior 364.72
        peripheral 364.73
    intrauterine (traumatic) 621.5
    posterior 364.71
    vulvae, congenital 752.49

Synesthesia (*see also* Disturbance,
    sensation▶782.0
Synodontia 520.2
Synophthalmus 759.89
Synorchidism 752.89
Synorchism 752.89
Synostosis (congenital) 756.59
    astragaloscaphoid 755.67
    radioulnar 755.53
    talonavicular (bar) 755.67
    tarsal 755.67
Synovial - *see* condition
Synovioma (M9040/3) - *see also*
    Neoplasm, connective tissue,
    malignant
    benign (M9040/0) - *see* Neoplasm,
        connective tissue, benign
Synoviosarcoma (M9040/3) - *see*
    Neoplasm, connective tissue,
    malignant
Synovitis (*see also* Tenosynovitis)
    727.00
    chronic crepitant, wrist 727.2
    due to crystals - *see* Arthritis, due to
        crystals
    gonococcal 098.51
    gouty 274.00   ◀▥
    specified NEC 727.09
    syphilitic 095.7
        congenital 090.0
    traumatic, current - *see* Sprain, by site
    tuberculous - *see* Tuberculosis,
        synovitis
    villonodular 719.20
        ankle 719.27
        elbow 719.22
        foot 719.27
        hand 719.24
        hip 719.25
        knee 719.26
        multiple sites 719.29
        pelvic region 719.25
        shoulder (region) 719.21
        specified site NEC 719.28
        wrist 719.23
Syphilide 091.3
    congenital 090.0
    newborn 090.0
    tubercular 095.8
        congenital 090.0
Syphilis, syphilitic (acquired) 097.9
    with lung involvement 095.1
    abdomen (late) 095.2
    acoustic nerve 094.86
    adenopathy (secondary) 091.4
    adrenal (gland) 095.8
        with cortical hypofunction 095.8
    age under 2 years NEC (*see also*
        Syphilis, congenital) 090.9
        acquired 097.9
    alopecia (secondary) 091.82
    anemia 095.8
    aneurysm (artery) (ruptured) 093.89
        aorta 093.0
        central nervous system 094.89
        congenital 090.5
    anus 095.8
        primary 091.1
        secondary 091.3
    aorta, aortic (arch) (abdominal)
        (insufficiency) (pulmonary)
        (regurgitation) (stenosis)
        (thoracic) 093.89
        aneurysm 093.0

Syphilis, syphilitic (*Continued*)
  arachnoid (adhesive) 094.2
  artery 093.89
    cerebral 094.89
    spinal 094.89
  arthropathy (neurogenic) (tabetic) 094.0
    [713.5]
  asymptomatic - *see* Syphilis, latent
  ataxia, locomotor (progressive) 094.0
  atrophoderma maculatum 091.3
  auricular fibrillation 093.89
  Bell's palsy 094.89
  bladder 095.8
  bone 095.5
    secondary 091.61
  brain 094.89
  breast 095.8
  bronchus 095.8
  bubo 091.0
  bulbar palsy 094.89
  bursa (late) 095.7
  cardiac decompensation 093.89
  cardiovascular (early) (late) (primary)
    (secondary) (tertiary) 093.9
    specified type and site NEC 093.89
  causing death under 2 years of age (*see
    also* Syphilis, congenital) 090.9
    stated to be acquired NEC 097.9
  central nervous system (any site) (early)
    (late) (latent) (primary) (recurrent)
    (relapse) (secondary) (tertiary)
    094.9
    with
      ataxia 094.0
      paralysis, general 094.1
        juvenile 090.40
      paresis (general) 094.1
        juvenile 090.40
      tabes (dorsalis) 094.0
        juvenile 090.40
      taboparesis 094.1
        juvenile 090.40
    aneurysm (ruptured) 094.87
    congenital 090.40
    juvenile 090.40
    remission in (sustained) 094.9
    serology doubtful, negative, or
      positive 094.9
    specified nature or site NEC 094.89
    vascular 094.89
  cerebral 094.89
    meningovascular 094.2
    nerves 094.89
    sclerosis 094.89
    thrombosis 094.89
  cerebrospinal 094.89
    tabetic 094.0
  cerebrovascular 094.89
  cervix 095.8
  chancre (multiple) 091.0
    extragenital 091.2
    Rollet's 091.2
  Charcôt's joint 094.0 [713.5]
  choked disc 094.89 [377.00]
  chorioretinitis 091.51
    congenital 090.0 [363.13]
    late 094.83
  choroiditis 091.51
    congenital 090.0 [363.13]
    late 094.83
    prenatal 090.0 [363.13]
  choroidoretinitis (secondary) 091.51
    congenital 090.0 [363.13]
    late 094.83

Syphilis, syphilitic (*Continued*)
  ciliary body (secondary) 091.52
    late 095.8 [364.11]
  colon (late) 095.8
  combined sclerosis 094.89
  complicating pregnancy, childbirth, or
    puerperium 647.0●
    affecting fetus or newborn 760.2
  condyloma (latum) 091.3
  congenital 090.9
    with
      encephalitis 090.41
      paresis (general) 090.40
      tabes (dorsalis) 090.40
      taborparesis 090.40
    chorioretinitis, choroiditis 090.0
      [363.13]
    early or less than 2 years after birth
      NEC 090.2
      with manifestations 090.0
      latent (without manifestations)
        090.1
        negative spinal fluid test
          090.1
        serology, positive 090.1
      symptomatic 090.0
    interstitial keratitis 090.3
    juvenile neurosyphilis 090.40
    late or 2 years or more after birth
      NEC 090.7
      chorioretinitis, choroiditis 090.5
        [363.13]
      interstitial keratitis 090.3
      juvenile neurosyphilis NEC
        090.40
      latent (without manifestations)
        090.6
        negative spinal fluid test
          090.6
        serology, positive 090.6
      symptomatic or with
        manifestations NEC 090.5
        interstitial keratitis 090.3
  conjugal 097.9
    tabes 094.0
  conjunctiva 095.8 [372.10]
  contact V01.6
  cord, bladder 094.0
  cornea, late 095.8 [370.59]
  coronary (artery) 093.89
    sclerosis 093.89
  coryza 095.8
    congenital 090.0
  cranial nerve 094.89
  cutaneous - *see* Syphilis, skin
  dacryocystitis 095.8
  degeneration, spinal cord 094.89
  d'emblée 095.8
  dementia 094.1
    paralytica 094.1
      juvenilis 090.40
  destruction of bone 095.5
  dilatation, aorta 093.0
  due to blood transfusion 097.9
  dura mater 094.89
  ear 095.8
    inner 095.8
      nerve (eighth) 094.86
      neurorecurrence 094.86
  early NEC 091.0
    cardiovascular 093.9
    central nervous system 094.9
      paresis 094.1
      tabes 094.0

Syphilis, syphilitic (*Continued*)
  early NEC (*Continued*)
    latent (without manifestations) (less
      than 2 years after infection)
      092.9
      negative spinal fluid test 092.9
      serological relapse following
        treatment 092.0
      serology positive 092.9
    paresis 094.1
    relapse (treated, untreated) 091.7
    skin 091.3
    symptomatic NEC 091.89
      extragenital chancre 091.2
      primary, except extragenital
        chancre 091.0
      secondary (*see also* Syphilis,
        secondary) 091.3
        relapse (treated, untreated)
          091.7
    tabes 094.0
    ulcer 091.3
  eighth nerve 094.86
  endemic, nonveneral 104.0
  endocarditis 093.20
    aortic 093.22
    mitral 093.21
    pulmonary 093.24
    tricuspid 093.23
  epididymis (late) 095.8
  epiglottis 095.8
  epiphysitis (congenital) 090.0
  esophagus 095.8
  Eustachian tube 095.8
  exposure to V01.6
  eye 095.8 [363.13]
    neuromuscular mechanism
      094.85
  eyelid 095.8 [373.5]
    with gumma 095.8 [373.5]
    ptosis 094.89
  fallopian tube 095.8
  fracture 095.5
  gallbladder (late) 095.8
  gastric 095.8
    crisis 094.0
    polyposis 095.8
  general 097.9
    paralysis 094.1
      juvenile 090.40
  genital (primary) 091.0
  glaucoma 095.8
  gumma (late) NEC 095.9
    cardiovascular system 093.9
    central nervous system 094.9
    congenital 090.5
    heart or artery 093.89
  heart 093.89
    block 093.89
    decompensation 093.89
    disease 093.89
    failure 093.89
    valve (*see also* Syphilis, endocarditis)
      093.20
  hemianesthesia 094.89
  hemianopsia 095.8
  hemiparesis 094.89
  hemiplegia 094.89
  hepatic artery 093.89
  hepatitis 095.3
  hepatomegaly 095.3
    congenital 090.0
  hereditaria tarda (*see also* Syphilis,
    congenital, late) 090.7

◀ New ◀▥ Revised ~~deleted~~ Deleted ● Use Additional Digit(s) ▥ Omit code

Syphilis, syphilitic (Continued)
hereditary (see also Syphilis, congenital)
090.9
interstitial keratitis 090.3
Hutchinson's teeth 090.5
hyalitis 095.8
inactive - see Syphilis, latent
infantum NEC (see also Syphilis,
congenital) 090.9
inherited - see Syphilis, congenital
internal ear 095.8
intestine (late) 095.8
iris, iritis (secondary) 091.52
late 095.8 [364.11]
joint (late) 095.8
keratitis (congenital) (early)
(interstitial) (late)
(parenchymatous) (punctata
profunda) 090.3
kidney 095.4
lacrimal apparatus 095.8
laryngeal paralysis 095.8
larynx 095.8
late 097.0
cardiovascular 093.9
central nervous system 094.9
latent or 2 years or more after
infection (without
manifestation) 096
negative spinal fluid test 096
serology positive 096
paresis 094.1
specified site NEC 095.8
symptomatic or with symptoms
095.9
tabes 094.0
latent 097.1
central nervous system 094.9
date of infection unspecified
097.1
early or less than 2 years after
infection 092.9
late or 2 years or more after infection
096
serology
doubtful
follow-up of latent syphilis
097.1
central nervous system
094.9
date of infection unspecified
097.1
early or less than 2 years
after infection 092.9
late or 2 years or more after
infection 096
positive, only finding 097.1
date of infection unspecified
097.1
early or less than 2 years after
infection 097.1
late or 2 years or more after
infection 097.1
lens 095.8
leukoderma 091.3
late 095.8
lienis 095.8
lip 091.3
chancre 091.2
late 095.8
primary 091.2
Lissauer's paralysis 094.1
liver 095.3
secondary 091.62

Syphilis, syphilitic (Continued)
locomotor ataxia 094.0
lung 095.1
lymphadenitis (secondary) 091.4
lymph gland (early) (secondary) 091.4
late 095.8
macular atrophy of skin 091.3
striated 095.8
maternal, affecting fetus or newborn
760.2
manifest syphilis in newborn - see
Syphilis, congenital
mediastinum (late) 095.8
meninges (adhesive) (basilar) (brain)
(spinal cord) 094.2
meningitis 094.2
acute 091.81
congenital 090.42
meningoencephalitis 094.2
meningovascular 094.2
congenital 090.49
mesarteritis 093.89
brain 094.89
spine 094.89
middle ear 095.8
mitral stenosis 093.21
monoplegia 094.89
mouth (secondary) 091.3
late 095.8
mucocutaneous 091.3
late 095.8
mucous
membrane 091.3
late 095.8
patches 091.3
congenital 090.0
mulberry molars 090.5
muscle 095.6
myocardium 093.82
myositis 095.6
nasal sinus 095.8
neonatorum NEC (see also Syphilis,
congenital) 090.9
nerve palsy (any cranial nerve)
094.89
nervous system, central 094.9
neuritis 095.8
acoustic nerve 094.86
neurorecidive of retina 094.83
neuroretinitis 094.85
newborn (see also Syphilis, congenital)
090.9
nodular superficial 095.8
nonvenereal, endemic 104.0
nose 095.8
saddle back deformity 090.5
septum 095.8
perforated 095.8
occlusive arterial disease 093.89
ophthalmic 095.8 [363.13]
ophthalmoplegia 094.89
optic nerve (atrophy) (neuritis)
(papilla) 094.84
orbit (late) 095.8
orchitis 095.8
organic 097.9
osseous (late) 095.5
osteochondritis (congenital) 090.0
osteoporosis 095.5
ovary 095.8
oviduct 095.8
palate 095.8
gumma 095.8
perforated 090.5

Syphilis, syphilitic (Continued)
pancreas (late) 095.8
pancreatitis 095.8
paralysis 094.89
general 094.1
juvenile 090.40
paraplegia 094.89
paresis (general) 094.1
juvenile 090.40
paresthesia 094.89
Parkinson's disease or syndrome
094.82
paroxysmal tachycardia 093.89
pemphigus (congenital) 090.0
penis 091.0
chancre 091.0
late 095.8
pericardium 093.81
perichondritis, larynx 095.8
periosteum 095.5
congenital 090.0
early 091.61
secondary 091.61
peripheral nerve 095.8
petrous bone (late) 095.5
pharynx 095.8
secondary 091.3
pituitary (gland) 095.8
placenta 095.8
pleura (late) 095.8
pneumonia, white 090.0
pontine (lesion) 094.89
portal vein 093.89
primary NEC 091.2
anal 091.1
and secondary (see also Syphilis,
secondary) 091.9
cardiovascular 093.9
central nervous system 094.9
extragenital chancre NEC 091.2
fingers 091.2
genital 091.0
lip 091.2
specified site NEC 091.2
tonsils 091.2
prostate 095.8
psychosis (intracranial gumma) 094.89
ptosis (eyelid) 094.89
pulmonary (late) 095.1
artery 093.89
pulmonum 095.1
pyelonephritis 095.4
recently acquired, symptomatic NEC
091.89
rectum 095.8
respiratory tract 095.8
retina
late 094.83
neurorecidive 094.83
retrobulbar neuritis 094.85
salpingitis 095.8
sclera (late) 095.0
sclerosis
cerebral 094.89
coronary 093.89
multiple 094.89
subacute 094.89
scotoma (central) 095.8
scrotum 095.8
secondary (and primary) 091.9
adenopathy 091.4
anus 091.3
bone 091.61
cardiovascular 093.9

Syphilis, syphilitic *(Continued)*
  secondary *(Continued)*
    central nervous system 094.9
    chorioretinitis, choroiditis 091.51
    hepatitis 091.62
    liver 091.62
    lymphadenitis 091.4
    meningitis, acute 091.81
    mouth 091.3
    mucous membranes 091.3
    periosteum 091.61
    periostitis 091.61
    pharynx 091.3
    relapse (treated) (untreated) 091.7
    skin 091.3
    specified form NEC 091.89
    tonsil 091.3
    ulcer 091.3
    viscera 091.69
    vulva 091.3
  seminal vesicle (late) 095.8
  seronegative
    with signs or symptoms - *see*
      Syphilis, by site and stage
  seropositive
    with signs or symptoms - *see*
      Syphilis, by site or stage
    follow-up of latent syphilis - *see*
      Syphilis, latent
    only finding - *see* Syphilis, latent
  seventh nerve (paralysis) 094.89
  sinus 095.8
  sinusitis 095.8
  skeletal system 095.5
  skin (early) (secondary) (with
    ulceration) 091.3
    late or tertiary 095.8
  small intestine 095.8
  spastic spinal paralysis 094.0
  spermatic cord (late) 095.8
  spinal (cord) 094.89
    with
      paresis 094.1
      tabes 094.0
  spleen 095.8
  splenomegaly 095.8
  spondylitis 095.5
  staphyloma 095.8
  stigmata (congenital) 090.5
  stomach 095.8
  synovium (late) 095.7

Syphilis, syphilitic *(Continued)*
  tabes dorsalis (early) (late) 094.0
    juvenile 090.40
  tabetic type 094.0
    juvenile 090.40
  taboparesis 094.1
    juvenile 090.40
  tachycardia 093.89
  tendon (late) 095.7
  tertiary 097.0
    with symptoms 095.8
    cardiovascular 093.9
    central nervous system 094.9
    multiple NEC 095.8
    specified site NEC 095.8
  testis 095.8
  thorax 095.8
  throat 095.8
  thymus (gland) 095.8
  thyroid (late) 095.8
  tongue 095.8
  tonsil (lingual) 095.8
    primary 091.2
    secondary 091.3
  trachea 095.8
  tricuspid valve 093.23
  tumor, brain 094.89
  tunica vaginalis (late) 095.8
  ulcer (any site) (early) (secondary)
    091.3
    late 095.9
    perforating 095.9
      foot 094.0
  urethra (stricture) 095.8
  urogenital 095.8
  uterus 095.8
  uveal tract (secondary) 091.50
    late 095.8 *[363.13]*
  uveitis (secondary) 091.50
    late 095.8 *[363.13]*
  uvula (late) 095.8
    perforated 095.8
  vagina 091.0
    late 095.8
  valvulitis NEC 093.20
  vascular 093.89
    brain or cerebral 094.89
  vein 093.89
    cerebral 094.89
  ventriculi 095.8
  vesicae urinariae 095.8

Syphilis, syphilitic *(Continued)*
  viscera (abdominal) 095.2
    secondary 091.69
  vitreous (hemorrhage) (opacities) 095.8
  vulva 091.0
    late 095.8
    secondary 091.3
Syphiloma 095.9
  cardiovascular system 093.9
  central nervous system 094.9
  circulatory system 093.9
  congenital 090.5
Syphilophobia 300.29
Syringadenoma (M8400/0) - *see also*
  Neoplasm, skin, benign
  papillary (M8406/0) - *see* Neoplasm,
    skin, benign
Syringobulbia 336.0
Syringocarcinoma (M8400/3) - *see*
  Neoplasm, skin, malignant
Syringocystadenoma (M8400/0) - *see also*
  Neoplasm, skin, benign
  papillary (M8406/0) - *see* Neoplasm,
    skin, benign
Syringocystoma (M8407/0) - *see*
  Neoplasm, skin, benign
Syringoma (M8407/0) - *see also*
  Neoplasm, skin, benign
  chondroid (M8940/0) - *see* Neoplasm,
    by site, benign
Syringomyelia 336.0
Syringomyelitis 323.9
  late effect - *see* category 326
Syringomyelocele (*see also* Spina bifida)
  741.9●
Syringopontia 336.0
System, systemic - *see also* condition
  disease, combined - *see* Degeneration,
    combined
  fibrosclerosing syndrome 710.8
  inflammatory response syndrome
    (SIRS) 995.90
    due to
      infectious process 995.91
        with acute organ dysfunction
          995.92
      non-infectious process 995.93
        with acute organ dysfunction
          995.94
  lupus erythematosus 710.0
    inhibitor 286.5

◄ New   ◄▥ Revised   ~~deleted~~ Deleted   ● Use Additional Digit(s)   ▨ Omit code

T

Tab - *see* Tag
Tabacism 989.84
Tabacosis 989.84
Tabardillo 080
  flea-borne 081.0
  louse-borne 080
Tabes, tabetic
  with
      central nervous system syphilis
        094.0
        Charcôt's joint 094.0 [713.5]
        cord bladder 094.0
        crisis, viscera (any) 094.0
        paralysis, general 094.1
        paresis (general) 094.1
        perforating ulcer 094.0
    arthropathy 094.0 [713.5]
    bladder 094.0
    bone 094.0
    cerebrospinal 094.0
    congenital 090.40
    conjugal 094.0
    dorsalis 094.0
      neurosyphilis 094.0
    early 094.0
    juvenile 090.40
    latent 094.0
    mesenterica (*see also* Tuberculosis)
      014.8●
    paralysis insane, general 094.1
    peripheral (nonsyphilitic) 799.89
    spasmodic 094.0
      not dorsal or dorsalis 343.9
    syphilis (cerebrospinal) 094.0
Taboparalysis 094.1
Taboparesis (remission) 094.1
  with
      Charcôt's joint 094.1 [713.5]
      cord bladder 094.1
      perforating ulcer 094.1
    juvenile 090.40
Tache noir 923.20
Tachyalimentation 579.3
Tachyarrhythmia, tachyrhythmia - *see also*
    Tachycardia
  paroxysmal with sinus bradycardia
    427.81
Tachycardia 785.0
  atrial 427.89
  auricular 427.89
  AV nodal re-entry (re-entrant)
    427.89
  junctional ectopic 427.0
  newborn 779.82
  nodal 427.89
    nonparoxysmal atrioventricular
      426.89
    nonparoxysmal atrioventricular (nodal)
      426.89
  nonsustained 427.2
  paroxysmal 427.2
    with sinus bradycardia 427.81
    atrial (PAT) 427.0
      psychogenic 316 [427.0]
    atrioventricular (AV) 427.0
      psychogenic 316 [427.0]
    essential 427.2
    junctional 427.0
    nodal 427.0
    psychogenic 316 [427.2]
      atrial 316 [427.0]
      supraventricular 316 [427.0]
      ventricular 316 [427.1]

Tachycardia (*Continued*)
  paroxysmal (*Continued*)
    supraventricular 427.0
      psychogenic 316 [427.0]
    ventricular 427.1
      psychogenic 316 [427.1]
  postoperative 997.1
  psychogenic 306.2
  sick sinus 427.81
  sinoauricular 427.89
  sinus 427.89
  supraventricular 427.89
  sustained 427.2
    supraventricular 427.0
    ventricular 427.1
  ventricular (paroxysmal) 427.1
    psychogenic 316 [427.1]
Tachygastria 536.8
Tachypnea 786.06
  hysterical 300.11
  newborn (idiopathic) (transitory) 770.6
  psychogenic 306.1
  transitory, of newborn 770.6
Taenia (infection) (infestation) (*see also*
    Infestation, taenia) 123.3
  diminuta 123.6
  echinococcal infestation (*see also*
    Echinococcus) 122.9
  nana 123.6
  saginata infestation 123.2
  solium (intestinal form) 123.0
    larval form 123.1
Taeniasis (intestine) (*see also* Infestation,
    taenia) 123.3
  saginata 123.2
  solium 123.0
Taenzer's disease 757.4
Tag (hypertrophied skin) (infected) 701.9
  adenoid 474.8
  anus 455.9
  endocardial (*see also* Endocarditis)
    424.90
  hemorrhoidal 455.9
  hymen 623.8
  perineal 624.8
  preauricular 744.1
  rectum 455.9
  sentinel 455.9
  skin 701.9
    accessory 757.39
    anus 455.9
    congenital 757.39
    preauricular 744.1
    rectum 455.9
  tonsil 474.8
  urethra, urethral 599.84
  vulva 624.8
Tahyna fever 062.5
Takayasu (-Onishi) disease or syndrome
    (pulseless disease) 446.7
Takotsubo syndrome 429.83
Talc granuloma 728.82
  in operation wound 998.7
Talcosis 502
Talipes (congenital) 754.70
  acquired NEC 736.79
    planus 734
  asymmetric 754.79
    acquired 736.79
  calcaneovalgus 754.62
    acquired 736.76
  calcaneovarus 754.59
    acquired 736.76
  calcaneus 754.79
    acquired 736.76

Talipes (*Continued*)
  cavovarus 754.59
    acquired 736.75
  cavus 754.71
    acquired 736.73
  equinovalgus 754.69
    acquired 736.72
  equinovarus 754.51
    acquired 736.71
  equinus 754.79
    acquired, NEC 736.72
  percavus 754.71
    acquired 736.73
  planovalgus 754.69
    acquired 736.79
  planus (acquired) (any degree) 734
    congenital 754.61
    due to rickets 268.1
  valgus 754.60
    acquired 736.79
  varus 754.50
    acquired 736.79
Talma's disease 728.85
Talon noir 924.20
  hand 923.20
  heel 924.20
  toe 924.3
Tamponade heart (Rose's) (*see also*
    Pericarditis) 423.3
Tanapox 059.21
Tangier disease (familial high-density
    lipoprotein deficiency) 272.5
Tank ear 380.12
Tantrum (childhood) (*see also* Disturbance,
    conduct) 312.1●
Tapeworm (infection) (infestation) (*see
    also* Infestation, tapeworm) 123.9
Tapia's syndrome 352.6
Tarantism 297.8
Target-oval cell anemia 282.49
Tarlov's cyst 355.9
Tarral-Besnier disease (pityriasis rubra
    pilaris) 696.4
Tarsalgia 729.2
Tarsal tunnel syndrome 355.5
Tarsitis (eyelid) 373.00
  syphilitic 095.8 [373.00]
  tuberculous (*see also* Tuberculosis)
    017.0● [373.4]
Tartar (teeth) 523.6
Tattoo (mark) 709.09
Taurodontism 520.2
Taussig-Bing defect, heart, or syndrome
    (transposition, aorta and overriding
    pulmonary artery) 745.11
Tay's choroiditis 363.41
Tay-Sachs
  amaurotic familial idiocy 330.1
  disease 330.1
Taybi's syndrome (otopalatodigital)
    759.89
Taylor's
  disease (diffuse idiopathic cutaneous
    atrophy) 701.8
  syndrome 625.5
TBI (traumatic brain injury) (*see also*
    Injury, intracranial) 854.0 ◄
  with skull fracture - *see* Fracture,
    skull, by site ◄
Tear, torn (traumatic) - *see also* Wound,
    open, by site
  anus, anal (sphincter) 863.89
    with open wound in cavity 863.99
    complicating delivery (healed) (old)
      654.8●
      with mucosa 664.3●

◄ New   ◄▥ Revised   ~~deleted~~ Deleted   ● Use Additional Digit(s)   ▨ Omit code

Tear, torn *(Continued)*
    anus, anal *(Continued)*
        complicating delivery *(Continued)*
            not associated with third-degree
                perineal laceration 664.6●
        nontraumatic, nonpuerperal
            (healed) (old) 569.43
    articular cartilage, old *(see also*
        Disorder, cartilage, articular)
        718.0●
    bladder
        with
            abortion - *see* Abortion, by type,
                with damage to pelvic
                organs
            ectopic pregnancy *(see also*
                categories 633.0–633.9)
                639.2
            molar pregnancy *(see also*
                categories 630–632) 639.2
        following
            abortion 639.2
            ectopic or molar pregnancy 639.2
        obstetrical trauma 665.5●
    bowel
        with
            abortion - *see* Abortion, by type,
                with damage to pelvic
                organs
            ectopic pregnancy *(see also*
                categories 633.0–633.9) 639.2
            molar pregnancy *(see also*
                categories 630–632) 639.2
        following
            abortion 639.2
            ectopic or molar pregnancy
                639.2
        obstetrical trauma 665.5●
    broad ligament
        with
            abortion - *see* Abortion, by type,
                with damage to pelvic
                organs
            ectopic pregnancy *(see also*
                categories 633.0–633.9)
                639.2
            molar pregnancy *(see also*
                categories 630–632) 639.2
        following
            abortion 639.2
            ectopic or molar pregnancy
                639.2
        obstetrical trauma 665.6●
    bucket handle (knee) (meniscus) - *see*
        Tear, meniscus
    capsule
        joint - *see* Sprain, by site
        spleen - *see* Laceration, spleen,
            capsule
    cartilage - *see also* Sprain, by site
        articular, old *(see also* Disorder,
            cartilage, articular) 718.0●
        knee - *see* Tear, meniscus
        semilunar (knee) (current injury) -
            see Tear, meniscus
    cervix
        with
            abortion - *see* Abortion, by type,
                with damage to pelvic
                organs
            ectopic pregnancy *(see also*
                categories 633.0–633.9)
                639.2
            molar pregnancy *(see also*
                categories 630–632) 639.2

Tear, torn *(Continued)*
    cervix *(Continued)*
        following
            abortion 639.2
            ectopic or molar pregnancy 639.2
        obstetrical trauma (current) 665.3●
        old 622.3
    dural 349.31
        accidental puncture or laceration
            during a procedure 349.31
        incidental (inadvertent) 349.31
        nontraumatic NEC 349.39
    internal organ (abdomen, chest, or
        pelvis) - *see* Injury, internal, by
        site
    ligament - *see also* Sprain, by site
        with open wound - *see* Wound,
            open, by site
    meniscus (knee) (current injury) 836.2
        bucket handle 836.0
            old 717.0
        lateral 836.1
            anterior horn 836.1
                old 717.42
            bucket handle 836.1
                old 717.41
            old 717.40
            posterior horn 836.1
                old 717.43
            specified site NEC 836.1
                old 717.49
        medial 836.0
            anterior horn 836.0
                old 717.1
            bucket handle 836.0
                old 717.0
            old 717.3
            posterior horn 836.0
                old 717.2
        old NEC 717.5
        site other than knee - *see* Sprain, by
            site
    muscle - *see also* Sprain, by site
        with open wound - *see* Wound,
            open, by site
    pelvic
        floor, complicating delivery 664.1●
        organ NEC
            with
                abortion - *see* Abortion, by
                    type, with damage to
                    pelvic organs
                ectopic pregnancy *(see also*
                    categories 633.0–633.9)
                    639.2
                molar pregnancy *(see also*
                    categories 630–632) 639.2
            following
                abortion 639.2
                ectopic or molar pregnancy
                    639.2
            obstetrical trauma 665.5●
    perineum - *see also* Laceration,
        perineum
        obstetrical trauma 665.5●
    periurethral tissue
        with
            abortion - *see* Abortion, by type,
                with damage to pelvic
                organs
            ectopic pregnancy *(see also*
                categories 633.0–633.9) 639.2
            molar pregnancy *(see also*
                categories 630–632) 639.2
        following
            abortion 639.2
            ectopic or molar pregnancy 639.2

Tear, torn *(Continued)*
    periurethral tissue *(Continued)*
        obstetrical trauma 665.5●
    rectovaginal septum - *see* Laceration,
        rectovaginal septum
    retina, retinal (recent) (with
        detachment) 361.00
        without detachment 361.30
        dialysis (juvenile) (with detachment)
            361.04
        giant (with detachment) 361.03
        horseshoe (without detachment)
            361.32
        multiple (with detachment) 361.02
            without detachment 361.33
        old
            delimited (partial) 361.06
            partial 361.06
            total or subtotal 361.07
        partial (without detachment)
            giant 361.03
            multiple defects 361.02
            old (delimited) 361.06
            single defect 361.01
        round hole (without detachment)
            361.31
        single defect (with detachment)
            361.01
        total or subtotal (recent) 361.05
            old 361.07
    rotator cuff (traumatic) 840.4
        current injury 840.4
        degenerative 726.10
        nontraumatic 727.61
    semilunar cartilage, knee *(see also* Tear,
        meniscus) 836.2
        old 717.5
    tendon - *see also* Sprain, by site
        with open wound - *see* Wound,
            open, by site
    tentorial, at birth 767.0
    umbilical cord
        affecting fetus or newborn 772.0
        complicating delivery 663.8●
    urethra
        with
            abortion - *see* Abortion, by type,
                with damage to pelvic
                organs
            ectopic pregnancy *(see also*
                categories 633.0–633.9) 639.2
            molar pregnancy *(see also*
                categories 630–632) 639.2
        following
            abortion 639.2
            ectopic or molar pregnancy
                639.2
        obstetrical trauma 665.5●
    uterus - *see* Injury, internal, uterus
    vagina - *see* Laceration, vagina
    vessel, from catheter 998.2
    vulva, complicating delivery
        664.0●
Tear stone 375.57
Teeth, tooth - *see also* condition
    grinding 306.8
    prenatal 520.6
Teething 520.7
    syndrome 520.7
Tegmental syndrome 344.89
Telangiectasia, telangiectasis (verrucous)
    448.9
    ataxic (cerebellar) 334.8
    familial 448.0
    hemorrhagic, hereditary (congenital)
        (senile) 448.0

◄ New   ◄▥ Revised   ~~deleted~~ Deleted   ● Use Additional Digit(s)   ▨ Omit code

Telangiectasia, telangiectasis (Continued)
  hereditary hemorrhagic 448.0
  retina 362.15
  spider 448.1
Telecanthus (congenital) 743.63
Telescoped bowel or intestine (see also
    Intussusception) 560.0
Teletherapy, adverse effect NEC 990
Telogen effluvium 704.02
Temperature
  body, high (of unknown origin) (see also
      Pyrexia) 780.60
  cold, trauma from 991.9
    newborn 778.2
    specified effect NEC 991.8
  high
    body (of unknown origin) (see also
        Pyrexia) 780.60
    trauma from - see Heat
Temper tantrum (childhood) (see also
    Disturbance, conduct) 312.1●
Temple - see condition
Temporal - see also condition
  lobe syndrome 310.0
Temporomandibular joint-pain-
    dysfunction syndrome 524.60
Temporosphenoidal - see condition
Tendency
  bleeding (see also Defect, coagulation)
      286.9
  homosexual, ego-dystonic
      302.0
  paranoid 301.0
  suicide 300.9
Tenderness
  abdominal (generalized) (localized)
      789.6●
  rebound 789.6●
  skin 782.0
Tendinitis, tendonitis (see also
    Tenosynovitis) 726.90
  Achilles 726.71
  adhesive 726.90
    shoulder 726.0
  calcific 727.82
    shoulder 726.11
  gluteal 726.5
  patellar 726.64
  peroneal 726.79
  pes anserinus 726.61
  psoas 726.5
  tibialis (anterior) (posterior) 726.72
  trochanteric 726.5
Tendon - see condition
Tendosynovitis - see Tenosynovitis
Tendovaginitis - see Tenosynovitis
Tenesmus 787.99
  rectal 787.99
  vesical 788.99
Tenia - see Taenia
Teniasis - see Taeniasis
Tennis elbow 726.32
Tenonitis - see also Tenosynovitis
  eye (capsule) 376.04
Tenontosynovitis - see Tenosynovitis
Tenontothecitis - see Tenosynovitis
Tenophyte 727.9
Tenosynovitis (see also Synovitis) 727.00
  adhesive 726.90
    shoulder 726.0
  ankle 727.06
  bicipital (calcifying) 726.12
  buttock 727.09
  due to crystals - see Arthritis, due to
      crystals
  elbow 727.09

Tenosynovitis (Continued)
  finger 727.05
  foot 727.06
  gonococcal 098.51
  hand 727.05
  hip 727.09
  knee 727.09
  radial styloid 727.04
  shoulder 726.10
    adhesive 726.0
  specified NEC 727.09
  spine 720.1
  supraspinatus 726.10
  toe 727.06
  tuberculous - see Tuberculosis,
      tenosynovitis
  wrist 727.05
Tenovaginitis - see Tenosynovitis
Tension
  arterial, high (see also Hypertension)
      401.9
    without diagnosis of hypertension
        796.2
  headache 307.81
  intraocular (elevated) 365.00
  nervous 799.21   ◀▥
  ocular (elevated) 365.00
  pneumothorax 512.0
    iatrogenic 512.1
    postoperative 512.1
    spontaneous 512.0
  premenstrual 625.4
  state 300.9
Tentorium - see condition
Teratencephalus 759.89
Teratism 759.7
Teratoblastoma (malignant)
    (M9080/3) - see Neoplasm,
    by site, malignant
Teratocarcinoma (M9081/3) - see also
    Neoplasm, by site, malignant
  liver 155.0
Teratoma (solid) (M9080/1) - see also
    Neoplasm, by site, uncertain
    behavior
  adult (cystic) (M9080/0) - see
      Neoplasm, by site, benign
  and embryonal carcinoma, mixed
      (M9081/3) - see Neoplasm, by
      site, malignant
  benign (M9080/0) - see Neoplasm, by
      site, benign
  combined with choriocarcinoma
      (M9101/3) - see Neoplasm, by
      site, malignant
  cystic (adult) (M9080/0) - see
      Neoplasm, by site, benign
  differentiated type (M9080/0) - see
      Neoplasm, by site, benign
  embryonal (M9080/3) - see also
      Neoplasm, by site, malignant
    liver 155.0
  fetal
    sacral, causing fetopelvic
        disproportion 653.7●
  immature (M9080/3) - see Neoplasm,
      by site, malignant
  liver (M9080/3) 155.0
    adult, benign, cystic, differentiated
        type, or mature (M9080/0)
        211.5
  malignant (M9080/3) - see also
      Neoplasm, by site, malignant
    anaplastic type (M9082/3) - see
        Neoplasm, by site, malignant

Teratoma (Continued)
  malignant (Continued)
    intermediate type (M9083/3) - see
        Neoplasm, by site, malignant
    liver (M9080/3) 155.0
    trophoblastic (M9102/3)
      specified site - see Neoplasm, by
          site, malignant
      unspecified site 186.9
    undifferentiated type (M9082/3) -
        see Neoplasm, by site,
        malignant
  mature (M9080/0) - see Neoplasm, by
      site, benign
  malignant (M9080/3) - see
      Neoplasm, by site,
      malignant
  ovary (M9080/0) 220
    embryonal, immature, or malignant
        (M9080/3) 183.0
  suprasellar (M9080/3) - see Neoplasm,
      by site, malignant
  testis (M9080/3) 186.9
    adult, benign, cystic, differentiated
        type or mature (M9080/0)
        222.0
    undescended 186.0
Terminal care V66.7
Termination
  anomalous - see also Malposition,
      congenital
    portal vein 747.49
    right pulmonary vein 747.42
  pregnancy (legal) (therapeutic) (see
      Abortion, legal) 635.9●
    fetus NEC 779.6
    illegal (see also Abortion, illegal)
        636.9●
Ternidens diminutus infestation 127.7
Terrors, night (child) 307.46
Terry's syndrome (see also Retinopathy
    of prematurity) 362.21
Tertiary - see condition
Tessellated fundus, retina (tigroid)
    362.89
Test(s)
  adequacy
    hemodialysis V56.31
    peritoneal dialysis V56.32
  AIDS virus V72.69   ◀▥
  allergen V72.7
  bacterial disease NEC (see also
      Screening, by name of disease)
      V74.9
  basal metabolic rate V72.69   ◀▥
  blood - alcohol V70.4   ◀▥
    alcohol V70.4   ◀
    drug V70.4   ◀
      for therapeutic drug monitoring
          V58.83   ◀
      for routine general physical
          examination V72.62   ◀
      prior to treatment or procedure
          V72.63   ◀
    typing V72.86   ◀
      Rh typing V72.86   ◀
  blood-drug V70.4
    for therapeutic drug monitoring
        V58.83
  blood typing V72.86
    Rh typing V72.86
  developmental, infant or child
      V20.2
  Dick V74.8
  fertility V26.21

Test(s) *(Continued)*
  genetic
    female V26.32
    for genetic disease carrier status
      female V26.31
      male V26.34
    male V26.39
  hearing V72.19
    following failed hearing screening
      V72.11
    routine, for infant and child V20.2 ◀
  HIV V72.69 ◀⫴
  human immunodeficiency virus
      V72.69 ◀⫴
  immunity status V72.61 ◀
  Kveim V82.89
  laboratory V72.60 ◀⫴
    for medicolegal reason V70.4
    ordered as part of a routine
        general medical
        examination V72.62 ◀
    pre-operative V72.63 ◀
    pre-procedural V72.63 ◀
    specified NEC V72.69 ◀
  male partner of habitual aborter V26.35
  Mantoux (for tuberculosis) V74.1
  mycotic organism V75.4
  nuchal translucency V28.89
  parasitic agent NEC V75.8
  paternity V70.4
  peritoneal equilibration V56.32
  pregnancy
    negative result V72.41
    positive result V72.42
      first pregnancy V72.42
    unconfirmed V72.40
  preoperative V72.84
    cardiovascular V72.81
    respiratory V72.82
    specified NEC V72.83
  procreative management NEC V26.29
    genetic disease carrier status
      female V26.31
      male V26.34
  Rh typing V72.86
  sarcoidosis V82.89
  Schick V74.3
  Schultz-Charlton V74.8
  skin, diagnostic
    allergy V72.7
    bacterial agent NEC *(see also*
        Screening, by name of
        disease) V74.9
    Dick V74.8
    hypersensitivity V72.7
    Kveim V82.89
    Mantoux V74.1
    mycotic organism V75.4
    parasitic agent NEC V75.8
    sarcoidosis V82.89
    Schick V74.3
    Schultz-Charlton V74.8
    tuberculin V74.1
  specified type NEC V72.85
  tuberculin V74.1
  vision V72.0
    routine, for infant and child
        V20.2 ◀
  Wassermann
    positive *(see also* Serology for
        syphilis, positive) 097.1
    false 795.6
Testicle, testicular, testis - *see also*
    condition
  feminization (syndrome) 259.51
Tetanus, tetanic (cephalic) (convulsions)
    037

Tetanus, tetanic *(Continued)*
  with
    abortion - *see* Abortion, by type,
        with sepsis
    ectopic pregnancy (*see also*
        categories 633.0–633.9) 639.0
    molar pregnancy (*see* categories
        630–632) 639.0
  following
    abortion 639.0
    ectopic or molar pregnancy 639.0
  inoculation V03.7
    reaction (due to serum) - *see*
        Complications, vaccination
  neonatorum 771.3
  puerperal, postpartum, childbirth
    670.8 ◀⫴
Tetany, tetanic 781.7
  alkalosis 276.3
  associated with rickets 268.0
  convulsions 781.7
    hysterical 300.11
  functional (hysterical) 300.11
  hyperkinetic 781.7
    hysterical 300.11
  hyperpnea 786.01
    hysterical 300.11
    psychogenic 306.1
  hyperventilation 786.01
    hysterical 300.11
    psychogenic 306.1
  hypocalcemic, neonatal 775.4
  hysterical 300.11
  neonatal 775.4
  parathyroid (gland) 252.1
  parathyroprival 252.1
  postoperative 252.1
  postthyroidectomy 252.1
  pseudotetany 781.7
    hysterical 300.11
  psychogenic 306.1
    specified as conversion reaction
        300.11
Tetralogy of Fallot 745.2
Tetraplegia - *see* Quadriplegia
Thailand hemorrhagic fever 065.4
Thalassanemia 282.49
Thalassemia (alpha) (beta) (disease)
    (Hb-C) (Hb-D) (Hb-E) (Hb-H)
    (Hb-I) (high fetal gene) (high fetal
    hemoglobin) (intermedia) (major)
    (minima) (minor) (mixed) (trait)
    (with other hemoglobinopathy)
    282.49
  Hb-S (without crisis) 282.41
    with
      crisis 282.42
      vaso-occlusive pain 282.42
  sickle-cell (without crisis) 282.41
    with
      crisis 282.42
      vaso-occlusive pain 282.42
Thalassemic variants 282.49
Thaysen-Gee disease (nontropical
    sprue) 579.0
Thecoma (M8600/0) 220
  malignant (M8600/3) 183.0
Thelarche, precocious 259.1
Thelitis 611.0
  puerperal, postpartum 675.0●
Therapeutic - *see* condition
Therapy V57.9
  blood transfusion, without reported
      diagnosis V58.2
  breathing V57.0
  chemotherapy, antineoplastic
      V58.11

Therapy *(Continued)*
  chemotherapy, *(Continued)*
    fluoride V07.31
    prophylactic NEC V07.39
  dialysis (intermittent) (treatment)
    extracorporeal V56.0
    peritoneal V56.8
    renal V56.0
    specified type NEC V56.8
  exercise NEC V57.1
    breathing V57.0
  extracorporeal dialysis (renal) V56.0
  fluoride prophylaxis V07.31
  hemodialysis V56.0
  hormone replacement
      (postmenopausal) V07.4
  immunotherapy antineoplastic V58.12
  long term oxygen therapy V46.2
  occupational V57.21
  orthoptic V57.4
  orthotic V57.81
  peritoneal dialysis V56.8
  physical NEC V57.1
  postmenopausal hormone replacement
      V07.4
  radiation V58.0
  speech (-language) V57.3 ◀⫴
  vocational V57.22
Thermalgesia 782.0
Thermalgia 782.0
Thermanalgesia 782.0
Thermanesthesia 782.0
Thermic - *see* condition
Thermography (abnormal) 793.99
  breast 793.89
Thermoplegia 992.0
Thesaurismosis
  amyloid 277.39
  bilirubin 277.4
  calcium 275.40
  cystine 270.0
  glycogen (*see also* Disease, glycogen
      storage) 271.0
  kerasin 272.7
  lipoid 272.7
  melanin 255.41
  phosphatide 272.7
  urate 274.9
Thiaminic deficiency 265.1
  with beriberi 265.0
Thibierge-Weissenbach syndrome
      (cutaneous systemic sclerosis)
      710.1
Thickened endometrium 793.5
Thickening
  bone 733.99
    extremity 733.99
  breast 611.79
  hymen 623.3
  larynx 478.79
  nail 703.8
    congenital 757.5
  periosteal 733.99
  pleura (*see also* Pleurisy) 511.0
  skin 782.8
  subepiglottic 478.79
  tongue 529.8
  valve, heart - *see* Endocarditis
Thiele syndrome 724.6
Thigh - *see* condition
Thinning vertebra (*see also* Osteoporosis)
      733.00
Thirst, excessive 783.5
  due to deprivation of water 994.3
Thomsen's disease 359.22
Thomson's disease (congenital
      poikiloderma) 757.33

◀ New   ◀⫴ Revised   ~~deleted~~ Deleted   ● Use Additional Digit(s)   ▬ Omit code

Thoracic - *see also* condition
  kidney 753.3
  outlet syndrome 353.0
  stomach - *see* Hernia, diaphragm
Thoracogastroschisis (congenital) 759.89
Thoracopagus 759.4
Thoracoschisis 756.3
Thoracoscopic surgical procedure
    converted to open procedure V64.42
Thorax - *see* condition
Thorn's syndrome (*see also* Disease, renal)
    593.9
Thornwaldt's, Tornwaldt's
  bursitis (pharyngeal) 478.29
  cyst 478.26
  disease (pharyngeal bursitis) 478.29
Thorson-Biörck syndrome (malignant
    carcinoid) 259.2
Threadworm (infection) (infestation) 127.4
Threatened
  abortion or miscarriage 640.0●
    with subsequent abortion (*see also*
      Abortion, spontaneous) 634.9●
      affecting fetus 762.1
  labor 644.1●
    affecting fetus or newborn 761.8
    premature 644.0●
  miscarriage 640.0●
    affecting fetus 762.1
  premature
    delivery 644.2●
      affecting fetus or newborn 761.8
    labor 644.0●
      before 22 completed weeks
        gestation 640.0●
Three-day fever 066.0
Threshers' lung 495.0
Thrix annulata (congenital) 757.4
Throat - *see* condition
Thrombasthenia (Glanzmann's)
    (hemorrhagic) (hereditary) 287.1
Thromboangiitis 443.1
  obliterans (general) 443.1
    cerebral 437.1
    vessels
      brain 437.1
      spinal cord 437.1
Thromboarteritis - *see* Arteritis
Thromboasthenia (Glanzmann's)
    (hemorrhagic) (hereditary) 287.1
Thrombocytasthenia (Glanzmann's) 287.1
Thrombocythemia (primary) (M9962/1)
    238.71
  essential 238.71
  hemorrhagic 238.71
  idiopathic (hemorrhagic) (M9962/1)
    238.71
Thrombocytopathy (dystrophic)
    (granulopenic) 287.1
Thrombocytopenia, thrombocytopenic
    287.5
  with
    absent radii (TAR) syndrome 287.33
    giant hemangioma 287.39
  amegakaryocytic, congenital 287.33
  congenital 287.33
  cyclic 287.39
  dilutional 287.4
  due to
    drugs 287.4
    extracorporeal circulation of blood
      287.4
    massive blood transfusion 287.4
    platelet alloimmunization 287.4
  essential 287.30
  fetal 678.0●
  heparin-induced (HIT) 289.84

Thrombocytopenia,
    thrombocytopenic (*Continued*)
  hereditary 287.33
  Kasabach-Merritt 287.39
  neonatal, transitory 776.1
    due to
      exchange transfusion 776.1
      idiopathic maternal
        thrombocytopenia 776.1
      isoimmunization 776.1
  primary 287.30
  puerperal, postpartum 666.3●
  purpura (*see also* Purpura,
    thrombocytopenic) 287.30
    thrombotic 446.6
  secondary 287.4
  sex-linked 287.39
Thrombocytosis 238.71
  essential 238.71
  primary 238.71
Thromboembolism - *see* Embolism
Thrombopathy (Bernard-Soulier)
    287.1
  constitutional 286.4
  Willebrand-Jürgens (angiohemophilia)
    286.4
Thrombopenia (*see also*
    Thrombocytopenia) 287.5
Thrombophlebitis 451.9
  antecubital vein 451.82
  antepartum (superficial) 671.2●
    affecting fetus or newborn 760.3
    deep 671.3●
  arm 451.89
    deep 451.83
    superficial 451.82
  breast, superficial 451.89
  cavernous (venous) sinus - *see*
    Thrombophlebitis, intracranial
    venous sinus
  cephalic vein 451.82
  cerebral (sinus) (vein) 325
    late effect - *see* category 326
    nonpyogenic 437.6
      in pregnancy or puerperium
        671.5●
      late effect - *see* Late effect(s) (of)
        cerebrovascular disease
  due to implanted device - *see*
    Complications, due to (presence
    of) any device, implant, or graft
    classified to 996.0-996.5 NEC
  during or resulting from a procedure
    NEC 997.2
  femoral 451.11
  femoropopliteal 451.19
  following infusion, perfusion, or
    transfusion 999.2
  hepatic (vein) 451.89
  idiopathic, recurrent 453.1
  iliac vein 451.81
  iliofemoral 451.11
  intracranial venous sinus (any) 325
    late effect - *see* category 326
    nonpyogenic 437.6
      in pregnancy or puerperium
        671.5
      late effect - *see* Late effect(s) (of)
        cerebrovascular disease
  jugular vein 451.89
  lateral (venous) sinus - *see*
    Thrombophlebitis, intracranial
    venous sinus
  leg 451.9
    deep (vessels) 451.19
      femoral vein 451.11
      specified vessel NEC 451.19

Thrombophlebitis (*Continued*)
  leg (*Continued*)
    superficial (vessels) 451.0
      femoral vein 451.11
  longitudinal (venous) sinus - *see*
    Thrombophlebitis, intracranial
    venous sinus
  lower extremity 451.2
    deep (vessels) 451.19
      femoral vein 451.11
      specified vessel NEC 451.19
    superficial (vessels) 451.0
  migrans, migrating 453.1
  pelvic
    with
      abortion - *see* Abortion, by type,
        with sepsis
      ectopic pregnancy (*see also*
        categories 633.0-633.9) 639.0
      molar pregnancy (*see also*
        categories 630-632) 639.0
    following
      abortion 639.0
      ectopic or molar pregnancy 639.0
    puerperal 671.4●
  popliteal vein 451.19
  portal (vein) 572.1
  postoperative 997.2
  pregnancy (superficial) 671.2●
    affecting fetus or newborn 760.3
    deep 671.3●
  puerperal, postpartum, childbirth
    (extremities) (superficial)
    671.2●
    deep 671.4●
    pelvic 671.4●
    septic 670.3
    specified site NEC 671.5●
  radial vein 451.82
  saphenous (greater) (lesser) 451.0
  sinus (intracranial) - *see*
    Thrombophlebitis, intracranial
    venous sinus
  specified site NEC 451.89
  tibial vein 451.19
Thrombosis, thrombotic (marantic)
    (multiple) (progressive) (vein)
    (vessel) 453.9
  with childbirth or during the
    puerperium - *see* Thrombosis,
    puerperal, postpartum
  antepartum - *see* Thrombosis,
    pregnancy
  aorta, aortic 444.1
    abdominal 444.0
    bifurcation 444.0
    saddle 444.0
    terminal 444.0
    thoracic 444.1
    valve - *see* Endocarditis, aortic
  apoplexy (*see also* Thrombosis, brain)
    434.0●
    late effect - *see* Late effect(s) (of)
      cerebrovascular disease
  appendix, septic - *see* Appendicitis,
    acute
  arteriolar-capillary platelet,
    disseminated 446.6
  artery, arteries (postinfectional) 444.9
    auditory, internal 433.8●
    basilar (*see also* Occlusion, artery,
      basilar) 433.0●
    carotid (common) (internal) (*see also*
      Occlusion, artery, carotid)
      433.1●
      with other precerebral artery
        433.3●

◀ ▬

Thrombosis, thrombotic *(Continued)*
    artery, arteries *(Continued)*
        cerebellar (anterior inferior)
            (posterior inferior) (superior)
            433.8●
        cerebral *(see also* Thrombosis, brain)
            434.0●
        choroidal (anterior) 433.8●
        communicating posterior 433.8●
        coronary *(see also* Infarct,
            myocardium) 410.9●
            without myocardial infarction
                411.81
            due to syphilis 093.89
            healed or specified as old 412
        extremities 444.22
            lower 444.22
            upper 444.21
        femoral 444.22
        hepatic 444.89
        hypophyseal 433.8●
        meningeal, anterior or posterior
            433.8●
        mesenteric (with gangrene) 557.0
        ophthalmic *(see also* Occlusion,
            retina) 362.30
        pontine 433.8●
        popliteal 444.22
        precerebral - *see* Occlusion, artery,
            precerebral NEC
        pulmonary 415.19
            iatrogenic 415.11
            personal history of V12.51 ◄
            postoperative 415.11
            septic 415.12
        renal 593.81
        retinal *(see also* Occlusion, retina)
            362.30
        specified site NEC 444.89
        spinal, anterior or posterior 433.8●
        traumatic (complication) (early) *(see*
            also Injury, blood vessel, by
            site) 904.9
        vertebral *(see also* Occlusion, artery,
            vertebral) 433.2●
            with other precerebral artery
                433.3●
    atrial (endocardial) 424.90
        without endocarditis 429.89
        due to syphilis 093.89
    auricular *(see also* Infarct, myocardium)
        410.9●
    axillary (acute) (vein) 453.84 ◄▮▮▮
        chronic 453.74 ◄
        personal history of V12.51 ◄
    basilar (artery) *(see also* Occlusion,
        artery, basilar) 433.0●
    bland NEC 453.9
    brain (artery) (stem) 434.0●
        due to syphilis 094.89
        iatrogenic 997.02
        late effect - *see* Late effect(s) (of)
            cerebrovascular disease
        postoperative 997.02
        puerperal, postpartum, childbirth
            674.0●
        sinus *(see also* Thrombosis,
            intracranial venous sinus)
            325
    capillary 448.9
        arteriolar, generalized 446.6
    cardiac *(see also* Infarct, myocardium)
        410.9●
        due to syphilis 093.89
        healed or specified as old 412
        valve - *see* Endocarditis

Thrombosis, thrombotic *(Continued)*
    carotid (artery) (common) (internal)
        (see also Occlusion, artery, carotid)
        433.1●
        with other precerebral artery
            433.3●
    cavernous sinus (venous) - *see*
        Thrombosis, intracranial venous
        sinus
    cerebellar artery (anterior inferior)
        (posterior inferior) (superior)
        433.8●
        late effect - *see* Late effect(s) (of)
            cerebrovascular disease
    cerebral (arteries) *(see also* Thrombosis,
        brain) 434.0●
        late effect - *see* Late effect(s) (of)
            cerebrovascular disease
    coronary (artery) *(see also* Infarct,
        myocardium) 410.9●
        without myocardial infarction
            411.81
        due to syphilis 093.89
        healed or specified as old 412
    corpus cavernosum 607.82
    cortical *(see also* Thrombosis, brain)
        434.0●
    due to (presence of) any device,
        implant, or graft classifiable to
        996.0–996.5 - *see* Complications,
        due to (presence of) any device,
        implant, or graft classified to
        996.0–996.5 NEC
    effort 453.89 ◄▮▮▮
    endocardial - *see* Infarct, myocardium
    eye *(see also* Occlusion, retina)
        362.30
    femoral (vein) 453.6 ◄▮▮▮
        with inflammation or phlebitis
            451.11
        artery 444.22
        deep 453.41
        personal history of V12.51 ◄
    genital organ, male 608.83
    heart (chamber) *(see also* Infarct,
        myocardium) 410.9●
    hepatic (vein) 453.0
        artery 444.89
        infectional or septic 572.1
    iliac (vein) 453.89 ◄▮▮▮
        with inflammation or phlebitis
            451.81
        artery (common) (external)
            (internal) 444.81
        personal history of V12.51 ◄
    inflammation, vein - *see*
        Thrombophlebitis
    internal carotid artery *(see also*
        Occlusion, artery, carotid)
        433.1●
        with other precerebral artery
            433.3●
    intestine (with gangrene) 557.0
    intracranial *(see also* Thrombosis, brain)
        434.0●
        venous sinus (any) 325
            nonpyogenic origin 437.6
            in pregnancy or puerperium
                671.5●
    intramural *(see also* Infarct,
        myocardium) 410.9●
        without
            cardiac condition 429.89
            coronary artery disease 429.89
            myocardial infarction 429.89
        healed or specified as old 412

Thrombosis, thrombotic *(Continued)*
    jugular (bulb) 453.8 ◄▮▮▮
        external ◄
            acute 453.89 ◄
            chronic 453.79 ◄
        internal ◄
            acute 453.86 ◄
            chronic 453.76 ◄
    kidney 593.81
        artery 593.81
    lateral sinus (venous) - *see* Thrombosis,
        intracranial venous sinus
    leg *(see also* Thrombosis, lower
        extremity) 453.6 ◄▮▮▮
        with inflammation or phlebitis - *see*
            Thrombophlebitis
        deep (vessels) 453.40
            acute 453.40 ◄
                lower (distal) 453.42 ◄
                upper (proximal) 453.41 ◄
            chronic 453.50 ◄
                lower (distal) 453.52 ◄
                upper (proximal) 453.51 ◄
            lower (distal) 453.42 ◄
            upper (proximal) 453.41 ◄
        personal history of V12.51 ◄
        superficial (vessels) 453.6 ◄▮▮▮
    liver (venous) 453.0
        artery 444.89
        infectional or septic 572.1
        portal vein 452
    longitudinal sinus (venous) - *see*
        Thrombosis, intracranial venous
        sinus
    lower extremity 453.8
        deep vessels 453.40
            acute 453.40 ◄
                calf 453.42 ◄
                distal (lower leg) 453.42 ◄
                femoral 453.41 ◄
                iliac 453.41 ◄
                lower leg 453.42 ◄
                peroneal 453.42 ◄
                popliteal 453.41 ◄
                proximal (upper leg) 453.41 ◄
                thigh 453.41 ◄
                tibial 453.42 ◄
            calf 453.42
            chronic 453.50 ◄
                calf 453.52 ◄
                distal (lower leg) 453.52 ◄
                femoral 453.51 ◄
                iliac 453.51 ◄
                lower leg 453.52 ◄
                peroneal 453.52 ◄
                popliteal 453.51 ◄
                proximal (upper leg) 453.51 ◄
                thigh 453.51 ◄
                tibial 453.52 ◄
            distal (lower leg) 453.42
            femoral 453.41
            iliac 453.41
            lower leg 453.42
            peroneal 453.42
            popliteal 453.41
            proximal (upper leg) 453.41
            thigh 453.41
            tibial 453.42
    personal history of V12.51 ◄
    saphenous (greater) (lesser) 453.6 ◄
    superficial 453.6 ◄
    lung 415.19
        iatrogenic 415.11
        personal history of V12.51 ◄
        postoperative 415.11
        septic 415.12
    marantic, dural sinus 437.6

◄ New   ◄▮▮▮ Revised   ~~deleted~~ Deleted   ● Use Additional Digit(s)   ▮▮▮ Omit code

Thrombosis, thrombotic (Continued)

meninges (brain) (see also Thrombosis, brain) 434.0●

mesenteric (artery) (with gangrene) 557.0

  vein (inferior) (superior) 557.0

mitral - see Insufficiency, mitral

mural (heart chamber) (see also Infarct, myocardium) 410.9●

  without

    cardiac condition 429.89

    coronary artery disease 429.89

    myocardial infarction 429.89

  due to syphilis 093.89

  following myocardial infarction 429.79

  healed or specified as old 412

omentum (with gangrene) 557.0

ophthalmic (artery) (see also Occlusion, retina) 362.30

pampiniform plexus (male) 608.83

  female 620.8

parietal (see also Infarct, myocardium) 410.9●

penis, penile 607.82

peripheral arteries 444.22

  lower 444.22

  upper 444.21

platelet 446.6

portal 452

  due to syphilis 093.89

  infectional or septic 572.1

precerebral artery - see also Occlusion, artery, precerebral NEC

pregnancy 671.2

  deep (vein) 671.3●

  superficial (vein) 671.2●

puerperal, postpartum, childbirth 671.2

  brain (artery) 674.0●

    venous 671.5●

  cardiac 674.8●

  cerebral (artery) 674.0●

    venous 671.5●

  deep (vein) 671.4●

  intracranial sinus (nonpyogenic) (venous) 671.5●

  pelvic 671.4●

  pulmonary (artery) 673.2●

  specified site NEC 671.5●

  superficial 671.2●

pulmonary (artery) (vein) 415.19

  iatrogenic 415.11

  personal history of V12.51

  postoperative 415.11

  septic 415.12

renal (artery) 593.81

  vein 453.3

resulting from presence of shunt or other internal prosthetic device - see Complications, due to (presence of) any device, implant, or graft classifiable to 996.0–996.5 NEC

retina, retinal (artery) 362.30

  arterial branch 362.32

  central 362.31

  partial 362.33

  vein

    central 362.35

    tributary (branch) 362.36

saphenous vein (greater) (lesser) 453.6

scrotum 608.83

seminal vesicle 608.83

Thrombosis, thrombotic (Continued)

sigmoid (venous) sinus (see Thrombosis, intracranial venous sinus) 325

silent NEC 453.9

sinus, intracranial (venous) (any) (see also Thrombosis, intracranial venous sinus) 325

softening, brain (see also Thrombosis, brain) 434.0●

specified site NEC (acute) 453.89

  chronic 453.79

spermatic cord 608.83

spinal cord 336.1

  due to syphilis 094.89

  in pregnancy or puerperium 671.5●

  pyogenic origin 324.1

    late effect - see category 326

spleen, splenic 289.59

  artery 444.89

testis 608.83

traumatic (complication) (early) (see also Injury, blood vessel, by site) 904.9

tricuspid - see Endocarditis, tricuspid

tumor - see Neoplasm, by site

tunica vaginalis 608.83

umbilical cord (vessels) 663.6●

  affecting fetus or newborn 762.6

upper extremity 453.83

  acute 453.83

    deep 453.82

    superficial 453.81

  chronic 453.73

    deep 453.72

    superficial 453.71

vas deferens 608.83

vein

  antecubital

    acute 453.81

    chronic 453.71

  axillary

    acute 453.84

    chronic 453.74

  basilic

    acute 453.81

    chronic 453.71

  brachial

    acute 453.82

    chronic 453.72

  brachiocephalic (innominate)

    acute 453.87

    chronic 453.77

  cephalic

    acute 453.81

    chronic 453.71

  deep 453.40

    personal history of V12.51

  internal jugular

    acute 453.86

    chronic 453.76

  lower extremity - see Thrombosis, lower extremity

  personal history of V12.51

  radial

    acute 453.82

    chronic 453.72

  saphenous (greater) (lesser) 453.6

  specified site NEC

    acute 453.89

    chronic 453.79

  subclavian

    acute 453.85

    chronic 453.75

Thrombosis, thrombotic (Continued)

vein (Continued)

  superior vena cava

    acute 453.87

    chronic 453.77

  thoracic

    acute 453.87

    chronic 453.77

  ulnar

    acute 453.82

    chronic 453.72

  upper extremity - see Thrombosis, upper extremity

vena cava (inferior) (superior) 453.2

  inferior 453.2

  personal history of V12.51

  superior

    acute 453.87

    chronic 453.77

Thrombus - see Thrombosis

Thrush 112.0

newborn 771.7

Thumb - see also condition

gamekeeper's 842.12

sucking (child problem) 307.9

Thygeson's superficial punctate keratitis 370.21

Thymergasia (see also Psychosis, affective) 296.80

Thymitis 254.8

Thymoma (benign) (M8580/0) 212.6

malignant (M8580/3) 164.0

Thymus, thymic (gland) - see condition

Thyrocele (see also Goiter) 240.9

Thyroglossal - see also condition

cyst 759.2

duct, persistent 759.2

Thyroid (body) (gland) - see also condition

hormone resistance 246.8

lingual 759.2

Thyroiditis 245.9

acute (pyogenic) (suppurative) 245.0

  nonsuppurative 245.0

autoimmune 245.2

chronic (nonspecific) (sclerosing) 245.8

  fibrous 245.3

  lymphadenoid 245.2

  lymphocytic 245.2

  lymphoid 245.2

complicating pregnancy, childbirth, or puerperium 648.1●

de Quervain's (subacute granulomatous) 245.1

fibrous (chronic) 245.3

giant (cell) (follicular) 245.1

granulomatous (de Quervain's) (subacute) 245.1

Hashimoto's (struma lymphomatosa) 245.2

iatrogenic 245.4

invasive (fibrous) 245.3

ligneous 245.3

lymphocytic (chronic) 245.2

lymphoid 245.2

lymphomatous 245.2

pseudotuberculous 245.1

pyogenic 245.0

radiation 245.4

Riedel's (ligneous) 245.3

subacute 245.1

suppurative 245.0

Thyroiditis (*Continued*)
  tuberculous (*see also* Tuberculosis)
    017.5●
  viral 245.1
  woody 245.3
Thyrolingual duct, persistent
  759.2
Thyromegaly 240.9
Thyrotoxic
  crisis or storm (*see also* Thyrotoxicosis)
    242.9●
  heart failure (*see also* Thyrotoxicosis)
    242.9● [*425.7*]
Thyrotoxicosis 242.9●

> **Note 68** Use the following fifth-digit
> subclassification with category 242:
>
> 0 without mention of thyrotoxic
>   crisis or storm
> 1 with mention of thyrotoxic crisis
>   or storm

  with
    goiter (diffuse) 242.0●
      adenomatous 242.3●
        multinodular 242.2●
        uninodular 242.1●
      nodular 242.3●
        multinodular 242.2●
        uninodular 242.1●
    infiltrative●
      dermopathy 242.0●
      ophthalmopathy 242.0●
      thyroid acropachy 242.0●
  complicating pregnancy, childbirth, or
    puerperium 648.1●
  due to
    ectopic thyroid nodule 242.4●
    ingestion of (excessive) thyroid
      material 242.8●
    specified cause NEC 242.8●
  factitia 242.8●
  heart 242.9● [*425.7*]
  neonatal (transient) 775.3
TIA (transient ischemic attack) 435.9
  with transient neurologic deficit
    435.9
  late effect - *see* Late effect(s) (of)
    cerebrovascular disease
Tibia vara 732.4
Tic 307.20
  breathing 307.20
  child problem 307.21
  compulsive 307.22
  convulsive 307.20
  degenerative (generalized) (localized)
    333.3
    facial 351.8
  douloureux (*see also* Neuralgia,
    trigeminal) 350.1
    atypical 350.2
  habit 307.20
    chronic (motor or vocal) 307.22
    transient (of childhood) 307.21
  lid 307.20
    transient (of childhood) 307.21
  motor-verbal 307.23
  occupational 300.89
  orbicularis 307.20
    transient (of childhood) 307.21
  organic origin 333.3
  postchoreic - *see* Chorea
  psychogenic 307.20
    compulsive 307.22
  salaam 781.0

Tic (*Continued*)
  spasm 307.20
    chronic (motor or vocal) 307.22
    transient (of childhood) 307.21
Tick (-borne) fever NEC 066.1
  American mountain 066.1
  Colorado 066.1
  hemorrhagic NEC 065.3
    Crimean 065.0
    Kyasanur Forest 065.2
    Omsk 065.1
  mountain 066.1
  nonexanthematous 066.1
Tick-bite fever NEC 066.1
  African 087.1
  Colorado (virus) 066.1
  Rocky Mountain 082.0
Tick paralysis 989.5
Tics and spasms, compulsive 307.22
Tietze's disease or syndrome 733.6
Tight, tightness
  anus 564.89
  chest 786.59
  fascia (lata) 728.9
  foreskin (congenital) 605
  hymen 623.3
  introitus (acquired) (congenital) 623.3
  rectal sphincter 564.89
  tendon 727.81
    Achilles (heel) 727.81
  urethral sphincter 598.9
Tilting vertebra 737.9
Timidity, child 313.21
Tinea (intersecta) (tarsi) 110.9
  amiantacea 110.0
  asbestina 110.0
  barbae 110.0
  beard 110.0
  black dot 110.0
  blanca 111.2
  capitis 110.0
  corporis 110.5
  cruris 110.3
  decalvans 704.09
  flava 111.0
  foot 110.4
  furfuracea 111.0
  imbricata (Tokelau) 110.5
  lepothrix 039.0
  manuum 110.2
  microsporic (*see also*
    Dermatophytosis) 110.9
  nigra 111.1
  nodosa 111.2
  pedis 110.4
  scalp 110.0
  specified site NEC 110.8
  sycosis 110.0
  tonsurans 110.0
  trichophytic (*see also*
    Dermatophytosis) 110.9
  unguium 110.1
  versicolor 111.0
Tingling sensation (*see also*
  Disturbance, sensation)
  782.0
Tin-miners' lung 503
Tinnitus (aurium) 388.30
  audible 388.32
  objective 388.32
  subjective 388.31
Tipped, teeth 524.33
Tipping
  pelvis 738.6
    with disproportion (fetopelvic)
      653.0●

Tipping (*Continued*)
  pelvis (*Continued*)
    with disproportion (*Continued*)
      affecting fetus or newborn 763.1
      causing obstructed labor
        660.1●
        affecting fetus or newborn
        763.1
  teeth 524.33
Tiredness 780.79
Tissue - *see* condition
Tobacco
  abuse (affecting health) NEC (*see also*
    Abuse, drugs, nondependent)
    305.1
  heart 989.84
  use disorder complicating pregnancy,
    childbirth, or the puerperium
    649.0●
Tobias' syndrome (carcinoma,
  pulmonary apex) (M8010/3)
  162.3
Tocopherol deficiency 269.1
Todd's
  cirrhosis - *see* Cirrhosis, biliary
  paralysis (postepileptic transitory
    paralysis) 344.89
Toe - *see* condition
Toilet, artificial opening (*see also*
  Attention to, artificial, opening)
  V55.9
Tokelau ringworm 110.5
Tollwut 071
Tolosa-Hunt syndrome 378.55
Tommaselli's disease
  correct substance properly
    administered 599.70
  overdose or wrong substance given or
    taken 961.4
Tongue - *see also* condition
  worms 134.1
Tongue tie 750.0
Toni-Fanconi syndrome (cystinosis)
  270.0
Tonic pupil 379.46
Tonsil - *see* condition
Tonsillitis (acute) (catarrhal) (croupous)
  (follicular) (gangrenous) (infective)
  (lacunar) (lingual) (malignant)
  (membranous) (phlegmonous)
  (pneumococcal)
  (pseudomembranous) (purulent)
  (septic) (staphylococcal) (subacute)
  (suppurative) (toxic) (ulcerative)
  (vesicular) (viral) 463
  with influenza, flu, or grippe 487.1
  chronic 474.00
  diphtheritic (membranous) 032.0
  hypertrophic 474.00
  influenzal 487.1
  parenchymatous 475
  streptococcal 034.0
  tuberculous (*see also* Tuberculosis)
    012.8●
  Vincent's 101
Tonsillopharyngitis 465.8
Tooth, teeth - *see* condition
Toothache 525.9
Topagnosis 782.0
Tophi (gouty) 274.03 ◀━
  ear 274.81
  heart 274.82
  specified site NEC 274.82
TORCH infection - (*see also* Infection,
  congenital) 760.2
Torn - *see* Tear, torn

◀ New   ◀▥ Revised   ~~deleted~~ Deleted   ● Use Additional Digit(s)   ▥ Omit code

Tornwaldt's bursitis (disease)
   (pharyngeal bursitis) 478.29
   cyst 478.26
Torpid liver 573.9
Torsion
   accessory tube 620.5
   adnexa (female) 620.5
   aorta (congenital) 747.29
      acquired 447.1
   appendix
      epididymis 608.24
      testis 608.23
   bile duct 576.8
      with calculus, choledocholithiasis
         or stones - see
         Choledocholithiasis
      congenital 751.69
   bowel, colon, or intestine 560.2
   cervix - see Malposition, uterus
   duodenum 537.3
   dystonia - see Dystonia, torsion
   epididymis 608.24
      appendix 608.24
   fallopian tube 620.5
   gallbladder (see also Disease,
         gallbladder) 575.8
      congenital 751.69
   gastric 537.89
   hydatid of Morgagni (female)
         620.5
   kidney (pedicle) 593.89
   Meckel's diverticulum (congenital)
         751.0
   mesentery 560.2
   omentum 560.2
   organ or site, congenital NEC - see
         Anomaly, specified type NEC
   ovary (pedicle) 620.5
      congenital 752.0
   oviduct 620.5
   penis 607.89
      congenital 752.69
   renal 593.89
   spasm - see Dystonia, torsion
   spermatic cord 608.22
      extravaginal 608.21
      intravaginal 608.22
   spleen 289.59
   testicle, testis 608.20
      appendix 608.23
   tibia 736.89
   umbilical cord - see Compression,
         umbilical cord
   uterus (see also Malposition, uterus)
         621.6
Torticollis (intermittent) (spastic) 723.5
   congenital 754.1
      sternomastoid 754.1
   due to birth injury 767.8
   hysterical 300.11
   ocular 781.93
   psychogenic 306.0
      specified as conversion reaction
         300.11
   rheumatic 723.5
   rheumatoid 714.0
   spasmodic 333.83
   traumatic, current NEC 847.0
Tortuous
   artery 447.1
   fallopian tube 752.19
   organ or site, congenital NEC - see
         Distortion
   renal vessel (congenital) 747.62
   retina vessel (congenital) 743.58
      acquired 362.17

Tortuous (Continued)
   ureter 593.4
   urethra 599.84
   vein - see Varicose, vein
Torula, torular (infection) 117.5
   histolytica 117.5
   lung 117.5
Torulosis 117.5
Torus
   fracture
      fibula 823.41
         with tibia 823.42
      humerus 812.49   ◀
      radius (alone) 813.45   ◀▮▮▮
         with ulna 813.47   ◀
      tibia 823.40
         with fibula 823.42
      ulna (alone) 813.46   ◀
         with radius 813.47   ◀
   mandibularis 526.81
   palatinus 526.81
Touch, vitreous 997.99
Touraine's syndrome (hereditary osteo-
      onychodysplasia) 756.89
Touraine-Solente-Golé syndrome
      (acropachyderma) 757.39
Tourette's disease (motor-verbal tic)
      307.23
Tower skull 756.0
   with exophthalmos 756.0
Toxemia 799.89
   with
      abortion - see Abortion, by type,
         with toxemia
      bacterial - see Septicemia
   biliary (see also Disease, biliary)
         576.8
   burn - see Burn, by site
   congenital NEC 779.89
   eclamptic 642.6●
      with pre-existing hypertension
         642.7●
   erysipelatous (see also Erysipelas) 035
   fatigue 799.89
   fetus or newborn NEC 779.89
   food (see also Poisoning, food) 005.9
   gastric 537.89
   gastrointestinal 558.2
   intestinal 558.2
   kidney (see also Disease, renal) 593.9
   lung 518.89
   malarial NEC (see also Malaria) 084.6
   maternal (of pregnancy), affecting fetus
         or newborn 760.0
   myocardial - see Myocarditis, toxic
   of pregnancy (mild) (pre-eclamptic)
         642.4●
      with
         convulsions 642.6●
         pre-existing hypertension
            642.7●
      affecting fetus or newborn 760.0
      severe 642.5●
   pre-eclamptic - see Toxemia, of
         pregnancy
   puerperal, postpartum - see Toxemia, of
         pregnancy
   pulmonary 518.89
   renal (see also Disease, renal) 593.9
   septic (see also Septicemia) 038.9
   small intestine 558.2
   staphylococcal 038.10
      aureus 038.11
      due to food 005.0
      specified organism NEC 038.19
   stasis 799.89

Toxemia (Continued)
   stomach 537.89
   uremic (see also Uremia) 586
   urinary 586
Toxemica cerebropathia psychica
      (nonalcoholic) 294.0
   alcoholic 291.1
Toxic (poisoning) - see also condition
   from drug or poison - see Table of
         Drugs and Chemicals
   oil syndrome 710.5
   shock syndrome 040.82
   thyroid (gland) (see also Thyrotoxicosis)
         242.9●
Toxicemia - see Toxemia
Toxicity
   dilantin
      asymptomatic 796.0
      symptomatic - see Table of Drugs
         and Chemicals
   drug
      asymptomatic 796.0
      symptomatic - see Table of Drugs
         and Chemicals
   fava bean 282.2
   from drug or poison
      asymptomatic 796.0
      symptomatic - see Table of Drugs
         and Chemicals
Toxicosis (see also Toxemia) 799.89
   capillary, hemorrhagic 287.0
Toxinfection 799.89
   gastrointestinal 558.2
Toxocariasis 128.0
Toxoplasma infection, generalized
      130.9
Toxoplasmosis (acquired) 130.9
   with pneumonia 130.4
   congenital, active 771.2
   disseminated (multisystemic) 130.8
   maternal
      with suspected damage to fetus
         affecting management of
         pregnancy 655.4●
      affecting fetus or newborn
         760.2
         manifest toxoplasmosis in fetus
            or newborn 771.2
   multiple sites 130.8
   multisystemic disseminated 130.8
   specified site NEC 130.7
Trabeculation, bladder 596.8
Trachea - see condition
Tracheitis (acute) (catarrhal) (infantile)
      (membranous) (plastic)
      (pneumococcal) (septic)
      (suppurative) (viral) 464.10
   with
      bronchitis 490
         acute or subacute 466.0
         chronic 491.8
         tuberculosis - see Tuberculosis,
            pulmonary
      laryngitis (acute) 464.20
         with obstruction 464.21
         chronic 476.1
         tuberculous (see also Tuberculosis,
            larynx) 012.3●
      obstruction 464.11
   chronic 491.8
      with
         bronchitis (chronic) 491.8
         laryngitis (chronic) 476.1
      due to external agent - see
         Condition, respiratory, chronic,
         due to

Tracheitis (Continued)
  diphtheritic (membranous) 032.3
    due to external agent - see
      Inflammation, respiratory,
      upper, due to
  edematous 464.11
  influenzal 487.1
  streptococcal 034.0
  syphilitic 095.8
  tuberculous (see also Tuberculosis)
    012.8●
Trachelitis (nonvenereal) (see also
    Cervicitis) 616.0
  trichomonal 131.09
Tracheobronchial - see condition
Tracheobronchitis (see also Bronchitis)
    490
  acute or subacute 466.0
    with bronchospasm or obstruction
      466.0
  chronic 491.8
  influenzal 487.1
  senile 491.8
Tracheobronchomegaly (congenital)
    748.3
  with bronchiectasis 494.0
    with (acute) exacerbation 494.1
  acquired 519.19
    with bronchiectasis 494.0
      with (acute) exacerbation
        494.1
Tracheobronchopneumonitis - see
    Pneumonia, broncho
Tracheocele (external) (internal) 519.19
  congenital 748.3
Tracheomalacia 519.19
  congenital 748.3
Tracheopharyngitis (acute) 465.8
  chronic 478.9
    due to external agent - see
      Condition, respiratory, chronic,
      due to
    due to external agent - see
      Inflammation, respiratory, upper,
      due to
Tracheostenosis 519.19
  congenital 748.3
Tracheostomy
  attention to V55.0
  complication 519.00
  granuloma 519.09
  hemorrhage 519.09
  infection 519.01
  malfunctioning 519.02
  obstruction 519.09
  sepsis 519.01
  status V44.0
  stenosis 519.02
Trachoma, trachomatous 076.9
  active (stage) 076.1
  contraction of conjunctiva 076.1
  dubium 076.0
  healed or late effect 139.1
  initial (stage) 076.0
  Türck's (chronic catarrhal laryngitis)
    476.0
Trachyphonia 784.49
Training
  insulin pump V65.46
  orthoptic V57.4
  orthotic V57.81
Train sickness 994.6
Trait
  hemoglobin
    abnormal NEC 282.7
      with thalassemia 282.49

Trait (Continued)
  hemoglobin (Continued)
    C (see also Disease, hemoglobin, C)
      282.7
      with elliptocytosis 282.7
    S (Hb-S) 282.5
    Lepore 282.49
      with other abnormal hemoglobin
        NEC 282.49
    paranoid 301.0
    sickle-cell 282.5
      with
        elliptocytosis 282.5
        spherocytosis 282.5
Traits, paranoid 301.0
Tramp V60.0
Trance 780.09
  hysterical 300.13
Transaminasemia 790.4
Transfusion, blood
  donor V59.01
    stem cells V59.02
  fetal twin to twin 678.0●
  incompatible 999.6   ◄▦
    ABO 999.6   ◄
    minor blood group 999.89   ◄
  reaction or complication - see
    Complications, transfusion
  related acute lung injury (TRALI) 518.7
  syndrome
    fetomaternal 772.0
    twin-to-twin
      blood loss (donor twin) 772.0
      recipient twin 776.4
  twin to twin fetal 678.0●
  without reported diagnosis V58.2
Transient - see also condition
  alteration of awareness 780.02
  blindness 368.12
  deafness (ischemic) 388.02
  global amnesia 437.7
  hyperglycemia (post-procedural)
    790.29   ◄
  hypoglycemia (post-procedural)
    251.2   ◄
  person (homeless) NEC V60.0
Transitional, lumbosacral joint of
    vertebra 756.19
Translocation
  autosomes NEC 758.5
    13–15 758.1
    16–18 758.2
    21 or 22 758.0
    balanced in normal individual 758.4
    D₁ 758.1
    E₃ 758.2
    G 758.0
  balanced autosomal in normal
    individual 758.4
  chromosomes NEC 758.89
  Down's syndrome 758.0
Translucency, iris 364.53
Transmission of chemical substances
    through the placenta (affecting fetus
    or newborn) 760.70
  alcohol 760.71
  anticonvulsants 760.77
  antifungals 760.74
  anti-infective agents 760.74
  antimetabolics 760.78
  cocaine 760.75
  "crack" 760.75
  diethylstilbestrol [DES] 760.76
  hallucinogenic agents 760.73
  medicinal agents NEC 760.79
  narcotics 760.72

Transmission of chemical
    substances (Continued)
  obstetric anesthetic or analgesic drug
    763.5
  specified agent NEC 760.79
  suspected, affecting management of
    pregnancy 655.5●
Transplant (ed)
  bone V42.4
    marrow V42.81
  complication - see also Complications,
    due to (presence of) any device,
    implant, or graft classified to
    996.0–996.5 NEC
    bone marrow 996.85
    corneal graft NEC 996.79
      infection or inflammation 996.69
      reaction 996.51
      rejection 996.51
    organ (failure) (immune or
      nonimmune cause) (infection)
      (rejection) 996.80
      bone marrow 996.85
      heart 996.83
      intestines 996.87
      kidney 996.81
      liver 996.82
      lung 996.84
      pancreas 996.86
      specified NEC 996.89
    previously removed due to
      complication, failure, rejection
      or infection V45.87
    removal status V45.87
    skin NEC 996.79
      infection or inflammation
        996.69
      rejection 996.52
      artificial 996.55
        decellularized allodermis
          996.55
  cornea V42.5
  hair V50.0
  heart V42.1
    valve V42.2
  intestine V42.84
  kidney V42.0
  liver V42.7
  lung V42.6
  organ V42.9
    specified NEC V42.89
  pancreas V42.83
  peripheral stem cells V42.82
  skin V42.3
  stem cells, peripheral V42.82
  tissue V42.9
    specified NEC V42.89
Transplants, ovarian, endometrial
    617.1
Transposed - see Transposition
Transposition (congenital) - see also
    Malposition, congenital
  abdominal viscera 759.3
  aorta (dextra) 745.11
  appendix 751.5
  arterial trunk 745.10
  colon 751.5
  great vessels (complete) 745.10
    both originating from right ventricle
      745.11
    corrected 745.12
    double outlet right ventricle
      745.11
    incomplete 745.11
    partial 745.11
    specified type NEC 745.19

◄ New   ◄▦ Revised   deleted Deleted   ● Use Additional Digit(s)   ▦ Omit code

Transposition *(Continued)*
  heart 746.87
    with complete transposition of
      viscera 759.3
    intestine (large) (small) 751.5
    pulmonary veins 747.49
    reversed jejunal (for bypass) (status)
      V45.3
    scrotal 752.81
    stomach 750.7
      with general transposition of viscera
        759.3
    teeth, tooth 524.30
    vessels (complete) 745.10
      partial 745.11
    viscera (abdominal) (thoracic) 759.3
Trans-sexualism 302.50
  with
    asexual history 302.51
    heterosexual history 302.53
    homosexual history 302.52
Transverse - *see also* condition
  arrest (deep), in labor 660.3●
    affecting fetus or newborn 763.1
  lie 652.3●
    before labor, affecting fetus or
      newborn 761.7
    causing obstructed labor 660.0●
      affecting fetus or newborn 763.1
    during labor, affecting fetus or
      newborn 763.1
Transvestism, transvestitism (transvestic
  fetishism) 302.3
Trapped placenta (with hemorrhage)
  666.0●
  without hemorrhage 667.0●
Trauma, traumatism *(see also* Injury, by
  site) 959.9
  birth - *see* Birth, injury NEC
  causing hemorrhage of pregnancy or
    delivery 641.8●
  complicating
    abortion - *see* Abortion, by type,
      with damage to pelvic organs
    ectopic pregnancy *(see also*
      categories 633.0–633.9) 639.2
    molar pregnancy *(see also* categories
      630–632) 639.2
  during delivery NEC 665.9●
  following
    abortion 639.2
    ectopic or molar pregnancy 639.2
  maternal, during pregnancy, affecting
    fetus or newborn 760.5
  neuroma - *see* Injury, nerve, by site
  previous major, affecting management
    of pregnancy, childbirth, or
    puerperium V23.89
  psychic (current) - *see also* Reaction,
    adjustment
    previous (history) V15.49
  psychologic, previous (affecting health)
    V15.49
  transient paralysis - *see* Injury, nerve,
    by site
Traumatic - *see also* condition   ◄▥
  brain injury (TBI) *(see also* Injury,
    intracranial) 854.0   ◄
    with skull fracture - *see* Fracture,
      skull, by site   ◄
Treacher Collins' syndrome (incomplete
  facial dysostosis) 756.0
Treitz's hernia - *see* Hernia, Treitz's
Trematode infestation NEC 121.9
Trematodiasis NEC 121.9
Trembles 988.8

Trembling paralysis *(see also*
  Parkinsonism) 332.0
Tremor 781.0
  essential (benign) 333.1
  familial 333.1
  flapping (liver) 572.8
  hereditary 333.1
  hysterical 300.11
  intention 333.1
  medication-induced postural 333.1
  mercurial 985.0
  muscle 728.85
  Parkinson's *(see also* Parkinsonism)
    332.0
  psychogenic 306.0
    specified as conversion reaction
      300.11
  senilis 797
  specified type NEC 333.1
Trench
  fever 083.1
  foot 991.4
  mouth 101
  nephritis - *see* Nephritis, acute
Treponema pallidum infection *(see also*
  Syphilis) 097.9
Treponematosis 102.9
  due to
    T. pallidum - *see* Syphilis
    T. pertenue (yaws) *(see also* Yaws)
      102.9
Triad
  Kartagener's 759.3
  Reiter's (complete) (incomplete)
    099.3
  Saint's *(see also* Hernia, diaphragm)
    553.3
Trichiasis 704.2
  cicatricial 704.2
  eyelid 374.05
    with entropion *(see also* Entropion)
      374.00
Trichinella spiralis (infection)
  (infestation) 124
Trichinelliasis 124
Trichinellosis 124
Trichiniasis 124
Trichinosis 124
Trichobezoar 938
  intestine 936
  stomach 935.2
Trichocephaliasis 127.3
Trichocephalosis 127.3
Trichocephalus infestation 127.3
Trichoclasis 704.2
Trichoepithelioma (M8100/0) - *see also*
  Neoplasm, skin, benign
  breast 217
  genital organ NEC - *see* Neoplasm, by
    site, benign
  malignant (M8100/3) - *see* Neoplasm,
    skin, malignant
Trichofolliculoma (M8101/0) - *see*
  Neoplasm, skin, benign
Tricholemmoma (M8102/0) - *see*
  Neoplasm, skin, benign
Trichomatosis 704.2
Trichomoniasis 131.9
  bladder 131.09
  cervix 131.09
  intestinal 007.3
  prostate 131.03
  seminal vesicle 131.09
  specified site NEC 131.8
  urethra 131.02
  urogenitalis 131.00

Trichomoniasis *(Continued)*
  vagina 131.01
  vulva 131.01
  vulvovaginal 131.01
Trichomycosis 039.0
  axillaris 039.0
  nodosa 111.2
  nodularis 111.2
  rubra 039.0
Trichonocardiosis (axillaris) (palmellina)
  039.0
Trichonodosis 704.2
Trichophytid, trichophyton infection *(see
  also* Dermatophytosis) 110.9
Trichophytide - *see* Dermatophytosis
Trichophytobezoar 938
  intestine 936
  stomach 935.2
Trichophytosis - *see* Dermatophytosis
Trichoptilosis 704.2
Trichorrhexis (nodosa) 704.2
Trichosporosis nodosa 111.2
Trichostasis spinulosa (congenital) 757.4
Trichostrongyliasis (small intestine) 127.6
Trichostrongylosis 127.6
Trichostrongylus (instabilis) infection
  127.6
Trichotillomania 312.39
Trichromat, anomalous (congenital)
  368.59
Trichromatopsia, anomalous (congenital)
  368.59
Trichuriasis 127.3
Trichuris trichiuria (any site) (infection)
  (infestation) 127.3
Tricuspid (valve) - *see* condition
Trifid - *see also* Accessory
  kidney (pelvis) 753.3
  tongue 750.13
Trigeminal neuralgia *(see also* Neuralgia,
  trigeminal) 350.1
Trigeminoencephaloangiomatosis 759.6
Trigeminy 427.89
  postoperative 997.1
Trigger finger (acquired) 727.03
  congenital 756.89
Trigonitis (bladder) (chronic)
  (pseudomembranous) 595.3
  tuberculous *(see also* Tuberculosis)
    016.1●
Trigonocephaly 756.0
Trihexosidosis 272.7
Trilobate placenta - *see* Placenta,
  abnormal
Trilocular heart 745.8
Trimethylaminuria 270.8
Tripartita placenta - *see* Placenta,
  abnormal
Triple - *see also* Accessory
  kidneys 753.3
  uteri 752.2
  X female 758.81
Triplegia 344.89
  congenital or infantile 343.8
Triplet
  affected by maternal complications of
    pregnancy 761.5
  healthy liveborn - *see* Newborn,
    multiple
  pregnancy (complicating delivery)
    NEC 651.1●
    with fetal loss and retention of one
      or more fetus(es) 651.4●
    following (elective) fetal reduction
      651.7●
Triplex placenta - *see* Placenta, abnormal

Triplication - *see* Accessory

Trismus 781.0
  neonatorum 771.3
  newborn 771.3
Trisomy (syndrome) NEC 758.5
  13 (partial) 758.1
  16–18 758.2
  18 (partial) 758.2
  21 (partial) 758.0
  22 758.0
  autosomes NEC 758.5
  D₁ 758.1
  E₃ 758.2
  G (group) 758.0
  group D₁ 758.1
  group E 758.2
  group G 758.0
Tritanomaly 368.53
Tritanopia 368.53
Troisier-Hanot-Chauffard syndrome
    (bronze diabetes) 275.0
Trombidiosis 133.8
Trophedema (hereditary) 757.0
  congenital 757.0
Trophoblastic disease (*see also*
    Hydatidiform mole) 630
  previous, affecting management of
    pregnancy V23.1
Tropholymphedema 757.0
Trophoneurosis NEC 356.9
  arm NEC 354.9
  disseminated 710.1
  facial 349.89
  leg NEC 355.8
  lower extremity NEC 355.8
  upper extremity NEC 354.9
Tropical - *see also* condition
  maceration feet (syndrome) 991.4
  wet foot (syndrome) 991.4
Trouble - *see also* Disease
  bowel 569.9
  heart - *see* Disease, heart
  intestine 569.9
  kidney (*see also* Disease, renal)
    593.9
  nervous 799.21   ◀▥
  sinus (*see also* Sinusitis) 473.9
Trousseau's syndrome (thrombophlebitis
    migrans) 453.1
Truancy, childhood - *see also* Disturbance,
    conduct
  socialized 312.2●
  undersocialized, unsocialized 312.1●
Truncus
  arteriosus (persistent) 745.0
  common 745.0
  communis 745.0
Trunk - *see* condition
Trychophytide - *see* Dermatophytosis
Trypanosoma infestation - *see*
    Trypanosomiasis
Trypanosomiasis 086.9
  with meningoencephalitis 086.9
    [323.2]
  African 086.5
    due to Trypanosoma 086.5
      gambiense 086.3
      rhodesiense 086.4
  American 086.2
    with
      heart involvement 086.0
      other organ involvement 086.1
    without mention of organ
      involvement 086.2
  Brazilian - *see* Trypanosomiasis,
    American

Trypanosomiasis (*Continued*)
  Chagas' - *see* Trypanosomiasis,
    American
  due to Trypanosoma
    cruzi - *see* Trypanosomiasis,
      American
    gambiense 086.3
    rhodesiense 086.4
  gambiensis, Gambian 086.3
  North American - *see* Trypanosomiasis,
    American
  rhodesiensis, Rhodesian 086.4
  South American - *see* Trypanosomiasis,
    American
T-shaped incisors 520.2
Tsutsugamushi fever 081.2
Tube, tubal, tubular - *see also* condition
  ligation, admission for V25.2
Tubercle - *see also* Tuberculosis
  brain, solitary 013.2●
  Darwin's 744.29
  epithelioid noncaseating 135
  Ghon, primary infection 010.0●
Tuberculid, tuberculide (indurating)
    (lichenoid) (miliary)
    (papulonecrotic) (primary) (skin)
    (subcutaneous) (*see also*
    Tuberculosis) 017.0●
Tuberculoma - *see also* Tuberculosis
  brain (any part) 013.2●
  meninges (cerebral) (spinal) 013.1●
  spinal cord 013.4●
Tuberculosis, tubercular, tuberculous
    (calcification) (calcified) (caseous)
    (chromogenic acid-fast bacilli)
    (congenital) (degeneration) (disease)
    (fibrocaseous) (fistula) (gangrene)
    (interstitial) (isolated circumscribed
    lesions) (necrosis) (parenchymatous)
    (ulcerative) 011.9●

Note 69   Use the following fifth-digit
subclassification with categories
010–018:

  0   unspecified
  1   bacteriological or histological
      examination not done
  2   bacteriological or histological
      examination unknown (at
      present)
  3   tubercle bacilli found (in sputum)
      by microscopy
  4   tubercle bacilli not found (in
      sputum) by microscopy, but
      found by bacterial culture
  5   tubercle bacilli not found by
      bacteriological examination,
      but tuberculosis confirmed
      histologically
  6   tubercle bacilli not found by
      bacteriological or
      histological examination,
      but tuberculosis confirmed
      by other methods
      [inoculation of animals]

For tuberculous conditions specified as
late effects or sequelae, *see* category 137.

---

  abdomen 014.8●
    lymph gland 014.8●
  abscess 011.9●
    arm 017.9
    bone (*see also* Osteomyelitis, due to,
      tuberculosis) 015.9● [730.8]●
      hip 015.1● [730.85]

Tuberculosis, tubercular, tuberculous
    (*Continued*)
  abscess (*Continued*)
    bone (*Continued*)
      knee 015.2● [730.86]
      sacrum 015.0● [730.88]
      specified site NEC 015.7●
        [730.88]
      spinal 015.0● [730.88]
      vertebra 015.0● [730.88]
    brain 013.3●
    breast 017.9●
    Cowper's gland 016.5●
    dura (mater) 013.8●
      brain 013.3●
      spinal cord 013.5●
    epidural 013.8●
      brain 013.3●
      spinal cord 013.5●
    frontal sinus - *see* Tuberculosis, sinus
    genital organs NEC 016.9●
      female 016.7●
      male 016.5●
    genitourinary NEC 016.9●
    gland (lymphatic) - *see* Tuberculosis,
      lymph gland
    hip 015.1●
    iliopsoas 015.0● [730.88]
    intestine 014.8●
    ischiorectal 014.8●
    joint 015.9●
      hip 015.1●
      knee 015.2●
      specified joint NEC 015.8●
      vertebral 015.0● [730.88]
    kidney 016.0● [590.81]
    knee 015.2●
    lumbar 015.0● [730.88]
    lung 011.2●
      primary, progressive 010.8●
    meninges (cerebral) (spinal) 013.0●
    pelvic 016.9●
      female 016.7●
      male 016.5●
    perianal 014.8●
      fistula 014.8●
    perinephritic 016.0● [590.81]
    perineum 017.9●
    perirectal 014.8●
    psoas 015.0● [730.88]
    rectum 014.8●
    retropharyngeal 012.8●
    sacrum 015.0● [730.88]
    scrofulous 017.2●
    scrotum 016.5●
    skin 017.0●
      primary 017.0●
    spinal cord 013.5●
    spine or vertebra (column) 015.0●
      [730.88]
    strumous 017.2●
    subdiaphragmatic 014.8●
    testis 016.5●
    thigh 017.9●
    urinary 016.3●
      kidney 016.0● [590.81]
    uterus 016.7●
  accessory sinus - *see* Tuberculosis, sinus
  Addison's disease 017.6●
  adenitis (*see also* Tuberculosis, lymph
    gland) 017.2●
  adenoids 012.8●
  adenopathy (*see also* Tuberculosis,
    lymph gland) 017.2●
    tracheobronchial 012.1●
      primary progressive 010.8●

◀ New   ◀▥ Revised   ~~deleted~~ Deleted   ● Use Additional Digit(s)   ▨ Omit code

Tuberculosis, tubercular, tuberculous
(Continued)
adherent pericardium 017.9● [420.0]
adnexa (uteri) 016.7●
adrenal (capsule) (gland) 017.6●
air passage NEC 012.8●
alimentary canal 014.8●
anemia 017.9●
ankle (joint) 015.8●
bone 015.5● [730.87]
anus 014.8●
apex (see also Tuberculosis, pulmonary)
011.9●
apical (see also Tuberculosis,
pulmonary) 011.9●
appendicitis 014.8●
appendix 014.8●
arachnoid 013.0●
artery 017.9●
arthritis (chronic) (synovial) 015.9●
[711.40]
ankle 015.8● [730.87]
hip 015.1● [711.45]
knee 015.2 [711.46]
specified site NEC 015.8 ● [711.48]
spine or vertebra (column) 015.0●
[720.81]
wrist 015.8● [730.83]
articular - see Tuberculosis, joint
ascites 014.0●
asthma (see also Tuberculosis,
pulmonary) 011.9●
axilla, axillary 017.2●
gland 017.2●
bilateral (see also Tuberculosis,
pulmonary) 011.9●
bladder 016.1●
bone (see also Osteomyelitis, due to,
tuberculosis) 015.9● [730.8]
hip 015.1● [730.85]
knee 015.2● [730.86]
limb NEC 015.5● [730.88]
sacrum 015.0● [730.88]
specified site NEC 015.7● [730.88]
spinal or vertebral column 015.0●
[730.88]
bowel 014.8●
miliary 018.9●
brain 013.2●
breast 017.9●
broad ligament 016.7●
bronchi, bronchial, bronchus 011.3●
ectasia, ectasis 011.5●
fistula 011.3●
primary, progressive 010.8●
gland 012.1●
primary, progressive 010.8●
isolated 012.2●
lymph gland or node 012.1●
primary, progressive 010.8●
bronchiectasis 011.5●
bronchitis 011.3●
bronchopleural 012.0●
bronchopneumonia,
bronchopneumonic 011.6●
bronchorrhagia 011.3●
bronchotracheal 011.3●
isolated 012.2●
bronchus - see Tuberculosis, bronchi
bronze disease (Addison's) 017.6●
buccal cavity 017.9●
bulbourethral gland 016.5●
bursa (see also Tuberculosis, joint)
015.9●
cachexia NEC (see also Tuberculosis,
pulmonary) 011.9●

Tuberculosis, tubercular, tuberculous
(Continued)
cardiomyopathy 017.9● [425.8]
caries (see also Tuberculosis, bone)
015.9● [730.8]●
cartilage (see also Tuberculosis, bone)
015.9● [730.8]●
intervertebral 015.0● [730.88]
catarrhal (see also Tuberculosis,
pulmonary) 011.9●
cecum 014.8●
cellular tissue (primary) 017.0●
cellulitis (primary) 017.0●
central nervous system 013.9●
specified site NEC 013.8●
cerebellum (current) 013.2●
cerebral (current) 013.2●
meninges 013.0●
cerebrospinal 013.6●
meninges 013.0●
cerebrum (current) 013.2●
cervical 017.2●
gland 017.2●
lymph nodes 017.2●
cervicitis (uteri) 016.7●
cervix 016.7●
chest (see also Tuberculosis, pulmonary)
011.9●
childhood type or first infection
010.0●
choroid 017.3● [363.13]
choroiditis 017.3● [363.13]
ciliary body 017.3● [364.11]
colitis 014.8●
colliers' 011.4●
colliquativa (primary) 017.0●
colon 014.8●
ulceration 014.8●
complex, primary 010.0●
complicating pregnancy, childbirth, or
puerperium 647.3●
affecting fetus or newborn 760.2
congenital 771.2
conjunctiva 017.3● [370.31]
connective tissue 017.9●
bone - see Tuberculosis, bone
contact V01.1
converter (tuberculin skin test)
(without disease) 795.5
cornea (ulcer) 017.3● [370.31]
Cowper's gland 016.5●
coxae 015.1● [730.85]
coxalgia 015.1● [730.85]
cul-de-sac of Douglas 014.8●
curvature, spine 015.0● [737.40]
cutis (colliquativa) (primary) 017.0●
cyst, ovary 016.6●
cystitis 016.1●
dacryocystitis 017.3● [375.32]
dactylitis 015.5●
diarrhea 014.8●
diffuse (see also Tuberculosis, miliary)
018.9●
lung - see Tuberculosis, pulmonary
meninges 013.0●
digestive tract 014.8●
disseminated (see also Tuberculosis,
miliary) 018.9●
meninges 013.0●
duodenum 014.8●
dura (mater) 013.9●
abscess 013.8●
cerebral 013.3●
spinal 013.5●
dysentery 014.8●

Tuberculosis, tubercular, tuberculous
(Continued)
ear (inner) (middle) 017.4●
bone 015.6●
external (primary) 017.0●
skin (primary) 017.0●
elbow 015.8●
emphysema - see Tuberculosis,
pulmonary
empyema 012.0●
encephalitis 013.6●
endarteritis 017.9●
endocarditis (any valve) 017.9●
[424.91]
endocardium (any valve) 017.9●
[424.91]
endocrine glands NEC 017.9●
endometrium 016.7●
enteric, enterica 014.8●
enteritis 014.8●
enterocolitis 014.8●
epididymis 016.4●
epididymitis 016.4●
epidural abscess 013.8●
brain 013.3●
spinal cord 013.5●
epiglottis 012.3●
episcleritis 017.3● [379.00]
erythema (induratum) (nodosum)
(primary) 017.1●
esophagus 017.8●
Eustachian tube 017.4●
exposure to V01.1
exudative 012.0●
primary, progressive 010.1●
eye 017.3●
eyelid (primary) 017.0●
lupus 017.0● [373.4]
fallopian tube 016.6●
fascia 017.9●
fauces 012.8●
finger 017.9●
first infection 010.0●
fistula, perirectal 014.8●
Florida 011.6●
foot 017.9●
funnel pelvis 137.3
gallbladder 017.9●
galloping (see also Tuberculosis,
pulmonary) 011.9●
ganglionic 015.9●
gastritis 017.9●
gastrocolic fistula 014.8●
gastroenteritis 014.8●
gastrointestinal tract 014.8●
general, generalized 018.9●
acute 018.0●
chronic 018.8●
genital organs NEC 016.9●
female 016.7●
male 016.5●
genitourinary NEC 016.9●
genu 015.2●
glandulae suprarenalis 017.6●
glandular, general 017.2●
glottis 012.3●
grinders' 011.4●
groin 017.2●
gum 017.9●
hand 017.9●
heart 017.9 [425.8]●
hematogenous - see Tuberculosis,
miliary

Tuberculosis, tubercular, tuberculous (Continued)

hemoptysis (see also Tuberculosis, pulmonary) 011.9●
hemorrhage NEC (see also Tuberculosis, pulmonary) 011.9●
hemothorax 012.0●
hepatitis 017.9●
hilar lymph nodes 012.1●
   primary, progressive 010.8●
hip (disease) (joint) 015.1●
   bone 015.1● [730.85]
hydrocephalus 013.8●
hydropneumothorax 012.0●
hydrothorax 012.0●
hypoadrenalism 017.6●
hypopharynx 012.8●
ileocecal (hyperplastic) 014.8●
ileocolitis 014.8●
ileum 014.8●
iliac spine (superior) 015.0● [730.88]
incipient NEC (see also Tuberculosis, pulmonary) 011.9●
indurativa (primary) 017.1●
infantile 010.0●
infection NEC 011.9●
   without clinical manifestation 010.0●
infraclavicular gland 017.2●
inguinal gland 017.2●
inguinalis 017.2●
intestine (any part) 014.8●
iris 017.3● [364.11]
iritis 017.3● [364.11]
ischiorectal 014.8●
jaw 015.7● [730.88]
jejunum 014.8●
joint 015.9●
   hip 015.1●
   knee 015.2●
   specified site NEC 015.8●
   vertebral 015.0● [730.88]
keratitis 017.3● [370.31]
   interstitial 017.3● [370.59]
keratoconjunctivitis 017.3● [370.31]
kidney 016.0●
knee (joint) 015.2●
kyphoscoliosis 015.0● [737.43]
kyphosis 015.0● [737.41]
lacrimal apparatus, gland 017.3●
laryngitis 012.3●
larynx 012.3●
leptomeninges, leptomeningitis (cerebral) (spinal) 013.0●
lichenoides (primary) 017.0●
linguae 017.9●
lip 017.9●
liver 017.9●
lordosis 015.0● [737.42]
lung - see Tuberculosis, pulmonary ●
luposa 017.0●
   eyelid 017.0● [373.4]
lymphadenitis - see Tuberculosis, lymph gland
lymphangitis - see Tuberculosis, lymph gland
lymphatic (gland) (vessel) - see Tuberculosis, lymph gland
lymph gland or node (peripheral) 017.2●
   abdomen 014.8●
   bronchial 012.1●
     primary, progressive 010.8●
   cervical 017.2●

Tuberculosis, tubercular, tuberculous (Continued)

lymph gland or node (Continued)
   hilar 012.1●
     primary, progressive 010.8●
   intrathoracic 012.1●
     primary, progressive 010.8●
   mediastinal 012.1●
     primary, progressive 010.8●
   mesenteric 014.8●
   peripheral 017.2●
   retroperitoneal 014.8●
   tracheobronchial 012.1●
     primary, progressive 010.8●
malignant NEC (see also Tuberculosis, pulmonary) 011.9●
mammary gland 017.9●
marasmus NEC (see also Tuberculosis, pulmonary) 011.9●
mastoiditis 015.6●
maternal, affecting fetus or newborn 760.2
mediastinal (lymph) gland or node 012.1●
   primary, progressive 010.8●
mediastinitis 012.8●
   primary, progressive 010.8●
mediastinopericarditis 017.9● [420.0]
mediastinum 012.8●
   primary, progressive 010.8●
medulla 013.9●
   brain 013.2●
   spinal cord 013.4●
melanosis, Addisonian 017.6●
membrane, brain 013.0●
meninges (cerebral) (spinal) 013.0●
meningitis (basilar) (brain) (cerebral) (cerebrospinal) (spinal) 013.0●
meningoencephalitis 013.0●
mesentery, mesenteric 014.8●
   lymph gland or node 014.8●
miliary (any site) 018.9●
   acute 018.0●
   chronic 018.8●
   specified type NEC 018.8●
millstone makers' 011.4●
miners' 011.4●
moulders' 011.4●
mouth 017.9●
multiple 018.9●
   acute 018.0●
   chronic 018.8●
muscle 017.9●
myelitis 013.6●
myocarditis 017.9● [422.0]
myocardium 017.9● [422.0]
nasal (passage) (sinus) 012.8●
nasopharynx 012.8●
neck gland 017.2●
nephritis 016.0● [583.81]
nerve 017.9●
nose (septum) 012.8●
ocular 017.3●
old NEC 137.0
   without residuals V12.01
omentum 014.8●
oophoritis (acute) (chronic) 016.6●
optic 017.3● [377.39]
   nerve trunk 017.3● [377.39]
   papilla, papillae 017.3● [377.39]
orbit 017.3●
orchitis 016.5● [608.81]
organ, specified NEC 017.9●

Tuberculosis, tubercular, tuberculous (Continued)

orificialis (primary) 017.0●
osseous (see also Tuberculosis, bone) 015.9● [730.8]
osteitis (see also Tuberculosis, bone) 015.9● [730.8]
osteomyelitis (see also Tuberculosis, bone) 015.9● [730.8]
otitis (media) 017.4●
ovaritis (acute) (chronic) 016.6●
ovary (acute) (chronic) 016.6●
oviducts (acute) (chronic) 016.6●
pachymeningitis 013.0●
palate (soft) 017.9●
pancreas 017.9●
papulonecrotic (primary) 017.0●
parathyroid glands 017.9●
paronychia (primary) 017.0●
parotid gland or region 017.9●
pelvic organ NEC 016.9●
   female 016.7●
   male 016.5●
pelvis (bony) 015.7● [730.85]
penis 016.5●
peribronchitis 011.3●
pericarditis 017.9● [420.0]
pericardium 017.9● [420.0]
perichondritis, larynx 012.3●
perineum 017.9●
periostitis (see also Tuberculosis, bone) 015.9● [730.8]
periphlebitis 017.9●
   eye vessel 017.3● [362.18]
   retina 017.3● [362.18]
perirectal fistula 014.8●
peritoneal gland 014.8●
peritoneum 014.0●
peritonitis 014.0●
pernicious NEC (see also Tuberculosis, pulmonary) 011.9●
pharyngitis 012.8●
pharynx 012.8●
phlyctenulosis (conjunctiva) 017.3● [370.31]
phthisis NEC (see also Tuberculosis, pulmonary) 011.9●
pituitary gland 017.9●
placenta 016.7●
pleura, pleural, pleurisy, pleuritis (fibrinous) (obliterative) (purulent) (simple plastic) (with effusion) 012.0●
   primary, progressive 010.1●
pneumonia, pneumonic 011.6●
pneumothorax 011.7●
polyserositis 018.9●
   acute 018.0●
   chronic 018.8●
potters' 011.4●
prepuce 016.5●
primary 010.9●
   complex 010.0●
   complicated 010.8●
     with pleurisy or effusion 010.1●
   progressive 010.8●
     with pleurisy or effusion 010.1●
   skin 017.0●
proctitis 014.8●
prostate 016.5● [601.4]
prostatitis 016.5● [601.4]
pulmonaris (see also Tuberculosis, pulmonary) 011.9●

◀ New   ◀▥ Revised   ~~deleted~~ Deleted   ● Use Additional Digit(s)   ▬ Omit code

Tuberculosis, tubercular, tuberculous
(Continued)
pulmonary (artery) (incipient)
(malignant) (multiple round foci)
(pernicious) (reinfection stage)
011.9●
cavitated or with cavitation 011.2●
primary, progressive 010.8●
childhood type or first infection
010.0●
chromogenic acid-fast bacilli 795.39
fibrosis or fibrotic 011.4●
infiltrative 011.0●
primary, progressive 010.9●
nodular 011.1●
specified NEC 011.8●
sputum positive only 795.39●
status following surgical collapse of
lung NEC 011.9●
pyelitis 016.0● [590.81]
pyelonephritis 016.0● [590.81]
pyemia - see Tuberculosis, miliary
pyonephrosis 016.0●
pyopneumothorax 012.0●
pyothorax 012.0●
rectum (with abscess) 014.8●
fistula 014.8●
reinfection stage (see also Tuberculosis,
pulmonary) 011.9●
renal 016.0●
renis 016.0●
reproductive organ 016.7●
respiratory NEC (see also Tuberculosis,
pulmonary) 011.9●
specified site NEC 012.8●
retina 017.3● [363.13]
retroperitoneal (lymph gland or node)
014.8●
gland 014.8●
retropharyngeal abscess 012.8●
rheumatism 015.9●
rhinitis 012.8●
sacroiliac (joint) 015.8●
sacrum 015.0● [730.88]
salivary gland 017.9●
salpingitis (acute) (chronic) 016.6●
sandblasters' 011.4●
sclera 017.3● [379.09]
scoliosis 015.0● [737.43]
scrofulous 017.2●
scrotum 016.5●
seminal tract or vesicle 016.5●
[608.81]
senile NEC (see also Tuberculosis,
pulmonary) 011.9●
septic NEC (see also Tuberculosis,
miliary) 018.9●
shoulder 015.8●
blade 015.7● [730.8]●
sigmoid 014.8●
sinus (accessory) (nasal) 012.8●
bone 015.7● [730.88]
epididymis 016.4●
skeletal NEC (see also Osteomyelitis,
due to tuberculosis) 015.9●
[730.8]●
skin (any site) (primary) 017.0●
small intestine 014.8●
soft palate 017.9●
spermatic cord 016.5●
spinal
column 015.0● [730.88]
cord 013.4●
disease 015.0● [730.88]

Tuberculosis, tubercular, tuberculous
(Continued)
spinal (Continued)
medulla 013.4●
membrane 013.0●
meninges 013.0●
spine 015.0● [730.88]
spleen 017.7●
splenitis 017.7●
spondylitis 015.0● [720.81]
spontaneous pneumothorax - see
Tuberculosis, pulmonary
sternoclavicular joint 015.8●
stomach 017.9●
stonemasons' 011.4●
struma 017.2●
subcutaneous tissue (cellular)
(primary) 017.0●
subcutis (primary) 017.0●
subdeltoid bursa 017.9●
submaxillary 017.9●
region 017.9●
supraclavicular gland 017.2●
suprarenal (capsule) (gland) 017.6●
swelling, joint (see also Tuberculosis,
joint) 015.9●
symphysis pubis 015.7● [730.88]
synovitis 015.9● [727.01]
hip 015.1● [727.01]
knee 015.2● [727.01]
specified site NEC 015.8●
[727.01]
spine or vertebra 015.0● [727.01]
systemic - see Tuberculosis, miliary
tarsitis (eyelid) 017.0● [373.4]
ankle (bone) 015.5● [730.87]
tendon (sheath) - see Tuberculosis,
tenosynovitis
tenosynovitis 015.9● [727.01]
hip 015.1● [727.01]
knee 015.2● [727.01]
specified site NEC 015.8● [727.01]
spine or vertebra 015.0● [727.01]
testis 016.5● [608.81]
throat 012.8●
thymus gland 017.9●
thyroid gland 017.5●
toe 017.9●
tongue 017.9●
tonsil (lingual) 012.8●
tonsillitis 012.8●
trachea, tracheal 012.8●
gland 012.1●
primary, progressive 010.8●
isolated 012.2●
tracheobronchial 011.3●
glandular 012.1●
primary, progressive 010.8●
isolated 012.2●
lymph gland or node 012.1●
primary, progressive 010.8●
tubal 016.6●
tunica vaginalis 016.5●
typhlitis 014.8●
ulcer (primary) (skin) 017.0●
bowel or intestine 014.8●
specified site NEC - see Tuberculosis,
by site
unspecified site - see Tuberculosis,
pulmonary
ureter 016.2●
urethra, urethral 016.3●
urinary organ or tract 016.3●
kidney 016.0●

Tuberculosis, tubercular, tuberculous
(Continued)
uterus 016.7●
uveal tract 017.3● [363.13]
uvula 017.9●
vaccination, prophylactic (against)
V03.2
vagina 016.7●
vas deferens 016.5●
vein 017.9●
verruca (primary) 017.0●
verrucosa (cutis) (primary) 017.0●
vertebra (column) 015.0● [730.88]
vesiculitis 016.5● [608.81]
viscera NEC 014.8●
vulva 016.7● [616.51]
wrist (joint) 015.8●
bone 015.5● [730.83]
Tuberculum
auriculae 744.29
occlusal 520.2
paramolare 520.2
Tuberosity
jaw, excessive 524.07
maxillary, entire 524.07
Tuberous sclerosis (brain) 759.5
Tubo-ovarian - see condition
Tuboplasty, after previous sterilization
V26.0
Tubotympanitis 381.10
Tularemia 021.9
with
conjunctivitis 021.3
pneumonia 021.2
bronchopneumonic 021.2
conjunctivitis 021.3
cryptogenic 021.1
disseminated 021.8
enteric 021.1
generalized 021.8
glandular 021.8
intestinal 021.1
oculoglandular 021.3
ophthalmic 021.3
pneumonia 021.2
pulmonary 021.2
specified NEC 021.8
typhoidal 021.1
ulceroglandular 021.0
vaccination, prophylactic (against)
V03.4
Tularensis conjunctivitis 021.3
Tumefaction - see also Swelling
liver (see also Hypertrophy, liver) 789.1
Tumor (M8000/1) - see also Neoplasm,
by site, unspecified nature
Abrikossov's (M9580/0) - see also
Neoplasm, connective tissue,
benign
malignant (M9580/3) - see
Neoplasm, connective tissue,
malignant
acinar cell (M8550/1) - see
Neoplasm, by site,
uncertain behavior
acinic cell (M8550/1) - see
Neoplasm, by site,
uncertain behavior
adenomatoid (M9054/0) - see also
Neoplasm, by site, benign
odontogenic (M9300/0) 213.1
upper jaw (bone) 213.0
adnexal (skin) (M8390/0) - see
Neoplasm, skin, benign

Tumor *(Continued)*
  adrenal
    cortical (benign) (M8370/0) 227.0
      malignant (M8370/3) 194.0
    rest (M8671/0) - *see* Neoplasm, by
      site, benign
  alpha cell (M8152/0)
    malignant (M8152/3)
      pancreas 157.4
      specified site NEC - *see*
        Neoplasm, by site,
        malignant
      unspecified site 157.4
    pancreas 211.7
    specified site NEC - *see* Neoplasm,
      by site, benign
    unspecified site 211.7
  aneurysmal (*see also* Aneurysm)
    442.9
  aortic body (M8691/1) 237.3
    malignant (M8691/3) 194.6
  argentaffin (M8241/1) - *see* Neoplasm,
    by site, uncertain behavior
  basal cell (M8090/1) - *see also*
    Neoplasm, skin, uncertain
    behavior
  benign (M8000/0) - *see* Neoplasm, by
    site, benign
  beta cell (M8151/0)
    malignant (M8151/3)
      pancreas 157.4
      specified site - *see* Neoplasm, by
        site, malignant
      unspecified site 157.4
    pancreas 211.7
    specified site NEC - *see* Neoplasm,
      by site, benign
    unspecified site 211.7
  blood - *see* Hematoma
  brenner (M9000/0) 220
    borderline malignancy (M9000/1)
      236.2
    malignant (M9000/3) 183.0
    proliferating (M9000/1) 236.2
  Brooke's (M8100/0) - *see* Neoplasm,
    skin, benign
  brown fat (M8880/0) - *see* Lipoma, by
    site
  Burkitt's (M9750/3) 200.2●
  calcifying epithelial odontogenic
    (M9340/0) 213.1
    upper jaw (bone) 213.0
  carcinoid (M8240/1) 209.60
    benign 209.60
      appendix 209.51
      ascending colon 209.53
      bronchus 209.61
      cecum 209.52
      colon 209.50
      descending colon 209.55
      duodenum 209.41
      foregut 209.65
      hindgut 209.67
      ileum 209.43
      jejunum 209.42
      kidney 209.64
      large intestine 209.50
      lung 209.61
      midgut 209.66
      rectum 209.57
      sigmoid colon 209.56
      small intestine 209.40
      specified NEC 209.69
      stomach 209.63

Tumor *(Continued)*
  carcinoid *(Continued)*
    benign *(Continued)*
      thymus 209.62
      transverse colon 209.54
    malignant (of) 209.20
      appendix 209.11
      ascending colon 209.13
      bronchus 209.21
      cecum 209.12
      colon 209.10
      descending colon 209.15
      duodenum 209.01
      foregut 209.25
      hindgut 209.27
      ileum 209.03
      jejunum 209.02
      kidney 209.24
      large intestine 209.10
      lung 209.21
      midgut 209.26
      rectum 209.17
      sigmoid colon 209.16
      small intestine 209.00
      specified NEC 209.29
      stomach 209.23
      thymus 209.22
      transverse colon 209.14
    secondary - *see* Tumor,
      neuroendocrine, secondary ◄
    neuroendocrine 209.60
      malignant poorly differentiated
        209.30
  carotid body (M8692/1) 237.3
    malignant (M8692/3) 194.5
  Castleman's (mediastinal lymph node
    hyperplasia) 785.6
  cells (M8001/1) - *see also* Neoplasm, by
    site, unspecified nature
    benign (M8001/0) - *see* Neoplasm,
      by site, benign
    malignant (M8001/3) - *see*
      Neoplasm, by site, malignant
    uncertain whether benign or
      malignant (M8001/1) - *see*
      Neoplasm, by site, uncertain
      nature
  cervix
    in pregnancy or childbirth 654.6●
      affecting fetus or newborn 763.89
      causing obstructed labor 660.2●
        affecting fetus or newborn
          763.1
  chondromatous giant cell (M9230/0) -
    see Neoplasm, bone, benign
  chromaffin (M8700/0) - *see also*
    Neoplasm, by site, benign
    malignant (M8700/3) - *see*
      Neoplasm, by site, malignant
  Cock's peculiar 706.2
  Codman's (benign chondroblastoma)
    (M9230/0) - *see* Neoplasm, bone,
    benign
  dentigerous, mixed (M9282/0) 213.1
    upper jaw (bone) 213.0
  dermoid (M9084/0) - *see* Neoplasm, by
    site, benign
    with malignant transformation
      (M9084/3) 183.0
  desmoid (extra-abdominal)
    (M8821/1) - *see also* Neoplasm,
    connective tissue, uncertain
    behavior
    abdominal (M8822/1) - *see*
      Neoplasm, connective tissue,
      uncertain behavior

Tumor *(Continued)*
  embryonal (mixed) (M9080/1) - *see also*
    Neoplasm, by site, uncertain
    behavior
    liver (M9080/3) 155.0
  endodermal sinus (M9071/3)
    specified site - *see* Neoplasm, by site,
      malignant
    unspecified site
      female 183.0
      male 186.9
  epithelial
    benign (M8010/0) - *see* Neoplasm,
      by site, benign
    malignant (M8010/3) - *see*
      Neoplasm, by site, malignant
  Ewing's (M9260/3) - *see* Neoplasm,
    bone, malignant
  fatty - *see* Lipoma
  fetal, causing disproportion 653.7●
    causing obstructed labor 660.1●
  fibroid (M8890/0) - *see* Leiomyoma
  G cell (M8153/1)
    malignant (M8153/3)
      pancreas 157.4
      specified site NEC - *see* Neoplasm,
        by site, malignant
      unspecified site 157.4
    specified site - *see* Neoplasm, by site,
      uncertain behavior
    unspecified site 235.5
  giant cell (type) (M8003/1) - *see also*
    Neoplasm, by site, unspecified
    nature
    bone (M9250/1) 238.0
      malignant (M9250/3) - *see*
        Neoplasm, bone, malignant
    chondromatous (M9230/0) - *see*
      Neoplasm, bone, benign
    malignant (M8003/3) - *see*
      Neoplasm, by site, malignant
    peripheral (gingiva) 523.8
    soft parts (M9251/1) - *see also*
      Neoplasm, connective tissue,
      uncertain behavior
      malignant (M9251/3) - *see*
        Neoplasm, connective
        tissue, malignant
    tendon sheath 727.02
  glomus (M8711/0) - *see also*
    Hemangioma, by site
    jugulare (M8690/1) 237.3
      malignant (M8690/3) 194.6
  gonadal stromal (M8590/1) - *see*
    Neoplasm, by site, uncertain
    behavior
  granular cell (M9580/0) - *see also*
    Neoplasm, connective tissue,
    benign
    malignant (M9580/3) - *see*
      Neoplasm, connective tissue,
      malignant
  granulosa cell (M8620/1) 236.2
    malignant (M8620/3) 183.0
  granulosa cell-theca cell (M8621/1) 236.2
    malignant (M8621/3) 183.0
  Grawitz's (hypernephroma) (M8312/3)
    189.0
  hazard-crile (M8350/3) 193
  hemorrhoidal - *see* Hemorrhoids
  hilar cell (M8660/0) 220
  Hürthle cell (benign) (M8290/0) 226
    malignant (M8290/3) 193
  hydatid (*see also* Echinococcus) 122.9

◄ New   ◄▥ Revised   deleted Deleted   ● Use Additional Digit(s)   ▨ Omit code

Tumor *(Continued)*
hypernephroid (M8311/1) - *see also* Neoplasm, by site, uncertain behavior
interstitial cell (M8650/1) - *see also* Neoplasm, by site, uncertain behavior
  benign (M8650/0) - *see* Neoplasm, by site, benign
  malignant (M8650/3) - *see* Neoplasm, by site, malignant
islet cell (M8150/0)
  malignant (M8150/3)
    pancreas 157.4
    specified site - *see* Neoplasm, by site, malignant
    unspecified site 157.4
  pancreas 211.7
  specified site NEC - *see* Neoplasm, by site, benign
  unspecified site 211.7
juxtaglomerular (M8361/1) 236.91
Krukenberg's (M8490/6) 198.6
Leydig cell (M8650/1)
  benign (M8650/0)
    specified site - *see* Neoplasm, by site, benign
    unspecified site
      female 220
      male 222.0
  malignant (M8650/3)
    specified site - *see* Neoplasm, by site, malignant
    unspecified site
      female 183.0
      male 186.9
  specified site - *see* Neoplasm, by site, uncertain behavior
  unspecified site
    female 236.2
    male 236.4
lipid cell, ovary (M8670/0) 220
lipoid cell, ovary (M8670/0) 220
lymphomatous, benign (M9590/0) - *see also* Neoplasm, by site, benign
lysis syndrome (following antineoplastic drug therapy) (spontaneous) 277.88 ◀
Malherbe's (M8110/0) - *see* Neoplasm, skin, benign
malignant (M8000/3) - *see also* Neoplasm, by site, malignant
  fusiform cell (type) (M8004/3) - *see* Neoplasm, by site, malignant
  giant cell (type) (M8003/3) - *see* Neoplasm, by site, malignant
  mixed NEC (M8940/3) - *see* Neoplasm, by site, malignant
  small cell (type) (M8002/3) - *see* Neoplasm, by site, malignant
  spindle cell (type) (M8004/3) - *see* Neoplasm, by site, malignant
mast cell (M9740/1) 238.5
  malignant (M9740/3) 202.6 ●
melanotic, neuroectodermal (M9363/0) - *see* Neoplasm, by site, benign
Merkel cell - *see* ~~Neoplasm, by site, malignant~~ Carcinoma, Merkel cell ◀▥
mesenchymal
  malignant (M8800/3) - *see* Neoplasm, connective tissue, malignant
  mixed (M8990/1) - *see* Neoplasm, connective tissue, uncertain behavior

Tumor *(Continued)*
mesodermal, mixed (M8951/3) - *see also* Neoplasm, by site, malignant
  liver 155.0
mesonephric (M9110/1) - *see also* Neoplasm, by site, uncertain behavior
  malignant (M9110/3) - *see* Neoplasm, by site, malignant
metastatic
  from specified site (M8000/3) - *see* Neoplasm, by site, malignant
  to specified site (M8000/6) - *see* Neoplasm, by site, malignant, secondary
mixed NEC (M8940/0) - *see also* Neoplasm, by site, benign
  malignant (M8940/3) - *see* Neoplasm, by site, malignant
mucocarcinoid, malignant (M8243/3) - *see* Neoplasm, by site, malignant
mucoepidermoid (M8430/1) - *see* Neoplasm, by site, uncertain behavior
Müllerian, mixed (M8950/3) - *see* Neoplasm, by site, malignant
myoepithelial (M8982/0) - *see* Neoplasm, by site, benign
neuroendocrine 209.60
  malignant poorly differentiated 209.30 ◀
  secondary 209.70 ◀
    bone 209.73 ◀
    distant lymph nodes 209.71 ◀
    liver 209.72 ◀
    peritoneum 209.74 ◀
    site specified NEC 209.79 ◀
neurogenic olfactory (M9520/3) 160.0
nonencapsulated sclerosing (M8350/3) 193
odontogenic (M9270/1) 238.0
  adenomatoid (M9300/0) 213.1
    upper jaw (bone) 213.0
  benign (M9270/0) 213.1
    upper jaw (bone) 213.0
  calcifying epithelial (M9340/0) 213.1
    upper jaw (bone) 213.0
  malignant (M9270/3) 170.1
    upper jaw (bone) 170.0
  squamous (M9312/0) 213.1
    upper jaw (bone) 213.0
ovarian stromal (M8590/1) 236.2
ovary
  in pregnancy or childbirth 654.4 ●
    affecting fetus or newborn 763.89
    causing obstructed labor 660.2 ●
      affecting fetus or newborn 763.1
pacinian (M9507/0) - *see* Neoplasm, skin, benign
Pancoast's (M8010/3) 162.3
papillary - *see* Papilloma
pelvic, in pregnancy or childbirth 654.9 ●
  affecting fetus or newborn 763.89
  causing obstructed labor 660.2 ●
    affecting fetus or newborn 763.1
phantom 300.11
plasma cell (M9731/1) 238.6
  benign (M9731/0) - *see* Neoplasm, by site, benign
  malignant (M9731/3) 203.8 ●

Tumor *(Continued)*
polyvesicular vitelline (M9071/3)
  specified site - *see* Neoplasm, by site, malignant
  unspecified site
    female 183.0
    male 186.9
Pott's puffy (*see also* Osteomyelitis) 730.2 ●
Rathke's pouch (M9350/1) 237.0
regaud's (M8082/3) - *see* Neoplasm, nasopharynx, malignant
rete cell (M8140/0) 222.0
retinal anlage (M9363/0) - *see* Neoplasm, by site, benign
Rokitansky's 620.2
salivary gland type, mixed (M8940/0) - *see also* Neoplasm, by site, benign
  malignant (M8940/3) - *see* Neoplasm, by site, malignant
Sampson's 617.1
Schloffer's (*see also* Peritonitis) 567.29
Schmincke (M8082/3) - *see* Neoplasm, nasopharynx, malignant
sebaceous (*see also* Cyst, sebaceous) 706.2
secondary (M8000/6) - *see* Neoplasm, by site, secondary
  carcinoid - *see* Tumor, neuroendocrine, secondary ◀
  neuroendocrine - *see* Tumor, neuroendocrine, secondary ◀
Sertoli cell (M8640/0)
  with lipid storage (M8641/0)
    specified site, - *see* Neoplasm, by site, benign
    unspecified site
      female 220
      male 222.0
  specified site - *see* Neoplasm, by site, benign
  unspecified site
    female 220
    male 222.0
Sertoli-Leydig cell (M8631/0)
  specified site - *see* Neoplasm, by site, benign
  unspecified site
    female 220
    male 222.0
sex cord (-stromal) (M8590/1) - *see* Neoplasm, by site, uncertain behavior
skin appendage (M8390/0) - *see* Neoplasm, skin, benign
soft tissue
  benign (M8800/0) - *see* Neoplasm, connective tissue, benign
  malignant (M8800/3) - *see* Neoplasm, connective tissue, malignant
sternomastoid 754.1
stromal
  abdomen
    benign 215.5
    malignant NEC 171.5
    uncertain behavior 238.1
  digestive system 238.1
    benign 215.5
    malignant NEC 171.5
    uncertain behavior 238.1

◀ New   ◀▥ Revised   ~~deleted~~ Deleted   ● Use Additional Digit(s)   ▥ Omit code

Tumor (Continued)
  stromal (Continued)
    gastric 238.1
      benign 215.5
      malignant 151.9
      uncertain behavior 238.1
    gastrointestinal 238.1
      benign 215.5
      malignant NEC 171.5
      uncertain behavior 238.1
    intestine (small) 238.1
      benign 215.5
      malignant 152.9
      uncertain behavior 238.1
    stomach 238.1
      benign 215.5
      malignant 151.9
      uncertain behavior 238.1
  superior sulcus (lung) (pulmonary)
    (syndrome) (M8010/3) 162.3
  suprasulcus (M8010/3) 162.3
  sweat gland (M8400/1) - see also
    Neoplasm, skin, uncertain
    behavior
    benign (M8400/0) - see Neoplasm,
      skin, benign
    malignant (M8400/3) - see
      Neoplasm, skin, malignant
  syphilitic brain 094.89
    congenital 090.49
  testicular stromal (M8590/1) 236.4
  theca cell (M8600/0) 220
  theca cell-granulosa cell (M8621/1)
    236.2
  theca-lutein (M8610/0) 220
  turban (M8200/0) 216.4
  uterus
    in pregnancy or childbirth 654.1●
      affecting fetus or newborn
        763.89
      causing obstructed labor
        660.2●
        affecting fetus or newborn
          763.1
  vagina
    in pregnancy or childbirth 654.7●
      affecting fetus or newborn
        763.89
      causing obstructed labor 660.2●
        affecting fetus or newborn
          763.1
  varicose (see also Varicose, vein) 454.9
  von Recklinghausen's (M9540/1)
    237.71
  vulva
    in pregnancy or childbirth 654.8●
      affecting fetus or newborn
        763.89
      causing obstructed labor
        660.2●
        affecting fetus or newborn
          763.1
  Warthin's (salivary gland) (M8561/0)
    210.2
  white - see also Tuberculosis, arthritis
  White-Darier 757.39
  Wilms' (nephroblastoma) (M8960/3)
    189.0
  yolk sac (M9071/3)
    specified site - see Neoplasm, by site,
      malignant
    unspecified site
      female 183.0
      male 186.9

Tumorlet (M8040/1) - see Neoplasm, by
  site, uncertain behavior
Tungiasis 134.1
Tunica vasculosa lentis 743.39
Tunnel vision 368.45
Turban tumor (M8200/0) 216.4
Türck's trachoma (chronic catarrhal
  laryngitis) 476.0
Türk's syndrome (ocular retraction
  syndrome) 378.71
Turner's
  hypoplasia (tooth) 520.4
  syndrome 758.6
  tooth 520.4
Turner-Kieser syndrome (hereditary
  osteo-onychodysplasia) 756.89
Turner-Varny syndrome 758.6
Turricephaly 756.0
Tussis convulsiva (see also Whooping
  cough) 033.9
Twiddler's syndrome (due to)
  automatic implantable defibrillator
    996.04
  pacemaker 996.01
Twin
  affected by maternal complications of
    pregnancy 761.5
  conjoined 759.4
    fetal 678.1●
  healthy liveborn - see Newborn, twin
  pregnancy (complicating delivery)
    NEC 651.0●
    with fetal loss and retention of one
      fetus 651.3●
    conjoined 678.1●
    following (elective) fetal reduction
      651.7●
Twinning, teeth 520.2
Twist, twisted
  bowel, colon, or intestine 560.2
  hair (congenital) 757.4
  mesentery 560.2
  omentum 560.2
  organ or site, congenital NEC - see
    Anomaly, specified type NEC
  ovarian pedicle 620.5
    congenital 752.0
  umbilical cord - see Compression,
    umbilical cord
Twitch 781.0
Tylosis 700
  buccalis 528.6
  gingiva 523.8
  linguae 528.6
  palmaris et plantaris 757.39
Tympanism 787.3
Tympanites (abdominal) (intestine)
  787.3
Tympanitis - see Myringitis
Tympanosclerosis 385.00
  involving
    combined sites NEC 385.09
      with tympanic membrane 385.03
    tympanic membrane 385.01
      with ossicles 385.02
        and middle ear 385.03
Tympanum - see condition
Tympany
  abdomen 787.3
  chest 786.7
Typhlitis (see also Appendicitis) 541
Typhoenteritis 002.0
Typhogastric fever 002.0

Typhoid (abortive) (ambulant) (any site)
  (fever) (hemorrhagic) (infection)
  (intermittent) (malignant)
  (rheumatic) 002.0
  with pneumonia 002.0 [484.8]
  abdominal 002.0
  carrier (suspected) of V02.1
  cholecystitis (current) 002.0
  clinical (Widal and blood test negative)
    002.0
  endocarditis 002.0 [421.1]
  inoculation reaction - see
    Complications, vaccination
  meningitis 002.0 [320.7]
  mesenteric lymph nodes 002.0
  myocarditis 002.0 [422.0]
  osteomyelitis (see also Osteomyelitis,
    due to, typhoid) 002.0 [730.8]●
  perichondritis, larynx 002.0 [478.71]
  pneumonia 002.0 [484.8]
  spine 002.0 [720.81]
  ulcer (perforating) 002.0
  vaccination, prophylactic (against)
    V03.1
  Widal negative 002.0
Typhomalaria (fever) (see also Malaria)
  084.6
Typhomania 002.0
Typhoperitonitis 002.0
Typhus (fever) 081.9
  abdominal, abdominalis 002.0
  African tick 082.1
  amarillic (see also Fever, Yellow)
    060.9
  brain 081.9
  cerebral 081.9
  classical 080
  endemic (flea-borne) 081.0
  epidemic (louse-borne) 080
  exanthematic NEC 080
  exanthematicus SAI 080
    brillii SAI 081.1
    Mexicanus SAI 081.0
    pediculo vestimenti causa 080
    typhus murinus 081.0
  flea-borne 081.0
  Indian tick 082.1
  Kenya tick 082.1
  louse-borne 080
  Mexican 081.0
    flea-borne 081.0
    louse-borne 080
    tabardillo 080
  mite-borne 081.2
  murine 081.0
  North Asian tick-borne 082.2
  petechial 081.9
  Queensland tick 082.3
  rat 081.0
  recrudescent 081.1
  recurrent (see also Fever, relapsing)
    087.9
  São Paulo 082.0
  scrub (China) (India) (Malaya) (New
    Guinea) 081.2
  shop (of Malaya) 081.0
  Siberian tick 082.2
  tick-borne NEC 082.9
  tropical 081.2
  vaccination, prophylactic (against)
    V05.8
Tyrosinemia 270.2
  neonatal 775.89
Tyrosinosis (Medes) (Sakai) 270.2
Tyrosinuria 270.2
Tyrosyluria 270.2

◀ New   ⬅ Revised   deleted Deleted   ● Use Additional Digit(s)   ▓ Omit code

U

Uehlinger's syndrome (acropachyderma) 757.39

Uhl's anomaly or disease (hypoplasia of myocardium, right ventricle) 746.84

Ulcer, ulcerated, ulcerating, ulceration, ulcerative 707.9
with gangrene 707.9 [785.4]
abdomen (wall) (see also Ulcer, skin) 707.8
ala, nose 478.19
alveolar process 526.5
amebic (intestine) 006.9
    skin 006.6
anastomotic - see Ulcer, gastrojejunal
anorectal 569.41
antral - see Ulcer, stomach
anus (sphincter) (solitary) 569.41
    varicose - see Varicose, ulcer, anus
aorta - see Aneurysm
aphthous (oral) (recurrent) 528.2
    genital organ(s)
        female 616.50
        male 608.89
    mouth 528.2
arm (see also Ulcer, skin) 707.8
arteriosclerotic plaque - see Arteriosclerosis, by site
artery NEC 447.2
    without rupture 447.8
atrophic NEC - see Ulcer, skin
Barrett's (chronic peptic ulcer of esophagus) 530.85
bile duct 576.8
bladder (solitary) (sphincter) 596.8
    bilharzial (see also Schistosomiasis) 120.9 [595.4]
    submucosal (see also Cystitis) 595.1
    tuberculous (see also Tuberculosis) 016.1●
bleeding NEC - see Ulcer, peptic, with hemorrhage
bone 730.9●
bowel (see also Ulcer, intestine) 569.82
breast 611.0
bronchitis 491.8
bronchus 519.19
buccal (cavity) (traumatic) 528.9
burn (acute) - see Ulcer, duodenum
Buruli 031.1
buttock (see also Ulcer, skin) 707.8
    decubitus (see also Ulcer, pressure) 707.00
cancerous (M8000/3) - see Neoplasm, by site, malignant
cardia - see Ulcer, stomach
cardio-esophageal (peptic) 530.20
    with bleeding 530.21
cecum (see also Ulcer, intestine) 569.82
cervix (uteri) (trophic) 622.0
    with mention of cervicitis 616.0
chancroidal 099.0
chest (wall) (see also Ulcer, skin) 707.8
Chiclero 085.4
chin (pyogenic) (see also Ulcer, skin) 707.8
chronic (cause unknown) - see also Ulcer, skin
    penis 607.89
Cochin-China 085.1
colitis - see Colitis, ulcerative
colon (see also Ulcer, intestine) 569.82

Ulcer, ulcerated, ulcerating, ulceration, ulcerative (Continued)
conjunctiva (acute) (postinfectional) 372.00
cornea (infectional) 370.00
    with perforation 370.06
    annular 370.02
    catarrhal 370.01
    central 370.03
    dendritic 054.42
    marginal 370.01
    mycotic 370.05
    phlyctenular, tuberculous (see also Tuberculosis) 017.3● [370.31]
    ring 370.02
    rodent 370.07
    serpent, serpiginous 370.04
    superficial marginal 370.01
    tuberculous (see also Tuberculosis) 017.3● [370.31]
corpus cavernosum (chronic) 607.89
crural - see Ulcer, lower extremity
Curling's - see Ulcer, duodenum
Cushing's - see Ulcer, peptic
cystitis (interstitial) 595.1
decubitus (unspecified site) (see also Ulcer, pressure) 707.00
    with gangrene 707.00 [785.4]
    ankle 707.06
    back
        lower 707.03
        upper 707.02
    buttock 707.05
    coccyx 707.03
    elbow 707.01
    head 707.09
    heel 707.07
    hip 707.04
    other site 707.09
    sacrum 707.03
    shoulder blades 707.02
dendritic 054.42
diabetes, diabetic (mellitus) 250.8● [707.9]
    due to secondary diabetes 249.8● [707.9]
    lower limb 250.8● [707.10]
        due to secondary diabetes 249.8● [707.10]
        ankle 250.8● [707.13]
            due to secondary diabetes 249.8● [707.13]
        calf 250.8● [707.12]
            due to secondary diabetes 249.8● [707.12]
        foot 250.8● [707.15]
            due to secondary diabetes 249.8● [707.15]
        heel 250.8● [707.14]
            due to secondary diabetes 249.8● [707.14]
        knee 250.8● [707.19]
            due to secondary diabetes 249.8● [707.19]
        specified site NEC 250.8● [707.19]
            due to secondary diabetes 249.8● [707.19]
        thigh 250.8● [707.11]
            due to secondary diabetes 249.8● [707.11]
        toes 250.8● [707.15]
            due to secondary diabetes 249.8● [707.15]

◀

Ulcer, ulcerated, ulcerating, ulceration, ulcerative (Continued)
diabetes, diabetic (Continued)
    lower limb (Continued)
        specified site NEC 250.8● [707.8]
            due to secondary diabetes 249.8● [707.8]
Dieulafoy - see Lesion, Dieulafoy
    due to
        infection NEC - see Ulcer, skin
        radiation, radium - see Ulcer, by site
        trophic disturbance (any region) - see Ulcer, skin
        x-ray - see Ulcer, by site
duodenum, duodenal (eroded) (peptic) 532.9●

> Note 70   Use the following fifth-digit subclassification with categories 531–534:
>
> 0   without mention of obstruction
> 1   with obstruction

    with
        hemorrhage (chronic) 532.4●
            and perforation 532.6●
        perforation (chronic) 532.5●
            and hemorrhage 532.6●
    acute 532.3●
        with
            hemorrhage 532.0●
                and perforation 532.2●
            perforation 532.1●
                and hemorrhage 532.2●
    bleeding (recurrent) - see Ulcer, duodenum, with hemorrhage
    chronic 532.7●
        with
            hemorrhage 532.4●
                and perforation 532.6●
            perforation 532.5●
                and hemorrhage 532.6●
    penetrating - see Ulcer, duodenum, with perforation
    perforating - see Ulcer, duodenum, with perforation
dysenteric NEC 009.0
elusive 595.1
endocarditis (any valve) (acute) (chronic) (subacute) 421.0
enteritis - see Colitis, ulcerative
enterocolitis 556.0
epiglottis 478.79
esophagus (peptic) 530.20
    with bleeding 530.21
    due to ingestion
        aspirin 530.20
        chemicals 530.20
        medicinal agents 530.20
    fungal 530.20
    infectional 530.20
    varicose (see also Varix, esophagus) 456.1
        bleeding (see also Varix, esophagus, bleeding) 456.0
eye NEC 360.00
    dendritic 054.42
eyelid (region) 373.01
face (see also Ulcer, skin) 707.8
fauces 478.29
Fenwick (-Hunner) (solitary) (see also Cystitis) 595.1

Ulcer, ulcerated, ulcerating, ulceration, ulcerative (Continued)
- fistulous NEC - see Ulcer, skin
- foot (indolent) (see also Ulcer, lower extremity) 707.15
  - perforating 707.15
    - leprous 030.1
    - syphilitic 094.0
  - trophic 707.15
  - varicose 454.0
    - inflamed or infected 454.2
- frambesial, initial or primary 102.0
- gallbladder or duct 575.8
- gall duct 576.8
- gangrenous (see also Gangrene) 785.4
- gastric - see Ulcer, stomach
- gastrocolic - see Ulcer, gastrojejunal
- gastroduodenal - see Ulcer, peptic
- gastroesophageal - see Ulcer, stomach
- gastrohepatic - see Ulcer, stomach
- gastrointestinal - see Ulcer, gastrojejunal
- gastrojejunal (eroded) (peptic) 534.9

Note 71   Use the following fifth-digit subclassification with categories 531–534:

0   without mention of obstruction
1   with obstruction

- with
  - hemorrhage (chronic) 534.4●
    - and perforation 534.6●
  - perforation 534.5●
    - and hemorrhage 534.6●
  - acute 534.3●
    - with
      - hemorrhage 534.0●
        - and perforation 534.2●
      - perforation 534.1●
        - and hemorrhage 534.2●
  - bleeding (recurrent) - see Ulcer, gastrojejunal, with hemorrhage
  - chronic 534.7●
    - with
      - hemorrhage 534.4●
        - and perforation 534.6●
      - perforation 534.5●
        - and hemorrhage 534.6●
  - penetrating - see Ulcer, gastrojejunal, with perforation
  - perforating - see Ulcer, gastrojejunal, with perforation
- gastrojejunocolic - see Ulcer, gastrojejunal
- genital organ
  - female 629.89
  - male 608.89
- gingiva 523.8
- gingivitis 523.10
- glottis 478.79
- granuloma of pudenda 099.2
- groin (see also Ulcer, skin) 707.8
- gum 523.8
- gumma, due to yaws 102.4
- hand (see also Ulcer, skin) 707.8
- hard palate 528.9
- heel (see also Ulcer, lower extremity) 707.14
  - decubitus (see also Ulcer, pressure) 707.07
- hemorrhoids 455.8
  - external 455.5
  - internal 455.2

Ulcer, ulcerated, ulcerating, ulceration, ulcerative (Continued)
- hip (see also Ulcer, skin) 707.8
  - decubitus (see also Ulcer, pressure) 707.04
- Hunner's 595.1
- hypopharynx 478.29
- hypopyon (chronic) (subacute) 370.04
- hypostaticum - see Ulcer, varicose
- ileocolitis 556.1
- ileum (see also Ulcer, intestine) 569.82
- intestine, intestinal NEC 569.82
  - with perforation 569.83
  - amebic 006.9
  - duodenal - see Ulcer, duodenum
  - granulocytopenic (with hemorrhage) 288.09
  - marginal 569.82
  - perforating 569.83
  - small, primary 569.82
  - stercoraceous 569.82
  - stercoral 569.82
  - tuberculous (see also Tuberculosis) 014.8●
  - typhoid (fever) 002.0
  - varicose 456.8
- ischemic 707.9
  - lower extremity (see also Ulcer, lower extremity) 707.10
    - ankle 707.13
    - calf 707.12
    - foot 707.15
    - heel 707.14
    - knee 707.19
    - specified site NEC 707.19
    - thigh 707.11
    - toes 707.15
- jejunum, jejunal - see Ulcer, gastrojejunal
- keratitis (see also Ulcer, cornea) 370.00
- knee - see Ulcer, lower extremity
- labium (majus) (minus) 616.50
- laryngitis (see also Laryngitis) 464.00
  - with obstruction 464.01
- larynx (aphthous) (contact) 478.79
  - diphtheritic 032.3
- leg - see Ulcer, lower extremity
- lip 528.5
- Lipschütz's 616.50
- lower extremity (atrophic) (chronic) (neurogenic) (perforating) (pyogenic) (trophic) (tropical) 707.10
  - with gangrene (see also Ulcer, lower extremity) 707.10 [785.4]
    - arteriosclerotic 440.24
  - ankle 707.13
  - arteriosclerotic 440.23
    - with gangrene 440.24
  - calf 707.12
  - decubitus (see also Ulcer, pressure) 707.00
    - with gangrene 707.00 [785.4]
    - ankle 707.06
    - buttock 707.05
    - heel 707.07
    - hip 707.04
  - foot 707.15
  - heel 707.14
  - knee 707.19
  - specified site NEC 707.19
  - thigh 707.11

Ulcer, ulcerated, ulcerating, ulceration, ulcerative (Continued)
- lower extremity (Continued)
  - toes 707.15
  - varicose 454.0
    - inflamed or infected 454.2
- luetic - see Ulcer, syphilitic
- lung 518.89
  - tuberculous (see also Tuberculosis) 011.2●
- malignant (M8000/3) - see Neoplasm, by site, malignant
- marginal NEC - see Ulcer, gastrojejunal
- meatus (urinarius) 597.89
- Meckel's diverticulum 751.0
- Meleney's (chronic undermining) 686.09
- Mooren's (cornea) 370.07
- mouth (traumatic) 528.9
- mycobacterial (skin) 031.1
- nasopharynx 478.29
- navel cord (newborn) 771.4
- neck (see also Ulcer, skin) 707.8
  - uterus 622.0
- neurogenic NEC - see Ulcer, skin
- nose, nasal (infectional) (passage) 478.19
  - septum 478.19
    - varicose 456.8
  - skin - see Ulcer, skin
  - spirochetal NEC 104.8
- oral mucosa (traumatic) 528.9
- palate (soft) 528.9
- penetrating NEC - see Ulcer, peptic, with perforation
- penis (chronic) 607.89
- peptic (site unspecified) 533.9

Note 72   Use the following fifth-digit subclassification with categories 531–534:

0   without mention of obstruction
1   with obstruction

- with
  - hemorrhage 533.4●
    - and perforation 533.6●
  - perforation (chronic) 533.5●
    - and hemorrhage 533.6●
  - acute 533.3●
    - with
      - hemorrhage 533.0●
        - and perforation 533.2●
      - perforation 533.1●
        - and hemorrhage 533.2●
  - bleeding (recurrent) - see Ulcer, peptic, with hemorrhage
  - chronic 533.7●
    - with
      - hemorrhage 533.4●
        - and perforation 533.6●
      - perforation 533.5●
        - and hemorrhage 533.6●
  - penetrating - see Ulcer, peptic, with perforation
  - perforating NEC (see also Ulcer, peptic, with perforation) 533.5●
- skin 707.9
- perineum (see also Ulcer, skin) 707.8
- peritonsillar 474.8
- phagedenic (tropical) NEC - see Ulcer, skin
- pharynx 478.29
- phlebitis - see Phlebitis

◀ New   ◀◀◀ Revised   ~~deleted~~ Deleted   ● Use Additional Digit(s)   ▓▓▓ Omit code

Ulcer, ulcerated, ulcerating, ulceration, ulcerative (*Continued*)
plaster (*see also* Ulcer, pressure) 707.00
popliteal space - *see* Ulcer, lower extremity
postpyloric - *see* Ulcer, duodenum
prepuce 607.89
prepyloric - *see* Ulcer, stomach
pressure 707.00
  with
    abrasion, blister, partial thickness skin loss involving epidermis and/or dermis 707.22
    full thickness skin loss involving damage or necrosis of subcutaneous tissue 707.23
    gangrene 707.00 [785.4]
    necrosis of soft tissues through to underlying muscle, tendon, or bone 707.24
  ankle 707.06
  back
    lower 707.03
    upper 707.02
  buttock 707.05
  coccyx 707.03
  elbow 707.01
  head 707.09
  healed - *omit code*
  healing - *code to* Ulcer, pressure, by stage
  heel 707.07
  hip 707.04
  other site 707.09
  sacrum 707.03
  shoulder blades 707.02
  stage
    I (healing) 707.21
    II (healing) 707.22
    III (healing) 707.23
    IV (healing) 707.24
    unspecified (healing) 707.20
  unstageable 707.25
primary of intestine 569.82
  with perforation 569.83
proctitis 556.2
  with ulcerative sigmoiditis 556.3
prostate 601.8
pseudopeptic - *see* Ulcer, peptic
pyloric - *see* Ulcer, stomach
rectosigmoid 569.82
  with perforation 569.83
rectum (sphincter) (solitary) 569.41
  stercoraceous, stercoral 569.41
  varicose - *see* Varicose, ulcer, anus
retina (*see also* Chorioretinitis) 363.20
rodent (M8090/3) - *see also* Neoplasm, skin, malignant
  cornea 370.07
round - *see* Ulcer, stomach
sacrum (region) (*see also* Ulcer, skin) 707.8
Saemisch's 370.04
scalp (*see also* Ulcer, skin) 707.8
sclera 379.09
scrofulous (*see also* Tuberculosis) 017.2●
scrotum 608.89
  tuberculous (*see also* Tuberculosis) 016.5●
  varicose 456.4
seminal vesicle 608.89

Ulcer, ulcerated, ulcerating, ulceration, ulcerative (*Continued*)
sigmoid 569.82
  with perforation 569.83
skin (atrophic) (chronic) (neurogenic) (non-healing) (perforating) (pyogenic) (trophic) 707.9
  with gangrene 707.9 [785.4]
  amebic 006.6
  decubitus (*see also* Ulcer, pressure) 707.00
    with gangrene 707.00 [785.4]
  in granulocytopenia 288.09
  lower extremity (*see also* Ulcer, lower extremity) 707.10
    with gangrene 707.10 [785.4]
      arteriosclerotic 440.24
    ankle 707.13
    arteriosclerotic 440.23
      with gangrene 440.24
    calf 707.12
    foot 707.15
    heel 707.14
    knee 707.19
    specified site NEC 707.19
    thigh 707.11
    toes 707.15
  mycobacterial 031.1
  syphilitic (early) (secondary) 091.3
  tuberculous (primary) (*see also* Tuberculosis) 017.0●
  varicose - *see* Ulcer, varicose
sloughing NEC - *see* Ulcer, skin
soft palate 528.9
solitary, anus or rectum (sphincter) 569.41
sore throat 462
  streptococcal 034.0
spermatic cord 608.89
spine (tuberculous) 015.0● [730.88]
stasis (leg) (venous) 454.0
  with varicose veins 454.0
  without varicose veins 459.81
  inflamed or infected 454.2
stercoral, stercoraceous 569.82
  with perforation 569.83
  anus or rectum 569.41
stoma, stomal - *see* Ulcer, gastrojejunal
stomach (eroded) (peptic) (round) 531.9●

Note 73 Use the following fifth-digit subclassification with categories 531–534:

  0 without mention of obstruction
  1 with obstruction

  with
    hemorrhage 531.4●
      and perforation 531.6●
    perforation (chronic) 531.5●
      and hemorrhage 531.6●
  acute 531.3●
    with
      hemorrhage 531.0●
        and perforation 531.2●
      perforation 531.1●
        and hemorrhage 531.2●
  bleeding (recurrent) - *see* Ulcer, stomach, with hemorrhage

Ulcer, ulcerated, ulcerating, ulceration, ulcerative (*Continued*)
stomach (*Continued*)
  chronic 531.7●
    with
      hemorrhage 531.4●
        and perforation 531.6●
      perforation 531.5●
        and hemorrhage 531.6●
  penetrating - *see* Ulcer, stomach, with perforation
  perforating - *see* Ulcer, stomach, with perforation
stomatitis 528.00
stress - *see* Ulcer, peptic
strumous (tuberculous) (*see also* Tuberculosis) 017.2●
submental (*see also* Ulcer, skin) 707.8
submucosal, bladder 595.1
syphilitic (any site) (early) (secondary) 091.3
  late 095.9
  perforating 095.9
    foot 094.0
testis 608.89
thigh - *see* Ulcer, lower extremity
throat 478.29
  diphtheritic 032.0
toe - *see* Ulcer, lower extremity
tongue (traumatic) 529.0
tonsil 474.8
  diphtheritic 032.0
trachea 519.19
trophic - *see* Ulcer, skin
tropical NEC (*see also* Ulcer, skin) 707.9
tuberculous - *see* Tuberculosis, ulcer
tunica vaginalis 608.89
turbinate 730.9●
typhoid (fever) 002.0
  perforating 002.0
umbilicus (newborn) 771.4
unspecified site NEC - *see* Ulcer, skin
urethra (meatus) (*see also* Urethritis) 597.89
uterus 621.8
  cervix 622.0
    with mention of cervicitis 616.0
  neck 622.0
    with mention of cervicitis 616.0
vagina 616.89
valve, heart 421.0
varicose (lower extremity, any part) 454.0
  anus - *see* Varicose, ulcer, anus
  broad ligament 456.5
  esophagus (*see also* Varix, esophagus) 456.1
    bleeding (*see also* Varix, esophagus, bleeding) 456.0
  inflamed or infected 454.2
  nasal septum 456.8
  perineum 456.6
  rectum - *see* Varicose, ulcer, anus
  scrotum 456.4
  specified site NEC 456.8
  sublingual 456.3
  vulva 456.6
vas deferens 608.89
vesical (*see also* Ulcer, bladder) 596.8
vulva (acute) (infectional) 616.50
  Behçet's syndrome 136.1 [616.51]
  herpetic 054.12
  tuberculous 016.7● [616.51]

Ulcer, ulcerated, ulcerating, ulceration, ulcerative (Continued)
vulvobuccal, recurring 616.50
x-ray - see Ulcer, by site
yaws 102.4
Ulcerosa scarlatina 034.1
Ulcus - see also Ulcer
cutis tuberculosum (see also
Tuberculosis) 017.0●
duodeni - see Ulcer, duodenum
durum 091.0
extragenital 091.2
gastrojejunale - see Ulcer, gastrojejunal
hypostaticum - see Ulcer, varicose
molle (cutis) (skin) 099.0
serpens corneae (pneumococcal)
370.04
ventriculi - see Ulcer, stomach
Ulegyria 742.4
Ulerythema
acneiforma 701.8
centrifugum 695.4
ophryogenes 757.4
Ullrich (-Bonnevie) (-Turner) syndrome
758.6
Ullrich-Feichtiger syndrome 759.89
Ulnar - see condition
Ulorrhagia 523.8
Ulorrhea 523.8
Umbilicus, umbilical - see also condition
cord necrosis, affecting fetus or
newborn 762.6
Unacceptable
existing dental restoration
contours 525.65
morphology 525.65
Unavailability of medical facilities (at)
V63.9
due to
investigation by social service
agency V63.8
lack of services at home V63.1
remoteness from facility V63.0
waiting list V63.2
home V63.1
outpatient clinic V63.0
specified reason NEC V63.8
Uncinaria americana infestation 126.1
Uncinariasis (see also Ancylostomiasis)
126.9
Unconscious, unconsciousness 780.09
Underdevelopment - see also
Undeveloped sexual 259.0
Underfill, endodontic 526.63
Undernourishment 269.9
Undernutrition 269.9
Under observation - see Observation
Underweight 783.22
for gestational age - see Light-for-dates
Underwood's disease (sclerema
neonatorum) 778.1
Undescended - see also Malposition,
congenital
cecum 751.4
colon 751.4
testis 752.51
Undetermined diagnosis or cause
799.9
Undeveloped, undevelopment - see also
Hypoplasia
brain (congenital) 742.1
cerebral (congenital) 742.1
fetus or newborn 764.9●
heart 746.89

Undeveloped, undevelopment
(Continued)
lung 748.5
testis 257.2
uterus 259.0
Undiagnosed (disease) 799.9
Undulant fever (see also Brucellosis) 023.9
Unemployment, anxiety concerning
V62.0
Unequal leg (acquired) (length) 736.81
congenital 755.30
Unerupted teeth, tooth 520.6
Unextracted dental root 525.3
Unguis incarnatus 703.0
Unicornis uterus 752.3
Unicorporeus uterus 752.3
Uniformis uterus 752.3
Unilateral - see also condition
development, breast 611.89
organ or site, congenital NEC - see
Agenesis
vagina 752.49
Unilateralis uterus 752.3
Unilocular heart 745.8
Uninhibited bladder 596.54
with cauda equina syndrome
344.61
neurogenic (see also Neurogenic,
bladder) 596.54
Union, abnormal - see also Fusion
divided tendon 727.89
larynx and trachea 748.3
Universal
joint, cervix 620.6
mesentery 751.4
Unknown
cause of death 799.9
diagnosis 799.9
Unna's disease (seborrheic dermatitis)
690.10
Unresponsiveness, adrenocorticotropin
(ACTH) 255.41
Unsatisfactory
cytology smear
anal 796.78
cervical 795.08
vaginal 795.18
restoration, tooth (existing) 525.60
specified NEC 525.69
Unsoundness of mind (see also Psychosis)
298.9
Unspecified cause of death 799.9
Unstable
back NEC 724.9
colon 569.89
joint - see Instability, joint
lie 652.0●
affecting fetus or newborn (before
labor) 761.7
causing obstructed labor 660.0●
affecting fetus or newborn
763.1
lumbosacral joint (congenital)
756.19
acquired 724.6
sacroiliac 724.6
spine NEC 724.9
Untruthfulness, child problem (see also
Disturbance, conduct) 312.0●
Unverricht (-Lundborg) disease,
syndrome, or epilepsy 345.1   ◄▥
Unverricht-Wagner syndrome
(dermatomyositis) 710.3
Upper respiratory - see condition

Upset
gastric 536.8
psychogenic 306.4
gastrointestinal 536.8
psychogenic 306.4
virus (see also Enteritis, viral)
008.8
intestinal (large) (small) 564.9
psychogenic 306.4
menstruation 626.9
mental 300.9
stomach 536.8
psychogenic 306.4
Urachus - see also condition
patent 753.7
persistent 753.7
Uratic arthritis 274.00   ◄▥
Urbach's lipoid proteinosis 272.8
Urbach-Oppenheim disease or syndrome
(necrobiosis lipoidica diabeticorum)
250.8● [709.3]
due to secondary diabetes 249.8●
[709.3]
Urbach-Wiethe disease or syndrome
(lipoid proteinosis) 272.8
Urban yellow fever 060.1
Urea, blood, high - see Uremia
Uremia, uremic (absorption) (amaurosis)
(amblyopia) (aphasia) (apoplexy)
(coma) (delirium) (dementia)
(dropsy) (dyspnea) (fever)
(intoxication) (mania) (paralysis)
(poisoning) (toxemia) (vomiting)
586
with
abortion - see Abortion, by type,
with renal failure
ectopic pregnancy (see also
categories 633.0–633.9) 639.3
hypertension (see also Hypertension,
kidney) 403.91
molar pregnancy (see also categories
630–632) 639.3
chronic 585.9
complicating
abortion 639.3
ectopic or molar pregnancy 639.3
hypertension (see also Hypertension,
kidney) 403.91
labor and delivery 669.3●
congenital 779.89
extrarenal 788.99
hypertensive (chronic) (see also
Hypertension, kidney)
403.91
maternal NEC, affecting fetus or
newborn 760.1
neuropathy 585.9 [357.4]
pericarditis 585.9 [420.0]
prerenal 788.99
pyelitic (see also Pyelitis) 590.80
Ureter, ureteral - see condition
Ureteralgia 788.0
Ureterectasis 593.89
Ureteritis 593.89
cystica 590.3
due to calculus 592.1
gonococcal (acute) 098.19
chronic or duration of 2 months or
over 098.39
nonspecific 593.89
Ureterocele (acquired) 593.89
congenital 753.23
Ureterolith 592.1

◄ New   ◄▥ Revised   ~~deleted~~ Deleted   ● Use Additional Digit(s)   ▬ Omit code

Ureterolithiasis 592.1
Ureterostomy status V44.6
　with complication 997.5
Urethra, urethral - *see* condition
Urethralgia 788.99
Urethritis (abacterial) (acute) (allergic)
　(anterior) (chronic) (nonvenereal)
　(posterior) (recurrent) (simple)
　(subacute) (ulcerative)
　(undifferentiated) 597.80
　diplococcal (acute) 098.0
　　chronic or duration of 2 months or
　　　over 098.2
　due to Trichomonas (vaginalis)
　　131.02
　gonococcal (acute) 098.0
　　chronic or duration of 2 months or
　　　over 098.2
　nongonococcal (sexually transmitted)
　　099.40
　　Chlamydia trachomatis 099.41
　　Reiter's 099.3
　　specified organism NEC 099.49
　nonspecific (sexually transmitted) (*see
　　also* Urethritis, nongonococcal)
　　099.40
　not sexually transmitted 597.80
　Reiter's 099.3
　trichomonal or due to Trichomonas
　　(vaginalis) 131.02
　tuberculous (*see also* Tuberculosis)
　　016.3●
　venereal NEC (*see also* Urethritis,
　　nongonococcal) 099.40
Urethrocele
　female 618.03
　　with uterine prolapse 618.4
　　　complete 618.3
　　　incomplete 618.2
　male 599.5
Urethrolithiasis 594.2
Urethro-oculoarticular syndrome
　099.3
Urethro-oculosynovial syndrome
　099.3
Urethrorectal - *see* condition
Urethrorrhagia 599.84
Urethrorrhea 788.7
Urethrostomy status V44.6
　with complication 997.5
Urethrotrigonitis 595.3
Urethrovaginal - *see* condition
Urhidrosis, uridrosis 705.89
Uric acid
　diathesis 274.9
　in blood 790.6
Uricacidemia 790.6
Uricemia 790.6
Uricosuria 791.9
Urination
　frequent 788.41
　painful 788.1
　urgency 788.63
Urine, urinary - *see also* condition
　abnormality NEC 788.69
　blood in (*see also* Hematuria)
　　599.70
　discharge, excessive 788.42
　enuresis 788.30
　　nonorganic origin 307.6
　extravasation 788.8
　frequency 788.41
　hesitancy 788.64

Urine, urinary (*Continued*)
　incontinence 788.30
　　active 788.30
　　female 788.30
　　　stress 625.6
　　　　and urge 788.33
　　male 788.30
　　　stress 788.32
　　　　and urge 788.33
　　mixed (stress and urge) 788.33
　　neurogenic 788.39
　　nonorganic origin 307.6
　　overflow 788.38
　　stress (female) 625.6
　　　male NEC 788.32
　intermittent stream 788.61
　pus in 791.9
　retention or stasis NEC 788.20
　　bladder, incomplete emptying
　　　788.21
　　psychogenic 306.53
　　specified NEC 788.29
　secretion
　　deficient 788.5
　　excessive 788.42
　　frequency 788.41
　strain 788.65
　stream
　　intermittent 788.61
　　slowing 788.62
　　splitting 788.61
　　weak 788.62
　urgency 788.63
Urinemia - *see* Uremia
Urinoma NEC 599.9
　bladder 596.8
　kidney 593.89
　renal 593.89
　ureter 593.89
　urethra 599.84
Uroarthritis, infectious 099.3
Urodialysis 788.5
Urolithiasis 592.9
Uronephrosis 593.89
Uropathy 599.9
　obstructive 599.60
Urosepsis 599.0
　meaning sepsis 995.91
　meaning urinary tract infection 599.0
Urticaria 708.9
　with angioneurotic edema 995.1
　　hereditary 277.6
　allergic 708.0
　cholinergic 708.5
　chronic 708.8
　cold, familial 708.2
　dermatographic 708.3
　due to
　　cold or heat 708.2
　　drugs 708.0
　　food 708.0
　　inhalants 708.0
　　plants 708.8
　　serum 999.5
　factitial 708.3
　giant 995.1
　　hereditary 277.6
　gigantea 995.1
　　hereditary 277.6
　idiopathic 708.1
　larynx 995.1
　　hereditary 277.6
　neonatorum 778.8

Urticaria (*Continued*)
　nonallergic 708.1
　papulosa (Hebra) 698.2
　perstans hemorrhagica 757.39
　pigmentosa 757.33
　recurrent periodic 708.8
　serum 999.5
　solare 692.72
　specified type NEC 708.8
　thermal (cold) (heat) 708.2
　vibratory 708.4
Urticarioides acarodermatitis 133.9
Use of
　methadone 304.00
　nonprescribed drugs (*see also* Abuse,
　　drugs, nondependent) 305.9●
　patent medicines (*see also* Abuse, drugs,
　　nondependent) 305.9●
Usher-Senear disease (pemphigus
　erythematosus) 694.4
Uta 085.5
Uterine size-date discrepancy 649.6●
Uteromegaly 621.2
Uterovaginal - *see* condition
Uterovesical - *see* condition
Uterus - *see* condition
Utriculitis (utriculus prostaticus) 597.89
Uveal - *see* condition
Uveitis (anterior) (*see also* Iridocyclitis)
　364.3
　acute or subacute 364.00
　　due to or associated with
　　　gonococcal infection 098.41
　　　herpes (simplex) 054.44
　　　zoster 053.22
　　primary 364.01
　　recurrent 364.02
　　secondary (noninfectious) 364.04
　　　infectious 364.03
　allergic 360.11
　chronic 364.10
　　due to or associated with
　　　sarcoidosis 135 [*364.11*]
　　　tuberculosis (*see also* Tuberculosis)
　　　　017.3● [*364.11*]
　due to
　　operation 360.11
　　toxoplasmosis (acquired) 130.2
　　　congenital (active) 771.2
　granulomatous 364.10
　heterochromic 364.21
　lens-induced 364.23
　nongranulomatous 364.00
　posterior 363.20
　　disseminated - *see* Chorioretinitis,
　　　disseminated
　　focal - *see* Chorioretinitis, focal
　recurrent 364.02
　sympathetic 360.11
　syphilitic (secondary) 091.50
　　congenital 090.0 [*363.13*]
　　late 095.8 [*363.13*]
　tuberculous (*see also* Tuberculosis)
　　017.3● [*364.11*]
Uveoencephalitis 363.22
Uveokeratitis (*see also* Iridocyclitis) 364.3
Uveoparotid fever 135
Uveoparotitis 135
Uvula - *see* condition
Uvulitis (acute) (catarrhal) (chronic)
　(gangrenous) (membranous)
　(suppurative) (ulcerative) 528.3

V

Vaccination
- complication or reaction - *see*
  - Complications, vaccination
- delayed V64.00
- not carried out V64.00
  - because of
    - acute illness V64.01
    - allergy to vaccine or component V64.04
    - caregiver refusal V64.05
    - chronic illness V64.02
    - guardian refusal V64.05
    - immune compromised state V64.03
    - parent refusal V64.05
    - patient had disease being vaccinated against V64.08
    - patient refusal V64.06
    - reason NEC V64.09
    - religious reasons V64.07
- prophylactic (against) V05.9
  - arthropod-borne viral
    - disease NEC V05.1
    - encephalitis V05.0
  - chicken pox V05.4
  - cholera (alone) V03.0
    - with typhoid-paratyphoid (cholera + TAB) V06.0
  - common cold V04.7
  - diphtheria (alone) V03.5
    - with
      - poliomyelitis (DTP + polio) V06.3
      - tetanus V06.5
        - pertussis combined [DTP] (DTaP) V06.1
        - typhoid-paratyphoid (DTP + TAB) V06.2
  - disease (single) NEC V05.9
    - bacterial NEC V03.9
      - specified type NEC V03.89
    - combination NEC V06.9
      - specified type NEC V06.8
    - specified type NEC V05.8
  - encephalitis, viral, arthropod-borne V05.0
  - Hemophilus influenzae, type B [Hib] V03.81
  - hepatitis, viral V05.3
  - influenza V04.81
    - with
      - Streptococcus pneumoniae [pneumococcus] V06.6
  - leishmaniasis V05.2
  - measles (alone) V04.2
    - with mumps-rubella (MMR) V06.4
  - mumps (alone) V04.6
    - with measles and rubella (MMR) V06.4
  - pertussis alone V03.6
  - plague V03.3
  - poliomyelitis V04.0
    - with diphtheria-tetanus-pertussis (DTP polio) V06.3
  - rabies V04.5
  - respiratory syncytial virus (RSV) V04.82
  - rubella (alone) V04.3
    - with measles and mumps (MMR) V06.4

Vaccination *(Continued)*
- prophylactic *(Continued)*
  - smallpox V04.1
  - Streptococcus pneumoniae [pneumococcus] V03.82
    - with
      - influenza V06.6
  - tetanus toxoid (alone) V03.7
    - with diphtheria [Td] [DT] V06.5
      - with
        - pertussis (DTP) (DTaP) V06.1
          - with poliomyelitis (DTP + polio) V06.3
  - tuberculosis (BCG) V03.2
  - tularemia V03.4
  - typhoid-paratyphoid (TAB) (alone) V03.1
    - with diphtheria-tetanus-pertussis (TAB + DTP) V06.2
  - varicella V05.4
  - viral
    - disease NEC V04.89
    - encephalitis, arthropod-borne V05.0
    - hepatitis V05.3
  - yellow fever V04.4
Vaccinia (generalized) 999.0
- congenital 771.2
- conjunctiva 999.39
- eyelids 999.0 *[373.5]*
- localized 999.39
- nose 999.39
- not from vaccination 051.02
  - eyelid 051.02 *[373.5]*
- sine vaccinatione 051.02
- without vaccination 051.02
Vacuum
- extraction of fetus or newborn 763.3
- in sinus (accessory) (nasal) (*see also* Sinusitis) 473.9
Vagabond V60.0
Vagabondage V60.0
Vagabonds' disease 132.1
Vagina, vaginal - *see also* condition
- high risk human papillomavirus (HPV) DNA test positive 795.15
- low risk human papillomavirus (HPV) DNA test positive 795.19
Vaginalitis (tunica) 608.4
Vaginismus (reflex) 625.1
- functional 306.51
- hysterical 300.11
- psychogenic 306.51
Vaginitis (acute) (chronic) (circumscribed) (diffuse) (emphysematous) (Hemophilus vaginalis) (nonspecific) (nonvenereal) (ulcerative) 616.10
- with
  - abortion - *see* Abortion, by type, with sepsis
  - ectopic pregnancy (*see also* categories 633.0–633.9) 639.0
  - molar pregnancy (*see also* categories 630–632) 639.0
- adhesive, congenital 752.49
- atrophic, postmenopausal 627.3
- bacterial 616.10
- blennorrhagic (acute) 098.0
  - chronic or duration of 2 months or over 098.2
- candidal 112.1

Vaginitis *(Continued)*
- chlamydial 099.53
- complicating pregnancy or puerperium 646.6●
  - affecting fetus or newborn 760.8
- congenital (adhesive) 752.49
- due to
  - C. albicans 112.1
  - Trichomonas (vaginalis) 131.01
- following
  - abortion 639.0
  - ectopic or molar pregnancy 639.0
- gonococcal (acute) 098.0
  - chronic or duration of 2 months or over 098.2
- granuloma 099.2
- Monilia 112.1
- mycotic 112.1
- pinworm 127.4 *[616.11]*
- postirradiation 616.10
- postmenopausal atrophic 627.3
- senile (atrophic) 627.3
- syphilitic (early) 091.0
  - late 095.8
- trichomonal 131.01
- tuberculous (*see also* Tuberculosis) 016.7●
- venereal NEC 099.8
Vaginosis - *see* Vaginitis
Vagotonia 352.3
Vagrancy V60.0
VAIN I (vaginal intraepithelial neoplasia I) 623.0
VAIN II (vaginal intraepithelial neoplasia II) 623.0
VAIN III (vaginal intraepithelial neoplasia III) 233.31
Vallecula - *see* condition
Valley fever 114.0
Valsuani's disease (progressive pernicious anemia, puerperal) 648.2●
Valve, valvular (formation) - *see also* condition
- cerebral ventricle (communicating) in situ V45.2
- cervix, internal os 752.49
- colon 751.5
- congenital NEC - *see* Atresia
- formation congenital NEC - *see* Atresia
- heart defect - *see* Anomaly, heart, valve
- ureter 753.29
  - pelvic junction 753.21
  - vesical orifice 753.22
- urethra 753.6
Valvulitis (chronic) (*see also* Endocarditis) 424.90
- rheumatic (chronic) (inactive) (with chorea) 397.9
  - active or acute (aortic) (mitral) (pulmonary) (tricuspid) 391.1
- syphilitic NEC 093.20
  - aortic 093.22
  - mitral 093.21
  - pulmonary 093.24
  - tricuspid 093.23
Valvulopathy - *see* Endocarditis
van Bogaert's leukoencephalitis (sclerosing) (subacute) 046.2
van Bogaert-Nijssen (-Peiffer) disease 330.0
van Buchem's syndrome (hyperostosis corticalis) 733.3

◀ New ◀‖‖ Revised ~~deleted~~ Deleted ● Use Additional Digit(s) ▨ Omit code

Vancomycin (glycopeptide)
  intermediate staphylococcus aureus
    (VISA/GISA) V09.8
  resistant
    enterococcus (VRE) V09.8
    staphylococcus aureus (VRSA/
      GRSA) V09.8
van Creveld-von Gierke disease
  (glycogenosis I) 271.0
van den Bergh's disease (enterogenous
  cyanosis) 289.7
van der Hoeve's syndrome (brittle bones
  and blue sclera, deafness) 756.51
van der Hoeve-Halbertsma-
  Waardenburg syndrome (ptosis-
  epicanthus) 270.2
van der Hoeve-Waardenburg-Gualdi
  syndrome (ptosis-epicanthus) 270.2
Vanillism 692.89
Vanishing lung 492.0
Vanishing twin 651.33
van Neck (-Odelberg) disease or
  syndrome (juvenile osteochondrosis)
  732.1
Vapor asphyxia or suffocation NEC 987.9
  specified agent - see Table of Drugs and
    Chemicals
Vaquez's disease (M9950/1) 238.4
Vaquez-Osler disease (polycythemia
  vera) (M9950/1) 238.4
Variance, lethal ball, prosthetic heart
  valve 996.02
Variants, thalassemic 282.49
Variations in hair color 704.3
Varicella 052.9
  with
    complication 052.8
      specified NEC 052.7
    pneumonia 052.1
  exposure to V01.71
  vaccination and inoculation (against)
    (prophylactic) V05.4
Varices - see Varix
Varicocele (scrotum) (thrombosed) 456.4
  ovary 456.5
  perineum 456.6
  spermatic cord (ulcerated) 456.4
Varicose
  aneurysm (ruptured) (see also
    Aneurysm) 442.9
  dermatitis (lower extremity) - see
    Varicose, vein, inflamed or
    infected
  eczema - see Varicose, vein
  phlebitis - see Varicose, vein, inflamed
    or infected
  placental vessel - see Placenta,
    abnormal
  tumor - see Varicose, vein
  ulcer (lower extremity, any part) 454.0
    anus 455.8
      external 455.5
      internal 455.2
    esophagus (see also Varix,
      esophagus) 456.1
      bleeding (see also Varix,
        esophagus, bleeding)
        456.0
    inflamed or infected 454.2
    nasal septum 456.8
    perineum 456.6
    rectum - see Varicose, ulcer, anus
    scrotum 456.4
    specified site NEC 456.8

Varicose (Continued)
  vein (lower extremity) (ruptured) (see
    also Varix) 454.9
    with
      complications NEC 454.8
      edema 454.8
      inflammation or infection 454.1
        ulcerated 454.2
      pain 454.8
      stasis dermatitis 454.1
        with ulcer 454.2
      swelling 454.8
      ulcer 454.0
        inflamed or infected 454.2
    anus - see Hemorrhoids
    broad ligament 456.5
    congenital (peripheral) 747.60
      gastrointestinal 747.61
      lower limb 747.64
      renal 747.62
      specified NEC 747.69
      upper limb 747.63
    esophagus (ulcerated (see also Varix,
      esophagus) 456.1
      bleeding (see also Varix,
        esophagus, bleeding)
        456.0
    inflamed or infected 454.1
      with ulcer 454.2
    in pregnancy or puerperium
      671.0●
      vulva or perineum 671.1●
    nasal septum (with ulcer) 456.8
    pelvis 456.5
    perineum 456.6
      in pregnancy, childbirth, or
        puerperium 671.1●
    rectum - see Hemorrhoids
    scrotum (ulcerated) 456.4
    specified site NEC 456.8
    sublingual 456.3
    ulcerated 454.0
      inflamed or infected 454.2
    umbilical cord, affecting fetus or
      newborn 762.6
    urethra 456.8
    vulva 456.6
      in pregnancy, childbirth, or
        puerperium 671.1●
  vessel - see also Varix
    placenta - see Placenta, abnormal
Varicosis, varicosities, varicosity (see also
  Varix) 454.9
Variola 050.9
  hemorrhagic (pustular) 050.0
  major 050.0
  minor 050.1
  modified 050.2
Varioloid 050.2
Variolosa, purpura 050.0
Varix (lower extremity) (ruptured)
  454.9
  with
    complications NEC 454.8
    edema 454.8
    inflammation or infection 454.1
      with ulcer 454.2
    pain 454.8
    stasis dermatitis 454.1
      with ulcer 454.2
    swelling 454.8
    ulcer 454.0
      with inflammation or infection
        454.2

Varix (Continued)
  aneurysmal (see also Aneurysm)
    442.9
  anus - see Hemorrhoids
  arteriovenous (congenital) (peripheral)
    NEC 747.60
    gastrointestinal 747.61
    lower limb 747.64
    renal 747.62
    specified NEC 747.69
    spinal 747.82
    upper limb 747.63
  bladder 456.5
  broad ligament 456.5
  congenital (peripheral) 747.60
  esophagus (ulcerated) 456.1
    bleeding 456.0
    in
      cirrhosis of liver 571.5
        [456.20]
      portal hypertension 572.3
        [456.20]
    congenital 747.69
    in
      cirrhosis of liver 571.5 [456.21]
        with bleeding 571.5 [456.20]
      portal hypertension 572.3 [456.21]
        with bleeding 572.3 [456.20]
  gastric 456.8
  inflamed or infected 454.1
    ulcerated 454.2
  in pregnancy or puerperium 671.0●
    perineum 671.1●
    vulva 671.1●
  labia (majora) 456.6
  orbit 456.8
    congenital 747.69
  ovary 456.5
  papillary 448.1
  pelvis 456.5
  perineum 456.6
    in pregnancy or puerperium
      671.1●
  pharynx 456.8
  placenta - see Placenta, abnormal
  prostate 456.8
  rectum - see Hemorrhoids
  renal papilla 456.8
  retina 362.17
  scrotum (ulcerated) 456.4
  sigmoid colon 456.8
  specified site NEC 456.8
  spinal (cord) (vessels) 456.8
  spleen, splenic (vein) (with phlebolith)
    456.8
  sublingual 456.3
  ulcerated 454.0
    inflamed or infected 454.2
  umbilical cord, affecting fetus or
    newborn 762.6
  uterine ligament 456.5
  vocal cord 456.8
  vulva 456.6
    in pregnancy, childbirth, or
      puerperium 671.1●
Vasa previa 663.5●
  affecting fetus or newborn 762.6
  hemorrhage from, affecting fetus or
    newborn 772.0
Vascular - see also condition
  loop on papilla (optic) 743.57
  sheathing, retina 362.13
  spasm 443.9
  spider 448.1

Vascularity, pulmonary, congenital 747.3
Vascularization
   choroid 362.16
   cornea 370.60
     deep 370.63
     localized 370.61
   retina 362.16
   subretinal 362.16
Vasculitis 447.6
   allergic 287.0
   cryoglobulinemic 273.2
   disseminated 447.6
   kidney 447.8
   leukocytoclastic 446.29
   nodular 695.2
   retinal 362.18
   rheumatic - see Fever, rheumatic
Vasculopathy
   cardiac allograft 996.83
Vas deferens - see condition
Vas deferentitis 608.4
Vasectomy, admission for V25.2
Vasitis 608.4
   nodosa 608.4
   scrotum 608.4
   spermatic cord 608.4
   testis 608.4
   tuberculous (see also Tuberculosis)
     016.5●
   tunica vaginalis 608.4
   vas deferens 608.4
Vasodilation 443.9
Vasomotor - see condition
Vasoplasty, after previous sterilization
   V26.0
Vasoplegia, splanchnic (see also
   Neuropathy, peripheral, autonomic)
   337.9
Vasospasm 443.9
   cerebral (artery) 435.9
     with transient neurologic deficit
       435.9
   coronary 413.1
   nerve
     arm NEC 354.9
     autonomic 337.9
     brachial plexus 353.0
     cervical plexus 353.2
     leg NEC 355.8
     lower extremity NEC 355.8
     peripheral NEC 335.9
     spinal NEC 355.9
     sympathetic 337.9
     upper extremity NEC 354.9
   peripheral NEC 443.9
   retina (artery) (see also Occlusion,
     retinal, artery) 362.30
Vasospastic - see condition
Vasovagal attack (paroxysmal) 780.2
   psychogenic 306.2
Vater's ampulla - see condition
VATER syndrome 759.89
vCJD (variant Creutzfeldt-Jakob disease)
   046.11
Vegetation, vegetative
   adenoid (nasal fossa) 474.2
   consciousness (persistent) 780.03
   endocarditis (acute) (any valve)
     (chronic) (subacute) 421.0
   heart (mycotic) (valve) 421.0
   state (persistent) 780.03
Veil
   Jackson's 751.4
   over face (causing asphyxia) 768.9

Vein, venous - see condition
Veldt sore (see also Ulcer, skin) 707.9
Velo-cardio-facial syndrome 758.32
Velpeau's hernia - see Hernia, femoral
Venereal
   balanitis NEC 099.8
   bubo 099.1
   disease 099.9
     specified nature or type NEC 099.8
   granuloma inguinale 099.2
   lymphogranuloma (Durand-Nicolas-
     Favre), any site 099.1
   salpingitis 098.37
   urethritis (see also Urethritis,
     nongonococcal) 099.40
   vaginitis NEC 099.8
   warts 078.11
Vengefulness, in child (see also
   Disturbance, conduct) 312.0●
Venofibrosis 459.89
Venom, venomous
   bite or sting (animal or insect) 989.5
   poisoning 989.5
Venous - see condition
Ventouse delivery NEC 669.5●
   affecting fetus or newborn 763.3
Ventral - see condition
Ventricle, ventricular - see also condition
   escape 427.69
   standstill (see also Arrest, cardiac)
     427.5
Ventriculitis, cerebral (see also Meningitis)
   322.9
Ventriculostomy status V45.2
Verbiest's syndrome (claudicatio
   intermittens spinalis) 435.1
Vernet's syndrome 352.6
Verneuil's disease (syphilitic bursitis)
   095.7
Verruca (filiformis) 078.10
   acuminata (any site) 078.11
   necrogenica (primary) (see also
     Tuberculosis) 017.0●
   peruana 088.0
   peruviana 088.0
   plana (juvenilis) 078.19
   plantaris 078.12
   seborrheica 702.19
     inflamed 702.11
   senilis 702.0
   tuberculosa (primary) (see also
     Tuberculosis) 017.0●
   venereal 078.11
   viral 078.10
     specified NEC 078.19
   vulgaris 078.10
Verrucosities (see also Verruca) 078.10
Verrucous endocarditis (acute) (any
   valve) (chronic) (subacute) 710.0
   [424.91]
   nonbacterial 710.0 [424.91]
Verruga
   peruana 088.0
   peruviana 088.0
Verse's disease (calcinosis
   intervertebralis) 275.49 [722.90]
Version
   before labor, affecting fetus or newborn
     761.7
   cephalic (correcting previous
     malposition) 652.1●
     affecting fetus or newborn
       763.1
   cervix - see Version, uterus

Version (Continued)
   uterus (postinfectional) (postpartal,
     old) (see also Malposition, uterus)
     621.6
     forward - see Anteversion, uterus
     lateral - see Lateroversion, uterus
Vertebra, vertebral - see condition
Vertigo 780.4
   auditory 386.19
   aural 386.19
   benign paroxysmal positional 386.11
   central origin 386.2
   cerebral 386.2
   Dix and Hallpike (epidemic) 386.12
   endemic paralytic 078.81
   epidemic 078.81
     Dix and Hallpike 386.12
     Gerlier's 078.81
     Pedersen's 386.12
     vestibular neuronitis 386.12
   epileptic - see Epilepsy
   Gerlier's (epidemic) 078.81
   hysterical 300.11
   labyrinthine 386.10
   laryngeal 786.2
   malignant positional 386.2
   Ménière's (see also Disease, Ménière's)
     386.00
   menopausal 627.2
   otogenic 386.19
   paralytic 078.81
   paroxysmal positional, benign
     386.11
   Pedersen's (epidemic) 386.12
   peripheral 386.10
     specified type NEC 386.19
   positional
     benign paroxysmal 386.11
     malignant 386.2
Verumontanitis (chronic) (see also
   Urethritis) 597.89
Vesania (see also Psychosis) 298.9
Vesical - see condition
Vesicle
   cutaneous 709.8
   seminal - see condition
   skin 709.8
Vesicocolic - see condition
Vesicoperineal - see condition
Vesicorectal - see condition
Vesicourethrorectal - see condition
Vesicovaginal - see condition
Vesicular - see condition
Vesiculitis (seminal) 608.0
   amebic 006.8
   gonorrheal (acute) 098.14
     chronic or duration of 2 months or
       over 098.34
   trichomonal 131.09
   tuberculous (see also Tuberculosis)
     016.5● [608.81]
Vestibulitis (ear) (see also Labyrinthitis)
   386.30
   nose (external) 478.19
   vulvar 625.71
Vestibulopathy, acute peripheral
   (recurrent) 386.12
Vestige, vestigial - see also Persistence
   branchial 744.41
   structures in vitreous 743.51
Vibriosis NEC 027.9
Vidal's disease (lichen simplex chronicus)
   698.3
Video display tube syndrome 723.8

◀ New   ⬅III Revised   deleted Deleted   ● Use Additional Digit(s)   Omit code

Vienna-type encephalitis 049.8
Villaret's syndrome 352.6
Villous - see condition
VIN I (vulvar intraepithelial neoplasia I) 624.01
VIN II (vulvar intraepithelial neoplasia II) 624.02
VIN III (vulvar intraepithelial neoplasia III) 233.32
Vincent's
  angina 101
  bronchitis 101
  disease 101
  gingivitis 101
  infection (any site) 101
  laryngitis 101
  stomatitis 101
  tonsillitis 101
Vinson-Plummer syndrome (sideropenic dysphagia) 280.8
Viosterol deficiency (see also Deficiency, calciferol) 268.9
Virchow's disease 733.99
Viremia 790.8
Virilism (adrenal) (female) NEC 255.2
  with
    3-beta-hydroxysteroid dehydrogenase defect 255.2
    11-hydroxylase defect 255.2
    21-hydroxylase defect 255.2
    adrenal
      hyperplasia 255.2
      insufficiency (congenital) 255.2
    cortical hyperfunction 255.2
Virilization (female) (suprarenal) (see also Virilism) 255.2
  isosexual 256.4
Virulent bubo 099.0
Virus, viral - see also condition
  infection NEC (see also Infection, viral) 079.99
  septicemia 079.99
  yaba monkey tumor 059.22
VISA (vancomycin intermediate staphylococcus aureus) V09.8
Viscera, visceral - see condition
Visceroptosis 569.89
Visible peristalsis 787.4
Vision, visual
  binocular, suppression 368.31
  blurred, blurring 368.8
    hysterical 300.11
  defect, defective (see also Impaired, vision) 369.9
  disorientation (syndrome) 368.16
  disturbance NEC (see also Disturbance, vision) 368.9
    hysterical 300.11
  examination V72.0
  field, limitation 368.40
  fusion, with defective steropsis 368.33
  hallucinations 368.16
  halos 368.16
  loss 369.9
    both eyes (see also Blindness, both eyes) 369.3
    complete (see also Blindness, both eyes) 369.00
    one eye 369.8
    sudden 368.16
  low (both eyes) 369.20
    one eye (other eye normal) (see also Impaired, vision) 369.70
      blindness, other eye 369.10

Vision, visual (Continued)
  perception, simultaneous without fusion 368.32
  tunnel 368.45
Vitality, lack or want of 780.79
  newborn 779.89
Vitamin deficiency NEC (see also Deficiency, vitamin) 269.2
Vitelline duct, persistent 751.0
Vitiligo 709.01
  due to pinta (carate) 103.2
  eyelid 374.53
  vulva 624.8
Vitium cordis - see Disease, heart
Vitreous - see also condition
  touch syndrome 997.99
VLCAD (long chain/very long chain acyl CoA dehydrogenase deficiency, LCAD) 277.85
Vocal cord - see condition
Vocational rehabilitation V57.22
Vogt's (Cecile) disease or syndrome 333.7
Vogt-Koyanagi syndrome 364.24
Vogt-Spielmeyer disease (amaurotic familial idiocy) 330.1
Voice
  change (see also Dysphonia) 784.49
  loss (see also Aphonia) 784.41
Volhard-Fahr disease (malignant nephrosclerosis) 403.00
Volhynian fever 083.1
Volkmann's ischemic contracture or paralysis (complicating trauma) 958.6
Voluntary starvation 307.1
Volvulus (bowel) (colon) (intestine) 560.2
  with
    hernia - see also Hernia, by site, with obstruction
      gangrenous - see Hernia, by site, with gangrene
    perforation 560.2
  congenital 751.5
  duodenum 537.3
  fallopian tube 620.5
  oviduct 620.5
  stomach (due to absence of gastrocolic ligament) 537.89
Vomiting 787.03
  with nausea 787.01
  allergic 535.4 ●
  asphyxia 933.1
  bilious (cause unknown) 787.04
    following gastrointestinal surgery 564.3
    newborn 779.32
  blood (see also Hematemesis) 578.0
  causing asphyxia, choking, or suffocation (see also Asphyxia, food) 933.1
  cyclical 536.2
    associated with migraine 346.2 ●
    psychogenic 306.4
  epidemic 078.82
  fecal matter 569.87
  following gastrointestinal surgery 564.3
  functional 536.8
    psychogenic 306.4
  habit 536.2
  hysterical 300.11
  nervous 306.4
  neurotic 306.4
  newborn 779.33
    bilous 779.32

Vomiting (Continued)
  of or complicating pregnancy 643.9 ●
    due to
      organic disease 643.8 ●
      specific cause NEC 643.8 ●
    early - see Hyperemesis, gravidarum
    late (after 22 completed weeks of gestation) 643.2 ●
  pernicious or persistent 536.2
    complicating pregnancy - see Hyperemesis, gravidarum
    psychogenic 306.4
  physiological 787.03
    bilious 787.04
  psychic 306.4
  psychogenic 307.54
  stercoral 569.89
  uncontrollable 536.2
    psychogenic 306.4
  uremic - see Uremia
  winter 078.82
von Bechterew (-Strümpell) disease or syndrome (ankylosing spondylitis) 720.0
von Bezold's abscess 383.01
von Economo's disease (encephalitis lethargica) 049.8
von Eulenburg's disease (congenital paramyotonia) 359.29
von Gierke's disease (glycogenosis I) 271.0
von Gies' joint 095.8
von Graefe's disease or syndrome 378.72
von Hippel (-Lindau) disease or syndrome (retinocerebral angiomatosis) 759.6
von Jaksch's anemia or disease (pseudoleukemia infantum) 285.8
von Recklinghausen's
  disease or syndrome (nerves) (skin) (M9540/1) 237.71
  bones (osteitis fibrosa cystica) 252.01
  tumor (M9540/1) 237.71
von Recklinghausen-Applebaum disease (hemochromatosis) 275.0
von Schroetter's syndrome (intermittent venous claudication) 453.89
von Willebrand (-Jürgens) (-Minot) disease or syndrome (angiohemophilia) 286.4
von Zambusch's disease (lichen sclerosus et atrophicus) 701.0
Voorhoeve's disease or dyschondroplasia 756.4
Vossius' ring 921.3
  late effect 366.21
Voyeurism 302.82
VRE (vancomycin resistant enterococcus) V09.8
Vrolik's disease (osteogenesis imperfecta) 756.51
VRSA (vancomycin resistant staphylococcus aureus) V09.8
Vulva - see condition
Vulvismus 625.1
Vulvitis (acute) (allergic) (chronic) (gangrenous) (hypertrophic) (intertriginous) 616.10
  with
    abortion - see Abortion, by type, with sepsis
    ectopic pregnancy (see also categories 633.0–633.9) 639.0
    molar pregnancy (see also categories 630–632) 639.0

Vulvitis *(Continued)*
  adhesive, congenital 752.49
  blennorrhagic (acute) 098.0
    chronic or duration of 2 months or
      over 098.2
  chlamydial 099.53
  complicating pregnancy or puerperium
    646.6●
  due to Ducrey's bacillus 099.0
  following
    abortion 639.0
    ectopic or molar pregnancy
      639.0

Vulvitis *(Continued)*
  gonococcal (acute) 098.0
    chronic or duration of
      2 months or over
      098.2
  herpetic 054.11
  leukoplakic 624.09
  monilial 112.1
  puerperal, postpartum, childbirth
    646.6●
  syphilitic (early) 091.0
    late 095.8
  trichomonal 131.01

Vulvodynia 625.70
  specified NEC 625.79
Vulvorectal - *see* condition
Vulvovaginitis *(see also* Vulvitis) 616.10
  amebic 006.8
  chlamydial 099.53
  gonococcal (acute) 098.0
    chronic or duration of 2 months or
      over 098.2
  herpetic 054.11
  monilial 112.1
  trichomonal (Trichomonas vaginalis)
    131.01

◀ New   ◀▥ Revised   ~~deleted~~ Deleted   ● Use Additional Digit(s)   ▨ Omit code

W

Waardenburg's syndrome 756.89
  meaning ptosis-epicanthus 270.2
Waardenburg-Klein syndrome (ptosis-epicanthus) 270.2
Wagner's disease (colloid milium) 709.3
Wagner (-Unverricht) syndrome (dermatomyositis) 710.3
Waiting list, person on V63.2
  undergoing social agency investigation V63.8
Wakefulness disorder (see also Hypersomnia) 780.54
  nonorganic origin 307.43
Waldenström's
  disease (osteochondrosis, capital femoral) 732.1
  hepatitis (lupoid hepatitis) 571.49
  hypergammaglobulinemia 273.0
  macroglobulinemia 273.3
  purpura, hypergammaglobulinemic 273.0
  syndrome (macroglobulinemia) 273.3
Waldenström-Kjellberg syndrome (sideropenic dysphagia) 280.8
Walking
  difficulty 719.7
    psychogenic 307.9
  sleep 307.46
    hysterical 300.13
Wall, abdominal - see condition
Wallenberg's syndrome (posterior inferior cerebellar artery) (see also Disease, cerebrovascular, acute) 436
Wallgren's
  disease (obstruction of splenic vein with collateral circulation) 459.89
  meningitis (see also Meningitis, aseptic) 047.9
Wandering
  acetabulum 736.39
  gallbladder 751.69
  kidney, congenital 753.3
  organ or site, congenital NEC - see Malposition, congenital
  pacemaker (atrial) (heart) 427.89
  spleen 289.59
Wardrop's disease (with lymphangitis) 681.9
  finger 681.02
  toe 681.11
War neurosis 300.16
Wart (digitate) (filiform) (infectious) (viral) 078.10
  common 078.19
  external genital organs (venereal) 078.11
  fig 078.19
  flat 078.19
  genital 078.11
  Hassall-Henle's (of cornea) 371.41
  Henle's (of cornea) 371.41
  juvenile 078.19
  moist 078.10
  Peruvian 088.0
  plantar 078.12
  prosector (see also Tuberculosis) 017.0●
  seborrheic 702.19
    inflamed 702.11
  senile 702.0

Wart (Continued)
  specified NEC 078.19
  syphilitic 091.3
  tuberculous (see also Tuberculosis) 017.0●
  venereal (female) (male) 078.11
Warthin's tumor (salivary gland) (M8561/0) 210.2
Washerwoman's itch 692.4
Wassilieff's disease (leptospiral jaundice) 100.0
Wasting
  disease 799.4
    due to malnutrition 261
  extreme (due to malnutrition) 261
  muscular NEC 728.2
  palsy, paralysis 335.21
  pelvic muscle 618.83
Water
  clefts 366.12
  deprivation of 994.3
  in joint (see also Effusion, joint) 719.0●
  intoxication 276.6
  itch 120.3
  lack of 994.3
  loading 276.6
  on
    brain - see Hydrocephalus
    chest 511.89
  poisoning 276.6
Waterbrash 787.1
Water-hammer pulse (see also Insufficiency, aortic) 424.1
Waterhouse (-Friderichsen) disease or syndrome 036.3
Water-losing nephritis 588.89
Watermelon stomach 537.82
  with hemorrhage 537.83
  without hemorrhage 537.82
Wax in ear 380.4
Waxy
  degeneration, any site 277.39
  disease 277.39
  kidney 277.39 [583.81]
  liver (large) 277.39
  spleen 277.39
Weak, weakness (generalized) 780.79
  arches (acquired) 734
    congenital 754.61
  bladder sphincter 596.59
  congenital 779.89
  eye muscle - see Strabismus
  facial 781.94
  foot (double) - see Weak, arches
  heart, cardiac (see also Failure, heart) 428.9
    congenital 746.9
  mind 317
  muscle (generalized) 728.87
  myocardium (see also Failure, heart) 428.9
  newborn 779.89
  pelvic fundus
    pubocervical tissue 618.81
    rectovaginal tissue 618.82
  pulse 785.9
  senile 797
  urinary stream 788.62
  valvular - see Endocarditis
Wear, worn, tooth, teeth (approximal) (hard tissues) (interproximal) (occlusal) - see also Attrition, teeth 521.10

Weather, weathered
  effects of
    cold NEC 991.9
      specified effect NEC 991.8
    hot (see also Heat) 992.9
  skin 692.74
Web, webbed (congenital) - see also Anomaly, specified type NEC
  canthus 743.63
  digits (see also Syndactylism) 755.10
  duodenal 751.5
  esophagus 750.3
  fingers (see also Syndactylism, fingers) 755.11
  larynx (glottic) (subglottic) 748.2
  neck (pterygium colli) 744.5
  Paterson-Kelly (sideropenic dysphagia) 280.8
  popliteal syndrome 756.89
  toes (see also Syndactylism, toes) 755.13
Weber's paralysis or syndrome 344.89
Weber-Christian disease or syndrome (nodular nonsuppurative panniculitis) 729.30
Weber-Cockayne syndrome (epidermolysis bullosa) 757.39
Weber-Dimitri syndrome 759.6
Weber-Gubler syndrome 344.89
Weber-Leyden syndrome 344.89
Weber-Osler syndrome (familial hemorrhagic telangiectasia) 448.0
Wedge-shaped or wedging vertebra (see also Osteoporosis) 733.00
Wegener's granulomatosis or syndrome 446.4
Wegner's disease (syphilitic osteochondritis) 090.0
Weight
  gain (abnormal) (excessive) 783.1
    during pregnancy 646.1●
      insufficient 646.8●
  less than 1000 grams at birth 765.0●
  loss (cause unknown) 783.21
Weightlessness 994.9
Weil's disease (leptospiral jaundice) 100.0
Weill-Marchesani syndrome (brachymorphism and ectopia lentis) 759.89
Weingarten's syndrome (tropical eosinophilia) 518.3
Weir Mitchell's disease (erythromelalgia) 443.82
Weiss-Baker syndrome (carotid sinus syncope) 337.01
Weissenbach-Thibierge syndrome (cutaneous systemic sclerosis) 710.1
Wen (see also Cyst, sebaceous) 706.2
Wenckebach's phenomenon, heart block (second degree) 426.13
Werdnig-Hoffmann syndrome (muscular atrophy) 335.0
Werlhof's disease (see also Purpura, thrombocytopenic) 287.39
Werlhof-Wichmann syndrome (see also Purpura, thrombocytopenic) 287.39
Wermer's syndrome or disease (polyendocrine adenomatosis) 258.01
Werner's disease or syndrome (progeria adultorum) 259.8
Werner-His disease (trench fever) 083.1

◄ New ◄ Revised deleted Deleted ● Use Additional Digit(s) Omit code

Werner-Schultz disease (agranulocytosis) 288.09
Wernicke's encephalopathy, disease, or syndrome (superior hemorrhagic polioencephalitis) 265.1
Wernicke-Korsakoff syndrome or psychosis (nonalcoholic) 294.0
  alcoholic 291.1
Wernicke-Posadas disease (*see also* Coccidioidomycosis) 114.9
Wesselsbron fever 066.3
West African fever 084.8
West Nile
  encephalitis 066.41
  encephalomyelitis 066.41
  fever 066.40
    with
      cranial nerve disorders 066.42
      encephalitis 066.41
      optic neuritis 066.42
      other complications 066.49
      other neurologic manifestations 066.42
      polyradiculitis 066.42
    virus 066.40
Westphal-Strümpell syndrome (hepatolenticular degeneration) 275.1
Wet
  brain (alcoholic) (*see also* Alcoholism) 303.9●
  feet, tropical (syndrome) (maceration) 991.4
  lung (syndrome)
    adult 518.5
    newborn 770.6
Wharton's duct - *see* condition
Wheal 709.8
Wheelchair confinement status V46.3
Wheezing 786.07
Whiplash injury or syndrome 847.0
Whipple's disease or syndrome (intestinal lipodystrophy) 040.2
Whipworm 127.3
"Whistling face" syndrome (craniocarpotarsal dystrophy) 759.89
White - *see also* condition
  kidney
    large - *see* Nephrosis
    small 582.9
  leg, puerperal, postpartum, childbirth 671.4●
    nonpuerperal 451.19
  mouth 112.0
  patches of mouth 528.6
  sponge nevus of oral mucosa 750.26
  spot lesions, teeth 521.01
White's disease (congenital) (keratosis follicularis) 757.39
Whitehead 706.2
Whitlow (with lymphangitis) 681.01
  herpetic 054.6
Whitmore's disease or fever (melioidosis) 025
Whooping cough 033.9
  with pneumonia 033.9 [*484.3*]
  due to
    Bordetella
      bronchoseptica 033.8
        with pneumonia 033.8 [*484.3*]
      parapertussis 033.1
        with pneumonia 033.1 [*484.3*]

Whooping cough (*Continued*)
  due to (*Continued*)
    Bordetella (*Continued*)
      pertussis 033.0
        with pneumonia 033.0 [*484.3*]
    specified organism NEC 033.8
      with pneumonia 033.8 [*484.3*]
  vaccination, prophylactic (against) V03.6
Wichmann's asthma (laryngismus stridulus) 478.75
Widal (-Abrami) syndrome (acquired hemolytic jaundice) 283.9
Widening aorta (*see also* Aneurysm, aorta) 441.9
  ruptured 441.5
Wilkie's disease or syndrome 557.1
Wilkinson-Sneddon disease or syndrome (subcorneal pustular dermatosis) 694.1
Willan's lepra 696.1
Willan-Plumbe syndrome (psoriasis) 696.1
Willebrand (-Jürgens) syndrome or thrombopathy (angiohemophilia) 286.4
Willi-Prader syndrome (hypogenital dystrophy with diabetic tendency) 759.81
Willis' disease (diabetes mellitus) (*see also* Diabetes) 250.0●
  due to secondary diabetes 249.0●
Wilms' tumor or neoplasm (nephroblastoma) (M8960/3) 189.0
Wilson's
  disease or syndrome (hepatolenticular degeneration) 275.1
  hepatolenticular degeneration 275.1
  lichen ruber 697.0
Wilson-Brocq disease (dermatitis exfoliativa) 695.89
Wilson-Mikity syndrome 770.7
Window - *see also* Imperfect, closure
  aorticopulmonary 745.0
Winged scapula 736.89
Winter - *see also* condition
  vomiting disease 078.82
Wise's disease 696.2
Wiskott-Aldrich syndrome (eczema-thrombocytopenia) 279.12
Withdrawal symptoms, syndrome
  alcohol 291.81
    delirium (acute) 291.0
      chronic 291.1
    newborn 760.71
  drug or narcotic 292.0
  newborn, infant of dependent mother 779.5
  steroid NEC
    correct substance properly administered 255.41
    overdose or wrong substance given or taken 962.0
Withdrawing reaction, child or adolescent 313.22
Witts' anemia (achlorhydric anemia) 280.9
Witzelsucht 301.9
Woakes' syndrome (ethmoiditis) 471.1
Wohlfart-Kugelberg-Welander disease 335.11
Woillez's disease (acute idiopathic pulmonary congestion) 518.5

Wolff-Parkinson-White syndrome (anomalous atrioventricular excitation) 426.7
Wolhynian fever 083.1
Wolman's disease (primary familial xanthomatosis) 272.7
Wood asthma 495.8
Woolly, wooly hair (congenital) (nevus) 757.4
Wool-sorters' disease 022.1
Word
  blindness (congenital) (developmental) 315.01
    secondary to organic lesion 784.61
  deafness (secondary to organic lesion) 784.69
  developmental 315.31
Worm(s) (colic) (fever) (infection) (infestation) (*see also* Infestation) 128.9
  guinea 125.7
  in intestine NEC 127.9
Worm-eaten soles 102.3
Worn out (*see also* Exhaustion) 780.79
  artificial heart valve 996.02 ◄
  cardiac defibrillator V53.32 ◄
  cardiac pacemaker lead or battery V53.31 ◄
  joint prosthesis (*see also* Complications, mechanical, device NEC, prosthetic NEC, joint) 996.46
"Worried well" V65.5
Wound, open (by cutting or piercing instrument) (by firearms) (cut) (dissection) (incised) (laceration) (penetration) (perforating) (puncture) (with initial hemorrhage, not internal) 879.8

> **Note 74** For fracture with open wound, see Fracture.
>
> For laceration, traumatic rupture, tear, or penetrating wound of internal organs, such as heart, lung, liver, kidney, pelvic organs, etc., whether or not accompanied by open wound or fracture in the same region, see Injury, internal. For contused wound, see Contusion. For crush injury, see Crush. For abrasion, insect bite (nonvenomous), blister, or scratch, see Injury, superficial.
>
> Complicated includes wounds with:
>
> delayed healing
> delayed treatment
> foreign body
> primary infection
>
> For late effect of open wound, see Late, effect, wound, open, by site.

  abdomen, abdominal (external) (muscle) 879.2
    complicated 879.3
    wall (anterior) 879.2
      complicated 879.3
      lateral 879.4
        complicated 879.5
  alveolar (process) 873.62
    complicated 873.72
  ankle 891.0
    with tendon involvement 891.2
    complicated 891.1
  anterior chamber, eye (*see also* Wound, open, intraocular) 871.9

◄ New　◄|||| Revised　~~deleted~~ Deleted　● Use Additional Digit(s)　▓ Omit code

Wound, open (Continued)
  anus 879.6
    complicated 879.7
  arm 884.0
    with tendon involvement 884.2
    complicated 884.1
    forearm 881.00
      with tendon involvement 881.20
      complicated 881.10
    multiple sites - see Wound, open,
        multiple, upper limb
    upper 880.03
      with tendon involvement
          880.23
      complicated 880.13
        multiple sites (with axillary or
            shoulder regions) 880.09
          with tendon involvement
              880.29
          complicated 880.19
  artery - see Injury, blood vessel, by site
  auditory
    canal (external) (meatus) 872.02
      complicated 872.12
    ossicles (incus) (malleus) (stapes)
        872.62
      complicated 872.72
  auricle, ear 872.01
    complicated 872.11
  axilla 880.02
    with tendon involvement 880.22
    complicated 880.12
      with tendon involvement
          880.29
    involving other sites of upper arm
        880.09
      complicated 880.19
  back 876.0
    complicated 876.1
  bladder - see Injury, internal, bladder
  blood vessel - see Injury, blood vessel,
      by site
  brain - see Injury, intracranial, with
      open intracranial wound
  breast 879.0
    complicated 879.1
  brow 873.42
    complicated 873.52
  buccal mucosa 873.61
    complicated 873.71
  buttock 877.0
    complicated 877.1
  calf 891.0
    with tendon involvement 891.2
    complicated 891.1
  canaliculus lacrimalis 870.8
    with laceration of eyelid 870.2
  canthus, eye 870.8
    laceration - see Laceration, eyelid
  cavernous sinus - see Injury,
      intracranial
  cerebellum - see Injury, intracranial
  cervical esophagus 874.4
    complicated 874.5
  cervix - see Injury, internal, cervix
  cheek(s) (external) 873.41
    complicated 873.51
    internal 873.61
      complicated 873.71
  chest (wall) (external) 875.0
    complicated 875.1
  chin 873.44
    complicated 873.54
  choroid 363.63
  ciliary body (eye) (see also Wound,
      open, intraocular) 871.9

Wound, open (Continued)
  clitoris 878.8
    complicated 878.9
  cochlea 872.64
    complicated 872.74
  complicated 879.9
  conjunctiva - see Wound, open,
      intraocular
  cornea (nonpenetrating) (see also
      Wound, open, intraocular)
      871.9
  costal region 875.0
    complicated 875.1
  Descemet's membrane (see also Wound,
      open, intraocular) 871.9
  digit(s)
    foot 893.0
      with tendon involvement
          893.2
      complicated 893.1
    hand 883.0
      with tendon involvement
          883.2
      complicated 883.1
  drumhead, ear 872.61
    complicated 872.71
  ear 872.8
    canal 872.02
      complicated 872.12
    complicated 872.9
    drum 872.61
      complicated 872.71
    external 872.00
      complicated 872.10
    multiple sites 872.69
      complicated 872.79
    ossicles (incus) (malleus) (stapes)
        872.62
      complicated 872.72
    specified part NEC 872.69
      complicated 872.79
  elbow 881.01
    with tendon involvement 881.21
    complicated 881.11
  epididymis 878.2
    complicated 878.3
  epigastric region 879.2
    complicated 879.3
  epiglottis 874.01
    complicated 874.11
  esophagus (cervical) 874.4
    complicated 874.5
    thoracic - see Injury, internal,
        esophagus
  Eustachian tube 872.63
    complicated 872.73
  extremity
    lower (multiple) NEC 894.0
      with tendon involvement 894.2
      complicated 894.1
    upper (multiple) NEC 884.0
      with tendon involvement 884.2
      complicated 884.1
  eye(s) (globe) - see Wound, open,
      intraocular
  eyeball NEC 871.9
    laceration (see also Laceration,
        eyeball) 871.4
    penetrating (see also Penetrating
        wound, eyeball) 871.7
  eyebrow 873.42
    complicated 873.52
  eyelid NEC 870.8
    laceration - see Laceration, eyelid

Wound, open (Continued)
  face 873.40
    complicated 873.50
    multiple sites 873.49
      complicated 873.59
    specified part NEC 873.49
      complicated 873.59
  fallopian tube - see Injury, internal,
      fallopian tube
  finger(s) (nail) (subungual) 883.0
    with tendon involvement 883.2
    complicated 883.1
  flank 879.4
    complicated 879.5
  foot (any part, except toe(s) alone)
      892.0
    with tendon involvement 892.2
    complicated 892.1
  forearm 881.00
    with tendon involvement 881.20
    complicated 881.10
  forehead 873.42
    complicated 873.52
  genital organs (external) NEC 878.8
    complicated 878.9
    internal - see Injury, internal, by site
  globe (eye) (see also Wound, open,
      eyeball) 871.9
  groin 879.4
    complicated 879.5
  gum(s) 873.62
    complicated 873.72
  hand (except finger(s) alone) 882.0
    with tendon involvement 882.2
    complicated 882.1
  head NEC 873.8
    with intracranial injury - see Injury,
        intracranial
      due to or associated with skull
          fracture - see Fracture,
          skull
    complicated 873.9
    scalp - see Wound, open, scalp
  heel 892.0
    with tendon involvement 892.2
    complicated 892.1
  high-velocity (grease gun) - see
      Wound, open, complicated,
      by site
  hip 890.0
    with tendon involvement 890.2
    complicated 890.1
  hymen 878.6
    complicated 878.7
  hypochondrium 879.4
    complicated 879.5
  hypogastric region 879.2
    complicated 879.3
  iliac (region) 879.4
    complicated 879.5
  incidental to
    dislocation - see Dislocation, open,
        by site
    fracture - see Fracture, open, by site
    intracranial injury - see Injury,
        intracranial, with open
        intracranial wound
    nerve injury - see Injury, nerve, by
        site
  inguinal region 879.4
    complicated 879.5
  instep 892.0
    with tendon involvement 892.2
    complicated 892.1

Wound, open *(Continued)*
  interscapular region 876.0
    complicated 876.1
  intracranial - *see* Injury, intracranial,
    with open intracranial wound
  intraocular 871.9
    with
      partial loss (of intraocular tissue)
        871.2
      prolapse or exposure (of
        intraocular tissue) 871.1
      laceration (*see also* Laceration,
        eyeball) 871.4
      penetrating 871.7
        with foreign body (nonmagnetic)
          871.6
          magnetic 871.5
      without prolapse (of intraocular
        tissue) 871.0
  iris (*see also* Wound, open, eyeball)
    871.9
  jaw (fracture not involved) 873.44
    with fracture - *see* Fracture, jaw
    complicated 873.54
  knee 891.0
    with tendon involvement 891.2
    complicated 891.1
  labium (majus) (minus) 878.4
    complicated 878.5
  lacrimal apparatus, gland, or sac
    870.8
    with laceration of eyelid 870.2
  larynx 874.01
    with trachea 874.00
      complicated 874.10
    complicated 874.11
  leg (multiple) 891.0
    with tendon involvement 891.2
    complicated 891.1
    lower 891.0
      with tendon involvement 891.2
      complicated 891.1
    thigh 890.0
      with tendon involvement 890.2
      complicated 890.1
    upper 890.0
      with tendon involvement 890.2
      complicated 890.1
  lens (eye) (alone) (*see also* Cataract,
    traumatic) 366.20
    with involvement of other eye
      structures - *see* Wound, open,
      eyeball
  limb
    lower (multiple) NEC 894.0
      with tendon involvement 894.2
      complicated 894.1
    upper (multiple) NEC 884.0
      with tendon involvement 884.2
      complicated 884.1
  lip 873.43
    complicated 873.53
  loin 876.0
    complicated 876.1
  lumbar region 876.0
    complicated 876.1
  malar region 873.41
    complicated 873.51
  mastoid region 873.49
    complicated 873.59
  mediastinum - *see* Injury, internal,
    mediastinum
  midthoracic region 875.0
    complicated 875.1

Wound, open *(Continued)*
  mouth 873.60
    complicated 873.70
    floor 873.64
      complicated 873.74
    multiple sites 873.69
      complicated 873.79
    specified site NEC 873.69
      complicated 873.79
  multiple, unspecified site(s) 879.8

> Note 75   Multiple open wounds of
> sites classifiable to the same four-digit
> category should be classified to that
> category unless they are in different
> limbs.
>
> Multiple open wounds of sites
> classifiable to different four-digit
> categories, or to different limbs, should
> be coded separately.

    complicated 879.9
    lower limb(s) (one or both) (sites
      classifiable to more than one
      three-digit category in 890–
      893) 894.0
      with tendon involvement 894.2
      complicated 894.1
    upper limb(s) (one or both) (sites
      classifiable to more than one
      three-digit category in 880–
      883) 884.0
      with tendon involvement
        884.2
      complicated 884.1
  muscle - *see* Sprain, by site
  nail
    finger(s) 883.0
      complicated 883.1
    thumb 883.0
      complicated 883.1
    toe(s) 893.0
      complicated 893.1
  nape (neck) 874.8
    complicated 874.9
    specified part NEC 874.8
      complicated 874.9
  nasal - *see also* Wound, open, nose
    cavity 873.22
      complicated 873.32
    septum 873.21
      complicated 873.31
    sinuses 873.23
      complicated 873.33
  nasopharynx 873.22
    complicated 873.32
  neck 874.8
    complicated 874.9
    nape 874.8
      complicated 874.9
    specified part NEC 874.8
      complicated 874.9
  nerve - *see* Injury, nerve, by site
  non-healing surgical 998.83
  nose 873.20
    complicated 873.30
    multiple sites 873.29
      complicated 873.39
    septum 873.21
      complicated 873.31
    sinuses 873.23
      complicated 873.33
  occipital region - *see* Wound, open,
    scalp

Wound, open *(Continued)*
  ocular NEC 871.9
    adnexa 870.9
      specified region NEC 870.8
    laceration (*see also* Laceration,
      ocular) 871.4
    muscle (extraocular) 870.3
      with foreign body 870.4
      eyelid 870.1
      intraocular - *see* Wound, open,
        eyeball
    penetrating (*see also* Penetrating
      wound, ocular) 871.7
  orbit 870.8
    penetrating 870.3
      with foreign body 870.4
  orbital region 870.9
  ovary - *see* Injury, internal, pelvic
    organs
  palate 873.65
    complicated 873.75
  palm 882.0
    with tendon involvement 882.2
    complicated 882.1
  parathyroid (gland) 874.2
    complicated 874.3
  parietal region - *see* Wound, open,
    scalp
  pelvic floor or region 879.6
    complicated 879.7
  penis 878.0
    complicated 878.1
  perineum 879.6
    complicated 879.7
  periocular area 870.8
    laceration of skin 870.0
  pharynx 874.4
    complicated 874.5
  pinna 872.01
    complicated 872.11
  popliteal space 891.0
    with tendon involvement 891.2
    complicated 891.1
  prepuce 878.0
    complicated 878.1
  pubic region 879.2
    complicated 879.3
  pudenda 878.8
    complicated 878.9
  rectovaginal septum 878.8
    complicated 878.9
  sacral region 877.0
    complicated 877.1
  sacroiliac region 877.0
    complicated 877.1
  salivary (ducts) (glands) 873.69
    complicated 873.79
  scalp 873.0
    complicated 873.1
  scalpel, fetus or newborn 767.8
  scapular region 880.01
    with tendon involvement 880.21
    complicated 880.11
    involving other sites of upper arm
      880.09
      with tendon involvement
        880.29
      complicated 880.19
  sclera (*see also* Wound, open,
    intraocular) 871.9
  scrotum 878.2
    complicated 878.3
  seminal vesicle - *see* Injury, internal,
    pelvic organs

◄ New   ⬅ Revised   ~~deleted~~ Deleted   ● Use Additional Digit(s)   ▓ Omit code

Wound, open (*Continued*)
  shin 891.0
    with tendon involvement 891.2
    complicated 891.1
  shoulder 880.00
    with tendon involvement 880.20
    complicated 880.10
    involving other sites of upper arm
        880.09
      with tendon involvement 880.29
      complicated 880.19
  skin NEC 879.8
    complicated 879.9
  skull - *see also* Injury, intracranial, with
        open intracranial wound
    with skull fracture - *see* Fracture,
        skull
  spermatic cord (scrotal) 878.2
    complicated 878.3
    pelvic region - *see* Injury, internal,
        spermatic cord
  spinal cord - *see* Injury, spinal
  sternal region 875.0
    complicated 875.1
  subconjunctival - *see* Wound, open,
        intraocular
  subcutaneous NEC 879.8
    complicated 879.9
  submaxillary region 873.44
    complicated 873.54
  submental region 873.44
    complicated 873.54
  subungual
    finger(s) (thumb) - *see* Wound, open,
        finger
    toe(s) - *see* Wound, open, toe
  supraclavicular region 874.8
    complicated 874.9
  supraorbital 873.42
    complicated 873.52

Wound, open (*Continued*)
  surgical, non-healing 998.83
  temple 873.49
    complicated 873.59
  temporal region 873.49
    complicated 873.59
  testis 878.2
    complicated 878.3
  thigh 890.0
    with tendon involvement 890.2
    complicated 890.1
  thorax, thoracic (external) 875.0
    complicated 875.1
  throat 874.8
    complicated 874.9
  thumb (nail) (subungual) 883.0
    with tendon involvement 883.2
    complicated 883.1
  thyroid (gland) 874.2
    complicated 874.3
  toe(s) (nail) (subungual) 893.0
    with tendon involvement 893.2
    complicated 893.1
  tongue 873.64
    complicated 873.74
  tonsil - *see* Wound, open, neck
  trachea (cervical region) 874.02
    with larynx 874.00
      complicated 874.10
    complicated 874.12
    intrathoracic - *see* Injury, internal,
        trachea
  trunk (multiple) NEC 879.6
    complicated 879.7
    specified site NEC 879.6
      complicated 879.7
  tunica vaginalis 878.2
    complicated 878.3
  tympanic membrane 872.61
    complicated 872.71

Wound, open (*Continued*)
  tympanum 872.61
    complicated 872.71
  umbilical region 879.2
    complicated 879.3
  ureter - *see* Injury, internal, ureter
  urethra - *see* Injury, internal, urethra
  uterus - *see* Injury, internal, uterus
  uvula 873.69
    complicated 873.79
  vagina 878.6
    complicated 878.7
  vas deferens - *see* Injury, internal, vas
        deferens
  vitreous (humor) 871.2
  vulva 878.4
    complicated 878.5
  wrist 881.02
    with tendon involvement 881.22
    complicated 881.12
Wright's syndrome (hyperabduction)
    447.8
  pneumonia 390 *[517.1]*
Wringer injury - *see* Crush injury, by site
Wrinkling of skin 701.8
Wrist - *see also* condition
  drop (acquired) 736.05
Wrong drug (given in error) NEC 977.9
  specified drug or substance - *see* Table
        of Drugs and Chemicals
Wry neck - *see also* Torticollis
  congenital 754.1
Wuchereria infestation 125.0
  bancrofti 125.0
  Brugia malayi 125.1
  malayi 125.1
Wuchereriasis 125.0
Wuchereriosis 125.0
Wuchernde struma langhans (M8332/3)
    193

X

Xanthelasma 272.2
  eyelid 272.2 [374.51]
  palpebrarum 272.2 [374.51]
Xanthelasmatosis (essential) 272.2
Xanthelasmoidea 757.33
Xanthine stones 277.2
Xanthinuria 277.2
Xanthofibroma (M8831/0) - see
    Neoplasm, connective tissue, benign
Xanthoma(s), xanthomatosis 272.2
  with
    hyperlipoproteinemia
      type I 272.3
      type III 272.2
      type IV 272.1
      type V 272.3
  bone 272.7
  craniohypophyseal 277.89
  cutaneotendinous 272.7
  diabeticorum 250.8● [272.2]
    due to secondary diabetes
      249.8● [272.2]
  disseminatum 272.7
  eruptive 272.2
  eyelid 272.2 [374.51]
  familial 272.7
  hereditary 272.7
  hypercholesterinemic 272.0

Xanthoma(s) (Continued)
  hypercholesterolemic 272.0
  hyperlipemic 272.4
  hyperlipidemic 272.4
  infantile 272.7
  joint 272.7
  juvenile 272.7
  multiple 272.7
  multiplex 272.7
  primary familial 272.7
  tendon (sheath) 272.7
  tuberosum 272.2
  tuberous 272.2
  tubo-eruptive 272.2
Xanthosis 709.09
  surgical 998.81
Xenophobia 300.29
Xeroderma (congenital) 757.39
  acquired 701.1
    eyelid 373.33
  eyelid 373.33
  pigmentosum 757.33
  vitamin A deficiency 264.8
Xerophthalmia 372.53
  vitamin A deficiency 264.7
Xerosis
  conjunctiva 372.53
    with Bitôt's spot 372.53
      vitamin A deficiency 264.1
    vitamin A deficiency 264.0

Xerosis (Continued)
  cornea 371.40
    with corneal ulceration
      370.00
      vitamin A deficiency
        264.3
    vitamin A deficiency
      264.2
  cutis 706.8
  skin 706.8
Xerostomia 527.7
Xiphodynia 733.90
Xiphoidalgia 733.90
Xiphoiditis 733.99
Xiphopagus 759.4
XO syndrome 758.6
X-ray
  effects, adverse, NEC 990
  of chest
    for suspected tuberculosis
      V71.2
    routine V72.5
XXX syndrome 758.81
XXXXY syndrome 758.81
XXY syndrome 758.7
Xyloketosuria 271.8
Xylosuria 271.8
Xylulosuria 271.8
XYY syndrome 758.81

◀ New   ◀ Revised   ~~deleted~~ Deleted   ● Use Additional Digit(s)   ▬ Omit code

Y

Yaba monkey tumor virus 059.22
Yawning 786.09
    psychogenic 306.1
Yaws 102.9
    bone or joint lesions 102.6
    butter 102.1
    chancre 102.0
    cutaneous, less than five years after
        infection 102.2
    early (cutaneous) (macular)
        (maculopapular) (micropapular)
        (papular) 102.2
      frambeside 102.2
      skin lesions NEC 102.2
    eyelid 102.9 [373.4]
    ganglion 102.6
    gangosis, gangosa 102.5
    gumma, gummata 102.4
      bone 102.6

Yaws (Continued)
    gummatous
      frambeside 102.4
      osteitis 102.6
      periostitis 102.6
    hydrarthrosis 102.6
    hyperkeratosis (early) (late) (palmar)
        (plantar) 102.3
    initial lesions 102.0
    joint lesions 102.6
    juxta-articular nodules 102.7
    late nodular (ulcerated) 102.4
    latent (without clinical
        manifestations) (with
        positive serology) 102.8
    mother 102.0
    mucosal 102.7
    multiple papillomata 102.1
    nodular, late (ulcerated) 102.4
    osteitis 102.6

Yaws (Continued)
    papilloma, papillomata (palmar)
        (plantar) 102.1
    periostitis (hypertrophic) 102.6
    ulcers 102.4
    wet crab 102.1
Yeast infection (see also Candidiasis)
    112.9
Yellow
    atrophy (liver) 570
      chronic 571.8
      resulting from administration of
        blood, plasma, serum, or other
        biological substance (within 8
        months of administration) - see
        Hepatitis, viral
    fever - see Fever, yellow
    jack (see also Fever, yellow) 060.9
    jaundice (see also Jaundice) 782.4
Yersinia septica 027.8

Z

Zagari's disease (xerostomia) 527.7
Zahorsky's disease (exanthema subitum)
   (*see also* Exanthem subitum)
   058.10
  syndrome (herpangina) 074.0
Zellweger syndrome 277.86
Zenker's diverticulum (esophagus) 530.6
Ziehen-Oppenheim disease 333.6

Zieve's syndrome (jaundice,
   hyperlipemia, and hemolytic
   anemia) 571.1
Zika fever 066.3
Zollinger-Ellison syndrome (gastric
   hypersecretion with pancreatic islet
   cell tumor) 251.5
Zona (*see also* Herpes, zoster) 053.9
Zoophilia (erotica) 302.1
Zoophobia 300.29

Zoster (herpes) (*see also* Herpes, zoster)
   053.9
Zuelzer (-Ogden) anemia or syndrome
   (nutritional megaloblastic anemia)
   281.2
Zygodactyly (*see also* Syndactylism)
   755.10
Zygomycosis 117.7
Zymotic - *see* condition

◀ New   ◀▥ Revised   ~~deleted~~ Deleted   ● Use Additional Digit(s)   ▨ Omit code

ALPHABETIC INDEX TO POISONING AND EXTERNAL CAUSES OF ADVERSE EFFECTS OF DRUGS AND OTHER CHEMICAL SUBSTANCES

This table contains a classification of drugs and other chemical substances to identify poisoning states and external causes of adverse effects.

Each of the listed substances in the table is assigned a code according to the poisoning classification (960–989). These codes are used when there is a statement of poisoning, overdose, wrong substance given or taken, or intoxication.

The table also contains a listing of external causes of adverse effects. An adverse effect is a pathologic manifestation due to ingestion or exposure to drugs or other chemical substances (e.g., dermatitis, hypersensitivity reaction, aspirin gastritis). The adverse effect is to be identified by the appropriate code found in Section I, Index to Diseases and Injuries. An external cause code can then be used to identify the circumstances involved. The table headings pertaining to external causes are defined below:

Accidental poisoning (E850–E869)-accidental overdose of drug, wrong substance given or taken, drug taken inadvertently, accidents in the usage of drugs and biologicals in medical and surgical procedures, and to show external causes of poisonings classifiable to 980–989.

Therapeutic use (E930–E949)-a correct substance properly administered in therapeutic or prophylactic dosage as the external cause of adverse effects.

Suicide attempt (E950–E952)-instances in which self-inflicted injuries or poisonings are involved.

Assault (E961–E962)-injury or poisoning inflicted by another person with the intent to injure or kill.

Undetermined (E980–E982)-to be used when the intent of the poisoning or injury cannot be determined whether it was intentional or accidental.

The American Hospital Formulary Service (AHFS) list numbers are included in the table to help classify new drugs not identified in the table by name. The AHFS list numbers are keyed to the continually revised AHFS (American Hospital Formulary Service, 2 vol. Washington, D.C.: American Society of Hospital Pharmacists, 1959-). These listings are found in the table under the main term **Drug.**

Excluded from the table are radium and other radioactive substances. The classification of adverse effects and complications pertaining to these substances will be found in Index to Diseases and Injuries, and Index to External Causes of Injuries.

Although certain substances are indexed with one or more subentries, the majority are listed according to one use or state. It is recognized that many substances may be used in various ways, in medicine and in industry, and may cause adverse effects whatever the state of the agent (solid, liquid, or fumes arising from a liquid). In cases in which the reported data indicate a use or state not in the table, or which is clearly different from the one listed, an attempt should be made to classify the substance in the form which most nearly expresses the reported facts.

Substance	Poisoning	External Cause (E Code)				
		Accident	Therapeutic Use	Suicide Attempt	Assault	Undetermined
1-propanol	980.3	E860.4	—	E950.9	E962.1	E980.9
2-propanol	980.2	E860.3	—	E950.9	E962.1	E980.9
2,4-D (dichlorophenoxyacetic acid)	989.4	E863.5	—	E950.6	E962.1	E980.7
2,4-toluene diisocyanate	983.0	E864.0	—	E950.7	E962.1	E980.6
2,4,5-T (trichlorophenoxyacetic acid)	989.2	E863.5	—	E950.6	E962.1	E980.7
14-hydroxydihydromorphinone	965.09	E850.2	E935.2	E950.0	E962.0	E980.0
ABOB	961.7	E857	E931.7	E950.4	E962.0	E980.4
Abrus (seed)	988.2	E865.3	—	E950.9	E962.1	E980.9
Absinthe	980.0	E860.1	—	E950.9	E962.1	E980.9
beverage	980.0	E860.0	—	E950.9	E962.1	E980.9
Acenocoumarin, acenocoumarol	964.2	E858.2	E934.2	E950.4	E962.0	E980.4
Acepromazine	969.1	E853.0	E939.1	E950.3	E962.0	E980.3
Acetal	982.8	E862.4	—	E950.9	E962.1	E980.9
Acetaldehyde (vapor)	987.8	E869.8	—	E952.8	E962.2	E982.8
liquid	989.89	E866.8	—	E950.9	E962.1	E980.9
Acetaminophen	965.4	E850.4	E935.4	E950.0	E962.0	E980.0
Acetaminosalol	965.1	E850.3	E935.3	E950.0	E962.0	E980.0
Acetanilid(e)	965.4	E850.4	E935.4	E950.0	E962.0	E980.0
Acetarsol, acetarsone	961.1	E857	E931.1	E950.4	E962.0	E980.4
Acetazolamide	974.2	E858.5	E944.2	E950.4	E962.0	E980.4
Acetic	—	—	—	—	—	—
acid	983.1	E864.1	—	E950.7	E962.1	E980.6
with sodium acetate (ointment)	976.3	E858.7	E946.3	E950.4	E962.0	E980.4
irrigating solution	974.5	E858.5	E944.5	E950.4	E962.0	E980.4
lotion	976.2	E858.7	E946.2	E950.4	E962.0	E980.4
anhydride	983.1	E864.1	—	E950.7	E962.1	E980.6
ether (vapor)	982.8	E862.4	—	E950.9	E962.1	E980.9
Acetohexamide	962.3	E858.0	E932.3	E950.4	E962.0	E980.4
Acetomenaphthone	964.3	E858.2	E934.3	E950.4	E962.0	E980.4
Acetomorphine	965.01	E850.0	E935.0	E950.0	E962.0	E980.0
Acetone (oils) (vapor)	982.8	E862.4	—	E950.9	E962.1	E980.9
Acetophenazine (maleate)	969.1	E853.0	E939.1	E950.3	E962.0	E980.3
Acetophenetidin	965.4	E850.4	E935.4	E950.0	E962.0	E980.0
Acetophenone	982.0	E862.4	—	E950.9	E962.1	E980.9
Acetorphine	965.09	E850.2	E935.2	E950.0	E962.0	E980.0
Acetosulfone (sodium)	961.8	E857	E931.8	E950.4	E962.0	E980.4
Acetrizoate (sodium)	977.8	E858.8	E947.8	E950.4	E962.0	E980.4
Acetylcarbromal	967.3	E852.2	E937.3	E950.2	E962.0	E980.2

◀ New   ◀━ Revised   ~~deleted~~ Deleted   ● Use Additional Digit(s)

Substance	Poisoning	External Cause (E Code)				
		Accident	Therapeutic Use	Suicide Attempt	Assault	Undetermined
Acetylcholine (chloride)	971.0	E855.3	E941.0	E950.4	E962.0	E980.4
Acetylcysteine	975.5	E858.6	E945.5	E950.4	E962.0	E980.4
Acetyldigitoxin	972.1	E858.3	E942.1	E950.4	E962.0	E980.4
Acetyldihydrocodeine	965.09	E850.2	E935.2	E950.0	E962.0	E980.0
Acetyldihydrocodeinone	965.09	E850.2	E935.2	E950.0	E962.0	E980.0
Acetylene (gas) (industrial)	987.1	E868.1	—	E951.8	E962.2	E981.8
incomplete combustion of - *see* Carbon monoxide, fuel, utility	—	—	—	—	—	—
tetrachloride (vapor)	982.3	E862.4	—	E950.9	E962.1	E980.9
Acetyliodosalicylic acid	965.1	E850.3	E935.3	E950.0	E962.0	E980.0
Acetylphenylhydrazine	965.8	E850.8	E935.8	E950.0	E962.0	E980.0
Acetylsalicylic acid	965.1	E850.3	E935.3	E950.0	E962.0	E980.0
Achromycin	960.4	E856	E930.4	E950.4	E962.0	E980.4
ophthalmic preparation	976.5	E858.7	E946.5	E950.4	E962.0	E980.4
topical NEC	976.0	E858.7	E946.0	E950.4	E962.0	E980.4
Acidifying agents	963.2	E858.1	E933.2	E950.4	E962.0	E980.4
Acids (corrosive) NEC	983.1	E864.1	—	E950.7	E962.1	E980.6
Aconite (wild)	988.2	E865.4	—	E950.9	E962.1	E980.9
Aconitine (liniment)	976.8	E858.7	E946.8	E950.4	E962.0	E980.4
Aconitum ferox	988.2	E865.4	—	E950.9	E962.1	E980.9
Acridine	983.0	E864.0	—	E950.7	E962.1	E980.6
vapor	987.8	E869.8	—	E952.8	E962.2	E982.8
Acriflavine	961.9	E857	E931.9	E950.4	E962.0	E980.4
Acrisorcin	976.0	E858.7	E946.0	E950.4	E962.0	E980.4
Acrolein (gas)	987.8	E869.8	—	E952.8	E962.2	E982.8
liquid	989.89	E866.8	—	E950.9	E962.1	E980.9
Actaea spicata	988.2	E865.4	—	E950.9	E962.1	E980.9
Acterol	961.5	E857	E931.5	E950.4	E962.0	E980.4
ACTH	962.4	E858.0	E932.4	E950.4	E962.0	E980.4
Acthar	962.4	E858.0	E932.4	E950.4	E962.0	E980.4
Actinomycin (C) (D)	960.7	E856	E930.7	E950.4	E962.0	E980.4
Adalin (acetyl)	967.3	E852.2	E937.3	E950.2	E962.0	E980.2
Adenosine (phosphate)	977.8	E858.8	E947.8	E950.4	E962.0	E980.4
Adhesives	989.89	E866.6	—	E950.9	E962.1	E980.9
ADH	962.5	E858.0	E932.5	E950.4	E962.0	E980.4
Adicillin	960.0	E856	E930.0	E950.4	E962.0	E980.4
Adiphenine	975.1	E855.6	E945.1	E950.4	E962.0	E980.4
Adjunct, pharmaceutical	977.4	E858.8	E947.4	E950.4	E962.0	E980.4

◀ New   ◀▥ Revised   ~~deleted~~ Deleted   ● Use Additional Digit(s)

Substance	External Cause (E Code)					
	Poisoning	Accident	Therapeutic Use	Suicide Attempt	Assault	Undetermined
Adrenal (extract, cortex or medulla) (glucocorticoids) (hormones) (mineralocorticoids)	962.0	E858.0	E932.0	E950.4	E962.0	E980.4
ENT agent	976.6	E858.7	E946.6	E950.4	E962.0	E980.4
ophthalmic preparation	976.5	E858.7	E946.5	E950.4	E962.0	E980.4
topical NEC	976.0	E858.7	E946.0	E950.4	E962.0	E980.4
Adrenalin	971.2	E855.5	E941.2	E950.4	E962.0	E980.4
Adrenergic blocking agents	971.3	E855.6	E941.3	E950.4	E962.0	E980.4
Adrenergics	971.2	E855.5	E941.2	E950.4	E962.0	E980.4
Adrenochrome (derivatives)	972.8	E858.3	E942.8	E950.4	E962.0	E980.4
Adrenocorticotropic hormone	962.4	E858.0	E932.4	E950.4	E962.0	E980.4
Adrenocorticotropin	962.4	E858.0	E932.4	E950.4	E962.0	E980.4
Adriamycin	960.7	E856	E930.7	E950.4	E962.0	E980.4
Aerosol spray - see Sprays	—	—	—	—	—	—
Aerosporin	960.8	E856	E930.8	E950.4	E962.0	E980.4
ENT agent	976.6	E858.7	E946.6	E950.4	E962.0	E980.4
ophthalmic preparation	976.5	E858.7	E946.5	E950.4	E962.0	E980.4
topical NEC	976.0	E858.7	E946.0	E950.4	E962.0	E980.4
Aethusa cynapium	988.2	E865.4	—	E950.9	E962.1	E980.9
Afghanistan black	969.6	E854.1	E939.6	E950.3	E962.0	E980.3
Aflatoxin	989.7	E865.9	—	E950.9	E962.1	E980.9
African boxwood	988.2	E865.4	—	E950.9	E962.1	E980.9
Agar (-agar)	973.3	E858.4	E943.3	E950.4	E962.0	E980.4
Agricultural agent NEC	989.89	E863.9	—	E950.6	E962.1	E980.7
Agrypnal	967.0	E851	E937.0	E950.1	E962.0	E980.1
Air contaminant(s), source or type not specified	—	—	—	—	—	—
specified type - see specific substance	987.9	E869.9	—	E952.9	E962.2	E982.9
Akee	988.2	E865.4	—	E950.9	E962.1	E980.9
Akrinol	976.0	E858.7	E946.0	E950.4	E962.0	E980.4
Alantolactone	961.6	E857	E931.6	E950.4	E962.0	E980.4
Albamycin	960.8	E856	E930.8	E950.4	E962.0	E980.4
Albumin (normal human serum)	964.7	E858.2	E934.7	E950.4	E962.0	E980.4
Albuterol	975.7	E858.6	E945.7	E950.4	E962.0	E980.4
Alcohol	980.9	E860.9	—	E950.9	E962.1	E980.9
absolute	980.0	E860.1	—	E950.9	E962.1	E980.9
beverage	980.0	E860.0	E947.8	E950.9	E962.1	E980.9
amyl	980.3	E860.4	—	E950.9	E962.1	E980.9
antifreeze	980.1	E860.2	—	E950.9	E962.1	E980.9
butyl	980.3	E860.4	—	E950.9	E962.1	E980.9

◀ New   ◀▥ Revised   deleted Deleted   ● Use Additional Digit(s)

Substance	Poisoning	External Cause (E Code)				
		Accident	Therapeutic Use	Suicide Attempt	Assault	Undetermined
Alcohol *(Continued)*						
dehydrated	980.0	E860.1	—	E950.9	E862.1	E980.9
beverage	980.0	E860.0	E947.8	E950.9	E962.1	E980.9
denatured	980.0	E860.1	—	E950.9	E962.1	E980.9
deterrents	977.3	E858.8	E947.3	E950.4	E962.0	E980.4
diagnostic (gastric function)	977.8	E858.8	E947.8	E950.4	E962.0	E980.4
ethyl	980.0	E860.1	—	E950.9	E962.1	E980.9
beverage	980.0	E860.0	E947.8	E950.9	E962.1	E980.9
grain	980.0	E860.1	—	E950.9	E962.1	E980.9
beverage	980.0	E860.0	E947.8	E950.9	E962.1	E980.9
industrial	980.9	E860.9	—	E950.9	E962.1	E980.9
isopropyl	980.2	E860.3	—	E950.9	E962.1	E980.9
methyl	980.1	E860.2	—	E950.9	E962.1	E980.9
preparation for consumption	980.0	E860.0	E947.8	E950.9	E962.1	E980.9
propyl	980.3	E860.4	—	E950.9	E962.1	E980.9
secondary	980.2	E860.3	—	E950.9	E962.1	E980.9
radiator	980.1	E860.2	—	E950.9	E962.1	E980.9
rubbing	980.2	E860.3	—	E950.9	E962.1	E980.9
specified type NEC	980.8	E860.8	—	E950.9	E962.1	E980.9
surgical	980.9	E860.9	—	E950.9	E962.1	E980.9
vapor (from any type of alcohol)	987.8	E869.8	—	E952.8	E962.2	E982.8
wood	980.1	E860.2	—	E950.9	E962.1	E980.9
Alcuronium chloride	975.2	E858.6	E945.2	E950.4	E962.0	E980.4
Aldactone	974.4	E858.5	E944.4	E950.4	E962.0	E980.4
Aldicarb	989.3	E863.2	—	E950.6	E962.1	E980.7
Aldomet	972.6	E858.3	E942.6	E950.4	E962.0	E980.4
Aldosterone	962.0	E858.0	E932.0	E950.4	E962.0	E980.4
Aldrin (dust)	989.2	E863.0	—	E950.6	E962.1	E980.7
Aleve - *see* Naproxen	—	—	—	—	—	—
Algeldrate	973.0	E858.4	E943.0	E950.4	E962.0	E980.4
Alidase	963.4	E858.1	E933.4	E950.4	E962.0	E980.4
Aliphatic thiocyanates	989.0	E866.8	—	E950.9	E962.1	E980.9
Alkaline antiseptic solution (aromatic)	976.6	E858.7	E946.6	E950.4	E962.0	E980.4
Alkalinizing agents (medicinal)	963.3	E858.1	E933.3	E950.4	E962.0	E980.4
Alkalis, caustic	983.2	E864.2	—	E950.7	E962.1	E980.6
Alkalizing agents (medicinal)	963.3	E858.1	E933.3	E950.4	E962.0	E980.4
Alka-seltzer	965.1	E850.3	E935.3	E950.0	E962.0	E980.0
Alkavervir	972.6	E858.3	E942.6	E950.4	E962.0	E980.4

◀ New　◀▥ Revised　~~deleted~~ Deleted　● Use Additional Digit(s)

TABLE OF DRUGS AND CHEMICALS

Substance	Poisoning	External Cause (E Code)				
		Accident	Therapeutic Use	Suicide Attempt	Assault	Undetermined
Allegron	969.05 ◀	E854.0	E939.0	E950.3	E962.0	E980.3
Allobarbital, allobarbitone	967.0	E851	E937.0	E950.1	E962.0	E980.1
Allopurinol	974.7	E858.5	E944.7	E950.4	E962.0	E980.4
Allylestrenol	962.2	E858.0	E932.2	E950.4	E962.0	E980.4
Allylisopropylacetylurea	967.8	E852.8	E937.8	E950.2	E962.0	E980.2
Allylisopropylmalonylurea	967.0	E851	E937.0	E950.1	E962.0	E980.1
Allyltribromide	967.3	E852.2	E937.3	E950.2	E962.0	E980.2
Aloe, aloes, aloin	973.1	E858.4	E943.1	E950.4	E962.0	E980.4
Alosetron	973.8	E858.4	E943.8	E950.4	E962.0	E980.4
Aloxidone	966.0	E855.0	E936.0	E950.4	E962.0	E980.4
Aloxiprin	965.1	E850.3	E935.3	E950.0	E962.0	E980.0
Alpha amylase	963.4	E858.1	E933.4	E950.4	E962.0	E980.4
Alpha-1 blockers	971.3	E855.6	E941.3	E950.4	E962.0	E980.4
Alphaprodine (hydrochloride)	965.09	E850.2	E935.2	E950.0	E962.0	E980.0
Alpha tocopherol	963.5	E858.1	E933.5	E950.4	E962.0	E980.4
Alseroxylon	972.6	E858.3	E942.6	E950.4	E962.0	E980.4
Alum (ammonium) (potassium)	983.2	E864.2	—	E950.7	E962.1	E980.6
medicinal (astringent) NEC	976.2	E858.7	E946.2	E950.4	E962.0	E980.4
Aluminium, aluminum (gel) (hydroxide)	973.0	E858.4	E943.0	E950.4	E962.0	E980.4
acetate solution	976.2	E858.7	E946.2	E950.4	E962.0	E980.4
aspirin	965.1	E850.3	E935.3	E950.0	E962.0	E980.0
carbonate	973.0	E858.4	E943.0	E950.4	E962.0	E980.4
glycinate	973.0	E858.4	E943.0	E950.4	E962.0	E980.4
nicotinate	972.2	E858.3	E942.2	E950.4	E962.0	E980.4
ointment (surgical) (topical)	976.3	E858.7	E946.3	E950.4	E962.0	E980.4
phosphate	973.0	E858.4	E943.0	E950.4	E962.0	E980.4
subacetate	976.2	E858.7	E946.2	E950.4	E962.0	E980.4
topical NEC	976.3	E858.7	E946.3	E950.4	E962.0	E980.4
Alurate	967.0	E851	E937.0	E950.1	E962.0	E980.1
Alverine (citrate)	975.1	E858.6	E945.1	E950.4	E962.0	E980.4
Alvodine	965.09	E850.2	E935.2	E950.0	E962.0	E980.0
Amanita phalloides	988.1	E865.5	—	E950.9	E962.1	E980.9
Amantadine (hydrochloride)	966.4	E855.0	E936.4	E950.4	E962.0	E980.4
Ambazone	961.9	E857	E931.9	E950.4	E962.0	E980.4
Ambenonium	971.0	E855.3	E941.0	E950.4	E962.0	E980.4
Ambutonium bromide	971.1	E855.4	E941.1	E950.4	E962.0	E980.4
Ametazole	977.8	E858.8	E947.8	E950.4	E962.0	E980.4
Amethocaine (infiltration) (topical)	968.5	E855.2	E938.5	E950.4	E962.0	E980.4
nerve block (peripheral) (plexus)	968.6	E855.2	E938.6	E950.4	E962.0	E980.4
spinal	968.7	E855.2	E938.7	E950.4	E962.0	E980.4

◀ New   ◀▦ Revised   ~~deleted~~ Deleted   ● Use Additional Digit(s)

Substance	Poisoning	External Cause (E Code)				
		Accident	Therapeutic Use	Suicide Attempt	Assault	Undetermined
Amethopterin	963.1	E858.1	E933.1	E950.4	E962.0	E980.4
Amfepramone	977.0	E858.8	E947.0	E950.4	E962.0	E980.4
Amidone	965.02	E850.1	E935.1	E950.0	E962.0	E980.0
Amidopyrine	965.5	E850.5	E935.5	E950.0	E962.0	E980.0
Aminacrine	976.0	E858.7	E946.0	E950.4	E962.0	E980.4
Aminitrozole	961.5	E857	E931.5	E950.4	E962.0	E980.4
Aminoacetic acid	974.5	E858.5	E944.5	E950.4	E962.0	E980.4
Amino acids	974.5	E858.5	E944.5	E950.4	E962.0	E980.4
Aminocaproic acid	964.4	E858.2	E934.4	E950.4	E962.0	E980.4
Aminoethylisothiourium	963.8	E858.1	E933.8	E950.4	E962.0	E980.4
Aminoglutethimide	966.3	E855.0	E936.3	E950.4	E962.0	E980.4
Aminometradine	974.3	E858.5	E944.3	E950.4	E962.0	E980.4
Aminopentamide	971.1	E855.4	E941.1	E950.4	E962.0	E980.4
Aminophenazone	965.5	E850.5	E935.5	E950.0	E962.0	E980.0
Aminophenol	983.0	E864.0	—	E950.7	E962.1	E980.6
Aminophenylpyridone	969.5	E853.8	E939.5	E950.3	E962.0	E980.3
Aminophylline	975.7	E858.6	E945.7	E950.4	E962.0	E980.4
Aminopterin	963.1	E858.1	E933.1	E950.4	E962.0	E980.4
Aminopyrine	965.5	E850.5	E935.5	E950.0	E962.0	E980.0
Aminosalicylic acid	961.8	E857	E931.8	E950.4	E962.0	E980.4
Amiphenazole	970.1	E854.3	E940.1	E950.4	E962.0	E980.4
Amiquinsin	972.6	E858.3	E942.6	E950.4	E962.0	E980.4
Amisometradine	974.3	E858.5	E944.3	E950.4	E962.0	E980.4
Amitriptyline	969.05 ◄	E854.0	E939.0	E950.3	E962.0	E980.3
Ammonia (fumes) (gas) (vapor)	987.8	E869.8	—	E952.8	E962.2	E982.8
liquid (household) NEC	983.2	E861.4	—	E950.7	E962.1	E980.6
spirit, aromatic	970.8	E854.3	E940.8	E950.4	E962.0	E980.4
Ammoniated mercury	976.0	E858.7	E946.0	E950.4	E962.0	E980.4
Ammonium	—	—	—	—	—	—
carbonate	983.2	E864.2	—	E950.7	E962.1	E980.6
chloride (acidifying agent)	963.2	E858.1	E933.2	E950.4	E962.0	E980.4
expectorant	975.5	E858.6	E945.5	E950.4	E962.0	E980.4
compounds (household) NEC	983.2	E861.4	—	E950.7	E962.1	E980.6
fumes (any usage)	987.8	E869.8	—	E952.8	E962.2	E982.8
industrial	983.2	E864.2	—	E950.7	E962.1	E980.6
ichthosulfonate	976.4	E858.7	E946.4	E950.4	E962.0	E980.4
mandelate	961.9	E857	E931.9	E950.4	E962.0	E980.4
Amobarbital	967.0	E851	E937.0	E950.1	E962.0	E980.1
Amodiaquin(e)	961.4	E857	E931.4	E950.4	E962.0	E980.4
Amopyroquin(e)	961.4	E857	E931.4	E950.4	E962.0	E980.4

◄ New   ◄▒ Revised   ~~deleted~~ Deleted   ● Use Additional Digit(s)

Substance	Poisoning	External Cause (E Code)				
		Accident	Therapeutic Use	Suicide Attempt	Assault	Undetermined
Amphenidone	969.5	E853.8	E939.5	E950.3	E962.0	E980.3
Amphetamine	969.72 ◀	E854.2	E939.7	E950.3	E962.0	E980.3
Amphomycin	960.8	E856	E930.8	E950.4	E962.0	E980.4
Amphotericin B	960.1	E856	E930.1	E950.4	E962.0	E980.4
topical	976.0	E858.7	E946.0	E950.4	E962.0	E980.4
Ampicillin	960.0	E856	E930.0	E950.4	E962.0	E980.4
Amprotropine	971.1	E855.4	E941.1	E950.4	E962.0	E980.4
Amygdalin	977.8	E858.8	E947.8	E950.4	E962.0	E980.4
Amyl	—	—	—	—	—	—
acetate (vapor)	982.8	E862.4	—	E950.9	E962.1	E980.9
alcohol	980.3	E860.4	—	E950.9	E962.1	E980.9
nitrite (medicinal)	972.4	E858.3	E942.4	E950.4	E962.0	E980.4
Amylase (alpha)	963.4	E858.1	E933.4	E950.4	E962.0	E980.4
Amylene hydrate	980.8	E860.8	—	E950.9	E962.1	E980.9
Amylobarbitone	967.0	E851	E937.0	E950.1	E962.0	E980.1
Amylocaine	968.9	E855.2	E938.9	E950.4	E962.0	E980.4
infiltration (subcutaneous)	968.5	E855.2	E938.5	E950.4	E962.0	E980.4
nerve block (peripheral) (plexus)	968.6	E855.2	E938.6	E950.4	E962.0	E980.4
spinal	968.7	E855.2	E938.7	E950.4	E962.0	E980.4
topical (surface)	968.5	E855.2	E938.5	E950.4	E962.0	E980.4
Amytal (sodium)	967.0	E851	E937.0	E950.1	E962.0	E980.1
Analeptics	970.0	E854.3	E940.0	E950.4	E962.0	E980.4
Analgesics	965.9	E850.9	E935.9	E950.0	E962.0	E980.0
aromatic NEC	965.4	E850.4	E935.4	E950.0	E962.0	E980.0
non-narcotic NEC	965.7	E850.7	E935.7	E950.0	E962.0	E980.0
specified NEC	965.8	E850.8	E935.8	E950.0	E962.0	E980.0
Anamirta cocculus	988.2	E865.3	—	E950.9	E962.1	E980.9
Ancillin	960.0	E856	E930.0	E950.4	E962.0	E980.4
Androgens (anabolic congeners)	962.1	E858.0	E932.1	E950.4	E962.0	E980.4
Androstalone	962.1	E858.0	E932.1	E950.4	E962.0	E980.4
Androsterone	962.1	E858.0	E932.1	E950.4	E962.0	E980.4
Anemone pulsatilia	988.2	E865.4	—	E950.9	E962.1	E980.9
Anesthesia, anesthetic (general) NEC	968.4	E855.1	E938.4	E950.4	E962.0	E980.4
block (nerve) (plexus)	968.6	E855.2	E938.6	E950.4	E962.0	E980.4
gaseous NEC	968.2	E855.1	E938.2	E950.4	E962.0	E980.4
halogenated hydrocarbon derivatives NEC	968.2	E855.1	E938.2	E950.4	E962.0	E980.4
infiltration (intradermal) (subcutaneous) (submucosal)	968.5	E855.2	E938.5	E950.4	E962.0	E980.4
intravenous	968.3	E855.1	E938.3	E950.4	E962.0	E980.4
local NEC	968.9	E855.2	E938.9	E950.4	E962.0	E980.4

◀ New　◀ⅢⅢ Revised　deleted Deleted　● Use Additional Digit(s)

Substance	Poisoning	External Cause (E Code)				
		Accident	Therapeutic Use	Suicide Attempt	Assault	Undetermined
Anesthesia *(Continued)*						
nerve blocking (peripheral) (plexus)	968.6	E855.2	E938.6	E950.4	E962.0	E980.4
rectal NEC	968.3	E855.1	E938.3	E950.4	E962.0	E980.4
spinal	968.7	E855.2	E938.7	E950.4	E962.0	E980.4
surface	968.5	E855.2	E938.5	E950.4	E962.0	E980.4
topical	968.5	E855.2	E938.5	E950.4	E962.0	E980.4
Aneurine	963.5	E858.1	E933.5	E950.4	E962.0	E980.4
Anginine - *see* Glyceryl trinitrate	971.2	E855.5	E941.2	E950.4	E962.0	E980.4
Angio-Conray	977.8	E858.8	E947.8	E950.4	E962.0	E980.4
Angiotensin	971.2	E855.5	E941.2	E950.4	E962.0	E980.4
Anhydrohydroxyprogesterone	962.2	E858.0	E932.2	E950.4	E962.0	E980.4
Anhydron	974.3	E858.5	E944.3	E950.4	E962.0	E980.4
Anileridine	965.09	E850.2	E935.2	E950.0	E962.0	E980.0
Aniline (dye) (liquid)	983.0	E864.0	—	E950.7	E962.1	E980.6
analgesic	965.4	E850.4	E935.4	E950.0	E962.0	E980.0
derivatives, therapeutic NEC	965.4	E850.4	E935.4	E950.0	E962.0	E980.0
vapor	987.8	E869.8	—	E952.8	E962.2	E982.8
Aniscoropine	971.1	E855.4	E941.1	E950.4	E962.0	E980.4
Anisindione	964.2	E858.2	E934.2	E950.4	E962.0	E980.4
Anorexic agents	977.0	E858.8	E947.0	E950.4	E962.0	E980.4
Ant (bite) (sting)	989.5	E905.5	—	E950.9	E962.1	E980.9
Antabuse	977.3	E858.8	E947.3	E950.4	E962.0	E980.4
Antacids	973.0	E858.4	E943.0	E950.4	E962.0	E980.4
Antazoline	963.0	E858.1	E933.0	E950.4	E962.0	E980.4
Anthelmintics	961.6	E857	E931.6	E950.4	E962.0	E980.4
Anthralin	976.4	E858.7	E946.4	E950.4	E962.0	E980.4
Anthramycin	960.7	E856	E930.7	E950.4	E962.0	E980.4
Antiadrenergics	971.3	E855.6	E941.3	E950.4	E962.0	E980.4
Antiallergic agents	963.0	E858.1	E933.0	E950.4	E962.0	E980.4
Antianemic agents NEC	964.1	E858.2	E934.1	E950.4	E962.0	E980.4
Antiaris toxicaria	988.2	E865.4	—	E950.9	E962.1	E980.9
Antiarteriosclerotic agents	972.2	E858.3	E942.2	E950.4	E962.0	E980.4
Antiasthmatics	975.7	E858.6	E945.7	E950.4	E962.0	E980.4
Antibiotics	960.9	E856	E930.9	E950.4	E962.0	E980.4
antifungal	960.1	E856	E930.1	E950.4	E962.0	E980.4
antimycobacterial	960.6	E856	E930.6	E950.4	E962.0	E980.4
antineoplastic	960.7	E856	E930.7	E950.4	E962.0	E980.4
cephalosporin (group)	960.5	E856	E930.5	E950.4	E962.0	E980.4
chloramphenicol (group)	960.2	E856	E930.2	E950.4	E962.0	E980.4
macrolides	960.3	E856	E930.3	E950.4	E962.0	E980.4

◀ New   ◀▥ Revised   ~~deleted~~ Deleted   ● Use Additional Digit(s)

Substance	Poisoning	External Cause (E Code)				
		Accident	Therapeutic Use	Suicide Attempt	Assault	Undetermined
Antibiotics *(Continued)*						
specified NEC	960.8	E856	E930.8	E950.4	E962.0	E980.4
tetracycline (group)	960.4	E856	E930.4	E950.4	E962.0	E980.4
Anticancer agents NEC	963.1	E858.1	E933.1	E950.4	E962.0	E980.4
antibiotics	960.7	E856	E930.7	E950.4	E962.0	E980.4
Anticholinergics	971.1	E855.4	E941.1	E950.4	E962.0	E980.4
Anticholinesterase (organophosphorus) (reversible)	971.0	E855.3	E941.0	E950.4	E962.0	E980.4
Anticoagulants	964.2	E858.2	E934.2	E950.4	E962.0	E980.4
antagonists	964.5	E858.2	E934.5	E950.4	E962.0	E980.4
Anti-common cold agents NEC	975.6	E858.6	E945.6	E950.4	E962.0	E980.4
Anticonvulsants NEC	966.3	E855.0	E936.3	E950.4	E962.0	E980.4
Antidepressants	969.00 ◄ⅲ	E854.0	E939.0	E950.3	E962.0	E980.3
monoamine oxidase inhibitors (MAOI)	969.01	E854.0	E939.0	E950.3	E962.0	E980.3 ◄
specified type NEC	969.09	E854.0	E939.0	E950.3	E962.0	E980.3 ◄
SSNRI (selective serotonin and norepinephrine reuptake inhibitors)	969.02	E854.0	E939.0	E950.3	E962.0	E980.3 ◄
SSRI (selective serotonin reuptake inhibitors)	969.03	E854.0	E939.0	E950.3	E962.0	E980.3 ◄
tetracyclic	969.04	E854.0	E939.0	E950.3	E962.0	E980.3 ◄
tricyclic	969.05	E854.0	E939.0	E950.3	E962.0	E980.3 ◄
Antidiabetic agents	962.3	E858.0	E932.3	E950.4	E962.0	E980.4
Antidiarrheal agents	973.5	E858.4	E943.5	E950.4	E962.0	E980.4
Antidiuretic hormone	962.5	E858.0	E932.5	E950.4	E962.0	E980.4
Antidotes NEC	977.2	E858.8	E947.2	E950.4	E962.0	E980.4
Antiemetic agents	963.0	E858.1	E933.0	E950.4	E962.0	E980.4
Antiepilepsy agent NEC	966.3	E855.0	E936.3	E950.4	E962.0	E980.4
Antifertility pills	962.2	E858.0	E932.2	E950.4	E962.0	E980.4
Antiflatulents	973.8	E858.4	E943.8	E950.4	E962.0	E980.4
Antifreeze	989.89	E866.8	—	E950.9	E962.1	E980.9
alcohol	980.1	E860.2	—	E950.9	E962.1	E980.9
ethylene glycol	982.8	E862.4	—	E950.9	E962.1	E980.9
Antifungals (nonmedicinal) (sprays)	989.4	E863.6	—	E950.6	E962.1	E980.7
medicinal NEC	961.9	E857	E931.9	E950.4	E962.0	E980.4
antibiotic	960.1	E856	E930.1	E950.4	E962.0	E980.4
topical	976.0	E858.7	E946.0	E950.4	E962.0	E980.4
Antigastric secretion agents	973.0	E858.4	E943.0	E950.4	E962.0	E980.4
Antihelmintics	961.6	E857	E931.6	E950.4	E962.0	E980.4
Antihemophilic factor (human)	964.7	E858.2	E934.7	E950.4	E962.0	E980.4
Antihistamine	963.0	E858.1	E933.0	E950.4	E962.0	E980.4
Antihypertensive agents NEC	972.6	E858.3	E942.6	E950.4	E962.0	E980.4

◄ New   ◄ⅲ Revised   ~~deleted~~ Deleted   ● Use Additional Digit(s)

Substance	Poisoning	External Cause (E Code)				
		Accident	Therapeutic Use	Suicide Attempt	Assault	Undetermined
Anti-infectives NEC	961.9	E857	E931.9	E950.4	E962.0	E980.4
antibiotics	960.9	E856	E930.9	E950.4	E962.0	E980.4
specified NEC	960.8	E856	E930.8	E950.4	E962.0	E980.4
anthelmintic	961.6	E857	E931.6	E950.4	E962.0	E980.4
antimalarial	961.4	E857	E931.4	E950.4	E962.0	E980.4
antimycobacterial NEC	961.8	E857	E931.8	E950.4	E962.0	E980.4
antibiotics	960.6	E856	E930.6	E950.4	E962.0	E980.4
antiprotozoal NEC	961.5	E857	E931.5	E950.4	E962.0	E980.4
blood	961.4	E857	E931.4	E950.4	E962.0	E980.4
antiviral	961.7	E857	E931.7	E950.4	E962.0	E980.4
arsenical	961.1	E857	E931.1	E950.4	E962.0	E980.4
ENT agents	976.6	E858.7	E946.6	E950.4	E962.0	E980.4
heavy metals NEC	961.2	E857	E931.2	E950.4	E962.0	E980.4
local	976.0	E858.7	E946.0	E950.4	E962.0	E980.4
ophthalmic preparation	976.5	E858.7	E946.5	E950.4	E962.0	E980.4
topical NEC	976.0	E858.7	E946.0	E950.4	E962.0	E980.4
Anti-inflammatory agents (topical)	976.0	E858.7	E946.0	E950.4	E962.0	E980.4
Antiknock (tetraethyl lead)	984.1	E862.1	—	E950.9	E962.1	E980.9
Antilipemics	972.2	E858.3	E942.2	E950.4	E962.0	E980.4
Antimalarials	961.4	E857	E931.4	E950.4	E962.0	E980.4
Antimony (compounds) (vapor) NEC	985.4	E866.2	—	E950.9	E962.1	E980.9
anti-infectives	961.2	E857	E931.2	E950.4	E962.0	E980.4
pesticides (vapor)	985.4	E863.4	—	E950.6	E962.2	E980.7
potassium tartrate	961.2	E857	E931.2	E950.4	E962.0	E980.4
tartrated	961.2	E857	E931.2	E950.4	E962.0	E980.4
Antimuscarinic agents	971.1	E855.4	E941.1	E950.4	E962.0	E980.4
Antimycobacterials NEC	961.8	E857	E931.8	E950.4	E962.0	E980.4
antibiotics	960.6	E856	E930.6	E950.4	E962.0	E980.4
Antineoplastic agents	963.1	E858.1	E933.1	E950.4	E962.0	E980.4
antibiotics	960.7	E856	E930.7	E950.4	E962.0	E980.4
Anti-Parkinsonism agents	966.4	E855.0	E936.4	E950.4	E962.0	E980.4
Antiphlogistics	965.69	E850.6	E935.6	E950.0	E962.0	E980.0
Antiprotozoals NEC	961.5	E857	E931.5	E950.4	E962.0	E980.4
blood	961.4	E857	E931.4	E950.4	E962.0	E980.4
Antipruritics (local)	976.1	E858.7	E946.1	E950.4	E962.0	E980.4
Antipsychotic agents NEC	969.3	E853.8	E939.3	E950.3	E962.0	E980.3
Antipyretics	965.9	E850.9	E935.9	E950.0	E962.0	E980.0
specified NEC	965.8	E850.8	E935.8	E950.0	E962.0	E980.0
Antipyrine	965.5	E850.5	E935.5	E950.0	E962.0	E980.0
Antirabies serum (equine)	979.9	E858.8	E949.9	E950.4	E962.0	E980.4

◄ New   ◄▬ Revised   ~~deleted~~ Deleted   ● Use Additional Digit(s)

Substance	Poisoning	External Cause (E Code)				
		Accident	Therapeutic Use	Suicide Attempt	Assault	Undetermined
Antirheumatics	965.69	E850.6	E935.6	E950.0	E962.0	E980.0
Antiseborrheics	976.4	E858.7	E946.4	E950.4	E962.0	E980.4
Antiseptics (external) (medicinal)	976.0	E858.7	E946.0	E950.4	E962.0	E980.4
Antistine	963.0	E858.1	E933.0	E950.4	E962.0	E980.4
Antithyroid agents	962.8	E858.0	E932.8	E950.4	E962.0	E980.4
Antitoxin, any	979.9	E858.8	E949.9	E950.4	E962.0	E980.4
Antituberculars	961.8	E857	E931.8	E950.4	E962.0	E980.4
antibiotics	960.6	E856	E930.6	E950.4	E962.0	E980.4
Antitussives	975.4	E858.6	E945.4	E950.4	E962.0	E980.4
Antivaricose agents (sclerosing)	972.7	E858.3	E942.7	E950.4	E962.0	E980.4
Antivenin (crotaline) (spider-bite)	979.9	E858.8	E949.9	E950.4	E962.0	E980.4
Antivert	963.0	E858.1	E933.0	E950.4	E962.0	E980.4
Antivirals NEC	961.7	E857	E931.7	E950.4	E962.0	E980.4
Ant poisons - *see* Pesticides	—	—	—	—	—	—
Antrol	989.4	E863.4	—	E950.6	E962.1	E980.7
fungicide	989.4	E863.6	—	E950.6	E962.1	E980.7
Apomorphine hydrochloride (emetic)	973.6	E858.4	E943.6	E950.4	E962.0	E980.4
Appetite depressants, central	977.0	E858.8	E947.0	E950.4	E962.0	E980.4
Apresoline	972.6	E858.3	E942.6	E950.4	E962.0	E980.4
Aprobarbital, aprobarbitone	967.0	E851	E937.0	E950.1	E962.0	E980.1
Apronalide	967.8	E852.8	E937.8	E950.2	E962.0	E980.2
Aqua fortis	983.1	E864.1	—	E950.7	E962.1	E980.6
Arachis oil (topical)	976.3	E858.7	E946.3	E950.4	E962.0	E980.4
cathartic	973.2	E858.4	E943.2	E950.4	E962.0	E980.4
Aralen	961.4	E857	E931.4	E950.4	E962.0	E980.4
Arginine salts	974.5	E858.5	E944.5	E950.4	E962.0	E980.4
Argyrol	976.0	E858.7	E946.0	E950.4	E962.0	E980.4
ENT agent	976.6	E858.7	E946.6	E950.4	E962.0	E980.4
ophthalmic preparation	976.5	E858.7	E946.5	E950.4	E962.0	E980.4
Aristocort	962.0	E858.0	E932.0	E950.4	E962.0	E980.4
ENT agent	976.6	E858.7	E946.6	E950.4	E962.0	E980.4
ophthalmic preparation	976.5	E858.7	E946.5	E950.4	E962.0	E980.4
topical NEC	976.0	E858.7	E946.0	E950.4	E962.0	E980.4
Aromatics, corrosive	983.0	E864.0	—	E950.7	E962.1	E980.6
disinfectants	983.0	E861.4	—	E950.7	E962.1	E980.6
Arsenate of lead (insecticide)	985.1	E863.4	—	E950.8	E962.1	E980.8
herbicide	985.1	E863.5	—	E950.8	E962.1	E980.8
Arsenic, arsenicals (compounds) (dust) (fumes) (vapor) NEC	985.1	E866.3	—	E950.8	E962.1	E980.8
anti-infectives	961.1	E857	E931.1	E950.4	E962.0	E980.4
pesticide (dust) (fumes)	985.1	E863.4	—	E950.8	E962.1	E980.8

◀ New ◀▥ Revised deleted Deleted ● Use Additional Digit(s)

Substance	Poisoning	External Cause (E Code)				
		Accident	Therapeutic Use	Suicide Attempt	Assault	Undetermined
Arsine (gas)	985.1	E866.3	—	E950.8	E962.1	E980.8
Arsphenamine (silver)	961.1	E857	E931.1	E950.4	E962.0	E980.4
Arsthinol	961.1	E857	E931.1	E950.4	E962.0	E980.4
Artane	971.1	E855.4	E941.1	E950.4	E962.0	E980.4
Arthropod (venomous) NEC	989.5	E905.5	—	E950.9	E962.1	E980.9
Asbestos	989.81	E866.8	—	E950.9	E962.1	E980.9
Ascaridole	961.6	E857	E931.6	E950.4	E962.0	E980.4
Ascorbic acid	963.5	E858.1	E933.5	E950.4	E962.0	E980.4
Asiaticoside	976.0	E858.7	E946.0	E950.4	E962.0	E980.4
Aspidium (oleoresin)	961.6	E857	E931.6	E950.4	E962.0	E980.4
Aspirin	965.1	E850.3	E935.3	E950.0	E962.0	E980.0
Astringents (local)	976.2	E858.7	E946.2	E950.4	E962.0	E980.4
Atabrine	961.3	E857	E931.3	E950.4	E962.0	E980.4
Ataractics	969.5	E853.8	E939.5	E950.3	E962.0	E980.3
Atonia drug, intestinal	973.3	E858.4	E943.3	E950.4	E962.0	E980.4
Atophan	974.7	E858.5	E944.7	E950.4	E962.0	E980.4
Atropine	971.1	E855.4	E941.1	E950.4	E962.0	E980.4
Attapulgite	973.5	E858.4	E943.5	E950.4	E962.0	E980.4
Attenuvax	979.4	E858.8	E949.4	E950.4	E962.0	E980.4
Aureomycin	960.4	E856	E930.4	E950.4	E962.0	E980.4
ophthalmic preparation	976.5	E858.7	E946.5	E950.4	E962.0	E980.4
topical NEC	976.0	E858.7	E946.0	E950.4	E962.0	E980.4
Aurothioglucose	965.69	E850.6	E935.6	E950.0	E962.0	E980.0
Aurothioglycanide	965.69	E850.6	E935.6	E950.0	E962.0	E980.0
Aurothiomalate	965.69	E850.6	E935.6	E950.0	E962.0	E980.0
Automobile fuel	981	E862.1	—	E950.9	E962.1	E980.9
Autonomic nervous system agents NEC	971.9	E855.9	E941.9	E950.4	E962.0	E980.4
Avlosulfon	961.8	E857	E931.8	E950.4	E962.0	E980.4
Avomine	967.8	E852.8	E937.8	E950.2	E962.0	E980.2
Azacyclonol	969.5	E853.8	E939.5	E950.3	E962.0	E980.3
Azapetine	971.3	E855.6	E941.3	E950.4	E962.0	E980.4
Azaribine	963.1	E858.1	E933.1	E950.4	E962.0	E980.4
Azaserine	960.7	E856	E930.7	E950.4	E962.0	E980.4
Azathioprine	963.1	E858.1	E933.1	E950.4	E962.0	E980.4
Azosulfamide	961.0	E857	E931.0	E950.4	E962.0	E980.4
Azulfidine	961.0	E857	E931.0	E950.4	E962.0	E980.4
Azuresin	977.8	E858.8	E947.8	E950.4	E962.0	E980.4
Bacimycin	976.0	E858.7	E946.0	E950.4	E962.0	E980.4
ophthalmic preparation	976.5	E858.7	E946.5	E950.4	E962.0	E980.4

◀ New　◀▥ Revised　~~deleted~~ Deleted　● Use Additional Digit(s)

Substance	Poisoning	External Cause (E Code)				
		Accident	Therapeutic Use	Suicide Attempt	Assault	Undetermined
Bacitracin	960.8	E856	E930.8	E950.4	E962.0	E980.4
ENT agent	976.6	E858.7	E946.6	E950.4	E962.0	E980.4
ophthalmic preparation	976.5	E858.7	E946.5	E950.4	E962.0	E980.4
topical NEC	976.0	E858.7	E946.0	E950.4	E962.0	E980.4
Baking soda	963.3	E858.1	E933.3	E950.4	E962.0	E980.4
BAL	963.8	E858.1	E933.8	E950.4	E962.0	E980.4
Bamethan (sulfate)	972.5	E858.3	E942.5	E950.4	E962.0	E980.4
Bamipine	963.0	E858.1	E933.0	E950.4	E962.0	E980.4
Baneberry	988.2	E865.4	—	E950.9	E962.1	E980.9
Banewort	988.2	E865.4	—	E950.9	E962.1	E980.9
Barbenyl	967.0	E851	E937.0	E950.1	E962.0	E980.1
Barbital, barbitone	967.0	E851	E937.0	E950.1	E962.0	E980.1
Barbiturates, barbituric acid	967.0	E851	E937.0	E950.1	E962.0	E980.1
anesthetic (intravenous)	968.3	E855.1	E938.3	E950.4	E962.0	E980.4
Barium (carbonate) (chloride) (sulfate)	985.8	E866.4	—	E950.9	E962.1	E980.9
diagnostic agent	977.8	E858.8	E947.8	E950.4	E962.0	E980.4
pesticide	985.8	E863.4	—	E950.6	E962.1	E980.7
rodenticide	985.8	E863.7	—	E950.6	E962.1	E980.7
Barrier cream	976.3	E858.7	E946.3	E950.4	E962.0	E980.4
Battery acid or fluid	983.1	E864.1	—	E950.7	E962.1	E980.6
Bay rum	980.8	E860.8	—	E950.9	E962.1	E980.9
BCG vaccine	978.0	E858.8	E948.0	E950.4	E962.0	E980.4
Bearsfoot	988.2	E865.4	—	E950.9	E962.1	E980.9
Beclamide	966.3	E855.0	E936.3	E950.4	E962.0	E980.4
Bee (sting) (venom)	989.5	E905.3	—	E950.9	E962.1	E980.9
Belladonna (alkaloids)	971.1	E855.4	E941.1	E950.4	E962.0	E980.4
Bemegride	970.0	E854.3	E940.0	E950.4	E962.0	E980.4
Benactyzine	969.8	E855.8	E939.8	E950.3	E962.0	E980.3
Benadryl	963.0	E858.1	E933.0	E950.4	E962.0	E980.4
Bendrofluazide	974.3	E858.5	E944.3	E950.4	E962.0	E980.4
Bendroflumethiazide	974.3	E858.5	E944.3	E950.4	E962.0	E980.4
Benemid	974.7	E858.5	E944.7	E950.4	E962.0	E980.4
Benethamine penicillin G	960.0	E856	E930.0	E950.4	E962.0	E980.4
Benisone	976.0	E858.7	E946.0	E950.4	E962.0	E980.4
Benoquin	976.8	E858.7	E946.8	E950.4	E962.0	E980.4
Benoxinate	968.5	E855.2	E938.5	E950.4	E962.0	E980.4
Bentonite	976.3	E858.7	E946.3	E950.4	E962.0	E980.4
Benzalkonium (chloride)	976.0	E858.7	E946.0	E950.4	E962.0	E980.4
ophthalmic preparation	976.5	E858.7	E946.5	E950.4	E962.0	E980.4
Benzamidosalicylate (calcium)	961.8	E857	E931.8	E950.4	E962.0	E980.4

◀ New　◀▥ Revised　deleted Deleted　● Use Additional Digit(s)

Substance	Poisoning	External Cause (E Code)				
		Accident	Therapeutic Use	Suicide Attempt	Assault	Undetermined
Benzathine penicillin	960.0	E856	E930.0	E950.4	E962.0	E980.4
Benzcarbimine	963.1	E858.1	E933.1	E950.4	E962.0	E980.4
Benzedrex	971.2	E855.5	E941.2	E950.4	E962.0	E980.4
Benzedrine (amphetamine)	969.72◀	E854.2	E939.7	E950.3	E962.0	E980.3
Benzene (acetyl) (dimethyl) (methyl) (solvent) (vapor)	982.0	E862.4	—	E950.9	E962.1	E980.9
hexachloride (gamma) (insecticide) (vapor)	989.2	E863.0	—	E950.6	E962.1	E980.7
Benzethonium	976.0	E858.7	E946.0	E950.4	E962.0	E980.4
Benzhexol (chloride)	966.4	E855.0	E936.4	E950.4	E962.0	E980.4
Benzilonium	971.1	E855.4	E941.1	E950.4	E962.0	E980.4
Benzin(e) - see Ligroin	—	—	—	—	—	—
Benziodarone	972.4	E858.3	E942.4	E950.4	E962.0	E980.4
Benzocaine	968.5	E855.2	E938.5	E950.4	E962.0	E980.4
Benzodiapin	969.4	E853.2	E939.4	E950.3	E962.0	E980.3
Benzodiazepines (tranquilizers) NEC	969.4	E853.2	E939.4	E950.3	E962.0	E980.3
Benzoic acid (with salicylic acid) (anti-infective)	976.0	E858.7	E946.0	E950.4	E962.0	E980.4
Benzoin	976.3	E858.7	E946.3	E950.4	E962.0	E980.4
Benzol (vapor)	982.0	E862.4	—	E950.9	E962.1	E980.9
Benzomorphan	965.09	E850.2	E935.2	E950.0	E962.0	E980.0
Benzonatate	975.4	E858.6	E945.4	E950.4	E962.0	E980.4
Benzothiadiazides	974.3	E858.5	E944.3	E950.4	E962.0	E980.4
Benzoylpas	961.8	E857	E931.8	E950.4	E962.0	E980.4
Benzperidol	969.5	E853.8	E939.5	E950.3	E962.0	E980.3
Benzphetamine	977.0	E858.8	E947.0	E950.4	E962.0	E980.4
Benzpyrinium	971.0	E855.3	E941.0	E950.4	E962.0	E980.4
Benzquinamide	963.0	E858.1	E933.0	E950.4	E962.0	E980.4
Benzthiazide	974.3	E858.5	E944.3	E950.4	E962.0	E980.4
Benztropine	971.1	E855.4	E941.1	E950.4	E962.0	E980.4
Benzyl	—	—	—	—	—	—
acetate	982.8	E862.4	—	E950.9	E962.1	E980.9
benzoate (anti-infective)	976.0	E858.7	E946.0	E950.4	E962.0	E980.4
morphine	965.09	E850.2	E935.2	E950.0	E962.0	E980.0
penicillin	960.0	E856	E930.0	E950.4	E962.0	E980.4
Bephenium	—	—	—	—	—	—
hydroxynapthoate	961.6	E857	E931.6	E950.4	E962.0	E980.4
Bergamot oil	989.89	E866.8	—	E950.9	E962.1	E980.9
Berries, poisonous	988.2	E865.3	—	E950.9	E962.1	E980.9
Beryllium (compounds) (fumes)	985.3	E866.4	—	E950.9	E962.1	E980.9
Beta-carotene	976.3	E858.7	E946.3	E950.4	E962.0	E980.4
Beta-Chlor	967.1	E852.0	E937.1	E950.2	E962.0	E980.2

◀ New　◀▥ Revised　~~deleted~~ Deleted　● Use Additional Digit(s)

Substance	Poisoning	External Cause (E Code)				
		Accident	Therapeutic Use	Suicide Attempt	Assault	Undetermined
Betamethasone	962.0	E858.0	E932.0	E950.4	E962.0	E980.4
topical	976.0	E858.7	E946.0	E950.4	E962.0	E980.4
Betazole	977.8	E858.8	E947.8	E950.4	E962.0	E980.4
Bethanechol	971.0	E855.3	E941.0	E950.4	E962.0	E980.4
Bethanidine	972.6	E858.3	E942.6	E950.4	E962.0	E980.4
Betula oil	976.3	E858.7	E946.3	E950.4	E962.0	E980.4
Bhang	969.6	E854.1	E939.6	E950.3	E962.0	E980.3
Bialamicol	961.5	E857	E931.5	E950.4	E962.0	E980.4
Bichloride of mercury - *see* Mercury, chloride	—	—	—	—	—	—
Bichromates (calcium) (crystals) (potassium) (sodium)	983.9	E864.3	—	E950.7	E962.1	E980.6
fumes	987.8	E869.8	—	E952.8	E962.2	E982.8
Biguanide derivatives, oral	962.3	E858.0	E932.3	E950.4	E962.0	E980.4
Biligrafin	977.8	E858.8	E947.8	E950.4	E962.0	E980.4
Bilopaque	977.8	E858.8	E947.8	E950.4	E962.0	E980.4
Bioflavonoids	972.8	E858.3	E942.8	E950.4	E962.0	E980.4
Biological substance NEC	979.9	E858.8	E949.9	E950.4	E962.0	E980.4
Biperiden	966.4	E855.0	E936.4	E950.4	E962.0	E980.4
Bisacodyl	973.1	E858.4	E943.1	E950.4	E962.0	E980.4
Bishydroxycoumarin	964.2	E858.2	E934.2	E950.4	E962.0	E980.4
Bismarsen	961.1	E857	E931.1	E950.4	E962.0	E980.4
Bismuth (compounds) NEC	985.8	E866.4	—	E950.9	E962.1	E980.9
anti-infectives	961.2	E857	E931.2	E950.4	E962.0	E980.4
subcarbonate	973.5	E858.4	E943.5	E950.4	E962.0	E980.4
sulfarsphenamine	961.1	E857	E931.1	E950.4	E962.0	E980.4
Bisphosphonates	—	—	—	—	—	—
intravenous	963.1	E858.1	E933.7	E950.4	E962.0	E980.4
oral	963.1	E858.1	E933.6	E950.4	E962.0	E980.4
Bithionol	961.6	E857	E931.6	E950.4	E962.0	E980.4
Bitter almond oil	989.0	E866.8	—	E950.9	E962.1	E980.9
Bittersweet	988.2	E865.4	—	E950.9	E962.1	E930.9
Black	—	—	—	—	—	—
flag	989.4	E863.4	—	E950.6	E962.1	E980.7
henbane	988.2	E865.4	—	E950.9	E962.1	E980.9
leaf (40)	989.4	E863.4	—	E950.6	E962.1	E980.7
widow spider (bite)	989.5	E905.1	—	E950.9	E962.1	E980.9
antivenin	979.9	E858.8	E949.9	E950.4	E962.0	E980.4
Blast furnace gas (carbon monoxide from)	986	E868.8	—	E952.1	E962.2	E982.1
Bleach NEC	983.9	E864.3	—	E950.7	E962.1	E980.6
Bleaching solutions	983.9	E864.3	—	E950.7	E962.1	E980.6
Bleomycin (sulfate)	960.7	E856	E930.7	E950.4	E962.0	E980.4

◀ New ◀⃪ Revised ~~deleted~~ Deleted ● Use Additional Digit(s)

Substance	Poisoning	External Cause (E Code) Accident	Therapeutic Use	Suicide Attempt	Assault	Undetermined
Blockain	968.9	E855.2	E938.9	E950.4	E962.0	E980.4
infiltration (subcutaneous)	968.5	E855.2	E938.5	E950.4	E962.0	E980.4
nerve block (peripheral) (plexus)	968.6	E855.2	E938.6	E950.4	E962.0	E980.4
topical (surface)	968.5	E855.2	E938.5	E950.4	E962.0	E980.4
Blood (derivatives) (natural) (plasma) (whole)	964.7	E858.2	E934.7	E950.4	E962.0	E980.4
affecting agent	964.9	E858.2	E934.9	E950.4	E962.0	E980.4
specified NEC	964.8	E858.2	E934.8	E950.4	E962.0	E980.4
substitute (macromolecular)	964.8	E858.2	E934.8	E950.4	E962.0	E980.4
Blue velvet	965.09	E850.2	E935.2	E950.0	E962.0	E980.0
Bone meal	989.89	E866.5	—	E950.9	E962.1	E980.9
Bonine	963.0	E858.1	E933.0	E950.4	E962.0	E980.4
Boracic acid	976.0	E858.7	E946.0	E950.4	E962.0	E980.4
ENT agent	976.6	E858.7	E946.6	E950.4	E962.0	E980.4
ophthalmic preparation	976.5	E858.7	E946.5	E950.4	E962.0	E980.4
Borate (cleanser) (sodium)	989.6	E861.3	—	E950.9	E962.1	E980.9
Borax (cleanser)	989.6	E861.3	—	E950.9	E962.1	E980.9
Boric acid	976.0	E858.7	E946.0	E950.4	E962.0	E980.4
ENT agent	976.6	E858.7	E946.6	E950.4	E962.0	E980.4
ophthalmic preparation	976.5	E858.7	E946.5	E950.4	E962.0	E980.4
Boron hydride NEC	989.89	E866.8	—	E950.9	E962.1	E980.9
fumes or gas	987.8	E869.8	—	E952.8	E962.2	E982.8
Botox	975.3	E858.6	E945.3	E950.4	E962.0	E980.4
Brake fluid vapor	987.8	E869.8	—	E952.8	E962.2	E982.8
Brass (compounds) (fumes)	985.8	E866.4	—	E950.9	E962.1	E980.9
Brasso	981	E861.3	—	E950.9	E962.1	E980.9
Bretylium (tosylate)	972.6	E858.3	E942.6	E950.4	E962.0	E980.4
Brevital (sodium)	968.3	E855.1	E938.3	E950.4	E962.0	E980.4
British antilewisite	963.8	E858.1	E933.8	E950.4	E962.0	E980.4
Bromal (hydrate)	967.3	E852.2	E937.3	E950.2	E962.0	E980.2
Bromelains	963.4	E858.1	E933.4	E950.4	E962.0	E980.4
Bromides NEC	967.3	E852.2	E937.3	E950.2	E962.0	E980.2
Bromine (vapor)	987.8	E869.8	—	E952.8	E962.2	E982.8
compounds (medicinal)	967.3	E852.2	E937.3	E950.2	E962.0	E980.2
Bromisovalum	967.3	E852.2	E937.3	E950.2	E962.0	E980.2
Bromobenzyl cyanide	987.5	E869.3	—	E952.8	E962.2	E982.8
Bromodiphenhydramine	963.0	E858.1	E933.0	E950.4	E962.0	E980.4
Bromoform	967.3	E852.2	E937.3	E950.2	E962.0	E980.2
Bromophenol blue reagent	977.8	E858.8	E947.8	E950.4	E962.0	E980.4
Bromosalicylhydroxamic acid	961.8	E857	E931.8	E950.4	E962.0	E980.4
Bromo-seltzer	965.4	E850.4	E935.4	E950.0	E962.0	E980.0

◀ New   ◀ⅲ Revised   deleted Deleted   ● Use Additional Digit(s)

	External Cause (E Code)					
Substance	Poisoning	Accident	Therapeutic Use	Suicide Attempt	Assault	Undetermined
Brompheniramine	963.0	E858.1	E933.0	E950.4	E962.0	E980.4
Bromural	967.3	E852.2	E937.3	E950.2	E962.0	E980.2
Brown spider (bite) (venom)	989.5	E905.1	—	E950.9	E962.1	E980.9
Brucia	988.2	E865.3	—	E950.9	E962.1	E980.9
Brucine	989.1	E863.7	—	E950.6	E962.1	E980.7
Brunswick green - see Copper	—	—	—	—	—	—
Bruten - see Ibuprofen	—	—	—	—	—	—
Bryonia (alba) (dioica)	988.2	E865.4	—	E950.9	E962.1	E980.9
Buclizine	969.5	E853.8	E939.5	E950.3	E962.0	E980.3
Bufferin	965.1	E850.3	E935.3	E950.0	E962.0	E980.0
Bufotenine	969.6	E854.1	E939.6	E950.3	E962.0	E980.3
Buphenine	971.2	E855.5	E941.2	E950.4	E962.0	E980.4
Bupivacaine	968.9	E855.2	E938.9	E950.4	E962.0	E980.4
infiltration (subcutaneous)	968.5	E855.2	E938.5	E950.4	E962.0	E980.4
nerve block (peripheral) (plexus)	968.6	E855.2	E938.6	E950.4	E962.0	E980.4
Busulfan	963.1	E858.1	E933.1	E950.4	E962.0	E980.4
Butabarbital (sodium)	967.0	E851	E937.0	E950.1	E962.0	E980.1
Butabarbitone	967.0	E851	E937.0	E950.1	E962.0	E980.1
Butabarpal	967.0	E851	E937.0	E950.1	E962.0	E980.1
Butacaine	968.5	E855.2	E938.5	E950.4	E962.0	E980.4
Butallylonal	967.0	E851	E937.0	E950.1	E962.0	E980.1
Butane (distributed in mobile container)	987.0	E868.0	—	E951.1	E962.2	E981.1
distributed through pipes	987.0	E867	—	E951.0	E962.2	E981.0
incomplete combustion of - see Carbon monoxide, butane	—	—	—	—	—	—
Butanol	980.3	E860.4	—	E950.9	E962.1	E980.9
Butanone	982.8	E862.4	—	E950.9	E962.1	E980.9
Butaperazine	969.1	E853.0	E939.1	E950.3	E962.0	E980.3
Butazolidin	965.5	E850.5	E935.5	E950.0	E962.0	E980.0
Butethal	967.0	E851	E937.0	E950.1	E962.0	E980.1
Butethamate	971.1	E855.4	E941.1	E950.4	E962.0	E980.4
Buthalitone (sodium)	968.3	E855.1	E938.3	E950.4	E962.0	E980.4
Butisol (sodium)	967.0	E851	E937.0	E950.1	E962.0	E980.1
Butobarbital, butobarbitone	967.0	E851	E937.0	E950.1	E962.0	E980.1
Butriptyline	969.05◄▥	E854.0	E939.0	E950.3	E962.0	E980.3
Buttercups	988.2	E865.4	—	E950.9	E962.1	E980.9
Butter of antimony - see Antimony	—	—	—	—	—	—
Butyl	—	—	—	—	—	—
acetate (secondary)	982.8	E862.4	—	E950.9	E962.1	E980.9
alcohol	980.3	E860.4	—	E950.9	E962.1	E980.9

◄ New   ◄▥ Revised   ~~deleted~~ Deleted   ● Use Additional Digit(s)

Substance	Poisoning	External Cause (E Code)				
		Accident	Therapeutic Use	Suicide Attempt	Assault	Undetermined
Butyl *(Continued)*						
carbinol	980.8	E860.8	—	E950.9	E962.1	E980.9
carbitol	982.8	E862.4	—	E950.9	E962.1	E980.9
cellosolve	982.8	E862.4	—	E950.9	E962.1	E980.9
chloral (hydrate)	967.1	E852.0	E937.1	E950.2	E962.0	E980.2
formate	982.8	E862.4	—	E950.9	E962.1	E980.9
scopolammonium bromide	971.1	E855.4	E941.1	E950.4	E962.0	E980.4
Butyn	968.5	E855.2	E938.5	E950.4	E962.0	E980.4
Butyrophenone (-based tranquilizers)	969.2	E853.1	E939.2	E950.3	E962.0	E980.3
Cacodyl, cacodylic acid - *see* Arsenic	—	—	—	—	—	—
Cactinomycin	960.7	E856	E930.7	E950.4	E962.0	E980.4
Cade oil	976.4	E858.7	E946.4	E950.4	E962.0	E980.4
Cadmium (chloride) (compounds) (dust) (fumes) (oxide)	985.5	E866.4	—	E950.9	E962.1	E980.9
sulfide (medicinal) NEC	976.4	E858.7	E946.4	E950.4	E962.0	E980.4
Caffeine	969.71◀▥	E854.2	E939.7	E950.3	E962.0	E980.3
Calabar bean	988.2	E865.4	—	E950.9	E962.1	E980.9
Caladium seguinium	988.2	E865.4	—	E950.9	E962.1	E980.9
Calamine (liniment) (lotion)	976.3	E858.7	E946.3	E950.4	E962.0	E980.4
Calciferol	963.5	E858.1	E933.5	E950.4	E962.0	E980.4
Calcium (salts) NEC	974.5	E858.5	E944.5	E950.4	E962.0	E980.4
acetylsalicylate	965.1	E850.3	E935.3	E950.0	E962.0	E980.0
benzamidosalicylate	961.8	E857	E931.8	E950.4	E962.0	E980.4
carbaspirin	965.1	E850.3	E935.3	E950.0	E962.0	E980.0
carbimide (citrated)	977.3	E858.8	E947.3	E950.4	E962.0	E980.4
carbonate (antacid)	973.0	E858.4	E943.0	E950.4	E962.0	E980.4
cyanide (citrated)	977.3	E858.8	E947.3	E950.4	E962.0	E980.4
dioctyl sulfosuccinate	973.2	E858.4	E943.2	E950.4	E962.0	E980.4
disodium edathamil	963.8	E858.1	E933.8	E950.4	E962.0	E980.4
disodium edetate	963.8	E858.1	E933.8	E950.4	E962.0	E980.4
EDTA	963.8	E858.1	E933.8	E950.4	E962.0	E980.4
hydrate, hydroxide	983.2	E864.2	—	E950.7	E962.1	E980.6
mandelate	961.9	E857	E931.9	E950.4	E962.0	E980.4
oxide	983.2	E864.2	—	E950.7	E962.1	E980.6
Calomel - *see* Mercury, chloride	—	—	—	—	—	—
Caloric agents NEC	974.5	E858.5	E944.5	E950.4	E962.0	E980.4
Calusterone	963.1	E858.1	E933.1	E950.4	E962.0	E980.4
Camoquin	961.4	E857	E931.4	E950.4	E962.0	E980.4
Camphor (oil)	976.1	E858.7	E946.1	E950.4	E962.0	E980.4
Candeptin	976.0	E858.7	E946.0	E950.4	E962.0	E980.4

◀ New   ◀▥ Revised   ~~deleted~~ Deleted   ● Use Additional Digit(s)

TABLE OF DRUGS AND CHEMICALS

Substance	Poisoning	External Cause (E Code)				
		Accident	Therapeutic Use	Suicide Attempt	Assault	Undetermined
Candicidin	976.0	E858.7	E946.0	E950.4	E962.0	E980.4
Cannabinols	969.6	E854.1	E939.6	E950.3	E962.0	E980.3
Cannabis (derivatives) (indica) (sativa)	969.6	E854.1	E939.6	E950.3	E962.0	E980.3
Canned heat	980.1	E860.2	—	E950.9	E962.1	E980.9
Cantharides, cantharidin, cantharis	976.8	E858.7	E946.8	E950.4	E962.0	E980.4
Capillary agents	972.8	E858.3	E942.8	E950.4	E962.0	E980.4
Capreomycin	960.6	E856	E930.6	E950.4	E962.0	E980.4
Captodiame, captodiamine	969.5	E853.8	E939.5	E950.3	E962.0	E980.3
Caramiphen (hydrochloride)	971.1	E855.4	E941.1	E950.4	E962.0	E980.4
Carbachol	971.0	E855.3	E941.0	E950.4	E962.0	E980.4
Carbacrylamine resins	974.5	E858.5	E944.5	E950.4	E962.0	E980.4
Carbamate (sedative)	967.8	E852.8	E937.8	E950.2	E962.0	E980.2
herbicide	989.3	E863.5	—	E950.6	E962.1	E980.7
insecticide	989.3	E863.2	—	E950.6	E962.1	E980.7
Carbamazepine	966.3	E855.0	E936.3	E950.4	E962.0	E980.4
Carbamic esters	967.8	E852.8	E937.8	E950.2	E962.0	E980.2
Carbamide	974.4	E858.5	E944.4	E950.4	E962.0	E980.4
topical	976.8	E858.7	E946.8	E950.4	E962.0	E980.4
Carbamylcholine chloride	971.0	E855.3	E941.0	E950.4	E962.0	E980.4
Carbarsone	961.1	E857	E931.1	E950.4	E962.0	E980.4
Carbaryl	989.3	E863.2	—	E950.6	E962.1	E980.7
Carbaspirin	965.1	E850.3	E935.3	E950.0	E962.0	E980.0
Carbazochrome	972.8	E858.3	E942.8	E950.4	E962.0	E980.4
Carbenicillin	960.0	E856	E930.0	E950.4	E962.0	E980.4
Carbenoxolone	973.8	E858.4	E943.8	E950.4	E962.0	E980.4
Carbetapentane	975.4	E858.6	E945.4	E950.4	E962.0	E980.4
Carbimazole	962.8	E858.0	E932.8	E950.4	E962.0	E980.4
Carbinol	980.1	E860.2	—	E950.9	E962.1	E980.9
Carbinoxamine	963.0	E858.1	E933.0	E950.4	E962.0	E980.4
Carbitol	982.8	E862.4	—	E950.9	E962.1	E980.9
Carbocaine	968.9	E855.2	E938.9	E950.4	E962.0	E980.4
infiltration (subcutaneous)	968.5	E855.2	E938.5	E950.4	E962.0	E980.4
nerve block (peripheral) (plexus)	968.6	E855.2	E938.6	E950.4	E962.0	E980.4
topical (surface)	968.5	E855.2	E938.5	E950.4	E962.0	E980.4
Carbol-fuchsin solution	976.0	E858.7	E946.0	E950.4	E962.0	E980.4
Carbolic acid (see also Phenol)	983.0	E864.0	—	E950.7	E962.1	E980.6
Carbomycin	960.8	E856	E930.8	E950.4	E962.0	E980.4
Carbon	—	—	—	—	—	—
bisulfide (liquid) (vapor)	982.2	E862.4	—	E950.9	E962.1	E980.9

◀ New   ◀▥ Revised   deleted Deleted   ● Use Additional Digit(s)

Substance	Poisoning	External Cause (E Code)				
		Accident	Therapeutic Use	Suicide Attempt	Assault	Undetermined
Carbon *(Continued)*						
dioxide (gas)	987.8	E869.8	—	E952.8	E962.2	E982.8
disulfide (liquid) (vapor)	982.2	E862.4	—	E950.9	E962.1	E980.9
monoxide (from incomplete combustion of) (in) NEC	986	E868.9	—	E952.1	E962.2	E982.1
blast furnace gas	986	E868.8	—	E952.1	E962.2	E982.1
butane (distributed in mobile container)	986	E868.0	—	E951.1	E962.2	E981.1
distributed through pipes	986	E867	—	E951.0	E962.2	E981.0
charcoal fumes	986	E868.3	—	E952.1	E962.2	E982.1
coal						
gas (piped)	986	E867	—	E951.0	E962.2	E981.0
solid (in domestic stoves, fireplaces)	986	E868.3	—	E952.1	E962.2	E982.1
coke (in domestic stoves, fireplaces)	986	E868.3	—	E952.1	E962.2	E982.1
exhaust gas (motor) not in transit	986	E868.2	—	E952.0	E962.2	E982.0
combustion engine, any not in watercraft	986	E868.2	—	E952.0	E962.2	E982.0
farm tractor, not in transit	986	E868.2	—	E952.0	E962.2	E982.0
gas engine	986	E868.2	—	E952.0	E962.2	E982.0
motor pump	986	E868.2	—	E952.0	E962.2	E982.0
motor vehicle, not in transit	986	E868.2	—	E952.0	E962.2	E982.0
fuel (in domestic use)	986	E868.3	—	E952.1	E962.2	E982.1
gas (piped)	986	E867	—	E951.0	E962.2	E981.0
in mobile container	986	E868.0	—	E951.1	E962.2	E981.1
utility	986	E868.1	—	E951.8	E962.2	E981.1
in mobile container	986	E868.0	—	E951.1	E962.2	E981.1
piped (natural)	986	E867	—	E951.0	E962.2	E981.0
illuminating gas	986	E868.1	—	E951.8	E962.2	E981.8
industrial fuels or gases, any	986	E868.8	—	E952.1	E962.2	E982.1
kerosene (in domestic stoves, fireplaces)	986	E868.3	—	E952.1	E962.2	E982.1
kiln gas or vapor	986	E868.8	—	E952.1	E962.2	E982.1
motor exhaust gas, not in transit	986	E868.2	—	E952.0	E962.2	E982.0
piped gas (manufactured) (natural)	986	E867	—	E951.0	E962.2	E981.0
producer gas	986	E868.8	—	E952.1	E962.2	E982.1
propane (distributed in mobile container)	986	E868.0	—	E951.1	E962.2	E981.1
distributed through pipes	986	E867	—	E951.0	E962.2	E981.0
specified source NEC	986	E868.8	—	E952.1	E962.2	E982.1
stove gas	986	E868.1	—	E951.8	E962.2	E981.8
piped	986	E867	—	E951.0	E962.2	E981.0
utility gas	986	E868.1	—	E951.8	E962.2	E981.8
piped	986	E867	—	E951.0	E962.2	E981.0

◀ New ⬅ Revised ~~deleted~~ Deleted ● Use Additional Digit(s)

Substance	Poisoning	External Cause (E Code)				
		Accident	Therapeutic Use	Suicide Attempt	Assault	Undetermined
Carbon *(Continued)*						
monoxide (from incomplete combustion of) (in) NEC *(Continued)*						
water gas	986	E868.1	—	E951.8	E962.2	E981.8
wood (in domestic stoves, fireplaces)	986	E868.3	—	E952.1	E962.2	E982.1
tetrachloride (vapor) NEC	987.8	E869.8	—	E952.8	E962.2	E982.8
liquid (cleansing agent) NEC	982.1	E861.3	—	E950.9	E962.1	E980.9
solvent	982.1	E862.4	—	E950.9	E962.1	E980.9
Carbonic acid (gas)	987.8	E869.8	—	E952.8	E962.2	E982.8
anhydrase inhibitors	974.2	E858.5	E944.2	E950.4	E962.0	E980.4
Carbowax	976.3	E858.7	E946.3	E950.4	E962.0	E980.4
Carbrital	967.0	E851	E937.0	E950.1	E962.0	E980.1
Carbromal (derivatives)	967.3	E852.2	E937.3	E950.2	E962.0	E980.2
Cardiac	—	—	—	—	—	—
depressants	972.0	E858.3	E942.0	E950.4	E962.0	E980.4
rhythm regulators	972.0	E858.3	E942.0	E950.4	E962.0	E980.4
Cardiografin	977.8	E858.8	E947.8	E950.4	E962.0	E980.4
Cardio-green	977.8	E858.8	E947.8	E950.4	E962.0	E980.4
Cardiotonic glycosides	972.1	E858.3	E942.1	E950.4	E962.0	E980.4
Cardiovascular agents NEC	972.9	E858.3	E942.9	E950.4	E962.0	E980.4
Cardrase	974.2	E858.5	E944.2	E950.4	E962.0	E980.4
Carfusin	976.0	E858.7	E946.0	E950.4	E962.0	E980.4
Carisoprodol	968.0	E855.1	E938.0	E950.4	E962.0	E980.4
Carmustine	963.1	E858.1	E933.1	E950.4	E962.0	E980.4
Carotene	963.5	E858.1	E933.5	E950.4	E962.0	E980.4
Carphenazine (maleate)	969.1	E853.0	E939.1	E950.3	E962.0	E980.3
Carter's Little Pills	973.1	E858.4	E943.1	E950.4	E962.0	E980.4
Cascara (sagrada)	973.1	E858.4	E943.1	E950.4	E962.0	E980.4
Cassava	988.2	E865.4	—	E950.9	E962.1	E980.9
Castellani's paint	976.0	E858.7	E946.0	E950.4	E962.0	E980.4
Castor	—	—	—	—	—	—
bean	988.2	E865.3	—	E950.9	E962.1	E980.9
oil	973.1	E858.4	E943.1	E950.4	E962.0	E980.4
Caterpillar (sting)	989.5	E905.5	—	E950.9	E962.1	E980.9
Catha (edulis)	970.8	E854.3	E940.8	E950.4	E962.0	E980.4
Cathartics NEC	973.3	E858.4	E943.3	E950.4	E962.0	E980.4
contact	973.1	E858.4	E943.1	E950.4	E962.0	E980.4
emollient	973.2	E858.4	E943.2	E950.4	E962.0	E980.4
intestinal irritants	973.1	E858.4	E943.1	E950.4	E962.0	E980.4
saline	973.3	E858.4	E943.3	E950.4	E962.0	E980.4
Cathomycin	960.8	E856	E930.8	E950.4	E962.0	E980.4

◀ New   ◀▥ Revised   ~~deleted~~ Deleted   ● Use Additional Digit(s)

Substance	Poisoning	External Cause (E Code)				
		Accident	Therapeutic Use	Suicide Attempt	Assault	Undetermined
Caustic(s)	983.9	E864.4	—	E950.7	E962.1	E980.6
alkali	983.2	E864.2	—	E950.7	E962.1	E980.6
hydroxide	983.2	E864.2	—	E950.7	E962.1	E980.6
potash	983.2	E864.2	—	E950.7	E962.1	E980.6
soda	983.2	E864.2	—	E950.7	E962.1	E980.6
specified NEC	983.9	E864.3	—	E950.7	E962.1	E980.6
Ceepryn	976.0	E858.7	E946.0	E950.4	E962.0	E980.4
ENT agent	976.6	E858.7	E946.6	E950.4	E962.0	E980.4
lozenges	976.6	E858.7	E946.6	E950.4	E962.0	E980.4
Celestone	962.0	E858.0	E932.0	E950.4	E962.0	E980.4
topical	976.0	E858.7	E946.0	E950.4	E962.0	E980.4
Cellosolve	982.8	E862.4	—	E950.9	E962.1	E980.9
Cell stimulants and proliferants	976.8	E858.7	E946.8	E950.4	E962.0	E980.4
Cellulose derivatives, cathartic	973.3	E858.4	E943.3	E950.4	E962.0	E980.4
nitrates (topical)	976.3	E858.7	E946.3	E950.4	E962.0	E980.4
Centipede (bite)	989.5	E905.4	—	E950.9	E962.1	E980.9
Central nervous system	—	—	—	—	—	—
depressants	968.4	E855.1	E938.4	E950.4	E962.0	E980.4
anesthetic (general) NEC	968.4	E855.1	E938.4	E950.4	E962.0	E980.4
gases NEC	968.2	E855.1	E938.2	E950.4	E962.0	E980.4
intravenous	968.3	E855.1	E938.3	E950.4	E962.0	E980.4
barbiturates	967.0	E851	E937.0	E950.1	E962.0	E980.1
bromides	967.3	E852.2	E937.3	E950.2	E962.0	E980.2
cannabis sativa	969.6	E854.1	E939.6	E950.3	E962.0	E980.3
chloral hydrate	967.1	E852.0	E937.1	E950.2	E962.0	E980.2
hallucinogenics	969.6	E854.1	E939.6	E950.3	E962.0	E980.3
hypnotics	967.9	E852.9	E937.9	E950.2	E962.0	E980.2
specified NEC	967.8	E852.8	E937.8	E950.2	E962.0	E980.2
muscle relaxants	968.0	E855.1	E938.0	E950.4	E962.0	E980.4
paraldehyde	967.2	E852.1	E937.2	E950.2	E962.0	E980.2
sedatives	967.9	E852.9	E937.9	E950.2	E962.0	E980.2
mixed NEC	967.6	E852.5	E937.6	E950.2	E962.0	E980.2
specified NEC	967.8	E852.8	E937.8	E950.2	E962.0	E980.2
muscle-tone depressants	968.0	E855.1	E938.0	E950.4	E962.0	E980.4
stimulants	970.9	E854.3	E940.9	E950.4	E962.0	E980.4
amphetamines	969.72 ◀▥	E854.2	E939.7	E950.3	E962.0	E980.3
analeptics	970.0	E854.3	E940.0	E950.4	E962.0	E980.4
antidepressants	969.00 ◀▥	E854.0	E939.0	E950.3	E962.0	E980.3
opiate antagonists	970.1	E854.3	E940.0	E950.4	E962.0	E980.4
specified NEC	970.8	E854.3	E940.8	E950.4	E962.0	E980.4

◀ New   ◀▥ Revised   ~~deleted~~ Deleted   ● Use Additional Digit(s)

Substance	Poisoning	External Cause (E Code)				
		Accident	Therapeutic Use	Suicide Attempt	Assault	Undetermined
Cephalexin	960.5	E856	E930.5	E950.4	E962.0	E980.4
Cephaloglycin	960.5	E856	E930.5	E950.4	E962.0	E980.4
Cephaloridine	960.5	E856	E930.5	E950.4	E962.0	E980.4
Cephalosporins NEC	960.5	E856	E930.5	E950.4	E962.0	E980.4
N (adicillin)	960.0	E856	E930.0	E950.4	E962.0	E980.4
Cephalothin (sodium)	960.5	E856	E930.5	E950.4	E962.0	E980.4
Cerbera (odallam)	988.2	E865.4	—	E950.9	E962.1	E980.9
Cerberin	972.1	E858.3	E942.1	E950.4	E962.0	E980.4
Cerebral stimulants	970.9	E854.3	E940.9	E950.4	E962.0	E980.4
psychotherapeutic	969.79◀▥	E854.2	E939.7	E950.3	E962.0	E980.3
specified NEC	970.8	E854.3	E940.8	E950.4	E962.0	E980.4
Cetalkonium (chloride)	976.0	E858.7	E946.0	E950.4	E962.0	E980.4
Cetoxime	963.0	E858.1	E933.0	E950.4	E962.0	E980.4
Cetrimide	976.2	E858.7	E946.2	E950.4	E962.0	E980.4
Cetylpyridinium	976.0	E858.7	E946.0	E950.4	E962.0	E980.4
ENT agent	976.6	E858.7	E946.6	E950.4	E962.0	E980.4
lozenges	976.6	E858.7	E946.6	E950.4	E962.0	E980.4
Cevadilla - see Sabadilla	—	—	—	—	—	—
Cevitamic acid	963.5	E858.1	E933.5	E950.4	E962.0	E980.4
Chalk, precipitated	973.0	E858.4	E943.0	E950.4	E962.0	E980.4
Charcoal	—	—	—	—	—	—
fumes (carbon monoxide)	986	E868.3	—	E952.1	E962.2	E982.1
industrial	986	E868.8	—	E952.1	E962.2	E982.1
medicinal (activated)	973.0	E858.4	E943.0	E950.4	E962.0	E980.4
Chelating agents NEC	977.2	E858.8	E947.2	E950.4	E962.0	E980.4
Chelidonium majus	988.2	E865.4	—	E950.9	E962.1	E980.9
Chemical substance	989.9	E866.9	—	E950.9	E962.1	E980.9
specified NEC	989.89	E866.8	—	E950.9	E962.1	E980.9
Chemotherapy, antineoplastic	963.1	E858.1	E933.1	E950.4	E962.0	E980.4
Chenopodium (oil)	961.6	E857	E931.6	E950.4	E962.0	E980.4
Cherry laurel	988.2	E865.4	—	E950.9	E962.1	E980.9
Chiniofon	961.3	E857	E931.3	E950.4	E962.0	E980.4
Chlophedianol	975.4	E858.6	E945.4	E950.4	E962.0	E980.4
Chloral (betaine) (formamide) (hydrate)	967.1	E852.0	E937.1	E950.2	E962.0	E980.2
Chloralamide	967.1	E852.0	E937.1	E950.2	E962.0	E980.2
Chlorambucil	963.1	E858.1	E933.1	E950.4	E962.0	E980.4
Chloramphenicol	960.2	E856	E930.2	E950.4	E962.0	E980.4
ENT agent	976.6	E858.7	E946.6	E950.4	E962.0	E980.4
ophthalmic preparation	976.5	E858.7	E946.5	E950.4	E962.0	E980.4
topical NEC	976.0	E858.7	E946.0	E950.4	E962.0	E980.4

◀ New   ◀▥ Revised   ~~deleted~~ Deleted   ● Use Additional Digit(s)

Substance	Poisoning	External Cause (E Code) Accident	Therapeutic Use	Suicide Attempt	Assault	Undetermined
Chlorate(s) (potassium) (sodium) NEC	983.9	E864.3	—	E950.7	E962.1	E980.6
herbicides	989.4	E863.5	—	E950.6	E962.1	E980.7
Chlorcyclizine	963.0	E858.1	E933.0	E950.4	E962.0	E980.4
Chlordan(e) (dust)	989.2	E863.0	—	E950.6	E962.1	E980.7
Chlordantoin	976.0	E858.7	E946.0	E950.4	E962.0	E980.4
Chlordiazepoxide	969.4	E853.2	E939.4	E950.3	E962.0	E980.3
Chloresium	976.8	E858.7	E946.8	E950.4	E962.0	E980.4
Chlorethiazol	967.1	E852.0	E937.1	E950.2	E962.0	E980.2
Chlorethyl - see Ethyl, chloride	—	—	—	—	—	—
Chloretone	967.1	E852.0	E937.1	E950.2	E962.0	E980.2
Chlorex	982.3	E862.4	—	E950.9	E962.1	E980.9
Chlorhexadol	967.1	E852.0	E937.1	E950.2	E962.0	E980.2
Chlorhexidine (hydrochloride)	976.0	E858.7	E946.0	E950.4	E962.0	E980.4
Chlorhydroxyquinolin	976.0	E858.7	E946.0	E950.4	E962.0	E980.4
Chloride of lime (bleach)	983.9	E864.3	—	E950.7	E962.1	E980.6
Chlorinated	—	—	—	—	—	—
camphene	989.2	E863.0	—	E950.6	E962.1	E980.7
diphenyl	989.89	E866.8	—	E950.9	E962.1	E980.9
hydrocarbons NEC	989.2	E863.0	—	E950.6	E962.1	E980.7
solvent	982.3	E862.4	—	E950.9	E962.1	E980.9
lime (bleach)	983.9	E864.3	—	E950.7	E962.1	E980.6
naphthalene - see Naphthalene	—	—	—	—	—	—
pesticides NEC	989.2	E863.0	—	E950.6	E962.1	E980.7
soda - see Sodium, hypochlorite	—	—	—	—	—	—
Chlorine (fumes) (gas)	987.6	E869.8	—	E952.8	E962.2	E982.8
bleach	983.9	E864.3	—	E950.7	E962.1	E980.6
compounds NEC	983.9	E864.3	—	E950.7	E962.1	E980.6
disinfectant	983.9	E861.4	—	E950.7	E962.1	E980.6
releasing agents NEC	983.9	E864.3	—	E950.7	E962.1	E980.6
Chlorisondamine	972.3	E858.3	E942.3	E950.4	E962.0	E980.4
Chlormadinone	962.2	E858.0	E932.2	E950.4	E962.0	E980.4
Chlormerodrin	974.0	E858.5	E944.0	E950.4	E962.0	E980.4
Chlormethiazole	967.1	E852.0	E937.1	E950.2	E962.0	E980.2
Chlormethylenecycline	960.4	E856	E930.4	E950.4	E962.0	E980.4
Chlormezanone	969.5	E853.8	E939.5	E950.3	E962.0	E980.3
Chloroacetophenone	987.5	E869.3	—	E952.8	E962.2	E982.8
Chloroaniline	983.0	E864.0	—	E950.7	E962.1	E980.6
Chlorobenzene, chlorobenzol	982.0	E862.4	—	E950.9	E962.1	E980.9
Chlorobutanol	967.1	E852.0	E937.1	E950.2	E962.0	E980.2

◀ New   ◀▥ Revised   ~~deleted~~ Deleted   ● Use Additional Digit(s)

Substance	External Cause (E Code)					
	Poisoning	Accident	Therapeutic Use	Suicide Attempt	Assault	Undetermined
Chlorodinitrobenzene	983.0	E864.0	—	E950.7	E962.1	E980.6
dust or vapor	987.8	E869.8	—	E952.8	E962.2	E982.8
Chloroethane - *see* Ethyl, chloride	—	—	—	—	—	—
Chloroform (fumes) (vapor)	987.8	E869.8	—	E952.8	E962.2	E982.8
anesthetic (gas)	968.2	E855.1	E938.2	E950.4	E962.0	E980.4
liquid NEC	968.4	E855.1	E938.4	E950.4	E962.0	E980.4
solvent	982.3	E862.4	—	E950.9	E962.1	E980.9
Chloroguanide	961.4	E857	E931.4	E950.4	E962.0	E980.4
Chloromycetin	960.2	E856	E930.2	E950.4	E962.0	E980.4
ENT agent	976.6	E858.7	E946.6	E950.4	E962.0	E980.4
ophthalmic preparation	976.5	E858.7	E946.5	E950.4	E962.0	E980.4
otic solution	976.6	E858.7	E946.6	E950.4	E962.0	E980.4
topical NEC	976.0	E858.7	E946.0	E950.4	E962.0	E980.4
Chloronitrobenzene	983.0	E864.0	—	E950.7	E962.1	E980.6
dust or vapor	987.8	E869.8	—	E952.8	E962.2	E982.8
Chlorophenol	983.0	E864.0	—	E950.7	E962.1	E980.6
Chlorophenothane	989.2	E863.0	—	E950.6	E962.1	E980.7
Chlorophyll (derivatives)	976.8	E858.7	E946.8	E950.4	E962.0	E980.4
Chloropicrin (fumes)	987.8	E869.8	—	E952.8	E962.2	E982.8
fumigant	989.4	E863.8	—	E950.6	E962.1	E980.7
fungicide	989.4	E863.6	—	E950.6	E962.1	E980.7
pesticide (fumes)	989.4	E863.4	—	E950.6	E962.1	E980.7
Chloroprocaine	968.9	E855.2	E938.9	E950.4	E962.0	E980.4
infiltration (subcutaneous)	968.5	E855.2	E938.5	E950.4	E962.0	E980.4
nerve block (peripheral) (plexus)	968.6	E855.2	E938.6	E950.4	E962.0	E980.4
Chloroptic	976.5	E858.7	E946.5	E950.4	E962.0	E980.4
Chloropurine	963.1	E858.1	E933.1	E950.4	E962.0	E980.4
Chloroquine (hydrochloride) (phosphate)	961.4	E857	E931.4	E950.4	E962.0	E980.4
Chlorothen	963.0	E858.1	E933.0	E950.4	E962.0	E980.4
Chlorothiazide	974.3	E858.5	E944.3	E950.4	E962.0	E980.4
Chlorotrianisene	962.2	E858.0	E932.2	E950.4	E962.0	E980.4
Chlorovinyldichloroarsine	985.1	E866.3	—	E950.8	E962.1	E980.8
Chloroxylenol	976.0	E858.7	E946.0	E950.4	E962.0	E980.4
Chlorphenesin (carbamate)	968.0	E855.1	E938.0	E950.4	E962.0	E980.4
topical (antifungal)	976.0	E858.7	E946.0	E950.4	E962.0	E980.4
Chlorpheniramine	963.0	E858.1	E933.0	E950.4	E962.0	E980.4
Chlorphenoxamine	966.4	E855.0	E936.4	E950.4	E962.0	E980.4
Chlorphentermine	977.0	E858.8	E947.0	E950.4	E962.0	E980.4
Chlorproguanil	961.4	E857	E931.4	E950.4	E962.0	E980.4

◀ New   ◀░ Revised   ~~deleted~~ Deleted   ● Use Additional Digit(s)

Substance	Poisoning	External Cause (E Code)				
		Accident	Therapeutic Use	Suicide Attempt	Assault	Undetermined
Chlorpromazine	969.1	E853.0	E939.1	E950.3	E962.0	E980.3
Chlorpropamide	962.3	E858.0	E932.3	E950.4	E962.0	E980.4
Chlorprothixene	969.3	E853.8	E939.3	E950.3	E962.0	E980.3
Chlorquinaldol	976.0	E858.7	E946.0	E950.4	E962.0	E980.4
Chlortetracycline	960.4	E856	E930.4	E950.4	E962.0	E980.4
Chlorthalidone	974.4	E858.5	E944.4	E950.4	E962.0	E980.4
Chlortrianisene	962.2	E858.0	E932.2	E950.4	E962.0	E980.4
Chlor-Trimeton	963.0	E858.1	E933.0	E950.4	E962.0	E980.4
Chlorzoxazone	968.0	E855.1	E938.0	E950.4	E962.0	E980.4
Choke damp	987.8	E869.8	—	E952.8	E962.2	E982.8
Cholebrine	977.8	E858.8	E947.8	E950.4	E962.0	E980.4
Cholera vaccine	978.2	E858.8	E948.2	E950.4	E962.0	E980.4
Cholesterol-lowering agents	972.2	E858.3	E942.2	E950.4	E962.0	E980.4
Cholestyramine (resin)	972.2	E858.3	E942.2	E950.4	E962.0	E980.4
Cholic acid	973.4	E858.4	E943.4	E950.4	E962.0	E980.4
Choline	—	—	—	—	—	—
dihydrogen citrate	977.1	E858.8	E947.1	E950.4	E962.0	E980.4
salicylate	965.1	E850.3	E935.3	E950.0	E962.0	E980.0
theophyllinate	974.1	E858.5	E944.1	E950.4	E962.0	E980.4
Cholinergics	971.0	E855.3	E941.0	E950.4	E962.0	E980.4
Cholografin	977.8	E858.8	E947.8	E950.4	E962.0	E980.4
Chorionic gonadotropin	962.4	E858.0	E932.4	E950.4	E962.0	E980.4
Chromates	983.9	E864.3	—	E950.7	E962.1	E980.6
dust or mist	987.8	E869.8	—	E952.8	E962.2	E982.8
lead	984.0	E866.0	—	E950.9	E962.1	E980.9
paint	984.0	E861.5	—	E950.9	E962.1	E980.9
Chromic acid	983.9	E864.3	—	E950.7	E962.1	E980.6
dust or mist	987.8	E869.8	—	E952.8	E962.2	E982.8
Chromium	985.6	E866.4	—	E950.9	E962.1	E980.9
compounds - *see* Chromates	—	—	—	—	—	—
Chromonar	972.4	E858.3	E942.4	E950.4	E962.0	E980.4
Chromyl chloride	983.9	E864.3	—	E950.7	E962.1	E980.6
Chrysarobin (ointment)	976.4	E858.7	E946.4	E950.4	E962.0	E980.4
Chrysazin	973.1	E858.4	E943.1	E950.4	E962.0	E980.4
Chymar	963.4	E858.1	E933.4	E950.4	E962.0	E980.4
ophthalmic preparation	976.5	E858.7	E946.5	E950.4	E962.0	E980.4
Chymotrypsin	963.4	E858.1	E933.4	E950.4	E962.0	E980.4
ophthalmic preparation	976.5	E858.7	E946.5	E950.4	E962.0	E980.4
Cicuta maculata or virosa	988.2	E865.4	—	E950.9	E962.1	E980.9

◀ New   ◀▥ Revised   ~~deleted~~ Deleted   ● Use Additional Digit(s)

Substance	Poisoning	External Cause (E Code)				
		Accident	Therapeutic Use	Suicide Attempt	Assault	Undetermined
Cigarette lighter fluid	981	E862.1	—	E950.9	E962.1	E980.9
Cinchocaine (spinal)	968.7	E855.2	E938.7	E950.4	E962.0	E980.4
topical (surface)	968.5	E855.2	E938.5	E950.4	E962.0	E980.4
Cinchona	961.4	E857	E931.4	E950.4	E962.0	E980.4
Cinchonine alkaloids	961.4	E857	E931.4	E950.4	E962.0	E980.4
Cinchophen	974.7	E858.5	E944.7	E950.4	E962.0	E980.4
Cinnarizine	963.0	E858.1	E933.0	E950.4	E962.0	E980.4
Citanest	968.9	E855.2	E938.9	E950.4	E962.0	E980.4
infiltration (subcutaneous)	968.5	E855.2	E938.5	E950.4	E962.0	E980.4
nerve block (peripheral) (plexus)	968.6	E855.2	E938.6	E950.4	E962.0	E980.4
Citric acid	989.89	E866.8	—	E950.9	E962.1	E980.9
Citrovorum factor	964.1	E858.2	E934.1	E950.4	E962.0	E980.4
Claviceps purpurea	988.2	E865.4	—	E950.9	E962.1	E980.9
Cleaner, cleansing agent NEC	989.89	E861.3	—	E950.9	E962.1	E980.9
of paint or varnish	982.8	E862.9	—	E950.9	E962.1	E980.9
Clematis vitalba	988.2	E865.4	—	E950.9	E962.1	E980.9
Clemizole	963.0	E858.1	E933.0	E950.4	E962.0	E980.4
penicillin	960.0	E856	E930.0	E950.4	E962.0	E980.4
Clidinium	971.1	E855.4	E941.1	E950.4	E962.0	E980.4
Clindamycin	960.8	E856	E930.8	E950.4	E962.0	E980.4
Cliradon	965.09	E850.2	E935.2	E950.0	E962.0	E980.0
Clocortolone	962.0	E858.0	E932.0	E950.4	E962.0	E980.4
Clofedanol	975.4	E858.6	E945.4	E950.4	E962.0	E980.4
Clofibrate	972.2	E858.3	E942.2	E950.4	E962.0	E980.4
Clomethiazole	967.1	E852.0	E937.1	E950.2	E962.0	E980.2
Clomiphene	977.8	E858.8	E947.8	E950.4	E962.0	E980.4
Clonazepam	969.4	E853.2	E939.4	E950.3	E962.0	E980.3
Clonidine	972.6	E858.3	E942.6	E950.4	E962.0	E980.4
Clopamide	974.3	E858.5	E944.3	E950.4	E962.0	E980.4
Clorazepate	969.4	E853.2	E939.4	E950.3	E962.0	E980.3
Clorexolone	974.4	E858.5	E944.4	E950.4	E962.0	E980.4
Clorox (bleach)	983.9	E864.3	—	E950.7	E962.1	E980.6
Clortermine	977.0	E858.8	E947.0	E950.4	E962.0	E980.4
Clotrimazole	976.0	E858.7	E946.0	E950.4	E962.0	E980.4
Cloxacillin	960.0	E856	E930.0	E950.4	E962.0	E980.4
Coagulants NEC	964.5	E858.2	E934.5	E950.4	E962.0	E980.4
Coal (carbon monoxide from) - see also Carbon, monoxide, coal	—	—	—	—	—	—
oil - see Kerosene	—	—	—	—	—	—

◀ New   ◀▥ Revised   ~~deleted~~ Deleted   ● Use Additional Digit(s)

Substance	Poisoning	External Cause (E Code)				
		Accident	Therapeutic Use	Suicide Attempt	Assault	Undetermined
Coal (carbon monoxide from) *(Continued)*						
tar NEC	983.0	E864.0	—	E950.7	E962.1	E980.6
fumes	987.8	E869.8	—	E952.8	E962.2	E982.8
medicinal (ointment)	976.4	E858.7	E946.4	E950.4	E962.0	E980.4
analgesics NEC	965.5	E850.5	E935.5	E950.0	E962.0	E980.0
naphtha (solvent)	981	E862.0	—	E950.9	E962.1	E980.9
Cobalt (fumes) (industrial)	985.8	E866.4	—	E950.9	E962.1	E980.9
Cobra (venom)	989.5	E905.0	—	E950.9	E962.1	E980.9
Coca (leaf)	970.8	E854.3	E940.8	E950.4	E962.0	E980.4
Cocaine (hydrochloride) (salt)	970.8	E854.3	E940.8	E950.4	E962.0	E980.4
topical anesthetic	968.5	E855.2	E938.5	E950.4	E962.0	E980.4
Coccidioidin	977.8	E858.8	E947.8	E950.4	E962.0	E980.4
Cocculus indicus	988.2	E865.3	—	E950.9	E962.1	E980.9
Cochineal	989.89	E866.8	—	E950.9	E962.1	E980.9
medicinal products	977.4	E858.8	E947.4	E950.4	E962.0	E980.4
Codeine	965.09	E850.2	E935.2	E950.0	E962.0	E980.0
Coffee	989.89	E866.8	—	E950.9	E962.1	E980.9
Cogentin	971.1	E855.4	E941.1	E950.4	E962.0	E980.4
Coke fumes or gas (carbon monoxide)	986	E868.3	—	E952.1	E962.2	E982.1
industrial use	986	E868.8	—	E952.1	E962.2	E982.1
Colace	973.2	E858.4	E943.2	E950.4	E962.0	E980.4
Colchicine	974.7	E858.5	E944.7	E950.4	E962.0	E980.4
Colchicum	988.2	E865.3	—	E950.9	E962.1	E980.9
Cold cream	976.3	E858.7	E946.3	E950.4	E962.0	E980.4
Colestipol	972.2	E858.3	E942.2	E950.4	E962.0	E980.4
Colistimethate	960.8	E856	E930.8	E950.4	E962.0	E980.4
Colistin	960.8	E856	E930.8	E950.4	E962.0	E980.4
Collagen	977.8	E866.8	E947.8	E950.9	E962.1	E980.9
Collagenase	976.8	E858.7	E946.8	E950.4	E962.0	E980.4
Collodion (flexible)	976.3	E858.7	E946.3	E950.4	E962.0	E980.4
Colocynth	973.1	E858.4	E943.1	E950.4	E962.0	E980.4
Coloring matter - *see* Dye(s)	—	—	—	—	—	—
Combustion gas - *see* Carbon, monoxide	—	—	—	—	—	—
Compazine	969.1	E853.0	E939.1	E950.3	E962.0	E980.3
Compound	—	—	—	—	—	—
42 (warfarin)	989.4	E863.7	—	E950.6	E962.1	E980.7
269 (endrin)	989.2	E863.0	—	E950.6	E962.1	E980.7
497 (dieldrin)	989.2	E863.0	—	E950.6	E962.1	E980.7

◀ New ◀▥ Revised ~~deleted~~ Deleted ● Use Additional Digit(s)

Substance	Poisoning	External Cause (E Code)				
		Accident	Therapeutic Use	Suicide Attempt	Assault	Undetermined
Compound *(Continued)*						
1080 (sodium fluoroacetate)	989.4	E863.7	—	E950.6	E962.1	E980.7
3422 (parathion)	989.3	E863.1	—	E950.6	E962.1	E980.7
3911 (phorate)	989.3	E863.1	—	E950.6	E962.1	E980.7
3956 (toxaphene)	989.2	E863.0	—	E950.6	E962.1	E980.7
4049 (malathion)	989.3	E863.1	—	E950.6	E962.1	E980.7
4124 (dicapthon)	989.4	E863.4	—	E950.6	E962.1	E980.7
E (cortisone)	962.0	E858.0	E932.0	E950.4	E962.0	E980.4
F (hydrocortisone)	962.0	E858.0	E932.0	E950.4	E962.0	E980.4
Congo red	977.8	E858.8	E947.8	E950.4	E962.0	E980.4
Coniine, conine	965.7	E850.7	E935.7	E950.0	E962.0	E980.0
Conium (maculatum)	988.2	E865.4	—	E950.9	E962.1	E980.9
Conjugated estrogens (equine)	962.2	E858.0	E932.2	E950.4	E962.0	E980.4
Contac	975.6	E858.6	E945.6	E950.4	E962.0	E980.4
Contact lens solution	976.5	E858.7	E946.5	E950.4	E962.0	E980.4
Contraceptives (oral)	962.2	E858.0	E932.2	E950.4	E962.0	E980.4
vaginal	976.8	E858.7	E946.8	E950.4	E962.0	E980.4
Contrast media (roentgenographic)	977.8	E858.8	E947.8	E950.4	E962.0	E980.4
Convallaria majalis	988.2	E865.4	—	E950.9	E962.1	E980.9
Copper (dust) (fumes) (salts) NEC	985.8	E866.4	—	E950.9	E962.1	E980.9
arsenate, arsenite	985.1	E866.3	—	E950.8	E962.1	E980.8
insecticide	985.1	E863.4	—	E950.8	E962.1	E980.8
emetic	973.6	E858.4	E943.6	E950.4	E962.0	E980.4
fungicide	985.8	E863.6	—	E950.6	E962.1	E980.7
insecticide	985.8	E863.4	—	E950.6	E962.1	E980.7
oleate	976.0	E858.7	E946.0	E950.4	E962.0	E980.4
sulfate	983.9	E864.3	—	E950.7	E962.1	E980.6
fungicide	983.9	E863.6	—	E950.7	E962.1	E980.6
cupric	973.6	E858.4	E943.6	E950.4	E962.0	E980.4
cuprous	983.9	E864.3	—	E950.7	E962.1	E980.6
Copperhead snake (bite) (venom)	989.5	E905.0	—	E950.9	E962.1	E980.9
Coral (sting)	989.5	E905.6	—	E950.9	E962.1	E980.9
snake (bite) (venom)	989.5	E905.0	—	E950.9	E962.1	E980.9
Cordran	976.0	E858.7	E946.0	E950.4	E962.0	E980.4
Corn cures	976.4	E858.7	E946.4	E950.4	E962.0	E980.4
Cornhusker's lotion	976.3	E858.7	E946.3	E950.4	E962.0	E980.4
Corn starch	976.3	E858.7	E946.3	E950.4	E962.0	E980.4
Corrosive	983.9	E864.4	—	E950.7	E962.1	E980.6
acids NEC	983.1	E864.1	—	E950.7	E962.1	E980.6

◄ New ◄ Revised ~~deleted~~ Deleted ● Use Additional Digit(s)

TABLE OF DRUGS AND CHEMICALS

Substance	Poisoning	External Cause (E Code)				
		Accident	Therapeutic Use	Suicide Attempt	Assault	Undetermined
Corrosive *(Continued)*						
aromatics	983.0	E864.0	—	E950.7	E962.1	E980.6
disinfectant	983.0	E861.4	—	E950.7	E962.1	E980.6
fumes NEC	987.9	E869.9	—	E952.9	E962.2	E982.9
specified NEC	983.9	E864.3	—	E950.7	E962.1	E980.6
sublimate - *see* Mercury, chloride	—	—	—	—	—	—
Cortate	962.0	E858.0	E932.0	E950.4	E962.0	E980.4
Cort-Dome	962.0	E858.0	E932.0	E950.4	E962.0	E980.4
ENT agent	976.6	E858.7	E946.6	E950.4	E962.0	E980.4
ophthalmic preparation	976.5	E858.7	E946.5	E950.4	E962.0	E980.4
topical NEC	976.0	E858.7	E946.0	E950.4	E962.0	E980.4
Cortef	962.0	E858.0	E932.0	E950.4	E962.0	E980.4
ENT agent	976.6	E858.7	E946.6	E950.4	E962.0	E980.4
ophthalmic preparation	976.5	E858.7	E946.5	E950.4	E962.0	E980.4
topical NEC	976.0	E858.7	E946.0	E950.4	E962.0	E980.4
Corticosteroids (fluorinated)	962.0	E858.0	E932.0	E950.4	E962.0	E980.4
ENT agent	976.6	E858.7	E946.6	E950.4	E962.0	E980.4
ophthalmic preparation	976.5	E858.7	E946.5	E950.4	E962.0	E980.4
topical NEC	976.0	E858.7	E946.0	E950.4	E962.0	E980.4
Corticotropin	962.4	E858.0	E932.4	E950.4	E962.0	E980.4
Cortisol	962.0	E858.0	E932.0	E950.4	E962.0	E980.4
ENT agent	976.6	E858.7	E946.6	E950.4	E962.0	E980.4
ophthalmic preparation	976.5	E858.7	E946.5	E950.4	E962.0	E980.4
topical NEC	976.0	E858.7	E946.0	E950.4	E962.0	E980.4
Cortisone derivatives (acetate)	962.0	E858.0	E932.0	E950.4	E962.0	E980.4
ENT agent	976.6	E858.7	E946.6	E950.4	E962.0	E980.4
ophthalmic preparation	976.5	E858.7	E946.5	E950.4	E962.0	E980.4
topical NEC	976.0	E858.7	E946.0	E950.4	E962.0	E980.4
Cortogen	962.0	E858.0	E932.0	E950.4	E962.0	E980.4
ENT agent	976.6	E858.7	E946.6	E950.4	E962.0	E980.4
ophthalmic preparation	976.5	E858.7	E946.5	E950.4	E962.0	E980.4
Cortone	962.0	E858.0	E932.0	E950.4	E962.0	E980.4
ENT agent	976.6	E858.7	E946.6	E950.4	E962.0	E980.4
ophthalmic preparation	976.5	E858.7	E946.5	E950.4	E962.0	E980.4
Cortril	962.0	E858.0	E932.0	E950.4	E962.0	E980.4
ENT agent	976.6	E858.7	E946.6	E950.4	E962.0	E980.4
ophthalmic preparation	976.5	E858.7	E946.5	E950.4	E962.0	E980.4
topical NEC	976.0	E858.7	E946.0	E950.4	E962.0	E980.4
Cosmetics	989.89	E866.7	—	E950.9	E962.1	E980.9

◀ New   ◀▥ Revised   ~~deleted~~ Deleted   ● Use Additional Digit(s)

Substance	Poisoning	External Cause (E Code)				
		Accident	Therapeutic Use	Suicide Attempt	Assault	Undetermined
Cosyntropin	977.8	E858.8	E947.8	E950.4	E962.0	E980.4
Cotarnine	964.5	E858.2	E934.5	E950.4	E962.0	E980.4
Cottonseed oil	976.3	E858.7	E946.3	E950.4	E962.0	E980.4
Cough mixtures (antitussives)	975.4	E858.6	E945.4	E950.4	E962.0	E980.4
containing opiates	965.09	E850.2	E935.2	E950.0	E962.0	E980.0
expectorants	975.5	E858.6	E945.5	E950.4	E962.0	E980.4
Coumadin	964.2	E858.2	E934.2	E950.4	E962.0	E980.4
rodenticide	989.4	E863.7	—	E950.6	E962.1	E980.7
Coumarin	964.2	E858.2	E934.2	E950.4	E962.0	E980.4
Coumetarol	964.2	E858.2	E934.2	E950.4	E962.0	E980.4
Cowbane	988.2	E865.4	—	E950.9	E962.1	E980.9
Cozyme	963.5	E858.1	E933.5	E950.4	E962.0	E980.4
Crack	970.8	E854.3	E940.8	E950.4	E962.0	E980.4
Creolin	983.0	E864.0	—	E950.7	E962.1	E980.6
disinfectant	983.0	E861.4	—	E950.7	E962.1	E980.6
Creosol (compound)	983.0	E864.0	—	E950.7	E962.1	E980.6
Creosote (beechwood) (coal tar)	983.0	E864.0	—	E950.7	E962.1	E980.6
medicinal (expectorant)	975.5	E858.6	E945.5	E950.4	E962.0	E980.4
syrup	975.5	E858.6	E945.5	E950.4	E962.0	E980.4
Cresol	983.0	E864.0	—	E950.7	E962.1	E980.6
disinfectant	983.0	E861.4	—	E950.7	E962.1	E980.6
Cresylic acid	983.0	E864.0	—	E950.7	E962.1	E980.6
Cropropamide	965.7	E850.7	E935.7	E950.0	E962.0	E980.0
with crotethamide	970.0	E854.3	E940.0	E950.4	E962.0	E980.4
Crotamiton	976.0	E858.7	E946.0	E950.4	E962.0	E980.4
Crotethamide	965.7	E850.7	E935.7	E950.0	E962.0	E980.0
with cropropamide	970.0	E854.3	E940.0	E950.4	E962.0	E980.4
Croton (oil)	973.1	E858.4	E943.1	E950.4	E962.0	E980.4
chloral	967.1	E852.0	E937.1	E950.2	E962.0	E980.2
Crude oil	981	E862.1	—	E950.9	E962.1	E980.9
Cryogenine	965.8	E850.8	E935.8	E950.0	E962.0	E980.0
Cryolite (pesticide)	989.4	E863.4	—	E950.6	E962.1	E980.7
Cryptenamine	972.6	E858.3	E942.6	E950.4	E962.0	E980.4
Crystal violet	976.0	E858.7	E946.0	E950.4	E962.0	E980.4
Cuckoopint	988.2	E865.4	—	E950.9	E962.1	E980.9
Cumetharol	964.2	E858.2	E934.2	E950.4	E962.0	E980.4
Cupric sulfate	973.6	E858.4	E943.6	E950.4	E962.0	E980.4
Cuprous sulfate	983.9	E864.3	—	E950.7	E962.1	E980.6
Curare, curarine	975.2	E858.6	E945.2	E950.4	E962.0	E980.4

◀ New　◀|||| Revised　~~deleted~~ Deleted　● Use Additional Digit(s)

Substance	Poisoning	External Cause (E Code)				
		Accident	Therapeutic Use	Suicide Attempt	Assault	Undetermined
Cyanic acid - *see* Cyanide(s)	—	—	—	—	—	—
Cyanide(s) (compounds) (hydrogen) (potassium) (sodium) NEC	989.0	E866.8	—	E950.9	E962.1	E980.9
dust or gas (inhalation) NEC	987.7	E869.8	—	E952.8	E962.2	E982.8
fumigant	989.0	E863.8	—	E950.6	E962.1	E980.7
mercuric - *see* Mercury	—	—	—	—	—	—
pesticide (dust) (fumes)	989.0	E863.4	—	E950.6	E962.1	E980.7
Cyanocobalamin	964.1	E858.2	E934.1	E950.4	E962.0	E980.4
Cyanogen (chloride) (gas)	—	—	—	—	—	—
NEC	987.8	E869.8	—	E952.8	E962.2	E982.8
Cyclaine	968.5	E855.2	E938.5	E950.4	E962.0	E980.4
Cyclamen europaeum	988.2	E865.4	—	E950.9	E962.1	E980.9
Cyclandelate	972.5	E858.3	E942.5	E950.4	E962.0	E980.4
Cyclazocine	965.09	E850.2	E935.2	E950.0	E962.0	E980.0
Cyclizine	963.0	E858.1	E933.0	E950.4	E962.0	E980.4
Cyclobarbital, cyclobarbitone	967.0	E851	E937.0	E950.1	E962.0	E980.1
Cycloguanil	961.4	E857	E931.4	E950.4	E962.0	E980.4
Cyclohexane	982.0	E862.4	—	E950.9	E962.1	E980.9
Cyclohexanol	980.8	E860.8	—	E950.9	E962.1	E980.9
Cyclohexanone	982.8	E862.4	—	E950.9	E962.1	E980.9
Cyclomethycaine	968.5	E855.2	E938.5	E950.4	E962.0	E980.4
Cyclopentamine	971.2	E855.5	E941.2	E950.4	E962.0	E980.4
Cyclopenthiazide	974.3	E858.5	E944.3	E950.4	E962.0	E980.4
Cyclopentolate	971.1	E855.4	E941.1	E950.4	E962.0	E980.4
Cyclophosphamide	963.1	E858.1	E933.1	E950.4	E962.0	E980.4
Cyclopropane	968.2	E855.1	E938.2	E950.4	E962.0	E980.4
Cycloserine	960.6	E856	E930.6	E950.4	E962.0	E980.4
Cyclothiazide	974.3	E858.5	E944.3	E950.4	E962.0	E980.4
Cycrimine	966.4	E855.0	E936.4	E950.4	E962.0	E980.4
Cymarin	972.1	E858.3	E942.1	E950.4	E962.0	E980.4
Cyproheptadine	963.0	E858.1	E933.0	E950.4	E962.0	E980.4
Cyprolidol	969.09 ◀ⅲ	E854.0	E939.0	E950.3	E962.0	E980.3
Cytarabine	963.1	E858.1	E933.1	E950.4	E962.0	E980.4
Cytisus	—	—	—	—	—	—
laburnum	988.2	E865.4	—	E950.9	E962.1	E980.9
scoparius	988.2	E865.4	—	E950.9	E962.1	E980.9
Cytomel	962.7	E858.0	E932.7	E950.4	E962.0	E980.4
Cytosine (antineoplastic)	963.1	E858.1	E933.1	E950.4	E962.0	E980.4
Cytoxan	963.1	E858.1	E933.1	E950.4	E962.0	E980.4
Dacarbazine	963.1	E858.1	E933.1	E950.4	E962.0	E980.4

◀ New   ◀ⅲ Revised   ~~deleted~~ Deleted   ● Use Additional Digit(s)

Substance	Poisoning	External Cause (E Code)				
		Accident	Therapeutic Use	Suicide Attempt	Assault	Undetermined
Dactinomycin	960.7	E856	E930.7	E950.4	E962.0	E980.4
DADPS	961.8	E857	E931.8	E950.4	E962.0	E980.4
Dakin's solution (external)	976.0	E858.7	E946.0	E950.4	E962.0	E980.4
Dalmane	969.4	E853.2	E939.4	E950.3	E962.0	E980.3
DAM	977.2	E858.8	E947.2	E950.4	E962.0	E980.4
Danilone	964.2	E858.2	E934.2	E950.4	E962.0	E980.4
Danthron	973.1	E858.4	E943.1	E950.4	E962.0	E980.4
Dantrolene	975.2	E858.6	E945.2	E950.4	E962.0	E980.4
Daphne (gnidium) (mezereum)	988.2	E865.4	—	E950.9	E962.1	E980.9
berry	988.2	E865.3	—	E950.9	E962.1	E980.9
Dapsone	961.8	E857	E931.8	E950.4	E962.0	E980.4
Daraprim	961.4	E857	E931.4	E950.4	E962.0	E980.4
Darnel	988.2	E865.3	—	E950.9	E962.1	E980.9
Darvon	965.8	E850.8	E935.8	E950.0	E962.0	E980.0
Daunorubicin	960.7	E856	E930.7	E950.4	E962.0	E980.4
DBI	962.3	E858.0	E932.3	E950.4	E962.0	E980.4
D-Con (rodenticide)	989.4	E863.7	—	E950.6	E962.1	E980.7
DDS	961.8	E857	E931.8	E950.4	E962.0	E980.4
DDT	989.2	E863.0	—	E950.6	E962.1	E980.7
Deadly nightshade	988.2	E865.4	—	E950.9	E962.1	E980.9
berry	988.2	E865.3	—	E950.9	E962.1	E980.9
Deanol	969.79 ◄▥	E854.2	E939.7	E950.3	E962.0	E980.3
Debrisoquine	972.6	E858.3	E942.6	E950.4	E962.0	E980.4
Decaborane	989.89	E866.8	—	E950.9	E962.1	E980.9
fumes	987.8	E869.8	—	E952.8	E962.2	E982.8
Decadron	962.0	E858.0	E932.0	E950.4	E962.0	E980.4
ENT agent	976.6	E858.7	E946.6	E950.4	E962.0	E980.4
ophthalmic preparation	976.5	E858.7	E946.5	E950.4	E962.0	E980.4
topical NEC	976.0	E858.7	E946.0	E950.4	E962.0	E980.4
Decahydronaphthalene	982.0	E862.4	—	E950.9	E962.1	E980.9
Decalin	982.0	E862.4	—	E950.9	E962.1	E980.9
Decamethonium	975.2	E858.6	E945.2	E950.4	E962.0	E980.4
Decholin	973.4	E858.4	E943.4	E950.4	E962.0	E980.4
sodium (diagnostic)	977.8	E858.8	E947.8	E950.4	E962.0	E980.4
Declomycin	960.4	E856	E930.4	E950.4	E962.0	E980.4
Deferoxamine	963.8	E858.1	E933.8	E950.4	E962.0	E980.4
Dehydrocholic acid	973.4	E858.4	E943.4	E950.4	E962.0	E980.4
DeKalin	982.0	E862.4	—	E950.9	E962.1	E980.9
Delalutin	962.2	E858.0	E932.2	E950.4	E962.0	E980.4

◄ New   ◄▥ Revised   ~~deleted~~ Deleted   ● Use Additional Digit(s)

Substance	Poisoning	External Cause (E Code)				
		Accident	Therapeutic Use	Suicide Attempt	Assault	Undetermined
Delphinium	988.2	E865.3	—	E950.9	E962.1	E980.9
Deltasone	962.0	E858.0	E932.0	E950.4	E962.0	E980.4
Deltra	962.0	E858.0	E932.0	E950.4	E962.0	E980.4
Delvinal	967.0	E851	E937.0	E950.1	E962.0	E980.1
Demecarium (bromide)	971.0	E855.3	E941.0	E950.4	E962.0	E980.4
Demeclocycline	960.4	E856	E930.4	E950.4	E962.0	E980.4
Demecolcine	963.1	E858.1	E933.1	E950.4	E962.0	E980.4
Demelanizing agents	976.8	E858.7	E946.8	E950.4	E962.0	E980.4
Demerol	965.09	E850.2	E935.2	E950.0	E962.0	E980.0
Demethylchlortetracycline	960.4	E856	E930.4	E950.4	E962.0	E980.4
Demethyltetracycline	960.4	E856	E930.4	E950.4	E962.0	E980.4
Demeton	989.3	E863.1	—	E950.6	E962.1	E980.7
Demulcents	976.3	E858.7	E946.3	E950.4	E962.0	E980.4
Demulen	962.2	E858.0	E932.2	E950.4	E962.0	E980.4
Denatured alcohol	980.0	E860.1	—	E950.9	E962.1	E980.9
Dendrid	976.5	E858.7	E946.5	E950.4	E962.0	E980.4
Dental agents, topical	976.7	E858.7	E946.7	E950.4	E962.0	E980.4
Deodorant spray (feminine hygiene)	976.8	E858.7	E946.8	E950.4	E962.0	E980.4
Deoxyribonuclease	963.4	E858.1	E933.4	E950.4	E962.0	E980.4
Depressants	—	—	—	—	—	—
appetite, central	977.0	E858.8	E947.0	E950.4	E962.0	E980.4
cardiac	972.0	E858.3	E942.0	E950.4	E962.0	E980.4
central nervous system (anesthetic)	968.4	E855.1	E938.4	E950.4	E962.0	E980.4
psychotherapeutic	969.5	E853.9	E939.5	E950.3	E962.0	E980.3
Dequalinium	976.0	E858.7	E946.0	E950.4	E962.0	E980.4
Dermolate	976.2	E858.7	E946.2	E950.4	E962.0	E980.4
DES	962.2	E858.0	E932.2	E950.4	E962.0	E980.4
Desenex	976.0	E858.7	E946.0	E950.4	E962.0	E980.4
Deserpidine	972.6	E858.3	E942.6	E950.4	E962.0	E980.4
Desipramine	969.05◄▥	E854.0	E939.0	E950.3	E962.0	E980.3
Deslanoside	972.1	E858.3	E942.1	E950.4	E962.0	E980.4
Desocodeine	965.09	E850.2	E935.2	E950.0	E962.0	E980.0
Desomorphine	965.09	E850.2	E935.2	E950.0	E962.0	E980.0
Desonide	976.0	E858.7	E946.0	E950.4	E962.0	E980.4
Desoxycorticosterone derivatives	962.0	E858.0	E932.0	E950.4	E962.0	E980.4
Desoxyephedrine	969.72◄▥	E854.2	E939.7	E950.3	E962.0	E980.3
DET	969.6	E854.1	E939.6	E950.3	E962.0	E980.3
Detergents (ingested) (synthetic)	989.6	E861.0	—	E950.9	E962.1	E980.9
external medication	976.2	E858.7	E946.2	E950.4	E962.0	E980.4

◄ New   ◄▥ Revised   ~~deleted~~ Deleted   ● Use Additional Digit(s)

TABLE OF DRUGS AND CHEMICALS

		External Cause (E Code)				
Substance	**Poisoning**	**Accident**	**Therapeutic Use**	**Suicide Attempt**	**Assault**	**Undetermined**
Deterrent, alcohol	977.3	E858.8	E947.3	E950.4	E962.0	E980.4
Detrothyronine	962.7	E858.0	E932.7	E950.4	E962.0	E980.4
Dettol (external medication)	976.0	E858.7	E946.0	E950.4	E962.0	E980.4
Dexamethasone	962.0	E858.0	E932.0	E950.4	E962.0	E980.4
ENT agent	976.6	E858.7	E946.6	E950.4	E962.0	E980.4
ophthalmic preparation	976.5	E858.7	E946.5	E950.4	E962.0	E980.4
topical NEC	976.0	E858.7	E946.0	E950.4	E962.0	E980.4
Dexamphetamine	969.72◀▥	E854.2	E939.7	E950.3	E962.0	E980.3
Dexedrine	969.72◀▥	E854.2	E939.7	E950.3	E962.0	E980.3
Dexpanthenol	963.5	E858.1	E933.5	E950.4	E962.0	E980.4
Dextran	964.8	E858.2	E934.8	E950.4	E962.0	E980.4
Dextriferron	964.0	E858.2	E934.0	E950.4	E962.0	E980.4
Dextroamphetamine	969.72◀▥	E854.2	E939.7	E950.3	E962.0	E980.3
Dextro calcium pantothenate	963.5	E858.1	E933.5	E950.4	E962.0	E980.4
Dextromethorphan	975.4	E858.6	E945.4	E950.4	E962.0	E980.4
Dextromoramide	965.09	E850.2	E935.2	E950.0	E962.0	E980.0
Dextro pantothenyl alcohol	963.5	E858.1	E933.5	E950.4	E962.0	E980.4
topical	976.8	E858.7	E946.8	E950.4	E962.0	E980.4
Dextropropoxyphene (hydrochloride)	965.8	E850.8	E935.8	E950.0	E962.0	E980.0
Dextrorphan	965.09	E850.2	E935.2	E950.0	E962.0	E980.0
Dextrose NEC	974.5	E858.5	E944.5	E950.4	E962.0	E980.4
Dextrothyroxine	962.7	E858.0	E932.7	E950.4	E962.0	E980.4
DFP	971.0	E855.3	E941.0	E950.4	E962.0	E980.4
DHE-45	972.9	E858.3	E942.9	E950.4	E962.0	E980.4
Diabinese	962.3	E858.0	E932.3	E950.4	E962.0	E980.4
Diacetyl monoxime	977.2	E858.8	E947.2	E950.4	E962.0	E980.4
Diacetylmorphine	965.01	E850.0	E935.0	E950.0	E962.0	E980.0
Diagnostic agents	977.8	E858.8	E947.8	E950.4	E962.0	E980.4
Dial (soap)	976.2	E858.7	E946.2	E950.4	E962.0	E980.4
sedative	967.0	E851	E937.0	E950.1	E962.0	E980.1
Diallylbarbituric acid	967.0	E851	E937.0	E950.1	E962.0	E980.1
Diaminodiphenyisulfone	961.8	E857	E931.8	E950.4	E962.0	E980.4
Diamorphine	965.01	E850.0	E935.0	E950.0	E962.0	E980.0
Diamox	974.2	E858.5	E944.2	E950.4	E962.0	E980.4
Diamthazole	976.0	E858.7	E946.0	E950.4	E962.0	E980.4
Diaphenyisulfone	961.8	E857	E931.8	E950.4	E962.0	E980.4
Diasone (sodium)	961.8	E857	E931.8	E950.4	E962.0	E980.4
Diazepam	969.4	E853.2	E939.4	E950.3	E962.0	E980.3
Diazinon	989.3	E863.1	—	E950.6	E962.1	E980.7

◀ New   ◀▥ Revised   ~~deleted~~ Deleted   ● Use Additional Digit(s)

Substance	Poisoning	External Cause (E Code)				
		Accident	Therapeutic Use	Suicide Attempt	Assault	Undetermined
Diazomethane (gas)	987.8	E869.8	—	E952.8	E962.2	E982.8
Diazoxide	972.5	E858.3	E942.5	E950.4	E962.0	E980.4
Dibenamine	971.3	E855.6	E941.3	E950.4	E962.0	E980.4
Dibenzheptropine	963.0	E858.1	E933.0	E950.4	E962.0	E980.4
Dibenzyline	971.3	E855.6	E941.3	E950.4	E962.0	E980.4
Diborane (gas)	987.8	E869.8	—	E952.8	E962.2	E982.8
Dibromomannitol	963.1	E858.1	E933.1	E950.4	E962.0	E980.4
Dibucaine (spinal)	968.7	E855.2	E938.7	E950.4	E962.0	E980.4
topical (surface)	968.5	E855.2	E938.5	E950.4	E962.0	E980.4
Dibunate sodium	975.4	E858.6	E945.4	E950.4	E962.0	E980.4
Dibutoline	971.1	E855.4	E941.1	E950.4	E962.0	E980.4
Dicapthon	989.4	E863.4	—	E950.6	E962.1	E980.7
Dichloralphenazone	967.1	E852.0	E937.1	E950.2	E962.0	E980.2
Dichlorodifluoromethane	987.4	E869.2	—	E952.8	E962.2	E982.8
Dichloroethane	982.3	E862.4	—	E950.9	E962.1	E980.9
Dichloroethylene	982.3	E862.4	—	E950.9	E962.1	E980.9
Dichloroethyl sulfide	987.8	E869.8	—	E952.8	E962.2	E982.8
Dichlorohydrin	982.3	E862.4	—	E950.9	E962.1	E980.9
Dichloromethane (solvent) (vapor)	982.3	E862.4	—	E950.9	E962.1	E980.9
Dichlorophen(e)	961.6	E857	E931.6	E950.4	E962.0	E980.4
Dichlorphenamide	974.2	E858.5	E944.2	E950.4	E962.0	E980.4
Dichlorvos	989.3	E863.1	—	E950.6	E962.1	E980.7
Diclofenac sodium	965.69	E850.6	E935.6	E950.0	E962.0	E980.0
Dicoumarin, dicumarol	964.2	E858.2	E934.2	E950.4	E962.0	E980.4
Dicyanogen (gas)	987.8	E869.8	—	E952.8	E962.2	E982.8
Dicyclomine	971.1	E855.4	E941.1	E950.4	E962.0	E980.4
Dieldrin (vapor)	989.2	E863.0	—	E950.6	E962.1	E980.7
Dienestrol	962.2	E858.0	E932.2	E950.4	E962.0	E980.4
Dietetics	977.0	E858.8	E947.0	E950.4	E962.0	E980.4
Diethazine	966.4	E855.0	E936.4	E950.4	E962.0	E980.4
Diethyl	—	—	—	—	—	—
barbituric acid	967.0	E851	E937.0	E950.1	E962.0	E980.1
carbamazine	961.6	E857	E931.6	E950.4	E962.0	E980.4
carbinol	980.8	E860.8	—	E950.9	E962.1	E980.9
carbonate	982.8	E862.4	—	E950.9	E962.1	E980.9
ether (vapor) - *see* Ether(s)	—	—	—	—	—	—
propion	977.0	E858.8	E947.0	E950.4	E962.0	E980.4
stilbestrol	962.2	E858.0	E932.2	E950.4	E962.0	E980.4

◀ New   ◀▥ Revised   ~~deleted~~ Deleted   ● Use Additional Digit(s)

Substance	Poisoning	External Cause (E Code)				
		Accident	Therapeutic Use	Suicide Attempt	Assault	Undetermined
Diethylene	—	—	—	—	—	—
dioxide	982.8	E862.4	—	E950.9	E962.1	E980.9
glycol (monoacetate) (monoethyl ether)	982.8	E862.4	—	E950.9	E962.1	E980.9
Diethylsulfone-diethylmethane	967.8	E852.8	E937.8	E950.2	E962.0	E980.2
Difencloxazine	965.09	E850.2	E935.2	E950.0	E962.0	E980.0
Diffusin	963.4	E858.1	E933.4	E950.4	E962.0	E980.4
Diflos	971.0	E855.3	E941.0	E950.4	E962.0	E980.4
Digestants	973.4	E858.4	E943.4	E950.4	E962.0	E980.4
Digitalin(e)	972.1	E858.3	E942.1	E950.4	E962.0	E980.4
Digitalis glycosides	972.1	E858.3	E942.1	E950.4	E962.0	E980.4
Digitoxin	972.1	E858.3	E942.1	E950.4	E962.0	E980.4
Digoxin	972.1	E858.3	E942.1	E950.4	E962.0	E980.4
Dihydrocodeine	965.09	E850.2	E935.2	E950.0	E962.0	E980.0
Dihydrocodeinone	965.09	E850.2	E935.2	E950.0	E962.0	E980.0
Dihydroergocristine	972.9	E858.3	E942.9	E950.4	E962.0	E980.4
Dihydroergotamine	972.9	E858.3	E942.9	E950.4	E962.0	E980.4
Dihydroergotoxine	972.9	E858.3	E942.9	E950.4	E962.0	E980.4
Dihydrohydroxycodeinone	965.09	E850.2	E935.2	E950.0	E962.0	E980.0
Dihydrohydroxymorphinone	965.09	E850.2	E935.2	E950.0	E962.0	E980.0
Dihydroisocodeine	965.09	E850.2	E935.2	E950.0	E962.0	E980.0
Dihydromorphine	965.09	E850.2	E935.2	E950.0	E962.0	E980.0
Dihydromorphinone	965.09	E850.2	E935.2	E950.0	E962.0	E980.0
Dihydrostreptomycin	960.6	E856	E930.6	E950.4	E962.0	E980.4
Dihydrotachysterol	962.6	E858.0	E932.6	E950.4	E962.0	E980.4
Dihydroxyanthraquinone	973.1	E858.4	E943.1	E950.4	E962.0	E980.4
Dihydroxycodeinone	965.09	E850.2	E935.2	E950.0	E962.0	E980.0
Diiodohydroxyquin	961.3	E857	E931.3	E950.4	E962.0	E980.4
topical	976.0	E858.7	E946.0	E950.4	E962.0	E980.4
Diiodohydroxyquinoline	961.3	E857	E931.3	E950.4	E962.0	E980.4
Dilantin	966.1	E855.0	E936.1	E950.4	E962.0	E980.4
Dilaudid	965.09	E850.2	E935.2	E950.0	E962.0	E980.0
Diloxanide	961.5	E857	E931.5	E950.4	E962.0	E980.4
Dimefline	970.0	E854.3	E940.0	E950.4	E962.0	E980.4
Dimenhydrinate	963.0	E858.1	E933.0	E950.4	E962.0	E980.4
Dimercaprol	963.8	E858.1	E933.8	E950.4	E962.0	E980.4
Dimercaptopropanol	963.8	E858.1	E933.8	E950.4	E962.0	E980.4
Dimetane	963.0	E858.1	E933.0	E950.4	E962.0	E980.4
Dimethicone	976.3	E858.7	E946.3	E950.4	E962.0	E980.4
Dimethindene	963.0	E858.1	E933.0	E950.4	E962.0	E980.4

◄ New   ◄▥ Revised   ~~deleted~~ Deleted   ● Use Additional Digit(s)

Substance	Poisoning	External Cause (E Code)				
		Accident	Therapeutic Use	Suicide Attempt	Assault	Undetermined
Dimethisoquin	968.5	E855.2	E938.5	E950.4	E962.0	E980.4
Dimethisterone	962.2	E858.0	E932.2	E950.4	E962.0	E980.4
Dimethoxanate	975.4	E858.6	E945.4	E950.4	E962.0	E980.4
Dimethyl	—	—	—	—	—	—
arsine, arsinic acid - *see* Arsenic	—	—	—	—	—	—
carbinol	980.2	E860.3	—	E950.9	E962.1	E980.9
diguanide	962.3	E858.0	E932.3	E950.4	E962.0	E980.4
ketone	982.8	E862.4	—	E950.9	E962.1	E980.9
vapor	987.8	E869.8	—	E952.8	E962.2	E982.8
meperidine	965.09	E850.2	E935.2	E950.0	E962.0	E980.0
parathion	989.3	E863.1	—	E950.6	E962.1	E980.7
polysiloxane	973.8	E858.4	E943.8	E950.4	E962.0	E980.4
sulfate (fumes)	987.8	E869.8	—	E952.8	E962.2	E982.8
liquid	983.9	E864.3	—	E950.7	E962.1	E980.6
sulfoxide NEC	982.8	E862.4	—	E950.9	E962.1	E980.9
medicinal	976.4	E858.7	E946.4	E950.4	E962.0	E980.4
triptamine	969.6	E854.1	E939.6	E950.3	E962.0	E980.3
tubocurarine	975.2	E858.6	E945.2	E950.4	E962.0	E980.4
Dindevan	964.2	E858.2	E934.2	E950.4	E962.0	E980.4
Dinitro (-ortho-) cresol (herbicide) (spray)	989.4	E863.5	—	E950.6	E962.1	E980.7
insecticide	989.4	E863.4	—	E950.6	E962.1	E980.7
Dinitrobenzene	983.0	E864.0	—	E950.7	E962.1	E980.6
vapor	987.8	E869.8	—	E952.8	E962.2	E982.8
Dinitro-orthocresol (herbicide)	989.4	E863.5	—	E950.6	E962.1	E980.7
insecticide	989.4	E863.4	—	E950.6	E962.1	E980.7
Dinitrophenol (herbicide) (spray)	989.4	E863.5	—	E950.6	E962.1	E980.7
insecticide	989.4	E863.4	—	E950.6	E962.1	E980.7
Dinoprost	975.0	E858.6	E945.0	E950.4	E962.0	E980.4
Dioctyl sulfosuccinate (calcium) (sodium)	973.2	E858.4	E943.2	E950.4	E962.0	E980.4
Diodoquin	961.3	E857	E931.3	E950.4	E962.0	E980.4
Dione derivatives NEC	966.3	E855.0	E936.3	E950.4	E962.0	E980.4
Dionin	965.09	E850.2	E935.2	E950.0	E962.0	E980.0
Dioxane	982.8	E862.4	—	E950.9	E962.1	E980.9
Dioxin - *see* herbicide	—	—	—	—	—	—
Dioxyline	972.5	E858.3	E942.5	E950.4	E962.0	E980.4
Dipentene	982.8	E862.4	—	E950.9	E962.1	E980.9
Diphemanil	971.1	E855.4	E941.1	E950.4	E962.0	E980.4
Diphenadione	964.2	E858.2	E934.2	E950.4	E962.0	E980.4
Diphenhydramine	963.0	E858.1	E933.0	E950.4	E962.0	E980.4

◀ New   ◀▥ Revised   ~~deleted~~ Deleted   ● Use Additional Digit(s)

TABLE OF DRUGS AND CHEMICALS

Substance	Poisoning	External Cause (E Code)				
		Accident	Therapeutic Use	Suicide Attempt	Assault	Undetermined
Diphenidol	963.0	E858.1	E933.0	E950.4	E962.0	E980.4
Diphenoxylate	973.5	E858.4	E943.5	E950.4	E962.0	E980.4
Diphenylchlorarsine	985.1	E866.3	—	E950.8	E962.1	E980.8
Diphenylhydantoin (sodium)	966.1	E855.0	E936.1	E950.4	E962.0	E980.4
Diphenylpyraline	963.0	E858.1	E933.0	E950.4	E962.0	E980.4
Diphtheria	—	—	—	—	—	—
antitoxin	979.9	E858.8	E949.9	E950.4	E962.0	E980.4
toxoid	978.5	E858.8	E948.5	E950.4	E962.0	E980.4
with tetanus toxoid	978.9	E858.8	E948.9	E950.4	E962.0	E980.4
with pertussis component	978.6	E858.8	E948.6	E950.4	E962.0	E980.4
vaccine	978.5	E858.8	E948.5	E950.4	E962.0	E980.4
Dipipanone	965.09	E850.2	E935.2	E950.0	E962.0	E980.0
Diplovax	979.5	E858.8	E949.5	E950.4	E962.0	E980.4
Diprophylline	975.1	E858.6	E945.1	E950.4	E962.0	E980.4
Dipyridamole	972.4	E858.3	E942.4	E950.4	E962.0	E980.4
Dipyrone	965.5	E850.5	E935.5	E950.0	E962.0	E980.0
Diquat	989.4	E863.5	—	E950.6	E962.1	E980.7
Disinfectant NEC	983.9	E861.4	—	E950.7	E962.1	E980.6
alkaline	983.2	E861.4	—	E950.7	E962.1	E980.6
aromatic	983.0	E861.4	—	E950.7	E962.1	E980.6
Disipal	966.4	E855.0	E936.4	E950.4	E962.0	E980.4
Disodium edetate	963.8	E858.1	E933.8	E950.4	E962.0	E980.4
Disulfamide	974.4	E858.5	E944.4	E950.4	E962.0	E980.4
Disulfanilamide	961.0	E857	E931.0	E950.4	E962.0	E980.4
Disulfiram	977.3	E858.8	E947.3	E950.4	E962.0	E980.4
Dithiazanine	961.6	E857	E931.6	E950.4	E962.0	E980.4
Dithioglycerol	963.8	E858.1	E933.8	E950.4	E962.0	E980.4
Dithranol	976.4	E858.7	E946.4	E950.4	E962.0	E980.4
Diucardin	974.3	E858.5	E944.3	E950.4	E962.0	E980.4
Diupres	974.3	E858.5	E944.3	E950.4	E962.0	E980.4
Diuretics NEC	974.4	E858.5	E944.4	E950.4	E962.0	E980.4
carbonic acid anhydrase inhibitors	974.2	E858.5	E944.2	E950.4	E962.0	E980.4
mercurial	974.0	E858.5	E944.0	E950.4	E962.0	E980.4
osmotic	974.4	E858.5	E944.4	E950.4	E962.0	E980.4
purine derivatives	974.1	E858.5	E944.1	E950.4	E962.0	E980.4
saluretic	974.3	E858.5	E944.3	E950.4	E962.0	E980.4
Diuril	974.3	E858.5	E944.3	E950.4	E962.0	E980.4
Divinyl ether	968.2	E855.1	E938.2	E950.4	E962.0	E980.4
D-lysergic acid diethylamide	969.6	E854.1	E939.6	E950.3	E962.0	E980.3

◀ New   ◀▥ Revised   deleted Deleted   ● Use Additional Digit(s)

Substance	Poisoning	External Cause (E Code)				
		Accident	Therapeutic Use	Suicide Attempt	Assault	Undetermined
DMCT	960.4	E856	E930.4	E950.4	E962.0	E980.4
DMSO	982.8	E862.4	—	E950.9	E962.1	E980.9
DMT	969.6	E854.1	E939.6	E950.3	E962.0	E980.3
DNOC	989.4	E863.5	—	E950.6	E962.1	E980.7
DOCA	962.0	E858.0	E932.0	E950.4	E962.0	E980.4
Dolophine	965.02	E850.1	E935.1	E950.0	E962.0	E980.0
Doloxene	965.8	E850.8	E935.8	E950.0	E962.0	E980.0
DOM	969.6	E854.1	E939.6	E950.3	E962.0	E980.3
Domestic gas - *see* Gas, utility	—	—	—	—	—	—
Domiphen (bromide) (lozenges)	976.6	E858.7	E946.6	E950.4	E962.0	E980.4
Dopa (levo)	966.4	E855.0	E936.4	E950.4	E962.0	E980.4
Dopamine	971.2	E855.5	E941.2	E950.4	E962.0	E980.4
Doriden	967.5	E852.4	E937.5	E950.2	E962.0	E980.2
Dormiral	967.0	E851	E937.0	E950.1	E962.0	E980.1
Dormison	967.8	E852.8	E937.8	E950.2	E962.0	E980.2
Dornase	963.4	E858.1	E933.4	E950.4	E962.0	E980.4
Dorsacaine	968.5	E855.2	E938.5	E950.4	E962.0	E980.4
Dothiepin hydrochloride	969.05 ◄▥	E854.0	E939.0	E950.3	E962.0	E980.3
Doxapram	970.0	E854.3	E940.0	E950.4	E962.0	E980.4
Doxepin	969.05 ◄▥	E854.0	E939.0	E950.3	E962.0	E980.3
Doxorubicin	960.7	E856	E930.7	E950.4	E962.0	E980.4
Doxycycline	960.4	E856	E930.4	E950.4	E962.0	E980.4
Doxylamine	963.0	E858.1	E933.0	E950.4	E962.0	E980.4
Dramamine	963.0	E858.1	E933.0	E950.4	E962.0	E980.4
Drano (drain cleaner)	983.2	E864.2	—	E950.7	E962.1	E980.6
Dromoran	965.09	E850.2	E935.2	E950.0	E962.0	E980.0
Dromostanolone	962.1	E858.0	E932.1	E950.4	E962.0	E980.4
Droperidol	969.2	E853.1	E939.2	E950.3	E962.0	E980.3
Drotrecogin alfa	964.2	E858.2	E934.2	E950.4	E962.0	E980.4
Drug	977.9	E858.9	E947.9	E950.5	E962.0	E980.5
specified NEC	977.8	E858.8	E947.8	E950.4	E962.0	E980.4
AHFS List	—	—	—	—	—	—
4:00 antihistamine drugs	963.0	E858.1	E933.0	E950.4	E962.0	E980.4
8:04 amebacides	961.5	E857	E931.5	E950.4	E962.0	E980.4
arsenical anti-infectives	961.1	E857	E931.1	E950.4	E962.0	E980.4
quinoline derivatives	961.3	E857	E931.3	E950.4	E962.0	E980.4
8:08 anthelmintics	961.6	E857	E931.6	E950.4	E962.0	E980.4
quinoline derivatives	961.3	E857	E931.3	E950.4	E962.0	E980.4
8:12.04 antifungal antibiotics	960.1	E856	E930.1	E950.4	E962.0	E980.4

◄ New   ◄▥ Revised   deleted Deleted   ● Use Additional Digit(s)

TABLE OF DRUGS AND CHEMICALS

Substance	Poisoning	External Cause (E Code)				
		Accident	Therapeutic Use	Suicide Attempt	Assault	Undetermined
Drug *(Continued)*						
8:12.06 cephalosporins	960.5	E856	E930.5	E950.4	E962.0	E980.4
8:12.08 chloramphenicol	960.2	E856	E930.2	E950.4	E962.0	E980.4
8:12.12 erythromycins	960.3	E856	E930.3	E950.4	E962.0	E980.4
8:12.16 penicillins	960.0	E856	E930.0	E950.4	E962.0	E980.4
8:12.20 streptomycins	960.6	E856	E930.6	E950.4	E962.0	E980.4
8:12.24 tetracyclines	960.4	E856	E930.4	E950.4	E962.0	E980.4
8:12.28 other antibiotics	960.8	E856	E930.8	E950.4	E962.0	E980.4
antimycobacterial	960.6	E856	E930.6	E950.4	E962.0	E980.4
macrolides	960.3	E856	E930.3	E950.4	E962.0	E980.4
8:16 antituberculars	961.8	E857	E931.8	E950.4	E962.0	E980.4
antibiotics	960.6	E856	E930.6	E950.4	E962.0	E980.4
8:18 antivirals	961.7	E857	E931.7	E950.4	E962.0	E980.4
8:20 plasmodicides (antimalarials)	961.4	E857	E931.4	E950.4	E962.0	E980.4
8:24 sulfonamides	961.0	E857	E931.0	E950.4	E962.0	E980.4
8:26 sulfones	961.8	E857	E931.8	E950.4	E962.0	E980.4
8:28 treponemicides	961.2	E857	E931.2	E950.4	E962.0	E980.4
8:32 trichomonacides	961.5	E857	E931.5	E950.4	E962.0	E980.4
quinoline derivatives	961.3	E857	E931.3	E950.4	E962.0	E980.4
nitrofuran derivatives	961.9	E857	E931.9	E950.4	E962.0	E980.4
8:36 urinary germicides	961.9	E857	E931.9	E950.4	E962.0	E980.4
quinoline derivatives	961.3	E857	E931.3	E950.4	E962.0	E980.4
8:40 other anti-infectives	961.9	E857	E931.9	E950.4	E962.0	E980.4
10:00 antineoplastic agents	963.1	E858.1	E933.1	E950.4	E962.0	E980.4
antibiotics	960.7	E856	E930.7	E950.4	E962.0	E980.4
progestogens	962.2	E858.0	E932.2	E950.4	E962.0	E980.4
12:04 parasympathomimetic (cholinergic) agents	971.0	E855.3	E941.0	E950.4	E962.0	E980.4
12:08 parasympatholytic (cholinergic-blocking) agents	971.1	E855.4	E941.1	E950.4	E962.0	E980.4
12:12 sympathomimetic (adrenergic) agents	971.2	E855.5	E941.2	E950.4	E962.0	E980.4
12:16 sympatholytic (adrenergic-blocking) agents	971.3	E855.6	E941.3	E950.4	E962.0	E980.4
12:20 skeletal muscle relaxants	—	—	—	—	—	—
central nervous system muscle-tone depressants	968.0	E855.1	E938.0	E950.4	E962.0	E980.4
myoneural blocking agents	975.2	E858.6	E945.2	E950.4	E962.0	E980.4
16:00 blood derivatives	964.7	E858.2	E934.7	E950.4	E962.0	E980.4
20:04 antianemia drugs	964.1	E858.2	E934.1	E950.4	E962.0	E980.4
20:04.04 iron preparations	964.0	E858.2	E934.0	E950.4	E962.0	E980.4
20:04.08 liver and stomach preparations	964.1	E858.2	E934.1	E950.4	E962.0	E980.4
20:12.04 anticoagulants	964.2	E858.2	E934.2	E950.4	E962.0	E980.4
20:12.08 antiheparin agents	964.5	E858.2	E934.5	E950.4	E962.0	E980.4

◀ New　◀▥▥ Revised　~~deleted~~ Deleted　● Use Additional Digit(s)

Substance	Poisoning	External Cause (E Code)				
		Accident	Therapeutic Use	Suicide Attempt	Assault	Undetermined
Drug *(Continued)*						
20:12.12 coagulants	964.5	E858.2	E934.5	E950.4	E962.0	E980.4
20:12.16 hemostatics NEC	964.5	E858.2	E934.5	E950.4	E962.0	E980.4
capillary active drugs	972.8	E858.3	E942.8	E950.4	E962.0	E980.4
24:04 cardiac drugs	972.9	E858.3	E942.9	E950.4	E962.0	E980.4
cardiotonic agents	972.1	E858.3	E942.1	E950.4	E962.0	E980.4
rhythm regulators	972.0	E858.3	E942.0	E950.4	E962.0	E980.4
24:06 antilipemic agents	972.2	E858.3	E942.2	E950.4	E962.0	E980.4
thyroid derivatives	962.7	E858.0	E932.7	E950.4	E962.0	E980.4
24:08 hypotensive agents	972.6	E858.3	E942.6	E950.4	E962.0	E980.4
adrenergic blocking agents	971.3	E855.6	E941.3	E950.4	E962.0	E980.4
ganglion blocking agents	972.3	E858.3	E942.3	E950.4	E962.0	E980.4
vasodilators	972.5	E858.3	E942.5	E950.4	E962.0	E980.4
24:12 vasodilating agents NEC	972.5	E858.3	E942.5	E950.4	E962.0	E980.4
coronary	972.4	E858.3	E942.4	E950.4	E962.0	E980.4
nicotinic acid derivatives	972.2	E858.3	E942.2	E950.4	E962.0	E980.4
24:16 sclerosing agents	972.7	E858.3	E942.7	E950.4	E962.0	E980.4
28:04 general anesthetics	968.4	E855.1	E938.4	E950.4	E962.0	E980.4
gaseous anesthetics	968.2	E855.1	E938.2	E950.4	E962.0	E980.4
halothane	968.1	E855.1	E938.1	E950.4	E962.0	E980.4
intravenous anesthetics	968.3	E855.1	E938.3	E950.4	E962.0	E980.4
28:08 analgesics and antipyretics	965.9	E850.9	E935.9	E950.0	E962.0	E980.0
antirheumatics	965.69	E850.6	E935.6	E950.0	E962.0	E980.0
aromatic analgesics	965.4	E850.4	E935.4	E950.0	E962.0	E980.0
non-narcotic NEC	965.7	E850.7	E935.7	E950.0	E962.0	E980.0
opium alkaloids	965.00	E850.2	E935.2	E950.0	E962.0	E980.0
heroin	965.01	E850.0	E935.0	E950.0	E962.0	E980.0
methadone	965.02	E850.1	E935.1	E950.0	E962.0	E980.0
specified type NEC	965.09	E850.2	E935.2	E950.0	E962.0	E980.0
pyrazole derivatives	965.5	E850.5	E935.5	E950.0	E962.0	E980.0
salicylates	965.1	E850.3	E935.3	E950.0	E962.0	E980.0
specified NEC	965.8	E850.8	E935.8	E950.0	E962.0	E980.0
28:10 narcotic antagonists	970.1	E854.3	E940.1	E950.4	E962.0	E980.4
28:12 anticonvulsants	966.3	E855.0	E936.3	E950.4	E962.0	E980.4
barbiturates	967.0	E851	E937.0	E950.1	E962.0	E980.1
benzodiazepine-based tranquilizers	969.4	E853.2	E939.4	E950.3	E962.0	E980.3
bromides	967.3	E852.2	E937.3	E950.2	E962.0	E980.2
hydantoin derivatives	966.1	E855.0	E936.1	E950.4	E962.0	E980.4
oxazolidine (derivatives)	966.0	E855.0	E936.0	E950.4	E962.0	E980.4
succinimides	966.2	E855.0	E936.2	E950.4	E962.0	E980.4

◀ New   ◀▥ Revised   ~~deleted~~ Deleted   ● Use Additional Digit(s)

Substance	Poisoning	External Cause (E Code)				
		Accident	Therapeutic Use	Suicide Attempt	Assault	Undetermined
Drug *(Continued)*						
28:16.04 antidepressants	969.00 ◄▬	E854.0	E939.0	E950.3	E962.0	E980.3
28:16.08 tranquilizers	969.5	E853.9	E939.5	E950.3	E962.0	E980.3
benzodiazepine-based	969.4	E853.2	E939.4	E950.3	E962.0	E980.3
butyrophenone-based	969.2	E853.1	E939.2	E950.3	E962.0	E980.3
major NEC	969.3	E853.8	E939.3	E950.3	E962.0	E980.3
phenothiazine-based	969.1	E853.0	E939.1	E950.3	E962.0	E980.3
28:16.12 other psychotherapeutic agents	969.8	E855.8	E939.8	E950.3	E962.0	E980.3
28:20 respiratory and cerebral stimulants	970.9	E854.3	E940.9	E950.4	E962.0	E980.4
analeptics	970.0	E854.3	E940.0	E950.4	E962.0	E980.4
anorexigenic agents	977.0	E858.8	E947.0	E950.4	E962.0	E980.4
psychostimulants	969.70 ◄▬	E854.2	E939.7	E950.3	E962.0	E980.3
specified NEC	970.8	E854.3	E940.8	E950.4	E962.0	E980.4
28:24 sedatives and hypnotics	967.9	E852.9	E937.9	E950.2	E962.0	E980.2
barbiturates	967.0	E851	E937.0	E950.1	E962.0	E980.1
benzodiazepine-based tranquilizers	969.4	E853.2	E939.4	E950.3	E962.0	E980.3
chloral hydrate (group)	967.1	E852.0	E937.1	E950.2	E962.0	E980.2
glutethimide group	967.5	E852.4	E937.5	E950.2	E962.0	E980.2
intravenous anesthetics	968.3	E855.1	E938.3	E950.4	E962.0	E980.4
methaqualone (compounds)	967.4	E852.3	E937.4	E950.2	E962.0	E980.2
paraldehyde	967.2	E852.1	E937.2	E950.2	E962.0	E980.2
phenothiazine-based tranquilizers	969.1	E853.0	E939.1	E950.3	E962.0	E980.3
specified NEC	967.8	E852.8	E937.8	E950.2	E962.0	E980.2
thiobarbiturates	968.3	E855.1	E938.3	E950.4	E962.0	E980.4
tranquilizer NEC	969.5	E853.9	E939.5	E950.3	E962.0	E980.3
36:04 to 36:88 diagnostic agents	977.8	E858.8	E947.8	E950.4	E962.0	E980.4
40:00 electrolyte, caloric, and water balance agents NEC	974.5	E858.5	E944.5	E950.4	E962.0	E980.4
40:04 acidifying agents	963.2	E858.1	E933.2	E950.4	E962.0	E980.4
40:08 alkalinizing agents	963.3	E858.1	E933.3	E950.4	E962.0	E980.4
40:10 ammonia detoxicants	974.5	E858.5	E944.5	E950.4	E962.0	E980.4
40:12 replacement solutions	974.5	E858.5	E944.5	E950.4	E962.0	E980.4
plasma expanders	964.8	E858.2	E934.8	E950.4	E962.0	E980.4
40:16 sodium-removing resins	974.5	E858.5	E944.5	E950.4	E962.0	E980.4
40:18 potassium-removing resins	974.5	E858.5	E944.5	E950.4	E962.0	E980.4
40:20 caloric agents	974.5	E858.5	E944.5	E950.4	E962.0	E980.4
40:24 salt and sugar substitutes	974.5	E858.5	E944.5	E950.4	E962.0	E980.4
40:28 diuretics NEC	974.4	E858.5	E944.4	E950.4	E962.0	E980.4
carbonic acid anhydrase inhibitors	974.2	E858.5	E944.2	E950.4	E962.0	E980.4

◄ New   ◄▬ Revised   ~~deleted~~ Deleted   ● Use Additional Digit(s)

TABLE OF DRUGS AND CHEMICALS

Substance	External Cause (E Code)					
	Poisoning	Accident	Therapeutic Use	Suicide Attempt	Assault	Undetermined
Drug *(Continued)*						
40:28 diuretics NEC *(Continued)*						
mercurials	974.0	E858.5	E944.0	E950.4	E962.0	E980.4
purine derivatives	974.1	E858.5	E944.1	E950.4	E962.0	E980.4
saluretics	974.3	E858.5	E944.3	E950.4	E962.0	E980.4
thiazides	974.3	E858.5	E944.3	E950.4	E962.0	E980.4
40:36 irrigating solutions	974.5	E858.5	E944.5	E950.4	E962.0	E980.4
40:40 uricosuric agents	974.7	E858.5	E944.7	E950.4	E962.0	E980.4
44:00 enzymes	963.4	E858.1	E933.4	E950.4	E962.0	E980.4
fibrinolysis-affecting agents	964.4	E858.2	E934.4	E950.4	E962.0	E980.4
gastric agents	973.4	E858.4	E943.4	E950.4	E962.0	E980.4
48:00 expectorants and cough preparations	—	—	—	—	—	—
antihistamine agents	963.0	E858.1	E933.0	E950.4	E962.0	E980.4
antitussives	975.4	E858.6	E945.4	E950.4	E962.0	E980.4
codeine derivatives	965.09	E850.2	E935.2	E950.0	E962.0	E980.0
expectorants	975.5	E858.6	E945.5	E950.4	E962.0	E980.4
narcotic agents NEC	965.09	E850.2	E935.2	E950.0	E962.0	E980.0
52:04 anti-infectives (EENT)	—	—	—	—	—	—
ENT agent	976.6	E858.7	E946.6	E950.4	E962.0	E980.4
ophthalmic preparation	976.5	E858.7	E946.5	E950.4	E962.0	E980.4
52:04.04 antibiotics (EENT)	—	—	—	—	—	—
ENT agent	976.6	E858.7	E946.6	E950.4	E962.0	E980.4
ophthalmic preparation	976.5	E858.7	E946.5	E950.4	E962.0	E980.4
52:04.06 antivirals (EENT)	—	—	—	—	—	—
ENT agent	976.6	E858.7	E946.6	E950.4	E962.0	E980.4
ophthalmic preparation	976.5	E858.7	E946.5	E950.4	E962.0	E980.4
52:04.08 sulfonamides (EENT)	—	—	—	—	—	—
ENT agent	976.6	E858.7	E946.6	E950.4	E962.0	E980.4
ophthalmic preparation	976.5	E858.7	E946.5	E950.4	E962.0	E980.4
52:04.12 miscellaneous anti-infectives (EENT)	—	—	—	—	—	—
ENT agent	976.6	E858.7	E946.6	E950.4	E962.0	E980.4
ophthalmic preparation	976.5	E858.7	E946.5	E950.4	E962.0	E980.4
52:08 anti-inflammatory agents (EENT)	—	—	—	—	—	—
ENT agent	976.6	E858.7	E946.6	E950.4	E962.0	E980.4
ophthalmic preparation	976.5	E858.7	E946.5	E950.4	E962.0	E980.4
52:10 carbonic anhydrase inhibitors	974.2	E858.5	E944.2	E950.4	E962.0	E980.4
52:12 contact lens solutions	976.5	E858.7	E946.5	E950.4	E962.0	E980.4
52:16 local anesthetics (EENT)	968.5	E855.2	E938.5	E950.4	E962.0	E980.4

◄ New   ◄▥ Revised   ~~deleted~~ Deleted   ● Use Additional Digit(s)

Substance	External Cause (E Code)					
	Poisoning	Accident	Therapeutic Use	Suicide Attempt	Assault	Undetermined
Drug *(Continued)*						
52:20 miotics	971.0	E855.3	E941.0	E950.4	E962.0	E980.4
52:24 mydriatics	—	—	—	—	—	—
adrenergics	971.2	E855.5	E941.2	E950.4	E962.0	E980.4
anticholinergics	971.1	E855.4	E941.1	E950.4	E962.0	E980.4
antimuscarinics	971.1	E855.4	E941.1	E950.4	E962.0	E980.4
parasympatholytics	971.1	E855.4	E941.1	E950.4	E962.0	E980.4
spasmolytics	971.1	E855.4	E941.1	E950.4	E962.0	E980.4
sympathomimetics	971.2	E855.5	E941.2	E950.4	E962.0	E980.4
52:28 mouth washes and gargles	976.6	E858.7	E946.6	E950.4	E962.0	E980.4
52:32 vasoconstrictors (EENT)	971.2	E855.5	E941.2	E950.4	E962.0	E980.4
52:36 unclassified agents (EENT)	—	—	—	—	—	—
ENT agent	976.6	E858.7	E946.6	E950.4	E962.0	E980.4
ophthalmic preparation	976.5	E858.7	E946.5	E950.4	E962.0	E980.4
56:04 antacids and adsorbents	973.0	E858.4	E943.0	E950.4	E962.0	E980.4
56:08 antidiarrhea agents	973.5	E858.4	E943.5	E950.4	E962.0	E980.4
56:10 antiflatulents	973.8	E858.4	E943.8	E950.4	E962.0	E980.4
56:12 cathartics NEC	973.3	E858.4	E943.3	E950.4	E962.0	E980.4
emollients	973.2	E858.4	E943.2	E950.4	E962.0	E980.4
irritants	973.1	E858.4	E943.1	E950.4	E962.0	E980.4
56:16 digestants	973.4	E858.4	E943.4	E950.4	E962.0	E980.4
56:20 emetics and antiemetics	—	—	—	—	—	—
antiemetics	963.0	E858.1	E933.0	E950.4	E962.0	E980.4
emetics	973.6	E858.4	E943.6	E950.4	E962.0	E980.4
56:24 lipotropic agents	977.1	E858.8	E947.1	E950.4	E962.0	E980.4
56:40 miscellaneous G.I. drugs	973.8	E858.4	E943.8	E950.4	E962.0	E980.4
60:00 gold compounds	965.69	E850.6	E935.6	E950.0	E962.0	E980.0
64:00 heavy metal antagonists	963.8	E858.1	E933.8	E950.4	E962.0	E980.4
68:04 adrenals	962.0	E858.0	E932.0	E950.4	E962.0	E980.4
68:08 androgens	962.1	E858.0	E932.1	E950.4	E962.0	E980.4
68:12 contraceptives, oral	962.2	E858.0	E932.2	E950.4	E962.0	E980.4
68:16 estrogens	962.2	E858.0	E932.2	E950.4	E962.0	E980.4
68:18 gonadotropins	962.4	E858.0	E932.4	E950.4	E962.0	E980.4
68:20 insulins and antidiabetic agents	962.3	E858.0	E932.3	E950.4	E962.0	E980.4
68:20.08 insulins	962.3	E858.0	E932.3	E950.4	E962.0	E980.4
68:24 parathyroid	962.6	E858.0	E932.6	E950.4	E962.0	E980.4
68:28 pituitary (posterior)	962.5	E858.0	E932.5	E950.4	E962.0	E980.4
anterior	962.4	E858.0	E932.4	E950.4	E962.0	E980.4
68:32 progestogens	962.2	E858.0	E932.2	E950.4	E962.0	E980.4

◀ New   ◀▥ Revised   ~~deleted~~ Deleted   ● Use Additional Digit(s)

Substance	Poisoning	External Cause (E Code)				
		Accident	Therapeutic Use	Suicide Attempt	Assault	Undetermined
Drug *(Continued)*						
68:34 other corpus luteum hormones NEC	962.2	E858.0	E932.2	E950.4	E962.0	E980.4
68:36 thyroid and antithyroid	—	—	—	—	—	—
antithyroid	962.8	E858.0	E932.8	E950.4	E962.0	E980.4
thyroid (derivatives)	962.7	E858.0	E932.7	E950.4	E962.0	E980.4
72:00 local anesthetics NEC	968.9	E855.2	E938.9	E950.4	E962.0	E980.4
topical (surface)	968.5	E855.2	E938.5	E950.4	E962.0	E980.4
infiltration (intradermal) (subcutaneous) (submucosal)	968.5	E855.2	E938.5	E950.4	E962.0	E980.4
nerve blocking (peripheral) (plexus) (regional)	968.6	E855.2	E938.6	E950.4	E962.0	E980.4
spinal	968.7	E855.2	E938.7	E950.4	E962.0	E980.4
76:00 oxytocics	975.0	E858.6	E945.0	E950.4	E962.0	E980.4
78:00 radioactive agents	990	—	—	—	—	—
80:04 serums NEC	979.9	E858.8	E949.9	E950.4	E962.0	E980.4
immune gamma globulin (human)	964.6	E858.2	E934.6	E950.4	E962.0	E980.4
80:08 toxoids NEC	978.8	E858.8	E948.8	E950.4	E962.0	E980.4
diphtheria	978.5	E858.8	E948.5	E950.4	E962.0	E980.4
and tetanus	978.9	E858.8	E948.9	E950.4	E962.0	E980.4
with pertussis component	978.6	E858.8	E948.6	E950.4	E962.0	E980.4
tetanus	978.4	E858.8	E948.4	E950.4	E962.0	E980.4
and diphtheria	978.9	E858.8	E948.9	E950.4	E962.0	E980.4
with pertussis component	978.6	E858.8	E948.6	E950.4	E962.0	E980.4
80:12 vaccines	979.9	E858.8	E949.9	E950.4	E962.0	E980.4
bacterial NEC	978.8	E858.8	E948.8	E950.4	E962.0	E980.4
with	—	—	—	—	—	—
other bacterial components	978.9	E858.8	E948.9	E950.4	E962.0	E980.4
pertussis component	978.6	E858.8	E948.6	E950.4	E962.0	E980.4
viral and rickettsial components	979.7	E858.8	E949.7	E950.4	E962.0	E980.4
rickettsial NEC	979.6	E858.8	E949.6	E950.4	E962.0	E980.4
with	—	—	—	—	—	—
bacterial component	979.7	E858.8	E949.7	E950.4	E962.0	E980.4
pertussis component	978.6	E858.8	E948.6	E950.4	E962.0	E980.4
viral component	979.7	E858.8	E949.7	E950.4	E962.0	E980.4
viral NEC	979.6	E858.8	E949.6	E950.4	E962.0	E980.4
with	—	—	—	—	—	—
bacterial component	979.7	E858.8	E949.7	E950.4	E962.0	E980.4
pertussis component	978.6	E858.8	E948.6	E950.4	E962.0	E980.4
rickettsial component	979.7	E858.8	E949.7	E950.4	E962.0	E980.4
84:04.04 antibiotics (skin and mucous membrane)	976.0	E858.7	E946.0	E950.4	E962.0	E980.4
84:04.08 fungicides (skin and mucous membrane)	976.0	E858.7	E946.0	E950.4	E962.0	E980.4

◀ New   ◀▥ Revised   ~~deleted~~ Deleted   ● Use Additional Digit(s)

Substance	Poisoning	External Cause (E Code)				
		Accident	Therapeutic Use	Suicide Attempt	Assault	Undetermined
Drug *(Continued)*						
84:04.12 scabicides and pediculicides (skin and mucous membrane)	976.0	E858.7	E946.0	E950.4	E962.0	E980.4
84:04.16 miscellaneous local anti-infectives (skin and mucous membrane)	976.0	E858.7	E946.0	E950.4	E962.0	E980.4
84:06 anti-inflammatory agents (skin and mucous membrane)	976.0	E858.7	E946.0	E950.4	E962.0	E980.4
84:08 antipruritics and local anesthetics	—	—	—	—	—	—
antipruritics	976.1	E858.7	E946.1	E950.4	E962.0	E980.4
local anesthetics	968.5	E855.2	E938.5	E950.4	E962.0	E980.4
84:12 astringents	976.2	E858.7	E946.2	E950.4	E962.0	E980.4
84:16 cell stimulants and proliferants	976.8	E858.7	E946.8	E950.4	E962.0	E980.4
84:20 detergents	976.2	E858.7	E946.2	E950.4	E962.0	E980.4
84:24 emollients, demulcents, and protectants	976.3	E858.7	E946.3	E950.4	E962.0	E980.4
84:28 keratolytic agents	976.4	E858.7	E946.4	E950.4	E962.0	E980.4
84:32 keratoplastic agents	976.4	E858.7	E946.4	E950.4	E962.0	E980.4
84:36 miscellaneous agents (skin and mucous membrane)	976.8	E858.7	E946.8	E950.4	E962.0	E980.4
86:00 spasmolytic agents	975.1	E858.6	E945.1	E950.4	E962.0	E980.4
antiasthmatics	975.7	E858.6	E945.7	E950.4	E962.0	E980.4
papaverine	972.5	E858.3	E942.5	E950.4	E962.0	E980.4
theophylline	974.1	E858.5	E944.1	E950.4	E962.0	E980.4
88:04 vitamin A	963.5	E858.1	E933.5	E950.4	E962.0	E980.4
88:08 vitamin B complex	963.5	E858.1	E933.5	E950.4	E962.0	E980.4
hematopoietic vitamin	964.1	E858.2	E934.1	E950.4	E962.0	E980.4
nicotinic acid derivatives	972.2	E858.3	E942.2	E950.4	E962.0	E980.4
88:12 vitamin C	963.5	E858.1	E933.5	E950.4	E962.0	E980.4
88:16 vitamin D	963.5	E858.1	E933.5	E950.4	E962.0	E980.4
88:20 vitamin E	963.5	E858.1	E933.5	E950.4	E962.0	E980.4
88:24 vitamin K activity	964.3	E858.2	E934.3	E950.4	E962.0	E980.4
88:28 multivitamin preparations	963.5	E858.1	E933.5	E950.4	E962.0	E980.4
92:00 unclassified therapeutic agents	977.8	E858.8	E947.8	E950.4	E962.0	E980.4
Duboisine	971.1	E855.4	E941.1	E950.4	E962.0	E980.4
Dulcolax	973.1	E858.4	E943.1	E950.4	E962.0	E980.4
Duponol (C) (EP)	976.2	E858.7	E946.2	E950.4	E962.0	E980.4
Durabolin	962.1	E858.0	E932.1	E950.4	E962.0	E980.4
Dyclone	968.5	E855.2	E938.5	E950.4	E962.0	E980.4
Dyclonine	968.5	E855.2	E938.5	E950.4	E962.0	E980.4
Dydrogesterone	962.2	E858.0	E932.2	E950.4	E962.0	E980.4
Dyes NEC	989.89	E866.8	—	E950.9	E962.1	E980.9
diagnostic agents	977.8	E858.8	E947.8	E950.4	E962.0	E980.4
pharmaceutical NEC	977.4	E858.8	E947.4	E950.4	E962.0	E980.4
Dyflos	971.0	E855.3	E941.0	E950.4	E962.0	E980.4

◀ New   ◀▥ Revised   deleted Deleted   ● Use Additional Digit(s)

Substance	Poisoning	External Cause (E Code)				
		Accident	Therapeutic Use	Suicide Attempt	Assault	Undetermined
Dymelor	962.3	E858.0	E932.3	E950.4	E962.0	E980.4
Dynamite	989.89	E866.8	—	E950.9	E962.1	E980.9
fumes	987.8	E869.8	—	E952.8	E962.2	E982.8
Dyphylline	975.1	E858.6	E945.1	E950.4	E962.0	E980.4
Ear preparations	976.6	E858.7	E946.6	E950.4	E962.0	E980.4
Echothiopate, ecotrhiopate	971.0	E855.3	E941.0	E950.4	E962.0	E980.4
Ecstasy	969.72◄▥	E854.2	E939.7	E950.3	E962.0	E980.3
Ectylurea	967.8	E852.8	E937.8	E950.2	E962.0	E980.2
Edathamil disodium	963.8	E858.1	E933.8	E950.4	E962.0	E980.4
Edecrin	974.4	E858.5	E944.4	E950.4	E962.0	E980.4
Edetate, disodium (calcium)	963.8	E858.1	E933.8	E950.4	E962.0	E980.4
Edrophonium	971.0	E855.3	E941.0	E950.4	E962.0	E980.4
Elase	976.8	E858.7	E946.8	E950.4	E962.0	E980.4
Elaterium	973.1	E858.4	E943.1	E950.4	E962.0	E980.4
Elder	988.2	E865.4	—	E950.9	E962.1	E980.9
berry (unripe)	988.2	E865.3	—	E950.9	E962.1	E980.9
Electrolytes NEC	974.5	E858.5	E944.5	E950.4	E962.0	E980.4
Electrolytic agent NEC	974.5	E858.5	E944.5	E950.4	E962.0	E980.4
Embramine	963.0	E858.1	E933.0	E950.4	E962.0	E980.4
Emetics	973.6	E858.4	E943.6	E950.4	E962.0	E980.4
Emetine (hydrochloride)	961.5	E857	E931.5	E950.4	E962.0	E980.4
Emollients	976.3	E858.7	E946.3	E950.4	E962.0	E980.4
Emylcamate	969.5	E853.8	E939.5	E950.3	E962.0	E980.3
Encyprate	969.09◄▥	E854.0	E939.0	E950.3	E962.0	E980.3
Endocaine	968.5	E855.2	E938.5	E950.4	E962.0	E980.4
Endrin	989.2	E863.0	—	E950.6	E962.1	E980.7
Enflurane	968.2	E855.1	E938.2	E950.4	E962.0	E980.4
Enovid	962.2	E858.0	E932.2	E950.4	E962.0	E980.4
ENT preparations (anti-infectives)	976.6	E858.7	E946.6	E950.4	E962.0	E980.4
Enzodase	963.4	E858.1	E933.4	E950.4	E962.0	E980.4
Enzymes NEC	963.4	E858.1	E933.4	E950.4	E962.0	E980.4
Epanutin	966.1	E855.0	E936.1	E950.4	E962.0	E980.4
Ephedra (tincture)	971.2	E855.5	E941.2	E950.4	E962.0	E980.4
Ephedrine	971.2	E855.5	E941.2	E950.4	E962.0	E980.4
Epiestriol	962.2	E858.0	E932.2	E950.4	E962.0	E980.4
Epilim - *see* Sodium valproate	—	—	—	—	—	—
Epinephrine	971.2	E855.5	E941.2	E950.4	E962.0	E980.4
Epsom salt	973.3	E858.4	E943.3	E950.4	E962.0	E980.4
Equanil	969.5	E853.8	E939.5	E950.3	E962.0	E980.3

◄ New   ◀▥ Revised   ~~deleted~~ Deleted   ● Use Additional Digit(s)

Substance	Poisoning	External Cause (E Code)				
		Accident	Therapeutic Use	Suicide Attempt	Assault	Undetermined
Equisetum (diuretic)	974.4	E858.5	E944.4	E950.4	E962.0	E980.4
Ergometrine	975.0	E858.6	E945.0	E950.4	E962.0	E980.4
Ergonovine	975.0	E858.6	E945.0	E950.4	E962.0	E980.4
Ergot NEC	988.2	E865.4	—	E950.9	E962.1	E980.9
medicinal (alkaloids)	975.0	E858.6	E945.0	E950.4	E962.0	E980.4
Ergotamine (tartrate) (for migraine) NEC	972.9	E858.3	E942.9	E950.4	E962.0	E980.4
Ergotrate	975.0	E858.6	E945.0	E950.4	E962.0	E980.4
Erythrityl tetranitrate	972.4	E858.3	E942.4	E950.4	E962.0	E980.4
Erythrol tetranitrate	972.4	E858.3	E942.4	E950.4	E962.0	E980.4
Erythromycin	960.3	E856	E930.3	E950.4	E962.0	E980.4
ophthalmic preparation	976.5	E858.7	E946.5	E950.4	E962.0	E980.4
topical NEC	976.0	E858.7	E946.0	E950.4	E962.0	E980.4
Eserine	971.0	E855.3	E941.0	E950.4	E962.0	E980.4
Eskabarb	967.0	E851	E937.0	E950.1	E962.0	E980.1
Eskalith	969.8	E855.8	E939.8	E950.3	E962.0	E980.3
Estradiol (cypionate) (dipropionate) (valerate)	962.2	E858.0	E932.2	E950.4	E962.0	E980.4
Estriol	962.2	E858.0	E932.2	E950.4	E962.0	E980.4
Estrogens (with progestogens)	962.2	E858.0	E932.2	E950.4	E962.0	E980.4
Estrone	962.2	E858.0	E932.2	E950.4	E962.0	E980.4
Etafedrine	971.2	E855.5	E941.2	E950.4	E962.0	E980.4
Ethacrynate sodium	974.4	E858.5	E944.4	E950.4	E962.0	E980.4
Ethacrynic acid	974.4	E858.5	E944.4	E950.4	E962.0	E980.4
Ethambutol	961.8	E857	E931.8	E950.4	E962.0	E980.4
Ethamide	974.2	E858.5	E944.2	E950.4	E962.0	E980.4
Ethamivan	970.0	E854.3	E940.0	E950.4	E962.0	E980.4
Ethamsylate	964.5	E858.2	E934.5	E950.4	E962.0	E980.4
Ethanol	980.0	E860.1	—	E950.9	E962.1	E980.9
beverage	980.0	E860.0	—	E950.9	E962.1	E980.9
Ethchlorvynol	967.8	E852.8	E937.8	E950.2	E962.0	E980.2
Ethebenecid	974.7	E858.5	E944.7	E950.4	E962.0	E980.4
Ether(s) (diethyl) (ethyl) (vapor)	987.8	E869.8	—	E952.8	E962.2	E982.8
anesthetic	968.2	E855.1	E938.2	E950.4	E962.0	E980.4
petroleum - see Ligroin solvent	982.8	E862.4	—	E950.9	E962.1	E980.9
Ethidine chloride (vapor)	987.8	E869.8	—	E952.8	E962.2	E982.8
liquid (solvent)	982.3	E862.4	—	E950.9	E962.1	E980.9
Ethinamate	967.8	E852.8	E937.8	E950.2	E962.0	E980.2
Ethinylestradiol	962.2	E858.0	E932.2	E950.4	E962.0	E980.4
Ethionamide	961.8	E857	E931.8	E950.4	E962.0	E980.4
Ethisterone	962.2	E858.0	E932.2	E950.4	E962.0	E980.4

◀ New　◀▥ Revised　deleted Deleted　● Use Additional Digit(s)

Substance	Poisoning	External Cause (E Code)				
		Accident	Therapeutic Use	Suicide Attempt	Assault	Undetermined
Ethobral	967.0	E851	E937.0	E950.1	E962.0	E980.1
Ethocaine (infiltration) (topical)	968.5	E855.2	E938.5	E950.4	E962.0	E980.4
nerve block (peripheral) (plexus)	968.6	E855.2	E938.6	E950.4	E962.0	E980.4
spinal	968.7	E855.2	E938.7	E950.4	E962.0	E980.4
Ethoheptazine (citrate)	965.7	E850.7	E935.7	E950.0	E962.0	E980.0
Ethopropazine	966.4	E855.0	E936.4	E950.4	E962.0	E980.4
Ethosuximide	966.2	E855.0	E936.2	E950.4	E962.0	E980.4
Ethotoin	966.1	E855.0	E936.1	E950.4	E962.0	E980.4
Ethoxazene	961.9	E857	E931.9	E950.4	E962.0	E980.4
Ethoxzolamide	974.2	E858.5	E944.2	E950.4	E962.0	E980.4
Ethyl	—	—	—	—	—	—
acetate (vapor)	982.8	E862.4	—	E950.9	E962.1	E980.9
alcohol	980.0	E860.1	—	E950.9	E962.1	E980.9
beverage	980.0	E860.0	—	E950.9	E962.1	E980.9
aldehyde (vapor)	987.8	E869.8	—	E952.8	E962.2	E982.8
liquid	989.89	E866.8	—	E950.9	E962.1	E980.9
aminobenzoate	968.5	E855.2	E938.5	E950.4	E962.0	E980.4
biscoumacetate	964.2	E858.2	E934.2	E950.4	E962.0	E980.4
bromide (anesthetic)	968.2	E855.1	E938.2	E950.4	E962.0	E980.4
carbamate (antineoplastic)	963.1	E858.1	E933.1	E950.4	E962.0	E980.4
carbinol	980.3	E860.4	—	E950.9	E962.1	E980.9
chaulmoograte	961.8	E857	E931.8	E950.4	E962.0	E980.4
chloride (vapor)	987.8	E869.8	—	E952.8	E962.2	E982.8
anesthetic (local)	968.5	E855.2	E938.5	E950.4	E962.0	E980.4
inhaled	968.2	E855.1	E938.2	E950.4	E962.0	E980.4
solvent	982.3	E862.4	—	E950.9	E962.1	E980.9
estranol	962.1	E858.0	E932.1	E950.4	E962.0	E980.4
ether - see Ether(s)	—	—	—	—	—	—
formate (solvent) NEC	982.8	E862.4	—	E950.9	E962.1	E980.9
iodoacetate	987.5	E869.3	—	E952.8	E962.2	E982.8
lactate (solvent) NEC	982.8	E862.4	—	E950.9	E962.1	E980.9
methylcarbinol	980.8	E860.8	—	E950.9	E962.1	E980.9
morphine	965.09	E850.2	E935.2	E950.0	E962.0	E980.0
Ethylene (gas)	987.1	E869.8	—	E952.8	E962.2	E982.8
anesthetic (general)	968.2	E855.1	E938.2	E950.4	E962.0	E980.4
chlorohydrin (vapor)	982.3	E862.4	—	E950.9	E962.1	E980.9
dichloride (vapor)	982.3	E862.4	—	E950.9	E962.1	E980.9
glycol(s) (any) (vapor)	982.8	E862.4	—	E950.9	E962.1	E980.9

◀ New ◀▦ Revised ~~deleted~~ Deleted ● Use Additional Digit(s)

			External Cause (E Code)			
Substance	**Poisoning**	**Accident**	**Therapeutic Use**	**Suicide Attempt**	**Assault**	**Undetermined**
Ethylidene	—	—	—	—	—	—
chloride NEC	982.3	E862.4	—	E950.9	E962.1	E980.9
diethyl ether	982.8	—	E862.4	E950.9	E962.1	E980.9
Ethynodiol	962.2	E858.0	E932.2	E950.4	E962.0	E980.4
Etidocaine	968.9	E855.2	E938.9	E950.4	E962.0	E980.4
infiltration (subcutaneous)	968.5	E855.2	E938.5	E950.4	E962.0	E980.4
nerve (peripheral) (plexus)	968.6	E855.2	E938.6	E950.4	E962.0	E980.4
Etilfen	967.0	E851	E937.0	E950.1	E962.0	E980.1
Etomide	965.7	E850.7	E935.7	E950.0	E962.0	E980.0
Etorphine	965.09	E850.2	E935.2	E950.0	E962.0	E980.0
Etoval	967.0	E851	E937.0	E950.1	E962.0	E980.1
Etryptamine	969.01 ◀▥▥	E854.0	E939.0	E950.3	E962.0	E980.3
Eucaine	968.5	E855.2	E938.5	E950.4	E962.0	E980.4
Eucalyptus (oil) NEC	975.5	E858.6	E945.5	E950.4	E962.0	E980.4
Eucatropine	971.1	E855.4	E941.1	E950.4	E962.0	E980.4
Eucodal	965.09	E850.2	E935.2	E950.0	E962.0	E980.0
Euneryl	967.0	E851	E937.0	E950.1	E962.0	E980.1
Euphthalmine	971.1	E855.4	E941.1	E950.4	E962.0	E980.4
Eurax	976.0	E858.7	E946.0	E950.4	E962.0	E980.4
Euresol	976.4	E858.7	E946.4	E950.4	E962.0	E980.4
Euthroid	962.7	E858.0	E932.7	E950.4	E962.0	E980.4
Evans blue	977.8	E858.8	E947.8	E950.4	E962.0	E980.4
Evipal	967.0	E851	E937.0	E950.1	E962.0	E980.1
sodium	968.3	E855.1	E938.3	E950.4	E962.0	E980.4
Evipan	967.0	E851	E937.0	E950.1	E962.0	E980.1
sodium	968.3	E855.1	E938.3	E950.4	E962.0	E980.4
Exalgin	965.4	E850.4	E935.4	E950.0	E962.0	E980.0
Excipients, pharmaceutical	977.4	E858.8	E947.4	E950.4	E962.0	E980.4
Exhaust gas - see Carbon, monoxide	—	—	—	—	—	—
Ex-Lax (phenolphthalein)	973.1	E858.4	E943.1	E950.4	E962.0	E980.4
Expectorants	975.5	E858.6	E945.5	E950.4	E962.0	E980.4
External medications (skin) (mucous membrane)	976.9	E858.7	E946.9	E950.4	E962.0	E980.4
dental agent	976.7	E858.7	E946.7	E950.4	E962.0	E980.4
ENT agent	976.6	E858.7	E946.6	E950.4	E962.0	E980.4
ophthalmic preparation	976.5	E858.7	E946.5	E950.4	E962.0	E980.4
specified NEC	976.8	E858.7	E946.8	E950.4	E962.0	E980.4
Eye agents (anti-infective)	976.5	E858.7	E946.5	E950.4	E962.0	E980.4
Factor IX complex (human)	964.5	E858.2	E934.5	E950.4	E962.0	E980.4
Fecal softeners	973.2	E858.4	E943.2	E950.4	E962.0	E980.4

◀ New　　◀▥▥ Revised　　~~deleted~~ Deleted　　● Use Additional Digit(s)

		External Cause (E Code)				
Substance	**Poisoning**	**Accident**	**Therapeutic Use**	**Suicide Attempt**	**Assault**	**Undetermined**
Fenbutrazate	977.0	E858.8	E947.0	E950.4	E962.0	E980.4
Fencamfamin	970.8	E854.3	E940.8	E950.4	E962.0	E980.4
Fenfluramine	977.0	E858.8	E947.0	E950.4	E962.0	E980.4
Fenoprofen	965.61	E850.6	E935.6	E950.0	E962.0	E980.0
Fentanyl	965.09	E850.2	E935.2	E950.0	E962.0	E980.0
Fentazin	969.1	E853.0	E939.1	E930.3	E962.0	E980.3
Fenticlor, fentichlor	976.0	E858.7	E946.0	E950.4	E962.0	E980.4
Fer de lance (bite) (venom)	989.5	E905.0	—	E950.9	E962.1	E980.9
Ferric - *see* Iron	—	—	—	—	—	—
Ferrocholinate	964.0	E858.2	E934.0	E950.4	E962.0	E980.4
Ferrous fumerate, gluconate, lactate, salt NEC, sulfate (medicinal)	964.0	E858.2	E934.0	E950.4	E962.0	E980.4
Ferrum - *see* Iron	—	—	—	—	—	—
Fertilizers NEC	989.89	E866.5	—	E950.9	E962.1	E980.4
with herbicide mixture	989.4	E863.5	—	E950.6	E962.1	E980.7
Fibrinogen (human)	964.7	E858.2	E934.7	E950.4	E962.0	E980.4
Fibrinolysin	964.4	E858.2	E934.4	E950.4	E962.0	E980.4
Fibrinolysis-affecting agents	964.4	E858.2	E934.4	E950.4	E962.0	E980.4
Filix mas	961.6	E857	E931.6	E950.4	E962.0	E980.4
Fiorinal	965.1	E850.3	E935.3	E950.0	E962.0	E980.0
Fire damp	987.1	E869.8	—	E952.8	E962.2	E982.8
Fish, nonbacterial or noxious	988.0	E865.2	—	E950.9	E962.1	E980.9
shell	988.0	E865.1	—	E950.9	E962.1	E980.9
Flagyl	961.5	E857	E931.5	E950.4	E962.0	E980.4
Flavoxate	975.1	E858.6	E945.1	E950.4	E962.0	E980.4
Flaxedil	975.2	E858.6	E945.2	E950.4	E962.0	E980.4
Flaxseed (medicinal)	976.3	E858.7	E946.3	E950.4	E962.0	E980.4
Flomax	971.3	E855.6	E941.3	E950.4	E962.0	E980.4
Florantyrone	973.4	E858.4	E943.4	E950.4	E962.0	E980.4
Floraquin	961.3	E857	E931.3	E950.4	E962.0	E980.4
Florinef	962.0	E858.0	E932.0	E950.4	E962.0	E980.4
ENT agent	976.6	E858.7	E946.6	E950.4	E962.0	E980.4
ophthalmic preparation	976.5	E858.7	E946.5	E950.4	E962.0	E980.4
topical NEC	976.0	E858.7	E946.0	E950.4	E962.0	E980.4
Flowers of sulfur	976.4	E858.7	E946.4	E950.4	E962.0	E980.4
Floxuridine	963.1	E858.1	E933.1	E950.4	E962.0	E980.4
Flucytosine	961.9	E857	E931.9	E950.4	E962.0	E980.4
Fludrocortisone	962.0	E858.0	E932.0	E950.4	E962.0	E980.4
ENT agent	976.6	E858.7	E946.6	E950.4	E962.0	E980.4
ophthalmic preparation	976.5	E858.7	E946.5	E950.4	E962.0	E980.4

◀ New   ◀▥▥ Revised   ~~deleted~~ Deleted   ● Use Additional Digit(s)

TABLE OF DRUGS AND CHEMICALS

Substance	Poisoning	External Cause (E Code)				
		Accident	Therapeutic Use	Suicide Attempt	Assault	Undetermined
Fludrocortisone *(Continued)*						
topical NEC	976.0	E858.7	E946.0	E950.4	E962.0	E980.4
Flumethasone	976.0	E858.7	E946.0	E950.4	E962.0	E980.4
Flumethiazide	974.3	E858.5	E944.3	E950.4	E962.0	E980.4
Flumidin	961.7	E857	E931.7	E950.4	E962.0	E980.4
Flunitrazepam	969.4	E853.2	E939.4	E950.3	E962.0	E980.3
Fluocinolone	976.0	E858.7	E946.0	E950.4	E962.0	E980.4
Fluocortolone	962.0	E858.0	E932.0	E950.4	E962.0	E980.4
Fluohydrocortisone	962.0	E858.0	E932.0	E950.4	E962.0	E980.4
ENT agent	976.6	E858.7	E946.6	E950.4	E962.0	E980.4
ophthalmic preparation	976.5	E858.7	E946.5	E950.4	E962.0	E980.4
topical NEC	976.0	E858.7	E946.0	E950.4	E962.0	E980.4
Fluonid	976.0	E858.7	E946.0	E950.4	E962.0	E980.4
Fluopromazine	969.1	E853.0	E939.1	E950.3	E962.0	E980.3
Fluoracetate	989.4	E863.7	—	E950.6	E962.1	E980.7
Fluorescein (sodium)	977.8	E858.8	E947.8	E950.4	E962.0	E980.4
Fluoride(s) (pesticides) (sodium) NEC	989.4	E863.4	—	E950.6	E962.1	E980.7
hydrogen - *see* Hydrofluoric acid	—	—	—	—	—	—
medicinal	976.7	E858.7	E946.7	E950.4	E962.0	E980.4
not pesticide NEC	983.9	E864.4	—	E950.7	E962.1	E980.6
stannous	976.7	E858.7	E946.7	E950.4	E962.0	E980.4
Fluorinated corticosteroids	962.0	E858.0	E932.0	E950.4	E962.0	E980.4
Fluorine (compounds) (gas)	987.8	E869.8	—	E952.8	E962.2	E982.8
salt - *see* Fluoride(s)	—	—	—	—	—	—
Fluoristan	976.7	E858.7	E946.7	E950.4	E962.0	E980.4
Fluoroacetate	989.4	E863.7	—	E950.6	E962.1	E980.7
Fluorodeoxyuridine	963.1	E858.1	E933.1	E950.4	E962.0	E980.4
Fluorometholone (topical) NEC	976.0	E858.7	E946.0	E950.4	E962.0	E980.4
ophthalmic preparation	976.5	E858.7	E946.5	E950.4	E962.0	E980.4
Fluorouracil	963.1	E858.1	E933.1	E950.4	E962.0	E980.4
Fluothane	968.1	E855.1	E938.1	E950.4	E962.0	E980.4
Fluoxetine hydrochloride	969.03◄ⅲ	E854.0	E939.0	E950.3	E962.0	E980.3
Fluoxymesterone	962.1	E858.0	E932.1	E950.4	E962.0	E980.4
Fluphenazine	969.1	E853.0	E939.1	E950.3	E962.0	E980.3
Fluprednisolone	962.0	E858.0	E932.0	E950.4	E962.0	E980.4
Flurandrenolide	976.0	E858.7	E946.0	E950.4	E962.0	E980.4
Flurazepam (hydrochloride)	969.4	E853.2	E939.4	E950.3	E962.0	E980.3
Flurbiprofen	965.61	E850.6	E935.6	E950.0	E962.0	E980.0

◄ New ◄ⅲ Revised ~~deleted~~ Deleted ● Use Additional Digit(s)

Substance	Poisoning	External Cause (E Code)				
		Accident	Therapeutic Use	Suicide Attempt	Assault	Undetermined
Flurobate	976.0	E858.7	E946.0	E950.4	E962.0	E980.4
Flurothyl	969.8	E855.8	E939.8	E950.3	E962.0	E980.3
Fluroxene	968.2	E855.1	E938.2	E950.4	E962.0	E980.4
Folacin	964.1	E858.2	E934.1	E950.4	E962.0	E980.4
Folic acid	964.1	E858.2	E934.1	E950.4	E962.0	E980.4
Follicle stimulating hormone	962.4	E858.0	E932.4	E950.4	E962.0	E980.4
Food, foodstuffs, nonbacterial or noxious	988.9	E865.9	—	E950.9	E962.1	E980.9
berries, seeds	988.2	E865.3	—	E950.9	E962.1	E980.9
fish	988.0	E865.2	—	E950.9	E962.1	E980.9
mushrooms	988.1	E865.5	—	E950.9	E962.1	E980.9
plants	988.2	E865.9	—	E950.9	E962.1	E980.9
specified type NEC	988.2	E865.4	—	E950.9	E962.1	E980.9
shellfish	988.0	E865.1	—	E950.9	E962.1	E980.9
specified NEC	988.8	E865.8	—	E950.9	E962.1	E980.9
Fool's parsley	988.2	E865.4	—	E950.9	E962.1	E980.9
Formaldehyde (solution)	989.89	E861.4	—	E950.9	E962.1	E980.9
fungicide	989.4	E863.6	—	E950.6	E962.1	E980.7
gas or vapor	987.8	E869.8	—	E952.8	E962.2	E982.8
Formalin	989.89	E861.4	—	E950.9	E962.1	E980.9
fungicide	989.4	E863.6	—	E950.6	E962.1	E980.7
vapor	987.8	E869.8	—	E952.8	E962.2	E982.8
Formic acid	983.1	E864.1	—	E950.7	E962.1	E980.6
vapor	987.8	E869.8	—	E952.8	E962.2	E982.8
Fowler's solution	985.1	E866.3	—	E950.8	E962.1	E980.8
Foxglove	988.2	E865.4	—	E950.9	E962.1	E980.9
Fox green	977.8	E858.8	E947.8	E950.4	E962.0	E980.4
Framycetin	960.8	E856	E930.8	E950.4	E962.0	E980.4
Frangula (extract)	973.1	E858.4	E943.1	E950.4	E962.0	E980.4
Frei antigen	977.8	E858.8	E947.8	E950.4	E962.0	E980.4
Freons	987.4	E869.2	—	E952.8	E962.2	E982.8
Fructose	974.5	E858.5	E944.5	E950.4	E962.0	E980.4
Frusemide	974.4	E858.5	E944.4	E950.4	E962.0	E980.4
FSH	962.4	E858.0	E932.4	E950.4	E962.0	E980.4
Fuel	—	—	—	—	—	—
automobile	981	E862.1	—	E950.9	E962.1	E980.9
exhaust gas, not in transit	986	E868.2	—	E952.0	E962.2	E982.0
vapor NEC	987.1	E869.8	—	E952.8	E962.2	E982.8

◀ New   ◀▥ Revised   ~~deleted~~ Deleted   ● Use Additional Digit(s)

TABLE OF DRUGS AND CHEMICALS

Substance	External Cause (E Code)					
	Poisoning	Accident	Therapeutic Use	Suicide Attempt	Assault	Undetermined
Fuel *(Continued)*						
gas (domestic use) - *see also* Carbon, monoxide, fuel	—	—	—	—	—	—
utility	987.1	E868.1	—	E951.8	E962.2	E981.8
incomplete combustion of - *see* Carbon, monoxide, fuel, utility	—	—	—	—	—	—
in mobile container	987.0	E868.0	—	E951.1	E962.2	E981.1
piped (natural)	987.1	E867	—	E951.0	E962.2	E981.0
industrial, incomplete combustion	986	E868.3	—	E952.1	E962.2	E982.1
Fugillin	960.8	E856	E930.8	E950.4	E962.0	E980.4
Fulminate of mercury	985.0	E866.1	—	E950.9	E962.1	E980.9
Fulvicin	960.1	E856	E930.1	E950.4	E962.0	E980.4
Fumadil	960.8	E856	E930.8	E950.4	E962.0	E980.4
Fumagillin	960.8	E856	E930.8	E950.4	E962.0	E980.4
Fumes (from)	987.9	E869.9	—	E952.9	E962.2	E982.9
carbon monoxide - *see* Carbon, monoxide	—	—	—	—	—	—
charcoal (domestic use)	986	E868.3	—	E952.1	E962.2	E982.1
chloroform - *see* Chloroform						
coke (in domestic stoves, fireplaces)	986	E868.3	—	E952.1	E962.2	E982.1
corrosive NEC	987.8	E869.8	—	E952.8	E962.2	E982.8
ether - *see* Ether(s)						
freons	987.4	E869.2	—	E952.8	E962.2	E982.8
hydrocarbons	987.1	E869.8	—	E952.8	E962.2	E982.8
petroleum (liquefied)	987.0	E868.0	—	E951.1	E962.2	E981.1
distributed through pipes (pure or mixed with air)	987.0	E867	—	E951.0	E962.2	E981.0
lead - *see* Lead	—	—	—	—	—	—
metals - *see* specified metal	—	—	—	—	—	—
nitrogen dioxide	987.2	E869.0	—	E952.8	E962.2	E982.8
pesticides - *see* Pesticides	—	—	—	—	—	—
petroleum (liquefied)	987.0	E868.0	—	E951.1	E962.2	E981.1
distributed through pipes (pure or mixed with air)	987.0	E867	—	E951.0	E962.2	E981.0
polyester	987.8	E869.8	—	E952.8	E962.2	E982.8
specified source, other (*see also* substance specified)	987.8	E869.8	—	E952.8	E962.2	E982.8
sulfur dioxide	987.3	E869.1	—	E952.8	E962.2	E982.8
Fumigants	989.4	E863.8	—	E950.6	E962.1	E980.7
Fungi, noxious, used as food	988.1	E865.5	—	E950.9	E962.1	E980.9
Fungicides (*see also* Antifungals)	989.4	E863.6	—	E950.6	E962.1	E980.7
Fungizone	960.1	E856	E930.1	E950.4	E962.0	E980.4
topical	976.0	E858.7	E946.0	E950.4	E962.0	E980.4
Furacin	976.0	E858.7	E946.0	E950.4	E962.0	E980.4

◄ New ◄▥ Revised ~~deleted~~ Deleted ● Use Additional Digit(s)

TABLE OF DRUGS AND CHEMICALS

Substance	Poisoning	External Cause (E Code)				
		Accident	Therapeutic Use	Suicide Attempt	Assault	Undetermined
Furadantin	961.9	E857	E931.9	E950.4	E962.0	E980.4
Furazolidone	961.9	E857	E931.9	E950.4	E962.0	E980.4
Furnace (coal burning) (domestic), gas from	986	E868.3	—	E952.1	E962.2	E982.1
industrial	986	E868.8	—	E952.1	E962.2	E982.1
Furniture polish	989.89	E861.2	—	E950.9	E962.1	E980.9
Furosemide	974.4	E858.5	E944.4	E950.4	E962.0	E980.4
Furoxone	961.9	E857	E931.9	E950.4	E962.0	E980.4
Fusel oil (amyl) (butyl) (propyl)	980.3	E860.4	—	E950.9	E962.1	E980.9
Fusidic acid	960.8	E856	E930.8	E950.4	E962.0	E980.4
Gallamine	975.2	E858.6	E945.2	E950.4	E962.0	E980.4
Gallotannic acid	976.2	E858.7	E946.2	E950.4	E962.0	E980.4
Gamboge	973.1	E858.4	E943.1	E950.4	E962.0	E980.4
Gamimune	964.6	E858.2	E934.6	E950.4	E962.0	E980.4
Gamma-benzene hexachloride (vapor)	989.2	E863.0	—	E950.6	E962.1	E980.7
Gamma globulin	964.6	E858.2	E934.6	E950.4	E962.0	E980.4
Gamma hydroxy butyrate (GHB)	968.4	E855.1	E938.4	E950.4	E962.0	E980.4
Gamulin	964.6	E858.2	E934.6	E950.4	E962.0	E980.4
Ganglionic blocking agents	972.3	E858.3	E942.3	E950.4	E962.0	E980.4
Ganja	969.6	E854.1	E939.6	E950.3	E962.0	E980.3
Garamycin	960.8	E856	E930.8	E950.4	E962.0	E980.4
ophthalmic preparation	976.5	E858.7	E946.5	E950.4	E962.0	E980.4
topical NEC	976.0	E858.7	E946.0	E950.4	E962.0	E980.4
Gardenal	967.0	E851	E937.0	E950.1	E962.0	E980.1
Gardepanyl	967.0	E851	E937.0	E950.1	E962.0	E980.1
Gas	987.9	E869.9	—	E952.9	E962.2	E982.9
acetylene	987.1	E868.1	—	E951.8	E962.2	E981.8
incomplete combustion of - *see* Carbon, monoxide, fuel, utility	—	—	—	—	—	—
air contaminants, source or type not specified	987.9	E869.9	—	E952.9	E962.2	E982.9
anesthetic (general) NEC	968.2	E855.1	E938.2	E950.4	E962.0	E980.4
blast furnace	986	E868.8	—	E952.1	E962.2	E982.1
butane - *see* Butane	—	—	—	—	—	—
carbon monoxide - *see* Carbon, monoxide, chlorine	987.6	E869.8	—	E952.8	E962.2	E982.8
coal - *see* Carbon, monoxide, coal	—	—	—	—	—	—
cyanide	987.7	E869.8	—	E952.8	E962.2	E982.8
dicyanogen	987.8	E869.8	—	E952.8	E962.2	E982.8
domestic - *see* Gas, utility	—	—	—	—	—	—
exhaust - *see* Carbon, monoxide, exhaust gas	—	—	—	—	—	—
from wood- or coal-burning stove or fireplace	986	E868.3	—	E952.1	E962.2	E982.1

Substance	Poisoning	External Cause (E Code)				
		Accident	Therapeutic Use	Suicide Attempt	Assault	Undetermined
Gas (Continued)						
fuel (domestic use) - see also Carbon, monoxide, fuel	—	—	—	—	—	—
industrial use	986	E868.8	—	E952.1	E962.2	E982.1
utility	987.1	E868.1	—	E951.8	E962.2	E981.8
incomplete combustion of - see Carbon, monoxide, fuel, utility	—	—	—	—	—	—
in mobile container	987.0	E868.0	—	E951.1	E962.2	E981.1
piped (natural)	987.1	E867	—	E951.0	E962.2	E981.0
garage	986	E868.2	—	E952.0	E962.2	E982.0
hydrocarbon NEC	987.1	E869.8	—	E952.8	E962.2	E982.8
incomplete combustion of - see Carbon, monoxide, fuel, utility	—	—	—	—	—	—
liquefied (mobile container)	987.0	E868.0	—	E951.1	E962.2	E981.1
piped	987.0	E867	—	E951.0	E962.2	E981.0
hydrocyanic acid	987.7	E869.8	—	E952.8	E962.2	E982.8
illuminating - see Gas, utility	—	—	—	—	—	—
incomplete combustion, any - see Carbon, monoxide	—	—	—	—	—	—
kiln	986	E868.8	—	E952.1	E962.2	E982.1
lacrimogenic	987.5	E869.3	—	E952.8	E962.2	E982.8
marsh	987.1	E869.8	—	E952.8	E962.2	E982.8
motor exhaust, not in transit	986	E868.8	—	E952.1	E962.2	E982.1
mustard - see Mustard, gas	—	—	—	—	—	—
natural	987.1	E867	—	E951.0	E962.2	E981.0
nerve (war)	987.9	E869.9	—	E952.9	E962.2	E982.9
oils	981	E862.1	—	E950.9	E962.1	E980.9
petroleum (liquefied) (distributed in mobile containers)	987.0	E868.0	—	E951.1	E962.2	E981.1
piped (pure or mixed with air)	987.0	E867	—	E951.1	E962.2	E981.1
piped (manufactured) (natural) NEC	987.1	E867	—	E951.0	E962.2	E981.0
producer	986	E868.8	—	E952.1	E962.2	E982.1
propane - see Propane	—	—	—	—	—	—
refrigerant (freon)	987.4	E869.2	—	E952.8	E962.2	E982.8
not freon	987.9	E869.9	—	E952.9	E962.2	E982.9
sewer	987.8	E869.8	—	E952.8	E962.2	E982.8
specified source NEC (see also substance specified)	987.8	E869.8	—	E952.8	E962.2	E982.8
stove - see Gas, utility	—	—	—	—	—	—
tear	987.5	E869.3	—	E952.8	E962.2	E982.8
utility (for cooking, heating, or lighting) (piped) NEC	987.1	E868.1	—	E951.8	E962.2	E981.8
incomplete combustion of - see Carbon, monoxide, fuel, utilty	—	—	—	—	—	—
in mobile container	987.0	E868.0	—	E951.1	E962.2	E981.1
piped (natural)	987.1	E867	—	E951.0	E962.2	E981.0
water	987.1	E868.1	—	E951.8	E962.2	E981.8
incomplete combustion of - see Carbon, monoxide, fuel, utility	—	—	—	—	—	—

◀ New   ◀▥ Revised   ~~deleted~~ Deleted   ● Use Additional Digit(s)

Substance	Poisoning	External Cause (E Code)				
		Accident	Therapeutic Use	Suicide Attempt	Assault	Undetermined
Gaseous substance - *see* Gas	—	—	—	—	—	—
Gasoline, gasolene	981	E862.1	—	E950.9	E962.1	E980.9
vapor	987.1	E869.8	—	E952.8	E962.2	E982.8
Gastric enzymes	973.4	E858.4	E943.4	E950.4	E962.0	E980.4
Gastrografin	977.8	E858.8	E947.8	E950.4	E962.0	E980.4
Gastrointestinal agents	973.9	E858.4	E943.9	E950.4	E962.0	E980.4
specified NEC	973.8	E858.4	E943.8	E950.4	E962.0	E980.4
Gaultheria procumbens	988.2	E865.4	—	E950.9	E962.1	E980.9
Gelatin (intravenous)	964.8	E858.2	E934.8	E950.4	E962.0	E980.4
absorbable (sponge)	964.5	E858.2	E934.5	E950.4	E962.0	E980.4
Gelfilm	976.8	E858.7	E946.8	E950.4	E962.0	E980.4
Gelfoam	964.5	E858.2	E934.5	E950.4	E962.0	E980.4
Gelsemine	970.8	E854.3	E940.8	E950.4	E962.0	E980.4
Gelsemium (sempervirens)	988.2	E865.4	—	E950.9	E962.1	E980.9
Gemonil	967.0	E851	E937.0	E950.1	E962.0	E980.1
Gentamicin	960.8	E856	E930.8	E950.4	E962.0	E980.4
ophthalmic preparation	976.5	E858.7	E946.5	E950.4	E962.0	E980.4
topical NEC	976.0	E858.7	E946.0	E950.4	E962.0	E980.4
Gentian violet	976.0	E858.7	E946.0	E950.4	E962.0	E980.4
Gexane	976.0	E858.7	E946.0	E950.4	E962.0	E980.4
Gila monster (venom)	989.5	E905.0	—	E950.9	E962.1	E980.9
Ginger, Jamaica	989.89	E866.8	—	E950.9	E962.1	E980.9
Gitalin	972.1	E858.3	E942.1	E950.4	E962.0	E980.4
Gitoxin	972.1	E858.3	E942.1	E950.4	E962.0	E980.4
Glandular extract (medicinal) NEC	977.9	E858.9	E947.9	E950.5	E962.0	E980.5
Glaucarubin	961.5	E857	E931.5	E950.4	E962.0	E980.4
Globin zinc insulin	962.3	E858.0	E932.3	E950.4	E962.0	E980.4
Glucagon	962.3	E858.0	E932.3	E950.4	E962.0	E980.4
Glucochloral	967.1	E852.0	E937.1	E950.2	E962.0	E980.2
Glucocorticoids	962.0	E858.0	E932.0	E950.4	E962.0	E980.4
Glucose	974.5	E858.5	E944.5	E950.4	E962.0	E980.4
oxidase reagent	977.8	E858.8	E947.8	E950.4	E962.0	E980.4
Glucosulfone sodium	961.8	E857	E931.8	E950.4	E962.0	E980.4
Glue(s)	989.89	E866.6	—	E950.9	E962.1	E980.9
Glutamic acid (hydrochloride)	973.4	E858.4	E943.4	E950.4	E962.0	E980.4
Glutaraldehyde	989.89	E861.4	—	E950.9	E962.1	E980.9
Glutathione	963.8	E858.1	E933.8	E950.4	E962.0	E980.4
Glutethimide (group)	967.5	E852.4	E937.5	E950.2	E962.0	E980.2
Glycerin (lotion)	976.3	E858.7	E946.3	E950.4	E962.0	E980.4
Glycerol (topical)	976.3	E858.7	E946.3	E950.4	E962.0	E980.4

 New   ◀▦ Revised   ~~deleted~~ Deleted   ● Use Additional Digit(s)

Substance	Poisoning	External Cause (E Code)				
		Accident	Therapeutic Use	Suicide Attempt	Assault	Undetermined
Glyceryl	—	—	—	—	—	—
guaiacolate	975.5	E858.6	E945.5	E950.4	E962.0	E980.4
triacetate (topical)	976.0	E858.7	E946.0	E950.4	E962.0	E980.4
trinitrate	972.4	E858.3	E942.4	E950.4	E962.0	E980.4
Glycine	974.5	E858.5	E944.5	E950.4	E962.0	E980.4
Glycobiarsol	961.1	E857	E931.1	E950.4	E962.0	E980.4
Glycols (ether)	982.8	E862.4	—	E950.9	E962.1	E980.9
Glycopyrrolate	971.1	E855.4	E941.1	E950.4	E962.0	E980.4
Glymidine	962.3	E858.0	E932.3	E950.4	E962.0	E980.4
Gold (compounds) (salts)	965.69	E850.6	E935.6	E950.0	E962.0	E980.0
Golden sulfide of antimony	985.4	E866.2	—	E950.9	E962.1	E980.9
Goldylocks	988.2	E865.4	—	E950.9	E962.1	E980.9
Gonadal tissue extract	962.9	E858.0	E932.9	E950.4	E962.0	E980.4
female	962.2	E858.0	E932.2	E950.4	E962.0	E980.4
male	962.1	E858.0	E932.1	E950.4	E962.0	E980.4
Gonadotropin	962.4	E858.0	E932.4	E950.4	E962.0	E980.4
Grain alcohol	980.0	E860.1	—	E950.9	E962.1	E980.9
beverage	980.0	E860.0	—	E950.9	E962.1	E980.9
Gramicidin	960.8	E856	E930.8	E950.4	E962.0	E980.4
Gratiola officinalis	988.2	E865.4	—	E950.9	E962.1	E980.9
Grease	989.89	E866.8	—	E950.9	E962.1	E980.9
Green hellebore	988.2	E865.4	—	E950.9	E962.1	E980.9
Green soap	976.2	E858.7	E946.2	E950.4	E962.0	E980.4
Grifulvin	960.1	E856	E930.1	E950.4	E962.0	E980.4
Griseofulvin	960.1	E856	E930.1	E950.4	E962.0	E980.4
Growth hormone	962.4	E858.0	E932.4	E950.4	E962.0	E980.4
Guaiacol	975.5	E858.6	E945.5	E950.4	E962.0	E980.4
Givaiac reagent	977.8	E858.8	E947.8	E950.4	E962.0	E980.4
Guaifenesin	975.5	E858.6	E945.5	E950.4	E962.0	E980.4
Guaiphenesin	975.5	E858.6	E945.5	E950.4	E962.0	E980.4
Guanatol	961.4	E857	E931.4	E950.4	E962.0	E980.4
Guanethidine	972.6	E858.3	E942.6	E950.4	E962.0	E980.4
Guano	989.89	E866.5	—	E950.9	E962.1	E980.9
Guanochlor	972.6	E858.3	E942.6	E950.4	E962.0	E980.4
Guanoctine	972.6	E858.3	E942.6	E950.4	E962.0	E980.4
Guanoxan	972.6	E858.3	E942.6	E950.4	E962.0	E980.4
Hair treatment agent NEC	976.4	E858.7	E946.4	E950.4	E962.0	E980.4
Halcinonide	976.0	E858.7	E946.0	E950.4	E962.0	E980.4
Halethazole	976.0	E858.7	E946.0	E950.4	E962.0	E980.4

◀ New　◀ Revised　deleted Deleted　● Use Additional Digit(s)

Substance	Poisoning	External Cause (E Code)				
		Accident	Therapeutic Use	Suicide Attempt	Assault	Undetermined
Hallucinogens	969.6	E854.1	E939.6	E950.3	E962.0	E980.3
Haloperidol	969.2	E853.1	E939.2	E950.3	E962.0	E980.3
Haloprogin	976.0	E858.7	E946.0	E950.4	E962.0	E980.4
Halotex	976.0	E858.7	E946.0	E950.4	E962.0	E980.4
Halothane	968.1	E855.1	E938.1	E950.4	E962.0	E980.4
Halquinols	976.0	E858.7	E946.0	E950.4	E962.0	E980.4
Hand sanitizer	976.0	E858.7	E946.0	E950.4	E962	E980.4
Harmonyl	972.6	E858.3	E942.6	E950.4	E962.0	E980.4
Hartmann's solution	974.5	E858.5	E944.5	E950.4	E962.0	E980.4
Hashish	969.6	E854.1	E939.6	E950.3	E962.0	E980.3
Hawaiian wood rose seeds	969.6	E854.1	E939.6	E950.3	E962.0	E980.3
Headache cures, drugs, powders NEC	977.9	E858.9	E947.9	E950.5	E962.0	E980.9
Heavenly Blue (morning glory)	969.6	E854.1	E939.6	E950.3	E962.0	E980.3
Heavy metal antagonists	963.8	E858.1	E933.8	E950.4	E962.0	E980.4
anti-infectives	961.2	E857	E931.2	E950.4	E962.0	E980.4
Hedaquinium	976.0	E858.7	E946.0	E950.4	E962.0	E980.4
Hedge hyssop	988.2	E865.4	—	E950.9	E962.1	E980.9
Heet	976.8	E858.7	E946.8	E950.4	E962.0	E980.4
Helenin	961.6	E857	E931.6	E950.4	E962.0	E980.4
Hellebore (black) (green) (white)	988.2	E865.4	—	E950.9	E962.1	E980.9
Hemlock	988.2	E865.4	—	E950.9	E962.1	E980.9
Hemostatics	964.5	E858.2	E934.5	E950.4	E962.0	E980.4
capillary active drugs	972.8	E858.3	E942.8	E950.4	E962.0	E980.4
Henbane	988.2	E865.4	—	E950.9	E962.1	E980.9
Heparin (sodium)	964.2	E858.2	E934.2	E950.4	E962.0	E980.4
Heptabarbital, heptabarbitone	967.0	E851	E937.0	E950.1	E962.0	E980.1
Heptachlor	989.2	E863.0	—	E950.6	E962.1	E980.7
Heptalgin	965.09	E850.2	E935.2	E950.0	E962.0	E980.0
Herbicides	989.4	E863.5	—	E950.6	E962.1	E980.7
Heroin	965.01	E850.0	E935.0	E950.0	E962.0	E980.0
Herplex	976.5	E858.7	E946.5	E950.4	E962.0	E980.4
HES	964.8	E858.2	E934.8	E950.4	E962.0	E980.4
Hetastarch	964.8	E858.2	E934.8	E950.4	E962.0	E980.7
Hexachlorocyclohexane	989.2	E863.0	—	E950.6	E962.1	E980.7
Hexachlorophene	976.2	E858.7	E946.2	E950.4	E962.0	E980.4
Hexadimethrine (bromide)	964.5	E858.2	E934.5	E950.4	E962.0	E980.4
Hexafluorenium	975.2	E858.6	E945.2	E950.4	E962.0	E980.4
Hexa-germ	976.2	E858.7	E946.2	E950.4	E962.0	E980.4
Hexahydrophenol	980.8	E860.8	—	E950.9	E962.1	E980.9

◀ New   ◀▥ Revised   deleted Deleted   ● Use Additional Digit(s)

Substance	Poisoning	External Cause (E Code)				
		Accident	Therapeutic Use	Suicide Attempt	Assault	Undetermined
Hexalen	980.8	E860.8	—	E950.9	E962.1	E980.9
Hexamethonium	972.3	E858.3	E942.3	E950.4	E962.0	E980.4
Hexamethylenamine	961.9	E857	E931.9	E950.4	E962.0	E980.4
Hexamine	961.9	E857	E931.9	E950.4	E962.0	E980.4
Hexanone	982.8	E862.4	—	E950.9	E962.1	E980.9
Hexapropymate	967.8	E852.8	E937.8	E950.2	E962.0	E980.2
Hexestrol	962.2	E858.0	E932.2	E950.4	E962.0	E980.4
Hexethal (sodium)	967.0	E851	E937.0	E950.1	E962.0	E980.1
Hexetidine	976.0	E858.7	E946.0	E950.4	E962.0	E980.4
Hexobarbital, hexobarbitone	967.0	E851	E937.0	E950.1	E962.0	E980.1
sodium (anesthetic)	968.3	E855.1	E938.3	E950.4	E962.0	E980.4
soluble	968.3	E855.1	E938.3	E950.4	E962.0	E980.4
Hexocyclium	971.1	E855.4	E941.1	E950.4	E962.0	E980.4
Hexoestrol	962.2	E858.0	E932.2	E950.4	E962.0	E980.4
Hexone	982.8	E862.4	—	E950.9	E962.1	E980.9
Hexylcaine	968.5	E855.2	E938.5	E950.4	E962.0	E980.4
Hexylresorcinol	961.6	E857	E931.6	E950.4	E962.0	E980.4
Hinkle's pills	973.1	E858.4	E943.1	E950.4	E962.0	E980.4
Histalog	977.8	E858.8	E947.8	E950.4	E962.0	E980.4
Histamine (phosphate)	972.5	E858.3	E942.5	E950.4	E962.0	E980.4
Histoplasmin	977.8	E858.8	E947.8	E950.4	E962.0	E980.4
Holly berries	988.2	E865.3	—	E950.9	E962.1	E980.9
Homatropine	971.1	E855.4	E941.1	E950.4	E962.0	E980.4
Homo-tet	964.6	E858.2	E934.6	E950.4	E962.0	E980.4
Hormones (synthetic substitute) NEC	962.9	E858.0	E932.9	E950.4	E962.0	E980.4
adrenal cortical steroids	962.0	E858.0	E932.0	E950.4	E962.0	E980.4
antidiabetic agents	962.3	E858.0	E932.3	E950.4	E962.0	E980.4
follicle stimulating	962.4	E858.0	E932.4	E950.4	E962.0	E980.4
gonadotropic	962.4	E858.0	E932.4	E950.4	E962.0	E980.4
growth	962.4	E858.0	E932.4	E950.4	E962.0	E980.4
ovarian (substitutes)	962.2	E858.0	E932.2	E950.4	E962.0	E980.4
parathyroid (derivatives)	962.6	E858.0	E932.6	E950.4	E962.0	E980.4
pituitary (posterior)	962.5	E858.0	E932.5	E950.4	E962.0	E980.4
anterior	962.4	E858.0	E932.4	E950.4	E962.0	E980.4
thyroid (derivative)	962.7	E858.0	E932.7	E950.4	E962.0	E980.4
Hornet (sting)	989.5	E905.3	—	E950.9	E962.1	E980.9
Horticulture agent NEC	989.4	E863.9	—	E950.6	E962.1	E980.7
Hyaluronidase	963.4	E858.1	E933.4	E950.4	E962.0	E980.4
Hyazyme	963.4	E858.1	E933.4	E950.4	E962.0	E980.4

◀ New   ◀▥ Revised   ~~deleted~~ Deleted   ● Use Additional Digit(s)

	External Cause (E Code)					
Substance	**Poisoning**	**Accident**	**Therapeutic Use**	**Suicide Attempt**	**Assault**	**Undetermined**
Hycodan	965.09	E850.2	E935.2	E950.0	E962.0	E980.0
Hydantoin derivatives	966.1	E855.0	E936.1	E950.4	E962.0	E980.4
Hydeltra	962.0	E858.0	E932.0	E950.4	E962.0	E980.4
Hydergine	971.3	E855.6	E941.3	E950.4	E962.0	E980.4
Hydrabamine penicillin	960.0	E856	E930.0	E950.4	E962.0	E980.4
Hydralazine, hydrallazine	972.6	E858.3	E942.6	E950.4	E962.0	E980.4
Hydrargaphen	976.0	E858.7	E946.0	E950.4	E962.0	E980.4
Hydrazine	983.9	E864.3	—	E950.7	E962.1	E980.6
Hydriodic acid	975.5	E858.6	E945.5	E950.4	E962.0	E980.4
Hydrocarbon gas	987.1	E869.8	—	E952.8	E962.2	E982.8
incomplete combustion of - *see* Carbon, monoxide, fuel, utility	—	—	—	—	—	—
liquefied (mobile container)	987.0	E868.0	—	E951.1	E962.2	E981.1
piped (natural)	987.0	E867	—	E951.0	E962.2	E981.0
Hydrochloric acid (liquid)	983.1	E864.1	—	E950.7	E962.1	E980.6
medicinal	973.4	E858.4	E943.4	E950.4	E962.0	E980.4
vapor	987.8	E869.8	—	E952.8	E962.2	E982.8
Hydrochlorothiazide	974.3	E858.5	E944.3	E950.4	E962.0	E980.4
Hydrocodone	965.09	E850.2	E935.2	E950.0	E962.0	E980.0
Hydrocortisone	962.0	E858.0	E932.0	E950.4	E962.0	E980.4
ENT agent	976.6	E858.7	E946.6	E950.4	E962.0	E980.4
ophthalmic preparation	976.5	E858.7	E946.5	E950.4	E962.0	E980.4
topical NEC	976.0	E858.7	E946.0	E950.4	E962.0	E980.4
Hydrocortone	962.0	E858.0	E932.0	E950.4	E962.0	E980.4
ENT agent	976.6	E858.7	E946.6	E950.4	E962.0	E980.4
ophthalmic preparation	976.5	E858.7	E946.5	E950.4	E962.0	E980.4
topical NEC	976.0	E858.7	E946.0	E950.4	E962.0	E980.4
Hydrocyanic acid - *see* Cyanide(s)	—	—	—	—	—	—
Hydroflumethiazide	974.3	E858.5	E944.3	E950.4	E962.0	E980.4
Hydrofluoric acid (liquid)	983.1	E864.1	—	E950.7	E962.1	E980.6
vapor	987.8	E869.8	—	E952.8	E962.2	E982.8
Hydrogen	987.8	E869.8	—	E952.8	E962.2	E982.8
arsenide	985.1	E866.3	—	E950.8	E962.1	E980.8
arseniurated	985.1	E866.3	—	E950.8	E962.1	E980.8
cyanide (salts)	989.0	E866.8	—	E950.9	E962.1	E980.9
gas	987.7	E869.8	—	E952.8	E962.2	E982.8
fluoride (liquid)	983.1	E864.1	—	E950.7	E962.1	E980.6
vapor	987.8	E869.8	—	E952.8	E962.2	E982.8
peroxide (solution)	976.6	E858.7	E946.6	E950.4	E962.0	E980.4
phosphorated	987.8	E869.8	—	E952.8	E962.2	E982.8

◀ New   ◀⫶⫶⫶ Revised   ~~deleted~~ Deleted   ● Use Additional Digit(s)

Substance	Poisoning	External Cause (E Code)				
		Accident	Therapeutic Use	Suicide Attempt	Assault	Undetermined
Hydrogen *(Continued)*						
sulfide (gas)	987.8	E869.8	—	E952.8	E962.2	E982.8
arseniurated	985.1	E866.3	—	E950.8	E962.1	E980.8
sulfureted	987.8	E869.8	—	E952.8	E962.2	E982.8
Hydromorphinol	965.09	E850.2	E935.2	E950.0	E962.0	E980.0
Hydromorphinone	965.09	E850.2	E935.2	E950.0	E962.0	E980.0
Hydromorphone	965.09	E850.2	E935.2	E950.0	E962.0	E980.0
Hydromox	974.3	E858.5	E944.3	E950.4	E962.0	E980.4
Hydrophilic lotion	976.3	E858.7	E946.3	E950.4	E962.0	E980.4
Hydroquinone	983.0	E864.0	—	E950.7	E962.1	E980.6
vapor	987.8	E869.8	—	E952.8	E962.2	E982.8
Hydrosulfuric acid (gas)	987.8	E869.8	—	E952.8	E962.2	E982.8
Hydrous wool fat (lotion)	976.3	E858.7	E946.3	E950.4	E962.0	E980.4
Hydroxide, caustic	983.2	E864.2	—	E950.7	E962.1	E980.6
Hydroxocobalamin	964.1	E858.2	E934.1	E950.4	E962.0	E980.4
Hydroxyamphetamine	971.2	E858.5	E941.2	E950.4	E962.0	E980.4
Hydroxychloroquine	961.4	E857	E931.4	E950.4	E962.0	E980.4
Hydroxydihydrocodeinone	965.09	E850.2	E935.2	E950.0	E962.0	E980.0
Hydroxyethyl starch	964.8	E858.2	E934.8	E950.4	E962.0	E980.4
Hydroxyphenamate	969.5	E853.8	E939.5	E950.3	E962.0	E980.3
Hydroxyphenylbutazone	965.5	E850.5	E935.5	E950.0	E962.0	E980.0
Hydroxyprogesterone	962.2	E858.0	E932.2	E950.4	E962.0	E980.4
Hydroxyquinoline derivatives	961.3	E857	E931.3	E950.4	E962.0	E980.4
Hydroxystilbamidine	961.5	E857	E931.5	E950.4	E962.0	E980.4
Hydroxyurea	963.1	E858.1	E933.1	E950.4	E962.0	E980.4
Hydroxyzine	969.5	E853.8	E939.5	E950.3	E962.0	E980.3
Hyoscine (hydrobromide)	971.1	E855.4	E941.1	E950.4	E962.0	E980.4
Hyoscyamine	971.1	E855.4	E941.1	E950.4	E962.0	E980.4
Hyoscyamus (albus) (niger)	988.2	E865.4	—	E950.9	E962.1	E980.9
Hypaque	977.8	E858.8	E947.8	E950.4	E962.0	E980.4
Hypertussis	964.6	E858.2	E934.6	E950.4	E962.0	E980.4
Hypnotics NEC	967.9	E852.9	E937.9	E950.2	E962.0	E980.2
Hypochlorites - *see* Sodium, hypochlorite	—	—	—	—	—	—
Hypotensive agents NEC	972.6	E858.3	E942.6	E950.4	E962.0	E980.4
Ibufenac	965.69	E850.6	E935.6	E950.0	E962.0	E980.0
Ibuprofen	965.61	E850.6	E935.6	E950.0	E962.0	E980.0
ICG	977.8	E858.8	E947.8	E950.4	E962.0	E980.4
Ichthammol	976.4	E858.7	E946.4	E950.4	E962.0	E980.4

◀ New   ◀ Revised   ~~deleted~~ Deleted   ● Use Additional Digit(s)

Substance	Poisoning	External Cause (E Code)				
		Accident	Therapeutic Use	Suicide Attempt	Assault	Undetermined
Ichthyol	976.4	E858.7	E946.4	E950.4	E962.0	E980.4
Idoxuridine	976.5	E858.7	E946.5	E950.4	E962.0	E980.4
IDU	976.5	E858.7	E946.5	E950.4	E962.0	E980.4
Iletin	962.3	E858.0	E932.3	E950.4	E962.0	E980.4
Ilex	988.2	E865.4	—	E950.9	E962.1	E980.9
Illuminating gas - see Gas, utility	—	—	—	—	—	—
Ilopan	963.5	E858.1	E933.5	E950.4	E962.0	E980.4
Ilotycin	960.3	E856	E930.3	E950.4	E962.0	E980.4
ophthalmic preparation	976.5	E858.7	E946.5	E950.4	E962.0	E980.4
topical NEC	976.0	E858.7	E946.0	E950.4	E962.0	E980.4
Imipramine	969.05◄▥	E854.0	E939.0	E950.3	E962.0	E980.3
Immu-G	964.6	E858.2	E934.6	E950.4	E962.0	E980.4
Immuglobin	964.6	E858.2	E934.6	E950.4	E962.0	E980.4
Immune serum globulin	964.6	E858.2	E934.6	E950.4	E962.0	E980.4
Immunosuppressive agents	963.1	E858.1	E933.1	E950.4	E962.0	E980.4
Immu-tetanus	964.6	E858.2	E934.6	E950.4	E962.0	E980.4
Indandione (derivatives)	964.2	E858.2	E934.2	E950.4	E962.0	E980.4
Inderal	972.0	E858.3	E942.0	E950.4	E962.0	E980.4
Indian	—	—	—	—	—	—
hemp	969.6	E854.1	E939.6	E950.3	E962.0	E980.3
tobacco	988.2	E865.4	—	E950.9	E962.1	E980.9
Indigo carmine	977.8	E858.8	E947.8	E950.4	E962.0	E980.4
Indocin	965.69	E850.6	E935.6	E950.0	E962.0	E980.0
Indocyanine green	977.8	E858.8	E947.8	E950.4	E962.0	E980.4
Indomethacin	965.69	E850.6	E935.6	E950.0	E962.0	E980.0
Industrial	—	—	—	—	—	—
alcohol	980.9	E860.9	—	E950.9	E962.1	E980.9
fumes	987.8	E869.8	—	E952.8	E962.2	E982.8
solvents (fumes) (vapors)	982.8	E862.9	—	E950.9	E962.1	E980.9
Influenza vaccine	979.6	E858.8	E949.6	E950.4	E962.0	E982.8
Ingested substances NEC	989.9	E866.9	—	E950.9	E962.1	E980.9
INH (isoniazid)	961.8	E857	E931.8	E950.4	E962.0	E980.4
Inhalation, gas (noxious) - see Gas	—	—	—	—	—	—
Ink	989.89	E866.8	—	E950.9	E962.1	E980.9
Innovar	967.6	E852.5	E937.6	E950.2	E962.0	E980.2
Inositol niacinate	972.2	E858.3	E942.2	E950.4	E962.0	E980.4
Inproquone	963.1	E858.1	E933.1	E950.4	E962.0	E980.4
Insect (sting), venomous	989.5	E905.5	—	E950.9	E962.1	E980.9

Substance	Poisoning	External Cause (E Code)				
		Accident	Therapeutic Use	Suicide Attempt	Assault	Undetermined
Insecticides (*see also* Pesticides)	989.4	E863.4	—	E950.6	E962.1	E980.7
chlorinated	989.2	E863.0	—	E950.6	E962.1	E980.7
mixtures	989.4	E863.3	—	E950.6	E962.1	E980.7
organochlorine (compounds)	989.2	E863.0	—	E950.6	E962.1	E980.7
organophosphorus (compounds)	989.3	E863.1	—	E950.6	E962.1	E980.7
Insular tissue extract	962.3	E858.0	E932.3	E950.4	E962.0	E980.4
Insulin (amorphous) (globin) (isophane) (Lente) (NPH) (Protamine) (Semilente) (Ultralente) (zinc)	962.3	E858.0	E932.3	E950.4	E962.0	E980.4
Intranarcon	968.3	E855.1	E938.3	E950.4	E962.0	E980.4
Inulin	977.8	E858.8	E947.8	E950.4	E962.0	E980.4
Invert sugar	974.5	E858.5	E944.5	E950.4	E962.0	E980.4
Inza - see Naproxen	—	—	—	—	—	—
Iodide NEC (*see also* Iodine)	976.0	E858.7	E946.0	E950.4	E962.0	E980.4
mercury (ointment)	976.0	E858.7	E946.0	E950.4	E962.0	E980.4
methylate	976.0	E858.7	E946.0	E950.4	E962.0	E980.4
potassium (expectorant) NEC	975.5	E858.6	E945.5	E950.4	E962.0	E980.4
Iodinated glycerol	975.5	E858.6	E945.5	E950.4	E962.0	E980.4
Iodine (antiseptic, external) (tincture) NEC	976.0	E858.7	E946.0	E950.4	E962.0	E980.4
diagnostic	977.8	E858.8	E947.8	E950.4	E962.0	E980.4
for thyroid conditions (antithyroid)	962.8	E858.0	E932.8	E950.4	E962.0	E980.4
vapor	987.8	E869.8	—	E952.8	E962.2	E982.8
Iodized oil	977.8	E858.8	E947.8	E950.4	E962.0	E980.4
Iodobismitol	961.2	E857	E931.2	E950.4	E962.0	E980.4
Iodochlorhydroxyquin	961.3	E857	E931.3	E950.4	E962.0	E980.4
topical	976.0	E858.7	E946.0	E950.4	E962.0	E980.4
Iodoform	976.0	E858.7	E946.0	E950.4	E962.0	E980.4
Iodopanoic acid	977.8	E858.8	E947.8	E950.4	E962.0	E980.4
Iodophthalein	977.8	E858.8	E947.8	E950.4	E962.0	E980.4
Ion exchange resins	974.5	E858.5	E944.5	E950.4	E962.0	E980.4
Iopanoic acid	977.8	E858.8	E947.8	E950.4	E962.0	E980.4
Iophendylate	977.8	E858.8	E947.8	E950.4	E962.0	E980.4
Iothiouracil	962.8	E858.0	E932.8	E950.4	E962.0	E980.4
Ipecac	973.6	E858.4	E943.6	E950.4	E962.0	E980.4
Ipecacuanha	973.6	E858.4	E943.6	E950.4	E962.0	E980.4
Ipodate	977.8	E858.8	E947.8	E950.4	E962.0	E980.4
Ipral	967.0	E851	E937.0	E950.1	E962.0	E980.1
Ipratropium	975.1	E858.6	E945.1	E950.4	E962.0	E980.4
Iproniazid	969.01 ◄▥	E854.0	E939.0	E950.3	E962.0	E980.3

◄ New　◄▥ Revised　deleted Deleted　● Use Additional Digit(s)

Substance	Poisoning	External Cause (E Code)				
		Accident	Therapeutic Use	Suicide Attempt	Assault	Undetermined
Iron (compounds) (medicinal) (preparations)	964.0	E858.2	E934.0	E950.4	E962.0	E980.4
dextran	964.0	E858.2	E934.0	E950.4	E962.0	E980.4
nonmedicinal (dust) (fumes) NEC	985.8	E866.4	—	E950.9	E962.1	E980.9
Irritant drug	977.9	E858.9	E947.9	E950.5	E962.0	E980.5
Ismelin	972.6	E858.3	E942.6	E950.4	E962.0	E980.4
Isoamyl nitrite	972.4	E858.3	E942.4	E950.4	E962.0	E980.4
Isobutyl acetate	982.8	E862.4	—	E950.9	E962.1	E980.9
Isocarboxazid	969.01◄	E854.0	E939.0	E950.3	E962.0	E980.3
Isoephedrine	971.2	E855.5	E941.2	E950.4	E962.0	E980.4
Isoetharine	971.2	E855.5	E941.2	E950.4	E962.0	E980.4
Isofluorophate	971.0	E855.3	E941.0	E950.4	E962.0	E980.4
Isoniazid (INH)	961.8	E857	E931.8	E950.4	E962.0	E980.4
Isopentaquine	961.4	E857	E931.4	E950.4	E962.0	E980.4
Isophane insulin	962.3	E858.0	E932.3	E950.4	E962.0	E980.4
Isopregnenone	962.2	E858.0	E932.2	E950.4	E962.0	E980.4
Isoprenaline	971.2	E855.5	E941.2	E950.4	E962.0	E980.4
Isopropamide	971.1	E855.4	E941.1	E950.4	E962.0	E980.4
Isopropanol	980.2	E860.3	—	E950.9	E962.1	E980.9
topical (germicide)	976.0	E858.7	E946.0	E950.4	E962.0	E980.4
Isopropyl	—	—	—	—	—	—
acetate	982.8	E862.4	—	E950.9	E962.1	E980.9
alcohol	980.2	E860.3	—	E950.9	E962.1	E980.9
topical (germicide)	976.0	E858.7	E946.0	E950.4	E962.0	E980.4
ether	982.8	E862.4	—	E950.9	E962.1	E980.9
Isoproterenol	971.2	E855.5	E941.2	E950.4	E962.0	E980.4
Isosorbide dinitrate	972.4	E858.3	E942.4	E950.4	E962.0	E980.4
Isothipendyl	963.0	E858.1	E933.0	E950.4	E962.0	E980.4
Isoxazolyl penicillin	960.0	E856	E930.0	E950.4	E962.0	E980.4
Isoxsuprine hydrochloride	972.5	E858.3	E942.5	E950.4	E962.0	E980.4
l-thyroxine sodium	962.7	E858.0	E932.7	E950.4	E962.0	E980.4
Jaborandi (pilocarpus) (extract)	971.0	E855.3	E941.0	E950.4	E962.0	E980.4
Jalap	973.1	E858.4	E943.1	E950.4	E962.0	E980.4
Jamaica	—	—	—	—	—	—
dogwood (bark)	965.7	E850.7	E935.7	E950.0	E962.0	E980.0
ginger	989.89	E866.8	—	E950.9	E962.1	E980.9
Jatropha	988.2	E865.4	—	E950.9	E962.1	E980.9
curcas	988.2	E865.3	—	E950.9	E962.1	E980.9
Jectofer	964.0	E858.2	E934.0	E950.4	E962.0	E980.4

◄ New　◄▥ Revised　deleted Deleted　● Use Additional Digit(s)

Substance	Poisoning	External Cause (E Code)				
		Accident	Therapeutic Use	Suicide Attempt	Assault	Undetermined
Jellyfish (sting)	989.5	E905.6	—	E950.9	E962.1	E980.9
Jequirity (bean)	988.2	E865.3	—	E950.9	E962.1	E980.9
Jimson weed	988.2	E865.4	—	E950.9	E962.1	E980.9
seeds	988.2	E865.3	—	E950.9	E962.1	E980.9
Juniper tar (oil) (ointment)	976.4	E858.7	E946.4	E950.4	E962.0	E980.4
Kallikrein	972.5	E858.3	E942.5	E950.4	E962.0	E980.4
Kanamycin	960.6	E856	E930.6	E950.4	E962.0	E980.4
Kantrex	960.6	E856	E930.6	E950.4	E962.0	E980.4
Kaolin	973.5	E858.4	E943.5	E950.4	E962.0	E980.4
Karaya (gum)	973.3	E858.4	E943.3	E950.4	E962.0	E980.4
Kemithal	968.3	E855.1	E938.3	E950.4	E962.0	E980.4
Kenacort	962.0	E858.0	E932.0	E950.4	E962.0	E980.4
Keratolytics	976.4	E858.7	E946.4	E950.4	E962.0	E980.4
Keratoplastics	976.4	E858.7	E946.4	E950.4	E962.0	E980.4
Kerosene, kerosine (fuel) (solvent) NEC	981	E862.1	—	E950.9	E962.1	E980.9
insecticide	981	E863.4	—	E950.6	E962.1	E980.7
vapor	987.1	E869.8	—	E952.8	E962.2	E982.8
Ketamine	968.3	E855.1	E938.3	E950.4	E962.0	E980.4
Ketobemidone	965.09	E850.2	E935.2	E950.0	E962.0	E980.0
Ketols	982.8	E862.4	—	E950.9	E962.1	E980.9
Ketone oils	982.8	E862.4	—	E950.9	E962.1	E980.9
Ketoprofen	965.61	E850.6	E935.6	E950.0	E962.0	E980.0
Kiln gas or vapor (carbon monoxide)	986	E868.8	—	E952.1	E962.2	E982.1
Konsyl	973.3	E858.4	E943.3	E950.4	E962.0	E980.4
Kosam seed	988.2	E865.3	—	E950.9	E962.1	E980.9
Krait (venom)	989.5	E905.0	—	E950.9	E962.1	E980.9
Kwell (insecticide)	989.2	E863.0	—	E950.6	E962.1	E980.7
anti-infective (topical)	976.0	E858.7	E946.0	E950.4	E962.0	E980.4
Laburnum (flowers) (seeds)	988.2	E865.3	—	E950.9	E962.1	E980.9
leaves	988.2	E865.4	—	E950.9	E962.1	E980.9
Lacquers	989.89	E861.6	—	E950.9	E962.1	E980.9
Lacrimogenic gas	987.5	E869.3	—	E952.8	E962.2	E982.8
Lactic acid	983.1	E864.1	—	E950.7	E962.1	E980.6
Lactobacillus acidophilus	973.5	E858.4	E943.5	E950.4	E962.0	E980.4
Lactoflavin	963.5	E858.1	E933.5	E950.4	E962.0	E980.4
Lactuca (virosa) (extract)	967.8	E852.8	E937.8	E950.2	E962.0	E980.2
Lactucarium	967.8	E852.8	E937.8	E950.2	E962.0	E980.2
Laevulose	974.5	E858.5	E944.5	E950.4	E962.0	E980.4
Lanatoside (C)	972.1	E858.3	E942.1	E950.4	E962.0	E980.4
Lanolin (lotion)	976.3	E858.7	E946.3	E950.4	E962.0	E980.4

◀ New   ◀▥ Revised   ~~deleted~~ Deleted   ● Use Additional Digit(s)

Substance	Poisoning	External Cause (E Code)				
		Accident	Therapeutic Use	Suicide Attempt	Assault	Undetermined
Largactil	969.1	E853.0	E939.1	E950.3	E962.0	E980.3
Larkspur	988.2	E865.3	—	E950.9	E962.1	E980.9
Laroxyl	969.05◀	E854.0	E939.0	E950.3	E962.0	E980.3
Lasix	974.4	E858.5	E944.4	E950.4	E962.0	E980.4
Latex	989.82	E866.8	—	E950.9	E962.1	E980.9
Lathyrus (seed)	988.2	E865.3	—	E950.9	E962.1	E980.9
Laudanum	965.09	E850.2	E935.2	E950.0	E962.0	E980.0
Laudexium	975.2	E858.6	E945.2	E950.4	E962.0	E980.4
Laurel, black or cherry	988.2	E865.4	—	E950.9	E962.1	E980.9
Laurolinium	976.0	E858.7	E946.0	E950.4	E962.0	E980.4
Lauryl sulfoacetate	976.2	E858.7	E946.2	E950.4	E962.0	E980.4
Laxatives NEC	973.3	E858.4	E943.3	E950.4	E962.0	E980.4
emollient	973.2	E858.4	E943.2	E950.4	E962.0	E980.4
L-dopa	966.4	E855.0	E936.4	E950.4	E962.0	E980.4
L-Tryptophan - *see* amino acid	—	—	—	—	—	—
Lead (dust) (fumes) (vapor) NEC	984.9	E866.0	—	E950.9	E962.1	E980.9
acetate (dust)	984.1	E866.0	—	E950.9	E962.1	E980.9
anti-infectives	961.2	E857	E931.2	E950.4	E962.0	E980.4
antiknock compound (tetra-ethyl)	984.1	E862.1	—	E950.9	E962.1	E980.9
arsenate, arsenite (dust) (insecticide) (vapor)	985.1	E863.4	—	E950.8	E962.1	E980.8
herbicide	985.1	E863.5	—	E950.8	E962.1	E980.8
carbonate	984.0	E866.0	—	E950.9	E962.1	E980.9
paint	984.0	E861.5	—	E950.9	E962.1	E980.9
chromate	984.0	E866.0	—	E950.9	E962.1	E980.9
paint	984.0	E861.5	—	E950.9	E962.1	E980.9
dioxide	984.0	E866.0	—	E950.9	E962.1	E980.9
inorganic (compound)	984.0	E866.0	—	E950.9	E962.1	E980.9
paint	984.0	E861.5	—	E950.9	E962.1	E980.9
iodide	984.0	E866.0	—	E950.9	E962.1	E980.9
pigment (paint)	984.0	E861.5	—	E950.9	E962.1	E980.9
monoxide (dust)	984.0	E866.0	—	E950.9	E962.1	E980.9
paint	984.0	E861.5	—	E950.9	E962.1	E980.9
organic	984.1	E866.0	—	E950.9	E962.1	E980.9
oxide	984.0	E866.0	—	E950.9	E962.1	E980.9
paint	984.0	E861.5	—	E950.9	E962.1	E980.9
paint	984.0	E861.5	—	E950.9	E962.1	E980.9
salts	984.0	E866.0	—	E950.9	E962.1	E980.9
specified compound NEC	984.8	E866.0	—	E950.9	E962.1	E980.9
tetra-ethyl	984.1	E862.1	—	E950.9	E962.1	E980.9
Lebanese red	969.6	E854.1	E939.6	E950.3	E962.0	E980.3

◀ New   ◀▥ Revised   ~~deleted~~ Deleted   ● Use Additional Digit(s)

Substance	Poisoning	External Cause (E Code)				
		Accident	Therapeutic Use	Suicide Attempt	Assault	Undetermined
Lente Iletin (insulin)	962.3	E858.0	E932.3	E950.4	E962.0	E980.4
Leptazol	970.0	E854.3	E940.0	E950.4	E962.0	E980.4
Leritine	965.09	E850.2	E935.2	E950.0	E962.0	E980.0
Letter	962.7	E858.0	E932.7	E950.4	E962.0	E980.4
Lettuce opium	967.8	E852.8	E937.8	E950.2	E962.0	E980.2
Leucovorin (factor)	964.1	E858.2	E934.1	E950.4	E962.0	E980.4
Leukeran	963.1	E858.1	E933.1	E950.4	E962.0	E980.4
Levalbuterol	975.7	E858.6	E945.7	E950.4	E962.0	E980.4
Levallorphan	970.1	E854.3	E940.1	E950.4	E962.0	E980.4
Levanil	967.8	E852.8	E937.8	E950.2	E962.0	E980.2
Levarterenol	971.2	E855.5	E941.2	E950.4	E962.0	E980.4
Levodopa	966.4	E855.0	E936.4	E950.4	E962.0	E980.4
Levo-dromoran	965.09	E850.2	E935.2	E950.0	E962.0	E980.0
Levoid	962.7	E858.0	E932.7	E950.4	E962.0	E980.4
Levo-iso-methadone	965.02	E850.1	E935.1	E950.0	E962.0	E980.0
Levomepromazine	967.8	E852.8	E937.8	E950.2	E962.0	E980.2
Levoprome	967.8	E852.8	E937.8	E950.2	E962.0	E980.2
Levopropoxyphene	975.4	E858.6	E945.4	E950.4	E962.0	E980.4
Levorphan, levophanol	965.09	E850.2	E935.2	E950.0	E962.0	E980.0
Levothyroxine (sodium)	962.7	E858.0	E932.7	E950.4	E962.0	E980.4
Levsin	971.1	E855.4	E941.1	E950.4	E962.0	E980.4
Levulose	974.5	E858.5	E944.5	E950.4	E962.0	E980.4
Lewisite (gas)	985.1	E866.3	—	E950.8	E962.1	E980.8
Librium	969.4	E853.2	E939.4	E950.3	E962.0	E980.3
Lidex	976.0	E858.7	E946.0	E950.4	E962.0	E980.4
Lidocaine (infiltration) (topical)	968.5	E855.2	E938.5	E950.4	E962.0	E980.4
nerve block (peripheral) (plexus)	968.6	E855.2	E938.6	E950.4	E962.0	E980.4
spinal	968.7	E855.2	E938.7	E950.4	E962.0	E980.4
Lighter fluid	981	E862.1	—	E950.9	E962.1	E980.9
Lignocaine (infiltration) (topical)	968.5	E855.2	E938.5	E950.4	E962.0	E980.4
nerve block (peripheral) (plexus)	968.6	E855.2	E938.6	E950.4	E962.0	E980.4
spinal	968.7	E855.2	E938.7	E950.4	E962.0	E980.4
Ligroin(e) (solvent)	981	E862.0	—	E950.9	E962.1	E980.9
vapor	987.1	E869.8	—	E952.8	E962.2	E982.8
Ligustrum vulgare	988.2	E865.3	—	E950.9	E962.1	E980.9
Lily of the valley	988.2	E865.4	—	E950.9	E962.1	E980.9
Lime (chloride)	983.2	E864.2	—	E950.7	E962.1	E980.6
solution, sulferated	976.4	E858.7	E946.4	E950.4	E962.0	E980.4
Limonene	982.8	E862.4	—	E950.9	E962.1	E980.9

◀ New　◀▥ Revised　deleted Deleted　● Use Additional Digit(s)

Substance	Poisoning	External Cause (E Code) Accident	Therapeutic Use	Suicide Attempt	Assault	Undetermined
Lincomycin	960.8	E856	E930.8	E950.4	E962.0	E980.4
Lindane (insecticide) (vapor)	989.2	E863.0	—	E950.6	E962.1	E980.7
anti-infective (topical)	976.0	E858.7	E946.0	E950.4	E962.0	E980.4
Liniments NEC	976.9	E858.7	E946.9	E950.4	E962.0	E980.4
Linoleic acid	972.2	E858.3	E942.2	E950.4	E962.0	E980.4
Liothyronine	962.7	E858.0	E932.7	E950.4	E962.0	E980.4
Liotrix	962.7	E858.0	E932.7	E950.4	E962.0	E980.4
Lipancreatin	973.4	E858.4	E943.4	E950.4	E962.0	E980.4
Lipo-Lutin	962.2	E858.0	E932.2	E950.4	E962.0	E980.4
Lipotropic agents	977.1	E858.8	E947.1	E950.4	E962.0	E980.4
Liquefied petroleum gases	987.0	E868.0	—	E951.1	E962.2	E981.1
piped (pure or mixed with air)	987.0	E867	—	E951.0	E962.2	E981.0
Liquid petrolatum	973.2	E858.4	E943.2	E950.4	E962.0	E980.4
substance	989.9	E866.9	—	E950.9	E962.1	E980.9
specified NEC	989.89	E866.8	—	E950.9	E962.1	E980.9
Lirugen	979.4	E858.8	E949.4	E950.4	E962.0	E980.4
Lithane	969.8	E855.8	E939.8	E950.3	E962.0	E980.3
Lithium	985.8	E866.4	—	E950.9	E962.1	E980.9
carbonate	969.8	E855.8	E939.8	E950.3	E962.0	E980.3
Lithonate	969.8	E855.8	E939.8	E950.3	E962.0	E980.3
Liver (extract) (injection) (preparations)	964.1	E858.2	E934.1	E950.4	E962.0	E980.4
Lizard (bite) (venom)	989.5	E905.0	—	E950.9	E962.1	E980.9
LMD	964.8	E858.2	E934.8	E950.4	E962.0	E980.4
Lobelia	988.2	E865.4	—	E950.9	E962.1	E980.9
Lobeline	970.0	E854.3	E940.0	E950.4	E962.0	E980.4
Locorten	976.0	E858.7	E946.0	E950.4	E962.0	E980.4
Lolium temulentum	988.2	E865.3	—	E950.9	E962.1	E980.9
Lomotil	973.5	E858.4	E943.5	E950.4	E962.0	E980.4
Lomustine	963.1	E858.1	E933.1	E950.4	E962.0	E980.4
Lophophora williamsii	969.6	E854.1	E939.6	E950.3	E962.0	E980.3
Lorazepam	969.4	E853.2	E939.4	E950.3	E962.0	E980.3
Lotions NEC	976.9	E858.7	E946.9	E950.4	E962.0	E980.4
Lotronex	973.8	E858.4	E943.8	E950.4	E962.0	E980.4
Lotusate	967.0	E851	E937.0	E950.1	E962.0	E980.1
Lowila	976.2	E858.7	E946.2	E950.4	E962.0	E980.4
Loxapine	969.3	E853.8	E939.3	E950.3	E962.0	E980.3
Lozenges (throat)	976.6	E858.7	E946.6	E950.4	E962.0	E980.4
LSD (25)	969.6	E854.1	E939.6	E950.3	E962.0	E980.3
Lubricating oil NEC	981	E862.2	—	E950.9	E962.1	E980.9

◀ New   ◀▥ Revised   ~~deleted~~ Deleted   ● Use Additional Digit(s)

Substance	Poisoning	External Cause (E Code)				
		Accident	Therapeutic Use	Suicide Attempt	Assault	Undetermined
Lucanthone	961.6	E857	E931.6	E950.4	E962.0	E980.4
Luminal	967.0	E851	E937.0	E950.1	E962.0	E980.1
Lung irritant (gas) NEC	987.9	E869.9	—	E952.9	E962.2	E982.9
Lutocylol	962.2	E858.0	E932.2	E950.4	E962.0	E980.4
Lutromone	962.2	E858.0	E932.2	E950.4	E962.0	E980.4
Lututrin	975.0	E858.6	E945.0	E950.4	E962.0	E980.4
Lye (concentrated)	983.2	E864.2	—	E950.7	E962.1	E980.6
Lygranum (skin test)	977.8	E858.8	E947.8	E950.4	E962.0	E980.4
Lymecycline	960.4	E856	E930.4	E950.4	E962.0	E980.4
Lymphogranuloma venereum antigen	977.8	E858.8	E947.8	E950.4	E962.0	E980.4
Lynestrenol	962.2	E858.0	E932.2	E950.4	E962.0	E980.4
Lyovac Sodium Edecrin	974.4	E858.5	E944.4	E950.4	E962.0	E980.4
Lypressin	962.5	E858.0	E932.5	E950.4	E962.0	E980.4
Lysergic acid (amide) (diethylamide)	969.6	E854.1	E939.6	E950.3	E962.0	E980.3
Lysergide	969.6	E854.1	E939.6	E950.3	E962.0	E980.3
Lysine vasopressin	962.5	E858.0	E932.5	E950.4	E962.0	E980.4
Lysol	983.0	E864.0	—	E950.7	E962.1	E980.6
Lytta (vitatta)	976.8	E858.7	E946.8	E950.4	E962.0	E980.4
Mace	987.5	E869.3	—	E952.8	E962.2	E982.8
Macrolides (antibiotics)	960.3	E856	E930.3	E950.4	E962.0	E980.4
Mafenide	976.0	E858.7	E946.0	E950.4	E962.0	E980.4
Magaldrate	973.0	E858.4	E943.0	E950.4	E962.0	E980.4
Magic mushroom	969.6	E854.1	E939.6	E950.3	E962.0	E980.3
Magnamycin	960.8	E856	E930.8	E950.4	E962.0	E980.4
Magnesia magma	973.0	E858.4	E943.0	E950.4	E962.0	E980.4
Magnesium (compounds) (fumes) NEC	985.8	E866.4	—	E950.9	E962.1	E980.9
antacid	973.0	E858.4	E943.0	E950.4	E962.0	E980.4
carbonate	973.0	E858.4	E943.0	E950.4	E962.0	E980.4
cathartic	973.3	E858.4	E943.3	E950.4	E962.0	E980.4
citrate	973.3	E858.4	E943.3	E950.4	E962.0	E980.4
hydroxide	973.0	E858.4	E943.0	E950.4	E962.0	E980.4
oxide	973.0	E858.4	E943.0	E950.4	E962.0	E980.4
sulfate (oral)	973.3	E858.4	E943.3	E950.4	E962.0	E980.4
intravenous	966.3	E855.0	E936.3	E950.4	E962.0	E980.4
trisilicate	973.0	E858.4	E943.0	E950.4	E962.0	E980.4
Malathion (insecticide)	989.3	E863.1	—	E950.6	E962.1	E980.7
Male fern (oleoresin)	961.6	E857	E931.6	E950.4	E962.0	E980.4
Mandelic acid	961.9	E857	E931.9	E950.4	E962.0	E980.4
Manganese compounds (fumes) NEC	985.2	E866.4	—	E950.9	E962.1	E980.9

◀ New   ◀▥ Revised   ~~deleted~~ Deleted   ● Use Additional Digit(s)

Substance	Poisoning	External Cause (E Code)				
		Accident	Therapeutic Use	Suicide Attempt	Assault	Undetermined
Mannitol (diuretic) (medicinal) NEC	974.4	E858.5	E944.4	E950.4	E962.0	E980.4
hexanitrate	972.4	E858.3	E942.4	E950.4	E962.0	E980.4
mustard	963.1	E858.1	E933.1	E950.4	E962.0	E980.4
Mannomustine	963.1	E858.1	E933.1	E950.4	E962.0	E980.4
MAO inhibitors	969.01 ◀ⅲ	E854.0	E939.0	E950.3	E962.0	E980.3
Mapharsen	961.1	E857	E931.1	E950.4	E962.0	E980.4
Marcaine	968.9	E855.2	E938.9	E950.4	E962.0	E980.4
infiltration (subcutaneous)	968.5	E855.2	E938.5	E950.4	E962.0	E980.4
nerve block (peripheral) (plexus)	968.6	E855.2	E938.6	E950.4	E962.0	E980.4
Marezine	963.0	E858.1	E933.0	E950.4	E962.0	E980.4
Marihuana, marijuana (derivatives)	969.6	E854.1	E939.6	E950.3	E962.0	E980.3
Marine animals or plants (sting)	989.5	E905.6	—	E950.9	E962.1	E980.9
Marplan	969.01 ◀ⅲ	E854.0	E939.0	E950.3	E962.0	E980.3
Marsh gas	987.1	E869.8	—	E952.8	E962.2	E982.8
Marsilid	969.01 ◀ⅲ	E854.0	E939.0	E950.3	E962.0	E980.3
Matulane	963.1	E858.1	E933.1	E950.4	E962.0	E980.4
Mazindol	977.0	E858.8	E947.0	E950.4	E962.0	E980.4
MDMA	969.72 ◀ⅲ	E854.2	E939.7	E950.3	E962.0	E980.3
Meadow saffron	988.2	E865.3	—	E950.9	E962.1	E980.9
Measles vaccine	979.4	E858.8	E949.4	E950.4	E962.0	E980.4
Meat, noxious or nonbacterial	988.8	E865.0	—	E950.9	E962.1	E980.9
Mebanazine	969.01 ◀ⅲ	E854.0	E939.0	E950.3	E962.0	E980.3
Mebaral	967.0	E851	E937.0	E950.1	E962.0	E980.1
Mebendazole	961.6	E857	E931.6	E950.4	E962.0	E980.4
Mebeverine	975.1	E858.6	E945.1	E950.4	E962.0	E980.4
Mebhydroline	963.0	E858.1	E933.0	E950.4	E962.0	E980.4
Mebrophenhydramine	963.0	E858.1	E933.0	E950.4	E962.0	E980.4
Mebutamate	969.5	E853.8	E939.5	E950.3	E962.0	E980.3
Mecamylamine (chloride)	972.3	E858.3	E942.3	E950.4	E962.0	E980.4
Mechlorethamine hydrochloride	963.1	E858.1	E933.1	E950.4	E962.0	E980.4
Meclizene (hydrochloride)	963.0	E858.1	E933.0	E950.4	E962.0	E980.4
Meclofenoxate	970.0	E854.3	E940.0	E950.4	E962.0	E980.4
Meclozine (hydrochloride)	963.0	E858.1	E933.0	E950.4	E962.0	E980.4
Medazepam	969.4	E853.2	E939.4	E950.3	E962.0	E980.3
Medicine, medicinal substance	977.9	E858.9	E947.9	E950.5	E962.0	E980.5
specified NEC	977.8	E858.8	E947.8	E950.4	E962.0	E980.4
Medinal	967.0	E851	E937.0	E950.1	E962.0	E980.1
Medomin	967.0	E851	E937.0	E950.1	E962.0	E980.1
Medroxyprogesterone	962.2	E858.0	E932.2	E950.4	E962.0	E980.4

◀ New   ◀ⅲ Revised   ~~deleted~~ Deleted   ● Use Additional Digit(s)

Substance	Poisoning	External Cause (E Code)				
		Accident	Therapeutic Use	Suicide Attempt	Assault	Undetermined
Medrysone	976.5	E858.7	E946.5	E950.4	E962.0	E980.4
Mefenamic acid	965.7	E850.7	E935.7	E950.0	E962.0	E980.0
Megahallucinogen	969.6	E854.1	E939.6	E950.3	E962.0	E980.3
Megestrol	962.2	E858.0	E932.2	E950.4	E962.0	E980.4
Meglumine	977.8	E858.8	E947.8	E950.4	E962.0	E980.4
Meladinin	976.3	E858.7	E946.3	E950.4	E962.0	E980.4
Melanizing agents	976.3	E858.7	E946.3	E950.4	E962.0	E980.4
Melarsoprol	961.1	E857	E931.1	E950.4	E962.0	E980.4
Melia azedarach	988.2	E865.3	—	E950.9	E962.1	E980.9
Mellaril	969.1	E853.0	E939.1	E950.3	E962.0	E980.3
Meloxine	976.3	E858.7	E946.3	E950.4	E962.0	E980.4
Melphalan	963.1	E858.1	E933.1	E950.4	E962.0	E980.4
Memantine hydrochloride	969.8	E854.8	E939.8	E950.3	E962.0	E980.3
Menadiol sodium diphosphate	964.3	E858.2	E934.3	E950.4	E962.0	E980.4
Menadione (sodium bisulfite)	964.3	E858.2	E934.3	E950.4	E962.0	E980.4
Menaphthone	964.3	E858.2	E934.3	E950.4	E962.0	E980.4
Meningococcal vaccine	978.8	E858.8	E948.8	E950.4	E962.0	E980.4
Menningovax-C	978.8	E858.8	E948.8	E950.4	E962.0	E980.4
Menotropins	962.4	E858.0	E932.4	E950.4	E962.0	E980.4
Menthol NEC	976.1	E858.7	E946.1	E950.4	E962.0	E980.4
Mepacrine	961.3	E857	E931.3	E950.4	E962.0	E980.4
Meparfynol	967.8	E852.8	E937.8	E950.2	E962.0	E980.2
Mepazine	969.1	E853.0	E939.1	E950.3	E962.0	E980.3
Mepenzolate	971.1	E855.4	E941.1	E950.4	E962.0	E980.4
Meperidine	965.09	E850.2	E935.2	E950.0	E962.0	E980.0
Mephenamin(e)	966.4	E855.0	E936.4	E950.4	E962.0	E980.4
Mephenesin (carbamate)	968.0	E855.1	E938.0	E950.4	E962.0	E980.4
Mephenoxalone	969.5	E853.8	E939.5	E950.3	E962.0	E980.3
Mephentermine	971.2	E855.5	E941.2	E950.4	E962.0	E980.4
Mephenytoin	966.1	E855.0	E936.1	E950.4	E962.0	E980.4
Mephobarbital	967.0	E851	E937.0	E950.1	E962.0	E980.1
Mepiperphenidol	971.1	E855.4	E941.1	E950.4	E962.0	E980.4
Mepivacaine	968.9	E855.2	E938.9	E950.4	E962.0	E980.4
infiltration (subcutaneous)	968.5	E855.2	E938.5	E950.4	E962.0	E980.4
nerve block (peripheral) (plexus)	968.6	E855.2	E938.6	E950.4	E962.0	E980.4
topical (surface)	968.5	E855.2	E938.5	E950.4	E962.0	E980.4
Meprednisone	962.0	E858.0	E932.0	E950.4	E962.0	E980.4
Meprobam	969.5	E853.8	E939.5	E950.3	E962.0	E980.3
Meprobamate	969.5	E853.8	E939.5	E950.3	E962.0	E980.3

◀ New   ◀ Revised   ~~deleted~~ Deleted   ● Use Additional Digit(s)

Substance	Poisoning	External Cause (E Code)				
		Accident	Therapeutic Use	Suicide Attempt	Assault	Undetermined
Mepyramine (maleate)	963.0	E858.1	E933.0	E950.4	E962.0	E980.4
Meralluride	974.0	E858.5	E944.0	E950.4	E962.0	E980.4
Merbaphen	974.0	E858.5	E944.0	E950.4	E962.0	E980.4
Merbromin	976.0	E858.7	E946.0	E950.4	E962.0	E980.4
Mercaptomerin	974.0	E858.5	E944.0	E950.4	E962.0	E980.4
Mercaptopurine	963.1	E858.1	E933.1	E950.4	E962.0	E980.4
Mercumatilin	974.0	E858.5	E944.0	E950.4	E962.0	E980.4
Mercuramide	974.0	E858.5	E944.0	E950.4	E962.0	E980.4
Mercuranin	976.0	E858.7	E946.0	E950.4	E962.0	E980.4
Mercurochrome	976.0	E858.7	E946.0	E950.4	E962.0	E980.4
Mercury, mercuric, mercurous (compounds) (cyanide) (fumes) (nonmedicinal) (vapor) NEC	985.0	E866.1	—	E950.9	E962.1	E980.9
ammoniated	976.0	E858.7	E946.0	E950.4	E962.0	E980.4
anti-infective	961.2	E857	E931.2	E950.4	E962.0	E980.4
topical	976.0	E858.7	E946.0	E950.4	E962.0	E980.4
chloride (antiseptic) NEC	976.0	E858.7	E946.0	E950.4	E962.0	E980.4
fungicide	985.0	E863.6	—	E950.6	E962.1	E980.7
diuretic compounds	974.0	E858.5	E944.0	E950.4	E962.0	E980.4
fungicide	985.0	E863.6	—	E950.6	E962.1	E980.7
organic (fungicide)	985.0	E863.6	—	E950.6	E962.1	E980.7
Merethoxylline	974.0	E858.5	E944.0	E950.4	E962.0	E980.4
Mersalyl	974.0	E858.5	E944.0	E950.4	E962.0	E980.4
Merthiolate (topical)	976.0	E858.7	E946.0	E950.4	E962.0	E980.4
ophthalmic preparation	976.5	E858.7	E946.5	E950.4	E962.0	E980.4
Meruvax	979.4	E858.8	E949.4	E950.4	E962.0	E980.4
Mescal buttons	969.6	E854.1	E939.6	E950.3	E962.0	E980.3
Mescaline (salts)	969.6	E854.1	E939.6	E950.3	E962.0	E980.3
Mesoridazine besylate	969.1	E853.0	E939.1	E950.3	E962.0	E980.3
Mestanolone	962.1	E858.0	E932.1	E950.4	E962.0	E980.4
Mestranol	962.2	E858.0	E932.2	E950.4	E962.0	E980.4
Metactesylacetate	976.0	E858.7	E946.0	E950.4	E962.0	E980.4
Metaldehyde (snail killer) NEC	989.4	E863.4	—	E950.6	E962.1	E980.7
Metals (heavy) (nonmedicinal) NEC	985.9	E866.4	—	E950.9	E962.1	E980.9
dust, fumes, or vapor NEC	985.9	E866.4	—	E950.9	E962.1	E980.9
light NEC	985.9	E866.4	—	E950.9	E962.1	E980.9
dust, fumes, or vapor NEC	985.9	E866.4	—	E950.9	E962.1	E980.9
pesticides (dust) (vapor)	985.9	E863.4	—	E950.6	E962.1	E980.7
Metamucil	973.3	E858.4	E943.3	E950.4	E962.0	E980.4
Metaphen	976.0	E858.7	E946.0	E950.4	E962.0	E980.4

◀ New　　◀▥ Revised　　deleted Deleted　　● Use Additional Digit(s)

Substance	Poisoning	External Cause (E Code)				
		Accident	Therapeutic Use	Suicide Attempt	Assault	Undetermined
Metaproterenol	975.1	E858.6	E945.1	E950.4	E962.0	E980.4
Metaraminol	972.8	E858.3	E942.8	E950.4	E962.0	E980.4
Metaxalone	968.0	E855.1	E938.0	E950.4	E962.0	E980.4
Metformin	962.3	E858.0	E932.3	E950.4	E962.0	E980.4
Methacycline	960.4	E856	E930.4	E950.4	E962.0	E980.4
Methadone	965.02	E850.1	E935.1	E950.0	E962.0	E980.0
Methallenestril	962.2	E858.0	E932.2	E950.4	E962.0	E980.4
Methamphetamine	969.72◄	E854.2	E939.7	E950.3	E962.0	E980.3
Methandienone	962.1	E858.0	E932.1	E950.4	E962.0	E980.4
Methandriol	962.1	E858.0	E932.1	E950.4	E962.0	E980.4
Methandrostenolone	962.1	E858.0	E932.1	E950.4	E962.0	E980.4
Methane gas	987.1	E869.8	—	E952.8	E962.2	E982.8
Methanol	980.1	E860.2	—	E950.9	E962.1	E980.9
vapor	987.8	E869.8	—	E952.8	E962.2	E982.8
Methantheline	971.1	E855.4	E941.1	E950.4	E962.0	E980.4
Methaphenilene	963.0	E858.1	E933.0	E950.4	E962.0	E980.4
Methapyrilene	963.0	E858.1	E933.0	E950.4	E962.0	E980.4
Methaqualone (compounds)	967.4	E852.3	E937.4	E950.2	E962.0	E980.2
Metharbital, metharbitone	967.0	E851	E937.0	E950.1	E962.0	E980.1
Methazolamide	974.2	E858.5	E944.2	E950.4	E962.0	E980.4
Methdilazine	963.0	E858.1	E933.0	E950.4	E962.0	E980.4
Methedrine	969.72◄	E854.2	E939.7	E950.3	E962.0	E980.3
Methenamine (mandelate)	961.9	E857	E931.9	E950.4	E962.0	E980.4
Methenolone	962.1	E858.0	E932.1	E950.4	E962.0	E980.4
Methergine	975.0	E858.6	E945.0	E950.4	E962.0	E980.4
Methiacil	962.8	E858.0	E932.8	E950.4	E962.0	E980.4
Methicillin (sodium)	960.0	E856	E930.0	E950.4	E962.0	E980.4
Methimazole	962.8	E858.0	E932.8	E950.4	E962.0	E980.4
Methionine	977.1	E858.8	E947.1	E950.4	E962.0	E980.4
Methisazone	961.7	E857	E931.7	E950.4	E962.0	E980.4
Methitural	967.0	E851	E937.0	E950.1	E962.0	E980.1
Methixene	971.1	E855.4	E941.1	E950.4	E962.0	E980.4
Methobarbital, methobarbitone	967.0	E851	E937.0	E950.1	E962.0	E980.1
Methocarbamol	968.0	E855.1	E938.0	E950.4	E962.0	E980.4
Methohexital, methohexitone (sodium)	968.3	E855.1	E938.3	E950.4	E962.0	E980.4
Methoin	966.1	E855.0	E936.1	E950.4	E962.0	E980.4
Methopholine	965.7	E850.7	E935.7	E950.0	E962.0	E980.0
Methorate	975.4	E858.6	E945.4	E950.4	E962.0	E980.4
Methoserpidine	972.6	E858.3	E942.6	E950.4	E962.0	E980.4

◄ New   ◄▥ Revised   deleted Deleted   ● Use Additional Digit(s)

Substance	Poisoning	External Cause (E Code)				
		Accident	Therapeutic Use	Suicide Attempt	Assault	Undetermined
Methotrexate	963.1	E858.1	E933.1	E950.4	E962.0	E980.4
Methotrimeprazine	967.8	E852.8	E937.8	E950.2	E962.0	E980.2
Methoxa-Dome	976.3	E858.7	E946.3	E950.4	E962.0	E980.4
Methoxamine	971.2	E855.5	E941.2	E950.4	E962.0	E980.4
Methoxsalen	976.3	E858.7	E946.3	E950.4	E962.0	E980.4
Methoxybenzyl penicillin	960.0	E856	E930.0	E950.4	E962.0	E980.4
Methoxychlor	989.2	E863.0	—	E950.6	E962.1	E980.7
Methoxyflurane	968.2	E855.1	E938.2	E950.4	E962.0	E980.4
Methoxyphenamine	971.2	E855.5	E941.2	E950.4	E962.0	E980.4
Methoxypromazine	969.1	E853.0	E939.1	E950.3	E962.0	E980.3
Methoxypsoralen	976.3	E858.7	E946.3	E950.4	E962.0	E980.4
Methscopolamine (bromide)	971.1	E855.4	E941.1	E950.4	E962.0	E980.4
Methsuximide	966.2	E855.0	E936.2	E950.4	E962.0	E980.4
Methyclothiazide	974.3	E858.5	E944.3	E950.4	E962.0	E980.4
Methyl	—	—	—	—	—	—
acetate	982.8	E862.4	—	E950.9	E962.1	E980.9
acetone II	982.8	E862.4	—	E950.9	E962.1	E980.9
alcohol	980.1	E860.2	—	E950.9	E962.1	E980.9
amphetamine	969.72 ◀ⅢⅢ	E854.2	E939.7	E950.3	E962.0	E980.3
androstanolone	962.1	E858.0	E932.1	E950.4	E962.0	E980.4
atropine	971.1	E855.4	E941.1	E950.4	E962.0	E980.4
benzene	982.0	E862.4	—	E950.9	E962.1	E980.9
bromide (gas)	987.8	E869.8	—	E952.8	E962.2	E982.8
fumigant	987.8	E863.8	—	E950.6	E962.2	E980.7
butanol	980.8	E860.8	—	E950.9	E962.1	E980.9
carbinol	980.1	E860.2	—	E950.9	E962.1	E980.9
cellosolve	982.8	E862.4	—	E950.9	E962.1	E980.9
cellulose	973.3	E858.4	E943.3	E950.4	E962.0	E980.4
chloride (gas)	987.8	E869.8	—	E952.8	E962.2	E982.8
cyclohexane	982.8	E862.4	—	E950.9	E962.1	E980.9
cyclohexanone	982.8	E862.4	—	E950.9	E962.1	E980.9
dihydromorphinone	965.09	E850.2	E935.2	E950.0	E962.0	E980.0
ergometrine	975.0	E858.6	E945.0	E950.4	E962.0	E980.4
ergonovine	975.0	E858.6	E945.0	E950.4	E962.0	E980.4
ethyl ketone	982.8	E862.4	—	E950.9	E962.1	E980.9
hydrazine	983.9	E864.3	—	E950.7	E962.1	E980.6
isobutyl ketone	982.8	E862.4	—	E950.9	E962.1	E980.9
morphine NEC	965.09	E850.2	E935.2	E950.0	E962.0	E980.0
parafynol	967.8	E852.8	E937.8	E950.2	E962.0	E980.2

◀ New ◀ⅢⅢ Revised ~~deleted~~ Deleted ● Use Additional Digit(s)

Substance	Poisoning	External Cause (E Code)				
		Accident	Therapeutic Use	Suicide Attempt	Assault	Undetermined
Methyl (Continued)						
parathion	989.3	E863.1	—	E950.6	E962.1	E980.7
pentynol NEC	967.8	E852.8	E937.8	E950.2	E962.0	E980.2
peridol	969.2	E853.1	E939.2	E950.3	E962.0	E980.3
phenidate	969.73◀▥	E854.2	E939.7	E950.3	E962.0	E980.3
prednisolone	962.0	E858.0	E932.0	E950.4	E962.0	E980.4
ENT agent	976.6	E858.7	E946.6	E950.4	E962.0	E980.4
ophthalmic preparation	976.5	E858.7	E946.5	E950.4	E962.0	E980.4
topical NEC	976.0	E858.7	E946.0	E950.4	E962.0	E980.4
propylcarbinol	980.8	E860.8	—	E950.9	E962.1	E980.9
rosaniline NEC	976.0	E858.7	E946.0	E950.4	E962.0	E980.4
salicylate NEC	976.3	E858.7	E946.3	E950.4	E962.0	E980.4
sulfate (fumes)	987.8	E869.8	—	E952.8	E962.2	E982.8
liquid	983.9	E864.3	—	E950.7	E962.1	E980.6
sulfonal	967.8	E852.8	E937.8	E950.2	E962.0	E980.2
testosterone	962.1	E858.0	E932.1	E950.4	E962.0	E980.4
thiouracil	962.8	E858.0	E932.8	E950.4	E962.0	E980.4
Methylated spirit	980.0	E860.1	—	E950.9	E962.1	E980.9
Methyldopa	972.6	E858.3	E942.6	E950.4	E962.0	E980.4
Methylene blue	961.9	E857	E931.9	E950.4	E962.0	E980.4
chloride or dichloride (solvent) NEC	982.3	E862.4	—	E950.9	E962.1	E980.9
Methylhexabital	967.0	E851	E937.0	E950.1	E962.0	E980.1
Methylparaben (ophthalmic)	976.5	E858.7	E946.5	E950.4	E962.0	E980.4
Methyprylon	967.5	E852.4	E937.5	E950.2	E962.0	E980.2
Methysergide	971.3	E855.6	E941.3	E950.4	E962.0	E980.4
Metoclopramide	963.0	E858.1	E933.0	E950.4	E962.0	E980.4
Metofoline	965.7	E850.7	E935.7	E950.0	E962.0	E980.0
Metopon	965.09	E850.2	E935.2	E950.0	E962.0	E980.0
Metronidazole	961.5	E857	E931.5	E950.4	E962.0	E980.4
Metycaine	968.9	E855.2	E938.9	E950.4	E962.0	E980.4
infiltration (subcutaneous)	968.5	E855.2	E938.5	E950.4	E962.0	E980.4
nerve block (peripheral) (plexus)	968.6	E855.2	E938.6	E950.4	E962.0	E980.4
topical (surface)	968.5	E855.2	E938.5	E950.4	E962.0	E980.4
Metyrapone	977.8	E858.8	E947.8	E950.4	E962.0	E980.4
Mevinphos	989.3	E863.1	—	E950.6	E962.1	E980.7
Mezereon (berries)	988.2	E865.3	—	E950.9	E962.1	E980.9
Micatin	976.0	E858.7	E946.0	E950.4	E962.0	E980.4
Miconazole	976.0	E858.7	E946.0	E950.4	E962.0	E980.4
Midol	965.1	E850.3	E935.3	E950.0	E962.0	E980.0

◀ New   ◀▥ Revised   deleted Deleted   ● Use Additional Digit(s)

Substance	Poisoning	External Cause (E Code)				
		Accident	Therapeutic Use	Suicide Attempt	Assault	Undetermined
Mifepristone	962.9	E858.0	E932.9	E950.4	E962.0	E980.4
Milk of magnesia	973.0	E858.4	E943.0	E950.4	E962.0	E980.4
Millipede (tropical) (venomous)	989.5	E905.4	—	E950.9	E962.1	E980.9
Miltown	969.5	E853.8	E939.5	E950.3	E962.0	E980.3
Mineral	—	—	—	—	—	—
oil (medicinal)	973.2	E858.4	E943.2	E950.4	E962.0	E980.4
nonmedicinal	981	E862.1	—	E950.9	E962.1	E980.9
topical	976.3	E858.7	E946.3	E950.4	E962.0	E980.4
salts NEC	974.6	E858.5	E944.6	E950.4	E962.0	E980.4
spirits	981	E862.0	—	E950.9	E962.1	E980.9
Minocycline	960.4	E856	E930.4	E950.4	E962.0	E980.4
Mithramycin (antineoplastic)	960.7	E856	E930.7	E950.4	E962.0	E980.4
Mitobronitol	963.1	E858.1	E933.1	E950.4	E962.0	E980.4
Mitomycin (antineoplastic)	960.7	E856	E930.7	E950.4	E962.0	E980.4
Mitotane	963.1	E858.1	E933.1	E950.4	E962.0	E980.4
Moderil	972.6	E858.3	E942.6	E950.4	E962.0	E980.4
Mogadon - *see* Nitrazepam	—	—	—	—	—	—
Molindone	969.3	E853.8	E939.3	E950.3	E962.0	E980.3
Monistat	976.0	E858.7	E946.0	E950.4	E962.0	E980.4
Monkshood	988.2	E865.4	—	E950.9	E962.1	E980.9
Monoamine oxidase inhibitors	969.01 ◂▥	E854.0	E939.0	E950.3	E962.0	E980.3
Monochlorobenzene	982.0	E862.4	—	E950.9	E962.1	E980.9
Monosodium glutamate	989.89	E866.8	—	E950.9	E962.1	E980.9
Monoxide, carbon - *see* Carbon, monoxide	—	—	—	—	—	—
Moperone	969.2	E853.1	E939.2	E950.3	E962.0	E980.3
Morning glory seeds	969.6	E854.1	E939.6	E950.3	E962.0	E980.3
Moroxydine (hydrochloride)	961.7	E857	E931.7	E950.4	E962.0	E980.4
Morphazinamide	961.8	E857	E931.8	E950.4	E962.0	E980.4
Morphinans	965.09	E850.2	E935.2	E950.0	E962.0	E980.0
Morphine NEC	965.09	E850.2	E935.2	E950.0	E962.0	E980.0
antagonists	970.1	E854.3	E940.1	E950.4	E962.0	E980.4
Morpholinylethyl morphine	965.09	E850.2	E935.2	E950.0	E962.0	E980.0
Morrhuate sodium	972.7	E858.3	E942.7	E950.4	E962.0	E980.4
Moth balls (*see also* Pesticides)	989.4	E863.4	—	E950.6	E962.1	E980.7
naphthalene	983.0	E863.4	—	E950.7	E962.1	E980.6
Motor exhaust gas - *see* Carbon, monoxide, exhaust gas	—	—	—	—	—	—
Mouth wash	976.6	E858.7	E946.6	E950.4	E962.0	E980.4
Mucolytic agent	975.5	E858.6	E945.5	E950.4	E962.0	E980.4
Mucomyst	975.5	E858.6	E945.5	E950.4	E962.0	E980.4

◀ New　　◂▥ Revised　　deleted Deleted　　● Use Additional Digit(s)

Substance	Poisoning	External Cause (E Code)				
		Accident	Therapeutic Use	Suicide Attempt	Assault	Undetermined
Mucous membrane agents (external)	976.9	E858.7	E946.9	E950.4	E962.0	E980.4
specified NEC	976.8	E858.7	E946.8	E950.4	E962.0	E980.4
Mumps	—	—	—	—	—	—
immune globulin (human)	964.6	E858.2	E934.6	E950.4	E962.0	E980.4
skin test antigen	977.8	E858.8	E947.8	E950.4	E962.0	E980.4
vaccine	979.6	E858.8	E949.6	E950.4	E962.0	E980.4
Mumpsvax	979.6	E858.8	E949.6	E950.4	E962.0	E980.4
Muriatic acid - *see* Hydrochloric acid	—	—	—	—	—	—
Muscarine	971.0	E855.3	E941.0	E950.4	E962.0	E980.4
Muscle affecting agents NEC	975.3	E858.6	E945.3	E950.4	E962.0	E980.4
oxytocic	975.0	E858.6	E945.0	E950.4	E962.0	E980.4
relaxants	975.3	E858.6	E945.3	E950.4	E962.0	E980.4
central nervous system	968.0	E855.1	E938.0	E950.4	E962.0	E980.4
skeletal	975.2	E858.6	E945.2	E950.4	E962.0	E980.4
smooth	975.1	E858.6	E945.1	E950.4	E962.0	E980.4
Mushrooms, noxious	988.1	E865.5	—	E950.9	E962.1	E980.9
Mussel, noxious	988.0	E865.1	—	E950.9	E962.1	E980.9
Mustard (emetic)	973.6	E858.4	E943.6	E950.4	E962.0	E980.4
gas	987.8	E869.8	—	E952.8	E962.2	E982.8
nitrogen	963.1	E858.1	E933.1	E950.4	E962.0	E980.4
Mustine	963.1	E858.1	E933.1	E950.4	E962.0	E980.4
M-vac	979.4	E858.8	E949.4	E950.4	E962.0	E980.4
Mycifradin	960.8	E856	E930.8	E950.4	E962.0	E980.4
topical	976.0	E858.7	E946.0	E950.4	E962.0	E980.4
Mycitracin	960.8	E856	E930.8	E950.4	E962.0	E980.4
ophthalmic preparation	976.5	E858.7	E946.5	E950.4	E962.0	E980.4
Mycostatin	960.1	E856	E930.1	E950.4	E962.0	E980.4
topical	976.0	E858.7	E946.0	E950.4	E962.0	E980.4
Mydriacyl	971.1	E855.4	E941.1	E950.4	E962.0	E980.4
Myelobromal	963.1	E858.1	E933.1	E950.4	E962.0	E980.4
Myleran	963.1	E858.1	E933.1	E950.4	E962.0	E980.4
Myochrysin(e)	965.69	E850.6	E935.6	E950.0	E962.0	E980.0
Myoneural blocking agents	975.2	E858.6	E945.2	E950.4	E962.0	E980.4
Myristica fragrans	988.2	E865.3	—	E950.9	E962.1	E980.9
Myristicin	988.2	E865.3	—	E950.9	E962.1	E980.9
Mysoline	966.3	E855.0	E936.3	E950.4	E962.0	E980.4
Nafcillin (sodium)	960.0	E856	E930.0	E950.4	E962.0	E980.4
Nail polish remover	982.8	E862.4	—	E950.9	E962.1	E980.9
Nalidixic acid	961.9	E857	E931.9	E950.4	E962.0	E980.4

◀ New ◀▪▪ Revised ~~deleted~~ Deleted ● Use Additional Digit(s)

Substance	Poisoning	External Cause (E Code)				
		Accident	Therapeutic Use	Suicide Attempt	Assault	Undetermined
Nalorphine	970.1	E854.3	E940.1	E950.4	E962.0	E980.4
Naloxone	970.1	E854.3	E940.1	E950.4	E962.0	E980.4
Namenda	969.8	E854.8	E939.8	E950.3	E962.0	E980.3
Nandrolone (decanoate) (phenpropionate)	962.1	E858.0	E932.1	E950.4	E962.0	E980.4
Naphazoline	971.2	E855.5	E941.2	E950.4	E962.0	E980.4
Naphtha (painter's) (petroleum)	981	E862.0	—	E950.9	E962.1	E980.9
solvent	981	E862.0	—	E950.9	E962.1	E980.9
vapor	987.1	E869.8	—	E952.8	E962.2	E982.8
Naphthalene (chlorinated)	983.0	E864.0	—	E950.7	E962.1	E980.6
insecticide or moth repellent	983.0	E863.4	—	E950.7	E962.1	E980.6
vapor	987.8	E869.8	—	E952.8	E962.2	E982.8
Naphthol	983.0	E864.0	—	E950.7	E962.1	E980.6
Naphthylamine	983.0	E864.0	—	E950.7	E962.1	E980.6
Naprosyn - *see* Naproxen	—	—	—	—	—	—
Naproxen	965.61	E850.6	E935.6	E950.0	E962.0	E980.0
Narcotic (drug)	967.9	E852.9	E937.9	E950.2	E962.0	E980.2
analgesic NEC	965.8	E850.8	E935.8	E950.0	E962.0	E980.0
antagonist	970.1	E854.3	E940.1	E950.4	E962.0	E980.4
specified NEC	967.8	E852.8	E937.8	E950.2	E962.0	E980.2
Narcotine	975.4	E858.6	E945.4	E950.4	E962.0	E980.4
Nardil	969.01◄ⅲ	E854.0	E939.0	E950.3	E962.0	E980.3
Natrium cyanide - *see* Cyanide(s)	—	—	—	—	—	—
Natural	—	—	—	—	—	—
blood (product)	964.7	E858.2	E934.7	E950.4	E962.0	E980.4
gas (piped)	987.1	E867	—	E951.0	E962.2	E981.0
incomplete combustion	986	E867	—	E951.0	E962.2	E981.0
Nealbarbital, nealbarbitone	967.0	E851	E937.0	E950.1	E962.0	E980.1
Nectadon	975.4	E858.6	E945.4	E950.4	E962.0	E980.4
Nematocyst (sting)	989.5	E905.6	—	E950.9	E962.1	E980.9
Nembutal	967.0	E851	E937.0	E950.1	E962.0	E980.1
Neoarsphenamine	961.1	E857	E931.1	E950.4	E962.0	E980.4
Neocinchophen	974.7	E858.5	E944.7	E950.4	E962.0	E980.4
Neomycin	960.8	E856	E930.8	E950.4	E962.0	E980.4
ENT agent	976.6	E858.7	E946.6	E950.4	E962.0	E980.4
ophthalmic preparation	976.5	E858.7	E946.5	E950.4	E962.0	E980.4
topical NEC	976.0	E858.7	E946.0	E950.4	E962.0	E980.4
Neonal	967.0	E851	E937.0	E950.1	E962.0	E980.1
Neoprontosil	961.0	E857	E931.0	E950.4	E962.0	E980.4
Neosalvarsan	961.1	E857	E931.1	E950.4	E962.0	E980.4

◄ New   ◄ⅲ Revised   ~~deleted~~ Deleted   ● Use Additional Digit(s)

Substance	Poisoning	External Cause (E Code)				
		Accident	Therapeutic Use	Suicide Attempt	Assault	Undetermined
Neosilversalvarsan	961.1	E857	E931.1	E950.4	E962.0	E980.4
Neosporin	960.8	E856	E930.8	E950.4	E962.0	E980.4
ENT agent	976.6	E858.7	E946.6	E950.4	E962.0	E980.4
ophthalmic preparation	976.5	E858.7	E946.5	E950.4	E962.0	E980.4
topical NEC	976.0	E858.7	E946.0	E950.4	E962.0	E980.4
Neostigmine	971.0	E855.3	E941.0	E950.4	E962.0	E980.4
Neraval	967.0	E851	E937.0	E950.1	E962.0	E980.1
Neravan	967.0	E851	E937.0	E950.1	E962.0	E980.1
Nerium oleander	988.2	E865.4	—	E950.9	E962.1	E980.9
Nerve gases (war)	987.9	E869.9	—	E952.9	E962.2	E982.9
Nesacaine	968.9	E855.2	E938.9	E950.4	E962.0	E980.4
infiltration (subcutaneous)	968.5	E855.2	E938.5	E950.4	E962.0	E980.4
nerve block (peripheral) (plexus)	968.6	E855.2	E938.6	E950.4	E962.0	E980.4
Neurobarb	967.0	E851	E937.0	E950.1	E962.0	E980.1
Neuroleptics NEC	969.3	E853.8	E939.3	E950.3	E962.0	E980.3
Neuroprotective agent	977.8	E858.8	E947.8	E950.4	E962.0	E980.4
Neutral spirits	980.0	E860.1	—	E950.9	E962.1	E980.9
beverage	980.0	E860.0	—	E950.9	E962.1	E980.9
Niacin, niacinamide	972.2	E858.3	E942.2	E950.4	E962.0	E980.4
Nialamide	969.01 ◀▥	E854.0	E939.0	E950.3	E962.0	E980.3
Nickle (carbonyl) (compounds) (fumes) (tetracarbonyl) (vapor)	985.8	E866.4	—	E950.9	E962.1	E980.9
Niclosamide	961.6	E857	E931.6	E950.4	E962.0	E980.4
Nicomorphine	965.09	E850.2	E935.2	E950.0	E962.0	E980.0
Nicotinamide	972.2	E858.3	E942.2	E950.4	E962.0	E980.4
Nicotine (insecticide) (spray) (sulfate) NEC	989.4	E863.4	—	E950.6	E962.1	E980.7
not insecticide	989.89	E866.8	—	E950.9	E962.1	E980.9
Nicotinic acid (derivatives)	972.2	E858.3	E942.2	E950.4	E962.0	E980.4
Nicotinyl alcohol	972.2	E858.3	E942.2	E950.4	E962.0	E980.4
Nicoumalone	964.2	E858.2	E934.2	E950.4	E962.0	E980.4
Nifenazone	965.5	E850.5	E935.5	E950.0	E962.0	E980.0
Nifuraldezone	961.9	E857	E931.9	E950.4	E962.0	E980.4
Nightshade (deadly)	988.2	E865.4	—	E950.9	E962.1	E980.9
Nikethamide	970.0	E854.3	E940.0	E950.4	E962.0	E980.4
Nilstat	960.1	E856	E930.1	E950.4	E962.0	E980.4
topical	976.0	E858.7	E946.0	E950.4	E962.0	E980.4
Nimodipine	977.8	E858.8	E947.8	E950.4	E962.0	E980.4
Niridazole	961.6	E857	E931.6	E950.4	E962.0	E980.4
Nisentil	965.09	E850.2	E935.2	E950.0	E962.0	E980.0
Nitrates	972.4	E858.3	E942.4	E950.4	E962.0	E980.4

◀ New   ◀▥ Revised   ~~deleted~~ Deleted   ● Use Additional Digit(s)

Substance	Poisoning	External Cause (E Code) Accident	Therapeutic Use	Suicide Attempt	Assault	Undetermined
Nitrazepam	969.4	E853.2	E939.4	E950.3	E962.0	E980.3
Nitric	—	—	—	—	—	—
acid (liquid)	983.1	E864.1	—	E950.7	E962.1	E980.6
vapor	987.8	E869.8	—	E952.8	E962.2	E982.8
oxide (gas)	987.2	E869.0	—	E952.8	E962.2	E982.8
Nitrite, amyl (medicinal) (vapor)	972.4	E858.3	E942.4	E950.4	E962.0	E980.4
Nitroaniline	983.0	E864.0	—	E950.7	E962.1	E980.6
vapor	987.8	E869.8	—	E952.8	E962.2	E982.8
Nitrobenzene, nitrobenzol	983.0	E864.0	—	E950.7	E962.1	E980.6
vapor	987.8	E869.8	—	E952.8	E962.2	E982.8
Nitrocellulose	976.3	E858.7	E946.3	E950.4	E962.0	E980.4
Nitrofuran derivatives	961.9	E857	E931.9	E950.4	E962.0	E980.4
Nitrofurantoin	961.9	E857	E931.9	E950.4	E962.0	E980.4
Nitrofurazone	976.0	E858.7	E946.0	E950.4	E962.0	E980.4
Nitrogen (dioxide) (gas) (oxide)	987.2	E869.0	—	E952.8	E962.2	E982.8
mustard (antineoplastic)	963.1	E858.1	E933.1	E950.4	E962.0	E980.4
Nitroglycerin, nitroglycerol (medicinal)	972.4	E858.3	E942.4	E950.4	E962.0	E980.4
nonmedicinal	989.89	E866.8	—	E950.9	E962.1	E980.9
fumes	987.8	E869.8	—	E952.8	E962.2	E982.8
Nitrohydrochloric acid	983.1	E864.1	—	E950.7	E962.1	E980.6
Nitromersol	976.0	E858.7	E946.0	E950.4	E962.0	E980.4
Nitronaphthalene	983.0	E864.0	—	E950.7	E962.2	E980.6
Nitrophenol	983.0	E864.0	—	E950.7	E962.2	E980.6
Nitrothiazol	961.6	E857	E931.6	E950.4	E962.0	E980.4
Nitrotoluene, nitrotoluol	983.0	E864.0	—	E950.7	E962.1	E980.6
vapor	987.8	E869.8	—	E952.8	E962.2	E982.8
Nitrous	968.2	E855.1	E938.2	E950.4	E962.0	E980.4
acid (liquid)	983.1	E864.1	—	E950.7	E962.1	E980.6
fumes	987.2	E869.0	—	E952.8	E962.2	E982.8
oxide (anesthetic) NEC	968.2	E855.1	E938.2	E950.4	E962.0	E980.4
Nitrozone	976.0	E858.7	E946.0	E950.4	E962.0	E980.4
Noctec	967.1	E852.0	E937.1	E950.2	E962.0	E980.2
Noludar	967.5	E852.4	E937.5	E950.2	E962.0	E980.2
Noptil	967.0	E851	E937.0	E950.1	E962.0	E980.1
Noradrenalin	971.2	E855.5	E941.2	E950.4	E962.0	E980.4
Noramidopyrine	965.5	E850.5	E935.5	E950.0	E962.0	E980.0
Norepinephrine	971.2	E855.5	E941.2	E950.4	E962.0	E980.4
Norethandrolone	962.1	E858.0	E932.1	E950.4	E962.0	E980.4
Norethindrone	962.2	E858.0	E932.2	E950.4	E962.0	E980.4

◀ New   ◀▥ Revised   ~~deleted~~ Deleted   ● Use Additional Digit(s)

TABLE OF DRUGS AND CHEMICALS

Substance	Poisoning	External Cause (E Code)				
		Accident	Therapeutic Use	Suicide Attempt	Assault	Undetermined
Norethisterone	962.2	E858.0	E932.2	E950.4	E962.0	E980.4
Norethynodrel	962.2	E858.0	E932.2	E950.4	E962.0	E980.4
Norlestrin	962.2	E858.0	E932.2	E950.4	E962.0	E980.4
Norlutin	962.2	E858.0	E932.2	E950.4	E962.0	E980.4
Normison - *see* Benzodiazepines	—	—	—	—	—	—
Normorphine	965.09	E850.2	E935.2	E950.0	E962.0	E980.0
Nortriptyline	969.05◄	E854.0	E939.0	E950.3	E962.0	E980.3
Noscapine	975.4	E858.6	E945.4	E950.4	E962.0	E980.4
Nose preparations	976.6	E858.7	E946.6	E950.4	E962.0	E980.4
Novobiocin	960.8	E856	E930.8	E950.4	E962.0	E980.4
Novocain (infiltration) (topical)	968.5	E855.2	E938.5	E950.4	E962.0	E980.4
nerve block (peripheral) (plexus)	968.6	E855.2	E938.6	E950.4	E962.0	E980.4
spinal	968.7	E855.2	E938.7	E950.4	E962.0	E980.4
Noxythiolin	961.9	E857	E931.9	E950.4	E962.0	E980.4
NPH Iletin (insulin)	962.3	E858.0	E932.3	E950.4	E962.0	E980.4
Numorphan	965.09	E850.2	E935.2	E950.0	E962.0	E980.0
Nunol	967.0	E851	E937.0	E950.1	E962.0	E980.1
Nupercaine (spinal anesthetic)	968.7	E855.2	E938.7	E950.4	E962.0	E980.4
topical (surface)	968.5	E855.2	E938.5	E950.4	E962.0	E980.4
Nutmeg oil (liniment)	976.3	E858.7	E946.3	E950.4	E962.0	E980.4
Nux vomica	989.1	E863.7	—	E950.6	E962.1	E980.7
Nydrazid	961.8	E857	E931.8	E950.4	E962.0	E980.4
Nylidrin	971.2	E855.5	E941.2	E950.4	E962.0	E980.4
Nystatin	960.1	E856	E930.1	E950.4	E962.0	E980.4
topical	976.0	E858.7	E946.0	E950.4	E962.0	E980.4
Nytol	963.0	E858.1	E933.0	E950.4	E962.0	E980.4
Oblivion	967.8	E852.8	E937.8	E950.2	E962.0	E980.2
Octyl nitrite	972.4	E858.3	E942.4	E950.4	E962.0	E980.4
Oestradiol (cypionate) (dipropionate) (valerate)	962.2	E858.0	E932.2	E950.4	E962.0	E980.4
Oestriol	962.2	E858.0	E932.2	E950.4	E962.0	E980.4
Oestrone	962.2	E858.0	E932.2	E950.4	E962.0	E980.4
Oil (of) NEC	989.89	E866.8	—	E950.9	E962.1	E980.9
bitter almond	989.0	E866.8	—	E950.9	E962.1	E980.9
camphor	976.1	E858.7	E946.1	E950.4	E962.0	E980.4
colors	989.89	E861.6	—	E950.9	E962.1	E980.9
fumes	987.8	E869.8	—	E952.8	E962.2	E982.8
lubricating	981	E862.2	—	E950.9	E962.1	E980.9
specified source, other - *see* substance specified	—	—	—	—	—	—

◄ New   ◄▥ Revised   deleted Deleted   ● Use Additional Digit(s)

Substance	Poisoning	External Cause (E Code)				
		Accident	Therapeutic Use	Suicide Attempt	Assault	Undetermined
Oil (of) NEC *(Continued)*						
vitriol (liquid)	983.1	E864.1	—	E950.7	E962.1	E980.6
fumes	987.8	E869.8	—	E952.8	E962.2	E982.8
wintergreen (bitter) NEC	976.3	E858.7	E946.3	E950.4	E962.0	E980.4
Ointments NEC	976.9	E858.7	E946.9	E950.4	E962.0	E980.4
Oleander	988.2	E865.4	—	E950.9	E962.1	E980.9
Oleandomycin	960.3	E856	E930.3	E950.4	E962.0	E980.4
Oleovitamin A	963.5	E858.1	E933.5	E950.4	E962.0	E980.4
Oleum ricini	973.1	E858.4	E943.1	E950.4	E962.0	E980.4
Olive oil (medicinal) NEC	973.2	E858.4	E943.2	E950.4	E962.0	E980.4
OMPA	989.3	E863.1	—	E950.6	E962.1	E980.7
Oncovin	963.1	E858.1	E933.1	E950.4	E962.0	E980.4
Ophthaine	968.5	E855.2	E938.5	E950.4	E962.0	E980.4
Ophthetic	968.5	E855.2	E938.5	E950.4	E962.0	E980.4
Opiates, opioids, opium NEC	965.00	E850.2	E935.2	E950.0	E962.0	E980.0
antagonists	970.1	E854.3	E940.1	E950.4	E962.0	E980.4
Oracon	962.2	E858.0	E932.2	E950.4	E962.0	E980.4
Oragrafin	977.8	E858.8	E947.8	E950.4	E962.0	E980.4
Oral contraceptives	962.2	E858.0	E932.2	E950.4	E962.0	E980.4
Orciprenaline	975.1	E858.6	E945.1	E950.4	E962.0	E980.4
Organidin	975.5	E858.6	E945.5	E950.4	E962.0	E980.4
Organophosphates	989.3	E863.1	—	E950.6	E962.1	E980.7
Orimune	979.5	E858.8	E949.5	E950.4	E962.0	E980.4
Orinase	962.3	E858.0	E932.3	E950.4	E962.0	E980.4
Orphenadrine	966.4	E855.0	E936.4	E950.4	E962.0	E980.4
Ortal (sodium)	967.0	E851	E937.0	E950.1	E962.0	E980.1
Orthoboric acid	976.0	E858.7	E946.0	E950.4	E962.0	E980.4
ENT agent	976.6	E858.7	E946.6	E950.4	E962.0	E980.4
ophthalmic preparation	976.5	E858.7	E946.5	E950.4	E962.0	E980.4
Orthocaine	968.5	E855.2	E938.5	E950.4	E962.0	E980.4
Ortho-Novum	962.2	E858.0	E932.2	E950.4	E962.0	E980.4
Orthotolidine (reagent)	977.8	E858.8	E947.8	E950.4	E962.0	E980.4
Osmic acid (liquid)	983.1	E864.1	—	E950.7	E962.1	E980.6
fumes	987.8	E869.8	—	E952.8	E962.2	E982.8
Osmotic diuretics	974.4	E858.5	E944.4	E950.4	E962.0	E980.4
Ouabain	972.1	E858.3	E942.1	E950.4	E962.0	E980.4
Ovarian hormones (synthetic substitutes)	962.2	E858.0	E932.2	E950.4	E962.0	E980.4
Ovral	962.2	E858.0	E932.2	E950.4	E962.0	E980.4

◀ New   ◀▥ Revised   ~~deleted~~ Deleted   ● Use Additional Digit(s)

Substance	Poisoning	External Cause (E Code)				
		Accident	Therapeutic Use	Suicide Attempt	Assault	Undetermined
Ovulation suppressants	962.2	E858.0	E932.2	E950.4	E962.0	E980.4
Ovulen	962.2	E858.0	E932.2	E950.4	E962.0	E980.4
Oxacillin (sodium)	960.0	E856	E930.0	E950.4	E962.0	E980.4
Oxalic acid	983.1	E864.1	—	E950.7	E962.1	E980.6
Oxanamide	969.5	E853.8	E939.5	E950.3	E962.0	E980.3
Oxandrolone	962.1	E858.0	E932.1	E950.4	E962.0	E980.4
Oxaprozin	965.61	E850.6	E935.6	E950.0	E962.0	E980.0
Oxazepam	969.4	E853.2	E939.4	E950.3	E962.0	E980.3
Oxazolidine derivatives	966.0	E855.0	E936.0	E950.4	E962.0	E980.4
Ox bile extract	973.4	E858.4	E943.4	E950.4	E962.0	E980.4
Oxedrine	971.2	E855.5	E941.2	E950.4	E962.0	E980.4
Oxeladin	975.4	E858.6	E945.4	E950.4	E962.0	E980.4
Oxethazaine NEC	968.5	E855.2	E938.5	E950.4	E962.0	E980.4
Oxidizing agents NEC	983.9	E864.3	—	E950.7	E962.1	E980.6
Oxolinic acid	961.3	E857	E931.3	E950.4	E962.0	E980.4
Oxophenarsine	961.1	E857	E931.1	E950.4	E962.0	E980.4
Oxsoralen	976.3	E858.7	E946.3	E950.4	E962.0	E980.4
Oxtriphylline	976.7	E858.6	E945.7	E950.4	E962.0	E980.4
Oxybuprocaine	968.5	E855.2	E938.5	E950.4	E962.0	E980.4
Oxybutynin	975.1	E858.6	E945.1	E950.4	E962.0	E980.4
Oxycodone	965.09	E850.2	E935.2	E950.0	E962.0	E980.0
Oxygen	987.8	E869.8	—	E952.8	E962.2	E982.8
Oxylone	976.0	E858.7	E946.0	E950.4	E962.0	E980.4
ophthalmic preparation	976.5	E858.7	E946.5	E950.4	E962.0	E980.4
Oxymesterone	962.1	E858.0	E932.1	E950.4	E962.0	E980.4
Oxymetazoline	971.2	E855.5	E941.2	E950.4	E962.0	E980.4
Oxymetholone	962.1	E858.0	E932.1	E950.4	E962.0	E980.4
Oxymorphone	965.09	E850.2	E935.2	E950.0	E962.0	E980.0
Oxypertine	969.09◀▥	E854.0	E939.0	E950.3	E962.0	E980.3
Oxyphenbutazone	965.5	E850.5	E935.5	E950.0	E962.0	E980.0
Oxyphencyclimine	971.1	E855.4	E941.1	E950.4	E962.0	E980.4
Oxyphenisatin	973.1	E858.4	E943.1	E950.4	E962.0	E980.4
Oxyphenonium	971.1	E855.4	E941.1	E950.4	E962.0	E980.4
Oxyquinoline	961.3	E857	E931.3	E950.4	E962.0	E980.4
Oxytetracycline	960.4	E856	E930.4	E950.4	E962.0	E980.4
Oxytocics	975.0	E858.6	E945.0	E950.4	E962.0	E980.4
Oxytocin	975.0	E858.6	E945.0	E950.4	E962.0	E980.4
Ozone	987.8	E869.8	—	E952.8	E962.2	E982.8
PABA	976.3	E858.7	E946.3	E950.4	E962.0	E980.4

◀ New   ◀▥ Revised   deleted Deleted   ● Use Additional Digit(s)

Substance	Poisoning	External Cause (E Code)				
		Accident	Therapeutic Use	Suicide Attempt	Assault	Undetermined
Packed red cells	964.7	E858.2	E934.7	E950.4	E962.0	E980.4
Paint NEC	989.89	E861.6	—	E950.9	E962.1	E980.9
cleaner	982.8	E862.9	—	E950.9	E962.1	E980.9
fumes NEC	987.8	E869.8	—	E952.8	E962.1	E982.8
lead (fumes)	984.0	E861.5	—	E950.9	E962.1	E980.9
solvent NEC	982.8	E862.9	—	E950.9	E962.1	E980.9
stripper	982.8	E862.9	—	E950.9	E962.1	E980.9
Palfium	965.09	E850.2	E935.2	E950.0	E962.0	E980.0
Palivizumab	979.9	E858.8	E949.6	E950.4	E962.0	E980.4
Paludrine	961.4	E857	E931.4	E950.4	E962.0	E980.4
PAM	977.2	E855.8	E947.2	E950.4	E962.0	E980.4
Pamaquine (napthoate)	961.4	E857	E931.4	E950.4	E962.0	E980.4
Pamprin	965.1	E850.3	E935.3	E950.0	E962.0	E980.0
Panadol	965.4	E850.4	E935.4	E950.0	E962.0	E980.0
Pancreatic dornase (mucolytic)	963.4	E858.1	E933.4	E950.4	E962.0	E980.4
Pancreatin	973.4	E858.4	E943.4	E950.4	E962.0	E980.4
Pancrelipase	973.4	E858.4	E943.4	E950.4	E962.0	E980.4
Pangamic acid	963.5	E858.1	E933.5	E950.4	E962.0	E980.4
Panthenol	963.5	E858.1	E933.5	E950.4	E962.0	E980.4
topical	976.8	E858.7	E946.8	E950.4	E962.0	E980.4
Pantopaque	977.8	E858.8	E947.8	E950.4	E962.0	E980.4
Pantopon	965.00	E850.2	E935.2	E950.0	E962.0	E980.0
Pantothenic acid	963.5	E858.1	E933.5	E950.4	E962.0	E980.4
Panwarfin	964.2	E858.2	E934.2	E950.4	E962.0	E980.4
Papain	973.4	E858.4	E943.4	E950.4	E962.0	E980.4
Papaverine	972.5	E858.3	E942.5	E950.4	E962.0	E980.4
Para-aminobenzoic acid	976.3	E858.7	E946.3	E950.4	E962.0	E980.4
Para-aminophenol derivatives	965.4	E850.4	E935.4	E950.0	E962.0	E980.0
Para-aminosalicylic acid (derivatives)	961.8	E857	E931.8	E950.4	E962.0	E980.4
Paracetaldehyde (medicinal)	967.2	E852.1	E937.2	E950.2	E962.0	E980.2
Paracetamol	965.4	E850.4	E935.4	E950.0	E962.0	E980.0
Paracodin	965.09	E850.2	E935.2	E950.0	E962.0	E980.0
Paradione	966.0	E855.0	E936.0	E950.4	E962.0	E980.4
Paraffin(s) (wax)	981	E862.3	—	E950.9	E962.1	E980.9
liquid (medicinal)	973.2	E858.4	E943.2	E950.4	E962.0	E980.4
nonmedicinal (oil)	981	E962.1	—	E950.9	E962.1	E980.9
Paraldehyde (medicinal)	967.2	E852.1	E937.2	E950.2	E962.0	E980.2
Paramethadione	966.0	E855.0	E936.0	E950.4	E962.0	E980.4
Paramethasone	962.0	E858.0	E932.0	E950.4	E962.0	E980.4

◀ New   ◀||| Revised   ~~deleted~~ Deleted   ● Use Additional Digit(s)

Substance	Poisoning	External Cause (E Code)				
		Accident	Therapeutic Use	Suicide Attempt	Assault	Undetermined
Paraquat	989.4	E863.5	—	E950.6	E962.1	E980.7
Parasympatholytics	971.1	E855.4	E941.1	E950.4	E962.0	E980.4
Parasympathomimetics	971.0	E855.3	E941.0	E950.4	E962.0	E980.4
Parathion	989.3	E863.1	—	E950.6	E962.1	E980.7
Parathormone	962.6	E858.0	E932.6	E950.4	E962.0	E980.4
Parathyroid (derivatives)	962.6	E858.0	E932.6	E950.4	E962.0	E980.4
Paratyphoid vaccine	978.1	E858.8	E948.1	E950.4	E962.0	E980.4
Paredrine	971.2	E855.5	E941.2	E950.4	E962.0	E980.4
Paregoric	965.00	E850.2	E935.2	E950.0	E962.0	E980.0
Pargyline	972.3	E858.3	E942.3	E950.4	E962.0	E980.4
Paris green	985.1	E866.3	—	E950.8	E962.1	E980.8
insecticide	985.1	E863.4	—	E950.8	E962.1	E980.8
Parnate	969.01◀▥	E854.0	E939.0	E950.3	E962.0	E980.3
Paromomycin	960.8	E856	E930.8	E950.4	E962.0	E980.4
Paroxypropione	963.1	E858.1	E933.1	E950.4	E962.0	E980.4
Parzone	965.09	E850.2	E935.2	E950.0	E962.0	E980.0
PAS	961.8	E857	E931.8	E950.4	E962.0	E980.4
PCBs	981	E862.3	—	E950.9	E962.1	E980.9
PCP (pentachlorophenol)	989.4	E863.6	—	E950.6	E962.1	E980.7
herbicide	989.4	E863.5	—	E950.6	E962.1	E980.7
insecticide	989.4	E863.4	—	E950.6	E962.1	E980.7
phencyclidine	968.3	E855.1	E938.3	E950.4	E962.0	E980.4
Peach kernel oil (emulsion)	973.2	E858.4	E943.2	E950.4	E962.0	E980.4
Peanut oil (emulsion) NEC	973.2	E858.4	E943.2	E950.4	E962.0	E980.4
topical	976.3	E858.7	E946.3	E950.4	E962.0	E980.4
Pearly Gates (morning glory seeds)	969.6	E854.1	E939.6	E950.3	E962.0	E980.3
Pecazine	969.1	E853.0	E939.1	E950.3	E962.0	E980.3
Pecilocin	960.1	E856	E930.1	E950.4	E962.0	E980.4
Pectin (with kaolin) NEC	973.5	E858.4	E943.5	E950.4	E962.0	E980.4
Pelletierine tannate	961.6	E857	E931.6	E950.4	E962.0	E980.4
Pemoline	969.79◀▥	E854.2	E939.7	E950.3	E962.0	E980.3
Pempidine	972.3	E858.3	E942.3	E950.4	E962.0	E980.4
Penamecillin	960.0	E856	E930.0	E950.4	E962.0	E980.4
Penethamate hydriodide	960.0	E856	E930.0	E950.4	E962.0	E980.4
Penicillamine	963.8	E858.1	E933.8	E950.4	E962.0	E980.4
Penicillin (any type)	960.0	E856	E930.0	E950.4	E962.0	E980.4
Penicillinase	963.4	E858.1	E933.4	E950.4	E962.0	E980.4
Pentachlorophenol (fungicide)	989.4	E863.6	—	E950.6	E962.1	E980.7
herbicide	989.4	E863.5	—	E950.6	E962.1	E980.7
insecticide	989.4	E863.4	—	E950.6	E962.1	E980.7

◀ New   ◀▥ Revised   ~~deleted~~ Deleted   ● Use Additional Digit(s)

Substance	Poisoning	External Cause (E Code)				
		Accident	Therapeutic Use	Suicide Attempt	Assault	Undetermined
Pentaerythritol	972.4	E858.3	E942.4	E950.4	E962.0	E980.4
chloral	967.1	E852.0	E937.1	E950.2	E962.0	E980.2
tetranitrate NEC	972.4	E858.3	E942.4	E950.4	E962.0	E980.4
Pentagastrin	977.8	E858.8	E947.8	E950.4	E962.0	E980.4
Pentalin	982.3	E862.4	—	E950.9	E962.1	E980.9
Pentamethonium (bromide)	972.3	E858.3	E942.3	E950.4	E962.0	E980.4
Pentamidine	961.5	E857	E931.5	E950.4	E962.0	E980.4
Pentanol	980.8	E860.8	—	E950.9	E962.1	E980.9
Pentaquine	961.4	E857	E931.4	E950.4	E962.0	E980.4
Pentazocine	965.8	E850.8	E935.8	E950.0	E962.0	E980.0
Penthienate	971.1	E855.4	E941.1	E950.4	E962.0	E980.4
Pentobarbital, pentobarbitone (sodium)	967.0	E851	E937.0	E950.1	E962.0	E980.1
Pentolinium (tartrate)	972.3	E858.3	E942.3	E950.4	E962.0	E980.4
Pentothal	968.3	E855.1	E938.3	E950.4	E962.0	E980.4
Pentylenetetrazol	970.0	E854.3	E940.0	E950.4	E962.0	E980.4
Pentylsalicylamide	961.8	E857	E931.8	E950.4	E962.0	E980.4
Pepsin	973.4	E858.4	E943.4	E950.4	E962.0	E980.4
Peptavlon	977.8	E858.8	E947.8	E950.4	E962.0	E980.4
Percaine (spinal)	968.7	E855.2	E938.7	E950.4	E962.0	E980.4
topical (surface)	968.5	E855.2	E938.5	E950.4	E962.0	E980.4
Perchloroethylene (vapor)	982.3	E862.4	—	E950.9	E962.1	E980.9
medicinal	961.6	E857	E931.6	E950.4	E962.0	E980.4
Percodan	965.09	E850.2	E935.2	E950.0	E962.0	E980.0
Percogesic	965.09	E850.2	E935.2	E950.0	E962.0	E980.0
Percorten	962.0	E858.0	E932.0	E950.4	E962.0	E980.4
Pergonal	962.4	E858.0	E932.4	E950.4	E962.0	E980.4
Perhexiline	972.4	E858.3	E942.4	E950.4	E962.0	E980.4
Periactin	963.0	E858.1	E933.0	E950.4	E962.0	E980.4
Periclor	967.1	E852.0	E937.1	E950.2	E962.0	E980.2
Pericyazine	969.1	E853.0	E939.1	E950.3	E962.0	E980.3
Peritrate	972.4	E858.3	E942.4	E950.4	E962.0	E980.4
Permanganates NEC	983.9	E864.3	—	E950.7	E962.1	E980.6
potassium (topical)	976.0	E858.7	E946.0	E950.4	E962.0	E980.4
Pernocton	967.0	E851	E937.0	E950.1	E962.0	E980.1
Pernoston	967.0	E851	E937.0	E950.1	E962.0	E980.1
Peronin(e)	965.09	E850.2	E935.2	E950.0	E962.0	E980.0
Perphenazine	969.1	E853.0	E939.1	E950.3	E962.0	E980.3
Pertofrane	969.05◀▦	E854	E939.0	E950.3	E962.0	E980.3

TABLE OF DRUGS AND CHEMICALS

Substance	Poisoning	External Cause (E Code) Accident	Therapeutic Use	Suicide Attempt	Assault	Undetermined
Pertussis	—	—	—	—	—	—
immune serum (human)	964.6	E858.2	E934.6	E950.4	E962.0	E980.4
vaccine (with diphtheria toxoid) (with tetanus toxoid)	978.6	E858.8	E948.6	E950.4	E962.0	E980.4
Peruvian balsam	976.8	E858.7	E946.8	E950.4	E962.0	E980.4
Pesticides (dust) (fumes) (vapor)	989.4	E863.4	—	E950.6	E962.1	E980.7
arsenic	985.1	E863.4	—	E950.8	E962.1	E980.8
chlorinated	989.2	E863.0	—	E950.6	E962.1	E980.7
cyanide	989.0	E863.4	—	E950.6	E962.1	E980.7
kerosene	981	E863.4	—	E950.6	E962.1	E980.7
mixture (of compounds)	989.4	E863.3	—	E950.6	E962.1	E980.7
naphthalene	983.0	E863.4	—	E950.7	E962.1	E980.6
organochlorine (compounds)	989.2	E863.0	—	E950.6	E962.1	E980.7
petroleum (distillate) (products) NEC	981	E863.4	—	E950.6	E962.1	E980.7
specified ingredient NEC	989.4	E863.4	—	E950.6	E962.1	E980.7
strychnine	989.1	E863.4	—	E950.6	E962.1	E980.7
thallium	985.8	E863.7	—	E950.6	E962.1	E980.7
Pethidine (hydrochloride)	965.09	E850.2	E935.2	E950.0	E962.0	E980.0
Petrichloral	967.1	E852.0	E937.1	E950.2	E962.0	E980.2
Petrol	981	E862.1	—	E950.9	E962.1	E980.9
vapor	987.1	E869.8	—	E952.8	E962.2	E982.8
Petrolatum (jelly) (ointment)	976.3	E858.7	E946.3	E950.4	E962.0	E980.4
hydrophilic	976.3	E858.7	E946.3	E950.4	E962.0	E980.4
liquid	973.2	E858.4	E943.2	E950.4	E962.0	E980.4
topical	976.3	E858.7	E946.3	E950.4	E962.0	E980.4
nonmedicinal	981	E862.1	—	E950.9	E962.1	E980.9
Petroleum (cleaners) (fuels) (products) NEC	981	E862.1	—	E950.9	E962.1	E980.9
benzin(e) - see Ligroin	—	—	—	—	—	—
ether - see Ligroin	—	—	—	—	—	—
jelly - see Petrolatum	—	—	—	—	—	—
aphtha - see Ligroin	—	—	—	—	—	—
pesticide	981	E863.4	—	E950.6	E962.1	E980.7
solids	981	E862.3	—	E950.9	E962.1	E980.9
solvents	981	E862.0	—	E950.9	E962.1	E980.9
vapor	987.1	E869.8	—	E952.8	E962.2	E982.8
Peyote	969.6	E854.1	E939.6	E950.3	E962.0	E980.3
Phanodorm, phanodorn	967.0	E851	E937.0	E950.1	E962.0	E980.1
Phanquinone, phanquone	961.5	E857	E931.5	E950.4	E962.0	E980.4
Pharmaceutical excipient or adjunct	977.4	E858.8	E947.4	E950.4	E962.0	E980.4
Phenacemide	966.3	E855.0	E936.3	E950.4	E962.0	E980.4

◀ New ◀▥ Revised ~~deleted~~ Deleted ● Use Additional Digit(s)

Substance	Poisoning	External Cause (E Code)				
		Accident	Therapeutic Use	Suicide Attempt	Assault	Undetermined
Phenacetin	965.4	E850.4	E935.4	E950.0	E962.0	E980.0
Phenadoxone	965.09	E850.2	E935.2	E950.0	E962.0	E980.0
Phenaglycodol	969.5	E853.8	E939.5	E950.3	E962.0	E980.3
Phenantoin	966.1	E855.0	E936.1	E950.4	E962.0	E980.4
Phenaphthazine reagent	977.8	E858.8	E947.8	E950.4	E962.0	E980.4
Phenazocine	965.09	E850.2	E935.2	E950.0	E962.0	E980.0
Phenazone	965.5	E850.5	E935.5	E950.0	E962.0	E980.0
Phenazopyridine	976.1	E858.7	E946.1	E950.4	E962.0	E980.4
Phenbenicillin	960.0	E856	E930.0	E950.4	E962.0	E980.4
Phenbutrazate	977.0	E858.8	E947.0	E950.4	E962.0	E980.4
Phencyclidine	968.3	E855.1	E938.3	E950.4	E962.0	E980.4
Phendimetrazine	977.0	E858.8	E947.0	E950.4	E962.0	E980.4
Phenelzine	969.01◄▦	E854.0	E939.0	E950.3	E962.0	E980.3
Phenergan	967.8	E852.8	E937.8	E950.2	E962.0	E980.2
Phenethicillin (potassium)	960.0	E856	E930.0	E950.4	E962.0	E980.4
Phenetsal	965.1	E850.3	E935.3	E950.0	E962.0	E980.0
Pheneturide	966.3	E855.0	E936.3	E950.4	E962.0	E980.4
Phenformin	962.3	E858.0	E932.3	E950.4	E962.0	E980.4
Phenglutarimide	971.1	E855.4	E941.1	E950.4	E962.0	E980.4
Phenicarbazide	965.8	E850.8	E935.8	E950.0	E962.0	E980.0
Phenindamine (tartrate)	963.0	E858.1	E933.0	E950.4	E962.0	E980.4
Phenindione	964.2	E858.2	E934.2	E950.4	E962.0	E980.4
Pheniprazine	969.01◄▦	E854.0	E939.0	E950.3	E962.0	E980.3
Pheniramine (maleate)	963.0	E858.1	E933.0	E950.4	E962.0	E980.4
Phenmetrazine	977.0	E858.8	E947.0	E950.4	E962.0	E980.4
Phenobal	967.0	E851	E937.0	E950.1	E962.0	E980.1
Phenobarbital	967.0	E851	E937.0	E950.1	E962.0	E980.1
Phenobarbitone	967.0	E851	E937.0	E950.1	E962.0	E980.1
Phenoctide	976.0	E858.7	E946.0	E950.4	E962.0	E980.4
Phenol (derivatives) NEC	983.0	E864.0	—	E950.7	E962.1	E980.6
disinfectant	983.0	E864.0	—	E950.7	E962.1	E980.6
pesticide	989.4	E863.4	—	E950.6	E962.1	E980.7
red	977.8	E858.8	E947.8	E950.4	E962.0	E980.4
Phenolphthalein	973.1	E858.4	E943.1	E950.4	E962.0	E980.4
Phenolsulfonphthalein	977.8	E858.8	E947.8	E950.4	E962.0	E980.4
Phenomorphan	965.09	E850.2	E935.2	E950.0	E962.0	E980.0
Phenonyl	967.0	E851	E937.0	E950.1	E962.0	E980.1
Phenoperidine	965.09	E850.2	E935.2	E950.0	E962.0	E980.0
Phenoquin	974.7	E858.5	E944.7	E950.4	E962.0	E980.4

◄ New   ◄▦ Revised   ~~deleted~~ Deleted   ● Use Additional Digit(s)

Substance	Poisoning	External Cause (E Code)				
		Accident	Therapeutic Use	Suicide Attempt	Assault	Undetermined
Phenothiazines (tranquilizers) NEC	969.1	E853.0	E939.1	E950.3	E962.0	E980.3
insecticide	989.3	E863.4	—	E950.6	E962.1	E980.7
Phenoxybenzamine	971.3	E855.6	E941.3	E950.4	E962.0	E980.4
Phenoxymethyl penicillin	960.0	E856	E930.0	E950.4	E962.0	E980.4
Phenprocoumon	964.2	E858.2	E934.2	E950.4	E962.0	E980.4
Phensuximide	966.2	E855.0	E936.2	E950.4	E962.0	E980.4
Phentermine	977.0	E858.8	E947.0	E950.4	E962.0	E980.4
Phentolamine	971.3	E855.6	E941.3	E950.4	E962.0	E980.4
Phenyl	—	—	—	—	—	—
butazone	965.5	E850.5	E935.5	E950.0	E962.0	E980.0
enediamine	983.0	E864.0	—	E950.7	E962.1	E980.6
hydrazine	983.0	E864.0	—	E950.7	E962.1	E980.6
antineoplastic	963.1	E858.1	E933.1	E950.4	E962.0	E980.4
mercuric compounds - see Mercury	—	—	—	—	—	—
salicylate	976.3	E858.7	E946.3	E950.4	E962.0	E980.4
Phenylephrine	971.2	E855.5	E941.2	E950.4	E962.0	E980.4
Phenylethylbiguanide	962.3	E858.0	E932.3	E950.4	E962.0	E980.4
Phenylpropanolamine	971.2	E855.5	E941.2	E950.4	E962.0	E980.4
Phenylsulfthion	989.3	E863.1	—	E950.6	E962.1	E980.7
Phenyramidol, phenyramidon	965.7	E850.7	E935.7	E950.0	E962.0	E980.0
Phenytoin	966.1	E855.0	E936.1	E950.4	E962.0	E980.4
pHisoHex	976.2	E858.7	E946.2	E950.4	E962.0	E980.4
Pholcodine	965.09	E850.2	E935.2	E950.0	E962.0	E980.0
Phorate	989.3	E863.1	—	E950.6	E962.1	E980.7
Phosdrin	989.3	E863.1	—	E950.6	E962.1	E980.7
Phosgene (gas)	987.8	E869.8	—	E952.8	E962.2	E982.8
Phosphate (tricresyl)	989.89	E866.8	—	E950.9	E962.1	E980.9
organic	989.3	E863.1	—	E950.6	E962.1	E980.7
solvent	982.8	E862.4	—	E950.9	E962.1	E980.9
Phosphine	987.8	E869.8	—	E952.8	E962.2	E982.8
fumigant	987.8	E863.8	—	E950.6	E962.2	E980.7
Phospholine	971.0	E855.3	E941.0	E950.4	E962.0	E980.4
Phosphoric acid	983.1	E864.1	—	E950.7	E962.1	E980.6
Phosphorus (compounds) NEC	983.9	E864.3	—	E950.7	E962.1	E980.6
rodenticide	983.9	E863.7	—	E950.7	E962.1	E980.6
Phthalimidoglutarimide	967.8	E852.8	E937.8	E950.2	E962.0	E980.2
Phthalylsulfathiazole	961.0	E857	E931.0	E950.4	E962.0	E980.4
Phylloquinone	964.3	E858.2	E934.3	E950.4	E962.0	E980.4
Physeptone	965.02	E850.1	E935.1	E950.0	E962.0	E980.0

◀ New   ◀▪▪ Revised   ~~deleted~~ Deleted   ● Use Additional Digit(s)

Substance	Poisoning	External Cause (E Code)				
		Accident	Therapeutic Use	Suicide Attempt	Assault	Undetermined
Physostigma venenosum	988.2	E865.4	—	E950.9	E962.1	E980.9
Physostigmine	971.0	E855.3	E941.0	E950.4	E962.0	E980.4
Phytolacca decandra	988.2	E865.4	—	E950.9	E962.1	E980.9
Phytomenadione	964.3	E858.2	E934.3	E950.4	E962.0	E980.4
Phytonadione	964.3	E858.2	E934.3	E950.4	E962.0	E980.4
Picric (acid)	983.0	E864.0	—	E950.7	E962.1	E980.6
Picrotoxin	970.0	E854.3	E940.0	E950.4	E962.0	E980.4
Pilocarpine	971.0	E855.3	E941.0	E950.4	E962.0	E980.4
Pilocarpus (jaborandi) extract	971.0	E855.3	E941.0	E950.4	E962.0	E980.4
Pimaricin	960.1	E856	E930.1	E950.4	E962.0	E980.4
Piminodine	965.09	E850.2	E935.2	E950.0	E962.0	E980.0
Pine oil, pinesol (disinfectant)	983.9	E861.4	—	E950.7	E962.1	E980.6
Pinkroot	961.6	E857	E931.6	E950.4	E962.0	E980.4
Pipadone	965.09	E850.2	E935.2	E950.0	E962.0	E980.0
Pipamazine	963.0	E858.1	E933.0	E950.4	E962.0	E980.4
Pipazethate	975.4	E858.6	E945.4	E950.4	E962.0	E980.4
Pipenzolate	971.1	E855.4	E941.1	E950.4	E962.0	E980.4
Piperacetazine	969.1	E853.0	E939.1	E950.3	E962.0	E980.3
Piperazine NEC	961.6	E857	E931.6	E950.4	E962.0	E980.4
estrone sulfate	962.2	E858.0	E932.2	E950.4	E962.0	E980.4
Piper cubeba	988.2	E865.4	—	E950.9	E962.1	E980.9
Piperidione	975.4	E858.6	E945.4	E950.4	E962.0	E980.4
Piperidolate	971.1	E855.4	E941.1	E950.4	E962.0	E980.4
Piperocaine	968.9	E855.2	E938.9	E950.4	E962.0	E980.4
infiltration (subcutaneous)	968.5	E855.2	E938.5	E950.4	E962.0	E980.4
nerve block (peripheral) (plexus)	968.6	E855.2	E938.6	E950.4	E962.0	E980.4
topical (surface)	968.5	E855.2	E938.5	E950.4	E962.0	E980.4
Pipobroman	963.1	E858.1	E933.1	E950.4	E962.0	E980.4
Pipradrol	970.8	E854.3	E940.8	E950.4	E962.0	E980.4
Piscidia (bark) (erythrina)	965.7	E850.7	E935.7	E950.0	E962.0	E980.0
Pitch	983.0	E864.0	—	E950.7	E962.1	E980.6
Pitkin's solution	968.7	E855.2	E938.7	E950.4	E962.0	E980.4
Pitocin	975.0	E858.6	E945.0	E950.4	E962.0	E980.4
Pitressin (tannate)	962.5	E858.0	E932.5	E950.4	E962.0	E980.4
Pituitary extracts (posterior)	962.5	E858.0	E932.5	E950.4	E962.0	E980.4
anterior	962.4	E858.0	E932.4	E950.4	E962.0	E980.4
Pituitrin	962.5	E858.0	E932.5	E950.4	E962.0	E980.4
Placental extract	962.9	E858.0	E932.9	E950.4	E962.0	E980.4
Placidyl	967.8	E852.8	E937.8	E950.2	E962.0	E980.2

◀ New   ◀ⅢⅢ Revised   ~~deleted~~ Deleted   ● Use Additional Digit(s)

Substance	Poisoning	External Cause (E Code)				
		Accident	Therapeutic Use	Suicide Attempt	Assault	Undetermined
Plague vaccine	978.3	E858.8	E948.3	E950.4	E962.0	E980.4
Plant foods or fertilizers NEC	989.89	E866.5	—	E950.9	E962.1	E980.9
mixed with herbicides	989.4	E863.5	—	E950.6	E962.1	E930.7
Plants, noxious, used as food	988.2	E865.9	—	E950.9	E962.1	E980.9
berries and seeds	988.2	E865.3	—	E950.9	E962.1	E980.9
specified type NEC	988.2	E865.4	—	E950.9	E962.1	E980.9
Plasma (blood)	964.7	E858.2	E934.7	E950.4	E962.0	E980.4
expanders	964.8	E858.2	E934.8	E950.4	E962.0	E980.4
Plasmanate	964.7	E858.2	E934.7	E950.4	E962.0	E980.4
Plegicil	969.1	E853.0	E939.1	E950.3	E962.0	E980.3
Podophyllin	976.4	E858.7	E946.4	E950.4	E962.0	E980.4
Podophyllum resin	976.4	E858.7	E946.4	E950.4	E962.0	E980.4
Poison NEC	989.9	E866.9	—	E950.9	E962.1	E980.9
Poisonous berries	988.2	E865.3	—	E950.9	E962.1	E980.9
Pokeweed (any part)	988.2	E865.4	—	E950.9	E962.1	E980.9
Poldine	971.1	E855.4	E941.1	E950.4	E962.0	E980.4
Poliomyelitis vaccine	979.5	E858.8	E949.5	E950.4	E962.0	E980.4
Poliovirus vaccine	979.5	E858.8	E949.5	E950.4	E962.0	E980.4
Polish (car) (floor) (furniture) (metal) (silver)	989.89	E861.2	—	E950.9	E962.1	E980.9
abrasive	989.89	E861.3	—	E950.9	E962.1	E980.9
porcelain	989.89	E861.3	—	E950.9	E962.1	E980.9
Poloxalkol	973.2	E858.4	E943.2	E950.4	E962.0	E980.4
Polyaminostyrene resins	974.5	E858.5	E944.5	E950.4	E962.0	E980.4
Polychlorinated biphenyl - *see* PCBs	—	—	—	—	—	—
Polycycline	960.4	E856	E930.4	E950.4	E962.0	E980.4
Polyester resin hardener	982.8	E862.4	—	E950.9	E962.1	E980.9
fumes	987.8	E869.8	—	E952.8	E962.2	E982.8
Polyestradiol (phosphate)	962.2	E858.0	E932.2	E950.4	E962.0	E980.4
Polyethanolamine alkyl sulfate	976.2	E858.7	E946.2	E950.4	E962.0	E980.4
Polyethylene glycol	976.3	E858.7	E946.3	E950.4	E962.0	E980.4
Polyferose	964.0	E858.2	E934.0	E950.4	E962.0	E980.4
Polymyxin B	960.8	E856	E930.8	E950.4	E962.0	E980.4
ENT agent	976.6	E858.7	E946.6	E950.4	E962.0	E980.4
ophthalmic preparation	976.5	E858.7	E946.5	E950.4	E962.0	E980.4
topical NEC	976.0	E858.7	E946.0	E950.4	E962.0	E980.4
Polynoxylin(e)	976.0	E858.7	E946.0	E950.4	E962.0	E980.4
Polyoxymethyleneurea	976.0	E858.7	E946.0	E950.4	E962.0	E980.4
Polytetrafluoroethylene (inhaled)	987.8	E869.8	—	E952.8	E962.2	E982.8
Polythiazide	974.3	E858.5	E944.3	E950.4	E962.0	E980.4

◀ New   ◀▦ Revised   ~~deleted~~ Deleted   ● Use Additional Digit(s)

Substance	Poisoning	External Cause (E Code)				
		Accident	Therapeutic Use	Suicide Attempt	Assault	Undetermined
Polyvinylpyrrolidone	964.8	E858.2	E934.8	E950.4	E962.0	E980.4
Pontocaine (hydrochloride) (infiltration) (topical)	968.5	E855.2	E938.5	E950.4	E962.0	E980.4
nerve block (peripheral) (plexus)	968.6	E855.2	E938.6	E950.4	E962.0	E980.4
spinal	968.7	E855.2	E938.7	E950.4	E962.0	E980.4
Pot	969.6	E854.1	E939.6	E950.3	E962.0	E980.3
Potash (caustic)	983.2	E864.2	—	E950.7	E962.1	E980.6
Potassic saline injection (lactated)	974.5	E858.5	E944.5	E950.4	E962.0	E980.4
Potassium (salts) NEC	974.5	E858.5	E944.5	E950.4	E962.0	E980.4
aminosalicylate	961.8	E857	E931.8	E950.4	E962.0	E980.4
arsenite (solution)	985.1	E866.3	—	E950.8	E962.1	E980.8
bichromate	983.9	E864.3	—	E950.7	E962.1	E980.6
bisulfate	983.9	E864.3	—	E950.7	E962.1	E980.6
bromide (medicinal) NEC	967.3	E852.2	E937.3	E950.2	E962.0	E980.2
carbonate	983.2	E864.2	—	E950.7	E962.1	E980.6
chlorate NEC	983.9	E864.3	—	E950.7	E962.1	E980.6
cyanide - see Cyanide	—	—	—	—	—	—
hydroxide	983.2	E864.2	—	E950.7	E962.1	E980.6
iodide (expectorant) NEC	975.5	E858.6	E945.5	E950.4	E962.0	E980.4
nitrate	989.89	E866.8	—	E950.9	E962.1	E980.9
oxalate	983.9	E864.3	—	E950.7	E962.1	E980.6
perchlorate NEC	977.8	E858.8	E947.8	E950.4	E962.0	E980.4
antithyroid	962.8	E858.0	E932.8	E950.4	E962.0	E980.4
permanganate	976.0	E858.7	E946.0	E950.4	E962.0	E980.4
nonmedicinal	983.9	E864.3	—	E950.7	E962.1	E980.6
Povidone-iodine (anti-infective) NEC	976.0	E858.7	E946.0	E950.4	E962.0	E980.4
Practolol	972.0	E858.3	E942.0	E950.4	E962.0	E980.4
Pralidoxime (chloride)	977.2	E858.8	E947.2	E950.4	E962.0	E980.4
Pramoxine	968.5	E855.2	E938.5	E950.4	E962.0	E980.4
Prazosin	972.6	E858.3	E942.6	E950.4	E962.0	E980.4
Prednisolone	962.0	E858.0	E932.0	E950.4	E962.0	E980.4
ENT agent	976.6	E858.7	E946.6	E950.4	E962.0	E980.4
ophthalmic preparation	976.5	E858.7	E946.5	E950.4	E962.0	E980.4
topical NEC	976.0	E858.7	E946.0	E950.4	E962.0	E980.4
Prednisone	962.0	E858.0	E932.0	E950.4	E962.0	E980.4
Pregnanediol	962.2	E858.0	E932.2	E950.4	E962.0	E980.4
Pregneninolone	962.2	E858.0	E932.2	E950.4	E962.0	E980.4
Preludin	977.0	E858.8	E947.0	E950.4	E962.0	E980.4
Premarin	962.2	E858.0	E932.2	E950.4	E962.0	E980.4
Prenylamine	972.4	E858.3	E942.4	E950.4	E962.0	E980.4

◀ New   ◀◀◀ Revised   ~~deleted~~ Deleted   ● Use Additional Digit(s)

TABLE OF DRUGS AND CHEMICALS

Substance	Poisoning	External Cause (E Code)				
		Accident	Therapeutic Use	Suicide Attempt	Assault	Undetermined
Preparation H	976.8	E858.7	E946.8	E950.4	E962.0	E980.4
Preservatives	989.89	E866.8	—	E950.9	E962.1	E980.9
Pride of China	988.2	E865.3	—	E950.9	E962.1	E980.9
Prilocaine	968.9	E855.2	E938.9	E950.4	E962.0	E980.4
infiltration (subcutaneous)	968.5	E855.2	E938.5	E950.4	E962.0	E980.4
nerve block (peripheral) (plexus)	968.6	E855.2	E938.6	E950.4	E962.0	E980.4
Primaquine	961.4	E857	E931.4	E950.4	E962.0	E980.4
Primidone	966.3	E855.0	E936.3	E950.4	E962.0	E980.4
Primula (veris)	988.2	E865.4	—	E950.9	E962.1	E980.9
Prinodol	965.09	E850.2	E935.2	E950.0	E962.0	E980.0
Priscol, Priscoline	971.3	E855.6	E941.3	E950.4	E962.0	E980.4
Privet	988.2	E865.4	—	E950.9	E962.1	E980.9
Privine	971.2	E855.5	E941.2	E950.4	E962.0	E980.4
Pro-Banthine	971.1	E855.4	E941.1	E950.4	E962.0	E980.4
Probarbital	967.0	E851	E937.0	E950.1	E962.0	E980.1
Probenecid	974.7	E858.5	E944.7	E950.4	E962.0	E980.4
Procainamide (hydrochloride)	972.0	E858.3	E942.0	E950.4	E962.0	E980.4
Procaine (hydrochloride) (infiltration) (topical)	968.5	E855.2	E938.5	E950.4	E962.0	E980.4
nerve block (periphreal) (plexus)	968.6	E855.2	E938.6	E950.4	E962.0	E980.4
penicillin G	960.0	E856	E930.0	E950.4	E962.0	E980.4
spinal	968.7	E855.2	E938.7	E950.4	E962.0	E980.4
Procalmidol	969.5	E853.8	E939.5	E950.3	E962.0	E980.3
Procarbazine	963.1	E858.1	E933.1	E950.4	E962.0	E980.4
Prochlorperazine	969.1	E853.0	E939.1	E950.3	E962.0	E980.3
Procyclidine	966.4	E855.0	E936.4	E950.4	E962.0	E980.4
Producer gas	986	E868.8	—	E952.1	E962.2	E982.1
Profenamine	966.4	E855.0	E936.4	E950.4	E962.0	E980.4
Profenil	975.1	E858.6	E945.1	E950.4	E962.0	E980.4
Progesterones	962.2	E858.0	E932.2	E950.4	E962.0	E980.4
Progestin	962.2	E858.0	E932.2	E950.4	E962.0	E980.4
Progestogens (with estrogens)	962.2	E858.0	E932.2	E950.4	E962.0	E980.4
Progestone	962.2	E858.0	E932.2	E950.4	E962.0	E980.4
Proguanil	961.4	E857	E931.4	E950.4	E962.0	E980.4
Prolactin	962.4	E858.0	E932.4	E950.4	E962.0	E980.4
Proloid	962.7	E858.0	E932.7	E950.4	E962.0	E980.4
Proluton	962.2	E858.0	E932.2	E950.4	E962.0	E980.4
Promacetin	961.8	E857	E931.8	E950.4	E962.0	E980.4
Promazine	969.1	E853.0	E939.1	E950.3	E962.0	E980.3
Promedrol	965.09	E850.2	E935.2	E950.0	E962.0	E980.0

◀ New   ◀ Revised   ~~deleted~~ Deleted   ● Use Additional Digit(s)

Substance	Poisoning	External Cause (E Code)				
		Accident	Therapeutic Use	Suicide Attempt	Assault	Undetermined
Promethazine	967.8	E852.8	E937.8	E950.2	E962.0	E980.2
Promine	961.8	E857	E931.8	E950.4	E962.0	E980.4
Pronestyl (hydrochloride)	972.0	E858.3	E942.0	E950.4	E962.0	E980.4
Pronetalol, pronethalol	972.0	E858.3	E942.0	E950.4	E962.0	E980.4
Prontosil	961.0	E857	E931.0	E950.4	E962.0	E980.4
Propamidine isethionate	961.5	E857	E931.5	E950.4	E962.0	E980.4
Propanal (medicinal)	967.8	E852.8	E937.8	E950.2	E962.0	E980.2
Propane (gas) (distributed in mobile container)	987.0	E868.0	—	E951.1	E962.2	E981.1
distributed through pipes	987.0	E867	—	E951.0	E962.2	E981.0
incomplete combustion of - *see* Carbon monoxide, Propane	—	—	—	—	—	—
Propanidid	968.3	E855.1	E938.3	E950.4	E962.0	E980.4
Propanol	980.3	E860.4	—	E950.9	E962.1	E980.9
Propantheline	971.1	E855.4	E941.1	E950.4	E962.0	E980.4
Proparacaine	968.5	E855.2	E938.5	E950.4	E962.0	E980.4
Propatyl nitrate	972.4	E858.3	E942.4	E950.4	E962.0	E980.4
Propicillin	960.0	E856	E930.0	E950.4	E962.0	E980.4
Propiolactone (vapor)	987.8	E869.8	—	E952.8	E962.2	E982.8
Propiomazine	967.8	E852.8	E937.8	E950.2	E962.0	E980.2
Propionaldehyde (medicinal)	967.8	E852.8	E937.8	E950.2	E962.0	E980.2
Propionate compound	976.0	E858.7	E946.0	E950.4	E962.0	E980.4
Propion gel	976.0	E858.7	E946.0	E950.4	E962.0	E980.4
Propitocaine	968.9	E855.2	E938.9	E950.4	E962.0	E980.4
infiltration (subcutaneous)	968.5	E855.2	E938.5	E950.4	E962.0	E980.4
nerve block (peripheral) (plexus)	968.6	E855.2	E938.6	E950.4	E962.0	E980.4
Propoxur	989.3	E863.2	—	E950.6	E962.1	E980.7
Propoxycaine	968.9	E855.2	E938.9	E950.4	E962.0	E980.4
infiltration (subcutaneous)	968.5	E855.2	E938.5	E950.4	E962.0	E980.4
nerve block (peripheral) (plexus)	968.6	E855.2	E938.6	E950.4	E962.0	E980.4
topical (surface)	968.5	E855.2	E938.5	E950.4	E962.0	E980.4
Propoxyphene (hydrochloride)	965.8	E850.8	E935.8	E950.0	E962.0	E980.0
Propranolol	972.0	E858.3	E942.0	E950.4	E962.0	E980.4
Propyl	—	—	—	—	—	—
alcohol	980.3	E860.4	—	E950.9	E962.1	E980.9
carbinol	980.3	E860.4	—	E950.9	E962.1	E980.9
hexadrine	971.2	E855.5	E941.2	E950.4	E962.0	E980.4
iodone	977.8	E858.8	E947.8	E950.4	E962.0	E980.4
thiouracil	962.8	E858.0	E932.8	E950.4	E962.0	E980.4
Propylene	987.1	E869.8	—	E952.8	E962.2	E982.8
Propylparaben (ophthalmic)	976.5	E858.7	E946.5	E950.4	E962.0	E980.4

 New   ◀▥ Revised   ~~deleted~~ Deleted   ● Use Additional Digit(s)

Substance	Poisoning	External Cause (E Code)				
		Accident	Therapeutic Use	Suicide Attempt	Assault	Undetermined
Proscillaridin	972.1	E858.3	E942.1	E950.4	E962.0	E980.4
Prostaglandins	975.0	E858.6	E945.0	E950.4	E962.0	E980.4
Prostigmin	971.0	E855.3	E941.0	E950.4	E962.0	E980.4
Protamine (sulfate)	964.5	E858.2	E934.5	E950.4	E962.0	E980.4
zinc insulin	962.3	E858.0	E932.3	E950.4	E962.0	E980.4
Protectants (topical)	976.3	E858.7	E946.3	E950.4	E962.0	E980.4
Protein hydrolysate	974.5	E858.5	E944.5	E950.4	E962.0	E980.4
Prothiaden - *see* Dothiepin hydrochloride	—	—	—	—	—	—
Prothionamide	961.8	E857	E931.8	E950.4	E962.0	E980.4
Prothipendyl	969.5	E853.8	E939.5	E950.3	E962.0	E980.3
Protokylol	971.2	E855.5	E941.2	E950.4	E962.0	E980.4
Protopam	977.2	E858.8	E947.2	E950.4	E962.0	E980.4
Protoveratrine(s) (A) (B)	972.6	E858.3	E942.6	E950.4	E962.0	E980.4
Protriptyline	969.05◀	E854.0	E939.0	E950.3	E962.0	E980.3
Provera	962.2	E858.0	E932.2	E950.4	E962.0	E980.4
Provitamin A	963.5	E858.1	E933.5	E950.4	E962.0	E980.4
Proxymetacaine	968.5	E855.2	E938.5	E950.4	E962.0	E980.4
Proxyphylline	975.1	E858.6	E945.1	E950.4	E962.0	E980.4
Prozac - *see* Fluoxetine hydrochloride	—	—	—	—	—	—
Prunus	—	—	—	—	—	—
laurocerasus	988.2	E865.4	—	E950.9	E962.1	E980.9
virginiana	988.2	E865.4	—	E950.9	E962.1	E980.9
Prussic acid	989.0	E866.8	—	E950.9	E962.1	E980.9
vapor	987.7	E869.8	—	E952.8	E962.2	E982.8
Pseudoephedrine	971.2	E855.5	E941.2	E950.4	E962.0	E980.4
Psilocin	969.6	E854.1	E939.6	E950.3	E962.0	E980.3
Psilocybin	969.6	E854.1	E939.6	E950.3	E962.0	E980.3
PSP	977.8	E858.8	E947.8	E950.4	E962.0	E980.4
Psychedelic agents	969.6	E854.1	E939.6	E950.3	E962.0	E980.3
Psychodysleptics	969.6	E854.1	E939.6	E950.3	E962.0	E980.3
Psychostimulants	969.70◀	E854.2	E939.7	E950.3	E962.0	E980.3
Psychotherapeutic agents	969.9	E855.9	E939.9	E950.3	E962.0	E980.3
antidepressants	969.00◀	E854.0	E939.0	E950.3	E962.0	E980.3
specified NEC	969.8	E855.8	E939.8	E950.3	E962.0	E980.3
tranquilizers NEC	969.5	E853.9	E939.5	E950.3	E962.0	E980.3
Psychotomimetic agents	969.6	E854.1	E939.6	E950.3	E962.0	E980.3
Psychotropic agents	969.9	E854.8	E939.9	E950.3	E962.0	E980.3
specified NEC	969.8	E854.8	E939.8	E950.3	E962.0	E980.3
Psyllium	973.3	E858.4	E943.3	E950.4	E962.0	E980.4

◀ New   ◀▥ Revised   ~~deleted~~ Deleted   ● Use Additional Digit(s)

Substance	Poisoning	External Cause (E Code)				
		Accident	Therapeutic Use	Suicide Attempt	Assault	Undetermined
Pteroylglutamic acid	964.1	E858.2	E934.1	E950.4	E962.0	E980.4
Pteroyltriglutamate	963.1	E858.1	E933.1	E950.4	E962.0	E980.4
PTFE	987.8	E869.8	—	E952.8	E962.2	E982.8
Pulsatilla	988.2	E865.4	—	E950.9	E962.1	E980.9
Purex (bleach)	983.9	E864.3	—	E950.7	E962.1	E980.6
Purine diuretics	974.1	E858.5	E944.1	E950.4	E962.0	E980.4
Purinethol	963.1	E858.1	E933.1	E950.4	E962.0	E980.4
PVP	964.8	E858.2	E934.8	E950.4	E962.0	E980.4
Pyrabital	965.7	E850.7	E935.7	E950.0	E962.0	E980.0
Pyramidon	965.5	E850.5	E935.5	E950.0	E962.0	E980.0
Pyrantel (pamoate)	961.6	E857	E931.6	E950.4	E962.0	E980.4
Pyrathiazine	963.0	E858.1	E933.0	E950.4	E962.0	E980.4
Pyrazinamide	961.8	E857	E931.8	E950.4	E962.0	E980.4
Pyrazinoic acid (amide)	961.8	E857	E931.8	E950.4	E962.0	E980.4
Pyrazole (derivatives)	965.5	E850.5	E935.5	E950.0	E962.0	E980.0
Pyrazolone (analgesics)	965.5	E850.5	E935.5	E950.0	E962.0	E980.0
Pyrethrins, pyrethrum	989.4	E863.4	—	E950.6	E962.1	E980.7
Pyribenzamine	963.0	E858.1	E933.0	E950.4	E962.0	E980.4
Pyridine (liquid) (vapor)	982.0	E862.4	—	E950.9	E962.1	E980.9
aldoxime chloride	977.2	E858.8	E947.2	E950.4	E962.0	E980.4
Pyridium	976.1	E858.7	E946.1	E950.4	E962.0	E980.4
Pyridostigmine	971.0	E855.3	E941.0	E950.4	E962.0	E980.4
Pyridoxine	963.5	E858.1	E933.5	E950.4	E962.0	E980.4
Pyrilamine	963.0	E858.1	E933.0	E950.4	E962.0	E980.4
Pyrimethamine	961.4	E857	E931.4	E950.4	E962.0	E980.4
Pyrogallic acid	983.0	E864.0	—	E950.7	E962.1	E980.6
Pyroxylin	976.3	E858.7	E946.3	E950.4	E962.0	E980.4
Pyrrobutamine	963.0	E858.1	E933.0	E950.4	E962.0	E980.4
Pyrrocitine	968.5	E855.2	E938.5	E950.4	E962.0	E980.4
Pyrvinium (pamoate)	961.6	E857	E931.6	E950.4	E962.0	E980.4
PZI	962.3	E858.0	E932.3	E950.4	E962.0	E980.4
Quaalude	967.4	E852.3	E937.4	E950.2	E962.0	E980.2
Quaternary ammonium derivatives	971.1	E855.4	E941.1	E950.4	E962.0	E980.4
Quicklime	983.2	E864.2	—	E950.7	E962.1	E980.6
Quinacrine	961.3	E857	E931.3	E950.4	E962.0	E980.4
Quinaglute	972.0	E858.3	E942.0	E950.4	E962.0	E980.4
Quinalbarbitone	967.0	E851	E937.0	E950.1	E962.0	E980.1
Quinestradiol	962.2	E858.0	E932.2	E950.4	E962.0	E980.4
Quinethazone	974.3	E858.5	E944.3	E950.4	E962.0	E980.4

◀ New　◀▥ Revised　deleted Deleted　● Use Additional Digit(s)

Substance	Poisoning	External Cause (E Code)				
		Accident	Therapeutic Use	Suicide Attempt	Assault	Undetermined
Quinidine (gluconate) (polygalacturonate) (salts) (sulfate)	972.0	E858.3	E942.0	E950.4	E962.0	E980.4
Quinine	961.4	E857	E931.4	E950.4	E962.0	E980.4
Quiniobine	961.3	E857	E931.3	E950.4	E962.0	E980.4
Quinolines	961.3	E857	E931.3	E950.4	E962.0	E980.4
Quotane	968.5	E855.2	E938.5	E950.4	E962.0	E980.4
Rabies	—	—	—	—	—	—
immune globulin (human)	964.6	E858.2	E934.6	E950.4	E962.0	E980.4
vaccine	979.1	E858.8	E949.1	E950.4	E962.0	E980.4
Racemoramide	965.09	E850.2	E935.2	E950.0	E962.0	E980.0
Racemorphan	965.09	E850.2	E935.2	E950.0	E962.0	E980.0
Radiator alcohol	980.1	E860.2	—	E950.9	E962.1	E980.9
Radio-opaque (drugs) (materials)	977.8	E858.8	E947.8	E950.4	E962.0	E980.4
Ranunculus	988.2	E865.4	—	E950.9	E962.1	E980.9
Rat poison	989.4	E863.7	—	E950.6	E962.1	E980.7
Rattlesnake (venom)	989.5	E905.0	—	E950.9	E962.1	E980.9
Raudixin	972.6	E858.3	E942.6	E950.4	E962.0	E980.4
Rautensin	972.6	E858.3	E942.6	E950.4	E962.0	E980.4
Rautina	972.6	E858.3	E942.6	E950.4	E962.0	E980.4
Rautotal	972.6	E858.3	E942.6	E950.4	E962.0	E980.4
Rauwiloid	972.6	E858.3	E942.6	E950.4	E962.0	E980.4
Rauwoldin	972.6	E858.3	E942.6	E950.4	E962.0	E980.4
Rauwolfia (alkaloids)	972.6	E858.3	E942.6	E950.4	E962.0	E980.4
Realgar	985.1	E866.3	—	E950.8	E962.1	E980.8
Red cells, packed	964.7	E858.2	E934.7	E950.4	E962.0	E980.4
Reducing agents, industrial NEC	983.9	E864.3	—	E950.7	E962.1	E980.6
Refrigerant gas (freon)	987.4	E869.2	—	E952.8	E962.2	E982.8
not freon	987.9	E869.9	—	E952.9	E962.2	E982.9
Regroton	974.4	E858.5	E944.4	E950.4	E962.0	E980.4
Rela	968.0	E855.1	E938.0	E950.4	E962.0	E980.4
Relaxants, skeletal muscle (autonomic)	975.2	E858.6	E945.2	E950.4	E962.0	E980.4
central nervous system	968.0	E855.1	E938.0	E950.4	E962.0	E980.4
Renese	974.3	E858.5	E944.3	E950.4	E962.0	E980.4
Renografin	977.8	E858.8	E947.8	E950.4	E962.0	E980.4
Replacement solutions	974.5	E858.5	E944.5	E950.4	E962.0	E980.4
Rescinnamine	972.6	E858.3	E942.6	E950.4	E962.0	E980.4
Reserpine	972.6	E858.3	E942.6	E950.4	E962.0	E980.4
Resorcin, resorcinol	976.4	E858.7	E946.4	E950.4	E962.0	E980.4
Respaire	975.5	E858.6	E945.5	E950.4	E962.0	E980.4
Respiratory agents NEC	975.8	E858.6	E945.8	E950.4	E962.0	E980.4

◀ New   ◀▥ Revised   ~~deleted~~ Deleted   ● Use Additional Digit(s)

TABLE OF DRUGS AND CHEMICALS

Substance	Poisoning	External Cause (E Code)				
		Accident	Therapeutic Use	Suicide Attempt	Assault	Undetermined
Retinoic acid	976.8	E858.7	E946.8	E950.4	E962.0	E980.4
Retinol	963.5	E858.1	E933.5	E950.4	E962.0	E980.4
Rh (D) immune globulin (human)	964.6	E858.2	E934.6	E950.4	E962.0	E980.4
Rhodine	965.1	E850.3	E935.3	E950.0	E962.0	E980.0
RhoGAM	964.6	E858.2	E934.6	E950.4	E962.0	E980.4
Riboflavin	963.5	E858.1	E933.5	E950.4	E962.0	E980.4
Ricin	989.89	E866.8	—	E950.9	E962.1	E980.9
Ricinus communis	988.2	E865.3	—	E950.9	E962.1	E980.9
Rickettsial vaccine NEC	979.6	E858.8	E949.6	E950.4	E962.0	E980.4
with viral and bacterial vaccine	979.7	E858.8	E949.7	E950.4	E962.0	E980.4
Rifampin	960.6	E856	E930.6	E950.4	E962.0	E980.4
Rimifon	961.8	E857	E931.8	E950.4	E962.0	E980.4
Ringer's injection (lactated)	974.5	E858.5	E944.5	E950.4	E962.0	E980.4
Ristocetin	960.8	E856	E930.8	E950.4	E962.0	E980.4
Ritalin	969.73◀▥	E854.2	E939.7	E950.3	E962.0	E980.3
Roach killers - *see* Pesticides	—	—	—	—	—	—
Rocky Mountain spotted fever vaccine	979.6	E858.8	E949.6	E950.4	E962.0	E980.4
Rodenticides	989.4	E863.7	—	E950.6	E962.1	E980.7
Rohypnol	969.4	E853.2	E939.4	E950.3	E962.0	E980.3
Rolaids	973.0	E858.4	E943.0	E950.4	E962.0	E980.4
Rolitetracycline	960.4	E856	E930.4	E950.4	E962.0	E980.4
Romilar	975.4	E858.6	E945.4	E950.4	E962.0	E980.4
Rose water ointment	976.3	E858.7	E946.3	E950.4	E962.0	E980.4
Rotenone	989.4	E863.7	—	E950.6	E962.1	E980.7
Rotoxamine	963.0	E858.1	E933.0	E950.4	E962.0	E980.4
Rough-on-rats	989.4	E863.7	—	E950.6	E962.1	E980.7
RU486	962.9	E858.0	E932.9	E950.4	E962.0	E980.4
Rubbing alcohol	980.2	E860.3	—	E950.9	E962.1	E980.9
Rubella virus vaccine	979.4	E858.8	E949.4	E950.4	E962.0	E980.4
Rubelogen	979.4	E858.8	E949.4	E950.4	E962.0	E980.4
Rubeovax	979.4	E858.8	E949.4	E950.4	E962.0	E980.4
Rubidomycin	960.7	E856	E930.7	E950.4	E962.0	E980.4
Rue	988.2	E865.4	—	E950.9	E962.1	E980.9
Ruta	988.2	E865.4	—	E950.9	E962.1	E980.9
Sabadilla (medicinal)	976.0	E858.7	E946.0	E950.4	E962.0	E980.4
pesticide	989.4	E863.4	—	E950.6	E962.1	E980.7
Sabin oral vaccine	979.5	E858.8	E949.5	E950.4	E962.0	E980.4
Saccharated iron oxide	964.0	E858.2	E934.0	E950.4	E962.0	E980.4
Saccharin	974.5	E858.5	E944.5	E950.4	E962.0	E980.4

◀ New   ◀▥ Revised   ~~deleted~~ Deleted   ● Use Additional Digit(s)

Substance	Poisoning	External Cause (E Code)				
		Accident	Therapeutic Use	Suicide Attempt	Assault	Undetermined
Safflower oil	972.2	E858.3	E942.2	E950.4	E962.0	E980.4
Salbutamol sulfate	975.7	E858.6	E945.7	E950.4	E962.0	E980.4
Salicylamide	965.1	E850.3	E935.3	E950.0	E962.0	E980.0
Salicylate(s)	965.1	E850.3	E935.3	E950.0	E962.0	E980.0
methyl	976.3	E858.7	E946.3	E950.4	E962.0	E980.4
theobromine calcium	974.1	E858.5	E944.1	E950.4	E962.0	E980.4
Salicylazosulfapyridine	961.0	E857	E931.0	E950.4	E962.0	E980.4
Salicylhydroxamic acid	976.0	E858.7	E946.0	E950.4	E962.0	E980.4
Salicylic acid (keratolytic) NEC	976.4	E858.7	E946.4	E950.4	E962.0	E980.4
congeners	965.1	E850.3	E935.3	E950.0	E962.0	E980.0
salts	965.1	E850.3	E935.3	E950.0	E962.0	E980.0
Saliniazid	961.8	E857	E931.8	E950.4	E962.0	E980.4
Salol	976.3	E858.7	E946.3	E950.4	E962.0	E980.4
Salt (substitute) NEC	974.5	E858.5	E944.5	E950.4	E962.0	E980.4
Saluretics	974.3	E858.5	E944.3	E950.4	E962.0	E980.4
Saluron	974.3	E858.5	E944.3	E950.4	E962.0	E980.4
Salvarsan 606 (neosilver) (silver)	961.1	E857	E931.1	E950.4	E962.0	E980.4
Sambucus canadensis	988.2	E865.4	—	E950.9	E962.1	E980.9
berry	988.2	E865.3	—	E950.9	E962.1	E980.9
Sandril	972.6	E858.3	E942.6	E950.4	E962.0	E980.4
Sanguinaria canadensis	988.2	E865.4	—	E950.9	E962.1	E980.9
Saniflush (cleaner)	983.9	E861.3	—	E950.7	E962.1	E980.6
Santonin	961.6	E857	E931.6	E950.4	E962.0	E980.4
Santyl	976.8	E858.7	E946.8	E950.4	E962.0	E980.4
Sarkomycin	960.7	E856	E930.7	E950.4	E962.0	E980.4
Saroten	969.05 ◀▥	E854.0	E939.0	E950.3	E962.0	E980.3
Saturnine - see Lead	—	—	—	—	—	—
Savin (oil)	976.4	E858.7	E946.4	E950.4	E962.0	E980.4
Scammony	973.1	E858.4	E943.1	E950.4	E962.0	E980.4
Scarlet red	976.8	E858.7	E946.8	E950.4	E962.0	E980.4
Scheele's green	985.1	E866.3	—	E950.8	E962.1	E980.8
insecticide	985.1	E863.4	—	E950.8	E962.1	E980.8
Schradan	989.3	E863.1	—	E950.6	E962.1	E980.7
Schweinfurt(h) green	985.1	E866.3	—	E950.8	E962.1	E980.8
insecticide	985.1	E863.4	—	E950.8	E962.1	E980.8
Scilla - see Squill	—	—	—	—	—	—
Sclerosing agents	972.7	E858.3	E942.7	E950.4	E962.0	E980.4
Scopolamine	971.1	E855.4	E941.1	E950.4	E962.0	E980.4
Scouring powder	989.89	E861.3	—	E950.9	E962.1	E980.9

◀ New   ◀▥ Revised   ~~deleted~~ Deleted   ● Use Additional Digit(s)

Substance	Poisoning	External Cause (E Code)				
		Accident	Therapeutic Use	Suicide Attempt	Assault	Undetermined
Sea	—	—	—	—	—	—
anemone (sting)	989.5	E905.6	—	E950.9	E962.1	E980.9
cucumber (sting)	989.5	E905.6	—	E950.9	E962.1	E980.9
snake (bite) (venom)	989.5	E905.0	—	E950.9	E962.1	E980.9
urchin spine (puncture)	989.5	E905.6	—	E950.9	E962.1	E980.9
Secbutabarbital	967.0	E851	E937.0	E950.1	E962.0	E980.1
Secbutabarbitone	967.0	E851	E937.0	E950.1	E962.0	E980.1
Secobarbital	967.0	E851	E937.0	E950.1	E962.0	E980.1
Seconal	967.0	E851	E937.0	E950.1	E962.0	E980.1
Secretin	977.8	E858.8	E947.8	E950.4	E962.0	E980.4
Sedatives, nonbarbiturate	967.9	E852.9	E937.9	E950.2	E962.0	E980.2
specified NEC	967.8	E852.8	E937.8	E950.2	E962.0	E980.2
Sedormid	967.8	E852.8	E937.8	E950.2	E962.0	E980.2
Seed (plant)	988.2	E865.3	—	E950.9	E962.1	E980.9
disinfectant or dressing	989.89	E866.5	—	E950.9	E962.1	E980.9
Selective serotonin and norepinephrine reuptake inhibitors (SSNRI)	969.02	E854.0	E939.0	E950.3	E962.0	E980.3 ◀
Selective serotonin reuptake inhibitors (SSRI)	969.03	E854.0	E939.0	E950.3	E962.0	E980.3 ◀
Selenium (fumes) NEC	985.8	E866.4	—	E950.9	E962.1	E980.9
disulfide or sulfide	976.4	E858.7	E946.4	E950.4	E962.0	E980.4
Selsun	976.4	E858.7	E946.4	E950.4	E962.0	E980.4
Senna	973.1	E858.4	E943.1	E950.4	E962.0	E980.4
Septisol	976.2	E858.7	E946.2	E950.4	E962.0	E980.4
Serax	969.4	E853.2	E939.4	E950.3	E962.0	E980.3
Serenesil	967.8	E852.8	E937.8	E950.2	E962.0	E980.2
Serenium (hydrochloride)	961.9	E857	E931.9	E950.4	E962.0	E980.4
Serepax - *see* Oxazepam	—	—	—	—	—	—
Sernyl	968.3	E855.1	E938.3	E950.4	E962.0	E980.4
Serotonin	977.8	E858.8	E947.8	E950.4	E962.0	E980.4
Serpasil	972.6	E858.3	E942.6	E950.4	E962.0	E980.4
Sewer gas	987.8	E869.8	—	E952.8	E962.2	E982.8
Shampoo	989.6	E861.0	—	E950.9	E962.1	E980.9
Shellfish, nonbacterial or noxious	988.0	E865.1	—	E950.9	E962.1	E980.9
Silicones NEC	989.83	E866.8	E947.8	E950.9	E962.1	E980.9
Silvadene	976.0	E858.7	E946.0	E950.4	E962.0	E980.4
Silver (compound) (medicinal) NEC	976.0	E858.7	E946.0	E950.4	E962.0	E980.4
anti-infectives	976.0	E858.7	E946.0	E950.4	E962.0	E980.4
arsphenamine	961.1	E857	E931.1	E950.4	E962.0	E980.4
nitrate	976.0	E858.7	E946.0	E950.4	E962.0	E980.4
ophthalmic preparation	976.5	E858.7	E946.5	E950.4	E962.0	E980.4
toughened (keratolytic)	976.4	E858.7	E946.4	E950.4	E962.0	E980.4

◀ New   ◀▥ Revised   ~~deleted~~ Deleted   ● Use Additional Digit(s)

Substance	Poisoning	Accident	Therapeutic Use	Suicide Attempt	Assault	Undetermined
Silver (compound) (medicinal) NEC *(Continued)*						
nonmedicinal (dust)	985.8	E866.4	—	E950.9	E962.1	E980.9
protein (mild) (strong)	976.0	E858.7	E946.0	E950.4	E962.0	E980.4
salvarsan	961.1	E857	E931.1	E950.4	E962.0	E980.4
Simethicone	973.8	E858.4	E943.8	E950.4	E962.0	E980.4
Sinequan	969.05 ◄ⅢⅢ	E854.0	E939.0	E950.3	E962.0	E980.3
Singoserp	972.6	E858.3	E942.6	E950.4	E962.0	E980.4
Sintrom	964.2	E858.2	E934.2	E950.4	E962.0	E980.4
Sitosterols	972.2	E858.3	E942.2	E950.4	E962.0	E980.4
Skeletal muscle relaxants	975.2	E858.6	E945.2	E950.4	E962.0	E980.4
Skin	—	—	—	—	—	—
agents (external)	976.9	E858.7	E946.9	E950.4	E962.0	E980.4
specified NEC	976.8	E858.7	E946.8	E950.4	E962.0	E980.4
test antigen	977.8	E858.8	E947.8	E950.4	E962.0	E980.4
Sleep-eze	963.0	E858.1	E933.0	E950.4	E962.0	E980.4
Sleeping draught (drug) (pill) (tablet)	967.9	E852.9	E937.9	E950.2	E962.0	E980.2
Smallpox vaccine	979.0	E858.8	E949.0	E950.4	E962.0	E980.4
Smelter fumes NEC	985.9	E866.4	—	E950.9	E962.1	E980.9
Smog	987.3	E869.1	—	E952.8	E962.2	E982.8
Smoke NEC	987.9	E869.9	—	E952.9	E962.2	E982.9
Smooth muscle relaxant	975.1	E858.6	E945.1	E950.4	E962.0	E980.4
Snail killer	989.4	E863.4	—	E950.6	E962.1	E980.7
Snake (bite) (venom)	989.5	E905.0	—	E950.9	E962.1	E980.9
Snuff	989.89	E866.8	—	E950.9	E962.1	E980.9
Soap (powder) (product)	989.6	E861.1	—	E950.9	E962.1	E980.9
medicinal, soft	976.2	E858.7	E946.2	E950.4	E962.0	E980.4
Soda (caustic)	983.2	E864.2	—	E950.7	E962.1	E980.6
bicarb	963.3	E858.1	E933.3	E950.4	E962.0	E980.4
chlorinated - *see* Sodium, hypochlorite	—	—	—	—	—	—
Sodium	—	—	—	—	—	—
acetosulfone	961.8	E857	E931.8	E950.4	E962.0	E980.4
acetrizoate	977.8	E858.8	E947.8	E950.4	E962.0	E980.4
amytal	967.0	E851	E937.0	E950.1	E962.0	E980.1
arsenate - *see* Arsenic	—	—	—	—	—	—
bicarbonate	963.3	E858.1	E933.3	E950.4	E962.0	E980.4
bichromate	983.9	E864.3	—	E950.7	E962.1	E980.6
biphosphate	963.2	E858.1	E933.2	E950.4	E962.0	E980.4
bisulfate	983.9	E864.3	—	E950.7	E962.1	E980.6
borate (cleanser)	989.6	E861.3	—	E950.9	E962.1	E980.9
bromide NEC	967.3	E852.2	E937.3	E950.2	E962.0	E980.2

◄ New   ◄ⅢⅢ Revised   ~~deleted~~ Deleted   ● Use Additional Digit(s)

Substance	Poisoning	External Cause (E Code)				
		Accident	Therapeutic Use	Suicide Attempt	Assault	Undetermined
Sodium *(Continued)*						
cacodylate (nonmedicinal) NEC	978.8	E858.8	E948.8	E950.4	E962.0	E980.4
anti-infective	961.1	E857	E931.1	E950.4	E962.0	E980.4
herbicide	989.4	E863.5	—	E950.6	E962.1	E980.7
calcium edetate	963.8	E858.1	E933.8	E950.4	E962.0	E980.4
carbonate NEC	983.2	E864.2	—	E950.7	E962.1	E980.6
chlorate NEC	983.9	E864.3	—	E950.7	E962.1	E980.6
herbicide	983.9	E863.5	—	E950.7	E962.1	E980.6
chloride NEC	974.5	E858.5	E944.5	E950.4	E962.0	E980.4
chromate	983.9	E864.3	—	E950.7	E962.1	E980.6
citrate	963.3	E858.1	E933.3	E950.4	E962.0	E980.4
cyanide - *see* Cyanide(s)	—	—	—	—	—	—
cyclamate	974.5	E858.5	E944.5	E950.4	E962.0	E980.4
diatrizoate	977.8	E858.8	E947.8	E950.4	E962.0	E980.4
dibunate	975.4	E858.6	E945.4	E950.4	E962.0	E980.4
dioctyl sulfosuccinate	973.2	E858.4	E943.2	E950.4	E962.0	E980.4
edetate	963.8	E858.1	E933.8	E950.4	E962.0	E980.4
ethacrynate	974.4	E858.5	E944.4	E950.4	E962.0	E980.4
fluoracetate (dust) (rodenticide)	989.4	E863.7	—	E950.6	E962.1	E980.7
fluoride - *see* Fluoride(s)	—	—	—	—	—	—
free salt	974.5	E858.5	E944.5	E950.4	E962.0	E980.4
glucosulfone	961.8	E857	E931.8	E950.4	E962.0	E980.4
hydroxide	983.2	E864.2	—	E950.7	E962.1	E980.6
hypochlorite (bleach) NEC	983.9	E864.3	—	E950.7	E962.1	E980.6
disinfectant	983.9	E861.4	—	E950.7	E962.1	E980.6
medicinal (anti-infective) (external)	976.0	E858.7	E946.0	E950.4	E962.0	E980.4
vapor	987.8	E869.8	—	E952.8	E962.2	E982.8
hyposulfite	976.0	E858.7	E946.0	E950.4	E962.0	E980.4
indigotindisulfonate	977.8	E858.8	E947.8	E950.4	E962.0	E980.4
iodide	977.8	E858.8	E947.8	E950.4	E962.0	E980.4
iothalamate	977.8	E858.8	E947.8	E950.4	E962.0	E980.4
iron edetate	964.0	E858.2	E934.0	E950.4	E962.0	E980.4
lactate	963.3	E858.1	E933.3	E950.4	E962.0	E980.4
lauryl sulfate	976.2	E858.7	E946.2	E950.4	E962.0	E980.4
L-triiodothyronine	962.7	E858.0	E932.7	E950.4	E962.0	E980.4
metrizoate	977.8	E858.8	E947.8	E950.4	E962.0	E980.4
monofluoracetate (dust) (rodenticide)	989.4	E863.7	—	E950.6	E962.1	E980.7
morrhuate	972.7	E858.3	E942.7	E950.4	E962.0	E980.4
nafcillin	960.0	E856	E930.0	E950.4	E962.0	E980.4

◀ New   ◀▥ Revised   ~~deleted~~ Deleted   ● Use Additional Digit(s)

Substance	Poisoning	External Cause (E Code)				
		Accident	Therapeutic Use	Suicide Attempt	Assault	Undetermined
Sodium (Continued)						
nitrate (oxidizing agent)	983.9	E864.3	—	E950.7	E962.1	E980.6
nitrite (medicinal)	972.4	E858.3	E942.4	E950.4	E962.0	E980.4
nitroferricyanide	972.6	E858.3	E942.6	E950.4	E962.0	E980.4
nitroprusside	972.6	E858.3	E942.6	E950.4	E962.0	E980.4
para-aminohippurate	977.8	E858.8	E947.8	E950.4	E962.0	E980.4
perborate (nonmedicinal) NEC	989.89	E866.8	—	E950.9	E962.1	E980.9
medicinal	976.6	E858.7	E946.6	E950.4	E962.0	E980.4
soap	989.6	E861.1	—	E950.9	E962.1	E980.9
percarbonate - see Sodium, perborate	—	—	—	—	—	—
phosphate	973.3	E858.4	E943.3	E950.4	E962.0	E980.4
polystyrene sulfonate	974.5	E858.5	E944.5	E950.4	E962.0	E980.4
propionate	976.0	E858.7	E946.0	E950.4	E962.0	E980.4
psylliate	972.7	E858.3	E942.7	E950.4	E962.0	E980.4
removing resins	974.5	E858.5	E944.5	E950.4	E962.0	E980.4
salicylate	965.1	E850.3	E935.3	E950.0	E962.0	E980.0
sulfate	973.3	E858.4	E943.3	E950.4	E962.0	E980.4
sulfoxone	961.8	E857	E931.8	E950.4	E962.0	E980.4
tetradecyl sulfate	972.7	E858.3	E942.7	E950.4	E962.0	E980.4
thiopental	968.3	E855.1	E938.3	E950.4	E962.0	E980.4
thiosalicylate	965.1	E850.3	E935.3	E950.0	E962.0	E980.0
thiosulfate	976.0	E858.7	E946.0	E950.4	E962.0	E980.4
tolbutamide	977.8	E858.8	E947.8	E950.4	E962.0	E980.4
tyropanoate	977.8	E858.8	E947.8	E950.4	E962.0	E980.4
valproate	966.3	E855.0	E936.3	E950.4	E962.0	E980.4
Solanine	977.8	E858.8	E947.8	E950.4	E962.0	E980.4
Solanum dulcamara	988.2	E865.4	—	E950.9	E962.1	E980.9
Solapsone	961.8	E857	E931.8	E950.4	E962.0	E980.4
Solasulfone	961.8	E857	E931.8	E950.4	E962.0	E980.4
Soldering fluid	983.1	E864.1	—	E950.7	E962.1	E980.6
Solid substance	989.9	E866.9	—	E950.9	E962.1	E980.9
specified NEC	989.9	E866.8	—	E950.9	E962.1	E980.9
Solvents, industrial	982.8	E862.9	—	E950.9	E962.1	E980.9
naphtha	981	E862.0	—	E950.9	E962.1	E980.9
petroleum	981	E862.0	—	E950.9	E962.1	E980.9
specified NEC	982.8	E862.4	—	E950.9	E962.1	E980.9
Soma	968.0	E855.1	E938.0	E950.4	E962.0	E980.4
Somatotropin	962.4	E858.0	E932.4	E950.4	E962.0	E980.4
Sominex	963.0	E858.1	E933.0	E950.4	E962.0	E980.4

◀ New   ◀■ Revised   deleted Deleted   ● Use Additional Digit(s)

Substance	Poisoning	External Cause (E Code)				
		Accident	Therapeutic Use	Suicide Attempt	Assault	Undetermined
Somnos	967.1	E852.0	E937.1	E950.2	E962.0	E980.2
Somonal	967.0	E851	E937.0	E950.1	E962.0	E980.1
Soneryl	967.0	E851	E937.0	E950.1	E962.0	E980.1
Soothing syrup	977.9	E858.9	E947.9	E950.5	E962.0	E980.5
Sopor	967.4	E852.3	E937.4	E950.2	E962.0	E980.2
Soporific drug	967.9	E852.9	E937.9	E950.2	E962.0	E980.2
specified type NEC	967.8	E852.8	E937.8	E950.2	E962.0	E980.2
Sorbitol NEC	977.4	E858.8	E947.4	E950.4	E962.0	E980.4
Sotradecol	972.7	E858.3	E942.7	E950.4	E962.0	E980.4
Spacoline	975.1	E858.6	E945.1	E950.4	E962.0	E980.4
Spanish fly	976.8	E858.7	E946.8	E950.4	E962.0	E980.4
Sparine	969.1	E853.0	E939.1	E950.3	E962.0	E980.3
Sparteine	975.0	E858.6	E945.0	E950.4	E962.0	E980.4
Spasmolytics	975.1	E858.6	E945.1	E950.4	E962.0	E980.4
anticholinergics	971.1	E855.4	E941.1	E950.4	E962.0	E980.4
Spectinomycin	960.8	E856	E930.8	E950.4	E962.0	E980.4
Speed	969.72 ◀▥	E854.2	E939.7	E950.3	E962.0	E980.3
Spermicides	976.8	E858.7	E946.8	E950.4	E962.0	E980.4
Spider (bite) (venom)	989.5	E905.1	—	E950.9	E962.1	E980.9
antivenin	979.9	E858.8	E949.9	E950.4	E962.0	E980.4
Spigelia (root)	961.6	E857	E931.6	E950.4	E962.0	E980.4
Spiperone	969.2	E853.1	E939.2	E950.3	E962.0	E980.3
Spiramycin	960.3	E856	E930.3	E950.4	E962.0	E980.4
Spirilene	969.5	E853.8	E939.5	E950.3	E962.0	E980.3
Spirit(s) (neutral) NEC	980.0	E860.1	—	E950.9	E962.1	E980.9
beverage	980.0	E860.0	—	E950.9	E962.1	E980.9
industrial	980.9	E860.9	—	E950.9	E962.1	E980.9
mineral	981	E862.0	—	E950.9	E962.1	E980.9
of salt - see Hydrochloric acid	—	—	—	—	—	—
surgical	980.9	E860.9	—	E950.9	E962.1	E980.9
Spironolactone	974.4	E858.5	E944.4	E950.4	E962.0	E980.4
Sponge, absorbable (gelatin)	964.5	E858.2	E934.5	E950.4	E962.0	E980.4
Sporostacin	976.0	E858.7	E946.0	E950.4	E962.0	E980.4
Sprays (aerosol)	989.89	E866.8	—	E950.9	E962.1	E980.9
cosmetic	989.89	E866.7	—	E950.9	E962.1	E980.9
medicinal NEC	977.9	E858.9	E947.9	E950.5	E962.0	E980.5
pesticides - see Pesticides	—	—	—	—	—	—
specified content - see substance specified	—	—	—	—	—	—
Spurge flax	988.2	E865.4	—	E950.9	E962.1	E980.9

◀ New　◀▥ Revised　~~deleted~~ Deleted　● Use Additional Digit(s)

685

TABLE OF DRUGS AND CHEMICALS

Substance	Poisoning	External Cause (E Code)				
		Accident	Therapeutic Use	Suicide Attempt	Assault	Undetermined
Spurges	988.2	E865.4	—	E950.9	E962.1	E980.9
Squill (expectorant) NEC	975.5	E858.6	E945.5	E950.4	E962.0	E980.4
rat poison	989.4	E863.7	—	E950.6	E962.1	E980.7
Squirting cucumber (cathartic)	973.1	E858.4	E943.1	E950.4	E962.0	E980.4
SSNRI (selective serotonin and norepinephrine reuptake inhibitors)	969.02	E854.0	E939.0	E950.3	E962.0	E980.3 ◄
SSRI (selective serotonin reuptake inhibitors)	969.03	E854.0	E939.0	E950.3	E962.0	E980.3 ◄
Stains	989.89	E866.8	—	E950.9	E962.1	E980.9
Stannous - see also Tin fluoride	976.7	E858.7	E946.7	E950.4	E962.0	E980.4
Stanolone	962.1	E858.0	E932.1	E950.4	E962.0	E980.4
Stanozolol	962.1	E858.0	E932.1	E950.4	E962.0	E980.4
Staphisagria or stavesacre (pediculicide)	976.0	E858.7	E946.0	E950.4	E962.0	E980.4
Stelazine	969.1	E853.0	E939.1	E950.3	E962.0	E980.3
Stemetil	969.1	E853.0	E939.1	E950.3	E962.0	E980.3
Sterculia (cathartic) (gum)	973.3	E858.4	E943.3	E950.4	E962.0	E980.4
Sternutator gas	987.8	E869.8	—	E952.8	E962.2	E982.8
Steroids NEC	962.0	E858.0	E932.0	E950.4	E962.0	E980.4
ENT agent	976.6	E858.7	E946.6	E950.4	E962.0	E980.4
ophthalmic preparation	976.5	E858.7	E946.5	E950.4	E962.0	E980.4
topical NEC	976.0	E858.7	E946.0	E950.4	E962.0	E980.4
Stibine	985.8	E866.4	—	E950.9	E962.1	E980.9
Stibophen	961.2	E857	E931.2	E950.4	E962.0	E980.4
Stilbamide, stilbamidine	961.5	E857	E931.5	E950.4	E962.0	E980.4
Stilbestrol	962.2	E858.0	E932.2	E950.4	E962.0	E980.4
Stimulants (central nervous system)	970.9	E854.3	E940.9	E950.4	E962.0	E980.4
analeptics	970.0	E854.3	E940.0	E950.4	E962.0	E980.4
opiate antagonist	970.1	E854.3	E940.1	E950.4	E962.0	E980.4
psychotherapeutic NEC	969.09 ◄	E854.0	E939.0	E950.3	E962.0	E980.3
specified NEC	970.8	E854.3	E940.8	E950.4	E962.0	E980.4
Storage batteries (acid) (cells)	983.1	E864.1	—	E950.7	E962.1	E980.6
Stovaine	968.9	E855.2	E938.9	E950.4	E962.0	E980.4
infiltration (subcutaneous)	968.5	E855.2	E938.5	E950.4	E962.0	E980.4
nerve block (peripheral) (plexus)	968.6	E855.2	E938.6	E950.4	E962.0	E980.4
spinal	968.7	E855.2	E938.7	E950.4	E962.0	E980.4
topical (surface)	968.5	E855.2	E938.5	E950.4	E962.0	E980.4
Stovarsal	961.1	E857	E931.1	E950.4	E962.0	E980.4
Stove gas - see Gas, utility	—	—	—	—	—	—
Stoxil	976.5	E858.7	E946.5	E950.4	E962.0	E980.4
STP	969.6	E854.1	E939.6	E950.3	E962.0	E980.3
Stramonium (medicinal) NEC	971.1	E855.4	E941.1	E950.4	E962.0	E980.4
natural state	988.2	E865.4	—	E950.9	E962.1	E980.9

◄ New   ◄ Revised   deleted Deleted   ● Use Additional Digit(s)

Substance	Poisoning	External Cause (E Code)				
		Accident	Therapeutic Use	Suicide Attempt	Assault	Undetermined
Streptodornase	964.4	E858.2	E934.4	E950.4	E962.0	E980.4
Streptoduocin	960.6	E856	E930.6	E950.4	E962.0	E980.4
Streptokinase	964.4	E858.2	E934.4	E950.4	E962.0	E980.4
Streptomycin	960.6	E856	E930.6	E950.4	E962.0	E980.4
Streptozocin	960.7	E856	E930.7	E950.4	E962.0	E980.4
Stripper (paint) (solvent)	982.8	E862.9	—	E950.9	E962.1	E980.9
Strobane	989.2	E863.0	—	E950.6	E962.1	E980.7
Strophanthin	972.1	E858.3	E942.1	E950.4	E962.0	E980.4
Strophanthus hispidus or kombe	988.2	E865.4	—	E950.9	E962.1	E980.9
Strychnine (rodenticide) (salts)	989.1	E863.7	—	E950.6	E962.1	E980.7
medicinal NEC	970.8	E854.3	E940.8	E950.4	E962.0	E980.4
Strychnos (ignatii) - *see* Strychnine	—	—	—	—	—	—
Styramate	968.0	E855.1	E938.0	E950.4	E962.0	E980.4
Styrene	983.0	E864.0	—	E950.7	E962.1	E980.6
Succinimide (anticonvulsant)	966.2	E855.0	E936.2	E950.4	E962.0	E980.4
mercuric - *see* Mercury	—	—	—	—	—	—
Succinylcholine	975.2	E858.6	E945.2	E950.4	E962.0	E980.4
Succinylsulfathiazole	961.0	E857	E931.0	E950.4	E962.0	E980.4
Sucrose	974.5	E858.5	E944.5	E950.4	E962.0	E980.4
Sulfacetamide	961.0	E857	E931.0	E950.4	E962.0	E980.4
ophthalmic preparation	976.5	E858.7	E946.5	E950.4	E962.0	E980.4
Sulfachlorpyridazine	961.0	E857	E931.0	E950.4	E962.0	E980.4
Sulfacytine	961.0	E857	E931.0	E950.4	E962.0	E980.4
Sulfadiazine	961.0	E857	E931.0	E950.4	E962.0	E980.4
silver (topical)	976.0	E858.7	E946.0	E950.4	E962.0	E980.4
Sulfadimethoxine	961.0	E857	E931.0	E950.4	E962.0	E980.4
Sulfadimidine	961.0	E857	E931.0	E950.4	E962.0	E980.4
Sulfaethidole	961.0	E857	E931.0	E950.4	E962.0	E980.4
Sulfafurazole	961.0	E857	E931.0	E950.4	E962.0	E980.4
Sulfaguanidine	961.0	E857	E931.0	E950.4	E962.0	E980.4
Sulfamerazine	961.0	E857.2	E931.0	E950.4	E962.0	E980.4
Sulfameter	961.0	E857	E931.0	E950.4	E962.0	E980.4
Sulfamethizole	961.0	E857	E931.0	E950.4	E962.0	E980.4
Sulfamethoxazole	961.0	E857	E931.0	E950.4	E962.0	E980.4
Sulfamethoxydiazine	961.0	E857	E931.0	E950.4	E962.0	E980.4
Sulfamethoxypyridazine	961.0	E857	E931.0	E950.4	E962.0	E980.4
Sulfamethylthiazole	961.0	E857	E931.0	E950.4	E962.0	E980.4
Sulfamylon	976.0	E858.7	E946.0	E950.4	E962.0	E980.4
Sulfan blue (diagnostic dye)	977.8	E858.8	E947.8	E950.4	E962.0	E980.4
Sulfanilamide	961.0	E857	E931.0	E950.4	E962.0	E980.4

◀ New   ◀▥ Revised   ~~deleted~~ Deleted   ● Use Additional Digit(s)

Substance	Poisoning	External Cause (E Code)				
		Accident	Therapeutic Use	Suicide Attempt	Assault	Undetermined
Sulfanilylguanidine	961.0	E857	E931.0	E950.4	E962.0	E980.4
Sulfaphenazole	961.0	E857	E931.0	E950.4	E962.0	E980.4
Sulfaphenylthiazole	961.0	E857	E931.0	E950.4	E962.0	E980.4
Sulfaproxyline	961.0	E857	E931.0	E950.4	E962.0	E980.4
Sulfapyridine	961.0	E857	E931.0	E950.4	E962.0	E980.4
Sulfapyrimidine	961.0	E857	E931.0	E950.4	E962.0	E980.4
Sulfarsphenamine	961.1	E857	E931.1	E950.4	E962.0	E980.4
Sulfasalazine	961.0	E857	E931.0	E950.4	E962.0	E980.4
Sulfasomizole	961.0	E857	E931.0	E950.4	E962.0	E980.4
Sulfasuxidine	961.0	E857	E931.0	E950.4	E962.0	E980.4
Sulfinpyrazone	974.7	E858.5	E944.7	E950.4	E962.0	E980.4
Sulfisoxazole	961.0	E857	E931.0	E950.4	E962.0	E980.4
ophthalmic preparation	976.5	E858.7	E946.5	E950.4	E962.0	E980.4
Sulfomyxin	960.8	E856	E930.8	E950.4	E962.0	E980.4
Sulfonal	967.8	E852.8	E937.8	E950.2	E962.0	E980.2
Sulfonamides (mixtures)	961.0	E857	E931.0	E950.4	E962.0	E980.4
Sulfones	961.8	E857	E931.8	E950.4	E962.0	E980.4
Sulfonethylmethane	967.8	E852.8	E937.8	E950.2	E962.0	E980.2
Sulfonmethane	967.8	E852.8	E937.8	E950.2	E962.0	E980.2
Sulfonphthal, sulfonphthol	977.8	E858.8	E947.8	E950.4	E962.0	E980.4
Sulfonylurea derivatives, oral	962.3	E858.0	E932.3	E950.4	E962.0	E980.4
Sulfoxone	961.8	E857	E931.8	E950.4	E962.0	E980.4
Sulfur, sulfureted, sulfuric, sulfurous, sulfuryl (compounds) NEC	989.89	E866.8	—	E950.9	E962.1	E980.9
acid	983.1	E864.1	—	E950.7	E962.1	E980.6
dioxide	987.3	E869.1	—	E952.8	E962.2	E982.8
ether - see Ether(s)	—	—	—	—	—	—
hydrogen	987.8	E869.8	—	E952.8	E962.2	E982.8
medicinal (keratolytic) (ointment) NEC	976.4	E858.7	E946.4	E950.4	E962.0	E980.4
pesticide (vapor)	989.4	E863.4	—	E950.6	E962.1	E980.7
vapor NEC	987.8	E869.8	—	E952.8	E962.2	E982.8
Sulkowitch's reagent	977.8	E858.8	E947.8	E950.4	E962.0	E980.4
Sulph - see also Sulf-	—	—	—	—	—	—
Sulphadione	961.8	E857	E931.8	E950.4	E962.0	E980.4
Sulthiame, sultiame	966.3	E855.0	E936.3	E950.4	E962.0	E980.4
Superinone	975.5	E858.6	E945.5	E950.4	E962.0	E980.4
Suramin	961.5	E857	E931.5	E950.4	E962.0	E980.4
Surfacaine	968.5	E855.2	E938.5	E950.4	E962.0	E980.4
Surital	968.3	E855.1	E938.3	E950.4	E962.0	E980.4
Sutilains	976.8	E858.7	E946.8	E950.4	E962.0	E980.4

◀ New   ◀▥ Revised   ~~deleted~~ Deleted   ● Use Additional Digit(s)

Substance	Poisoning	External Cause (E Code)				
		Accident	Therapeutic Use	Suicide Attempt	Assault	Undetermined
Suxamethonium (bromide) (chloride) (iodide)	975.2	E858.6	E945.2	E950.4	E962.0	E980.4
Suxethonium (bromide)	975.2	E858.6	E945.2	E950.4	E962.0	E980.4
Sweet oil (birch)	976.3	E858.7	E946.3	E950.4	E962.0	E980.4
Sym-dichloroethyl ether	982.3	E862.4	—	E950.9	E962.1	E980.9
Sympatholytics	971.3	E855.6	E941.3	E950.4	E962.0	E980.4
Sympathomimetics	971.2	E855.5	E941.2	E950.4	E962.0	E980.4
Synagis	979.6	E858.8	E949.6	E950.4	E962.0	E980.4
Synalar	976.0	E858.7	E946.0	E950.4	E962.0	E980.4
Synthroid	962.7	E858.0	E932.7	E950.4	E962.0	E980.4
Syntocinon	975.0	E858.6	E945.0	E950.4	E962.0	E950.4
Syrosingopine	972.6	E858.3	E942.6	E950.4	E962.0	E980.4
Systemic agents (primarily)	963.9	E858.1	E933.9	E950.4	E962.0	E980.4
specified NEC	963.8	E858.1	E933.8	E950.4	E962.0	E980.4
Tablets (*see also* specified substance)	977.9	E858.9	E947.9	E950.5	E962.0	E980.5
Tace	962.2	E858.0	E932.2	E950.4	E962.0	E980.4
Tacrine	971.0	E855.3	E941.0	E950.4	E962.0	E980.4
Talbutal	967.0	E851	E937.0	E950.1	E962.0	E980.1
Talc	976.3	E858.7	E946.3	E950.4	E962.0	E980.4
Talcum	976.3	E858.7	E946.3	E950.4	E962.0	E980.4
Tamsulosin	971.3	E855.6	E941.3	E950.4	E962.0	E980.4
Tandearil, tanderil	965.5	E850.5	E935.5	E950.0	E962.0	E980.0
Tannic acid	983.1	E864.1	—	E950.7	E962.1	E980.6
medicinal (astringent)	976.2	E858.7	E946.2	E950.4	E962.0	E980.4
Tannin - *see* Tannic acid	—	—	—	—	—	—
Tansy	988.2	E865.4	—	E950.9	E962.1	E980.9
TAO	960.3	E856	E930.3	E950.4	E962.0	E980.4
Tapazole	962.8	E858.0	E932.8	E950.4	E962.0	E980.4
Tar NEC	983.0	E864.0	—	E950.7	E962.1	E980.6
camphor - *see* Naphthalene	—	—	—	—	—	—
fumes	987.8	E869.8	—	E952.8	E962.2	E982.8
Taractan	969.3	E853.8	E939.3	E950.3	E962.0	E980.3
Tarantula (venomous)	989.5	E905.1	—	E950.9	E962.1	E980.9
Tartar emetic (anti-infective)	961.2	E857	E931.2	E950.4	E962.0	E980.4
Tartaric acid	983.1	E864.1	—	E950.7	E962.1	E980.6
Tartrated antimony (anti-infective)	961.2	E857	E931.2	E950.4	E962.0	E980.4
TCA - *see* Trichloroacetic acid	—	—	—	—	—	—
TDI	983.0	E864.0	—	E950.7	E962.1	E980.6
vapor	987.8	E869.8	—	E952.8	E962.2	E982.8
Tear gas	987.5	E869.3	—	E952.8	E962.2	E982.8

◀ New   ◀▥ Revised   ~~deleted~~ Deleted   ● Use Additional Digit(s)

TABLE OF DRUGS AND CHEMICALS

Substance	Poisoning	External Cause (E Code)				
		Accident	Therapeutic Use	Suicide Attempt	Assault	Undetermined
Teclothiazide	974.3	E858.5	E944.3	E950.4	E962.0	E980.4
Tegretol	966.3	E855.0	E936.3	E950.4	E962.0	E980.4
Telepaque	977.8	E858.8	E947.8	E950.4	E962.0	E980.4
Tellurium	985.8	E866.4	—	E950.9	E962.1	E980.9
fumes	985.8	E866.4	—	E950.9	E962.1	E980.9
TEM	963.1	E858.1	E933.1	E950.4	E962.0	E980.4
Temazepam - see Benzodiazepines	—	—	—	—	—	—
TEPA	963.1	E858.1	E933.1	E950.4	E962.0	E980.4
TEPP	989.3	E863.1	—	E950.6	E962.1	E980.7
Terbutaline	971.2	E855.5	E941.2	E950.4	E962.0	E980.4
Teroxalene	961.6	E857	E931.6	E950.4	E962.0	E980.4
Terpin hydrate	975.5	E858.6	E945.5	E950.4	E962.0	E980.4
Terramycin	960.4	E856	E930.4	E950.4	E962.0	E980.4
Tessalon	975.4	E858.6	E945.4	E950.4	E962.0	E980.4
Testosterone	962.1	E858.0	E932.1	E950.4	E962.0	E980.4
Tetanus (vaccine)	978.4	E858.8	E948.4	E950.4	E962.0	E980.4
antitoxin	979.9	E858.8	E949.9	E950.4	E962.0	E980.4
immune globulin (human)	964.6	E858.2	E934.6	E950.4	E962.0	E980.4
toxoid	978.4	E858.8	E948.4	E950.4	E962.0	E980.4
with diphtheria toxoid	978.9	E858.8	E948.9	E950.4	E962.0	E980.4
with pertussis	978.6	E858.8	E948.6	E950.4	E962.0	E980.4
Tetrabenazine	969.5	E853.8	E939.5	E950.3	E962.0	E980.3
Tetracaine (infiltration) (topical)	968.5	E855.2	E938.5	E950.4	E962.0	E980.4
nerve block (peripheral) (plexus)	968.6	E855.2	E938.6	E950.4	E962.0	E980.4
spinal	968.7	E855.2	E938.7	E950.4	E962.0	E980.4
Tetrachlorethvlene - see Tetrachloroethylene	—	—	—	—	—	—
Tetrachlormethiazide	974.3	E858.5	E944.3	E950.4	E962.0	E980.4
Tetrachloroethane (liquid) (vapor)	982.3	E862.4	—	E950.9	E962.1	E980.9
paint or varnish	982.3	E861.6	—	E950.9	E962.1	E980.9
Tetrachloroethylene (liquid) (vapor)	982.3	E862.4	—	E950.9	E962.1	E980.9
medicinal	961.6	E857	E931.6	E950.4	E962.0	E980.4
Tetrachloromethane - see Carbon, tetrachloride	—	—	—	—	—	—
Tetracycline	960.4	E856	E930.4	E950.4	E962.0	E980.4
ophthalmic preparation	976.5	E858.7	E946.5	E950.4	E962.0	E980.4
topical NEC	976.0	E858.7	E946.0	E950.4	E962.0	E980.4
Tetraethylammonium chloride	972.3	E858.3	E942.3	E950.4	E962.0	E980.4
Tetraethyl lead (antiknock compound)	984.1	E862.1	—	E950.9	E962.1	E980.9
Tetraethyl pyrophosphate	989.3	E863.1	—	E950.6	E962.1	E980.7
Tetraethylthiuram disulfide	977.3	E858.8	E947.3	E950.4	E962.0	E980.4

◀ New ◀▥ Revised ~~deleted~~ Deleted ● Use Additional Digit(s)

Substance	Poisoning	External Cause (E Code)				
		Accident	Therapeutic Use	Suicide Attempt	Assault	Undetermined
Tetrahydroaminoacridine	971.0	E855.3	E941.0	E950.4	E962.0	E980.4
Tetrahydrocannabinol	969.6	E854.1	E939.6	E950.3	E962.0	E980.3
Tetrahydronaphthalene	982.0	E862.4	—	E950.9	E962.1	E980.9
Tetrahydrozoline	971.2	E855.5	E941.2	E950.4	E962.0	E980.4
Tetralin	982.0	E862.4	—	E950.9	E962.1	E980.9
Tetramethylthiuram (disulfide) NEC	989.4	E863.6	—	E950.6	E962.1	E980.7
medicinal	976.2	E858.7	E946.2	E950.4	E962.0	E980.4
Tetronal	967.8	E852.8	E937.8	E950.2	E962.0	E980.2
Tetryl	983.0	E864.0	—	E950.7	E962.1	E980.6
Thalidomide	967.8	E852.8	E937.8	E950.2	E962.0	E980.2
Thallium (compounds) (dust) NEC	985.8	E866.4	—	E950.9	E962.1	E980.9
pesticide (rodenticide)	985.8	E863.7	—	E950.6	E962.1	E980.7
THC	969.6	E854.1	E939.6	E950.3	E962.0	E980.3
Thebacon	965.09	E850.2	E935.2	E950.0	E962.0	E980.0
Thebaine	965.09	E850.2	E935.2	E950.0	E962.0	E980.0
Theobromine (calcium salicylate)	974.1	E858.5	E944.1	E950.4	E962.0	E980.4
Theophylline (diuretic)	974.1	E858.5	E944.1	E950.4	E962.0	E980.4
ethylenediamine	975.7	E858.6	E945.7	E950.4	E962.0	E980.4
Thiabendazole	961.6	E857	E931.6	E950.4	E962.0	E980.4
Thialbarbital, thialbarbitone	968.3	E855.1	E938.3	E950.4	E962.0	E980.4
Thiamine	963.5	E858.1	E933.5	E950.4	E962.0	E980.4
Thiamylal (sodium)	968.3	E855.1	E938.3	E950.4	E962.0	E980.4
Thiazesim	969.09 ◀▥	E854.0	E939.0	E950.3	E962.0	E980.3
Thiazides (diuretics)	974.3	E858.5	E944.3	E950.4	E962.0	E980.4
Thiethylperazine	963.0	E858.1	E933.0	E950.4	E962.0	E980.4
Thimerosal (topical)	976.0	E858.7	E946.0	E950.4	E962.0	E980.4
ophthalmic preparation	976.5	E858.7	E946.5	E950.4	E962.0	E980.4
Thioacetazone	961.8	E857	E931.8	E950.4	E962.0	E980.4
Thiobarbiturates	968.3	E855.1	E938.3	E950.4	E962.0	E980.4
Thiobismol	961.2	E857	E931.2	E950.4	E962.0	E980.4
Thiocarbamide	962.8	E858.0	E932.8	E950.4	E962.0	E980.4
Thiocarbarsone	961.1	E857	E931.1	E950.4	E962.0	E980.4
Thiocarlide	961.8	E857	E931.8	E950.4	E962.0	E980.4
Thioguanine	963.1	E858.1	E933.1	E950.4	E962.0	E980.4
Thiomercaptomerin	974.0	E858.5	E944.0	E950.4	E962.0	E980.4
Thiomerin	974.0	E858.5	E944.0	E950.4	E962.0	E980.4
Thiopental, thiopentone (sodium)	968.3	E855.1	E938.3	E950.4	E962.0	E980.4
Thiopropazate	969.1	E853.0	E939.1	E950.3	E962.0	E980.3
Thioproperazine	969.1	E853.0	E939.1	E950.3	E962.0	E980.3

◀ New   ◀▥ Revised   ~~deleted~~ Deleted   ● Use Additional Digit(s)

Substance	Poisoning	External Cause (E Code)				
		Accident	Therapeutic Use	Suicide Attempt	Assault	Undetermined
Thioridazine	969.1	E853.0	E939.1	E950.3	E962.0	E980.3
Thio-TEPA, thiotepa	963.1	E858.1	E933.1	E950.4	E962.0	E980.4
Thiothixene	969.3	E853.8	E939.3	E950.3	E962.0	E980.3
Thiouracil	962.8	E858.0	E932.8	E950.4	E962.0	E980.4
Thiourea	962.8	E858.0	E932.8	E950.4	E962.0	E980.4
Thiphenamil	971.1	E855.4	E941.1	E950.4	E962.0	E980.4
Thiram NEC	989.4	E863.6	—	E950.6	E962.1	E980.7
medicinal	976.2	E858.7	E946.2	E950.4	E962.0	E980.4
Thonzylamine	963.0	E858.1	E933.0	E950.4	E962.0	E980.4
Thorazine	969.1	E853.0	E939.1	E950.3	E962.0	E980.3
Thornapple	988.2	E865.4	—	E950.9	E962.1	E980.9
Throat preparation (lozenges) NEC	976.6	E858.7	E946.6	E950.4	E962.0	E980.4
Thrombin	964.5	E858.2	E934.5	E950.4	E962.0	E980.4
Thrombolysin	964.4	E858.2	E934.4	E950.4	E962.0	E980.4
Thymol	983.0	E864.0	—	E950.7	E962.1	E980.6
Thymus extract	962.9	E858.0	E932.9	E950.4	E962.0	E980.4
Thyroglobulin	962.7	E858.0	E932.7	E950.4	E962.0	E980.4
Thyroid (derivatives) (extract)	962.7	E858.0	E932.7	E950.4	E962.0	E980.4
Thyrolar	962.7	E858.0	E932.7	E950.4	E962.0	E980.4
Thyrotrophin, thyrotropin	977.8	E858.8	E947.8	E950.4	E962.0	E980.4
Thyroxin(e)	962.7	E858.0	E932.7	E950.4	E962.0	E980.4
Tigan	963.0	E858.1	E933.0	E950.4	E962.0	E980.4
Tigloidine	968.0	E855.1	E938.0	E950.4	E962.0	E980.4
Tin (chloride) (dust) (oxide) NEC	985.8	E866.4	—	E950.9	E962.1	E980.9
anti-infectives	961.2	E857	E931.2	E950.4	E962.0	E980.4
Tinactin	976.0	E858.7	E946.0	E950.4	E962.0	E980.4
Tincture, iodine - see Iodine	—	—	—	—	—	—
Tindal	969.1	E853.0	E939.1	E950.3	E962.0	E980.3
Titanium (compounds) (vapor)	985.8	E866.4	—	E950.9	E962.1	E980.9
ointment	976.3	E858.7	E946.3	E950.4	E962.0	E980.4
Titroid	962.7	E858.0	E932.7	E950.4	E962.0	E980.4
TMTD - see Tetramethylthiuram disulfide	—	—	—	—	—	—
TNT	989.89	E866.8	—	E950.9	E962.1	E980.9
fumes	987.8	E869.8	—	E952.8	E962.2	E982.8
Toadstool	988.1	E865.5	—	E950.9	E962.1	E980.9
Tobacco NEC	989.84	E866.8	—	E950.9	E962.1	E980.9
Indian	988.2	E865.4	—	E950.9	E962.1	E980.9
smoke, second-hand	987.8	E869.4	—	—	—	—

◀ New ◀▥ Revised ~~deleted~~ Deleted ● Use Additional Digit(s)

TABLE OF DRUGS AND CHEMICALS

Substance	Poisoning	External Cause (E Code)				
		Accident	Therapeutic Use	Suicide Attempt	Assault	Undetermined
Tocopherol	963.5	E858.1	E933.5	E950.4	E962.0	E980.4
Tocosamine	975.0	E858.6	E945.0	E950.4	E962.0	E980.4
Tofranil	969.05◀	E854.0	E939.0	E950.3	E962.0	E980.3
Toilet deodorizer	989.89	E866.8	—	E950.9	E962.1	E980.9
Tolazamide	962.3	E858.0	E932.3	E950.4	E962.0	E980.4
Tolazoline	971.3	E855.6	E941.3	E950.4	E962.0	E980.4
Tolbutamide	962.3	E858.0	E932.3	E950.4	E962.0	E980.4
sodium	977.8	E858.8	E947.8	E950.4	E962.0	E980.4
Tolmetin	965.69	E850.6	E935.6	E950.0	E962.0	E980.0
Tolnaftate	976.0	E858.7	E946.0	E950.4	E962.0	E980.4
Tolpropamine	976.1	E858.7	E946.1	E950.4	E962.0	E980.4
Tolserol	968.0	E855.1	E938.0	E950.4	E962.0	E980.4
Toluene (liquid) (vapor)	982.0	E862.4	—	E950.9	E962.1	E980.9
diisocyanate	983.0	E864.0	—	E950.7	E962.1	E980.6
Toluidine	983.0	E864.0	—	E950.7	E962.1	E980.6
vapor	987.8	E869.8	—	E952.8	E962.2	E982.8
Toluol (liquid) (vapor)	982.0	E862.4	—	E950.9	E962.1	E980.9
Tolylene-2,4-diisocyanate	983.0	E864.0	—	E950.7	E962.1	E980.6
Tonics, cardiac	972.1	E858.3	E942.1	E950.4	E962.0	E980.4
Toxaphene (dust) (spray)	989.2	E863.0	—	E950.6	E962.1	E980.7
Toxoids NEC	978.8	E858.8	E948.8	E950.4	E962.0	E980.4
Tractor fuel NEC	981	E862.1	—	E950.9	E962.1	E980.9
Tragacanth	973.3	E858.4	E943.3	E950.4	E962.0	E980.4
Tramazoline	971.2	E855.5	E941.2	E950.4	E962.0	E980.4
Tranquilizers	969.5	E853.9	E939.5	E950.3	E962.0	E980.3
benzodiazepine-based	969.4	E853.2	E939.4	E950.3	E962.0	E980.3
butyrophenone-based	969.2	E853.1	E939.2	E950.3	E962.0	E980.3
major NEC	969.3	E853.8	E939.3	E950.3	E962.0	E980.3
phenothiazine-based	969.1	E853.0	E939.1	E950.3	E962.0	E980.3
specified NEC	969.5	E853.8	E939.5	E950.3	E962.0	E980.3
Trantoin	961.9	E857	E931.9	E950.4	E962.0	E980.4
Tranxene	969.4	E853.2	E939.4	E950.3	E962.0	E980.3
Tranylcypromine (sulfate)	969.01◀	E854.0	E939.0	E950.3	E962.0	E980.3
Trasentine	975.1	E858.6	E945.1	E950.4	E962.0	E980.4
Travert	974.5	E858.5	E944.5	E950.4	E962.0	E980.4
Trecator	961.8	E857	E931.8	E950.4	E962.0	E980.4
Tretinoin	976.8	E858.7	E946.8	E950.4	E962.0	E980.4
Triacetin	976.0	E858.7	E946.0	E950.4	E962.0	E980.4

◀ New   ◀▥ Revised   ~~deleted~~ Deleted   ● Use Additional Digit(s)

Substance	Poisoning	External Cause (E Code)				
		Accident	Therapeutic Use	Suicide Attempt	Assault	Undetermined
Triacetyloleandomycin	960.3	E856	E930.3	E950.4	E962.0	E980.4
Triamcinolone	962.0	E858.0	E932.0	E950.4	E962.0	E980.4
ENT agent	976.6	E858.7	E946.6	E950.4	E962.0	E980.4
ophthalmic preparation	976.5	E858.7	E946.5	E950.4	E962.0	E980.4
topical NEC	976.0	E858.7	E946.0	E950.4	E962.0	E980.4
Triamterene	974.4	E858.5	E944.4	E950.4	E962.0	E980.4
Triaziquone	963.1	E858.1	E933.1	E950.4	E962.0	E980.4
Tribromacetaldehyde	967.3	E852.2	E937.3	E950.2	E962.0	E980.2
Tribromoethanol	968.2	E855.1	E938.2	E950.4	E962.0	E980.4
Tribromomethane	967.3	E852.2	E937.3	E950.2	E962.0	E980.2
Trichlorethane	982.3	E862.4	—	E950.9	E962.1	E980.9
Trichlormethiazide	974.3	E858.5	E944.3	E950.4	E962.0	E980.4
Trichloroacetic acid	983.1	E864.1	—	E950.7	E962.1	E980.6
medicinal (keratolytic)	976.4	E858.7	E946.4	E950.4	E962.0	E980.4
Trichloroethanol	967.1	E852.0	E937.1	E950.2	E962.0	E980.2
Trichloroethylene (liquid) (vapor)	982.3	E862.4	—	E950.9	E962.1	E980.9
anesthetic (gas)	968.2	E855.1	E938.2	E950.4	E962.0	E980.4
Trichloroethyl phosphate	967.1	E852.0	E937.1	E950.2	E962.0	E980.2
Trichlorofluoromethane NEC	987.4	E869.2	—	E952.8	E962.2	E982.8
Trichlorotriethylamine	963.1	E858.1	E933.1	E950.4	E962.0	E980.4
Trichomonacides NEC	961.5	E857	E931.5	E950.4	E962.0	E980.4
Trichomycin	960.1	E856	E930.1	E950.4	E962.0	E980.4
Triclofos	967.1	E852.0	E937.1	E950.2	E962.0	E980.2
Tricresyl phosphate	989.89	E866.8	—	E950.9	E962.1	E980.9
solvent	982.8	E862.4	—	E950.9	E962.1	E980.9
Tricyclamol	966.4	E855.0	E936.4	E950.4	E962.0	E980.4
Tridesilon	976.0	E858.7	E946.0	E950.4	E962.0	E980.4
Tridihexethyl	971.1	E855.4	E941.1	E950.4	E962.0	E980.4
Tridione	966.0	E855.0	E936.0	E950.4	E962.0	E980.4
Triethanolamine NEC	983.2	E864.2	—	E950.7	E962.1	E980.6
detergent	983.2	E861.0	—	E950.7	E962.1	E980.6
trinitrate	972.4	E858.3	E942.4	E950.4	E962.0	E980.4
Triethanomelamine	963.1	E858.1	E933.1	E950.4	E962.0	E980.4
Triethylene melamine	963.1	E858.1	E933.1	E950.4	E962.0	E980.4
Triethylenephosphoramide	963.1	E858.1	E933.1	E950.4	E962.0	E980.4
Triethylenethiophosphoramide	963.1	E858.1	E933.1	E950.4	E962.0	E980.4
Trifluoperazine	969.1	E853.0	E939.1	E950.3	E962.0	E980.3
Trifluperidol	969.2	E853.1	E939.2	E950.3	E962.0	E980.3
Triflupromazine	969.1	E853.0	E939.1	E950.3	E962.0	E980.3

◀ New ◀ᴵᴵᴵ Revised ~~deleted~~ Deleted ● Use Additional Digit(s)

Substance	Poisoning	External Cause (E Code)				
		Accident	Therapeutic Use	Suicide Attempt	Assault	Undetermined
Trihexyphenidyl	971.1	E855.4	E941.1	E950.4	E962.0	E980.4
Triiodothyronine	962.7	E858.0	E932.7	E950.4	E962.0	E980.4
Trilene	968.2	E855.1	E938.2	E950.4	E962.0	E980.4
Trimeprazine	963.0	E858.1	E933.0	E950.4	E962.0	E980.4
Trimetazidine	972.4	E858.3	E942.4	E950.4	E962.0	E980.4
Trimethadione	966.0	E855.0	E936.0	E950.4	E962.0	E980.4
Trimethaphan	972.3	E858.3	E942.3	E950.4	E962.0	E980.4
Trimethidinium	972.3	E858.3	E942.3	E950.4	E962.0	E980.4
Trimethobenzamide	963.0	E858.1	E933.0	E950.4	E962.0	E980.4
Trimethylcarbinol	980.8	E860.8	—	E950.9	E962.1	E980.9
Trimethylpsoralen	976.3	E858.7	E946.3	E950.4	E962.0	E980.4
Trimeton	963.0	E858.1	E933.0	E950.4	E962.0	E980.4
Trimipramine	969.05 ◀▥	E854.0	E939.0	E950.3	E962.0	E980.3
Trimustine	963.1	E858.1	E933.1	E950.4	E962.0	E980.4
Trinitrin	972.4	E858.3	E942.4	E950.4	E962.0	E980.4
Trinitrophenol	983.0	E864.0	—	E950.7	E962.1	E980.6
Trinitrotoluene	989.89	E866.8	—	E950.9	E962.1	E980.9
fumes	987.8	E869.8	—	E952.8	E962.2	E982.8
Trional	967.8	E852.8	E937.8	E950.2	E962.0	E980.2
Trioxide of arsenic - *see* Arsenic	—	—	—	—	—	—
Trioxsalen	976.3	E858.7	E946.3	E950.4	E962.0	E980.4
Tripelennamine	963.0	E858.1	E933.0	E950.4	E962.0	E980.4
Triperidol	969.2	E853.1	E939.2	E950.3	E962.0	E980.3
Triprolidine	963.0	E858.1	E933.0	E950.4	E962.0	E980.4
Trisoralen	976.3	E858.7	E946.3	E950.4	E962.0	E980.4
Troleandomycin	960.3	E856	E930.3	E950.4	E962.0	E980.4
Trolnitrate (phosphate)	972.4	E858.3	E942.4	E950.4	E962.0	E980.4
Trometamol	963.3	E858.1	E933.3	E950.4	E962.0	E980.4
Tromethamine	963.3	E858.1	E933.3	E950.4	E962.0	E980.4
Tronothane	968.5	E855.2	E938.5	E950.4	E962.0	E980.4
Tropicamide	971.1	E855.4	E941.1	E950.4	E962.0	E980.4
Troxidone	966.0	E855.0	E936.0	E950.4	E962.0	E980.4
Tryparsamide	961.1	E857	E931.1	E950.4	E962.0	E980.4
Trypsin	963.4	E858.1	E933.4	E950.4	E962.0	E980.4
Tryptizol	969.05 ◀▥	E854.0	E939.0	E950.3	E962.0	E980.3
Tuaminoheptane	971.2	E855.5	E941.2	E950.4	E962.0	E980.4
Tuberculin (old)	977.8	E858.8	E947.8	E950.4	E962.0	E980.4
Tubocurare	975.2	E858.6	E945.2	E950.4	E962.0	E980.4
Tubocurarine	975.2	E858.6	E945.2	E950.4	E962.0	E980.4

TABLE OF DRUGS AND CHEMICALS

◀ New   ◀▥ Revised   deleted Deleted   ● Use Additional Digit(s)

Substance	Poisoning	External Cause (E Code)				
		Accident	Therapeutic Use	Suicide Attempt	Assault	Undetermined
Turkish green	969.6	E854.1	E939.6	E950.3	E962.0	E980.3
Turpentine (spirits of) (liquid) (vapor)	982.8	E862.4	—	E950.9	E962.1	E980.9
Tybamate	969.5	E853.8	E939.5	E950.3	E962.0	E980.3
Tyloxapol	975.5	E858.6	E945.5	E950.4	E962.0	E980.4
Tymazoline	971.2	E855.5	E941.2	E950.4	E962.0	E980.4
Typhoid vaccine	978.1	E858.8	E948.1	E950.4	E962.0	E980.4
Typhus vaccine	979.2	E858.8	E949.2	E950.4	E962.0	E980.4
Tyrothricin	976.0	E858.7	E946.0	E950.4	E962.0	E980.4
ENT agent	976.6	E858.7	E946.6	E950.4	E962.0	E980.4
ophthalmic preparation	976.5	E858.7	E946.5	E950.4	E962.0	E980.4
Undecenoic acid	976.0	E858.7	E946.0	E950.4	E962.0	E980.4
Undecylenic acid	976.0	E858.7	E946.0	E950.4	E962.0	E980.4
Unna's boot	976.3	E858.7	E946.3	E950.4	E962.0	E980.4
Uracil mustard	963.1	E858.1	E933.1	E950.4	E962.0	E980.4
Uramustine	963.1	E858.1	E933.1	E950.4	E962.0	E980.4
Urari	975.2	E858.6	E945.2	E950.4	E962.0	E980.4
Urea	974.4	E858.5	E944.4	E950.4	E962.0	E980.4
topical	976.8	E858.7	E946.8	E950.4	E962.0	E980.4
Urethan(e) (antineoplastic)	963.1	E858.1	E933.1	E950.4	E962.0	E980.4
Urginea (maritima) (scilla) - see Squill	—	—	—	—	—	—
Uric acid metabolism agents NEC	974.7	E858.5	E944.7	E950.4	E962.0	E980.4
Urokinase	964.4	E858.2	E934.4	E950.4	E962.0	E980.4
Urokon	977.8	E858.8	E947.8	E950.4	E962.0	E980.4
Urotropin	961.9	E857	E931.9	E950.4	E962.0	E980.4
Urtica	988.2	E865.4	—	E950.9	E962.1	E980.9
Utility gas - see Gas, utility	—	—	—	—	—	—
Vaccine NEC	979.9	E858.8	E949.9	E950.4	E962.0	E980.4
bacterial NEC	978.8	E858.8	E948.8	E950.4	E962.0	E980.4
with	—	—	—	—	—	—
other bacterial component	978.9	E858.8	E948.9	E950.4	E962.0	E980.4
pertussis component	978.6	E858.8	E948.6	E950.4	E962.0	E980.4
viral-rickettsial component	979.7	E858.8	E949.7	E950.4	E962.0	E980.4
mixed NEC	978.9	E858.8	E948.9	E950.4	E962.0	E980.4
BCG	978.0	E858.8	E948.0	E950.4	E962.0	E980.4
cholera	978.2	E858.8	E948.2	E950.4	E962.0	E980.4
diphtheria	978.5	E858.8	E948.5	E950.4	E962.0	E980.4
influenza	979.6	E858.8	E949.6	E950.4	E962.0	E980.4

◀ New ◀▥ Revised ~~deleted~~ Deleted ● Use Additional Digit(s)

Substance	Poisoning	External Cause (E Code)				
		Accident	Therapeutic Use	Suicide Attempt	Assault	Undetermined
Vaccine NEC *(Continued)*						
measles	979.4	E858.8	E949.4	E950.4	E962.0	E980.4
meningococcal	978.8	E858.8	E948.8	E950.4	E962.0	E980.4
mumps	979.6	E858.8	E949.6	E950.4	E962.0	E980.4
paratyphoid	978.1	E858.8	E948.1	E950.4	E962.0	E980.4
pertussis (with diphtheria toxoid) (with tetanus toxoid)	978.6	E858.8	E948.6	E950.4	E962.0	E980.4
plague	978.3	E858.8	E948.3	E950.4	E962.0	E980.4
poliomyelitis	979.5	E858.8	E949.5	E950.4	E962.0	E980.4
poliovirus	979.5	E858.8	E949.5	E950.4	E962.0	E980.4
rabies	979.1	E858.8	E949.1	E950.4	E962.0	E980.4
respiratory syncytial virus	979.6	E858.8	E949.6	E950.4	E962.0	E980.4
rickettsial NEC	979.6	E858.8	E949.6	E950.4	E962.0	E980.4
with	—	—	—	—	—	—
bacterial component	979.7	E858.8	E949.7	E950.4	E962.0	E980.4
pertussis component	978.6	E858.8	E948.6	E950.4	E962.0	E980.4
viral component	979.7	E858.8	E949.7	E950.4	E962.0	E980.4
Rocky Mountain spotted fever	979.6	E858.8	E949.6	E950.4	E962.0	E980.4
rotavirus	979.6	E858.8	E949.6	E950.4	E962.0	E980.4
rubella virus	979.4	E858.8	E949.4	E950.4	E962.0	E980.4
sabin oral	979.5	E858.8	E949.5	E950.4	E962.0	E980.4
smallpox	979.0	E858.8	E949.0	E950.4	E962.0	E980.4
tetanus	978.4	E858.8	E948.4	E950.4	E962.0	E980.4
typhoid	978.1	E858.8	E948.1	E950.4	E962.0	E980.4
typhus	979.2	E858.8	E949.2	E950.4	E962.0	E980.4
viral NEC	979.6	E858.8	E949.6	E950.4	E962.0	E980.4
with	—	—	—	—	—	—
bacterial component	979.7	E858.8	E949.7	E950.4	E962.0	E980.4
pertussis component	978.6	E858.8	E948.6	E950.4	E962.0	E980.4
rickettsial component	979.7	E858.8	E949.7	E950.4	E962.0	E980.4
yellow fever	979.3	E858.8	E949.3	E950.4	E962.0	E980.4
Vaccinia immune globulin (human)	964.6	E858.2	E934.6	E950.4	E962.0	E980.4
Vaginal contraceptives	976.8	E858.7	E946.8	E950.4	E962.0	E980.4
Valethamate	971.1	E855.4	E941.1	E950.4	E962.0	E980.4
Valisone	976.0	E858.7	E946.0	E950.4	E962.0	E980.4
Valium	969.4	E853.2	E939.4	E950.3	E962.0	E980.3
Valmid	967.8	E852.8	E937.8	E950.2	E962.0	E980.2
Vanadium	985.8	E866.4	—	E950.9	E962.1	E980.9
Vancomycin	960.8	E856	E930.8	E950.4	E962.0	E980.4

◀ New   ◀▥ Revised   ~~deleted~~ Deleted   ● Use Additional Digit(s)

Substance	External Cause (E Code)					
	Poisoning	Accident	Therapeutic Use	Suicide Attempt	Assault	Undetermined
Vapor (*see also* Gas)	987.9	E869.9	—	E952.9	E962.2	E982.9
kiln (carbon monoxide)	986	E868.8	—	E952.1	E962.2	E982.1
lead - *see* Lead	—	—	—	—	—	—
specified source NEC - (*see also* specific substance)	987.8	E869.8	—	E952.8	E962.2	E982.8
Varidase	964.4	E858.2	E934.4	E950.4	E962.0	E980.4
Varnish	989.89	E861.6	—	E950.9	E962.1	E980.9
cleaner	982.8	E862.9	—	E950.9	E962.1	E980.9
Vaseline	976.3	E858.7	E946.3	E950.4	E962.0	E980.4
Vasodilan	972.5	E858.3	E942.5	E950.4	E962.0	E980.4
Vasodilators NEC	972.5	E858.3	E942.5	E950.4	E962.0	E980.4
coronary	972.4	E858.3	E942.4	E950.4	E962.0	E980.4
Vasopressin	962.5	E858.0	E932.5	E950.4	E962.0	E980.4
Vasopressor drugs	962.5	E858.0	E932.5	E950.4	E962.0	E980.4
Venom, venomous (bite) (sting)	989.5	E905.9	—	E950.9	E962.1	E980.9
arthropod NEC	989.5	E905.5	—	E950.9	E962.1	E980.9
bee	989.5	E905.3	—	E950.9	E962.1	E980.9
centipede	989.5	E905.4	—	E950.9	E962.1	E980.9
hornet	989.5	E905.3	—	E950.9	E962.1	E980.9
lizard	989.5	E905.0	—	E950.9	E962.1	E980.9
marine animals or plants	989.5	E905.6	—	E950.9	E962.1	E980.9
millipede (tropical)	989.5	E905.4	—	E950.9	E962.1	E980.9
plant NEC	989.5	E905.7	—	E950.9	E962.1	E980.9
marine	989.5	E905.6	—	E950.9	E962.1	E980.9
scorpion	989.5	E905.2	—	E950.9	E962.1	E980.9
snake	989.5	E905.0	—	E950.9	E962.1	E980.9
specified NEC	989.5	E905.8	—	E950.9	E962.1	E980.9
spider	989.5	E905.1	—	E950.9	E962.1	E980.9
wasp	989.5	E905.3	—	E950.9	E962.1	E980.9
Ventolin - *see* Salbutamol sulfate	—	—	—	—	—	—
Veramon	967.0	E851	E937.0	E950.1	E962.0	E980.1
Veratrum	—	—	—	—	—	—
album	988.2	E865.4	—	E950.9	E962.1	E980.9
alkaloids	972.6	E858.3	E942.6	E950.4	E962.0	E980.4
viride	988.2	E865.4	—	E950.9	E962.1	E980.9
Verdigris (*see also* Copper)	985.8	E866.4	—	E950.9	E962.1	E980.9
Veronal	967.0	E851	E937.0	E950.1	E962.0	E980.1
Veroxil	961.6	E857	E931.6	E950.4	E962.0	E980.4
Versidyne	965.7	E850.7	E935.7	E950.0	E962.0	E980.0
Viagra	972.5	E858.3	E942.5	E950.4	E962.0	E980.4

◀ New   ◀▥ Revised   deleted Deleted   ● Use Additional Digit(s)

Substance	Poisoning	External Cause (E Code)				
		Accident	Therapeutic Use	Suicide Attempt	Assault	Undetermined
Vienna	—	—	—	—	—	—
green	985.1	E866.3	—	E950.8	E962.1	E980.8
insecticide	985.1	E863.4	—	E950.6	E962.1	E980.7
red	989.89	E866.8	—	E950.9	E962.1	E980.9
pharmaceutical dye	977.4	E858.8	E947.4	E950.4	E962.0	E980.4
Vinbarbital, vinbarbitone	967.0	E851	E937.0	E950.1	E962.0	E980.1
Vinblastine	963.1	E858.1	E933.1	E950.4	E962.0	E980.4
Vincristine	963.1	E858.1	E933.1	E950.4	E962.0	E980.4
Vinesthene, vinethene	968.2	E855.1	E938.2	E950.4	E962.0	E980.4
Vinyl	—	—	—	—	—	—
bital	967.0	E851	E937.0	E950.1	E962.0	E980.1
ether	968.2	E855.1	E938.2	E950.4	E962.0	E980.4
Vioform	961.3	E857	E931.3	E950.4	E962.0	E980.4
topical	976.0	E858.7	E946.0	E950.4	E962.0	E980.4
Viomycin	960.6	E856	E930.6	E950.4	E962.0	E980.4
Viosterol	963.5	E858.1	E933.5	E950.4	E962.0	E980.4
Viper (venom)	989.5	E905.0	—	E950.9	E962.1	E980.9
Viprynium (embonate)	961.6	E857	E931.6	E950.4	E962.0	E980.4
Virugon	961.7	E857	E931.7	E950.4	E962.0	E980.4
Visine	976.5	E858.7	E946.5	E950.4	E962.0	E980.4
Vitamins NEC	963.5	E858.1	E933.5	E950.4	E962.0	E980.4
B₁₂	964.1	E858.2	E934.1	E950.4	E962.0	E980.4
hematopoietic	964.1	E858.2	E934.1	E950.4	E962.0	E980.4
K	964.3	E858.2	E934.3	E950.4	E962.0	E980.4
Vleminckx's solution	976.4	E858.7	E946.4	E950.4	E962.0	E980.4
Voltaren - see Diclofenac sodium	—	—	—	—	—	—
Warfarin (potassium) (sodium)	964.2	E858.2	E934.2	E950.4	E962.0	E980.4
rodenticide	989.4	E863.7	—	E950.6	E962.1	E980.7
Wasp (sting)	989.5	E905.3	—	E950.9	E962.1	E980.9
Water	—	—	—	—	—	—
balance agents NEC	974.5	E858.5	E944.5	E950.4	E962.0	E980.4
gas	987.1	E868.1	—	E951.8	E962.2	E981.8
incomplete combustion of - see Carbon, monoxide, fuel, utility	—	—	—	—	—	—
hemlock	988.2	E865.4	—	E950.9	E962.1	E980.9
moccasin (venom)	989.5	E905.0	—	E950.9	E962.1	E980.9
Wax (paraffin) (petroleum)	981	E862.3	—	E950.9	E962.1	E980.9
automobile	989.89	E861.2	—	E950.9	E962.1	E980.9
floor	981	E862.0	—	E950.9	E962.1	E980.9
Weed killers NEC	989.4	E863.5	—	E950.6	E962.1	E980.7

◄ New   ◄▦ Revised   ~~deleted~~ Deleted   ● Use Additional Digit(s)

TABLE OF DRUGS AND CHEMICALS

Substance	Poisoning	External Cause (E Code)				
		Accident	Therapeutic Use	Suicide Attempt	Assault	Undetermined
Welldorm	967.1	E852.0	E937.1	E950.2	E962.0	E980.2
White	—	—	—	—	—	—
arsenic - *see* Arsenic	—	—	—	—	—	—
hellebore	988.2	E865.4	—	E950.9	E962.1	E980.9
lotion (keratolytic)	976.4	E858.7	E946.4	E950.4	E962.0	E980.4
spirit	981	E862.0	—	E950.9	E962.1	E980.9
Whitewashes	989.89	E861.6	—	E950.9	E962.1	E980.9
Whole blood	964.7	E858.2	E934.7	E950.4	E962.0	E980.4
Wild	—	—	—	—	—	—
black cherry	988.2	E865.4	—	E950.9	E962.1	E980.9
poisonous plants NEC	988.2	E865.4	—	E950.9	E962.1	E980.9
Window cleaning fluid	989.89	E861.3	—	E950.9	E962.1	E980.9
Wintergreen (oil)	976.3	E858.7	E946.3	E950.4	E962.0	E980.4
Witch hazel	976.2	E858.7	E946.2	E950.4	E962.0	E980.4
Wood	—	—	—	—	—	—
alcohol	980.1	E860.2	—	E950.9	E962.1	E980.9
spirit	980.1	E860.2	—	E950.9	E962.1	E980.9
Woorali	975.2	E858.6	E945.2	E950.4	E962.0	E980.4
Wormseed, American	961.6	E857	E931.6	E950.4	E962.0	E980.4
Xanthine diuretics	974.1	E858.5	E944.1	E950.4	E962.0	E980.4
Xanthocillin	960.0	E856	E930.0	E950.4	E962.0	E980.4
Xanthotoxin	976.3	E858.7	E946.3	E950.4	E962.0	E980.4
Xigris	964.2	E858.2	E934.2	E950.4	E962.0	E980.4
Xylene (liquid) (vapor)	982.0	E862.4	—	E950.9	E962.1	E980.9
Xylocaine (infiltration) (topical)	968.5	E855.2	E938.5	E950.4	E962.0	E980.4
nerve block (peripheral) (plexus)	968.6	E855.2	E938.6	E950.4	E962.0	E980.4
spinal	968.7	E855.2	E938.7	E950.4	E962.0	E980.4
Xylol (liquid) (vapor)	982.0	E862.4	—	E950.9	E962.1	E980.9
Xylometazoline	971.2	E855.5	E941.2	E950.4	E962.0	E980.4
Yellow	—	—	—	—	—	—
fever vaccine	979.3	E858.8	E949.3	E950.4	E962.0	E980.4
jasmine	988.2	E865.4	—	E950.9	E962.1	E980.9
Yew	988.2	E865.4	—	E950.9	E962.1	E980.9
Zactane	965.7	E850.7	E935.7	E950.0	E962.0	E980.0
Zaroxolyn	974.3	E858.5	E944.3	E950.4	E962.0	E980.4
Zephiran (topical)	976.0	E858.7	E946.0	E950.4	E962.0	E980.4
ophthalmic preparation	976.5	E858.7	E946.5	E950.4	E962.0	E980.4
Zerone	980.1	E860.2	—	E950.9	E962.1	E980.9

◀ New   ◀▦ Revised   ~~deleted~~ Deleted   ● Use Additional Digit(s)

Substance	Poisoning	External Cause (E Code)				
		Accident	Therapeutic Use	Suicide Attempt	Assault	Undetermined
Zinc (compounds) (fumes) (salts) (vapor) NEC	985.8	E866.4	—	E950.9	E962.1	E980.9
anti-infectives	976.0	E858.7	E946.0	E950.4	E962.0	E980.4
antivaricose	972.7	E858.3	E942.7	E950.4	E962.0	E980.4
bacitracin	976.0	E858.7	E946.0	E950.4	E962.0	E980.4
chloride	976.2	E858.7	E946.2	E950.4	E962.0	E980.4
gelatin	976.3	E858.7	E946.3	E950.4	E962.0	E980.4
oxide	976.3	E858.7	E946.3	E950.4	E962.0	E980.4
peroxide	976.0	E858.7	E946.0	E950.4	E962.0	E980.4
pesticides	985.8	E863.4	—	E950.6	E962.1	E980.7
phosphide (rodenticide)	985.8	E863.7	—	E950.6	E962.1	E980.7
stearate	976.3	E858.7	E946.3	E950.4	E962.0	E980.4
sulfate (antivaricose)	972.7	E858.3	E942.7	E950.4	E962.0	E980.4
ENT agent	976.6	E858.7	E946.6	E950.4	E962.0	E980.4
ophthalmic solution	976.5	E858.7	E946.5	E950.4	E962.0	E980.4
topical NEC	976.0	E858.7	E946.0	E950.4	E962.0	E980.4
undecylenate	976.0	E858.7	E946.0	E950.4	E962.0	E980.4
Zovant	964.2	E858.2	E934.2	E950.4	E962.0	E980.4
Zoxazolamine	968.0	E855.1	E938.0	E950.4	E962.0	E980.4
Zygadenus (venenosus)	988.2	E865.4	—	E950.9	E962.1	E980.9

◀ New   ◀▥ Revised   ~~deleted~~ Deleted   ● Use Additional Digit(s)

SECTION III

INDEX TO EXTERNAL CAUSES OF INJURY (E CODE)

This section contains the index to the codes which classify environmental events, circumstances, and other conditions as the cause of injury and other adverse effects. Where a code from the section Supplementary Classification of External Causes of Injury and Poisoning (E800–E998) is applicable, it is intended that the E code shall be used in addition to a code from the main body of the classification, Chapters 1 to 17.

The alphabetic index to the E codes is organized by main terms which describe the accident, circumstance, event, or specific agent which caused the injury or other adverse effect.

Note   Transport accidents (E800–E848) include accidents involving:

> aircraft and spacecraft (E840–E845)
> watercraft (E830–E838)
> motor vehicle (E810–E825)
> railway (E800–E807)
> other road vehicles (E826–E829)

For definitions and examples related to transport accidents - see Supplementary Classification of External Causes of Injury and Poisoning (E800–E999).

The fourth-digit subdivisions for use with categories E800–E848 to identify the injured person are found at the end of this section.

For identifying the place in which an accident or poisoning occurred (circumstances classifiable to categories E850–E869 and E880–E928) - see the listing in this section under "Accident, occurring."

See the Table of Drugs and Chemicals (Section 2 of this volume) for identifying the specific agent involved in drug overdose or a wrong substance given or taken in error, and for intoxication or poisoning by a drug or other chemical substance.

The specific adverse effect, reaction, or localized toxic effect to a correct drug or substance properly administered in therapeutic or prophylactic dosage should be classified according to the nature of the adverse effect (e.g., allergy, dermatitis, tachycardia) listed in Section I of this volume.

A

Abandonment
  causing exposure to weather
    conditions - *see* Exposure
  child, with intent to injure or kill
    E968.4
  helpless person, infant, newborn
    E904.0
    with intent to injure or kill E968.4
Abortion, criminal, injury to child
  E968.8
Abuse (alleged) (suspected)
  adult
    by
        child E967.4
        ex-partner E967.3
        ex-spouse E967.3
        father E967.0
        grandchild E967.7
        grandparent E967.6
        mother E967.2
        non-related caregiver E967.8
        other relative E967.7
        other specified person E967.1
        partner E967.3
        sibling E967.5
        spouse E967.3
        stepfather E967.0
        stepmother E967.2
        unspecified person E967.9
  child
    by
        boyfriend of parent or guardian
          E967.0
        child E967.4
        father E967.0
        female partner of parent or
          guardian E967.2
        girlfriend of parent or guardian
          E967.2
        grandchild E967.7
        grandparent E967.6
        male partner of parent or
          guardian E967.0
        mother E967.2
        non-related caregiver E967.8
        other relative E967.7
        other specified person(s) E967.1
        sibling E967.5
        stepfather E967.0
        stepmother E967.2
        unspecified person E967.9
Accident (to) E928.9
  aircraft (in transit) (powered) E841●
    at landing, take-off E840●
    due to, caused by cataclysm - *see*
      categories E908, E909
    late effect of E929.1
    unpowered (*see also* Collision,
      aircraft, unpowered) E842●
    while alighting, boarding E843●
  amphibious vehicle
    on
        land - *see* Accident, motor
          vehicle
        water - *see* Accident, watercraft
  animal, ridden NEC E828●
  animal-drawn vehicle NEC E827●
  balloon (*see also* Collision, aircraft,
    unpowered) E842●
  caused by, due to
    abrasive wheel (metalworking)
      E919.3

Accident (*Continued*)
  caused by, due to (*Continued*)
    animal NEC E906.9
      being ridden (in sport or
        transport) E828●
    avalanche NEC E909.2
    band saw E919.4
    bench saw E919.4
    bore, earth-drilling or mining (land)
      (seabed) E919.1
    bulldozer E919.7
    cataclysmic
      earth surface movement or
        eruption E909.9
      storm E908.9
    chain
      hoist E919.2
        agricultural operations E919.0
        mining operations E919.1
      saw E920.1
    circular saw E919.4
    cold (excessive) (*see also* Cold,
      exposure to) E901.9
    combine E919.0
      conflagration - *see* Conflagration
    corrosive liquid, substance NEC
      E924.1
    cotton gin E919.8
    crane E919.2
      agricultural operations E919.0
      mining operations E919.1
    cutting or piercing instrument (*see
      also* Cut) E920.9
    dairy equipment E919.8
    derrick E919.2
      agricultural operations E919.0
      mining operations E919.1
    drill E920.1
      earth (land) (seabed) E919.1
      hand (powered) E920.1
        not powered E920.4
      metalworking E919.3
      woodworking E919.4
    earth(-)
      drilling machine E919.1
      moving machine E919.7
      scraping machine E919.7
    electric
      current (*see also* Electric shock)
        E925.9
      motor - *see also* Accident,
        machine, by type of
        machine
        current (of) - *see* Electric shock
    elevator (building) (grain) E919.2
      agricultural operations E919.0
      mining operations E919.1
    environmental factors NEC E928.9
    excavating machine E919.7
    explosive material (*see also*
      Explosion) E923.9
    farm machine E919.0
    fire, flames - *see also* Fire
      conflagration - *see* Conflagration
    firearm missile - *see* Shooting
    forging (metalworking) machine
      E919.3
    forklift (truck) E919.2
      agricultural operations E919.0
      mining operations E919.1
    gas turbine E919.5
    harvester E919.0
    hay derrick, mower, or rake
      E919.0

Accident (*Continued*)
  caused by, due to (*Continued*)
    heat (excessive) (*see also* Heat)
      E900.9
    hoist (*see also* Accident, caused by,
      due to, lift) E919.2
      chain - *see* Accident, caused by,
        due to, chain
      shaft E919.1
    hot
      liquid E924.0
        caustic or corrosive E924.1
      object (not producing fire or
        flames) E924.8
      substance E924.9
        caustic or corrosive E924.1
        liquid (metal) NEC E924.0
        specified type NEC E924.8
    human bite E928.3
    ignition - *see* Ignition E919.4
    internal combustion engine
      E919.5
    landslide NEC E909.2
    lathe (metalworking) E919.3
      turnings E920.8
      woodworking E919.4
    lift, lifting (appliances) E919.2
      agricultural operations
        E919.0
      mining operations E919.1
      shaft E919.1
    lightning NEC E907
    machine, machinery - *see also*
      Accident, machine
      drilling, metal E919.3
      manufacturing, for manufacture
        of steam
        beverages E919.8
        clothing E919.8
        foodstuffs E919.8
        paper E919.8
        textiles E919.8
      milling, metal E919.3
      moulding E919.4
      power press, metal E919.3
      printing E919.8
      rolling mill, metal E919.3
      sawing, metal E919.3
      specified type NEC E919.8
      spinning E919.8
      weaving E919.8
    natural factor NEC E928.9
    overhead plane E919.4
    plane E920.4
      overhead E919.4
    powered
      hand tool NEC E920.1
      saw E919.4
        hand E920.1
    printing machine E919.8
    pulley (block) E919.2
      agricultural operations
        E919.0
      mining operations E919.1
      transmission E919.6
    radial saw E919.4
    radiation - *see* Radiation
    reaper E919.0
    road scraper E919.7
      when in transport under its own
        power - *see* categories
        E810–E825
    roller, coaster E919.8
    sander E919.4

E CODES

Accident *(Continued)*
 caused by, due to *(Continued)*
  saw E920.4
   band E919.4
   bench E919.4
   chain E920.1
   circular E919.4
   hand E920.4
    powered E920.1
   powered, except hand E919.4
   radial E919.4
  sawing machine, metal E919.3
  shaft
   hoist E919.1
   lift E919.1
   transmission E919.6
  shears E920.4
   hand E920.4
    powered E920.1
   mechanical E919.3
  shovel E920.4
   steam E919.7
  spinning machine E919.8
  steam - *see also* Burning, steam
   engine E919.5
   shovel E919.7
  thresher E919.0
  thunderbolt NEC E907
  tractor E919.0
   when in transport under its own
    power - *see* categories
    E810–E825
  transmission belt, cable, chain, gear,
   pinion, pulley, shaft E919.6
  turbine (gas) (water driven) E919.5
  under-cutter E919.1
  weaving machine E919.8
  winch E919.2
   agricultural operations E919.0
   mining operations E919.1
 diving E883.0
  with insufficient air supply E913.2
 glider (hang) (*see also* Collision,
  aircraft, unpowered) E842●
 hovercraft
  on
   land - *see* Accident, motor
    vehicle
   water - *see* Accident, watercraft
 ice yacht (*see also* Accident, vehicle
  NEC) E848
 in
  medical, surgical procedure
   as, or due to misadventure - *see*
    Misadventure
   causing an abnormal reaction or
    later complication without
    mention of misadventure - *see*
    Reaction, abnormal
 kite carrying a person (*see also* Collision,
  involving aircraft, unpowered)
  E842●
 land yacht (*see also* Accident, vehicle
  NEC) E848
 late effect of - *see* Late effect
 launching pad E845●
 machine, machinery (*see also* Accident,
  caused by, due to, by specific type
  of machine) E919.9
  agricultural including animal-
   powered premises E919.0
  earth-drilling E919.1
  earth moving or scraping E919.7
  excavating E919.7

Accident *(Continued)*
 machine, machinery *(Continued)*
  involving transport under own
   power on highway or transport
   vehicle - *see* categories E810-
   E825, E840-E845
  lifting (appliances) E919.2
  metalworking E919.3
  mining E919.1
  prime movers, except electric
   motors E919.5
   electric motors - *see* Accident,
    machine, by specific type of
    machine
  recreational E919.8
  specified type NEC E919.8
  transmission E919.6
  watercraft (deck) (engine room)
   (galley) (laundry) (loading)
   E836●
  woodworking or forming E919.4
 motor vehicle (on public highway)
  (traffic) E819●
  due to cataclysm - *see* categories
   E908, E909
  involving
   collision (*see also* Collision, motor
    vehicle) E812●
  nontraffic, not on public highway -
   see categories E820–E825
  not involving collision - *see*
   categories E816–E819
 nonmotor vehicle NEC E829●
  nonroad - *see* Accident, vehicle NEC
  road, except pedal cycle, animal-
   drawn vehicle, or animal being
   ridden E829●
 nonroad vehicle NEC - *see* Accident,
  vehicle NEC
 not elsewhere classifiable involving
  cable car (not on rails) E847
   on rails E829●
  coal car in mine E846
  hand truck - *see* Accident, vehicle
   NEC
  logging car E846
  sled(ge), meaning snow or ice
   vehicle E848
  tram, mine or quarry E846
  truck
   mine or quarry E846
   self-propelled, industrial E846
   station baggage E846
  tub, mine or quarry E846
  vehicle NEC E848
   snow and ice E848
   used only on industrial premises
    E846
  wheelbarrow E848
 occurring (at) (in)
  apartment E849.0
  baseball field, diamond E849.4
  construction site, any E849.3
  dock E849.8
   yard E849.3
  dormitory E849.7
  factory (building) (premises) E849.3
  farm E849.1
   buildings E849.1
   house E849.0
  football field E849.4
  forest E849.8
  garage (place of work) E849.3
   private (home) E849.0

Accident *(Continued)*
 occurring *(Continued)*
  gravel pit E849.2
  gymnasium E849.4
  highway E849.5
  home (private) (residential) E849.0
   institutional E849.7
  hospital E849.7
  hotel E849.6
  house (private) (residential) E849.0
   movie E849.6
   public E849.6
  institution, residential E849.7
  jail E849.7
  mine E849.2
  motel E849.6
  movie house E849.6
  office (building) E849.6
  orphanage E849.7
  park (public) E849.4
   mobile home E849.8
   trailer E849.8
  parking lot or place E849.8
  place
   industrial NEC E849.3
   parking E849.8
   public E849.8
    specified place NEC E849.5
   recreational NEC E849.4
   sport NEC E849.4
  playground (park) (school) E849.4
  prison E849.6
  public building NEC E849.6
  quarry E849.2
  railway
   line NEC E849.8
   yard E849.3
  residence
   home (private) E849.0
  resort (beach) (lake) (mountain)
   (seashore) (vacation) E849.4
  restaurant E849.6
  sand pit E849.2
  school (building) (private) (public)
   (state) E849.6
   reform E849.7
   riding E849.4
  seashore E849.8
   resort E849.4
  shop (place of work) E849.3
   commercial E849.6
  skating rink E849.4
  sports palace E849.4
  stadium E849.4
  store E849.6
  street E849.5
  swimming pool (public) E849.4
   private home or garden E849.0
  tennis court E849.4 public
  theatre, theater E849.6
  trailer court E849.8
  tunnel E849.8
   under construction E849.2
  warehouse E849.3
  yard
   dock E849.3
   industrial E849.3
   private (home) E849.0
   railway E849.3
 off-road type motor vehicle (not on
  public highway) NEC E821●
 on public highway - *see* categories
  E810–E819
 pedal cycle E826●

◀ New   ⬅ Revised   ~~deleted~~ Deleted   ● Use Additional Digit(s)   ▬ Omit code

E CODES

Accident *(Continued)*
railway E807●
  due to cataclysm - *see* categories
    E908, E909
  involving
    burning by engine, locomotive,
      train *(see also* Explosion,
      railway engine) E803●
    collision *(see also* Collision,
      railway) E800●
    derailment *(see also* Derailment,
      railway) E802●
    explosion *(see also* Explosion,
      railway engine) E803●
    fall *(see also* Fall, from, railway
      rolling stock) E804●
    fire *(see also* Explosion, railway
      engine) E803●
    hitting by, being struck by
      object falling in, on, from,
        rolling stock, train,
        vehicle E806●
      rolling stock, train, vehicle
        E805●
    overturning, railway rolling
      stock, train, vehicle *(see also*
      Derailment, railway) E802●
    running off rails, railway *(see also*
      Derailment, railway) E802●
    specified circumstances NEC
      E806●
    train or vehicle hit by
      avalanche E909.2
      falling object (earth, rock, tree)
        E806●
        due to cataclysm - *see*
          categories E908, E909
      landslide E909.2
  roller skate E885.1
  scooter (nonmotorized) E885.0
  skateboard E885.2
  ski(ing) E885.3
    jump E884.9
    lift or tow (with chair or gondola) E847
  snow vehicle, motor driven (not on
    public highway) E820●
    on public highway - *see* categories
      E810–E819
  snowboard E885.4
  spacecraft E845●
  specified cause NEC E928.8
  street car E829●
  traffic NEC E819●
  vehicle NEC (with pedestrian) E848
    battery powered
      airport passenger vehicle E846
      truck (baggage) (mail) E846
    powered commercial or industrial
      (with other vehicle or object
      within commercial or
      industrial premises) E846
  watercraft E838●
    with
      drowning or submersion
        resulting from
        accident other than to
          watercraft E832●
        accident to watercraft E830●
      injury, except drowning or
        submersion, resulting from
        accident other than to
          watercraft - *see* categories
          E833–E838
        accident to watercraft E831●

Accident *(Continued)*
  watercraft *(Continued)*
    due to, caused by cataclysm - *see*
      categories E908, E909
    machinery E836●
Acid throwing E961
Acosta syndrome E902.0
Activity (involving) E030 ◄
  aerobic and step exercise (class)
    E009.2 ◄
  alpine skiing E003.2 ◄
  animal care NEC E019.9 ◄
  arts and handcrafts NEC E012.9 ◄
  athletics NEC E008.9 ◄
    played
      as a team or group NEC E007.9 ◄
      individually NEC E006.9 ◄
  baking E015.2 ◄
  ballet E005.0 ◄
  barbells E010.2 ◄
  BASE (Building, Antenna, Span,
    Earth) jumping E004.2 ◄
  baseball E007.3 ◄
  basketball E007.6 ◄
  bathing (personal) E013.0 ◄
  beach volleyball E007.7 ◄
  bike riding E006.4 ◄
  boogie boarding E002.7 ◄
  bowling E006.3 ◄
  boxing E008.0 ◄
  brass instrument playing E018.3 ◄
  building and construction E016.2 ◄
  bungee jumping E004.3 ◄
  calisthenics E009.1 ◄
  canoeing (in calm and turbulent
    water) E002.5 ◄
  capture the flag E007.8 ◄
  cardiorespiratory exercise
    NEC E009.9 ◄
  caregiving (providing) NEC E014.9 ◄
    bathing E014.0 ◄
    lifting E014.1 ◄
  cellular
    communication device E011.1 ◄
    telephone E011.1 ◄
  challenge course E009.4 ◄
  cheerleading E005.4 ◄
  circuit training E009.3 ◄
  cleaning
    floor E013.4 ◄
  climbing NEC E004.9 ◄
    mountain E004.0 ◄
    rock E004.0 ◄
    wall climbing E004.0 ◄
  combatives E008.4 ◄
  computer
    keyboarding E011.0 ◄
    technology NEC E011.9 ◄
  confidence course E009.4 ◄
  construction (building) E016.2 ◄
  cooking and baking E015.2 ◄
  cooking and grilling NEC E015.9 ◄
  cool down exercises E009.1 ◄
  cricket E007.9 ◄
  crocheting E012.0 ◄
  cross country skiing E003.3 ◄
  dancing (all types) E005.0 ◄
  digging
    dirt E016.0 ◄
  dirt digging E016.0 ◄
  dishwashing E015.0 ◄
  diving (platform) (springboard)
    E002.1 ◄
    underwater E002.4 ◄

Activity *(Continued)*
  dodge ball E007.8 ◄
  downhill skiing E003.2 ◄
  drum playing E018.1 ◄
  dumbbells E010.2 ◄
  electronic
    devices NEC E011.9 ◄
      hand held interactive E011.1 ◄
    game playing (using) (with)
      interactive device E011.1 ◄
      keyboard or other stationary
        device E011.0 ◄
  elliptical machine E009.0 ◄
  exercise(s)
    machines ((primarily) for)
      cardiorespiratory conditioning
        E009.0 ◄
      muscle strengthening E010.0 ◄
    muscle strengthening
      (non-machine) NEC
      E010.9 ◄
  external motion NEC E017.9 ◄
    rollercoaster E017.0 ◄
  field hockey E007.4 ◄
  figure skating (pairs) (singles)
    E003.0 ◄
  flag football E007.1 ◄
  floor mopping and cleaning E013.4 ◄
  food preparation and clean up
    E015.0 ◄
  football (American) NOS E007.0 ◄
    flag E007.1 ◄
    tackle E007.0 ◄
    touch E007.1 ◄
  four square E007.8 ◄
  free weights E010.2 ◄
  frisbee (ultimate) E008.3 ◄
  furniture
    building E012.2 ◄
    finishing E012.2 ◄
    repair E012.2 ◄
  game playing (electronic)
    using
      interactive device E011.1 ◄
      keyboard or other stationary
        device E011.0 ◄
  gardening E016.1 ◄
  golf E006.2 ◄
  grass drills E009.5 ◄
  grilling and smoking food
    E015.1 ◄
  grooming and shearing an animal
    E019.2 ◄
  guerilla drills E009.5 ◄
  gymnastics (rhythmic) E005.2 ◄
  handball E008.2 ◄
  handcrafts NEC E012.9 ◄
  hand held interactive electronic
    device E011.1 ◄
  hang gliding E004.4 ◄
  hiking (on level or elevated
    terrain) E001.0 ◄
  hockey (ice) E003.1 ◄
    field E007.4 ◄
  horseback riding E006.1 ◄
  household maintenance
    NEC E013.9 ◄
  ice NEC E003.9 ◄
    dancing E003.0 ◄
    hockey E003.1 ◄
    skating E003.0 ◄
  inline roller skating E006.0 ◄
  ironing E013.3 ◄
  judo E008.4 ◄

E CODES

◄ New   ◄▥ Revised   ~~deleted~~ Deleted   ● Use Additional Digit(s)   ▬ Omit code

Asphyxia, asphyxiation
by
chemical
in
terrorism E979.7
war operations E997.2
explosion - *see* Explosion E965.8
food (bone) (regurgitated food)
(seed) E911
foreign object, except food E912
fumes
in
terrorism (chemical weapons)
E979.7
war operations E997.2
gas - *see also* Table of Drugs and
Chemicals
in
terrorism E979.7
war operations E997.2
legal
execution E978
intervention (tear) E972
tear E972
mechanical means (*see also*
Suffocation) E913.9
from
conflagration - *see* Conflagration
fire - *see also* Fire E899
in
terrorism E979.3
war operations E990.9
ignition - *see* Ignition
Aspiration
foreign body - *see* Foreign body,
aspiration
mucus, not of newborn (with asphyxia,
obstruction respiratory passage,
suffocation) E912
phlegm (with asphyxia, obstruction
respiratory passage, suffocation)
E912
vomitus (with asphyxia, obstruction
respiratory passage, suffocation)
(*see also* Foreign body, aspiration,
food) E911
Assassination (attempt) (*see also* Assault)
E968.9
Assault (homicidal) (by) (in) E968.9
acid E961
swallowed E962.1
air gun E968.6
BB gun E968.6
bite NEC E968.8
of human being E968.7
bomb ((placed in) car or house) E965.8
antipersonnel E965.5
letter E965.7
petrol E965.6
brawl (hand) (fists) (foot) E960.0
burning, burns (by fire) E968.0
acid E961
swallowed E962.1
caustic, corrosive substance E961
swallowed E962.1
chemical from swallowing caustic,
corrosive substance NEC
E962.1
hot liquid E968.3
scalding E968.3
vitriol E961
swallowed E962.1
caustic, corrosive substance E961
swallowed E962.1
cut, any part of body E966

Assault (*Continued*)
dagger E966
drowning E964
explosives E965.9
bomb (*see also* Assault, bomb) E965.8
dynamite E965.8
fight (hand) (fists) (foot) E960.0
with weapon E968.9
blunt or thrown E968.2
cutting or piercing E966
firearm - *see* Shooting, homicide
fire E968.0
firearm(s) - *see* Shooting, homicide
garrotting E963
gunshot (wound) - *see* Shooting,
homicide
hanging E963
injury NEC E968.9
knife E966
late effect of E969
ligature E963
poisoning E962.9
drugs or medicinals E962.0
gas(es) or vapors, except drugs and
medicinals E962.2
solid or liquid substances, except
drugs and medicinals
E962.1
puncture, any part of body E966
pushing
before moving object, train, vehicle
E968.5
from high place E968.1
rape E960.1
scalding E968.3
shooting - *see* Shooting, homicide
sodomy E960.1
stab, any part of body E966
strangulation E963
submersion E964
suffocation E963
transport vehicle E968.5
violence NEC E968.9
vitriol E961
swallowed E962.1
weapon E968.9
blunt or thrown E968.2
cutting or piercing E966
firearm - *see* Shooting, homicide
wound E968.9
cutting E966
gunshot - *see* Shooting, homicide
knife E966
piercing E966
puncture E966
stab E966
Attack by animal NEC E906.9
Avalanche E909.2
falling on or hitting
motor vehicle (in motion) (on public
highway) E909.2
railway train E909.2
Aviators' disease E902.1

B

**Barotitis, barodontalgia, berosinusitis,
barotrauma** (otitic) (sinus) - *see*
Effects of, air pressure
Battered
baby or child (syndrome) - *see* Abuse,
child; category E967
person other than baby or child - *see*
Assault

Bayonet wound (*see also* Cut, by bayonet)
E920.3
in
legal intervention E974
terrorism E979.8
war operations E995.2
Bean in nose E912
Bed set on fire NEC E898.0
Beheading (by guillotine)
homicide E966
legal execution E978
Bending, injury in E927.8
Bends E902.0
Bite
animal NEC E906.5
other specified (except arthropod)
E906.3
venomous NEC E905.9
arthropod (nonvenomous) NEC E906.4
venomous - *see* Sting
black widow spider E905.1
cat E906.3
centipede E905.4
cobra E905.0
copperhead snake E905.0
coral snake E905.0
dog E906.0
fer de lance E905.0
gila monster E905.0
human being
accidental E928.3
assault E968.7
insect (nonvenomous) E906.4
venomous - *see* Sting
krait E905.0
late effect of - *see* Late effect
lizard E906.2
venomous E905.0
mamba E905.0
marine animal
nonvenomous E906.3
snake E906.2
venomous E905.6
snake E905.0
millipede E906.4
venomous E905.4
moray eel E906.3
rat E906.1
rattlesnake E905.0
rodent, except rat E906.3
serpent - *see* Bite, snake
shark E906.3
snake (venomous) E905.0
nonvenomous E906.2
sea E905.0
spider E905.1
nonvenomous E906.4
tarantula (venomous) E905.1
venomous NEC E905.9
by specific animal - *see* category
E905
viper E905.0
water moccasin E905.0
Blast (air)
in
terrorism E979.2
from nuclear explosion E979.5
underwater E979.0
war operations E993.9
from nuclear explosion (*see
also* War operations,
injury due to, nuclear
weapons) E996.0
underwater E992.9
Blizzard E908.3

◀ New   ⇐ Revised   ~~deleted~~ Deleted   ● Use Additional Digit(s)   ▨ Omit code

E CODES

Blow E928.9
  by law-enforcing agent, police (on
    duty) E975
    with blunt object (baton)
      (nightstick) (stave)
      (truncheon) E973
Blowing up (*see also* Explosion) E923.9
Brawl (hand) (fists) (foot) E960.0
Breakage (accidental)
  cable of cable car not on rails E847
  ladder (causing fall) E881.0
  part (any) of
    animal-drawn vehicle E827●
    ladder (causing fall) E881.0
    motor vehicle
      in motion (on public highway)
        E818●
      not on public highway
        E825●
    nonmotor road vehicle, except
      animal-drawn vehicle or pedal
      cycle E829●
    off-road type motor vehicle (not
      on public highway)
      NEC E821●
      on public highway E818●
    pedal cycle E826●
    scaffolding (causing fall) E881.1
    snow vehicle, motor-driven (not on
      public highway) E820●
      on public highway E818●
    vehicle NEC - *see* Accident, vehicle
Broken
  glass
    fall on E888.0
    injury by E920.8
  power line (causing electric shock)
    E925.1
Bumping against, into (accidentally)
  object (moving) E917.9
    caused by crowd E917.1
      with subsequent fall E917.6
    furniture E917.3
      with subsequent fall E917.7
    in
      running water E917.2
      sports E917.0
        with subsequent fall E917.5
    stationary E917.4
      with subsequent fall E917.8
  person(s) E917.9
    with fall E886.9
      in sports E886.0
    as, or caused by, a crowd E917.1
      with subsequent fall E917.6
    in sports E917.0
      with fall E886.0
Burning, burns (accidental) (by) (from)
  (on) E899
  acid (any kind) E924.1
    swallowed - *see* Table of Drugs and
      Chemicals
  airgun E928.7 ◄
  bedclothes (*see also* Fire, specified NEC)
    E898.0
  blowlamp (*see also* Fire, specified NEC)
    E898.1
  blowtorch (*see also* Fire, specified NEC)
    E898.1
  boat, ship, watercraft - *see* categories
    E830, E831, E837
  bonfire (controlled) E897
    uncontrolled E892
  candle (*see also* Fire, specified NEC)
    E898.1

Burning, burns (*Continued*)
  caustic liquid, substance E924.1
    swallowed - *see* Table of Drugs and
      Chemicals
  chemical E924.1
    from swallowing caustic, corrosive
      substance - *see* Table of Drugs
      and Chemicals
    in
      terrorism E979.7
      war operations E997.2
  cigar(s) or cigarette(s) (*see also* Fire,
    specified NEC) E898.1
  clothes, clothing, nightdress - *see*
    Ignition, clothes
    with conflagration - *see*
      Conflagration
  conflagration - *see* Conflagration
  corrosive liquid, substance
    E924.1
    swallowed - *see* Table of Drugs
      and Chemicals
  electric current (*see also* Electric shock)
    E925.9
  fire, flames (*see also* Fire) E899
  firearm E928.7 ◄
  flare, Verey pistol E922.8
  heat
    from appliance (electrical) E924.8
    in local application, or packing
      during medical or surgical
      procedure E873.5
  homicide (attempt) (*see also* Assault,
    burning) E968.0
  hot
    liquid E924.0
      caustic or corrosive E924.1
    object (not producing fire or flames)
      E924.8
    substance E924.9
      caustic or corrosive E924.1
      liquid (metal) NEC E924.0
      specified type NEC E924.8
    tap water E924.2
  ignition - *see also* Ignition
    clothes, clothing, nightdress - *see also*
      Ignition, clothes
      with conflagration - *see*
        Conflagration
    highly inflammable material
      (benzine) (fat) (gasoline)
      (kerosine) (paraffin) (petrol)
      E894
  inflicted by other person
    stated as
      homicidal, intentional (*see also*
        Assault, burning) E968.0
      undetermined whether
        accidental or intentional
        (*see also* Burn, stated as
        undetermined whether
        accidental or intentional)
        E988.1
  internal, from swallowed caustic,
    corrosive liquid, substance - *see*
    Table of Drugs and Chemicals
  in
    terrorism E979.3
      from nuclear explosion E979.5
      petrol bomb E979.3
    war operations (from fire-producing
      device or conventional
      weapon) E990.9
      from nuclear explosion (*see*
       also War operations,
       injury due to, nuclear
       weapons) E996.2 ◄

Burning, burns (*Continued*)
  in (*Continued*)
    war operations (*Continued*)
      incendiary bomb E990.0 ◄
      petrol bomb E990.0
    lamp (*see also* Fire, specified NEC)
      E898.1
    late effect of NEC E929.4
    lighter (cigar) (cigarette) (*see also* Fire,
      specified NEC) E898.1
    lightning E907
    liquid (boiling) (hot) (molten)
      E924.0
      caustic, corrosive (external)
        E924.1
        swallowed - *see* Table of Drugs
          and Chemicals
    local application of externally applied
      substance in medical or surgical
      care E873.5
    machinery - *see* Accident, machine
    matches (*see also* Fire, specified NEC)
      E898.1
    medicament, externally applied
      E873.5
    metal, molten E924.0
    object (hot) E924.8
      producing fire or flames - *see* Fire
    oven (electric) (gas) E924.8
    pipe (smoking) (*see also* Fire, specified
      NEC) E898.1
    radiation - *see* Radiation
    railway engine, locomotive, train (*see*
      also Explosion, railway engine)
      E803●
    self-inflicted (unspecified whether
      accidental or intentional)
      E988.1
    caustic or corrosive substance NEC
      E988.7
    stated as intentional, purposeful
      E958.1
      caustic or corrosive substance
        NEC E958.7
    stated as undetermined whether
      accidental or intentional
      E988.1
      caustic or corrosive substance NEC
        E988.7
    steam E924.0
      pipe E924.8
    substance (hot) E924.9
      boiling or molten E924.0
      caustic, corrosive (external)
        E924.1
        swallowed - *see* Table of Drugs
          and Chemicals
    suicidal (attempt) NEC E958.1
      caustic substance E958.7
      late effect of E959
    tanning bed E926.2
    therapeutic misadventure
      overdose of radiation E873.2
    torch, welding (*see also* Fire, specified
      NEC) E898.1
    trash fire (*see also* Burning, bonfire)
      E897
    vapor E924.0
    vitriol E924.1
    x-rays E926.3
      in medical, surgical procedure - *see*
        Misadventure, failure, in
        dosage, radiation
        operations
Butted by animal E906.8

◄ New   ◄▦ Revised   ~~deleted~~ Deleted   ● Use Additional Digit(s)   ▦ Omit code

E CODES

C

Cachexia, lead or saturnine E866.0
  from pesticide NEC (*see also* Table
    of Drugs and Chemicals)
    E863.4
Caisson disease E902.2
Capital punishment (any means) E978
Car sickness E903
Casualty (not due to war) NEC E928.9
  terrorism E979.8
  war (*see also* War operations) E995.9 ◄▥
Cat
  bite E906.3
  scratch E906.8
Cataclysmic (any injury)
  earth surface movement or eruption
    E909.9
    specified type NEC E909.8
  storm or flood resulting from storm
    E908.9
    specified type NEC E909.8
Catching fire - *see* Ignition
Caught
  between
    objects (moving) (stationary and
      moving) E918
      and machinery - *see* Accident,
        machine
  by cable car, not on rails E847
  in
    machinery (moving parts of) - *see*
      Accident, machine
    object E918
Cave-in (causing asphyxia, suffocation
  (by pressure)) (*see also* Suffocation,
  due to, cave-in) E913.3
  with injury other than asphyxia or
    suffocation E916
    with asphyxia or suffocation (*see
      also* Suffocation, due to,
      cave-in) E913.3
  struck or crushed by E916
    with asphyxia or suffocation (*see also*
      Suffocation, due to, cave-in)
      E913.3
Change(s) in air pressure - *see also* Effects
  of, air pressure
  sudden, in aircraft (ascent) (descent)
    (causing aeroneurosis or aviators'
    disease) E902.1
Chilblains E901.0
  due to manmade conditions E901.1
Choking (on) (any object except food or
  vomitus) E912
  apple E911
  bone E911
  food, any type (regurgitated) E911
  mucus or phlegm E912
  seed E911
Civil insurrection - *see* War operations
Cloudburst E908.8
Cold, exposure to (accidental) (excessive)
  (extreme) (place) E901.9
  causing chilblains or immersion foot
    E901.0
  due to
    manmade conditions E901.1
    specified cause NEC E901.8
    weather (conditions) E901.0
  late effect of NEC E929.5
  self-inflicted (undetermined whether
    accidental or intentional)
    E988.3
    suicidal E958.3
  suicide E958.3

Colic, lead, painters', or saturnine - *see*
  category E866
Collapse
  building E916
    burning (uncontrolled fire) E891.8
      in terrorism E979.3
      private E890.8
  dam E909.3
  due to heat - *see* Heat
  machinery - *see* Accident, machine or
    vehicle
  man-made structure E909.3
  postoperative NEC E878.9
  structure
    burning (uncontrolled fire) NEC
      E891.8
      in terrorism E979.3
Collision (accidental)

> **Note 80** In the case of collisions
> between different types of vehicles,
> persons and objects, priority in
> classification is in the following order:
>
>   Aircraft
>   Watercraft
>   Motor vehicle
>   Railway vehicle
>   Pedal cycle
>   Animal-drawn vehicle
>   Animal being ridden
>   Streetcar or other
>   nonmotor road vehicle
>   Other vehicle
>   Pedestrian or person using
>   pedestrian conveyance
>   Object (except where falling from
>   or set in motion by vehicle,
>   etc. listed above)
>
> In the listing below, the combinations
> are listed only under the vehicle, etc.,
> having priority. For definitions, *see*
> Supplementary Classification of
> External Causes of Injury and
> Poisoning (E800–E999).

  aircraft (with object or vehicle) (fixed)
    (movable) (moving) E841●
    with
      person (while landing, taking off)
        (without accident to
        aircraft) E844●
    powered (in transit) (with
      unpowered aircraft) E841●
      while landing, taking off E840●
    unpowered E842●
      while landing, taking off E840●
  animal being ridden (in sport or
    transport) E828●
    and
      animal (being ridden) (herded)
        (unattended) E828●
      nonmotor road vehicle, except
        pedal cycle or animal-
        drawn vehicle E828●
      object (fallen) (fixed) (movable)
        (moving) not falling from or
        set in motion by vehicle of
        higher priority E828●
      pedestrian (conveyance or
        vehicle) E828●
  animal-drawn vehicle E827●
    and
      animal (being ridden) (herded)
        (unattended) E827●

Collision (*Continued*)
  animal-drawn vehicle (*Continued*)
    and (*Continued*)
      nonmotor road vehicle, except
        pedal cycle E827●
      object (fallen) (fixed) (movable)
        (moving) not falling from or
        set in motion by vehicle of
        higher priority E827●
      pedestrian (conveyance or
        vehicle) E827●
      streetcar E827●
  motor vehicle (on public highway)
    (traffic accident) E812●
    after leaving, running off, public
      highway (without antecedent
      collision) (without re-entry)
      E816●
    with antecedent collision on
      public highway - *see*
      categories E810–E815
    with re-entrance collision with
      another motor vehicle
      E811●
    and
      abutment (bridge) (overpass)
        E815●
      animal (herded) (unattended)
        E815●
        carrying person, property
          E813●
      animal-drawn vehicle E813●
      another motor vehicle
        (abandoned) (disabled)
        (parked) (stalled) (stopped)
        E812●
        with, involving re-entrance (on
          same roadway) (across
          median strip) E811●
      any object, person, or vehicle off
        the public highway
        resulting from a
        noncollision motor vehicle
        nontraffic accident E816●
      avalanche, fallen or not moving
        E815●
        falling E909.2
      boundary fence E815●
      culvert E815●
      fallen
        stone E815●
        tree E815●
      guard post or guard rail E815●
      inter-highway divider E815●
      landslide, fallen or not moving
        E815●
        moving E909.2
      machinery (road) E815●
      nonmotor road vehicle NEC
        E813●
      object (any object, person, or
        vehicle off the public
        highway resulting from a
        noncollision motor vehicle
        nontraffic accident) E815●
      off, normally not on, public
        highway resulting from a
        noncollision motor
        vehicle traffic accident
        E816●
      pedal cycle E813●
      pedestrian (conveyance)
        E814●
      person (using pedestrian
        conveyance) E814●

E CODES

Collision (*Continued*)
  motor vehicle (*Continued*)
    and (*Continued*)
      post or pole (lamp) (light) (signal)
        (telephone) (utility) E815●
      railway rolling stock, train,
        vehicle E810●
      safety island E815●
      street car E813●
      traffic signal, sign, or marker
        (temporary) E815●
      tree E815●
      tricycle E813●
      wall of cut made for road E815●
    due to cataclysm - *see* categories
      E908, E909
    not on public highway, nontraffic
      accident E822●
    and
      animal (carrying person,
        property) (herded)
        (unattended) E822●
      animal-drawn vehicle E822●
      another motor vehicle
        (moving), except off-road
        motor vehicle E822●
        stationary E823●
      avalanche, fallen, not moving
        NEC E823●
        moving E909.2
      landslide, fallen, not moving
        E823●
        moving E909.2
      nonmotor vehicle (moving)
        E822●
        stationary E823●
      object (fallen) ((normally)
        (fixed) (movable but not
        in motion) (stationary)
        E823●
        moving, except when
          falling from, set in
          motion by, aircraft or
          cataclysm E822●
      pedal cycle (moving) E822●
        stationary E823●
      pedestrian (conveyance)
        E822●
      person (using pedestrian
        conveyance) E822●
      railway rolling stock, train,
        vehicle (moving)
        E822●
        stationary E823●
      road vehicle (any) (moving)
        E822●
        stationary E823●
      tricycle (moving) E822●
        stationary E823●
  off-road type motor vehicle (not on
    public highway) E821●
    and
      animal (being ridden) (-drawn
        vehicle) E821●
      another off-road motor vehicle,
        except snow vehicle
        E821●
      other motor vehicle, not on public
        highway E821●
      other object or vehicle NEC, fixed
        or movable, not set in
        motion by aircraft, motor
        vehicle on highway, or
        snow vehicle, motor-driven
        E821●

Collision (*Continued*)
  off-road type motor vehicle
    (*Continued*)
    and (*Continued*)
      pedal cycle E821●
      pedestrian (conveyance)
        E821●
      railway train E821●
    on public highway - *see* Collision,
      motor vehicle
  pedal cycle E826●
    and
      animal (carrying person,
        property) (herded)
        (unherded) E826●
      animal-drawn vehicle E826●
      another pedal cycle E826●
      nonmotor road vehicle
        E826●
      object (fallen) (fixed) (movable)
        (moving) not falling from
        or set in motion by
        aircraft, motor vehicle,
        or railway train NEC
        E826●
      pedestrian (conveyance)
        E826●
      person (using pedestrian
        conveyance) E826●
      street car E826●
  pedestrian(s) (conveyance) E917.9
    with fall E886.9
      in sports E886.0
    and
      crowd, human stampede
        E917.1
        with subsequent fall E917.6
      furniture E917.3
        with subsequent fall E917.7
      machinery - *see* Accident,
        machine
      object (fallen) (moving) not
        falling from or set in
        motion by any vehicle
        classifiable to E800–E848,
        E917.9
      caused by a crowd E917.1
        with subsequent fall
          E917.6
      furniture E917.3
        with subsequent fall
          E917.7
      in
        running water E917.2
          with drowning or
            submersion - *see*
            Submersion
        sports E917.0
          with subsequent fall
            E917.5
        stationary E917.4
          with subsequent fall
            E917.8
      vehicle, nonmotor, nonroad
        E848
    in
      running water E917.2
        with drowning or
          submersion - *see*
          Submersion
      sports E917.0
        with fall E886.0
  person(s) (using pedestrian
    conveyance) (*see also* Collision,
    pedestrian) E917.9

Collision (*Continued*)
  railway (rolling stock) (train) (vehicle)
    (with (subsequent) derailment,
    explosion, fall or fire) E800●
    with antecedent derailment
      E802●
    and
      animal (carrying person)
        (herded) (unattended)
        E801●
      another railway train or vehicle
        E800●
      buffers E801●
      fallen tree on railway E801●
      farm machinery, nonmotor (in
        transport) (stationary)
        E801●
      gates E801●
      nonmotor vehicle E801●
      object (fallen) (fixed) (movable)
        (movable) (moving) not
        falling from, set in motion
        by, aircraft or motor vehicle
        NEC E801●
      pedal cycle E801●
      pedestrian (conveyance)
        E805●
      person (using pedestrian
        conveyance) E805●
      platform E801●
      rock on railway E801●
      street car E801●
  snow vehicle, motor-driven (not on
    public highway) E820●
    and
      animal (being ridden) (-drawn
        vehicle) E820●
      another off-road motor vehicle
        E820●
      other motor vehicle, not on public
        highway E820●
      other object or vehicle NEC,
        fixed or movable, not set in
        motion by aircraft or motor
        vehicle on highway E820●
      pedal cycle E820●
      pedestrian (conveyance) E820●
      railway train E820●
    on public highway - *see* Collision,
      motor vehicle
  street car(s) E829●
    and
      animal, herded, not being ridden,
        unattended E829●
      nonmotor road vehicle NEC
        E829●
      object (fallen) (fixed) (movable)
        (moving) not falling from or
        set in motion by aircraft,
        animal-drawn vehicle,
        animal being ridden, motor
        vehicle, pedal cycle, or
        railway train E829●
      pedestrian (conveyance)
        E829●
      person (using pedestrian
        conveyance) E829●
  vehicle
    animal-drawn - *see* Collision,
      animal-drawn vehicle
    motor - *see* Collision, motor vehicle
    nonmotor
      nonroad E848
      and
        another nonmotor, nonroad
          vehicle E848

◀ New   ◀❙❙❙ Revised   ~~deleted~~ Deleted   ● Use Additional Digit(s)   ▨ Omit code

E CODES

Collision *(Continued)*
  vehicle *(Continued)*
    nonmotor *(Continued)*
      nonroad *(Continued)*
        and *(Continued)*
          object (fallen) (fixed)
            (movable) (moving)
            not falling from or set
            in motion by aircraft,
            animal-drawn vehicle,
            animal being ridden,
            motor vehicle,
            nonmotor road
            vehicle, pedal cycle,
            railway train, or
            streetcar E848
      road, except animal being ridden,
        animal-drawn vehicle, or
        pedal cycle E829●
        and
          animal, herded, not being
            ridden, unattended
            E829
          another nonmotor road
            vehicle, except animal
            being ridden, animal-
            drawn vehicle, or
            pedal cycle E829●
          object (fallen) (fixed)
            (movable) (moving)
            not falling from or set
            in motion by, aircraft,
            animal-drawn vehicle,
            animal being ridden,
            motor vehicle, pedal
            cycle, or railway train
            E829●
          pedestrian (conveyance)
            E829●
          person (using pedestrian
            conveyance) E829●
          vehicle, nonmotor, nonroad
            E829●
  watercraft E838●
    and
      person swimming or water skiing
        E838●
    causing
      drowning, submersion E830●
      injury except drowning,
        submersion E831
Combustion, spontaneous - *see* Ignition
Complication of medical or surgical
    procedure or treatment
  as an abnormal reaction - *see* Reaction,
    abnormal
  delayed, without mention of
    misadventure - *see* Reaction,
    abnormal
  due to misadventure - *see*
    Misadventure
Compression
  divers' squeeze E902.2
  trachea by
    food E911
    foreign body, except food E912
Conflagration
  building or structure, except private
    dwelling (barn) (church)
    (convalescent or residential
    home) (factory) (farm
    outbuilding) (hospital) (hotel) or
    (institution (educational)
    (dormitory) (residential))
    (school) (shop) (store) (theatre)
    E891.9

Conflagration *(Continued)*
  building or structure, except private
    dwelling *(Continued)*
    with or causing (injury due to)
      accident or injury NEC E891.9
        specified circumstance NEC
          E891.8
      burns, burning E891.3
      carbon monoxide E891.2
      fumes E891.2
      polyvinylchloride (PVC) or
        similar material E891.1
      smoke E891.2
    causing explosion E891.0
    in terrorism E979.3
  not in building or structure E892
  private dwelling (apartment) (boarding
    house) (camping place) (caravan)
    (farmhouse) (home (private))
    (house) (lodging house) (private
    garage) (rooming house)
    (tenement) E890.9
    with or causing (injury due to)
      accident or injury NEC E890.9
        specified circumstance NEC
          E890.8
      burns, burning E890.3
      carbon monoxide E890.2
      fumes E890.2
        polyvinylchloride (PVC) or
          similar material E890.1
      smoke E890.2
    causing explosion E890.0
Constriction, external
  caused by
    hair E928.4
    other object E928.5
Contact with
  dry ice E901.1
  liquid air, hydrogen, nitrogen E901.1
Cramp(s)
  heat - *see* Heat
  swimmers (*see also* category E910) 910.2
    not in recreation or sport E910.3
Cranking (car) (truck) (bus) (engine)
  injury by E917.9
Crash
  aircraft (in transit) (powered) E841●
    at landing, take-off E840●
    in
      terrorism E979.1
      war operations E994.9 ◀▥
    on runway NEC E840●
    stated as
      homicidal E968.8
      suicidal E958.6
      undetermined whether
        accidental or intentional
        E988.6
    unpowered E842●
  glider E842●
  motor vehicle - *see also* Accident, motor
    vehicle
    homicidal E968.5
    suicidal E958.5
    undetermined whether accidental
      or intentional E988.5
Crushed (accidentally) E928.9
  between
    boat(s), ship(s), watercraft (and
      dock or pier) (without
      accident to watercraft)
      E838●
      after accident to, or collision,
        watercraft E831●
    objects (moving) (stationary and
      moving) E918

Crushed *(Continued)*
  by
    avalanche NEC E909.2
    boat, ship, watercraft after accident
      to, collision, watercraft
      E831●
    cave-in E916
      with asphyxiation or suffocation
        (*see also* Suffocation, due to,
        cave-in) E913.3
    crowd, human stampede E917.1
    falling
      aircraft (*see also* Accident, aircraft)
        E841●
        in
          terrorism E979.1
          war operations E994.8 ◀▥
      earth, material E916
        with asphyxiation or
          suffocation (*see also*
          Suffocation, due to,
          cave-in) E913.3
      object E916
        on ship, watercraft E838●
        while loading, unloading
          watercraft E838●   ◀
    firearm E928.7
    landslide NEC E909.2
    lifeboat after abandoning ship
      E831●
    machinery - *see* Accident, machine
    railway rolling stock, train, vehicle
      (part of) E805●
    slide trigger mechanism, scope or
      other part of the gun E928.7 ◀
    street car E829●
    vehicle NEC - *see* Accident, vehicle
      NEC
  in
    machinery - *see* Accident, machine
    object E918
    transport accident - *see* categories
      E800–E848
  late effect of NEC E929.9
Cut, cutting (any part of body)
    (accidental) E920.9
  by
    arrow E920.8
    axe E920.4
    bayonet (*see also* Bayonet wound)
      E920.3
      in war operations E995.2   ◀
    blender E920.2
    broken glass E920.8
      following fall E888.0
    can opener E920.4
      powered E920.2
    chisel E920.4
    circular saw E919.4
    cutting or piercing instrument - *see
      also* category E920
      following fall E888.0
      late effect of E929.8
    dagger E920.3
    dart E920.8
    drill - *see* Accident, caused by drill
    edge of stiff paper E920.8
    electric
      beater E920.2
      fan E920.2
      knife E920.2
      mixer E920.2
    firearm component E928.7   ◀
    fork E920.4
    garden fork E920.4

E CODES

◄ New   ◄▓ Revised   ~~deleted~~ Deleted   ● Use Additional Digit(s)   ▓ Omit code

E CODES

Electric shock, electrocution *(Continued)*
electric power generating plant,
distribution station E925.1
electroshock gun (taser) (stun gun)
E925.8
caused by other person E968.8
legal intervention E975
stated as accidental E925.8
stated as intentional E968.8
due to legal intervention E975
stated as intentional self-harm
(suicidal (attempt)) E958.4
stated as undetermined whether
accidental or intentional
E988.4
suicide (attempt) E958.4
homicidal (attempt) E968.8
legal execution E978
lightning E907
machinery E925.9
domestic E925.0
factory E925.2
farm E925.8
home E925.0
misadventure in medical or surgical
procedure
in electroshock therapy E873.4
self-inflicted (undetermined whether
accidental or intentional)
E988.4
stated as intentional E958.4
stated as undetermined whether
accidental or intentional
E988.4
suicidal (attempt) E958.4
transmission line E925.1
Electrocution - *see* Electric shock
Embolism E921.1
air (traumatic) NEC - *see* Air, embolism
Encephalitis
lead or saturnine E866.0
from pesticide NEC E863.4
Entanglement
in
bedclothes, causing suffocation
E913.0
wheel of pedal cycle E826●
Entry of foreign body, material, any - *see*
Foreign body
Execution, legal (any method) E978
Exertion, excessive physical, from
prolonged activity E927.2
Exhaustion
cold - *see* Cold, exposure to
due to excessive exertion E927.8
heat - *see* Heat
Explosion (accidental) (in) (of) (on) E923.9
acetylene E923.2
aerosol can E921.8
aircraft (in transit) (powered) E841●
at landing, take-off E840●
in
terrorism E979.1
war operations E994 ◀▦
from ◀
enemy fire or explosive(s)
(device placed on
aircraft) E994.0 ◀
own onboard explosives
E994.1 ◀
unpowered E842●
air tank (compressed) (in machinery)
E921.1
anesthetic gas in operating theatre
E923.2

Explosion *(Continued)*
automobile tire NEC E921.8
causing transport accident - *see*
categories E810-E825
blasting (cap) (materials) E923.1
boiler (machinery), not on transport
vehicle E921.0
steamship - *see* Explosion, watercraft
bomb E923.8
in
terrorism E979.2
war operations E993.8 ◀▦
after cessation of hostilities
E998.1 ◀▦
atom, hydrogen or nuclear
(*see also* War operations,
injury due to, nuclear
weapons) E996.9 ◀▦
injury by fragments from
E991.9
antipersonnel bomb E991.3
butane E923.2
caused by
other person
stated as
intentional, homicidal - *see*
Assault, explosive
undetermined whether
accidental or homicidal
E985.5
coal gas E923.2
detonator E923.1
dynamite E923.1
explosive (material) NEC E923.9
gas(es) E923.2
missile E923.8
in
terrorism E979.2
war operations E993.1 ◀▦
injury by fragments from
E991.9
antipersonnel bomb
E991.3
used in blasting operations E923.1
fire-damp E923.2
fireworks E923.0
gas E923.2
cylinder (in machinery) E921.1
pressure tank (in machinery)
E921.1
gasoline (fumes) (tank) not in moving
motor vehicle E923.2
grain store (military) (munitions)
E923.8
grenade E923.8
in
terrorism E979.2
war operations E993.8 ◀▦
injury by fragments from
E991.4 ◀▦
homicide (attempt) - *see* Assault,
explosive
hot water heater, tank (in machinery)
E921.0
in mine (of explosive gases) NEC
E923.2
late effect of NEC E929.8
machinery - *see also* Accident, machine
pressure vessel - *see* Explosion,
pressure vessel
methane E923.2
missile E923.8
in
terrorism E979.2
war operations E993.1 ◀▦
injury by fragments from
E991.4 ◀▦

Explosion *(Continued)*
motor vehicle (part of)
in motion (on public highway)
E818●
not on public highway E825●
munitions (dump) (factory) E923.8
in
terrorism E979.2
war operations E993.9 ◀▦
of mine E923.8
in
terrorism
at sea or in harbor E979.0
land E979.2
marine E979.0
war operations
after cessation of hostilities
E998.0 ◀▦
at sea or in harbor E992.2 ◀▦
land E993.8 ◀▦
after cessation of hostilities
E998.0 ◀▦
injury by fragments from
E991.4 ◀▦
marine E992.2 ◀▦
own weapons
in
terrorism (*see also* Suicide)
E979.2
war operations E993.7 ◀▦
injury by fragments from
E991.9
antipersonnel bomb
E991.3
pressure
cooker E921.8
gas tank (in machinery) E921.1
vessel (in machinery) E921.9
on transport vehicle - *see*
categories E800-E848
specified type NEC E921.8
propane E923.2
railway engine, locomotive, train
(boiler) (with subsequent
collision, derailment, fall)
E803●
with
collision (antecedent) (*see also*
Collision, railway)
E800●
derailment (antecedent) E802●
fire (without antecedent collision
or derailment) E803●
secondary fire resulting from - *see* Fire
self-inflicted (unspecified whether
accidental or intentional) E985.5
stated as intentional, purposeful
E955.5
shell (artillery) E923.8
in
terrorism E979.2
war operations E993.2 ◀▦
injury by fragments from
E991.4 ◀▦
stated as undetermined whether
caused accidentally or purposely
inflicted E985.5
steam or water lines (in machinery)
E921.0
suicide (attempted) E955.5
terrorism - *see* Terrorism, explosion
torpedo E923.8
in
terrorism E979.0
war operations E992.0 ◀▦

◀ New   ◀▦ Revised   ~~deleted~~ Deleted   ● Use Additional Digit(s)   ▦ Omit code   713

Explosion (*Continued*)
  transport accident - *see* categories
    E800–E848
  war operations - *see* War operations,
    explosion
  watercraft (boiler) E837●
    causing drowning, submersion
      (after jumping from
      watercraft) E830●
Exposure (weather) (conditions) (rain)
    (wind) E904.3
  with homicidal intent E968.4
  environmental
    to
      algae bloom E928.6
      blue-green algae bloom
        E928.6
      brown tide E928.6
      cyanobacteria bloom E928.6
      Florida red tide E928.6
      harmful algae
        and toxins E928.6
        bloom E928.6
      pfiesteria piscicida E928.6
      red tide E928.6
  excessive E904.3
    cold (*see also* Cold, exposure to)
      E901.9
      self-inflicted - *see* Cold, exposure
        to, self-inflicted
    heat (*see also* Heat) E900.9
  helpless person, infant, newborn
      due to abandonment or neglect
      E904.0
  noise E928.1
  prolonged in deep-freeze unit or
    refrigerator E901.1
  radiation - *see* Radiation
  resulting from transport accident - *see*
    categories E800–E848
  smoke from, due to
    fire - *see* Fire
    tobacco, second-hand E869.4
  vibration E928.2
External cause status E000.9 ◀
  civilian ◀
    done for ◀
      financial or other
        compensation E000.0 ◀
      pay or income E000.0 ◀
  for income E000.0 ◀
  hobby or leisure E000.8 ◀
    off duty military E000.8 ◀
  military E000.1 ◀
    off duty E000.8 ◀
  recreation E000.8 ◀
  specified NEC E000.8 ◀
  sport not for income E000.8 ◀
  student E000.8 ◀
  volunteer E000.8 ◀

F

Fall, falling (accidental) E888.9
  building E916
    burning E891.8
      private E890.8
  down
    escalator E880.0
    ladder E881.0
      in boat, ship, watercraft
        E833●
    staircase E880.9
    stairs, steps - *see* Fall, from, stairs

Fall, falling (*Continued*)
  earth (with asphyxia or suffocation (by
    pressure)) (*see also* Earth, falling)
    E913.3
  from, off
    aircraft (at landing, take-off)
      (in-transit) (while alighting,
      boarding) E843●
      resulting from accident to
        aircraft - *see* categories
        E840–E842
    animal (in sport or transport) E828●
    animal-drawn vehicle E827●
    balcony E882
    bed E884.4
    bicycle E826●
    boat, ship, watercraft (into water)
      E832
      after accident to, collision, fire on
        E830●
        and subsequently struck by
          (part of) boat E831●
        and subsequently struck by (part
          of) while alighting, boat
          E838●
      burning, crushed, sinking E830●
        and subsequently struck by
          (part of) boat E831●
    bridge E882
    building E882
      burning (uncontrolled fire) E891.8
        in terrorism E979.3
      private E890.8
    bunk in boat, ship, watercraft
      E834●
      due to accident to watercraft
        E831●
    cable car (not on rails) E847
      on rails E829●
    car - *see* Fall from motor vehicle
      E884.9
    chair E884.2
    cliff E884.1
    commode E884.6
    curb (sidewalk) E880.1
    elevation aboard ship E834●
      due to accident to ship E831●
    embankment E884.9
    escalator E880.0
    fire escape E882
    flagpole E882
    furniture NEC E884.5
    gangplank (into water) (*see also* Fall,
      from, boat) E832●
      to deck, dock E834●
    hammock on ship E834●
      due to accident to watercraft
        E831●
    haystack E884.9
    heelies E885.1
    high place NEC E884.9
      stated as undetermined whether
        accidental or intentional -
        see Jumping, from, high
        place
    horse (in sport or transport) E828●
    in-line skates E885.1
    ladder E881.0
      in boat, ship, watercraft E833●
        due to accident to watercraft
          E831●
    machinery - *see also* Accident,
      machine
      not in operation E884.9

Fall, falling (*Continued*)
  from, off (*Continued*)
    motor vehicle (in motion) (on public
      highway) E818●
      not on public highway E825●
        stationary, except while
          alighting, boarding,
          entering, leaving E884.9
        while alighting, boarding,
          entering, leaving E824●
      stationary, except while alighting,
        boarding, entering, leaving
        E884.9
      while alighting, boarding,
        entering, leaving, except
        off-road type motor vehicle
        E817●
      off-road type - *see* Fall, from,
        off-road type motor
        vehicle
    nonmotor road vehicle (while
      alighting, boarding) NEC
      E829●
      stationary, except while alighting,
        boarding, entering, leaving
        E884.9
    off road type motor vehicle (not
      on public highway) NEC
      E821●
      on public highway E818●
        while alighting, boarding,
          entering, leaving
          E817●
    snow vehicle - *see* Fall from snow
      vehicle, motor-driven
    one
      deck to another on ship E834●
        due to accident to ship
          E831●
      level to another NEC E884.9
        boat, ship, or watercraft
          E834●
          due to accident to
            watercraft E831●
    pedal cycle E826●
    playground equipment E884.0
    railway rolling stock, train, vehicle
      (while alighting, boarding)
      E804●
      with
        collision (*see also* Collision,
          railway) E800●
        derailment (*see also*
          Derailment, railway)
          E802●
        explosion (*see also* Explosion,
          railway engine) E803●
    rigging (aboard ship) E834●
      due to accident to watercraft
        E831●
    roller skates E885.1
    scaffolding E881.1
    scooter (nonmotorized) E885.0
    sidewalk (curb) E880.1
      moving E885.9
    skateboard E885.2
    skis E885.3
    snow vehicle, motor-driven (not on
      public highway) E820●
      on public highway E818●
        while alighting, boarding,
          entering, leaving
          E817●
    snowboard E885.4

◀ New   ◀═ Revised   ~~deleted~~ Deleted   ● Use Additional Digit(s)   ▦ Omit code

E CODES

Fall, falling *(Continued)*
  from, off *(Continued)*
    stairs, steps E880.9
      boat, ship, watercraft E833●
      due to accident to watercraft
          E831●
      motor bus, motor vehicle - *see*
          Fall, from, motor vehicle,
          while alighting, boarding
      street car E829●
    stationary vehicle NEC E884.9
    stepladder E881.0
    street car (while boarding, alighting)
        E829●
      stationary, except while boarding
          or alighting E884.9
    structure NEC E882
      burning (uncontrolled fire)
          E891.8
        in terrorism E979.3
    table E884.9
    toilet E884.6
    tower E882
    tree E884.9
    turret E882
    vehicle NEC - *see also* Accident,
        vehicle NEC
      stationary E884.9
    viaduct E882
    wall E882
    wheelchair E884.3
    wheelies E885.1
    window E882
  in, on
    aircraft (at landing, take-off)
        (in-transit) E843●
      resulting from accident to
          aircraft - *see* categories
          E840–E842
    boat, ship, watercraft E835●
      due to accident to watercraft
          E831●
      one level to another NEC
          E834●
      on ladder, stairs E833●
    cutting or piercing instrument
        machine E888.0
    deck (of boat, ship, watercraft)
        E835●
      due to accident to watercraft
          E831●
    escalator E880.0
    gangplank E835●
    glass, broken E888.0
    knife E888.0
    ladder E881.0
      in boat, ship, watercraft E833●
      due to accident to watercraft
          E831●
    object
      edged, pointed or sharp E888.0
      other E888.1
    pitchfork E888.0
    railway rolling stock, train, vehicle
        (while alighting, boarding)
        E804●
      with
        collision (*see also* Collision,
            railway) E800●
        derailment (*see also*
            Derailment, railway)
            E802●
        explosion (*see also* Explosion,
            railway engine) E803●

Fall, falling *(Continued)*
  in, on *(Continued)*
    scaffolding E881.1
    scissors E888.0
    staircase, stairs, steps (*see also* Fall,
        from, stairs) E880.9
    street car E829●
    water transport (*see also* Fall, in,
        boat) E835●
  into
    cavity E883.9
    dock E883.9
      from boat, ship, watercraft (*see
          also* Fall, from, boat)
          E832●
    hold (of ship) E834●
      due to accident to watercraft
          E831●
    hole E883.9
    manhole E883.2
    moving part of machinery - *see*
        Accident, machine
    opening in surface NEC E883.9
    pit E883.9
    quarry E883.9
    shaft E883.9
    storm drain E883.2
    tank E883.9
    water (with drowning or
        submersion) E910.9
    well E883.1
  late effect of NEC E929.3
  object (*see also* Hit by, object, falling)
      E916
  other E888.8
  over
    animal E885.9
    cliff E884.1
    embankment E884.9
    small object E885.9
  overboard (*see also* Fall, from, boat)
      E832●
  resulting in striking against object
      E888.1
    sharp E888.0
  rock E916
  same level NEC E888.9
    aircraft (any kind) E843●
      resulting from accident to
          aircraft - *see* categories
          E840–E842
    boat, ship, watercraft E835●
      due to accident to, collision,
          watercraft E831●
    from
      collision, pushing, shoving, by
          or with other person(s)
          E886.9
        as, or caused by, a crowd
            E917.6
        in sports E886.0
      in-line skates E885.1
      roller skates E885.1
      scooter (nonmotorized)
          E885.0
      skateboard E885.2
      skis E885.3
      slipping, stumbling, tripping
          E885.9
      snowboard E885.4
  snowslide E916
    as avalanche E909.2
  stone E916

Fall, falling *(Continued)*
  through
    hatch (on ship) E834●
      due to accident to watercraft
          E831●
    roof E882
    window E882
  timber E916
  while alighting from, boarding,
      entering, leaving
    aircraft (any kind) E843●
    motor bus, motor vehicle - *see* Fall,
        from, motor vehicle, while
        alighting, boarding
    nonmotor road vehicle NEC E829●
    railway train E804●
    street car E829●
Fallen on by
  animal (horse) (not being ridden)
      E906.8
    being ridden (in sport or transport)
        E828●
**Fell or jumped from high place, so
    stated** - *see* Jumping, from, high
    place
Felo-de-se (*see also* Suicide) E958.9
Fever
  heat - *see* Heat
  thermic - *see* Heat
Fight (hand) (fist) (foot) (*see also* Assault,
    fight) E960.0
Fire (accidental) (caused by great heat
    from appliance (electrical), hot
    object, or hot substance) (secondary,
    resulting from explosion) E899
  conflagration - *see* Conflagration E892
  controlled, normal (in brazier,
      fireplace, furnace, or stove)
      (charcoal) (coal) (coke) (electric)
      (gas) (wood)
    bonfire E897
    brazier, not in building or structure
        E897
    in building or structure, except
        private dwelling (barn) (church)
        (convalescent or residential
        home) (factory) (farm
        outbuilding) (hospital) (hotel)
        (institution (educational)
        (dormitory) (residential)
        (private garage) (school) (shop)
        (store) (theatre) E896
    in private dwelling (apartment)
        (boarding house) (camping
        place) (caravan) (farmhouse)
        (home (private) (house)
        (lodging house) (rooming
        house) (tenement) E895
    not in building or structure E897
    trash E897
  forest (uncontrolled) E892
  grass (uncontrolled) E892
  hay (uncontrolled) E892
  homicide (attempt) E968.0
    late effect of E969
  in, of, on, starting in E892
    aircraft (in transit) (powered) E841●
      at landing, take-off E840●
      stationary E892
      unpowered (balloon) (glider)
          E842●
    balloon E842●
    boat, ship, watercraft - *see* categories
        E830, E831, E837

E CODES

Fire *(Continued)*
  in, of, on, starting in *(Continued)*
    building or structure, except private
      dwelling (barn) (church)
      (convalescent or residential
      home) (factory) (farm
      outbuilding) (hospital) (hotel)
      (institution) (educational)
      (dormitory) (residential))
      (school) (shop) (store) (theatre)
      (see also Conflagration, building
      or structure, except private
      dwelling) E891.9
    forest (uncontrolled) E892
    glider E842●
    grass (uncontrolled) E892
    hay (uncontrolled) E892
    lumber (uncontrolled) E892
    machinery - *see* Accident, machine
    mine (uncontrolled) E892
    motor vehicle (in motion) (on
      public highway) E818●
      not on public highway E825●
      stationary E892
    prairie (uncontrolled) E892
    private dwelling (apartment)
      (boarding house) (camping
      place) (caravan) (farmhouse)
      (home (private)) (house)
      (lodging house) (private
      garage) (rooming house)
      (tenement) *(see also*
      Conflagration, private
      dwelling) E890.9
    railway rolling stock, train, vehicle
      (see also Explosion, railway
      engine) E803●
      stationary E892
    room NEC E898.1
    street car (in motion) E829●
      stationary E892
    terrorism (by fire-producing
      device) E979.3
      fittings or furniture (burning
        building) (uncontrolled
        fire) E979.3
      from nuclear explosion
        E979.5
    transport vehicle, stationary
      NEC E892
    tunnel (uncontrolled) E892
    war operations (by fire-producing
      device or conventional
      weapon) E990.9
      from nuclear explosion *(see
        also* War operations, injury
        due to, nuclear weapons)
        E996.2 ◀▥
      incendiary bomb E990.0 ◀
      petrol bomb E990.0
    late effect of NEC E929.4
    lumber (uncontrolled) E892
    mine (uncontrolled) E892
    prairie (uncontrolled) E892
    self-inflicted (unspecified whether
      accidental or intentional) E988.1
      stated as intentional, purposeful
        E958.1
    specified NEC E898.1
      with
        conflagration - *see* Conflagration
        ignition (of)
          clothing - *see* Ignition, clothes
          highly inflammable material
            (benzine) (fat) (gasoline)
            (kerosene) (paraffin)
            (petrol) E894

Fire *(Continued)*
  started by other person
    stated as
      with intent to injure or kill
        E968.0
      undetermined whether or not
        with intent to injure or kill
        E988.1
  suicide (attempted) E958.1
    late effect of E959
  tunnel (uncontrolled) E892
Fireball effects from nuclear explosion
  in
    terrorism E979.5
    war operations *(see also* War
      operations, injury due to,
      nuclear weapons) E996.2 ◀▥
Fireworks (explosion) E923.0
Flash burns from explosion *(see also*
  Explosion) E923.9
Flood (any injury) (resulting from storm)
  E908.2
  caused by collapse of dam or manmade
    structure E909.3
Forced landing (aircraft) E840●
Foreign body, object or material
  (entrance into (accidental))
  air passage (causing injury) E915
    with asphyxia, obstruction,
      suffocation E912
      food or vomitus E911
    nose (with asphyxia, obstruction,
      suffocation) E912
      causing injury without asphyxia,
        obstruction, suffocation
        E915
  alimentary canal (causing injury)
    (with obstruction) E915
    with asphyxia, obstruction
      respiratory passage,
      suffocation E912
      food E911
    mouth E915
      with asphyxia, obstruction,
        suffocation E912
        food E911
    pharynx E915
      with asphyxia, obstruction,
        suffocation E912
        food E911
  aspiration (with asphyxia, obstruction
    respiratory passage, suffocation)
    E912
    causing injury without asphyxia,
      obstruction respiratory
      passage, suffocation E915
    food (regurgitated) (vomited)
      E911
      causing injury without asphyxia,
        obstruction respiratory
        passage, suffocation E915
    mucus (not of newborn) E912
    phlegm E912
  bladder (causing injury or obstruction)
    E915
  bronchus, bronchi - *see* Foreign body,
    air passages
  conjunctival sac E914
  digestive system - *see* Foreign body,
    alimentary canal
  ear (causing injury or obstruction) E915
  esophagus (causing injury or
    obstruction) *(see also* Foreign
    body, alimentary canal) E915
  eye (any part) E914
  eyelid E914

Foreign body, object or
  material *(Continued)*
    hairball (stomach) (with obstruction)
      E915
    ingestion - *see* Foreign body, alimentary
      canal
    inhalation - *see* Foreign body, aspiration
    intestine (causing injury or obstruction)
      E915
    iris E914
    lacrimal apparatus E914
    larynx - *see* Foreign body, air passage
    late effect of NEC E929.8
    lung - *see* Foreign body, air passage
    mouth - *see* Foreign body, alimentary
      canal, mouth
    nasal passage - *see* Foreign body, air
      passage, nose
    nose - *see* Foreign body, air passage,
      nose
    ocular muscle E914
    operation wound (left in) - *see*
      Misadventure, foreign object
    orbit E914
    pharynx - *see* Foreign body, alimentary
      canal, pharynx
    rectum (causing injury or obstruction)
      E915
    stomach (hairball) (causing injury or
      obstruction) E915
    tear ducts or glands E914
    trachea - *see* Foreign body, air
      passage
    urethra (causing injury or obstruction)
      E915
    vagina (causing injury or obstruction)
      E915
Found dead, injured
  from exposure (to) - *see* Exposure
  on
    public highway E819●
    railway right of way E807●
Fracture (circumstances unknown or
  unspecified) E887
  due to specified external means - *see*
    manner of accident
  late effect of NEC E929.3
  occurring in water transport NEC
    E835●
Freezing - *see* Cold, exposure to
Frostbite E901.0
  due to manmade conditions E901.1
Frozen - *see* Cold, exposure to

G

Garrotting, homicidal (attempted) E963
Gored E906.8
Gunshot wound *(see also* Shooting)
  E922.9

H

Hailstones, injury by E904.3
Hairball (stomach) (with obstruction)
  E915
Hanged himself *(see also* Hanging, self-
  inflicted) E983.0
Hang gliding E842●
Hanging (accidental) E913.8
  caused by other person
    in accidental circumstances
      E913.8

◀ New   ◀▥ Revised   ~~deleted~~ Deleted   ● Use Additional Digit(s)   ▥ Omit code

E CODES

Hanging (Continued)
  caused by other person (Continued)
    stated as
      intentional, homicidal E963
      undetermined whether accidental
        or intentional E983.0
  homicide (attempt) E963
  in bed or cradle E913.0
  legal execution E978
  self-inflicted (unspecified whether
    accidental or intentional)
    E983.0
    in accidental circumstances E913.8
    stated as intentional, purposeful
      E953.0
  stated as undetermined whether
    accidental or intentional E983.0
  suicidal (attempt) E953.0
Heat (apoplexy) (collapse) (cramps)
  (effects of) (excessive) (exhaustion)
  (fever) (prostration) (stroke) E900.9
  due to
    manmade conditions (as listed in
      E900.1, except boat, ship,
      watercraft) E900.1
    weather (conditions) E900.0
  from
    electric heating apparatus causing
      burning E924.8
    nuclear explosion
    in
      terrorism E979.5
      war operations (see also War
        operations, injury due
        to, nuclear weapons)
        E996.2 ⬅▥
  generated in, boiler, engine,
    evaporator, fire room of boat,
    ship, watercraft E838 ●
  inappropriate in local application or
    packing in medical or surgical
    procedure E873.5
  late effect of NEC E989
Hemorrhage
  delayed following medical or surgical
    treatment without mention of
    misadventure - see Reaction,
    abnormal
  during medical or surgical treatment as
    misadventure - see Misadventure,
    cut
High
  altitude, effects E902.9
  level of radioactivity, effects - see
    Radiation
  pressure effects - see also Effects of, air
    pressure
    from rapid descent in water
      (causing caisson or divers'
      disease, palsy, or paralysis)
      E902.2
  temperature, effects - see Heat
Hit, hitting (accidental) by
  aircraft (propeller) (without accident to
    aircraft) E844 ●
    unpowered E842 ●
  avalanche E909.2
  being thrown against object in or
    part of
    motor vehicle (in motion) (on public
      highway) E818 ●
      not on public highway E825 ●
    nonmotor road vehicle NEC
      E829 ●
    street car E829 ●

Hit, hitting (Continued)
  boat, ship, watercraft
    after fall from watercraft E838 ●
    damaged, involved in accident
      E831 ●
    while swimming, water skiing
      E838 ●
  bullet (see also Shooting) E922.9
    from air gun E922.4
    in
      terrorism E979.4
    war operations E991.2
      rubber E991.0
  flare, Verey pistol (see also Shooting)
    E922.8
  hailstones E904.3
  landslide E909.2
  law-enforcing agent (on duty) E975
    with blunt object (baton) (night
      stick) (stave) (truncheon)
      E973
  machine - see Accident, machine
  missile
    firearm (see also Shooting)
      E922.9
    in
      terrorism - see Terrorism,
        missile
      war operations - see War
        operations, missile
  motor vehicle (on public highway)
    (traffic accident) E814 ●
    not on public highway, nontraffic
      accident E822 ●
  nonmotor road vehicle NEC E829 ●
  object
    falling E916
      from, in, on
      aircraft E844 ●
        due to accident to aircraft -
          see categories
          E840–E842
        unpowered E842 ●
      boat, ship, watercraft E838 ●
        due to accident to
          watercraft E831 ●
      building E916
        burning E891.8
          in terrorism E979.3
          private E890.8
      cataclysmic
        earth surface movement or
          eruption E909.9
        storm E908.9
      cave-in E916
        with asphyxiation or
          suffocation (see also
          Suffocation, due to,
          cave-in) E913.3
      earthquake E909.0
      motor vehicle (in motion)
        (on public highway)
        E818 ●
        not on public highway
          E825 ●
        stationary E916
      nonmotor road vehicle NEC
        E829 ●
      pedal cycle E826 ●
      railway rolling stock, train,
        vehicle E806 ●
      street car E829 ●
      structure, burning NEC
        E891.8
      vehicle, stationary E916

Hit, hitting (Continued)
  object (Continued)
    moving NEC - see Striking against,
      object
    projected NEC - see Striking against,
      object
    set in motion by
      compressed air or gas, spring,
        striking, throwing - see
        Striking against, object
      explosion - see Explosion
    thrown into, on, or towards
      motor vehicle (in motion) (on
        public highway) E818 ●
        not on public highway E825 ●
      nonmotor road vehicle NEC
        E829 ●
      pedal cycle E826 ●
      street car E829 ●
    off-road type motor vehicle (not on
      public highway) E821 ●
      on public highway E814 ●
    other person(s) E917.9
      with blunt or thrown object
        E917.9
      in sports E917.0
        with subsequent fall E917.5
      intentionally, homicidal E968.2
      as, or caused by, a crowd E917.1
        with subsequent fall E917.6
      in sports E917.0
    pedal cycle E826 ●
    police (on duty) E975
      with blunt object (baton)
        (nightstick) (stave)
        (truncheon) E973
    railway, rolling stock, train, vehicle
      (part of) E805 ●
    shot - see Shooting
    snow vehicle, motor-driven (not on
      public highway) E820 ●
      on public highway E814 ●
    street car E829 ●
    vehicle NEC - see Accident, vehicle
      NEC
Homicide, homicidal (attempt)
  (justifiable) (see also Assault) E968.9
Hot
  liquid, object, substance, accident
    caused by - see also Accident,
    caused by, hot, by type of
    substance
    late effect of E929.8
  place, effects - see Heat
  weather, effects E900.0
Humidity, causing problem E904.3
Hunger E904.1
  resulting from
    abandonment or neglect E904.0
    transport accident - see categories
      E800–E848
Hurricane (any injury) E908.0
Hypobarism, hypobaropathy - see Effects
  of, air pressure
Hypothermia - see Cold, exposure to

I

Ictus
  caloris - see Heat
  solaris E900.0
Ignition (accidental)
  anesthetic gas in operating theatre
    E923.2

E CODES

Ignition (Continued)
  bedclothes
    with
      conflagration - see Conflagration
      ignition (of)
        clothing - see Ignition, clothes
        highly inflammable material
          obstruction (benzine)
          (fat) (gasoline) (kerosene)
          (paraffin) (petrol) E894
  benzine E894
  clothes, clothing (from controlled fire)
    (in building) E893.9
    with conflagration - see
      Conflagration
    from
      bonfire E893.2
      highly inflammable material
        E894
      sources or material as listed in
        E893.8
      trash fire E893.2
      uncontrolled fire - see
        Conflagration
    in
      private dwelling E893.0
      specified building or structure,
        except of private dwelling
        E893.1
  not in building or structure E893.2
  explosive material - see Explosion
  fat E894
  gasoline E894
  kerosene E894
  material
    explosive - see Explosion
    highly inflammable E894
      with conflagration - see
        Conflagration
      with explosion E923.2
  nightdress - see Ignition, clothes
  paraffin E894
  petrol E894
Immersion - see Submersion
Implantation of quills of porcupine
  E906.8
Inanition (from) E904.9
  hunger - see Lack of, food
  resulting from homicidal intent
    E968.4
  thirst - see Lack of, water
Inattention after, at birth E904.0
  homicidal, infanticidal intent E968.4
Infanticide (see also Assault)
Ingestion
  foreign body (causing injury) (with
    obstruction) - see Foreign body,
    alimentary canal
  poisonous substance NEC - see Table of
    Drugs and Chemicals
Inhalation
  excessively cold substance, manmade
    E901.1
  foreign body - see Foreign body,
    aspiration
  liquid air, hydrogen, nitrogen E901.1
  mucus, not of newborn (with asphyxia,
    obstruction respiratory passage,
    suffocation) E912
  phlegm (with asphyxia, obstruction
    respiratory passage, suffocation)
    E912
  poisonous gas - see Table of Drugs and
    Chemicals

Inhalation (Continued)
  smoke from, due to
    fire - see Fire
    tobacco, second-hand E869.4
  vomitus (with asphyxia, obstruction
    respiratory passage, suffocation)
    E911
Injury, injured (accidental(ly)) NEC
  E928.9
  by, caused by, from
    air rifle (B-B gun) E922.4
    animal (not being ridden) NEC
      E906.9
      being ridden (in sport or
        transport) E828●
    assault (see also Assault) E968.9
    avalanche E909.2
    bayonet (see also Bayonet wound)
      E920.3
    being thrown against some part of,
      or object in
      motor vehicle (in motion) (on
        public highway) E818●
        not on public highway E825●
      nonmotor road vehicle NEC
        E829●
      off-road motor vehicle NEC
        E821●
      railway train E806●
      snow vehicle, motor-driven
        E820●
      street car E829●
    bending E927.8
    bite, human E928.3
    broken glass E920.8
    bullet - see Shooting
    cave-in (see also Suffocation, due to,
      cave-in) E913.3
      earth surface movement or
        eruption E909.9
      storm E908.9
      without asphyxiation or
        suffocation E916
    cloudburst E908.8
    component of firearm or air gun
      E928.7 ◀
    cutting or piercing instrument (see
      also Cut) E920.9
    cyclone E908.1
    earth surface movement or eruption
      E909.9
    earthquake E909.0
    electric current (see also Electric
      shock) E925.9
    explosion (see also Explosion) E923.9
      of gun part E928.7 ◀
    fire - see Fire
    flare, Verey pistol E922.8
    flood E908.2
    foreign body - see Foreign body
    gun recoil E928.7 ◀
    hailstones E904.3
    hurricane E908.0
    landslide E909.2
    law-enforcing agent, police, in
      course of legal intervention -
      see Legal intervention
    lightning E907
    live rail or live wire - see Electric
      shock
    machinery - see also Accident,
      machine aircraft, without
      accident to aircraft E844●
      boat, ship, watercraft (deck)
        (engine room) (galley)
        (laundry) (loading) E836●

Injury, injured (Continued)
  by, caused by, from (Continued)
    mechanism of firearm or air gun
      E928.7 ◀
    missile
      explosive E923.8
      firearm - see Shooting
      in
        terrorism - see Terrorism,
          missile
        war operations - see War
          operations, missile
    moving part of motor vehicle (in
      motion) (on public highway)
      E818●
      not on public highway, nontraffic
        accident E825●
      while alighting, boarding,
        entering, leaving - see Fall,
        from, motor vehicle, while
        alighting, boarding
    nail E920.8
    needle (sewing) E920.4
      hypodermic E920.5
    noise E928.1
    object
      fallen on
        motor vehicle (in motion) (on
          public highway) E818●
        not on public highway
          E825●
      falling - see Hit by, object, falling
    paintball gun E922.5
    radiation - see Radiation
    railway rolling stock, train, vehicle
      (part of) E805●
      door or window E806●
    recoil of firearm E938.7 ◀
    rotating propeller, aircraft E844●
    rough landing of off-road type
      motor vehicle (after leaving
      ground or rough terrain)
      E821●
    snow vehicle E820●
    saber (see also Wound, saber)
      E920.3
    shot - see Shooting
    sound waves E928.1
    splinter or sliver, wood E920.8
    straining E927.8
    street car (door) E829●
    suicide (attempt) E958.9
    sword E920.3
    terrorism - see Terrorism
    third rail - see Electric shock
    thunderbolt E907
    tidal wave E909.4
      caused by storm E908.0
    tornado E908.1
    torrential rain E908.2
    twisting E927.8
    vehicle NEC - see Accident, vehicle
      NEC
    vibration E928.2
    volcanic eruption E909.1
    weapon burst, in war operations
      E993.9 ◀▬
    weightlessness (in spacecraft, real or
      simulated) E928.0
    wood splinter or sliver E920.8
  due to
    civil insurrection - see War
      operations
      occurring after cessation of
        hostilities E998.9 ◀▬
    terrorism - see Terrorism

◀ New   ◀▬ Revised   ~~deleted~~ Deleted   ● Use Additional Digit(s)   ▨ Omit code

E CODES

Injury, injured *(Continued)*
 due to *(Continued)*
  war operations - *see* War operations
   occurring after cessation of
    hostilities E998.9 ◀▥
  weapon of mass destruction
   [WMD] E997.3 ◀
 homicidal *(see also* Assault) E968.9
 in, on
  civil insurrection - *see* War
   operations
  fight E960.0
  parachute descent (voluntary)
   (without accident to aircraft)
   E844●
    with accident to aircraft - *see*
     categories E840-E842
  public highway E819●
  railway right of way E807●
  terrorism - *see* Terrorism
  war operations - *see* War operations
 inflicted (by)
  in course of arrest (attempted),
   suppression of disturbance,
   maintenance of order, by law
   enforcing agents - *see* Legal
   intervention
  law-enforcing agent (on duty) - *see*
   Legal intervention
  other person
   stated as
    accidental E928.9
    homicidal, intentional - *see*
     Assault
    undetermined whether
     accidental or intentional -
     see Injury, stated as
     undetermined
  police (on duty) - *see* Legal
   intervention
 late effect of E929.9
 purposely (inflicted) by other
  person(s) - *see* Assault
 self-inflicted (unspecified whether
  accidental or intentional) E988.9
  stated as
   accidental E928.9
   intentionally, purposely E958.9
 specified cause NEC E928.8
 stated as
  undetermined whether accidentally
   or purposely inflicted (by)
   E988.9
   cut (any part of body) E986
   cutting or piercing instrument
    (classifiable to E920) E986
   drowning E984
   explosive(s) (missile) E985.5
   falling from high place E987.9
    manmade structure, except
     residential E987.1
    natural site E987.2
    residential premises E987.0
   hanging E983.0
   knife E986
   late effect of E989
   puncture (any part of body) E986
   shooting - *see* Shooting, stated as
    undetermined whether
    accidental or intentional
   specified means NEC E988.8
   stab (any part of body) E986
   strangulation - *see* Suffocation,
    stated as undetermined
    whether accidental or
    intentional

Injury, injured *(Continued)*
 stated as *(Continued)*
  submersion E984
  suffocation - *see* Suffocation, stated
   as undetermined whether
   accidental or intentional
  to child due to criminal abortion
   E968.8
Insufficient nourishment - *see also* Lack
 of, food
 homicidal intent E968.4
Insulation, effects - *see* Heat
Interruption of respiration by
 food lodged in esophagus E911
 foreign body, except food, in
  esophagus E912
Intervention, legal - *see* Legal
 intervention
Intoxication, drug or poison - *see* Table
 of Drugs and Chemicals
Irradiation - *see* Radiation

J

Jammed (accidentally)
 between objects (moving) (stationary
  and moving) E918
 in object E918
Jumped or fell from high place, so
 stated - *see* Jumping, from, high
 place, stated as
 in undetermined circumstances
Jumping
 before train, vehicle or other moving
  object (unspecified whether
  accidental or intentional)
  E988.0
  stated as
   intentional, purposeful
    E958.0
   suicidal (attempt) E958.0
 from
  aircraft
   by parachute (voluntarily)
    (without accident to
    aircraft) E844●
   due to accident to aircraft - *see*
    categories E840–E842
  boat, ship, watercraft (into water)
   after accident to, fire on,
    watercraft E830●
    and subsequently struck by
     (part of) boat E831●
   burning, crushed, sinking
    E830●
    and subsequently struck by
     (part of) boat E831●
   voluntarily, without accident (to
    boat) with injury other than
    drowning or submersion
    E883.0
  building - *see also* Jumping, from,
   high place
   burning (uncontrolled fire)
    E891.8
    in terrorism E979.3
    private E890.8
  cable car (not on rails) E847
   on rails E829●
  high place
   in accidental circumstances or
    in sport - *see* categories
    E880–E884

Jumping *(Continued)*
 from *(Continued)*
  high place *(Continued)*
   stated as
    with intent to injure self E957.9
     man-made structures NEC
      E957.1
     natural sites E957.2
     residential premises E957.0
    in undetermined
     circumstances E987.9
     man-made structures NEC
      E987.1
     natural sites E987.2
     residential premises E987.0
    suicidal (attempt) E957.9
     man-made structures NEC
      E957.1
     natural sites E957.1
     residential premises E957.0
  motor vehicle (in motion) (on public
   highway) - *see* Fall, from,
   motor vehicle
  nonmotor road vehicle NEC E829●
  street car E829●
  structure - *see also* Jumping, from,
   high place
   burning NEC (uncontrolled fire)
    E891.8
    in terrorism E979.3
 into water
  with injury other than drowning or
   submersion E883.0
  drowning or submersion - *see*
   Submersion
 from, off, watercraft - *see* Jumping,
  from, boat
Justifiable homicide - *see* Assault

K

Kicked by
 animal E906.8
 person(s) (accidentally) E917.9
  with intent to injure or kill E960.0
  as, or caused by a crowd E917.1
   with subsequent fall E917.6
  in fight E960.0
  in sports E917.0
   with subsequent fall E917.5
Kicking against
 object (moving) E917.9
  in sports E917.0
   with subsequent fall E917.5
  stationary E917.4
   with subsequent fall E917.8
 person - *see* Striking against, person
Killed, killing (accidentally) NEC *(see also*
 Injury) E928.9
 in
  action - *see* War operations
  brawl, fight (hand) (fists) (foot)
   E960.0
  by weapon - *see also* Assault
   cutting, piercing E966
   firearm - *see* Shooting,
    homicide
 self
  stated as
   accident E928.9
   suicide - *see* Suicide
  unspecified whether accidental or
   suicidal E988.9

E CODES

Knocked down (accidentally) (by) NEC E928.9
  animal (not being ridden) E906.8
    being ridden (in sport or transport) E828●
  blast from explosion (see also Explosion) E923.9
  crowd, human stampede E917.6
  late effect of - see Late effect
  person (accidentally) E917.9
    in brawl, fight E960.0
    in sports E917.5
  transport vehicle - see vehicle involved under Hit by
  while boxing E917.5

L

Laceration NEC E928.9
Lack of
  air (refrigerator or closed place), suffocation by E913.2
  care (helpless person) (infant) (newborn) E904.0
    homicidal intent E968.4
  food except as result of transport accident E904.1
    helpless person, infant, newborn due to abandonment or neglect E904.0
  water except as result of transport accident E904.2
    helpless person, infant, newborn due to abandonment or neglect E904.0
Landslide E909.2
  falling on, hitting
    motor vehicle (any) (in motion) (on or off public highway) E909.2
    railway rolling stock, train, vehicle E909.2
Late effect of
  accident NEC (accident classifiable to E928.9) E929.9
    specified NEC (accident classifiable to E910–E928.8) E929.8
  assault E969
  fall, accidental (accident classifiable to E880–E888) E929.3
  fire, accident caused by (accident classifiable to E890–E899) E929.4
  homicide, attempt (any means) E969
  injury due to terrorism E999.1
  injury undetermined whether accidentally or purposely inflicted (injury classifiable to E980–E988) E989
  legal intervention (injury classifiable to E970–E976) E977
  medical or surgical procedure, test or therapy
    as, or resulting in, or from
      abnormal or delayed reaction or complication - see Reaction, abnormal
      misadventure - see Misadventure
  motor vehicle accident (accident classifiable to E810–E825) E929.0
  natural or environmental factor, accident due to (accident classifiable to E900–E909) E929.5

Late effect of (Continued)
  poisoning, accidental (accident classifiable to E850–E858, E860–E869) E929.2
  suicide, attempt (any means) E959
  transport accident NEC (accident classifiable to E800–E807, E826–E838, E840–E848) E929.1
  war operations, injury due to (injury classifiable to E990–E998) E999.0
Launching pad accident E845●
Legal
  execution, any method E978
  intervention (by) (injury from) E976
    baton E973
    bayonet E974
    blow E975
    blunt object (baton) (nightstick) (stave) (truncheon) E973
    cutting or piercing instrument E974
    dynamite E971
    execution, any method E973
    explosive(s) (shell) E971
    firearm(s) E970
    gas (asphyxiation) (poisoning) (tear) E972
    grenade E971
    late effect of E977
    machine gun E970
    manhandling E975
    mortar bomb E971
    nightstick E973
    revolver E970
    rifle E970
    specified means NEC E975
    stabbing E974
    stave E973
    truncheon E973
Lifting, injury in E927.8
Lightning (shock) (stroke) (struck by) E907
Liquid (noncorrosive) in eye E914
  corrosive E924.1
Loss of control
  motor vehicle (on public highway) (without antecedent collision) E816●
    with
      antecedent collision on public highway - see Collision, motor vehicle
      involving any object, person or vehicle not on public highway E816●
      on public highway - see Collision, motor vehicle
      not on public highway, nontraffic accident E825●
        with antecedent collision - see Collision, motor vehicle, not on public highway
    off-road type motor vehicle (not on public highway) E821●
      on public highway - see Loss of control, motor vehicle
    snow vehicle, motor-driven (not on public highway) E820●
      on public highway - see Loss of control, motor vehicle

Lost at sea E832●
  with accident to watercraft E830● ⬅
  in war operations E995.8
Low
  pressure, effects - see Effects of, air pressure
  temperature, effects - see Cold exposure to
Lying before train, vehicle or other moving object (unspecified whether accidental or intentional) E988.0
  stated as intentional, purposeful, suicidal (attempt) E958.0
Lynching (see also Assault) E968.9

M

Malfunction, atomic power plant in water transport E838●
Mangled (accidentally) NEC E928.9
Manhandling (in brawl, fight) E960.0
  legal intervention E975
Manslaughter (nonaccidental) - see Assault
Marble in nose E912
Mauled by animal E906.8
Medical procedure, complication of
  delayed or as an abnormal reaction without mention of misadventure - see Reaction, abnormal
  due to or as a result of misadventure - see Misadventure
Melting of fittings and furniture in burning
  in terrorism E979.3
Minamata disease E865.2
Misadventure(s) to patient(s) during surgical or medical care E876.9
  contaminated blood, fluid, drug or biological substance (presence of agents and toxins as listed in E875) E875.9
    administered (by) NEC E875.9
      infusion E875.0
      injection E875.1
      specified means NEC E875.2
      transfusion E875.0
      vaccination E875.1
  cut, cutting, puncture, perforation or hemorrhage (accidental) (inadvertent) (inappropriate) (during) E870.9
    aspiration of fluid or tissue (by puncture or catheterization, except heart) E870.5
    biopsy E870.8
      needle (aspirating) E870.5
    blood sampling E870.5
    catheterization E870.5
      heart E870.6
    dialysis (kidney) E870.2
    endoscopic examination E870.4
    enema E870.7
    infusion E870.1
    injection E870.3
    lumbar puncture E870.5
    needle biopsy E870.5
    paracentesis, abdominal E870.5
    perfusion E870.2
    specified procedure NEC E870.8
    surgical operation E870.0

E CODES

Misadventure(s) to patient(s) during surgical or medical care *(Continued)*
cut, cutting, puncture, perforation or hemorrhage *(Continued)*
thoracentesis E870.5
transfusion E870.1
vaccination E870.3
excessive amount of blood or other fluid during transfusion or infusion E873.0
failure
in dosage E873.9
electroshock therapy E873.4
inappropriate temperature (too hot or too cold) in local application and packing E873.5
infusion
excessive amount of fluid E873.0
incorrect dilution of fluid E873.1
insulin-shock therapy E873.4
nonadministration of necessary drug or medicinal E873.6
overdose - *see also* Overdose radiation, in therapy E873.2
radiation
inadvertent exposure of patient (receiving radiation for test or therapy) E873.3
not receiving radiation for test or therapy - *see* Radiation
overdose E873.2
specified procedure NEC E873.8
transfusion
excessive amount of blood E873.0
mechanical, of instrument or apparatus (during procedure) E874.9
aspiration of fluid or tissue (by puncture or catheterization, except of heart) E874.4
biopsy E874.8
needle (aspirating) E874.4
blood sampling E874.4
catheterization E874.4
heart E874.5
dialysis (kidney) E874.2
endoscopic examination E874.3
enema E874.8
infusion E874.1
injection E874.8
lumbar puncture E874.4
needle biopsy E874.4
paracentesis, abdominal E874.4
perfusion E874.2
specified procedure NEC E874.8
surgical operation E874.0
thoracentesis E874.4
transfusion E874.1
vaccination E874.8
sterile precautions (during procedure) E872.9
aspiration of fluid or tissue (by puncture or catheterization, except heart) E872.5
biopsy E872.8
needle (aspirating) E872.5

Misadventure(s) to patient(s) during surgical or medical care *(Continued)*
failure *(Continued)*
sterile precautions *(Continued)*
blood sampling E872.5
catheterization E872.5
heart E872.6
dialysis (kidney) E872.2
endoscopic examination E872.4
enema E872.8
infusion E872.1
injection E872.3
lumbar puncture E872.5
needle biopsy E872.5
paracentesis, abdominal E872.5
perfusion E872.2
removal of catheter or packing E872.8
specified procedure NEC E872.8
surgical operation E872.0
thoracentesis E872.5
transfusion E872.1
vaccination E872.3
suture or ligature during surgical procedure E876.2
to introduce or to remove tube or instrument E876.4
foreign object left in body - *see* Misadventure, foreign object
foreign object left in body (during procedure) E871.9
aspiration of fluid or tissue (by puncture or catheterization, except heart) E871.5
biopsy E871.8
needle (aspirating) E871.5
blood sampling E871.5
catheterization E871.5
heart E871.6
dialysis (kidney) E871.2
endoscopic examination E871.4
enema E871.8
infusion E871.1
injection E871.3
lumbar puncture E871.5
needle biopsy E871.5
paracentesis, abdominal E871.5
perfusion E871.2
removal of catheter or packing E871.7
specified procedure NEC E871.8
surgical operation E871.0
thoracentesis E871.5
transfusion E871.1
vaccination E871.3
hemorrhage - *see* Misadventure, cut
inadvertent exposure of patient to radiation (being received for test or therapy) E873.3
inappropriate
operation performed E876.5
temperature (too hot or too cold) in local application or packing E873.5
infusion - *see also* Misadventure, by specific type, infusion
excessive amount of fluid E873.0
incorrect dilution of fluid E873.1
wrong fluid E876.1
mismatched blood in transfusion E876.0

Misadventure(s) to patient(s) during surgical or medical care *(Continued)*
nonadministration of necessary drug or medicinal E873.6
overdose - *see also* Overdose radiation, in therapy E873.2
perforation - *see* Misadventure, cut
performance of correct operation (procedure) on wrong ◄
body part E876.7 ◄
side E876.7 ◄
site E876.7 ◄
performance of operation (procedure) ◄
intended for another patient E876.6 ◄
on patient not scheduled for surgery E876.6 ◄
on wrong patient E876.6 ◄
performance of ~~inappropriate~~ wrong operation on correct patient E876.5 ◄⦙⦙
puncture - *see* Misadventure, cut
specified type NEC E876.8
failure
suture or ligature during surgical operation E876.2
to introduce or to remove tube or instrument E876.4
foreign object left in body E871.9
infusion of wrong fluid E876.1
~~performance of inappropriate operation E876.5~~
transfusion of mismatched blood E876.0
wrong
device implanted into correct surgical site E876.5 ◄
fluid in infusion E876.1
placement of endotracheal tube during anesthetic procedure E876.3
procedure (operation) performed on the correct patient E876.5 ◄
transfusion - *see also* Misadventure, by specific type, transfusion
excessive amount of blood E873.0
mismatched blood E876.0
wrong
drug given in error - *see* Table of Drugs and Chemicals
fluid in infusion E876.1
placement of endotracheal tube during anesthetic procedure E876.3
Motion (effects) E903
sickness E903
Mountain sickness E902.0
Mucus aspiration or inhalation, not of newborn (with asphyxia, obstruction respiratory passage, suffocation) E912
Mudslide of cataclysmic nature E909.2
Murder (attempt) (*see also* Assault) E968.9

N

Nail, injury by E920.8
Needlestick (sewing needle) E920.4
hypodermic E920.5

E CODES

Neglect - *see also* Privation
  criminal E968.4
  homicidal intent E968.4
Noise (causing injury) (pollution)
    E928.1
Nuclear weapon (*see also* War
    operations, injury due to,
    nuclear weapons) E996.9 ◀

O

Object
  falling
    from, in, on, hitting
      aircraft E844●
        due to accident to aircraft - *see*
            categories E840–E842
      machinery - *see also* Accident,
          machine
        not in operation E916
      motor vehicle (in motion) (on
          public highway) E818●
        not on public highway E825●
        stationary E916
      nonmotor road vehicle NEC
          E829●
      pedal cycle E826●
      person E916
      railway rolling stock, train,
          vehicle E806●
      street car E829●
      watercraft E838●
        due to accident to
            watercraft E831●
  set in motion by
    accidental explosion of pressure
        vessel - *see* category E921
    firearm - *see* category E922
    machine(ry) - *see* Accident,
        machine
    transport vehicle - *see* categories
        E800–E848
  thrown from, in, on, towards
    aircraft E844●
    cable car (not on rails) E847
      on rails E829●
    motor vehicle (in motion) (on public
        highway) E818●
      not on public highway
          E825●
    nonmotor road vehicle NEC E829●
    pedal cycle E826●
    street car E829●
    vehicle NEC - *see* Accident, vehicle
        NEC
Obstruction
  air passages, larynx, respiratory
      passages
    by
      external means NEC - *see*
          Suffocation
      food, any type (regurgitated)
          (vomited) E911
      material or object, except food
          E912
      mucus E912
      phlegm E912
      vomitus E911
  digestive tract, except mouth or
      pharynx
    by
      food, any type E915
      foreign body (any) E915

Obstruction (*Continued*)
  esophagus
    food E911
    foreign body, except food E912
    without asphyxia or obstruction of
        respiratory passage E915
  mouth or pharynx
    by
      food, any type E911
      material or object, except food
          E912
  respiration - *see* Obstruction, air
      passages
Oil in eye E914
Overdose
  anesthetic (drug) - *see* Table of Drugs
      and Chemicals
  drug - *see* Table of Drugs and
      Chemicals
Overexertion E927.9
  from
    lifting E927.8
    maintaining prolonged positions
        E927.1
      holding E927.1
      sitting E927.1
      standing E927.1
    prolonged static position E927.1
    pulling E927.8
    pushing E927.8
    sudden strenuous movement
        E927.0
Overexposure (accidental) (to)
  cold (*see also* Cold, exposure to)
      E901.9
    due to manmade conditions
        E901.1
  heat (*see also* Heat) E900.9
  radiation - *see* Radiation
  radioactivity - *see* Radiation
  sun, except sunburn E900.0
  weather - *see* Exposure
  wind - *see* Exposure
Overheated (*see also* Heat) E900.9
Overlaid E913.0
Overturning (accidental)
  animal-drawn vehicle E827●
  boat, ship, watercraft
    causing
      drowning, submersion E830●
      injury except drowning,
          submersion E831●
  machinery - *see* Accident, machine
  motor vehicle (*see also* Loss of control,
      motor vehicle) E816●
    with antecedent collision on public
        highway - *see* Collision, motor
        vehicle
    not on public highway, nontraffic
        accident E825●
      with antecedent collision - *see*
          Collision, motor vehicle, not
          on public highway
  nonmotor road vehicle NEC E829●
  off-road type motor vehicle - *see* Loss of
      control, off-road type motor
      vehicle
  pedal cycle E826●
  railway rolling stock, train, vehicle
      (*see also* Derailment, railway)
      E802●
  street car E829●
  vehicle NEC - *see* Accident, vehicle
      NEC

P

Palsy, divers' E902.2
Parachuting (voluntary) (without
    accident to aircraft) E844●
  due to accident to aircraft - *see*
      categories E840–E842
Paralysis
  divers' E902.2
  lead or saturnine E866.0
    from pesticide NEC E863.4
Pecked by bird E906.8
Performance of correct operation
    (procedure) on wrong
  body part E876.7 ◀
  side E876.7 ◀
  site E876.7 ◀
Performance of operation
    (procedure) ◀
  intended for another patient
      E876.6 ◀
  on patient not scheduled for
      surgery E876.6 ◀
  on wrong patient E876.6 ◀
Performance of wrong operation on
    correct patient E876.5 ◀
Phlegm aspiration or inhalation (with
    asphyxia, obstruction respiratory
    passage, suffocation) E912
Piercing (*see also* Cut) E920.9
  by slide trigger mechanism, scope
      or other part of gun E928.7 ◀
Pinched
  between objects (moving) (stationary
      and moving) E918
  by slide trigger mechanism, scope
      or other part of gun E928.7 ◀
  in object E918
Pinned under
  machine(ry) - *see* Accident, machine
Place of occurrence of accident - *see*
    Accident (to), occurring (at) (in)
Plumbism E866.0
  from insecticide NEC E863.4
Poisoning (accidental) (by) - *see also* Table
    of Drugs and Chemicals
  carbon monoxide
    generated by
      aircraft in transit E844●
      motor vehicle
        in motion (on public highway)
            E818●
        not on public highway
            E825●
      watercraft (in transit) (not in
          transit) E838●
  caused by injection of poisons or toxins
      into or through skin by plant
      thorns, spines, or other
      mechanism E905.7
  marine or sea plants E905.6
  fumes or smoke due to
    conflagration - *see* Conflagration
    explosion or fire - *see* Fire
    ignition - *see* Ignition
  gas
    in legal intervention E972
    legal execution, by E978
    on watercraft E838●
    used as anesthetic - *see* Table of
        Drugs and Chemicals
  in
    terrorism (chemical weapons) E979.7
    war operations E997.2

◀ New   ◀▦ Revised   ~~deleted~~ Deleted   ● Use Additional Digit(s)   ▦ Omit code

E CODES

Poisoning *(Continued)*
  late effect of - *see* Late effect
  legal
    execution E978
    intervention
      by gas E972
Pressure, external, causing asphyxia, suffocation *(see also* Suffocation*)* E913.9
Privation E904.9
  food *(see also* Lack of, food*)* E904.1
  helpless person, infant, newborn due to abandonment or neglect E904.0
  late effect of NEC E929.5
  resulting from transport accident - *see* categories E800–E848
  water *(see also* Lack of, water*)* E904.2
Projected objects, striking against or struck by - *see* Striking against, object
Prolonged stay in
  high altitude (causing conditions as listed in E902.0) E902.0
  weightless environment E928.0
Prostration
  heat - *see* Heat
Pulling, injury in E927.8
Puncture, puncturing *(see also* Cut*)* E920.9
  by
    plant thorns or spines E920.8
      toxic reaction E905.7
        marine or sea plants E905.6
    sea-urchin spine E905.6
Pushing (injury in) (overexertion) E927.8
  by other person(s) (accidental) E917.9
    as, or caused by, a crowd, human stampede E917.1
      with subsequent fall E917.6
    before moving vehicle or object
      stated as
        intentional, homicidal E968.5
        undetermined whether accidental or intentional E988.8
    from
      high place
        in accidental circumstances - *see* categories E880–E884
        stated as
          intentional, homicidal E968.1
          undetermined whether accidental or intentional E987.9
          man-made structure, except residential E987.1
          natural site E987.2
          residential E987.0
      motor vehicle *(see also* Fall, from, motor vehicle*)* E818 ●
        stated as
          intentional, homicidal E968.5
          undetermined whether accidental or intentional E988.8
  in sports E917.0
    with fall E886.0
  with fall E886.9
    in sports E886.0

R

Radiation (exposure to) E926.9
  abnormal reaction to medical test or therapy E879.2
  arc lamps E926.2
  atomic power plant (malfunction) NEC E926.9
    in water transport E838 ●
  electromagnetic, ionizing E926.3
  gamma rays E926.3
  in
    terrorism (from or following nuclear explosion) (direct) (secondary) E979.5
      laser E979.8
    war operations ~~(from or following nuclear explosion) (direct) (secondary)~~ *(see also* War operations, injury due to, nuclear weapons) E996.3 ◀▥
      laser(s) E997.0
    water transport E838 ●
  inadvertent exposure of patient (receiving test or therapy) E873.3
  infrared (heaters and lamps) E926.1
    excessive heat E900.1
  ionized, ionizing (particles, artificially accelerated) E926.8
    electromagnetic E926.3
  isotopes, radioactive - *see* Radiation, radioactive isotopes
  laser(s) E926.4
    in
      terrorism E979.8
      war operations E997.0
    misadventure in medical care - *see* Misadventure, failure, in dosage, radiation
  late effect of NEC E929.8
    excessive heat from - *see* Heat
  light sources (visible) (ultraviolet) E926.2
  misadventure in medical or surgical procedure - *see* Misadventure, failure, in dosage, radiation
  overdose (in medical or surgical pacemaker procedure) E873.2
  radar E926.0
  radioactive isotopes E926.5
    atomic power plant malfunction E926.5
    in water transport E838 ●
    misadventure in medical or surgical treatment - *see* Misadventure, failure, in dosage, radiation
  radiobiologicals - *see* Radiation, radioactive isotopes
  radiofrequency E926.0
  radiopharmaceuticals - *see* Radiation, radioactive isotopes
  radium NEC E926.9
  sun E926.2
    excessive heat from E900.0
  tanning bed E926.2
  welding arc or torch E926.2
    excessive heat from E900.1
  x-rays (hard) (soft) E926.3
    misadventure in medical or surgical treatment - *see* Misadventure, failure, in dosage, radiation

Rape E960.1
Reaction, abnormal to or following (medical or surgical procedure) E879.9
  amputation (of limbs) E878.5
  anastomosis (arteriovenous) (blood vessel) (gastrojejunal) (skin) (tendon) (natural, artificial material, tissue) E878.2
    external stoma, creation of E878.3
  aspiration (of fluid) E879.4
    tissue E879.8
  biopsy E879.8
  blood
    sampling E879.7
    transfusion
      procedure E879.8
  bypass - *see* Reaction, abnormal, anastomosis
  catheterization
    cardiac E879.0
    urinary E879.6
  colostomy E878.3
  cystostomy E878.3
  dialysis (kidney) E879.1
  drugs or biologicals - *see* Table of Drugs and Chemicals
  duodenostomy E878.3
  electroshock therapy E879.3
  formation of external stoma E878.3
  gastrostomy E878.3
  graft - *see* Reaction, abnormal, anastomosis
  hypothermia E879.8
  implant, implantation (of)
    artificial
      internal device (cardiac pacemaker) (electrodes in brain) (heart valve prosthesis) (orthopedic) E878.1
      material or tissue (for anastomosis or bypass) E878.2
        with creation of external stoma E878.3
    natural tissues (for anastomosis or bypass) E878.2
      as transplantion - *see* Reaction, abnormal, transplant
      with creation of external stoma E878.3
  infusion
    procedure E879.8
  injection
    procedure E879.8
  insertion of gastric or duodenal sound E879.5
  insulin-shock therapy E879.3
  lumbar puncture E879.4
  perfusion E879.1
  procedures other than surgical operation *(see also* Reaction, abnormal, by specific type of procedure) E879.9
    specified procedure NEC E879.8
  radiological procedure or therapy E879.2
  removal of organ (partial) (total) NEC E878.6
    with
      anastomosis, bypass or graft E878.2
      formation of external stoma E878.3

E CODES

Reaction, abnormal to or following *(Continued)*
  removal of organ NEC *(Continued)*
    with *(Continued)*
      implant of artificial internal device E878.1
      transplant(ation)
        partial organ E878.4
        whole organ E878.0
  sampling
    blood E879.7
    fluid NEC E879.4
    tissue E879.8
  shock therapy E879.3
  surgical operation *(see also* Reaction, abnormal, by specified type of operation) E878.9
    restorative NEC E878.4
      with
        anastomosis, bypass or graft E878.2
        formation of external stoma E878.3
        implant(ation) - *see* Reaction, abnormal, implant
        transplantation - *see* Reaction, abnormal, transplant
    specified operation NEC E878.8
  thoracentesis E879.4
  transfusion
    procedure E879.8
  transplant, transplantation (heart) (kidney) (liver) E878.0
    partial organ E878.4
  ureterostomy E878.3
  vaccination E879.8
Reduction in
  atmospheric pressure - *see also* Effects of, air pressure
    while surfacing from
      deep water diving causing caisson or divers' disease, palsy or paralysis E902.2
      underground E902.8
Residual (effect) - *see* Late effect
Rock falling on or hitting (accidentally)
  motor vehicle (in motion) (on public highway) E818●
    not on public highway E825●
  nonmotor road vehicle NEC E829●
  pedal cycle E826●
  person E916
  railway rolling stock, train, vehicle E806●
Running off, away
  animal (being ridden) (in sport or transport) E828●
    not being ridden E906.8
  animal-drawn vehicle E827●
  rails, railway *(see also* Derailment) E802●
  roadway
    motor vehicle (without antecedent collision) E816●
      nontraffic accident E825●
        with antecedent collision - *see* categories Collision, motor vehicle, not on public highway

Running off, away *(Continued)*
  roadway *(Continued)*
    motor vehicle *(Continued)*
      with
        antecedent collision - *see* Collision motor vehicle
        subsequent collision
          involving any object, person or vehicle not on public highway E816●
          on public highway E811●
    nonmotor road vehicle NEC E829●
    pedal cycle E826●
Run over (accidentally) (by)
  animal (not being ridden) E906.8
    being ridden (in sport or transport) E828●
  animal-drawn vehicle E827●
  machinery - *see* Accident, machine
  motor vehicle (on public highway) - *see* Hit by, motor vehicle
  nonmotor road vehicle NEC E829●
  railway train E805●
  street car E829●
  vehicle NEC E848

S

Saturnism E866.0
  from insecticide NEC E863.4
Scald, scalding (accidental) (by) (from) (in) E924.0
  acid - *see* Scald, caustic
  boiling tap water E924.2
  caustic or corrosive liquid, substance E924.1
    swallowed - *see* Table of Drugs and Chemicals
  homicide (attempt) - *see* Assault, burning
  inflicted by other person
    stated as
      intentional or homicidal E968.3
      undetermined whether accidental or intentional E988.2
  late effect of NEC E929.8
  liquid (boiling) (hot) E924.0
  local application of externally applied substance in medical or surgical care E873.5
  molten metal E924.0
  self-inflicted (unspecified whether accidental or intentional) E988.2
    stated as intentional, purposeful E958.2
  stated as undetermined whether accidental or intentional E988.2
  steam E924.0
  tap water (boiling) E924.2
  transport accident - *see* categories E800–E848
  vapor E924.0
Scratch, cat E906.8
Sea
  sickness E903
Self-mutilation - *see* Suicide
Sequelae (of)
  in
    terrorism E999.1
    war operations E999.0

Shock
  anaphylactic *(see also* Table of Drugs and Chemicals) E947.9
    due to
      bite (venomous) - *see* Bite, venomous NEC
      sting - *see* Sting
  electric *(see also* Electric shock) E925.9
  from electric appliance or current *(see also* Electric shock) E925.9
Shooting, shot (accidental(ly)) E922.9
  air gun E922.4
  BB gun E922.4
  hand gun (pistol) (revolver) E922.0
  himself *(see also* Shooting, self-inflicted) E985.4
    hand gun (pistol) (revolver) E985.0
    military firearm, except hand gun E985.3
      hand gun (pistol) (revolver) E985.0
    rifle (hunting) E985.2
      military E985.3
    shotgun (automatic) E985.1
    specified firearm NEC E985.4
    Verey pistol E985.4
  homicide (attempt) E965.4
    air gun E968.6
    BB gun E968.6
    hand gun (pistol) (revolver) E965.0
    military firearm, except hand gun E965.3
      hand gun (pistol) (revolver) E965.0
    paintball gun E965.4
    rifle (hunting) E965.2
      military E965.3
    shotgun (automatic) E965.1
    specified firearm NEC E965.4
    Verey pistol E965.4
  inflicted by other person
    in accidental circumstances E922.9
      hand gun (pistol) (revolver) E922.0
      military firearm, except hand gun E922.3
        hand gun (pistol) (revolver) E922.0
      rifle (hunting) E922.2
        military E922.3
      shotgun (automatic) E922.1
      specified firearm NEC E922.8
      Verey pistol E922.8
    stated as
      intentional, homicidal E965.4
        hand gun (pistol) (revolver) E965.0
        military firearm, except hand gun E965.3
          hand gun (pistol) (revolver) E965.0
        paintball gun E965.4
        rifle (hunting) E965.2
          military E965.3
        shotgun (automatic) E965.1
        specified firearm E965.4
        Verey pistol E965.4
      undetermined whether accidental or intentional E985.4
        air gun E985.6
        BB gun E985.6
        hand gun (pistol) (revolver) E985.0
        military firearm, except hand gun E985.3

◀ New   ◀▥ Revised   ~~deleted~~ Deleted   ● Use Additional Digit(s)   ▨ Omit code

E CODES

Shooting, shot (*Continued*)
  inflicted by other person (*Continued*)
    stated as (*Continued*)
      undetermined whether accidental
        or intentional (*Continued*)
          hand gun (pistol) (revolver)
            E985.0
          paintball gun E985.7
          rifle (hunting) E985.2
          shotgun (automatic) E985.1
          specified firearm NEC
            E985.4
          Verey pistol E985.4
  in
    terrorism - *see* Terrorism, shooting
    war operations - *see* War operations,
      shooting
  legal
    execution E978
    intervention E970
  military firearm, except hand gun
    E922.3
    hand gun (pistol) (revolver)
      E922.0
  paintball gun E922.5
  rifle (hunting) E922.2
    military E922.3
  self-inflicted (unspecified whether
    accidental or intentional)
    E985.4
    air gun E985.6
    BB gun E985.6
    hand gun (pistol) (revolver)
      E985.0
    military firearm, except hand gun
      E985.3
      hand gun (pistol) (revolver)
        E985.0
    paintball gun E985.7
    rifle (hunting) E985.2
      military E985.3
    shotgun (automatic) E985.1
    specified firearm NEC E985.4
  stated as
    accidental E922.9
      hand gun (pistol) (revolver)
        E922.0
      military firearm, except hand
        gun E922.3
        hand gun (pistol) (revolver)
          E922.0
      paintball gun E922.5
      rifle (hunting) E922.2
        military E922.3
      shotgun (automatic) E922.1
      specified firearm NEC
        E922.8
      Verey pistol E922.8
    intentional, purposeful E955.4
      hand gun (pistol) (revolver)
        E955.0
      military firearm, except hand
        gun E955.3
        hand gun (pistol) (revolver)
          E955.0
      paintball gun E955.7
      rifle (hunting) E955.2
        military E955.3
      shotgun (automatic) E955.1
      specified firearm NEC
        E955.4
      Verey pistol E955.4
  shotgun (automatic) E922.1
  specified firearm NEC E922.8

Shooting, shot (*Continued*)
  stated as undetermined whether
    accidental or intentional E985.4
    hand gun (pistol) (revolver)
      E985.0
    military firearm, except hand gun
      E985.3
      hand gun (pistol) (revolver)
        E985.0
    paintball gun E985.7
    rifle (hunting) E985.2
      military E985.3
    shotgun (automatic) E985.1
    specified firearm NEC E985.4
    Verey pistol E985.4
  suicidal (attempt) E955.4
    air gun E985.6
    BB gun E985.6
    hand gun (pistol) (revolver)
      E955.0
    military firearm, except hand gun
      E955.3
      hand gun (pistol) (revolver)
        E955.0
    paintball gun E955.7
    rifle (hunting) E955.2
      military E955.3
    shotgun (automatic) E955.1
    specified firearm NEC E955.4
    Verey pistol E955.4
Shoving (accidentally) by other person
  (*see also* Pushing by other person)
  E917.9
Sickness
  air E903
  alpine E902.0
  car E903
  motion E903
  mountain E902.0
  sea E903
  travel E903
Sinking (accidental)
  boat, ship, watercraft (causing
    drowning, submersion)
    E830●
    causing injury except drowning,
      submersion E831●
Siriasis E900.0
Skydiving E844●
Slashed wrists (*see also* Cut, self-inflicted)
  E986
Slipping (accidental)
  on
    deck (of boat, ship, watercraft) (icy)
      (oily) (wet) E835●
    ice E885.9
    ladder of ship E833●
      due to accident to watercraft
        E831●
    mud E885.9
    oil E885.9
    snow E885.9
    stairs of ship E833●
      due to accident to watercraft
        E831●
    surface
      slippery E885.9
      wet E885.9
Sliver, wood, injury by E920.8
Smothering, smothered (*see also*
  Suffocation) E913.9
Smouldering building or structure in
  terrorism E979.3

Sodomy (assault) E960.1
Solid substance in eye (any part) or
  adnexa E914
Sound waves (causing injury) E928.1
Splinter, injury by E920.8
Stab, stabbing E966
  accidental - *see* Cut
Starvation E904.1
  helpless person, infant, newborn - *see*
    Lack of food
  homicidal intent E968.4
  late effect of NEC E929.5
  resulting from accident connected
    with transport - *see* categories
    E800–E848
Stepped on
  by
    animal (not being ridden) E906.8
      being ridden (in sport or
        transport) E828●
    crowd E917.1
    person E917.9
      in sports E917.0
  in sports E917.0
Stepping on
  object (moving) E917.9
    in sports E917.0
      with subsequent fall E917.5
    stationary E917.4
      with subsequent fall E917.8
  person E917.9
    as, or caused by a crowd E917.1
      with subsequent fall E917.6
    in sports E917.0
Sting E905.9
  ant E905.5
  bee E905.3
  caterpillar E905.5
  coral E905.6
  hornet E905.3
  insect NEC E905.5
  jelly fish E905.6
  marine animal or plant E905.6
  nematocysts E905.6
  scorpion E905.2
  sea anemone E905.6
  sea cucumber E905.6
  wasp E905.3
  yellow jacket E905.3
Storm E908.9
  specified type NEC E908.8
Straining, injury in E927.8
Strangling - *see* Suffocation
Strangulation - *see* Suffocation
Strenuous movements (in recreational or
  other activities) E927.8
Striking against
  bottom (when jumping or diving into
    water) E883.0
  object (moving) E917.9
    caused by crowd E917.1
      with subsequent fall E917.6
    furniture E917.3
      with subsequent fall E917.7
    in
      running water E917.2
        with drowning or
          submersion - *see*
          Submersion
      sports E917.0
        with subsequent fall E917.5
    stationary E917.4
      with subsequent fall E917.8

E CODES

◀ New   ⬅ Revised   ~~deleted~~ Deleted   ● Use Additional Digit(s)   ▭ Omit code

E CODES

Suffocation (Continued)
in (Continued)
plastic bag (Continued)
suicidal, purposely self-inflicted
E953.1
refrigerator E913.2
self-inflicted - see also Suffocation,
stated as undetermined whether
accidental or intentional E953.9
in accidental circumstances - see
category E913
stated as intentional, purposeful - see
Suicide, suffocation
stated as undetermined whether
accidental or intentional E983.9
by, in
hanging E983.0
plastic bag E983.1
specified means NEC E983.8
suicidal - see Suicide, suffocation
war operations E995.3 ◄
Suicide, suicidal (attempted) (by)
E958.9
burning, burns E958.1
caustic substance E958.7
poisoning E950.7
swallowed E950.7
cold, extreme E958.3
cut (any part of body) E956
cutting or piercing instrument
(classifiable to E920) E956
drowning E954
electrocution E958.4
explosive(s) (classifiable to E923)
E955.5
fire E958.1
firearm (classifiable to E922) - see
Shooting, suicidal
hanging E953.0
jumping
before moving object, train, vehicle
E958.0
from high place - see Jumping,
from, high place, stated as,
suicidal
knife E956
late effect of E959
motor vehicle, crashing of E958.5
poisoning - see Table of Drugs and
Chemicals
puncture (any part of body) E956
scald E958.2
shooting - see Shooting, suicidal
specified means NEC E958.8
stab (any part of body) E956
strangulation - see Suicide,
suffocation
submersion E954
suffocation E953.9
by, in
hanging E953.0
plastic bag E953.1
specified means NEC E953.8
wound NEC E958.9
Sunburn E926.2
Sunstroke E900.0
Supersonic waves (causing injury)
E928.1
Surgical procedure, complication of
delayed or as an abnormal reaction
without mention of
misadventure, see Reaction,
abnormal
due to or as a result of misadventure -
see Misadventure

Swallowed, swallowing
foreign body - see Foreign body,
alimentary canal
poison - see Table of Drugs and
Chemicals
substance
caustic - see Table of Drugs and
Chemicals drugs
corrosive - see Table of Drugs and
Chemicals
poisonous - see Table of Drugs and
Chemicals
Swimmers' cramp (see also category
E910) E910.2
not in recreation or sport E910.3
Syndrome, battered
baby or child - see Abuse, child
wife - see Assault

T

Tackle in sport E886.0
Terrorism (by) (in) (injury) E979.8
air blast E979.2
aircraft burned, destroyed, exploded,
shot down E979.1
used as a weapon E979.1
anthrax E979.6
asphyxia from
chemical (weapons) E979.7
fire, conflagration (caused by fire-
producing device) E979.3
from nuclear explosion
E979.5
gas or fumes E979.7
bayonet E979.8
biological agents E979.6
blast (air) (effects) E979.2
from nuclear explosion E979.5
underwater E979.0
bomb (antipersonnel) (mortar)
(explosion) (fragments)
E979.2
bullet(s) (from carbine, machine gun,
pistol, rifle, shotgun)
E979.4
burn from
chemical E979.7
fire, conflagration (caused by fire-
producing device) E979.3
from nuclear explosion E979.5
gas E979.7
burning aircraft E979.1
chemical E979.7
cholera E979.6
conflagration E979.3
crushed by falling aircraft E979.1
depth-charge E979.0
destruction of aircraft E979.1
disability, as sequelae one year or more
after injury E999.1
drowning E979.8
effect
of nuclear weapon (direct)
(secondary) E979.5
secondary NEC E979.9
sequelae E999.1
explosion (artillery shell) (breech-
block) (cannon block) E979.2
aircraft E979.1
bomb (antipersonnel) (mortar)
E979.2
nuclear (atom) (hydrogen)
E979.5

Terrorism (Continued)
explosion (Continued)
depth-charge E979.0
grenade E979.2
injury by fragments from E979.2
land-mine E979.2
marine weapon E979.0
mine (land) E979.2
at sea or in harbor E979.0
marine E979.0
missile (explosive) NEC E979.2
munitions (dump) (factory)
E979.2
nuclear (weapon) E979.5
other direct and secondary effects
of E979.5
sea-based artillery shell
E979.0
torpedo E979.0
exposure to ionizing radiation from
nuclear explosion E979.5
falling aircraft E979.1
fire or fire-producing device E979.3
firearms E979.4
fireball effects from nuclear explosion
E979.5
fragments from artillery shell, bomb
NEC, grenade, guided missile,
land-mine, rocket, shell, shrapnel
E979.2
gas or fumes E979.7
grenade (explosion) (fragments)
E979.2
guided missile (explosion) (fragments)
E979.2
nuclear E979.5
heat from nuclear explosion E979.5
hot substances E979.3
hydrogen cyanide E979.7
land-mine (explosion) (fragments)
E979.2
laser(s) E979.8
late effect of E999.1
lewisite E979.7
lung irritant (chemical) (fumes) (gas)
E979.7
marine mine E979.0
mine E979.2
at sea E979.0
in harbor E979.0
land (explosion) (fragments)
E979.2
marine E979.0
missile (explosion) (fragments)
(guided) E979.2
marine E979.0
nuclear weapons E979.5
mortar bomb (explosion) (fragments)
E979.2
mustard gas E979.7
nerve gas E979.7
nuclear weapons E979.5
pellets (shotgun) E979.4
petrol bomb E979.3
phosgene E979.7
piercing object E979.8
poisoning (chemical) (fumes) (gas)
E979.7
radiation, ionizing from nuclear
explosion E979.5
rocket (explosion) (fragments)
E979.2
saber, sabre E979.8
sarin E979.7
screening smoke E979.7

E CODES

Terrorism (*Continued*)
  sequelae effect (of) E999.1
  shell (aircraft) (artillery) (cannon)
    (land-based) (explosion)
    (fragments) E979.2
    sea-based E979.0
  shooting E979.4
    bullet(s) E979.4
    pellet(s) (rifle) (shotgun)
      E979.4
  shrapnel E979.2
  smallpox E979.7
  stabbing object(s) E979.8
  submersion E979.8
  torpedo E979.0
  underwater blast E979.0
  vesicant (chemical) (fumes) (gas)
    E979.7
  weapon burst E979.2
Thermic fever E900.9
Thermoplegia E900.9
Thirst - *see also* Lack of water
  resulting from accident connected
    with transport - *see* categories
    E800–E848
Thrown (accidentally)
  against object in or part of vehicle
    by motion of vehicle
      aircraft E844●
      boat, ship, watercraft E838●
      motor vehicle (on public
        highway) E818●
        not on public highway
          E825●
        off-road type (not on public
          highway) E821●
        on public highway
          E818●
        snow vehicle E820●
          on public highway
            E818●
      nonmotor road vehicle NEC
        E829●
      railway rolling stock, train, vehicle
        E806●
      street car E829●
  from
    animal (being ridden) (in sport or
      transport) E828●
    high place, homicide (attempt)
      E968.1
    machinery - *see* Accident,
      machine
    vehicle NEC - *see* Accident, vehicle
      NEC
  off - *see* Thrown, from
  overboard (by motion of boat, ship,
    watercraft) E832●
    by accident to boat, ship, watercraft
      E830●
Thunderbolt NEC E907
Tidal wave (any injury) E909.4
  caused by storm E908.0
Took
  overdose of drug - *see* Table of Drugs
    and Chemicals
  poison - *see* Table of Drugs and
    Chemicals
Tornado (any injury) E908.1
Torrential rain (any injury) E908.2
Traffic accident NEC E819●
Trampled by animal E906.8
  being ridden (in sport or transport)
    E828●

Trapped (accidentally)
  between
    objects (moving) (stationary and
      moving) E918
  by
    door of
      elevator E918
      motor vehicle (on public
        highway)
        (while alighting, boarding) -
          see Fall, from, motor
          vehicle, while alighting
      railway train (underground)
        E806●
      street car E829●
      subway train E806●
  in object E918
Trauma
  cumulative
    from
      repetitive
        impact E927.4
        motion or movements E927.3

  sudden from strenuous movement
    E927.0
Travel (effects) E903
  sickness E903
Tree
  falling on or hitting E916
    motor vehicle (in motion) (on public
      highway) E818●
      not on public highway E825●
    nonmotor road vehicle NEC
      E829●
    pedal cycle E826●
    person E916
    railway rolling stock, train, vehicle
      E806●
    street car E829●
Trench foot E901.0
Tripping over animal, carpet, curb, rug,
  or small object (with fall) E885.9
  without fall - *see* Striking against, object
Tsunami E909.4
Twisting, injury in E927.8

V

Violence, nonaccidental (*see also* Assault)
  E968.9
Volcanic eruption (any injury)
  E909.1
Vomitus in air passages (with asphyxia,
  obstruction or suffocation)
  E911

W

War operations (during hostilities)
  (injury) (by) (in) E995.9 ◄▦
  after cessation of hostilities, injury
    due to E998.9 ◄▦
  air blast E993.9 ◄▦
  aircraft burned, destroyed, exploded,
    shot down E991.9
  asphyxia from
    chemical E997.2
    fire, conflagration (caused by
      fire-producing device or
      conventional weapon)
      E990.9

War operations (*Continued*)
  asphyxia from (*Continued*)
    fire, conflagration (*Continued*)
      from nuclear explosion (*see also*
        War operations, injury due
        to, nuclear weapons)
        E996.8 ◄▦
      incendiary bomb E990.0 ◄
      petrol bomb E990.0
    fumes E997.2
    gas E997.2
  baton (nightstick) E995.1 ◄
  battle wound NEC E995.8 ◄▦
  bayonet E995.2 ◄▦
  biological warfare agents E997.1
  blast (air) (effects) E993.9 ◄▦
    from nuclear explosion (*see also*
      War operations, injury due
      to, nuclear weapons) E996.1 ◄▦
    underwater E992.9 ◄▦
  bomb (mortar) (explosion) E993.2 ◄▦
    after cessation of hostilities
      E998.1 ◄▦
    fragments, injury by E991.4 ◄▦
      antipersonnel E991.3
  bullet(s) (from carbine, machine gun,
    pistol, rifle, shotgun) E991.2
    rubber E991.0
  burn from
    chemical E997.2
    fire, conflagration (caused by
      fire-producing device or
      conventional weapon)
      E990.9
      from ~~nuclear explosion E996~~ ◄▦
      conventional weapon
        E990.3 ◄
      flamethrower E990.1 ◄
      incendiary bomb E990.0 ◄
      incendiary bullet E990.2 ◄
      nuclear explosion E996.2 ◄
      petrol bomb E990.0
    gas E997.2
  burning aircraft E994.3 ◄▦
  chemical E997.2
  chlorine E997.2
  conventional warfare, specified form
    NEC E995.8 ◄▦
  crushing by falling aircraft
    E994.8 ◄▦
  depth charge E992.1 ◄▦
  destruction of aircraft E994.9 ◄▦
  detonation of own munitions
    (ammunition) (artillery)
    (mortars), unintentional E993.6 ◄
  disability as sequela one year or more
    after injury E999.0
  discharge of own munitions launch
    device (autocannons) (automatic
    grenade launchers) (missile
    launchers) (small arms),
    unintentional E993.7 ◄
  drowning E995.4 ◄▦
  effect ~~(direct) (secondary)~~ nuclear
    weapon (*see also* War
    operations, injury due to,
    nuclear weapons) E996.9 ◄▦
  explosion ~~(artillery shell)~~ (breech
    block) (cannon shell) E993.9 ◄▦
    after cessation of hostilities ~~of bomb,~~
      ~~mine placed in war E998~~ ◄▦
    bomb placed in war E998.1 ◄
    mine placed in war E998.0 ◄
    aircraft E994.1 ◄▦

◄ New   ◄▦ Revised   ~~deleted~~ Deleted   ● Use Additional Digit(s)   � Omit code

E CODES

War operations *(Continued)*
  explosion *(Continued)*
    aircraft *(Continued)*
      due to ◄
        enemy fire or explosives
          E994.0 ◄
        own onboard explosives
          E994.1 ◄
    artillery shell E993.2 ◄
    bomb (mortar) E993.2 ◄▥
      aerial E993.0 ◄
      atom *(see also* War operations,
        injury due to, nuclear
        weapons) E996.9 ◄▥
      hydrogen *(see also* War
        operations, injury due to,
        nuclear weapons) E996.9 ◄▥
      injury by fragments from
        E991.4 ◄▥
        antipersonnel E991.3
      nuclear *(see also* War operations,
        injury due to, nuclear
        weapons) E996.9 ◄▥
    depth charge E992.1 ◄▥
    injury by fragments from E991.4 ◄▥
      antipersonnel E991.3
    marine weapon NEC E992.8 ◄▥
    mine
      at sea or in harbor E992.2 ◄▥
      land E993.8 ◄▥
        injury by fragments from
          E991.4 ◄▥
      marine E992.2 ◄▥
    missile, guided E993.1 ◄
    mortar E993.2 ◄
    munitions (accidental) (being used
      in war) (dump) (factory)
      E993.9 ◄▥
      own E993.7 ◄
        launch device (autocannons)
          (automatic grenade
          launchers) (missile
          launchers) (small arms)
          E993.7 ◄
    nuclear (weapon) *(see also* War
      operations, injury due to,
      nuclear weapons) E996.9 ◄▥
    own weapons (accidental) E993.7 ◄▥
      injury by fragments from E991.9
        antipersonnel E991.3
    sea-based artillery shell E992.3 ◄▥
    specified NEC E993.8 ◄
    torpedo E992.0 ◄▥
  exposure to ionizing radiation from
    nuclear explosion *(see also* War
    operations, injury due to, nuclear
    weapons) E996.3 ◄▥
  falling aircraft E994.8 ◄
  fire or fire-producing device E990.9
    flamethrower E990.1 ◄
    incendiary bomb E990.0 ◄
    incendiary bullet E990.2 ◄
    indirectly caused from conventional
      weapon E990.3 ◄
    petrol bomb E990.0 ◄
  fireball effects from nuclear explosion
    E996.2 ◄▥
  fragments from
    antipersonnel bomb E991.3
    artillery shell, ~~bomb NEC, grenade,~~
      ~~guided missile, land mine,~~
      ~~rocket, shell, shrapnel~~
      ~~E991.9~~ E991.4 ◄▥
    bomb NEC E991.4 ◄
    grenade E991.4 ◄
    guided missile E991.4 ◄

War operations *(Continued)*
  fragments from *(Continued)*
    land mine E991.4 ◄
    rocket E991.4 ◄
    shell E991.4 ◄
    shrapnel E991.9 ◄
  fumes E997.2
  gas E997.2
  grenade (explosion) E993.8 ◄▥
    fragments, injury by E991.4 ◄▥
  guided missile (explosion) E993.1 ◄▥
    fragments, injury by E991.4 ◄▥
  nuclear *(see also* War operations,
    injury due to, nuclear
    weapons) E996.9 ◄▥
  heat from nuclear explosion
    E996.2 ◄▥
  injury due to, ~~but occurring after~~
    ~~cessation of hostilities E998~~
    aerial bomb E993.0 ◄
    air blast E993.9 ◄
    aircraft shot down E994.0 ◄
    artillery shell E993.2 ◄
    blast E993.9 ◄
      wave E993.9 ◄
      wind E993.9 ◄
    bomb E998.8 ◄
    but occurring after cessation of
      hostilities ◄
      explosion of bombs E998.1 ◄
      explosion of mines E998.0 ◄
      specified NEC E998.8 ◄
    conventional warfare E995.9 ◄
      specified form NEC E995.8 ◄
    depth charge E992.1 ◄
    destruction of aircraft E994.9 ◄
      due to ◄
        air to air missile E994.0 ◄
        collision with other aircraft
          E994.2 ◄
        enemy fire or explosives
          E994.0 ◄
        on board explosion
          (explosives) E994.1 ◄
        on board fire E994.3 ◄
        rocket propelled grenade
          [RPG] E994.0 ◄
        small arms fire E994.0 ◄
        surface to air missile E994.0 ◄
      specified NEC E994.8 ◄
    dirty bomb *(see also* War
      operations, injury due to,
      nuclear weapons) E996.9 ◄
    drowning E995.4 ◄
    explosion (direct pressure)
      (indirect pressure)
      (due to) E993.9 ◄
      depth charge E992.1 ◄
      improvised explosive device
        [IED] ◄
        person borne E993.3 ◄
        roadside E993.5 ◄
        specified NEC E993.5 ◄
        transport vehicle (air) (land)
          (water) borne E993.4 ◄
        vehicle (air) (land) (water)
          borne E993.4 ◄
      marine mines (in harbor)
        (at sea) E992.2 ◄
      marine weapons E992.9 ◄
        specified NEC E992.8 ◄
      sea based artillery shell
        E992.3 ◄
      specified NEC E993.8 ◄
      torpedo E992.0 ◄

War operations *(Continued)*
  injury due to, *(Continued)*
    explosion *(Continued)*
      unintentional (of own) ◄
        autocannons E993.7 ◄
        automatic grenade launchers
          E993.7 ◄
        launch device discharge
          E993.7 ◄
        munitions detonation
          (ammunition) (artillery)
          (mortars) E993.6 ◄
        missile launchers E993.7 ◄
        small arms E993.7 ◄
    fragments (from) E991.9 ◄
      artillery E991.8 ◄
      artillery shells E991.4 ◄
      autocannons E991.8 ◄
      automatic grenade launchers
        [AGL] E991.8 ◄
      bombs E991.4 ◄
        antipersonnel E991.3 ◄
      detonation of unexploded
        ordnance [UXO] E991.4 ◄
      grenade E991.4 ◄
      guided missile E991.4 ◄
      improvised explosive device
        [IED] ◄
        person borne E991.5 ◄
        roadside E991.7 ◄
        specified NEC E991.7 ◄
        transport vehicle (air) (land)
          (water) borne E991.6 ◄
        vehicle (air) (land) (water)
          borne E991.6 ◄
      land mine E991.4 ◄
      missile launchers E991.8 ◄
      mortars E991.8 ◄
      munitions (artillery shells)
        (bombs) (grenades)
        (rockets) (shells) E991.4 ◄
      rockets E991.4 ◄
      shells E991.4 ◄
      small arms E991.8 ◄
      specified NEC E991.9 ◄
      weapons (artillery)
        (autocannons) (mortars)
        (small arms) E991.8 ◄
    grenade E993.8 ◄
    guided missile E993.1 ◄
    hand to hand combat,
      unarmed E995.0 ◄
    improvised explosive device
      [IED] ◄
      person borne E993.3 ◄
      roadside E993.5 ◄
      specified NEC E993.5 ◄
      transport vehicle (air) (land)
        (water) borne E993.4 ◄
      vehicle (air) (land) (water) borne
        E993.4 ◄
    inability to surface or obtain air
      E995.4 ◄
    land mine E993.8 ◄
    marine mines (in harbor) (at sea)
      E992.2 ◄
    marine weapons E992.9 ◄
      specified NEC E992.8 ◄
    mortar E993.2 ◄
    nuclear weapons E996.9 ◄
      beta burns E996.3 ◄
      blast debris E996.1 ◄
      blast pressure E996.0 ◄
      burns due to thermal radiation
        E996.2 ◄

◄ New   ◄▥ Revised   ~~deleted~~ Deleted   ● Use Additional Digit(s)   � Omit code

War operations *(Continued)*
  injury due to, *(Continued)*
    nuclear weapons *(Continued)*
      direct blast effect E996.0 ◀
      fallout exposure E996.3 ◀
      fireball effect E996.2 ◀
      flash burns E996.2 ◀
      heat effect E996.2 ◀
      indirect blast effect E996.1 ◀
      nuclear radiation effects
        E996.3 ◀
      radiation exposure (acute)
        E996.3 ◀
      radiation sickness E996.3 ◀
      secondary effects E996.3 ◀
      specified effects NEC E996.8 ◀
      thermal radiation effect E996.2 ◀
    piercing object E995.2 ◀
    restriction of airway, intentional
      E995.3 ◀
    sea based artillery shell E992.3 ◀
    shrapnel E991.9 ◀
    stave E995.1 ◀
    strangulation E995.3 ◀
    strike by blunt object (baton)
      (nightstick) (stave) E995.1 ◀
    submersion (accidental)
      (unintentional) E995.4 ◀
      intentional E995.3 ◀
    suffocation E995.3 ◀
      accidental E995.4 ◀
    torpedo E992.0 ◀
    underwater blast E992.9 ◀
    weapon of mass destruction
      [WMD] E997.3 ◀
  knife E995.2 ◀
  lacrimator (gas) (chemical) E997.2
  land mine (explosion) E993.8 ⬅
    after cessation of hostilities
      E998.0 ⬅
    fragments, injury by E991.4 ⬅
  laser(s) E997.0
  late effect of E999.0
  lewisite E997.2
  lung irritant (chemical) (fumes)
    (gas) E997.2
  marine mine E992.2 ⬅
  mine
    after cessation of hostilities
      E998.0 ⬅
    at sea E992.2 ⬅
    in harbor E992.2 ⬅

War operations *(Continued)*
  mine *(Continued)*
    land (explosion) E993.8 ⬅
      fragments, injury by E991.4 ⬅
    marine E992.2 ⬅
  missile (guided) (explosion) E993.1 ⬅
    fragments, injury by E991.4 ⬅
    marine E992.8 ⬅
    nuclear (*see also* War operations,
      injury due to, nuclear
      weapons) E996.9 ⬅
  mortar bomb (explosion) E993.2 ⬅
    fragments, injury by E991.4 ⬅
  mustard gas E997.2
  nerve gas E997.2
  phosgene E997.2
  piercing object E995.2 ◀
  poisoning (chemical) (fumes) (gas)
    E997.2
  radiation, ionizing from nuclear
    explosion (*see also* War
    operations, injury due to,
    nuclear weapons) E996.3 ⬅
  rocket (explosion) E993.8 ⬅
    fragments, injury by E991.4 ⬅
  saber, sabre E995.2 ⬅
  screening smoke E997.8
  shell (aircraft) (artillery) (cannon)
    (land based) (explosion)
    E993.2 ⬅
    fragments, injury by E991.4 ⬅
    sea-based E992.3 ⬅
  shooting E991.2
    after cessation of hostilities
      E998.8 ⬅
    bullet(s) E991.2
      rubber E991.0
    pellet(s) (rifle) E991.1
    shrapnel E991.9
  stave E995.2 ◀
  strike by blunt object (baton)
    (nightstick) (stave) E995.1 ◀
  submersion E995.4 ⬅
  intentional E995.3 ◀
  sword E995.2 ◀
  torpedo E992.0 ⬅
  unconventional warfare, except by
    nuclear weapon E997.9
    biological (warfare) E997.1
    gas, fumes, chemicals E997.2
    laser(s) E997.0

War operations *(Continued)*
  unconventional warfare *(Continued)*
    specified type NEC E997.8
    underwater blast E992.9 ⬅
    vesicant (chemical) (fumes) (gas)
      E997.2
    weapon burst E993.9 ⬅
Washed
  away by flood - *see* Flood
  away by tidal wave - *see* Tidal wave
  off road by storm (transport vehicle)
    E908.9
  overboard E832●
Weapon of mass destruction [WMD]
  E997.3 ◀
Weather exposure - *see also* Exposure
  cold E901.0
  hot E900.0
Weightlessness (causing injury) (effects
  of) (in spacecraft, real or simulated)
  E928.0
Wound (accidental) NEC (*see also* Injury)
  E928.9
  battle (*see also* War operations)
    E995.9 ⬅
  bayonet E920.3
    in
      legal intervention E974
      war operations E995.2 ⬅
  gunshot - *see* Shooting
  incised - *see* Cut
  saber, sabre E920.3
    in war operations E995.2 ⬅
Wrong
  body part, performance of correct
    operation (procedure) on
    E876.7 ◀
  device implanted into correct
    surgical site E876.5 ◀
  patient, performance of operation
    (procedure) on E876.6 ◀
  procedure (operation) performed
    on correct patient E876.5 ◀
  side, performance of correct operation
    (procedure) on E876.7 ◀
  site, performance of correct operation
    (procedure) on E876.7 ◀

◀ New   ⬅ Revised   ~~deleted~~ Deleted   ● Use Additional Digit(s)   ▓ Omit code

E CODES

PART III

Diseases: Tabular List Volume 1

1. INFECTIOUS AND PARASITIC DISEASES (001–139)

Note: Categories for "late effects" of infectious and parasitic diseases are to be found at 137–139.

Includes   diseases generally recognized as communicable or transmissible as well as a few diseases of unknown but possibly infectious origin

Excludes   *acute respiratory infections (460–466)*
carrier or suspected carrier of infectious organism (V02.0–V02.9)
certain localized infections
influenza (487.0–487.8, 488.0–488.1) ◀▥

INTESTINAL INFECTIOUS DISEASES (001–009)

Excludes   *helminthiases (120.0–129)*
Diseases or infestations caused by parasitic worms

● **001 Cholera**
A serious, often deadly, infectious disease of the small intestine

001.0 Due to Vibrio cholerae 🦠
   (Ex) 001.0-001.9

001.1 Due to Vibrio cholerae el tor 🦠
   (Ex) 001.0-001.9

001.9 Cholera, unspecified 🦠
   (Ex) 001.0-001.9

● **002 Typhoid and paratyphoid fevers**
Caused by Salmonella typhi and Salmonella paratyphi A, B, and C bacteria

002.0 Typhoid fever 🦠
Typhoid (fever) (infection) [any site]
   (Ex) 002.0-002.9

002.1 Paratyphoid fever A 🦠
   (Ex) 002.0-002.9

002.2 Paratyphoid fever B 🦠
   (Ex) 002.0-002.9

002.3 Paratyphoid fever C 🦠
   (Ex) 002.0-002.9

002.9 Paratyphoid fever, unspecified 🦠
   (Ex) 002.0-002.9

Item 1-1 Salmonella is a bacterium that lives in the intestines of fowl and mammals and can spread to humans through improper food preparation and cooking. Salmonellosis is an infection with the bacterium. Symptoms include diarrhea, fever, and abdominal cramps 12 to 72 hours after infection. The illness usually lasts 4 to 7 days, and most persons recover without treatment. The diarrhea may be so severe that the patient needs to be hospitalized. Patients with immunocompromised systems in chronic, ill health are more likely to have the infection invade their bloodstream with life-threatening results. For example, patients with sickle cell disease are more prone to salmonella osteomyelitis than others.

● **003 Other salmonella infections**

Includes   infection or food poisoning by Salmonella [any serotype]

003.0 Salmonella gastroenteritis 🦠
Salmonellosis
   (Ex) 002.0, 002.9-003.0, 004.9-005.2, 007.5, 008.00-009.0, 040.41-040.42, 536.8, 558.2-558.9, 564.1, 567.21, 567.23, 567.31-567.39, 567.89, 777.50-777.53, 777.8

003.1 Salmonella septicemia 🦠
   (Ex) 003.1, 020.2, 022.3, 036.2, 038.0-038.9, 040.89-041.85, 041.89-041.9, 054.5, 139.8, 771.81, 771.83-771.89, 995.90-995.94, V09.0-V09.91

● **003.2 Localized salmonella infections**

003.20 Localized salmonella infection, unspecified
Specified in the documentation as localized, but unspecified as to type

003.21 Salmonella meningitis 🦠
Specified as localized in the meninges
   (Ex) 003.21, 013.00-013.16, 036.0, 047.0-047.9, 049.0-049.1, 072.1, 078.88-078.89, 079.81, 079.88-079.99, 090.42, 091.81, 094.2, 098.89, 100.81, 112.83, 114.2, 115.01, 115.11, 115.91, 130.0, 139.8, 320.0-322.9, 349.89-349.9

003.22 Salmonella pneumonia 🦠
Specified as localized in the lungs
   (Ex) 003.22, 011.00-012.16, 012.80-012.86, 017.90-017.96, 020.3-020.5, 021.3, 022.1, 031.0, 039.1, 073.0, 115.05, 115.15, 115.95, 122.1, 130.4, 136.3, 480.0-480.2, 480.8-487.1, 488, 495.0-495.7, 500, 502-508.9, 517.1, 517.8, 518.89, 519.8-519.9

N Newborn Age: 0   **P** Pediatric Age: 0–17   **M** Maternity Age: 12–55   **A** Adult Age: 15–124   ♀ Females Only   ♂ Males Only

(Ex) CC Exclusions   🦠 Complication\Comorbidity   🦠 Major C\C   🦠 Present on Admission Requirement   🦠 Hospital-Acquired Condition   **731**

INFECTIOUS AND PARASITIC DISEASES (001–139)

003.23 Salmonella arthritis 🅒
Specified as localized in the joints
(Ex) 003.23, 015.80-015.96, 036.82, 056.71, 098.50-098.51,
098.59, 098.89, 711.00-714.0, 715.00, 715.09-715.10,
715.18-716.99, 718.00-718.08, 719.00-719.10,
719.18-719.69, 719.80-719.99

003.24 Salmonella osteomyelitis 🅒
Specified as localized in bone
(Ex) 003.24, 015.50-015.56, 015.70-015.76, 015.90-015.96,
730.00-730.39, 730.80-730.99

003.29 Other 🅒
*Specified as localized (because it is still under
localized heading) but does not assign into
any of the above codes*
(Ex) 003.29

003.8 Other specified salmonella infections 🅒
*Any specified salmonella infection which does NOT
assign into any of the above codes (not specified as
localized)*
(Ex) 003.8

003.9 Salmonella infection, unspecified 🅒
*Unspecified in the documentation as to specific type of
salmonella*
(Ex) 003.9

● **004 Shigellosis**
An infectious disease caused by a group of bacteria (Shigella)
Includes bacillary dysentery

004.0 Shigella dysenteriae 🅒
Infection by group A Shigella (Schmitz) (Shiga)
(Ex) 001.1, 002.0, 002.9-003.0, 004.0, 004.9-005.2, 006.0-006.2, 006.9,
007.1-007.9, 008.1-008.3, 008.5, 008.8-009.0, 014.80-014.86,
040.41-040.42, 112.85, 129, 487.8, 536.3, 536.8, 555.0-557.9,
558.9-558.9, 5641, 775.0-775.7, 775.9, 777.50-777.53, 777.8

004.1 Shigella flexneri
Infection by group B Shigella

004.2 Shigella boydii
Infection by group C Shigella

004.3 Shigella sonnei
Infection by group D Shigella

004.8 Other specified shigella infections

004.9 Shigellosis, unspecified

● **005 Other food poisoning (bacterial)**
See Table A, Table of Bacterial Food Poisoning, pg. 1230
Excludes *salmonella infections (003.0–003.9)
toxic effect of:
food contaminants (989.7)
noxious foodstuffs (988.0–988.9)*

005.0 Staphylococcal food poisoning 🅒
Staphylococcal toxemia specified as due to food
(Ex) 001.0-009.3, 040.41-040.42

005.1 Botulism food poisoning 🅒
Botulism NOS
Food poisoning due to Clostridium botulinum
Excludes *infant botulism (040.41)
wound botulism (040.42)*
(Ex) 005.0-005.2, 008.45-008.46, 040.41-040.42

**005.2 Food poisoning due to Clostridium perfringens
[C. welchii]** 🅒
Enteritis necroticans
(Ex) 003.0, 004.9-005.2, 007.5, 008.00-009.0, 040.41-040.42, 487.8, 536.3,
536.8, 558.2-558.9, 564.1, 567.21, 567.23, 567.31-567.39, 567.89,
777.50-777.53, 777.8

005.3 Food poisoning due to other Clostridia 🅒
(Ex) 001.0-009.3, 040.41-040.42

005.4 Food poisoning due to Vibrio parahaemolyticus 🅒
(Ex) 001.0-009.3, 040.41-040.42

● **005.8 Other bacterial food poisoning**
Excludes *salmonella food poisoning (003.0–003.9)*

005.81 Food poisoning due to Vibrio vulnificus 🅒
(Ex) 001.0-009.3, 040.41-040.42

005.89 Other bacterial food poisoning 🅒
Food poisoning due to Bacillus cereus
(Ex) 001.0-009.3, 040.41-040.42

005.9 Food poisoning, unspecified

● **006 Amebiasis**
*An intestinal illness caused by the microscopic parasite
Entamoeba histolytica*
Includes infection due to Entamoeba histolytica
Excludes *amebiasis due to organisms other than Entamoeba
histolytica (007.8)*

**006.0 Acute amebic dysentery without mention
of abscess** 🅒
Acute amebiasis
(Ex) 006.0-0061, 007.5

**006.1 Chronic intestinal amebiasis without mention of
abscess** 🅒
Chronic:
amebiasis
amebic dysentery
(Ex) 006.0-006.1, 007.5

006.2 Amebic nondysenteric colitis 🅒
(Ex) 003.0, 004.9-005.0, 005.2, 006.0-006.2, 006.9, 007.1-009.0, 129, 487.8,
536.3, 536.8, 555.0-557.9, 558.2-558.9, 564.1, 777.50-777.53, 777.8

006.3 Amebic liver abscess 🅒
Hepatic amebiasis
(Ex) 006.3, 572.0

006.4 Amebic lung abscess 🅒
Amebic abscess of lung (and liver)
(Ex) 006.4, 513.0

006.5 Amebic brain abscess 🅒
Amebic abscess of brain (and liver) (and lung)
(Ex) 006.5, 324.0

006.6 Amebic skin ulceration
Cutaneous amebiasis

006.8 Amebic infection of other sites 🅒
Amebic:
appendicitis
balanitis
Ameboma
Excludes *specific infections by free-living amebae
(136.21–136.29)*
(Ex) 006.0-006.5, 006.8

006.9 Amebiasis, unspecified
Amebiasis NOS

● **007 Other protozoal intestinal diseases**
Includes protozoal:
colitis
diarrhea
dysentery

007.0 Balantidiasis
Infection by Balantidium coli

◀ New   ◀▥ Revised   ~~deleted~~ Deleted   ● Unacceptable Principal Diagnosis   ● Use Additional Digit(s)
▸ Manifestation Code   **OGCR** Official Guidelines   **Coding Clinic**   Excludes   Includes   Use additional   Code first   Omit code

007.1 Giardiasis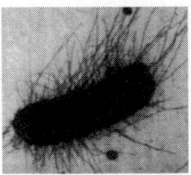
Infection by Giardia lamblia
Lambliasis
(Ex) 003.0, 004.9-005.0, 005.2, 006.0-006.2, 006.9, 007.1-009.0, 129, 487.8, 536.3, 536.8, 558.2-558.9, 5641

007.2 Coccidiosis
Infection by Isospora belli and Isospora hominis
Isosporiasis
(Ex) 003.0, 004.9-005.0, 005.2, 006.0-006.2, 006.9, 007.1-009.0, 129, 487.8, 536.3, 536.8, 558.2-558.9, 564.1

007.3 Intestinal trichomoniasis

007.4 Cryptosporidiosis
(Ex) 003.0, 004.9-005.0, 005.2, 006.0-006.2, 006.9, 007.1-009.0, 129, 487.8, 536.3, 536.8, 558.2-558.9, 564.1
Coding Clinic: 1997, Q4, P30-31

007.5 Cyclosporiasis
(Ex) 003.0, 004.9-005.0, 005.2, 006.0-006.2, 006.9, 007.1-009.0, 129, 487.8, 536.3, 536.8, 558.2-558.9, 564.1, 567.21, 567.23, 567.31-567.39, 567.89

007.8 Other specified protozoal intestinal diseases
Amebiasis due to organisms other than Entamoeba histolytica
(Ex) 003.0, 004.9-005.0, 005.2, 006.0-006.2, 006.9, 007.1-009.0, 129, 487.8, 536.3, 536.8, 558.2-558.9, 564.1

007.9 Unspecified protozoal intestinal disease
Flagellate diarrhea
Protozoal dysentery NOS
(Ex) 003.0, 004.9-005.0, 005.2, 006.0-006.2, 006.9, 007.1-009.0, 129, 487.8, 536.3, 536.8, 558.2-558.9, 564.1

Figure 1-1 Electron micrograph of escherichia coli *(E. coli)* expressing P fimbriae. (From Mandell, Bennett, & Dolin: Principles and Practice of Infectious Diseases, 6th ed. 2005, Churchill Livingstone, An Imprint of Elsevier.)

Item 1-2 *Escherichia coli [E. coli]* is a gram-negative bacterium found in the intestinal tracts of humans and animals and is usually nonpathogenic. Pathogenic strains can cause diarrhea or pyogenic (pus-producing) infections. Can be a threat to food safety.

● **008 Intestinal infections due to other organisms**

Includes any condition classifiable to 009.0–009.3 with mention of the responsible organisms

Excludes *food poisoning by these organisms (005.0–005.9)*

● **008.0 Escherichia coli [E. coli]**
Coding Clinic: 1988, Q2, P10

008.00 E. coli, unspecified
E. coli enteritis NOS
(Ex) 003.0, 004.9-005.0, 005.2, 007.5, 008.00-009.0, 487.8, 536.3, 536.8, 558.2-558.9, 564.1, 567.21, 567.23, 567.31-567.39, 567.89, 777.50-777.53, 777.8

008.01 Enteropathogenic E. coli
(Ex) 003.0, 004.9-005.0, 005.2, 007.5, 008.00-009.0, 487.8, 536.3, 536.8, 558.2-558.9, 564.1, 567.21, 567.23, 567.31-567.39, 567.89, 777.50-777.53, 777.8

008.02 Enterotoxigenic E. coli
(Ex) 003.0, 004.9-005.0, 005.2, 007.5, 008.00-009.0, 487.8, 536.3, 536.8, 558.2-558.9, 564.1, 567.21, 567.23, 567.31-567.39, 567.89, 777.50-777.53, 777.8

008.03 Enteroinvasive E. coli
(Ex) 003.0, 004.9-005.0, 005.2, 007.5, 008.00-009.0, 487.8, 536.3, 536.8, 558.2-558.9, 564.1, 567.21, 567.23, 567.31-567.39, 567.89, 777.50-777.53, 777.8

008.04 Enterohemorrhagic E. coli
(Ex) 003.0, 004.9-005.0, 005.2, 007.5, 008.00-009.0, 487.8, 536.3, 536.8, 558.2-558.9, 564.1, 567.21, 567.23, 567.31-567.39, 567.89, 777.50-777.53, 777.8

008.09 Other intestinal E. coli infections
(Ex) 003.0, 004.9-005.0, 005.2, 007.5, 008.00-009.0, 487.8, 536.3, 536.8, 558.2-558.9, 564.1, 567.21, 567.23, 567.31-567.39, 567.89, 777.50-777.53, 777.8

008.1 Arizona group of paracolon bacilli
(Ex) 003.0, 004.9-005.0, 005.2, 007.5, 008.00-009.0, 487.8, 536.3, 536.8, 558.2-558.9, 564.1, 567.21, 567.23, 567.31-567.39, 567.89, 777.50-777.53, 777.8

008.2 Aerobacter aerogenes
Enterobacter aerogenes
(Ex) 003.0, 004.9-005.0, 005.2, 007.5, 008.00-009.0, 487.8, 536.3, 536.8, 558.2-558.9, 564.1, 567.21, 567.23, 567.31-567.39, 567.89, 777.50-777.53, 777.8

008.3 Proteus (mirabilis) (morganii)
(Ex) 003.0, 004.9-005.0, 005.2, 007.5, 008.00-009.0, 487.8, 536.3, 536.8, 558.2-558.9, 564.1, 567.21, 567.23, 567.31-567.39, 567.89, 777.50-777.53, 777.8

● **008.4 Other specified bacteria**

008.41 Staphylococcus
Staphylococcal enterocolitis
(Ex) 001.1, 002.0, 002.9-003.0, 004.9-005.2, 006.0-006.2, 006.9, 007.1-009.0, 014.80-014.86, 040.41-040.42, 112.85, 129, 487.8, 536.3, 536.8, 555.0-557.9, 558.2-558.9, 564.1, 775.0-775.7, 775.9, 777.50-777.53, 777.8

008.42 Pseudomonas
(Ex) 001.1, 002.0, 002.9-003.0, 004.9-005.2, 006.0-006.2, 006.9, 007.1-009.0, 014.80-014.86, 040.41-040.42, 112.85, 129, 487.8, 536.3, 536.8, 555.0-557.9, 558.2-558.9, 564.1, 775.0-775.7, 775.9, 777.50-777.53, 777.8
Coding Clinic: 1989, Q2, P10

008.43 Campylobacter
(Ex) 001.1, 002.0, 002.9-003.0, 004.9-005.2, 006.0-006.2, 006.9, 007.1-009.0, 014.80-014.86, 040.41-040.42, 112.85, 129, 487.8, 536.3, 536.8, 555.0-557.9, 558.2-558.9, 564.1, 775.0-775.7, 775.9, 777.50-777.53, 777.8

008.44 Yersinia enterocolitica
(Ex) 001.1, 002.0, 002.9-003.0, 004.9-005.2, 006.0-006.2, 006.9, 007.1-009.0, 014.80-014.86, 040.41-040.42, 112.85, 129, 487.8, 536.3, 536.8, 555.0-557.9, 558.2-558.9, 564.1, 775.0-775.7, 775.9, 777.50-777.53, 777.8

008.45 Clostridium difficile
Pseudomembranous colitis
(Ex) 001.1, 002.0, 002.9-003.0, 004.9-005.2, 006.0-006.2, 006.9, 007.1-009.0, 014.80-014.86, 040.41-040.42, 112.85, 129, 487.8, 536.3, 536.8, 555.0-557.9, 558.2-558.9, 564.1, 775.0-775.7, 775.9, 777.50-777.53, 777.8

N Newborn Age: 0   **P** Pediatric Age: 0–17   **M** Maternity Age: 12–55   **A** Adult Age: 15–124   ♀ Females Only   ♂ Males Only
(Ex) CC Exclusions   Complication\Comorbidity   Major C\C   Present on Admission Requirement   Hospital-Acquired Condition

733

INFECTIOUS AND PARASITIC DISEASES (001–139)

008.46   Other anaerobes 🔏
    Anaerobic enteritis NOS
    Bacteroides (fragilis)
    Gram-negative anaerobes
    (Ex:) 001.1, 002.0, 002.9-003.0, 004.9-005.2, 006.0-006.2, 006.9,
        007.1-009.0, 014.80-014.86, 040.41-040.42, 112.88, 129,
        487.8, 536.3, 536.8, 555.0-557.9, 558.2-558.9, 564.1,
        775.0-775.7, 775.9, 777.50-777.53, 777.8

008.47   Other gram-negative bacteria 🔏
    Gram-negative enteritis NOS
    Excludes   *gram-negative anaerobes (008.46)*
    (Ex:) 001.1, 002.0, 002.9-003.0, 004.9-005.2, 006.0-006.2, 006.9,
        007.1-009.0, 014.80-014.86, 040.41-040.42, 112.85, 129,
        487.8, 536.3, 536.8, 555.0-557.9, 558.2-558.9, 564.1,
        775.0-775.7, 775.9, 777.50-777.53, 777.8

008.49   Other 🔏
    (Ex:) 001.1, 002.0, 002.9-003.0, 004.9-005.2 006.0-006.2, 006.9,
        007.1-009.0, 014.80-014.86, 040.41-040.42, 112.85, 129,
        487.8, 536.3, 536.8, 555.0-557.9, 558.2-558.9, 564.1,
        775.0-775.7, 775.9, 777.50-777.53, 777.8
    Coding Clinic: 1989, Q2, P10

008.5   Bacterial enteritis, unspecified 🔏
    (Ex:) 001.1, 002.0, 002.9-003.0, 004.9-005.0, 005.2, 006.0-006.2, 006.9,
        007.1-009.0 014.80-014.86, 112.85, 129, 487.8, 536.3, 536.8,
        558.2-558.9, 564.1, 567.21, 567.23, 567.31-567.39, 567.89,
        777.50-777.53, 777.8

● **008.6   Enteritis due to specified virus**

008.61   Rotavirus 🔏
    (Ex:) 003.0, 004.9-005.0, 005.2, 006.0-006.2, 006.9, 0071-009.0,
        014.80-014.86, 112.85, 129, 487.8, 536.3, 536.8,
        558.2-558.9, 564.1, 567.21, 567.23, 567.31-567.39, 567.89,
        777.50-777.53, 777.8

008.62   Adenovirus 🔏
    (Ex:) 003.0, 004.9-005.0, 005.2, 006.0-006.2, 006.9, 007.1-009.0,
        014.80-014.86, 112.85, 129, 487.8, 536.3, 536.8,
        558.2-558.9, 564.1, 567.21, 567.23, 567.31-567.39, 567.89,
        777.50-777.53, 777.8

008.63   Norwalk virus 🔏   ◀
    Norovirus
    Norwalk-like agent
    (Ex:) 003.0, 004.9-005.0, 005.2, 006.0-006.2, 006.9, 007.1-009.0,
        0148.0-014.86, 112.85, 129, 487.8, 536.3, 536.8,
        558.2-558.9, 564.1, 567.21, 567.23, 567.31-567.39, 567.89,
        777.50-777.53, 777.8

008.64   Other small round viruses [SRV's] 🔏
    Small round virus NOS
    (Ex:) 003.0, 004.9-005.0, 005.2, 006.0-006.2, 006.9, 007.1-009.0,
        014.80-014.86, 112.85, 129, 487.8, 536.3, 536.8,
        558.2-558.9, 564.1, 567.21, 567.23, 567.31-567.39, 567.89,
        777.50-777.53, 777.8

008.65   Calicivirus 🔏   ◀▥
    (Ex:) 003.0, 004.9-005.0, 005.2, 006.0-006.2, 006.9, 007.1-009.0,
        014.80-014.86, 112.85, 129, 487.8, 536.3, 536.8,
        558.2-558.9, 564.1, 567.21, 567.23, 567.31-567.39, 567.89,
        777.50-777.53, 777.8

008.66   Astrovirus 🔏
    (Ex:) 003.0, 004.9-005.0, 005.2, 006.0-006.2, 006.9, 007.1-009.0,
        014.80-014.86, 112.85, 129, 487.8, 536.3, 536.8,
        558.2-558.9, 564.1, 567.21, 567.23, 567.31-567.39, 567.89,
        777.50-777.53, 777.8

008.67   Enterovirus NEC 🔏
    Coxsackie virus
    Echovirus
    Excludes   *poliovirus (045.0–045.9)*
    (Ex:) 003.0, 004.9-005.0, 005.2, 006.0-006.2, 006.9, 007.1-009.0,
        014.80-014.86, 112.85, 129, 487.8, 536.3, 536.8,
        558.2-558.9, 564.1, 567.21, 567.23, 567.31-567.39, 567.89,
        777.50-777.53, 777.8

008.69   Other viral enteritis 🔏
    Torovirus
    (Ex:) 003.0, 004.9-005.0, 005.2, 006.0-006.2, 006.9, 007.1-009.0,
        014.80-014.86, 112.85, 129, 4878, 536.3, 536.8,
        558.2-558.9, 564.1, 567.21, 567.23, 567.31-567.39, 567.89,
        777.50-777.53, 777.8
    Coding Clinic: 2003, Q1, P10-11

008.8   Other organism, not elsewhere classified
    Viral:
       enteritis NOS
       gastroenteritis
    Excludes   *influenza with involvement of*
                  gastrointestinal tract (487.8)

● **009   Ill-defined intestinal infections**
    Excludes   *diarrheal disease or intestinal infection due to*
                  specified organism (001.0–008.8)
                  diarrhea following gastrointestinal surgery (564.4)
                  intestinal malabsorption (579.0–579.9)
                  ischemic enteritis (557.0–557.9)
                  other noninfectious gastroenteritis and colitis
                     (558.1–558.9)
                  regional enteritis (555.0–555.9)
                  ulcerative colitis (556)

009.0   Infectious colitis, enteritis, and gastroenteritis 🔏
    Colitis (septic)
    Dysentery:
       NOS
       catarrhal
       hemorrhagic
    Enteritis (septic)
    Gastroenteritis (septic)
    (Ex:) 001.0-009.3, 040.41-040.42
    Coding Clinic: 1988, Q2, P10

009.1   Colitis, enteritis, and gastroenteritis of presumed infectious origin 🔏
    Excludes   *colitis NOS (558.9)*
                  enteritis NOS (558.9)
                  gastroenteritis NOS (558.9)
    (Ex:) 009.1
    Coding Clinic: 1999, Q3, P6-7

009.2   Infectious diarrhea 🔏
    Diarrhea:
       dysenteric
       epidemic
    Infectious diarrheal disease NOS
    (Ex:) 001.0-009.3, 040.41-040.42

009.3   Diarrhea of presumed infectious origin 🔏
    Excludes   *diarrhea NOS (787.91)*
    (Ex:) 009.3
    Coding Clinic: 1987, Nov-Dec, P7

◀ New   ◀▥ Revised   ~~deleted~~ Deleted   ● Unacceptable Principal Diagnosis   ● Use Additional Digit(s)
▶ Manifestation Code   **OGCR** Official Guidelines   **Coding Clinic**   Excludes   Includes   Use additional   Code first   Omit code

Figure 1–2 Far advanced bilateral pulmonary tuberculosis before and after 8 months of treatment with streptomycin, PAS, and isoniazid. (From Hinshaw HC, Garland LH: Diseases of the Chest, 2nd ed. Philadelphia, WB Saunders, 1963, p. 538.)

Item 1-3 Tuberculosis is a common and deadly infectious disease caused by the *Mycobacterium tuberculosis* organism. The first tuberculosis infection is called the **primary infection** and most commonly attacks the lungs but can affect the central nervous system, lymphatic system, circulatory system, genitourinary system, bones, joints, and even the skin. A **Ghon** lesion is the **initial lesion**. A **secondary lesion** occurs when the tubercle bacilli are carried to other areas.

TUBERCULOSIS (010–018)

Includes infection by Mycobacterium tuberculosis
(human) (bovine)

Excludes *congenital tuberculosis (771.2)*
late effects of tuberculosis (137.0–137.4)

The following fifth-digit subclassification is for use with categories 010–018:

> 0 unspecified
> 1 bacteriological or histological examination not done
> 2 bacteriological or histological examination unknown (at present)
> 3 tubercle bacilli found (in sputum) by microscopy
> 4 tubercle bacilli not found (in sputum) by microscopy, but found by bacterial culture
> 5 tubercle bacilli not found by bacteriological examination, but tuberculosis confirmed histologically
> 6 tubercle bacilli not found by bacteriological or histological examination, but tuberculosis confirmed by other methods [inoculation of animals]

● 010 **Primary tuberculous infection**

Requires fifth digit. See beginning of section 010–018 for codes and definitions.

● 010.0 **Primary tuberculous infection** 🦠
[0-6]   **Excludes** *nonspecific reaction to tuberculin skin test without active tuberculosis (795.5)*
positive PPD (795.5)
positive tuberculin skin test without active tuberculosis (795.5)
(Ex:) 010.00-018.96

● 010.1 **Tuberculous pleurisy in primary progressive**
[0-6] **tuberculosis** 🦠
(Ex:) 010.00-018.96

● 010.8 **Other primary progressive tuberculosis** 🦠
[0-6]   **Excludes** *tuberculous erythema nodosum (017.1)*
(Ex:) 010.00-018.96

● 010.9 **Primary tuberculous infection, unspecified** 🦠
[0-6]   (Ex:) 010.00-018.96

● 011 **Pulmonary tuberculosis**

Requires fifth digit. See beginning of section 010–018 for codes and definitions.

Use additional code to identify any associated silicosis (502)

● 011.0 **Tuberculosis of lung, infiltrative** 🦠
[0-6] (Ex:) 011.00-012.86, 017.90-018.96, 031.0, 031.2-031.9, 041.81-041.9, 137.0, 139.8, 480.0-480.2, 480.8-487.1, 488, 494.0-508.9, 517.1, 518.89

● 011.1 **Tuberculosis of lung, nodular** 🦠
[0-6] (Ex:) 011.00-012.86, 017.90-018.96, 031.0, 031.2-031.9, 041.81-041.9, 137.0, 139.8, 480.0-480.2, 480.8-487.1, 488, 494.0-508.9, 517.1, 518.89

● 011.2 **Tuberculosis of lung with cavitation** 🦠
[0-6] *Cavitation = pitting*
(Ex:) 011.00-012.86, 017.90-018.96, 031.0, 031.2-031.9, 041.81-041.9, 137.0, 139.8, 480.0-480.2, 480.8-487.1, 488, 494.0-508.9, 517.1, 518.89
Coding Clinic: 1994, Q4, P36

● 011.3 **Tuberculosis of bronchus** 🦠
[0-6]   **Excludes** *isolated bronchial tuberculosis (012.2)*
(Ex:) 011.00-012.86, 017.90-018.96, 031.0, 031.2-031.9, 041.81-041.9, 137.0, 139.8, 480.0-480.2, 480.8-487.1, 488, 494.0-508.9, 517.1, 518.89

● 011.4 **Tuberculous fibrosis of lung** 🦠
[0-6] (Ex:) 011.00-012.86, 017.90-018.96, 031.0, 031.2-031.9, 041.81-041.9, 137.0, 139.8, 480.0-480.2, 480.8-487.1, 488, 494.0-508.9, 517.1, 518.89

● 011.5 **Tuberculous bronchiectasis** 🦠
[0-6] (Ex:) 011.00-012.86, 017.90-018.96, 031.0, 031.2-031.9, 041.81-041.9, 137.0, 139.8, 480.0-480.2, 480.8-487.1, 488, 494.0-508.9, 517.1, 518.89

● 011.6 **Tuberculous pneumonia [any form]** 🦠
[0-6] (Ex:) 011.00-012.86, 017.90-018.96, 031.0, 031.2-031.9, 041.81-041.9, 137.0, 139.8, 480.0-480.2, 480.8-487.1, 488, 494.0-508.9, 517.1, 518.89

● 011.7 **Tuberculous pneumothorax** 🦠
[0-6] (Ex:) 011.00-012.86, 017.90-018.96, 031.2-031.9, 041.81-041.9, 137.0, 139.8, 480.0-480.2, 480.8-487.1, 488, 494.0-508.9, 517.1, 518.89

● 011.8 **Other specified pulmonary tuberculosis** 🦠
[0-6] (Ex:) 011.00-012.86, 017.90-018.96, 031.0, 031.2-031.9, 041.81-041.9, 137.0, 139.8, 480.0-480.2, 480.8-487.1, 488, 494.0-508.9, 517.1, 518.89

● 011.9 **Pulmonary tuberculosis, unspecified** 🦠
[0-6] Respiratory tuberculosis NOS
Tuberculosis of lung NOS
(Ex:) 011.00-012.86, 017.90-018.96, 031.0, 031.2-031.9, 041.81-041.9, 137.0, 139.8, 480.0-480.2, 480.8-487.1, 488, 494.0-508.9, 517.1, 518.89

N Newborn Age: 0   **P** Pediatric Age: 0–17   **M** Maternity Age: 12–55   **A** Adult Age: 15–124   ♀ Females Only   ♂ Males Only
(Ex:) CC Exclusions   🦠 Complication\Comorbidity   🦠 Major C\C   🦠 Present on Admission Requirement   🦠 Hospital-Acquired Condition

735

INFECTIOUS AND PARASITIC DISEASES (001–139)

● **012   Other respiratory tuberculosis**

> Requires fifth digit. See beginning of section 010–018 for codes and definitions.
>
> > **Excludes**   *respiratory tuberculosis, unspecified (011.9)*

● **012.0   Tuberculous pleurisy**🔖

  [0-6]   Tuberculosis of pleura
            Tuberculous empyema
            Tuberculous hydrothorax

> > **Excludes**   *pleurisy with effusion without mention of cause (511.9)*
> > *tuberculous pleurisy in primary progressive tuberculosis (010.1)*

        (Ex:) 011.00-012.86, 017.90-018.96, 031.0 031.2-031.9, 041.81-041.9, 137.0, 139.8 480.0-480.2, 480.8-487.1, 488, 494.0-508.9, 517.1, 518.89

● **012.1   Tuberculosis of intrathoracic lymph nodes**🔖

  [0-6]   Tuberculosis of lymph nodes:
            hilar
            mediastinal
            tracheobronchial
            Tuberculous tracheobronchial adenopathy

> > **Excludes**   *that specified as primary (010.0–010.9)*

        (Ex:) 011.00-012.86, 017.90-018.96, 031.0, 031.2-031.9, 041.81-041.9, 137.0, 139.8, 480.0-480.2, 480.8-487.1, 488, 494.0-508.9, 517.1, 518.89

● **012.2   Isolated tracheal or bronchial tuberculosis**🔖

  [0-6]   (Ex:) 010.00-014.86, 018.00-018.96

● **012.3   Tuberculous laryngitis**🔖

  [0-6]   Tuberculosis of glottis
        (Ex:) 010.00-014.86, 018.00-018.96

● **012.8   Other specified respiratory tuberculosis**🔖

  [0-6]   Tuberculosis of:
            mediastinum
            nasopharynx
            nose (septum)
            sinus [any nasal]
        (Ex:) 010.00-014.86, 018.00-018.96

● **013   Tuberculosis of meninges and central nervous system**

> Requires fifth digit. See beginning of section 010–018 for codes and definitions.

● **013.0   Tuberculous meningitis**🔖

  [0-6]   Tuberculosis of meninges (cerebral) (spinal)
            Tuberculous:
              leptomeningitis
              meningoencephalitis

> > **Excludes**   *tuberculoma of meninges (013.1)*

        (Ex:) 003.21, 013.00-013.16, 013.40-013.56, 013.80-013.96, 017.90-017.96, 031.2-031.9, 036.0, 041.81-041.9, 047.0-047.9, 049.0-049.1, 053.0, 054.72, 072.1, 090.42, 091.81, 094.2, 098.89, 100.81, 112.83, 114.2, 115.01, 115.11, 115.91, 130.0, 137.1, 139.8, 320.0-322.9, 349.89-349.9, 357.0

Item 1–4   Although it primarily affects the lungs, the bacteria ***Mycobacterium tuberculosis*** can travel from the pulmonary circulation to virtually any organ in the body, much as a cancer metastasizes to a secondary site. If the immune system becomes compromised by age or disease, what would otherwise be a self-limiting primary tuberculosis in the lungs will develop in other organs. These are known as extrapulmonary sites.

● **013.1   Tuberculoma of meninges**🔖

  [0-6]   (Ex:) 003.21, 013.00-013.16, 013.40-013.56, 013.80-013.96, 017.90-017.96, 031.2-031.9, 036.0, 041.81-041.9, 047.0-047.9, 049.0-049.1, 053.0, 054.72, 072.1, 090.42, 091.81, 094.2, 098.89, 100.81, 112.83, 114.2, 115.01, 115.11, 115.91, 130.0, 137.1, 139.8, 320.0-322.9, 349.89-349.9, 357.0

● **013.2   Tuberculoma of brain**🔖

  [0-6]   Tuberculosis of brain (current disease)
        (Ex:) 013.20-013.36, 013.60-013.96, 017.90-017.96, 031.2-031.9, 041.81-041.9, 137.1, 139.8

● **013.3   Tuberculous abscess of brain**🔖

  [0-6]   (Ex:) 013.20-013.36, 013.60-013.96, 017.90-017.96, 031.2-031.9, 041.81-041.9, 137.1, 139.8

● **013.4   Tuberculoma of spinal cord**🔖

  [0-6]   (Ex:) 013.00-013.16, 013.40-013.56, 013.80-013.96, 017.90-017.96, 031.2-031.9, 041.81-041.9, 137.1, 139.8

● **013.5   Tuberculous abscess of spinal cord**🔖

  [0-6]   (Ex:) 013.00-013.16, 013.40-013.56, 013.80-013.96, 017.90-017.96, 031.2-031.9, 041.81-041.9, 137.1, 139.8

● **013.6   Tuberculous encephalitis or myelitis**🔖

  [0-6]   (Ex:) 013.20-013.36, 013.60-013.96, 017.90-017.96, 031.2-031.9, 041.81-041.9, 137.1, 139.8

● **013.8   Other specified tuberculosis of central nervous**
  [0-6]   **system**🔖
        (Ex:) 013.80-013.96, 017.90-017.96, 031.2-031.9, 041.81-041.9, 137.1, 139.8

● **013.9   Unspecified tuberculosis of central nervous**
  [0-6]   **system**🔖
        Tuberculosis of central nervous system NOS
        (Ex:) 013.80-013.96, 017.90-017.96, 031.2-031.9, 041.81-041.9, 137.1, 139.8

● **014   Tuberculosis of intestines, peritoneum, and mesenteric glands**

> Requires fifth digit. See beginning of section 010–018 for codes and definitions.

● **014.0   Tuberculous peritonitis**🔖

  [0-6]   Tuberculous ascites
        (Ex:) 014.00-014.86, 017.90-017.96, 031.2-031.9, 041.81-041.9, 139.8

● **014.8   Other**🔖

  [0-6]   Tuberculosis (of):
            anus
            intestine (large) (small)
            mesenteric glands
            rectum
            retroperitoneal (lymph nodes)
        Tuberculous enteritis
        (Ex:) 014.00-014.86, 017.90-017.96, 031.2-031.9, 041.81-041.9, 139.8

◀ New   ◀≡ Revised   ~~deleted~~ Deleted   ● Unacceptable Principal Diagnosis   ● Use Additional Digit(s)
▶ Manifestation Code   **OGCR** Official Guidelines   **Coding Clinic**   Excludes   Includes   Use additional   Code first   Omit code

● **015   Tuberculosis of bones and joints**

> Requires fifth digit. See beginning of section 010–018 for codes and definitions.

> Use additional code to identify manifestation, as:
> tuberculous:
> > arthropathy (711.4)
> > necrosis of bone (730.8)
> > osteitis (730.8)
> > osteomyelitis (730.8)
> > synovitis (727.01)
> > tenosynovitis (727.01)

● **015.0   Vertebral column** 🦠
[0-6]   Pott's disease

> Use additional code to identify manifestation, as:
> > curvature of spine [Pott's] (737.4)
> > kyphosis (737.4)
> > spondylitis (720.81)
> (Ex) 015.00-015.06

● **015.1   Hip** 🦠
[0-6]   (Ex) 015.10-015.16

● **015.2   Knee** 🦠
[0-6]   (Ex) 015.20-015.26

● **015.5   Limb bones** 🦠
[0-6]   Tuberculous dactylitis
> (Ex) 015.10-015.56

● **015.6   Mastoid** 🦠
[0-6]   Tuberculous mastoiditis
> (Ex) 015.60-015.66

● **015.7   Other specified bone** 🦠
[0-6]   (Ex) 015.00-015.70

● **015.8   Other specified joint** 🦠
[0-6]   (Ex) 015.80-015.86

● **015.9   Tuberculosis of unspecified bones and joints** 🦠
[0-6]   (Ex) 015.00-015.66, 015.80-015.96

● **016   Tuberculosis of genitourinary system**

> Requires fifth digit. See beginning of section 010–018 for codes and definitions.

● **016.0   Kidney** 🦠
[0-6]   Renal tuberculosis

> Use additional code to identify manifestation, as:
> tuberculous:
> > nephropathy (583.81)
> > pyelitis (590.81)
> > pyelonephritis (590.81)
> (Ex) 016.00-016.36, 016.90-016.96, 017.90-017.96, 031.2-031.9, 041.81-041.9, 137.2, 139.8

● **016.1   Bladder** 🦠
[0-6]   (Ex) 016.00-016.36, 016.90-016.96, 017.90-017.96, 031.2-031.9, 041.81-041.9, 137.2, 139.8

● **016.2   Ureter** 🦠
[0-6]   (Ex) 016.00-016.36, 016.90-016.96, 017.90-017.96, 031.2-031.9, 041.81-041.9, 137.2, 139.8

● **016.3   Other urinary organs** 🦠
[0-6]   (Ex) 016.00-016.36, 016.90-016.96, 017.90-017.96, 031.2-031.9, 041.81-041.9, 137.2, 139.8

● **016.4   Epididymis** ♂ 🦠
[0-6]   (Ex) 016.40-165.6, 016.90-016.96, 017.90-017.96, 031.2-031.9, 041.81-041.9, 137.2, 139.8

● **016.5   Other male genital organs** ♂ 🦠
[0-6]
> Use additional code to identify manifestation, as:
> tuberculosis of:
> > prostate (601.4)
> > seminal vesicle (608.81)
> > testis (608.81)
> (Ex) 016.40-016.56, 016.90-016.96, 017.90-017.96, 031.2-031.9, 041.81-041.9, 137.2, 139.8

● **016.6   Tuberculous oophoritis and salpingitis** ♀ 🦠
[0-6]   *Oophoritis = inflammation of ovary*
> *Salpingitis = inflammation of fallopian tube*
> (Ex) 016.60-016.96, 017.90-017.96, 031.2-031.9, 041.81-041.9, 137.2, 139.8

● **016.7   Other female genital organs** ♀ 🦠
[0-6]   Tuberculous:
> > cervicitis
> > endometritis
> (Ex) 016.60-016.96, 017.90-017.96, 031.2-031.9, 041.81-041.9, 137.2, 139.8

● **016.9   Genitourinary tuberculosis, unspecified** 🦠
[0-6]   (Ex) 016.90-016.96, 017.90-017.96, 031.2-031.9, 041.81-041.9, 137.2, 139.8

● **017   Tuberculosis of other organs**

> Requires fifth digit. See beginning of section 010–018 for codes and definitions.

● **017.0   Skin and subcutaneous cellular tissue** 🦠
[0-6]

Lupus:	Tuberculosis:
exedens	colliquativa
vulgaris	cutis
Scrofuloderma	lichenoides
	papulonecrotica
	verrucosa cutis

> **Excludes**   *lupus erythematosus (695.4)*
> > *disseminated (710.0)*
> *lupus NOS (710.0)*
> *nonspecific reaction to tuberculin skin test*
> > *without active tuberculosis (795.5)*
> *positive PPD (795.5)*
> *positive tuberculin skin test without active*
> > *tuberculosis (795.5)*
> (Ex) 010.00-018.96

● **017.1   Erythema nodosum with hypersensitivity reaction in**
[0-6] **tuberculosis**
> Bazin's disease
> Erythema:
> > induratum
> > nodosum, tuberculous
> Tuberculosis indurativa
> **Excludes**   *erythema nodosum NOS (695.2)*

N Newborn Age: 0   **P** Pediatric Age: 0–17   **M** Maternity Age: 12–55   **A** Adult Age: 15–124   ♀ Females Only   ♂ Males Only

(Ex) CC Exclusions   🦠 Complication\Comorbidity   🦠 Major C\C   🦠 Present on Admission Requirement   🦠 Hospital-Acquired Condition

737

INFECTIOUS AND PARASITIC DISEASES (001–139)

● **017.2 Peripheral lymph nodes** 🔒
[0-6]   Scrofula
      Scrofulous abscess
      Tuberculous adenitis

> **Excludes**   *tuberculosis of lymph nodes:*
>   *bronchial and mediastinal (012.1)*
>   *mesenteric and retroperitoneal (014.8)*
>   *tuberculous tracheobronchial adenopathy*
>   *(012.1)*

(Ex) 017.20-017.26, 017.90-017.96, 031.2-031.9, 041.81-041.9, 139.8

● **017.3 Eye** 🔒
[0-6]
Use additional code to identify manifestation, as:
     tuberculous:
       episcleritis (379.09)
       interstitial keratitis (370.59)
       iridocyclitis, chronic (364.11)
       keratoconjunctivitis (phlyctenular) (370.31)

(Ex) 017.30-017.36, 017.90-017.96, 031.2-031.9, 041.81-041.9, 139.8

● **017.4 Ear** 🔒
[0-6]   Tuberculosis of ear
      Tuberculous otitis media

> **Excludes**   *tuberculous mastoiditis (015.6)*

(Ex) 017.40-017.46, 017.90-017.96, 031.2-031.9, 041.81-041.9, 139.8

● **017.5 Thyroid gland** 🔒
[0-6]   (Ex) 017.50-017.56, 017.90-017.96, 031.2-031.9, 041.81-041.9, 139.8

● **017.6 Adrenal glands** 🔒
[0-6]   Addison's disease, tuberculous
      (Ex) 017.60-017.66, 017.90-017.96, 031.2-031.9, 041.81-041.9, 139.8

● **017.7 Spleen** 🔒
[0-6]   (Ex) 017.70-017.76, 017.90-017.96, 031.2-031.9, 041.81-041.9, 139.8

● **017.8 Esophagus** 🔒
[0-6]   (Ex) 017.80-017.96, 031.2-031.9, 041.81-041.9, 139.8

● **017.9 Other specified organs** 🔒
[0-6]
Use additional code to identify manifestation, as:
     tuberculosis of:
       endocardium [any valve] (424.91)
       myocardium (422.0)
       pericardium (420.0)

(Ex) 017.90-017.96, 031.2-031.9, 041.81-041.9, 139.8

SCRUB TYPHUS
(R. tsutsugamushi)

MURINE TYPHUS
(R. moosen)

RICKETTSIAL POX
(R. akari)

LOUSE–BORNE TYPHUS
(R. prowazekii)

Q FEVER
(Coxiella burnetii)

TRENCH FEVER
(R. quintana)

SPOTTED FEVER
(R. rickettsii)

Man / Fleas / Chigger / Mites / Man / Field Rodents / Domestic Rat / SMALL MAMMAL HOST / House Mice / Cattle/Sheep / Man / Aerosol ? / Flying Squirrel / Field Mice / Cottontail / ARTHROPOD VECTORS / Ticks / Man / Lice / Man / DOMESTIC EXTENSIONS / Aerosol ? / Dog / Man / DISEASE AND TYPICAL AMBIANCE / Airborne dust Placenta, Milk?

Figure 1–3   Schematic summary of some major interactions between rickettsial organisms and their small animal hosts and arthropod vectors, the participation of domestic animals, and examples of the typical ambiance under which each rickettsial infection is contacted by humans. (From Strickland GT: Hunter's Tropical Medicine, 7th ed. Philadelphia, WB Saunders, 1991, p. 261. Courtesy of Dr. J. K. Frenkel, University of New Mexico, Albuquerque, N.M.)

◀ New   ◀▦ Revised   ~~deleted~~ Deleted   ● Unacceptable Principal Diagnosis   ● Use Additional Digit(s)

▶ Manifestation Code   **OGCR** Official Guidelines   **Coding Clinic**   Excludes   Includes   Use additional   Code first   Omit code

Item 1–5   Miliary tuberculosis can be a life-threatening condition. If a tuberculous lesion enters a blood vessel, immense dissemination of tuberculous organisms can occur if the immune system is weak. High-risk populations—children under 4 years of age, the elderly, or the immunocompromised—are particularly prone to this type of infection. The lesions will have a millet seed-like appearance on chest x-ray. Bronchial washings and biopsy may aid in diagnosis.

● **018   Miliary tuberculosis**

> Requires fifth digit. See beginning of section 010–018 for codes and definitions.

> **Includes**   tuberculosis:
> > disseminated
> > generalized
> > miliary, whether of a single specified site, multiple sites, or unspecified site
> > polyserositis

● **018.0   Acute miliary tuberculosis** 🦠
[0-6]   (Ex) 017.90-018.96, 031.2-031.9, 041.81-041.9, 139.8

● **018.8   Other specified miliary tuberculosis** 🦠
[0-6]   (Ex) 017.90-018.96, 031.2-031.9, 041.81-041.9, 139.8

● **018.9   Miliary tuberculosis, unspecified** 🦠
[0-6]   (Ex) 017.90-018.96, 031.2-031.9, 041.81-041.9, 139.8

ZOONOTIC BACTERIAL DISEASES (020–027)

● **020   Plague**

> *Infectious disease caused by Yersinia pestis bacterium, transmitted by rodent flea bite or handling infected animal*

> **Includes**   infection by Yersinia [Pasteurella] pestis

020.0   Bubonic 🦠
> (Ex) 020.0-020.9

020.1   Cellulocutaneous 🦠
> (Ex) 020.0-020.9

020.2   Septicemic 🦠
> (Ex) 020.0-020.9, 771.81, 771.83-771.89, 995.90-995.94

020.3   Primary pneumonic 🦠
> (Ex) 011.00-012.16, 012.80-012.86, 017.90-017.96, 020.0-020.9, 021.3, 022.1, 031.0, 039.1, 073.0, 115.05, 115.15, 115.95, 122.1, 130.4, 136.3, 480.0-487.1, 488, 495.0-495.9, 500-502

020.4   Secondary pneumonic 🦠
> (Ex) 011.73-011.93, 480.3

020.5   Pneumonic, unspecified 🦠
> (Ex) 020.5, 480.3

020.8   Other specified types of plague 🦠
> Abortive plague
> Ambulatory plague
> Pestis minor
> (Ex) 020.8

020.9   Plague, unspecified 🦠
> (Ex) 020.9

● **021   Tularemia**

> *Caused by Francisella tularensis bacterium found in rodents, rabbits, and hares; transmitted by contact with infected animal tissues or ticks, biting flies, and mosquitoes*

> **Includes**   deerfly fever
> > infection by Francisella [Pasteurella] tularensis
> > rabbit fever

021.0   Ulceroglandular tularemia 🦠
> (Ex) 021.0

021.1   Enteric tularemia 🦠
> Tularemia:
> > cryptogenic
> > intestinal
> > typhoidal
> (Ex) 021.1

021.2   Pulmonary tularemia 🦠
> Bronchopneumonic tularemia
> (Ex) 482.49-487.1, 488, 495.0-495.9, 500-508.9, 517.1, 517.8, 518.89, 519.8-519.9

021.3   Oculoglandular tularemia 🦠
> (Ex) 021.3, 480.3

021.8   Other specified tularemia 🦠
> Tularemia:
> > generalized or disseminated
> > glandular
> (Ex) 021.0-021.9

021.9   Unspecified tularemia 🦠
> (Ex) 021.0-021.9

● **022   Anthrax**

> *An acute infectious disease caused by the spore-forming Bacillus anthracis; it may occur in humans exposed to infected animals or tissue from infected animals*

022.0   Cutaneous anthrax 🦠
> Malignant pustule
> (Ex) 022.0

022.1   Pulmonary anthrax 🦠
> Respiratory anthrax
> Wool-sorters' disease
> (Ex) 011.00-012.16, 012.80-012.86, 017.90-017.96, 020.3-020.5, 021.3, 022.1, 031.0, 039.1, 073.0, 115.05, 115.15, 115.95, 122.1, 130.4, 136.3, 480.0-487.1, 488, 494.0-495.9, 500-508.9, 517.1, 517.8, 518.89, 519.8-519.9

022.2   Gastrointestinal anthrax 🦠
> (Ex) 022.2

022.3   Anthrax septicemia 🦠
> (Ex) 003.1, 020.2, 022.3, 036.2, 038.0-038.9, 040.89-041.9, 054.5, 139.8, 771.81, 771.83-771.89, 995.90-995.94, V09.0-V09.91

022.8   Other specified manifestations of anthrax 🦠
> (Ex) 022.8

022.9   Anthrax, unspecified 🦠
> (Ex) 022.0-022.9

INFECTIOUS AND PARASITIC DISEASES (001–139)

N   Newborn Age: 0   **P**   Pediatric Age: 0–17   **M**   Maternity Age: 12–55   **A**   Adult Age: 15–124   ♀ Females Only   ♂ Males Only

(Ex) CC Exclusions   🦠 Complication\Comorbidity   🦠 Major C\C   🦠 Present on Admission Requirement   🦠 Hospital-Acquired Condition

739

● **023 Brucellosis**

Infectious disease caused by bacterium Brucella. Humans are infected by contact with contaminated animals or animal products. Brucellosis symptoms are similar to flu.

    Includes fever:
                 Malta
                 Mediterranean
                 undulant
                     Rising and falling

023.0 Brucella melitensis

023.1 Brucella abortus

023.2 Brucella suis

023.3 Brucella canis

023.8 Other brucellosis🗪
    Infection by more than one organism
    (Ex:) 023.0-023.9

023.9 Brucellosis, unspecified🗪
    (Ex:) 023.0-023.9

024 Glanders🗪
    Infection by:
         Actinobacillus mallei
         Malleomyces mallei
         Pseudomonas mallei
         Farcy
         Malleus
    (Ex:) 024

025 Melioidosis🗪
    Infection by:
         Malleomyces pseudomallei
         Pseudomonas pseudomallei
         Whitmore's bacillus
    Pseudoglanders
    (Ex:) 025

● **026 Rat-bite fever**

RBF is an infectious disease caused by Streptobacillus moniliformis or Spirillum minus.

026.0 Spirillary fever🗪
    Rat-bite fever due to Spirillum minor [S. minus]
    Sodoku
    (Ex:) 026.0-026.9

026.1 Streptobacillary fever🗪
    Epidemic arthritic erythema
    Haverhill fever
    Rat-bite fever due to Streptobacillus moniliformis
    (Ex:) 026.0-026.9

026.9 Unspecified rat-bite fever🗪
    (Ex:) 026.0-026.9

● **027 Other zoonotic bacterial diseases**

027.0 Listeriosis🗪
    Infection by Listeria monocytogenes
    Septicemia by Listeria monocytogenes

    Use additional code to identify manifestations, as
         meningitis (320.7)

    Excludes *congenital listeriosis (771.2)*
    (Ex:) 027.0-027.9

027.1 Erysipelothrix infection
    Erysipeloid (of Rosenbach)
    Infection by Erysipelothrix insidiosa
         [E. rhusiopathiae]
    Septicemia by Erysipelothrix insidiosa
         [E. rhusiopathiae]

027.2 Pasteurellosis🗪
    Pasteurella pseudotuberculosis infection by
         Pasteurella multocida [P. septica]
    Mesenteric adenitis by Pasteurella multocida
         [P. septica]
    Septic infection (cat bite) (dog bite) by Pasteurella
         multocida [P. septica]

    Excludes *infection by:*
             Francisella [Pasteurella] tularensis
                (021.0–021.9)
             Yersinia [Pasteurella] pestis
                (020.0–020.9)
    (Ex:) 027.0-027.9

027.8 Other specified zoonotic bacterial diseases🗪
    (Ex:) 027.0-027.9

027.9 Unspecified zoonotic bacterial disease🗪
    (Ex:) 027.0-027.9

OTHER BACTERIAL DISEASES (030–041)

    Excludes *bacterial venereal diseases (098.0–099.9)*
                 bartonellosis (088.0)

● **030 Leprosy**

Also known as Hansen's disease; chronic infectious disease attacking skin, peripheral nerves, and mucous membranes

    Includes Hansen's disease
                 infection by Mycobacterium leprae

030.0 Lepromatous [type L]🗪
    Lepromatous leprosy (macular) (diffuse)
         (infiltrated) (nodular) (neuritic)
    (Ex:) 030.0

030.1 Tuberculoid [type T]🗪
    Tuberculoid leprosy (macular) (maculoanesthetic)
         (major) (minor) (neuritic)
    (Ex:) 030.1

030.2 Indeterminate [group I]🗪
    Indeterminate [uncharacteristic] leprosy (macular)
         (neuritic)
    (Ex:) 030.2

030.3 Borderline [group B]🗪
    Borderline or dimorphous leprosy (infiltrated)
         (neuritic)
    (Ex:) 030.3

030.8 Other specified leprosy🗪
    (Ex:) 030.8

030.9 Leprosy, unspecified🗪
    (Ex:) 030.9

● **031 Diseases due to other mycobacteria**

031.0 Pulmonary🗪
    Battey disease
    Infection by Mycobacterium:
         avium
         intracellulare [Battey bacillus]
         kansasii
    (Ex:) 011.00-012.86, 017.90-017.96, 030.0, 031.2-031.9, 041.81-041.9, 137.0,
               139.8, 480.0-480.2, 480.8-487.1, 488, 494.0-508.9, 517.1, 518.89

◀ New   ◀▥ Revised   ~~deleted~~ Deleted   ● Unacceptable Principal Diagnosis   ● Use Additional Digit(s)

▶ Manifestation Code   **OGCR** Official Guidelines   **Coding Clinic**   Excludes   Includes   Use additional   Code first   Omit code

031.1 Cutaneous 🗪
Buruli ulcer
Infection by Mycobacterium:
    marinum [M. balnei]
    ulcerans
(Ex:) 031.0-031.9

031.2 Disseminated 🗪
Disseminated mycobacterium avium-intracellulare
    complex (DMAC)
Mycobacterium avium-intracellulare complex
    (MAC) bacteremia
(Ex:) 031.0-031.9
Coding Clinic: 1997, Q4, P31

031.8 Other specified mycobacterial diseases 🗪
(Ex:) 031.0-031.9

031.9 Unspecified diseases due to mycobacteria 🗪
Atypical mycobacterium infection NOS
(Ex:) 031.0-031.9

⬤ **032 Diphtheria**
*Highly contagious bacterial disease that results in formation
of an adherent membrane in the throat that may lead to
suffocation. It may attack the heart and lungs. The exact
location is specified in the codes.*

Includes infection by Corynebacterium diphtheriae

032.0 Faucial diphtheria 🗪
Membranous angina, diphtheritic
(Ex:) 032.0-032.9

032.1 Nasopharyngeal diphtheria 🗪
(Ex:) 032.0-032.9

032.2 Anterior nasal diphtheria 🗪
(Ex:) 032.0-032.9

032.3 Laryngeal diphtheria 🗪
Laryngotracheitis, diphtheritic
(Ex:) 032.0-032.9

⬤ **032.8 Other specified diphtheria**

032.81 Conjunctival diphtheria 🗪
Pseudomembranous diphtheritic
    conjunctivitis
(Ex:) 032.0-032.9

032.82 Diphtheritic myocarditis 🗪
(Ex:) 032.82, 074.20, 074.22-074.23, 093.82, 390, 391.2-391.9,
398.0-398.90, 398.99, 422.0-422.99, 429.0, 429.71-429.79,
459.89-459.9

032.83 Diphtheritic peritonitis 🗪
(Ex:) 014.00-014.06, 032.83, 090.0, 095.2, 098.86, 099.56,
540.0-540.1, 567.0-567.1, 567.22, 567.29, 567.81, 567.9,
569.89-569.9, 577.8, 614.5-614.7, 639.0, 670.00-670.04,
777.6, 998.7

032.84 Diphtheritic cystitis 🗪
(Ex:) 032.0-032.9

032.85 Cutaneous diphtheria 🗪
(Ex:) 032.0-032.9

032.89 Other 🗪
(Ex:) 032.0-032.9

032.9 Diphtheria, unspecified 🗪
(Ex:) 032.0-032.9

⬤ **033 Whooping cough**
*Pertussis (whooping cough) is a highly contagious disease
caused by the bacterium Bordetella pertussis and results
in a whooping sound.*

Includes pertussis

Use additional code to identify any associated
    pneumonia (484.3)

033.0 Bordetella pertussis [B. pertussis] 🗪
(Ex:) 033.0-033.9

033.1 Bordetella parapertussis [B. parapertussis] 🗪
(Ex:) 033.0-033.9

033.8 Whooping cough due to other specified organism 🗪
Bordetella bronchiseptica [B. bronchiseptica]
(Ex:) 033.0-033.9

033.9 Whooping cough, unspecified organism 🗪
(Ex:) 033.0-033.9

Item 1-6 034.0 is the common **"strep throat"** (sore throat
with strep infection). It is grouped in the same three-digit category
with scarlet fever. If a patient has both scarlet fever and the strep
throat, use both codes. "Streptococcal" must be indicated on
the laboratory report to use 034.0; otherwise use 462 for "sore
throat" (pharyngitis).

⬤ **034 Streptococcal sore throat and scarlet fever**

034.0 Streptococcal sore throat
Septic: Streptococcal:
    angina   angina
    sore throat   laryngitis
                                     pharyngitis
                                     tonsillitis
Coding Clinic: 1985, Sept-Oct, P9

034.1 Scarlet fever 🗪
Scarlatina
Excludes *parascarlatina (057.8)*
(Ex:) 034.0-035

035 Erysipelas
Excludes *postpartum or puerperal erysipelas (670.8)* ⬅

⬤ **036 Meningococcal infection**
*Most commonly caused by bacteria Streptococcus pneumoniae
and Neisseria meningitidis*

036.0 Meningococcal meningitis 🗪
Cerebrospinal fever (meningococcal)
Meningitis:
    cerebrospinal
    epidemic
(Ex:) 003.21, 013.00-013.16, 036.0, 036.89-036.9, 041.81-041.9, 047.0-047.9,
049.0-049.1, 053.0, 054.72, 072.1, 090.42, 091.81, 094.2, 098.89,
100.81, 112.83, 114.2, 115.01, 115.11, 115.91, 130.0, 139.8,
320.0-322.9, 349.89-349.9, 357.0

036.1 Meningococcal encephalitis 🗪
(Ex:) 036.1, 036.89-036.9, 041.81-041.9, 139.8

036.2 Meningococcemia 🗪
Meningococcal septicemia
(Ex:) 003.1, 020.2, 036.2, 036.89-036.9, 038.0-038.9, 041.81-041.9, 054.5,
139.8, 995.90-995.94

036.3 Waterhouse-Friderichsen syndrome, meningococcal 🗪
Meningococcal hemorrhagic adrenalitis
Meningococcic adrenal syndrome
Waterhouse-Friderichsen syndrome NOS
(Ex:) 036.3, 036.89-036.9, 041.81-041.9, 139.8

INFECTIOUS AND PARASITIC DISEASES (001–139)

N Newborn Age: 0   **P** Pediatric Age: 0–17   **M** Maternity Age: 12–55   **A** Adult Age: 15–124   ♀ Females Only   ♂ Males Only
(Ex:) CC Exclusions   🗪 Complication\Comorbidity   🗪 Major C\C   Present on Admission Requirement   Hospital-Acquired Condition

741

● **036.4 Meningococcal carditis**

    036.40 Meningococcal carditis, unspecified 🔖
      (Ex:) 036.40, 036.89-036.9, 041.81-041.9, 139.8

    036.41 Meningococcal pericarditis 🔖
      (Ex:) 036.41, 036.89-036.9, 041.81-041.9, 139.8

    036.42 Meningococcal endocarditis 🔖
      (Ex:) 036.42, 036.89-036.9, 041.81-041.9, 139.8

    036.43 Meningococcal myocarditis 🔖
      (Ex:) 036.43, 041.81-041.9, 139.8

● **036.8 Other specified meningococcal infections**

    036.81 Meningococcal optic neuritis 🔖
      (Ex:) 036.81, 036.89-036.9, 041.81-041.9, 139.8

    036.82 Meningococcal arthropathy 🔖
      (Ex:) 036.82-036.9, 041.81-041.9, 139.8

    036.89 Other 🔖
      (Ex:) 036.89-036.9, 041.81-041.9, 139.8

036.9 Meningococcal infection, unspecified 🔖
  Meningococcal infection NOS
  (Ex:) 036.89-036.9, 041.81-041.9, 139.8

037 Tetanus 🔖
  Also indexed as "lockjaw." Do not confuse tetanus with tetany,
  which is severe muscle twitches, cramps, and spasms
  (781.7).

  | Excludes | *tetanus:*
      complicating:
        abortion (634–638 with .0, 639.0)
        ectopic or molar pregnancy (639.0)
      neonatorum (771.3)
      puerperal (670.8) ⏴▬
  (Ex:) 037, 139.8

● **038 Septicemia**
  Blood poisoning/bacteremia, often associated with serious
  illness.

  Note: Use additional code for systemic inflammatory
  response syndrome (SIRS) (995.91–995.92).

  | Excludes | *bacteremia (790.7)*
      septicemia (sepsis) of newborn (771.81)
  Coding Clinic: 2004, Q2, P16; 1994, Q2, P13; 1993, Q3, P6; 1988, Q2, P12

  038.0 Streptococcal septicemia 🔖
    (Ex:) 003.1, 020.2, 036.2, 038.0-038.9, 040.82-041.9, 139.8,
      995.90-995.94, V09.0-V09.91
    Coding Clinic: 1996, Q2, P5

● **038.1 Staphylococcal septicemia**

    038.10 Staphylococcal septicemia, unspecified 🔖
      (Ex:) 003.1, 020.2, 036.2, 038.0-038.9, 040.82-041.9, 054.5, 139.8,
        995.90-995.94, V09.0-V09.91

    038.11 Methicillin susceptible Staphylococcus
       aureus septicemia 🔖
      MSSA septicemia
      Staphylococcus aureus septicemia NOS
      (Ex:) 003.1, 020.2, 036.2, 038.0-038.9, 040.82-041.9, 054.5, 139.8,
        995.90-995.94, V09.0-V09.91
      Coding Clinic: 2008, Q4, P69-73; 1998, Q4, P41-42

    038.12 Methicillin resistant Staphylococcus aureus
       septicemia 🔖
      (Ex:) 003.1, 020.2, 036.2, 038.0-038.9, 040.82-041.9, 054.5, 139.8,
        995.90-995.94, V09.0-V09.91
      Coding Clinic: 2008, Q4, P69-73

    038.19 Other staphylococcal septicemia 🔖
      (Ex:) 003.1, 020.2, 036.2, 038.0-038.9, 040.82-041.9, 054.5, 139.8,
        995.90-995.94, V09.0-V09.91

038.2 Pneumococcal septicemia [Streptococcus
  pneumoniae septicemia] 🔖
  (Ex:) 003.1, 020.2, 036.2, 038.0-038.9, 040.82-041.9, 054.5, 139.8,
    995.90-995.94, V09.0-V09.91
  Coding Clinic: 1996, Q2, P5; 1991, Q1, P13

038.3 Septicemia due to anaerobes 🔖
  Septicemia due to bacteroides

  | Excludes | *gas gangrene (040.0)*
      that due to anaerobic streptococci (038.0)
  (Ex:) 003.1, 020.2, 036.2, 038.0-038.9, 040.82-041.9, 054.5, 139.8,
    995.90-995.94, V09.0-V09.91

● **038.4 Septicemia due to other gram-negative organisms**

    038.40 Gram-negative organism, unspecified 🔖
      Gram-negative septicemia NOS
      (Ex:) 003.1, 020.2, 036.2, 038.0-038.9, 040.82-041.9, 054.5, 139.8,
        995.90-995.94, V09.0-V09.91
      Coding Clinic: 2007, Q4, P84-86

    038.41 Hemophilus influenzae [H. influenzae] 🔖
      (Ex:) 003.1, 020.2, 036.2, 038.0-038.9, 040.82-041.9, 054.5, 139.8,
        995.90-995.94, V09.0-V09.91

    038.42 Escherichia coli [E. coli] 🔖
      (Ex:) 003.1, 020.2, 036.2, 038.0-038.9 040.82-041.9, 054.5, 139.8,
        995.90-995.94, V09.0-V09.91
      Coding Clinic: 2003, Q4, P73

    038.43 Pseudomonas 🔖
      (Ex:) 003.1, 020.2, 036.2, 038.0-038.9, 040.82-041.9, 054.5, 139.8,
        995.90-995.94, V09.0-V09.91

    038.44 Serratia 🔖
      (Ex:) 003.1, 020.2, 036.2, 038.0-038.9, 040.82-041.9, 054.5, 139.8,
        995.90-995.94, V09.0-V09.91

    038.49 Other 🔖
      (Ex:) 003.1, 020.2, 036.2, 038.0-038.9, 040.82-041.9, 054.5, 139.8,
        995.90-995.94, V09.0-V09.91

038.8 Other specified septicemias 🔖

  | Excludes | *septicemia (due to):*
      anthrax (022.3)
      gonococcal (098.89)
      herpetic (054.5)
      meningococcal (036.2)
    septicemic plague (020.2)
  (Ex:) 003.1, 020.2, 036.2, 038.0-038.9, 040.82-041.9, 054.5, 139.8,
    995.90-995.94, V09.0-V09.91

038.9 Unspecified septicemia 🔖
  Septicemia NOS

  | Excludes | *bacteremia NOS (790.7)*
  (Ex:) 003.1, 020.2, 036.2, 038.0-038.9, 040.82-041.9, 054.5, 139.8,
    995.90-995.94, V09.0-V09.91
  Coding Clinic: 2007, Q4, P96-97; 2005, Q2, P18-20; 2004, Q2, P16;
    1999, Q3, P9; Q3, P5-6; 1998, Q1, P5; 1996, Q3, P16; Q2,
    P6; 1995, Q2, P7

● **039 Actinomycotic infections**

  | Includes | actinomycotic mycetoma
    infection by Actinomycetales, such as
      species of Actinomyces, Actinomadura,
      Nocardia, Streptomyces
    maduromycosis (actinomycotic)
    schizomycetoma (actinomycotic)

  039.0 Cutaneous 🔖
    Erythrasma
    Trichomycosis axillaris
    (Ex:) 039.0, 039.8-039.9

◀ New   ⏴▬ Revised   ~~deleted~~ Deleted   ● Unacceptable Principal Diagnosis   ● Use Additional Digit(s)
▶ Manifestation Code   **OGCR** Official Guidelines   **Coding Clinic** | Excludes | Includes   Use additional   Code first   Omit code

INFECTIOUS AND PARASITIC DISEASES (001–139)

039.1 Pulmonary 🔴
Thoracic actinomycosis
(Ex) 039.1, 039.8-039.9, 480.3

039.2 Abdominal 🔴
(Ex) 039.2, 039.8-039.9

039.3 Cervicofacial 🔴
(Ex) 039.3, 039.8-039.9

039.4 Madura foot 🔴
Excludes madura foot due to mycotic infection (117.4)
(Ex) 039.4-039.9

039.8 Of other specified sites 🔴
(Ex) 039.0-039.9

039.9 Of unspecified site 🔴
Actinomycosis NOS
Maduromycosis NOS
Nocardiosis NOS
(Ex) 039.0-039.9

Item 1–7 Gas gangrene is a necrotizing subcutaneous infection that will cause tissue death. Patients with poor circulation (e.g., diabetes, peripheral nephropathy) will have low oxygen content in their tissues (hypoxia), which allows the Clostridium bacteria to flourish. Gas gangrene often occurs at the site of a surgical wound or trauma. Onset is sudden and dramatic. Treatment can include debridement, amputation, and/or hyperbaric oxygen treatments.

●**040 Other bacterial diseases**
Excludes bacteremia NOS (790.7)
bacterial infection NOS (041.9)

040.0 Gas gangrene 🔴
Gas bacillus infection or gangrene
Infection by Clostridium:
histolyticum
oedematiens
perfringens [welchii]
septicum
sordellii
Malignant edema
Myonecrosis, clostridial
Myositis, clostridial
(Ex) 040.0, 139.8
Coding Clinic: 1995, Q1, P11

040.1 Rhinoscleroma

040.2 Whipple's disease 🔴
Intestinal lipodystrophy
(Ex) 040.2

040.3 Necrobacillosis 🔴
(Ex) No Exclusions
Coding Clinic: 2007, Q4, P84-86

●**040.4 Other specified botulism**
Non-foodborne intoxication due to toxins of Clostridium botulinum [C. botulinum]
Excludes botulism NOS (005.1)
food poisoning due to toxins of Clostridium botulinum (005.1)

040.41 Infant botulism 🔴   P
(Ex) 005.0-005.2, 008.45-008.46, 040.41-040.42
Coding Clinic: 2007, Q4, P60-61

040.42 Wound botulism 🔴
Non-foodborne botulism NOS
Use additional code to identify complicated open wound
(Ex) 005.0-005.2, 008.45-008.46, 040.41-040.42
Coding Clinic: 2007, Q4, P60-61; 2006, Q2, P7

●**040.8 Other specified bacterial diseases**
040.81 Tropical pyomyositis 🔴
(Ex) 040.81, 040.89

040.82 Toxic shock syndrome 🔴
Use additional code to identify the organism
(Ex) 040.82, 338.0-338.4, 780.64-780.65, 780.91-780.99, 785.50-785.59, 785.9, 799.81-799.89
Coding Clinic: 2002, Q4, P44

040.89 Other
Coding Clinic: 1986, Nov-Dec, P7

●**041 Bacterial infection in conditions classified elsewhere and of unspecified site**
Note: This category is provided to be used as an additional code to identify the bacterial agent in diseases classified elsewhere. This category will also be used to classify bacterial infections of unspecified nature or site.
Code the disease first, then the bacterium.
Excludes septicemia (038.0–038.9)
Coding Clinic: 2001, Q2, P12; 1984, July-Aug, P19

●**041.0 Streptococcus**
Gram-positive bacteria that is the primary cause of strep throat
041.00 Streptococcus, unspecified
Specified in documentation as streptococcus, but unspecified as to Group

041.01 Group A
Specified as Group A
Coding Clinic: 2002, Q1, P3-4

041.02 Group B
Specified as Group B

041.03 Group C
Specified as Group C

041.04 Group D [Enterococcus]
Specified as Group D

041.05 Group G
Specified as Group G

041.09 Other Streptococcus
Streptococcus that is documented but not specified as Group A, B, C, D, or G

●**041.1 Staphylococcus**
"Staph" infections caused by **Staphylococcus aureus** bacteria and range from common skin infections (pimples and boils) to serious infection of surgical wounds, bloodstream infections, and pneumonia.
Coding Clinic: 1987, Jan-Feb, P14-15

041.10 Staphylococcus, unspecified
Coding Clinic: 2006, Q2, P15

INFECTIOUS AND PARASITIC DISEASES (001–139)

041.11 Methicillin susceptible Staphylococcus aureus
MSSA
Staphylococcus aureus NOS
Coding Clinic: 2008, Q4, P69-73; 2006, Q2, P16-17; 2003, Q4, P104-107; 2001, Q2, P11; 1998, Q4, P42-44, 54.55; 1994, Q3, P6

041.12 Methicillin resistant Staphylococcus aureus
Methicillin-resistant staphylococcus aureus (MRSA)
Coding Clinic: 2008, Q4, P69-73

041.19 Other Staphylococcus
Coding Clinic: 2008, Q2, P3

041.2 Pneumococcus

041.3 ~~Friedländer's bacillus~~ Klebsiella pneumoniae ◀▥
~~Infection by Klebsiella pneumoniae~~
Coding Clinic: 2008, Q4, P148-149

041.4 Escherichia coli [E.coli]
Coding Clinic: 1984, July-Aug, P19

041.5 Hemophilus influenzae [H. influenzae]

041.6 Proteus (mirabilis) (morganii)

041.7 Pseudomonas
Coding Clinic: 1988, Q4, P10

● **041.8 Other specified bacterial infections**

041.81 Mycoplasma
Eaton's agent
Pleuropneumonia-like organisms [PPLO]

041.82 Bacteroides fragilis

041.83 Clostridium perfringens

041.84 Other anaerobes
Gram-negative anaerobes
| Excludes | *Helicobacter pylori (041.86)* |

041.85 Other gram-negative organisms
Aerobacter aerogenes
Gram-negative bacteria NOS
Mima polymorpha
Serratia
| Excludes | *gram-negative anaerobes (041.84)* |
Coding Clinic: 1994, Q1, P18

041.86 Helicobacter pylori ~~(H. pylori)~~ [H. pylori] ◀▥

041.89 Other specified bacteria
Coding Clinic: 2006, Q2, P7; 2003, Q2, P7-8

041.9 Bacterial infection, unspecified
Coding Clinic: 1991, Q2, P9

Item 1–8   AIDS (acquired immune deficiency syndrome) is caused by **HIV** (human immunodeficiency virus). HIV affects certain white blood cells (T-4 lymphocytes) and destroys the ability of the cells to fight infections, making patients susceptible to a host of infectious diseases (e.g., ***Pneumocystis carinii* pneumonia (PCP), Kaposi's sarcoma,** and **lymphoma**). **AIDS-related complex (ARC)** is an early stage of AIDS in which tests for HIV are positive but the symptoms are mild.

Figure 1–4   Kaposi's sarcoma. There are large confluent hyperpigmented patch-stage lesions with lymphedema. (From Cohen & Powderly: Infectious Diseases, 2nd ed. 2004, Mosby, An Imprint of Elsevier)

OGCR   Section I.C.2.a. and b.
If a patient is admitted for an HIV-related condition, the principal diagnosis should be 042, followed by additional diagnosis codes for all reported HIV-related conditions. If a patient with HIV disease is admitted for an unrelated condition (such as a traumatic injury), the code for the unrelated condition (e.g., the nature of injury code) should be the principal diagnosis. Other diagnoses would be 042 followed by additional diagnosis codes for all reported HIV-related conditions.

HUMAN IMMUNODEFICIENCY VIRUS (HIV) INFECTION (042)

042 Human immunodeficiency virus [HIV] disease🅠
Acquired immune deficiency syndrome
Acquired immunodeficiency syndrome
AIDS
AIDS-like syndrome
AIDS-related complex
ARC
HIV infection, symptomatic

Use additional code(s) to identify all manifestations of HIV

Use additional code to identify HIV-2 infection (079.53)

Excludes	*asymptomatic HIV infection status (V08)*
	exposure to HIV virus (V01.79)
	nonspecific serologic evidence of HIV (795.71)

(Ex:) 042, 139.8
Coding Clinic: 2007, Q4, P61-64; 2006, Q3, P14-15; 2004, Q2, P11-12; Q1, P5; 2003, Q1, P10-11,15; 1999, Q1, P14; 1997, Q4, P30-31; 1994, Q4, P35-36x2; 1993, Q3, P9; Q1, P20-22; 1990, Q3, P17; 1989, Q1, P9

INFECTIOUS AND PARASITIC DISEASES (001–139)

◀ New   ◀▥ Revised   ~~deleted~~ Deleted   ● Unacceptable Principal Diagnosis   ● Use Additional Digit(s)
▶ Manifestation Code   **OGCR** Official Guidelines   **Coding Clinic** | Excludes | Includes   Use additional   Code first   Omit code

POLIOMYELITIS AND OTHER NON-ARTHROPOD-BORNE VIRAL DISEASES
AND PRION DISEASES OF CENTRAL NERVOUS SYSTEM (045–049)

● **045 Acute poliomyelitis**
Also called infantile paralysis caused by poliovirus, which
enters the body orally and infects the intestinal wall and
then enters the bloodstream and central nervous system,
causing muscle weakness and paralysis.

| **Excludes** | *late effects of acute poliomyelitis (138)* |

The following fifth-digit subclassification is for use with
category 045:

> 0 poliovirus, unspecified type
> 1 poliovirus type I
> 2 poliovirus type II
> 3 poliovirus type III

● **045.0 Acute paralytic poliomyelitis specified as bulbar**
[0-3] Infantile paralysis (acute) specified as bulbar
Poliomyelitis (acute) (anterior) specified as bulbar
Polioencephalitis (acute) (bulbar)
Polioencephalomyelitis (acute) (anterior) (bulbar)
Ex: 045.00-045.13

● **045.1 Acute poliomyelitis with other paralysis**
[0-3] Paralysis:
acute atrophic, spinal
infantile, paralytic
Poliomyelitis (acute) with paralysis except bulbar
anterior with paralysis except bulbar
epidemic with paralysis except bulbar
Ex: 045.00-045.13

● **045.2 Acute nonparalytic poliomyelitis**
[0-3] Poliomyelitis (acute) specified as nonparalytic
anterior specified as nonparalytic
epidemic specified as nonparalytic

● **045.9 Acute poliomyelitis, unspecified**
[0-3] Infantile paralysis unspecified whether paralytic or
nonparalytic
Poliomyelitis (acute) unspecified whether paralytic
or nonparalytic
anterior unspecified whether paralytic or
nonparalytic
epidemic unspecified whether paralytic or
nonparalytic

● **046 Slow virus infections and prion diseases of central**
nervous system
046.0 Kuru
Ex: 046.0-046.9
● **046.1 Jakob-Creutzfeldt disease** *(JCD)*
Use additional code to identify dementia: ◀
with behavioral disturbance (294.11) ◀
without behavioral disturbance (294.10) ◀

046.11 Variant Creutzfeldt-Jakob disease
vCJD
Ex: 013.60-013.66, 046.0-046.9, 048-049.0, 049.8, 052.0, 052.2,
054.3, 054.74, 056.01, 057.8-058.29, 059.00-059.9,
062.0-064, 066.2-066.3, 072.2, 073.7, 079.99, 081.9, 083.9,
090.41, 094.81, 117.5, 124, 130.0, 290.12, 323.01-323.9,
341.1, 487.8, 771.2, 984.9

046.19 Other and unspecified Creutzfeldt-Jakob
disease
CJD
Familial Creutzfeldt-Jakob disease
Iatrogenic Creutzfeldt-Jakob disease
Jakob-Creutzfeldt disease, unspecified
Sporadic Creutzfeldt-Jakob disease
Subacute spongiform encephalopathy

| **Excludes** | *variant Creutzfeldt-Jakob disease* |
| | *(vCJD) (046.11)* |

Ex: 013.60-013.66, 046.0-046.9, 048-049.0, 049.8, 052.0, 052.2,
054.3, 054.74, 056.01, 057.8-058.29, 059.00-059.9,
062.0-064, 066.2-066.3, 072.2, 073.7, 079.99, 081.9, 083.9,
090.41, 094.81, 117.5, 124, 130.0, 290.12, 323.01-323.9,
341.1, 487.8, 77.12, 984.9

046.2 Subacute sclerosing panencephalitis
Dawson's inclusion body encephalitis
Van Bogaert's sclerosing leukoencephalitis
Ex: 046.2, 139.8

046.3 Progressive multifocal leukoencephalopathy
Multifocal leukoencephalopathy NOS
Ex: 013.60-013.66, 046.0-046.9, 048-049.0, 049.8, 052.0, 052.2, 054.3,
054.74, 056.01, 057.8-058.29, 059.00-059.9, 062.0-064, 066.2-066.3,
072.2, 073.7, 075, 081.9, 083.9, 090.41, 094.81, 117.5, 124, 130.0,
290.12, 323.01-323.9, 341.1, 487.8, 771.2, 984.9

● **046.7 Other specified prion diseases of central nervous**
system

Excludes	*Creutzfeldt-Jakob disease*
	(046.11-046.19)
	Jakob-Creutzfeldt disease
	(046.11-046.19)
	kuru (046.0)
	variant Creutzfeldt-Jakob disease
	(vCJD) (046.11)

046.71 Gerstmann-Sträussler-Scheinker
syndrome
GSS syndrome
Ex: 046.0-046.9, 066.40-066.49, 079.82

046.72 Fatal familial insomnia
FFI
Ex: 046.0-046.9, 066.40-066.49, 079.82

046.79 Other and unspecified prion disease of
central nervous system
Ex: 046.0-046.9, 066.40-066.49, 079.82

046.8 Other specified slow virus infection of central
nervous system
Ex: 046.0-046.9, 066.40-066.49, 079.82

046.9 Unspecified slow virus infection of central nervous
system
Ex: 046.0-046.9

N Newborn Age: 0   P Pediatric Age: 0–17   M Maternity Age: 12–55   A Adult Age: 15–124   ♀ Females Only   ♂ Males Only
Ex: CC Exclusions   Complication\Comorbidity   Major C\C   Present on Admission Requirement   Hospital-Acquired Condition

● **047　Meningitis due to enterovirus**

    Includes　meningitis:
        abacterial
        aseptic
        viral

    Excludes　*meningitis due to:*
        adenovirus (049.1)
        arthropod-borne virus (060.0–066.9)
        leptospira (100.81)
        virus of:
          herpes simplex (054.72)
          herpes zoster (053.0)
          lymphocytic choriomeningitis (049.0)
          mumps (072.1)
          poliomyelitis (045.0–045.9)
          any other infection specifically classified
            elsewhere

  047.0　Coxsackie virus 🦠
    Ⓔⓧ 003.21, 013.00-013.16, 036.0, 047.0-047.9, 049.0-049.1, 072.1,
    078.88-078.89, 079.81, 079.88-079.99, 090.42, 091.81, 094.2, 098.89,
    100.81, 112.83, 114.2, 115.01, 115.11, 115.91, 130.0, 139.8,
    320.0-322.9, 349.89-349.9, 357.0

  047.1　ECHO virus 🦠
    Meningo-eruptive syndrome
    Ⓔⓧ 003.21, 013.00-013.16, 036.0, 047.0-047.9, 049.0-049.1, 072.1,
    078.88-078.89, 079.81, 079.88-079.99, 090.42, 091.81, 094.2, 098.89,
    100.81, 112.83, 114.2, 115.01, 115.11, 115.91, 130.0, 139.8,
    320.0-322.9, 349.89-349.9, 357.0

  047.8　Other specified viral meningitis 🦠
    Ⓔⓧ 003.21, 013.00-013.16, 036.0, 047.0-047.9, 049.0-049.1, 072.1,
    078.88-078.89, 079.81, 079.88-079.99, 090.42, 091.81, 094.2, 098.89,
    100.81, 112.83, 114.2, 115.01, 115.11, 115.91, 130.0, 139.8,
    320.0-322.9, 349.89-349.9, 357.0

  047.9　Unspecified viral meningitis 🦠
    Viral meningitis NOS
    Ⓔⓧ 003.21, 013.00-013.16, 036.0, 047.0-047.9, 049.0-049.1, 072.1,
    078.88-078.89, 079.81, 079.88-079.99, 090.42, 091.81, 094.2, 098.89,
    100.81, 112.83, 114.2, 115.01, 115.11, 115.91, 130.0, 139.8,
    320.0-322.9, 349.89-349.9, 357.0

048　Other enterovirus diseases of central nervous system 🦠
  Boston exanthem
  Ⓔⓧ 013.60-013.66, 046.2, 046.71-046.8, 048-049.0, 049.8, 052.0, 052.2, 054.3, 054.74,
  056.01, 057.8-058.29, 059.00-059.9, 062.0-064, 066.2-066.49, 072.2, 073.7,
  075, 079.82, 079.99, 081.9, 083.9, 090.41, 094.81, 117.5, 124, 130.0, 290.12,
  323.01-323.9, 341.1, 487.8, 771.2, 984.9

● **049　Other non-arthropod-borne viral diseases of central nervous system**

    Excludes　*late effects of viral encephalitis (139.0)*

  049.0　Lymphocytic choriomeningitis 🦠
    Lymphocytic:
      meningitis (serous) (benign)
      meningoencephalitis (serous) (benign)
    Ⓔⓧ 003.21, 013.00-013.16, 036.0, 047.0-047.9, 049.0-049.1, 066.40-066.49,
    072.1, 078.88-078.89, 079.81-079.82, 079.88-079.99, 090.42, 091.81,
    094.2, 098.89, 100.81, 112.83, 114.2, 115.01, 115.11, 115.91, 130.0,
    139.8, 320.0-322.9, 349.89-349.9, 357.0

  049.1　Meningitis due to adenovirus 🦠
    Ⓔⓧ 003.21, 013.00-013.16, 036.0, 047.0-047.9, 049.0-049.1, 072.1,
    078.88-078.89, 079.81, 079.88-079.99, 090.42, 091.81, 094.2, 098.89,
    100.81, 112.83, 114.2, 115.01, 115.11, 115.91, 130.0, 139.8,
    320.0-322.9, 349.89-349.9, 357.0

  049.8　Other specified non-arthropod-borne viral diseases of central nervous system 🦠
    Encephalitis:
      acute:
        inclusion body
        necrotizing
      epidemic
      lethargica
      Rio Bravo
    von Economo's disease

    Excludes　*human herpesvirus 6 encephalitis (058.21)*
      other human herpesvirus encephalitis
        (058.29)
    Ⓔⓧ 013.60-013.66, 046.2, 046.71-046.8, 048-049.0, 049.8, 052.0, 052.2,
    054.3, 054.74, 056.01, 057.8-058.29, 059.00-059.9, 062.0-064,
    066.2-066.49, 072.2, 073.7, 075, 079.82, 079.99, 081.9, 083.9, 090.41,
    094.81, 117.5, 124, 130.0, 290.12, 323.01-323.9, 341.1, 382.4, 487.8,
    710.0, 771.2, 984.9

  049.9　Unspecified non-arthropod-borne viral diseases of central nervous system 🦠
    Viral encephalitis NOS
    Ⓔⓧ 013.60-013.66, 046.2, 046.71-046.8, 048-049.0, 049.8-049.9, 052.0,
    052.2, 054.3, 054.74, 056.01, 057.8-058.29, 059.00-059.9, 062.0-064,
    066.2-066.3, 072.2, 073.7, 075, 079.99, 081.9, 083.9, 090.41, 094.81,
    117.5, 124, 130.0, 290.12, 323.01-323.9, 341.1, 382.4, 487.8, 710.0,
    771.2, 984.9

VIRAL DISEASES GENERALLY ACCOMPANIED BY EXANTHEM (050–059) ◀▥

    Excludes　*arthropod-borne viral diseases (060.0–066.9)*
      Boston exanthem (048)

● **050　Smallpox**
  Caused by variola virus and is a serious, contagious, and
  sometimes fatal infectious disease

  050.0　Variola major 🦠
    Hemorrhagic (pustular) smallpox
    Malignant smallpox
    Purpura variolosa
    Ⓔⓧ 050.0-052.9

  050.1　Alastrim 🦠
    Variola minor
    Ⓔⓧ 050.0-052.9

  050.2　Modified smallpox 🦠
    Varioloid
    Ⓔⓧ 050.0-052.9

  050.9　Smallpox, unspecified 🦠
    Ⓔⓧ 050.0-052.9

● **051　Cowpox and paravaccinia**

  ● **051.0　Cowpox and vaccinia not from vaccination**
    Coding Clinic: 2008, Q4, P76-78

    051.01　Cowpox

    051.02　Vaccinia not from vaccination

      Excludes　*vaccinia (generalized) (from*
        vaccination) (999.0)

  051.1　Pseudocowpox
    Milkers' node

  051.2　Contagious pustular dermatitis
    Ecthyma contagiosum
    Orf

  051.9　Paravaccinia, unspecified

● 052 **Chickenpox**
> *Very contagious disease caused by varicella zoster virus; results in itchy outbreak of skin blisters (varicella). The same virus causes shingles (zoster). The Varicella zoster virus is a member of the herpes virus family.*

  052.0 **Postvaricella encephalitis**
      Postchickenpox encephalitis
      (Ex:) 051.9-052.0, 052.2-052.9, 078.88-078.89, 079.81, 079.88-079.99, 139.8

  052.1 **Varicella (hemorrhagic) pneumonitis** 🅲
      (Ex:) 051.9, 052.1-052.9, 078.88-078.89, 079.81, 079.88-079.99, 139.8

  052.2 **Postvaricella myelitis** 🅲
      Postchickenpox myelitis
      (Ex:) 051.9, 052.2-052.9, 053.14, 054.74, 078.88-078.89, 079.81, 079.88-079.99, 139.8, 323.01-323.02, 323.41-323.82, 341.20-341.22

  052.7 **With other specified complications** 🅲
      (Ex:) 051.9, 052.2-052.9, 078.88-078.89, 079.81, 079.88-079.99, 139.8
      Coding Clinic: 2002, Q1, P3-4

  052.8 **With unspecified complication** 🅲
      (Ex:) 051.9, 052.2-052.9, 078.88-078.89, 079.81, 079.88-079.99, 139.8

  052.9 **Varicella without mention of complication** 🅲
      Chickenpox NOS
      Varicella NOS
      (Ex:) 051.9, 052.2-052.9, 078.88-078.89, 079.81, 079.88-079.99, 139.8

Figure 1-5 Primary herpes simplex in and around the mouth. The infection is usually acquired from siblings or parents and is readily transmitted to other direct contacts. (From Forbes, Jackson: Colour Atlas and Text of Clinical Medicine, International Edition. 2002, Mosby)

Item 1-9 **Herpes** is a viral disease for which there is no cure. There are two types of the herpes simplex virus: **Type I** causes **cold sores** or **fever blisters,** and **Type II** causes **genital herpes.** The virus can be spread from a sore on the lips to the genitals or from the genitals to the lips.

● 053 **Herpes zoster**
> *Also known as **shingles,** caused by same virus as chickenpox. After exposure, the virus lies dormant in nerve tissue and is activated by factors including aging, stress, suppression of the immune system, and certain medication. Begins as a unilateral rash that leads to blisters and sores on skin. Chickenpox NOS is reported with 052.9.*

  Includes shingles
                zona

  053.0 **With meningitis** 🅲
      (Ex:) 003.21, 013.00-013.16, 036.0, 047.0-047.9, 049.0-049.1, 053.0-053.19, 053.79-053.9, 054.72, 054.74-054.9, 058.81-058.89, 072.1, 078.88-078.89, 079.81, 079.88-079.99, 090.42, 091.81, 094.2, 098.89, 100.81, 112.83, 114.2, 115.01, 115.11, 115.91, 130.0, 139.8, 320.0-322.9, 349.89-349.9, 357.0

● 053.1 **With other nervous system complications**

  053.10 **With unspecified nervous system complication** 🅲
      (Ex:) 053.0-053.19, 053.79-053.9, 054.72, 054.74-054.9, 058.81-058.89, 078.88-078.89, 079.81, 079.88-079.99, 139.8

  053.11 **Geniculate herpes zoster** 🅲
      Herpetic geniculate ganglionitis
      (Ex:) 053.0-053.19, 053.79-053.9, 054.72, 054.74-054.9, 058.81-058.89, 078.88-078.89, 079.81, 079.88-079.99, 139.8

  053.12 **Postherpetic trigeminal neuralgia** 🅲
      (Ex:) 053.0-053.19, 053.79-053.9, 054.72, 054.74-054.9, 058.81-058.89, 078.88-078.89, 079.81, 079.88-079.99, 139.8

  053.13 **Postherpetic polyneuropathy** 🅲
      (Ex:) 053.0-053.19, 053.79-053.9, 054.72, 054.74-054.9, 058.81-058.89, 078.88-078.89, 079.81, 079.88-079.99, 139.8'

  053.14 **Herpes zoster myelitis** 🅲
      (Ex:) 052.2, 053.0-053.19, 053.79-053.9, 054.72, 054.74-054.9, 058.81-058.89, 078.88-078.89, 079.81, 079.88-079.99, 139.8, 323.01-323.02, 323.41-323.82, 341.20-341.22

  053.19 **Other** 🅲
      (Ex:) 053.0-053.19, 053.79-053.9, 054.72, 054.74-054.9, 058.81-058.89, 078.88-078.89, 079.81, 079.88-079.99, 139.8

● 053.2 **With ophthalmic complications**
      (Ex:) 053.20-053.29

  053.20 **Herpes zoster dermatitis of eyelid** 🅲
      Herpes zoster ophthalmicus

  053.21 **Herpes zoster keratoconjunctivitis** 🅲
      (Ex:) 053.20-053.29

  053.22 **Herpes zoster iridocyclitis** 🅲
      (Ex:) 053.20-053.29

  053.29 **Other** 🅲
      (Ex:) 053.20-053.29

● 053.7 **With other specified complications**

  053.71 **Otitis externa due to herpes zoster** 🅲
      (Ex:) 053.71

  053.79 **Other** 🅲
      (Ex:) 053.0-054.71, 054.73-054.9, 058.21-058.89, 078.88-078.89, 079.81, 079.88-079.99, 139.8

  053.8 **With unspecified complication** 🅲
      (Ex:) 053.0-054.71, 054.73-054.9, 058.21-058.89, 078.88-078.89, 079.81, 079.88-079.99, 139.8

  053.9 **Herpes zoster without mention of complication**
      Herpes zoster NOS

● 054 **Herpes simplex**
  Excludes *congenital herpes simplex (771.2)*

  054.0 **Eczema herpeticum**
      Kaposi's varicelliform eruption

● 054.1 **Genital herpes**

  054.10 **Genital herpes, unspecified**
      Herpes progenitalis
      Coding Clinic: 2007, Q4, P61-64; 1985, Jan-Feb, P15-16

  054.11 **Herpetic vulvovaginitis** ♀

  054.12 **Herpetic ulceration of vulva** ♀

  054.13 **Herpetic infection of penis** ♂

  054.19 **Other**

  054.2 **Herpetic gingivostomatitis** 🅲
      (Ex:) 054.2

  054.3 **Herpetic meningoencephalitis** 🅲
      Herpes encephalitis   Simian B disease
      Excludes *human herpesvirus 6 encephalitis (058.21)*
                other human herpesvirus encephalitis (058.29)
      (Ex:) 054.3, 054.74-054.9, 058.21-058.89, 139.8

INFECTIOUS AND PARASITIC DISEASES (001-139)

N Newborn Age: 0   P Pediatric Age: 0-17   M Maternity Age: 12-55   A Adult Age: 15-124   ♀ Females Only   ♂ Males Only

(Ex:) CC Exclusions   🅲 Complication\Comorbidity   🅼 Major C\C   Present on Admission Requirement   Hospital-Acquired Condition   **747**

● 054.4   **With ophthalmic complications**

     054.40   **With unspecified ophthalmic complication** 🔧
         Ⓔⓧ 054.40-054.49, 054.79-054.9, 058.81-058.89

     054.41   **Herpes simplex dermatitis of eyelid** 🔧
         Ⓔⓧ 054.40-054.49, 054.79-054.9, 058.81-058.89

     054.42   **Dendritic keratitis** 🔧
         Ⓔⓧ 054.40-054.49, 054.79-054.9, 058.81-058.89

     054.43   **Herpes simplex disciform keratitis** 🔧
         Ⓔⓧ 054.40-054.49, 054.79-054.9, 058.81-058.89

     054.44   **Herpes simplex iridocyclitis** 🔧
         Ⓔⓧ 054.40-054.49, 054.79-054.9, 058.81-058.89

     054.49   **Other** 🔧
         Ⓔⓧ 054.40-054.49, 054.79-054.9, 058.81-058.89

054.5   **Herpetic septicemia** 🔧
     Ⓔⓧ 003.1, 020.2, 036.2, 038.0-038.9, 054.5, 054.74-054.9, 058.81-058.89, 139.8, 995.90-995.94

054.6   **Herpetic whitlow**
     Herpetic felon

● 054.7   **With other specified complications**

     054.71   **Visceral herpes simplex** 🔧
         Ⓔⓧ 054.71-054.72, 054.74-054.9, 058.81-058.89, 139.8

     054.72   **Herpes simplex meningitis** 🔧
         Ⓔⓧ 003.21, 013.00-013.16, 036.0, 047.0-047.9, 049.0-049.1, 053.0, 054.72, 054.74-054.9, 058.81-058.89, 072.1, 090.42, 091.81, 094.2, 098.89, 100.81, 112.83, 114.2, 115.01, 115.11, 115.91, 130.0, 139.8, 320.0-322.9, 349.89-349.9, 357.0

     054.73   **Herpes simplex otitis externa**

     054.74   **Herpes simplex myelitis** 🔧
         Ⓔⓧ 052.2, 053.14, 054.74-054.9, 058.81-058.89, 078.88-078.89, 079.81, 079.88-079.99, 139.8, 323.01-323.02, 323.41-323.82, 341.20-341.22

     054.79   **Other** 🔧
         Ⓔⓧ 054.74-054.9, 058.81-058.89, 078.88-078.89, 079.81, 079.88-079.99, 139.8

054.8   **With unspecified complication**

054.9   **Herpes simplex without mention of complication**

Item 1–10   **Rubeola** (055) and **rubella** (056) are medical terms for two different strains of measles. The MMR (measles, mumps, and rubella) vaccination is an attempt to eradicate these childhood diseases.

● 055   **Measles**

     Includes   morbilli
               rubeola
     The first four combination codes specify condition(s)/ complication(s) manifesting after measles.

055.0   **Postmeasles encephalitis** 🔧
     Ⓔⓧ 055.0, 055.79-055.9, 078.88-078.89, 079.81, 079.88-079.99, 139.8

055.1   **Postmeasles pneumonia** 🔧
     Ⓔⓧ 055.1, 055.79-055.9, 078.88-078.89, 079.81, 079.88-079.99, 139.8

055.2   **Postmeasles otitis media**

● 055.7   **With other specified complications**

     055.71   **Measles keratoconjunctivitis** 🔧
         Measles keratitis
         Ⓔⓧ 055.71-055.9, 078.88-078.89, 079.81, 079.88-079.99, 139.8

     055.79   **Other** 🔧
         Ⓔⓧ 055.79-055.9, 078.88-078.89, 079.81, 079.88-079.99, 139.8

055.8   **With unspecified complication**

055.9   **Measles without mention of complication**

● 056   **Rubella**

     Includes   German measles
     Excludes   *congenital rubella (771.0)*

● 056.0   **With neurological complications**

     056.00   **With unspecified neurological complication** 🔧
         Ⓔⓧ 056.00-056.09, 056.79-056.9, 078.88-078.89, 079.81, 079.88-079.99, 139.8

     056.01   **Encephalomyelitis due to rubella** 🔧
         Encephalitis due to rubella
         Meningoencephalitis due to rubella
         Ⓔⓧ 056.00-056.09, 056.79-056.9, 078.88-078.89, 079.81, 079.88-079.99, 139.8

     056.09   **Other** 🔧
         Ⓔⓧ 056.00-056.09, 056.79-056.9, 078.88-078.89, 079.81, 079.88-079.99, 139.8

● 056.7   **With other specified complications**

     056.71   **Arthritis due to rubella** 🔧
         Ⓔⓧ 056.71-056.9, 078.88-078.89, 079.81, 079.88-079.99, 139.8

     056.79   **Other** 🔧
         Ⓔⓧ 056.00-056.09, 056.79-056.9, 078.88-078.89, 079.81, 079.88-079.99, 139.8

056.8   **With unspecified complications**

056.9   **Rubella without mention of complication**

● 057   **Other viral exanthemata**

057.0   **Erythema infectiosum [fifth disease]** 🔧
     Ⓔⓧ 057.0, 079.83

057.8   **Other specified viral exanthemata**
     Dukes (-Filatow) disease   Parascarlatina
     Fourth disease   Pseudoscarlatina
     Excludes   *exanthema subitum [sixth disease] (058.10–058.12)*
                 roseola infantum (058.10–058.12)

057.9   **Viral exanthem, unspecified**

● 058   **Other human herpesvirus**

     Excludes   *congenital herpes (771.2)*
                 cytomegalovirus (078.5)
                 Epstein-Barr virus (075)
                 herpes NOS (054.0–054.9)
                 herpes simplex (054.0–054.9)
                 herpes zoster (053.0–053.9)
                 human herpesvirus NOS (054.0–054.9)
                 human herpesvirus 1 (054.0–054.9)
                 human herpesvirus 2 (054.0–054.9)
                 human herpesvirus 3 (052.0–053.9)
                 human herpesvirus 4 (075)
                 human herpesvirus 5 (078.5)
                 varicella (052.0–052.9)
                 varicella-zoster virus (052.0–053.9)

● 058.1   **Roseola infantum**
     Exanthema subitum [sixth disease]

     058.10   **Roseola infantum, unspecified**   P
         Exanthema subitum [sixth disease], unspecified

     058.11   **Roseola infantum due to human herpesvirus 6**   P
         Exanthema subitum [sixth disease] due to human herpesvirus 6

     058.12   **Roseola infantum due to human herpesvirus 7**   P
         Exanthema subitum [sixth disease] due to human herpesvirus 7

● 058.2   **Other human herpesvirus encephalitis**

     Excludes   *herpes encephalitis NOS (054.3)*
         herpes simplex encephalitis (054.3)
         human herpesvirus encephalitis NOS
           (054.3)
         simian B herpes virus encephalitis (054.3)

     Coding Clinic: 2007, Q4, P61-64

     058.21   **Human herpesvirus 6 encephalitis** 🗞
         (Ex:) 054.3, 054.74-054.9, 058.21-058.89, 139.8

     058.29   **Other human herpesvirus encephalitis** 🗞
         Human herpesvirus 7 encephalitis
         (Ex:) 054.3, 054.74-054.9, 058.21-058.89, 139.8

● 058.8   **Other human herpesvirus infections**

     058.81   **Human herpesvirus 6 infection**

     058.82   **Human herpesvirus 7 infection**

     058.89   **Other human herpesvirus infection**
         Human herpesvirus 8 infection
         Kaposi's sarcoma-associated herpesvirus
           infection
         Coding Clinic: 2007, Q4, P61-64

● 059   **Other poxvirus infections**

     Excludes   *contagious pustular dermatitis (051.2)*
         cowpox (051.01)
         ecthyma contagiosum (051.2)
         milker's nodule (051.1)
         orf (051.2)
         paravaccinia NOS (051.9)
         pseudocowpox (051.1)
         smallpox (050.0-050.9)
         vaccinia (generalized) (from vaccination)
           (999.0)
         vaccinia not from vaccination (051.02)

     Coding Clinic: 2008, Q4, P76-78

● 059.0   **Other orthopoxvirus infections**

     059.00   **Orthopoxvirus infection, unspecified**

     059.01   **Monkeypox** 🗞
         (Ex:) 051.01-051.02, 057.0-057.9, 059.00-059.9

     059.09   **Other orthopoxvirus infection**

● 059.1   **Other parapoxvirus infections**

     059.10   **Parapoxvirus infection, unspecified**

     059.11   **Bovine stomatitis**

     059.12   **Sealpox**

     059.19   **Other parapoxvirus infections**

● 059.2   **Yatapoxvirus infections**

     059.20   **Yatapoxvirus infection, unspecified**

     059.21   **Tanapox** 🗞
         (Ex:) 051.01-051.02, 057.0-057.9, 059.00-059.9

     059.22   **Yaba monkey tumor virus**

     059.8   **Other poxvirus infections**

     059.9   **Poxvirus infections, unspecified**

ARTHROPOD-BORNE VIRAL DISEASES (060–066)

Use additional code to identify any associated meningitis
(321.2)

     Excludes   *late effects of viral encephalitis (139.0)*

● 060   **Yellow fever**

     060.0   **Sylvatic** 🗞
         Yellow fever:
           jungle
           sylvan
         (Ex:) 060.0-060.9

     060.1   **Urban** 🗞
         (Ex:) 060.0-060.9

     060.9   **Yellow fever, unspecified** 🗞
         (Ex:) 060.0-060.9

● 061   **Dengue** 🗞
     Breakbone fever

     Excludes   *hemorrhagic fever caused by dengue virus (065.4)*

     (Ex:) 061

● 062   **Mosquito-borne viral encephalitis**
     Inflammation of the brain caused most commonly by Herpes
       Simplex virus. It may be a complication of Lyme disease
       and is often transmitted by mosquitoes, ticks, or rabid
       animals.

     062.0   **Japanese encephalitis** 🗞
         Japanese B encephalitis
         (Ex:) 013.60-013.66, 046.2, 046.71-046.8, 048-049.0, 049.8, 052.0, 052.2, 054.3,
           054.74, 056.01, 057.8-058.29, 059.00-059.9, 062.0-064, 066.2-066.49,
           072.2, 073.7, 075, 079.82, 079.99, 081.9, 083.9, 090.41, 094.81, 117.5,
           124, 130.0, 290.12, 323.01-323.9, 341.1, 487.8, 771.2, 984.9

     062.1   **Western equine encephalitis** 🗞
         (Ex:) 013.60-013.66, 046.2, 046.71-046.8, 048-049.0, 049.8, 052.0, 052.2, 054.3,
           054.74, 056.01, 057.8-058.29, 059.00-059.9, 062.0-064, 066.2-066.49,
           072.2, 073.7, 075, 079.82, 079.99, 081.9, 083.9, 090.41, 094.81, 117.5,
           124, 130.0, 290.12, 323.01-323.9, 341.1, 487.8, 771.2, 984.9

     062.2   **Eastern equine encephalitis** 🗞

         Excludes   *Venezuelan equine encephalitis (066.2)*

         (Ex:) 013.60-013.66, 046.2, 046.71-046.8, 048-049.0, 049.8, 052.0, 052.2, 054.3,
           054.74, 056.01, 057.8-058.29, 059.00-059.9, 062.0-064, 066.2-066.49,
           072.2, 073.7, 075, 079.82, 079.99, 081.9, 083.9, 090.41, 094.81, 117.5,
           124, 130.0, 290.12, 323.01-323.9, 341.1, 487.8, 771.2, 984.9

     062.3   **St. Louis encephalitis** 🗞
         (Ex:) 013.60-013.66, 046.2, 046.71-046.8, 048-049.0, 049.8, 052.0, 052.2, 054.3,
           054.74, 056.01, 057.8-058.29, 059.00-059.9, 062.0-064, 066.2-066.49,
           072.2, 073.7, 075, 079.82, 079.99, 081.9, 083.9, 090.41, 094.81, 117.5,
           124, 130.0, 290.12, 323.01-323.9, 341.1, 487.8, 771.2, 984.9

     062.4   **Australian encephalitis** 🗞
         Australian arboencephalitis
         Australian X disease
         Murray Valley encephalitis
         (Ex:) 013.60-013.66, 046.2, 046.71-046.8, 048-049.0, 049.8, 052.0, 052.2, 054.3,
           054.74, 056.01, 057.8-058.29, 059.00-059.9, 062.0-064, 066.2-066.49,
           072.2, 073.7, 075, 079.82, 079.99, 081.9, 083.9, 090.41, 094.81, 117.5,
           124, 130.0, 290.12, 323.01-323.9, 341.1, 487.8, 771.2, 984.9

INFECTIOUS AND PARASITIC DISEASES (001–139)

062.5 California virus encephalitis ✿

Encephalitis: Encephalitis:
  California   Tahyna fever
  La Crosse

Ex: 013.60-013.66, 046.2, 046.71-046.8, 048-049.0, 049.8, 052.0, 052.2, 054.3, 054.74, 056.01, 057.8-058.29, 059.00-059.9, 062.0-064, 066.2-066.49, 072.2, 073.7, 075, 079.82, 079.99, 081.9, 083.9, 090.41, 094.81, 117.5, 124, 130.0, 290.12, 323.01-323.9, 341.1, 487.8, 771.2, 984.9

062.8 Other specified mosquito-borne viral encephalitis ✿

Encephalitis by Ilheus virus

> **Excludes** *West Nile virus (066.40–066.49)*

Ex: 013.60-013.66, 046.2, 046.71-046.8, 048-049.0, 049.8, 052.0, 052.2, 054.3, 054.74, 056.01, 057.8-058.29, 059.00-059.9, 062.0-064, 066.2-066.49, 072.2, 073.7, 075, 079.82, 079.99, 081.9, 083.9, 090.41, 094.81, 117.5, 124, 130.0, 290.12, 323.01-323.9, 341.1, 487.8, 771.2, 984.9

062.9 Mosquito-borne viral encephalitis, unspecified ✿

Ex: 013.60-013.66, 046.2, 046.71-046.8, 048-049.0, 049.8, 052.0, 052.2, 054.3, 054.74, 056.01, 057.8-058.29, 059.00-059.9, 062.0-064, 066.2-066.49, 072.2, 073.7, 075, 079.82, 079.99, 081.9, 083.9, 090.41, 094.81, 117.5, 124, 130.0, 290.12, 323.01-323.9, 341.1, 487.8, 771.2, 984.9

● **063   Tick-borne viral encephalitis**

> **Includes**   diphasic meningoencephalitis

063.0 Russian spring-summer [taiga] encephalitis ✿

Ex: 013.60-013.66, 046.2, 046.71-046.8, 048-049.0, 049.8, 052.0, 052.2, 054.3, 054.74, 056.01, 057.8-058.29, 059.00-059.9, 062.0-064, 066.2-066.49, 072.2, 073.7, 075, 079.82, 079.99, 081.9, 083.9, 090.41, 094.81, 117.5, 124, 130.0, 290.12, 323.01-323.9, 341.1, 487.8, 771.2, 984.9

063.1 Louping ill ✿

Ex: 013.60-013.66, 046.2, 046.71-046.8, 048-049.0, 049.8, 052.0, 052.2, 054.3, 054.74, 056.01, 057.8-058.29, 059.00-059.9, 062.0-064, 066.2-066.49, 072.2, 073.7, 075, 079.82, 079.99, 081.9, 083.9, 090.41, 094.81, 117.5, 124, 130.0, 290.12, 323.01-323.9, 341.1, 487.8, 771.2, 984.9

063.2 Central European encephalitis ✿

Ex: 013.60-013.66, 046.2, 046.71-046.8, 048-049.0, 049.8, 052.0, 052.2, 054.3, 054.74, 056.01, 057.8-058.29, 059.00-059.9, 062.0-064, 066.2-066.49, 072.2, 073.7, 075, 079.82, 079.99, 081.9, 083.9, 090.41, 094.81, 117.5, 124, 130.0, 290.12, 323.01-323.9, 341.1, 487.8, 771.2, 984.9

063.8 Other specified tick-borne viral encephalitis ✿

Langat encephalitis
Powassan encephalitis

Ex: 013.60-013.66, 046.2, 046.71-046.8, 048-049.0, 049.8, 052.0, 052.2, 054.3, 054.74, 056.01, 057.8-058.29, 059.00-059.9, 062.0-064, 066.2-066.49, 072.2, 073.7, 075, 079.82, 079.99, 081.9, 083.9, 090.41, 094.81, 117.5, 124, 130.0, 290.12, 323.01-323.9, 341.1, 487.8, 771.2, 984.9

063.9 Tick-borne viral encephalitis, unspecified ✿

Ex: 013.60-013.66, 046.2, 046.71-046.8, 048-049.0, 049.8, 052.0, 052.2, 054.3, 054.74, 056.01, 057.8-058.29, 059.00-059.9, 062.0-064, 066.2-066.49, 072.2, 073.7, 075, 079.82, 079.99, 081.9, 083.9, 090.41, 094.81, 117.5, 124, 130.0, 290.12, 323.01-323.9, 341.1, 487.8, 771.2, 984.9

064   Viral encephalitis transmitted by other and unspecified arthropods ✿

Arthropod-borne viral encephalitis, vector unknown
Negishi virus encephalitis

> **Excludes** *viral encephalitis NOS (049.9)*

Ex: 013.60-013.66, 046.2, 046.71-046.8, 048-049.0, 049.8, 052.2, 054.3, 054.74, 056.01, 057.8-058.29, 059.00-059.9, 062.0-064, 066.2-066.49, 072.2, 073.7, 075, 079.82, 079.99, 081.9, 083.9, 090.41, 094.81, 117.5, 124, 130.0, 290.12, 323.01-323.9, 341.1, 487.8, 771.2, 984.9

● **065   Arthropod-borne hemorrhagic fever**

065.0 Crimean hemorrhagic fever [CHF Congo virus] ✿

Central Asian hemorrhagic fever
Ex: 065.0-066.9

065.1 Omsk hemorrhagic fever ✿

Ex: 065.0-066.9

065.2 Kyasanur Forest disease ✿

Ex: 065.0-066.9

065.3 Other tick-borne hemorrhagic fever ✿

Ex: 065.0-066.9

065.4 Mosquito-borne hemorrhagic fever ✿

Chikungunya hemorrhagic fever
Dengue hemorrhagic fever

> **Excludes** *Chikungunya fever (066.3)*
> *dengue (061)*
> *yellow fever (060.0–060.9)*

Ex: 065.0-066.9

065.8 Other specified arthropod-borne hemorrhagic fever ✿

Mite-borne hemorrhagic fever
Ex: 065.0-066.9

065.9 Arthropod-borne hemorrhagic fever, unspecified ✿

Arbovirus hemorrhagic fever NOS
Ex: 065.0-066.9

● **066   Other arthropod-borne viral diseases**

066.0 Phlebotomus fever ✿

Changuinola fever
Sandfly fever
Ex: 065.0-066.9

066.1 Tick-borne fever ✿

Nairobi sheep disease
Tick fever:
  American mountain
  Colorado
  Kemerovo
  Quaranfil
Ex: 065.0-066.9

066.2 Venezuelan equine fever ✿

Venezuelan equine encephalitis
Ex: 013.60-013.66, 046.2, 046.71-046.8, 048-049.0, 049.8, 052.0, 052.2, 054.3, 054.74, 056.01, 057.8-058.29, 059.00-059.9, 062.0-066.9, 072.2, 073.7, 075, 079.82, 079.99, 081.9, 083.9, 090.41, 094.81, 117.5, 124, 130.0, 290.12, 323.01-323.9, 341.1, 487.8, 771.2, 984.9

066.3 Other mosquito-borne fever ✿

Fever (viral):   Fever (viral):
  Bunyamwera   Oropouche
  Bwamba   Pixuna
  Chikungunya   Rift valley
  Guama   Ross river
  Mayaro   Wesselsbron
  Mucambo   Zika
  O' Nyong-Nyong

> **Excludes** *dengue (061)*
> *yellow fever (060.0–060.9)*

Ex: 013.60-013.66, 046.2, 046.71-046.8, 048-049.0, 049.8, 052.0, 052.2, 054.3, 054.74, 056.01, 057.8-058.29, 059.00-059.9, 062.0-066.9, 072.2, 073.7, 075, 079.82, 079.99, 081.9, 083.9, 090.41, 094.81, 117.5, 124, 130.0, 290.12, 323.01-323.9, 341.1, 487.8, 771.2, 984.9

● **066.4 West Nile fever**

Also indexed as West Nile virus
Coding Clinic: 2004, Q4, P50-52; 2002, Q4, P44

066.40 West Nile fever, unspecified ✿

West Nile fever NOS
West Nile fever without complications
West Nile virus NOS
Ex: 013.60-013.66, 046.2, 046.71-046.8, 048-049.0, 049.8, 052.0, 052.2, 054.3, 054.74, 056.01, 057.8-058.29, 059.00-059.9, 062.0-064, 066.8-066.9, 072.2, 073.7, 075, 079.99, 081.9, 083.9, 090.41, 094.81, 117.5, 124, 130.0, 323.01-323.9, 341.1, 487.8, 771.2

066.41 West Nile fever with encephalitis ✿

West Nile encephalitis
West Nile encephalomyelitis
Ex: 013.60-013.66, 046.2, 046.71-046.8, 048-049.0, 049.8, 052.0, 052.2, 054.3, 054.74, 056.01, 057.8-058.29, 059.00-059.9, 062.0-066.3, 066.8-066.9, 072.2, 073.7, 075, 079.99, 081.9, 083.9, 090.41, 094.81, 117.5, 124, 130.0, 323.01-323.9, 341.1, 487.8, 771.2

◀ New   ◀▥ Revised   ~~deleted~~ Deleted   ● Unacceptable Principal Diagnosis   ● Use Additional Digit(s)
▶ Manifestation Code   **OGCR** Official Guidelines   **Coding Clinic**   Excludes   Includes   Use additional   Code first   Omit code

INFECTIOUS AND PARASITIC DISEASES (001–139)

066.42 West Nile fever with other neurologic manifestation 🖐
  Use additional code to specify the neurologic manifestation
  (Ex:) 013.60-013.66, 046.2, 046.71-046.8, 048-049.0, 049.8, 052.0, 052.2, 054.3, 054.74, 056.01, 057.8-058.29, 059.00-059.9, 062.0-066.3, 066.8-066.9, 072.2, 073.7, 075, 079.99, 081.9, 083.9, 090.41, 094.81, 117.5, 124, 130.0, 323.01-323.9, 341.1, 487.8, 771.2

066.49 West Nile fever with other complications 🖐
  Use additional code to specify the other conditions
  (Ex:) 013.60-013.66, 046.2, 046.71-046.8, 048-049.0, 049.8, 052.0, 052.2, 054.3, 054.74, 056.01, 057.8-058.29, 059.00-059.9, 062.0-066.3, 066.8-066.9, 072.2, 073.7, 075, 079.99, 081.9, 083.9, 090.41, 094.81, 117.5, 124, 130.0, 323.01-323.9, 341.1, 487.8, 771.2

066.8 Other specified arthropod-borne viral diseases 🖐
  Chandipura fever
  Piry fever
  (Ex:) 065.0-066.9

066.9 Arthropod-borne viral disease, unspecified 🖐
  Arbovirus infection NOS
  (Ex:) 065.0-066.9

Figure 1-6 Hepatitis B viral infection. **A.** Liver parenchyma showing hepatocytes with diffuse granular cytoplasm, so-called ground glass hepatocytes (H&E). **B.** Immunoperoxidase stains from the same case, showing cytoplasmic inclusions of viral particles. (From Kumar: Robbins and Cotran: Pathologic Basis of Disease, 7th ed. 2005, Saunders, An Imprint of Elsevier)

Item 1-11 Hepatitis A (HAV) was formerly called epidemic, infectious, short-incubation, or acute catarrhal jaundice hepatitis. The primary transmission mode is the oral–fecal route. **Hepatitis B (HBV)** was formerly called long-incubation period, serum, or homologous serum hepatitis. Transmission modes are through blood from infected persons and from body fluids of infected mother to neonate. **Hepatitis C (HCV),** caused by the hepatitis C virus, is primarily transfusion associated. **Hepatitis D (HDV),** also called delta hepatitis, is caused by the hepatitis D virus in patients formerly or currently infected with hepatitis B. **Hepatitis E (HEV)** is also called enterically transmitted non-A, non-B hepatitis. The primary transmission mode is the oral–fecal route, usually through contaminated water.

OTHER DISEASES DUE TO VIRUSES AND CHLAMYDIAE (070–079)

070 Viral hepatitis
  Includes viral hepatitis (acute) (chronic)
  Excludes *cytomegalic inclusion virus hepatitis (078.5)*
  The following fifth-digit subclassification is for use with categories 070.2 and 070.3:

  > 0 acute or unspecified, without mention of hepatitis delta
  > 1 acute or unspecified, with hepatitis delta
  > 2 chronic, without mention of hepatitis delta
  > 3 chronic, with hepatitis delta

  Coding Clinic: 2007, Q2, P6-7x3; 2004, Q4, P52-53

070.0 Viral hepatitis A with hepatic coma 🖐
  (Ex:) 070.0-070.9, 078.88-078.89, 079.81, 079.88-079.99, 139.8

070.1 Viral hepatitis A without mention of hepatic coma 🖐
  Infectious hepatitis
  (Ex:) 070.0-070.9, 078.88-078.89, 079.81, 079.88-079.99, 139.8

070.2 Viral hepatitis B with hepatic coma 🖐
[0-3] (Ex:) 070.0-070.9, 078.88-078.89, 079.81, 079.88-079.99, 139.8

070.3 Viral hepatitis B without mention of hepatic coma 🖐
[0-3] Serum hepatitis
  (Ex:) 070.0-070.9, 078.88-078.89, 079.81, 079.88-079.99, 139.8
  Coding Clinic: 1993, Q1, P28

070.4 Other specified viral hepatitis with hepatic coma
  070.41 Acute hepatitis C with hepatic coma 🖐
    (Ex:) 070.0-070.9, 078.88-078.89, 079.81, 079.88-079.99, 139.8

  070.42 Hepatitis delta without mention of active hepatitis B disease with hepatic coma 🖐
    Hepatitis delta with hepatitis B carrier state
    (Ex:) 070.0-070.9, 078.88-078.89, 079.81, 079.88-079.99, 139.8

  070.43 Hepatitis E with hepatic coma 🖐
    (Ex:) 070.0-070.9, 078.88-078.89, 079.81, 079.88-079.99, 139.8

  070.44 Chronic hepatitis C with hepatic coma 🖐
    (Ex:) 070.0-070.9, 078.88-078.89, 079.81, 079.88-079.99, 139.8

  070.49 Other specified viral hepatitis with hepatic coma 🖐
    (Ex:) 070.0-070.9, 078.88-078.89, 079.81, 079.88-079.99, 139.8

070.5 Other specified viral hepatitis without mention of hepatic coma
  070.51 Acute hepatitis C without mention of hepatic coma 🖐
    (Ex:) 070.0-070.9, 078.88-078.89, 079.81, 079.88-079.99, 139.8

  070.52 Hepatitis delta without mention of active hepatitis B disease or hepatic coma 🖐
    (Ex:) 070.0-070.9, 078.88-078.89, 079.81, 079.88-079.99, 139.8

  070.53 Hepatitis E without mention of hepatic coma 🖐
    (Ex:) 070.0-070.9, 078.88-078.89, 079.81, 079.88-079.99, 139.8

  070.54 Chronic hepatitis C without mention of hepatic coma
    Coding Clinic: 2008, Q4, P120; 2007, Q3, P9; 2006, Q2, P13

  070.59 Other specified viral hepatitis without mention of hepatic coma 🖐
    (Ex:) 070.0-070.9, 078.88-078.89, 079.81, 079.88-079.99, 139.8

070.6 Unspecified viral hepatitis with hepatic coma 🖐
  Excludes *unspecified viral hepatitis C with hepatic coma (070.71)*
  (Ex:) 070.0-070.9, 078.88-078.89, 079.81, 079.88-079.99, 139.8

070.7 Unspecified viral hepatitis C
  070.70 Unspecified viral hepatitis C without hepatic coma
    Unspecified viral hepatitis C NOS

  070.71 Unspecified viral hepatitis C with hepatic coma 🖐
    (Ex:) 070.0-070.9, 078.88-078.89, 079.81, 079.88-079.99, 139.8

070.9 Unspecified viral hepatitis without mention of hepatic coma 🖐
  Viral hepatitis NOS
  Excludes *unspecified viral hepatitis C without hepatic coma (070.70)*
  (Ex:) 070.0-070.9, 078.88-078.89, 079.81, 079.88-079.99, 139.8

N Newborn Age: 0   **P** Pediatric Age: 0–17   **M** Maternity Age: 12–55   **A** Adult Age: 15–124   ♀ Females Only   ♂ Males Only
(Ex:) CC Exclusions   🖐 Complication\Comorbidity   🖐 Major C\C   🖐 Present on Admission Requirement   🖐 Hospital-Acquired Condition

751

INFECTIOUS AND PARASITIC DISEASES (001–139)

071 Rabies 🦠
Viral disease affecting central nervous system and transmitted from infected mammals.
Hydrophobia
Lyssa
Ⓔⓧ 071

● **072 Mumps**
An acute, contagious, viral disease that causes painful enlargement of the salivary or parotid glands and is spread by respiratory droplets or direct contact. The following combination codes are specific diseases as an existing complication of mumps.

072.0 Mumps orchitis ♂ 🦠
Ⓔⓧ 072.0, 072.79-072.9, 078.88-078.89, 079.81, 079.88-079.99, 139.8

072.1 Mumps meningitis 🦠
Ⓔⓧ 003.21, 013.00-013.16, 036.0, 047.0-047.9, 049.0-049.1, 053.0, 054.72, 072.1, 072.79-072.9, 078.88-078.89, 079.81, 079.88-079.99, 090.42, 091.81, 094.2, 098.89, 100.81, 112.83, 114.2, 115.01, 115.11, 115.91, 130.0, 139.8, 320.0-322.9, 349.89-349.9, 357.0

072.2 Mumps encephalitis 🦠
Mumps meningoencephalitis
Ⓔⓧ 072.2, 072.79-072.9, 078.88-078.89, 079.81, 079.88-079.99, 139.8

072.3 Mumps pancreatitis 🦠
Ⓔⓧ 072.3, 072.79-072.9, 078.88-078.89, 079.81, 079.88-079.99, 139.8

● **072.7 Mumps with other specified complications**

072.71 Mumps hepatitis 🦠
Ⓔⓧ 072.71, 072.79-072.9, 078.88-078.89, 079.81, 079.88-079.99, 139.8

072.72 Mumps polyneuropathy 🦠
Ⓔⓧ 072.72-072.9, 078.88-078.89, 079.81, 079.88-079.99, 139.8

072.79 Other 🦠
Ⓔⓧ 072.79-072.9, 078.88-078.89, 079.81, 079.88-079.99, 139.8

072.8 Mumps with unspecified complication 🦠
Ⓔⓧ 072.79-072.9, 078.88-078.89, 079.81, 079.88-079.99

072.9 Mumps without mention of complication
Epidemic parotitis
Infectious parotitis

● **073 Ornithosis**

Includes   parrot fever
psittacosis

073.0 With pneumonia 🦠
Lobular pneumonitis due to ornithosis
Ⓔⓧ 011.00-012.16, 012.80-012.86, 017.90-017.96, 020.3-020.5, 021.3, 022.1, 031.0, 039.1, 073.0, 073.8-073.9, 115.05, 115.15, 115.95, 122.1, 130.4, 136.3, 480.0-487.1, 488, 495.0-495.9, 500-508.9, 517.1, 517.8, 518.89, 519.8-519.9

073.7 With other specified complications 🦠
Ⓔⓧ 013.60-013.66, 046.2, 046.71-046.8, 048-049.0, 049.8, 052.0, 052.2, 054.3, 054.74, 056.01, 057.8-058.29, 059.00-059.9, 062.0-064, 066.2-066.49, 072.2, 073.0-073.9, 079.82, 079.99, 081.9, 083.9, 090.41, 094.81, 117.5, 124, 130.0, 290.12, 323.01-323.9, 341.1, 487.8, 771.2, 984.9

073.8 With unspecified complication 🦠
Ⓔⓧ 073.0, 073.8-073.9

073.9 Ornithosis, unspecified 🦠
Ⓔⓧ 073.0, 073.8-073.9

● **074 Specific diseases due to Coxsackie virus**

Excludes   *Coxsackie virus:*
infection NOS (079.2)
meningitis (047.0)

074.0 Herpangina
Vesicular pharyngitis

074.1 Epidemic pleurodynia
Bornholm disease
Devil's grip
Epidemic:
myalgia
myositis

● **074.2 Coxsackie carditis**

074.20 Coxsackie carditis, unspecified 🦠
Ⓔⓧ 074.20, 074.22-074.23, 093.82, 390, 391.2-391.9, 398.0-398.90, 398.99, 422.0-422.99, 429.0, 429.71-429.79, 459.89-459.9

074.21 Coxsackie pericarditis 🦠
Ⓔⓧ 074.21, 093.81, 391.0, 393, 420.0-420.99, 423.3-423.9, 459.89-459.9

074.22 Coxsackie endocarditis 🦠
Ⓔⓧ 002.0, 036.42, 074.22, 083.0, 093.20-093.24, 098.84, 112.81, 115.94, 116.0, 390, 391.1, 391.8-392.0, 394.0-395.9, 396.9-397.9, 398.90, 398.99, 421.0-421.9, 424.0-424.99, 425.3, 459.89-459.9, 746.09, 746.89, 996.61

074.23 Coxsackie myocarditis 🦠
Aseptic myocarditis of newborn
Ⓔⓧ 074.20, 074.22-074.23, 093.82, 390, 391.2-391.9, 398.0-398.90, 398.99, 422.0-422.99, 429.0, 429.71-429.79, 459.89-459.9

074.3 Hand, foot, and mouth disease
Vesicular stomatitis and exanthem
Check your documentation—this code is HAND, foot, and mouth disease. Code 078.4 is foot and mouth disease.

074.8 Other specified diseases due to Coxsackie virus
Acute lymphonodular pharyngitis

075 Infectious mononucleosis
Glandular fever
Pfeiffer's disease
Monocytic angina
Coding Clinic: 2001, Q3, P13-14x2

● **076 Trachoma**

Excludes   *late effect of trachoma (139.1)*

076.0 Initial stage
Trachoma dubium

076.1 Active stage
Granular conjunctivitis (trachomatous)
Trachomatous:
follicular conjunctivitis
pannus

076.9 Trachoma, unspecified
Trachoma NOS

● **077 Other diseases of conjunctiva due to viruses and Chlamydiae**

Excludes   *ophthalmic complications of viral diseases classified elsewhere*

077.0 Inclusion conjunctivitis
Paratrachoma
Swimming pool conjunctivitis

Excludes   *inclusion blennorrhea (neonatal) (771.6)*

077.1 Epidemic keratoconjunctivitis
Shipyard eye

077.2 Pharyngoconjunctival fever
Viral pharyngoconjunctivitis

INFECTIOUS AND PARASITIC DISEASES (001–139)

◀ New   ◀◀◀ Revised   ~~deleted~~ Deleted   ● Unacceptable Principal Diagnosis   ● Use Additional Digit(s)
▶ Manifestation Code   **OGCR** Official Guidelines   **Coding Clinic**   Excludes   Includes   Use additional   Code first   Omit code

077.3 Other adenoviral conjunctivitis
Acute adenoviral follicular conjunctivitis

077.4 Epidemic hemorrhagic conjunctivitis
Apollo:
conjunctivitis
disease
Conjunctivitis due to enterovirus type 70
Hemorrhagic conjunctivitis (acute) (epidemic)

077.8 Other viral conjunctivitis
Newcastle conjunctivitis

● **077.9 Unspecified diseases of conjunctiva due to viruses and Chlamydiae**

077.98 Due to Chlamydiae

077.99 Due to viruses
Viral conjunctivitis NOS

● **078 Other diseases due to viruses and Chlamydiae**

Excludes viral infection NOS (079.0–079.9)
viremia NOS (790.8)

078.0 Molluscum contagiosum

● **078.1 Viral warts**
Viral warts due to human papillomavirus
Coding Clinic: 1997, Q2, P9

078.10 Viral warts, unspecified
Verruca:
NOS
Vulgaris
Warts (infectious)

078.11 Condyloma acuminatum
Condyloma NOS
Genital warts NOS

078.12 Plantar wart
Verruca plantaris
Coding Clinic: 2008, Q4, P78-79

078.19 Other specified viral warts
Common wart
Flat wart
Verruca plana

078.2 Sweating fever
Miliary fever
Sweating disease

078.3 Cat-scratch disease
Benign lymphoreticulosis (of inoculation)
Cat-scratch fever
(Ex) 078.3, 079.82

078.4 Foot and mouth disease
Aphthous fever
Epizootic:
aphthae
stomatitis
Check your documentation. Code 074.3 is for HAND,
foot, and mouth disease.

078.5 Cytomegaloviral disease
Cytomegalic inclusion disease
Salivary gland virus disease
Use additional code to identify manifestation, as:
cytomegalic inclusion virus:
hepatitis (573.1)
pneumonia (484.1)
Excludes congenital cytomegalovirus infection
(771.1)
(Ex) 078.5-078.7, 078.89-079.50, 079.59, 079.81-079.82, 079.89, 079.99
Coding Clinic: 2003, Q1, P11; 1993, Q3, P13; Q2, P11; Q1, P24; 1989,
Q1, P9

078.6 Hemorrhagic nephrosonephritis
Hemorrhagic fever:
epidemic
Korean
Russian with renal syndrome
(Ex) 016.00-016.06, 016.30-016.36, 016.90-016.96, 017.90-017.96, 078.6,
079.82, 098.10, 098.19, 098.30-098.31, 098.89, 112.2, 131.00,
131.8-131.9, 249.40-249.41, 249.80-249.91, 250.40-250.43,
250.80-250.93, 274.10, 274.19, 580.0-584.9, 586-591, 593.0-593.2,
593.89-593.9, 599.70-599.9

078.7 Arenaviral hemorrhagic fever
Hemorrhagic fever:
Argentine
Bolivian
Junin virus
Machupo virus
(Ex) 078.5-079.82, 079.88-079.99

● **078.8 Other specified diseases due to viruses and Chlamydiae**

Excludes epidemic diarrhea (009.2)
lymphogranuloma venereum (099.1)

078.81 Epidemic vertigo

078.82 Epidemic vomiting syndrome
Winter vomiting disease

078.88 Other specified diseases due to Chlamydiae

078.89 Other specified diseases due to viruses
Epidemic cervical myalgia
Marburg disease
~~Tanapox~~

Item 1–12 Retrovirus develops by copying its RNA,
genetic materials, into the DNA, which then produces new virus
particles. It is from the Retroviridae virus family.
Human T-cell lymphotropic virus, Type I (HTLV-I) is
also called human T-cell leukemia virus, Type I, and is a retrovirus
thought to cause T-cell leukemia/lymphoma.
Human T-cell lymphotropic virus, Type II (HTLV-II), is
also called human T-cell leukemia virus, Type II, and is a retrovirus
associated with hematologic disorders.
HIV-2 is one of the serotypes of HIV and is usually confined to
West Africa, whereas HIV-1 is found worldwide.

● **079 Viral and chlamydial infection in conditions classified elsewhere and of unspecified site**
Note: This category is provided to be used as an
additional code to identify the viral agent in
diseases classifiable elsewhere. This category
will also be used to classify virus infection of
unspecified nature or site.

079.0 Adenovirus

079.1 ECHO virus

079.2 Coxsackie virus

079.3 Rhinovirus

079.4 Human papillomavirus
Coding Clinic: 1997, Q2, P9

● **079.5 Retrovirus**

Excludes human immunodeficiency virus, type 1
[HIV-1] (042)
human T-cell lymphotrophic virus, type III
[HTLV-III] (042)
lymphadenopathy-associated virus [LAV]
(042)

079.50 Retrovirus, unspecified

**079.51 Human T-cell lymphotrophic virus, type I
[HTLV-I]**
(Ex) 079.51-079.59, 079.81-079.82, 079.88-079.99

N Newborn Age: 0   P Pediatric Age: 0–17   M Maternity Age: 12–55   A Adult Age: 15–124   ♀ Females Only   ♂ Males Only
(Ex) CC Exclusions   ● Complication\Comorbidity   ● Major C\C   ● Present on Admission Requirement   ● Hospital-Acquired Condition

753

079.52 Human T-cell lymphotrophic virus, type II [HTLV-II] 🐾
  (Ex:) 079.50-079.59, 079.81-079.82, 079.88-079.99

079.53 Human immunodeficiency virus, type 2 [HIV-2] 🐾
  (Ex:) 042, 079.50-079.59, 079.81-079.82, 079.88-079.99

079.59 Other specified retrovirus

079.6 Respiratory syncytial virus (RSV)
  Coding Clinic: 1996, Q4, P27-28

● **079.8 Other specified viral and chlamydial infections**
  Coding Clinic: 1988, Q1, P12; Q1, P12

079.81 Hantavirus 🐾
  (Ex:) 070.70-070.71, 078.5-079.82, 079.88-079.99

079.82 SARS-associated coronavirus 🐾
  (Ex:) 011.00-012.16, 012.80-012.86, 017.90-017.96, 021.2, 031.0, 039.1, 079.82-079.89, 115.05, 115.15, 115.95, 122.1, 130.4, 136.3, 480.0-480.2, 480.8-487.1, 488, 494.0-508.9, 517.1, 517.8, 518.89, 519.8-519.9, 748.61
  Coding Clinic: 2003, Q4, P46-48

079.83 Parvovirus B19 🐾
  Human parvovirus
  Parvovirus NOS
  | Excludes | erythema infectiosum [fifth disease] (057.0)
  (Ex:) 057.0, 079.83
  Coding Clinic: 2007, Q4, P64

079.88 Other specified chlamydial infection

079.89 Other specified viral infection
  Coding Clinic: 1995, Q1, P7

● **079.9 Unspecified viral and chlamydial infections**
  | Excludes | viremia NOS (790.8)
  Coding Clinic: 1988, Q4, P10; 1987, Jan-Feb, P16

079.98 Unspecified chlamydial infection
  Chlamydial infection NOS

079.99 Unspecified viral infection
  Viral infection NOS
  Coding Clinic: 1991, Q2, P8

Item 1–13 Rickettsioses are diseases spread from ticks, lice, fleas, or mites to humans.
Typhus is spread to humans chiefly by the fleas of rats.
Endemic identifies a disease as being present in low numbers of humans at all times, whereas **epidemic** identifies a disease as being present in high numbers of humans at a specific time. Morbidity (death) is higher in epidemic diseases.
Brill's disease, also known as **Brill-Zinsser disease,** is spread from human to human by body lice and also from the lice of flying squirrels. **Scrub typhus** is spread in the same ways as Brill's disease.
Malaria is spread to humans by mosquitoes.

RICKETTSIOSES AND OTHER ARTHROPOD-BORNE DISEASES (080–088)

  | Excludes | arthropod-borne viral diseases (060.0–066.9)

080 Louse-borne [epidemic] typhus 🐾
  Typhus (fever):
    classical
    epidemic
      Infecting a large number of individuals at the same time
    exanthematic NOS
    louse-borne
  (Ex:) 080-083.9, 085.0-088.9

● **081 Other typhus**

081.0 Murine [endemic] typhus 🐾
  Typhus (fever):
    endemic
      Restricted to a particular region
    flea-borne
  (Ex:) 080-083.9, 085.0-088.9

081.1 Brill's disease 🐾
  Brill-Zinsser disease
  Recrudescent typhus (fever)
  (Ex:) 080-083.9, 085.0-088.9

081.2 Scrub typhus 🐾
  Japanese river fever
  Kedani fever
  Mite-borne typhus
  Tsutsugamushi
  (Ex:) 080-083.9, 085.0-088.9

081.9 Typhus, unspecified 🐾
  Typhus (fever) NOS
  (Ex:) 013.60-013.66, 046.2, 046.71-046.8, 048-049.0, 049.8, 052.0, 052.2, 054.3, 054.74, 056.01, 057.8-058.29, 059.00-059.9, 062.0-064, 066.2-066.49, 072.2, 073.7, 079.82, 079.99-084.0, 085.0-088.9, 090.41, 094.81, 117.5, 124, 130.0, 290.12, 323.01-323.9, 341.1, 487.8, 771.2, 984.9

● **082 Tick-borne rickettsioses**

082.0 Spotted fevers 🐾
  Rocky mountain spotted fever
  Sao Paulo fever
  (Ex:) 080-083.9, 085.0-088.9

082.1 Boutonneuse fever 🐾
  African tick typhus
  India tick typhus
  Kenya tick typhus
  Marseilles fever
  Mediterranean tick fever
  (Ex:) 080-083.9, 085.0-088.9

082.2 North Asian tick fever 🐾
  Siberian tick typhus
  (Ex:) 080-083.9, 085.0-088.9

082.3 Queensland tick typhus 🐾
  (Ex:) 080-083.9, 085.0-088.9

● **082.4 Ehrlichiosis**

082.40 Ehrlichiosis, unspecified 🐾
  (Ex:) 080-083.9, 085.0-088.9

082.41 Ehrlichiosis chaffeensis [E. chaffeensis] 🐾
  (Ex:) 080-083.9, 085.0-088.9

082.49 Other ehrlichiosis 🐾
  (Ex:) 080-083.9, 085.0-088.9

082.8 Other specified tick-borne rickettsioses 🐾
  Lone star fever
  (Ex:) 080-083.9, 085.0-088.9
  Coding Clinic: 1999, Q4, P19

082.9 Tick-borne rickettsiosis, unspecified 🐾
  Tick-borne typhus NOS
  (Ex:) 080-083.9, 085.0-088.9

● **083 Other rickettsioses**

083.0 Q fever 🐾
  (Ex:) 080-083.9, 085.0-088.9

083.1 Trench fever 🐾
  Quintan fever
  Wolhynian fever
  (Ex:) 080-083.9, 085.0-088.9

◄ New   ⬅ Revised   ~~deleted~~ Deleted   ● Unacceptable Principal Diagnosis   ● Use Additional Digit(s)
◗ Manifestation Code   **OGCR** Official Guidelines   **Coding Clinic** | Excludes | Includes   Use additional   Code first   Omit code

083.2 Rickettsialpox 🦠
    Vesicular rickettsiosis
    (Ex:) 082.0-083.9

083.8 Other specified rickettsioses 🦠
    (Ex:) 082.0-083.9

083.9 Rickettsiosis, unspecified 🦠
    (Ex:) 082.0-083.9

● **084 Malaria**
    Mosquito-borne disease caused by parasite. Left untreated,
    severe complications and death may result.

    Note: Subcategories 084.0–084.6 exclude the
    listed conditions with mention of pernicious
    complications (084.8–084.9).

    Excludes | congenital malaria (771.2)

084.0 Falciparum malaria [malignant tertian] 🦠
    Malaria (fever):
        by Plasmodium falciparum
        subtertian
    (Ex:) 084.0-086.9

084.1 Vivax malaria [benign tertian] 🦠
    Malaria (fever) by Plasmodium vivax
    (Ex:) 084.0-088.9

084.2 Quartan malaria 🦠
    Malaria (fever) by Plasmodium malariae
    Malariae malaria
    (Ex:) 084.0-086.9

084.3 Ovale malaria 🦠
    Malaria (fever) by Plasmodium ovale
    (Ex:) 084.0-086.9

084.4 Other malaria 🦠
    Monkey malaria
    (Ex:) 084.0-086.9

084.5 Mixed malaria 🦠
    Malaria (fever) by more than one parasite
    (Ex:) 084.0-086.9

084.6 Malaria, unspecified 🦠
    Malaria (fever) NOS
    (Ex:) 079.82, 084.0-086.9

084.7 Induced malaria 🦠
    Therapeutically induced malaria

    Excludes | *accidental infection from syringe, blood*
                transfusion, etc. (084.0–084.6, above,
                according to parasite species)
                transmission from mother to child during
                delivery (771.2)
    (Ex:) 084.1-086.9

084.8 Blackwater fever 🦠
    Hemoglobinuric:
        fever (bilious)
        malaria
    Malarial hemoglobinuria
    (Ex:) 084.0-086.9

084.9 Other pernicious complications of malaria 🦠
    Algid malaria
    Cerebral malaria

    Use additional code to identify complication, as:
        malarial:
            hepatitis (573.2)
            nephrosis (581.81)
    (Ex:) 084.0-086.9

● **085 Leishmaniasis**

085.0 Visceral [kala-azar] 🦠
    Dumdum fever
    Infection by Leishmania:
        donovani
        infantum
    Leishmaniasis:
        dermal, post-kala-azar
        Mediterranean
        visceral (Indian)
    (Ex:) 080-088.9

085.1 Cutaneous, urban 🦠
    Aleppo boil
    Baghdad boil
    Delhi boil
    Infection by Leishmania tropica (minor)
    Leishmaniasis, cutaneous:
        dry form
        late
        recurrent
        ulcerating
    Oriental sore
    (Ex:) 080-088.9

085.2 Cutaneous, Asian desert 🦠
    Infection by Leishmania tropica major
    Leishmaniasis, cutaneous:
        acute necrotizing
        rural
        wet form
        zoonotic form
    (Ex:) 080-088.9

085.3 Cutaneous, Ethiopian 🦠
    Infection by Leishmania ethiopica
    Leishmaniasis, cutaneous:
        diffuse
        lepromatous
    (Ex:) 080-088.9

085.4 Cutaneous, American 🦠
    Chiclero ulcer
    Infection by Leishmania mexicana
    Leishmaniasis tegumentaria diffusa
    (Ex:) 080-088.9

085.5 Mucocutaneous (American) 🦠
    Espundia
    Infection by Leishmania braziliensis
    Uta
    (Ex:) 080-088.9

085.9 Leishmaniasis, unspecified 🦠
    (Ex:) 080-088.9

● **086 Trypanosomiasis**
    Human African trypanosomiasis (HAT) is transmitted by fly
    bites that transmit either Trypanosoma brucei gambiense
    (causes a chronic infection lasting years) or Trypanosoma
    brucei rhodesiense (causes acute illness lasting several
    weeks).

    Use additional code to identify manifestations, as:
        trypanosomiasis:
            encephalitis (323.2)
            meningitis (321.3)

086.0 Chagas' disease with heart involvement 🦠
    American trypanosomiasis with heart involvement
    Infection by Trypanosoma cruzi with heart
        involvement
    Any condition classifiable to 086.2 with heart
        involvement
    (Ex:) 086.0, 139.8

INFECTIOUS AND PARASITIC DISEASES (001–139)

086.1 Chagas' disease with other organ involvement 🦠
American trypanosomiasis with involvement of
organ other than heart
Infection by Trypanosoma cruzi with involvement
of organ other than heart
Any condition classifiable to 086.2 with
involvement of organ other than heart
(Ex:) 080-088.9

**086.2 Chagas' disease without mention of organ
involvement** 🦠
American trypanosomiasis
Infection by Trypanosoma cruzi
(Ex:) 080-088.9

086.3 Gambian trypanosomiasis 🦠
Gambian sleeping sickness
(Ex:) 080-088.9
Infection by Trypanosoma gambiense

086.4 Rhodesian trypanosomiasis 🦠
Infection by Trypanosoma rhodesiense
Rhodesian sleeping sickness
(Ex:) 080-088.9

086.5 African trypanosomiasis, unspecified 🦠
Sleeping sickness NOS
(Ex:) 080-088.9

086.9 Trypanosomiasis, unspecified 🦠
(Ex:) 013.60-013.66, 046.2, 046.71-046.8, 048-049.0, 049.8, 052.0, 052.2, 054.3,
054.74, 056.01, 057.8-058.29, 059.00-059.9, 062.0-064, 066.2-066.3,
072.2, 073.7, 075, 078.3, 079.99-088.9, 090.41, 094.81, 117.5, 124,
130.0, 290.12, 323.01-323.9, 341.1, 382.4, 487.8, 771.2, 984.9

● **087 Relapsing fever**
> **Includes** recurrent fever

087.0 Louse-borne 🦠
(Ex:) 080-083.9, 085.0-088.9

087.1 Tick-borne 🦠
(Ex:) 080-083.9, 085.0-088.9

087.9 Relapsing fever, unspecified 🦠
(Ex:) 080-083.9, 085.0-088.9

● **088 Other arthropod-borne diseases**

088.0 Bartonellosis 🦠
Carrión's disease
Oroya fever
Verruga peruana
(Ex:) 080-083.9, 085.0-088.9

● **088.8 Other specified arthropod-borne diseases**

088.81 Lyme disease 🦠
Erythema chronicum migrans
(Ex:) 080-083.9, 085.0-088.9
Coding Clinic: 1990, Q3, P14; 1989, Q2, P10

088.82 Babesiosis 🦠
Babesiasis
(Ex:) 080-088.9

088.89 Other

088.9 Arthropod-borne disease, unspecified

Figure 1-7 Chancre of primary syphilis. (From Mandell, Bennett, & Dolin: Principles and Practice of Infectious Diseases, 6th ed. 2005, Churchill Livingstone, An Imprint of Elsevier)

Item 1-14 Syphilis, also known as lues, is the most serious of the venereal diseases caused by *Treponema pallidum*. The **primary** stage is characterized by an ulceration known as **chancre,** which usually appears on the genitals but can also develop on the anus, lips, tonsils, breasts, or fingers. Syphilis is easy to cure in its early stages. A single intramuscular injection of penicillin will usually cure a person who has had syphilis for less than a year.
The **secondary** stage is characterized by a rash that can affect any area of the body. **Latent** syphilis is divided into **early,** which is diagnosed within two years of infection, and **late,** which is diagnosed two years or more after infection. Additional doses of penicillin or another antibiotic are needed to treat someone who has had syphilis for longer than a year. For those allergic to penicillin, there are other antibiotic treatments. **Congenital** syphilis is also labeled **early** or **late** based on the time of diagnosis.

SYPHILIS AND OTHER VENEREAL DISEASES (090–099)

> **Excludes** nonvenereal endemic syphilis (104.0)
> urogenital trichomoniasis (131.0)

● **090 Congenital syphilis**

090.0 Early congenital syphilis, symptomatic 🦠
Congenital syphilitic:
choroiditis
coryza (chronic)
hepatomegaly
mucous patches
periostitis
splenomegaly
Syphilitic (congenital):
epiphysitis
osteochondritis
pemphigus
Any congenital syphilitic condition specified as early
or manifest less than two years after birth
(Ex:) 090.0-097.9

090.1 Early congenital syphilis, latent
Congenital syphilis without clinical manifestations,
with positive serological reaction and
negative spinal fluid test, less than two years
after birth

090.2 Early congenital syphilis, unspecified 🦠
Congenital syphilis NOS, less than two years after
birth
(Ex:) 090.0-099.9, 139.8

090.3 Syphilitic interstitial keratitis 🦠
Syphilitic keratitis:
parenchymatous
punctata profunda
> **Excludes** interstitial keratitis NOS (370.50)
(Ex:) 090.0-097.9

INFECTIOUS AND PARASITIC DISEASES (001–139)

◀ New   ◀◀ Revised   ~~deleted~~ Deleted   ● Unacceptable Principal Diagnosis   ● Use Additional Digit(s)
▶ Manifestation Code   **OGCR** Official Guidelines   **Coding Clinic**   Excludes   Includes   Use additional   Code first   Omit code

● 090.4 **Juvenile neurosyphilis**
     Use additional code to identify any associated
          mental disorder

     090.40 **Juvenile neurosyphilis, unspecified**🍖
          Congenital neurosyphilis
          Dementia paralytica juvenilis
          Juvenile:
               general paresis
               tabes
               taboparesis
          (Ex) 090.0-097.9, 999.40-099.9, 139.8

     090.41 **Congenital syphilitic encephalitis**🍖
          (Ex) 090.0-097.9, 099.40-099.9, 139.8

     090.42 **Congenital syphilitic meningitis**🍖
          (Ex) 003.21, 013.00-013.16, 036.0, 047.0-047.9, 049.0-049.1,
               053.0, 054.72, 072.1, 090.0-097.9, 098.89, 099.40-099.9,
               100.81, 112.83, 114.2, 115.01, 115.11, 115.91, 130.0,
               139.8, 320.0-322.9, 349.89-349.9, 357.0

     090.49 **Other**🍖
          (Ex) 090.0-097.9, 099.40-099.9, 139.8

090.5 **Other late congenital syphilis, symptomatic**🍖
     Gumma due to congenital syphilis
     Hutchinson's teeth
     Syphilitic saddle nose
     Any congenital syphilitic condition specified as late
          or manifest two years or more after birth
     (Ex) 090.0-097.9

090.6 **Late congenital syphilis, latent**
     Congenital syphilis without clinical manifestations,
          with positive serological reaction and
          negative spinal fluid test, two years or more
          after birth

090.7 **Late congenital syphilis, unspecified**
     Congenital syphilis NOS, two years or more after
          birth

090.9 **Congenital syphilis, unspecified**

● 091 **Early syphilis, symptomatic**
     Excludes *early cardiovascular syphilis (093.0–093.9)*
                  early neurosyphilis (094.0–094.9)

     091.0 **Genital syphilis (primary)**
          Genital chancre

     091.1 **Primary anal syphilis**

     091.2 **Other primary syphilis**
          Primary syphilis of:
               breast
               fingers
               lip
               tonsils

     091.3 **Secondary syphilis of skin or mucous membranes**🍖
          Condyloma latum
          Secondary syphilis of:
               anus
               mouth
               pharynx
               skin
               tonsils
               vulva
          (Ex) 090.0-097.9

     091.4 **Adenopathy due to secondary syphilis**🍖
          Syphilitic adenopathy (secondary)
          Syphilitic lymphadenitis (secondary)
          (Ex) 090.0-097.9

Item 1–15 Notice the placement of 091.4 combination
code in with the Infectious and Parasitic Disease codes
(syphilis). This uveitis does not appear in the eye code
section because it is a manifestation of the underlying
disease of syphilis.

● 091.5 **Uveitis due to secondary syphilis**
     091.50 **Syphilitic uveitis, unspecified**🍖
          (Ex) 090.0-097.9

     091.51 **Syphilitic chorioretinitis (secondary)**🍖
          (Ex) 090.0-097.9

     091.52 **Syphilitic iridocyclitis (secondary)**🍖
          (Ex) 090.0-097.9

● 091.6 **Secondary syphilis of viscera and bone**
     091.61 **Secondary syphilitic periostitis**🍖
          (Ex) 015.90-015.96, 090.0-099.9, 102.6, 730.10-730.19,
               730.30-730.39, 733.99

     091.62 **Secondary syphilitic hepatitis**🍖
          Secondary syphilis of liver
          (Ex) 090.0-099.9, 571.42-571.9, 573.1-573.3, 573.8-573.9

     091.69 **Other viscera**🍖
          (Ex) 090.0-099.9, 139.8

091.7 **Secondary syphilis, relapse**🍖
     Secondary syphilis, relapse (treated) (untreated)
     (Ex) 090.0-099.9, 139.8

● 091.8 **Other forms of secondary syphilis**
     091.81 **Acute syphilitic meningitis (secondary)**🍖
          (Ex) 003.21, 013.00-013.16, 036.0, 047.0-047.9, 049.0-049.1,
               072.1, 078.88-078.89, 079.81, 079.88-079.99, 090.0-099.9,
               100.81, 112.83, 114.2, 115.01, 115.11, 115.91, 130.0,
               139.8, 320.0-322.9, 349.89-349.9, 357.0

     091.82 **Syphilitic alopecia**🍖
          (Ex) 090.0-099.9

     091.89 **Other**🍖
          (Ex) 090.0-099.9, 139.8

091.9 **Unspecified secondary syphilis**🍖
     (Ex) 090.0-099.9, 139.8

● 092 **Early syphilis, latent**
     Early syphilis is the disease, latent is the characteristic.

     Includes syphilis (acquired) without clinical
                   manifestations, with positive serological
                   reaction and negative spinal fluid test,
                   less than two years after infection

     092.0 **Early syphilis, latent, serological relapse after
          treatment**

     092.9 **Early syphilis, latent, unspecified**

● 093 **Cardiovascular syphilis**
     093.0 **Aneurysm of aorta, specified as syphilitic**🍖
          Dilatation of aorta, specified as syphilitic
          (Ex) 090.0-097.9, 099.40-099.9, 139.8

     093.1 **Syphilitic aortitis**🍖
          (Ex) 090.0-097.9, 099.40-099.9, 139.8

● 093.2 **Syphilitic endocarditis**
     *Check documentation for documentation of a specific
          valve.*

     093.20 **Valve, unspecified**🍖
          Syphilitic ostial coronary disease
          (Ex) 090.0-097.9, 099.40-099.9, 139.8

     093.21 **Mitral valve**🍖
          (Ex) 090.0-097.9, 099.40-099.9, 139.8

INFECTIOUS AND PARASITIC DISEASES (001–139)

093.22 Aortic valve🖑
  Syphilitic aortic incompetence or stenosis
  (Ex:) 090.0-097.9, 099.40-099.9, 139.8

093.23 Tricuspid valve🖑
  (Ex:) 090.0-097.9, 099.40-099.9, 139.8

093.24 Pulmonary valve🖑
  (Ex:) 090.0-097.9, 099.40-099.9, 139.8

● **093.8 Other specified cardiovascular syphilis**

  093.81 Syphilitic pericarditis🖑
    (Ex:) 090.0-097.9, 099.40-099.9, 139.8

  093.82 Syphilitic myocarditis🖑
    (Ex:) 090.0-097.9, 099.40-099.9, 139.8

  093.89 Other🖑
    (Ex:) 090.0-097.9, 099.40-099.9, 139.8

093.9 Cardiovascular syphilis, unspecified🖑
  (Ex:) 090.0-097.9, 099.40-099.9, 139.8

● **094 Neurosyphilis**

  Use additional code to identify any associated mental disorder

  094.0 Tabes dorsalis🖑
    Locomotor ataxia (progressive)
    Posterior spinal sclerosis (syphilitic)
    Tabetic neurosyphilis

    Use additional code to identify manifestation, as:
      neurogenic arthropathy [Charcot's joint disease] (713.5)
    (Ex:) 090.0-097.9, 099.40-099.9, 139.8

  094.1 General paresis🖑
    Dementia paralytica
    General paralysis (of the insane) (progressive)
    Paretic neurosyphilis
    Taboparesis
    (Ex:) 090.0-097.9, 099.40-099.9, 139.8

  094.2 Syphilitic meningitis🖑
    Meningovascular syphilis

    Excludes *acute syphilitic meningitis (secondary) (091.81)*
    (Ex:) 003.21, 013.00-013.16, 036.0, 047.0-047.9, 049.0-049.1, 053.0, 054.72, 072.1, 090.0-097.9, 098.89, 099.40-099.9, 100.81, 112.83, 114.2, 115.01, 115.11, 115.91, 130.0, 139.8, 320.0-322.9, 349.89-349.9, 357.0

  094.3 Asymptomatic neurosyphilis🖑
    (Ex:) 090.0-097.9, 099.40-099.9, 139.8

● **094.8 Other specified neurosyphilis**

  094.81 Syphilitic encephalitis🖑
    (Ex:) 090.0-097.9, 099.40-099.9, 139.8

  094.82 Syphilitic Parkinsonism🖑
    (Ex:) 090.0-099.9, 332.0-333.0

  094.83 Syphilitic disseminated retinochoroiditis🖑
    (Ex:) 017.30-017.36, 090.0-099.9, 115.02, 115.12, 362.01, 362.12-362.13, 362.29, 362.41, 362.52, 362.76, 363.00, 363.05-363.10, 363.13-363.15, 646.80-646.84, 679.12, 679.14

  094.84 Syphilitic optic atrophy🖑
    (Ex:) 090.0-099.9

  094.85 Syphilitic retrobulbar neuritis🖑
    (Ex:) 090.0-099.9, 377.32

  094.86 Syphilitic acoustic neuritis🖑
    (Ex:) 090.0-099.9, 388.5

  094.87 Syphilitic ruptured cerebral aneurysm🖑
    (Ex:) 090.0-097.9, 099.40-099.9, 139.8

  094.89 Other🖑
    (Ex:) 090.0-097.9, 099.40-099.9, 139.8

094.9 Neurosyphilis, unspecified🖑
  Gumma (syphilitic) of central nervous system NOS
  Syphilis (early) (late) of central nervous system NOS
  Syphiloma of central nervous system NOS
  (Ex:) 090.0-097.9, 099.40-099.9, 139.8

● **095 Other forms of late syphilis, with symptoms**

  In the late stages, syphilis can damage organs and body systems.

  Includes   gumma (syphilitic)
    Destructive lesions of syphilis
    tertiary, or unspecified stage

  095.0 Syphilitic episcleritis🖑
    (Ex:) 017.30-017.36, 090.0-099.9, 379.00-379.02, 379.09

  095.1 Syphilis of lung🖑
    (Ex:) 090.0-099.9

  095.2 Syphilitic peritonitis🖑
    (Ex:) 014.00-014.06, 032.83, 090.0-099.9, 540.0-540.1, 567.0-567.1, 567.22, 567.29, 567.81, 567.9, 569.89-569.9, 577.8, 614.5-614.7, 639.0, 670.00-670.04, 777.6, 998.7

  095.3 Syphilis of liver🖑
    (Ex:) 090.0-099.9

  095.4 Syphilis of kidney🖑
    (Ex:) 090.0-099.9

  095.5 Syphilis of bone🖑
    (Ex:) 090.0-099.9

  095.6 Syphilis of muscle🖑
    Syphilitic myositis
    (Ex:) 090.0-099.9

  095.7 Syphilis of synovium, tendon, and bursa🖑
    Syphilitic:
      bursitis
      synovitis
    (Ex:) 090.0-099.9

  095.8 Other specified forms of late symptomatic syphilis🖑
    Excludes *cardiovascular syphilis (093.0–093.9)*
      neurosyphilis (094.0–094.9)

  095.9 Late symptomatic syphilis, unspecified🖑
    (Ex:) 090.0-099.9

096 Late syphilis, latent
  Syphilis (acquired) without clinical manifestations, with positive serological reaction and negative spinal fluid test, two years or more after infection

● **097 Other and unspecified syphilis**

  097.0 Late syphilis, unspecified

  097.1 Latent syphilis, unspecified
    Positive serological reaction for syphilis

  097.9 Syphilis, unspecified
    Syphilis (acquired) NOS

    Excludes *syphilis NOS causing death under two years of age (090.9)*

◀ New   ◀▥ Revised   ~~deleted~~ Deleted   ● Unacceptable Principal Diagnosis   ● Use Additional Digit(s)
▶ Manifestation Code   OGCR Official Guidelines   Coding Clinic   Excludes   Includes   Use additional   Code first   Omit code

INFECTIOUS AND PARASITIC DISEASES (001–139)

● **098 Gonococcal infections**

STD (sexually transmitted disease) caused by Neisseria gonorrhoeae that flourishes in the warm, moist areas of the reproductive tract. Untreated gonorrhea spreads to other parts of the body, causing inflammation of the testes or prostate or pelvic inflammatory disease (PID).

098.0 Acute, of lower genitourinary tract 🦠

Gonococcal:
Bartholinitis (acute)
Female only: Bartholin gland
urethritis (acute)
vulvovaginitis (acute)
Gonorrhea (acute):
NOS
genitourinary (tract) NOS
Ⓔ 098.0-098.39, 098.89, 099.40-099.9 139.8

● **098.1 Acute, of upper genitourinary tract**

098.10 Gonococcal infection (acute) of upper genitourinary tract, site unspecified 🦠
Ⓔ 098.0-098.39, 098.89, 099.40-099.9 139.8

098.11 Gonococcal cystitis (acute) 🦠
Gonorrhea (acute) of bladder
Ⓔ 098.0-098.39, 098.89, 099.40-099.9 139.8

098.12 Gonococcal prostatitis (acute) ♂ 🦠
Ⓔ 098.0-098.39, 098.89, 099.40-099.9 139.8

098.13 Gonococcal epididymo-orchitis (acute) ♂ 🦠
Gonococcal orchitis (acute)
Ⓔ 098.0-098.39, 098.89, 099.40-099.9 139.8

098.14 Gonococcal seminal vesiculitis (acute) ♂ 🦠
Gonorrhea (acute) of seminal vesicle
Ⓔ 098.0-098.39, 098.89, 099.40-099.9 139.8

098.15 Gonococcal cervicitis (acute) ♀ 🦠
Gonorrhea (acute) of cervix
Ⓔ 098.0-098.39, 098.89, 099.40-099.9 139.8

098.16 Gonococcal endometritis (acute) ♀ 🦠
Gonorrhea (acute) of uterus
Ⓔ 098.0-098.39, 098.89, 099.40-099.9 139.8

098.17 Gonococcal salpingitis, specified as acute ♀ 🦠
Ⓔ 098.0-098.39, 098.89, 099.40-099.9 139.8

098.19 Other 🦠
Ⓔ 098.0-098.39, 098.89, 099.40-099.9 139.8

098.2 Chronic, of lower genitourinary tract

Gonococcal specified as chronic or with duration of two months or more:
Bartholinitis specified as chronic or with duration of two months or more
urethritis specified as chronic or with duration of two months or more
vulvovaginitis specified as chronic or with duration of two months or more
Gonorrhea specified as chronic or with duration of two months or more:
NOS specified as chronic or with duration of two months or more
genitourinary (tract) specified as chronic or with duration of two months or more
Any condition classifiable to 098.0 specified as chronic or with duration of two months or more

● **098.3 Chronic, of upper genitourinary tract**

Any condition classifiable to 098.1 stated as chronic or with a duration of two months or more

098.30 Chronic gonococcal infection of upper genitourinary tract, site unspecified

098.31 Gonococcal cystitis, chronic
Any condition classifiable to 098.11, specified as chronic
Gonorrhea of bladder, chronic

098.32 Gonococcal prostatitis, chronic ♂
Any condition classifiable to 098.12, specified as chronic

098.33 Gonococcal epididymo-orchitis, chronic ♂
Any condition classifiable to 098.13, specified as chronic
Chronic gonococcal orchitis

098.34 Gonococcal seminal vesiculitis, chronic ♂
Any condition classifiable to 098.14, specified as chronic
Gonorrhea of seminal vesicle, chronic

098.35 Gonococcal cervicitis, chronic ♀
Any condition classifiable to 098.15, specified as chronic
Gonorrhea of cervix, chronic

098.36 Gonococcal endometritis, chronic ♀
Any condition classifiable to 098.16, specified as chronic

098.37 Gonococcal salpingitis (chronic) ♀

098.39 Other

● **098.4 Gonococcal infection of eye**

098.40 Gonococcal conjunctivitis (neonatorum) 🦠
Neonate = newborn
Gonococcal ophthalmia (neonatorum)
Ⓔ 090.0-099.9

098.41 Gonococcal iridocyclitis 🦠
Ⓔ 090.0-099.9

098.42 Gonococcal endophthalmia 🦠
Ⓔ 090.0-099.9

098.43 Gonococcal keratitis 🦠
Ⓔ 090.0-099.9

098.49 Other 🦠
Ⓔ 090.0-099.9

● **098.5 Gonococcal infection of joint**

098.50 Gonococcal arthritis 🦠
Gonococcal infection of joint NOS
Ⓔ 003.23, 015.80, 015.96, 017.90-017.96, 036.82, 056.71, 090.0-099.9, 711.00-714.0, 715.00, 715.09-715.10 715.18-716.99, 718.00-718.08, 719.00-719.10, 719.18-719.69, 719.80-719.99

098.51 Gonococcal synovitis and tenosynovitis 🦠
Ⓔ 003.23, 015.80-015.96, 017.90-017.96, 036.82, 056.71, 090.0-099.9, 711.00-714.0, 715.00, 715.09-715.10, 715.18-716.99, 718.00-718.08, 719.00-719.10, 719.18-719.69, 719.80-719.99

098.52 Gonococcal bursitis 🦠
Ⓔ 003.23, 015.80-015.96, 017.90-017.96, 036.82, 056.71, 090.0-099.9, 711.00-714.0, 715.00, 715.09-715.10, 715.18-716.99, 718.00-718.08, 719.00-719.10, 719.18-719.69, 719.80-719.99

N Newborn Age: 0   **P** Pediatric Age: 0–17   **M** Maternity Age: 12–55   **A** Adult Age: 15–124   ♀ Females Only   ♂ Males Only
Ⓔ CC Exclusions   🦠 Complication\Comorbidity   🦠 Major C\C   Present on Admission Requirement   Hospital-Acquired Condition

759

INFECTIOUS AND PARASITIC DISEASES (001–139)

098.53 Gonococcal spondylitis (Ex)
   (Ex:) 003.23, 015.80-015.96, 017.90-017.96, 036.82, 056.71,
      090.0-099.9, 711.00-714.0, 715.00, 715.09-715.10,
      715.18-716.99, 718.00-718.08, 719.00-719.10,
      719.18-719.69, 719.80-719.99

098.59 Other (Ex)
   Gonococcal rheumatism
   (Ex:) 003.23, 015.80-015.96, 017.90-017.96, 036.82, 056.71,
      090.0-099.9, 711.00-714.0, 715.00, 715.09-715.10,
      715.18-716.99, 718.00-718.08, 719.00-719.10,
      719.18-719.69, 719.80-719.99

098.6 Gonococcal infection of pharynx

098.7 Gonococcal infection of anus and rectum
   Gonococcal proctitis

● **098.8 Gonococcal infection of other specified sites**

098.81 Gonococcal keratosis (blennorrhagica) (Ex)
   (Ex:) 098.40-098.49, 098.81

098.82 Gonococcal meningitis (Ex)
   (Ex:) 003.21, 013.00-013.16, 036.0, 047.0-047.9, 049.0-049.1,
      072.1, 078.88-078.89, 079.81, 079.88-079.99, 090.0-099.9,
      100.81, 112.83, 114.2, 115.01, 115.11, 115.91, 130.0,
      139.8, 320.0-322.9, 349.89-349.9, 357.0

098.83 Gonococcal pericarditis (Ex)
   (Ex:) 074.21, 090.0-099.9, 391.0, 393, 420.0-420.99, 423.3-423.9,
      459.89-459.9

098.84 Gonococcal endocarditis (Ex)
   (Ex:) 002.0, 036.42, 074.22, 083.0, 090.0-099.9, 112.81, 115.94,
      116.0, 390, 391.1, 391.8-392.0, 394.0-395.9, 396.9-397.9,
      398.90, 398.99, 421.0-421.9, 424.0-424.99, 425.3,
      459.89-459.9, 711.00, 711.08-711.09, 746.09, 746.89,
      996.61

098.85 Other gonococcal heart disease (Ex)
   (Ex:) 002.0, 036.42, 074.20, 074.22-074.23, 083.0, 090.0-099.9,
      112.81, 115.94, 116.0, 390, 391.1-392.0, 394.0-395.9,
      396.9-398.90, 398.99, 421.0-422.99, 424.0-424.99, 425.3,
      429.0, 429.71-429.79, 459.89-459.9, 711.00,
      711.08-711.09, 746.09, 746.89, 996.61

098.86 Gonococcal peritonitis (Ex)
   (Ex:) 014.00-014.06, 032.83, 090.0-099.9, 540.0-540.1, 567.0-567.1,
      567.22, 567.29, 567.81, 567.9, 569.89-569.9, 577.8,
      614.5-614.7, 639.0, 670.00-670.04, 777.6, 998.7

098.89 Other (Ex)
   Gonococcemia
   Blood condition
   (Ex:) 090.0-099.9, 588.81-588.89

● **099 Other venereal diseases**

099.0 Chancroid
   Sexually transmitted infection caused by bacteria
     (Haemophilus ducreyi).
   Bubo (inguinal):
     chancroidal
     due to Hemophilus ducreyi
   Chancre:
     Ducrey's simple soft
   Ulcus molle (cutis) (skin)

099.1 Lymphogranuloma venereum
   Climatic or tropical bubo
   (Durand-) Nicolas-Favre disease
   Esthiomene
   Lymphogranuloma inguinale

099.2 Granuloma inguinale
   Donovanosis
   Granuloma pudendi (ulcerating)
   Granuloma venereum
   Pudendal ulcer

099.3 Reiter's disease
   Reiter's syndrome
   Use additional code for associated:
     arthropathy (711.1)
     conjunctivitis (372.33)

● **099.4 Other nongonococcal urethritis [NGU]**

099.40 Unspecified
   Nonspecific urethritis

099.41 Chlamydia trachomatis

099.49 Other specified organism

● **099.5 Other venereal diseases due to Chlamydia trachomatis**

   Excludes *Chlamydia trachomatis infection of*
     conjunctiva (076.0–076.9, 077.0,
     077.9)
     Lymphogranuloma venereum (099.1)

099.50 Unspecified site

099.51 Pharynx

099.52 Anus and rectum

099.53 Lower genitourinary sites

   Excludes *urethra (099.41)*
   Use additional code to specify site of
     infection, such as:
     bladder (595.4)
     cervix (616.0)
     vagina and vulva (616.11)

099.54 Other genitourinary sites

   Use additional code to specify site of
     infection, such as:
     pelvic inflammatory disease NOS (614.9)
     testis and epididymis (604.91)

099.55 Unspecified genitourinary site

099.56 Peritoneum (Ex)
   Perihepatitis
   (Ex:) 014.00-014.06, 032.83, 090.0-099.9, 540.0-540.1, 567.0-567.1,
      567.22, 567.29, 567.81, 567.9, 569.89-569.9, 577.8,
      614.5-614.7, 639.0, 670.00-670.04, 777.6, 998.7

099.59 Other specified site

099.8 Other specified venereal diseases

099.9 Venereal disease, unspecified

OTHER SPIROCHETAL DISEASES (100–104)

● **100 Leptospirosis**

● **100.0 Leptospirosis icterohemorrhagica** (Ex)
   Leptospiral or spirochetal jaundice (hemorrhagic)
   Weil's disease
   (Ex:) 100.0-100.9

● **100.8 Other specified leptospiral infections**

100.81 Leptospiral meningitis (aseptic) (Ex)
   (Ex:) 003.21, 013.00-013.16, 036.0, 047.0-047.9, 049.0-049.1, 072.1
      078.88-078.89, 079.81, 079.88-079.99, 090.42, 091.81,
      094.2, 098.89, 100.0-100.9, 112.83, 114.2, 115.01, 115.11,
      115.91, 130.0, 139.8, 320.0-322.9, 349.89-349.9, 357.0

◀ New　　◀ Revised　　deleted Deleted　　● Unacceptable Principal Diagnosis　　● Use Additional Digit(s)
▶ Manifestation Code　　**OGCR** Official Guidelines　　**Coding Clinic**　　Excludes　　Includes　　Use additional　　Code first　　Omit code

100.89 Other 🅒
Fever:
    Fort Bragg
    pretibial
    swamp
Infection by Leptospira:
    australis
    bataviae
    pyrogenes
    (Ex) 100.0-100.9

100.9 Leptospirosis, unspecified 🅒
    (Ex) 100.0-100.9

101 Vincent's angina 🅒
Acute necrotizing ulcerative:
    gingivitis
    stomatitis
Fusospirochetal pharyngitis
Spirochetal stomatitis
Trench mouth
Vincent's:
    gingivitis
    infection [any site]
    (Ex) 101

● **102 Yaws**

    Includes   frambesia
              pian

102.0 Initial lesions
Chancre of yaws
Frambesia, initial or primary
Initial frambesial ulcer
Mother yaw

102.1 Multiple papillomata and wet crab yaws
Butter yaws
Frambesioma
Pianoma
Plantar or palmar papilloma of yaws

102.2 Other early skin lesions
Cutaneous yaws, less than five years after infection
Early yaws (cutaneous) (macular) (papular)
    (maculopapular) (micropapular)
Frambeside of early yaws

102.3 Hyperkeratosis
Ghoul hand
Hyperkeratosis, palmar or plantar (early) (late) due
    to yaws
Worm-eaten soles

102.4 Gummata and ulcers
Nodular late yaws (ulcerated)
Gummatous frambeside

102.5 Gangosa
Rhinopharyngitis mutilans

102.6 Bone and joint lesions
Goundou of yaws (late)
Gumma, bone of yaws (late)
Gummatous osteitis or periostitis of yaws (late)
Hydrarthrosis of yaws (early) (late)
Osteitis of yaws (early) (late)
Periostitis (hypertrophic) of yaws (early) (late)

102.7 Other manifestations
Juxta-articular nodules of yaws
Mucosal yaws

102.8 Latent yaws
Yaws without clinical manifestations, with positive
    serology

102.9 Yaws, unspecified

● **103 Pinta**

103.0 Primary lesions
Chancre (primary) of pinta [carate]
Papule (primary) of pinta [carate]
Pintid of pinta [carate]

103.1 Intermediate lesions
Erythematous plaques of pinta [carate]
Hyperchromic lesions of pinta [carate]
Hyperkeratosis of pinta [carate]

103.2 Late lesions
Cardiovascular lesions of pinta [carate]
Skin lesions of pinta [carate]:
    achromic of pinta [carate]
    cicatricial of pinta [carate]
    dyschromic of pinta [carate]
Vitiligo of pinta [carate]

103.3 Mixed lesions
Achromic and hyperchromic skin lesions of pinta
    [carate]

103.9 Pinta, unspecified

● **104 Other spirochetal infection**

104.0 Nonvenereal endemic syphilis
Bejel
Njovera

104.8 Other specified spirochetal infections
    Excludes   *relapsing fever (087.0–087.9)*
                  syphilis (090.0–097.9)

104.9 Spirochetal infection, unspecified

MYCOSES (110–118)

Use additional code to identify manifestation, as:
arthropathy (711.6)
meningitis (321.0–321.1)
otitis externa (380.15)

    Excludes   *infection by Actinomycetales, such as species of*
                  Actinomyces, Actinomadura, Nocardia,
                  Streptomyces (039.0–039.9)

● **110 Dermatophytosis**
*Also known as tinea or ringworm; condition of scalp, glabrous
skin, and/or nails. Caused by fungi (dermatophytes).*

    Includes   infection by species of Epidermophyton,
                Microsporum, and Trichophyton
                tinea, any type except those in 111

110.0 Of scalp and beard
Kerion
Sycosis, mycotic
Trichophytic tinea [black dot tinea], scalp

110.1 Of nail
Dermatophytic onychia
Onychomycosis
Tinea unguium

110.2 Of hand
Tinea manuum

110.3 Of groin and perianal area
Dhobie itch
Eczema marginatum
Tinea cruris

110.4 Of foot
Athlete's foot
Tinea pedis

N Newborn Age: 0   **P** Pediatric Age: 0–17   **M** Maternity Age: 12–55   **A** Adult Age: 15–124   ♀ Females Only   ♂ Males Only

(Ex) CC Exclusions   🅒 Complication\Comorbidity   🅒 Major C\C   Present on Admission Requirement   🅒 Hospital-Acquired Condition

761

INFECTIOUS AND PARASITIC DISEASES (001–139)

INFECTIOUS AND PARASITIC DISEASES (001–139)

110.5 Of the body
Herpes circinatus
Tinea imbricata [Tokelau]

110.6 Deep seated dermatophytosis
Granuloma trichophyticum
Majocchi's granuloma

110.8 Of other specified sites

110.9 Of unspecified site
Favus NOS
Microsporic tinea NOS
Ringworm NOS

● **111 Dermatomycosis, other and unspecified**

111.0 Pityriasis versicolor
Infection by Malassezia [Pityrosporum] furfur
Tinea flava
Tinea versicolor

111.1 Tinea nigra
Infection by Cladosporium species
Keratomycosis nigricans
Microsporosis nigra
Pityriasis nigra
Tinea palmaris nigra

111.2 Tinea blanca
Infection by Trichosporon (beigelii) cutaneum
White piedra

111.3 Black piedra
Infection by Piedraia hortai

111.8 Other specified dermatomycoses

111.9 Dermatomycosis, unspecified

Figure 1–8 Oral candidiasis (thrush). *(Courtesy of Stephen Raffanti, MD, MPH.)* (From Mandell, Bennett, & Dolin: Principles and Practice of Infectious Diseases, 6th ed. 2005, Churchill Livingstone, An Imprint of Elsevier)

Item 1–16 Candidiasis, also called oidiomycosis or moniliasis, is a fungal infection. It most often appears on moist cutaneous areas of the body but can also be responsible for a variety of systemic infections such as endocarditis, meningitis, arthritis, and myositis. Antifungal medications cure most yeast infections.

● **112 Candidiasis**

Includes   infection by Candida species
moniliasis

Excludes   *neonatal monilial infection (771.7)*

112.0 Of mouth 🦠
Thrush (oral)
(Ex:) 112.0-112.9, 117.9, 139.8

112.1 Of vulva and vagina ♀
Candidal vulvovaginitis
Monilial vulvovaginitis
Coding Clinic: 1994, Q1, P21

112.2 Of other urogenital sites 🦠 🦠
Candidal balanitis
Male condition only
(Ex:) 112.2, 112.4-112.9, 588.81-588.89
Coding Clinic: 2003, Q4, P105-106; 1996, Q4, P33

112.3 Of skin and nails
Candidal intertrigo
Candidal onychia
Candidal perionyxis [paronychia]

112.4 Of lung 🦠
Candidal pneumonia
(Ex:) 112.0-112.9, 117.9, 139.8
Coding Clinic: 1998, Q2, P7

112.5 Disseminated 🦠
Systemic candidiasis
(Ex:) 112.0-112.9, 117.9, 139.8
Coding Clinic: 1989, Q2, P10

● **112.8 Of other specified sites**

112.81 Candidal endocarditis 🦠
(Ex:) 112.0-112.9, 117.9, 139.8

112.82 Candidal otitis externa 🦠
Otomycosis in moniliasis
(Ex:) 112.0-112.9, 117.9, 139.8

112.83 Candidal meningitis 🦠
(Ex:) 003.21, 013.00-013.16, 036.0, 047.0-047.9, 049.0-049.1, 053.0, 054.72, 072.1, 090.42, 091.81, 094.2, 098.89, 100.81, 112.0-112.9, 114.2, 115.01, 115.11, 115.91, 117.9, 130.0, 139.8, 320.0-322.9, 349.89-349.9, 357.0

112.84 Candidal esophagitis 🦠
(Ex:) 112.0-112.9, 117.9, 139.8

112.85 Candidal enteritis 🦠
(Ex:) 112.0-112.9, 117.9, 139.8

112.89 Other 🦠
(Ex:) 112.4-112.9
Coding Clinic: 1992, Q1, P17; 1991, Q3, P20

112.9 Of unspecified site
Coding Clinic: 1996, Q4, P33

● **114 Coccidioidomycosis**

Includes   infection by Coccidioides (immitis)
Posada-Wernicke disease

114.0 Primary coccidioidomycosis (pulmonary) 🦠
Acute pulmonary coccidioidomycosis
Coccidioidomycotic pneumonitis
Desert rheumatism
Pulmonary coccidioidomycosis
San Joaquin Valley fever
(Ex:) 114.0, 114.3-114.9, 117.9, 139.8

114.1 Primary extrapulmonary coccidioidomycosis 🦠
Chancriform syndrome
Primary cutaneous coccidioidomycosis
(Ex:) 114.0-114.9

114.2 Coccidioidal meningitis 🦠
(Ex:) 003.21, 013.00-013.16, 036.0, 047.0-047.9, 049.0-049.1, 053.0, 054.72, 072.1, 090.42, 091.81, 094.2, 098.89, 100.81, 112.83, 114.2-114.3, 114.9, 115.01, 115.11, 115.91, 117.9, 130.0, 139.8, 320.0-322.9, 349.89-349.9, 357.0

114.3 Other forms of progressive coccidioidomycosis 🦠
Coccidioidal granuloma
Disseminated coccidioidomycosis
(Ex:) 114.3, 114.9, 117.9, 139.8

114.4 Chronic pulmonary coccidioidomycosis 🦠
(Ex:) 114.0-115.99

114.5 Pulmonary coccidioidomycosis, unspecified 🦠
(Ex:) 114.0-115.99

114.9 Coccidioidomycosis, unspecified 🦠
(Ex:) 114.3, 114.9, 117.9, 139.8

◄ New   ◄▥ Revised   ~~deleted~~ Deleted   ● Unacceptable Principal Diagnosis   🦠 Use Additional Digit(s)
▶ Manifestation Code   **OGCR** Official Guidelines   **Coding Clinic**   Excludes   Includes   Use additional   Code first   Omit code

Item 1–17 Bird and bat droppings that fall into the soil give rise to a fungus that can spread airborne spores. When inhaled into the lungs, these spores divide and multiply into lesions. Histoplasmosis capsulatum takes three forms: primary (lodged in the lungs only), chronic (resembles TB), and disseminated (infection has moved to other organs). This is an opportunistic infection in immunosuppressed patients.

● **115   Histoplasmosis**
The following fifth-digit subclassification is for use with category 115:

> 0 **without mention of manifestation**
> 1 **meningitis**
> 2 **retinitis**
> 3 **pericarditis**
> 4 **endocarditis**
> 5 **pneumonia**
> 9 **other**

● **115.0 Infection by Histoplasma capsulatum 2,9🔹, 1,3-5🔹**
[0-5,9]   American histoplasmosis
Darling's disease
Reticuloendothelial cytomycosis
Small form histoplasmosis
For code **115.01**: (Ex) 003.21, 013.00-013.16, 036.0, 047.0-047.9, 049.0-049.1, 053.0, 054.72, 072.1, 090.42, 091.81, 094.2, 098.89, 100.81, 112.83, 114.2, 115.00-115.01, 115.09, 115.11, 115.90-115.91, 115.99, 117.9, 130.0, 139.8, 320.0-322.9, 349.89-349.9, 357.0;
For code **115.02**: (Ex) 115.00, 115.02, 115.09, 115.90, 115.92, 115.99, 117.9, 139.8;
For code **115.03**: (Ex) 115.00, 115.03, 115.09, 115.90, 115.93, 115.99, 117.9, 139.8;
For code **115.04**: (Ex) 115.00, 115.04, 115.09, 115.90, 115.94, 115.99, 117.9, 139 8;
For code **115.05**: (Ex) 115.00, 115.05-115.09, 115.90, 115.95-115.99, 117.9, 139.8, 480.0-480.2, 480.8-487.1, 488, 494.0-508.9, 517.1, 518.89;
For code **115.09**: (Ex) 114.0-115.09

● **115.1 Infection by Histoplasma duboisii 2,9🔹, 1, 3-5🔹**
[0-5,9]   African histoplasmosis
Large form histoplasmosis
For code **115.11**: (Ex) 003.21, 013.00-013.16, 036.0, 047.0-047.9, 049.0-049.1, 053.0, 054.72, 072.1, 090.42, 091.81, 094.2, 098.89, 100.81, 112.83, 114.2, 115.01, 115.10-115.11, 115.19-115.91, 115.99, 117.9, 130.0, 139.8, 320.0-322.9, 349.89-349.9, 357.0;
For code **115.12**: (Ex) 115.10, 115.12, 115.19-115.90, 115.92, 115.99, 117.9, 139.8;
For code **115.13**: (Ex) 115.10, 115.13, 115.19-115.90, 115.93, 115.99, 117.9, 139.8;
For code **115.14**: (Ex) 115.10, 115.14, 115.19-115.90, 115.94, 115.99, 117.9, 139.8;
For code **115.15**: (Ex) 115.05, 115.10, 115.15-115.90, 115.95-115.99, 117.9, 139.8, 480.0-480.2, 480.8-487.1, 488, 494.0-508.9, 517.1, 518.89;
For code **115.19**: (Ex) 115.10, 115.19-115.90, 115.99, 117.9, 139.8

● **115.9 Histoplasmosis, unspecified 2🔹, 1, 3-5🔹**
[0-5,9]   Histoplasmosis NOS
For code **115.91**: (Ex) 003.21, 013.00-013.16, 036.0, 047.0-047.9, 049.0-049.1, 053.0, 054.72, 072.1, 090.42, 091.81, 094.2, 098.89, 100.81, 112.83, 114.2, 115.01, 115.11, 115.91, 115.99, 117.9, 130.0, 139.8, 320.0-322.9, 349.89-349.9, 357.0;
For code **115.92**: (Ex) 115.92, 115.99, 117.9, 139.8;
For code **115.93**: (Ex) 115.93, 115.99, 117.9, 139.8;
For code **115.94**: (Ex) 115.94, 115.99, 117.9, 139.8;
For code **115.95**: (Ex) 115.05, 115.15, 115.95-115.99, 117.9, 139.8

● **116   Blastomycotic infection**
Rare and potentially fatal infections caused by fungus B. dermatitidis inhaled and found in moist soil in temperate climates.

116.0 Blastomycosis 🔹
Blastomycotic dermatitis
Chicago disease
Cutaneous blastomycosis
Disseminated blastomycosis
Gilchrist's disease
Infection by Blastomyces [Ajellomyces] dermatitidis
North American blastomycosis
Primary pulmonary blastomycosis
(Ex) 116.0, 111.79, 139.8

116.1 Paracoccidioidomycosis 🔹
Brazilian blastomycosis
Infection by Paracoccidioides [Blastomyces] brasiliensis
Lutz-Splendore-Almeida disease
Mucocutaneous-lymphangitic paracoccidioidomycosis
Pulmonary paracoccidioidomycosis
South American blastomycosis
Visceral paracoccidioidomycosis
(Ex) 116.1, 117.9, 139.8

116.2 Lobomycosis
Infections by Loboa [Blastomyces] loboi
Keloidal blastomycosis
Lobo's disease

● **117   Other mycoses**
117.0 Rhinosporidiosis
Infection by Rhinosporidium seeberi

117.1 Sporotrichosis
Cutaneous sporotrichosis
Disseminated sporotrichosis
Infection by Sporothrix [Sporotrichum] schenckii
Lymphocutaneous sporotrichosis
Pulmonary sporotrichosis
Sporotrichosis of the bones

117.2 Chromoblastomycosis
Chromomycosis
Infection by Cladosporidium carrionii, Fonsecaea compactum, Fonsecaea pedrosoi, Phialophora verrucosa

117.3 Aspergillosis 🔹
Infection by Aspergillus species, mainly A. fumigatus, A. flavus group, A. terreus group
(Ex) 117.3, 117.9, 139.8
Coding Clinic: 1997, Q4, P40

117.4 Mycotic mycetomas 🔹
Infection by various genera and species of Ascomycetes and Deuteromycetes, such as Acremonium [Cephalosporium] falciforme, Neotestudina rosatii, Madurella grisea, Madurella mycetomii, Pyrenochaeta romeroi, Zopfia [Leptosphaeria] senegalensis
Madura foot, mycotic
Maduromycosis, mycotic

| Excludes | *actinomycotic mycetomas (039.0–039.9)* |

(Ex) 117.4, 117.9, 139.8

N Newborn Age: 0   **P** Pediatric Age: 0–17   **M** Maternity Age: 12–55   **A** Adult Age: 15–124   ♀ Females Only   ♂ Males Only
(Ex) CC Exclusions   🔹 Complication\Comorbidity   🔹 Major C\C   🔹 Present on Admission Requirement   🔹 Hospital-Acquired Condition

117.5 Cryptococcosis 🔵
> Busse-Buschke's disease
> European cryptococcosis
> Infection by Cryptococcus neoformans
> Pulmonary cryptococcosis
> Systemic cryptococcosis
> Torula
> (Ex) 117.5, 117.9, 139.8

117.6 Allescheriosis [Petriellidosis] 🔵
> Infections by Allescheria [Petriellidium] boydii [Monosporium apiospermum]
>
> **Excludes** *mycotic mycetoma (117.4)*
>
> (Ex) 117.6, 117.9, 139.8

117.7 Zygomycosis [Phycomycosis or Mucormycosis] 🔵
> Infection by species of Absidia, Basidiobolus, Conidiobolus, Cunninghamella, Entomophthora, Mucor, Rhizopus, Saksenaea
> (Ex) 117.7, 117.9, 139.8

117.8 Infection by dematiacious fungi [Phaehyphomycosis] 🔵
> Infection by dematiacious fungi, such as Cladosporium trichoides [bantianum], Dreschlera hawaiiensis, Phialophora gougerotii, Phialophora jeanselmi
> (Ex) 117.8-117.9

117.9 Other and unspecified mycoses 🔵
> (Ex) 117.8-117.9
> **Coding Clinic: 1995, Q2, P7**

118 Opportunistic mycoses 🔵
> Infection of skin, subcutaneous tissues, and/or organs by a wide variety of fungi generally considered to be pathogenic to compromised hosts only (e.g., infection by species of Alternaria, Dreschlera, Fusarium)
>
> Use additional code to identify manifestation, such as: keratitis (370.8)
> (Ex) 117.9-118, 139.8

HELMINTHIASES (120–129)

120 Schistosomiasis [bilharziasis]
> *Parasitic disease (worm induced) that leads to chronic illness*

120.0 Schistosoma haematobium 🔵
> Vesical schistosomiasis NOS
> (Ex) 120.0-120.9

120.1 Schistosoma mansoni 🔵
> Intestinal schistosomiasis NOS
> (Ex) 120.0-120.9

120.2 Schistosoma japonicum 🔵
> Asiatic schistosomiasis NOS
> Katayama disease or fever
> (Ex) 120.0-120.9

120.3 Cutaneous 🔵
> Cercarial dermatitis
> Infection by cercariae of Schistosoma
> Schistosome dermatitis
> Swimmers' itch
> (Ex) 120.0-120.9

120.8 Other specified schistosomiasis 🔵
> Infection by Schistosoma:
>   bovis
>   intercalatum
>   mattheii
> Infection by Schistosoma spindale
> Schistosomiasis chestermani
> (Ex) 120.0-120.9

120.9 Schistosomiasis, unspecified 🔵
> Blood flukes NOS   Hemic distomiasis
> (Ex) 120.0-120.9

● **121 Other trematode infections**

121.0 Opisthorchiasis 🔵
> Infection by:
>   cat liver fluke
>   Opisthorchis (felineus) (tenuicollis) (viverrini)
> (Ex) 121.0-121.9

121.1 Clonorchiasis 🔵
> Biliary cirrhosis due to clonorchiasis
> Chinese liver fluke disease
> Hepatic distomiasis due to Clonorchis sinensis
> Oriental liver fluke disease
> (Ex) 121.0-121.9

121.2 Paragonimiasis 🔵
> Infection by Paragonimus
> Lung fluke disease (oriental)
> Pulmonary distomiasis
> (Ex) 121.0-121.9

121.3 Fascioliasis 🔵
> Infection by Fasciola:
>   gigantica
>   hepatica
> Liver flukes NOS
> Sheep liver fluke infection
> (Ex) 121.0-121.9

121.4 Fasciolopsiasis 🔵
> Infection by Fasciolopsis (buski)
> Intestinal distomiasis
> (Ex) 121.0-121.9

121.5 Metagonimiasis 🔵
> Infection by Metagonimus yokogawai
> (Ex) 121.0-121.9

121.6 Heterophyiasis 🔵
> Infection by:
>   Heterophyes heterophyes
>   Stellantchasmus falcatus
> (Ex) 121.0-121.9

121.8 Other specified trematode infections 🔵
> Infection by:
>   Dicrocoelium dendriticum
>   Echinostoma ilocanum
>   Gastrodiscoides hominis
> (Ex) 121.0-121.9

121.9 Trematode infection, unspecified
> Distomiasis NOS
> Fluke disease NOS

● **122 Echinococcosis**
> *Also known as hydatid disease; caused by Echinococcus granulosus, E. multilocularis, and E. vogeli tapeworms; and is contracted from infected food.*
>
> **Includes**   echinococciasis
>   hydatid disease
>   hydatidosis

122.0 Echinococcus granulosus infection of liver 🔵
> (Ex) 122.0, 122.8-122.9

122.1 Echinococcus granulosus infection of lung 🔵
> (Ex) 122.1, 122.8-122.9, 480.3

122.2 Echinococcus granulosus infection of thyroid 🔵
> (Ex) 122.2, 122.8-122.9

122.3 Echinococcus granulosus infection, other 🔵
> (Ex) 122.3, 122.8-122.9

122.4 Echinococcus granulosus infection, unspecified 🔵
> (Ex) 122.4, 122.8-122.9

◀ New   ◀ⅢⅢ Revised   ~~deleted~~ Deleted   ● Unacceptable Principal Diagnosis   ● Use Additional Digit(s)
▶ Manifestation Code   **OGCR** Official Guidelines   **Coding Clinic**   Excludes   Includes   Use additional   Code first   Omit code

INFECTIOUS AND PARASITIC DISEASES (001–139)

122.5 **Echinococcus multilocularis infection of liver**🦠
Ⓔ 122.5, 122.8-122.9

122.6 **Echinococcus multilocularis infection, other**🦠
Ⓔ 122.6, 122.8-122.9

122.7 **Echinococcus multilocularis infection, unspecified**🦠
Ⓔ 122.7-122.9

122.8 **Echinococcosis, unspecified, of liver**🦠
Ⓔ 122.8-122.9

122.9 **Echinococcosis, other and unspecified**🦠
Ⓔ 122.8-122.9

● 123 **Other cestode infection**

123.0 **Taenia solium infection, intestinal form**🦠
Pork tapeworm (adult) (infection)
Ⓔ 001.1, 002.0, 002.9-003.0, 004.9-005.2, 006.0-006.2, 006.9, 007.1-009.0,
014.80-0148.6, 040.41-040.42, 112.85, 123.0-123.9, 129, 487.8,
536.3, 536.8, 558.2-558.9, 564.1, 777.50-777.53, 777.8

123.1 **Cysticercosis**🦠
Cysticerciasis
Infection by Cysticercus cellulosae [larval form of
Taenia solium]
Ⓔ 123.0-123.9
Coding Clinic: 1997, Q2, P8

123.2 **Taenia saginata infection**🦠
Beef tapeworm (infection)
Infection by Taeniarhynchus saginatus
Ⓔ 123.0-123.9

123.3 **Taeniasis, unspecified**🦠
Ⓔ 123.0-123.9

123.4 **Diphyllobothriasis, intestinal**🦠
Diphyllobothrium (adult) (latum) (pacificum)
infection
Fish tapeworm (infection)
Ⓔ 123.0-123.9

123.5 **Sparganosis [larval diphyllobothriasis]**🦠
Infection by:
Diphyllobothrium larvae
Sparganum (mansoni) (proliferum)
Spirometra larvae
Ⓔ 123.0-123.9

123.6 **Hymenolepiasis**🦠
Dwarf tapeworm (infection)
Hymenolepis (diminuta) (nana) infection
Rat tapeworm (infection)
Ⓔ 123.0-123.9

123.8 **Other specified cestode infection**🦠
Diplogonoporus (grandis) infection
Dipylidium (caninum) infection
Dog tapeworm (infection)
Ⓔ 123.0-123.9

123.9 **Cestode infection, unspecified**
Tapeworm (infection) NOS

124 **Trichinosis**🦠
Trichinella spiralis infection
Trichinellosis
Trichiniasis
Ⓔ 013.60-013.66, 046.2, 046.71-046.8, 048-049.0, 049.8, 052.0, 052.2, 054.3, 054.74,
056.01, 057.8-058.29, 059.00-059.9, 062.0-064, 066.2-066.49, 072.2, 073.7,
079.82, 079.99, 081.9, 083.9, 090.41, 094.81, 117.5, 124, 130.0, 290.12,
323.01-323.9, 341.1, 487.8, 771.2, 984.9

● 125 **Filarial infection and dracontiasis**

125.0 **Bancroftian filariasis**🦠
Chyluria due to Wuchereria bancrofti
Elephantiasis due to Wuchereria bancrofti
Infection due to Wuchereria bancrofti
Lymphadenitis due to Wuchereria bancrofti
Lymphangitis due to Wuchereria bancrofti
Wuchereriasis
Ⓔ 125.0-125.9

125.1 **Malayan filariasis**🦠
Brugia filariasis due to Brugia [Wuchereria] malayi
Chyluria due to Brugia [Wuchereria] malayi
Elephantiasis due to Brugia [Wuchereria] malayi
Infection due to Brugia [Wuchereria] malayi
Lymphadenitis due to Brugia [Wuchereria] malayi
Lymphangitis due to Brugia [Wuchereria] malayi
Ⓔ 125.0-125.9

125.2 **Loiasis**🦠
Eyeworm disease of Africa
Loa loa infection
Ⓔ 125.0-125.9

125.3 **Onchocerciasis**🦠
Onchocerca volvulus infection
Onchocercosis
125.0-125.9

125.4 **Dipetalonemiasis**🦠
Infection by:
Acanthocheilonema perstans
Dipetalonema perstans
Ⓔ 125.0-125.9

125.5 **Mansonella ozzardi infection**🦠
Filariasis ozzardi
Ⓔ 125.0-125.9

125.6 **Other specified filariasis**🦠
Dirofilaria infection
Infection by:
Acanthocheilonema streptocerca
Dipetalonema streptocerca
Ⓔ 125.0-125.9

125.7 **Dracontiasis**🦠
Guinea-worm infection
Infection by Dracunculus medinensis
Ⓔ 125.0-125.9

125.9 **Unspecified filariasis**🦠
Ⓔ 125.0-125.9

● 126 **Ancylostomiasis and necatoriasis**

Includes cutaneous larva migrans due to Ancylostoma
hookworm (disease) (infection)
uncinariasis

126.0 **Ancylostoma duodenale**🦠
Ⓔ 126.0-126.9

126.1 **Necator americanus**🦠
Ⓔ 126.0-126.9

126.2 **Ancylostoma braziliense**🦠
Ⓔ 126.0-126.9

126.3 **Ancylostoma ceylanicum**🦠
Ⓔ 126.0-126.9

126.8 **Other specified Ancylostoma**🦠
Ⓔ 126.0-126.9

126.9 **Ancylostomiasis and necatoriasis, unspecified**🦠
Creeping eruption NOS
Cutaneous larva migrans NOS
Ⓔ 126.0-126.9

INFECTIOUS AND PARASITIC DISEASES (001–139)

N Newborn Age: 0   **P** Pediatric Age: 0–17   **M** Maternity Age: 12–55   **A** Adult Age: 15–124   ♀ Females Only   ♂ Males Only
Ⓔ CC Exclusions   🦠 Complication\Comorbidity   🦠 Major C\C   🦠 Present on Admission Requirement   🦠 Hospital-Acquired Condition

765

INFECTIOUS AND PARASITIC DISEASES (001–139)

● 127   **Other intestinal helminthiases**

   127.0   **Ascariasis** ⦿
      Ascaridiasis
      Infection by Ascaris lumbricoides
      Roundworm infection
      (Ex) 127.0-127.9

   127.1   **Anisakiasis** ⦿
      Infection by Anisakis larva
      (Ex) 127.0-127.9

   127.2   **Strongyloidiasis** ⦿
      Infection by Strongyloides stercoralis
      Excludes   *trichostrongyliasis (127.6)*
      (Ex) 127.0-127.9

   127.3   **Trichuriasis** ⦿
      Infection by Trichuris trichiura
      Trichocephaliasis
      Whipworm (disease) (infection)
      (Ex) 127.0-127.9

   127.4   **Enterobiasis** ⦿
      Infection by Enterobius vermicularis
      Oxyuriasis
      Oxyuris vermicularis infection
      Pinworm (disease) (infection)
      Threadworm infection
      (Ex) 127.0-127.9

   127.5   **Capillariasis** ⦿
      Infection by Capillaria philippinensis
      Excludes   *infection by Capillaria hepatica (128.8)*
      (Ex) 127.0-127.9

   127.6   **Trichostrongyliasis** ⦿
      Infection by Trichostrongylus species
      (Ex) 127.0-127.9

   127.7   **Other specified intestinal helminthiasis** ⦿
      Infection by:
        Oesophagostomum apiostomum and related
          species
        Ternidens diminutus
        other specified intestinal helminth
      Physalopteriasis
      (Ex) 127.0-129

   127.8   **Mixed intestinal helminthiasis** ⦿
      Infection by intestinal helminths classified to more
        than one of the categories 120.0–127.7
      Mixed helminthiasis NOS
      (Ex) 127.0-129

   127.9   **Intestinal helminthiasis, unspecified** ⦿
      (Ex) 127.0-129

● 128   **Other and unspecified helminthiases**

   128.0   **Toxocariasis**
      Larva migrans visceralis
      Toxocara (canis) (cati) infection
      Visceral larva migrans syndrome

   128.1   **Gnathostomiasis**
      Infection by Gnathostoma spinigerum and related
        species

   128.8   **Other specified helminthiasis**
      Infection by:
        Angiostrongylus cantonensis
        Capillaria hepatica
        other specified helminth

   128.9   **Helminth infection, unspecified**
      Helminthiasis NOS
      Worms NOS

129   **Intestinal parasitism, unspecified**

Item 1–18   **Toxoplasmosis** is caused by the protozoa **Toxoplasma gondii,** of which the house cat can be a host. Human infection occurs when contact is made with materials containing the pathogen, such as feces, contaminated soil, or ingestion of infected lamb, goat, or pork. Of the infected, very few have symptoms because a healthy person's immune system keeps the parasite from causing illness. When the immune system is compromised, symptoms may occur. Clinical symptoms include flu-like symptoms, but the disease progresses to include the eyes and the brain in babies.

OTHER INFECTIOUS AND PARASITIC DISEASES (130–136)

● 130   **Toxoplasmosis**
      Includes   infection by toxoplasma gondii
                 toxoplasmosis (acquired)
      Excludes   *congenital toxoplasmosis (771.2)*

   130.0   **Meningoencephalitis due to toxoplasmosis** ⦿
      Encephalitis due to acquired toxoplasmosis
      (Ex) 130.0, 130.7-130.9, 139.8

   130.1   **Conjunctivitis due to toxoplasmosis** ⦿
      (Ex) 130.1, 130.7-130.9, 139.8

   130.2   **Chorioretinitis due to toxoplasmosis** ⦿
      Focal retinochoroiditis due to acquired toxoplasmosis
      (Ex) 130.2, 130.7-130.9, 139.8

   130.3   **Myocarditis due to toxoplasmosis** ⦿
      (Ex) 130.3, 130.7-130.9, 139.8

   130.4   **Pneumonitis due to toxoplasmosis** ⦿
      (Ex) 130.4, 130.7-130.9, 139.8, 480.0-480.2, 480.8-487.1, 488, 494.0-508.9,
        517.1 518.89

   130.5   **Hepatitis due to toxoplasmosis** ⦿
      (Ex) 130.5-130.9, 139.8

   130.7   **Toxoplasmosis of other specified sites** ⦿
      (Ex) 130.7-130.9, 139.8

   130.8   **Multisystemic disseminated toxoplasmosis** ⦿
      Toxoplasmosis of multiple sites
      (Ex) 130.7-130.9, 139.8

   130.9   **Toxoplasmosis, unspecified** ⦿
      (Ex) 130.9

● 131   **Trichomoniasis**
      A common STD caused by a parasite, Trichomonas vaginalis,
        affecting both women and men.
      Includes   infection due to Trichomonas (vaginalis)

  ● 131.0   **Urogenital trichomoniasis**

     131.00   **Urogenital trichomoniasis, unspecified**
        Fluor (vaginalis) trichomonal or due to
          Trichomonas (vaginalis)
        Leukorrhea (vaginalis) trichomonal or due
          to Trichomonas (vaginalis)

     131.01   **Trichomonal vulvovaginitis** ♀
        Vaginitis, trichomonal or due to
          Trichomonas (vaginalis)

     131.02   **Trichomonal urethritis**

     131.03   **Trichomonal prostatitis** ♂

     131.09   **Other**

   131.8   **Other specified sites**
      Excludes   *intestinal (007.3)*

   131.9   **Trichomoniasis, unspecified**

◀ New   ◀▦ Revised   ~~deleted~~ Deleted   ● Unacceptable Principal Diagnosis   ● Use Additional Digit(s)
▶ Manifestation Code   **OGCR** Official Guidelines   **Coding Clinic**   Excludes   Includes   Use additional   Code first   Omit code

● 132   **Pediculosis and phthirus infestation**
  Infestation of lice, Pediculus humanus, specifically capitis
   infest the head, corporis infest the body-trunk area, and
   pubis infest the pubic region.

 132.0   Pediculus capitis [head louse]

 132.1   Pediculus corporis [body louse]

 132.2   Phthirus pubis [pubic louse]
   Pediculus pubis

 132.3   Mixed infestation
   This is a combination code.
   Infestation classifiable to more than one of the
    categories 132.0–132.2

 132.9   Pediculosis, unspecified

● 133   **Acariasis**

 133.0   Scabies
   Infestation by Sarcoptes scabiei
   Norwegian scabies
   Sarcoptic itch

 133.8   Other acariasis
   Chiggers
   Infestation by:
    Demodex folliculorum
    Trombicula

 133.9   Acariasis, unspecified
   Infestation by mites NOS

● 134   **Other infestation**

 134.0   Myiasis
   Infestation by:
    Dermatobia (hominis)
    fly larvae
    Gasterophilus (intestinalis)
    maggots
    Oestrus ovis

 134.1   Other arthropod infestation
   Infestation by:
    chigoe
    Jigger disease
    sand flea
    Scarabiasis
    Tunga penetrans
    Tungiasis

 134.2   Hirudiniasis
   Hirudiniasis (external) (internal)
   Leeches (aquatic) (land)

 134.8   Other specified infestations

 134.9   Infestation, unspecified
   Infestation (skin) NOS
   Skin parasites NOS

 135   **Sarcoidosis**
  Symptom of an inflammation producing tiny lumps of cells
   (granulomas) in various organs, most commonly the
   lungs and lymph nodes, that affect organ function.
   Besnier-Boeck-Schaumann disease
   Lupoid (miliary) of Boeck
   Lupus pernio (Besnier)
   Lymphogranulomatosis, benign (Schaumann's)
   Sarcoid (any site):
    NOS
    Boeck
    Darier-Roussy
   Uveoparotid fever

● 136   **Other and unspecified infectious and parasitic diseases**

 136.0   Ainhum
   Dactylolysis spontanea

 136.1   Behçet's syndrome

● **136.2   Specific infections by free-living amebae**

  136.21   Specific infection due to acanthamoeba
   Use additional code to identify
    manifestation, such as:
    keratitis (370.8)
   Coding Clinic: 2008, Q4, P79-81

  **136.29   Other specific infections by free-living
   amebae** 🦠
   Meningoencephalitis due to Naegleria
   (Ex) 136.0-136.9
   Coding Clinic: 2008, Q4, P79-81

 136.3   Pneumocystosis 🦠
   Pneumonia due to Pneumocystis carinii
   Pneumonia due to Pneumocystis jiroveci
   (Ex) 136.3, 139.8, 480.0-480.2, 480.8-487.1, 488, 494.0-508.9, 517.1, 518.89
   Coding Clinic: 2003, Q1, P15; 1987, Nov-Dec, P5-6

 136.4   Psorospermiasis 🦠
   (Ex) 136.0-136.9

 136.5   Sarcosporidiosis 🦠
   Infection by Sarcocystis lindemanni
   (Ex) 136.0-136.9

 136.8   Other specified infectious and parasitic diseases
   Candiru infestation

 136.9   Unspecified infectious and parasitic diseases
   Infectious disease NOS
   Parasitic disease NOS
   Coding Clinic: 1991, Q2, P8

LATE EFFECTS OF INFECTIOUS AND PARASITIC DISEASES (137–139)

Item 1–19   Before you use the late code 137.X, check your
documentation. The original problem (tuberculosis, TB) that
is causing the current late effect (necrosis) must have been
attributable to categories 010–018. A patient who originally
had TB of a joint (015.2X) now has a late effect (137.3), which is
necrosis of bone (730.8). Because there is no active TB, 015.2X
is not coded but serves as an authorization to use the late effect
code. Remember to code the manifestation of the late effect,
which is the current problem (necrosis).

● 137   **Late effects of tuberculosis**
 Note: This category is to be used to indicate conditions
   classifiable to 010–018 as the cause of late effects,
   which are themselves classified elsewhere. The
   "late effects" include those specified as such, as
   sequelae, or as due to old or inactive tuberculosis,
   without evidence of active disease.

 **137.0   Late effects of respiratory or unspecified
   tuberculosis** 🦠

 **137.1   Late effects of central nervous system
   tuberculosis** 🦠

 137.2   Late effects of genitourinary tuberculosis 🦠

 137.3   Late effects of tuberculosis of bones and joints 🦠

 **137.4   Late effects of tuberculosis of other specified
   organs** 🦠

INFECTIOUS AND PARASITIC DISEASES (001–139)

| **N** Newborn Age: 0 | **P** Pediatric Age: 0–17 | **M** Maternity Age: 12–55 | **A** Adult Age: 15–124 | ♀ Females Only | ♂ Males Only |
| (Ex) CC Exclusions | 🦠 Complication\Comorbidity | 🦠 Major C\C | 🦠 Present on Admission Requirement | 🦠 Hospital-Acquired Condition |

767

INFECTIOUS AND PARASITIC DISEASES (001–139)

138 Late effects of acute poliomyelitis 🔖

    Note: This category is to be used to indicate conditions classifiable to 045 as the cause of late effects, which are themselves classified elsewhere. The "late effects" include conditions specified as such, or as sequelae, or as due to old or inactive poliomyelitis, without evidence of active disease.

● **139 Late effects of other infectious and parasitic diseases**

    Note: This category is to be used to indicate conditions classifiable to categories 001–009, 020–041, 046–136 as the cause of late effects, which are themselves classified elsewhere. The "late effects" include conditions specified as such; they also include sequela of diseases classifiable to the above categories if there is evidence that the disease itself is no longer present.

139.0 Late effects of viral encephalitis 🔖

    Late effects of conditions classifiable to 049.8–049.9, 062–064

139.1 Late effects of trachoma 🔖

    Late effects of conditions classifiable to 076

139.8 Late effects of other and unspecified infectious and parasitic diseases 🔖

    Coding Clinic: 2006, Q2, P17-18; 1990, Q3, P14

◄ New   ◄▦ Revised   ~~deleted~~ Deleted   ● Unacceptable Principal Diagnosis   ● Use Additional Digit(s)

▶ Manifestation Code   **OGCR** Official Guidelines   **Coding Clinic**   Excludes   Includes   Use additional   Code first   Omit code

Item 2-1 Neoplasm: Neo = new, plasm = growth, development, formation. This new growth (mass, tumor) can be malignant or benign, which is confirmed by the pathology report. Do not assign a code to a neoplasm until you review the pathology report. Certain CPT codes will specify benign or malignant lesion, so be certain the diagnosis code supports the procedure code.

2. NEOPLASMS (140–239)

1. Content:
   This chapter contains the following broad groups:
   140–195 Malignant neoplasms, stated or presumed to be primary, of specified sites, except of lymphatic and hematopoietic tissue
   196–198 Malignant neoplasms, stated or presumed to be secondary, of specified sites
   199 Malignant neoplasms, without specification of site
   200–208 Malignant neoplasms, stated or presumed to be primary, of lymphatic and hematopoietic tissue
   209 Neuroendocrine tumors
   210–229 Benign neoplasms
   230–234 Carcinoma in situ
   235–238 Neoplasms of uncertain behavior [see Note, at beginning of section 235–238]
   239 Neoplasms of unspecified nature

2. Functional activity
   All neoplasms are classified in this chapter, whether or not functionally active. An additional code from Chapter 3 may be used to identify such functional activity associated with any neoplasm, e.g.:
   catecholamine-producing malignant pheochromocytoma of adrenal:
   code 194.0, additional code 255.6
   basophil adenoma of pituitary with Cushing's syndrome: code 227.3, additional code 255.0

3. Morphology [Histology]
   For those wishing to identify the histological type of neoplasms, a comprehensive coded nomenclature, which comprises the morphology rubrics of the ICD-Oncology, is given after the E-code chapter.

4. Malignant neoplasms overlapping site boundaries
   Categories 140–195 are for the classification of primary malignant neoplasms according to their point of origin. A malignant neoplasm that overlaps two or more subcategories within a three-digit rubric and whose point of origin cannot be determined should be classified to the subcategory .8 "Other." For example, "carcinoma involving tip and ventral surface of tongue" should be assigned to 141.8. On the other hand, "carcinoma of tip of tongue, extending to involve the ventral surface" should be coded to 141.2, as the point of origin, the tip, is known. Three subcategories (149.8, 159.8, 165.8) have been provided for malignant neoplasms that overlap the boundaries of three-digit rubrics within certain systems. Overlapping malignant neoplasms that cannot be classified as indicated above should be assigned to the appropriate subdivision of category 195 (Malignant neoplasm of other and ill-defined sites).

MALIGNANT NEOPLASM OF LIP, ORAL CAVITY, AND PHARYNX (140–149)

> **Excludes** *carcinoma in situ (230.0)*

● **140 Malignant neoplasm of lip**
   Malignant neoplasm is a general term used to describe a cancerous growth or tumor.

> **Excludes** *skin of lip (173.0)*

140.0 Upper lip, vermilion border
   Upper lip: Upper lip:
     NOS   lipstick area
     external

140.1 Lower lip, vermilion border
   Lower lip: Lower lip:
     NOS   lipstick area
     external

140.3 Upper lip, inner aspect
   Upper lip: Upper lip:
     buccal aspect   mucosa
     frenulum   oral aspect

140.4 Lower lip, inner aspect
   Lower lip: Lower lip:
     buccal aspect   mucosa
     frenulum   oral aspect

140.5 Lip, unspecified, inner aspect
   Lip, not specified whether upper or lower:
     buccal aspect
     frenulum
     mucosa
     oral aspect

140.6 Commissure of lip
   Labial commissure

140.8 Other sites of lip
   Malignant neoplasm of contiguous or overlapping sites of lip whose point of origin cannot be determined

140.9 Lip, unspecified, vermilion border
   Lip, not specified as upper or lower:
     NOS
     external
     lipstick area

● **141 Malignant neoplasm of tongue**

141.0 Base of tongue
   Dorsal surface of base of tongue
   Fixed part of tongue NOS
   Coding Clinic: 2006, Q4, P88-91

141.1 Dorsal surface of tongue
   Anterior two-thirds of tongue, dorsal surface
   Dorsal tongue NOS
   Midline of tongue

> **Excludes** *dorsal surface of base of tongue (141.0)*

141.2 Tip and lateral border of tongue

Figure 2-1 Anatomical structures of the mouth and lips. **A.** Transitional or vermilion borders. Lips are connected to the gums by frenulum. **B.** Dorsal surface. **C.** Ventral surface.

Transitional or vermilion surfaces

Lips are connected to
A the gums by frenulum

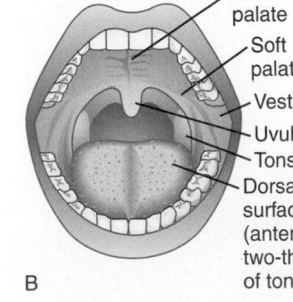

Hard palate
Soft palate
Vestibule
Uvula
Tonsil
Dorsal surface (anterior two-thirds of tongue)
B

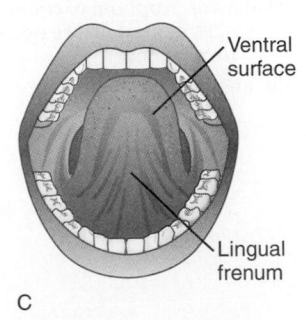

Ventral surface
Lingual frenum
C

N Newborn Age: 0   P Pediatric Age: 0–17   M Maternity Age: 12–55   A Adult Age: 15–124   ♀ Females Only   ♂ Males Only

Ⓔⓧ CC Exclusions   Ⓒ Complication\Comorbidity   Ⓜ Major C\C   Ⓟ Present on Admission Requirement   Ⓗ Hospital-Acquired Condition

769

NEOPLASMS (140–239)

141.3 Ventral surface of tongue
Anterior two-thirds of tongue, ventral surface
Frenulum linguae

141.4 Anterior two-thirds of tongue, part unspecified
Mobile part of tongue NOS

141.5 Junctional zone
Border of tongue at junction of fixed and mobile parts at insertion of anterior tonsillar pillar

141.6 Lingual tonsil

141.8 Other sites of tongue
Malignant neoplasm of contiguous or overlapping sites of tongue whose point of origin cannot be determined

141.9 Tongue, unspecified
Tongue NOS

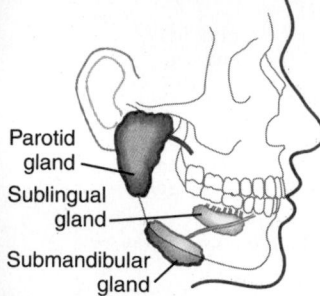

Figure 2–2 Major salivary glands.

Parotid gland
Sublingual gland
Submandibular gland

● **142 Malignant neoplasm of major salivary glands**
   Includes salivary ducts
   Excludes *malignant neoplasm of minor salivary glands:*
       NOS (145.9)
       buccal mucosa (145.0)
       soft palate (145.3)
       tongue (141.0–141.9)
       tonsil, palatine (146.0)

142.0 Parotid gland

142.1 Submandibular gland
Submaxillary gland

142.2 Sublingual gland

142.8 Other major salivary glands
Malignant neoplasm of contiguous or overlapping sites of salivary glands and ducts whose point of origin cannot be determined

142.9 Salivary gland, unspecified
Salivary gland (major) NOS

● **143 Malignant neoplasm of gum**
   Includes alveolar (ridge) mucosa
          gingiva (alveolar) (marginal)
          interdental papillae
   Excludes *malignant odontogenic neoplasms (170.0–170.1)*

143.0 Upper gum

143.1 Lower gum

143.8 Other sites of gum
Malignant neoplasm of contiguous or overlapping sites of gum whose point of origin cannot be determined

143.9 Gum, unspecified

● **144 Malignant neoplasm of floor of mouth**

144.0 Anterior portion
Anterior to the premolar-canine junction

144.1 Lateral portion

144.8 Other sites of floor of mouth
Malignant neoplasm of contiguous or overlapping sites of floor of mouth whose point of origin cannot be determined

144.9 Floor of mouth, part unspecified

● **145 Malignant neoplasm of other and unspecified parts of mouth**
   Excludes *mucosa of lips (140.0–140.9)*

145.0 Cheek mucosa
Buccal mucosa
Cheek, inner aspect

145.1 Vestibule of mouth
Buccal sulcus (upper) (lower)
Labial sulcus (upper) (lower)

145.2 Hard palate

145.3 Soft palate
   Excludes *nasopharyngeal [posterior] [superior] surface of soft palate (147.3)*
   Coding Clinic: 1993, 5th Issue, P16

145.4 Uvula

145.5 Palate, unspecified
Junction of hard and soft palate
Roof of mouth

145.6 Retromolar area

145.8 Other specified parts of mouth
Malignant neoplasm of contiguous or overlapping sites of mouth whose point of origin cannot be determined

145.9 Mouth, unspecified
Buccal cavity NOS
Minor salivary gland, unspecified site
Oral cavity NOS

● **146 Malignant neoplasm of oropharynx**

146.0 Tonsil
Tonsil: Tonsil:
  NOS   palatine
  faucial
   Excludes *lingual tonsil (141.6)*
           pharyngeal tonsil (147.1)
   Coding Clinic: 1987, Sept-Oct, P8

146.1 Tonsillar fossa

146.2 Tonsillar pillars (anterior) (posterior)
Faucial pillar
Glossopalatine fold
Palatoglossal arch
Palatopharyngeal arch

146.3 Vallecula
Anterior and medial surface of the pharyngoepiglottic fold

146.4 Anterior aspect of epiglottis
Epiglottis, free border [margin]
Glossoepiglottic fold(s)
   Excludes *epiglottis:*
       NOS (161.1)
       suprahyoid portion (161.1)

◀ New   ◀▦ Revised   ~~deleted~~ Deleted   ● Unacceptable Principal Diagnosis   ● Use Additional Digit(s)
▶ Manifestation Code   **OGCR** Official Guidelines   **Coding Clinic**   Excludes   Includes   Use additional   Code first   Omit code

146.5 Junctional region
　　Junction of the free margin of the epiglottis, the aryepiglottic fold, and the pharyngoepiglottic fold

146.6 Lateral wall of oropharynx

146.7 Posterior wall of oropharynx

146.8 Other specified sites of oropharynx
　　Branchial cleft
　　Malignant neoplasm of contiguous or overlapping sites of oropharynx whose point of origin cannot be determined

146.9 Oropharynx, unspecified
　　Coding Clinic: 2002, Q2, P6

● **147 Malignant neoplasm of nasopharynx**

　147.0 Superior wall
　　Roof of nasopharynx

　147.1 Posterior wall
　　Adenoid　　　　　　　Pharyngeal tonsil

　147.2 Lateral wall
　　Fossa of Rosenmüller　　Pharyngeal recess
　　Opening of auditory tube

　147.3 Anterior wall
　　Floor of nasopharynx
　　Nasopharyngeal [posterior] [superior] surface of soft palate
　　Posterior margin of nasal septum and choanae

　147.8 Other specified sites of nasopharynx
　　Malignant neoplasm of contiguous or overlapping sites of nasopharynx whose point of origin cannot be determined

　147.9 Nasopharynx, unspecified
　　Nasopharyngeal wall NOS

● **148 Malignant neoplasm of hypopharynx**

　148.0 Postcricoid region
　　Behind the cricoid cartilage of neck

　148.1 Pyriform sinus
　　Pyriform fossa

　148.2 Aryepiglottic fold, hypopharyngeal aspect
　　Aryepiglottic fold or interarytenoid fold:
　　　NOS
　　　marginal zone
　　Excludes　*aryepiglottic fold or interarytenoid fold, laryngeal aspect (161.1)*

　148.3 Posterior hypopharyngeal wall

　148.8 Other specified sites of hypopharynx
　　Malignant neoplasm of contiguous or overlapping sites of hypopharynx whose point of origin cannot be determined

　148.9 Hypopharynx, unspecified
　　Hypopharyngeal wall NOS
　　Hypopharynx NOS

● **149 Malignant neoplasm of other and ill-defined sites within the lip, oral cavity, and pharynx**

　149.0 Pharynx, unspecified

　149.1 Waldeyer's ring

　149.8 Other
　　Malignant neoplasms of lip, oral cavity, and pharynx whose point of origin cannot be assigned to any one of the categories 140–148
　　Excludes　*"book leaf" neoplasm [ventral surface of tongue and floor of mouth] (145.8)*

　149.9 Ill-defined

CERVICAL ESOPHAGUS
Left subclavian artery
First rib
Arch of aorta
Diaphragm
THORACIC ESOPHAGUS
ABDOMINAL ESOPHAGUS
Stomach

Figure 2–3　The esophagus is the muscular tube that connects the pharynx and the stomach. The 10 inch (25 cm) long esophagus is divided into three parts: **cervical, thoracic,** and **abdominal.**

MALIGNANT NEOPLASM OF DIGESTIVE ORGANS AND PERITONEUM (150–159)

Excludes　*carcinoma in situ (230.1–230.9)*

● **150 Malignant neoplasm of esophagus**

　150.0 Cervical esophagus 🦠
　　(Ex:) 150.0-150.9, 159.0, 159.8-159.9, 176.3, 195.8, 199.0-199.2, 209.20, 209.29-209.30, 239.0, 239.8-239.9

　150.1 Thoracic esophagus 🦠
　　(Ex:) 150.0-150.9, 159.0, 159.8-159.9, 176.3, 195.8, 199.0-199.2, 209.20, 209.29-209.30, 239.0, 239.8-239.9

　150.2 Abdominal esophagus 🦠
　　Excludes　*adenocarcinoma (151.0)*
　　　　　　　cardio-esophageal junction (151.0)
　　(Ex:) 150.0-150.9, 159.0, 159.8-159.9, 176.3, 195.8, 199.0-199.2, 209.20, 209.29-209.30, 239.0, 239.8-239.9

　150.3 Upper third of esophagus 🦠
　　Proximal third of esophagus
　　(Ex:) 150.0-150.9, 159.0, 159.8-159.9, 176.3, 195.8, 199.0-199.2, 209.20, 209.29-209.30, 239.0, 239.8-239.9

　150.4 Middle third of esophagus 🦠
　　(Ex:) 150.0-150.9, 159.0, 159.8-159.9, 176.3, 195.8, 199.0-199.2, 209.20, 209.29-209.30, 239.0, 239.8-239.9

　150.5 Lower third of esophagus 🦠
　　Distal third of esophagus
　　Excludes　*adenocarcinoma (151.0)*
　　　　　　　cardio-esophageal junction (151.0)
　　(Ex:) 150.0-150.9, 159.0, 159.8-159.9, 176.3, 195.8, 199.0-199.2, 209.20, 209.29-209.30, 239.0, 239.8-239.9

　150.8 Other specified part 🦠
　　Malignant neoplasm of contiguous or overlapping sites of esophagus whose point of origin cannot be determined
　　(Ex:) 150.0-150.9, 159.0, 159.8-159.9, 176.3, 195.8, 199.0-199.2, 209.20, 209.29-209.30, 239.0, 239.8-239.9

　150.9 Esophagus, unspecified 🦠
　　(Ex:) 150.0-150.9, 159.0, 159.8-159.9, 176.3, 195.8, 199.0-199.2, 209.20, 209.29-209.30, 239.0, 239.8-239.9

N Newborn Age: 0　　**P** Pediatric Age: 0–17　　**M** Maternity Age: 12–55　　**A** Adult Age: 15–124　　♀ Females Only　　♂ Males Only

(Ex:) CC Exclusions　　🦠 Complication\Comorbidity　　Major C\C　　Present on Admission Requirement　　Hospital-Acquired Condition

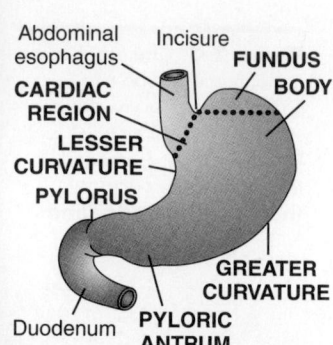

Figure 2–4   Parts of the stomach.

Abdominal esophagus   Incisure
FUNDUS
CARDIAC REGION   **BODY**
LESSER CURVATURE
PYLORUS
Duodenum   **PYLORIC ANTRUM**
GREATER CURVATURE

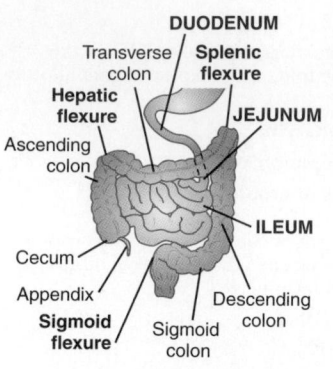

Figure 2–5   Small intestine and colon.

DUODENUM
Transverse colon   **Splenic flexure**
Hepatic flexure   **JEJUNUM**
Ascending colon
Cecum
Appendix
Sigmoid flexure   Sigmoid colon
ILEUM
Descending colon

Item 2–2   The esophagus opens into the stomach through the **cardiac orifice**, also called the **cardioesophageal junction.** The **cardia** is adjacent to the cardiac orifice. The stomach widens into the **greater** and **lesser curvatures.** The **pyloric antrum** precedes the **pylorus,** which opens to the duodenum.

● **151 Malignant neoplasm of stomach**

> Excludes   *benign carcinoid tumor of stomach (209.63)*
> *malignant carcinoid tumor of stomach (209.23)*

151.0 Cardia 🦠
Cardiac orifice
Cardio-esophageal junction

> Excludes   *squamous cell carcinoma (150.2, 150.5)*

(Ex:) 151.0-151.9, 159.0, 159.8-159.9, 176.3, 195.8, 199.0-199.2, 209.20, 209.23, 209.25-209.30, 239.0, 239.8-239.9

151.1 Pylorus 🦠
Prepylorus
Pyloric canal
(Ex:) 151.0-151.9, 159.0, 159.8-159.9, 176.3, 195.8, 199.0-199.2, 209.20, 209.23, 209.25-209.30, 239.0, 239.8-239.9

151.2 Pyloric antrum 🦠
Antrum of stomach NOS
(Ex:) 151.0-151.9, 159.0, 159.8-159.9, 176.3, 195.8, 199.0-199.2, 209.20, 209.23, 209.25-209.30, 239.0, 239.8-239.9

151.3 Fundus of stomach 🦠
(Ex:) 151.0-151.9, 159.0, 159.8-159.9, 176.3, 195.8, 199.0-199.2, 209.20, 209.23, 209.25-209.30, 239.0, 239.8-239.9

151.4 Body of stomach 🦠
(Ex:) 151.0-151.9, 159.0, 159.8-159.9, 176.3, 195.8, 199.0-199.2, 209.20, 209.23, 209.25-209.30, 239.0, 239.8-239.9

151.5 Lesser curvature, unspecified 🦠
Lesser curvature, not classifiable to 151.1–151.4
(Ex:) 151.0-151.9, 159.0, 159.8-159.9, 176.3, 195.8, 199.0-199.2, 209.20, 209.23, 209.25-209.30, 239.0, 239.8-239.9

151.6 Greater curvature, unspecified 🦠
Greater curvature, not classifiable to 151.0–151.4
(Ex:) 151.0-151.9, 159.0, 159.8-159.9, 176.3, 195.8, 199.0-199.2, 209.20, 209.23, 209.25-209.30, 239.0, 239.8-239.9

151.8 Other specified sites of stomach 🦠
Anterior wall, not classifiable to 151.0–151.4
Posterior wall, not classifiable to 151.0–151.4
Malignant neoplasm of contiguous or overlapping sites of stomach whose point of origin cannot be determined
(Ex:) 151.0-151.9, 159.0, 159.8-159.9, 176.3, 195.8, 199.0-199.2, 209.20, 209.23, 209.25-209.30, 239.0, 239.8-239.9

151.9 Stomach, unspecified 🦠
Carcinoma ventriculi
Gastric cancer
(Ex:) 151.0-151.9, 159.0, 159.8-159.9, 176.3, 195.8, 199.0-199.2, 209.20, 209.23, 209.25-209.30, 239.0, 239.8-239.9
Coding Clinic: 2001, Q2, P17-18; 1988, Q2, P11

● **152 Malignant neoplasm of small intestine, including duodenum**

> Excludes   *benign carcinoid tumor of small intestine and duodenum (209.40-209.43)*
> *malignant carcinoid tumor of small intestine and duodenum (209.00-209.03)*

152.0 Duodenum 🦠
(Ex:) 152.0, 152.8-152.9, 159.0, 159.8-159.9, 176.3, 195.8, 199.0-199.2, 209.00-209.01, 209.20, 209.29-209.30, 239.0, 239.8-239.9

152.1 Jejunum 🦠
(Ex:) 152.1, 152.8-152.9, 159.0, 159.8-159.9, 176.3, 195.8, 199.0-199.2, 209.00, 209.02, 209.20, 209.29-209.30, 239.0, 239.8-239.9

152.2 Ileum 🦠

> Excludes   *ileocecal valve (153.4)*

(Ex:) 152.2, 152.8-152.9, 159.0, 159.8-159.9 176.3, 195.8, 199.0-199.2, 209.00, 209.03 209.20, 209.29-209.30, 239.0, 239.8-239.9

152.3 Meckel's diverticulum 🦠
(Ex:) 152.3-152.9, 159.0, 159.8-159.9, 176.3 195.8, 199.0-199.2, 209.00, 209.20, 209.29-209.30, 239.0, 239.8-239.9

152.8 Other specified sites of small intestine 🦠
Duodenojejunal junction
Malignant neoplasm of contiguous or overlapping sites of small intestine whose point of origin cannot be determined
(Ex:) 152.8-152.9, 159.0, 159.8-159.9, 176.3, 195.8, 199.0-199.2, 209.00, 209.20, 209.29-209.30, 239.0, 239.8-239.9

152.9 Small intestine, unspecified 🦠
(Ex:) 152.8-152.9, 159.0, 159.8-159.9, 176.3 195.8, 199.0-199.2, 209.00, 209.20, 209.29-209.30, 239.0, 239.8-239.9

● 153 **Malignant neoplasm of colon**

> **Excludes** *benign carcinoid tumor of colon (209.50-*
> *209.56)*
> *malignant carcinoid tumor of colon*
> *(209.10-209.16)*

153.0 Hepatic flexure🖢

Flexure is a bending in a structure or organ. Note the three flexures illustrated in Figure 2–5. Hepatic = liver, sigmoid = colon, splenic = spleen.

(Ex:) 153.0, 153.8-153.9, 159.0, 159.8-159.9, 176.3, 195.8, 199.0-199.2, 209.10, 209.20, 209.29-209.30, 239.0, 239.8-239.9

153.1 Transverse colon🖢

(Ex:) 153.1, 153.8-153.9, 159.0, 159.8-159.9, 176.3, 195.8, 199.0-199.2, 209.10, 209.14, 209.20, 209.29-209.30, 239.0, 239.8-239.9

153.2 Descending colon🖢

Left colon

(Ex:) 153.2, 153.8-153.9, 159.0, 159.8-159.9, 176.3, 195.8, 199.0-199.2, 209.10, 209.15, 209.20, 209.29-209.30, 239.0, 239.8-239.9

Coding Clinic: 1995, Q1, P4

153.3 Sigmoid colon🖢

Sigmoid (flexure)

> **Excludes** *rectosigmoid junction (154.0)*

Flexure is a bending in a structure or organ. Note the three flexures illustrated in Figure 2–5. Hepatic = liver, sigmoid = colon, splenic = spleen.

(Ex:) 153.3, 153.8-153.9, 159.0, 159.8-159.9, 176.3, 195.8, 199.0-199.2, 209.10, 209.16, 209.20, 209.29-209.30, 239.0, 239.8-239.9

153.4 Cecum🖢

Ileocecal valve

(Ex:) 153.4, 153.8-153.9, 159.0, 159.8-159.9, 176.3, 195.8, 199.0-199.2, 209.10, 209.12, 209.20, 209.29-209.30, 239.0, 239.8-239.9

153.5 Appendix🖢

(Ex:) 153.5, 153.8-153.9, 159.0, 159.8-159.9, 176.3, 195.8, 199.0-199.2, 209.10-209.11, 209.20, 209.29-209.30, 239.0, 239.8-239.9

153.6 Ascending colon🖢

Right colon

(Ex:) 153.6, 153.8-153.9, 159.0, 159.8-159.9, 176.3, 195.8, 199.0-199.2, 209.10, 209.13, 209.20, 209.29-209.30, 239.0, 239.8-239.9

153.7 Splenic flexure🖢

Flexure is a bending in a structure or organ. Note the three flexures illustrated in Figure 2–5. Hepatic = liver, sigmoid = colon, splenic = spleen.

(Ex:) 153.7-153.9, 159.0, 159.8-159.9, 176.3, 195.8, 199.0-199.2, 209.10, 209.20, 209.29-209.30, 239.0, 239.8-239.9

153.8 Other specified sites of large intestine🖢

Malignant neoplasm of contiguous or overlapping sites of colon whose point of origin cannot be determined

> **Excludes** *ileocecal valve (153.4)*
> *rectosigmoid junction (154.0)*

(Ex:) 153.8-153.9, 159.0, 159.8-159.9, 176.3, 195.8, 199.0-199.2, 209.10, 209.20, 209.29-209.30, 239.0, 239.8-239.9

153.9 Colon, unspecified🖢

Large intestine NOS

(Ex:) 153.8-153.9, 159.0, 159.8-159.9, 176.3, 195.8, 199.0-199.2, 209.10, 209.20, 209.29-209.30, 239.0, 239.8-239.9

● 154 **Malignant neoplasm of rectum, rectosigmoid junction, and anus**

> **Excludes** *benign carcinoid tumor of rectum (209.57)*
> *malignant carcinoid tumor of rectum (209.17)*

154.0 Rectosigmoid junction🖢

Colon with rectum
Rectosigmoid (colon)

(Ex:) 154.0, 154.8, 159.0, 159.8-159.9, 176.3, 195.8, 199.0-199.2, 209.20, 209.29-209.30, 239.0, 239.8-239.9

154.1 Rectum🖢

Rectal ampulla

(Ex:) 154.1, 154.8, 159.0, 159.8-159.9, 176.3, 195.8, 199.0-199.2, 209.17-209.20, 209.29-209.30, 239.0, 239.8-239.9

154.2 Anal canal🖢

Anal sphincter

> **Excludes** *skin of anus (172.5, 173.5)*

(Ex:) 154.2-154.8, 159.0, 159.8-159.9, 176.3, 195.8, 199.0-199.2, 209.20, 209.29-209.30, 239.0, 239.8-239.9

Coding Clinic: 2001, Q1, P8

154.3 Anus, unspecified🖢

> **Excludes** *anus:*
> *margin (172.5, 173.5)*
> *skin (172.5, 173.5)*
> *perianal skin (172.5, 173.5)*

(Ex:) 154.2-154.8, 159.0, 159.8-159.9, 176.3, 195.8, 199.0-199.2, 209.20, 209.29-209.30, 239.0, 239.8-239.9

154.8 Other🖢

Anorectum
Cloacogenic zone
Malignant neoplasm of contiguous or overlapping sites of rectum, rectosigmoid junction, and anus whose point of origin cannot be determined

(Ex:) 154.8, 159.0, 159.8-159.9, 176.3, 195.8, 199.0-199.2, 209.20, 209.29-209.30, 239.0, 239.8-239.9

● 155 **Malignant neoplasm of liver and intrahepatic bile ducts**

155.0 Liver, primary🖢

Carcinoma:
liver, specified as primary
hepatocellular
liver cell
Hepatoblastoma

(Ex:) 155.0-155.2, 159.0, 159.8-159.9, 176.3, 195.8, 199.0-199.2, 209.20, 209.29-209.30, 239.0, 239.8-239.9

Coding Clinic: 2008, Q4, P82-83

N Newborn Age: 0   P Pediatric Age: 0–17   M Maternity Age: 12–55   A Adult Age: 15–124   ♀ Females Only   ♂ Males Only

(Ex:) CC Exclusions   🖢 Complication\Comorbidity   🖢 Major C\C   🖢 Present on Admission Requirement   🖢 Hospital-Acquired Condition

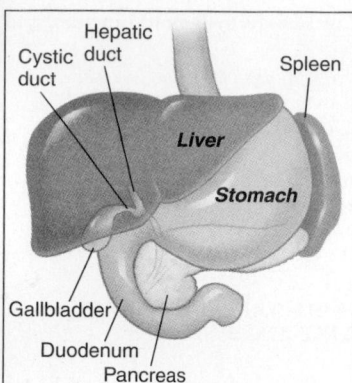

Figure 2-6 Diagram of liver, gallbladder, hepatic duct, pancreas, and spleen. (From Thibodeau and Patton: Anatomy and Physiology, 6th ed. 2007, Mosby)

155.1 Intrahepatic bile ducts 🖐
Canaliculi biliferi
Interlobular:
  bile ducts
  biliary canals
Intrahepatic:
  biliary passages
  canaliculi
  gall duct
> Excludes hepatic duct (156.1)

Ex: 155.0-155.2, 159.0, 159.8-159.9, 176.3, 195.8, 199.0-199.2, 209.20, 209.29-209.30, 239.0, 239.8-239.9

155.2 Liver, not specified as primary or secondary 🖐
Stated as a liver neoplasm, but not specific as to type
Ex: 155.0-155.2, 159.0, 159.8-159.9, 176.3, 195.8, 199.0-199.2, 209.20, 209.29-209.30, 239.0, 239.8-239.9

● **156 Malignant neoplasm of gallbladder and extrahepatic bile ducts**
Extrahepatic = outside the liver

156.0 Gallbladder 🖐
Ex: 156.0, 156.8-156.9, 159.0, 159.8-159.9, 176.3, 195.8, 199.0-199.2, 209.20, 209.29-209.30, 239.0, 239.8-239.9

156.1 Extrahepatic bile ducts 🖐
Biliary duct or passage
NOS
Common bile duct
Cystic duct
Hepatic duct
Sphincter of Oddi
Ex: 156.1, 156.8-156.9, 159.0, 159.8-159.9, 176.3, 195.8, 199.0-199.2, 209.20, 209.29-209.30, 239.0, 239.8-239.9

156.2 Ampulla of Vater 🖐
Ex: 156.2-156.9, 159.0, 159.8-159.9, 176.3, 195.8, 199.0-199.2, 209.20, 209.29-209.30, 239.0, 239.8-239.9

156.8 Other specified sites of gallbladder and extrahepatic bile ducts 🖐
Malignant neoplasm of contiguous or overlapping sites of gallbladder and extrahepatic bile ducts whose point of origin cannot be determined
Ex: 156.8-156.9, 159.0, 159.8-159.9, 176.3, 195.8, 199.0-199.2, 209.20, 209.29-209.30, 239.0, 239.8-239.9

156.9 Biliary tract, part unspecified 🖐
Malignant neoplasm involving both intrahepatic and extrahepatic bile ducts
Intra = inside; extra = outside
Ex: 156.8-156.9, 159.0, 159.8-159.9, 176.3, 195.8, 199.0-199.2, 209.20, 209.29-209.30, 239.0, 239.8-239.9

● **157 Malignant neoplasm of pancreas**
Check documentation for specific site.

157.0 Head of pancreas 🖐
Ex: 157.0-157.9, 159.0, 159.8-159.9, 176.3, 195.8, 199.0-199.2, 209.20, 209.29-209.30, 239.0, 239.8-239.9
Coding Clinic: 2005, Q2, P9-10; 2000, Q4, P39-40

157.1 Body of pancreas 🖐
Ex: 157.0-157.9, 159.0, 159.8-159.9, 176.3, 195.8, 199.0-199.2, 209.20, 209.29-209.30, 239.0, 239.8-239.9

157.2 Tail of pancreas 🖐
Ex: 157.0-157.9, 159.0, 159.8-159.9, 176.3, 195.8, 199.0-199.2, 209.20, 209.29-209.30, 239.0, 239.8-239.9

157.3 Pancreatic duct 🖐
Duct of:
  Santorini
  Wirsung
Ex: 157.0-157.9, 159.0, 159.8-159.9, 176.3, 195.8, 199.0-199.2, 209.20, 209.29-209.30, 239.0, 239.8-289.9

Item 2-3 Islets of Langerhans (endocrine producing cells comprising 1% to 2% of the pancreatic mass) make and secrete hormones that regulate the body's production of insulin, glucagon, and stomach acid. Breakdown of the insulin-producing cells can cause diabetes mellitus.
Islet cell tumors can be benign or malignant and include glucagonomas, insulinomas, gastrinomas, and neuroendocrine tumor. The neoplasm table must be consulted for the correct neoplasm code.

157.4 Islets of Langerhans 🖐
Islets of Langerhans, any part of pancreas
Use additional code to identify any functional activity
Ex: 157.0-157.9, 159.0, 159.8-159.9, 176.3, 195.8, 199.0-199.2, 209.20, 209.29- 209.30, 239.0, 239.8-239.9
Coding Clinic: 2007, Q4, P70-72

157.8 Other specified sites of pancreas 🖐
Ectopic pancreatic tissue
Malignant neoplasm of contiguous or overlapping sites of pancreas whose point of origin cannot be determined
Ex: 157.0-157.9, 159.0, 159.8-159.9, 176.3, 195.8, 199.0-199.2, 209.20, 209.29-209.30, 239.0, 239.8-239.9

157.9 Pancreas, part unspecified 🖐
Ex: 157.0-157.9, 159.0, 159.8-159.9, 176.3, 195.8, 199.0-199.2, 209.20, 209.29-209.30, 239.0, 239.8-239.9
Coding Clinic: 1989, Q4, P11

● **158 Malignant neoplasm of retroperitoneum and peritoneum**

158.0 Retroperitoneum 🖐
Periadrenal tissue
Perinephric tissue
Perirenal tissue
Retrocecal tissue
Ex: 158.0, V58.0

158.8 Specified parts of peritoneum 🖐
Cul-de-sac (of Douglas)
Mesentery
Mesocolon
Omentum
Peritoneum:
  parietal
  pelvic
Rectouterine pouch
Malignant neoplasm of contiguous or overlapping sites of retroperitoneum and peritoneum whose point of origin cannot be determined
Ex: 158.0-158.9, V58.0

158.9 Peritoneum, unspecified 🖐
Ex: 158.0-158.9, V58.0

NEOPLASMS (140-239)

◄ New   ◄▮▮▮ Revised   ~~deleted~~ Deleted   ● Unacceptable Principal Diagnosis   ● Use Additional Digit(s)
▶ Manifestation Code   **OGCR** Official Guidelines   **Coding Clinic**   Excludes   Includes   Use additional   Code first   Omit code

●**159 Malignant neoplasm of other and ill-defined sites within the digestive organs and peritoneum**

159.0 Intestinal tract, part unspecified
Intestine NOS

159.1 Spleen, not elsewhere classified
Angiosarcoma of spleen
Fibrosarcoma of spleen

| Excludes | *Hodgkin's disease (201.0–201.9)*
lymphosarcoma (200.1)
reticulosarcoma (200.0) |

159.8 Other sites of digestive system and intra-abdominal organs
Malignant neoplasm of digestive organs and peritoneum whose point of origin cannot be assigned to any one of the categories 150–158

| Excludes | *anus and rectum (154.8)*
cardio-esophageal junction (151.0)
colon and rectum (154.0) |

159.9 Ill-defined
Alimentary canal or tract NOS
Gastrointestinal tract NOS

| Excludes | *abdominal NOS (195.2)*
intra-abdominal NOS (195.2) |

MALIGNANT NEOPLASM OF RESPIRATORY AND INTRATHORACIC ORGANS (160–165)

| Excludes | *carcinoma in situ (231.0–231.9)* |

●**160 Malignant neoplasm of nasal cavities, middle ear, and accessory sinuses**

160.0 Nasal cavities
Cartilage of nose
Conchae, nasal
Internal nose
Septum of nose
Vestibule of nose

| Excludes | *nasal bone (170.0)*
nose NOS (195.0)
olfactory bulb (192.0)
posterior margin of septum and choanae (147.3)
skin of nose (172.3, 173.3)
turbinates (170.0) |

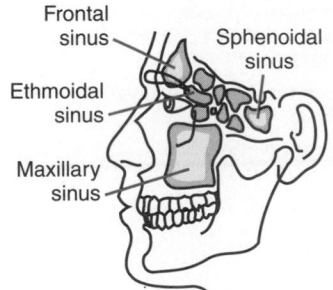

Frontal sinus
Sphenoidal sinus
Ethmoidal sinus
Maxillary sinus

Figure 2–7 Paranasal sinuses. (From Buck CJ: Step-by-Step Medical Coding, 2006 ed. Philadelphia, WB Saunders, 2006.)

160.1 Auditory tube, middle ear, and mastoid air cells
Antrum tympanicum
Eustachian tube
Tympanic cavity

| Excludes | *auditory canal (external) (172.2, 173.2)*
bone of ear (meatus) (170.0)
cartilage of ear (171.0)
ear (external) (skin) (172.2, 173.2) |

160.2 Maxillary sinus
Antrum (Highmore) (maxillary)

160.3 Ethmoidal sinus

160.4 Frontal sinus

160.5 Sphenoidal sinus

160.8 Other
Malignant neoplasm of contiguous or overlapping sites of nasal cavities, middle ear, and accessory sinuses whose point of origin cannot be determined

160.9 Accessory sinus, unspecified

●**161 Malignant neoplasm of larynx**

161.0 Glottis
Intrinsic larynx
Laryngeal commissure (anterior) (posterior)
True vocal cord
True vocal cords (lower vocal folds) produce vocalization when air from lungs passes between them. Check your documentation. Code 161.1 is for malignant neoplasm of false vocal cords.
Vocal cord NOS

161.1 Supraglottis
Aryepiglottic fold or interarytenoid fold, laryngeal aspect
Epiglottis (suprahyoid portion) NOS
Extrinsic larynx
False vocal cords
False vocal cords (upper vocal folds) are not involved in vocalization. Check your documentation. Code 161.0 is for true vocal cords.
Posterior (laryngeal) surface of epiglottis
Ventricular bands

| Excludes | *anterior aspect of epiglottis (146.4)*
aryepiglottic fold or interarytenoid fold:
NOS (148.2)
hypopharyngeal aspect (148.2)
marginal zone (148.2) |

161.2 Subglottis

161.3 Laryngeal cartilages
Cartilage: Cartilage:
arytenoid   cuneiform
cricoid   thyroid

161.8 Other specified sites of larynx
Malignant neoplasm of contiguous or overlapping sites of larynx whose point of origin cannot be determined
Coding Clinic: 2007, Q3, P8-9

161.9 Larynx, unspecified

N Newborn Age: 0   P Pediatric Age: 0–17   M Maternity Age: 12–55   A Adult Age: 15–124   ♀ Females Only   ♂ Males Only
(Ex) CC Exclusions   🔵 Complication\Comorbidity   🔵 Major C\C   🔵 Present on Admission Requirement   🔵 Hospital-Acquired Condition

775

NEOPLASMS (140–239)

● **162 Malignant neoplasm of trachea, bronchus, and lung**

> **Excludes** *benign carcinoid tumor of bronchus (209.61)*
> *malignant carcinoid tumor of bronchus (209.21)*

Coding Clinic: 2006, Q3, P7-8

162.0 Trachea
Cartilage of trachea
Mucosa of trachea
Ex: 162.0-162.9, 165.8-165.9, 176.4, 195.1, 195.8, 197.0-197.1, 197.3, 199.0-199.2, 209.20-209.21, 209.29-209.30, 239.1, 239.8-239.9

162.2 Main bronchus
Carina
Hilus of lung
Ex: 162.2, 162.8-162.9, 165.8-165.9, 176.4, 195.8, 199.0-199.2, 209.20-209.21, 209.29-209.30, 239.1, 239.8-239.9

162.3 Upper lobe, bronchus or lung
Ex: 162.3, 162.8-162.9, 165.8-165.9, 176.4, 195.8, 199.0-199.2, 209.20-209.21, 209.29-209.30, 239.1, 239.8-239.9

Coding Clinic: 2004, Q1, P4-5

162.4 Middle lobe, bronchus or lung
Ex: 162.4, 162.8-162.9, 165.8-165.9, 176.4, 195.8, 199.0-199.2, 209.20-209.21, 209.29-209.30, 239.1, 239.8-239.9

162.5 Lower lobe, bronchus or lung
Ex: 162.5-162.9, 165.8-165.9, 176.4, 195.8, 199.0-199.2, 209.20-209.21, 209.29-209.30, 239.1, 239.8-239.9

162.8 Other parts of bronchus or lung
Malignant neoplasm of contiguous or overlapping sites of bronchus or lung whose point of origin cannot be determined
Ex: 162.8-162.9, 165.8-165.9, 176.4, 195.8, 199.0-199.2, 209.20-209.21, 209.29-209.30, 239.1, 239.8-239.9

Coding Clinic: 2006, Q3, P7-8

162.9 Bronchus and lung, unspecified
Ex: 162.8-162.9, 165.8-165.9, 176.4, 195.8, 199.0-199.2, 209.20-209.21, 209.29-209.30, 239.1, 239.8-239.9

Coding Clinic: 2006, Q3, P14-15; 1997, Q2, P3; 1996, Q4, P47-48; 1993, Q4, P 36;1988, Q2, P10; 1984, May-June, P11, 14

● **163 Malignant neoplasm of pleura**
Pleura are comprised of serous membrane that lines thoracic cavity (parietal) and covers lungs (visceral).

163.0 Parietal pleura
Ex: 163.0-163.9, 165.8-165.9, 195.8, 199.0-199.2, 209.20, 209.29-209.30, 239.1, 239.8-239.9

163.1 Visceral pleura
Ex: 163.0-163.9, 165.8-165.9, 195.8, 199.0-199.2, 209.20, 209.29-209.30, 239.1, 239.8-239.9

163.8 Other specified sites of pleura
Malignant neoplasm of contiguous or overlapping sites of pleura whose point of origin cannot be determined
Ex: 163.0-163.9, 165.8-165.9, 195.8, 199.0-199.2, 209.20, 209.29-209.30, 239.1, 239.8-239.9

163.9 Pleura, unspecified
Ex: 163.0-163.9, 165.8-165.9, 195.8, 199.0-199.2, 209.20, 209.29-209.30, 239.1, 239.8-239.9

● **164 Malignant neoplasm of thymus, heart, and mediastinum**

164.0 Thymus

> **Excludes** *benign carcinoid tumor of the thymus (209.62)*
> *malignant carcinoid tumor of the thymus (209.22)*

Ex: 164.0, 209.22

164.1 Heart
Endocardium   Myocardium
Epicardium   Pericardium

> **Excludes** *great vessels (171.4)*

Ex: 164.1

164.2 Anterior mediastinum
Ex: 164.2-164.9, 165.8-165.9, 195.8, 199.0-199.2, 209.20, 209.29-209.30, 239.1, 239.8-239.9

164.3 Posterior mediastinum
Ex: 164.2-164.9, 165.8-165.9, 195.8, 199.0-199.2, 209.20, 209.29-209.30, 239.1, 239.8-239.9

164.8 Other
Malignant neoplasm of contiguous or overlapping sites of thymus, heart, and mediastinum whose point of origin cannot be determined
Ex: 164.2-164.9, 165.8-165.9, 195.8, 199.0-199.2, 209.20, 209.29-209.30, 239.1, 239.8-239.9

164.9 Mediastinum, part unspecified
Ex: 164.2-164.9, 165.8-165.9, 195.8, 199.0-199.2, 209.20, 209.29-209.30, 239.1, 239.8-239.9

● **165 Malignant neoplasm of other and ill-defined sites within the respiratory system and intrathoracic organs**

165.0 Upper respiratory tract, part unspecified

165.8 Other
Malignant neoplasm of respiratory and intrathoracic organs whose point of origin cannot be assigned to any one of the categories 160–164

165.9 Ill-defined sites within the respiratory system
Respiratory tract NOS

> **Excludes** *intrathoracic NOS (195.1)*
> *thoracic NOS (195.1)*

◀ New   ◀▦ Revised   ~~deleted~~ Deleted   ● Unacceptable Principal Diagnosis   ● Use Additional Digit(s)
▸ Manifestation Code   **OGCR** Official Guidelines   **Coding Clinic**   Excludes   Includes   Use additional   Code first   Omit code

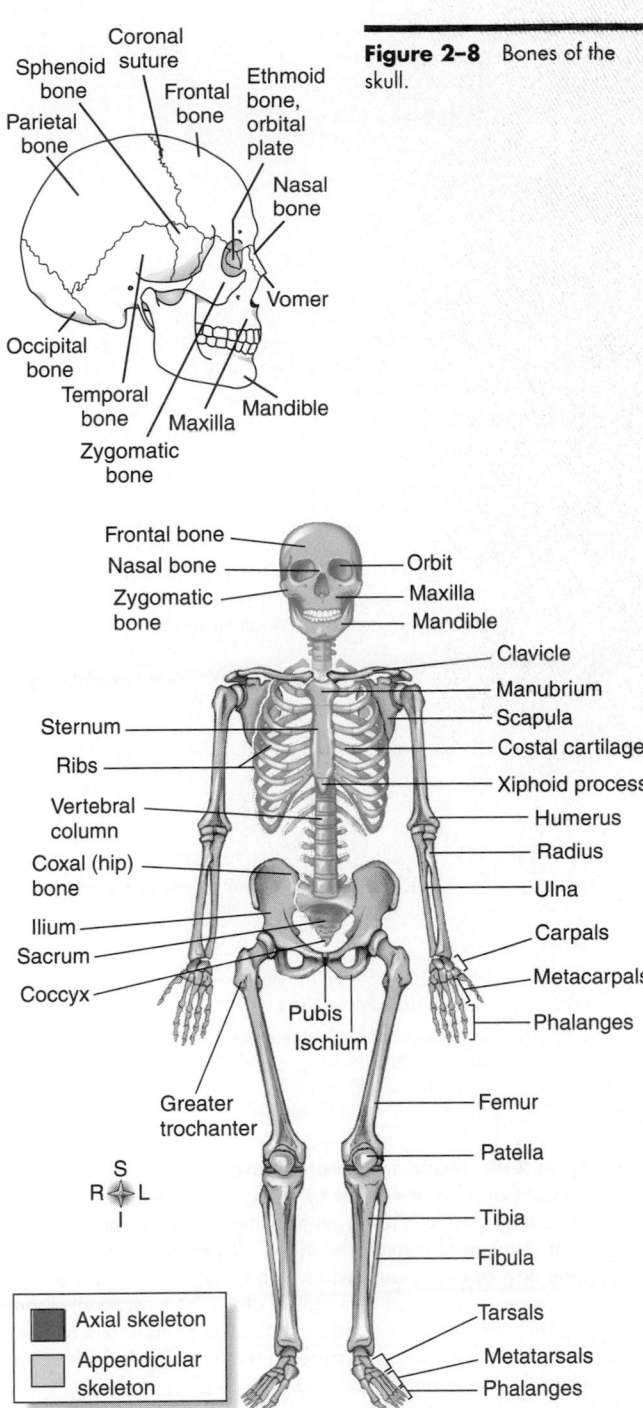

Figure 2-8 Bones of the skull.

Figure 2-9 Diagram of skeleton of trunk and limbs with bones labeled. (From Thibodeau and Patton: Anatomy and Physiology, 6th ed. 2007, Mosby)

MALIGNANT NEOPLASM OF BONE, CONNECTIVE TISSUE, SKIN, AND BREAST (170–176)

> **Excludes** *carcinoma in situ:*
> *breast (233.0)*
> *skin (232.0–232.9)*

● **170 Malignant neoplasm of bone and articular cartilage**

> **Includes** cartilage (articular) (joint)
> periosteum

> **Excludes** *bone marrow NOS (202.9)*
> *cartilage:*
> *ear (171.0)*
> *eyelid (171.0)*
> *larynx (161.3)*
> *nose (160.0)*
> *synovia (171.0–171.9)*

170.0 Bones of skull and face, except mandible🔖

> *Mandible = lower jaw*

Bone:
  ethmoid
  frontal
  malar
  nasal
  occipital
  orbital
  parietal

Bone:
  sphenoid
  temporal
  zygomatic
  Maxilla (superior)
  Turbinate
  Upper jaw bone
  Vomer

> **Excludes** *carcinoma, any type except intraosseous or odontogenic:*
> *maxilla, maxillary (sinus) (160.2)*
> *upper jaw bone (143.0)*
> *jaw bone (lower) (170.1)*

(Ex) 170.0, 170.9, V58.0

170.1 Mandible🔖
Inferior maxilla
Jaw bone NOS
Lower jaw bone

> **Excludes** *carcinoma, any type except intraosseous or odontogenic:*
> *jaw bone NOS (143.9)*
> *lower (143.1)*
> *upper jaw bone (170.0)*

(Ex) 170.1, 170.9, V58.0

170.2 Vertebral column, excluding sacrum and coccyx🔖
Spinal column
Spine
Vertebra

> **Excludes** *sacrum and coccyx (170.6)*

(Ex) 170.2, 170.9, V58.0

170.3 Ribs, sternum, and clavicle🔖
Costal cartilage
Costovertebral joint
Xiphoid process
(Ex) 170.3, 170.9, V58.0

170.4 Scapula and long bones of upper limb🔖
Acromion   Radius
Bones NOS of upper limb   Ulna
Humerus
(Ex) 170.4, 170.9, V58.0
Coding Clinic: 1999, Q2, P9

170.5 Short bones of upper limb🔖
Carpal   Scaphoid (of hand)
Cuneiform, wrist   Semilunar or lunate
Metacarpal   Trapezium
Navicular, of hand   Trapezoid
Phalanges of hand   Unciform
Pisiform
(Ex) 170.5, 170.9, V58.0

N Newborn Age: 0   P Pediatric Age: 0–17   M Maternity Age: 12–55   A Adult Age: 15–124   ♀ Females Only   ♂ Males Only
(Ex) CC Exclusions   🔖 Complication\Comorbidity   🔖 Major C\C   🔖 Present on Admission Requirement   🔖 Hospital-Acquired Condition

777

NEOPLASMS (140–239)

170.6 Pelvic bones, sacrum, and coccyx🔍

    Coccygeal vertebra   Pubic bone
    Ilium   Sacral vertebra
    Ischium
    (Ex:) 170.6, 170.9, V58.0

170.7 Long bones of lower limb🔍

    Bones NOS of lower limb   Fibula
    Femur   Tibia
    (Ex:) 170.7, 170.9, V58.0

170.8 Short bones of lower limb🔍

    Astragalus [talus]   Navicular (of ankle)
    Calcaneus   Patella
    Cuboid   Phalanges of foot
    Cuneiform, ankle   Tarsal
    Metatarsal
    (Ex:) 170.8-170.9, V58.0

170.9 Bone and articular cartilage, site unspecified🔍

    (Ex:) 170.0-170.9, V58.0

● **171   Malignant neoplasm of connective and other soft tissue**

    Includes   blood vessel
                     bursa
                     fascia
                     fat
                     ligament, except uterine
                     muscle
                     peripheral, sympathetic, and parasympathetic
                         nerves and ganglia
                     synovia
                     tendon (sheath)

    Excludes   *cartilage (of):*
                articular (170.0–170.9)
                larynx (161.3)
                nose (160.0)
            connective tissue:
                breast (174.0–175.9)
                internal organs—code to malignant neoplasm of
                   the site [e.g., leiomyosarcoma of stomach,
                   151.9]
                   heart (164.1)
                uterine ligament (183.4)

171.0 Head, face, and neck🔍

    Cartilage of:
        ear
        eyelid
    (Ex:) V58.0
    Coding Clinic: 1999, Q2, P6-7

171.2 Upper limb, including shoulder🔍

    Arm
    Finger
    Forearm
    Hand
    (Ex:) V58.0

171.3 Lower limb, including hip🔍

    Foot
    Leg
    Popliteal space
       Popliteal space = popliteal cavity, popliteal fossa.
         Depression in posterior aspect of knee (behind
         knee).
    Thigh
    Toe
    (Ex:) V58.0

171.4 Thorax🔍

    Axilla
    Diaphragm
    Great vessels

    Excludes   *heart (164.1)*
             mediastinum (164.2–164.9)
             thymus (164.0)
    (Ex:) V58.0

171.5 Abdomen🔍

    Abdominal wall
    Hypochondrium

    Excludes   *peritoneum (158.8)*
             retroperitoneum (158.0)
    (Ex:) V58.0

171.6 Pelvis🔍

    Buttock
    Groin
    Inguinal region
    Perineum

    Excludes   *pelvic peritoneum (158.8)*
             retroperitoneum (158.0)
             uterine ligament, any (183.3–183.5)
    (Ex:) V58.0

171.7 Trunk, unspecified🔍

    Back NOS
    Flank NOS
    (Ex:) V58.0

171.8 Other specified sites of connective and other soft tissue🔍

    Malignant neoplasm of contiguous or overlapping
        sites of connective tissue whose point of
        origin cannot be determined
    (Ex:) V58.0

171.9 Connective and other soft tissue, site unspecified🔍

    (Ex:) V58.0

● **172   Malignant melanoma of skin**

    Includes   melanocarcinoma
                     melanoma in situ of skin
                     melanoma (skin) NOS

    Excludes   *skin of genital organs (184.0–184.9, 187.1–187.9)*
            sites other than skin - code to malignant neoplasm
              of the site

172.0 Lip

    Excludes   *vermilion border of lip (140.0–140.1, 140.9)*

172.1 Eyelid, including canthus

172.2 Ear and external auditory canal

    Auricle (ear)
    Auricular canal, external
    External [acoustic] meatus
    Pinna

Item 2–4   Malignant melanoma is a serious form of skin cancer that affects the melanocytes (pigment-forming cells) and is caused by ultraviolet (UV) rays from the sun that damage skin. It is most commonly seen in the 40- to 60-year-olds with fair skin, blue or green eyes, and red or blond hair who sunburn easily. Melanoma can spread very rapidly and is the most deadly form of skin cancer. It is less common than other types of skin cancer. The rate of melanoma is increasing and currently is the leading cause of death from skin disease.

Figure 2–10 Malignant melanoma of skin. (From Goldman: Cecil Textbook of Medicine, 22nd ed. 2004, Saunders)

◀ New   ⧏ Revised   ~~deleted~~ Deleted   ● Unacceptable Principal Diagnosis   ● Use Additional Digit(s)
▶ Manifestation Code   **OGCR** Official Guidelines   **Coding Clinic**   Excludes   Includes   Use additional   Code first   Omit code

NEOPLASMS (140–239)

172.3 Other and unspecified parts of face

Cheek (external)	Forehead
Chin	Nose, external
Eyebrow	Temple

172.4 Scalp and neck

172.5 Trunk, except scrotum

Axilla	Perianal skin
Breast	Perineum
Buttock	Umbilicus
Groin	

> **Excludes** *anal canal (154.2)*
> *anus NOS (154.3)*
> *scrotum (187.7)*

172.6 Upper limb, including shoulder

Arm	Forearm
Finger	Hand

172.7 Lower limb, including hip

Ankle	Leg
Foot	Popliteal area
Heel	Thigh
Knee	Toe

172.8 Other specified sites of skin
Malignant melanoma of contiguous or overlapping sites of skin whose point of origin cannot be determined

172.9 Melanoma of skin, site unspecified

● **173 Other malignant neoplasm of skin**

> **Includes** malignant neoplasm of:
> sebaceous glands
> sudoriferous, sudoriparous glands
> sweat glands

> **Excludes** *Kaposi's sarcoma (176.0–176.9)*
> *malignant melanoma of skin (172.0–172.9)*
> *skin of genital organs (184.0–184.9, 187.1–187.9)*

Coding Clinic: 2000, Q1, P8; 1996, Q2, P12

173.0 Skin of lip

> **Excludes** *vermilion border of lip (140.0–140.1, 140.9)*

173.1 Eyelid, including canthus

> **Excludes** *cartilage of eyelid (171.0)*

173.2 Skin of ear and external auditory canal
Auricle (ear)
Auricular canal, external
External meatus
Pinna

> **Excludes** *cartilage of ear (171.0)*

173.3 Skin of other and unspecified parts of face
Cheek, external
Chin
Eyebrow
Forehead
Nose, external
Temple
Coding Clinic: 2000, Q1, P3

173.4 Scalp and skin of neck

173.5 Skin of trunk, except scrotum
Axillary fold
Perianal skin
Skin of:
  abdominal wall
  anus
  back
  breast
  buttock
  chest wall
  groin
  perineum
Umbilicus

> **Excludes** *anal canal (154.2)*
> *anus NOS (154.3)*
> *skin of scrotum (187.7)*

Coding Clinic: 2001, Q1, P8

173.6 Skin of upper limb, including shoulder
Arm
Finger
Forearm
Hand

173.7 Skin of lower limb, including hip
Ankle
Foot
Heel
Knee
Leg
Popliteal area
Thigh
Toe

173.8 Other specified sites of skin
Malignant neoplasm of contiguous or overlapping sites of skin whose point of origin cannot be determined

173.9 Skin, site unspecified

● **174 Malignant neoplasm of female breast**
This code is for female breast; see 175 for male breast.

> **Includes** breast (female)
> connective tissue
> soft parts
> Paget's disease of:
> breast
> nipple

> **Use additional** code to identify estrogen receptor status (V86.0, V86.1)

> **Excludes** *skin of breast (172.5, 173.5)*

174.0 Nipple and areola ♀

174.1 Central portion ♀

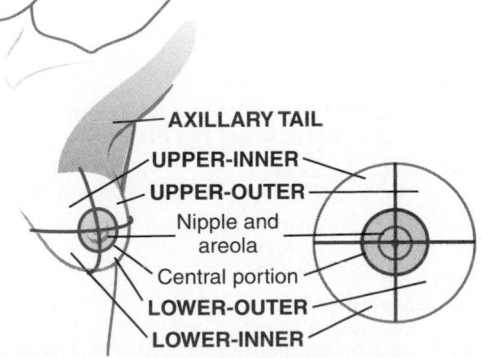

Figure 2–11 Female breast quadrants and axillary tail.

N Newborn Age: 0   P Pediatric Age: 0–17   M Maternity Age: 12–55   A Adult Age: 15–124   ♀ Females Only   ♂ Males Only   779

(Ex) CC Exclusions   ● Complication\Comorbidity   ● Major C\C   ● Present on Admission Requirement   ● Hospital-Acquired Condition

NEOPLASMS (140–239)

174.2 Upper-inner quadrant ♀
Coding Clinic: 1989, Q4, P11

174.3 Lower-inner quadrant ♀
Coding Clinic: 1989, Q4, P11

174.4 Upper-outer quadrant ♀
Coding Clinic: 2008, Q4, P152-155; 2004, Q1, P3-4; 1997, Q3, P8;
1984, May-June, P11

174.5 Lower-outer quadrant ♀

174.6 Axillary tail ♀

174.8 Other specified sites of female breast ♀
Ectopic sites
Inner breast
Lower breast
Malignant neoplasm of contiguous or overlapping
    sites of breast whose point of origin cannot be
    determined
Midline of breast
Outer breast
Upper breast
Coding Clinic: 1985, July-Aug, P11

174.9 Breast (female), unspecified ♀
Coding Clinic: 2005, Q3, P11-12; 1994, Q2, P10x2

● **175 Malignant neoplasm of male breast**
Use additional code to identify estrogen receptor status
    (V86.0, V86.1)
Excludes skin of breast (172.5, 173.5)

175.0 Nipple and areola ♂

175.9 Other and unspecified sites of male breast ♂
Ectopic breast tissue, male

Item 2–5 Kaposi's sarcoma is a cancer that causes
patches of abnormal tissue to grow under the skin; in the
lining of the mouth, nose, and throat; or in other organs, often
beginning and spreading to other organs. Patients who have
had organ transplants or patients with AIDS are at high risk for
this malignancy.

● **176 Kaposi's sarcoma**
176.0 Skin 🦠
(Ex) 176.0, 176.8-176.9, V58.0
Coding Clinic: 2007, Q4, P61-64

176.1 Soft tissue 🦠
Blood vessel   Ligament
Connective tissue   Lymphatic(s) NEC
Fascia   Muscle
Excludes lymph glands and nodes (176.5)
(Ex) 176.1, 176.8-176.9, V58.0

176.2 Palate 🦠
(Ex) 176.2, 176.8-176.9, V58.0

176.3 Gastrointestinal sites 🦠
(Ex) 176.3, 176.8-176.9, V58.0

176.4 Lung 🦠
(Ex) 162.8-162.9, 165.8-165.9, 176.4, 195.8 199.0-199.2, 209.20-209.21,
209.29-209.30, 239.1, 239.8-239.9

176.5 Lymph nodes 🦠
(Ex) 176.5, 195.8-196.9, 199.0-199.2, 209.20 209.29-209.30, 239.8-239.9

176.8 Other specified sites 🦠
Oral cavity NEC
(Ex) 176.0-176.9, V58.0

176.9 Unspecified 🦠
Viscera NOS
(Ex) 176.0-192.9, 195.0-199.2, 209.20, 209.24 209.29-209.30, 230.0-237.6,
237.9-238.3 238.8-239.9, V58.0

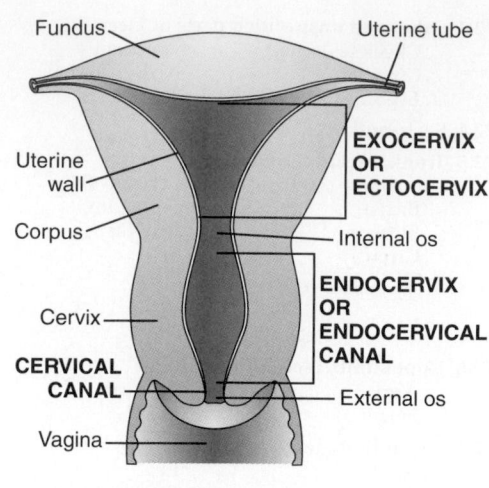

Fundus · Uterine tube · EXOCERVIX OR ECTOCERVIX · Uterine wall · Corpus · Internal os · ENDOCERVIX OR ENDOCERVICAL CANAL · Cervix · CERVICAL CANAL · External os · Vagina

Figure 2–12 Cervix uteri.

MALIGNANT NEOPLASM OF GENITOURINARY ORGANS (179–189)

Excludes carcinoma in situ (233.1–233.9)

179 Malignant neoplasm of uterus, part unspecified ♀

● **180 Malignant neoplasm of cervix uteri**
Includes invasive malignancy [carcinoma]
Excludes carcinoma in situ (233.1)

180.0 Endocervix ♀
Inside the cervix
Cervical canal NOS
Endocervical canal
Endocervical gland

180.1 Exocervix ♀
Outside the cervix

180.8 Other specified sites of cervix ♀
Cervical stump
Squamocolumnar junction of cervix
Malignant neoplasm of contiguous or overlapping
    sites of cervix uteri whose point of origin
    cannot be determined

180.9 Cervix uteri, unspecified ♀

181 Malignant neoplasm of placenta ♀
Choriocarcinoma NOS
Chorioepithelioma NOS
Excludes chorioadenoma (destruens) (236.1)
          hydatidiform mole (630)
              malignant (236.1)
          invasive mole (236.1)
          male choriocarcinoma NOS (186.0–186.9)

● **182 Malignant neoplasm of body of uterus**
Excludes carcinoma in situ (233.2)

182.0 Corpus uteri, except isthmus ♀
Cornu
Endometrium
Fundus
Myometrium

182.1 Isthmus ♀
Lower uterine segment

182.8 Other specified sites of body of uterus ♀
Malignant neoplasm of contiguous or overlapping
    sites of body of uterus whose point of origin
    cannot be determined
Excludes uterus NOS (179)

◄ New   ◄▥ Revised   deleted Deleted   ● Unacceptable Principal Diagnosis   ● Use Additional Digit(s)
▶ Manifestation Code   **OGCR** Official Guidelines   **Coding Clinic**   Excludes   Includes   Use additional   Code first   Omit code

● **183   Malignant neoplasm of ovary and other uterine adnexa**

> **Excludes**   *Douglas' cul-de-sac (158.8)*

183.0   Ovary ♀ 🔵

> Use additional code to identify any functional activity
>
> (Ex) 183.0-183.9, 195.3, 198.6, 199.0-199.2, 209.20, 209.29-209.30
>
> Coding Clinic: 2007, Q4, P95-96

183.2   Fallopian tube ♀
> Oviduct
> Uterine tube

183.3   Broad ligament ♀
> Mesovarium
> Parovarian region

183.4   Parametrium ♀
> Uterine ligament NOS
> Uterosacral ligament

183.5   Round ligament ♀

183.8   Other specified sites of uterine adnexa ♀
> Tubo-ovarian
> Utero-ovarian
> Malignant neoplasm of contiguous or overlapping sites of ovary and other uterine adnexa whose point of origin cannot be determined

183.9   Uterine adnexa, unspecified ♀

● **184   Malignant neoplasm of other and unspecified female genital organs**

> **Excludes**   *carcinoma in situ (233.30–233.39)*

184.0   Vagina ♀
> Gartner's duct   Vaginal vault

184.1   Labia majora ♀
> Greater vestibular [Bartholin's] gland

184.2   Labia minora ♀

184.3   Clitoris ♀

184.4   Vulva, unspecified ♀
> External female genitalia NOS
> Pudendum

184.8   Other specified sites of female genital organs ♀
> Malignant neoplasm of contiguous or overlapping sites of female genital organs whose point of origin cannot be determined

184.9   Female genital organ, site unspecified ♀
> Female genitourinary tract NOS

185   Malignant neoplasm of prostate ♂

> **Excludes**   *seminal vesicles (187.8)*
>
> Coding Clinic: 2003, Q3, P13; 1999, Q3, P5; 1994, Q1, P20; 1992, Q3, P7

● **186   Malignant neoplasm of testis**

> Use additional code to identify any functional activity

186.0   Undescended testis ♂
> Ectopic testis   Retained testis

186.9   Other and unspecified testis ♂
> Testis: Testis:
>   NOS   scrotal
>   descended

● **187   Malignant neoplasm of penis and other male genital organs**

187.1   Prepuce ♂
> Foreskin

187.2   Glans penis ♂

187.3   Body of penis ♂
> Corpus cavernosum

187.4   Penis, part unspecified ♂
> Skin of penis NOS

187.5   Epididymis ♂

187.6   Spermatic cord ♂
> Vas deferens

Figure 2–13   Penis and other male genital organs.

187.7   Scrotum ♂
> Skin of scrotum

187.8   Other specified sites of male genital organs ♂
> Seminal vesicle
> Tunica vaginalis
> Malignant neoplasm of contiguous or overlapping sites of penis and other male genital organs whose point of origin cannot be determined

187.9   Male genital organ, site unspecified ♂
> Male genital organ or tract NOS

● **188   Malignant neoplasm of bladder**

> **Excludes**   *carcinoma in situ (233.7)*

188.0   Trigone of urinary bladder

188.1   Dome of urinary bladder

188.2   Lateral wall of urinary bladder

188.3   Anterior wall of urinary bladder

188.4   Posterior wall of urinary bladder

188.5   Bladder neck
> Internal urethral orifice

188.6   Ureteric orifice

188.7   Urachus

188.8   Other specified sites of bladder
> Malignant neoplasm of contiguous or overlapping sites of bladder whose point of origin cannot be determined

188.9   Bladder, part unspecified
> Bladder wall NOS
> Coding Clinic: 2000, Q1, P5

● **189   Malignant neoplasm of kidney and other and unspecified urinary organs**

> **Excludes**   *benign carcinoid tumor of kidney (209.64)*
>   *malignant carcinoid tumor of kidney (209.24)*

189.0   Kidney, except pelvis 🔵
> Kidney NOS   Kidney parenchyma
> (Ex) 189.0-189.1, 189.8-189.9, 195.8, 199.0-199.2, 209.20, 209.24, 209.29-209.30, 239.5, 239.8-239.9
> Coding Clinic: 2005, Q2, P4-5; 2004, Q2, P4

189.1   Renal pelvis 🔵
> Renal calyces   Ureteropelvic junction
> (Ex) 189.0-189.1, 189.8-189.9, 195.8, 199.0-199.2, 209.20, 209.24, 209.29-209.30, 239.5, 239.8-239.9

189.2   Ureter 🔵

> **Excludes**   *ureteric orifice of bladder (188.6)*
>
> (Ex) 189.2, 189.8-189.9, 195.8, 199.0-199.2, 209.20, 209.29-209.30, 239.5, 239.8-239.9

N   Newborn Age: 0   P   Pediatric Age: 0–17   M   Maternity Age: 12–55   A   Adult Age: 15–124   ♀   Females Only   ♂   Males Only   **781**

(Ex)   CC Exclusions   🔵   Complication\Comorbidity   🔵   Major C\C   🔵   Present on Admission Requirement   🔵   Hospital-Acquired Condition

NEOPLASMS (140–239)

189.3 Urethra 🦠
> **Excludes**   *urethral orifice of bladder (188.5)*
> Ⓔ⟨ 189.3-189.9, 198.82

189.4 Paraurethral glands 🦠
> Ⓔ⟨ 189.3-189.9, 198.82

189.8 Other specified sites of urinary organs 🦠
> Malignant neoplasm of contiguous or overlapping
> sites of kidney and other urinary organs
> whose point of origin cannot be determined
> Ⓔ⟨ 189.0-189.9, 195.3, 198.0-198.1, 209.24

189.9 Urinary organ, site unspecified 🦠
> Urinary system NOS

MALIGNANT NEOPLASM OF OTHER AND UNSPECIFIED SITES (190–199)

> **Excludes**   *carcinoma in situ (234.0–234.9)*
> Ⓔ⟨ 189.0-189.9, 195.3, 198.0-198.1, 209.24

● **190   Malignant neoplasm of eye**
> **Excludes**   *carcinoma in situ (234.0)*
> *dark area on retina and choroid (239.81)* ◀
> *eyelid (skin) (172.1, 173.1)*
>   *cartilage (171.0)*
> *optic nerve (192.0)*
> *orbital bone (170.0)*
> *retinal freckle (239.81)* ◀

190.0 Eyeball, except conjunctiva, cornea, retina, and choroid
> *Note the use of "except" in this code.*
> Ciliary body
> Crystalline lens
> Iris
> Sclera
> Uveal tract

190.1 Orbit
> Connective tissue of orbit
> Extraocular muscle
> Retrobulbar
> **Excludes**   *bone of orbit (170.0)*

190.2 Lacrimal gland

190.3 Conjunctiva

190.4 Cornea

190.5 Retina

190.6 Choroid

190.7 Lacrimal duct
> Lacrimal sac
> Nasolacrimal duct

190.8 Other specified sites of eye
> Malignant neoplasm of contiguous or overlapping
> sites of eye whose point of origin cannot be
> determined

190.9 Eye, part unspecified

● **191   Malignant neoplasm of brain**
> **Excludes**   *cranial nerves (192.0)*
> *retrobulbar area (190.1)*

191.0 Cerebrum, except lobes and ventricles 🦠
> Basal ganglia
> Cerebral cortex
> Corpus striatum
> Globus pallidus
> Hypothalamus
> Thalamus
> Ⓔ⟨ 191.0-192.1, 192.8-192.9, 195.8, 199.0-199.2, 209.20, 209.29-209.30, 239.6-239.9

191.1 Frontal lobe 🦠
> Ⓔ⟨ 191.0-192.1, 192.8-192.9, 195.8, 199.0-199.2, 209.20, 209.29-209.30, 239.6-239.9
> **Coding Clinic:** 2005, Q4, P117-119; 1993, Q4, P33

191.2 Temporal lobe 🦠
> Hippocampus
> Uncus
> Ⓔ⟨ 191.0-192.1, 192.8-192.9, 195.8, 199.0-199.2, 209.20, 209.29-209.30, 239.6-239.9
> **Coding Clinic:** 2006, Q4, P122-123

191.3 Parietal lobe 🦠
> Ⓔ⟨ 191.0-192.1, 192.8-192.9, 195.8, 199.0-199.2, 209.20, 209.29-209.30, 239.6-239.9

191.4 Occipital lobe 🦠
> Ⓔ⟨ 191.0-192.1, 192.8-192.9, 195.8, 199.0-199.2, 209.20, 209.29-209.30, 239.6-239.9

191.5 Ventricles 🦠
> Choroid plexus
> Floor of ventricle
> Ⓔ⟨ 191.0-192.1, 192.8-192.9, 195.8, 199.0-199.2, 209.20, 209.29-209.30, 239.6-239.9

191.6 Cerebellum NOS 🦠
> Cerebellopontine angle
> Ⓔ⟨ 191.0-192.1, 192.8-192.9, 195.8, 199.0-199.2, 209.20, 209.29-209.30, 239.6-239.9

191.7 Brain stem 🦠
> Cerebral peduncle
> Medulla oblongata
> Midbrain
> Pons
> Ⓔ⟨ 191.0-192.1, 192.8-192.9, 195.8, 199.0-199.2, 209.20, 209.29-209.30, 239.6-239.9

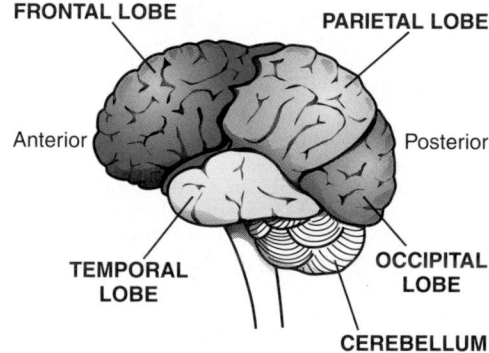

Figure 2–14   The brain.

191.8 Other parts of brain 🦠
> Corpus callosum
> Tapetum
> Malignant neoplasm of contiguous or overlapping
> sites of brain whose point of origin cannot be
> determined
> Ⓔ⟨ 191.0-192.1, 192.8-192.9, 195.8, 199.0-199.2, 209.20, 209.29-209.30, 239.6-239.9
> **Coding Clinic:** 2007, Q4, P103-104

191.9 Brain, unspecified 🦠
> Cranial fossa NOS
> Ⓔ⟨ 191.0-192.1, 192.8-192.9, 195.8, 199.0-199.2, 209.20, 209.29-209.30, 239.6-239.9
> **Coding Clinic:** 1994, Q2, P8

NEOPLASMS (140–239)

◀ New   ◀⫴ Revised   ~~deleted~~ Deleted   ● Unacceptable Principal Diagnosis   ● Use Additional Digit(s)
▶ Manifestation Code   **OGCR** Official Guidelines   **Coding Clinic**   Excludes   Includes   Use additional   Code first   Omit code

● 192 **Malignant neoplasm of other and unspecified parts of nervous system**

> **Excludes** | *peripheral, sympathetic, and parasympathetic nerves and ganglia (171.0–171.9)*

192.0 **Cranial nerves** 🦠
Olfactory bulb
Ⓔⓧ 192.0, 192.8-192.9, 195.8, 199.0-199.2, 209.20, 209.29-209.30, 239.6-239.9

192.1 **Cerebral meninges** 🦠
Dura (mater)
Falx (cerebelli) (cerebri)
Meninges NOS
Tentorium
Ⓔⓧ 192.1, 192.8-192.9, 195.8, 199.0-199.2, 209.20, 209.29-209.30, 239.6-239.9

192.2 **Spinal cord** 🦠
Cauda equina
Ⓔⓧ 192.2, 192.8-192.9, 195.8, 199.0-199.2, 209.20, 209.29-209.30, 239.6-239.9

192.3 **Spinal meninges** 🦠
Ⓔⓧ 192.3-192.9, 195.8, 199.0-199.2, 209.20, 209.29-209.30, 239.6-239.9

192.8 **Other specified sites of nervous system** 🦠
Malignant neoplasm of contiguous or overlapping sites of other parts of nervous system whose point of origin cannot be determined
Ⓔⓧ 191.0-192.9, 195.8, 199.0-199.2, 209.20, 209.29-209.30, 239.6-239.9

192.9 **Nervous system, part unspecified** 🦠
Nervous system (central) NOS

> **Excludes** | *meninges NOS (192.1)*

Ⓔⓧ 191.0-192.9, 195.8, 198.3-198.4, 199.0-199.2, 209.20, 209.29-209.30, 239.6-239.9

193 **Malignant neoplasm of thyroid gland**
Thyroglossal duct

Use additional code to identify any functional activity

● 194 **Malignant neoplasm of other endocrine glands and related structures**

> **Excludes** | *islets of Langerhans (157.4)*
> *neuroendocrine tumors (209.00–209.69)*
> *ovary (183.0)*
> *testis (186.0–186.9)*
> *thymus (164.0)*

194.0 **Adrenal gland** 🦠
Adrenal cortex
Adrenal medulla
Suprarenal gland
Ⓔⓧ 194.0, 194.9, 195.2, 195.8, 198.7, 199.0-199.2, 209.20, 209.29-209.30

194.1 **Parathyroid gland** 🦠
Ⓔⓧ 194.1, 194.8-194.9

194.3 **Pituitary gland and craniopharyngeal duct** 🦠
Craniobuccal pouch
Hypophysis
Rathke's pouch
Sella turcica
Ⓔⓧ 194.3, V58.0
Coding Clinic: 1985, July-Aug, P9

194.4 **Pineal gland** 🦠
Ⓔⓧ 194.4, V58.0

194.5 **Carotid body** 🦠
Ⓔⓧ 194.5, 194.8-194.9

194.6 **Aortic body and other paraganglia** 🦠
Coccygeal body
Glomus jugulare
Para-aortic body
Ⓔⓧ 194.5-194.9

194.8 **Other** 🦠
Pluriglandular involvement NOS

Note: If the sites of multiple involvements are known, they should be coded separately.
Ⓔⓧ 194.0-194.9

194.9 **Endocrine gland, site unspecified** 🦠
Ⓔⓧ 194.0-194.9

● 195 **Malignant neoplasm of other and ill-defined sites**

> **Includes** malignant neoplasms of contiguous sites, not elsewhere classified, whose point of origin cannot be determined

> **Excludes** | *malignant neoplasm:*
> *lymphatic and hematopoietic tissue (200.0–208.9)*
> *secondary sites (196.0–198.8)*
> *unspecified site (199.0–199.1)*

195.0 **Head, face, and neck**
Cheek NOS
Jaw NOS
Nose NOS
Supraclavicular region NOS
Coding Clinic: 2003, Q4, P107

195.1 **Thorax**
Axilla
Chest (wall) NOS
Intrathoracic NOS

195.2 **Abdomen**
Intra-abdominal NOS
Coding Clinic: 1997, Q2, P3

195.3 **Pelvis**
Groin
Inguinal region NOS
Presacral region
Sacrococcygeal region
Sites overlapping systems within pelvis, as:
rectovaginal (septum)
rectovesical (septum)

195.4 **Upper limb**

195.5 **Lower limb**

195.8 **Other specified sites**
Back NOS
Flank NOS
Trunk NOS

(See Plate 315 on page NAP-1.)

● 196 **Secondary and unspecified malignant neoplasm of lymph nodes**

> **Excludes** | *any malignant neoplasm of lymph nodes, specified as primary (200.0–202.9)*
> *Hodgkin's disease (201.0–201.9)*
> *lymphosarcoma (200.1)*
> *other forms of lymphoma (202.0–202.9)*
> *reticulosarcoma (200.0)*
> *secondary neuroendocrine tumor of (distant) lymph nodes (209.71)* ◀

Coding Clinic: 1992, Q2, P3-4

196.0 **Lymph nodes of head, face, and neck** 🦠
Cervical   Scalene
Cervicofacial   Supraclavicular
Ⓔⓧ 176.5, 195.8-196.9, 199.0-199.2, 209.20, 209.29-209.30, 239.8-239.9
Coding Clinic: 2007, Q3, P8-9

196.1 **Intrathoracic lymph nodes** 🦠
Bronchopulmonary   Mediastinal
Intercostal   Tracheobronchial
Ⓔⓧ 176.5, 195.8-196.9, 199.0-199.2, 209.20, 209.29-209.30, 239.8-239.9
Coding Clinic: 2006, Q3, P7-8

N Newborn Age: 0   **P** Pediatric Age: 0–17   **M** Maternity Age: 12–55   **A** Adult Age: 15–124   ♀ Females Only   ♂ Males Only
Ⓔⓧ CC Exclusions   🦠 Complication\Comorbidity   🦠 Major C\C   🦠 Present on Admission Requirement   🦠 Hospital-Acquired Condition

783

NEOPLASMS (140–239)

196.2 Intra-abdominal lymph nodes 🔾
Intestinal   Retroperitoneal
Mesenteric
ⒺⓍ 176.5, 195.8-196.9, 199.0-199.2, 209.20, 209.29-209.30, 239.8-239.9
Coding Clinic: 2003, Q4, P111

196.3 Lymph nodes of axilla and upper limb 🔾
Brachial   Infraclavicular
Epitrochlear   Pectoral
ⒺⓍ 176.5, 195.8-196.9, 199.0-199.2, 209.20, 209.29-209.30, 239.8-239.9

196.5 Lymph nodes of inguinal region and lower limb 🔾
Femoral   Popliteal
Groin   Tibial
ⒺⓍ 176.5, 195.8-196.9, 199.0-199.2, 209.20, 209.29-209.30, 239.8-239.9

196.6 Intrapelvic lymph nodes 🔾
Hypogastric   Obturator
Iliac   Parametrial
ⒺⓍ 176.5, 195.8-196.9, 199.0-199.2, 209.20, 209.29-209.30, 239.8-239.9

196.8 Lymph nodes of multiple sites 🔾
ⒺⓍ 176.5, 195.8-196.9, 199.0-199.2, 209.20, 209.29-209.30, 239.8-239.9

196.9 Site unspecified 🔾
Lymph nodes NOS
ⒺⓍ 176.5, 195.8-196.9, 199.0-199.2, 209.20, 209.29-209.30, 239.8-239.9

● **197 Secondary malignant neoplasm of respiratory and digestive systems**

> Excludes | lymph node metastasis (196.0–196.9)
> secondary neuroendocrine tumor of liver
> (209.72) ◀
> secondary neuroendocrine tumor
> of respiratory organs (209.79) ◀

197.0 Lung 🔾
Bronchus
ⒺⓍ 195.8, 197.0, 197.3, 198.89-199.2, 209.20, 209.29-209.30, 239.8-239.9
Coding Clinic: 2006, Q1, P4-5; 1999, Q2, P9

197.1 Mediastinum 🔾
ⒺⓍ 195.8, 197.1, 197.3, 198.89-199.2, 209.20, 209.29-209.30, 239.8-239.9
Coding Clinic: 2006, Q3, P7-8

197.2 Pleura 🔾
ⒺⓍ 195.8, 197.2-197.3, 198.89-199.2, 209.20, 209.29-209.30, 239.8-239.9, 511.81
Coding Clinic: 2008, Q1, P16-17; 2007, Q3, P3; 2003, Q4, P110; 1989, Q4, P11

197.3 Other respiratory organs 🔾
Trachea
ⒺⓍ 195.8, 197.0-197.3, 198.89-199.2, 209.20, 209.29-209.30, 239.8-239.9

197.4 Small intestine, including duodenum 🔾
ⒺⓍ 195.8, 197.4, 197.8, 198.89-199.2, 209.20, 209.29-209.30, 239.8-239.9

197.5 Large intestine and rectum 🔾
ⒺⓍ 195.8, 197.5, 197.8, 198.89-199.2, 209.20, 209.29-209.30, 239.8-239.9

197.6 Retroperitoneum and peritoneum 🔾
ⒺⓍ 195.8, 197.6, 197.8, 198.89-199.2, 209.20, 209.29-209.30, 239.8-239.9
Coding Clinic: 2004, Q2, P4; 1989, Q4, P11

197.7 Liver, specified as secondary 🔾
ⒺⓍ 195.8, 197.7-197.8, 198.89-199.2, 209.20, 209.29-209.30, 239.8-239.9
Coding Clinic: 2006, Q1, P4-5; 2005, Q2, P9-10; 1984, May-June, P11

197.8 Other digestive organs and spleen 🔾
ⒺⓍ 195.8, 197.4-197.8, 198.89-199.2, 209.20, 209.29-209.30, 239.8-239.9
Coding Clinic: 1997, Q2, P3

● **198 Secondary malignant neoplasm of other specified sites**

> Excludes | lymph node metastasis (196.0–196.9)
> secondary neuroendocrine tumor of other
> specified sites (209.79) ◀

198.0 Kidney 🔾
ⒺⓍ 195.8, 198.0-198.1, 198.89-199.2, 209.20, 209.29-209.30, 239.8-239.9

198.1 Other urinary organs 🔾
ⒺⓍ 195.8, 198.0-198.1, 198.89-199.2, 209.20, 209.29-209.30, 239.8-239.9

198.2 Skin 🔾
Skin of breast
ⒺⓍ 195.8, 198.2, 198.89-199.2, 209.20, 209.29- 209.30, 239.8-239.9

198.3 Brain and spinal cord 🔾
ⒺⓍ 195.8, 198.3, 198.89-199.2, 209.20, 209.29-209.30, 239.8-239.9
Coding Clinic: 2007, Q3, P4; 1999, Q3, P7-8; 1984, May-June, P14

198.4 Other parts of nervous system 🔾
Meninges (cerebral) (spinal)
ⒺⓍ 195.8, 198.4, 198.89-199.2, 209.20, 209.29-209.30, 239.8-239.9

198.5 Bone and bone marrow 🔾
ⒺⓍ 195.8, 198.5, 198.89-199.2, 209.20, 209.29-209.30, 239.8-239.9
Coding Clinic: 2007, Q1, P3-8; 2003, Q4, P110; 1999, Q3, P5; 1989, Q4, P12; 1984, May-June, P14

198.6 Ovary ♀ 🔾
ⒺⓍ 195.8, 198.6, 198.89-199.2, 209.20, 209.29-209.30, 239.8-239.9

198.7 Adrenal gland 🔾
Suprarenal gland
ⒺⓍ 195.8, 198.7, 198.89-199.2, 209.20, 209.29-209.30, 239.8-239.9
Coding Clinic: 1988, Q2, P10

● **198.8 Other specified sites**

198.81 Breast 🔾

> Excludes | skin of breast (198.2)

ⒺⓍ 195.8, 198.81, 198.89-199.2, 209.20, 209.29-209.30, 239.8-239.9

198.82 Genital organs 🔾
ⒺⓍ 195.8, 198.82-199.2, 209.20, 209.29-209.30, 239.8-239.9

198.89 Other 🔾

> Excludes | retroperitoneal lymph nodes (196.2)

ⒺⓍ 195.8, 198.89-199.2, 209.20, 209.29-209.30, 239.8-239.9
Coding Clinic: 2005, Q2, P4-5; 1997, Q2, P4

● **199 Malignant neoplasm without specification of site**

> Excludes | malignant carcinoid tumor of unknown primary
> site (209.20)
> malignant (poorly differentiated) neuroendocrine
> carcinoma, any site (209.30) ◀
> malignant (poorly differentiated)
> neuroendocrine tumor, any site (209.30) ◀⫴
> neuroendocrine carcinoma (high grade), any
> site (209.30) ◀⫴

199.0 Disseminated 🔾
Carcinomatosis unspecified site (primary)
(secondary)
Generalized:
cancer unspecified site (primary) (secondary)
malignancy unspecified site (primary)
(secondary)
Multiple cancer unspecified site (primary)
(secondary)
ⒺⓍ 195.8, 198.89-199.2, 209.20, 209.29-209.30, 239.8-239.9
Coding Clinic: 1989, Q4, P10; 1988, Q2, P11

199.1 Other
Cancer unspecified site (primary) (secondary)
Carcinoma unspecified site (primary) (secondary)
Malignancy unspecified site (primary) (secondary)
Coding Clinic: 2006, Q3, P14-15; Q1, P4-5

● **199.2 Malignant neoplasm associated with transplanted organ** 🔾

> *Code first* complication of transplanted organ
> (996.80-996.89)

> Use additional code for specific malignancy
> ~~site~~ ◀⫴

ⒺⓍ 195 8, 198.89-199.2, 209.20, 209.29-209.30, 239.8-239.9
Coding Clinic: 2008, Q4, P82-83

NEOPLASMS (140–239)

Item 2–6 Lymphosarcoma, also known as malignant lymphoma, is a cancer of the lymph system exhibiting abnormal cells encompassing an entire lymph node creating a diffuse pattern without any definite organization. Diffuse pattern lymphoma has a more unfavorable survival outlook than those with a follicular or nodular pattern. Reticulosarcoma is the most common aggressive form of non-Hodgkin's lymphoma.

MALIGNANT NEOPLASM OF LYMPHATIC AND HEMATOPOIETIC TISSUE (200–208)

Excludes	autoimmune lymphoproliferative
	syndrome (279.41) ◄
	secondary neoplasm of:
	bone marrow (198.5)
	spleen (197.8)
	secondary and unspecified neoplasm of lymph
	nodes (196.0–196.9)

The following fifth-digit subclassification is for use with categories 200–202:

> **0** unspecified site, extranodal and solid organ sites
> **1** lymph nodes of head, face, and neck
> **2** intrathoracic lymph nodes
> **3** intra-abdominal lymph nodes
> **4** lymph nodes of axilla and upper limb
> **5** lymph nodes of inguinal region and lower limb
> **6** intrapelvic lymph nodes
> **7** spleen
> **8** lymph nodes of multiple sites

● **200** **Lymphosarcoma and reticulosarcoma and other specified malignant tumors of lymphatic tissue**

> Requires fifth digit. See note before section 200 for codes and definitions.
> **Coding Clinic: 2007, Q4, P65-67**

● **200.0** **Reticulosarcoma** 🅒
[0-8]   Lymphoma (malignant):
        histiocytic (diffuse):
           nodular
           pleomorphic cell type
        reticulum cell type
    Reticulum cell sarcoma:
        NOS
        pleomorphic cell type
For code **200.00:** (Ex) 200.00-200.08, 239.8-239.9;
For code **200.01:** (Ex) 200.00-200.01, 200.08, 239.8-239.9;
For code **200.02:** (Ex) 200.00, 200.02, 200.08, 239.8-239.9;
For code **200.03:** (Ex) 200.00, 200.03, 200.08, 239.8-239.9;
For code **200.04:** (Ex) 200.00, 200.04, 200.08, 239.8-239.9;
For code **200.05:** (Ex) 200.00, 200.05, 200.08, 239.8-239.9;
For code **200.06:** (Ex) 200.00, 200.06, 200.08, 239.8-239.9;
For code **200.07:** (Ex) 200.00, 200.07-200.08, 239.8-239.9;
For code **200.08:** (Ex) 200.00-200.08, 239.8-239.9
Coding Clinic: 2006, Q4, P135-136; 2001, Q3, P12-13

● **200.1** **Lymphosarcoma** 🅒
[0-8]   Lymphoblastoma (diffuse)
    Lymphoma (malignant):
        lymphoblastic (diffuse)
        lymphocytic (cell type) (diffuse)
        lymphosarcoma type
    Lymphosarcoma:
        NOS
        diffuse NOS
        lymphoblastic (diffuse)
        lymphocytic (diffuse)
        prolymphocytic

Excludes	lymphosarcoma:
	follicular or nodular (202.0)
	mixed cell type (200.8)
	lymphosarcoma cell leukemia (207.8)

For code **200.10:** (Ex) 200.10-200.18, 239.8-239.9 (Ex) 200.10-200.11, 200.18, 239.8-239.9;
For code **200.12:** (Ex) 200.10, 200.12, 200.18, 239.8-239.9;
For code **200.13:** (Ex) 200.10, 200.13, 200.18, 239.8-239.9;
For code **200.14:** (Ex) 200.10, 200.14, 200.18, 239.8-239.9;
For code **200.15:** (Ex) 200.10, 200.15, 200.18, 239.8-239.9;
For code **200.16:** (Ex) 200.10, 200.16, 200.18, 239.8-239.9;
For code **200.17:** (Ex) 200.10, 200.17-200.18, 239.8-239.9;
For code **200.18:** (Ex) 200.10-200.18, 239.8-239.9

● **200.2** **Burkitt's tumor or lymphoma** 🅒
[0-8]   Malignant lymphoma, Burkitt's type
For code **200.20:** (Ex) 200.20-200.28, 239.8-239.9;
For code **200.21:** (Ex) 200.20-200.21, 200.28, 239.8-239.9;
For code **200.22:** (Ex) 200.20, 200.22, 200.28, 239.8-239.9;
For code **200.23:** (Ex) 200.20, 200.23, 200.28, 239.8-239.9;
For code **200.24:** (Ex) 200.20, 200.24, 200.28, 239.8-239.9;
For code **200.25:** (Ex) 200.20, 200.25, 200.28, 239.8-239.9;
For code **200.26:** (Ex) 200.20, 200.26, 200.28, 239.8-239.9;
For code **200.27:** (Ex) 200.20, 200.27-200.28, 239.8-239.9;
For code **200.28:** (Ex) 200.20-200.28, 239.8-239.9

● **200.3** **Marginal zone lymphoma** 🅒
[0-8]   Extranodal marginal zone B-cell lymphoma
    Mucosa associated lymphoid tissue [MALT]
    Nodal marginal zone B-cell lymphoma
    Splenic marginal zone B-cell lymphoma
For code **200.30:** (Ex) 200.30-200.78, 20270-20290, 239.8-239.9;
For code **200.31:** (Ex) 200.30-200.31, 200.38-200.41, 200.48-200.51, 200.58-200.61, 200.68-200.71, 200.78, 202.70-202.71 202.78-202.81, 202.88, 202.91, 239.8-239.9;
For code **200.32:** (Ex) 200.30, 200.32, 200.38-200.40, 200.42 200.48-200.50, 200.52, 200.58-200.60 200.62, 200.68-200.70, 200.72, 200.78, 202.70, 202.72, 202.78-202.80, 202.82 202.88, 202.92, 239.8-239.9;
For code **200.33:** (Ex) 200.30, 200.33, 200.38-200.40, 200.43, 200.48-200.50, 200.53, 200.58-200.60, 200.63, 200.68-200.70, 200.73, 200.78, 202.70, 202.73, 202.78-202.80, 202.83, 202.88, 202.93, 239.8-239.9;
For code **200.34:** (Ex) 200.30, 200.34, 200.38-200.40, 200.44, 200.48-200.50, 200.54, 200.58-200.60, 200.64, 200.68-200.70, 200.74, 200.78, 202.70, 202.74, 202.78-202.80, 202.84, 202.88, 202.94, 239.8-239.9;
For code **200.35:** (Ex) 200.30, 200.35, 200.38-200.40, 200.45, 200.48-200.50, 200.55, 200.58-200.60, 200.65, 200.68-200.70, 200.75, 200.78, 202.70, 202.75, 202.78-202.80, 202.85, 202.88, 202.95, 239.8-239.9;
For code **200.36:** (Ex) 200.30, 200.36, 200.38-200.40, 200.46, 200.48-200.50, 200.56, 200.58-200.60, 200.66, 200.68-200.70, 200.76, 200.78, 202.70, 202.76, 202.78-202.80, 202.86, 202.88, 202.96, 239.8-239.9;
For code **200.37:** (Ex) 200.30, 200.37-200.40, 200.47-200.50, 200.57-200.60, 200.67-200.70, 200.77-200.78, 202.70, 202.77-202.80, 202.87-202.88, 202.97, 239.8-239.9;
For code **200.38:** (Ex) 200.30-200.78, 202.70-202.88, 202.98, 239.8-239.9

N Newborn Age: 0   **P** Pediatric Age: 0–17   **M** Maternity Age: 12–55   **A** Adult Age: 15–124   ♀ Females Only   ♂ Males Only

(Ex) CC Exclusions   🅒 Complication\Comorbidity   Major C\C   Present on Admission Requirement   Hospital-Acquired Condition   785

NEOPLASMS (140–239)

● **200.4   Mantle cell lymphoma** 🍷
[0-8]   For code **200.40:** (Ex:) 200.30-200.78, 202.70-202.90, 239.8-239.9;
     For code **200.41:** (Ex:) 200.30-200.31, 200.38-200.41, 200.48-200.51,
         200.58-200.61, 200.68-200.71, 200.78, 202.70-202.71, 202.78-202.81,
         202.88, 202.91, 239.8-239.9;vv
     For code **200.42:** (Ex:) 200.30, 200.32, 200.38-200.40, 200.42, 200.48-200.50,
         200.52, 200.58-200.60, 200.62, 200.68-200.70, 200.72, 200.78, 202.70,
         202.72, 202.78-202.80, 202.82, 202.88, 202.92, 239.8-239.9;
     For code **200.43:** (Ex:) 200.30, 200.33, 200.38-200.40, 200.43, 200.48-200.50,
         200.53, 200.58-200.60, 200.63, 200.68-200.70, 200.73, 200.78, 202.70,
         202.73, 202.78-202.80, 202.83, 202.88, 202.93, 239.8-239.9;
     For code **200.44:** (Ex:) 200.30, 200.34, 200.38-200.40, 200.44, 200.48-200.50,
         200.54, 200.58-200.60, 200.64, 200.68-200.70, 200.74, 200.78, 202.70,
         202.74, 202.78-202.80, 202.84, 202.88, 202.94, 239.8-239.9;
     For code **200.45:** (Ex:) 200.30, 200.35, 200.38-200.40, 200.45, 200.48-200.50,
         200.55, 200.58-200.60, 200.65, 200.68-200.70, 200.75, 200.78, 202.70,
         202.75, 202.78-202.80, 202.85, 202.88, 202.95, 239.8-239.9;
     For code **200.46:** (Ex:) 200.30, 200.36, 200.38-200.40, 200.46, 200.48-200.50,
         200.56, 200.58-200.60, 200.66, 200.68-200.70, 200.76, 200.78, 202.70,
         202.76, 202.78-202.80, 202.86, 202.88, 202.96, 239.8-239.9;
     For code **200.47:** (Ex:) 200.30, 200.37-200.40, 200.47-200.50, 200.57-200.60,
         200.67-200.70, 200.77-200.78, 202 70, 202.77-202.80, 202.87-202.88,
         202.97, 239.8-239.9;
     For code **200.48:** (Ex:) 200.30-200.78, 202.70-202.88, 202.98, 239.8-239.9

● **200.5   Primary central nervous system lymphoma** 🍷
[0-8]   For code **200.50:** (Ex:) 200.30-200.78, 202.70-202.90, 239.8-239.9;
     For code **200.51:** (Ex:) 200.30-200.31, 200.38-200.41, 200.48-200.51,
         200.58-200.61, 200.68-200.71, 200.78, 202.70-202.71, 202.78-202.81,
         202.88, 202.91, 239.8-239.9;
     For code **200.52:** (Ex:) 200.30, 200.32, 200.38-200.40, 200.42, 200.48-200.50,
         200.52, 200.58-200.60, 200.62, 200.68-200.70, 200.72, 200.78, 202.70,
         202.72, 202.78-202.80, 202.82, 202.88, 202.92, 239.8-239.9;
     For code **200.53:** (Ex:) 200.30, 200.33, 200.38-200.40, 200.43, 200.48-200.50,
         200.53, 200.58-200.60, 200.63, 200.68-200.70, 200.73, 200.78, 202.70,
         202.73, 202.78-202.80, 202.83, 202.88, 202.93, 239.8-239.9;
     For code **200.54:** (Ex:) 200.30, 200.34, 200.38-200.40, 200.44, 200.48-200.50,
         200.54, 200.58-200.60, 200.64, 200.68-200.70, 200.74, 200.78, 202.70,
         202.74, 202.78-202.80, 202.84, 202.88, 202.94, 239.8-239.9;
     For code **200.55:** (Ex:) 200.30, 200.35, 200.38-200.40, 200.45, 200.48-200.50,
         200.55, 200.58-200.60, 200.65, 200.68-200.70, 200.75, 200.78, 202.70,
         202.75, 202.78-202.80, 202.85, 202.88, 202.95, 239.8-239.9;
     For code **200.56:** (Ex:) 200.30, 200.36, 200.38-200.40, 200.46, 200.48-200.50,
         200.56, 200.58-200.60, 200.66, 200.68-200.70, 200.76, 200.78, 202.70,
         202.76, 202.78-202.80, 202.86, 202.88, 202.96, 239.8-239.9;
     For code **200.57:** (Ex:) 200.30, 200.37-200.40, 200.47-200.50, 200.57-200.60,
         200.67-200.70, 200.77-200.78, 202.70, 202.77-202.80, 202.87-202.88,
         202.97, 239.8-239.9;
     For code **200.58:** (Ex:) 200.30-200.78, 202.70-202.88, 202.98, 239.8-239.9

● **200.6   Anaplastic large cell lymphoma** 🍷
[0-8]   For code **200.60:** (Ex:) 200.30-200.78, 202.70-202.90, 239.8-239.9;
     For code **200.61:** (Ex:) 200.30-200.31, 200.38-200.41, 200.48-200.51,
         200.58-200.61, 200.68-200.71, 200.78, 202.70-202.71, 202.78-202.81,
         202.88, 202.91, 239.8-239.9;
     For code **200.62:** (Ex:) 200.30, 200.32, 200.38-200.40, 200.42, 200.48-200.50,
         200.52, 200.58-200.60, 200.62, 200.68-200.70, 200.72, 200.78, 202.70,
         202.72, 202.78-202.80, 202.82, 202.88, 202.92, 239.8-239.9;
     For code **200.63:** (Ex:) 200.30, 200.33, 200.38-200.40, 200.43, 200.48-200.50,
         200.53, 200.58-200.60, 200.63, 200.68-200.70, 200.73, 200.78, 202.70,
         202.73, 202.78-202.80, 202.83, 202.88, 202.93, 239.8-239.9;
     For code **200.64:** (Ex:) 200.30, 200.34, 200.38-200.40, 200.44, 200.48-200.50,
         200.54, 200.58-200.60, 200.64, 200.68-200.70, 200.74, 200.78,
         202.70, 202.74, 202.78-202.80, 202.84, 202.88, 202.94, 239.8-239.9;
     For code **200.65:** (Ex:) 200.30, 200.35, 200.38-200.40, 200.45, 200.48-200.50,
         200.55, 200.58-200.60, 200.65, 200.68-200.70, 200.75, 200.78, 202.70,
         202.75, 202.78-202.80, 202.85, 202.88, 202.95, 239.8-239.9;
     For code **200.66:** (Ex:) 200.30, 200.36, 200.38-200.40, 200.46, 200.48-200.50,
         200.56, 200.58-200.60, 200.66, 200.68-200.70, 200.76, 200.78, 202.70,
         202.76, 202.78-202.80, 202.86, 202.88, 202.96, 239.8-239.9;
     For code **200.67:** (Ex:) 200.30, 200.37-200.40, 200.47-200.50, 200.57-200.60,
         200.67-200.70, 200.77-200.78, 202.70, 202.77-202.80, 202.87-202.88,
         202.97, 239.8-239.9;
     For code **200.68:** (Ex:) 200.30-200.78, 202.70-202.88, 202.98, 239.8-239.9

● **200.7   Large cell lymphoma** 🍷
[0-8]   For code **200.70:** (Ex:) 200.30-200.78, 202.70-202.90, 239.8-239.9;
     For code **200.71:** (Ex:) 200.30-200.31, 200.38-200.41, 200.48-200.51,
         200.58-200.61, 200.68-200.71, 200.78, 202.70-202.71, 202.78-202.81,
         202.88, 202.91, 239.8-239.9;
     For code **200.72:** (Ex:) 200.30, 200.32, 200.38-200.40, 200.42, 200.48-200.50,
         200.52, 200.58-200.60, 200.62, 200.68-200.70, 200.72, 200.78, 202.70,
         202.72, 202.78-202.80, 202.82, 202.88, 202.92, 239.8-239.9;
     For code **200.73:** (Ex:) 200.30, 200.33, 200.38-200.40, 200.43, 200.48-200.50,
         200.53, 200.58-200.60, 200.63, 200.68-200.70, 200.73, 200.78, 202.70,
         202.73, 202.78-202.80, 202.83, 202.88, 202.93, 239.8-239.9;
     For code **200.74:** (Ex:) 200.30, 200.34, 200.38-200.40, 200.44, 200.48-200.50,
         200.54, 200.58-200.60, 200.64, 200.68-200.70, 200.74, 200.78, 202.70,
         202.74, 202.78-202.80, 202.84, 202.88, 202.94, 239.8-239.9;
     For code **200.75:** (Ex:) 200.30, 200.35, 200.38-200.40, 200.45, 200.48-200.50,
         200.55, 200.58-200.60, 200.65, 200.68-200.70, 200.75, 200.78, 202.70,
         202.75, 202.78-202.80, 202.85, 202.88, 202.95, 239.8-239.9;
     For code **200.76:** (Ex:) 200.30, 200.36, 200.38-200.40, 200.46, 200.48-200.50,
         200.56, 200.58-200.60, 200.66, 200.68-200.70, 200.76, 200.78, 202.70,
         202.76, 202.78-202.80, 202.86, 202.88, 202.96, 239.8-239.9;
     For code **200.77:** (Ex:) 200.30, 200.37-200.40, 200.47-200.50, 200.57-200.60,
         200.67-200.70, 200.77-200.78, 202.70, 202.77-202.80, 202.87-202.88,
         202.97, 239.8-239.9;
     For code **200.78:** (Ex:) 200.30-200.78, 202.70-202.88, 202.98, 239.8-239.9

● **200.8   Other named variants** 🍷
[0-8]   Lymphoma (malignant):
         lymphoplasmacytoid type
         mixed lymphocytic-histiocytic (diffuse)
     Lymphosarcoma, mixed cell type (diffuse)
     Reticulolymphosarcoma (diffuse)
     For code **200.80:** (Ex:) 200.80-200.88, 239.8-239.9;
     For code **200.81:** (Ex:) 200.80-200.81, 200.88, 239.8-239.9;
     For code **200.82:** (Ex:) 200.80, 200.82, 200.88, 239.8-239.9;
     For code **200.83:** (Ex:) 200.80, 200.83, 200.88, 239.8-239.9;
     For code **200.84:** (Ex:) 200.80, 200.84, 200.88, 239.8-239.9;
     For code **200.85:** (Ex:) 200.80, 200.85, 200.88, 239.8-239.9;
     For code **200.86:** (Ex:) 200.80, 200.86, 200.88, 239.8-239.9;
     For code **200.87:** (Ex:) 200.80, 200.87-200.88, 239.8-239.9;
     For code **200.88:** (Ex:) 200.80-200.88, 239.8-239.9

● **201   Hodgkin's disease**
     Also known as malignant lymphoma/lymphosarcoma and is
     cancer of the lymphatic system including the lymph
     nodes and related structures

     Requires fifth digit. See note before section 200 for codes
     and definitions.

● **201.0   Hodgkin's paragranuloma** 🍷
[0-8]   For code **201.00:** (Ex:) 201.00-201.08, 201.90, 239.8-239.9;
     For code **201.01:** (Ex:) 201.00-201.01, 201.08, 201.90-201.91, 239.8-239.9 ;
     For code **201.02:** (Ex:) 201.00, 201.02, 201.08, 201.90, 201.92 239.8-239.9 ;
     For code **201.03:** (Ex:) 201.00, 201.03, 201.08, 201.90, 201.93 239.8-239.9 ;
     For code **201.04:** (Ex:) 201.00, 201.04, 201.08, 201.90, 201.94 239.8-239.9 ;
     For code **201.05:** (Ex:) 201.00, 201.05, 201.08, 201.90, 201.95, 239.8-239.9;
     For code **201.06:** (Ex:) 201.00, 201.06, 201.08, 201.90, 201.96, 239.8-239.9;
     For code **201.07:** (Ex:) 201.00, 201.07-201.08, 201.90, 201.97, 239.8-239.9;
     For code **201.08:** (Ex:) 201.00-201.08, 201.90, 201.98, 239.8-239.9

● **201.1   Hodgkin's granuloma** 🍷
[0-8]   For code **201.10:** (Ex:) 201.10-201.18, 201.90, 201.98, 239.8-239.9;
     For code **201.11:** (Ex:) 201.10-201.11, 201.18, 201.90-201.91, 201.98,
         239.8-239.9;
     For code **201.12:** (Ex:) 201.10, 201.12, 201.18, 201.90, 201.92, 201.98,
         239.8-239.9;
     For code **201.13:** (Ex:) 201.10, 201.13, 201.18, 201.90, 201.93, 201.98,
         239.8-239.9;
     For code **201.14:** (Ex:) 201.10, 201.14, 201.18, 201.90, 201.94, 201.98,
         239.8-239.9;
     For code **201.15:** (Ex:) 201.10, 201.15, 201.18, 201.90, 201.95, 201.98,
         239.8-239.9;
     For code **201.16:** (Ex:) 201.10, 201.16, 201.18, 201.90, 201.96, 201.98,
         239.8-239.9;
     For code **201.17:** (Ex:) 201.10, 201.17-201.18, 201.90, 201.97-201.98,
         239.8-239.9;
     For code **201.18:** (Ex:) 201.10-201.18, 201.90, 201.98, 239.8-239.9

◀ New   ◀▥ Revised   ~~deleted~~ Deleted   ● Unacceptable Principal Diagnosis   ● Use Additional Digit(s)
▶ Manifestation Code   **OGCR** Official Guidelines   **Coding Clinic**   Excludes   Includes   Use additional   Code first   Omit code

● **201.2 Hodgkin's sarcoma** 🕿
[0-8]   For code **201.20:** (Ex) 201.20-201.28, 201.90, 201.98, 239.8-239.9;
       For code **201.21:** (Ex) 201.20-201.21, 201.28, 201.90-201.91, 201.98, 239.8-239.9;
       For code **201.22:** (Ex) 201.20, 201.22, 201.28, 201.90, 201.92, 201.98, 239.8-239.9;
       For code **201.23:** (Ex) 201.20, 201.23, 201.28, 201.90, 201.93, 201.98, 239.8-239.9;
       For code **201.24:** (Ex) 201.20, 201.24, 201.28, 201.90, 201.94, 201.98, 239.8-239.9;
       For code **201.25:** (Ex) 201.20, 201.25, 201.28, 201.90, 201.95, 201.98, 239.8-239.9;
       For code **201.26:** (Ex) 201.20, 201.26, 201.28, 201.90, 201.96, 201.98, 239.8-239.9;
       For code **201.27:** (Ex) 201.20, 201.27-201.28, 201.90, 201.97-201.98, 239.8-239.9;
       For code **201.28:** (Ex) 201.20-201.28, 201.90, 201.98, 239.8-239.9

● **201.4 Lymphocytic-histiocytic predominance** 🕿
[0-8]   For code **201.40:** (Ex) 201.40-201.48, 201.90, 201.98, 239.8-239.9;
       For code **201.41:** (Ex) 201.40-201.41, 201.48, 201.90-201.91, 201.98, 239.8-239.9;
       For code **201.42:** (Ex) 201.40, 201.42, 201.48, 201.90, 201.92, 201.98, 239.8-239.9;
       For code **201.43:** (Ex) 201.40, 201.43, 201.48, 201.90, 201.93, 201.98, 239.8-239.9;
       For code **201.44:** (Ex) 201.40, 201.44, 201.48, 201.90, 201.94, 201.98, 239.8-239.9;
       For code **201.45:** (Ex) 201.40, 201.45, 201.48, 201.90, 201.95, 201.98, 239.8-239.9;
       For code **201.46:** (Ex) 201.40, 201.46, 201.48, 201.90, 201.96, 201.98, 239.8-239.9;
       For code **201.47:** (Ex) 201.40, 201.47-201.48, 201.90, 201.97-201.98, 239.8-239.9;
       For code **201.48:** (Ex) 201.40-201.48, 201.90, 201.98, 239.8-239.9

● **201.5 Nodular sclerosis** 🕿
[0-8]   Hodgkin's disease, nodular sclerosis:
       NOS
       cellular phase
       For code **201.50:** (Ex) 201.50-201.58, 201.90, 201.98, 239.8-239.9;
       For code **201.51:** (Ex) 201.50-201.51, 201.58, 201.90-201.91, 201.98, 239.8-239.9;
       For code **201.52:** (Ex) 201.50, 201.52, 201.58, 201.90, 201.92, 201.98, 239.8-239.9;
       For code **201.53:** (Ex) 201.50, 201.53, 201.58, 201.90, 201.93, 201.98, 239.8-239.9;
       For code **201.54:** (Ex) 201.50, 201.54, 201.58, 201.90, 201.94, 201.98, 239.8-239.9;
       For code **201.55:** (Ex) 201.50, 201.55, 201.58, 201.90, 201.95, 201.98, 239.8-239.9;
       For code **201.56:** (Ex) 201.50, 201.56, 201.58, 201.90, 201.96, 201.98, 239.8-239.9;
       For code **201.57:** (Ex) 201.50, 201.57-201.58, 201.90, 201.97 -201.98, 239.8-239.9;
       For code **201.58:** (Ex) 201.50-201.58, 201.90, 201.98, 239.8-239.9

● **201.6 Mixed cellularity** 🕿
[0-8]   For code **201.60:** (Ex) 201.60-201.68, 201.90, 201.98, 239.8-239.9;
       For code **201.61:** (Ex) 201.60-201.61, 201.68, 201.90-201.91, 201.98, 239.8-239.9;
       For code **201.62:** (Ex) 201.60, 201.62, 201.68, 201.90, 201.92, 201.98, 239.8-239.9;
       For code **201.63:** (Ex) 201.60, 201.63, 201.68, 201.90, 201.93, 201.98, 239.8-239.9;
       For code **201.64:** (Ex) 201.60, 201.64, 201.68, 201.90, 201.94, 201.98, 239.8-239.9;
       For code **201.65:** (Ex) 201.60, 201.65, 201.68, 201.90, 201.95, 201.98, 239.8-239.9;
       For code **201.66:** (Ex) 201.60, 201.66, 201.68, 201.90, 201.96, 201.98, 239.8-239.9;
       For code **201.67:** (Ex) 201.60, 201.67-201.68, 201.90, 201.97-201.98, 239.8-239.9;
       For code **201.68:** (Ex) 201.60-201.68, 201.90, 201.98, 239.8-239.9

● **201.7 Lymphocytic depletion** 🕿
[0-8]   Hodgkin's disease, lymphocytic depletion:
       NOS
       diffuse fibrosis
       reticular type
       For code **201.70:** (Ex) 201.70-201.90, 201.98, 239.8-239.9;
       For code **201.71:** (Ex) 201.70-201.71, 201.78, 201.91, 201.98, 239.8-239.9;
       For code **201.72:** (Ex) 201.70, 201.72, 201.78, 201.92, 201.98 239.8-239.9;
       For code **201.73:** (Ex) 201.70, 201.73, 201.78, 201.93, 201.98, 239.8-239.9;
       For code **201.74:** (Ex) 201.70, 201.74, 201.78, 201.94, 201.98, 239.8-239.9;
       For code **201.75:** (Ex) 201.70, 201.75, 201.78, 201.95, 201.98, 239.8-239.9;
       For code **201.76:** (Ex) 201.70, 201.76, 201.78, 201.96, 201.98, 239.8-239.9;
       For code **201.77:** (Ex) 201.70, 201.77-201.78, 201.97-201.98, 239.8-239.9;
       For code **201.78:** (Ex) 201.70-201.78, 201.98, 239.8-239.9

● **201.9 Hodgkin's disease, unspecified** 🕿
[0-8]   Hodgkin's:
       disease NOS
       lymphoma NOS
       Malignant:
       lymphogranuloma
       lymphogranulomatosis
       For code **201.90:** (Ex) 201.90-201.98, 239.8-239.9;
       For code **201.91:** (Ex) 201.90-201.91, 201.98, 239.8-239.9;
       For code **201.92:** (Ex) 201.90, 201.92, 201.98, 239.8-239.9;
       For code **201.93:** (Ex) 201.90, 201.93, 201.98, 239.8-239.9;
       For code **201.94:** (Ex) 201.90, 201.94, 201.98, 239.8-239.9:
       For code **201.95:** (Ex) 201.90, 201.95, 201.98, 239.8-239.9;
       For code **201.96:** (Ex) 201.90, 201.96, 201.98, 239.8-239.9;
       For code **201.97:** (Ex) 201.90, 201.97-201.98, 239.8-239.9;
       For code **201.98:** (Ex) 201.90-201.98, 239.8-239.9

● **202   Other malignant neoplasms of lymphoid and histiocytic tissue**
       Requires fifth digit. See note before section 200 for codes and definitions.

● **202.0 Nodular lymphoma** 🕿
[0-8]   Brill-Symmers disease
       Lymphoma:
       follicular (giant) (large cell)   ◀▥
       lymphocytic, nodular
       Lymphosarcoma:
       follicular (giant)
       nodular
       For code **202.00:** (Ex) 200.30, 200.40, 200.50, 200.60, 200.70, 202.00-202.08, 202.70, 202.80, 202.90, 239.8-239.9;
       For code **202.01:** (Ex) 200.31, 200.41, 200.51, 200.61, 200.71, 202.00-202.01, 202.08, 202.71, 202.81, 202.91, 239.8-239.9;
       For code **202.02:** (Ex) 200.32, 200.42, 200.52, 200.62, 200.72, 202.00, 202.02, 202.08, 202.72, 202.82, 202.92, 239.8-239.9;
       For code **202.03:** (Ex) 200.33, 200.43, 200.53, 200.63, 200.73, 202.00, 202.03, 202.08, 202.73, 202.83, 202.93, 239.8-239.9;
       For code **202.04:** (Ex) 200.34, 200.44, 200.54, 200.64, 200.74, 202.00, 202.04, 202.08, 202.74, 202.84, 202.94, 239.8-239.9;
       For code **202.05:** (Ex) 200.35, 200.45, 200.55, 200.65, 200.75, 202.00, 202.05, 202.08, 202.75, 202.85, 202.95, 239.8-239.9;
       For code **202.06:** (Ex) 200.36, 200.46, 200.56, 200.66, 200.76, 202.00, 202.06, 202.08, 202.76, 202.86, 202.96, 239.8-239.9;
       For code **202.07:** (Ex) 200.37, 200.47, 200.57, 200.67, 200.77, 202.00, 202.07-202.08, 202.77, 202.87, 202.97, 239.8-239.9;
       For code **202.08:** (Ex) 200.38, 200.48, 200.58, 200.68, 200.78, 202.00-202.08, 202.78, 202.88, 202.98, 239.8-239.9

N Newborn Age: 0   **P** Pediatric Age: 0–17   **M** Maternity Age: 12–55   **A** Adult Age: 15–124   ♀ Females Only   ♂ Males Only

(Ex) CC Exclusions   🕿 Complication\Comorbidity   Major C\C   Present on Admission Requirement   Hospital-Acquired Condition   **787**

NEOPLASMS (140–239)

● **202.1 Mycosis fungoides** 🔖
[0-8]

Excludes *peripheral T-cell lymphoma (202.7)* ◀

For code **202.10:** (Ex:) 200.30, 200.40, 200.50, 200.60, 200.70, 202.10-202.18, 202.70, 202.80, 202.90, 239.8-239.9;

For code **202.11:** (Ex:) 200.31, 200.41, 200.51, 200.61, 200.71, 202.10-202.11, 202.18, 202.71, 202.81, 202.91, 239.8-239.9;

For code **202.12:** (Ex:) 200.32, 200.42, 200.52, 200.62, 200.72 202.10, 202.12, 202.18, 202.72, 202.82 202.92, 239.8-239.9;

For code **202.13:** (Ex:) 200.33, 200.43, 200.53, 200.63, 200.73 202.10, 202.13, 202.18, 202.73, 202.83 202.93, 239.8-239.9;

For code **202.14:** (Ex:) 200.34, 200.44, 200.54, 200.64, 200.74 202.10, 202.14, 202.18, 202.74, 202.84 202.94, 239.8-239.9;

For code **202.15:** (Ex:) 200.35, 200.45, 200.55, 200.65, 200.75, 202.10, 202.15, 202.18, 202.75, 202.85, 202.95, 239.8-239.9;

For code **202.16:** (Ex:) 200.36, 200.46, 200.56, 200.66, 200.76, 202.10, 202.16, 202.18, 202.76, 202.86, 202.96, 239.8-239.9;

For code **202.17:** (Ex:) 200.37, 200.47, 200.57, 200.67, 200.77, 202.10, 202.17-202.18, 202.77, 202.87, 202.97, 239.8-239.9;

For code **202.18:** (Ex:) 200.38, 200.48, 200.58, 200.68, 200.78, 202.10-202.18, 202.78, 202.88, 202.98, 239.8-239.9

Coding Clinic: 1999, Q2, P7-8; 1992, Q2, P4

● **202.2 Sézary's disease** 🔖
[0-8]

For code **202.20:** (Ex:) 200.30, 200.40, 200.50, 200.60, 200.70, 202.20-202.28, 202.70, 202.80, 202.90, 239.8-239.9;

For code **202.21:** (Ex:) 200.31, 200.41, 200.51, 200.61, 200.71, 202.20-202.21, 202.28, 202.71, 202.81, 202.91, 239.8-239.9;

For code **202.22:** (Ex:) 200.32, 200.42, 200.52, 200.62, 200.72, 202.20, 202.22, 202.28, 202.72, 202.82, 202.92, 239.8-239.9;

For code **202.23:** (Ex:) 200.33, 200.43, 200.53, 200.63, 200.73, 202.20, 202.23, 202.28, 202.73, 202.83, 202.93, 239.8-239.9;

For code **202.24:** (Ex:) 200.34, 200.44, 200.54, 200.64, 200.74, 202.20, 202.24, 202.28, 202.74, 202.84, 202.94, 239.8-239.9;

For code **202.25:** (Ex:) 200.35, 200.45, 200.55, 200.65, 200.75, 202.20, 202.25, 202.28, 202.75, 202.85, 202.95, 239.8-239.9;

For code **202.26:** (Ex:) 200.36, 200.46, 200.56, 200.66, 200.76, 202.20, 202.26, 202.28, 202.76, 202.86, 202.96, 239.8-239.9;

For code **202.27:** (Ex:) 200.37, 200.47, 200.57, 200.67, 200.77, 202.20, 202.27-202.28, 202.77, 202.87, 202.97, 239.8-239.9;

For code **202.28:** (Ex:) 200.38, 200.48, 200.58, 200.68, 200.78, 202.20-202.28, 202.78, 202.88, 202.98, 239.8-239.9

Coding Clinic: 1999, Q2, P7-8

● **202.3 Malignant histiocytosis** 🔖
[0-8]
Histiocytic medullary reticulosis
Malignant:
    reticuloendotheliosis
    reticulosis

For code **202.30:** (Ex:) 200.30, 200.40, 200.50, 200.60, 200.70, 202.30-202.38, 202.70, 202.80, 202.90, 239.8-239.9;

For code **202.31:** (Ex:) 200.31, 200.41, 200.51, 200.61, 200.71, 202.30-202.31, 202.38, 202.71, 202.81, 202.91, 239.8-239.9;

For code **202.32:** (Ex:) 200.32, 200.42, 200.52, 200.62, 200.72, 202.30, 202.32, 202.38, 202.72, 202.82, 202.92, 239.8-239.9;

For code **202.33:** (Ex:) 200.33, 200.43, 200.53, 200.63, 200.73, 202.30, 202.33, 202.38, 202.73, 202.83, 202.93, 239.8-239.9;

For code **202.34:** (Ex:) 200.34, 200.44, 200.54, 200.64, 200.74, 202.30, 202.34, 202.38, 202.74, 202.84, 202.94, 239.8-239.9;

For code **202.35:** (Ex:) 200.35, 200.45, 200.55, 200.65, 200.75, 202.30, 202.35, 202.38, 202.75, 202.85, 202.95, 239.8-239.9;

For code **202.36:** (Ex:) 200.36, 200.46, 200.56, 200.66, 200.76, 202.30, 202.36, 202.38, 202.76, 202.86, 202.96, 239.8-239.9;

For code **202.37:** (Ex:) 200.37, 200.47, 200.57, 200.67, 200.77, 202.30, 202.37-202.38, 202.77, 202.87, 202.97, 239.8-239.9;

For code **202.38:** (Ex:) 200.38, 200.48, 200.58, 200.68, 200.78, 202.30-202.38, 202.78, 202.88, 202.98, 239.8-239.9

● **202.4 Leukemic reticuloendotheliosis** 🔖
[0-8]
Hairy-cell leukemia

For code **202.40:** (Ex:) 200.30, 200.40, 200.50, 200.60, 200.70, 202.40-202.48, 202.70, 202.80, 202.90, 239.8-239.9 ;

For code **202.41:** (Ex:) 200.31, 200.41, 200.51, 200.61, 200.71, 202.40-202.41, 202.48, 202.71, 202.81, 202.91, 239.8-239.9;

For code **202.42:** (Ex:) 200.32, 200.42, 200.52, 200.62, 200.72, 202.40, 202.42, 202.48, 202.72, 202.82, 202.92, 239.8-239.9;

For code **202.43:** (Ex:) 200.33, 200.43, 200.53, 200.63, 200.73, 202.40, 202.43, 202.48, 202.73, 202.83, 202.93, 239.8-239.9;

For code **202.44:** (Ex:) 200.34, 200.44, 200.54, 200.64, 200.74, 202.40, 202.44, 202.48, 202.74, 202.84, 202.94, 239.8-239.9;

For code **202.45:** (Ex:) 200.35, 200.45, 200.55, 200.65, 200.75, 202.40, 202.45, 202.48, 202.75, 202.85, 202.95, 239.8-239.9;

For code **202.46:** (Ex:) 200.36, 200.46, 200.56, 200.66, 200.76, 202.40, 202.46, 202.48, 202.76, 202.86, 202.96, 239.8-239.9;

For code **202.47:** (Ex:) 200.37, 200.47, 200.57, 200.67, 200.77, 202.40, 202.47-202.48, 202.77, 202.87, 202.97, 239.8-239.9;

For code **202.48:** (Ex:) 200.38, 200.48, 200.58, 200.68, 200.78, 202.40-202.48, 202.78, 202.88, 202.98, 239.8-239.9

● **202.5 Letterer-Siwe disease** 🔖
[0-8]
Acute:
    differentiated progressive histiocytosis
    histiocytosis X (progressive)
    infantile reticuloendotheliosis
    reticulosis of infancy

Excludes *Hand-Schüller-Christian disease (277.89)*
histiocytosis (acute) (chronic) (277.89)
histiocytosis X (chronic) (277.89)

For code **202.50:** (Ex:) 200.30, 200.40, 200.50, 200.60, 200.70, 202.50-202.58, 202.70, 202.80, 202.90, 239.8-239.9;

For code **202.51:** (Ex:) 200.31, 200.41, 200.51, 200.61, 200.71, 202.50-202.51, 202.58, 202.71, 202.81, 202.91, 239.8-239.9;

For code **202.52:** (Ex:) 200.32, 200.42, 200.52, 200.62, 200.72, 202.50, 202.52, 202.58, 202.72, 202.82, 202.92, 239.8-239.9;

For code **202.53:** (Ex:) 200.33, 200.43, 200.53, 200.63, 200.73, 202.50, 202.53, 202.58, 202.73, 202.83, 202.93, 239.8-239.9;

For code **202.54:** (Ex:) 200.34, 200.44, 200.54, 200.64, 200.74, 202.50, 202.54, 202.58, 202.74, 202.84, 202.94, 239.8-239.9;

For code **202.55:** (Ex:) 200.35, 200.45, 200.55, 200.65, 200.75, 202.50, 202.55, 202.58, 202.75, 202.85, 202.95, 239.8-239.9;

For code **202.56:** (Ex:) 200.36, 200.46, 200.56, 200.66, 200.76, 202.50, 202.56, 202.58, 202.76, 202.86, 202.96, 239.8-239.9;

For code **202.57:** (Ex:) 200.37, 200.47, 200.57, 200.67, 200.77, 202.50, 202.57-202.58, 202.77, 202.87, 202.97, 239.8-239.9;

For code **202.58:** (Ex:) 200.38, 200.48, 200.58, 200.68, 200.78, 202.50-202.58, 202.78, 202.88, 202.98, 239.8-239.9

● **202.6 Malignant mast cell tumors** 🔖
[0-8]
Malignant:
    mastocytoma
    mastocytosis
Mast cell sarcoma
Systemic tissue mast cell disease

Excludes *mast cell leukemia (207.8)*

For code **202.60:** (Ex:) 200.30, 200.40, 200.50, 200.60, 200.70, 202.60-202.70, 202.80, 202.90, 239.8-239.9;

For code **202.61:** (Ex:) 200.31, 200.41, 200.51, 200.61, 200.71, 202.60-202.61, 202.68, 202.71, 202.81, 202.91, 239.8-239.9;

For code **202.62:** (Ex:) 200.32, 200.42, 200.52, 200.62, 200.72, 202.60, 202.62, 202.68, 202.72, 202.82, 202.92, 239.8-239.9;

For code **202.63:** (Ex:) 200.33, 200.43, 200.53, 200.63, 200.73, 202.60, 202.63, 202.68, 202.73, 202.83, 202.93, 239.8-239.9;

For code **202.64:** (Ex:) 200.34, 200.44, 200.54, 200.64, 200.74, 202.60, 202.64, 202.68, 202.74, 202.84, 202.94, 239.8-239.9;

For code **202.65:** (Ex:) 200.35, 200.45, 200.55, 200.65, 200.75, 202.60, 202.65, 202.68, 202.75, 202.85, 202.95, 239.8-239.9;

For code **202.66:** (Ex:) 200.36, 200.46, 200.56, 200.66, 200.76, 202.60, 202.66, 202.68, 202.76, 202.86, 202.96, 239.8-239.9;

For code **202.67:** (Ex:) 200.37, 200.47, 200.57, 200.67, 200.77, 202.60, 202.67-202.68, 202.77, 202.87, 202.97, 239.8-239.9;

For code **202.68:** (Ex:) 200.38, 200.48, 200.58, 200.68, 200.78, 202.60-202.68, 202.78, 202.88, 202.98, 239.8-239.9

◀ New   ◀◀ Revised   ~~deleted~~ Deleted   ● Unacceptable Principal Diagnosis   ● Use Additional Digit(s)
▶ Manifestation Code   **OGCR** Official Guidelines   **Coding Clinic**   Excludes   Includes   Use additional   Code first   Omit code

● 202.7 **Peripheral T cell lymphoma** 🅒
[0-8]   For code **202.70:** (Ex:) 200.30-200.78, 202.70-202.90, 239.8-239.9;
      For code **202.71:** (Ex:) 200.30-200.31, 200.38-200.41, 200.48-200.51,
           200.58-200.61, 200.68-200.71, 200.78, 202.70-202.71, 202.78-202.81,
           202.88, 202.91, 239.8-239.9;
      For code **202.72:** (Ex:) 200.30, 200.32, 200.38-200.40, 200.42, 200.48-200.50,
           200.52, 200.58-200.60, 200.62, 200.68-200.70, 200.72, 200.78,
           202.70, 202.72, 202.78-202.80, 202.82, 202.88, 202.92, 239.8-239.9;
      For code **202.73:** (Ex:) 200.30, 200.33, 200.38-200.40, 200.43, 200.48-200.50,
           200.53, 200.58-200.60, 200.63, 200.68-200.70, 200.73, 200.78,
           202.70, 202.73, 202.78-202.80, 202.83, 202.88, 202.93, 239.8-239.9;
      For code **202.74:** (Ex:) 200.30, 200.34, 200.38-200.40, 200.44, 200.48-200.50,
           200.54, 200.58-200.60, 200.64, 200.68-200.70, 200.74, 200.78,
           202.70, 202.74, 202.78-202.80, 202.84, 202.88, 202.94, 239.8-239.9;
      For code **202.75:** (Ex:) 200.30, 200.35, 200.38-200.40, 200.45, 200.48-200.50,
           200.55, 200.58-200.60, 200.65, 200.68-200.70, 200.75, 200.78,
           202.70, 202.75, 202.78-202.80, 202.85, 202.88, 202.95, 239.8-239.9;
      For code **202.76:** (Ex:) 200.30, 200.36, 200.38-200.40, 200.46, 200.48-200.50,
           200.56, 200.58-200.60, 200.66, 200.68-200.70, 200.76, 200.78,
           202.70, 202.76, 202.78-202.80, 202.86, 202.88, 202.96, 239.8-239.9;
      For code **202.77:** (Ex:) 200.30, 200.37-200.40, 200.47-200.50, 200.57-200.60,
           200.67-200.70, 200.77-200.78, 202.70, 202.77-202.80, 202.87-202.88,
           202.97, 239.8-239.9;
      For code **202.78:** (Ex:) 200.30-200.78, 202.70-202.88, 202.98, 239.8-239.9

● 202.8 **Other lymphomas** 🅒
[0-8]   Lymphoma (malignant):
        NOS
        diffuse
      Excludes   benign lymphoma (229.0)
      For code **202.80:** (Ex:) 200.30-200.78, 202.70-202.90, 239.8-239.9;
      For code **202.81:** (Ex:) 200.30-200.31, 200.38-200.41 200.48-200.51,
           200.58-200.61 200.68-200.71, 200.78, 202.70-202.71 202.78-202.81,
           202.88, 202.91, 239.8-239.9;
      For code **202.82:** (Ex:) 200.30, 200.32, 200.38-200.40, 200.42, 200.48-200.50,
           200.52, 200.58-200.60 200.62, 200.68-200.70, 200.72, 200.78, 202.70,
           202.72, 202.78-202.80, 202.82 202.88, 202.92, 239.8-239.9 ;
      For code **202.83:** (Ex:) 200.30, 200.33, 200.38-200.40, 200.43 200.48-200.50,
           200.53, 200.58-200.60 200.63, 200.68-200.70, 200.73, 200.78 202.70,
           202.73, 202.78-202.80, 202.83 202.88, 202.93, 239.8-239.9 ;
      For code **202.84:** (Ex:) 200.30, 200.34, 200.38-200.40, 200.44 200.48-200.50,
           200.54, 200.58-200.60 200.64, 200.68-200.70, 200.74, 200.78 202.70,
           202.74, 202.78-202.80, 202.84, 202.88, 202.94, 239.8-239.9;
      For code **202.85:** (Ex:) 200.30, 200.35, 200.38-200.40, 200.45, 200.48-200.50,
           200.55, 200.58-200.60, 200.65, 200.68-200.70, 200.75, 200.78,
           202.70, 202.75, 202.78-202.80, 202.85, 202.88, 202.95, 239.8-239.9;
      For code **202.86:** (Ex:) 200.30, 200.36, 200.38-200.40, 200.46, 200.48-200.50,
           200.56, 200.58-200.60, 200.66, 200.68-200.70, 200.76, 200.78,
           202.70, 202.76, 202.78-202.80, 202.86, 202.88, 202.96, 239.8-239.9;
      For code **202.87:** (Ex:) 200.30, 200.37-200.40, 200.47-200.50, 200.57-200.60,
           200.67-200.70, 200.77-200.78, 202.70, 202.77-202.80, 202.87-202.88,
           202.97, 239.8-239.9;
      For code **202.88:** (Ex:) 200.30-200.78, 202.70-202.88, 202.98, 239.8-239.9
      Coding Clinic: 2008, Q4, P82-83; Q1, P16-17; 2007, Q3, P3; 2006,
          Q4, P135-136; Q2, P20-22; 1993, Q4, P33; 1992, Q2, P3-4

● 202.9 **Other and unspecified malignant neoplasms of**
[0-8] **lymphoid and histiocytic tissue** 🅒
        Follicular dendritic cell sarcoma
        Interdigitating dendritic cell sarcoma
        Langerhans cell sarcoma
        Malignant neoplasm of bone marrow NOS
      For code **202.90:** (Ex:) 202.90-202.98, 239.8-239.9;
      For code **202.91:** (Ex:) 202.90-202.91, 202.98, 239.8-239.9;
      For code **202.92:** (Ex:) 202.90, 202.92, 202.98, 239.8-239.9;
      For code **202.93:** (Ex:) 202.90, 202.93, 202.98, 239.8-239.9;
      For code **202.94:** (Ex:) 202.90, 202.94, 202.98, 239.8-239.9;
      For code **202.95:** (Ex:) 202.90, 202.95, 202.98, 239.8-239.9;
      For code **202.96:** (Ex:) 202.90, 202.96, 202.98, 239.8-239.9;
      For code **202.97:** (Ex:) 202.90, 202.97-202.98, 239.8-239.9;
      For code **202.98:** (Ex:) 202.90-202.98, 239.8-239.9

● 203 **Multiple myeloma and immunoproliferative neoplasms**
Multiple myeloma is cancer of plasma cell (type of white blood cell) and is incurable but treatable disease. Immunoproliferative neoplasm is term for diseases (mostly cancers) in which immune system cells proliferate.

The following fifth-digit subclassification is for use with category 203:

> 0   **without mention of having achieved remission**
>   **failed remission**
> 1   **in remission**
> 2   **in relapse**

     Coding Clinic: 2008, Q4, P83-85

● 203.0 **Multiple myeloma** 🅒
[0-2]   Kahler's disease   Myelomatosis
      Excludes   solitary myeloma (238.6)
      (Ex:) 203.00-208.92, 239.8-239.9
      Coding Clinic: 2008, Q4, P90-91; 2007, Q2, P9-10; 1999, Q4, P10;
          1996, Q1, P16

● 203.1 **Plasma cell leukemia** 🅒
[0-2]   Plasmacytic leukemia
      (Ex:) 203.00-208.92, 239.8-239.9

● 203.8 **Other immunoproliferative neoplasms** 🅒
[0-2]   (Ex:) 203.00-208.92, 239.8-239.9
      Coding Clinic: 1990, Q4, P26

Item 2-7 Leukemia is a cancer (acute or chronic) of the blood-forming tissues of the bone marrow. Blood cells all start out as stem cells. They mature and become red cells, white cells, or platelets. There are three main types of leukocytes (white cells that fight infection): monocytes, lymphocytes, and granulocytes. **Acute monocytic leukemia** (AML) affects monocytes. **Acute lymphoid leukemia** (ALL) affects lymphocytes, and **acute myeloid leukemia** (AML) affects cells that typically develop into white blood cells (not lymphocytes), though it may develop in other blood cells.

● 204 **Lymphoid leukemia**
     Includes   leukemia: leukemia:
               lymphatic   lymphocytic
               lymphoblastic   lymphogenous

The following fifth-digit subclassification is for use with category 204:

> 0   **without mention of having achieved remission**
>   **failed remission**
> 1   **in remission**
> 2   **in relapse**

     Coding Clinic: 2008, Q4, P83-85

● 204.0 **Acute** 🅒
[0-2]   **Excludes**   acute exacerbation of chronic lymphoid
                     leukemia (204.1)
      (Ex:) 203.00-208.92, 239.8-239.9
      Coding Clinic: 1999, Q3, P4, 6-7; 1993, Q3, P4x2; 1985, May-June,
          P18-19

● 204.1 **Chronic** 🅒
[0-2]   (Ex:) 203.00-208.92, 239.8-239.9

N   Newborn Age: 0   **P**   Pediatric Age: 0-17   **M**   Maternity Age: 12-55   **A**   Adult Age: 15-124   ♀   Females Only   ♂   Males Only   789
(Ex:)   CC Exclusions   🅒   Complication\Comorbidity   Major C\C   Present on Admission Requirement   Hospital-Acquired Condition

NEOPLASMS (140-239)

● **204.2 Subacute** 🕮
[0-2]   (Ex:) 203.00-208.92, 239.8-239.9

● **204.8 Other lymphoid leukemia** 🕮
[0-2]   Aleukemic leukemia:
       lymphatic
       lymphocytic
       lymphoid
       (Ex:) 203.00-208.92, 239.8-239.9

● **204.9 Unspecified lymphoid leukemia** 🕮
[0-2]   (Ex:) 203.00-208.92, 239.8-239.9

● **205 Myeloid leukemia**

    Includes   leukemia: leukemia:
            granulocytic   myelomonocytic
            myeloblastic   myelosclerotic
            myelocytic   myelosis
            myelogenous

The following fifth-digit subclassification is for use with category 205:

> **0 without mention of having achieved remission**
>   **failed remission**
> **1 in remission**
> **2 in relapse**

     Coding Clinic: 2008, Q4, P83-85

● **205.0 Acute** 🕮
[0-2]   Acute promyelocytic leukemia

> **Excludes**   *acute exacerbation of chronic myeloid*
>   *leukemia (205.1)*
>   (Ex:) 203.00-208.92, 239.8-239.9
>   Coding Clinic: 2006, Q2, P20-22; 2002, Q1, P11-12; 1993, Q3,
>   P3-4x2

● **205.1 Chronic** 🕮
[0-2]   Eosinophilic leukemia
       Neutrophilic leukemia
       (Ex:) 203.00-208.92, 239.8-239.9
       Coding Clinic: 2008, Q4, P140-143; 2000, Q1, P6; 1995, Q2, P12;
         1985, July-Aug, P13

● **205.2 Subacute** 🕮
[0-2]   (Ex:) 203.00-208.92, 239.8-239.9

● **205.3 Myeloid sarcoma** 🕮
[0-2]   Chloroma
       Granulocytic sarcoma
       (Ex:) 203.00-208.92, 239.8-239.9

● **205.8 Other myeloid leukemia** 🕮
[0-2]   Aleukemic leukemia:
       granulocytic
       myelogenous
       myeloid
       Aleukemic myelosis
       (Ex:) 203.00-208.92, 239.8-239.9

● **205.9 Unspecified myeloid leukemia** 🕮
[0-2]   (Ex:) 203.00-208.92, 239.8-239.9
       Coding Clinic: 1985, May-June, P18-19

● **206 Monocytic leukemia**

    Includes   leukemia:
            histiocytic
            monoblastic
            monocytoid

The following fifth-digit subclassification is for use with category 206:

> **0 without mention of having achieved remission**
>   **failed remission**
> **1 in remission**
> **2 in relapse**

     Coding Clinic: 2008, Q4, P83-85

● **206.0 Acute** 🕮
[0-2]   **Excludes**   *acute exacerbation of chronic monocytic*
               leukemia (206.1)
       (Ex:) 203.00-208.92, 239.8-239.9

● **206.1 Chronic** 🕮
[0-2]   (Ex:) 203.00-208.92, 239.8-239.9

● **206.2 Subacute** 🕮
[0-2]   (Ex:) 203.00-208.92, 239.8-239.9

● **206.8 Other monocytic leukemia** 🕮
[0-2]   Aleukemic:
       monocytic leukemia
       monocytoid leukemia
       (Ex:) 203.00-208.92, 239.8-239.9

● **206.9 Unspecified monocytic leukemia** 🕮
[0-2]

● **207 Other specified leukemia**

    Excludes   *leukemic reticuloendotheliosis (202.4)*
             plasma cell leukemia (203.1)

The following fifth-digit subclassification is for use with category 207:

> **0 without mention of having achieved remission**
>   **failed remission**
> **1 in remission**
> **2 in relapse**

     (Ex:) 203.00-208.92, 239.8-239.9
     Coding Clinic: 2008, Q4, P83-85

● **207.0 Acute erythremia and erythroleukemia** 🕮
[0-2]   Acute erythremic myelosis
       Di Guglielmo's disease
       Erythremic myelosis
       (Ex:) 203.00-208.92, 239.8-239.9

● **207.1 Chronic erythremia** 🕮
[0-2]   Heilmeyer-Schöner disease
       (Ex:) 203.00-208.92, 239.8-239.9

● **207.2 Megakaryocytic leukemia** 🕮
[0-2]   Megakaryocytic myelosis
       Thrombocytic leukemia
       (Ex:) 203.00-208.92, 239.8-239.9

● **207.8 Other specified leukemia** 🕮
[0-2]   Lymphosarcoma cell leukemia
       (Ex:) 203.00-208.92, 239.8-239.9

◄ New   ◄ Revised   ~~deleted~~ Deleted   ● Unacceptable Principal Diagnosis   ● Use Additional Digit(s)
▶ Manifestation Code   **OGCR** Official Guidelines   **Coding Clinic**   Excludes   Includes   Use additional   Code first   Omit code

● **208   Leukemia of unspecified cell type**

The following fifth-digit subclassification is for use with category 208:

> **0   without mention of having achieved remission**
>   **failed remission**
> **1   in remission**
> **2   in relapse**

Coding Clinic: 2008, Q4, P83-85

● **208.0   Acute** 🦠
[0-2]   Acute leukemia NOS
      Blast cell leukemia
      Stem cell leukemia

> **Excludes**   *acute exacerbation of chronic unspecified leukemia (208.1)*

Ⓔ 203.00-208.92, 239.8-239.9
Coding Clinic: 1987, Mar-April, P12

● **208.1   Chronic** 🦠
[0-2]   Chronic leukemia NOS
      Ⓔ 203.00-208.92, 239.8-239.9

● **208.2   Subacute** 🦠
[0-2]   *Somewhat acute, between acute and chronic*
      Subacute leukemia NOS
      Ⓔ 203.00-208.92, 239.8-239.9

● **208.8   Other leukemia of unspecified cell type** 🦠
[0-2]   Ⓔ 203.00-208.92, 239.8-239.9
      Coding Clinic: 1987, Mar-April, P12

● **208.9   Unspecified leukemia** 🦠
[0-2]   Leukemia NOS
      Ⓔ 203.00-208.92, 239.8-239.9

NEUROENDOCRINE TUMORS (209)

● **209   Neuroendocrine tumors**

> **Code first** *any associated multiple endocrine neoplasia syndrome (258.01-258.03)*

> **Use additional** code to identify associated endocrine syndrome, such as:
> carcinoid syndrome (259.2)

> **Excludes**   *benign pancreatic islet cell tumors (211.7)* ◀
>   *malignant pancreatic islet cell tumors (157.4)* ◀

Coding Clinic: 2008, Q4, P85-90

● **209.0   Malignant carcinoid tumors of the small intestine**

   ● **209.00   Malignant carcinoid tumor of the small intestine, unspecified portion** 🦠
        Ⓔ 152.8-152.9, 159.0, 159.8-159.9, 176.3, 195.8, 199.0-199.2, 209.00-209.30, 239.0, 239.8-239.9

   ● **209.01   Malignant carcinoid tumor of the duodenum** 🦠
        Ⓔ 152.0, 152.8-152.9, 159.0, 159.8-159.9, 176.3, 195.8, 199.0-199.2, 209.00-209.30, 239.0, 239.8-239.9

   ● **209.02   Malignant carcinoid tumor of the jejunum** 🦠
        Ⓔ 152.1, 152.8-152.9, 159.0, 159.8-159.9, 176.3, 195.8, 199.0-199.2, 209.00-209.30, 239.0, 239.8-239.9

   ● **209.03   Malignant carcinoid tumor of the ileum** 🦠
        Ⓔ 152.2, 152.8-152.9, 159.0, 159.8-159.9, 176.3, 195.8, 199.0-199.2, 209.00-209.30, 239.0, 239.8-239.9

● **209.1   Malignant carcinoid tumors of the appendix, large intestine, and rectum**

   ● **209.10   Malignant carcinoid tumor of the large intestine, unspecified portion** 🦠
        Malignant carcinoid tumor of the colon NOS
        Ⓔ 153.8-153.9, 159.0, 159.8-159.9, 176.3, 195.8, 199.0-199.2, 209.00-209.30, 239.0, 239.8-239.9

   ● **209.11   Malignant carcinoid tumor of the appendix** 🦠
        Ⓔ 153.5, 153.8-153.9, 159.0, 159.8-159.9, 176.3, 195.8, 199.0-199.2, 209.00-209.30, 239.0, 239.8-239.9

   ● **209.12   Malignant carcinoid tumor of the cecum** 🦠
        Ⓔ 153.4, 153.8-153.9, 159.0, 159.8-159.9 176.3, 195.8, 199.0-199.2, 209.00-209.30 239.0, 239.8-239.9

   ● **209.13   Malignant carcinoid tumor of the ascending colon** 🦠
        Ⓔ 153.6, 153.8-153.9, 159.0, 159.8-159.9, 176.3, 195.8, 199.0-199.2, 209.00-209.30 239.0, 239.8-239.9

   ● **209.14   Malignant carcinoid tumor of the transverse colon** 🦠
        Ⓔ 153.1, 153.8-153.9, 159.0, 159.8-159.9 176.3, 195.8, 199.0-199.2, 209.00, 209.30 239.0, 239.8-239.9

   ● **209.15   Malignant carcinoid tumor of the descending colon** 🦠
        Ⓔ 153.2, 153.8, 153.9, 159.0, 159.8-159.9 176.3, 195.8, 199.0-199.2, 209.00-209.30, 239.0, 239.8-239.9

   ● **209.16   Malignant carcinoid tumor of the sigmoid colon** 🦠
        Ⓔ 153.3, 153.8-153.9, 159.0, 159.8-159.9, 176.3, 195.8, 199.0, 199.2, 209.00-209.30 239.0, 239.8-239.9

   ● **209.17   Malignant carcinoid tumor of the rectum** 🦠
        Ⓔ 154.1, 154.8, 159.0, 159.8-159.9, 176.3, 195.8, 199.0-199.2, 209.00-209.30, 239.0, 239.8-239.9

● **209.2   Malignant carcinoid tumors of other and unspecified sites**

   ● **209.20   Malignant carcinoid tumor of unknown primary site** 🦠
        Ⓔ 195.8, 198.89-199.2, 209.00-209.30, 239.8-239.9

   ● **209.21   Malignant carcinoid tumor of the bronchus and lung** 🦠
        Ⓔ 162.8-162.9, 165.8-165.9, 176.4, 195.8, 199.0-199.2, 209.00-209.30, 239.1, 239.8-239.9

   ● **209.22   Malignant carcinoid tumor of the thymus** 🦠
        Ⓔ 164.0, 209.00-209.30

   ● **209.23   Malignant carcinoid tumor of the stomach** 🦠
        Ⓔ 151.0-151.9, 159.0, 159.8-159.9, 176.3, 195.8, 199.0-199.2, 209.00-209.30, 239.0, 239.8-239.9
        Coding Clinic: 2008, Q4, P85-90

   ● **209.24   Malignant carcinoid tumor of the kidney** 🦠
        Ⓔ 189.0-189.1, 189.8-189.9, 195.8, 199.0-199.2, 209.00-209.30, 239.5, 239.8-239.9

   ● **209.25   Malignant carcinoid tumor of the foregut NOS** 🦠
        Ⓔ 151.0-151.9, 159.0, 159.8-159.9, 176.3, 195.8, 199.0-199.2, 209.00-209.30, 239.0, 239.8-239.9

   ● **209.26   Malignant carcinoid tumor of the midgut NOS** 🦠
        Ⓔ 151.0-151.9, 159.0, 159.8-159.9, 176.3, 195.8, 199.0-199.2, 209.00-209.30, 239.0, 239.8-239.9

   ● **209.27   Malignant carcinoid tumor of the hindgut NOS** 🦠
        Ⓔ 151.0-151.9, 159.0, 159.8-159.9, 176.3, 195.8, 199.0-199.2, 209.00-209.30, 239.0, 239.8-239.9

   ● **209.29   Malignant carcinoid tumors of other sites** 🦠
        Ⓔ 195.8, 198.89-199.2, 209.00-209.30, 239.8-239.9

● **209.3 Malignant poorly differentiated neuroendocrine tumors**

   ● **209.30 Malignant poorly differentiated neuroendocrine carcinoma, any site** ◀▦▦
      High grade neuroendocrine carcinoma, any site
      Malignant poorly differentiated neuroendocrine tumor NOS

      | **Excludes** | *Merkel cell carcinoma (209.31-209.36)* | ◀

      (Ex) 195.8, 198.89-199.2, 209.00-209.30, 239.8-239.9

   209.31 Merkel cell carcinoma of the face ◀
      Merkel cell carcinoma of the ear ◀
      Merkel cell carcinoma of the eyelid, including canthus ◀
      Merkel cell carcinoma of the lip ◀

   209.32 Merkel cell carcinoma of the scalp and neck ◀

   209.33 Merkel cell carcinoma of the upper limb ◀

   209.34 Merkel cell carcinoma of the lower limb ◀

   209.35 Merkel cell carcinoma of the trunk ◀

   209.36 Merkel cell carcinoma of other sites ◀
      Merkel cell carcinoma of the buttock ◀
      Merkel cell carcinoma of the genitals ◀
      Merkel cell carcinoma NOS ◀

● **209.4 Benign carcinoid tumors of the small intestine**

   ● **209.40 Benign carcinoid tumor of the small intestine, unspecified portion**

   ● **209.41 Benign carcinoid tumor of the duodenum**

   ● **209.42 Benign carcinoid tumor of the jejunum**

   ● **209.43 Benign carcinoid tumor of the ileum**

● **209.5 Benign carcinoid tumors of the appendix, large intestine, and rectum**

   ● **209.50 Benign carcinoid tumor of the large intestine, unspecified portion**
      Benign carcinoid tumor of the colon NOS

   ● **209.51 Benign carcinoid tumor of the appendix**

   ● **209.52 Benign carcinoid tumor of the cecum**

   ● **209.53 Benign carcinoid tumor of the ascending colon**

   ● **209.54 Benign carcinoid tumor of the transverse colon**

   ● **209.55 Benign carcinoid tumor of the descending colon**

   ● **209.56 Benign carcinoid tumor of the sigmoid colon**

   ● **209.57 Benign carcinoid tumor of the rectum**

● **209.6 Benign carcinoid tumors of other and unspecified sites**

   ● **209.60 Benign carcinoid tumor of unknown primary site**
      Carcinoid tumor NOS
      Neuroendocrine tumor NOS

   ● **209.61 Benign carcinoid tumor of the bronchus and lung**

   ● **209.62 Benign carcinoid tumor of the thymus**

   ● **209.63 Benign carcinoid tumor of the stomach**

   ● **209.64 Benign carcinoid tumor of the kidney**

   ● **209.65 Benign carcinoid tumor of the foregut NOS**

   ● **209.66 Benign carcinoid tumor of the midgut NOS**

   ● **209.67 Benign carcinoid tumor of the hindgut NOS**

   ● **209.69 Benign carcinoid tumors of other sites**

● **209.7 Secondary neuroendocrine tumors** ◀
   Secondary carcinoid tumors ◀

   209.70 Secondary neuroendocrine tumor, unspecified site ◀

   209.71 Secondary neuroendocrine tumor of distant lymph nodes ◀
      Mesentery metastasis of neuroendocrine tumor ◀

   209.72 Secondary neuroendocrine tumor of liver ◀

   209.73 Secondary neuroendocrine tumor of bone ◀

   209.74 Secondary neuroendocrine tumor of peritoneum ◀

   209.75 Secondary Merkel cell carcinoma ◀
      Merkel cell carcinoma nodal presentation ◀
      Merkel cell carcinoma visceral metastatic presentation ◀
      Secondary Merkel cell carcinoma, any site ◀

   209.79 Secondary neuroendocrine tumor of other sites ◀

BENIGN NEOPLASMS (210–229)

Benign neoplasm: Tumor that does not metastasize to other parts of body and is caused by cell overgrowth, differentiating it from cyst or abscess

● **210 Benign neoplasm of lip, oral cavity, and pharynx**

   | **Excludes** | *cyst (of):*
      jaw (526.0–526.2, 526.89)
      oral soft tissue (528.4)
      radicular (522.8)

   210.0 Lip
      Frenulum labii
      Lip (inner aspect) (mucosa) (vermilion border)

      | **Excludes** | *labial commissure (210.4)*
      skin of lip (216.0)

   210.1 Tongue
      Lingual tonsil

   210.2 Major salivary glands
      Gland: Gland:
        parotid   submandibular
        sublingual

      | **Excludes** | *benign neoplasms of minor salivary glands:*
      NOS (210.4)
      buccal mucosa (210.4)
      lips (210.0)
      palate (hard) (soft) (210.4)
      tongue (210.1)
      tonsil, palatine (210.5)

   210.3 Floor of mouth

   210.4 Other and unspecified parts of mouth
      Gingiva
      Gum (upper) (lower)
      Labial commissure
      Oral cavity NOS
      Oral mucosa
      Palate (hard) (soft)
      Uvula

      | **Excludes** | *benign odontogenic neoplasms of bone (213.0–213.1)*
      developmental odontogenic cysts (526.0)
      mucosa of lips (210.0)
      nasopharyngeal [posterior] [superior] surface of soft palate (210.7)

◀ New   ◀▦▦ Revised ~~deleted~~ Deleted ● Unacceptable Principal Diagnosis ● Use Additional Digit(s)
▶ Manifestation Code **OGCR** Official Guidelines **Coding Clinic** Excludes Includes Use additional Code first Omit code

210.5 Tonsil
Tonsil (faucial) (palatine)

> **Excludes** *lingual tonsil (210.1)*
> *pharyngeal tonsil (210.7)*
> *tonsillar:*
> *fossa (210.6)*
> *pillars (210.6)*

210.6 Other parts of oropharynx
Branchial cleft or vestiges
Epiglottis, anterior aspect
Fauces NOS
Mesopharynx NOS
Tonsillar:
fossa
pillars
Vallecula

> **Excludes** *epiglottis:*
> *NOS (212.1)*
> *suprahyoid portion (212.1)*

210.7 Nasopharynx
Adenoid tissue   Pharyngeal tonsil
Lymphadenoid tissue   Posterior nasal septum

210.8 Hypopharynx
Arytenoid fold   Postcricoid region
Laryngopharynx   Pyriform fossa

210.9 Pharynx, unspecified
Throat NOS

● **211 Benign neoplasm of other parts of digestive system**

> **Excludes** *benign stromal tumors of digestive system (215.5)*

211.0 Esophagus

211.1 Stomach
Body of stomach
Cardia of stomach
Fundus of stomach
Cardiac orifice
Pylorus

> **Excludes** *benign carcinoid tumors of the stomach*
> *(209.63)*

211.2 Duodenum, jejunum, and ileum
Small intestine NOS

> **Excludes** *ampulla of Vater (211.5)*
> *benign carcinoid tumors of the small*
> *intestine (209.40-209.43)*
> *ileocecal valve (211.3)*

211.3 Colon
Appendix   Ileocecal valve
Cecum   Large intestine NOS

> **Excludes** *benign carcinoid tumors of the large*
> *intestine (209.50-209.56)*
> *rectosigmoid junction (211.4)*

Coding Clinic: 2005, Q3, P17-18; Q2, P16-17; 2001, Q4, P55-56x2;
1995, Q1, P4; 1992, Q3, P11

211.4 Rectum and anal canal
Anal canal or sphincter
Anus NOS
Rectosigmoid junction

> **Excludes** *anus:*
> *margin (216.5)*
> *perianal skin (216.5)*
> *skin (216.5)*
> *benign carcinoid tumors of the rectum*
> *(209.57)*

211.5 Liver and biliary passages
Ampulla of Vater   Gallbladder
Common bile duct   Hepatic duct
Cystic duct   Sphincter of Oddi

211.6 Pancreas, except islets of Langerhans

211.7 Islets of Langerhans
Islet cell tumor

> Use additional code to identify any functional
> activity

211.8 Retroperitoneum and peritoneum
Mesentery   Omentum
Mesocolon   Retroperitoneal tissue

211.9 Other and unspecified site
Alimentary tract NOS
Digestive system NOS
Gastrointestinal tract NOS
Intestinal tract NOS
Intestine NOS
Spleen, not elsewhere classified

● **212 Benign neoplasm of respiratory and intrathoracic organs**

212.0 Nasal cavities, middle ear, and accessory sinuses
Cartilage of nose
Eustachian tube
Nares
Septum of nose
Sinus: Sinus:
ethmoidal   maxillary
frontal   sphenoidal

> **Excludes** *auditory canal (external) (216.2)*
> *bone of:*
> *ear (213.0)*
> *nose [turbinates] (213.0)*
> *cartilage of ear (215.0)*
> *ear (external) (skin) (216.2)*
> *nose NOS (229.8)*
> *skin (216.3)*
> *olfactory bulb (225.1)*
> *polyp of:*
> *accessory sinus (471.8)*
> *ear (385.30–385.35)*
> *nasal cavity (471.0)*
> *posterior margin of septum and choanae*
> *(210.7)*

Coding Clinic: 2000, Q3, P10-11

212.1 Larynx
Cartilage:
arytenoid
cricoid
cuneiform
thyroid
Epiglottis (suprahyoid portion) NOS
Glottis
Vocal cords (false) (true)

> **Excludes** *epiglottis, anterior aspect (210.6)*
> *polyp of vocal cord or larynx (478.4)*

212.2 Trachea

212.3 Bronchus and lung
Carina
Hilus of lung

> **Excludes** *benign carcinoid tumors of bronchus and*
> *lung (209.61)*

212.4 Pleura

212.5 Mediastinum

212.6 Thymus

> **Excludes** *benign carcinoid tumors of thymus (209.62)*

212.7 Heart

> **Excludes** *great vessels (215.4)*

212.8 Other specified sites

212.9 Site unspecified
Respiratory organ NOS
Upper respiratory tract NOS

> **Excludes** *intrathoracic NOS (229.8)*
> *thoracic NOS (229.8)*

N Newborn Age: 0   **P** Pediatric Age: 0–17   **M** Maternity Age: 12–55   **A** Adult Age: 15–124   ♀ Females Only   ♂ Males Only

(Ex.) CC Exclusions   🔵 Complication\Comorbidity   🔵 Major C\C   🔵 Present on Admission Requirement   🔵 Hospital-Acquired Condition   793

NEOPLASMS (140–239)

● **213 Benign neoplasm of bone and articular cartilage**

    Includes cartilage (articular) (joint)
                  periosteum

    Excludes *cartilage of:*
                ear (215.0)
                eyelid (215.0)
                larynx (212.1)
                nose (212.0)
            exostosis NOS (726.91)
            synovia (215.0–215.9)

  213.0 Bones of skull and face

      Excludes *lower jaw bone (213.1)*

  213.1 Lower jaw bone

  213.2 Vertebral column, excluding sacrum and coccyx

  213.3 Ribs, sternum, and clavicle

  213.4 Scapula and long bones of upper limb

  213.5 Short bones of upper limb

  213.6 Pelvic bones, sacrum, and coccyx

  213.7 Long bones of lower limb

  213.8 Short bones of lower limb

  213.9 Bone and articular cartilage, site unspecified

● **214 Lipoma**

    Slow growing benign tumors (discrete rubbery masses) of mature fat cells enclosed in a thin fibrous capsule found in subcutaneous tissues of trunk and proximal extremities and in internal organs

    Includes angiolipoma
               fibrolipoma
               hibernoma
               lipoma (fetal) (infiltrating) (intramuscular)
               myelolipoma
               myxolipoma

  214.0 Skin and subcutaneous tissue of face

  214.1 Other skin and subcutaneous tissue

  214.2 Intrathoracic organs

  214.3 Intra-abdominal organs

  214.4 Spermatic cord ♂

  214.8 Other specified sites
      Coding Clinic: 1994, Q3, P7

  214.9 Lipoma, unspecified site

● **215 Other benign neoplasm of connective and other soft tissue**

    Includes blood vessel
               bursa
               fascia
               ligament
               muscle
               peripheral, sympathetic, and parasympathetic
                    nerves and ganglia
               synovia
               tendon (sheath)

    Excludes *cartilage:*
                articular (213.0–213.9)
                larynx (212.1)
                nose (212.0)
            connective tissue of:
                breast (217)
                internal organ, except lipoma and
                    hemangioma-code to benign neoplasm
                    of the site
            lipoma (214.0–214.9)

  215.0 Head, face, and neck

  215.2 Upper limb, including shoulder

  215.3 Lower limb, including hip

  215.4 Thorax

      Excludes *heart (212.7)*
                  mediastinum (212.5)
                  thymus (212.6)

  215.5 Abdomen
      Abdominal wall
      Benign stromal tumors of abdomen
      Hypochondrium

  215.6 Pelvis
      Buttock   Inguinal region
      Groin   Perineum

      Excludes *uterine:*
                  leiomyoma (218.0–218.9)
                  ligament, any (221.0)

  215.7 Trunk, unspecified
      Back NOS
      Flank NOS

  215.8 Other specified sites

  215.9 Site unspecified

● **216 Benign neoplasm of skin**

    Includes blue nevus
               dermatofibroma
               hydrocystoma
               pigmented nevus
               syringoadenoma
               syringoma

    Excludes *skin of genital organs (221.0–222.9)*
    Coding Clinic: 2000, Q1, P21-22

  216.0 Skin of lip

      Excludes *vermilion border of lip (210.0)*

  216.1 Eyelid, including canthus

      Excludes *cartilage of eyelid (215.0)*

  216.2 Ear and external auditory canal
      Auricle (ear)
      Auricular canal, external
      External meatus
      Pinna

      Excludes *cartilage of ear (215.0)*

  216.3 Skin of other and unspecified parts of face
      Cheek, external
      Eyebrow
      Nose, external
      Temple

  216.4 Scalp and skin of neck

  216.5 Skin of trunk, except scrotum
      Axillary fold
      Perianal skin
      Skin of: Skin of:
        abdominal wall   chest wall
        anus   groin
        back   perineum
        breast
        buttock
      Umbilicus

      Excludes *anal canal (211.4)*
                  anus NOS (211.4)
                  skin of scrotum (222.4)

  216.6 Skin of upper limb, including shoulder

  216.7 Skin of lower limb, including hip

  216.8 Other specified sites of skin

  216.9 Skin, site unspecified

NEOPLASMS (140–239)

◄ New   ◄ Revised   ~~deleted~~ Deleted   ● Unacceptable Principal Diagnosis   ● Use Additional Digit(s)
▶ Manifestation Code   **OGCR** Official Guidelines   **Coding Clinic**   Excludes   Includes   Use additional   Code first   Omit code

217 Benign neoplasm of breast

Note no gender difference for this code.

Breast (male) (female)
   connective tissue
   glandular tissue
   soft parts

Excludes *adenofibrosis (610.2)*
   benign cyst of breast (610.0)
   fibrocystic disease (610.1)
   skin of breast (216.5)

Coding Clinic: 2000, Q1, P4

● **218 Uterine leiomyoma**

Benign tumors or nodules of the uterine wall

Includes   fibroid (bleeding) (uterine)
   uterine:
     fibromyoma
     myoma

218.0 Submucous leiomyoma of uterus ♀

218.1 Intramural leiomyoma of uterus ♀
   Interstitial leiomyoma of uterus

218.2 Subserous leiomyoma of uterus ♀
   Subperitoneal leiomyoma of uterus

218.9 Leiomyoma of uterus, unspecified ♀
   Coding Clinic: 2003, Q1, P4-5; 1995, Q4, P50

● **219 Other benign neoplasm of uterus**

219.0 Cervix uteri ♀

219.1 Corpus uteri ♀
   Endometrium   Myometrium
   Fundus

219.8 Other specified parts of uterus ♀

219.9 Uterus, part unspecified ♀

220 Benign neoplasm of ovary ♀

Use additional code to identify any functional activity
   (256.0–256.1)

Excludes *cyst:*
     corpus albicans (620.2)
     corpus luteum (620.1)
     endometrial (617.1)
     follicular (atretic) (620.0)
     graafian follicle (620.0)
     ovarian NOS (620.2)
     retention (620.2)

Item 2–8   Teratoma: terat = monster, oma = mass, tumor. Alternate terms: dermoid cyst of the ovary, ovarian teratoma. Teratomas are neoplasms and arise from germ cells (ovaries in female and testes in male) and can be benign or malignant. Teratomas have been known to contain hair, nails, and teeth, giving them a bizarre ("monster") appearance.

● **221 Benign neoplasm of other female genital organs**

Includes   adenomatous polyp
   benign teratoma

Excludes *cyst:*
     epoophoron (752.11)
     fimbrial (752.11)
     Gartner's duct (752.11)
     parovarian (752.11)

221.0 Fallopian tube and uterine ligaments ♀
   Oviduct
   Parametrium
   Uterine ligament (broad) (round) (uterosacral)
   Uterine tube

221.1 Vagina ♀

221.2 Vulva ♀
   Clitoris
   External female genitalia NOS
   Greater vestibular [Bartholin's] gland
   Labia (majora) (minora)
   Pudendum

Excludes *Bartholin's (duct) (gland) cyst (616.2)*

221.8 Other specified sites of female genital organs ♀

221.9 Female genital organ, site unspecified ♀
   Female genitourinary tract NOS

● **222 Benign neoplasm of male genital organs**

222.0 Testis ♂

Use additional code to identify any functional activity

222.1 Penis ♂
   Corpus cavernosum
   Glans penis
   Prepuce

222.2 Prostate ♂

Excludes *adenomatous hyperplasia of prostate*
     (600.20–600.21)
   prostatic:
     adenoma (600.20–600.21)
     enlargement (600.00–600.01)
     hypertrophy (600.00–600.01)

222.3 Epididymis ♂

222.4 Scrotum ♂
   Skin of scrotum

222.8 Other specified sites of male genital organs ♂
   Seminal vesicle
   Spermatic cord

222.9 Male genital organ, site unspecified ♂
   Male genitourinary tract NOS

● **223 Benign neoplasm of kidney and other urinary organs**

223.0 Kidney, except pelvis
   Kidney NOS

Excludes *benign carcinoid tumors of kidney*
     (209.64)
   renal:
     calyces (223.1)
     pelvis (223.1)

223.1 Renal pelvis

223.2 Ureter

Excludes *ureteric orifice of bladder (223.3)*

223.3 Bladder

● **223.8 Other specified sites of urinary organs**

223.81 Urethra

Excludes *urethral orifice of bladder (223.3)*

223.89 Other
   Paraurethral glands

223.9 Urinary organ, site unspecified
   Urinary system NOS

N Newborn Age: 0   **P** Pediatric Age: 0–17   **M** Maternity Age: 12–55   **A** Adult Age: 15–124   ♀ Females Only   ♂ Males Only

(Ex:) CC Exclusions   Complication\Comorbidity   Major C\C   Present on Admission Requirement   Hospital-Acquired Condition

795

NEOPLASMS (140–239)

● **224 Benign neoplasm of eye**

> **Excludes** *cartilage of eyelid (215.0)*
> *eyelid (skin) (216.1)*
> *optic nerve (225.1)*
> *orbital bone (213.0)*

224.0 Eyeball, except conjunctiva, cornea, retina, and choroid
Ciliary body
Iris
Sclera
Uveal tract

224.1 Orbit

> **Excludes** *bone of orbit (213.0)*

224.2 Lacrimal gland

224.3 Conjunctiva

224.4 Cornea

224.5 Retina

> **Excludes** *hemangioma of retina (228.03)*

224.6 Choroid

224.7 Lacrimal duct
Lacrimal sac
Nasolacrimal duct

224.8 Other specified parts of eye

224.9 Eye, part unspecified

● **225 Benign neoplasm of brain and other parts of nervous system**

> **Excludes** *hemangioma (228.02)*
> *neurofibromatosis (237.7)*
> *peripheral, sympathetic, and parasympathetic*
>   *nerves and ganglia (215.0–215.9)*
> *retrobulbar (224.1)*

225.0 Brain

225.1 Cranial nerves
Coding Clinic: 2004, Q4, P111-113

225.2 Cerebral meninges
Meninges NOS
Meningioma (cerebral)

225.3 Spinal cord
Cauda equina

225.4 Spinal meninges
Spinal meningioma

225.8 Other specified sites of nervous system

225.9 Nervous system, part unspecified
Nervous system (central) NOS

> **Excludes** *meninges NOS (225.2)*

226 Benign neoplasm of thyroid glands
Use additional code to identify any functional activity

● **227 Benign neoplasm of other endocrine glands and related structures**
Use additional code to identify any functional activity

> **Excludes** *ovary (220)*
> *pancreas (211.6)*
> *testis (222.0)*

227.0 Adrenal gland
Suprarenal gland

227.1 Parathyroid gland

227.3 Pituitary gland and craniopharyngeal duct (pouch)
Craniobuccal pouch
Hypophysis
Rathke's pouch
Sella turcica

227.4 Pineal gland
Pineal body

227.5 Carotid body

227.6 Aortic body and other paraganglia
Coccygeal body
Glomus jugulare
Para-aortic body
Coding Clinic: 1984, Nov-Dec, P17

227.8 Other

227.9 Endocrine gland, site unspecified

● **228 Hemangioma and lymphangioma, any site**

> **Includes** angioma (benign) (cavernous) (congenital)
>   NOS
> cavernous nevus
> glomus tumor
> hemangioma (benign) (congenital)

> **Excludes** *benign neoplasm of spleen, except hemangioma and*
>   *lymphangioma (211.9)*
> *glomus jugulare (227.6)*
> *nevus:*
>   *NOS (216.0–216.9)*
>   *blue or pigmented (216.0–216.9)*
>   *vascular (757.32)*

● **228.0 Hemangioma, any site**
Coding Clinic: 2001, Q1, P18; 1999, Q2, P9

228.00 Of unspecified site

228.01 Of skin and subcutaneous tissue
Coding Clinic: 1988, Q4, P6

228.02 Of intracranial structures
Coding Clinic: 1988, Q4, P6; 1985, Jan-Feb, P15

228.03 Of retina

228.04 Of intra-abdominal structures
Peritoneum
Retroperitoneal tissue
Coding Clinic: 1988, Q4, P6

228.09 Of other sites
Systemic angiomatosis
Coding Clinic: 1991, Q3, P20

228.1 Lymphangioma, any site
Congenital lymphangioma
Lymphatic nevus

Item 2–9   Hemangiomas are abnormally dense collections of dilated capillaries that occur on the skin or in internal organs. Hemangiomas are both deep and superficial and undergo a rapid growth phase when the size increases rapidly, followed by a rest phase, in which the tumor changes very little, followed by an involutional phase in which the tumor begins to and can disappear altogether. **Lymphangiomas** or cystic hygroma are benign collections of overgrown lymph vessels and, although rare, may occur anywhere but most commonly on the head and neck of children and infants. Visceral organs, lungs, and gastrointestinal tract may also be involved.

Figure 2–15 Hemangioma of skin and subcutaneous tissue. (From Yanoff: Ophthalmology, 2nd ed. 2004, Mosby, Inc.)

◀ New   ⬅ Revised   ~~deleted~~ Deleted   ● Unacceptable Principal Diagnosis   ● Use Additional Digit(s)
▶ Manifestation Code   **OGCR** Official Guidelines   **Coding Clinic**   Excludes   Includes   Use additional   Code first   Omit code

NEOPLASMS (140–239)

● **229 Benign neoplasm of other and unspecified sites**

229.0 Lymph nodes

   Excludes | *lymphangioma (228.1)*

229.8 Other specified sites
   Intrathoracic NOS
   Thoracic NOS

229.9 Site unspecified

CARCINOMA IN SITU (230–234)

   Includes   Bowen's disease
   erythroplasia
   Queyrat's erythroplasia

   Excludes | *leukoplakia - see Alphabetic Index*

● **230 Carcinoma in situ of digestive organs**
   *Cancer involving cells in localized tissues that has not spread
   to nearby tissues*

230.0 Lip, oral cavity, and pharynx
   Gingiva
   Hypopharynx
   Mouth [any part]
   Nasopharynx
   Oropharynx
   Salivary gland or duct
   Tongue

   Excludes | *aryepiglottic fold or interarytenoid fold,
      laryngeal aspect (231.0)*
   epiglottis:
      NOS (231.0)
      suprahyoid portion (231.0)
   skin of lip (232.0)

230.1 Esophagus

230.2 Stomach
   Body of stomach
   Cardia of stomach
   Fundus of stomach
   Cardiac orifice
   Pylorus

230.3 Colon
   Appendix
   Cecum
   Ileocecal valve
   Large intestine NOS

   Excludes | *rectosigmoid junction (230.4)*

230.4 Rectum
   Rectosigmoid junction

230.5 Anal canal
   Anal sphincter

230.6 Anus, unspecified

   Excludes | *anus:*
      margin (232.5)
      skin (232.5)
      perianal skin (232.5)

230.7 Other and unspecified parts of intestine
   Duodenum
   Ileum
   Jejunum
   Small intestine NOS

   Excludes | *ampulla of Vater (230.8)*

230.8 Liver and biliary system
   Ampulla of Vater
   Common bile duct
   Cystic duct
   Gallbladder
   Hepatic duct
   Sphincter of Oddi

230.9 Other and unspecified digestive organs
   Digestive organ NOS
   Gastrointestinal tract NOS
   Pancreas
   Spleen

● **231 Carcinoma in situ of respiratory system**

231.0 Larynx
   Cartilage: Epiglottis:
      arytenoid   NOS
      cricoid   posterior surface
      cuneiform   suprahyoid portion
      thyroid   Vocal cords (false) (true)

   Excludes | *aryepiglottic fold or interarytenoid fold:*
      NOS (230.0)
      hypopharyngeal aspect (230.0)
      marginal zone (230.0)

231.1 Trachea

231.2 Bronchus and lung
   Carina
   Hilus of lung

231.8 Other specified parts of respiratory system
   Accessory sinuses   Nasal cavities
   Middle ear   Pleura

   Excludes | *ear (external) (skin) (232.2)*
      nose NOS (234.8)
      skin (232.3)

231.9 Respiratory system, part unspecified
   Respiratory organ NOS

● **232 Carcinoma in situ of skin**

   Includes   pigment cells

   Excludes | *melanoma in situ of skin (172.0-172.9)*

232.0 Skin of lip

   Excludes | *vermilion border of lip (230.0)*

232.1 Eyelid, including canthus

232.2 Ear and external auditory canal

232.3 Skin of other and unspecified parts of face

232.4 Scalp and skin of neck

232.5 Skin of trunk, except scrotum
   Anus, margin   Skin of:
   Axillary fold   breast
   Perianal skin   buttock
   Skin of: chest wall
      abdominal wall   groin
      anus   perineum
      back   Umbilicus

   Excludes | *anal canal (230.5)*
      anus NOS (230.6)
      *skin of genital organs (233.30–233.39,
         233.5–233.6)*

232.6 Skin of upper limb, including shoulder

232.7 Skin of lower limb, including hip

232.8 Other specified sites of skin

232.9 Skin, site unspecified

N Newborn Age: 0   **P** Pediatric Age: 0–17   **M** Maternity Age: 12–55   **A** Adult Age: 15–124   ♀ Females Only   ♂ Males Only

(Ex) CC Exclusions   Complication\Comorbidity   Major C\C   Present on Admission Requirement   Hospital-Acquired Condition

797

● 233 **Carcinoma in situ of breast and genitourinary system**
This category incorporates specific male and female genitourinary designations (233.0–233.6), while codes 233.7 and 233.9 apply to either male or female organs.

233.0 **Breast**

Excludes	*Paget's disease (174.0–174.9)*
	skin of breast (232.5)

233.1 **Cervix uteri** ♀
Adenocarcinoma in situ of cervix
Cervical intraepithelial glandular neoplasia, grade III
Cervical intraepithelial neoplasia III [CIN III]
Severe dysplasia of cervix

Excludes	*cervical intraepithelial neoplasia II [CIN II] (622.12)*
	cytologic evidence of malignancy without histologic confirmation (795.06)
	high grade squamous intraepithelial lesion (HGSIL) (795.04)
	moderate dysplasia of cervix (622.12)

Coding Clinic: 1992, Q3, P7-8; 1991, Q1, P11

233.2 **Other and unspecified parts of uterus** ♀

● 233.3 **Other and unspecified female genital organs**
Coding Clinic: 2007, Q4, P67-68

233.30 **Unspecified female genital organ** ♀

233.31 **Vagina** ♀
Severe dysplasia of vagina
Vaginal intraepithelial neoplasia [VAIN III]

233.32 **Vulva** ♀
Severe dysplasia of vulva
Vulvar intraepithelial neoplasia [VIN III]
Coding Clinic: 1995, Q1, P8

233.39 **Other female genital organ** ♀

233.4 **Prostate** ♂

233.5 **Penis** ♂

233.6 **Other and unspecified male genital organs** ♂

233.7 **Bladder**

233.9 **Other and unspecified urinary organs**

● 234 **Carcinoma in situ of other and unspecified sites**

234.0 **Eye**

Excludes	*cartilage of eyelid (234.8)*
	eyelid (skin) (232.1)
	optic nerve (234.8)
	orbital bone (234.8)

234.8 **Other specified sites**
Endocrine gland [any]

234.9 **Site unspecified**
Carcinoma in situ NOS

NEOPLASMS OF UNCERTAIN BEHAVIOR (235–238)

Note: Categories 235–238 classify by site certain histo-morphologically well-defined neoplasms, the subsequent behavior of which cannot be predicted from the present appearance.

● 235 **Neoplasm of uncertain behavior of digestive and respiratory systems**

Excludes	*stromal tumors of uncertain behavior of digestive system (238.1)*

235.0 **Major salivary glands**
Gland:
parotid
sublingual
submandibular

Excludes	*minor salivary glands (235.1)*

235.1 **Lip, oral cavity, and pharynx**
Gingiva
Hypopharynx
Minor salivary glands
Mouth
Nasopharynx
Oropharynx
Tongue

Excludes	*aryepiglottic fold or interarytenoid fold, laryngeal aspect (235.6)*
	epiglottis:
	NOS (235.6)
	suprahyoid portion (235.6)
	skin of lip (238.2)

235.2 **Stomach, intestines, and rectum**

235.3 **Liver and biliary passages**
Ampulla of Vater   Gallbladder
Bile ducts [any]   Liver

235.4 **Retroperitoneum and peritoneum**

235.5 **Other and unspecified digestive organs**
Anal: Esophagus
 canal   Pancreas
 sphincter   Spleen
Anus NOS

Excludes	*anus:*
	margin (238.2)
	skin (238.2)
	perianal skin (238.2)

235.6 **Larynx**

Excludes	*aryepiglottic fold or interarytenoid fold:*
	NOS (235.1)
	hypopharyngeal aspect (235.1)
	marginal zone (235.1)

235.7 **Trachea, bronchus, and lung**

235.8 **Pleura, thymus, and mediastinum**

235.9 **Other and unspecified respiratory organs**
Accessory sinuses
Middle ear
Nasal cavities
Respiratory organ NOS

Excludes	*ear (external) (skin) (238.2)*
	nose (238.8)
	skin (238.2)

NEOPLASMS (140–239)

● **236 Neoplasm of uncertain behavior of genitourinary organs**

236.0 Uterus ♀

236.1 Placenta ♀
　Chorioadenoma (destruens)
　Invasive mole
　Malignant hydatid(iform) mole

236.2 Ovary ♀
　Use additional code to identify any functional
　　activity

236.3 Other and unspecified female genital organs ♀

236.4 Testis ♂
　Use additional code to identify any functional
　　activity

236.5 Prostate ♂

236.6 Other and unspecified male genital organs ♂

236.7 Bladder

● **236.9 Other and unspecified urinary organs**

　　236.90 Urinary organ, unspecified

　　236.91 Kidney and ureter

　　236.99 Other

● **237 Neoplasm of uncertain behavior of endocrine glands and nervous system**

237.0 Pituitary gland and craniopharyngeal duct
　Use additional code to identify any functional
　　activity

237.1 Pineal gland

237.2 Adrenal gland
　Suprarenal gland
　Use additional code to identify any functional
　　activity
　*Pair of glands situated on top of or above each kidney
　("suprarenal") responsible for regulating stress
　response through corticosteroids.*

237.3 Paraganglia
　Aortic body
　Carotid body
　Coccygeal body
　Glomus jugulare
　Coding Clinic: 1984, Nov-Dec, P17

237.4 Other and unspecified endocrine glands
　Parathyroid gland
　Thyroid gland

237.5 Brain and spinal cord

237.6 Meninges
　Meninges:
　　NOS
　　cerebral
　　spinal

● **237.7 Neurofibromatosis**
　*Disorder of nervous system that causes tumors to grow
　around nerves.*
　von Recklinghausen's disease

　　237.70 Neurofibromatosis, unspecified

　　237.71 Neurofibromatosis, type 1 [von Recklinghausen's disease]

　　237.72 Neurofibromatosis, type 2 [acoustic neurofibromatosis]

237.9 Other and unspecified parts of nervous system
　Cranial nerves
　| Excludes | *peripheral, sympathetic, and
　　parasympathetic nerves and ganglia
　　(238.1)* |

● **238 Neoplasm of uncertain behavior of other and unspecified sites and tissues**

238.0 Bone and articular cartilage
　| Excludes | *cartilage:
　　ear (238.1)
　　eyelid (238.1)
　　larynx (235.6)
　　nose (235.9)
　　synovia (238.1)* |
　Coding Clinic: 2004, Q4, P128-129

238.1 Connective and other soft tissue
　Peripheral, sympathetic, and parasympathetic
　　nerves and ganglia
　Stromal tumors of digestive system
　| Excludes | *cartilage (of):
　　articular (238.0)
　　larynx (235.6)
　　nose (235.9)
　connective tissue of breast (238.3)* |

238.2 Skin
　| Excludes | *anus NOS (235.5)
　　skin of genital organs (236.3, 236.6)
　　vermilion border of lip (235.1)* |

238.3 Breast
　| Excludes | *skin of breast (238.2)* |

238.4 Polycythemia vera
　*Primary polycythemia. Secondary polycythemia is 289.0.
　Check your documentation. Polycythemia is caused
　by too many red blood cells, which increase thickness
　of blood (viscosity). This can cause engorgement
　of the spleen (splenomegaly) with extra RBCs and
　potential clot formation.*

238.5 Histiocytic and mast cells 🅒
　Mast cell tumor NOS
　Mastocytoma NOS
　(Ex) 238.4-238.76, 238.79, 289.83, V58.0

238.6 Plasma cells 🅒
　Plasmacytoma NOS
　Solitary myeloma
　(Ex) 238.4-238.76, 238.79, 289.83, V58.0

● **238.7 Other lymphatic and hematopoietic tissues**
　| Excludes | *acute myelogenous leukemia (205.0)
　　chronic myelomonocytic leukemia (205.1)
　　myelosclerosis NOS (289.89)
　　myelosis:
　　　NOS (205.9)
　　　megakaryocytic (207.2)* |
　Coding Clinic: 2006, Q4, P63-66; 2001, Q3, P13-14; 1997, Q1, P5-6

　　238.71 Essential thrombocythemia
　　　Essential hemorrhagic thrombocythemia
　　　Essential thrombocytosis
　　　Idiopathic (hemorrhagic)
　　　　thrombocythemia
　　　Primary thrombocytosis
　　　Coding Clinic: 2006, Q4, P64

238.72 Low grade myelodysplastic syndrome lesions
    Refractory anemia with excess blasts-1 (RAEB-1) ◀
    Refractory anemia (RA)
    Refractory anemia with ringed sideroblasts (RARS)
    Refractory cytopenia with multilineage dysplasia (RCMD)
    Refractory cytopenia with multilineage dysplasia and ringed sideroblasts (RCMD-RS)

238.73 High grade myelodysplastic syndrome lesions 🅖
    ~~Refractory anemia with excess blasts-1 (RAEB-1)~~
    Refractory anemia with excess blasts-2 (RAEB-2)
    Ⓔˣ 202.40-202.48, 203.10-203.11, 203.80-203.81, 204.00-208.92, 238.4-238.76, 238.79-238.9

238.74 Myelodysplastic syndrome with 5q deletion 🅖
    5q minus syndrome NOS
    Excludes *constitutional 5q deletion (758.39)*
              high grade myelodysplastic syndrome with 5q deletion (238.73)
    Ⓔˣ 202.40-202.48, 203.10-203.11, 203.80-203.81, 204.00-208.92, 238.4-238.76, 238.79-238.9

238.75 Myelodysplastic syndrome, unspecified

238.76 Myelofibrosis with myeloid metaplasia 🅖
    Agnogenic myeloid metaplasia
    Idiopathic myelofibrosis (chronic)
    Myelosclerosis with myeloid metaplasia
    Primary myelofibrosis
    Excludes *myelofibrosis NOS (289.83)*
              myelophthisic anemia (284.2)
              myelophthisis (284.2)
              secondary myelofibrosis (289.83)
    Ⓔˣ 202.40-202.48, 203.10-203.11 203.80-203.81, 204.00-208.92, 238.4-238.76, 238.79-238.9

● **238.77 Post-transplant lymphoproliferative disorder (PTLD)** 🅖
    Code first complications of transplant (996.80-996.89)
    Ⓔˣ 238.77, 996.80, 996.87, 997.91-997.99
    Coding Clinic: 2008, Q4, P90-91

238.79 Other lymphatic and hematopoietic tissues 🅖
    Lymphoproliferative disease (chronic) NOS
    Megakaryocytic myelosclerosis
    Myeloproliferative disease (chronic) NOS
    Panmyelosis (acute)
    Ⓔˣ 202.40-202.48, 203.10-203.11, 203.80-203.81, 204.00-208.92, 238.4-238.76, 238.79-238.9

238.8 Other specified sites
    Eye
    Heart
    Excludes *eyelid (skin) (238.2)*
              cartilage (238.1)

238.9 Site unspecified

NEOPLASMS OF UNSPECIFIED NATURE (239)

● **239 Neoplasms of unspecified nature**
    Note: Category 239 classifies by site neoplasms of unspecified morphology and behavior. The term "mass," unless otherwise stated, is not to be regarded as a neoplastic growth.
    Includes "growth" NOS
              neoplasm NOS
              new growth NOS
              tumor NOS

239.0 Digestive system
    Excludes *anus:*
              margin (239.2)
              skin (239.2)
              perianal skin (239.2)

239.1 Respiratory system

239.2 Bone, soft tissue, and skin
    Excludes *anal canal (239.0)*
              anus NOS (239.0)
              bone marrow (202.9)
              cartilage:
                  larynx (239.1)
                  nose (239.1)
              connective tissue of breast (239.3)
              skin of genital organs (239.5)
              vermilion border of lip (239.0)

239.3 Breast
    Excludes *skin of breast (239.2)*

239.4 Bladder

239.5 Other genitourinary organs

239.6 Brain
    Excludes *cerebral meninges (239.7)*
              cranial nerves (239.7)

239.7 Endocrine glands and other parts of nervous system
    Excludes *peripheral, sympathetic, and parasympathetic nerves and ganglia (239.2)*

● **239.8 Other specified sites** ◀ⁱⁱⁱ
    Excludes *eyelid (skin) (239.2)*
              cartilage (239.2)
              great vessels (239.2)
              optic nerve (239.7)

    239.81 Retina and choroid ◀
        Dark area on retina ◀
        Retinal freckle ◀
    239.89 Other specified sites ◀

239.9 Site unspecified

◀ New   ◀ⁱⁱⁱ Revised   ~~deleted~~ Deleted   ● Unacceptable Principal Diagnosis   ● Use Additional Digit(s)
▶ Manifestation Code   **OGCR** Official Guidelines   **Coding Clinic**   Excludes   Includes   Use additional   Code first   Omit code

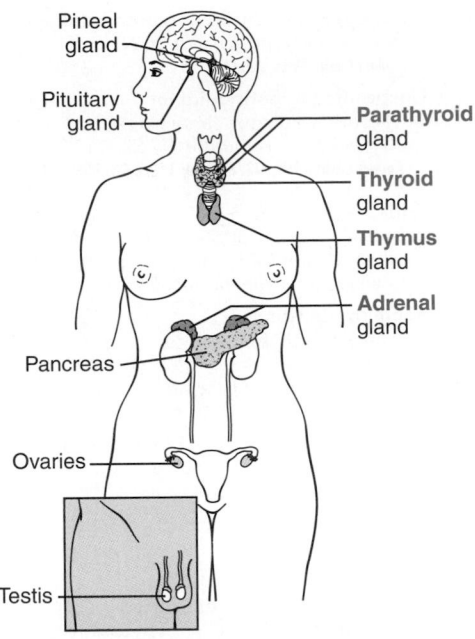

Figure 3-1 The endocrine system. (From Buck CJ: Step-by-Step Medical Coding, 2006 ed. Philadelphia, WB Saunders, 2006.)

Item 3-1 Simple goiter indicates no nodules are present. The most common type of goiter is a **diffuse colloidal,** also called a **nontoxic** or **endemic** goiter. Goiters classifiable to 240.0 or 240.9 are those goiters without mention of nodules.

Figure 3-2 Goiter is an enlargement of the thyroid gland.

3. ENDOCRINE, NUTRITIONAL AND METABOLIC DISEASES, AND IMMUNITY DISORDERS (240–279)

| Excludes | endocrine and metabolic disturbances specific to the fetus and newborn (775.0–775.9) |

Note: All neoplasms, whether functionally active or not, are classified in Chapter 2. Codes in Chapter 3 (i.e., 242.8, 246.0, 251–253, 255–259) may be used to identify such functional activity associated with any neoplasm, or by ectopic endocrine tissue.

DISORDERS OF THYROID GLAND (240–246)

● **240 Simple and unspecified goiter**

240.0 Goiter, specified as simple
Any condition classifiable to 240.9, specified as simple

240.9 Goiter, unspecified
Enlargement of thyroid   Goiter or struma:
Goiter or struma: hyperplastic
   NOS   nontoxic (diffuse)
   diffuse colloid   parenchymatous
   endemic   sporadic

| Excludes | congenital (dyshormonogenic) goiter (246.1) |

Figure 3-3 Graves' disease. In Graves' disease, exophthalmos often looks more pronounced than it actually is because of the extreme lid retraction that may occur. This patient, for instance, had minimal proptosis of the left eye but marked lid retraction. (Courtesy Dr. HG Scheie. From Yanoff M, Fine BS: Ocular Pathology, ed 5. St. Louis, Mosby, 2002.)

Item 3-2 Thyrotoxicosis is a condition caused by excessive amounts of the thyroid hormone thyroxine production or hyperthyroidism. **Graves' disease is associated with hyperthyroidism** (known as **Basedow's disease** in Europe).

● **241 Nontoxic nodular goiter**

| Excludes | adenoma of thyroid (226) |
| | cystadenoma of thyroid (226) |

241.0 Nontoxic uninodular goiter
Thyroid nodule
Uninodular goiter (nontoxic)

241.1 Nontoxic multinodular goiter
Multinodular goiter (nontoxic)

241.9 Unspecified nontoxic nodular goiter
Adenomatous goiter
Nodular goiter (nontoxic) NOS
Struma nodosa (simplex)

● **242 Thyrotoxicosis with or without goiter**

| Excludes | neonatal thyrotoxicosis (775.3) |

The following fifth-digit subclassification is for use with category 242:

> **0 without mention of thyrotoxic crisis or storm**
> **1 with mention of thyrotoxic crisis or storm** 🔖

● **242.0 Toxic diffuse goiter**
[0-1]   Basedow's disease
        Exophthalmic or toxic goiter NOS
        Graves' disease
        Primary thyroid hyperplasia
        (Ex:) 017.50-017.56, 017.90-017.96, 240.0-246.9, 259.50-259.9

● **242.1 Toxic uninodular goiter**
[0-1]   Thyroid nodule, toxic or with hyperthyroidism
        Uninodular goiter, toxic or with hyperthyroidism
        (Ex:) 017.50-017.56, 017.90-017.96, 240.0-246.9, 259.50-259.9

● **242.2 Toxic multinodular goiter**
[0-1]   Secondary thyroid hyperplasia
        (Ex:) 017.50-017.56, 017.90-017.96, 240.0-246.9, 259.50-259.9

● **242.3 Toxic nodular goiter, unspecified**
[0-1]   Adenomatous goiter, toxic or with hyperthyroidism
        Nodular goiter, toxic or with hyperthyroidism
        Struma nodosa, toxic or with hyperthyroidism
        Any condition classifiable to 241.9 specified as toxic or with hyperthyroidism
        (Ex:) 017.50-017.56, 017.90-017.96, 240.0-246.9, 259.50-259.9

● **242.4 Thyrotoxicosis from ectopic thyroid nodule**
[0-1]   (Ex:) 017.50-017.56, 017.90-017.96, 240.0-246.9, 259.50-259.9

N Newborn Age: 0   P Pediatric Age: 0–17   M Maternity Age: 12–55   A Adult Age: 15–124   ♀ Females Only   ♂ Males Only

(Ex:) CC Exclusions   ✱ Complication\Comorbidity   🔖 Major C\C   ◷ Present on Admission Requirement   ⟳ Hospital-Acquired Condition

801

ENDOCRINE, NUTRITIONAL AND METABOLIC DISEASES, AND IMMUNITY DISORDERS (240–279)

ENDOCRINE, NUTRITIONAL AND METABOLIC DISEASES, AND IMMUNITY DISORDERS (240–279)

Figure 3–4 Typical appearance of patients with moderately severe primary hypothyroidism or myxedema. (From Larsen: Williams Textbook of Endocrinology, 10th ed. 2003, Saunders, An Imprint of Elsevier)

Item 3–3   Hypothyroidism is a condition in which there are insufficient levels of thyroxine.
Cretinism is congenital hypothyroidism, which can result in mental and physical retardation.

● **242.8 Thyrotoxicosis of other specified origin**
[0-1]   Overproduction of thyroid-stimulating hormone [TSH]
           Thyrotoxicosis:
               factitia from ingestion of excessive thyroid material
           Use additional E code to identify cause, if drug-induced
           (Ex) 017.50-017.56, 017.90-017.96, 240.0-246.9, 259.50-259.9

● **242.9 Thyrotoxicosis without mention of goiter or other**
[0-1] **cause**
           Hyperthyroidism NOS
           Thyrotoxicosis NOS
           Thyrotoxicosis is also known as thyroid storm.
           (Ex) 017.50-017.56, 017.90-017.96, 240.0-246.9, 259.50-259.9

243 Congenital hypothyroidism
           Congenital thyroid insufficiency
           Cretinism (athyrotic) (endemic)
           Use additional code to identify associated mental retardation
           Excludes   congenital (dyshormonogenic) goiter (246.1)

● **244 Acquired hypothyroidism**
           Includes   athyroidism (acquired)
                       hypothyroidism (acquired)
                       myxedema (adult) (juvenile)
                       thyroid (gland) insufficiency (acquired)

244.0 Postsurgical hypothyroidism

244.1 Other postablative hypothyroidism
           Hypothyroidism following therapy, such as irradiation

244.2 Iodine hypothyroidism
           Hypothyroidism resulting from administration or ingestion of iodide
           Use additional E code to identify drug

244.3 Other iatrogenic hypothyroidism
           Hypothyroidism resulting from:
               P-aminosalicylic acid [PAS]
               Phenylbutazone
               Resorcinol
           Iatrogenic hypothyroidism NOS
           Use additional E code to identify drug

244.8 Other specified acquired hypothyroidism
           Secondary hypothyroidism NEC
           Coding Clinic: 1985, July-Aug, P9

244.9 Unspecified hypothyroidism
           Hypothyroidism, primary or NOS
           Myxedema, primary or NOS
           Coding Clinic: 1999, Q3, P19-20; 1996, Q4, P29

● **245 Thyroiditis**
           Inflammation of thyroid gland, results in inability to convert iodine into thyroid hormone. Common types are autoimmune or chronic lymphatic thyroiditis.

245.0 Acute thyroiditis 🔗
           Abscess of thyroid
           Thyroiditis: Thyroiditis:
               nonsuppurative, acute   suppurative
               pyogenic
           Use additional code to identify organism
           (Ex) 245.0-245.9

245.1 Subacute thyroiditis
           Thyroiditis: Thyroiditis:
               de Quervain's   granulomatous
               giant cell   viral

245.2 Chronic lymphocytic thyroiditis
           Hashimoto's disease   Thyroiditis:
           Struma lymphomatosa   autoimmune
                                            lymphocytic (chronic)

245.3 Chronic fibrous thyroiditis
           Struma fibrosa
           Thyroiditis: Thyroiditis:
               invasive (fibrous)   Riedel's
               ligneous

245.4 Iatrogenic thyroiditis
           Use additional E to identify cause

245.8 Other and unspecified chronic thyroiditis
           Chronic thyroiditis:
               NOS
               nonspecific

245.9 Thyroiditis, unspecified
           Thyroiditis NOS

● **246 Other disorders of thyroid**

246.0 Disorders of thyrocalcitonin secretion
           Hypersecretion of calcitonin or thyrocalcitonin

246.1 Dyshormonogenic goiter
           Congenital (dyshormonogenic) goiter
           Goiter due to enzyme defect in synthesis of thyroid hormone
           Goitrous cretinism (sporadic)

246.2 Cyst of thyroid
           Excludes   cystadenoma of thyroid (226)

246.3 Hemorrhage and infarction of thyroid 🔗
           (Ex) 246.3

246.8 Other specified disorders of thyroid
           Abnormality of thyroid-binding globulin
           Atrophy of thyroid
           Hyper-TBG-nemia
           Hypo-TBG-nemia
           Coding Clinic: 2006, Q2, P5

246.9 Unspecified disorder of thyroid

◄ New   ◄▥ Revised   deleted Deleted   ● Unacceptable Principal Diagnosis   ● Use Additional Digit(s)
▶ Manifestation Code   **OGCR** Official Guidelines   **Coding Clinic**   Excludes   Includes   Use additional   Code first   Omit code

DISEASES OF OTHER ENDOCRINE GLANDS (249–259)

OGCR Section I.C.3.a.2
If the type of diabetes mellitus is not documented in the medical record the default is type II.

● **249 Secondary diabetes mellitus**

> **Includes**   diabetes mellitus (due to) (in) (secondary) (with):
> drug-induced or chemical induced infection

> **Excludes**   *gestational diabetes (648.8)*
> *hyperglycemia NOS (790.29)*
> *neonatal diabetes mellitus (775.1)*
> *nonclinical diabetes (790.29)*
> *Type I diabetes – see category 250*
> *Type II diabetes – see category 250*

The following fifth-digit subclassification is for use with category 249:

> **0 not stated as uncontrolled, or unspecified**
> **1 uncontrolled**

> Use additional code to identify any associated insulin use (V58.67)
> Coding Clinic: 2008, Q4, P91-95

● **249.0 Secondary diabetes mellitus without mention of**
[0-1] **complication**
> Secondary diabetes mellitus without mention of complication or manifestation classifiable to 249.1-249.9
> Secondary diabetes mellitus NOS

● **249.1 Secondary diabetes mellitus with ketoacidosis** 🅒🅒 🅒🅒
[0-1]   Secondary diabetes mellitus with diabetic acidosis without mention of coma
> Secondary diabetes mellitus with diabetic ketosis without mention of coma
> (Ex) 249.00-251.3, 259.8-259.9

● **249.2 Secondary diabetes mellitus with**
[0-1] **hyperosmolarity** 🅒🅒 🅒🅒
> Secondary diabetes mellitus with hyperosmolar (nonketotic) coma
> (Ex) 249.00-251.3, 259.8-259.9

● **249.3 Secondary diabetes mellitus with other coma** 🅒🅒
[0-1]   Secondary diabetes mellitus with diabetic coma (with ketoacidosis)
> Secondary diabetes mellitus with diabetic hypoglycemic coma
> Secondary diabetes mellitus with insulin coma NOS

> **Excludes**   *secondary diabetes mellitus with hyperosmolar coma (249.2)*
> (Ex) 249.00-251.3, 259.8-259.9

● **249.4 Secondary diabetes mellitus with renal**
[0-1] **manifestations**
> Use additional code to identify manifestation, as:
> chronic kidney disease (585.1-585.9)
> diabetic nephropathy NOS (583.81)
> diabetic nephrosis (581.81)
> intercapillary glomerulosclerosis (581.81)
> Kimmelstiel-Wilson syndrome (581.81)

● **249.5 Secondary diabetes mellitus with ophthalmic**
[0-1] **manifestations**
> Use additional code to identify manifestation, as:
> diabetic blindness (369.00-369.9)
> diabetic cataract (366.41)
> diabetic glaucoma (365.44)
> diabetic macular edema (362.07)
> diabetic retinal edema (362.07)
> diabetic retinopathy (362.01-362.07)

● **249.6 Secondary diabetes mellitus with neurological**
[0-1] **manifestations**
> Use additional code to identify manifestation, as:
> diabetic amyotrophy (353.5)
> diabetic gastroparalysis (536.3)
> diabetic gastroparesis (536.3)
> diabetic mononeuropathy (354.0-355.9)
> diabetic neurogenic arthropathy (713.5)
> diabetic peripheral autonomic neuropathy (337.1)
> diabetic polyneuropathy (357.2)
> Coding Clinic: 2008, Q4, P91-95

● **249.7 Secondary diabetes mellitus with peripheral**
[0-1] **circulatory disorders**
> Use additional code to identify manifestation, as:
> diabetic gangrene (785.4)
> diabetic peripheral angiopathy (443.81)

● **249.8 Secondary diabetes mellitus with other specified**
[0-1] **manifestations**
> Secondary diabetic hypoglycemia in diabetes mellitus
> Secondary hypoglycemic shock in diabetes mellitus

> Use additional code to identify manifestation, as:
> any associated ulceration (707.10-707.9)
> diabetic bone changes (731.8)

●● **249.9 Secondary diabetes mellitus with unspecified**
[0-1] **complication**

N   Newborn Age: 0   **P**   Pediatric Age: 0–17   **M**   Maternity Age: 12–55   **A**   Adult Age: 15–124   ♀   Females Only   ♂   Males Only

(Ex) CC Exclusions   🅒 Complication\Comorbidity   🅒🅒 Major C\C   🅟 Present on Admission Requirement   🅗🅒 Hospital-Acquired Condition   **803**

ENDOCRINE, NUTRITIONAL AND METABOLIC DISEASES, AND IMMUNITY DISORDERS (240–279)

ENDOCRINE, NUTRITIONAL AND METABOLIC DISEASES, AND IMMUNITY DISORDERS (240–279)

● 250 **Diabetes mellitus**

Metabolic disease that results in persistent hyperglycemia.
The three primary forms of diabetes mellitus are
differentiated by patterns of pancreatic failure—type 1,
type 2 and 3.

Excludes	*gestational diabetes (648.8)*
	hyperglycemia NOS (790.29)
	neonatal diabetes mellitus (775.1)
	nonclinical diabetes (790.29)
	secondary diabetes (249.0–249.9)

The following fifth-digit subclassification is for use with
category 250:

> **0 type II or unspecified type, not stated as**
> **uncontrolled**
> Fifth-digit 0 is for use for type II patients, even if
> the patient requires insulin
> Use additional code, if applicable, for associated
> long-term (current) insulin use V58.67
> **1 type I [juvenile type], not stated as uncontrolled**
> **2 type II or unspecified type, uncontrolled**
> Fifth-digit 2 is for use for type II patients, even if
> the patient requires insulin
> Use additional code, if applicable, for associated
> long-term (current) insulin use V58.67
> **3 type I [juvenile type], uncontrolled**

Coding Clinic: 2006, Q1, P14; 1996, Q3, P5

OGCR Section I.C.3.a.3

If the documentation in a medical record does not
indicate the type of diabetes but does indicate that
the patient uses insulin, the appropriate fifth-digit for
type II must be used.

● 250.0 **Diabetes mellitus without mention of complication**
[0-3]   Diabetes mellitus without mention of complication
or manifestation classifiable to 250.1–250.9
Diabetes (mellitus) NOS
Coding Clinic: 2005, Q2, P21-22; Q1, P15; 2004, Q2, P17; 2003,
Q4, P105-106, 108-109, P110; Q2, P6-7, 16; Q1, P5; 2002,
Q2, P13; Q1, P7-8; 2001, Q2, P16; 1997, Q4, P33; 1994,
Q1, P16-17, 21; 1993, Q4, P42; 5th Issue, P15; 1992, Q2,
P15; 1990, Q2, P22; 1985, Nov-Dec, P11; Sept-Oct, P11;
Mar-April, P12

MCE: Questionable admission, principal diagnosis
only, 250.00

● 250.1 **Diabetes with ketoacidosis** 🔹🔹
[0-3]   Diabetic:
acidosis without mention of coma
ketosis without mention of coma
Ⓔⓧ 249.00-251.3, 259.8-259.9
Coding Clinic: 2006, Q2, P19-20; 2003, Q4, P81-82; 1987, Jan-Feb,
P15

● 250.2 **Diabetes with hyperosmolarity** 🔹🔹
[0-3]   Hyperosmolar (nonketotic) coma
Ⓔⓧ 249.00-251.3, 259.8-259.9

● 250.3 **Diabetes with other coma** 🔹
[0-3]   Diabetic coma (with ketoacidosis)
Diabetic hypoglycemic coma
Insulin coma NOS

> | Excludes | *diabetes with hyperosmolar coma (250.2)* |
> | --- | --- |

Ⓔⓧ 249.00-251.3, 259.8-259.9

● 250.4 **Diabetes with renal manifestations**
[0-3]   Use additional code to identify manifestation, as:
chronic kidney disease (585.1–585.9) diabetic:
nephropathy NOS (583.81)
nephrosis (581.81)
intercapillary glomerulosclerosis (581.81)
Kimmelstiel-Wilson syndrome (581.81)
Coding Clinic: 2003, Q1, P20-21; 1987, Sept-Oct, P9

● 250.5 **Diabetes with ophthalmic manifestations**
[0-3]   Use additional code to identify manifestation, as:
diabetic:
blindness (369.00–369.9)
cataract (366.41)
glaucoma (365.44)
macular edema (362.07)
retinal edema (362.07)
retinopathy (362.01–362.07)
Coding Clinic: 2005, Q4, P65-67; 1993, Q4, P38; 1985, Sept-Oct, P11

● 250.6 **Diabetes with neurological manifestations**
[0-3]   Use additional code to identify manifestation, as:
diabetic:
amyotrophy (353.5)
gastroparalysis (536.3)
gastroparesis (536.3)
mononeuropathy (354.0–355.9)
neurogenic arthropathy (713.5)
peripheral autonomic neuropathy (337.1)
polyneuropathy (357.2)
Coding Clinic: 2009, Q2, P10; 2008, Q3, P5-6; 2004, Q2, P7; 2003,
Q4, P105; 1993, Q2, P6; 5th Issue, P15; 1984, Nov-Dec, P9

● 250.7 **Diabetes with peripheral circulatory disorders**
[0-3]   Use additional code to identify manifestation, as:
diabetic:
gangrene (785.4)
peripheral angiopathy (443.81)
Coding Clinic: 2004, Q1, P14-15; 2002, Q1, P7-8; 1996, Q1, P10;
1994, Q3, P5; Q2, P17; 1990, Q3, P15; 1986, Mar-April, P12

● 250.8 **Diabetes with other specified manifestations**
[0-3]   Diabetic hypoglycemia NOS
Hypoglycemic shock NOS

Use additional code to identify manifestation, as:
any associated ulceration (707.10–707.9)
diabetic bone changes (731.8)
Coding Clinic: 1997, Q4, P43; 1994, Q2, P13

● 250.9 **Diabetes with unspecified complication**
[0-3]   **Coding Clinic: 2006, Q1, P14; 1993, Q4, P38; 5th Issue, P15; 5th**
Issue, P11; 1985, Nov-Dec, P11

● 251 **Other disorders of pancreatic internal secretion**

251.0 **Hypoglycemic coma** 🔹🔹
Iatrogenic hyperinsulinism
Non-diabetic insulin coma

Use additional E code to identify cause, if
drug-induced

> | Excludes | *hypoglycemic coma in diabetes mellitus* |
> | --- | --- |
> | | *(249.3, 250.3)* |

Ⓔⓧ 249.00-251.3, 259.50-259.9
Coding Clinic: 1985, Mar-April, P8-9

◀ New   ◀▥ Revised   ~~deleted~~ Deleted   ● Unacceptable Principal Diagnosis   ● Use Additional Digit(s)
▶ Manifestation Code   OGCR Official Guidelines   Coding Clinic   Excludes   Includes   Use additional   Code first   Omit code

251.1 Other specified hypoglycemia
Hyperinsulinism:
    NOS
    ectopic
    functional
Hyperplasia of pancreatic islet beta cells NOS

> **Excludes**   *hypoglycemia in diabetes mellitus*
>   *(249.8, 250.8)*
> *hypoglycemia in infant of diabetic*
>   *mother (775.0)*
> *hypoglycemic coma (251.0)*
> *neonatal hypoglycemia (775.6)*

Use additional E code to identify cause, if
    drug-induced
Coding Clinic: 2003, Q1, P10

251.2 Hypoglycemia, unspecified
Hypoglycemia:
    NOS
    reactive
    spontaneous

> **Excludes**   *hypoglycemia:*
>   *with coma (251.0)*
>   *in diabetes mellitus (249.8, 250.8)*
>   *leucine-induced (270.3)*

Coding Clinic: 1985, Mar-April, P8-9

251.3 Postsurgical hypoinsulinemia 🔖
Hypoinsulinemia following complete or partial
    pancreatectomy
Postpancreatectomy hyperglycemia

Use additional code to identify (any associated): ◀
    acquired absence of pancreas (V45.79) ◀
    insulin use (V58.67) ◀
    secondary diabetes mellitus (249.00-249.91) ◀

> **Excludes**   *transient hyperglycemia post procedure*
>   *(790.29)* ◀
> *transient hypoglycemia post procedure*
>   *(251.2)* ◀

(Ex) 249.00-251.3, 259.50-259.9

251.4 Abnormality of secretion of glucagon
Hyperplasia of pancreatic islet alpha cells with
    glucagon excess

251.5 Abnormality of secretion of gastrin
Hyperplasia of pancreatic alpha cells with gastrin
    excess
Zollinger-Ellison syndrome

**251.8 Other specified disorders of pancreatic internal
secretion**
Coding Clinic: 1998, Q2, P15

251.9 Unspecified disorder of pancreatic internal secretion
Islet cell hyperplasia NOS

● **252 Disorders of parathyroid gland**

> **Excludes**   *hungry bone syndrome (275.5)*

● **252.0 Hyperparathyroidism**

> **Excludes**   *ectopic hyperparathyroidism (259.3)*

Coding Clinic: 2004, Q4, P57-59

252.00 Hyperparathyroidism, unspecified

252.01 Primary hyperparathyroidism
Hyperplasia of parathyroid

252.02 Secondary hyperparathyroidism, non-renal

> **Excludes**   *secondary hyperparathyroidism (of*
>   *renal origin) (588.81)*

252.08 Other hyperparathyroidism
Tertiary hyperparathyroidism

Figure 3–5 Tetany caused by
hypoparathyroidism.

Item 3–4 Hyperparathyroidism is an overactive
parathyroid gland that secretes excessive parathormone, causing
increased levels of circulating calcium. This results in a loss of
calcium in the bone (osteoporosis).
Hypoparathyroidism is an underactive parathyroid gland
that results in decreased levels of circulating calcium. The primary
manifestation is **tetany,** a continuous muscle spasm.

252.1 Hypoparathyroidism
Parathyroiditis (autoimmune)
Tetany:
    parathyroid
    parathyroprival

> **Excludes**   *pseudohypoparathyroidism (275.49)*
> *pseudopseudohypoparathyroidism (275.49)*
> *tetany NOS (781.7)*
> *transitory neonatal hypoparathyroidism*
>   *(775.4)*

252.8 Other specified disorders of parathyroid gland
Cyst of parathyroid gland
Hemorrhage of parathyroid gland

252.9 Unspecified disorder of parathyroid gland

● **253 Disorders of the pituitary gland and its hypothalamic
control**

> **Includes**   the listed conditions whether the disorder is in
>   the pituitary or the hypothalamus

> **Excludes**   *Cushing's syndrome (255.0)*

253.0 Acromegaly and gigantism
Overproduction of growth hormone

**253.1 Other and unspecified anterior pituitary
hyperfunction** 🔖
Forbes-Albright syndrome

> **Excludes**   *overproduction of:*
>   *ACTH (255.3)*
>   *thyroid-stimulating hormone [TSH]*
>   *(242.8)*

(Ex) 253.1, 253.4, 253.6
Coding Clinic: 1985, July-Aug, P9

253.2 Panhypopituitarism 🔖
Cachexia, pituitary
Necrosis of pituitary (postpartum)
Pituitary insufficiency NOS
Sheehan's syndrome
Simmonds' disease

> **Excludes**   *iatrogenic hypopituitarism (253.7)*

(Ex) 253.0-253.9, 259.50-259.9

253.3 Pituitary dwarfism
Isolated deficiency of (human) growth hormone
    [HGH]
Lorain-Levi dwarfism

253.4 Other anterior pituitary disorders
Isolated or partial deficiency of an anterior
    pituitary hormone, other than growth
    hormone
Prolactin deficiency
Coding Clinic: 1985, July-Aug, P9

ENDOCRINE, NUTRITIONAL AND METABOLIC DISEASES, AND IMMUNITY DISORDERS (240—279)

253.5 Diabetes insipidus 🅦
Vasopressin deficiency

> **Excludes**   *nephrogenic diabetes insipidus (588.1)*

Ⓔ 253.1-253.2, 253.4-253.9, 259.50-259.9

253.6 Other disorders of neurohypophysis 🅦
Syndrome of inappropriate secretion of antidiuretic hormone [ADH]

> **Excludes**   *ectopic antidiuretic hormone secretion (259.3)*

Ⓔ 253.0-253.9, 259.8-259.9
Coding Clinic: 1993, 5th Issue, P8

253.7 Iatrogenic pituitary disorders
Hypopituitarism:
   hormone-induced
   hypophysectomy-induced
   postablative
   radiotherapy-induced

> Use additional E code to identify cause

253.8 Other disorders of the pituitary and other syndromes of diencephalohypophyseal origin
Abscess of pituitary
Adiposogenital dystrophy
Cyst of Rathke's pouch
Fröhlich's syndrome

> **Excludes**   *craniopharyngioma (237.0)*

253.9 Unspecified
Dyspituitarism

● **254   Diseases of thymus gland**

> **Excludes**   *aplasia or dysplasia with immunodeficiency (279.2)*
> *hypoplasia with immunodeficiency (279.2)*
> *myasthenia gravis (358.00–358.01)*

254.0 Persistent hyperplasia of thymus
Hypertrophy of thymus

254.1 Abscess of thymus 🅦
Ⓔ 254.0-254.9, 259.50-259.9

254.8 Other specified diseases of thymus gland
Atrophy of thymus
Cyst of thymus

> **Excludes**   *thymoma (212.6)*

254.9 Unspecified disease of thymus gland

● **255   Disorders of adrenal glands**

> **Includes**   the listed conditions whether the basic disorder is in the adrenals or is pituitary-induced

255.0 Cushing's syndrome 🅦
Adrenal hyperplasia due to excess ACTH
Cushing's syndrome:
   NOS
   iatrogenic
   idiopathic
   pituitary-dependent
Ectopic ACTH syndrome
Iatrogenic syndrome of excess cortisol
Overproduction of cortisol

> Use additional E code to identify cause, if drug-induced

Ⓔ 255.0-255.2, 259.50-259.9

> **Excludes**   *congenital adrenal hyperplasia (255.2)*

Figure 3–6   Centripetal and generalized obesity and dorsal kyphosis in a 30-year-old woman with Cushing's disease. (From Larsen: Williams Textbook of Endocrinology, 10th ed. 2003, Saunders, An Imprint of Elsevier)

Item 3–5   Hyperadrenalism is overactivity of the adrenal cortex, which secretes corticosterioid hormones. Excessive glucocorticoid hormone results in hyperglycemia (**Cushing's syndrome**), and excessive aldosterone results in **Conn's syndrome**. **Adrenogenital syndrome** is the result of excessive secretion of androgens, male hormones, which stimulates premature sexual development. **Hypoadrenalism, Addison's disease,** is a condition in which the adrenal glands atrophy.

● **255.1 Hyperaldosteronism**
   Coding Clinic: 2003, Q4, P48-50

> **255.10 Hyperaldosteronism, unspecified**
> Aldosteronism NOS
> Primary aldosteronism, unspecified
>
> > **Excludes**   *Conn's syndrome (255.12)*
>
> **255.11 Glucocorticoid-remediable aldosteronism**
> Familial aldosteronism type I
>
> > **Excludes**   *Conn's syndrome (255.12)*
>
> **255.12 Conn's syndrome**
>
> **255.13 Bartter's syndrome**
>
> **255.14 Other secondary aldosteronism**
>   **Coding Clinic: 2006, Q3, P24**

255.2 Adrenogenital disorders
Achard-Thiers syndrome
Adrenogenital syndromes, virilizing or feminizing, whether acquired or associated with congenital adrenal hyperplasia consequent on inborn enzyme defects in hormone synthesis
Congenital adrenal hyperplasia
Female adrenal pseudohermaphroditism
Male:
   macrogenitosomia praecox
   sexual precocity with adrenal hyperplasia
Virilization (female) (suprarenal)

> **Excludes**   *adrenal hyperplasia due to excess ACTH (255.0)*
> *isosexual virilization (256.4)*

255.3 Other corticoadrenal overactivity 🅦
Acquired benign adrenal androgenic overactivity
Overproduction of ACTH
Ⓔ 017.60-0176.6, 017.90-017.96, 255.3-255.9, 259.50-259.9

ENDOCRINE, NUTRITIONAL AND METABOLIC DISEASES, AND IMMUNITY DISORDERS (240–279)

● **255.4 Corticoadrenal insufficiency**

> **Excludes** | *tuberculous Addison's disease (017.6)*
>
> Coding Clinic: 2006, Q3, P24; 1985, July-Aug, P8

255.41 Glucocorticoid deficiency◔
Addisonian crisis
Addison's disease NOS
Adrenal atrophy (autoimmune)
Adrenal calcification
Adrenal crisis
Adrenal hemorrhage
Adrenal infarction
Adrenal insufficiency NOS
Combined glucocorticoid and
    mineralocorticoid deficiency
Corticoadrenal insufficiency NOS
Ⓔⓧ 017.60-0176.6, 017.90-017.96, 255.3-255.9, 259.50-259.9
Coding Clinic: 2007, Q4, P68-70

255.42 Mineralocorticoid deficiency◔
Hypoaldosteronism

> **Excludes** | *combined glucocorticoid and*
> *mineralocorticoid deficiency*
> *(255.41)*
> Ⓔⓧ 017.60-017.66, 017.90-017.96, 255.3-255.9, 259.50-259.9
> Coding Clinic: 2006, Q3, P24

255.5 Other adrenal hypofunction◔
Adrenal medullary insufficiency

> **Excludes** | *Waterhouse-Friderichsen syndrome*
> *(meningococcal) (036.3)*
> Ⓔⓧ 017.60-017.66, 017.90-017.96, 255.3-255.9, 259.50-259.9

255.6 Medulloadrenal hyperfunction◔
Catecholamine secretion by pheochromocytoma
Ⓔⓧ 017.60-017.66, 017.90-017.96, 255.3-255.9, 259.50-259.9

255.8 Other specified disorders of adrenal glands
Abnormality of cortisol-binding globulin
Coding Clinic: 1985, July-Aug, P8

255.9 Unspecified disorder of adrenal glands

● **256 Ovarian dysfunction**

256.0 Hyperestrogenism ♀

256.1 Other ovarian hyperfunction ♀
Hypersecretion of ovarian androgens
Coding Clinic: 1995, Q3, P15

256.2 Postablative ovarian failure ♀
Ovarian failure:
    iatrogenic
    postirradiation
    postsurgical

> Use additional code for states associated with
> artificial menopause (627.4)
>
> **Excludes** | *acquired absence of ovary (V45.77)*
> *asymptomatic age-related (natural)*
> *postmenopausal status (V49.81)*
> Coding Clinic: 2002, Q2, P12-13

● **256.3 Other ovarian failure**

> Use additional code for states associated with
> natural menopause (627.4)
>
> **Excludes** | *asymptomatic age-related (natural)*
> *postmenopausal status (V49.81)*

256.31 Premature menopause ♀   **A**

256.39 Other ovarian failure ♀
Delayed menarche
Ovarian hypofunction
Primary ovarian failure NOS

256.4 Polycystic ovaries ♀
Isosexual virilization Stein-Leventhal syndrome

256.8 Other ovarian dysfunction ♀

256.9 Unspecified ovarian dysfunction ♀

● **257 Testicular dysfunction**

257.0 Testicular hyperfunction ♂
Hypersecretion of testicular hormones

257.1 Postablative testicular hypofunction ♂
Testicular hypofunction:
    iatrogenic
    postirradiation
    postsurgical

257.2 Other testicular hypofunction
Defective biosynthesis of testicular androgen
Eunuchoidism:
    NOS
    hypogonadotropic
Failure:
    Leydig's cell, adult
    seminiferous tubule, adult
Testicular hypogonadism

> **Excludes** | *azoospermia (606.0)*

257.8 Other testicular dysfunction

> **Excludes** | *androgen insensitivity syndrome*
> *(259.50–259.52)*

257.9 Unspecified testicular dysfunction ♂

● **258 Polyglandular dysfunction and related disorders**

● **258.0 Polyglandular activity in multiple endocrine
adenomatosis**
Multiple endocrine neoplasia [MEN] syndromes

> Use additional codes to identify any malignancies
> and other conditions associated with the
> syndromes

**258.01 Multiple endocrine neoplasia [MEN]
type I**
Wermer's syndrome
Coding Clinic: 2008, Q4, P85-90; 2007, Q4, P70-72

**258.02 Multiple endocrine neoplasia [MEN]
type IIA**
Sipple's syndrome

**258.03 Multiple endocrine neoplasia [MEN]
type IIB**

258.1 Other combinations of endocrine dysfunction
Lloyd's syndrome
Schmidt's syndrome

258.8 Other specified polyglandular dysfunction

258.9 Polyglandular dysfunction, unspecified

ENDOCRINE, NUTRITIONAL AND METABOLIC DISEASES, AND IMMUNITY DISORDERS (240–279)

● **259 Other endocrine disorders**

259.0 Delay in sexual development and puberty, not elsewhere classified
Delayed puberty

259.1 Precocious sexual development and puberty, not elsewhere classified   P
Sexual precocity:
NOS
constitutional
cryptogenic
idiopathic

259.2 Carcinoid syndrome 🔖
Hormone secretion by carcinoid tumors
(Ex:) 259.2-259.3, 259.50-259.9
Coding Clinic: 2008, Q4, P85-90

259.3 Ectopic hormone secretion, not elsewhere classified
Ectopic:
antidiuretic hormone secretion [ADH]
hyperparathyroidism
| Excludes | ectopic ACTH syndrome (255.0) |

259.4 Dwarfism, not elsewhere classified
Dwarfism:
NOS
constitutional
| Excludes | dwarfism: |
achondroplastic (756.4)
intrauterine (759.7)
nutritional (263.2)
pituitary (253.3)
renal (588.0)
progeria (259.8)

● **259.5 Androgen insensitivity syndrome**
Coding Clinic: 2008, Q4, P95-96; 2005, Q4, P53-54

259.50 Androgen insensitivity, unspecified

259.51 Androgen insensitivity syndrome
Complete androgen insensitivity
de Quervain's syndrome
Goldberg-Maxwell Syndrome

259.52 Partial androgen insensitivity
Partial androgen insensitivity syndrome
Reifenstein syndrome

259.8 Other specified endocrine disorders
Pineal gland dysfunction
Progeria
Werner's syndrome

259.9 Unspecified endocrine disorder
Disturbance:
endocrine NOS
hormone NOS
Infantilism NOS

NUTRITIONAL DEFICIENCIES (260–269)

| Excludes | deficiency anemias (280.0–281.9) |

260 Kwashiorkor 🔖
Nutritional edema with dyspigmentation of skin and hair
(Ex:) 260-263.9

261 Nutritional marasmus 🔖
Nutritional atrophy
Severe calorie deficiency
Severe malnutrition NOS
(Ex:) 260-263.9
Coding Clinic: 2007, Q4, P96-97; 2006, Q3, P14-15; Q2, P12

262 Other severe protein-calorie malnutrition 🔖
Nutritional edema without mention of dyspigmentation of skin and hair
(Ex:) 260-263.9
Coding Clinic: 1985, July-Aug, P12-13

● **263 Other and unspecified protein-calorie malnutrition**

263.0 Malnutrition of moderate degree
Coding Clinic: 1985, July-Aug, P12-13

263.1 Malnutrition of mild degree
Coding Clinic: 1985, July-Aug, P12-13

263.2 Arrested development following protein-calorie malnutrition 🔖
Nutritional dwarfism
Physical retardation due to malnutrition
(Ex:) 260-263.9

263.8 Other protein-calorie malnutrition 🔖
(Ex:) 260-263.9

263.9 Unspecified protein-calorie malnutrition 🔖
Dystrophy due to malnutrition
Malnutrition (calorie) NOS
| Excludes | nutritional deficiency NOS (269.9) |
(Ex:) 260-263.9
Coding Clinic: 2006, Q2, P12; 2003, Q4, P109-110; 1984, Nov-Dec, P19

Figure 3–7   Bitot's spot on the conjunctiva.

Item 3–6 Bitot's spots are the result of a buildup of keratin debris found on the superficial surface the conjunctiva; oval, triangular, or irregular in shape; and a sign of vitamin A deficiency and associated with night blindness. The disease may progress to **keratomalacia,** which can result in eventual prolapse of the iris and loss of the lens.

Figure 3–8   The sharply demarcated, characteristic scaling dermatitis of pellagra. (From Kumar: Robbins and Cotran: Pathologic Basis of Disease, 7th ed. 2005, Saunders, An Imprint of Elsevier)

Item 3–7 Pellagra is associated with a deficiency of niacin and its precursor, **tryptophan.** Characteristics of the condition include diarrhea, dermatitis on exposed skin surfaces, dementia, and death. It is prevalent in developing countries where nutrition is inadequate. **Beriberi** is associated with thiamine deficiency.

● **264 Vitamin A deficiency**

264.0 With conjunctival xerosis

264.1 With conjunctival xerosis and Bitot's spot
Bitot's spot in the young child

264.2 With corneal xerosis

264.3 With corneal ulceration and xerosis

264.4 With keratomalacia

264.5 With night blindness

264.6 With xerophthalmic scars of cornea

264.7 Other ocular manifestations of vitamin A deficiency
Xerophthalmia due to vitamin A deficiency

264.8 Other manifestations of vitamin A deficiency
Follicular keratosis due to vitamin A deficiency
Xeroderma due to vitamin A deficiency

264.9 Unspecified vitamin A deficiency
Hypovitaminosis A NOS

◀ New   ◀▥ Revised   ~~deleted~~ Deleted   ● Unacceptable Principal Diagnosis   ● Use Additional Digit(s)
▸ Manifestation Code   **OGCR** Official Guidelines   **Coding Clinic** | Excludes | Includes   Use additional   Code first   Omit code

● **265   Thiamine and niacin deficiency states**

    265.0   Beribéri 🖤
       Ⓔₓ 265.0-266.9, 269.1-269.9

    265.1   Other and unspecified manifestations of thiamine deficiency 🖤
       Other vitamin B_1 deficiency states
       Ⓔₓ 265.0-266.9, 269.1-269.9

    265.2   Pellagra
       Deficiency:
          niacin (-tryptophan)
          nicotinamide
          nicotinic acid
          vitamin PP
       Pellagra (alcoholic)

● **266   Deficiency of B-complex components**

    266.0   Ariboflavinosis 🖤
       Riboflavin [vitamin B_2] deficiency
       Ⓔₓ 265.0-266.9, 269.1-269.9
       Coding Clinic: 1986, Sept-Oct, P10

    266.1   Vitamin B_6 deficiency
       Deficiency:
          pyridoxal
          pyridoxamine
          pyridoxine
       Vitamin B_6 deficiency syndrome
       | **Excludes** | *vitamin B_6-responsive sideroblastic anemia (285.0)*

    266.2   Other B-complex deficiencies
       Deficiency:
          cyanocobalamin
          folic acid
          vitamin B_{12}
       | **Excludes** | *combined system disease with anemia (281.0–281.1)*
            deficiency anemias (281.0–281.9)
            subacute degeneration of spinal cord with anemia (281.0–281.1)

    266.9   Unspecified vitamin B deficiency

267   Ascorbic acid deficiency
       Deficiency of vitamin C
       Scurvy
       | **Excludes** | *scorbutic anemia (281.8)*

● **268   Vitamin D deficiency**
       | **Excludes** | *vitamin D-resistant:*
            osteomalacia (275.3)
            rickets (275.3)

    268.0   Rickets, active 🖤
       | **Excludes** | *celiac rickets (579.0)*
            renal rickets (588.0)
       Ⓔₓ 268.0-269.9

    268.1   Rickets, late effect 🖤
       Any condition specified as due to rickets and stated to be a late effect or sequela of rickets
       Code first the nature of late effect

    268.2   Osteomalacia, unspecified
       Softening of bone

    268.9   Unspecified vitamin D deficiency
       Avitaminosis D

● **269   Other nutritional deficiencies**

    269.0   Deficiency of vitamin K
       | **Excludes** | *deficiency of coagulation factor due to vitamin K deficiency (286.7)*
            vitamin K deficiency of newborn (776.0)

    269.1   Deficiency of other vitamins
       Deficiency:
          vitamin E
          vitamin P

    269.2   Unspecified vitamin deficiency
       Multiple vitamin deficiency NOS

    269.3   Mineral deficiency, not elsewhere classified
       Deficiency:
          calcium, dietary
          iodine
       | **Excludes** | *deficiency:*
            calcium NOS (275.40)
            potassium (276.8)
            sodium (276.1)

    269.8   Other nutritional deficiency
       | **Excludes** | *adult failure to thrive (783.7)*
            failure to thrive in childhood (783.41)
            feeding problems (783.3)
            newborn (779.31–779.34) ◀▥

    269.9   Unspecified nutritional deficiency

OTHER METABOLIC AND IMMUNITY DISORDERS (270–279)

Use additional code to identify any associated mental retardation

● **270   Disorders of amino-acid transport and metabolism**
       | **Excludes** | *abnormal findings without manifest disease (790.0–796.9)*
            disorders of purine and pyrimidine metabolism (277.1–277.2)
            gout (274.00–274.9) ◀▥

    270.0   Disturbances of amino-acid transport 🖤
       Cystinosis
       Cystinuria
       Fanconi (-de Toni) (-Debré) syndrome
       Glycinuria (renal)
       Hartnup disease
       Ⓔₓ 270.0-273.3, 273.8-273.9

    270.1   Phenylketonuria [PKU] 🖤
       Hyperphenylalaninemia
       Ⓔₓ 270.0-273.3, 273.8-273.9

    270.2   Other disturbances of aromatic amino-acid metabolism 🖤
       Albinism
       Alkaptonuria
       Alkaptonuric ochronosis
       Disturbances of metabolism of tyrosine and tryptophan
       Homogentisic acid defects
       Hydroxykynureninuria
       Hypertyrosinemia
       Indicanuria
       Kynureninase defects
       Oasthouse urine disease
       Ochronosis
       Tyrosinosis
       Tyrosinuria
       Waardenburg syndrome
       | **Excludes** | *vitamin B_6-deficiency syndrome (266.1)*
       Ⓔₓ 270.0-273.3, 273.8-273.9
       Coding Clinic: 1999, Q3, P20-21

N   Newborn Age: 0   P   Pediatric Age: 0–17   M   Maternity Age: 12–55   A   Adult Age: 15–124   ♀   Females Only   ♂   Males Only

Ⓔₓ   CC Exclusions   🖤 Complication\Comorbidity   🖤 Major C\C   🖤 Present on Admission Requirement   🖤 Hospital-Acquired Condition   **809**

270.3 Disturbances of branched-chain amino-acid metabolism %

Disturbances of metabolism of leucine, isoleucine, and valine
Hypervalinemia
Intermittent branched-chain ketonuria
Leucine-induced hypoglycemia
Leucinosis
Maple syrup urine disease
Ex: 270.0-273.3, 273.8-273.9
Coding Clinic: 2000, Q3, P8

270.4 Disturbances of sulphur-bearing amino-acid metabolism %

Cystathioninemia
Cystathioninuria
Disturbances of metabolism of methionine, homocystine, and cystathionine
Homocystinuria
Hypermethioninemia
Methioninemia
Ex: 270.0-273.3, 273.8-273.9
Coding Clinic: 2007, Q2, P9; 2004, Q1, P6

270.5 Disturbances of histidine metabolism %

Carnosinemia   Hyperhistidinemia
Histidinemia   Imidazole
                    aminoaciduria
Ex: 270.0-273.3, 273.8-273.9

270.6 Disorders of urea cycle metabolism %

Argininosuccinic aciduria
Citrullinemia
Disorders of metabolism of ornithine, citrulline, argininosuccinic acid, arginine, and ammonia
Hyperammonemia
Hyperornithinemia
Ex: 270.0-273.3, 273.8-273.9

270.7 Other disturbances of straight-chain amino-acid metabolism %

Glucoglycinuria
Glycinemia (with methylmalonic acidemia)
Hyperglycinemia
Hyperlysinemia
Pipecolic acidemia
Saccharopinuria
Other disturbances of metabolism of glycine, threonine, serine, glutamine, and lysine
Ex: 270.0-273.3, 273.8-273.9
Coding Clinic: 2000, Q3, P8

Item 3–8 Any term ending with "emia" will be a blood condition. Any term ending with "uria" will have to do with urine. A term ending with "opathy" is a disease condition. Check for laboratory work.

270.8 Other specified disorders of amino-acid metabolism %

Alaninemia   Iminoacidopathy
Ethanolaminuria   Prolinemia
Glycoprolinuria   Prolinuria
Hydroxyprolinemia   Sarcosinemia
Hyperprolinemia
Ex: 270.0-273.3, 273.8-273.9

270.9 Unspecified disorder of amino-acid metabolism %

Ex: 270.0-273.3, 273.8-273.9

● 271 Disorders of carbohydrate transport and metabolism

Excludes   abnormality of secretion of glucagon (251.4)
            diabetes mellitus (249.0–249.9, 250.0–250.9)
            hypoglycemia NOS (251.2)
            mucopolysaccharidosis (277.5)

271.0 Glycogenosis %

Amylopectinosis
Glucose-6-phosphatase deficiency
Glycogen storage disease
McArdle's disease
Pompe's disease
von Gierke's disease
Ex: 270.0-273.3, 273.8-273.9
Coding Clinic: 1998, Q1, P5-6

271.1 Galactosemia %

Galactose-1-phosphate uridyl transferase deficiency
Galactosuria
Ex: 270.0-273.3, 273.8-273.9

271.2 Hereditary fructose intolerance

Essential benign fructosuria
Fructosemia

271.3 Intestinal disaccharidase deficiencies and disaccharide malabsorption

Intolerance or malabsorption (congenital) (of):
    glucose-galactose
    lactose
    sucrose-isomaltose

271.4 Renal glycosuria

Renal diabetes

271.8 Other specified disorders of carbohydrate transport and metabolism %

Essential benign pentosuria   Mannosidosis
Fucosidosis   Oxalosis
Glycolic aciduria   Xylosuria
Hyperoxaluria (primary)   Xylulosuria
Ex: 270.0-273.3, 273.8-273.9

271.9 Unspecified disorder of carbohydrate transport and metabolism

● 272 Disorders of lipoid metabolism

Excludes   localized cerebral lipidoses (330.1)

272.0 Pure hypercholesterolemia

Familial hypercholesterolemia
Fredrickson Type IIa hyperlipoproteinemia
Hyperbetalipoproteinemia
Hyperlipidemia, Group A
Low-density-lipoid-type [LDL] hyperlipoproteinemia
Coding Clinic: 2005, Q4, P68-69

272.1 Pure hyperglyceridemia

Endogenous hyperglyceridemia
Fredrickson Type IV hyperlipoproteinemia
Hyperlipidemia, Group B
Hyperprebetalipoproteinemia
Hypertriglyceridemia, essential
Very-low-density-lipoid-type [VLDL] hyperlipoproteinemia
Coding Clinic: 1985, Jan-Feb, P15

272.2 Mixed hyperlipidemia

Broad- or floating-betalipoproteinemia
Combined hyperlipidemia   ◄
Elevated cholesterol with elevated triglycerides ◄
    NEC
Fredrickson Type IIb or III hyperlipoproteinemia
Hypercholesterolemia with endogenous hyperglyceridemia
Hyperbetalipoproteinemia with prebetalipoproteinemia
Tubo-eruptive xanthoma
Xanthoma tuberosum

◄ New   ◄▦ Revised   ~~deleted~~ Deleted   ● Unacceptable Principal Diagnosis   ● Use Additional Digit(s)
▶ Manifestation Code   OGCR Official Guidelines   Coding Clinic   Excludes   Includes   Use additional   Code first   Omit code

272.3 Hyperchylomicronemia
Bürger-Grütz syndrome
Fredrickson type I or V hyperlipoproteinemia
Hyperlipidemia, Group D
Mixed hyperglyceridemia

272.4 Other and unspecified hyperlipidemia
Alpha-lipoproteinemia
~~Combined hyperlipidemia~~
Hyperlipidemia NOS
Hyperlipoproteinemia NOS
Coding Clinic: 2005, Q1, P17

272.5 Lipoprotein deficiencies
Abetalipoproteinemia
Bassen-Kornzweig syndrome
High-density lipoid deficiency
Hypoalphalipoproteinemia
Hypobetalipoproteinemia (familial)

272.6 Lipodystrophy
Barraquer-Simons disease
Progressive lipodystrophy

Use additional E code to identify cause, if
iatrogenic

Excludes   *intestinal lipodystrophy (040.2)*

272.7 Lipidoses
Chemically induced lipidosis
Disease:
Anderson's
Fabry's
Gaucher's
I cell [mucolipidosis I]
lipoid storage NOS
Niemann-Pick
pseudo-Hurler's or mucolipidosis III
triglyceride storage, Type I or II
Wolman's or triglyceride storage, Type III
Mucolipidosis II
Primary familial xanthomatosis

Excludes   *cerebral lipidoses (330.1)*
Tay-Sachs disease (330.1)

272.8 Other disorders of lipoid metabolism
Hoffa's disease or liposynovitis prepatellaris
Launois-Bensaude's lipomatosis
Lipoid dermatoarthritis

272.9 Unspecified disorder of lipoid metabolism

●**273 Disorders of plasma protein metabolism**

Excludes   *agammaglobulinemia and*
hypogammaglobulinemia (279.0–279.2)
coagulation defects (286.0–286.9)
hereditary hemolytic anemias (282.0–282.9)

273.0 Polyclonal hypergammaglobulinemia
Hypergammaglobulinemic purpura:
benign primary
Waldenström's

273.1 Monoclonal paraproteinemia
Benign monoclonal hypergammaglobulinemia
[BMH]
Monoclonal gammopathy:
NOS
associated with lymphoplasmacytic dyscrasias
benign
Paraproteinemia:
benign (familial)
secondary to malignant or inflammatory disease

273.2 Other paraproteinemias
Cryoglobulinemic:
purpura
vasculitis
Mixed cryoglobulinemia
Coding Clinic: 2008, Q2, P17

273.3 Macroglobulinemia
Macroglobulinemia (idiopathic) (primary)
Waldenström's macroglobulinemia

273.4 Alpha-1-antitrypsin deficiency
AAT deficiency
Coding Clinic: 2004, Q4, P59-60

273.8 Other disorders of plasma protein metabolism
Abnormality of transport protein
Bisalbuminemia
Coding Clinic: 1998, Q2, P11

273.9 Unspecified disorder of plasma protein metabolism
Coding Clinic: 1998, Q2, P11

●**274 Gout**
Result of accumulation of uric acid caused by either too much
production, or insufficient natural removal of uric acid
from body. Results in swollen, red, hot, painful, stiff
joints. Also called gouty arthritis.

Excludes   *lead gout (984.0–984.9)*

●**274.0 Gouty arthropathy** ◀▥

    274.00 Gouty arthropathy, unspecified ◀

    274.01 Acute gouty arthropathy ◀
Acute gout ◀
Gout attack ◀
Gout flare ◀
Podagra ◀

    274.02 Chronic gouty arthropathy without mention
of tophus (tophi) ◀
Chronic gout ◀

    274.03 Chronic gouty arthropathy with tophus
(tophi) ◀
Chronic tophaceous gout ◀
Gout with tophi NOS

●**274.1 Gouty nephropathy**

    274.10 Gouty nephropathy, unspecified
Coding Clinic: 1985, Nov-Dec, P15

    274.11 Uric acid nephrolithiasis ◐
(Ex) 016.00-016.06, 016.30-016.36, 016.90-016.96, 017.90-017.96,
078.6, 098.10, 098.19, 098.30-098.31, 098.89, 112.2,
131.00, 131.8-131.9, 249.40-249.41, 249.80-249.91,
250.40-250.43, 250.80-250.93, 274.10-274.19, 274.89,
580.0-584.9, 586-588.1, 588.9-591, 593.0-593.2,
593.89-593.9, 599.60-599.9

    274.19 Other

●**274.8 Gout with other specified manifestations**
Tophi = chalky deposit of sodium urate occurring in
gout

    274.81 Gouty tophi of ear

    274.82 Gouty tophi of other sites
Gouty tophi of heart

Excludes   *gout with tophi NOS (274.03)* ◀
gouty arthropathy with tophi
(274.03) ◀

    274.89 Other

Use additional code to identify
manifestations, as:
gouty:
iritis (364.11)
neuritis (357.4)

    274.9 Gout, unspecified

ENDOCRINE, NUTRITIONAL AND METABOLIC DISEASES, AND IMMUNITY DISORDERS (240–279)

● **275　Disorders of mineral metabolism**

> **Excludes**　*abnormal findings without manifest disease (790.0–796.9)*

275.0　Disorders of iron metabolism
　　Bronzed diabetes
　　Hemochromatosis
　　Pigmentary cirrhosis (of liver)

> **Excludes**　*anemia:*
> 　　*iron deficiency (280.0–280.9)*
> 　　*sideroblastic (285.0)*

　　Coding Clinic: 1997, Q2, P11

275.1　Disorders of copper metabolism
　　Hepatolenticular degeneration
　　Wilson's disease

275.2　Disorders of magnesium metabolism
　　Hypermagnesemia
　　Hypomagnesemia

275.3　Disorders of phosphorus metabolism
　　Familial hypophosphatemia
　　Hypophosphatasia
　　Vitamin D-resistant:
　　　osteomalacia
　　　rickets

● **275.4　Disorders of calcium metabolism**

> **Excludes**　*hungry bone syndrome (275.5)*
> 　　*parathyroid disorders (252.00–252.9)*
> 　　*vitamin D deficiency (268.0–268.9)*

　275.40　Unspecified disorder of calcium metabolism

　275.41　Hypocalcemia
　　　Coding Clinic: 2007, Q3, P5-6

　275.42　Hypercalcemia
　　　Coding Clinic: 2003, Q4, P110

　275.49　Other disorders of calcium metabolism
　　　Nephrocalcinosis
　　　Pseudohypoparathyroidism
　　　Pseudopseudohypoparathyroidism

275.5　Hungry bone syndrome
　　Coding Clinic: 2008, Q4, P96-97

275.8　Other specified disorders of mineral metabolism

275.9　Unspecified disorder of mineral metabolism

● **276　Disorders of fluid, electrolyte, and acid-base balance**

> **Excludes**　*diabetes insipidus (253.5)*
> 　　*familial periodic paralysis (359.3)*

276.0　Hyperosmolality and/or hypernatremia🅒
　　Sodium [Na] excess
　　Sodium [Na] overload
　　(Ex:) 276.0-276.9

276.1　Hyposmolality and/or hyponatremia🅒
　　Sodium [Na] deficiency
　　(Ex:) 276.0-276.9

276.2　Acidosis🅒
　　Acidosis:
　　　NOS　　　　　　metabolic
　　　lactic　　　　　respiratory

> **Excludes**　*diabetic acidosis (249.1, 250.1)*

　　(Ex:) 276.0-276.9
　　Coding Clinic: 1987, Jan-Feb, P15

276.3　Alkalosis🅒
　　Alkalosis:
　　　NOS
　　　metabolic
　　　respiratory
　　(Ex:) 276.0-276.9

276.4　Mixed acid-base balance disorder🅒
　　Hypercapnia with mixed acid-base disorder
　　(Ex:) 276.0-276.9

Item 3–9　Circulating fluid volume is regulated by the amount of water and sodium ingested, excreted by the kidneys into the urine, and lost through the gastrointestinal tract, lungs, and skin. To maintain blood volume within a normal range, the kidneys regulate the amount of water and sodium lost into the urine. Too much **(fluid overload)** or too little fluid volume **(volume depletion)** will affect blood pressure. Severe cases of vomiting, diarrhea, bleeding, and burns (fluid loss through exposed burn surface area) can contribute to fluid loss. Internal body environment must maintain a precise balance (homeostasis) between too much fluid and too little fluid. This complex balancing mechanism is critical to good health.

● **276.5　Volume depletion**

> **Excludes**　*hypovolemic shock:*
> 　　*postoperative (998.0)*
> 　　*traumatic (958.4)*

　Coding Clinic: 2005, Q4, P54-55; Q2, P9-10; 2003, Q1, P5, 20-22;
　　2002, Q3, P21x2; 1997, Q4, P30-31; 1993, 5th Issue, P1;
　　1988, Q2, P9-11; 1984, July-Aug, P19-20

　276.50　Volume depletion, unspecified

　276.51　Dehydration
　　　Coding Clinic: 2008, Q1, P10-11

　276.52　Hypovolemia
　　　Depletion of volume of plasma

276.6　Fluid overload
　　Fluid retention

> **Excludes**　*ascites (789.51–789.59)*
> 　　*localized edema (782.3)*

　　Coding Clinic: 2007, Q3, P11; 2006, Q4, P136; 1987, Sept-Oct, P9

276.7　Hyperpotassemia
　　Hyperkalemia
　　Potassium [K]:　　　　Potassium [K]:
　　　excess　　　　　　　overload
　　　intoxication
　　Coding Clinic: 2005, Q1, P9-10; 2001, Q2, P12-13

276.8　Hypopotassemia
　　Hypokalemia
　　Potassium [K] deficiency

276.9　Electrolyte and fluid disorders not elsewhere classified
　　Electrolyte imbalance
　　Hyperchloremia
　　Hypochloremia

> **Excludes**　*electrolyte imbalance:*
> 　　*associated with hyperemesis gravidarum (643.1)*
> 　　*complicating labor and delivery (669.0)*
> 　　*following abortion and ectopic or molar pregnancy (634–638 with .4, 639.4)*

　　Coding Clinic: 1987, Jan-Feb, P15

◀ New　　◀▥▥ Revised　　~~deleted~~ Deleted　　● Unacceptable Principal Diagnosis　　● Use Additional Digit(s)
▶ Manifestation Code　　**OGCR** Official Guidelines　　**Coding Clinic**　　Excludes　　Includes　　Use additional　　Code first　　Omit code

● **277   Other and unspecified disorders of metabolism**

  ● **277.0   Cystic fibrosis**

       Fibrocystic disease of the pancreas
       Mucoviscidosis
       Coding Clinic: 2002, Q4, P45-46; 1994, Q3, P7; 1990, Q3, P18

       277.00   Without mention of meconium ileus 🕭
           Cystic fibrosis NOS
           (Ex) 277.00-277.09
           Coding Clinic: 2003, Q2, P12

       277.01   With meconium ileus 🕭   **N**
           Meconium:
              ileus (of newborn)
              obstruction of intestine in mucoviscidosis
           (Ex) 277.00-277.09

       277.02   With pulmonary manifestations 🕭
           Cystic fibrosis with pulmonary exacerbation
           Use additional code to identify any
              infectious organism present, such as:
              pseudomonas (041.7)
           (Ex) 277.00-277.09
           Coding Clinic: 2002, Q4, P46

       277.03   With gastrointestinal manifestations 🕭
           Excludes   *with meconium ileus (277.01)*
           (Ex) 277.00-277.09

       277.09   With other manifestations 🕭
           (Ex) 277.00-277.09

  277.1   Disorders of porphyrin metabolism 🕭
       Hematoporphyria   Porphyrinuria
       Hematoporphyrinuria   Protocoproporphyria
       Hereditary coproporphyria   Protoporphyria
       Porphyria   Pyrroloporphyria
       (Ex) 277.1-277.2, 277.4-277.7

  277.2   Other disorders of purine and pyrimidine metabolism 🕭
       Hypoxanthine-guanine-phosphoribosyltransferase
           deficiency [HG-PRT deficiency]
       Lesch-Nyhan syndrome
       Xanthinuria
       (Ex) 277.1-277.2, 277.4-277.7
       Excludes   *gout (274.00–274.9)*   ◀▩
                   orotic aciduric anemia (281.4)

  ● **277.3   Amyloidosis**
       *Disorder resulting from abnormal deposition of
           particular protein (amyloid) into tissues.*
       Coding Clinic: 2006, Q4, P66-67; 1997, Q2, P12-13; 1996, Q1, P16;
           1985, July-Aug, P9

       277.30   Amyloidosis, unspecified 🕭
           Amyloidosis NOS
           (Ex) 277.30-277.39, 277.7

       277.31   Familial Mediterranean fever 🕭
           Benign paroxysmal peritonitis
           Hereditary amyloid nephropathy
           Periodic familial polyserositis
           Recurrent polyserositis
           (Ex) 277.30-277.39, 277.7

       277.39   Other amyloidosis 🕭
           Hereditary cardiac amyloidosis
           Inherited systemic amyloidosis
           Neuropathic (Portuguese) (Swiss)
              amyloidosis
           Secondary amyloidosis
           (Ex) 277.30-277.39, 277.7
           Coding Clinic: 2009, Q1, P17; 2008, Q2, P8-9

  277.4   Disorders of bilirubin excretion
       Hyperbilirubinemia:
           congenital
           constitutional
       Syndrome:
           Crigler-Najjar
           Dubin-Johnson
           Gilbert's
           Rotor's
       Excludes   *hyperbilirubinemias specific to the perinatal
                 period (774.0–774.7)*

  277.5   Mucopolysaccharidosis 🕭
       Gargoylism
       Hunter's syndrome
       Hurler's syndrome
       Lipochondrodystrophy
       Maroteaux-Lamy syndrome
       Morquio-Brailsford disease
       Osteochondrodystrophy
       Sanfilippo's syndrome
       Scheie's syndrome
       (Ex) 277.1-277.31, 277.4-277.7

  277.6   Other deficiencies of circulating enzymes
       Hereditary angioedema
       Coding Clinic: 2004, Q4, P59-60

  277.7   Dysmetabolic syndrome X
       Use additional code for associated manifestation,
           such as:
           cardiovascular disease (414.00–414.07)
           obesity (278.00–278.01)
       Coding Clinic: 2001, Q4, P42

  ● **277.8   Other specified disorders of metabolism**
       Coding Clinic: 2003, Q4, P50-51; 2001, Q2, P18-20

       277.81   Primary carnitine deficiency

       277.82   Carnitine deficiency due to inborn errors of metabolism

       277.83   Iatrogenic carnitine deficiency
           Carnitine deficiency due to:
              Hemodialysis
              Valproic acid therapy

       277.84   Other secondary carnitine deficiency

       277.85   Disorders of fatty acid oxidation 🕭
           Carnitine palmitoyltransferase deficiencies
              (CPT1, CPT2)
           Glutaric aciduria type II (type IIA, IIB, IIC)
           Long chain 3-hydroxyacyl CoA
              dehydrogenase deficiency (LCHAD)
           Long chain/very long chain acyl CoA
              dehydrogenase deficiency (LCAD,
              VLCAD)
           Medium chain acyl CoA dehydrogenase
              deficiency (MCAD)
           Short chain acyl CoA dehydrogenase
              deficiency (SCAD)
           Excludes   *primary carnitine deficiency
                 (277.81)*
           (Ex) 277.81-277.84, 277.86-277.89
           Coding Clinic: 2004, Q4, P60-61

       277.86   Peroxisomal disorders 🕭
           Adrenomyeloneuropathy
           Neonatal adrenoleukodystrophy
           Rhizomelic chondrodysplasia punctata
           X-linked adrenoleukodystrophy
           Zellweger syndrome
           Excludes   *infantile Refsum disease (356.3)*
           (Ex) 277.4, 277.81-277.85, 277.87-277.89
           Coding Clinic: 2004, Q4, P61-62

N   Newborn Age: 0   **P**   Pediatric Age: 0–17   **M**   Maternity Age: 12–55   **A**   Adult Age: 15–124   ♀   Females Only   ♂   Males Only

(Ex)   CC Exclusions   🕭   Complication\Comorbidity   🕭   Major C\C   🕭   Present on Admission Requirement   🕭   Hospital-Acquired Condition

ENDOCRINE, NUTRITIONAL AND METABOLIC DISEASES, AND IMMUNITY DISORDERS (240–279)

ENDOCRINE, NUTRITIONAL AND METABOLIC DISEASES, AND IMMUNITY DISORDERS (240–279)

277.87　Disorders of mitochondrial metabolism 🦠
　　Kearns-Sayre syndrome
　　Mitochondrial Encephalopathy, Lactic
　　　　Acidosis and Stroke-like episodes
　　　　(MELAS syndrome)
　　Mitochondrial Neurogastrointestinal
　　　　Encephalopathy syndrome (MNGIE)
　　Myoclonus with Epilepsy and with Ragged
　　　　Red Fibers (MERRF syndrome)
　　Neuropathy, Ataxia and Retinitis
　　　　Pigmentosa (NARP syndrome)

　　Use additional code for associated
　　　　conditions

　　Excludes　disorders of pyruvate metabolism
　　　　　　　　(271.8)
　　　　　　　Leber's optic atrophy (377.16)
　　　　　　　Leigh's subacute necrotizing
　　　　　　　　encephalopathy (330.8)
　　　　　　　Reye's syndrome (331.81)
　　Ex: 277.4, 277.81-277.86, 277.89
　　Coding Clinic: 2004, Q4, P62-63

277.88　Tumor lysis syndrome 🦠　　　◄
　　Spontaneous tumor lysis syndrome　　◄
　　Tumor lysis syndrome following
　　　　antineoplastic drug therapy　　◄

　　Use additional E code to identify cause,
　　　　if drug-induced　　◄

277.89　Other specified disorders of metabolism 🦠
　　Hand-Schüller-Christian disease
　　Histiocytosis (acute) (chronic)
　　Histiocytosis X (chronic)

　　Excludes　histiocytosis:
　　　　　　　　acute differentiated progressive
　　　　　　　　　(202.5)
　　　　　　　　X, acute (progressive) (202.5)
　　Ex: 277.4, 277.81-277.87

277.9　Unspecified disorder of metabolism
　　Enzymopathy NOS
　　Coding Clinic: 1987, Sept-Oct, P9

● **278　Overweight, obesity and other hyperalimentation**

　　Excludes　hyperalimentation NOS (783.6)
　　　　　　　poisoning by vitamins NOS (963.5)
　　　　　　　polyphagia (783.6)

● **278.0　Overweight and obesity**

　　Excludes　adiposogenital dystrophy (253.8)
　　　　　　　obesity of endocrine origin NOS (259.9)

　　Use additional code to identify Body Mass Index
　　　　(BMI), if known (V85.0–V85.54)
　　Coding Clinic: 2005, Q4, P55

278.00　Obesity, unspecified
　　Obesity NOS
　　Coding Clinic: 2001, Q4, P42; 1999, Q1, P5-6
　　MCE: Questionable admission, principal
　　　　diagnosis only

278.01　Morbid obesity 🦠
　　Severe obesity
　　HAC: Principal Diagnosis 278.01, 998.59
　　　　(CC), and one of the following procedure
　　　　codes: 44.38, 44.39, or 44.95
　　Coding Clinic: 2009, Q2, P10; 2006, Q2, P5-6;
　　　　2003, Q3, P3-8

278.02　Overweight

278.1　Localized adiposity
　　Fat pad
　　Coding Clinic: 2006, Q2, P10-11

278.2　Hypervitaminosis A

278.3　Hypercarotinemia

278.4　Hypervitaminosis D

278.8　Other hyperalimentation
　　Coding Clinic: 2009, Q2, P10

● **279　Disorders involving the immune mechanism**

● **279.0　Deficiency of humoral immunity**

279.00　Hypogammaglobulinemia, unspecified 🦠
　　Agammaglobulinemia NOS
　　Ex: 279.00-279.4, 279.8-279.9

279.01　Selective IgA immunodeficiency 🦠
　　Ex: 279.00-279.4, 279.8-279.9

279.02　Selective IgM immunodeficiency 🦠
　　Ex: 279.02-279.4, 279.8-279.9

**279.03　Other selective immunoglobulin
　　　　deficiencies** 🦠
　　Selective deficiency of IgG
　　Ex: 279.02-279.4, 279.8-279.9

279.04　Congenital hypogammaglobulinemia 🦠
　　Agammaglobulinemia:
　　　　Bruton's type
　　　　X-linked
　　Ex: 279.02-279.4, 279.8-279.9

279.05　Immunodeficiency with increased IgM 🦠
　　Immunodeficiency with hyper-IgM:
　　　　autosomal recessive
　　　　X-linked
　　Ex: 279.02-279.4, 279.8-279.9

279.06　Common variable immunodeficiency 🦠
　　Dysgammaglobulinemia (acquired)
　　　　(congenital) (primary)
　　Hypogammaglobulinemia:
　　　　acquired primary
　　　　congenital non-sex-linked
　　　　sporadic
　　Ex: 279.02-279.4, 279.8-279.9

279.09　Other 🦠
　　Transient hypogammaglobulinemia of
　　　　infancy
　　Ex: 279.02-279.4, 279.8-279.9

● **279.1　Deficiency of cell-mediated immunity**

**279.10　Immunodeficiency with predominant T-cell
　　　　defect, unspecified** 🦠
　　Ex: 279.02-279.4, 279.8-279.9
　　Coding Clinic: 1987, Sept-Oct, P10; 1985, Mar-April, P7

279.11　DiGeorge's syndrome 🦠
　　Pharyngeal pouch syndrome
　　Thymic hypoplasia
　　Ex: 279.02-279.4, 279.8-279.9

279.12　Wiskott-Aldrich syndrome 🦠
　　Ex: 279.02-279.4, 279.8-279.9

279.13　Nezelof's syndrome 🦠
　　Cellular immunodeficiency with abnormal
　　　　immunoglobulin deficiency
　　Ex: 279.02-279.4, 279.8-279.9

279.19　Other 🦠
　　Excludes　ataxia-telangiectasia (334.8)
　　Ex: 279.02-279.4, 279.8-279.9
　　Coding Clinic: 1985, Mar-April, P7

279.2　Combined immunity deficiency 🦠
　　Agammaglobulinemia:
　　　　autosomal recessive
　　　　Swiss-type
　　　　X-linked recessive
　　Severe combined immunodeficiency [SCID]
　　Thymic:
　　　　alymphoplasia
　　　　aplasia or dysplasia with immunodeficiency

　　Excludes　thymic hypoplasia (279.11)
　　Ex: 279.02-279.4, 279.8-279.9

◄ New　　◄▥ Revised　　deleted Deleted　　● Unacceptable Principal Diagnosis　　🦠 Use Additional Digit(s)
▶ Manifestation Code　　OGCR Official Guidelines　　Coding Clinic　　Excludes　　Includes　　Use additional　　Code first　　Omit code

279.3 Unspecified immunity deficiency 🅒
     Ⓔⓧ 279.02-279.4, 279.8-279.9

●**279.4 Autoimmune disease, not elsewhere classified** ◀Ⅲ
     ~~Autoimmune disease NOS~~

     | **Excludes** | *transplant failure or rejection*
                         (996.80–996.89)
     Coding Clinic: 2008, Q3, P5

     **279.41 Autoimmune lymphoproliferative
              syndrome** ◀
              ALPS ◀

     **279.49 Autoimmune disease, not elsewhere
              classified** ◀
              Autoimmune disease NOS ◀

●**279.5 Graft-versus-host disease**

     Code first underlying cause, such as:
         complication of blood transfusion (999.89) ◀Ⅲ
         complication of transplanted organ ~~(bone
         marrow)~~ (996.80-996.89) ◀Ⅲ

     Use additional code to identify associated
         manifestations, such as:
     desquamative dermatitis (695.89)
     diarrhea (787.91)
     elevated bilirubin (782.4)
     hair loss (704.09)
     Coding Clinic: 2008, Q4, P97-100

●**279.50 Graft-versus-host disease, unspecified** 🅒
     Ⓔⓧ 279.50-279.53, 996.85, 997.91-997.99

● **279.51 Acute graft-versus-host disease** 🅒
     Ⓔⓧ 279.50-279.53, 996.85, 997.91-997.99

● **279.52 Chronic graft-versus-host disease** 🅒
     Ⓔⓧ 279.50-279.53, 996.85, 997.91-997.99

● **279.53 Acute on chronic graft-versus-host
             disease** 🅒
     Ⓔⓧ 279.50-279.53, 996.85, 997.91-997.99

**279.8 Other specified disorders involving the immune
       mechanism**
     Single complement [C_1-C_9] deficiency or dysfunction

279.9 Unspecified disorder of immune mechanism
     Coding Clinic: 1996, Q2, P12; 1992, Q3, P13-14

ENDOCRINE, NUTRITIONAL AND METABOLIC DISEASES, AND IMMUNITY DISORDERS (240–279)

4. DISEASES OF THE BLOOD AND BLOOD-FORMING ORGANS (280–289)

● **280 Iron deficiency anemias**

Disease characterized by decrease in number of red cells (hemoglobin) in blood, diminishing body's ability to carry adequate amounts of oxygen to cells.

Includes   anemia:
    asiderotic
    hypochromic-microcytic
    sideropenic

Excludes   *familial microcytic anemia (282.49)*

280.0 Secondary to blood loss (chronic)
    Normocytic anemia due to blood loss

    Excludes   *acute posthemorrhagic anemia (285.1)*

    Coding Clinic: 1993, Q4, P34; 1985, July-Aug, P13

280.1 Secondary to inadequate dietary iron intake

280.8 Other specified iron deficiency anemias
    Paterson-Kelly syndrome
    Plummer-Vinson syndrome
    Sideropenic dysphagia

280.9 Iron deficiency anemia, unspecified
    Anemia:
        achlorhydric
        chlorotic
        idiopathic hypochromic
        iron [Fe] deficiency NOS

● **281 Other deficiency anemias**

281.0 Pernicious anemia
    Anemia:
        Addison's
        Biermer's
        congenital pernicious
    Congenital intrinsic factor [Castle's] deficiency

    Excludes   *combined system disease without mention of anemia (266.2)*
            subacute degeneration of spinal cord without mention of anemia (266.2)

281.1 Other vitamin B_{12} deficiency anemia
    Anemia:
        vegan's
        vitamin B_{12} deficiency (dietary)
        due to selective vitamin B_{12} malabsorption with proteinuria
    Syndrome:
        Imerslund's
        Imerslund-Gräsbeck

    Excludes   *combined system disease without mention of anemia (266.2)*
            subacute degeneration of spinal cord without mention of anemia (266.2)

281.2 Folate-deficiency anemia
    Congenital folate malabsorption
    Folate or folic acid deficiency anemia:
        NOS
        dietary
        drug-induced
    Goat's milk anemia
    Nutritional megaloblastic anemia (of infancy)

    Use additional E code to identify drug

281.3 Other specified megaloblastic anemias, not elsewhere classified
    Combined B_{12} and folate-deficiency anemia

281.4 Protein-deficiency anemia
    Amino-acid-deficiency anemia

281.8 Anemia associated with other specified nutritional deficiency
    Scorbutic anemia

281.9 Unspecified deficiency anemia
    Anemia:
        dimorphic
        macrocytic
        megaloblastic NOS
        nutritional NOS
        simple chronic
    Coding Clinic: 1984, Sept-Oct, P16

● **282 Hereditary hemolytic anemias**

Genetic condition in which bone marrow is unable to compensate for premature destruction of red blood cells

282.0 Hereditary spherocytosis
    Acholuric (familial) jaundice
    Congenital hemolytic anemia (spherocytic)
    Congenital spherocytosis
    Minkowski-Chauffard syndrome
    Spherocytosis (familial)

    Excludes   *hemolytic anemia of newborn (773.0–773.5)*

282.1 Hereditary elliptocytosis
    Elliptocytosis (congenital)
    Ovalocytosis (congenital) (hereditary)

282.2 Anemias due to disorders of glutathione metabolism
    Anemia:
        6-phosphogluconic dehydrogenase deficiency
        enzyme deficiency, drug-induced
        erythrocytic glutathione deficiency
        glucose-6-phosphate dehydrogenase [G-6-PD] deficiency
        glutathione-reductase deficiency
        hemolytic nonspherocytic (hereditary), type I
    Disorder of pentose phosphate pathway
    Favism

282.3 Other hemolytic anemias due to enzyme deficiency
    Anemia:
        hemolytic nonspherocytic (hereditary), type II
        hexokinase deficiency
        pyruvate kinase [PK] deficiency
        triosephosphate isomerase deficiency

● **282.4 Thalassemias**

Hereditary disorders characterized by low production of hemoglobin or excessive destruction of red blood cells

    Excludes   *sickle-cell:*
        disease (282.60–282.69)
        trait (282.5)

    Coding Clinic: 2003, Q4, P51-56

282.41 Sickle-cell thalassemia without crisis
    Sickle-cell thalassemia NOS
    Thalassemia Hb-S disease without crisis

◀ New   ⬅ Revised   ~~deleted~~ Deleted   ● Unacceptable Principal Diagnosis   ● Use Additional Digit(s)

▶ Manifestation Code   **OGCR** Official Guidelines   **Coding Clinic**   Excludes   Includes   Use additional   Code first   Omit code

282.42 Sickle-cell thalassemia with crisis🌑
Sickle-cell thalassemia with vaso-occlusive pain
Thalassemia Hb-S disease with crisis

Use additional code for type of crisis, such as:
Acute chest syndrome (517.3)
Splenic sequestration (289.52)
Occurs when sickled red blood cells become entrapped in spleen, causing splenomegaly (enlargement) and decreased circulating blood volume.
Ⓔⓧ 280.0-285.9, 289.81-289.83, 289.89-289.9, 517.3

282.49 Other thalassemia
Cooley's anemia
Hb-Bart's disease
Hereditary leptocytosis
Mediterranean anemia (with other hemoglobinopathy)
Microdrepanocytosis
Thalassemia (alpha) (beta) (intermedia) (major) (minima) (minor) (mixed) (trait) (with other hemoglobinopathy)
Thalassemia NOS

282.5 Sickle-cell trait
Hb-AS genotype
Hemoglobin S [Hb-S] trait
Heterozygous:
hemoglobin S
Hb-S

Excludes *that with other hemoglobinopathy (282.60–282.69)*
that with thalassemia (282.49)
Coding Clinic: 2003, Q4, P51-56

● **282.6 Sickle-cell disease**
Inherited disease in which red blood cells, normally disc-shaped, become crescent shaped. Small blood clots form, resulting in painful episodes called sickle cell pain crises.
Sickle-cell anemia

Excludes *sickle-cell thalassemia (282.41–282.42)*
sickle-cell trait (282.5)

282.60 Sickle-cell disease, unspecified
Sickle-cell anemia NOS
Coding Clinic: 1997, Q2, P11

282.61 Hb-SS disease without crisis
Coding Clinic: 2007, Q2, P9-10

282.62 Hb-SS disease with crisis🌑
Hb-SS disease with vaso-occlusive pain
Sickle-cell crisis NOS

Use additional code for type of crisis, such as:
Acute chest syndrome (517.3)
Splenic sequestration (289.52)
Ⓔⓧ 280.0-285.9, 289.81-289.83, 289.89-289.9, 517.3
Coding Clinic: 2003, Q4, P51-56; 1998, Q2, P8; 1991, Q2, P15

282.63 Sickle-cell/Hb-C disease without crisis
Hb-S/Hb-C disease without crisis

282.64 Sickle-cell/Hb-C disease with crisis🌑
Hb-S/Hb-C disease with crisis
Sickle-cell/Hb-C disease with vaso-occlusive pain

Use additional code for types of crisis, such as:
Acute chest syndrome (517.3)
Splenic sequestration (289.52)
Ⓔⓧ 280.0-285.9, 289.81-289.83, 289.89-289.9, 517.3

282.68 Other sickle-cell disease without crisis
Hb-S/Hb-D disease without crisis
Hb-S/Hb-E disease without crisis
Sickle-cell/Hb-D disease without crisis
Sickle-cell/Hb-E disease without crisis

282.69 Other sickle-cell disease with crisis🌑
Hb-S/Hb-D disease with crisis
Hb-S/Hb-E disease with crisis
Other sickle-cell disease with vaso-occlusive pain
Sickle-cell/Hb-D disease with crisis
Sickle-cell/Hb-E disease with crisis

Use additional code for type of crisis, such as:
Acute chest syndrome (517.3)
Splenic sequestration (289.52)
Ⓔⓧ 280.0-285.9, 289.81-289.83, 289.89-289.9, 517.3

282.7 Other hemoglobinopathies
Abnormal hemoglobin NOS
Congenital Heinz-body anemia
Disease:
hemoglobin C [Hb-C]
hemoglobin D [Hb-D]
hemoglobin E [Hb-E]
hemoglobin Zurich [Hb-Zurich]
Hemoglobinopathy NOS
Hereditary persistence of fetal hemoglobin [HPFH]
Unstable hemoglobin hemolytic disease

Excludes *familial polycythemia (289.6)*
hemoglobin M [Hb-M] disease (289.7)
high-oxygen-affinity hemoglobin (289.0)

282.8 Other specified hereditary hemolytic anemias🌑
Stomatocytosis
Ⓔⓧ 280.0-285.9, 289.9, 517.3, 776.5-776.6

282.9 Hereditary hemolytic anemia, unspecified🌑
Hereditary hemolytic anemia NOS
Ⓔⓧ 280.0-285.9, 289.9, 517.3, 776.5-776.6

DISEASES OF THE BLOOD AND BLOOD-FORMING ORGANS (280–289)

● **283   Acquired hemolytic anemias**

*Also known as autoimmune hemolytic or Coombs positive
hemolytic anemia. The red blood cells produced are
healthy but are destroyed when trapped in the spleen by
infection or certain drugs.*

     283.0   Autoimmune hemolytic anemias 🖝

       Autoimmune hemolytic disease (cold type) (warm
         type)
       Chronic cold hemagglutinin disease
       Cold agglutinin disease or hemoglobinuria
       Hemolytic anemia:
         cold type (secondary) (symptomatic)
         drug-induced
         warm type (secondary) (symptomatic)

       Use additional E code to identify cause, if
         drug-induced

       Excludes   *Evans' syndrome (287.32)*
          hemolytic disease of newborn (773.0–773.5)

       (Ex:) 280.0-285.9, 289.81-289.83, 289.89-289.9, 517.3

       Coding Clinic: 2008, Q3, P5

● **283.1   Non-autoimmune hemolytic anemias**

     **283.10   Non-autoimmune hemolytic anemia,
         unspecified** 🖝
         (Ex:) 280.0-285.9, 289.81-289.83, 289.89-289.9, 517.3

     283.11   Hemolytic-uremic syndrome 🖝
         (Ex:) 280.0-285.9, 289.81-289.83, 289.89-289.9, 517.3

     283.19   Other non-autoimmune hemolytic anemias 🖝
         Hemolytic anemia:
           mechanical
           microangiopathic
           toxic

         Use additional E code to identify cause
         (Ex:) 280.0-285.9, 289.81-289.83, 289.89-289.9, 517.3

     **283.2   Hemoglobinuria due to hemolysis from external
       causes**

       Acute intravascular hemolysis
       Hemoglobinuria:
         from exertion
         march
         paroxysmal (cold) (nocturnal)
         due to other hemolysis
       Marchiafava-Micheli syndrome

       Use additional E code to identify cause

     283.9   Acquired hemolytic anemia, unspecified 🖝
       Acquired hemolytic anemia NOS
       Chronic idiopathic hemolytic anemia
       (Ex:) 280.0-285.9, 289.81-289.83, 289.89-289.9, 517.3

● **284   Aplastic anemia and other bone marrow failure
    syndromes**
     Coding Clinic: 2006, Q4, P67-69

   ● **284.0   Constitutional aplastic anemia**
       Coding Clinic: 1991, Q1, P14

     284.01   Constitutional red blood cell aplasia 🖝
         Aplasia, (pure) red cell:
           congenital
           of infants
           primary
         Blackfan-Diamond syndrome
         Familial hypoplastic anemia
         (Ex:) 280.0-284.09, 284.81-285.9, 289.9, 776.5-776.6

     284.09   Other constitutional aplastic anemia 🖝
         Fanconi's anemia
         Pancytopenia with malformations
         (Ex:) 280.0-284.09, 284.81-285.9, 287.30-287.39, 289.9,
           776.5-776.6

     284.1   Pancytopenia 🖝

       *Marked deficiency of all the blood elements: Red blood
       cells (erythrocytes), white blood cells (leukocytes),
       and platelets (thrombocytes). Check laboratory
       results.*

       Excludes   *pancytopenia (due to) (with):*
         aplastic anemia NOS (284.9)
         bone marrow infiltration (284.2)
         *constitutional red blood cell aplasia
           (284.01)*
         drug induced (284.89)
         hairy cell leukemia (202.4)
         *human immunodeficiency virus disease
           (042)*
         leukoerythroblastic anemia (284.2)
         malformations (284.09)
         *myelodysplastic syndromes
           (238.72–238.75)*
         myeloproliferative disease (238.79)
         *other constitutional aplastic anemia
           (284.09)*

       (Ex:) 284.2-285.9, 288.00-288.09, 288.4-288.62, 288.66-288.69, 289.9, 776.6
       Coding Clinic: 2005, Q3, P11-12

▶ **284.2   Myelophthisis** 🖝
       Leukoerythroblastic anemia
       Myelophthisic anemia

       Code first *the underlying disorder, such as:*
         malignant neoplasm of breast (174.0–174.9,
           175.0–175.9)
         tuberculosis (015.0–015.9)

       Excludes   *idiopathic myelofibrosis (238.76)*
         myelofibrosis NOS (289.83)
         *myelofibrosis with myeloid metaplasia
           (238.76)*
         primary myelofibrosis (238.76)
         secondary myelofibrosis (289.83)
       (Ex:) 284.1-285.9, 288.00-288.09, 288.4-288.62, 288.66-288.69, 289.9, 776.6

● **284.8   Other specified aplastic anemias**
     **Coding Clinic: 2007, Q4, P72-73; 2005, Q3, P11-12; 1997, Q1, P5-6;
       1991, Q1, P14; 1984, Sept-Oct, P16**

     **284.81   Red cell aplasia (acquired) (adult) (with
         thymoma)** 🖝
         Red cell aplasia NOS
         (Ex:) 280.0-285.9, 289.81-289.83, 289.89-289.9, 517.3

     284.89   Other specified aplastic anemias 🖝
         Aplastic anemia (due to):
           chronic systemic disease
           drugs
           infection
           radiation
           toxic (paralytic)

         Use additional E code to identify cause
         (Ex:) 280.0-285.9, 289.81-289.83, 289.89-289.9, 517.3
         Coding Clinic: 2009, Q1, P17; 2008, Q2, P6

     284.9   Aplastic anemia, unspecified 🖝
       Anemia:
         aplastic (idiopathic) NOS
         aregenerative
         hypoplastic NOS
         nonregenerative
       Medullary hypoplasia

       Excludes   *refractory anemia (238.72)*
       (Ex:) 280.0-285.9, 289.81-289.83, 289.89-289.9, 517.3

◀ New   ◀═ Revised   ~~deleted~~ Deleted   ● Unacceptable Principal Diagnosis   ● Use Additional Digit(s)

▶ Manifestation Code   **OGCR** Official Guidelines   **Coding Clinic**   Excludes   Includes   Use additional   Code first   Omit code

DISEASES OF THE BLOOD AND BLOOD-FORMING ORGANS (280–289)

● **285   Other and unspecified anemias**
     Coding Clinic: 1990, Q3, P17

   285.0   Sideroblastic anemia
     Anemia:
       hypochromic with iron loading
       sideroachrestic
       sideroblastic:
         acquired
         congenital
         hereditary
         primary
         secondary (drug-induced) (due to disease)
         sex-linked hypochromic
         vitamin B_6-responsive
     Pyridoxine-responsive (hypochromic) anemia

     Excludes   *refractory sideroblastic anemia (238.72)*

     Use additional E code to identify cause, if
       drug-induced

   285.1   Acute posthemorrhagic anemia 🅒
     Anemia due to acute blood loss

     Excludes   *anemia due to chronic blood loss (280.0)*
                blood loss anemia NOS (280.0)
     (Ex:) 280.0-285.9, 289.81-289.83, 289.89-289.9, 517.3, 958.2
     Coding Clinic: 2007, Q1, P19; 2004, Q3, P4; 1993, Q4, P34; 1992,
       Q2, P15-16

● **285.2   Anemia of chronic disease**
     Anemia in (due to) (with) chronic illness   ⬅||||

     285.21   Anemia in chronic kidney disease
         Anemia in end stage renal disease
         Erythropoietin-resistant anemia (EPO
           resistant anemia)
         Coding Clinic: 2000, Q4, P39-40

     285.22   Anemia in neoplastic disease

         Excludes   *anemia due to antineoplastic*
                 chemotherapy (285.3)   ◄
         Coding Clinic: 2008, Q2, P6; 2000, Q4, P39-40

         OGCR Section I.C.4.a.2
         When assigning code 285.22, Anemia in
         neoplastic disease, it is also necessary to
         assign the neoplasm code that is responsible
         for the anemia. Code 285.22 is for use for
         anemia that is due to the malignancy, not for
         anemia due to antineoplastic chemotherapy
         drugs, which is an adverse effect.

     285.29   Anemia of other chronic disease
         Anemia in other chronic illness

   285.3   Antineoplastic chemotherapy induced anemia   ◄
     Anemia due to antineoplastic chemotherapy   ◄

     Excludes   *anemia due to drug NEC – code to*   ◄
              type of anemia   ◄
            anemia in neoplastic disease (285.22)   ◄
            aplastic anemia due to antineoplastic
              chemotherapy (284.89)   ◄

   285.8   Other specified anemias
     Anemia:
       dyserythropoietic (congenital)
       dyshematopoietic (congenital)
       von Jaksch's
     Infantile pseudoleukemia

   285.9   Anemia, unspecified
     Anemia:
       NOS
       essential
       normocytic, not due to blood loss
       profound
       progressive
       secondary
     Oligocythemia

     Excludes   *anemia (due to):*
               blood loss:
                  acute (285.1)
                  chronic or unspecified (280.0)
              iron deficiency (280.0–280.9)
     Coding Clinic: 2009, Q1, P17x2; 2007, Q1, P19; 2002, Q1, P14; 1992,
       Q2, P15-16; 1985, Mar-April, P13

● **286   Coagulation defects**
     Can be acquired or genetic and results in inability to control
     blood clotting. Most common genetic coagulation
     disorder is hemophilia.
     Coding Clinic: 2006, Q2, P17; 1992, Q3, P15

   286.0   Congenital factor VIII disorder 🅜🅒
     Antihemophilic globulin [AHG] deficiency
     Factor VIII (functional) deficiency
     Hemophilia:
       NOS
       A
       classical
       familial
       hereditary
     Subhemophilia

     Excludes   *factor VIII deficiency with vascular defect*
              (286.4)
     (Ex:) 286.0-287.9, 289.81-289.9

   286.1   Congenital factor IX disorder 🅜🅒
     Christmas disease
     Deficiency:
       factor IX (functional)
       plasma thromboplastin component [PTC]
     Hemophilia B
     (Ex:) 286.0-287.9, 289.81-289.9

   286.2   Congenital factor XI deficiency 🅒
     Hemophilia C
     Plasma thromboplastin antecedent [PTA] deficiency
     Rosenthal's disease
     (Ex:) 286.0-287.9, 289.81-289.9

   286.3   Congenital deficiency of other clotting factors 🅒
     Congenital afibrinogenemia
     Deficiency:
       AC globulin factor:
         I [fibrinogen]
         II [prothrombin]
         V [labile]
         VII [stable]
         X [Stuart-Prower]
         XII [Hageman]
         XIII [fibrin stabilizing]
       Laki-Lorand factor
       proaccelerin
     Disease:
       Owren's
       Stuart-Prower
     Dysfibrinogenemia (congenital)
     Dysprothrombinemia (constitutional)
     Hypoproconvertinemia
     Hypoprothrombinemia (hereditary)
     Parahemophilia
     (Ex:) 286.0-287.9, 289.81-289.9

DISEASES OF THE BLOOD AND BLOOD-FORMING ORGANS (280–289)

286.4 von Willebrand's disease 🔒
    Angiohemophilia (A) (B)
    Constitutional thrombopathy
    Factor VIII deficiency with vascular defect
    Pseudohemophilia type B
    Vascular hemophilia
    von Willebrand's (-Jürgens') disease

> **Excludes** *factor VIII deficiency:*
>   *NOS (286.0)*
>   *with functional defect (286.0)*
>   *hereditary capillary fragility (287.8)*

(Ex:) 286.0-287.9, 289.81-289.9

286.5 Hemorrhagic disorder due to intrinsic circulating anticoagulants 🔒
    Antithrombinemia
    Antithromboplastinemia
    Antithromboplastino-genemia
    Hyperheparinemia
    Increase in:
        anti-VIIIa
        anti-IXa
        anti-Xa
        anti-XIa
        antithrombin
    Secondary hemophilia
    Systemic lupus erythematosus [SLE] inhibitor

(Ex:) 286.0-287.9, 289.81-289.9

Coding Clinic: 2004, Q3, P7; 1994, Q1, P22; 1993, 5th Issue, P16; 1992, Q3, P15-16; 1990, Q3, P14

286.6 Defibrination syndrome 🔒🔒
    Afibrinogenemia, acquired
    Consumption coagulopathy
    Diffuse or disseminated intravascular coagulation [DIC syndrome]
    Fibrinolytic hemorrhage, acquired
    Hemorrhagic fibrinogenolysis
    Pathologic fibrinolysis
    Purpura:
        fibrinolytic
        fulminans

> **Excludes** *that complicating:*
>   *abortion (634–638 with .1, 639.1)*
>   *pregnancy or the puerperium*
>   *(641.3, 666.3)*
>   *disseminated intravascular coagulation in*
>   *newborn (776.2)*

(Ex:) 286.0-287.9, 289.81-289.9

286.7 Acquired coagulation factor deficiency 🔒
    Deficiency of coagulation factor due to:
        liver disease
        vitamin K deficiency
    Hypoprothrombinemia, acquired

> **Excludes** *vitamin K deficiency of newborn (776.0)*

Use additional E-code to identify cause, if drug-induced

(Ex:) 286.0-287.9, 289.81-289.9

286.9 Other and unspecified coagulation defects 🔒
    Defective coagulation NOS
    Deficiency, coagulation factor NOS
    Delay, coagulation
    Disorder:
        coagulation
        hemostasis

> **Excludes** *abnormal coagulation profile (790.92)*
>   *hemorrhagic disease of newborn (776.0)*
>   *that complicating:*
>   *abortion (634–638 with .1, 639.1)*
>   *pregnancy or the puerperium*
>   *(641.3, 666.3)*

(Ex:) 286.0-287.9, 289.81-289.9

Coding Clinic: 1999, Q4, P22-23

● **287 Purpura and other hemorrhagic conditions**

> **Excludes** *hemorrhagic thrombocythemia (238.79)*
>   *purpura fulminans (286.6)*

287.0 Allergic purpura 🔒
    Peliosis rheumatica
    Purpura:
        anaphylactoid
        autoimmune
        Henoch's
        nonthrombocytopenic:
            hemorrhagic
            idiopathic
        rheumatica
        Schönlein-Henoch
        vascular
    Vasculitis, allergic

> **Excludes** *hemorrhagic purpura (287.39)*
>   *purpura annularis telangiectodes (709.1)*

(Ex:) 286.0-287.9, 289.81-289.9

287.1 Qualitative platelet defects
    Thrombasthenia (hemorrhagic) (hereditary)
    Thrombocytasthenia
    Thrombocytopathy (dystrophic)
    Thrombopathy (Bernard-Soulier)

> **Excludes** *von Willebrand's disease (286.4)*

287.2 Other nonthrombocytopenic purpuras
    Purpura:
        NOS
        senile
        simplex

● **287.3 Primary thrombocytopenia**
    Also known as idiopathic thrombocytopenia, may be acquired or congenital and is a common cause of coagulation disorders.

> **Excludes** *thrombotic thrombocytopenic purpura*
>   *(446.6)*
>   *transient thrombocytopenia of newborn*
>   *(776.1)*
>   *Thrombo = clot forming, cyto = cell,*
>   *penia = deficiency of: deficiency of*
>   *platelets.*

287.30 Primary thrombocytopenia unspecified
    Megakaryocytic hypoplasia

287.31 Immune thrombocytopenic purpura 🔒
    Idiopathic thrombocytopenic purpura
    Tidal platelet dysgenesis
    (Ex:) 286.0-287.9, 289.81-289.9
    Coding Clinic: 2005, Q4, P56-57

287.32 Evans' syndrome 🔒
    (Ex:) 286.0-287.9, 289.81-289.9

287.33 Congenital and hereditary thrombocytopenic purpura 🔒
    Congenital and hereditary
        thrombocytopenia
    Thrombocytopenia with absent radii (TAR)
        syndrome

> **Excludes** *Wiskott-Aldrich syndrome (279.12)*

(Ex:) 286.0-287.9, 289.81-289.9

287.39 Other primary thrombocytopenia

◀ New   ◀▥ Revised   ~~deleted~~ Deleted   ● Unacceptable Principal Diagnosis   ● Use Additional Digit(s)
▷ Manifestation Code   **OGCR** Official Guidelines   **Coding Clinic**   Excludes   Includes   Use additional   Code first   Omit code

287.4 Secondary thrombocytopenia
Posttransfusion purpura
Thrombocytopenia (due to):
  dilutional
  drugs
  extracorporeal circulation of blood
  massive blood transfusion
  platelet alloimmunization

Use additional E code to identify cause

Excludes   *heparin-induced thrombocytopenia (HIT)*
(289.84)
transient thrombocytopenia of newborn
(776.1)

Coding Clinic: 1985, July-Aug, P13; Mar-April, P14

287.5 Thrombocytopenia, unspecified

287.8 Other specified hemorrhagic conditions
Capillary fragility (hereditary)
Vascular pseudohemophilia
Coding Clinic: 1985, Mar-April, P14

287.9 Unspecified hemorrhagic conditions
Hemorrhagic diathesis (familial)

● **288   Diseases of white blood cells**

Excludes   *leukemia (204.0–208.9)*

● **288.0 Neutropenia**
Decreased Absolute Neutrophil Count (ANC)

Use additional code for any associated:
  fever (780.61)
  mucositis (478.11, 528.00–528.09, 538, 616.81)

Excludes   *neutropenic splenomegaly (289.53)*
transitory neonatal neutropenia (776.7)

Coding Clinic: 2005, Q3, P11-12; 1999, Q3, P6-7; 1996, Q3, P16; Q2, P6; 1985, Mar-April, P14

288.00 Neutropenia, unspecified

288.01 Congenital neutropenia
Congenital agranulocytosis
Infantile genetic agranulocytosis
Kostmann's syndrome

288.02 Cyclic neutropenia
Cyclic hematopoiesis
Periodic neutropenia

288.03 Drug induced neutropenia
Use additional E code to identify drug
Coding Clinic: 2006, Q4, P69-73

288.04 Neutropenia due to infection

288.09 Other neutropenia
Agranulocytosis
Neutropenia:
  immune
  toxic

288.1 Functional disorders of polymorphonuclear neutrophils
Chronic (childhood) granulomatous disease
Congenital dysphagocytosis
Job's syndrome
Lipochrome histiocytosis (familial)
Progressive septic granulomatosis

288.2 Genetic anomalies of leukocytes
Anomaly (granulation) (granulocyte) or syndrome:
  Alder's (-Reilly)
  Chédiak-Steinbrinck (-Higashi)
  Jordan's
  May-Hegglin
  Pelger-Huet
Hereditary:
  hypersegmentation
  hyposegmentation
  leukomelanopathy

288.3 Eosinophilia
Eosinophilia
  allergic
  hereditary
  idiopathic
  secondary
Eosinophilic leukocytosis

Excludes   *Löffler's syndrome (518.3)*
pulmonary eosinophilia (518.3)

Coding Clinic: 2000, Q3, P11

288.4 Hemophagocytic syndromes 🔗
Familial hemophagocytic lymphohistiocytosis
Familial hemophagocytic reticulosis
Hemophagocytic syndrome, infection-associated
Histiocytic syndromes
Macrophage activation syndrome
Ⓔⓧ 284.1-284.9, 286.6, 287.30-288.09, 288.50, 288.59, 289.84, 289.9

● **288.5 Decreased white blood cell count**

Excludes   *neutropenia (288.01–288.09)*

288.50 Leukocytopenia, unspecified
Decreased leukocytes, unspecified
Decreased white blood cell count,
  unspecified
Leukopenia NOS

288.51 Lymphocytopenia
Decreased lymphocytes

288.59 Other decreased white blood cell count
Basophilic leukopenia
Eosinophilic leukopenia
Monocytopenia
Plasmacytopenia

● **288.6 Elevated white blood cell count**

Excludes   *eosinophilia (288.3)*

288.60 Leukocytosis, unspecified
Elevated leukocytes, unspecified
Elevated white blood cell count,
  unspecified

288.61 Lymphocytosis (symptomatic)
Elevated lymphocytes

288.62 Leukemoid reaction
Basophilic leukemoid reaction
Lymphocytic leukemoid reaction
Monocytic leukemoid reaction
Myelocytic leukemoid reaction
Neutrophilic leukemoid reaction

288.63 Monocytosis (symptomatic)

Excludes   *infectious mononucleosis (075)*

288.64 Plasmacytosis

288.65 Basophilia

N Newborn Age: 0   **P** Pediatric Age: 0–17   **M** Maternity Age: 12–55   **A** Adult Age: 15–124   ♀ Females Only   ♂ Males Only
Ⓔⓧ CC Exclusions   🔗 Complication\Comorbidity   🔗 Major C\C   🔗 Present on Admission Requirement   🔗 Hospital-Acquired Condition

288.66 Bandemia

Bandemia without diagnosis of specific infection

Excludes confirmed infection – code to infection
leukemia (204.00–208.9)
Coding Clinic: 2007, Q4, P73-74

288.69 Other elevated white blood cell count

288.8 Other specified disease of white blood cells

Excludes decreased white blood cell counts (288.50–288.59)
elevated white blood cell counts (288.60–288.69)
immunity disorders (279.0–279.9)
Coding Clinic: 1987, Mar-April, P12

288.9 Unspecified disease of white blood cells

● **289 Other diseases of blood and blood-forming organs**

289.0 Polycythemia, secondary

See 238.4 for primary polycythemia (polycythemia vera)
High-oxygen-affinity hemoglobin
Polycythemia:
acquired
benign
due to:
fall in plasma volume
high altitude
emotional
erythropoietin
hypoxemic
nephrogenous
relative
spurious
stress

Excludes polycythemia:
neonatal (776.4)
primary (238.4)
vera (238.4)

289.1 Chronic lymphadenitis

Chronic:
adenitis any lymph node, except mesenteric
lymphadenitis any lymph node, except mesenteric

Excludes acute lymphadenitis (683)
mesenteric (289.2)
enlarged glands NOS (785.6)

289.2 Nonspecific mesenteric lymphadenitis

Mesenteric lymphadenitis (acute) (chronic)

289.3 Lymphadenitis, unspecified, except mesenteric
Coding Clinic: 1992, Q2, P8

289.4 Hypersplenism

"Big spleen" syndrome
Dyssplenism
Hypersplenia

Excludes primary splenic neutropenia (289.53)

● **289.5 Other diseases of spleen**

289.50 Disease of spleen, unspecified

289.51 Chronic congestive splenomegaly

▶ **289.52 Splenic sequestration**

Code first sickle-cell disease in crisis (282.42, 282.62, 282.64, 282.69)
Coding Clinic: 2003, Q4, P51-56

289.53 Neutropenic splenomegaly

289.59 Other

Lien migrans   Splenic:
Perisplenitis   fibrosis
Splenic: infarction
abscess   rupture, nontraumatic
atrophy   Splenitis
cyst   Wandering spleen

Excludes bilharzial splenic fibrosis (120.0–120.9)
hepatolienal fibrosis (571.5)
splenomegaly NOS (789.2)

289.6 Familial polycythemia

Familial:
benign polycythemia
erythrocytosis

289.7 Methemoglobinemia

Congenital NADH [DPNH]-methemoglobin-reductase deficiency
Hemoglobin M [Hb-M] disease
Methemoglobinemia:
NOS
acquired (with sulfhemoglobinemia)
hereditary
toxic
Stokvis' disease
Sulfhemoglobinemia

Use additional E code to identify cause
(Ex:) 282.7-283.10, 283.19-283.9, 285.8-285.9, 289.7, 289.9

● **289.8 Other specified diseases of blood and blood-forming organs**
Coding Clinic: 2003, Q4, P56-57; 2002, Q1, P16-17; 1987, Mar-April, P12

289.81 Primary hypercoagulable state

Activated protein C resistance
Antithrombin III deficiency
Factor V Leiden mutation
Lupus anticoagulant
Protein C deficiency
Protein S deficiency
Prothrombin gene mutation
(Ex:) 288.00-288.9, 289.53, 289.81-289.83, 289.89-289.9
Coding Clinic: 2008, Q3, P16-17

289.82 Secondary hypercoagulable state

Excludes heparin-induced thrombocytopenia (HIT) (289.84)
(Ex:) 288.00-288.9, 289.53, 289.81-289.83, 289.89-289.9
Coding Clinic: 2008, Q3, P16-17

DISEASES OF THE BLOOD AND BLOOD-FORMING ORGANS (280–289)

◀ New ◀▥ Revised ~~deleted~~ Deleted ● Unacceptable Principal Diagnosis ● Use Additional Digit(s)
▶ Manifestation Code OGCR Official Guidelines Coding Clinic Excludes Includes Use additional Code first Omit code

▶ *289.83* *Myelofibrosis*🔵
    Myelofibrosis NOS
    Secondary myelofibrosis

    Code first the underlying disorder, such as:
        malignant neoplasm of breast
            (174.0–174.9, 175.0–175.9)

    | Excludes | *idiopathic myelofibrosis (238.76)*
                  leukoerythroblastic anemia (284.2)
                  myelofibrosis with myeloid
                     metaplasia (238.76)
                  myelophthisic anemia (284.2)
                  myelophthisis (284.2)
                  primary myelofibrosis (238.76)

    Use additional code for associated
        therapy-related myelodysplastic
        syndrome, if applicable (238.72,
        238.73)

    Use additional external cause code if
        due to anti-neoplastic chemotherapy
        (E933.1)
    (Ex) 202.40-202.48, 203.10-203.11, 203.80-203.81, 204.00-208.92,
        238.4-238.76, 238.79-238.9

289.84 **Heparin-induced thrombocytopenia**
        (HIT)
        Coding Clinic: 2008, Q4, P100-101

289.89 **Other specified diseases of blood and**
        blood-forming organs
        Hypergammaglobulinemia
        Pseudocholinesterase deficiency

289.9 **Unspecified diseases of blood and blood-forming**
  organs
        Blood dyscrasia NOS
        Erythroid hyperplasia
        Coding Clinic: 1985, Mar-April, P14

DISEASES OF THE BLOOD AND BLOOD-FORMING ORGANS (280–289)

5. MENTAL DISORDERS (290–319)

Item 5-1 Psychosis was a term formerly applied to any mental disorder but is now restricted to disturbances of a great magnitude in which there is a personality disintegration and loss of contact with reality.

PSYCHOSES (290–299)

Excludes *mental retardation (317–319)*

ORGANIC PSYCHOTIC CONDITIONS (290–294)

Includes psychotic organic brain syndrome

Excludes *nonpsychotic syndromes of organic etiology (310.0–310.9)*
psychoses classifiable to 295–298 and without impairment of orientation, comprehension, calculation, learning capacity, and judgment, but associated with physical disease, injury, or condition affecting the brain [e.g., following childbirth] (295.0–298.8)

● **290 Dementias**
Progressive decline in cognition along with a short- and long-term memory loss due to brain damage/disease.

Code first the associated neurological condition

Excludes *dementia due to alcohol (291.0–291.2)*
dementia due to drugs (292.82)
dementia not classified as senile, presenile, or arteriosclerotic (294.10–294.11)
psychoses classifiable to 295–298 occurring in the senium without dementia or delirium (295.0–298.8)
senility with mental changes of nonpsychotic severity (310.1)
transient organic psychotic conditions (293.0–293.9)

290.0 Senile dementia, uncomplicated   A
Senile dementia:
NOS
simple type

Excludes *mild memory disturbances, not amounting to dementia, associated with senile brain disease (310.8)* ⬅
senile dementia with:
delirium or confusion (290.3)
delusional [paranoid] features (290.20)
depressive features (290.21)
Coding Clinic: 1999, Q4, P4-5; 1994, Q1, P21

● **290.1 Presenile dementia**
Brain syndrome with presenile brain disease

Excludes *arteriosclerotic dementia (290.40–290.43)*
dementia associated with other cerebral conditions (294.10–294.11)

290.10 Presenile dementia, uncomplicated   A
Presenile dementia:
NOS
simple type
Coding Clinic: 1984, Nov-Dec, P20

290.11 Presenile dementia with delirium 🦠   A
Presenile dementia with acute confusional state
(Ex:) 290.0-290.12, 290.20-290.3, 290.8-290.9, 292.81, 293.0, V62.84
Coding Clinic: 1984, Nov-Dec, P20

290.12 Presenile dementia with delusional features 🦠   A
Presenile dementia, paranoid type
(Ex:) 079.82, 290.0-290.12, 290.20-290.3, 290.8-290.9, 292.81, 293.0
Coding Clinic: 1984, Nov-Dec, P20

290.13 Presenile dementia with depressive features 🦠   A
Presenile dementia, depressed type
(Ex:) 290.0, 290.13-290.3, 296.21-296.24, 296.30-296.34, 296.43-296.44, 296.53-296.54, 296.63-296.64
Coding Clinic: 1984, Nov-Dec, P20

● **290.2 Senile dementia with delusional or depressive features**

Excludes *senile dementia:*
NOS (290.0)
with delirium and/or confusion (290.3)

290.20 Senile dementia with delusional features 🦠 A
Senile dementia, paranoid type
Senile psychosis NOS
(Ex:) 290.0-290.20, 290.3

290.21 Senile dementia with depressive features 🦠 A
(Ex:) 290.13, 290.21

290.3 Senile dementia with delirium 🦠   A
Senile dementia with acute confusional state

Excludes *senile:*
dementia NOS (290.0)
psychosis NOS (290.20)
(Ex:) 290.10-290.20, 290.3, V62.84

● **290.4 Vascular dementia**
Multi-infarct dementia or psychosis

Use additional code to identify cerebral atherosclerosis (437.0)

Excludes *suspected cases with no clear evidence of arteriosclerosis (290.9)*

290.40 Vascular dementia, uncomplicated   A
Arteriosclerotic dementia:
NOS
simple type

290.41 Vascular dementia with delirium 🦠   A
Arteriosclerotic dementia with acute confusional state
(Ex:) 290.11-290.12, 290.20, 290.3, 290.41

290.42 Vascular dementia with delusions 🦠   A
Arteriosclerotic dementia, paranoid type
(Ex:) 290.42

290.43 Vascular dementia with depressed mood 🦠   A
Arteriosclerotic dementia, depressed type
(Ex:) 290.43

290.8 Other specified senile psychotic conditions 🦠
Presbyophrenic psychosis
(Ex:) 290.8-291.0, 292.11, 292.81-292.82, 295.00-295.04, 295.10-295.14, 295.21-295.24, 295.31, 295.33-295.34, 295.40-295.44, 295.53-295.54, 295.63-295.64, 295.71, 295.73-295.74, 295.80-295.84, 295.91, 295.93-295.94, 296.21-296.24, 296.30-296.34

290.9 Unspecified senile psychotic condition 🦠   A
(Ex:) 290.8-291.0, 292.11, 292.81-292.82, 295.00-295.04, 295.10-295.14, 295.21-295.24, 295.31, 295.33-295.34, 295.40-295.44, 295.53-295.54, 295.63-295.64, 295.71, 295.73-295.74, 295.80-295.84, 295.91, 295.93-295.94, 296.21-296.24, 296.30-296.34

◀ New   ⬅ Revised   ~~deleted~~ Deleted   ● Unacceptable Principal Diagnosis   ● Use Additional Digit(s)
▶ Manifestation Code   **OGCR** Official Guidelines   **Coding Clinic**   Excludes   Includes   Use additional   Code first   Omit code

● **291   Alcohol-induced mental disorders**

> **Excludes** *alcoholism without psychosis (303.0–303.9)*

291.0   Alcohol withdrawal delirium🆚
Alcoholic delirium
Delirium tremens

> **Excludes** *alcohol withdrawal (291.81)*

> Ⓔⓧ 291.0-294.9, 303.00-305.03, 305.20-305.93, 790.3

291.1   Alcohol-induced persisting amnestic disorder
Alcoholic polyneuritic psychosis
Korsakoff's psychosis, alcoholic
Wernicke-Korsakoff syndrome (alcoholic)

291.2   Alcohol-induced persisting dementia🆚
Alcoholic dementia NOS
Alcoholism associated with dementia NOS
Chronic alcoholic brain syndrome
Ⓔⓧ 291.0-294.9, 303.00-305.03, 305.20-305.93, 790.3

291.3   Alcohol-induced psychotic disorder with hallucinations🆚
Alcoholic:
hallucinosis (acute)
psychosis with hallucinosis

> **Excludes** *alcohol withdrawal with delirium (291.0)*
> *schizophrenia (295.0–295.9) and paranoid*
> *states (297.0–297.9) taking the form*
> *of chronic hallucinosis with clear*
> *consciousness in an alcoholic*

> Ⓔⓧ 291.0-294.9, 303.00-305.03, 305.20-305.93, 790.3

291.4   Idiosyncratic alcohol intoxication
Pathologic:
alcohol intoxication
drunkenness

> **Excludes** *acute alcohol intoxication (305.0)*
> *in alcoholism (303.0)*
> *simple drunkenness (305.0)*

291.5   Alcohol-induced psychotic disorder with delusions
Alcoholic:
paranoia
psychosis, paranoid type

> **Excludes** *nonalcoholic paranoid states (297.0–297.9)*
> *schizophrenia, paranoid type (295.3)*

● **291.8   Other specified alcohol-induced mental disorders**
Coding Clinic: 1989, Q2, P9

291.81   Alcohol withdrawal🆚
Alcohol:
abstinence syndrome or symptoms
withdrawal syndrome or symptoms

> **Excludes** *alcohol withdrawal:*
> *delirium (291.0)*
> *hallucinosis (291.3)*
> *delirium tremens (291.0)*

> Ⓔⓧ 291.0-294.9, 303.00-305.03, 305.20-305.93, 790.3
> Coding Clinic: 1985, July-Aug, P10

291.82   Alcohol induced sleep disorders
Alcohol induced circadian rhythm sleep
disorders
Alcohol induced hypersomnia
Alcohol induced insomnia
Alcohol induced parasomnia

291.89   Other🆚
Alcohol-induced anxiety disorder
Alcohol-induced mood disorder
Alcohol-induced sexual dysfunction
Ⓔⓧ 291.0-294.9, 303.00-305.03, 305.20-305.93, 790.3

291.9   Unspecified alcohol-induced mental disorders🆚
Alcoholic:
mania NOS
psychosis NOS
Alcoholism (chronic) with psychosis
Alcohol-related disorder NOS
Ⓔⓧ 291.0-294.9, 303.00-305.03, 305.20-305.93, 790.3

● **292   Drug-induced mental disorders**

> **Includes** organic brain syndrome associated with
> consumption of drugs

> **Use additional** code for any associated drug dependence
> (304.0–304.9)

> **Use additional** E code to identify drug
> Coding Clinic: 2004, Q3, P8

292.0   Drug withdrawal🆚
Drug:
abstinence syndrome or symptoms
withdrawal syndrome or symptoms
Ⓔⓧ 291.0-294.9, 303.00-305.03, 305.20-305.93, 790.3
Coding Clinic: 1997, Q1, P12-13

● **292.1   Drug-induced psychotic disorders**

292.11   Drug-induced psychotic disorder with delusions🆚
Paranoid state induced by drugs
Ⓔⓧ 291.0-294.9, 303.00-305.03, 305.20-305.93, 790.3

292.12   Drug-induced psychotic disorder with hallucinations🆚
Hallucinatory state induced by drugs

> **Excludes** *states following LSD or other*
> *hallucinogens, lasting only a*
> *few days or less ["bad trips"]*
> *(305.3)*

> Ⓔⓧ 291.0-294.9, 303.00-305.03, 305.20-305.93, 790.3
> Coding Clinic: 2004, Q3, P8

292.2   Pathological drug intoxication
Drug reaction resulting in brief psychotic states
NOS
idiosyncratic
pathologic

> **Excludes** *expected brief psychotic reactions to*
> *hallucinogens ["bad trips"] (305.3)*
> *physiological side-effects of drugs (e.g.,*
> *dystonias)*

● **292.8   Other specified drug-induced mental disorders**

292.81   Drug-induced delirium🆚
Ⓔⓧ 291.0-294.9, 303.00-305.03, 305.20-305.93, 790.3

292.82   Drug-induced persisting dementia🆚
Ⓔⓧ 291.0-294.9, 303.00-305.03, 305.20-305.93, 790.3
Coding Clinic: 2004, Q3, P8

292.83   Drug-induced persisting amnestic disorder

292.84   Drug-induced mood disorder
Depressive state induced by drugs

292.85   Drug induced sleep disorders
Drug induced circadian rhythm sleep
disorder
Drug induced hypersomnia
Drug induced insomnia
Drug induced parasomnia

292.89   Other
Drug-induced anxiety disorder
Drug-induced organic personality
syndrome
Drug-induced sexual dysfunction
Drug intoxication

292.9   Unspecified drug-induced mental disorder
Drug-related disorder NOS
Organic psychosis NOS due to or associated with
drugs

MENTAL DISORDERS (290–319)

N Newborn Age: 0   **P** Pediatric Age: 0–17   **M** Maternity Age: 12–55   **A** Adult Age: 15–124   ♀ Females Only   ♂ Males Only
Ⓔⓧ CC Exclusions   🆚 Complication\Comorbidity   🆚 Major C\C   Ⓟⓞⓐ Present on Admission Requirement   🆚 Hospital-Acquired Condition

● **293 Transient mental disorders due to conditions classified elsewhere**

  Includes transient organic mental disorders not associated with alcohol or drugs

  Code first the associated physical or neurological condition

  Excludes *confusional state or delirium superimposed on senile dementia (290.3)*
    dementia due to:
     alcohol (291.0–291.9)
     arteriosclerosis (290.40–290.43)
     drugs (292.82)
     senility (290.0)

 293.0 Delirium due to conditions classified elsewhere
  Acute:
   confusional state
   infective psychosis
   organic reaction
   posttraumatic organic psychosis
   psycho-organic syndrome
  Acute psychosis associated with endocrine, metabolic, or cerebrovascular disorder
  Epileptic:
   confusional state
   twilight state
  (Ex) 290.11, 290.3, 293.0, V62.84
  Coding Clinic: 1993, Q3, P11

 293.1 Subacute delirium
  Subacute:
   confusional state
   infective psychosis
   organic reaction
   posttraumatic organic psychosis
   psycho-organic syndrome
   psychosis associated with endocrine or metabolic disorder
  (Ex) 293.0-293.1, 293.89-293.9

● **293.8 Other specified transient mental disorders due to conditions classified elsewhere**

 293.81 Psychotic disorder with delusions in conditions classified elsewhere
  Transient organic psychotic condition, paranoid type
  (Ex) 291.0-294.9, 303.00-305.03, 305.20-305.93, 790.3

 293.82 Psychotic disorder with hallucinations in conditions classified elsewhere
  Transient organic psychotic condition, hallucinatory type
  (Ex) 291.0-294.9, 303.00-305.03, 305.20-305.93, 790.3

 293.83 Mood disorder in conditions classified elsewhere
  Transient organic psychotic condition, depressive type

 293.84 Anxiety disorder in conditions classified elsewhere
  Coding Clinic: 1996, Q4, P29

 293.89 Other
  Catatonic disorder in conditions classified elsewhere

 293.9 Unspecified transient mental disorder in conditions classified elsewhere
  Organic psychosis:
   infective NOS
   posttraumatic NOS
   transient NOS
  Psycho-organic syndrome
  (Ex) 291.0-294.9, 303.00-305.03, 305.20-305.93, 790.3

● **294 Persistent mental disorders due to conditions classified elsewhere**

  Includes organic psychotic brain syndromes (chronic), not elsewhere classified

 294.0 Amnestic disorder in conditions classified elsewhere
  Korsakoff's psychosis or syndrome (nonalcoholic)

  Code first underlying condition

  Excludes *alcoholic:*
    amnestic syndrome (291.1)
    Korsakoff's psychosis (291.1)

● **294.1 Dementia in conditions classified elsewhere**
  Dementia of the Alzheimer's type

  Code first any underlying physical condition as:
  dementia in:
   Alzheimer's disease (331.0)
   cerebral lipidoses (330.1)
   dementia with Lewy bodies (331.82)
   dementia with Parkinsonism (331.82)
   epilepsy (345.0–345.9)
   frontal dementia (331.19)
   frontotemporal dementia (331.19)
   general paresis [syphilis] (094.1)
   hepatolenticular degeneration (275.1)
   Huntington's chorea (333.4)
   Jakob-Creutzfeldt disease (046.11–046.19) ◀▥
   multiple sclerosis (340)
   Pick's disease of the brain (331.11)
   polyarteritis nodosa (446.0)
   syphilis (094.1)

  Excludes *dementia:*
    arteriosclerotic (290.40–290.43)
    presenile (290.10–290.13)
    senile (290.0)
    epileptic psychosis NOS (294.8)
  Coding Clinic: 1999, Q1, P14; 1985, Sept-Oct, P12

 ▌ **294.10 *Dementia in conditions classified elsewhere without behavioral disturbance***
  Dementia in conditions classified elsewhere NOS

 ▌ **294.11 *Dementia in conditions classified elsewhere with behavioral disturbance***
  Aggressive behavior
  Combative behavior
  Violent behavior
  Wandering off
  (Ex) 294.11
  Coding Clinic: 2000, Q4, P40-41

 294.8 Other persistent mental disorders due to conditions classified elsewhere
  Amnestic disorder NOS
  Dementia NOS
  Epileptic psychosis NOS
  Mixed paranoid and affective organic psychotic states

  Use additional code for associated epilepsy (345.0–345.9)

  Excludes *mild memory disturbances, not amounting to dementia (310.8)* ◀▥
  Coding Clinic: 2003, Q3, P14

 294.9 Unspecified persistent mental disorders due to conditions classified elsewhere
  Cognitive disorder NOS
  Organic psychosis (chronic)
  Coding Clinic: 2007, Q2, P5

OTHER PSYCHOSES (295–299)

Use additional code to identify any associated physical disease, injury, or condition affecting the brain with psychoses classifiable to 295–298

● 295 **Schizophrenic disorders**

Personality disorders characterized by multiple mental and behavioral irregularities.

Includes schizophrenia of the types described in 295.0–295.9 occurring in children

Excludes *childhood type schizophrenia (299.9)*
infantile autism (299.0)

The following fifth-digit subclassification is for use with category 295:

> 0 unspecified
> 1 subchronic
> 2 chronic
> 3 subchronic with acute exacerbation
> 4 chronic with acute exacerbation
> 5 in remission

● 295.0 **Simple type 0-4** 🖝
[0-5] Schizophrenia simplex

Excludes *latent schizophrenia (295.5)*

For codes **295.00-295.04:** (Ex) 295.00-301.9, 306.0-319, 339.10-339.12, 388.45

● 295.1 **Disorganized type 0-4** 🖝
[0-5] Hebephrenia
Hebephrenic type schizophrenia
For codes **295.10-295.14:** (Ex) 295.00-301.9, 306.0-319, 339.10-339.12, 388.45

● 295.2 **Catatonic type 0-4** 🖝
[0-5] Catatonic (schizophrenia):
agitation
excitation
excited type
stupor
withdrawn type
Schizophrenic:
catalepsy
catatonia
flexibilitas cerea
For codes **295.20-295.24:** (Ex) 295.00-301.9, 306.0-319, 339.10-339.12, 388.45

● 295.3 **Paranoid type 0-4** 🖝
[0-5] Paraphrenic schizophrenia

Excludes *involutional paranoid state (297.2)*
paranoia (297.1)
paraphrenia (297.2)

For codes **295.30-295.34:** (Ex) 295.00-301.9, 306.0-319, 339.10-339.12, 388.45

● 295.4 **Schizophreniform disorder 0-4** 🖝
[0-5] Oneirophrenia
Schizophreniform:
attack
psychosis, confusional type

Excludes *acute forms of schizophrenia of:*
catatonic type (295.2)
hebephrenic type (295.1)
paranoid type (295.3)
simple type (295.0)
undifferentiated type (295.8)

For codes **295.40-295.44:** (Ex) 295.00-301.9, 306.0-319, 339.10-339.12, 388.45

● 295.5 **Latent schizophrenia 3-4** 🖝
[0-5] Latent schizophrenic reaction
Schizophrenia: Schizophrenia:
borderline   prodromal
incipient   pseudoneurotic
prepsychotic   pseudopsychopathic

Excludes *schizoid personality (301.20–301.22)*

For codes **295.53-595.54:** (Ex) 295.00-295.04, 295.10-295.14, 295.21-295.24, 295.31, 295.33-295.34, 295.40-295.44, 295.53-295.54, 295.63-295.64, 295.71, 295.73-295.74, 295.80-295.84, 295.91, 295.93-295.94

● 295.6 **Residual type 0-4** 🖝
[0-5] Chronic undifferentiated schizophrenia
Restzustand (schizophrenic)
Schizophrenic residual state
For codes **295.60-295.64:** (Ex) 295.00-301.9, 306.0-319, 339.10-339.12, 388.45

Coding Clinic: 2006, Q4, P76-78

● 295.7 **Schizoaffective disorder 1-4** 🖝
[0-5] Cyclic schizophrenia
Mixed schizophrenic and affective psychosis
Schizo-affective psychosis
Schizophreniform psychosis, affective type
For codes **295.71-295.74:** (Ex) 295.00-301.9, 306.0-319, 339.10-339.12, 388.45

● 295.8 **Other specified types of schizophrenia 0-4** 🖝
[0-5] Acute (undifferentiated) schizophrenia
Atypical schizophrenia
Cenesthopathic schizophrenia

Excludes *infantile autism (299.0)*

For codes **295.80-295.84:** (Ex) 295.00-301.9, 306.0-319, 339.10-339.12, 388.45

● 295.9 **Unspecified schizophrenia 1-4** 🖝
[0-5] Schizophrenia: Schizophrenia:
NOS   undifferentiated NOS
mixed NOS   undifferentiated type
Schizophrenic reaction NOS
Schizophreniform psychosis NOS
For codes **295.91-295.94:** (Ex) 295.00-301.9, 306.0-319, 339.10-339.12, 388.45

Coding Clinic: 1995, Q3, P6

MENTAL DISORDERS (290–319)

N Newborn Age: 0   **P** Pediatric Age: 0–17   **M** Maternity Age: 12–55   **A** Adult Age: 15–124   ♀ Females Only   ♂ Males Only

(Ex) CC Exclusions   🖝 Complication\Comorbidity   🖝 Major C\C   🖝 Present on Admission Requirement   🖝 Hospital-Acquired Condition

827

● **296 Episodic mood disorders**

> **Includes** episodic affective disorders
>
> **Excludes** *neurotic depression (300.4)*
> *reactive depressive psychosis (298.0)*
> *reactive excitation (298.1)*

Coding Clinic: 1985, Mar-April, P14

The following fifth-digit subclassification is for use with categories 296.0–296.6:

> 0 unspecified
> 1 mild
> 2 moderate
> 3 severe, without mention of psychotic behavior
> 4 severe, specified as with psychotic behavior
> 5 in partial or unspecified remission
> 6 in full remission

● **296.0 Bipolar I disorder, single manic episode 0-4**

[0-6] *Manic depressive disorder, characterized by moods that swing between periods of exaggerated euphoria, irritability, or both (manic) and episodes of depression.*

Hypomania (mild) NOS single episode or unspecified
Hypomanic psychosis single episode or unspecified
Mania (monopolar) NOS single episode or unspecified
Manic-depressive psychosis or reaction, single episode or unspecified:
hypomanic, single episode or unspecified
manic, single episode or unspecified

> **Excludes** *circular type, if there was a previous attack of depression (296.4)*

For codes **296.00-296.02:** (Ex:) 295.00-301.9, 306.0-319, 339.10-339.12, 388.45;
For code **296.03:** (Ex:) 296.03-296.04, 296.13-296.14, 296.43-296.44, 296.53-296.54, 296.63-296.64;
For code **296.04:** (Ex:) 295.00-301.9, 306.0-319, 339.10-339.12, 388.45

● **296.1 Manic disorder, recurrent episode 0-4**

[0-6] Any condition classifiable to 296.0, stated to be recurrent

> **Excludes** *circular type, if there was a previous attack of depression (296.4)*

For codes **296.10-296.12 and 296.14:** (Ex:) 295.00-301.9, 306.0-319, 339.10-339.12, 388.45;
For code **296.13:** (Ex:) 296.13-296.14, 296.43-296.44, 296.53-296.54, 296.63-296.64;

● **296.2 Major depressive disorder, single episode 0-4**

[0-6] Depressive psychosis, single episode or unspecified
Endogenous depression, single episode or unspecified
Involutional melancholia, single episode or unspecified
Manic-depressive psychosis or reaction, depressed type, single episode or unspecified
Monopolar depression, single episode or unspecified
Psychotic depression, single episode or unspecified

> **Excludes** *circular type, if previous attack was of manic type (296.5)*
> *depression NOS (311)*
> *reactive depression (neurotic) (300.4)*
> *psychotic (298.0)*

For code **296.20:** (Ex:) 295.00-301.9, 306.0-319, 339.10-339.12, 388.45;
For codes **296.21-296.24:** (Ex:) 296.21-296.24, 296.30-296.34

● **296.3 Major depressive disorder, recurrent episode 0-4**

[0-6] Any condition classifiable to 296.2, stated to be recurrent

> **Excludes** *circular type, if previous attack was of manic type (296.5)*
> *depression NOS (311)*
> *reactive depression (neurotic) (300.4)*
> *psychotic (298.0)*

For codes **296.30-296.33:** (Ex:) 296.21-296.24, 296.30-296.34;
For code **296.34:** (Ex:) 295.00-301.9, 306.0-319, 339.10-339.12, 388.45

● **296.4 Bipolar I disorder, most recent episode (or current)**
[0-6] **manic 0-4**

Bipolar disorder, now manic
Manic-depressive psychosis, circular type but currently manic

> **Excludes** *brief compensatory or rebound mood swings (296.99)*

For codes **296.40-296.42 and 296.44:** (Ex:) 295.00-301.9, 306.0-319, 339.10-339.12, 388.45;
For code **296.43:** (Ex:) 296.43-296.44, 296.63-296.64

● **296.5 Bipolar I disorder, most recent episode (or current)**
[0-6] **depressed 0-4**

Bipolar disorder, now depressed
Manic-depressive psychosis, circular type but currently depressed

> **Excludes** *brief compensatory or rebound mood swings (296.99)*

For codes **296.50-296.52 and 293.54:** (Ex:) 295.00-301.9, 306.0-319, 339.10-339.12, 388.45;
For code **296.53:** (Ex:) 296.43-296.44, 296.53-296.54, 296.63-296.64
Coding Clinic: 2006, Q1, P10

● **296.6 Bipolar I disorder, most recent episode (or current)**
[0-6] **mixed 0-4**

Manic-depressive psychosis, circular type, mixed
For codes **296.60-296.62 and 296.64:** (Ex:) 295.00-301.9, 306.0-319, 339.10-339.12, 388.45;
For code **296.63:** (Ex:) 296.43-296.44, 296.53-296.54, 296.63-296.64

296.7 Bipolar I disorder, most recent episode (or current) unspecified

Atypical bipolar affective disorder NOS
Manic-depressive psychosis, circular type, current condition not specified as either manic or depressive

● **296.8 Other and unspecified bipolar disorders**

296.80 Bipolar disorder, unspecified
Bipolar disorder NOS
Manic-depressive:
reaction NOS
syndrome NOS

296.81 Atypical manic disorder

296.82 Atypical depressive disorder

296.89 Other
Bipolar II disorder
Manic-depressive psychosis, mixed type
(Ex:) 295.00-301.9, 306.0-319, 339.10-339.12, 388.45

● **296.9 Other and unspecified episodic mood disorder**

> **Excludes** *psychogenic affective psychoses (298.0–298.8)*

296.90 Unspecified episodic mood disorder
Affective psychosis NOS
Melancholia NOS
Mood disorder NOS
Coding Clinic: 1985, Mar-April, P14

◄ New ◄▥ Revised ~~deleted~~ Deleted ● Unacceptable Principal Diagnosis ● Use Additional Digit(s)
▶ Manifestation Code **OGCR** Official Guidelines **Coding Clinic** Excludes Includes Use additional Code first Omit code

296.99 Other specified episodic mood disorder 🗘
Mood swings:
brief compensatory
rebound
Ⓔ 295.00-301.9, 306.0-319, 339.10-339.12, 388.45

● **297 Delusional disorders**

Includes paranoid disorders

Excludes *acute paranoid reaction (298.3)*
alcoholic jealousy or paranoid state (291.5)
paranoid schizophrenia (295.3)

297.0 Paranoid state, simple

297.1 Delusional disorder
Chronic paranoid psychosis
Sander's disease
Systematized delusions

Excludes *paranoid personality disorder (301.0)*

297.2 Paraphrenia
Involutional paranoid state
Late paraphrenia
Paraphrenia (involutional)

297.3 Shared psychotic disorder
Folie à deux
Induced psychosis or paranoid disorder

297.8 Other specified paranoid states
Paranoia querulans
Sensitiver Beziehungswahn

Excludes *acute paranoid reaction or state (298.3)*
senile paranoid state (290.20)

297.9 Unspecified paranoid state
Paranoid:
disorder NOS
psychosis NOS
reaction NOS
state NOS

● **298 Other nonorganic psychoses**

Includes psychotic conditions due to or provoked by:
emotional stress
environmental factors as major part of
etiology

298.0 Depressive type psychosis 🗘
Psychogenic depressive psychosis
Psychotic reactive depression
Reactive depressive psychosis

Excludes *manic-depressive psychosis, depressed type*
(296.2–296.3)
neurotic depression (300.4)
reactive depression NOS (300.4)
Ⓔ 295.00-301.9, 306.0-319, 339.10-339.12, 388.45

298.1 Excitative type psychosis 🗘
Acute hysterical psychosis
Psychogenic excitation
Reactive excitation

Excludes *manic-depressive psychosis, manic type*
(296.0–296.1)
Ⓔ 295.00-301.9, 306.0-319, 339.10-339.12, 388.45

298.2 Reactive confusion
Psychogenic confusion
Psychogenic twilight state

Excludes *acute confusional state (293.0)*

298.3 Acute paranoid reaction 🗘
Acute psychogenic paranoid psychosis
Bouffée délirante

Excludes *paranoid states (297.0–297.9)*
Ⓔ 295.00-301.9, 306.0-319, 339.10-339.12, 388.45

298.4 Psychogenic paranoid psychosis 🗘
Protracted reactive paranoid psychosis
Ⓔ 295.00-301.9, 306.0-319, 339.10-339.12, 388.45

298.8 Other and unspecified reactive psychosis
Brief psychotic disorder
Brief reactive psychosis NOS
Hysterical psychosis
Psychogenic psychosis NOS
Psychogenic stupor

Excludes *acute hysterical psychosis (298.1)*

298.9 Unspecified psychosis
Atypical psychosis
Psychosis NOS
Psychotic disorder NOS
Coding Clinic: 2006, Q3, P22; 1993, Q3, P11

● **299 Pervasive developmental disorders**

Excludes *adult type psychoses occurring in childhood, as:*
affective disorders (296.0–296.9)
manic-depressive disorders (296.0–296.9)
schizophrenia (295.0–295.9)

The following fifth-digit subclassification is for use with
category 299:

0 current or active state
1 residual state

● **299.0 Autistic disorder** 🗘
[0-1] Childhood autism
Infantile psychosis
Kanner's syndrome

Excludes *disintegrative psychosis (299.1)*
Heller's syndrome (299.1)
schizophrenic syndrome of childhood (299.9)
Ⓔ 295.00-301.9, 306.0-319, 339.10-339.12, 388.45

● **299.1 Childhood disintegrative disorder** 🗘
[0-1] Heller's syndrome

Use additional code to identify any associated
neurological disorder

Excludes *infantile autism (299.0)*
schizophrenic syndrome of childhood (299.9)
Ⓔ 295.00-301.9, 306.0-319, 339.10-339.12, 388.45

● **299.8 Other specified pervasive developmental**
[0-1] **disorders** 🗘
Asperger's disorder
Atypical childhood psychosis
Borderline psychosis of childhood

Excludes *simple stereotypes without psychotic*
disturbance (307.3)
Ⓔ 295.00-301.9, 306.0-319, 339.10-339.12, 388.45

● **299.9 Unspecified pervasive developmental disorder** 🗘
[0-1] Child psychosis NOS
Pervasive developmental disorder NOS
Schizophrenia, childhood type NOS
Schizophrenic syndrome of childhood NOS

Excludes *schizophrenia of adult type occurring in*
childhood (295.0–295.9)
Ⓔ 295.00-301.9, 306.0-319, 339.10-339.12, 388.45

MENTAL DISORDERS (290–319)

N Newborn Age: 0   **P** Pediatric Age: 0–17   **M** Maternity Age: 12–55   **A** Adult Age: 15–124   ♀ Females Only   ♂ Males Only

Ⓔ CC Exclusions   🗘 Complication\Comorbidity   Major C\C   Present on Admission Requirement   Hospital-Acquired Condition

829

Item 5-2 Anxiety is also known as **generalized disorder** and is evidenced by persistent, excessive, and unrealistic worry about everyday things. **Dissociative disorders** are characterized by a persistent disruption in the integration of memory, consciousness, or identity and a lack of mental connectedness to events. **Somatoform disorders** are characterized by unusual physical symptoms in the absence of any known physical pathology and may lead to unnecessary medical treatments.

NEUROTIC DISORDERS, PERSONALITY DISORDERS, AND OTHER NONPSYCHOTIC MENTAL DISORDERS (300–316)

● 300 **Anxiety, dissociative and somatoform disorders**

  ● 300.0 **Anxiety states**

    | Excludes | anxiety in:
        acute stress reaction (308.0)
        transient adjustment reaction (309.24)
        neurasthenia (300.5)
        psychophysiological disorders (306.0–306.9)
        separation anxiety (309.21)

    300.00 **Anxiety state, unspecified**
      Anxiety:
        neurosis
        reaction
        state (neurotic)
      Atypical anxiety disorder

    300.01 **Panic disorder without agoraphobia**
      Panic:
        attack
        state

      | Excludes | *panic disorder with agoraphobia (300.21)*

    300.02 **Generalized anxiety disorder**

    300.09 **Other**

  ● 300.1 **Dissociative, conversion and factitious disorders**

    | Excludes | *adjustment reaction (309.0–309.9)*
        anorexia nervosa (307.1)
        gross stress reaction (308.0–308.9)
        hysterical personality (301.50–301.59)
        psychophysiologic disorders (306.0–306.9)

    300.10 **Hysteria, unspecified**

    300.11 **Conversion disorder**
      Astasia-abasia, hysterical
      Conversion hysteria or reaction
      Hysterical:
        blindness
        deafness
        paralysis
      Coding Clinic: 1985, Nov-Dec, P15

    300.12 **Dissociative amnesia**
      Hysterical amnesia

    300.13 **Dissociative fugue**
      Hysterical fugue

    300.14 **Dissociative identity disorder**

    300.15 **Dissociative disorder or reaction, unspecified**

    300.16 **Factitious disorder with predominantly psychological signs and symptoms**
      Compensation neurosis
      Ganser's syndrome, hysterical

    300.19 **Other and unspecified factitious illness**
      Factitious disorder (with combined psychological and physical signs and symptoms) (with predominantly physical signs and symptoms) NOS

      | Excludes | *multiple operations or hospital addiction syndrome (301.51)*

  ● 300.2 **Phobic disorders**
    Irrational fear with avoidance of the feared subject, activity, or situation. Divided into 3 types: specific phobias, social phobias, and agoraphobia.

    | Excludes | *anxiety state not associated with a specific situation or object (300.00–300.09)*
        obsessional phobias (300.3)

    300.20 **Phobia, unspecified**
      Anxiety-hysteria NOS
      Phobia NOS

    300.21 **Agoraphobia with panic disorder**
      Fear of:
        open spaces with panic attacks
        streets with panic attacks
        travel with panic attacks
      Panic disorder with agoraphobia

      | Excludes | *agoraphobia without panic disorder (300.22)*
        panic disorder without agoraphobia (300.01)

    300.22 **Agoraphobia without mention of panic attacks**
      Any condition classifiable to 300.21 without mention of panic attacks

    300.23 **Social phobia**
      Fear of:
        eating in public
        public speaking
        washing in public

    300.29 **Other isolated or specific phobias**
      Acrophobia
        Fear of heights
      Animal phobias
      Claustrophobia
        Fear of closed spaces
      Fear of crowds

  300.3 **Obsessive-compulsive disorders** *(OCD)*
    Anancastic neurosis
    Compulsive neurosis
    Obsessional phobia [any]

    | Excludes | *obsessive-compulsive symptoms occurring in:*
        endogenous depression (296.2–296.3)
        organic states (e.g., encephalitis)
        schizophrenia (295.0–295.9)

  300.4 **Dysthymic disorder**
    Anxiety depression
    Depression with anxiety
    Depressive reaction
    Neurotic depressive state
    Reactive depression

    | Excludes | *adjustment reaction with depressive symptoms (309.0–309.1)*
        depression NOS (311)
        manic-depressive psychosis, depressed type (296.2–296.3)
        reactive depressive psychosis (298.0)

◀ New   ◀◀ Revised   ~~deleted~~ Deleted   ● Unacceptable Principal Diagnosis   ● Use Additional Digit(s)
▶ Manifestation Code   OGCR Official Guidelines   **Coding Clinic** | Excludes | | Includes | | Use additional | | Code first | | Omit code |

300.5 Neurasthenia
    Fatigue neurosis
    Nervous debility
    Psychogenic:
      asthenia
      general fatigue
    Use additional code to identify any associated
      physical disorder

> **Excludes**   *anxiety state (300.00–300.09)*
> *neurotic depression (300.4)*
> *psychophysiological disorders (306.0–306.9)*
> *specific nonpsychotic mental disorders*
>   *following organic brain damage*
>   *(310.0–310.9)*

300.6 Depersonalization disorder
    Derealization (neurotic)
    Neurotic state with depersonalization episode

> **Excludes**   *depersonalization associated with:*
> *anxiety (300.00–300.09)*
> *depression (300.4)*
> *manic-depressive disorder or psychosis*
>   *(296.0–296.9)*
> *schizophrenia (295.0–295.9)*

300.7 Hypochondriasis
    Hypochondriac
    Body dysmorphic disorder

> **Excludes**   *hypochondriasis in:*
> *hysteria (300.10–300.19)*
> *manic-depressive psychosis, depressed*
>   *type (296.2–296.3)*
> *neurasthenia (300.5)*
> *obsessional disorder (300.3)*
> *schizophrenia (295.0–295.9)*

● **300.8 Somatoform disorders**

  300.81 Somatization disorder
    Briquet's disorder
    Severe somatoform disorder

  300.82 Undifferentiated somatoform disorder
    Atypical somatoform disorder
    Somatoform disorder NOS

  300.89 Other somatoform disorders
    Occupational neurosis, including writers'
      cramp
    Psychasthenia
    Psychasthenic neurosis

  300.9 Unspecified nonpsychotic mental disorder
    Psychoneurosis NOS

● **301 Personality disorders**
    Long-term patterns of thoughts and behaviors causing serious
    problems with relationships and work.

> **Includes**   character neurosis

    Use additional code to identify any associated neurosis
      or psychosis, or physical condition

> **Excludes**   *nonpsychotic personality disorder associated with*
> *organic brain syndromes (310.0–310.9)*

301.0 Paranoid personality disorder
    Fanatic personality
    Paranoid personality (disorder)
    Paranoid traits

> **Excludes**   *acute paranoid reaction (298.3)*
> *alcoholic paranoia (291.5)*
> *paranoid schizophrenia (295.3)*
> *paranoid states (297.0–297.9)*

● **301.1 Affective personality disorder**

> **Excludes**   *affective psychotic disorders (296.0–296.9)*
> *neurasthenia (300.5)*
> *neurotic depression (300.4)*

  301.10 Affective personality disorder, unspecified

  301.11 Chronic hypomanic personality disorder
    Chronic hypomanic disorder
    Hypomanic personality

  301.12 Chronic depressive personality disorder
    Chronic depressive disorder
    Depressive character or personality

  301.13 Cyclothymic disorder
    Cycloid personality
    Cyclothymia
    Cyclothymic personality

● **301.2 Schizoid personality disorder**

> **Excludes**   *schizophrenia (295.0–295.9)*

  301.20 Schizoid personality disorder, unspecified

  301.21 Introverted personality

  301.22 Schizotypal personality disorder

301.3 Explosive personality disorder
    Aggressive:
      personality
      reaction
    Aggressiveness
    Emotional instability (excessive)
    Pathological emotionality
    Quarrelsomeness

> **Excludes**   *dyssocial personality (301.7)*
> *hysterical neurosis (300.10–300.19)*

301.4 Obsessive-compulsive personality disorder
    Anancastic personality
    Obsessional personality

> **Excludes**   *obsessive-compulsive disorder (300.3)*
> *phobic state (300.20–300.29)*

● **301.5 Histrionic personality disorder**

> **Excludes**   *hysterical neurosis (300.10–300.19)*

  301.50 Histrionic personality disorder, unspecified
    Hysterical personality NOS

  **301.51 Chronic factitious illness with physical
    symptoms** 🅒
    Hospital addiction syndrome
    Multiple operations syndrome
    Munchausen syndrome
    Ⓔⓧ 295.00-301.9, 306.0-319, 339.10-339.12, 388.45

  301.59 Other histrionic personality disorder
    Personality: Personality:
      emotionally unstable   psychoinfantile
      labile

MENTAL DISORDERS (290–319)

301.6 Dependent personality disorder
Asthenic personality
Inadequate personality
Passive personality

Excludes	*neurasthenia (300.5)*
	passive-aggressive personality (301.84)

301.7 Antisocial personality disorder
Amoral personality
Asocial personality
Dyssocial personality
Personality disorder with predominantly
    sociopathic or asocial manifestation

Excludes	*disturbance of conduct without specifiable*
	personality disorder (312.0–312.9)
	explosive personality (301.3)

Coding Clinic: 1984, Sept-Oct, P16

● **301.8 Other personality disorders**

301.81 Narcissistic personality disorder

301.82 Avoidant personality disorder

301.83 Borderline personality disorder

301.84 Passive-aggressive personality

301.89 Other
Personality: Personality:
   eccentric   masochistic
   "haltlose" type   psychoneurotic
   immature

Excludes	*psychoinfantile personality (301.59)*

301.9 Unspecified personality disorder
Pathological personality NOS
Personality disorder NOS
Psychopathic:
   constitutional state
   personality (disorder)

● **302 Sexual and gender identity disorders**

Excludes	*sexual disorder manifest in:*
	organic brain syndrome (290.0–294.9,
	310.0–310.9)
	psychosis (295.0–298.9)

302.0 Ego-dystonic sexual orientation
Ego-dystonic lesbianism
Sexual orientation conflict disorder

Excludes	*homosexual pedophilia (302.2)*

302.1 Zoophilia
Bestiality

302.2 Pedophilia

302.3 Transvestic fetishism

Excludes	*trans-sexualism (302.5)*

302.4 Exhibitionism

● **302.5 Trans-sexualism**
Sex reassignment surgery status

Excludes	*transvestism (302.3)*

302.50 With unspecified sexual history

302.51 With asexual history

302.52 With homosexual history

302.53 With heterosexual history

302.6 Gender identity disorder in children
Check age: adolescents and adults separately classified
under 302.85.
Feminism in boys
Gender identity disorder NOS

Excludes	*gender identity disorder in adult (302.85)*
	trans-sexualism (302.50–302.53)
	transvestism (302.3)

● **302.7 Psychosexual dysfunction**

Excludes	*decreased sexual desire NOS (799.81)*
	impotence of organic origin (607.84)
	normal transient symptoms from ruptured
	hymen
	transient or occasional failures of erection
	due to fatigue, anxiety, alcohol, or
	drugs

302.70 Psychosexual dysfunction, unspecified
Sexual dysfunction NOS

302.71 Hypoactive sexual desire disorder

Excludes	*decreased sexual desire NOS*
	(799.81)

302.72 With inhibited sexual excitement
Female sexual arousal disorder
Frigidity
Impotence
Male erectile disorder

302.73 Female orgasmic disorder ♀

302.74 Male orgasmic disorder ♂

302.75 Premature ejaculation ♂

302.76 Dyspareunia, psychogenic ♀

302.79 With other specified psychosexual
dysfunctions
Sexual aversion disorder

● **302.8 Other specified psychosexual disorders**

302.81 Fetishism

302.82 Voyeurism

302.83 Sexual masochism

302.84 Sexual sadism

302.85 Gender identity disorder in adolescents or
adults

Use additional code to identify sex
   reassignment surgery status (302.5)

Excludes	*gender identity disorder NOS*
	(302.6)
	gender identity disorder in children
	(302.6)

302.89 Other
Frotteurism
Nymphomania
Satyriasis

302.9 Unspecified psychosexual disorder
Paraphilia NOS
Pathologic sexuality NOS
Sexual deviation NOS
Sexual disorder NOS

MENTAL DISORDERS (290–319)

◀ New   ◀▒ Revised   ~~deleted~~ Deleted   ● Unacceptable Principal Diagnosis   ● Use Additional Digit(s)
▶ Manifestation Code   **OGCR** Official Guidelines   **Coding Clinic**   Excludes   Includes   Use additional   Code first   Omit code

● **303 Alcohol dependence syndrome**

Use additional code to identify any associated
   condition, as:
   alcoholic psychoses (291.0–291.9)
   drug dependence (304.0–304.9)
   physical complications of alcohol, such as:
       cerebral degeneration (331.7)
       cirrhosis of liver (571.2)
       epilepsy (345.0–345.9)
       gastritis (535.3)
       hepatitis (571.1)
       liver damage NOS (571.3)

Excludes *drunkenness NOS (305.0)*

Coding Clinic: 1995, Q3, P6

The following fifth-digit subclassification is for use with
category 303:

0 **unspecified**
1 **continuous**
2 **episodic**
3 **in remission**

● **303.0 Acute alcoholic intoxication**
[0-3]   Acute drunkenness in alcoholism
        Coding Clinic: 1985, July-Aug, P15

● **303.9 Other and unspecified alcohol dependence**
[0-3]   Chronic alcoholism
        Dipsomania
        Coding Clinic: 2002, Q2, P4; Q1, P3-4; 1989, Q2, P9; 1985, Nov-Dec,
            P14

● **304 Drug dependence**
    *For some "dependence" codes there is a corresponding "abuse"
    code. There is a point at which drug use crosses from
    "dependence" to "abuse." Check documentation or query
    provider for patient status.*

Excludes *nondependent abuse of drugs (305.1–305.9)*

The following fifth-digit subclassification is for use with
category 304:

0 **unspecified**
1 **continuous**
2 **episodic**
3 **in remission**

● **304.0 Opioid type dependence 1**🅒
[0-3]   Heroin
        Meperidine
        Methadone
        Morphine
        Opium
        Opium alkaloids and their derivatives
        Synthetics with morphine-like effects
        For code **304.01:** (Ex) 291.0-292.9, 303.00-305.03, 305.20-305.93, 790.3
        Coding Clinic: 2006, Q2, P7; 1988, Q4, P8

● **304.1 Sedative, hypnotic or anxiolytic dependence 1**🅒
[0-3]   Barbiturates
        Nonbarbiturate sedatives and tranquilizers with a
            similar effect:
            chlordiazepoxide
            diazepam
            glutethimide
            meprobamate
            methaqualone
        For code **304.11:** (Ex) 291.0-292.9, 303.00-305.03, 305.20-305.93, 790.3

● **304.2 Cocaine dependence 1**🅒
[0-3]   Coca leaves and derivatives
        For code **304.21:** (Ex) 291.0-292.9, 303.00-305.03, 305.20-305.93, 790.3

● **304.3 Cannabis dependence**
[0-3]   *Code 305.2 is for abuse of cannabis.*
        Hashish
        Hemp
        Marihuana

● **304.4 Amphetamine and other psychostimulant**
[0-3]   **dependence 1**🅒
        Methylphenidate
        Phenmetrazine
        For code **304.41:** (Ex) 291.0-292.9, 303.00-305.03, 305.20-305.93, 790.3

● **304.5 Hallucinogen dependence 1**🅒
[0-3]   Dimethyltryptamine [DMT]
        Lysergic acid diethylamide [LSD] and derivatives
        Mescaline
        Psilocybin
        For code **304.51:** (Ex) 291.0-292.9, 303.00-305.03, 305.20-305.93, 790.3

● **304.6 Other specified drug dependence 1**🅒
[0-3]   Absinthe addiction
        Glue sniffing
        Inhalant dependence
        Phencyclidine dependence

        Excludes *tobacco dependence (305.1)*

        For code **304.61:** (Ex) 291.0-292.9, 303.00-305.03, 305.20-305.93, 790.3

● **304.7 Combinations of opioid type drug with any other 1**🅒
[0-3]   For code **304.71:** (Ex) 291.0-292.9, 303.00-305.03, 305.20-305.93, 790.3
        Coding Clinic: 1986, Mar-April, P12

● **304.8 Combinations of drug dependence excluding opioid**
[0-3]   **type drug 1**🅒
        For code **304.81:** (Ex) 291.0-292.9, 303.00-305.03, 305.20-305.93, 790.3
        Coding Clinic: 1986, Mar-April, P12

● **304.9 Unspecified drug dependence 1**🅒
[0-3]   Drug addiction NOS
        Drug dependence NOS
        For code **304.91:** (Ex) 291.0-292.9, 303.00-305.03, 305.20-305.93, 790.3
        Coding Clinic: 2003, Q4, P103-104

N Newborn Age: 0   **P** Pediatric Age: 0–17   **M** Maternity Age: 12–55   **A** Adult Age: 15–124   ♀ Females Only   ♂ Males Only   **833**

(Ex) CC Exclusions   🅒 Complication\Comorbidity   Major C\C   Present on Admission Requirement   Hospital-Acquired Condition

MENTAL DISORDERS (290–319)

● **305 Nondependent abuse of drugs**

Note: Includes cases where a person, for whom no other diagnosis is possible, has come under medical care because of the maladaptive effect of a drug on which he is not dependent and that he has taken on his own initiative (*self-medicating*) to the detriment of his health or social functioning.

Excludes	*alcohol dependence syndrome (303.0–303.9)*
	drug dependence (304.0–304.9)
	drug withdrawal syndrome (292.0)
	poisoning by drugs or medicinal substances (960.0–979.9)

The following fifth-digit subclassification is for use with codes 305.0–305.9:

> 0 **unspecified**
> 1 **continuous**
> 2 **episodic**
> 3 **in remission**

● **305.0 Alcohol abuse**
[0-3]   Drunkenness NOS
       Excessive drinking of alcohol NOS
       "Hangover" (alcohol)
       Inebriety NOS

Excludes	*acute alcohol intoxication in alcoholism (303.0)*
	alcoholic psychoses (291.0–291.9)

Coding Clinic: 1996, Q3, P16; 1985, July-Aug, P15

● **305.1 Tobacco use disorder**
[0-3]   Tobacco dependence   ⬅

Excludes	*history of tobacco use (V15.82)*
	smoking complicating pregnancy (649.0)
	tobacco use disorder complicating pregnancy (649.0)

Coding Clinic: 2009, Q1, P8; 1996, Q2, P10; 1984, Nov-Dec, P12

● **305.2 Cannabis abuse**
[0-3]   *Code 304.3 is for cannabis dependence.*

● **305.3 Hallucinogen abuse**
[0-3]   Acute intoxication from hallucinogens ["bad trips"]
       LSD reaction

● **305.4 Sedative, hypnotic or anxiolytic abuse**
[0-3]

● **305.5 Opioid abuse**
[0-3]

● **305.6 Cocaine abuse**
[0-3]   **Coding Clinic: 1993, Q1, P25; Q1, P25; 1988, Q4, P8**

● **305.7 Amphetamine or related acting sympathomimetic abuse**
[0-3]
       Coding Clinic: 2003, Q2, P10,11x2

● **305.8 Antidepressant type abuse**
[0-3]

● **305.9 Other, mixed, or unspecified drug abuse**
[0-3]   Caffeine intoxication
       Inhalant abuse
       "Laxative habit"
       Misuse of drugs NOS
       Nonprescribed use of drugs or patent medicinals
       Phencyclidine abuse
Coding Clinic: 1999, Q3, P20; 1994, Q4, P36

● **306 Physiological malfunction arising from mental factors**

Includes	psychogenic:
	physical symptoms not involving tissue damage
	physiological manifestations not involving tissue damage

Excludes	*hysteria (300.11–300.19)*
	physical symptoms secondary to a psychiatric disorder classified elsewhere
	psychic factors associated with physical conditions involving tissue damage classified elsewhere (316)
	specific nonpsychotic mental disorders following organic brain damage (310.0–310.9)

306.0 Musculoskeletal
       Psychogenic paralysis
       Psychogenic torticollis

Excludes	*Gilles de la Tourette's syndrome (307.23)*
	paralysis as hysterical or conversion reaction (300.11)
	tics (307.20–307.22)

306.1 Respiratory
Psychogenic: Psychogenic:
   air hunger   hyperventilation
   cough   yawning
   hiccough

Excludes	*psychogenic asthma (316 and 493.9)*

306.2 Cardiovascular
       Cardiac neurosis
       Cardiovascular neurosis
       Neurocirculatory asthenia
       Psychogenic cardiovascular disorder

Excludes	*psychogenic paroxysmal tachycardia (316 and 427.2)*

Coding Clinic: 1985, July-Aug, P14

306.3 Skin
       Psychogenic pruritus

Excludes	*psychogenic:*
	alopecia (316 and 704.00)
	dermatitis (316 and 692.9)
	eczema (316 and 691.8 or 692.9)
	urticaria (316 and 708.0–708.9)

306.4 Gastrointestinal
       Aerophagy
       Cyclical vomiting, psychogenic
       Diarrhea, psychogenic
       Nervous gastritis
       Psychogenic dyspepsia

Excludes	*cyclical vomiting NOS (536.2)*
	associated with migraine (346.2)
	globus hystericus (300.11)
	mucous colitis (316 and 564.9)
	psychogenic:
	cardiospasm (316 and 530.0)
	duodenal ulcer (316 and 532.0–532.9)
	gastric ulcer (316 and 531.0–531.9)
	peptic ulcer NOS (316 and 533.0–533.9)
	vomiting NOS (307.54)

Coding Clinic: 1989, Q2, P11

◀ New   ⬅ Revised   ~~deleted~~ Deleted   ● Unacceptable Principal Diagnosis   ● Use Additional Digit(s)
▶ Manifestation Code   **OGCR** Official Guidelines   **Coding Clinic**   Excludes   Includes   Use additional   Code first   Omit code

● **306.5 Genitourinary**

> | Excludes | *enuresis, psychogenic (307.6)*
> *frigidity (302.72)*
> *impotence (302.72)*
> *psychogenic dyspareunia (302.76)*

306.50 Psychogenic genitourinary malfunction, unspecified

306.51 Psychogenic vaginismus ♀
　Functional vaginismus

306.52 Psychogenic dysmenorrhea ♀

306.53 Psychogenic dysuria

306.59 Other

306.6 Endocrine

306.7 Organs of special sense

> | Excludes | *hysterical blindness or deafness (300.11)*
> *psychophysical visual disturbances (368.16)*

306.8 Other specified psychophysiological malfunction
　Bruxism
　　Sleep-related bruxism, 327.53
　Teeth grinding

306.9 Unspecified psychophysiological malfunction
　Psychophysiologic disorder NOS
　Psychosomatic disorder NOS

● **307 Special symptoms or syndromes, not elsewhere classified**

> **Note:** This category is intended for use if the psychopathology is manifested by a single specific symptom or group of symptoms which is not part of an organic illness or other mental disorder classifiable elsewhere.

> | Excludes | *those due to mental disorders classified elsewhere*
> *those of organic origin*

307.0 Stuttering

> | Excludes | *dysphasia (784.59)*
> *lisping or lalling (307.9)*
> *retarded development of speech (315.31–315.39)*
> *stuttering (fluency disorder) due to late effect of cerebrovascular accident (438.14)*

307.1 Anorexia nervosa

> | Excludes | *eating disturbance NOS (307.50)*
> *feeding problem (783.3)*
> *of nonorganic origin (307.59)*
> *loss of appetite (783.0)*
> *of nonorganic origin (307.59)*

> (Ex) 306.4, 306.8–306.9, 307.1, 307.50–307.59, 309.22
> **Coding Clinic: 2006, Q2, P12; 1989, Q4, P11**

● **307.2 Tics**

> | Excludes | *nail-biting or thumb-sucking (307.9)*
> *stereotypes occurring in isolation (307.3)*
> *tics of organic origin (333.3)*

307.20 Tic disorder, unspecified
　Tic disorder NOS

307.21 Transient tic disorder

307.22 Chronic motor or vocal tic disorder

307.23 Tourette's disorder
　Motor-verbal tic disorder

307.3 Stereotypic movement disorder
　Body-rocking
　Head banging
　Spasmus nutans
　Stereotypes NOS

> | Excludes | *tics (307.20–307.23)*
> *of organic origin (333.3)*

● **307.4 Specific disorders of sleep of nonorganic origin**

> | Excludes | *narcolepsy (347.00–347.11)*
> *organic hypersomnia (327.10–327.19)*
> *organic insomnia (327.00–327.09)*
> *those of unspecified cause (780.50–780.59)*

307.40 Nonorganic sleep disorder, unspecified

307.41 Transient disorder of initiating or maintaining sleep
　Adjustment insomnia
　Hyposomnia associated with acute or intermittent emotional reactions or conflicts
　Insomnia associated with acute or intermittent emotional reactions or conflicts
　Sleeplessness associated with acute or intermittent emotional reactions or conflicts

307.42 Persistent disorder of initiating or maintaining sleep
　Hyposomnia, insomnia, or sleeplessness associated with:
　　anxiety
　　conditioned arousal
　　depression (major) (minor)
　　psychosis
　Idiopathic insomnia
　Paradoxical insomnia
　Primary insomnia
　Psychophysiological insomnia

307.43 Transient disorder of initiating or maintaining wakefulness
　Hypersomnia associated with acute or intermittent emotional reactions or conflicts

307.44 Persistent disorder of initiating or maintaining wakefulness
　Hypersomnia associated with depression (major) (minor)
　Insufficient sleep syndrome
　Primary hypersomnia

> | Excludes | *sleep deprivation (V69.4)*

307.45 Circadian rhythm sleep disorder of nonorganic origin

307.46 Sleep arousal disorder
　Night terror disorder
　Night terrors
　Sleep terror disorder
　Sleepwalking
　Somnambulism

307.47 Other dysfunctions of sleep stages or arousal from sleep
　Nightmare disorder
　Nightmares:
　　NOS
　　REM-sleep type
　Sleep drunkenness

307.48 Repetitive intrusions of sleep
　Repetitive intrusion of sleep with:
　　atypical polysomnographic features
　　environmental disturbances
　　repeated REM-sleep interruptions

307.49 Other
　"Short-sleeper"
　Subjective insomnia complaint

N Newborn Age: 0　　**P** Pediatric Age: 0–17　　**M** Maternity Age: 12–55　　**A** Adult Age: 15–124　　♀ Females Only　　♂ Males Only

(Ex) CC Exclusions　　Complication\Comorbidity　　Major C\C　　Present on Admission Requirement　　Hospital-Acquired Condition　　　835

MENTAL DISORDERS (290–319)

● **307.5 Other and unspecified disorders of eating**

Excludes *anorexia:*
      nervosa (307.1)
      of unspecified cause (783.0)
    overeating, of unspecified cause (783.6)
    vomiting:
      NOS (787.03)
      cyclical (536.2)
        associated with migraine (346.2)
        psychogenic (306.4)

307.50 Eating disorder, unspecified
Eating disorder NOS

307.51 Bulimia nervosa 🔗
Overeating of nonorganic origin
Ⓔⓧ 307.1, 307.50-307.51, 307.53-307.59

307.52 Pica
Perverted appetite of nonorganic origin
Craving and eating substances such as paint, clay, or dirt to replace a nutritional deficit in the body.

307.53 Rumination disorder
Regurgitation, of nonorganic origin, of food with reswallowing

Excludes *obsessional rumination (300.3)*

307.54 Psychogenic vomiting

307.59 Other
Feeding disorder of infancy or early childhood of nonorganic origin
Infantile feeding disturbances of nonorganic origin
Loss of appetite of nonorganic origin

Item 5–3 Enuresis: Bed wetting by children at night. Causes can be either psychological or medical (diabetes, urinary tract infections, or abnormalities). **Encopresis**: Overflow incontinence of bowels sometimes resulting from chronic constipation or fecal impaction. Check the documentation for additional diagnoses.

307.6 Enuresis
Enuresis (primary) (secondary) of nonorganic origin

Excludes *enuresis of unspecified cause (788.3)*

307.7 Encopresis
Encopresis (continuous) (discontinuous) of nonorganic origin

Excludes *encopresis of unspecified cause (787.6)*

● **307.8 Pain disorders related to psychological factors**

307.80 Psychogenic pain, site unspecified

307.81 Tension headache

Excludes *headache:*
    migraine (346.0–346.9)
    NOS (784.0)
    syndromes (339.00–339.89)
    tension type (339.10–339.12)
Coding Clinic: 1985, Nov-Dec, P16

307.89 Other
Code first *to type or site of pain*

Excludes *pain disorder exclusively attributed to psychological factors (307.80)*
    psychogenic pain (307.80)

307.9 Other and unspecified special symptoms or syndromes, not elsewhere classified
Communication disorder NOS
Hair plucking
Lalling
Lisping
Masturbation
Nail-biting
Thumb-sucking

● **308 Acute reaction to stress**

Includes catastrophic stress
combat fatigue
gross stress reaction (acute)
transient disorders in response to exceptional physical or mental stress which usually subside within hours or days

Excludes *adjustment reaction or disorder (309.0–309.9)*
chronic stress reaction (309.1–309.9)

308.0 Predominant disturbance of emotions
Anxiety as acute reaction to exceptional [gross] stress
Emotional crisis as acute reaction to exceptional [gross] stress
Panic state as acute reaction to exceptional [gross] stress

308.1 Predominant disturbance of consciousness
Fugues as acute reaction to exceptional [gross] stress

308.2 Predominant psychomotor disturbance
Agitation states as acute reaction to exceptional [gross] stress
Stupor as acute reaction to exceptional [gross] stress

308.3 Other acute reactions to stress
Acute situational disturbance
Acute stress disorder

Excludes *prolonged posttraumatic emotional disturbance (309.81)*

308.4 Mixed disorders as reaction to stress

308.9 Unspecified acute reaction to stress

● **309 Adjustment reaction**

Includes adjustment disorders
reaction (adjustment) to chronic stress

Excludes *acute reaction to major stress (308.0–308.9)*
neurotic disorders (300.0–300.9)

309.0 Adjustment disorder with depressed mood
Grief reaction

Excludes *affective psychoses (296.0–296.9)*
neurotic depression (300.4)
prolonged depressive reaction (309.1)
psychogenic depressive psychosis (298.0)

309.1 Prolonged depressive reaction

Excludes *affective psychoses (296.0–296.9)*
brief depressive reaction (309.0)
neurotic depression (300.4)
psychogenic depressive psychosis (298.0)

● **309.2 With predominant disturbance of other emotions**

309.21 Separation anxiety disorder

309.22 Emancipation disorder of adolescence and early adult life

309.23 Specific academic or work inhibition

309.24 Adjustment disorder with anxiety

309.28 Adjustment disorder with mixed anxiety and depressed mood
Adjustment reaction with anxiety and depression

309.29 Other
Culture shock

309.3 Adjustment disorder with disturbance of conduct
Conduct disturbance as adjustment reaction
Destructiveness as adjustment reaction

Excludes	*destructiveness in child (312.9)*
	disturbance of conduct NOS (312.9)
	dyssocial behavior without manifest psychiatric disorder (V71.01–V71.02)
	personality disorder with predominantly sociopathic or asocial manifestations (301.7)

309.4 Adjustment disorder with mixed disturbance of emotions and conduct

● **309.8 Other specified adjustment reactions**

309.81 Posttraumatic stress disorder
Chronic posttraumatic stress disorder
Concentration camp syndrome
Posttraumatic stress disorder NOS
Post-Traumatic Stress Disorder (PTSD)

Excludes	*acute stress disorder (308.3)*
	posttraumatic brain syndrome:
	nonpsychotic (310.2)
	psychotic (293.0–293.9)

309.82 Adjustment reaction with physical symptoms

309.83 Adjustment reaction with withdrawal
Elective mutism as adjustment reaction
Hospitalism (in children) NOS

309.89 Other

309.9 Unspecified adjustment reaction
Adaptation reaction NOS
Adjustment reaction NOS

● **310 Specific nonpsychotic mental disorders due to brain damage**

Excludes	*neuroses, personality disorders, or other nonpsychotic conditions occurring in a form similar to that seen with functional disorders but in association with a physical condition (300.0–300.9, 301.0–301.9)*

310.0 Frontal lobe syndrome
Lobotomy syndrome
Postleucotomy syndrome [state]

Excludes	*postcontusion syndrome (310.2)*

310.1 Personality change due to conditions classified elsewhere
Cognitive or personality change of other type, of nonpsychotic severity
Organic psychosyndrome of nonpsychotic severity
Presbyophrenia NOS
Senility with mental changes of nonpsychotic severity

Excludes	~~*memory loss of unknown cause (780.93)*~~ ◄
	mild cognitive impairment (331.83)
	postconcussion syndrome (310.2) ◄
	signs and symptoms involving emotional state (799.21-799.29) ◄

Coding Clinic: 2005, Q2, P6-7

310.2 Postconcussion syndrome
Postcontusion syndrome or encephalopathy
Posttraumatic brain syndrome, nonpsychotic
Status postcommotio cerebri

Excludes	*any organic psychotic conditions following head injury (293.0–294.0)*
	frontal lobe syndrome (310.0)
	postencephalitic syndrome (310.8)

Use additional code to identify associated post-traumatic headache, if applicable (339.20-339.22)

310.8 Other specified nonpsychotic mental disorders following organic brain damage
Mild memory disturbance
Postencephalitic syndrome
Other focal (partial) organic psychosyndromes

Excludes	*memory loss of unknown cause (780.93)* ◄

310.9 Unspecified nonpsychotic mental disorder following organic brain damage
Coding Clinic: 2003, Q4, P103-104

311 Depressive disorder, not elsewhere classified
Depressive disorder NOS
Depressive state NOS
Depression NOS

Excludes	*acute reaction to major stress with depressive symptoms (308.0)*
	affective personality disorder (301.10–301.13)
	affective psychoses (296.0–296.9)
	brief depressive reaction (309.0)
	depressive states associated with stressful events (309.0–309.1)
	disturbance of emotions specific to childhood and adolescence, with misery and unhappiness (313.1)
	mixed adjustment reaction with depressive symptoms (309.4)
	neurotic depression (300.4)
	prolonged depressive adjustment reaction (309.1)
	psychogenic depressive psychosis (298.0)

Coding Clinic: 2003, Q4, P75-76

● **312 Disturbance of conduct, not elsewhere classified**

Excludes	*adjustment reaction with disturbance of conduct (309.3)*
	drug dependence (304.0–304.9)
	dyssocial behavior without manifest psychiatric disorder (V71.01–V71.02)
	personality disorder with predominantly sociopathic or asocial manifestations (301.7)
	sexual deviations (302.0–302.9)

The following fifth-digit subclassification is for use with categories 312.0–312.2:

0	unspecified
1	mild
2	moderate
3	severe

● **312.0 Undersocialized conduct disorder, aggressive type**
[0-3]   Aggressive outburst
Anger reaction
Unsocialized aggressive disorder

● **312.1 Undersocialized conduct disorder, unaggressive type**
[0-3]   Childhood truancy, unsocialized
Solitary stealing
Tantrums

MENTAL DISORDERS (290–319)

N Newborn Age: 0   **P** Pediatric Age: 0–17   **M** Maternity Age: 12–55   **A** Adult Age: 15–124   ♀ Females Only   ♂ Males Only   837

(Ex) CC Exclusions   🔵 Complication\Comorbidity   🔵 Major C\C   🔵 Present on Admission Requirement   🔵 Hospital-Acquired Condition

● **312.2 Socialized conduct disorder**
[0-3]   Childhood truancy, socialized
Group delinquency

> **Excludes** *gang activity without manifest psychiatric disorder (V71.01)*

● **312.3 Disorders of impulse control, not elsewhere classified**

     312.30 Impulse control disorder, unspecified

     312.31 Pathological gambling

     312.32 Kleptomania *(stealing)*

     312.33 Pyromania *(setting fires)*

     312.34 Intermittent explosive disorder

     312.35 Isolated explosive disorder

     312.39 Other
         Trichotillomania
         Pulling or twisting hair until it falls out

312.4 Mixed disturbance of conduct and emotions
     Neurotic delinquency

> **Excludes** *compulsive conduct disorder (312.3)*

● **312.8 Other specified disturbances of conduct, not elsewhere classified**

     312.81 Conduct disorder, childhood onset type

     312.82 Conduct disorder, adolescent onset type

     312.89 Other conduct disorder
         Conduct disorder of unspecified onset

312.9 Unspecified disturbance of conduct
     Delinquency (juvenile)
     Disruptive behavior disorder NOS

● **313 Disturbance of emotions specific to childhood and adolescence**

> **Excludes** *adjustment reaction (309.0–309.9)*
> *emotional disorder of neurotic type (300.0–300.9)*
> *masturbation, nail-biting, thumb-sucking, and other isolated symptoms (307.0–307.9)*

313.0 Overanxious disorder
     Anxiety and fearfulness of childhood and adolescence
     Overanxious disorder of childhood and adolescence

> **Excludes** *abnormal separation anxiety (309.21)*
> *anxiety states (300.00–300.09)*
> *hospitalism in children (309.83)*
> *phobic state (300.20–300.29)*

313.1 Misery and unhappiness disorder

> **Excludes** *depressive neurosis (300.4)*

● **313.2 Sensitivity, shyness, and social withdrawal disorder**

> **Excludes** *infantile autism (299.0)*
> *schizoid personality (301.20–301.22)*
> *schizophrenia (295.0–295.9)*

     313.21 Shyness disorder of childhood
         Sensitivity reaction of childhood or adolescence

     313.22 Introverted disorder of childhood
         Social withdrawal of childhood or adolescence
         Withdrawal reaction of childhood or adolescence

     313.23 Selective mutism

> **Excludes** *elective mutism as adjustment reaction (309.83)*

313.3 Relationship problems
     Sibling jealousy

> **Excludes** *relationship problems associated with aggression, destruction, or other forms of conduct disturbance (312.0–312.9)*

● **313.8 Other or mixed emotional disturbances of childhood or adolescence**

     313.81 Oppositional defiant disorder

     313.82 Identity disorder
         Identity problem

     313.83 Academic underachievement disorder

     313.89 Other   P
         Reactive attachment disorder of infancy or early childhood

313.9 Unspecified emotional disturbance of childhood or adolescence   P
     Mental disorder of infancy, childhood or adolescence NOS

● **314 Hyperkinetic syndrome of childhood**

> **Excludes** *hyperkinesis as symptom of underlying disorder-code the underlying disorder*

● **314.0 Attention deficit disorder** *(ADD)*
     Adult
     Child

     314.00 Without mention of hyperactivity
         Predominantly inattentive type
         Coding Clinic: 1997, Q1, P8-9

     314.01 With hyperactivity
         Attention deficit disorder with hyperactivity = ADHD
         Combined type
         Overactivity NOS
         Predominantly hyperactive/impulsive type
         Simple disturbance of attention with overactivity
         Coding Clinic: 1997, Q1, P8-9

314.1 Hyperkinesis with developmental delay
     Developmental disorder of hyperkinesis

> **Use additional** code to identify any associated neurological disorder

314.2 Hyperkinetic conduct disorder
     Hyperkinetic conduct disorder without developmental delay

> **Excludes** *hyperkinesis with significant delays in specific skills (314.1)*

314.8 Other specified manifestations of hyperkinetic syndrome

314.9 Unspecified hyperkinetic syndrome
     Hyperkinetic reaction of childhood or adolescence NOS
     Hyperkinetic syndrome NOS

● **315 Specific delays in development**

> **Excludes** *that due to a neurological disorder (320.0–389.9)*

● **315.0 Specific reading disorder**

     315.00 Reading disorder, unspecified

     315.01 Alexia

     315.02 Developmental dyslexia

     315.09 Other
         Specific spelling difficulty

315.1 Mathematics disorder
     Dyscalculia

315.2 Other specific learning difficulties
     Disorder of written expression

> **Excludes** *specific arithmetical disorder (315.1)*
> *specific reading disorder (315.00–315.09)*

MENTAL DISORDERS (290–319)

◀ New   ◀▥ Revised   ~~deleted~~ Deleted   ● Unacceptable Principal Diagnosis   ● Use Additional Digit(s)

▶ Manifestation Code   **OGCR** Official Guidelines   **Coding Clinic**   Excludes   Includes   Use additional   Code first   Omit code

● **315.3 Developmental speech or language disorder**

     315.31 Expressive language disorder
         Developmental aphasia
         Word deafness

         | Excludes | *acquired aphasia (784.3)*
                    elective mutism (309.83, 313.0,
                       313.23)

     315.32 Mixed receptive-expressive language disorder
         Central auditory processing disorder

         | Excludes | *acquired auditory processing*
                    disorder (388.45)
         Coding Clinic: 2005, Q2, P5-6

     315.34 Speech and language developmental delay
         due to hearing loss
         Coding Clinic: 2007, Q4, P80-81

     315.39 Other
         Developmental articulation disorder
         Dyslalia
         Phonological disorder

         | Excludes | *lisping and lalling (307.9)*
                    stammering and stuttering (307.0)
         Coding Clinic: 2007, Q3, P9-10

315.4 Developmental coordination disorder
     Clumsiness syndrome
     Dyspraxia syndrome
     Specific motor development disorder

315.5 Mixed development disorder
     Coding Clinic: 2002, Q2, P11

315.8 Other specified delays in development

315.9 Unspecified delay in development
     Developmental disorder NOS
     Learning disorder NOS

316 Psychic factors associated with diseases classified elsewhere
     Psychologic factors in physical conditions classified
         elsewhere

     Use additional code to identify the associated physical
         condition, as:
     psychogenic:
         asthma (493.9)
         dermatitis (692.9)
         duodenal ulcer (532.0–532.9)
         eczema (691.8, 692.9)
         gastric ulcer (531.0–531.9)
         mucous colitis (564.9)
         paroxysmal tachycardia (427.2)
         ulcerative colitis (556)
         urticaria (708.0–708.9)
     psychosocial dwarfism (259.4)

     | Excludes | *physical symptoms and physiological*
                   malfunctions, not involving tissue damage,
                   of mental origin (306.0–306.9)

MENTAL RETARDATION (317–319)

Use additional code(s) to identify any associated
     psychiatric or physical condition(s)

317 Mild mental retardation
     High-grade defect
     IQ 50–70
     Mild mental subnormality

● **318 Other specified mental retardation**

     318.0 Moderate mental retardation
         IQ 35–49
         Moderate mental subnormality

     318.1 Severe mental retardation 🗲
         IQ 20–34
         Severe mental subnormality
         (Ex) 318.1-318.2

     318.2 Profound mental retardation 🗲
         IQ under 20
         Profound mental subnormality
         (Ex) 318.1-318.2

319 Unspecified mental retardation
     Mental deficiency NOS
     Mental subnormality NOS

N Newborn Age: 0   **P** Pediatric Age: 0–17   **M** Maternity Age: 12–55   **A** Adult Age: 15–124   ♀ Females Only   ♂ Males Only

(Ex) CC Exclusions   🗲 Complication\Comorbidity   🗲 Major C\C   Present on Admission Requirement   Hospital-Acquired Condition   839

MENTAL DISORDERS (290–319)

(See Plate 164 on page NAP-2.)

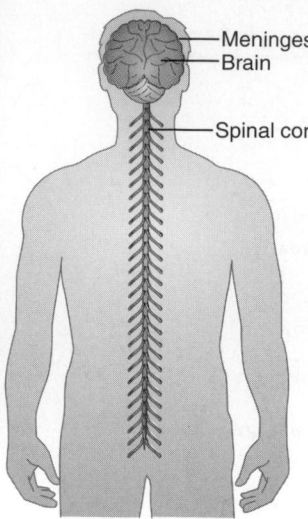

Meninges
Brain
Spinal cord

Figure 6–1 The brain and spinal cord make up the central nervous system.

Item 6–1 The two major classifications of the nervous system are the peripheral nervous system and the central nervous system (CNS). The central nervous system is comprised of the brain and the spinal cord. The peripheral nervous system is comprised of the parasympathetic and sympathetic systems. **Encephalitis** is the swelling of the brain. **Meningitis** is swelling of the covering of the brain, the meninges. Types and causes of brain infections are:

Type	Cause
purulent	bacterial
aseptic/abacterial	viral
chronic meningitis	mycobacterial and fungal

6. DISEASES OF THE NERVOUS SYSTEM AND SENSE ORGANS (320–389)

INFLAMMATORY DISEASES OF THE CENTRAL NERVOUS SYSTEM (320–326)

● **320 Bacterial meningitis**
Infection of cerebrospinal fluid surrounding spinal cord and brain

Includes arachnoiditis bacterial
leptomeningitis bacterial
meningitis bacterial
meningoencephalitis bacterial
meningomyelitis bacterial
pachymeningitis bacterial

320.0 Hemophilus meningitis
Meningitis due to Hemophilus influenzae [H. influenzae]
Ex: 003.21, 013.00-013.16, 036.0, 047.0-047.9, 049.0-049.1, 053.0, 054.72, 072.1, 090.42, 091.81, 094.2, 098.89, 100.81, 112.83, 114.2, 115.01, 115.11, 115.91, 130.0, 249.60-249.61, 249.80-249.91, 250.60-250.63, 250.80-250.93, 320.0-322.9, 349.89-349.9, 357.0

320.1 Pneumococcal meningitis
Ex: 003.21, 013.00-013.16, 036.0, 047.0-047.9, 049.0-049.1, 053.0, 054.72, 072.1, 090.42, 091.81, 094.2, 098.89, 100.81, 112.83, 114.2, 115.01, 115.11, 115.91, 130.0, 249.60-249.61, 249.80-249.91, 250.60-250.63, 250.80-250.93, 320.0-322.9, 349.89-349.9, 357.0

320.2 Streptococcal meningitis
Ex: 003.21, 013.00-013.16, 036.0, 047.0-047.9, 049.0-049.1, 053.0, 054.72, 072.1, 090.42, 091.81, 094.2, 098.89, 100.81, 112.83, 114.2, 115.01, 115.11, 115.91, 130.0, 249.60-249.61, 249.80-249.91, 250.60-250.63, 250.80-250.93, 320.0-322.9, 349.89-349.9, 357.0

320.3 Staphylococcal meningitis
Ex: 003.21, 013.00-013.16, 036.0, 047.0-047.9, 049.0-049.1, 053.0, 054.72, 072.1, 090.42, 091.81, 094.2, 098.89, 100.81, 112.83, 114.2, 115.01, 115.11, 115.91, 130.0, 249.60-249.61, 249.80-249.91, 250.60-250.63, 250.80-250.93, 320.0-322.9, 349.89-349.9, 357.0

▶ *320.7 Meningitis in other bacterial diseases classified elsewhere*

Code first underlying disease as:
actinomycosis (039.8)
listeriosis (027.0)
typhoid fever (002.0)
whooping cough (033.0–033.9)

Excludes *meningitis (in):*
epidemic (036.0)
gonococcal (098.82)
meningococcal (036.0)
salmonellosis (003.21)
syphilis:
NOS (094.2)
congenital (090.42)
meningovascular (094.2)
secondary (091.81)
tuberculosis (013.0)
Ex: 003.21, 013.00-013.16, 036.0, 047.0-047.9, 049.0-049.1, 053.0, 054.72, 072.1, 090.42, 091.81, 094.2, 098.89, 100.81, 112.83, 114.2, 115.01, 115.11, 115.91, 130.0, 249.60-249.61, 249.80-249.91, 250.60-250.63, 250.80-250.93, 320.0-322.9, 349.89-349.9, 357.0

● **320.8 Meningitis due to other specified bacteria**

320.81 Anaerobic meningitis
Bacteroides (fragilis)
Gram-negative anaerobes
Ex: 003.21, 013.00-013.16, 036.0, 047.0-047.9, 049.0-049.1, 053.0, 054.72, 072.1, 090.42, 091.81, 094.2, 098.89, 100.81, 112.83, 114.2, 115.01, 115.11, 115.91, 130.0, 249.60-249.61, 249.80-249.91, 250.60-250.63, 250.80-250.93, 320.0-322.9, 349.89-349.9, 357.0

320.82 Meningitis due to gram-negative bacteria, not elsewhere classified
Aerobacter aerogenes
Escherichia coli [E. coli]
Friedlander bacillus
Klebsiella pneumoniae
Proteus morganii
Pseudomonas

Excludes *gram-negative anaerobes (320.81)*
Ex: 003.21, 013.00-013.16, 036.0, 047.0-047.9, 049.0-049.1, 053.0, 054.72, 072.1, 090.42, 091.81, 094.2, 098.89, 100.81, 112.83, 114.2, 115.01, 115.11, 115.91, 130.0, 249.60-249.61, 249.80-249.91, 250.60-250.63, 250.80-250.93, 320.0-322.9, 349.89-349.9, 357.0

320.89 Meningitis due to other specified bacteria
Bacillus pyocyaneus
Ex: 003.21, 013.00-013.16, 036.0, 047.0-047.9, 049.0-049.1, 053.0, 054.72, 072.1, 090.42, 091.81, 094.2, 098.89, 100.81, 112.83, 114.2, 115.01, 115.11, 115.91, 130.0, 249.60-249.61, 249.80-249.91, 250.60-250.63, 250.80-250.93, 320.0-322.9, 349.89-349.9, 357.0

◀ New   ◀◀ Revised   ~~deleted~~ Deleted   ● Unacceptable Principal Diagnosis   ● Use Additional Digit(s)
▶ Manifestation Code   OGCR Official Guidelines   Coding Clinic   Excludes   Includes   Use additional   Code first   Omit code

320.9 Meningitis due to unspecified bacterium 🔵

Meningitis: Meningitis:
bacterial NOS   pyogenic NOS
purulent NOS   suppurative NOS

Ⓔⓧ 003.21, 013.00-013.16, 036.0, 047.0-047.9, 049.0-049.1, 053.0, 054.72, 072.1, 090.42, 091.81, 094.2, 098.89, 100.81, 112.83, 114.2, 115.01, 115.11, 115.91, 130.0, 249.60-249.61, 249.80-249.91, 250.60-250.63, 250.80-250.93, 320.0-322.9, 349.89-349.9, 357.0

● **321   Meningitis due to other organisms**

Includes   arachnoiditis due to organisms other than bacteria
leptomeningitis due to organisms other than bacteria
meningitis due to organisms other than bacteria
pachymeningitis due to organisms other than bacteria

▸ **321.0   Cryptococcal meningitis** 🔵

Code first underlying disease (117.5)

Ⓔⓧ 003.21, 013.00-013.16, 036.0, 047.0-047.9, 049.0-049.1, 053.0, 054.72, 072.1, 090.42, 091.81, 094.2, 098.89, 100.81, 112.83, 114.2, 115.01, 115.11, 115.91, 130.0, 249.60-249.61, 249.80-249.91, 250.60-250.63, 250.80-250.93, 320.0-322.9, 349.89-349.9, 357.0

▸ **321.1   Meningitis in other fungal diseases** 🔵

Code first underlying disease (110.0–118)

Excludes   meningitis in:
candidiasis (112.83)
coccidioidomycosis (114.2)
histoplasmosis (115.01, 115.11, 115.91)

Ⓔⓧ 003.21, 013.00-013.16, 036.0, 047.0-047.9, 049.0-049.1, 053.0, 054.72, 072.1, 090.42, 091.81, 094.2, 098.89, 100.81, 112.83, 114.2, 115.01, 115.11, 115.91, 130.0, 249.60-249.61, 249.80-249.91, 250.60-250.63, 250.80-250.93, 320.0-322.9, 349.89-349.9, 357.0

▸ **321.2   Meningitis due to viruses not elsewhere classified** 🔵

Code first underlying disease, as:
meningitis due to arbovirus (060.0–066.9)

Excludes   meningitis (due to):
abacterial (047.0–047.9)
adenovirus (049.1)
aseptic NOS (047.9)
Coxsackie (virus) (047.0)
ECHO virus (047.1)
enterovirus (047.0–047.9)
herpes simplex virus (054.72)
herpes zoster virus (053.0)
lymphocytic choriomeningitis virus (049.0)
mumps (072.1)
viral NOS (047.9)
meningo-eruptive syndrome (047.1)

Ⓔⓧ 003.21, 013.00-013.16, 036.0, 047.0-047.9, 049.0-049.1, 053.0, 054.72, 072.1, 090.42, 091.81, 094.2, 098.89, 100.81, 112.83, 114.2, 115.01, 115.11, 115.91, 130.0, 320.0-322.9, 349.89-349.9, 357.0

Coding Clinic: 2004, Q4, P50-52

▸ **321.3   Meningitis due to trypanosomiasis** 🔵

Code first underlying disease (086.0–086.9)

Ⓔⓧ 003.21, 013.00-013.16, 036.0, 047.0-047.9, 049.0-049.1, 053.0, 054.72, 072.1, 090.42, 091.81, 094.2, 098.89, 100.81, 112.83, 114.2, 115.01, 115.11, 115.91, 130.0, 249.60-249.61, 249.80-249.91, 250.60-250.63, 250.80-250.93, 320.0-322.9, 349.89-349.9, 357.0

▸ **321.4   Meningitis in sarcoidosis** 🔵

Code first underlying disease (135)

Ⓔⓧ 003.21, 013.00-013.16, 036.0, 047.0-047.9, 049.0-049.1, 053.0, 054.72, 072.1, 090.42, 091.81, 094.2, 098.89, 100.81, 112.83, 114.2, 115.01, 115.11, 115.91, 130.0, 249.60-249.61, 249.80-249.91, 250.60-250.63, 250.80-250.93, 320.0-322.9, 349.89-349.9, 357.0

▸ **321.8   Meningitis due to other nonbacterial organisms classified elsewhere** 🔵

Code first underlying disease

Excludes   leptospiral meningitis (100.81)

Ⓔⓧ 003.21, 013.00-013.16, 036.0, 047.0-047.9, 049.0-049.1, 053.0, 054.72, 072.1, 090.42, 091.81, 094.2, 098.89, 100.81, 112.83, 114.2, 115.01, 115.11, 115.91, 130.0, 249.60-249.61, 249.80-249.91, 250.60-250.63, 250.80-250.93, 320.0-322.9, 349.89-349.9, 357.0

● **322   Meningitis of unspecified cause**

Includes   arachnoiditis with no organism specified as cause
leptomeningitis with no organism specified as cause
meningitis with no organism specified as cause
pachymeningitis with no organism specified as cause

322.0   Nonpyogenic meningitis 🔵
Meningitis with clear cerebrospinal fluid

Ⓔⓧ 003.21, 013.00-013.16, 036.0, 047.0-047.9, 049.0-049.1, 053.0, 054.72, 0721, 090.42, 091.81, 094.2, 098.89, 100.81, 112.83, 114.2, 115.01, 115.11, 115.91, 130.0, 249.60-249.61, 249.80-249.91, 250.60-250.63, 250.80-250.93, 320.0-322.9, 349.89-349.9, 357.0

322.1   Eosinophilic meningitis 🔵

Ⓔⓧ 003.21, 013.00-013.16, 036.0, 047.0-047.9, 049.0-049.1, 053.0, 054.72, 072.1, 090.42, 091.81, 094.2, 098.89, 100.81, 112.83, 114.2, 115.01, 115.11, 115.91, 130.0, 249.60-249.61, 249.80-249.91, 250.60-250.63, 250.80-250.93, 320.0-322.9, 349.89-349.9, 357.0

322.2   Chronic meningitis 🔵

Ⓔⓧ 003.21, 013.00-013.16, 036.0, 047.0-047.9, 049.0-049.1, 053.0, 054.72, 072.1, 090.42, 091.81, 094.2, 098.89, 100.81, 112.83, 114.2, 115.01, 115.11, 115.91, 130.0, 249.60-249.61, 249.80-249.91, 250.60-250.63, 250.80-250.93, 320.0-322.9, 349.89-349.9, 357.0

322.9   Meningitis, unspecified 🔵

Ⓔⓧ 003.21, 013.00-013.16, 036.0, 047.0-047.9, 049.0-049.1, 053.0, 054.72, 072.1, 090.42, 091.81, 094.2, 098.89, 100.81, 112.83, 114.2, 115.01, 115.11, 115.91, 130.0, 249.60-249.61, 249.80-249.91, 250.60-250.63, 250.80-250.93, 320.0-322.9, 349.89-349.9, 357.0

DISEASES OF THE NERVOUS SYSTEM AND SENSE ORGANS (320–389)

N Newborn Age: 0   **P** Pediatric Age: 0–17   **M** Maternity Age: 12–55   **A** Adult Age: 15–124   ♀ Females Only   ♂ Males Only

Ⓔⓧ CC Exclusions   🔵 Complication\Comorbidity   🔵 Major C\C   🔵 Present on Admission Requirement   🔵 Hospital-Acquired Condition   **841**

Item 6-2 **Encephalitis** is an inflammation of the brain most often caused by a virus but may also be caused by a bacteria and most commonly transmitted by a mosquito. **Myelitis** is an inflammation of the spinal cord that may disrupt CNS function. Untreated myelitis may rapidly lead to permanent damage to the spinal cord. **Encephalomyelitis** is a general term for an inflammation of the brain and spinal cord.

● **323** **Encephalitis, myelitis, and encephalomyelitis**

> **Includes** acute disseminated encephalomyelitis
> meningoencephalitis, except bacterial
> meningomyelitis, except bacterial
> myelitis:
> ascending
> transverse

> **Excludes** *acute transverse myelitis NOS (341.20)*
> *acute transverse myelitis in conditions classified*
> *elsewhere (341.21)*
> *bacterial:*
> *meningoencephalitis (320.0–320.9)*
> *meningomyelitis (320.0–320.9)*
> *idiopathic transverse myelitis (341.22)*

> **Coding Clinic: 2006, Q4, P58-63**

● **323.0** **Encephalitis, myelitis, and encephalomyelitis in viral diseases classified elsewhere**

> *Code first* underlying disease, as:
> cat-scratch disease (078.3)
> infectious mononucleosis (075)
> ornithosis (073.7)

> ▌ **323.01** *Encephalitis and encephalomyelitis in viral diseases classified elsewhere*🔖

> > **Excludes** *encephalitis (in):*
> > *arthropod-borne viral*
> > *(062.0–064)*
> > *herpes simplex (054.3)*
> > *mumps (072.2)*
> > *other viral diseases of central*
> > *nervous system*
> > *(049.8–049.9)*
> > *poliomyelitis (045.0–045.9)*
> > *rubella (056.01)*
> > *slow virus infections of*
> > *central nervous system*
> > *(046.0–046.9)*
> > *viral NOS (049.9)*
> > *West Nile (066.41)*

> > (Ex:) 003.21, 013.00-013.16, 013.60-013.66, 036.0, 046.2, 046 71
> > -046.8, 047.0-049.8, 051.9-052.0, 052.7-053.13, 053.19,
> > 053.79-053.9, 054.3, 054.72, 054.79-054.9, 056.01,
> > 057.8-059.9, 062.0-064, 066.2-066.49, 072.1-072.2, 073.7,
> > 075, 078.89, 079.81-079.82, 079.89, 079.99,
> > 090.41-090.42, 091.81, 094.2, 094.81, 098.89, 100.81,
> > 112.83, 114.2, 115.01, 115.11, 115.91, 130.0, 139.8,
> > 290.12, 320.0-323.9, 341.1, 349.89-349.9, 357.0, 487.8,
> > 771.2

> ▌ **323.02** *Myelitis in viral diseases classified elsewhere*🔖

> > **Excludes** *myelitis (in):*
> > *herpes simplex (054.74)*
> > *herpes zoster (053.14)*
> > *other viral diseases of central*
> > *nervous system*
> > *(049.8–049.9)*
> > *poliomyelitis (045.0–045.9)*
> > *rubella (056.01)*

> > (Ex:) 003.21, 013.00-013.16, 013.60-013.66, 036.0, 046.2,
> > 046.71-046.8, 047.0-049.8, 051.9-052.0, 052.7-053.13,
> > 053.19, 053.79-053.9, 054.3, 054.72, 054.79-054.9, 056.01,
> > 057.8-059.9, 062.0-064, 066.2-066.49, 072.1-072.2, 073.7,
> > 075, 078.89, 079.81-079.82, 079.89, 079.99,
> > 090.41-090.42, 091.81, 094.2, 094.81, 098.89, 100.81,
> > 112.83, 114.2, 115.01, 115.11, 115.91, 130.0, 139.8,
> > 290.12, 320.0-323.9, 341.1, 349.89-349.9, 357.0, 487.8,
> > 771.2

> ▌ **323.1** *Encephalitis, myelitis, and encephalomyelitis in rickettsial diseases classified elsewhere*🔖

> > *Code first* underlying disease (080–083.9)

> > (Ex:) 013.60-013.66, 046.2, 046.71-04.68 048-049.0, 049.8, 052.0, 052.2, 054.3
> > 054.74, 056.01, 057.8-058.29, 059.00-059.9, 062.0-064, 066.2-066.49
> > 072.2, 073.7, 079.82, 079.99, 081.9 083.9, 090.41, 094.81, 117.5,
> > 124, 130.0 290.12, 323.01-323.9, 341.1, 487.8, 771.2 984.9

> ▌ **323.2** *Encephalitis, myelitis, and encephalomyelitis in protozoal diseases classified elsewhere*🔖

> > *Code first* underlying disease, as:
> > malaria (084.0–084.9)
> > trypanosomiasis (086.0–086.9)

> > (Ex:) 013.60-013.66, 046.2, 046.71-046.8 048-049.0, 049.8, 052.0, 052.2, 054.3
> > 054.74, 056.01, 057.8-058.29, 059.00-059.9, 062.0-064, 066.2-066.49
> > 072.2, 073.7, 079.82, 079.99, 081.9, 083.9, 084.6, 090.41, 094.81,
> > 117.5, 124, 130.0, 290.12, 323.01-323.9, 341.1, 487.8 771.2, 984.9

● **323.4** **Other encephalitis, myelitis, and encephalomyelitis due to infection classified elsewhere**

> *Code first* underlying disease

> ▌ **323.41** *Other encephalitis and encephalomyelitis due to infection classified elsewhere*🔖

> > **Excludes** *encephalitis (in):*
> > *meningococcal (036.1)*
> > *syphilis:*
> > *NOS (094.81)*
> > *congenital (090.41)*
> > *toxoplasmosis (130.0)*
> > *tuberculosis (013.6)*
> > *meningoencephalitis due to*
> > *free-living ameba [Naegleria]*
> > *(136.29)*

> > (Ex:) 003.21, 013.00-013.16, 013.60-013.66 036.0, 046.2,
> > 046.71-046.8, 047.0-049.8 051.9-052.0, 052.7-053.13,
> > 053.19, 053.79-053.9, 054.3, 054.72, 054.79-054.9,
> > 056.01, 057.8-059.9, 062.0-064, 066.2-066.49,
> > 072.1-072.2, 073.7, 075, 078.89, 079.81-079.82, 079.89,
> > 079.99, 090.41-090.42, 091.81, 094.2, 094.81, 098.89,
> > 100.81, 112.83, 114.2, 115.01, 115.11, 115.91, 130.0,
> > 139.8, 290.12, 320.0-323.9, 341.1, 349.89-349.9, 357.0,
> > 487.8, 771.2

◀ New ◀▥ Revised ~~deleted~~ Deleted ● Unacceptable Principal Diagnosis ● Use Additional Digit(s)
▌ Manifestation Code **OGCR** Official Guidelines **Coding Clinic** Excludes Includes Use additional Code first Omit code

▶ **323.42** *Other myelitis due to infection classified elsewhere* 🔖

     Excludes | myelitis (in):
            syphilis (094.89)
            tuberculosis (013.6)

     (Ex:) 003.21, 013.00-013.16, 013.60-013.66, 036.0, 046.2, 046.71-046.8, 047.0-049.8, 051.9-052.0, 052.7-053.13, 053.19, 053.79-053.9, 054.3, 054.72, 054.79-054.9, 056.01, 057.8-059.9, 062.0-064, 066.2-066.49, 072.1-072.2, 073.7, 075, 078.89, 079.81-079.82, 079.89, 079.99, 090.41-090.42, 091.81, 094.2, 094.81, 098.89, 100.81, 112.83, 114.2, 115.01, 115.11, 115.91, 130.0, 139.8, 290.12, 320.0-323.9, 341.1, 349.89-349.9, 357.0, 487.8, 771.2

● **323.5 Encephalitis, myelitis, and encephalomyelitis following immunization procedures**

     Use additional E code to identify vaccine

     323.51 Encephalitis and encephalomyelitis following immunization procedures 🔖

         Encephalitis postimmunization or postvaccinal
         Encephalomyelitis postimmunization or postvaccinal

         (Ex:) 003.21, 013.00-013.16, 013.60-013.66, 036.0, 046.2, 046.71-046.8, 047.0-049.8, 051.9-052.0, 052.7-053.13, 053.19, 053.79-053.9, 054.3, 054.72, 054.79-054.9, 056.01, 057.8-059.9, 062.0-064, 066.2-066.49, 072.1-072.2, 073.7, 075, 078.89, 079.81-079.82, 079.89, 079.99, 090.41-090.42, 091.81, 094.2, 094.81, 098.89, 100.81, 112.83, 114.2, 115.01, 115.11, 115.91, 130.0, 139.8, 290.12, 320.0-323.9, 341.1, 349.89-349.9, 357.0, 487.8, 771.2

     323.52 Myelitis following immunization procedures 🔖

         Myelitis postimmunization or postvaccinal

         (Ex:) 003.21, 013.00-013.16, 013.60-013.66, 036.0, 046.2, 046.71-046.8, 047.0-049.8, 051.9-052.0, 052.7-053.13, 053.19, 053.79-053.9, 054.3, 054.72, 054.79-054.9, 056.01, 057.8-059.9, 062.0-064, 066.2-066.49, 072.1-072.2, 073.7, 075, 078.89, 079.81-079.82, 079.89, 079.99, 090.41-090.42, 091.81, 094.2, 094.81, 098.89, 100.81, 112.83, 114.2, 115.01, 115.11, 115.91, 130.0, 139.8, 290.12, 320.0-323.9, 341.1, 349.89-349.9, 357.0, 487.8, 771.2

● **323.6 Postinfectious encephalitis, myelitis, and encephalomyelitis**

     Code first underlying disease

     ▶ **323.61** *Infectious acute disseminated encephalomyelitis (ADEM)* 🔖

         Acute necrotizing hemorrhagic encephalopathy

         Excludes | noninfectious acute disseminated encephalomyelitis (323.81)

         (Ex:) 003.21, 013.00-013.16, 013.60-013.66, 036.0, 046.2, 046.71-046.8, 047.0-049.8, 051.9-052.0, 052.7-053.13, 053.19, 053.79-053.9, 054.3, 054.72, 054.79-054.9, 056.01, 057.8-059.9, 062.0-064, 066.2-066.49, 072.1-072.2, 073.7, 075, 078.89, 079.81-079.82, 079.89, 079.99, 090.41-090.42, 091.81, 094.2, 094.81, 098.89, 100.81, 112.83, 114.2, 115.01, 115.11, 115.91, 130.0, 139.8, 290.12, 320.0-323.9, 341.1, 349.89-349.9, 357.0, 487.8, 771.2

▶ **323.62** *Other postinfectious encephalitis and encephalomyelitis* 🔖

     Excludes | encephalitis:
            postchickenpox (052.0)
            postmeasles (055.0)

     (Ex:) 003.21, 013.00-013.16, 013.60-013.66, 036.0, 046.2, 046.71-046.8, 047.0-049.8, 051.9-052.0, 052.7-053.13, 053.19, 053.79-053.9, 054.3, 054.72, 054.79-054.9, 056.01, 057.8-059.9, 062.0-064, 066.2-066.49, 072.1-072.2, 073.7, 075, 078.89, 079.81-079.82, 079.89, 079.99, 090.41-090.42, 091.81, 094.2, 094.81, 098.89, 100.81, 112.83, 114.2, 115.01, 115.11, 115.91, 130.0, 139.8, 290.12, 320.0-323.9, 341.1, 349.89-349.9, 357.0, 487.8, 771.2

▶ **323.63** *Postinfectious myelitis* 🔖

     (Ex:) 003.21, 013.00-013.16, 013.60-013.66, 036.0, 046.2, 046.71-046.8, 047.0-049.8, 051.9-052.0, 052.7-053.13, 053.19, 053.79-053.9, 054.3, 054.72, 054.79-054.9, 056.01, 057.8-059.9, 062.0-064, 066.2-066.49, 072.1-072.2, 073.7, 075, 078.89, 079.81-079.82, 079.89, 079.99, 090.41-090.42, 091.81, 094.2, 094.81, 098.89, 100.81, 112.83, 114.2, 115.01, 115.11, 115.91, 130.0, 139.8, 290.12, 320.0-323.9, 341.1, 349.89-349.9, 357.0, 487.8, 771.2

● **323.7 Toxic encephalitis, myelitis, and encephalomyelitis**

     Code first underlying cause, as:
         carbon tetrachloride (982.1)
         hydroxyquinoline derivatives (961.3)
         lead (984.0–984.9)
         mercury (985.0)
         thallium (985.8)

     ▶ **323.71** *Toxic encephalitis and encephalomyelitis* 🔖

         (Ex:) 003.21, 013.00-013.16, 013.60-013.66, 036.0, 046.2, 046.71-046.8, 047.0-049.8, 051.9-052.0, 052.7-053.13, 053.19, 053.79-053.9, 054.3, 054.72, 054.79-054.9, 056.01, 057.8-059.9, 062.0-064, 066.2-066.49, 072.1-072.2, 073.7, 075, 078.89, 079.81-079.82, 079.89, 079.99, 090.41-090.42, 091.81, 094.2, 094.81, 098.89, 100.81, 112.83, 114.2, 115.01, 115.11, 115.91, 130.0, 139.8, 290.12, 320.0-323.9, 341.1, 349.89-349.9, 357.0, 487.8, 771.2

     ▶ **323.72** *Toxic myelitis* 🔖

         (Ex:) 003.21, 013.00-013.16, 013.60-013.66, 036.0, 046.2, 046.71-046.8, 047.0-049.8, 051.9-052.0, 052.7-053.13, 053.19, 053.79-053.9, 054.3, 054.72, 054.79-054.9, 056.01, 057.8-059.9, 062.0-064, 066.2-066.49, 072.1-072.2, 073.7, 075, 078.89, 079.81-079.82, 079.89, 079.99, 090.41-090.42, 091.81, 094.2, 094.81, 098.89, 100.81, 112.83, 114.2, 115.01, 115.11, 115.91, 130.0, 139.8, 290.12, 320.0-323.9, 341.1, 349.89-349.9, 357.0, 487.8, 771.2

● **323.8 Other causes of encephalitis, myelitis, and encephalomyelitis**

     Coding Clinic: 1997, Q2, P8-9

     323.81 Other causes of encephalitis and encephalomyelitis 🔖

         Noninfectious acute disseminated encephalomyelitis (ADEM)

         (Ex:) 003.21, 013.00-013.16, 013.60-013.66, 036.0, 046.2, 046.71-046.8, 047.0-049.8, 051.9-052.0, 052.7-053.13, 053.19, 053.79-053.9, 054.3, 054.72, 054.79-054.9, 056.01, 057.8-059.9, 062.0-064, 066.2-066.49, 072.1-072.2, 073.7, 075, 078.89, 079.81-079.82, 079.89, 079.99, 090.41-090.42, 091.81, 094.2, 094.81, 098.89, 100.81, 112.83, 114.2, 115.01, 115.11, 115.91, 130.0, 139.8, 290.12, 320.0-323.9, 341.1, 349.89-349.9, 357.0, 487.8, 771.2

DISEASES OF THE NERVOUS SYSTEM AND SENSE ORGANS (320–389)

N   Newborn Age: 0   P   Pediatric Age: 0–17   M   Maternity Age: 12–55   A   Adult Age: 15–124   ♀   Females Only   ♂   Males Only

(Ex:)   CC Exclusions   🔖   Complication\Comorbidity   🔖   Major C\C   🔖   Present on Admission Requirement   🔖   Hospital-Acquired Condition   **843**

323.82 Other causes of myelitis 🕷
Transverse myelitis NOS
(Ex:) 003.21, 013.00-013.16, 013.60-013.66, 036.0, 046.2, 046.71-046.8, 047.0-049.8, 051.9-052.0, 052.7-053.13, 053.19, 053.79-053.9, 054.3, 054.72, 054.79-054.9, 056.01, 057.8-059.9, 062.0-064, 066.2-066.49, 072.1-072.2, 073.7, 075, 078.89, 079.81-079.82, 079.89, 079.99, 090.41-090.42, 091.81, 094.2, 094.81, 098.89, 100.81, 112.83, 114.2, 115.01, 115.11, 115.91, 130.0, 139.8, 290.12, 320.0-323.9, 341.1, 349.89-349.9, 357.0, 487.8, 771.2

323.9 Unspecified cause of encephalitis, myelitis, and encephalomyelitis 🕷
(Ex:) 013.60-013.66, 046.2, 046.71-046.8, 048-049.0, 049.8, 052.0, 052.2, 054.3, 054.74, 056.01, 057.8-058.29, 059.00-059.9, 062.0-064, 066.2-066.49, 072.2, 073.7, 075, 078.3, 079.82, 079.99, 081.9, 083.9, 084.6, 090.41, 094.81, 117.5, 124, 130.0, 290.12, 323.01-323.9, 341.1, 382.4, 487.8, 710.0, 771.2, 984.9
Coding Clinic: 2006, Q1, P8

● **324 Intracranial and intraspinal abscess**
Accumulation of pus in either brain or spinal cord

324.0 Intracranial abscess 🕷
Abscess (embolic):
   cerebellar
   cerebral
Abscess (embolic) of brain [any part]:
   epidural
   extradural
   otogenic
   subdural
   | **Excludes** | *tuberculous (013.3)* |
(Ex:) 006.5, 013.20-013.36, 249.60-249.61, 249.80-249.91, 250.60-250.63, 250.80-250.93, 324.0-325, 348.8-348.9

324.1 Intraspinal abscess 🕷
Abscess (embolic) of spinal cord [any part]:
   epidural
   extradural
   subdural
(Ex:) 006.5, 013.20-013.36, 249.60-249.61, 249.80-249.91, 250.60-250.63, 250.80-250.93, 324.1
   | **Excludes** | *tuberculous (013.5)* |

324.9 Of unspecified site 🕷
Extradural or subdural abscess NOS
(Ex:) 006.5, 013.20-013.36, 249.60-249.61, 249.80-249.91, 250.60-250.63, 250.80-250.93, 324.0-325

● **325 Phlebitis and thrombophlebitis of intracranial venous sinuses** 🕷
Embolism of cavernous, lateral, or other intracranial or unspecified intracranial venous sinus
Endophlebitis of cavernous, lateral, or other intracranial or unspecified intracranial venous sinus
Phlebitis, septic or suppurative of cavernous, lateral, or other intracranial or unspecified intracranial venous sinus
Thrombophlebitis of cavernous, lateral, or other intracranial or unspecified intracranial venous sinus
Thrombosis of cavernous, lateral, or other intracranial or unspecified intracranial venous sinus
| **Excludes** | *that specified as:* |
     complicating pregnancy, childbirth, or the puerperium (671.5)
     of nonpyogenic origin (437.6)
(Ex:) 006.5, 013.20-013.36, 249.60-249.61, 249.80-249.91, 250.60-250.63, 250.80-250.93, 324.0-325

● **326 Late effects of intracranial abscess or pyogenic infection** 🕷

Note: This category is to be used to indicate conditions whose primary classification is to 320–325 [excluding 320.7, 321.0–321.8, 323.01–323.42, 323.61–323.72] as the cause of late effects, themselves classifiable elsewhere. The "late effects" include conditions specified as such, or as sequelae, which may occur at any time after the resolution of the causal condition.

Use additional code to identify condition, as:
   hydrocephalus (331.4)
   paralysis (342.0–342.9, 344.0–344.9)

ORGANIC SLEEP DISORDERS (327)

● **327 Organic sleep disorders**
Involve difficulties of sleep at all levels, including difficulty falling or staying asleep, falling asleep at inappropriate times, excessive total sleep time, or abnormal behaviors associated with sleep

● **327.0 Organic disorders of initiating and maintaining sleep [Organic insomnia]**
| **Excludes** | *insomnia NOS (780.52)* |
     insomnia not due to a substance or known physiological condition (307.41–307.42)
     insomnia with sleep apnea NOS (780.51)

327.00 Organic insomnia, unspecified

▶ **327.01 *Insomnia due to medical condition classified elsewhere***
   Code first underlying condition
   | **Excludes** | *insomnia due to mental disorder (327.02)* |

▶ **327.02 *Insomnia due to mental disorder***
   Code first mental disorder
   | **Excludes** | *alcohol induced insomnia (291.82)* |
     drug induced insomnia (292.85)

327.09 Other organic insomnia

● **327.1 Organic disorder of excessive somnolence [Organic hypersomnia]**
| **Excludes** | *hypersomnia NOS (780.54)* |
     hypersomnia not due to a substance or known physiological condition (307.43–307.44)
     hypersomnia with sleep apnea NOS (780.53)

327.10 Organic hypersomnia, unspecified

327.11 Idiopathic hypersomnia with long sleep time

327.12 Idiopathic hypersomnia without long sleep time

327.13 Recurrent hypersomnia
Kleine-Levin syndrome
Menstrual related hypersomnia

▶ **327.14 *Hypersomnia due to medical condition classified elsewhere***
   Code first underlying condition
   | **Excludes** | *hypersomnia due to mental disorder (327.15)* |

▶ **327.15 *Hypersomnia due to mental disorder***
   Code first mental disorder
   | **Excludes** | *alcohol induced insomnia (291.82)* |
     drug induced insomnia (292.85)

327.19 Other organic hypersomnia

◀ New   ◀ Revised   ~~deleted~~ Deleted   ● Unacceptable Principal Diagnosis   ● Use Additional Digit(s)
▶ Manifestation Code   **OGCR** Official Guidelines   **Coding Clinic** | Excludes | | Includes | | Use additional | | Code first | | Omit code |

DISEASES OF THE NERVOUS SYSTEM AND SENSE ORGANS (320–389)

● **327.2　Organic sleep apnea**
　　Characterized by episodes in which breathing stops
　　during sleep, resulting in a lack of prolonged deep
　　sleep and excessive daytime sleepiness

　　　| **Excludes** | *Cheyne-Stokes breathing (786.04)*
　　　hypersomnia with sleep apnea NOS
　　　　(780.53)
　　　insomnia with sleep apnea NOS (780.51)
　　　sleep apnea in newborn (770.81–770.82)
　　　sleep apnea NOS (780.57)

　　327.20　Organic sleep apnea, unspecified

　　327.21　Primary central sleep apnea

　　327.22　High altitude periodic breathing

　　327.23　Obstructive sleep apnea (adult) (pediatric)

　　327.24　Idiopathic sleep related nonobstructive
　　　　alveolar hypoventilation
　　　　Sleep related hypoxia

　　327.25　Congenital central alveolar hypoventilation
　　　　syndrome

　▸ **327.26　*Sleep related hypoventilation/hypoxemia in***
　　　　conditions classifiable elsewhere
　　　　　Code first underlying condition

　▸ **327.27　*Central sleep apnea in conditions classified***
　　　　elsewhere
　　　　　Code first underlying condition

　　327.29　Other organic sleep apnea

● **327.3　Circadian rhythm sleep disorder**
　　Involves one of the sleep/wake regulating hormones. The
　　inability to sleep results from a mismatch between
　　the body's internal clock and the external 24-hour
　　schedule.
　　Organic disorder of sleep wake cycle
　　Organic disorder of sleep wake schedule

　　　| **Excludes** | *alcohol induced circadian rhythm sleep*
　　　　disorder (291.82)
　　　circadian rhythm sleep disorder of
　　　　nonorganic origin (307.45)
　　　disruption of 24 hour sleep wake cycle NOS
　　　　(780.55)
　　　drug induced circadian rhythm sleep
　　　　disorder (292.85)

　　327.30　Circadian rhythm sleep disorder,
　　　　unspecified

　　327.31　Circadian rhythm sleep disorder, delayed
　　　　sleep phase type

　　327.32　Circadian rhythm sleep disorder, advanced
　　　　sleep phase type

　　327.33　Circadian rhythm sleep disorder, irregular
　　　　sleep-wake type

　　327.34　Circadian rhythm sleep disorder,
　　　　free-running type

　　327.35　Circadian rhythm sleep disorder, jet lag type

　　327.36　Circadian rhythm sleep disorder, shift work
　　　　type

　▸ **327.37　*Circadian rhythm sleep disorder in conditions***
　　　　classified elsewhere
　　　　　Code first underlying condition

　　327.39　Other circadian rhythm sleep disorder

● **327.4　Organic parasomnia**

　　　| **Excludes** | *alcohol induced parasomnia (291.82)*
　　　drug induced parasomnia (292.85)
　　　parasomnia not due to a known
　　　　physiological condition (307.47)

　　327.40　Organic parasomnia, unspecified

　　327.41　Confusional arousals

　　327.42　REM sleep behavior disorder

　　327.43　Recurrent isolated sleep paralysis

　▸ **327.44　*Parasomnia in conditions classified***
　　　　elsewhere
　　　　　Code first underlying condition

　　327.49　Other organic parasomnia

● **327.5　Organic sleep related movement disorders**

　　　| **Excludes** | *restless legs syndrome (333.94)*
　　　sleep related movement disorder NOS
　　　　(780.58)

　　327.51　Periodic limb movement disorder
　　　　Periodic limb movement sleep disorder

　　327.52　Sleep related leg cramps

　　327.53　Sleep related bruxism

　　327.59　Other organic sleep related movement
　　　　disorders

　　327.8　Other organic sleep disorders
　　　　Coding Clinic: 2007, Q2, P7-8

Item 6–3　Leukodystrophy is characterized by degeneration and/or failure of the myelin formation of the central nervous system and sometimes of the peripheral nervous system. The disease is inherited and progressive.

HEREDITARY AND DEGENERATIVE DISEASES OF THE CENTRAL NERVOUS SYSTEM (330–337)

　　　| **Excludes** | *hepatolenticular degeneration (275.1)*
　　　multiple sclerosis (340)
　　　other demyelinating diseases of central nervous
　　　　system (341.0–341.9)

● **330　Cerebral degenerations usually manifest in childhood**
　　Use additional code to identify associated mental
　　　retardation

　　330.0　Leukodystrophy 🔴
　　　　Krabbe's disease
　　　　Leukodystrophy:
　　　　　NOS
　　　　　globoid cell
　　　　　metachromatic
　　　　　sudanophilic
　　　　Pelizaeus-Merzbacher disease
　　　　Sulfatide lipidosis
　　　　(Ex) 330.0-330.9, 331.7, 348.8-348.9, 349.89-349.9

　　330.1　Cerebral lipidoses 🔴
　　　　Amaurotic (familial) idiocy
　　　　Disease:
　　　　　Batten
　　　　　Jansky-Bielschowsky
　　　　　Kufs'
　　　　　Spielmeyer-Vogt
　　　　　Tay-Sachs
　　　　Gangliosidosis
　　　　(Ex) 330.1-331.2, 331.7, 331.83-331.9

N　Newborn Age: 0　　**P**　Pediatric Age: 0–17　　**M**　Maternity Age: 12–55　　**A**　Adult Age: 15–124　　♀　Females Only　　♂　Males Only　　　**845**

(Ex)　CC Exclusions　　🔴　Complication\Comorbidity　　🔴　Major C\C　　🔴　Present on Admission Requirement　　🔴　Hospital-Acquired Condition

DISEASES OF THE NERVOUS SYSTEM AND SENSE ORGANS (320–389)

▶ **330.2 Cerebral degeneration in generalized lipidoses** ✪

> Code first underlying disease, as:
> Fabry's disease (272.7)
> Gaucher's disease (272.7)
> Niemann-Pick disease (272.7)
> sphingolipidosis (272.7)
>
> Ⓔ 330.1-331.2, 331.7, 331.83-331.9

▶ **330.3 Cerebral degeneration of childhood in other diseases classified elsewhere** ✪

> Code first underlying disease, as:
> Hunter's disease (277.5)
> mucopolysaccharidosis (277.5)
>
> Ⓔ 330.1-331.2, 331.7, 331.83-331.9

330.8 Other specified cerebral degenerations in childhood ✪
Alpers' disease or gray-matter degeneration
Infantile necrotizing encephalomyelopathy
Leigh's disease
Subacute necrotizing encephalopathy or
    encephalomyelopathy
Ⓔ 330.1-331.2, 331.7, 331.83-331.9
Coding Clinic: 1995, Q1, P9

330.9 Unspecified cerebral degeneration in childhood ✪
Ⓔ 330.1-331.2, 331.7, 331.83-331.9

Item 6–4   Pick's disease is the atrophy of the frontal and temporal lobes, causing dementia; **Alzheimer's** is characterized by a more diffuse cerebral atrophy.

● **331 Other cerebral degenerations**

> Use additional code, where applicable, to identify
>   dementia:
> with behavioral disturbance (294.11)
> without behavioral disturbance (294.10)

331.0 Alzheimer's disease
Coding Clinic: 2000, Q4, P40-41; 1999, Q4, P7; 1994, Q2, P10-11;
    Q1, P21; 1984, Nov-Dec, P20

● **331.1 Frontotemporal dementia**

331.11 Pick's disease
Coding Clinic: 2003, Q4, P57-58

331.19 Other frontotemporal dementia
Frontal dementia
Coding Clinic: 2003, Q4, P57-58

331.2 Senile degeneration of brain
> **Excludes**   senility NOS (797)

331.3 Communicating hydrocephalus ✪
Secondary normal pressure hydrocephalus

> **Excludes**   congenital hydrocephalus (742.3)
> idiopathic normal pressure hydrocephalus
>   (331.5)
> normal pressure hydrocephalus (331.5)
> spina bifida with hydrocephalus (741.0)
>
> Ⓔ 331.3-331.5
Coding Clinic: 2007, Q4, P74-75; 1985, Sept-Oct, P12

331.4 Obstructive hydrocephalus ✪
Acquired hydrocephalus NOS

> **Excludes**   congenital hydrocephalus (742.3)
> idiopathic normal pressure hydrocephalus
>   (331.5)
> normal pressure hydrocephalus (331.5)
> spina bifida with hydrocephalus (741.0)
>
> Ⓔ 249.60-249.61, 249.80-249.91, 250.60-250.63, 250.80-250.93,
>   331.3-331.7, 331.82-331.9, 348.8-348.9, 741.00-741.03, 742.3-742.4,
>   742.59-742.9
Coding Clinic: 2007, Q4, P74-75; 2003, Q4, P106-107; 1999, Q1,
    P9-10

331.5 Idiopathic normal pressure hydrocephalus (INPH) ✪
Normal pressure hydrocephalus NOS

> **Excludes**   congenital hydrocephalus (742.3)
> secondary normal pressure hydrocephalus
>   (331.3)
> spina bifida with hydrocephalus (741.0)
Coding Clinic: 2007, Q4, P74-75
Ⓔ 331.3-331.5

▶ **331.7 Cerebral degeneration in diseases classified elsewhere**

> Code first underlying disease, as:
> alcoholism (303.0–303.9)
> beriberi (265.0)
> cerebrovascular disease (430–438)
> congenital hydrocephalus (741.0, 742.3)
> neoplastic disease (140.0–239.9)
> myxedema (244.0–244.9)
> vitamin B12 deficiency (266.2)

> **Excludes**   cerebral degeneration in:
> Jakob-Creutzfeldt disease
>   (046.11–046.19) ◀▥
> progressive multifocal
>   leukoencephvalopathy (046.3)
> subacute spongiform encephalopathy
>   (046.1)

● **331.8 Other cerebral degeneration**

331.81 Reye's syndrome ✪   P
Ⓔ 331.81

331.82 Dementia with Lewy bodies
Dementia with Parkinsonism
Lewy body dementia
Lewy body disease
Coding Clinic: 2003, Q4, P57-58

331.83 Mild cognitive impairment, so stated

> **Excludes**   altered mental status (780.97)
> cerebral degeneration (331.0–331.9)
> change in mental status (780.97)
> cognitive deficits following (late
>   effects of) cerebral hemorrhage
>   or infarction (438.0)
> cognitive impairment due to
>   intracranial or head injury
>   (850–854, 959.01)
> cognitive impairment due to late
>   effect of intracranial injury
>   (907.0)
> cognitive impairment due to
>   skull fracture (800-801,
>   803-804) ◀
> dementia (290.0–290.43, 294.8)
> mild memory disturbance (310.8)
> neurologic neglect syndrome
>   (781.8)
> personality change, nonpsychotic
>   (310.1)
>
Coding Clinic: 2006, Q4, P75-76

331.89 Other
Cerebral ataxia

331.9 Cerebral degeneration, unspecified

● **332 Parkinson's disease**
Movement disorder (chronic or progressive); cause unknown, and no cure.

> **Excludes**   dementia with Parkinsonism (331.82)

332.0 Paralysis agitans
Parkinsonism or Parkinson's disease:
    NOS
    idiopathic
    primary

◀ New   ◀▥ Revised   ~~deleted~~ Deleted   ● Unacceptable Principal Diagnosis   ● Use Additional Digit(s)
▶ Manifestation Code   OGCR Official Guidelines   Coding Clinic   Excludes   Includes   Use additional   Code first   Omit code

332.1 Secondary Parkinsonism 🔖
> Neuroleptic-induced Parkinsonism
> Parkinsonism due to drugs
>
> **Use additional** E code to identify drug, if
> drug-induced
>
>> **Excludes**   *Parkinsonism (in):*
>>> *Huntington's disease (333.4)*
>>> *progressive supranuclear palsy (333.0)*
>>> *Shy-Drager syndrome (333.0)*
>>> *syphilitic (094.82)*
>
> (Ex:) 332.0-332.1

● **333   Other extrapyramidal disease and abnormal movement disorders**
> **Includes**   other forms of extrapyramidal, basal ganglia, or striatopallidal disease
>
>> **Excludes**   *abnormal movements of head NOS (781.0)*
>>> *sleep related movement disorders (327.51–327.59)*

333.0   Other degenerative diseases of the basal ganglia 🔖
> Atrophy or degeneration:
>> olivopontocerebellar [Déjérine-Thomas syndrome]
>> pigmentary pallidal [Hallervorden-Spatz disease] striatonigral
> Parkinsonian syndrome associated with:
>> idiopathic orthostatic hypotension
>> symptomatic orthostatic hypotension
> Progressive supranuclear ophthalmoplegia
> Shy-Drager syndrome
>
> (Ex:) 332.0-332.1, 335.23, 337.00-337.09, 348.30-348.39
> **Coding Clinic: 1996, Q2, P8-9**

333.1   Essential and other specified forms of tremor
> Benign essential tremor
> Familial tremor
> Medication-induced postural tremor
>
>> **Use additional** E code to identify drug, if
>> drug-induced
>>
>>> **Excludes**   *tremor NOS (781.0)*

333.2   Myoclonus
> Familial essential myoclonus
> Palatal myoclonus   ◄
> ~~Progressive myoclonic epilepsy~~
> ~~Unverricht-Lundborg disease~~
>
>> **Excludes**   *progressive myoclonic epilepsy (345.1)* ◄
>>> *Unverricht-Lundborg disease (345.1)* ◄
>
>> **Use additional** E code to identify drug, if
>> drug-induced
> **Coding Clinic: 1997, Q3, P5; 1987, Mar-April, P12**

333.3   Tics of organic origin
>> **Excludes**   *Gilles de la Tourette's syndrome (307.23)*
>>> *habit spasm (307.22)*
>>> *tic NOS (307.20)*
>
>> **Use additional** E code to identify drug, if
>> drug-induced

> **Item 6–5   Huntington's chorea** is an inherited degenerative disorder of the central nervous system and is characterized by ceaseless, jerky movements and progressive cognitive and behavioral deterioration.

333.4   Huntington's chorea 🔖
> (Ex:) 332.0-332.1, 340-341.1, 341.8-341.9, 343.0-344.2, 348.1, 348.30-348.9,
> 349.1, 349.82-349.9, 780.72

333.5   Other choreas
> Hemiballism(us)
> Paroxysmal choreo-athetosis
>
>> **Excludes**   *Sydenham's or rheumatic chorea*
>>> *(392.0–392.9)*
>
>> **Use additional** E code to identify drug, if
>> drug-induced

333.6   Genetic torsion dystonia
> Dystonia:
>> deformans progressiva
>> musculorum deformans
>> (Schwalbe-) Ziehen-Oppenheim disease
> **Coding Clinic: 2006, Q4, P76-78**

● **333.7   Acquired torsion dystonia**
> **Coding Clinic: 2006, Q4, P76-78**
>
> **333.71   Athetoid cerebral palsy** 🔖
>> Double athetosis (syndrome)
>> Vogt's disease
>>
>>> **Excludes**   *infantile cerebral palsy*
>>>> *(343.0–343.9)*
>>
>> (Ex:) 332.0-332.1, 333.71, 333.90, 333.99, 343.0-343.9,
>> 348.30-348.39
>
> **333.72   Acute dystonia due to drugs** 🔖
>> Acute dystonic reaction due to drugs
>> Neuroleptic-induced acute dystonia
>>
>>> **Use additional** E code to identify drug
>>>
>>>> **Excludes**   *blepharospasm due to drugs*
>>>>> *(333.85)*
>>>>> *orofacial dyskinesia due to drugs*
>>>>> *(333.85)*
>>>>> *secondary Parkinsonism (332.1)*
>>>>> *subacute dyskinesia due to drugs*
>>>>> *(333.85)*
>>>>> *tardive dyskinesia (333.85)*
>>>> (Ex:) 332.0-332.1, 333.71, 333.90, 333.99, 348.30-348.39
>
> **333.79   Other acquired torsion dystonia** 🔖
>> (Ex:) 332.0-332.1, 333.71, 333.90, 333.99, 348.30-348.39

● **333.8   Fragments of torsion dystonia**
> **Use additional** E code to identify drug, if
> drug-induced
>
> **333.81   Blepharospasm**
>>> **Excludes**   *blepharospasm due to drugs*
>>>> *(333.85)*
>
> **333.82   Orofacial dyskinesia**
>>> **Excludes**   *orofacial dyskinesia due to drugs*
>>>> *(333.85)*
>
> **333.83   Spasmodic torticollis**
>>> **Excludes**   *torticollis:*
>>>> *NOS (723.5)*
>>>> *hysterical (300.11)*
>>>> *psychogenic (306.0)*
>
> **333.84   Organic writers' cramp**
>>> **Excludes**   *psychogenic (300.89)*
>
> **333.85   Subacute dyskinesia due to drugs**
>> Blepharospasm due to drugs
>> Orofacial dyskinesia due to drugs
>> Tardive dyskinesia
>>
>>> **Use additional** E code to identify drug
>>>
>>>> **Excludes**   *acute dystonia due to drugs*
>>>>> *(333.72)*
>>>>> *acute dystonic reaction due to drugs*
>>>>> *(333.72)*
>>>>> *secondary Parkinsonism (332.1)*
>>> **Coding Clinic: 2006, Q4, P76-78**
>
> **333.89   Other**

N Newborn Age: 0   **P** Pediatric Age: 0–17   **M** Maternity Age: 12–55   **A** Adult Age: 15–124   ♀ Females Only   ♂ Males Only

(Ex:) CC Exclusions   🔖 Complication\Comorbidity   🔖 Major C\C   🔖 Present on Admission Requirement   🔖 Hospital-Acquired Condition   847

DISEASES OF THE NERVOUS SYSTEM AND SENSE ORGANS (320–389)

● 333.9 **Other and unspecified extrapyramidal diseases and abnormal movement disorders**

  333.90 **Unspecified extrapyramidal disease and abnormal movement disorder**🔒
    Medication-induced movement disorders NOS
    Use additional E code to identify drug, if drug-induced
    Ex: 332.0-332.1, 333.1-333.83, 333.85-333.93, 333.99, 335.22-335.23, 340-341.1, 341.8-341.9, 343.0-344.2, 348.1, 348.30-348.9, 349.1, 349.82-349.9, 780.72

  333.91 **Stiff-man syndrome**🔒
    Ex: 332.0-332.1, 333.1-333.83, 333.85-333.93, 333.99, 335.22-335.23, 340-341.1, 341.8-341.9, 343.0-344.2, 348.1, 348.30-348.9, 349.1, 349.82-349.9, 780.72

  333.92 **Neuroleptic malignant syndrome**🔒
    Use additional E code to identify drug
    Excludes neuroleptic induced Parkinsonism (332.1)
    Ex: 333.0-333.93, 333.99, 342.00-342.92, 348.2-348.39

  333.93 **Benign shuddering attacks**

  333.94 **Restless legs syndrome (RLS)**
    Coding Clinic: 2006, Q4, P79

  333.99 **Other**
    Neuroleptic-induced acute akathisia
    Use additional E code to identify drug, if drug-induced
    Coding Clinic: 2004, Q2, P12

● 334 **Spinocerebellar disease**
  Group of degenerative disorders in which primary symptom is progressive ataxia (jerky, uncoordinated movements)
    Excludes *olivopontocerebellar degeneration (333.0)*
    peroneal muscular atrophy (356.1)

  334.0 **Friedreich's ataxia**🔒
    Ex: 334.0-334.9, 348.30-348.39

  334.1 **Hereditary spastic paraplegia**🔒
    Ex: 333.0-333.93, 333.99-337.9, 340-344.9, 348.1, 348.30-348.39, 348.8-349.2, 349.82-349.9, 780.72

  334.2 **Primary cerebellar degeneration**🔒
    Cerebellar ataxia:
      Marie's
      Sanger-Brown
    Dyssynergia cerebellaris myoclonica
    Primary cerebellar degeneration:
      NOS
      hereditary
      sporadic
    Ex: 333.0-333.93, 333.99-337.9, 340-344.9, 348.0-348.1, 348.30-348.39, 348.8-348.9, 349.82-349.9, 780.72
    Coding Clinic: 1987, Mar-April, P9

  334.3 **Other cerebellar ataxia**🔒
    Cerebellar ataxia NOS
    Use additional E code to identify drug, if drug-induced
    Ex: 333.0-333.93, 333.99-337.9, 340-344.9, 348.0-348.1, 348.30-348.39, 348.8-348.9, 349.82-349.9, 780.72

▶ 334.4 *Cerebellar ataxia in diseases classified elsewhere*🔒
    Code first underlying disease, as:
      alcoholism (303.0–303.9)
      myxedema (244.0–244.9)
      neoplastic disease (140.0–239.9)
    Ex: 333.0-333.93, 333.99-337.9, 340-344.9 348.0-348.1, 348.30-348.39, 348.8-348.9 349.82-349.9, 780.72

  334.8 **Other spinocerebellar diseases**🔒
    Ataxia-telangiectasia [Louis-Bar syndrome]
    Corticostriatal-spinal degeneration
    Ex: 333.0-333.93, 333.99-337.9, 340-344.9 348.0-348.1, 348.30-348.39, 348.8-348.9 349.82-349.9, 780.72

  334.9 **Spinocerebellar disease, unspecified**🔒
    Ex: 334.0-334.9

● 335 **Anterior horn cell disease**

  335.0 **Werdnig-Hoffmann disease**🔒
    Infantile spinal muscular atrophy
    Progressive muscular atrophy of infancy
    Ex: 249.60-249.61, 249.80-249.91, 250.60-250.63, 250.80-250.93, 334.8-337.9, 349.89-349.9

● 335.1 **Spinal muscular atrophy**

  335.10 **Spinal muscular atrophy, unspecified**🔒
    Ex: 249.60-249.61, 249.80-249.91, 250.60-250.63, 250.80-250.93, 334.8-337.9, 349.89-349.9

  335.11 **Kugelberg-Welander disease**🔒
    Spinal muscular atrophy:
      familial
      juvenile
    Ex: 249.60-249.61, 249.80-249.91, 250.60-250.63, 250.80-250.93, 334.8-337.9, 349.89-349.9

  335.19 **Other**🔒
    Adult spinal muscular atrophy
    Ex: 249.60-249.61, 249.80-249.91, 250.60-250.63, 250.80-250.93, 334.8-337.9, 349.89-349.9

● 335.2 **Motor neuron disease**

  335.20 **Amyotrophic lateral sclerosis**🔒   A
    Also listed in the Index as "Lou Gehrig's disease" (ALS)
    Motor neuron disease (bulbar) (mixed type)
    Ex: 249.60-249.61, 249.80-249.91, 250.60-250.63, 250.80-250.93, 334.8-337.9, 349.89-349.9
    Coding Clinic: 1995, Q4, P81

  335.21 **Progressive muscular atrophy**🔒
    Duchenne-Aran muscular atrophy
    Progressive muscular atrophy (pure)
    Ex: 249.60-249.61, 249.80-249.91, 250.60-250.63, 250.80-250.93, 334.8-337.9, 349.89-349.9

  335.22 **Progressive bulbar palsy**🔒
    Ex: 249.60-249.61, 249.80-249.91, 250.60-250.63, 250.80-250.93, 334.8-337.9, 349.89-349.9

  335.23 **Pseudobulbar palsy**🔒
    Ex: 249.60-249.61, 249.80-249.91, 250.60-250.63, 250.80-250.93, 334.8-337.9, 349.89-349.9

  335.24 **Primary lateral sclerosis**🔒
    Ex: 249.60-249.61, 249.80-249.91, 250.60-250.63, 250.80-250.93, 334.8-337.9, 349.89-349.9

  335.29 **Other**🔒
    Ex: 249.60-249.61, 249.80-249.91, 250.60-250.63, 250.80-250.93, 334.8-337.9, 349.89-349.9

  335.8 **Other anterior horn cell diseases**🔒
    Ex: 249.60-249.61, 249.80-249.91, 250.60-250.63, 250.80-250.93, 334.8-337.9, 349.89-349.9
    Coding Clinic: 2006, Q4, P76-78

  335.9 **Anterior horn cell disease, unspecified**🔒
    Ex: 249.60-249.61, 249.80-249.91, 250.60-250.63, 250.80-250.93, 334.8-337.9, 349.89-349.9

DISEASES OF THE NERVOUS SYSTEM AND SENSE ORGANS (320–389)

◀ New   ◀▥ Revised   ~~deleted~~ Deleted   ● Unacceptable Principal Diagnosis   ● Use Additional Digit(s)
▶ Manifestation Code   **OGCR** Official Guidelines   **Coding Clinic**   Excludes   Includes   Use additional   Code first   Omit code

● **336 Other diseases of spinal cord**

336.0 Syringomyelia and syringobulbia 🐾
> (Ex:) 334.8-337.9, 340-344.9, 348.30-348.39, 348.8-349.2, 349.89-349.9, 780.72
>
> **Coding Clinic: 1989, Q1, P10**

336.1 Vascular myelopathies 🐾
> Acute infarction of spinal cord (embolic) (nonembolic)
> Arterial thrombosis of spinal cord
> Edema of spinal cord
> Hematomyelia
> Subacute necrotic myelopathy
> (Ex:) 249.60-249.61, 250.60-250.63, 334.8-337.9, 340-344.9, 348.1, 348.30-348.39, 349.0-349.2, 349.89-349.9, 780.72

▶ **336.2 Subacute combined degeneration of spinal cord in diseases classified elsewhere** 🐾
> Code first underlying disease, as:
> pernicious anemia (281.0)
> other vitamin B12 deficiency anemia (281.1)
> vitamin B12 deficiency (266.2)
> (Ex:) 334.8-337.9, 340 -344.9, 348.1, 348.30-348.39, 349.0-349.2, 349.89-349.9, 780.72

▶ **336.3 Myelopathy in other diseases classified elsewhere** 🐾
> Code first underlying disease, as:
> myelopathy in neoplastic disease (140.0–239.9)
>
> | **Excludes** | myelopathy in: |
> intervertebral disc disorder (722.70–722.73)
> spondylosis (721.1, 721.41–721.42, 721.91)
> (Ex:) 249.60-249.61, 250.60-250.63, 334.8-337.9, 340-344.9, 348.1, 348.30-348.39, 349.0-349.2, 349.89-349.9, 780.72
>
> **Coding Clinic: 1999, Q3, P5**

336.8 Other myelopathy 🐾
> Myelopathy:
> drug-induced
> radiation-induced
>
> Use additional E code to identify cause
> (Ex:) 249.60-249.61, 250.60-250.63, 334.8-337.9, 340-344.9, 348.1, 348.30-348.39, 349.0-349.2, 349.89-349.9, 780.72

336.9 Unspecified disease of spinal cord 🐾
> Cord compression NOS
> Myelopathy NOS
>
> | **Excludes** | myelitis (323.02, 323.1, 323.2, 323.42, 323.52, 323.63, 323.72, 323.82, 323.9)
> spinal (canal) stenosis (723.0, 724.00–724.09)
> (Ex:) 249.60-249.61, 250.60-250.63, 334.1, 334.8-337.9, 340-344.9, 348.1, 348.30-348.39, 349.0-349.2, 349.89-349.9, 780.72

● **337 Disorders of the autonomic nervous system**
> **Includes** disorders of peripheral autonomic, sympathetic, parasympathetic, or vegetative system
>
> **Excludes** familial dysautonomia [Riley-Day syndrome] (742.8)

● **337.0 Idiopathic peripheral autonomic neuropathy**

337.00 Idiopathic peripheral autonomic neuropathy, unspecified

337.01 Carotid sinus syndrome
> Carotid sinus syncope
> **Coding Clinic: 2008, Q4, P101-102**

337.09 Other idiopathic peripheral autonomic neuropathy
> Cervical sympathetic dystrophy or paralysis

▶ **337.1 Peripheral autonomic neuropathy in disorders classified elsewhere** 🐾
> Code first underlying disease, as:
> amyloidosis (277.30–277.39)
> diabetes (249.6, 250.6)
> (Ex:) 337.00-337.29, 337.9, 348.30-348.39
> **Coding Clinic: 2009, Q2, P10; 1993, Q2, P6; 1984, Nov-Dec, P9**

● **337.2 Reflex sympathetic dystrophy**

337.20 Reflex sympathetic dystrophy, unspecified 🐾
> Complex regional pain syndrome type I, unspecified
> (Ex:) 337.20-337.29

337.21 Reflex sympathetic dystrophy of the upper limb 🐾
> Complex regional pain syndrome type I of the upper limb
> (Ex:) 249.60-249.61, 250.60-250.63, 334.8-337.9, 340-344.9, 348.1, 348.30-348.39, 349.0-349.2, 349.89-349.9, 780.72

337.22 Reflex sympathetic dystrophy of the lower limb 🐾
> Complex regional pain syndrome type I of the lower limb
> (Ex:) 249.60-249.61, 250.60-250.63, 334.8-337.9, 340-344.9, 348.1, 348.30-348.39, 349.0-349.2, 349.89-349.9, 780.72

337.29 Reflex sympathetic dystrophy of other specified site 🐾
> Complex regional pain syndrome type I of other specified site
> (Ex:) 249.60-249.61, 250.60-250.63, 334.8-337.9, 340-344.9, 348.1, 348.30-348.39, 349.0-349.2, 349.89-349.9, 780.72

337.3 Autonomic dysreflexia
> Use additional code to identify the cause, such as:
> fecal impaction (560.39)
> pressure ulcer (707.00–707.09)
> urinary tract infection (599.0)
> **Coding Clinic: 1998, Q4, P37-38**

337.9 Unspecified disorder of autonomic nervous system

N Newborn Age: 0   **P** Pediatric Age: 0–17   **M** Maternity Age: 12–55   **A** Adult Age: 15–124   ♀ Females Only   ♂ Males Only

(Ex:) CC Exclusions   🐾 Complication\Comorbidity   🐾 Major C\C   🐾 Present on Admission Requirement   🐾 Hospital-Acquired Condition

849

DISEASES OF THE NERVOUS SYSTEM AND SENSE ORGANS (320–389)

● **338   Pain, not elsewhere classified**

Use additional code to identify:
pain associated with psychological factors (307.89)

Excludes *generalized pain (780.96)*
headache syndromes (339.00-339.89)
localized pain, unspecified type - code to pain by
site
migraines (346.0-346.9)
pain disorder exclusively attributed to
psychological factors (307.80)
vulvar vestibulitis (625.71)
vulvodynia (625.70-625.79)

338.0   Central pain syndrome
Déjérine-Roussy syndrome
Myelopathic pain syndrome
Thalamic pain syndrome (hyperesthetic)

● **338.1   Acute pain**

338.11   Acute pain due to trauma
Coding Clinic: 2007, Q1, P3-8

338.12   Acute post-thoracotomy pain
Post-thoracotomy pain NOS

338.18   Other acute postoperative pain
Postoperative pain NOS
Coding Clinic: 2007, Q2, P13-15; 2003, Q1, P4-5, 8

338.19   Other acute pain
Excludes *neoplasm related acute pain (338.3)*
Coding Clinic: 2007, Q2, P13-15

● **338.2   Chronic pain**
Excludes *causalgia (355.9)*
lower limb (355.71)
upper limb (354.4)
chronic pain syndrome (338.4)
myofascial pain syndrome (729.1)
neoplasm related chronic pain (338.3)
reflex sympathetic dystrophy
(337.20–337.29)
Coding Clinic: 2008, Q3, P4

338.21   Chronic pain due to trauma

338.22   Chronic post-thoracotomy pain

338.28   Other chronic postoperative pain
Coding Clinic: 2007, Q2, P13-15

338.29   Other chronic pain
Coding Clinic: 2007, Q2, P13-15

338.3   Neoplasm related pain (acute) (chronic)
Cancer associated pain
Pain due to malignancy (primary) (secondary)
Tumor associated pain
Coding Clinic: 2007, Q2, P13-15

338.4   Chronic pain syndrome
Chronic pain associated with significant
psychosocial dysfunction
Coding Clinic: 2007, Q2, P13-15

● **339   Other headache syndromes**
Excludes *headache:*
NOS (784.0)
due to lumbar puncture (349.0)
migraine (346.0-346.9)
Coding Clinic: 2008, Q4, P102-109

● **339.0   Cluster headaches and other trigeminal autonomic**
cephalgias
TACS

339.00   Cluster headache syndrome, unspecified
Ciliary neuralgia
Cluster headache NOS
Histamine cephalgia
Lower half migraine
Migrainous neuralgia

339.01   Episodic cluster headache

339.02   Chronic cluster headache

339.03   Episodic paroxysmal hemicrania
Paroxysmal hemicrania NOS

339.04   Chronic paroxysmal hemicrania

339.05   Short lasting unilateral neuralgiform
headache with conjunctival injection and
tearing
SUNCT

339.09   Other trigeminal autonomic cephalgias

● **339.1   Tension type headache**
Excludes *tension headache NOS (307.81)*
tension headache related to psychological
factors (307.81)

339.10   Tension type headache, unspecified

339.11   Episodic tension type headache

339.12   Chronic tension type headache

● **339.2   Post-traumatic headache**

339.20   Post-traumatic headache, unspecified
Coding Clinic: 2008, Q4, P102-109

339.21   Acute post-traumatic headache
Coding Clinic: 2008, Q4, P102-109

339.22   Chronic post-traumatic headache

339.3   Drug induced headache, not elsewhere classified
Medication overuse headache
Rebound headache

● **339.4   Complicated headache syndromes**

339.41   Hemicrania continua

339.42   New daily persistent headache
NDPH

339.43   Primary thunderclap headache

339.44   Other complicated headache syndrome

● **339.8   Other specified headache syndromes**

339.81   Hypnic headache

339.82   Headache associated with sexual activity
Orgasmic headache
Preorgasmic headache

339.83   Primary cough headache

339.84   Primary exertional headache

339.85   Primary stabbing headache

339.89   Other specified headache syndromes

DISEASES OF THE NERVOUS SYSTEM AND SENSE ORGANS (320–389)

◀ New   ◀ᴵᴵᴵ Revised   ~~deleted~~ Deleted   ● Unacceptable Principal Diagnosis   ● Use Additional Digit(s)
▶ Manifestation Code   OGCR Official Guidelines   Coding Clinic   Excludes   Includes   Use additional   Code first   Omit code

Item 6-6 Multiple sclerosis (MS) is a nervous system disease affecting the brain and spinal cord by damaging the myelin sheath surrounding and protecting nerve cells. The damage slows down/blocks messages between the brain and body. Symptoms are: visual disturbances, muscle weakness, coordination and balance issues, numbness, prickling, thinking and memory problems. The cause is unknown, though it is thought that it may be an autoimmune disease. It affects women more than men, between 20 and 40 years of age. MS can be mild, but it may cause the loss of ability to write, walk, and speak. There is no cure, but medication may slow or control symptoms.

OTHER DISORDERS OF THE CENTRAL NERVOUS SYSTEM (340–349)

340 Multiple sclerosis (MS)
> Disseminated or multiple sclerosis:
> NOS   cord
> brain stem   generalized

● **341 Other demyelinating diseases of central nervous system**

341.0 Neuromyelitis optica 🐾
> Ⓔ 341.0, 348.30-348.39

341.1 Schilder's disease 🐾
> Balo's concentric sclerosis
> Encephalitis periaxialis:
>> concentrica [Balo's]
>> diffusa [Schilder's]
> Ⓔ 066.40-066.49, 079.82, 348.30-348.39

● **341.2 Acute (transverse) myelitis**

> **Excludes** *acute (transverse) myelitis (in) (due to):*
>> *following immunization procedures (323.52)*
>> *infection classified elsewhere (323.42)*
>> *postinfectious (323.63)*
>> *protozoal diseases classified elsewhere (323.2)*
>> *rickettsial diseases classified elsewhere (323.1)*
>> *toxic (323.72)*
>> *viral diseases classified elsewhere (323.02)*
>> *transverse myelitis NOS (323.82)*

341.20 Acute (transverse) myelitis NOS 🐾
> Ⓔ 003.21, 013.00-013.16, 036.0, 047.0-047.9, 049.0-049.1,
> 053.0-053.13, 053.19, 053.79-053.9, 054.72, 054.79-054.9,
> 058.81-058.89, 072.1, 078.89, 079.81, 079.89, 079.99,
> 090.42, 091.81, 094.2, 098.89, 100.81, 112.83, 114.2,
> 115.01, 115.11, 115.91, 130.0, 139.8, 249.60-249.61,
> 250.60-250.63, 320.0-322.9, 334.8-337.9, 340-341.1,
> 341.8-344.9, 348.1, 348.30-348.39, 349.0-349.2,
> 349.89-349.9, 357.0, 780.72

▶ **341.21 Acute (transverse) myelitis in conditions classified elsewhere** 🐾
> *Code first underlying condition*
> Ⓔ 003.21, 013.00-013.16, 036.0, 047.0-047.9, 049.0-049.1,
> 053.0-053.13, 053.19, 053.79-053.9, 054.72, 054.79-054.9,
> 058.81, 058.89, 072.1, 078.89, 079.81, 079.89, 079.99,
> 090.42, 091.81, 094.2, 098.89, 100.81, 112.83, 114.2,
> 115.01, 115.11, 115.91, 130.0, 139.8, 249.60-249.61,
> 250.60-250.63, 320.0-322.9, 334.8-337.9, 340-341.1,
> 341.8-344.9, 348.1, 348.30-348.39, 349.0-349.2,
> 349.89-349.9, 357.0, 780.72

341.22 Idiopathic transverse myelitis 🐾
> Ⓔ 003.21, 013.00-013.16, 036.0, 047.0-047.9, 049.0-049.1,
> 053.0-053.13, 053.19, 053.79-053.9, 054.72, 054.79-054.9,
> 058.81-058.89, 072.1, 078.89, 079.81, 079.89, 079.99,
> 090.42, 091.81, 094.2, 098.89, 100.81, 112.83, 114.2,
> 115.01, 115.11, 115.91, 130.0, 139.8, 249.60-249.61,
> 250.60-250.63, 320.0-322.9, 334.8-337.9, 340-341.1,
> 341.8-344.9, 348.1, 348.30-348.39, 349.0-349.2,
> 349.89-349.9, 357.0, 780.72

341.8 Other demyelinating diseases of central nervous system 🐾
> Central demyelination of corpus callosum
> Central pontine myelinosis
> Marchiafava (-Bignami) disease
> Ⓔ 333.1-333.93, 333.99-337.9, 340-344.9, 348.30-348.39, 348.8-348.9,
> 349.82-349.9, 780.72
> **Coding Clinic: 1987, Nov-Dec, P6**

341.9 Demyelinating disease of central nervous system, unspecified 🐾
> Ⓔ 333.1-333.93, 333.99-337.9, 340-344.9, 348.30-348.39, 348.8-348.9,
> 349.82-349.9, 780.72

● **342 Hemiplegia and hemiparesis**

> **Note:** This category is to be used when hemiplegia (complete) (incomplete) is reported without further specification, or is stated to be old or long-standing but of unspecified cause. The category is also for use in multiple coding to identify these types of hemiplegia resulting from any cause.

> **Excludes** *congenital (343.1)*
>> *hemiplegia due to late effect of cerebrovascular accident (438.20–438.22)*
>> *infantile NOS (343.4)*

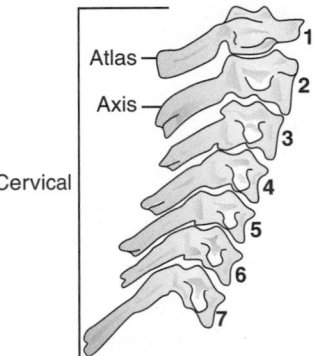

Figure 6–2 Cervical vertebrae.

Atlas — 1
Axis — 2
— 3
Cervical — 4
— 5
— 6
— 7

Item 6–7 Hemiplegia is complete paralysis of one side of the body—arm, leg, and trunk. **Hemiparesis** is a generalized weakness or incomplete paralysis of one side of the body. If most activities (eating, writing) are performed with the right hand, the right is the dominant side, and the left is the nondominant side. **Quadriplegia,** also called tetraplegia, is the complete paralysis of all four limbs. **Quadriparesis** is the incomplete paralysis of all four limbs. Nerve damage in C1–C4 is associated with lower limb paralysis, and C5–C7 damage is associated with upper limb paralysis. **Diplegia** is the paralysis of the upper limbs. **Monoplegia** is the complete paralysis of one limb. There are separate codes for upper (344.4x) and lower (344.3x) limb. Dominant, nondominant, or unspecified side becomes the fifth digit. Dominant side (right/left) is the side that a person leads with for movement, such as in writing and sports.
Cauda equina syndrome is due to pressure on the roots of the spinal nerves and causes paresthesia (abnormal sensations).

DISEASES OF THE NERVOUS SYSTEM AND SENSE ORGANS (320–389)

The following fifth-digits are for use with codes 342.0–342.9

> 0   affecting unspecified side
> 1   affecting dominant side
> 2   affecting nondominant side

● **342.0   Flaccid hemiplegia**🔴
[0-2]   (Ex:) 334.0-337.9, 340-344.9, 348.30-348.39, 348.8-348.9, 349.82-349.9, 780.72

● **342.1   Spastic hemiplegia**🔴
[0-2]   (Ex:) 334.0-337.9, 340-344.9, 348.30-348.39, 348.8-348.9, 349.82-349.9, 780.72

● **342.8   Other specified hemiplegia**🔴
[0-2]   (Ex:) 334.0-337.9, 340-344.9, 348.30-348.39, 348.8-348.9, 349.82-349.9, 780.72

● **342.9   Hemiplegia, unspecified**🔴
[0-2]   (Ex:) 334.0-337.9, 340-344.9, 348.30-348.39, 348.8-348.9, 349.82-349.9, 780.72
Coding Clinic: 2006, Q3, P5; 1998, Q4, P87

● **343   Infantile cerebral palsy**
Includes   cerebral:
     palsy NOS
     spastic infantile paralysis
   congenital spastic paralysis (cerebral)
   Little's disease
   paralysis (spastic) due to birth injury:
     intracranial
     spinal

Excludes   *athetoid cerebral palsy (333.71)*
   hereditary cerebral paralysis, such as:
     hereditary spastic paraplegia (334.1)
     Vogt's disease (333.71)
   spastic paralysis specified as noncongenital or
     noninfantile (344.0–344.9)

343.0   Diplegic🔴
Congenital diplegia
Congenital paraplegia
(Ex:) 343.0, 348.30-348.39

343.1   Hemiplegic🔴
Congenital hemiplegia
Excludes   *infantile hemiplegia NOS (343.4)*
(Ex:) 343.1, 348.30-348.39

343.2   Quadriplegic🔴
Tetraplegic
(Ex:) 249.60-249.61, 249.80-249.91, 250.60-250.63, 250.80-250.93, 342.00-344.9, 348.8-348.9, 349.89-349.9, 742.59-742.9, 780.72

343.3   Monoplegic

343.4   Infantile hemiplegia🔴
Infantile hemiplegia (postnatal) NOS
(Ex:) 334.0-337.9, 340-344.9, 348.30-348.39, 348.8-348.9, 349.82-349.9, 780.72

343.8   Other specified infantile cerebral palsy

343.9   Infantile cerebral palsy, unspecified
Cerebral palsy NOS
Coding Clinic: 2005, Q4, P89-90

● **344   Other paralytic syndromes**
Note: This category is to be used when the listed conditions are reported without further specification or are stated to be old or long-standing but of unspecified cause. The category is also for use in multiple coding to identify these conditions resulting from any cause.

Includes   paralysis (complete) (incomplete), except as classifiable to 342 and 343

Excludes   *congenital or infantile cerebral palsy (343.0–343.9)*
   hemiplegia (342.0–342.9)
     congenital or infantile (343.1, 343.4)

● **344.0   Quadriplegia and quadriparesis**

344.00   Quadriplegia, unspecified🔴
(Ex:) 249.60-249.61, 249.80-249.91, 250.60-250.63, 250.80-250.93, 342.00-344.9, 348.8-348.9, 349.89-349.9, 742.59-742.9, 780.72
Coding Clinic: 2003, Q4, P103-104; 1998, Q4, P37-38

344.01   C$_1$-C$_4$, complete🔴
(Ex:) 249.60-249.61, 249.80-249.91, 250.60-250.63, 250.80-250.93, 342.00-344.9, 348.8-348.9, 349.89-349.9, 742.59-742.9, 780.72

344.02   C$_1$-C$_4$, incomplete🔴
(Ex:) 249.60-249.61, 249.80-249.91, 250.60-250.63, 250.80-250.93, 342.00-344.9, 348.8-348.9, 349.89-349.9, 742.59-742.9, 780.72

344.03   C$_5$-C$_7$, complete🔴
(Ex:) 249.60-249.61, 249.80-249.91, 250.60-250.63, 250.80-250.93, 342.00-344.9, 348.8-348.9, 349.89-349.9, 742.59-742.9, 780.72

344.04   C$_5$-C$_7$, incomplete🔴
(Ex:) 249.60-249.61, 249.80-249.91, 250.60-250.63, 250.80-250.93, 342.00-344.9, 348.8-348.9, 349.89-349.9, 742.59-742.9, 780.72

344.09   Other🔴
(Ex:) 249.60-249.61, 249.80-249.91, 250.60-250.63, 250.80-250.93, 342.00-344.9, 348.8-348.9, 349.89-349.9, 742.59-742.9, 780.72
Coding Clinic: 2001, Q1, P12; 1998, Q4, P39-40

344.1   Paraplegia🔴
Paralysis of both lower limbs
Paraplegia (lower)
(Ex:) 334.0-337.9, 340-344.9, 348.30-348.39, 348.8-348.9, 349.82-349.9, 780.72
Coding Clinic: 2003, Q4, P110; 1987, Mar-April, P10-11

344.2   Diplegia of upper limbs🔴
Diplegia (upper)
Paralysis of both upper limbs
(Ex:) 344.00-344.09, 344.2, 344.81-344.9, 349.89-349.9, 780.72

● **344.3   Monoplegia of lower limb**
Paralysis of lower limb
Excludes   *monoplegia of lower limb due to late*
     effect of cerebrovascular accident
     (438.40–438.42)

344.30   Affecting unspecified side

344.31   Affecting dominant side

344.32   Affecting nondominant side

● **344.4   Monoplegia of upper limb**
Paralysis of upper limb
Excludes   *monoplegia of upper limb due to late*
     effect of cerebrovascular accident
     (438.30–438.32)

344.40   Affecting unspecified side

344.41   Affecting dominant side

344.42   Affecting nondominant side

◀ New   ◀▬ Revised   ~~deleted~~ Deleted   ● Unacceptable Principal Diagnosis   ● Use Additional Digit(s)
▶ Manifestation Code   **OGCR** Official Guidelines   **Coding Clinic**   Excludes   Includes   Use additional   Code first   Omit code

344.5 Unspecified monoplegia

● **344.6 Cauda equina syndrome**

    344.60 Without mention of neurogenic bladder🅒
        Ⓔⅹ 344.00-344.1, 344.30-344.32, 344.60-344.9, 349.89-349.9, 780.72

    344.61 With neurogenic bladder🅒
        Acontractile bladder
        Autonomic hyperreflexia of bladder
        Cord bladder
        Detrusor hyperreflexia
        Ⓔⅹ 334.0-337.9, 340-344.9, 348.30-348.39, 348.8-348.9, 349.82-349.9, 599.60-599.69, 780.72
        Coding Clinic: 1987, Mar-April, P10-11

● **344.8 Other specified paralytic syndromes**

    344.81 Locked-in state🅒
        Ⓔⅹ 342.00-344.9, 348.30-348.39, 348.8-348.9, 349.82-349.9, 780.72

    344.89 Other specified paralytic syndrome
        Coding Clinic: 1999, Q2, P4

    344.9 Paralysis, unspecified
        Coding Clinic: 1994, Q3, P4

● **345 Epilepsy and recurrent seizures**

The following fifth-digit subclassification is for use with categories 345.0, .1, .4–.9:

> **0 without mention of intractable epilepsy**
> **1 with intractable epilepsy**
>   **pharmacoresistant (pharmacologically resistant)** ◄
>   **poorly controlled** ◄
>   **refractory (medically)** ◄
>   **treatment resistant** ◄

    Excludes *hippocampal sclerosis (348.81)* ◄
                   mesial temporal sclerosis (348.81) ◄
                   progressive myoclonic epilepsy (333.2)
                   temporal sclerosis (348.81) ◄

● **345.0 Generalized nonconvulsive epilepsy 1**🅒
  [0-1]   Absences:
            atonic
            typical
        Minor epilepsy
        Petit mal
        Pykno-epilepsy
        Seizures:
            akinetic
            atonic
        For code **345.01**: Ⓔⅹ 249.60-249.61, 250.60-250.63, 345.00-345.91, 348.8-348.9, 349.89-349.9
        Coding Clinic: 2004, Q1, P18; 1992, Q2, P8

● **345.1 Generalized convulsive epilepsy 1**🅒
  [0-1]   Epileptic seizures:
            clonic
            myoclonic
            tonic
            tonic-clonic
        Grand mal
        Major epilepsy
        Progressive myoclonic epilepsy ◄
        Unverricht-Lundborg disease ◄
        Excludes *convulsions:*
                    NOS (780.39)
                    infantile (780.39)
                    newborn (779.0)
             infantile spasms (345.6)
        For code **345.11**: Ⓔⅹ 249.60-249.61, 250.60-250.63, 345.00-345.91, 348.8-348.9, 349.89-349.9
        Coding Clinic: 1997, Q3, P5; 1994, Q3, P9

345.2 Petit mal status🅒
    Epileptic absence status
    Temporary disturbance of brain function caused by abnormal electrical activity.
    Ⓔⅹ 249.60-249.61, 249.80-249.91, 250.60-250.63, 258.80-258.93, 345.00-345.91, 348.8-348.9, 349.89-349.9

345.3 Grand mal status🅒
    Status epilepticus NOS
    Grand mal seizure is a generalized tonic-clonic seizure involving the entire body, which involves muscle rigidity, violent muscle contractions, and loss of consciousness.
    Excludes *epilepsia partialis continua (345.7) status:*
                    psychomotor (345.7)
                    temporal lobe (345.7)
    Ⓔⅹ 249.60-249.61, 249.80-249.91, 250.60-250.63, 250.88-258.93, 345.00-345.91, 348.8-348.9, 349.89-349.9
    Coding Clinic: 2005, Q3, P12-13

● **345.4 Localization-related (focal) (partial) epilepsy and**
  [0-1] **epileptic syndromes with complex partial seizures**🅒
        Epilepsy:
            limbic system
            partial:
                secondarily generalized
                with impairment of consciousness
                with memory and ideational disturbances
                psychomotor
                psychosensory
                temporal lobe
        Epileptic automatism
        For code **345.40**: Ⓔⅹ 345.00-345.91, 348.30-348.39, 348.9 349.89-349.9;
        For code **345.41**: 249.60-249.61, 250.60-250.63, 345.00-345.91, 348.8-348.9, 349.89-349.9

● **345.5 Localization-related (focal) (partial) epilepsy and**
  [0-1] **epileptic syndromes with simple partial seizures**🅒
        Epilepsy:
            Bravais-Jacksonian NOS
            focal (motor) NOS
            Jacksonian NOS
            motor partial
            partial NOS
                without mention of impairment of consciousness
            sensory-induced
            somatomotor
            somatosensory
            visceral
            visual
        For code **345.50**: Ⓔⅹ 345.00-345.91, 348.30-348.39, 348.9, 349.89-349.9;
        For code **345.51**: Ⓔⅹ 249.60-249.61, 250.60-250.63, 345.00-345.91, 348.8-348.9, 349.89-349.9

● **345.6 Infantile spasms**🅒
  [0-1]   Hypsarrhythmia
        Lightning spasms
        Salaam attacks
        Excludes *salaam tic (781.0)*
        For code **345.60**: Ⓔⅹ 345.00-345.91, 348.30-348.39, 348.9, 349.89-349.9;
        For code **345.61**: Ⓔⅹ 249.60-249.61, 250.60-250.63, 345.00-345.91, 348.8-348.9, 349.89-349.9
        Coding Clinic: 1984, Nov-Dec, P11

● **345.7 Epilepsia partialis continua 0**🅒**, 1**🅒
  [0-1]   Kojevnikov's epilepsy
        Ⓔⅹ 249.60-249.61, 250.60-250.63, 345.00-345.91, 348.8-348.9, 349.89-349.9

● **345.8 Other forms of epilepsy and recurrent seizures** 🔾
[0-1]   Epilepsy:
        cursive [running]
        gelastic
    Recurrent seizures NOS
    Seizure disorder NOS
    (Ex:) 249.60-249.61, 250.60-250.63, 345.00-345.91, 348.8-348.9, 349.89-349.9

● **345.9 Epilepsy, unspecified 1** 🔾
[0-1]   Epileptic convulsions, fits, or seizures NOS
    Recurrent seizures NOS
    Seizure disorder NOS

> **Excludes**   *convulsion (convulsive) disorder (780.39)*
>   *convulsive seizure or fit NOS (780.39)*
>   *recurrent convulsions (780.39)*

    For code **345.91:** (Ex:) 249.60-249.61, 250.60-250.63, 345.00-345.91, 348.8-348.9, 349.89-349.9

    Coding Clinic: 2009, Q2, P11; 2008, Q1, P17; 1993, Q1, P24; 1987, Nov-Dec, P12

Item 6-8   Migraine headache is described as an intense pulsing or throbbing pain in one area of the head. It can be accompanied by extreme sensitivity to light (photophoic) and sound and is three times more common in women than in men. Symptoms include nausea and vomiting. Research indicates migraine headaches are caused by inherited abnormalities in genes that control the activities of certain cell populations in the brain.

● **346 Migraine**

> **Excludes**   *headache:*
>   *NOS (784.0)*
>   *syndromes (339.00-339.89)*

The following fifth-digit subclassification is for use with category 346:
    Coding Clinic: 2008, Q4, P102-109

> 0   **without mention of intractable migraine without mention of status migrainosus**
> 1   **with intractable migraine, so stated, without mention of status migrainosus**
> 2   **without mention of intractable migraine with status migrainosus**
> 3   **with intractable migraine, so stated, with status migrainosus**

Intractable migraine: Not easily cured or managed; relentless pain from a migraine

● **346.0 Migraine with aura**
[0-3]   Basilar migraine
    Classic migraine
    Migraine preceded or accompanied by transient focal neurological phenomena
    Migraine triggered seizures
    Migraine with acute-onset aura
    Migraine with aura without headache (migraine equivalents)
    Migraine with prolonged aura
    Migraine with typical aura
    Retinal migraine

> **Excludes**   *persistent migraine aura (346.5, 346.6)*

● **346.1 Migraine without aura**
[0-3]   Common migraine

● **346.2 Variants of migraine, not elsewhere classified**
[0-3]   Abdominal migraine
    Cyclical vomiting associated with migraine
    Ophthalmoplegic migraine
    Periodic headache syndromes in child or adolescent

> **Excludes**   *cyclical vomiting NOS (536.2)*
>   *psychogenic cyclical vomiting (306.4)*

● **346.3 Hemiplegic migraine**
[0-3]   Familial migraine
    Sporadic migraine

● **346.4 Menstrual migraine** ♀
[0-3]   Menstrual headache
    Menstrually related migraine
    Premenstrual headache
    Premenstrual migraine
    Pure menstrual migraine

● **346.5 Persistent migraine aura without cerebral**
[0-3] **infarction**
    Persistent migraine aura NOS

● **346.6 Persistent migraine aura with cerebral**
[0-3] **infarction** 🔾
    For code **346.60:** (Ex:) 346.60-346.63, 433.00-434.91;
    For codes **346.61-346.63:** (Ex:) 346.60-346.63, 433.00-434.91, 436

● **346.7 Chronic migraine without aura**
[0-3]   Transformed migraine without aura

● **346.8 Other forms of migraine**
[0-3]

● **346.9 Migraine, unspecified**
[0-3]   **Coding Clinic: 1985, Nov-Dec, P16**

● **347 Cataplexy and narcolepsy**
    Cataplexy is a disorder evidenced by seizures. **Narcolepsy** *is difficulty remaining awake during daytime.*
    Coding Clinic: 2004, Q4, P74-75

● **347.0 Narcolepsy**

    347.00 Without cataplexy
        Narcolepsy NOS

    347.01 With cataplexy

● **347.1 Narcolepsy in conditions classified elsewhere**
    Code first underlying condition

▶ **347.10 Without cataplexy**

▶ **347.11 With cataplexy**

◀ New   ◀▥ Revised   ~~deleted~~ Deleted   ● Unacceptable Principal Diagnosis   ● Use Additional Digit(s)
▶ Manifestation Code   **OGCR** Official Guidelines   **Coding Clinic**   Excludes   Includes   Use additional   Code first   Omit code

● **348   Other conditions of brain**

  348.0   Cerebral cysts
     Arachnoid cyst   Porencephaly, acquired
     Porencephalic cyst   Pseudoporencephaly

  348.1   Anoxic brain damage🔾
     Brain permanently damaged by lack of oxygen perfusion
     through brain tissues. This is the result of another
     problem, so use an additional E code to identify
     the cause.

     | **Excludes** | *that occurring in:*
         abortion (634–638 with .7, 639.8)
         ectopic or molar pregnancy (639.8)
         labor or delivery (668.2, 669.4)
         that of newborn (767.0, 768.0–768.9,
         772.1–772.2)

     Use additional E code to identify cause
     (Ex) 249.60-249.61, 249.80-249.91, 250.60-250.63, 250.80-250.93,
     348.1-348.2, 349.89-349.9

  348.2   Benign intracranial hypertension
     Pseudotumor cerebri

     | **Excludes** | *hypertensive encephalopathy (437.2)*

● **348.3   Encephalopathy, not elsewhere classified**
     A general term for any degenerative brain disease
     Coding Clinic: 2003, Q4, P58-59; 1997, Q3, P5

    348.30   Encephalopathy, unspecified🔾
       (Ex) 333.92, 344.81, 348.31-348.39

    348.31   Metabolic encephalopathy🔾
       Septic encephalopathy

       | **Excludes** | *toxic metabolic encephalopathy*
         (349.82)
       (Ex) 333.92, 344.81, 348.30, 348.39

    348.39   Other encephalopathy🔾

       | **Excludes** | *encephalopathy:*
         alcoholic (291.2)
         hepatic (572.2)
         hypertensive (437.2)
         toxic (349.82)
       (Ex) 333.92, 344.81, 348.30-348.31

  348.4   Compression of brain🔾
     Compression brain (stem)
     Herniation brain (stem)
     Posterior fossa compression syndrome
     (Ex) 342.90

  348.5   Cerebral edema🔾
     (Ex) 348.5

● **348.8   Other conditions of brain**   ◀▥
     ~~Cerebral:~~
       ~~calcification~~
       ~~fungus~~
     Coding Clinic: 1992, Q3, P8; 1987, Sept-Oct, P9

    348.81   Temporal sclerosis   ◀
       Hippocampal sclerosis   ◀
       Mesial temporal sclerosis   ◀

    348.89   Other conditions of brain   ◀
       Cerebral: ◀
         calcification   ◀
         fungus   ◀

  348.9   Unspecified condition of brain

● **349   Other and unspecified disorders of the nervous system**

  349.0   Reaction to spinal or lumbar puncture
     Headache following lumbar puncture
     Cerebral spinal fluid (CSF) maintains a specific level
     of pressure inside brain and spinal cord. If
     this pressure does not return to normal after a
     puncture, headache will result.
     Coding Clinic: 1999, Q2, P9-10; 1990, Q3, P18

  349.1   Nervous system complications from surgically
     implanted device🔾

     | **Excludes** | *immediate postoperative complications*
         (997.00–997.09)
         mechanical complications of nervous system
         device (996.2)
     (Ex) 249.60-249.61, 249.80-249.91, 250.60-250.63, 250.80-250.93, 349.1,
     349.89-349.9

  349.2   Disorders of meninges, not elsewhere classified
     Adhesions, meningeal (cerebral) (spinal)
     Cyst, spinal meninges
     Meningocele, acquired
     Pseudomeningocele, acquired
     Coding Clinic: 2006, Q1, P15-16; 1998, Q2, P18; 1994, Q3, P4; Q1,
     P22-23

● **349.3   Dural tear**
     Coding Clinic: 2008, Q4, P109-110

    349.31   Accidental puncture or laceration of dura
       during a procedure🔾
       Incidental (inadvertent) durotomy
       (Ex) 349.31-349.39, 997.91-997.99, 998.2, 998.81, 998.83-998.9

    349.39   Other dural tear🔾
       (Ex) 349.31-349.39, 997.91-997.99, 998.2, 998.81, 998.83-998.9

● **349.8   Other specified disorders of nervous system**

    349.81   Cerebrospinal fluid rhinorrhea🔾

       | **Excludes** | *cerebrospinal fluid otorrhea (388.61)*
       (Ex) 249.60-249.61, 249.80-249.91, 250.60-250.63, 250.80-250.93,
       349.81, 349.89-349.9

    349.82   Toxic encephalopathy🔾
       Toxic metabolic encephalopathy

       Use additional E code to identify cause
       (Ex) 013.60-013.66, 017.90-017.96, 036.1, 049.8-049.9, 052.0,
       054.3, 058.21-058.29, 062.0-063.9, 072.2, 090.41, 094.81,
       130.0, 249.60-249.61, 249.80-249.91, 250.60-250.63,
       250.80-250.93, 323.01-323.9, 341.20-341.22,
       348.30-348.39, 348.8-348.9, 349.82-349.9

    349.89   Other

  349.9   Unspecified disorders of nervous system
     Disorder of nervous system (central) NOS

DISEASES OF THE NERVOUS SYSTEM AND SENSE ORGANS (320–389)

Item 6–9 The **peripheral nervous system** consists of 31 pairs of spinal nerves, 12 pairs of cranial nerves, and the autonomic nerves, which are divided into the parasympathetic and sympathetic nerves. The cranial nerves are: olfactory (I), optic (II), oculomotor (III), trochlear (IV), trigeminal (V), abducens (VI), facial (VII), vestibulocochlear (VIII), glossopharyngeal (IX), vagus (X), accessory (XI), and hypoglossal (XII).

Item 6-10 Trigeminal neuralgia, tic douloureux, is a pain syndrome diagnosed from the patient's history alone. The condition is characterized by pain and a brief facial spasm or tic. Pain is unilateral and follows the sensory distribution of cranial nerve V, typically radiating to the maxillary (V2) or mandibular (V3) area.

DISORDERS OF THE PERIPHERAL NERVOUS SYSTEM (350–359)

Excludes *diseases of:*
> *acoustic [8th] nerve (388.5)*
> *oculomotor [3rd, 4th, 6th] nerves (378.0–378.9)*
> *optic [2nd] nerve (377.0–377.9)*
> *peripheral autonomic nerves (337.0–337.9)*
> *neuralgia NOS or "rheumatic" (729.2)*
> *neuritis NOS or "rheumatic" (729.2)*
> *radiculitis NOS or "rheumatic" (729.2)*
> *peripheral neuritis in pregnancy (646.4)*

● **350   Trigeminal nerve disorders**
Includes   disorders of 5th cranial nerve

350.1   Trigeminal neuralgia
Tic douloureux
Trifacial neuralgia
Trigeminal neuralgia NOS
Excludes   *postherpetic (053.12)*

350.2   Atypical face pain

350.8   Other specified trigeminal nerve disorders

350.9   Trigeminal nerve disorder, unspecified

● **351   Facial nerve disorders**
Includes   disorders of 7th cranial nerve
Excludes   *that in newborn (767.5)*

351.0   Bell's palsy
Facial palsy

351.1   Geniculate ganglionitis
Geniculate ganglionitis NOS
Excludes   *herpetic (053.11)*

Coding Clinic: 2002, Q2, P8

Item 6-11 The most common facial nerve disorder is **Bell's Palsy,** which occurs suddenly and results in facial drooping unilaterally. This disorder is the result of a reaction to a virus that causes the facial nerve in the ear to swell resulting in pressure in the bony canal.

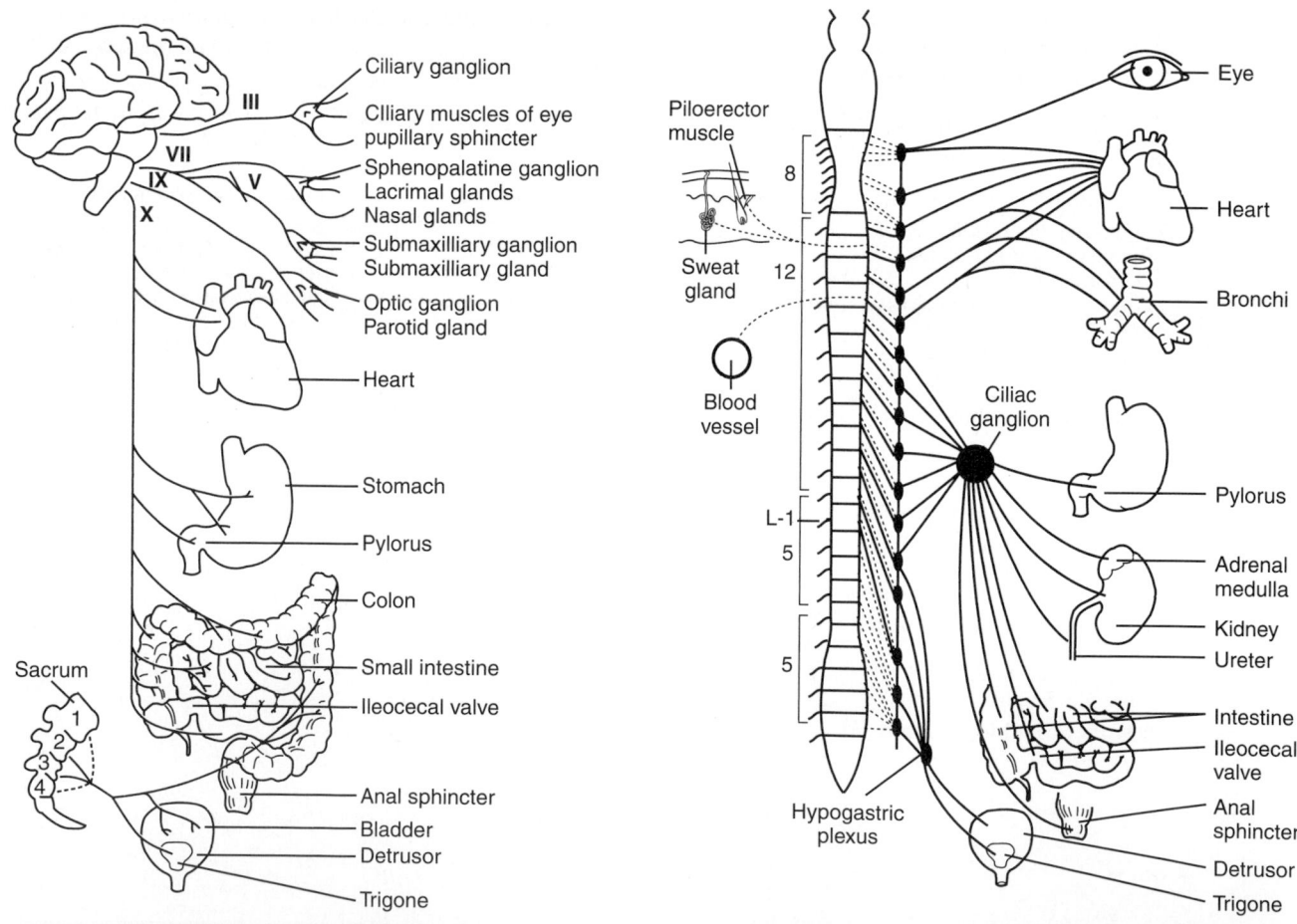

Figure 6–3   **A.** Parasympathetic nervous system. **B.** Sympathetic nervous system. (From Buck CJ: Step-by-Step Medical Coding, 2nd ed. Philadelphia, WB Saunders, 1998, pp 186 and 187.)

◀ New   ◀▥ Revised   ~~deleted~~ Deleted   ● Unacceptable Principal Diagnosis   ● Use Additional Digit(s)
▶ Manifestation Code   **OGCR** Official Guidelines   **Coding Clinic**   Excludes   Includes   Use additional   Code first   Omit code

351.8 Other facial nerve disorders
Facial myokymia
Melkersson's syndrome
Coding Clinic: 2002, Q3, P12-13

351.9 Facial nerve disorder, unspecified

● **352 Disorders of other cranial nerves**

352.0 Disorders of olfactory [1st] nerve

352.1 Glossopharyngeal neuralgia
Coding Clinic: 1987, Jan-Feb, P14

352.2 Other disorders of glossopharyngeal [9th] nerve

352.3 Disorders of pneumogastric [10th] nerve
Disorders of vagal nerve
| **Excludes** | *paralysis of vocal cords or larynx (478.30–478.34)* |

352.4 Disorders of accessory [11th] nerve

352.5 Disorders of hypoglossal [12th] nerve

352.6 Multiple cranial nerve palsies
Collet-Sicard syndrome
Polyneuritis cranialis

352.9 Unspecified disorder of cranial nerves

● **353 Nerve root and plexus disorders**
| **Excludes** | *conditions due to:* |
intervertebral disc disorders (722.0–722.9)
spondylosis (720.0–721.9)
vertebrogenic disorders (723.0–724.9)

353.0 Brachial plexus lesions
Cervical rib syndrome
Costoclavicular syndrome
Scalenus anticus syndrome
Thoracic outlet syndrome
| **Excludes** | *brachial neuritis or radiculitis NOS (723.4)* |
that in newborn (767.6)
Coding Clinic: 2006, Q3, P12

353.1 Lumbosacral plexus lesions

353.2 Cervical root lesions, not elsewhere classified

● **353.3 Thoracic root lesions, not elsewhere classified**

353.4 Lumbosacral root lesions, not elsewhere classified

353.5 Neuralgic amyotrophy
Parsonage-Aldren-Turner syndrome
Phantom limb syndrome: Patients with amputated limbs feel sensations in a limb that no longer exists. There is no separate code for phantom limb pain, and the pain can be part of the syndrome.

Code first *any associated underlying disease, such as:*
diabetes mellitus (249.6, 250.6)

353.6 Phantom limb (syndrome)

353.8 Other nerve root and plexus disorders

353.9 Unspecified nerve root and plexus disorder

● **354 Mononeuritis of upper limb and mononeuritis multiplex**

354.0 Carpal tunnel syndrome *(CTS)*
Of the wrist
Median nerve entrapment
Partial thenar atrophy

354.1 Other lesion of median nerve
Median nerve neuritis

354.2 Lesion of ulnar nerve
Cubital tunnel syndrome
Tardy ulnar nerve palsy

354.3 Lesion of radial nerve
Acute radial nerve palsy
Coding Clinic: 1987, Nov-Dec, P6

354.4 Causalgia of upper limb
Complex regional pain syndrome type II of the upper limb
| **Excludes** | *causalgia:* |
NOS (355.9)
lower limb (355.71)
complex regional pain syndrome type II of the lower limb (355.71)

354.5 Mononeuritis multiplex
Combinations of single conditions classifiable to 354 or 355

354.8 Other mononeuritis of upper limb

354.9 Mononeuritis of upper limb, unspecified

● **355 Mononeuritis of lower limb**
Coding Clinic: 1989, Q2, P12

355.0 Lesion of sciatic nerve
| **Excludes** | *sciatica NOS (724.3)* |
Coding Clinic: 1989, Q2, P12

355.1 Meralgia paresthetica
Lateral cutaneous femoral nerve of thigh compression or syndrome

355.2 Other lesion of femoral nerve

355.3 Lesion of lateral popliteal nerve
Lesion of common peroneal nerve

355.4 Lesion of medial popliteal nerve

355.5 Tarsal tunnel syndrome
Of the ankle

355.6 Lesion of plantar nerve
Morton's metatarsalgia, neuralgia, or neuroma

● **355.7 Other mononeuritis of lower limb**

355.71 Causalgia of lower limb
| **Excludes** | *causalgia:* |
NOS (355.9)
upper limb (354.4)
complex regional pain syndrome type II of the upper limb (354.4)

355.79 Other mononeuritis of lower limb

355.8 Mononeuritis of lower limb, unspecified

355.9 Mononeuritis of unspecified site
Causalgia NOS
Complex regional pain syndrome NOS
| **Excludes** | *causalgia:* |
lower limb (355.71)
upper limb (354.4)
complex regional pain syndrome:
lower limb (355.71)
upper limb (354.4)

DISEASES OF THE NERVOUS SYSTEM AND SENSE ORGANS (320–389)

N Newborn Age: 0   P Pediatric Age: 0–17   M Maternity Age: 12–55   A Adult Age: 15–124   ♀ Females Only   ♂ Males Only

ⒺⓍ CC Exclusions   🔖 Complication\Comorbidity   🔖 Major C\C   🔖 Present on Admission Requirement   🔖 Hospital-Acquired Condition   857

● 356 **Hereditary and idiopathic peripheral neuropathy**
Any disease that affects nervous system and of an unknown cause.

     356.0 **Hereditary peripheral neuropathy**
         Déjérine-Sottas disease

     356.1 **Peroneal muscular atrophy**
         Charcot-Marie-Tooth disease
         Neuropathic muscular atrophy

     356.2 **Hereditary sensory neuropathy**

     356.3 **Refsum's disease** 🔊
         Heredopathia atactica polyneuritiformis
         (Ex) 350.1-357.9

     356.4 **Idiopathic progressive polyneuropathy**

     356.8 **Other specified idiopathic peripheral neuropathy**
         Supranuclear paralysis

     356.9 **Unspecified**

● 357 **Inflammatory and toxic neuropathy**

     357.0 **Acute infective polyneuritis** 🔊
         Guillain-Barre syndrome
         Postinfectious polyneuritis
         (Ex) 003.21, 013.00-013.16, 036.0, 036.89-036.9, 041.81-041.9, 047.0-047.9, 049.0-049.1, 053.0, 054.72, 072.1, 090.42, 091.81, 094.2, 098.89, 100.81, 112.83, 114.2, 115.01, 115.11, 115.91, 130.0, 139.8, 320.0-322.9, 349.89-349.9, 357.0
         Coding Clinic: 1998, Q2, P12

     ▶ *357.1* ***Polyneuropathy in collagen vascular disease***

         Code first *underlying disease, as:*
            disseminated lupus erythematosus (710.0)
            polyarteritis nodosa (446.0)
            rheumatoid arthritis (714.0)

     ▶ *357.2* ***Polyneuropathy in diabetes***

         Code first *underlying disease (249.6, 250.6)*
         Coding Clinic: 2009, Q2, P11; 2008, Q3, P5-6; 2003, Q4, P105; 1992, Q2, P15

     ▶ *357.3* ***Polyneuropathy in malignant disease***

         Code first *underlying disease (140.0–208.9)*

     ▶ *357.4* ***Polyneuropathy in other diseases classified elsewhere***

         Code first *underlying disease, as:*
            amyloidosis (277.30–277.39)
            beriberi (265.0)
            chronic uremia (585.9)
            deficiency of B vitamins (266.0–266.9)
            diphtheria (032.0–032.9)
            hypoglycemia (251.2)
            pellagra (265.2)
            porphyria (277.1)
            sarcoidosis (135)
            uremia NOS (586)

         Excludes *polyneuropathy in:*
            herpes zoster (053.13)
            mumps (072.72)
         Coding Clinic: 2008, Q2, P8-9; 1998, Q2, P15

     357.5 **Alcoholic polyneuropathy**

     357.6 **Polyneuropathy due to drugs**
         Use additional E code to identify drug

     357.7 **Polyneuropathy due to other toxic agents**
         Use additional E code to identify toxic agent

   ● 357.8 **Other**
         Coding Clinic: 2002, Q4, P47-48; 1998, Q2, P12

         357.81 **Chronic inflammatory demyelinating polyneuritis** 🔊
            (Ex) 351.0-353.5, 353.8-356.9, 357.81-357.89

         357.82 **Critical illness polyneuropathy** 🔊
            Acute motor neuropathy
            (Ex) 351.0-353.5, 353.8-356.9, 357.81-357.9
            Coding Clinic: 2003, Q4, P111

         357.89 **Other inflammatory and toxic neuropathy**

     357.9 **Unspecified**

● 358 **Myoneural disorders**

   ● 358.0 **Myasthenia gravis**
         Acquired and results in fatigable muscle weakness exacerbated by activity and improved with rest. Caused by autoimmune assault against nerve-muscle junction.
         Coding Clinic: 2003, Q4, P59-60

         358.00 **Myasthenia gravis without (acute) exacerbation**

         358.01 **Myasthenia gravis with acute exacerbation** 🔊
            Myasthenia gravis in crisis
            (Ex) 249.60-249.61, 249.80-249.91, 250.60-250.63, 250.80-250.93, 349.89-349.9, 358.00-358.1
            Coding Clinic: 2007, Q4, P108-109; 2004, Q4, P139

     ▶ *358.1* ***Myasthenic syndromes in diseases classified elsewhere*** 🔊
         Eaton-Lambert syndrome from stated cause classified elsewhere

         Code first *underlying disease, as:*
            botulism (005.1, 040.41–040.42)
            hypothyroidism (244.0–244.9)
            malignant neoplasm (140.0–208.9)
            pernicious anemia (281.0)
            thyrotoxicosis (242.0–242.9)
         (Ex) 249.60-249.61, 249.80-249.91, 250.60-250.63, 250.80-250.93, 349.89-349.9, 358.00-358.1

     358.2 **Toxic myoneural disorders**
         Use additional E code to identify toxic agent

     358.8 **Other specified myoneural disorders**

     358.9 **Myoneural disorders, unspecified**
         Coding Clinic: 2002, Q2, P16

◀ New   ◀‖‖ Revised   ~~deleted~~ Deleted   ● Unacceptable Principal Diagnosis   ● Use Additional Digit(s)
▶ Manifestation Code   OGCR Official Guidelines   **Coding Clinic**   Excludes   Includes   Use additional   Code first   Omit code

Item 6-12 Muscular dystrophies (MD) are a group of rare inherited muscle diseases. Voluntary muscles become progressively weaker. In the late stages of MD, fat and connective tissue replace muscle fibers. In some types of muscular dystrophy, heart muscles, other involuntary muscles, and other organs are affected. **Myopathies** is a general term for neuromuscular diseases in which the muscle fibers dysfunction for any one of many reasons, resulting in muscular weakness.

● **359 Muscular dystrophies and other myopathies**

> **Excludes** *idiopathic polymyositis (710.4)*

359.0 Congenital hereditary muscular dystrophy 🅒
>   Benign congenital myopathy
>   Central core disease
>   Centronuclear myopathy
>   Myotubular myopathy
>   Nemaline body disease

> **Excludes** *arthrogryposis multiplex congenita (754.89)*

> Ⓔ 249.60-249.61, 249.80-249.91, 250.60-250.63, 250.80-250.93, 349.89-349.9, 359.0-359.1

359.1 Hereditary progressive muscular dystrophy 🅒
>   Muscular dystrophy:
>   NOS
>   distal
>   Duchenne
>   Erb's
>   fascioscapulohumeral
>   Gower's
>   Landouzy-Déjérine
>   limb-girdle
>   ocular
>   oculopharyngeal
> Ⓔ 249.60-249.61, 249.80-249.91, 250.60-250.63, 250.80-250.93, 349.89-349.9, 359.0-359.1

● **359.2 Myotonic disorders**

> **Excludes** *periodic paralysis (359.3)*

> **Coding Clinic: 2007, Q4, P75-77**

359.21 Myotonic muscular dystrophy
>   Dystrophia myotonica
>   Myotonia atrophica
>   Myotonic dystrophy
>   Proximal myotonic myopathy (PROMM)
>   Steinert's disease

359.22 Myotonia congenita
>   Acetazolamide responsive myotonia
>   congenita
>   Dominant form (Thomsen's disease)
>   Myotonia levior   ◀
>   Recessive form (Becker's disease)

359.23 Myotonic chondrodystrophy
>   Congenital myotonic
>   chondrodystrophy
>   Schwartz-Jampel disease

359.24 Drug-induced myotonia
>   Use additional E code to identify drug

359.29 Other specified myotonic disorder
>   Myotonia fluctuans
>   ~~Myotonia levior~~
>   Myotonia permanens
>   Paramyotonia congenita
>   (of von Eulenburg)

359.3 Periodic paralysis
>   Familial periodic paralysis
>   Hyperkalemic periodic paralysis
>   Hypokalemic familial periodic paralysis
>   Hypokalemic periodic paralysis
>   Potassium sensitive periodic paralysis

> **Excludes** *paramyotonia congenita (of von Eulenburg) (359.29)*

359.4 Toxic myopathy 🅒
>   Use additional E code to identify toxic agent
> Ⓔ 349.89-349.9, 358.00-359.9

▸ **359.5 *Myopathy in endocrine diseases classified elsewhere***

> *Code first* underlying disease, as:
>   Addison's disease (255.41)
>   Cushing's syndrome (255.0)
>   hypopituitarism (253.2)
>   myxedema (244.0–244.9)
>   thyrotoxicosis (242.0–242.9)

▸ **359.6 *Symptomatic inflammatory myopathy in diseases classified elsewhere*** 🅒

> *Code first* underlying disease, as:
>   amyloidosis (277.30–277.39)
>   disseminated lupus erythematosus (710.0)
>   malignant neoplasm (140.0–208.9)
>   polyarteritis nodosa (446.0)
>   rheumatoid arthritis (714.0)
>   sarcoidosis (135)
>   scleroderma (710.1)
>   Sjögren's disease (710.2)
> Ⓔ 249.60-249.61, 249.80-249.91, 250.60-250.63, 250.80-250.93, 349.89-349.9, 358.00-359.9

● **359.7 Inflammatory and immune myopathies, NEC**   ◀

359.71 Inclusion body myositis   ◀
>   IBM

359.79 Other inflammatory and immune   ◀
>   **myopathies, NEC**   ◀
>   Inflammatory myopathy NOS

● **359.8 Other myopathies**
> **Coding Clinic: 2002, Q4, P47-48; 1990, Q3, P17**

359.81 Critical illness myopathy 🅒
>   Acute necrotizing myopathy
>   Acute quadriplegic myopathy
>   Intensive care (ICU) myopathy
>   Myopathy of critical illness
> Ⓔ 358.1-359.9

359.89 Other myopathies

359.9 Myopathy, unspecified

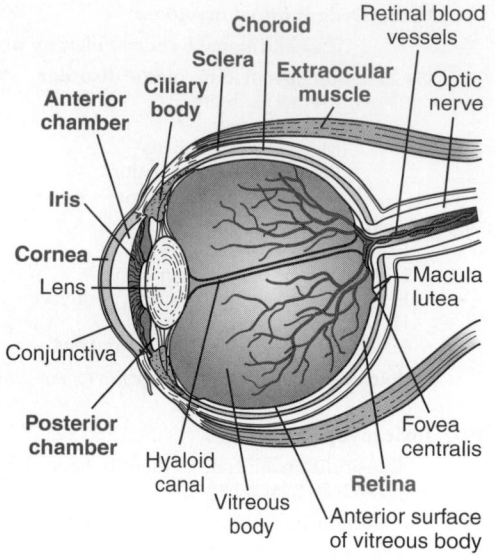

Figure 6–4 Eye and ocular adnexa. (From Buck CJ: Step-by-Step Medical Coding, 2005 ed. Philadelphia, WB Saunders, 2005.)

DISORDERS OF THE EYE AND ADNEXA (360–379)

Use additional external cause code, if applicable, to identify the cause of the eye condition

●360 **Disorders of the globe**

 Includes disorders affecting multiple structures of eye

●360.0 **Purulent endophthalmitis**

 Excludes bleb associated endophthalmitis (379.63)

 360.00 **Purulent endophthalmitis, unspecified** ✇
  (Ex:) 360.00-360.04, 360.13, 360.19, 364.05

 360.01 **Acute endophthalmitis** ✇
  (Ex:) 360.00-360.04, 360.13, 360.19, 364.05

 360.02 **Panophthalmitis** ✇
  (Ex:) 360.00-360.04, 360.13, 360.19, 364.05

 360.03 **Chronic endophthalmitis**

 360.04 **Vitreous abscess** ✇
  (Ex:) 360.00-360.19

●360.1 **Other endophthalmitis**

 Excludes bleb associated endophthalmitis (379.63)

 360.11 **Sympathetic uveitis** ✇
  (Ex:) 360.11-360.12

 360.12 **Panuveitis** ✇
  (Ex:) 360.11-360.12

 360.13 **Parasitic endophthalmitis NOS** ✇
  (Ex:) 360.00-360.04, 360.13, 360.19, 364.05

 360.14 **Ophthalmia nodosa**

 360.19 **Other** ✇
  Phacoanaphylactic endophthalmitis
  (Ex:) 360.00-360.04, 360.13, 360.19, 364.05

●360.2 **Degenerative disorders of globe**

 360.20 **Degenerative disorder of globe, unspecified**

 360.21 **Progressive high (degenerative) myopia**
  Malignant myopia

 360.23 **Siderosis**

 360.24 **Other metallosis**
  Chalcosis

 360.29 **Other**
  Excludes xerophthalmia (264.7)

●360.3 **Hypotony of eye**

 360.30 **Hypotony, unspecified**

 360.31 **Primary hypotony**

 360.32 **Ocular fistula causing hypotony**

 360.33 **Hypotony associated with other ocular disorders**

 360.34 **Flat anterior chamber**

●360.4 **Degenerated conditions of globe**

 360.40 **Degenerated globe or eye, unspecified**

 360.41 **Blind hypotensive eye**
  Atrophy of globe
  Phthisis bulbi

 360.42 **Blind hypertensive eye**
  Absolute glaucoma

 360.43 **Hemophthalmos, except current injury**
  Excludes traumatic (871.0–871.9,
   921.0–921.9)

 360.44 **Leucocoria**

●360.5 **Retained (old) intraocular foreign body, magnetic**

 Excludes current penetrating injury with magnetic
  foreign body (871.5)
  retained (old) foreign body of orbit (376.6)

 360.50 **Foreign body, magnetic, intraocular, unspecified**

 360.51 **Foreign body, magnetic, in anterior chamber**

 360.52 **Foreign body, magnetic, in iris or ciliary body**

 360.53 **Foreign body, magnetic, in lens**

 360.54 **Foreign body, magnetic, in vitreous**

 360.55 **Foreign body, magnetic, in posterior wall**

 360.59 **Foreign body, magnetic, in other or multiple sites**

●360.6 **Retained (old) intraocular foreign body, nonmagnetic**
  Retained (old) foreign body:
  NOS
  nonmagnetic

 Excludes current penetrating injury with
  (nonmagnetic) foreign body (871.6)
  retained (old) foreign body in orbit (376.6)

 360.60 **Foreign body, intraocular, unspecified**

 360.61 **Foreign body in anterior chamber**

 360.62 **Foreign body in iris or ciliary body**

 360.63 **Foreign body in lens**

 360.64 **Foreign body in vitreous**

 360.65 **Foreign body in posterior wall**

 360.69 **Foreign body in other or multiple sites**

●360.8 **Other disorders of globe**

 360.81 **Luxation of globe**

 360.89 **Other**

 360.9 **Unspecified disorder of globe**

◀ New ⬅ Revised deleted Deleted ● Unacceptable Principal Diagnosis ● Use Additional Digit(s)
▶ Manifestation Code **OGCR** Official Guidelines **Coding Clinic** Excludes Includes Use additional Code first Omit code

DISEASES OF THE NERVOUS SYSTEM AND SENSE ORGANS (320–389)

Item 6-13 Retinal detachments and defects are conditions of the eye in which the retina separates from the underlying tissue. Initial detachment may be localized, requiring rapid treatment (medical emergency) to avoid the entire retina from detaching, which leads to vision loss and blindness.

NON-RHEGMATOGENOUS RETINAL DETACHMENT

- Vitreous
- Retina
- Protein-rich fluid in sub-retinal space
- Retinal pigment epithelium

VITREOUS DETACHMENT

- Vitreous
- Posterior hyaloid
- Internal limiting membrane

RHEGMATOGENOUS RETINAL DETACHMENT

- Blood
- Vitreous
- Posterior hyaloid
- Retina
- Retinal tear
- Liquified vitreous
- Retinal pigment epithelium

Figure 6–5 Retinal detachment. (From Kumar: Robbins and Cotran: Pathologic Basis of Disease, 7th ed. 2005, Saunders)

● **361   Retinal detachments and defects**

● **361.0   Retinal detachment with retinal defect**
  Rhegmatogenous retinal detachment

  Excludes *detachment of retinal pigment epithelium (362.42–362.43)*
  retinal detachment (serous) (without defect) (361.2)

  Coding Clinic: 1994, Q1, P17

  361.00   Retinal detachment with retinal defect, unspecified

361.01   Recent detachment, partial, with single defect

361.02   Recent detachment, partial, with multiple defects

361.03   Recent detachment, partial, with giant tear

361.04   Recent detachment, partial, with retinal dialysis
  Dialysis (juvenile) of retina (with detachment)

361.05   Recent detachment, total or subtotal

361.06   Old detachment, partial
  Delimited old retinal detachment

361.07   Old detachment, total or subtotal

● **361.1   Retinoschisis and retinal cysts**

  Excludes *juvenile retinoschisis (362.73)*
  microcystoid degeneration of retina (362.62)
  parasitic cyst of retina (360.13)

  361.10   Retinoschisis, unspecified

  361.11   Flat retinoschisis

  361.12   Bullous retinoschisis

  361.13   Primary retinal cysts

  361.14   Secondary retinal cysts

  361.19   Other
  Pseudocyst of retina

361.2   Serous retinal detachment🅒
  Retinal detachment without retinal defect

  Excludes *central serous retinopathy (362.41)*
  retinal pigment epithelium detachment (362.42–362.43)

  (Ex) 361.00-361.9, 362.40-362.43

● **361.3   Retinal defects without detachment**

  Excludes *chorioretinal scars after surgery for detachment (363.30–363.35)*
  peripheral retinal degeneration without defect (362.60–362.66)

  361.30   Retinal defect, unspecified
  Retinal break(s) NOS

  361.31   Round hole of retina without detachment

  361.32   Horseshoe tear of retina without detachment
  Operculum of retina without mention of detachment

  361.33   Multiple defects of retina without detachment

● **361.8   Other forms of retinal detachment**

  361.81   Traction detachment of retina🅒
  (Ex) 361.00-361.9, 362.40-362.43
  Traction detachment with vitreoretinal organization

  361.89   Other🅒
  (Ex) 361.00-361.9, 362.40-362.43
  Coding Clinic: 1999, Q3, P12

  361.9   Unspecified retinal detachment🅒
  (Ex) 361.00-361.9, 362.40-362.43
  Coding Clinic: 1987, Nov-Dec, P10

DISEASES OF THE NERVOUS SYSTEM AND SENSE ORGANS (320–389)

● **362 Other retinal disorders**

| Excludes | chorioretinal scars (363.30–363.35)
chorioretinitis (363.0–363.2)

● **362.0 Diabetic retinopathy**

Code first diabetes (249.5, 250.5)

Most common diabetic eye disease and leading cause of blindness in adults. Caused by changes in the blood vessels of retina in which the blood vessels swell and leak fluid into retinal surface.

▶ **362.01 Background diabetic retinopathy**
Diabetic retinal microaneurysms
Diabetic retinopathy NOS

▶ **362.02 Proliferative diabetic retinopathy**
Coding Clinic: 1996, Q3, P5

▶ **362.03 Nonproliferative diabetic retinopathy NOS**

▶ **362.04 Mild nonproliferative diabetic retinopathy**

▶ **362.05 Moderate nonproliferative diabetic retinopathy**

▶ **362.06 Severe nonproliferative diabetic retinopathy**
Coding Clinic: 2005, Q4, P65-67

▶ **362.07 Diabetic macular edema**
Diabetic retinal edema

Note: Code 362.07 must be used with a code for diabetic retinopathy (362.01–362.06)

● **362.1 Other background retinopathy and retinal vascular changes**

362.10 Background retinopathy, unspecified
Coding Clinic: 2006, Q1, P12

362.11 Hypertensive retinopathy
OGCR Section I.C.7.a.6

Two codes are necessary to identify the condition. First assign the code from subcategory 362.11, Hypertensive retinopathy, then the appropriate code from categories 401–405 to indicate the type of hypertension.

362.12 Exudative retinopathy
Coats' syndrome
Coding Clinic: 1999, Q3, P12

362.13 Changes in vascular appearance
Vascular sheathing of retina
Use additional code for any associated atherosclerosis (440.8)

362.14 Retinal microaneurysms NOS

362.15 Retinal telangiectasia

362.16 Retinal neovascularization NOS
Neovascularization:
choroidal
subretinal

362.17 Other intraretinal microvascular abnormalities
Retinal varices

362.18 Retinal vasculitis
Eales' disease
Retinal:
arteritis
endarteritis
perivasculitis
phlebitis

● **362.2 Other proliferative retinopathy**

362.20 Retinopathy of prematurity, unspecified
Retinopathy of prematurity NOS
Coding Clinic: 2008, Q4, P110-111

362.21 Retrolental fibroplasia
Cicatricial retinopathy of prematurity

362.22 Retinopathy of prematurity, stage 0

362.23 Retinopathy of prematurity, stage 1

362.24 Retinopathy of prematurity, stage 2

362.25 Retinopathy of prematurity, stage 3

362.26 Retinopathy of prematurity, stage 4

362.27 Retinopathy of prematurity, stage 5

362.29 Other nondiabetic proliferative retinopathy
Coding Clinic: 1996, Q3, P5

● **362.3 Retinal vascular occlusion**
Blockage in vessel of the retina

362.30 Retinal vascular occlusion, unspecified 🔾
(Ex) 362.30-362.37

362.31 Central retinal artery occlusion 🔾
(Ex) 362.30-362.37

362.32 Arterial branch occlusion 🔾
(Ex) 362.30-362.37

362.33 Partial arterial occlusion 🔾
Hollenhorst plaque
Retinal microembolism
(Ex) 362.30-362.37

362.34 Transient arterial occlusion 🔾
Amaurosis fugax
(Ex) 362.30-362.37
Coding Clinic: 2000, Q1, P16

362.35 Central retinal vein occlusion 🔾
(Ex) 362.30-362.37
Coding Clinic: 1993, Q2, P6

362.36 Venous tributary (branch) occlusion

362.37 Venous engorgement
Occlusion:
of retinal vein
incipient of retinal vein
partial of retinal vein

● **362.4 Separation of retinal layers**

| Excludes | retinal detachment (serous) (361.2)
rhegmatogenous (361.00–361.07)

362.40 Retinal layer separation, unspecified 🔾
(Ex) 361.00-361.9, 362.40-362.43

362.41 Central serous retinopathy

362.42 Serous detachment of retinal pigment epithelium 🔾
Exudative detachment of retinal pigment epithelium
(Ex) 361.00-361.9, 362.40-362.43

362.43 Hemorrhagic detachment of retinal pigment epithelium 🔾
(Ex) 361.00-361.9, 362.40-362.43

◀ New　◀▥ Revised　deleted Deleted　● Unacceptable Principal Diagnosis　● Use Additional Digit(s)
▶ Manifestation Code　OGCR Official Guidelines　Coding Clinic　Excludes　Includes　Use additional　Code first　Omit code

DISEASES OF THE NERVOUS SYSTEM AND SENSE ORGANS (320–389)

Item 6-14 Macular degeneration is typically age-related, chronic, and is evidenced by deterioration of the macula (the part of the retina that provides for central field vision), resulting in blurred vision or a blind spot in the center of visual field while not affecting peripheral vision.

● **362.5 Degeneration of macula and posterior pole**

> **Excludes** degeneration of optic disc (377.21–377.24)
> hereditary retinal degeneration [dystrophy] (362.70–362.77)

362.50 Macular degeneration (senile), unspecified

362.51 Nonexudative senile macular degeneration
Senile macular degeneration:
atrophic
dry

362.52 Exudative senile macular degeneration
Kuhnt-Junius degeneration
Senile macular degeneration:
disciform
wet

362.53 Cystoid macular degeneration
Cystoid macular edema

362.54 Macular cyst, hole, or pseudohole

362.55 Toxic maculopathy

> Use additional E code to identify drug, if drug induced

362.56 Macular puckering
Preretinal fibrosis

362.57 Drusen (degenerative)

● **362.6 Peripheral retinal degenerations**

> **Excludes** hereditary retinal degeneration [dystrophy] (362.70–362.77)
> retinal degeneration with retinal defect (361.00–361.07)

362.60 Peripheral retinal degeneration, unspecified

362.61 Paving stone degeneration

362.62 Microcystoid degeneration
Blessig's cysts
Iwanoff's cysts

362.63 Lattice degeneration
Palisade degeneration of retina

362.64 Senile reticular degeneration

362.65 Secondary pigmentary degeneration
Pseudoretinitis pigmentosa

362.66 Secondary vitreoretinal degenerations

● **362.7 Hereditary retinal dystrophies**

362.70 Hereditary retinal dystrophy, unspecified

▶ *362.71 Retinal dystrophy in systemic or cerebroretinal lipidoses*

> Code first underlying disease, as:
> cerebroretinal lipidoses (330.1)
> systemic lipidoses (272.7)

▶ *362.72 Retinal dystrophy in other systemic disorders and syndromes*

> Code first underlying disease, as:
> Bassen-Kornzweig syndrome (272.5)
> Refsum's disease (356.3)

362.73 Vitreoretinal dystrophies
Juvenile retinoschisis

362.74 Pigmentary retinal dystrophy
Retinal dystrophy, albipunctate
Retinitis pigmentosa

362.75 Other dystrophies primarily involving the sensory retina
Progressive cone (-rod) dystrophy
Stargardt's disease

362.76 Dystrophies primarily involving the retinal pigment epithelium
Fundus flavimaculatus
Vitelliform dystrophy

362.77 Dystrophies primarily involving Bruch's membrane
Dystrophy:
hyaline
pseudoinflammatory foveal
Hereditary drusen

● **362.8 Other retinal disorders**

> **Excludes** chorioretinal inflammations (363.0–363.2)
> chorioretinal scars (363.30–363.35)

362.81 Retinal hemorrhage
Hemorrhage:
preretinal
retinal (deep) (superficial)
subretinal
Coding Clinic: 1996, Q4, P43-44

362.82 Retinal exudates and deposits

362.83 Retinal edema
Retinal:
cotton wool spots
edema (localized) (macular) (peripheral)

362.84 Retinal ischemia 🔴
(Ex) 362.81-362.89

362.85 Retinal nerve fiber bundle defects

362.89 Other retinal disorders

362.9 Unspecified retinal disorder

● **363 Chorioretinal inflammations, scars, and other disorders of choroid**

● **363.0 Focal chorioretinitis and focal retinochoroiditis**

> **Excludes** focal chorioretinitis or retinochoroiditis in:
> histoplasmosis (115.02, 115.12, 115.92)
> toxoplasmosis (130.2)
> congenital infection (771.2)

363.00 Focal chorioretinitis, unspecified
Focal:
choroiditis or chorioretinitis NOS
retinitis or retinochoroiditis NOS

363.01 Focal choroiditis and chorioretinitis, juxtapapillary

363.03 Focal choroiditis and chorioretinitis of other posterior pole

363.04 Focal choroiditis and chorioretinitis, peripheral

363.05 Focal retinitis and retinochoroiditis, juxtapapillary
Neuroretinitis

363.06 Focal retinitis and retinochoroiditis, macular or paramacular

363.07 Focal retinitis and retinochoroiditis of other posterior pole

363.08 Focal retinitis and retinochoroiditis, peripheral

N Newborn Age: 0　　P Pediatric Age: 0–17　　M Maternity Age: 12–55　　A Adult Age: 15–124　　♀ Females Only　　♂ Males Only
(Ex) CC Exclusions　　🔴 Complication\Comorbidity　　🔴 Major C\C　　🔴 Present on Admission Requirement　　🔴 Hospital-Acquired Condition

863

● **363.1   Disseminated chorioretinitis and disseminated retinochoroiditis**

> **Excludes**   *disseminated choroiditis or chorioretinitis in secondary syphilis (091.51)*
> *neurosyphilitic disseminated retinitis or retinochoroiditis (094.83)*
> *retinal (peri) vasculitis (362.18)*

     363.10   Disseminated chorioretinitis, unspecified ✪
         Disseminated:
           choroiditis or chorioretinitis NOS
           retinitis or retinochoroiditis NOS
         Ⓔⓧ 363.00-363.22

     363.11   Disseminated choroiditis and chorioretinitis, posterior pole ✪
         Ⓔⓧ 363.00-363.22

     363.12   Disseminated choroiditis and chorioretinitis, peripheral ✪
         Ⓔⓧ 363.00-363.22

     363.13   Disseminated choroiditis and chorioretinitis, generalized ✪

> Code first *any underlying disease, as:*
> tuberculosis (017.3)

         Ⓔⓧ 363.00-363.22

     363.14   Disseminated retinitis and retinochoroiditis, metastatic ✪
         Ⓔⓧ 363.00-363.22

     363.15   Disseminated retinitis and retinochoroiditis, pigment epitheliopathy ✪
         Acute posterior multifocal placoid pigment epitheliopathy
         Ⓔⓧ 363.00-363.22

● **363.2   Other and unspecified forms of chorioretinitis and retinochoroiditis**

> **Excludes**   *panophthalmitis (360.02)*
> *sympathetic uveitis (360.11)*
> *uveitis NOS (364.3)*

     363.20   Chorioretinitis, unspecified ✪
         Choroiditis NOS
         Retinitis NOS
         Uveitis, posterior NOS
         Ⓔⓧ 363.00-363.22

     363.21   Pars planitis
         Posterior cyclitis

     363.22   Harada's disease

● **363.3   Chorioretinal scars**
     Scar (postinflammatory) (postsurgical) (posttraumatic):
       choroid
       retina

     363.30   Chorioretinal scar, unspecified

     363.31   Solar retinopathy

     363.32   Other macular scars

     363.33   Other scars of posterior pole

     363.34   Peripheral scars

     363.35   Disseminated scars

● **363.4   Choroidal degenerations**

     363.40   Choroidal degeneration, unspecified
         Choroidal sclerosis NOS

     363.41   Senile atrophy of choroid

     363.42   Diffuse secondary atrophy of choroid

     363.43   Angioid streaks of choroid

● **363.5   Hereditary choroidal dystrophies**
     Hereditary choroidal atrophy:
       partial [choriocapillaris]
       total [all vessels]

     363.50   Hereditary choroidal dystrophy or atrophy, unspecified

     363.51   Circumpapillary dystrophy of choroid, partial

     363.52   Circumpapillary dystrophy of choroid, total
         Helicoid dystrophy of choroid

     363.53   Central dystrophy of choroid, partial
         Dystrophy, choroidal:
           central areolar
           circinate

     363.54   Central choroidal atrophy, total
         Dystrophy, choroidal:
           central gyrate
           serpiginous

     363.55   Choroideremia

     363.56   Other diffuse or generalized dystrophy, partial
         Diffuse choroidal sclerosis

     363.57   Other diffuse or generalized dystrophy, total
         Generalized gyrate atrophy, choroid

● **363.6   Choroidal hemorrhage and rupture**

     363.61   Choroidal hemorrhage, unspecified

     363.62   Expulsive choroidal hemorrhage

     363.63   Choroidal rupture ✪
         Ⓔⓧ 363.61-363.9

● **363.7   Choroidal detachment**

     363.70   Choroidal detachment, unspecified ✪
         Ⓔⓧ 363.61-363.9

     363.71   Serous choroidal detachment ✪
         Ⓔⓧ 363.61-363.9

     363.72   Hemorrhagic choroidal detachment ✪
         Ⓔⓧ 363.61-363.9

     363.8   Other disorders of choroid
         Coding Clinic: 2006, Q1, P12

     363.9   Unspecified disorder of choroid

● **364   Disorders of iris and ciliary body**

● **364.0   Acute and subacute iridocyclitis**
     Anterior uveitis, acute, subacute
     Cyclitis, acute, subacute
     Iridocyclitis, acute, subacute
     Iritis, acute, subacute

> **Excludes**   *gonococcal (098.41)*
> *herpes simplex (054.44)*
> *herpes zoster (053.22)*

     364.00   Acute and subacute iridocyclitis, unspecified ✪
         Ⓔⓧ 364.00-364.3

     364.01   Primary iridocyclitis ✪
         Ⓔⓧ 364.00-364.3

     364.02   Recurrent iridocyclitis ✪
         Ⓔⓧ 364.00-364.3

     364.03   Secondary iridocyclitis, infectious ✪
         Ⓔⓧ 364.00-364.3

     364.04   Secondary iridocyclitis, noninfectious
         Aqueous:
           cells
           fibrin
           flare

     364.05   Hypopyon

DISEASES OF THE NERVOUS SYSTEM AND SENSE ORGANS (320–389)

◄ New   ◄▬ Revised   ~~deleted~~ Deleted   ● Unacceptable Principal Diagnosis   ✪ Use Additional Digit(s)
▶ Manifestation Code   **OGCR** Official Guidelines   **Coding Clinic**   Excludes   Includes   Use additional   Code first   Omit code

● **364.1 Chronic iridocyclitis**

　　Excludes *posterior cyclitis (363.21)*

　　364.10 Chronic iridocyclitis, unspecified

　▶ **364.11 Chronic iridocyclitis in diseases classified elsewhere**

　　　Code first underlying disease, as:
　　　　sarcoidosis (135)
　　　　tuberculosis (017.3)

　　　Excludes *syphilitic iridocyclitis (091.52)*

● **364.2 Certain types of iridocyclitis**

　　Excludes *posterior cyclitis (363.21)*
　　　　　sympathetic uveitis (360.11)

　　364.21 Fuchs' heterochromic cyclitis

　　364.22 Glaucomatocyclitic crises 🔵
　　　　(Ex:) 364.00-364.3

　　364.23 Lens-induced iridocyclitis

　　364.24 Vogt-Koyanagi syndrome

　364.3 Unspecified iridocyclitis 🔵
　　　Uveitis NOS
　　　(Ex:) 364.00-364.3

● **364.4 Vascular disorders of iris and ciliary body**

　　364.41 Hyphema
　　　　Hemorrhage of iris or ciliary body

　　364.42 Rubeosis iridis
　　　　Neovascularization of iris or ciliary body

● **364.5 Degenerations of iris and ciliary body**

　　364.51 Essential or progressive iris atrophy

　　364.52 Iridoschisis

　　364.53 Pigmentary iris degeneration
　　　　Acquired heterochromia of iris
　　　　Pigment dispersion syndrome of iris
　　　　Translucency of iris

　　364.54 Degeneration of pupillary margin
　　　　Atrophy of sphincter of iris
　　　　Ectropion of pigment epithelium of iris

　　364.55 Miotic cysts of pupillary margin

　　364.56 Degenerative changes of chamber angle

　　364.57 Degenerative changes of ciliary body

　　364.59 Other iris atrophy
　　　　Iris atrophy (generalized) (sector shaped)

● **364.6 Cysts of iris, ciliary body, and anterior chamber**

　　Excludes *miotic pupillary cyst (364.55)*
　　　　　parasitic cyst (360.13)

　　364.60 Idiopathic cysts

　　364.61 Implantation cysts
　　　　Epithelial down-growth, anterior chamber
　　　　Implantation cysts (surgical) (traumatic)

　　364.62 Exudative cysts of iris or anterior chamber

　　364.63 Primary cyst of pars plana

　　364.64 Exudative cyst of pars plana

● **364.7 Adhesions and disruptions of iris and ciliary body**

　　Excludes *flat anterior chamber (360.34)*

　　364.70 Adhesions of iris, unspecified
　　　　Synechiae (iris) NOS

　　364.71 Posterior synechiae

　　364.72 Anterior synechiae

　　364.73 Goniosynechiae
　　　　Peripheral anterior synechiae

　　364.74 Pupillary membranes
　　　　Iris bombé
　　　　Pupillary:
　　　　　occlusion
　　　　　seclusion

　　364.75 Pupillary abnormalities
　　　　Deformed pupil
　　　　Ectopic pupil
　　　　Rupture of sphincter, pupil

　　364.76 Iridodialysis
　　　　Coding Clinic: 1985, July-Aug, P16

　　364.77 Recession of chamber angle

● **364.8 Other disorders of iris and ciliary body**
　　　Coding Clinic: 2007, Q2, P11

　　364.81 Floppy iris syndrome
　　　　Intraoperative floppy iris syndrome (IFIS)

　　　Use additional E code to identify cause,
　　　　such as:
　　　　sympatholytics [antiadrenergics] causing
　　　　　adverse effect in therapeutic use
　　　　　(E941.3)
　　　　Coding Clinic: 2007, Q4, P77-79

　　364.82 Plateau iris syndrome
　　　　Coding Clinic: 2008, Q4, P112

　　364.89 Other disorders of iris and ciliary body
　　　　Prolapse of iris NOS

　　　Excludes *prolapse of iris in recent wound*
　　　　　(871.1)

　　364.9 Unspecified disorder of iris and ciliary body

● **365 Glaucoma**
　　　Intraocular pressure (IOP) is too high. IOP is the result of too
　　　much aqueous humor because of excess production or
　　　inadequate drainage. Leads to optic nerve damage and
　　　vision loss.

　　Excludes *blind hypertensive eye [absolute glaucoma]*
　　　　　(360.42)
　　　　　congenital glaucoma (743.20–743.22)

● **365.0 Borderline glaucoma [glaucoma suspect]**

　　365.00 Preglaucoma, unspecified
　　　　Coding Clinic: 1990, Q1, P8

　　365.01 Open angle with borderline findings
　　　　Open angle with:
　　　　　borderline intraocular pressure
　　　　　cupping of optic discs

　　365.02 Anatomical narrow angle

　　365.03 Steroid responders

　　365.04 Ocular hypertension

● **365.1 Open-angle glaucoma**

　　365.10 Open-angle glaucoma, unspecified
　　　　Wide-angle glaucoma NOS

　　365.11 Primary open angle glaucoma
　　　　Chronic simple glaucoma

　　365.12 Low tension glaucoma

　　365.13 Pigmentary glaucoma

　　365.14 Glaucoma of childhood
　　　　Infantile or juvenile glaucoma

　　365.15 Residual stage of open angle glaucoma

N Newborn Age: 0　　**P** Pediatric Age: 0–17　　**M** Maternity Age: 12–55　　**A** Adult Age: 15–124　　♀ Females Only　　♂ Males Only

(Ex:) CC Exclusions　　🔵 Complication\Comorbidity　　🔵 Major C\C　　🔵 Present on Admission Requirement　　🔵 Hospital-Acquired Condition　　865

● **365.2 Primary angle-closure glaucoma**

  365.20 Primary angle-closure glaucoma, unspecified

  365.21 Intermittent angle-closure glaucoma
  Angle-closure glaucoma:
    interval
    subacute

  365.22 Acute angle-closure glaucoma 🔊
  Ex: 365.22

  365.23 Chronic angle-closure glaucoma
  Coding Clinic: 1998, Q2, P16

  365.24 Residual stage of angle-closure glaucoma

● **365.3 Corticosteroid-induced glaucoma**

  365.31 Glaucomatous stage

  365.32 Residual stage

● **365.4 Glaucoma associated with congenital anomalies, dystrophies, and systemic syndromes**

  ▶ *365.41 Glaucoma associated with chamber angle anomalies*

  ▶ *365.42 Glaucoma associated with anomalies of iris*

  ▶ *365.43 Glaucoma associated with other anterior segment anomalies*

  ▶ *365.44 Glaucoma associated with systemic syndromes*
  Code first associated disease, as:
    neurofibromatosis (237.7)
    Sturge-Weber (-Dimitri) syndrome (759.6)

● **365.5 Glaucoma associated with disorders of the lens**

  365.51 Phacolytic glaucoma

  365.52 Pseudoexfoliation glaucoma

  365.59 Glaucoma associated with other lens disorders

● **365.6 Glaucoma associated with other ocular disorders**

  365.60 Glaucoma associated with unspecified ocular disorder

  365.61 Glaucoma associated with pupillary block

  365.62 Glaucoma associated with ocular inflammations

  365.63 Glaucoma associated with vascular disorders

  365.64 Glaucoma associated with tumors or cysts

  365.65 Glaucoma associated with ocular trauma

● **365.8 Other specified forms of glaucoma**

  365.81 Hypersecretion glaucoma

  365.82 Glaucoma with increased episcleral venous pressure

  365.83 Aqueous misdirection
  Malignant glaucoma
  Coding Clinic: 2002, Q4, P48

  365.89 Other specified glaucoma
  Coding Clinic: 1998, Q2, P16

365.9 Unspecified glaucoma
Coding Clinic: 2003, Q3, P14; 2001, Q2, P16-17

● **366 Cataract**

  Excludes   *congenital cataract (743.30–743.34)*

● **366.0 Infantile, juvenile, and presenile cataract**

  366.00 Nonsenile cataract, unspecified
  Coding Clinic: 1987, Mar-April, P9

  366.01 Anterior subcapsular polar cataract

  366.02 Posterior subcapsular polar cataract

  366.03 Cortical, lamellar, or zonular cataract

  366.04 Nuclear cataract

  366.09 Other and combined forms of nonsenile cataract

Figure 6–6   Age-related cataract. Nuclear sclerosis and cortical lens opacities are present. (From Yanoff: Ophthalmology, 2nd ed. 2004, Mosby, Inc.)

Item 6–15   Senile cataracts are linked to the aging process. The most common area for the formation of a cataract is the cortical area of the lens. **Polar cataracts** can be either anterior or posterior. **Anterior polar cataracts** are more common and are small, white, capsular cataracts located on the anterior portion of the lens. **Total cataracts,** also called **complete** or **mature,** cause an opacity of all fibers of the lens. **Hypermature** describes a mature cataract with a swollen, milky cortex that covers the entire lens. **Immature,** also called **incipient,** cataracts have a clear cortex and are only slightly opaque. Treatment for all cataracts is the removal of the lens.

● **366.1 Senile cataract**

  366.10 Senile cataract, unspecified   A
  Coding Clinic: 2003, Q1, P5

  366.11 Pseudoexfoliation of lens capsule   A

  366.12 Incipient cataract   A
  Cataract:
    coronary
    immature NOS
    punctate
  Water clefts

  366.13 Anterior subcapsular polar senile cataract   A

  366.14 Posterior subcapsular polar senile cataract A

  366.15 Cortical senile cataract   A

  366.16 Nuclear sclerosis   A
  Cataracta brunescens
  Nuclear cataract
  Coding Clinic: 2007, Q4, P77-79; 1985, Sept-Oct, P11

  366.17 Total or mature cataract   A

  366.18 Hypermature cataract   A
  Morgagni cataract

  366.19 Other and combined forms of senile cataract   A

◀ New   ◀▥▥ Revised   ~~deleted~~ Deleted   ● Unacceptable Principal Diagnosis   ● Use Additional Digit(s)
▶ Manifestation Code   **OGCR** Official Guidelines   **Coding Clinic**   Excludes   Includes   Use additional   Code first   Omit code

DISEASES OF THE NERVOUS SYSTEM AND SENSE ORGANS (320–389)

Figure 6–7 Corneal perforation. Preoperative appearance of a patient who has a small, 1.5 mm corneal perforation at the 10 o'clock limbus. *(Courtesy of Dr RK Forster.)* (From Yanoff: Ophthalmology, 2nd ed. 2004, Mosby, Inc.)

Item 6–16 Vossius' ring is the result of contusion-type traumatic injury and results in a ring of iris pigment pressed onto the anterior lens capsule.

● **366.2 Traumatic cataract**

     366.20 Traumatic cataract, unspecified

     366.21 Localized traumatic opacities
         Vossius' ring

     366.22 Total traumatic cataract

     366.23 Partially resolved traumatic cataract

● **366.3 Cataract secondary to ocular disorders**

     366.30 Cataracta complicata, unspecified

     366.31 Glaucomatous flecks (subcapsular)
         Code first underlying glaucoma (365.0–365.9)

     366.32 Cataract in inflammatory disorders
         Code first underlying condition, as:
         chronic choroiditis (363.0–363.2)

     366.33 Cataract with neovascularization
         Code first underlying condition, as:
         chronic iridocyclitis (364.10)

     366.34 Cataract in degenerative disorders
         Sunflower cataract
         Code first underlying condition, as:
         chalcosis (360.24)
         degenerative myopia (360.21)
         pigmentary retinal dystrophy (362.74)

● **366.4 Cataract associated with other disorders**

     ▸ *366.41 Diabetic cataract*
         Code first diabetes (249.5, 250.5)
         Coding Clinic: 1985, Sept-Oct, P11

     ▸ *366.42 Tetanic cataract*
         Code first underlying disease as:
         calcinosis (275.40)
         hypoparathyroidism (252.1)

     ▸ *366.43 Myotonic cataract*
         Code first underlying disorder (359.21, 359.23)

     ▸ *366.44 Cataract associated with other syndromes*
         Code first underlying condition, as:
         craniofacial dysostosis (756.0)
         galactosemia (271.1)

     366.45 Toxic cataract
         Drug-induced cataract
         Use additional E code to identify drug or other toxic substance
         Coding Clinic: 1995, Q4, P51

     366.46 Cataract associated with radiation and other physical influences
         Use additional E code to identify cause

● **366.5 After-cataract**

     366.50 After-cataract, unspecified
         Secondary cataract NOS

     366.51 Soemmering's ring

     366.52 Other after-cataract, not obscuring vision

     366.53 After-cataract, obscuring vision

   366.8 Other cataract
     Calcification of lens
     Coding Clinic: 1994, Q1, P16

   366.9 Unspecified cataract
     Coding Clinic: 1985, Sept-Oct, P10

● **367 Disorders of refraction and accommodation**

   367.0 Hypermetropia
     Far-sightedness
     Hyperopia

   367.1 Myopia
     Near-sightedness

● **367.2 Astigmatism**

     367.20 Astigmatism, unspecified

     367.21 Regular astigmatism

     367.22 Irregular astigmatism

● **367.3 Anisometropia and aniseikonia**

     367.31 Anisometropia

     367.32 Aniseikonia

   367.4 Presbyopia

● **367.5 Disorders of accommodation**

     367.51 Paresis of accommodation
         Cycloplegia

     367.52 Total or complete internal ophthalmoplegia

     367.53 Spasm of accommodation

● **367.8 Other disorders of refraction and accommodation**

     367.81 Transient refractive change

     367.89 Other
         Drug-induced disorders of refraction and accommodation
         Toxic disorders of refraction and accommodation

   367.9 Unspecified disorder of refraction and accommodation

Item 6–17 Disorders of refraction: **Hypermetropia**, or far-sightedness, means focus at a distance is adequate but not on close objects. **Myopia** is near-sightedness or short-sightedness and means the focus on nearby objects is clear but distant objects appear blurred. **Astigmatism** is warping of the curvature of the cornea so light rays entering do not meet a single focal point, resulting in a distorted image. **Anisometropia** is unequal refractive power in which one eye may be myopic (near-sighted) and the other hyperopic (far-sighted). **Presbyopia** is the loss of focus on near objects, which occurs with age because the lens loses elasticity.

DISEASES OF THE NERVOUS SYSTEM AND SENSE ORGANS (320–389)

N Newborn Age: 0   **P** Pediatric Age: 0–17   **M** Maternity Age: 12–55   **A** Adult Age: 15–124   ♀ Females Only   ♂ Males Only

(Ex) CC Exclusions   Complication\Comorbidity   Major C\C   Present on Admission Requirement   Hospital-Acquired Condition

867

● **368 Visual disturbances**

> **Excludes** *electrophysiological disturbances (794.11–794.14)*

● **368.0 Amblyopia ex anopsia**

    368.00 Amblyopia, unspecified

    368.01 Strabismic amblyopia
        Suppression amblyopia

    368.02 Deprivation amblyopia

    368.03 Refractive amblyopia

● **368.1 Subjective visual disturbances**

    368.10 Subjective visual disturbance, unspecified

    368.11 Sudden visual loss 🔖
        (Ex:) 368.10-368.12, 368.16

    368.12 Transient visual loss 🔖
        Concentric fading
        Scintillating scotoma
        (Ex:) 368.10-368.12, 368.16

    368.13 Visual discomfort
        Asthenopia
        Eye strain
        Photophobia

    368.14 Visual distortions of shape and size
        Macropsia
        Metamorphopsia
        Micropsia

    368.15 Other visual distortions and entoptic phenomena
        Photopsia
        Refractive:
            diplopia
            polyopia
        Visual halos

    368.16 Psychophysical visual disturbances
        Prosopagnosia
        Visual:
            agnosia
            disorientation syndrome
            hallucinations
            object agnosia

368.2 Diplopia
    Double vision

● **368.3 Other disorders of binocular vision**

    368.30 Binocular vision disorder, unspecified

    368.31 Suppression of binocular vision

    368.32 Simultaneous visual perception without fusion

    368.33 Fusion with defective stereopsis

    368.34 Abnormal retinal correspondence

● **368.4 Visual field defects**

    368.40 Visual field defect, unspecified

    368.41 Scotoma involving central area
        Scotoma:
            central
            centrocecal
            paracentral

    368.42 Scotoma of blind spot area
        Enlarged:
            angioscotoma
            blind spot
        Paracecal scotoma

    368.43 Sector or arcuate defects
        Scotoma:
            arcuate
            Bjerrum
            Seidel

    368.44 Other localized visual field defect
        Scotoma:
            NOS
            ring
        Visual field defect:
            nasal step
            peripheral

    368.45 Generalized contraction or constriction

    368.46 Homonymous bilateral field defects
        Hemianopsia (altitudinal) (homonymous)
        Quadrant anopia

    368.47 Heteronymous bilateral field defects
        Hemianopsia:
            binasal
            bitemporal

● **368.5 Color vision deficiencies**
    Color blindness

    368.51 Protan defect
        Protanomaly
        Protanopia

    368.52 Deutan defect
        Deuteranomaly
        Deuteranopia

    368.53 Tritan defect
        Tritanomaly
        Tritanopia

    368.54 Achromatopsia
        Monochromatism (cone) (rod)

    368.55 Acquired color vision deficiencies

    368.59 Other color vision deficiencies

● **368.6 Night blindness**

    368.60 Night blindness, unspecified

    368.61 Congenital night blindness
        Hereditary night blindness
        Oguchi's disease

    368.62 Acquired night blindness

        > **Excludes** *that due to vitamin A deficiency (264.5)*

    368.63 Abnormal dark adaptation curve
        Abnormal threshold of cones or rods
        Delayed adaptation of cones or rods

    368.69 Other night blindness

368.8 Other specified visual disturbances
    Blurred vision NOS
    Coding Clinic: 2002, Q4, P56

368.9 Unspecified visual disturbance
    Coding Clinic: 2006, Q3, P22

◀ New   ◀▥ Revised   ~~deleted~~ Deleted   ● Unacceptable Principal Diagnosis   ● Use Additional Digit(s)

▶ Manifestation Code   **OGCR** Official Guidelines   **Coding Clinic**   Excludes   Includes   Use additional   Code first   Omit code

●369 **Blindness and low vision**

> **Excludes** *correctable impaired vision due to refractive errors (367.0–367.9)*

> **Note:** Visual impairment refers to a functional limitation of the eye (e.g., limited visual acuity or visual field). It should be distinguished from visual disability, indicating a limitation of the abilities of the individual (e.g., limited reading skills, vocational skills), and from visual handicap, indicating a limitation of personal and socioeconomic independence (e.g., limited mobility, limited employability).

The levels of impairment defined in the table after 369.9 are based on the recommendations of the WHO Study Group on Prevention of Blindness (Geneva, November 6–10, 1972; WHO Technical Report Series 518), and of the International Council of Ophthalmology (1976).

Note that definitions of blindness vary in different settings.

For international reporting, WHO defines blindness as profound impairment. This definition can be applied to blindness of one eye (369.1, 369.6) and to blindness of the individual (369.0).

For determination of benefits in the U.S.A., the definition of legal blindness as severe impairment is often used. This definition applies to blindness of the individual only.

●369.0 **Profound impairment, both eyes**

369.00 **Impairment level not further specified**
Blindness:
NOS according to WHO definition
both eyes

369.01 **Better eye: total impairment; lesser eye: total impairment**

369.02 **Better eye: near-total impairment; lesser eye: not further specified**

369.03 **Better eye: near-total impairment; lesser eye: total impairment**

369.04 **Better eye: near-total impairment; lesser eye: near-total impairment**

369.05 **Better eye: profound impairment; lesser eye: not further specified**

369.06 **Better eye: profound impairment; lesser eye: total impairment**

369.07 **Better eye: profound impairment; lesser eye: near-total impairment**

369.08 **Better eye: profound impairment; lesser eye: profound impairment**

●369.1 **Moderate or severe impairment, better eye, profound impairment lesser eye**

369.10 **Impairment level not further specified**
Blindness, one eye, low vision other eye

369.11 **Better eye: severe impairment; lesser eye: blind, not further specified**

369.12 **Better eye: severe impairment; lesser eye: total impairment**

369.13 **Better eye: severe impairment; lesser eye: near-total impairment**

369.14 **Better eye: severe impairment; lesser eye: profound impairment**

369.15 **Better eye: moderate impairment; lesser eye: blind, not further specified**

369.16 **Better eye: moderate impairment; lesser eye: total impairment**

369.17 **Better eye: moderate impairment; lesser eye: near-total impairment**

369.18 **Better eye: moderate impairment; lesser eye: profound impairment**

●369.2 **Moderate or severe impairment, both eyes**

369.20 **Impairment level not further specified**
Low vision, both eyes NOS

369.21 **Better eye: severe impairment; lesser eye: not further specified**

369.22 **Better eye: severe impairment; lesser eye: severe impairment**

369.23 **Better eye: moderate impairment; lesser eye: not further specified**

369.24 **Better eye: moderate impairment; lesser eye: severe impairment**

369.25 **Better eye: moderate impairment; lesser eye: moderate impairment**

369.3 **Unqualified visual loss, both eyes**

> **Excludes** *blindness NOS:*
> *legal [U.S.A. definition] (369.4)*
> *WHO definition (369.00)*

369.4 **Legal blindness, as defined in U.S.A.**
Blindness NOS according to U.S.A. definition

> **Excludes** *legal blindness with specification of impairment level (369.01–369.08, 369.11–369.14, 369.21–369.22)*

●369.6 **Profound impairment, one eye**
Coding Clinic: 2002, Q3, P20-21

369.60 **Impairment level not further specified**
Blindness, one eye

369.61 **One eye: total impairment; other eye: not specified**

369.62 **One eye: total impairment; other eye: near-normal vision**

369.63 **One eye: total impairment; other eye: normal vision**

369.64 **One eye: near-total impairment; other eye: not specified**

369.65 **One eye: near-total impairment; other eye: near-normal vision**

369.66 **One eye: near-total impairment; other eye: normal vision**

369.67 **One eye: profound impairment; other eye: not specified**

369.68 **One eye: profound impairment; other eye: near-normal vision**

369.69 **One eye: profound impairment; other eye: normal vision**

N Newborn Age: 0   **P** Pediatric Age: 0–17   **M** Maternity Age: 12–55   **A** Adult Age: 15–124   ♀ Females Only   ♂ Males Only

(Ex.) CC Exclusions   Complication\Comorbidity   Major C\C   Present on Admission Requirement   Hospital-Acquired Condition

869

DISEASES OF THE NERVOUS SYSTEM AND SENSE ORGANS (320–389)

DISEASES OF THE NERVOUS SYSTEM AND SENSE ORGANS (320–389)

● **369.7 Moderate or severe impairment, one eye**

  369.70 Impairment level not further specified
Low vision, one eye

  369.71 One eye: severe impairment; other eye: not specified

  369.72 One eye: severe impairment; other eye: near-normal vision

  369.73 One eye: severe impairment; other eye: normal vision

  369.74 One eye: moderate impairment; other eye: not specified

  369.75 One eye: moderate impairment; other eye: near-normal vision

  369.76 One eye: moderate impairment; other eye: normal vision

369.8 Unqualified visual loss, one eye

369.9 Unspecified visual loss

Classification		Levels of Visual Impairment	Additional Descriptors Which May Be Encountered
"Legal"	WHO	Visual Acuity and/or Visual Field Limitation (Whichever Is Worse)	
	(Near-)normal vision	Range of Normal Vision 20/10 20/13 20/16 20/20 20/25 2.0 1.6 1.25 1.0 0.8	
		Near-Normal Vision 20/30 20/40 20/50 20/60 0.7 0.6 0.5 0.4 0.3	
	Low vision	Moderate Visual Impairment 20/70 20/80 20/100 20/125 20/160 0.25 0.20 0.16 0.12	Moderate low vision
Legal Blindness (U.S.A.) both eyes	Blindness (WHO) one or both eyes	Severe Visual Impairment 20/200 20/250 20/320 20/400 0.10 0.08 0.06 0.05 Visual field: 20 degrees or less	Severe low vision, "Legal" blindness
		Profound Visual Impairment 20/500 20/630 20/800 20/1000 0.04 0.03 0.025 0.02 Count fingers at: less than 3 m (10 ft) Visual field: 10 degrees or less	Profound low vision, Moderate blindness
		Near-Total Visual Impairment Visual acuity: less than 0.02 (20/1000) Count fingers: 1 m (3 ft) or less Hand movements: 5 m (15 ft) or less Light projection, light perception Visual field: 5 degrees or less	Severe blindness, Near-total blindness
		Total Visual Impairment No light perception (NLP)	Total blindness

Visual acuity refers to best achievable acuity with correction.
Non-listed Snellen fractions may be classified by converting to the nearest decimal equivalent, e.g., 10/200 = 0.05, 6/30 = 0.20.
CF (count fingers) without designation of distance, may be classified to profound impairment.
HM (hand motion) without designation of distance, may be classified to near-total impairment.
Visual field measurements refer to the largest field diameter for a 1/100 white test object.

370 Keratitis

● **370.0 Corneal ulcer**

  Excludes   *that due to vitamin A deficiency (264.3)*

  370.00 Corneal ulcer, unspecified

  370.01 Marginal corneal ulcer

  370.02 Ring corneal ulcer

  370.03 Central corneal ulcer

  370.04 Hypopyon ulcer
Serpiginous ulcer

  370.05 Mycotic corneal ulcer

  370.06 Perforated corneal ulcer

  370.07 Mooren's ulcer

● **370.2 Superficial keratitis without conjunctivitis**

  Excludes   *dendritic [herpes simplex] keratitis (054.42)*

  370.20 Superficial keratitis, unspecified

  370.21 Punctate keratitis
Thygeson's superficial punctate keratitis

Marginal (catarrhal) ulcer   Ring ulcer

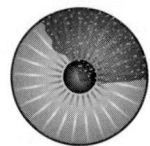

Central corneal ulcer   Rosacea ulcer   Mooren's (rodent) ulcer

Figure 6–8   Corneal ulcers: marginal, ring, central corneal, rosacea, and Mooren's.

Item 6–18 An infected ulcer is usually called a **serpiginous** or **hypopyon** ulcer which is a pus sac in the anterior chamber of the eye.

Marginal ulcers are usually asymptomatic, not primary, and are often superficial and simple. More severe marginal ulcers spread to form a ring ulcer. **Ring** ulcers can extend around the entire corneal periphery.

Central corneal ulcers develop when there is an abrasion to the epithelium and an infection develops in the eroded area.

The **pyocyaneal** ulcer is the most serious corneal infection, which, if left untreated, can lead to loss of the eye.

◀ New   ◀▦ Revised   ~~deleted~~ Deleted   ● Unacceptable Principal Diagnosis   ● Use Additional Digit(s)
▶ Manifestation Code   OGCR Official Guidelines   Coding Clinic   Excludes   Includes   Use additional   Code first   Omit code

370.22 Macular keratitis
     Keratitis: Keratitis:
       areolar   stellate
       nummular   striate

370.23 Filamentary keratitis

370.24 Photokeratitis
     Snow blindness
     Welders' keratitis
     Coding Clinic: 1996, Q3, P6

● **370.3 Certain types of keratoconjunctivitis**

370.31 Phlyctenular keratoconjunctivitis
     Phlyctenulosis
     Use additional code for any associated
       tuberculosis (017.3)

370.32 Limbal and corneal involvement in vernal conjunctivitis
     Use additional code for vernal
       conjunctivitis (372.13)

370.33 Keratoconjunctivitis sicca, not specified as Sjögren's
     Excludes   *Sjögren's syndrome (710.2)*

370.34 Exposure keratoconjunctivitis
     Coding Clinic: 1996, Q3, P6

370.35 Neurotrophic keratoconjunctivitis

● **370.4 Other and unspecified keratoconjunctivitis**

370.40 Keratoconjunctivitis, unspecified
     Superficial keratitis with conjunctivitis NOS

▶ **370.44 *Keratitis or keratoconjunctivitis in exanthema***
     Code first underlying condition (050.0–052.9)
     Excludes   *herpes simplex (054.43)*
                   herpes zoster (053.21)
                    measles (055.71)

370.49 Other
     Excludes   *epidemic keratoconjunctivitis*
                   (077.1)

● **370.5 Interstitial and deep keratitis**

370.50 Interstitial keratitis, unspecified

370.52 Diffuse interstitial keratitis
     Cogan's syndrome

370.54 Sclerosing keratitis

370.55 Corneal abscess

370.59 Other
     Excludes   *disciform herpes simplex keratitis*
                   (054.43)
                   syphilitic keratitis (090.3)

● **370.6 Corneal neovascularization**

370.60 Corneal neovascularization, unspecified

370.61 Localized vascularization of cornea

370.62 Pannus (corneal)
     Coding Clinic: 2002, Q3, P20-21

370.63 Deep vascularization of cornea

370.64 Ghost vessels (corneal)

● **370.8 Other forms of keratitis**
     Code first underlying condition, such as:
     Acanthamoeba (136.21)
     Fusarium (118)
     Coding Clinic: 2008, Q4, P79-81; 1994, Q3, P5

370.9 Unspecified keratitis

● **371 Corneal opacity and other disorders of cornea**

● **371.0 Corneal scars and opacities**
     Excludes   *that due to vitamin A deficiency (264.6)*

371.00 Corneal opacity, unspecified
     Corneal scar NOS

371.01 Minor opacity of cornea
     Corneal nebula

371.02 Peripheral opacity of cornea
     Corneal macula not interfering with central
       vision

371.03 Central opacity of cornea
     Corneal:
       leucoma interfering with central vision
       macula interfering with central vision

371.04 Adherent leucoma

▶ **371.05 *Phthisical cornea***
     Code first underlying tuberculosis (017.3)

● **371.1 Corneal pigmentations and deposits**

371.10 Corneal deposit, unspecified

371.11 Anterior pigmentations
     Stähli's lines

371.12 Stromal pigmentations
     Hematocornea

371.13 Posterior pigmentations
     Krukenberg spindle

371.14 Kayser-Fleischer ring

371.15 Other deposits associated with metabolic disorders

371.16 Argentous deposits

● **371.2 Corneal edema**

371.20 Corneal edema, unspecified

371.21 Idiopathic corneal edema

371.22 Secondary corneal edema

371.23 Bullous keratopathy

371.24 Corneal edema due to wearing of contact lenses

● **371.3 Changes of corneal membranes**

371.30 Corneal membrane change, unspecified

371.31 Folds and rupture of Bowman's membrane

371.32 Folds in Descemet's membrane

371.33 Rupture in Descemet's membrane

● **371.4 Corneal degenerations**

371.40 Corneal degeneration, unspecified

371.41 Senile corneal changes
     Arcus senilis   Hassall-Henle bodies

371.42 Recurrent erosion of cornea
     Excludes   *Mooren's ulcer (370.07)*

371.43 Band-shaped keratopathy

371.44 Other calcerous degenerations of cornea

371.45 Keratomalacia NOS
     Excludes   *that due to vitamin A deficiency*
                   (264.4)

371.46 Nodular degeneration of cornea
     Salzmann's nodular dystrophy

371.48 Peripheral degenerations of cornea
     Marginal degeneration of cornea [Terrien's]

371.49 Other
     Discrete colliquative keratopathy

DISEASES OF THE NERVOUS SYSTEM AND SENSE ORGANS (320–389)

● **371.5 Hereditary corneal dystrophies**

    371.50 Corneal dystrophy, unspecified

    371.51 Juvenile epithelial corneal dystrophy

    371.52 Other anterior corneal dystrophies
Corneal dystrophy:
    microscopic cystic
    ring-like

    371.53 Granular corneal dystrophy

    371.54 Lattice corneal dystrophy

    371.55 Macular corneal dystrophy

    371.56 Other stromal corneal dystrophies
Crystalline corneal dystrophy

    371.57 Endothelial corneal dystrophy
Combined corneal dystrophy
Cornea guttata
Fuchs' endothelial dystrophy

    371.58 Other posterior corneal dystrophies
Polymorphous corneal dystrophy

● **371.6 Keratoconus**

    371.60 Keratoconus, unspecified

    371.61 Keratoconus, stable condition

    371.62 Keratoconus, acute hydrops

● **371.7 Other corneal deformities**

    371.70 Corneal deformity, unspecified

    371.71 Corneal ectasia

    371.72 Descemetocele

    371.73 Corneal staphyloma

● **371.8 Other corneal disorders**

    371.81 Corneal anesthesia and hypoesthesia

    371.82 Corneal disorder due to contact lens

        | Excludes | *corneal edema due to contact lens (371.24)*

    371.89 Other
Coding Clinic: 1999, Q3, P12

371.9 Unspecified corneal disorder

Figure 6-9   Lateral view of the displacement of the cone apex in keratoconus. (From Yanoff: Ophthalmology, 2nd ed. 2004, Mosby, Inc.)

Item 6-19   Keratoconus results in corneal degeneration that begins in childhood, gradually changes the cornea from a round to cone shape, decreasing visual acuity. Treatment includes contact lenses. In severe cases the need for corneal transplant may be the treatment of choice; however, newer technologies may use high frequency radio energy to shrink the edges of the cornea, pulling the central area back to a more normal shape. It can help delay or avoid the need for a corneal transplantation.

● **372 Disorders of conjunctiva**

    | Excludes | *keratoconjunctivitis (370.3–370.4)*

● **372.0 Acute conjunctivitis**

    372.00 Acute conjunctivitis, unspecified

    372.01 Serous conjunctivitis, except viral

        | Excludes | *viral conjunctivitis NOS (077.9)*
        Coding Clinic: 2008, Q3, P6-7

    372.02 Acute follicular conjunctivitis
Conjunctival folliculosis NOS

        | Excludes | *conjunctivitis:*
            adenoviral (acute follicular) (077.3)
            epidemic hemorrhagic (077.4)
            inclusion (077.0)
            Newcastle (077.8)
            epidemic keratoconjunctivitis (077.1)
            pharyngoconjunctival fever (077.2)

    372.03 Other mucopurulent conjunctivitis
Catarrhal conjunctivitis

        | Excludes | *blennorrhea neonatorum (gonococcal) (098.40)*
            neonatal conjunctivitis (771.6)
            ophthalmia neonatorum NOS (771.6)

    372.04 Pseudomembranous conjunctivitis
Membranous conjunctivitis

        | Excludes | *diphtheritic conjunctivitis (032.81)*

    372.05 Acute atopic conjunctivitis

    372.06 Acute chemical conjunctivitis ◄
Acute toxic conjunctivitis ◄

        Use additional E code to identify the chemical or toxic agent ◄

        | Excludes | *burn of eye and adnexa (940.0–940.9)* ◄
            chemical corrosion injury of eye (940.2-940.3) ◄

● **372.1 Chronic conjunctivitis**

    372.10 Chronic conjunctivitis, unspecified

    372.11 Simple chronic conjunctivitis

    372.12 Chronic follicular conjunctivitis

    372.13 Vernal conjunctivitis
Coding Clinic: 1996, Q3, P8

    372.14 Other chronic allergic conjunctivitis
Coding Clinic: 1996, Q3, P8

  ▶ **372.15 *Parasitic conjunctivitis***

        Code first *underlying disease as:*
          filariasis (125.0–125.9)
          mucocutaneous leishmaniasis (085.5)

● **372.2 Blepharoconjunctivitis**

    372.20 Blepharoconjunctivitis, unspecified

    372.21 Angular blepharoconjunctivitis

    372.22 Contact blepharoconjunctivitis

● **372.3 Other and unspecified conjunctivitis**

    372.30 Conjunctivitis, unspecified

  ▶ **372.31 *Rosacea conjunctivitis***

        Code first *underlying rosacea dermatitis (695.3)*

  ▶ **372.33 *Conjunctivitis in mucocutaneous disease***

        Code first *underlying disease as:*
          erythema multiforme (695.10–695.19)
          Reiter's disease (099.3)

        | Excludes | *ocular pemphigoid (694.61)*

◄ New   ◄▦ Revised   ~~deleted~~ Deleted   ● Unacceptable Principal Diagnosis   ● Use Additional Digit(s)
▶ Manifestation Code   **OGCR** Official Guidelines   **Coding Clinic** | Excludes | Includes   Use additional   Code first   Omit code

Figure 6-10 Double pterygium. Note both nasal and temporal pterygia in a 57-year-old farmer. (From Yanoff: Ophthalmology, 2nd ed. 2004, Mosby, Inc.)

Figure 6-11 Photograph of eyelids with marginal blepharitis. (From Mandell, Bennett, & Dolin: Principles and Practice of Infectious Diseases, 6th ed. 2005, Churchill Livingstone, An Imprint of Elsevier)

Item 6-20　Pterygium is Greek for batlike. The condition is characterized by a membrane that extends from the limbus to the center of the cornea and resembles a wing.

372.34　Pingueculitis
> **Excludes** *pinguecula (372.51)* ◀
> Coding Clinic: 2008, Q4, P112-113

372.39　Other
> Coding Clinic: 2007, Q2, P11

● **372.4　Pterygium**
> **Excludes** *pseudopterygium (372.52)*

372.40　Pterygium, unspecified

372.41　Peripheral pterygium, stationary

372.42　Peripheral pterygium, progressive

372.43　Central pterygium

372.44　Double pterygium

372.45　Recurrent pterygium

● **372.5　Conjunctival degenerations and deposits**

372.50　Conjunctival degeneration, unspecified

372.51　Pinguecula
> **Excludes** *pingueculitis (372.34)* ◀

372.52　Pseudopterygium

372.53　Conjunctival xerosis
> **Excludes** *conjunctival xerosis due to vitamin A deficiency (264.0, 264.1, 264.7)*

372.54　Conjunctival concretions

372.55　Conjunctival pigmentations
> Conjunctival argyrosis

372.56　Conjunctival deposits

● **372.6　Conjunctival scars**

372.61　Granuloma of conjunctiva

372.62　Localized adhesions and strands of conjunctiva

372.63　Symblepharon
> Extensive adhesions of conjunctiva

372.64　Scarring of conjunctiva
> Contraction of eye socket (after enucleation)

● **372.7　Conjunctival vascular disorders and cysts**

372.71　Hyperemia of conjunctiva

372.72　Conjunctival hemorrhage
> Hyposphagma
> Subconjunctival hemorrhage

372.73　Conjunctival edema
> Chemosis of conjunctiva
> Subconjunctival edema

372.74　Vascular abnormalities of conjunctiva
> Aneurysm(ata) of conjunctiva

372.75　Conjunctival cysts

● **372.8　Other disorders of conjunctiva**

372.81　Conjunctivochalasis
> Coding Clinic: 2000, Q4, P41

372.89　Other disorders of conjunctiva

372.9　Unspecified disorder of conjunctiva

Item 6-21　Blepharitis is a common condition in which the eyelid is swollen and yellow scaling and conjunctivitis develop. Usually the hair on the scalp and brow is involved.

● **373　Inflammation of eyelids**

● **373.0　Blepharitis**
> **Excludes** *blepharoconjunctivitis (372.20–372.22)*

373.00　Blepharitis, unspecified

373.01　Ulcerative blepharitis

373.02　Squamous blepharitis

● **373.1　Hordeolum and other deep inflammation of eyelid**
> *Bacterial infection (staphylococcus) of sebaceous gland of eyelid (stye)*

373.11　Hordeolum externum
> Hordeolum NOS
> Stye

373.12　Hordeolum internum
> Infection of meibomian gland

373.13　Abscess of eyelid
> Furuncle of eyelid

373.2　Chalazion
> *Most often caused by accumulation of meibomian gland secretions resulting from blockage of duct.*
> Meibomian (gland) cyst
> **Excludes** *infected meibomian gland (373.12)*

● **373.3　Noninfectious dermatoses of eyelid**

373.31　Eczematous dermatitis of eyelid

373.32　Contact and allergic dermatitis of eyelid

373.33　Xeroderma of eyelid

373.34　Discoid lupus erythematosus of eyelid

▶ **373.4　*Infective dermatitis of eyelid of types resulting in deformity***
> Code first underlying disease, as:
> leprosy (030.0–030.9)
> lupus vulgaris (tuberculous) (017.0)
> yaws (102.0–102.9)

▶ **373.5　*Other infective dermatitis of eyelid***
> Code first underlying disease, as:
> actinomycosis (039.3)
> impetigo (684)
> mycotic dermatitis (110.0–111.9)
> vaccinia (051.0)
> postvaccination (999.0)
> **Excludes** *herpes:*
> *simplex (054.41)*
> *zoster (053.20)*

▶ **373.6　*Parasitic infestation of eyelid***
> Code first underlying disease, as:
> leishmaniasis (085.0–085.9)
> loiasis (125.2)
> onchocerciasis (125.3)
> pediculosis (132.0)

373.8　Other inflammations of eyelids

373.9　Unspecified inflammation of eyelid

DISEASES OF THE NERVOUS SYSTEM AND SENSE ORGANS (320–389)

N Newborn Age: 0　**P** Pediatric Age: 0–17　**M** Maternity Age: 12–55　**A** Adult Age: 15–124　♀ Females Only　♂ Males Only

(Ex.) CC Exclusions　　🔖 Complication\Comorbidity　　🔖 Major C\C　　🔖 Present on Admission Requirement　　🔖 Hospital-Acquired Condition　　873

Figure 6–12 Right lower eyelid entropion. Note the inward rotation of the tarsal plate about the horizontal axis and the resultant contact between the mucocutaneous junction and ocular surface. (From Yanoff: Ophthalmology, 2nd ed. 2004, Mosby, Inc.)

● **374 Other disorders of eyelids**

  ● **374.0 Entropion and trichiasis of eyelid**

    374.00 Entropion, unspecified

    374.01 Senile entropion   A

    374.02 Mechanical entropion

    374.03 Spastic entropion

    374.04 Cicatricial entropion

    374.05 Trichiasis without entropion

  ● **374.1 Ectropion**

    374.10 Ectropion, unspecified

    374.11 Senile ectropion   A

    374.12 Mechanical ectropion

    374.13 Spastic ectropion

    374.14 Cicatricial ectropion

  ● **374.2 Lagophthalmos**

    374.20 Lagophthalmos, unspecified

    374.21 Paralytic lagophthalmos

    374.22 Mechanical lagophthalmos

    374.23 Cicatricial lagophthalmos

  ● **374.3 Ptosis of eyelid**

    Falling forward, drooping, sagging of eyelid

    374.30 Ptosis of eyelid, unspecified
        Coding Clinic: 1996, Q2, P11

    374.31 Paralytic ptosis

    374.32 Myogenic ptosis

    374.33 Mechanical ptosis

    374.34 Blepharochalasis
        Pseudoptosis

  ● **374.4 Other disorders affecting eyelid function**

    | **Excludes** | *blepharoclonus (333.81)* |
    blepharospasm (333.81)
    facial nerve palsy (351.0)
    third nerve palsy or paralysis
      (378.51–378.52)
    tic (psychogenic) (307.20–307.23)
      organic (333.3)

    374.41 Lid retraction or lag

Item 6-22 Ptosis of eyelid is drooping of the upper eyelid over the pupil when the eyes are fully opened resulting from nerve or muscle damage, which may require surgical correction.

Figure 6–13 Ptosis of eyelid. (From Yanoff: Ophthalmology, 2nd ed. 2004, Mosby, Inc.)

    374.43 Abnormal innervation syndrome
        Jaw-blinking
        Paradoxical facial movements

    374.44 Sensory disorders

    374.45 Other sensorimotor disorders
        Deficient blink reflex

    374.46 Blepharophimosis
        Ankyloblepharon

  ● **374.5 Degenerative disorders of eyelid and periocular area**

    374.50 Degenerative disorder of eyelid, unspecified

    ▶ **374.51 *Xanthelasma***
        Xanthoma (planum) (tuberosum) of eyelid
        Code first underlying condition (272.0–272.9)

    374.52 Hyperpigmentation of eyelid
        Chloasma
        Dyspigmentation

    374.53 Hypopigmentation of eyelid
        Vitiligo of eyelid

    374.54 Hypertrichosis of eyelid

    374.55 Hypotrichosis of eyelid
        Madarosis of eyelid

    374.56 Other degenerative disorders of skin affecting eyelid

  ● **374.8 Other disorders of eyelid**

    374.81 Hemorrhage of eyelid

      | **Excludes** | *black eye (921.0)* |

    374.82 Edema of eyelid
        Hyperemia of eyelid
        Coding Clinic: 2008, Q4, P128-131

    374.83 Elephantiasis of eyelid

    374.84 Cysts of eyelids
        Sebaceous cyst of eyelid

    374.85 Vascular anomalies of eyelid

    374.86 Retained foreign body of eyelid

    374.87 Dermatochalasis

    374.89 Other disorders of eyelid

    374.9 Unspecified disorder of eyelid

● **375 Disorders of lacrimal system**

  ● **375.0 Dacryoadenitis**

    375.00 Dacryoadenitis, unspecified

    375.01 Acute dacryoadenitis

    375.02 Chronic dacryoadenitis

    375.03 Chronic enlargement of lacrimal gland

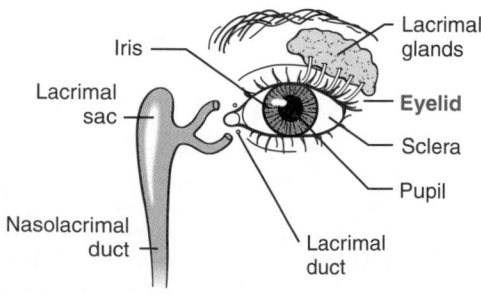

Figure 6–14 Lacrimal apparatus. (From Buck CJ: Step-by-Step Medical Coding. Philadelphia, WB Saunders, 2006, p 302.)

DISEASES OF THE NERVOUS SYSTEM AND SENSE ORGANS (320–389)

◀ New   ◀▥ Revised   ~~deleted~~ Deleted   ● Unacceptable Principal Diagnosis   ● Use Additional Digit(s)
▶ Manifestation Code   **OGCR** Official Guidelines   **Coding Clinic**   Excludes   Includes   Use additional   Code first   Omit code

● **375.1 Other disorders of lacrimal gland**

     375.11 Dacryops

     375.12 Other lacrimal cysts and cystic degeneration

     375.13 Primary lacrimal atrophy

     375.14 Secondary lacrimal atrophy

     375.15 Tear film insufficiency, unspecified
         Dry eye syndrome
         Coding Clinic: 1996, Q3, P6

     375.16 Dislocation of lacrimal gland

● **375.2 Epiphora**

     375.20 Epiphora, unspecified as to cause

     375.21 Epiphora due to excess lacrimation

     375.22 Epiphora due to insufficient drainage

● **375.3 Acute and unspecified inflammation of lacrimal passages**

         Excludes   *neonatal dacryocystitis (771.6)*

     375.30 Dacryocystitis, unspecified

     375.31 Acute canaliculitis, lacrimal

     375.32 Acute dacryocystitis
         Acute peridacryocystitis

     375.33 Phlegmonous dacryocystitis

● **375.4 Chronic inflammation of lacrimal passages**

     375.41 Chronic canaliculitis

     375.42 Chronic dacryocystitis

     375.43 Lacrimal mucocele

● **375.5 Stenosis and insufficiency of lacrimal passages**

     375.51 Eversion of lacrimal punctum

     375.52 Stenosis of lacrimal punctum

     375.53 Stenosis of lacrimal canaliculi

     375.54 Stenosis of lacrimal sac

     375.55 Obstruction of nasolacrimal duct, neonatal
         Excludes   *congenital anomaly of nasolacrimal duct (743.65)*

     375.56 Stenosis of nasolacrimal duct, acquired

     375.57 Dacryolith

● **375.6 Other changes of lacrimal passages**

     375.61 Lacrimal fistula

     375.69 Other

● **375.8 Other disorders of lacrimal system**

     375.81 Granuloma of lacrimal passages

     375.89 Other

     375.9 Unspecified disorder of lacrimal system

● **376 Disorders of the orbit**

● **376.0 Acute inflammation of orbit**

     376.00 Acute inflammation of orbit, unspecified

     376.01 Orbital cellulitis ✪
         Abscess of orbit
         (Ex:) 376.00-376.04

     376.02 Orbital periostitis ✪
         (Ex:) 003.24, 015.50-015.56, 015.70-015.76, 015.90-015.96,
             017.90-017.96, 376.02, 730.00-730.39, 730.80-730.99

     376.03 Orbital osteomyelitis ✪
         (Ex:) 003.24, 015.50-015.56, 015.70-015.76, 015.90-015.96,
             017.90-017.96, 376.03, 730.00-730.39, 730.80-730.99

     376.04 Tenonitis

● **376.1 Chronic inflammatory disorders of orbit**

     376.10 Chronic inflammation of orbit, unspecified

     376.11 Orbital granuloma
         Pseudotumor (inflammatory) of orbit

     376.12 Orbital myositis

▶   376.13 *Parasitic infestation of orbit*
         Code first underlying disease, as:
         hydatid infestation of orbit (122.3,
             122.6, 122.9)
         myiasis of orbit (134.0)

● **376.2 Endocrine exophthalmos**
         Code first underlying thyroid disorder (242.0–242.9)

▶   376.21 *Thyrotoxic exophthalmos*

▶   376.22 *Exophthalmic ophthalmoplegia*

● **376.3 Other exophthalmic conditions**

     376.30 Exophthalmos, unspecified

     376.31 Constant exophthalmos

     376.32 Orbital hemorrhage

     376.33 Orbital edema or congestion

     376.34 Intermittent exophthalmos

     376.35 Pulsating exophthalmos

     376.36 Lateral displacement of globe

● **376.4 Deformity of orbit**

     376.40 Deformity of orbit, unspecified

     376.41 Hypertelorism of orbit

     376.42 Exostosis of orbit

     376.43 Local deformities due to bone disease

     376.44 Orbital deformities associated with craniofacial deformities

     376.45 Atrophy of orbit

     376.46 Enlargement of orbit

     376.47 Deformity due to trauma or surgery

● **376.5 Enophthalmos**

     376.50 Enophthalmos, unspecified as to cause

     376.51 Enophthalmos due to atrophy of orbital tissue

     376.52 Enophthalmos due to trauma or surgery

     376.6 Retained (old) foreign body following penetrating wound of orbit
         Retrobulbar foreign body

● **376.8 Other orbital disorders**

     376.81 Orbital cysts
         Encephalocele of orbit
         Coding Clinic: 1999, Q3, P13

     376.82 Myopathy of extraocular muscles

     376.89 Other

     376.9 Unspecified disorder of orbit

● **377 Disorders of optic nerve and visual pathways**

● **377.0 Papilledema**

     377.00 Papilledema, unspecified ✪
         (Ex:) 017.30-017.36, 017.90-017.96, 036.81, 249.50-249.51,
             249.80-249.91, 250.50-250.53, 250.80-250.93,
             377.00-377.03, 377.14, 377.24, 379.60-379.90, 379.99,
             743.8-743.9

DISEASES OF THE NERVOUS SYSTEM AND SENSE ORGANS (320–389)

N Newborn Age: 0   **P** Pediatric Age: 0–17   **M** Maternity Age: 12–55   **A** Adult Age: 15–124   ♀ Females Only   ♂ Males Only

(Ex:) CC Exclusions   ✪ Complication\Comorbidity   Major C\C   Present on Admission Requirement   Hospital-Acquired Condition   **875**

Item 6-23 Papilledema is swelling of the optic disc caused by increased intracranial pressure. It is most often bilateral and occurs quickly (hours) or over weeks of time. It is a common symptom of a brain tumor. The term should not be used to describe optic disc swelling with underlying infectious, infiltrative, or inflammatory etiologies.

Figure 6–15 Papilledema. (From Behrman: Nelson Textbook of Pediatrics, 17th ed. 2004, Saunders)

377.01 **Papilledema associated with increased intracranial pressure** 🔗
      Ex: 017.30-017.36, 017.90-017.96, 036.81, 249.50-249.51, 249.80-249.91, 250.50-250.53, 250.80-250.93, 377.00-377.03, 377.14, 377.24, 379.60-379.90, 379.99, 743.8-743.9

377.02 **Papilledema associated with decreased ocular pressure**

377.03 **Papilledema associated with retinal disorder**

377.04 **Foster-Kennedy syndrome**

● 377.1 **Optic atrophy**

377.10 **Optic atrophy, unspecified**

377.11 **Primary optic atrophy**
      | Excludes | *neurosyphilitic optic atrophy (094.84)*

377.12 **Postinflammatory optic atrophy**

377.13 **Optic atrophy associated with retinal dystrophies**

377.14 **Glaucomatous atrophy [cupping] of optic disc**

377.15 **Partial optic atrophy**
      Temporal pallor of optic disc

377.16 **Hereditary optic atrophy**
      Optic atrophy:
        dominant hereditary
        Leber's

● 377.2 **Other disorders of optic disc**

377.21 **Drusen of optic disc**

377.22 **Crater-like holes of optic disc**

377.23 **Coloboma of optic disc**

377.24 **Pseudopapilledema**

● 377.3 **Optic neuritis**
      | Excludes | *meningococcal optic neuritis (036.81)*

377.30 **Optic neuritis, unspecified** 🔗
      Ex: 377.30-377.39

377.31 **Optic papillitis** 🔗
      Ex: 377.30-377.39

377.32 **Retrobulbar neuritis (acute)** 🔗
      | Excludes | *syphilitic retrobulbar neuritis (094.85)*
      Ex: 377.30-377.39

377.33 **Nutritional optic neuropathy**

377.34 **Toxic optic neuropathy**
      Toxic amblyopia

377.39 **Other** 🔗
      | Excludes | *ischemic optic neuropathy (377.41)*
      Ex: 377.30-377.39

● 377.4 **Other disorders of optic nerve**

377.41 **Ischemic optic neuropathy**

377.42 **Hemorrhage in optic nerve sheaths**

377.43 **Optic nerve hypoplasia**
      Coding Clinic: 2006, Q4, P81-82

377.49 **Other**
      Compression of optic nerve

● 377.5 **Disorders of optic chiasm**

377.51 **Associated with pituitary neoplasms and disorders** 🔗
      Ex: 377.51-377.63

377.52 **Associated with other neoplasms** 🔗
      Ex: 377.51-377.63

377.53 **Associated with vascular disorders** 🔗
      Ex: 377.51-377.63

377.54 **Associated with inflammatory disorders** 🔗
      Ex: 377.51-377.63

● 377.6 **Disorders of other visual pathways**

377.61 **Associated with neoplasms** 🔗
      Ex: 377.51-377.63

377.62 **Associated with vascular disorders** 🔗
      Ex: 377.51-377.63

377.63 **Associated with inflammatory disorders** 🔗
      Ex: 377.51-377.63

● 377.7 **Disorders of visual cortex**
      | Excludes | *visual:*
        agnosia (368.16)
        hallucinations (368.16)
        halos (368.15)

377.71 **Associated with neoplasms** 🔗
      Ex: 377.71-377.9

377.72 **Associated with vascular disorders** 🔗
      Ex: 377.71-377.9

377.73 **Associated with inflammatory disorders** 🔗
      Ex: 377.71-377.9

377.75 **Cortical blindness**

377.9 **Unspecified disorder of optic nerve and visual pathways**

DISEASES OF THE NERVOUS SYSTEM AND SENSE ORGANS (320–389)

◀ New   ◀▥ Revised   ~~deleted~~ Deleted   ● Unacceptable Principal Diagnosis   ● Use Additional Digit(s)
▶ Manifestation Code   **OGCR** Official Guidelines   **Coding Clinic** | Excludes | Includes   Use additional   Code first   Omit code

Item 6-24 Strabismus or esotropia (crossed eyes) is a condition of the extraocular eye muscles, resulting in an inability of the eyes to focus and also affects depth perception.

A

B

Figure 6–16 **A.** Image of strabismus. **B.** Exotropia. (**A** from Yanoff: Ophthalmology, 2nd ed. 2004, Mosby, Inc. **B** from Rakel: Textbook of Family Practice, 7th ed. 2007, Saunders)

● **378 Strabismus and other disorders of binocular eye movements**

> **Excludes** *nystagmus and other irregular eye movements (379.50–379.59)*

● **378.0 Esotropia**
Convergent concomitant strabismus

> **Excludes** *intermittent esotropia (378.20–378.22)*

378.00 Esotropia, unspecified

378.01 Monocular esotropia

378.02 Monocular esotropia with A pattern

378.03 Monocular esotropia with V pattern

378.04 Monocular esotropia with other noncomitancies
Monocular esotropia with X or Y pattern

378.05 Alternating esotropia

378.06 Alternating esotropia with A pattern

378.07 Alternating esotropia with V pattern

378.08 Alternating esotropia with other noncomitancies
Alternating esotropia with X or Y pattern

● **378.1 Exotropia**
Misalignment in which one eye deviates outward (away from nose) while other fixates normally
Divergent concomitant strabismus

> **Excludes** *intermittent exotropia (378.20, 378.23–378.24)*

378.10 Exotropia, unspecified

378.11 Monocular exotropia

378.12 Monocular exotropia with A pattern

378.13 Monocular exotropia with V pattern

378.14 Monocular exotropia with other noncomitancies
Monocular exotropia with X or Y pattern

378.15 Alternating exotropia

378.16 Alternating exotropia with A pattern

378.17 Alternating exotropia with V pattern

378.18 Alternating exotropia with other noncomitancies
Alternating exotropia with X or Y pattern

● **378.2 Intermittent heterotropia**
Displacement of an organ or part of an organ from normal position

> **Excludes** *vertical heterotropia (intermittent) (378.31)*

378.20 Intermittent heterotropia, unspecified
Intermittent:
esotropia NOS
exotropia NOS

378.21 Intermittent esotropia, monocular

378.22 Intermittent esotropia, alternating

378.23 Intermittent exotropia, monocular

378.24 Intermittent exotropia, alternating

● **378.3 Other and unspecified heterotropia**

378.30 Heterotropia, unspecified

378.31 Hypertropia
Vertical heterotropia (constant) (intermittent)

378.32 Hypotropia

378.33 Cyclotropia

378.34 Monofixation syndrome
Microtropia

378.35 Accommodative component in esotropia

● **378.4 Heterophoria**
Condition in which one or both eyes wander away from position where both eyes are looking

378.40 Heterophoria, unspecified

378.41 Esophoria
Eye deviates inward (toward nose)

378.42 Exophoria
Eye deviates outward (toward ear)

378.43 Vertical heterophoria

378.44 Cyclophoria

378.45 Alternating hyperphoria

● **378.5 Paralytic strabismus**

378.50 Paralytic strabismus, unspecified

378.51 Third or oculomotor nerve palsy, partial

378.52 Third or oculomotor nerve palsy, total

378.53 Fourth or trochlear nerve palsy
Coding Clinic: 2001, Q2, P21

378.54 Sixth or abducens nerve palsy

378.55 External ophthalmoplegia
Coding Clinic: 1989, Q2, P12

378.56 Total ophthalmoplegia

● **378.6 Mechanical strabismus**

378.60 Mechanical strabismus, unspecified

378.61 Brown's (tendon) sheath syndrome

378.62 Mechanical strabismus from other musculofascial disorders

378.63 Limited duction associated with other conditions

● **378.7 Other specified strabismus**

378.71 Duane's syndrome

378.72 Progressive external ophthalmoplegia

378.73 Strabismus in other neuromuscular disorders

● **378.8 Other disorders of binocular eye movements**

> **Excludes** *nystagmus (379.50–379.56)*

378.81 **Palsy of conjugate gaze**

378.82 **Spasm of conjugate gaze**

378.83 **Convergence insufficiency or palsy**

378.84 **Convergence excess or spasm**

378.85 **Anomalies of divergence**

378.86 **Internuclear ophthalmoplegia**

378.87 **Other dissociated deviation of eye movements**
Skew deviation

378.9 **Unspecified disorder of eye movements**
Ophthalmoplegia NOS
Strabismus NOS
Coding Clinic: 2001, Q2, P21

● **379 Other disorders of eye**

● **379.0 Scleritis and episcleritis**

> *Inflammation of white (sclera and episclera) of eye.*
> *Autoimmune disorders are most common cause.*

> **Excludes** *syphilitic episcleritis (095.0)*

379.00 **Scleritis, unspecified**
Episcleritis NOS

379.01 **Episcleritis periodica fugax**

379.02 **Nodular episcleritis**

379.03 **Anterior scleritis**

379.04 **Scleromalacia perforans**

379.05 **Scleritis with corneal involvement**
Scleroperikeratitis

379.06 **Brawny scleritis**

379.07 **Posterior scleritis**
Sclerotenonitis

379.09 **Other**
Scleral abscess

● **379.1 Other disorders of sclera**

> **Excludes** *blue sclera (743.47)*

379.11 **Scleral ectasia**
Scleral staphyloma NOS

379.12 **Staphyloma posticum**

379.13 **Equatorial staphyloma**

379.14 **Anterior staphyloma, localized**

379.15 **Ring staphyloma**

379.16 **Other degenerative disorders of sclera**

379.19 **Other**

● **379.2 Disorders of vitreous body**

379.21 **Vitreous degeneration**
Vitreous:
cavitation
detachment
liquefaction

379.22 **Crystalline deposits in vitreous**
Asteroid hyalitis
Synchysis scintillans

379.23 **Vitreous hemorrhage**
Coding Clinic: 1991, Q3, P15-16

379.24 **Other vitreous opacities**
Vitreous floaters
Small clumps of cells that float in vitreous of
the eye, appearing as black specks or dots
in field of vision.
Coding Clinic: 1994, Q1, P16

379.25 **Vitreous membranes and strands**

379.26 **Vitreous prolapse**

379.29 **Other disorders of vitreous**

> **Excludes** *vitreous abscess (360.04)*

Coding Clinic: 1999, Q1, P11

● **379.3 Aphakia and other disorders of lens**

> **Excludes** *after-cataract (366.50–366.53)*

379.31 **Aphakia**

> **Excludes** *cataract extraction status (V45.61)*

379.32 **Subluxation of lens**
Coding Clinic: 1994, Q1, P16-17

379.33 **Anterior dislocation of lens**

379.34 **Posterior dislocation of lens**

379.39 **Other disorders of lens**

● **379.4 Anomalies of pupillary function**

379.40 **Abnormal pupillary function, unspecified**

379.41 **Anisocoria**

379.42 **Miosis (persistent), not due to miotics**

379.43 **Mydriasis (persistent), not due to mydriatics**

379.45 **Argyll Robertson pupil, atypical**
Argyll Robertson phenomenon or pupil,
nonsyphilitic

> **Excludes** *Argyll Robertson pupil (syphilitic)*
> *(094.89)*

379.46 **Tonic pupillary reaction**
Adie's pupil or syndrome

379.49 **Other**
Hippus
Pupillary paralysis

● **379.5 Nystagmus and other irregular eye movements**
Nystagmus is rapid, involuntary movements of eyes in
horizontal or vertical direction.

379.50 **Nystagmus, unspecified**
Coding Clinic: 2002, Q4, P68; 2001, Q2, P21

379.51 **Congenital nystagmus**

379.52 **Latent nystagmus**

379.53 **Visual deprivation nystagmus**

379.54 **Nystagmus associated with disorders of the
vestibular system**

379.55 **Dissociated nystagmus**

379.56 **Other forms of nystagmus**

379.57 **Deficiencies of saccadic eye movements**
Abnormal optokinetic response

379.58 **Deficiencies of smooth pursuit movements**

379.59 **Other irregularities of eye movements**
Opsoclonus

DISEASES OF THE NERVOUS SYSTEM AND SENSE ORGANS (320–389)

◀ New   ◀▥ Revised   ~~deleted~~ Deleted   ● Unacceptable Principal Diagnosis   ● Use Additional Digit(s)

▶ Manifestation Code   OGCR Official Guidelines   **Coding Clinic**   Excludes   Includes   Use additional   Code first   Omit code

● **379.6 Inflammation (infection) of postprocedural bleb**
Postprocedural blebitis

379.60 Inflammation (infection) of postprocedural bleb, unspecified

379.61 Inflammation (infection) of postprocedural bleb, stage 1

379.62 Inflammation (infection) of postprocedural bleb, stage 2
Coding Clinic: 2006, Q4, P82-83

379.63 Inflammation (infection) of postprocedural bleb, stage 3
Bleb associated endophthalmitis

379.8 Other specified disorders of eye and adnexa

● **379.9 Unspecified disorder of eye and adnexa**

379.90 Disorder of eye, unspecified

379.91 Pain in or around eye

379.92 Swelling or mass of eye

379.93 Redness or discharge of eye

379.99 Other ill-defined disorders of eye
| Excludes | *blurred vision NOS (368.8)*

DISEASES OF THE EAR AND MASTOID PROCESS (380–389)

Use additional external cause code, if applicable, to identify the cause of the ear condition

● **380 Disorders of external ear**

● **380.0 Perichondritis and chondritis of pinna**
Chondritis of auricle
Perichondritis of auricle

380.00 Perichondritis of pinna, unspecified

380.01 Acute perichondritis of pinna

380.02 Chronic perichondritis of pinna

380.03 Chondritis of pinna
Coding Clinic: 2004, Q4, P75-76

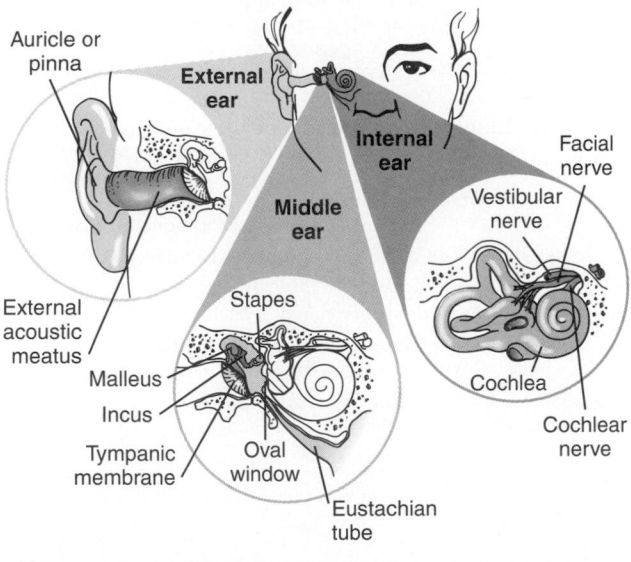

Figure 6–17 Auditory system. (From Buck CJ: Step-by-Step Medical Coding, 2009 ed. Philadelphia, WB Saunders, 2009.)

● **380.1 Infective otitis externa**

380.10 Infective otitis externa, unspecified
Otitis externa (acute):
NOS
circumscribed
diffuse
hemorrhagica
infective NOS

380.11 Acute infection of pinna
| Excludes | *furuncular otitis externa (680.0)*

380.12 Acute swimmers' ear
Beach ear
Tank ear

▶ **380.13 Other acute infections of external ear**
Code first underlying disease, as:
erysipelas (035)
impetigo (684)
seborrheic dermatitis (690.10–690.18)
| Excludes | *herpes simplex (054.73)*
herpes zoster (053.71)

380.14 Malignant otitis externa 🔵
(Ex) 380.14, 383.00-383.1

▶ **380.15 Chronic mycotic otitis externa**
Code first underlying disease, as:
aspergillosis (117.3)
otomycosis NOS (111.9)
| Excludes | *candidal otitis externa (112.82)*

380.16 Other chronic infective otitis externa
Chronic infective otitis externa NOS

● **380.2 Other otitis externa**

380.21 Cholesteatoma of external ear
Keratosis obturans of external ear (canal)
| Excludes | *cholesteatoma NOS*
(385.30–385.35)
postmastoidectomy (383.32)

380.22 Other acute otitis externa
Acute otitis externa:
actinic
chemical
contact
eczematoid
reactive

380.23 Other chronic otitis externa
Chronic otitis externa NOS

● **380.3 Noninfectious disorders of pinna**

380.30 Disorder of pinna, unspecified

380.31 Hematoma of auricle or pinna

380.32 Acquired deformities of auricle or pinna
| Excludes | *cauliflower ear (738.7)*
Coding Clinic: 2003, Q3, P12-13

380.39 Other
| Excludes | *gouty tophi of ear (274.81)*

380.4 Impacted cerumen
Wax in ear
MCE: Questionable admission, principal diagnosis only

● **380.5 Acquired stenosis of external ear canal**
Collapse of external ear canal

380.50 Acquired stenosis of external ear canal, unspecified as to cause

380.51 Secondary to trauma

380.52 Secondary to surgery

380.53 Secondary to inflammation

N Newborn Age: 0   P Pediatric Age: 0–17   M Maternity Age: 12–55   A Adult Age: 15–124   ♀ Females Only   ♂ Males Only
(Ex) CC Exclusions   🔵 Complication\Comorbidity   🔵 Major C\C   🔵 Present on Admission Requirement   🔵 Hospital-Acquired Condition

879

● **380.8 Other disorders of external ear**

    380.81 Exostosis of external ear canal

    380.89 Other

380.9 Unspecified disorder of external ear

● **381 Nonsuppurative otitis media and Eustachian tube disorders**
    Nonsuppurative: not producing pus.

● **381.0 Acute nonsuppurative otitis media**
    Acute tubotympanic catarrh
    Otitis media, acute or subacute:
      catarrhal
      exudative
      transudative
      with effusion

    Excludes *otitic barotrauma (993.0)*

    381.00 Acute nonsuppurative otitis media, unspecified

    381.01 Acute serous otitis media
      Acute or subacute secretory otitis media

    381.02 Acute mucoid otitis media
      Acute or subacute seromucinous otitis media
      Blue drum syndrome

    381.03 Acute sanguinous otitis media

    381.04 Acute allergic serous otitis media

    381.05 Acute allergic mucoid otitis media

    381.06 Acute allergic sanguinous otitis media

● **381.1 Chronic serous otitis media**
    Chronic tubotympanic catarrh

    381.10 Chronic serous otitis media, simple or unspecified

    381.19 Other
      Serosanguinous chronic otitis media

● **381.2 Chronic mucoid otitis media**
    Glue ear
    Excludes *adhesive middle ear disease (385.10–385.19)*

    381.20 Chronic mucoid otitis media, simple or unspecified

    381.29 Other
      Mucosanguinous chronic otitis media

381.3 Other and unspecified chronic nonsuppurative otitis media
    Otitis media, chronic: Otitis media, chronic:
      allergic   seromucinous
      exudative   transudative
      secretory   with effusion

381.4 Nonsuppurative otitis media, not specified as acute or chronic
    Otitis media: Otitis media:
      allergic   seromucinous
      catarrhal   serous
      exudative   transudative
      mucoid   with effusion
      secretory

● **381.5 Eustachian salpingitis**

    381.50 Eustachian salpingitis, unspecified

    381.51 Acute Eustachian salpingitis

    381.52 Chronic Eustachian salpingitis

● **381.6 Obstruction of Eustachian tube**
    Stenosis of Eustachian tube
    Stricture of Eustachian tube

    381.60 Obstruction of Eustachian tube, unspecified

    381.61 Osseous obstruction of Eustachian tube
      Obstruction of Eustachian tube from cholesteatoma, polyp, or other osseous lesion

    381.62 Intrinsic cartilaginous obstruction of Eustachian tube

    381.63 Extrinsic cartilaginous obstruction of Eustachian tube
      Compression of Eustachian tube

381.7 Patulous Eustachian tube

● **381.8 Other disorders of Eustachian tube**

    381.81 Dysfunction of Eustachian tube

    381.89 Other

381.9 Unspecified Eustachian tube disorder

● **382 Suppurative and unspecified otitis media**

● **382.0 Acute suppurative otitis media**
    Suppurative: Discharging pus
    Otitis media, acute:
      necrotizing NOS
      purulent
      pus-filled

    382.00 Acute suppurative otitis media without spontaneous rupture of ear drum

    382.01 Acute suppurative otitis media with spontaneous rupture of ear drum

   ▸ **382.02 Acute suppurative otitis media in diseases classified elsewhere**

      Code first underlying disease, as:
      influenza (487.8)
      scarlet fever (034.1)

      Excludes *postmeasles otitis (055.2)*

382.1 Chronic tubotympanic suppurative otitis media
    Benign chronic suppurative otitis media (with anterior perforation of ear drum)
    Chronic tubotympanic disease (with anterior perforation of ear drum)

382.2 Chronic atticoantral suppurative otitis media
    Chronic atticoantral disease (with posterior or superior marginal perforation of ear drum)
    Persistent mucosal disease (with posterior or superior marginal perforation of ear drum)

382.3 Unspecified chronic suppurative otitis media
    Chronic purulent otitis media
    Excludes *tuberculous otitis media (017.4)*

382.4 Unspecified suppurative otitis media
    Purulent otitis media NOS

382.9 Unspecified otitis media
    Otitis media:
      NOS
      acute NOS
      chronic NOS

DISEASES OF THE NERVOUS SYSTEM AND SENSE ORGANS (320–389)

◀ New   ◀▥ Revised   ~~deleted~~ Deleted   ● Unacceptable Principal Diagnosis   ● Use Additional Digit(s)
▸ Manifestation Code   **OGCR** Official Guidelines   **Coding Clinic**   Excludes   Includes   Use additional   Code first   Omit code

Item 6-25 Mastoiditis is an infection of the portion of the temporal bone of the skull that is behind the ear (mastoid process) caused by an untreated otitis media, leading to an infection of the surrounding structures which may include the brain.

● **383   Mastoiditis and related conditions**

  ● **383.0   Acute mastoiditis**
       Abscess of mastoid
       Empyema of mastoid

     383.00   Acute mastoiditis without complications 🅒
         (Ex) 015.60-015.66, 017.40-017.46, 017.90-017.96, 383.00-383.9,
             388.71-388.9, 744.00, 744.02, 744.09 744.29-744.3

     383.01   Subperiosteal abscess of mastoid 🅒
         (Ex) 015.60-015.66, 017.40-017.46, 017.90-017.96, 383.00-383.9,
             388.71-388.9, 744.00, 744.02, 744.09 744.29-744.3

     383.02   Acute mastoiditis with other complications 🅒
         Gradenigo's syndrome
         (Ex) 015.60-015.66, 017.40-017.46, 017.90-017.96, 383.00-383.9,
             388.71-388.9, 744.00, 744.02, 744.09, 744.29-744.3

   383.1   Chronic mastoiditis
       Caries of mastoid
       Fistula of mastoid

     Excludes   *tuberculous mastoiditis (015.6)*

  ● **383.2   Petrositis**
       Coalescing osteitis of petrous bone
       Inflammation of petrous bone
       Osteomyelitis of petrous bone

     383.20   Petrositis, unspecified

     383.21   Acute petrositis

     383.22   Chronic petrositis

  ● **383.3   Complications following mastoidectomy**

     383.30   Postmastoidectomy complication, unspecified

     383.31   Mucosal cyst of postmastoidectomy cavity

     383.32   Recurrent cholesteatoma of postmastoidectomy cavity

     383.33   Granulations of postmastoidectomy cavity
         Chronic inflammation of
            postmastoidectomy cavity

  ● **383.8   Other disorders of mastoid**

     383.81   Postauricular fistula

     383.89   Other

   383.9   Unspecified mastoiditis

● **384   Other disorders of tympanic membrane**

  ● **384.0   Acute myringitis without mention of otitis media**

     384.00   Acute myringitis, unspecified
         Acute tympanitis NOS

     384.01   Bullous myringitis
         Myringitis bullosa hemorrhagica

     384.09   Other

   384.1   Chronic myringitis without mention of otitis media
       Chronic tympanitis

● **384.2   Perforation of tympanic membrane**
       Perforation of ear drum:
       NOS
       persistent posttraumatic
       postinflammatory

     Excludes   *otitis media with perforation of tympanic*
            membrane (382.00–382.9)
            traumatic perforation [current injury]
            (872.61)

     384.20   Perforation of tympanic membrane, unspecified

     384.21   Central perforation of tympanic membrane

     384.22   Attic perforation of tympanic membrane
         Pars flaccida

     384.23   Other marginal perforation of tympanic membrane

     384.24   Multiple perforations of tympanic membrane

     384.25   Total perforation of tympanic membrane

  ● **384.8   Other specified disorders of tympanic membrane**

     384.81   Atrophic flaccid tympanic membrane
         Healed perforation of ear drum

     384.82   Atrophic nonflaccid tympanic membrane

   384.9   Unspecified disorder of tympanic membrane

● **385   Other disorders of middle ear and mastoid**

     Excludes   *mastoiditis (383.0–383.9)*

  ● **385.0   Tympanosclerosis**

     385.00   Tympanosclerosis, unspecified as to involvement

     385.01   Tympanosclerosis involving tympanic membrane only

     385.02   Tympanosclerosis involving tympanic membrane and ear ossicles

     385.03   Tympanosclerosis involving tympanic membrane, ear ossicles, and middle ear

     385.09   Tympanosclerosis involving other combination of structures

  ● **385.1   Adhesive middle ear disease**
       Adhesive otitis
       Otitis media: Otitis media:
         chronic adhesive   fibrotic

     Excludes   *glue ear (381.20–381.29)*

     385.10   Adhesive middle ear disease, unspecified as to involvement

     385.11   Adhesions of drum head to incus

     385.12   Adhesions of drum head to stapes

     385.13   Adhesions of drum head to promontorium

     385.19   Other adhesions and combinations

DISEASES OF THE NERVOUS SYSTEM AND SENSE ORGANS (320–389)

N   Newborn Age: 0   **P**   Pediatric Age: 0–17   **M**   Maternity Age: 12–55   **A**   Adult Age: 15–124   ♀   Females Only   ♂   Males Only   **881**

(Ex)   CC Exclusions   🅒   Complication\Comorbidity   Major C\C   Present on Admission Requirement   Hospital-Acquired Condition

● **385.2 Other acquired abnormality of ear ossicles**

    385.21 Impaired mobility of malleus
        Ankylosis of malleus

    385.22 Impaired mobility of other ear ossicles
        Ankylosis of ear ossicles, except malleus

    385.23 Discontinuity or dislocation of ear ossicles

    385.24 Partial loss or necrosis of ear ossicles

● **385.3 Cholesteatoma of middle ear and mastoid**
    Cholesterosis of (middle) ear
    Epidermosis of (middle) ear
    Keratosis of (middle) ear
    Polyp of (middle) ear

    | Excludes | *cholesteatoma:* |
        external ear canal (380.21)
        recurrent of postmastoidectomy cavity
        (383.32)

    385.30 Cholesteatoma, unspecified

    385.31 Cholesteatoma of attic

    385.32 Cholesteatoma of middle ear

    385.33 Cholesteatoma of middle ear and mastoid
        Coding Clinic: 2000, Q3, P10-11

    385.35 Diffuse cholesteatosis

● **385.8 Other disorders of middle ear and mastoid**

    385.82 Cholesterin granuloma

    385.83 Retained foreign body of middle ear
        Coding Clinic: 1987, Nov-Dec, P9

    385.89 Other

    385.9 Unspecified disorder of middle ear and mastoid

● **386 Vertiginous syndromes and other disorders of vestibular system**

    | Excludes | *vertigo NOS (780.4)* |
    Coding Clinic: 1985, Mar-April, P12

● **386.0 Méniére's disease**
    Vestibular disorder that produces recurring symptoms
    including severe and intermittent hearing loss
    including feeling of ear pressure or pain.
    Endolymphatic hydrops
    Lermoyez's syndrome
    Méniére's syndrome or vertigo

    386.00 Méniére's disease, unspecified
        Méniére's disease (active)
        Coding Clinic: 1985, Mar-April, P12

    386.01 Active Méniére's disease, cochleovestibular

    386.02 Active Méniére's disease, cochlear

    386.03 Active Méniére's disease, vestibular

    386.04 Inactive Méniére's disease
        Méniére's disease in remission

● **386.1 Other and unspecified peripheral vertigo**

    | Excludes | *epidemic vertigo (078.81)* |

    386.10 Peripheral vertigo, unspecified

    386.11 Benign paroxysmal positional vertigo
        Benign paroxysmal positional nystagmus

    386.12 Vestibular neuronitis
        Acute (and recurrent) peripheral
        vestibulopathy

    386.19 Other
        Aural vertigo   Otogenic vertigo

    386.2 Vertigo of central origin
        Central positional nystagmus
        Malignant positional vertigo

● **386.3 Labyrinthitis**
    Balance disorder that follows a URI or head injury. The
    inflammatory process affects the labyrinth that
    houses vestibular system (senses changes in head
    position) of inner ear.

    386.30 Labyrinthitis, unspecified

    386.31 Serous labyrinthitis
        Diffuse labyrinthitis

    386.32 Circumscribed labyrinthitis
        Focal labyrinthitis

    386.33 Suppurative labyrinthitis
        Purulent labyrinthitis

    386.34 Toxic labyrinthitis

    386.35 Viral labyrinthitis

● **386.4 Labyrinthine fistula**

    386.40 Labyrinthine fistula, unspecified

    386.41 Round window fistula

    386.42 Oval window fistula

    386.43 Semicircular canal fistula

    386.48 Labyrinthine fistula of combined sites

● **386.5 Labyrinthine dysfunction**

    386.50 Labyrinthine dysfunction, unspecified

    386.51 Hyperactive labyrinth, unilateral

    386.52 Hyperactive labyrinth, bilateral

    386.53 Hypoactive labyrinth, unilateral

    386.54 Hypoactive labyrinth, bilateral

    386.55 Loss of labyrinthine reactivity, unilateral

    386.56 Loss of labyrinthine reactivity, bilateral

    386.58 Other forms and combinations

    386.8 Other disorders of labyrinth

    386.9 Unspecified vertiginous syndromes and labyrinthine disorders

● **387 Otosclerosis**
    Inherited middle ear spongelike bone growth causing hearing
    loss because growth prevents vibration from sound waves
    required for hearing.

    | Includes | otospongiosis |

    387.0 Otosclerosis involving oval window, nonobliterative

    387.1 Otosclerosis involving oval window, obliterative

    387.2 Cochlear otosclerosis
        Otosclerosis involving:
        otic capsule
        round window

    387.8 Other otosclerosis

    387.9 Otosclerosis, unspecified

● **388 Other disorders of ear**

● **388.0 Degenerative and vascular disorders of ear**

    388.00 Degenerative and vascular disorders, unspecified

    388.01 Presbyacusis

    388.02 Transient ischemic deafness

◀ New   ◀▥ Revised   ~~deleted~~ Deleted   ● Unacceptable Principal Diagnosis   ● Use Additional Digit(s)

▶ Manifestation Code   **OGCR** Official Guidelines   **Coding Clinic**   Excludes   Includes   Use additional   Code first   Omit code

DISEASES OF THE NERVOUS SYSTEM AND SENSE ORGANS (320–389)

● **388.1   Noise effects on inner ear**

    388.10   Noise effects on inner ear, unspecified

    388.11   Acoustic trauma (explosive) to ear
        Otitic blast injury

    388.12   Noise-induced hearing loss

388.2   Sudden hearing loss, unspecified

● **388.3   Tinnitus**
    Perception of sound in absence of external noise and may
    affect one or both ears and/or head

    388.30   Tinnitus, unspecified

    388.31   Subjective tinnitus

    388.32   Objective tinnitus

● **388.4   Other abnormal auditory perception**

    388.40   Abnormal auditory perception, unspecified

    388.41   Diplacusis

    388.42   Hyperacusis

    388.43   Impairment of auditory discrimination

    388.44   Recruitment

    388.45   Acquired auditory processing disorder
        Auditory processing disorder NOS

        Excludes *central auditory processing disorder*
             (315.32)
        Coding Clinic: 2007, Q4, P79

388.5   Disorders of acoustic nerve
    Acoustic neuritis
    Degeneration of acoustic or eighth nerve
    Disorder of acoustic or eighth nerve

    Excludes *acoustic neuroma (225.1)*
            syphilitic acoustic neuritis (094.86)
    Coding Clinic: 1987, Mar-April, P8

● **388.6   Otorrhea**

    388.60   Otorrhea, unspecified
        Discharging ear NOS

    388.61   Cerebrospinal fluid otorrhea🔖

        Excludes *cerebrospinal fluid rhinorrhea*
             (349.81)

        (Ex) 388.61-388.69

    388.69   Other
        Otorrhagia

● **388.7   Otalgia**

    388.70   Otalgia, unspecified
        Earache NOS

    388.71   Otogenic pain

    388.72   Referred pain
        Pain from a diseased area of the body that is not
            felt directly in that area, but in another
            part of the body.

388.8   Other disorders of ear

388.9   Unspecified disorder of ear

● **389   Hearing loss**

● **389.0   Conductive hearing loss**
    Conductive deafness

    Excludes *mixed conductive and sensorineural hearing*
            loss (389.20–389.22)

    389.00   Conductive hearing loss, unspecified

    389.01   Conductive hearing loss, external ear

    389.02   Conductive hearing loss, tympanic
          membrane

    389.03   Conductive hearing loss, middle ear

    389.04   Conductive hearing loss, inner ear

    389.05   Conductive hearing loss, unilateral

    389.06   Conductive hearing loss, bilateral
        Coding Clinic: 2007, Q4, P80-81

    389.08   Conductive hearing loss of combined types

● **389.1   Sensorineural hearing loss**
    Perceptive hearing loss or deafness

    Excludes *abnormal auditory perception*
            (388.40–388.44)
         mixed conductive and sensorineural hearing
            loss (389.20–389.22)
         psychogenic deafness (306.7)
    Coding Clinic: 2007, Q4, P80-81; 2006, Q4, P84

    389.10   Sensorineural hearing loss, unspecified
        Coding Clinic: 1993, Q1, P29

    389.11   Sensory hearing loss, bilateral

    389.12   Neural hearing loss, bilateral

    389.13   Neural hearing loss, unilateral

    389.14   Central hearing loss

    389.15   Sensorineural hearing loss, unilateral

    389.16   Sensorineural hearing loss, asymmetrical

    389.17   Sensory hearing loss, unilateral

    389.18   Sensorineural hearing loss, bilateral

● **389.2   Mixed conductive and sensorineural hearing loss**
    Deafness or hearing loss of type classifiable
        to 389.00–389.08 with type classifiable to
        389.10–389.18
    Coding Clinic: 2007, Q4, P80-81

    389.20   Mixed hearing loss, unspecified

    389.21   Mixed hearing loss, unilateral

    389.22   Mixed hearing loss, bilateral

389.7   Deaf nonspeaking, not elsewhere classifiable

389.8   Other specified forms of hearing loss

389.9   Unspecified hearing loss
    Deafness NOS
    Coding Clinic: 2004, Q1, P15-16

DISEASES OF THE NERVOUS SYSTEM AND SENSE ORGANS (320–389)

N   Newborn Age: 0   P   Pediatric Age: 0–17   M   Maternity Age: 12–55   A   Adult Age: 15–124   ♀   Females Only   ♂   Males Only

(Ex)   CC Exclusions   🔖   Complication\Comorbidity   🔖   Major C\C   🔖   Present on Admission Requirement   🔖   Hospital-Acquired Condition   **883**

Figure 7–1 Cardiovascular valves.

Item 7–1 Rheumatic fever is the inflammation of the valve(s) of the heart, usually the mitral or aortic, which leads to valve damage. Rheumatic heart inflammations are usually **pericarditis** (sac surrounding heart), **endocarditis** (heart cavity), or **myocarditis** (heart muscle).

7.   DISEASES OF THE CIRCULATORY SYSTEM (390–459)

ACUTE RHEUMATIC FEVER (390–392)

390   Rheumatic fever without mention of heart involvement
     Arthritis, rheumatic, acute or subacute
     Rheumatic fever (active) (acute)
     Rheumatism, articular, acute or subacute
     Excludes   *that with heart involvement (391.0–391.9)*

● **391   Rheumatic fever with heart involvement**
     Excludes   *chronic heart diseases of rheumatic origin (393–398.99) unless rheumatic fever is also present or there is evidence of recrudescence or activity of the rheumatic process*

    391.0   Acute rheumatic pericarditis 🍰
       Rheumatic:
         fever (active) (acute) with pericarditis
         pericarditis (acute)
       Any condition classifiable to 390 with pericarditis
       Excludes   *that not specified as rheumatic (420.0–420.9)*
       (Ex:) 074.21, 093.81, 391.0, 393, 420.0-420.99, 423.3-423.9, 459.89-459.9

    391.1   Acute rheumatic endocarditis 🍰
       Rheumatic:
         endocarditis, acute
         fever (active) (acute) with endocarditis or valvulitis
         valvulitis acute
       Any condition classifiable to 390 with endocarditis or valvulitis
       (Ex:) 002.0, 036.42, 074.22, 083.0, 093.20-093.24, 098.84, 112.81, 115.94, 390, 391.1, 391.8-392.0, 394.0-395.9, 396.9-397.9, 398.90, 398.99, 421.0-421.9, 424.0-424.99, 425.3, 459.89-459.9, 746.09, 746.89, 996.61

    391.2   Acute rheumatic myocarditis 🍰
       Rheumatic fever (active) (acute) with myocarditis
       Any condition classifiable to 390 with myocarditis
       (Ex:) 074.20, 074.22-074.23, 093.82, 390, 391.2-391.9, 398.0-398.90, 398.99, 422.0-422.99, 429.0, 429.71-429.79, 459.89-459.9

391.8   Other acute rheumatic heart disease 🍰
     Rheumatic:
       fever (active) (acute) with other or multiple types of heart involvement
       pancarditis, acute
     Any condition classifiable to 390 with other or multiple types of heart involvement
     (Ex:) 391.0-398.99, 428.20-428.43

391.9   Acute rheumatic heart disease, unspecified 🍰
     Rheumatic:
       carditis, acute
       fever (active) (acute) with unspecified type of heart involvement
       heart disease, active or acute
     Any condition classifiable to 390 with unspecified type of heart involvement
     (Ex:) 391.0-398.99

● **392   Rheumatic chorea**
     Includes   Sydenham's chorea
     Excludes   *chorea:*
         NOS (333.5)
         Huntington's (333.4)

    392.0   With heart involvement 🍰
       Rheumatic chorea with heart involvement of any type classifiable to 391
       (Ex:) 391.0-398.99, 428.20-428.43

    392.9   Without mention of heart involvement 🍰
       (Ex:) 391.0-398.99

Item 7–2   Rheumatic chorea, also called Sydenham's, juvenile, minor, simple, or St. Vitus' dance, is a major symptom of rheumatic fever and is characterized by ceaseless, involuntary, jerky, purposeless movements.

CHRONIC RHEUMATIC HEART DISEASE (393–398)

393   Chronic rheumatic pericarditis 🍰
     Adherent pericardium, rheumatic
     Chronic rheumatic:
       mediastinopericarditis
       myopericarditis
     Excludes   *pericarditis NOS or not specified as rheumatic (423.0–423.9)*
     (Ex:) 074.21, 093.81, 391.0, 393, 420.0-420.99, 423.3-423.9, 459.89-459.9

● **394   Diseases of mitral valve**
     Excludes   *that with aortic valve involvement (396.0–396.9)*

    394.0   Mitral stenosis
       Mitral (valve):
         obstruction (rheumatic)
         stenosis NOS

Item 7–3   Mitral stenosis is the narrowing of the mitral valve separating the left atrium from the left ventricle. **Mitral insufficiency** is the improper closure of the mitral valve which may lead to enlargement (hypertrophy) of the left atrium.

◀ New   ◀☰ Revised   ~~deleted~~ Deleted   ● Unacceptable Principal Diagnosis   ● Use Additional Digit(s)
▶ Manifestation Code   **OGCR** Official Guidelines   **Coding Clinic**   Excludes   Includes   Use additional   Code first   Omit code

DISEASES OF THE CIRCULATORY SYSTEM (390–459)

394.1 Rheumatic mitral insufficiency
Rheumatic mitral:
indent incompetence
indent regurgitation

> **Excludes** *that not specified as rheumatic (424.0)*

Coding Clinic: 2005, Q2, P14-15

394.2 Mitral stenosis with insufficiency
Mitral stenosis with incompetence or regurgitation
Coding Clinic: 2007, Q2, P11-12

394.9 Other and unspecified mitral valve diseases
Mitral (valve):
indent disease (chronic)
indent failure

Item 7–4 Aortic stenosis is the narrowing of the aortic valve located between the left ventricle and the aorta. **Aortic insufficiency** is the improper closure of the aortic valve which may lead to enlargement (hypertrophy) of the left ventricle.

● **395 Diseases of aortic valve**

> **Excludes** *that not specified as rheumatic (424.1)*
> *that with mitral valve involvement (396.0–396.9)*

395.0 Rheumatic aortic stenosis
Rheumatic aortic (valve) obstruction
Coding Clinic: 1988, Q4, P8

395.1 Rheumatic aortic insufficiency
Rheumatic aortic:
indent incompetence
indent regurgitation

395.2 Rheumatic aortic stenosis with insufficiency
Rheumatic aortic stenosis with incompetence or regurgitation

395.9 Other and unspecified rheumatic aortic diseases
Rheumatic aortic (valve) disease

Item 7–5 Mitral and aortic valve stenosis is the narrowing of these valves, which leads to enlargement (hypertrophy) of the left atrium and left ventricle respectively, while **mitral and aortic insufficiency** is the improper closure of the mitral and aortic valves resulting in the same outcome as stenosis.

● **396 Diseases of mitral and aortic valves**

> **Includes** involvement of both mitral and aortic valves, whether specified as rheumatic or not

396.0 Mitral valve stenosis and aortic valve stenosis
Atypical aortic (valve) stenosis
Mitral and aortic (valve) obstruction (rheumatic)

396.1 Mitral valve stenosis and aortic valve insufficiency

396.2 Mitral valve insufficiency and aortic valve stenosis
Coding Clinic: 2009, Q2, P11; 2000, Q2, P16-17; 1987, Nov-Dec, P8

396.3 Mitral valve insufficiency and aortic valve insufficiency
Mitral and aortic (valve):
indent incompetence
indent regurgitation
Coding Clinic: 2009, Q2, P11; Q1, P8; 1995, Q1, P6

396.8 Multiple involvement of mitral and aortic valves
Stenosis and insufficiency of mitral or aortic valve with stenosis or insufficiency, or both, of the other valve

396.9 Mitral and aortic valve diseases, unspecified

● **397 Diseases of other endocardial structures**
Affects thin serous endothelial tissue that lines inside of heart

397.0 Diseases of tricuspid valve
Tricuspid (valve) (rheumatic):
indent disease
indent insufficiency
indent obstruction
indent regurgitation
indent stenosis
Coding Clinic: 2006, Q3, P7; 2000, Q2, P16-17

397.1 Rheumatic diseases of pulmonary valve

> **Excludes** *that not specified as rheumatic (424.3)*

397.9 Rheumatic diseases of endocardium, valve unspecified
Rheumatic:
indent endocarditis (chronic)
indent valvulitis (chronic)

> **Excludes** *that not specified as rheumatic (424.90–424.99)*

● **398 Other rheumatic heart disease**

398.0 Rheumatic myocarditis 🄒
Rheumatic degeneration of myocardium

> **Excludes** *myocarditis not specified as rheumatic (429.0)*

Ex: 390, 391.2-391.9, 398.0-398.90, 398.99, 422.0-422.99, 429.0, 429.71-429.79, 459.89-459.9

● **398.9 Other and unspecified rheumatic heart diseases**

398.90 Rheumatic heart disease, unspecified
Rheumatic:
indent carditis
indent heart disease NOS

> **Excludes** *carditis not specified as rheumatic (429.89)*
> *heart disease NOS not specified as rheumatic (429.9)*

398.91 Rheumatic heart failure (congestive) 🄒
Rheumatic left ventricular failure
Ex: 398.90-398.99, 402.01, 402.11, 402.91, 428.0-428.9, 459.89-459.9
Coding Clinic: 2005, Q2, P14-15; 1995, Q1, P6

398.99 Other

Item 7–6 Hypertension is caused by high arterial blood pressure in the arteries. **Essential, primary,** or **idiopathic** hypertension occurs without identifiable organic cause.
Secondary hypertension is that which has an organic cause.
Malignant hypertension is severely elevated blood pressure.
Benign hypertension is mildly elevated blood pressure.

HYPERTENSIVE DISEASE (401–405)

Excludes   *that complicating pregnancy, childbirth, or the*
      puerperium (642.0–642.9)
      that involving coronary vessels (410.00–414.9)

● **401   Essential hypertension**

Includes   high blood pressure
     hyperpiesia
     hyperpiesis
     hypertension (arterial) (essential) (primary)
       (systemic)
     hypertensive vascular:
      degeneration
      disease

Excludes   *elevated blood pressure without diagnosis of*
      hypertension (796.2)
      pulmonary hypertension (416.0–416.9)
      that involving vessels of:
       brain (430–438)
       eye (362.11)
Coding Clinic: 1992, Q2, P5

401.0   Malignant🔾
    (Ex) 401.0-405.99, 459.89-459.9
    Coding Clinic: 1993, Q4, P37; 5th Issue, P9-10

401.1   Benign
    MCE: Questionable admission, principal diagnosis
     only

401.9   Unspecified
    Coding Clinic: 2009, Q1, P6; 2008, Q2, P16; 2005, Q4, P68-69; Q3,
     P3-9; 2004, Q4, P77-78; 2003, Q4, P105-106,108, 111; Q3,
     P14-15; Q2, P16; 1997, Q4, P35-37; 1989, Q2, P12; 1987,
     Sept-Oct, P11

OGCR   Section I.C.7.a.2
    Heart conditions (425.8, 429.0-429.3, 429.8, 429.9)
    are assigned to a code from category 402 when a
    causal relationship is stated (due to hypertension)
    or implied (hypertensive). Use an additional
    code from category 428 to identify the type of
    heart failure in those patients with heart failure.
    More than one code from category 428 may be
    assigned if the patient has systolic or diastolic
    failure and congestive heart failure. The same
    heart conditions (425.8, 429.0-429.3, 429.8, 429.9)
    with hypertension, but without a stated causal
    relationship, are coded separately. Sequence
    according to the circumstances of the admission/
    encounter.

● **402   Hypertensive heart disease**

Includes   hypertensive:
     cardiomegaly
     cardiopathy
     cardiovascular disease
     heart (disease) (failure)
    any condition classifiable to 429.0–429.3, 429.8,
     429.9 due to hypertension

Use additional code to specify type of heart failure
    (428.0–428.43), if known
Coding Clinic: 1993, Q2, P9; 1987, Nov-Dec, P9

● **402.0   Malignant**
    402.00   Without heart failure🔾
      (Ex) 401.0-405.99, 459.89-459.9
      Coding Clinic: 2008, Q4, P177-180

    402.01   With heart failure🔾
      (Ex) 398.91, 401.0-405.99, 428.0-428.9, 459.89-459.9

● **402.1   Benign**
    402.10   Without heart failure
    402.11   With heart failure

● **402.9   Unspecified**
    Coding Clinic: 1993, Q2, P9
    402.90   Without heart failure
    402.91   With heart failure
      Coding Clinic: 2002, Q4, P52; 1993, Q1, P19-20; 1989, Q2,
      P12; 1984, Nov-Dec, P18

OGCR   Section I.C.7.a.3
    Assign codes from category 403, Hypertensive
    kidney disease, when conditions classified
    to categories 585-587 are present. Unlike
    hypertension with heart disease, ICD-9-CM
    presumes a cause-and-effect relationship and
    classifies renal failure with hypertension as
    hypertensive kidney disease.

● **403   Hypertensive chronic kidney disease**

Includes   arteriolar nephritis
     arteriosclerosis of:
      kidney
      renal arterioles
     arteriosclerotic nephritis (chronic) (interstitial)
     hypertensive:
      nephropathy
      renal failure
      uremia (chronic)
     nephrosclerosis
     renal sclerosis with hypertension
     any condition classifiable to 585 with any
      condition classifiable to 401

Excludes   *acute ~~renal~~ kidney failure (584.5–584.9)* ◀▥
     renal disease stated as not due to hypertension
     renovascular hypertension (405.0–405.9 with
      fifth-digit 1)
Coding Clinic: 2003, Q1, P20-21; 1992, Q2, P5

The following fifth-digit subclassification is for use with
category 403:

> **0   with chronic kidney disease stage I through stage**
>   **IV, or unspecified**
>   Use additional code to identify the stage of chronic
>   kidney disease (585.1–585.4, 585.9)
>
> **1   with chronic kidney disease stage V or end stage**
>   **renal disease**
>   Use additional code to identify the stage of chronic
>   kidney disease (585.5, 585.6)

● **403.0   Malignant**🔾
   [0-1]   (Ex) 401.0-405.99, 459.89-459.9

● **403.1   Benign 1**🔾
   [0-1]   For code **403.11:** (Ex) 401.0-405.99, 459.89-459.9

● **403.9   Unspecified 1**🔾
   [0-1]   For code **403.91:** (Ex) 401.0-405.99, 459.89-459.9
      Coding Clinic: 2008, Q1, P7-8, 10-11; 2007, Q2, P3; 2006, Q4,
      P84-86; 2005, Q4, P68-69; 2004, Q1, P14-15; 2001, Q2,
      P11; 1987, Sept-Oct, P9, 11; 1985, Nov-Dec, P15

◀ New   ◀▥ Revised   ~~deleted~~ Deleted   ● Unacceptable Principal Diagnosis   ● Use Additional Digit(s)
▶ Manifestation Code   OGCR Official Guidelines   Coding Clinic   Excludes   Includes   Use additional   Code first   Omit code

OGCR Section I.C.7.a.4

> Assign codes from combination category 404
> when both hypertensive kidney disease and
> hypertensive heart disease are stated in the
> diagnosis. Assume a relationship between the
> hypertension and the kidney disease, whether
> or not the condition is so designated. Assign an
> additional code from category 428, to identify the
> type of heart failure. More than one code from
> category 428 may be assigned if the patient has
> systolic or diastolic failure and congestive heart
> failure.

● **404   Hypertensive heart and chronic kidney disease**

> **Includes**   disease:
> cardiorenal
> cardiovascular renal
> any condition classifiable to 402 with any
> condition classifiable to 403

Use additional code to specify type of heart failure
(428.0–428.43), if known
Coding Clinic: 2006, Q4, P84-86; 2005, Q4, P68-69

The following fifth-digit subclassification is for use with
category 404:

> **0   without heart failure and with chronic kidney
> disease stage I through stage IV, or unspecified**
> Use additional code to identify the stage of chronic
> kidney disease (585.1–585.4, 585.9)
>
> **1   with heart failure and with chronic kidney disease
> stage I through stage IV, or unspecified**
> Use additional code to identify the stage of chronic
> kidney disease (585.1–585.4, 585.9)
>
> **2   without heart failure and with chronic kidney
> disease stage V or end stage renal disease**
> Use additional code to identify the stage of chronic
> kidney disease (585.5, 585.6)
>
> **3   with heart failure and chronic kidney disease stage
> V or end stage renal disease**
> Use additional code to identify the stage of chronic
> kidney disease (585.5, 585.6)

● **404.0 Malignant** 🝙
  [0-3]   (Ex) 401.0-405.99, 459.89-459.9
● **404.1 Benign 1-3** 🝙
  [0-3]   For codes **404.11-404.13:** (Ex) 401.0-405.99, 459.89-459.9
● **404.9 Unspecified 1-3** 🝙
  [0-3]   For codes **404.91-404.93:** (Ex) 401.0-405.99, 459.89-459.9

● **405   Secondary hypertension**
  ● **405.0 Malignant**
      405.01 Renovascular 🝙
              (Ex) 401.0-405.99, 459.89-459.9
      405.09 Other 🝙
              (Ex) 401.0-405.99, 459.89-459.9
  ● **405.1 Benign**
      405.11 Renovascular
      405.19 Other
  ● **405.9 Unspecified**
      405.91 Renovascular
      405.99 Other
      Coding Clinic: 2000, Q3, P4-5; 1987, Sept-Oct, P9, 11

Figure 7-2   Myocardial
infarction.

—Zone of
injury
—Zone of
infarction
—Zone of
ischemia

Item 7-7   Myocardial infarction is a sudden decrease in
the coronary artery blood flow that results in death of the heart
muscle. Classifications are based on the affected heart tissue.

OGCR Section I.C.7.e.1

> The codes for acute myocardial infarction (AMI) identify
> the site, such as anterolateral wall or true posterior wall.
> Subcategories 410.0-410.6 and 410.8 are used for ST
> elevation myocardial infarction (STEMI).

ISCHEMIC HEART DISEASE (410–414)

Includes   that with mention of hypertension
Use additional code to identify presence of hypertension
(401.0–405.9)

● **410   Acute myocardial infarction**

> **Includes**   cardiac infarction
> coronary (artery):
> embolism
> occlusion
> rupture
> thrombosis
> infarction of heart, myocardium, or ventricle
> rupture of heart, myocardium, or ventricle
> ST elevation (STEMI) and non-ST elevation
> (NSTEMI) myocardial infarction
> any condition classifiable to 414.1–414.9
> specified as acute or with a stated
> duration of 8 weeks or less
> Coding Clinic: 2006, Q2, P9; 1997, Q4, P37; 1994, Q4, P55; 1993, Q4,
> P39-41; 1992, Q1, P10; 1991, Q3, P18; 1986, Nov-Dec, P12

The following fifth-digit subclassification is for use with
category 410:

> **0   episode of care unspecified**
> Use when the source document does not contain
> sufficient information for the assignment of
> fifth-digit 1 or 2.
> **1   initial episode of care**
> Use fifth-digit 1 to designate the first episode of
> care (regardless of facility site) for a newly
> diagnosed myocardial infarction. The
> fifth-digit 1 is assigned regardless of the
> number of times a patient may be transferred
> during the initial episode of care.
> **2   subsequent episode of care**
> Use fifth-digit 2 to designate an episode of care
> following the initial episode when the patient
> is admitted for further observation, evaluation
> or treatment for a myocardial infarction that
> has received initial treatment, but is still less
> than 8 weeks old.

● **410.0 Of anterolateral wall 1** 🝙
  [0-2]   ST elevation myocardial infarction (STEMI) of
          anterolateral wall
          For code **410.01:** (Ex) 410.00-410.92, 459.89-459.9
          Coding Clinic: 2008, Q4, P69-73; 2001, Q3, P21; 1998, Q3, P15;
          1993, 5th Issue, P14, 17-24

DISEASES OF THE CIRCULATORY SYSTEM (390–459)

N   Newborn Age: 0   P   Pediatric Age: 0–17   M   Maternity Age: 12–55   A   Adult Age: 15–124   ♀   Females Only   ♂   Males Only
(Ex) CC Exclusions   🝙 Complication\Comorbidity   🝙 Major C\C   🝙 Present on Admission Requirement   🝙 Hospital-Acquired Condition

● **410.1 Of other anterior wall** 1 🐾
[0-2]   Infarction:
         anterior (wall) NOS (with contiguous portion of
            intraventricular septum)
         anteroapical (with contiguous portion of
            intraventricular septum)
         anteroseptal (with contiguous portion of
            intraventricular septum)
         ST elevation myocardial infarction (STEMI) of other
            anterior wall
         For code **410.11:** (Ex) 410.00-410.92, 459.89-459.9
         Coding Clinic: 2003, Q3, P10-11

● **410.2 Of inferolateral wall** 1 🐾
[0-2]   ST elevation myocardial infarction (STEMI) of
         inferolateral wall
         For code **410.31:** (Ex) 410.00-410.92, 459.89-459.9
         Coding Clinic: 1993, 5th Issue, P17-24

● **410.3 Of inferoposterior wall** 1 🐾
[0-2]   ST elevation myocardial infarction (STEMI) of
         inferoposterior wall
         For code **410.31:** (Ex) 410.00-410.92, 459.89-459.9

● **410.4 Of other inferior wall** 1 🐾
[0-2]   Infarction:
         diaphragmatic wall NOS (with contiguous
            portion of intraventricular septum)
         inferior (wall) NOS (with contiguous portion of
            intraventricular septum)
         ST elevation myocardial infarction (STEMI) of other
            inferior wall
         For code **410.41:** (Ex) 410.00-410.92, 459.89-459.9
         Coding Clinic: 2006, Q3, P8-9; 2001, Q2, P8-9; 2000, Q1, P7; 1997,
            Q3, P10; 1993, 5th Issue, P13-14x2

● **410.5 Of other lateral wall** 1 🐾
[0-2]   Infarction:
         apical-lateral
         basal-lateral
         high lateral
         posterolateral
         ST elevation myocardial infarction (STEMI) of other
            lateral wall
         For code **410.51:** (Ex) 410.00-410.92, 459.89-459.9

● **410.6 True posterior wall infarction** 1 🐾
[0-2]   Infarction:
         posterobasal
         strictly posterior
         ST elevation myocardial infarction (STEMI) of true
            posterior wall
         For code **410.61:** (Ex) 410.00-410.92, 459.89-459.9

● **410.7 Subendocardial infarction** 1 🐾
[0-2]   Non-ST elevation myocardial infarction (NSTEMI)
         Nontransmural infarction
         For code **410.71:** (Ex) 410.00-410.92, 459.89-459.9
         Coding Clinic: 2005, Q4, P69-72; Q2, P19-20; 2000, Q1, P7

OGCR Section I.C.7.e.1

The ICD-9-CM codes for acute myocardial
infarction (AMI) identify the site, such as
anterolateral wall or true posterior wall.
Subcategories 410.0–410.6 and 410.8 are used
for ST elevtion myocardial infarction (STEMI).
Subcategory 410.7, Subendocardial infarction, is
used for non ST elevation myocardial infarction
(NSTEMI) and nontransmural MIs.

● **410.8 Of other specified sites** 1 🐾
[0-2]   Infarction of:
         atrium
         papillary muscle
         septum alone
         ST elevation myocardial infarction (STEMI) of other
            specified sites
         For code **410.81:** (Ex) 410.00-410.92, 459.89-459.9

● **410.9 Unspecified site** 1 🐾
[0-2]   Acute myocardial infarction NOS
         Coronary occlusion NOS
         Myocardial infarction NOS
         For code **410.91:** (Ex) 410.00-410.92, 459.89-459.9
         Coding Clinic: 2005, Q2, P18-19; 2002, Q3, P5; 1999, Q4, P9; 1993,
            5th Issue, P13

OGCR Section I.C.7.e.2

Subcategory 410.9 is the default for the
unspecified term acute myocardial infarction. If
only STEMI or transmural MI without the site is
documented, query the provider as to the site, or
assign a code from subcategory 410.9.

● **411 Other acute and subacute forms of ischemic heart disease**
         Coding Clinic: 1994, Q4, P55

    411.0 Postmyocardial infarction syndrome 🐾
         Dressler's syndrome
         (Ex) 411.0, 411.81-411.89, 459.89-459.9

    411.1 Intermediate coronary syndrome 🐾
         Impending infarction
         Preinfarction angina
         Preinfarction syndrome
         Unstable angina

         | **Excludes** | *angina (pectoris) (413.9)*
                       decubitus (413.0)
         (Ex) 398.91, 402.01, 402.11, 402.91, 404.01, 404.03, 404.11, 404.13, 404.91,
            404.93, 410.00-410.92, 411.1-411.89, 413.0-414.00, 414.2-414.9,
            428.0-428.1, 428.9, 459.89-459.9, 785.50-785.51
         Coding Clinic: 2005, Q4, P103-106; 2004, Q2, P3-4; 2003, Q1,
            P12-13; 2001, Q3, P15; Q2, P7-9; 1998, Q4, P85-86; 1996,
            Q2, P10; 1995, Q2, P18-19; 1993, Q4, P39-40; 5th Issue,
            P17-24; 1991, Q1, P14; 1989, Q4, P10

◀ New   ◀≡ Revised   ~~deleted~~ Deleted   ● Unacceptable Principal Diagnosis   ● Use Additional Digit(s)
▶ Manifestation Code   **OGCR** Official Guidelines   **Coding Clinic**   Excludes   Includes   Use additional   Code first   Omit code

● **411.8 Other**

     411.81 Acute coronary occlusion without myocardial infarction 🍎

         Acute coronary (artery):
            embolism without or not resulting in myocardial infarction
            obstruction without or not resulting in myocardial infarction
            occlusion without or not resulting in myocardial infarction
            thrombosis without or not resulting in myocardial infarction

         | **Excludes** | *obstruction without infarction due to atherosclerosis (414.00–414.07)* |
         | | *occlusion without infarction due to atherosclerosis (414.00–414.07)* |

         (Ex) 410.00-411.89, 413.0-413.9, 414.8-414.9, 459.89-459.9
         Coding Clinic: 2001, Q2, P7-8; 1991, Q3, P18; Q1, P14

     411.89 Other 🍎
         Coronary insufficiency (acute)
         Subendocardial ischemia
         (Ex) 410.00-411.89, 413.0-413.9, 414.8-414.9, 459.89-459.9
         Coding Clinic: 2001, Q3, P14; 1992, Q1, P9-10; 1991, Q3, P18

Item 7-8 "Old" (healed) myocardial infarction: Code 412 cannot be used if the patient is experiencing current ischemic heart disease symptoms. Recent infarctions still under care cannot be coded to 412. This code is only assigned if infarction has some impact on the current episode of care—essentially, it is a history of (H/O) a past, healed MI. (There is no V code for this status/post MI.)

412 Old myocardial infarction 🔖
     Healed myocardial infarction
     Past myocardial infarction diagnosed on ECG [EKG] or other special investigation, but currently presenting no symptoms
     Coding Clinic: 2003, Q2, P10; 2001, Q3, P21; Q2, P9; 1998, Q3, P15; 1993, 5th Issue, P17-24

● **413 Angina pectoris**
     Chest pain/discomfort due to lack of oxygen to heart muscle. Principal symptom of myocardial infarction.

     413.0 Angina decubitus 🍎
         Nocturnal angina
         (Ex) 410.00-410.92, 411.1-411.89, 413.0-413.9, 414.8-414.9, 459.89-459.9

     413.1 Prinzmetal angina 🍎
         Variant angina pectoris
         (Ex) 410.00-410.92, 411.1-411.89, 413.0-413.9, 414.8-414.9, 459.89-459.9
         Coding Clinic: 2006, Q3, P23

     413.9 Other and unspecified angina pectoris
         Angina:
            NOS
            cardiac
            equivalent ◄
            of effort
         Anginal syndrome
         Status anginosus
         Stenocardia
         Syncope anginosa

         | **Excludes** | *preinfarction angina (411.1)* |

         Use additional code(s) for symptoms associated with angina equivalent ◄
         Coding Clinic: 2008, Q2, P16; 2003, Q1, P12-13; 2002, Q3, P4-5; 1995, Q2, P18; 1993, 5th Issue, P17-24; 1991, Q3, P16; 1985, Sept-Oct, P9

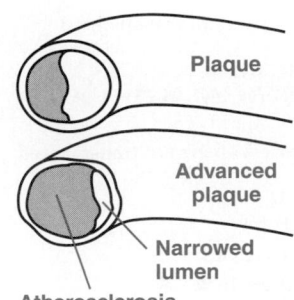

Figure 7-3 Atherosclerosis. (From Buck CJ: Step-by-Step Medical Coding, 2008 ed. Philadelphia, WB Saunders, 2008.)

Item 7-9 Classification is based on the location of the atherosclerosis. **"Of native coronary artery"** indicates the atherosclerosis is within an original heart artery. **"Of autologous vein bypass graft"** indicates that the atherosclerosis is within a vein graft that was taken from within the patient. **"Of nonautologous biological bypass graft"** indicates the atherosclerosis is within a vessel grafted from other than the patient. **"Of artery bypass graft"** indicates the atherosclerosis is within an artery that was grafted from within the patient.

● **414 Other forms of chronic ischemic heart disease**
     | **Excludes** | *arteriosclerotic cardiovascular disease [ASCVD] (429.2)* |
     | | *cardiovascular:* |
     | | *arteriosclerosis or sclerosis (429.2)* |
     | | *degeneration or disease (429.2)* |

● **414.0 Coronary atherosclerosis**
     Arteriosclerotic heart disease [ASHD]
     Atherosclerotic heart disease
     Coronary (artery):
         arteriosclerosis
         arteritis or endarteritis
         atheroma
         sclerosis
         stricture

     Use additional code, if applicable, to identify chronic total occlusion of coronary artery (414.2)

     | **Excludes** | *embolism of graft (996.72)* |
     | | *occlusion NOS of graft (996.72)* |
     | | *thrombus of graft (996.72)* |
     Coding Clinic: 2002, Q3, P3-9; 1994, Q2, P13, 15; Q1, P6-7; 1993, Q1, P20; 5th Issue, P17-24; 5th Issue, P14; 1984, Nov-Dec, P18

     414.00 Of unspecified type of vessel, native or graft A
         Coding Clinic: 2003, Q2, P16; 2001, Q3, P15; 1997, Q3, P15; 1996, Q4, P31

     414.01 Of native coronary artery   A
         Coding Clinic: 2008, Q3, P10-11; Q2, P16; 2006, Q3, P25; 2005, Q4, P68-69; 2004, Q2, P3-4; 2003, Q4, P105-106, 108-109; Q3, P9.10, 14; 2001, Q3, P15-16; Q2, P8-9; 1997, Q3, P15; 1996, Q2, P10; 1995, Q2, P17-19

     414.02 Of autologous biological bypass graft 🍎 A
         (Ex) 414.00-414.05, 414.07, 414.2-414.3
         Coding Clinic: 1995, Q2, P18-19

     414.03 Of nonautologous biological bypass graft 🍎 A
         (Ex) 414.00-414.05, 414.07, 414.2-414.3

     414.04 Of artery bypass graft 🍎   A
         Internal mammary artery
         (Ex) 414.00-414.05, 414.07, 414.2-414.3

     414.05 Of unspecified type of bypass graft   A
         Bypass graft NOS
         Coding Clinic: 1997, Q3, P15; 1996, Q4, P31

N Newborn Age: 0   P Pediatric Age: 0–17   M Maternity Age: 12–55   A Adult Age: 15–124   ♀ Females Only   ♂ Males Only

(Ex) CC Exclusions   🍎 Complication\Comorbidity   🍎 Major C\C   Present on Admission Requirement   🍎 Hospital-Acquired Condition

889

DISEASES OF THE CIRCULATORY SYSTEM (390–459)

414.06 Of native coronary artery of transplanted heart 🔖
> (Ex:) 414.00-414.07, 414.2-414.3
> **Coding Clinic:** 2003, Q4, P60; 2002, Q4, P53-54; Q4, P53-54

414.07 Of bypass graft (artery) (vein) of transplanted heart 🔖   A
> (Ex:) 414.00-414.06, 414.2-414.3
> **Coding Clinic:** 2003, Q4, P60

● **414.1 Aneurysm and dissection of heart**

414.10 Aneurysm of heart (wall) 🔖
> Aneurysm (arteriovenous):
>   mural
>   ventricular
> (Ex:) 414.10-414.11, 414.19

414.11 Aneurysm of coronary vessels
> Aneurysm (arteriovenous) of coronary vessels
> **Coding Clinic:** 1999, Q1, P17-18

414.12 Dissection of coronary artery 🔖
> (Ex:) 414.12, 443.29, 447.2, 447.5-447.9
> **Coding Clinic:** 2002, Q4, P54-55

414.19 Other aneurysm of heart 🔖
> Arteriovenous fistula, acquired, of heart
> (Ex:) 414.10-414.11, 414.19

● **414.2 Chronic total occlusion of coronary artery**
> Complete occlusion of coronary artery
> Total occlusion of coronary artery
>
> *Code first* coronary atherosclerosis (414.00–414.07)
>
> **Excludes** *acute coronary occlusion with myocardial infarction (410.00–410.92)*
>   *acute coronary occlusion without myocardial infarction (411.81)*
> **Coding Clinic:** 2007, Q4, P82

● **414.3 Coronary atherosclerosis due to lipid rich plaque**   A
> *Code first* coronary atherosclerosis (414.00-414.07)
> **Coding Clinic:** 2008, Q4, P113

414.8 Other specified forms of chronic ischemic heart disease
> Chronic coronary insufficiency
> Ischemia, myocardial (chronic)
> Any condition classifiable to 410 specified as chronic, or presenting with symptoms after 8 weeks from date of infarction
>
> **Excludes** *coronary insufficiency (acute) (411.89)*
> **Coding Clinic:** 2003, Q2, P10; 2001, Q3, P15-16; 1992, Q1, P10; 1990, Q3, P15; Q2, P19; 1986, Nov-Dec, P12

414.9 Chronic ischemic heart disease, unspecified
> Ischemic heart disease NOS
> **Coding Clinic:** 2001, Q3, P15-16

Item 7-10 Pulmonary heart disease or cor pulmonale is right ventricle hypertrophy or RVH as a result of a respiratory disorder increasing back flow pressure to the right ventricle. Left untreated, cor pulmonale leads to right-heart failure and death.

DISEASES OF PULMONARY CIRCULATION (415–417)

● **415 Acute pulmonary heart disease**

415.0 Acute cor pulmonale 🔖
> **Excludes** *cor pulmonale NOS (416.9)*
> (Ex:) 415.0, 416.8-416.9, 459.89-459.9

● **415.1 Pulmonary embolism and infarction**
> Pulmonary (artery) (vein):
>   apoplexy   infarction (hemorrhagic)
>   embolism   thrombosis
>
> **Excludes** *chronic pulmonary embolism (416.2)* ◀
>   *personal history of pulmonary embolism (V12.51)* ◀
>   *that complicating:*
>   *abortion (634–638 with .6, 639.6)*
>   *ectopic or molar pregnancy (639.6)*
>   *pregnancy, childbirth, or the puerperium (673.0–673.8)*

415.11 Iatrogenic pulmonary embolism and infarction 🔖 🔖
> **Use additional** code for associated septic pulmonary embolism, if applicable, 415.12
>
> HAC: And one of the following procedure codes: 00.85-00.87, 81.51-81.52, 81.54
> (Ex:) 415.11-415.19, 459.89-459.9
> **Coding Clinic:** 1990, Q4, P25

● **415.12 Septic pulmonary embolism** 🔖
> Septic embolism NOS
>
> *Code first* underlying infection, such as:
>   septicemia (038.0–038.9)
>
> **Excludes** *septic arterial embolism (449)*
> (Ex:) 415.11-415.19, 459.89-459.9
> **Coding Clinic:** 2007, Q4, P84-86

415.19 Other 🔖 🔖
> HAC: And one of the following procedure codes: 00.85-00.87, 81.51-81.52, 81.54
> (Ex:) 415.11-415.19, 459.89-459.9
> **Coding Clinic:** 1998, Q2, P8

● **416 Chronic pulmonary heart disease**

416.0 Primary pulmonary hypertension 🔖
> Idiopathic pulmonary arteriosclerosis
> Pulmonary hypertension (essential) (idiopathic) (primary)
> (Ex:) 416.0, 416.8-416.9, 417.8-417.9, 459.89-459.9

416.1 Kyphoscoliotic heart disease 🔖
> (Ex:) 416.0-416.9

416.2 Chronic pulmonary embolism 🔖   ◀
> **Use additional** code, if applicable, for associated long-term (current) use of anticoagulants (V58.61) ◀
>
> **Excludes** *personal history of pulmonary embolism (V12.51)* ◀

416.8 Other chronic pulmonary heart diseases
> Pulmonary hypertension, secondary

416.9 Chronic pulmonary heart disease, unspecified
> Chronic cardiopulmonary disease
> Cor pulmonale (chronic) NOS

● **417 Other diseases of pulmonary circulation**

417.0 Arteriovenous fistula of pulmonary vessels 🔖
> **Excludes** *congenital arteriovenous fistula (747.3)*
> (Ex:) 417.0-417.9

417.1 Aneurysm of pulmonary artery 🔖
> **Excludes** *congenital aneurysm (747.3)*
> (Ex:) 417.0-417.9

◀ New   ◀≡ Revised   ~~deleted~~ Deleted   ● Unacceptable Principal Diagnosis   ● Use Additional Digit(s)
▶ Manifestation Code   **OGCR** Official Guidelines   **Coding Clinic**   Excludes   Includes   Use additional   Code first   Omit code

417.8 Other specified diseases of pulmonary circulation
Pulmonary:
    arteritis
    endarteritis
Rupture of pulmonary vessel
Stricture of pulmonary vessel

417.9 Unspecified disease of pulmonary circulation

OTHER FORMS OF HEART DISEASE (420–429)

● **420 Acute pericarditis**
Inflammation of the sac surrounding the heart caused by infection. The chest pain is significant on inspiration, and onset is sudden and worst when lying down.

Includes   acute:
                mediastinopericarditis
                myopericarditis
                pericardial effusion
                pleuropericarditis
                pneumopericarditis

Excludes   acute rheumatic pericarditis (391.0)
                postmyocardial infarction syndrome [Dressler's]
                    (411.0)

▶ **420.0 Acute pericarditis in diseases classified elsewhere** ⚉
Code first underlying disease, as:
    actinomycosis (039.8)
    amebiasis (006.8)
    chronic uremia (585.9)
    nocardiosis (039.8)
    tuberculosis (017.9)
    uremia NOS (586)

Excludes   pericarditis (acute) (in):
                Coxsackie (virus) (074.21)
                gonococcal (098.83)
                histoplasmosis (115.0–115.9 with
                    fifth-digit 3)
                meningococcal infection (036.41)
                syphilitic (093.81)
ⒺⓍ 391.0, 393, 420.0-420.99, 423.3-423.9, 459.89-459.9

● **420.9 Other and unspecified acute pericarditis**

420.90 Acute pericarditis, unspecified ⚉
Pericarditis (acute):
    NOS
    infective NOS
    sicca
ⒺⓍ 391.0, 393, 420.0-420.99, 423.3-423.9, 459.89-459.9
Coding Clinic: 1989, Q2, P12

420.91 Acute idiopathic pericarditis ⚉
Pericarditis, acute:
    benign
    nonspecific
    viral
ⒺⓍ 391.0, 393, 420.0-420.99, 423.3-423.9, 459.89-459.9

420.99 Other ⚉
Pericarditis (acute):
    pneumococcal
    purulent
    staphylococcal
    streptococcal
    suppurative
Pneumopyopericardium
Pyopericardium

Excludes   pericarditis in diseases classified
                elsewhere (420.0)
ⒺⓍ 391.0, 393, 420.0-420.99, 423.3-423.9, 459.89-459.9

● **421 Acute and subacute endocarditis**
Inflammation/infection of lining of heart, affecting heart valves, usually caused by bacterial infection

421.0 Acute and subacute bacterial endocarditis ⚉
Endocarditis (acute) (chronic) (subacute):
    bacterial
    infective NOS
    lenta
    malignant
    purulent
    septic
    ulcerative
    vegetative
Infective aneurysm
Subacute bacterial endocarditis [SBE]

Use additional code, if desired, to identify
    infectious organism [e.g., Streptococcus 041.0,
    Staphylococcus 041.1]
ⒺⓍ 391.1, 397.9, 421.0-421.9, 424.90-424.99, 459.89-459.9
Coding Clinic: 2008, Q4, P69-73; 2006, Q2, P16-17; 1999, Q1, P12; 1991, Q1, P15

▶ **421.1 Acute and subacute infective endocarditis in diseases classified elsewhere** ⚉
Code first underlying disease, as:
    blastomycosis (116.0)
    Q fever (083.0)
    typhoid (fever) (002.0)

Excludes   endocarditis (in):
                Coxsackie (virus) (074.22)
                gonococcal (098.84)
                histoplasmosis (115.0–115.9 with
                    fifth-digit 4)
                meningococcal infection (036.42)
                monilial (112.81)
ⒺⓍ 391.1, 397.9, 421.0-421.9, 424.90-424.99, 459.89-459.9

421.9 Acute endocarditis, unspecified ⚉
Endocarditis, acute or subacute
Myoendocarditis, acute or subacute
Periendocarditis, acute or subacute

Excludes   acute rheumatic endocarditis (391.1)
ⒺⓍ 391.1, 397.9, 421.0-421.9, 424.90-424.99, 459.89-459.9

● **422 Acute myocarditis**
An inflammation of the heart muscle due to an infection (viral/bacterial).

Excludes   acute rheumatic myocarditis (391.2)

▶ **422.0 Acute myocarditis in diseases classified elsewhere** ⚉
Code first underlying disease, as:
    myocarditis (acute):
        influenzal (487.8)
        tuberculous (017.9)

Excludes   myocarditis (acute) (due to):
                aseptic, of newborn (074.23)
                Coxsackie (virus) (074.23)
                diphtheritic (032.82)
                meningococcal infection (036.43)
                syphilitic (093.82)
                toxoplasmosis (130.3)
ⒺⓍ 391.2, 398.0, 422.0-422.99, 429.0, 429.71-429.79, 459.89-459.9

DISEASES OF THE CIRCULATORY SYSTEM (390–459)

● **422.9   Other and unspecified acute myocarditis**

     422.90   Acute myocarditis, unspecified 🔎

         Acute or subacute (interstitial) myocarditis

         Ⓔⓧ 391.2, 398.0, 422.0-422.99, 429.0, 429.71-429.79, 459.89-459.9

     422.91   Idiopathic myocarditis 🔎

         Myocarditis (acute or subacute):

           Fiedler's

           giant cell

           isolated (diffuse) (granulomatous)

           nonspecific granulomatous

         Ⓔⓧ 391.2, 398.0, 422.0-422.99, 429.0, 429.71-429.79, 459.89-459.9

     422.92   Septic myocarditis 🔎

         Myocarditis, acute or subacute:

           pneumococcal

           staphylococcal

         Use additional code to identify infectious organism [e.g., Staphylococcus 041.1]

         Excludes   *myocarditis, acute or subacute:*

           in bacterial diseases classified elsewhere (422.0)

           streptococcal (391.2)

         Ⓔⓧ 391.2, 398.0, 422.0-422.99, 429.0, 429.71-429.79, 459.89-459.9

     422.93   Toxic myocarditis 🔎

         Ⓔⓧ 391.2, 398.0, 422.0-422.99, 429.0, 429.71-429.79, 459.89-459.9

     422.99   Other 🔎

         Ⓔⓧ 391.2, 398.0, 422.0-422.99, 429.0, 429.71-429.79, 459.89-459.9

● **423   Other diseases of pericardium**

     Excludes   *that specified as rheumatic (393)*

     423.0   Hemopericardium 🔎

         Ⓔⓧ 423.0-423.9, 459.89-459.9

     423.1   Adhesive pericarditis 🔎

         Adherent pericardium

         Fibrosis of pericardium

         Milk spots

         Pericarditis:

           adhesive

           obliterative

         Soldiers' patches

         Ⓔⓧ 423.0-423.9, 459.89-459.9

     423.2   Constrictive pericarditis 🔎

         Concato's disease

         Pick's disease of heart (and liver)

         Ⓔⓧ 423.0-423.9, 459.89-459.9

●   **423.3   Cardiac tamponade** 🔎

         Code first the underlying cause

         Ⓔⓧ 074.21, 093.81, 391.0, 393, 420.0-420.99, 423.3-423.9, 459.89-459.9

         Coding Clinic: 2007, Q4, P86-87; 2007, Q2, P11-12

     423.8   Other specified diseases of pericardium 🔎

         Calcification of pericardium

         Fistula of pericardium

         Ⓔⓧ 074.21, 093.81, 391.0, 393, 420.0-420.99, 423.3-423.9, 459.89-459.9

         Coding Clinic: 1989, Q2, P12

     423.9   Unspecified disease of pericardium 🔎

         Ⓔⓧ 074.21, 093.81, 391.0, 393, 420.0-420.99, 423.3-423.9, 459.89-459.9

         Coding Clinic: 2007, Q2, P11-12

● **424   Other diseases of endocardium**

     Excludes   *bacterial endocarditis (421.0–421.9)*

         rheumatic endocarditis (391.1, 394.0–397.9)

         syphilitic endocarditis (093.20–093.24)

     424.0   Mitral valve disorders

         Mitral (valve):

           incompetence NOS of specified cause, except rheumatic

           insufficiency NOS of specified cause, except rheumatic

           regurgitation NOS of specified cause, except rheumatic

         Excludes   *mitral (valve):*

           disease (394.9)

           failure (394.9)

           stenosis (394.0)

           the listed conditions:

           specified as rheumatic (394.1)

           unspecified as to cause but with mention of:

           diseases of aortic valve (396.0–396.9)

           mitral stenosis or obstruction (394.2)

         Coding Clinic: 2006, Q3, P7; 2000, Q2, P16-17; 1998, Q3, P11; 1987, Nov-Dec, P8

     424.1   Aortic valve disorders

         Aortic (valve):

           incompetence NOS of specified cause, except rheumatic

           insufficiency NOS of specified cause, except rheumatic

           regurgitation NOS of specified cause, except rheumatic

           stenosis NOS of specified cause, except rheumatic

         Excludes   *hypertrophic subaortic stenosis (425.1)*

           that specified as rheumatic (395.0–395.9)

           that of unspecified cause but with mention of diseases of mitral valve (396.0–396.9)

         Coding Clinic: 2008, Q4, P177-180; 1988, Q4, P8; 1987, Nov-Dec, P8

     424.2   Tricuspid valve disorders, specified as nonrheumatic

         Tricuspid valve:

           incompetence of specified cause, except rheumatic

           insufficiency of specified cause, except rheumatic

           regurgitation of specified cause, except rheumatic

           stenosis of specified cause, except rheumatic

         Excludes   *rheumatic or of unspecified cause (397.0)*

     424.3   Pulmonary valve disorders

         Pulmonic:

           incompetence NOS

           insufficiency NOS

           regurgitation NOS

           stenosis NOS

         Excludes   *that specified as rheumatic (397.1)*

DISEASES OF THE CIRCULATORY SYSTEM (390–459)

◀ New   ◀▥ Revised   ~~deleted~~ Deleted   ● Unacceptable Principal Diagnosis   ● Use Additional Digit(s)

▶ Manifestation Code   **OGCR** Official Guidelines   **Coding Clinic**   Excludes   Includes   Use additional   Code first   Omit code

● **424.9 Endocarditis, valve unspecified**

    424.90 Endocarditis, valve unspecified, unspecified cause 🅒

        Endocarditis (chronic):
           NOS
           nonbacterial thrombotic
        Valvular:
           incompetence of unspecified valve, unspecified cause
           insufficiency of unspecified valve, unspecified cause
           regurgitation of unspecified valve, unspecified cause
           stenosis of unspecified valve, unspecified cause
        Valvulitis (chronic)
        Ⓔⓧ 424.90-424.99, 459.89-459.9

▸ **424.91 *Endocarditis in diseases classified elsewhere*** 🅒

        Code first underlying disease, as:
           atypical verrucous endocarditis [Libman-Sacks] (710.0)
           disseminated lupus erythematosus (710.0)
           tuberculosis (017.9)

        | **Excludes** | syphilitic (093.20–093.24) |

        Ⓔⓧ 424.90-424.99, 459.89-459.9

    424.99 Other 🅒

        Any condition classifiable to 424.90 with specified cause, except rheumatic

        | **Excludes** | endocardial fibroelastosis (425.3) |
        | | that specified as rheumatic (397.9) |

        Ⓔⓧ 424.90-424.99, 459.89-459.9

● **425 Cardiomyopathy**

    Disease of the heart muscle resulting in abnormally enlarged, weakened, thickened, and/or stiffened muscle causing an inability to pump blood normally and leads to CHF.

    | **Includes** | myocardiopathy |

    425.0 Endomyocardial fibrosis 🅒
        Ⓔⓧ 398.91, 402.01, 402.11, 402.91, 404.01, 404.03, 404.11, 404.13, 404.91, 404.93, 414.00-414.07, 414.2-414.9, 425.0-425.9, 426.10-426.13, 426.50-426.54, 426.81-426.89, 427.31-427.42, 427.60-427.89, 428.0-428.1, 428.9, 459.89-459.9, 746.86, 785.0-785.1, 785.50-785.51

    425.1 Hypertrophic obstructive cardiomyopathy 🅒
        Hypertrophic subaortic stenosis (idiopathic)
        Ⓔⓧ 398.91, 402.01, 402.11, 402.91, 404.01, 404.03, 404.11, 404.13, 404.91, 404.93, 414.00-414.07, 414.2-414.9, 425.0-425.9, 426.10-426.13, 426.50-426.54, 426.81-426.89, 427.31-427.42, 427.60-427.89, 428.0-428.1, 428.9, 459.89-459.9, 746.86, 785.0-785.1, 785.50-785.51

    425.2 Obscure cardiomyopathy of Africa 🅒
        Becker's disease
        Idiopathic mural endomyocardial disease
        Ⓔⓧ 398.91, 402.01, 402.11, 402.91, 404.01, 404.03, 404.11, 404.13, 404.91, 404.93, 414.00-414.07, 414.2-414.9, 425.0-425.9, 426.10-426.13, 426.50-426.54, 426.81-426.89, 427.31-427.42, 427.60-427.89, 428.0-428.1, 428.9, 459.89-459.9, 746.86, 785.0-785.1, 785.50-785.51

    425.3 Endocardial fibroelastosis 🅒
        Elastomyofibrosis
        Ⓔⓧ 398.91, 402.01, 402.11, 402.91, 404.01, 404.03, 404.11, 404.13, 404.91, 404.93, 414.00-414.07, 414.2-414.9, 425.0-425.9, 426.10-426.13, 426.50-426.54, 426.81-426.89, 427.31-427.42, 427.60-427.89, 428.0-428.1, 428.9, 459.89-459.9, 746.86, 785.0-785.1, 785.50-785.51

425.4 Other primary cardiomyopathies 🅒
    Cardiomyopathy:
        NOS
        congestive
        constrictive
        familial
        hypertrophic
        idiopathic
        nonobstructive
        obstructive
        restrictive
    Cardiovascular collagenosis
    Ⓔⓧ 398.91, 402.01, 402.11, 402.91, 404.01, 404.03, 404.11, 404.13, 404.91, 404.93, 414.00-414.07, 414.2-414.9, 425.0-425.9, 426.10-426.13, 426.50-426.54, 426.81-426.89, 427.31-427.42, 427.60-427.89, 428.0-428.1, 428.9, 746.86, 785.0-785.1, 785.50-785.51
    Coding Clinic: 2007, Q1, P20; 2005, Q2, P14-15; 2000, Q1, P22; 1997, Q4, P54-55; 1990, Q2, P19; 1985, Sept-Oct, P15

425.5 Alcoholic cardiomyopathy 🅒
    Ⓔⓧ 398.91, 402.01, 402.11, 402.91, 404.01, 404.03, 404.11, 404.13, 404.91, 404.93, 414.00-414.07, 414.2-414.9, 425.0-425.9 426.10-426.13, 426.50-426.54, 426.81-426.89, 427.31-427.42, 427.60-427.89, 428.0-428.1, 428.9, 459.89-459.9, 746.86, 785.0-785.1, 785.50-785.51
    Coding Clinic: 1985, Sept-Oct, P15; July-Aug, P15

▸ **425.7 *Nutritional and metabolic cardiomyopathy*** 🅒

    Code first underlying disease, as:
        amyloidosis (277.30–277.39)
        beriberi (265.0)
        cardiac glycogenosis (271.0)
        mucopolysaccharidosis (277.5)
        thyrotoxicosis (242.0–242.9)

    | **Excludes** | gouty tophi of heart (274.82) |

    Ⓔⓧ 398.91, 402.01, 402.11, 402.91, 404.01, 404.03, 404.11, 404.13, 404.91, 404.93, 414.00-414.07, 414.2-414.9, 425.0-425.9, 426.10-426.13, 426.50-426.54, 426.81-426.89, 427.31-427.42, 427.60-427.89, 428.0-428.1, 428.9, 459.89-459.9, 746.86, 785.0-785.1, 785.50-785.51

▸ **425.8 *Cardiomyopathy in other diseases classified elsewhere*** 🅒

    Code first underlying disease, as:
        Friedreich's ataxia (334.0)
        myotonia atrophica (359.21)
        progressive muscular dystrophy (359.1)
        sarcoidosis (135)

    | **Excludes** | cardiomyopathy in Chagas' disease (086.0) |

    Ⓔⓧ 398.91, 402.01, 402.11, 402.91, 404.01, 404.03, 404.11, 404.13, 404.91, 404.93, 414.00-414.07, 414.2-414.9, 425.0-425.9, 426.10-426.13, 426.50-426.54, 426.81-426.89, 427.31-427.42, 427.60-427.89, 428.0-428.1, 428.9, 459.89-459.9, 746.86, 785.0-785.1, 785.50-785.51
    Coding Clinic: 1993, Q2, P9

425.9 Secondary cardiomyopathy, unspecified 🅒
    Ⓔⓧ 398.91, 402.01, 402.11, 402.91, 404.01, 404.03, 404.11, 404.13, 404.91, 404.93, 414.00-414.07, 414.2-414.9, 425.0-425.9, 426.10-426.13, 426.50-426.54, 426.81-426.89, 427.31-427.42, 427.60-427.89, 428.0-428.1, 428.9, 459.89-459.9, 746.86, 785.0-785.1, 785.50-785.51

N Newborn Age: 0   **P** Pediatric Age: 0–17   **M** Maternity Age: 12–55   **A** Adult Age: 15–124   ♀ Females Only   ♂ Males Only

Ⓔⓧ CC Exclusions   🅒 Complication\Comorbidity   🅜 Major C\C   Present on Admission Requirement   Hospital-Acquired Condition

893

● **426   Conduction disorders**

Heart block or atrioventricular block (AV block) caused by conduction problem resulting in arrhythmias/ dysrhythmias due to lack of electrical impulses being transmitted normally through heart.

426.0   Atrioventricular block, complete 🐾
Third degree atrioventricular block
   Ⓔ 426.0-427.5, 427.89, 459.89-459.9
   Coding Clinic: 2006, Q2, P14

● **426.1   Atrioventricular block, other and unspecified**

426.10   Atrioventricular block, unspecified
Atrioventricular [AV] block (incomplete) (partial)

426.11   First degree atrioventricular block
Incomplete atrioventricular block, first degree
Prolonged P-R interval NOS
   Coding Clinic: 2006, Q2, P14

426.12   Mobitz (type) II atrioventricular block 🐾
Incomplete atrioventricular block:
   Mobitz (type) II
   second degree, Mobitz (type) II
   Ⓔ 426.0-427.5, 427.89, 459.89-459.9
   Coding Clinic: 2006, Q2, P14

426.13   Other second degree atrioventricular block
Incomplete atrioventricular block:
   Mobitz (type) I [Wenckebach's]
   second degree:
     NOS
     Mobitz (type) I
     with 2:1 atrioventricular response [block]
   Wenckebach's phenomenon

426.2   Left bundle branch hemiblock
Block:
   left anterior fascicular
   left posterior fascicular
MCE: Questionable admission, principal diagnosis only

426.3   Other left bundle branch block
Left bundle branch block:
   NOS
   anterior fascicular with posterior fascicular
   complete
   main stem
MCE: Questionable admission, principal diagnosis only

426.4   Right bundle branch block
MCE: Questionable admission, principal diagnosis only
   Coding Clinic: 2000, Q3, P3

● **426.5   Bundle branch block, other and unspecified**

426.50   Bundle branch block, unspecified

426.51   Right bundle branch block and left posterior fascicular block

426.52   Right bundle branch block and left anterior fascicular block

426.53   Other bilateral bundle branch block 🐾
Bifascicular block NOS
Bilateral bundle branch block NOS
Right bundle branch with left bundle branch block (incomplete) (main stem)
   Ⓔ 426.0-427.5, 427.89, 459.89-459.9

426.54   Trifascicular block 🐾
   Ⓔ 426.0-427.5, 427.89, 459.89-459.9

426.6   Other heart block
Intraventricular block:
   NOS
   diffuse
   myofibrillar
Sinoatrial block
Sinoauricular block

426.7   Anomalous atrioventricular excitation
Atrioventricular conduction:
   accelerated
   accessory
   pre-excitation
Ventricular pre-excitation
Wolff-Parkinson-White syndrome

● **426.8   Other specified conduction disorders**

426.81   Lown-Ganong-Levine syndrome
Syndrome of short P-R interval, normal QRS complexes, and supraventricular tachycardias

426.82   Long QT syndrome
   Coding Clinic: 2005, Q4, P72-73

426.89   Other 🐾
Dissociation:
   atrioventricular [AV]
   interference
   isorhythmic
Nonparoxysmal AV nodal tachycardia
   Ⓔ 426.0-427.5, 427.89, 459.89-459.9

426.9   Conduction disorder, unspecified
Heart block NOS
Stokes-Adams syndrome

● **427   Cardiac dysrhythmias**

Abnormality in rate, regularity, or sequence of cardiac activation.

> **Excludes**   *that complicating:*
>   *abortion (634–638 with .7, 639.8)*
>   *ectopic or molar pregnancy (639.8)*
>   *labor or delivery (668.1, 669.4)*

427.0   Paroxysmal supraventricular tachycardia 🐾
Paroxysmal tachycardia:
   atrial [PAT]   junctional
   atrioventricular [AV]   nodal
   Ⓔ 426.0-427.5, 427.89, 459.89-459.9

427.1   Paroxysmal ventricular tachycardia 🐾
Ventricular tachycardia (paroxysmal)
   Ⓔ 426.0-427.5, 427.89, 459.89-459.9
   Coding Clinic: 2008, Q1, P14-15; 2006, Q2, P15-16; 1995, Q3, P9; Q1, P8; 1986, Mar-April, P11-12; 1985, July-Aug, P15

427.2   Paroxysmal tachycardia, unspecified
Bouveret-Hoffmann syndrome
Paroxysmal tachycardia:
   NOS
   essential

● **427.3   Atrial fibrillation and flutter**

427.31   Atrial fibrillation
Most common abnormal heart rhythm (arrhythmia) presenting as irregular, rapid beating (tachycardia) of the heart's upper chamber.
   Coding Clinic: 2008, Q4, P134-136; 2005, Q3, P3-9; 2004, Q4, P77-78, 121-122; Q3, P7; 2003, Q4, P93-95, 105-106; Q1, P8; 1999, Q2, P17; 1996, Q2, P7x2; 1995, Q3, P8; 1994, Q1, P22; 1985, July-Aug, P15

427.32   Atrial flutter 🐾
Rapid contractions of the upper heart chamber, but regular, rather than irregular, beats.
   Ⓔ 426.0-427.5, 427.89, 459.89-459.9
   Coding Clinic: 2003, Q4, P93-95

◀ New   ◀▥ Revised   ~~deleted~~ Deleted   ● Unacceptable Principal Diagnosis   ● Use Additional Digit(s)
▶ Manifestation Code   **OGCR** Official Guidelines   **Coding Clinic**   Excludes   Includes   Use additional   Code first   Omit code

● **427.4** **Ventricular fibrillation and flutter**

     427.41 **Ventricular fibrillation**🅫
         MCC only for patients discharged alive
         (Ex:) 426.0-427.5, 427.89, 459.89-459.9
         Coding Clinic: 2002, Q3, P5

     427.42 **Ventricular flutter**🅫
         (Ex:) 426.0-427.5, 427.89, 459.89-459.9

   427.5 **Cardiac arrest**🅫
         Cardiorespiratory arrest
         MCC only for patients discharged alive
         (Ex:) 427.0-427.5, 459.89-459.9
         Coding Clinic: 2002, Q3, P5; 2000, Q2, P12; 1995, Q3, P9

● **427.6** **Premature beats**

     427.60 **Premature beats, unspecified**
         Ectopic beats
         Extrasystoles
         Extrasystolic arrhythmia
         Premature contractions or systoles NOS

     427.61 **Supraventricular premature beats**
         Atrial premature beats, contractions, or
             systoles
         Coding Clinic: 1994, Q1, P20

     427.69 **Other**
         Ventricular premature beats, contractions,
             or systoles
         Coding Clinic: 1993, Q4, P42-43

● **427.8** **Other specified cardiac dysrhythmias**

     427.81 **Sinoatrial node dysfunction**
         Sinus bradycardia:
             persistent
             severe
         Syndrome:
             sick sinus
             tachycardia-bradycardia

         | **Excludes** | *sinus bradycardia NOS (427.89)*

     427.89 **Other**
         Rhythm disorder:
             coronary sinus
             ectopic
             nodal
         Wandering (atrial) pacemaker

         | **Excludes** | *carotid sinus syncope (337.0)*
                      neonatal bradycardia (779.81)
                      neonatal tachycardia (779.82)
                      reflex bradycardia (337.0)
                      tachycardia NOS (785.0)
         Coding Clinic: 2000, Q3, P8-9; 1985, July-Aug, P15

   427.9 **Cardiac dysrhythmia, unspecified**
         Arrhythmia (cardiac) NOS
         Coding Clinic: 1989, Q2, P10

Item 7–11 Congestive heart failure (CHF) is a condition in which the left ventricle of the heart cannot pump enough blood to the body. The blood flow from the heart slows or returns to the heart from the venous system back flow resulting in congestion (fluid accumulation) particularly in the abdomen. Most commonly, fluid collects in the lungs and results in shortness of breath, especially when in a reclining position.

● **428** **Heart failure**
     Code, if applicable, heart failure due to hypertension
         first (402.0–402.9, with fifth-digit 1 or 404.0–404.9
         with fifth-digit 1 or 3)

     | **Excludes** | *rheumatic (398.91)*
                that complicating:
                     abortion (634–638 with .7, 639.8)
                     ectopic or molar pregnancy (639.8)
                     labor or delivery (668.1, 669.4)
     Coding Clinic: 2005, Q2, P14-15; 2002, Q4, P49-53

   428.0 **Congestive heart failure, unspecified**
         Congestive heart disease
         Right heart failure (secondary to left heart failure)

         | **Excludes** | *fluid overload NOS (276.6)*

     Coding Clinic: 2009, Q1, P6x2; 2008, Q4, P69-73, 177-182; Q3, P12-13x2; 2007, Q3, P11; Q1, P20; 2006, Q3, P7; 2005, Q4, P119-120; Q3, P3-9; Q1, P9; 2004, Q4, P140; Q3, P7; 2003, Q4, P109-110; Q1, P9; 2002, Q4, P52-53; 2001, Q2, P13; 2000, Q4, P47-48; Q2, P16-17; Q1, P22; 1999, Q4, P13-14; Q1, P11, 1998, Q3, P5; 1997, Q4, P54-55; Q3, P10; 1996, Q3, P9; 1991, Q3, P18-20; 1990, Q2, P19; 1989, Q2, P12; 1987, Sept-Oct, P11; 1985, Sept-Oct, P15; Nov-Dec, P14

   428.1 **Left heart failure**🅫
         Acute edema of lung with heart disease NOS or
             heart failure
         Acute pulmonary edema with heart disease NOS
             or heart failure
         Cardiac asthma
         Left ventricular failure
         (Ex:) 398.91, 402.01, 402.11, 402.91, 428.0-428.9, 459.89-459.9
         Coding Clinic: 1990, Q2, P19

● **428.2** **Systolic heart failure**

         | **Excludes** | *combined systolic and diastolic heart failure*
                      (428.40–428.43)

     428.20 **Unspecified** 🅫
         (Ex:) 398.91, 402.01, 402.11, 402.91, 428.0-428.9, 459.89-459.9, 518.4

     428.21 **Acute**🅫
         Presenting a short and relatively severe episode
         (Ex:) 398.91, 402.01, 402.11, 402.91, 428.0-428.9, 459.89-459.9, 518.4

     428.22 **Chronic**🅫
         Long-lasting, presenting over time
         (Ex:) 398.91, 402.01, 402.11, 402.91, 428.0-428.9, 459.89-459.9, 518.4
         Coding Clinic: 2005, Q4, P119-120

     428.23 **Acute on chronic**🅫
         Combination code. What was a chronic
             condition now has an acute exacerbation
             (to make more severe). Because two
             conditions are now present, the
             combination code reports both.
         (Ex:) 398.91, 402.01, 402.11, 402.91, 428.0-428.9, 459.89-459.9, 518.4
         Coding Clinic: 2009, Q1, P10; 2003, Q1, P9

DISEASES OF THE CIRCULATORY SYSTEM (390–459)

● **428.3 Diastolic heart failure**

> **Excludes** *combined systolic and diastolic heart failure (428.40–428.43)*

  428.30 Unspecified 🔖
> Ex: 398.91, 402.01, 402.11, 402.91, 428.0-428.9, 459.89-459.9, 518.4
> **Coding Clinic:** 2002, Q4, P52

  428.31 Acute 🔖
> Ex: 398.91, 402.01, 402.11, 402.91, 428.0-428.9, 459.89-459.9, 518.4

  428.32 Chronic 🔖
> Ex: 398.91, 402.01, 402.11, 402.91, 428.0-428.9, 459.89-459.9, 518.4
> **Coding Clinic:** 2008, Q3, P12-13

  428.33 Acute on chronic 🔖
> Ex: 398.91, 402.01, 402.11, 402.91, 428.0-428.9, 459.89-459.9, 518.4
> **Coding Clinic:** 2008, Q3, P12; 2007, Q1, P20

● **428.4 Combined systolic and diastolic heart failure**

  428.40 Unspecified 🔖
> Ex: 398.91, 402.01, 402.11, 402.91, 428.0-428.9, 459.89-459.9, 518.4

  428.41 Acute 🔖
> Ex: 398.91, 402.01, 402.11, 402.91, 428.0-428.9, 459.89-459.9, 518.4
> **Coding Clinic:** 2004, Q4, P140

  428.42 Chronic 🔖
> Ex: 398.91, 402.01, 402.11, 402.91, 428.0-428.9, 459.89-459.9, 518.4

  428.43 Acute on chronic 🔖
> Ex: 398.91, 402.01, 402.11, 402.91, 428.0-428.9, 459.89-459.9, 518.4
> **Coding Clinic:** 2006, Q3, P7; 2002, Q4, P52-53

428.9 Heart failure, unspecified
Cardiac failure NOS
Heart failure NOS
Myocardial failure NOS
Weak heart
Coding Clinic: 1989, Q2, P10; 1985, Nov-Dec, P14

● **429 Ill-defined descriptions and complications of heart disease**

429.0 Myocarditis, unspecified
Myocarditis (with mention of arteriosclerosis):
  NOS (with mention of arteriosclerosis)
  chronic (interstitial) (with mention of arteriosclerosis)
  fibroid (with mention of arteriosclerosis)
  senile (with mention of arteriosclerosis)

> Use additional code to identify presence of arteriosclerosis

> **Excludes** *acute or subacute (422.0–422.9)*
> *rheumatic (398.0)*
> * acute (391.2)*
> *that due to hypertension (402.0–402.9)*

429.1 Myocardial degeneration
Degeneration of heart or myocardium (with mention of arteriosclerosis):
  fatty (with mention of arteriosclerosis)
  mural (with mention of arteriosclerosis)
  muscular (with mention of arteriosclerosis)
Myocardial (with mention of arteriosclerosis):
  degeneration (with mention of arteriosclerosis)
  disease (with mention of arteriosclerosis)

> Use additional code to identify presence of arteriosclerosis

> **Excludes** *that due to hypertension (402.0–402.9)*

429.2 Cardiovascular disease, unspecified
Arteriosclerotic cardiovascular disease [ASCVD]
Cardiovascular arteriosclerosis
Cardiovascular:
  degeneration (with mention of arteriosclerosis)
  disease (with mention of arteriosclerosis)
  sclerosis (with mention of arteriosclerosis)

> Use additional code to identify presence of arteriosclerosis

> **Excludes** *that due to hypertension (402.0–402.9)*

429.3 Cardiomegaly
Cardiac:
  dilatation
  hypertrophy
Ventricular dilatation

> **Excludes** *that due to hypertension (402.0–402.9)*

429.4 Functional disturbances following cardiac surgery
Cardiac insufficiency following cardiac surgery or due to prosthesis
Heart failure following cardiac surgery or due to prosthesis
Postcardiotomy syndrome
Postvalvulotomy syndrome

> **Excludes** *cardiac failure in the immediate postoperative period (997.1)*

> **Coding Clinic:** 2002, Q2, P12-13

429.5 Rupture of chordae tendineae 🔖
> Ex: 429.5, 429.71-429.79, 459.89-459.9

429.6 Rupture of papillary muscle 🔖
> Ex: 429.6-429.81, 459.89-459.9

● **429.7 Certain sequelae of myocardial infarction, not elsewhere classified**

> Use additional code to identify the associated myocardial infarction:
> with onset of 8 weeks or less (410.00–410.92)
> with onset of more than 8 weeks (414.8)

> **Excludes** *congenital defects of heart (745, 746)*
> *coronary aneurysm (414.11)*
> *disorders of papillary muscle (429.6, 429.81)*
> *postmyocardial infarction syndrome (411.0)*
> *rupture of chordae tendineae (429.5)*

  429.71 Acquired cardiac septal defect 🔖   A

> > **Excludes** *acute septal infarction (410.00–410.92)*
> > Ex: 422.0-422.99, 429.0, 429.4-429.82, 459.89-459.9, 745.0-745.9, 746.89-746.9, 747.83-747.9, 759.7-759.89

  429.79 Other 🔖   A
Mural thrombus (atrial) (ventricular)
  acquired, following myocardial infarction
> Ex: 422.0-422.99, 429.0, 429.4-429.82, 459.89-459.9, 745.0-745.9, 746.89-746.9, 747.83-747.9, 759.7-759.89
> **Coding Clinic:** 1992, Q1, P10

◀ New   ◀▥ Revised   ~~deleted~~ Deleted   ● Unacceptable Principal Diagnosis   ● Use Additional Digit(s)
▶ Manifestation Code   **OGCR** Official Guidelines   **Coding Clinic**   Excludes   Includes   Use additional   Code first   Omit code

DISEASES OF THE CIRCULATORY SYSTEM (390–459)

● **429.8 Other ill-defined heart diseases**

429.81 Other disorders of papillary muscle 🔒

Papillary muscle:
  atrophy
  degeneration
  dysfunction
  incompetence
  incoordination
  scarring
  ⒺⓍ 429.6-429.81, 459.89-459.9

429.82 Hyperkinetic heart disease 🔒
  ⒺⓍ 429.71-429.79, 429.82, 459.89-459.9

429.83 Takotsubo syndrome 🔒
  Broken heart syndrome
  Reversible left ventricular dysfunction
    following sudden emotional stress
  Stress induced cardiomyopathy
  Transient left ventricular apical ballooning
    syndrome
  ⒺⓍ 398.91, 402.01, 402.11, 402.91, 428.0-428.9, 429.83, 429.9,
    459.89-459.9
  Coding Clinic: 2006, Q4, P87

429.89 Other
  Carditis
  ┌──────────┐
  │ **Excludes** │ *that due to hypertension*
  └──────────┘   *(402.0–402.9)*
  Coding Clinic: 2006, Q2, P18-19; 2005, Q3, P14; 1992,
    Q1, P10

429.9 Heart disease, unspecified
  Heart disease (organic) NOS
  Morbus cordis NOS
  ┌──────────┐
  │ **Excludes** │ *that due to hypertension (402.0–402.9)*
  └──────────┘
  Coding Clinic: 2009, Q1, P10x2; 1993, Q1, P19-20

───────────────────────────────
CEREBROVASCULAR DISEASE (430–438)

┌──────────┐
│ **Includes** │ with mention of hypertension (conditions
└──────────┘   classifiable to 401–405)

Use additional code to identify presence of hypertension
┌──────────┐
│ **Excludes** │ *any condition classifiable to 430–434, 436, 437*
└──────────┘   *occurring during pregnancy, childbirth, or*
               the puerperium, or specified as puerperal
               (674.0)
               iatrogenic cerebrovascular infarction or
               hemorrhage (997.02)

OGCR Section I.C.7.a.5
First assign codes from 430-438, Cerebrovascular
disease, then the appropriate hypertension code from
categories 401-405.

430 Subarachnoid hemorrhage 🔒
  Meningeal hemorrhage
  Ruptured:
    berry aneurysm
    (congenital) cerebral aneurysm NOS
  ┌──────────┐
  │ **Excludes** │ *syphilitic ruptured cerebral aneurysm (094.87)*
  └──────────┘
  ⒺⓍ 430-432.9, 459.89-459.9, 780.01-780.09, 800.00-801.99, 803.00-804.96,
    850.0-852.19, 852.21-854.19
  Coding Clinic: 2000, Q3, P16; 1991, Q3, P15-16

431 Intracerebral hemorrhage 🔒
  Hemorrhage (of):
    basilar
    bulbar
    cerebellar
    cerebral
    cerebromeningeal
    cortical
    internal capsule
    intrapontine
    pontine
    subcortical
    ventricular
  Rupture of blood vessel in brain
  ⒺⓍ 430-432.9, 459.89-459.9, 780.01-780.09, 800.00-801.99, 803.00-804.96,
    850.0-852.19, 852.21-854.19
  Coding Clinic: 2007, Q3, P4; 1997, Q3, P11

● **432 Other and unspecified intracranial hemorrhage**

432.0 Nontraumatic extradural hemorrhage 🔒
  Nontraumatic epidural hemorrhage
  ⒺⓍ 430-432.9, 459.89-459.9, 780.01-780.09, 800.00-801.99, 803.00-804.96,
    850.0-852.19, 852.21-854.19

432.1 Subdural hemorrhage 🔒
  Subdural hematoma, nontraumatic
  ⒺⓍ 430-432.9, 459.89-459.9, 780.01-780.09, 800.00-801.99, 803.00-804.96,
    850.0-852.19, 852.21-854.19

432.9 Unspecified intracranial hemorrhage 🔒
  Intracranial hemorrhage NOS
  ⒺⓍ 430-432.9, 459.89-459.9, 780.01-780.09, 800.00-801.99, 803.00-804.96,
    850.0-852.19, 852.21-854.19

● **433 Occlusion and stenosis of precerebral arteries**

The following fifth-digit subclassification is for use with
category 433:

┌──┐
│ 0 **without mention of cerebral infarction** │
│ 1 **with cerebral infarction**   │
└──┘

┌──────────┐
│ **Includes** │ embolism of basilar, carotid, and vertebral
└──────────┘   arteries
               narrowing of basilar, carotid, and vertebral
                 arteries
               obstruction of basilar, carotid, and vertebral
                 arteries
               thrombosis of basilar, carotid, and vertebral
                 arteries
┌──────────┐
│ **Excludes** │ *insufficiency NOS of precerebral arteries*
└──────────┘   *(435.0–435.9)*

Use additional code, if applicable, to identify status post
  administration of tPA (rtPA) in a different facility
  within the last 24 hours prior to admission to
  current facility (V45.88)
  Coding Clinic: 1995, Q2, P16; 1993, Q4, P38-39

● **433.0 Basilar artery** 1 🔒
  [0-1]   For code **433.01:** ⒺⓍ 249.70-249.91, 250.70-250.93, 346.60-346.63,
             433.00-433.91, 435.0, 459.89-459.9

● **433.1 Carotid artery** 1 🔒
  [0-1]   For code **433.11:** ⒺⓍ 249.70-249.91, 250.70-250.93, 346.60-346.63,
             433.00-433.91, 459.89-459.9
           Coding Clinic: 2006, Q1, P17; 2002, Q1, P7-8, 10-11; 2000, Q1, P16;
             1995, Q2, P16

DISEASES OF THE CIRCULATORY SYSTEM (390–459)

● **433.2 Vertebral artery 1**🔇
[0-1]   For code **433.21:** (Ex:) 249.70-249.91, 250.70-250.93, 346.60-346.63,
               433.00-433.91, 435.1, 459.89-459.9

● **433.3 Multiple and bilateral 1**🔇
[0-1]   For code **433.31:** (Ex:) 249.70-249.91, 250.70-250.93, 346.60-346.63,
               433.00-433.91, 459.89-459.9
         Coding Clinic: 2006, Q1, P17; 2002, Q1, P10-11

● **433.8 Other specified precerebral artery 1**🔇
[0-1]   For code **433.81:** (Ex:) 249.70-249.91, 250.70-250.93, 346.60-346.63,
               433.00-433.91, 435.0, 459.89-459.9

● **433.9 Unspecified precerebral artery 1**🔇
[0-1]   Precerebral artery NOS
        For code **433.91:** (Ex:) 249.70-249.91, 250.70-250.93, 346.60-346.63,
               433.00-433.91, 435.0, 459.89-459.9

● **434 Occlusion of cerebral arteries**

The following fifth-digit subclassification is for use with category 434:

> **0   without mention of cerebral infarction**
> **1   with cerebral infarction**

Use additional code, if applicable, to identify status post administration of tPA (rtPA) in a different facility within the last 24 hours prior to admission to current facility (V45.88)
Coding Clinic: 2007, Q3, P12; 1995, Q2, P16; 1993, Q4, P38-39

● **434.0 Cerebral thrombosis 1**🔇
[0-1]   Thrombosis of cerebral arteries
        For code **434.01:** (Ex:) 249.70-249.91, 250.70-250.93, 346.60-346.63,
               434.00-434.91, 436, 459.89-459.9

● **434.1 Cerebral embolism 1**🔇
[0-1]   For code **434.11:** (Ex:) 249.70-249.91, 250.70-250.93, 346.60-346.63,
               434.00-434.91, 436, 459.89-459.9
         Coding Clinic: 1997, Q3, P11

● **434.9 Cerebral artery occlusion, unspecified 1**🔇
[0-1]   For code **434.91:** (Ex:) 249.70-249.91, 250.70-250.93, 346.60-346.63,
               434.00-434.91, 436, 459.89-459.9
         Coding Clinic: 2008, Q4, P102-109; 2007, Q1, P23-24; 2004, Q4, P77-78; 1998, Q4, P87; 1996, Q2, P5

OGCR   Section I.C.7.b

The terms stroke and CVA are often used interchangeably to refer to a cerebral vascular infarction. The terms stroke, CVA, and cerebral infarction NOS are all indexed to the default code 434.91, Cerebral artery occlusion, unspecified, with infarction. Code 436, Acute, but ill-defined, cerebrovascular disease, should not be used when the documentation states stroke or CVA.

● **435 Transient cerebral ischemia**

Includes   cerebrovascular insufficiency (acute) with transient focal neurological signs and symptoms
             insufficiency of basilar, carotid, and vertebral arteries
             spasm of cerebral arteries

Excludes *acute cerebrovascular insufficiency NOS (437.1)*
           that due to any condition classifiable to 433 (433.0–433.9)

435.0 Basilar artery syndrome🔇
     (Ex:) 249.70-249.91, 250.70-250.93, 433.00-433.91, 435.0-435.9, 459.89-459.9

435.1 Vertebral artery syndrome🔇
     (Ex:) 249.70-249.91, 250.70-250.93, 433.00-433.91, 435.0-435.9, 459.89-459.9

435.2 Subclavian steal syndrome🔇
     (Ex:) 249.70-249.91, 250.70-250.93, 433.00-433.91, 435.0-435.9, 459.89-459.9

435.3 Vertebrobasilar artery syndrome🔇
     (Ex:) 249.70-249.91, 250.70-250.93, 433.00-433.91, 435.0-435.9, 459.89-459.9

435.8 Other specified transient cerebral ischemias🔇
     (Ex:) 249.70-249.91, 250.70-250.93, 433.00-433.91, 435.0-435.9, 459.89-459.9

435.9 Unspecified transient cerebral ischemia🔇
     Impending cerebrovascular accident
     Intermittent cerebral ischemia
     Transient ischemic attack [TIA]
     (Ex:) 249.70-249.91, 250.70-250.93, 433.00-433.91, 435.0-435.9, 459.89-459.9
     Coding Clinic: 1985, Nov-Dec, P12

● **436 Acute, but ill-defined, cerebrovascular disease**🔇
     Apoplexy, apoplectic:
       NOS
       attack
       cerebral
       seizure
     Cerebral seizure

Excludes   *any condition classifiable to categories 430–435*
          cerebrovascular accident (434.91)
          CVA (ischemic) (434.91)
            embolic (434.11)
            hemorrhagic (430, 431, 432.0–432.9)
            thrombotic (434.01)
          postoperative cerebrovascular accident (997.02)
          stroke (ischemic) (434.91)
            embolic (434.11)
            hemorrhagic (430, 431, 432.0–432.9)
            thrombotic (434.01)
   (Ex:) 249.70-249.91, 250.70-250.93, 346.60-346.63, 430-432.9, 434.00-434.91, 436, 459.89-459.9, 780.01-780.09, 800.00-801.99, 803.00-804.96, 850.0-852.19, 852.21-854.19
   Coding Clinic: 2004, Q4, P77-78; 1999, Q4, P3-4; 1993, Q4, P38-39; Q1, P27

OGCR   Section I.C.7.b

The terms stroke and CVA are often used interchangeably to refer to a cerebral vascular infarction. The terms stroke, CVA, and cerebral infarction NOS are all indexed to the default code 434.91, Cerebral artery occlusion, unspecified, with infarction. Code 436, Acute, but ill-defined, cerebrovascular disease, should not be used when the documentation states stroke or CVA.

● **437 Other and ill-defined cerebrovascular disease**

437.0 Cerebral atherosclerosis   A
     Atheroma of cerebral arteries
     Cerebral arteriosclerosis

437.1 Other generalized ischemic cerebrovascular disease🔇
     Acute cerebrovascular insufficiency NOS
     Cerebral ischemia (chronic)
     (Ex:) 249.70-249.91, 250.70-250.93, 430-432.9, 434.00-436, 437.1, 459.89-459.9
     Coding Clinic: 2009, Q1, P10

437.2 Hypertensive encephalopathy🔇
     (Ex:) 249.70-249.91, 250.70-250.93, 437.2, 459.89-459.9

437.3 Cerebral aneurysm, nonruptured
     Internal carotid artery, intracranial portion
     Internal carotid artery NOS

Excludes   *congenital cerebral aneurysm, nonruptured (747.81)*
          internal carotid artery, extracranial portion (442.81)
     Coding Clinic: 2009, Q2, P11

437.4 Cerebral arteritis🔇
     (Ex:) 249.70-249.91, 250.70-250.93, 437.4, 459.89-459.9
     Coding Clinic: 1999, Q4, P21-22

◀ New   ◀▥ Revised   ~~deleted~~ Deleted   ● Unacceptable Principal Diagnosis   ● Use Additional Digit(s)
▶ Manifestation Code   **OGCR** Official Guidelines   **Coding Clinic**   Excludes   Includes   Use additional   Code first   Omit code

437.5 Moyamoya disease 🖑
> (Ex) 249.70-249.91, 250.70-250.93, 437.5, 459.89-459.9

437.6 Nonpyogenic thrombosis of intracranial venous sinus 🖑
> | Excludes | *pyogenic (325)*
>
> (Ex) 249.70-249.91, 250.70-250.93, 437.6, 459.89-459.9

437.7 Transient global amnesia

437.8 Other

437.9 Unspecified
> Cerebrovascular disease or lesion NOS
>
> **OGCR** Section I.C.7.d.3
> Assign code V12.54, Transient ischemic attack (TIA), and cerebral infarction without residual deficits (and not a code from category 438) as an additional code for history of cerebrovascular disease when no neurologic deficits are present.
>
> Coding Clinic: 2009, Q1, P16; 1986, Nov-Dec, P12

● **438   Late effects of cerebrovascular disease**
> **Note:** This category is to be used to indicate conditions in 430–437 as the cause of late effects. The "late effects" include conditions specified as such, or as sequelae, which may occur at any time after the onset of the causal condition.
>
> | Excludes | *personal history of:*
> *cerebral infarction without residual deficits (V12.54)*
> *PRIND (Prolonged reversible ischemic neurologic deficit) (V12.54)*
> *RIND (Reversible ischemic neurological deficit) (V12.54)*
> *transient ischemic attack (TIA) (V12.54)*
> Coding Clinic: 2006, Q3, P3-4, 6; 1999, Q4, P6-8x2; Q4, P4-5; 1994, Q1, P22-23; 1993, Q1, P27

438.0 Cognitive deficits 🖑
> Coding Clinic: 2007, Q2, P5

● **438.1 Speech and language deficits**

     438.10 Speech and language deficit, unspecified 🖑

     438.11 Aphasia 🖑
> Coding Clinic: 2003, Q4, P105-106; 1997, Q4, P35-37

     438.12 Dysphasia 🖑
> Coding Clinic: 1999, Q4, P9; Q4, P3-4

     438.13 Dysarthria ◄

     438.14 Fluency disorder ◄
> Stuttering ◄

     438.19 Other speech and language deficits 🖑

● **438.2 Hemiplegia/hemiparesis**
> Coding Clinic: 2005, Q1, P13

     438.20 Hemiplegia affecting unspecified side 🖑 🖑
> (Ex) 438.20
> Coding Clinic: 2007, Q4, P92-95; 2003, Q4, P105-106; 1999, Q4, P9; Q4, P3-4

     438.21 Hemiplegia affecting dominant side 🖑 🖑
> (Ex) 438.21

     438.22 Hemiplegia affecting nondominant side 🖑 🖑
> (Ex) 438.22
> Coding Clinic: 2003, Q4, P105; 2002, Q1, P16

● **438.3 Monoplegia of upper limb**

     438.30 Monoplegia of upper limb affecting unspecified side 🖑

     438.31 Monoplegia of upper limb affecting dominant side 🖑

     438.32 Monoplegia of upper limb affecting nondominant side 🖑

● **438.4 Monoplegia of lower limb**

     438.40 Monoplegia of lower limb affecting unspecified side 🖑

     438.41 Monoplegia of lower limb affecting dominant side 🖑

     438.42 Monoplegia of lower limb affecting nondominant side 🖑

● **438.5 Other paralytic syndrome**
> Use additional code to identify type of paralytic syndrome, such as:
> locked-in state (344.81)
> quadriplegia (344.00–344.09)
>
> | Excludes | *late effects of cerebrovascular accident with:*
> *hemiplegia/hemiparesis (438.20–438.22)*
> *monoplegia of lower limb (438.40–438.42)*
> *monoplegia of upper limb (438.40–438.42)*

     438.50 Other paralytic syndrome affecting unspecified side 🖑

     438.51 Other paralytic syndrome affecting dominant side 🖑

     438.52 Other paralytic syndrome affecting nondominant side 🖑

     438.53 Other paralytic syndrome, bilateral 🖑
> Coding Clinic: 1998, Q4, P39-40

438.6 Alterations of sensations 🖑
> Use additional code to identify the altered sensation
> Coding Clinic: 2002, Q4, P56

438.7 Disturbances of vision 🖑
> Use additional code to identify the visual disturbance
> Coding Clinic: 2002, Q4, P56

● **438.8 Other late effects of cerebrovascular disease**
> Coding Clinic: 2005, Q1, P13; 2002, Q4, P56

     438.81 Apraxia 🖑

     438.82 Dysphagia 🖑
> Use additional code to identify the type of dysphagia, if known (787.20–787.29)
> Coding Clinic: 2007, Q4, P92-95

     438.83 Facial weakness 🖑
> Facial droop

     438.84 Ataxia 🖑

     438.85 Vertigo 🖑
> Coding Clinic: 2002, Q4, P56

     438.89 Other late effects of cerebrovascular disease 🖑
> Use additional code to identify the late effect
> Coding Clinic: 2009, Q2, P11; 2005, Q1, P13; 1998, Q4, P39-40

438.9 Unspecified late effects of cerebrovascular disease 🖑

N Newborn Age: 0   **P** Pediatric Age: 0–17   **M** Maternity Age: 12–55   **A** Adult Age: 15–124   ♀ Females Only   ♂ Males Only   **899**

(Ex) CC Exclusions   🖑 Complication\Comorbidity   🖑 Major C\C   🖑 Present on Admission Requirement   🖑 Hospital-Acquired Condition

DISEASES OF THE CIRCULATORY SYSTEM (390–459)

Figure 7-4 Atherosclerotic plaque.

Atherosclerotic plaque (atheromas)

DISEASES OF ARTERIES, ARTERIOLES, AND CAPILLARIES (440–449)

● 440 **Atherosclerosis**
Disease in which fatty deposits form on walls of arteries

Includes arteriolosclerosis
arteriosclerosis (obliterans) (senile)
arteriosclerotic vascular disease
atheroma
degeneration:
    arterial
    arteriovascular
    vascular
endarteritis deformans or obliterans
senile:
    arteritis
    endarteritis

Excludes *atheroembolism (445.01–445.89)*
atherosclerosis of bypass graft of the extremities (440.30–440.32)

440.0 **Of aorta**   A
Coding Clinic: 1993, Q2, P7-8; 1988, Q4, P8

440.1 **Of renal artery**   A
Excludes *atherosclerosis of renal arterioles (403.00–403.91)*

●440.2 **Of native arteries of the extremities**
Use additional code, if applicable, to identify chronic total occlusion of artery of the extremities (440.4)
Excludes *atherosclerosis of bypass graft of the extremities (440.30–440.32)*
Coding Clinic: 1994, Q3, P5; 1990, Q3, P15

440.20 **Atherosclerosis of the extremities, unspecified**   A

440.21 **Atherosclerosis of the extremities with intermittent claudication**   A

440.22 **Atherosclerosis of the extremities with rest pain**   A
Any condition classifiable to 440.21

440.23 **Atherosclerosis of the extremities with ulceration**   A
Any condition classifiable to 440.21–440.22
Use additional code for any associated ulceration (707.10–707.9)

440.24 **Atherosclerosis of the extremities with gangrene**🔒
Any condition classifiable to 440.21, 440.22, and 440.23 with ischemic gangrene 785.4
Use additional code for any associated ulceration (707.10–707.9)
Excludes *gas gangrene 040.0*
(Ex) 338.0-338.4, 440.24, 780.64-780.65, 780.91-780.99, 785.4, 799.81-799.89
Coding Clinic: 2003, Q4, P109-110; Q3, P14x2; 1995, Q1, P11; 1994, Q3, P5

440.29 **Other**   A
Coding Clinic: 1995, Q1, P11

●440.3 **Of bypass graft of the extremities**
Excludes *atherosclerosis of native artery of the extremity (440.21–440.24)*
embolism [occlusion NOS] [thrombus] of graft (996.74)

440.30 **Of unspecified graft**   A

440.31 **Of autologous vein bypass graft**   A

440.32 **Of nonautologous vein bypass graft**   A

● 440.4 **Chronic total occlusion of artery of the extremities**
Complete occlusion of artery of the extremities
Total occlusion of artery of the extremities
Code first atherosclerosis of arteries of the extremities (440.20–440.29, 440.30–440.32)
Excludes *acute occlusion of artery of extremity (444.21–444.22)*
Coding Clinic: 2007, Q4, P82-83

440.8 **Of other specified arteries**   A
Excludes *basilar (433.0)*
carotid (433.1)
cerebral (437.0)
coronary (414.00–414.07)
mesenteric (557.1)
precerebral (433.0–433.9)
pulmonary (416.0)
vertebral (433.2)

440.9 **Generalized and unspecified atherosclerosis** A
Arteriosclerotic vascular disease NOS
Excludes *arteriosclerotic cardiovascular disease [ASCVD] (429.2)*

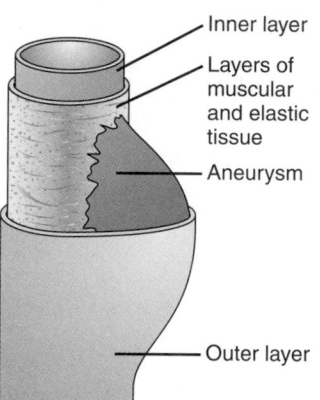

Inner layer
Layers of muscular and elastic tissue
Aneurysm
Outer layer

Figure 7-5 An aneurysm is an enclosed swelling on the wall of the vessel.

Item 7-12 Rupture is the tearing of the aneurysm.

●441 **Aortic aneurysm and dissection**
Excludes *syphilitic aortic aneurysm (093.0)*
traumatic aortic aneurysm (901.0, 902.0)

●441.0 **Dissection of aorta**
Coding Clinic: 1989, Q4, P10

441.00 **Unspecified site**🔒
(Ex) 249.70-249.91, 250.70-250.93, 441.00-441.9, 459.89-459.9

441.01 **Thoracic**🔒
(Ex) 249.70-249.91, 250.70-250.93, 441.00-441.9, 459.89-459.9
Coding Clinic: 2009, Q1, P16; 2007, Q4, P86-87

441.02 **Abdominal**🔒
(Ex) 249.70-249.91, 250.70-250.93, 441.00-441.9, 459.89-459.9

441.03 **Thoracoabdominal**🔒
(Ex) 249.70-249.91, 250.70-250.93, 441.00-441.9, 459.89-459.9

◄ New ◄▥ Revised ~~deleted~~ Deleted ● Unacceptable Principal Diagnosis ● Use Additional Digit(s)
▶ Manifestation Code **OGCR** Official Guidelines **Coding Clinic** Excludes Includes Use additional Code first Omit code

441.1 Thoracic aneurysm, ruptured 🐞
  (Ex) 249.70-249.91, 250.70-250.93, 441.00-441.9, 459.89-459.9
  Coding Clinic: 1994, Q2, P15

441.2 Thoracic aneurysm without mention of rupture
  Coding Clinic: 1992, Q3, P10-11

441.3 Abdominal aneurysm, ruptured 🐞
  (Ex) 249.70-249.91, 250.70-250.93, 441.00-441.9, 459.89-459.9

441.4 Abdominal aneurysm without mention of rupture
  Coding Clinic: 2000, Q4, P63-64; 1999, Q1, P15-17x2; 1992, Q3, P10-11

441.5 Aortic aneurysm of unspecified site, ruptured 🐞
  Rupture of aorta NOS
  (Ex) 249.70-249.91, 250.70-250.93, 441.00-441.9, 459.89-459.9

441.6 Thoracoabdominal aneurysm, ruptured 🐞
  (Ex) 249.70-249.91, 250.70-250.93, 441.00-441.9, 459.89-459.9

441.7 Thoracoabdominal aneurysm, without mention of rupture
  Coding Clinic: 2006, Q2, P16-17

441.9 Aortic aneurysm of unspecified site without mention of rupture
  Aneurysm
  Dilatation of aorta
  Hyaline necrosis of aorta
  Coding Clinic: 1992, Q3, P10-11

● **442 Other aneurysm**
  Includes aneurysm (ruptured) (cirsoid) (false) (varicose)
    aneurysmal varix

  Excludes arteriovenous aneurysm or fistula:
    acquired (447.0)
    congenital (747.60–747.69)
    traumatic (900.0–904.9)

442.0 Of artery of upper extremity

442.1 Of renal artery

442.2 Of iliac artery
  Coding Clinic: 1999, Q1, P16-17

442.3 Of artery of lower extremity
  Aneurysm:
    femoral artery
    popliteal artery
  Coding Clinic: 2008, Q2, P13; 2002, Q3, P24-27; 1999, Q1, P16

● **442.8 Of other specified artery**

  442.81 Artery of neck
    Aneurysm of carotid artery (common) (external) (internal, extracranial portion)
    Excludes internal carotid artery, intracranial portion (437.3)

  442.82 Subclavian artery

  442.83 Splenic artery

  442.84 Other visceral artery
    Aneurysm:
      celiac artery
      gastroduodenal artery
      gastroepiploic artery
      hepatic artery
      pancreaticoduodenal artery
      superior mesenteric artery

  442.89 Other
    Aneurysm: Aneurysm:
      mediastinal artery   spinal artery
    Excludes cerebral (nonruptured) (437.3)
      congenital (747.81)
        ruptured (430)
      coronary (414.11)
      heart (414.10)
      pulmonary (417.1)

442.9 Of unspecified site

● **443 Other peripheral vascular disease**

  443.0 Raynaud's syndrome
    Resulting from a diminishing oxygen supply to fingers, toes, nose, and ears when exposed to temperature changes or stress with symptoms of pallor, numbness, and feeling cold
    Raynaud's:
      disease
      phenomenon (secondary)
    Use additional code to identify gangrene (785.4)

  443.1 Thromboangiitis obliterans [Buerger's disease]
    Inflammatory occlusive disease resulting in poor circulation to legs, feet, and sometimes hands due to progressive inflammatory narrowing of the small arteries
    Presenile gangrene

● **443.2 Other arterial dissection**
    Excludes dissection of aorta (441.00–441.03)
      dissection of coronary arteries (414.12)
    Coding Clinic: 2002, Q4, P54-55

  443.21 Dissection of carotid artery 🐞
    (Ex) 447.2, 447.5-447.9

  443.22 Dissection of iliac artery 🐞
    (Ex) 447.2, 447.5-447.9

  443.23 Dissection of renal artery 🐞
    (Ex) 447.2, 447.5-447.9

  443.24 Dissection of vertebral artery 🐞
    (Ex) 447.2, 447.5-447.9

  443.29 Dissection of other artery 🐞
    (Ex) 447.2, 447.5-447.9

● **443.8 Other specified peripheral vascular diseases**

  ▶ **443.81 Peripheral angiopathy in diseases classified elsewhere**
    Code first underlying disease, as:
      diabetes mellitus (249.7, 250.7)
    Coding Clinic: 2004, Q1, P14-15; 1996, Q1, P10

  443.82 Erythromelalgia
    Coding Clinic: 2005, Q4, P73-74

  443.89 Other
    Acrocyanosis
    Acroparesthesia:
      simple [Schultze's type]
      vasomotor [Nothnagel's type]
    Erythrocyanosis
    Excludes chilblains (991.5)
      frostbite (991.0–991.3)
      immersion foot (991.4)
    Coding Clinic: 2007, Q4, P124

  443.9 Peripheral vascular disease, unspecified
    Intermittent claudication NOS
    Peripheral:
      angiopathy NOS
      vascular disease NOS
    Spasm of artery
    Excludes atherosclerosis of the arteries of the extremities (440.20–440.22)
      spasm of cerebral artery (435.0–435.9)

DISEASES OF THE CIRCULATORY SYSTEM (390–459)

N Newborn Age: 0   P Pediatric Age: 0–17   M Maternity Age: 12–55   A Adult Age: 15–124   ♀ Females Only   ♂ Males Only

(Ex) CC Exclusions   🐞 Complication\Comorbidity   🐞 Major C\C   🐞 Present on Admission Requirement   🐞 Hospital-Acquired Condition

901

Figure 7-6 An arterial embolus.

Item 7-13 An **embolus** is a mass of undissolved matter present in the blood that is transported by the blood current. A **thrombus** is a blood clot that occludes or shuts off a vessel. When a thrombus is dislodged, it becomes an embolus.

● **444 Arterial embolism and thrombosis**

  Includes infarction:
      embolic
      thrombotic
      occlusion

  Excludes *atheroembolism (445.01–445.89)*
    septic arterial embolism (449)
    that complicating:
      abortion (634–638 with .6, 639.6)
      ectopic or molar pregnancy (639.6)
      pregnancy, childbirth, or the puerperium (673.0–673.8)
  Coding Clinic: 2003, Q1, P16-18x2; 1992, Q2, P10-11

444.0 Of abdominal aorta
  Aortic bifurcation syndrome
  Aortoiliac obstruction
  Leriche's syndrome
  Saddle embolus
  (Ex:) 249.70-249.91, 250.70-250.93, 444.0, 444.89-444.9, 449, 459.89-459.9
  Coding Clinic: 1990, Q4, P27

444.1 Of thoracic aorta
  Embolism or thrombosis of aorta (thoracic)
  (Ex:) 249.70-249.91, 250.70-250.93, 444.1, 444.89-444.9, 449, 459.89-459.9

● **444.2 Of arteries of the extremities**

  444.21 Upper extremity
    (Ex:) 249.70-249.91, 250.70-250.93, 444.21, 444.89-444.9, 449, 459.89-459.9
    Coding Clinic: 1990, Q3, P16

  444.22 Lower extremity
    Arterial embolism or thrombosis:
      femoral   popliteal
      peripheral NOS
    Excludes *iliofemoral (444.81)*
    (Ex:) 249.70-249.91, 250.70-250.93, 444.22, 444.89-444.9, 449, 459.89-459.9
    Coding Clinic: 2007, Q4, P84-86; 2003, Q3, P10

● **444.8 Of other specified artery**

  444.81 Iliac artery
    (Ex:) 249.70-249.91, 250.70-250.93, 444.81-444.9, 449, 459.89-459.9
    Coding Clinic: 2003, Q1, P16-17

  444.89 Other
    Excludes *basilar (433.0)*
      carotid (433.1)
      cerebral (434.0–434.9)
      coronary (410.00–410.92)
      mesenteric (557.0)
      ophthalmic (362.30–362.34)
      precerebral (433.0–433.9)
      pulmonary (415.19)
      renal (593.81)
      retinal (362.30–362.34)
      vertebral (433.2)
    (Ex:) 249.70-249.91, 250.70-250.93, 444.89-444.9, 449, 459.89-459.9

444.9 Of unspecified artery
  (Ex:) 249.70-249.91, 250.70-250.93, 444.89-444.9, 449, 459.89-459.9

● **445 Atheroembolism**
  Includes Atherothrombotic microembolism
    Cholesterol embolism
  Coding Clinic: 2002, Q4, P57-58

● **445.0 Of extremities**

  445.01 Upper extremity
    (Ex:) 249.70-249.91, 250.70-250.93, 444.89-445.01, 449, 459.89-459.9

  445.02 Lower extremity
    (Ex:) 249.70-249.91, 250.70-250.93, 444.89-444.9, 445.02, 449, 459.89-459.9

● **445.8 Of other sites**

  445.81 Kidney
    Use additional code for any associated acute renal kidney failure or chronic kidney disease (584, 585)
    (Ex:) 249.70-249.91, 250.70-250.93, 444.89-444.9, 445.81, 449, 459.89-459.9

  445.89 Other site
    (Ex:) 249.70-249.91, 250.70-250.93, 444.89-444.9, 445.89, 449, 459.89-459.9

● **446 Polyarteritis nodosa and allied conditions**

  446.0 Polyarteritis nodosa
    Disseminated necrotizing periarteritis
    Necrotizing angiitis
    Panarteritis (nodosa)
    Periarteritis (nodosa)
    (Ex:) 249.70-249.91, 250.70-250.93, 446.0-446.7, 459.89-459.9

  446.1 Acute febrile mucocutaneous lymph node syndrome [MCLS]
    Kawasaki disease
    (Ex:) 446.0-446.29, 446.4-446.7, 459.89-459.9

● **446.2 Hypersensitivity angiitis**
  Excludes *antiglomerular basement membrane disease without pulmonary hemorrhage (583.89)*

  446.20 Hypersensitivity angiitis, unspecified
    (Ex:) 249.70-249.91, 250.70-250.93, 446.0-446.7, 459.89-459.9

  446.21 Goodpasture's syndrome
    Antiglomerular basement membrane antibody-mediated nephritis with pulmonary hemorrhage
    Use additional code to identify renal disease (583.81)
    (Ex:) 249.70-249.91, 250.70-250.93, 446.0-446.7, 459.89-459.9

  446.29 Other specified hypersensitivity angiitis
    (Ex:) 249.70-249.91, 250.70-250.93, 446.0-446.7, 459.89-459.9
    Coding Clinic: 1995, Q1, P3

  446.3 Lethal midline granuloma
    Malignant granuloma of face
    (Ex:) 249.70-249.91, 250.70-250.93, 446.0-446.7, 459.89-459.9

  446.4 Wegener's granulomatosis
    Necrotizing respiratory granulomatosis
    Wegener's syndrome
    (Ex:) 249.70-249.91, 250.70-250.93, 446.0-446.7, 459.89-459.9
    Coding Clinic: 2000, Q3, P11

  446.5 Giant cell arteritis
    Cranial arteritis
    Horton's disease
    Temporal arteritis

  446.6 Thrombotic microangiopathy
    Moschcowitz's syndrome
    Thrombotic thrombocytopenic purpura
    (Ex:) 249.70-249.91, 250.70-250.93, 446.0-446.7, 459.89-459.9

  446.7 Takayasu's disease
    Aortic arch arteritis
    Pulseless disease
    (Ex:) 249.70-249.91, 250.70-250.93, 446.0-446.7, 459.89-459.9

◀ New   ◀ Revised   deleted Deleted   ● Unacceptable Principal Diagnosis   ● Use Additional Digit(s)
▶ Manifestation Code   OGCR Official Guidelines   Coding Clinic   Excludes   Includes   Use additional   Code first   Omit code

● 447 **Other disorders of arteries and arterioles**

447.0 Arteriovenous fistula, acquired
Arteriovenous aneurysm, acquired
Excludes *cerebrovascular (437.3)*
coronary (414.19)
pulmonary (417.0)
surgically created arteriovenous shunt or
fistula:
complication (996.1, 996.61–996.62)
status or presence (V45.11)
traumatic (900.0–904.9)

447.1 Stricture of artery
Coding Clinic: 1993, Q2, P8; 1987, Jan-Feb, P14

447.2 Rupture of artery🔹
Erosion of artery
Fistula, except arteriovenous of artery
Ulcer of artery
Excludes *traumatic rupture of artery (900.0–904.9)*
(Ex) 414.12, 443.22-443.29, 447.2

447.3 Hyperplasia of renal artery
Fibromuscular hyperplasia of renal artery

447.4 Celiac artery compression syndrome🔹
Celiac axis syndrome
Marable's syndrome
(Ex) 447.4

447.5 Necrosis of artery🔹
(Ex) 447.5

447.6 Arteritis, unspecified
Aortitis NOS
Endarteritis NOS
Excludes *arteritis, endarteritis:*
aortic arch (446.7)
cerebral (437.4)
coronary (414.00–414.07)
deformans (440.0–440.9)
obliterans (440.0–440.9)
pulmonary (417.8)
senile (440.0–440.9)
polyarteritis NOS (446.0)
syphilitic aortitis (093.1)
Coding Clinic: 1999, Q4, P21-22

447.8 Other specified disorders of arteries and arterioles
Fibromuscular hyperplasia of arteries, except renal

447.9 Unspecified disorders of arteries and arterioles

● 448 **Disease of capillaries**

448.0 Hereditary hemorrhagic telangiectasia
Rendu-Osler-Weber disease

448.1 Nevus, non-neoplastic
Nevus:
araneus
senile
spider
stellar
Excludes *neoplastic (216.0–216.9)*
port wine (757.32)
strawberry (757.32)

448.9 Other and unspecified capillary diseases
Capillary:
hemorrhage
hyperpermeability
thrombosis
Excludes *capillary fragility (hereditary) (287.8)*

● 449 **Septic arterial embolism**🔹
Code first underlying infection, such as:
infective endocarditis (421.0)
lung abscess (513.0)
Use additional code to identify the site of the embolism
(433.0–433.9, 444.0–444.9)
Excludes *septic pulmonary embolism (415.12)*
(Ex) 249.70-249.91, 250.70-250.93, 444.89-444.9, 449, 459.89-459.9
Coding Clinic: 2007, Q4, P84-86

**DISEASES OF VEINS AND LYMPHATICS, AND OTHER DISEASES
OF CIRCULATORY SYSTEM (451–459)**

● 451 **Phlebitis and thrombophlebitis**
*Inflammation of vein with infiltration of walls (phlebitis)
and, usually, formation of clot (thrombus) in vein
(thrombophlebitis)*
Includes endophlebitis
inflammation, vein
periphlebitis
suppurative phlebitis
Use additional E code to identify drug if drug-induced
Excludes *that complicating:*
abortion (634–638 with .7, 639.8)
ectopic or molar pregnancy (639.8)
pregnancy, childbirth, or the puerperium
(671.0–671.9)
that due to or following:
implant or catheter device (996.61–996.62)
infusion, perfusion, or transfusion (999.2)
Coding Clinic: 2004, Q4, P78-80; 1993, Q1, P26; 1992, Q1, P15-16

451.0 Of superficial vessels of lower extremities
Saphenous vein (greater) (lesser)

● **451.1 Of deep vessels of lower extremities**
Coding Clinic: 1991, Q3, P16

451.11 Femoral vein (deep) (superficial)🔹
(Ex) 249.70-249.91, 250.70-250.93, 451.0-451.9, 459.89-459.9

451.19 Other🔹
Femoropopliteal vein
Popliteal vein
Tibial vein
(Ex) 249.70-249.91, 250.70-250.93, 451.0-451.9, 459.89-459.9

451.2 Of lower extremities, unspecified
Coding Clinic: 2004, Q4, P78-80

● **451.8 Of other sites**
Excludes *intracranial venous sinus (325)*
nonpyogenic (437.6)
portal (vein) (572.1)

451.81 Iliac vein🔹
(Ex) 249.70-249.91, 250.70-250.93, 451.0-451.9, 459.89-459.9

451.82 Of superficial veins of upper extremities
Antecubital vein
Basilic vein
Cephalic vein

451.83 Of deep veins of upper extremities🔹
Brachial vein
Radial vein
Ulnar vein
(Ex) 451.0-451.2, 451.83, 451.89-451.9

451.84 Of upper extremities, unspecified

451.89 Other🔹
Axillary vein
Jugular vein
Subclavian vein
Thrombophlebitis of breast (Mondor's disease)
(Ex) 451.0-451.2, 451.89-451.9

451.9 Of unspecified site

N Newborn Age: 0   **P** Pediatric Age: 0–17   **M** Maternity Age: 12–55   **A** Adult Age: 15–124   ♀ Females Only   ♂ Males Only
(Ex) CC Exclusions   🔹 Complication\Comorbidity   🔹 Major C\C   Present on Admission Requirement   🔹 Hospital-Acquired Condition

DISEASES OF THE CIRCULATORY SYSTEM (390–459)

452 Portal vein thrombosis 🔵
Portal (vein) obstruction

> **Excludes** *hepatic vein thrombosis (453.0)*
> *phlebitis of portal vein (572.1)*
> (Ex) 249.70-249.91, 250.70-250.93, 452, 453.40-453.9, 459.89-459.9

● **453 Other venous embolism and thrombosis**

> **Excludes** *that complicating:*
> *abortion (634–638 with .7, 639.8)*
> *ectopic or molar pregnancy (639.8)*
> *pregnancy, childbirth, or the puerperium*
> *(671.0–671.9)*
> ~~*that with inflammation, phlebitis, and*~~
> ~~*thrombophlebitis (451.0–451.9)*~~

Coding Clinic: 2004, Q4, P78-80; 1992, Q1, P15-16

453.0 Budd-Chiari syndrome 🔵
Hepatic vein thrombosis
(Ex) 249.70-249.91, 250.70-250.93, 453.0, 453.40-453.9, 459.89-459.9

453.1 Thrombophlebitis migrans 🔵
"White leg" is the other term used to describe a
migrating thrombus.
(Ex) 249.70-249.91, 250.70-250.93, 453.1, 453.40-453.9, 459.89-459.9

453.2 Of inferior vena cava 🔵 ◀▥
(Ex) 249.70-249.91, 250.70-250.93, 453.2, 453.40-453.9, 459.89-459.9

453.3 Of renal vein 🔵
(Ex) 249.70-249.91, 250.70-250.93, 453.3-453.9, 459.89-459.9

● **453.4 Acute ~~V~~venous embolism and thrombosis of deep**
vessels of lower extremity ◀▥

453.40 Acute ~~V~~venous embolism and thrombosis of
unspecified deep vessels of lower
extremity 🔵 🔵 ◀▥
Deep vein thrombosis NOS
DVT NOS
HAC: And one of the following procedure
codes: 00.85-00.87, 81.51-81.52,
81.54
(Ex) 249.70-249.91, 250.70-250.93, 453.40-453.9, 459.89-459.9

453.41 Acute ~~V~~venous embolism and thrombosis
of deep vessels of proximal lower
extremity 🔵 🔵 ◀▥
Femoral
Iliac
Popliteal
Thigh
Upper leg NOS
HAC: And one of the following procedure
codes: 00.85-00.87, 81.51-81.52,
81.54
(Ex) 249.70-249.91, 250.70-250.93, 453.40-453.9, 459.89-459.9
Coding Clinic: 2004, Q4, P78-80

453.42 Acute ~~V~~venous embolism and thrombosis of
deep vessels of distal lower extremity 🔵 🔵 ◀▥
Calf
Lower leg NOS
Peroneal
Tibial
HAC: And one of the following procedure
codes: 00.85-00.87, 81.51-81.52,
81.54
(Ex) 249.70-249.91, 250.70-250.93, 453.40-453.9, 459.89-459.9

● **453.5 Chronic venous embolism and thrombosis of deep**
vessels of lower extremity ◀

> **Use additional** code, if applicable, for associated
> long-term (current) use of anticoagulants
> (V58.61) ◀

> **Excludes** *personal history of venous thrombosis*
> *and embolism (V12.51)* ◀

453.50 Chronic venous embolism and thrombosis
of unspecified deep vessels of lower
extremity 🔵 ◀

453.51 Chronic venous embolism and thrombosis of
deep vessels of proximal lower extremity 🔵 ◀

453.52 Chronic venous embolism and thrombosis of
deep vessels of distal lower extremity 🔵 ◀

453.6 Venous embolism and thrombosis of superficial
vessels of lower extremity 🔵 ◀
Saphenous vein (greater) (lesser) ◀

● **453.7 Chronic venous embolism and thrombosis of other**
specified vessels ◀

> **Use additional** code, if applicable, for associated
> long-term (current) use of anticoagulants
> (V58.61) ◀

> **Excludes** *personal history of venous thrombosis*
> *and embolism (V12.51)* ◀

453.71 Chronic venous embolism and thrombosis
of superficial veins of upper extremity 🔵 ◀
Antecubital vein ◀
Basilic vein ◀
Cephalic vein ◀

453.72 Chronic venous embolism and thrombosis
of deep veins of upper extremity 🔵 ◀
Brachial vein ◀
Radial vein ◀
Ulnar vein ◀

453.73 Chronic venous embolism and thrombosis
of upper extremity, unspecified 🔵 ◀

453.74 Chronic venous embolism and thrombosis
of axillary veins 🔵 ◀

453.75 Chronic venous embolism and thrombosis
of subclavian veins 🔵 ◀

453.76 Chronic venous embolism and thrombosis
of internal jugular veins 🔵 ◀

453.77 Chronic venous embolism and
thrombosis of other thoracic veins 🔵 ◀
Brachiocephalic (innominate) ◀
Superior vena cava ◀

453.79 Chronic venous embolism and
thrombosis of other specified veins 🔵 ◀

453.8 Acute venous embolism and thrombosis ⊖of other
specified veins ◀▥

> **Excludes** *cerebral (434.0–434.9)*
> *coronary (410.00–410.92)*
> *intracranial venous sinus (325)*
> *nonpyogenic (437.6)*
> *mesenteric (557.0)*
> *portal (452)*
> *precerebral (433.0–433.9)*
> *pulmonary (415.19)*
> (Ex) 249.70-249.91, 250.70-250.93, 453.40-453.9, 459.89-459.9
> **Coding Clinic: 2004, Q4, P78-80; 1992, Q1, P15-16**

453.81 Acute venous embolism and thrombosis of
superficial veins of upper extremity 🔵 ◀
Antecubital vein ◀
Basilic vein ◀
Cephalic vein ◀

453.82   Acute venous embolism and thrombosis of deep veins of upper extremity 🔓
Brachial vein ◀
Radial vein ◀
Ulnar vein ◀

453.83   Acute venous embolism and thrombosis of upper extremity, unspecified 🔓 ◀

453.84   Acute venous embolism and thrombosis of axillary veins 🔓 ◀

453.85   Acute venous embolism and thrombosis of subclavian veins 🔓 ◀

453.86   Acute venous embolism and thrombosis of internal jugular veins 🔓 ◀

453.87   Acute venous embolism and thrombosis of other thoracic veins 🔓 ◀
Brachiocephalic (innominate) ◀
Superior vena cava ◀

453.89   Acute venous embolism and thrombosis of other specified veins 🔓 ◀

453.9   Of unspecified site 🔓
Embolism of vein
Thrombosis (vein)
    (Ex:) 249.70-249.91, 250.70-250.93, 453.40-453.9, 459.89-459.9

Item 7–14   Varicose/Varicosities (varix = singular, varices = plural): Enlarged, engorged, tortuous, twisted vascular vessels (veins, arteries, lymphatics). As such, the condition can present in various parts of the body, although the most familiar locations are the lower extremities. A common complication of varices is thrombophlebitis. Varicosities of the anus and rectum are called hemorrhoids. There are additional codes for esophageal, sublingual (under the tongue), scrotal, pelvic, vulval, and nasal varices as well.

Figure 7–7   Varicose veins of the legs. (From Goldman: Cecil Medicine, 23rd ed. 2008, Saunders)

🔵**454   Varicose veins of lower extremities**
    Excludes   *that complicating pregnancy, childbirth, or the puerperium (671.0)*

454.0   With ulcer   A
Varicose ulcer (lower extremity, any part)
Varicose veins with ulcer of lower extremity [any part] or of unspecified site
Any condition classifiable to 454.9 with ulcer or specified as ulcerated
    Coding Clinic: 1999, Q4, P18

454.1   With inflammation   A
Stasis dermatitis
Varicose veins with inflammation of lower extremity [any part] or of unspecified site
Any condition classifiable to 454.9 with inflammation or specified as inflamed
    Coding Clinic: 1991, Q2, P20

454.2   With ulcer and inflammation 🔓   A
Varicose veins with ulcer and inflammation of lower extremity [any part] or of unspecified site
Any condition classifiable to 454.9 with ulcer and inflammation
    (Ex:) 454.0-454.2, 454.9
    Coding Clinic: 2004, Q3, P5-6; 1991, Q2, P20

454.8   With other complications
Edema
Pain
Swelling
    Coding Clinic: 2002, Q4, P58-60

454.9   Asymptomatic varicose veins   A
Phlebectasia of lower extremity [any part] or of unspecified site
Varicose veins NOS
Varicose veins of lower extremity [any part] or of unspecified site
Varix of lower extremity [any part] or of unspecified site

🔵**455   Hemorrhoids**
    Includes   hemorrhoids (anus) (rectum)
          piles
          varicose veins, anus or rectum
    Excludes   *that complicating pregnancy, childbirth, or the puerperium (671.8)*

455.0   Internal hemorrhoids without mention of complication
    Coding Clinic: 2005, Q3, P17

455.1   Internal thrombosed hemorrhoids

455.2   Internal hemorrhoids with other complication
Internal hemorrhoids:
    bleeding
    prolapsed
    strangulated
    ulcerated
    Coding Clinic: 2005, Q3, P17; 2003, Q1, P8

455.3   External hemorrhoids without mention of complication
    Coding Clinic: 2007, Q1, P13

455.4   External thrombosed hemorrhoids

455.5   External hemorrhoids with other complication
External hemorrhoids:
    bleeding
    prolapsed
    strangulated
    ulcerated
    Coding Clinic: 2005, Q3, P17; 2003, Q1, P8

455.6   Unspecified hemorrhoids without mention of complication
Hemorrhoids NOS

455.7   Unspecified thrombosed hemorrhoids
Thrombosed hemorrhoids, unspecified whether internal or external

455.8   Unspecified hemorrhoids with other complication
Hemorrhoids, unspecified whether internal or external:
    bleeding
    prolapsed
    strangulated
    ulcerated

455.9   Residual hemorrhoidal skin tags
Skin tags, anus or rectum

DISEASES OF THE CIRCULATORY SYSTEM (390–459)

● 456 **Varicose veins of other sites**

    456.0 **Esophageal varices with bleeding** 🔧
        Ⓔⓧ 25.15, 456.0, 456.20, 459.89-459.9, 530.20-530.21, 530.7, 530.82,
        530.85, 531.00-534.91, 535.01, 535.11, 535.21, 535.31, 535.41,
        535.51, 535.61, 535.71, 537.83, 562.02-562.03, 562.12-562.13, 569.3,
        569.85, 578.0-578.9

    456.1 **Esophageal varices without mention of bleeding** 🔧
        Ⓔⓧ 251.5, 456.0-456.20, 459.89-459.9, 530.7, 530.82, 531.00-534.91, 535.01,
        535.11, 535.21, 535.31, 535.41, 535.51, 535.61, 535.71, 537.83,
        578.0-578.9

  ● 456.2 **Esophageal varices in diseases classified elsewhere**
      Code first *underlying disease, as:*
      cirrhosis of liver (571.0–571.9)
      portal hypertension (572.3)

    ▶ 456.20 **With bleeding** 🔧
        Ⓔⓧ 456.0, 456.20, 459.89-459.9, 530.82
        Coding Clinic: 1985, Nov-Dec, P14

    ▶ 456.21 **Without mention of bleeding** 🔧
        Ⓔⓧ 251.5, 456.0, 456.20-456.21, 459.89-459.9, 530.7, 530.82,
        531.00-534.91, 535.01, 535.11, 535.21, 535.31, 535.41,
        535.51, 535.61, 535.71, 537.83, 578.0-578.9
        Coding Clinic: 2005, Q3, P15-16; 2002, Q2, P4

    456.3 **Sublingual varices**

    456.4 **Scrotal varices** ♂
      Varicocele

    456.5 **Pelvic varices**
      Varices of broad ligament

    456.6 **Vulval varices** ♀
      Varices of perineum
        Excludes *that complicating pregnancy, childbirth, or*
          the puerperium (671.1)

    456.8 **Varices of other sites**
      Varicose veins of nasal septum (with ulcer)
        Excludes *placental varices (656.7)*
          retinal varices (362.17)
          varicose ulcer of unspecified site (454.0)
          varicose veins of unspecified site (454.9)
      Coding Clinic: 2002, Q2, P4

● 457 **Noninfectious disorders of lymphatic channels**

    457.0 **Postmastectomy lymphedema syndrome**   A
      Elephantiasis due to mastectomy
      Obliteration of lymphatic vessel due to mastectomy
      Coding Clinic: 2002, Q2, P12-13

    457.1 **Other lymphedema**
      Elephantiasis (nonfilarial) NOS
      Lymphangiectasis
      Lymphedema:
        acquired (chronic)
        praecox
        secondary
      Obliteration, lymphatic vessel
        Excludes *elephantiasis (nonfilarial):*
          congenital (757.0)
          eyelid (374.83)
          vulva (624.8)
      Coding Clinic: 2004, Q3, P5-6

    457.2 **Lymphangitis**
      Lymphangitis:
        NOS
        chronic
        subacute
        Excludes *acute lymphangitis (682.0–682.9)*

    457.8 **Other noninfectious disorders of lymphatic channels**
      Chylocele (nonfilarial)
      Chylous:
        ascites
        cyst
      Lymph node or vessel:
        fistula
        infarction
        rupture
        Excludes *chylocele:*
          filarial (125.0–125.9)
          tunica vaginalis (nonfilarial) (608.84)
      Coding Clinic: 2004, Q1, P5; 2003, Q3, P16-17

    457.9 **Unspecified noninfectious disorder of lymphatic channels**

● 458 **Hypotension**
    Subnormal arterial blood pressure
    Includes hypopiesis
    Excludes *cardiovascular collapse (785.50)*
        maternal hypotension syndrome (669.2)
        shock (785.50–785.59)
        Shy-Drager syndrome (333.0)
    Coding Clinic: 1994, Q3, P9; 1993, 5th Issue, P6-7

    458.0 **Orthostatic hypotension**
      Hypotension:
        orthostatic (chronic)
        postural
        Moving from sitting or reclining position to
          standing position precipitates sudden drop
          in blood pressure.
      Coding Clinic: 2000, Q3, P8-9

    458.1 **Chronic hypotension**
      Permanent idiopathic hypotension

    458.2 **Iatrogenic hypotension**
      Coding Clinic: 2002, Q3, P12; 1993, Q4, P41-42

      458.21 **Hypotension of hemodialysis**
        Intra-dialytic hypotension
        Coding Clinic: 2003, Q4, P60-61

      458.29 **Other iatrogenic hypotension**
        Postoperative hypotension
        Coding Clinic: 1993, Q4, P41-42

    458.8 **Other specified hypotension**
      Coding Clinic: 1997. Q4, P37

    458.9 **Hypotension, unspecified**
      Hypotension (arterial) NOS

DISEASES OF THE CIRCULATORY SYSTEM (390–459)

◀ New   ⬅ Revised   deleted Deleted   ● Unacceptable Principal Diagnosis   ● Use Additional Digit(s)
▶ Manifestation Code   OGCR Official Guidelines   Coding Clinic   Excludes   Includes   Use additional   Code first   Omit code

● **459   Other disorders of circulatory system**

    459.0   Hemorrhage, unspecified

        Rupture of blood vessel NOS

        Spontaneous hemorrhage NEC

        | Excludes | *hemorrhage:*

            gastrointestinal NOS (578.9)

            in newborn NOS (772.9)

            nontraumatic hematoma of soft tissue

                (729.92)

            secondary or recurrent following trauma

                (958.2)

            traumatic rupture of blood vessel

                (900.0–904.9)

        Coding Clinic:1999, Q4, P18

● **459.1 Postphlebitic syndrome**

        Chronic venous hypertension due to deep vein

          thrombosis

        | Excludes | *chronic venous hypertension without*

              deep vein thrombosis (459.30–459.39)

        Coding Clinic: 2002, Q4, P58-60; 1991, Q2, P20

    459.10 Postphlebitic syndrome without

        complications

        Asymptomatic postphlebitic syndrome

        Postphlebitic syndrome NOS

    459.11 Postphlebitic syndrome with ulcer 🌑

        (Ex) 451.0-451.9

    459.12 Postphlebitic syndrome with inflammation

    459.13 Postphlebitic syndrome with ulcer and

        inflammation 🌑

        (Ex) 451.0-451.9

    459.19 Postphlebitic syndrome with other

        complication

    459.2 Compression of vein 🌑

        Stricture of vein

        Vena cava syndrome (inferior) (superior)

        (Ex) 459.2

● **459.3 Chronic venous hypertension (idiopathic)**

        Stasis edema

        | Excludes | *chronic venous hypertension due to deep*

              vein thrombosis (459.10–459.19)

              varicose veins (454.0–454.9)

        Coding Clinic: 2002, Q4, P58-60

    459.30 Chronic venous hypertension without

        complications

        Asymptomatic chronic venous hypertension

        Chronic venous hypertension NOS

    459.31 Chronic venous hypertension with ulcer 🌑

        (Ex) 454.0-454.2, 454.9, 459.81-459.9

    459.32 Chronic venous hypertension with

        inflammation

    459.33 Chronic venous hypertension with ulcer and

        inflammation 🌑

        (Ex) 454.0-454.2, 454.9, 459.81-459.9

    459.39 Chronic venous hypertension with other

        complication

● **459.8 Other specified disorders of circulatory system**

    459.81 Venous (peripheral) insufficiency,

        unspecified

        Chronic venous insufficiency NOS

        Use additional code for any associated

          ulceration (707.10–707.9)

        Coding Clinic: 2004, Q3, P5-6; 1991, Q2, P20

    459.89 Other

        Collateral circulation (venous), any site

        Phlebosclerosis

        Venofibrosis

    459.9 Unspecified circulatory system disorder

N Newborn Age: 0   **P** Pediatric Age: 0–17   **M** Maternity Age: 12–55   **A** Adult Age: 15–124   ♀ Females Only   ♂ Males Only   **907**

(Ex) CC Exclusions   🌑 Complication\Comorbidity   🌑 Major C\C   🌑 Present on Admission Requirement   🌑 Hospital-Acquired Condition

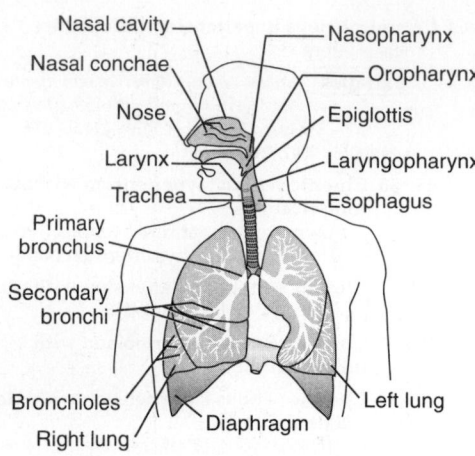

Figure 8–1   Respiratory system. (From Buck CJ: Step-by-Step Medical Coding, 2006 ed. Philadelphia, WB Saunders, 2006.)

8.   DISEASES OF THE RESPIRATORY SYSTEM (460–519)

Use additional code to identify infectious organism

ACUTE RESPIRATORY INFECTIONS (460–466)

> **Excludes**   *pneumonia and influenza (480.0–488)*

460   Acute nasopharyngitis [common cold]
Coryza (acute)
Nasal catarrh, acute
Nasopharyngitis: Rhinitis:
   NOS   acute
   acute   infective
   infective NOS

> **Excludes**   *nasopharyngitis, chronic (472.2)*
> *pharyngitis:*
>   *acute or unspecified (462)*
>   *chronic (472.1)*
> *rhinitis:*
>   *allergic (477.0–477.9)*
>   *chronic or unspecified (472.0)*
> *sore throat:*
>   *acute or unspecified (462)*
>   *chronic (472.1)*

Coding Clinic: 1988, Q1, P12

● 461   Acute sinusitis
Code to specific sinus if indicated in documentation.

> **Includes**   abscess, acute, of sinus (accessory) (nasal)
> empyema, acute, of sinus (accessory) (nasal)
> infection, acute, of sinus (accessory) (nasal)
> inflammation, acute, of sinus (accessory)
>   (nasal)
> suppuration, acute, of sinus (accessory) (nasal)

> **Excludes**   *chronic or unspecified sinusitis (473.0–473.9)*

461.0   Maxillary
Acute antritis

461.1   Frontal

461.2   Ethmoidal

461.3   Sphenoidal

461.8   Other acute sinusitis
Acute pansinusitis

461.9   Acute sinusitis, unspecified
Acute sinusitis NOS

Figure 8–2   Paranasal sinuses. (From Buck CJ: Step-by-Step Medical Coding, 2006 ed. Philadelphia, WB Saunders, 2006.)

Item 8-1   Pharyngitis is painful inflammation of the pharynx (sore throat). Ninety percent of the infections are caused by a virus with the remaining being bacterial and rarely a fungus (candidiasis). Other irritants such as pollutants, chemicals, or smoke may cause similar symptoms.

462   Acute pharyngitis
Acute sore throat NOS
Pharyngitis (acute):
   NOS
   gangrenous
   infective
   phlegmonous
   pneumococcal
   staphylococcal
   suppurative
   ulcerative
Sore throat (viral) NOS
Viral pharyngitis

> **Excludes**   *abscess:*
>   *peritonsillar [quinsy] (475)*
>   *pharyngeal NOS (478.29)*
>   *retropharyngeal (478.24)*
> *chronic pharyngitis (472.1)*
> *infectious mononucleosis (075)*
> *that specified as (due to):*
>   *Coxsackie (virus) (074.0)*
>   *gonococcus (098.6)*
>   *herpes simplex (054.79)*
>   *influenza (487.1)*
>   *septic (034.0)*
>   *streptococcal (034.0)*

Coding Clinic: 1985, Sept-Oct, P9

463   Acute tonsillitis
Inflammation of pharyngeal tonsils caused by virus/bacteria
Tonsillitis (acute):   Tonsillitis (acute):
   NOS   septic
   follicular   staphylococcal
   gangrenous   suppurative
   infective   ulcerative
   pneumococcal   viral

> **Excludes**   *chronic tonsillitis (474.0)*
> *hypertrophy of tonsils (474.1)*
> *peritonsillar abscess [quinsy] (475)*
> *sore throat:*
>   *acute or NOS (462)*
>   *septic (034.0)*
> *streptococcal tonsillitis (034.0)*

Coding Clinic: 1984, Nov-Dec, P16

◀ New   ◀ Revised   ~~deleted~~ Deleted   ● Unacceptable Principal Diagnosis   ● Use Additional Digit(s)
▶ Manifestation Code   OGCR Official Guidelines   **Coding Clinic**   Excludes   Includes   Use additional   Code first   Omit code

Item 8-2   **Laryngitis** is an inflammation of the larynx (voice box) resulting in hoarse voice or the complete loss of the voice. **Tracheitis** is an inflammation of the trachea (often following a URI) commonly caused by *staphylococcus aureus* resulting in inspiratory stridor (crowing sound on inspiration) and a croup like cough.

● **464**   **Acute laryngitis and tracheitis**

   Excludes   *that associated with influenza (487.1)*
                that due to Streptococcus (034.0)

● **464.0**   **Acute laryngitis**
     Laryngitis (acute):
       NOS
       edematous
       Hemophilus influenzae [H. influenzae]
       pneumococcal
       septic
       suppurative
       ulcerative

     Excludes   *chronic laryngitis (476.0–476.1)*
                influenzal laryngitis (487.1)

     464.00   **Without mention of obstruction**
     464.01   **With obstruction** ⬤
         Ⓔ 012.20-012.86, 464.00-464.31, 519.8-519.9

● **464.1**   **Acute tracheitis**
     Tracheitis (acute):   Tracheitis (acute):
       NOS   viral
       catarrhal

     Excludes   *chronic tracheitis (491.8)*

     464.10   **Without mention of obstruction**
     464.11   **With obstruction** ⬤
         Ⓔ 012.20-012.86, 017.90-017.96, 464.10-464.31, 519.8-519.9

● **464.2**   **Acute laryngotracheitis**
     Laryngotracheitis (acute)
     Tracheitis (acute) with laryngitis (acute)

     Excludes   *chronic laryngotracheitis (476.1)*

     464.20   **Without mention of obstruction**
     464.21   **With obstruction** ⬤
         Ⓔ 012.20-012.86, 017.90-017.96, 464.10-464.31, 519.8-519.9

● **464.3**   **Acute epiglottitis**
     Viral epiglottitis

     Excludes   *epiglottitis, chronic (476.1)*

     464.30   **Without mention of obstruction** ⬤
         Ⓔ 464.01, 464.30-464.31, 464.51

     464.31   **With obstruction** ⬤
         Ⓔ 012.20-012.86, 017.90-017.96, 464.10-464.31, 519.8-519.9

   464.4   **Croup**
     Croup syndrome

● **464.5**   **Supraglottitis, unspecified**

     464.50   **Without mention of obstruction**
         Coding Clinic: 2001, Q4, P42-43

     464.51   **With obstruction** ⬤
         Ⓔ 012.20-012.86, 017.90-017.96, 464.00-464.31, 519.8-519.9

● **465**   **Acute upper respiratory infections of multiple or unspecified sites**

   Excludes   *upper respiratory infection due to:*
                 influenza (487.1)
                 Streptococcus (034.0)

   465.0   **Acute laryngopharyngitis**

   465.8   **Other multiple sites**
     Multiple URI
     Coding Clinic: 2007, Q4, P84-86

   465.9   **Unspecified site**
     Acute URI NOS
     Upper respiratory infection (acute)
     Coding Clinic: 1990, Q1, P19

● **466**   **Acute bronchitis and bronchiolitis**

   Includes   that with:
                bronchospasm
                obstruction

   466.0   **Acute bronchitis**
     Inflammation/irritation of bronchial tubes lasting 2-3
       weeks, which is most commonly caused by a virus
     Bronchitis, acute or   Bronchitis, acute or
       subacute: subacute:
       fibrinous   septic
       membranous   viral
       pneumococcal   with tracheitis
       purulent
     Croupous bronchitis
     Tracheobronchitis, acute

     Excludes   *acute bronchitis with chronic obstructive*
                pulmonary disease (491.22)
     Coding Clinic: 2004, Q4, P81-82,137; Q1, P3; 2002, Q4, P46; 1996,
         Q4, P27-28; 1993, 5th Issue, P4x2; 1991, Q3, P17-18; 1988,
         Q1, P12

     OGCR   Section I.C.8.b.1

     Acute bronchitis, 466.0, is due to an infectious organism. When acute bronchitis is documented with COPD, code 491.22, Obstructive chronic bronchitis with acute bronchitis, should be assigned. It is not necessary to also assign code 466.0. If a medical record documents acute bronchitis with COPD with acute exacerbation, only code 491.22 should be assigned. The acute bronchitis included in code 491.22 supersedes the acute exacerbation. If a medical record documents COPD with acute exacerbation without mention of acute bronchitis, only code 491.21 should be assigned.

● **466.1**   **Acute bronchiolitis**
     Bronchiolitis (acute)
     Capillary pneumonia
     Coding Clinic: 1988, Q1, P12

     466.11   **Acute bronchiolitis due to respiratory syncytial virus (RSV)** ⬤
         Ⓔ 466.11
         Coding Clinic: 2005, Q1, P10; 1996, Q4, P27-28

     466.19   **Acute bronchiolitis due to other infectious organisms** ⬤
         Use additional code to identify organism
         Ⓔ 466.0-466.19

DISEASES OF THE RESPIRATORY SYSTEM (460–519)

N   Newborn Age: 0   **P**   Pediatric Age: 0–17   **M**   Maternity Age: 12–55   **A**   Adult Age: 15–124   ♀   Females Only   ♂   Males Only

Ⓔ   CC Exclusions   ⬤   Complication\Comorbidity   ⬤   Major C\C   ⬤   Present on Admission Requirement   ⬤   Hospital-Acquired Condition   **909**

Deviated septal cartilage

Figure 8–3   Deviated nasal septum.

Item 8-3   A deviated nasal septum is the displacement of the septal cartilage that separates the nares. This displacement causes obstructed air flow through the nasal passages. A child can be born with this displacement (congenital), or the condition may be acquired through trauma, such as a sports injury. Symptoms include nasal block, sinusitis, and related secondary infections. Septoplasty is surgical repair of this condition.

Item 8-4   **Nasal polyps** are an abnormal growth of tissue (tumor) projecting from a mucous membrane and attached to the surface by a narrow elongated stalk (pedunculated). Nasal polyps usually originate in the ethmoid sinus but also may occur in the maxillary sinus. Symptoms are nasal block, sinusitis, anosmia, and secondary infections.

OTHER DISEASES OF THE UPPER RESPIRATORY TRACT (470–478)

470   Deviated nasal septum
    Deflected septum (nasal) (acquired)
    Excludes   *congenital (754.0)*

471   Nasal polyps
    Excludes   *adenomatous polyps (212.0)*

    471.0   Polyp of nasal cavity
       Polyp:
         choanal
         nasopharyngeal

    471.1   Polypoid sinus degeneration
       Woakes' syndrome or ethmoiditis

    471.8   Other polyp of sinus
       Polyp of sinus:
         accessory
         ethmoidal
         maxillary
         sphenoidal

    471.9   Unspecified nasal polyp
       Nasal polyp NOS

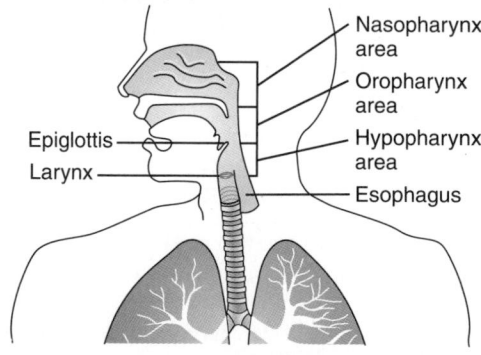

Nasopharynx area
Oropharynx area
Hypopharynx area
Esophagus
Epiglottis
Larynx

Figure 8–4   The pharynx.

Item 8-5   The **pharynx** is the passage for both food and air between the mouth and the esophagus and is divided into three areas: nasopharynx, oropharynx, and hypopharynx. The hypopharynx branches into the esophagus and the voice box.

472   Chronic pharyngitis and nasopharyngitis
    472.0   Chronic rhinitis
       Ozena
       Rhinitis: Rhinitis:
         NOS   obstructive
         atrophic   purulent
         granulomatous   ulcerative
         hypertrophic
       Excludes   *allergic rhinitis (477.0–477.9)*

    472.1   Chronic pharyngitis
       Chronic sore throat
       Pharyngitis: Pharyngitis:
         atrophic   hypertrophic
         granular (chronic)

    472.2   Chronic nasopharyngitis
       Excludes   *acute or unspecified nasopharyngitis (460)*

473   Chronic sinusitis
    Includes   abscess (chronic) of sinus (accessory) (nasal)
              empyema (chronic) of sinus (accessory) (nasal)
              infection (chronic) of sinus (accessory) (nasal)
              suppuration (chronic) of sinus (accessory)
                (nasal)
    Excludes   *acute sinusitis (461.0–461.9)*

    473.0   Maxillary
       Antritis (chronic)

    473.1   Frontal

    473.2   Ethmoidal
       Excludes   *Woakes' ethmoiditis (471.1)*

    473.3   Sphenoidal

    473.8   Other chronic sinusitis
       Pansinusitis (chronic)

    473.9   Unspecified sinusitis (chronic)
       Sinusitis (chronic) NOS

474   Chronic disease of tonsils and adenoids
    474.0   Chronic tonsillitis and adenoiditis
       Excludes   *acute or unspecified tonsillitis (463)*

       474.00   Chronic tonsillitis
           Coding Clinic: 1984, Nov-Dec, P16

       474.01   Chronic adenoiditis

       474.02   Chronic tonsillitis and adenoiditis

    474.1   Hypertrophy of tonsils and adenoids
       Enlargement of tonsils or adenoids
       Hyperplasia of tonsils or adenoids
       Hypertrophy of tonsils or adenoids
       Excludes   *that with:*
           adenoiditis (474.01)
           adenoiditis and tonsillitis (474.02)
           tonsillitis (474.00)

       474.10   Tonsils with adenoids
           Coding Clinic: 2005, Q2, P16

       474.11   Tonsils alone
           Coding Clinic: 1984, Nov-Dec, P16

       474.12   Adenoids alone

    474.2   Adenoid vegetations

    474.8   Other chronic disease of tonsils and adenoids
       Amygdalolith
       Calculus, tonsil
       Cicatrix of tonsil (and adenoid)
       Tonsillar tag
       Ulcer, tonsil

    474.9   Unspecified chronic disease of tonsils and adenoids
       Disease (chronic) of tonsils (and adenoids)

◀ New   ⬅ Revised   ~~deleted~~ Deleted   ● Unacceptable Principal Diagnosis   ● Use Additional Digit(s)

▶ Manifestation Code   **OGCR** Official Guidelines   **Coding Clinic**   Excludes   Includes   Use additional   Code first   Omit code

475 **Peritonsillar abscess**🏷
     Abscess of tonsil
     Peritonsillar cellulitis
     Quinsy
     | **Excludes** | *tonsillitis:*
                acute or NOS (463)
                chronic (474.0)
     (Ex) 475, 519.8-519.9

● 476 **Chronic laryngitis and laryngotracheitis**
     476.0 **Chronic laryngitis**
         Laryngitis: Laryngitis:
           catarrhal   sicca
           hypertrophic
     476.1 **Chronic laryngotracheitis**
         Laryngitis, chronic, with tracheitis (chronic)
         Tracheitis, chronic, with laryngitis
         | **Excludes** | *chronic tracheitis (491.8)*
                       laryngitis and tracheitis, acute or
                          unspecified (464.00–464.51)

● 477 **Allergic rhinitis**
     | **Includes** | allergic rhinitis (nonseasonal) (seasonal)
                hay fever
                spasmodic rhinorrhea
     | **Excludes** | *allergic rhinitis with asthma (bronchial) (493.0)*
     477.0 **Due to pollen**
         Pollinosis
     477.1 **Due to food**
     477.2 **Due to animal (cat) (dog) hair and dander**
     477.8 **Due to other allergen**
     477.9 **Cause unspecified**
         Coding Clinic: 1997, Q2, P9-10

● 478 **Other diseases of upper respiratory tract**
     478.0 **Hypertrophy of nasal turbinates**
  ● 478.1 **Other diseases of nasal cavity and sinuses**
         | **Excludes** | *varicose ulcer of nasal septum (456.8)*
         Coding Clinic: 1995, Q4, P50; 1990, Q1, P8
       478.11 **Nasal mucositis (ulcerative)**
           Use additional E code to identify adverse
              effects of therapy, such as:
              antineoplastic and immunosuppressive
                drugs (E930.7, E933.1)
              radiation therapy (E879.2)
           Coding Clinic: 2006, Q4, P88-91
       478.19 **Other disease of nasal cavity and sinuses**
           Abscess of nose (septum)
           Cyst or mucocele of sinus (nasal)
           Necrosis of nose (septum)
           Rhinolith
           Ulcer of nose (septum)
  ● 478.2 **Other diseases of pharynx, not elsewhere classified**
       478.20 **Unspecified disease of pharynx**
       478.21 **Cellulitis of pharynx or nasopharynx**🏷
           (Ex) 478.20-478.24, 519.8-519.9
       478.22 **Parapharyngeal abscess**🏷
           (Ex) 478.20-478.24, 519.8-519.9
       478.24 **Retropharyngeal abscess**🏷
           (Ex) 478.20-478.24, 519.8-519.9
       478.25 **Edema of pharynx or nasopharynx**
       478.26 **Cyst of pharynx or nasopharynx**
       478.29 **Other**
           Abscess of pharynx or nasopharynx
           | **Excludes** | *ulcerative pharyngitis (462)*

● 478.3 **Paralysis of vocal cords or larynx**
     478.30 **Paralysis, unspecified**
         Laryngoplegia
         Paralysis of glottis
     478.31 **Unilateral, partial**
     478.32 **Unilateral, complete**
     478.33 **Bilateral, partial**
     478.34 **Bilateral, complete**🏷
         (Ex) 478.30-478.34, 478.5, 478.70, 519.8-519.9
     478.4 **Polyp of vocal cord or larynx**
         | **Excludes** | *adenomatous polyps (212.1)*

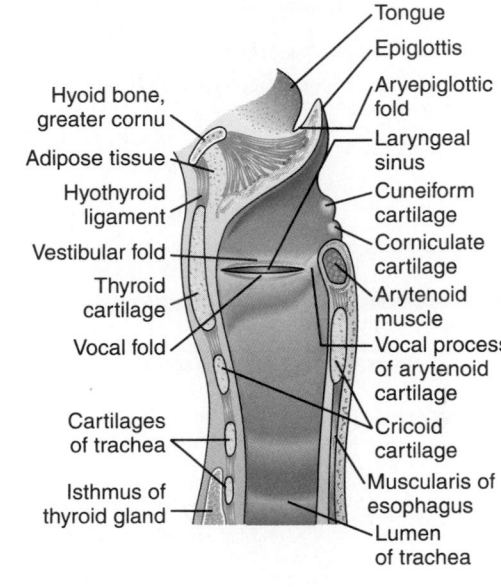

Figure 8–5   Coronal section of the larynx.

Item 8–6 The **larynx** extends from the tongue to the trachea and is divided into an upper and lower portion separated by folds. The framework of the larynx is cartilage composed of the single cricoid, thyroid, and epiglottic cartilages, and the paired arytenoid, cuneiform, and corniculate cartilages.

     478.5 **Other diseases of vocal cords**
         Abscess of vocal cords
         Cellulitis of vocal cords
         Granuloma of vocal cords
         Leukoplakia of vocal cords
         Chorditis (fibrinous) (nodosa) (tuberosa)
         Singers' nodes
     478.6 **Edema of larynx**
         Edema (of):
           glottis
           subglottic
           supraglottic

DISEASES OF THE RESPIRATORY SYSTEM (460–519)

● 478.7   **Other diseases of larynx, not elsewhere classified**

   478.70   **Unspecified disease of larynx**

   478.71   **Cellulitis and perichondritis of larynx**◐
       Ex: 478.70-478.71, 478.79

   478.74   **Stenosis of larynx**

   478.75   **Laryngeal spasm**
       Laryngismus (stridulus)

   478.79   **Other**
       Abscess of larynx
       Necrosis of larynx
       Obstruction of larynx
       Pachyderma of larynx
       Ulcer of larynx

       | Excludes | *ulcerative laryngitis (464.00–464.01)*

       Coding Clinic: 1991, Q3, P20

478.8   **Upper respiratory tract hypersensitivity reaction, site unspecified**

       | Excludes | *hypersensitivity reaction of lower respiratory tract, as:*
          extrinsic allergic alveolitis (495.0–495.9)
          pneumoconiosis (500–505)

478.9   **Other and unspecified diseases of upper respiratory tract**
       Abscess of trachea
       Cicatrix of trachea

PNEUMONIA AND INFLUENZA (480–488)

       | Excludes | *pneumonia:*
          allergic or eosinophilic (518.3)
          aspiration:
             NOS (507.0)
             newborn (770.18)
             solids and liquids (507.0–507.8)
          congenital (770.0)
          lipoid (507.1)
          passive (514)
          rheumatic (390)
          ventilator-associated (997.31)

Item 8-7   Pneumonia is an infection of the lungs, caused by a variety of microorganisms, including viruses, most commonly the *Streptococcus pneumoniae* (pneumococcus) bacteria, fungi, and parasites. Pneumonia occurs when the immune system is weakened, often by a URI or influenza.

● 480   **Viral pneumonia**

   480.0   **Pneumonia due to adenovirus**◐
       Ex: 011.00-012.16, 012.80-012.86, 017.90-017.96, 020.3-020.5, 021.3, 022.1, 031.0, 039.1, 073.0, 115.05, 115.15, 115.95, 122.1, 130.4, 136.3, 480.0-487.1, 488, 495.0-495.9, 500-508.9, 517.1, 517.8, 518.89, 519.8-519.9

   480.1   **Pneumonia due to respiratory syncytial virus**◐
       Ex: 011.00-012.16, 012.80-012.86, 017.90-017.96, 020.3-020.5, 021.3, 022.1, 031.0, 039.1, 073.0, 115.05, 115.15, 115.95, 122.1, 130.4, 136.3, 480.0-487.1, 488, 495.0-495.9, 500-508.9, 517.1, 517.8, 518.89, 519.8-519.9
       Coding Clinic: 1996, Q4, P27-28; 1988, Q1, P12

   480.2   **Pneumonia due to parainfluenza virus**◐
       Ex: 011.00-012.16, 012.80-012.86, 017.90-017.96, 020.3-020.5, 021.3, 022.1, 031.0, 039.1, 073.0, 115.05, 115.15, 115.95, 122.1, 130.4, 136.3, 480.0-487.1, 488, 495.0-495.9, 500-508.9, 517.1, 517.8, 518.89, 519.8-519.9

   480.3   **Pneumonia due to SARS-associated coronavirus**◐
       Ex: 011.00-012.16, 012.80-012.86, 017.90-017.96, 021.2, 031.0, 039.1, 115.05, 115.15, 115.95, 122.1, 130.4, 136.3, 480.0-487.1, 488, 494.0-508.9, 517.1, 517.8, 518.89, 519.8-519.9, 748.61
       Coding Clinic: 2003, Q4, P46-48

   480.8   **Pneumonia due to other virus not elsewhere classified**◐

       | Excludes | *congenital rubella pneumonitis (771.0)*
          influenza with pneumonia, any form (487.0)
          pneumonia complicating viral diseases classified elsewhere (484.1–484.8)
       Ex: 011.00-012.16, 012.80-012.86, 017.90-017.96, 020.3-020.5, 021.3, 022.1, 031.0, 039.1, 073.0, 115.05, 115.15, 115.95, 122.1, 130.4, 136.3, 480.0-487.1, 488, 495.0-495.9, 500-508.9, 517.1, 517.8, 518.89, 519.8-519.9

   480.9   **Viral pneumonia, unspecified**◐
       Ex: 011.00-012.16, 012.80-012.86, 017.90-017.96, 020.3-020.5, 021.3, 022.1, 031.0, 039.1, 073.0, 115.05, 115.15, 115.95, 122.1, 130.4, 136.3, 480.0-487.1, 488, 495.0-495.9, 500-508.9, 517.1, 517.8, 518.89, 519.8-519.9
       Coding Clinic: 1998, Q3, P5

481   **Pneumococcal pneumonia [Streptococcus pneumoniae pneumonia]**◐
       Lobar pneumonia, organism unspecified
       Ex: 011.00-0121.6, 012.80-012.86, 017.90-017.96, 021.2, 031.0, 039.1, 115.05, 115.15, 115.95, 122.1, 130.4, 136.3, 480.0-480.2, 480.8-487.1, 488, 494.0-508.9, 517.1, 517.8, 518.89, 519.8-519.9, 748.61
       Coding Clinic: 1998, Q2, P7; 1991, Q1, P13; 1988, Q1, P13; 1985, Mar-April, P6

● 482   **Other bacterial pneumonia**

   482.0   **Pneumonia due to Klebsiella pneumoniae**◐
       Ex: 011.00-012.16, 012.80-012.86, 017.90-017.96, 021.2, 031.0, 039.1, 115.05, 115.15, 115.95, 122.1, 130.4, 136.3, 480.0-480.2, 480.8-487.1, 488, 494.0-508.9, 517.1, 517.8, 518.89, 519.8-519.9, 748.61

   482.1   **Pneumonia due to Pseudomonas**◐
       Ex: 011.00-012.16, 012.80-012.86, 017.90-017.96, 021.2, 031.0, 039.1, 115.05, 115.15, 115.95, 122.1, 130.4, 136.3, 480.0-480.2, 480.8-487.1, 488, 494.0-508.9, 517.1, 517.8, 518.89, 519.8-519.9, 748.61

   482.2   **Pneumonia due to Hemophilus influenzae [H. influenzae]**◐
       Ex: 011.00-012.16, 012.80-012.86, 017.90-017.96, 021.2, 031.0, 039.1, 115.05, 115.15, 115.95, 122.1, 130.4 136.3, 480.0-480.2, 480.8-487.1, 488, 494.0-508.9, 517.1, 517.8, 518.89, 519.8-519.9, 748.61
       Coding Clinic: 2005, Q2, P19-20; 1993, Q4, P39

● 482.3   **Pneumonia due to Streptococcus**

       | Excludes | *Streptococcus pneumoniae pneumonia (481)*
       Coding Clinic: 1988, Q1, P13

   482.30   **Streptococcus, unspecified**◐
       Ex: 011.00-012.16, 012.80-012.86, 017.90-017.96, 021.2, 031.0, 039.1, 115.05, 115.15, 115.95, 122.1, 130.4, 136.3, 480.0-480.2, 480.8-487.1, 488, 494.0-508.9, 517.1, 517.8, 518.89, 519.8-519.9, 748.61

   482.31   **Group A**◐
       Ex: 011.00-012.16, 012.80-012.86, 017.90-017.96, 021.2, 031.0, 039.1, 115.05, 115.15, 115.95, 122.1, 130.4, 136.3, 480.0-480.2, 480.8-487.1, 488, 494.0-508.9, 517.1, 517.8, 518.89, 519.8-519.9, 748.61

   482.32   **Group B**◐
       Ex: 011.00-012.16, 012.80-012.86, 017.90-017.96, 021.2, 031.0, 039.1, 115.05, 115.15, 115.95, 122.1, 130.4, 136.3, 480.0-480.2, 480.8-487.1, 488, 494.0-508.9, 517.1, 517.8, 518.89, 519.8-519.9, 748.61

DISEASES OF THE RESPIRATORY SYSTEM (460–519)

◀ New   ◀ Revised   ~~deleted~~ Deleted   ● Unacceptable Principal Diagnosis   ● Use Additional Digit(s)

▶ Manifestation Code   OGCR Official Guidelines   Coding Clinic | Excludes | | Includes | Use additional   Code first   Omit code

482.39 Other Streptococcus ⊛
(Ex:) 011.00-012.16, 012.80-012.86, 017.90-017.96, 021.2, 031.0,
039.1, 115.05, 115.15, 115.95, 122.1, 130.4, 136.3,
480.0-480.2, 480.8-487.1, 488, 494.0-508.9, 517.1, 517.8,
518.89, 519.8-519.9, 748.61

● **482.4 Pneumonia due to Staphylococcus**
Coding Clinic: 1991, Q3, P16-17

**482.40 Pneumonia due to Staphylococcus,
unspecified** ⊛
(Ex:) 011.00-012.16, 012.80-012.86, 017.90-017.96, 021.2, 031.0,
039.1, 115.05, 115.15, 115.95, 122.1, 130.4, 136.3,
480.0-480.2, 480.8-487.1, 488, 494.0-508.9, 517.1, 517.8,
518.89, 519.8-519.9, 748.61

**482.41 Methicillin susceptible pneumonia due to
Staphylococcus aureus** ⊛
MSSA pneumonia
Pneumonia due to Staphylococcus aureus
NOS
(Ex:) 011.00-0121.6, 012.80-012.86, 017.90-017.96, 021.2, 031.0,
039.1, 115.05, 115.15, 115.95, 122.1, 130.4, 136.3,
480.0-480.2, 480.8-487.1, 488, 494.0-508.9, 517.1, 517.8,
518.89, 519.8-519.9, 748.61

Coding Clinic: 2008, Q4, P69-73

**482.42 Methicillin resistant pneumonia due to
Staphylococcus aureus** ⊛
(Ex:) 011.00-012.16, 012.80-012.86, 017.90-017.96, 021.2, 031.0,
039.1, 115.05, 115.15, 115.95, 122.1, 130.4, 136.3,
480.0-480.2, 480.8-487.1, 488, 494.0-508.9, 517.1, 517.8,
518.89, 519.8-519.9, 748.61

Coding Clinic: 2008, Q4, P69-73

482.49 Other Staphylococcus pneumonia ⊛
(Ex:) 011.00-012.16, 012.80-012.86, 017.90-017.96, 021.2, 031.0,
039.1, 115.05, 115.15, 115.95, 122.1, 130.4, 136.3,
480.0-480.2, 480.8-487.1, 488, 494.0-508.9, 517.1, 517.8,
518.89, 519.8-519.9, 748.61

● **482.8 Pneumonia due to other specified bacteria**

| **Excludes** | *pneumonia complicating infectious disease
classified elsewhere (484.1–484.8)* |

Coding Clinic: 1988, Q3, P11

482.81 Anaerobes ⊛
Bacteroides (melaninogenicus)
Gram-negative anaerobes
(Ex:) 011.00-012.16, 012.80-012.86, 017.90-017.96, 021.2, 031.0,
039.1, 115.05, 115.16, 115.95, 122.1, 130.4, 136.3,
480.0-480.2, 480.8-487.1, 488, 494.0-508.9, 517.1, 517.8,
518.89, 519.8-519.9, 748.61

482.82 Escherichia coli [E. coli] ⊛
(Ex:) 011.00-012.16, 012.80-012.86, 017.90-017.96, 021.2, 031.0,
039.1, 115.05, 115.15, 115.95, 122.1, 130.4, 136.3,
480.0-480.2, 480.8-487.1, 488, 494.0-508.9, 517.1, 517.8,
518.89, 519.8-519.9, 748.61

482.83 Other gram-negative bacteria ⊛
Gram-negative pneumonia NOS
Proteus
Serratia marcescens

| **Excludes** | *gram-negative anaerobes (482.81)
Legionnaires' disease (482.84)* |

(Ex:) 011.00-012.16, 012.80-012.86, 017.90-017.96, 021.2, 031.0,
039.1, 115.05, 115.15, 115.95, 122.1, 130.4, 136.3,
480.0-480.2, 480.8-487.1, 488, 494.0-508.9, 517.1, 517.8,
518.89, 519.8-519.9, 748.61

Coding Clinic: 1998, Q2, P5; 1994, Q3, P9; 1993, Q4, P39

482.84 Legionnaires' disease ⊛
(Ex:) 011.00-012.16, 012.80-012.86, 017.90-017.96, 021.2, 031.0,
039.1, 115.05, 115.15, 115.95, 122.1, 130.4, 136.3,
480.0-480.2, 480.8-487.1, 488, 494.0-508.9, 517.1, 517.8,
518.89, 519.8-519.9, 748.61

482.89 Other specified bacteria ⊛
(Ex:) 011.00-012.16, 012.80-012.86, 017.90-017.96, 021.2, 031.0,
039.1, 115.05, 115.15, 115.95, 122.1, 130.4, 136.3,
480.0-480.2, 480.8-487.1, 488, 494.0-508.9, 517.1, 517.8,
518.89, 519.8-519.9, 748.61
Coding Clinic: 1998, Q2, P6; 1997, Q2, P6; 1994, Q1,
P17-18

482.9 Bacterial pneumonia unspecified ⊛
(Ex:) 011.00-012.16, 012.80-012.86, 017.90-017.96, 021.2, 031.0, 039.1,
115.05, 115.15, 115.95, 122.1, 130.4, 136.3, 480.0-480.2, 480.8-487.1,
488, 494.0-508.9, 517.1, 517.8, 518.89, 519.8-519.9, 748.61
Coding Clinic: 1998, Q2, P4, 6X2; 1997, Q2, P6; 1994, Q1, P17-18

● **483 Pneumonia due to other specified organism**

483.0 Mycoplasma pneumoniae ⊛
Eaton's agent
Pleuropneumonia-like organisms [PPLO]
(Ex:) 011.00-012.16, 012.80-012.86, 017.90-017.96, 021.2, 031.0, 039.1,
115.05, 115.15, 115.95, 122.1, 130.4, 136.3, 480.0-480.2, 480.8-487.1,
488, 494.0-508.9, 517.1, 517.8, 518.89, 519.8-519.9, 748.61

Coding Clinic: 1987, Nov-Dec, P5-6

483.1 Chlamydia ⊛
(Ex:) 011.00-012.16, 012.80-012.86, 017.90-017.96, 021.2, 031.0, 039.1,
115.05, 115.15, 115.95, 122.1, 130.4, 136.3, 480.0-480.2, 480.8-487.1,
488, 494.0-508.9, 517.1, 517.8, 518.89, 519.8-519.9, 748.61

483.8 Other specified organism ⊛
(Ex:) 011.00-012.16, 012.80-012.86, 017.90-017.96, 021.2, 031.0, 039.1,
115.05, 115.15, 115.95, 122.1, 130.4, 136.3, 480.0-480.2, 480.8-487.1,
488, 494.0-508.9, 517.1, 517.8, 518.89, 519.8-519.9, 748.61

● **484 Pneumonia in infectious diseases classified elsewhere**

| **Excludes** | *influenza with pneumonia, any form (487.0)* |

▶ **484.1 Pneumonia in cytomegalic inclusion disease** ⊛
Code first underlying disease, as: (078.5)
(Ex:) 011.00-012.16, 012.80-012.86, 017.90-017.96, 021.2, 031.0, 039.1,
115.05, 115.15, 115.95, 122.1, 130.4, 136.3, 480.0-480.2, 480.8-487.1,
488, 494.0-508.9, 517.1, 517.8, 518.89, 519.8-519.9, 748.61

▶ **484.3 Pneumonia in whooping cough** ⊛
Code first underlying disease, as: (033.0–033.9)
(Ex:) 011.00-012.16, 012.80-012.86, 017.90-017.96, 021.2, 031.0, 039.1,
115.05, 115.15, 115.95, 122.1, 130.4, 136.3, 480.0-480.2, 480.8-487.1,
488, 494.0-508.9, 517.1, 517.8, 518.89, 519.8-519.9, 748.61

▶ **484.5 Pneumonia in anthrax** ⊛
Code first underlying disease (022.1)
(Ex:) 011.00-012.16, 012.80-012.86, 017.90-017.96, 021.2, 031.0, 039.1,
115.05, 115.15, 115.95, 122.1, 130.4, 136.3, 480.0-480.2, 480.8-487.1,
488, 494.0-508.9, 517.1, 517.8, 518.89, 519.8-519.9, 748.61

▶ **484.6 Pneumonia in aspergillosis** ⊛
Code first underlying disease (117.3)
(Ex:) 011.00-012.16, 012.80-012.86, 017.90-017.96, 021.2, 031.0, 039.1,
115.05, 115.15, 115.95, 122.1, 130.4, 136.3, 480.0-480.2, 480.8-487.1,
488, 494.0-508.9, 517.1, 517.8, 518.89, 519.8-519.9, 748.61
Coding Clinic: 1997, Q4, P40

▶ **484.7 Pneumonia in other systemic mycoses** ⊛
Code first underlying disease

| **Excludes** | *pneumonia in:
   candidiasis (112.4)
   coccidioidomycosis (114.0)
   histoplasmosis (115.0–115.9 with
     fifth-digit 5)* |

(Ex:) 011.00-012.16, 012.80-012.86, 017.90-017.96, 021.2, 031.0, 039.1,
115.05, 115.15, 115.95, 122.1, 130.4, 136.3, 480.0-480.2, 480.8-487.1,
488, 494.0-508.9, 517.1, 517.8, 518.89, 519.8-519.9, 748.61

DISEASES OF THE RESPIRATORY SYSTEM (460–519)

▶ **484.8 Pneumonia in other infectious diseases classified elsewhere** 🔒

Code first underlying disease, as:
Q fever (083.0)
typhoid fever (002.0)

Excludes pneumonia in:
actinomycosis (039.1)
measles (055.1)
nocardiosis (039.1)
ornithosis (073.0)
Pneumocystis carinii (136.3)
salmonellosis (003.22)
toxoplasmosis (130.4)
tuberculosis (011.6)
tularemia (021.2)
varicella (052.1)

Ex: 011.00-012.16, 012.80-012.86, 017.90-017.96, 021.2, 031.0, 039.1, 115.05, 115.15, 115.95, 122.1, 130.4, 136.3, 480.0-480.2, 480.8-487.1, 488, 494.0-508.9, 517.1, 517.8, 518.89, 519.8-519.9, 748.61

485 Bronchopneumonia, organism unspecified 🔒

Bronchopneumonia:
hemorrhagic
terminal
Pleurobronchopneumonia

Pneumonia:
lobular
segmental

Excludes bronchiolitis (acute) (466.11–466.19)
chronic (491.8)
lipoid pneumonia (507.1)

Ex: 011.00-012.16, 012.80-012.86, 017.90-017.96, 021.2, 031.0, 039.1, 115.05, 115.15, 115.95, 122.1, 130.4, 136.3, 480.0-480.2, 480.8-487.1, 488, 494.0-508.9, 517.1, 517.8, 518.89, 519.8-519.9, 748.61

486 Pneumonia, organism unspecified 🔒

Excludes hypostatic or passive pneumonia (514)
influenza with pneumonia, any form (487.0)
inhalation or aspiration pneumonia due to foreign materials (507.0–507.8)
pneumonitis due to fumes and vapors (506.0)

Ex: 011.00-012.16, 012.80-012.86, 017.90-017.96, 021.2, 031.0, 039.1, 115.05, 115.15, 115.95, 122.1, 130.4, 136.3, 480.0-480.2, 480.8-487.1, 488, 494.0-508.9, 517.1, 517.8, 518.89, 519.8-519.9, 748.61

Coding Clinic: 2008, Q4, P140-143; 2006, Q2, P20; 1999, Q4, P6; Q3, P9; 1998, Q3, P7; Q2, P4-5; Q1, P8; 1997, Q3, P9; 1995, Q4, P52; 1994, Q1, P17-18; 1993, Q3, P9; Q1, P21; 1985, Mar-April, P6

● **487 Influenza**

Influenza caused by unspecified virus ◀

Excludes Hemophilus influenzae [H. influenzae]:
infection NOS (041.5)
laryngitis (464.00–464.01)
meningitis (320.0)
influenza due to 2009 H1N1 [swine] influenza virus (488.1) ◀
influenza due to identified avian influenza virus (488.0) ◀▥
influenza due to identified novel H1N1 influenza (488.1) ◀

487.0 With pneumonia 🔒
Influenza with pneumonia, any form
Influenzal:
bronchopneumonia
pneumonia

Use additional code to identify the type of pneumonia (480.0–480.9, 481, 482.0–482.9, 483.0–483.8, 485)

Ex: 011.00-012.16, 012.80-012.86, 017.90-017.96, 021.2, 031.0, 039.1, 115.05, 115.15, 115.95, 122.1, 130.4, 136.3, 480.0-480.2, 480.8-487.1, 488, 494.0-508.9, 517.1, 517.8, 519.8-519.9, 748.61

Coding Clinic: 2005, Q2, P18-19

487.1 With other respiratory manifestations
Influenza NOS
Influenzal:
laryngitis
pharyngitis
respiratory infection (upper) (acute)

Coding Clinic: 2005, Q2, P18-19; 1999, Q4, P26; 1987, Jan-Feb, P16

487.8 With other manifestations
Encephalopathy due to influenza
Influenza with involvement of gastrointestinal tract

Excludes "intestinal flu" [viral gastroenteritis] (008.8)

● **488 Influenza due to certain identified ~~avian~~ influenza viruses** ◀▥

~~Note: Influenza caused by influenza viruses that normally infect only birds and, less commonly, other animals~~

Excludes influenza caused by ~~other~~ unspecified influenza viruses (487.0–487.8) ◀▥

Coding Clinic: 2007, Q4, P87-88

488.0 Influenza due to identified avian influenza virus ◀
Avian influenza ◀
Bird flu ◀
Influenza A/H5N1 ◀

488.1 Influenza due to identified novel H1N1 influenza virus ◀
2009 H1N1 [swine] influenza virus ◀
Novel 2009 influenza H1N1 ◀
Novel H1N1 influenza ◀
Novel influenza A/H1N1 ◀
Swine flu

Item 8–8   Chronic bronchitis is usually defined as being present in any patient who has persistent cough with sputum production for at least three months in at least two consecutive years. **Simple chronic bronchitis** is marked by a productive cough but no pathological airflow obstruction. **Chronic obstructive pulmonary disease (COPD)** is a group of conditions—bronchitis, emphysema, asthma, bronchiectasis, allergic alveolitis—marked by dyspnea. **Catarrhal** bronchitis is an acute form of bronchitis marked by profuse mucus and pus production (**mucopurulent** discharge). **Croupous** bronchitis, also known as pseudomembranous, fibrinous, plastic, exudative, or membranous, is marked by a violent cough and dyspnea.

CHRONIC OBSTRUCTIVE PULMONARY DISEASE AND ALLIED CONDITIONS (490–496)

490 Bronchitis, not specified as acute or chronic
Bronchitis NOS:
catarrhal
Tracheobronchitis NOS

Bronchitis NOS:
with tracheitis NOS

Excludes bronchitis:
allergic NOS (493.9)
asthmatic NOS (493.9)
due to fumes and vapors (506.0)

● **491 Chronic bronchitis**

Excludes chronic obstructive asthma (493.2)

491.0 Simple chronic bronchitis
Catarrhal bronchitis, chronic
Smokers' cough

491.1 Mucopurulent chronic bronchitis
Bronchitis (chronic) (recurrent):
fetid   purulent
mucopurulent

Coding Clinic: 1988, Q2, P11

◀ New   ◀▥ Revised   ~~deleted~~ Deleted   ● Unacceptable Principal Diagnosis   ● Use Additional Digit(s)
▶ Manifestation Code   OGCR Official Guidelines   Coding Clinic   Excludes   Includes   Use additional   Code first   Omit code

● **491.2 Obstructive chronic bronchitis**
Bronchitis:
  emphysematous
  obstructive (chronic) (diffuse)
Bronchitis with:
  chronic airway obstruction
  emphysema

| **Excludes** | *asthmatic bronchitis (acute) (NOS) 493.9* |
| | *chronic obstructive asthma 493.2* |

Coding Clinic: 2004, Q4, P81-82; 2002, Q3, P18, 19x2; 1991, Q2, P21; 1984, Nov-Dec, P17

491.20 Without exacerbation
Emphysema with chronic bronchitis
Coding Clinic: 1997, Q3, P9

491.21 With (acute) exacerbation 🅒
Acute exacerbation of chronic obstructive
  pulmonary disease [COPD]
Decompensated chronic obstructive
  pulmonary disease [COPD]
Decompensated chronic obstructive
  pulmonary disease [COPD] with
  exacerbation

| **Excludes** | *chronic obstructive asthma with* |
| | *acute exacerbation 493.22* |

(Ex) 491.1-491.9, 493.20-493.21
Coding Clinic: 2004, Q1, P3; 1996, Q2, P10; 1993, 5th
    Issue, P5x2

491.22 With acute bronchitis 🅒
(Ex) 491.1-491.9, 493.20-493.21
Coding Clinic: 2006, Q3, P20; 2004, Q4, P80-81; Q1, P3
OGCR Section I.C.8.b.1
  When acute bronchitis, 466.0, is
  documented with COPD, code 491.22
  should be assigned. It is not necessary to
  also assign code 466.0. If a medical record
  documents acute bronchitis with COPD
  with acute exacerbation, only code 491.22
  should be assigned. The acute bronchitis
  included in code 491.22 supersedes the
  acute exacerbation. If a medical record
  documents COPD with acute exacerbation
  without mention of acute bronchitis, only
  code 491.21 should be assigned.

491.8 Other chronic bronchitis
Chronic: Chronic:
  tracheitis   tracheobronchitis

491.9 Unspecified chronic bronchitis
Coding Clinic: 1991, Q3, P17-18

● **492 Emphysema**
Coding Clinic: 1991, Q2, P21; 1984, Nov-Dec, P19

492.0 Emphysematous bleb
Giant bullous emphysema
Ruptured emphysematous bleb
Tension pneumatocele
Vanishing lung

492.8 Other emphysema

Emphysema (lung or	Emphysema (lung or
pulmonary):	pulmonary):
NOS	panacinar
centriacinar	panlobular
centrilobular	unilateral
obstructive	vesicular

MacLeod's syndrome
Swyer-James syndrome
Unilateral hyperlucent lung

Excludes	*emphysema:*
	with chronic bronchitis 491.20–491.22)
	compensatory (518.2)
	due to fumes and vapors (506.4)
	interstitial (518.1)
	newborn (770.2)
	mediastinal (518.1)
	surgical (subcutaneous) (998.81)
	traumatic (958.7)

Coding Clinic: 2008, Q4, P174-175; 1993, Q4, P41; 5th Issue, P4

● **493 Asthma**

| **Excludes** | *wheezing NOS (786.07)* |

Coding Clinic: 2003, Q4, P62, 137; 1991, Q1, P13; 1985, July-Aug, P8

The following fifth-digit subclassification is for use with
category 493.0–493.2, 493.9:

0	unspecified
1	with status asthmaticus
2	with (acute) exacerbation

● **493.0 Extrinsic asthma 1-2** 🅒
[0-2]   Asthma:
      allergic with stated cause
      atopic
      childhood
      hay
      platinum
  Hay fever with asthma

Excludes	*asthma:*
	allergic NOS (493.9)
	detergent (507.8)
	miners' (500)
	wood (495.8)

For codes 493.01-493.02: (Ex) 493.00-493.92, 517.8, 518.89, 519.8-519.9
Coding Clinic: 1990, Q2, P20

Item 8–9 Asthma is a bronchial condition marked by airway
obstruction, hyper-responsiveness, and inflammation. **Extrinsic**
asthma, also known as allergic asthma, is characterized by the
same symptoms that occur with exposure to allergens and is
divided into the following types: **atopic, occupational, and
allergic bronchopulmonary aspergillosis. Intrinsic**
asthma occurs in patients who have no history of allergy or
sensitivities to allergens and is divided into the following types:
nonreaginic and pharmacologic. Status asthmaticus
is the most severe form of asthma attack and can last for days
or weeks.

DISEASES OF THE RESPIRATORY SYSTEM (460–519)

DISEASES OF THE RESPIRATORY SYSTEM (460–519)

● **493.1 Intrinsic asthma 1-2** 🚫
[0-2]   Late-onset asthma
For codes **493.11-493.12**: (Ex:) 493.00-493.92, 517.8, 518.89, 519.8-519.9
Coding Clinic: 1990, Q2, P20

● **493.2 Chronic obstructive asthma 1-2** 🚫
[0-2]   Asthma with chronic obstructive pulmonary
disease [COPD]
Chronic asthmatic bronchitis

> **Excludes** *acute bronchitis (466.0)*
> *chronic obstructive bronchitis*
> *(491.20–491.22)*

For code **493.21**: (Ex:) 491.1-493.92, 517.8, 518.89, 519.8-519.9;
For code **493.22**: (Ex:) 493.00-493.92, 517.8, 518.89, 519.8-519.9
**Coding Clinic: 2009, Q1, P16; 2006, Q3, P20; 2003, Q4, P108; 1993,
5th Issue, P4; 1991, Q2, P21; 1990, Q2, P20**

● **493.8 Other forms of asthma**

493.81 Exercise induced bronchospasm
Coding Clinic: 2003, Q4, P62

493.82 Cough variant asthma
Coding Clinic: 2003, Q4, P62

● **493.9 Asthma, unspecified 1-2** 🚫
[0-2]   Asthma (bronchial) (allergic NOS)
Bronchitis:
  allergic
  asthmatic
For codes **493.91-493.92**: (Ex:) 493.00-493.92, 517.8, 518.89, 519.8-519.9
**Coding Clinic: 2004, Q4, P137; 2003, Q4, P108-109; Q1, P9; 1999,
Q4, P25; 1997, Q4, P39-40; Q1, P7; 1996, Q3, P20; 1993,
Q4, P32; 1992, Q1, P15; 1990, Q2, P20; 1984, Nov-Dec, P17**

● **494 Bronchiectasis**
Bronchiectasis (fusiform) (postinfectious) (recurrent)
Bronchiolectasis

> **Excludes** *congenital (748.61)*
> *tuberculous bronchiectasis (current disease) (011.5)*

494.0 Bronchiectasis without acute exacerbation

494.1 Bronchiectasis with acute exacerbation 🚫
(Ex:) 017.90-017.96, 487.1, 488, 494.1, 496, 506.1, 506.4-506.9, 748.61

● **495 Extrinsic allergic alveolitis**

> **Includes** allergic alveolitis and pneumonitis due to
> inhaled organic dust particles of fungal,
> thermophilic actinomycete, or other
> origin

495.0 Farmers' lung

495.1 Bagassosis

495.2 Bird-fanciers' lung
Budgerigar-fanciers' disease or lung
Pigeon-fanciers' disease or lung

495.3 Suberosis
Cork-handlers' disease or lung

495.4 Malt workers' lung
Alveolitis due to Aspergillus clavatus

495.5 Mushroom workers' lung

495.6 Maple bark-strippers' lung
Alveolitis due to Cryptostroma corticale

495.7 "Ventilation" pneumonitis 🚫
Allergic alveolitis due to fungal, thermophilic
actinomycete, and other organisms growing
in ventilation [air conditioning] systems
(Ex:) 011.00-012.16, 012.80-012.86, 017.90-017.96, 021.2, 031.0, 039.1,
115.05, 115.15, 115.95, 122.1, 130.4, 136.3, 480.0-480.2, 480.8-487.1,
488, 494.0-508.9, 517.1, 517.8, 518.89, 519.8-519.9, 748.61

495.8 Other specified allergic alveolitis and pneumonitis 🚫
Cheese-washers' lung
Coffee workers' lung
Fish-meal workers' lung
Furriers' lung
Grain-handlers' disease or lung
Pituitary snuff-takers' disease
Sequoiosis or red-cedar asthma
Wood asthma
(Ex:) 011.00-012.16, 012.80-012.86, 017.90-017.96, 021.2, 031.0, 039.1,
115.05, 115.15, 115.95, 122.1, 130.4, 136.3, 480.0-480.2, 480.8-487.1,
488, 494.0-508.9, 517.1, 517.8, 518.89, 519.8-519.9, 748.61

495.9 Unspecified allergic alveolitis and pneumonitis 🚫
Alveolitis, allergic (extrinsic)
Hypersensitivity pneumonitis
(Ex:) 011.00-012.16, 012.80-012.86, 017.90-017.96, 021.2, 031.0, 039.1,
115.05, 115.15, 115.95, 122.1, 130.4, 136.3, 480.0-480.2, 480.8-487.1,
488, 494.0-508.9, 517.1, 517.8, 518.89, 519.8-519.9, 748.61

496 Chronic airway obstruction, not elsewhere classified
Chronic:
  nonspecific lung disease
  obstructive lung disease
  obstructive pulmonary disease [COPD] NOS

> **Note:** This code is not to be used with any code from
> categories 491–493.

> **Excludes** *chronic obstructive lung disease [COPD] specified*
> *(as) (with):*
> *allergic alveolitis (495.0–495.9)*
> *asthma (493.2)*
> *bronchiectasis (494.0–494.1)*
> *bronchitis (491.20–491.22)*
> *with emphysema (491.20–491.22)*
> *decompensated (491.21)*
> *emphysema (492.0–492.8)*

**Coding Clinic: 2009, Q1, P16; 2006, Q3, P20; 2003, Q4, P109-110; 2000, Q2,
P15; 1994, Q1, P19; 1993, Q4, P 43; 1992, Q2, P16-17; 1991, Q2,
P21; 1988, Q2, P12**

OGCR Section I.C.8.a.2

> Code 496 is a nonspecific code that should only be used
> when the documentation in a medical record does not
> specify the type of COPD being treated.

◀ New   ⬅ Revised   ~~deleted~~ Deleted   ● Unacceptable Principal Diagnosis   ● Use Additional Digit(s)
▶ Manifestation Code   **OGCR** Official Guidelines   **Coding Clinic**   Excludes   Includes   Use additional   Code first   Omit code

Figure 8–6 Progressive massive fibrosis superimposed on coal workers' pneumoconiosis. The large, blackened scars are located principally in the upper lobe. (From Cotran R, Kumar V, Collins T: Robbins Pathologic Basis of Disease, 6th ed. Philadelphia, WB Saunders, 1999, p 730. Courtesy of Dr. Warner Laquer, Dr. Jerome Kleinerman, and the National Institute of Occupational Safety and Health, Morgantown, WV.)

Item 8–10 Pneumoconiosis refers to a lung condition resulting from exposure to inorganic or organic airborne particles, such as coal dust or moldy hay, as well as chemical fumes and vapors, such as insecticides. In this condition, the lungs retain the airborne particles.

PNEUMOCONIOSES AND OTHER LUNG DISEASES DUE TO EXTERNAL AGENTS (500–508)

500 Coal workers' pneumoconiosis A
  Anthracosilicosis   Coal workers' lung
  Anthracosis   Miners' asthma
  Black lung disease

501 Asbestosis A

502 Pneumoconiosis due to other silica or silicates
  Pneumoconiosis due to talc
  Silicotic fibrosis (massive) of lung
  Silicosis (simple) (complicated)

503 Pneumoconiosis due to other inorganic dust
  Aluminosis (of lung)
  Bauxite fibrosis (of lung)
  Berylliosis
  Graphite fibrosis (of lung)
  Siderosis
  Stannosis

504 Pneumonopathy due to inhalation of other dust
  Byssinosis
  Cannabinosis
  Flax-dressers' disease

Excludes	*allergic alveolitis (495.0–495.9)*
	asbestosis (501)
	bagassosis (495.1)
	farmers' lung (495.0)

505 Pneumoconiosis, unspecified

● **506 Respiratory conditions due to chemical fumes and vapors**
  Use additional E code to identify cause

  506.0 Bronchitis and pneumonitis due to fumes and vapors 🗝
    Chemical bronchitis (acute)
    (Ex) 011.00-012.16, 012.80-012.86, 017.90-017.96, 021.2, 031.0, 039.1, 115.05, 115.15, 115.95, 122.1, 130.4, 136.3, 480.0-480.2, 480.8-487.1, 488, 494.0-508.9, 517.1, 517.8, 518.89, 519.8-519.9, 748.61
    Coding Clinic: 2008, Q3, P6-7

506.1 Acute pulmonary edema due to fumes and vapors 🗝
  Chemical pulmonary edema (acute)

  | Excludes | *acute pulmonary edema NOS (518.4)* |
  | | *chronic or unspecified pulmonary edema (514)* |

  (Ex) 011.00-012.16, 012.80-012.86, 017.90-017.96, 021.2, 031.0, 039.1, 115.05, 115.15, 115.95, 122.1, 130.4, 136.3, 480.0-480.2, 480.8-487.1, 488, 494.0-508.9, 517.1, 517.8, 518.89, 519.8-519.9, 748.61

506.2 Upper respiratory inflammation due to fumes and vapors
  Coding Clinic: 2005, Q3, P10

506.3 Other acute and subacute respiratory conditions due to fumes and vapors

506.4 Chronic respiratory conditions due to fumes and vapors
  Emphysema (diffuse) (chronic) due to inhalation of chemical fumes and vapors
  Obliterative bronchiolitis (chronic) (subacute) due to inhalation of chemical fumes and vapors
  Pulmonary fibrosis (chronic) due to inhalation of chemical fumes and vapors

506.9 Unspecified respiratory conditions due to fumes and vapors
  Silo-fillers' disease

● **507 Pneumonitis due to solids and liquids**

  | Excludes | *fetal aspiration pneumonitis (770.18)* |

  Coding Clinic: 1993, Q2, P9-10

  507.0 Due to inhalation of food or vomitus 🗝
    Aspiration pneumonia (due to):
    NOS   milk
    food (regurgitated)   saliva
    gastric secretions   vomitus
    (Ex) 011.00-012.16, 012.80-012.86, 017.90-017.96, 021.2, 031.0, 039.1 115.05, 115.15, 115.95, 122.1, 130.4 136.3, 480.0-480.2, 480.8-487.1, 488, 494.0-508.9, 517.1, 517.8, 518.89, 519.8-519.9, 748.61
    Coding Clinic: 2008, Q1, P18-19; Q1, P18-19; 1991, Q3, P16-17; 1989, Q1, P10

  507.1 Due to inhalation of oils and essences 🗝
    Lipoid pneumonia (exogenous)

    | Excludes | *endogenous lipoid pneumonia (516.8)* |

    (Ex) 011.00-012.16, 012.80-012.86, 017.90-017.96, 021.2, 031.0, 039.1 115.05, 115.15, 115.95, 122.1, 130.4, 136.3, 480.0-480.2, 480.8-487.1, 488, 494.0-508.9, 517.1, 517.8, 518.89, 519.8-519.9, 748.61
    Coding Clinic: 1991, Q3, P16-17

  507.8 Due to other solids and liquids 🗝
    Detergent asthma
    (Ex) 011.00-012.16, 012.80-012.86, 017.90-017.96, 021.2, 031.0, 039.1, 115.05, 115.15, 115.95, 122.1, 130.4, 136.3, 480.0-480.2, 480.8-487.1, 488, 494.0-508.9, 517.1, 517.8, 518.89, 519.8-519.9, 748.61
    Coding Clinic: 1991, Q3, P16-17

● **508 Respiratory conditions due to other and unspecified external agents**

> Use additional E code to identify cause

508.0 Acute pulmonary manifestations due to radiation 🔍
Radiation pneumonitis
(Ex:) 011.00-012.16, 012.80-0128.6, 017.90-017.96, 021.2, 031.0, 039.1, 115.05, 115.15, 115.95, 122.1, 130.4, 136.3, 480.0-480.2, 480.8-487.1, 488, 494.0-508.9, 517.1, 517.8, 518.89, 519.8-519.9, 748.61

508.1 Chronic and other pulmonary manifestations due to radiation 🔍
Fibrosis of lung following radiation
(Ex:) 011.00-012.16, 012.80-012.86, 017.90-017.96, 021.2, 031.0, 039.1, 115.05, 115.15, 115.95, 122.1, 130.4, 136.3, 480.0-480.2, 480.8-487.1, 488, 494.0-508.9, 517.1, 517.8, 518.89, 519.8-519.9, 748.61

508.8 Respiratory conditions due to other specified external agents

508.9 Respiratory conditions due to unspecified external agent

Figure 8–7 Bullous emphysema with large subpleural bullae *(upper left)*. (From Kumar: Robbins and Cotran: Pathologic Basis of Disease, 7th ed. 2005, Saunders, An Imprint of Elsevier)

Item 8–11 Empyema is a condition in which pus accumulates in a body cavity. Empyema **with fistula** occurs when the pus passes from one cavity to another organ or structure.

OTHER DISEASES OF RESPIRATORY SYSTEM (510–519)

● **510 Empyema**

> Use additional code to identify infectious organism (041.0–041.9)

> **Excludes** *abscess of lung (513.0)*

510.0 With fistula 🔍
Fistula:
  bronchocutaneous
  bronchopleural
  hepatopleural
  mediastinal
  pleural
  thoracic
Any condition classifiable to 510.9 with fistula
(Ex:) 510.0-510.9, 517.8, 518.89, 519.8-519.9

510.9 Without mention of fistula 🔍
Abscess:
  pleura
  thorax
Empyema (chest) (lung) (pleura)
Fibrinopurulent pleurisy
Pleurisy:
  purulent
  septic
  seropurulent
  suppurative
Pyopneumothorax
Pyothorax
(Ex:) 510.0-510.9, 517.8, 518.89, 519.8-519.9
Coding Clinic: 2007, Q4, P109-113; 1994, Q3, P6

● **511 Pleurisy**
Occurs when double membrane (pleura) lining chest cavity and lung surface becomes inflamed causing sharp pain on inspiration and expiration.

> **Excludes** *pleurisy with mention of tuberculosis, current disease (012.0)*

511.0 Without mention of effusion or current tuberculosis
Adhesion, lung or pleura
Calcification of pleura
Pleurisy (acute) (sterile):
  diaphragmatic
  fibrinous
  interlobar
Pleurisy:
  NOS
  pneumococcal
  staphylococcal
  streptococcal
Thickening of pleura
Coding Clinic: 1994, Q3, P5

511.1 With effusion, with mention of a bacterial cause other than tuberculosis 🔍
Pleurisy with effusion (exudative) (serous):
  pneumococcal
  staphylococcal
  streptococcal
  other specified nontuberculous bacterial cause
(Ex:) 011.00-012.16, 012.80-012.86, 017.90-017.96, 511.0-511.9, 517.8, 518.89, 519.8-519.9

● **511.8 Other specified forms of effusion, except tuberculous**

> **Excludes** *traumatic (860.2–860.5, 862.29, 862.39)*

Coding Clinic: 2008, Q1, P16-17; 1997, Q1, P10

511.81 Malignant pleural effusion 🔍

> *Code first malignant neoplasm, if known*

(Ex:) 195.8, 197.2-197.3, 198.89-199.2, 209.20, 209.29-209.30, 239.8-239.9, 511.81-511.89
Coding Clinic: 2008, Q4, P113-114

511.89 Other specified forms of effusion, except tuberculous 🔍
Encysted pleurisy
Hemopneumothorax
Hemothorax
Hydropneumothorax
Hydrothorax
(Ex:) 011.00-012.16, 012.80-012.86, 017.90-017.96, 511.0-511.9, 517.8, 518.89, 519.8-519.9

511.9 Unspecified pleural effusion 🔍
Pleural effusion NOS
Pleurisy:
  exudative
  serofibrinous
  serous
  with effusion NOS
(Ex:) 011.00-012.16, 012.80-012.86, 017.90-017.96, 511.0-511.9, 517.8, 518.89, 519.8-519.9
Coding Clinic: 2003, Q2, P7-8; 1991, Q3, P19-20; 1989, Q4, P11; 1988, Q1, P9

● **512 Pneumothorax**
Collapsed lung

512.0 Spontaneous tension pneumothorax 🔍
Tension pneumothorax (most serious type) occurs when air (positive pressure) collects in the pleural space
(Ex:) 512.0-512.8, 517.8, 518.89, 519.8-519.9

512.1 Iatrogenic pneumothorax 🔍
Postoperative pneumothorax
(Ex:) 512.0-512.8, 517.8, 518.89, 519.8-519.9
Coding Clinic: 2003, Q3, P19

◀ New   ◀▦ Revised   ~~deleted~~ Deleted   ● Unacceptable Principal Diagnosis   🔍 Use Additional Digit(s)
▶ Manifestation Code   OGCR Official Guidelines   Coding Clinic Coding Clinic   Excludes Excludes   Includes Includes   Use additional Use additional   Code first Code first   Omit code Omit code

512.8 Other spontaneous pneumothorax🍡

    Pneumothorax: Pneumothorax:
      NOS   chronic
      acute

> **Excludes** *pneumothorax:*
>   *congenital (770.2)*
>   *traumatic (860.0–860.1, 860.4–860.5)*
>   *tuberculous, current disease (011.7)*

   (Ex:) 512.0-512.8, 517.8, 518.89, 519.8-519.9
   Coding Clinic: 1993, Q2, P3

● **513 Abscess of lung and mediastinum**

513.0 Abscess of lung🍡

    Abscess (multiple) of lung
    Gangrenous or necrotic pneumonia
    Pulmonary gangrene or necrosis
   (Ex:) 006.4, 011.00-012.16, 012.80-012.86, 017.90-017.96, 513.0, 519.8-519.9
   Coding Clinic: 2007, Q4, P84-86; 2005, Q2, P14-15; 1998, Q2, P7

513.1 Abscess of mediastinum🍡
   (Ex:) 513.1, 519.8-519.9,

514 Pulmonary congestion and hypostasis🍡

    Hypostatic:
      bronchopneumonia
      pneumonia
    Passive pneumonia
    Pulmonary congestion (chronic) (passive)
    Pulmonary edema:
      NOS
      chronic

> **Excludes** *acute pulmonary edema:*
>   *NOS (518.4)*
>   *with mention of heart disease or failure (428.1)*
>   *hypostatic pneumonia due to or specified as a*
>   *specific type of pneumonia - code to the*
>   *type of pneumonia (480.0–480.9, 481,*
>   *482.0–482.9, 483.0–483.8, 485, 486, 487.0)*

   (Ex:) 514, 517.8, 518.89, 519.8-519.9
   Coding Clinic: 1998, Q2, P6-7

515 Postinflammatory pulmonary fibrosis

    Cirrhosis of lung chronic or unspecified
    Fibrosis of lung (atrophic) (confluent) (massive)
      (perialveolar) (peribronchial) chronic or unspecified
    Induration of lung chronic or unspecified

● **516 Other alveolar and parietoalveolar pneumonopathy**

516.0 Pulmonary alveolar proteinosis🍡
   (Ex:) 011.00-012.16, 012.80-012.86, 017.90-017.96, 494.0-508.9, 515-516.9,
      517.2, 517.8, 518.89, 519.8-519.9, 748.61

▶ **516.1 *Idiopathic pulmonary hemosiderosis***🍡
    Essential brown induration of lung
    Code first underlying disease (275.0)
   (Ex:) 011.00-012.16, 012.80-012.86, 017.90-017.96, 494.0-508.9, 515-516.9,
      517.2, 517.8, 518.89, 519.8-519.9, 748.61

516.2 Pulmonary alveolar microlithiasis🍡
   (Ex:) 011.00-012.16, 012.80-012.86, 017.90-017.96, 494.0-508.9, 515-516.9,
      517.2, 517.8, 518.89, 519.8-519.9, 748.61

516.3 Idiopathic fibrosing alveolitis🍡
    Alveolar capillary block
    Diffuse (idiopathic) (interstitial) pulmonary
      fibrosis
    Hamman-Rich syndrome
   (Ex:) 011.00-012.16, 012.80-012.86, 017.90-017.96, 494.0-508.9, 515-516.9,
      517.2, 517.8, 518.89, 519.8-519.9, 748.61

516.8 Other specified alveolar and parietoalveolar pneumonopathies🍡
    Endogenous lipoid pneumonia
    Interstitial pneumonia (desquamative) (lymphoid)

> **Excludes** *lipoid pneumonia, exogenous or unspecified*
>   *(507.1)*

   (Ex:) 011.00-012.16, 012.80-012.86, 017.90-017.96, 494.0-508.9, 515-516.9,
      517.2, 517.8, 518.89, 519.8-519.9, 748.61
   Coding Clinic: 2006, Q2, P20; 1992, Q1, P12

516.9 Unspecified alveolar and parietoalveolar pneumonopathy🍡
   (Ex:) 011.00-012.16, 012.80-012.86, 017.90-017.96, 494.0-508.9, 515-516.9,
      517.2, 517.8, 518.89, 519.8-519.9, 748.61

● **517 Lung involvement in conditions classified elsewhere**

> **Excludes** *rheumatoid lung (714.81)*

▶ **517.1 *Rheumatic pneumonia***🍡
    Code first underlying disease (390)
   (Ex:) 011.00-012.16, 012.80-012.86, 017.90-017.96, 480.0-480.2, 480.8-487.1,
      488, 494.0-508.9, 515-517.2, 517.8, 518.89, 519.8-519.9, 748.61

▶ **517.2 *Lung involvement in systemic sclerosis***🍡
    Code first underlying disease (710.1)
   (Ex:) 011.00-012.16, 012.80-012.86, 017.90-017.96, 494.0-508.9, 515-516.9,
      517.2, 517.8, 518.89, 519.8-519.9, 748.61

▶ **517.3 *Acute chest syndrome***🍡
    Code first sickle-cell disease in crisis (282.42, 282.62,
      282.64, 282.69)
   (Ex:) 280.0-282.3, 282.5-282.63, 282.69-285.9, 289.9, 776.5-776.6
   Coding Clinic: 2003, Q4, P51-56; 1998, Q2, P8

▶ **517.8 *Lung involvement in other diseases classified elsewhere***

    Code first underlying disease, as:
      amyloidosis (277.30–277.39)
      polymyositis (710.4)
      sarcoidosis (135)
      Sjögren's disease (710.2)
      systemic lupus erythematosus (710.0)

> **Excludes** *syphilis (095.1)*

   Coding Clinic: 2003, Q2, P7-8

● **518 Other diseases of lung**

518.0 Pulmonary collapse🍡
    Atelectasis
    Collapse of lung
    Middle lobe syndrome

> **Excludes** *atelectasis:*
>   *congenital (partial) (770.5)*
>   *primary (770.4)*
>   *tuberculous, current disease (011.8)*

   (Ex:) 518.0, 519.8-519.9
   Coding Clinic: 1990, Q4, P25

518.1 Interstitial emphysema
    Mediastinal emphysema

> **Excludes** *surgical (subcutaneous) emphysema*
>   *(998.81)*
>   *that in fetus or newborn (770.2)*
>   *traumatic emphysema (958.7)*

518.2 Compensatory emphysema

N Newborn Age: 0   **P** Pediatric Age: 0–17   **M** Maternity Age: 12–55   **A** Adult Age: 15–124   ♀ Females Only   ♂ Males Only

(Ex:) CC Exclusions   🍡 Complication\Comorbidity   🍡 Major C\C   🍡 Present on Admission Requirement   🍡 Hospital-Acquired Condition   **919**

DISEASES OF THE RESPIRATORY SYSTEM (460–519)

518.3   Pulmonary eosinophilia 🔖
Eosinophilic asthma
Löffler's syndrome
Pneumonia:
   allergic
   eosinophilic
Tropical eosinophilia
Ⓔ 011.00-012.16, 012.80-012.86, 017.90-017.96, 020.3-020.5, 021.3, 022.1, 031.0, 039.1, 073.0, 115.05, 115.15, 115.95, 122.1, 130.4, 136.3, 480.0-480.2, 480.8-487.1, 488, 494.0-495.9, 500-508.9, 517.1, 517.8, 518.3, 518.89, 519.8-519.9, 748.61

518.4   Acute edema of lung, unspecified 🔖
Acute pulmonary edema NOS
Pulmonary edema, postoperative

Excludes	pulmonary edema:

              acute, with mention of heart disease or
                    failure (428.1)
              chronic or unspecified (514)
              due to external agents (506.0–508.9)
Ⓔ 398.91, 428.0-428.9, 518.4, 519.8-519.9

518.5   Pulmonary insufficiency following trauma and surgery 🔖
Adult respiratory distress syndrome
Pulmonary insufficiency following:
   shock
   surgery
   trauma
Shock lung

Excludes	adult respiratory distress syndrome

              associated with other conditions
                 (518.82)
             pneumonia:
                aspiration (507.0)
                hypostatic (514)
             respiratory failure in other conditions
                 (518.81, 518.83–518.84)
Ⓔ 518.5, 519.8-519.9
Coding Clinic: 2004, Q4, P139

518.6   Allergic bronchopulmonary aspergillosis 🔖
Ⓔ 518.6, 519.8-519.9
Coding Clinic: 1997, Q4, P39-40

518.7   Transfusion related acute lung injury (TRALI) 🔖
Ⓔ 518.7, 997.31-997.39, 997.91-997.99, 998.81, 998.83-998.9
Coding Clinic: 2006, Q4, P91-92

● **518.8   Other diseases of lung**

   518.81   Acute respiratory failure 🔖
       Respiratory failure NOS

Excludes	acute and chronic respiratory failure

               (518.84)
             acute respiratory distress (518.82)
             chronic respiratory failure (518.83)
             respiratory arrest (799.1)
             respiratory failure, newborn
                (770.84)
     Ⓔ 518.81-518.84, 519.8-519.9, 799.1
     Coding Clinic: 2009, Q2, P13; 2008, Q1, P18-19; 2007, Q3, P7-8; 2005, Q2, P19-20; Q1, P3-8; 2004, Q4, P139; 2003, Q2, P21-22; Q1, P15; 1993, Q1, P25; 1991, Q3, P14; 1990, Q4, P25; 1987, Nov-Dec, P5-6

518.82   Other pulmonary insufficiency, not elsewhere classified 🔖
Acute respiratory distress
Acute respiratory insufficiency
Adult respiratory distress syndrome NEC

Excludes	adult respiratory distress syndrome

              associated with trauma or
                surgery (518.5)
             pulmonary insufficiency following
                trauma or surgery (518.5)
             respiratory distress:
               NOS (786.09)
               newborn (770.89)
               syndrome, newborn (769)
               shock lung (518.5)
Ⓔ 518.81-518.84, 519.8-519.9, 799.1
Coding Clinic: 2003, Q4, P105-106; 1995, Q1, P7; 1991, Q2, P21

518.83   Chronic respiratory failure 🔖
Ⓔ 518.81-518.84, 519.8-519.9, 799.1
Coding Clinic: 2003, Q4, P103-104, 111

518.84   Acute and chronic respiratory failure 🔖
Acute on chronic respiratory failure
Ⓔ 518.81-518.84, 519.8-519.9, 799.1

518.89   Other diseases of lung, not elsewhere classified
Broncholithiasis
Calcification of lung
Lung disease NOS
Pulmolithiasis
Coding Clinic: 1988, Q4, P6; 1987, Nov-Dec, P8; 1986, Sept-Oct, P10

● **519   Other diseases of respiratory system**

  ● **519.0   Tracheostomy complications**
     These complications do not appear in the usual complication range of 996–999.

   519.00   Tracheostomy complication, unspecified 🔖
     Ⓔ 519.00-519.19, 519.8-519.9

   519.01   Infection of tracheostomy 🔖

     Use additional code to identify type of infection, such as:
       abscess or cellulitis of neck (682.1)
       septicemia (038.0–038.9)

     Use additional code to identify organism (041.00–041.9)
     Ⓔ 519.00-519.19, 519.8-519.9
     Coding Clinic: 1998, Q4, P41-42

   519.02   Mechanical complication of tracheostomy 🔖
     Tracheal stenosis due to tracheostomy
     Ⓔ 519.00-519.19, 519.8-519.9

   519.09   Other tracheostomy complications 🔖
     Hemorrhage due to tracheostomy
     Tracheoesophageal fistula due to tracheostomy
     Ⓔ 519.00-519.19, 519.8-519.9

◄ New   ◄▥ Revised   ~~deleted~~ Deleted   ● Unacceptable Principal Diagnosis   ● Use Additional Digit(s)
▶ Manifestation Code   **OGCR** Official Guidelines   **Coding Clinic**   Excludes   Includes   Use additional   Code first   Omit code

DISEASES OF THE RESPIRATORY SYSTEM (460–519)

● **519.1 Other diseases of trachea and bronchus, not elsewhere classified**
   Coding Clinic: 2002, Q3, P18

   519.11 Acute bronchospasm
      Bronchospasm NOS

Excludes	*acute bronchitis with bronchospasm (466.0)*
	asthma (493.00–493.92)
	exercise induced bronchospasm (493.81)

      Coding Clinic: 2006, Q4, P92-93

   519.19 Other diseases of trachea and bronchus
      Calcification of bronchus or trachea
      Stenosis of bronchus or trachea
      Ulcer of bronchus or trachea

519.2 Mediastinitis 🔖 🔖
   HAC: And one of the following procedure codes:
      36.10-36.19
      (Ex) 519.2-519.3, 519.8-519.9

519.3 Other diseases of mediastinum, not elsewhere classified
   Fibrosis of mediastinum
   Hernia of mediastinum
   Retraction of mediastinum

519.4 Disorders of diaphragm
   Diaphragmitis
   Paralysis of diaphragm
   Relaxation of diaphragm

Excludes	*congenital defect of diaphragm (756.6)*
	diaphragmatic hernia (551–553 with .3)
	congenital (756.6)

519.8 Other diseases of respiratory system, not elsewhere classified
   Coding Clinic: 1989, Q4, P12

519.9 Unspecified disease of respiratory system
   Respiratory disease (chronic) NOS

N Newborn Age: 0   **P** Pediatric Age: 0–17   **M** Maternity Age: 12–55   **A** Adult Age: 15–124   ♀ Females Only   ♂ Males Only   **921**

(Ex) CC Exclusions   🔖 Complication\Comorbidity   🔖 Major C\C   🔖 Present on Admission Requirement   🔖 Hospital-Acquired Condition

DISEASES OF THE RESPIRATORY SYSTEM (460–519)

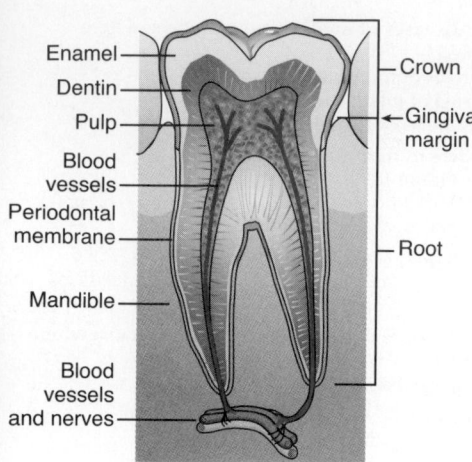

Figure 9–1
Anatomy of
a tooth.

Enamel
Dentin
Pulp
Blood
vessels
Periodontal
membrane
Mandible
Blood
vessels
and nerves

Crown
Gingival
margin
Root

Item 9–1 Anodontia is the congenital absence of teeth.
Hypodontia is partial anodontia. **Oligodontia** is the
congenital absence of some teeth, whereas **supernumerary** is
having more teeth than the normal number. **Mesiodens** are small
extra teeth that often appear in pairs, although single small teeth
are not uncommon.

9. DISEASES OF THE DIGESTIVE SYSTEM (520–579)

DISEASES OF ORAL CAVITY, SALIVARY GLANDS, AND JAWS (520–529)

● **520 Disorders of tooth development and eruption**

520.0 Anodontia
Absence of teeth (complete) (congenital) (partial)
Hypodontia
Oligodontia
> **Excludes** *acquired absence of teeth (525.10–525.19)*

520.1 Supernumerary teeth
Distomolar
Fourth molar
Mesiodens
Paramolar
Supplemental teeth
> **Excludes** *supernumerary roots (520.2)*

520.2 Abnormalities of size and form
Concrescence of teeth
Fusion of teeth
Gemination of teeth
Dens evaginatus
Dens in dente
Dens invaginatus
Enamel pearls
Macrodontia
Microdontia
Peg-shaped [conical] teeth
Supernumerary roots
Taurodontism
Tuberculum paramolare
> **Excludes** *that due to congenital syphilis (090.5)*
> *tuberculum Carabelli, which is regarded as*
> *a normal variation*

520.3 Mottled teeth
Dental fluorosis
Mottling of enamel
Nonfluoride enamel opacities

520.4 Disturbances of tooth formation
Aplasia and hypoplasia of cementum
Dilaceration of tooth
Enamel hypoplasia (neonatal) (postnatal) (prenatal)
Horner's teeth
Hypocalcification of teeth
Regional odontodysplasia
Turner's tooth
> **Excludes** *Hutchinson's teeth and mulberry molars in*
> *congenital syphilis (090.5)*
> *mottled teeth (520.3)*

520.5 Hereditary disturbances in tooth structure, not elsewhere classified
Amelogenesis imperfecta
Dentinogenesis imperfecta
Odontogenesis imperfecta
Dentinal dysplasia
Shell teeth

520.6 Disturbances in tooth eruption
Teeth:
embedded
impacted
natal
neonatal
prenatal
primary [deciduous]:
persistent
shedding, premature
Tooth eruption:
late
obstructed
premature
> **Excludes** *exfoliation of teeth (attributable to disease of*
> *surrounding tissues) (525.0–525.19)*
> **Coding Clinic: 2006, Q1, P18; 2005, Q2, P15-16; 2004, Q1, P17**

520.7 Teething syndrome

520.8 Other specified disorders of tooth development and eruption
Color changes during tooth formation
Pre-eruptive color changes
> **Excludes** *posteruptive color changes (521.7)*

520.9 Unspecified disorder of tooth development and eruption

◀ New   ◀◁ Revised   ~~deleted~~ Deleted   ● Unacceptable Principal Diagnosis   ● Use Additional Digit(s)
▶ Manifestation Code   **OGCR** Official Guidelines   **Coding Clinic**   Excludes   Includes   Use additional   Code first   Omit code

DISEASES OF THE DIGESTIVE SYSTEM (520–579)

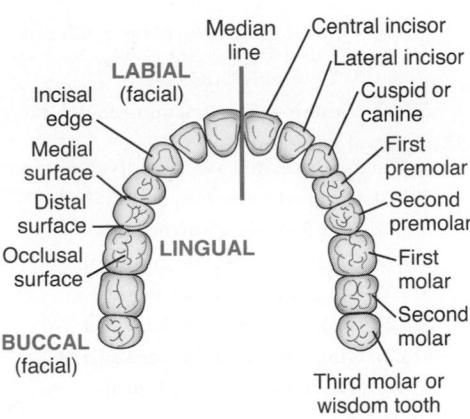

Figure 9-2 The permanent teeth within the dental arch.

Item 9-2 Each dental arch (jaw) normally contains 16 teeth. Tooth decay or **dental caries** is a disease of the enamel, dentin, and cementum of the tooth and can result in a cavity.

● 521 **Diseases of hard tissues of teeth**

  ● 521.0 **Dental caries**

    521.00 Dental caries, unspecified

    521.01 Dental caries limited to enamel
      Initial caries
      White spot lesion

    521.02 Dental caries extending into dentin

    521.03 Dental caries extending into pulp

    521.04 Arrested dental caries

    521.05 Odontoclasia
      Infantile melanodontia
      Melanodontoclasia

      Excludes *internal and external resorption of teeth (521.40–521.49)*

    521.06 Dental caries pit and fissure
      Primary dental caries, pit and fissure origin

    521.07 Dental caries of smooth surface
      Primary dental caries, smooth surface origin

    521.08 Dental caries of root surface
      Primary dental caries, root surface

    521.09 Other dental caries
      Coding Clinic: 2002, Q3, P14

  ● 521.1 **Excessive attrition (approximal wear) (occlusal wear)**

    521.10 Excessive attrition, unspecified

    521.11 Excessive attrition, limited to enamel

    521.12 Excessive attrition, extending into dentine

    521.13 Excessive attrition, extending into pulp

    521.14 Excessive attrition, localized

    521.15 Excessive attrition, generalized

● 521.2 **Abrasion**
    Abrasion of teeth:
      dentifrice
      habitual
      occupational
      ritual
      traditional
    Wedge defect NOS of teeth

    521.20 Abrasion, unspecified

    521.21 Abrasion, limited to enamel

    521.22 Abrasion, extending into dentine

    521.23 Abrasion, extending into pulp

    521.24 Abrasion, localized

    521.25 Abrasion, generalized

● 521.3 **Erosion**
    Erosion of teeth:
      NOS
      due to:
        medicine
        persistent vomiting
      idiopathic
      occupational

    521.30 Erosion, unspecified

    521.31 Erosion, limited to enamel

    521.32 Erosion, extending into dentine

    521.33 Erosion, extending into pulp

    521.34 Erosion, localized

    521.35 Erosion, generalized

● 521.4 **Pathological resorption**

    521.40 Pathological resorption, unspecified

    521.41 Pathological resorption, internal

    521.42 Pathological resorption, external

    521.49 Other pathological resorption
      Internal granuloma of pulp

  521.5 **Hypercementosis**
    Cementation hyperplasia

  521.6 **Ankylosis of teeth**

  521.7 **Intrinsic posteruptive color changes**
    Staining [discoloration] of teeth:
      NOS
      due to:
        drugs
        metals
      pulpal bleeding

    Excludes *accretions [deposits] on teeth (523.6)*
        extrinsic color changes (523.6)
        pre-eruptive color changes (520.8)

● 521.8 **Other specified diseases of hard tissues of teeth**

    521.81 Cracked tooth

      Excludes *asymptomatic craze lines in enamel - omit code*
        broken tooth due to trauma (873.63, 873.73)
        fractured tooth due to trauma (873.63, 873.73)

    521.89 Other specified diseases of hard tissues of teeth
      Irradiated enamel
      Sensitive dentin

  521.9 **Unspecified disease of hard tissues of teeth**

N Newborn Age: 0   **P** Pediatric Age: 0–17   **M** Maternity Age: 12–55   **A** Adult Age: 15–124   ♀ Females Only   ♂ Males Only
(Ex) CC Exclusions   Complication\Comorbidity   Major C\C   Present on Admission Requirement   Hospital-Acquired Condition

923

DISEASES OF THE DIGESTIVE SYSTEM (520–579)

● 522   Diseases of pulp and periapical tissues

522.0   Pulpitis 🔵

Pulpal:
   abscess
   polyp
Pulpitis:
   acute
   chronic (hyperplastic) (ulcerative)
   suppurative
   Ex 520.0-525.9

522.1   Necrosis of the pulp
Pulp gangrene

522.2   Pulp degeneration
Denticles   Pulp calcifications
Pulp stones

522.3   Abnormal hard tissue formation in pulp
Secondary or irregular dentin

522.4   Acute apical periodontitis of pulpal origin 🔵
   Ex 520.0-525.9

522.5   Periapical abscess without sinus
Abscess:
   dental
   dentoalveolar

> **Excludes**   *periapical abscess with sinus (522.7)*

522.6   Chronic apical periodontitis
Apical or periapical granuloma
Apical periodontitis NOS

522.7   Periapical abscess with sinus
Fistula:
   alveolar process
   dental

522.8   Radicular cyst
Cyst:
   apical (periodontal)
   periapical
   radiculodental
   residual radicular

> **Excludes**   *lateral developmental or lateral periodontal cyst (526.0)*

522.9   Other and unspecified diseases of pulp and periapical tissues

> **Item 9–3   Acute gingivitis,** also known as orilitis or ulitis, is the short-term, severe inflammation of the gums (gingiva) caused by bacteria. **Chronic gingivitis** is persistent inflammation of the gums. When the gingivitis moves into the periodontium it is called periodontitis, also known as paradentitis.

● 523   Gingival and periodontal diseases

● 523.0   Acute gingivitis

> **Excludes**   *acute necrotizing ulcerative gingivitis (101)*
> *herpetic gingivostomatitis (054.2)*

523.00   Acute gingivitis, plaque induced
Acute gingivitis NOS

523.01   Acute gingivitis, non-plaque induced

● 523.1   Chronic gingivitis
Gingivitis (chronic):
   desquamative
   hyperplastic
   simple marginal
   ulcerative

> **Excludes**   *herpetic gingivostomatitis (054.2)*

523.10   Chronic gingivitis, plaque induced
Chronic gingivitis NOS
Gingivitis NOS

523.11   Chronic gingivitis, non-plaque induced

● 523.2   Gingival recession
Gingival recession (postinfective) (postoperative)

523.20   Gingival recession, unspecified

523.21   Gingival recession, minimal

523.22   Gingival recession, moderate

523.23   Gingival recession, severe

523.24   Gingival recession, localized

523.25   Gingival recession, generalized

● 523.3   Aggressive and acute periodontitis
Acute:
   pericementitis
   pericoronitis

> **Excludes**   *acute apical periodontitis (522.4)*
> *periapical abscess (522.5, 522.7)*

523.30   Aggressive periodontitis, unspecified

523.31   Aggressive periodontitis, localized
Periodontal abscess

523.32   Aggressive periodontitis, generalized

523.33   Acute periodontitis

● 523.4   Chronic periodontitis
Chronic pericoronitis
Pericementitis (chronic)
Periodontitis:
   NOS
   complex
   simplex

> **Excludes**   *chronic apical periodontitis (522.6)*

523.40   Chronic periodontitis, unspecified

523.41   Chronic periodontitis, localized

523.42   Chronic periodontitis, generalized

523.5   Periodontosis

523.6   Accretions on teeth
Dental calculus:
   subgingival
   supragingival
Deposits on teeth:
   betel
   materia alba
   soft
   tartar
   tobacco
Extrinsic discoloration of teeth

> **Excludes**   *intrinsic discoloration of teeth (521.7)*

523.8   Other specified periodontal diseases
Giant cell:
   epulis
   peripheral granuloma
Gingival:
   cysts
   enlargement NOS
   fibromatosis
Gingival polyp
Periodontal lesions due to traumatic occlusion
Peripheral giant cell granuloma

> **Excludes**   *leukoplakia of gingiva (528.6)*

523.9   Unspecified gingival and periodontal disease
Coding Clinic: 2002, Q3, P14

◀ New   ◀▥ Revised   ~~deleted~~ Deleted   ● Unacceptable Principal Diagnosis   ⬤ Use Additional Digit(s)
▶ Manifestation Code   **OGCR** Official Guidelines   **Coding Clinic**   Excludes   Includes   Use additional   Code first   Omit code

Figure 9–3 Dentofacial malocclusion.

Item 9–4 Hyperplasia is a condition of overdevelopment, whereas **hypoplasia** is a condition of underdevelopment. **Macrogenia** is overdevelopment of the chin, whereas microgenia is underdevelopment of the chin.

● **524 Dentofacial anomalies, including malocclusion**

● **524.0 Major anomalies of jaw size**

| Excludes | hemifacial atrophy or hypertrophy (754.0) unilateral condylar hyperplasia or hypoplasia of mandible |

524.00 Unspecified anomaly

524.01 Maxillary hyperplasia

524.02 Mandibular hyperplasia

524.03 Maxillary hypoplasia

524.04 Mandibular hypoplasia

524.05 Macrogenia

524.06 Microgenia

524.07 Excessive tuberosity of jaw
Entire maxillary tuberosity

524.09 Other specified anomaly

● **524.1 Anomalies of relationship of jaw to cranial base**

524.10 Unspecified anomaly
Prognathism   Retrognathism

524.11 Maxillary asymmetry

524.12 Other jaw asymmetry

524.19 Other specified anomaly

● **524.2 Anomalies of dental arch relationship**
Anomaly of dental arch

| Excludes | hemifacial atrophy or hypertrophy (754.0) soft tissue impingement (524.81–524.82) unilateral condylar hyperplasia or hypoplasia of mandible (526.89) |

524.20 Unspecified anomaly of dental arch relationship

524.21 Malocclusion, Angle's class I
Neutro-occlusion

524.22 Malocclusion, Angle's class II
Disto-occlusion Division I
Disto-occlusion Division II

524.23 Malocclusion, Angle's class III
Mesio-occlusion

524.24 Open anterior occlusal relationship
Anterior open bite

524.25 Open posterior occlusal relationship
Posterior open bite

524.26 Excessive horizontal overlap
Excessive horizontal overjet

524.27 Reverse articulation
Anterior articulation
Crossbite
Posterior articulation

524.28 Anomalies of interarch distance
Excessive interarch distance
Inadequate interarch distance

524.29 Other anomalies of dental arch relationship
Other anomalies of dental arch

● **524.3 Anomalies of tooth position of fully erupted teeth**

| Excludes | impacted or embedded teeth with abnormal position of such teeth or adjacent teeth (520.6) |

Coding Clinic: 2004, Q1, P17

524.30 Unspecified anomaly of tooth position
Diastema of teeth NOS
Displacement of teeth NOS
Transposition of teeth NOS

524.31 Crowding of teeth

524.32 Excessive spacing of teeth

524.33 Horizontal displacement of teeth
Tipped teeth
Tipping of teeth

524.34 Vertical displacement of teeth
Extruded tooth
Infraeruption of teeth
Intruded tooth
Supraeruption of teeth

524.35 Rotation of tooth/teeth

524.36 Insufficient interocclusal distance of teeth (ridge)
Lack of adequate intermaxillary vertical dimension

524.37 Excessive interocclusal distance of teeth
Excessive intermaxillary vertical dimension
Loss of occlusal vertical dimension

524.39 Other anomalies of tooth position

524.4 Malocclusion, unspecified

● **524.5 Dentofacial functional abnormalities**

524.50 Dentofacial functional abnormality, unspecified

524.51 Abnormal jaw closure

524.52 Limited mandibular range of motion

524.53 Deviation in opening and closing of the mandible

524.54 Insufficient anterior guidance
Insufficient anterior occlusal guidance

524.55 Centric occlusion maximum intercuspation discrepancy
Centric occlusion of teeth discrepancy

524.56 Non-working side interference
Balancing side interference

524.57 Lack of posterior occlusal support

524.59 Other dentofacial functional abnormalities
Abnormal swallowing
Mouth breathing
Sleep postures
Tongue, lip, or finger habits

DISEASES OF THE DIGESTIVE SYSTEM (520–579)

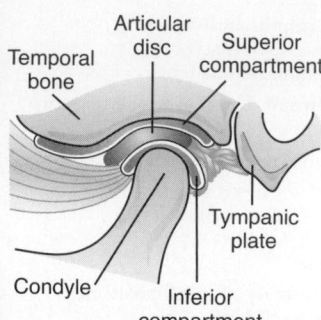

Temporal bone

Articular disc

Superior compartment

Tympanic plate

Condyle

Inferior compartment

Figure 9–4
Temporomandibular joint.

Item 9–5 Dysfunction of the temporomandibular joint is termed **temporomandibular joint (TMJ) syndrome** and is characterized by pain and tenderness/spasm of the muscles of mastication, joint noise, and in the later stages, limited mandibular movement.

● **524.6 Temporomandibular joint disorders**

> **Excludes** *current temporomandibular joint:*
> *dislocation (830.0–830.1)*
> *strain (848.1)*

524.60 Temporomandibular joint disorders, unspecified
Temporomandibular joint-pain-dysfunction syndrome [TMJ]

524.61 Adhesions and ankylosis (bony or fibrous)

524.62 Arthralgia of temporomandibular joint

524.63 Articular disc disorder (reducing or nonreducing)

524.64 Temporomandibular joint sounds on opening and/or closing the jaw

524.69 Other specified temporomandibular joint disorders

● **524.7 Dental alveolar anomalies**

524.70 Unspecified alveolar anomaly

524.71 Alveolar maxillary hyperplasia

524.72 Alveolar mandibular hyperplasia

524.73 Alveolar maxillary hypoplasia

524.74 Alveolar mandibular hypoplasia

524.75 Vertical displacement of alveolus and teeth
Extrusion of alveolus and teeth

524.76 Occlusal plane deviation

524.79 Other specified alveolar anomaly

● **524.8 Other specified dentofacial anomalies**

524.81 Anterior soft tissue impingement

524.82 Posterior soft tissue impingement

524.89 Other specified dentofacial anomalies

524.9 Unspecified dentofacial anomalies

● **525 Other diseases and conditions of the teeth and supporting structures**

525.0 Exfoliation of teeth due to systemic causes

● **525.1 Loss of teeth due to trauma, extraction, or periodontal disease**

> *Code first* class of edentulism (525.40–525.44, 525.50–525.54)

▶ **525.10 Acquired absence of teeth, unspecified**
Tooth extraction status, NOS

▶ **525.11 Loss of teeth due to trauma**
Check for E code assignment.

▶ **525.12 Loss of teeth due to periodontal disease**

▶ **525.13 Loss of teeth due to caries**

▶ **525.19 Other loss of teeth**

● **525.2 Atrophy of edentulous alveolar ridge**

525.20 Unspecified atrophy of edentulous alveolar ridge
Atrophy of the mandible NOS
Atrophy of the maxilla NOS

525.21 Minimal atrophy of the mandible

525.22 Moderate atrophy of the mandible

525.23 Severe atrophy of the mandible

525.24 Minimal atrophy of the maxilla

525.25 Moderate atrophy of the maxilla

525.26 Severe atrophy of the maxilla

525.3 Retained dental root

● **525.4 Complete edentulism**

> *Use additional* code to identify cause of edentulism (525.10–525.19)

525.40 Complete edentulism, unspecified
Edentulism NOS

525.41 Complete edentulism, class I

525.42 Complete edentulism, class II

525.43 Complete edentulism, class III

525.44 Complete edentulism, class IV

● **525.5 Partial edentulism**

> *Use additional* code to identify cause of edentulism (525.10–525.19)

525.50 Partial edentulism, unspecified

525.51 Partial edentulism, class I

525.52 Partial edentulism, class II

525.53 Partial edentulism, class III

525.54 Partial edentulism, class IV

● **525.6 Unsatisfactory restoration of tooth**
Defective bridge, crown, fillings
Defective dental restoration

> **Excludes** *dental restoration status (V45.84)*
> *unsatisfactory endodontic treatment (526.61–526.69)*

525.60 Unspecified unsatisfactory restoration of tooth
Unspecified defective dental restoration

525.61 Open restoration margins
Dental restoration failure of marginal integrity
Open margin on tooth restoration

525.62 Unrepairable overhanging of dental restorative materials
Overhanging of tooth restoration

525.63 Fractured dental restorative material without loss of material

> **Excludes** *cracked tooth (521.81)*
> *fractured tooth (873.63, 873.73)*

525.64 Fractured dental restorative material with loss of material

> **Excludes** *cracked tooth (521.81)*
> *fractured tooth (873.63, 873.73)*

◀ New   ◀▥ Revised   ~~deleted~~ Deleted   ● Unacceptable Principal Diagnosis   ● Use Additional Digit(s)
▶ Manifestation Code   **OGCR** Official Guidelines   **Coding Clinic**   Excludes   Includes   Use additional   Code first   Omit code

525.65 Contour of existing restoration of tooth biologically incompatible with oral health
Dental restoration failure of periodontal anatomical integrity
Unacceptable contours of existing restoration
Unacceptable morphology of existing restoration

525.66 Allergy to existing dental restorative material
Use additional code to identify the specific type of allergy

525.67 Poor aesthetics of existing restoration
Dental restoration aesthetically inadequate or displeasing

525.69 Other unsatisfactory restoration of existing tooth

● **525.7 Endosseous dental implant failure**

525.71 Osseointegration failure of dental implant
Failure of dental implant due to infection
Failure of dental implant due to unintentional loading
Failure of dental implant osseointegration due to premature loading
Failure of dental implant to osseointegrate prior to intentional prosthetic loading
Hemorrhagic complications of dental implant placement
Iatrogenic osseointegration failure of dental implant
Osseointegration failure of dental implant due to complications of systemic disease
Osseointegration failure of dental implant due to poor bone quality
Pre-integration failure of dental implant NOS
Pre-osseointegration failure of dental implant

525.72 Post-osseointegration biological failure of dental implant
Failure of dental implant due to lack of attached gingiva
Failure of dental implant due to occlusal trauma (caused by poor prosthetic design)
Failure of dental implant due to parafunctional habits
Failure of dental implant due to periodontal infection (peri-implantitis)
Failure of dental implant due to poor oral hygiene
Failure of dental implant to osseointegrate following intentional prosthetic loading
Iatrogenic post-osseointegration failure of dental implant
Post-osseointegration failure of dental implant due to complications of systemic disease

525.73 Post-osseointegration mechanical failure of dental implant
Failure of dental prosthesis causing loss of dental implant
Fracture of dental implant
Mechanical failure of dental implant NOS
| **Excludes** | *cracked tooth (521.81)* |

fractured dental restorative material with loss of material (525.64)
fractured dental restorative material without loss of material (525.63)
fractured tooth (873.63, 873.73)

525.79 Other endosseous dental implant failure
Dental implant failure NOS

525.8 Other specified disorders of the teeth and supporting structures
Enlargement of alveolar ridge NOS
Irregular alveolar process

525.9 Unspecified disorder of the teeth and supporting structures

● **526 Diseases of the jaws**

526.0 Developmental odontogenic cysts
Cyst:
dentigerous
eruption
follicular
lateral developmental
lateral periodontal
primordial
Keratocyst
| **Excludes** | *radicular cyst (522.8)* |

526.1 Fissural cysts of jaw
Cyst:
globulomaxillary
incisor canal
median anterior maxillary
median palatal
nasopalatine
palatine of papilla
| **Excludes** | *cysts of oral soft tissues (528.4)* |

526.2 Other cysts of jaws
Cyst of jaw: Cyst of jaw:
NOS   hemorrhagic
aneurysmal   traumatic

526.3 Central giant cell (reparative) granuloma
| **Excludes** | *peripheral giant cell granuloma (523.8)* |

526.4 Inflammatory conditions
Abscess of jaw (acute) (chronic) (suppurative)
Osteitis of jaw (acute) (chronic) (suppurative)
Osteomyelitis (neonatal) of jaw (acute) (chronic) (suppurative)
Periostitis of jaw (acute) (chronic) (suppurative)
Sequestrum of jaw bone
| **Excludes** | *alveolar osteitis (526.5)* |
| | *osteonecrosis of jaw (733.45)* |

526.5 Alveolitis of jaw
Alveolar osteitis
Dry socket

● **526.6 Periradicular pathology associated with previous endodontic treatment**

526.61 Perforation of root canal space

526.62 Endodontic overfill

526.63 Endodontic underfill

526.69 Other periradicular pathology associated with previous endodontic treatment

● **526.8 Other specified diseases of the jaws**

526.81 Exostosis of jaw
Torus mandibularis
Torus palatinus

526.89 Other
Cherubism
Fibrous dysplasia of jaw(s)
Latent bone cyst of jaw(s)
Osteoradionecrosis of jaw(s)
Unilateral condylar hyperplasia or hypoplasia of mandible

526.9 Unspecified disease of the jaws

N Newborn Age: 0   **P** Pediatric Age: 0–17   **M** Maternity Age: 12–55   **A** Adult Age: 15–124   ♀ Females Only   ♂ Males Only

(Ex) CC Exclusions   ◐ Complication\Comorbidity   ◐ Major C\C   ◐ Present on Admission Requirement   ◐ Hospital-Acquired Condition

927

Figure 9–5 Major salivary glands.

Parotid gland

Sublingual gland

Submandibular gland

Item 9–6 Atrophy is wasting away of a tissue or organ, whereas **hypertrophy** is overdevelopment or enlargement of a tissue or organ. **Sialoadenitis** is salivary gland inflammation. **Parotitis** is the inflammation of the parotid gland. In the epidemic form, parotitis is also known as mumps. **Sialolithiasis** is the formation of calculus within a salivary gland. **Mucocele** is a polyp composed of mucus.

● **527 Diseases of the salivary glands**

527.0 Atrophy

527.1 Hypertrophy

527.2 Sialoadenitis

Parotitis: Sialoangitis
     NOS   Sialodochitis
     allergic
     toxic

    Excludes *epidemic or infectious parotitis (072.0–072.9)*
                uveoparotid fever (135)

527.3 Abscess 🗝
    ⒺⓍ 527.0-527.9, 537.89-538

527.4 Fistula 🗝
    Excludes *congenital fistula of salivary gland (750.24)*
    ⒺⓍ 527.0-527.9, 537.89-538

527.5 Sialolithiasis
    Calculus of salivary gland or duct
    Stone of salivary gland or duct
    Sialodocholithiasis

527.6 Mucocele
    Mucous:
       extravasation cyst of salivary gland
       retention cyst of salivary gland
    Ranula

527.7 Disturbance of salivary secretion
    Hyposecretion
    Ptyalism
    Sialorrhea
    Xerostomia

527.8 Other specified diseases of the salivary glands
    Benign lymphoepithelial lesion of salivary gland
    Sialectasia
    Sialosis
    Stenosis of salivary duct
    Stricture of salivary duct

527.9 Unspecified disease of the salivary glands

Item 9–7 Stomatitis is the inflammation of the oral mucosa. **Cancrum oris**, also known as **noma** or **gangrenous stomatitis**, begins as an ulcer of the gingiva and results in a progressive gangrenous process. Mucositis is the inflammation of the mucous membranes lining the digestive tract from the mouth to the anus. It is a common side effect of chemotherapy and of radiotherapy that involves any part of the digestive tract.

● **528 Diseases of the oral soft tissues, excluding lesions specific for gingiva and tongue**

● **528.0 Stomatitis and mucositis (ulcerative)**

    Excludes *Stevens-Johnson syndrome (695.13)*
            stomatitis:
               acute necrotizing ulcerative (101)
               aphthous (528.2)
               cellulitis and abscess of mouth (528.3)
               diphtheritic stomatitis (032.0)
               epizootic stomatitis (078.4)
               gangrenous (528.1)
               gingivitis (523.0–523.1)
               herpetic (054.2)
               oral thrush (112.0)
               Vincent's (101)
    Coding Clinic: 1999, Q2, P9

528.00 Stomatitis and mucositis, unspecified
    Mucositis NOS
    Ulcerative mucositis NOS
    Ulcerative stomatitis NOS
    Vesicular stomatitis NOS

528.01 Mucositis (ulcerative) due to antineoplastic therapy
    Use additional E code to identify adverse
       effects of therapy, such as:
       antineoplastic and immunosuppressive
          drugs (E930.7, E933.1)
       radiation therapy (E879.2)
    Coding Clinic: 2006, Q4, P88-91

528.02 Mucositis (ulcerative) due to other drugs
    Use additional E code to identify drug

528.09 Other stomatitis and mucositis (ulcerative)

528.1 Cancrum oris
    Gangrenous stomatitis
    Noma

528.2 Oral aphthae
    Aphthous stomatitis
    Canker sore
    Periadenitis mucosa necrotica recurrens
    Recurrent aphthous ulcer
    Stomatitis herpetiformis
    Excludes *herpetic stomatitis (054.2)*

528.3 Cellulitis and abscess 🗝
    Cellulitis of mouth (floor)
    Ludwig's angina
    Oral fistula
    Excludes *abscess of tongue (529.0)*
            cellulitis or abscess of lip (528.5)
            fistula (of):
               dental (522.7)
               lip (528.5)
            gingivitis (523.00–523.11)
    ⒺⓍ 528.00-528.09, 528.3, 529.0, 529.2

DISEASES OF THE DIGESTIVE SYSTEM (520–579)

◀ New   ◀▥ Revised   ~~deleted~~ Deleted   ● Unacceptable Principal Diagnosis   ● Use Additional Digit(s)

▶ Manifestation Code   **OGCR** Official Guidelines   **Coding Clinic**   Excludes   Includes   Use additional   Code first   Omit code

528.4 Cysts
　　Dermoid cyst of mouth
　　Epidermoid cyst of mouth
　　Epstein's pearl of mouth
　　Lymphoepithelial cyst of mouth
　　Nasoalveolar cyst of mouth
　　Nasolabial cyst of mouth

　　　Excludes *cyst:*
　　　　　　　gingiva (523.8)
　　　　　　　tongue (529.8)

528.5 Diseases of lips
　　Abscess of lip(s)
　　Cellulitis of lip(s)
　　Fistula of lip(s)
　　Hypertrophy of lip(s)
　　Cheilitis:
　　　NOS
　　　angular
　　Cheilodynia
　　Cheilosis

　　　Excludes *actinic cheilitis (692.79)*
　　　　　　　congenital fistula of lip (750.25)
　　　　　　　leukoplakia of lips (528.6)

　　Coding Clinic: 1986, Sept-Oct, P10

528.6 Leukoplakia of oral mucosa, including tongue
　　Considered precancerous and evidenced by thickened
　　　　white patches of epithelium on mucous membranes
　　Leukokeratosis of oral mucosa
　　Leukoplakia of:
　　　gingiva
　　　lips
　　　tongue

　　　Excludes *carcinoma in situ (230.0, 232.0)*
　　　　　　　leukokeratosis nicotina palati (528.79)

●**528.7 Other disturbances of oral epithelium, including tongue**

　　　Excludes *carcinoma in situ (230.0, 232.0)*
　　　　　　　leukokeratosis NOS (702.8)

　　528.71 Minimal keratinized residual ridge mucosa
　　　　Minimal keratinization of alveolar ridge
　　　　　mucosa

　　528.72 Excessive keratinized residual ridge mucosa
　　　　Excessive keratinization of alveolar ridge
　　　　　mucosa

　　528.79 Other disturbances of oral epithelium, including tongue
　　　　Erythroplakia of mouth or tongue
　　　　Focal epithelial hyperplasia of mouth or
　　　　　tongue
　　　　Leukoedema of mouth or tongue
　　　　Leukokeratosis nicotina palati
　　　　Other oral epithelium disturbances

528.8 Oral submucosal fibrosis, including of tongue

528.9 Other and unspecified diseases of the oral soft tissues
　　Cheek and lip biting
　　Denture sore mouth
　　Denture stomatitis
　　Melanoplakia
　　Papillary hyperplasia of palate
　　Eosinophilic granuloma of oral mucosa
　　Irritative hyperplasia of oral mucosa
　　Pyogenic granuloma of oral mucosa
　　Ulcer (traumatic) of oral mucosa

Figure 9-6 Oral leukoplakia and associated squamous carcinoma. (From Feldman: Sleisenger & Fordtran's Gastrointestinal and Liver Disease, 8th ed. 2006, Saunders, An Imprint of Elsevier)

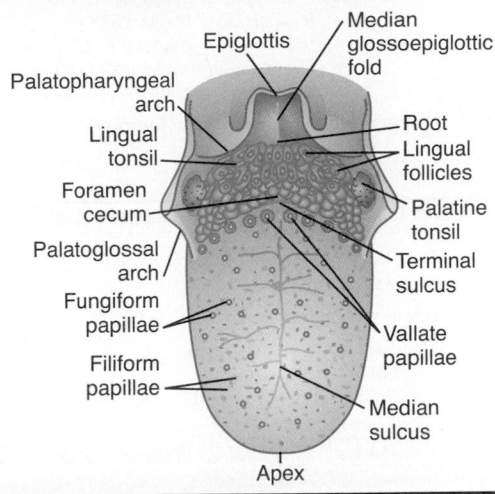

Figure 9-7 Structure of the tongue.

●**529 Diseases and other conditions of the tongue**

　529.0 Glossitis
　　Abscess of tongue
　　Ulceration (traumatic) of tongue

　　　Excludes *glossitis:*
　　　　　　　benign migratory (529.1)
　　　　　　　Hunter's (529.4)
　　　　　　　median rhomboid (529.2)
　　　　　　　Moeller's (529.4)

　529.1 Geographic tongue
　　Benign migratory glossitis
　　Glossitis areata exfoliativa

　529.2 Median rhomboid glossitis

　529.3 Hypertrophy of tongue papillae
　　Black hairy tongue
　　Coated tongue
　　Hypertrophy of foliate papillae
　　Lingua villosa nigra

　529.4 Atrophy of tongue papillae
　　Bald tongue
　　Glazed tongue
　　Glossitis:
　　　Hunter's
　　　Moeller's
　　Glossodynia exfoliativa
　　Smooth atrophic tongue

　529.5 Plicated tongue
　　Fissured tongue　　　　Scrotal tongue
　　Furrowed tongue

　　　Excludes *fissure of tongue, congenital (750.13)*

　529.6 Glossodynia
　　Glossopyrosis　　　　　Painful tongue

　　　Excludes *glossodynia exfoliativa (529.4)*

Labels in Figure 9-7:
Epiglottis
Median glossoepiglottic fold
Palatopharyngeal arch
Lingual tonsil
Root
Lingual follicles
Foramen cecum
Palatine tonsil
Palatoglossal arch
Terminal sulcus
Fungiform papillae
Vallate papillae
Filiform papillae
Median sulcus
Apex

DISEASES OF THE DIGESTIVE SYSTEM (520–579)

N Newborn Age: 0　　**P** Pediatric Age: 0–17　　**M** Maternity Age: 12–55　　**A** Adult Age: 15–124　　♀ Females Only　　♂ Males Only
(Ex) CC Exclusions　　◐ Complication\Comorbidity　　◑ Major C\C　　◐ Present on Admission Requirement　　◑ Hospital-Acquired Condition

929

529.8   Other specified conditions of the tongue
Atrophy (of) tongue
Crenated (of) tongue
Enlargement (of) tongue
Hypertrophy (of) tongue
Glossocele
Glossoptosis

> **Excludes**   *erythroplasia of tongue (528.79)*
> *leukoplakia of tongue (528.6)*
> *macroglossia (congenital) (750.15)*
> *microglossia (congenital) (750.16)*
> *oral submucosal fibrosis (528.8)*

529.9   Unspecified condition of the tongue

DISEASES OF ESOPHAGUS, STOMACH, AND DUODENUM (530–538)

● **530   Diseases of esophagus**

> **Excludes**   *esophageal varices (456.0–456.2)*

530.0   Achalasia and cardiospasm
Achalasia (of cardia)
Aperistalsis of esophagus
Megaesophagus

> **Excludes**   *congenital cardiospasm (750.7)*

CERVICAL ESOPHAGUS
Left subclavian artery
First rib
Arch of aorta
Diaphragm
THORACIC ESOPHAGUS
ABDOMINAL ESOPHAGUS
Stomach

Figure 9–8   The esophagus is the muscular tube that connects the pharynx and the stomach. The 10 inch (25 cm) long esophagus is divided into three parts: **cervical, thoracic,** and **abdominal.**

Item 9–8   Achalasia is a condition in which the smooth muscle fibers of the esophagus do not relax. Most frequently, this condition occurs at the esophagogastric sphincter. **Cardiospasm,** also known as **megaesophagus,** is achalasia of the thoracic esophagus.

Item 9–9   Dyskinesia is difficulty in moving, and **diverticulum** is a sac or pouch.

● **530.1   Esophagitis**
Esophagitis: Esophagitis:
  chemical   postoperative
  peptic   regurgitant

> Use additional E code to identify cause, if induced by chemical

> **Excludes**   *tuberculous esophagitis (017.8)*

Coding Clinic: 1985, Sept-Oct, P9

530.10   Esophagitis, unspecified
Esophagitis NOS
Coding Clinic: 2005, Q3, P17-18

530.11   Reflux esophagitis
Coding Clinic: 1995, Q4, P82

530.12   Acute esophagitis 🕭
Ex: 530.10-530.21, 530.4, 530.7, 530.82, 530.85-530.89

530.13   Eosinophilic esophagitis
Coding Clinic: 2008, Q4, P115-116

530.19   Other esophagitis
Abscess of esophagus
Coding Clinic: 2001, Q3, P15

A   B

C

Figure 9–9   A. Ulcer. **B.** Perforated ulcer. **C.** Laparoscopic view of a perforated duodenal ulcer *(arrow)* with fibrinous exudate on the adjacent peritoneum. (**C** from Feldman: Sleisenger & Fordtran's Gastrointestinal and Liver Disease, 8th ed. 2006, Saunders, An Imprint of Elsevier)

Item 9–10   Gastric ulcers are lesions of the stomach that result in the death of the tissue and a defect of the surface. **Perforated ulcers** are those in which the lesion penetrates the gastric wall, leaving a hole. **Peptic ulcers** are lesions of the stomach or the duodenum. **Peptic** refers to the gastric juice, pepsin.

● **530.2   Ulcer of esophagus**
Ulcer of esophagus
  fungal
  peptic
Ulcer of esophagus due to ingestion of:
  aspirin
  chemicals
  medicines

> Use additional E code to identify cause, if induced by chemical or drug

530.20   Ulcer of esophagus without bleeding 🕭
Ulcer of esophagus NOS
Ex: 530.21, 530.89-530.9, 537.84

530.21   Ulcer of esophagus with bleeding 🕭

> **Excludes**   *bleeding esophageal varices (456.0, 456.20)*

Ex: 251.5, 456.0, 530.20-530.21, 530.7, 530.82, 530.85, 531.00-534.91, 535.01, 535.11, 535.21, 535.31, 535.41, 535.51, 535.61, 535.71, 537.83, 537.89-538, 562.02-562.03, 562.12-562.13, 569.3, 569.85, 578.0-578.9

◄ New   ◄ Revised   ~~deleted~~ Deleted   ● Unacceptable Principal Diagnosis   ● Use Additional Digit(s)
▷ Manifestation Code   OGCR Official Guidelines   Coding Clinic   Excludes   Includes   Use additional   Code first   Omit code

530.3 Stricture and stenosis of esophagus
Compression of esophagus
Obstruction of esophagus

> **Excludes** *congenital stricture of esophagus (750.3)*

Coding Clinic: 2001, Q2, P4; 1997, Q2, P3; 1988, Q1, P13

530.4 Perforation of esophagus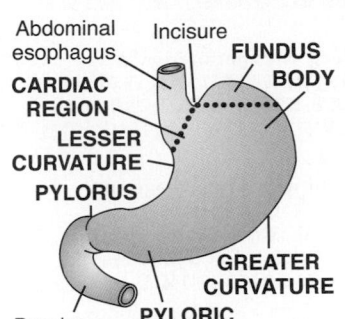
Rupture of esophagus

> **Excludes** *traumatic perforation of esophagus (862.22, 862.32, 874.4–874.5)*

(Ex:) 530.4, 530.7-530.81, 530.83-530.84, 530.89-530.9

530.5 Dyskinesia of esophagus
Corkscrew esophagus
Curling esophagus
Esophagospasm
Spasm of esophagus

> **Excludes** *cardiospasm (530.0)*

Coding Clinic: 1988, Q1, P13; 1984, Nov-Dec, P19

530.6 Diverticulum of esophagus, acquired
Diverticulum, acquired:
   epiphrenic
   pharyngoesophageal
   pulsion
   subdiaphragmatic
   traction
   Zenker's (hypopharyngeal)
Esophageal pouch, acquired
Esophagocele, acquired

> **Excludes** *congenital diverticulum of esophagus (750.4)*

Coding Clinic: 1985, Mar-April, P15

530.7 Gastroesophageal laceration-hemorrhage syndrome
Mallory-Weiss syndrome
(Ex:) 251.5, 456.0, 530.20-530.21, 530.4, 530.7-530.85, 530.89-534.91, 535.01, 535.11, 535.21, 535.31, 535.41, 535.51, 535.61, 535.71, 537.83, 562.02-562.03, 562.12-562.13, 569.3, 569.85, 578.0-578.9

● **530.8 Other specified disorders of esophagus**

    530.81 Esophageal reflux
Gastroesophageal reflux

> **Excludes** *reflux esophagitis (530.11)*

Coding Clinic: 2001, Q2, P4; 1995, Q1, P7

    530.82 Esophageal hemorrhage

> **Excludes** *hemorrhage due to esophageal varices (456.0–456.2)*

(Ex:) 251.5, 456.0, 456.20, 459.89-459.9, 530.20-530.21, 530.7, 530.82, 530.85, 531.00-534.91, 535.01, 535.11, 535.21, 535.31, 535.41, 535.51, 535.61, 535.71, 537.83, 562.02-562.03, 562.12-562.13, 569.3, 569.85, 578.0-578.9

Coding Clinic: 2005, Q1, P17-18

    530.83 Esophageal leukoplakia

    530.84 Tracheoesophageal fistula

> **Excludes** *congenital tracheoesophageal fistula (750.3)*

(Ex:) 530.4, 530.7-530.81, 530.83-530.84, 530.89-530.9

    530.85 Barrett's esophagus
Coding Clinic: 2003, Q4, P63

    530.86 Infection of esophagostomy

> Use additional code to specify infection
>
> (Ex:) 530.86-530.87, 536.40-536.49, 997.4, 997.71, 997.91-997.99, 998.81, 998.83-998.9
>
> Coding Clinic: 2004, Q4, P83

    530.87 Mechanical complication of esophagostomy
Malfunction of esophagostomy
(Ex:) 530.86-530.87, 536.40-536.49, 997.4, 997.71, 997.91-997.99, 998.81, 998.83-998.9
Coding Clinic: 2004, Q4, P83

    530.89 Other

> **Excludes** *Paterson-Kelly syndrome (280.8)*

530.9 Unspecified disorder of esophagus

Figure 9–10 Parts of the stomach.

Item 9–11 Esophageal reflux is the return flow of the contents of the stomach to the esophagus and is referred to as GERD and/or "heartburn." **Gastroesophageal reflux** is the return flow of the contents of the stomach and duodenum to the esophagus. **Esophageal leukoplakia** are white areas on the mucous membrane of the esophagus for which no specific cause can be identified.

● **531 Gastric ulcer**

> **Includes** ulcer (peptic):
>   prepyloric
>   pylorus
>   stomach
>
> Use additional E code to identify drug, if drug-induced
>
> **Excludes** *peptic ulcer NOS (533.0–533.9)*
>
> Coding Clinic: 1990, Q4, P27

The following fifth-digit subclassification is for use with category 531:

0	**without mention of obstruction**
1	**with obstruction**

● **531.0 Acute with hemorrhage**
[0-1] (Ex:) 251.5, 456.0, 530.20-530.21, 530.7, 530.82, 530.85, 531.00-534.91, 535.01, 535.11, 535.21, 535.31, 535.41, 535.51, 535.61, 535.71, 537.83, 537.89-538, 562.02-562.03, 562.12-562.13, 569.3, 569.85, 578.0-578.9

Coding Clinic: 1984, Nov-Dec, P15

● **531.1 Acute with perforation**
[0-1] (Ex:) 251.5, 456.0, 530.20-530.21, 530.7, 530.82, 530.85, 531.00-534.91, 535.01, 535.11, 535.21, 535.31, 535.41, 535.51, 535.61, 535.71, 537.83, 537.89-538, 562.02-562.03, 562.12-562.13, 569.3, 569.85, 578.0-578.9

● **531.2 Acute with hemorrhage and perforation**
[0-1] (Ex:) 251.5, 456.0, 530.20-530.21, 530.7, 530.82, 530.85, 531.00-534.91, 535.01, 535.11, 535.21, 535.31, 535.41, 535.51, 535.61, 535.71, 537.83, 537.89-538, 562.02-562.03, 562.12-562.13, 569.3, 569.85, 578.0-578.9

N Newborn Age: 0   **P** Pediatric Age: 0–17   **M** Maternity Age: 12–55   **A** Adult Age: 15–124   ♀ Females Only   ♂ Males Only

(Ex:) CC Exclusions   Complication\Comorbidity   Major C\C   Present on Admission Requirement   Hospital-Acquired Condition

931

DISEASES OF THE DIGESTIVE SYSTEM (520–579)

●**531.3 Acute without mention of hemorrhage or**
[0-1]   **perforation** 0🔖, 1🔖
      (Ex:) 251.5, 456.0, 530.20-530.21, 530.7, 530.82, 530.85, 531.00-534.91,
      535.01, 535.11, 535.21, 535.31, 535.41, 535.51, 535.61, 535.71,
      537.83, 537.89-538, 562.02-562.03, 562.12-562.13, 569.3, 569.85,
      578.0-578.9

●**531.4 Chronic or unspecified with hemorrhage**🔖
[0-1]   (Ex:) 251.5, 456.0, 530.20-530.21, 530.7, 530.82, 530.85, 531.00-534.91,
      535.01, 535.11, 535.21, 535.31, 535.41, 535.51, 535.61, 535.71,
      537.83, 537.89-538, 562.02-562.03, 562.12-562.13, 569.3, 569.85,
      578.0-578.9

●**531.5 Chronic or unspecified with perforation**🔖
[0-1]   (Ex:) 251.5, 456.0, 530.20-530.21, 530.7, 530.82, 530.85, 531.00-534.91,
      535.01 535.11, 535.21, 535.31, 535.41, 535.51, 535.61, 535.71,
      537.83, 537.89-538, 562.02-562.03, 562.12-562.13, 569.3, 569.85,
      578.0-578.9

●**531.6 Chronic or unspecified with hemorrhage and**
[0-1]   **perforation**🔖
      (Ex:) 251.5, 456.0, 530.20-530.21, 530.7, 530.82, 530.85, 531.00-534.91,
      535.01, 535.11, 535.21, 535.31, 535.41, 535.51, 535.61, 535.71,
      537.83, 537.89-538, 562.02-562.03, 562.12-562.13, 569.3, 569.85,
      578.0-578.9

●**531.7 Chronic without mention of hemorrhage or**
[0-1]   **perforation** 1🔖
      For code **531.71**: (Ex:) 251.5, 456.0, 530.20-530.21, 530.7, 530.82, 530.85,
      531.00-534.91, 535.01, 535.11, 535.21, 535.31, 535.41, 535.51,
      535.61, 535.71, 537.83, 537.89-538, 562.02-562.03, 562.12-562.13,
      569.3, 569.85, 578.0-578.9

●**531.9 Unspecified as acute or chronic, without mention of**
[0-1]   **hemorrhage or perforation** 1🔖
      For code **531.91**: (Ex:) 251.5, 456.0, 530.20-530.21, 530.7, 530.82, 530.85,
      531.00-534.91, 535.01, 535.11, 535.21, 535.31, 535.41, 535.51,
      535.61, 535.71, 537.83, 537.89-538, 562.02-562.03, 562.12-562.13,
      569.3, 569.85, 578.0-578.9

●**532 Duodenal ulcer**

  Includes   erosion (acute) of duodenum
      ulcer (peptic):
          duodenum
          postpyloric

  Use additional E code to identify drug, if drug-induced

  Excludes *peptic ulcer NOS (533.0–533.9)*

  Coding Clinic: 1990, Q4, P27

  The following fifth-digit subclassification is for use with category 532:

0	without mention of obstruction
1	with obstruction

●**532.0 Acute with hemorrhage**🔖
[0-1]   (Ex:) 251.5, 456.0, 530.20-530.21, 530.7, 530.82, 530.85, 531.00-534.91,
      535.01, 535.11, 535.21, 535.31, 535.41, 535.51, 535.61, 535.71,
      537.3, 537.83, 537.89-538, 562.02-562.03, 562.12-562.13, 569.3,
      569.85, 578.0-578.9

●**532.1 Acute with perforation**🔖
[0-1]   (Ex:) 251.5, 456.0, 530.20-530.21, 530.7, 530.82, 530.85, 531.00-534.91,
      535.01, 535.11, 535.21, 535.31, 535.41, 535.51, 535.61, 535.71,
      537.3, 537.83, 537.89-538, 562.02-562.03, 562.12-562.13, 569.3,
      569.85, 578.0-578.9

●**532.2 Acute with hemorrhage and perforation**🔖
[0-1]   (Ex:) 251.5, 456.0, 530.20-530.21, 530.7, 530.82, 530.85, 531.00-534.91,
      535.01, 535.11, 535.21, 535.31, 535.41, 535.51, 535.61, 535.71,
      537.3, 537.83, 537.89-538, 562.02-562.03, 562.12-562.13, 569.3,
      569.85, 578.0-578.9

●**532.3 Acute without mention of hemorrhage or**
[0-1]   **perforation** 0🔖, 1🔖
      For code **532.30**: (Ex:) 251.5, 456.0, 530.7, 530.82, 531.00-534.91, 535.01,
      535.11, 535.21, 535.31, 535.41, 535.51, 535.61, 535.71, 537.3,
      537.83-538, 562.02-562.03, 562.12-562.13, 569.3, 569.85,
      578.0-578.9;
      For code **532.31**: (Ex:) 251.5, 456.0, 530.20-530.21, 530.7, 530.82, 530.85,
      531.00-534.91, 535.01, 535.11, 535.21, 535.31, 535.41, 535.51,
      535.61, 535.71, 537.3, 537.83, 537.89-538, 562.02-562.03,
      562.12-562.13, 569.3, 569.85, 578.0-578.9

●**532.4 Chronic or unspecified with hemorrhage**🔖
[0-1]   (Ex:) 251.5, 456.0, 530.20-530.21, 530.7, 530.82, 530.85, 531.00-534.91,
      535.01, 535.11, 535.21, 535.31, 535.41, 535.51, 535.61, 535.71,
      537.3, 537.83, 537.89-538, 562.02-562.03, 562.12-562.13, 569.3,
      569.85, 578.0-578.9

●**532.5 Chronic or unspecified with perforation**🔖
[0-1]   (Ex:) 251.5, 456.0, 530.20-530.21, 530.7, 530.82, 530.85, 531.00-534.91,
      535.01, 535.11, 535.21, 535.31, 535.41, 535.51, 535.61, 535.71,
      537.3, 537.83, 537.89-538, 562.02-562.03, 562.12-562.13, 569.3,
      569.85, 578.0-578.9

●**532.6 Chronic or unspecified with hemorrhage and**
[0-1]   **perforation**🔖
      (Ex:) 251.5, 456.0, 530.20-530.21, 530.7, 530.82, 530.85, 531.00-534.91,
      535.01, 535.11, 535.21, 535.31, 535.41, 535.51, 535.61, 535.71,
      537.3, 537.83, 537.89-538, 562.02-562.03, 562.12-562.13, 569.3,
      569.85, 578.0-578.9

●**532.7 Chronic without mention of hemorrhage or**
[0-1]   **perforation** 1🔖
      (Ex:) 251.5, 456.0, 530.20-530.21, 530.7, 530.82, 530.85, 531.00-534.91,
      535.01, 535.11, 535.21, 535.31, 535.41, 535.51, 535.61, 535.71,
      537.3, 537.83, 537.89-538, 562.02-562.03, 562.12-562.13, 569.3,
      569.85, 578.0-578.9

●**532.9 Unspecified as acute or chronic, without mention of**
[0-1]   **hemorrhage or perforation** 1🔖
      (Ex:) 251.5, 456.0, 530.20-530.21, 530.7, 530.82, 530.85, 531.00-534.91,
      535.01, 535.11, 535.21, 535.31, 535.41, 535.51, 535.61, 535.71,
      537.3, 537.83, 537.89-538, 562.02-562.03, 562.12-562.13, 569.3,
      569.85, 578.0-578.9

●**533 Peptic ulcer, site unspecified**

  Includes   gastroduodenal ulcer NOS
      peptic ulcer NOS
      stress ulcer NOS

  Use additional E code to identify drug, if drug-induced

  Excludes *peptic ulcer:*
      duodenal (532.0–532.9)
      gastric (531.0–531.9)

  Coding Clinic: 1990, Q4, P27

  The following fifth-digit subclassification is for use with category 533:

0	without mention of obstruction
1	with obstruction

●**533.0 Acute with hemorrhage**🔖
[0-1]   (Ex:) 251.5, 456.0, 530.20-530.21, 530.7, 530.82, 530.85, 531.00-534.91,
      535.01, 535.11, 535.21, 535.31, 535.41, 535.51, 535.61, 535.71,
      537.3, 537.83, 537.89-538, 562.02-562.03, 562.12-562.13, 569.3,
      569.85, 578.0-578.9

●**533.1 Acute with perforation**🔖
[0-1]   (Ex:) 251.5, 456.0, 530.20-530.21, 530.7, 530.82, 530.85, 531.00-534.91,
      535.01, 535.11, 535.21, 535.31, 535.41, 535.51, 535.61, 535.71,
      537.3, 537.83, 537.89-538, 562.02-562.03, 562.12-56-13, 569.3,
      569.85, 578.0-578.9

◄ New   ◄▪▪▪ Revised   ~~deleted~~ Deleted   ● Unacceptable Principal Diagnosis   ● Use Additional Digit(s)
▶ Manifestation Code   **OGCR** Official Guidelines   **Coding Clinic**   Excludes   Includes   Use additional   Code first   Omit code

● **533.2 Acute with hemorrhage and perforation** 🗞
[0-1]   (Ex) 251.5, 456.0, 530.20-530.21, 530.7, 530.82, 530.85, 531.00-534.91, 535.01, 535.11, 535.21, 535.31, 535.41, 535.51, 535.61, 535.71, 537.3, 537.83, 537.89-538, 562.02-562.03, 562.12-562.13, 569.3, 569.85, 578.0-578.9

● **533.3 Acute without mention of hemorrhage and**
[0-1] **perforation 0** 🗞**, 1** 🗞
(Ex) 251.5, 456.0, 530.20-530.21, 530.7, 530.82, 530.85, 531.00-534.91, 535.01, 535.11, 535.21, 535.31, 535.41, 535.51, 535.61, 535.71, 537.3, 537.83, 537.89-538, 562.02-562.03, 562.12-562.13, 569.3, 569.85, 578.0-578.9

● **533.4 Chronic or unspecified with hemorrhage** 🗞
[0-1]   (Ex) 251.5, 456.0, 530.20-530.21, 530.7, 530.82, 530.85, 531.00-534.91, 535.01, 535.11, 535.21, 535.31, 535.41, 535.51, 535.61, 535.71, 537.3, 537.83, 537.89-538, 562.02-562.03, 562.12-562.13, 569.3, 569.85, 578.0-578.9

● **533.5 Chronic or unspecified with perforation** 🗞
[0-1]   (Ex) 251.5, 456.0, 530.20-530.21, 530.7 530.82, 530.85, 531.00-534.91, 535.01 535.11, 535.21, 535.31, 535.41, 535.51, 535.61, 535.71, 537.3, 537.83, 537.89-538, 562.02-562.03, 562.12-562.13, 569.3, 569.85, 578.0-578.9

● **533.6 Chronic or unspecified with hemorrhage and**
[0-1] **perforation** 🗞
(Ex) 251.5, 456.0, 530.20-530.21, 530.7, 530.82, 530.85, 531.00-534.91, 535.01 535.11, 535.21, 535.31, 535.41, 535.51, 535.61, 535.71, 537.3, 537.83, 537.89-538, 562.02-562.03, 562.12-562.13, 569.3, 569.85, 578.0-578.9

● **533.7 Chronic without mention of hemorrhage or**
[0-1] **perforation 1** 🗞
For code **533.71:** (Ex) 251.5, 456.0, 530.20-530.21, 530.7, 530.82, 530.85, 531.00-534.91, 535.01, 535.11, 535.21, 535.31, 535.41, 535.51, 535.61, 535.71, 537.3, 537.83, 537.89-538, 562.02-562.03, 562.12-562.13, 569.3, 569.85, 578.0-578.9

Coding Clinic: 1989, Q2, P16

● **533.9 Unspecified as acute or chronic, without mention of**
[0-1] **hemorrhage or perforation 1** 🗞
For code **533.91:** (Ex) 251.5, 456.0, 530.20-530.21, 530.7, 530.82, 530.85, 531.00-534.91, 535.01, 535.11, 535.21, 535.31, 535.41, 535.51, 535.61, 535.71, 537.3, 537.83, 537.89-538, 562.02-562.03, 562.12-562.13, 569.3, 569.85, 578.0-578.9

● **534 Gastrojejunal ulcer**
| **Includes** | ulcer (peptic) or erosion: |

        anastomotic
        gastrocolic
        gastrointestinal
        gastrojejunal
        jejunal
        marginal
        stomal

| **Excludes** | *primary ulcer of small intestine (569.82)* |

Coding Clinic: 1990, Q4, P27

The following fifth-digit subclassification is for use with category 534:

| **0** | **without mention of obstruction** |
| **1** | **with obstruction** |

● **534.0 Acute with hemorrhage** 🗞
[0-1]   (Ex) 251.5, 456.0, 530.20-530.21, 530.7, 530.82, 530.85, 531.00-534.91, 535.01, 535.11, 535.21, 535.31, 535.41, 535.51, 535.61, 535.71, 537.83, 537.89-538, 562.02-562.03, 562.12-562.13, 569.3, 569.85, 578.0-578.9

● **534.1 Acute with perforation** 🗞
[0-1]   (Ex) 251.5, 4560, 530.20-530.21, 530.7, 530.82, 530.85, 531.00-534.91, 535.01, 535.11, 535.21, 535.31, 535.41, 535.51, 535.61, 535.71, 537.83, 537.89-538, 562.02-562.03, 562.12-562.13, 569.3, 569.85, 578.0-578.9

● **534.2 Acute with hemorrhage and perforation** 🗞
[0-1]   (Ex) 251.5, 456.0, 530.20-530.21, 530.7, 530.82, 530.85, 531.00-534.91, 535.01, 535.11, 535.21, 535.31, 535.41, 535.51, 535.61, 535.71, 537.83, 537.89-538, 562.02-562.03, 562.12-562.13, 569.3, 569.85, 578.0-578.9

● **534.3 Acute without mention of hemorrhage or**
[0-1] **perforation 0** 🗞**, 1** 🗞
(Ex) 251.5, 456.0, 530.20-530.21, 530.7, 530.82, 530.85, 531.00-534.91, 535.01, 535.11, 535.21, 535.31, 535.41, 535.51, 535.61, 535.71, 537.83, 537.89-538, 562.02-562.03, 562.12-562.13, 569.3, 569.85, 578.0-578.9

● **534.4 Chronic or unspecified with hemorrhage** 🗞
[0-1]   (Ex) 251.5, 456.0, 530.20-530.21, 530.7, 530.82, 530.85, 531.00-534.91, 535.01, 535.11, 535.21, 535.31, 535.41, 535.51, 535.61, 535.71, 537.83, 537.89-538, 562.02-562.03, 562.12-562.13, 569.3, 569.85, 578.0-578.9

● **534.5 Chronic or unspecified with perforation** 🗞
[0-1]   (Ex) 251.5, 456.0, 530.20-530.21, 530.7, 530.82, 530.85, 531.00-534.91, 535.01, 535.11, 535.21, 535.31, 535.41, 535.51, 535.61, 535.71, 537.83, 537.89-538, 562.02-562.03, 562.12-562.13, 569.3, 569.85, 578.0-578.9

DISEASES OF THE DIGESTIVE SYSTEM (520–579)

● **534.6 Chronic or unspecified with hemorrhage and**
[0-1] **perforation**🔍
Ⓔⓧ 251.5, 456.0, 530.20-530.21, 530.7, 530.82, 530.85, 531.00-534.91, 535.01, 535.11, 535.21, 535.31, 535.41, 535.51, 535.61, 535.71, 537.83, 537.89-538, 562.02-562.03, 562.12-562.13, 569.3, 569.85, 578.0-578.9

● **534.7 Chronic without mention of hemorrhage or**
[0-1] **perforation** 1🔍
For code **534.71:** Ⓔⓧ 251.5, 456.0, 530.20-530.21, 530.7, 530.82, 530.85, 531.00-534.91, 535.01, 535.11, 535.21, 535.31, 535.41, 535.51, 535.61, 535.71, 537.83, 537.89-538, 562.02-562.03, 562.12-562.13, 569.3, 569.85, 578.0-578.9

● **534.9 Unspecified as acute or chronic, without mention of**
[0-1] **hemorrhage or perforation** 1🔍
For code **534.91:** Ⓔⓧ 251.5, 456.0, 530.20-530.21, 530.7, 530.82, 530.85, 531.00-534.91, 535.01, 535.11, 535.21, 535.31, 535.41, 535.51, 535.61, 535.71, 537.83, 537.89-538, 562.02-562.03, 562.12-562.13, 569.3, 569.85, 578.0-578.9

Item 9–12 Gastritis is a severe inflammation of the stomach. **Atrophic gastritis** is a chronic inflammation of the stomach that results in destruction of the cells of the mucosa of the stomach. Duodenitis is an inflammation of the duodenum, the first section of the small intestine.

● **535 Gastritis and duodenitis**
Coding Clinic: 2007, Q2, P13; 2005, Q3, P17-18

The following fifth-digit subclassification is for use with category 535:

> **0 without mention of hemorrhage**
> **1 with hemorrhage**

● **535.0 Acute gastritis** 1🔍
[0-1] For code **535.01:** Ⓔⓧ 251.5, 456.0, 530.20-530.21, 530.7, 530.82, 530.85, 531.00-534.91, 535.01, 535.11, 535.21, 535.31, 535.41, 535.51, 535.61, 535.71, 537.83, 562.02-562.03, 562.12-562.13, 569.3, 569.85, 578.0-578.9
Coding Clinic: 1992, Q2, P8-9; 1986, Nov-Dec, P9

● **535.1 Atrophic gastritis** 1🔍
[0-1] Gastritis:
atrophic-hyperplastic   chronic (atrophic)
For code **535.11:** Ⓔⓧ 251.5, 456.0, 530.20-530.21, 530.7, 530.82, 530.85, 531.00-534.91, 535.01, 535.11, 535.21, 535.31, 535.41, 535.51, 535.61, 535.71, 537.83, 562.02-562.03, 562.12-562.13, 569.3, 569.85, 578.0-578.9
Coding Clinic: 1994, Q1, P18

● **535.2 Gastric mucosal hypertrophy** 1🔍
[0-1] Hypertrophic gastritis
For code **535.21:** Ⓔⓧ 251.5, 456.0, 530.20-530.21, 530.7, 530.82, 530.85, 531.00-534.91, 535.01, 535.11, 535.21, 535.31, 535.41, 535.51, 535.61, 535.71, 537.83, 562.02-562.03, 562.12-562.13, 569.3, 569.85, 578.0-578.9

● **535.3 Alcoholic gastritis** 1🔍
[0-1] For code **535.31:** Ⓔⓧ 251.5, 456.0, 530.20-530.21, 530.7, 530.82, 530.85, 531.00-534.91, 535.01, 535.11, 535.21, 535.31, 535.41, 535.51, 535.61, 535.71, 537.83, 562.02-562.03, 562.12-562.13, 569.3, 569.85, 578.0-578.9

● **535.4 Other specified gastritis** 1🔍
[0-1] Gastritis:
allergic
bile induced
irritant
superficial
toxic

> **Excludes** *eosinophilic gastritis (535.7)*

For code **535.41:** Ⓔⓧ 251.5, 456.0, 530.20-530.21, 530.7, 530.82, 530.85, 531.00-534.91, 535.01, 535.11, 535.21, 535.31, 535.41, 535.51, 535.61, 535.71, 537.83, 562.02-562.03, 562.12-562.13, 569.3, 569.85, 578.0-578.9
Coding Clinic: 1990, Q4, P27

● **535.5 Unspecified gastritis and gastroduodenitis** 1🔍
[0-1] For code **535.51:** Ⓔⓧ 251.5, 456.0, 530.20-530.21, 530.7, 530.82, 530.85, 531.00-534.91, 535.01, 535.11, 535.21, 535.31, 535.41, 535.51, 535.61, 535.71, 537.83, 562.02-562.03, 562.12-562.13, 569.3, 569.85, 578.0-578.9
Coding Clinic: 2005, Q3, P17-18; 1999, Q4, P25-26; 1992, Q3, P15

● **535.6 Duodenitis** 1🔍
[0-1] For code **535.61:** Ⓔⓧ 251.5, 456.0, 530.20-530.21, 530.7, 530.82, 530.85, 531.00-534.91, 535.01, 535.11, 535.21, 535.31, 535.41, 535.51, 535.61, 535.71, 537.83, 562.02-562.03, 562.12-562.13, 569.3, 569.85, 578.0-578.9
Coding Clinic: 2005, Q3, P17-18

● **535.7 Eosinophilic gastritis** 1🔍
[0-1] For code **535.71:** Ⓔⓧ 251.5, 456.0, 530.20-530.21, 530.7, 530.82, 530.85, 531.00-534.91, 535.01, 535.11, 535.21, 535.31, 535.41, 535.51, 535.61-535.71, 537.83, 558.41, 562.02-562.03, 562.12-562.13, 569.3, 569.85, 578.0-578.9
Coding Clinic: 2008, Q4, P115-116

● **536 Disorders of function of stomach**

> **Excludes** *functional disorders of stomach specified as psychogenic (306.4)*

536.0 Achlorhydria

536.1 Acute dilatation of stomach🔍
Acute distention of stomach
Ⓔⓧ 536.1

536.2 Persistent vomiting
Cyclical vomiting
Habit vomiting
Persistent vomiting [not of pregnancy]
Uncontrollable vomiting

> **Excludes** *bilious emesis (vomiting) (787.04)* ◀
> *excessive vomiting in pregnancy (643.0–643.9)*
> *vomiting NOS (787.03)*
> *cyclical, associated with migraine (346.2)*
> *vomiting fecal matter (569.87)* ◀

536.3 Gastroparesis
Gastroparalysis

> *Code first* underlying disease, such as:
> diabetes mellitus (249.6, 250.6)
> Coding Clinic: 2004, Q2, P7-8x2; 2001, Q2, P4

Item 9–13 Achlorhydria, also known as gastric anacidity, is the absence of gastric acid. **Gastroparesis** is paralysis of the stomach.

◀ New   ◀▥ Revised   ~~deleted~~ Deleted   ● Unacceptable Principal Diagnosis   ● Use Additional Digit(s)
▶ Manifestation Code   **OGCR** Official Guidelines   **Coding Clinic**   Excludes   Includes   Use additional   Code first   Omit code

DISEASES OF THE DIGESTIVE SYSTEM (520–579)

● **536.4 Gastrostomy complications**

　536.40 Gastrostomy complication, unspecified

　536.41 Infection of gastrostomy🦠

　　Use additional code to identify type of
　　　infection, such as:
　　　abscess or cellulitis of abdomen (682.2)
　　　septicemia (038.0–038.9)

　　Use additional code to identify organism
　　　(041.00–041.9)

　　Ⓔₓ 530.86-530.87, 536.40-536.49, 997.4, 997.71, 997.91-997.99,
　　　998.81, 998.83-998.9
　　Coding Clinic: 1998, Q4, P42-44

　536.42 Mechanical complication of gastrostomy🦠
　　Ⓔₓ 530.86-530.87, 536.40-536.49, 997.4, 997.71, 997.91-997.99,
　　　998.81, 998.83-998.9

　536.49 Other gastrostomy complications
　　Coding Clinic: 1998, Q4, P42-44

**536.8 Dyspepsia and other specified disorders of function
　　of stomach**

Achylia gastrica	Hyperchlorhydria
Hourglass contraction	Hypochlorhydria
of stomach	Indigestion
Hyperacidity	Tachygastria

　　Excludes | *achlorhydria (536.0)*
　　　　　　　heartburn (787.1)
　　Coding Clinic: 1993, Q2, P6; 1989, Q2, P16; 1984, Nov-Dec, P9

536.9 Unspecified functional disorder of stomach
　　Functional gastrointestinal:
　　　disorder
　　　disturbance
　　　irritation
　　Coding Clinic: 2007, Q1, P19

● **537 Other disorders of stomach and duodenum**

　537.0 Acquired hypertrophic pyloric stenosis🦠
　　Constriction of pylorus, acquired or adult
　　Obstruction of pylorus, acquired or adult
　　Stricture of pylorus, acquired or adult

　　Excludes | *congenital or infantile pyloric stenosis*
　　　　　　　(750.5)
　　Ⓔₓ 536.3, 536.8-537.0, 537.3, 750.5, 750.8-750.9, 751.1, 751.5
　　Coding Clinic: 2001, Q2, P17-18; 1985, Jan-Feb, P14-15

　537.1 Gastric diverticulum

　　Excludes | *congenital diverticulum of stomach (750.7)*

　537.2 Chronic duodenal ileus

　537.3 Other obstruction of duodenum🦠
　　Cicatrix of duodenum
　　　Cicatrix = scar
　　Stenosis of duodenum
　　　Stenosis = narrowing
　　Stricture of duodenum
　　　Stricture = narrowing
　　Volvulus of duodenum
　　　Volvulus = twisting/knotting

　　Excludes | *congenital obstruction of duodenum (751.1)*
　　Ⓔₓ 537.3, 750.8-750.9, 751.1, 751.5

537.4 Fistula of stomach or duodenum🦠
　　Gastrocolic fistula
　　Gastrojejunocolic fistula
　　Ⓔₓ 537.4, 750.8-750.9, 751.5

537.5 Gastroptosis

537.6 Hourglass stricture or stenosis of stomach
　　Cascade stomach

　　Excludes | *congenital hourglass stomach (750.7)*
　　　　　　　hourglass contraction of stomach (536.8)

● **537.8 Other specified disorders of stomach and duodenum**

　537.81 Pylorospasm

　　Excludes | *congenital pylorospasm (750.5)*

　**537.82 Angiodysplasia of stomach and duodenum
　　　without mention of hemorrhage**
　　Coding Clinic: 2007, Q2, P9; 1996, Q3, P10

　**537.83 Angiodysplasia of stomach and duodenum
　　　with hemorrhage**🦠
　　Ⓔₓ 251.5, 456.0, 530.20-530.21, 530.7, 530.82, 530.85,
　　　531.00-534.91, 535.01, 535.11, 535.21, 535.31, 535.41,
　　　535.51, 535.61, 535.71, 537.83, 562.02-562.03,
　　　562.12-562.13, 569.3, 569.85, 578.0-578.9
　　Coding Clinic: 2007, Q2, P9

　**537.84 Dieulafoy lesion (hemorrhagic) of stomach
　　　and duodenum**🦠
　　Ⓔₓ 251.5, 456.0, 530.20-530.21, 530.7, 530.82, 530.85,
　　　531.00-534.91, 535.01, 535.11, 535.21, 535.31, 535.41,
　　　535.51, 535.61, 535.71, 537.83-537.84, 562.02-562.03,
　　　562.12-562.13, 569.3, 569.85, 578.0-578.9
　　Coding Clinic: 2002, Q4, P60-61

　537.89 Other
　　Gastric or duodenal:
　　　prolapse
　　　rupture
　　Intestinal metaplasia of gastric mucosa
　　Passive congestion of stomach

　　Excludes | *diverticula of duodenum*
　　　　　　　(562.00–562.01)
　　　　　　　gastrointestinal hemorrhage
　　　　　　　(578.0–578.9)
　　Coding Clinic: 2005, Q3, P15-16

537.9 Unspecified disorder of stomach and duodenum

538 Gastrointestinal mucositis (ulcerative)🦠

　　Use additional E code to identify adverse effects of
　　　therapy, such as:
　　antineoplastic and immunosuppressive drugs (E930.7,
　　　E933.1)
　　radiation therapy (E879.2)

　　Excludes | *mucositis (ulcerative) of mouth and oral soft*
　　　　　　　tissue (528.00–528.09)
　　Ⓔₓ 251.5, 456.0, 530.20-530.21, 530.7, 530.82, 530.85, 531.00-534.91, 535.01,
　　　535.11, 535.21, 535.31, 535.41, 535.51, 535.61, 535.71, 537.83, 537.89-538,
　　　562.02-562.03, 562.12-562.13, 569.3, 569.85, 578.0-578.9

DISEASES OF THE DIGESTIVE SYSTEM (520–579)

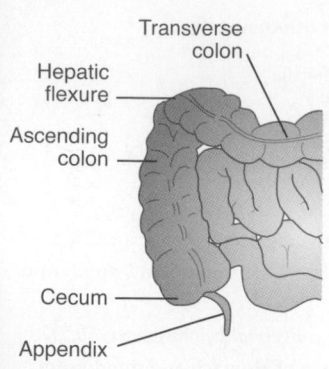

Figure 9–11 Acute appendicitis is the inflammation of the appendix, usually associated with obstruction. Most often this is a disease of adolescents and young adults.

Transverse colon
Hepatic flexure
Ascending colon
Cecum
Appendix

APPENDICITIS (540–543)

● **540 Acute appendicitis**

    540.0 With generalized peritonitis🔱
      Appendicitis (acute) with: perforation, peritonitis (generalized), rupture:
        fulminating
        gangrenous
        obstructive
      Cecitis (acute) with: perforation, peritonitis (generalized), rupture
      Rupture of appendix

        Excludes   *acute appendicitis with peritoneal abscess (540.1)*

        (Ex:) 537.89-543.9
        Coding Clinic: 1984, Nov-Dec, P19

    540.1 With peritoneal abscess🔱
      Abscess of appendix
        With generalized peritonitis
      (Ex:) 537.89-543.9,
      Coding Clinic: 1984, Nov-Dec, P19

    540.9 Without mention of peritonitis🔱
      Acute:
        appendicitis without mention of perforation, peritonitis, or rupture:
          fulminating
          gangrenous
          inflamed
          obstructive
        cecitis without mention of perforation, peritonitis, or rupture
      (Ex:) 537.89-543.9
      Coding Clinic: 2001, Q1, P15-16; 1997, Q4, P52

  541 Appendicitis, unqualified
    Coding Clinic: 1990, Q2, P26

  542 Other appendicitis
    Appendicitis:
      chronic
      recurrent
      relapsing
      subacute

      Excludes   *hyperplasia (lymphoid) of appendix (543.0)*
    Coding Clinic: 2001, Q1, P15-16

● **543 Other diseases of appendix**

    543.0 Hyperplasia of appendix (lymphoid)

    543.9 Other and unspecified diseases of appendix
      Appendicular or appendiceal:
        colic
        concretion
        fistula
      Diverticulum of appendix
      Fecalith of appendix
      Intussusception of appendix
      Mucocele of appendix
      Stercolith of appendix

Right Lumbar | Umbilical | Left Lumbar
RIGHT INGUINAL OR ILIAC | Hypogastric or pubic | LEFT INGUINAL OR ILIAC

Figure 9–12 Inguinal hernias are those that are located in the inguinal or iliac areas of the abdomen.

Item 9–14 Hernias of the groin are the most common type, accounting for 80 percent of all hernias. There are two major types of inguinal hernias: indirect (oblique) affecting men only and direct. **Indirect inguinal hernias** result when the intestines emerge through the abdominal wall in an indirect fashion through the inguinal canal. **Direct inguinal hernias** penetrate through the abdominal wall in a direct fashion. **Femoral hernias** occur at the femoral ring where the femoral vessels enter the thigh and is most common in women. An abdominal wall hernia is also called a ventral or epigastric hernia and occurs in both sexes. Classification is based on location of the hernia and whether there is obstruction or gangrene.

HERNIA OF ABDOMINAL CAVITY (550–553)

    Includes   hernia:
        acquired
        congenital, except diaphragmatic or hiatal

● **550 Inguinal hernia**
    Includes   bubonocele
        inguinal hernia (direct) (double) (indirect) (oblique) (sliding)
        scrotal hernia

The following fifth-digit subclassification is for use with category 550:

> 0 **unilateral or unspecified (not specified as recurrent)**
>   **Unilateral NOS**
> 1 **unilateral or unspecified, recurrent**
> 2 **bilateral (not specified as recurrent)**
>   **Bilateral NOS**
> 3 **bilateral, recurrent**

● **550.0 Inguinal hernia, with gangrene**🔱
  [0-3]   Inguinal hernia with gangrene (and obstruction)
        (Ex:) 537.89-538, 550.00-550.93, 552.8-552.9, 553.8-553.9

● **550.1 Inguinal hernia, with obstruction, without mention**
  [0-3] **of gangrene**🔱
      Inguinal hernia with mention of incarceration, irreducibility, or strangulation
      (Ex:) 537.89-538, 550.00-550.93, 552.8-552.9, 553.8-553.9

◀ New   ◀▥ Revised   ~~deleted~~ Deleted   ● Unacceptable Principal Diagnosis   ● Use Additional Digit(s)
▶ Manifestation Code   **OGCR** Official Guidelines   **Coding Clinic**   [Excludes]   Includes   Use additional   Code first   Omit code

● **550.9** **Inguinal hernia, without mention of obstruction or**
[0-3] **gangrene**
     Inguinal hernia NOS
       Coding Clinic: 2003, Q3, P10-11; 2003, Q1, P4; 1985, Nov-Dec, P12;
       1984, May-June, P11

● **551** **Other hernia of abdominal cavity, with gangrene**
    Includes   that with gangrene (and obstruction)

● **551.0** **Femoral hernia with gangrene**

     551.00 **Unilateral or unspecified (not specified as**
         recurrent) 🔓
         Femoral hernia NOS with gangrene
         (Ex:) 537.89-538, 551.00-551.03, 552.8-553.03, 553.8-553.9

     551.01 **Unilateral or unspecified, recurrent** 🔓
         (Ex:) 537.89-538, 551.00-551.03, 552.8-553.03, 553.8-553.9

     551.02 **Bilateral (not specified as recurrent)** 🔓
         (Ex:) 537.89-538, 551.00-551.03, 552.8-553.03, 553.8-553.9

     551.03 **Bilateral, recurrent** 🔓
         (Ex:) 537.89-538, 551.00-551.03, 552.8-553.03, 553.8-553.9

● **551.1** **Umbilical hernia with gangrene** 🔓
     Parumbilical hernia specified as gangrenous
     (Ex:) 537.89-538, 551.1-551.29, 552.1-552.29, 552.8-55.29, 553.1-553.29,
     553.8-553.9

● **551.2** **Ventral hernia with gangrene**

     551.20 **Ventral, unspecified, with gangrene** 🔓
         (Ex:) 537.89-538, 551.1-551.29, 552.1-552.29, 552.8-552.9,
         553.1-553.29, 553.8-553.9

     551.21 **Incisional, with gangrene** 🔓
         Hernia:
            postoperative specified as gangrenous
            recurrent, ventral specified as
               gangrenous
         (Ex:) 537.89-538, 551.1-551.29, 552.1-552.29, 552.8-552.9,
         553.1-553.29, 553.8-553.9

     551.29 **Other** 🔓
         Epigastric hernia specified as gangrenous
         (Ex:) 537.89-538, 551.1-551.29, 552.1-552.29, 552.8-552.9,
         553.1-553.29, 553.8-553.9

● **551.3** **Diaphragmatic hernia with gangrene** 🔓
     Hernia:
        hiatal (esophageal) (sliding) specified as
           gangrenous
        paraesophageal specified as gangrenous
     Thoracic stomach specified as gangrenous
     Excludes *congenital diaphragmatic hernia (756.6)*
     (Ex:) 551.3, 552.3-552.9, 553.3-553.9

● **551.8** **Hernia of other specified sites, with gangrene** 🔓
     Any condition classifiable to 553.8 if specified as
        gangrenous
     (Ex:) 537.89-538, 550.00-553.9

● **551.9** **Hernia of unspecified site, with gangrene** 🔓
     Any condition classifiable to 553.9 if specified as
        gangrenous
     (Ex:) 537.89-538, 550.00-553.9

● **552** **Other hernia of abdominal cavity, with obstruction, but**
without mention of gangrene
    Excludes   *that with mention of gangrene (551.0–551.9)*

● **552.0** **Femoral hernia with obstruction**
     Femoral hernia specified as incarcerated, irreducible,
        strangulated, or causing obstruction

     552.00 **Unilateral or unspecified (not specified as**
         recurrent) 🔓
         (Ex:) 537.89-538, 551.00-551.03, 552.00-552.03, 552.8-553.03,
         553.8-553.9

     552.01 **Unilateral or unspecified, recurrent** 🔓
         (Ex:) 537.89-538, 551.00-551.03, 552.00-552.03, 552.8-553.03,
         553.8-553.9

     552.02 **Bilateral (not specified as recurrent)** 🔓
         (Ex:) 53.789-538, 551.00-551.03, 552.00-552.03, 552.8-553.03,
         553.8-553.9

     552.03 **Bilateral, recurrent** 🔓
         (Ex:) 537.89-538, 551.00-551.03, 552.00-552.03, 552.8-553.03,
         553.8-553.9

● **552.1** **Umbilical hernia with obstruction** 🔓
     (Ex:) 551.1-551.29, 552.1-552.29, 552.8-552.9, 553.8-553.9
     Parumbilical hernia specified as incarcerated,
        irreducible, strangulated, or causing
        obstruction

● **552.2** **Ventral hernia with obstruction**
     Ventral hernia specified as incarcerated, irreducible,
        strangulated, or causing obstruction

     552.20 **Ventral, unspecified, with obstruction** 🔓
         (Ex:) 551.1-551.29, 552.1-552.29, 552.8-552.9, 553.8-553.9

     552.21 **Incisional, with obstruction** 🔓
         Hernia:
            postoperative specified as incarcerated,
               irreducible, strangulated, or
               causing obstruction
            recurrent, ventral specified as
               incarcerated, irreducible,
               strangulated, or causing
               obstruction
         (Ex:) 551.1-551.29, 552.1-552.29, 552.8-552.9, 553.8-553.9
         Coding Clinic: 2003, Q3, P11

     552.29 **Other** 🔓
         Epigastric hernia specified as incarcerated,
            irreducible, strangulated, or causing
            obstruction
         (Ex:) 551.1-551.29, 552.1-552.29, 552.8-552.9, 553.8-553.9

Item 9-15 Ventral, epigastric, or incisional hernia occurs on the abdominal surface caused by musculature weakness or a tear at a previous surgical site and is evidenced by a bulge that changes in size, becoming larger with exertion. An **incarcerated** hernia is one in which the intestines become trapped in the hernia. A **strangulated** hernia is one in which the blood supply to the intestines is lost. Hiatal hernia occurs when a loop of the stomach protrudes upward through the small opening in the diaphragm through which the esophagus passes, leaving the abdominal cavity and entering the chest. It occurs in both sexes.

N Newborn Age: 0   **P** Pediatric Age: 0–17   **M** Maternity Age: 12–55   **A** Adult Age: 15–124   ♀ Females Only   ♂ Males Only

(Ex:) CC Exclusions   🔓 Complication\Comorbidity   🔓 Major C\C   🔓 Present on Admission Requirement   🔓 Hospital-Acquired Condition   937

DISEASES OF THE DIGESTIVE SYSTEM (520–579)

552.3 Diaphragmatic hernia with obstruction 🔍
   Hernia:
     hiatal (esophageal) (sliding) specified as incarcerated, irreducible, strangulated, or causing obstruction
     paraesophageal specified as incarcerated, irreducible, strangulated, or causing obstruction
     Thoracic stomach specified as incarcerated, irreducible, strangulated, or causing obstruction

> **Excludes**   *congenital diaphragmatic hernia (756.6)*

   (Ex:) 551.3, 552.3-552.9, 553.3-553.9

552.8 Hernia of other specified sites, with obstruction 🔍
   Any condition classifiable to 553.8 if specified as incarcerated, irreducible, strangulated, or causing obstruction

> **Excludes**   *hernia due to adhesion with obstruction (560.81)*

   (Ex:) 550.00-553.9
   Coding Clinic: 2004, Q1, P10-11

552.9 Hernia of unspecified site, with obstruction 🔍
   Any condition classifiable to 553.9 if specified as incarcerated, irreducible, strangulated, or causing obstruction

   (Ex:) 550.00-553.9

● **553   Other hernia of abdominal cavity without mention of obstruction or gangrene**

> **Excludes**   *the listed conditions with mention of:*
>   *gangrene (and obstruction) (551.0–551.9)*
>   *obstruction (552.0–552.9)*

● **553.0 Femoral hernia**

   553.00 Unilateral or unspecified (not specified as recurrent)
     Femoral hernia NOS

   553.01 Unilateral or unspecified, recurrent

   553.02 Bilateral (not specified as recurrent)

   553.03 Bilateral, recurrent

553.1 Umbilical hernia
   Parumbilical hernia

● **553.2 Ventral hernia**

   553.20 Ventral, unspecified
     Coding Clinic: 2006, Q2, P10-11; 2003, Q3, P6-7; 1996, Q3, P15

   553.21 Incisional
     Hernia:
       postoperative
       recurrent, ventral
     Coding Clinic: 2003, Q3, P6

   553.29 Other
     Hernia:
       epigastric
       spigelian

553.3 Diaphragmatic hernia
   Hernia:
     hiatal (esophageal) (sliding)
     paraesophageal
   Thoracic stomach

> **Excludes**   *congenital:*
>   *diaphragmatic hernia (756.6)*
>   *hiatal hernia (750.6)*
>   *esophagocele (530.6)*

   Coding Clinic: 2001, Q2, P6; 2000, Q1, P6

553.8 Hernia of other specified sites
   Hernia:
     ischiatic
     ischiorectal
     lumbar
     obturator
     pudendal
     retroperitoneal
     sciatic
   Other abdominal hernia of specified site

> **Excludes**   *vaginal enterocele (618.6)*

553.9 Hernia of unspecified site
   Enterocele
   Epiplocele
   Hernia:
     NOS
     interstitial
     intestinal
     intra-abdominal
   Rupture (nontraumatic)
   Sarcoepiplocele

NONINFECTIOUS ENTERITIS AND COLITIS (555–558)

● **555   Regional enteritis**

> **Includes**   Crohn's disease
>   Granulomatous enteritis

> **Excludes**   *ulcerative colitis (556)*

555.0 Small intestine 🔍
   Ileitis:
     regional
     segmental
     terminal
   Regional enteritis or Crohn's disease of:
     duodenum
     ileum
     jejunum
   (Ex:) 555.0-556.9

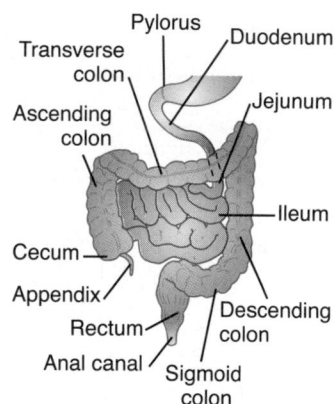

Figure 9–13   Small and large intestines.

Item 9–16   Crohn's disease, also known as **regional enteritis,** is a chronic inflammatory disease of the intestines. Classification is based on location in the small (duodenum, ileum, jejunum) or large (cecum, colon, rectum, anal canal) intestine.

◄ New   ◄▥ Revised   ~~deleted~~ Deleted   ● Unacceptable Principal Diagnosis   ● Use Additional Digit(s)
▶ Manifestation Code   OGCR Official Guidelines   Coding Clinic   Excludes   Includes   Use additional   Code first   Omit code

555.1 Large intestine 🦠
    Colitis:
       granulomatous
       regional
       transmural
    Regional enteritis or Crohn's disease of:
       colon
       large bowel
       rectum
    Ⓔ 555.0-556.9
    Coding Clinic: 1999, Q3, P8

555.2 Small intestine with large intestine 🦠
    Regional ileocolitis
    Ⓔ 555.0-556.9
    Coding Clinic: 2003, Q1, P18

555.9 Unspecified site 🦠
    Crohn's disease NOS
    Regional enteritis NOS
    Ⓔ 555.0-555.9
    Coding Clinic: 2009, Q1, P20; 2005, Q2, P11-12; 1999, Q3, P8-9;
        1997, Q4, P37; Q2, P3; 1996, Q1, P13; 1988, Q2, P9-10

● **556 Ulcerative colitis**

556.0 Ulcerative (chronic) enterocolitis 🦠
    Ⓔ 555.0-556.9

556.1 Ulcerative (chronic) ileocolitis 🦠
    Ⓔ 555.0-556.9

556.2 Ulcerative (chronic) proctitis 🦠
    Ⓔ 555.0-556.9

> **Item 9–17 Ulcerative colitis** attacks the colonic mucosa and forms abscesses. The disease involves the intestines. Classification is based on the location:
>   Enterocolitis: large and small intestine
>   Ileocolitis: ileum and colon
>   Proctitis: rectum
>   Proctosigmoiditis: sigmoid colon and rectum

556.3 Ulcerative (chronic) proctosigmoiditis 🦠
    Ⓔ 555.0-556.9

556.4 Pseudopolyposis of colon 🦠
    Ⓔ 555.0-556.9

556.5 Left-sided ulcerative (chronic) colitis 🦠
    Ⓔ 555.0-556.9

556.6 Universal ulcerative (chronic) colitis 🦠
    Pancolitis
    Ⓔ 555.0-556.9

556.8 Other ulcerative colitis 🦠
    Ⓔ 555.0-556.9

556.9 Ulcerative colitis, unspecified 🦠
    Ulcerative enteritis NOS
    Ⓔ 556.0-556.9
    Coding Clinic: 2003, Q1, P10-11

● **557 Vascular insufficiency of intestine**

> **Excludes**   *necrotizing enterocolitis of the newborn*
>   *(777.50–777.53)*

557.0 Acute vascular insufficiency of intestine 🦠
    Acute:
       hemorrhagic enterocolitis
       ischemic colitis, enteritis, or enterocolitis
       massive necrosis of intestine
    Bowel infarction
    Embolism of mesenteric artery
    Fulminant enterocolitis
    Hemorrhagic necrosis of intestine
    Infarction of appendices epiploicae
    Intestinal gangrene
    Intestinal infarction (acute) (agnogenic)
       (hemorrhagic) (nonocclusive)
    Mesenteric infarction (embolic) (thrombotic)
    Necrosis of intestine
    Terminal hemorrhagic enteropathy
    Thrombosis of mesenteric artery
    Ⓔ 557.0-557.1
    Coding Clinic: 2008, Q2, P15-16

557.1 Chronic vascular insufficiency of intestine 🦠
    Angina, abdominal
    Chronic ischemic colitis, enteritis, or enterocolitis
    Ischemic stricture of intestine
    Mesenteric:
       angina
       artery syndrome (superior)
       vascular insufficiency
    Ⓔ 557.0-557.9
    Coding Clinic: 1996, Q3, P9-10; 1986, Nov-Dec, P11; 1985,
        Sept-Oct, P9

557.9 Unspecified vascular insufficiency of intestine 🦠
    Alimentary pain due to vascular insufficiency
    Ischemic colitis, enteritis, or enterocolitis NOS
    Ⓔ 557.0-557.9

N Newborn Age: 0   **P** Pediatric Age: 0–17   **M** Maternity Age: 12–55   **A** Adult Age: 15–124   ♀ Females Only   ♂ Males Only

Ⓔ CC Exclusions   🦠 Complication\Comorbidity   🦠 Major C\C   🦠 Present on Admission Requirement   🦠 Hospital-Acquired Condition   **939**

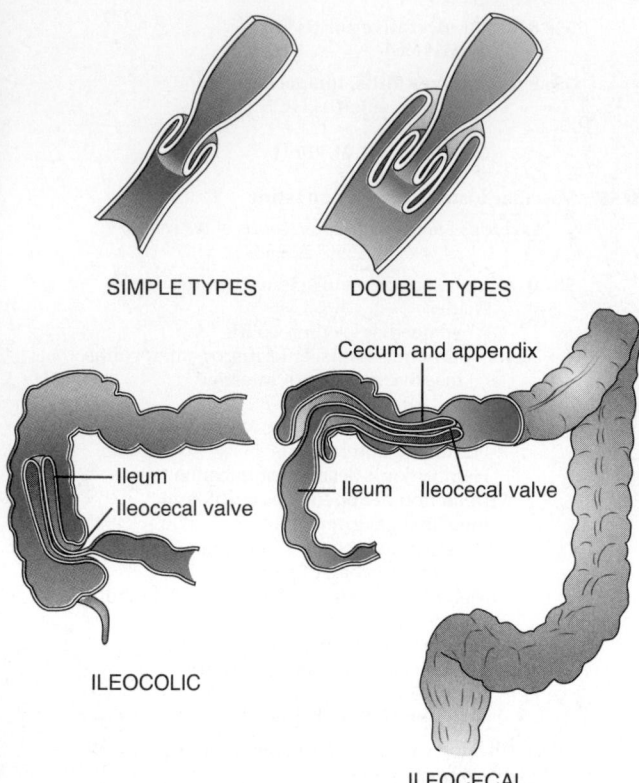

SIMPLE TYPES   DOUBLE TYPES

Cecum and appendix

Ileum
Ileocecal valve

Ileum   Ileocecal valve

ILEOCOLIC

ILEOCECAL

Figure 9–14 Types of intussusception.

● **558 Other and unspecified noninfectious gastroenteritis and colitis**

| Excludes | infectious:
colitis, enteritis, or gastroenteritis
(009.0–009.1)
diarrhea (009.2–009.3)

558.1 Gastroenteritis and colitis due to radiation🐾
Radiation enterocolitis
Ⓔ 558.1

558.2 Toxic gastroenteritis and colitis🐾
| Use additional | E code to identify cause
Ⓔ 558.2
Coding Clinic: 2008, Q2, P10-11

558.3 Allergic gastroenteritis and colitis
| Use additional | code to identify type of food allergy
(V15.01–V15.05)
Coding Clinic: 2008, Q4, P115-116; 2003, Q1, P12

● **558.4 Eosinophilic gastroenteritis and colitis**

558.41 Eosinophilic gastroenteritis
Eosinophilic enteritis
Coding Clinic: 2008, Q4, P115-116

558.42 Eosinophilic colitis
Coding Clinic: 2008, Q4, P115-116

558.9 Other and unspecified noninfectious gastroenteritis and colitis
Colitis, NOS, dietetic, or noninfectious
Enteritis, NOS, dietetic, or noninfectious
Gastroenteritis, NOS, dietetic, or noninfectious
Ileitis, NOS, dietetic or noninfectious
Jejunitis, NOS, dietetic, or noninfectious
Sigmoiditis, NOS, dietetic, or noninfectious
Coding Clinic: 2008, Q2, P10-11; Q1, P10-12; 1999, Q3, P4-7; 1987, Nov-Dec, P7-8; 1984, July-Aug, P19-20

Item 9–18 Intussusception is the prolapse (telescoping) of a part of the intestine into another adjacent part of the intestine. Intussusception may be enteric (ileoileal, jejunoileal, jejunojejunal), colic (colocolic), or intracolic (ileocecal, ileocolic).

Item 9–19 Volvulus is the twisting of a segment of the intestine, resulting in obstruction. Paralytic ileus is paralysis of the intestine. It need not be a complete paralysis, but it must prohibit the passage of food through the intestine and lead to intestinal blockage. It is a common aftermath of some types of surgery.

OTHER DISEASES OF INTESTINES AND PERITONEUM (560–569)

● **560 Intestinal obstruction without mention of hernia**

| Excludes | duodenum (537.2–537.3)
inguinal hernia with obstruction (550.1)
intestinal obstruction complicating hernia
(552.0–552.9)
mesenteric:
embolism (557.0)
infarction (557.0)
thrombosis (557.0)
neonatal intestinal obstruction (277.01,
777.1–777.2, 777.4)

560.0 Intussusception🐾
Intussusception (colon) (intestine) (rectum)
Invagination of intestine or colon

| Excludes | intussusception of appendix (543.9)
Ⓔ 560.0-560.9, 569.89-569.9
Coding Clinic: 1998, Q4, P82-83

560.1 Paralytic ileus🐾
Adynamic ileus
Ileus (of intestine) (of bowel) (of colon)
Paralysis of intestine or colon

| Excludes | gallstone ileus (560.31)
Ⓔ 560.0-560.9, 569.89-569.9
Coding Clinic: 1987, Jan-Feb, P13-14

560.2 Volvulus🐾
Knotting of intestine, bowel, or colon
Strangulation of intestine, bowel, or colon
Torsion of intestine, bowel, or colon
Twist of intestine, bowel, or colon
Ⓔ 560.0-560.9, 569.89-569.9

● **560.3 Impaction of intestine**

560.30 Impaction of intestine, unspecified🐾
Impaction of colon
Ⓔ 560.0-560.9, 569.89-569.9

560.31 Gallstone ileus🐾
Obstruction of intestine by gallstone
Ⓔ 560.0-560.9, 569.89-569.9

560.39 Other🐾
Concretion of intestine
Enterolith
Fecal impaction
Ⓔ 560.0-560.9, 569.89-569.9
Coding Clinic: 1998, Q4, P37-38

◄ New   ◄▭ Revised   ~~deleted~~ Deleted   ● Unacceptable Principal Diagnosis   ● Use Additional Digit(s)
▶ Manifestation Code   OGCR Official Guidelines   Coding Clinic   Excludes   Includes   Use additional   Code first   Omit code

DISEASES OF THE DIGESTIVE SYSTEM (520–579)

● **560.8 Other specified intestinal obstruction**

     560.81 Intestinal or peritoneal adhesions with obstruction (postoperative) (postinfection) 🅒

       Excludes *adhesions without obstruction (568.0)*

       Ⓔⓧ 560.0-560.9, 569.89-569.9
       Coding Clinic: 1995, Q3, P6; 1987, Nov-Dec, P9

     560.89 Other 🅒
       Acute pseudo-obstruction of intestine
       Mural thickening causing obstruction

       Excludes *ischemic stricture of intestine (557.1)*

       Ⓔⓧ 560.0-560.9, 569.89-569.9
       Coding Clinic: 1997, Q2, P3

     560.9 Unspecified intestinal obstruction 🅒
       Enterostenosis
       Obstruction of intestine or colon
       Occlusion of intestine or colon
       Stenosis of intestine or colon
       Stricture of intestine or colon

       Excludes *congenital stricture or stenosis of intestine (751.1–751.2)*

       Ⓔⓧ 560.0-560.9, 569.89-569.9

Item 9–20 Diverticula of the intestines are acquired herniations of the mucosa. Diverticulum (singular): Pocket or pouch that bulges outward through a weak spot (herniation) in the colon. Diverticula (plural). **Diverticulosis** is the condition of having diverticula. **Diverticulitis** is inflammation of these pouches or herniations. Classification is based on location (small intestine or colon) and whether it occurs with or without hemorrhage.

● **562 Diverticula of intestine**

     Use additional code to identify any associated:
     peritonitis (567.0–567.9)

     Excludes *congenital diverticulum of colon (751.5)*
                diverticulum of appendix (543.9)
                Meckel's diverticulum (751.0)

● **562.0 Small intestine**

     562.00 Diverticulosis of small intestine (without mention of hemorrhage)
       Diverticulosis:
         duodenum without mention of diverticulitis
         ileum without mention of diverticulitis
         jejunum without mention of diverticulitis

     562.01 Diverticulitis of small intestine (without mention of hemorrhage) 🅒
       Diverticulitis (with diverticulosis):
         duodenum
         ileum
         jejunum
         small intestine
       Ⓔⓧ 562.00-562.03

     562.02 Diverticulosis of small intestine with hemorrhage 🅒🅒
       Ⓔⓧ 251.5, 456.0, 530.20-530.21, 530.7, 530.82, 530.85,
         531.00-534.91, 535.01, 535.11, 535.21, 535.31, 535.41,
         535.51, 535.61, 535.71, 537.83, 562.02-562.03,
         562.12-562.13, 569.3, 569.85, 578.0-578.9

     562.03 Diverticulitis of small intestine with hemorrhage 🅒🅒
       Ⓔⓧ 251.5, 456.0, 530.20-530.21, 530.7, 530.82, 530.85,
         531.00-534.91, 535.01, 535.11, 535.21, 535.31, 535.41,
         535.51, 535.61, 535.71, 537.83, 562.02-562.03,
         562.12-562.13, 569.3, 569.85, 578.0-578.9

● **562.1 Colon**

     562.10 Diverticulosis of colon (without mention of hemorrhage)
       Diverticulosis without mention of diverticulitis:
         NOS
         intestine (large) without mention of diverticulitis
       Diverticular disease (colon) without mention of diverticulitis
       Coding Clinic: 2005, Q3, P17-18; 2002, Q3, P14-15

     562.11 Diverticulitis of colon without mention of hemorrhage 🅒
       Diverticulitis (with diverticulosis):
         NOS
         colon
         intestine (large)
       Ⓔⓧ 562.10-562.13
       Coding Clinic: 1996, Q1, P13-14

     562.12 Diverticulosis of colon with hemorrhage 🅒🅒
       Ⓔⓧ 251.5, 456.0, 530.20-530.21, 530.7, 530.82, 530.85,
         531.00-534.91, 535.01, 535.11, 535.21, 535.31, 535.41,
         535.51, 535.61, 535.71, 537.83, 562.02-562.03,
         562.12-562.13, 569.3, 569.85, 578.0-578.9

     562.13 Diverticulitis of colon with hemorrhage 🅒🅒
       Ⓔⓧ 251.5, 456.0, 530.20-530.21, 530.7, 530.82, 530.85,
         531.00-534.91, 535.01, 535.11, 535.21, 535.31, 535.41,
         535.51, 535.61, 535.71, 537.83, 562.02-562.03,
         562.12-562.13, 569.3, 569.85, 578.0-578.9

● **564 Functional digestive disorders, not elsewhere classified**

     Excludes *functional disorders of stomach (536.0–536.9)*
                those specified as psychogenic (306.4)

● **564.0 Constipation**

     Excludes *psychogenic constipation (306.4)*

     564.00 Constipation, unspecified

     564.01 Slow transit constipation

     564.02 Outlet dysfunction constipation

     564.09 Other constipation

     564.1 Irritable bowel syndrome
       Irritable colon
       Spastic colon

     564.2 Postgastric surgery syndromes
       Dumping syndrome
       Jejunal syndrome
       Postgastrectomy syndrome
       Postvagotomy syndrome

       Excludes *malnutrition following gastrointestinal surgery (579.3)*
                     postgastrojejunostomy ulcer (534.0–534.9)
       Coding Clinic: 1995, Q1, P11

     564.3 Vomiting following gastrointestinal surgery
       Vomiting (bilious) following gastrointestinal surgery

DISEASES OF THE DIGESTIVE SYSTEM (520–579)

N Newborn Age: 0   **P** Pediatric Age: 0–17   **M** Maternity Age: 12–55   **A** Adult Age: 15–124   ♀ Females Only   ♂ Males Only

Ⓔⓧ CC Exclusions   🅒 Complication\Comorbidity   🅒🅒 Major C\C   🅒 Present on Admission Requirement   🅒 Hospital-Acquired Condition   **941**

564.4 Other postoperative functional disorders
Diarrhea following gastrointestinal surgery

> **Excludes** *colostomy and enterostomy complications (569.60–569.69)*

564.5 Functional diarrhea

> **Excludes** *diarrhea:*
> *NOS (787.91)*
> *psychogenic (306.4)*

Coding Clinic: 1988, Q2, P9-10

564.6 Anal spasm
Proctalgia fugax

564.7 Megacolon, other than Hirschsprung's 🔵
Dilatation of colon

> **Excludes** *megacolon:*
> *congenital [Hirschsprung's] (751.3)*
> *toxic (556)*

(Ex:) 564.1-564.9

● **564.8 Other specified functional disorders of intestine**

> **Excludes** *malabsorption (579.0–579.9)*

564.81 Neurogenic bowel 🔵
(Ex:) 564.1-564.9
Coding Clinic: 2001, Q1, P12

564.89 Other functional disorders of intestine
Atony of colon

564.9 Unspecified functional disorder of intestine

Item 9–21 A **fissure** is a groove in the surface, whereas a **fistula** is an abnormal passage. An abscess is an accumulation of pus in a tissue cavity resulting from a bacterial or parasitic infection.

● **565 Anal fissure and fistula**

565.0 Anal fissure

> **Excludes** *anal sphincter tear (healed) (non-traumatic) (old) (569.43)*
> *traumatic (863.89, 863.99)*

565.1 Anal fistula
Fistula:
anorectal
rectal
rectum to skin

> **Excludes** *fistula of rectum to internal organs - see Alphabetic Index*
> *ischiorectal fistula (566)*
> *rectovaginal fistula (619.1)*

Coding Clinic: 2007, Q1, P13

566 Abscess of anal and rectal regions 🔵

Abscess:
ischiorectal
perianal
perirectal

Cellulitis:
anal
perirectal
rectal
Ischiorectal fistula

(Ex:) 566
Coding Clinic: 1999, Q3, P8-9

Item 9-22 Peritonitis is an inflammation of the lining (peritoneum) of the abdominal cavity and surface of the intestines. **Retroperitoneal infections** occur between the posterior parietal peritoneum and posterior abdominal wall where the kidneys, adrenal glands, ureters, duodenum, ascending colon, descending colon, pancreas, and the large vessels and nerves are located. Both are caused by bacteria, parasites, injury, bleeding, or diseases such as systemic lupus erythematosus.

● **567 Peritonitis and retroperitoneal infections**

> **Excludes** *peritonitis:*
> *benign paroxysmal (277.31)*
> *pelvic, female (614.5, 614.7)*
> *periodic familial (277.31)*
> *puerperal (670.8)* ◀▥
> *with or following:*
> *abortion (634–638 with .0, 639.0)*
> *appendicitis (540.0–540.1)*
> *ectopic or molar pregnancy (639.0)*

▶ **567.0 Peritonitis in infectious diseases classified elsewhere** 🔵

Code first underlying disease

> **Excludes** *peritonitis:*
> *gonococcal (098.86)*
> *syphilitic (095.2)*
> *tuberculous (014.0)*

(Ex:) 567.0-567.29, 567.38-567.9, 569.89-569.9

567.1 Pneumococcal peritonitis 🔵
(Ex:) 567.0-567.29, 567.38-567.9, 569.89-569.9

● **567.2 Other suppurative peritonitis**
Coding Clinic: 2005, Q4, P74-77; 1998, Q2, P19-20; 1996, Q1, P13-14; 1987, Jan-Feb, P14-15

567.21 Peritonitis (acute) generalized 🔵
Pelvic peritonitis, male
(Ex:) 567.0-567.29, 567.38-56.79, 569.89-569.9

567.22 Peritoneal abscess 🔵

Abscess (of):
abdominopelvic
mesenteric
omentum
peritoneum

Abscess (of):
retrocecal
subdiaphragmatic
subhepatic
subphrenic

(Ex:) 567.0-567.29, 567.38-567.9, 569.89-569.9

567.23 Spontaneous bacterial peritonitis 🔵

> **Excludes** *bacterial peritonitis NOS (567.29)*

(Ex:) 567.0-567.29, 567.38-567.9, 569.89-569.9

567.29 Other suppurative peritonitis 🔵
Subphrenic peritonitis
(Ex:) 567.0-567.29, 567.38-567.9, 569.89-569.9
Coding Clinic: 2001, Q2, P11-12; 1999, Q3, P9; 1995, Q3, P5

● **567.3 Retroperitoneal infections**

567.31 Psoas muscle abscess 🔵
(Ex:) 567.31, 728.0, 728.11-728.3, 728.81, 728.86

567.38 Other retroperitoneal abscess 🔵
(Ex:) 567.0-567.29, 567.38-567.9, 569.89-569.9
Coding Clinic: 2005, Q4, P74-77; 1998, Q2, P19-20

567.39 Other retroperitoneal infections 🔵
(Ex:) 567.0-567.29, 567.38-567.9, 569.89-569.9

DISEASES OF THE DIGESTIVE SYSTEM (520–579)

◀ New ◀▥ Revised ~~deleted~~ Deleted ● Unacceptable Principal Diagnosis ● Use Additional Digit(s)
▶ Manifestation Code OGCR Official Guidelines Coding Clinic Excludes Includes Use additional Code first Omit code

● **567.8 Other specified peritonitis**

    567.81 Choleperitonitis 🔖
        Peritonitis due to bile
        Ⓔₓ 567.0-567.29, 567.38-567.9, 569.89-569.9

    567.82 Sclerosing mesenteritis 🔖
        Fat necrosis of peritoneum
        (Idiopathic) sclerosing mesenteric fibrosis
        Mesenteric lipodystrophy
        Mesenteric panniculitis
        Retractile mesenteritis
        Ⓔₓ 567.0-567.29, 567.38-567.9, 569.89-569.9
        Coding Clinic: 2005, Q4, P74-77

    567.89 Other specified peritonitis 🔖
        Chronic proliferative peritonitis
        Mesenteric saponification
        Peritonitis due to urine
        Ⓔₓ 567.0-567.29, 567.38-567.9, 569.89-569.9

567.9 Unspecified peritonitis 🔖
    Peritonitis: Peritonitis:
      NOS   of unspecified cause
    Ⓔₓ 567.0-567.29, 567.38-567.9, 569.89-569.9
    Coding Clinic: 2004, Q1, P10-11

● **568 Other disorders of peritoneum**

    568.0 Peritoneal adhesions (postoperative) (postinfection)
        Adhesions (of):   Adhesions (of):
          abdominal (wall)   mesenteric
          diaphragm   omentum
          intestine   stomach
          male pelvis
        Adhesive bands
        Excludes *adhesions:*
               pelvic, female (614.6)
               with obstruction:
                 duodenum (537.3)
                 intestine (560.81)
        Coding Clinic: 2003, Q3, P7&11; 1995, Q3, P7; 1985, Sept-Oct, P11

● **568.8 Other specified disorders of peritoneum**

    568.81 Hemoperitoneum (nontraumatic) 🔖
        Ⓔₓ 568.81

    568.82 Peritoneal effusion (chronic) 🔖
        Excludes *ascites NOS (789.51–789.59)*
        Ⓔₓ 568.82

    568.89 Other
        Peritoneal: Peritoneal:
          cyst   granuloma

568.9 Unspecified disorder of peritoneum

● **569 Other disorders of intestine**

    569.0 Anal and rectal polyp
        Anal and rectal polyp NOS
        Excludes *adenomatous anal and rectal polyp (211.4)*

    569.1 Rectal prolapse
        Procidentia: Prolapse:
          anus (sphincter)   anal canal
          rectum (sphincter)   rectal mucosa
        Proctoptosis
        Excludes *prolapsed hemorrhoids (455.2, 455.5)*

    569.2 Stenosis of rectum and anus
        Stricture of anus (sphincter)

569.3 Hemorrhage of rectum and anus 🔖
    Excludes *gastrointestinal bleeding NOS (578.9)*
               melena (578.1)
    Ⓔₓ 251.5, 456.0, 530.20-530.21, 530.7, 530.82, 530.85, 531.00-534.91,
        535.01, 535.11, 535.21, 535.31, 535.41, 535.51, 535.61, 535.71,
        537.83, 562.02-562.03, 562.12-562.13, 569.3, 569.85, 578.0-578.9
    Coding Clinic: 2005, Q3, P17

● **569.4 Other specified disorders of rectum and anus**

    569.41 Ulcer of anus and rectum 🔖
        Solitary ulcer of anus (sphincter) or rectum
          (sphincter)
        Stercoral ulcer of anus (sphincter) or rectum
          (sphincter)
        Ⓔₓ 569.41

    569.42 Anal or rectal pain
        Coding Clinic: 2003, Q1, P8; 1996, Q1, P13

    569.43 Anal sphincter tear (healed) (old)
        Tear of anus, nontraumatic
        Use additional code for any associated fecal
          incontinence (787.6)
        Excludes *anal fissure (565.0)*
               anal sphincter tear (healed) (old)
                 complicating delivery (654.8)

    569.44 Dysplasia of anus
        Anal intraepithelial neoplasia I and II
          (AIN I and II) (histologically
          confirmed)
        Dysplasia of anus NOS
        Mild and moderate dysplasia of anus
          (histologically confirmed)
        Excludes *abnormal results from anal*
               cytologic examination
               without histologic
               confirmation (796.70-
               796.79)
              anal intraepithelial neoplasia III
                 (230.5, 230.6)
              carcinoma in situ of anus
                 (230.5, 230.6)
              HGSIL of anus (796.74)
               severe dysplasia of anus
                 (230.5, 230.6)
        Coding Clinic: 2008, Q4, P117-119

    569.49 Other
        Granuloma of rectum (sphincter)
        Rupture of rectum (sphincter)
        Hypertrophy of anal papillae
        Proctitis NOS
        Excludes *fistula of rectum to:*
               internal organs - see Alphabetic
                 Index
              skin (565.1)
              hemorrhoids (455.0–455.9)
             incontinence of sphincter ani
                 (787.6)

569.5 Abscess of intestine 🔖
    Excludes *appendiceal abscess (540.1)*
    Ⓔₓ 569.5
    Coding Clinic: 1996, Q1, P13-14

DISEASES OF THE DIGESTIVE SYSTEM (520–579)

● **569.6 Colostomy and enterostomy complications**

569.60 Colostomy and enterostomy complication, unspecified

569.61 Infection of colostomy and enterostomy 🗝

Use additional code to specify type of infection, such as:
  abscess or cellulitis of abdomen (682.2)
  septicemia (038.0–038.9)

Use additional code to identify organism (041.00–041.9)

(Ex:) 569.60-569.69

569.62 Mechanical complication of colostomy and enterostomy 🗝

Malfunction of colostomy and enterostomy
(Ex:) 530.86-530.87, 536.40-536.49, 569.60-569.69, 997.4, 997.71, 997.91-997.99, 998.81, 998.83-998.9
Coding Clinic: 2005, Q2, P11-12; 2003, Q1, P10

569.69 Other complication 🗝
Fistula   Prolapse
Hernia
(Ex:) 569.60-569.69

● **569.7 Complications of intestinal pouch** ◄

569.71 Pouchitis 🗝 ◄
Inflammation of internal ileoanal pouch ◄

569.79 Other complications of intestinal pouch 🗝 ◄

● **569.8 Other specified disorders of intestine**

569.81 Fistula of intestine, excluding rectum and anus 🗝
Fistula:
  abdominal wall
  enterocolic
  enteroenteric
  ileorectal

Excludes   *fistula of intestine to internal organs - see Alphabetic Index*
persistent postoperative fistula (998.6)

(Ex:) 569.81
Coding Clinic: 1999, Q3, P8

569.82 Ulceration of intestine 🗝
Primary ulcer of intestine
Ulceration of colon

Excludes   *that with perforation (569.83)*

(Ex:) 569.82

569.83 Perforation of intestine 🗝
(Ex:) 569.83

569.84 Angiodysplasia of intestine (without mention of hemorrhage)
Coding Clinic: 1996, Q3, P9-10

569.85 Angiodysplasia of intestine with hemorrhage 🗝
(Ex:) 251.5, 456.0, 530.20-530.21, 530.7, 530.82, 530.85, 531.00-534.91, 535.01, 535.11, 535.21, 535.31, 535.41, 535.51 535.61, 535.71, 537.83, 562.02-562.03, 562.12-562.13, 569.3, 569.85-569.86, 578.0-578.9
Coding Clinic: 1996, Q3, P9-10

569.86 Dieulafoy lesion (hemorrhagic) of intestine 🗝
(Ex:) 251.5, 456.0, 530.20-530.21, 530.7, 530.82, 530.85, 531.00-534.91, 535.01, 535.11, 535.21, 535.31, 535.41, 535.51 535.61, 535.71, 537.83, 562.02-562.03, 562.12-562.13, 569.3, 569.85-569.86, 578.0-578.9
Coding Clinic: 2002, Q4, P60-61

569.87 Vomiting of fecal matter ◄

569.89 Other
Enteroptosis   Pericolitis
Granuloma of intestine   Perisigmoiditis
Prolapse of intestine   Visceroptosis

Excludes   *gangrene of intestine, mesentery, or omentum (557.0)*
hemorrhage of intestine NOS (578.9)
obstruction of intestine (560.0–560.9)

569.9 Unspecified disorder of intestine

OTHER DISEASES OF DIGESTIVE SYSTEM (570–579)

570 Acute and subacute necrosis of liver 🗝
Acute hepatic failure
Acute or subacute hepatitis, not specified as infective
Necrosis of liver (acute) (diffuse) (massive) (subacute)
Parenchymatous degeneration of liver
Yellow atrophy (liver) (acute) (subacute)

Excludes   *icterus gravis of newborn (773.0–773.2)*
serum hepatitis (070.2–070.3)
that with:
  abortion (634–638 with .7, 639.8)
  ectopic or molar pregnancy (639.8)
  pregnancy, childbirth, or the puerperium (646.7)
  viral hepatitis (070.0–070.9)

(Ex:) 570, 573.4-573.9
Coding Clinic: 2005, Q2, P9-10; 2000, Q1, P22

● **571 Chronic liver disease and cirrhosis**

571.0 Alcoholic fatty liver   A

571.1 Acute alcoholic hepatitis   A
Acute alcoholic liver disease
Coding Clinic: 2002, Q2, P4

571.2 Alcoholic cirrhosis of liver   A
Florid cirrhosis
Laennec's cirrhosis (alcoholic)
Coding Clinic: 2007, Q3, P9; Q2, P6-7x2; 2002, Q2, P4; Q1, P3; 1985, Nov-Dec, P14

571.3 Alcoholic liver damage, unspecified   A

● **571.4 Chronic hepatitis**
Excludes   *viral hepatitis (acute) (chronic) (070.0–070.9)*

571.40 Chronic hepatitis, unspecified

571.41 Chronic persistent hepatitis

571.42 Autoimmune hepatitis
Coding Clinic: 2008, Q4, P120

571.49 Other
Chronic hepatitis:
  active
  aggressive
Recurrent hepatitis
Coding Clinic: 1999, Q3, P19

◄ New   ◄ⅲ Revised   ~~deleted~~ Deleted   ● Unacceptable Principal Diagnosis   ● Use Additional Digit(s)
▶ Manifestation Code   **OGCR** Official Guidelines   **Coding Clinic**   Excludes   Includes   Use additional   Code first   Omit code

DISEASES OF THE DIGESTIVE SYSTEM (520–579)

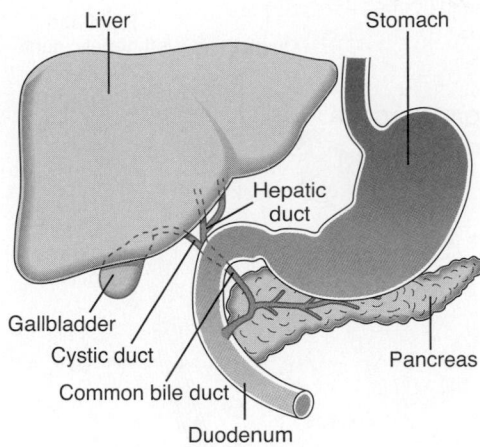

Figure 9-15   Liver and bile ducts.

Item 9-23   Cirrhosis is the progressive fibrosis of the liver resulting in loss of liver function. The main causes of cirrhosis of the liver are alcohol abuse, chronic hepatitis (inflammation of the liver), biliary disease, and excessive amounts of iron. **Alcoholic cirrhosis of the liver** is also called portal, Laënnec's, or fatty nutritional cirrhosis.

571.5   Cirrhosis of liver without mention of alcohol

Cirrhosis of liver:	Cirrhosis of liver:
NOS	micronodular
cryptogenic	posthepatitic
macronodular	postnecrotic

  Healed yellow atrophy (liver)
  Portal cirrhosis

> *Code first, if applicable, viral hepatitis (acute) (chronic) (070.0-070.9)*
> **Coding Clinic: 2007, Q3, P9**

571.6   Biliary cirrhosis
  Chronic nonsuppurative destructive cholangitis
  Cirrhosis:
    cholangitic
    cholestatic

571.8   Other chronic nonalcoholic liver disease
  Chronic yellow atrophy (liver)
  Fatty liver, without mention of alcohol
  Coding Clinic: 1996, Q2, P12

571.9   Unspecified chronic liver disease without mention of alcohol

● **572   Liver abscess and sequelae of chronic liver disease**

572.0   Abscess of liver 🕭
> **Excludes**   *amebic liver abscess (006.3)*
> Ⓔ 006.3, 572.0-572.1, 573.8-573.9

572.1   Portal pyemia 🕭
  Phlebitis of portal vein
  Portal thrombophlebitis
  Pylephlebitis
  Pylethrombophlebitis
  Ⓔ 006.3, 572.0-572.1, 573.8-573.9

572.2   Hepatic ~~coma~~ **encephalopathy** 🕭   ◀▥
  ~~Hepatic encephalopathy~~   ◀
  Hepatic coma
  Hepatocerebral intoxication
  Portal-systemic encephalopathy
> **Excludes**   *hepatic coma associated with viral hepatitis - see category 070*
> Ⓔ 572.2, 573.8-573.9
> **Coding Clinic: 2007, Q2, P6; 2005, Q2, P9-10; 2002, Q1, P3; 1995, Q3, P14**

572.3   Portal hypertension 🕭
> Ⓔ 572.2-572.3, 573.8-573.9
> **Coding Clinic: 2005, Q3, P15-16**

572.4   Hepatorenal syndrome 🕭
> **Excludes**   *that following delivery (674.8)*
> Ⓔ 572.4, 573.8-573.9
> **Coding Clinic: 1992, Q3, P15**

572.8   Other sequelae of chronic liver disease

● **573   Other disorders of liver**
> **Excludes**   *amyloid or lardaceous degeneration of liver (277.39)*
>   *congenital cystic disease of liver (751.62)*
>   *glycogen infiltration of liver (271.0)*
>   *hepatomegaly NOS (789.1)*
>   *portal vein obstruction (452)*

573.0   Chronic passive congestion of liver

▶ **573.1   *Hepatitis in viral diseases classified elsewhere*** 🕭
> *Code first* underlying disease, as:
>   Coxsackie virus disease (074.8)
>   cytomegalic inclusion virus disease (078.5)
>   infectious mononucleosis (075)
> **Excludes**   *hepatitis (in):*
>   *mumps (072.71)*
>   *viral (070.0-070.9)*
>   *yellow fever (060.0-060.9)*
> Ⓔ 573.1-573.3, 573.8-573.9

▶ **573.2   *Hepatitis in other infectious diseases classified elsewhere*** 🕭
> *Code first* underlying disease, as:
>   malaria (084.9)
> **Excludes**   *hepatitis in:*
>   *late syphilis (095.3)*
>   *secondary syphilis (091.62)*
>   *toxoplasmosis (130.5)*
> Ⓔ 573.1-573.3, 573.8-573.9

573.3   Hepatitis, unspecified
  Toxic (noninfectious) hepatitis
> Use additional E code to identify cause
> **Coding Clinic: 1998, Q3, P4; 1990, Q4, P26**

573.4   Hepatic infarction 🕭
> Ⓔ 570, 573.4-573.9

573.8   Other specified disorders of liver
  Hepatoptosis

573.9   Unspecified disorder of liver

N   Newborn Age: 0   P   Pediatric Age: 0–17   M   Maternity Age: 12–55   A   Adult Age: 15–124   ♀   Females Only   ♂   Males Only

Ⓔ   CC Exclusions   🕭   Complication\Comorbidity   🕭   Major C\C   🕭   Present on Admission Requirement   🕭   Hospital-Acquired Condition   **945**

DISEASES OF THE DIGESTIVE SYSTEM (520–579)

● **574   Cholelithiasis**
Presence or formation of gallstones
Coding Clinic: 1990, Q1, P19

The following fifth-digit subclassification is for use with category 574:

> 0   **without mention of obstruction**
> 1   **with obstruction**

Check documentation for acute/chronic gallbladder/common bile duct either with or without obstruction.

● **574.0   Calculus of gallbladder with acute cholecystitis** 🦠
[0-1]   Biliary calculus with acute cholecystitis
       Calculus of cystic duct with acute cholecystitis
       Cholelithiasis with acute cholecystitis
       Any condition classifiable to 574.2 with acute cholecystitis
       For code **574.00:** (Ex) 574.00-574.21, 574.40, 574.60-574.61, 574.80-574.81, 575.0-575.12, 575.9, 576.8-576.9;
       For code **574.01:** (Ex) 574.00-574.21, 574.60-574.61, 574.80-574.81, 575.0-575.12, 575.9, 576.8-576.9
       Coding Clinic: 1996, Q4, P32; 1984, Nov-Dec, P18

● **574.1   Calculus of gallbladder with other cholecystitis** 🦠
[0-1]   Biliary calculus with cholecystitis
       Calculus of cystic duct with cholecystitis
       Cholelithiasis with cholecystitis
       Cholecystitis with cholelithiasis NOS
       Any condition classifiable to 574.2 with cholecystitis (chronic)
       (Ex) 574.00-574.21, 574.60-574.61, 574.80-574.81, 575.0-575.12, 575.9, 576.8-576.9
       Coding Clinic: 2003, Q1, P5; 1999, Q3, P9; 1996, Q4, P69; Q2, P13-15; Q1, P7

● **574.2   Calculus of gallbladder without mention of**
[0-1] **cholecystitis 1** 🦠
       Biliary:
           calculus NOS
           colic NOS
       Calculus of cystic duct
       Cholelithiasis NOS
       Colic (recurrent) of gallbladder
       Gallstone (impacted)
       For code **574.21:** (Ex) 574.00-574.21, 574.60-574.61, 574.80-574.81, 575.0-575.12, 575.9, 576.8-576.9
       Coding Clinic: 1995, Q4, P51-52; 1988, Q1, P14

● **574.3   Calculus of bile duct with acute cholecystitis** 🦠
[0-1]   Calculus of bile duct [any] with acute cholecystitis
       Choledocholithiasis with acute cholecystitis
       Any condition classifiable to 574.5 with acute cholecystitis
       (Ex) 574.30-575.12, 576.8-576.9

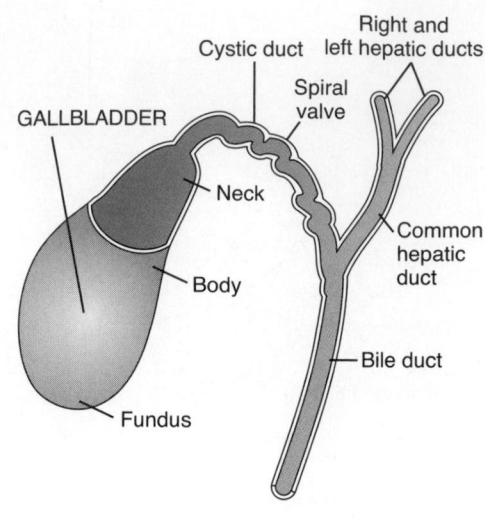

Figure 9–16   *Gallbladder and bile ducts.*

● **574.4   Calculus of bile duct with other cholecystitis** 🦠
[0-1]   Calculus of bile duct [any] with cholecystitis (chronic)
       Choledocholithiasis with cholecystitis (chronic)
       Any condition classifiable to 574.5 with cholecystitis (chronic)
       (Ex) 574.30-575.12, 576.8-576.9
       Coding Clinic: 1996, Q1, P7

● **574.5   Calculus of bile duct without mention of**
[0-1] **cholecystitis 1** 🦠

Calculus of:	Choledocholithiasis
bile duct [any]	Hepatic:
common duct	colic (recurrent)
hepatic duct	lithiasis

       For code **574.51:** (Ex) 574.30-575.12, 576.8-576.9
       Coding Clinic: 1996, Q2, P13-15; 1994, Q3, P11

● **574.6   Calculus of gallbladder and bile duct with acute**
[0-1] **cholecystitis** 🦠
       Any condition classifiable to 574.0 and 574.3
       (Ex) 574.60-574.61, 575.0-575.12, 575.9, 576.8-576.9

● **574.7   Calculus of gallbladder and bile duct with other**
[0-1] **cholecystitis** 🦠
       Any condition classifiable to 574.1 and 574.4
       (Ex) 574.30-575.12, 576.8-576.9

● **574.8   Calculus of gallbladder and bile duct with acute and**
[0-1] **chronic cholecystitis 0** 🦠**, 1** 🦠
       Any condition classifiable to 574.6 and 574.7
       (Ex) 574.80-574.81, 575.0-575.12, 575.9, 576.8-576.9
       Coding Clinic: 1996, Q4, P32

● **574.9   Calculus of gallbladder and bile duct without**
[0-1] **cholecystitis 1** 🦠
       Any condition classifiable to 574.2 and 574.5
       For code **574.91:** (Ex) 574.30-575.12, 576.8-576.9

DISEASES OF THE DIGESTIVE SYSTEM (520–579)

◀ New   ◀▥ Revised   ~~deleted~~ Deleted   ● Unacceptable Principal Diagnosis   ● Use Additional Digit(s)
▶ Manifestation Code   **OGCR** Official Guidelines   **Coding Clinic**   Excludes   Includes   Use additional   Code first   Omit code

● **575   Other disorders of gallbladder**
Cholecystitis is chronic or acute inflammation of gallbladder.

575.0   Acute cholecystitis 🍋
Abscess of gallbladder without mention of calculus
Angiocholecystitis without mention of calculus
Cholecystitis without mention of calculus:
    emphysematous (acute)
    gangrenous
    suppurative
Empyema of gallbladder without mention of
    calculus
Gangrene of gallbladder without mention of
    calculus

Excludes	*that with:*

        acute and chronic cholecystitis (575.12)
        choledocholithiasis (574.3)
        choledocholithiasis and cholelithiasis
          (574.6)
        cholelithiasis (574.0)
    (Ex) 574.60-574.61, 574.80-574.81, 575.0-575.12, 575.9, 576.8-576.9
    Coding Clinic: 1991, Q3, P17-18

● **575.1   Other cholecystitis**
Cholecystitis without mention of calculus:
    NOS without mention of calculus
    chronic without mention of calculus

Excludes	*that with:*

        choledocholithiasis (574.4)
        choledocholithiasis and cholelithiasis
          (574.8)
        cholelithiasis (574.1)
    Coding Clinic: 1991, Q3, P17-18

    575.10   Cholecystitis, unspecified
       Cholecystitis NOS

    575.11   Chronic cholecystitis

    575.12   Acute and chronic cholecystitis 🍋
        (Ex) 575.0-575.12, 575.9, 576.8-576.9
        Coding Clinic: 1997, Q4, P52; 1996, Q4, P32

575.2   Obstruction of gallbladder 🍋
Occlusion of cystic duct or gallbladder without
    mention of calculus
Stenosis of cystic duct or gallbladder without
    mention of calculus
Stricture of cystic duct or gallbladder without
    mention of calculus
    (Ex) 575.2-575.9, 576.8-576.9

575.3   Hydrops of gallbladder 🍋
Mucocele of gallbladder
    (Ex) 575.2-575.9, 576.8-576.9

575.4   Perforation of gallbladder 🍋
Rupture of cystic duct or gallbladder
    (Ex) 575.2-575.9, 576.8-576.9

575.5   Fistula of gallbladder 🍋
Fistula: Fistula:
    cholecystoduodenal   cholecystoenteric
    (Ex) 575.2-575.9, 576.8-576.9

575.6   Cholesterolosis of gallbladder
Strawberry gallbladder

575.8   Other specified disorders of gallbladder
Adhesions (of) cystic duct gallbladder
Atrophy (of) cystic duct gallbladder
Cyst (of) cystic duct gallbladder
Hypertrophy (of) cystic duct gallbladder
Nonfunctioning (of) cystic duct gallbladder
Ulcer (of) cystic duct gallbladder
Biliary dyskinesia

Excludes	*Hartmann's pouch of intestine (V44.3)*
	nonvisualization of gallbladder (793.3)

    Coding Clinic: 1989, Q2, P13

575.9   Unspecified disorder of gallbladder

● **576   Other disorders of biliary tract**

Excludes	*that involving the:*
	cystic duct (575.0–575.9)
	gallbladder (575.0–575.9)

576.0   Postcholecystectomy syndrome
    Coding Clinic: 1988, Q1, P10

576.1   Cholangitis 🍋
Cholangitis: Cholangitis:
    NOS   recurrent
    acute   sclerosing
    ascending   secondary
    chronic   stenosing
    primary   suppurative
    (Ex) 576.1, 576.8-576.9
    Coding Clinic: 1999, Q2, P13-14; 1995, Q2, P7

576.2   Obstruction of bile duct 🍋
Occlusion of bile duct, except cystic duct, without
    mention of calculus
Stenosis of bile duct, except cystic duct, without
    mention of calculus
Stricture of bile duct, except cystic duct, without
    mention of calculus

Excludes	*congenital (751.61)*
	that with calculus (574.3–574.5 with
	fifth-digit 1)

    (Ex) 574.31, 574.41, 574.51, 576.2, 576.8-576.9, 751.61
    Coding Clinic: 2003, Q3, P17-18; 2001, Q1, P8-9; 1999, Q2, P13-14

576.3   Perforation of bile duct 🍋
Rupture of bile duct, except cystic duct
    (Ex) 576.3-576.4, 576.8-576.9

576.4   Fistula of bile duct 🍋
Choledochoduodenal fistula
    (Ex) 576.3-576.4, 576.8-576.9

576.5   Spasm of sphincter of Oddi

576.8   Other specified disorders of biliary tract
Adhesions of bile duct [any]
Atrophy of bile duct [any]
Cyst of bile duct [any]
Hypertrophy of bile duct [any]
Stasis of bile duct [any]
Ulcer of bile duct [any]

Excludes	*congenital choledochal cyst (751.69)*

    Coding Clinic: 2003, Q3, P17-18; 1999, Q2, P14

576.9   Unspecified disorder of biliary tract

DISEASES OF THE DIGESTIVE SYSTEM (520–579)

N   Newborn Age: 0   **P**   Pediatric Age: 0–17   **M**   Maternity Age: 12–55   **A**   Adult Age: 15–124   ♀   Females Only   ♂   Males Only

(Ex)   CC Exclusions   🍋   Complication\Comorbidity   🍋   Major C\C   ⊗   Present on Admission Requirement   🍋   Hospital-Acquired Condition   **947**

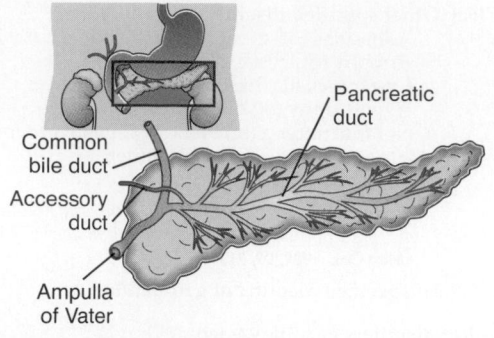

Figure 9–17   Pancreatic ductal system.

● 577   Diseases of pancreas

Pancreatitis is inflammatory process that may be acute or chronic.

577.0   Acute pancreatitis 🔏
Abscess of pancreas
Necrosis of pancreas:
acute
infective
Pancreatitis:
NOS
acute (recurrent)
apoplectic
hemorrhagic
subacute
suppurative

Excludes   *mumps pancreatitis (072.3)*

Ex: 577.0-577.1, 577.8-577.9
Coding Clinic: 1999, Q3, P9; 1998, Q2, P19-20; 1996, Q2, P13-15; 1989, Q2, P9

577.1   Chronic pancreatitis 🔏
Chronic pancreatitis: Pancreatitis:
NOS   painless
infectious   recurrent
interstitial   relapsing
Ex: 251.8, 577.0-577.9
Coding Clinic: 2001, Q1, P8-9; 1996, Q2, P13-15; 1994, Q3, P11

577.2   Cyst and pseudocyst of pancreas 🔏
Ex: 577.2-577.9

577.8   Other specified diseases of pancreas
Atrophy of pancreas
Calculus of pancreas
Cirrhosis of pancreas
Fibrosis of pancreas
Pancreatic:
infantilism
necrosis:
NOS
aseptic
fat
Pancreatolithiasis

Excludes   *fibrocystic disease of pancreas*
(277.00–277.09)
islet cell tumor of pancreas (211.7)
pancreatic steatorrhea (579.4)
Coding Clinic: 2001, Q1, P8-9

577.9   Unspecified disease of pancreas

● 578   Gastrointestinal hemorrhage

Excludes   *that with mention of:*
angiodysplasia of stomach and duodenum
(537.83)
angiodysplasia of intestine (569.85)
diverticulitis, intestine:
large (562.13)
small (562.03)
diverticulosis, intestine:
large (562.12)
small (562.02)
gastritis and duodenitis (535.0–535.6)
ulcer:
duodenal, gastric, gastrojejunal, or peptic
(531.00–534.91)
Coding Clinic: 2007, Q2, P13; 1992, Q2, P9-10; Q2, P8-9

578.0   Hematemesis 🔏
Vomiting of blood
Ex: 251.5, 456.0, 530.20-530.21, 530.7, 530.82, 530.85, 531.00-534.91,
535.01, 535.11, 535.21, 535.31, 535.41, 535.51, 535.61, 535.71,
537.83, 562.02-562.03, 562.12-562.13, 569.3, 569.85, 578.0-578.9
Coding Clinic: 2002, Q2, P4

578.1   Blood in stool 🔏
Melena

Excludes   *melena of the newborn (772.4, 777.3)*
occult blood (792.1)
Ex: 251.5, 456.0, 530.20-530.21, 530.7, 530.82, 530.85, 531.00-534.91,
535.01, 535.11, 535.21, 535.31, 535.41, 535.51, 535.61, 535.71,
537.83, 562.02-562.03, 562.12-562.13, 569.3, 569.85, 578.0-578.9
Coding Clinic: 2006, Q2, P17; 1992, Q2, P8-9

578.9   Hemorrhage of gastrointestinal tract, unspecified 🔏
Gastric hemorrhage   Intestinal hemorrhage
Ex: 251.5, 456.0, 530.20-530.21, 530.7, 530.82, 530.85, 531.00-534.91,
535.01, 535.11, 535.21, 535.31, 535.41, 535.51, 535.61, 535.71,
537.83, 562.02-562.03, 562.12-562.13, 569.3, 569.85, 578.0-578.9
Coding Clinic: 2008, Q2, P15-16; 2006, Q4, P91-92; 2005, Q3,
P17-18; 1986, Nov-Dec, P9; 1985, Sept-Oct, P9

● 579   Intestinal malabsorption

579.0   Celiac disease
Celiac: Gee (-Herter) disease
crisis   Gluten enteropathy
infantilism   Idiopathic steatorrhea
rickets   Nontropical sprue

579.1   Tropical sprue 🔏
Sprue:
NOS
tropical
Tropical steatorrhea
Ex: 277.03, 579.0-579.9

579.2   Blind loop syndrome 🔏
Postoperative blind loop syndrome
Ex: 277.03, 579.0-579.9

579.3   Other and unspecified postsurgical nonabsorption 🔏
Hypoglycemia following gastrointestinal surgery
Malnutrition following gastrointestinal surgery
Ex: 579.3-579.9
Coding Clinic: 2003, Q4, P104-105

579.4   Pancreatic steatorrhea 🔏
Ex: 277.03, 579.0-579.9

579.8   Other specified intestinal malabsorption 🔏
Enteropathy:
exudative
protein-losing
Steatorrhea (chronic)
Ex: 277.03, 579.0-579.9
Coding Clinic: 2003, Q1, P12

579.9   Unspecified intestinal malabsorption 🔏
Malabsorption syndrome NOS
Ex: 277.03, 579.0-579.9
Coding Clinic: 2004, Q4, P57-59

DISEASES OF THE DIGESTIVE SYSTEM (520–579)

◀ New   ◀▦ Revised   ~~deleted~~ Deleted   ● Unacceptable Principal Diagnosis   ● Use Additional Digit(s)
▶ Manifestation Code   **OGCR** Official Guidelines   **Coding Clinic**   Excludes   Includes   Use additional   Code first   Omit code

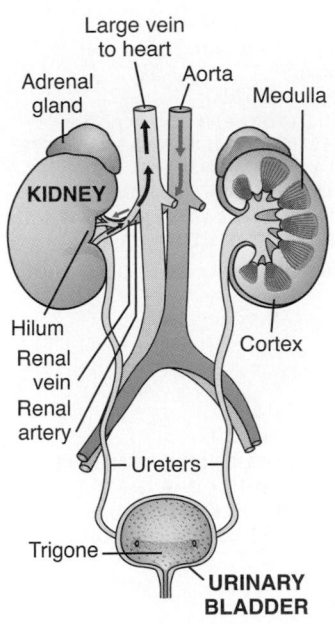

Figure 10-1   Kidneys within the urinary system.

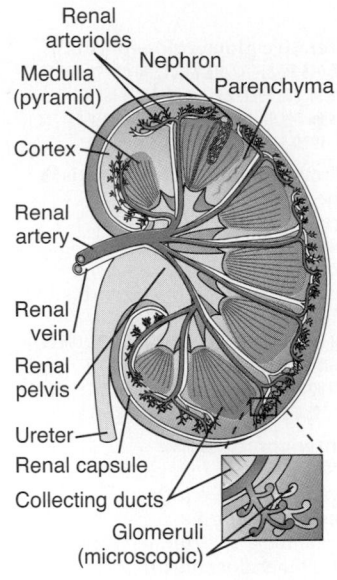

Figure 10-2   Kidney cross section.

Item 10-1   Glomerulonephritis is nephritis accompanied by inflammation of the glomeruli of the kidney, resulting in the degeneration of the glomeruli and the nephrons.
Acute glomerulonephritis primarily affects children and young adults and is usually a result of a streptococcal infection.
Proliferative glomerulonephritis is the acute form of the disease resulting from a streptococcal infection.
Rapidly progressive glomerulonephritis, also known as **crescentic** or **malignant glomerulonephritis,** is the acute form of the disease, which leads quickly to rapid and progressive decline in renal function.

10.   DISEASES OF THE GENITOURINARY SYSTEM (580–629)

NEPHRITIS, NEPHROTIC SYNDROME, AND NEPHROSIS (580–589)

Excludes	*hypertensive chronic kidney disease (403.00–403.91, 404.00–404.93)*

● **580   Acute glomerulonephritis**

   Includes   acute nephritis

580.0   With lesion of proliferative glomerulonephritis 🅒
    Acute (diffuse) proliferative glomerulonephritis
    Acute poststreptococcal glomerulonephritis
    (Ex:) 016.00-016.06, 016.30-016.36, 016.90-016.96, 017.90-017.96, 098.10, 098.19, 098.30-098.31, 098.89, 112.2, 131.00, 131.8-131.9, 249.40-249.41, 249.80-249.91, 250.40-250.43, 250.80-250.93, 274.10, 274.19, 580.0-591, 593.0-593.2, 593.89-593.9, 599.70-599.9

580.4   With lesion of rapidly progressive glomerulonephritis 🅒
    Acute nephritis with lesion of necrotizing glomerulitis
    (Ex:) 016.00-016.06, 016.30-016.36, 016.90-016.96, 017.90-017.96, 098.10, 098.19, 098.30-098.31, 098.89, 112.2, 131.00, 131.8-131.9, 249.40-249.41, 249.80-249.91, 250.40-250.43, 250.80-250.93, 274.10, 274.19, 580.0-591, 593.0-593.2, 593.89-593.9, 599.70-599.9

Item 10-2   Nephrotic syndrome (NS) is marked by massive proteinuria (protein in the urine) and water retention. Patients with NS are particularly vulnerable to staphylococcal and pneumococcal infections. NS with lesion of proliferative glomerulonephritis results from a streptococcal infection. NS with lesion of membranous glomerulonephritis results in thickening of the capillary walls. NS with lesion of minimal change glomerulonephritis is usually a benign disorder that occurs mostly in children and requires electron microscopy (biopsy) to verify changes in the glomeruli.

● **580.8   With other specified pathological lesion in kidney**

▶ *580.81   Acute glomerulonephritis in diseases classified elsewhere* 🅒

     Code first underlying disease, as:
       infectious hepatitis (070.0–070.9)
       mumps (072.79)
       subacute bacterial endocarditis (421.0)
       typhoid fever (002.0)
     (Ex:) 016.00-016.06, 016.30-016.36, 016.90-016.96, 017.90-017.96, 098.10, 098.19, 098.30-098.31, 098.89, 112.2, 131.00, 131.8-131.9, 249.40-249.41, 249.80-249.91, 250.40-250.43, 250.80-250.93, 274.10, 274.19, 580.0-591, 593.0-593.2, 593.89-593.9, 599.70-599.9

   580.89   Other 🅒
     Glomerulonephritis, acute, with lesion of:
       exudative nephritis
       interstitial (diffuse) (focal) nephritis
     (Ex:) 016.00-016.06, 016.30-016.36, 016.90-016.96, 017.90-017.96, 098.10, 098.19, 098.30-098.31, 098.89, 112.2, 131.00, 131.8-131.9, 274.10, 274.19, 580.0-591, 593.0-593.2, 593.89-593.9, 599.70-599.9

580.9   Acute glomerulonephritis with unspecified pathological lesion in kidney 🅒
    Glomerulonephritis: specified as acute
     NOS specified as acute
     hemorrhagic specified as acute
    Nephritis specified as acute
    Nephropathy specified as acute
    (Ex:) 016.00-016.06, 016.30-016.36, 016.90-016.96, 017.90-017.96, 098.10, 098.19, 098.30-098.31, 098.89, 112.2, 131.00, 131.8-131.9, 249.40-249.41, 249.80-249.91, 250.40-250.43, 250.80-250.93, 274.10, 274.19, 580.0-591, 593.0-593.2, 593.89-593.9, 599.70-599.9

N   Newborn Age: 0   **P**   Pediatric Age: 0–17   **M**   Maternity Age: 12–55   **A**   Adult Age: 15–124   ♀ Females Only   ♂ Males Only   **949**

(Ex:) CC Exclusions   🅒 Complication\Comorbidity   🅒 Major C\C   ⊘ Present on Admission Requirement   🅒 Hospital-Acquired Condition

● **581 Nephrotic syndrome**

581.0 With lesion of proliferative glomerulonephritis ⊘
(Ex:) 016.00-016.06, 016.30-016.36, 016.90-016.96, 017.90-017.96, 098.10, 098.19, 098.30-098.31, 098.89, 112.2, 131.00, 131.8-131.9, 249.40-249.41, 249.80-249.91, 250.40-250.43, 250.80-250.93, 274.10, 274.19, 580.0-591, 593.0-593.2, 593.89-593.9, 599.0-599.9

581.1 With lesion of membranous glomerulonephritis ⊘
Epimembranous nephritis
Idiopathic membranous glomerular disease
Nephrotic syndrome with lesion of:
    focal glomerulosclerosis
    sclerosing membranous glomerulonephritis
    segmental hyalinosis
(Ex:) 016.00-016.06, 016.30-016.36, 016.90-016.96, 017.90-017.96, 098.10, 098.19, 098.30-098.31, 098.89, 112.2, 131.00, 131.8-131.9, 249.40-249.41, 249.80-249.91, 250.40-250.43, 250.80-250.93, 274.10, 274.19, 580.0-591, 593.0-593.2, 593.89-593.9, 599.70-599.9

581.2 With lesion of membranoproliferative glomerulonephritis ⊘
Nephrotic syndrome with lesion (of):
    endothelial glomerulonephritis
    hypocomplementemic glomerulonephritis
        persistent glomerulonephritis
    lobular glomerulonephritis
    mesangiocapillary glomerulonephritis
    mixed membranous and proliferative
        glomerulonephritis
(Ex:) 016.00-016.06, 016.30-016.36, 016.90-016.96, 017.90-017.96, 098.10, 098.19, 098.30-098.31, 098.89, 112.2, 131.00, 131.8-131.9, 249.40-249.41, 249.80-249.91, 250.40-250.43, 250.80-250.93, 274.10, 274.19, 580.0-591, 593.0-593.2, 593.89-593.9, 599.70-599.9

581.3 With lesion of minimal change glomerulonephritis ⊘
Foot process disease
Lipoid nephrosis
Minimal change:
    glomerular disease
    glomerulitis
    nephrotic syndrome
(Ex:) 016.00-016.06, 016.30-016.36, 016.90-016.96, 017.90-017.96, 098.10, 098.19, 098.30-098.31, 098.89, 112.2, 131.00, 131.8-131.9, 249.40-249.41, 249.80-249.91, 250.40-250.43, 250.80-250.93, 274.10, 274.19, 580.0-591, 593.0-593.2, 593.89-593.9, 599.70-599.9
Coding Clinic: 2007, Q1, P23

● **581.8 With other specified pathological lesion in kidney**

▸ *581.81 Nephrotic syndrome in diseases classified elsewhere* ⊘

    Code first underlying disease, as:
        amyloidosis (277.30–277.39)
        diabetes mellitus (249.4, 250.4)
        malaria (084.9)
        polyarteritis (446.0)
        systemic lupus erythematosus (710.0)

    | **Excludes** | *nephrosis in epidemic hemorrhagic fever (078.6)* |

    (Ex:) 016.00-016.06, 016.30-016.36, 016.90-016.96, 017.90-017.96, 098.10, 098.19, 098.30-098.31, 098.89, 112.2, 131.00, 131.8-131.9, 249.40-249.41, 249.80-249.91, 250.40-250.43, 250.80-250.93, 274.10, 274.19, 580.0-591, 593.0-593.2, 593.89-593.9, 599.70-599.9

581.89 Other ⊘
Glomerulonephritis with edema and
    lesion of:
        exudative nephritis
        interstitial (diffuse) (focal) nephritis
(Ex:) 016.00-016.06, 016.30-016.36, 016.90-016.96, 017.90-017.96, 098.10, 098.19, 098.30-098.31, 098.89, 112.2, 131.00, 131.8-131.9, 249.40-249.41, 249.80-249.91, 250.40-250.43, 250.80-250.93, 274.10, 274.19, 580.0-591, 593.0-593.2, 593.89-593.9, 599.70-599.9

581.9 Nephrotic syndrome with unspecified pathological lesion in kidney ⊘
Glomerulonephritis with edema NOS
Nephritis:
    nephrotic NOS
    with edema NOS
Nephrosis NOS
Renal disease with edema NOS
(Ex:) 016.00-016.06, 016.30-016.36, 016.90-016.96, 017.90-017.96, 098.10, 098.19, 098.30-098.31, 098.89, 112.2, 131.00, 131.8-131.9, 249.40-249.41, 249.80-249.91, 250.40-250.43, 250.80-250.93, 274.10, 274.19, 580.0-591, 593.0-593.2, 593.89-593.9, 599.70-599.9

● **582 Chronic glomerulonephritis**

| **Includes** | chronic nephritis |

582.0 With lesion of proliferative glomerulonephritis ⊘
Chronic (diffuse) proliferative glomerulonephritis
(Ex:) 016.00-016.06, 016.30-016.36, 016.90-016.96, 017.90-017.96, 078.6, 098.10, 098.19, 098.30-098.31, 098.89, 112.2, 131.00, 131.8-131.9, 249.40-249.41, 249.80-249.91, 250.40-250.43, 250.80-250.93, 274.10, 274.19, 580.0-584.9, 586-591, 593.0-593.2, 593.89-593.9, 599.70-599.9

582.1 With lesion of membranous glomerulonephritis ⊘
Chronic glomerulonephritis:
    membranous
    sclerosing
Focal glomerulosclerosis
Segmental hyalinosis
(Ex:) 016.00-016.06, 016.30 -016.36, 016.90-016.96, 017.90-017.96, 078.6, 098.10, 098.19, 098.30-098.31, 098.89, 112.2, 131.00, 131.8-131.9, 249.40-249.41, 249.80-249.91, 250.40-250.43, 250.80-250.93, 274.10, 274.19, 580.0-584.9, 586-591, 593.0-593.2, 593.89-593.9, 599.70-599.9
Coding Clinic: 1984, Sept-Oct, P16

Item 10–3 Chronic glomerulonephritis (GN) persists over a period of years, with remissions and exacerbation.
Chronic GN with lesion of proliferative glomerulonephritis results from a streptococcal infection.
Chronic GN with lesion of membranous glomerulonephritis, also known as membranous nephropathy, is characterized by deposits along the epithelial side of the basement membrane.
Chronic GN with lesion of membranoproliferative glomerulonephritis (MPGN) is a group of disorders characterized by alterations in the basement membranes of the kidney and the glomerular cells.
Chronic GN with lesion of rapidly progressive glomerulonephritis is characterized by necrosis, endothelial proliferation, and mesangial proliferation. The condition is marked by rapid and progressive decline in renal function.

DISEASES OF THE GENITOURINARY SYSTEM (580–629)

◀ New   ◀▥ Revised   ~~deleted~~ Deleted   ● Unacceptable Principal Diagnosis   ● Use Additional Digit(s)
▸ Manifestation Code   **OGCR** Official Guidelines   **Coding Clinic** | Excludes | | Includes | | Use additional | | Code first | | Omit code |

582.2 With lesion of membranoproliferative glomerulonephritis 🅖

Chronic glomerulonephritis:
    endothelial
    hypocomplementemic persistent
    lobular
    membranoproliferative
    mesangiocapillary
    mixed membranous and proliferative

Ⓔⓧ 016.00-016.06, 016.30-016.36, 016.90-016.96, 017.90-017.96, 078.6, 098.10, 098.19, 098.30-098.31, 098.89, 112.2, 131.00, 131.8-131.9, 249.40-249.41, 249.80-249.91, 250.40-250.43, 250.80-250.93, 274.10, 274.19, 580.0-584.9, 586-591, 593.0-593.2, 593.89-593.9, 599.70-599.9

582.4 With lesion of rapidly progressive glomerulonephritis 🅖

Chronic nephritis with lesion of necrotizing glomerulitis

Ⓔⓧ 016.00-016.06, 016.30-016.36, 016.90-016.96, 017.90-017.96, 078.6, 098.10, 098.19, 098.30-098.31, 098.89, 112.2, 131.00, 131.8-131.9, 249.40-249.41, 249.80-249.91, 250.40-250.43, 250.80-250.93, 274.10, 274.19, 580.0-584.9, 586-591, 593.0-593.2, 593.89-593.9, 599.70-599.9

● **582.8 With other specified pathological lesion in kidney**

▸ **582.81 Chronic glomerulonephritis in diseases classified elsewhere** 🅖

Code first underlying disease, as:
    amyloidosis (277.30–277.39)
    systemic lupus erythematosus (710.0)

Ⓔⓧ 016.00-016.06, 016.30-016.36, 016.90-016.96, 017.90-017.96, 078.6, 098.10, 098.19, 098.30-098.31, 098.89, 112.2, 131.00, 131.8-131.9, 249.40-249.41, 249.80-249.91, 250.40-250.43, 250.80-250.93, 274.10, 274.19, 580.0-584.9, 586-591, 593.0-593.2, 593.89-593.9, 599.70-599.9

582.89 Other 🅖

Chronic glomerulonephritis with lesion of:
    exudative nephritis
    interstitial (diffuse) (focal) nephritis

Ⓔⓧ 016.00-016.06, 016.30-016.36, 016.90-016.96, 017.90-017.96, 078.6, 098.10, 098.19, 098.30-098.31, 098.89, 112.2, 131.00, 131.8-131.9, 249.40-249.41, 249.80-249.91, 250.40-250.43, 250.80-250.93, 274.10, 274.19, 580.0-584.9, 586-591, 593.0-593.2, 593.89-593.9, 599.70-599.9

582.9 Chronic glomerulonephritis with unspecified pathological lesion in kidney 🅖

Glomerulonephritis: specified as chronic
    NOS specified as chronic
    hemorrhagic specified as chronic
Nephritis specified as chronic
Nephropathy specified as chronic

Ⓔⓧ 016.00-016.06, 016.30-016.36, 016.90-016.96, 017.90-017.96, 078.6, 098.10, 098.19, 098.30-098.31, 098.89, 112.2, 131.00, 131.8-131.9, 249.40-249.41, 249.80-249.91, 250.40-250.43, 250.80-250.93, 274.10, 274.19, 580.0-584.9, 586-591, 593.0-593.2, 593.89-593.9, 599.70-599.9

Coding Clinic: 2001, Q2, P12

Item 10–4 **Nephritis** (inflammation) or **nephropathy** (disease) **with lesion of proliferative glomerulonephritis** results from a streptococcal infection.

Nephritis (inflammation) or **nephropathy** (disease) **with lesion of membranous glomerulonephritis** is characterized by deposits along the epithelial side of the basement membrane.

Nephritis (inflammation) or **nephropathy** (disease) **with lesion of membranoproliferative glomerulonephritis** is characterized by alterations in the basement membranes of the kidney and the glomerular cells.

Nephritis (inflammation) or **nephropathy** (disease) **with lesion of rapidly progressive glomerulonephritis** is characterized by rapid and progressive decline in renal function.

Nephritis (inflammation) or **nephropathy** (disease) **with lesion of renal cortical necrosis** is characterized by death of the cortical tissues.

Nephritis (inflammation) or **nephropathy** (disease) **with lesion of renal medullary necrosis** is characterized by death of the tissues that collect urine.

● **583 Nephritis and nephropathy, not specified as acute or chronic**

    Includes   "renal disease" so stated, not specified as acute or chronic but with stated pathology or cause

583.0 With lesion of proliferative glomerulonephritis 🅖

Proliferative:
    glomerulonephritis (diffuse) NOS
    nephritis NOS
    nephropathy NOS

Ⓔⓧ 016.00-016.06, 016.30-016.36, 016.90-016.96, 017.90-017.96, 078.6, 098.10, 098.19, 098.30-098.31, 098.89, 112.2, 131.00, 131.8-131.9, 249.40-249.41, 249.80-249.91, 250.40-250.43, 250.80-250.93, 274.10, 274.19, 580.0-584.9, 586-591, 593.0-593.2, 593.89-593.9, 599.70-599.9

583.1 With lesion of membranous glomerulonephritis 🅖

Membranous:
    glomerulonephritis NOS
    nephritis NOS
Membranous nephropathy NOS

Ⓔⓧ 016.00-016.06, 016.30-016.36, 016.90-016.96, 017.90-017.96, 078.6, 098.10, 098.19, 098.30-098.31, 098.89, 112.2, 131.00, 131.8-131.9, 249.40-249.41, 249.80-249.91, 250.40-250.43, 250.80-250.93, 274.10, 274.19, 580.0-584.9, 586-591, 593.0-593.2, 593.89-593.9, 599.70-599.9

DISEASES OF THE GENITOURINARY SYSTEM (580–629)

N Newborn Age: 0   **P** Pediatric Age: 0–17   **M** Maternity Age: 12–55   **A** Adult Age: 15–124   ♀ Females Only   ♂ Males Only   **951**

Ⓔⓧ CC Exclusions   🅒 Complication\Comorbidity   🅜 Major C\C   🅟 Present on Admission Requirement   🅗 Hospital-Acquired Condition

583.2 With lesion of membranoproliferative glomerulonephritis 🔹

Membranoproliferative:
  glomerulonephritis NOS
  nephritis NOS
  nephropathy NOS
Nephritis NOS, with lesion of:
  hypocomplementemic persistent
    glomerulonephritis
  lobular glomerulonephritis
  mesangiocapillary glomerulonephritis
  mixed membranous and proliferative
    glomerulonephritis

Ex: 016.00-016.06, 016.30-016.36, 016.90-016.96, 017.90-017.96, 078.6, 098.10, 098.19, 098.30-098.31, 098.89, 112.2, 131.00, 131.8-131.9, 249.40-249.41, 249.80-249.91, 250.40-250.43, 250.80-250.93, 274.10, 274.19, 580.0-584.9, 586-591, 593.0-593.2, 593.89-593.9, 599.70-599.9

583.4 With lesion of rapidly progressive glomerulonephritis 🔹

Necrotizing or rapidly progressive:
  glomerulitis NOS
  glomerulonephritis NOS
  nephritis NOS
  nephropathy NOS
Nephritis, unspecified, with lesion of necrotizing
  glomerulitis

Ex: 016.00-016.06, 016.30-016.36, 016.90-016.96, 017.90-017.96, 098.10, 098.19, 098.30-098.31, 098.89, 112.2, 131.00, 131.8-131.9, 249.40-249.41, 249.80-249.91, 250.40-250.43, 250.80-250.93, 274.10, 274.19, 580.0-591, 593.0-593.2, 593.89-593.9, 599.70-599.9

583.6 With lesion of renal cortical necrosis 🔹

Nephritis NOS with (renal) cortical necrosis
Nephropathy NOS with (renal) cortical necrosis
Renal cortical necrosis NOS

Ex: 583.6, 588.81 -588.89

583.7 With lesion of renal medullary necrosis 🔹

Nephritis NOS with (renal) medullary [papillary] necrosis
Nephropathy NOS with (renal) medullary [papillary] necrosis

Ex: 583.7, 588.81-588.89

● **583.8 With other specified pathological lesion in kidney**

▶ *583.81 Nephritis and nephropathy, not specified as acute or chronic, in diseases classified elsewhere*

Code first *underlying disease, as:*
  amyloidosis (277.30–277.39)
  diabetes mellitus (249.4, 250.4)
  gonococcal infection (098.19)
  Goodpasture's syndrome (446.21)
  systemic lupus erythematosus (710.0)
  tuberculosis (016.0)

Excludes *gouty nephropathy (274.10)*
      syphilitic nephritis (095.4)

Coding Clinic: 2003, Q2, P7

583.89 Other

Glomerulitis with lesion of:
  exudative nephritis
  interstitial nephritis
Glomerulonephritis with lesion of:
  exudative nephritis
  interstitial nephritis
Nephritis with lesion of:
  exudative nephritis
  interstitial nephritis
Nephropathy with lesion of:
  exudative nephritis
  interstitial nephritis
Renal disease with lesion of:
  exudative nephritis
  interstitial nephritis

583.9 With unspecified pathological lesion in kidney

Glomerulitis NOS   Nephritis NOS
Glomerulonephritis NOS   Nephropathy NOS

Excludes *nephropathy complicating pregnancy, labor, or the puerperium (642.0–642.9, 646.2)*
      renal disease NOS with no stated cause (593.9)

Coding Clinic: 1994, Q4, P35

Item 10–5 Decreased blood flow is the usual cause of **acute renal failure** that offers a good prognosis for recovery. **Chronic renal failure** is usually the result of long-standing kidney disease and is a very serious condition that generally results in death.

● **584 Acute ~~renal~~ kidney failure** ◀▬

Includes   Acute renal failure   ◀

Excludes *following labor and delivery (669.3)*
    posttraumatic (958.5)
    that complicating:
      abortion (634–638 with .3, 639.3)
      ectopic or molar pregnancy (639.3)

Coding Clinic: 1992, Q2, P5x2

584.5 Acute kidney failure ~~W~~with lesion of tubular necrosis 🔹 ◀▬

Lower nephron nephrosis
Renal failure with (acute) tubular necrosis
Tubular necrosis:
  NOS
  acute

Ex: 249.40-249.41, 249.80-249.91, 250.40-250.43, 250.80-250.93, 274.10, 274.19, 580.0-591, 593.0-593.2, 593.89-593.9, 599.70-599.9, 753.0-753.3, 753.9

584.6 Acute kidney failure ~~W~~with lesion of renal cortical necrosis 🔹 ◀▬

Ex: 249.40-249.41, 249.80-249.91, 250.40-250.43, 250.80-250.93, 274.10, 274.19, 580.0-591, 593.0-593.2, 593.89-593.9, 599.70-599.9, 753.0-753.3, 753.9

584.7 Acute kidney failure ~~W~~with lesion of renal medullary [papillary] necrosis 🔹 ◀▬

Necrotizing renal papillitis

Ex: 249.40-249.41, 249.80-249.91, 250.40-250.43, 250.80-250.93, 274.10, 274.19, 580.0-591, 593.0-593.2, 593.89-593.9, 599.70-599.9, 753.0-753.3, 753.9

584.8 Acute kidney failure ~~W~~with other specified pathological lesion in kidney 🔹 ◀▬

Ex: 249.40-249.41, 249.80-249.91, 250.40-250.43, 250.80-250.93, 274.10, 274.19, 580.0-591, 593.0-593.2, 593.89-593.9, 599.70-599.9

584.9 Acute ~~renal~~ kidney failure, unspecified ◄▥
Acute kidney injury (nontraumatic)

> **Excludes** *traumatic kidney injury (866.00-866.13)*

(Ex:) 249.40-249.41, 249.80-249.91, 250.40-250.43, 250.80-250.93, 274.10, 274.19, 580.0-591, 593.0-593.2, 593.89-593.9, 599.70-599.9, 753.0-753.3, 753.9

Coding Clinic: 2008, Q4, P192-193; 2007, Q4, P96-97; 2005, Q2, P18-19; 2003, Q2, P7; 2003, Q1, P22; 2002, Q3, P21x2, 28x2; 2001, Q2, P14x2; 2000, Q3, P9; 2000, Q1, P22; 1996, Q3, P9; 1993, Q4, P34

OGCR Section I.C.10.a.1
> The ICD-9-CM classifies CKD based on severity. The severity of CKD is designated by stages I-V. Stage II, code 585.2, equates to mild CKD; stage III, code 585.3, equates to moderate CKD; and stage IV, code 585.4, equates to severe CKD. Code 585.6, End stage renal disease (ESRD), is assigned when the provider has documented end-stage-renal disease (ESRD). If both a stage of CKD and ESRD are documented, assign code 585.6 only.

● **585 Chronic kidney disease (CKD)**

> **Includes** Chronic uremia

Code first hypertensive chronic kidney disease, if applicable, (403.00–403.91, 404.00–404.93)

Use additional code to identify:
kidney transplant status, if applicable (V42.0)
manifestation as:
   uremic:
      neuropathy (357.4)
      pericarditis (420.0)

585.1 Chronic kidney disease, Stage I

585.2 Chronic kidney disease, Stage II (mild)

585.3 Chronic kidney disease, Stage III (moderate)
Coding Clinic: 2005, Q4, P68-69

585.4 Chronic kidney disease, Stage IV (severe) ▥
(Ex:) 249.40-249.41, 249.80-249.91, 250.40-250.43, 250.80-250.93, 274.10, 274.19, 580.0-591, 593.0-593.2, 593.89-593.9, 599.70-599.9, 753.0-753.3, 753.9

585.5 Chronic kidney disease, Stage V ▥

> **Excludes** *chronic kidney disease, stage V requiring chronic dialysis (585.6)*

(Ex:) 249.40-249.41, 249.80-249.91, 250.40-250.43, 250.80-250.93, 274.10, 274.19, 580.0-591, 593.0-593.2, 593.89-593.9, 599.70-599.9, 753.0-753.3, 753.9

585.6 End stage renal disease ▥
Chronic kidney disease, stage V requiring chronic dialysis
(Ex:) 249.40-249.41, 249.80-249.91, 250.40-250.43, 250.80-250.93, 274.10, 274.19, 580.0-591, 593.0-593.2, 593.89-593.9, 599.70-599.9, 753.0-753.3, 753.9

Coding Clinic: 2008, Q4, P193; Q1, P7-8; 2007, Q4, P84-86; Q3, P5-6; Q3, P11; 2006, Q4, P136; 2004, Q1, P5

585.9 Chronic kidney disease, unspecified
Chronic renal disease
Chronic renal failure NOS
Chronic renal insufficiency
Coding Clinic: 2008, Q1, P7-8, 19; 2007, Q2, P3; 2006, Q4, P84-86; 2003, Q4, P60-61,111-112; 2001, Q2, P11-13x2; Q1, P3; 2000, Q4, P39-40; 1998, Q4, P54-55; Q3, P6-7; Q2, P20-21; 1996, Q3, P9; 1995, Q2, P10; 1987, Sept-Oct, P10; 1985, Nov-Dec, P15

586 Renal failure, unspecified

> **Includes** Uremia NOS

> **Excludes** *following labor and delivery (669.3)*
> *posttraumatic renal failure (958.5)*
> *that complicating:*
>   *abortion (634–638 with .3, 639.3)*
>   *ectopic or molar pregnancy (639.3)*
> *uremia:*
>   *extrarenal (788.9)*
>   *prerenal (788.9)*

Coding Clinic: 1998, Q3, P6; 1984, Sept-Oct, P16

587 Renal sclerosis, unspecified ◄

> **Includes** Atrophy of kidney
> Contracted kidney
> Renal:
>   ~~Atropy of kidney~~
>   cirrhosis
>   fibrosis

● **588 Disorders resulting from impaired renal function**

588.0 Renal osteodystrophy
Azotemic osteodystrophy
Phosphate-losing tubular disorders
Renal:
   dwarfism
   infantilism
   rickets

588.1 Nephrogenic diabetes insipidus ▥

> **Excludes** *diabetes insipidus NOS (253.5)*

(Ex:) 016.00-016.06, 016.30-016.36, 016.90 -016.96, 017.90-017.96, 078.6, 098.10, 098.19, 098.30-098.31, 098.89, 112.2, 131.00, 131.8-131.9, 249.40-249.41, 249.80-249.91, 250.40-250.43, 250.80-250.93, 274.10, 274.19, 580.0-584.9, 585.3-585.6, 586-591, 593.0-593.2, 593.89-593.9, 599.70-599.9

● **588.8 Other specified disorders resulting from impaired renal function**

> **Excludes** *secondary hypertension (405.0–405.9)*

Coding Clinic: 2004, Q4, P57-59

588.81 Secondary hyperparathyroidism (of renal origin) ▥
Secondary hyperparathyroidism NOS
(Ex:) 016.00-016.06, 016.30-016.36, 016.90-016.96, 017.90-017.96, 078.6, 098.10, 098.19, 098.30-098.31, 098.89, 112.2, 131.00, 131.8-131.9, 249.40-249.41, 249.80-249.91, 250.40-250.43, 250.80-250.93, 274.10, 274.19, 580.0-584.9, 586-588.1, 588.89-591, 593.0-593.2, 593.89-593.9, 599.70-599.9

588.89 Other specified disorders resulting from impaired renal function
Hypokalemic nephropathy

588.9 Unspecified disorder resulting from impaired renal function

● **589 Small kidney of unknown cause**

589.0 Unilateral small kidney

589.1 Bilateral small kidneys

589.9 Small kidney, unspecified

DISEASES OF THE GENITOURINARY SYSTEM (580–629)

OTHER DISEASES OF URINARY SYSTEM (590–599)

● **590 Infections of kidney**

Use additional code to identify organism, such as Escherichia coli [E. coli] (041.4)

● **590.0 Chronic pyelonephritis**
Chronic pyelitis
Chronic pyonephrosis

Code, if applicable, any causal condition first

590.00 Without lesion of renal medullary necrosis

590.01 With lesion of renal medullary necrosis 🅴
Ex: 016.00-016.06, 016.30-016.36, 016.90-016.96, 017.90-017.96, 078.6, 098.10, 098.19, 098.30-098.31, 098.89, 112.2, 131.00, 131.8-131.9, 249.40-249.41, 249.80-249.91, 250.40-250.43, 250.80-250.93, 274.10, 274.19, 580.0-584.9, 586-591, 593.0-593.2, 593.89-593.9, 599.70-599.9, 646.61-646.64

● **590.1 Acute pyelonephritis**
Acute pyelitis
Acute pyonephrosis

590.10 Without lesion of renal medullary necrosis 🅴 🅴
Ex: 016.00-016.06, 016.30-016.36, 016.90-016.96, 017.90-017.96, 098.10, 098.19, 098.30-098.31, 098.89, 112.2, 131.00, 131.8-131.9, 249.40-249.41, 249.80-249.91, 250.40-250.43, 250.80-250.93, 274.10, 274.19, 580.0-591, 593.0-593.2, 593.89-593.9, 599.0, 599.70-599.9

590.11 With lesion of renal medullary necrosis 🅴 🅴
Ex: 016.00-016.06, 016.30-016.36, 016.90-016.96, 017.90-017.96, 098.10, 098.19, 098.30-098.31, 098.89, 112.2, 131.00, 131.8-131.9, 249.40-249.41, 249.80- 249.91, 250.40-250.43, 250.80-250.93, 274.10, 274.19, 580.0-591, 593.0-593.2, 593.89-593.9, 599.0, 599.70-599.9

590.2 Renal and perinephric abscess 🅴 🅴
Abscess:
  kidney
  nephritic
  perirenal
Carbuncle of kidney
Ex: 016.00-016.06, 016.30-016.36, 016.90- 016.96, 017.90-017.96, 098.10, 098.19, 098.30-098.31, 098.89, 112.2, 131.00, 131.8-131.9, 249.40-249.41, 249.80-249.91, 250.40-250.43, 250.80-250.93, 274.10, 274.19, 580.0-591, 593.0-593.2, 593.89-593.9, 599.0, 599.70-599.9

590.3 Pyeloureteritis cystica 🅴 🅴
Infection of renal pelvis and ureter
Ureteritis cystica
Cystica is an infection of the urinary bladder.
Ex: 016.00-016.06, 016.30-016.36, 016.90-016.96, 017.90-017.96, 098.10, 098.19, 098.30-098.31, 098.89, 112.2, 131.00, 131.8-131.9, 274.10, 274.19, 580.0-591, 593.0-593.2, 593.89-593.9, 599.0, 599.70-599.9

● **590.8 Other pyelonephritis or pyonephrosis, not specified as acute or chronic**

590.80 Pyelonephritis, unspecified 🅴 🅴
Pyelitis NOS
Pyelonephritis NOS
Ex: 016.00-016.06, 016.30-016.36, 016.90-016.96, 017.90-017.96, 098.10, 098.19, 098.30-098.31, 098.89, 112.2, 131.00, 131.8-131.9, 274.10, 274.19, 580.0-591, 593.0-593.2, 593.89-593.9, 599.0, 599.70-599.9
Coding Clinic: 1997, Q4, P40

▶ *590.81 Pyelitis or pyelonephritis in diseases classified elsewhere* 🅴 🅴

Code first underlying disease, as:
tuberculosis (016.0)
Ex: 016.00-016.06, 016.30-016.36, 016.90-016.96, 017.90-017.96, 098.10, 098.19, 098.30-098.31, 098.89, 112.2, 131.00, 131.8-131.9, 274.10, 274.19, 580.0-591, 593.0-593.2, 593.89-593.9, 599.0, 599.70-599.9

590.9 Infection of kidney, unspecified

Excludes *urinary tract infection NOS (599.0)*

● **591 Hydronephrosis** 🅴
Hydrocalycosis
Hydronephrosis
Hydroureteronephrosis

Excludes *congenital hydronephrosis (753.29)*
hydroureter (593.5)
Ex: 016.00-016.06, 016.30-016.36, 016.90-016.96, 017.90-017.96, 098.10, 098.19, 098.30-098.31, 098.89, 112.2, 131.00, 131.8-131.9, 274.10, 274.19, 580.0-591, 593.0-593.2, 593.89-593.9, 599.0, 599.70-599.9
Coding Clinic: 1998, Q2, P9

● **592 Calculus of kidney and ureter**

Excludes *nephrocalcinosis (275.49)*

592.0 Calculus of kidney
Nephrolithiasis NOS
Renal calculus or stone
Staghorn calculus
Stone in kidney

Excludes *uric acid nephrolithiasis (274.11)*
Coding Clinic: 2000, Q1, P4; 1993, Q2, P3

592.1 Calculus of ureter 🅴
Ureteric stone
Ureterolithiasis
Ex: 592.0-592.9, 593.3-593.5, 593.89-594.9, 599.60-599.9
Coding Clinic: 1998, Q2, P9; 1991, Q1, P11

592.9 Urinary calculus, unspecified
Coding Clinic: 1997, Q4, P40

◀ New   ◀▥ Revised   ~~deleted~~ Deleted   ● Unacceptable Principal Diagnosis   ● Use Additional Digit(s)
▶ Manifestation Code   OGCR Official Guidelines   Coding Clinic   Excludes   Includes   Use additional   Code first   Omit code

Figure 10–3 Acute pyelonephritis. Cortical surface exhibits grayish white areas of inflammation and abscess formation. (From Kumar: Robbins and Cotran: Pathologic Basis of Disease, 7th ed. 2005, Saunders, An Imprint of Elsevier)

Item 10-6 Pyelonephritis is an infection of the kidneys and ureters and may be chronic or acute in one or both kidneys.

Figure 10–4 Hydronephrosis of the kidney, with marked dilatation of pelvis and calyces and thinning of renal parenchyma. (From Kumar: Robbins and Cotran: Pathologic Basis of Disease, 7th ed. 2005, Saunders, An Imprint of Elsevier)

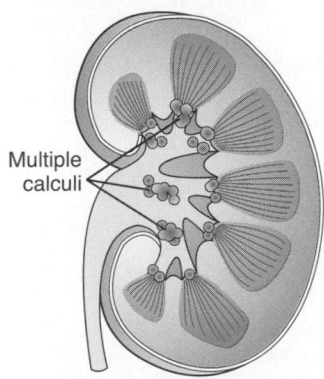

Multiple calculi

Figure 10–5 Multiple urinary calculi.

● **593   Other disorders of kidney and ureter**

593.0 Nephroptosis
Floating kidney   Mobile kidney

593.1 Hypertrophy of kidney

593.2 Cyst of kidney, acquired
Cyst (multiple) (solitary) of kidney, not congenital
Peripelvic (lymphatic) cyst
Excludes calyceal or pyelogenic cyst of kidney (591)
congenital cyst of kidney (753.1)
polycystic (disease of) kidney (753.1)

593.3 Stricture or kinking of ureter
Angulation of ureter (postoperative)
Constriction of ureter (postoperative)
Stricture of pelviureteric junction
Coding Clinic: 1994, Q3, P8

593.4 Other ureteric obstruction 🅒
Idiopathic retroperitoneal fibrosis
Occlusion NOS of ureter
Excludes that due to calculus (592.1)
(Ex) 593.3-593.5, 593.89-593.9, 595.0-595.9, 596.8-596.9, 599.0, 599.60-599.9, 753.4-75.35, 753.9, V45.74
Coding Clinic: 1997, Q2, P4

593.5 Hydroureter 🅒
Excludes congenital hydroureter (753.22)
hydroureteronephrosis (591)
(Ex) 593.3-593.5, 593.89-593.9, 595.0-595.9, 596.8-596.9, 599.0, 599.60-599.9, 753.4-753.5, 753.9

593.6 Postural proteinuria
Benign postural proteinuria
Orthostatic proteinuria
Excludes proteinuria NOS (791.0)

● **593.7 Vesicoureteral reflux**
Occurs when urine flows from bladder back into ureters
593.70 Unspecified or without reflux nephropathy
593.71 With reflux nephropathy, unilateral
593.72 With reflux nephropathy, bilateral
593.73 With reflux nephropathy NOS

● **593.8 Other specified disorders of kidney and ureter**
593.81 Vascular disorders of kidney 🅒
Renal (artery):
embolism
hemorrhage
thrombosis
Renal infarction
(Ex) 593.70-593.81, 593.9
593.82 Ureteral fistula 🅒
Intestinoureteral fistula
Excludes fistula between ureter and female genital tract (619.0)
(Ex) 593.82-593.9
593.89 Other
Adhesions, kidney or ureter
Periureteritis
Polyp of ureter
Pyelectasia
Ureterocele
Excludes tuberculosis of ureter (016.2)
ureteritis cystica (590.3)
Coding Clinic: 1984, Nov-Dec, P17

593.9 Unspecified disorder of kidney and ureter
Acute renal disease
Acute renal insufficiency
Renal disease NOS
Salt-losing nephritis or syndrome
Excludes chronic renal insufficiency (585.9)
cystic kidney disease (753.1)
nephropathy, so stated (583.0–583.9)
renal disease:
arising in pregnancy or the puerperium (642.1–642.2, 642.4–642.7, 646.2)
not specified as acute or chronic, but with stated pathology or cause (583.0–583.9)
Coding Clinic: 2005, Q4, P79-80; 1998, Q2, P9

DISEASES OF THE GENITOURINARY SYSTEM (580–629)

● **594 Calculus of lower urinary tract**

    594.0 Calculus in diverticulum of bladder

    594.1 Other calculus in bladder

        Urinary bladder stone

        | **Excludes** | *staghorn calculus (592.0)* |

    594.2 Calculus in urethra

    594.8 Other lower urinary tract calculus

        Coding Clinic: 1985, Jan-Feb, P16

    594.9 Calculus of lower urinary tract, unspecified

        | **Excludes** | *calculus of urinary tract NOS (592.9)* |

● **595 Cystitis**

    A general term used to describe an infection of the bladder and irritations in the lower urinary tract

    | **Excludes** | *prostatocystitis (601.3)* |

    Use additional code to identify organism, such as Escherichia coli [E. coli] (041.4)

    595.0 Acute cystitis 🏵 🏵

        | **Excludes** | *trigonitis (595.3)* |

        (Ex) 016.10-016.16, 016.30-016.36, 016.90-016.96, 017.90-017.96, 098.0, 098.11, 098.2, 098.39, 098.89, 112.2, 131.00, 131.8-131.9, 593.3-593.5, 593.89-593.9, 595.0-595.9, 596.8-596.9, 599.0, 599.60-599.9

        Coding Clinic: 1999, Q2, P15-16; 1984, Nov-Dec, P15

    595.1 Chronic interstitial cystitis

        Describes an ongoing infection of the kidney glomeruli and tubules

        Hunner's ulcer

        Panmural fibrosis of bladder

        Submucous cystitis

    595.2 Other chronic cystitis

        Chronic cystitis NOS

        Subacute cystitis

        | **Excludes** | *trigonitis (595.3)* |

    595.3 Trigonitis

        Inflammation of triangular area of bladder (where ureters and urethra come together)

        Follicular cystitis

        Trigonitis (acute) (chronic)

        Urethrotrigonitis

▶ **595.4 Cystitis in diseases classified elsewhere**

        Code first underlying disease, as:

            actinomycosis (039.8)

            amebiasis (006.8)

            bilharziasis (120.0–120.9)

            Echinococcus infestation (122.3, 122.6)

        | **Excludes** | *cystitis:* |

                diphtheritic (032.84)

                gonococcal (098.11, 098.31)

                monilial (112.2)

                trichomonal (131.09)

                tuberculous (016.1)

    595.8 Other specified types of cystitis

    595.81 Cystitis cystica

    595.82 Irradiation cystitis 🏵

        Use additional E code to identify cause

        (Ex) 016.10-016.16, 016.30-016.36, 016.90-016.96, 017.90-017.96, 098.0, 098.11, 098.2, 098.39, 098.89, 112.2, 131.00, 131.8-131.9, 593.3-593.5, 593.89-593.9, 595.0-595.9, 596.8-596.9, 599.0, 599.60-599.9

    595.89 Other

        Abscess of bladder

        Cystitis:

            bullous

            emphysematous

            glandularis

    595.9 Cystitis, unspecified

● **596 Other disorders of bladder**

    Use additional code to identify urinary incontinence (625.6, 788.30–788.39)

    596.0 Bladder neck obstruction

        Contracture (acquired) of bladder neck or vesicourethral orifice

        Obstruction (acquired) of bladder neck or vesicourethral orifice

        Stenosis (acquired) of bladder neck or vesicourethral orifice

        | **Excludes** | *congenital (753.6)* |

        Coding Clinic: 2002, Q3, P28; 2001, Q2, P14; 1994, Q3, P12

    596.1 Intestinovesical fistula 🏵

        Passage between bladder and the intestine

        Fistula: Fistula:

            enterovesical   vesicoenteric

            vesicocolic   vesicorectal

        (Ex) 098.0, 098.2, 098.39, 098.89, 596.1-596.2, 596.8-596.9, 599.70-599.9, 788.1

    596.2 Vesical fistula, not elsewhere classified 🏵

        Fistula: Fistula:

            bladder NOS   vesicocutaneous

            urethrovesical   vesicoperineal

        | **Excludes** | *fistula between bladder and female genital tract (619.0)* |

        (Ex) 098.0, 098.2, 098.39, 098.89, 596.1-596.2, 596.8-596.9, 599.70-599.9, 788.1

    596.3 Diverticulum of bladder

        Formation of a sac from a herniation of the wall of the bladder

        Diverticulitis of bladder

        Diverticulum (acquired) (false) of bladder

        | **Excludes** | *that with calculus in diverticulum of bladder (594.0)* |

    596.4 Atony of bladder

        Diminished tone of bladder muscle

        High compliance bladder

        Hypotonicity of bladder

        Inertia of bladder

        | **Excludes** | *neurogenic bladder (596.54)* |

◀ New   ◀▥ Revised   ~~deleted~~ Deleted   ● Unacceptable Principal Diagnosis   ● Use Additional Digit(s)

▶ Manifestation Code   **OGCR** Official Guidelines   **Coding Clinic**   Excludes   Includes   Use additional   Code first   Omit code

● **596.5 Other functional disorders of bladder**

> | **Excludes** | *cauda equina syndrome with neurogenic bladder (344.61)* |

  596.51 Hypertonicity of bladder
     Hyperactivity
     Overactive bladder

  596.52 Low bladder compliance

  596.53 Paralysis of bladder

  596.54 Neurogenic bladder NOS
     Coding Clinic: 2001, Q1, P12

  596.55 Detrusor sphincter dyssynergia

  596.59 Other functional disorder of bladder
     Detrusor instability
     Coding Clinic: 1995, Q4, P72-73

596.6 Rupture of bladder, nontraumatic 🔾
   Ⓔ 596.6-596.9, 599.70-599.9, 788.1

596.7 Hemorrhage into bladder wall 🔾
   Hyperemia of bladder

> | **Excludes** | *acute hemorrhagic cystitis (595.0)* |

   Ⓔ 596.6-596.9, 599.70-599.9, 788.1

596.8 Other specified disorders of bladder
   Calcified
   Contracted
   Hemorrhage
   Hypertrophy

> | **Excludes** | *cystocele, female (618.01–618.02, 618.09, 618.2–618.4)* |
> | | *hernia or prolapse of bladder, female (618.01–618.02, 618.09, 618.2–618.4)* |

596.9 Unspecified disorder of bladder

● **597 Urethritis, not sexually transmitted, and urethral syndrome**
Inflammation of urethra caused by bacteria or virus

> | **Excludes** | *nonspecific urethritis, so stated (099.4)* |

597.0 Urethral abscess 🔾 🔾
   Abscess of:
     bulbourethral gland
     Cowper's gland
     Littré's gland
   Abscess:
     periurethral
     urethral (gland)
   Periurethral cellulitis

> | **Excludes** | *urethral caruncle (599.3)* |

   Ⓔ 098.0, 098.2, 098.39, 098.89, 099.40-099.49, 112.2, 131.00, 131.02 131.8-131.9, 597.0-598.01, 598.8-599.0, 599.60-599.9, 607.1-607.83, 607.85-607.9, 608.4-608.81, 608.85, 608.87-608.89, 752.61-752.69, 752.81-75.29, 753.6-753.9, 788.1

● **597.8 Other urethritis**

  597.80 Urethritis, unspecified

  597.81 Urethral syndrome NOS

  597.89 Other
     Adenitis, Skene's glands
     Cowperitis
     Meatitis, urethral
     Ulcer, urethra (meatus)
     Verumontanitis

> | **Excludes** | *trichomonal (131.02)* |

● **598 Urethral stricture**
Narrowing of lumen of urethra caused by scarring from an infection or injury, which results in functional obstruction

> | **Includes** | pinhole meatus |
> | | stricture of urinary meatus |

Use additional code to identify urinary incontinence (625.6, 788.30–788.39)

> | **Excludes** | *congenital stricture of urethra and urinary meatus (753.6)* |

● **598.0 Urethral stricture due to infection**

  598.00 Due to unspecified infection

  ▶ **598.01 Due to infective diseases classified elsewhere**
     Code first underlying disease, as:
      gonococcal infection (098.2)
      schistosomiasis (120.0–120.9)
      syphilis (095.8)

598.1 Traumatic urethral stricture
   Stricture of urethra:
     late effect of injury
     postobstetric

> | **Excludes** | *postoperative following surgery on genitourinary tract (598.2)* |

598.2 Postoperative urethral stricture
   Postcatheterization stricture of urethra
   Coding Clinic: 1997, Q3, P6

598.8 Other specified causes of urethral stricture
   Coding Clinic: 1984, Nov-Dec, P9

598.9 Urethral stricture, unspecified

● **599 Other disorders of urethra and urinary tract**

599.0 Urinary tract infection, site not specified 🔾 🔾

> | **Excludes** | *Candidiasis of urinary tract (112.2)* |
> | | *urinary tract infection of newborn (771.82)* |

Use additional code to identify organism, such as Escherichia coli [E. coli] (041.4)
   Ⓔ 098.2, 098.39, 098.89, 099.40-099.49, 112.2, 131.00, 131.8-131.9, 590.10-591 593.89-593.9, 595.0-595.9, 599.0, 599.60-599.9, 788.1, 996.64
   Coding Clinic: 2005, Q3, P12-13; 2004, Q2, P13; 1999, Q4, P6; Q2, P15-16; 1998, Q1, P5; 1996, Q4, P33; 1995, Q2, P7; 1994, Q1, P21; 1992, Q1, P13; 1988, Q4, P10; 1984, Nov-Dec, P15; July-Aug, P19

599.1 Urethral fistula 🔾
   Fistula:
     urethroperineal
     urethrorectal
   Urinary fistula NOS

> | **Excludes** | *fistula:* |
> | | *urethroscrotal (608.89)* |
> | | *urethrovaginal (619.0)* |
> | | *urethrovesicovaginal (619.0)* |

   Ⓔ 597.0-598.9, 599.1-599.9, 607.1-607.83 607.85-607.9, 608.4-608.81, 608.85, 608.87-608.89, 752.61-752.69, 752.81-752.9, 753.9, 788.1
   Coding Clinic: 1997, Q3, P6

599.2 Urethral diverticulum

599.3 Urethral caruncle
   Polyp of urethra

599.4 Urethral false passage

N Newborn Age: 0   **P** Pediatric Age: 0–17   **M** Maternity Age: 12–55   **A** Adult Age: 15–124   ♀ Females Only   ♂ Males Only

Ⓔ CC Exclusions   🔾 Complication\Comorbidity   🔾 Major C\C   🔾 Present on Admission Requirement   🔾 Hospital-Acquired Condition   **957**

DISEASES OF THE GENITOURINARY SYSTEM (580–629)

599.5 Prolapsed urethral mucosa
Prolapse of urethra
Urethrocele

> | Excludes | *urethrocele, female (618.03, 618.09, 618.2–618.4)*

● **599.6 Urinary obstruction**

> Use additional code to identify urinary
> incontinence (625.6, 788.30–788.39)

> | Excludes | *obstructive nephropathy NOS (593.89)*

Coding Clinic: 2005, Q4, P80-81

599.60 Urinary obstruction, unspecified
Obstructive uropathy NOS
Urinary (tract) obstruction NOS

599.69 Urinary obstruction, not elsewhere classified
Code, if applicable, any causal condition first,
such as:
hyperplasia of prostate (600.0–600.9 with
fifth-digit 1)

● **599.7 Hematuria**
Hematuria (benign) (essential)

> | Excludes | *hemoglobinuria (791.2)*

Coding Clinic: 2008, Q4, P121; 2000, Q1, P5; 1995, Q3, P8; 1993, Q1,
P26; 5th Issue, P16; 1985, Nov-Dec, P15

599.70 Hematuria, unspecified

599.71 Gross hematuria

599.72 Microscopic hematuria

● **599.8 Other specified disorders of urethra and urinary tract**

> Use additional code to identify urinary
> incontinence (625.6, 788.30–788.39)

> | Excludes | *symptoms and other conditions classifiable*
> *to 788.0–788.2, 788.4–788.9,*
> *791.0–791.9*

599.81 Urethral hypermobility

599.82 Intrinsic (urethral) sphincter deficiency [ISD]

599.83 Urethral instability

599.84 Other specified disorders of urethra
Rupture of urethra (nontraumatic)
Urethral:
cyst
granuloma
Coding Clinic: 2009, Q1, P20

599.89 Other specified disorders of urinary tract

599.9 Unspecified disorder of urethra and urinary tract

(See Plate 366B, 387 on pages NAP-3 and NAP-5.)

DISEASES OF MALE GENITAL ORGANS (600–608)

● **600 Hyperplasia of prostate**
Benign prostatic hyperplasia (BPH) and is an enlargement of
prostate gland usually occurring with age and causing
obstructed urine flow

> | Includes | Enlarged prostate

Coding Clinic: 2005, Q3, P20; 2003, Q4, P63-64; 2002, Q3, P28; 1994, Q3,
P12-13; 1992, Q3, P7; 1986, Sept-Oct, P12; Nov-Dec, P10; 1984,
Nov-Dec, P9

● **600.0 Hypertrophy (benign) of prostate**
Benign prostatic hypertrophy
Enlargement of prostate
Smooth enlarged prostate
Soft enlarged prostate
Coding Clinic: 2003, Q1, P6; 2001, Q2, P14

600.00 Hypertrophy (benign) of prostate without
urinary obstruction and other lower urinary
tract symptoms (LUTS) ♂   A
Hypertrophy (benign) of prostate NOS

600.01 Hypertrophy (benign) of prostate with
urinary obstruction and other lower urinary
tract symptoms (LUTS) ♂   A
Hypertrophy (benign) of prostate with
urinary retention

> Use additional code to identify symptoms:
> incomplete bladder emptying (788.21)
> nocturia (788.43)
> straining on urination (788.65)
> urinary frequency (788.41)
> urinary hesitancy (788.64)
> urinary incontinence (788.30–788.39)
> urinary obstruction (599.69)
> urinary retention (788.20)
> urinary urgency (788.63)
> weak urinary stream (788.62)
> Coding Clinic: 2006, Q4, P93-95

● **600.1 Nodular prostate**
Hard, firm prostate
Multinodular prostate

> | Excludes | *malignant neoplasm of prostate (185)*

600.10 Nodular prostate without urinary
obstruction ♂   A
Nodular prostate NOS

600.11 Nodular prostate with urinary obstruction ♂   A
Nodular prostate with urinary retention

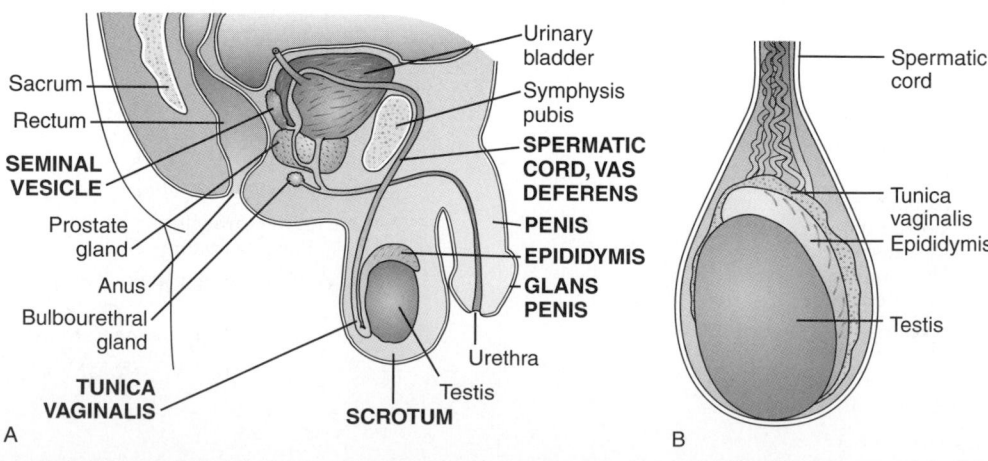

Figure 10–6 **A.** Male genital system. **B.** Testis.

◀ New   ◀▥ Revised   ~~deleted~~ Deleted   ● Unacceptable Principal Diagnosis   ● Use Additional Digit(s)
▶ Manifestation Code   **OGCR** Official Guidelines   **Coding Clinic** | Excludes | Includes   Use additional   Code first   Omit code

● **600.2   Benign localized hyperplasia of prostate**
Adenofibromatous hypertrophy of prostate
Adenoma of prostate
Fibroadenoma of prostate
Fibroma of prostate
Myoma of prostate
Polyp of prostate

> Excludes   *benign neoplasms of prostate (222.2)*
> *hypertrophy of prostate (600.00–600.01)*
> *malignant neoplasm of prostate (185)*

600.20   Benign localized hyperplasia of prostate without urinary obstruction and other lower urinary tract symptoms (LUTS) ♂   A
Benign localized hyperplasia of prostate NOS

600.21   Benign localized hyperplasia of prostate with urinary obstruction and other lower urinary tract symptoms (LUTS) ♂   A
Benign localized hyperplasia of prostate with urinary retention

> Use additional code to identify symptoms:
> incomplete bladder emptying (788.21)
> nocturia (788.43)
> straining on urination (788.65)
> urinary frequency (788.41)
> urinary hesitancy (788.64)
> urinary incontinence (788.30–788.39)
> urinary obstruction (599.69)
> urinary retention (788.20)
> urinary urgency (788.63)
> weak urinary stream (788.62)

600.3   Cyst of prostate ♂   A

● **600.9   Hyperplasia of prostate, unspecified**
Median bar
Prostatic obstruction NOS

600.90   Hyperplasia of prostate, unspecified, without urinary obstruction and other lower urinary tract symptoms (LUTS) ♂   A
Hyperplasia of prostate NOS

600.91   Hyperplasia of prostate, unspecified, with urinary obstruction and other lower urinary tract symptoms (LUTS) ♂   A
Hyperplasia of prostate, unspecified, with urinary retention

> Use additional code to identify symptoms:
> incomplete bladder emptying (788.21)
> nocturia (788.43)
> straining on urination (788.65)
> urinary frequency (788.41)
> urinary hesitancy (788.64)
> urinary incontinence (788.30–788.39)
> urinary obstruction (599.69)
> urinary retention (788.20)
> urinary urgency (788.63)
> weak urinary stream (788.62)

● **601   Inflammatory diseases of prostate**

> Use additional code to identify organism, such as Staphylococcus (041.1), or Streptococcus (041.0)

601.0   Acute prostatitis ♂ 🦠   A
(Ex:) 098.12, 098.32, 098.89, 112.2, 131.00, 131.03, 131.8-131.9, 600.00-602.9

601.1   Chronic prostatitis ♂   A

601.2   Abscess of prostate ♂ 🦠   A
(Ex:) 098.12, 098.32, 098.89, 112.2, 131.00, 131.03, 131.8-131.9, 600.00-602.9

601.3   Prostatocystitis ♂   A

▷ **601.4   *Prostatitis in diseases classified elsewhere* ♂**   A

> *Code first* underlying disease, as:
> actinomycosis (039.8)   syphilis (095.8)
> blastomycosis (116.0)   tuberculosis (016.5)

> Excludes   *prostatitis:*
> *gonococcal (098.12, 098.32)*
> *monilial (112.2)*
> *trichomonal (131.03)*

601.8   Other specified inflammatory diseases of prostate ♂   A
Prostatitis:
   cavitary   granulomatous
   diverticular

601.9   Prostatitis, unspecified ♂   A
Prostatitis NOS

● **602   Other disorders of prostate**

602.0   Calculus of prostate ♂   A
Prostatic stone

602.1   Congestion or hemorrhage of prostate ♂   A

602.2   Atrophy of prostate ♂   A

602.3   Dysplasia of prostate ♂
Prostatic intraepithelial neoplasia I (PIN I)
Prostatic intraepithelial neoplasia II (PIN II)

> Excludes   *prostatic intraepithelial neoplasia III (PIN III) (233.4)*

602.8   Other specified disorders of prostate ♂   A
Fistula of prostate
Infarction of prostate
Stricture of prostate
Periprostatic adhesions

602.9   Unspecified disorder of prostate ♂   A

● **603   Hydrocele**

> Includes   hydrocele of spermatic cord, testis, or tunica vaginalis

> Excludes   *congenital (778.6)*

603.0   Encysted hydrocele

603.1   Infected hydrocele 🦠

> Use additional code to identify organism
> (Ex:) 112.2, 131.00, 131.8-131.9, 603.0-603.9

603.8   Other specified types of hydrocele

603.9   Hydrocele, unspecified

DISEASES OF THE GENITOURINARY SYSTEM (580–629)

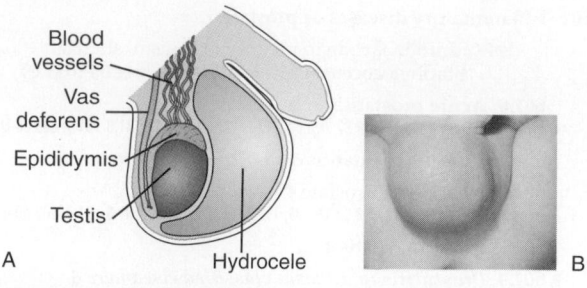

Figure 10–7 **A.** Hydrocele. **B.** Newborn with large right hydrocele. (**B** from Behrman: Nelson Textbook of Pediatrics, 17th ed. 2004, Saunders, An Imprint of Elsevier)

> **Item 10–7** **Hydrocele** is a sac of fluid accumulating in the testes membrane.

● **604 Orchitis and epididymitis**

An inflammation of one or both testes as a result of mumps or other infection, trauma, or metastasis. **Epididymitis** *is an inflammation of the epididymis (the tubular structure that connects testicle with vas deferens).*

Use additional code to identify organism such as Escherichia coli [E. coli] (041.4), Staphylococcus (041.1), or Streptococcus (041.0)

604.0 Orchitis, epididymitis, and epididymo-orchitis, with abscess ♂ 🕮

Abscess of epididymis or testis

Ⓔ 072.0, 098.13-098.14, 098.33-098.34, 098.89, 112.2, 131.00, 131.8-131.9, 604.0-604.99

● **604.9 Other orchitis, epididymitis, and epididymo-orchitis, without mention of abscess**

604.90 Orchitis and epididymitis, unspecified ♂

▶ **604.91 Orchitis and epididymitis in diseases classified elsewhere** ♂

Code first underlying disease, as:
diphtheria (032.89)
filariasis (125.0–125.9)
syphilis (095.8)

| Excludes | orchitis:
gonococcal (098.13, 098.33)
mumps (072.0)
tuberculous (016.5)
tuberculous epididymitis (016.4)

604.99 Other ♂

605 Redundant prepuce and phimosis ♂

Adherent prepuce
Paraphimosis
Phimosis (congenital)
Tight foreskin
Coding Clinic: 2008, Q3, P9

> **Item 10-8** Male infertility is the inability of the female sex partner to conceive after one year of unprotected intercourse. **Azoospermia** is no sperm ejaculated and **oligospermia** is few sperm ejaculated—both resulting in infertility. Extratesticular causes such as injury, infections, radiation, and chemotherapy may also cause male infertility.

● **606 Infertility, male**
Coding Clinic: 1996, Q2, P9

606.0 Azoospermia ♂   A

Absolute infertility
Infertility due to:
germinal (cell) aplasia
spermatogenic arrest (complete)

606.1 Oligospermia ♂   A

Infertility due to:
germinal cell desquamation
hypospermatogenesis
incomplete spermatogenic arrest

606.8 Infertility due to extratesticular causes ♂   A

Infertility due to:
drug therapy
infection
obstruction of efferent ducts
radiation
systemic disease

606.9 Male infertility, unspecified ♂   A

● **607 Disorders of penis**

| Excludes | phimosis (605)

607.0 Leukoplakia of penis ♂

Kraurosis of penis

| Excludes | carcinoma in situ of penis (233.5)
erythroplasia of Queyrat (233.5)

607.1 Balanoposthitis ♂

Balanitis

Use additional code to identify organism

607.2 Other inflammatory disorders of penis ♂

Abscess of corpus cavernosum or penis
Boil of corpus cavernosum or penis
Carbuncle of corpus cavernosum or penis
Cellulitis of corpus cavernosum or penis
Cavernitis (penis)

Use additional code to identify organism

| Excludes | herpetic infection (054.13)

607.3 Priapism ♂ 🕮

Painful erection
Ⓔ 607.0-607.9

● **607.8 Other specified disorders of penis**

607.81 Balanitis xerotica obliterans ♂

Induratio penis plastica

607.82 Vascular disorders of penis ♂ 🕮

Embolism of corpus cavernosum or penis
Hematoma (nontraumatic) of corpus cavernosum or penis
Hemorrhage of corpus cavernosum or penis
Thrombosis of corpus cavernosum or penis
Ⓔ 607.82-607.83

607.83 Edema of penis ♂

607.84 Impotence of organic origin ♂   A

> **Excludes** *nonorganic (302.72)*

Coding Clinic: 1985, July-Aug, P9

607.85 Peyronie's disease ♂

Coding Clinic: 2003, Q4, P64-65

607.89 Other ♂

Atrophy of corpus cavernosum or penis
Fibrosis of corpus cavernosum or penis
Hypertrophy of corpus cavernosum or
  penis
Ulcer (chronic) of corpus cavernosum or
  penis

607.9 Unspecified disorder of penis ♂

● **608 Other disorders of male genital organs**

608.0 Seminal vesiculitis ♂

Abscess of seminal vesicle
Cellulitis of seminal vesicle
Vesiculitis (seminal)

> Use additional code to identify organism

> **Excludes** *gonococcal infection (098.14, 098.34)*

608.1 Spermatocele ♂

● **608.2 Torsion of testis**

Coding Clinic: 2006, Q4, P95-96

608.20 Torsion of testis, unspecified ♂🗝
(Ex) 608.20-608.24

608.21 Extravaginal torsion of spermatic cord ♂🗝
(Ex) 608.20-608.24

608.22 Intravaginal torsion of spermatic cord ♂🗝
Torsion of spermatic cord NOS
(Ex) 608.20-608.24

Rotation of
spermatic cord

Epididymis

Testis

A   B

Figure 10–8   A. Torsion of testis. **B.** Torsion of the testis. (**B** from
Kumar: Robbins and Cotran: Pathologic Basis of Disease, 7th ed.
2005, Saunders, An Imprint of Elsevier)

Item 10–9 Seminal vesiculitis is an inflammation of the
seminal vesicle. Spermatocele is a benign cystic accumulation
of sperm arising from the head of the epididymis. Torsion of the
testis is a medical emergency occurring most commonly in boys
7 to 12 years of age and results from a congenital abnormality
of the covering of the testis allowing the testis to twist within its
sac and cutting off the blood supply to the testis.

608.23 Torsion of appendix testis ♂🗝
(Ex) 608.20-608.24

608.24 Torsion of appendix epididymis ♂🗝
(Ex) 608.20-608.24

608.3 Atrophy of testis ♂

**608.4 Other inflammatory disorders of male genital
organs** ♂

Abscess of scrotum, spermatic cord, testis [except
  abscess], tunica vaginalis, or vas deferens
Boil of scrotum, spermatic cord, testis [except
  abscess], tunica vaginalis, or vas deferens
Carbuncle of scrotum, spermatic cord, testis [except
  abscess], tunica vaginalis, or vas deferens
Cellulitis of scrotum, spermatic cord, testis [except
  abscess], tunica vaginalis, or vas deferens
Vasitis

> Use additional code to identify organism

> **Excludes** *abscess of testis (604.0)*

● **608.8 Other specified disorders of male genital organs**

▶ *608.81 Disorders of male genital organs in diseases
  classified elsewhere* ♂

> *Code first* underlying disease, as:
  filariasis (125.0–125.9)
  tuberculosis (016.5)

608.82 Hematospermia ♂

608.83 Vascular disorders ♂

Hematoma (nontraumatic) of seminal
  vesicle, spermatic cord, testis, scrotum,
  tunica vaginalis, or vas deferens
Hemorrhage of seminal vesicle, spermatic
  cord, testis, scrotum, tunica vaginalis,
  or vas deferens
Thrombosis of seminal vesicle, spermatic
  cord, testis, scrotum, tunica vaginalis,
  or vas deferens
Hematocele NOS, male

Coding Clinic: 2003, Q4, P110

608.84 Chylocele of tunica vaginalis ♂

608.85 Stricture ♂

Stricture of: Stricture of:
  spermatic cord   vas deferens
  tunica vaginalis

608.86 Edema ♂

608.87 Retrograde ejaculation ♂

608.89 Other ♂

Atrophy of seminal vesicle, spermatic cord,
  testis, scrotum tunica vaginalis, or vas
  deferens
Fibrosis of seminal vesicle, spermatic cord,
  testis, scrotum tunica vaginalis, or vas
  deferens
Hypertrophy of seminal vesicle, spermatic
  cord, testis, scrotum tunica vaginalis,
  or vas deferens
Ulcer of seminal vesicle, spermatic cord,
  testis, scrotum tunica vaginalis, or vas
  deferens

> **Excludes** *atrophy of testis (608.3)*

608.9 Unspecified disorder of male genital organs ♂

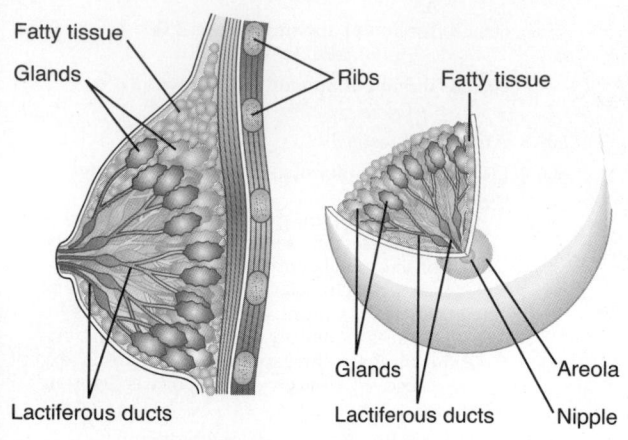

Figure 10–9   Breast.

DISORDERS OF BREAST (610–612)

● **610   Benign mammary dysplasias**
Benign lumpiness of the breast.

610.0   Solitary cyst of breast
Cyst (solitary) of breast

610.1   Diffuse cystic mastopathy   A
Chronic cystic mastitis
Cystic breast
Fibrocystic disease of breast
Coding Clinic: 2006, Q2, P10

610.2   Fibroadenosis of breast
Fibroadenosis of breast:	Fibroadenosis of breast:
NOS	diffuse
chronic	periodic
cystic	segmental

610.3   Fibrosclerosis of breast

610.4   Mammary duct ectasia
Comedomastitis
Duct ectasia
Mastitis:
   periductal
   plasma cell

610.8   Other specified benign mammary dysplasias
Mazoplasia
Sebaceous cyst of breast
Coding Clinic: 2009, Q2, P8

610.9   Benign mammary dysplasia, unspecified

● **611   Other disorders of breast**
Excludes   *that associated with lactation or the puerperium*
(675.0–676.9)

611.0   Inflammatory disease of breast
Abscess (acute) (chronic) (nonpuerperal) of:
   areola
   breast
Mammillary fistula
Mastitis (acute) (subacute) (nonpuerperal):
   NOS
   infective
   retromammary
   submammary

Excludes   *carbuncle of breast (680.2)*
chronic cystic mastitis (610.1)
neonatal infective mastitis (771.5)
thrombophlebitis of breast [Mondor's
disease] (451.89)

611.1   Hypertrophy of breast
Gynecomastia
Hypertrophy of breast:
   NOS
   massive pubertal
Excludes   *breast engorgement in newborn (778.7)*
disproportion of reconstructed breast
(612.1)

611.2   Fissure of nipple

● **611.3   Fat necrosis of breast**
Fat necrosis (segmental) of breast
Code first breast necrosis due to breast graft (996.79)

611.4   Atrophy of breast

611.5   Galactocele

611.6   Galactorrhea not associated with childbirth
Excessive or spontaneous flow of milk
Coding Clinic: 1985, July-Aug, P9

● **611.7   Signs and symptoms in breast**

611.71   Mastodynia
Pain in breast

611.72   Lump or mass in breast
Coding Clinic: 2003, Q2, P3-5

611.79   Other
Induration of breast
Inversion of nipple
Nipple discharge
Retraction of nipple

● **611.8   Other specified disorders of breast**
Coding Clinic: 2008, Q4, P121-122

611.81   Ptosis of breast   A
Excludes   *ptosis of native breast in relation to*
reconstructed breast (612.1)

611.82   Hypoplasia of breast   A
Micromastia
Excludes   *congenital absence of breast* ◀
(757.6)
hypoplasia of native breast in
relation to reconstructed
breast (612.1)

611.83   Capsular contracture of breast implant   A

611.89   Other specified disorders of breast
Hematoma (nontraumatic) of breast
Infarction of breast
Occlusion of breast duct
Subinvolution of breast (postlactational)
   (postpartum)

611.9   Unspecified breast disorder

● **612   Deformity and disproportion of reconstructed breast**
Coding Clinic: 2008, Q4, P123

612.0   Deformity of reconstructed breast   A
Contour irregularity in reconstructed breast
Excess tissue in reconstructed breast
Misshapen reconstructed breast

612.1   Disproportion of reconstructed breast   A
Breast asymmetry between native breast and
   reconstructed breast
Disproportion between native breast and
   reconstructed breast

DISEASES OF THE GENITOURINARY SYSTEM (580–629)

◀ New   ◀▥ Revised   ~~deleted~~ Deleted   ● Unacceptable Principal Diagnosis   ● Use Additional Digit(s)
▶ Manifestation Code   **OGCR** Official Guidelines   **Coding Clinic**   Excludes   Includes   Use additional   Code first   Omit code

(See Plate 366A on page NAP-3.)

Item 10-10 Salpingitis is an infection of one or both fallopian tubes. **Oophoritis** is an infection of one or both ovaries.

INFLAMMATORY DISEASE OF FEMALE PELVIC ORGANS (614–616)

Use additional code to identify organism, such as Staphylococcus (041.1), or Streptococcus (041.0)

Excludes *that associated with pregnancy, abortion, childbirth, or the puerperium (630–676.9)*

● **614 Inflammatory disease of ovary, fallopian tube, pelvic cellular tissue, and peritoneum**

Excludes *endometritis (615.0–615.9)*
major infection following delivery (670.0-670.8) ◀▥
that complicating:
    abortion (634–638 with .0, 639.0)
    ectopic or molar pregnancy (639.0)
    pregnancy or labor (646.6)

614.0 Acute salpingitis and oophoritis ♀ 🔖

Any condition classifiable to 614.2, specified as acute or subacute

Ⓔ 016.60-016.96, 017.90-017.96, 098.15-098.17, 098.35-098.37, 098.89, 112.2, 131.00, 131.8-131.9, 614.0-615.9, 616.81-616.9, 625.70, 625.79-625.9, 629.20-629.9, 752.81-752.9

614.1 Chronic salpingitis and oophoritis ♀

Hydrosalpinx
Salpingitis:
    follicularis
    isthmica nodosa
Any condition classifiable to 614.2, specified as chronic

614.2 Salpingitis and oophoritis not specified as acute, subacute, or chronic ♀

Abscess (of):
    fallopian tube
    ovary
    tubo-ovarian
Oophoritis
Perioophoritis
Perisalpingitis
Pyosalpinx
Salpingitis
Salpingo-oophoritis
Tubo-ovarian inflammatory disease

Excludes *gonococcal infection (chronic) (098.37)*
acute (098.17)
tuberculous (016.6)

614.3 Acute parametritis and pelvic cellulitis ♀ 🔖

Acute inflammatory pelvic disease
Any condition classifiable to 614.4, specified as acute

Ⓔ 016.60-016.96, 017.90-017.96, 098.15-098.17, 098.35-098.37, 098.89, 112.2, 131.00, 131.8-131.9, 614.0-615.9, 616.81-616.9, 625.70, 625.79-625.9, 629.20-629.9, 752.81-752.9

614.4 Chronic or unspecified parametritis and pelvic cellulitis ♀

Abscess (of):
    broad ligament chronic or NOS
    parametrium chronic or NOS
    pelvis, female chronic or NOS
    pouch of Douglas chronic or NOS
Chronic inflammatory pelvic disease
Pelvic cellulitis, female

Excludes *tuberculous (016.7)*

614.5 Acute or unspecified pelvic peritonitis, female ♀ 🔖

Ⓔ 016.60-016.96, 017.90-017.96, 098.15-098.17, 098.35-098.37, 098.89, 112.2, 131.00, 131.8-131.9, 614.0-615.9, 616.81-616.9, 625.70, 625.79-625.9, 629.20-629.9, 752.81-752.9

614.6 Pelvic peritoneal adhesions, female (postoperative) (postinfection) ♀

Adhesions:
    peritubal
    tubo-ovarian

Use additional code to identify any associated infertility (628.2)

Coding Clinic: 2003, Q3, P6-7; Q1, P4-5; 1995, Q3, P7

614.7 Other chronic pelvic peritonitis, female ♀ 🔖

Excludes *tuberculous (016.7)*

Ⓔ 016.60-016.96, 017.90-017.96, 098.15-098.17, 098.35-098.37, 098.89, 112.2, 131.00, 131.8-131.9, 614.0-615.9, 616.81-616.9, 625.70, 625.79-625.9, 629.20-629.9, 752.81-752.9

614.8 Other specified inflammatory disease of female pelvic organs and tissues ♀

614.9 Unspecified inflammatory disease of female pelvic organs and tissues ♀

Pelvic infection or inflammation, female NOS
Pelvic inflammatory disease [PID]

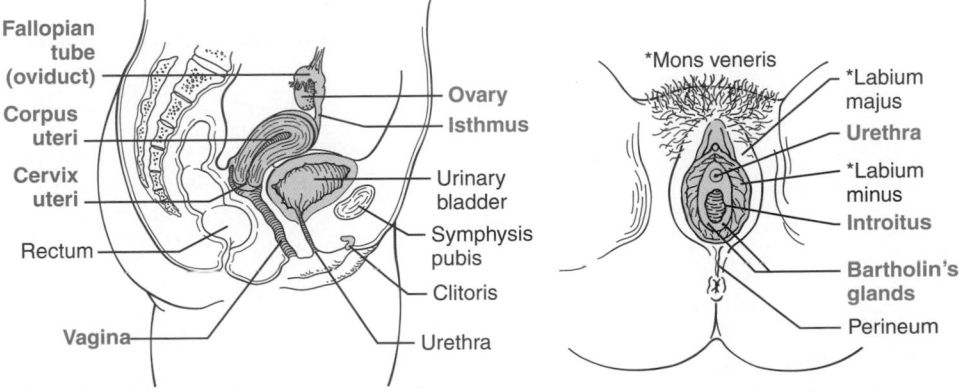

A   Female Genital System   B   *The three parts of the **vulva**

Figure 10–10 A. Female genital system. **B.** External female genital system. (From Buck CJ: Step-by-Step Medical Coding, 2006 ed. Philadelphia, WB Saunders, 2006.)

N Newborn Age: 0   **P** Pediatric Age: 0–17   **M** Maternity Age: 12–55   **A** Adult Age: 15–124   ♀ Females Only   ♂ Males Only

Ⓔ CC Exclusions   🔖 Complication\Comorbidity   Major C\C   Present on Admission Requirement   Hospital-Acquired Condition   **963**

DISEASES OF THE GENITOURINARY SYSTEM (580–629)

● **615 Inflammatory diseases of uterus, except cervix**

> | Excludes | *following delivery (670.0-670.8)* ◀▥
> | --- | --- |
> | | *hyperplastic endometritis (621.30-621.35)* ◀▥ |
> | | *that complicating:* |
> | | *abortion (634–638 with .0, 639.0)* |
> | | *ectopic or molar pregnancy (639.0)* |
> | | *pregnancy or labor (646.6)* |

  615.0 Acute ♀ 🕮

    Any condition classifiable to 615.9, specified as acute or subacute

    Ⓔⓧ 016.60-016.96, 017.90-017.96, 098.15-098.17, 098.35-098.37, 098.89, 112.2, 131.00, 131.8-131.9, 614.0-616.0, 616.81-616.9, 621.8-621.9, 625.70, 625.79-625.9, 629.20-629.9, 752.81-752.9

  615.1 Chronic ♀

    Any condition classifiable to 615.9, specified as chronic

  615.9 Unspecified inflammatory disease of uterus ♀

Endometritis	Perimetritis
Endomyometritis	Pyometra
Metritis	Uterine abscess
Myometritis	

● **616 Inflammatory disease of cervix, vagina, and vulva**

> | Excludes | *that complicating:* |
> | --- | --- |
> | | *abortion (634–638 with .0, 639.0)* |
> | | *ectopic or molar pregnancy (639.0)* |
> | | *pregnancy, childbirth, or the puerperium* |
> | | *(646.6)* |

  616.0 Cervicitis and endocervicitis ♀

    Cervicitis with or without mention of erosion or ectropion

    Endocervicitis with or without mention of erosion or ectropion

    Nabothian (gland) cyst or follicle

> | Excludes | *erosion or ectropion without mention of* |
> | --- | --- |
> | | *cervicitis (622.0)* |

● **616.1 Vaginitis and vulvovaginitis**

> | Excludes | *vulvar vestibulitis (625.71)* |
> | --- | --- |

  616.10 Vaginitis and vulvovaginitis, unspecified ♀

    Vaginitis:

      NOS

      postirradiation

    Vulvitis NOS

    Vulvovaginitis NOS

    Use additional code to identify organism, such as Escherichia coli [E. coli] (041.4), Staphylococcus (041.1), or Streptococcus (041.0)

> | Excludes | *noninfective leukorrhea (623.5)* |
> | --- | --- |
> | | *postmenopausal or senile vaginitis* |
> | | *(627.3)* |

▌ **616.11 *Vaginitis and vulvovaginitis in diseases classified elsewhere ♀***

    Code first underlying disease, as:

      pinworm vaginitis (127.4)

> | Excludes | *herpetic vulvovaginitis (054.11)* |
> | --- | --- |
> | | *monilial vulvovaginitis (112.1)* |
> | | *trichomonal vaginitis or* |
> | | *vulvovaginitis (131.01)* |

  616.2 Cyst of Bartholin's gland ♀

    Cysts filled with liquid or semisolid material.

    Bartholin's duct cyst

  616.3 Abscess of Bartholin's gland ♀ 🕮

    Localized collection of pus

    Vulvovaginal gland abscess

    Ⓔⓧ 016.70-016.96, 017.90-017.96, 112.1-112.2, 131.00-131.01, 131.8-131.9, 616.10-616.9, 624.3-624.9, 625.70-625.9, 629.20-629.9, 752.81-752.9

  616.4 Other abscess of vulva ♀ 🕮

    Abscess of vulva

    Carbuncle of vulva

    Furuncle of vulva

    Ⓔⓧ 016.70-016.96, 017.90-017.96, 112.1-112.2, 131.00-131.01, 131.8-131.9, 616.10-616.9, 624.3-624.9, 625.70-625.9, 629.20-629.9, 752.81-752.9

● **616.5 Ulceration of vulva**

  616.50 Ulceration of vulva, unspecified ♀

    Ulcer NOS of vulva

▌ **616.51 *Ulceration of vulva in diseases classified elsewhere ♀***

    Code first underlying disease, as:

      Behçet's syndrome (136.1)

      tuberculosis (016.7)

> | Excludes | *vulvar ulcer (in):* |
> | --- | --- |
> | | *gonococcal (098.0)* |
> | | *herpes simplex (054.12)* |
> | | *syphilitic (091.0)* |

● **616.8 Other specified inflammatory diseases of cervix, vagina, and vulva**

> | Excludes | *noninflammatory disorders of:* |
> | --- | --- |
> | | *cervix (622.0–622.9)* |
> | | *vagina (623.0–623.9)* |
> | | *vulva (624.0–624.9)* |

  616.81 Mucositis (ulcerative) of cervix, vagina, and vulva ♀ 🕮

    Use additional E code to identify adverse effects of therapy, such as:

      antineoplastic and immunosuppressive drugs (E930.7, E933.1)

      radiation therapy (E879.2)

    Ⓔⓧ 616.0, 616.81-616.9

  616.89 Other inflammatory disease of cervix, vagina and vulva ♀

    Caruncle, vagina or labium

    Ulcer, vagina

  616.9 Unspecified inflammatory disease of cervix, vagina, and vulva ♀

◀ New	◀▥ Revised	~~deleted~~ Deleted	● Unacceptable Principal Diagnosis	● Use Additional Digit(s)
▌ Manifestation Code	**OGCR** Official Guidelines	**Coding Clinic**	Excludes Includes Use additional Code first Omit code	

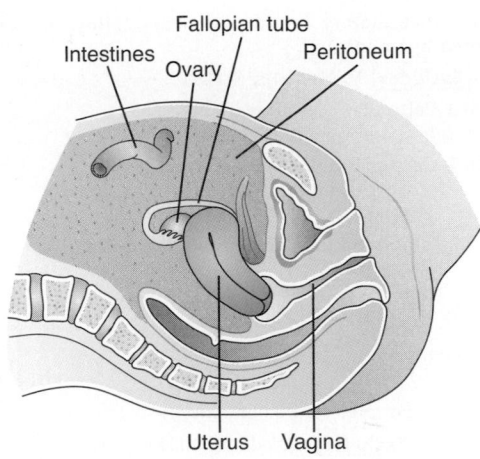

Figure 10-11 Sites of potential endometrial implants.

Item 10-11 Endometriosis is a condition for which no clear cause has been identified. Endometrial tissue is expelled from the uterus into the abdominal cavity and can implant onto a variety of organs. Classification is based on the site of implant of the endometrial tissue.

OTHER DISORDERS OF FEMALE GENITAL TRACT (617–629)

● **617 Endometriosis**
Coding Clinic: 1995, Q1, P7

617.0 Endometriosis of uterus ♀
Adenomyosis
Endometriosis:
  cervix
  internal
  myometrium
  Excludes *stromal endometriosis (236.0)*
Coding Clinic: 1992, Q3, P7-8

617.1 Endometriosis of ovary ♀
Chocolate cyst of ovary
Endometrial cystoma of ovary

617.2 Endometriosis of fallopian tube ♀

617.3 Endometriosis of pelvic peritoneum ♀
Endometriosis:
  broad ligament
  cul-de-sac (Douglas')
  parametrium
  round ligament

617.4 Endometriosis of rectovaginal septum and vagina ♀

617.5 Endometriosis of intestine ♀
Endometriosis:
  appendix
  colon
  rectum

617.6 Endometriosis in scar of skin ♀

617.8 Endometriosis of other specified sites ♀
Endometriosis:
  bladder
  lung
  umbilicus
  vulva

617.9 Endometriosis, site unspecified ♀

● **618 Genital prolapse**
Use additional code to identify urinary incontinence (625.6, 788.31, 788.33–788.39)
  Excludes *that complicating pregnancy, labor, or delivery (654.4)*

● **618.0 Prolapse of vaginal walls without mention of uterine prolapse**
  Excludes *that with uterine prolapse (618.2–618.4)*
    enterocele (618.6)
    vaginal vault prolapse following hysterectomy (618.5)
Coding Clinic: 2004, Q4, P83-85

618.00 Unspecified prolapse of vaginal walls ♀
Vaginal prolapse NOS

618.01 Cystocele, midline ♀
Cystocele NOS

618.02 Cystocele, lateral ♀
Paravaginal

618.03 Urethrocele ♀

618.04 Rectocele ♀
Proctocele

618.05 Perineocele ♀

618.09 Other prolapse of vaginal walls without mention of uterine prolapse ♀
Cystourethrocele

A

B   C

Figure 10-12 Three stages of uterine prolapse. **A.** Uterus is prolapsed. **B.** Vagina and uterus are prolapsed (incomplete uterovaginal prolapse). **C.** Vagina and uterus are completely prolapsed and are exposed through the external genitalia (complete uterovaginal prolapse).

DISEASES OF THE GENITOURINARY SYSTEM (580–629)

N Newborn Age: 0   **P** Pediatric Age: 0–17   **M** Maternity Age: 12–55   **A** Adult Age: 15–124   ♀ Females Only   ♂ Males Only

 CC Exclusions   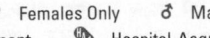 Complication\Comorbidity   Major C\C   Present on Admission Requirement   Hospital-Acquired Condition   **965**

618.1 Uterine prolapse without mention of vaginal wall prolapse ♀
Descensus uteri
Uterine prolapse:
  NOS
  complete
  first degree
  second degree
  third degree

> **Excludes** *that with mention of cystocele, urethrocele, or rectocele (618.2–618.4)*

618.2 Uterovaginal prolapse, incomplete ♀

618.3 Uterovaginal prolapse, complete ♀

618.4 Uterovaginal prolapse, unspecified ♀

618.5 Prolapse of vaginal vault after hysterectomy ♀

618.6 Vaginal enterocele, congenital or acquired ♀
Pelvic enterocele, congenital or acquired

618.7 Old laceration of muscles of pelvic floor ♀

● **618.8 Other specified genital prolapse**

618.81 Incompetence or weakening of pubocervical tissue ♀

618.82 Incompetence or weakening of rectovaginal tissue ♀

618.83 Pelvic muscle wasting ♀
Disuse atrophy of pelvic muscles and anal sphincter

618.84 Cervical stump prolapse ♀

618.89 Other specified genital prolapse ♀

618.9 Unspecified genital prolapse ♀

● **619 Fistula involving female genital tract**

> **Excludes** *vesicorectal and intestinovesical fistula (596.1)*

619.0 Urinary-genital tract fistula, female ♀ 🕮
Fistula:
  cervicovesical
  ureterovaginal
  urethrovaginal
  urethrovesicovaginal
  uteroureteric
  uterovesical
  vesicocervicovaginal
  vesicovaginal
Ⓔⓧ 619.0-619.9

619.1 Digestive-genital tract fistula, female ♀ 🕮
Fistula: Fistula:
  intestinouterine   rectovulval
  intestinovaginal   sigmoidovaginal
  rectovaginal   uterorectal
Ⓔⓧ 619.0-619.9

619.2 Genital tract-skin fistula, female ♀ 🕮
Fistula:
  uterus to abdominal wall
  vaginoperineal
Ⓔⓧ 619.0-619.9

619.8 Other specified fistulas involving female genital tract ♀ 🕮
Fistula:
  cervix
  cul-de-sac (Douglas')
  uterus
  vagina
Ⓔⓧ 619.0-619.9

619.9 Unspecified fistula involving female genital tract ♀ 🕮
Ⓔⓧ 619.0-619.9

● **620 Noninflammatory disorders of ovary, fallopian tube, and broad ligament**

> **Excludes** *hydrosalpinx (614.1)*

620.0 Follicular cyst of ovary ♀
Cyst of graafian follicle

620.1 Corpus luteum cyst or hematoma ♀
Corpus luteum hemorrhage or rupture
Lutein cyst

620.2 Other and unspecified ovarian cyst ♀
Cyst of ovary:
  NOS
  corpus albicans
  retention NOS
  serous
  theca-lutein
Simple cystoma of ovary

> **Excludes** *cystadenoma (benign) (serous) (220)*
> *developmental cysts (752.0)*
> *neoplastic cysts (220)*
> *polycystic ovaries (256.4)*
> *Stein-Leventhal syndrome (256.4)*

620.3 Acquired atrophy of ovary and fallopian tube ♀
Senile involution of ovary

620.4 Prolapse or hernia of ovary and fallopian tube ♀
Displacement of ovary and fallopian tube
Salpingocele

620.5 Torsion of ovary, ovarian pedicle, or fallopian tube ♀ 🕮
Torsion:
  accessory tube
  hydatid of Morgagni
Ⓔⓧ 620.0-620.9

620.6 Broad ligament laceration syndrome ♀
Masters-Allen syndrome

620.7 Hematoma of broad ligament ♀
Hematocele, broad ligament

620.8 Other noninflammatory disorders of ovary, fallopian tube, and broad ligament ♀
Cyst of broad ligament or fallopian tube
Polyp of broad ligament or fallopian tube
Infarction of ovary or fallopian tube
Rupture of ovary or fallopian tube
Hematosalpinx of ovary or fallopian tube

> **Excludes** *hematosalpinx in ectopic pregnancy (639.2)*
> *peritubal adhesions (614.6)*
> *torsion of ovary, ovarian pedicle, or fallopian tube (620.5)*

620.9 Unspecified noninflammatory disorder of ovary, fallopian tube, and broad ligament ♀

● **621 Disorders of uterus, not elsewhere classified**

621.0 Polyp of corpus uteri ♀
Polyp:
  endometrium
  uterus NOS

> **Excludes** *cervical polyp NOS (622.7)*

621.1 Chronic subinvolution of uterus ♀

> **Excludes** *puerperal (674.8)*

621.2 Hypertrophy of uterus ♀
Bulky or enlarged uterus

> **Excludes** *puerperal (674.8)*

◀ New   ◀═ Revised   ~~deleted~~ Deleted   ● Unacceptable Principal Diagnosis   ● Use Additional Digit(s)
▶ Manifestation Code   **OGCR** Official Guidelines   **Coding Clinic**   Excludes   Includes   Use additional   Code first   Omit code

● **621.3   Endometrial hyperplasia**
~~Hyperplasia (adenomatous) (cystic) (glandular) of endometrium~~
~~Hyperplastic endometritis~~
Coding Clinic: 2004, Q4, P85-86

    621.30   Endometrial hyperplasia, unspecified ♀
Endometrial hyperplasia NOS
Hyperplasia (adenomatous) (cystic) (glandular) of endometrium ◄
Hyperplastic endometritis ◄

    621.31   Simple endometrial hyperplasia without atypia ♀

      Excludes   *benign endometrial hyperplasia (621.34)* ◄

    621.32   Complex endometrial hyperplasia without atypia ♀

      Excludes   *benign endometrial hyperplasia (621.34)* ◄

    621.33   Endometrial hyperplasia with atypia ♀

      Excludes   *endometrial intraepithelial neoplasia [EIN] (621.35)* ◄

    621.34   Benign endometrial hyperplasia ◄

    621.35   Endometrial intraepithelial neoplasia [EIN] ◄

      Excludes   *malignant neoplasm of endometrium with endometrium intraepithelial neoplasia [EIN] (182.0)* ◄

   621.4   Hematometra ♀
Hemometra

     Excludes   *that in congenital anomaly (752.2–752.3)*

   621.5   Intrauterine synechiae ♀
Adhesions of uterus   Band(s) of uterus

   621.6   Malposition of uterus ♀
Anteversion of uterus
Retroflexion of uterus
Retroversion of uterus

     Excludes   *malposition complicating pregnancy, labor, or delivery (654.3–654.4)*
prolapse of uterus (618.1–618.4)

   621.7   Chronic inversion of uterus ♀

     Excludes   *current obstetrical trauma (665.2)*
prolapse of uterus (618.1–618.4)

   621.8   Other specified disorders of uterus, not elsewhere classified ♀
Atrophy, acquired of uterus
Cyst of uterus
Fibrosis NOS of uterus
Old laceration (postpartum) of uterus
Ulcer of uterus

     Excludes   *bilharzial fibrosis (120.0–120.9)*
endometriosis (617.0)
fistulas (619.0–619.8)
inflammatory diseases (615.0–615.9)

   621.9   Unspecified disorder of uterus ♀

● **622   Noninflammatory disorders of cervix**

     Excludes   *abnormality of cervix complicating pregnancy, labor, or delivery (654.5–654.6)*
fistula (619.0–619.8)

   622.0   Erosion and ectropion of cervix ♀
Eversion of cervix
Ulcer of cervix

     Excludes   *that in chronic cervicitis (616.0)*

● **622.1   Dysplasia of cervix (uteri)**

     Excludes   *abnormal results from cervical cytologic examination without histologic confirmation (795.00–795.09)*
carcinoma in situ of cervix (233.1)
cervical intraepithelial neoplasia III [CIN III] (233.1)
HGSIL of cervix (795.04)
Coding Clinic: 2004, Q4, P86-88; 1991, Q1, P11

    622.10   Dysplasia of cervix, unspecified ♀
Anaplasia of cervix
Cervical atypism
Cervical dysplasia NOS

    622.11   Mild dysplasia of cervix ♀
Cervical intraepithelial neoplasia I [CIN I]

    622.12   Moderate dysplasia of cervix ♀
Cervical intraepithelial neoplasia II [CIN II]

      Excludes   *carcinoma in situ of cervix (233.1)*
cervical intraepithelial neoplasia III [CIN III] (233.1)
severe dysplasia (233.1)

   622.2   Leukoplakia of cervix (uteri) ♀

     Excludes   *carcinoma in situ of cervix (233.1)*

   622.3   Old laceration of cervix ♀
Adhesions of cervix
Band(s) of cervix
Cicatrix (postpartum) of cervix

     Excludes   *current obstetrical trauma (665.3)*

   622.4   Stricture and stenosis of cervix ♀
Atresia (acquired) of cervix
Contracture of cervix
Occlusion of cervix
Pinpoint os uteri

     Excludes   *congenital (752.49)*
that complicating labor (654.6)

   622.5   Incompetence of cervix ♀

     Excludes   *complicating pregnancy (654.5)*
that affecting fetus or newborn (761.0)

   622.6   Hypertrophic elongation of cervix ♀

   622.7   Mucous polyp of cervix ♀
Polyp NOS of cervix

     Excludes   *adenomatous polyp of cervix (219.0)*

   622.8   Other specified noninflammatory disorders of cervix ♀
Atrophy (senile) of cervix
Cyst of cervix
Fibrosis of cervix
Hemorrhage of cervix

     Excludes   *endometriosis (617.0)*
fistula (619.0–619.8)
inflammatory diseases (616.0)

   622.9   Unspecified noninflammatory disorder of cervix ♀

DISEASES OF THE GENITOURINARY SYSTEM (580–629)

N Newborn Age: 0   **P** Pediatric Age: 0–17   **M** Maternity Age: 12–55   **A** Adult Age: 15–124   ♀ Females Only   ♂ Males Only

ⒺⓍ CC Exclusions   🄲 Complication\Comorbidity   🄼🄲 Major C\C   Present on Admission Requirement   Hospital-Acquired Condition   **967**

DISEASES OF THE GENITOURINARY SYSTEM (580–629)

● **623 Noninflammatory disorders of vagina**

> Excludes | abnormality of vagina complicating pregnancy,
>   labor, or delivery (654.7)
>   congenital absence of vagina (752.49)
>   congenital diaphragm or bands (752.49)
>   fistulas involving vagina (619.0–619.8)

623.0 Dysplasia of vagina ♀
Mild and moderate dysplasia of vagina
Vaginal intraepithelial neoplasia I and II [VAIN I and II]

> Excludes | abnormal results from vaginal cytological
>   examination without histologic
>   confirmation (795.10-795.19)
>   carcinoma in situ of vagina (233.31)
>   HGSIL of vagina (795.14)
>   severe dysplasia of vagina (233.31)
>   vaginal intraepithelial neoplasia III [VAIN
>   III] (233.31)

623.1 Leukoplakia of vagina ♀

623.2 Stricture or atresia of vagina ♀
Adhesions (postoperative) (postradiation) of vagina
Occlusion of vagina
Stenosis, vagina

> Use additional E code to identify any external cause

> Excludes | congenital atresia or stricture (752.49)

623.3 Tight hymenal ring ♀
Rigid hymen acquired or congenital
Tight hymenal ring acquired or congenital
Tight introitus acquired or congenital

> Excludes | imperforate hymen (752.42)

623.4 Old vaginal laceration ♀

> Excludes | old laceration involving muscles of pelvic
>   floor (618.7)

623.5 Leukorrhea, not specified as infective ♀
Leukorrhea NOS of vagina
Vaginal discharge NOS

> Excludes | trichomonal (131.00)

623.6 Vaginal hematoma ♀

> Excludes | current obstetrical trauma (665.7)

623.7 Polyp of vagina ♀

623.8 Other specified noninflammatory disorders of vagina ♀
Cyst of vagina
Hemorrhage of vagina

623.9 Unspecified noninflammatory disorder of vagina ♀

● **624 Noninflammatory disorders of vulva and perineum**

> Excludes | abnormality of vulva and perineum complicating
>   pregnancy, labor, or delivery (654.8)
>   condyloma acuminatum (078.11) ◀▥
>   fistulas involving:
>   perineum - see Alphabetic Index
>   vulva (619.0–619.8)
>   vulval varices (456.6)
>   vulvar involvement in skin conditions (690–709.9)

● **624.0 Dystrophy of vulva**

> Excludes | carcinoma in situ of vulva (233.32)
>   severe dysplasia of vulva (233.32)
>   vulvar intraepithelial neoplasia III [VIN III]
>   (233.32)

624.01 Vulvar intraepithelial neoplasia I [VIN I] ♀
Mild dysplasia of vulva

624.02 Vulvar intraepithelial neoplasia II [VIN II] ♀
Moderate dysplasia of vulva
Coding Clinic: 2007, Q4, P90-91

624.09 Other dystrophy of vulva ♀
Kraurosis of vulva
Leukoplakia of vulva

624.1 Atrophy of vulva ♀

624.2 Hypertrophy of clitoris ♀

> Excludes | that in endocrine disorders (255.2, 256.1)

624.3 Hypertrophy of labia ♀
Hypertrophy of vulva NOS

624.4 Old laceration or scarring of vulva ♀

624.5 Hematoma of vulva ♀

> Excludes | that complicating delivery (664.5)

624.6 Polyp of labia and vulva ♀

624.8 Other specified noninflammatory disorders of vulva and perineum ♀
Cyst of vulva
Edema of vulva
Stricture of vulva
Coding Clinic: 2003, Q1, P13-14; 1995, Q1, P8

624.9 Unspecified noninflammatory disorder of vulva and perineum ♀

● **625 Pain and other symptoms associated with female genital organs**

625.0 Dyspareunia ♀
Painful intercourse/coitus

> Excludes | psychogenic dyspareunia (302.76)

625.1 Vaginismus ♀
Colpospasm
Vulvismus

> Excludes | psychogenic vaginismus (306.51)

625.2 Mittelschmerz ♀
Intermenstrual pain
Ovulation pain

625.3 Dysmenorrhea ♀
Painful menstruation

> Excludes | psychogenic dysmenorrhea (306.52)

Coding Clinic: 1994, Q2, P12

625.4 Premenstrual tension syndromes ♀
Menstrual molimen
Premenstrual dysphoric disorder
Premenstrual syndrome
Premenstrual tension NOS

> Excludes | menstrual migraine (346.4)

Coding Clinic: 2003, Q4, P116

625.5 Pelvic congestion syndrome ♀
Congestion-fibrosis syndrome
Taylor's syndrome

625.6 Stress incontinence, female ♀

> Excludes | mixed incontinence (788.33)
>   stress incontinence, male (788.32)

● **625.7 Vulvodynia**
Coding Clinic: 2008, Q4, P124

625.70 Vulvodynia, unspecified ♀
Vulvodynia NOS

625.71 Vulvar vestibulitis ♀

625.79 Other vulvodynia ♀

625.8 Other specified symptoms associated with female genital organs ♀
Coding Clinic: 1985, Nov-Dec, P16

625.9 Unspecified symptom associated with female genital organs ♀
Coding Clinic: 2006, Q4, P109-110; 1994, Q2, P12; 1985, Nov-Dec, P16

◀ New   ◀▥ Revised   ~~deleted~~ Deleted   ● Unacceptable Principal Diagnosis   ● Use Additional Digit(s)
▶ Manifestation Code   **OGCR** Official Guidelines   **Coding Clinic**   Excludes   Includes   Use additional   Code first   Omit code

● **626 Disorders of menstruation and other abnormal bleeding from female genital tract**

| Excludes | menopausal and premenopausal bleeding (627.0) pain and other symptoms associated with menstrual cycle (625.2–625.4) postmenopausal bleeding (627.1) |

626.0 Absence of menstruation ♀
Amenorrhea (primary) (secondary)
Coding Clinic: 1985, July-Aug, P9

626.1 Scanty or infrequent menstruation ♀
Hypomenorrhea
Oligomenorrhea

626.2 Excessive or frequent menstruation ♀

| Heavy periods | Menorrhagia |
| Menometrorrhagia | Polymenorrhea |

| Excludes | premenopausal (627.0) that in puberty (626.3) |

Coding Clinic: 2006, Q4, P97-98; 2004, Q4, P88-90; 1994, Q2, P12

626.3 Puberty bleeding ♀
Excessive bleeding associated with onset of menstrual periods
Pubertal menorrhagia

626.4 Irregular menstrual cycle ♀

Irregular:	Irregular:
bleeding NOS	periods
menstruation	

626.5 Ovulation bleeding ♀
Regular intermenstrual bleeding

626.6 Metrorrhagia ♀
Bleeding unrelated to menstrual cycle
Irregular intermenstrual bleeding

626.7 Postcoital bleeding ♀

626.8 Other ♀
Dysfunctional or functional uterine hemorrhage NOS

| Menstruation: | Menstruation: |
| retained | suppression of |

626.9 Unspecified ♀

● **627 Menopausal and postmenopausal disorders**

| Excludes | asymptomatic age-related (natural) postmenopausal status (V49.81) |

627.0 Premenopausal menorrhagia ♀
Excessive bleeding associated with onset of menopause

Menorrhagia:	Menorrhagia:
climacteric	preclimacteric
menopausal	

627.1 Postmenopausal bleeding ♀

627.2 Symptomatic menopausal or female climacteric states ♀
Symptoms, such as flushing, sleeplessness, headache, lack of concentration, associated with the menopause

627.3 Postmenopausal atrophic vaginitis ♀
Senile (atrophic) vaginitis

627.4 Symptomatic states associated with artificial menopause ♀
Postartificial menopause syndromes
Any condition classifiable to 627.1, 627.2, or 627.3 which follows induced menopause

627.8 Other specified menopausal and postmenopausal disorders ♀

| Excludes | premature menopause NOS (256.31) |

627.9 Unspecified menopausal and postmenopausal disorder ♀

● **628 Infertility, female**

| Includes | primary and secondary sterility |

Coding Clinic: 1996, Q2, P9; 1995, Q1, P7

628.0 Associated with anovulation ♀
Anovulatory cycle

Use additional code for any associated Stein-Leventhal syndrome (256.4)

▶ **628.1 Of pituitary-hypothalamic origin ♀**

Code first underlying disease, as:
adiposogenital dystrophy (253.8)
anterior pituitary disorder (253.0–253.4)

628.2 Of tubal origin ♀
Infertility associated with congenital anomaly of tube

Tubal:	Tubal:
block	stenosis
occlusion	

Use additional code for any associated peritubal adhesions (614.6)

628.3 Of uterine origin ♀
Infertility associated with congenital anomaly of uterus
Nonimplantation

Use additional code for any associated tuberculous endometritis (016.7)

628.4 Of cervical or vaginal origin ♀
Infertility associated with:
anomaly or cervical mucus
congenital structural anomaly
dysmucorrhea

628.8 Of other specified origin ♀

628.9 Of unspecified origin ♀

N Newborn Age: 0   **P** Pediatric Age: 0–17   **M** Maternity Age: 12–55   **A** Adult Age: 15–124   ♀ Females Only   ♂ Males Only

Ⓔⓧ CC Exclusions   🔵 Complication\Comorbidity   🔵 Major C\C   🔵 Present on Admission Requirement   🔵 Hospital-Acquired Condition

969

● **629 Other disorders of female genital organs**

629.0 Hematocele, female, not elsewhere classified ♀

> Excludes hematocele or hematoma:
> broad ligament (620.7)
> fallopian tube (620.8)
> that associated with ectopic pregnancy
> (633.00–633.91)
> uterus (621.4)
> vagina (623.6)
> vulva (624.5)

629.1 Hydrocele, canal of Nuck ♀
Cyst of canal of Nuck (acquired)

> Excludes congenital (752.41)

● **629.2 Female genital multilation status**
Female circumcision status
Female genital cutting

629.20 Female genital mutilation status, unspecified ♀
Female genital cutting status, unspecified
Female genital mutilation status NOS

629.21 Female genital mutilation Type I status ♀
Clitorectomy status
Female genital cutting Type I status

629.22 Female genital mutilation Type II status ♀
Clitorectomy with excision of labia minora status
Female genital cutting Type II status
Coding Clinic: 2004, Q4, P88-90

629.23 Female genital mutilation Type III status ♀
Female genital cutting Type III status
Infibulation status

629.29 Other female genital mutilation status ♀
Female genital cutting Type IV status
Female genital mutilation Type IV status
Other female genital cutting status

● **629.8 Other specified disorders of female genital organs**

629.81 Habitual aborter without current pregnancy ♀

> Excludes habitual aborter with current
> pregnancy (646.3)
> Coding Clinic: 2006, Q4, P98

629.89 Other specified disorders of female genital organs ♀

629.9 Unspecified disorder of female genital organs ♀

◀ New ◀▦ Revised ~~deleted~~ Deleted ● Unacceptable Principal Diagnosis ● Use Additional Digit(s)
▶ Manifestation Code **OGCR** Official Guidelines **Coding Clinic** Excludes Includes Use additional Code first Omit code

(See Plate 375 on page NAP-4.)

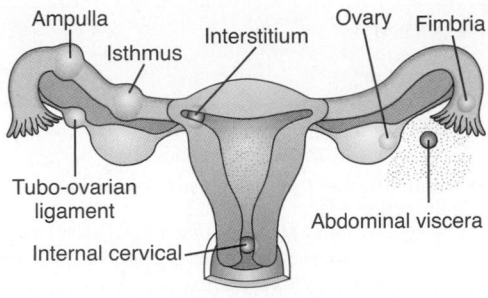

Figure 11-1   Implantation sites of ectopic pregnancy.

Item 11-1   Ectopic pregnancy most often occurs in the fallopian tube. Pregnancy outside the uterus may end in a life-threatening rupture.

Item 11-2   A hydatidiform mole is a benign tumor of the placenta. The tumor secretes a hormone, chorionic gonadotropic hormone (CGH), that indicates a positive pregnancy test.

OGCR   Section I.C.11.a

> Chapter 11 codes have sequencing priority over codes from other chapters. Additional codes from other chapters may be used in conjunction with chapter 11 codes to further specify conditions. Should the provider document that the pregnancy is incidental to the encounter, then code V22.2 should be used in place of any chapter 11 codes. It is the provider's responsibility to state that the condition being treated is not affecting the pregnancy. Chapter 11 codes are to be used only on the maternal record, never on the record of the newborn.

11.   COMPLICATIONS OF PREGNANCY, CHILDBIRTH, AND THE PUERPERIUM (630–679)

ECTOPIC AND MOLAR PREGNANCY (630–633)

Use additional code from category 639 to identify any complications

630   Hydatidiform mole ♀   M
Trophoblastic disease NOS
Vesicular mole
> **Excludes**   *chorioadenoma (destruens) (236.1)*
> *chorionepithelioma (181)*
> *malignant hydatidiform mole (236.1)*

631   Other abnormal product of conception ♀   M
Blighted ovum
Mole:
    NOS
    carneous
    fleshy
    stone

632   Missed abortion ♀   M
Early fetal death before completion of 22 weeks' gestation with retention of dead fetus
Retained products of conception, not following spontaneous or induced abortion or delivery
> **Excludes**   *failed induced abortion (638.0–638.9)*
> *fetal death (intrauterine) (late) (656.4)*
> *missed delivery (656.4)*
> *that with abnormal product of conception (630, 631)*

Coding Clinic: 2001, Q1, P5

● **633   Ectopic pregnancy**
> **Includes**   ruptured ectopic pregnancy

Coding Clinic: 2002, Q4, P61-62

● **633.0   Abdominal pregnancy**
Intraperitoneal pregnancy

    633.00   Abdominal pregnancy without intrauterine pregnancy ♀ ⬤   M
       Ⓔ 633.01, 633.11-633.91

    633.01   Abdominal pregnancy with intrauterine pregnancy ♀ ⬤   M
       Ⓔ 633.00-633.91

● **633.1   Tubal pregnancy**
Fallopian pregnancy
Rupture of (fallopian) tube due to pregnancy
Tubal abortion

    633.10   Tubal pregnancy without intrauterine pregnancy ♀ ⬤   M
       Ⓔ 633.00-633.91

    633.11   Tubal pregnancy with intrauterine pregnancy ♀ ⬤   M
       Ⓔ 633.00-633.91

● **633.2   Ovarian pregnancy**

    633.20   Ovarian pregnancy without intrauterine pregnancy ♀ ⬤   M
       Ⓔ 633.00-633.91

    633.21   Ovarian pregnancy with intrauterine pregnancy ♀ ⬤   M
       Ⓔ 633.00-633.91

● **633.8   Other ectopic pregnancy**
Pregnancy:
    cervical
    combined
    cornual
    intraligamentous
    mesometric
    mural

    633.80   Other ectopic pregnancy without intrauterine pregnancy ♀ ⬤   M
       Ⓔ 633.00-633.91

    633.81   Other ectopic pregnancy with intrauterine pregnancy ♀ ⬤   M
       Ⓔ 633.00-633.91

● **633.9   Unspecified ectopic pregnancy**

    633.90   Unspecified ectopic pregnancy without intrauterine pregnancy ♀ ⬤   M
       Ⓔ 633.00-633.91

    633.91   Unspecified ectopic pregnancy with intrauterine pregnancy ♀ ⬤   M
       Ⓔ 633.00-633.91

OTHER PREGNANCY WITH ABORTIVE OUTCOME (634–639)

The following fourth digit subdivisions are for use with categories 634–638:

0 Complicated by genital tract and pelvic infection
    Endometritis
    Salpingo-oophoritis
    Sepsis NOS
    Septicemia NOS
    Any condition classifiable to 639.0, with condition
        classifiable to 634–638
    Excludes *urinary tract infection (634–638 with .7)*

1 Complicated by delayed or excessive hemorrhage
    Afibrinogenemia
    Defibrination syndrome
    Intravascular hemolysis
    Any condition classifiable to 639.1, with condition
        classifiable to 634–638

2 Complicated by damage to pelvic organs and tissues
    Laceration, perforation, or tear of:
        bladder
        uterus
    Any condition classifiable to 639.2, with condition
        classifiable to 634–638

3 Complicated by renal failure
    Oliguria
    Uremia
    Any condition classifiable to 639.3, with condition
        classifiable to 634–638

4 Complicated by metabolic disorder
    Electrolyte imbalance with conditions classifiable to
        634–638

5 Complicated by shock
    Circulatory collapse
    Shock (postoperative) (septic)
    Any condition classifiable to 639.5, with condition
        classifiable to 634–638

6 Complicated by embolism
    Embolism:
        NOS
        amniotic fluid
        pulmonary
    Any condition classifiable to 639.6, with condition
        classifiable to 634–638

7 With other specified complications
    Cardiac arrest or failure
    Urinary tract infection
    Any condition classifiable to 639.8, with condition
        classifiable to 634–638

8 With unspecified complications

9 Without mention of complication

OGCR Section I.C.10.k.1

Fifth-digits are required for abortion categories 634-637. Fifth-digit 1, incomplete, indicates that all of the products of conception have not been expelled from the uterus. Fifth-digit 2, complete, indicates that all products of conception have been expelled from the uterus.

OGCR Section I.C.10.k.5

Subsequent admissions for retained products of conception following a spontaneous or legally induced abortion are assigned the appropriate code from category 634, Spontaneous abortion, or 635 Legally induced abortion, with a fifth digit of "1" (incomplete). This advice is appropriate even when the patient was discharged previously with a discharge diagnosis of complete abortion.

● **634 Spontaneous abortion**

Requires fifth digit to identify stage:

> **0 unspecified**
> **1 incomplete**
> **2 complete**

Includes   miscarriage
               spontaneous abortion

● **634.0 Complicated by genital tract and pelvic**
  [0-2] **infection** ♀ 🐾   M
         (Ex:) 634.00-638.9, 640.00-641.23, 646.80-646.93, 648.90-649.64, 650,
         669.40-669.44, 669.80-669.94, 679.00-679.04, 679.12, 679.14

● **634.1 Complicated by delayed or excessive hemorrhage** ♀ M
  [0-2] Coding Clinic: 2003, Q1, P6

● **634.2 Complicated by damage to pelvic organs or**
  [0-2] **tissues** ♀ 🐾   M
         (Ex:) 634.00-638.9, 640.00-641.23, 646.80-646.93, 648.90-649.64, 650,
         669.40-669.44, 669.80-669.94, 679.00-679.04, 679.12, 679.14

● **634.3 Complicated by renal failure** ♀ 🐾   M
  [0-2] (Ex:) 634.00-638.9, 640.00-641.23, 646.80-646.93, 648.90-649.64, 650,
         669.40-669.44, 669.80-669.94, 679.00-679.04, 679.12, 679.14

● **634.4 Complicated by metabolic disorder** ♀ 🐾   M
  [0-2] (Ex:) 634.00-638.9, 640.00-641.23, 646.80-646.93, 648.90-649.64, 650,
         669.40-669.44, 669.80-669.94, 679.00-679.04, 679.12, 679.14

● **634.5 Complicated by shock** ♀ 🐾   M
  [0-2] (Ex:) 634.00-638.9, 640.00-641.23, 646.80-646.93, 648.90-649.64, 650,
         669.40-669.44, 669.80-669.94, 679.00-679.04, 679.12, 679.14

● **634.6 Complicated by embolism** ♀ 0🐾, 1,2🐾   M
  [0-2] (Ex:) 634.00-638.9, 640.00-641.23, 646.80-646.93, 648.90-649.64, 650,
         669.40-669.44, 669.80-669.94, 679.00-679.04, 679.12, 679.14

● **634.7 With other specified complications** ♀ 🐾   M
  [0-2] (Ex:) 634.00-638.9, 640.00-641.23, 646.80-646.93, 648.90-649.64, 650,
         669.40-669.44, 669.80-669.94, 679.00-679.04, 679.12, 679.14

● **634.8 With unspecified complication** ♀ 🐾   M
  [0-2] (Ex:) 634.00-638.9, 640.00-641.23, 646.80-646.93, 648.90-649.64, 650,
         669.40-669.44, 669.80-669.94, 679.00-679.04, 679.12, 679.14

● **634.9 Without mention of complication** ♀   M
  [0-2]

◄ New   ◄▦ Revised   ~~deleted~~ Deleted   ● Unacceptable Principal Diagnosis   ● Use Additional Digit(s)
▶ Manifestation Code   **OGCR** Official Guidelines   **Coding Clinic**   Excludes   Includes   Use additional   Code first   Omit code

● **635 Legally induced abortion**

Requires fifth digit to identify stage:

0   unspecified
1   incomplete
2   complete

Includes   abortion or termination of pregnancy:
    elective
    legal
    therapeutic

Excludes *menstrual extraction or regulation (V25.3)*

● **635.0 Complicated by genital tract and pelvic**
[0-2] **infection** ♀ 🦠   M
    (Ex:) 634.00-635.02, 635.20-635.22, 635.70-638.9, 640.00-641.23,
    646.80-646.93, 648.90-649.64, 650, 669.40-669.44, 669.80-669.94,
    679.00-679.04, 679.12, 679.14

● **635.1 Complicated by delayed or excessive hemorrhage** ♀ M
[0-2]

● **635.2 Complicated by damage to pelvic organs or**
[0-2] **tissues** ♀ 🦠   M
    For code **635.20:** (Ex:) 634.00-638.9, 640.00-641.23, 646.80-646.93,
    648.90-649.64, 650, 669.40-669.44, 669.80-669.94, 679.00-679.04,
    679.12, 679.14;
    For code **635.21:** (Ex:) 634.00-635.62, 638.5-638.9, 640.00-641.00;
    For code **635.22:** (Ex:) 635.22

● **635.3 Complicated by renal failure** ♀ 🦠   M
[0-2] For code **635.30:** (Ex:) 635.30-635.32;
    For code **635.31:** (Ex:) 635.30-635.32, 637.11-638.9, 640.00-641.23,
    646.80-646.93, 648.90-649.64, 650, 669.40-669.44, 669.80-669.94,
    679.00-679.04, 679.12, 679.14;
    For code **635.32:** (Ex:) 634.00-634.92, 635.30-635.32, 635.70-638.9,
    640.00-641.23, 646.80-646.93, 648.90-649.64, 650, 669.40-669.44,
    669.80-669.94, 679.00-679.04, 679.12, 679.14

● **635.4 Complicated by metabolic disorder** ♀ 🦠   M
[0-2] (Ex:) 634.00-638.9, 640.00-641.23, 646.80-646.93, 648.90-649.64, 650,
    669.40-669.44, 669.80-669.94, 679.00-679.04, 679.12, 679.14

● **635.5 Complicated by shock** ♀ 🦠   M
[0-2] (Ex:) 634.00 -634.92, 635.50-635.52, 635.70-638.9, 640.00-641.23,
    646.80-646.93, 648.90-649.64, 650, 669.40-669.44, 669.80-669.94,
    679.00-679.04, 679.12, 679.14

● **635.6 Complicated by embolism** ♀ 🦠   M
[0-2] (Ex:) 634.00-634.92, 635.60-638.9, 640.00-641.23, 646.80-646.93,
    648.90-649.64, 650, 669.40 669.44, 669.80-669.94, 679.00-679.04,
    679.12, 679.14

● **635.7 With other specified complications** ♀ 🦠   M
[0-2] (Ex:) 634.00-638.9, 640.00-641.23, 646.80-646.93, 648.90-649.64, 650,
    669.40-669.44, 669.80-669.94, 679.00-679.04, 679.12, 679.14

● **635.8 With unspecified complication** ♀ 🦠   M
[0-2] (Ex:) 634.00-638.9, 640.00-641.23, 646.80-646.93, 648.90-649.64, 650,
    669.40-669.44, 669.80-669.94, 679.00-679.04, 679.12, 679.14

● **635.9 Without mention of complication** ♀   M
[0-2] **Coding Clinic: 1994, Q2, P14**

● **636 Illegally induced abortion**

Requires fifth digit to identify stage:

0   unspecified
1   incomplete
2   complete

Includes   abortion:
    criminal
    illegal
    self-induced

● **636.0 Complicated by genital tract and pelvic**
[0-2] **infection** ♀ 🦠   M
    (Ex:) 634.00-636.02, 636.70-638.9, 640.00-641.23, 646.80-646.93,
    648.90-649.64, 650, 669.40-669.44, 669.80-669.94, 679.00-679.04,
    679.12, 679.14

● **636.1 Complicated by delayed or excessive hemorrhage** ♀ M
[0-2]

● **636.2 Complicated by damage to pelvic organs or**
[0-2] **tissues** ♀ 🦠   M
    (Ex:) 634.00-638.9, 640.00-641.23, 646.80-646.93, 648.90-649.64, 650,
    669.40-669.44, 669.80-669.94, 679.00-679.04, 679.12, 679.14

● **636.3 Complicated by renal failure** ♀ 🦠   M
[0-2] (Ex:) 634.00-635.92, 636.30-636.32, 636.70-638.9, 640.00-641.23,
    646.80-646.93, 648.90-649.64, 650, 669.40-669.44, 669.80-669.94,
    679.00-679.04, 679.12, 679.14

● **636.4 Complicated by metabolic disorder** ♀ 🦠   M
[0-2] (Ex:) 634.00-638.9, 640.00-641.23, 646.80-646.93, 648.90-649.64, 650,
    669.40-669.44, 669.80-669.94, 679.00-679.04, 679.12, 679.14

● **636.5 Complicated by shock** ♀ 🦠   M
[0-2] For codes **635.50-635.51:** (Ex:) 634.00-635.92, 636.50-636.52, 636.70-638.9,
    640.00-641.23, 646.80-646.93, 648.90-649.64, 650, 669.40-669.44,
    669.80-669.94, 679.00-679.04, 679.12, 679.14;
    For code **636.52:** (Ex:) 634.00-635.92, 636.50-636.52, 636.70-636.92,
    637.50-637.52, 637.70-637.92, 638.5, 638.7-638.9, 640.00-641.23,
    646.80-646.93, 648.90-649.64, 650, 669.40-669.44, 669.80-669.94,
    679.00-679.04, 679.12, 679.14

● **636.6 Complicated by embolism** ♀ 🦠   M
[0-2] (Ex:) 634.00-635.92, 636.60-638.9, 640.00-641.23, 646.80-646.93,
    648.90-649.64, 650, 669.40-669.44, 669.80-669.94, 679.00-679.04,
    679.12, 679.14

● **636.7 With other specified complications** ♀ 🦠   M
[0-2] (Ex:) 634.00-638.9, 640.00-641.23, 646.80-646.93, 648.90-649.64, 650,
    669.40-669.44, 669.80-669.94, 679.00-679.04, 679.12, 679.14

● **636.8 With unspecified complication** ♀ 🦠   M
[0-2] (Ex:) 634.00-638.9, 640.00-641.23, 646.80-646.93, 648.90-649.64, 650,
    669.40-669.44, 669.80-669.94, 679.00-679.04, 679.12, 679.14

● **636.9 Without mention of complication** ♀   M
[0-2]

N Newborn Age: 0   **P** Pediatric Age: 0–17   **M** Maternity Age: 12–55   **A** Adult Age: 15–124   ♀ Females Only   ♂ Males Only
(Ex:) CC Exclusions   🦠 Complication\Comorbidity   🦠 Major C\C   🦠 Present on Admission Requirement   🦠 Hospital-Acquired Condition

● **637   Unspecified abortion**
Requires following fifth digit to identify stage:
Coding Clinic: 1994, Q2, P14

> 0   unspecified
> 1   incomplete
> 2   complete

Includes   abortion NOS
retained products of conception following
abortion, not classifiable elsewhere

● **637.0   Complicated by genital tract and pelvic**
[0-2]   **infection** ♀ 🕮   M
Ex: 634.00-637.02, 637.70-638.9, 640.00-641.23, 646.80-646.93,
648.90-649.64, 650, 669.40-669.44, 669.80-669.94, 679.00-679.04,
679.12, 679.14

● **637.1   Complicated by delayed or excessive hemorrhage** ♀ M
[0-2]

● **637.2   Complicated by damage to pelvic organs or**
[0-2]   **tissues** ♀ 🕮   M
Ex: 634.00-638.9, 640.00-641.23, 646.80-646.93, 648.90-649.64, 650,
669.40-669.44, 669.80-669.94, 679.00-679.04, 679.12, 679.14

● **637.3   Complicated by renal failure** ♀ 🕮   M
[0-2]   Ex: 634.00-636.92, 637.30-637.32, 637.70-638.9, 640.00-641.23,
646.80-646.93, 648.90-649.64, 650, 669.40-669.44, 669.80-669.94,
679.00-679.04, 679.12, 679.14

● **637.4   Complicated by metabolic disorder** ♀ 🕮   M
[0-2]   Ex: 634.00-638.9, 640.00-641.23, 646.80-646.93, 648.90-649.64, 650,
669.40-669.44, 669.80-669.94, 679.00-679.04, 679.12, 679.14

● **637.5   Complicated by shock** ♀ 🕮   M
[0-2]   Ex: 634.00-636.92, 637.50-637.52, 637.70-638.9, 640.00-641.23,
646.80-646.93, 648.90-649.64, 650, 669.40-669.44, 669.80-669.94,
679.00-679.04, 679.12, 679.14

● **637.6   Complicated by embolism** ♀ 🕮   M
[0-2]   For codes **637.60-637.61:** Ex: 634.00-636.92, 637.60-638.9, 640.00-641.23,
646.80-646.93, 648.90-649.64, 650, 669.40-669.44, 669.80-669.94,
679.00-679.04, 679.12, 679.14;
For code **637.62:** Ex: 634.00-636.02, 636.11-636.92, 637.60-638.9,
640.00-641.23, 646.80-646.93, 648.90-649.64, 650, 669.40-669.44,
669.80-669.94, 679.00-679.04, 679.12, 679.14

● **637.7   With other specified complications** ♀ 🕮   M
[0-2]   Ex: 634.00-638.9, 640.00-641.23, 646.80-646.93, 648.90-649.64, 650,
669.40-669.44, 669.80-669.94, 679.00-679.04, 679.12, 679.14

● **637.8   With unspecified complication** ♀ 🕮   M
[0-2]   Ex: 634.00-638.9, 640.00-641.23, 646.80-646.93, 648.90-649.64, 650,
669.40-669.44, 669.80-669.94, 679.00-679.04, 679.12, 679.14

● **637.9   Without mention of complication** ♀   M
[0-2]

● **638   Failed attempted abortion**
Includes   failure of attempted induction of (legal)
abortion
Excludes   *incomplete abortion (634.0–637.9)*

638.0   Complicated by genital tract and pelvic
infection ♀ 🕮   M
Ex: 634.00-638.0, 638.7-638.9, 640.00-641.23, 646.80-646.93, 648.90-649.64,
650, 669.40-669.44, 669.80-669.94, 679.00-679.04, 679.12, 679.14

638.1   Complicated by delayed or excessive
hemorrhage ♀ 🕮   M
Ex: 634.00-637.92, 638.1, 638.7-638.9, 640.00-641.23, 646.80-646.93,
648.90-649.64, 650, 669.40-669.44, 669.80-669.94, 679.00-679.04,
679.12, 679.14

638.2   Complicated by damage to pelvic organs or
tissues ♀ 🕮   M
Ex: 634.00-637.92, 638.2, 638.7-638.9, 640.00-641.23, 646.80-646.93,
648.90-649.64, 650, 669.40-669.44, 669.80-669.94, 679.00-679.04,
679.12, 679.14

638.3   Complicated by renal failure ♀ 🕮   M
Ex: 634.00-637.92, 638.3, 638.7-638.9, 640.00-641.23, 646.80-646.93,
648.90-649.64, 650, 669.40-669.44, 669.80-669.94, 679.00-679.04,
679.12, 679.14

638.4   Complicated by metabolic disorder ♀ 🕮   M
Ex: 634.00-638.9, 640.00-641.23, 646.80-646.93, 648.90-649.64, 650,
669.40-669.44, 669.80-669.94, 679.00-679.04, 679.12, 679.14

638.5   Complicated by shock ♀ 🕮   M
Ex: 634.00-637.12, 637.21-637.92, 638.4-638.5, 638.7-638.9, 640.00-641.23,
646.80-646.93, 648.90-649.64, 650, 669.40-669.44, 669.80-669.94,
679.00-679.04, 679.12, 679.14

638.6   Complicated by embolism ♀ 🕮   M
Ex: 634.00-637.92, 638.6-638.9, 640.00-641.23, 646.80-646.93,
648.90-649.64, 650, 669.40-669.44, 669.80-669.94, 679.00-679.04,
679.12, 679.14

638.7   With other specified complications ♀ 🕮   M
Ex: 634.00-638.9, 640.00-641.23, 646.80-646.93, 648.90-649.64, 650,
669.40-669.44, 669.80-669.94, 679.00-679.04, 679.12, 679.14

638.8   With unspecified complication ♀ 🕮   M
Ex: 634.00-638.9, 640.00-641.23, 646.80-646.93, 648.90-649.64, 650,
669.40-669.44, 669.80-669.94, 679.00-679.04, 679.12, 679.14

638.9   Without mention of complication ♀   M

● **639   Complications following abortion and ectopic and molar**
pregnancies

> **Note:** This category is provided for use when it is
> required to classify separately the complications
> classifiable to the fourth digit level in categories
> 634–638; for example:
> a) when the complication itself was responsible
> for an episode of medical care, the abortion,
> ectopic or molar pregnancy itself having been
> dealt with at a previous episode
> b) when these conditions are immediate
> complications of ectopic or molar pregnancies
> classifiable to 630–633 where they cannot be
> identified at fourth digit level.

OGCR   Section I.C.10.k.3

Code 639 is to be used for all complications following
abortion. Code 639 cannot be assigned with codes from
categories 634-638.

◀ New   ◀▥▥ Revised   ~~deleted~~ Deleted   ● Unacceptable Principal Diagnosis   ● Use Additional Digit(s)
▶ Manifestation Code   **OGCR** Official Guidelines   **Coding Clinic**   Excludes   Includes   Use additional   Code first   Omit code

639.0 Genital tract and pelvic infection ♀ 🦠   **M**

Endometritis following conditions classifiable to 630–638

Parametritis following conditions classifiable to 630–638

Pelvic peritonitis following conditions classifiable to 630–638

Salpingitis following conditions classifiable to 630–638

Salpingo-oophoritis following conditions classifiable to 630–638

Sepsis NOS following conditions classifiable to 630–638

Septicemia NOS following conditions classifiable to 630–638

Excludes *urinary tract infection (639.8)*

Ex: 639.0, 639.2-641.23, 646.80-646.93, 648.90-649.64, 650, 669.40-669.44, 669.80-669.94, 679.00-679.04, 679.12, 679.14

639.1 Delayed or excessive hemorrhage ♀ 🦠   **M**

Afibrinogenemia following conditions classifiable to 630–638

Defibrination syndrome following conditions classifiable to 630–638

Intravascular hemolysis following conditions classifiable to 630–638

Ex: 639.1-641.23, 646.80-646.93, 648.90-649.64, 650, 669.40-669.44, 669.80-669.94, 679.00-679.04, 679.12, 679.14

639.2 Damage to pelvic organs and tissues ♀ 🦠   **M**

Laceration, perforation, or tear of:

bladder following conditions classifiable to 630–638

bowel following conditions classifiable to 630–638

broad ligament following conditions classifiable to 630–638

cervix following conditions classifiable to 630–638

periurethral tissue following conditions classifiable to 630–638

uterus following conditions classifiable to 630–638

vagina following conditions classifiable to 630–638

Ex: 639.2-641.23, 646.80-646.93, 648.90-649.64, 650, 669.40-669.44, 669.80-669.94, 679.00-679.04, 679.12, 679.14

639.3 ~~Renal~~ Kidney failure ♀ 🦠   **M** ◄‖‖‖

Oliguria following conditions classifiable to 630–638

Renal (kidney):   ◄‖‖‖

failure (acute) following conditions classifiable to 630–638

shutdown following conditions classifiable to 630–638

tubular necrosis following conditions classifiable to 630–638

Uremia following conditions classifiable to 630–638

Ex: 639.2-641.23, 646.80-646.93, 648.90-649.64, 650, 669.40-669.44, 669.80-669.94, 679.00-679.04, 679.12, 679.14

639.4 Metabolic disorders ♀ 🦠   **M**

Electrolyte imbalance following conditions classifiable to 630–638

Ex: 639.2-641.23, 646.80-646.93, 648.90-649.64, 650, 669.40-669.44, 669.80-669.94, 679.00-679.04, 679.12, 679.14

639.5 Shock ♀ 🦠   **M**

Circulatory collapse following conditions classifiable to 630–638

Shock (postoperative) (septic) following conditions classifiable to 630–638

Ex: 639.2-641.23, 646.80-646.93, 648.90-649.64, 650, 669.40-669.44, 669.80-669.94, 679.00-679.04, 679.12, 679.14

639.6 Embolism ♀ 🦠   **M**

Embolism:

NOS following conditions classifiable to 630–638

air following conditions classifiable to 630–638

amniotic fluid following conditions classifiable to 630–638

blood-clot following conditions classifiable to 630–638

fat following conditions classifiable to 630–638

pulmonary following conditions classifiable to 630–638

pyemic following conditions classifiable to 630–638

septic following conditions classifiable to 630–638

soap following conditions classifiable to 630–638

Ex: 639.2-641.23, 646.80-646.93, 648.90-649.64, 650, 669.40-669.44, 669.80-669.94, 679.00-679.04, 679.12, 679.14

639.8 Other specified complications following abortion or ectopic and molar pregnancy ♀ 🦠   **M**

Acute yellow atrophy or necrosis of liver following conditions classifiable to 630–638

Cardiac arrest or failure following conditions classifiable to 630–638

Cerebral anoxia following conditions classifiable to 630–638

Urinary tract infection following conditions classifiable to 630–638

Ex: 639.2-641.23, 646.80-646.93, 648.90-649.64, 650, 669.40-669.44, 669.80-669.94, 679.00-679.04, 679.12, 679.14

639.9 Unspecified complication following abortion or ectopic and molar pregnancy ♀ 🦠   **M**

Complication(s) not further specified following conditions classifiable to 630–638

Ex: 639.2-641.23, 646.80-646.93, 648.90-649.64, 650, 669.40-669.44, 669.80-669.94, 679.00-679.04, 679.12, 679.14

COMPLICATIONS OF PREGNANCY, CHILDBIRTH, AND THE PUERPERIUM (630–679)

N Newborn Age: 0   P Pediatric Age: 0–17   M Maternity Age: 12–55   A Adult Age: 15–124   ♀ Females Only   ♂ Males Only   975

Ex CC Exclusions   🦠 Complication\Comorbidity   🦠 Major C\C   🦠 Present on Admission Requirement   🦠 Hospital-Acquired Condition

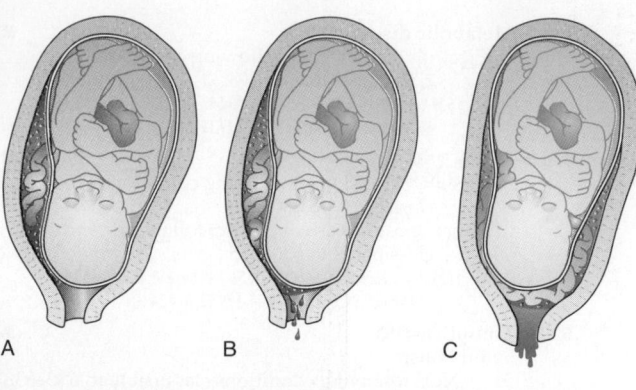

Figure 11–2 A. Marginal placenta previa. **B.** Partial placenta previa. **C.** Total placenta previa.

Item 11–3 Placenta previa is a condition in which the opening of the cervix is obstructed by the displaced placenta. The three types, marginal, partial, and total, are varying degrees of placenta displacement. Placenta abruption is the premature breaking away of the placenta from the site of the uterine implant before the delivery of the fetus.

OGCR Section I.C.10.k.2

A code from categories 640-648 and 651-659 may be used as additional codes with an abortion code to indicate the complication leading to the abortion. Fifth digit 3 is assigned with codes from these categories when used with an abortion code because the other fifth digits will not apply. Codes from the 660-669 series are not to be used for complications of abortion.

COMPLICATIONS MAINLY RELATED TO PREGNANCY (640–649)

Includes   the listed conditions even if they arose or were present during labor, delivery, or the puerperium

The following fifth-digit subclassification is for use with categories 640–649 to denote the current episode of care:

> **0   unspecified as to episode of care or not applicable**
> **1   delivered, with or without mention of antepartum condition**
> > Antepartum condition with delivery
> > Delivery NOS (with mention of antepartum complication during current episode of care)
> > Intrapartum
> > > obstetric condition (with mention of antepartum complication during current episode of care)
> >
> > Pregnancy, delivered (with mention of antepartum complication during current episode of care)
>
> **2   delivered, with mention of postpartum complication**
> > Delivery with mention of puerperal complication during current episode of care
>
> **3   antepartum condition or complication**
> > Antepartum obstetric condition, not delivered during the current episode of care
>
> **4   postpartum condition or complication**
> > Postpartum or puerperal obstetric condition or complication following delivery that occurred:
> > > during previous episode of care
> > > outside hospital, with subsequent admission for observation or care

● **640   Hemorrhage in early pregnancy**

Requires fifth digit; valid digits are in [brackets] under each code. See beginning of section 640–649 for definitions.

Includes   hemorrhage before completion of 22 weeks' gestation

● **640.0   Threatened abortion** ♀ 1,3 🕭   M
    [0,1,3]   For codes **640.01 and 640.03:** (Ex) 640.00-641.13, 646.80-646.93, 648.90-649.64, 650, 669.40-669.64, 669.80-669.94, 679.00-679.04, 679.12, 679.14

● **640.8   Other specified hemorrhage in early pregnancy** ♀   M
    [0,1,3]

● **640.9   Unspecified hemorrhage in early pregnancy** ♀ 3 🕭   M
    [0,1,3]   For code **640.93:** (Ex) 640.00-641.13, 646.80-646.93, 648.90-649.64, 650, 669.40-669.44, 669.80-669.94, 679.00-679.04, 679.12, 679.14

● **641   Antepartum hemorrhage, abruptio placentae, and placenta previa**

Requires fifth digit; valid digits are in [brackets] under each code. See beginning of section 640–649 for definitions.

● **641.0   Placenta previa without hemorrhage** ♀ 1,3 🕭   M
    [0,1,3]   Low implantation of placenta without hemorrhage
         Placenta previa noted:
            during pregnancy without hemorrhage
            before labor (and delivered by cesarean delivery) without hemorrhage
         For codes **641.01 and 641.03:** (Ex) 640.00-641.13, 646.80-646.93, 648.90-649.64, 650, 669.40-669.94, 669.80-669.94, 679.00-679.04, 679.12, 679.14

● **641.1   Hemorrhage from placenta previa** ♀ 1,3 🕭   M
    [0,1,3]   Low-lying placenta NOS or with hemorrhage (intrapartum)
         Placenta previa:
            incomplete NOS or with hemorrhage (intrapartum)
            marginal NOS or with hemorrhage (intrapartum)
            partial NOS or with hemorrhage (intrapartum)
            total NOS or with hemorrhage (intrapartum)

       Excludes   *hemorrhage from vasa previa (663.5)*

         For codes **641.11 and 641.13:** (Ex) 640.00-641.13, 646.80-646.93, 648.90-649.64, 650, 669.40-669.44, 669.80-669.94, 679.00-679.04, 679.12, 679.14

● **641.2   Premature separation of placenta** ♀ 3 🕭, 1 🕭   M
    [0,1,3]   Ablatio placentae
         Abruptio placentae
         Accidental antepartum hemorrhage
         Couvelaire uterus
         Detachment of placenta (premature)
         Premature separation of normally implanted placenta
         For codes **641.21 and 641.23:** (Ex) 640.00-641.13, 641.21, 646.80-646.93, 648.90-649.64, 650, 669.40-669.44, 669.80-669.94, 679.00-679.04, 679.12, 679.14

◀ New   ◀▥ Revised   ~~deleted~~ Deleted   ● Unacceptable Principal Diagnosis   ● Use Additional Digit(s)
◗ Manifestation Code   **OGCR** Official Guidelines   **Coding Clinic**   [Excludes]   Includes   Use additional   Code first   Omit code

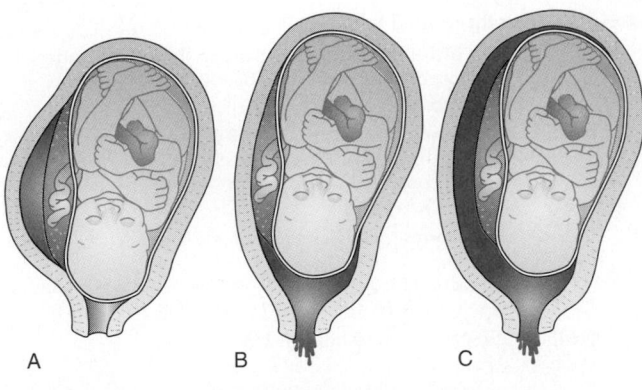

Figure 11–3 Abruptio placentae is classified according to the grade of separation of the placenta from the uterine wall. **A.** Mild separation in which hemorrhage is internal. **B.** Moderate separation in which there is external hemorrhage. **C.** Severe separation in which there is external hemorrhage and extreme separation.

● **641.3 Antepartum hemorrhage associated with coagulation** M
[0,1,3] **defects** ♀ 1,3 ◔

Antepartum or intrapartum hemorrhage associated with:
afibrinogenemia
hyperfibrinolysis
hypofibrinogenemia

> **Excludes** *coagulation defects not associated with antepartum hemorrhage (649.3)*

For codes **641.31 and 641.33:** (Ex) 641.30-641.93, 646.80-646.93, 648.90-649.64, 650, 669.40-669.44, 669.80-669.94, 679.00-679.04, 679.12, 679.14

● **641.8 Other antepartum hemorrhage** ♀ M
[0,1,3] Antepartum or intrapartum hemorrhage associated with:
trauma
uterine leiomyoma

● **641.9 Unspecified antepartum hemorrhage** ♀ M
[0,1,3] Hemorrhage:
antepartum NOS
intrapartum NOS
of pregnancy NOS

● **642 Hypertension complicating pregnancy, childbirth, and the puerperium**

Requires fifth digit; valid digits are in [brackets] under each code. See beginning of section 640–649 for definitions.

● **642.0 Benign essential hypertension complicating**
[0-4] **pregnancy, childbirth, and the puerperium** ♀ 1-3 ◔ M
Hypertension:
benign essential specified as complicating, or as a reason for obstetric care during pregnancy, childbirth, or the puerperium
chronic NOS specified as complicating, or as a reason for obstetric care during pregnancy, childbirth, or the puerperium
essential specified as complicating, or as a reason for obstetric care during pregnancy, childbirth, or the puerperium
pre-existing NOS specified as complicating, or as a reason for obstetric care during pregnancy, childbirth, or the puerperium

For codes **642.01-642.03:** (Ex) 642.00-642.94, 646.10-646.14, 646.80-646.93, 648.90-649.64, 650, 669.40-669.44, 669.80-669.94, 679.00-679.04, 679.12, 679.14

● **642.1 Hypertension secondary to renal disease,**
[0-4] **complicating pregnancy, childbirth, and the puerperium** ♀ 3,4 ◔, 1,2 ◔ M
Hypertension secondary to renal disease, specified as complicating, or as a reason for obstetric care during pregnancy, childbirth, or the puerperium

For codes **641.11-642.14:** (Ex) 642.00-642.94, 646.10-646.14, 646.80-646.93, 648.90-649.64, 650, 669.40-669.44, 669.80-669.94, 679.00-679.04, 679.12, 679.14

● **642.2 Other pre-existing hypertension complicating**
[0-4] **pregnancy, childbirth, and the puerperium** ♀ M
Hypertensive:
chronic kidney disease specified as complicating, or as a reason for obstetric care during pregnancy, childbirth, or the puerperium
heart and chronic kidney disease specified as complicating, or as a reason for obstetric care during pregnancy, childbirth, or the puerperium
heart disease specified as complicating, or as a reason for obstetric care during pregnancy, childbirth, or the puerperium
Malignant hypertension specified as complicating, or as a reason for obstetric care during pregnancy, childbirth, or the puerperium

● **642.3 Transient hypertension of pregnancy** ♀ 1,2 ◔ M
[0-4] Gestational hypertension
Transient hypertension, so described, in pregnancy, childbirth, or the puerperium

For codes **642.31-642.32:** (Ex) 642.00-642.94, 646.10-646.14, 646.80-646.93, 648.90-649.64, 650, 669.40-669.44, 669.80-669.94, 679.00-679.04, 679.12, 679.14

> **OGCR** Section I.C.7.a.8
> Assign code 796.2, Elevated blood pressure reading without diagnosis of hypertension, unless patient has an established diagnosis of hypertension. Assign code 642.3x for transient hypertension of pregnancy.

● **642.4 Mild or unspecified pre-eclampsia** ♀ 1,3,4 ◔, 2 ◔ M
[0-4] Hypertension in pregnancy, childbirth, or the puerperium, not specified as pre-existing, with either albuminuria or edema, or both; mild or unspecified
Pre-eclampsia:
NOS
mild
Toxemia (pre-eclamptic):
NOS
mild

> **Excludes** *albuminuria in pregnancy, without mention of hypertension (646.2)*
> *edema in pregnancy, without mention of hypertension (646.1)*

For codes **642.41-642.44:** (Ex) 642.00-642.94, 646.10-646.14, 646.80-646.93, 648.90-649.64, 650, 669.40-669.44, 669.80-669.94, 679.00-679.04, 679.12, 679.14

● **642.5 Severe pre-eclampsia** ♀ 1-4 ◔ M
[0-4] Hypertension in pregnancy, childbirth, or the puerperium, not specified as pre-existing, with either albuminuria or edema, or both; specified as severe
Pre-eclampsia, severe
Toxemia (pre-eclamptic), severe

For codes **642.51-642.54:** (Ex) 642.00-642.94, 646.10-646.14, 646.80-646.93, 648.90-649.64, 650, 669.40-669.44, 669.80-669.94, 679.00-679.04, 679.12, 679.14

COMPLICATIONS OF PREGNANCY, CHILDBIRTH, AND THE PUERPERIUM (630–679)

N Newborn Age: 0 **P** Pediatric Age: 0–17 **M** Maternity Age: 12–55 **A** Adult Age: 15–124 ♀ Females Only ♂ Males Only
(Ex) CC Exclusions ◔ Complication\Comorbidity ◔ Major C\C ◔ Present on Admission Requirement ◔ Hospital-Acquired Condition

977

● **642.6 Eclampsia** ♀ 1-4   M
[0-4]   Toxemia:
       eclamptic
       with convulsions
     For codes **642.61-642.64:** (Ex:) 642.00-642.94, 646.10-646.14,
       646.80-646.93, 648.90-649.64, 650, 669.40-669.44, 669.80-669.94,
       679.00-679.04, 679.12, 679.14

● **642.7 Pre-eclampsia or eclampsia superimposed on pre-**   M
[0-4]   **existing hypertension** ♀ 1-4
       Conditions classifiable to 642.4–642.6, with
       conditions classifiable to 642.0–642.2
     For codes **642.71-642.74:** (Ex:) 642.00-642.94, 646.10-646.14,
       646.80-646.93, 648.90-649.64, 650, 669.40-669.44, 669.80-669.94,
       679.00-679.04, 679.12, 679.14

● **642.9 Unspecified hypertension complicating pregnancy,**   M
[0-4]   **childbirth, or the puerperium** ♀ 1-4
       Hypertension NOS, without mention of
       albuminuria or edema, complicating
       pregnancy, childbirth, or the puerperium
     For codes **642.91-642.92:** (Ex:) 642.00-642.94, 646.10-646.14,
       646.80-646.93, 648.90-649.64, 650, 669.40-669.44, 669.80-669.94,
       679.00-679.04, 679.12, 679.14;
     For codes **642.93-642.94:** (Ex:) 642.01-642.44, 642.61-642.94
     Coding Clinic: 2009, Q1, P18

● **643 Excessive vomiting in pregnancy**
     Requires fifth digit; valid digits are in [brackets] under
     each code. See beginning of section 640–649 for
     definitions.

   Includes   hyperemesis arising during pregnancy
            vomiting:
                persistent arising during pregnancy
                vicious arising during pregnancy
                hyperemesis gravidarum

● **643.0 Mild hyperemesis gravidarum** ♀   M
[0,1,3]   Hyperemesis gravidarum, mild or unspecified,
       starting before the end of the 22nd week of
       gestation

● **643.1 Hyperemesis gravidarum with metabolic**   M
[0,1,3]   **disturbance** ♀
       Hyperemesis gravidarum, starting before the end
       of the 22nd week of gestation, with metabolic
       disturbance, such as:
       carbohydrate depletion
       dehydration
       electrolyte imbalance

● **643.2 Late vomiting of pregnancy** ♀   M
[0,1,3]   Excessive vomiting starting after 22 completed
       weeks of gestation

● **643.8 Other vomiting complicating pregnancy** ♀   M
[0,1,3]   Vomiting due to organic disease or other cause,
       specified as complicating pregnancy, or as a
       reason for obstetric care during pregnancy

   Use additional code to specify cause

● **643.9 Unspecified vomiting of pregnancy** ♀   M
[0,1,3]   Vomiting as a reason for care during pregnancy,
       length of gestation unspecified

● **644 Early or threatened labor**
     Requires fifth digit; valid digits are in [brackets] under
     each code. See beginning of section 640–649 for
     definitions.

● **644.0 Threatened premature labor** ♀ 3   M
[0,3]   Premature labor after 22 weeks, but before 37
       completed weeks of gestation without
       delivery

   Excludes   *that occurring before 22 completed weeks of*
          gestation (640.0)
     For code **644.03:** (Ex:) 644.00-644.21, 646.80-646.93, 648.90-649.64, 650,
       669.40-669.44, 669.80-669.94, 679.00-679.04, 679.12, 679.14

● **644.1 Other threatened labor** ♀ 3   M
[0,3]   False labor:
       NOS without delivery
       after 37 completed weeks of gestation without
         delivery
       Threatened labor NOS without delivery
     For code **644.13:** (Ex:) 644.00-644.21, 646.80-646.93, 648.90-649.64, 650,
       669.40-669.44, 669.80-669.94, 679.00-679.04, 679.12, 679.14

● **644.2 Early onset of delivery** ♀ 0, 1   M
[0-1]   Onset (spontaneous) of delivery before 37
       completed weeks of gestation
       Premature labor with onset of delivery before 37
       completed weeks of gestation
     (Ex:) 644.00-644.21, 646.80-646.93, 648.90-649.64, 650, 669.40-669.44,
       669.80-669.94, 679.00-679.04, 679.12, 679.14
     Coding Clinic: 1991, Q2, P16

   OGCR   Section I.C.10.k.4
     When an attempted termination of pregnancy
     results in a liveborn fetus assign code 644.21 with
     an appropriate code from category V27, Outcome
     of Delivery. The procedure code for the attempted
     termination of pregnancy should also be assigned.

● **645 Late pregnancy**
     Requires fifth digit; valid digits are in [brackets] under
     each code. See beginning of section 640–649 for
     definitions.
     Coding Clinic: 2000, Q1, P17-18

● **645.1 Post term pregnancy** ♀   M
[0,1,3]   Pregnancy over 40 completed weeks to 42
       completed weeks gestation

● **645.2 Prolonged pregnancy** ♀   M
[0,1,3]   Pregnancy which has advanced beyond 42
       completed weeks of gestation

● **646 Other complications of pregnancy, not elsewhere**
    classified

   Use additional code(s) to further specify complication

     Requires fifth digit; valid digits are in [brackets] under
     each code. See beginning of section 640–649 for
     definitions.

● **646.0 Papyraceous fetus** ♀   M
[0,1,3]

● **646.1 Edema or excessive weight gain in pregnancy,**   M
[0-4]   **without mention of hypertension** ♀
       Gestational edema
       Maternal obesity syndrome

   Excludes   *that with mention of hypertension*
          (642.0–642.9)

◄ New   ◄▦ Revised   ~~deleted~~ Deleted   ● Unacceptable Principal Diagnosis   ● Use Additional Digit(s)
▸ Manifestation Code   **OGCR** Official Guidelines   **Coding Clinic**   Excludes   Includes   Use additional   Code first   Omit code

● **646.2 Unspecified renal disease in pregnancy, without**
[0-4] **mention of hypertension** ♀ 1-4 🕭   M
     Albuminuria in pregnancy or the puerperium,
     without mention of hypertension
     Nephropathy NOS in pregnancy or the
     puerperium, without mention of
     hypertension
     Renal disease NOS in pregnancy or the
     puerperium, without mention of
     hypertension
     Uremia in pregnancy or the puerperium, without
     mention of hypertension
     Gestational proteinuria in pregnancy or
     the puerperium, without mention of
     hypertension

> **Excludes** *that with mention of hypertension*
> *(642.0–642.9)*

For codes **646.21-646.24:** (Ex) 646.21-646.24

● **646.3 Habitual aborter** ♀ 1 🕭   M
[0,1,3]
> **Excludes** *with current abortion (634.0–634.9)*
> *without current pregnancy (629.81)*

For code **646.31:** (Ex) 646.31

● **646.4 Peripheral neuritis in pregnancy** ♀   M
[0-4]

● **646.5 Asymptomatic bacteriuria in pregnancy** ♀   M
[0-4]

● **646.6 Infections of genitourinary tract in**
[0-4] **pregnancy** ♀ 1-4 🕭   M
     Conditions classifiable to 590, 595, 597, 599.0, 616
     complicating pregnancy, childbirth, or the
     puerperium
     Conditions classifiable to 614.0–614.5, 614.7–614.9,
     615 complicating pregnancy or labor

> **Excludes** *major puerperal infection (670.0–670.8)* ◀▥

For codes **646.61-646.64:** (Ex) 646.60-646.64, 646.80-646.93,
648.90-649.64, 650, 669.40-669.44, 669.80-669.94, 679.00-679.04,
679.12, 679.14

Coding Clinic: 2004, Q4, P88-90

OGCR Section I.C.2.g.

During pregnancy, childbirth or the puerperium,
a patient admitted (or presenting for a health
care encounter) because of an HIV-related illness
should receive a principal diagnosis code of
647.6X, Other specified infectious and parasitic
diseases in the mother classifiable elsewhere, but
complicating the pregnancy, childbirth or the
puerpium, followed by 042 and the code(s) for
the HIV-related illness(es). Codes from Chapter
15 always take sequencing priority. Patients with
asymptomatic HIV infection status admitted (or
presenting for a health care encounter) during
pregnancy, childbirth, or the puerperium should
receive codes of 647.6X and V08.

● **646.7 Liver disorders in pregnancy** ♀ 1,3 🕭   M
[0,1,3]   Acute yellow atrophy of liver (obstetric) (true) of
     pregnancy
     Icterus gravis of pregnancy
     Necrosis of liver of pregnancy

> **Excludes** *hepatorenal syndrome following delivery*
> *(674.8)*
> *viral hepatitis (647.6)*

For codes **646.71 and 646.73:** (Ex) 646.70-646.93, 648.90-649.64, 650,
669.40-669.44, 669.80-669.94, 679.00-679.04, 679.12, 679.14

● **646.8 Other specified complications of pregnancy** ♀   M
[0-4]   Fatigue during pregnancy
     Herpes gestationis
     Insufficient weight gain of pregnancy
     Coding Clinic: 1998, Q3, P16; 1985, Jan-Feb, P15-16

● **646.9 Unspecified complication of pregnancy** ♀   M
[0,1,3]

● **647 Infectious and parasitic conditions in the mother**
classifiable elsewhere, but complicating pregnancy,
childbirth, or the puerperium

     Use additional code(s) to further specify complication

     Requires fifth digit; valid digits are in [brackets] under
     each code. See beginning of section 640–649 for
     definitions.

> **Includes** the listed conditions when complicating
> the pregnant state, aggravated by the
> pregnancy, or when a main reason for
> obstetric care

> **Excludes** *those conditions in the mother known or suspected*
> *to have affected the fetus (655.0–655.9)*

● **647.0 Syphilis** ♀ 1-4 🕭   M
[0-4]   Conditions classifiable to 090–097
     For codes **647.01-647.04:** (Ex) 646.81-647.24, 679.12, 679.14

● **647.1 Gonorrhea** ♀ 1-4 🕭   M
[0-4]   Conditions classifiable to 098
     For codes **647.11-647.14:** (Ex) 646.81-647.24, 679.12, 679.14

● **647.2 Other venereal diseases** ♀ 1-4 🕭   M
[0-4]   Conditions classifiable to 099
     For codes **647.21-647.24:** (Ex) 646.81-647.24, 679.12, 679.14

● **647.3 Tuberculosis** ♀ 1-4 🕭   M
[0-4]   Conditions classifiable to 010–018
     For codes **647.31-647.34:** (Ex) 646.80-646.93, 647.30-647.34,
     648.90-649.64, 650, 669.40-669.44, 669.80-669.94, 679.00-679.04,
     679.12 679.14

● **647.4 Malaria** ♀ 1-4 🕭   M
[0-4]   Conditions classifiable to 084
     For codes **647.41-647.44:** (Ex) 646.80-646.93, 647.40-647.44,
     648.90-649.64, 650, 669.40-669.44, 669.80-669.94, 679.00-679.04,
     679.12, 679.14

● **647.5 Rubella** ♀ 1-4 🕭   M
[0-4]   Conditions classifiable to 056
     For codes **647.51-647.54:** (Ex) 647.51-647.94

● **647.6 Other viral diseases** ♀ 1-4 🕭   M
[0-4]   Conditions classifiable to 042, 050-055, 057-079,
     795.05, 795.15, 796.75
     For codes **647.61-647.64:** (Ex) 647.51-647.94
     Coding Clinic: 1985, Jan-Feb, P15-16

● **647.8 Other specified infectious and parasitic**
[0-4] **diseases** ♀ 1-4 🕭   M
     For codes **647.81-647.84:** (Ex) 647.51-647.94

● **647.9 Unspecified infection or infestation** ♀ 1-4 🕭   M
[0-4]   For codes **647.91-647.94:** (Ex) 647.51-647.94

● **648 Other current conditions in the mother classifiable**
elsewhere, but complicating pregnancy, childbirth,
or the puerperium

     Use additional code(s) to identify the condition

     Requires fifth digit; valid digits are in [brackets] under
     each code. See beginning of section 640–649 for
     definitions.

> **Includes** the listed conditions when complicating
> the pregnant state, aggravated by the
> pregnancy, or when a main reason for
> obstetric care

> **Excludes** *those conditions in the mother known or suspected*
> *to have affected the fetus (655.0–655.9)*

● **648.0 Diabetes mellitus** ♀ 0,3,4 🕭, 1-2 🕭   M
[0-4]   Conditions classifiable to 249, 250

> **Excludes** *gestational diabetes (648.8)*

     (Ex) 646.80-646.93, 648.00-648.04, 648.90-649.64, 650, 669.40-669.44,
     669.80-669.94, 679.00-679.04, 679.12, 679.14

N Newborn Age: 0   **P** Pediatric Age: 0–17   **M** Maternity Age: 12–55   **A** Adult Age: 15–124   ♀ Females Only   ♂ Males Only

(Ex) CC Exclusions   🕭 Complication\Comorbidity   🕭 Major C\C   🕭 Present on Admission Requirement   🕭 Hospital-Acquired Condition   **979**

COMPLICATIONS OF PREGNANCY, CHILDBIRTH, AND THE PUERPERIUM (630–679)

● **648.1 Thyroid dysfunction** ♀ M
[0-4]   Conditions classifiable to 240–246

● **648.2 Anemia** ♀ M
[0-4]   Conditions classifiable to 280–285
  Coding Clinic: 2002, Q1, P14

● **648.3 Drug dependence** ♀ 1-4 ⚫ M
[0-4]   Conditions classifiable to 304
  For codes **648.31-648.34:** (Ex) 646.80-646.93, 648.30-648.34,
    648.90-649.64, 650, 669.40-669.44, 669.80-669.94, 679.00-679.04,
    679.12, 679.14
  Coding Clinic: 1998, Q2, P13-14; 1988, Q4, P8

● **648.4 Mental disorders** ♀ M
[0-4]   Conditions classifiable to 290–303, 305.0,
    305.2–305.9, 306–316, 317–319
  Coding Clinic: 1998, Q2, P13-14

● **648.5 Congenital cardiovascular disorders** ♀ 1-4 ⚫ M
[0-4]   Conditions classifiable to 745–747
  For codes **648.51-648.54:** (Ex) 646.80-646.93, 648.50-648.64,
    648.90-649.64, 650, 669.40-669.44, 669.80-669.94, 679.00-679.04,
    679.12, 679.14

● **648.6 Other cardiovascular diseases** ♀ 1-4 ⚫ M
[0-4]   Conditions classifiable to 390–398, 410–429

  | Excludes | *cerebrovascular disorders in the puerperium*
  | | *(674.0)*
  | | *peripartum cardiomyopathy (674.5)*
  | | *venous complications (671.0–671.9)*
  For codes **648.61-648.64:** (Ex) 646.80-646.93, 648.50-648.64,
    648.90-649.64, 650, 669.40-669.44, 669.80-669.94, 679.00-679.04,
    679.12, 679.14
  Coding Clinic: 1998, Q3, P11

● **648.7 Bone and joint disorders of back, pelvis, and lower**
[0-4] **limbs** ♀ 1-4 ⚫ M
    Conditions classifiable to 720–724, and those
    classifiable to 711–719 or 725–738, specified as
    affecting the lower limbs
  For codes **648.71-648.74:** (Ex) 648.71-648.74

● **648.8 Abnormal glucose tolerance** ♀ M
[0-4]   Conditions classifiable to 790.21–790.29
    Gestational diabetes

    Use additional code, if applicable, for associated
    long-term (current) insulin use V58.67
  Coding Clinic: 2004, Q4, P53-56

● **648.9 Other current conditions classifiable elsewhere** ♀ M
[0-4]   Conditions classifiable to 440–459, 795.01–795.04,
    795.06, 795.10–795.14, 795.16, 796.70–796.74,
    796.76
    Nutritional deficiencies [conditions classifiable to
    260–269]
  Coding Clinic: 2009, Q1, P17; 2006, Q3, P14; 2004, Q4, P88-90;
    2002, Q1, P14-15; 1984, Nov-Dec, P18

● **649 Other conditions or status of the mother complicating**
pregnancy, childbirth, or the puerperium

    Requires fifth digit; valid digits are in [brackets] under
    each code. See beginning of section 640-649 for
    definitions.

● **649.0 Tobacco use disorder complicating pregnancy,**
[0-4] **childbirth, or the puerperium** ♀ M
    Smoking complicating pregnancy, childbirth, or
    the puerperium

● **649.1 Obesity complicating pregnancy, childbirth, or the**
[0-4] **puerperium** ♀ M

    Use additional code to identify the obesity (278.00,
    278.01)

● **649.2 Bariatric surgery status complicating pregnancy,**
[0-4] **childbirth, or the puerperium** ♀ M
    Gastric banding status complicating pregnancy,
    childbirth, or the puerperium
    Gastric bypass status for obesity complicating
    pregnancy, childbirth, or the puerperium
    Obesity surgery status complicating pregnancy,
    childbirth, or the puerperium

● **649.3 Coagulation defects complicating pregnancy,**
[0-4] **childbirth, or the puerperium** ♀ ⚫ M ◀▥
    Conditions classifiable to 286, 287, 289 ◀▥

    Use additional code to identify the specific
    coagulation defect (286.0–286.9,
    287.0–287.9, 289.0–289.9) ◀▥

  | Excludes | *coagulation defects causing antepartum*
  | | *hemorrhage (641.3)*
  (Ex) 648.90

● **649.4 Epilepsy complicating pregnancy, childbirth, or the**
[0-4] **puerperium** ♀ 1-4 ⚫ M
    Conditions classifiable to 345

    Use additional code to identify the specific type of
    epilepsy (345.00–345.91)

  | Excludes | *eclampsia (642.6)*
  For codes **649.41-649.44:** (Ex) 648.91-648.94

● **649.5 Spotting complicating pregnancy** ♀ M
[0,1,3] | Excludes | *antepartum hemorrhage (641.0–641.9)*
          | | *hemorrhage in early pregnancy*
          | | *(640.0–640.9)*

● **649.6 Uterine size date discrepancy** ♀ M
[0-4] | Excludes | *suspected problem with fetal growth not*
        | | *found (V89.04)*

● **649.7 Cervical shortening** ♀ ⚫ M
[0,1,3] | Excludes | *suspected cervical shortening not found*
          | | *(V89.05)*
  For codes **649.70, 649.71, and 649.73:** (Ex) 649.70-649.73, 654.51-654.54
  Coding Clinic: 2008, Q4, P124-125

COMPLICATIONS OF PREGNANCY, CHILDBIRTH, AND THE PUERPERIUM (630–679)

◀ New ◀▥ Revised ~~deleted~~ Deleted ● Unacceptable Principal Diagnosis ● Use Additional Digit(s)
▶ Manifestation Code **OGCR** Official Guidelines **Coding Clinic** | Excludes | Includes Use additional Code first Omit code

Figure 11–4 The four stages of normal delivery: **I.** Lightening, which occurs 2 to 4 weeks before birth, at which time the fetus turns with head toward the vagina. **II.** Regular contractions begin, the amniotic sac ruptures, and dilation is complete. **III.** Delivery of the head and rotation. **IV.** Expulsion of placenta.

OGCR Section I.C.10.h.1

Code 650 is for use in cases when a woman is admitted for a full-term normal delivery and delivers a single, healthy infant without any complications antepartum, during the delivery, or postpartum during the delivery episode. Code 650 is always a principal diagnosis. It is not to be used if any other code from chapter 11 is needed to describe a current complication of the antenatal, delivery, or perinatal period. Additional codes from other chapters may be used with code 650 if they are not related to or are in any way complicating the pregnancy.

OGCR Section I.C.10.h.2

Code 650 may be used if the patient had a complication at some point during her pregnancy, but the complication is not present at the time of the admission for delivery.

OGCR Section I.C.10.h.3

V27.0, Single liveborn, is the only outcome of delivery code appropriate for use with 650.

OGCR Section I.C.10.i.1

The postpartum period begins immediately after delivery and continues for six weeks following delivery. The peripartum period is defined as the last month of pregnancy to five months postpartum.

NORMAL DELIVERY, AND OTHER INDICATIONS FOR CARE IN PREGNANCY, LABOR, AND DELIVERY (650–659)

The following fifth-digit subclassification is for use with categories 651–659 to denote the current episode of care:

> 0   unspecified as to episode of care or not applicable
> 1   delivered, with or without mention of antepartum condition
> 2   delivered, with mention of postpartum complication
> 3   antepartum condition or complication
> 4   postpartum condition or complication

650 Normal delivery ♀ 🖥   **M**

Delivery requiring minimal or no assistance, with or without episiotomy, without fetal manipulation [e.g., rotation version] or instrumentation [forceps] of a spontaneous, cephalic, vaginal, full-term, single, live-born infant. This code is for use as a single diagnosis code and is not to be used with any other code in the range 630–676.

> Use additional code to indicate outcome of delivery (V27.0)

> **Excludes**   *breech delivery (assisted) (spontaneous) NOS (652.2)*
> *delivery by vacuum extractor, forceps, cesarean section, or breech extraction, without specified complication (669.5–669.7)*

Coding Clinic: 2002, Q2, P10; 2001, Q3, P12; 2000, Q3, P5

● **651 Multiple gestation**

Requires fifth digit; valid digits are in [brackets] under each code. See beginning of section 650–659 for definitions.

> **Excludes** *fetal conjoined twins (678.1)*

● **651.0 Twin pregnancy** ♀ 1🖥   **M**
[0,1,3]
> **Excludes** *fetal conjoined twins (678.1)*
> For code **651.01**: Ⓔⅹ: 650-651.63, 651.71-652.20, 652.23-652.93
> Coding Clinic: 2006, Q3, P16-18; 1992, Q3, P10

● **651.1 Triplet pregnancy** ♀ 1,3🖥   **M**
[0,1,3]   For codes **651.11 and 651.13**: Ⓔⅹ: 650-651.63, 651.71-652.93

● **651.2 Quadruplet pregnancy** ♀ 1,3🖥   **M**
[0,1,3]   For codes **651.21 and 651.23**: Ⓔⅹ: 650-651.63, 651.71-652.93

● **651.3 Twin pregnancy with fetal loss and retention of one**
[0,1,3] **fetus** ♀   **M**

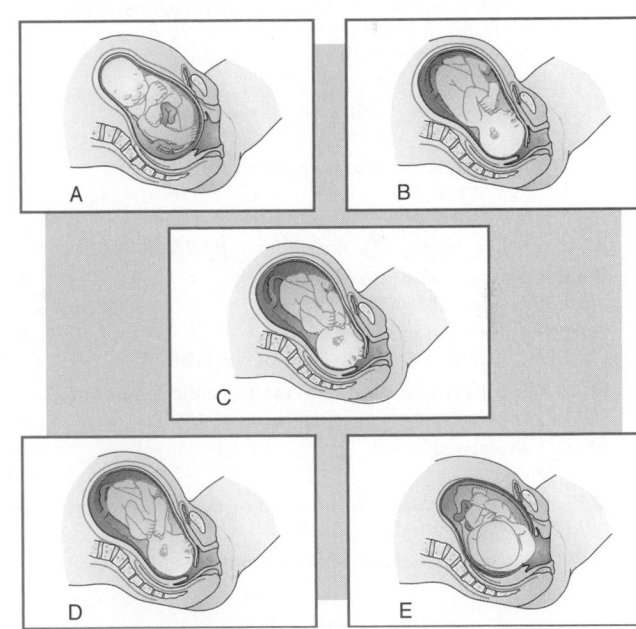

Figure 11–5 Five types of malposition and malpresentation of the fetus: **A.** Breech. **B.** Vertex. **C.** Face. **D.** Brow. **E.** Shoulder.

OGCR Section I.C.10.k.2

A code from categories 640-648 and 651-659 may be used as additional codes with an abortion code to indicate the complication leading to the abortion. Fifth digit 3 is assigned with codes from these categories when used with an abortion code because the other fifth digits will not apply. Codes from the 660-669 series are not to be used for complications of abortion.

● **651.4 Triplet pregnancy with fetal loss and retention of**
[0,1,3] **one or more fetus(es) ♀ 1,3** 🔾   M
    For codes 654.41 and 651.43: ⓔⓧ 650-651.63, 651.71-652.93

● **651.5 Quadruplet pregnancy with fetal loss and retention**
[0,1,3] **of one or more fetus(es) ♀ 1,3** 🔾   M
    For codes 651.51 and 651.53: ⓔⓧ 650-651.63, 651.71-652.93

● **651.6 Other multiple pregnancy with fetal loss and**
[0,1,3] **retention of one or more fetus(es) ♀**   M

● **651.7 Multiple gestation following (elective) fetal**
[0,1,3] **reduction ♀**   M
    Fetal reduction of multiple fetuses reduced to
      single fetus
    Coding Clinic: 2006, Q3, P16-18; 2005, Q4, P81

● **651.8 Other specified multiple gestation ♀ 1,3** 🔾   M
[0,1,3]   For codes 651.81 and 651.83: ⓔⓧ 650-651.63, 651.71-652.93

● **651.9 Unspecified multiple gestation ♀**   M
[0,1,3]

● **652 Malposition and malpresentation of fetus**
    Requires fifth digit; valid digits are in [brackets] under
      each code. See beginning of section 650–659 for
      definitions.

    Code first any associated obstructed labor (660.0)

    Coding Clinic: 1995, Q3, P10

● **652.0 Unstable lie ♀**   M
[0,1,3]

● **652.1 Breech or other malpresentation successfully**
[0,1,3] **converted to cephalic presentation ♀**   M
    Cephalic version NOS

● **652.2 Breech presentation without mention of version ♀** M
[0,1,3]   Breech delivery (assisted) (spontaneous) NOS
    Buttocks presentation
    Complete breech
    Frank breech

      Excludes *footling presentation (652.8)*
                incomplete breech (652.8)

● **652.3 Transverse or oblique presentation ♀**   M
[0,1,3]   Oblique lie
    Transverse lie

      Excludes *transverse arrest of fetal head (660.3)*

● **652.4 Face or brow presentation ♀**   M
[0,1,3]   Mentum presentation

● **652.5 High head at term ♀**   M
[0,1,3]   Failure of head to enter pelvic brim

● **652.6 Multiple gestation with malpresentation of one**
[0,1,3] **fetus or more ♀**   M

● **652.7 Prolapsed arm ♀**   M
[0,1,3]

● **652.8 Other specified malposition or malpresentation ♀** M
[0,1,3]   Compound presentation

● **652.9 Unspecified malposition or malpresentation ♀** M
[0,1,3]

Figure 11–6 Hydrocephalic fetus causing disproportion.

● **653 Disproportion**
    Requires fifth digit; valid digits are in [brackets] under
      each code. See beginning of section 650–659 for
      definitions.

    Code first any associated obstructed labor (660.1)

    Coding Clinic: 1995, Q3, P10

● **653.0 Major abnormality of bony pelvis, not further**
[0,1,3] **specified ♀**   M
    Pelvic deformity NOS

● **653.1 Generally contracted pelvis ♀**   M
[0,1,3]   Contracted pelvis NOS

● **653.2 Inlet contraction of pelvis ♀**   M
[0,1,3]   Inlet contraction (pelvis)

● **653.3 Outlet contraction of pelvis ♀**   M
[0,1,3]   Outlet contraction (pelvis)

● **653.4 Fetopelvic disproportion ♀**   M
[0,1,3]   Cephalopelvic disproportion NOS
    Disproportion of mixed maternal and fetal origin,
      with normally formed fetus

● **653.5 Unusually large fetus causing disproportion ♀**   M
[0,1,3]   Disproportion of fetal origin with normally formed
      fetus
    Fetal disproportion NOS

      Excludes *that when the reason for medical care was*
                concern for the fetus (656.6)

● **653.6 Hydrocephalic fetus causing disproportion ♀**   M
[0,1,3]   **Excludes** *that when the reason for medical care was*
                concern for the fetus (655.0)

● **653.7 Other fetal abnormality causing disproportion ♀**   M
[0,1,3]   Fetal: Fetal:
      ascites   sacral teratoma
      hydrops   tumor
      myelomeningocele

      Excludes *conjoined twins causing disporportion*
                (678.1)

● **653.8 Disproportion of other origin ♀**   M
[0,1,3]   **Excludes** *shoulder (girdle) dystocia (660.4)*

● **653.9 Unspecified disproportion ♀**   M
[0,1,3]

COMPLICATIONS OF PREGNANCY, CHILDBIRTH, AND THE PUERPERIUM (630–679)

◀ New   ⬅ Revised   ~~deleted~~ Deleted   ● Unacceptable Principal Diagnosis   ● Use Additional Digit(s)
▶ Manifestation Code   OGCR Official Guidelines   Coding Clinic   Excludes   Includes   Use additional   Code first   Omit code

● **654 Abnormality of organs and soft tissues of pelvis**

> Requires fifth digit; valid digits are in [brackets] under each code. See beginning of section 650–659 for definitions.
>
> > **Includes** the listed conditions during pregnancy, childbirth, or the puerperium
>
> *Code first any associated obstructed labor (660.2)*
>
> > **Excludes** *trauma to perineum and vulva complicating current delivery (664.0–664.9)*
>
> Coding Clinic: 1995, Q3, P10

● **654.0 Congenital abnormalities of uterus ♀**   M
  [0-4]   Double uterus
           Uterus bicornis

● **654.1 Tumors of body of uterus ♀**   M
  [0-4]   Uterine fibroids
           Coding Clinic: 1994, Q2, P14

● **654.2 Previous cesarean delivery ♀**   M
  [0,1,3] Uterine scar from previous cesarean delivery

● **654.3 Retroverted and incarcerated gravid uterus ♀**   M
  [0-4]

● **654.4 Other abnormalities in shape or position of**
  [0-4] **gravid uterus and of neighboring structures ♀**   M
           Cystocele
           Pelvic floor repair
           Pendulous abdomen
           Prolapse of gravid uterus
           Rectocele
           Rigid pelvic floor

● **654.5 Cervical incompetence ♀ 1-4** 🔖   M
  [0-4]   Presence of Shirodkar suture with or without
              mention of cervical incompetence
           For codes **654.51-654.54**: (Ex) 649.70-649.73, 654.51-654.54

● **654.6 Other congenital or acquired abnormality of**
  [0-4] **cervix ♀**   M
           Cicatricial cervix
           Polyp of cervix
           Previous surgery to cervix
           Rigid cervix (uteri)
           Stenosis or stricture of cervix
           Tumor of cervix

● **654.7 Congenital or acquired abnormality of vagina ♀**   M
  [0-4]   Previous surgery to vagina
           Septate vagina
           Stenosis of vagina (acquired) (congenital)
           Stricture of vagina
           Tumor of vagina

● **654.8 Congenital or acquired abnormality of vulva ♀**   M
  [0-4]   Anal sphincter tear (healed) (old) complicating
              delivery
           Fibrosis of perineum
           Persistent hymen
           Previous surgery to perineum or vulva
           Rigid perineum
           Tumor of vulva

> > **Excludes** *anal sphincter tear (healed) (old) not associated with delivery (569.43)*
> > *varicose veins of vulva (671.1)*
>
> Coding Clinic: 2003, Q1, P14

● **654.9 Other and unspecified ♀**   M
  [0-4]   Uterine scar NEC

OGCR Section I.C.10.a.2

In cases when in utero surgery is performed on the fetus, a code from category 655 should be assigned identifying the fetal condition. Procedure code 75.36, Correction of fetal defect, should be assigned on the hospital inpatient record. No code from Chapter 15, the perinatal codes, should be used on the mother's record to identify fetal conditions. Surgery performed in utero on a fetus is still to be coded as an obstetric encounter.

● **655 Known or suspected fetal abnormality affecting management of mother**

> Requires fifth digit; valid digits are in [brackets] under each code. See beginning of section 650–659 for definitions.
>
> > **Includes** the listed conditions in the fetus as a reason for observation or obstetrical care of the mother, or for termination of pregnancy

● **655.0 Central nervous system malformation in fetus ♀**   M
  [0,1,3] Fetal or suspected fetal:
              anencephaly
              hydrocephalus
              spina bifida (with myelomeningocele)

● **655.1 Chromosomal abnormality in fetus ♀**   M
  [0,1,3]

● **655.2 Hereditary disease in family possibly affecting**
  [0,1,3] **fetus ♀**   M

● **655.3 Suspected damage to fetus from viral disease in the**
  [0,1,3] **mother ♀**   M
           Suspected damage to fetus from maternal rubella

● **655.4 Suspected damage to fetus from other disease in the**
  [0,1,3] **mother ♀**   M
           Suspected damage to fetus from maternal:
              alcohol addiction
              listeriosis
              toxoplasmosis

● **655.5 Suspected damage to fetus from drugs ♀**   M
  [0,1,3]

● **655.6 Suspected damage to fetus from radiation ♀**   M
  [0,1,3]

● **655.7 Decreased fetal movements ♀**   M
  [0,1,3] Coding Clinic: 1997, Q4, P41

● **655.8 Other known or suspected fetal abnormality, not**
  [0,1,3] **elsewhere classified ♀**   M
           Suspected damage to fetus from:
              environmental toxins
              intrauterine contraceptive device
           Coding Clinic: 2006, Q3, P16-18x2

● **655.9 Unspecified ♀**   M
  [0,1,3]

N Newborn Age: 0   **P** Pediatric Age: 0–17   **M** Maternity Age: 12–55   **A** Adult Age: 15–124   ♀ Females Only   ♂ Males Only

(Ex) CC Exclusions   🔖 Complication\Comorbidity   🔖 Major C\C   🔖 Present on Admission Requirement   🔖 Hospital-Acquired Condition

● 656 **Other known or suspected fetal and placental problems affecting management of mother**

Requires fifth digit; valid digits are in [brackets] under each code. See beginning of section 650–659 for definitions.

Excludes   *fetal hematologic conditions (678.0)*
suspected placental problems not found (V89.02)

● 656.0 **Fetal-maternal hemorrhage** ♀   M
[0,1,3]   Leakage (microscopic) of fetal blood into maternal circulation

● 656.1 **Rhesus isoimmunization** ♀ 3   M
[0,1,3]   Anti-D [Rh] antibodies
Rh incompatibility
For code **656.13:** (Ex) 656.11-656.13

● 656.2 **Isoimmunization from other and unspecified blood-group incompatibility** ♀   M
[0,1,3]   ABO isoimmunization
Coding Clinic: 2006, Q4, P135

● 656.3 **Fetal distress** ♀ 1   M
[0,1,3]   Fetal metabolic acidemia

Excludes   *abnormal fetal acid-base balance (656.8)*
abnormality in fetal heart rate or rhythm (659.7)
fetal bradycardia (659.7)
fetal tachycardia (659.7)
meconium in liquor (656.8)
For code **656.31:** (Ex) 656.31-656.33, 659.71, 763.82

● 656.4 **Intrauterine death** ♀ 1,3   M
[0,1,3]   Fetal death:
    NOS
    after completion of 22 weeks' gestation
    late
Missed delivery

Excludes   *missed abortion (632)*
For codes **656.41 and 656.43:** (Ex) 656.41-656.43

● 656.5 **Poor fetal growth** ♀ 1   M
[0,1,3]   "Light-for-dates"
"Placental insufficiency"
"Small-for-dates"
For code **656.51:** (Ex) 656.51-656.53

● 656.6 **Excessive fetal growth** ♀   M
[0,1,3]   "Large-for-dates"

● 656.7 **Other placental conditions** ♀   M
[0,1,3]   Abnormal placenta
Placental infarct

Excludes   *placental polyp (674.4)*
placentitis (658.4)

● 656.8 **Other specified fetal and placental problems** ♀   M
[0,1,3]   Abnormal acid-base balance
Intrauterine acidosis
Lithopedian
Meconium in liquor
Subchorionic hematoma

● 656.9 **Unspecified fetal and placental problem** ♀   M
[0,1,3]

● 657 **Polyhydramnios** ♀ 1   M
[0,1,3]   Hydramnios

Requires fifth digit; valid digits are in [brackets] under each code. See beginning of section 650–659 for definitions.

Use 0 as fourth digit for category 657

Excludes   *suspected polyhydramnios not found (V89.01)*

For code **657.01:** (Ex) 657.01-657.03
Coding Clinic: 2006, Q3, P16-18

● 658 **Other problems associated with amniotic cavity and membranes**

Requires fifth digit; valid digits are in [brackets] under each code. See beginning of section 650–659 for definitions.

Excludes   *amniotic fluid embolism (673.1)*
suspected problems with amniotic cavity and membranes not found (V89.01)

● 658.0 **Oligohydramnios** ♀ 1,3   M
[0,1,3]   Oligohydramnios without mention of rupture of membranes
For codes **658.01 and 658.03:** (Ex) 658.01-658.03
Coding Clinic: 2006, Q3, P16-18

● 658.1 **Premature rupture of membranes** ♀   M
[0,1,3]   Rupture of amniotic sac less than 24 hours prior to the onset of labor
Coding Clinic: 2001, Q1, P5; 1998, Q4, P76-77

● 658.2 **Delayed delivery after spontaneous or unspecified rupture of membranes** ♀   M
[0,1,3]   Prolonged rupture of membranes NOS
Rupture of amniotic sac 24 hours or more prior to the onset of labor

● 658.3 **Delayed delivery after artificial rupture of membranes** ♀   M
[0,1,3]

● 658.4 **Infection of amniotic cavity** ♀ 1,3   M
[0,1,3]   Amnionitis
Chorioamnionitis
Membranitis
Placentitis
For codes **658.41 and 658.43:** (Ex) 658.41-658.43

● 658.8 **Other** ♀ 1   M
[0,1,3]   Amnion nodosum
Amniotic cyst
For code **658.81:** (Ex) 658.81

● 658.9 **Unspecified** ♀   M
[0,1,3]

● 659 **Other indications for care or intervention related to labor and delivery, not elsewhere classified**

Requires fifth digit; valid digits are in [brackets] under each code. See beginning of section 650–659 for definitions.

● 659.0 **Failed mechanical induction** ♀   M
[0,1,3]   Failure of induction of labor by surgical or other instrumental methods

● 659.1 **Failed medical or unspecified induction** ♀   M
[0,1,3]   Failed induction NOS
Failure of induction of labor by medical methods, such as oxytocic drugs

● 659.2 **Maternal pyrexia during labor, unspecified** ♀ 1   M
[0,1,3]   For code **659.21:** (Ex) 659.21-659.23

● 659.3 **Generalized infection during labor** ♀ 1,3   M
[0,1,3]   Septicemia during labor
For codes **659.31 and 659.33:** (Ex) 646.80-646.93, 648.90-649.64, 650, 659.30-659.33, 669.40-669.44, 669.80-669.94, 679.00-679.04, 679.12, 679.14

● 659.4 **Grand multiparity** ♀   M
[0,1,3]   Excludes   *supervision only, in pregnancy (V23.3)*
without current pregnancy (V61.5)

● 659.5 **Elderly primigravida** ♀   M
[0,1,3]   First pregnancy in a woman who will be 35 years of age or older at expected date of delivery

Excludes   *supervision only, in pregnancy (V23.81)*

Coding Clinic: 2001, Q3, P12

◄ New   ◄▬ Revised   ~~deleted~~ Deleted   ● Unacceptable Principal Diagnosis   ● Use Additional Digit(s)
▶ Manifestation Code   **OGCR** Official Guidelines   **Coding Clinic**   Excludes   Includes   Use additional   Code first   Omit code

● **659.6 Elderly multigravida** ♀   M
[0,1,3]   Second or more pregnancy in a woman who will
       be 35 years of age or older at expected date of
       delivery

     | **Excludes** | *elderly primigravida (659.5)* |
                      supervision only, in pregnancy (V23.82)
     Coding Clinic: 2001, Q3, P12

● **659.7 Abnormality in fetal heart rate or rhythm** ♀   M
[0,1,3]   Depressed fetal heart tones
     Fetal:
       bradycardia
       tachycardia
     Fetal heart rate decelerations
     Non-reassuring fetal heart rate or rhythm
     Coding Clinic: 1998, Q4, P47-48

● **659.8 Other specified indications for care or intervention**
[0,1,3] **related to labor and delivery** ♀   M
     Pregnancy in a female less than 16 years of age at
       expected date of delivery
     Very young maternal age
     Coding Clinic: 2001, Q3, P12

● **659.9 Unspecified indication for care or intervention**
[0,1,3] **related to labor and delivery** ♀   M

   OGCR   Section I.C.10.k.2
     Codes from the 660-669 series are not to be used for
     complications of abortion.

COMPLICATIONS OCCURRING MAINLY IN THE COURSE OF LABOR AND DELIVERY (660–669)

The following fifth-digit subclassification is for use with
categories 660–669 to denote the current episode of care:

> 0   unspecified as to episode of care or not applicable
> 1   delivered, with or without mention of antepartum
>   condition
> 2   delivered, with mention of postpartum complication
> 3   antepartum condition or complication
> 4   postpartum condition or complication

● **660   Obstructed labor**
     Requires fifth digit; valid digits are in [brackets] under
       each code. See beginning of section 660–669 for
       definitions.
     Coding Clinic: 1995, Q3, P10

● **660.0 Obstruction caused by malposition of fetus at onset**
[0,1,3] **of labor** ♀ 3 ◔   M
     Any condition classifiable to 652, causing
       obstruction during labor
     Use additional code from 652.0–652.9 to identify
       condition
     For code **660.03**: ⓔⓧ 646.80-646.93, 648.90-649.64, 650 655.70-655.73,
       660.03, 665.00-665.11 665.50-665.54, 665.80-665.94, 669.40-669.44,
       669.80-669.94, 679.00-679.04, 679.12, 679.14
     Coding Clinic: 1995, Q3, P10

● **660.1 Obstruction by bony pelvis** ♀   M
[0,1,3]   Any condition classifiable to 653, causing
       obstruction during labor
     Use additional code from 653.0–653.9 to identify
       condition
     Coding Clinic: 1995, Q3, P10

● **660.2 Obstruction by abnormal pelvic soft tissues** ♀   M
[0,1,3]   Prolapse of anterior lip of cervix
     Any condition classifiable to 654, causing
       obstruction during labor
     Use additional code from 654.0–654.9 to identify
       condition
     Coding Clinic: 1995, Q3, P10

● **660.3 Deep transverse arrest and persistent occipito-**
[0,1,3] **posterior position** ♀   M

● **660.4 Shoulder (girdle) dystocia** ♀   M
[0,1,3]   Impacted shoulders

● **660.5 Locked twins** ♀   M
[0,1,3]

● **660.6 Failed trial of labor, unspecified** ♀   M
[0,1,3]   Failed trial of labor, without mention of condition
       or suspected condition

● **660.7 Failed forceps or vacuum extractor, unspecified** ♀ ◔ M
[0,1,3]   Application of ventouse or forceps, without
       mention of condition

● **660.8 Other causes of obstructed labor** ♀   M
[0,1,3]   Use additional code to identify condition

● **660.9 Unspecified obstructed labor** ♀   M
[0,1,3]   Dystocia:
       NOS
       fetal NOS
       maternal NOS

● **661   Abnormality of forces of labor**
     Requires fifth digit; valid digits are in [brackets] under
       each code. See beginning of section 660–669 for
       definitions.

● **661.0 Primary uterine inertia** ♀   M
[0,1,3]   Failure of cervical dilation
     Hypotonic uterine dysfunction, primary
     Prolonged latent phase of labor
     Coding Clinic: 1985, July-Aug, P11

● **661.1 Secondary uterine inertia** ♀   M
[0,1,3]   Arrested active phase of labor
     Hypotonic uterine dysfunction, secondary
     Coding Clinic: 1985, July-Aug, P11

● **661.2 Other and unspecified uterine inertia** ♀   M
[0,1,3]   Atony of uterus without hemorrhage
     Desultory labor
     Irregular labor
     Poor contractions
     Slow slope active phase of labor

     | **Excludes** | *atony of uterus with hemorrhage (666.1)* |
                      postpartum atony of uterus without
                      hemorrhage (669.8)
     Coding Clinic: 1985, July-Aug, P11

● **661.3 Precipitate labor** ♀   M
[0,1,3]

● **661.4 Hypertonic, incoordinate, or prolonged uterine**
[0,1,3] **contractions** ♀   M
     Cervical spasm
     Contraction ring (dystocia)
     Dyscoordinate labor
     Hourglass contraction of uterus
     Hypertonic uterine dysfunction
     Incoordinate uterine action
     Retraction ring (Bandl's) (pathological)
     Tetanic contractions
     Uterine dystocia NOS
     Uterine spasm

● **661.9 Unspecified abnormality of labor** ♀   M
[0,1,3]

N Newborn Age: 0   **P** Pediatric Age: 0–17   **M** Maternity Age: 12–55   **A** Adult Age: 15–124   ♀ Females Only   ♂ Males Only
ⓔⓧ CC Exclusions   ◔ Complication\Comorbidity   ◔ Major C\C   ◔ Present on Admission Requirement   ◔ Hospital-Acquired Condition

COMPLICATIONS OF PREGNANCY, CHILDBIRTH, AND THE PUERPERIUM (630–679)

● **662   Long labor**

     Requires fifth digit; valid digits are in [brackets] under each code. See beginning of section 660–669 for definitions.

● **662.0   Prolonged first stage** ♀   **M**
[0,1,3]

● **662.1   Prolonged labor, unspecified** ♀ 1 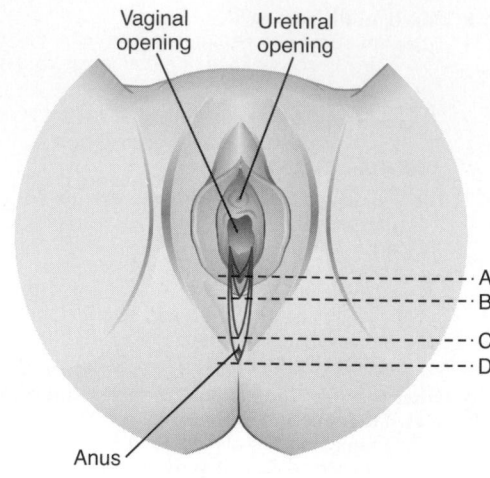   **M**
[0,1,3]   For code **662.11:** (Ex) 646.80-646.93, 648.90-649.64, 650, 655.70-655.73, 662.11, 665.00-665.11 665.50-665.54, 665.80-665.94, 669.40-669.44, 669.80-669.94, 679.00-679.04, 679.12, 679.14

● **662.2   Prolonged second stage** ♀   **M**
[0,1,3]

● **662.3   Delayed delivery of second twin, triplet, etc.** ♀   **M**
[0,1,3]

● **663   Umbilical cord complications**

     Requires fifth digit; valid digits are in [brackets] under each code. See beginning of section 660–669 for definitions.

● **663.0   Prolapse of cord** ♀   **M**
[0,1,3]   Presentation of cord

● **663.1   Cord around neck, with compression** ♀   **M**
[0,1,3]   Cord tightly around neck

● **663.2   Other and unspecified cord entanglement, with**
[0,1,3]   **compression** ♀   **M**
     Entanglement of cords of twins in mono-amniotic sac
     Knot in cord (with compression)

● **663.3   Other and unspecified cord entanglement, without**
[0,1,3]   **mention of compression** ♀   **M**
     Coding Clinic: 2003, Q2, P9

● **663.4   Short cord** ♀   **M**
[0,1,3]

● **663.5   Vasa previa** ♀   **M**
[0,1,3]

● **663.6   Vascular lesions of cord** ♀   **M**
[0,1,3]   Bruising of cord
     Hematoma of cord
     Thrombosis of vessels of cord

● **663.8   Other umbilical cord complications** ♀   **M**
[0,1,3]   Velamentous insertion of umbilical cord

● **663.9   Unspecified umbilical cord complication** ♀   **M**
[0,1,3]

● **664   Trauma to perineum and vulva during delivery**

     Requires fifth digit; valid digits are in [brackets] under each code. See beginning of section 660–669 for definitions.

     Includes   damage from instruments
              that from extension of episiotomy
     Coding Clinic: 2008, Q4, P192; 1992, Q1, P10-11

● **664.0   First-degree perineal laceration** ♀   **M**
[0,1,4]   Perineal laceration, rupture, or tear involving:
       fourchette
       hymen
       labia vulva
       skin
       vagina
     Coding Clinic: 1984, Nov-Dec, P10

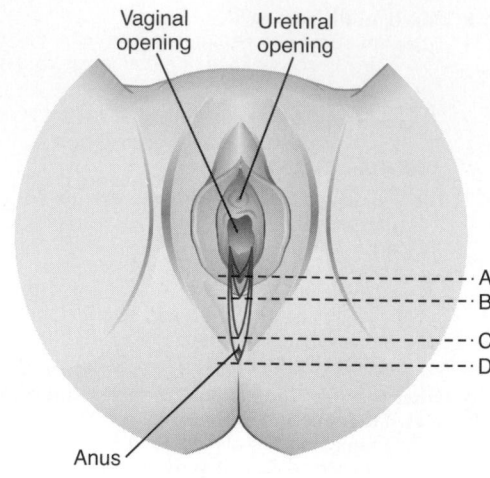

Figure 11–7   Perineal lacerations: **A.** First-degree is laceration of superficial tissues. **B.** Second-degree is limited to the pelvic floor and may involve the perineal or vaginal muscles. **C.** Third-degree involves the anal sphincter. **D.** Fourth-degree involves anal or rectal mucosa.

● **664.1   Second-degree perineal laceration** ♀   **M**
[0,1,4]   Perineal laceration, rupture, or tear (following episiotomy) involving:
       pelvic floor
       perineal muscles
       vaginal muscles

     Excludes   *that involving anal sphincter (664.2)*
     Coding Clinic: 2008, Q4, P192; 1984, Nov-Dec, P10

● **664.2   Third-degree perineal laceration** ♀ 1 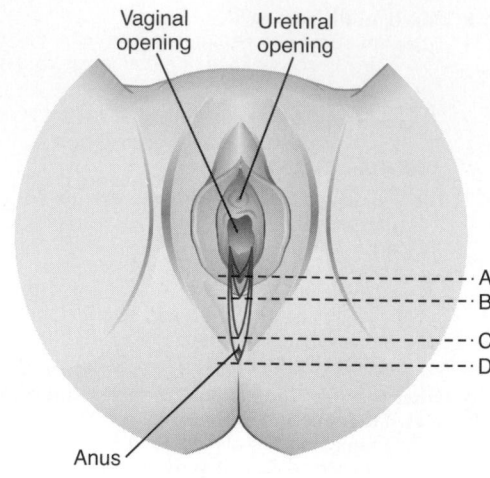   **M**
[0,1,4]   Perineal laceration, rupture, or tear (following episiotomy) involving:
       anal sphincter
       rectovaginal septum
       sphincter NOS

     Excludes   *anal sphincter tear during delivery not associated with third-degree perineal laceration (664.6)*
             that with anal or rectal mucosal laceration (664.3)
     For code **664.21:** (Ex) 646.80-646.93, 648.90-649.64, 650, 655.70-655.73, 664.21, 664.61, 665.00-665.11, 665.50-665.54, 665.80-665.94, 669.40-669.44, 669.80-669.94, 679.00-679.04, 679.12, 679.14
     Coding Clinic: 1984, Nov-Dec, P10

● **664.3   Fourth-degree perineal laceration** ♀ 1 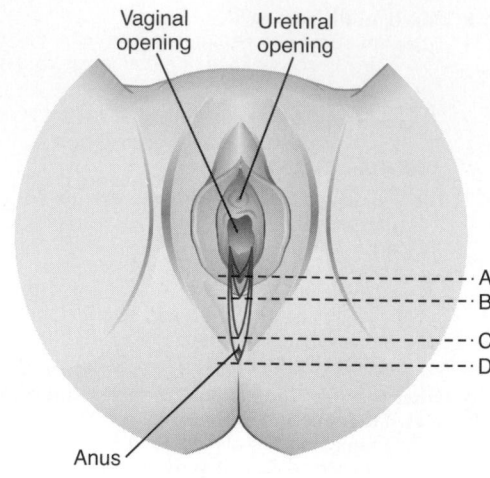   **M**
[0,1,4]   Perineal laceration, rupture, or tear as classifiable to 664.2 and involving also:
       anal mucosa
       rectal mucosa
     For code **664.31:** (Ex) 646.80-646.93, 648.90-649.64, 650, 655.70-655.73, 664.31, 665.00-665.11, 665.50-665.54, 665.80-665.94, 669.40-669.44, 669.80-669.94, 679.00-679.04, 679.12, 679.14
     Coding Clinic: 1984, Nov-Dec, P10

● **664.4   Unspecified perineal laceration** ♀   **M**
[0,1,4]   Central laceration

◀ New   ◀◁◁ Revised   ~~deleted~~ Deleted   ● Unacceptable Principal Diagnosis   ● Use Additional Digit(s)

▶ Manifestation Code   **OGCR** Official Guidelines   **Coding Clinic**   Excludes   Includes   Use additional   Code first   Omit code

● **664.5** **Vulval and perineal hematoma** ♀   M
[0,1,4]   **Coding Clinic: 1984, Nov-Dec, P10**

● **664.6** **Anal sphincter tear complicating delivery, not**
[0,1,4]   **associated with third-degree perineal**
     laceration ♀ **1,4** 🦠   M

> **Excludes**   *third-degree perineal laceration (664.2)*

For codes **664.61 and 664.64:** Ⓔⓧ 646.80-646.93, 648.90-649.64, 650,
655.70-655.73, 664.21, 664.60-664.64, 665.00-665.11, 665.50-665.54,
665.80-665.94, 669.40-669.44, 669.80-669.94, 679.00-679.04, 679.12,
679.14

Coding Clinic: 2007, Q4, P88-90

● **664.8** **Other specified trauma to perineum and vulva** ♀   M
[0,1,4]   **Coding Clinic: 2007, Q4, P125**

● **664.9** **Unspecified trauma to perineum and vulva** ♀   M
[0,1,4]

● **665** **Other obstetrical trauma**

Requires fifth digit; valid digits are in [brackets] under
each code. See beginning of section 660–669 for
definitions.

> **Includes**   damage from instruments

● **665.0** **Rupture of uterus before onset of labor** ♀ **1,3** 🦠   M
[0,1,3]   For codes **665.01 and 665.03:** Ⓔⓧ 646.80-646.93, 648.90-649.64, 650,
655.70-655.73, 665.00-665.11, 665.50-665.54, 665.80-665.94,
669.40-669.44, 669.80-669.94, 679.00-679.04, 679.12, 679.14

● **665.1** **Rupture of uterus during labor** ♀ **1** 🦠   M
[0,1]   Rupture of uterus NOS
For code **665.11:** Ⓔⓧ 646.80-646.93, 648.90-649.64, 650, 655.70-655.73,
665.00-665.11, 665.50-665.54, 665.80-665.94, 669.40-669.44,
669.80-669.94, 679.00-679.04, 679.12, 679.14

● **665.2** **Inversion of uterus** ♀ **2** 🦠   M
[0,2,4]   For code **665.22:** Ⓔⓧ 646.80-646.93, 648.90-649.64, 650, 655.70-655.73,
665.00-665.11, 665.22, 665.50-665.54, 665.80-665.94, 669.40-669.44,
669.80-669.94, 679.00-679.04, 679.12, 679.14

● **665.3** **Laceration of cervix** ♀ **1** 🦠   M
[0,1,4]   For code **665.31:** Ⓔⓧ 646.80-646.93, 648.90-649.64, 650, 655.70-655.73,
665.00-665.11, 665.31, 665.50-665.54, 665.80-665.94, 669.40-669.44,
669.80-669.94, 679.00-679.04, 679.12, 679.14
Coding Clinic: 1984, Nov-Dec, P10

● **665.4** **High vaginal laceration** ♀ **1** 🦠   M
[0,1,4]   Laceration of vaginal wall or sulcus without
     mention of perineal laceration
For code **664.41:** Ⓔⓧ 646.80-646.93, 648.90-649.64, 650, 655.70-655.73,
665.00-665.11, 665.41, 665.50-665.54, 665.80-665.94, 669.40-669.44,
669.80-669.94, 679.00-679.04, 679.12, 679.14
Coding Clinic: 1984, Nov-Dec, P10

● **665.5** **Other injury to pelvic organs** ♀ **1** 🦠   M
[0,1,4]   Injury to:
     bladder
     urethra
For code **665.51:** Ⓔⓧ 646.80-646.93, 648.90-649.64, 650, 655.70-655.73,
665.00-665.11, 665.50-665.54, 665.80-665.94, 669.40-669.44,
669.80-669.94, 679.00-679.04, 679.12, 679.14
Coding Clinic: 1984, Nov-Dec, P10, 12

● **665.6** **Damage to pelvic joints and ligaments** ♀ **1** 🦠   M
[0,1,4]   Avulsion of inner symphyseal cartilage
     Damage to coccyx
     Separation of symphysis (pubis)
For code **665.61:** Ⓔⓧ 646.80-646.93, 648.90-649.64, 650, 655.70-655.73,
665.00-665.11, 665.50-665.54, 665.61, 665.80-665.94, 669.40-669.44,
669.80-669.94, 679.00-679.04, 679.12, 679.14

● **665.7** **Pelvic hematoma** ♀ **1,2** 🦠   M
[0-2,4]   Hematoma of vagina
For codes **665.71-665.72:** Ⓔⓧ 646.80-646.93, 648.90-649.64, 650,
655.70-655.73, 665.00-665.11, 665.50-665.54, 665.71, 665.80-665.94,
669.40-669.44, 669.80-669.94, 679.00-679.04, 679.12, 679.14
Coding Clinic: 1984, Nov-Dec, P10

● **665.8** **Other specified obstetrical trauma** ♀   M
[0-4]

● **665.9** **Unspecified obstetrical trauma** ♀   M
[0-4]

● **666** **Postpartum hemorrhage**

Requires fifth digit; valid digits are in [brackets] under
each code. See beginning of section 660–669 for
definitions.

● **666.0** **Third-stage hemorrhage** ♀ **2,4** 🦠   M
[0,2,4]   Hemorrhage associated with retained, trapped, or
     adherent placenta
     Retained placenta NOS
For codes **666.02 and 666.04:** Ⓔⓧ 646.80-646.93, 648.90-649.64, 650,
655.70-655.73, 665.00-665.11, 665.50-665.54, 665.80-665.94, 666.02,
669.40-669.44, 669.80-669.94, 679.00-679.04, 679.12, 679.14
Coding Clinic: 1988, Q1, P14

● **666.1** **Other immediate postpartum hemorrhage** ♀ **2,4** 🦠   M
[0,2,4]   Atony of uterus with hemorrhage
     Hemorrhage within the first 24 hours following
     delivery of placenta
     Postpartum atony of uterus with hemorrhage
     Postpartum hemorrhage (atonic) NOS

> **Excludes**   *atony of uterus without hemorrhage (661.2)*
>   *postpartum atony of uterus without*
>   *hemorrhage (669.8)*

For code **666.12:** Ⓔⓧ 646.80-646.93, 648.90-649.64, 650, 655.70-655.73,
665.00-665.11, 665.50-665.54, 665.80-665.94, 666.12, 669.40-669.44,
669.80-669.94, 679.00-679.04, 679.12, 679.14;
For code **666.14:** Ⓔⓧ 666.10-666.14
Coding Clinic: 1988, Q1, P14

● **666.2** **Delayed and secondary postpartum**
[0,2,4] **hemorrhage** ♀ **2,4** 🦠   M
     Hemorrhage:
       after the first 24 hours following delivery
       associated with retained portions of placenta or
         membranes
     Postpartum hemorrhage specified as delayed or
       secondary
     Retained products of conception NOS, following
       delivery
For code **666.22:** Ⓔⓧ 646.80-646.93, 648.90-649.64, 650, 655.70-655.73,
665.00-665.11, 665.50-665.54, 665.80-665.94, 666.22, 669.40-669.44,
669.80-669.94, 679.00-679.04, 679.12, 679.14;
For code **666.24:** Ⓔⓧ 666.20-666.24
Coding Clinic: 1988, Q1, P14

● **666.3** **Postpartum coagulation defects** ♀ **2** 🦠   M
[0,2,4]   Postpartum:
     afibrinogenemia
     fibrinolysis
For code **666.32:** Ⓔⓧ 646.80-646.93, 648.90-649.64, 650, 666.00-666.34,
669.40-669.44, 669.80-669.94, 679.00-679.04, 679.12, 679.14

COMPLICATIONS OF PREGNANCY, CHILDBIRTH, AND THE PUERPERIUM (630–679)

N Newborn Age: 0	**P** Pediatric Age: 0–17	**M** Maternity Age: 12–55	**A** Adult Age: 15–124	♀ Females Only	♂ Males Only
Ⓔⓧ CC Exclusions	🦠 Complication\Comorbidity	🦠 Major C\C	Present on Admission Requirement	🦠 Hospital-Acquired Condition	

987

● **667 Retained placenta without hemorrhage**

Requires fifth digit; valid digits are in [brackets] under each code. See beginning of section 660–669 for definitions.

● **667.0 Retained placenta without hemorrhage ♀**   M
[0,2,4]   Placenta accreta without hemorrhage
Retained placenta:
    NOS without hemorrhage
    total without hemorrhage
   Coding Clinic: 1988, Q1, P14

● **667.1 Retained portions of placenta or membranes,**
[0,2,4] **without hemorrhage ♀**   M
Retained products of conception following delivery, without hemorrhage
   Coding Clinic: 1988, Q1, P14

● **668 Complications of the administration of anesthetic or other sedation in labor and delivery**

Use additional code(s) to further specify complication

Requires fifth digit; valid digits are in [brackets] under each code. See beginning of section 660–669 for definitions.

Includes   complications arising from the administration of a general or local anesthetic, analgesic, or other sedation in labor and delivery

Excludes   *reaction to spinal or lumbar puncture (349.0)*
spinal headache (349.0)

● **668.0 Pulmonary complications ♀**   M
[0-4]   Inhalation [aspiration] of stomach contents or secretions following anesthesia or other sedation in labor or delivery
Mendelson's syndrome following anesthesia or other sedation in labor or delivery
Pressure collapse of lung following anesthesia or other sedation in labor or delivery

● **668.1 Cardiac complications ♀**   M
[0-4]   Cardiac arrest or failure following anesthesia or other sedation in labor and delivery

● **668.2 Central nervous system complications ♀**   M
[0-4]   Cerebral anoxia following anesthesia or other sedation in labor and delivery

● **668.8 Other complications of anesthesia or other sedation**
[0-4] **in labor and delivery ♀**   M
   Coding Clinic: 1999, Q2, P9-10

● **668.9 Unspecified complication of anesthesia and other**
[0-4] **sedation ♀**   M

● **669 Other complications of labor and delivery, not elsewhere classified**

Requires fifth digit; valid digits are in [brackets] under each code. See beginning of section 660–669 for definitions.

● **669.0 Maternal distress ♀**   M
[0-4]   Metabolic disturbance in labor and delivery

● **669.1 Shock during or following labor and**
[0-4] **delivery ♀ 1-4** Ⓦ   M
Obstetric shock
For codes **669.11-669.14:** Ⓔ 646.80-646.93, 648.90-649.64, 650, 669.10-669.14, 669.40-669.44, 669.80-669.94, 679.00-679.04, 679.12, 679.14

● **669.2 Maternal hypotension syndrome ♀ 4**Ⓦ**, 1,2**Ⓦ   M
[0-4]   For codes **669.21, 669.22, and 669.24:** Ⓔ 646.80-646.93, 648.90-649.64, 650, 669.10-669.14, 669.21, 669.40-669.44, 669.80-669.94, 679.00-679.04, 679.12, 679.14

● **669.3 Acute ~~renal~~ kidney failure following labor and**
[0,2,4] **delivery ♀ 2,4**Ⓦ   M ◀▥
For codes **669.32 and 669.34:** Ⓔ 646.80-646.93, 648.90-649.64, 650, 669.30-669.44, 669.80-669.94, 679.00-679.04, 679.12, 679.14

● **669.4 Other complications of obstetrical surgery and**
[0-4] **procedures ♀**   M
Cardiac:
   arrest following cesarean or other obstetrical surgery or procedure, including delivery NOS
   failure following cesarean or other obstetrical surgery or procedure, including delivery NOS
Cerebral anoxia following cesarean or other obstetrical surgery or procedure, including delivery NOS

Excludes   *complications of obstetrical surgical wounds (674.1–674.3)*

● **669.5 Forceps or vacuum extractor delivery without**
[0,1] **mention of indication ♀**   M
Delivery by ventouse, without mention of indication

● **669.6 Breech extraction, without mention of indication ♀ M**
[0,1]   **Excludes**   *breech delivery NOS (652.2)*

● **669.7 Cesarean delivery, without mention of indication ♀ M**
[0,1]   **Coding Clinic: 2001, Q1, P11-12**

● **669.8 Other complications of labor and delivery ♀**   M
[0-4]   **Coding Clinic: 2006, Q4, P135**

● **669.9 Unspecified complication of labor and delivery ♀**   M
[0-4]

COMPLICATIONS OF THE PUERPERIUM (670–677)

Note: Categories 671 and 673–676 include the listed conditions even if they occur during pregnancy or childbirth.

The following fifth-digit subclassification is for use with categories 670–676 to denote the current episode of care:

0   unspecified as to episode of care or not applicable
1   delivered, with or without mention of antepartum condition
2   delivered, with mention of postpartum complication
3   antepartum condition or complication
4   postpartum condition or complication

● **670** **Major puerperal infection** ♀
[0,2,4]   Puerperal: Puerperal:
    endometritis   peritonitis
    fever (septic)   pyemia
    pelvic: salpingitis
      cellulitis   septicemia
    sepsis

    Requires fifth digit; valid digits are in [brackets] under each code. See beginning of section 670–676 for definitions.
    Use 0 as fourth digit for category 670

> **Excludes** *infection following abortion (639.0)*
> *minor genital tract infection following delivery (646.6)*
> *puerperal fever NOS (672)*
> *puerperal pyrexia NOS (672)*
> *puerperal pyrexia of unknown origin (672)*
> *urinary tract infection following delivery (646.6)*

    For codes **670.02 and 670.04:** (Ex) 646.80-646.93, 648.90-649.64, 650, 669.40-669.44, 669.80-670.04, 679.00-679.04, 679.12, 679.14
    Coding Clinic: 2007, Q3, P10

    670.0 **Major puerpal infection, unspecified** ♀ 0 , 2,4 M
    [0,2,4]

    670.1 **Puerpal endometritis** ♀ 0,2,4 M
    [0,2,4]

    670.2 **Puerpal sepsis** ♀ 0 M
    [0,2,4]   Puerpal pyemia ♀

    670.3 **Puerpal septic thrombophlebitis** ♀ 0 , 2,4 M
    [0,2,4]

    670.8 **Other major puerpal infection** ♀ M
    [0,2,4]   Puerpal:
          pelvic cellulitis
          peritonitis
          salpingitis

● **671** **Venous complications in pregnancy and the puerperium**

> **Excludes** *personal history of venous complications prior to pregnancy such as:*
> *thrombophlebitis (V12.52)*
> *thrombosis and embolism (V12.51)*

    Requires fifth digit; valid digits are in [brackets] under each code. See beginning of section 670–676 for definitions.

● **671.0** **Varicose veins of legs** ♀ M
    [0-4]   Varicose veins NOS

● **671.1** **Varicose veins of vulva and perineum** ♀ M
    [0-4]

● **671.2** **Superficial thrombophlebitis** ♀ M
    [0-4]   Phlebitis NOS
          Thrombophlebitis (superficial)
          Thrombosis NOS
    (Ex) 646.80-646.93, 648.90-649.64, 650, 669.40-669.44, 669.80-669.94, 671.20-671.94, 679.00-679.04, 679.12, 679.14

● **671.3** **Deep phlebothrombosis, antepartum** ♀ 0 , 1,3 M
    [0,1,3]   Use additional code to identify the deep vein thrombosis (453.40-453.42, 453.50-453.52, 453.72-453.79, 453.82-453.89)
          Use additional code for long-term (current) use of anticoagulants if applicable (V58.61)
          Deep-vein thrombosis, antepartum
    For codes **671.30, 671.31, and 671.33:** (Ex) 646.80-646.93, 648.90-649.64, 650, 669.40-669.44, 669.80-669.94, 671.20-671.94, 679.00-679.04, 679.12, 679.14

● **671.4** **Deep phlebothrombosis, postpartum** ♀ 0 , 2,4 M
    [0,2,4]   Deep-vein thrombosis, postpartum
          Pelvic thrombophlebitis, postpartum
          Phlegmasia alba dolens (puerperal)
          Use additional code to identify the deep vein thrombosis (453.40-453.42, 453.50-453.52, 453.72-453.79, 453.82-453.89)
          Use additional code for long-term (current) use of anticoagulants if applicable (V58.61)
    For codes **671.40, 671.42, and 671.44:** (Ex) 646.80-646.93, 648.90-649.64, 650, 669.40-669.44, 669.80-669.94, 671.20-671.94, 679.00-679.04, 679.12, 679.14

● **671.5** **Other phlebitis and thrombosis** ♀ M
    [0-4]   Cerebral venous thrombosis
          Thrombosis of intracranial venous sinus
    (Ex) 646.80-646.93, 648.90-649.64, 650, 669.40-669.44, 669.80-669.94, 671.20-671.94, 679.00-679.04, 679.12, 679.14

● **671.8** **Other venous complications** ♀ M
    [0-4]   Hemorrhoids
    For codes **671.80-671.83:** (Ex) 646.80-646.93, 648.90-649.64, 650, 669.40-669.44, 669.80-669.94, 671.20-671.94, 679.00-679.04, 679.12, 679.14;
    For code **671.84:** (Ex) 671.80-671.84

● **671.9** **Unspecified venous complication** ♀ 0-2 M
    [0-4]   Phlebitis NOS
          Thrombosis NOS
    For codes **671.90-671.92:** (Ex) 646.80-646.93, 648.90-649.64, 650, 669.40-669.44, 669.80-669.94, 671.20-671.94, 679.00-679.04, 679.12, 679.14

● **672** **Pyrexia of unknown origin during the**
[0,2,4] **puerperium** ♀ 2,4 M
    Postpartum fever NOS
    Puerperal fever NOS
    Puerperal pyrexia NOS

    Requires fifth digit; valid digits are in [brackets] under each code. See beginning of section 670–676 for definitions.

    Use 0 as fourth digit for category 672
    For code **672.02:** (Ex) 646.80-646.93, 648.90-649.64, 650, 669.40-669.44, 669.80-669.94, 671.20, 671.23-671.30, 671.33-671.40, 671.50, 671.53-671.80, 671.83-671.90, 671.93-671.94, 672.02, 679.00-679.04, 679.12, 679.14;
    For code **672.04:** (Ex) 672.02-672.04

COMPLICATIONS OF PREGNANCY, CHILDBIRTH, AND THE PUERPERIUM (630–679)

● **673 Obstetrical pulmonary embolism**

> Requires fifth digit; valid digits are in [brackets] under each code. See beginning of section 670–676 for definitions.

> **Includes** pulmonary emboli in pregnancy, childbirth, or the puerperium, or specified as puerperal

> **Excludes** *embolism following abortion (639.6)*

● **673.0 Obstetrical air embolism** ♀ 1-4 🔖   M
[0-4]   For codes **673.01-673.04:** (Ex) 646.80-646.93, 648.90-649.64, 650, 669.40-669.44, 669.80-669.94, 673.00-673.84, 679.00-679.04, 679.12, 679.14

● **673.1 Amniotic fluid embolism** ♀ 1-4 🔖   M
[0-4]   For codes **673.11-673.14:** (Ex) 646.80-646.93, 648.90-649.64, 650, 669.40-669.44, 669.80-669.94, 673.00-673.84, 679.00-679.04, 679.12, 679.14

● **673.2 Obstetrical blood-clot embolism** ♀ 1-4 🔖   M
[0-4]   Puerperal pulmonary embolism NOS
           For codes **673.21-673.24:** (Ex) 646.80-646.93, 648.90-649.64, 650, 669.40-669.44, 669.80-669.94, 673.00-673.84, 679.00-679.04, 679.12, 679.14

● **673.3 Obstetrical pyemic and septic**
[0-4] **embolism** ♀ 0 🔖, 1-4 🔖   M
           (Ex) 646.80-646.93, 648.90-649.64, 650, 669.40-669.44, 669.80-669.94, 673.00-673.84, 679.00-679.04, 679.12, 679.14

● **673.8 Other pulmonary embolism** ♀ 1-4 🔖   M
[0-4]   Fat embolism
           For codes **673.81-673.84:** (Ex) 646.80-646.93, 648.90-649.64, 650, 669.40-669.44, 669.80-669.94, 673.00-673.84, 679.00-679.04, 679.12, 679.14

● **674 Other and unspecified complications of the puerperium, not elsewhere classified**

> Requires fifth digit; valid digits are in [brackets] under each code. See beginning of section 670–676 for definitions.

● **674.0 Cerebrovascular disorders in the**
[0-4] **puerperium** ♀ 2-4 🔖, 1 🔖   M
           Any condition classifiable to 430–434, 436–437 occurring during pregnancy, childbirth, or the puerperium, or specified as puerperal

> **Excludes** *intracranial venous sinus thrombosis (671.5)*

           For codes **674.01-674.04:** (Ex) 646.80-646.93, 648.90-649.64, 650, 669.40-669.44, 669.80-669.94, 674.00-674.04, 674.50-674.54, 679.00-679.04, 679.12, 679.14

● **674.1 Disruption of cesarean wound** ♀   M
[0,2,4]   Dehiscence or disruption of uterine wound

> **Excludes** *uterine rupture before onset of labor (665.0) uterine rupture during labor (665.1)*

● **674.2 Disruption of perineal wound** ♀   M
[0,2,4]   Breakdown of perineum
           Disruption of wound of:
             episiotomy
             perineal laceration
           Secondary perineal tear
           Coding Clinic: 1997, Q1, P9-10

● **674.3 Other complications of obstetrical surgical**
[0,2,4] **wounds** ♀   M
           Hematoma of cesarean section or perineal wound
           Hemorrhage of cesarean section or perineal wound
           Infection of cesarean section or perineal wound

> **Excludes** *damage from instruments in delivery (664.0–665.9)*

● **674.4 Placental polyp** ♀   M
[0,2,4]

● **674.5 Peripartum cardiomyopathy** ♀ 🔖   M
[0-4]   Postpartum cardiomyopathy
           (Ex) 646.80-646.93, 648.90-649.64, 650, 669.40-669.44, 669.80-669.94, 674.00-674.04, 674.50-674.54, 679.00-679.04, 679.12, 679.14
           Coding Clinic: 2003, Q4, P65

● **674.8 Other** ♀   M
[0,2,4]   Hepatorenal syndrome, following delivery
           Postpartum:
             subinvolution of uterus
             uterine hypertrophy
           Coding Clinic: 1998, Q3, P16

● **674.9 Unspecified** ♀   M
[0,2,4]   Sudden death of unknown cause during the puerperium

● **675 Infections of the breast and nipple associated with childbirth**

> Requires fifth digit; valid digits are in [brackets] under each code. See beginning of section 670–676 for definitions.

> **Includes** the listed conditions during pregnancy, childbirth, or the puerperium

● **675.0 Infections of nipple** ♀   M
[0-4]   Abscess of nipple

● **675.1 Abscess of breast** ♀ 1,2 🔖   M
[0-4]   Abscess:
             mammary
             subareolar
             submammary
           Mastitis:
             purulent
             retromammary
             submammary
           For codes **675.11-675.12:** (Ex) 646.80-646.93, 648.90-649.64, 650, 669.40-669.44, 669.80-669.94, 675.00-675.94, 679.00-679.04, 679.12, 679.14

● **675.2 Nonpurulent mastitis** ♀   M
[0-4]   Lymphangitis of breast
           Mastitis:
             NOS
             interstitial
             parenchymatous

● **675.8 Other specified infections of the breast and**
[0-4] **nipple** ♀   M

● **675.9 Unspecified infection of the breast and nipple** ♀   M
[0-4]

◄ New   ◄▏▏ Revised   deleted Deleted   ● Unacceptable Principal Diagnosis   ● Use Additional Digit(s)
▶ Manifestation Code   OGCR Official Guidelines   Coding Clinic   Excludes   Includes   Use additional   Code first   Omit code

● **676 Other disorders of the breast associated with childbirth and disorders of lactation**

Requires fifth digit; valid digits are in [brackets] under each code. See beginning of section 670–676 for definitions.

Includes the listed conditions during pregnancy, the puerperium, or lactation

● **676.0 Retracted nipple** ♀   M
[0-4]

● **676.1 Cracked nipple** ♀   M
[0-4]   Fissure of nipple

● **676.2 Engorgement of breasts** ♀   M
[0-4]

● **676.3 Other and unspecified disorder of breast** ♀   M
[0-4]

● **676.4 Failure of lactation** ♀   M
[0-4]   Agalactia

● **676.5 Suppressed lactation** ♀   M
[0-4]

● **676.6 Galactorrhea** ♀   M
[0-4]   **Excludes** *galactorrhea not associated with childbirth (611.6)*
           Coding Clinic: 1985, July-Aug, P9

● **676.8 Other disorders of lactation** ♀   M
[0-4]   Galactocele

● **676.9 Unspecified disorder of lactation** ♀   M
[0-4]

OGCR Section I.C.10.j.1-3

Code 677, Late effect of complication of pregnancy, childbirth, and the puerpium is for use in those cases when an initial complication of a pregnancy develops a sequelae requiring care or treatment at a future date. This code may be used at any time after the initial postpartum period and like all late effect codes, is to be sequenced following the code describing the sequelae of the complication.

677 Late effect of complication of pregnancy, childbirth, and the puerperium ♀ 🔖

Note: This category is to be used to indicate conditions in 632–648.9 and 651–676.9 as the cause of the late effect, themselves classifiable elsewhere. The "late effects " include conditions specified as such, or as sequelae, which may occur at any time after the puerperium.

Code first any sequelae

Coding Clinic: 1997, Q1, P9-10

OTHER MATERNAL AND FETAL COMPLICATIONS (678-679)

The following fifth-digit subclassification is for use with categories 678-679 to denote the current episode of care:

> 0 unspecified as to episode of care or not applicable
> 1 delivered, with or without mention of antepartum condition
> 2 delivered, with mention of postpartum complication
> 3 antepartum condition or complication
> 4 postpartum condition or complication

● **678 Other fetal conditions**

Requires fifth digit; valid digits are in [brackets] under each code. See beginning of section 678-679 for definitions.
Coding Clinic: 2008, Q4, P125-127

● **678.0 Fetal hematologic conditions** ♀   M
[0,1,3]   Fetal anemia
           Fetal thrombocytopenia
           Fetal twin to twin transfusion

           Excludes *fetal and neonatal hemorrhage (772.0-772.9)*
           fetal hematologic disorders affecting newborn (776.0-776.9)
           fetal-maternal hemorrhage (656.00-656.03)
           isoimmunization incompatibility (656.10-656.13, 656.20-656.23)

● **678.1 Fetal conjoined twins** ♀   M
[0,1,3]

● **679 Complications of in utero procedures**

Requires fifth digit; valid digits are in [brackets] under each code. See beginning of section 678-679 for definitions.
Coding Clinic: 2008, Q4, P127-128

● **679.0 Maternal complications from in utero procedure** ♀ M
[0-4]   **Excludes** *maternal history of in utero procedure during previous pregnancy (V23.86)*

● **679.1 Fetal complications from in utero procedure** ♀   M
[0-4]   Fetal complications from amniocentesis

           Excludes *newborn affected by in utero procedure (760.61-760.64)*

COMPLICATIONS OF PREGNANCY, CHILDBIRTH, AND THE PUERPERIUM (630–679)

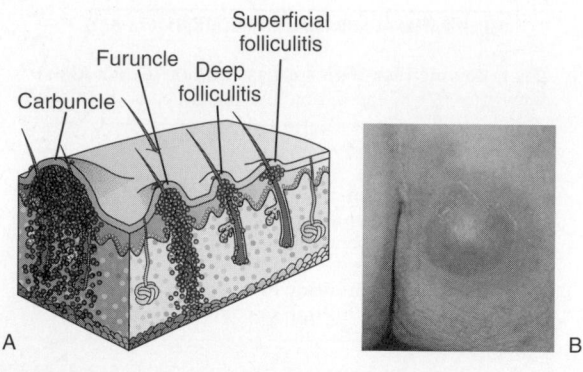

Figure 12–1 Furuncle, also known as a boil, is a staphylococcal infection. The organism enters the body through a hair follicle and so furuncles usually appear in hairy areas of the body. A cluster of furuncles is known as a carbuncle and involves infection into the deep subcutaneous fascia. These usually appear on the back and neck. (**B** from Habif: Clinical Dermatology, 4th ed. 2004, Mosby)

12.   DISEASES OF THE SKIN AND SUBCUTANEOUS TISSUE (680–709)

INFECTIONS OF SKIN AND SUBCUTANEOUS TISSUE (680–686)

Excludes *certain infections of skin classified under "Infectious and Parasitic Diseases," such as:*
    erysipelas (035)
    erysipeloid of Rosenbach (027.1)
    herpes:
       simplex (054.0–054.9)
       zoster (053.0–053.9)
    molluscum contagiosum (078.0)
    viral warts (078.10-078.19) ⬅

● **680   Carbuncle and furuncle**

Includes   boil
             furunculosis

680.0 Face
    Ear [any part]   Nose (septum)
    Face [any part, except eye] Temple (region)
    Excludes *eyelid (373.13)*
             lacrimal apparatus (375.31)
             orbit (376.01)

680.1 Neck

680.2 Trunk
    Abdominal wall
    Back [any part, except buttocks]
    Breast
    Chest wall
    Flank
    Groin
    Pectoral region
    Perineum
    Umbilicus
    Excludes *buttocks (680.5)*
             external genital organs:
                female (616.4)
                male (607.2, 608.4)

680.3 Upper arm and forearm
    Arm [any part, except hand]
    Axilla
    Shoulder

680.4 Hand
    Finger [any]   Wrist
    Thumb

680.5 Buttock
    Anus   Gluteal region

680.6 Leg, except foot
    Ankle   Knee
    Hip   Thigh

680.7 Foot
    Heel
    Toe

680.8 Other specified sites
    Head [any part, except face]
    Scalp
    Excludes *external genital organs:*
                female (616.4)
                male (607.2, 608.4)

680.9 Unspecified site
    Boil NOS   Furuncle NOS
    Carbuncle NOS

Item 12-1   Cellulitis is an acute spreading bacterial infection below the surface of the skin characterized by redness (erythema), warmth, swelling, pain, fever, chills, and enlarged lymph nodes ("swollen glands"). **Abscess** is a localized collection of pus in tissues or organs and is a sign of infection resulting in swelling and inflammation. **Onychia** is an inflammation of the tissue surrounding the nail with pus accumulation and loss of the nail, resulting from microscopic pathogens entering through small wounds. **Paronychia** is a nail disease also known as felon or whitlow and is a bacterial or fungal infection.

● **681   Cellulitis and abscess of finger and toe**

Includes   that with lymphangitis

Use additional code to identify organism, such as:
    Staphylococcus (041.1)

● **681.0   Finger**

  681.00 Cellulitis and abscess, unspecified

  681.01 Felon
       Pulp abscess   Whitlow
       Excludes *herpetic whitlow (054.6)*

  681.02 Onychia and paronychia of finger
       Panaritium of finger
       Perionychia of finger

● **681.1   Toe**

  681.10 Cellulitis and abscess, unspecified
       Coding Clinic: 2005, Q1, P14

  681.11 Onychia and paronychia of toe
       Panaritium of toe
       Perionychia of toe

● **681.9   Cellulitis and abscess of unspecified digit**
    Infection of nail NOS

◀ New   ⬅ Revised   deleted Deleted   ● Unacceptable Principal Diagnosis   ● Use Additional Digit(s)
▶ Manifestation Code   **OGCR** Official Guidelines   **Coding Clinic**   Excludes   Includes   Use additional   Code first   Omit code

● **682 Other cellulitis and abscess**

> **Includes** abscess (acute) (with lymphangitis) except of finger or toe
> cellulitis (diffuse) (with lymphangitis) except of finger or toe
> lymphangitis, acute (with lymphangitis) except of finger or toe

Use additional code to identify organism, such as:
Staphylococcus (041.1)

> **Excludes** lymphangitis (chronic) (subacute) (457.2)

682.0 Face 🦠
This code reports forehead but not head (682.8).

Cheek, external	Nose, external
Chin	Submandibular
Forehead	Temple (region)

> **Excludes** ear [any part] (380.10–380.16)
> eyelid (373.13)
> lacrimal apparatus (375.31)
> lip (528.5)
> mouth (528.3)
> nose (internal) (478.1)
> orbit (376.01)

Ⓔⓧ 017.00-017.06, 017.90-017.96, 040.82-041.9, 682.0, 682.8-682.9, 686.00-686.9, 705.83, 709.8, V09.0-V09.91

682.1 Neck 🦠
Ⓔⓧ 017.00-017.06, 017.90-017.96, 040.82-041.9, 682.1, 682.8-682.9, 686.00-686.9, 705.83, 709.8, V09.0-V09.91

682.2 Trunk 🦠
Abdominal wall
Back [any part, except buttock]
Buttocks see 682.5
Chest wall
Flank
Groin
Pectoral region
Perineum
Umbilicus, except newborn

> **Excludes** anal and rectal regions (566)
> breast:
> NOS (611.0)
> puerperal (675.1)
> external genital organs:
> female (616.3–616.4)
> male (604.0, 607.2, 608.4)
> umbilicus, newborn (771.4)

Ⓔⓧ 017.00-017.06, 017.90-017.96, 040.82-041.9, 682.2, 682.8-682.9, 686.00-686.9, 705.83, 709.8, V09.0-V09.91
Coding Clinic: 1993, Q1, P26

682.3 Upper arm and forearm 🦠
Arm [any part, except hand]
Axilla
Shoulder

> **Excludes** hand (682.4)

Ⓔⓧ 017.00-017.06, 017.90-017.96, 040.82-041.9, 682.3, 682.8-682.9, 686.00-686.9, 705.83, 709.8, V09.0-V09.91
Coding Clinic: 2003, Q2, P7-8; 1998, Q4, P42-44

682.4 Hand, except fingers and thumb 🦠
Wrist

> **Excludes** finger and thumb (681.00–681.02)

Ⓔⓧ 017.00-017.06, 017.90-017.96, 040.82-041.9, 682.4, 682.8-682.9, 686.00-686.9, 705.83, 709.8, V09.0-V09.91

682.5 Buttock 🦠
Gluteal region

> **Excludes** anal and rectal regions (566)

Ⓔⓧ 017.00-017.06, 017.90-017.96, 040.82-041.9, 682.5, 682.8-682.9, 686.00-686.9, 705.83, 709.8, V09.0-V09.91

682.6 Leg, except foot 🦠
Ankle
Hip
Knee
Thigh

Ⓔⓧ 017.00-017.06, 017.90-017.96, 040.82-041.9, 682.5, 682.8-682.9, 686.00-686.9, 705.83, 709.8, V09.0-V09.91
Coding Clinic: 2009, Q1, P18x2; 2004, Q3, P5-6; 2003, Q4, P108; 1995, Q1, P3

682.7 Foot, except toes 🦠
Heel

> **Excludes** toe (681.10–681.11)

Ⓔⓧ 017.00-017.06, 017.90-017.96, 040.82-041.9, 682.7-682.9, 686.00-686.9, 705.83, 709.8, V09.0-V09.91

682.8 Other specified sites 🦠
Head [except face]
Scalp

> **Excludes** face (682.0)

Ⓔⓧ 017.00-017.06, 017.90-017.96, 040.82-041.9, 682.8-682.9, 686.00-686.9 705.83, 709.8, V09.0-V09.91

682.9 Unspecified site 🦠
Abscess NOS
Cellulitis NOS
Lymphangitis, acute NOS

> **Excludes** lymphangitis NOS (457.2)

Ⓔⓧ 017.00-017.06, 017.90-017.96, 040.82-041.9, 682.8-682.9, 686.00-686.9 705.83, 709.8, V09.0-V09.91

683 Acute lymphadenitis
Short term inflammation of lymph nodes which can be regionalized to involve a given area of lymph system or systemic involvement
Abscess (acute) lymph gland or node, except mesenteric
Adenitis, acute lymph gland or node, except mesenteric
Lymphadenitis, acute lymph gland or node, except mesenteric

Use additional code to identify organism such as
Staphylococcus (041.1)

> **Excludes** enlarged glands NOS (785.6)
> lymphadenitis:
> chronic or subacute, except mesenteric (289.1)
> mesenteric (acute) (chronic) (subacute) (289.2)
> unspecified (289.3)

Figure 12-2 Impetigo. A thick, honey-yellow adherent crust covers the entire eroded surface. (From Habif: Clinical Dermatology, 4th ed. 2004, Mosby, Inc.)

Item 12-2 Pilonidal cyst, also called a coccygeal cyst, is the result of a disorder called pilonidal disease. The cyst usually contains hair and pus.

684 Impetigo

Contagious skin infection caused by streptococcus or staphylococcus aureus that produces blisters or sores on the face and hands

Impetiginization of other dermatoses
Impetigo (contagiosa) [any site] [any organism]:
    bullousneonatorum
    circinate
    simplex
Pemphigus neonatorum

> **Excludes** *impetigo herpetiformis (694.3)*

● 685 Pilonidal cyst

> **Includes** fistula, coccygeal or pilonidal
> sinus, coccygeal or pilonidal

685.0 With abscess 🔾
> (Ex:) 685.0-685.1, 709.8

685.1 Without mention of abscess

● 686 Other local infections of skin and subcutaneous tissue

> **Use additional** code to identify any infectious organism (041.0–041.8)

● 686.0 Pyoderma
Dermatitis:
    purulent
    septic
    suppurative

686.00 Pyoderma, unspecified

686.01 Pyoderma gangrenosum 🔾
> (Ex:) 686.00-686.09
> **Coding Clinic: 1997, Q4, P42**

686.09 Other pyoderma

686.1 Pyogenic granuloma
Granuloma:
    septic
    suppurative
    telangiectaticum

> **Excludes** *pyogenic granuloma of oral mucosa (528.9)*

686.8 Other specified local infections of skin and subcutaneous tissue
Bacterid (pustular)
Dermatitis vegetans
Ecthyma
Perlèche

> **Excludes** *dermatitis infectiosa eczematoides (690.8)*
> *panniculitis (729.30–729.39)*

Figure 12-3 Seborrheic dermatitis. (From Cohen BA: Atlas of Pediatric Dermatology. St. Louis, Mosby, 1993.)

Item 12-3 Seborrheic dermatitis is characterized by greasy, scaly, red patches and is associated with oily skin and scalp.

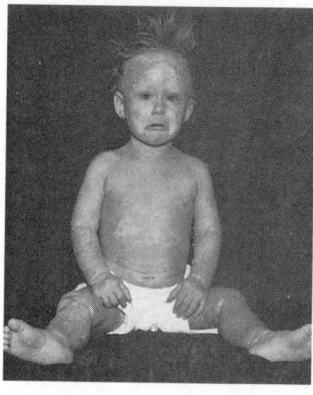

Figure 12-4 Atopic dermatitis. (From Moschella SL, Hurley HJ: Dermatology, 2nd ed. Philadelphia, WB Saunders, 1985, p 336.)

Item 12-4 Atopic dermatitis, also known as atopic eczema, infantile eczema, disseminated neurodermatitis, flexural eczema, and *prurigo diathesique* (Besnier), is characterized by intense itching and is often hereditary.

686.9 Unspecified local infection of skin and subcutaneous tissue
Fistula of skin NOS
Skin infection NOS

> **Excludes** *fistula to skin from internal organs—see Alphabetic Index*

OTHER INFLAMMATORY CONDITIONS OF SKIN AND SUBCUTANEOUS TISSUE (690–698)

> **Excludes** *panniculitis (729.30–729.39)*

● 690 Erythematosquamous dermatosis

> **Excludes** *eczematous dermatitis of eyelid (373.31)*
> *parakeratosis variegata (696.2)*
> *psoriasis (696.0–696.1)*
> *seborrheic keratosis (702.11–702.19)*

● 690.1 Seborrheic dermatitis

690.10 Seborrheic dermatitis, unspecified
Seborrheic dermatitis NOS

690.11 Seborrhea capitis   P
Cradle cap

690.12 Seborrheic infantile dermatitis   P

690.18 Other seborrheic dermatitis

690.8 Other erythematosquamous dermatosis

◀ New   ◀▥ Revised   ~~deleted~~ Deleted   ● Unacceptable Principal Diagnosis   ● Use Additional Digit(s)
▶ Manifestation Code   **OGCR** Official Guidelines   **Coding Clinic**   Excludes   Includes   Use additional   Code first   Omit code

● **691 Atopic dermatitis and related conditions**

  691.0 Diaper or napkin rash
      Ammonia dermatitis
      Diaper or napkin:
        dermatitis
        erythema
        rash
      Psoriasiform napkin eruption

  691.8 Other atopic dermatitis and related conditions
      Atopic dermatitis
      Besnier's prurigo
      Eczema:
        atopic
        flexural
        intrinsic (allergic)
      Neurodermatitis:
        atopic
        diffuse (of Brocq)

● **692 Contact dermatitis and other eczema**

  Includes   dermatitis:
        NOS
        contact
        occupational
        venenata
      eczema (acute) (chronic):
        NOS
        allergic
        erythematous
        occupational

  Excludes   *allergy NOS (995.3)*
      contact dermatitis of eyelids (373.32)
      dermatitis due to substances taken internally
        (693.0–693.9)
      eczema of external ear (380.22)
      perioral dermatitis (695.3)
      urticarial reactions (708.0–708.9, 995.1)

  692.0 Due to detergents

  692.1 Due to oils and greases

  692.2 Due to solvents
      Dermatitis due to solvents of:
        chlorocompound group
        cyclohexane group
        ester group
        glycol group
        hydrocarbon group
        ketone group

  692.3 Due to drugs and medicines in contact with skin
      Dermatitis (allergic) (contact) due to:
        arnica
        fungicides
        iodine
        keratolytics
        mercurials
        neomycin
        pediculocides
        phenols
        scabicides
        any drug applied to skin
      Dermatitis medicamentosa due to drug applied to
        skin

    Use additional E code to identify drug

    Excludes   *allergy NOS due to drugs (995.27)*
        dermatitis due to ingested drugs (693.0)
        dermatitis medicamentosa NOS (693.0)

  692.4 Due to other chemical products

Dermatitis due to:	Dermatitis due to:
acids	insecticide
adhesive plaster	nylon
alkalis	plastic
caustics	rubber
dichromate	

    Coding Clinic: 2008, Q3, P6-7; 1989, Q2, P16

  692.5 Due to food in contact with skin
      Dermatitis, contact, due to:
        cereals
        fish
        flour
        fruit
        meat
        milk

    Excludes   *dermatitis due to:*
        dyes (692.89)
        ingested foods (693.1)
        preservatives (692.89)

  692.6 Due to plants [except food]
      Dermatitis due to:
        lacquer tree [Rhus verniciflua]
        poison:
          ivy [Rhus toxicodendron]
          oak [Rhus diversiloba]
          sumac [Rhus venenata]
          vine [Rhus radicans]
        primrose [Primula]
        ragweed [Senecio jacobae]
        other plants in contact with the skin

    Excludes   *allergy NOS due to pollen (477.0)*
        nettle rash (708.8)

● **692.7 Due to solar radiation**

    Excludes   *sunburn due to other ultraviolet radiation*
        exposure (692.82)

  692.70 Unspecified dermatitis due to sun

  692.71 Sunburn
      First degree sunburn
        See codes 692.76 and 692.77 for second and
          third degrees.
      Sunburn NOS

  692.72 Acute dermatitis due to solar radiation
      Berloque dermatitis
      Photoallergic response
      Phototoxic response
      Polymorphous light eruption
      Acute solar skin damage NOS

    Excludes   *sunburn (692.71, 692.76–692.77)*

    Use additional E code to identify drug, if
        drug induced

  692.73 Actinic reticuloid and actinic granuloma

  **692.74 Other chronic dermatitis due to solar
      radiation**
      Chronic solar skin damage NOS
      Solar elastosis

    Excludes   *actinic [solar] keratosis (702.0)*

  **692.75 Disseminated superficial actinic
      porokeratosis (DSAP)**

DISEASES OF THE SKIN AND SUBCUTANEOUS TISSUE (680–709)

N Newborn Age: 0   **P** Pediatric Age: 0–17   **M** Maternity Age: 12–55   **A** Adult Age: 15–124   ♀ Females Only   ♂ Males Only

(Ex) CC Exclusions   ⓒ Complication\Comorbidity   ⓜ Major C\C   Present on Admission Requirement   Hospital-Acquired Condition   **995**

692.76 Sunburn of second degree

692.77 Sunburn of third degree

692.79 Other dermatitis due to solar radiation
Hydroa aestivale
Photodermatitis (due to sun)
Photosensitiveness (due to sun)
Solar skin damage NOS

● **692.8 Due to other specified agents**

692.81 Dermatitis due to cosmetics

692.82 Dermatitis due to other radiation
Infrared rays
Light, except from sun
Radiation NOS
Tanning bed
Ultraviolet rays, except from sun
X-rays
> **Excludes** *that due to solar radiation*
> *(692.70–692.79)*
> Coding Clinic: 2000, Q3, P5

692.83 Dermatitis due to metals
Jewelry

692.84 Due to animal (cat) (dog) dander
Due to animal (cat) (dog) hair
Coding Clinic: 2004, Q4, P90-91

692.89 Other
Dermatitis due to:
cold weather
dyes
hot weather
preservatives
> **Excludes** *allergy (NOS) (rhinitis) due to*
> *animal hair or dander (477.2)*
> *allergy to dust (477.8)*
> *sunburn (692.71, 692.76–692.77)*

692.9 Unspecified cause
Dermatitis:
NOS
contact NOS
venenata NOS
Eczema NOS

● **693 Dermatitis due to substances taken internally**
> **Excludes** *adverse effect NOS of drugs and medicines*
> *(995.20)*
> *allergy NOS (995.3)*
> *contact dermatitis (692.0–692.9)*
> *urticarial reactions (708.0–708.9, 995.1)*

693.0 Due to drugs and medicines
Dermatitis medicamentosa NOS
Use additional E code to identify drug
> **Excludes** *that due to drugs in contact with skin*
> *(692.3)*
> Coding Clinic: 2007, Q2, P9-10

693.1 Due to food

693.8 Due to other specified substances taken internally

693.9 Due to unspecified substance taken internally
> **Excludes** *dermatitis NOS (692.9)*

Figure 12–5 Dermatitis herpetiformis. (From Arnold HL, Odom RB, James WD: Andrews' Diseases of the Skin, Clinical Dermatology, 8th ed. Philadelphia, WB Saunders, 1990, p 553.)

Item 12–5 Dermatitis herpetiformis, also known as Duhring's disease, is a systemic disease characterized by small blisters (3 to 5 mm) and occasionally large bullae (+5 mm).

● **694 Bullous dermatoses**

694.0 Dermatitis herpetiformis
Dermatosis herpetiformis
Duhring's disease
Hydroa herpetiformis
> **Excludes** *herpes gestationis (646.8)*
> *dermatitis herpetiformis:*
> *juvenile (694.2)*
> *senile (694.5)*

694.1 Subcorneal pustular dermatosis
Sneddon-Wilkinson disease or syndrome

694.2 Juvenile dermatitis herpetiformis
Juvenile pemphigoid

694.3 Impetigo herpetiformis

694.4 Pemphigus 🔖
Pemphigus:
NOS
erythematosus
foliaceus
malignant
vegetans
vulgaris
> **Excludes** *pemphigus neonatorum (684)*
> Ⓔⓧ 694.4-694.9, 709.8

694.5 Pemphigoid 🔖
Benign pemphigus NOS
Bullous pemphigoid
Herpes circinatus bullosus
Senile dermatitis herpetiformis
Ⓔⓧ 694.4-694.9, 709.8

DISEASES OF THE SKIN AND SUBCUTANEOUS TISSUE (680–709)

◀ New   ◀═ Revised   ~~deleted~~ Deleted   ● Unacceptable Principal Diagnosis   ● Use Additional Digit(s)
▶ Manifestation Code   **OGCR** Official Guidelines   **Coding Clinic**   Excludes   Includes   Use additional   Code first   Omit code

● **694.6 Benign mucous membrane pemphigoid**
Cicatricial pemphigoid
Mucosynechial atrophic bullous dermatitis

     694.60 Without mention of ocular involvement

     694.61 With ocular involvement
         Ocular pemphigus

     694.8 Other specified bullous dermatoses
         Excludes   *herpes gestationis (646.8)*

     694.9 Unspecified bullous dermatoses

● **695 Erythematous conditions**

     695.0 Toxic erythema 🦠
         Erythema venenatum
         (Ex) 695.0-695.4, 709.8

● **695.1 Erythema multiforme**
         Use additional code to identify associated
         manifestations, such as:
         arthropathy associated with dermatological
           disorders (713.3)
         conjunctival edema (372.73)
         conjunctivitis (372.04, 372.33)
         corneal scars and opacities (371.00-371.05)
         corneal ulcer (370.00-370.07)
         edema of eyelid (374.82)
         inflammation of eyelid (373.8)
         keratoconjunctivitis sicca (370.33)
         mechanical lagophthalmos (374.22)
         mucositis (478.11, 528.00, 538, 616.81)
         stomatitis (528.00)
         symblepharon (372.63)
         Use additional E-code to identify drug, if drug-
         induced
         Use additional code to identify percentage of skin
         exfoliation (695.50–695.59)
         Excludes   *(staphylococcal) scalded skin syndrome*
           (695.81)
         Coding Clinic: 2008, Q4, P128-131

     695.10 Erythema multiforme, unspecified
         Erythema iris
         Herpes iris

     695.11 Erythema multiforme minor

     695.12 Erythema multiforme major 🦠
         (Ex) 695.0-695.4, 695.81-695.9, 709.8

     695.13 Stevens-Johnson syndrome 🦠
         (Ex) 695.0-695.4, 695.81-695.9, 709.8

     695.14 Stevens-Johnson syndrome-toxic epidermal
         necrolysis overlap syndrome 🦠
         SJS-TEN overlap syndrome
         (Ex) 695.0-695.4, 695.81-695.9, 709.8
         Coding Clinic: 2008, Q4, P128-131

     695.15 Toxic epidermal necrolysis 🦠
         Lyell's syndrome
         (Ex) 695.0-695.4, 695.81-695.9, 709.8

     695.19 Other erythema multiforme

     695.2 Erythema nodosum
         Excludes   *tuberculous erythema nodosum (017.1)*

     695.3 Rosacea
         Acne:
           erythematosa
           rosacea
         Perioral dermatitis
         Rhinophyma

     695.4 Lupus erythematosus
         See 710.0 for designated as systemic lupus
         erythematosus (SLE).
         Lupus:
           erythematodes (discoid)
           erythematosus (discoid), not disseminated
         Excludes   *lupus (vulgaris) NOS (017.0)*
           systemic [disseminated] lupus
           erythematosus (710.0)

● **695.5 Exfoliation due to erythematous conditions**
     according to extent of body surface involved
         Code first *erythematous condition causing*
         exfoliation, such as:
         Ritter's disease (695.81)
         (Staphylococcal) scalded skin syndrome
           (695.81)
         Stevens-Johnson syndrome (695.13)
         Stevens-Johnson syndrome-toxic epidermal
           necrolysis overlap syndrome (695.14)
         toxic epidermal necrolysis (695.15)

●   **695.50 Exfoliation due to erythematous condition**
         involving less than 10 percent of body
         surface
         Exfoliation due to erythematous condition
           NOS

●   **695.51 Exfoliation due to erythematous condition**
         involving 10-19 percent of body surface

●   **695.52 Exfoliation due to erythematous condition**
         involving 20-29 percent of body surface

●   **695.53 Exfoliation due to erythematous condition**
         involving 30-39 percent of body surface 🦠
         (Ex) 695.53
         Coding Clinic: 2008, Q4, P128-131

●   **695.54 Exfoliation due to erythematous condition**
         involving 40-49 percent of body surface 🦠
         (Ex) 695.54

●   **695.55 Exfoliation due to erythematous condition**
         involving 50-59 percent of body surface 🦠
         (Ex) 695.55

●   **695.56 Exfoliation due to erythematous condition**
         involving 60-69 percent of body surface 🦠
         (Ex) 695.56

●   **695.57 Exfoliation due to erythematous condition**
         involving 70-79 percent of body surface 🦠
         (Ex) 695.57

●   **695.58 Exfoliation due to erythematous condition**
         involving 80-89 percent of body surface 🦠
         (Ex) 695.58

●   **695.59 Exfoliation due to erythematous condition**
         involving 90 percent or more of body
         surface 🦠
         (Ex) 695.59

● **695.8 Other specified erythematous conditions**

     695.81 Ritter's disease
         Dermatitis exfoliativa neonatorum
         (Staphylococcal) Scalded skin syndrome
         Use additional code to identify percentage
         of skin exfoliation (695.50-695.59)

     695.89 Other
         Erythema intertrigo
         Intertrigo
         Pityriasis rubra (Hebra)
         Excludes   *mycotic intertrigo (111.0–111.9)*
         Coding Clinic: 1986, Sept-Oct, P10

     695.9 Unspecified erythematous condition
         Erythema NOS
         Erythroderma (secondary)

DISEASES OF THE SKIN AND SUBCUTANEOUS TISSUE (680–709)

N Newborn Age: 0   **P** Pediatric Age: 0–17   **M** Maternity Age: 12–55   **A** Adult Age: 15–124   ♀ Females Only   ♂ Males Only

(Ex) CC Exclusions   🦠 Complication\Comorbidity   🦠 Major C\C   🦠 Present on Admission Requirement   🦠 Hospital-Acquired Condition

Figure 12–6 Erythematous plaques with silvery scales in a patient with psoriasis. (From Goldman: Cecil Textbook of Medicine, 22nd ed. 2004, Saunders)

Item 12–6 Psoriasis is a chronic, recurrent inflammatory skin disease characterized by small patches covered with thick silvery scales. **Parapsoriasis** is a treatment-resistant erythroderma. **Pityriasis rosea** is characterized by a herald patch that is a single large lesion and that usually appears on the trunk and is followed by scattered, smaller lesions.

● **696 Psoriasis and similar disorders**

    696.0 Psoriatic arthropathy

    696.1 Other psoriasis
        Acrodermatitis continua
        Dermatitis repens
        Psoriasis:
          NOS
          any type, except arthropathic
        | Excludes | *psoriatic arthropathy (696.0)* |

        Coding Clinic: 1996, Q2, P12

    696.2 Parapsoriasis
        Parakeratosis variegata
        Parapsoriasis lichenoides chronica
        Pityriasis lichenoides et varioliformis

    696.3 Pityriasis rosea
        Pityriasis circinata (et maculata)

    696.4 Pityriasis rubra pilaris
        Devergie's disease
        Lichen ruber acuminatus
        | Excludes | *pityriasis rubra (Hebra) (695.89)* |

    696.5 Other and unspecified pityriasis
        Pityriasis:
          NOS
          alba
          streptogenes
        | Excludes | *pityriasis:* |
                  simplex (690.18)
                  versicolor (111.0)

    696.8 Other

● **697 Lichen**
    | Excludes | *lichen:* |
          obtusus corneus (698.3)
          pilaris (congenital) (757.39)
          ruber acuminatus (696.4)
          sclerosus et atrophicus (701.0)
          scrofulosus (017.0)
          simplex chronicus (698.3)
          spinulosus (congenital) (757.39)
          urticatus (698.2)

    697.0 Lichen planus
        Lichen:
          planopilaris
          ruber planus

    697.1 Lichen nitidus
        Pinkus' disease

    697.8 Other lichen, not elsewhere classified
        Lichen:
          ruber moniliforme
          striata

    697.9 Lichen, unspecified

● **698 Pruritus and related conditions**
    | Excludes | *pruritus specified as psychogenic (306.3)* |

    698.0 Pruritus ani
        Perianal itch

    698.1 Pruritus of genital organs

    698.2 Prurigo
        Lichen urticatus
        Prurigo: Prurigo:
          NOS   mitis
          Hebra's   simplex
        Urticaria papulosa (Hebra)
        | Excludes | *prurigo nodularis (698.3)* |

    698.3 Lichenification and lichen simplex chronicus
        Hyde's disease
        Neurodermatitis (circumscripta) (local)
        Prurigo nodularis
        | Excludes | *neurodermatitis, diffuse (of Brocq) (691.8)* |

    698.4 Dermatitis factitia [artefacta]
        Dermatitis ficta
        Neurotic excoriation
        Use additional code to identify any associated
          mental disorder

    698.8 Other specified pruritic conditions
        Pruritus:
          hiemalis
          senilis
        Winter itch

    698.9 Unspecified pruritic disorder
        Itch NOS
        Pruritus NOS

DISEASES OF THE SKIN AND SUBCUTANEOUS TISSUE (680–709)

◀ New   ◀▥ Revised   ~~deleted~~ Deleted   ● Unacceptable Principal Diagnosis   ● Use Additional Digit(s)
▶ Manifestation Code   **OGCR** Official Guidelines   **Coding Clinic** | Excludes | Includes   Use additional   Code first   Omit code

Item 12–7   Scleroderma means hard skin. It is a group of diseases that causes abnormal growth of connective tissues that support the skin and organs. There are two types: localized scleroderma affecting the skin and systemic scleroderma affecting blood vessels and internal organs and the skin. **Keratoderma** is characterized by firm horny papules that have a cobblestone appearance. **Keratoderma climactericum,** also known as endocrine keratoderma, is hyperkeratosis located on the palms and soles.

OTHER DISEASES OF SKIN AND SUBCUTANEOUS TISSUE (700–709)

> **Excludes**   *conditions confined to eyelids (373.0–374.9)*
> *congenital conditions of skin, hair, and nails*
> *(757.0–757.9)*

700   Corns and callosities
     Callus
     Clavus

● **701   Other hypertrophic and atrophic conditions of skin**

> **Excludes**   *dermatomyositis (710.3)*
> *hereditary edema of legs (757.0)*
> *scleroderma (generalized) (710.1)*

701.0   Circumscribed scleroderma
     Addison's keloid
     Dermatosclerosis, localized
     Lichen sclerosus et atrophicus
     Morphea
     Scleroderma, circumscribed or localized

701.1   Keratoderma, acquired
     Acquired:
         ichthyosis
         keratoderma palmaris et plantaris
     Elastosis perforans serpiginosa
     Hyperkeratosis:
         NOS
         follicularis in cutem penetrans
         palmoplantaris climacterica
     Keratoderma:
         climactericum
         tylodes, progressive
     Keratosis (blennorrhagica)

> **Excludes**   *Darier's disease [keratosis follicularis]*
> *(congenital) (757.39)*
> *keratosis:*
> *arsenical (692.4)*
> *gonococcal (098.81)*

701.2   Acquired acanthosis nigricans
     Keratosis nigricans

701.3   Striae atrophicae
     Atrophic spots of skin
     Atrophoderma maculatum
     Atrophy blanche (of Milian)
     Degenerative colloid atrophy
     Senile degenerative atrophy
     Striae distensae

701.4   Keloid scar
     Cheloid
     Hypertrophic scar
     Keloid
     Coding Clinic: 1995, Q3, P14

701.5   Other abnormal granulation tissue
     Excessive granulation

701.8   Other specified hypertrophic and atrophic conditions of skin
     Acrodermatitis atrophicans chronica
     Atrophia cutis senilis
     Atrophoderma neuriticum
     Confluent and reticulate papillomatosis
     Cutis laxa senilis
     Elastosis senilis
     Folliculitis ulerythematosa reticulata
     Gougerot-Carteaud syndrome or disease
     Coding Clinic: 2008, Q1, P7-8

701.9   Unspecified hypertrophic and atrophic conditions of skin
     Atrophoderma

● **702   Other dermatoses**

> **Excludes**   *carcinoma in situ (232.0–232.9)*

702.0   Actinic keratosis

● **702.1   Seborrheic keratosis**

     702.11   Inflamed seborrheic keratosis

     702.19   Other seborrheic keratosis
         Seborrheic keratosis NOS

702.8   Other specified dermatoses

● **703   Diseases of nail**

> **Excludes**   *congenital anomalies (757.5)*
> *onychia and paronychia (681.02, 681.11)*

703.0   Ingrowing nail
     Ingrowing nail with infection
     Unguis incarnatus

> **Excludes**   *infection, nail NOS (681.9)*

DISEASES OF THE SKIN AND SUBCUTANEOUS TISSUE (680–709)

N   Newborn Age: 0   **P**   Pediatric Age: 0–17   **M**   Maternity Age: 12–55   **A**   Adult Age: 15–124   ♀   Females Only   ♂   Males Only

(Ex)   CC Exclusions   🔹   Complication\Comorbidity   🔹   Major C\C   🔹   Present on Admission Requirement   🔹   Hospital-Acquired Condition   **999**

Figure 12–7 Male pattern alopecia.

Item 12–8 Alopecia is lack of hair and takes many forms. The most common is male pattern alopecia, also known as **androgenetic alopecia. Telogen effluvium** is early and excessive loss of hair resulting from a trauma to the hair follicle (fever, drugs, surgery, etc.).

703.8 Other specified diseases of nail
    Dystrophia unguium
    Hypertrophy of nail
    Koilonychia
    Leukonychia (punctata) (striata)
    Onychauxis
    Onychogryposis
    Onycholysis

703.9 Unspecified disease of nail

● **704 Diseases of hair and hair follicles**
    Excludes *congenital anomalies (757.4)*

  ● **704.0 Alopecia**
    Excludes *madarosis (374.55)*
             syphilitic alopecia (091.82)

    704.00 Alopecia, unspecified
        Baldness   Loss of hair

    704.01 Alopecia areata
        Ophiasis

    704.02 Telogen effluvium

    704.09 Other
        Folliculitis decalvans
        Hypotrichosis:
          NOS
          postinfectional NOS
        Pseudopelade

704.1 Hirsutism
    Excessive growth of hair
    Hypertrichosis:
      NOS
      lanuginosa, acquired
    Polytrichia
    Excludes *hypertrichosis of eyelid (374.54)*

704.2 Abnormalities of the hair
    Atrophic hair   Trichiasis:
    Clastothrix   NOS
    Fragilitas crinium   cicatrical
                     Trichorrhexis (nodosa)
    Excludes *trichiasis of eyelid (374.05)*
    Coding Clinic: 2004, Q4, P91-92

704.3 Variations in hair color
    Canities (premature)
    Grayness, hair (premature)
    Heterochromia of hair
    Poliosis:
      NOS
      circumscripta, acquired

704.8 Other specified diseases of hair and hair follicles
    Folliculitis:
      NOS
      abscedens et suffodiens
      pustular
    Perifolliculitis:
      NOS
      capitis abscedens et suffodiens
      scalp
    Sycosis:
      NOS
      barbae [not parasitic]
      lupoid
      vulgaris

704.9 Unspecified disease of hair and hair follicles

● **705 Disorders of sweat glands**

  705.0 Anhidrosis
    Hypohidrosis   Oligohidrosis

  705.1 Prickly heat
    Heat rash   Sudamina
    Miliaria rubra (tropicalis)

  ● **705.2 Focal hyperhidrosis**
    Excludes *generalized (secondary) hyperhidrosis*
                    (780.8)

    705.21 Primary focal hyperhidrosis
        Focal hyperhidrosis NOS
        Hyperhidrosis NOS
        Hyperhidrosis of:
          axilla   palms
          face   soles

    705.22 Secondary focal hyperhidrosis
        Frey's syndrome

DISEASES OF THE SKIN AND SUBCUTANEOUS TISSUE (680–709)

◀ New   ⬅ Revised   ~~deleted~~ Deleted   ● Unacceptable Principal Diagnosis   ● Use Additional Digit(s)
▶ Manifestation Code   **OGCR** Official Guidelines   **Coding Clinic**   Excludes   Includes   Use additional   Code first   Omit code

● **705.8 Other specified disorders of sweat glands**

　705.81 Dyshidrosis
　　· Cheiropompholyx
　　Pompholyx

　705.82 Fox-Fordyce disease

　705.83 Hidradenitis
　　Hidradenitis suppurativa

　705.89 Other
　　Bromhidrosis　　Granulosis rubra nasi
　　Chromhidrosis　　Urhidrosis

　　| **Excludes** | hidrocystoma (216.0–216.9) |
　　　　　generalized hyperhidrosis (780.8)

　705.9 Unspecified disorder of sweat glands
　　Disorder of sweat glands NOS

● **706 Diseases of sebaceous glands**

　706.0 Acne varioliformis
　　Acne:
　　　frontalis
　　　necrotica

　706.1 Other acne
　　Acne:
　　　NOS
　　　conglobata
　　　cystic
　　　pustular
　　　vulgaris
　　Blackhead
　　Comedo

　　| **Excludes** | acne rosacea (695.3) |

　706.2 Sebaceous cyst
　　Atheroma, skin
　　Keratin cyst
　　Wen

　706.3 Seborrhea

　　| **Excludes** | seborrhea: |
　　　　　capitis (690.11)
　　　　　sicca (690.18)
　　　　seborrheic
　　　　　dermatitis (690.10)
　　　　　keratosis (702.11–702.19)

　706.8 Other specified diseases of sebaceous glands
　　Asteatosis (cutis)
　　Xerosis cutis

　706.9 Unspecified disease of sebaceous glands

● **707 Chronic ulcer of skin**

　　| **Includes** | non-infected sinus of skin
　　non-healing ulcer

　　| **Excludes** | varicose ulcer (454.0, 454.2) |

● **707.0 Pressure ulcer**
　　Bed sore
　　Decubitus ulcer
　　Plaster ulcer

　　Use additional code to identify pressure ulcer
　　　stage (707.20–707.25)
　　Coding Clinic: 2004, Q4, P92-93; Q1, P14-15; 2003, Q4, P110; 1999,
　　　Q4, P20; 1996, Q1, P15; 1990, Q3, P15; 1987, Nov-Dec, P9

　707.00 Unspecified site

　707.01 Elbow

　707.02 Upper back
　　Shoulder blades

　707.03 Lower back　　　　　　　　　◀
　　Coccyx
　　Sacrum
　　Coding Clinic: 2008, Q3, P17; 2005, Q1, P16

　707.04 Hip

　707.05 Buttock

　707.06 Ankle

　707.07 Heel
　　Coding Clinic: 2005, Q1, P16

　707.09 Other site
　　Head
　　Coding Clinic: 2008, Q3, P17

● **707.1 Ulcer of lower limbs, except pressure ulcer**
　　Ulcer, chronic, of lower limb:
　　　neurogenic of lower limb
　　　trophic of lower limb
　　Code if applicable, any causal condition first:
　　　atherosclerosis of the extremities with ulceration
　　　　(440.23)
　　　chronic venous hypertension with ulcer (459.31)
　　　chronic venous hypertension with ulcer and
　　　　inflammation (459.33)
　　　diabetes mellitus (249.80–249.81, 250.80–250.83)
　　　postphlebitic syndrome with ulcer (459.11)
　　　postphlebitic syndrome with ulcer and
　　　　inflammation (459.13)
　　Coding Clinic: 2004, Q1, P14-15; 1999, Q4, P15; 1996, Q1, P10

　707.10 Ulcer of lower limb, unspecified 🦠
　　Ex: 440.23, 707.10-707.19, 707.8-707.9, 709.8
　　Coding Clinic: 2004, Q3, P5-6

　707.11 Ulcer of thigh 🦠
　　Ex: 440.23, 707.10-707.19, 707.8-707.9, 709.8

　707.12 Ulcer of calf 🦠
　　Ex: 440.23, 707.10-707.19, 707.8-707.9, 709.8

　707.13 Ulcer of ankle 🦠
　　Ex: 440.23, 707.10-707.19, 707.8-707.9, 709.8

　707.14 Ulcer of heel and midfoot 🦠
　　Plantar surface of midfoot
　　Ex: 440.23, 707.10-707.19, 707.8-707.9, 709.8

　707.15 Ulcer of other part of foot
　　Toes

　707.19 Ulcer of other part of lower limb 🦠
　　Ex: 440.23, 707.10-707.19, 707.8-707.9, 709.8

● **707.2 Pressure ulcer stages**

Code first site of pressure ulcer (707.00-707.09)

Coding Clinic: 2008, Q4, P132-134

707.20 Pressure ulcer, unspecified stage
Healing pressure ulcer NOS
Healing pressure ulcer, unspecified stage

707.21 Pressure ulcer stage I
Healing pressure ulcer, stage I
Pressure pre-ulcer skin changes limited to persistent focal erythema

707.22 Pressure ulcer stage II
Healing pressure ulcer, stage II
Pressure ulcer with abrasion, blister, partial thickness skin loss involving epidermis and/or dermis

707.23 Pressure ulcer stage III
Healing pressure ulcer, stage III
Pressure ulcer with full thickness skin loss involving damage or necrosis of subcutaneous tissue
(Ex) 707.00-707.9

707.24 Pressure ulcer stage IV
Healing pressure ulcer, stage IV
Pressure ulcer with necrosis of soft tissues through to underlying muscle, tendon, or bone
(Ex) 707.00-707.9

707.25 Pressure ulcer, unstageable

707.8 Chronic ulcer of other specified sites
Ulcer, chronic, of other specified sites:
neurogenic of other specified sites
trophic of other specified sites

707.9 Chronic ulcer of unspecified site
Chronic ulcer NOS   Tropical ulcer NOS
Trophic ulcer NOS   Ulcer of skin NOS

● **708 Urticaria**
Excludes edema:
angioneurotic (995.1)
Quincke's (995.1)
hereditary angioedema (277.6)
urticaria:
giant (995.1)
papulosa (Hebra) (698.2)
pigmentosa (juvenile) (congenital) (757.33)

708.0 Allergic urticaria
Coding Clinic: 1984, May-June, P11

708.1 Idiopathic urticaria

708.2 Urticaria due to cold and heat
Thermal urticaria

708.3 Dermatographic urticaria
Dermatographia
Factitial urticaria

708.4 Vibratory urticaria

708.5 Cholinergic urticaria
Coding Clinic: 1995, Q4, P50

708.8 Other specified urticaria
Nettle rash
Urticaria:
chronic
recurrent periodic

708.9 Urticaria, unspecified
Hives NOS

Figure 12–8 Urticaria (hives). *(Courtesy of David Effron, MD.)* (From Marx: Rosen's Emergency Medicine: Concepts and Clinical Practice, 6th ed. 2006, Mosby, Inc.)

Item 12–9 Urticaria is a vascular reaction in which wheals surrounded by a red halo appear and cause severe itching. The causes of urticaria or hives are extensive and varied (e.g., food, heat, cold, drugs, stress, infections). Dyschromia is any disorder of the pigmentation of the skin or hair.

● **709 Other disorders of skin and subcutaneous tissue**
● **709.0 Dyschromia**
Excludes albinism (270.2)
pigmented nevus (216.0–216.9)
that of eyelid (374.52–374.53)

709.00 Dyschromia, unspecified

709.01 Vitiligo

709.09 Other

709.1 Vascular disorders of skin
Angioma serpiginosum
Purpura (primary) annularis telangiectodes

709.2 Scar conditions and fibrosis of skin
Adherent scar (skin)
Cicatrix
Disfigurement (due to scar)
Fibrosis, skin NOS
Scar NOS
Excludes keloid scar (701.4)
Coding Clinic: 1984, Nov-Dec, P19

709.3 Degenerative skin disorders
Calcinosis:
circumscripta
cutis
Colloid milium
Degeneration, skin
Deposits, skin
Senile dermatosis NOS
Subcutaneous calcification

709.4 Foreign body granuloma of skin and subcutaneous tissue
Excludes residual foreign body without granuloma of skin and subcutaneous tissue (729.6)
that of muscle (728.82)

709.8 Other specified disorders of skin
Epithelial hyperplasia
Menstrual dermatosis
Vesicular eruption
Coding Clinic: 1987, Nov-Dec, P6

709.9 Unspecified disorder of skin and subcutaneous tissue
Dermatosis NOS

◄ New   ◄ Revised   ~~deleted~~ Deleted   ● Unacceptable Principal Diagnosis   ● Use Additional Digit(s)
▶ Manifestation Code   OGCR Official Guidelines   Coding Clinic   Excludes   Includes   Use additional   Code first   Omit code

13. **DISEASES OF THE MUSCULOSKELETAL SYSTEM AND CONNECTIVE TISSUE (710–739)**

Use additional external cause code, if applicable, to identify the cause of the musculoskeletal condition

The following fifth-digit subclassification is for use with categories 711–712, 715–716, 718–719, and 730:

> 0 **site unspecified**
> 1 **shoulder region**
>   Acromioclavicular joint(s)
>   Clavicle
>   Glenohumeral joint(s)
>   Scapula
>   Sternoclavicular joint(s)
> 2 **upper arm**
>   Elbow joint
>   Humerus
> 3 **forearm**
>   Radius
>   Ulna
>   Wrist joint
> 4 **hand**
>   Carpus
>   Metacarpus
>   Phalanges [fingers]
> 5 **pelvic region and thigh**
>   Buttock
>   Femur
>   Hip (joint)
> 6 **lower leg**
>   Fibula
>   Knee joint
>   Patella
>   Tibia
> 7 **ankle and foot**
>   Ankle joint
>   Digits [toes]
>   Metatarsus
>   Phalanges, foot
>   Tarsus
>   Other joints in foot
> 8 **other specified sites**
>   Head
>   Neck
>   Ribs
>   Skull
>   Trunk
>   Vertebral column
> 9 **multiple sites**

ARTHROPATHIES AND RELATED DISORDERS (710–719)

Excludes *disorders of spine (720.0–724.9)*

● **710 Diffuse diseases of connective tissue**

Includes all collagen diseases whose effects are not mainly confined to a single system

Excludes *those affecting mainly the cardiovascular system, i.e., polyarteritis nodosa and allied conditions (446.0–446.7)*

710.0 Systemic lupus erythematosus
Autoimmune inflammatory connective tissue disease of unknown cause that occurs most often in women. See 695.4 for nonsystemic.
Disseminated lupus erythematosus
Libman-Sacks disease

Use additional code to identify manifestation, as:
   endocarditis (424.91)
   nephritis (583.81)
      chronic (582.81)
   nephrotic syndrome (581.81)

Excludes *lupus erythematosus (discoid) NOS (695.4)*

Coding Clinic: 2003, Q2, P7x2; 1997, Q2, P8-9; 1987, Sept-Oct, P8

710.1 Systemic sclerosis
Acrosclerosis
CRST syndrome
Progressive systemic sclerosis
Scleroderma

Use additional code to identify manifestation, as:
   lung involvement (517.2)
   myopathy (359.6)

Excludes *circumscribed scleroderma (701.0)*

710.2 Sicca syndrome
Keratoconjunctivitis sicca
Sjögren's disease

710.3 Dermatomyositis ⦿
Poikilodermatomyositis
Polymyositis with skin involvement
(Ex) 710.3

710.4 Polymyositis ⦿
(Ex) 710.4

710.5 Eosinophilia myalgia syndrome ⦿
Toxic oil syndrome

Use additional E code to identify drug, if drug induced
(Ex) 292.0-293.9, 710.5

710.8 Other specified diffuse diseases of connective tissue ⦿
Multifocal fibrosclerosis (idiopathic) NEC
Systemic fibrosclerosing syndrome
(Ex) 710.8
Coding Clinic: 1987, Mar-April, P12

710.9 Unspecified diffuse connective tissue disease
Collagen disease NOS

DISEASES OF THE MUSCULOSKELETAL SYSTEM AND CONNECTIVE TISSUE (710–739)

N Newborn Age: 0   **P** Pediatric Age: 0–17   **M** Maternity Age: 12–55   **A** Adult Age: 15–124   ♀ Females Only   ♂ Males Only

(Ex) CC Exclusions   ⦿ Complication\Comorbidity   ⦿ Major C\C   ⦿ Present on Admission Requirement   ⦿ Hospital-Acquired Condition

1003

● **711**   **Arthropathy associated with infections**
    Abnormality of a joint

    Includes   arthritis associated with conditions classifiable
                 below
            arthropathy associated with conditions
                 classifiable below
            polyarthritis associated with conditions
                 classifiable below
            polyarthropathy associated with conditions
                 classifiable below

    Excludes   *rheumatic fever (390)*

    Coding Clinic: 1992, Q1, P16-17

The following fifth-digit subclassification is for use with
category 711; valid digits are in [brackets] under each code.
See list at beginning of chapter for definitions:

> 0   site unspecified
> 1   shoulder region
> 2   upper arm
> 3   forearm
> 4   hand
> 5   pelvic region and thigh
> 6   lower leg
> 7   ankle and foot
> 8   other specified sites
> 9   multiple sites

● **711.0**   **Pyogenic arthritis** 🔒
  [0-9]   Arthritis or polyarthritis (due to):
            coliform [Escherichia coli]
            Hemophilus influenzae [H. influenzae]
            pneumococcal
            Pseudomonas
            staphylococcal
            streptococcal
       Pyarthrosis

       Use additional code to identify infectious organism
       (041.0–041.8)

    For codes **711.00, 711.08-711.09:** (Ex) 015.80-015.96, 017.90-017.96,
    036.82, 056.71, 098.50-098.51, 098.59, 098.89, 711.00-714.0, 715.00,
    715.09-715.10, 715.18-716.99, 718.00-718.08, 719.00-719.10,
    719.18-719.99;

    For code **711.01:** (Ex) 015.80-015.96, 017.90-017.96, 036.82, 056.71,
    098.50-098.51, 098.59, 098.89, 711.00-711.01, 711.08-711.11,
    711.18-711.21, 711.28-711.31, 711.38-711.41, 711.48-711.51,
    711.58-711.61, 711.68-711.71, 711.78-711.81, 711.88-711.91,
    711.98-712.11, 712.18-712.21, 712.28-712.31, 712.38-712.81,
    712.88-712.91, 712.98-714.0, 715.00, 715.09-715.11, 715.18-715.21,
    715.28-715.31, 715.38-715.91, 715.98-716.01, 716.08-716.11,
    716.18-716.21, 716.28-716.31, 716.38-716.41, 716.48-716.51,
    716.58-716.61, 716.68-716.81, 716.88-716.91, 716.98-716.99,
    718.00-718.01, 718.08, 719.00-719.01, 719.08-719.11, 719.18-719.21,
    719.28-719.31, 719.38-719.41, 719.48-719.51, 719.58-719.61,
    719.68-719.81, 719.88-719.91, 719.98-719.99;

    For code **711.02:** (Ex) 015.80-015.96, 017.90-017.96, 036.82, 056.71,
    098.50-098.51, 098.59, 098.89, 711.00, 711.02, 711.08-711.10, 711.12,
    711.18-711.20, 711.22, 711.28-711.30, 711.32, 711.38-711.40, 711.42,
    711.48-711.50, 711.52, 711.58-711.60, 711.62, 711.68-711.70, 711.72,
    711.78-711.80, 711.82, 711.88-711.90, 711.92, 711.98-712.10, 712.12,
    712.18-712.20, 712.22, 712.28-712.30, 712.32, 712.38-712.80, 712.82,
    712.88-712.90, 712.92, 712.98-714.0, 715.00, 715.09-715.10, 715.12,
    715.18-715.20, 715.22, 715.28-715.30, 715.32, 715.38-715.90, 715.92,
    715.98-716.00, 716.02, 716.08-716.10, 716.12, 716.18-716.20, 716.22,
    716.28-716.30, 716.32, 716.38-716.40, 716.42, 716.48-716.50, 716.52,
    716.58-716.60, 716.62, 716.68-716.80, 716.82, 716.88-716.90, 716.92,
    716.98-716.99, 718.00, 718.02, 718.08, 719.00, 719.02, 719.08-719.10,
    719.12, 719.18-719.20, 719.22, 719.28-719.30, 719.32, 719.38-719.40,
    719.42, 719.48-719.50, 719.52, 719.58-719.60, 719.62, 719.68-719.80,
    719.82, 719.88-719.90, 719.92, 719.98-719.99;

    For code **711.03:** (Ex) 015.80-015.96, 017.90-017.96, 036.82, 056.71,
    098.50-098.51, 098.59, 098.89, 711.00, 711.03, 711.08-711.10, 711.13,
    711.18-711.20, 711.23, 711.28-711.30, 711.33, 711.38-711.40, 711.43,
    711.48-711.50, 711.53, 711.58-711.60, 711.63, 711.68-711.70, 711.73,
    711.78-711.80, 711.83, 711.88-711.90, 711.93, 711.98-712.10, 712.13,
    712.18-712.20, 712.23, 712.28-712.30, 712.33, 712.38-712.80, 712.83,

    712.88-712.90, 712.93, 712.98-714.0, 715.00, 715.09-715.10, 715.13,
    715.18-715.20, 715.23, 715.28-715.30, 715.33, 715.38-715.90, 715.93,
    715.98-716.00, 716.03, 716.08-716.10, 716.13, 716.18-716.20, 716.23,
    716.28-716.30, 716.33, 716.38-716.40, 716.43, 716.48-716.50, 716.53,
    716.58-716.60, 716.63, 716.68-716.80, 716.83, 716.88-716.90, 716.93,
    716.98-716.99, 718.00, 718.03, 718.08, 719.00, 719.03, 719.08-719.10,
    719.13, 719.18-719.20, 719.23, 719.28-719.30, 719.33, 719.38-719.40,
    719.43, 719.48-719.50, 719.53, 719.58-719.60, 719.63, 719.68-719.80,
    719.83, 719.88-719.90, 719.93, 719.98-719.99;

    For code **711.04:** (Ex) 015.80-015.96, 017.90-017.96, 036.82, 056.71,
    098.50-098.51, 098.59, 098.89, 711.00, 711.04, 711.08-711.10, 711.14,
    711.18-711.20, 711.24, 711.28-711.30, 711.34, 711.38-711.40, 711.44,
    711.48-711.50, 711.54, 711.58-711.60, 711.64, 711.68-711.70, 711.74,
    711.78-711.80, 711.84, 711.88-711.90, 711.94, 711.98-712.10, 712.14,
    712.18-712.20, 712.24, 712.28-712.30, 712.34, 712.38-712.80, 712.84,
    712.88-712.90, 712.94, 712.98-714.0, 715.00-715.10, 715.14,
    715.18-715.20, 715.24, 715.28 -715.30, 715.34, 715.38-715.90, 715.94,
    715.98-716.00, 716.04, 716.08-716.10, 716.14, 716.18-716.20, 716.24,
    716.28-716.30, 716.34, 716.38-716.40, 716.44, 716.48-716.50, 716.54,
    716.58-716.60, 716.64, 716.68-716.80, 716.84, 716.88-716.90, 716.94,
    716.98-716.99, 718.00, 718.04, 718.08, 719.00, 719.04, 719.08-719.10,
    719.14, 719.18-719.20, 719.24, 719.28-719.30, 719.34, 719.38-719.40,
    719.44, 719.48-719.50, 719.54, 719.58-719.60, 719.64, 719.68-719.80,
    719.84, 719.88-719.90, 719.94, 719.98-719.99;

    For code **711.05:** (Ex) 015.80-015.96, 017.90-017.96, 036.82, 056.71,
    098.50-098.51, 098.59, 098.89, 711.00, 711.05, 711.08-711.10, 711.15,
    711.18-711.20, 711.25, 711.28-711.30, 711.35, 711.38-711.40, 711.45,
    711.48-711.50, 711.55, 711.58-711.60, 711.65, 711.68-711.70, 711.75,
    711.78-711.80, 711.85, 711.88-711.90, 711.95, 711.98-712.10, 712.15,
    712.18-712.20, 712.25, 712.28-712.30, 712.35, 712.38-712.80, 712.85,
    712.88-712.90, 712.95, 712.98-714.0, 715.00, 715.09-715.10, 715.15,
    715.18--715.20, 715.25, 715.28-715.30, 715.35, 715.38-715.90, 715.95,
    715.98-716.00, 716.05, 716.08-716.10, 716.15, 716.18-716.20, 716.25,
    716.28-716.30, 716.35, 716.38-716.40, 716.45, 716.48-716.50, 716.55,
    716.58-716.60, 716.65, 716.68-716.80, 716.85, 716.88-716.90, 716.95,
    716.98-716.99, 718.00, 718.05, 718.08, 719.00, 719.05, 719.08-719.10,
    719.15, 719.18-719.20, 719.25, 719.28-719.30, 719.35, 719.38-719.40,
    719.45, 719.48-719.50, 719.55, 719.58-719.60, 719.65, 719.68-719.80,
    719.85, 719.88-719.90, 719.95, 719.98-719.99;

    For code **711.06:** (Ex) 015.80-015.96, 017.90-017.96, 036.82, 056.71,
    098.50-098.51, 098.59, 098.89, 711.00, 711.06, 711.08-711.10, 711.16,
    711.18-711.20, 711.26, 711.28-711.30, 711.36, 711.38-711.40, 711.46,
    711.48-711.50, 711.56, 711.58-711.60, 711.66, 711.68-711.70, 711.76,
    711.78-711.80, 711.86, 711.88-711.90, 711.96, 711.98-712.10, 712.16,
    712.18-712.20, 712.26, 712.28-712.30, 712.36, 712.38-712.80, 712.86,
    712.88-712.90, 712.96, 712.98-714.0, 715.00, 715.09-715.10, 715.16,
    715.18-715.20, 715.26, 715.28-715.30, 715.36, 715.38-715.90, 715.96,
    715.98-716.00, 716.06, 716.08-716.10, 716.16, 716.18-716.20, 716.26,
    716.28-716.30, 716.36, 716.38-716.40, 716.46, 716.48-716.50, 716.56,
    716.58-716.60, 716.66, 716.68-716.80, 716.86, 716.88-716.90, 716.96,
    716.98-716.99, 718.00, 718.08, 719.00, 719.06, 719.08-719.10, 719.16,
    719.18-719.20, 719.26, 719.28-719.30, 719.36, 719.38-719.40, 719.46,
    719.48-719.50, 719.56, 719.58-719.60, 719.66, 719.68-719.80, 719.86,
    719.88-719.90, 719.96, 719.98-719.99;

    For code **711.07:** (Ex) 015.80-015.96, 017.90-017.96, 036.82, 056.71,
    098.50-098.51, 098.59, 098.89, 711.00, 711.07-711.10, 711.17-711.20,
    711.27-7113.0, 711.37-711.40, 711.47-711.50, 711.57-711.60,
    711.67-711.70, 711.77-711.80, 711.87-711.90, 711.97-712.10,
    712.17-712.20, 712.27-712.30, 712.37-712.80, 712.87-712.90,
    712.97-714.0, 715.00, 715.09-715.10, 715.17-715.20, 715.27-715.30,
    715.37-715.90, 715.97-716.00, 716.07-716.10, 716.17-716.20,
    716.27-716.30, 716.37-716.40, 716.47-716.50, 716.57-716.60,
    716.67-716.80, 716.87-716.90, 716.97-716.99, 718.00, 718.07-718.08,
    719.00, 719.07-719.10, 719.17-719.20, 719.27-719.30, 719.37-719.40,
    719.47-719.50, 719.57-719.60, 719.67-719.80, 719.87-719.90,
    719.97-719.99

    Coding Clinic: 1992, Q1, P16-17; 1991, Q1, P15

● ▸ **711.1**   **Arthropathy associated with Reiter's disease and**
  [0-9]   **nonspecific urethritis** 🔒

    Code first underlying disease, as:
       nonspecific urethritis (099.4)
       Reiter's disease (099.3)

    (Ex) 003.23, 015.80-015.96, 017.90-017.96, 036.82, 056.71, 098.50-098.51,
    098.59, 098.89, 711.00-714.0, 715.00, 715.09-715.10, 715.18-716.99,
    718.00-718.08, 719.00-719.10, 719.18-719.69, 719.80-719.99

◀ New   ◀ Revised   ~~deleted~~ Deleted   ● Unacceptable Principal Diagnosis   ● Use Additional Digit(s)
▸ Manifestation Code   **OGCR** Official Guidelines   **Coding Clinic**   Excludes   Includes   Use additional   Code first   Omit code

DISEASES OF THE MUSCULOSKELETAL SYSTEM AND CONNECTIVE TISSUE (710–739)

● ▶ **711.2 Arthropathy in Behçet's syndrome** 🦠
[0-9]   *Code first* underlying disease (136.1)

       (Ex) 003.23, 015.80-015.96, 017.90-017.96, 036.82, 056.71, 098.50-098.51,
       098.59, 098.89, 711.00-714.0, 715.00, 715.09-715.10, 715.18-716.99,
       718.00-718.08, 719.00-719.10, 719.18-719.69, 719.80-719.99

● ▶ **711.3 Postdysenteric arthropathy** 🦠
[0-9]   *Code first* underlying disease, as:
       dysentery (009.0)
       enteritis, infectious (008.0–009.3)
       paratyphoid fever (002.1–002.9)
       typhoid fever (002.0)

       Excludes   *salmonella arthritis (003.23)*

       For codes **711.30-711.35, 711.37, and 711.39:** (Ex) 003.23,
       015.80-015.96, 017.90-017.96, 036.82, 056.71, 098.50-098.51,
       098.59, 098.89, 711.00-714.0, 715.00, 715.09-715.10, 715.18-716.99,
       718.00-718.08, 719.00-719.10, 719.18-719.69, 719.80-719.99;
       For code **711.36:** (Ex) 003.23, 015.80-015.96, 017.90-017.96, 036.82, 056.71,
       098.50-098.51, 098.59, 098.89, 711.00-714.0, 715.00, 715.09-715.10,
       715.18-716.07, 716.09-716.99, 718.00-718.08, 719.00-719.10,
       719.18-719.69, 719.80-719.99;
       For code **711.38:** (Ex) 003.23, 015.80-015.96, 017.90-017.96, 036.82, 056.71,
       098.50-098.51, 098.59, 098.89, 711.00-714.0, 715.00, 715.09-715.10,
       715.18-716.57, 716.59-716.99, 718.00-718.08, 719.00-719.10,
       719.18-719.69, 719.80-719.99

● ▶ **711.4 Arthropathy associated with other bacterial**
[0-9] **diseases** 🦠
       Code first underlying disease, as:
       diseases classifiable to 010–040, 090–099, except
         as in 711.1, 711.3, and 713.5
       leprosy (030.0–030.9)
       tuberculosis (015.0–015.9)

       Excludes   *gonococcal arthritis (098.50)*
                      meningococcal arthritis (036.82)

       For codes **711.40, 711.42-711.49:** ◯Ex: 003.23, 015.80-015.96,
       017.90-017.96, 036.82, 056.71, 098.50-098.51, 098.59, 098.89,
       711.00-714.0, 715.00, 715.09-715.10, 715.18-716.99, 718.00-718.08,
       719.00-719.10, 719.18-719.69, 719.80-719.99;
       For code **711.41:** (Ex) 003.23, 015.80-015.96, 017.90-017.96, 036.82, 056.71,
       098.50-098.51, 098.59, 098.89, 711.00-714.0, 715.00, 715.09-715.10,
       715.18-716.99, 718.00-718.08, 719.00-719.10, 719.18-719.39, 719.41
       -719.69, 719.80-719.99

● ▶ **711.5 Arthropathy associated with other viral diseases** 🦠
[0-9]   *Code first* underlying disease, as:
       diseases classifiable to 045–049, 050–079, 480, 487
       O'nyong-nyong (066.3)

       Excludes   *that due to rubella (056.71)*

       (Ex) 003.23, 015.80-015.96, 017.90-017.96, 036.82, 056.71, 098.50-098.51,
       098.59, 098.89, 711.00-714.0, 715.00, 715.09-715.10, 715.18-716.99,
       718.00-718.08, 719.00-719.10, 719.18-719.69, 719.80-719.99

● ▶ **711.6 Arthropathy associated with mycoses** 🦠
[0-9]   *Code first* underlying disease (110.0–118)
       For codes **711.60, 711.68-711.69:** (Ex) 015.80-015.96, 017.90-017.96, 036.82,
       056.71, 098.50-098.51, 098.59, 098.89, 711.00-714.0, 715.00,
       715.09-715.10, 715.18-716.99, 718.00-718.08, 719.00-719.10,
       719.18-719.99;
       For code **711.61:** (Ex) 015.80-015.96, 017.90-017.96, 036.82, 056.71,
       098.50-098.51, 098.59, 098.89, 711.00-711.01, 711.08-711.11,
       711.18-711.21, 711.28-711.31, 711.38-711.41, 711.48-711.51,
       711.58-711.61, 711.68-711.71, 711.78-711.81, 711.88-711.91,
       711.98-712.11, 712.18-712.21, 712.28-712.31, 712.38-712.81,
       712.88-712.91, 712.98-714.0, 715.00, 715.09-715.11, 715.18-715.21,
       715.28-715.31, 715.38-715.91, 715.98-716.01, 716.08-716.11,
       716.18-716.21, 716.28-716.31, 716.38-716.41, 716.48-716.51,
       716.58-716.61, 716.68-716.81, 716.88-716.91, 716.98-716.99,
       718.00-718.01, 718.08, 719.00-719.01, 719.08-719.11, 719.18-719.21,
       719.28-719.31, 719.38-719.41, 719.48-719.51, 719.58-719.61,
       719.68-719.81, 719.88-719.91, 719.98-719.99;
       For code **711.62:** (Ex) 015.80-015.96, 017.90-017.96, 036.82, 056.71,
       098.50-098.51, 098.59, 098.89, 711.00, 711.02, 711.08-711.10, 711.12,

711.18-711.20, 711.22, 711.28-711.30, 711.32, 711.38-711.40, 711.42, 711.48-711.50,
711.52, 711.58-711.60, 711.62, 711.68-711.70, 711.72, 711.78-711.80, 711.82,
711.88-711.90, 711.92, 711.98-712.10, 712.12, 712.18-712.20, 712.22, 712.28-712.30,
712.32, 712.38-712.80, 712.82, 712.88-712.90, 712.92, 712.98-714.0, 715.00,
715.09-715.10, 715.12, 715.18-715.20, 715.22, 715.28-715.30, 715.32, 715.38-715.90,
715.92, 715.98-716.00, 716.02, 716.08-716.10, 716.12, 716.18-716.20, 716.22,
716.28-716.30, 716.32, 716.38-716.40, 716.42, 716.48-716.50, 716.52, 716.58-716.60,
716.62, 716.68-716.80, 716.82, 716.88-716.90, 716.92, 716.98-716.99, 718.00,
718.02, 718.08, 719.00, 719.02, 719.08-719.10, 719.12, 719.18-719.20, 719.22,
719.28-719.30, 719.32, 719.38-719.40, 719.42, 719.48-719.50, 719.52, 719.58-719.60,
719.62, 719.68-719.80, 719.82, 719.88-719.90, 719.92, 719.98-719.99;

For code **711.63:** (Ex) 015.80-015.96, 017.90-017.96, 036.82, 056.71, 098.50-098.51, 098.59,
098.89, 711.00, 711.03, 711.08-711.10, 711.13, 711.18-711.20, 711.23,
711.28-711.30, 711.33, 711.38-711.40, 711.43, 711.48-711.50, 711.53, 711.58-711.60,
711.63, 711.68-711.70, 711.73, 711.78-711.80, 711.83, 711.88-711.90, 711.93,
711.98-712.10, 712.13, 712.18-712.20, 712.23, 712.28-712.30, 712.33, 712.38-712.80,
712.83, 712.88-712.90, 712.93, 712.98-714.0, 715.00, 715.09-715.10, 715.13,
715.18-715.20, 715.23, 715.28-715.30, 715.33, 715.38-715.90, 715.93, 715.98-716.00,
716.03, 716.08-716.10, 716.13, 716.18-716.20, 716.23, 716.28-716.30, 716.33,
716.38-716.40, 716.43, 716.48-716.50, 716.53, 716.58-716.60, 716.63, 716.68-716.80,
716.83, 716.88-716.90, 716.93, 716.98-716.99, 718.00, 718.03, 718.08, 719.00,
719.03, 719.08-719.10, 719.13, 719.18-719.20, 719.23, 719.28-719.30, 719.33,
719.38-719.40, 719.43, 719.48-719.50, 719.53, 719.58-719.60, 719.63, 719.68-719.80,
719.83, 719.88-719.90, 719.93, 719.98-719.99;

For code **711.64:** (Ex) 015.80-015.96, 017.90-017.96, 036.82, 056.71, 098.50-098.51, 098.59,
098.89, 711.00, 711.04, 711.08-711.10, 711.14, 711.18-711.20, 711.24,
711.28-711.30, 711.34, 711.38-711.40, 711.44, 711.48-711.50, 711.54, 711.58-711.60,
711.64, 711.68-711.70, 711.74, 711.78-711.80, 711.84, 711.88-711.90, 711.94,
711.98-712.10, 712.14, 712.18-712.20, 712.24, 712.28-712.30, 712.34, 712.38-712.80,
712.84, 712.88-712.90, 712.94, 712.98-714.0, 715.00-715.10, 715.14, 715.18-715.20,
715.24, 715.28-715.30, 715.34, 715.38-715.90, 715.94, 715.98-716.00, 716.04,
716.08-716.10, 716.14, 716.18-716.20, 716.24, 716.28-716.30, 716.34, 716.38-716.40,
716.44, 716.48-716.50, 716.54, 716.58-716.60, 716.64, 716.68-716.80, 716.84,
716.88-716.90, 716.94, 716.98-716.99, 718.00, 718.04, 718.08, 719.00, 719.04,
719.08-719.10, 719.14, 719.18-719.20, 719.24, 719.28-719.30, 719.34, 719.38-719.40,
719.44, 719.48-719.50, 719.54, 719.58-719.60, 719.64, 719.68-719.80, 719.84,
719.88-719.90, 719.94, 719.98-719.99;

For code **711.65:** (Ex) 015.80-015.96, 017.90-017.96, 036.82, 056.71, 098.50-098.51, 098.59,
098.89, 711.00, 711.05, 711.08-711.10, 711.15, 711.18-711.20, 711.25,
711.28-711.30, 711.35, 711.38-711.40, 711.45, 711.48-711.50, 711.55, 711.58-711.60,
711.65, 711.68-711.70, 711.75, 711.78-711.80, 711.85, 711.88-711.90 711.95,
711.98-712.10, 712.15, 712.18-712.20, 712.25, 712.28-712.30 712.35, 712.38-712.80,
712.85, 712.88-712.90, 712.95, 712.98-714.0 715.00, 715.09-715.10, 715.15,
715.18-715.20, 715.25, 715.28-715.30, 715.35, 715.38-715.90, 715.95, 715.98-716.00,
716.05, 716.08-716.10, 716.15, 716.18-716.20, 716.25, 716.28-716.30, 716.35,
716.38-716.40, 716.45, 716.48-716.50, 716.55, 716.58-716.60, 716.65, 716.68-716.80,
716.85, 716.88-716.90, 716.95, 716.98-716.99, 718.00, 718.05, 718.08, 719.00,
719.05, 719.08-719.10, 719.15, 719.18-719.20, 719.25, 719.28-719.30, 719.35,
719.38-719.40, 719.45, 719.48-719.50, 719.55, 719.58-719.60, 719.65, 719.68-719.80,
719.85, 719.88-719.90, 719.95, 719.98-719.99;

For code **711.66:** (Ex) 015.80-015.96, 017.90-017.96, 036.82, 056.71, 098.50-098.51, 098.59,
098.89, 711.00, 711.06, 711.08-711.10, 711.16, 711.18-711.20, 711.26,
711.28-711.30, 711.36, 711.38-711.40, 711.46, 711.48-711.50, 711.56, 711.58-711.60,
711.66, 711.68-711.70, 711.76, 711.78-711.80, 711.86, 711.88-711.90, 711.96,
711.98-712.10, 712.16, 712.18-712.20, 712.26, 712.28-712.30, 712.36, 712.38-712.80,
712.86, 712.88-712.90, 712.96, 712.98-714.0, 715.00, 715.09-715.10, 715.16,
715.18-715.20, 715.26, 715.28-715.30, 715.36, 715.38-715.90, 715.96, 715.98-716.00,
716.06, 716.08-716.10, 716.16, 716.18-716.20, 716.26, 716.28-716.30, 716.36,
716.38-716.40, 716.46, 716.48-716.50, 716.56, 716.58-716.60, 716.66, 716.68-716.80,
716.86, 716.88-716.90, 716.96, 716.98-716.99, 718.00, 718.08, 719.00, 719.06,
719.08-719.10, 719.16, 719.18-719.20, 719.26, 719.28-719.30, 719.36, 719.38-719.40,
719.46, 719.48-719.50, 719.56, 719.58-719.60, 719.66, 719.68-719.80, 719.86,
719.88-719.90, 719.96, 719.98-719.99;

For code **711.67:** (Ex) 015.80-015.96, 017.90-017.96, 036.82, 056.71, 098.50-098.51, 098.59,
098.89, 711.00, 711.07-711.10, 711.17-711.20, 711.27-711.30, 711.37 -711.40,
711.47-711.50, 711.57-711.60, 711.67-711.70, 711.77-711.80, 711.87-711.90,
711.97-712.10, 712.17-712.20, 712.27-712.30, 712.37-712.80, 712.87-712.90,
712.97-714.0, 715.00, 715.09-715.10, 715.17-715.20, 715.27-715.30, 715.37-715.90,
715.97-716.00, 716.07-716.10, 716.17-716.20, 716.27-716.30, 716.37-716.40,
716.47-716.50, 716.57-716.60, 716.67-716.80, 716.87-716.90, 716.97-716.99, 718.00,
718.07-718.08, 719.00, 719.07-719.10, 719.17-719.20, 719.27-719.30, 719.37-719.40,
719.47-719.50, 719.57-719.60, 719.67-719.80, 719.87-719.90, 719.97-719.99

N   Newborn Age: 0   **P**   Pediatric Age: 0–17   **M**   Maternity Age: 12–55   **A**   Adult Age: 15–124   ♀   Females Only   ♂   Males Only   **1005**

(Ex)   CC Exclusions   🦠 Complication\Comorbidity   🦠 Major C\C   🦠 Present on Admission Requirement   🦠 Hospital-Acquired Condition

DISEASES OF THE MUSCULOSKELETAL SYSTEM AND CONNECTIVE TISSUE (710-739)

711.7 Arthropathy associated with helminthiasis 🔖
[0-9]   Code first underlying disease, as:
       filariasis (125.0–125.9)
      For codes **711.70-711.14, 711.76, 711.78-711.79:** (Ex:) 003.23,
       015.80-015.96, 017.90-017.96, 036.82, 056.71, 098.50-098.51,
       098.59, 098.89, 711.00-714.0, 715.00, 715.09-715.10, 715.18-716.99,
       718.00-718.08, 719.00-719.10, 719.18-719.69, 719.80-719.99;
      For code **711.75:** (Ex:) 003.23, 015.80-015.96, 017.90-017.96, 036.82, 056.71,
       098.50-098.51, 098.59, 098.89, 711.00-714.0, 715.00, 715.09-7 15.10,
       715.18-716.99, 718.00-718.08, 719.00-719.10, 719.18-719.43,
       719.45-719.69, 719.80-719.99;
      For code **711.77:** (Ex:) 003.23, 015.80-015.96, 017.90-017.96, 036.82, 056.71,
       098.50-098.51, 098.59, 098.89, 711.00-714.0, 715.00, 715.09-715.10,
       715.18-716.99, 718.00-718.08, 719.00-719.10, 719.18-719.69,
       719.80-719.97, 719.99

711.8 Arthropathy associated with other infectious and
[0-9] **parasitic diseases** 🔖
    Code first underlying disease, as:
       diseases classifiable to 080–088, 100–104,
       130–136

    Excludes arthropathy associated with sarcoidosis
       (713.7)
      For codes: **711.80, 711.82-711.89:** (Ex:) 003.23, 015.80-015.96,
       017.90-017.96, 036.82, 056.71, 098.50-098.51, 098.59, 098.89,
       711.00-714.0, 715.00, 715.09-715.10, 715.18-716.99, 718.00-718.08,
       719.00-719.10, 719.18-719.69, 719.80-719.99;
      For code **711.81:** (Ex:) 003.23, 015.80-015.96, 017.90-017.96, 036.82, 056.71,
       098.50-098.51, 098.59, 098.89, 711.00-711.41, 711.43-714.0, 715.00,
       715.09-715.10, 715.18-716.99, 718.00-718.08, 719.00-719.10,
       719.18-719.69, 719.80-719.99

    Coding Clinic: 1990, Q3, P14

711.9 Unspecified infective arthritis 🔖
[0-9]   Infective arthritis or polyarthritis (acute) (chronic)
       (subacute) NOS
      (Ex:) 003.23, 015.80-015.96, 017.90-017.96, 036.82, 056.71, 098.50-098.51,
       098.59, 098.89, 711.00-714.0, 715.00, 715.09-715.10, 715.18-716.99,
       718.00-718.08, 719.00-719.10, 719.18-719.69, 719.80-719.99

712 Crystal arthropathies

    Includes crystal-induced arthritis and synovitis
    Excludes gouty arthropathy (274.00-274.03)   ◄▥

    The following fifth-digit subclassification is for use with
    category 712; valid digits are in [brackets] under each code.
    See list at beginning of chapter for definitions:

     0   site unspecified
     1   shoulder region
     2   upper arm
     3   forearm
     4   hand
     5   pelvic region and thigh
     6   lower leg
     7   ankle and foot
     8   other specified sites
     9   multiple sites

712.1 Chondrocalcinosis due to dicalcium phosphate
[0-9] **crystals**
       Chondrocalcinosis due to dicalcium phosphate
       crystals (with other crystals)
       Code first underlying disease (275.49)

712.2 Chondrocalcinosis due to pyrophosphate crystals
[0-9]   Code first underlying disease (275.49)

712.3 Chondrocalcinosis, unspecified
[0-9]   Code first underlying disease (275.49)

712.8 Other specified crystal arthropathies
[0-9]

712.9 Unspecified crystal arthropathy
[0-9]

---

713 Arthropathy associated with other disorders classified elsewhere

    Includes arthritis associated with conditions classifiable
       below
       arthropathy associated with conditions
       classifiable below
       polyarthritis associated with conditions
       classifiable below
       polyarthropathy associated with conditions
       classifiable below

713.0 Arthropathy associated with other endocrine and metabolic disorders

    Code first underlying disease, as:
       acromegaly (253.0)
       hemochromatosis (275.0)
       hyperparathyroidism (252.00–252.08)
       hypogammaglobulinemia (279.00–279.09)
       hypothyroidism (243–244.9)
       lipoid metabolism disorder (272.0–272.9)
       ochronosis (270.2)

    Excludes arthropathy associated with:
       amyloidosis (713.7)
       crystal deposition disorders, except gout
       (712.1–712.9)
       diabetic neuropathy (713.5)
       gouty arthropathy (274.00-274.03)   ◄▥

713.1 Arthropathy associated with gastrointestinal conditions other than infections

    Code first underlying disease, as:
       regional enteritis (555.0–555.9)
       ulcerative colitis (556)

713.2 Arthropathy associated with hematological disorders

    Code first underlying disease, as:
       hemoglobinopathy (282.4–282.7)
       hemophilia (286.0–286.2)
       leukemia (204.0–208.9)
       malignant reticulosis (202.3)
       multiple myelomatosis (203.0)

    Excludes arthropathy associated with
       Henoch-Schönlein purpura (713.6)

713.3 Arthropathy associated with dermatological disorders

    Code first underlying disease, as:
       erythema multiforme (695.10–695.19)
       erythema nodosum (695.2)

    Excludes psoriatic arthropathy (696.0)

713.4 Arthropathy associated with respiratory disorders

    Code first underlying disease, as:
       diseases classifiable to 490–519

    Excludes arthropathy associated with respiratory
       infections (711.0, 711.4–711.8)

713.5 Arthropathy associated with neurological disorders

    Charcot's arthropathy associated with diseases
       classifiable elsewhere
    Neuropathic arthritis associated with diseases
       classifiable elsewhere

    Code first underlying disease, as:
       neuropathic joint disease [Charcot's joints]:
       NOS (094.0)
       diabetic (249.6, 250.6)
       syringomyelic (336.0)
       tabetic [syphilitic] (094.0)

DISEASES OF THE MUSCULOSKELETAL SYSTEM AND CONNECTIVE TISSUE (710–739)

    ◄ New   ◄▥ Revised   ~~deleted~~ Deleted   ● Unacceptable Principal Diagnosis   ● Use Additional Digit(s)
    ▶ Manifestation Code   **OGCR** Official Guidelines   **Coding Clinic**   Excludes   Includes   Use additional   Code first   Omit code

▶ **713.6** *Arthropathy associated with hypersensitivity reaction*

> Code first *underlying disease, as:*
> Henoch-Schönlein purpura (287.0)
> serum sickness (999.5)
>
> **Excludes** *allergic arthritis NOS (716.2)*

▶ **713.7** *Other general diseases with articular involvement*

> Code first *underlying disease, as:*
> amyloidosis (277.30–277.39)
> familial Mediterranean fever (277.31)
> sarcoidosis (135)
> **Coding Clinic: 1997, Q2, P12-13**

▶ **713.8** *Arthropathy associated with other conditions classifiable elsewhere*

> Code first *underlying disease, as:*
> conditions classifiable elsewhere except as in 711.1–711.8, 712, and 713.0–713.7

Item 13-1   Rheumatoid arthritis (RA) is a chronic systemic inflammatory disease of undetermined etiology involving primarily the synovial membranes and articular structures of multiple joints. The disease is often progressive and results in pain, stiffness, and swelling of joints. In late stages, deformity, ankylosis, and other **inflammatory polyarthropathies** develop.

● **714 Rheumatoid arthritis and other inflammatory polyarthropathies**

> **Excludes** *rheumatic fever (390)*
> *rheumatoid arthritis of spine NOS (720.0)*

714.0 Rheumatoid arthritis
> Arthritis or polyarthritis:
> atrophic
> rheumatic (chronic)
>
> Use additional code to identify manifestation, as:
> myopathy (359.6)
> polyneuropathy (357.1)
>
> **Excludes** *juvenile rheumatoid arthritis NOS (714.30)*
>
> **Coding Clinic: 2006, Q2, P20; 1995, Q4, P51**

714.1 Felty's syndrome
> Rheumatoid arthritis with splenoadenomegaly and leukopenia

714.2 Other rheumatoid arthritis with visceral or systemic involvement
> Rheumatoid carditis

● **714.3 Juvenile chronic polyarthritis**

> **714.30 Polyarticular juvenile rheumatoid arthritis, chronic or unspecified**
> Juvenile rheumatoid arthritis NOS
> Still's disease
>
> **714.31 Polyarticular juvenile rheumatoid arthritis, acute** 🔖
> (Ex) 036.82, 056.71, 711.00-714.4, 715.00, 715.09-715.10, 715.18-716.99, 718.00-718.08, 719.00-719.10, 719.18-719.99
>
> **714.32 Pauciarticular juvenile rheumatoid arthritis**
>
> **714.33 Monoarticular juvenile rheumatoid arthritis**

714.4 Chronic postrheumatic arthropathy
> Chronic rheumatoid nodular fibrositis
> Jaccoud's syndrome

●**714.8 Other specified inflammatory polyarthropathies**

> **714.81 Rheumatoid lung**
> Caplan's syndrome
> Diffuse interstitial rheumatoid disease of lung
> Fibrosing alveolitis, rheumatoid
>
> **714.89 Other**

714.9 Unspecified inflammatory polyarthropathy
> Inflammatory polyarthropathy or polyarthritis NOS
>
> **Excludes** *polyarthropathy NOS (716.5)*

● **715 Osteoarthrosis and allied disorders**
> *Degenerative joint disease with breaking down the cartilage causing pain, swelling, and reduced motion in the joints, affecting any joint.*
>
> **Note:** Localized, in the subcategories below, includes bilateral involvement of the same site.
>
> **Includes** arthritis or polyarthritis:
> degenerative
> hypertrophic
> degenerative joint disease
> osteoarthritis
>
> **Excludes** *Marie-Strümpell spondylitis (720.0)*
> *osteoarthrosis [osteoarthritis] of spine (721.0–721.9)*

The following fifth-digit subclassification is for use with category 715; valid digits are in [brackets] under each code. See list at beginning of chapter for definitions:

> 0   site unspecified
> 1   shoulder region
> 2   upper arm
> 3   forearm
> 4   hand
> 5   pelvic region and thigh
> 6   lower leg
> 7   ankle and foot
> 8   other specified sites
> 9   multiple sites

●**715.0 Osteoarthrosis, generalized**
[0,4,9]   Degenerative joint disease, involving multiple joints
> Primary generalized hypertrophic osteoarthrosis
> **Coding Clinic: 1995, Q2, P5**

●**715.1 Osteoarthrosis, localized, primary**
[0-8]   Localized osteoarthropathy, idiopathic

●**715.2 Osteoarthrosis, localized, secondary**
[0-8]   Coxae malum senilis

●**715.3 Osteoarthrosis, localized, not specified whether**
[0-8] **primary or secondary**
> Otto's pelvis
> **Coding Clinic: 2004, Q2, P15; 2003, Q2, P18; 1995, Q2, P5**

●**715.8 Osteoarthrosis involving, or with mention of more**
[0,9] **than one site, but not specified as generalized**
> **Coding Clinic: 1995, Q2, P5**

●**715.9 Osteoarthrosis, unspecified whether generalized or**
[0-8] **localized**
> **Coding Clinic: 2003, Q2, P18; 1997, Q2, P12-13; 1996, Q1, P16; 1995, Q2, P5**

DISEASES OF THE MUSCULOSKELETAL SYSTEM AND CONNECTIVE TISSUE (710–739)

● **716   Other and unspecified arthropathies**

> **Excludes** *cricoarytenoid arthropathy (478.79)*

The following fifth-digit subclassification is for use with category 716; valid digits are in [brackets] under each code. See list at beginning of chapter for definitions:

> 0   site unspecified
> 1   shoulder region
> 2   upper arm
> 3   forearm
> 4   hand
> 5   pelvic region and thigh
> 6   lower leg
> 7   ankle and foot
> 8   other specified sites
> 9   multiple sites

● **716.0   Kaschin-Beck disease**
[0-9]   Endemic polyarthritis

● **716.1   Traumatic arthropathy**
[0-9]   Coding Clinic: 2009, Q2, P13; 2002, Q1, P9-10

● **716.2   Allergic arthritis**
[0-9]
> **Excludes** *arthritis associated with Henoch-Schönlein purpura or serum sickness (713.6)*

● **716.3   Climacteric arthritis ♀**
[0-9]   Menopausal arthritis

● **716.4   Transient arthropathy**
[0-9]
> **Excludes** *palindromic rheumatism (719.3)*

● **716.5   Unspecified polyarthropathy or polyarthritis**
[0-9]

● **716.6   Unspecified monoarthritis**
[0-8]   Coxitis

● **716.8   Other specified arthropathy**
[0-9]

● **716.9   Arthropathy, unspecified**
[0-9]   Arthritis (acute) (chronic) (subacute)
Arthropathy (acute) (chronic) (subacute)
Articular rheumatism (chronic)
Inflammation of joint NOS

● **717   Internal derangement of knee**

> **Includes**   degeneration of articular cartilage or meniscus of knee
> rupture, old of articular cartilage or meniscus of knee
> tear, old of articular cartilage or meniscus of knee

> **Excludes** *acute derangement of knee (836.0–836.6)*
> *ankylosis (718.5)*
> *contracture (718.4)*
> *current injury (836.0–836.6)*
> *deformity (736.4–736.6)*
> *recurrent dislocation (718.3)*

717.0   Old bucket handle tear of medial meniscus
Old bucket handle tear of unspecified cartilage

717.1   Derangement of anterior horn of medial meniscus

717.2   Derangement of posterior horn of medial meniscus

717.3   Other and unspecified derangement of medial meniscus
Degeneration of internal semilunar cartilage

● **717.4   Derangement of lateral meniscus**

717.40   Derangement of lateral meniscus, unspecified

717.41   Bucket handle tear of lateral meniscus

717.42   Derangement of anterior horn of lateral meniscus

717.43   Derangement of posterior horn of lateral meniscus

717.49   Other

717.5   Derangement of meniscus, not elsewhere classified
Congenital discoid meniscus
Cyst of semilunar cartilage
Derangement of semilunar cartilage NOS

717.6   Loose body in knee
Joint mice, knee
Rice bodies, knee (joint)

717.7   Chondromalacia of patella
Chondromalacia patellae
Degeneration [softening] of articular cartilage of patella
Coding Clinic: 1985, July-Aug, P14; 1984, Nov-Dec, P9

● **717.8   Other internal derangement of knee**

717.81   Old disruption of lateral collateral ligament

717.82   Old disruption of medial collateral ligament

717.83   Old disruption of anterior cruciate ligament

717.84   Old disruption of posterior cruciate ligament

717.85   Old disruption of other ligaments of knee
Capsular ligament of knee

717.89   Other
Old disruption of ligaments of knee NOS

717.9   Unspecified internal derangement of knee
Derangement NOS of knee

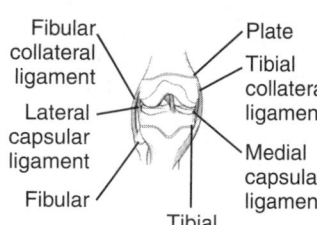

Figure 13–1 Collateral and cruciate ligament of knee. (From DeLee: DeLee and Drez's Orthopaedic Sports Medicine, 2nd ed. 2002, Saunders)

Fibular collateral ligament
Lateral capsular ligament
Fibular
Plate
Tibial collateral ligament
Medial capsular ligament
Tibial

DISEASES OF THE MUSCULOSKELETAL SYSTEM AND CONNECTIVE TISSUE (710–739)

◀ New   ◀▥ Revised   deleted Deleted   ● Unacceptable Principal Diagnosis   ● Use Additional Digit(s)
▷ Manifestation Code   **OGCR** Official Guidelines   **Coding Clinic**   Excludes   Includes   Use additional   Code first   Omit code

● 718 **Other derangement of joint**

> **Excludes** *current injury (830.0–848.9)*
> *jaw (524.60–524.69)*

The following fifth-digit subclassification is for use with category 718; valid digits are in [brackets] under each code. See list at beginning of chapter for definitions:

> 0 site unspecified
> 1 shoulder region
> 2 upper arm
> 3 forearm
> 4 hand
> 5 pelvic region and thigh
> 6 lower leg
> 7 ankle and foot
> 8 other specified sites
> 9 multiple sites

● 718.0 **Articular cartilage disorder**
[0-5,7-9]   Meniscus:
                disorder
                rupture, old
                tear, old
            Old rupture of ligament(s) of joint NOS

> **Excludes** *articular cartilage disorder:*
> *in ochronosis (270.2)*
> *knee (717.0–717.9)*
> *chondrocalcinosis (275.49)*
> *metastatic calcification (275.40)*

● 718.1 **Loose body in joint**
[0-5,7-9]   Joint mice

> **Excludes** *knee (717.6)*

> **Coding Clinic: 2001, Q2, P14-15**

● 718.2 **Pathological dislocation**
[0-9]   Dislocation or displacement of joint, not recurrent and not current

● 718.3 **Recurrent dislocation of joint**
[0-9]   **Coding Clinic: 1987, Nov-Dec, P7**

● 718.4 **Contracture of joint**
[0-9]   **Coding Clinic: 1998, Q4, P39-40**

● 718.5 **Ankylosis of joint**
[0-9]   Ankylosis of joint (fibrous) (osseous)

> **Excludes** *spine (724.9)*
> *stiffness of joint without mention of ankylosis (719.5)*

> **Coding Clinic: 1995, Q1, P10**

● 718.6 **Unspecified intrapelvic protrusion of acetabulum**
[0,5]   Protrusio acetabuli, unspecified

● 718.7 **Developmental dislocation of joint**
[0-9]   **Excludes** *congenital dislocation of joint (754.0–755.8)*
> *traumatic dislocation of joint (830–839)*

● 718.8 **Other joint derangement, not elsewhere classified**
[0-9]   Flail joint (paralytic)
            Instability of joint

> **Excludes** *deformities classifiable to 736 (736.0–736.9)*

> **Coding Clinic: 2000, Q2, P14-15**

● 718.9 **Unspecified derangement of joint**
[0-5,7-9]   **Excludes** *knee (717.9)*

● 719 **Other and unspecified disorders of joint**

> **Excludes** *jaw (524.60–524.69)*

The following fifth-digit subclassification is for use with codes 719.0–719.6, 719.8–719.9; valid digits are in [brackets] under each code. See list at beginning of chapter for definitions:

> 0 site unspecified
> 1 shoulder region
> 2 upper arm
> 3 forearm
> 4 hand
> 5 pelvic region and thigh
> 6 lower leg
> 7 ankle and foot
> 8 other specified sites
> 9 multiple sites

● 719.0 **Effusion of joint**
[0-9]   Hydrarthrosis
            Swelling of joint, with or without pain

> **Excludes** *intermittent hydrarthrosis (719.3)*

● 719.1 **Hemarthrosis** 🔗
[0-9]   **Excludes** *current injury (840.0–848.9)*

> For codes **719.10, 719.15, 719.18-719.19:** (Ex) 719.10-719.19, 958.91-958.92;
> For code **719.11:** (Ex) 719.10-719.13, 719.18-719.19, 958.91;
> For code **719.12:** (Ex) 719.10-719.12, 719.18-719.19, 958.91;
> For code **719.13:** (Ex) 719.10, 719.12-719.14, 719.18-719.19, 958.91;
> For code **719.14:** (Ex) 719.10, 719.13-719.14, 719.18-719.19, 958.91;
> For codes **719.16-719.17:** (Ex) 719.10, 719.16-719.19, 958.92

● 719.2 **Villonodular synovitis**
[0-9]

● 719.3 **Palindromic rheumatism**
[0-9]   Hench-Rosenberg syndrome
            Intermittent hydrarthrosis

● 719.4 **Pain in joint**
[0-9]   Arthralgia
            Coding Clinic: 2001, Q1, P3-4

● 719.5 **Stiffness of joint, not elsewhere classified**
[0-9]

● 719.6 **Other symptoms referable to joint**
[0-9]   Joint crepitus
            Snapping hip
            Coding Clinic: 2007, Q2, P7; 1984, Sept-Oct, P15-16

719.7 **Difficulty in walking**

> **Excludes** *abnormality of gait (781.2)*

> **Coding Clinic: 2004, Q2, P15**

● 719.8 **Other specified disorders of joint**
[0-9]   Calcification of joint
            Fistula of joint

> **Excludes** *temporomandibular joint-pain-dysfunction syndrome [Costen's syndrome] (524.60)*

● 719.9 **Unspecified disorder of joint**
[0-9]

N Newborn Age: 0   **P** Pediatric Age: 0–17   **M** Maternity Age: 12–55   **A** Adult Age: 15–124   ♀ Females Only   ♂ Males Only
(Ex) CC Exclusions   🔗 Complication\Comorbidity   🔗 Major C\C   🔗 Present on Admission Requirement   🔗 Hospital-Acquired Condition

1009

DISEASES OF THE MUSCULOSKELETAL SYSTEM AND CONNECTIVE TISSUE (710–739)

Item 13-2 **Ankylosis** or arthrokleisis is a consolidation of a joint due to disease, injury, or surgical procedure. Spondylosis is the degeneration of the vertebral processes and formation of osteophytes and commonly occurs with age. **Spondylitis** or ankylosing spondylitis is a type of arthritis that affects the spine or backbone causing back pain and stiffness.

DORSOPATHIES (720–724)

> **Excludes**   curvature of spine (737.0–737.9)
> osteochondrosis of spine (juvenile) (732.0) adult
> (732.8)

● **720 Ankylosing spondylitis and other inflammatory spondylopathies**

     720.0 Ankylosing spondylitis
         Rheumatoid arthritis of spine NOS
         Spondylitis:
            Marie-Strümpell
            rheumatoid

     720.1 Spinal enthesopathy
         Disorder of peripheral ligamentous or muscular attachments of spine
         Romanus lesion

     720.2 Sacroiliitis, not elsewhere classified
         Inflammation of sacroiliac joint NOS

     ● **720.8 Other inflammatory spondylopathies**

        ▶ *720.81 Inflammatory spondylopathies in diseases classified elsewhere*

            Code first underlying disease, as:
               tuberculosis (015.0)

        720.89 Other

     720.9 Unspecified inflammatory spondylopathy
         Spondylitis NOS

● **721 Spondylosis and allied disorders**
     Coding Clinic: 1989, Q2, P14

     721.0 Cervical spondylosis without myelopathy
         Cervical or cervicodorsal:
            arthritis
            osteoarthritis
            spondylarthritis

     721.1 Cervical spondylosis with myelopathy 🔖
         Anterior spinal artery compression syndrome
         Spondylogenic compression of cervical spinal cord
         Vertebral artery compression syndrome
         (Ex:) 721.0-721.1

     721.2 Thoracic spondylosis without myelopathy
         Thoracic:
            arthritis
            osteoarthritis
            spondylarthritis

     721.3 Lumbosacral spondylosis without myelopathy
         Lumbar or lumbosacral:
            arthritis
            osteoarthritis
            spondylarthritis
         Coding Clinic: 2002, Q4, P107-108

● **721.4 Thoracic or lumbar spondylosis with myelopathy**

     721.41 Thoracic region 🔖
         Spondylogenic compression of thoracic spinal cord
         (Ex:) 721.41

     721.42 Lumbar region 🔖
         Spondylogenic compression of lumbar spinal cord
         (Ex:) 721.3, 721.42, 722.10, 722.2, 722.32, 722.52-722.70, 722.73, 722.83-722.90, 722.93

     721.5 Kissing spine
         Baastrup's syndrome

     721.6 Ankylosing vertebral hyperostosis

     721.7 Traumatic spondylopathy 🔖
         Kümmell's disease or spondylitis
         (Ex:) 721.7

     721.8 Other allied disorders of spine

● **721.9 Spondylosis of unspecified site**

     721.90 Without mention of myelopathy
         Spinal:
            arthritis (deformans) (degenerative) (hypertrophic)
            osteoarthritis NOS
            Spondylarthrosis NOS

     721.91 With myelopathy 🔖
         Spondylogenic compression of spinal cord NOS
         (Ex:) 721.0-721.91

● **722 Intervertebral disc disorders**
     Coding Clinic: 1989, Q2, P14

     722.0 Displacement of cervical intervertebral disc without myelopathy
         Neuritis (brachial) or radiculitis due to displacement or rupture of cervical intervertebral disc
         Any condition classifiable to 722.2 of the cervical or cervicothoracic intervertebral disc
         Coding Clinic: 1988, Q1, P10

● **722.1 Displacement of thoracic or lumbar intervertebral disc without myelopathy**

     722.10 Lumbar intervertebral disc without myelopathy
         Lumbago or sciatica due to displacement of intervertebral disc
         Neuritis or radiculitis due to displacement or rupture of lumbar intervertebral disc
         Any condition classifiable to 722.2 of the lumbar or lumbosacral intervertebral disc
         Coding Clinic: 2008, Q4, P183-184; 2007, Q1, P9; 2003, Q3, P12; Q1, P7; 2002, Q4, P107-108; 1994, Q3, P14

     722.11 Thoracic intervertebral disc without myelopathy
         Any condition classifiable to 722.2 of thoracic intervertebral disc

◀ New   ◀▥ Revised   ~~deleted~~ Deleted   ● Unacceptable Principal Diagnosis   ● Use Additional Digit(s)
▶ Manifestation Code   OGCR Official Guidelines   Coding Clinic   Excludes   Includes   Use additional   Code first   Omit code

722.2 Displacement of intervertebral disc, site unspecified, without myelopathy
Discogenic syndrome NOS
Herniation of nucleus pulposus NOS
Intervertebral disc NOS:
    extrusion
    prolapse
    protrusion
    rupture
Neuritis or radiculitis due to displacement or
    rupture of intervertebral disc
Coding Clinic: 1988, Q1, P10

● **722.3 Schmorl's nodes**

    722.30 Unspecified region

    722.31 Thoracic region

    722.32 Lumbar region

    722.39 Other

722.4 Degeneration of cervical intervertebral disc
Degeneration of cervicothoracic intervertebral disc

● **722.5 Degeneration of thoracic or lumbar intervertebral disc**

    722.51 Thoracic or thoracolumbar intervertebral disc

    722.52 Lumbar or lumbosacral intervertebral disc
    Coding Clinic: 2006, Q2, P18; 2004, Q4, P129-133

722.6 Degeneration of intervertebral disc, site unspecified
Degenerative disc disease NOS
Narrowing of intervertebral disc or space NOS

● **722.7 Intervertebral disc disorder with myelopathy**

    722.70 Unspecified region

    722.71 Cervical region 🔴
      (Ex:) 722.0, 722.71

    722.72 Thoracic region 🔴
      (Ex:) 722.11, 722.72

    722.73 Lumbar region 🔴
      (Ex:) 722.11, 722.73

● **722.8 Postlaminectomy syndrome**

    722.80 Unspecified region

    722.81 Cervical region

    722.82 Thoracic region

    722.83 Lumbar region
    Coding Clinic: 1997, Q2, P15x2

● **722.9 Other and unspecified disc disorder**
Calcification of intervertebral cartilage or disc
Discitis

    722.90 Unspecified region
    Coding Clinic: 1984, Nov-Dec, P19

    722.91 Cervical region

    722.92 Thoracic region

    722.93 Lumbar region

● **723 Other disorders of cervical region**

    Excludes *conditions due to:*
        intervertebral disc disorders (722.0–722.9)
        spondylosis (721.0–721.9)
    Coding Clinic: 1989, Q2, P14

    723.0 Spinal stenosis of cervical region
    Coding Clinic: 2003, Q4, P99-101

    723.1 Cervicalgia
    Pain in neck

    723.2 Cervicocranial syndrome
    Barré-Liéou syndrome
    Posterior cervical sympathetic syndrome

    723.3 Cervicobrachial syndrome (diffuse)
    Coding Clinic: 1985, Nov-Dec, P12

    723.4 Brachia neuritis or radiculitis NOS
    Cervical radiculitis
    Radicular syndrome of upper limbs

    723.5 Torticollis, unspecified
    Contracture of neck

        Excludes *congenital (754.1)*
            due to birth injury (767.8)
            hysterical (300.11)
            ocular torticollis (781.93)
            psychogenic (306.0)
            spasmodic (333.83)
            traumatic, current (847.0)
    Coding Clinic: 2001, Q2, P21; 1995, Q1, P7

    723.6 Panniculitis specified as affecting neck

    723.7 Ossification of posterior longitudinal ligament in cervical region

    723.8 Other syndromes affecting cervical region
    Cervical syndrome NEC
    Klippel's disease
    Occipital neuralgia
    Coding Clinic: 2000, Q1, P7-8

    723.9 Unspecified musculoskeletal disorders and symptoms referable to neck
    Cervical (region) disorder NOS

● **724 Other and unspecified disorders of back**

    Excludes *collapsed vertebra (code to cause, e.g., osteoporosis, 733.00–733.09)*
        conditions due to:
            intervertebral disc disorders (722.0–722.9)
            spondylosis (721.0–721.9)
    Coding Clinic: 1989, Q2, P14

● **724.0 Spinal stenosis, other than cervical**

    724.00 Spinal stenosis, unspecified region

    724.01 Thoracic region

    724.02 Lumbar region
    Coding Clinic: 2008, Q4, P109-110; 2007, Q4, P116-120; Q1, P20-21; 1999, Q4, P13-14; 1994, Q3, P14

    724.09 Other

N Newborn Age: 0   **P** Pediatric Age: 0–17   **M** Maternity Age: 12–55   **A** Adult Age: 15–124   ♀ Females Only   ♂ Males Only

(Ex:) CC Exclusions   🔴 Complication\Comorbidity   🔴 Major C\C   Present on Admission Requirement   🔴 Hospital-Acquired Condition   **1011**

DISEASES OF THE MUSCULOSKELETAL SYSTEM AND CONNECTIVE TISSUE (710–739)

724.1 Pain in thoracic spine

724.2 Lumbago

Low back pain   Lumbalgia

Low back syndrome

Coding Clinic: 2007, Q2, P13-15; 1985, Nov-Dec, P12

724.3 Sciatica

Neuralgia or neuritis of sciatic nerve

Excludes | *specified lesion of sciatic nerve (355.0)*

Coding Clinic: 1989, Q2, P12

724.4 Thoracic or lumbosacral neuritis or radiculitis, unspecified

Radicular syndrome of lower limbs

Coding Clinic: 1999, Q2, P3-4

724.5 Backache, unspecified

Vertebrogenic (pain) syndrome NOS

724.6 Disorders of sacrum

Ankylosis, lumbosacral or sacroiliac (joint)

Instability, lumbosacral or sacroiliac (joint)

● **724.7 Disorders of coccyx**

724.70 Unspecified disorder of coccyx

724.71 Hypermobility of coccyx

724.79 Other

Coccygodynia

724.8 Other symptoms referable to back

Ossification of posterior longitudinal ligament NOS

Panniculitis specified as sacral or affecting back

724.9 Other unspecified back disorders

Ankylosis of spine NOS

Compression of spinal nerve root NEC

Spinal disorder NOS

Excludes | *sacroiliitis (720.2)*

Item 13-3 Polymyalgia rheumatica is a syndrome characterized by aching and morning stiffness and is related to aging and hereditary predisposition.

RHEUMATISM, EXCLUDING THE BACK (725–729)

Includes   disorders of muscles and tendons and their attachments, and of other soft tissues

725 Polymyalgia rheumatica

● **726 Peripheral enthesopathies and allied syndromes**

Note: Enthesopathies are disorders of peripheral ligamentous or muscular attachments.

Excludes | *spinal enthesopathy (720.1)*

726.0 Adhesive capsulitis of shoulder

● **726.1 Rotator cuff syndrome of shoulder and allied disorders**

726.10 Disorders of bursae and tendons in shoulder region, unspecified

Rotator cuff syndrome NOS

Supraspinatus syndrome NOS

Coding Clinic: 2001, Q2, P12

726.11 Calcifying tendinitis of shoulder

726.12 Bicipital tenosynovitis

726.19 Other specified disorders

Excludes | *complete rupture of rotator cuff, nontraumatic (727.61)*

Coding Clinic: 2002, Q1, P9-10

726.2 Other affections of shoulder region, not elsewhere classified

Periarthritis of shoulder

Scapulohumeral fibrositis

● **726.3 Enthesopathy of elbow region**

726.30 Enthesopathy of elbow, unspecified

726.31 Medial epicondylitis

726.32 Lateral epicondylitis

Epicondylitis NOS   Tennis elbow

Golfers' elbow

726.33 Olecranon bursitis

Bursitis of elbow

726.39 Other

726.4 Enthesopathy of wrist and carpus

Bursitis of hand or wrist

Periarthritis of wrist

726.5 Enthesopathy of hip region

Bursitis of hip   Psoas tendinitis

Gluteal tendinitis   Trochanteric tendinitis

Iliac crest spur

● **726.6 Enthesopathy of knee**

726.60 Enthesopathy of knee, unspecified

Bursitis of knee NOS

726.61 Pes anserinus tendinitis or bursitis

726.62 Tibial collateral ligament bursitis

Pellegrini-Stieda syndrome

726.63 Fibular collateral ligament bursitis

726.64 Patellar tendinitis

726.65 Prepatellar bursitis

Coding Clinic: 2006, Q2, P15

726.69 Other

Bursitis:

infrapatellar

subpatellar

● **726.7 Enthesopathy of ankle and tarsus**

726.70 Enthesopathy of ankle and tarsus, unspecified

Metatarsalgia NOS

Excludes | *Morton's metatarsalgia (355.6)*

726.71 Achilles bursitis or tendinitis

726.72 Tibialis tendinitis

Tibialis (anterior) (posterior) tendinitis

726.73 Calcaneal spur

726.79 Other

Peroneal tendinitis

726.8 Other peripheral enthesopathies

● **726.9 Unspecified enthesopathy**

726.90 Enthesopathy of unspecified site

Capsulitis NOS   Tendinitis NOS

Periarthritis NOS

726.91 Exostosis of unspecified site

Bone spur NOS

Coding Clinic: 2001, Q2, P13-15

◀ New   ◀▮▮ Revised   ~~deleted~~ Deleted   ● Unacceptable Principal Diagnosis   ● Use Additional Digit(s)

▶ Manifestation Code   OGCR Official Guidelines   Coding Clinic   Excludes   Includes   Use additional   Code first   Omit code

Item 13-4 Synovitis is an inflammation of a synovial membrane resulting in pain on motion and is characterized by fluctuating swelling due to effusion in a synovial sac. **Tenosynovitis** is an inflammation of a tendon sheath and occurs most commonly in the wrists, hands, and feet. Bursitis is inflammation of a bursa (fluid filled sac) caused by repetitive use, trauma, infection, or systemic inflammatory disease. Bursae act as protectors and facilitate movement between bones and overlapping muscles (deep bursae) or between bones and tendons/skin (superficial bursae).

● **727   Other disorders of synovium, tendon, and bursa**

  ● **727.0   Synovitis and tenosynovitis**

      727.00   Synovitis and tenosynovitis, unspecified
         Synovitis NOS
         Tenosynovitis NOS

     ▶ **727.01   *Synovitis and tenosynovitis in diseases classified elsewhere***
         Code first underlying disease, as:
           tuberculosis (015.0–015.9)
         | **Excludes** | *crystal-induced (275.49)*
               gonococcal (098.51)
               gouty (274.00-274.03) ◀
               syphilitic (095.7)

      727.02   Giant cell tumor of tendon sheath

      727.03   Trigger finger (acquired)

      727.04   Radial styloid tenosynovitis
         de Quervain's disease

      727.05   Other tenosynovitis of hand and wrist

      727.06   Tenosynovitis of foot and ankle

      727.09   Other

   727.1   Bunion

   727.2   Specific bursitides often of occupational origin
      Beat:
        elbow
        hand
        knee
      Chronic crepitant synovitis of wrist
      Miners':
        elbow
        knee

   727.3   Other bursitis
      Bursitis NOS
      | **Excludes** | *bursitis:*
            gonococcal (098.52)
            subacromial (726.19)
            subcoracoid (726.19)
            subdeltoid (726.19)
            syphilitic (095.7)
            "frozen shoulder" (726.0)

  ● **727.4   Ganglion and cyst of synovium, tendon, and bursa**

      727.40   Synovial cyst, unspecified
         | **Excludes** | *that of popliteal space (727.51)*
         Coding Clinic: 1997, Q2, P6

      727.41   Ganglion of joint

      727.42   Ganglion of tendon sheath

      727.43   Ganglion, unspecified

      727.49   Other
         Cyst of bursa

● **727.5   Rupture of synovium**

      727.50   Rupture of synovium, unspecified

      727.51   Synovial cyst of popliteal space
         Baker's cyst (knee)

      727.59   Other

● **727.6   Rupture of tendon, nontraumatic**

      727.60   Nontraumatic rupture of unspecified tendon

      727.61   Complete rupture of rotator cuff

      727.62   Tendons of biceps (long head)

      727.63   Extensor tendons of hand and wrist

      727.64   Flexor tendons of hand and wrist

      727.65   Quadriceps tendon

      727.66   Patellar tendon

      727.67   Achilles tendon

      727.68   Other tendons of foot and ankle

      727.69   Other

● **727.8   Other disorders of synovium, tendon, and bursa**

      727.81   Contracture of tendon (sheath)
         Short Achilles tendon (acquired)

      727.82   Calcium deposits in tendon and bursa
         Calcification of tendon NOS
         Calcific tendinitis NOS
         | **Excludes** | *peripheral ligamentous or muscular*
                  attachments (726.0–726.9)

      727.83   Plica syndrome
         Plica knee

      727.89   Other
         Abscess of bursa or tendon
         | **Excludes** | *xanthomatosis localized to tendons*
                  (272.7)
         Coding Clinic: 1989, Q2, P15; 1985, July-Aug, P14; 1984, Nov-Dec, P9

   727.9   Unspecified disorder of synovium, tendon, and bursa

● **728   Disorders of muscle, ligament, and fascia**
      | **Excludes** | *enthesopathies (726.0–726.9)*
            muscular dystrophies (359.0–359.1)
            myoneural disorders (358.00–358.9)
            myopathies (359.2–359.9)
            nontraumatic hematoma of muscle (729.92)
            old disruption of ligaments of knee (717.81–717.89)

   728.0   Infective myositis 🦠
      Myositis:
        purulent
        suppurative
      | **Excludes** | *myositis:*
           epidemic (074.1)
           interstitial (728.81)
           myoneural disorder (358.00–358.9)
           syphilitic (095.6)
           tropical (040.81)
      (Ex) 567.31, 728.0, 728.11-728.3, 728.81, 728.86

● **728.1   Muscular calcification and ossification**

      728.10   Calcification and ossification, unspecified
         Massive calcification (paraplegic)

      728.11   Progressive myositis ossificans

      728.12   Traumatic myositis ossifications
         Myositis ossificans (circumscripta)

      728.13   Postoperative heterotopic calcification

      728.19   Other
         Polymyositis ossificans

DISEASES OF THE MUSCULOSKELETAL SYSTEM AND CONNECTIVE TISSUE (710–739)

DISEASES OF THE MUSCULOSKELETAL SYSTEM AND CONNECTIVE TISSUE (710–739)

728.2   Muscular wasting and disuse atrophy, not elsewhere classified
Amyotrophia NOS
Myofibrosis

> **Excludes**   *neuralgic amyotrophy (353.5)*
> *pelvic muscle wasting and disuse atrophy (618.83)*
> *progressive muscular atrophy (335.0–335.9)*

728.3   Other specific muscle disorders
Arthrogryposis
Immobility syndrome (paraplegic)

> **Excludes**   *arthrogryposis multiplex congenita (754.89)*
> *stiff-man syndrome (333.91)*

728.4   Laxity of ligament

728.5   Hypermobility syndrome

728.6   Contracture of palmar fascia   A
Dupuytren's contracture

● **728.7   Other fibromatoses**

     728.71   Plantar fascial fibromatosis
         Contracture of plantar fascia
         Plantar fasciitis (traumatic)

     728.79   Other
         Garrod's or knuckle pads
         Nodular fasciitis
         Pseudosarcomatous Fibromatosis
           (proliferative) (subcutaneous)

● **728.8   Other disorders of muscle, ligament, and fascia**

     728.81   Interstitial myositis

     728.82   Foreign body granuloma of muscle
         Talc granuloma of muscle

     728.83   Rupture of muscle, nontraumatic

     728.84   Diastasis of muscle
         Diastasis recti (abdomen)

> **Excludes**   *diastasis recti complicating pregnancy, labor, and delivery (665.8)*

     728.85   Spasm of muscle

     728.86   Necrotizing fasciitis 🔘

> **Use additional** code to identify:
> infectious organism (041.00–041.89)
> gangrene (785.4), if applicable
> (Ex) 567.31, 728.0, 728.11-728.3, 728.81, 728.86

     728.87   Muscle weakness (generalized)

> **Excludes**   *generalized weakness (780.79)*

         Coding Clinic: 2005, Q1, P13

     728.88   Rhabdomyolysis 🔘
         (Ex) 567.31, 728.0, 728.11-728.3, 728.81, 728.86, 728.88
         Coding Clinic: 2003, Q4, P66-67; 2001, Q2, P14

     728.89   Other
         Eosinophilic fasciitis

> **Use additional** E code to identify drug, if drug induced

         Coding Clinic: 2006, Q3, P13; 2002, Q3, P28; 2001, Q2, P15

728.9   Unspecified disorder of muscle, ligament, and fascia

● **729   Other disorders of soft tissues**

> **Excludes**   *acroparesthesia (443.89)*
> *carpal tunnel syndrome (354.0)*
> *disorders of the back (720.0–724.9)*
> *entrapment syndromes (354.0–355.9)*
> *palindromic rheumatism (719.3)*
> *periarthritis (726.0–726.9)*
> *psychogenic rheumatism (306.0)*

Coding Clinic: 1984, Nov-Dec, P17

729.0   Rheumatism, unspecified and fibrositis

729.1   Myalgia and myositis, unspecified
Fibromyositis NOS
Coding Clinic: 1984, Nov-Dec, P17

729.2   Neuralgia, neuritis, and radiculitis, unspecified

> **Excludes**   *brachia radiculitis (723.4)*
> *cervical radiculitis (723.4)*
> *lumbosacral radiculitis (724.4)*
> *mononeuritis (354.0–355.9)*
> *radiculitis due to intervertebral disc involvement (722.0–722.2, 722.7)*
> *sciatica (724.3)*

● **729.3   Panniculitis, unspecified**
Inflammation of adipose tissue of heel pad

     729.30   Panniculitis, unspecified site
         Weber-Christian disease

     729.31   Hypertrophy of fat pad, knee
         Hypertrophy of infrapatellar fat pad

     729.39   Other site

> **Excludes**   *panniculitis specified as (affecting):*
> *back (724.8)*
> *neck (723.6)*
> *sacral (724.8)*

729.4   Fasciitis, unspecified

> **Excludes**   *necrotizing fasciitis (728.86)*
> *nodular fasciitis (728.79)*

Coding Clinic: 1994, Q2, P13

729.5   Pain in limb
Coding Clinic: 2007, Q2, P13-15

729.6   Residual foreign body in soft tissue

> **Excludes**   *foreign body granuloma:*
> *muscle (728.82)*
> *skin and subcutaneous tissue (709.4)*

● **729.7   Nontraumatic compartment syndrome**

> **Excludes**   *compartment syndrome NOS (958.90)*
> *traumatic compartment syndrome (958.90–958.99)*

Code first, if applicable, postprocedural complication (998.89)

     729.71   Nontraumatic compartment syndrome of upper extremity 🔘
         Nontraumatic compartment syndrome of shoulder, arm, forearm, wrist, hand and fingers
         (Ex) 729.81, 729.89-729.99, 903.8, 904.9
         Coding Clinic: 2006, Q4, P100-102

     729.72   Nontraumatic compartment syndrome of lower extremity 🔘
         Nontraumatic compartment syndrome of hip, buttock, thigh, leg, foot and toes
         (Ex) 729.81, 729.89-729.99, 904.7, 904.9

     729.73   Nontraumatic compartment syndrome of abdomen 🔘
         (Ex) 863.0-867.3, 867.5-868.14, 869.0-869.1, 879.2-879.9, 929.0-929.9, 958.8, 959.8-959.9

     729.79   Nontraumatic compartment syndrome of other sites 🔘
         (Ex) 868.03-868.10, 868.13-869.1

● **729.8   Other musculoskeletal symptoms referable to limbs**

     729.81   Swelling of limb
         Coding Clinic: 1988, Q4, P6

     729.82   Cramp

     729.89   Other

> **Excludes**   *abnormality of gait (781.2)*
> *tetany (781.7)*
> *transient paralysis of limb (781.4)*

         Coding Clinic: 1988, Q4, P12

◀ New   ◀◀ Revised   ~~deleted~~ Deleted   ● Unacceptable Principal Diagnosis   ● Use Additional Digit(s)
▶ Manifestation Code   **OGCR** Official Guidelines   **Coding Clinic**   Excludes   Includes   Use additional   Code first   Omit code

● **729.9 Other and unspecified disorders of soft tissue**
    Coding Clinic: 2008, Q4, P134-136

    729.90 Disorders of soft tissue, unspecified

    729.91 Post-traumatic seroma

      Excludes   *seroma complicating a procedure (998.13)*

    729.92 Nontraumatic hematoma of soft tissue
      Nontraumatic hematoma of muscle

    729.99 Other disorders of soft tissue
      Polyalgia

OSTEOPATHIES, CHONDROPATHIES, AND ACQUIRED MUSCULOSKELETAL DEFORMITIES (730–739)

● **730 Osteomyelitis, periostitis, and other infections involving bone**

      Excludes   *jaw (526.4–526.5)*
               petrous bone (383.2)

      Use additional code to identify organism, such as:
      Staphylococcus (041.1)
      Coding Clinic: 1997, Q4, P43; 1993, 5th Issue, P3

The following fifth-digit subclassification is for use with category 730; valid digits are in [brackets] under each code. See list at beginning of chapter for definitions:

> 0   site unspecified
> 1   shoulder region
> 2   upper arm
> 3   forearm
> 4   hand
> 5   pelvic region and thigh
> 6   lower leg
> 7   ankle and foot
> 8   other specified sites
> 9   multiple sites

Figure 13–2   Osteomyelitis of the spine. A lateral view of the lower thoracic spine demonstrates destruction of the disk space *(arrow)* as well as destruction of the adjoining vertebral bodies. (From Mettler: Essentials of Radiology, 2nd ed. 2005, Saunders, An Imprint of Elsevier)

Item 13–5   Osteomyelitis is an inflammation of the bone. **Acute osteomyelitis** is a rapidly destructive, pus-producing infection capable of causing severe bone destruction. **Chronic osteomyelitis** can remain long after the initial acute episode has passed and may lead to a recurrence of the acute phase. **Brodie's abscess** is an encapsulated focal abscess that must be surgically drained. Periostitis is an inflammation of the periosteum, a dense membrane composed of fibrous connective tissue that closely wraps all bone, except those with articulating surfaces in joints, which are covered by synovial membranes.

● **730.0 Acute osteomyelitis** 🖐
   [0-9]   Abscess of any bone except accessory sinus, jaw, or mastoid
        Acute or subacute osteomyelitis, with or without mention of periostitis

        Use additional code to identify major osseous defect, if applicable (731.3)
        For code **730.00:** (Ex:) 015.50-015.56, 015.70-015.76, 015.90-015.96, 017.90-017.96, 730.00-730.39, 730.80-730.99;
        For code **730.01:** (Ex:) 015.50-015.56, 015.70-015.76, 015.90-015.96, 017.90-017.96, 730.00, 730.08-730.11, 730.18-730.21, 730.28-730.31, 730.38-730.39, 730.80-730.81, 730.88-730.91, 730.98-730.99;
        For code **730.02:** (Ex:) 015.50-015.56, 015.70-015.76, 015.90-015.96, 017.90-017.96, 730.00, 730.08-730.10, 730.12, 730.18-730.20, 730.22, 730.28-730.30, 730.32, 730.38-730.39, 730.80, 730.82, 730.88-730.90, 730.92, 730.98-730.99;
        For code **730.03:** (Ex:) 015.50-015.56, 015.70-015.76, 015.90-015.96, 017.90-017.96, 730.00, 730.08-730.10, 730.13, 730.18-730.20, 730.23, 730.28-730.30, 730.33, 730.38-730.39, 730.80, 730.83, 730.88-730.90, 730.93, 730.98-730.99;
        For code **730.04:** (Ex:) 015.50-015.56, 015.70-015.76, 015.90-015.96, 017.90-017.96, 730.00, 730.08-730.10, 730.14, 730.18-730.20, 730.24, 730.28-730.30, 730.34, 730.38-730.39, 730.80, 730.84, 730.88-730.90, 730.94, 730.98-730.99;
        For code **730.05:** (Ex:) 015.10-015.16, 015.50-015.56, 015.70-015.76, 015.90-015.96, 017.90-017.96, 730.00, 730.08-730.10, 730.15, 730.18-730.20, 730.25, 730.28-730.30, 730.35, 730.38-730.39, 730.80, 730.85, 730.88-730.90, 730.95, 730.98-730.99;
        For code **730.06:** (Ex:) 015.20-015.56, 015.70-015.76, 015.90-015.96, 017.90-017.96, 730.00, 730.08-730.10, 730.16, 730.18-730.20, 730.26, 730.28-730.30, 730.36, 730.38-730.39, 730.80, 730.86, 730.88-730.90, 730.96, 730.98-730.99;
        For code **730.07:** (Ex:) 015.50-015.56, 015.70-015.76, 015.90-015.96, 017.90-017.96, 730.00, 730.08 -730.10, 730.17-730.20, 730.27-730.30, 730.37-730.39, 730.80, 730.87-730.90, 730.97-730.99;
        For code **730.08:** (Ex:) 015.00-015.06, 015.50-015.56, 015.70-015.76, 015.90-015.96, 017.90-017.96, 730.00-730.39, 730.80-730.99;
        For code **730.09:** (Ex:) 015.50-015.56, 015.70-015.76, 015.90-015.96, 017.90-017.96, 730.00-730.39, 730.80-730.99
        Coding Clinic: 2004, Q1, P14-15; 2002, Q1, P3-4

● **730.1 Chronic osteomyelitis** 🖐
   [0-9]   Brodie's abscess
        Chronic or old osteomyelitis, with or without mention of periostitis
        Sequestrum
        Sclerosing osteomyelitis of Garré

        Use additional code to identify major osseous defect, if applicable (731.3)

        Excludes   *aseptic necrosis of bone (733.40–733.49)*

        For code **730.10:** (Ex:) 730.10-730.39, 730.80-731.1;
        For codes **730.11-730.19:** (Ex:) 003.24, 015.50-015.56, 015.70-015.76, 015.90-015.96, 017.90-017.96, 730.00-730.39, 730.80-730.99
        Coding Clinic: 2000, Q3, P4

● **730.2 Unspecified osteomyelitis** 🖐
   [0-9]   Osteitis or osteomyelitis NOS, with or without mention of periostitis

        Use additional code to identify major osseous defect, if applicable (731.3)
        For code **730.20:** (Ex:) 730.10-730.39, 730.80-731.1;
        For codes **730.21-730.29:** (Ex:) 003.24, 015.50-015.56, 015.70-015.76, 015.90-015.96, 017.90-017.96, 730.00-730.39, 730.80-730.99

● **730.3 Periostitis without mention of osteomyelitis**
   [0-9]   Abscess of periosteum, without mention of osteomyelitis
        Periostosis, without mention of osteomyelitis

        Excludes   *that in secondary syphilis (091.61)*

N Newborn Age: 0   **P** Pediatric Age: 0–17   **M** Maternity Age: 12–55   **A** Adult Age: 15–124   ♀ Females Only   ♂ Males Only   **1015**

(Ex:) CC Exclusions   🖐 Complication\Comorbidity   🖐 Major C\C   🖐 Present on Admission Requirement   🖐 Hospital-Acquired Condition

DISEASES OF THE MUSCULOSKELETAL SYSTEM AND CONNECTIVE TISSUE (710–739)

730.7 *Osteopathy resulting from poliomyelitis*
[0-9]   Code first *underlying disease (045.0–045.9)*

730.8 *Other infections involving bone in disease classified*
[0-9] *elsewhere*

     Code first *underlying disease, as:*
        tuberculosis (015.0–015.9)
        typhoid fever (002.0)

     Excludes   *syphilitis of bone NOS (095.5)*

For codes **730.80, 730.89:** (Ex) 015.50-015.56, 015.70-015.76,
     015.90-015.96, 017.90-017.96, 730.00-730.39, 730.80-730.99;
For code **730.81:** (Ex) 015.50-015.56, 015.70-015.76, 015.90-015.96,
     017.90-017.96, 730.00-730.01, 730.08-730.11, 730.18-730.21,
     730.28-730.31, 730.38-730.39, 730.80, 730.88-730.91 730.98-730.99;
For code **730.82:** (Ex) 015.50-015.56, 015.70-015.76, 015.90-015.96,
     017.90-017.96, 730.00, 730.02, 730.08-730.10, 730.12,
     730.18-730.20, 730.22, 730.28-730.30 730.32, 730.38-730.39, 730.80
     730.88 -730.90, 730.92, 730.98-730.99;
For code **730.83:** (Ex) 015.50-015.56, 015.70-015.76, 015.90-015.96,
     017.90-017.96, 730.00, 730.03, 730.08-730.10, 730.13, 730.18
     -730.20, 730.23, 730.28-730.30, 730.33, 730.38-730.39, 730.80,
     730.88-730.90, 730.93, 730.98-730.99;
For code **730.84:** (Ex) 015.50-015.56, 015.70-015.76, 015.90-015.96,
     017.90-017.96, 730.00, 730.04, 730.08-730.10, 730.14, 730.18-730.20,
     730.24, 730.28-730.30, 730.34, 730.38-730.39, 730.80, 730.88-730.90,
     730.94, 730.98-730.99;
For code **730.85:** (Ex) 015.10-015.16, 015.50-015.56, 015.70-015.76,
     015.90-015.96, 017.90-017.96, 730.00, 730.05, 730.08-730.10,
     730.15, 730.18-730.20, 730.25, 730.28-730.30, 730.35,
     730.38-730.39, 730.80, 730.88-730.90, 730.95, 730.98-730.99;
For code **730.86:** (Ex) 015.20 -015.56, 015.70-015.76, 015.90-015.96,
     017.90-017.96, 730.00, 730.06, 730.08-730.10, 730.16, 730.18-730.20,
     730.26, 730.28-730.30, 730.36, 730.38-730.39, 730.80, 730.88-730.90,
     730.96, 730.98-730.99;
For code **730.87:** (Ex) 015.50-015.56, 015.70-015.76, 015.90-015.96,
     017.90-017.96, 730.00, 730.07-730.10, 730.17-730.20, 730.27-730.30,
     730.37-730.39, 730.80, 730.88-730.90, 730.97-730.99;
For code **730.88:** (Ex) 015.00-015.06, 015.50-015.56, 015.70-015.76,
     015.90-015.96, 017.90-017.96, 730.00-730.39, 730.80-730.99

730.9 Unspecified infection of bone
[0-9]   For codes **730.90, 730.99:** (Ex) 015.50-015.56, 015.70-015.76,
     015.90-015.96, 017.90-017.96, 730.00-730.39, 730.80 -730.99;
For code **730.91:** (Ex) 015.50-015.56, 015.70-015.76, 015.90-015.96,
     017.90-017.96, 730.00-730.01, 730.08-730.11, 730.18-730.21,
     730.28-730.31, 730.38-730.39, 730.80-730.81, 730.88-730.90,
     730.98-730.99;
For code **730.92:** (Ex) 015.50-015.56, 015.70-015.76, 015.90-015.96,
     017.90-017.96, 730.00, 730.02, 730.08-730.10, 730.12, 730.18-730.20,
     730.22, 730.28-730.30, 730.32, 730.38-730.39, 730.80, 730.82,
     730.88-730.90, 730.98-730.99;
For code **730.93:** (Ex) 015.50-015.56, 015.70-015.76, 015.90-015.96,
     017.90-017.96, 730.00, 730.03, 730.08-730.10, 730.13, 730.18-730.20,
     730.23, 730.28-730.30, 730.33, 730.38-730.39, 730.80, 730.83,
     730.88-730.90, 730.98-730.99;
For code **730.94:** (Ex) 015.50-015.56, 015.70-015.76, 015.90-015.96,
     017.90-017.96, 730.00, 730.04, 730.08-730.10, 730.14, 730.18-730.20,
     730.24, 730.28-730.30, 730.34, 730.38-730.39, 730.80, 730.84,
     730.88-730.90, 730.98-730.99;
For code **730.95:** (Ex) 015.10-015.16, 015.50-015.56, 015.70-015.76, 015.90
     -015.96, 017.90-017.96, 730.00, 730.05, 730.08-730.10, 730.15,
     730.18-730.20, 730.25, 730.28-730.30, 730.35, 730.38-730.39,
     730.80, 730.85, 730.88-730.90, 730.98-730.99;
For code **730.96:** (Ex) 015.20-015.56, 015.70-015.76, 015.90-015.96,
     017.90-017.96, 730.00, 730.06, 730.08-730.10, 730.16, 730.18-730.20,
     730.26, 730.28-730.30, 730.36, 730.38-730.39, 730.80, 730.86,
     730.88-730.90, 730.98-730.99;
For code **730.97:** (Ex) 015.50-015.56, 015.70-015.76, 015.90-015.96,
     017.90-017.96, 730.00, 730.07-730.10, 730.17-730.20,
     730.27-730.30, 730.37-730.39, 730.80, 730.87-730.90, 730.98-730.99;
For code **730.98:** (Ex) 015.00-015.06, 015.50-015.56, 015.70-015.76,
     015.90-015.96, 017.90-017.96, 730.00-730.39, 730.80-730.99

**731 Osteitis deformans and osteopathies associated with
other disorders classified elsewhere**
     *Also known as Paget's Disease; chronic disorder that results in
enlarged and deformed bones. The excessive breakdown
and formation of bone tissue causes bones to weaken and
results in bone pain, arthritis, deformities, and fractures.
Osteopathy describes bone pathologies of unknown
cause.*

**731.0 Osteitis deformans without mention of bone
tumor**
     Paget's disease of bone
     Coding Clinic: 1994, Q2, P6-7

731.1 *Osteitis deformans in diseases classified elsewhere*

     Code first *underlying disease, as:*
        malignant neoplasm of bone (170.0–170.9)

731.2 Hypertrophic pulmonary osteoarthropathy
     Bamberger-Marie disease

731.3 Major osseous defects

     Code first *underlying disease, if known, such as:*
        aseptic necrosis (733.40–733.49)
        malignant neoplasm of bone (170.0–170.9)
        osteomyelitis (730.00–730.29)
        osteoporosis (733.00–733.09)
        peri-prosthetic osteolysis (996.45)
     Coding Clinic: 2006, Q4, P103-104

731.8 *Other bone involvement in diseases classified
elsewhere*

     Code first *underlying disease, as:*
        diabetes mellitus (249.8, 250.8)

     Use additional *code to specify bone condition,*
        such as:
        acute osteomyelitis (730.00–730.09)
     Coding Clinic: 2004, Q1, P14-115; 1997, Q4, P43

732 Osteochondropathies

732.0 Juvenile osteochondrosis of spine
     Juvenile osteochondrosis (of):
        marginal or vertebral ephiphysis (of
           Scheuermann) spine NOS
     Vertebral epiphysitis

     Excludes   *adolescent postural kyphosis (737.0)*

732.1 Juvenile osteochondrosis of hip and pelvis
     Coxa plana
     Ischiopubic synchondrosis (of van Neck)
     Osteochondrosis (juvenile) of:
        acetabulum
        head of femur (of Legg-Calvé-Perthes)
        iliac crest (of Buchanan)
        symphysis pubis (of Pierson)
     Pseudocoxalgia

732.2 Nontraumatic slipped upper femoral epiphysis
     Slipped upper femoral epiphysis NOS

732.3 Juvenile osteochondrosis of upper extremity
     Osteochondrosis (juvenile) of:
        capitulum of humerus (of Panner)
        carpal lunate (of Kienbock)
        hand NOS
        head of humerus (of Haas)
        heads of metacarpals (of Mauclaire)
        lower ulna (of Burns)
        radial head (of Brailsford)
        upper extremity NOS

DISEASES OF THE MUSCULOSKELETAL SYSTEM AND CONNECTIVE TISSUE (710–739)

◄ New   ◄■■ Revised   ~~deleted~~ Deleted   ● Unacceptable Principal Diagnosis   ● Use Additional Digit(s)
▶ Manifestation Code   **OGCR** Official Guidelines   **Coding Clinic**   Excludes   Includes   Use additional   Code first   Omit code

732.4 Juvenile osteochondrosis of lower extremity, excluding foot

Osteochondrosis (juvenile) of:
  lower extremity NOS
  primary patellar center (of Köhler)
  proximal tibia (of Blount)
  secondary patellar center (of Sinding-Larsen)
  tibial tubercle (of Osgood-Schlatter)
Tibia vara

732.5 Juvenile osteochondrosis of foot

Calcaneal apophysitis
Epiphysitis, os calcis
Osteochondrosis (juvenile) of:
  astragalus (of Diaz)
  calcaneum (of Sever)
  foot NOS
  metatarsal:
    second (of Freiberg)
    fifth (of Iselin)
  os tibiale externum (of Haglund)
  tarsal navicular (of Köhler)

732.6 Other juvenile osteochondrosis

Apophysitis specified as juvenile, of other site, or site NOS
Epiphysitis specified as juvenile, of other site, or site NOS
Osteochondritis specified as juvenile, of other site, or site NOS
Osteochondrosis specified as juvenile, of other site, or site NOS

732.7 Osteochondritis dissecans

732.8 Other specified forms of osteochondropathy

Adult osteochondrosis of spine

732.9 Unspecified osteochondropathy

Apophysitis
  NOS
  not specified as adult or juvenile, of unspecified site
Epiphysitis
  NOS
  not specified as adult or juvenile, of unspecified site
Osteochondritis
  NOS
  not specified as adult or juvenile, of unspecified site
Osteochondrosis
  NOS
  not specified as adult or juvenile, of unspecified site

● **733 Other disorders of bone and cartilage**

Excludes	bone spur (726.91)
	cartilage of, or loose body in, joint (717.0–717.9, 718.0–718.9)
	giant cell granuloma of jaw (526.3)
	osteitis fibrosa cystica generalisata (252.01)
	osteomalacia (268.2)
	polyostotic fibrous dysplasia of bone (756.54)
	prognathism, retrognathism (524.1)
	xanthomatosis localized to bone (272.7)

● **733.0 Osteoporosis**

Condition of excessive skeletal fragility (porous bone) resulting in bone fractures

Use additional code to identify:
  major osseous defect, if applicable (731.3)
  personal history of pathologic (healed) fracture (V13.51)
Coding Clinic: 1993, Q4, P25-26

733.00 Osteoporosis, unspecified
Wedging of vertebra NOS
Coding Clinic: 2007, Q4, P91-92; Q1, P22; 2001, Q3, P19; 1998, Q2, P12

733.01 Senile osteoporosis
Postmenopausal osteoporosis
Coding Clinic: 2007, Q1, P3-8

733.02 Idiopathic osteoporosis

733.03 Disuse osteoporosis

733.09 Other
Drug-induced osteoporosis
Use additional E code to identify drug
Coding Clinic: 2003, Q4, P108-109

● **733.1 Pathologic fracture**
Chronic fracture
Spontaneous fracture

Excludes	stress fracture (733.93–733.95)
	traumatic fractures (800–829)

Coding Clinic: 1986, Nov-Dec, P10; 1985, Nov-Dec, P16

733.10 Pathologic fracture, unspecified site 🦠
Ex: 733.10-733.19, 733.93-733.98

733.11 Pathologic fracture of humerus 🦠
Ex: 733.10-733.19, 733.93 -733.98

733.12 Pathologic fracture of distal radius and ulna 🦠
Wrist NOS
Ex: 733.10-733.19, 733.93-733.98

733.13 Pathologic fracture of vertebrae 🦠
Collapse of vertebra NOS
Ex: 733.10-733.19, 733.93-733.98
Coding Clinic: 2008, Q3, P4; 2007, Q1, P3-8,22; 1999, Q3, P5

733.14 Pathologic fracture of neck of femur 🦠
Femur NOS
Hip NOS
Ex: 733.10-733.19, 733.93-733.98
Coding Clinic: 2001, Q1, P10-11; 1996, Q1, P16; 1993, Q4, P25-26

733.15 Pathologic fracture of other specified part of femur 🦠
Ex: 733.10-733.19, 733.93-733.98
Coding Clinic: 1998, Q2, P12; 1994, Q2, P6-7

733.16 Pathologic fracture of tibia and fibula 🦠
Ankle NOS
Ex: 733.10-733.19, 733.93-733.98

733.19 Pathologic fracture of other specified site 🦠
Ex: 733.10-733.19, 733.93-733.98

N Newborn Age: 0   **P** Pediatric Age: 0–17   **M** Maternity Age: 12–55   **A** Adult Age: 15–124   ♀ Females Only   ♂ Males Only

Ex: CC Exclusions   🦠 Complication\Comorbidity   Major C\C   Present on Admission Requirement   Hospital-Acquired Condition

1017

● **733.2 Cyst of bone**

    733.20 Cyst of bone (localized), unspecified

    733.21 Solitary bone cyst
        Unicameral bone cyst

    733.22 Aneurysmal bone cyst

    733.29 Other
        Fibrous dysplasia (monostotic)

        | **Excludes** | *cyst of jaw (526.0–526.2, 526.89)* |
                     osteitis fibrosa cystica (252.01)
                     polyostotic fibrous dysplasia of bone (756.54)

733.3 Hyperostosis of skull
    Hyperostosis interna frontalis
    Leontiasis ossium

● **733.4 Aseptic necrosis of bone**

    Use additional code to identify major osseous defect, if applicable (731.3)

    | **Excludes** | *osteochondropathies (732.0–732.9)* |

    Coding Clinic: 2007, Q4, P116-120

    733.40 Aseptic necrosis of bone, site unspecified 🔘
        Ex: 733.40-733.49

    733.41 Head of humerus 🔘
        Ex: 733.40-733.41, 733.45-733.49

    733.42 Head and neck of femur 🔘
        Femur NOS

        | **Excludes** | *Legg-Calvé-Perthes disease (732.1)* |
        Ex: 733.40, 733.42, 733.45-733.49

    733.43 Medial femoral condyle 🔘
        Ex: 733.40, 733.43, 733.45-733.49

    733.44 Talus 🔘
        Ex: 733.40, 733.44-733.49

    733.45 Jaw 🔘

        Use additional E code to identify drug, if drug-induced

        | **Excludes** | *osteoradionecrosis of jaw (526.89)* |
        Ex: 733.40-733.49
        Coding Clinic: 2007, Q4, P91-92

    733.49 Other 🔘
        Ex: 733.40-733.49

733.5 Osteitis condensans
    Piriform sclerosis of ilium

733.6 Tietze's disease
    Costochondral junction syndrome
    Costochondritis

733.7 Algoneurodystrophy
    Disuse atrophy of bone
    Sudeck's atrophy

● **733.8 Malunion and nonunion of fracture**

    733.81 Malunion of fracture 🔘
        Fracture ends do not heal together correctly.
        Ex: 733.81-733.82

    733.82 Nonunion of fracture 🔘
        Total failure of fracture healing
        Pseudoarthrosis (bone)
        Ex: 733.81-733.82
        Coding Clinic: 1994, Q2, P7; 1987, Jan-Feb, P13; 1984, Nov-Dec, P18

● **733.9 Other and unspecified disorders of bone and cartilage**
    Coding Clinic: 2008, Q4, P136-137

    733.90 Disorder of bone and cartilage, unspecified

    733.91 Arrest of bone development or growth
        Epiphyseal arrest

    733.92 Chondromalacia
        Chondromalacia:
          NOS
          localized, except patella
          systemic
          tibial plateau

        | **Excludes** | *chondromalacia of patella (717.7)* |

    733.93 Stress fracture of tibia or fibula
        Stress reaction of tibia or fibula

        Use additional external cause code(s) to identify the cause of the stress fracture

    733.94 Stress fracture of the metatarsals
        Stress reaction of metatarsals

        Use additional external cause code(s) to identify the cause of the stress fracture
        Coding Clinic: 2001, Q4, P48-49

    733.95 Stress fracture of other bone
        Stress reaction of other bone

        Use additional external cause code(s) to identify the cause of the stress fracture

        | **Excludes** | *stress fracture of:* |
             femoral neck (733.96)
             fibula (733.93)
             metatarsals (733.94)
             pelvis (733.98)
             shaft of femur (733.97)
             tibia (733.93)

    733.96 Stress fracture of femoral neck
        Stress reaction of femoral neck

        Use additional external cause code(s) to identify the cause of the stress fracture

    733.97 Stress fracture of shaft of femur
        Stress reaction of shaft of femur

        Use additional external cause code(s) to identify the cause of the stress fracture

    733.98 Stress fracture of pelvis
        Stress reaction of pelvis

        Use additional external cause code(s) to identify the cause of the stress fracture

    733.99 Other
        Diaphysitis
        Hypertrophy of bone
        Relapsing polychondritis
        Coding Clinic: 2000, Q3, P4; 1987, Jan-Feb, P14

734 Flat foot
    Pes planus (acquired)
    Talipes planus (acquired)

    | **Excludes** | *congenital (754.61)* |
            rigid flat foot (754.61)
            spastic (everted) flat foot (754.61)

Figure 13–3 **A.** Claw toes, right foot, secondary to medial and lateral plantar nerve laceration. **B.** Metatarsophalangeal joints of second and third toes could not be flexed to neutral position and none could be flexed past neutral. **C.** Extension posture of claw toes increases plantar pressure on metatarsal heads. (From Canale: Campbell's Operative Orthopaedics, 10th ed. 2003, Mosby, Inc.)

Item 13–6 **Claw toe** is caused by a contraction of the flexor tendon producing a flexion deformity characterized by hyperextension of the big toe.

Figure 13–4   Hallux valgus or bunion.

Item 13–7 **Hallux valgus, or bunion,** is a bursa usually found along the medial aspect of the big toe. It is most often attributed to heredity or poorly fitted shoes.

Item 13-8 **Hallux valgus** or bunion is a sometimes painful structural deformity caused by an inflammation of the bursal sac at the base of the metatarsophalangeal joint (big toe). **Hallus varus** is a deviation of the great toe to the inner side of the foot or away from the next toe.

● **735** **Acquired deformities of toe**
    Excludes *congenital (754.60–754.69, 755.65–755.66)*
    735.0 **Hallux valgus (acquired)**
    735.1 **Hallux varus (acquired)**
    735.2 **Hallux rigidus**
    735.3 **Hallux malleus**
    735.4 **Other hammer toe (acquired)**
    735.5 **Claw toe (acquired)**
       Coding Clinic: 2007, Q4, P123
    735.8 **Other acquired deformities of toe**
    735.9 **Unspecified acquired deformity of toe**

Item 13-9 Cubitus valgus is a deformity of the elbow resulting in an increased carrying angle in which the arm extends at the side and the palm faces forward, which results in the forearm and hand extended at greater than 15 degrees. Cubitus varus is a deformity of the elbow resulting in the arm extended at the side and the palm facing forward so that the forearm and hand are held at less than 5 degrees, decreasing the carrying angle.

● **736** **Other acquired deformities of limbs**
    Excludes *congenital (754.3–755.9)*
 ● **736.0** **Acquired deformities of forearm, excluding fingers**
    736.00 **Unspecified deformity**
       Deformity of elbow, forearm, hand, or wrist (acquired) NOS
    736.01 **Cubitus valgus (acquired)**
    736.02 **Cubitus varus (acquired)**
    736.03 **Valgus deformity of wrist (acquired)**
    736.04 **Varus deformity of wrist (acquired)**
    736.05 **Wrist drop (acquired)**
    736.06 **Claw hand (acquired)**
    736.07 **Club hand (acquired)**
    736.09 **Other**
    736.1 **Mallet finger**
 ● **736.2** **Other acquired deformities of finger**
    736.20 **Unspecified deformity**
       Deformity of finger (acquired) NOS
    736.21 **Boutonniere deformity**
    736.22 **Swan-neck deformity**
    736.29 **Other**
       Excludes *trigger finger (727.03)*
       Coding Clinic: 2005, Q2, P7; 1989, Q2, P13
 ● **736.3** **Acquired deformities of hip**
       Coding Clinic: 2008, Q2, P3-4
    736.30 **Unspecified deformity**
       Deformity of hip (acquired) NOS
    736.31 **Coxa valga (acquired)**
    736.32 **Coxa vara (acquired)**
    736.39 **Other**
 ● **736.4** **Genu valgum or varum (acquired)**
    736.41 **Genu valgum (acquired)**
    736.42 **Genu varum (acquired)**
    736.5 **Genu recurvatum (acquired)**
    736.6 **Other acquired deformities of knee**
       Deformity of knee (acquired) NOS

DISEASES OF THE MUSCULOSKELETAL SYSTEM AND CONNECTIVE TISSUE (710–739)

Figure 13–5 Supination and cavus deformity of forefoot. *(Courtesy Jay Cummings, MD.)* *(From Canale: Campbell's Operative Orthopaedics, 10th ed. 2003, Mosby, Inc.)*

Item 13–10 Equinus foot is a term referring to the hoof of a horse. The deformity is usually congenital or spastic. Talipes equinovarus is referred to as clubfoot. The foot tends to be smaller than normal, with the heel pointing downward and the forefoot turning inward. The heel cord (Achilles tendon) is tight, causing the heel to be drawn up toward the leg.

● **736.7 Other acquired deformities of ankle and foot**

> **Excludes** *deformities of toe (acquired) (735.0–735.9)*
> *pes planus (acquired) (734)*

736.70 Unspecified deformity of ankle and foot, acquired

736.71 Acquired equinovarus deformity
Clubfoot, acquired

> **Excludes** *clubfoot not specified as acquired (754.5–754.7)*

736.72 Equinus deformity of foot, acquired

736.73 Cavus deformity of foot

> **Excludes** *that with claw foot (736.74)*

736.74 Claw foot, acquired

736.75 Cavovarus deformity of foot, acquired

736.76 Other calcaneus deformity

736.79 Other
Acquired:
    pes not elsewhere classified
    talipes not elsewhere classified

● **736.8 Acquired deformities of other parts of limbs**
736.81 Unequal leg length (acquired)
Coding Clinic: 1995, Q1, P10

736.89 Other
Deformity (acquired):
    arm or leg, not elsewhere classified
    shoulder
Coding Clinic: 2008, Q2, P5-6

736.9 Acquired deformity of limb, site unspecified
Coding Clinic: 2008, Q2, P3-4

● **737 Curvature of spine**

> **Excludes** *congenital (754.2)*

737.0 Adolescent postural kyphosis

> **Excludes** *osteochondrosis of spine (juvenile) (732.0)*
> *adult (732.8)*

● **737.1 Kyphosis (acquired)**
737.10 Kyphosis (acquired) (postural)
737.11 Kyphosis due to radiation
737.12 Kyphosis, postlaminectomy
737.19 Other

> **Excludes** *that associated with conditions*
> *classifiable elsewhere (737.41)*

Coding Clinic: 2007, Q1, P20-21

● **737.2 Lordosis (acquired)**
Abnormal increase in normal curvature of lumbar spine (sway back)

737.20 Lordosis (acquired) (postural)
737.21 Lordosis, postlaminectomy
737.22 Other postsurgical lordosis
737.29 Other

> **Excludes** *that associated with conditions*
> *classifiable elsewhere (737.42)*

Item 13–11 Kyphosis is an abnormal curvature of the spine. **Senile kyphosis** is a result of disc degeneration causing ossification (turning to bone). **Adolescent** or **juvenile kyphosis** is also known as **Scheuermann's disease,** a condition in which the discs of the lower thoracic spine herniate, causing the disc space to narrow and the spine to tilt forward. This condition is attributed to poor posture. Lordosis or swayback is an abnormal curvature of the spine resulting in an inward curve of the lumbar spine just above the buttocks. Scoliosis causes a sideways curve to the spine. The curves are S- or C-shaped, and it is most commonly acquired in late childhood and early teen years, when growth is fast.

Item 13–12 Spondylolisthesis is a condition caused by the slipping forward of one disc over another.

Figure 13–6 Scoliosis is a lateral curvature of the spine.

DISEASES OF THE MUSCULOSKELETAL SYSTEM AND CONNECTIVE TISSUE (710–739)

◀ New   ◀▥ Revised   ~~deleted~~ Deleted   ● Unacceptable Principal Diagnosis   ● Use Additional Digit(s)
▶ Manifestation Code   **OGCR** Official Guidelines   **Coding Clinic**   Excludes   Includes   Use additional   Code first   Omit code

● 737.3 **Kyphoscoliosis and scoliosis**

     737.30 **Scoliosis [and kyphoscoliosis], idiopathic**
         Coding Clinic: 2003, Q3, P19x2

     737.31 **Resolving infantile idiopathic scoliosis**

     737.32 **Progressive infantile idiopathic scoliosis**
         Coding Clinic: 2002, Q3, P12

     737.33 **Scoliosis due to radiation**

     737.34 **Thoracogenic scoliosis**

     737.39 **Other**
         Excludes *that associated with conditions*
                 classifiable elsewhere (737.43)
                 that in kyphoscoliotic heart disease
                 (416.1)
         Coding Clinic: 2002, Q2, P16

● 737.4 **Curvature of spine associated with other conditions**

     Code first associated condition, as:
         Charcot-Marie-Tooth disease (356.1)
         mucopolysaccharidosis (277.5)
         neurofibromatosis (237.7)
         osteitis deformans (731.0)
         osteitis fibrosa cystica (252.01)
         osteoporosis (733.00–733.09)
         poliomyelitis (138)
         tuberculosis [Pott's curvature] (015.0)

     ▶ 737.40 *Curvature of spine, unspecified*

     ▶ 737.41 *Kyphosis*

     ▶ 737.42 *Lordosis*

     ▶ 737.43 *Scoliosis*

     737.8 **Other curvatures of spine**

     737.9 **Unspecified curvature of spine**
         Curvature of spine (acquired) (idiopathic) NOS
         Hunchback, acquired
         Excludes *deformity of spine NOS (738.5)*

● 738 **Other acquired deformity**
     Excludes *congenital (754.0–756.9, 758.0–759.9)*
                 dentofacial anomalies (524.0–524.9)

     738.0 **Acquired deformity of nose**
         Deformity of nose (acquired)
         Overdevelopment of nasal bones
         Excludes *deflected or deviated nasal septum (470)*

● 738.1 **Other acquired deformity of head**

     738.10 **Unspecified deformity**

     738.11 **Zygomatic hyperplasia**

     738.12 **Zygomatic hypoplasia**

     738.19 **Other specified deformity**
         Coding Clinic: 2006, Q1, P6-7; 2003, Q2, P13

     738.2 **Acquired deformity of neck**

     738.3 **Acquired deformity of chest and rib**
         Deformity:
            chest (acquired)
            rib (acquired)
         Pectus:
            carinatum, acquired
            excavatum, acquired

     738.4 **Acquired spondylolisthesis**
         Degenerative spondylolisthesis
         Spondylolysis, acquired
         Excludes *congenital (756.12)*
         Coding Clinic: 2007, Q4, P116-120

     738.5 **Other acquired deformity of back or spine**
         Deformity of spine NOS
         Excludes *curvature of spine (737.0–737.9)*
         Coding Clinic: 2007, Q4, P116-120

     738.6 **Acquired deformity of pelvis**
         Pelvic obliquity
         Excludes *intrapelvic protrusion of acetabulum (718.6)*
                 that in relation to labor and delivery
                 (653.0–653.4, 653.8–653.9)

     738.7 **Cauliflower ear**

     738.8 **Acquired deformity of other specified site**
         Deformity of clavicle
         Coding Clinic: 2001, Q2, P14-15

     738.9 **Acquired deformity of unspecified site**

● 739 **Nonallopathic lesions, not elsewhere classified**
     Includes segmental dysfunction
                   somatic dysfunction
     Coding Clinic: 1995, Q4, P51; 1990, Q1, P18

     739.0 **Head region**
         Occipitocervical region

     739.1 **Cervical region**
         Cervicothoracic region

     739.2 **Thoracic region**
         Thoracolumbar region

     739.3 **Lumbar region**
         Lumbosacral region

     739.4 **Sacral region**
         Sacrococcygeal region
         Sacroiliac region

     739.5 **Pelvic region**
         Hip region
         Pubic region

     739.6 **Lower extremities**

     739.7 **Upper extremities**
         Acromioclavicular region
         Sternoclavicular region

     739.8 **Rib cage**
         Costochondral region
         Costovertebral region
         Sternochondral region

     739.9 **Abdomen and other**

DISEASES OF THE MUSCULOSKELETAL SYSTEM AND CONNECTIVE TISSUE (710–739)

N Newborn Age: 0   **P** Pediatric Age: 0–17   **M** Maternity Age: 12–55   **A** Adult Age: 15–124   ♀ Females Only   ♂ Males Only

Ⓔ⒳ CC Exclusions   ◕ Complication\Comorbidity   ◔ Major C\C   ◔ Present on Admission Requirement   ◔ Hospital-Acquired Condition   **1021**

Figure 14–1 Generalized craniosynostosis in a 4-year-old girl without symptoms or signs of increased intracranial pressure. (From Bell WE, McCormick WF: Increased Intracranial Pressure in Children, 2nd ed. Philadelphia, WB Saunders, 1978, p 116.)

Item 14–1 **Anencephalus** is a congenital deformity of the cranial vault. **Craniosynostosis**, also known as craniostenosis and stenocephaly, signifies any form of congenital deformity of the skull that results from the premature closing of the sutures of the skull. **Iniencephaly** is a deformity in which the head and neck are flexed backward to a great extent and the head is very large in comparison to the shortened body.

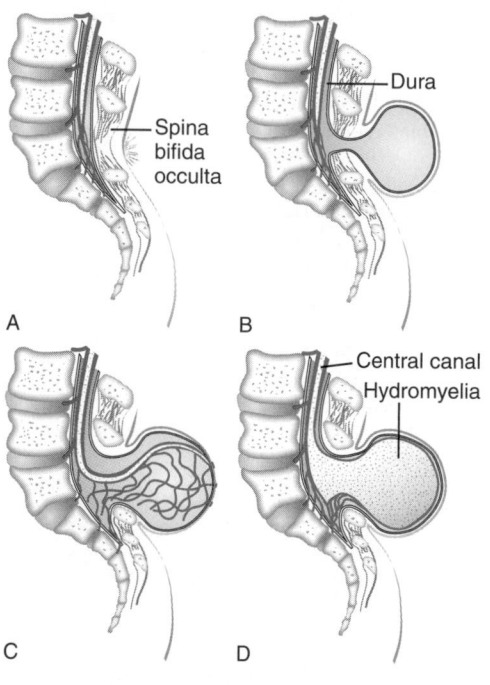

Figure 14–2 **A.** Spina bifida occulta. **B.** Meningocele. **C.** Myelomeningocele. **D.** Myelocystocele (syringomyelocele) or hydromyelia.

Item 14–2 **Spina bifida** is a midline spinal defect in which one or more vertebrae fail to fuse, leaving an opening in the vertebral canal. When the defect is not visible, it is called spina bifida occulta, and when it is visible, it is called spina bifida cystica.

Figure 14–3 An infant with a large occipital encephalocele. The large skin-covered encephalocele is visible. (From Townsend: Sabiston Textbook of Surgery, 17th ed. 2004, Saunders, An Imprint of Elsevier)

14.   CONGENITAL ANOMALIES (740–759)

● **740   Anencephalus and similar anomalies**

    740.0   Anencephalus 🔖
       Acrania
       Amyelencephalus
       Hemianencephaly
       Hemicephaly
       Ⓔx 740.0-740.2

    740.1   Craniorachischisis 🔖
       Ⓔx 740.0-740.2

    740.2   Iniencephaly 🔖
       740.0-740.2

● **741   Spina bifida**

    Ⓔ**Excludes**   *spina bifida occulta (756.17)*

    Coding Clinic: 1994, Q3, P7

    The following fifth-digit subclassification is for use with category 741:

    0   unspecified region
    1   cervical region
    2   dorsal (thoracic) region
    3   lumbar region

●   **741.0   With hydrocephalus** 🔖
    [0-3]   Arnold-Chiari syndrome, type II
         Any condition classifiable to 741.9 with any condition classifiable to 742.3
         Chiari malformation, type II
         Ⓔx 741.00-741.93, 742.59-742.9, 759.7-759.89
         Coding Clinic: 1997, Q4, P51; 1987, Sept-Oct, P10

●   **741.9   Without mention of hydrocephalus**
    [0-3]   Hydromeningocele (spinal)
         Hydromyelocele
         Meningocele (spinal)
         Meningomyelocele
         Myelocele
         Myelocystocele
         Rachischisis
         Spina bifida (aperta)
         Syringomyelocele
         Coding Clinic: 1987, Sept-Oct, P10

● **742   Other congenital anomalies of nervous system**

    Ⓔ**Excludes**   *congenital central alveolar hypoventilation syndrome (327.25)*

    742.0   Encephalocele 🔖
      Sac-like protrusions of brain and membranes visible through an opening in various locations in skull
       Encephalocystocele
       Encephalomyelocele
       Hydroencephalocele
       Hydromeningocele, cranial
       Meningocele, cerebral
       Meningoencephalocele
       Ⓔx 742.0-742.2, 742.4

    742.1   Microcephalus
      Describes head size that measures significantly below normal based on standardized charts for age and sex
       Hydromicrocephaly
       Micrencephaly

◀ New   ◀ Revised   ~~deleted~~ Deleted   ● Unacceptable Principal Diagnosis   ● Use Additional Digit(s)
▶ Manifestation Code   **OGCR** Official Guidelines   **Coding Clinic**   Excludes   Includes   Use additional   Code first   Omit code

742.2 Reduction deformities of brain
    Absence of part of brain
    Agenesis of part of brain
    Agyria
    Aplasia of part of brain
    Arhinencephaly
    Holoprosencephaly
    Hypoplasia of part of brain
    Microgyria
    (Ex) 742.0-742.2, 742.4
    Coding Clinic: 2003, Q3, P15-16

742.3 Congenital hydrocephalus
    An accumulation of cerebrospinal fluid in ventricles
        resulting in swelling and enlargement
    Aqueduct of Sylvius:
      anomaly
      obstruction, congenital
      stenosis
    Atresia of foramina of Magendie and Luschka
    Hydrocephalus in newborn

    | **Excludes** | *hydrocephalus:* |
             acquired (331.3–331.4)
             due to congenital toxoplasmosis (771.2)
             with any condition classifiable to 741.9
                 (741.0)

    Coding Clinic: 2005, Q4, P82-83

742.4 Other specified anomalies of brain
    Congenital cerebral cyst
    Macroencephaly
    Macrogyria
    Megalencephaly
    Multiple anomalies of brain NOS
    Porencephaly
    Ulegyria
    (Ex) 742.4
    Coding Clinic: 1999, Q1, P9-10; 1992, Q3, P12

742.5 Other specified anomalies of spinal cord

    742.51 Diastematomyelia

    742.53 Hydromyelia
        Hydrorhachis

    742.59 Other
        Amyelia
        Atelomyelia
        Congenital anomaly of spinal meninges
        Defective development of cauda equina
        Hypoplasia of spinal cord
        Myelatelia
        Myelodysplasia
        Coding Clinic: 1991, Q2, P14; 1989, Q1, P10

742.8 Other specified anomalies of nervous system
    Agenesis of nerve
    Displacement of brachial plexus
    Familial dysautonomia
    Jaw-winking syndrome
    Marcus-Gunn syndrome
    Riley-Day syndrome

    | **Excludes** | *neurofibromatosis (237.7)* |

742.9 Unspecified anomaly of brain, spinal cord, and nervous system
    Anomaly of brain, nervous system, and spinal cord
    Congenital, of brain, nervous system, and spinal cord:
      disease of brain, nervous system, and spinal
        cord
      lesion of brain, nervous system, and spinal cord
    Deformity of brain, nervous system, and spinal cord

● **743 Congenital anomalies of eye**

● **743.0 Anophthalmos**
    Absence of eye and optic pit

    743.00 Clinical anophthalmos, unspecified
        Agenesis
        Congenital absence of eye
        Anophthalmos NOS

    743.03 Cystic eyeball, congenital

    743.06 Cryptophthalmos

● **743.1 Microphthalmos**
    Partial absence of eye and optic pit
    Dysplasia of eye
    Hypoplasia of eye
    Rudimentary eye

    743.10 Microphthalmos, unspecified

    743.11 Simple microphthalmos

    743.12 Microphthalmos associated with other anomalies of eye and adnexa

Figure 14–4   Bilateral congenital **hydrophthalmia,** in which the eyes are very large in comparison to the other facial features due to glaucoma.

● **743.2 Buphthalmos**
    Also known as Sturge-Weber Syndrome and is
        congenital syndrome characterized by a port-wine
        nevus covering portions of face and cranium
    Glaucoma:
      congenital
      newborn
    Hydrophthalmos

    | **Excludes** | *glaucoma of childhood (365.14)* |
             traumatic glaucoma due to birth injury
                 (767.8)

    743.20 Buphthalmos, unspecified

    743.21 Simple buphthalmos

    743.22 Buphthalmos associated with other ocular anomalies
        Keratoglobus, congenital, associated with
          buphthalmos
        Megalocornea associated with buphthalmos

● **743.3 Congenital cataract and lens anomalies**

    | **Excludes** | *infantile cataract (366.00–366.09)* |

    743.30 Congenital cataract, unspecified

    743.31 Capsular and subcapsular cataract

    743.32 Cortical and zonular cataract

CONGENITAL ANOMALIES (740–759)

743.33 Nuclear cataract

743.34 Total and subtotal cataract, congenital

743.35 Congenital aphakia
Congenital absence of lens

743.36 Anomalies of lens shape
Microphakia
Spherophakia

743.37 Congenital ectopic lens

743.39 Other

● **743.4 Coloboma and other anomalies of anterior segment**

743.41 Anomalies of corneal size and shape
Microcornea

| Excludes | *that associated with buphthalmos (743.22)* |

743.42 Corneal opacities, interfering with vision, congenital

743.43 Other corneal opacities, congenital

743.44 Specified anomalies of anterior chamber, chamber angle, and related structures
Anomaly:
Axenfeld's
Peters'
Rieger's

743.45 Aniridia
Coding Clinic: 2002, Q3, P20-21

743.46 Other specified anomalies of iris and ciliary body
Anisocoria, congenital
Atresia of pupil
Coloboma of iris
Corectopia

743.47 Specified anomalies of sclera

743.48 Multiple and combined anomalies of anterior segment

743.49 Other

● **743.5 Congenital anomalies of posterior segment**

743.51 Vitreous anomalies
Congenital vitreous opacity

743.52 Fundus coloboma

743.53 Chorioretinal degeneration, congenital

743.54 Congenital folds and cysts of posterior segment

743.55 Congenital macular changes

743.56 Other retinal changes, congenital
Coding Clinic: 1999, Q3, P12

743.57 Specified anomalies of optic disc
Coloboma of optic disc (congenital)

743.58 Vascular anomalies
Congenital retinal aneurysm

743.59 Other

● **743.6 Congenital anomalies of eyelids, lacrimal system, and orbit**

743.61 Congenital ptosis

743.62 Congenital deformities of eyelids
Ablepharon
Absence of eyelid
Accessory eyelid
Congenital:
ectropion
entropion
Coding Clinic: 2000, Q1, P22-23

743.63 Other specified congenital anomalies of eyelid
Absence, agenesis, of cilia

743.64 Specified congenital anomalies of lacrimal gland

743.65 Specified congenital anomalies of lacrimal passages
Absence, agenesis of:
lacrimal apparatus
punctum lacrimale
Accessory lacrimal canal

743.66 Specified congenital anomalies of orbit

743.69 Other
Accessory eye muscles

743.8 Other specified anomalies of eye

Excludes	*congenital nystagmus (379.51)*
	ocular albinism (270.2)
	optic nerve hypoplasia (377.43)
	retinitis pigmentosa (362.74)

743.9 Unspecified anomaly of eye
Congenital:
anomaly NOS of eye [any part]
deformity NOS of eye [any part]

● **744 Congenital anomalies of ear, face, and neck**

Excludes	*anomaly of:*
	cervical spine (754.2, 756.10–756.19)
	larynx (748.2–748.3)
	nose (748.0–748.1)
	parathyroid gland (759.2)
	thyroid gland (759.2)
	cleft lip (749.10–749.25)

● **744.0 Anomalies of ear causing impairment of hearing**

| Excludes | *congenital deafness without mention of cause (380.0–389.9)* |

744.00 Unspecified anomaly of ear with impairment of hearing

744.01 Absence of external ear
Absence of:
auditory canal (external)
auricle (ear) (with stenosis or atresia of auditory canal)

744.02 Other anomalies of external ear with impairment of hearing
Atresia or stricture of auditory canal (external)

744.03 Anomaly of middle ear, except ossicles
Atresia or stricture of osseous meatus (ear)

744.04 Anomalies of ear ossicles
Fusion of ear ossicles

744.05 Anomalies of inner ear
Congenital anomaly of:
membranous labyrinth
organ of Corti

744.09 Other
Absence of ear, congenital

◀ New   ◀╍ Revised   ~~deleted~~ Deleted   ● Unacceptable Principal Diagnosis   ● Use Additional Digit(s)
▶ Manifestation Code   **OGCR** Official Guidelines   **Coding Clinic**   Excludes   Includes   Use additional   Code first   Omit code

744.1 Accessory auricle
　　Accessory tragus
　　Polyotia
　　Preauricular appendage
　　Supernumerary:
　　　　ear
　　　　lobule

● **744.2 Other specified anomalies of ear**
　　| **Excludes** | *that with impairment of hearing*
　　　　　　　　　(744.00–744.09)

　　744.21 Absence of ear lobe, congenital

　　744.22 Macrotia
　　　　Enlarged ear

　　744.23 Microtia
　　　　Abnormally small ear

　　744.24 Specified anomalies of Eustachian tube
　　　　Absence of Eustachian tube

　　744.29 Other
　　　　Bat ear
　　　　Darwin's tubercle
　　　　Pointed ear
　　　　Prominence of auricle
　　　　Ridge ear
　　　　| **Excludes** | *preauricular sinus (744.46)*

744.3 Unspecified anomaly of ear
　　Congenital:
　　　　anomaly NOS of ear, NEC
　　　　deformity NOS of ear, NEC

● **744.4 Branchial cleft cyst or fistula; preauricular sinus**

　　744.41 Branchial cleft sinus or fistula
　　　　Branchial:
　　　　　　sinus (external) (internal)
　　　　　　vestige

　　744.42 Branchial cleft cyst

　　744.43 Cervical auricle

　　744.46 Preauricular sinus or fistula

　　744.47 Preauricular cyst

　　744.49 Other
　　　　Fistula (of):
　　　　　　auricle, congenital
　　　　　　cervicoaural

744.5 Webbing of neck
　　Pterygium colli

● **744.8 Other specified anomalies of face and neck**

　　744.81 Macrocheilia
　　　　Hypertrophy of lip, congenital

　　744.82 Microcheilia

　　744.83 Macrostomia
　　　　Abnormally large mouth

　　744.84 Microstomia

　　744.89 Other
　　　　| **Excludes** | *congenital fistula of lip (750.25)*
　　　　　　　　　musculoskeletal anomalies
　　　　　　　　　　(754.0–754.1, 756.0)

744.9 Unspecified anomalies of face and neck
　　Congenital:
　　　　anomaly NOS of face [any part] or neck [any part]
　　　　deformity NOS of face [any part] or neck [any part]

● **745 Bulbus cordis anomalies and anomalies of cardiac septal closure**

　　745.0 Common truncus ℃
　　　　Absent septum between aorta and pulmonary artery
　　　　Communication (abnormal) between aorta and pulmonary artery
　　　　Aortic septal defect
　　　　Common aortopulmonary trunk
　　　　Persistent truncus arteriosus
　　　　(Ex) 429.71 -429.79, 745.0-745.9, 746.89-746.9, 747.83-747.9, 759.7-759.89

● **745.1 Transposition of great vessels**

　　745.10 Complete transposition of great vessels ℃
　　　　Transposition of great vessels:
　　　　　　NOS
　　　　　　classical
　　　　(Ex) 429.71-429.79, 745.0-745.9, 746.89 -746.9, 747.83-747.9, 759.7-759.89

　　745.11 Double outlet right ventricle ℃
　　　　Dextrotransposition of aorta
　　　　Incomplete transposition of great vessels
　　　　Origin of both great vessels from right ventricle
　　　　Taussig-Bing syndrome or defect
　　　　(Ex) 429.71-429.79, 745.0-745.9, 746.89-746.9, 747.83-747.9, 759.7-759.89

　　745.12 Corrected transposition of great vessels ℃
　　　　(Ex) 429.71-429.79, 745.0-745.9, 746.89-746.9, 747.83-747.9, 759.7-759.89

　　745.19 Other ℃
　　　　(Ex) 429.71-429.79, 745.0-745.9, 746.89-746.9, 747.83-747.9, 759.7-759.89

　　745.2 Tetralogy of Fallot ℃
　　　　Fallot's pentalogy
　　　　Ventricular septal defect with pulmonary stenosis or atresia, dextroposition of aorta, and hypertrophy of right ventricle
　　　　| **Excludes** | *Fallot's triad (746.09)*
　　　　(Ex) 429.71-429.79, 745.0-745.9, 746.89-746.9, 747.83-747.9, 759.7-759.89

　　745.3 Common ventricle ℃
　　　　Cor triloculare biatriatum
　　　　Single ventricle
　　　　(Ex) 429.71-429.79, 745.0-745.9, 746.89-746.9, 747.83-747.9, 759.7-759.89

　　745.4 Ventricular septal defect ℃
　　　　Eisenmenger's defect or complex
　　　　Gerbode defect
　　　　Interventricular septal defect
　　　　Left ventricular-right atrial communication
　　　　Roger's disease
　　　　| **Excludes** | *common atrioventricular canal type*
　　　　　　　　　(745.69)
　　　　　　　　　single ventricle (745.3)
　　　　(Ex) 429.71-429.79, 745.0-745.9, 746.89-746.9, 747.83-747.9, 759.7-759.89

　　745.5 Ostium secundum type atrial septal defect ℃
　　　　Defect:　　　　　　　　　Patent or persistent:
　　　　　　atrium secundum　　　　foramen ovale
　　　　　　fossa ovalis　　　　　　ostium secundum
　　　　Lutembacher's syndrome
　　　　(Ex) 429.71-429.79, 745.0-745.3, 745.5-745.9, 746.89-746.9, 747.89-747.9, 759.7, 759.89

CONGENITAL ANOMALIES (740–759)

CONGENITAL ANOMALIES (740–759)

● **745.6 Endocardial cushion defects**

  745.60 Endocardial cushion defect, unspecified type🔓
    Ex: 429.71-429.79, 745.0-745.9, 746.89-746.9, 747.83-747.9, 759.7-759.89

  745.61 Ostium primum defect🔓
    Persistent ostium primum
    Ex: 429.71-429.79, 745.0-745.3, 745.5-745.9, 746.89-746.9, 747.89-747.9, 759.7, 759.89

  745.69 Other🔓
    Absence of atrial septum
    Atrioventricular canal type ventricular septal defect
    Common atrioventricular canal
    Common atrium
    Ex: 429.71-429.79, 745.0-745.9, 746.89-746.9, 747.83-747.9, 759.7-759.89

745.7 Cor biloculare🔓
  Absence of atrial and ventricular septa
  Ex: 429.71-429.79, 745.0-745.9, 746.89-746.9, 747.83-747.9, 759.7-759.89

745.8 Other

745.9 Unspecified defect of septal closure
  Septal defect NOS

● **746 Other congenital anomalies of heart**
  Excludes *endocardial fibroelastosis (425.3)*
  Coding Clinic: 2004, Q3, P4-5

● **746.0 Anomalies of pulmonary valve**
  Excludes *infundibular or subvalvular pulmonic stenosis (746.83)*
  tetralogy of Fallot (745.2)

  746.00 Pulmonary valve anomaly, unspecified🔓
    Ex: 746.00-746.09, 746.89-746.9, 747.89-747.9, 759.7, 759.89

  746.01 Atresia, congenital🔓
    Congenital absence of pulmonary valve
    Ex: 746.00-746.09, 746.89-746.9, 747.83-747.9, 759.7-759.89

  746.02 Stenosis, congenital🔓
    Ex: 746.00-746.09, 746.89-746.9, 747.83-747.9, 759.7-759.89
    Coding Clinic: 2004, Q1, P16-17

  746.09 Other🔓
    Congenital insufficiency of pulmonary valve
    Fallot's triad or trilogy
    Ex: 746.00-746.09, 746.89-746.9, 747.89-747.9, 759.7, 759.89

746.1 Tricuspid atresia and stenosis, congenital🔓
  Absence of tricuspid valve
  Ex: 746.1-746.7, 7468.9-746.9, 747.83-747.9, 759.7-759.89

746.2 Ebstein's anomaly🔓
  Ex: 746.1-746.7, 746.89-746.9, 747.83-747.9, 759.7-759.89

746.3 Congenital stenosis of aortic valve🔓
  Congenital aortic stenosis
  Excludes *congenital:*
    subaortic stenosis (746.81)
    supravalvular aortic stenosis (747.22)
  Ex: 746.1-746.7, 746.89-746.9, 747.83-747.9, 759.7-759.89
  Coding Clinic: 1988, Q4, P8

746.4 Congenital insufficiency of aortic valve🔓
  Bicuspid aortic valve
  Congenital aortic insufficiency
  Ex: 746.1-746.7, 746.89-746.9, 747.83-747.9, 759.7-759.89

746.5 Congenital mitral stenosis🔓
  Fused commissure of mitral valve
  Parachute deformity of mitral valve
  Supernumerary cusps of mitral valve
  Ex: 746.1-746.7, 746.89-746.9, 747.83-747.9, 759.7-759.89
  Coding Clinic: 2007, Q3, P3

746.6 Congenital mitral insufficiency🔓
  Ex: 746.1-746.7, 746.89-746.9, 747.83-747.9, 759.7-759.89

746.7 Hypoplastic left heart syndrome🔓
  Atresia, or marked hypoplasia, of aortic orifice or valve, with hypoplasia of ascending aorta and defective development of left ventricle (with mitral valve atresia)
  Ex: 746.1-746.7, 746.89-746.9, 747.83-747.9, 759.7-759.89

● **746.8 Other specified anomalies of heart**

  746.81 Subaortic stenosis🔓
    Ex: 746.81-746.84, 746.89-746.9, 747.83-747.9, 759.7-759.89
    Coding Clinic: 2007, Q3, P3

  746.82 Cor triatriatum🔓
    Ex: 746.81-746.84, 746.89-746.9, 747.83-747.9, 759.7-759.89

  746.83 Infundibular pulmonic stenosis🔓
    Subvalvular pulmonic stenosis
    Ex: 746.81-746.84, 746.89-746.9, 747.83-747.9, 759.7-759.89

  746.84 Obstructive anomalies of heart, NEC🔓
    Shone's syndrome
    Uhl's disease
    Use additional code for associated anomalies, such as:
      coarctation of aorta (747.10)
      congenital mitral stenosis (746.5)
      subaortic stenosis (746.81)
    Ex: 746.81-746.84, 746.89-746.9, 747.83-747.9, 759.7-759.89

  746.85 Coronary artery anomaly🔓
    Anomalous origin or communication of coronary artery
    Arteriovenous malformation of coronary artery
    Coronary artery:
      absence
      arising from aorta or pulmonary trunk
      single
    Ex: 746.85, 746.89-746.9

  746.86 Congenital heart block🔓
    Complete or incomplete atrioventricular [AV] block
    Ex: 746.86, 746.89-746.9, 747.83-747.9, 759.7-759.89

  746.87 Malposition of heart and cardiac apex🔓
    Abdominal heart
    Dextrocardia
    Ectopia cordis
    Levocardia (isolated)
    Mesocardia
    Excludes *dextrocardia with complete transposition of viscera (759.3)*
    Ex: 746.81-746.84, 746.87-746.9, 747.89-747.9, 759.7, 759.89

  746.89 Other
    Atresia of cardiac vein
    Hypoplasia of cardiac vein
    Congenital:
      cardiomegaly
      diverticulum, left ventricle
      pericardial defect
    Coding Clinic: 2000, Q3, P3; 1999, Q1, P11; 1995, Q1, P8

746.9 Unspecified anomaly of heart
  Congenital:
    anomaly of heart NOS
    heart disease NOS

◀ New   ◀▥ Revised   ~~deleted~~ Deleted   ● Unacceptable Principal Diagnosis   ● Use Additional Digit(s)
▶ Manifestation Code   **OGCR** Official Guidelines   **Coding Clinic**   Excludes   Includes   Use additional   Code first   Omit code

● **747   Other congenital anomalies of circulatory system**

  747.0   Patent ductus arteriosus *(PDA)* 🌑
      Patent ductus Botalli
      Persistent ductus arteriosus
      (Ex:) 747.0, 747.89

● **747.1   Coarctation of aorta**

  747.10   Coarctation of aorta (preductal) (postductal) 🌑
      Hypoplasia of aortic arch
      (Ex:) 747.10-747.22, 747.89-747.9, 759.7, 759.89
      Coding Clinic: 2007, Q3, P3; 1999, Q1, P11; 1988, Q4, P8

  747.11   Interruption of aortic arch 🌑
      (Ex:) 747.10-747.22, 747.83-747.9, 759.7-759.89

● **747.2   Other anomalies of aorta**

  747.20   Anomaly of aorta, unspecified 🌑
      (Ex:) 747.10-747.22, 747.89-747.9, 759.7, 759.89

  747.21   Anomalies of aortic arch 🌑
      Anomalous origin, right subclavian artery
      Dextroposition of aorta
      Double aortic arch
      Kommerell's diverticulum
      Overriding aorta
      Persistent:
        convolutions, aortic arch
        right aortic arch
      Vascular ring

      | **Excludes** | *hypoplasia of aortic arch (747.10)* |

      (Ex:) 747.10-747.22, 747.89-747.9, 759.7, 759.89
      Coding Clinic: 2003, Q1, P15-16

  747.22   Atresia and stenosis of aorta 🌑
      Absence of aorta
      Aplasia of aorta
      Hypoplasia of aorta
      Stricture of aorta
      Supra (valvular)-aortic stenosis

      | **Excludes** | *congenital aortic (valvular) stenosis or stricture, so stated (746.3)* |
      | | *hypoplasia of aorta in hypoplastic left heart syndrome (746.7)* |

      (Ex:) 747.10-747.22, 747.83-747.9, 759.7-759.89
      Coding Clinic: 1988, Q4, P8

  747.29   Other 🌑
      Aneurysm of sinus of Valsalva
      Congenital: Congenital:
        aneurysm of aorta   dilation of aorta
      (Ex:) 747.10-747.29, 747.89-747.9, 759.7, 759.89

  747.3   Anomalies of pulmonary artery 🌑
      Agenesis of pulmonary artery
      Anomaly of pulmonary artery
      Atresia of pulmonary artery
      Coarctation of pulmonary artery
      Hypoplasia of pulmonary artery
      Stenosis of pulmonary artery
      Pulmonary arteriovenous aneurysm
      (Ex:) 747.3, 747.89-747.9
      Coding Clinic: 2004, Q1, P16-17; 1994, Q1, P15

● **747.4   Anomalies of great veins**

  747.40   Anomaly of great veins, unspecified 🌑
      Anomaly NOS of: Anomaly NOS of:
        pulmonary veins   vena cava
      (Ex:) 747.40, 747.89-747.9

  747.41   Total anomalous pulmonary venous connection 🌑
      Total anomalous pulmonary venous return
        [TAPVR]:
        subdiaphragmatic
        supradiaphragmatic
      (Ex:) 747.41, 747.89-747.9

  747.42   Partial anomalous pulmonary venous connection 🌑
      Partial anomalous pulmonary venous
        return
      (Ex:) 747.42, 747.89-747.9

  747.49   Other anomalies of great veins 🌑
      Absence of vena cava (inferior) (superior)
      Congenital stenosis of vena cava (inferior)
        (superior)
      Persistent:
        left posterior cardinal vein
        left superior vena cava
      Scimitar syndrome
      Transposition of pulmonary veins NOS
      (Ex:) 747.49, 747.89-747.9

  747.5   Absence or hypoplasia of umbilical artery
      Single umbilical artery

● **747.6   Other anomalies of peripheral vascular system**
      Absence of artery or vein, NEC
      Anomaly of artery or vein, NEC
      Atresia of artery or vein, NEC
      Arteriovenous aneurysm (peripheral)
      Arteriovenous malformation of the peripheral
        vascular system
      Congenital: Congenital:
        aneurysm (peripheral)   stricture, artery
        phlebectasia   varix
      Multiple renal arteries

      | **Excludes** | *anomalies of:* |
      | | *cerebral vessels (747.81)* |
      | | *pulmonary artery (747.3)* |
      | | *congenital retinal aneurysm (743.58)* |
      | | *hemangioma (228.00–228.09)* |
      | | *lymphangioma (228.1)* |

  747.60   Anomaly of the peripheral vascular system, unspecified site

  747.61   Gastrointestinal vessel anomaly
      Coding Clinic: 1996, Q3, P10

  747.62   Renal vessel anomaly

  747.63   Upper limb vessel anomaly

  747.64   Lower limb vessel anomaly

  747.69   Anomalies of other specified sites of peripheral vascular system

CONGENITAL ANOMALIES (740–759)

● **747.8   Other specified anomalies of circulatory system**

     747.81   Anomalies of cerebrovascular system🅱

         Arteriovenous malformation of brain
         Cerebral arteriovenous aneurysm,
            congenital
         Congenital anomalies of cerebral vessels

         | Excludes | *ruptured cerebral (arteriovenous)*
                       aneurysm (430)

         (Ex:) 747.81, 747.89-747.9
         Coding Clinic: 1985, Jan-Feb, P15

     747.82   Spinal vessel anomaly🅱

         Arteriovenous malformation of spinal
            vessel

         (Ex:) 747.82, 747.89-747.9
         Coding Clinic: 1995, Q3, P5-6

     747.83   Persistent fetal circulation🅱   **N**

         Persistent pulmonary hypertension
         Primary pulmonary hypertension of
            newborn

         (Ex:) 416.0, 416.8-416.9
         Coding Clinic: 2002, Q4, P62-63

     747.89   Other🅱

         Aneurysm, congenital, specified site not
            elsewhere classified

         | Excludes | *congenital aneurysm:*
                       coronary (746.85)
                       peripheral (747.6)
                       pulmonary (747.3)
                       retinal (743.58)

         (Ex:) 745.0-745.9, 747.89

    747.9   Unspecified anomaly of circulatory system🅱

         (Ex:) 745.0-747.82, 747.89-747.9

● **748   Congenital anomalies of respiratory system**

    | Excludes | *congenital central alveolar hypoventilation*
                syndrome (327.25)
                congenital defect of diaphragm (756.6)

   748.0   Choanal atresia

       Atresia of nares (anterior) (posterior)
       Congenital stenosis of nares (anterior) (posterior)

   748.1   Other anomalies of nose

       Absent nose
       Accessory nose
       Cleft nose
       Deformity of wall of nasal sinus
       Congenital:
          deformity of nose
          notching of tip of nose
          perforation of wall of nasal sinus

       | Excludes | *congenital deviation of nasal septum (754.0)*

   748.2   Web of larynx

       Web of larynx: Web of larynx:
         NOS   subglottic
         glottic

748.3   Other anomalies of larynx, trachea, and bronchus🅱

       Absence or agenesis of:
         bronchus
         larynx
         trachea
       Anomaly (of):   Anomaly (of):
         cricoid cartilage   thyroid cartilage
         epiglottis   tracheal cartilage
       Atresia (of):   Atresia (of):
         epiglottis   larynx
         glottis   trachea
       Cleft thyroid, cartilage, congenital
       Congenital:
         dilation, trachea
         stenosis:
           larynx
           trachea
         tracheocele
       Diverticulum:
         bronchus
         trachea
       Fissure of epiglottis
       Laryngocele
       Posterior cleft of cricoid cartilage (congenital)
       Rudimentary tracheal bronchus
       Stridor, laryngeal, congenital

       (Ex:) 493.81, 519.19, 748.3, 748.8-748.9
       Coding Clinic: 1999, Q1, P14

748.4   Congenital cystic lung🅱

       Disease, lung:
         cystic, congenital
         polycystic, congenital
       Honeycomb lung, congenital

       | Excludes | *acquired or unspecified cystic lung (518.89)*

       (Ex:) 748.4-748.9

748.5   Agenesis, hypoplasia, and dysplasia of lung🅱

       Absence of lung (fissures) (lobe)
       Aplasia of lung
       Hypoplasia of lung (lobe)
       Sequestration of lung

       (Ex:) 748.4-748.9

● **748.6   Other anomalies of lung**

     748.60   Anomaly of lung, unspecified

     748.61   Congenital bronchiectasis🅱

         (Ex:) 494.0-494.1, 496, 506.1, 506.4-506.9, 748.61

     748.69   Other

         Accessory lung (lobe)
         Azygos lobe (fissure), lung

748.8   Other specified anomalies of respiratory system

       Abnormal communication between pericardial and
         pleural sacs
       Anomaly, pleural folds
       Atresia of nasopharynx
       Congenital cyst of mediastinum

748.9   Unspecified anomaly of respiratory system

       Anomaly of respiratory system NOS

CONGENITAL ANOMALIES (740–759)

◄ New   ◄ᴵᴵᴵ Revised   ~~deleted~~ Deleted   ● Unacceptable Principal Diagnosis   ● Use Additional Digit(s)
▶ Manifestation Code   **OGCR** Official Guidelines   **Coding Clinic** | Excludes | Includes   Use additional   Code first   Omit code

Figure 14–5 Cleft palate.

● **749 Cleft palate and cleft lip**

  ● **749.0 Cleft palate**

    749.00 Cleft palate, unspecified

    749.01 Unilateral, complete

    749.02 Unilateral, incomplete
      Cleft uvula

    749.03 Bilateral, complete

    749.04 Bilateral, incomplete

  ● **749.1 Cleft lip**
    Cheiloschisis   Harelip
    Congenital fissure of lip   Labium leporinum

    749.10 Cleft lip, unspecified

    749.11 Unilateral, complete

    749.12 Unilateral, incomplete

    749.13 Bilateral, complete

    749.14 Bilateral, incomplete

  ● **749.2 Cleft palate with cleft lip**
    Cheilopalatoschisis

    749.20 Cleft palate with cleft lip, unspecified

    749.21 Unilateral, complete

    749.22 Unilateral, incomplete

    749.23 Bilateral, complete
      Coding Clinic: 1996, Q1, P14

    749.24 Bilateral, incomplete

    749.25 Other combinations

● **750 Other congenital anomalies of upper alimentary tract**
    Excludes *dentofacial anomalies (524.0–524.9)*

  750.0 Tongue tie
    Ankyloglossia

  ● **750.1 Other anomalies of tongue**

    750.10 Anomaly of tongue, unspecified

    750.11 Aglossia

    750.12 Congenital adhesions of tongue

    750.13 Fissure of tongue
      Bifid tongue
      Double tongue

    750.15 Macroglossia
      Congenital hypertrophy of tongue

    750.16 Microglossia
      Hypoplasia of tongue

    750.19 Other

  ● **750.2 Other specified anomalies of mouth and pharynx**

    750.21 Absence of salivary gland

    750.22 Accessory salivary gland

    750.23 Atresia, salivary gland
      Imperforate salivary duct

    750.24 Congenital fistula of salivary gland

    750.25 Congenital fistula of lip
      Congenital (mucus) lip pits

    750.26 Other specified anomalies of mouth
      Absence of uvula

    750.27 Diverticulum of pharynx
      Pharyngeal pouch

    750.29 Other specified anomalies of pharynx
      Imperforate pharynx

  750.3 Tracheoesophageal fistula, esophageal atresia and stenosis 🔾
    Absent esophagus
    Atresia of esophagus
    Congenital:
      esophageal ring
      stenosis of esophagus
      stricture of esophagus
    Congenital fistula:
      esophagobronchial
      esophagotracheal
    Imperforate esophagus
    Webbed esophagus
    (Ex) 530.84, 750.3-750.4, 751.8-751.9

  750.4 Other specified anomalies of esophagus 🔾
    Dilatation, congenital, of esophagus
    Displacement, congenital, of esophagus
    Diverticulum of esophagus
    Duplication of esophagus
    Esophageal pouch
    Giant esophagus
    Excludes *congenital hiatus hernia (750.6)*
    (Ex) 750.4, 751.8-751.9

Item 14-3 A muscle thickening and pyloric stenosis overgrows the pyloric sphincter, resulting in a narrowing of the outlet between the stomach and small intestine. Infants with pyloric stenosis have projectile vomiting, leading to dehydration and electrolyte imbalance.

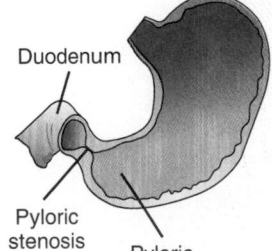

Figure 14–6 Pyloric stenosis.

Duodenum

Pyloric stenosis

Pyloric part of stomach

  750.5 Congenital hypertrophic pyloric stenosis
    Congenital or infantile:
      constriction of pylorus
      hypertrophy of pylorus
      spasm of pylorus
      stenosis of pylorus
      stricture of pylorus

  750.6 Congenital hiatus hernia
    Displacement of cardia through esophageal hiatus
    Excludes *congenital diaphragmatic hernia (756.6)*

N Newborn Age: 0   **P** Pediatric Age: 0–17   **M** Maternity Age: 12–55   **A** Adult Age: 15–124   ♀ Females Only   ♂ Males Only

(Ex) CC Exclusions   🔾 Complication\Comorbidity   🔾 Major C\C   🔾 Present on Admission Requirement   🔾 Hospital-Acquired Condition

CONGENITAL ANOMALIES (740–759)

1029

750.7   Other specified anomalies of stomach
Congenital:
    cardiospasm
    hourglass stomach
Displacement of stomach
Diverticulum of stomach, congenital
Duplication of stomach
Megalogastria
Microgastria
Transposition of stomach

750.8   Other specified anomalies of upper alimentary tract

750.9   Unspecified anomaly of upper alimentary tract
Congenital:
    anomaly NOS of upper alimentary tract [any
        part, except tongue]
    deformity NOS of upper alimentary tract [any
        part, except tongue]

● **751   Other congenital anomalies of digestive system**

751.0   Meckel's diverticulum
Meckel's diverticulum (displaced) (hypertrophic)
Persistent:
    omphalomesenteric duct
    vitelline duct
Coding Clinic: 2004, Q1, P10-11

751.1   Atresia and stenosis of small intestine 🗝   P
Atresia of:
    duodenum
    ileum
    intestine NOS
Congenital:
    absence of small intestine or intestine NOS
    obstruction of small intestine or intestine NOS
    stenosis of small intestine or intestine NOS
    stricture of small intestine or intestine NOS
Imperforate jejunum
Ⓔ⒳ 751.1, 751.8-751.9

751.2   Atresia and stenosis of large intestine, rectum, and anal canal 🗝   P
Absence:
    anus (congenital)
    appendix, congenital
    large instestine, congenital
    rectum
Atresia of:
    anus
    colon
    rectum
Congenital or infantile:
    obstruction of large intestine
    occlusion of anus
    stricture of anus
Imperforate:
    anus
    rectum
Stricture of rectum, congenital
Ⓔ⒳ 751.2, 751.8-751.9
Coding Clinic: 1998, Q2, P16-17

751.3   Hirschsprung's disease and other congenital functional disorders of colon 🗝
Absence of ganglion cells in distal colon resulting in functional obstruction.
Aganglionosis
Congenital dilation of colon
Congenital megacolon
Macrocolon
Ⓔ⒳ 751.3, 751.8-751.9

751.4   Anomalies of intestinal fixation 🗝
Congenital adhesions:
    omental, anomalous
    peritoneal
Jackson's membrane
Malrotation of colon
Rotation of cecum or colon:
    failure of
    incomplete
    insufficient
Universal mesentery
Ⓔ⒳ 751.4-751.5
Coding Clinic: 1985, Sept-Oct, P11

751.5   Other anomalies of intestine 🗝
Congenital diverticulum,	Megaloappendix
colon	Megaloduodenum
Dolichocolon	Microcolon
Duplication of:	Persistent cloaca
anus	Transposition of:
appendix	appendix
cecum	colon
intestine	intestine
Ectopic anus	

Ⓔ⒳ 751.0-751.5
Coding Clinic: 2002, Q3, P11; 2001, Q3, P8-9

● **751.6   Anomalies of gallbladder, bile ducts, and liver**

751.60   Unspecified anomaly of gallbladder, bile ducts, and liver 🗝
Ⓔ⒳ 751.60

751.61   Biliary atresia 🗝   P
Congenital:
    absence of bile duct (common) or passage
    hypoplasia of bile duct (common) or
        passage
    obstruction of bile duct (common) or
        passage
    stricture of bile duct (common) or
        passage
Ⓔ⒳ 751.61, 751.8-751.9
Coding Clinic: 1987, Sept-Oct, P8

751.62   Congenital cystic disease of liver 🗝
Congenital polycystic disease of liver
Fibrocystic disease of liver
Ⓔ⒳ 751.62-751.69

751.69   Other anomalies of gallbladder, bile ducts, and liver 🗝
Absence of:
    gallbladder, congenital
    liver (lobe)
Accessory:
    hepatic ducts
    liver
Congenital:
    choledochal cyst
    hepatomegaly

Duplication of:	Duplication of:
biliary duct	gallbladder
cystic duct	liver
Floating:	Floating:
gallbladder	liver

Intrahepatic gallbladder
Ⓔ⒳ 751.60-751.69
Coding Clinic: 1987, Sept-Oct, P8

◄ New   ◄▥ Revised   ̶d̶e̶l̶e̶t̶e̶d̶ Deleted   ● Unacceptable Principal Diagnosis   ● Use Additional Digit(s)
▶ Manifestation Code   **OGCR** Official Guidelines   **Coding Clinic**   Excludes   Includes   Use additional   Code first   Omit code

751.7 Anomalies of pancreas 🍇
    Absence of pancreas
    Accessory pancreas
    Agenesis of pancreas
    Annular pancreas
    Ectopic pancreatic tissue
    Hypoplasia of pancreas
    Pancreatic heterotopia

> **Excludes**   *diabetes mellitus (249.0–249.9,*
>   *(250.0–250.9)*
>   *fibrocystic disease of pancreas*
>   *(277.00–277.09)*
>   *neonatal diabetes mellitus (775.1)*

(Ex) 751.7-751.9

751.8 Other specified anomalies of digestive system
    Absence (complete) (partial) of alimentary tract NOS
    Duplication of digestive organs NOS
    Malposition, congenital of digestive organs NOS

> **Excludes**   *congenital diaphragmatic hernia (756.6)*
>   *congenital hiatus hernia (750.6)*

751.9 Unspecified anomaly of digestive system
    Congenital:
        anomaly NOS of digestive system NOS
        deformity NOS of digestive system NOS

● **752 Congenital anomalies of genital organs**

> **Excludes**   *syndromes associated with anomalies in the*
>   *number and form of chromosomes*
>   *(758.0–758.9)*

752.0 Anomalies of ovaries ♀
    Absence, congenital, of ovary
    Accessory ovary
    Ectopic ovary
    Streak of ovary

● **752.1 Anomalies of fallopian tubes and broad ligaments**

    752.10 Unspecified anomaly of fallopian tubes and broad ligaments ♀

    752.11 Embryonic cyst of fallopian tubes and broad ligaments ♀
        Cyst:
           epoophoron
           fimbrial
           parovarian
        Coding Clinic: 1985, Sept-Oct, P13

    752.19 Other ♀
        Absence of fallopian tube or broad ligament
        Accessory fallopian tube or broad ligament
        Atresia of fallopian tube or broad ligament

752.2 Doubling of uterus ♀
    Didelphic uterus
    Doubling of uterus [any degree] (associated with doubling of cervix and vagina)

752.3 Other anomalies of uterus ♀
    Absence, congenital, of uterus
    Agenesis of uterus
    Aplasia of uterus
    Bicornuate uterus
    Uterus unicornis
    Uterus with only one functioning horn
    Coding Clinic: 2006, Q3, P18-19

● **752.4 Anomalies of cervix, vagina, and external female genitalia**

    752.40 Unspecified anomaly of cervix, vagina, and external female genitalia ♀

    752.41 Embryonic cyst of cervix, vagina, and external female genitalia ♀
        Cyst of:
           canal of Nuck, congenital
           Gartner's duct
           vagina, embryonal
           vulva, congenital

    752.42 Imperforate hymen ♀

    752.49 Other anomalies of cervix, vagina, and external female genitalia ♀
        Absence of cervix, clitoris, vagina, or vulva
        Agenesis of cervix, clitoris, vagina, or vulva
        Congenital stenosis or stricture of:
           cervical canal
           vagina

> **Excludes**   *double vagina associated with total*
>   *duplication (752.2)*

    Coding Clinic: 2006, Q3, P18-19

● **752.5 Undescended and retractile testicle**

    752.51 Undescended testis ♂
        Cryptorchism
        Ectopic testis

    752.52 Retractile testis ♂

● **752.6 Hypospadias and epispadias and other penile anomalies**

    752.61 Hypospadias ♂
        Coding Clinic: 2003, Q4, P67-68; 1997, Q3, P6; Q3, P6; 1996, Q4, P34-35

    752.62 Epispadias ♂
        Anaspadias

ECTOPIC TESTES	CRYPTORCHID TESTES
Penile	Abdominal
Superficial inguinal (most common)	Inguinal
Femoral	Prepubic (most common)

Figure 14–7   Undescended testes and the positions of the testes in various types of cryptorchidism or abnormal paths of descent.

Item 14–4   Testes form in the abdomen of the male and only descend into the scrotum during normal embryonic development. "Ectopic" testes are out of their normal place or "retained" (left behind) in the abdomen. Crypto (hidden) orchism (testicle) is a major risk factor for testicular cancer.

CONGENITAL ANOMALIES (740–759)

752.63 Congenital chordee ♂
Coding Clinic: 1996, Q4, P34-35

752.64 Micropenis ♂

752.65 Hidden penis ♂

752.69 Other penile anomalies ♂

752.7 Indeterminate sex and pseudohermaphroditism
Condition in which internal reproductive organs are opposite external physical characteristics.
Gynandrism
Hermaphroditism
Ovotestis
Pseudohermaphroditism (male) (female)
Pure gonadal dysgenesis

Excludes *androgen insensitivity (259.50–259.52)*
pseudohermaphroditism:
    female, with adrenocortical disorder
      (255.2)
    male, with gonadal disorder (257.8)
    with specified chromosomal anomaly
      (758.0–758.9)
testicular feminization syndrome
    (259.50–259.52)

● **752.8 Other specified anomalies of genital organs**

Excludes *congenital hydrocele (778.6)*
penile anomalies (752.61–752.69)
phimosis or paraphimosis (605)

752.81 Scrotal transposition ♂
Coding Clinic: 2003, Q4, P67-68

752.89 Other specified anomalies of genital organs
Absence of:
Check Index for V codes for acquired or congenital.
    prostate
    spermatic cord
    vas deferens
Anorchism
Aplasia (congenital) of:
    prostate
    round ligament
    testicle
Atresia of:
    ejaculatory duct
    vas deferens
Fusion of testes
Hypoplasia of testis
Monorchism
Polyorchism

752.9 Unspecified anomaly of genital organs
Congenital:
    anomaly NOS of genital organ, NEC
    deformity NOS of genital organ, NEC

● **753 Congenital anomalies of urinary system**

753.0 Renal agenesis and dysgenesis ✆
Atrophy of kidney:
    congenital
    infantile
Congenital absence of kidney(s)
Hypoplasia of kidney(s)
Ex: 599.60-599.69, 753.0

● **753.1 Cystic kidney disease**

Excludes *acquired cyst of kidney (593.2)*

753.10 Cystic kidney disease, unspecified ✆
Ex: 599.60-599.69, 753.10

753.11 Congenital single renal cyst ✆
Ex: 599.60-599.69, 753.11

753.12 Polycystic kidney, unspecified type ✆
PKD (polycystic kidney disease)
Ex: 599.60-599.69, 753.12-753.14

753.13 Polycystic kidney, autosomal dominant ✆
Ex: 599.60-599.69, 753.12-753.14

753.14 Polycystic kidney, autosomal recessive ✆
Ex: 599.60-599.69, 753.12-753.14

753.15 Renal dysplasia ✆
Ex: 599.60-599.69, 753.15

753.16 Medullary cystic kidney ✆
Nephronophthisis
Ex: 599.60-599.69, 753.16-753.19

753.17 Medullary sponge kidney ✆
Ex: 599.60-599.69, 753.16-753.19

753.19 Other specified cystic kidney disease ✆
Multicystic kidney
Ex: 599.60-599.69, 753.16-753.19

● **753.2 Obstructive defects of renal pelvis and ureter**

753.20 Unspecified obstructive defect of renal pelvis and ureter ✆
Ex: 599.60-599.69, 753.20-753.22, 753.29

753.21 Congenital obstruction of ureteropelvic junction ✆
Ex: 599.60-599.69, 753.20-753.22, 753.29

753.22 Congenital obstruction of ureterovesical junction ✆
Adynamic ureter
Congenital hydroureter
Ex: 599.60-599.69, 753.20-753.22, 753.29

753.23 Congenital ureterocele ✆
Ex: 599.60-599.69, 753.20-753.22, 753.29

753.29 Other ✆
Ex: 599.60-599.69, 753.20-753.22, 753.29

753.3 Other specified anomalies of kidney
Accessory kidney
Congenital:
    calculus of kidney
    displaced kidney
Discoid kidney
Double kidney with double pelvis
Ectopic kidney
Fusion of kidneys
Giant kidney
Horseshoe kidney
Hyperplasia of kidney
Lobulation of kidney
Malrotation of kidney
Trifid kidney (pelvis)
Coding Clinic: 2007, Q1, P23

753.4 Other specified anomalies of ureter
Absent ureter
Accessory ureter
Deviaton of ureter
Displaced ureteric orifice
Double ureter
Ectopic ureter
Implantation, anomalous, of ureter

◀ New   ◀▥ Revised   deleted Deleted   ● Unacceptable Principal Diagnosis   ● Use Additional Digit(s)
▶ Manifestation Code   OGCR Official Guidelines   Coding Clinic   Excludes   Includes   Use additional   Code first   Omit code

753.5 Exstrophy of urinary bladder🌀
  Ectopia vesicae
  Extroversion of bladder
  (Ex) 599.60-599.69, 753.5, 753.9

753.6 Atresia and stenosis of urethra and bladder neck🌀
  Congenital obstruction:
    bladder neck
    urethra
  Congenital stricture of:
    urethra (valvular)
    urinary meatus
    vesicourethral orifice
  Imperforate urinary meatus
  Impervious urethra
  Urethral valve formation
  (Ex) 599.60-599.69, 753.6, 753.9

753.7 Anomalies of urachus
  Cyst (of) urachus
  Fistula (of) urachus
  Patent (of) urachus
  Persistent umbilical sinus

753.8 Other specified anomalies of bladder and urethra
  Absence, congenital of:
    bladder
    urethra
  Accessory:
    bladder
    urethra
  Congenital:
    diverticulum of bladder
    hernia of bladder
  Congenital urethrorectal fistula
  Congenital prolapse of:
    bladder (mucosa)
    urethra
  Double:
    urethra
    urinary meatus

753.9 Unspecified anomaly of urinary system
  Congenital:
    anomaly NOS of urinary system [any part,
      except urachus]
    deformity NOS of urinary system [any part,
      except urachus]

●**754 Certain congenital musculoskeletal deformities**
  Includes nonteratogenic deformities which are
              considered to be due to intrauterine
              malposition and pressure

754.0 Of skull, face, and jaw
  Asymmetry of face
  Compression facies
  Depressions in skull
  Deviation of nasal septum, congenital
  Dolichocephaly
  Plagiocephaly
  Potter's facies
  Squashed or bent nose, congenital
  Excludes *dentofacial anomalies (524.0–524.9)*
              syphilitic saddle nose (090.5)

754.1 Of sternocleidomastoid muscle
  Congenital sternomastoid torticollis
  Congenital wryneck
  Contracture of sternocleidomastoid (muscle)
  Sternomastoid tumor

754.2 Of spine🌀
  Congenital postural:
    lordosis
    scoliosis
    (Ex) 754.2

●**754.3 Congenital dislocation of hip**
  754.30 Congenital dislocation of hip, unilateral
    Congenital dislocation of hip NOS

  754.31 Congenital dislocation of hip, bilateral

  754.32 Congenital subluxation of hip, unilateral
    Congenital flexion deformity, hip or thigh
    Predislocation status of hip at birth
    Preluxation of hip, congenital

  754.33 Congenital subluxation of hip, bilateral

  **754.35 Congenital dislocation of one hip with
          subluxation of other hip**

●**754.4 Congenital genu recurvatum and bowing of long
         bones of leg**
  754.40 Genu recurvatum
    *Hyperextension of knee resulting from
      hypermobility*

  **754.41 Congenital dislocation of knee (with genu
          recurvatum)**

  754.42 Congenital bowing of femur

  754.43 Congenital bowing of tibia and fibula

  **754.44 Congenital bowing of unspecified long bones
          of leg**

●**754.5 Varus deformities of feet**
  *Foot deformity (pes equino varus) also known as club
    foot in which there is an inward angulation of
    distal segment of a bone or joint*
  Excludes *acquired (736.71, 736.75, 736.79)*

  754.50 Talipes varus
    Congenital varus deformity of foot,
      unspecified
    Pes varus

  754.51 Talipes equinovarus
    Equinovarus (congenital)

  754.52 Metatarsus primus varus

  754.53 Metatarsus varus

  754.59 Other
    Talipes calcaneovarus

●**754.6 Valgus deformities of feet**
  Inward angulation
  Excludes *valgus deformity of foot (acquired) (736.79)*

  754.60 Talipes valgus
    Congenital valgus deformity of foot,
      unspecified

Figure 14–8 Mild to moderate inbowing of the lower leg. (From Jones KL: Smith's Recognizable Patterns of Human Malformation, 4th ed. Philadelphia, Saunders, 1988, p 671.)

N Newborn Age: 0   **P** Pediatric Age: 0–17   **M** Maternity Age: 12–55   **A** Adult Age: 15–124   ♀ Females Only   ♂ Males Only
(Ex) CC Exclusions   🌀 Complication\Comorbidity   🌀 Major C\C   🌀 Present on Admission Requirement   🌀 Hospital-Acquired Condition   1033

CONGENITAL ANOMALIES (740–759)

754.61 Congenital pes planus
Congenital rocker bottom flat foot
Flat foot, congenital
Excludes | pes planus (acquired) (734)

754.62 Talipes calcaneovalgus

754.69 Other
Talipes:
   equinovalgus
   planovalgus

● **754.7 Other deformities of feet**
Excludes | acquired (736.70–736.79)

754.70 Talipes, unspecified
Congenital deformity of foot NOS

754.71 Talipes cavus
Cavus foot (congenital)

754.79 Other
Asymmetric talipes
Talipes:
   calcaneus
   equinus

● **754.8 Other specified nonteratogenic anomalies**

754.81 Pectus excavatum
Congenital funnel chest

754.82 Pectus carinatum
Congenital pigeon chest [breast]

754.89 Other ✇
Club hand (congenital)
Congenital:
   deformity of chest wall
   dislocation of elbow
Generalized flexion contractures of lower
   limb joints, congenital
Spade-like hand (congenital)
Ex: 754.81-754.89

● **755 Other congenital anomalies of limbs**
Excludes | those deformities classifiable to 754.0–754.8

● **755.0 Polydactyly**
Also known as hyperdactyly, consists of duplicate
fingers or toes

755.00 Polydactyly, unspecified digits
Supernumerary digits

755.01 Of fingers
Accessory fingers

755.02 Of toes
Accessory toes

Figure 14–9 Polydactyly, congenital duplicated thumb. (From DeLee: DeLee and Drez's Orthopaedic Sports Medicine, 2nd ed. 2003, Saunders, An Imprint of Elsevier)

● **755.1 Syndactyly**
Symphalangy
Webbing of digits

755.10 Of multiple and unspecified sites

755.11 Of fingers without fusion of bone

755.12 Of fingers with fusion of bone

755.13 Of toes without fusion of bone

755.14 Of toes with fusion of bone

● **755.2 Reduction deformities of upper limb**

755.20 Unspecified reduction deformity of upper limb
Ectromelia NOS of upper limb
Gross hypoplasia or aplasia of one or more
long bones of one or more limbs
Hemimelia NOS of upper limb
Absence of one-half of long bone
Shortening of arm, congenital

755.21 Transverse deficiency of upper limb
Amelia of upper limb
Congenital absence of:
   fingers, all (complete or partial)
   forearm, including hand and fingers
   upper limb, complete
Congenital amputation of upper limb
Transverse hemimelia of upper limb

755.22 Longitudinal deficiency of upper limb, NEC
Phocomelia NOS of upper limb
Absence/shortening of long bones primarily
as a result of thalidomide
Rudimentary arm

755.23 Longitudinal deficiency, combined, involving humerus, radius, and ulna (complete or incomplete)
Congenital absence of arm and forearm
   (complete or incomplete) with or
   without metacarpal deficiency and/or
   phalangeal deficiency, incomplete
Phocomelia, complete, of upper limb

755.24 Longitudinal deficiency, humeral, complete or partial (with or without distal deficiencies, incomplete)
Congenital absence of humerus (with or
   without absence of some [but not all]
   distal elements)
Proximal phocomelia of upper limb

755.25 Longitudinal deficiency, radioulnar, complete or partial (with or without distal deficiencies, incomplete)
Congenital absence of radius and ulna (with
   or without absence of some [but not
   all] distal elements)
Distal phocomelia of upper limb

755.26 Longitudinal deficiency, radial, complete or partial (with or without distal deficiencies, incomplete)
Agenesis of radius
Congenital absence of radius (with or
   without absence of some [but not all]
   distal elements)

755.27 Longitudinal deficiency, ulnar, complete or partial (with or without distal deficiencies, incomplete)
Agenesis of ulna
Congenital absence of ulna (with or without
   absence of some [but not all] distal
   elements)

755.28 Longitudinal deficiency, carpals or metacarpals, complete or partial (with or without incomplete phalangeal deficiency)

755.29 Longitudinal deficiency, phalanges, complete or partial
Absence of finger, congenital
Aphalangia of upper limb, terminal,
   complete or partial
Excludes | terminal deficiency of all five digits
          (755.21)
          transverse deficiency of phalanges
          (755.21)

◀ New   ◀▦ Revised   ~~deleted~~ Deleted   ● Unacceptable Principal Diagnosis   ● Use Additional Digit(s)
▶ Manifestation Code   OGCR Official Guidelines   Coding Clinic   Excludes   Includes   Use additional   Code first   Omit code

● **755.3 Reduction deformities of lower limb**

    755.30 Unspecified reduction deformity of lower limb
       Ectromelia NOS of lower limb
       Hemimelia NOS of lower limb
       Shortening of leg, congenital

    755.31 Transverse deficiency of lower limb
       Amelia of lower limb
       Congenital absence of:
          foot
             leg, including foot and toes
             lower limb, complete
             toes, all, complete
       Transverse hemimelia of lower limb

    755.32 Longitudinal deficiency of lower limb, NEC
       Phocomelia NOS of lower limb

    755.33 Longitudinal deficiency, combined, involving femur, tibia, and fibula (complete or incomplete)
       Congenital absence of thigh and (lower) leg (complete or incomplete) with or without metacarpal deficiency and/or phalangeal deficiency, incomplete
       Phocomelia, complete, of lower limb

    755.34 Longitudinal deficiency, femoral, complete or partial (with or without distal deficiencies, incomplete)
       Congenital absence of femur (with or without absence of some [but not all] distal elements)
       Proximal phocomelia of lower limb

    755.35 Longitudinal deficiency, tibiofibular, complete or partial (with or without distal deficiencies, incomplete)
       Congenital absence of tibia and fibula (with or without absence of some [but not all] distal elements)
       Distal phocomelia of lower limb

    755.36 Longitudinal deficiency, tibia, complete or partial (with or without distal deficiencies, incomplete)
       Agenesis of tibia
       Congenital absence of tibia (with or without absence of some [but not all] distal elements)

    755.37 Longitudinal deficiency, fibular, complete or partial (with or without distal deficiencies, incomplete)
       Agenesis of fibula
       Congenital absence of fibula (with or without absence of some [but not all] distal elements)

    755.38 Longitudinal deficiency, tarsals or metatarsals, complete or partial (with or without incomplete phalangeal deficiency)

    755.39 Longitudinal deficiency, phalanges, complete or partial
       Absence of toe, congenital
       Aphalangia of lower limb, terminal, complete or partial
       Excludes *terminal deficiency of all five digits (755.31)*
                  transverse deficiency of phalanges (755.31)

755.4 Reduction deformities, unspecified limb
       Absence, congenital (complete or partial) of limb NOS
       Amelia of unspecified limb
       Ectromelia of unspecified limb
       Hemimelia of unspecified limb
       Phocomelia of unspecified limb

● **755.5 Other anomalies of upper limb, including shoulder girdle**

    755.50 Unspecified anomaly of upper limb

    755.51 Congenital deformity of clavicle

    755.52 Congenital elevation of scapula
       Sprengel's deformity

    755.53 Radioulnar synostosis

    755.54 Madelung's deformity

    755.55 Acrocephalosyndactyly 🦠
       Apert's syndrome
       (Ex) 755.50, 755.55, 755.59

    755.56 Accessory carpal bones

    755.57 Macrodactylia (fingers)

    755.58 Cleft hand, congenital
       Lobster-claw hand

    755.59 Other
       Cleidocranial dysostosis
       Cubitus:
          valgus, congenital
          varus, congenital
       Excludes *club hand (congenital) (754.89)*
                  congenital dislocation of elbow (754.89)

● **755.6 Other anomalies of lower limb, including pelvic girdle**

    755.60 Unspecified anomaly of lower limb

    755.61 Coxa valga, congenital

    755.62 Coxa vara, congenital

    755.63 Other congenital deformity of hip (joint)
       Congenital anteversion of femur (neck)
       Excludes *congenital dislocation of hip (754.30–754.35)*

    755.64 Congenital deformity of knee (joint)
       Congenital:
          absence of patella
          genu valgum [knock-knee]
          genu varum [bowleg]
       Rudimentary patella
       Coding Clinic: 1985, July-Aug, P14; 1984, Nov-Dec, P9

    755.65 Macrodactylia of toes

    755.66 Other anomalies of toes
       Congenital:
          hallux valgus
          hallux varus
          hammer toe

    755.67 Anomalies of foot, NEC
       Astragaloscaphoid synostosis
       Calcaneonavicular bar
       Coalition of calcaneus
       Talonavicular synostosis
       Tarsal coalitions

    755.69 Other
       Congenital:
          angulation of tibia
          deformity (of):
             ankle (joint)
             sacroiliac (joint)
          fusion of sacroiliac joint

CONGENITAL ANOMALIES (740–759)

N Newborn Age: 0   **P** Pediatric Age: 0–17   **M** Maternity Age: 12–55   **A** Adult Age: 15–124   ♀ Females Only   ♂ Males Only

(Ex) CC Exclusions   🦠 Complication\Comorbidity   🦠 Major C\C   Present on Admission Requirement   🦠 Hospital-Acquired Condition   **1035**

755.8   Other specified anomalies of unspecified limb

755.9   Unspecified anomaly of unspecified limb
Congenital:
     anomaly NOS of unspecified limb
     deformity NOS of unspecified limb

> **Excludes**   *reduction deformity of unspecified limb (755.4)*

● **756   Other congenital musculoskeletal anomalies**

> **Excludes**   *congenital myotonic chondrodystrophy (359.23)*
> *those deformities classifiable to 754.0–754.8*

756.0   Anomalies of skull and face bones
Absence of skull bones
Acrocephaly
Congenital deformity of forehead
Craniosynostosis
Crouzon's disease
Hypertelorism
Imperfect fusion of skull
Oxycephaly
Platybasia
Premature closure of cranial sutures
Tower skull
Trigonocephaly

> **Excludes**   *acrocephalosyndactyly [Apert's syndrome]*
> *(755.55)*
> *dentofacial anomalies (524.0–524.9)*
> *skull defects associated with brain*
> *anomalies, such as:*
> *anencephalus (740.0)*
> *encephalocele (742.0)*
> *hydrocephalus (742.3)*
> *microcephalus (742.1)*

Coding Clinic: 1998, Q3, P9-10; 1996, Q3, P15

● **756.1   Anomalies of spine**

756.10   Anomaly of spine, unspecified

756.11   Spondylolysis, lumbosacral region
Prespondylolisthesis (lumbosacral)

756.12   Spondylolisthesis

756.13   Absence of vertebra, congenital 🅖
(Ex:) 756.10-756.19

756.14   Hemivertebra

756.15   Fusion of spine [vertebra], congenital

756.16   Klippel-Feil syndrome

756.17   Spina bifida occulta

> **Excludes**   *spina bifida (aperta) (741.0–741.9)*

756.19   Other
Platyspondylia
Supernumerary vertebra

756.2   Cervical rib
Supernumerary rib in the cervical region

756.3   Other anomalies of ribs and sternum 🅖
Congenital absence of:
     rib
     sternum
Congenital:
     fissure of sternum
     fusion of ribs
Sternum bifidum

> **Excludes**   *nonteratogenic deformity of chest wall*
> *(754.81–754.89)*

(Ex:) 756.2-756.3

756.4   Chondrodystrophy
Skeletal dysplasia (dwarfism) is caused by genetic
mutations affecting hyaline cartilage capping long
bones and vertebrae
Achondroplasia   Enchondromatosis
Chondrodystrophia (fetalis)   Ollier's disease
Dyschondroplasia

> **Excludes**   *congenital myotonic chondrodystrophy*
> *(359.23)*
> *lipochondrodystrophy [Hurler's syndrome]*
> *(277.5)*
> *Morquio's disease (277.5)*

Coding Clinic: 2002, Q2, P16-17; 1987, Sept-Oct, P10

● **756.5   Osteodystrophies**
Defective bone development; most commonly caused
by renal disease or disturbances in calcium and
phosphorus metabolism

756.50   Osteodystrophy, unspecified

756.51   Osteogenesis imperfecta 🅖
Fragilitas ossium
Osteopsathyrosis
(Ex:) 756.50-756.59

756.52   Osteopetrosis 🅖
(Ex:) 756.50-756.59

756.53   Osteopoikilosis

756.54   Polyostotic fibrous dysplasia of bone

756.55   Chondroectodermal dysplasia
Ellis-van Creveld syndrome

756.56   Multiple epiphyseal dysplasia

756.59   Other
Albright (-McCune)-Sternberg syndrome

756.6   Anomalies of diaphragm 🅖
Absence of diaphragm
Congenital hernia:
     diaphragmatic
     foramen of Morgagni
Eventration of diaphragm

> **Excludes**   *congenital hiatus hernia (750.6)*

(Ex:) 750.6, 756.6

● **756.7   Anomalies of abdominal wall**

756.70   Anomaly of abdominal wall, unspecified 🅖
(Ex:) 756.70-756.79

756.71   Prune belly syndrome 🅖
Eagle-Barrett syndrome
Prolapse of bladder mucosa
(Ex:) 756.70-756.79

756.72   Omphalocele 🅖   ◄
Exomphalos   ◄

756.73   Gastroschisis 🅖   ◄

756.79   Other congenital anomalies of abdominal wall 🅖
~~Exomphalos~~   ~~Omphalocele~~
~~Gastroschisis~~

> **Excludes**   *umbilical hernia (551–553 with .1)*

(Ex:) 756.70-756.79

● **756.8   Other specified anomalies of muscle, tendon, fascia, and connective tissue**

756.81   Absence of muscle and tendon
Absence of muscle (pectoral)

756.82   Accessory muscle

756.83   Ehlers-Danlos syndrome 🅖
(Ex:) 756.83-756.89

◄ New   ◄▥ Revised   ~~deleted~~ Deleted   ● Unacceptable Principal Diagnosis   🅖 Use Additional Digit(s)
▶ Manifestation Code   **OGCR** Official Guidelines   **Coding Clinic**   Excludes   Includes   Use additional   Code first   Omit code

756.89 Other
Amyotrophia congenita
Congenital shortening of tendon
Coding Clinic: 1999, Q3, P16-17

756.9 Other and unspecified anomalies of musculoskeletal system
Congenital:
anomaly NOS of musculoskeletal system, NEC
deformity NOS of musculoskeletal system, NEC

● **757 Congenital anomalies of the integument**
Includes anomalies of skin, subcutaneous tissue, hair, nails, and breast
Excludes *hemangioma (228.00–228.09)*
pigmented nevus (216.0–216.9)

757.0 Hereditary edema of legs
Congenital lymphedema
Hereditary trophedema
Milroy's disease

757.1 Ichthyosis congenita
Congenital ichthyosis
Harlequin fetus
Ichthyosiform erythroderma

757.2 Dermatoglyphic anomalies
Abnormal palmar creases

● **757.3 Other specified anomalies of skin**

757.31 Congenital ectodermal dysplasia

757.32 Vascular hamartomas
Birthmarks
Port-wine stain
Strawberry nevus

757.33 Congenital pigmentary anomalies of skin
Congenital poikiloderma
Urticaria pigmentosa
Xeroderma pigmentosum
Excludes *albinism (270.2)*

757.39 Other
Accessory skin tags, congenital
Congenital scar
Epidermolysis bullosa
Keratoderma (congenital)
Excludes *pilonidal cyst (685.0–685.1)*

757.4 Specified anomalies of hair
Congenital:
alopecia
atrichosis
beaded hair
hypertrichosis
monilethrix
Persistent lanugo

757.5 Specified anomalies of nails
Anonychia
Congenital:
clubnail
koilonychia
leukonychia
onychauxis
pachyonychia

757.6 Specified congenital anomalies of breast ⬅||||
Congenital a~~A~~bsent breast or nipple ⬅||||
Accessory breast or nipple
Supernumerary breast or nipple
Excludes *absence of pectoral muscle (756.81)*
hypoplasia of breast (611.82)
micromastia (611.82) ◀

757.8 Other specified anomalies of the integument

757.9 Unspecified anomaly of the integument
Congenital:
anomaly NOS of integument
deformity NOS of integument

● **758 Chromosomal anomalies**
Includes syndromes associated with anomalies in the number and form of chromosomes
Use additional codes for conditions associated with the chromosomal anomalies

758.0 Down's syndrome
Mongolism
Translocation Down's syndrome
Trisomy:
21 or 22
G

758.1 Patau's syndrome 🅲
Trisomy:
13
D$_1$
(Ex) 758.0-758.9

758.2 Edward's syndrome 🅲
Trisomy:
18
E$_3$
(Ex) 758.0-758.9

● **758.3 Autosomal deletion syndromes**
Coding Clinic: 2004, Q4, P93-95; 1995, Q2, P6-7, 11

758.31 Cri-du-chat syndrome 🅲
Deletion 5p
(Ex) 758.0-758.2, 758.32-758.9

758.32 Velo-cardio-facial syndrome 🅜🅒
Deletion 22q11.2
(Ex) 758.0-758.31, 758.33-758.9

758.33 Other microdeletions 🅲
Miller-Dieker syndrome
Smith-Magenis syndrome
(Ex) 758.0-758.32, 758.39-758.9

758.39 Other autosomal deletions 🅲
(Ex) 758.0-758.33, 758.4-758.9

758.4 Balanced autosomal translocation in normal individual

758.5 Other conditions due to autosomal anomalies
Accessory autosomes NEC

758.6 Gonadal dysgenesis
Ovarian dysgenesis
Turner's syndrome
XO syndrome
Excludes *pure gonadal dysgenesis (752.7)*

758.7 Klinefelter's syndrome ♂
XXY syndrome

● **758.8 Other conditions due to chromosome anomalies**

758.81 Other conditions due to sex chromosome anomalies

758.89 Other

758.9 Conditions due to anomaly of unspecified chromosome

● **759   Other and unspecified congenital anomalies**

    759.0 Anomalies of spleen 🔾

        Aberrant spleen   Congenital splenomegaly

        Absent spleen   Ectopic spleen

        Accessory spleen   Lobulation of spleen

        (Ex) 759.0, 759.9

    759.1 Anomalies of adrenal gland

        Aberrant adrenal gland

        Absent adrenal gland

        Accessory adrenal gland

        | Excludes | *adrenogenital disorders (255.2)*
                              congenital disorders of steroid metabolism (255.2)

    759.2 Anomalies of other endocrine glands

        Absent parathyroid gland

        Accessory thyroid gland

        Persistent thyroglossal or thyrolingual duct

        Thyroglossal (duct) cyst

        | Excludes | *congenital:*
                           goiter (246.1)
                           hypothyroidism (243)

    759.3 Situs inversus 🔾

        Situs inversus or transversus:

          abdominalis

          thoracis

        Transposition of viscera:

          abdominal

          thoracic

        | Excludes | *dextrocardia without mention of complete transposition (746.87)*

        (Ex) 759.3, 759.7, 759.9

    759.4 Conjoined twins 🔾

        Craniopagus

        Dicephalus

        Pygopagus

        Thoracopagus

        Xiphopagus

        (Ex) 759.4, 759.7, 759.9

    759.5 Tuberous sclerosis 🔾

        Bourneville's disease

        Epiloia

        (Ex) 759.5-759.7, 759.9

    759.6 Other hamartoses, NEC 🔾

        Syndrome:

          Peutz-Jeghers

          Sturge-Weber (-Dimitri)

          von Hippel-Lindau

        | Excludes | *neurofibromatosis (237.7)*

        (Ex) 759.6, 759.9

        Coding Clinic: 1992, Q3, P11

    759.7 Multiple congenital anomalies, so described 🔾

        Congenital:

          anomaly, multiple NOS

          deformity, multiple NOS

        (Ex) 759.3, 759.7, 759.9

●   **759.8 Other specified anomalies**

        759.81 Prader-Willi syndrome 🔾

              (Ex) 759.6-759.9

        759.82 Marfan syndrome 🔾

              (Ex) 759.6-759.9

              Coding Clinic: 1993, Q3, P11

        759.83 Fragile X syndrome

        759.89 Other 🔾

              Index directs coder to this code for Noonan's syndrome.

              Congenital malformation syndromes affecting multiple systems, NEC

              Laurence-Moon-Biedl syndrome

              (Ex) 759.81-759.89

              Coding Clinic: 2008, Q3, P3-4; 2006, Q3, P21; 2005, Q2, P17; 2004, Q2, P12; 2001, Q1, P3; 1999, Q3, P17-19x2; 1998, Q3, P8; 1987, Sept-Oct, P9; 1985, Sept-Oct, P11

    759.9 Congenital anomaly, unspecified

◀ New   ◀‖‖ Revised   ~~deleted~~ Deleted   ● Unacceptable Principal Diagnosis   ● Use Additional Digit(s)

▶ Manifestation Code   **OGCR** Official Guidelines   **Coding Clinic**   Excludes   Includes   Use additional   Code first   Omit code

OGCR Section I.C.15

The perinatal period is defined as before birth through the 28th day following birth.

OGCR Section I.C.15.a.1

Chapter 15 codes are never for use on the maternal record. Codes from Chapter 11, the obstetric chapter, are never permitted on the newborn record. Chapter 15 code may be used throughout the life of the patient if the condition is still present.

OGCR Section I.C.15.a.2

Generally, codes from Chapter 15 should be sequenced as the principal/first-listed diagnosis on the newborn record, with the exception of the appropriate V30 code for the birth episode, followed by codes from any other chapter that provide additional detail.

OGCR Section I.C.15.a.3

If a newborn has a condition that may be either due to the birth process or community acquired and the documentation does not indicate which it is, the default is due to the birth process and the code from Chapter 15 should be used. If the condition is community-acquired, a code from Chapter 15 should not be assigned.

15.   CERTAIN CONDITIONS ORIGINATING IN THE PERINATAL PERIOD (760–779)

> **Includes**   conditions which have their origin in the perinatal period, before birth through the first 28 days after birth, even though death or morbidity occurs later

Use additional code(s) to further specify condition

MATERNAL CAUSES OF PERINATAL MORBIDITY AND MORTALITY (760–763)

● **760   Fetus or newborn affected by maternal conditions which may be unrelated to present pregnancy**

> **Includes**   the listed maternal conditions only when specified as a cause of mortality or morbidity of the fetus or newborn

> **Excludes**   *maternal endocrine and metabolic disorders affecting fetus or newborn (775.0–775.9)*

Coding Clinic: 1992, Q2, P12

760.0   Maternal hypertensive disorders
Fetus or newborn affected by maternal conditions classifiable to 642

760.1   Maternal renal and urinary tract diseases
Fetus or newborn affected by maternal conditions classifiable to 580–599

760.2   Maternal infections
Fetus or newborn affected by maternal infectious disease classifiable to 001–136 and 487, but fetus or newborn not manifesting that disease

> **Excludes**   *congenital infectious diseases (771.0–771.8)*
> *maternal genital tract and other localized infections (760.8)*

760.3   Other chronic maternal circulatory and respiratory diseases
Fetus or newborn affected by chronic maternal conditions classifiable to 390–459, 490–519, 745–748

760.4   Maternal nutritional disorders
Fetus or newborn affected by:
maternal disorders classifiable to 260–269
maternal malnutrition NOS

> **Excludes**   *fetal malnutrition (764.10–764.29)*

760.5   Maternal injury
Fetus or newborn affected by maternal conditions classifiable to 800–995

● **760.6   Surgical operation on mother and fetus**

> **Excludes**   *cesarean section for present delivery (763.4)*
> *damage to placenta from amniocentesis, cesarean section, or surgical induction (762.1)*

Coding Clinic: 2008, Q4, P137-138

760.61   Newborn affected by amniocentesis

> **Excludes**   *fetal complications from amniocentesis (679.1)*

760.62   Newborn affected by other in utero procedure

> **Excludes**   *fetal complications of in utero procedure (679.1)*

760.63   Newborn affected by other surgical operations on mother during pregnancy

> **Excludes**   *newborn affected by previous surgical procedure on mother not associated with pregnancy (760.64)*

760.64   Newborn affected by previous surgical procedure on mother not associated with pregnancy

● **760.7   Noxious influences affecting fetus or newborn via placenta or breast milk**
Fetus or newborn affected by noxious substance transmitted via placenta or breast milk

> **Excludes**   *anesthetic and analgesic drugs administered during labor and delivery (763.5)*
> *drug withdrawal syndrome in newborn (779.5)*

Coding Clinic: 1991, Q3, P21

760.70   Unspecified noxious substance
Fetus or newborn affected by:
drug NEC

760.71   Alcohol
Fetal alcohol syndrome

760.72   Narcotics

760.73   Hallucinogenic agents

760.74   Anti-infectives
Antibiotics
Antifungals

760.75   Cocaine
Coding Clinic: 1994, Q3, P6; 1992, Q2, P12

760.76   Diethylstilbestrol [DES]

760.77   Anticonvulsants   N
Carbamazepine
Phenobarbital
Phenytoin
Valproic acid
Coding Clinic: 2005, Q4, P82-83

760.78   Antimetabolic agents   N
Methotrexate
Retinoic acid
Statins
Coding Clinic: 2005, Q4, P82-83

760.79   Other
Fetus or newborn affected by:
immune sera transmitted via placenta or breast milk
medicinal agents NEC transmitted via placenta or breast milk
toxic substance NEC transmitted via placenta or breast milk

N Newborn Age: 0   **P** Pediatric Age: 0–17   **M** Maternity Age: 12–55   **A** Adult Age: 15–124   ♀ Females Only   ♂ Males Only   **1039**

(Ex) CC Exclusions   🍎 Complication\Comorbidity   🍎 Major C\C   🍎 Present on Admission Requirement   🍎 Hospital-Acquired Condition

760.8 Other specified maternal conditions affecting fetus or newborn

Maternal genital tract and other localized infection affecting fetus or newborn, but fetus or newborn not manifesting that disease

> **Excludes** *maternal urinary tract infection affecting fetus or newborn (760.1)*

760.9 Unspecified maternal condition affecting fetus or newborn

● **761 Fetus or newborn affected by maternal complications of pregnancy**

> **Includes** the listed maternal conditions only when specified as a cause of mortality or morbidity of the fetus or newborn

761.0 Incompetent cervix

761.1 Premature rupture of membranes

761.2 Oligohydramnios

Scant volume of amniotic fluid

> **Excludes** *that due to premature rupture of membranes (761.1)*

761.3 Polyhydramnios

Overabundance of amniotic fluid
Hydramnios (acute) (chronic)

761.4 Ectopic pregnancy

Pregnancy:
    abdominal
    intraperitoneal
    tubal

761.5 Multiple pregnancy

Triplet (pregnancy)
Twin (pregnancy)

761.6 Maternal death

761.7 Malpresentation before labor

Breech presentation before labor
External version before labor
Oblique lie before labor
Transverse lie before labor
Unstable lie before labor

761.8 Other specified maternal complications of pregnancy affecting fetus or newborn

Spontaneous abortion, fetus

761.9 Unspecified maternal complication of pregnancy affecting fetus or newborn

● **762 Fetus or newborn affected by complications of placenta, cord, and membranes**

> **Includes** the listed maternal conditions only when specified as a cause of mortality or morbidity in the fetus or newborn

762.0 Placenta previa   N

762.1 Other forms of placental separation and hemorrhage   N

Abruptio placentae
Antepartum hemorrhage
Damage to placenta from amniocentesis, cesarean section, or surgical induction
Maternal blood loss
Premature separation of placenta
Rupture of marginal sinus

762.2 Other and unspecified morphological and functional abnormalities of placenta   N

Placental:
    dysfunction
    infarction
    insufficiency

762.3 Placental transfusion syndromes   N

Placental and cord abnormality resulting in twin-to-twin or other transplacental transfusion

> Use additional code to indicate resultant condition in ~~fetus or~~ newborn: ◄▥
>   fetal blood loss (772.0)
>   polycythemia neonatorum (776.4)

762.4 Prolapsed cord   N

Cord presentation

762.5 Other compression of umbilical cord   N

Cord around neck
Entanglement of cord
Knot in cord
Torsion of cord

Coding Clinic: 2003, Q2, P9

762.6 Other and unspecified conditions of umbilical cord N

Short cord
Thrombosis of umbilical cord
Varices of umbilical cord
Velamentous insertion of umbilical cord
Vasa previa

> **Excludes** *infection of umbilical cord (771.4)*
>   *single umbilical artery (747.5)*

762.7 Chorioamnionitis   N

Amnionitis
Membranitis
Placentitis

762.8 Other specified abnormalities of chorion and amnion N

762.9 Unspecified abnormality of chorion and amnion   N

● **763 Fetus or newborn affected by other complications of labor and delivery**

> **Includes** the listed conditions only when specified as a cause of mortality or morbidity in the fetus or newborn

> **Excludes** *newborn affected by surgical procedures on mother (760.61-760.64)*

763.0 Breech delivery and extraction   N

763.1 Other malpresentation, malposition, and disproportion during labor and delivery   N

Fetus or newborn affected by:
    abnormality of bony pelvis
    contracted pelvis
    persistent occipitoposterior position
    shoulder presentation
    transverse lie
    conditions classifiable to 652, 653, and 660

763.2 Forceps delivery   N

Fetus or newborn affected by forceps extraction

763.3 Delivery by vacuum extractor   N

763.4 Cesarean delivery   N

> **Excludes** *placental separation or hemorrhage from cesarean section (762.1)*

763.5 Maternal anesthesia and analgesia   N

Reactions and intoxications from maternal opiates and tranquilizers during labor and delivery

> **Excludes** *drug withdrawal syndrome in newborn (779.5)*

763.6 Precipitate delivery   N

Rapid second stage

◀ New   ◀▥ Revised   ~~deleted~~ Deleted   ● Unacceptable Principal Diagnosis   ● Use Additional Digit(s)
▶ Manifestation Code   **OGCR** Official Guidelines   **Coding Clinic**   Excludes   Includes   Use additional   Code first   Omit code

763.7 Abnormal uterine contractions   N
Fetus or newborn affected by:
contraction ring
hypertonic labor
hypotonic uterine dysfunction
uterine inertia or dysfunction
conditions classifiable to 661, except 661.3

●**763.8 Other specified complications of labor and delivery affecting fetus or newborn**

763.81 Abnormality in fetal heart rate or rhythm before the onset of labor   N

763.82 Abnormality in fetal heart rate or rhythm during labor   N
Coding Clinic: 1998, Q4, P46-47

763.83 Abnormality in fetal heart rate or rhythm, unspecified as to time of onset   N

763.84 Meconium passage during delivery   N

Excludes   meconium aspiration (770.11, 770.12)
meconium staining (779.84)
Coding Clinic: 2005, Q4, P83-89

763.89 Other specified complications of labor and delivery affecting fetus or newborn   N
Fetus or newborn affected by:
abnormality of maternal soft tissues
destructive operation on live fetus to facilitate delivery
induction of labor (medical)
other conditions classifiable to 650–669
other procedures used in labor and delivery

763.9 Unspecified complication of labor and delivery affecting fetus or newborn   N

OTHER CONDITIONS ORIGINATING IN THE PERINATAL PERIOD (764–779)

The following fifth-digit subclassification is for use with category 764 and codes 765.0 and 765.1 to denote birthweight:

0	unspecified [weight]
1	less than 500 grams
2	500–749 grams
3	750–999 grams
4	1,000–1,249 grams
5	1,250–1,499 grams
6	1,500–1,749 grams
7	1,750–1,999 grams
8	2,000–2,499 grams
9	2,500 grams and over

●**764 Slow fetal growth and fetal malnutrition**
Requires fifth digit. See beginning of section 764–779 for codes and definitions.
Coding Clinic: 2009, Q1, P7; 2004, Q3, P4-5; 1994, Q1, P15; 1989, Q2, P15
OGCR Section I.C.15.i
The 5th digit assignment for category 764 codes is based on the recorded birth weight and estimated gestational age

●**764.0 "Light-for-dates" without mention of fetal**
[0-9] **malnutrition**   N
Infants underweight for gestational age
"Small-for-dates"

●**764.1 "Light-for-dates" with signs of fetal malnutrition**   N
[0-9]   Infants "light-for-dates" classifiable to 764.0, who in addition show signs of fetal malnutrition, such as dry peeling skin and loss of subcutaneous tissue

●**764.2 Fetal malnutrition without mention of**
[0-9] **"light-for-dates"**   N
Infants, not underweight for gestational age, showing signs of fetal malnutrition, such as dry peeling skin and loss of subcutaneous tissue
Intrauterine malnutrition

●**764.9 Fetal growth retardation, unspecified**   N
[0-9]   Intrauterine growth retardation
Coding Clinic: 1997, Q1, P6

●**765 Disorders relating to short gestation and low birthweight**
Requires fifth digit. See beginning of section 764–779 for codes and definitions.

Includes   the listed conditions, without further specification, as causes of mortality, morbidity, or additional care, in fetus or newborn
Coding Clinic: 2002, Q4, P63-64; 1994, Q1, P15; 1991, Q2, P19, 1989, Q2, P15

●**765.0 Extreme immaturity**   N
[0-9]   **Note:** Usually implies a birthweight of less than 1,000 grams

Use additional code for weeks of gestation (765.20–765.29)
Coding Clinic: 2009, Q1, P12; 2004, Q3, P4-5; 2001, Q4, P50-51

OGCR Section I.C.15.i
Providers utilize different criteria in determining prematurity. A code for prematurity should not be assigned unless it is documented. The 5th digit assignment for codes from subcategory 765.0 should be based on the recorded birth weight and estimated gestational age.

●**765.1 Other preterm infants**   N
[0-9]   Prematurity NOS
Prematurity or small size, not classifiable to 765.0 or as "light-for-dates" in 764
Note: Usually implies birthweight of 1,000–2,499 grams

Use additional code for weeks of gestation (765.20–765.29)
Coding Clinic: 2009, Q1, P12; 2008, Q4, P138-140; 2004, Q3, P4-5; 2002, Q4, P64; 1997, Q1, P6; 1994, Q1, P14

OGCR Section I.C.15.i
Providers utilize different criteria in determining prematurity. A code for prematurity should not be assigned unless it is documented. The 5th digit assignment for codes from subcategory 765.1 should be based on the recorded birth weight and estimated gestational age.

CERTAIN CONDITIONS ORIGINATING IN THE PERINATAL PERIOD (760–779)

● **765.2 Weeks of gestation**
Coding Clinic: 2004, Q3, P4-5

OGCR Section I.C.15.i
A code from subcategory 765.2, Weeks of gestation, should be assigned as an additional code with category 764 and codes from 765.0 and 765.1 to specify weeks of gestation as documented by the provider in the record.

765.20   Unspecified weeks of gestation   N

765.21   Less than 24 completed weeks of gestation   N

765.22   24 weeks of gestation   N

765.23   25–26 weeks of gestation   N
Coding Clinic: 2009, Q1, P6

765.24   27–28 weeks of gestation   N

765.25   29–30 weeks of gestation   N

765.26   31–32 weeks of gestation   N
Coding Clinic: 2008, Q4, P138-140

765.27   33–34 weeks of gestation   N

765.28   35–36 weeks of gestation   N
Coding Clinic: 2002, Q4, P64

765.29   37 or more weeks of gestation   N

● **766   Disorders relating to long gestation and high birthweight**

Includes   the listed conditions, without further specification, as causes of mortality, morbidity, or additional care, in fetus or newborn

766.0   Exceptionally large baby   N

Note: Usually implies a birthweight of 4,500 grams or more.

766.1   Other "heavy-for-dates" infants   N
Other fetus or infant "heavy-" or "large-for-dates" regardless of period of gestation

● **766.2   Late infant, not "heavy-for-dates"**
Coding Clinic: 2006, Q2, P12-13; 2003, Q4, P69

766.21   **Post-term infant**   N
Infant with gestation period over 40 completed weeks to 42 completed weeks
Coding Clinic: 2009, Q1, P6; 2006, Q2, P12-13

766.22   **Prolonged gestation of infant**   N
Infant with gestation period over 42 completed weeks
Postmaturity NOS
Coding Clinic: 2009, Q1, P6; 2006, Q2, P12-13

● **767   Birth trauma**

767.0   Subdural and cerebral hemorrhage 🔊   N
Subdural and cerebral hemorrhage, whether described as due to birth trauma or to intrapartum anoxia or hypoxia
Subdural hematoma (localized)
Tentorial tear

Use additional code to identify cause

Excludes   *intraventricular hemorrhage (772.10–772.14)*
subarachnoid hemorrhage (772.2)
(Ex) 767.0, 767.8-767.9, 779.81-779.84, 779.89

● **767.1   Injuries to scalp**
Coding Clinic: 2003, Q4, P69-70

767.11   **Epicranial subaponeurotic hemorrhage (massive)** 🔊   N
Subgaleal hemorrhage
(Ex) 767.0-767.11, 767.8-767.9, 779.81-779.84, 779.89

767.19   **Other injuries to scalp**   N
Caput succedaneum
Cephalhematoma
Chignon (from vacuum extraction)

767.2   Fracture of clavicle   N

767.3   Other injuries to skeleton   N
Fracture of:
long bones
skull

Excludes   *congenital dislocation of hip (754.30–754.35)*
fracture of spine, congenital (767.4)

767.4   Injury to spine and spinal cord   N
Dislocation of spine or spinal cord due to birth trauma
Fracture of spine or spinal cord due to birth trauma
Laceration of spine or spinal cord due to birth trauma
Rupture of spine or spinal cord due to birth trauma

767.5   Facial nerve injury   N
Facial palsy

767.6   Injury to brachial plexus   N
Palsy or paralysis:
brachial
Erb (-Duchenne)
Klumpke (-Déjérine)

767.7   Other cranial and peripheral nerve injuries   N
Phrenic nerve paralysis

767.8   Other specified birth trauma   N
Eye damage
Hematoma of:
liver (subcapsular)
testes
vulva
Rupture of:
liver
spleen
Scalpel wound
Traumatic glaucoma

Excludes   *hemorrhage classifiable to 772.0–772.9*

767.9   Birth trauma, unspecified   N
Birth injury NOS

● **768   Intrauterine hypoxia and birth asphyxia**
Use only when associated with newborn morbidity classifiable elsewhere

Excludes   *acidemia NOS of newborn (775.81)*
acidosis NOS of newborn (775.81)
cerebral ischemia NOS (779.2)
hypoxia NOS of newborn (770.88)
mixed metabolic and respiratory acidosis of newborn (775.81)
respiratory arrest of newborn (770.87)

768.0   Fetal death from asphyxia or anoxia before onset of labor or at unspecified time   N

◀ New   ◀▥ Revised   ~~deleted~~ Deleted   ● Unacceptable Principal Diagnosis   ● Use Additional Digit(s)
▶ Manifestation Code   **OGCR** Official Guidelines   **Coding Clinic**   Excludes   Includes   Use additional   Code first   Omit code

768.1 Fetal death from asphyxia or anoxia during labor N

768.2 Fetal distress before onset of labor, in liveborn infant N
Fetal metabolic acidemia before onset of labor, in liveborn infant

768.3 Fetal distress first noted during labor and delivery, in liveborn infant N
Fetal metabolic acidemia first noted during labor and delivery, in liveborn infant

768.4 Fetal distress, unspecified as to time of onset, in liveborn infant N
Fetal metabolic acidemia unspecified as to time of onset, in liveborn infant
Coding Clinic: 1986, Nov-Dec, P10

768.5 Severe birth asphyxia N
Birth asphyxia with neurologic involvement

> **Excludes** *hypoxic-ischemic encephalopathy (HIE) (768.70-768.73)* ◄

(Ex) 768.5-768.6, 768.9-770.86, 770.89-770.9, 779.81-779.84, 779.89

768.6 Mild or moderate birth asphyxia N
Other specified birth asphyxia (without mention of neurologic involvement)

> **Excludes** *hypoxic-ischemic encephalopathy (HIE) (768.70-768.73)* ◄

●**768.7 Hypoxic-ischemic encephalopathy (HIE)** N ◄
(Ex) 768.5-768.6, 768.9
Coding Clinic: 2006, Q4, P104-106

   768.70 Hypoxic-ischemic encephalopathy, unspecified ◄

   768.71 Mild hypoxic-ischemic encephalopathy ◄

   768.72 Moderate hypoxic-ischemic encephalopathy ◄

   768.73 Severe hypoxic-ischemic encephalopathy ◄

768.9 Unspecified birth asphyxia in liveborn infant N
Anoxia NOS, in liveborn infant
Asphyxia NOS, in liveborn infant

769 Respiratory distress syndrome N
Cardiorespiratory distress syndrome of newborn
Hyaline membrane disease (pulmonary)
Idiopathic respiratory distress syndrome [IRDS or RDS] of newborn
Pulmonary hypoperfusion syndrome

> **Excludes** *transient tachypnea of newborn (770.6)*

(Ex) 768.5-768.6, 768.9-770.86, 770.89-770.9, 779.81-779.84, 779.89
Coding Clinic: 1989, Q1, P10

●**770 Other respiratory conditions of fetus and newborn**

770.0 Congenital pneumonia N
Infective pneumonia acquired prenatally

> **Excludes** *pneumonia from infection acquired after birth (480.0–486)*

(Ex) 768.5-768.6, 768.9-770.86, 770.89-770.9, 779.81-779.84, 779.89
Coding Clinic: 2005, Q1, P10-11

●**770.1 Fetal and newborn aspiration**

> **Excludes** *aspiration of postnatal stomach contents (770.85, 770.86)*
> *meconium passage during delivery (763.84)*
> *meconium staining (779.84)*

Coding Clinic: 2005, Q4, P83-89

   770.10 Fetal and newborn aspiration, unspecified N

   770.11 Meconium aspiration without respiratory symptoms N
Meconium aspiration NOS

   770.12 Meconium aspiration with respiratory symptoms N
Meconium aspiration pneumonia
Meconium aspiration pneumonitis
Meconium aspiration syndrome NOS

> Use additional code to identify any secondary pulmonary hypertension (416.8), if applicable

(Ex) 768.5-768.6, 768.9-770.86, 770.89-770.9, 779.81-779.84, 779.89

   770.13 Aspiration of clear amniotic fluid without respiratory symptoms N
Aspiration of clear amniotic fluid NOS

   770.14 Aspiration of clear amniotic fluid with respiratory symptoms N
Aspiration of clear amniotic fluid with pneumonia
Aspiration of clear amniotic fluid with pneumonitis

> Use additional code to identify any secondary pulmonary hypertension (416.8), if applicable

(Ex) 768.5-768.6, 768.9-770.86, 770.89-770.9, 779.81-779.84, 779.89

   770.15 Aspiration of blood without respiratory symptoms N
Aspiration of blood NOS

   770.16 Aspiration of blood with respiratory symptoms N
Aspiration of blood with pneumonia
Aspiration of blood with pneumonitis

> Use additional code to identify any secondary pulmonary hypertension (416.8), if applicable

(Ex) 768.5-768.6, 768.9-770.86, 770.89-770.9, 779.81-779.84, 779.89

   770.17 Other fetal and newborn aspiration without respiratory symptoms N

   770.18 Other fetal and newborn aspiration with respiratory symptoms N
Other aspiration pneumonia
Other aspiration pneumonitis

> Use additional code to identify any secondary pulmonary hypertension (416.8), if applicable

(Ex) 768.5-768.6, 768.9-770.86, 770.89-770.9, 779.81-779.84, 779.89

770.2 Interstitial emphysema and related conditions N
Pneumomediastinum originating in the perinatal period
Pneumopericardium originating in the perinatal period
Pneumothorax originating in the perinatal period
(Ex) 768.5-768.6, 768.9-770.86, 770.89-770.9, 779.81-779.84, 779.89

770.3 Pulmonary hemorrhage N
Hemorrhage:
alveolar (lung) originating in the perinatal period
intra-alveolar (lung) originating in the perinatal period
massive pulmonary originating in the perinatal period
(Ex) 768.5-768.6, 768.9-770.86, 770.89-770.9, 779.81-779.84, 779.89

N Newborn Age: 0 P Pediatric Age: 0–17 M Maternity Age: 12–55 A Adult Age: 15–124 ♀ Females Only ♂ Males Only
(Ex) CC Exclusions ⬥ Complication\Comorbidity ⬥ Major C\C ⬥ Present on Admission Requirement ⬥ Hospital-Acquired Condition

1043

CERTAIN CONDITIONS ORIGINATING IN THE PERINATAL PERIOD (760–779)

CERTAIN CONDITIONS ORIGINATING IN THE PERINATAL PERIOD (760–779)

770.4 Primary atelectasis 🔵   N
Failure of lungs to expand properly at birth
Pulmonary immaturity NOS
(Ex:) 768.5-768.6, 768.9-770.86, 770.89-770.9, 779.81-779.84, 779.89

770.5 Other and unspecified atelectasis 🔵   N
Atelectasis:
    NOS originating in the perinatal period
    partial originating in the perinatal period
    secondary originating in the perinatal period
Pulmonary collapse originating in the perinatal
    period
(Ex:) 768.5-768.6, 768.9-770.86, 770.89-770.9, 779.81-779.84, 779.89

770.6 Transitory tachypnea of newborn   N
Idiopathic tachypnea of newborn
Wet lung syndrome

> **Excludes**   *respiratory distress syndrome (769)*

Coding Clinic: 1993, Q3, P7x2; 1989, Q1, P10

770.7 Chronic respiratory disease arising in the perinatal period 🔵   N
Bronchopulmonary dysplasia
Interstitial pulmonary fibrosis of prematurity
Wilson-Mikity syndrome
(Ex:) 768.5-768.6, 768.9-770.86, 770.89-770.9, 779.81-779.84, 779.89
Coding Clinic: 1991, Q2, P19; 1986, Nov-Dec, P11-12

● **770.8 Other respiratory problems after birth**

> **Excludes**   *mixed metabolic and respiratory acidosis of newborn (775.81)*

Coding Clinic: 2005, Q4, P83-89; 2002, Q4, P65-66; 1998, Q2, P10; 1996, Q2, P10-11

770.81 Primary apnea of newborn 🔵   N
Apneic spells of newborn NOS
Essential apnea of newborn
Sleep apnea of newborn
(Ex:) 770.82-770.83, 770.87-770.9, 786.03

770.82 Other apnea of newborn 🔵   N
Obstructive apnea of newborn
(Ex:) 770.81-770.83, 770.87-770.9, 786.03

770.83 Cyanotic attacks of newborn 🔵   N
(Ex:) 770.81-770.83, 770.87-770.9, 782.5, 786.03

770.84 Respiratory failure of newborn 🔵   N

> **Excludes**   *respiratory distress syndrome (769)*

(Ex:) 768.5-768.6, 768.9-770.86, 770.89-770.9, 779.81-779.84, 779.89

770.85 Aspiration of postnatal stomach contents without respiratory symptoms   N
Aspiration of postnatal stomach contents NOS

770.86 Aspiration of postnatal stomach contents with respiratory symptoms 🔵   N
Aspiration of postnatal stomach contents
    with pneumonia
Aspiration of postnatal stomach contents
    with pneumonitis

> Use additional code to identify any
> secondary pulmonary hypertension
> (416.8), if applicable

(Ex:) 768.5-768.6, 768.9-770.86, 770.89-770.9, 779.81-779.84, 779.89

770.87 Respiratory arrest of newborn 🔵   N
(Ex:) 770.11, 770.13, 770.15, 770.17, 770.6, 770.81-770.85, 770.88-770.9, 779.85, 786.03, 799.1

770.88 Hypoxemia of newborn   N
Hypoxia NOS, in liveborn infant

770.89 Other respiratory problems after birth   N

770.9 Unspecified respiratory condition of fetus and newborn   N

● **771 Infections specific to the perinatal period**

> **Includes**   infections acquired before or during birth or
> via the umbilicus or during the first 28
> days after birth

> **Excludes**   *congenital pneumonia (770.0)*
> *congenital syphilis (090.0–090.9)*
> *infant botulism (040.41)*
> *maternal infectious disease as a cause of mortality*
> *or morbidity in fetus or newborn, but fetus*
> *or newborn not manifesting the disease*
> *(760.2)*
> *ophthalmia neonatorum due to gonococcus*
> *(098.40)*
> *other infections not specifically classified to this*
> *category*

Coding Clinic: 2005, Q1, P10

771.0 Congenital rubella 🔵   N
Congenital rubella pneumonitis
(Ex:) 771.0-771.2, 779.81-779.84, 779.89

771.1 Congenital cytomegalovirus infection 🔵   N
Congenital cytomegalic inclusion disease
(Ex:) 771.0-771.2, 779.81-779.84, 779.89

771.2 Other congenital infections 🔵   N
Congenital: Congenital:
  herpes simplex   toxoplasmosis
  listeriosis   tuberculosis
  malaria
(Ex:) 013.60-013.66, 046.2, 046.71-046.8, 048-049.0, 049.8, 052.0, 052.2, 054.3, 054.74, 056.01, 057.8-058.29, 059.00-059.9, 062.0-064, 066.2-066.49, 072.2, 073.7, 075, 078.3, 079.82, 079.99, 081.9, 083.9, 084.6, 090.41, 094.81, 117.5, 124, 130.0, 290.12, 323.01-323.9, 341.1, 382.4, 487.8, 710.0, 771.2, 984.9

771.3 Tetanus neonatorum 🔵   N
Tetanus omphalitis

> **Excludes**   *hypocalcemic tetany (775.4)*

(Ex:) 771.3, 779.81-779.84, 779.89

771.4 Omphalitis of the newborn 🔵   N
Infection: Infection:
  navel cord   umbilical stump

> **Excludes**   *tetanus omphalitis (771.3)*

(Ex:) 771.89

771.5 Neonatal infective mastitis 🔵   N

> **Excludes**   *noninfective neonatal mastitis (778.7)*

(Ex:) 771.89

771.6 Neonatal conjunctivitis and dacryocystitis   N
Ophthalmia neonatorum NOS

> **Excludes**   *ophthalmia neonatorum due to gonococcus*
> *(098.40)*

771.7 Neonatal Candida infection   N
Neonatal moniliasis
Thrush in newborn

● **771.8 Other infections specific to the perinatal period**

> Use additional code to identify organism
> (041.00–041.9)

771.81 Septicemia [sepsis] of newborn 🔵   N

> Use additional code to identify
> severe sepsis (995.92) and any
> associated acute organ dysfunction,
> if applicable

(Ex:) 771.4-771.89, 776.0-776.9, 779.81 -779.84, 779.89

◀ New   ◀▦ Revised   ~~deleted~~ Deleted   ● Unacceptable Principal Diagnosis   ● Use Additional Digit(s)
▶ Manifestation Code   **OGCR** Official Guidelines   **Coding Clinic** Coding Clinic   Excludes   Includes   Use additional   Code first   Omit code

OGCR Section I.C.15.j

> 771.81 should be assigned with a secondary code from category 041, Bacterial infections in conditions classified elsewhere and of unspecified site, to identify the organism.

771.82 Urinary tract infection of newborn   N
    (Ex) 041.9, 590.00-590.9, 593.89-593.9, 595.0 -595.81,
      595.89-595.9, 599.0, 599.9 771.89, 788.1, 996.64

771.83 Bacteremia of newborn   N
    (Ex) 771.4-771.89, 776.0-776.9, 779.81-779.84, 779.89

771.89 Other infections specific to the perinatal period   N
    Intra-amniotic infection of fetus NOS
    Infection of newborn NOS
    (Ex) 003.1, 020.2, 022.3, 036.2, 038.0-038.9, 040.89-041.9, 054.5,
      139.8, 771.82 -771.89, 779.9, 790.7
    Coding Clinic: 2005, Q1, P10

● **772 Fetal and neonatal hemorrhage**

    Excludes   *fetal hematologic conditions complicating pregnancy (678.0)*
      hematological disorders of fetus and newborn (776.0–776.9)

772.0 Fetal blood loss affecting newborn   N
    Fetal blood loss from:
      cut end of co-twin's cord
      placenta
      ruptured cord
      vasa previa
    Fetal exsanguination
    Fetal hemorrhage into:
      co-twin
      mother's circulation

● **772.1 Intraventricular hemorrhage**
    Intraventricular hemorrhage from any perinatal cause
    Coding Clinic: 1992, Q3, P8; 1988, Q4, P8

772.10 Unspecified grade   N
    (Ex) 772.0-772.2, 772.8-772.9, 776.0-776.9, 779.81-779.84, 779.89

772.11 Grade I   N
    Bleeding into germinal matrix
    (Ex) 772.0-772.2, 772.8-772.9, 776.0-776.9, 779.81 -779.84, 779.89

772.12 Grade II   N
    Bleeding into ventricle
    (Ex) 772.0 -772.2, 772.8-772.9, 776.0-776.9, 779.81-779.84, 779.89

772.13 Grade III   N
    Bleeding with enlargement of ventricle
    (Ex) 772.0-772.2, 772.8-772.9, 776.0-776.9, 779.81-779.84, 779.89
    Coding Clinic: 2001, Q4, P50-51

772.14 Grade IV   N
    Bleeding into cerebral cortex
    (Ex) 772.0 -772.2, 772.8-772.9, 776.0-776.9, 779.81-779.84, 779.89

772.2 Subarachnoid hemorrhage   N
    Subarachnoid hemorrhage from any perinatal cause

    Excludes   *subdural and cerebral hemorrhage (767.0)*
    (Ex) 772.0-772.2, 772.8-772.9, 776.0-776.9, 779.7-779.84, 779.89

772.3 Umbilical hemorrhage after birth   N
    Slipped umbilical ligature

772.4 Gastrointestinal hemorrhage   N
    Excludes   *swallowed maternal blood (777.3)*
    (Ex) 772.0, 772.4-772.5, 772.8-772.9, 776.0-776.9, 779.81-779.84, 779.89

772.5 Adrenal hemorrhage   N
    772.0, 772.4-772.5, 772.8-772.9, 776.0-776.9, 779.81-779.84, 779.89

772.6 Cutaneous hemorrhage   N
    Bruising in fetus or newborn
    Ecchymoses in fetus or newborn
    Petechiae in fetus or newborn
    Superficial hematoma in fetus or newborn

772.8 Other specified hemorrhage of fetus or newborn   N
    Excludes   *hemorrhagic disease of newborn (776.0)*
      pulmonary hemorrhage (770.3)

772.9 Unspecified hemorrhage of newborn   N

● **773 Hemolytic disease of fetus or newborn, due to isoimmunization**
    Also known as erythroblastosis fetalis as a result of Rh blood factor incompatibilities between mother (Rh negative) and fetus (Rh positive)

773.0 Hemolytic disease due to Rh isoimmunization   N
    Anemia due to RH:
      antibodies
      isoimmunization
      maternal/fetal incompatibility
    Erythroblastosis (fetalis) due to RH:
      antibodies
      isoimmunization
      maternal/fetal incompatibility
    Hemolytic disease (fetus) (newborn) due to RH:
      antibodies
      isoimmunization
      maternal/fetal incompatibility
    Jaundice due to RH:
      antibodies
      isoimmunization
      maternal/fetal incompatibility
    Rh hemolytic disease
    Rh isoimmunization

773.1 Hemolytic disease due to ABO isoimmunization   N
    ABO hemolytic disease
    ABO isoimmunization
    Anemia due to ABO:
      antibodies
      isoimmunization
      maternal/fetal incompatibility
    Erythroblastosis (fetalis) due to ABO:
      antibodies
      isoimmunization
      maternal/fetal incompatibility
    Hemolytic disease (fetus) (newborn) due to ABO:
      antibodies
      isoimmunization
      maternal/fetal incompatibility
    Jaundice due to ABO:
      antibodies
      isoimmunization
      maternal/fetal incompatibility
    Coding Clinic: 2003, Q2, P14-15; 1992, Q3, P8-9

773.2 Hemolytic disease due to other and unspecified isoimmunization   N
    Erythroblastosis (fetalis) (neonatorum) NOS
    Hemolytic disease (fetus) (newborn) NOS
    Jaundice or anemia due to other and unspecified blood-group incompatibility
    Coding Clinic: 1994, Q1, P13

773.3 Hydrops fetalis due to isoimmunization   N
    Use additional code, if desired, to identify type of isoimmunization (773.0–773.2)
    (Ex) 773.0-773.5, 779.81 -779.84, 779.89

N Newborn Age: 0   **P** Pediatric Age: 0–17   **M** Maternity Age: 12–55   **A** Adult Age: 15–124   ♀ Females Only   ♂ Males Only   **1045**

(Ex) CC Exclusions   Complication\Comorbidity   Major C\C   Present on Admission Requirement   Hospital-Acquired Condition

CERTAIN CONDITIONS ORIGINATING IN THE PERINATAL PERIOD (760–779)

773.4 Kernicterus due to isoimmunization 🔖   N

Use additional code, if desired, to identify type of isoimmunization (773.0–773.2)

(Ex:) 773.0-773.5, 779.81-779.84, 779.89

773.5 Late anemia due to isoimmunization   N

● **774 Other perinatal jaundice**

▶ **774.0 Perinatal jaundice from hereditary hemolytic anemias**   N

Code first underlying disease (282.0–282.9)

774.1 Perinatal jaundice from other excessive hemolysis   N

Fetal or neonatal jaundice from:
  bruising
  drugs or toxins transmitted from mother
  infection
  polycythemia
  swallowed maternal blood

Use additional code to identify cause

Excludes | jaundice due to isoimmunization (773.0–773.2)

774.2 Neonatal jaundice associated with preterm delivery   N

Hyperbilirubinemia of prematurity
Jaundice due to delayed conjugation associated with preterm delivery

Coding Clinic: 1994, Q1, P13; 1991, Q3, P21

● **774.3 Neonatal jaundice due to delayed conjugation from other causes**

    774.30 Neonatal jaundice due to delayed conjugation, cause unspecified   N

▶   **774.31 Neonatal jaundice due to delayed conjugation in diseases classified elsewhere**   N

Code first underlying diseases, as:
  congenital hypothyroidism (243)
  Crigler-Najjar syndrome (277.4)
  Gilbert's syndrome (277.4)

    774.39 Other   N

Jaundice due to delayed conjugation from causes, such as:
  breast milk inhibitors
  delayed development of conjugating system

774.4 Perinatal jaundice due to hepatocellular damage 🔖   N

Fetal or neonatal hepatitis
Giant cell hepatitis
Inspissated bile syndrome

(Ex:) 774.0-774.7, 779.81 -779.84, 779.89

▶ **774.5 Perinatal jaundice from other causes**   N

Code first underlying cause, as:
  congenital obstruction of bile duct (751.61)
  galactosemia (271.1)
  mucoviscidosis (277.00–277.09)

774.6 Unspecified fetal and neonatal jaundice   N

Icterus neonatorum
Neonatal hyperbilirubinemia (transient)
Physiologic jaundice NOS in newborn

Excludes | that in preterm infants (774.2)

Coding Clinic: 1994, Q1, P13

774.7 Kernicterus not due to isoimmunization 🔖   N

Bilirubin encephalopathy
Kernicterus of newborn NOS

Excludes | kernicterus due to isoimmunization (773.4)

(Ex:) 774.0-774.7, 779.81-779.84, 779.89

● **775 Endocrine and metabolic disturbances specific to the fetus and newborn**

Includes   transitory endocrine and metabolic disturbances caused by the infant's response to maternal endocrine and metabolic factors, its removal from them, or its adjustment to extrauterine existence

775.0 Syndrome of "infant of a diabetic mother"   N

Maternal diabetes mellitus affecting fetus or newborn (with hypoglycemia)

Coding Clinic: 2004, Q1, P7-8x3

775.1 Neonatal diabetes mellitus 🔖   N

Diabetes mellitus syndrome in newborn infant

(Ex:) 775.0-775.7, 775.9, 779.81-779.84, 779.89

775.2 Neonatal myasthenia gravis 🔖   N

(Ex:) 775.0-775.7, 775.9, 779.81-779.84, 779.89

775.3 Neonatal thyrotoxicosis 🔖   N

Neonatal hyperthyroidism (transient)

(Ex:) 775.0-775.7, 775.9, 779.81-779.84, 779.89

775.4 Hypocalcemia and hypomagnesemia of newborn 🔖   N

Cow's milk hypocalcemia
Hypocalcemic tetany, neonatal
Neonatal hypoparathyroidism
Phosphate-loading hypocalcemia

(Ex:) 775.0-775.7, 775.9, 779.81-779.84, 779.89

775.5 Other transitory neonatal electrolyte disturbances   N

Dehydration, neonatal

Coding Clinic: 2008, Q4, P139-140; 2005, Q1, P9-10

775.6 Neonatal hypoglycemia   N

Excludes | infant of mother with diabetes mellitus (775.0)

775.7 Late metabolic acidosis of newborn 🔖   N

(Ex:) 775.0-775.7, 775.9, 779.81-779.84, 779.89

● **775.8 Other neonatal endocrine and metabolic disturbances**

    775.81 Other acidosis of newborn 🔖   N

Acidemia NOS of newborn
Acidosis of newborn NOS
Mixed metabolic and respiratory acidosis of newborn

(Ex:) 775.5, 775.7, 775.9

    775.89 Other neonatal endocrine and metabolic disturbances 🔖   N

Amino-acid metabolic disorders described as transitory

(Ex:) 775.0-775.7, 775.9

775.9 Unspecified endocrine and metabolic disturbances specific to the fetus and newborn   N

● **776 Hematological disorders of newborn**

Includes   disorders specific to the ~~fetus or~~ newborn though possibly originating in utero ◀▥

Excludes | fetal hematologic conditions (678.0)

776.0 Hemorrhagic disease of newborn 🔖   N

Hemorrhagic diathesis of newborn
Vitamin K deficiency of newborn

Excludes | fetal or neonatal hemorrhage (772.0–772.9)

(Ex:) 776.0-776.9, 779.81-779.84, 779.89

◀ New   ◀▥ Revised   ~~deleted~~ Deleted   ● Unacceptable Principal Diagnosis   🔖 Use Additional Digit(s)

▶ Manifestation Code   OGCR Official Guidelines   Coding Clinic   Excludes   Includes   Use additional   Code first   Omit code

776.1 Transient neonatal thrombocytopenia 🔹 N
Lack of sufficient numbers of circulating thrombocytes (platelets)
Neonatal thrombocytopenia due to:
  exchange transfusion
  idiopathic maternal thrombocytopenia
  isoimmunization
Ex: 776.0-776.9, 779.81-779.84, 779.89

776.2 Disseminated intravascular coagulation in newborn 🔹 N
Ex: 776.0-776.9, 779.81-779.84, 779.89

776.3 Other transient neonatal disorders of coagulation 🔹 N
Transient coagulation defect, newborn
Ex: 776.0-776.9, 779.81-779.84, 779.89

776.4 Polycythemia neonatorum N
Excess number of thrombocytes (platelets)
Plethora of newborn
Polycythemia due to:
  donor twin transfusion
  maternal-fetal transfusion

776.5 Congenital anemia 🔹 N
Anemia following fetal blood loss
> **Excludes** *anemia due to isoimmunization*
> *(773.0–773.2, 773.5)*
> *hereditary hemolytic anemias (282.0–282.9)*
Ex: 280.0-282.3, 282.5-285.9, 289.9, 517.3, 776.5-776.6

776.6 Anemia of prematurity 🔹 N
Ex: 280.0-282.3, 282.5-285.9, 289.9, 517.3, 776.5-776.6

776.7 Transient neonatal neutropenia 🔹 N
Isoimmune neutropenia
Low levels of granulocytic neutrophilic white blood cells
Maternal transfer neutropenia
> **Excludes** *congenital neutropenia (nontransient)*
> *(288.01)*
Ex: 280.1-281.9, 282.5-282.63, 282.69-282.7, 283.0, 283.11, 284.01-285.0, 285.21-285.9, 289.9, 776.7-776.9

776.8 Other specified transient hematological disorders N

776.9 Unspecified hematological disorder specific to ~~fetus or~~ newborn N ◀

● **777 Perinatal disorders of digestive system**
> **Includes** disorders specific to the fetus and newborn
> **Excludes** *intestinal obstruction classifiable to 560.0–560.9*

777.1 Meconium obstruction N
Congenital fecaliths
Stoney feces formations
Delayed passage of meconium
Meconium ileus NOS
Meconium plug syndrome
> **Excludes** *meconium ileus in cystic fibrosis (277.01)*

777.2 Intestinal obstruction due to inspissated milk N
Being thickened, dried, or made less fluid

777.3 Hematemesis and melena due to swallowed maternal blood N
Swallowed blood syndrome in newborn
> **Excludes** *that not due to swallowed maternal blood (772.4)*

777.4 Transitory ileus of newborn 🔹 N
> **Excludes** *Hirschsprung's disease (751.3)*
Ex: 777.1-777.9

● **777.5 Necrotizing enterocolitis in newborn**
~~Pseudomembranous enterocolitis in newborn~~

777.50 Necrotizing enterocolitis in newborn, unspecified 🔹 N
Necrotizing enterocolitis in newborn, NOS
Ex: 777.1-777.9, 779.81-779.84, 779.89

777.51 Stage I necrotizing enterocolitis in newborn 🔹 N
Necrotizing enterocolitis without pneumatosis, without perforation ◀
Ex: 777.1-777.9, 779.81-779.84, 779.89

777.52 Stage II necrotizing enterocolitis in newborn 🔹 N
Necrotizing enterocolitis with pneumatosis, without perforation
Ex: 777.1-777.9, 779.81 -779.84, 779.89

777.53 Stage III necrotizing enterocolitis in newborn 🔹 N
Necrotizing enterocolitis with perforation
Necrotizing enterocolitis with pneumatosis and perforation
Ex: 777.1-777.9, 779.81 -779.84, 779.89
Coding Clinic: 2008, Q4, P138-140

777.6 Perinatal intestinal perforation 🔹 N
Meconium peritonitis
Ex: 777.1-777.9, 779.81-779.84, 779.89

777.8 Other specified perinatal disorders of digestive system N

777.9 Unspecified perinatal disorder of digestive system N

● **778 Conditions involving the integument and temperature regulation of fetus and newborn**

778.0 Hydrops fetalis not due to isoimmunization 🔹 N
Idiopathic hydrops
Severe, life-threatening problem of edema (swelling) in fetus and newborn
> **Excludes** *hydrops fetalis due to isoimmunization (773.3)*
Ex: 778.0, 779.81-779.84, 779.89

778.1 Sclerema neonatorum 🔹 N
Ex: 778.1, 778.5

778.2 Cold injury syndrome of newborn N

778.3 Other hypothermia of newborn N

778.4 Other disturbances of temperature regulation of newborn N
Dehydration fever in newborn
Environmentally induced pyrexia
Hyperthermia in newborn
Transitory fever of newborn

778.5 Other and unspecified edema of newborn 🔹 N
Edema neonatorum
Ex: 778.1-778.5

778.6 Congenital hydrocele N
Congenital hydrocele of tunica vaginalis

778.7 Breast engorgement in newborn N
Noninfective mastitis of newborn
> **Excludes** *infective mastitis of newborn (771.5)*

778.8 Other specified conditions involving the integument of fetus and newborn N
Urticaria neonatorum
Skin rash
> **Excludes** *impetigo neonatorum (684)*
> *pemphigus neonatorum (684)*

778.9 Unspecified condition involving the integument and temperature regulation of fetus and newborn N

N Newborn Age: 0   **P** Pediatric Age: 0–17   **M** Maternity Age: 12–55   **A** Adult Age: 15–124   ♀ Females Only   ♂ Males Only
Ex: CC Exclusions 🔹 Complication\Comorbidity 🔹 Major C\C 🔹 Present on Admission Requirement 🔹 Hospital-Acquired Condition

● **779 Other and ill-defined conditions originating in the perinatal period**

779.0 Convulsions in newborn 🔖   N
> Fits in newborn
> Seizures in newborn
> (Ex:) 779.0-779.1, 779.81-779.84, 779.89
> **Coding Clinic: 1984, Nov-Dec, P11**

779.1 Other and unspecified cerebral irritability in newborn   N

779.2 Cerebral depression, coma, and other abnormal cerebral signs 🔖   N
> Cerebral ischemia NOS of newborn
> CNS dysfunction in newborn NOS
> | Excludes | cerebral ischemia due to birth trauma (767.0)
> intrauterine cerebral ischemia (768.2–768.9)
> intraventricular hemorrhage (772.10–772.14)
> (Ex:) 779.0-779.2

● **779.3 Disorder of stomach function and ~~F~~feeding problems in newborn**   N ◀◀
> ~~Regurgitation of food in newborn~~
> ~~Slow feeding in newborn~~
> ~~Vomiting in newborn~~
> **Coding Clinic: 1989, Q2, P15**

  779.31 Feeding problems in newborn ◀
> Slow feeding in newborn ◀
> | Excludes | feeding problem in child over 28 days old (783.3) ◀

  779.32 Bilious vomiting in newborn 🔖 ◀
> | Excludes | bilious vomiting in child over 28 days old (787.04) ◀

  779.33 Other vomiting in newborn ◀
> Regurgitation of food in newborn ◀
> | Excludes | vomiting in child over 28 days old (536.2, 787.01-787.03, 787.04) ◀

  779.34 Failure to thrive in newborn ◀
> | Excludes | failure to thrive in child over 28 days old (783.41) ◀

779.4 Drug reactions and intoxications specific to newborn 🔖   N
> Gray syndrome from chloramphenicol administration in newborn
> | Excludes | fetal alcohol syndrome (760.71)
> reactions and intoxications from maternal opiates and tranquilizers (763.5)
> (Ex:) 779.4-779.5

779.5 Drug withdrawal syndrome in newborn 🔖   N
> Drug withdrawal syndrome in infant of dependent mother
> | Excludes | fetal alcohol syndrome (760.71)
> (Ex:) 779.4-779.5
> **Coding Clinic: 1994, Q3, P6**

779.6 Termination of pregnancy (fetus)   N
> Fetal death due to:
> induced abortion
> termination of pregnancy
> | Excludes | spontaneous abortion (fetus) (761.8)

779.7 Periventricular leukomalacia 🔖
> (Ex:) 772.0-772.2, 772.8-772.9, 776.0-776.9, 779.7-779.84, 779.89
> **Coding Clinic: 2001, Q4, P50-51**

● **779.8 Other specified conditions originating in the perinatal period**
> **Coding Clinic: 2006, Q1, P18; 2002, Q4, P67; 1994, Q1, P15**

  779.81 Neonatal bradycardia   N
> | Excludes | abnormality in fetal heart rate or rhythm complicating labor and delivery (763.81–763.83)
> bradycardia due to birth asphyxia (768.5–768.9)

  779.82 Neonatal tachycardia   N
> | Excludes | abnormality in fetal heart rate or rhythm complicating labor and delivery (763.81–763.83)

  779.83 Delayed separation of umbilical cord   N
> **Coding Clinic: 2003, Q4, P71**

  779.84 Meconium staining   N
> | Excludes | meconium aspiration (770.11, 770.12)
> meconium passage during delivery (763.84)
> **Coding Clinic: 2005, Q4, P83-89x2**

  779.85 Cardiac arrest of newborn 🔖   N
> (Ex:) 779.85

  779.89 Other specified conditions originating in the perinatal period   N
> Use additional code to specify condition
> **Coding Clinic: 2005, Q2, P15-16; Q1, P9**
> **OGCR** Section I.C.15.a.2
> If the index does not provide a specific code for a perinatal condition, assign code 779.89 followed by the code from another chapter that specifies the condition.

779.9 Unspecified condition originating in the perinatal period   N
> Congenital debility NOS
> Stillbirth NEC

◀ New   ◀◀ Revised   ~~deleted~~ Deleted   ● Unacceptable Principal Diagnosis   ● Use Additional Digit(s)
▶ Manifestation Code   **OGCR** Official Guidelines   **Coding Clinic**   Excludes   Includes   Use additional   Code first   Omit code

16. SYMPTOMS, SIGNS, AND ILL-DEFINED CONDITIONS (780–799)

This section includes symptoms, signs, abnormal results of laboratory or other investigative procedures, and ill-defined conditions regarding which no diagnosis classifiable elsewhere is recorded.

Signs and symptoms that point rather definitely to a given diagnosis are assigned to some category in the preceding part of the classification. In general, categories 780–796 include the more ill-defined conditions and symptoms that point with perhaps equal suspicion to two or more diseases or to two or more systems of the body, and without the necessary study of the case to make a final diagnosis. Practically all categories in this group could be designated as "not otherwise specified," or as "unknown etiology," or as "transient." The Alphabetic Index should be consulted to determine which symptoms and signs are to be allocated here and which to more specific sections of the classification; the residual subcategories numbered .9 are provided for other relevant symptoms which cannot be allocated elsewhere in the classification.

The conditions and signs or symptoms included in categories 780–796 consist of: (a) cases for which no more specific diagnosis can be made even after all facts bearing on the case have been investigated; (b) signs or symptoms existing at the time of initial encounter that proved to be transient and whose causes could not be determined; (c) provisional diagnoses in a patient who failed to return for further investigation or care; (d) cases referred elsewhere for investigation or treatment before the diagnosis was made; (e) cases in which a more precise diagnosis was not available for any other reason; (f) certain symptoms which represent important problems in medical care and which it might be desired to classify in addition to a known cause.

SYMPTOMS (780–789)

● **780 General symptoms**

● **780.0 Alteration of consciousness**

Excludes	*alteration of consciousness due to:* ◄
	intracranial injuries (850.0–854.19) ◄
	skull fractures (800.00-801.99, ◄
	803.00-804.99)
	coma:
	diabetic (249.2–249.3, 250.2–250.3)
	hepatic (572.2)
	originating in the perinatal period
	(779.2)

780.01 Coma ⬗

Ⓔⓧ 070.0-070.9, 249.00-251.3, 338.0-338.4, 348.8-348.9,
349.89-349.9, 430-432.9, 572.2, 780.01-780.09, 780.2,
780.4, 780.64-780.65, 780.91-780.99, 799.81-799.89,
800.00-801.99, 803.00-804.96, 850.0-852.19,
852.21-854.19

Coding Clinic: 1996, Q3, P16

780.02 Transient alteration of awareness

780.03 Persistent vegetative state ⬗

Ⓔⓧ 070.0-070.9, 249.00-251.3, 338.0-338.4, 348.8-348.9,
349.89-349.9, 430-432.9, 572.2, 780.01-780.09, 780.2,
780.4, 780.64-780.65, 780.91-780.99, 799.81-799.89,
800.00-801.99, 803.00-804.96, 850.0-852.19,
852.21-854.19

780.09 Other

Drowsiness	Somnolence
Semicoma	Stupor
	Unconsciousness

780.1 Hallucinations ⬗

Hallucinations:
  NOS
  auditory
  gustatory
  olfactory
  tactile

Excludes	*those associated with mental disorders, as*
	functional psychoses (295.0–298.9)
	organic brain syndromes (290.0–294.9,
	310.0–310.9)
	visual hallucinations (368.16)

Ⓔⓧ 338.0-338.4, 780.1, 780.4, 780.64-780.65, 780.91-780.99, 799.81 -799.89

780.2 Syncope and collapse

Blackout	(Near) (Pre)syncope
Fainting	Vasovagal attack

Excludes	*carotid sinus syncope (337.0)*
	heat syncope (992.1)
	neurocirculatory asthenia (306.2)
	orthostatic hypotension (458.0)
	shock NOS (785.50)

Coding Clinic: 2002, Q1, P6; 2000, Q3, P12; 1995, Q4, P50-51; Q3, P14; 1992, Q3, P16; 1990, Q1, P9; 1985, Nov-Dec, P12

● 780.3 Convulsions

Excludes	*convulsions:*
	epileptic (345.10–345.91)
	in newborn (779.0)

Coding Clinic: 1984, Nov-Dec, P11

780.31 Febrile convulsions (simple), unspecified ⬗

Febrile seizures NOS

Ⓔⓧ 338.0-338.4, 345.00 -345.91, 348.8-348.9, 349.89-349.9,
779.0-779.1, 780.31 -780.39, 780.64-780.65,
780.91-780.99, 799.81-799.89

Coding Clinic: 2005, Q3, P12-13; 1987, Nov-Dec, P11

780.32 Complex febrile convulsions ⬗

Febrile seizure:
  atypical
  complex
  complicated

Excludes	*status epilepticus (345.3)*

Ⓔⓧ 338.0-338.4, 345.00 -345.91, 348.8-348.9, 349.89 -349.9,
779.0-779.1, 780.31-780.39, 780.64-780.65,
780.91-780.99, 799.81-799.89

Coding Clinic: 2006, Q4, P106-107

780.39 Other convulsions

Convulsive disorder NOS
Fits NOS
Recurrent convulsions NOS
Seizure NOS
Seizures NOS

Coding Clinic: 2008, Q1, P17; 2006, Q3, P22; 2004, Q4, P50-52; 2003, Q1, P7; 1998, Q4, P39-40; 1997, Q2, P8; Q1, P12-13; 1994, Q3, P9; 1993, Q1, P24; 1987, Nov-Dec, P12; 1985, July-Aug, P10; 1984, May-June, P14

780.4 Dizziness and giddiness

Light-headedness
Vertigo NOS

Excludes	*Méniére's disease and other specified*
	vertiginous syndromes
	(386.0–386.9)

Coding Clinic: 2003, Q2, P11; 2000, Q3, P12; 1997, Q2, P9-10; 1991, Q2, P17

SYMPTOMS, SIGNS, AND ILL-DEFINED CONDITIONS (780–799)

N Newborn Age: 0   P Pediatric Age: 0–17   M Maternity Age: 12–55   A Adult Age: 15–124   ♀ Females Only   ♂ Males Only   1049

Ⓔⓧ CC Exclusions   ⬗ Complication\Comorbidity   ⬗ Major C\C   ⬗ Present on Admission Requirement   ⬗ Hospital-Acquired Condition
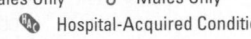

● **780.5　Sleep disturbances**

> | Excludes | circadian rhythm sleep disorders
> (327.30–327.39)
> organic hypersomnia (327.10–327.19)
> organic insomnia (327.00–327.09)
> organic sleep apnea (327.20–327.29)
> organic sleep related movement disorders
> (327.51–327.59)
> parasomnias (327.40–327.49)
> that of nonorganic origin (307.40–307.49)

780.50　Sleep disturbance, unspecified

780.51　Insomnia with sleep apnea, unspecified
　　　　Coding Clinic: 1993, Q1, P28-29

780.52　Insomnia, unspecified

780.53　Hypersomnia with sleep apnea, unspecified
　　　　Coding Clinic: 1993, Q1, P28-29

780.54　Hypersomnia, unspecified

780.55　Disruptions of 24 hour sleep wake cycle,
　　　　unspecified

780.56　Dysfunctions associated with sleep stages or
　　　　arousal from sleep

780.57　Unspecified sleep apnea
　　　　Coding Clinic: 2001, Q1, P6-7; 1997, Q1, P5; 1993, Q1,
　　　　P28-29

780.58　Sleep related movement disorder, unspecified

> | Excludes | restless legs syndrome (333.94)

　　　　Coding Clinic: 2004, Q4, P95-96

780.59　Other

● **780.6　Fever and other physiologic disturbances of
temperature regulation**

> | Excludes | effects of reduced environmental
> temperature (991.0-991.9)
> effects of heat and light (992.0-992.9)
> fever, chills or hypothermia associated
> with confirmed infection – code to
> infection

　　Coding Clinic: 2008, Q4, P140-143; 2005, Q3, P16-17; 2000, Q3,
　　P13; 1991, Q2, P8x2; 1990, Q1, P8; 1985, July-Aug, P13

780.60　Fever, unspecified
　　　　Chills with fever
　　　　Fever NOS
　　　　Fever of unknown origin (FUO)
　　　　Hyperpyrexia NOS
　　　　Pyrexia NOS
　　　　Pyrexia of unknown origin

> | Excludes | chills without fever (780.64)
> neonatal fever (778.4)
> pyrexia of unknown origin
> (during):
> in newborn (778.4)
> labor (659.2)
> the puerperium (672)

▶ 780.61　*Fever presenting with conditions classified
elsewhere*

> Code first *underlying condition when associated
> fever is present, such as with:*
> leukemia (conditions classifiable to
> 204-208)
> neutropenia (288.00-288.09)
> sickle-cell disease (282.60-282.69)

　　　　Coding Clinic: 2008, Q4, P140-143

780.62　Postprocedural fever

> | Excludes | postvaccination fever (780.63)

780.63　Postvaccination fever
　　　　Postimmunization fever

780.64　Chills (without fever)
　　　　Chills NOS

> | Excludes | chills with fever (780.60)

780.65　Hypothermia not associated with low
　　　　environmental temperature

> | Excludes | hypothermia:
> associated with low
> environmental temperature
> (991.6)
> due to anesthesia (995.89)
> of newborn (778.2, 778.3)

● **780.7　Malaise and fatigue**

> | Excludes | debility, unspecified (799.3)
> fatigue (during):
> combat (308.0–308.9)
> heat (992.6)
> pregnancy (646.8)
> neurasthenia (300.5)
> senile asthenia (797)

780.71　Chronic fatigue syndrome
　　　　Coding Clinic: 1998, Q4, P48-49

780.72　Functional quadriplegia 🔁
　　　　Complete immobility due to severe physical
　　　　disability or frailty

> | Excludes | hysterical paralysis (300.11)
> immobility syndrome (728.3)
> neurologic quadriplegia
> (344.00-344.09)
> quadriplegia NOS (344.00)

　　Ⓔx 249.60-249.61, 249.80-249.91, 250.60-250.63, 250.80-250.93,
　　342.00-344.9, 348.8-348.9, 349.89-349.9, 742.59-742.9,
　　780.72

　　　　Coding Clinic: 2008, Q4, P143

780.79　Other malaise and fatigue
　　　　Asthenia NOS
　　　　Lethargy
　　　　Postviral (asthenic) syndrome
　　　　Tiredness
　　　　Coding Clinic: 2004, Q4, P77-78; 2000, Q1, P6

780.8　Generalized hyperhidrosis
　　　　Diaphoresis
　　　　Excessive sweating
　　　　Secondary hyperhidrosis

> | Excludes | focal (localized) (primary) (secondary)
> hyperhidrosis (705.21–705.22)
> Frey's syndrome (705.22)

● **780.9　Other general symptoms**

> | Excludes | hypothermia:
> NOS (accidental) (991.6)
> due to anesthesia (995.89)
> memory disturbance as part of a pattern
> of mental disorder
> of newborn (778.2–778.3)

　　　Coding Clinic: 2002, Q4, P67-68

780.91　Fussy infant (baby)　　　　　　　　　　　P

780.92　Excessive crying of infant (baby)　　　　N

> | Excludes | excessive crying of child, adolescent
> or adult (780.95)

　　　　Coding Clinic: 2005, Q4, P89-90

◀ New　　◀▥ Revised　　~~deleted~~ Deleted　　● Unacceptable Principal Diagnosis　　● Use Additional Digit(s)
▶ Manifestation Code　　**OGCR** Official Guidelines　　**Coding Clinic**　　Excludes　　Includes　　Use additional　　Code first　　Omit code

SYMPTOMS, SIGNS, AND ILL-DEFINED CONDITIONS (780–799)

780.93 Memory loss
Amnesia (retrograde)
Memory loss NOS

| Excludes | *memory loss due to:* ◄
intracranial injuries ◄
(850.0-854.19)
skull fractures (800.00-801.99, ◄
803.00-804.99)
mild memory disturbance due to
organic brain damage
(310.8) ◄
transient global amnesia (437.7)

Coding Clinic: 2003, Q4, P71

780.94 Early satiety
Coding Clinic: 2003, Q4, P72

780.95 Excessive crying of child, adolescent, or adult

| Excludes | *excessive crying of infant (baby)*
(780.92)

Coding Clinic: 2005, Q4, P89-90

780.96 Generalized pain
Pain NOS

780.97 Altered mental status
Change in mental status

| Excludes | *altered level of consciousness*
(780.01–780.09)
altered mental status due to known
condition - code to condition
delirium NOS (780.09)

Coding Clinic: 2006, Q4, P107-108; 1993, Q3, P11

780.99 Other general symptoms
Coding Clinic: 2003, Q4, P103-104; 1999, Q4, P10; 1985, Nov-Dec, P12

● **781 Symptoms involving nervous and musculoskeletal systems**

| Excludes | *depression NOS (311)*
disorders specifically relating to:
back (724.0–724.9)
hearing (388.0–389.9)
joint (718.0–719.9)
limb (729.0–729.9)
neck (723.0–723.9)
vision (368.0–369.9)
pain in limb (729.5)

781.0 Abnormal involuntary movements
Abnormal head movements
Fasciculation
Spasms NOS
Tremor NOS

| Excludes | *abnormal reflex (796.1)*
chorea NOS (333.5)
infantile spasms (345.60–345.61)
spastic paralysis (342.1, 343.0–344.9)
specified movement disorders classifiable to
333 (333.0–333.9)
that of nonorganic origin (307.2–307.3)

781.1 Disturbances of sensation of smell and taste
Anosmia   Parosmia
Parageusia

781.2 Abnormality of gait
Gait:
ataxic
paralytic
spastic
staggering

| Excludes | *ataxia:*
NOS (781.3)
difficulty in walking (719.7)
locomotor (progressive) (094.0)

Coding Clinic: 2005, Q2, P6-7; 2004, Q2, P15

781.3 Lack of coordination
Ataxia NOS
Muscular incoordination

| Excludes | *ataxic gait (781.2)*
cerebellar ataxia (334.0–334.9)
difficulty in walking (719.7)
vertigo NOS (780.4)

Coding Clinic: 2004, Q4, P50-52; 1997, Q3, P12-13

781.4 Transient paralysis of limb 🦠
Monoplegia, transient NOS

| Excludes | *paralysis (342.0–344.9)*

(Ex) 781.4, 781.94

781.5 Clubbing of fingers

781.6 Meningismus 🦠
Dupre's syndrome   Meningism
(Ex) 781.6, 781.94
Coding Clinic: 2000, Q3, P13

781.7 Tetany 🦠
Carpopedal spasm

| Excludes | *tetanus neonatorum (771.3)*
tetany:
hysterical (300.11)
newborn (hypocalcemic) (775.4)
parathyroid (252.1)
psychogenic (306.0)

(Ex) 037, 332.0-333.93, 333.99-334.4, 338.0-338.4, 342.10-342.12, 771.3,
780.64-780.65, 780.91-780.99, 781.7, 799.81-799.89

781.8 Neurologic neglect syndrome 🦠
Asomatognosia   Left-sided neglect
Hemi-akinesia   Sensory extinction
Hemi-inattention   Sensory neglect
Hemispatial neglect   Visuospatial neglect
(Ex) 781.8-781.92, 781.94-781.99

● **781.9 Other symptoms involving nervous and musculoskeletal systems**

781.91 Loss of height

| Excludes | *osteoporosis (733.00–733.09)*

781.92 Abnormal posture

781.93 Ocular torticollis
Coding Clinic: 2002, Q4, P68; Q4, P68

781.94 Facial weakness
Facial droop

| Excludes | *facial weakness due to late effect*
of cerebrovascular accident
(438.83)

Coding Clinic: 2003, Q4, P72

781.99 Other symptoms involving nervous and musculoskeletal systems

● **782 Symptoms involving skin and other integumentary tissue**

| Excludes | *symptoms relating to breast (611.71–611.79)*

782.0 Disturbance of skin sensation
Anesthesia of skin
Burning or prickling sensation
Hyperesthesia
Hypoesthesia
Numbness
Paresthesia
Tingling

782.1 Rash and other nonspecific skin eruption
Exanthem

| Excludes | *vesicular eruption (709.8)*

SYMPTOMS, SIGNS, AND ILL-DEFINED CONDITIONS (780–799)

782.2   Localized superficial swelling, mass, or lump
Subcutaneous nodules

> **Excludes**   *localized adiposity (278.1)*

782.3   Edema
Anasarca
Dropsy
Localized edema NOS

> **Excludes**   *ascites (789.51–789.59)*
> *edema of:*
>   *newborn NOS (778.5)*
>   *pregnancy (642.0–642.9, 646.1)*
> *fluid retention (276.6)*
> *hydrops fetalis (773.3, 778.0)*
> *hydrothorax (511.81–511.89)*
> *nutritional edema (260, 262)*

Coding Clinic: 2000, Q2, P18

782.4   Jaundice, unspecified, not of newborn 📞
Cholemia NOS
Icterus NOS

> **Excludes**   *due to isoimmunization (773.0–773.2,*
>   *773.4)*
> *jaundice in newborn (774.0–774.7)*

(Ex) 774.0-774.7, 782.4, 782.9

782.5   Cyanosis

> **Excludes**   *newborn (770.83)*

● **782.6   Pallor and flushing**

   782.61   Pallor

   782.62   Flushing
     Excessive blushing

782.7   Spontaneous ecchymoses
Petechiae

> **Excludes**   *ecchymosis in fetus or newborn (772.6)*
> *purpura (287.0–287.9)*

782.8   Changes in skin texture
Induration of skin
Thickening of skin

782.9   Other symptoms involving skin and integumentary tissues

● **783   Symptoms concerning nutrition, metabolism, and development**

783.0   Anorexia
Loss of appetite

> **Excludes**   *anorexia nervosa (307.1)*
> *loss of appetite of nonorganic origin*
>   *(307.59)*

783.1   Abnormal weight gain

> **Excludes**   *excessive weight gain in pregnancy (646.1)*
> *obesity (278.00)*
>   *morbid (278.01)*

● **783.2   Abnormal loss of weight and underweight**

> Use additional code to identify Body Mass Index (BMI), if known (V85.0–V85.54)

   783.21   Loss of weight

   783.22   Underweight

783.3   Feeding difficulties and mismanagement
Feeding problem (elderly) (infant)

> **Excludes**   *feeding disturbance or problems:*
>   *in newborn (779.31-779.34)* ◀▥
>   *of nonorganic origin (307.50–307.59)*

Coding Clinic: 1997, Q3, P12-13; 1994, Q2, P10-11

● **783.4   Lack of expected normal physiological development in childhood**

> **Excludes**   *delay in sexual development and puberty*
>   *(259.0)*
> *gonadal dysgenesis (758.6)*
> *pituitary dwarfism (253.3)*
> *slow fetal growth and fetal malnutrition*
>   *(764.00–764.99)*
> *specific delays in mental development*
>   *(315.0–315.9)*

Coding Clinic: 1997, Q3, P5

   783.40   Lack of normal physiological development, unspecified
     Inadequate development
     Lack of development

   783.41   Failure to thrive   P
     Failure to gain weight

> **Excludes**   *failure to thrive in*
>   *newborn (779.34)* ◀

Coding Clinic: 2003, Q1, P12

   783.42   Delayed milestones   P
     Late talker
     Late walker

   783.43   Short stature
     Growth failure
     Growth retardation
     Lack of growth
     Physical retardation
     Coding Clinic: 2004, Q2, P3

783.5   Polydipsia
Excessive thirst

783.6   Polyphagia
Excessive eating
Hyperalimentation NOS

> **Excludes**   *disorders of eating of nonorganic origin*
>   *(307.50–307.59)*

783.7   Adult failure to thrive   A

783.9   Other symptoms concerning nutrition, metabolism, and development
Hypometabolism

> **Excludes**   *abnormal basal metabolic rate (794.7)*
> *dehydration (276.51)*
> *other disorders of fluid, electrolyte, and*
>   *acid-base balance (276.0–276.9)*

Coding Clinic: 2004, Q2, P3

● **784   Symptoms involving head and neck**

> **Excludes**   *encephalopathy NOS (348.30)*
> *specific symptoms involving neck classifiable to*
>   *723 (723.0–723.9)*

784.0   Headache
Facial pain
Pain in head NOS

> **Excludes**   *atypical face pain (350.2)*
> *migraine (346.0–346.9)*
> *tension headache (307.81)*

Coding Clinic: 2006, Q3, P22; Q2, P17-18; 2000, Q3, P13; 1992, Q3, P14; 1990, Q1, P9

784.1   Throat pain

> **Excludes**   *dysphagia (787.20–787.29)*
> *neck pain (723.1)*
> *sore throat (462)*
>   *chronic (472.1)*

784.2   Swelling, mass, or lump in head and neck
Space-occupying lesion, intracranial NOS
Coding Clinic: 2003, Q1, P8

◀ New   ◀▥ Revised   ~~deleted~~ Deleted   ● Unacceptable Principal Diagnosis   ● Use Additional Digit(s)
▶ Manifestation Code   **OGCR** Official Guidelines   **Coding Clinic**   Excludes   Includes   Use additional   Code first   Omit code

SYMPTOMS, SIGNS, AND ILL-DEFINED CONDITIONS (780–799)

● **784.3 Aphasia** 🗝

     Excludes *aphasia due to late effects of cerebrovascular disease (438.11)*
         developmental aphasia (315.31)
     (Ex:) 315.31, 432.0-434.91, 436, 784.3-784.5
     Coding Clinic: 2004, Q4, P77-78; 1998, Q4, P87; 1997, Q3, P12-13

● **784.4 Voice** ~~disturbance~~ **and resonance disorders**

     784.40 Voice ~~disturbance~~ **and resonance disorder, unspecified**

     784.41 Aphonia
         Loss of voice

     784.42 Dysphonia
         Hoarseness

     784.43 Hypernasality

     784.44 Hyponasality

     784.49 Other voice and resonance disorders
         Change in voice
         ~~Dysphonia~~
         ~~Hoarseness~~
         ~~Hypernasality~~
         ~~Hyponasality~~

● **784.5 Other speech disturbance**
     ~~Dysarthria~~
     ~~Dysphasia~~
     ~~Slurred speech~~

     Excludes *speech disorder due to late effect of cerebrovascular accident (438.10-438.19)*
         stammering and stuttering (307.0)
         that of nonorganic origin (307.0, 307.9)

     784.51 Dysarthria

         Excludes *dysarthria due to late effect of cerebrovascular accident (438.13)*

     784.59 Other speech disturbance
         Dysphasia
         Slurred speech
         Speech disturbance NOS

● **784.6 Other symbolic dysfunction**

     Excludes *developmental learning delays (315.0–315.9)*

     784.60 Symbolic dysfunction, unspecified

     784.61 Alexia and dyslexia
         Alexia (with agraphia)
         Loss of ability to read

     784.69 Other
         Acalculia
         Difficulty performing simple mathematical tasks
         Agnosia
         Loss of ability to recognize objects, persons, sounds, shapes, or smells
         Agraphia NOS
         Apraxia
         Loss of the ability to execute or carry out movements

784.7 Epistaxis
     Hemorrhage from nose
     Nosebleed
     Coding Clinic: 2004, Q3, P7; 1995, Q1, P5

784.8 Hemorrhage from throat
     Excludes *hemoptysis (786.3)*
         Spitting blood

● **784.9 Other symptoms involving head and neck**

     784.91 Postnasal drip

     784.99 Other symptoms involving head and neck
         Choking sensation
         Feeling of foreign body in throat
         Halitosis
            Bad breath
         Mouth breathing
         Sneezing

         Excludes *foreign body in throat (933.0)*

● **785 Symptoms involving cardiovascular system**

     Excludes *heart failure NOS (428.9)*

     785.0 Tachycardia, unspecified
         Rapid heart beat

         Excludes *neonatal tachycardia (779.82)*
            paroxysmal tachycardia (427.0–427.2)
         Coding Clinic: 2003, Q2, P11

     785.1 Palpitations
         Awareness of heart beat

         Excludes *specified dysrhythmias (427.0–427.9)*

     785.2 Undiagnosed cardiac murmurs
         Heart murmur NOS

     785.3 Other abnormal heart sounds
         Cardiac dullness, increased or decreased
         Friction fremitus, cardiac
         Precordial friction

     785.4 Gangrene 🗝
         Gangrene:
            NOS
            spreading cutaneous
         Gangrenous cellulitis
         Phagedena
         Rapidly spreading destructive ulceration of soft tissue

         Code first *any associated underlying condition*

         Excludes *gangrene of certain sites-see Alphabetic Index*
            gangrene with atherosclerosis of the extremities (440.24)
            gas gangrene (040.0)
         (Ex:) 338.0-338.4, 440.24, 780.64-780.65, 780.91 -780.99, 785.4, 799.81-799.89
         Coding Clinic: 2004, Q1, P14-15; 1994, Q3, P5; 1990, Q3, P15; 1986, Mar-April, P12

● **785.5 Shock without mention of trauma**

     785.50 Shock, unspecified 🗝
         Failure of peripheral circulation
         Resulting in significant blood pressure drop
         (Ex:) 338.0-338.4, 780.64-780.65, 780.91 -780.99, 785.50-785.59, 785.9, 799.81-799.89

     785.51 Cardiogenic shock 🗝
         MCC only for patients discharged alive
         (Ex:) 338.0-338.4, 780.64-780.65, 780.91 -780.99, 785.50-785.59, 785.9, 799.81-799.89
         Coding Clinic: 2008, Q4, P180-182; 2005, Q3, P14

SYMPTOMS, SIGNS, AND ILL-DEFINED CONDITIONS (780–799)

N Newborn Age: 0   **P** Pediatric Age: 0–17   **M** Maternity Age: 12–55   **A** Adult Age: 15–124   ♀ Females Only   ♂ Males Only

 CC Exclusions   Complication\Comorbidity   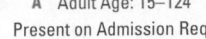 Major C\C   Present on Admission Requirement   Hospital-Acquired Condition   **1053**

▶ **785.52 Septic shock** 🔲
Endotoxic
Gram-negative

Code first:
  systemic inflammatory response
    syndrome due to infectious process
    with organ dysfunction (995.92)
(Ex:) 338.0-338.4, 780.64-780.65, 780.91-780.99, 785.50-785.59,
785.9, 799.81-799.89
Coding Clinic: 2005, Q3, P23; Q2, P18-20x2; 2003, Q4,
P73,79-81

785.59 Other 🔲
Shock:
  hypovolemic
    Decreased blood volume

  Excludes *shock (due to):*
    anesthetic (995.4)
    anaphylactic (995.0)
    due to serum (999.4)
    electric (994.8)
    following abortion (639.5)
    lightning (994.0)
    obstetrical (669.1)
    postoperative (998.0)
    traumatic (958.4)
MCC only for patients discharged alive
(Ex:) 338.0-338.4, 780.64-780.65, 780.91-780.99, 785.50-785.59,
785.9, 799.81-799.89
Coding Clinic: 2008, Q4, P97-100

785.6 Enlargement of lymph nodes
Lymphadenopathy
"Swollen glands"

  Excludes *lymphadenitis (chronic) (289.1–289.3)*
    acute (683)

785.9 Other symptoms involving cardiovascular system
Bruit (arterial)   Weak pulse

● **786 Symptoms involving respiratory system and other chest symptoms**

● **786.0 Dyspnea and respiratory abnormalities**

786.00 Respiratory abnormality, unspecified

786.01 Hyperventilation

  Excludes *hyperventilation, psychogenic*
    (306.1)

786.02 Orthopnea

786.03 Apnea

  Excludes *apnea of newborn (770.81, 770.82)*
    sleep apnea (780.51, 780.53,
    780.57)
  Coding Clinic: 1998, Q2, P10

786.04 Cheyne-Stokes respiration 🔲
Abnormal pattern of breathing with gradually
increasing and decreasing tidal volume
with some periods of apnea
(Ex:) 518.81-518.84, 519.8-519.9, 786.03-786.04, 799.1

786.05 Shortness of breath
Coding Clinic: 1999, Q4, P25; Q1, P6

786.06 Tachypnea

  Excludes *transitory tachypnea of newborn*
    (770.6)

786.07 Wheezing

  Excludes *asthma (493.00–493.92)*

786.09 Other
Respiratory:
  distress
  insufficiency

  Excludes *respiratory distress:*
    following trauma and surgery
    (518.5)
    newborn (770.89)
    respiratory failure (518.81,
    518.83–518.84)
    newborn (770.84)
    syndrome (newborn) (769)
    adult (518.5)
  Coding Clinic: 1990, Q1, P9

786.1 Stridor

  Excludes *congenital laryngeal stridor (748.3)*

786.2 Cough

  Excludes *cough:*
    psychogenic (306.1)
    smokers' (491.0)
    with hemorrhage (786.3)
  Coding Clinic: 1995, Q4, P50; 1990, Q1, P8

786.3 Hemoptysis 🔲
Cough with hemorrhage
Pulmonary hemorrhage NOS

  Excludes *pulmonary hemorrhage of newborn (770.3)*
  (Ex:) 338.0-338.4, 780.64-780.65, 780.91-780.99, 786.3-786.4, 786.9,
  799.81-799.89
  Coding Clinic: 2006, Q2, P17

786.4 Abnormal sputum
Abnormal:
  amount of sputum
  color of sputum
  odor of sputum
Excessive sputum

● **786.5 Chest pain**

786.50 Chest pain, unspecified
Coding Clinic: 2007, Q1, P19; 2006, Q2, P7-8; 2003, Q1,
P6-7; 2002, Q1, P4-5; 1999, Q4, P25-26; 1993,
Q1, P25

786.51 Precordial pain
Coding Clinic: 1984, May-June, P11

786.52 Painful respiration
Pain:
  anterior chest wall
  pleuritic
  Pleurodynia

  Excludes *epidemic pleurodynia (074.1)*

  Coding Clinic: 1984, Nov-Dec, P17

786.59 Other
Discomfort in chest
Pressure in chest
Tightness in chest

  Excludes *pain in breast (611.71)*

  Coding Clinic: 2007, Q1, P19; 2002, Q1, P6

786.6 Swelling, mass, or lump in chest

  Excludes *lump in breast (611.72)*

◀ New   ◀|||| Revised   ~~deleted~~ Deleted   ● Unacceptable Principal Diagnosis   ● Use Additional Digit(s)
▶ Manifestation Code   **OGCR** Official Guidelines   **Coding Clinic**   Excludes   Includes   Use additional   Code first   Omit code

786.7 Abnormal chest sounds
Abnormal percussion, chest
Friction sounds, chest
Rales
   *Wet rattling, clicking, crackling sounds on
    auscultation*
Tympany, chest
Excludes *wheezing (786.07)*

786.8 Hiccough
Excludes *psychogenic hiccough (306.1)*

786.9 Other symptoms involving respiratory system and chest
Breath-holding spell

●**787 Symptoms involving digestive system**
Excludes *constipation (564.0–564.9)*
        pylorospasm (537.81)
        congenital (750.5)

●**787.0 Nausea and vomiting**
Emesis
Excludes *hematemesis NOS (578.0)*
      vomiting:
        bilious, following gastrointestinal surgery
          (564.3)
        cyclical (536.2)
          associated with migraine (346.2)
          psychogenic (306.4)
        excessive, in pregnancy (643.0–643.9) ◄
        fecal matter (569.87)
        habit (536.2)
        of newborn (779.32, 779.33) ◄▥
        persistent (536.2) ◄
        psychogenic NOS (307.54)

   787.01 Nausea with vomiting
     Concurrent conditions
     Coding Clinic: 2003, Q1, P5

   787.02 Nausea alone
     Separate condition
     Coding Clinic: 2000, Q3, P12; 1997, Q2, P9-10

   787.03 Vomiting alone
     Separate condition
     Coding Clinic: 1985, Mar-April, P11

   787.04 Bilious emesis ◄
     Bilious vomiting ◄
     Excludes *bilious emesis (vomiting) in*
          newborn (779.32) ◄

787.1 Heartburn
Pyrosis
Waterbrash
Excludes *dyspepsia or indigestion (536.8)*
Coding Clinic: 2001, Q2, P6

●**787.2 Dysphagia**
*Code first, if applicable, dysphagia due to late effect of
   cerebrovascular accident (438.82)*
**Coding Clinic: 2007, Q3, P8-9; 2003, Q4, P103-104, 109-110; 2001,
   Q2, P4-6; 1993, 5th Issue, P16; 1986, Nov-Dec, P10**

   787.20 Dysphagia, unspecified
     Difficulty in swallowing NOS

   787.21 Dysphagia, oral phase

   787.22 Dysphagia, oropharyngeal phase
     Coding Clinic: 2007, Q4, P92-95

   787.23 Dysphagia, pharyngeal phase

   787.24 Dysphagia, pharyngoesophageal phase

   787.29 Other dysphagia
     Cervical dysphagia
     Neurogenic dysphagia

787.3 Flatulence, eructation, and gas pain
Abdominal distention (gaseous)
Bloating
Tympanites (abdominal) (intestinal)
Excludes *aerophagy (306.4)*

787.4 Visible peristalsis
Hyperperistalsis

787.5 Abnormal bowel sounds
Absent bowel sounds
Hyperactive bowel sounds

787.6 Incontinence of feces
Encopresis NOS
Incontinence of sphincter ani
Excludes *that of nonorganic origin (307.7)*
Coding Clinic: 1997, Q1, P9-10

787.7 Abnormal feces
Bulky stools
Excludes *abnormal stool content (792.1)*
       melena:
        NOS (578.1)
        newborn (772.4, 777.3)

●**787.9 Other symptoms involving digestive system**
Excludes *gastrointestinal hemorrhage (578.0–578.9)*
       intestinal obstruction (560.0–560.9)
       specific functional digestive disorders:
        esophagus (530.0–530.9)
        stomach and duodenum (536.0–536.9)
        those not elsewhere classified
         (564.0–564.9)

   787.91 Diarrhea
     Diarrhea NOS
     Coding Clinic: 2008, Q4, P97-100

   787.99 Other
     Change in bowel habits
     Tenesmus (rectal)

●**788 Symptoms involving urinary system**
Excludes *hematuria (599.70–599.72)*
       nonspecific findings on examination of the urine
        (791.0–791.9)
       small kidney of unknown cause (589.0–589.9)
       uremia NOS (586)
       urinary obstruction (599.60, 599.69)

788.0 Renal colic
Colic (recurrent) of:
   kidney
   ureter
Coding Clinic: 2004, Q3, P8

788.1 Dysuria
Painful urination
Strangury

●**788.2 Retention of urine**
*Code first, if applicable, hyperplasia of prostate
   (600.0–600.9 with fifth-digit 1)*
Coding Clinic: 2003, Q3, P13; 1994, Q1, P20; 1986, Sept-Oct, P12

   788.20 Retention of urine, unspecified
     **Coding Clinic: 2006, Q4, P93-95; 2004, Q2, P18; 2003, Q3,
     P12; Q1, P6; 1996, Q3, P10-11; 1994, Q3, P13**

   788.21 Incomplete bladder emptying

   788.29 Other specified retention of urine

SYMPTOMS, SIGNS, AND ILL-DEFINED CONDITIONS (780–799)

● **788.3 Urinary incontinence**

    Excludes *functional urinary incontinence (788.91)*
      that of nonorganic origin (307.6)
      urinary incontinence associated with
        cognitive impairment (788.91)
    Code, if applicable, any causal condition first,
      such as:
      congenital ureterocele (753.23)
      genital prolapse (618.00–618.9)
      hyperplasia of prostate (600.0–600.9 with
        fifth-digit 1)
    Coding Clinic: 2005, Q3, P20

  788.30 Urinary incontinence, unspecified
    Enuresis NOS
    Coding Clinic: 2009, Q1, P18; 1995, Q4, P72-73

  788.31 Urge incontinence
    Coding Clinic: 2000, Q1, P19-20

  788.32 Stress incontinence, male ♂
    Excludes *stress incontinence, female (625.6)*
    Coding Clinic: 1995, Q4, P72-73

  788.33 Mixed incontinence (female) (male)
    Urge and stress

  788.34 Incontinence without sensory awareness

  788.35 Post-void dribbling

  788.36 Nocturnal enuresis

  788.37 Continuous leakage

  788.38 Overflow incontinence
    Coding Clinic: 2004, Q4, P96

  788.39 Other urinary incontinence

● **788.4 Frequency of urination and polyuria**

    Code first, if applicable, hyperplasia of prostate
      (600.0–600.9 with fifth-digit 1)

  788.41 Urinary frequency
    Frequency of micturition

  788.42 Polyuria

  788.43 Nocturia

  788.5 Oliguria and anuria
    Deficient secretion of urine
    Suppression of urinary secretion

    Excludes *that complicating:*
      abortion (634–638 with .3, 639.3)
      ectopic or molar pregnancy (639.3)
      pregnancy, childbirth, or the puerperium
        (642.0–642.9, 646.2)

● **788.6 Other abnormality of urination**

    Code first, if applicable, hyperplasia of prostate
      (600.0–600.9 with fifth-digit 1)

  788.61 Splitting of urinary stream
    Intermittent urinary stream

  788.62 Slowing of urinary stream
    Weak stream

  788.63 Urgency of urination
    Excludes *urge incontinence (788.31, 788.33)*
    Coding Clinic: 2003, Q4, P74

  788.64 Urinary hesitancy

  788.65 Straining on urination

  788.69 Other

788.7 Urethral discharge
  Penile discharge
  Urethrorrhea

788.8 Extravasation of urine 🔗
  Leakage, discharge
  (Ex) 788.8-788.99

● **788.9 Other symptoms involving urinary system**
  Coding Clinic: 2005, Q1, P12-13

  788.91 Functional urinary incontinence
    Urinary incontinence due to cognitive
      impairment, or severe physical
      disability or immobility

    Excludes *urinary incontinence due to*
      physiologic condition
      (788.30-788.39)
    Coding Clinic: 2008, Q4, P144-145

  788.99 Other symptoms involving urinary system
    Extrarenal uremia
    Vesical:
      pain
      tenesmus

● **789 Other symptoms involving abdomen and pelvis**

  The following fifth-digit subclassification is to be used for
  codes 789.0, 789.3, 789.4, 789.6

    0 **unspecified site**
    1 **right upper quadrant**
    2 **left upper quadrant**
    3 **right lower quadrant**
    4 **left lower quadrant**
    5 **periumbilic**
    6 **epigastric**
    7 **generalized**
    9 **other specified site**
       multiple sites

  Excludes *symptoms referable to genital organs:*
    female (625.0–625.9)
    male (607.0–608.9)
    psychogenic (302.70–302.79)

● **789.0 Abdominal pain**
[0-7,9]   ~~Colic:~~
    ~~NOS~~
    ~~infantile~~
    Cramps, abdominal
    Excludes ~~renal colic (788.0)~~
    Coding Clinic: 2002, Q1, P5; 1995, Q1, P3; 1990, Q2, P26

  789.1 Hepatomegaly
    Enlargement of liver

  789.2 Splenomegaly
    Enlargement of spleen

● **789.3 Abdominal or pelvic swelling, mass, or lump**
[0-7,9]   Diffuse or generalized swelling or mass:
    abdominal NOS
    umbilical
    Excludes *abdominal distention (gaseous) (787.3)*
    ascites (789.51–789.59)

● **789.4 Abdominal rigidity**
[0-7,9]

◀ New   ◀ Revised   ~~deleted~~ Deleted   ● Unacceptable Principal Diagnosis   ● Use Additional Digit(s)
▶ Manifestation Code   OGCR Official Guidelines   Coding Clinic   Excludes   Includes   Use additional   Code first   Omit code

SYMPTOMS, SIGNS, AND ILL-DEFINED CONDITIONS (780–799)

● **789.5   Ascites**
     Fluid in peritoneal cavity
     Coding Clinic: 2008, Q1, P16-18; 2007, Q4, P95-96; 2005, Q2, P8;
         1989, Q4, P11

   ● **789.51   Malignant ascites** 🔵
         Code first malignancy, such as:
         malignant neoplasm of ovary (183.0)
         secondary malignant neoplasm of
           retroperitoneum and peritoneum
           (197.6)
         (Ex:) 338.0-338.4, 780.64-780.65, 780.91-780.99, 789.30-789.59,
           789.9, 799.81-799.89
         Coding Clinic: 2008, Q1, P16-17

   789.59   Other ascites 🔵
         (Ex:) 338.0-338.4, 780.64-780.65, 780.91-780.99, 789.30-789.59,
           789.9, 799.81-799.89

● **789.6   Abdominal tenderness**
[0-7,9]   Rebound tenderness

   789.7   Colic ◄
     Colic NOS ◄
     Infantile colic ◄
     Excludes   *colic in adult and child over
           12 months old (789.0)* ◄
           renal colic (788.0) ◄

   789.9   Other symptoms involving abdomen and pelvis
     Umbilical: Umbilical:
       bleeding   discharge

NONSPECIFIC ABNORMAL FINDINGS (790–796)

● **790   Nonspecific findings on examination of blood**
     Excludes   *abnormality of:*
           platelets (287.0–287.9)
           thrombocytes (287.0–287.9)
           white blood cells (288.00–288.9)

● **790.0   Abnormality of red blood cells**
     Excludes   *anemia:*
           congenital (776.5)
           *newborn, due to isoimmunization
             (773.0–773.2, 773.5)*
           of premature infant (776.6)
           other specified types (280.0–285.9)
           hemoglobin disorders (282.5–282.7)
           polycythemia:
           familial (289.6)
           neonatorum (776.4)
           secondary (289.0)
           vera (238.4)

   790.01   Precipitous drop in hematocrit 🔵
     Drop in hematocrit
     Drop in hemoglobin ◄
       Decrease in red blood cells
     (Ex:) 285.1, 285.8-285.9

   790.09   Other abnormality of red blood cells
     Abnormal red cell morphology NOS
     Abnormal red cell volume NOS
     Anisocytosis
       Red blood cells of unequal size
     Poikilocytosis
       Red blood cells of abnormal shape

   790.1   Elevated sedimentation rate

● **790.2   Abnormal glucose**
     Excludes   *diabetes mellitus (249.00–249.91,
           250.00–250.93)*
           dysmetabolic syndrome X (277.7)
           gestational diabetes (648.8)
           glycosuria (791.5)
           hypoglycemia (251.2)
           *that complicating pregnancy, childbirth, or
             the puerperium (648.8)*
     Coding Clinic: 2003, Q4, P74-75

   790.21   Impaired fasting glucose
     Elevated fasting glucose

   790.22   Impaired glucose tolerance test (oral)
     Elevated glucose tolerance test

   790.29   Other abnormal glucose
     Abnormal glucose NOS
     Abnormal non-fasting glucose
     Hyperglycemia NOS
     Pre-diabetes NOS
     Coding Clinic: 2005, Q2, P21-22; 2004, Q4, P53-56

   790.3   Excessive blood level of alcohol
     Elevated blood-alcohol

   **790.4   Nonspecific elevation of levels of transaminase or
     lactic acid dehydrogenase [LDH]**

   790.5   Other nonspecific abnormal serum enzyme levels
     Abnormal serum level of:
       acid phosphatase
       alkaline phosphatase
       amylase
       lipase
     Excludes   *deficiency of circulating enzymes (277.6)*

● **790.6   Other abnormal blood chemistry**
     Abnormal blood levels of:
       cobalt
       copper
       iron
       lead
       lithium
       magnesium
       mineral
       zinc
     Excludes   *abnormality of electrolyte or acid-base
           balance (276.0–276.9)*
           hypoglycemia NOS (251.2)
           lead poisoning (984.0–984.9)
           *specific finding indicating abnormality of:
             amino-acid transport and metabolism
               (270.0–270.9)
             carbohydrate transport and metabolism
               (271.0–271.9)*
           lipid metabolism (272.0–272.9)
           uremia NOS (586)

   790.7   Bacteremia 🔵
     Excludes   *bacteremia of newborn (771.83)*
           septicemia (038)
     Use additional code to identify organism (041)
     (Ex:) 338.0-338.4, 780.64-780.65, 780.91-780.99, 790.7-790.99, 799.81-799.89
     Coding Clinic: 2003, Q2, P7-8

   790.8   Viremia, unspecified
     Coding Clinic: 1988, Q4, P10

SYMPTOMS, SIGNS, AND ILL-DEFINED CONDITIONS (780–799)

● **790.9 Other nonspecific findings on examination of blood**

    790.91 Abnormal arterial blood gases

    790.92 Abnormal coagulation profile
        Abnormal or prolonged:
          bleeding time
          coagulation time
          partial thromboplastin time [PTT]
          prothrombin time [PT]

        Excludes *coagulation (hemorrhagic) disorders (286.0–286.9)*
        Coding Clinic: 1994, Q1, P22

    790.93 Elevated prostate specific antigen [PSA] ♂   A
        MCE: Questionable admission, principal diagnosis only

    790.94 Euthyroid sick syndrome

    790.95 Elevated C-reactive protein (CRP)
        Coding Clinic: 2004, Q4, P96-97

    790.99 Other

● **791 Nonspecific findings on examination of urine**

    Excludes *hematuria NOS (599.70–599.72)*
        specific findings indicating abnormality of:
          amino-acid transport and metabolism (270.0–270.9)
          carbohydrate transport and metabolism (271.0–271.9)

    791.0 Proteinuria
        Albuminuria
        Bence-Jones proteinuria

        Excludes *postural proteinuria (593.6)*
            that arising during pregnancy or the puerperium (642.0–642.9, 646.2)

    791.1 Chyluria 🔓
        White milky urine

        Excludes *filarial (125.0–125.9)*

        (Ex:) 338.0-338.4, 780.64-780.65, 780.91-780.99, 791.1, 791.9, 799.81-799.89

    791.2 Hemoglobinuria

    791.3 Myoglobinuria 🔓
        (Ex:) 338.0-338.4, 780.64-780.65, 780.91-780.99, 791.2-791.3, 791.9, 799.81-799.89

    791.4 Biliuria

    791.5 Glycosuria

        Excludes *renal glycosuria (271.4)*

    791.6 Acetonuria
        Ketonuria

    791.7 Other cells and casts in urine

● **791.9 Other nonspecific findings on examination of urine**
        Crystalluria
        Elevated urine levels of:
          17-ketosteroids
          catecholamines
          indolacetic acid
          vanillylmandelic acid [VMA]
        Melanuria
        Coding Clinic: 2005, Q1, P12

● **792 Nonspecific abnormal findings in other body substances**

    Excludes *that in chromosomal analysis (795.2)*

    792.0 Cerebrospinal fluid

    792.1 Stool contents
        Abnormal stool color
        Fat in stool
        Mucus in stool
        Occult blood
        Pus in stool

        Excludes *blood in stool [melena] (578.1)*
            newborn (772.4, 777.3)
        Coding Clinic: 1992, Q2, P9-10; Q2, P9

    792.2 Semen ♂
        Abnormal spermatozoa

        Excludes *azoospermia (606.0)*
            oligospermia (606.1)

    792.3 Amniotic fluid ♀   M

    792.4 Saliva

        Excludes *that in chromosomal analysis (795.2)*

    792.5 Cloudy (hemodialysis) (peritoneal) dialysis effluent

    792.9 Other nonspecific abnormal findings in body substances
        Peritoneal fluid
        Pleural fluid
        Synovial fluid
        Vaginal fluids

● **793 Nonspecific (abnormal) findings on radiological and other examination of body structure** ◀▥

    Includes nonspecific abnormal findings of:
        thermography
        ultrasound examination [echogram]
        x-ray examination

    Excludes *abnormal results of function studies and radioisotope scans (794.0–794.9)*

    793.0 Skull and head

        Excludes *nonspecific abnormal echoencephalogram (794.01)*
        Coding Clinic: 2006, Q3, P22

    793.1 Lung field
        Coin lesion lung
        Shadow, lung

    793.2 Other intrathoracic organ
        Abnormal:
          echocardiogram
          heart shadow
          ultrasound cardiogram
        Mediastinal shift

    793.3 Biliary tract
        Nonvisualization of gallbladder

    793.4 Gastrointestinal tract

    793.5 Genitourinary organs
        Filling defect:
          bladder
          kidney
          ureter

    793.6 Abdominal area, including retroperitoneum

    793.7 Musculoskeletal system

◀ New   ◀▥ Revised   ~~deleted~~ Deleted   ● Unacceptable Principal Diagnosis   ● Use Additional Digit(s)
▶ Manifestation Code   **OGCR** Official Guidelines   **Coding Clinic**   Excludes   Includes   Use additional   Code first   Omit code

● **793.8 Breast**

    793.80 Abnormal mammogram, unspecified

    793.81 Mammographic microcalcification

        | **Excludes** | *mammographic calcification (793.89)*
        mammographic calculus (793.89)

    793.82 Inconclusive mammogram ◀
        Dense breasts NOS ◀
        Inconclusive mammogram NEC ◀
        Inconclusive mammography due to dense
            breasts ◀
        Inconclusive mammography NEC ◀

    793.89 Other (abnormal) findings on radiological
        examination of breast ◀▥
        Mammographic calcification
        Mammographic calculus

● **793.9 Other**

    | **Excludes** | *abnormal finding by radioisotope*
        localization of placenta (794.9)

    793.91 Image test inconclusive due to excess
        body fat
        Use additional code to identify Body Mass
            Index (BMI), if known (V85.0–V85.54)
        Coding Clinic: 2006, Q4, P109-110

    793.99 Other nonspecific (abnormal) findings on
        radiological and other examinations of body
        structure ◀▥
        Abnormal:
           placental finding by x-ray or ultrasound
              method
           radiological findings in skin and
              subcutaneous tissue

● **794 Nonspecific abnormal results of function studies**

    | **Includes** | radioisotope:
        scans
          uptake studies
        scintiphotography

● **794.0 Brain and central nervous system**

    794.00 Abnormal function study, unspecified

    794.01 Abnormal echoencephalogram

    794.02 Abnormal electroencephalogram [EEG]

    794.09 Other
        Abnormal brain scan

● **794.1 Peripheral nervous system and special senses**

    794.10 Abnormal response to nerve stimulation,
        unspecified

    794.11 Abnormal retinal function studies
        Abnormal electroretinogram [ERG]

    794.12 Abnormal electro-oculogram [EOG]

    794.13 Abnormal visually evoked potential

    794.14 Abnormal oculomotor studies

    794.15 Abnormal auditory function studies
        Coding Clinic: 2004, Q1, P15-16

    794.16 Abnormal vestibular function studies

    794.17 Abnormal electromyogram [EMG]

        | **Excludes** | *that of eye (794.14)*

    794.19 Other

● **794.2 Pulmonary**
    Abnormal lung scan
    Reduced:
        ventilatory capacity
        vital capacity

● **794.3 Cardiovascular**

    794.30 Abnormal function study, unspecified

    794.31 Abnormal electrocardiogram [ECG] [EKG]

        | **Excludes** | *long QT syndrome (426.82)*

        Coding Clinic: 1985, Mar-April, P13

    794.39 Other
        Abnormal:
           ballistocardiogram
           phonocardiogram
           vectorcardiogram

    794.4 Kidney
        Abnormal renal function test

    794.5 Thyroid
        Abnormal thyroid:
           scan
           uptake

    794.6 Other endocrine function study

    794.7 Basal metabolism
        Abnormal basal metabolic rate [BMR]

    794.8 Liver
        Abnormal liver scan

    794.9 Other
        Bladder
        Pancreas
        Placenta
        Spleen

● **795 Other and nonspecific abnormal cytological, histological, immunological, and DNA test findings**

    | **Excludes** | *abnormal cytologic smear of anus and anal HPV (796.70-796.79)*
        nonspecific abnormalities of red blood cells (790.01–790.09)

    Coding Clinic: 2002, Q4, P69-70

● **795.0 Abnormal Papanicolaou smear of cervix and cervical HPV**
    Abnormal thin preparation smear of cervix
    Abnormal cervical cytology

    | **Excludes** | *abnormal cytologic smear of vagina and*
        vaginal HPV (795.10-795.19)
        carcinoma in situ of cervix (233.1) ◀▥
        cervical intraepithelial neoplasia I (CIN I)
        (622.11)
        cervical intraepithelial neoplasia II (CIN II)
        (622.12)
        cervical intraepithelial neoplasia III (CIN
        III) (233.1)
        dysplasia (histologically confirmed) of
        cervix (uteri) NOS (622.10)
        mild cervical dysplasia (histologically
        confirmed) (622.11)
        moderate cervical dysplasia (histologically
        confirmed) (622.12)
        severe cervical dysplasia (histologically
        confirmed) (233.1)

    Coding Clinic: 2008, Q4, P145-148; 2004, Q4, P97-99

    795.00 Abnormal glandular Papanicolaou smear of
        cervix ♀
        Atypical endocervical cells NOS
        Atypical endometrial cells NOS
        Atypical cervical glandular cells NOS

    795.01 Papanicolaou smear of cervix with atypical
        squamous cells of undetermined significance
        (ASC-US) ♀
        Coding Clinic: 2006, Q2, P3,4

N Newborn Age: 0   P Pediatric Age: 0–17   M Maternity Age: 12–55   A Adult Age: 15–124   ♀ Females Only   ♂ Males Only

Ⓔ CC Exclusions   ● Complication\Comorbidity   Major C\C   Present on Admission Requirement   Hospital-Acquired Condition   **1059**

SYMPTOMS, SIGNS, AND ILL-DEFINED CONDITIONS (780–799)

795.02 Papanicolaou smear of cervix with atypical squamous cells cannot exclude high grade squamous intraepithelial lesion (ASC-H) ♀

795.03 Papanicolaou smear of cervix with low grade squamous intraepithelial lesion (LGSIL) ♀

795.04 Papanicolaou smear of cervix with high grade squamous intraepithelial lesion (HGSIL) ♀

795.05 Cervical high risk human papillomavirus (HPV) DNA test positive ♀

795.06 Papanicolaou smear of cervix with cytologic evidence of malignancy ♀

795.07 Satisfactory cervical smear but lacking transformation zone ♀

795.08 Unsatisfactory cervical cytology smear ♀
    Inadequate cervical cytology sample
    Coding Clinic: 2006, Q2, P3,4

795.09 Other abnormal Papanicolaou smear of cervix and cervical HPV ♀
    Cervical low risk human papillomavirus (HPV) DNA test positive

    Use additional code for associated human papillomavirus (079.4)

    Excludes encounter for Papanicolaou cervical smear to confirm findings of recent normal smear following initial abnormal smear (V72.32)

● **795.1 Abnormal Papanicolaou smear of vagina and vaginal HPV**
    Abnormal thin preparation smear of vagina NOS
    Abnormal vaginal cytology NOS

    Use additional code to identify acquired absence of uterus and cervix, if applicable (V88.01-V88.03)

    Excludes abnormal cytologic smear of cervix and cervical HPV (795.00-795.09)
            carcinoma in situ of vagina (233.31)
            carcinoma in situ of vulva (233.32)
            dysplasia (histologically confirmed) of vagina NOS (623.0, 233.31)
            dysplasia (histologically confirmed) of vulva NOS (624.01, 624.02, 233.32)
            mild vaginal dysplasia (histologically confirmed) (623.0)
            mild vulvar dysplasia (histologically confirmed) (624.01)
            moderate vaginal dysplasia (histologically confirmed) (623.0)
            moderate vulvar dysplasia (histologically confirmed) (624.02)
            severe vaginal dysplasia (histologically confirmed) (233.31)
            severe vulvar dysplasia (histologically confirmed) (233.32)
            vaginal intraepithelial neoplasia I (VAIN I) (623.0)
            vaginal intraepithelial neoplasia II (VAIN II) (623.0)
            vaginal intraepithelial neoplasia III (VAIN III) (233.31)
            vulvar intraepithelial neoplasia I (VIN I) (624.01)
            vulvar intraepithelial neoplasia II (VIN II) (624.02)
            vulvar intraepithelial neoplasia III (VIN III) (233.32)
    Coding Clinic: 2008, Q4, P145-148

795.10 Abnormal glandular Papanicolaou smear of vagina ♀
    Atypical vaginal glandular cells NOS

795.11 Papanicolaou smear of vagina with atypical squamous cells of undetermined significance (ASC-US) ♀

795.12 Papanicolaou smear of vagina with atypical squamous cells cannot exclude high grade squamous intraepithelial lesion (ASC-H) ♀

795.13 Papanicolaou smear of vagina with low grade squamous intraepithelial lesion (LGSIL) ♀

795.14 Papanicolaou smear of vagina with high grade squamous intraepithelial lesion (HGSIL) ♀

795.15 Vaginal high risk human papillomavirus (HPV) DNA test positive ♀

    Excludes condyloma acuminatum (078.11)
            genital warts (078.11)

795.16 Papanicolaou smear of vagina with cytologic evidence of malignancy ♀
    Coding Clinic: 2004, Q2, P11

795.18 Unsatisfactory vaginal cytology smear ♀
    Inadequate vaginal cytology sample

795.19 Other abnormal Papanicolaou smear of vagina and vaginal HPV ♀
    Vaginal low risk human papillomavirus (HPV) DNA test positive

    Use additional code for associated human papillomavirus (079.4)

795.2 Nonspecific abnormal findings on chromosomal analysis
    Abnormal karyotype

● **795.3 Nonspecific positive culture findings**
    Positive culture findings in:
        nose
        sputum
        throat
        wound

    Excludes that of:
            blood (790.7–790.8)
            urine (791.9)

795.31 Nonspecific positive findings for anthrax
    Positive findings by nasal swab
    Coding Clinic: 2002, Q4, P70

795.39 Other nonspecific positive culture findings

    Excludes colonization status (V02.0-V02.9) ◄

795.4 Other nonspecific abnormal histological findings

795.5 Nonspecific reaction to tuberculin skin test without active tuberculosis
    Abnormal result of Mantoux test
    PPD positive
    Tuberculin (skin test):
        positive
        reactor

795.6 False positive serological test for syphilis
    False positive Wassermann reaction

◄ New   ◄▥ Revised   deleted Deleted   ● Unacceptable Principal Diagnosis   ● Use Additional Digit(s)
▶ Manifestation Code   OGCR Official Guidelines   Coding Clinic   Excludes   Includes   Use additional   Code first   Omit code

SYMPTOMS, SIGNS, AND ILL-DEFINED CONDITIONS (780–799)

● **795.7 Other nonspecific immunological findings**

> Excludes   *abnormal tumor markers (795.81–795.89)*
> *elevated prostate specific antigen [PSA]*
>   *(790.93)*
> *elevated tumor associated antigens*
>   *(795.81–795.89)*
> *isoimmunization, in pregnancy*
>   *(656.1–656.2)*
> *affecting fetus or newborn (773.0–773.2)*

795.71 Nonspecific serologic evidence of human immunodeficiency virus [HIV]

Inconclusive human immunodeficiency virus [HIV] test (adult) (infant)

Note: This code is ONLY to be used when a test finding is reported as nonspecific. Asymptomatic positive findings are coded to V08. If any HIV infection symptom or condition is present, see code 042. Negative findings are not coded.

> Excludes   *acquired immunodeficiency*
>   *syndrome [AIDS] (042)*
> *asymptomatic human*
>   *immunodeficiency virus*
>   *[HIV] infection status (V08)*
> *HIV infection, symptomatic (042)*
> *human immunodeficiency virus*
>   *[HIV] disease (042)*
> *positive (status) NOS (V08)*

OGCR Section I.C.2.e.

Patients with inconclusive HIV serology, but no definitive diagnosis or manifestations of the illness, may be assigned code 795.71, Inconclusive serologic test for Human Immunodeficiency Virus [HIV].

795.79 Other and unspecified nonspecific immunological findings

Raised antibody titer
Raised level of immunoglobulins
Coding Clinic: 1993, Q2, P6

● **795.8 Abnormal tumor markers**

Elevated tumor associated antigens [TAA]
Elevated tumor specific antigens [TSA]

> Excludes   *elevated prostate specific antigen*
>   *[PSA] (790.93)*

Coding Clinic: 2006, Q4, P111-112; 1993, Q1, P21-22; 1992, Q2, P11

795.81 Elevated carcinoembryonic antigen [CEA]

795.82 Elevated cancer antigen 125 [CA 125] ♀

795.89 Other abnormal tumor markers

● **796 Other nonspecific abnormal findings**

796.0 Nonspecific abnormal toxicological findings

Abnormal levels of heavy metals or drugs in blood, urine, or other tissue

> Excludes   *excessive blood level of alcohol (790.3)*

Coding Clinic: 1997, Q1, P16

796.1 Abnormal reflex

796.2 Elevated blood pressure reading without diagnosis of hypertension

Note: This category is to be used to record an episode of elevated blood pressure in a patient in whom no formal diagnosis of hypertension has been made, or as an incidental finding.

MCE: Questionable admission, principal diagnosis only

Coding Clinic: 2003, Q2, P11; 1993, 5th Issue, P6-7

OGCR Section I.C.7.a.8

Assign code 796.2, Elevated blood pressure reading without diagnosis of hypertension, unless patient has an established diagnosis of hypertension. Assign code 642.3x for transient hypertension of pregnancy.

796.3 Nonspecific low blood pressure reading

796.4 Other abnormal clinical findings
Coding Clinic: 1995, Q3, P13

796.5 Abnormal finding on antenatal screening ♀   M

796.6 Abnormal findings on neonatal screening   N

> Excludes   *nonspecific serologic evidence of human*
>   *immunodeficiency virus [HIV]*
>   *(795.71)*

Coding Clinic: 2004, Q4, P99-100

● **796.7 Abnormal cytologic smear of anus and anal HPV**

> Excludes   *abnormal cytologic smear of cervix and*
>   *cervical HPV (795.00-795.09)*
> *abnormal cytologic smear of vagina and*
>   *vaginal HPV (795.10-795.19)*
> *anal intraepithelial neoplasia I (AIN I)*
>   *(569.44)*
> *anal intraepithelial neoplasia II (AIN II)*
>   *(569.44)*
> *anal intraepithelial neoplasia III (AIN III)*
>   *(230.5, 230.6)*
> *carcinoma in situ of anus (230.5, 230.6)*
> *dysplasia (histologically confirmed) of*
>   *anus NOS (569.44)*
> *mild anal dysplasia (histologically*
>   *confirmed) (569.44)*
> *moderate anal dysplasia (histologically*
>   *confirmed) (569.44)*
> *severe anal dysplasia (histologically*
>   *confirmed) (230.5, 230.6)* ◀

Coding Clinic: 2008, Q4, P117-119

796.70 Abnormal glandular Papanicolaou smear of anus

Atypical anal glandular cells NOS

796.71 Papanicolaou smear of anus with atypical squamous cells of undetermined significance (ASC-US)

796.72 Papanicolaou smear of anus with atypical squamous cells cannot exclude high grade squamous intraepithelial lesion (ASC-H)

796.73 Papanicolaou smear of anus with low grade squamous intraepithelial lesion (LGSIL)

796.74 Papanicolaou smear of anus with high grade squamous intraepithelial lesion (HGSIL)

796.75 Anal high risk human papillomavirus (HPV) DNA test positive

796.76 Papanicolaou smear of anus with cytologic evidence of malignancy

796.77 Satisfactory anal smear but lacking transformation zone

796.78 Unsatisfactory anal cytology smear
Inadequate anal cytology sample

796.79 Other abnormal Papanicolaou smear of anus and anal HPV

Anal low risk human papillomavirus (HPV) DNA test positive

Use additional code for associated human papillomavirus (079.4)

796.9 Other

N Newborn Age: 0   P Pediatric Age: 0–17   M Maternity Age: 12–55   A Adult Age: 15–124   ♀ Females Only   ♂ Males Only   **1061**

Ex CC Exclusions   🔁 Complication\Comorbidity   🔁 Major C\C   🔁 Present on Admission Requirement   🔁 Hospital-Acquired Condition

SYMPTOMS, SIGNS, AND ILL-DEFINED CONDITIONS (780–799)

ILL-DEFINED AND UNKNOWN CAUSES OF MORBIDITY AND MORTALITY (797–799)

797   **Senility without mention of psychosis**
    Frailty
    Old age
    Senescence
    Senile asthenia
    Senile:
       debility
       exhaustion

    Excludes   *senile psychoses (290.0–290.9)*

● 798   **Sudden death, cause unknown**

    798.0   Sudden infant death syndrome *(SIDS)*   P
       Cot death
       Crib death
       Sudden death of nonspecific cause in infancy

   ● **798.1   Instantaneous death**

   ● **798.2   Death occurring in less than 24 hours from onset of symptoms, not otherwise explained**
       Death known not to be violent or instantaneous, for which no cause could be discovered
       Died without sign of disease

   ● **798.9   Unattended death**
       Death in circumstances where the body of the deceased was found and no cause could be discovered
       Found dead

● 799   **Other ill-defined and unknown causes of morbidity and mortality**

   ● **799.0   Asphyxia and hypoxemia**

      Excludes   *asphyxia and hypoxemia (due to):*
          carbon monoxide (986)
          hypercapnia (786.09)
          inhalation of food or foreign body (932–934.9)
          newborn (768.0–768.9)
          traumatic (994.7)
      Coding Clinic: 2005, Q4, P90; 1990, Q1, P20

      799.01   Asphyxia
          (Ex:) 338.0-338.4, 518.81-518.84, 780.64-780.65, 780.91-780.99, 798.0, 799.01-799.1, 799.81-799.89

      799.02   Hypoxemia
          Coding Clinic: 2006, Q2, P24,25

   799.1   Respiratory arrest
       Cardiorespiratory failure

      Excludes   *cardiac arrest (427.5)*
          failure of peripheral circulation (785.50)
          respiratory distress:
             NOS (786.09)
             acute (518.82)
             following trauma or surgery (518.5)
             newborn (770.89)
             syndrome (newborn) (769)
                adult (following trauma or surgery) (518.5)
                other (518.82)
          respiratory failure (518.81, 518.83–518.84)
             newborn (770.84)
          respiratory insufficiency (786.09)
             acute (518.82)
       MCC only for patients discharged alive
       (Ex:) 338.0-338.4, 518.81-518.84, 780.64-780.65, 780.91-780.99, 798.0, 799.01-799.1, 799.81-799.89

   ● **799.2   ~~Nervousness~~ Signs and symptoms involving emotional state**
       ~~"Nerves"~~

      Excludes   *anxiety (293.84, 300.00-300.09)*
          depression (311)

      799.21   Nervousness
          Nervous

      799.22   Irritability
          Irritable

      799.23   Impulsiveness
          Impulsive

        Excludes   *impulsive neurosis (300.3)*

      799.24   Emotional lability

      799.25   Demoralization and apathy
          Apathetic

      799.29   Other signs and symptoms involving emotional state

   799.3   Debility, unspecified

      Excludes   *asthenia (780.79)*
          nervous debility (300.5)
          neurasthenia (300.5)
          senile asthenia (797)
      Coding Clinic: 1997, Q3, P11-12

   799.4   Cachexia
       Wasting disease

      Code first underlying condition, if known

       (Ex:) 338.0-338.4, 780.64-780.65, 780.91-780.99, 799.3-799.89
       Coding Clinic: 2006, Q3, P14-15x2; 1990, Q3, P17

   ● **799.8   Other ill-defined conditions**

      799.81   Decreased libido   A
          Decreased sexual desire

        Excludes   *psychosexual dysfunction with inhibited sexual desire (302.71)*
         Coding Clinic: 2003, Q4, P75-76; Q4, P75-76

      799.82   Apparent life threatening event in infant
          ALTE
          Apparent life threatening event in newborn and infant

        Use additional code(s) for associated signs and symptoms

        Excludes   *signs and symptoms associated with a confirmed diagnosis--code to confirmed diagnosis*

      799.89   Other ill-defined conditions

   799.9   Other unknown and unspecified cause
       Undiagnosed disease, not specified as to site or system involved
       Unknown cause of morbidity or mortality
       Coding Clinic: 1998, Q1, P4; 1990, Q1, P22

◄ New   ◄▥ Revised   ~~deleted~~ Deleted   ● Unacceptable Principal Diagnosis   ● Use Additional Digit(s)
▶ Manifestation Code   OGCR Official Guidelines   Coding Clinic   Excludes   Includes   Use additional   Code first   Omit code

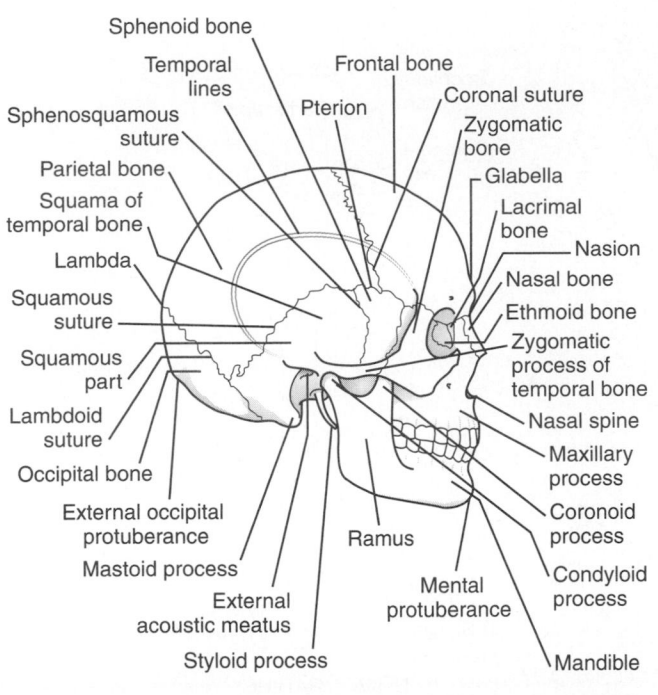

Figure 17–1 Lateral view of skull.

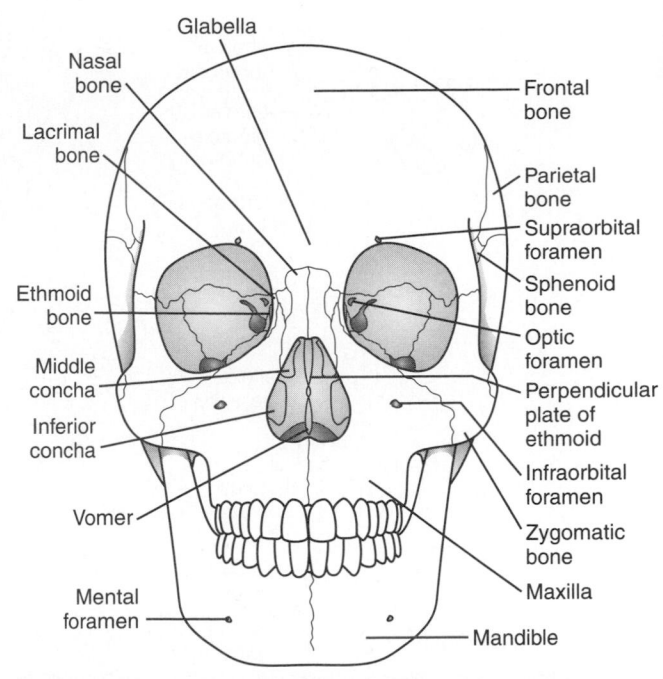

Figure 17–2 Frontal view of skull.

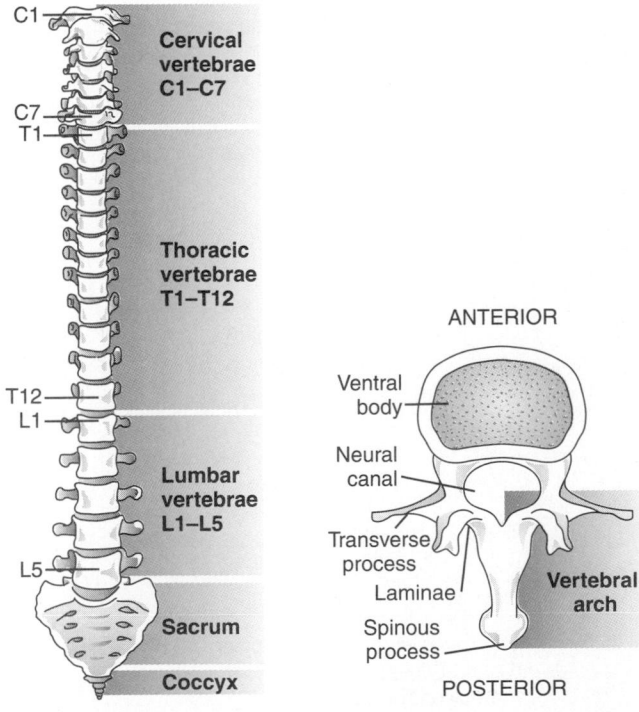

Figure 17–3 Anterior view of vertebral column.

Figure 17–4 Vertebra viewed from above.

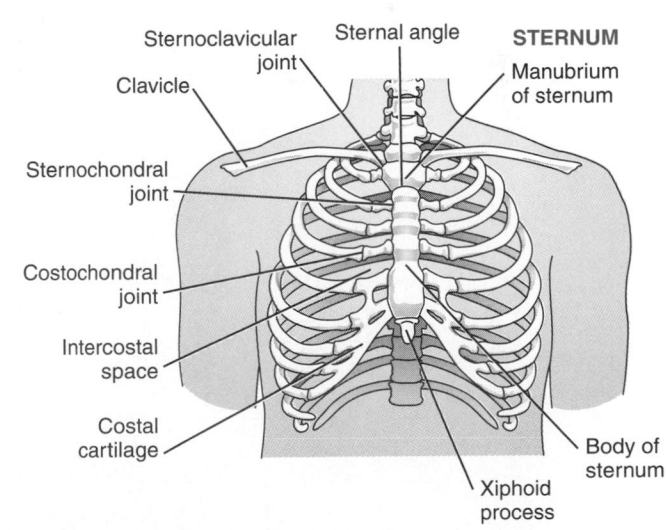

Figure 17–5 Anterior view of rib cage.

N Newborn Age: 0 **P** Pediatric Age: 0–17 **M** Maternity Age: 12–55 **A** Adult Age: 15–124 ♀ Females Only ♂ Males Only

(Ex) CC Exclusions Complication\Comorbidity Major C\C Present on Admission Requirement Hospital-Acquired Condition

INJURY AND POISONING (800–999)

1063

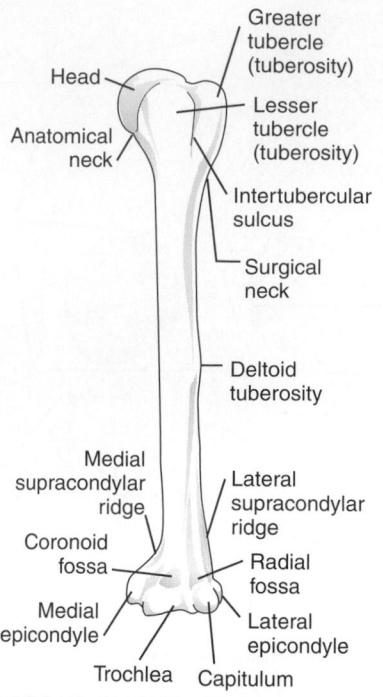

Figure 17–6 ▶ Anterior aspect of left humerus.

Figure 17–7 ▶ Anterior aspect of left radius and ulna.

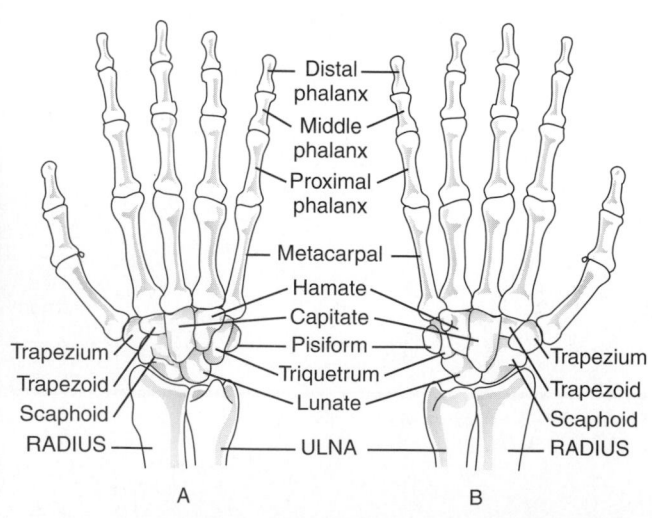

Figure 17–8 ▶ Right hand and wrist: **A.** Dorsal surface. **B.** Palmar surface.

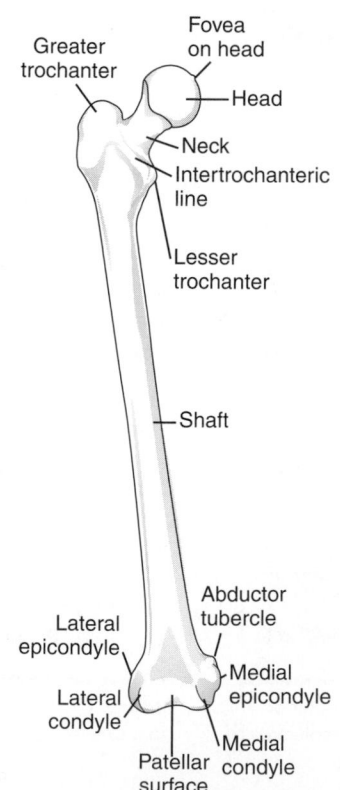

Figure 17–9 ▶ Anterior aspect of right femur.

INJURY AND POISONING (800–999)

◀ New ⬅ Revised ~~deleted~~ Deleted ● Unacceptable Principal Diagnosis ● Use Additional Digit(s)
▶ Manifestation Code **OGCR** Official Guidelines **Coding Clinic** Excludes Includes Use additional Code first Omit code

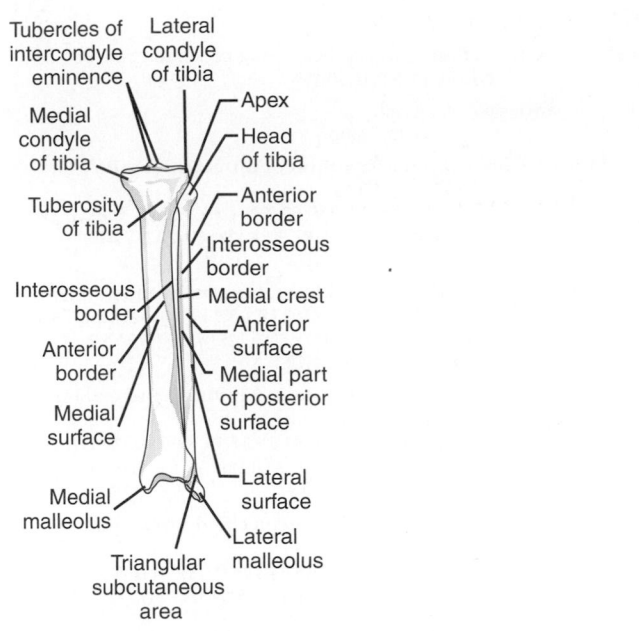

Figure 17–10 Anterior aspect of left tibia and fibula.

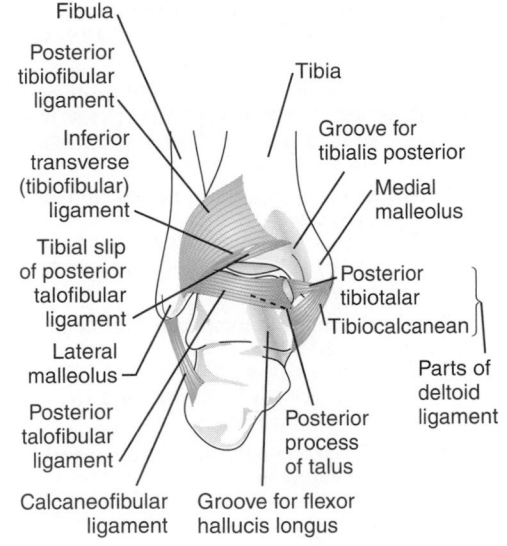

Figure 17–11 Posterior aspect of the left ankle joint.

Figure 17–12 Right foot viewed from above.

OGCR Section I.C.17.a

When coding injuries, assign separate codes for each injury unless a combination code is provided, in which case the combination code is assigned. Multiple injury codes are provided in ICD-9-CM, but should not be assigned unless information for a more specific code is not available. These codes are not to be used for normal, healing surgical wounds or to identify complications of surgical wounds.

The code for the most serious injury, as determined by the provider and the focus of treatment, is sequenced first.

1) **Superficial injuries:** Superficial injuries such as abrasions or contusions are not coded when associated with more severe injuries of the same site.

2) **Primary injury with damage to nerves/blood vessels:** When a primary injury results in minor damage to peripheral nerves or blood vessels, the primary injury is sequenced first with additional code(s) from categories 950-957, Injury to nerves and spinal cord, and/or 900-904, Injury to blood vessels. When the primary injury is to the blood vessels or nerves, that injury should be sequenced first.

17.   INJURY AND POISONING (800–999)

Use E code(s) to identify the cause and intent of the injury or poisoning (E800–E999)

Note:

1. The principle of multiple coding of injuries should be followed wherever possible. Combination categories for multiple injuries are provided for use when there is insufficient detail as to the nature of the individual conditions, or for primary tabulation purposes when it is more convenient to record a single code; otherwise, the component injuries should be coded separately.

   Where multiple sites of injury are specified in the titles, the word "with" indicates involvement of both sites, and the word "and" indicates involvement of either or both sites. The word "finger" includes thumb.

2. Categories for "late effect" of injuries are to be found at 905–909.

N Newborn Age: 0   **P** Pediatric Age: 0–17   **M** Maternity Age: 12–55   **A** Adult Age: 15–124   ♀ Females Only   ♂ Males Only   **1065**
Ex: CC Exclusions   Complication\Comorbidity   Major C\C   Present on Admission Requirement   Hospital-Acquired Condition

INJURY AND POISONING (800–999)

FRACTURES (800–829)

Excludes *malunion (733.81)*
nonunion (733.82)
pathologic or spontaneous fracture
(733.10–733.19)
stress fracture (733.93–733.95)

The terms "condyle," "coronoid process," "ramus," and "symphysis" indicate the portion of the bone fractured, not the name of the bone involved.

The descriptions "closed" and "open" used in the fourth-digit subdivisions include the following terms:
closed (with or without delayed healing):
comminuted
depressed
elevated
fissured
fracture NOS
greenstick
impacted
linear
simple
slipped epiphysis
spiral
open (with or without delayed healing):
compound
infected
missile
puncture
with foreign body

Note: A fracture not indicated as closed or open should be classified as closed.

FRACTURE OF SKULL (800–804)

Includes *traumatic brain injury due to fracture of*
skull   ◀

The following fifth-digit subclassification is for use with the appropriate codes in categories 800, 801, 803, and 804:

0 unspecified state of consciousness
1 with no loss of consciousness
2 with brief [less than one hour] loss of consciousness
3 with moderate [1–24 hours] loss of consciousness
4 with prolonged [more than 24 hours] loss of consciousness and return to pre-existing conscious level
5 with prolonged [more than 24 hours] loss of consciousness, without return to pre-existing conscious level
    Use fifth-digit 5 to designate when a patient is unconscious and dies before regaining consciousness, regardless of the duration of the loss of consciousness
6 with loss of consciousness of unspecified duration
9 with concussion, unspecified

● 800 **Fracture of vault of skull**
Requires fifth digit. See beginning of section 800–804 for codes and definitions.

Includes frontal bone
parietal bone

● 800.0 **Closed without mention of intracranial injury**
[0-6,9] 0-2,6,9 ✎ ✎, 3-5 ✎ ✎
Ex: 800.00-801.99, 803.00-804.99, 829.0-829.1, 850.0-852.19, 852.21-854.19, 873.8-873.9, 879.8-879.9, 905.0, 925.1-925.2, 929.0-929.9, 958.8-959.09, 959.8-959.9

● 800.1 **Closed with cerebral laceration and contusion** ✎ ✎
[0-6,9] Ex: 800.00-801.99, 803.00-804.99, 829.0-829.1, 850.0-852.19, 852.21-854.19, 873.8-873.9, 879.8-879.9, 905.0, 925.1-925.2, 929.0-929.9, 958.8-959.09, 959.8-959.9

● 800.2 **Closed with subarachnoid, subdural, and extradural**
[0-6,9] **hemorrhage** ✎ ✎
Ex: 800.00-801.99, 803.00-804.99, 829.0-829.1, 850.0-852.19, 852.21-854.19, 873.8-873.9, 879.8-879.9, 905.0, 925.1-925.2, 929.0-929.9, 958.8-959.09, 959.8-959.9

● 800.3 **Closed with other and unspecified intracranial**
[0-6,9] **hemorrhage** ✎ ✎
Ex: 800.00-801.99, 803.00-804.99, 829.0-829.1, 850.0-852.19, 852.21-854.19, 873.8-873.9, 879.8-879.9, 905.0, 925.1-925.2, 929.0-929.9, 958.8-959.09, 959.8-959.9

● 800.4 **Closed with intracranial injury of other and**
[0-6,9] **unspecified nature** 0-2,6,9 ✎ ✎, 3-5 ✎ ✎
Ex: 800.00-801.99, 803.00-804.99, 829.0-829.1, 850.0-852.19, 852.21-854.19, 873.8-873.9, 879.8-879.9, 905.0, 925.1-925.2, 929.0-929.9, 958.8-959.09, 959.8-959.9

● 800.5 **Open without mention of intracranial injury** ✎ ✎
[0-6,9] Ex: 800.00-801.99, 803.00-804.99, 829.0-829.1, 850.0-852.19, 852.21-854.19, 873.8-873.9, 879.8-879.9, 905.0, 925.1-925.2, 929.0-929.9, 958.8-959.09, 959.8-959.9

● 800.6 **Open with cerebral laceration and contusion** ✎ ✎
[0-6,9] Ex: 800.00-801.99, 803.00-804.99, 829.0-829.1, 850.0-852.19, 852.21-854.19, 873.8-873.9, 879.8-879.9, 905.0, 925.1-925.2, 929.0-929.9, 958.8-959.09, 959.8-959.9

● 800.7 **Open with subarachnoid, subdural, and extradural**
[0-6,9] **hemorrhage** ✎ ✎
Ex: 800.00-801.99, 803.00-804.99, 829.0-829.1, 850.0-852.19, 852.21-854.19, 873.8-873.9, 879.8-879.9, 905.0, 925.1-925.2, 929.0-929.9, 958.8-959.09, 959.8-959.9

● 800.8 **Open with other and unspecified intracranial**
[0-6,9] **hemorrhage** ✎ ✎
Ex: 800.00-801.99, 803.00-804.99, 829.0-829.1, 850.0-852.19, 852.21-854.19, 873.8-873.9, 879.8-879.9, 905.0, 925.1-925.2, 929.0-929.9, 958.8-959.09, 959.8-959.9

● 800.9 **Open with intracranial injury of other and**
[0-6,9] **unspecified nature** ✎ ✎
Ex: 800.00-801.99, 803.00-804.99, 829.0-829.1, 850.0-852.19, 852.21-854.19, 873.8-873.9, 879.8-879.9, 905.0, 925.1-925.2, 929.0-929.9, 958.8-959.09, 959.8-959.9

◀ New   ◀▥ Revised   ~~deleted~~ Deleted   ● Unacceptable Principal Diagnosis   ● Use Additional Digit(s)
▶ Manifestation Code   **OGCR** Official Guidelines   **Coding Clinic**   Excludes   Includes   Use additional   Code first   Omit code

● 801   **Fracture of base of skull**

> Requires fifth digit. See beginning of section 800–804 for codes and definitions.

> **Includes**   fossa:
> > anterior
> > middle
> > posterior
> > occiput bone
> > orbital roof
> > sinus:
> > > ethmoid
> > > frontal
> > sphenoid bone
> > temporal bone

● 801.0   **Closed without mention of intracranial**
[0-6,9]   **injury 0-2,6,9** 🅒 🅜, **3-5** 🅒 🅜
> (Ex:) 800.00-801.99, 803.00-804.99, 829.0-829.1, 850.0-852.19, 852.21-854.19, 873.8-873.9, 879.8-879.9, 905.0, 925.1-925.2, 929.0-929.9, 958.8-959.09, 959.8-959.9

● 801.1   **Closed with cerebral laceration and contusion** 🅒 🅜
[0-6,9]   (Ex:) 800.00-801.99, 803.00-804.99, 829.0-829.1, 850.0-852.19, 852.21-854.19, 873.8-873.9, 879.8-879.9, 905.0, 925.1-925.2, 929.0-929.9, 958.8-959.09, 959.8-959.9
> **Coding Clinic: 1996, Q4, P36.37**

● 801.2   **Closed with subarachnoid, subdural, and extradural**
[0-6,9]   **hemorrhage** 🅒 🅜
> (Ex:) 800.00-801.99, 803.00-804.99, 829.0-829.1, 850.0-852.19, 852.21-854.19, 873.8-873.9, 879.8-879.9, 905.0, 925.1-925.2, 929.0-929.9, 958.8-959.09, 959.8-959.9

● 801.3   **Closed with other and unspecified intracranial**
[0-6,9]   **hemorrhage** 🅒 🅜
> (Ex:) 800.00-801.99, 803.00-804.99, 829.0-829.1, 850.0-852.19, 852.21-854.19, 873.8-873.9, 879.8-879.9, 905.0, 925.1-925.2, 929.0-929.9, 958.8-959.09, 959.8-959.9

● 801.4   **Closed with intracranial injury of other and**
[0-6,9]   **unspecified nature 0-2,6,9** 🅒 🅜, **3-5** 🅒 🅜
> (Ex:) 800.00-801.99, 803.00-804.99, 829.0-829.1, 850.0-852.19, 852.21-854.19, 873.8-873.9, 879.8-879.9, 905.0, 925.1-925.2, 929.0-929.9, 958.8-959.09, 959.8-959.9

● 801.5   **Open without mention of intracranial injury** 🅒 🅜
[0-6,9]   (Ex:) 800.00-801.99, 803.00-804.99, 829.0-829.1, 850.0-852.19, 852.21-854.19, 873.8-873.9, 879.8-879.9, 905.0, 925.1-925.2, 929.0-929.9, 958.8-959.09, 959.8-959.9

● 801.6   **Open with cerebral laceration and contusion** 🅒 🅜
[0-6,9]   (Ex:) 800.00-801.99, 803.00-804.99, 829.0-829.1, 850.0-852.19, 852.21-854.19, 873.8-873.9, 879.8-879.9, 905.0, 925.1-925.2, 929.0-929.9, 958.8-959.09, 959.8-959.9

● 801.7   **Open with subarachnoid, subdural, and extradural**
[0-6,9]   **hemorrhage** 🅒 🅜
> (Ex:) 800.00-801.99, 803.00-804.99, 829.0-829.1, 850.0-852.19, 852.21-854.19, 873.8-873.9, 879.8-879.9, 905.0, 925.1-925.2, 929.0-929.9, 958.8-959.09, 959.8-959.9

● 801.8   **Open with other and unspecified intracranial**
[0-6,9]   **hemorrhage** 🅒 🅜
> (Ex:) 800.00-801.99, 803.00 -804.99, 829.0-829.1, 850.0-852.19, 852.21-854.19, 873.8-873.9, 879.8-879.9, 905.0, 925.1 -925.2, 929.0-929.9, 958.8-959.09, 959.8-959.9

● 801.9   **Open with intracranial injury of other and**
[0-6,9]   **unspecified nature** 🅒 🅜
> (Ex:) 800.00-801.99, 803.00 -804.99, 829.0-829.1, 850.0-852.19, 852.21-854.19, 873.8-873.9, 879.8-879.9, 905.0, 925.1 -925.2, 929.0-929.9, 958.8-959.09, 959.8-959.9

● 802   **Fracture of face bones**

    802.0   **Nasal bones, closed** 🅜

    802.1   **Nasal bones, open** 🅒 🅜
> (Ex:) 800.00-802.1, 803.00-804.99, 829.0-829.1, 850.0-852.19, 852.21-854.19, 873.8-873.9, 879.8-879.9, 905.0, 925.1-925.2, 929.0-929.9, 958.8-959.09, 959.8-959.9

● 802.2   **Mandible, closed**
       Inferior maxilla
       Lower jaw (bone)

    802.20   **Unspecified site** 🅒 🅜
> (Ex:) 800.00-801.99, 802.20-802.5, 803.00-804.99, 829.0-830.1, 850.0-852.19, 852.21-854.19, 873.8-873.9, 879.8-879.9, 905.0, 925.1-925.2, 929.0-929.9, 958.8-959.09, 959.8-959.9

    802.21   **Condylar process** 🅒 🅜
> (Ex:) 800.00-801.99, 802.20-802.5, 803.00-804.99, 829.0-830.1, 850.0-852.19, 852.21-854.19, 873.8-873.9, 879.8-879.9, 905.0, 925.1-925.2, 929.0-929.9, 958.8-959.09, 959.8-959.9

    802.22   **Subcondylar** 🅒 🅜
> (Ex:) 800.00-801.99, 802.20-802.5, 803.00-804.99, 829.0-830.1, 850.0-852.19, 852.21-854.19, 873.8-873.9, 879.8-879.9, 905.0, 925.1-925.2, 929.0-929.9, 958.8-959.09, 959.8-959.9

    802.23   **Coronoid process** 🅒 🅜
> (Ex:) 800.00-801.99, 802.20-802.5, 803.00-804.99, 829.0-830.1, 850.0-852.19, 852.21-854.19, 873.8-873.9, 879.8-879.9, 905.0, 925.1-925.2, 929.0-929.9, 958.8-959.09, 959.8-959.9

    802.24   **Ramus, unspecified** 🅒 🅜
> (Ex:) 800.00-801.99, 802.20-802.5, 803.00-804.99, 829.0-830.1, 850.0-852.19, 852.21-854.19, 873.8-873.9, 879.8-879.9, 905.0, 925.1-925.2, 929.0-929.9, 958.8-959.09, 959.8-959.9

    802.25   **Angle of jaw** 🅒 🅜
> (Ex:) 800.00-801.99, 802.20-802.5, 803.00-804.99, 829.0-830.1, 850.0-852.19, 852.21-854.19, 873.8-873.9, 879.8-879.9, 905.0, 925.1-925.2, 929.0-929.9, 958.8-959.09, 959.8-959.9

    802.26   **Symphysis of body** 🅒 🅜
> (Ex:) 800.00-801.99, 802.20-802.5, 803.00-804.99, 829.0-830.1, 850.0-852.19, 852.21-854.19, 873.8-873.9, 879.8-879.9, 905.0, 925.1-925.2, 929.0-929.9, 958.8-959.09, 959.8-959.9

    802.27   **Alveolar border of body** 🅒 🅜
> (Ex:) 800.00-801.99, 802.20-802.5, 803.00-804.99, 829.0-830.1, 850.0-852.19, 852.21-854.19, 873.8-873.9, 879.8-879.9, 905.0, 925.1-925.2, 929.0-929.9, 958.8-959.09, 959.8-959.9

    802.28   **Body, other and unspecified** 🅒 🅜
> (Ex:) 800.00-801.99, 802.20-802.5, 803.00-804.99, 829.0-830.1, 850.0-852.19, 852.21-854.19, 873.8-873.9, 879.8-879.9, 905.0, 925.1-925.2, 929.0-929.9, 958.8-959.09, 959.8-959.9

    802.29   **Multiple sites** 🅒 🅜
> (Ex:) 800.00-801.99, 802.20-802.5, 803.00-804.99, 829.0-830.1, 850.0-852.19, 852.21-854.19, 873.8-873.9, 879.8-879.9, 905.0, 925.1-925.2, 929.0-929.9, 958.8-959.09, 959.8-959.9

N Newborn Age: 0   **P** Pediatric Age: 0–17   **M** Maternity Age: 12–55   **A** Adult Age: 15–124   ♀ Females Only   ♂ Males Only

(Ex:) CC Exclusions   🅒 Complication\Comorbidity   🅜 Major C\C   Present on Admission Requirement   Hospital-Acquired Condition   **1067**

INJURY AND POISONING (800–999)

● **802.3　Mandible, open**

    802.30　Unspecified site 🦠 🦠
        Ex: 800.00-801.99, 802.20-802.5, 803.00-804.99, 829.0-830.1,
        850.0-852.19, 852.21-854.19, 873.8-873.9, 879.8-879.9,
        905.0, 925.1-925.2, 929.0-929.9, 958.8-959.09,
        959.8-959.9

    802.31　Condylar process 🦠 🦠
        Ex: 800.00-801.99, 802.20-802.5, 803.00-804.99, 829.0-830.1,
        850.0-852.19, 852.21-854.19, 873.8-873.9, 879.8-879.9,
        905.0, 925.1-925.2, 929.0-929.9, 958.8-959.09,
        959.8-959.9

    802.32　Subcondylar 🦠 🦠
        Ex: 800.00-801.99, 802.20-802.5, 803.00-804.99, 829.0-830.1,
        850.0-852.19, 852.21-854.19, 873.8-873.9, 879.8-879.9,
        905.0, 925.1-925.2, 929.0-929.9, 958.8-959.09,
        959.8-959.9

    802.33　Coronoid process 🦠 🦠
        Ex: 800.00-801.99, 802.20-802.5, 803.00-804.99, 829.0-830.1,
        850.0-852.19, 852.21-854.19, 873.8-873.9, 879.8-879.9,
        905.0, 925.1-925.2, 929.0-929.9, 958.8-959.09,
        959.8-959.9

    802.34　Ramus, unspecified 🦠 🦠
        Ex: 800.00-801.99, 802.20-802.5, 803.00-804.99, 829.0-830.1,
        850.0-852.19, 852.21-854.19, 873.8-873.9, 879.8-879.9,
        905.0, 925.1-925.2, 929.0-929.9, 958.8-959.09,
        959.8-959.9

    802.35　Angle of jaw 🦠 🦠
        Ex: 800.00-801.99, 802.20-802.5, 803.00-804.99, 829.0-830.1,
        850.0-852.19, 852.21-854.19, 873.8-873.9, 879.8-879.9,
        905.0, 925.1-925.2, 929.0-929.9, 958.8-959.09,
        959.8-959.9

    802.36　Symphysis of body 🦠 🦠
        Ex: 800.00-801.99, 802.20-802.5, 803.00-804.99, 829.0-830.1,
        850.0-852.19, 852.21-854.19, 873.8-873.9, 879.8-879.9,
        905.0, 925.1-925.2, 929.0-929.9, 958.8-959.09,
        959.8-959.9

    802.37　Alveolar border of body 🦠 🦠
        Ex: 800.00-801.99, 802.20-802.5, 803.00-804.99, 829.0-830.1,
        850.0-852.19, 852.21-854.19, 873.8-873.9, 879.8-879.9,
        905.0, 925.1-925.2, 929.0-929.9, 958.8-959.09,
        959.8-959.9

    802.38　Body, other and unspecified 🦠 🦠
        Ex: 800.00-801.99, 802.20-802.5, 803.00-804.99, 829.0-830.1,
        850.0-852.19, 852.21-854.19, 873.8-873.9, 879.8-879.9,
        905.0, 925.1-925.2, 929.0-929.9, 958.8-959.09,
        959.8-959.9

    802.39　Multiple sites 🦠 🦠
        Ex: 800.00-801.99, 802.20-802.5, 803.00-804.99, 829.0-830.1,
        850.0-852.19, 852.21-854.19, 873.8-873.9, 879.8-879.9,
        905.0, 925.1-925.2, 929.0-929.9, 958.8-959.09,
        959.8-959.9

● **802.4　Malar and maxillary bones, closed** 🦠 🦠
    Superior maxilla
    Upper jaw (bone)
    Zygoma
    Zygomatic arch
    Ex: 800.00-801.99, 802.20-802.5, 803.00-804.99, 829.0-830.1, 850.0-852.19,
    852.21-854.19, 873.8-873.9, 879.8-879.9, 905.0, 925.1-925.2,
    929.0-929.9, 958.8-959.09, 959.8-959.9

● **802.5　Malar and maxillary bones, open** 🦠 🦠
    Ex: 800.00-801.99, 802.20-802.5, 803.00-804.99, 829.0-830.1, 850.0-852.19,
    852.21-854.19, 873.8-873.9, 879.8-879.9, 905.0, 925.1-925.2,
    929.0-929.9, 958.8-959.09, 959.8-959.9

● **802.6　Orbital floor (blow-out), closed** 🦠 🦠
    Ex: 800.00-801.99, 802.6-804.99, 829.0-829.1, 850.0-852.19, 852.21-854.19,
    873.8-873.9, 879.8-879.9, 905.0, 925.1-925.2, 929.0-929.9,
    958.8-959.09, 959.8-959.9

● **802.7　Orbital floor (blow-out), open** 🦠 🦠
    Ex: 800.00-801.99, 802.6-804.99, 829.0-829.1, 850.0-852.19, 852.21-854.19,
    873.8-873.9, 879.8-879.9, 905.0, 925.1-925.2, 929.0-929.9,
    958.8-959.09, 959.8-959.9

● **802.8　Other facial bones, closed** 🦠 🦠
    Alveolus
    Orbit:
      NOS
      part other than roof or floor
    Palate

    Excludes　*orbital:*
          floor (802.6)
          roof (801.0–801.9)
    Ex: 800.00-801.99, 802.6-804.99, 829.0-829.1, 850.0-852.19, 852.21-854.19,
    873.8-873.9, 879.8-879.9, 905.0, 925.1-925.2, 929.0-929.9,
    958.8-959.09, 959.8-959.9

● **802.9　Other facial bones, open** 🦠 🦠
    Ex: 800.00-801.99, 802.6-804.99, 829.0-829.1, 850.0-852.19, 852.21-854.19,
    873.8-873.9, 879.8-879.9, 905.0, 925.1-925.2, 929.0-929.9,
    958.8-959.09, 959.8-959.9

● **803　Other and unqualified skull fractures**

    Requires fifth digit. See beginning of section 800–804 for
      codes and definitions.

    Includes　skull NOS
           skull multiple NOS

● **803.0　Closed without mention of intracranial injury**
  [0-6,9]　0-2,6,9 🦠 🦠, 3-5 🦠 🦠
    Ex: 800.00-801.99, 802.6-804.99, 829.0-829.1, 850.0-852.19, 852.21-854.19,
    873.8-873.9, 879.8-879.9, 905.0, 925.1-925.2, 929.0-929.9,
    958.8-959.09, 959.8-959.9

● **803.1　Closed with cerebral laceration and contusion** 🦠 🦠
  [0-6,9]　Ex: 800.00-801.99, 802.6-804.99, 829.0-829.1, 850.0-852.19, 852.21-854.19,
    873.8-873.9, 879.8-879.9, 905.0, 925.1-925.2, 929.0-929.9,
    958.8-959.09, 959.8-959.9

● **803.2　Closed with subarachnoid, subdural, and extradural**
  [0-6,9]　**hemorrhage** 🦠 🦠
    Ex: 800.00-801.99, 802.6-804.99, 829.0-829.1, 850.0-852.19, 852.21-854.19,
    873.8-873.9, 879.8-879.9, 905.0, 925.1-925.2, 929.0-929.9,
    958.8-959.09, 959.8-959.9

● **803.3　Closed with other and unspecified intracranial**
  [0-6,9]　**hemorrhage** 🦠 🦠
    Ex: 800.00-801.99, 802.6-804.99, 829.0-829.1, 850.0-852.19, 852.21-854.19,
    873.8-873.9, 879.8-879.9, 905.0, 925.1-925.2, 929.0-929.9,
    958.8-959.09, 959.8-959.9

● **803.4　Closed with intracranial injury of other and**
  [0-6,9]　**unspecified nature 0-2,6,9** 🦠 🦠, **3-5** 🦠 🦠
    Ex: 800.00-801.99, 802.6-804.99, 829.0-829.1, 850.0-852.19, 852.21-854.19,
    873.8-873.9, 879.8-879.9, 905.0, 925.1-925.2, 929.0-929.9,
    958.8-959.09, 959.8-959.9

● **803.5　Open without mention of intracranial injury** 🦠 🦠
  [0-6,9]　Ex: 800.00-801.99, 802.6-804.99, 829.0-829.1, 850.0-852.19, 852.21-854.19,
    873.8-873.9, 879.8-879.9, 905.0, 925.1-925.2, 929.0-929.9,
    958.8-959.09, 959.8-959.9

INJURY AND POISONING (800–999)

◀ New　　◀▥ Revised　　deleted Deleted　　● Unacceptable Principal Diagnosis　　● Use Additional Digit(s)
▶ Manifestation Code　　OGCR Official Guidelines　　Coding Clinic　　Excludes　　Includes　　Use additional　　Code first　　Omit code

● **803.6   Open with cerebral laceration and contusion** 🔹 🔹
[0-6,9]   Ex: 800.00-801.99, 802.6-804.99, 829.0-829.1, 850.0-852.19, 852.21-854.19,
      873.8-873.9, 879.8-879.9, 905.0, 925.1-925.2, 929.0-929.9,
      958.8-959.09, 959.8-959.9

● **803.7   Open with subarachnoid, subdural, and extradural**
[0-6,9]   **hemorrhage** 🔹 🔹
   Ex: 800.00-801.99, 802.6-804.99, 829.0-829.1, 850.0-852.19, 852.21-854.19,
      873.8-873.9, 879.8-879.9, 905.0, 925.1-925.2, 929.0-929.9,
      958.8-959.09, 959.8-959.9

● **803.8   Open with other and unspecified intracranial**
[0-6,9]   **hemorrhage** 🔹 🔹
   Ex: 800.00-801.99, 802.6-804.99, 829.0-829.1, 850.0-852.19, 852.21-854.19,
      873.8-873.9, 879.8-879.9, 905.0, 925.1-925.2, 929.0-929.9,
      958.8-959.09, 959.8-959.9

● **803.9   Open with intracranial injury of other and**
[0-6,9]   **unspecified nature** 🔹 🔹
   Ex: 800.00-801.99, 802.6-804.99, 829.0-829.1, 850.0-852.19, 852.21-854.19,
      873.8-873.9, 879.8-879.9, 905.0, 925.1-925.2, 929.0-929.9,
      958.8-959.09, 959.8-959.9

● **804   Multiple fractures involving skull or face with other bones**
     Requires fifth digit. See beginning of section 800–804 for
     codes and definitions.

● **804.0   Closed without mention of intracranial injury**
[0-6,9]   0-2,6,9 🔹 🔹, 3-5 🔹 🔹
   Ex: 800.00-801.99, 802.6-804.99, 829.0-829.1, 850.0-852.19, 852.21-854.19,
      873.8-873.9, 879.8-879.9, 905.0, 925.1-925.2, 929.0-929.9,
      958.8-959.09, 959.8-959.9

● **804.1   Closed with cerebral laceration and contusion** 🔹 🔹
[0-6,9]   Ex: 800.00-801.99, 802.6-804.99, 829.0-829.1, 850.0-852.19, 852.21-854.19,
      873.8-873.9, 879.8-879.9, 905.0, 925.1-925.2, 929.0-929.9,
      958.8-959.09, 959.8-959.9

     Coding Clinic: 2006, Q1, P6-7

● **804.2   Closed with subarachnoid, subdural, and extradural**
[0-6,9]   **hemorrhage** 🔹 🔹
   Ex: 800.00-801.99, 802.6-804.99, 829.0-829.1, 850.0-852.19, 852.21-854.19,
      873.8-873.9, 879.8-879.9, 905.0, 925.1-925.2, 929.0-929.9,
      958.8-959.09, 959.8-959.9

● **804.3   Closed with other and unspecified intracranial**
[0-6,9]   **hemorrhage** 🔹 🔹
   Ex: 800.00-801.99, 802.6-804.99, 829.0-829.1, 850.0-852.19, 852.21-854.19,
      873.8-873.9, 879.8-879.9, 905.0, 925.1-925.2, 929.0-929.9,
      958.8-959.09, 959.8-959.9

● **804.4   Closed with intracranial injury of other and**
[0-6,9]   **unspecified nature** 0-2,6,9 🔹 🔹, 3-5 🔹 🔹
   Ex: 800.00-801.99, 802.6-804.99, 829.0-829.1, 850.0-852.19, 852.21-854.19,
      873.8-873.9, 879.8-879.9, 905.0, 925.1-925.2, 929.0-929.9,
      958.8-959.09, 959.8-959.9

● **804.5   Open without mention of intracranial injury**
[0-6,9]   0-2,6,9 🔹 🔹, 3-5 🔹 🔹
   Ex: 800.00-801.99, 802.6-804.99, 829.0-829.1, 850.0-852.19, 852.21-854.19,
      873.8-873.9, 879.8-879.9, 905.0, 925.1-925.2, 929.0-929.9,
      958.8-959.09, 959.8-959.9

● **804.6   Open with cerebral laceration and contusion** 🔹 🔹
[0-6,9]   Ex: 800.00-801.99, 802.6-804.99, 829.0-829.1, 850.0-852.19, 852.21-854.19,
      873.8-873.9, 879.8-879.9, 905.0, 925.1-925.2, 929.0-929.9,
      958.8-959.09, 959.8-959.9

● **804.7   Open with subarachnoid, subdural, and extradural**
[0-6,9]   **hemorrhage** 🔹 🔹
   Ex: 800.00-801.99, 802.6-804.99, 829.0-829.1, 850.0-852.19, 852.21-854.19,
      873.8-873.9, 879.8-879.9, 905.0, 925.1-925.2, 929.0-929.9,
      958.8-959.09, 959.8-959.9

● **804.8   Open with other and unspecified intracranial**
[0-6,9]   **hemorrhage** 🔹 🔹
   Ex: 800.00-801.99, 802.6-804.99, 829.0-829.1, 850.0-852.19, 852.21-854.19,
      873.8-873.9, 879.8-879.9, 905.0, 925.1-925.2, 929.0-929.9,
      958.8-959.09, 959.8-959.9

● **804.9   Open with intracranial injury of other and**
[0-6,9]   **unspecified nature** 0-2,6,9 🔹 🔹, 3-5 🔹 🔹
   Ex: 800.00-801.99, 802.6-804.99, 829.0-829.1, 850.0-852.19, 852.21-854.19,
      873.8-873.9, 879.8-879.9, 905.0, 925.1-925.2, 929.0-929.9,
      958.8-959.09, 959.8-959.9

FRACTURE OF NECK AND TRUNK (805–809)

● **805   Fracture of vertebral column without mention of spinal cord injury**

   Includes   neural arch
            spine
            spinous process
            transverse process
            vertebra

   Coding Clinic: 1985, Nov-Dec, P16

The following fifth-digit subclassification is for use with codes 805.0–805.1:

> 0   cervical vertebra, unspecified level
> 1   first cervical vertebra
> 2   second cervical vertebra
> 3   third cervical vertebra
> 4   fourth cervical vertebra
> 5   fifth cervical vertebra
> 6   sixth cervical vertebra
> 7   seventh cervical vertebra
> 8   multiple cervical vertebrae

● **805.0   Cervical, closed** 🔹 🔹
[0-8]   Atlas
      Axis
   Ex: 805.00-805.18, 805.8-806.19, 806.8-806.9, 829.0-829.1, 839.00-839.18,
      839.40, 839.49-839.50, 839.59, 839.69, 839.79-839.9, 847.0, 847.9,
      848.8-848.9, 879.8-879.9, 905.1, 926.11, 929.0-929.9, 952.00-952.09,
      952.8-952.9, 958.8-958.99, 959.11-959.19, 959.8-959.9

● **805.1   Cervical, open** 🔹 🔹
[0-8]   Ex: 805.00-805.18, 805.8-806.19, 806.8-806.9, 829.0-829.1, 839.00-839.18,
      839.40, 839.49-839.50, 839.59, 839.69, 839.79-839.9, 847.0, 847.9,
      848.8-848.9, 879.8-879.9, 905.1, 926.11, 929.0-929.9, 952.00-952.09,
      952.8-952.9, 958.8-958.99, 959.11-959.19, 959.8-959.9

   805.2   Dorsal [thoracic], closed 🔹 🔹
     Ex: 805.2-805.3, 805.8-805.9, 806.20-806.9, 806.8-806.9, 829.0-829.1,
       839.21, 839.31-839.40, 839.49-839.50, 839.59, 839.69, 839.79-839.9,
       847.1, 847.9, 848.8-848.9, 879.8-879.9, 905.1, 926.11, 929.0-929.9,
       952.10-952.19, 952.8-952.9, 958.8-958.99, 959.11-959.19,
       959.8-959.9

INJURY AND POISONING (800-999)

805.3 Dorsal [thoracic], open 🔖 🔖
> (Ex:) 805.2-805.3, 805.8-805.9, 806.20-806.39, 806.8-806.9, 829.0-829.1, 839.21, 839.31-839.40, 839.49-839.50, 839.59, 839.69, 839.79-839.9, 847.1, 847.9, 848.8-848.9, 879.8-879.9, 905.1, 926.11, 929.0-929.9, 952.10-952.19, 952.8-952.9, 958.8-958.99, 959.11-959.19, 959.8-959.9

805.4 Lumbar, closed 🔖 🔖
> (Ex:) 805.4-805.5, 805.8-805.9, 806.4-806.5, 806.8-806.9, 829.0-829.1, 839.20, 839.30, 839.40, 839.49-839.50, 839.59, 839.69, 839.79-839.9, 847.2, 847.9, 848.8-848.9, 879.8-879.9, 905.1, 926.11, 929.0-929.9, 952.2, 952.8-952.9, 958.8-958.99, 959.11-959.19, 959.8-959.9

Coding Clinic: 2007, Q1, P3-8

805.5 Lumbar, open 🔖 🔖
> (Ex:) 805.4-805.5, 805.8-805.9, 806.4-806.5, 806.8-806.9, 829.0-829.1, 839.20, 839.30, 839.40, 839.49-839.50, 839.59, 839.69, 839.79-839.9, 847.2, 847.9, 848.8-848.9, 879.8-879.9, 905.1, 926.11, 929.0-929.9, 952.2, 952.8-952.9, 958.8-958.99, 959.11-959.19, 959.8-959.9

805.6 Sacrum and coccyx, closed 🔖 🔖
> (Ex:) 805.6-805.9, 806.60-806.9, 829.0-829.1, 839.40-839.59, 839.69, 839.79-839.9, 846.0-846.9, 847.3-847.9, 848.5-848.9, 879.8-879.9, 905.1, 926.11, 929.0-929.9, 952.3-952.9, 958.8-958.99, 959.11-959.19, 959.8-959.9

805.7 Sacrum and coccyx, open 🔖 🔖
> (Ex:) 805.6-805.9, 806.60-806.9, 829.0-829.1, 839.40-839.59, 839.69, 839.79-839.9, 846.0-846.9, 847.3-847.9, 848.5-848.9, 879.8-879.9, 905.1, 926.11, 929.0-929.9, 952.3-952.9, 958.8-958.99, 959.11-959.19, 959.8-959.9

805.8 Unspecified, closed 🔖 🔖
> (Ex:) 733.10-733.19, 733.93-733.98, 805.00-806.9, 829.0-829.1, 839.00-839.59, 839.69, 839.79-839.9, 846.0-847.9, 848.5-848.9, 879.8-879.9, 905.1, 926.11, 929.0-929.9, 952.00-952.9, 958.8-958.99, 959.11-959.19, 959.8-959.9

805.9 Unspecified, open 🔖 🔖
> (Ex:) 733.10-733.19, 733.93-733.98, 805.00-806.9, 829.0-829.1, 839.00-839.59, 839.69, 839.79-839.9, 846.0-847.9, 848.5-848.9, 879.8-879.9, 905.1, 926.11, 929.0-929.9, 952.00-952.9, 958.8-958.99, 959.11-959.19, 959.8-959.9

● **806 Fracture of vertebral column with spinal cord injury**

Includes   any condition classifiable to 805 with:
> complete or incomplete transverse lesion (of cord)
> hematomyelia
> injury to:
> > cauda equina
> > nerve
>
> paralysis
> paraplegia
> quadriplegia
> spinal concussion

● **806.0 Cervical, closed**

806.00 C_1-C_4 level with unspecified spinal cord injury 🔖 🔖
> Cervical region NOS with spinal cord injury NOS
> (Ex:) 733.10-733.19, 733.93-733.98, 805.00-805.18, 805.8-806.19, 806.8-806.9, 829.0-829.1, 839.00-839.18, 839.40, 839.49-839.50, 839.59, 839.69, 839.79-839.9, 847.9, 848.8-848.9, 879.8-879.9, 905.1, 926.11, 929.0-929.9, 952.00-952.09, 952.8-952.9, 958.8-958.99, 959.11-959.19, 959.8-959.9

806.01 C_1-C_4 level with complete lesion of cord 🔖 🔖
> (Ex:) 733.10-733.19, 733.93-733.98, 805.00-805.18, 805.8-806.19, 806.8-806.9, 829.0-829.1, 839.00-839.18, 839.40, 839.49-839.50, 839.59, 839.69, 839.79-839.9, 847.9, 848.8-848.9, 879.8-879.9, 905.1, 926.11, 929.0-929.9, 952.00-952.09, 952.8-952.9, 958.8-958.99, 959.11-959.19, 959.8-959.9

806.02 C_1-C_4 level with anterior cord syndrome 🔖 🔖
> (Ex:) 733.10-733.19, 733.93-733.98, 805.00-805.18, 805.8-806.19, 806.8-806.9, 829.0-829.1, 839.00-839.18, 839.40, 839.49-839.50, 839.59, 839.69, 839.79-839.9, 847.9, 848.8-848.9, 879.8-879.9, 905.1, 926.11, 929.0-929.9, 952.00-952.09, 952.8-952.9, 958.8-958.99, 959.11-959.19, 959.8-959.9

806.03 C_1-C_4 level with central cord syndrome 🔖 🔖
> (Ex:) 733.10-733.19, 733.93-733.98, 805.00-805.18, 805.8-806.19, 806.8-806.9, 829.0-829.1, 839.00-839.18, 839.40, 839.49-839.50, 839.59, 839.69, 839.79-839.9, 847.9, 848.8-848.9, 879.8-879.9, 905.1, 926.11, 929.0-929.9, 952.00-952.09, 952.8-952.9, 958.8-958.99, 959.11-959.19, 959.8-959.9

806.04 C_1-C_4 level with other specified spinal cord injury 🔖 🔖
> C_1-C_4 level with:
> > incomplete spinal cord lesion NOS
> > posterior cord syndrome
>
> (Ex:) 733.10-733.19, 733.93-733.98, 805.00-805.18, 805.8-806.19, 806.8-806.9, 829.0-829.1, 839.00-839.18, 839.40, 839.49-839.50, 839.59, 839.69, 839.79-839.9, 847.9, 848.8-848.9, 879.8-879.9, 905.1, 926.11, 929.0-929.9, 952.00-952.09, 952.8-952.9, 958.8-958.99, 959.11-959.19, 959.8-959.9

806.05 C_5-C_7 level with unspecified spinal cord injury 🔖 🔖
> (Ex:) 733.10-733.19, 733.93-733.98, 805.00-805.18, 805.8-806.19, 806.8-806.9, 829.0-829.1, 839.00-839.18, 839.40, 839.49-839.50, 839.59, 839.69, 839.79-839.9, 847.9, 848.8-848.9, 879.8-879.9, 905.1, 926.11, 929.0-929.9, 952.00-952.09, 952.8-952.9, 958.8-958.99, 959.11-959.19, 959.8-959.9

806.06 C_5-C_7 level with complete lesion of cord 🔖 🔖
> (Ex:) 733.10-733.19, 733.93-733.98, 805.00-805.18, 805.8-806.19, 806.8-806.9, 829.0-829.1, 839.00-839.18, 839.40, 839.49-839.50, 839.59, 839.69, 839.79-839.9, 847.9, 848.8-848.9, 879.8-879.9, 905.1, 926.11, 929.0-929.9, 952.00-952.09, 952.8-952.9, 958.8-958.99, 959.11-959.19, 959.8-959.9

806.07 C_5-C_7 level with anterior cord syndrome 🔖 🔖
> (Ex:) 733.10-733.19, 733.93-733.98, 805.00-805.18, 805.8-806.19, 806.8-806.9, 829.0-829.1, 839.00-839.18, 839.40, 839.49-839.50, 839.59, 839.69, 839.79-839.9, 847.9, 848.8-848.9, 879.8-879.9, 905.1, 926.11, 929.0-929.9, 952.00-952.09, 952.8-952.9, 958.8-958.99, 959.11-959.19, 959.8-959.9

806.08 C_5-C_7 level with central cord syndrome 🔖 🔖
> (Ex:) 733.10-733.19, 733.93-733.98, 805.00-805.18, 805.8-806.19, 806.8-806.9, 829.0-829.1, 839.00-839.18, 839.40, 839.49-839.50, 839.59, 839.69, 839.79-839.9, 847.9, 848.8-848.9, 879.8-879.9, 905.1, 926.11, 929.0-929.9, 952.00-952.09, 952.8-952.9, 958.8-958.99, 959.11-959.19, 959.8-959.9

◀ New   ◀▦ Revised   ~~deleted~~ Deleted   ● Unacceptable Principal Diagnosis   ● Use Additional Digit(s)
▶ Manifestation Code   OGCR Official Guidelines   **Coding Clinic**   Excludes   Includes   Use additional   Code first   Omit code

806.09 C$_5$-C$_7$ level with other specified spinal cord injury ⬟ ⬟

  C$_5$-C$_7$ level with:
    incomplete spinal cord lesion NOS
    posterior cord syndrome
    (Ex) 733.10-733.19, 733.93-733.98, 805.00-805.18, 805.8-806.19,
    806.8-806.9, 829.0-829.1, 839.00-839.18, 839.40,
    839.49-839.50, 839.59, 839.69, 839.79-839.9, 847.9,
    848.8-848.9, 879.8-879.9, 905.1, 926.11, 929.0-929.9,
    952.00-952.09, 952.8-952.9, 958.8-958.99, 959.11-959.19,
    959.8-959.9

● 806.1 Cervical, open

806.10 C$_1$-C$_4$ level with unspecified spinal cord injury ⬟ ⬟

  (Ex) 733.10-733.19, 733.93-733.98, 805.00-805.18, 805.8-806.19,
  806.8-806.9, 829.0-829.1, 839.00-839.18, 839.40,
  839.49-839.50, 839.59, 839.69, 839.79-839.9, 847.9,
  848.8-848.9, 879.8-879.9, 905.1, 926.11, 929.0-929.9,
  952.00-952.09, 952.8-952.9, 958.8-958.99, 959.11-959.19,
  959.8-959.9

806.11 C$_1$-C$_4$ level with complete lesion of cord ⬟ ⬟

  (Ex) 733.10-733.19, 733.93-733.98, 805.00-805.18, 805.8-806.19,
  806.8-806.9, 829.0-829.1, 839.00-839.18, 839.40,
  839.49-839.50, 839.59, 839.69, 839.79-839.9, 847.9,
  848.8-848.9, 879.8-879.9, 905.1, 926.11, 929.0-929.9,
  952.00-952.09, 952.8-952.9, 958.8-958.99, 959.11-959.19,
  959.8-959.9

806.12 C$_1$-C$_4$ level with anterior cord syndrome ⬟ ⬟

  (Ex) 733.10-733.19, 733.93-733.98, 805.00-805.18, 805.8-806.19,
  806.8-806.9, 829.0-829.1, 839.00-839.18, 839.40,
  839.49-839.50, 839.59, 839.69, 839.79-839.9, 847.9,
  848.8-848.9, 879.8-879.9, 905.1, 926.11, 929.0-929.9,
  952.00-952.09, 952.8-952.9, 958.8-958.99, 959.11-959.19,
  959.8-959.9

806.13 C$_1$-C$_4$ level with central cord syndrome ⬟ ⬟

  (Ex) 733.10-733.19, 733.93-733.98, 805.00-805.18, 805.8-806.19,
  806.8-806.9, 829.0-829.1, 839.00-839.18, 839.40,
  839.49-839.50, 839.59, 839.69, 839.79-839.9, 847.9,
  848.8-848.9, 879.8-879.9, 905.1, 926.11, 929.0-929.9,
  952.00-952.09, 952.8-952.9, 958.8-958.99, 959.11-959.19,
  959.8-959.9

806.14 C$_1$-C$_4$ level with other specified spinal cord injury ⬟ ⬟

  C$_1$-C$_4$ level with:
    incomplete spinal cord lesion NOS
    posterior cord syndrome
    (Ex) 733.10-733.19, 733.93-733.98, 805.00-805.18, 805.8-806.19,
    806.8-806.9, 829.0-829.1, 839.00-839.18, 839.40,
    839.49-839.50, 839.59, 839.69, 839.79-839.9, 847.9,
    848.8-848.9, 879.8-879.9, 905.1, 926.11, 929.0-929.9,
    952.00-952.09, 952.8-952.9, 958.8-958.99, 959.11-959.19,
    959.8-959.9

806.15 C$_5$-C$_7$ level with unspecified spinal cord injury ⬟ ⬟

  (Ex) 733.10-733.19, 733.93-733.98, 805.00-805.18, 805.8-806.19,
  806.8-806.9, 829.0-829.1, 839.00-839.18, 839.40,
  839.49-839.50, 839.59, 839.69, 839.79-839.9, 847.9,
  848.8-848.9, 879.8-879.9, 905.1, 926.11, 929.0-929.9,
  952.00-952.09, 952.8-952.9, 958.8-958.99, 959.11-959.19,
  959.8-959.9

806.16 C$_5$-C$_7$ level with complete lesion of cord ⬟ ⬟

  (Ex) 733.10-733.19, 733.93-733.98, 805.00-805.18, 805.8-806.19,
  806.8-806.9, 829.0-829.1, 839.00-839.18, 839.40,
  839.49-839.50, 839.59, 839.69, 839.79-839.9, 847.9,
  848.8-848.9, 879.8-879.9, 905.1, 926.11, 929.0-929.9,
  952.00-952.09, 952.8-952.9, 958.8-958.99, 959.11-959.19,
  959.8-959.9

806.17 C$_5$-C$_7$ level with anterior cord syndrome ⬟ ⬟

  (Ex) 733.10-733.19, 733.93-733.98, 805.00-805.18, 805.8-806.19,
  806.8-806.9, 829.0-829.1, 839.00-839.18, 839.40,
  839.49-839.50, 839.59, 839.69, 839.79-839.9, 847.9,
  848.8-848.9, 879.8-879.9, 905.1, 926.11, 929.0-929.9,
  952.00-952.09, 952.8-952.9, 958.8-958.99, 959.11-959.19,
  959.8-959.9

806.18 C$_5$-C$_7$ level with central cord syndrome ⬟ ⬟

  (Ex) 733.10-733.19, 733.93-733.98, 805.00-805.18, 805.8-806.19,
  806.8-806.9, 829.0-829.1, 839.00-839.18, 839.40,
  839.49-839.50, 839.59, 839.69, 839.79-839.9, 847.9,
  848.8-848.9, 879.8-879.9, 905.1, 926.11, 929.0-929.9,
  952.00-952.09, 952.8-952.9, 958.8-958.99, 959.11-959.19,
  959.8-959.9

806.19 C$_5$-C$_7$ level with other specified spinal cord injury ⬟ ⬟

  C$_5$-C$_7$ level with:
    incomplete spinal cord lesion NOS
    posterior cord syndrome
    (Ex) 733.10-733.19, 733.93-733.98, 805.00-805.18, 805.8-806.19,
    806.8-806.9, 829.0-829.1, 839.00-839.18, 839.40,
    839.49-839.50, 839.59, 839.69, 839.79-839.9, 847.9,
    848.8-848.9, 879.8-879.9, 905.1, 926.11, 929.0-929.9,
    952.00-952.09, 952.8-952.9, 958.8-958.99, 959.11-959.19,
    959.8-959.9

● 806.2 Dorsal [thoracic], closed

806.20 T$_1$-T$_6$ level with unspecified spinal cord injury ⬟ ⬟

  Thoracic region NOS with spinal cord injury NOS
    (Ex) 733.10-733.19, 733.93-733.98, 805.2-805.3, 805.8-805.9,
    806.20-806.39, 806.8-806.9, 829.0-829.1, 839.21,
    839.31-839.40, 839.49-839.50, 839.59, 839.69,
    839.79-839.9, 847.1, 847.9, 848.8-848.9, 879.8-879.9,
    905.1, 926.11, 929.0-929.9, 952.10-952.19, 952.8-952.9,
    958.8-958.99, 959.11-959.19, 959.8-959.9

806.21 T$_1$-T$_6$ level with complete lesion of cord ⬟ ⬟

  (Ex) 733.10-733.19, 733.93-733.98, 805.2-805.3, 805.8-805.9,
  806.20-806.39, 806.8-806.9, 829.0-829.1, 839.21,
  839.31-839.40, 839.49-839.50, 839.59, 839.69,
  839.79-839.9, 847.1, 847.9, 848.8-848.9, 879.8-879.9,
  905.1, 926.11, 929.0-929.9, 952.10-952.19, 952.8-952.9,
  958.8-958.99, 959.11-959.19, 959.8-959.9

806.22 T$_1$-T$_6$ level with anterior cord syndrome ⬟ ⬟

  (Ex) 733.10-733.19, 733.93-733.98, 805.2-805.3, 805.8-805.9,
  806.20-806.39, 806.8-806.9, 829.0-829.1, 839.21,
  839.31-839.40, 839.49-839.50, 839.59, 839.69,
  839.79-839.9, 847.1, 847.9, 848.8-848.9, 879.8-879.9,
  905.1, 926.11, 929.0-929.9, 952.10-952.19, 952.8-952.9,
  958.8-958.99, 959.11-959.19, 959.8-959.9

806.23 T$_1$-T$_6$ level with central cord syndrome ⬟ ⬟

  (Ex) 733.10-733.19, 733.93-733.98, 805.2-805.3, 805.8-805.9,
  806.20-806.39, 806.8-806.9, 829.0-829.1, 839.21,
  839.31-839.40, 839.49-839.50, 839.59, 839.69,
  839.79-839.9, 847.1, 847.9, 848.8-848.9, 879.8-879.9,
  905.1, 926.11, 929.0-929.9, 952.10-952.19, 952.8-952.9,
  958.8-958.99, 959.11-959.19, 959.8-959.9

N Newborn Age: 0   P Pediatric Age: 0–17   M Maternity Age: 12–55   A Adult Age: 15–124   ♀ Females Only   ♂ Males Only   1071
(Ex) CC Exclusions   ⬟ Complication\Comorbidity   ⬟ Major C\C   ⬟ Present on Admission Requirement   ⬟ Hospital-Acquired Condition

INJURY AND POISONING (800–999)

806.24 T₁-T₆ level with other specified spinal cord injury 🔵 🔵

T₁-T₆ level with:
    incomplete spinal cord lesion NOS
    posterior cord syndrome
(Ex:) 733.10-733.19, 733.93-733.98, 805.2-805.3, 805.8-805.9,
806.20-806.39, 806.8-806.9, 829.0-829.1, 839.21,
839.31-839.40, 839.49-839.50, 839.59, 839.69,
839.79-839.9, 847.1, 847.9, 848.8-848.9, 879.8-879.9,
905.1, 926.11, 929.0-929.9, 952.10-952.19, 952.8-952.9,
958.8-958.99, 959.11-959.19, 959.8-959.9

806.25 T₇-T₁₂ level with unspecified spinal cord injury 🔵 🔵

(Ex:) 733.10-733.19, 733.93-733.98, 805.2-805.3, 805.8-805.9,
806.20-806.39, 806.8-806.9, 829.0-829.1, 839.21,
839.31-839.40, 839.49-839.50, 839.59, 839.69,
839.79-839.9, 847.1, 847.9, 848.8-848.9, 879.8-879.9,
905.1, 926.11, 929.0-929.9, 952.10-952.19, 952.8-952.9,
958.8-958.99, 959.11-959.19, 959.8-959.9

806.26 T₇-T₁₂ level with complete lesion of cord 🔵 🔵

(Ex:) 733.10-733.19, 733.93-733.98, 805.2-805.3, 805.8-805.9,
806.20-806.39, 806.8-806.9, 829.0-829.1, 839.21,
839.31-839.40, 839.49-839.50, 839.59, 839.69,
839.79-839.9, 847.1, 847.9, 848.8-848.9, 879.8-879.9,
905.1, 926.11, 929.0-929.9, 952.10-952.19, 952.8-952.9,
958.8-958.99, 959.11-959.19, 959.8-959.9

806.27 T₇-T₁₂ level with anterior cord syndrome 🔵 🔵

(Ex:) 733.10-733.19, 733.93-733.98, 805.2-805.3, 805.8-805.9,
806.20-806.39, 806.8-806.9, 829.0-829.1, 839.21,
839.31-839.40, 839.49-839.50, 839.59, 839.69,
839.79-839.9, 847.1, 847.9, 848.8-848.9, 879.8-879.9,
905.1, 926.11, 929.0-929.9, 952.10-952.19, 952.8-952.9,
958.8-958.99, 959.11-959.19, 959.8-959.9

806.28 T₇-T₁₂ level with central cord syndrome 🔵 🔵

(Ex:) 733.10-733.19, 733.93-733.98, 805.2-805.3, 805.8-805.9,
806.20-806.39, 806.8-806.9, 829.0-829.1, 839.21,
839.31-839.40, 839.49-839.50, 839.59, 839.69,
839.79-839.9, 847.1, 847.9, 848.8-848.9, 879.8-879.9,
905.1, 926.11, 929.0-929.9, 952.10-952.19, 952.8-952.9,
958.8-958.99, 959.11-959.19, 959.8-959.9

806.29 T₇-T₁₂ level with other specified spinal cord injury 🔵 🔵

T₇-T₁₂ level with:
    incomplete spinal cord lesion NOS
    posterior cord syndrome
(Ex:) 733.10-733.19, 733.93-733.98, 805.2-805.3, 805.8-805.9,
806.20-806.39, 806.8-806.9, 829.0-829.1, 839.21,
839.31-839.40, 839.49-839.50, 839.59, 839.69,
839.79-839.9, 847.1, 847.9, 848.8-848.9, 879.8-879.9,
905.1, 926.11, 929.0-929.9, 952.10-952.19, 952.8-952.9,
958.8-958.99, 959.11-959.19, 959.8-959.9

● **806.3 Dorsal [thoracic], open**

806.30 T₁-T₆ level with unspecified spinal cord injury 🔵 🔵

(Ex:) 733.10-733.19, 733.93-733.98, 805.2-805.3, 805.8-805.9,
806.20-806.39, 806.8-806.9, 829.0-829.1, 839.21,
839.31-839.40, 839.49-839.50, 839.59, 839.69,
839.79-839.9, 847.1, 847.9, 848.8-848.9, 879.8-879.9,
905.1, 926.11, 929.0-929.9, 952.10-952.19, 952.8-952.9,
958.8-958.99, 959.11-959.19, 959.8-959.9

806.31 T₁-T₆ level with complete lesion of cord 🔵 🔵

(Ex:) 733.10-733.19, 733.93-733.98, 805.2-805.3, 805.8-805.9,
806.20-806.39, 806.8-806.9, 829.0-829.1, 839.21,
839.31-839.40, 839.49-839.50, 839.59, 839.69,
839.79-839.9, 847.1, 847.9, 848.8-848.9, 879.8-879.9,
905.1, 926.11, 929.0-929.9, 952.10-952.19, 952.8-952.9,
958.8-958.99, 959.11-959.19, 959.8-959.9

806.32 T₁-T₆ level with anterior cord syndrome 🔵 🔵

(Ex:) 733.10-733.19, 733.93-733.98, 805.2-805.3, 805.8-805.9,
806.20-806.39, 806.8-806.9, 829.0-829.1, 839.21,
839.31-839.40, 839.49-839.50, 839.59, 839.69,
839.79-839.9, 847.1, 847.9, 848.8-848.9, 879.8-879.9,
905.1, 926.11, 929.0-929.9, 952.10-952.19, 952.8-952.9,
958.8-958.99, 959.11-959.19, 959.8-959.9

806.33 T₁-T₆ level with central cord syndrome 🔵 🔵

(Ex:) 733.10-733.19, 733.93-733.98, 805.2-805.3, 805.8-805.9,
806.20-806.39, 806.8-806.9, 829.0-829.1, 839.21,
839.31-839.40, 839.49-839.50, 839.59, 839.69,
839.79-839.9, 847.1, 847.9, 848.8-848.9, 879.8-879.9,
905.1, 926.11, 929.0-929.9, 952.10-952.19, 952.8-952.9,
958.8-958.99, 959.11-959.19, 959.8-959.9

806.34 T₁-T₆ level with other specified spinal cord injury 🔵 🔵

T₁-T₆ level with:
    incomplete spinal cord lesion NOS
    posterior cord syndrome
(Ex:) 733.10-733.19, 733.93-733.98, 805.2-805.3, 805.8-805.9,
806.20-806.39, 806.8-806.9, 829.0-829.1, 839.21,
839.31-839.40, 839.49-839.50, 839.59, 839.69,
839.79-839.9, 847.1, 847.9, 848.8-848.9, 879.8-879.9,
905.1, 926.11, 929.0-929.9, 952.10-952.19, 952.8-952.9,
958.8-958.99, 959.11-959.19, 959.8-959.9

806.35 T₇-T₁₂ level with unspecified spinal cord injury 🔵 🔵

(Ex:) 733.10-733.19, 733.93-733.98, 805.2-805.3, 805.8-805.9,
806.20-806.39, 806.8-806.9, 829.0-829.1, 839.21,
839.31-839.40, 839.49-839.50, 839.59, 839.69,
839.79-839.9, 847.1, 847.9, 848.8-848.9, 879.8-879.9,
905.1, 926.11, 929.0-929.9, 952.10-952.19, 952.8-952.9,
958.8-958.99, 959.11-959.19, 959.8-959.9

806.36 T₇-T₁₂ level with complete lesion of cord 🔵 🔵

(Ex:) 733.10-733.19, 733.93-733.98, 805.2-805.3, 805.8-805.9,
806.20-806.39, 806.8-806.9, 829.0-829.1, 839.21,
839.31-839.40, 839.49-839.50, 839.59, 839.69,
839.79-839.9, 847.1, 847.9, 848.8-848.9, 879.8-879.9,
905.1, 926.11, 929.0-929.9, 952.10-952.19, 952.8-952.9,
958.8-958.99, 959.11-959.19, 959.8-959.9

806.37 T₇-T₁₂ level with anterior cord syndrome 🔵 🔵

(Ex:) 733.10-733.19, 733.93-733.98, 805.2-805.3, 805.8-805.9,
806.20-806.39, 806.8-806.9, 829.0-829.1, 839.21,
839.31-839.40, 839.49-839.50, 839.59, 839.69,
839.79-839.9, 847.1, 847.9, 848.8-848.9, 879.8-879.9,
905.1, 926.11, 929.0-929.9, 952.10-952.19, 952.8-952.9,
958.8-958.99, 959.11-959.19, 959.8-959.9

806.38 T₇-T₁₂ level with central cord syndrome 🔵 🔵

(Ex:) 733.10-733.19, 733.93-733.98, 805.2-805.3, 805.8-805.9,
806.20-806.39, 806.8-806.9, 829.0-829.1, 839.21,
839.31-839.40, 839.49-839.50, 839.59, 839.69,
839.79-839.9, 847.1, 847.9, 848.8-848.9, 879.8-879.9,
905.1, 926.11, 929.0-929.9, 952.10-952.19, 952.8-952.9,
958.8-958.99, 959.11-959.19, 959.8-959.9

806.39 T₇-T₁₂ level with other specified spinal cord injury 🔵 🔵

T₇-T₁₂ level with:
    incomplete spinal cord lesion NOS
    posterior cord syndrome
(Ex:) 733.10-733.19, 733.93-733.98, 805.2-805.3, 805.8-805.9,
806.20-806.39, 806.8-806.9, 829.0-829.1, 839.21,
839.31-839.40, 839.49-839.50, 839.59, 839.69,
839.79-839.9, 847.1, 847.9, 848.8-848.9, 879.8-879.9,
905.1, 926.11, 929.0-929.9, 952.10-952.19, 952.8-952.9,
958.8-958.99, 959.11-959.19, 959.8-959.9

◀ New   ◀▥ Revised   ~~deleted~~ Deleted   ● Unacceptable Principal Diagnosis   ● Use Additional Digit(s)

▶ Manifestation Code   **OGCR** Official Guidelines   **Coding Clinic**   Excludes   Includes   Use additional   Code first   Omit code

806.4 Lumbar, closed 🔵 🔵
    (Ex:) 733.10-733.19, 733.93-733.98, 805.4-805.5, 805.8-805.9, 806.4-806.5,
    806.8-806.9, 829.0-829.1, 839.20, 839.30, 839.40, 839.49-839.50,
    839.59, 839.69, 839.79-839.9, 847.2, 847.9, 848.8-848.9, 879.8-879.9,
    905.1, 926.11, 929.0-929.9, 952.2, 952.8-952.9, 958.8-958.99,
    959.11-959.19, 959.8-959.9

    Coding Clinic: 1999, Q4, P11-13

806.5 Lumbar, open 🔵 🔵
    (Ex:) 733.10-733.19, 733.93-733.98, 805.4-805.5, 805.8-805.9, 806.4-806.5,
    806.8-806.9, 829.0-829.1, 839.20, 839.30, 839.40, 839.49-839.50,
    839.59, 839.69, 839.79-839.9, 847.2, 847.9, 848.8-848.9, 879.8-879.9,
    905.1, 926.11, 929.0-929.9, 952.2, 952.8-952.9, 958.8-958.99,
    959.11-959.19, 959.8-959.9

● **806.6 Sacrum and coccyx, closed**

   806.60 With unspecified spinal cord injury 🔵 🔵
     (Ex:) 733.10-733.19, 733.93-733.98, 805.6-805.9, 806.60-806.9,
     829.0-829.1, 839.40-839.59, 839.69, 839.79-839.9,
     846.0-847.0, 847.3-847.9, 848.5-848.9, 879.8-879.9, 905.1,
     926.11, 929.0-929.9, 952.3-952.9, 958.8-958.99,
     959.11-959.19, 959.8-959.9

   806.61 With complete cauda equina lesion 🔵 🔵
     (Ex:) 733.10-733.19, 733.93-733.98, 805.6-805.9, 806.60-806.9,
     829.0-829.1, 839.40-839.59, 839.69, 839.79-839.9,
     846.0-847.0, 847.3-847.9, 848.5-848.9, 879.8-879.9, 905.1,
     926.11, 929.0-929.9, 952.3-952.9, 958.8-958.99,
     959.11-959.19, 959.8-959.9

   806.62 With other cauda equina injury 🔵 🔵
     (Ex:) 733.10-733.19, 733.93-733.98, 805.6-805.9, 806.60-806.9,
     829.0-829.1, 839.40-839.59, 839.69, 839.79-839.9,
     846.0-847.0, 847.3-847.9, 848.5-848.9, 879.8-879.9, 905.1,
     926.11, 929.0-929.9, 952.3-952.9, 958.8-958.99,
     959.11-959.19, 959.8-959.9

   806.69 With other spinal cord injury 🔵 🔵
     (Ex:) 733.10-733.19, 733.93-733.98, 805.6-805.9, 806.60-806.9,
     829.0-829.1, 839.40-839.59, 839.69, 839.79-839.9,
     846.0-847.0, 847.3-847.9, 848.5-848.9, 879.8-879.9, 905.1,
     926.11, 929.0-929.9, 952.3-952.9, 958.8-958.99,
     959.11-959.19, 959.8-959.9

● **806.7 Sacrum and coccyx, open**

   806.70 With unspecified spinal cord injury 🔵 🔵
     (Ex:) 733.10-733.19, 733.93-733.98, 805.6-805.9, 806.60-806.9,
     829.0-829.1, 839.40-839.59, 839.69, 839.79-839.9,
     846.0-847.0, 847.3-847.9, 848.5-848.9, 879.8-879.9, 905.1,
     926.11, 929.0-929.9, 952.3-952.9, 958.8-958.99,
     959.11-959.19, 959.8-959.9

   806.71 With complete cauda equina lesion 🔵 🔵
     (Ex:) 733.10-733.19, 733.93-733.98, 805.6-805.9, 806.60-806.9,
     829.0-829.1, 839.40-839.59, 839.69, 839.79-839.9,
     846.0-847.0, 847.3-847.9, 848.5-848.9, 879.8-879.9, 905.1,
     926.11, 929.0-929.9, 952.3-952.9, 958.8-958.99,
     959.11-959.19, 959.8-959.9

   806.72 With other cauda equina injury 🔵 🔵
     (Ex:) 733.10-733.19, 733.93-733.98, 805.6-805.9, 806.60-806.9,
     829.0-829.1, 839.40-839.59, 839.69, 839.79-839.9,
     846.0-847.0, 847.3-847.9, 848.5-848.9, 879.8-879.9, 905.1,
     926.11, 929.0-929.9, 952.3-952.9, 958.8-958.99,
     959.11-959.19, 959.8-959.9

   806.79 With other spinal cord injury 🔵 🔵
     (Ex:) 733.10-733.19, 733.93-733.98, 805.6-805.9, 806.60-806.9,
     829.0-829.1, 839.40-839.59, 839.69, 839.79-839.9,
     846.0-847.0, 847.3-847.9, 848.5-848.9, 879.8-879.9, 905.1,
     926.11, 929.0-929.9, 952.3-952.9, 958.8-958.99,
     959.11-959.19, 959.8-959.9

806.8 Unspecified, closed 🔵 🔵
    (Ex:) 733.10-733.19, 733.93-733.98, 805.00-806.9, 829.0-829.1, 839.00-839.59,
    839.69, 839.79-839.9, 846.0-847.9, 848.5-848.9, 879.8-879.9, 905.1,
    926.11, 929.0-929.9, 952.00-952.9, 958.8-958.99, 959.11-959.19,
    959.8-959.9

806.9 Unspecified, open 🔵 🔵
    (Ex:) 733.10-733.19, 733.93-733.98, 805.00-806.9, 829.0-829.1, 839.00-839.59,
    839.69, 839.79-839.9, 846.0-847.9, 848.5-848.9, 879.8-879.9, 905.1,
    926.11, 929.0-929.9, 952.00-952.9, 958.8-958.99, 959.11-959.19,
    959.8-959.9

● **807 Fracture of rib(s), sternum, larynx, and trachea**

The following fifth-digit subclassification is for use with
codes 807.0–807.1:

> 0 rib(s), unspecified
> 1 one rib
> 2 two ribs
> 3 three ribs
> 4 four ribs
> 5 five ribs
> 6 six ribs
> 7 seven ribs
> 8 eight or more ribs
> 9 multiple ribs, unspecified

● **807.0 Rib(s), closed** 🔵 🔵
   [0-9]   For codes **807.00-807.02:** (Ex:) 807.00-807.4, 819.0-819.1, 828.0-829.1,
         848.8-848.9, 879.8-879.9, 929.0-929.9, 958.8-958.99, 959.8-959.9;
       For code **807.03:** (Ex:) 807.00-807.19, 807.4, 819.0-819.1, 828.0-829.1,
         848.8-848.9, 879.8-879.9, 929.0-929.9, 958.8, 959.8-959.9;
       For codes **807.04-807.09:** (Ex:) 807.00-807.19, 807.4, 819.0-819.1,
         828.0-829.1, 848.8-848.9, 879.8-879.9, 929.0-929.9, 958.8-958.99,
         959.8-959.9

● **807.1 Rib(s), open** 🔵 🔵
   [0-9]   (Ex:) 807.00-807.19, 807.4, 819.0-819.1, 828.0-829.1, 848.8-848.9,
       879.8-879.9, 929.0-929.9, 958.8-958.99, 959.8-959.9

807.2 Sternum, closed 🔵 🔵
    (Ex:) 807.2-807.4, 829.0-829.1, 848.8-848.9, 879.8-879.9, 929.0-929.9,
    958.8-958.99, 959.8-959.9

807.3 Sternum, open 🔵 🔵
    (Ex:) 807.2-807.4, 829.0-829.1, 848.8-848.9, 879.8-879.9, 929.0-929.9,
    958.8-958.99, 959.8-959.9

807.4 Flail chest 🔵 🔵
    Unstable chest due to sternum and/or rib fracture
    (Ex:) 807.00-807.4, 829.0-829.1, 848.8-848.9, 879.8-879.9, 929.0-929.9,
    958.8-958.99, 959.8-959.9599

807.5 Larynx and trachea, closed 🔵 🔵
    Hyoid bone
    Thyroid cartilage
    Trachea
    (Ex:) 807.5-807.6, 829.0-829.1, 848.8-848.9, 879.8-879.9, 929.0-929.9,
    958.8-958.99, 959.8-959.9

807.6 Larynx and trachea, open 🔵 🔵
    (Ex:) 807.5-807.6, 829.0-829.1, 848.8-848.9, 879.8-879.9, 929.0-929.9,
    958.8-958.99, 959.8-959.9

INJURY AND POISONING (800–999)

N Newborn Age: 0   **P** Pediatric Age: 0–17   **M** Maternity Age: 12–55   **A** Adult Age: 15–124   ♀ Females Only   ♂ Males Only
(Ex:) CC Exclusions   🔵 Complication\Comorbidity   🔵 Major C\C   🔵 Present on Admission Requirement   🔵 Hospital-Acquired Condition

- **808 Fracture of pelvis**

  808.0 **Acetabulum, closed** 🅖 🅖
  > (Ex:) 733.10-733.19, 733.93-733.98, 808.0-808.1, 808.43-808.49, 808.53-809.1, 829.0-829.1, 835.00-835.13, 843.0-843.9, 846.0-846.9, 848.5-848.9, 879.8-879.9, 929.0-929.9, 958.8-958.99, 959.6, 959.8-959.9

  808.1 **Acetabulum, open** 🅖 🅖
  > (Ex:) 808.0-808.1, 808.43-808.49, 808.53-809.1, 829.0-829.1, 835.00-835.13, 843.0-843.9, 846.0-846.9, 848.5-848.9, 879.8-879.9, 929.0-929.9, 958.8-958.99, 959.6, 959.8-959.9

  808.2 **Pubis, closed** 🅖 🅖
  > (Ex:) 733.10-733.19, 733.93-733.98, 808.2-808.3, 808.43-808.49, 808.53-809.1, 829.0-829.1, 835.00-835.13, 843.0-843.9, 846.0-846.9, 848.5-848.9, 879.8-879.9, 929.0-929.9, 958.8-958.99, 959.6, 959.8-959.9
  >
  > **Coding Clinic: 2008, Q1, P9-10**

  808.3 **Pubis, open** 🅖 🅖
  > (Ex:) 733.10-733.19, 733.93-733.98, 808.2-808.3, 808.43-808.49, 808.53-809.1, 829.0-829.1, 835.00-835.13, 843.0-843.9, 846.0-846.9, 848.5-848.9, 879.8-879.9, 929.0-929.9, 958.8-958.99, 959.6, 959.8-959.9

- 808.4 **Other specified part, closed**

  808.41 **Ilium** 🅖 🅖
  > (Ex:) 733.10, 733.19, 808.0-809.1, 829.0-829.1, 835.00-835.13, 843.0-843.9, 846.0-846.9, 848.5-848.9, 879.8-879.9, 929.0-929.9, 958.8, 958.99, 959.6, 959.8-959.9

  808.42 **Ischium** 🅖 🅖
  > (Ex:) 808.42

  808.43 **Multiple pelvic fractures with disruption of pelvic circle** 🅖 🅖
  > (Ex:) 733.10-733.19, 733.93-733.98, 808.0-809.1, 829.0-829.1, 835.00-835.13, 843.0-843.9, 846.0-846.9, 848.5-848.9, 879.8-879.9, 929.0-929.9, 958.8-958.99, 959.6, 959.8-959.9
  >
  > **Coding Clinic: 2008, Q1, P9-10**

  808.49 **Other** 🅖 🅖
  > Innominate bone
  > Pelvic rim
  > (Ex:) 733.10-733.19, 733.93-733.98, 808.0-809.1, 829.0-829.1, 835.00-835.13, 843.0-843.9, 846.0-846.9, 848.5-848.9, 879.8-879.9, 929.0-929.9, 958.8-958.99, 959.6, 959.8-959.9

- 808.5 **Other specified part, open**

  808.51 **Ilium** 🅖 🅖
  > (Ex:) 733.10-733.19, 733.93-733.98, 808.41, 808.43-808.51, 808.53-809.1 829.0-829.1, 835.00-835.13, 843.0-843.9, 846.0-846.9, 848.5-848.9, 879.8-879.9, 929.0-929.9, 958.8-958.99, 959.6, 959.8-959.9

  808.52 **Ischium** 🅖 🅖
  > (Ex:) 733.10-733.19, 733.93-733.98, 808.42-808.49, 808.52-809.1, 829.0-829.1, 835.00-835.13, 843.0-843.9, 846.0-846.9, 848.5-848.9, 879.8-879.9, 929.0-929.9, 958.8-958.99, 959.6, 959.8-959.9

  808.53 **Multiple pelvic fractures with disruption of pelvic circle** 🅖 🅖
  > (Ex:) 733.10-733.19, 733.93-733.98, 808.0-809.1, 829.0-829.1, 835.00-835.13, 843.0-843.9, 846.0-846.9, 848.5-848.9, 879.8-879.9, 929.0-929.9, 958.8-958.99, 959.6, 959.8-959.9

  808.59 **Other** 🅖 🅖
  > (Ex:) 733.10-733.19, 733.93-733.98, 808.0-809.1, 829.0-829.1, 835.00-835.13, 843.0-843.9, 846.0-846.9, 848.5-848.9, 879.8-879.9, 929.0-929.9, 958.8-958.99, 959.6, 959.8-959.9

  808.8 **Unspecified, closed** 🅖 🅖
  > (Ex:) 733.10-733.19, 733.93-733.98, 808.0-809.1, 829.0-829.1, 835.00-835.13, 843.0-843.9, 846.0-846.9, 848.5-848.9, 879.8-879.9, 929.0-929.9, 958.8-958.99, 959.6, 959.8-959.9

  808.9 **Unspecified, open** 🅖 🅖
  > (Ex:) 733.10-733.19, 733.93-733.98, 808.0-809.1, 829.0-829.1, 835.00-835.13, 843.0-843.9, 846.0-846.9, 848.5-848.9, 879.8-879.9, 929.0-929.9, 958.8-958.99, 959.6, 959.8-959.9

- **809 Ill-defined fractures of bones of trunk**

Includes	bones of trunk with other bones except those of skull and face
	multiple bones of trunk

Excludes	*multiple fractures of:*
	pelvic bones alone (808.0–808.9)
	ribs alone (807.0–807.1, 807.4)
	ribs or sternum with limb bones (819.0–819.1, 828.0–828.1)
	skull or face with other bones (804.0–804.9)

  809.0 **Fracture of bones of trunk, closed** 🅖 🅖
  > (Ex:) 733.10, 733.19, 808.0-809.1, 829.0-829.1, 835.00-835.13, 843.0-843.9, 846.0-846.9, 848.5-848.9, 879.8-879.9, 929.0-929.9, 958.8, 958.99, 959.6, 959.8-959.9

  809.1 **Fracture of bones of trunk, open** 🅖 🅖
  > (Ex:) 733.10, 733.19, 808.0-809.1, 829.0-829.1, 835.00-835.13, 843.0-843.9, 846.0-846.9, 848.5-848.9, 879.8-879.9, 929.0-929.9, 958.8, 958.99, 959.6, 959.8-959.9

FRACTURE OF UPPER LIMB (810–819)

- **810 Fracture of clavicle**

Includes	collar bone
	interligamentous part of clavicle

  The following fifth-digit subclassification is for use with category 810:

  > 0 **unspecified part**
  >   Clavicle NOS
  > 1 **sternal end of clavicle**
  > 2 **shaft of clavicle**
  > 3 **acromial end of clavicle**

- 810.0 **Closed** 🅖
  [0-3]

- 810.1 **Open** 🅖 🅖
  [0-3]   (Ex:) 810.00-810.13, 818.0-819.1

- **811 Fracture of scapula**

Includes	shoulder blade

  The following fifth-digit subclassification is for use with category 811:

  > 0 **unspecified part**
  > 1 **acromial process**
  >   Acromion (process)
  > 2 **coracoid process**
  > 3 **glenoid cavity and neck of scapula**
  > 9 **other**

- 811.0 **Closed** 🅖
  [0-3,9]

- 811.1 **Open** 🅖 🅖
  [0-3,9]   (Ex:) 811.00-811.19, 818.0-819.1

● **812 Fracture of humerus**
  ● **812.0 Upper end, closed**
     812.00 Upper end, unspecified part
       Proximal end
       Shoulder
       (Ex) 812.00-812.59, 819.0-819.1

     812.01 Surgical neck
       Neck of humerus NOS
       (Ex) 812.00-812.59, 819.0-819.1

     812.02 Anatomical neck
       (Ex) 812.00-812.59, 819.0-819.1

     812.03 Greater tuberosity
       (Ex) 812.00-812.59, 819.0-819.1

     812.09 Other
       Head
       Upper epiphysis
       (Ex) 812.00-812.59, 819.0-819.1

  ● **812.1 Upper end, open**
     812.10 Upper end, unspecified part
       (Ex) 812.10-812.59, 818.0-819.1

     812.11 Surgical neck
       (Ex) 812.10-812.59, 818.0-819.1

     812.12 Anatomical neck
       (Ex) 812.10-812.59, 818.0-819.1

     812.13 Greater tuberosity
       (Ex) 812.10-812.59, 818.0-819.1

     812.19 Other
       (Ex) 812.10-812.59, 818.0-819.1

  ● **812.2 Shaft or unspecified part, closed**
     812.20 Unspecified part of humerus
       Humerus NOS
       Upper arm NOS
       (Ex) 812.10-812.59, 818.0-819.1

     812.21 Shaft of humerus
       (Ex) 812.21
       Coding Clinic: 2005, Q4, P127-129; 1999, Q3, P14-15

  ● **812.3 Shaft or unspecified part, open**
     812.30 Unspecified part of humerus
       (Ex) 812.10-812.59, 818.0-819.1

     812.31 Shaft of humerus
       (Ex) 812.10-812.59, 818.0-819.1

  ● **812.4 Lower end, closed**
     Distal end of humerus
     Elbow
     812.40 Lower end, unspecified part
       (Ex) 812.00-812.59, 819.0-819.1

     812.41 Supracondylar fracture of humerus
       (Ex) 812.00-812.59, 819.0-819.1

     812.42 Lateral condyle
       External condyle
       (Ex) 812.00-812.59, 819.0-819.1

     812.43 Medial condyle
       Internal epicondyle
       (Ex) 812.00-812.59, 819.0-819.1

     812.44 Condyle(s), unspecified
       Articular process NOS
       Lower epiphysis
       (Ex) 812.00-812.59, 819.0-819.1

     812.49 Other
       Multiple fractures of lower end
       Trochlea
       (Ex) 812.00-812.59, 819.0-819.1

● **812.5 Lower end, open**
     812.50 Lower end, unspecified part
       (Ex) 812.00-812.59, 819.0-819.1

     812.51 Supracondylar fracture of humerus
       (Ex) 812.10-812.59, 818.0-819.1

     812.52 Lateral condyle
       (Ex) 812.10-812.59, 818.0-819.1

     812.53 Medial condyle
       (Ex) 812.10-812.59, 818.0-819.1

     812.54 Condyle(s), unspecified
       (Ex) 812.10-812.59, 818.0-819.1

     812.59 Other
       (Ex) 812.10-812.59, 818.0-819.1

● **813 Fracture of radius and ulna**
  ● **813.0 Upper end, closed**
     Proximal end
     813.00 Upper end of forearm, unspecified

     813.01 Olecranon process of ulna

     813.02 Coronoid process of ulna

     813.03 Monteggia's fracture

     813.04 Other and unspecified fractures of proximal end of ulna (alone)
       Multiple fractures of ulna, upper end

     813.05 Head of radius

     813.06 Neck of radius

     813.07 Other and unspecified fractures of proximal end of radius (alone)
       Multiple fractures of radius, upper end

     813.08 Radius with ulna, upper end [any part]

  ● **813.1 Upper end, open**
     813.10 Upper end of forearm, unspecified
       (Ex) 813.10-813.44, 813.50-813.93, 818.0-819.1

     813.11 Olecranon process of ulna
       (Ex) 813.10-813.40, 813.42-813.44, 813.50-813.93, 818.0-819.1

     813.12 Coronoid process of ulna
       (Ex) 813.10-813.44, 813.50-813.93, 818.0-819.1

     813.13 Monteggia's fracture
       (Ex) 813.10-813.44, 813.50-813.93, 818.0-819.1

     813.14 Other and unspecified fractures of proximal end of ulna (alone)
       (Ex) 813.10-813.44, 813.50-813.93, 818.0-819.1

     813.15 Head of radius
       (Ex) 813.10-813.44, 813.50-813.93, 818.0-819.1

     813.16 Neck of radius
       (Ex) 813.10-813.44, 813.50-813.93, 818.0-819.1

     813.17 Other and unspecified fractures of proximal end of radius (alone)
       (Ex) 813.10-813.44, 813.50-813.93, 818.0-819.1

     813.18 Radius with ulna, upper end [any part]
       (Ex) 813.10-813.44, 813.50-813.93, 818.0-819.1

  ● **813.2 Shaft, closed**
     813.20 Shaft, unspecified
       (Ex) 813.00-813.93, 819.0-819.1

     813.21 Radius (alone)
       (Ex) 813.00-813.93, 819.0-819.1

     813.22 Ulna (alone)
       (Ex) 813.00-813.93, 819.0-819.1

     813.23 Radius with ulna
       (Ex) 813.00-813.93, 819.0-819.1

INJURY AND POISONING (800–999)

● 813.3   **Shaft, open**

    813.30   **Shaft, unspecified**🔍🔍
       Ⓔ 813.10-813.44, 813.50-813.93, 818.0-819.1

    813.31   **Radius (alone)**🔍🔍
       Ⓔ 813.10-813.44, 813.50-813.93, 818.0-819.1

    813.32   **Ulna (alone)**🔍🔍
       Ⓔ 813.10-813.44, 813.50-813.93, 818.0-819.1

    813.33   **Radius with ulna**🔍🔍
       Ⓔ 813.10-813.44, 813.50-813.93, 818.0-819.1

● 813.4   **Lower end, closed**
     Distal end

    813.40   **Lower end of forearm, unspecified**🔍🔍
       Ⓔ 813.00-813.93, 819.0-819.1

    813.41   **Colles' fracture**🔍🔍
       Smith's fracture
       Ⓔ 813.00-813.93, 819.0-819.1

    813.42   **Other fractures of distal end of radius (alone)**🔍🔍
       Dupuytren's fracture, radius
       Radius, lower end
       Ⓔ 813.00-813.93, 819.0-819.1

    813.43   **Distal end of ulna (alone)**🔍🔍
       Ulna: Ulna:
       head   lower epiphysis
       lower end   styloid process
       Ⓔ 813.00-813.93, 819.0-819.1

    813.44   **Radius with ulna, lower end**🔍🔍
       Ⓔ 813.00-813.93, 819.0-819.1
       Coding Clinic: 2007, Q1, P3-8

    813.45   **Torus fracture of radius (alone)**🔍🔍 ⬅
       Excludes   torus fracture of radius and ulna (813.47) ◀
       Ⓔ 813.00-813.93, 819.0-819.1
       Coding Clinic: 2002, Q4, P70-71

    813.46   **Torus fracture of ulna (alone)**🔍🔍 ◀
       Excludes   torus fracture of radius and ulna (813.47) ◀

    813.47   **Torus fracture of radius and ulna**🔍🔍 ◀

● 813.5   **Lower end, open**

    813.50   **Lower end of forearm, unspecified**🔍🔍
       Ⓔ 813.10-813.44, 813.50-813.93, 818.0-819.1

    813.51   **Colles' fracture**🔍🔍
       Ⓔ 813.10-813.44, 813.50-813.93, 818.0-819.1

    813.52   **Other fractures of distal end of radius (alone)**🔍🔍
       Ⓔ 813.10-813.44, 813.50-813.93, 818.0-819.1

    813.53   **Distal end of ulna (alone)**🔍🔍
       Ⓔ 813.10-813.44, 813.50-813.93, 818.0-819.1

    813.54   **Radius with ulna, lower end**🔍🔍
       Ⓔ 813.10-813.44, 813.50-813.93, 818.0-819.1

● 813.8   **Unspecified part, closed**

    813.80   **Forearm, unspecified**🔍🔍
       Ⓔ 813.00-813.93, 819.0-819.1

    813.81   **Radius (alone)**🔍
       Coding Clinic: 1998, Q2, P19

    813.82   **Ulna (alone)**🔍🔍
       Ⓔ 813.00-813.93, 819.0-819.1

    813.83   **Radius with ulna**🔍🔍
       Ⓔ 813.00-813.93, 819.0-819.1

● 813.9   **Unspecified part, open**

    813.90   **Forearm, unspecified**🔍🔍
       Ⓔ 813.10-813.44, 813.50-813.93, 818.0-819.1

    813.91   **Radius (alone)**🔍🔍
       Ⓔ 813.10-813.44, 813.50-813.93, 818.0-819.1

    813.92   **Ulna (alone)**🔍🔍
       Ⓔ 813.10-813.44, 813.50-813.93, 818.0-819.1

    813.93   **Radius with ulna**🔍🔍
       Ⓔ 813.10-813.44, 813.50-813.93, 818.0-819.1

● 814   **Fracture of carpal bone(s)**

    The following fifth-digit subclassification is for use with category 814:

> 0   carpal bone, unspecified
>   Wrist NOS
> 1   navicular [scaphoid] of wrist
> 2   lunate [semilunar] bone of wrist
> 3   triquetral [cuneiform] bone of wrist
> 4   pisiform
> 5   trapezium bone [larger multangular]
> 6   trapezoid bone [smaller multangular]
> 7   capitate bone [os magnum]
> 8   hamate [unciform] bone
> 9   other

● 814.0   **Closed**🔍
    [0-9]

● 814.1   **Open**🔍🔍
    [0-9]   Ⓔ 814.00-814.19, 819.0-819.1

● 815   **Fracture of metacarpal bone(s)**

    Includes   hand [except finger]
                metacarpus

    The following fifth-digit subclassification is for use with category 815:

> 0   metacarpal bone(s), site unspecified
> 1   base of thumb [first] metacarpal
>   Bennett's fracture
> 2   base of other metacarpal bone(s)
> 3   shaft of metacarpal bone(s)
> 4   neck of metacarpal bone(s)
> 9   multiple sites of metacarpus

● 815.0   **Closed**🔍
    [0-4,9]   **Coding Clinic: 1994, Q2, P6**

● 815.1   **Open**🔍🔍
    [0-4,9]   Ⓔ 815.00-815.19, 817.0-817.1

● 816   **Fracture of one or more phalanges of hand**

    Includes   finger(s)
                thumb

    The following fifth-digit subclassification is for use with category 816:

> 0   phalanx or phalanges, unspecified
> 1   middle or proximal phalanx or phalanges
> 2   distal phalanx or phalanges
> 3   multiple sites

● 816.0   **Closed**🔍
    [0-3]

● 816.1   **Open**🔍🔍
    [0-3]   For codes **816.10-816.12**: Ⓔ 816.00-817.1;
              For code **816.13**: Ⓔ 816.00-816.13, 818.0-819.1
              Coding Clinic: 2003, Q4, P76-78

INJURY AND POISONING (800–999)

◀ New   ⬅ Revised   ~~deleted~~ Deleted   ● Unacceptable Principal Diagnosis   ● Use Additional Digit(s)

▶ Manifestation Code   **OGCR** Official Guidelines   **Coding Clinic**   Excludes   Includes   Use additional   Code first   Omit code

● **817   Multiple fractures of hand bones**

> **Includes**   metacarpal bone(s) with phalanx or phalanges of same hand

817.0   Closed 🔩

817.1   Open 🔩 🔩
> (Ex:) 814.00-819.1

● **818   Ill-defined fractures of upper limb**

> **Includes**   arm NOS
> multiple bones of same upper limb

> **Excludes**   *multiple fractures of:*
> *metacarpal bone(s) with phalanx or phalanges*
> *(817.0–817.1)*
> *phalanges of hand alone (816.0–816.1)*
> *radius with ulna (813.0–813.9)*

818.0   Closed 🔩

818.1   Open 🔩 🔩
> (Ex:) 812.00-813.44, 813.50-819.1

OGCR   Section I.C.17.b.3
Multiple fracture category 819 classifies bilateral fractures of both upper limbs, but without any detail at the fourth-digit level other than open and closed type of fractures.

● **819   Multiple fractures involving both upper limbs, and upper limb with rib(s) and sternum**

> **Includes**   arm(s) with rib(s) or sternum
> both arms [any bones]

819.0   Closed 🔩 🔩
> (Ex:) 807.00-807.4, 812.00-813.44, 813.50-819.1

819.1   Open 🔩 🔩
> (Ex:) 807.00-807.4, 812.00-813.44, 813.50-819.1

FRACTURE OF LOWER LIMB (820–829)

● **820   Fracture of neck of femur**

● **820.0   Transcervical fracture, closed**

820.00   Intracapsular section, unspecified 🔩 🔩
> (Ex:) 733.10-733.19, 733.93-733.98, 820.00-821.39, 827.0-829.1,
> 843.0-843.9, 848.8-848.9, 879.8-879.9, 929.0-929.9,
> 958.8-958.99, 959.6, 959.8-959.9

820.01   Epiphysis (separation) (upper) 🔩 🔩
Transepiphyseal
Fracture and separation across growth plate
> (Ex:) 733.10-733.19, 733.93-733.98, 820.00-821.39, 827.0-829.1,
> 843.0-843.9, 848.8-848.9, 879.8-879.9, 929.0-929.9,
> 958.8-958.99, 959.6, 959.8-959.9

820.02   Midcervical section 🔩 🔩
Transcervical NOS
> (Ex:) 733.10-733.19, 733.93-733.98, 820.00-821.39, 827.0-829.1,
> 843.0-843.9, 848.8-848.9, 879.8-879.9, 929.0-929.9,
> 958.8-958.99, 959.6, 959.8-959.9

Coding Clinic: 2003, Q3, P12-13

820.03   Base of neck 🔩 🔩
Cervicotrochanteric section
> (Ex:) 733.10-733.19, 733.93-733.98, 820.00-821.39, 827.0-829.1,
> 843.0-843.9, 848.8-848.9, 879.8-879.9, 929.0-929.9,
> 958.8-958.99, 959.6, 959.8-959.9

820.09   Other 🔩 🔩
Head of femur
Subcapital
> (Ex:) 733.10-733.19, 733.93-733.98, 820.00-821.39, 827.0-829.1,
> 843.0-843.9, 848.8-848.9, 879.8-879.9, 929.0-929.9,
> 958.8-958.99, 959.6, 959.8-959.9

● **820.1   Transcervical fracture, open**

820.10   Intracapsular section, unspecified 🔩 🔩
> (Ex:) 733.10-733.19, 733.93-733.98, 820.00-821.39, 827.0-829.1,
> 843.0-843.9, 848.8-848.9, 879.8-879.9, 929.0-929.9,
> 958.8-958.99, 959.6, 959.8-959.9

820.11   Epiphysis (separation) (upper) 🔩 🔩
> (Ex:) 733.10-733.19, 733.93-733.98, 820.00-821.39, 827.0-829.1,
> 843.0-843.9, 848.8-848.9, 879.8-879.9, 929.0-929.9,
> 958.8-958.99, 959.6, 959.8-959.9

820.12   Midcervical section 🔩 🔩
> (Ex:) 733.10-733.19, 733.93-733.98, 820.00-821.39, 827.0-829.1,
> 843.0-843.9, 848.8-848.9, 879.8-879.9, 929.0-929.9,
> 958.8-958.99, 959.6, 959.8-959.9

820.13   Base of neck 🔩 🔩
> (Ex:) 733.10-733.19, 733.93-733.98, 820.00-821.39, 827.0-829.1,
> 843.0-843.9, 848.8-848.9, 879.8-879.9, 929.0-929.9,
> 958.8-958.99, 959.6, 959.8-959.9

820.19   Other 🔩 🔩
> (Ex:) 733.10-733.19, 733.93-733.98, 820.00-821.39, 827.0-829.1,
> 843.0-843.9, 848.8-848.9, 879.8-879.9, 929.0-929.9,
> 958.8-958.99, 959.6, 959.8-959.9

● **820.2   Pertrochanteric fracture, closed**

820.20   Trochanteric section, unspecified 🔩 🔩
Trochanter:
   NOS
   greater
   lesser
> (Ex:) 733.10-733.19, 733.93-733.98, 820.00-821.39, 827.0-829.1,
> 843.0-843.9, 848.8-848.9, 879.8-879.9, 929.0-929.9,
> 958.8-958.99, 959.6, 959.8-959.9

820.21   Intertrochanteric section 🔩 🔩
> (Ex:) 733.10-733.19, 733.93-733.98, 820.00-821.39, 827.0-829.1,
> 843.0-843.9, 848.8-848.9, 879.8-879.9, 929.0-929.9,
> 958.8-958.99, 959.6, 959.8-959.9

Coding Clinic: 1994, Q2, P6; 1984, May-June, P11

820.22   Subtrochanteric section 🔩 🔩
> (Ex:) 733.10-733.19, 733.93-733.98, 820.00-821.39, 827.0-829.1,
> 843.0-843.9, 848.8-848.9, 879.8-879.9, 929.0-929.9,
> 958.8-958.99, 959.6, 959.8-959.9

● **820.3   Pertrochanteric fracture, open**

820.30   Trochanteric section, unspecified 🔩 🔩
> (Ex:) 733.10-733.19, 733.93-733.98, 820.00-821.39, 827.0-829.1,
> 843.0-843.9, 848.8-848.9, 879.8-879.9, 929.0-929.9,
> 958.8-958.99, 959.6, 959.8-959.9

820.31   Intertrochanteric section 🔩 🔩
> (Ex:) 733.10-733.19, 733.93-733.98, 820.00-821.39, 827.0-829.1,
> 843.0-843.9, 848.8-848.9, 879.8-879.9, 929.0-929.9,
> 958.8-958.99, 959.6, 959.8-959.9

820.32   Subtrochanteric section 🔩 🔩
> (Ex:) 733.10-733.19, 733.93-733.98, 820.00-821.39, 827.0-829.1,
> 843.0-843.9, 848.8-848.9, 879.8-879.9, 929.0-929.9,
> 958.8-958.99, 959.6, 959.8-959.9

820.8   Unspecified part of neck of femur, closed 🔩 🔩
Hip NOS
Neck of femur NOS
> (Ex:) 733.10-733.19, 733.93-733.98, 820.00-821.39, 827.0-829.1, 843.0-843.9,
> 848.8-848.9, 879.8-879.9, 929.0-929.9, 958.8-958.99, 959.6,
> 959.8-959.9

Coding Clinic: 1994, Q2, P9; 1985, Nov-Dec, P16

820.9   Unspecified part of neck of femur, open 🔩 🔩
> (Ex:) 733.10-733.19, 733.93-733.98, 820.00-821.39, 827.0-829.1, 843.0-843.9,
> 848.8-848.9, 879.8-879.9, 929.0-929.9, 958.8-958.99, 959.6,
> 959.8-959.9

N   Newborn Age: 0   **P**   Pediatric Age: 0–17   **M**   Maternity Age: 12–55   **A**   Adult Age: 15–124   ♀ Females Only   ♂ Males Only   **1077**
(Ex:) CC Exclusions   🔩 Complication\Comorbidity   🔩 Major C\C   🔩 Present on Admission Requirement   🔩 Hospital-Acquired Condition

INJURY AND POISONING (800–999)

● **821 Fracture of other and unspecified parts of femur**

● **821.0 Shaft or unspecified part, closed**

821.00 Unspecified part of femur 🦕 🦕

Thigh   Upper leg

Excludes	*hip NOS (820.8)*

(Ex:) 733.10-733.19, 733.93-733.98, 820.00-821.39, 827.0-829.1, 843.0-843.9, 848.8-848.9, 879.8-879.9, 929.0-929.9, 958.8-958.99, 959.6, 959.8-959.9

821.01 Shaft 🦕 🦕

(Ex:) 733.10-733.19, 733.93-733.98, 820.00-821.39, 827.0-829.1, 843.0-843.9, 848.8-848.9, 879.8-879.9, 929.0-929.9, 958.8-958.99, 959.6, 959.8-959.9

Coding Clinic: 2007, Q1, P3-8; 1999, Q1, P5

● **821.1 Shaft or unspecified part, open**

821.10 Unspecified part of femur 🦕 🦕

(Ex:) 733.10-733.19, 733.93-733.98, 820.00-821.39, 827.0-829.1, 843.0-843.9, 848.8-848.9, 879.8-879.9, 929.0-929.9, 958.8-958.99, 959.6, 959.8-959.9

821.11 Shaft 🦕 🦕

(Ex:) 733.10-733.19, 733.93-733.98, 820.00-821.39, 827.0-829.1, 843.0-843.9, 848.8-848.9, 879.8-879.9, 929.0-929.9, 958.8-958.99, 959.6, 959.8-959.9

● **821.2 Lower end, closed**

Distal end

821.20 Lower end, unspecified part 🦕 🦕

(Ex:) 733.10, 733.14-733.15, 733.19, 820.00-821.39, 827.0-829.1, 843.0-843.9, 848.8-848.9, 879.8-879.9, 929.0-929.9, 958.8, 958.99, 959.6, 959.8-959.9

821.21 Condyle, femoral 🦕 🦕

(Ex:) 733.10, 733.14-733.15, 733.19, 820.00-821.39, 827.0-829.1, 843.0-843.9, 848.8-848.9, 879.8-879.9, 929.0-929.9, 958.8, 958.99, 959.6, 959.8-959.9

821.22 Epiphysis, lower (separation) 🦕 🦕

(Ex:) 733.10, 733.14-733.15, 733.19, 820.00-821.39, 827.0-829.1, 843.0-843.9, 848.8-848.9, 879.8-879.9, 929.0-929.9, 958.8, 958.99, 959.6, 959.8-959.9

821.23 Supracondylar fracture of femur 🦕 🦕

(Ex:) 733.10, 733.14-733.15, 733.19, 820.00-821.39, 827.0-829.1, 843.0-843.9, 848.8-848.9, 879.8-879.9, 929.0-929.9, 958.8, 958.99, 959.6, 959.8-959.9

821.29 Other 🦕 🦕

Multiple fractures of lower end

(Ex:) 733.10, 733.14-733.15, 733.19, 820.00-821.39, 827.0-829.1, 843.0-843.9, 848.8-848.9, 879.8-879.9, 929.0-929.9, 958.8, 958.99, 959.6, 959.8-959.9

● **821.3 Lower end, open**

821.30 Lower end, unspecified part 🦕 🦕

(Ex:) 733.10, 733.14-733.15, 733.19, 820.00-821.39, 827.0-829.1, 843.0-843.9, 848.8-848.9, 879.8-879.9, 929.0-929.9, 958.8, 958.99, 959.6, 959.8-959.9

821.31 Condyle, femoral 🦕 🦕

(Ex:) 733.10, 733.14-733.15, 733.19, 820.00-821.39, 827.0-829.1, 843.0-843.9, 848.8-848.9, 879.8-879.9, 929.0-929.9, 958.8, 958.99, 959.6, 959.8-959.9

821.32 Epiphysis, lower (separation) 🦕 🦕

(Ex:) 733.10, 733.14-733.15, 733.19, 820.00-821.39, 827.0-829.1, 843.0-843.9, 848.8-848.9, 879.8-879.9, 929.0-929.9, 958.8, 958.99, 959.6, 959.8-959.9

821.33 Supracondylar fracture of femur 🦕 🦕

(Ex:) 733.10, 733.14-733.15, 733.19, 820.00-821.39, 827.0-829.1, 843.0-843.9, 848.8-848.9, 879.8-879.9, 929.0-929.9, 958.8, 958.99, 959.6, 959.8-959.9

821.39 Other 🦕 🦕

(Ex:) 733.10, 733.14-733.15, 733.19, 821.39-822.1, 827.0-829.1, 843.0-843.9, 848.8-848.9, 879.8-879.9, 929.0-929.9, 958.8, 958.99, 959.6, 959.8-959.9

● **822 Fracture of patella**

822.0 Closed 🦕 🦕

(Ex:) 822.0-822.1, 828.0-828.1

822.1 Open 🦕 🦕

(Ex:) 733.10, 733.19, 822.1-823.32, 823.80-823.92, 827.0-829.1, 843.0-843.9, 848.8-848.9, 879.8-879.9, 929.0-929.9, 958.8, 958.99, 959.6, 959.8-959.9

● **823 Fracture of tibia and fibula**

Excludes	*Dupuytren's fracture (824.4–824.5)*
	ankle (824.4–824.5)
	radius (813.42, 813.52)
	Pott's fracture (824.4–824.5)
	that involving ankle (824.0–824.9)

The following fifth-digit subclassification is for use with category 823:

> **0 tibia alone**
> **1 fibula alone**
> **2 fibula with tibia**

● **823.0 Upper end, closed 0,2** 🦕 🦕

[0-2]   Head

Proximal end

Tibia:

    condyles

    tuberosity

For codes **823.00 and 823.02:** (Ex:) 733.10, 733.16-733.19, 823.00-823.32, 823.80-823.92, 827.0-829.1, 843.0-843.9, 848.8-848.9, 879.8-879.9, 929.0-929.9, 958.8, 958.99, 959.6, 959.8-959.9

● **823.1 Upper end, open** 🦕 🦕

[0-2]   (Ex:) 733.10, 733.16-733.19, 823.00-823.32, 823.80-823.92, 827.0-829.1, 843.0-843.9, 848.8-848.9, 879.8-879.9, 929.0-929.9, 958.8, 958.99, 959.6, 959.8-959.9

● **823.2 Shaft, closed 0,2** 🦕 🦕

[0-2]   For codes **823.20 and 823.22:** (Ex:) 733.10, 733.16-733.19, 823.00-823.32, 823.80-823.92, 827.0-829.1, 843.0-843.9, 848.8-848.9, 879.8-879.9, 929.0-929.9, 958.8, 958.99, 959.6, 959.8-959.9

● **823.3 Shaft, open** 🦕 🦕

[0-2]   (Ex:) 733.10, 733.16-733.19, 823.00-823.32, 823.80-823.92, 827.0-829.1, 843.0-843.9, 848.8-848.9, 879.8-879.9, 929.0-929.9, 958.8, 958.99, 959.6, 959.8-959.9

● **823.4 Torus fracture 0,2** 🦕 🦕

[0-2]   For code **823.40 and 823.42:** (Ex:) 823.00-823.92

Coding Clinic: 2002, Q4, P70-71

● **823.8 Unspecified part, closed 0,2** 🦕 🦕

[0-2]   Lower leg NOS

For code **823.80:** (Ex:) 823.00-823.92;

For code **823.82:** (Ex:) 733.10, 733.16-733.19, 823.00-823.32, 823.80-823.92, 827.0-829.1, 843.0-843.9, 848.8-848.9, 879.8-879.9, 929.0-929.9, 958.8, 958.99, 959.6, 959.8-959.9

Coding Clinic: 1997, Q1, P8

● **823.9 Unspecified part, open** 🦕 🦕

[0-2]   (Ex:) 733.10, 733.16-733.19, 823.00-823.32, 823.80-823.92, 827.0-829.1, 843.0-843.9, 848.8-848.9, 879.8-879.9, 929.0-929.9, 958.8, 958.99, 959.6, 959.8-959.9

◀ New   ◀|||| Revised   ~~deleted~~ Deleted   ● Unacceptable Principal Diagnosis   ● Use Additional Digit(s)

▶ Manifestation Code   **OGCR** Official Guidelines   **Coding Clinic**   Excludes   Includes   Use additional   Code first   Omit code

INJURY AND POISONING (800–999)

● **824 Fracture of ankle**

824.0 Medial malleolus, closed] 🕮
   Tibia involving:
     ankle
     malleolus
   Coding Clinic: 2004, Q1, P9

824.1 Medial malleolus, open 🕮 🕮
   (Ex:) 733.10, 733.16-733.19, 824.1-824.9, 827.0-829.1, 843.0-843.9,
     848.8-848.9, 879.8-879.9, 929.0-929.9, 958.8, 958.99, 959.6,
     959.8-959.9

824.2 Lateral malleolus, closed 🕮
   Fibula involving:
     ankle
     malleolus
   Coding Clinic: 2002, Q2, P3

824.3 Lateral malleolus, open 🕮 🕮
   (Ex:) 733.10, 733.16-733.19, 824.1-824.9, 827.0-829.1, 843.0-843.9,
     848.8-848.9, 879.8-879.9, 929.0-929.9, 958.8, 958.99, 959.6,
     959.8-959.9

824.4 Bimalleolar, closed 🕮
   Dupuytren's fracture, fibula
   Pott's fracture

824.5 Bimalleolar, open 🕮 🕮
   (Ex:) 733.10, 733.16-733.19, 824.1-824.9, 827.0-829.1, 843.0-843.9,
     848.8-848.9, 879.8-879.9, 929.0-929.9, 958.8, 958.99, 959.6,
     959.8-959.9

824.6 Trimalleolar, closed 🕮
   Lateral and medial malleolus with anterior or
     posterior lip of tibia

824.7 Trimalleolar, open 🕮 🕮
   (Ex:) 733.10, 733.16-733.19, 824.1-824.9, 827.0-829.1, 843.0-843.9,
     848.8-848.9, 879.8-879.9, 929.0-929.9, 958.8, 958.99, 959.6,
     959.8-959.9

824.8 Unspecified, closed 🕮
   Ankle NOS
   Coding Clinic: 2000, Q3, P12; 1994, Q2, P7

824.9 Unspecified, open 🕮 🕮
   (Ex:) 733.10, 733.16-733.19, 824.1-824.9, 827.0-829.1, 843.0-843.9,
     848.8-848.9, 879.8-879.9, 929.0-929.9, 958.8, 958.99, 959.6,
     959.8-959.9

● **825 Fracture of one or more tarsal and metatarsal bones**

825.0 Fracture of calcaneus, closed 🕮
   Heel bone
   Os calcis

825.1 Fracture of calcaneus, open 🕮 🕮
   (Ex:) 733.10, 733.16-733.19, 825.1-825.39, 827.0-829.1, 843.0-843.9,
     848.8-848.9, 879.8-879.9, 929.0-929.9, 958.8, 958.99, 959.6,
     959.8-959.9

● **825.2 Fracture of other tarsal and metatarsal bones, closed**

825.20 Unspecified bone(s) of foot [except toes] 🕮
   Instep

825.21 Astragalus 🕮
   Talus

825.22 Navicular [scaphoid], foot 🕮

825.23 Cuboid 🕮

825.24 Cuneiform, foot 🕮

825.25 Metatarsal bone(s) 🕮

825.29 Other 🕮
   Tarsal with metatarsal bone(s) only
     Excludes | calcaneus (825.0)
   Coding Clinic: 1994, Q2, P5

● **825.3 Fracture of other tarsal and metatarsal bones, open**

825.30 Unspecified bone(s) of foot [except toes] 🕮 🕮
   (Ex:) 825.0-826.1

825.31 Astragalus 🕮 🕮
   (Ex:) 733.10, 733.19, 825.1-825.39, 827.0-829.1, 843.0-843.9,
     848.8-848.9, 879.8-879.9, 929.0-929.9, 958.8, 958.99,
     959.6, 959.8-959.9

825.32 Navicular [scaphoid], foot 🕮 🕮
   (Ex:) 733.10, 733.19, 825.1-825.39, 827.0-829.1, 843.0-843.9,
     848.8-848.9, 879.8-879.9, 929.0-929.9, 958.8, 958.99,
     959.6, 959.8-959.9

825.33 Cuboid 🕮 🕮
   (Ex:) 733.10, 733.19, 825.1-825.39, 827.0-829.1, 843.0-843.9,
     848.8-848.9, 879.8-879.9, 929.0-929.9, 958.8, 958.99,
     959.6, 959.8-959.9

825.34 Cuneiform, foot 🕮 🕮
   (Ex:) 733.10, 733.19, 825.1-825.39, 827.0-829.1, 843.0-843.9,
     848.8-848.9, 879.8-879.9, 929.0-929.9, 958.8, 958.99,
     959.6, 959.8-959.9

825.35 Metatarsal bone(s) 🕮 🕮
   (Ex:) 733.10, 733.19, 825.1-825.39, 827.0-829.1, 843.0-843.9,
     848.8-848.9 879.8-879.9, 929.0-929.9, 958.8, 958.99,
     959.6, 959.8-959.9

825.39 Other 🕮 🕮
   (Ex:) 825.0-826.1

● **826 Fracture of one or more phalanges of foot**
   Includes   toe(s)

826.0 Closed 🕮

826.1 Open 🕮

● **827 Other, multiple, and ill-defined fractures of lower limb**
   Includes   leg NOS
     multiple bones of same lower limb

   Excludes | *multiple fractures of:*
     ankle bones alone (824.4–824.9)
     phalanges of foot alone (826.0–826.1)
     tarsal with metatarsal bones (825.29, 825.39)
     tibia with fibula (823.0–823.9 with fifth-digit 2)

827.0 Closed 🕮

827.1 Open 🕮 🕮
   (Ex:) 820.00-823.32, 823.80-829.1

● **828 Multiple fractures involving both lower limbs, lower with upper limb, and lower limb(s) with rib(s) and sternum**
   Includes   arm(s) with leg(s) [any bones]
     both legs [any bones]
     leg(s) with rib(s) or sternum
   OGCR Section I.C.17.b.3

   Multiple fracture category 828 classifies bilateral fractures of both upper limbs, but without any detail at the fourth-digit level other than open and closed type of fractures.

828.0 Closed 🕮 🕮
   (Ex:) 820.00-823.32, 823.80-829.1

828.1 Open 🕮 🕮
   (Ex:) 820.00-823.32, 823.80-829.1

● **829 Fracture of unspecified bones**

829.0 Unspecified bone, closed 🕮

829.1 Unspecified bone, open 🕮

N Newborn Age: 0   **P** Pediatric Age: 0–17   **M** Maternity Age: 12–55   **A** Adult Age: 15–124   ♀ Females Only   ♂ Males Only

(Ex:) CC Exclusions   🕮 Complication\Comorbidity   🕮 Major C\C   🕮 Present on Admission Requirement   🕮 Hospital-Acquired Condition

1079

INJURY AND POISONING (800–999)

A   B

Figure 17–13 Dislocation including displacement and subluxation. (From Grainger & Allison's Diagnostic Radiology: A Textbook of Medical Imaging, 4th ed. 2001, Churchill Livingstone)

DISLOCATION (830–839)

Includes	displacement
	subluxation
	Out of position

Excludes	*congenital dislocation (754.0–755.8)*
	pathological dislocation (718.2)
	recurrent dislocation (718.3)

The descriptions "closed" and "open," used in the fourth-digit subdivisions, include the following terms:

closed:
    complete
    dislocation NOS
    partial
    simple
    uncomplicated
open:
    compound
    infected
    with foreign body

Note: A dislocation not indicated as closed or open should be classified as closed.

● **830 Dislocation of jaw**

Includes	jaw (cartilage) (meniscus)
	mandible
	maxilla (inferior)
	temporomandibular (joint)

● **830.0 Closed dislocation** 🔾

● **830.1 Open dislocation** 🔾 🔾
    (Ex:) 830.0-830.1, 839.69, 839.79-839.9

● **831 Dislocation of shoulder**

Excludes	*sternoclavicular joint (839.61, 839.71)*
	sternum (839.61, 839.71)

The following fifth-digit subclassification is for use with category 831:

> 0 **shoulder, unspecified**
>   Humerus NOS
> 1 **anterior dislocation of humerus**
> 2 **posterior dislocation of humerus**
> 3 **inferior dislocation of humerus**
> 4 **acromioclavicular (joint)**
>   Clavicle
> 9 **other**
>   Scapula

● **831.0 Closed dislocation** 🔾
[0-4,9]   **Coding Clinic: 1987, Nov-Dec, P7**

● **831.1 Open dislocation** 🔾 🔾
[0-4,9]   For code **831.10:** (Ex:) 831.10, 839.69, 839.79-839.9;
        For code **831.11:** (Ex:) 831.11, 839.69, 839.79-839.9;
        For code **831.12:** (Ex:) 831.12, 839.69, 839.79-839.9;
        For code **831.13:** (Ex:) 831.13, 839.69, 839.79-839.9;
        For code **831.14:** (Ex:) 831.14, 839.69, 839.79-839.9;
        For code **831.19:** (Ex:) 831.19, 839.69, 839.79-839.9

● **832 Dislocation of elbow**

The following fifth-digit subclassification is for use with ~~category 832~~ subcategories 832.0 and 832.1: ◀━━

> 0 **elbow unspecified**
> 1 **anterior dislocation of elbow**
> 2 **posterior dislocation of elbow**
> 3 **medial dislocation of elbow**
> 4 **lateral dislocation of elbow**
> 9 **other**

● **832.0 Closed dislocation** 🔾
[0-4,9]

● **832.1 Open dislocation** 🔾 🔾
[0-4,9]   For code **832.10:** (Ex:) 832.10;
        For code **832.11:** (Ex:) 832.11;
        For code **832.12:** (Ex:) 832.12;
        For code **832.13:** (Ex:) 832.13;
        For code **832.14:** (Ex:) 832.14;
        For code **832.19:** (Ex:) 832.19

    832.2 Nursemaid's elbow 🔾   ◀
        Subluxation of radial head   ◀

● **833 Dislocation of wrist**

The following fifth-digit subclassification is for use with category 833:

> 0 **wrist, unspecified part**
>   Carpal (bone)
>   Radius, distal end
> 1 **radioulnar (joint), distal**
> 2 **radiocarpal (joint)**
> 3 **midcarpal (joint)**
> 4 **carpometacarpal (joint)**
> 5 **metacarpal (bone), proximal end**
> 9 **other**
>   Ulna, distal end

● **833.0 Closed dislocation** 🔾
[0-5,9]

● **833.1 Open dislocation** 🔾 🔾
[0-5,9]   For codes **833.10, 833.13-833.19:** (Ex:) 833.00-833.19;
        For code **833.11:** (Ex:) 833.11;
        For code **833.12:** (Ex:) 833.12

◀ New   ◀━ Revised   ~~deleted~~ Deleted   ● Unacceptable Principal Diagnosis   🔾 Use Additional Digit(s)

▶ Manifestation Code   **OGCR** Official Guidelines   **Coding Clinic**   Excludes   Includes   Use additional   Code first   Omit code

INJURY AND POISONING (800–999)

● 834　Dislocation of finger

Includes finger(s)
phalanx of hand
thumb

The following fifth-digit subclassification is for use with category 834:

> 0　finger, unspecified part
> 1　metacarpophalangeal (joint)
> 　　Metacarpal (bone), distal end
> 2　interphalangeal (joint), hand

● 834.0　Closed dislocation ⊛
[0-2]

● 834.1　Open dislocation ⊛
[0-2]

● 835　Dislocation of hip

The following fifth-digit subclassification is for use with category 835:

> 0　dislocation of hip, unspecified
> 1　posterior dislocation
> 2　obturator dislocation
> 3　other anterior dislocation

● 835.0　Closed dislocation ⊛ ⊛
[0-3]　For code **835.00:** (Ex) 835.00, 839.69, 839.79-839.9;
　　　For code **835.01:** (Ex) 835.01, 839.69, 839.79-839.9;
　　　For code **835.02:** (Ex) 835.02, 839.69, 839.79-839.9;
　　　For code **835.03:** (Ex) 835.03, 839.69, 839.79-839.9

● 835.1　Open dislocation ⊛ ⊛
[0-3]　For code **835.10:** (Ex) 835.10, 839.69, 839.79-839.9;
　　　For code **835.11:** (Ex) 835.11, 839.69, 839.79-839.9;
　　　For code **835.12:** (Ex) 835.12, 839.69, 839.79-839.9;
　　　For code **835.13:** (Ex) 835.13, 839.69, 839.79-839.9

● 836　Dislocation of knee

Excludes dislocation of knee:
old or pathological (718.2)
recurrent (718.3)
internal derangement of knee joint (717.0–717.5,
717.8–717.9)
old tear of cartilage or meniscus of knee
(717.0–717.5, 717.8–717.9)

836.0　Tear of medial cartilage or meniscus of knee, current ⊛
Bucket handle tear:
NOS current injury
medial meniscus current injury

836.1　Tear of lateral cartilage or meniscus of knee, current ⊛

836.2　Other tear of cartilage or meniscus of knee, current ⊛
Tear of:
cartilage (semilunar) current injury, not specified
as medial or lateral
meniscus current injury, not specified as medial
or lateral

836.3　Dislocation of patella, closed ⊛

836.4　Dislocation of patella, open ⊛ ⊛
(Ex) 836.3-836.4

● 836.5　Other dislocation of knee, closed

836.50　Dislocation of knee, unspecified ⊛

836.51　Anterior dislocation of tibia, proximal end ⊛
Posterior dislocation of femur, distal end

836.52　Posterior dislocation of tibia, proximal end ⊛
Anterior dislocation of femur, distal end

836.53　Medial dislocation of tibia, proximal end ⊛

836.54　Lateral dislocation of tibia, proximal end ⊛

836.59　Other ⊛

● 836.6　Other dislocation of knee, open

836.60　Dislocation of knee, unspecified ⊛ ⊛
(Ex) 717.0-717.9, 718.26, 718.36, 836.60, 839.69, 839.79-839.9

836.61　Anterior dislocation of tibia, proximal end ⊛ ⊛
(Ex) 836.61, 839.69, 839.79-839.9

836.62　Posterior dislocation of tibia, proximal end ⊛ ⊛
(Ex) 836.62, 839.69, 839.79-839.9

836.63　Medial dislocation of tibia, proximal end ⊛ ⊛
(Ex) 836.63, 839.69, 839.79-839.9

836.64　Lateral dislocation of tibia, proximal end ⊛ ⊛
(Ex) 836.64, 839.69, 839.79-839.9

836.69　Other ⊛ ⊛
(Ex) 836.69, 839.69, 839.79-839.9

● 837　Dislocation of ankle

Includes astragalus　　　　scaphoid, foot
fibula, distal end　tibia, distal end
navicular, foot

837.0　Closed dislocation ⊛

837.1　Open dislocation ⊛ ⊛
(Ex) 837.1, 839.69, 839.79-839.9

● 838　Dislocation of foot

The following fifth-digit subclassification is for use with category 838:

> 0　foot, unspecified
> 1　tarsal (bone), joint unspecified
> 2　midtarsal (joint)
> 3　tarsometatarsal (joint)
> 4　metatarsal (bone), joint unspecified
> 5　metatarsophalangeal (joint)
> 6　interphalangeal (joint), foot
> 9　other
> 　　Phalanx of foot
> 　　Toe(s)

● 838.0　Closed dislocation ⊛
[0-6,9]

● 838.1　Open dislocation ⊛
[0-6,9]

INJURY AND POISONING (800–999)

● **839 Other, multiple, and ill-defined dislocations**
Coding Clinic: 1995, Q4, P51

● **839.0 Cervical vertebra, closed**
Cervical spine
Neck

839.00 Cervical vertebra, unspecified 🔾 🔾
(Ex:) 805.00-805.18, 806.00-806.19, 806.8-806.9, 839.00-839.18,
847.0, 848.8-848.9, 879.8-879.9, 929.0-929.9,
952.00-952.09, 958.8-958.99, 959.8-959.9

839.01 First cervical vertebra 🔾 🔾
(Ex:) 805.00-805.18, 806.00-806.19, 806.8-806.9, 839.00-839.18,
847.0, 848.8-848.9, 879.8-879.9, 929.0-929.9,
952.00-952.09, 958.8-958.99, 959.8-959.9

839.02 Second cervical vertebra 🔾 🔾
(Ex:) 805.00-805.18, 806.00-806.19, 806.8-806.9, 839.00-839.18,
847.0, 848.8-848.9, 879.8-879.9, 929.0-929.9,
952.00-952.09, 958.8-958.99, 959.8-959.9

839.03 Third cervical vertebra 🔾 🔾
(Ex:) 805.00-805.18, 806.00-806.19, 806.8-806.9, 839.00-839.18,
847.0, 848.8-848.9, 879.8-879.9, 929.0-929.9,
952.00-952.09, 958.8-958.99, 959.8-959.9

839.04 Fourth cervical vertebra 🔾 🔾
(Ex:) 805.00-805.18, 806.00-806.19, 806.8-806.9, 839.00-839.18,
847.0, 848.8-848.9, 879.8-879.9, 929.0-929.9,
952.00-952.09, 958.8-958.99, 959.8-959.9

839.05 Fifth cervical vertebra 🔾 🔾
(Ex:) 805.00-805.18, 806.00-806.19, 806.8-806.9, 839.00-839.18,
847.0, 848.8-848.9, 879.8-879.9, 929.0-929.9,
952.00-952.09, 958.8-958.99, 959.8-959.9

839.06 Sixth cervical vertebra 🔾 🔾
(Ex:) 805.00-805.18, 806.00-806.19, 806.8-806.9, 839.00-839.18,
847.0, 848.8-848.9, 879.8-879.9, 929.0-929.9,
952.00-952.09, 958.8-958.99, 959.8-959.9

839.07 Seventh cervical vertebra 🔾 🔾
(Ex:) 805.00-805.18, 806.00-806.19, 806.8-806.9, 839.00-839.18,
847.0, 848.8-848.9, 879.8-879.9, 929.0-929.9,
952.00-952.09, 958.8-958.99, 959.8-959.9

839.08 Multiple cervical vertebrae 🔾 🔾
(Ex:) 805.00-805.18, 806.00-806.19, 806.8-806.9, 839.00-839.18,
847.0, 848.8-848.9, 879.8-879.9, 929.0-929.9,
952.00-952.09, 958.8-958.99, 959.8-959.9

● **839.1 Cervical vertebra, open**

839.10 Cervical vertebra, unspecified 🔾 🔾
(Ex:) 805.00-805.18, 806.00-806.19, 806.8-806.9, 839.00-839.18,
847.0, 848.8-848.9, 879.8-879.9, 929.0-929.9,
952.00-952.09, 958.8-958.99, 959.8-959.9

839.11 First cervical vertebra 🔾 🔾
(Ex:) 805.00-805.18, 806.00-806.19, 806.8-806.9, 839.00-839.18,
847.0, 848.8-848.9, 879.8-879.9, 929.0-929.9,
952.00-952.09, 958.8-958.99, 959.8-959.9

839.12 Second cervical vertebra 🔾 🔾
(Ex:) 805.00-805.18, 806.00-806.19, 806.8-806.9, 839.00-839.18,
847.0, 848.8-848.9, 879.8-879.9, 929.0-929.9,
952.00-952.09, 958.8-958.99, 959.8-959.9

839.13 Third cervical vertebra 🔾 🔾
(Ex:) 805.00-805.18, 806.00-806.19, 806.8-806.9, 839.00-839.18,
847.0, 848.8-848.9, 879.8-879.9, 929.0-929.9,
952.00-952.09, 958.8-958.99, 959.8-959.9

839.14 Fourth cervical vertebra 🔾 🔾
(Ex:) 805.00-805.18, 806.00-806.19, 806.8-806.9, 839.00-839.18,
847.0, 848.8-848.9, 879.8-879.9, 929.0-929.9,
952.00-952.09, 958.8-958.99, 959.8-959.9

839.15 Fifth cervical vertebra 🔾 🔾
(Ex:) 805.00-805.18, 806.00-806.19, 806.8-806.9, 839.00-839.18,
847.0, 848.8-848.9, 879.8-879.9, 929.0-929.9,
952.00-952.09, 958.8-958.99, 959.8-959.9

839.16 Sixth cervical vertebra 🔾 🔾
(Ex:) 805.00-805.18, 806.00-806.19, 806.8-806.9, 839.00-839.18,
847.0, 848.8-848.9, 879.8-879.9, 929.0-929.9,
952.00-952.09, 958.8-958.99, 959.8-959.9

839.17 Seventh cervical vertebra 🔾 🔾
(Ex:) 805.00-805.18, 806.00-806.19, 806.8-806.9, 839.00-839.18,
847.0, 848.8-848.9, 879.8-879.9, 929.0-929.9,
952.00-952.09, 958.8-958.99, 959.8-959.9

839.18 Multiple cervical vertebrae 🔾 🔾
(Ex:) 805.00-805.18, 806.00-806.19, 806.8-806.9, 839.00-839.18,
847.0, 848.8-848.9, 879.8-879.9, 929.0-929.9,
952.00-952.09, 958.8-958.99, 959.8-959.9

● **839.2 Thoracic and lumbar vertebra, closed**

839.20 Lumbar vertebra 🔾

839.21 Thoracic vertebra 🔾
Dorsal [thoracic] vertebra

● **839.3 Thoracic and lumbar vertebra, open**

839.30 Lumbar vertebra 🔾 🔾
(Ex:) 839.30

839.31 Thoracic vertebra 🔾 🔾
(Ex:) 839.21, 839.31

● **839.4 Other vertebra, closed**

839.40 Vertebra, unspecified site 🔾
Spine NOS

839.41 Coccyx 🔾

839.42 Sacrum 🔾
Sacroiliac (joint)

839.49 Other 🔾

● **839.5 Other vertebra, open**

839.50 Vertebra, unspecified site 🔾 🔾
(Ex:) 839.10-839.18, 839.30-839.31, 839.50-839.59, 839.79, 839.9

839.51 Coccyx 🔾 🔾
(Ex:) 839.51

839.52 Sacrum 🔾 🔾
(Ex:) 839.52

839.59 Other 🔾 🔾
(Ex:) 839.10-839.18, 839.30-839.31, 839.50-839.59, 839.79, 839.9

● **839.6 Other location, closed**

839.61 Sternum 🔾 🔾
Sternoclavicular joint
(Ex:) 839.61, 839.71

839.69 Other 🔾
Pelvis

● **839.7 Other location, open**

839.71 Sternum 🔾 🔾
(Ex:) 839.61, 839.71

839.79 Other 🔾 🔾
(Ex:) 830.1, 831.10-831.19, 832.10-832.19, 833.10-833.19,
834.10-834.12, 835.10-835.13, 836.4, 836.60-836.69,
837.1, 838.10-838.19, 839.10-839.18, 839.30-839.31,
839.50-839.59, 839.71-839.79, 839.9

INJURY AND POISONING (800–999)

◀ New   ◀⁞⁞⁞ Revised   ~~deleted~~ Deleted   ● Unacceptable Principal Diagnosis   🔾 Use Additional Digit(s)
▶ Manifestation Code   OGCR Official Guidelines   Coding Clinic   Excludes   Includes   Use additional   Code first   Omit code

839.8　Multiple and ill-defined, closed 🅌
　　Arm
　　Back
　　Hand
　　Multiple locations, except fingers or toes alone
　　Other ill-defined locations
　　Unspecified location

839.9　Multiple and ill-defined, open 🅒 🅌
　　Ⓔ𝔁 830.1, 831.10-831.19, 832.10-832.19, 833.10-833.19, 834.10-834.12,
　　835.10-835.13, 836.4, 836.60-836.69, 837.1, 838.10-838.19,
　　839.10-839.18, 839.30-839.31, 839.50-839.59, 839.71-839.79, 839.9

SPRAINS AND STRAINS OF JOINTS AND ADJACENT MUSCLES (840–848)

Includes　avulsion of joint capsule, ligament, muscle,
　　　　　　　tendon
　　　　　　hemarthrosis of joint capsule, ligament,
　　　　　　　muscle, tendon
　　　　　　　Bleeding into joint space
　　　　　　laceration of joint capsule, ligament, muscle,
　　　　　　　tendon
　　　　　　rupture of joint capsule, ligament, muscle,
　　　　　　　tendon
　　　　　　sprain of joint capsule, ligament, muscle,
　　　　　　　tendon
　　　　　　strain of joint capsule, ligament, muscle,
　　　　　　　tendon
　　　　　　tear of joint capsule, ligament, muscle, tendon

Excludes　*laceration of tendon in open wounds (880–884 and
　　　　　　890–894 with .2)*

● **840　Sprains and strains of shoulder and upper arm**
　　　　　*Sprains are an injury to ligaments when one or more is
　　　　　stretched/torn and strains are caused by twisting or
　　　　　pulling a muscle(s) or tendon.*

　　840.0　Acromioclavicular (joint) (ligament)

　　840.1　Coracoclavicular (ligament)

　　840.2　Coracohumeral (ligament)

　　840.3　Infraspinatus (muscle) (tendon)

　　840.4　Rotator cuff (capsule)
　　　　　Excludes　*complete rupture of rotator cuff,
　　　　　　　　　　　　nontraumatic (727.61)*

　　840.5　Subscapularis (muscle)

　　840.6　Supraspinatus (muscle) (tendon)

　　840.7　Superior glenoid labrum lesion
　　　　　SLAP lesion
　　　　　Coding Clinic: 2001, Q4, P52

　　840.8　Other specified sites of shoulder and upper arm

　　840.9　Unspecified site of shoulder and upper arm
　　　　　Arm NOS
　　　　　Shoulder NOS

● **841　Sprains and strains of elbow and forearm**

　　841.0　Radial collateral ligament

　　841.1　Ulnar collateral ligament

　　841.2　Radiohumeral (joint)

　　841.3　Ulnohumeral (joint)

　　841.8　Other specified sites of elbow and forearm

　　841.9　Unspecified site of elbow and forearm
　　　　　Elbow NOS

● **842　Sprains and strains of wrist and hand**

　● **842.0　Wrist**

　　842.00　Unspecified site

　　842.01　Carpal (joint)

　　842.02　Radiocarpal (joint) (ligament)

　　842.09　Other
　　　　　Radioulnar joint, distal

　● **842.1　Hand**

　　842.10　Unspecified site

　　842.11　Carpometacarpal (joint)

　　842.12　Metacarpophalangeal (joint)

　　842.13　Interphalangeal (joint)

　　842.19　Other
　　　　　Midcarpal (joint)

● **843　Sprains and strains of hip and thigh**

　　843.0　Iliofemoral (ligament)

　　843.1　Ischiocapsular (ligament)

　　843.8　Other specified sites of hip and thigh

　　843.9　Unspecified site of hip and thigh
　　　　　Hip NOS
　　　　　Thigh NOS

● **844　Sprains and strains of knee and leg**

　　844.0　Lateral collateral ligament of knee

　　844.1　Medial collateral ligament of knee

　　844.2　Cruciate ligament of knee

　　844.3　Tibiofibular (joint) (ligament), superior

　　844.8　Other specified sites of knee and leg

　　844.9　Unspecified site of knee and leg
　　　　　Knee NOS
　　　　　Leg NOS

● **845　Sprains and strains of ankle and foot**

　● **845.0　Ankle**

　　845.00　Unspecified site
　　　　　Coding Clinic: 2002, Q2, P3

　　845.01　Deltoid (ligament), ankle
　　　　　Internal collateral (ligament), ankle

　　845.02　Calcaneofibular (ligament)

　　845.03　Tibiofibular (ligament), distal
　　　　　Coding Clinic: 2004, Q1, P9

　　845.09　Other
　　　　　Achilles tendon

　● **845.1　Foot**

　　845.10　Unspecified site

　　845.11　Tarsometatarsal (joint) (ligament)

　　845.12　Metatarsophalangeal (joint)

　　845.13　Interphalangeal (joint), toe

　　845.19　Other

● 846   **Sprains and strains of sacroiliac region**

    846.0   Lumbosacral (joint) (ligament)

    846.1   Sacroiliac ligament

    846.2   Sacrospinatus (ligament)

    846.3   Sacrotuberous (ligament)

    846.8   Other specified sites of sacroiliac region

    846.9   Unspecified site of sacroiliac region

● 847   **Sprains and strains of other and unspecified parts of back**

    Excludes   *lumbosacral (846.0)*

    847.0   Neck

       Anterior longitudinal (ligament), cervical
       Atlanto-axial (joints)
       Atlanto-occipital (joints)
       Whiplash injury

       Excludes   *neck injury NOS (959.09)*
                    thyroid region (848.2)

    847.1   Thoracic

    847.2   Lumbar

    847.3   Sacrum

       Sacrococcygeal (ligament)

    847.4   Coccyx

    847.9   Unspecified site of back

       Back NOS

● 848   **Other and ill-defined sprains and strains**

    848.0   Septal cartilage of nose

    848.1   Jaw

       Temporomandibular (joint) (ligament)

    848.2   Thyroid region

       Cricoarytenoid (joint) (ligament)
       Cricothyroid (joint) (ligament)
       Thyroid cartilage

    848.3   Ribs

       Chondrocostal (joint) without mention of injury to sternum
       Costal cartilage without mention of injury to sternum

● 848.4   Sternum

    848.40   Unspecified site

    848.41   Sternoclavicular (joint) (ligament)

    848.42   Chondrosternal (joint)

    848.49   Other

         Xiphoid cartilage

    848.5   Pelvis

       Symphysis pubis

       Excludes   *that in childbirth (665.6)*

    848.8   Other specified sites of sprains and strains

    848.9   Unspecified site of sprain and strain

INTRACRANIAL INJURY, EXCLUDING THOSE WITH SKULL FRACTURE (850–854)

Includes   traumatic brain injury without skull fracture ◀

Excludes   *intracranial injury with skull fracture (800–801 and 803–804, except .0 and .5)*
open wound of head without intracranial injury (870.0–873.9)
skull fracture alone (800–801 and 803–804 with .0, .5)

Note: The description "with open intracranial wound," used in the fourth-digit subdivisions, includes those specified as open or with mention of infection or foreign body.

The following fifth-digit subclassification is for use with categories 851–854:

> 0   unspecified state of consciousness
> 1   with no loss of consciousness
> 2   with brief [less than one hour] loss of consciousness
> 3   with moderate [1–24 hours] loss of consciousness
> 4   with prolonged [more than 24 hours] loss of consciousness and return to pre-existing conscious level
> 5   with prolonged [more than 24 hours] loss of consciousness without return to pre-existing conscious level
>
>   Use fifth-digit 5 to designate when a patient is unconscious and dies before regaining consciousness, regardless of the duration of the loss of consciousness
>
> 6   with loss of consciousness of unspecified duration
> 9   with concussion, unspecified

● 850   **Concussion**

    Includes   commotio cerebri

    Excludes   *concussion with:*
              cerebral laceration or contusion (851.0–851.9)
              cerebral hemorrhage (852–853)
        head injury NOS (959.01)

    Coding Clinic: 1993, Q1, P22-23

    850.0   With no loss of consciousness 🖇

       Concussion with mental confusion or disorientation, without loss of consciousness
       Coding Clinic: 1992, Q2, P5-6

● 850.1   With brief loss of consciousness

       Loss of consciousness for less than one hour
       Coding Clinic: 2003, Q4, P76; 1999, Q1, P10; 1992, Q2, P5-6

    850.11   With loss of consciousness of 30 minutes or less 🖇 🖇

         Ⓔⓧ 800.00-801.99, 803.00-804.99, 850.0-852.19, 852.21-854.19, 873.8-873.9, 879.8-879.9, 905.0, 925.1-925.2, 929.0-929.9, 958.8-959.09, 959.8-959.9

    850.12   With loss of consciousness from 31 to 59 minutes 🖇 🖇

         Ⓔⓧ 800.00-801.99, 803.00-804.99, 850.0-852.19, 852.21-854.19, 873.8-873.9, 879.8-879.9, 905.0, 925.1-925.2, 929.0-929.9, 958.8-959.09, 959.8-959.9

    850.2   With moderate loss of consciousness 🖇 🖇

       Loss of consciousness for 1–24 hours
       Ⓔⓧ 800.00-801.99, 803.00-804.99, 850.0-852.19, 852.21-854.19, 873.8-873.9, 879.8-879.9, 905.0, 925.1-925.2, 929.0-929.9, 958.8-959.09, 959.8-959.9

INJURY AND POISONING (800–999)

850.3 With prolonged loss of consciousness and return to pre-existing conscious level 🟢 🟢
> Loss of consciousness for more than 24 hours with complete recovery
> (Ex:) 800.00-801.99, 803.00-804.99, 850.0-852.19, 852.21-854.19, 873.8-873.9, 879.8-879.9, 905.0, 925.1-925.2, 929.0-929.9, 958.8-959.09, 959.8-959.9

850.4 With prolonged loss of consciousness, without return to pre-existing conscious level 🟢 🟢
> (Ex:) 800.00-801.99, 803.00-804.99, 850.0-852.19, 852.21-854.19, 873.8-873.9, 879.8-879.9, 905.0, 925.1-925.2, 929.0-929.9, 958.8-959.09, 959.8-959.9

850.5 With loss of consciousness of unspecified duration 🟢 🟢
> (Ex:) 800.00-801.99, 803.00-804.99, 850.0-852.19, 852.21-854.19, 873.8-873.9, 879.8-879.9, 905.0, 925.1-925.2, 929.0-929.9, 958.8-959.09, 959.8-959.9

850.9 Concussion, unspecified 🟢

● **851 Cerebral laceration and contusion**
> *Cerebral lacerations* are tears in brain tissue. *Cerebral contusions* are bruises on brain.
>
> Requires fifth digit. See beginning of section 850–854 for codes and definitions.
> **Coding Clinic:** 1993, Q1, P22-23

● **851.0 Cortex (cerebral) contusion without mention of open**
[0-6,9] **intracranial wound 2-4,6** 🟢 🟢, **5** 🟢 🟢, **0-1,9** 🟢
> For codes **851.02-851.06:** (Ex:) 800.00-801.99, 803.00-804.99, 850.0-852.19, 852.21-854.19, 873.8-873.9, 879.8-879.9, 905.0, 925.1-925.2, 929.0-929.9, 958.8-959.09, 959.8-959.9

● **851.1 Cortex (cerebral) contusion with open intracranial**
[0-6,9] **wound** 🟢 🟢
> (Ex:) 800.00-801.99, 803.00-804.99, 850.0-852.19, 852.21-854.19, 873.8-873.9, 879.8-879.9, 905.0, 925.1-925.2, 929.0-929.9, 958.8-959.09, 959.8-959.9

● **851.2 Cortex (cerebral) laceration without mention of open**
[0-6,9] **intracranial wound** 🟢 🟢
> (Ex:) 800.00-801.99, 803.00-804.99, 850.0-852.19, 852.21-854.19, 873.8-873.9, 879.8-879.9, 905.0, 925.1-925.2, 929.0-929.9, 958.8-959.09, 959.8-959.9

● **851.3 Cortex (cerebral) laceration with open intracranial**
[0-6,9] **wound** 🟢 🟢
> (Ex:) 800.00-801.99, 803.00-804.99, 850.0-852.19, 852.21-854.19, 873.8-873.9, 879.8-879.9, 905.0, 925.1-925.2, 929.0-929.9, 958.8-959.09, 959.8-959.9

● **851.4 Cerebellar or brain stem contusion without mention**
[0-6,9] **of open intracranial wound 2-4,6** 🟢, **5** 🟢, **0-1,9** 🟢
> For codes **851.42-851.46:** (Ex:) 800.00-801.99, 803.00-804.99, 850.0-852.19, 852.21-854.19, 873.8-873.9, 879.8-879.9, 905.0, 925.1-925.2, 929.0-929.9, 958.8-959.09, 959.8-959.9

● **851.5 Cerebellar or brain stem contusion with open**
[0-6,9] **intracranial wound** 🟢 🟢
> (Ex:) 800.00-801.99, 803.00-804.99, 850.0-852.19, 852.21-854.19, 873.8-873.9, 879.8-879.9, 905.0, 925.1-925.2, 929.0-929.9, 958.8-959.09, 959.8-959.9

● **851.6 Cerebellar or brain stem laceration without mention**
[0-6,9] **of open intracranial wound** 🟢 🟢
> (Ex:) 800.00-801.99, 803.00-804.99, 850.0-852.19, 852.21-854.19, 873.8-873.9, 879.8-879.9, 905.0, 925.1-925.2, 929.0-929.9, 958.8-959.09, 959.8-959.9

● **851.7 Cerebellar or brain stem laceration with open**
[0-6,9] **intracranial wound** 🟢 🟢
> (Ex:) 800.00-801.99, 803.00-804.99, 850.0-852.19, 852.21-854.19, 873.8-873.9, 879.8-879.9, 905.0, 925.1-925.2, 929.0-929.9, 958.8-959.09, 959.8-959.9

● **851.8 Other and unspecified cerebral laceration and**
[0-6,9] **contusion, without mention of open intracranial wound** 🟢 🟢
> Brain (membrane) NOS
> (Ex:) 800.00-801.99, 803.00-804.99, 850.0-852.19, 852.21-854.19, 873.8-873.9, 879.8-879.9, 905.0, 925.1-925.2, 929.0-929.9, 958.8-959.09, 959.8-959.9
> **Coding Clinic:** 1996, Q4, P36.37

● **851.9 Other and unspecified cerebral laceration and**
[0-6,9] **contusion, with open intracranial wound** 🟢 🟢
> (Ex:) 800.00-801.99, 803.00-804.99, 850.0-852.19, 852.21-854.19, 873.8-873.9, 879.8-879.9, 905.0, 925.1-925.2, 929.0-929.9, 958.8-959.09, 959.8-959.9

● **852 Subarachnoid, subdural, and extradural hemorrhage, following injury**
> Requires fifth digit. See beginning of section 850–854 for codes and definitions.
>
> | **Excludes** | *cerebral contusion or laceration (with hemorrhage) (851.0–851.9)* |

● **852.0 Subarachnoid hemorrhage following injury without**
[0-6,9] **mention of open intracranial wound** 🟢 🟢
> Middle meningeal hemorrhage following injury
> (Ex:) 800.00-801.99, 803.00-804.99, 850.0-852.19, 852.21-854.19, 873.8-873.9, 879.8-879.9, 905.0, 925.1-925.2, 929.0-929.9, 958.8-959.09, 959.8-959.9
> **Coding Clinic:** 1991, Q3, P15-16

● **852.1 Subarachnoid hemorrhage following injury with**
[0-6,9] **open intracranial wound** 🟢 🟢
> (Ex:) 800.00-801.99, 803.00-804.99, 850.0-852.19, 852.21-854.19, 873.8-873.9, 879.8-879.9, 905.0, 925.1-925.2, 929.0-929.9, 958.8-959.09, 959.8-959.9
> **Coding Clinic:** 1991, Q3, P15-16

● **852.2 Subdural hemorrhage following injury without**
[0-6,9] **mention of open intracranial wound** 🟢 🟢
> For codes **852.20:** (Ex:) 800.00-801.99, 803.00-804.99, 850.0-854.19, 873.8-873.9, 879.8-879.9, 905.0, 925.1-925.2, 929.0-929.9, 958.8-959.09, 959.8-959.9;
> For codes **852.21-852.29:** (Ex:) 800.00-801.99, 803.00-804.99, 850.0-852.19, 852.21-854.19, 873.8-873.9, 879.8-879.9, 905.0, 925.1-925.2, 929.0-929.9, 958.8-959.09, 959.8-959.9
> **Coding Clinic:** 2007, Q4, P105-107; 1996, Q4, P43-44

● **852.3 Subdural hemorrhage following injury with open**
[0-6,9] **intracranial wound** 🔖 🔖
   Ⓔ 800.00-801.99, 803.00-804.99, 850.0-852.19, 852.21-854.19, 873.8-873.9,
   879.8-879.9, 905.0, 925.1-925.2, 929.0-929.9, 958.8-959.09,
   959.8-959.9

● **852.4 Extradural hemorrhage following injury without**
[0-6,9] **mention of open intracranial wound** 🔖 🔖
   Epidural hematoma following injury
   Ⓔ 800.00-801.99, 803.00-804.99, 850.0-852.19, 852.21-854.19, 873.8-873.9,
   879.8-879.9, 905.0, 925.1-925.2, 929.0-929.9, 958.8-959.09,
   959.8-959.9

● **852.5 Extradural hemorrhage following injury with open**
[0-6,9] **intracranial wound** 🔖 🔖
   Ⓔ 800.00-801.99, 803.00-804.99, 850.0-852.19, 852.21-854.19, 873.8-873.9,
   879.8-879.9, 905.0, 925.1-925.2, 929.0-929.9, 958.8-959.09,
   959.8-959.9

● **853 Other and unspecified intracranial hemorrhage following**
injury
   Requires fifth digit. See beginning of section 850–854 for
   codes and definitions.

● **853.0 Without mention of open intracranial wound** 🔖 🔖
[0-6,9]   Cerebral compression due to injury
   Intracranial hematoma following injury
   Traumatic cerebral hemorrhage
   Ⓔ 800.00-801.99, 803.00-804.99, 850.0-852.19, 852.21-854.19, 873.8-873.9,
   879.8-879.9, 905.0, 925.1-925.2, 929.0-929.9, 958.8-959.09,
   959.8-959.9
   Coding Clinic: 1990, Q3, P14

● **853.1 With open intracranial wound** 🔖 🔖
[0-6,9]   Ⓔ 800.00-801.99, 803.00-804.99, 850.0-852.19, 852.21-854.19, 873.8-873.9,
   879.8-879.9, 905.0, 925.1-925.2, 929.0-929.9, 958.8-959.09,
   959.8-959.9

● **854 Intracranial injury of other and unspecified nature**
   Requires fifth digit. See beginning of section 850-854 for
   codes and definitions.

   Includes   injury: ◀▥▥
                  brain injury NOS   ◀▥▥
                  cavernous sinus
                  intracranial injury   ◀▥▥
                  traumatic brain NOS   ◀

   Excludes   *any condition classifiable to 850–853*
                  head injury NOS (959.01)
   Coding Clinic: 1999, Q1, P10; 1992, Q2, P5-6

● **854.0 Without mention of open intracranial wound**
[0-6,9]   **2-4,6** 🔖 **5** 🔖 🔖 **0-1,9** 🔖
   For codes **854.02-854.06:** Ⓔ 800.00-801.99, 803.00-804.99, 850.0-852.19,
   852.21-854.19, 873.8-873.9, 879.8-879.9, 905.0, 925.1-925.2,
   929.0-929.9, 958.8-959.09, 959.8-959.9
   Coding Clinic: 2005, Q2, P6-7

● **854.1 With open intracranial wound** 🔖 🔖
[0-6,9]   Ⓔ 800.00-801.99, 803.00-804.99, 850.0-852.19, 852.21-854.19, 873.8-873.9,
   879.8-879.9, 905.0, 925.1-925.2, 929.0-929.9, 958.8-959.09,
   959.8-959.9

Item 17-1 Pneumothorax is a collection of gas (positive
air pressure) in the pleural space resulting in the lung collapsing.
A tension pneumothorax is life-threatening and is a result of air
in the pleural space causing a displacement in the mediastinal
structures and cardiopulmonary function compromise. A
traumatic pneumothorax results from blunt or penetrating injury
that disrupts the parietal/visceral pleura. **Hemothorax** is blood
or bloody fluid in the pleural cavity as a result of traumatic blood
vessel rupture or inflammation of the lungs from pneumonia.

INTERNAL INJURY OF THORAX, ABDOMEN, AND PELVIS (860–869)

   Includes   blast injuries of internal organs
                  blunt trauma of internal organs
                  bruise of internal organs
                  concussion injuries (except cerebral) of
                      internal organs
                  crushing of internal organs
                  hematoma of internal organs
                  laceration of internal organs
                  puncture of internal organs
                  tear of internal organs
                  traumatic rupture of internal organs

   Excludes   *concussion NOS (850.0–850.9)*
                  flail chest (807.4)
                  foreign body entering through orifice
                      (930.0–939.9)
                  injury to blood vessels (901.0–902.9)

Note: The description "with open wound," used in
   the fourth-digit subdivisions, includes those with
   mention of infection or foreign body.

● **860 Traumatic pneumothorax and hemothorax**

   860.0 Pneumothorax without mention of open wound into
   thorax 🔖
      Ⓔ 860.0-860.5, 861.20-861.32, 862.29, 862.39-862.9, 875.0-875.1,
      879.8-879.9, 929.0-929.9, 958.7-958.99, 959.8-959.9
      Coding Clinic: 1993, Q2, P4-5

   860.1 Pneumothorax with open wound into thorax 🔖
      Ⓔ 860.0-860.5, 861.20-861.32, 862.29, 862.39-862.9, 875.0-875.1,
      879.8-879.9, 929.0-929.9, 958.7-958.99, 959.8-959.9
      Coding Clinic: 1995, Q3, P17; 1993, Q2, P4-5

   860.2 Hemothorax without mention of open wound into
   thorax 🔖
      Ⓔ 860.0-860.5, 861.20-861.32, 862.29, 862.39-862.9, 875.0-875.1,
      879.8-879.9, 929.0-929.9, 958.7-958.99, 959.8-959.9

   860.3 Hemothorax with open wound into thorax 🔖
      Ⓔ 860.0-860.5, 861.20-861.32, 862.29, 862.39-862.9, 875.0-875.1,
      879.8-879.9, 929.0-929.9, 958.7-958.99, 959.8-959.9
      Coding Clinic: 1995, Q3, P17

   860.4 Pneumohemothorax without mention of open
   wound into thorax 🔖
      Ⓔ 860.0-860.5, 861.20-861.32, 862.29, 862.39-862.9, 875.0-875.1,
      879.8-879.9, 929.0-929.9, 958.7-958.99, 959.8-959.9

   860.5 Pneumohemothorax with open wound into thorax 🔖
      Ⓔ 860.0-860.5, 861.20-861.32, 862.29, 862.39-862.9, 875.0-875.1,
      879.8-879.9, 929.0-929.9, 958.7-958.99, 959.8-959.9
      Coding Clinic: 1995, Q3, P17

◀ New   ◀▥▥ Revised   ~~deleted~~ Deleted   ● Unacceptable Principal Diagnosis   🔖 Use Additional Digit(s)
▶ Manifestation Code   **OGCR** Official Guidelines   **Coding Clinic**   Excludes   Includes   Use additional   Code first   Omit code

● 861　**Injury to heart and lung**

> **Excludes**　*injury to blood vessels of thorax (901.0–901.9)*

> Coding Clinic: 1992, Q1, P9-10

　● 861.0　**Heart, without mention of open wound into thorax**

　　　861.00　**Unspecified injury**🦠
　　　　　Ⓔⓧ 861.00-861.13, 862.29, 862.39-862.9, 959.9

　　　861.01　**Contusion**🦠
　　　　　Cardiac contusion
　　　　　Myocardial contusion
　　　　　Ⓔⓧ 861.00-861.13, 862.29, 862.39-862.9, 875.0-875.1,
　　　　　　879.8-879.9, 929.0-929.9, 958.7-958.99, 959.8-959.9

　　　861.02　**Laceration without penetration of heart chambers**🦠
　　　　　Ⓔⓧ 861.00-861.13, 862.29, 862.39-862.9, 875.0-875.1,
　　　　　　879.8-879.9, 929.0-929.9, 958.7-958.99, 959.8-959.9

　　　861.03　**Laceration with penetration of heart chambers**🦠
　　　　　Ⓔⓧ 861.00-861.13, 862.29, 862.39-862.9, 875.0-875.1,
　　　　　　879.8-879.9, 929.0-929.9, 958.7-958.99, 959.8-959.9

　● 861.1　**Heart, with open wound into thorax**

　　　861.10　**Unspecified injury**🦠
　　　　　Ⓔⓧ 861.00-861.13, 862.29, 862.39-862.9, 875.0-875.1,
　　　　　　879.8-879.9, 929.0-929.9, 958.7-958.99, 959.8-959.9

　　　861.11　**Contusion**🦠
　　　　　Ⓔⓧ 861.00-861.13, 862.29, 862.39-862.9, 875.0-875.1,
　　　　　　879.8-879.9, 929.0-929.9, 958.7-958.99, 959.8-959.9

　　　861.12　**Laceration without penetration of heart chambers**🦠
　　　　　Ⓔⓧ 861.00-861.13, 862.29, 862.39-862.9, 875.0-875.1,
　　　　　　879.8-879.9, 929.0-929.9, 958.7-958.99, 959.8-959.9

　　　861.13　**Laceration with penetration of heart chambers**🦠
　　　　　Ⓔⓧ 861.00-861.13, 862.29, 862.39-862.9, 875.0-875.1,
　　　　　　879.8-879.9, 929.0-929.9, 958.7-958.99, 959.8-959.9

　● 861.2　**Lung, without mention of open wound into thorax**

　　　861.20　**Unspecified injury**🦠
　　　　　Ⓔⓧ 861.00-861.13, 862.29, 862.39-862.9, 875.0-875.1,
　　　　　　879.8-879.9, 929.0-929.9, 958.7-958.99, 959.8-959.9

　　　861.21　**Contusion**🦠
　　　　　Ⓔⓧ 861.00-861.13, 862.29, 862.39-862.9, 875.0-875.1,
　　　　　　879.8-879.9, 929.0-929.9, 958.7-958.99, 959.8-959.9

　　　861.22　**Laceration**🦠
　　　　　Ⓔⓧ 861.00-861.13, 862.29, 862.39-862.9, 875.0-875.1,
　　　　　　879.8-879.9, 929.0-929.9, 958.7-958.99, 959.8-959.9

　● 861.3　**Lung, with open wound into thorax**

　　　861.30　**Unspecified injury**🦠
　　　　　Ⓔⓧ 861.00-861.13, 862.29, 862.39-862.9, 875.0-875.1,
　　　　　　879.8-879.9, 929.0-929.9, 958.7-958.99, 959.8-959.9

　　　861.31　**Contusion**🦠
　　　　　Ⓔⓧ 861.00-861.13, 862.29, 862.39-862.9, 875.0-875.1,
　　　　　　879.8-879.9, 929.0-929.9, 958.7-958.99, 959.8-959.9

　　　861.32　**Laceration**🦠
　　　　　Ⓔⓧ 861.00-861.13, 862.29, 862.39-862.9, 875.0-875.1,
　　　　　　879.8-879.9, 929.0-929.9, 958.7-958.99, 959.8-959.9

● 862　**Injury to other and unspecified intrathoracic organs**

> **Excludes**　*injury to blood vessels of thorax (901.0–901.9)*

　　862.0　**Diaphragm, without mention of open wound into cavity**🦠
　　　　Ⓔⓧ 862.0-862.1, 862.29, 862.39-862.9, 875.0-875.1, 879.8-879.9, 929.0-929.9
　　　　　958.7-958.8, 958.99, 959.8-959.9

　　862.1　**Diaphragm, with open wound into cavity**🦠
　　　　Ⓔⓧ 862.0-862.1, 862.29, 862.39-862.9, 875.0-875.1, 879.8-879.9,
　　　　　929.0-929.9, 958.7-958.99, 959.8-959.9

　● 862.2　**Other specified intrathoracic organs, without mention of open wound into cavity**

　　　862.21　**Bronchus**🦠
　　　　　Ⓔⓧ 862.0-862.1, 862.29, 862.39-862.9, 875.0-875.1, 879.8-879.9,
　　　　　　929.0-929.9 958.7-958.8, 958.99, 959.8-959.9

　　　862.22　**Esophagus**🦠
　　　　　Ⓔⓧ 862.0-862.1, 862.29, 862.39-862.9, 875.0-875.1, 879.8-879.9,
　　　　　　929.0-929.9 958.7-958.8, 958.99, 959.8-959.9

　　　862.29　**Other**🦠
　　　　　Pleura
　　　　　Thymus gland
　　　　　Ⓔⓧ 862.29, 862.39-862.9, 875.0-875.1, 879.8-879.9, 929.0-929.9,
　　　　　　958.7-958.99, 959.8-959.9

　● 862.3　**Other specified intrathoracic organs, with open wound into cavity**

　　　862.31　**Bronchus**🦠
　　　　　Ⓔⓧ 862.0-862.1, 862.29, 862.39-862.9, 875.0-875.1, 879.8-879.9,
　　　　　　929.0-929.9 958.7-958.8, 958.99, 959.8-959.9

　　　862.32　**Esophagus**🦠
　　　　　Ⓔⓧ 862.22-862.29, 862.32-862.9, 875.0-875.1, 879.8-879.9,
　　　　　　929.0-929.9, 958.7-958.99, 959.8-959.9

　　　862.39　**Other**🦠
　　　　　Ⓔⓧ 862.29, 862.39-862.9, 875.0-875.1, 879.8-879.9, 929.0-929.9,
　　　　　　958.7-958.99, 959.8-959.9

　　862.8　**Multiple and unspecified intrathoracic organs, without mention of open wound into cavity**🦠
　　　　Crushed chest
　　　　Multiple intrathoracic organs
　　　　Ⓔⓧ 862.29, 862.39-862.9, 875.0-875.1, 879.8-879.9, 929.0-929.9,
　　　　　958.7-958.8, 958.93-958.99, 959.8-959.9

　　862.9　**Multiple and unspecified intrathoracic organs, with open wound into cavity**🦠
　　　　Ⓔⓧ 862.29, 862.39-862.9, 875.0-875.1, 879.8-879.9, 929.0-929.9,
　　　　　958.7-958.99, 959.8-959.9

● 863　**Injury to gastrointestinal tract**
　　　Trauma to any structure from the stomach to the anus

> **Excludes**　*anal sphincter laceration during delivery (664.2)*
> 　　　　　　*bile duct (868.0–868.1 with fifth-digit 2)*
> 　　　　　　*gallbladder (868.0–868.1 with fifth-digit 2)*

　　863.0　**Stomach, without mention of open wound into cavity**🦠
　　　　Ⓔⓧ 729.73, 863.0-863.1, 863.80, 863.89-863.90, 863.99, 868.00,
　　　　　868.03-868.10, 868.13-869.1, 879.2-879.9, 929.0-929.9, 958.8,
　　　　　958.93-958.99, 959.8-959.9

　　863.1　**Stomach, with open wound into cavity**🦠
　　　　Ⓔⓧ 863.0-863.1, 863.80, 863.89-863.90, 863.99, 868.00, 868.03-868.10,
　　　　　868.13-869.1, 879.2-879.9, 929.0-929.9, 958.8-958.99, 959.8-959.9

● 863.2 Small intestine, without mention of open wound into cavity

　863.20 Small intestine, unspecified site 🐾
　　Ex: 729.73, 863.0-863.1, 863.80, 863.89-863.90, 863.99, 868.00, 868.03-868.10, 868.13-869.1, 879.2-879.9, 929.0-929.9, 958.8, 958.93-958.99, 959.8-959.9

　863.21 Duodenum 🐾
　　Ex: 729.73, 863.20-863.39, 863.80, 863.89-863.90, 863.99, 868.00, 868.03-868.10, 868.13-869.1, 879.2-879.9, 929.0-929.9, 958.8, 958.93-958.99, 959.8-959.9

　863.29 Other 🐾
　　Ex: 729.73, 863.20-863.39, 863.80, 863.89-863.90, 863.99, 868.00, 868.03-868.10, 868.13-869.1, 879.2-879.9, 929.0-929.9, 958.8, 958.93-958.99, 959.8-959.9

● 863.3 Small intestine, with open wound into cavity

　863.30 Small intestine, unspecified site 🐾
　　Ex: 863.20-863.39, 863.80, 863.89-863.90, 863.99, 868.00, 868.03-868.10, 868.13-869.1, 879.2-879.9, 929.0-929.9, 958.8-958.99, 959.8-959.9

　863.31 Duodenum 🐾
　　Ex: 863.21, 863.31-863.39, 863.80, 863.89-863.90, 863.99, 868.00, 868.03-868.10, 868.13-869.1, 879.2-879.9, 929.0-929.9, 958.8-959.9

　863.39 Other 🐾
　　Ex: 863.20-863.39, 863.80, 863.89-863.90, 863.99, 868.00, 868.03-868.10, 868.13-869.1, 879.2-879.9, 929.0-929.9, 958.8-958.99, 959.8-959.9

● 863.4 Colon or rectum, without mention of open wound into cavity

　863.40 Colon, unspecified site 🐾
　　Ex: 729.73, 863.40-863.80, 863.89-863.90, 863.99, 868.00, 868.03-868.10, 868.13-869.1, 879.2-879.9, 929.0-929.9, 958.8, 958.93-958.99, 959.8-959.9

　863.41 Ascending [right] colon 🐾
　　Ex: 729.73, 863.40-863.80, 863.89-863.90, 863.99, 868.00, 868.03-868.10, 868.13-869.1, 879.2-879.9, 929.0-929.9, 958.8, 958.93-958.99, 959.8-959.9

　863.42 Transverse colon 🐾
　　Ex: 729.73, 863.40-863.80, 863.89-863.90, 863.99, 868.00, 868.03-868.10, 868.13-869.1, 879.2-879.9, 929.0-929.9, 958.8, 958.93-958.99, 959.8-959.9

　863.43 Descending [left] colon 🐾
　　Ex: 729.73, 863.40-863.80, 863.89-863.90, 863.99, 868.00, 868.03-868.10, 868.13-869.1, 879.2-879.9, 929.0-929.9, 958.8, 958.93-958.99, 959.8-959.9

　863.44 Sigmoid colon 🐾
　　Ex: 729.73, 863.40-863.80, 863.89-863.90, 863.99, 868.00, 868.03-868.10, 868.13-869.1, 879.2-879.9, 929.0-929.9, 958.8, 958.93-958.99, 959.8-959.9

　863.45 Rectum 🐾
　　Ex: 729.73, 863.40-863.80, 863.89-863.90, 863.99, 868.00, 868.03-868.10, 868.13-869.1, 879.2-879.9, 929.0-929.9, 958.8, 958.93-958.99, 959.8-959.9

　863.46 Multiple sites in colon and rectum 🐾
　　Ex: 729.73, 863.40-863.80, 863.89-863.90, 863.99, 868.00, 868.03-868.10, 868.13-869.1, 879.2-879.9, 929.0-929.9, 958.8, 958.93-958.99, 959.8-959.9

　863.49 Other 🐾
　　Ex: 729.73, 863.40-863.80, 863.89-863.90, 863.99, 868.00, 868.03-868.10, 868.13-869.1, 879.2-879.9, 929.0-929.9, 958.8, 958.93-958.99, 959.8-959.9

● 863.5 Colon or rectum, with open wound into cavity

　863.50 Colon, unspecified site 🐾
　　Ex: 863.40-863.80, 863.89-863.90, 863.99, 868.00, 868.03-868.10, 868.13-869.1, 879.2-879.9, 929.0-929.9, 958.8-958.99, 959.8-959.9

　863.51 Ascending [right] colon 🐾
　　Ex: 863.40-863.80, 863.89-863.90, 863.99, 868.00, 868.03-868.10, 868.13-869.1, 879.2-879.9, 929.0-929.9, 958.8-958.99, 959.8-959.9

　863.52 Transverse colon 🐾
　　Ex: 863.40-863.80, 863.89-863.90, 863.99, 868.00, 868.03-868.10, 868.13-869.1, 879.2-879.9, 929.0-929.9, 958.8-958.99, 959.8-959.9

　863.53 Descending [left] colon 🐾
　　Ex: 863.40-863.80, 863.89-863.90, 863.99, 868.00, 868.03-868.10, 868.13-869.1, 879.2-879.9, 929.0-929.9, 958.8-958.99, 959.8-959.9

　863.54 Sigmoid colon 🐾
　　Ex: 863.40-863.80, 863.89-863.90, 863.99, 868.00, 868.03-868.10, 868.13-869.1, 879.2-879.9, 929.0-929.9, 958.8-958.99, 959.8-959.9

　863.55 Rectum 🐾
　　Ex: 863.40-863.80, 863.89-863.90, 863.99, 868.00, 868.03-868.10, 868.13-869.1, 879.2-879.9, 929.0-929.9, 958.8-958.99, 959.8-959.9

　863.56 Multiple sites in colon and rectum 🐾
　　Ex: 863.40-863.80, 863.89-863.90, 863.99, 868.00, 868.03-868.10, 868.13-869.1, 879.2-879.9, 929.0-929.9, 958.8-958.99, 959.8-959.9

　863.59 Other 🐾
　　Ex: 863.40-863.80, 863.89-863.90, 863.99, 868.00, 868.03-868.10, 868.13-869.1, 879.2-879.9, 929.0-929.9, 958.8-958.99, 959.8-959.9

● 863.8 Other and unspecified gastrointestinal sites, without mention of open wound into cavity

　863.80 Gastrointestinal tract, unspecified site 🐾
　　Ex: 729.73, 863.0-863.80, 863.89-863.90, 863.99, 868.00, 868.03-868.10, 868.13-869.1, 879.2-879.9, 929.0-929.9, 958.8, 958.93-958.99, 959.8-959.9

　863.81 Pancreas, head 🐾
　　Ex: 729.73, 863.80-863.84, 863.91-863.94, 863.99, 868.00, 868.03-868.10, 868.13-869.1, 879.2-879.9, 929.0-929.9, 958.8, 958.93-958.99, 959.8-959.9

　863.82 Pancreas, body 🐾
　　Ex: 729.73, 863.80-863.84, 863.91-863.94, 863.99, 868.00, 868.03-868.10, 868.13-869.1, 879.2-879.9, 929.0-929.9, 958.8, 958.93-958.99, 959.8-959.9

　863.83 Pancreas, tail 🐾
　　Ex: 729.73, 863.80-863.84, 863.91-863.94, 863.99, 868.00, 868.03-868.10, 868.13-869.1, 879.2-879.9, 929.0-929.9, 958.8, 958.93-958.99, 959.8-959.9

　863.84 Pancreas, multiple and unspecified sites 🐾
　　Ex: 729.73, 863.80-863.84, 863.91-863.94, 863.99, 868.00, 868.03-868.10, 868.13-869.1, 879.2-879.9, 929.0-929.9, 958.8, 958.93-958.99, 959.8-959.9

　863.85 Appendix 🐾
　　Ex: 729.73, 863.80-863.84, 863.91-863.94, 863.99, 868.00, 868.03-868.10, 868.13-869.1, 879.2-879.9, 929.0-929.9, 958.8, 958.93-958.99, 959.8-959.9

　863.89 Other 🐾
　　Intestine NOS
　　Ex: 729.73, 863.80-863.84, 863.91-863.94, 863.99, 868.00, 868.03-868.10, 868.13-869.1, 879.2-879.9, 929.0-929.9, 958.8, 958.93-958.99, 959.8-959.9

◀ New　◀▥ Revised　deleted Deleted　● Unacceptable Principal Diagnosis　● Use Additional Digit(s)
▶ Manifestation Code　OGCR Official Guidelines　Coding Clinic　Excludes　Includes　Use additional　Code first　Omit code

INJURY AND POISONING (800–999)

● 863.9 **Other and unspecified gastrointestinal sites, with open wound into cavity**

  863.90 **Gastrointestinal tract, unspecified site**
      (Ex:) 863.80-863.84, 863.89-863.94, 863.99, 868.00, 868.03-868.10, 868.13-869.1, 879.2-879.9, 929.0-929.9, 958.8-958.99, 959.8-959.9

  863.91 **Pancreas, head**
      (Ex:) 863.80-863.84, 863.89-863.94, 863.99, 868.00, 868.03-868.10, 868.13-869.1, 879.2-879.9, 929.0-929.9, 958.8-958.99, 959.8-959.9

  863.92 **Pancreas, body**
      (Ex:) 863.80-863.84, 863.89-863.94, 863.99, 868.00, 868.03-868.10, 868.13-869.1, 879.2-879.9, 929.0-929.9, 958.8-958.99, 959.8-959.9

  863.93 **Pancreas, tail**
      (Ex:) 863.80-863.84, 863.89-863.94, 863.99, 868.00, 868.03-868.10, 868.13-869.1, 879.2-879.9, 929.0-929.9, 958.8-958.99, 959.8-959.9

  863.94 **Pancreas, multiple and unspecified sites**
      (Ex:) 863.80-863.84, 863.89-863.94, 863.99, 868.00, 868.03-868.10, 868.13-869.1, 879.2-879.9, 929.0-929.9, 958.8-958.99, 959.8-959.9

  863.95 **Appendix**
      (Ex:) 863.80, 863.85, 863.95-863.99, 868.00, 868.03-868.10, 868.13-869.1, 879.2-879.9, 929.0-929.9, 958.8-958.99, 959.8-959.9

  863.99 **Other**
      (Ex:) 863.80, 863.99, 868.00, 868.03-868.10, 868.13-869.1, 879.2-879.9, 929.0-929.9, 958.8-958.99, 959.8-959.9

● 864 **Injury to liver**

  The following fifth-digit subclassification is for use with category 864:

  > 0 **unspecified injury**
  > 1 **hematoma and contusion**
  > 2 **laceration, minor**
  >   Laceration involving capsule only, or without significant involvement of hepatic parenchyma [i.e., less than 1 cm deep]
  > 3 **laceration, moderate**
  >   Laceration involving parenchyma but without major disruption of parenchyma [i.e., less than 10 cm long and less than 3 cm deep]
  > 4 **laceration, major**
  >   Laceration with significant disruption of hepatic parenchyma [i.e., 10 cm long and 3 cm deep]
  >   Multiple moderate lacerations, with or without hematoma
  >   Stellate lacerations of liver
  > 5 **laceration, unspecified**
  > 9 **other**

● 864.0 **Without mention of open wound into**
  [0-5,9] **cavity 0-2,5,9, 3,4**
      (Ex:) 863.80, 863.85, 863.95-863.99, 868.00, 868.03-868.10, 868.13-869.1, 879.2-879.9, 929.0-929.9, 958.8-958.99, 959.8-959.9

● 864.1 **With open wound into cavity**
  [0-5,9] (Ex:) 863.80, 863.85, 863.95-863.99, 868.00, 868.03-868.10, 868.13-869.1, 879.2-879.9, 929.0-929.9, 958.8-958.99, 959.8-959.9

● 865 **Injury to spleen**

  The following fifth-digit subclassification is for use with category 865:

  > 0 **unspecified injury**
  > 1 **hematoma without rupture of capsule**
  > 2 **capsular tears, without major disruption of parenchyma**
  > 3 **laceration extending into parenchyma**
  > 4 **massive parenchymal disruption**
  > 9 **other**

● 865.0 **Without mention of open wound into**
  [0-4,9] **cavity 0-2,9, 3,4**
      (Ex:) 865.00-865.19, 868.00, 868.03-868.10, 868.13-869.1, 879.2-879.9, 929.0-929.9, 958.8-958.99, 959.8-959.9

● 865.1 **With open wound into cavity**
  [0-4,9] (Ex:) 865.00-865.19, 868.00, 868.03-868.10, 868.13-869.1, 879.2-879.9, 929.0-929.9, 958.8-958.99, 959.8-959.9

● 866 **Injury to kidney**

  The following fifth-digit subclassification is for use with category 866:

  > 0 **unspecified injury**
  > 1 **hematoma without rupture of capsule**
  > 2 **laceration**
  > 3 **complete disruption of kidney parenchyma**

  Excludes *acute kidney injury (nontraumatic) (584.9)*

● 866.0 **Without mention of open wound into cavity 0-2, 3**
  [0-3] (Ex:) 866.00-866.13, 868.00, 868.03-868.10, 868.13-869.1, 879.2-879.9, 929.0-929.9, 958.8-958.99, 959.8-959.9
      Coding Clinic: 2008, Q4, P192-193

● 866.1 **With open wound into cavity**
  [0-3] (Ex:) 866.00-866.13, 868.00, 868.03-868.10, 868.13-869.1, 879.2-879.9, 929.0-929.9, 958.8-958.99, 959.8-959.9

● 867 **Injury to pelvic organs**

  Excludes *injury during delivery (664.0–665.9)*

  867.0 **Bladder and urethra, without mention of open wound into cavity**
      (Ex:) 867.0-867.1, 867.6-868.00, 868.03-868.10, 868.13-869.1, 879.2-879.9, 929.0-929.9, 958.8-958.99, 959.8-959.9
      Coding Clinic: 2009, Q1, P8; 1985, Nov-Dec, P15; 1984, Nov-Dec, P15

  867.1 **Bladder and urethra, with open wound into cavity**
      (Ex:) 867.0-867.1, 867.6-868.00, 868.03-868.10, 868.13-869.1, 879.2-879.9, 929.0-929.9, 958.8-958.99, 959.8-959.9
      Coding Clinic: 1984, Nov-Dec, P12

  867.2 **Ureter, without mention of open wound into cavity**
      (Ex:) 867.2-867.3, 867.6-868.00, 868.03-868.10, 868.13-86.91, 879.2-879.9, 929.0-929.9, 958.8-958.99, 959.8-959.9

  867.3 **Ureter, with open wound into cavity**
      (Ex:) 867.2-867.3, 867.6-868.00, 868.03-868.10, 868.13-869.1, 879.2-879.9, 929.0-929.9, 958.8-958.99, 959.8-959.9

  867.4 **Uterus, without mention of open wound into cavity ♀**
      (Ex:) 867.4-868.00, 868.03-868.10, 868.13-869.1, 879.2-879.9, 929.0-929.9, 958.8-958.99, 959.8-959.9

INJURY AND POISONING (800–999)

867.5 Uterus, with open wound into cavity ♀ ⚲
(Ex:) 867.4-868.00, 868.03-868.10, 868.13-869.1, 879.2-879.9, 929.0-929.9, 958.8-958.99, 959.8-959.9

867.6 Other specified pelvic organs, without mention of open wound into cavity ⚲
Fallopian tube
Ovary
Prostate
Seminal vesicle
Vas deferens
(Ex:) 867.6-868.00, 868.03-868.10, 868.13-869.1, 879.2-879.9, 929.0-929.9, 958.8-958.99, 959.8-959.9

867.7 Other specified pelvic organs, with open wound into cavity ⚲
(Ex:) 867.6-868.00, 868.03-868.10, 868.13-869.1, 879.2-879.9, 929.0-929.9, 958.8-958.99, 959.8-959.9

867.8 Unspecified pelvic organ, without mention of open wound into cavity ⚲
(Ex:) 867.6-868.00, 868.03-868.10, 868.13-869.1, 879.2-879.9, 929.0-929.9, 958.8-958.99, 959.8-959.9

867.9 Unspecified pelvic organ, with open wound into cavity ⚲
(Ex:) 867.6-868.00, 868.03-868.10, 868.13-869.1, 879.2-879.9, 929.0-929.9, 958.8-958.99, 959.8-959.9

● **868 Injury to other intra-abdominal organs**

The following fifth-digit subclassification is for use with category 868:

> 0   unspecified intra-abdominal organ
> 1   adrenal gland
> 2   bile duct and gallbladder
> 3   peritoneum
> 4   retroperitoneum
> 9   other and multiple intra-abdominal organs

● **868.0 Without mention of open wound into cavity ⚲**
[0-4,9]   For codes **868.00, 868.03-868.09:** (Ex:) 868.00, 868.03-868.10, 868.13-869.1, 879.2-879.9, 929.0-929.9, 958.8-958.99, 959.8-959.9;
For code **868.01:** (Ex:) 868.00-868.01, 868.03-868.11, 868.13-869.1, 879.2-879.9, 929.0-929.9, 958.8-958.99, 959.8-959.9;
For code **868.02:** (Ex:) 868.00, 868.02-868.10, 868.13-869.1, 879.2-879.9, 929.0-929.9, 958.8-958.99, 959.8-959.9

● **868.1 With open wound into cavity ⚲**
[0-4,9]   For codes **868.10, 868.13-868.19:** (Ex:) 868.00, 868.03-868.10, 868.13-869.1, 879.2-879.9, 929.0-929.9, 958.8-958.99, 959.8-959.9;
For code **868.11:** (Ex:) 868.00-868.01, 868.03-868.11, 868.13-86.91, 879.2-879.9, 929.0-929.9, 958.8-958.99, 959.8-959.9;
For code **868.12:** (Ex:) 868.00, 868.03-868.10, 868.12-86.91, 879.2-879.9, 929.0-929.9, 958.8-958.99, 959.8-959.9

● **869 Internal injury to unspecified or ill-defined organs**

Includes	internal injury NOS
	multiple internal injury NOS

869.0 Without mention of open wound into cavity ⚲
(Ex:) 868.00, 868.03-868.10, 868.13-869.1, 879.2-879.9, 929.0-929.9, 958.8-958.99, 959.8-959.9

869.1 With open wound into cavity ⚲
(Ex:) 868.00, 868.03-868.10, 868.13-869.1, 879.2-879.9, 929.0-929.9, 958.8-958.99, 959.8-959.9

OPEN WOUNDS (870–897)

Includes	animal bite
	avulsion
	cut
	laceration
	puncture wound
	traumatic amputation

Excludes	*burn (940.0–949.5)*
	crushing (925–929.9)
	puncture of internal organs (860.0–869.1)
	superficial injury (910.0–919.9)
	that incidental to:
	dislocation (830.0–839.9)
	fracture (800.0–829.1)
	internal injury (860.0–869.1)
	intracranial injury (851.0–854.1)

Note: The description "complicated" used in the fourth-digit subdivisions includes those with mention of delayed healing, delayed treatment, foreign body, or infection.

~~Use additional code to identify infection~~

OPEN WOUND OF HEAD, NECK, AND TRUNK (870–879)

● **870 Open wound of ocular adnexa**

870.0 Laceration of skin of eyelid and periocular area

870.1 Laceration of eyelid, full-thickness, not involving lacrimal passages

870.2 Laceration of eyelid involving lacrimal passages ⚲
(Ex:) 870.0-871.9, 879.8-879.9, 929.0-929.9, 958.8, 959.8-959.9

870.3 Penetrating wound of orbit, without mention of foreign body ⚲
(Ex:) 870.0-871.9, 879.8-879.9, 929.0-929.9, 958.8-958.99, 959.8-959.9

870.4 Penetrating wound of orbit with foreign body ⚲

Excludes	*retained (old) foreign body in orbit (376.6)*

(Ex:) 870.0-871.9, 879.8-879.9, 929.0-929.9, 958.8-958.99, 959.8-959.9

870.8 Other specified open wounds of ocular adnexa ⚲
(Ex:) 870.0-871.9, 879.8-879.9, 929.0-929.9, 958.8-958.99, 959.8-959.9

870.9 Unspecified open wound of ocular adnexa ⚲
(Ex:) 870.0-871.9, 879.8-879.9, 929.0-929.9, 958.8-958.99, 959.8-959.9

● **871 Open wound of eyeball**

Excludes	*2nd cranial nerve [optic] injury (950.0–950.9)*
	3rd cranial nerve [oculomotor] injury (951.0)

871.0 Ocular laceration without prolapse of intraocular tissue ⚲
(Ex:) 870.0-871.9, 879.8-879.9, 929.0-929.9, 958.8-958.99, 959.8-959.9
Coding Clinic: 1996, Q3, P7

871.1 Ocular laceration with prolapse or exposure of intraocular tissue ⚲
(Ex:) 870.0-871.9, 879.8-879.9, 929.0-929.9, 958.8-958.99, 959.8-959.9

871.2 Rupture of eye with partial loss of intraocular tissue ⚲
(Ex:) 870.0-871.9, 879.8-879.9, 929.0-929.9, 958.8-958.99, 959.8-959.9

871.3 Avulsion of eye ⚲
Traumatic enucleation
(Ex:) 870.0-871.9, 879.8-879.9, 929.0-929.9, 958.8-958.99, 959.8-959.9

871.4 Unspecified laceration of eye

◀ New   ⬅ Revised   ~~deleted~~ Deleted   ● Unacceptable Principal Diagnosis   ⚲ Use Additional Digit(s)
▶ Manifestation Code   **OGCR** Official Guidelines   **Coding Clinic**   Excludes   Includes   Use additional   Code first   Omit code

871.5   **Penetration of eyeball with magnetic foreign body** ⬥

> | **Excludes** | *retained (old) magnetic foreign body in globe (360.50–360.59)* |
> | --- | --- |

     ⒺⓍ 870.0-871.9, 879.8-879.9, 929.0-929.9, 958.8-958.99, 959.8-959.9

871.6   **Penetration of eyeball with (nonmagnetic) foreign body** ⬥

> | **Excludes** | *retained (old) (nonmagnetic) foreign body in globe (360.60–360.69)* |
> | --- | --- |

     ⒺⓍ 870.0-871.9, 879.8-879.9, 929.0-929.9, 958.8-958.99, 959.8-959.9

871.7   **Unspecified ocular penetration**

871.9   **Unspecified open wound of eyeball** ⬥

     ⒺⓍ 870.0-871.9, 879.8-879.9, 929.0-929.9, 958.8-958.99, 959.8-959.9

● 872   **Open wound of ear**

   ● 872.0   **External ear, without mention of complication**

     872.00   External ear, unspecified site

     872.01   Auricle, ear
          Pinna

     872.02   Auditory canal

   ● 872.1   **External ear, complicated**

     872.10   External ear, unspecified site

     872.11   Auricle, ear

     872.12   Auditory canal ⬥
         ⒺⓍ 872.00-872.9, 879.8-879.9, 929.0-929.9, 958.8, 959.8-959.9

   ● 872.6   **Other specified parts of ear, without mention of complication**

     872.61   Ear drum ⬥
          Drumhead
          Tympanic membrane
         ⒺⓍ 872.00-872.9, 879.8-879.9, 929.0-929.9, 958.8, 959.8-959.9

     872.62   Ossicles ⬥
         ⒺⓍ 872.00-872.9, 879.8-879.9, 929.0-929.9, 958.8, 959.8-959.9

     872.63   Eustachian tube ⬥
         ⒺⓍ 872.00-872.9, 879.8-879.9, 929.0-929.9, 958.8, 959.8-959.9

     872.64   Cochlea ⬥
         ⒺⓍ 872.00-872.9, 879.8-879.9, 929.0-929.9, 958.8, 959.8-959.9

     872.69   Other and multiple sites ⬥
         ⒺⓍ 872.00-872.9, 879.8-879.9, 929.0-929.9, 958.8, 959.8-959.9

   ● 872.7   **Other specified parts of ear, complicated**

     872.71   Ear drum ⬥
         ⒺⓍ 872.00-872.9, 879.8-879.9, 929.0-929.9, 958.8, 959.8-959.9

     872.72   Ossicles ⬥
         ⒺⓍ 872.00-872.9, 879.8-879.9, 929.0-929.9, 958.8-958.99, 959.8-959.9

     872.73   Eustachian tube ⬥
         ⒺⓍ 872.00-872.9, 879.8-879.9, 929.0-929.9, 958.8-958.99, 959.8-959.9

     872.74   Cochlea ⬥
         ⒺⓍ 872.00-872.9, 879.8-879.9, 929.0-929.9, 958.8-958.99, 959.8-959.9

     872.79   Other and multiple sites ⬥
         ⒺⓍ 872.00-872.9, 879.8-879.9, 929.0-929.9, 958.8, 959.8-959.9

   872.8   **Ear, part unspecified, without mention of complication**
       Ear NOS

   872.9   **Ear, part unspecified, complicated**

● 873   **Other open wound of head**

   873.0   **Scalp, without mention of complication**

   873.1   **Scalp, complicated**

   ● 873.2   **Nose, without mention of complication**

     873.20   Nose, unspecified site

     873.21   Nasal septum

     873.22   Nasal cavity

     873.23   Nasal sinus ⬥
         ⒺⓍ 873.20-873.39, 879.8-879.9, 929.0-929.9, 958.8, 959.8-959.9

     873.29   Multiple sites

   ● 873.3   **Nose, complicated**

     873.30   Nose, unspecified site

     873.31   Nasal septum

     873.32   Nasal cavity

     873.33   Nasal sinus ⬥
         ⒺⓍ 873.20-873.39, 879.8-879.9, 929.0-929.9, 958.8-958.99, 959.8-959.9

     873.39   Multiple sites

   ● 873.4   **Face, without mention of complication**

     873.40   Face, unspecified site

     873.41   Cheek

     873.42   Forehead
          Eyebrow
          Coding Clinic: 1996, Q4, P43-44

     873.43   Lip

     873.44   Jaw

     873.49   Other and multiple sites

   ● 873.5   **Face, complicated**

     873.50   Face, unspecified site

     873.51   Cheek

     873.52   Forehead

     873.53   Lip

     873.54   Jaw

     873.59   Other and multiple sites

   ● 873.6   **Internal structures of mouth, without mention of complication**

     873.60   Mouth, unspecified site

     873.61   Buccal mucosa

     873.62   Gum (alveolar process)

     873.63   Tooth (broken) (fractured) (due to trauma)

> | **Excludes** | *cracked tooth (521.81)* |
> | --- | --- |

         Coding Clinic: 2004, Q1, P17

     873.64   Tongue and floor of mouth

     873.65   Palate

     873.69   Other and multiple sites

N Newborn Age: 0   **P** Pediatric Age: 0–17   **M** Maternity Age: 12–55   **A** Adult Age: 15–124   ♀ Females Only   ♂ Males Only

ⒺⓍ CC Exclusions   ⬥ Complication\Comorbidity   ⬥ Major C\C   ⬥ Present on Admission Requirement   ⬥ Hospital-Acquired Condition

1091

INJURY AND POISONING (800–999)

● **873.7 Internal structures of mouth, complicated**

    873.70 Mouth, unspecified site

    873.71 Buccal mucosa

    873.72 Gum (alveolar process)

    873.73 Tooth (broken) (fractured) (due to trauma)

         | Excludes | *cracked tooth (521.81)*

         Coding Clinic: 2004, Q1, P17

    873.74 Tongue and floor of mouth

    873.75 Palate

    873.79 Other and multiple sites

  873.8 Other and unspecified open wound of head without mention of complication

    Head NOS

  873.9 Other and unspecified open wound of head, complicated

● **874 Open wound of neck**

  ● **874.0 Larynx and trachea, without mention of complication**

    874.00 Larynx with trachea 🕊
         (Ex:) 847.0, 874.00-874.12, 874.8-874.9, 879.8-879.9, 929.0-929.9, 958.8-958.99, 959.8-959.9

    874.01 Larynx 🕊
         (Ex:) 847.0, 874.00-874.12, 874.8-874.9, 879.8-879.9, 929.0-929.9, 958.8-958.99, 959.8-959.9

    874.02 Trachea 🕊
         (Ex:) 847.0, 874.00-874.12, 874.8-874.9, 879.8-879.9, 929.0-929.9, 958.8-958.99, 959.8-959.9

  ● **874.1 Larynx and trachea, complicated**

    874.10 Larynx with trachea 🕊
         (Ex:) 847.0, 874.00-874.12, 874.8-874.9, 879.8-879.9, 929.0-929.9, 958.8-958.99, 959.8-959.9

    874.11 Larynx 🕊
         (Ex:) 847.0, 874.00-874.12, 874.8-874.9, 879.8-879.9, 929.0-929.9, 958.8-958.99, 959.8-959.9

    874.12 Trachea 🕊
         (Ex:) 847.0, 874.00-874.12, 874.8-874.9, 879.8-879.9, 929.0-929.9, 958.8-958.99, 959.8-959.9

  874.2 Thyroid gland, without mention of complication 🕊
     (Ex:) 847.0, 874.2-874.3, 874.8-874.9, 879.8-879.9, 929.0-929.9, 958.8, 959.8-959.9

  874.3 Thyroid gland, complicated 🕊
     (Ex:) 847.0, 874.2-874.3, 874.8-874.9, 879.8-879.9, 929.0-929.9, 958.8-958.99, 959.8-959.9

  874.4 Pharynx, without mention of complication 🕊
    Cervical esophagus
     (Ex:) 847.0, 874.4-874.9, 879.8-879.9, 929.0-929.9, 958.8, 959.8-959.9

  874.5 Pharynx, complicated 🕊
     (Ex:) 847.0, 874.4-874.9, 879.8-879.9, 929.0-929.9, 958.8-958.99, 959.8-959.9

  874.8 Other and unspecified parts, without mention of complication

    Nape of neck   Throat NOS
    Supraclavicular region

  874.9 Other and unspecified parts, complicated

● **875 Open wound of chest (wall)**

  | Excludes | *open wound into thoracic cavity (860.0–862.9)*
         traumatic pneumothorax and hemothorax (860.1, 860.3, 860.5)

  Coding Clinic: 1995, Q3, P17

  875.0 Without mention of complication 🕊
     (Ex:) 847.1, 862.29, 862.39-862.9, 875.0-875.1, 879.8-879.9, 929.0-929.9, 958.7-958.99, 959.8-959.9

  875.1 Complicated 🕊
     (Ex:) 847.1, 862.29, 862.39-862.9, 875.0-875.1, 879.8-879.9, 929.0-929.9, 958.7-958.99, 959.8-959.9

● **876 Open wound of back**

  | Includes | loin
                lumbar region

  | Excludes | *open wound into thoracic cavity (860.0–862.9)*
         traumatic pneumothorax and hemothorax (860.1, 860.3, 860.5)

  Coding Clinic: 1995, Q3, P17

  876.0 Without mention of complication
    Coding Clinic: 1993, Q2, P4-5

  876.1 Complicated

● **877 Open wound of buttock**

  | Includes | sacroiliac region

  877.0 Without mention of complication

  877.1 Complicated

● **878 Open wound of genital organs (external), including traumatic amputation**

  | Excludes | *injury during delivery (664.0–665.9)*
         internal genital organs (867.0–867.9)

  878.0 Penis, without mention of complication ♂

  878.1 Penis, complicated ♂

  878.2 Scrotum and testes, without mention of complication ♂

  878.3 Scrotum and testes, complicated ♂

  878.4 Vulva, without mention of complication ♀
    Labium (majus) (minus)

  878.5 Vulva, complicated ♀

  878.6 Vagina, without mention of complication ♀

  878.7 Vagina, complicated ♀

  878.8 Other and unspecified parts, without mention of complication

  878.9 Other and unspecified parts, complicated

● **879 Open wound of other and unspecified sites, except limbs**

  879.0 Breast, without mention of complication

  879.1 Breast, complicated

  879.2 Abdominal wall, anterior, without mention of complication

    Abdominal wall NOS   Pubic region
    Epigastric region   Umbilical region
    Hypogastric region

  879.3 Abdominal wall, anterior, complicated

INJURY AND POISONING (800–999)

◀ New   ◀▥ Revised   ~~deleted~~ Deleted   ● Unacceptable Principal Diagnosis   ● Use Additional Digit(s)
▶ Manifestation Code   **OGCR** Official Guidelines   **Coding Clinic** | Excludes | Includes   Use additional   Code first   Omit code

879.4 Abdominal wall, lateral, without mention of complication
Flank	Iliac (region)
Groin	Inguinal region
Hypochondrium	

879.5 Abdominal wall, lateral, complicated

879.6 Other and unspecified parts of trunk, without mention of complication
Pelvic region	Trunk NOS
Perineum	

879.7 Other and unspecified parts of trunk, complicated

879.8 Open wound(s) (multiple) of unspecified site(s) without mention of complication
Multiple open wounds NOS
Open wound NOS

879.9 Open wound(s) (multiple) of unspecified site(s), complicated

OPEN WOUND OF UPPER LIMB (880–887)

● **880 Open wound of shoulder and upper arm**

The following fifth-digit subclassification is for use with category 880:

> 0   shoulder region
> 1   scapular region
> 2   axillary region
> 3   upper arm
> 9   multiple sites

● **880.0 Without mention of complication**
[0-3,9]

● **880.1 Complicated**
[0-3,9]   **Coding Clinic: 2006, Q2, P7**

● **880.2 With tendon involvement**🕭
[0-3,9]   (Ex:) 880.00-880.29

● **881 Open wound of elbow, forearm, and wrist**

The following fifth-digit subclassification is for use with category 881:

> 0   forearm
> 1   elbow
> 2   wrist

● **881.0 Without mention of complication**
[0-2]

● **881.1 Complicated**
[0-2]

● **881.2 With tendon involvement**🕭
[0-2]   (Ex:) 881.00-881.22

● **882 Open wound of hand except finger(s) alone**

882.0 Without mention of complication

882.1 Complicated
    Coding Clinic: 2008, Q4, P149-152

882.2 With tendon involvement🕭
    (Ex:) 882.0-882.2

● **883 Open wound of finger(s)**

   Includes   fingernail
              thumb (nail)

883.0 Without mention of complication
Avulsion of fingernail reported with this code

883.1 Complicated

883.2 With tendon involvement🕭
    (Ex:) 883.0-883.2

● **884 Multiple and unspecified open wound of upper limb**

   Includes   arm NOS
              multiple sites of one upper limb
              upper limb NOS

884.0 Without mention of complication

884.1 Complicated

884.2 With tendon involvement🕭
    (Ex:) 884.0-884.2

● **885 Traumatic amputation of thumb (complete) (partial)**

   Includes   thumb(s) (with finger(s) of either hand)

885.0 Without mention of complication
    Coding Clinic: 2003, Q1, P7

885.1 Complicated

● **886 Traumatic amputation of other finger(s) (complete) (partial)**

   Includes   finger(s) of one or both hands, without
                 mention of thumb(s)

886.0 Without mention of complication

886.1 Complicated

● **887 Traumatic amputation of arm and hand (complete) (partial)**

887.0 Unilateral, below elbow, without mention of complication🕭
    (Ex:) 880.00-887.7, 929.0-929.9, 958.8-958.99, 959.8-959.9

887.1 Unilateral, below elbow, complicated🕭
    (Ex:) 880.00-887.7, 929.0-929.9, 958.8-958.99, 959.8-959.9

887.2 Unilateral, at or above elbow, without mention of complication🕭
    (Ex:) 880.00-887.7, 929.0-929.9, 958.8-958.99, 959.8-959.9

887.3 Unilateral, at or above elbow, complicated🕭
    (Ex:) 880.00-887.7, 929.0-929.9, 958.8-958.99, 959.8-959.9

887.4 Unilateral, level not specified, without mention of complication🕭
    (Ex:) 880.00-887.7, 929.0-929.9, 958.8-958.99, 959.8-959.9

887.5 Unilateral, level not specified, complicated🕭
    (Ex:) 880.00-887.7, 929.0-929.9, 958.8-958.99, 959.8-959.9

887.6 Bilateral [any level], without mention of complication🕭
One hand and other arm
    (Ex:) 880.00-887.7, 929.0-929.9, 958.8-958.99, 959.8-959.9

887.7 Bilateral [any level], complicated🕭
    (Ex:) 880.00-887.7, 929.0-929.9, 958.8-958.99, 959.8-959.9,

N Newborn Age: 0	**P** Pediatric Age: 0–17	**M** Maternity Age: 12–55	**A** Adult Age: 15–124	♀ Females Only	♂ Males Only

(Ex:) CC Exclusions   🕭 Complication\Comorbidity   🕭 Major C\C   🕭 Present on Admission Requirement   🕭 Hospital-Acquired Condition   **1093**

INJURY AND POISONING (800–999)

OPEN WOUND OF LOWER LIMB (890–897)

● **890　Open wound of hip and thigh**

890.0　Without mention of complication

890.1　Complicated

890.2　With tendon involvement ✿
　　　Ex: 890.0–890.2

● **891　Open wound of knee, leg [except thigh], and ankle**

Includes	leg NOS
	multiple sites of leg, except thigh

Excludes	that of thigh (890.0–890.2)
	with multiple sites of lower limb (894.0–894.2)

891.0　Without mention of complication

891.1　Complicated
　　　Coding Clinic: 2008, Q4, P69-73

891.2　With tendon involvement ✿
　　　Ex: 891.0–891.2

● **892　Open wound of foot except toe(s) alone**

Includes	heel

892.0　Without mention of complication

892.1　Complicated
　　　Coding Clinic: 1985, Sept-Oct, P10

892.2　With tendon involvement ✿
　　　Ex: 892.0–892.2

● **893　Open wound of toe(s)**

Includes	toenail

893.0　Without mention of complication

893.1　Complicated
　　　Coding Clinic: 2008, Q4, P69-73

893.2　With tendon involvement ✿
　　　Ex: 893.0–893.2

● **894　Multiple and unspecified open wound of lower limb**

Includes	lower limb NOS
	multiple sites of one lower limb, with thigh

894.0　Without mention of complication

894.1　Complicated

894.2　With tendon involvement ✿
　　　Ex: 894.0–894.2

● **895　Traumatic amputation of toe(s) (complete) (partial)**

Includes	toe(s) of one or both feet

895.0　Without mention of complication

895.1　Complicated

● **896　Traumatic amputation of foot (complete) (partial)**

896.0　Unilateral, without mention of complication ✿
　　　Ex: 890.0–897.7, 929.0–929.9, 958.8–958.99, 959.8–959.9

896.1　Unilateral, complicated ✿
　　　Ex: 890.0–897.7, 929.0–929.9, 958.8–958.99, 959.8–959.9

896.2　Bilateral, without mention of complication ✿

Excludes	one foot and other leg (897.6–897.7)

　　　Ex: 890.0–897.7, 929.0–929.9, 958.8–958.99, 959.8–959.9

896.3　Bilateral, complicated ✿
　　　Ex: 890.0–897.7, 929.0–929.9, 958.8–958.99, 959.8–959.9

● **897　Traumatic amputation of leg(s) (complete) (partial)**

897.0　Unilateral, below knee, without mention of complication ✿
　　　Ex: 890.0–897.7, 929.0–929.9, 958.8–958.99, 959.8–959.9

897.1　Unilateral, below knee, complicated ✿
　　　Ex: 890.0–897.7, 929.0–929.9, 958.8–958.99, 959.8–959.9

897.2　Unilateral, at or above knee, without mention of complication ✿
　　　Ex: 890.0–897.7, 929.0–929.9, 958.8–958.99, 959.8–959.9

897.3　Unilateral, at or above knee, complicated ✿
　　　Ex: 890.0–897.7, 929.0–929.9, 958.8–958.99, 959.8–959.9

897.4　Unilateral, level not specified, without mention of complication ✿
　　　Ex: 890.0–897.7, 929.0–929.9, 958.8–958.99, 959.8–959.9

897.5　Unilateral, level not specified, complicated ✿
　　　Ex: 890.0–897.7, 929.0–929.9, 958.8–958.99, 959.8–959.9

897.6　Bilateral [any level], without mention of complication ✿
　　　One foot and other leg
　　　Ex: 890.0–897.7, 929.0–929.9, 958.8–958.99, 959.8–959.9

897.7　Bilateral [any level], complicated ✿
　　　Ex: 890.0–897.7, 929.0–929.9, 958.8–958.99, 959.8–959.9

INJURY TO BLOOD VESSELS (900–904)

Includes	arterial hematoma of blood vessel, secondary to other injuries, e.g., fracture or open wound
	avulsion of blood vessel, secondary to other injuries, e.g., fracture or open wound
	cut of blood vessel, secondary to other injuries, e.g., fracture or open wound
	laceration of blood vessel, secondary to other injuries, e.g., fracture or open wound
	rupture of blood vessel, secondary to other injuries, e.g., fracture or open wound
	traumatic aneurysm or fistula (arteriovenous) of blood vessel, secondary to other injuries, e.g., fracture or open wound

Excludes	accidental puncture or laceration during medical procedure (998.2)
	intracranial hemorrhage following injury (851.0–854.1)

● **900　Injury to blood vessels of head and neck**

● 900.0　Carotid artery

900.00　Carotid artery, unspecified ✿
　　　Ex: 900.00, 900.82–900.9, 904.9, 929.0–929.9, 958.8–958.99, 959.8–959.9

900.01　Common carotid artery ✿
　　　Ex: 900.00, 900.82–900.9, 904.9, 929.0–929.9, 958.8–958.99, 959.8–959.9

900.02　External carotid artery ✿
　　　Ex: 900.00, 900.82–900.9, 904.9, 929.0–929.9, 958.8–958.99, 959.8–959.9

900.03　Internal carotid artery ✿
　　　Ex: 900.00, 900.82–900.9, 904.9, 929.0–929.9, 958.8–958.99, 959.8–959.9

900.1　Internal jugular vein ✿
　　　Ex: 900.82–900.9, 904.9, 929.0–929.9, 958.8–958.99, 959.8–959.9

◀ New　　◀≡ Revised　　deleted Deleted　　● Unacceptable Principal Diagnosis　　● Use Additional Digit(s)

▶ Manifestation Code　　OGCR Official Guidelines　　Coding Clinic　　Excludes　　Includes　　Use additional　　Code first　　Omit code

● **900.8 Other specified blood vessels of head and neck**

    900.81 External jugular vein 🔴
       Jugular vein NOS
       (Ex:) 900.82-900.9, 904.9, 929.0-929.9, 958.8-958.99, 959.8-959.9

    900.82 Multiple blood vessels of head and neck 🔴
       (Ex:) 900.82-900.9, 904.9, 929.0-929.9, 958.8-958.99, 959.8-959.9

    900.89 Other 🔴
       (Ex:) 900.82-900.9, 904.9, 929.0-929.9, 958.8-958.99, 959.8-959.9

    900.9 Unspecified blood vessel of head and neck 🔴
       (Ex:) 900.82-900.9, 904.9, 929.0-929.9, 958.8-958.99, 959.8-959.9

● **901 Injury to blood vessels of thorax**

    Excludes *traumatic hemothorax (860.2–860.5)*

    901.0 Thoracic aorta 🔴
       (Ex:) 901.0, 904.9, 929.0-929.9, 958.8-958.99, 959.8-959.9

    901.1 Innominate and subclavian arteries 🔴
       (Ex:) 901.1, 904.9, 929.0-929.9, 958.8-958.99, 959.8-959.9

    901.2 Superior vena cava 🔴
       (Ex:) 901.2, 904.9, 929.0-929.9, 958.8-958.99, 959.8-959.9

    901.3 Innominate and subclavian veins 🔴
       (Ex:) 901.3, 904.9, 929.0-929.9, 958.8-958.99, 959.8-959.9

● **901.4 Pulmonary blood vessels**

    901.40 Pulmonary vessel(s), unspecified 🔴
       (Ex:) 901.40-901.41, 904.9, 929.0-929.9, 958.8-958.90, 958.99, 959.8-959.9

    901.41 Pulmonary artery 🔴
       (Ex:) 901.40-901.41, 904.9, 929.0-929.9, 958.8-958.99, 959.8-959.9

    901.42 Pulmonary vein 🔴
       (Ex:) 901.40, 901.42, 904.9, 929.0-929.9, 958.8-958.99, 959.8-959.9

● **901.8 Other specified blood vessels of thorax**

    901.81 Intercostal artery or vein 🔴
       (Ex:) 901.81, 901.83-901.89

    901.82 Internal mammary artery or vein 🔴
       (Ex:) 901.82-901.89

    901.83 Multiple blood vessels of thorax 🔴
       (Ex:) 904.9, 929.0-929.9, 958.8-958.99, 959.8-959.9

    901.89 Other 🔴
       Azygos vein
       Hemiazygos vein
       (Ex:) 901.0-901.9

    901.9 Unspecified blood vessel of thorax 🔴
       (Ex:) 901.0-901.9

● **902 Injury to blood vessels of abdomen and pelvis**

    902.0 Abdominal aorta 🔴
       (Ex:) 902.0, 902.87-902.9, 904.9, 929.0-929.9, 958.8-958.99, 959.8-959.9

● **902.1 Inferior vena cava**

    902.10 Inferior vena cava, unspecified 🔴
       (Ex:) 902.10, 902.87-902.9, 904.9, 929.0-929.9 958.8-958.99, 959.8-959.9

    902.11 Hepatic veins 🔴
       (Ex:) 902.11, 902.87-902.9, 904.9, 929.0-929.9 958.8-958.99, 959.8-959.9

    902.19 Other 🔴
       (Ex:) 902.19, 902.87-902.9, 904.9, 929.0-929.9 958.8-958.99, 959.8-959.9

● **902.2 Celiac and mesenteric arteries**

    902.20 Celiac and mesenteric arteries, unspecified 🔴
       (Ex:) 902.20, 902.87-902.9, 904.9, 929.0-929.9 958.8-958.99, 959.8-959.9

    902.21 Gastric artery 🔴
       (Ex:) 902.21, 902.87-902.9, 904.9, 929.0-929.9, 958.8-958.90, 958.93-958.99, 959.8-959.9

    902.22 Hepatic artery 🔴
       (Ex:) 902.22, 902.87-902.9, 904.9, 929.0-929.9, 958.8-958.99, 959.8-959.9

    902.23 Splenic artery 🔴
       (Ex:) 902.23, 902.87-902.9, 904.9, 929.0-929.9, 958.8-958.99, 959.8-959.9

    902.24 Other specified branches of celiac axis 🔴
       (Ex:) 902.24, 902.87-902.9, 904.9, 929.0-929.9, 958.8-958.99, 959.8-959.9

    902.25 Superior mesenteric artery (trunk) 🔴
       (Ex:) 902.25, 902.87-902.9, 904.9, 929.0-929.9, 958.8-958.99, 959.8-959.9

    902.26 Primary branches of superior mesenteric artery 🔴
       Ileo-colic artery
       (Ex:) 902.26, 902.87-902.9, 904.9, 929.0-929.9, 958.8-958.99, 959.8-959.9

    902.27 Inferior mesenteric artery 🔴
       (Ex:) 902.27, 902.87-902.9, 904.9, 929.0-929.9, 958.8-958.99, 959.8-959.9

    902.29 Other 🔴
       (Ex:) 902.29, 902.87-902.9, 904.9, 929.0-929.9, 958.8-958.99, 959.8-959.9

● **902.3 Portal and splenic veins**

    902.31 Superior mesenteric vein and primary subdivisions 🔴
       Ileo-colic vein
       (Ex:) 902.31, 902.87-902.9, 904.9, 929.0-929.9, 958.8-958.99, 959.8-959.9

    902.32 Inferior mesenteric vein 🔴
       (Ex:) 902.32, 902.87-902.9, 904.9, 929.0-929.9, 958.8-958.99, 959.8-959.9

    902.33 Portal vein 🔴
       (Ex:) 902.33, 902.87-902.9, 904.9, 929.0-929.9, 958.8-958.99, 959.8-959.9

    902.34 Splenic vein 🔴
       (Ex:) 902.34, 902.87-902.9, 904.9, 929.0-929.9, 958.8-958.99, 959.8-959.9

    902.39 Other 🔴
       Cystic vein
       Gastric vein
       (Ex:) 902.39, 902.87-902.9, 904.9, 929.0-929.9, 958.8-958.99, 959.8-959.9

● **902.4 Renal blood vessels**

    902.40 Renal vessel(s), unspecified 🔴
       (Ex:) 902.40, 902.87-902.9, 904.9, 929.0-929.9, 958.8-958.99, 959.8-959.9

    902.41 Renal artery 🔴
       (Ex:) 902.41, 902.87-902.9, 904.9, 929.0-929.9, 958.8-958.99, 959.8-959.9

    902.42 Renal vein 🔴
       (Ex:) 902.42, 902.87-902.9, 904.9, 929.0-929.9, 958.8-958.99, 959.8-959.9

    902.49 Other 🔴
       Suprarenal arteries
       (Ex:) 902.49, 902.87-902.9, 904.9, 929.0-929.9, 958.8-958.99, 959.8-959.9

N Newborn Age: 0   **P** Pediatric Age: 0–17   **M** Maternity Age: 12–55   **A** Adult Age: 15–124   ♀ Females Only   ♂ Males Only

(Ex:) CC Exclusions   🔴 Complication\Comorbidity   🔴 Major C\C   🔴 Present on Admission Requirement   🔴 Hospital-Acquired Condition

● **902.5 Iliac blood vessels**

  902.50 Iliac vessel(s), unspecified 🐾
    (Ex:) 902.50, 902.53-902.54, 902.59, 902.87-902.9, 904.9,
    929.0-929.9, 958.8-958.99, 959.8-959.9

  902.51 Hypogastric artery 🐾
    (Ex:) 902.51, 902.87-902.9, 904.9, 929.0-929.9, 958.8-958.99,
    959.8-959.9

  902.52 Hypogastric vein 🐾
    (Ex:) 902.52, 902.87-902.9, 904.9, 929.0-929.9, 958.8-958.99,
    959.8-959.9

  902.53 Iliac artery 🐾
    (Ex:) 902.50, 902.53, 902.59, 902.87-902.9, 904.9, 929.0-929.9,
    958.8-958.99, 959.8-959.9

  902.54 Iliac vein 🐾
    (Ex:) 902.50, 902.54, 902.59, 902.87-902.9, 904.9, 929.0-929.9,
    958.8-958.99, 959.8-959.9

  902.55 Uterine artery ♀ 🐾
    (Ex:) 902.55, 902.59, 902.87-902.9, 904.9, 929.0-929.9,
    958.8-958.90, 958.93-958.99, 959.8-959.9

  902.56 Uterine vein ♀ 🐾
    (Ex:) 902.56-902.59, 902.87-902.9, 904.9, 929.0-929.9,
    958.8-958.90, 958.93-958.99, 959.8-959.9

  902.59 Other 🐾
    (Ex:) 902.50, 902.53-902.54, 902.59, 902.87-902.9, 904.9,
    929.0-929.9, 958.8-958.99, 959.8-959.9

● **902.8 Other specified blood vessels of abdomen and pelvis**

  902.81 Ovarian artery ♀ 🐾
    (Ex:) 902.81, 902.87-902.9, 904.9, 929.0-929.9, 958.8-958.90,
    958.93-958.99, 959.8-959.9

  902.82 Ovarian vein ♀ 🐾
    (Ex:) 902.82-902.9, 904.9, 929.0-929.9, 958.8-958.90,
    958.93-958.99, 959.8-959.9

  902.87 Multiple blood vessels of abdomen and pelvis 🐾
    (Ex:) 902.87-902.9, 904.9, 929.0-929.9, 958.8-958.99, 959.8-959.9

  902.89 Other 🐾
    (Ex:) 902.87-902.9, 904.9, 929.0-929.9, 958.8-958.90,
    958.93-958.99, 959.8-959.9

902.9 Unspecified blood vessel of abdomen and pelvis 🐾
  (Ex:) 902.0-902.9, 904.9, 929.0-929.9, 958.8-958.90, 958.93-958.99,
  959.8-959.9

● **903 Injury to blood vessels of upper extremity**

 ● **903.0 Axillary blood vessels**

  903.00 Axillary vessel(s), unspecified 🐾
    (Ex:) 903.00-903.02, 903.8-903.9, 904.9

  903.01 Axillary artery 🐾
    (Ex:) 903.00-903.01, 903.8-903.9, 904.9

  903.02 Axillary vein 🐾
    (Ex:) 903.00, 903.02, 903.8-903.9, 904.9

 903.1 Brachial blood vessels 🐾
  (Ex:) 903.1, 903.8-903.9, 904.9

 903.2 Radial blood vessels 🐾
  (Ex:) 903.2, 903.8-903.9, 904.9

 903.3 Ulnar blood vessels 🐾
  (Ex:) 903.3, 903.8-903.9, 904.9

 903.4 Palmar artery 🐾
  (Ex:) 903.4, 903.8-903.9, 904.9

 903.5 Digital blood vessels 🐾
  (Ex:) 903.5-903.9, 904.9

 903.8 Other specified blood vessels of upper extremity 🐾
  Multiple blood vessels of upper extremity
  (Ex:) 903.3-903.9, 904.9

 903.9 Unspecified blood vessel of upper extremity 🐾
  (Ex:) 903.3-903.9, 904.9

● **904 Injury to blood vessels of lower extremity and unspecified sites**

 904.0 Common femoral artery 🐾
  Femoral artery above profunda origin
   Profunda = deep and posterior
  (Ex:) 904.0, 904.7-904.9

 904.1 Superficial femoral artery 🐾
  (Ex:) 904.1, 904.7-904.9

 904.2 Femoral veins 🐾
  (Ex:) 904.2, 904.7-904.9

 904.3 Saphenous veins 🐾
  Saphenous vein (greater) (lesser)
  (Ex:) 904.3, 904.7-904.9

 ● **904.4 Popliteal blood vessels**

  904.40 Popliteal vessel(s), unspecified 🐾
    (Ex:) 904.40, 904.7-904.9

  904.41 Popliteal artery 🐾
    (Ex:) 904.41, 904.7-904.9

  904.42 Popliteal vein 🐾
    (Ex:) 904.42, 904.7-904.9

 ● **904.5 Tibial blood vessels**

  904.50 Tibial vessel(s), unspecified 🐾
    (Ex:) 904.50, 904.7-904.9

  904.51 Anterior tibial artery 🐾
    (Ex:) 904.51, 904.7-904.9

  904.52 Anterior tibial vein 🐾
    (Ex:) 904.52, 904.7-904.9

  904.53 Posterior tibial artery 🐾
    (Ex:) 904.53, 904.7-904.9

  904.54 Posterior tibial vein 🐾
    (Ex:) 904.54, 904.7-904.9

 904.6 Deep plantar blood vessels 🐾
  (Ex:) 904.6-904.9

 904.7 Other specified blood vessels of lower extremity 🐾
  Multiple blood vessels of lower extremity
  (Ex:) 729.72, 904.0-904.9

 904.8 Unspecified blood vessel of lower extremity 🐾
  (Ex:) 729.72, 904.0-904.9

 904.9 Unspecified site 🐾
  Injury to blood vessel NOS
  (Ex:) 729.71-729.72, 900.00-904.9

◄ New   ◄▥ Revised   ~~deleted~~ Deleted   ● Unacceptable Principal Diagnosis   ◐ Use Additional Digit(s)
▶ Manifestation Code   **OGCR** Official Guidelines   **Coding Clinic**   Excludes   Includes   Use additional   Code first   Omit code

INJURY AND POISONING (800–999)

LATE EFFECTS OF INJURIES, POISONINGS, TOXIC EFFECTS, AND OTHER EXTERNAL CAUSES (905–909)

Note: These categories are to be used to indicate conditions classifiable to 800–999 as the cause of late effects, which are themselves classified elsewhere. The "late effects" include those specified as such, or as sequelae, which may occur at any time after the acute injury.

● **905 Late effects of musculoskeletal and connective tissue injuries**

905.0 Late effect of fracture of skull and face bones 🔍
Late effect of injury classifiable to 800–804
Coding Clinic: 1997, Q3, P12-13

905.1 Late effect of fracture of spine and trunk without mention of spinal cord lesion 🔍
Late effects of injury classifiable to 805, 807-809
Coding Clinic: 2007, Q1, P20-21

905.2 Late effect of fracture of upper extremities 🔍
Late effect of injury classifiable to 810–819

905.3 Late effect of fracture of neck of femur 🔍
Late effect of injury classifiable to 820

905.4 Late effect of fracture of lower extremities 🔍
Late effect of injury classifiable to 821–827
Coding Clinic: 1995, Q1, P10; 1994, Q2, P7

905.5 Late effect of fracture of multiple and unspecified bones 🔍
Late effect of injury classifiable to 828–829

905.6 Late effect of dislocation 🔍
Late effect of injury classifiable to 830–839

905.7 Late effect of sprain and strain without mention of tendon injury 🔍
Late effect of injury classifiable to 840–848, except tendon injury

905.8 Late effect of tendon injury 🔍
Late effect of tendon injury due to:
open wound [injury classifiable to 880–884 with .2, 890–894 with .2]
sprain and strain [injury classifiable to 840–848]
Coding Clinic: 1989, Q2, P15; Q2, P13

905.9 Late effect of traumatic amputation 🔍
Late effect of injury classifiable to 885–887, 895–897

Excludes | *late amputation stump complication (997.60–997.69)*

● **906 Late effects of injuries to skin and subcutaneous tissues**

906.0 Late effect of open wound of head, neck, and trunk 🔍
Late effect of injury classifiable to 870–879

906.1 Late effect of open wound of extremities without mention of tendon injury 🔍
Late effect of injury classifiable to 880–884, 890–894 except .2
Coding Clinic: 1993, 5th Issue, P3

906.2 Late effect of superficial injury 🔍
Late effect of injury classifiable to 910–919

906.3 Late effect of contusion 🔍
Late effect of injury classifiable to 920–924

906.4 Late effect of crushing 🔍
Late effect of injury classifiable to 925–929

906.5 Late effect of burn of eye, face, head, and neck 🔍
Late effect of injury classifiable to 940–941
Coding Clinic: 2004, Q4, P75-76

906.6 Late effect of burn of wrist and hand 🔍
Late effect of injury classifiable to 944

906.7 Late effect of burn of other extremities 🔍
Late effect of injury classifiable to 943 or 945

906.8 Late effect of burns of other specified sites 🔍
Late effect of injury classifiable to 942, 946–947

906.9 Late effect of burn of unspecified site 🔍
Late effect of injury classifiable to 948–949

OGCR Section I.C.17.c.7
Encounters for the treatment of the late effects of burns (i.e., scars or joint contractures) should be coded to the residual condition (sequelae) followed by the appropriate late effect code (906.5-906.9). A late effect E code may also be used, if desired.

● **907 Late effects of injuries to the nervous system**

907.0 Late effect of intracranial injury without mention of skull fracture 🔍
Late effect of injury classifiable to 850–854
Coding Clinic: 2008, Q4, P102-109; 2003, Q4, P103-104; 1987, Nov-Dec, P12

907.1 Late effect of injury to cranial nerve 🔍
Late effect of injury classifiable to 950–951

907.2 Late effect of spinal cord injury 🔍
Late effect of injury classifiable to 806, 952
Coding Clinic: 2003, Q4, P103-104; 1998, Q4, P37-38; 1994, Q3, P4

907.3 Late effect of injury to nerve root(s), spinal plexus(es), and other nerves of trunk 🔍
Late effect of injury classifiable to 953–954
Coding Clinic: 2007, Q2, P13-15

907.4 Late effect of injury to peripheral nerve of shoulder girdle and upper limb 🔍
Late effect of injury classifiable to 955

907.5 Late effect of injury to peripheral nerve of pelvic girdle and lower limb 🔍
Late effect of injury classifiable to 956

907.9 Late effect of injury to other and unspecified nerve 🔍
Late effect of injury classifiable to 957

● **908 Late effects of other and unspecified injuries**

908.0 Late effect of internal injury to chest 🔍
Late effect of injury classifiable to 860–862

908.1 Late effect of internal injury to intra-abdominal organs 🔍
Late effect of injury classifiable to 863–866, 868

908.2 Late effect of internal injury to other internal organs 🔍
Late effect of injury classifiable to 867 or 869

908.3 Late effect of injury to blood vessel of head, neck, and extremities 🔍
Late effect of injury classifiable to 900, 903–904

908.4 Late effect of injury to blood vessel of thorax, abdomen, and pelvis 🔍
Late effect of injury classifiable to 901–902

908.5 Late effect of foreign body in orifice 🔍
Late effect of injury classifiable to 930–939

908.6 Late effect of certain complications of trauma 🔍
Late effect of complications classifiable to 958

908.9 Late effect of unspecified injury 🔍
Late effect of injury classifiable to 959
Coding Clinic: 2000, Q3, P4

INJURY AND POISONING (800–999)

N Newborn Age: 0   P Pediatric Age: 0–17   M Maternity Age: 12–55   A Adult Age: 15–124   ♀ Females Only   ♂ Males Only

(Ex) CC Exclusions   🔍 Complication\Comorbidity   🔍 Major C\C   🔍 Present on Admission Requirement   🔍 Hospital-Acquired Condition

1097

● **909 Late effects of other and unspecified external causes**

909.0 Late effect of poisoning due to drug, medicinal or biological substance 🔍
Late effect of conditions classifiable to 960–979

> **Excludes** *Late effect of adverse effect of drug, medicinal or biological substance (909.5)*

Coding Clinic: 2003, Q4, P103-104; 1984, Sept-Oct, P16

909.1 Late effect of toxic effects of nonmedical substances 🔍
Late effect of conditions classifiable to 980–989

909.2 Late effect of radiation 🔍
Late effect of conditions classifiable to 990
Coding Clinic: 1984, Nov-Dec, P19

909.3 Late effect of complications of surgical and medical care 🔍
Late effect of conditions classifiable to 996–999
Coding Clinic: 1993, Q1, P29

909.4 Late effect of certain other external causes 🔍
Late effect of conditions classifiable to 991–994

909.5 Late effect of adverse effect of drug, medicinal or biological substance 🔍

> **Excludes** *late effect of poisoning due to drug, medicinal or biological substances (909.0)*

909.9 Late effect of other and unspecified external causes 🔍

SUPERFICIAL INJURY (910–919)

> **Excludes** *burn (blisters) (940.0–949.5)*
> *contusion (920–924.9)*
> *foreign body:*
>   *granuloma (728.82)*
>   *inadvertently left in operative wound (998.4)*
>   *residual, in soft tissue (729.6)*
>   *insect bite, venomous (989.5)*
>   *open wound with incidental foreign body (870.0–897.7)*

● **910 Superficial injury of face, neck, and scalp except eye**

> **Includes**   cheek   lip
>   ear   nose
>   gum   throat

> **Excludes** *eye and adnexa (918.0–918.9)*

910.0 Abrasion or friction burn without mention of infection

910.1 Abrasion or friction burn, infected

910.2 Blister without mention of infection

910.3 Blister, infected

910.4 Insect bite, nonvenomous, without mention of infection

910.5 Insect bite, nonvenomous, infected

910.6 Superficial foreign body (splinter) without major open wound and without mention of infection

910.7 Superficial foreign body (splinter) without major open wound, infected

910.8 Other and unspecified superficial injury of face, neck, and scalp without mention of infection

910.9 Other and unspecified superficial injury of face, neck, and scalp, infected

● **911 Superficial injury of trunk**

> **Includes**   abdominal wall   interscapular region
>   anus   labium (majus) (minus)
>   back   penis
>   breast   perineum
>   buttock   scrotum
>   chest wall   testis
>   flank   vagina
>   groin   vulva

> **Excludes** *hip (916.0–916.9)*
> *scapular region (912.0–912.9)*

911.0 Abrasion or friction burn without mention of infection
Coding Clinic: 2001, Q3, P10

911.1 Abrasion or friction burn, infected

911.2 Blister without mention of infection

911.3 Blister, infected

911.4 Insect bite, nonvenomous, without mention of infection

911.5 Insect bite, nonvenomous, infected

911.6 Superficial foreign body (splinter) without major open wound and without mention of infection

911.7 Superficial foreign body (splinter) without major open wound, infected

911.8 Other and unspecified superficial injury of trunk without mention of infection

911.9 Other and unspecified superficial injury of trunk, infected

● **912 Superficial injury of shoulder and upper arm**

> **Includes**   axilla
>   scapular region

912.0 Abrasion or friction burn without mention of infection

912.1 Abrasion or friction burn, infected

912.2 Blister without mention of infection

912.3 Blister, infected

912.4 Insect bite, nonvenomous, without mention of infection

912.5 Insect bite, nonvenomous, infected

912.6 Superficial foreign body (splinter) without major open wound and without mention of infection

912.7 Superficial foreign body (splinter) without major open wound, infected

912.8 Other and unspecified superficial injury of shoulder and upper arm without mention of infection

912.9 Other and unspecified superficial injury of shoulder and upper arm, infected

● **913 Superficial injury of elbow, forearm, and wrist**

913.0 Abrasion or friction burn without mention of infection

913.1 Abrasion or friction burn, infected

913.2 Blister without mention of infection

913.3 Blister, infected

913.4 Insect bite, nonvenomous, without mention of infection

913.5 Insect bite, nonvenomous, infected

913.6 Superficial foreign body (splinter) without major open wound and without mention of infection

◀ New   ◀▥ Revised   ~~deleted~~ Deleted   ● Unacceptable Principal Diagnosis   ● Use Additional Digit(s)
▶ Manifestation Code   **OGCR** Official Guidelines   **Coding Clinic**   Excludes   Includes   Use additional   Code first   Omit code

913.7 **Superficial foreign body (splinter) without major open wound, infected**

913.8 **Other and unspecified superficial injury of elbow, forearm, and wrist without mention of infection**

913.9 **Other and unspecified superficial injury of elbow, forearm, and wrist, infected**

● 914 **Superficial injury of hand(s) except finger(s) alone**

914.0 **Abrasion or friction burn without mention of infection**

914.1 **Abrasion or friction burn, infected**

914.2 **Blister without mention of infection**

914.3 **Blister, infected**

914.4 **Insect bite, nonvenomous, without mention of infection**

914.5 **Insect bite, nonvenomous, infected**

914.6 **Superficial foreign body (splinter) without major open wound and without mention of infection**

914.7 **Superficial foreign body (splinter) without major open wound, infected**

914.8 **Other and unspecified superficial injury of hand without mention of infection**

914.9 **Other and unspecified superficial injury of hand, infected**

● 915 **Superficial injury of finger(s)**

     Includes   fingernail
                   thumb (nail)

915.0 **Abrasion or friction burn without mention of infection**

915.1 **Abrasion or friction burn, infected**

915.2 **Blister without mention of infection**

915.3 **Blister, infected**

915.4 **Insect bite, nonvenomous, without mention of infection**

915.5 **Insect bite, nonvenomous, infected**

915.6 **Superficial foreign body (splinter) without major open wound and without mention of infection**

915.7 **Superficial foreign body (splinter) without major open wound, infected**

915.8 **Other and unspecified superficial injury of fingers without mention of infection**
     Coding Clinic: 2001, Q3, P10

915.9 **Other and unspecified superficial injury of fingers, infected**

● 916 **Superficial injury of hip, thigh, leg, and ankle**

916.0 **Abrasion or friction burn without mention of infection**
     Coding Clinic: 2000, Q4, P61

916.1 **Abrasion or friction burn, infected**

916.2 **Blister without mention of infection**

916.3 **Blister, infected**

916.4 **Insect bite, nonvenomous, without mention of infection**

916.5 **Insect bite, nonvenomous, infected**

916.6 **Superficial foreign body (splinter) without major open wound and without mention of infection**

916.7 **Superficial foreign body (splinter) without major open wound, infected**

916.8 **Other and unspecified superficial injury of hip, thigh, leg, and ankle without mention of infection**

916.9 **Other and unspecified superficial injury of hip, thigh, leg, and ankle, infected**

● 917 **Superficial injury of foot and toe(s)**

     Includes   heel
                   toenail

917.0 **Abrasion or friction burn without mention of infection**

917.1 **Abrasion or friction burn, infected**

917.2 **Blister without mention of infection**

917.3 **Blister, infected**

917.4 **Insect bite, nonvenomous, without mention of infection**

917.5 **Insect bite, nonvenomous, infected**

917.6 **Superficial foreign body (splinter) without major open wound and without mention of infection**

917.7 **Superficial foreign body (splinter) without major open wound, infected**

917.8 **Other and unspecified superficial injury of foot and toes without mention of infection**
     Coding Clinic: 2003, Q1, P13

917.9 **Other and unspecified superficial injury of foot and toes, infected**
     Coding Clinic: 2003, Q1, P13

● 918 **Superficial injury of eye and adnexa**

     Excludes   *burn (940.0–940.9)*
                   foreign body on external eye (930.0–930.9)

918.0 **Eyelids and periocular area**
Abrasion
Insect bite
Superficial foreign body (splinter)

918.1 **Cornea**
Corneal abrasion
Superficial laceration
     Excludes   *corneal injury due to contact lens (371.82)*

918.2 **Conjunctiva**

918.9 **Other and unspecified superficial injuries of eye**
Eye (ball) NOS

● 919 **Superficial injury of other, multiple, and unspecified sites**

     Excludes   *multiple sites classifiable to the same three-digit category (910.0–918.9)*

919.0 **Abrasion or friction burn without mention of infection**

919.1 **Abrasion or friction burn, infected**

919.2 **Blister without mention of infection**

919.3 **Blister, infected**

919.4 **Insect bite, nonvenomous, without mention of infection**

919.5 **Insect bite, nonvenomous, infected**

919.6 **Superficial foreign body (splinter) without major open wound and without mention of infection**

919.7 **Superficial foreign body (splinter) without major open wound, infected**

919.8 **Other and unspecified superficial injury without mention of infection**

919.9 **Other and unspecified superficial injury, infected**

INJURY AND POISONING (800–999)

CONTUSION WITH INTACT SKIN SURFACE (920–924)

| **Includes** | bruise without fracture or open wound |
| | hematoma without fracture or open wound |

Excludes	concussion (850.0–850.9)
	hemarthrosis (840.0–848.9)
	internal organs (860.0–869.1)
	that incidental to:
	crushing injury (925–929.9)
	dislocation (830.0–839.9)
	fracture (800.0–829.1)
	internal injury (860.0–869.1)
	intracranial injury (850.0–854.1)
	nerve injury (950.0–957.9)
	open wound (870.0–897.7)

920   Contusion of face, scalp, and neck except eye(s)

Cheek	Mandibular joint area
Ear (auricle)	Nose
Gum	Throat
Lip	

● **921   Contusion of eye and adnexa**

921.0   Black eye, NOS

921.1   Contusion of eyelids and periocular area

921.2   Contusion of orbital tissues

921.3   Contusion of eyeball
     Coding Clinic: 1985, July-Aug, P16

921.9   Unspecified contusion of eye
     Injury of eye NOS

● **922   Contusion of trunk**

922.0   Breast

922.1   Chest wall

922.2   Abdominal wall
     Flank
     Groin

● **922.3   Back**

922.31   Back

| **Excludes** | interscapular region (922.33) |
     Coding Clinic: 1999, Q3, P14-15

922.32   Buttock

922.33   Interscapular region

| **Excludes** | scapular region (923.01) |

922.4   Genital organs

Labium (majus) (minus)	Testis
Penis	Vagina
Perineum	Vulva
Scrotum	

922.8   Multiple sites of trunk

922.9   Unspecified part
     Trunk NOS

● **923   Contusion of upper limb**

● **923.0   Shoulder and upper arm**

923.00   Shoulder region

923.01   Scapular region

923.02   Axillary region

923.03   Upper arm

923.09   Multiple sites

● **923.1   Elbow and forearm**

923.10   Forearm

923.11   Elbow

● **923.2   Wrist and hand(s), except finger(s) alone**

923.20   Hand(s)

923.21   Wrist

923.3   Finger
     Fingernail
     Thumb (nail)

923.8   Multiple sites of upper limb

923.9   Unspecified part of upper limb
     Arm NOS

● **924   Contusion of lower limb and of other and unspecified sites**

● **924.0   Hip and thigh**

924.00   Thigh
     Coding Clinic: 2009, Q1, P10x2

924.01   Hip

● **924.1   Knee and lower leg**

924.10   Lower leg

924.11   Knee

● **924.2   Ankle and foot, excluding toe(s)**

924.20   Foot
     Heel

924.21   Ankle

924.3   Toe
     Toenail

924.4   Multiple sites of lower limb

924.5   Unspecified part of lower limb
     Leg NOS

924.8   Multiple sites, not elsewhere classified
     Coding Clinic: 2003, Q1, P7

924.9   Unspecified site

◀ New   ◀▥ Revised   ~~deleted~~ Deleted   ● Unacceptable Principal Diagnosis   ● Use Additional Digit(s)

▶ Manifestation Code   **OGCR** Official Guidelines   **Coding Clinic**   Excludes   Includes   Use additional   Code first   Omit code

CRUSHING INJURY (925–929)

Use additional code to identify any associated injuries,
such as:
fractures (800–829)
internal injuries (860.0–869.1)
intracranial injury (850.0–854.1)

● **925 Crushing injury of face, scalp, and neck**
Cheek
Ear
Larynx
Pharynx
Throat
Coding Clinic: 2003, Q4, P76-78

925.1 Crushing injury of face and scalp 🌑 🌑
Cheek
Ear
(Ex) 873.8-873.9, 905.0, 925.1-925.2, 929.0-929.9, 958.8-959.09, 959.8-959.9

925.2 Crushing injury of neck 🌑 🌑
Larynx
Throat
Pharynx
(Ex) 873.8-873.9, 905.0, 925.1-925.2, 929.0-929.9, 958.8-959.09, 959.8-959.9

● **926 Crushing injury of trunk**
Coding Clinic: 2003, Q4, P76-78

926.0 External genitalia 🌑
Labium (majus) (minus)
Penis
Scrotum
Testis
Vulva

● **926.1 Other specified sites**
926.11 Back 🌑
926.12 Buttock 🌑
926.19 Other 🌑
Breast

926.8 Multiple sites of trunk 🌑
926.9 Unspecified site 🌑
Trunk NOS

● **927 Crushing injury of upper limb**
● **927.0 Shoulder and upper arm**
927.00 Shoulder region 🌑
927.01 Scapular region 🌑
927.02 Axillary region 🌑
927.03 Upper arm 🌑
927.09 Multiple sites 🌑

● **927.1 Elbow and forearm**
927.10 Forearm 🌑
927.11 Elbow 🌑

● **927.2 Wrist and hand(s), except finger(s) alone**
927.20 Hand(s) 🌑
927.21 Wrist 🌑

927.3 Finger(s)
Coding Clinic: 2003, Q4, P76-78

927.8 Multiple sites of upper limb 🌑
927.9 Unspecified site 🌑
Arm NOS

● **928 Crushing injury of lower limb**
Coding Clinic: 2003, Q4, P76-78

● **928.0 Hip and thigh**
928.00 Thigh 🌑 🌑
(Ex) 928.00, 928.8-929.9

928.01 Hip 🌑 🌑
(Ex) 928.01, 928.8-929.9

● **928.1 Knee and lower leg**
928.10 Lower leg 🌑
928.11 Knee 🌑

● **928.2 Ankle and foot, excluding toe(s) alone**
928.20 Foot 🌑
Heel
928.21 Ankle 🌑

928.3 Toe(s) 🌑
928.8 Multiple sites of lower limb 🌑
928.9 Unspecified site 🌑
Leg NOS

● **929 Crushing injury of multiple and unspecified sites**
Coding Clinic: 2003, Q4, P76-78

929.0 Multiple sites, not elsewhere classified 🌑
929.9 Unspecified site 🌑

EFFECTS OF FOREIGN BODY ENTERING THROUGH ORIFICE (930–939)

Excludes foreign body:
granuloma (728.82)
inadvertently left in operative wound (998.4,
998.7)
in open wound (800–839, 851–897)
residual, in soft tissues (729.6)
superficial without major open wound
(910–919 with .6 or .7)

● **930 Foreign body on external eye**

Excludes foreign body in penetrating wound of:
eyeball (871.5–871.6)
retained (old) (360.5–360.6)
ocular adnexa (870.4)
retained (old) (376.6)

930.0 Corneal foreign body
930.1 Foreign body in conjunctival sac
930.2 Foreign body in lacrimal punctum
930.8 Other and combined sites
930.9 Unspecified site
External eye NOS

931 Foreign body in ear
Auditory canal
Auricle

932 Foreign body in nose
Nasal sinus
Nostril

N Newborn Age: 0 **P** Pediatric Age: 0–17 **M** Maternity Age: 12–55 **A** Adult Age: 15–124 ♀ Females Only ♂ Males Only

(Ex) CC Exclusions 🌑 Complication\Comorbidity 🌑 Major C\C 🌑 Present on Admission Requirement 🌑 Hospital-Acquired Condition 1101

INJURY AND POISONING (800–999)

● **933   Foreign body in pharynx and larynx**

   933.0 Pharynx
       Nasopharynx
       Throat NOS

   933.1 Larynx
       Asphyxia due to foreign body
       Choking due to:
          food (regurgitated)
          phlegm

● **934   Foreign body in trachea, bronchus, and lung**

   934.0 Trachea 🔧
       (Ex:) 934.0

   934.1 Main bronchus 🔧
       (Ex:) 934.0-934.9

   934.8 Other specified parts 🔧
       Bronchioles
       Lung
       (Ex:) 934.0-934.9

   934.9 Respiratory tree, unspecified
       Inhalation of liquid or vomitus, lower respiratory
         tract NOS

● **935   Foreign body in mouth, esophagus, and stomach**

   935.0 Mouth

   935.1 Esophagus
       Coding Clinic: 1988, Q1, P13

   935.2 Stomach
       Coding Clinic: 1985, Jan-Feb, P14-15

  936   Foreign body in intestine and colon

  937   Foreign body in anus and rectum
       Rectosigmoid (junction)

  938   Foreign body in digestive system, unspecified
       Alimentary tract NOS
       Swallowed foreign body

● **939   Foreign body in genitourinary tract**

   939.0 Bladder and urethra

   939.1 Uterus, any part ♀

      | **Excludes** | *intrauterine contraceptive device:*
                 complications from (996.32, 996.65)
                 presence of (V45.51)

   939.2 Vulva and vagina ♀

   939.3 Penis ♂

   939.9 Unspecified site

Figure 17–14 A. 2nd degree burn. **B.** 3rd degree burn. (From Cummings: Otolaryngology: Head & Neck Surgery, 4th ed. 2005, Mosby)

BURNS (940–949)

OGCR   Section I.C.17.c
Current burns (940-948) are classified by depth, extent and by agent (E code). Burns are classified by depth as first degree (erythema), second degree (blistering), and third degree (full-thickness involvement).

OGCR   Section I.C.17.c.1
Sequence first the code that reflects the highest degree of burn when more than one burn is present.

OGCR   Section I.C.17.c.2
Classify burns of the same local site (three-digit category level, 940-947) but of different degrees to the subcategory identifying the highest degree recorded in the diagnosis.

| **Includes** | burns from:
          electrical heating appliance
          electricity
          flame
          hot object
          lightning
          radiation
       chemical burns (external) (internal)
       scalds

| **Excludes** | *friction burns (910–919 with .0, .1)*
           sunburn (692.71, 692.76–692.77)

● **940   Burn confined to eye and adnexa**

   940.0 Chemical burn of eyelids and periocular area 🔧

   940.1 Other burns of eyelids and periocular area 🔧

   940.2 Alkaline chemical burn of cornea and conjunctival sac 🔧

   940.3 Acid chemical burn of cornea and conjunctival sac 🔧

   940.4 Other burn of cornea and conjunctival sac 🔧

   940.5 Burn with resulting rupture and destruction of eyeball 🔧🔧
       (Ex:) No Exclusions

   940.9 Unspecified burn of eye and adnexa 🔧

INJURY AND POISONING (800–999)

◀ New   ◀▥ Revised   ~~deleted~~ Deleted   ● Unacceptable Principal Diagnosis   ● Use Additional Digit(s)
▸ Manifestation Code   **OGCR** Official Guidelines   **Coding Clinic**   Excludes   Includes   Use additional   Code first   Omit code

● **941   Burn of face, head, and neck**

    Excludes   mouth (947.0)

The following fifth-digit subclassification is for use with category 941:

> 0   face and head, unspecified site
> 1   ear [any part]
> 2   eye (with other parts of face, head, and neck)
> 3   lip(s)
> 4   chin
> 5   nose (septum)
> 6   scalp [any part]
>   Temple (region)
> 7   forehead and cheek
> 8   neck
> 9   multiple sites [except with eye] of face, head, and neck

● **941.0   Unspecified degree** 🦠
    [0-9]

● **941.1   Erythema [first degree]** 🦠
    [0-9]   Coding Clinic: 2005, Q3, P10-11

● **941.2   Blisters, epidermal loss [second degree]** 🦠
    [0-9]

● **941.3   Full-thickness skin loss [third degree NOS]** 🦠 🦠
    [0-9]   For code **941.30:** (Ex) 941.30, 941.39;
             For code **941.31:** (Ex) 941.31, 941.39;
             For code **941.32:** (Ex) 914.32, 914.39;
             For code **941.33:** (Ex) 941.33, 941.39;
             For code **941.34:** (Ex) 941.34, 941.39;
             For code **941.35:** (Ex) 941.35, 941.39;
             For code **941.36:** (Ex) 941.36, 941.39;
             For code **941.37:** (Ex) 941.37, 941.39;
             For code **941.38:** (Ex) 941.38-941.39;
             For code **941.39:** (Ex) 941.30-941.39

● **941.4   Deep necrosis of underlying tissues [deep third**
    [0-9]   **degree] without mention of loss of a body part** 🦠 🦠
             For codes **941.40, 941.49:** (Ex) 941.40, 941.49;
             For code **941.41:** (Ex) 941.40-941.41, 941.49;
             For code **941.42:** (Ex) 941.40, 941.42, 941.49;
             For code **941.43:** (Ex) 941.40, 941.43, 941.49;
             For code **941.44:** (Ex) 941.40, 941.44, 941.49;
             For code **941.45:** (Ex) 941.40, 941.45, 941.49;
             For code **941.46:** (Ex) 941.40, 941.46, 941.49;
             For code **941.47:** (Ex) 941.40, 941.47, 941.49;
             For code **941.48:** (Ex) 941.40, 941.48-941.49

● **941.5   Deep necrosis of underlying tissues [deep third**
    [0-9]   **degree] with loss of a body part** 🦠 🦠
             For codes **941.50, 941.59:** (Ex) 941.50, 941.59;
             For code **941.51:** (Ex) 941.50-941.51, 941.59;
             For code **941.52:** (Ex) 941.50, 941.52, 941.59;
             For code **941.53:** (Ex) 941.50, 941.53, 941.59;
             For code **941.54:** (Ex) 941.50, 941.54, 941.59;
             For code **941.55:** (Ex) 941.50, 941.55, 941.59;
             For code **941.56:** (Ex) 941.50, 941.56, 941.59;
             For code **941.57:** (Ex) 941.50, 941.57, 941.59;
             For code **941.58:** (Ex) 941.50, 941.58-941.59

● **942   Burn of trunk**

    Excludes   scapular region (943.0–943.5 with fifth-digit 6)

The following fifth-digit subclassification is for use with category 942:

> 0   trunk, unspecified site
> 1   breast
> 2   chest wall, excluding breast and nipple
> 3   abdominal wall
>   Flank
>   Groin
> 4   back [any part]
>   Buttock
>   Interscapular region
> 5   genitalia
>   Labium (majus) (minus)   Scrotum
>   Penis   Testis
>   Perineum   Vulva
> 9   other and multiple sites of trunk

● **942.0   Unspecified degree** 🦠
    [0-5,9]

● **942.1   Erythema [first degree]** 🦠
    [0-5,9]

● **942.2   Blisters, epidermal loss [second degree]** 🦠
    [0-5,9]   Coding Clinic: 1984, Nov-Dec, P13

● **942.3   Full-thickness skin loss [third degree NOS]** 🦠 🦠
    [0-5,9]   For codes **942.30, 942.39:** (Ex) 942.30, 942.39;
             For code **942.31:** (Ex) 942.30-942.31, 942.39;
             For code **942.32:** (Ex) 942.30, 942.32, 942.39;
             For code **942.33:** (Ex) 942.30, 942.33, 942.39;
             For code **942.34:** (Ex) 942.30, 942.34, 942.39;
             For code **942.35:** (Ex) 942.30, 942.35-942.39

● **942.4   Deep necrosis of underlying tissues [deep third**
    [0-5,9]   **degree] without mention of loss of a body part** 🦠 🦠
             For codes **942.40:** (Ex) 942.40, 942.49;
             For code **942.41:** (Ex) 942.40-942.41, 942.49;
             For code **942.42:** (Ex) 942.40, 942.42, 942.49;
             For code **942.43:** (Ex) 942.40, 942.43, 942.49;
             For code **942.44:** (Ex) 942.40, 942.44, 942.49;
             For code **942.45:** (Ex) 942.40, 942.45-942.49;
             For code **942.49:** (Ex) 942.40-942.49

● **942.5   Deep necrosis of underlying tissues [deep third**
    [0-5,9]   **degree] with loss of a body part** 🦠 🦠
             For codes **942.50:** (Ex) 942.50-942.59;
             For code **942.51:** (Ex) 942.50-942.51, 942.59;
             For code **942.52:** (Ex) 942.50, 942.52, 942.59;
             For code **942.53:** (Ex) 942.50, 942.53, 942.59;
             For code **942.54:** (Ex) 942.50, 942.54, 942.59;
             For code **942.55:** (Ex) 942.50, 942.55-942.59;
             For code **942.59:** (Ex) 942.50, 942.59

N Newborn Age: 0   **P** Pediatric Age: 0–17   **M** Maternity Age: 12–55   **A** Adult Age: 15–124   ♀ Females Only   ♂ Males Only   **1103**

(Ex) CC Exclusions   🦠 Complication\Comorbidity   🦠 Major C\C   🦠 Present on Admission Requirement   🦠 Hospital-Acquired Condition

INJURY AND POISONING (800–999)

● 943   Burn of upper limb, except wrist and hand

The following fifth-digit subclassification is for use with category 943:

> 0   upper limb, unspecified site
> 1   forearm
> 2   elbow
> 3   upper arm
> 4   axilla
> 5   shoulder
> 6   scapular region
> 9   multiple sites of upper limb, except wrist and hand

● 943.0   Unspecified degree ◐
[0-6,9]

● 943.1   Erythema [first degree] ◐
[0-6,9]

● 943.2   Blisters, epidermal loss [second degree] ◐
[0-6,9]

● 943.3   Full-thickness skin loss [third degree NOS] ◐ ◐
[0-6,9]   For codes **943.30, 943.39:** (Ex:) 943.30, 943.39;
         For code **943.31:** (Ex:) 943.30-943.31, 943.39;
         For code **943.32:** (Ex:) 943.30, 943.32, 943.39;
         For code **943.33:** (Ex:) 943.30, 943.33, 943.39;
         For code **943.34:** (Ex:) 943.30, 943.34, 943.39;
         For code **943.35:** (Ex:) 943.30, 943.35, 943.39;
         For code **943.36:** (Ex:) 943.30, 943.36-943.39

● 943.4   Deep necrosis of underlying tissues [deep third
[0-6,9]   degree] without mention of loss of a body part ◐ ◐
         For codes **943.40, 943.49:** (Ex:) 943.40, 943.49;
         For code **943.41:** (Ex:) 943.40-943.41, 943.49;
         For code **943.42:** (Ex:) 943.40, 943.42, 943.49;
         For code **943.43:** (Ex:) 943.40, 943.43, 943.49;
         For code **943.44:** (Ex:) 943.40, 943.44, 943.49;
         For code **943.45:** (Ex:) 943.40, 943.45, 943.49;
         For code **943.46:** (Ex:) 943.40, 943.46-943.49

● 943.5   Deep necrosis of underlying tissues [deep third
[0-6,9]   degree] with loss of a body part ◐ ◐
         For codes **943.50, 943.59:** (Ex:) 943.50, 943.59;
         For code **943.51:** (Ex:) 943.50-943.51, 943.59;
         For code **943.52:** (Ex:) 943.50, 943.52, 943.59;
         For code **943.53:** (Ex:) 943.50, 943.53, 943.59;
         For code **943.54:** (Ex:) 943.50, 943.54, 943.59;
         For code **943.55:** (Ex:) 943.50, 943.55, 943.59;
         For code **943.56:** (Ex:) 843.50, 943.56-943.59

● 944   Burn of wrist(s) and hand(s)

The following fifth-digit subclassification is for use with category 944:

> 0   hand, unspecified site
> 1   single digit [finger (nail)] other than thumb
> 2   thumb (nail)
> 3   two or more digits, not including thumb
> 4   two or more digits including thumb
> 5   palm
> 6   back of hand
> 7   wrist
> 8   multiple sites of wrist(s) and hand(s)

● 944.0   Unspecified degree ◐
[0-8]

● 944.1   Erythema [first degree] ◐
[0-8]

● 944.2   Blisters, epidermal loss [second degree] ◐
[0-8]

● 944.3   Full-thickness skin loss [third degree NOS] ◐ ◐
[0-8]   For codes **944.30, 944.38:** (Ex:) 944.30, 944.38;
         For code **944.31:** (Ex:) 944.30-944.31, 944.38;
         For code **944.32:** (Ex:) 944.30, 944.32, 944.38;
         For code **944.33:** (Ex:) 944.30, 944.33, 944.38;
         For code **944.34:** (Ex:) 944.30, 944.34, 944.38;
         For code **944.35:** (Ex:) 944.30, 944.35, 944.38;
         For code **944.36:** (Ex:) 944.30, 944.36, 944.38;
         For code **944.37:** (Ex:) 944.30, 944.37-944.38

● 944.4   Deep necrosis of underlying tissues [deep third
[0-8]   degree] without mention of loss of a body part ◐ ◐
         For codes **944.40, 944.48:** (Ex:) 944.40, 944.48;
         For code **944.41:** (Ex:) 944.40-944.41, 944.48;
         For code **944.42:** (Ex:) 944.40, 944.42, 944.48;
         For code **944.43:** (Ex:) 944.40, 944.43, 944.48;
         For code **944.44:** (Ex:) 944.40, 944.44, 944.48;
         For code **944.45:** (Ex:) 944.40, 944.45, 944.48;
         For code **944.46:** (Ex:) 944.40, 944.46, 944.48;
         For code **944.47:** (Ex:) 944.40, 944.47-944.48

● 944.5   Deep necrosis of underlying tissues [deep third
[0-8]   degree] with loss of a body part ◐ ◐
         For codes **944.50, 944.58:** (Ex:) 944.50, 944.58;
         For code **944.51:** (Ex:) 944.50-944.51, 944.58;
         For code **944.52:** (Ex:) 944.50, 944.52, 944.58;
         For code **944.53:** (Ex:) 944.50, 944.53, 944.58;
         For code **944.54:** (Ex:) 944.50, 944.54, 944.58;
         For code **944.55:** (Ex:) 944.50, 944.55, 944.58;
         For code **944.56:** (Ex:) 944.50, 944.56, 944.58;
         For code **944.57:** (Ex:) 944.50, 944.57-944.58

● 945   Burn of lower limb(s)

The following fifth-digit subclassification is for use with category 945:

> 0   lower limb [leg], unspecified site
> 1   toe(s) (nail)
> 2   foot
> 3   ankle
> 4   lower leg
> 5   knee
> 6   thigh [any part]
> 9   multiple sites of lower limb(s)

● 945.0   Unspecified degree ◐   ◀▥
[0-6,9]

● 945.1   Erythema [first degree] ◐   ◀▥
[0-6,9]

● 945.2   Blisters, epidermal loss [second degree] ◐   ◀▥
[0-6,9]

● 945.3   Full-thickness skin loss [third degree NOS] ◐ ◐   ◀▥
[0-6,9]   For codes **945.30, 945.39:** (Ex:) 945.30, 945.39;
         For code **945.31:** (Ex:) 945.30-945.31, 945.39;
         For code **945.32:** (Ex:) 945.30, 945.32, 945.39;
         For code **945.33:** (Ex:) 945.30, 945.33, 945.39;
         For code **945.34:** (Ex:) 945.30, 945.34, 945.39;
         For code **945.35:** (Ex:) 945.30, 945.35, 945.39;
         For code **945.36:** (Ex:) 945.30, 945.36-945.39

● 945.4   Deep necrosis of underlying tissues [deep third
[0-6,9]   degree] without mention of loss of a body
         part ◐ ◐   ◀▥
         For codes **945.40, 945.49:** (Ex:) 945.40, 945.49;
         For code **945.41:** (Ex:) 945.40-945.41, 945.49;
         For code **945.42:** (Ex:) 945.40, 945.42, 945.49;
         For code **945.43:** (Ex:) 945.40, 945.43, 945.49;
         For code **945.44:** (Ex:) 945.40, 945.44, 945.49;
         For code **945.45:** (Ex:) 945.40, 945.45, 945.49;
         For code **945.46:** (Ex:) 945.40, 945.46-945.49

◀ New   ◀▥ Revised   ~~deleted~~ Deleted   ● Unacceptable Principal Diagnosis   ● Use Additional Digit(s)

▶ Manifestation Code   **OGCR** Official Guidelines   **Coding Clinic**   Excludes   Includes   Use additional   Code first   Omit code

● **948.6 60–69 percent of body surface** 0 🌑 🐾, 1-6 🌑 🐾
[0-6]   (Ex:) 948.00-948.99

● **948.7 70–79 percent of body surface** 0 🌑 🐾, 1-7 🌑 🐾
[0-7]   (Ex:) 948.00-948.99

● **948.8 80–89 percent of body surface** 0 🌑 🐾, 1-8 🌑 🐾
[0-8]   (Ex:) 948.00-948.99

● **948.9 90 percent or more of body surface** 0 🌑 🐾, 1-9 🌑 🐾
[0-9]   (Ex:) 948.00-948.99

OGCR   Section I.C.17.c.5

> When coding burns, assign separate codes for each burn site. Category 949, Burn, unspecified, is extremely vague and should rarely be used.

● **949   Burn, unspecified**

Includes   burn NOS
              multiple burns NOS

Excludes   *burn of unspecified site but with statement of the extent of body surface involved (948.0–948.9)*

949.0 Unspecified degree 🐾

949.1 Erythema [first degree] 🐾

949.2 Blisters, epidermal loss [second degree] 🐾

949.3 Full-thickness skin loss [third degree NOS] 🌑 🐾
   (Ex:) 941.30-941.39, 942.30-942.39, 944.30-944.38, 945.30-945.39, 946.3, 949.3

949.4 Deep necrosis of underlying tissues [deep third degree] without mention of loss of a body part 🌑 🐾
   (Ex:) 941.40-941.49, 942.40-942.49, 944.40-944.48, 945.40-945.49, 946.4, 949.4

949.5 Deep necrosis of underlying tissues [deep third degree] with loss of a body part 🌑 🐾

INJURY TO NERVES AND SPINAL CORD (950–957)

Includes   division of nerve
              lesion in continuity (with open wound)
              traumatic neuroma (with open wound)
              traumatic transient paralysis (with open wound)

Excludes   *accidental puncture or laceration during medical procedure (998.2)*
   (Ex:) 946.5, 949.5

● **950   Injury to optic nerve and pathways**

950.0 Optic nerve injury 🌑
Second cranial nerve
(Ex:) 950.0-950.9, 951.8-951.9

950.1 Injury to optic chiasm 🌑
(Ex:) 950.0-950.9, 951.8-951.9

950.2 Injury to optic pathways 🌑
(Ex:) 950.0-950.9, 951.8-951.9

950.3 Injury to visual cortex 🌑
(Ex:) 950.0-950.9, 951.8-951.9

950.9 Unspecified 🌑
Traumatic blindness NOS
(Ex:) 950.0-950.9, 951.8-951.9

● **951   Injury to other cranial nerve(s)**

951.0 Injury to oculomotor nerve 🌑
Third cranial nerve
(Ex:) 951.0, 951.8-951.9

951.1 Injury to trochlear nerve 🌑
Fourth cranial nerve
(Ex:) 951.1, 951.8-951.9

951.2 Injury to trigeminal nerve 🌑
Fifth cranial nerve
(Ex:) 951.2, 951.8-951.9

951.3 Injury to abducens nerve 🌑
Sixth cranial nerve
(Ex:) 951.3, 951.8-951.9

951.4 Injury to facial nerve 🌑
Seventh cranial nerve
(Ex:) 951.4, 951.8-951.9

951.5 Injury to acoustic nerve 🌑
Auditory nerve
Eighth cranial nerve
Traumatic deafness NOS
(Ex:) 951.5, 951.8-951.9

951.6 Injury to accessory nerve 🌑
Eleventh cranial nerve
(Ex:) 951.6, 951.8-951.9

951.7 Injury to hypoglossal nerve 🌑
Twelfth cranial nerve
(Ex:) 951.7-951.9

951.8 Injury to other specified cranial nerves 🌑
Glossopharyngeal [9th cranial] nerve
Olfactory [1st cranial] nerve
Pneumogastric [10th cranial] nerve
Traumatic anosmia NOS
Vagus [10th cranial] nerve
(Ex:) 951.8-951.9

951.9 Injury to unspecified cranial nerve 🌑
(Ex:) 951.8-951.9

● **952   Spinal cord injury without evidence of spinal bone injury**

● **952.0 Cervical**

952.00 C_1-C_4 level with unspecified spinal cord injury 🌑
Spinal cord injury, cervical region NOS
(Ex:) 805.00-805.18, 805.8-806.19, 806.8-806.9, 839.00-839.18, 839.40, 839.49-839.50, 839.59, 839.69, 839.79-839.9, 847.9, 905.1, 926.11, 952.00-952.09, 952.8-952.9, 958.8-958.99, 959.11-959.19, 959.8-959.9

952.01 C_1-C_4 level with complete lesion of spinal cord 🌑
(Ex:) 805.00-805.18, 805.8-806.19, 806.8-806.9, 839.00-839.18, 839.40, 839.49-839.50, 839.59, 839.69, 839.79-839.9, 847.9, 905.1, 926.11, 952.00-952.09, 952.8-952.9, 958.8-958.99, 959.11-959.19, 959.8-959.9

952.02 C_1-C_4 level with anterior cord syndrome 🌑
(Ex:) 805.00-805.18, 805.8-806.19, 806.8-806.9, 839.00-839.18, 839.40, 839.49-839.50, 839.59, 839.69, 839.79-839.9, 847.9, 905.1, 926.11, 952.00-952.09, 952.8-952.9, 958.8-958.99, 959.11-959.19, 959.8-959.9

● **945.5 Deep necrosis of underlying tissues [deep third**
[0-6,9] **degree] with loss of a body part**
     For codes **945.50, 945.59:** (Ex) 945.50, 945.59;
     For code **945.51:** (Ex) 945.50-945.51, 945.59;
     For code **945.52:** (Ex) 945.50, 945.52, 945.59;
     For code **945.53:** (Ex) 945.50, 945.53, 945.59;
     For code **945.54:** (Ex) 945.50, 945.54, 945.59;
     For code **945.55:** (Ex) 945.50, 945.55, 945.59;
     For code **945.56:** (Ex) 945.50, 945.56-945.59

● 946 **Burns of multiple specified sites**
     Documented as multiple sites but not specified as to location

     Includes   burns of sites classifiable to more than one
         three-digit category in 940–945

     Excludes   *multiple burns NOS (949.0–949.5)*

     946.0 Unspecified degree

     946.1 Erythema [first degree]

     946.2 Blisters, epidermal loss [second degree]

     946.3 Full-thickness skin loss [third degree NOS]
         (Ex) 946.3

     946.4 Deep necrosis of underlying tissues [deep third
         degree] without mention of loss of a body part
         (Ex) 946.4

     946.5 Deep necrosis of underlying tissues [deep third
         degree] with loss of a body part
         (Ex) 946.5

     OGCR   Section I.C.17.c.5

     When coding burns, assign separate codes for each burn
     site. Category 946 should only be used if the location of
     the burns are not documented.

A

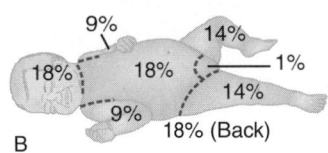

B

Figure 17–15   Rule of
nines: percentages of total
body area. (From Marx:
Rosen's Emergency Medicine:
Concepts and Clinical Practice,
6th ed. 2006, Mosby)

● 947 **Burn of internal organs**

     Includes   burns from chemical agents (ingested)

     947.0 Mouth and pharynx
         Gum
         Tongue

     947.1 Larynx, trachea, and lung
         (Ex) 947.1, 947.8-947.9

     947.2 Esophagus
         (Ex) 947.2, 947.8-947.9

     947.3 Gastrointestinal tract
         Colon
         Rectum
         Small intestine
         Stomach
         (Ex) 947.3, 947.8-947.9

     947.4 Vagina and uterus ♀
         (Ex) 947.4-947.9

     947.8 Other specified sites

     947.9 Unspecified site

     OGCR   Section I.C.17.c.6

     Fourth-digit identifies percentage of **total body surface**
     involved in a burn (all degrees). **Fifth-digit** identifies
     the percentage of body surface involved in **third-degree**
     burn with zero (0) assigned when less than 10 percent or
     when no body surface is involved in a third-degree burn.
     Category 948 is based on the classic "rule of nines"
     in estimating body surface involved: head and neck are
     assigned nine percent, each arm nine percent, each leg
     18 percent, the anterior trunk 18 percent, posterior trunk
     18 percent, and genitalia one percent.

● 948 **Burns classified according to extent of body surface involved**

     Excludes   *sunburn (692.71, 692.76–692.77)*

     Note: This category is to be used when the site of the
         burn is unspecified, or with categories 940–947
         when the site is specified.
     Coding Clinic: 1984, Nov-Dec, P13

     The following fifth-digit subclassification is for use with
     category 948 to indicate the percent of body surface with third
     degree burn; valid digits are in [brackets] under each code:

     0   **less than 10 percent or unspecified**
     1   **10–19%**
     2   **20–29%**
     3   **30–39%**
     4   **40–49%**
     5   **50–59%**
     6   **60–69%**
     7   **70–79%**
     8   **80–89%**
     9   **90% or more of body surface**

● **948.0 Burn [any degree] involving less than 10 percent of**
[0]   **body surface**

● **948.1 10–19 percent of body surface**
[0-1]   (Ex) 948.00-948.99
       Coding Clinic: 1984, Nov-Dec, P13

● **948.2 20–29 percent of body surface** 0, 1,2
[0-2]   (Ex) 948.00-948.99
       Coding Clinic: 1984, Nov-Dec, P13

● **948.3 30–39 percent of body surface** 0, 1-3
[0-3]   (Ex) 948.00-948.99

● **948.4 40–49 percent of body surface** 0, 1-4
[0-4]   (Ex) 948.00-948.99

● **948.5 50–59 percent of body surface** 0, 1-5
[0-5]   (Ex) 948.00-948.99

INJURY AND POISONING (800–999)

952.03 C_1-C_4 level with central cord syndrome 🔓
   (Ex:) 805.00-805.18, 805.8-806.19, 806.8-806.9, 839.00-839.18,
   839.40, 839.49-839.50, 839.59, 839.69, 839.79-839.9,
   847.9, 905.1, 926.11, 952.00-952.09, 952.8-952.9,
   958.8-958.99, 959.11-959.19, 959.8-959.9

952.04 C_1-C_4 level with other specified spinal cord injury 🔓
   Incomplete spinal cord lesion at C_1-C_4 level:
    NOS
     with posterior cord syndrome
   (Ex:) 805.00-805.18, 805.8-806.19, 806.8-806.9, 839.00-839.18,
   839.40, 839.49-839.50, 839.59, 839.69, 839.79-839.9,
   847.9, 905.1, 926.11, 952.00-952.09, 952.8-952.9,
   958.8-958.99, 959.11-959.19, 959.8-959.9

952.05 C_5-C_7 level with unspecified spinal cord injury 🔓
   (Ex:) 805.00-805.18, 805.8-806.19, 806.8-806.9, 839.00-839.18,
   839.40, 839.49-839.50, 839.59, 839.69, 839.79-839.9,
   847.9, 905.1, 926.11, 952.00-952.09, 952.8-952.9,
   958.8-958.99, 959.11-959.19, 959.8-959.9

952.06 C_5-C_7 level with complete lesion of spinal cord 🔓
   (Ex:) 805.00-805.18, 805.8-806.19, 806.8-806.9, 839.00-839.18,
   839.40, 839.49-839.50, 839.59, 839.69, 839.79-839.9,
   847.9, 905.1, 926.11, 952.00-952.09, 952.8-952.9,
   958.8-958.99, 959.11-959.19, 959.8-959.9

952.07 C_5-C_7 level with anterior cord syndrome 🔓
   (Ex:) 805.00-805.18, 805.8-806.19, 806.8-806.9, 839.00-839.18,
   839.40, 839.49-839.50, 839.59, 839.69, 839.79-839.9,
   847.9, 905.1, 926.11, 952.00-952.09, 952.8-952.9,
   958.8-958.99, 959.11-959.19, 959.8-959.9

952.08 C_5-C_7 level with central cord syndrome 🔓
   (Ex:) 805.00-805.18, 805.8-806.19, 806.8-806.9, 839.00-839.18,
   839.40, 839.49-839.50, 839.59, 839.69, 839.79-839.9,
   847.9, 905.1, 926.11, 952.00-952.09, 952.8-952.9,
   958.8-958.99, 959.11-959.19, 959.8-959.9

952.09 C_5-C_7 level with other specified spinal cord injury 🔓
   Incomplete spinal cord lesion at C_5-C_7 level:
    NOS
     with posterior cord syndrome
   (Ex:) 805.00-805.18, 805.8-806.19, 806.8-806.9, 839.00-839.18,
   839.40, 839.49-839.50, 839.59, 839.69, 839.79-839.9,
   847.9, 905.1, 926.11, 952.00-952.09, 952.8-952.9,
   958.8-958.99, 959.11-959.19, 959.8-959.9

● **952.1 Dorsal [thoracic]**

952.10 T_1-T_6 level with unspecified spinal cord injury 🔓
   Spinal cord injury, thoracic region NOS
   (Ex:) 805.8-805.9, 806.20-806.39, 839.40, 839.49-839.50, 839.59,
   839.69, 839.79-839.9, 847.9, 905.1, 926.11, 952.10-952.19,
   952.8-952.9, 958.8-958.99, 959.11-959.19, 959.8-959.9

952.11 T_1-T_6 level with complete lesion of spinal cord 🔓
   (Ex:) 805.8-805.9, 806.20-806.39, 839.40, 839.49-839.50, 839.59,
   839.69, 839.79-839.9, 847.9, 905.1, 926.11, 952.10-952.19,
   952.8-952.9, 958.8-958.99, 959.11-959.19, 959.8-959.9

952.12 T_1-T_6 level with anterior cord syndrome 🔓
   (Ex:) 805.8-805.9, 806.20-806.39, 839.40, 839.49-839.50, 839.59,
   839.69, 839.79-839.9, 847.9, 905.1, 926.11, 952.10 952.19,
   952.8-952.9, 958.8-958.99, 959.11-959.19, 959.8-959.9

952.13 T_1-T_6 level with central cord syndrome 🔓
   (Ex:) 805.8-805.9, 806.20-806.39, 839.40, 839.49-839.50, 839.59,
   839.69, 839.79-839.9, 847.9, 905.1, 926.11, 952.10-952.19,
   952.8-952.9, 958.8-958.99, 959.11-959.19, 959.8-959.9

952.14 T_1-T_6 level with other specified spinal cord injury 🔓
   Incomplete spinal cord lesion at T_1-T_6 level:
    NOS
     with posterior cord syndrome
   (Ex:) 805.8-805.9, 806.20-806.39, 839.40, 839.49-839.50, 839.59,
   839.69, 839.79-839.9, 847.9, 905.1, 926.11, 952.10-952.19,
   952.8-952.9, 958.8-958.99, 959.11-959.19, 959.8-959.9

952.15 T_7-T_{12} level with unspecified spinal cord injury 🔓
   (Ex:) 805.8-805.9, 806.20-806.39, 839.40, 839.49-839.50, 839.59,
   839.69, 839.79-839.9, 847.9, 905.1, 926.11, 952.10-952.19,
   952.8-952.9, 958.8-958.99, 959.11-959.19, 959.8-959.9

952.16 T_7-T_{12} level with complete lesion of spinal cord 🔓
   (Ex:) 805.8-805.9, 806.20-806.39, 839.40, 839.49-839.50, 839.59,
   839.69, 839.79-839.9, 847.9, 905.1, 926.11, 952.10-952.19,
   952.8-952.9, 958.8-958.99, 959.11-959.19, 959.8-959.9

952.17 T_7-T_{12} level with anterior cord syndrome 🔓
   (Ex:) 805.8-805.9, 806.20-806.39, 839.40, 839.49-839.50, 839.59,
   839.69, 839.79-839.9, 847.9, 905.1, 926.11, 952.10-952.19,
   952.8-952.9, 958.8-958.99, 959.11-959.19, 959.8-959.9

952.18 T_7-T_{12} level with central cord syndrome 🔓
   (Ex:) 805.8-805.9, 806.20-806.39, 839.40, 839.49-839.50, 839.59,
   839.69, 839.79-839.9, 847.9, 905.1, 926.11, 952.10-952.19,
   952.8-952.9, 958.8-958.99, 959.11-959.19, 959.8-959.9

952.19 T_7-T_{12} level with other specified spinal cord injury 🔓
   Incomplete spinal cord lesion at T_7-T_{12} level:
    NOS
     with posterior cord syndrome
   (Ex:) 805.8-805.9, 806.20-806.39, 839.40, 839.49-839.50, 839.59,
   839.69, 839.79-839.9, 847.9, 905.1, 926.11, 952.10-952.19,
   952.8-952.9, 958.8-958.99, 959.11-959.19, 959.8-959.9

952.2 Lumbar 🔓
   (Ex:) 805.8-805.9, 806.4-806.5, 839.40, 839.49-839.50, 839.59, 839.69,
   839.79-839.9, 847.9, 905.1, 926.11, 952.2, 952.8-952.9, 958.8-958.99,
   959.11-959.19, 959.8-959.9

952.3 Sacral 🔓
   (Ex:) 805.8-805.9, 806.60-806.79, 839.40, 839.49-839.50, 839.59, 839.69,
   839.79-839.9, 847.9, 905.1, 926.11, 952.3-952.9, 958.8-958.99,
   959.11-959.19, 959.8-959.9

952.4 Cauda equina 🔓
   (Ex:) 805.8-805.9, 806.60-806.79, 839.40, 839.49-839.50, 839.59, 839.69,
   839.79-839.9, 847.9, 905.1, 926.11, 952.3-952.9, 958.8-958.99,
   959.11-959.19, 959.8-959.9

952.8 Multiple sites of spinal cord 🔓
   (Ex:) 805.8-805.9, 839.40, 839.49-839.50, 839.59, 839.69, 839.79-839.9, 847.9,
   905.1, 926.11, 952.8-952.9, 958.8-958.99, 959.11-959.19, 959.8-959.9

952.9 Unspecified site of spinal cord

● **953 Injury to nerve roots and spinal plexus**

953.0 Cervical root

953.1 Dorsal root

953.2 Lumbar root

953.3 Sacral root

953.4 Brachial plexus

953.5 Lumbosacral plexus

953.8 Multiple sites

953.9 Unspecified site

N Newborn Age: 0   P Pediatric Age: 0–17   M Maternity Age: 12–55   A Adult Age: 15–124   ♀ Females Only   ♂ Males Only
(Ex:) CC Exclusions   🔓 Complication\Comorbidity   🔓 Major C\C   🔓 Present on Admission Requirement   🔓 Hospital-Acquired Condition   **1107**

INJURY AND POISONING (800–999)

● **954 Injury to other nerve(s) of trunk, excluding shoulder and pelvic girdles**

  954.0 Cervical sympathetic

  954.1 Other sympathetic
      Celiac ganglion or plexus   Splanchnic nerve(s)
      Inferior mesenteric plexus   Stellate ganglion

  954.8 Other specified nerve(s) of trunk

  954.9 Unspecified nerve of trunk

● **955 Injury to peripheral nerve(s) of shoulder girdle and upper limb**

  955.0 Axillary nerve

  955.1 Median nerve

  955.2 Ulnar nerve

  955.3 Radial nerve

  955.4 Musculocutaneous nerve

  955.5 Cutaneous sensory nerve, upper limb

  955.6 Digital nerve

  955.7 Other specified nerve(s) of shoulder girdle and upper limb

  955.8 Multiple nerves of shoulder girdle and upper limb

  955.9 Unspecified nerve of shoulder girdle and upper limb

● **956 Injury to peripheral nerve(s) of pelvic girdle and lower limb**

  956.0 Sciatic nerve

  956.1 Femoral nerve

  956.2 Posterior tibial nerve

  956.3 Peroneal nerve

  956.4 Cutaneous sensory nerve, lower limb

  956.5 Other specified nerve(s) of pelvic girdle and lower limb

  956.8 Multiple nerves of pelvic girdle and lower limb

  956.9 Unspecified nerve of pelvic girdle and lower limb

● **957 Injury to other and unspecified nerves**

  957.0 Superficial nerves of head and neck

  957.1 Other specified nerve(s)

  957.8 Multiple nerves in several parts
      Multiple nerve injury NOS

  957.9 Unspecified site
      Nerve injury NOS

CERTAIN TRAUMATIC COMPLICATIONS AND UNSPECIFIED INJURIES (958–959)

● **958 Certain early complications of trauma**

  Excludes   *adult respiratory distress syndrome (518.5)*
      flail chest (807.4)
      post-traumatic seroma (729.91)
      shock lung (518.5)
      that occurring during or following medical procedures (996.0–999.9)

  958.0 Air embolism
      Pneumathemia

    Excludes   *that complicating:*
        abortion (634–638 with .6, 639.6)
        ectopic or molar pregnancy (639.6)
        pregnancy, childbirth, or the puerperium (673.0)
    (Ex:) 958.0, 958.8-958.99, 959.8-959.9, 997.91-997.99, 998.81, 998.83-998.9, 999.1

958.1 Fat embolism

  Excludes   *that complicating:*
      abortion (634–638 with .6, 639.6)
      pregnancy, childbirth, or the puerperium (673.8)
  (Ex:) 958.1, 958.8-958.99, 959.8-959.9, 997.91-997.99, 998.81, 998.83-998.9

958.2 Secondary and recurrent hemorrhage
  (Ex:) 958.2, 958.8-958.99, 959.8-959.9, 997.91-997.99, 998.81, 998.83-998.9

958.3 Posttraumatic wound infection, not elsewhere classified

  Excludes   *infected open wounds - code to complicated open wound of site*
  (Ex:) 958.3, 958.8-958.99, 959.8-959.9, 997.91-997.99, 998.81, 998.83-998.9
  Coding Clinic: 1993, 5th Issue, P3; 1985, Sept-Oct, P10; 1984, Nov-Dec, P20

  OGCR   Section I.C.17.c.4
  Assign code 958.3 as an additional code for any documented infected burn site.

958.4 Traumatic shock
  Shock (immediate) (delayed) following injury

  Excludes   *shock:*
      anaphylactic (995.0)
        due to serum (999.4)
      anesthetic (995.4)
      electric (994.8)
      following abortion (639.5)
      lightning (994.0)
      nontraumatic NOS (785.50)
      obstetric (669.1)
      postoperative (998.0)
  (Ex:) 958.4, 958.8-958.99, 959.8-959.9, 997.91-997.99, 998.81, 998.83-998.9

958.5 Traumatic anuria
  Crush syndrome
  Renal failure following crushing

  Excludes   *that due to a medical procedure (997.5)*
  (Ex:) 958.5, 958.8-958.99, 959.8-959.9, 995.4, 997.91-998.13, 998.81, 998.83-998.9

958.6 Volkmann's ischemic contracture
  Posttraumatic muscle contracture

958.7 Traumatic subcutaneous emphysema

  Excludes   *subcutaneous emphysema resulting from a procedure (998.81)*
  (Ex:) 860.0-860.5, 861.20-862.1, 862.29-862.9, 875.0-875.1, 958.7-958.99, 959.8-959.9, 997.91-997.99, 998.81, 998.83-998.9

958.8 Other early complications of trauma
  Coding Clinic: 1992, Q2, P13

● **958.9 Traumatic compartment syndrome**

  Excludes   *nontraumatic compartment syndrome (729.71–729.79)*

  958.90 Compartment syndrome, unspecified
    (Ex:) 868.03-868.10, 868.13-869.1

  958.91 Traumatic compartment syndrome of upper extremity
    Traumatic compartment syndrome of shoulder, arm, forearm, wrist, hand, and fingers
    (Ex:) 729.81, 729.89-729.99

  958.92 Traumatic compartment syndrome of lower extremity
    Traumatic compartment syndrome of hip, buttock, thigh, leg, foot, and toes
    (Ex:) 729.81, 729.89-729.99

◄ New   ◄▓ Revised   ~~deleted~~ Deleted   ● Unacceptable Principal Diagnosis   ● Use Additional Digit(s)
▶ Manifestation Code   OGCR Official Guidelines   Coding Clinic   Excludes   Includes   Use additional   Code first   Omit code

958.93   Traumatic compartment syndrome of abdomen 🕮
> (Ex:) 863.0-867.3, 867.5-869.1, 879.2-879.9, 929.0-929.9, 958.8, 959.8-959.9
>
> Coding Clinic: 2006, Q4, P100-102

958.99   Traumatic compartment syndrome of other sites 🕮
> (Ex:) 868.03-868.10, 868.13-869.1

● **959   Injury, other and unspecified**

> **Includes**   injury NOS
>
> **Excludes**   *injury NOS of:*
> > *blood vessels (900.0–904.9)*
> > *eye (921.0–921.9)*
> > *internal organs (860.0–869.1)*
> > *intracranial sites (854.0–854.1)*
> > *nerves (950.0–951.9, 953.0–957.9)*
> > *spinal cord (952.0–952.9)*
>
> Coding Clinic: 1984, Nov-Dec, P9

● **959.0   Head, face, and neck**

> **959.01   Head injury, unspecified**
>
> > **Excludes**   *concussion (850.0–850.9)*
> > > *with head injury NOS (850.0–850.9)*
> > > *head injury NOS with loss of consciousness (850.1–850.5)*
> > > *specified head injuries (850.0–854.1)*
> >
> > Coding Clinic: 2008, Q4, P102-109; 1999, Q1, P10
>
> **959.09   Injury of face and neck**

● **959.1   Trunk**

> **Excludes**   *scapular region (959.2)*
>
> **959.11   Other injury of chest wall**
>
> **959.12   Other injury of abdomen**
>
> **959.13   Fracture of corpus cavernosum penis** ♂
>
> **959.14   Other injury of external genitals**
>
> **959.19   Other injury of other sites of trunk**
> > Injury of trunk NOS

959.2   Shoulder and upper arm
> Axilla
> Scapular region

959.3   Elbow, forearm, and wrist
> Coding Clinic: 1997, Q1, P8

959.4   Hand, except finger

959.5   Finger
> Fingernail
> Thumb (nail)

959.6   Hip and thigh
> Upper leg

959.7   Knee, leg, ankle, and foot

959.8   Other specified sites, including multiple
> **Excludes**   *multiple sites classifiable to the same four-digit category (959.0–959.7)*

959.9   Unspecified site
> Coding Clinic: 1984, Nov-Dec, P9

OGCR   Section I.C.17.e.1

Poisoning: An **error** was made in drug prescription or in the administration of the drug by provider, nurse, patient, or other person, use the appropriate poisoning code from the 960-979 series. If an overdose of a drug was **intentionally** taken or administered and resulted in drug toxicity, it would be coded as a poisoning (960-979 series). If a **nonprescribed** drug or medicinal agent was taken in combination with a correctly prescribed and properly administered drug, any drug toxicity or other reaction resulting from the interaction of the two drugs would be classified as a poisoning.

When a reaction results from the interaction of a drug(s) and alcohol, this would be classified as poisoning.

Sequencing of poisoning: When coding a poisoning or reaction to the improper use of a medication (e.g., wrong dose, wrong substance, wrong route of administration) the poisoning code is sequenced first, followed by a code for the manifestation. If there is also a diagnosis of drug abuse or dependence to the substance, the abuse or dependence is coded as an additional code.

See Section I.C.3.a.6.b. if poisoning is the result of insulin pump malfunctions and Section I.C.19 for general use of E-codes.

POISONING BY DRUGS, MEDICINAL AND BIOLOGICAL SUBSTANCES (960–979)

> **Includes**   overdose of these substances
> > wrong substance given or taken in error
>
> **Excludes**   *adverse effects ["hypersensitivity," "reaction," etc.] of correct substance properly administered. Such cases are to be classified according to the nature of the adverse effect, such as:*
> > *adverse effect NOS (995.20)*
> > *allergic lymphadenitis (289.3)*
> > *aspirin gastritis (535.4)*
> > *blood disorders (280.0–289.9)*
> > *dermatitis:*
> > > *contact (692.0–692.9)*
> > > *due to ingestion (693.0–693.9)*
> > *nephropathy (583.9)*
> > *[The drug giving rise to the adverse effect may be identified by use of categories E930–E949.]*
> > *drug dependence (304.0–304.9)*
> > *drug reaction and poisoning affecting the newborn (760.0–779.9)*
> > *nondependent abuse of drugs (305.0–305.9)*
> > *pathological drug intoxication (292.2)*
>
> **Use additional** code to specify the effects of the poisoning

● **960   Poisoning by antibiotics**

> **Excludes**   *antibiotics:*
> > *ear, nose, and throat (976.6)*
> > *eye (976.5)*
> > *local (976.0)*

960.0   Penicillins
> Ampicillin
> Carbenicillin
> Cloxacillin
> Penicillin G

N   Newborn Age: 0   P   Pediatric Age: 0–17   M   Maternity Age: 12–55   A   Adult Age: 15–124   ♀   Females Only   ♂   Males Only

(Ex:)   CC Exclusions   🕮   Complication\Comorbidity   🕮   Major C\C   🕮   Present on Admission Requirement   🕮   Hospital-Acquired Condition   **1109**

INJURY AND POISONING (800–999)

960.1 Antifungal antibiotics
    Amphotericin B
    Griseofulvin
    Nystatin
    Trichomycin

    Excludes *preparations intended for topical use (976.0–976.9)*

960.2 Chloramphenicol group
    Chloramphenicol
    Thiamphenicol

960.3 Erythromycin and other macrolides
    Oleandomycin
    Spiramycin

960.4 Tetracycline group
    Doxycycline
    Minocycline
    Oxytetracycline

960.5 Cephalosporin group
    Cephalexin   Cephaloridine
    Cephaloglycin   Cephalothin

960.6 Antimycobacterial antibiotics
    Cycloserine
    Kanamycin
    Rifampin
    Streptomycin

960.7 Antineoplastic antibiotics
    Actinomycin such as:
        Bleomycin   Dactinomycin
        Cactinomycin   Daunorubicin
                         Mitomycin

960.8 Other specified antibiotics

960.9 Unspecified antibiotic

● **961 Poisoning by other anti-infectives**

    Excludes *anti-infectives:*
        ear, nose, and throat (976.6)
        eye (976.5)
        local (976.0)

961.0 Sulfonamides
    Sulfadiazine
    Sulfafurazole
    Sulfamethoxazole

961.1 Arsenical anti-infectives

961.2 Heavy metal anti-infectives
    Compounds of: Compounds of:
      antimony   lead
      bismuth   mercury

    Excludes *mercurial diuretics (974.0)*

961.3 Quinoline and hydroxyquinoline derivatives
    Chiniofon
    Diiodohydroxyquin

    Excludes *antimalarial drugs (961.4)*

961.4 Antimalarials and drugs acting on other blood protozoa
    Chloroquine
    Cycloguanil
    Primaquine
    Proguanil [chloroguanide]
    Pyrimethamine
    Quinine

961.5 Other antiprotozoal drugs
    Emetine

961.6 Anthelmintics
    Hexylresorcinol   Thiabendazole
    Piperazine

961.7 Antiviral drugs
    Methisazone

    Excludes *amantadine (966.4)*
         cytarabine (963.1)
         idoxuridine (976.5)

961.8 Other antimycobacterial drugs
    Ethambutol
    Ethionamide
    Isoniazid
    Para-aminosalicylic acid derivatives
    Sulfones

961.9 Other and unspecified anti-infectives
    Flucytosine
    Nitrofuran derivatives

● **962 Poisoning by hormones and synthetic substitutes**

    Excludes *oxytocic hormones (975.0)*

962.0 Adrenal cortical steroids
    Cortisone derivatives
    Desoxycorticosterone derivatives
    Fluorinated corticosteroids

962.1 Androgens and anabolic congeners
    Methandriol
    Nandrolone
    Oxymetholone
    Testosterone

962.2 Ovarian hormones and synthetic substitutes
    Contraceptives, oral
    Estrogens
    Estrogens and progestogens, combined
    Progestogens

962.3 Insulins and antidiabetic agents
    Acetohexamide
    Biguanide derivatives, oral
    Chlorpropamide
    Glucagon
    Insulin
    Phenformin
    Sulfonylurea derivatives, oral
    Tolbutamide

962.4 Anterior pituitary hormones
    Corticotropin
    Gonadotropin
    Somatotropin [growth hormone]

962.5 Posterior pituitary hormones
    Vasopressin

    Excludes *oxytocic hormones (975.0)*

962.6 Parathyroid and parathyroid derivatives

962.7 Thyroid and thyroid derivatives
    Dextrothyroxin
    Levothyroxine sodium
    Liothyronine
    Thyroglobulin

962.8 Antithyroid agents
    Iodides
    Thiouracil
    Thiourea

962.9 Other and unspecified hormones and synthetic substitutes

◀ New   ◀◀◀ Revised   ~~deleted~~ Deleted   ● Unacceptable Principal Diagnosis   ● Use Additional Digit(s)
▶ Manifestation Code   **OGCR** Official Guidelines   **Coding Clinic**   Excludes   Includes   Use additional   Code first   Omit code

● **963 Poisoning by primarily systemic agents**

963.0 Antiallergic and antiemetic drugs
Antihistamines
Chlorpheniramine
Diphenhydramine
Diphenylpyraline
Thonzylamine
Tripelennamine

Excludes phenothiazine-based tranquilizers (969.1)

963.1 Antineoplastic and immunosuppressive drugs
Azathioprine
Busulfan
Chlorambucil
Cyclophosphamide
Cytarabine
Fluorouracil
Mercaptopurine
thio-TEPA

Excludes antineoplastic antibiotics (960.7)

963.2 Acidifying agents

963.3 Alkalizing agents

963.4 Enzymes, not elsewhere classified
Penicillinase

963.5 Vitamins, not elsewhere classified
Vitamin A
Vitamin D

Excludes nicotinic acid (972.2)
vitamin K (964.3)

963.8 Other specified systemic agents
Heavy metal antagonists

963.9 Unspecified systemic agent

● **964 Poisoning by agents primarily affecting blood constituents**

964.0 Iron and its compounds
Ferric salts
Ferrous sulfate and other ferrous salts

964.1 Liver preparations and other antianemic agents
Folic acid

964.2 Anticoagulants
Coumarin
Heparin
Phenindione
Warfarin sodium
Coding Clinic: 1994, Q1, P22

964.3 Vitamin K [phytonadione]

964.4 Fibrinolysis-affecting drugs
Aminocaproic acid
Streptodornase
Streptokinase
Urokinase

964.5 Anticoagulant antagonists and other coagulants
Hexadimethrine
Protamine sulfate

964.6 Gamma globulin

964.7 Natural blood and blood products
Blood plasma   Packed red cells
Human fibrinogen   Whole blood

Excludes transfusion reactions (999.4–999.8)

964.8 Other specified agents affecting blood constituents
Macromolecular blood substitutes
Plasma expanders

964.9 Unspecified agents affecting blood constituents

● **965 Poisoning by analgesics, antipyretics, and antirheumatics**
Use additional code to identify:
drug dependence (304.0–304.9)
nondependent abuse (305.0–305.9)

● **965.0 Opiates and related narcotics**

965.00 Opium (alkaloids), unspecified
Coding Clinic: 2007, Q3, P7-8

965.01 Heroin
Diacetylmorphine

965.02 Methadone

965.09 Other
Codeine [methylmorphine]
Meperidine [pethidine]
Morphine
Coding Clinic: 2007, Q3, P7-8

965.1 Salicylates
Acetylsalicylic acid [aspirin]
Salicylic acid salts
Coding Clinic: 1984, Nov-Dec, P15

965.4 Aromatic analgesics, not elsewhere classified
Acetanilid
Paracetamol [acetaminophen]
Phenacetin [acetophenetidin]

965.5 Pyrazole derivatives
Aminophenazone [aminopyrine]
Phenylbutazone

● **965.6 Antirheumatics [antiphlogistics]**

Excludes salicylates (965.1)
steroids (962.0–962.9)

965.61 Propionic acid derivatives
Fenoprofen
Flurbiprofen
Ibuprofen
Ketoprofen
Naproxen
Oxaprozin
Coding Clinic: 1998, Q4, P42-44

965.69 Other antirheumatics
Gold salts
Indomethacin

965.7 Other non-narcotic analgesics
Pyrabital

965.8 Other specified analgesics and antipyretics
Pentazocine

965.9 Unspecified analgesic and antipyretic

● **966 Poisoning by anticonvulsants and anti-Parkinsonism drugs**

966.0 Oxazolidine derivatives
Paramethadione
Trimethadione

966.1 Hydantoin derivatives
Phenytoin

966.2 Succinimides
Ethosuximide
Phensuximide

966.3 Other and unspecified anticonvulsants
Primidone

Excludes barbiturates (967.0)
sulfonamides (961.0)

966.4 Anti-Parkinsonism drugs
Amantadine
Ethopropazine [profenamine]
Levodopa [L-dopa]

INJURY AND POISONING (800–999)

● **967 Poisoning by sedatives and hypnotics**

Use additional code to identify:
drug dependence (304.0–304.9)
nondependent abuse (305.0–305.9)

967.0 Barbiturates
Amobarbital [amylobarbitone]
Barbital [barbitone]
Butabarbital [butabarbitone]
Pentobarbital [pentobarbitone]
Phenobarbital [phenobarbitone]
Secobarbital [quinalbarbitone]

Excludes thiobarbiturate anesthetics (968.3)

967.1 Chloral hydrate group

967.2 Paraldehyde

967.3 Bromine compounds
Bromide
Carbromal (derivatives)

967.4 Methaqualone compounds

967.5 Glutethimide group

967.6 Mixed sedatives, not elsewhere classified

967.8 Other sedatives and hypnotics

967.9 Unspecified sedative or hypnotic
Sleeping: Sleeping:
   drug NOS   tablet NOS
   pill NOS

● **968 Poisoning by other central nervous system depressants and anesthetics**

Use additional code to identify:
drug dependence (304.0–304.9)
nondependent abuse (305.0–305.9)

968.0 Central nervous system muscle-tone depressants
Chlorphenesin (carbamate)
Mephenesin
Methocarbamol

968.1 Halothane

968.2 Other gaseous anesthetics
Ether
Halogenated hydrocarbon derivatives, except halothane
Nitrous oxide

968.3 Intravenous anesthetics
Ketamine
Methohexital [methohexitone]
Thiobarbiturates, such as thiopental sodium

968.4 Other and unspecified general anesthetics

968.5 Surface [topical] and infiltration anesthetics
Cocaine   Procaine
Lidocaine [lignocaine]   Tetracaine
Coding Clinic: 1993, Q1, P25

968.6 Peripheral nerve- and plexus-blocking anesthetics

968.7 Spinal anesthetics

968.9 Other and unspecified local anesthetics

● **969 Poisoning by psychotropic agents**

Use additional code to identify:
drug dependence (304.0–304.9)
nondependent abuse (305.0–305.9)

● **969.0 Antidepressants** ◄▥
~~Amitriptyline~~
~~Imipramine~~
~~Monoamine oxidase [MAO] inhibitors~~
Coding Clinic: 2007, Q3, P7-8; 1991, Q3, P14

969.00 Antidepressant, unspecified ◄

969.01 Monoamine oxidase inhibitors ◄
MAOI ◄

969.02 Selective serotonin and norepinephrine reuptake inhibitors ◄
SSNRI antidepressants ◄

969.03 Selective serotonin reuptake inhibitors ◄
SSRI antidepressants ◄

969.04 Tetracyclic antidepressants ◄

969.05 Tricyclic antidepressants ◄

969.09 Other antidepressants ◄

969.1 Phenothiazine-based tranquilizers
Chlorpromazine
Fluphenazine
Prochlorperazine
Promazine

969.2 Butyrophenone-based tranquilizers
Haloperidol   Trifluperidol
Spiperone

969.3 Other antipsychotics, neuroleptics, and major tranquilizers

969.4 Benzodiazepine-based tranquilizers
Chlordiazepoxide   Lorazepam
Diazepam   Medazepam
Flurazepam   Nitrazepam
Coding Clinic: 1991, Q3, P14

969.5 Other tranquilizers
Hydroxyzine
Meprobamate

969.6 Psychodysleptics [hallucinogens]
Cannabis (derivatives)
Lysergide [LSD]
Marihuana (derivatives)
Marijuana
Mescaline
Psilocin
Psilocybin

● **969.7 Psychostimulants** ◄▥
~~Amphetamine~~
~~Caffeine~~

Excludes central appetite depressants (977.0)
Coding Clinic: 2003, Q2, P11

969.70 Psychostimulant, unspecified ◄

969.71 Caffeine ◄

969.72 Amphetamines ◄
Methamphetamines ◄

969.73 Methylphenidate ◄

969.79 Other psychostimulants ◄

969.8 Other specified psychotropic agents

969.9 Unspecified psychotropic agent

● **970 Poisoning by central nervous system stimulants**

970.0 Analeptics
Lobeline
Nikethamide

970.1 Opiate antagonists
Levallorphan
Nalorphine
Naloxone

970.8 Other specified central nervous system stimulants

970.9 Unspecified central nervous system stimulant

◄ New   ◄▥ Revised   ~~deleted~~ Deleted   ● Unacceptable Principal Diagnosis   ● Use Additional Digit(s)
▶ Manifestation Code   **OGCR** Official Guidelines   **Coding Clinic**   Excludes   Includes   Use additional   Code first   Omit code

● **971   Poisoning by drugs primarily affecting the autonomic nervous system**

    971.0   Parasympathomimetics [cholinergics]
       Acetylcholine
       Anticholinesterase:
         organophosphorus
         reversible
       Pilocarpine

    971.1   Parasympatholytics [anticholinergics and antimuscarinics] and spasmolytics
       Atropine
       Homatropine
       Hyoscine [scopolamine]
       Quaternary ammonium derivatives
       Excludes   *papaverine (972.5)*

    971.2   Sympathomimetics [adrenergics]
       Epinephrine [adrenalin]
       Levarterenol [noradrenalin]

    971.3   Sympatholytics [antiadrenergics]
       Phenoxybenzamine
       Tolazoline hydrochloride

    971.9   Unspecified drug primarily affecting autonomic nervous system

● **972   Poisoning by agents primarily affecting the cardiovascular system**

    972.0   Cardiac rhythm regulators
       Practolol
       Procainamide
       Propranolol
       Quinidine
       Excludes   *lidocaine (968.5)*

    972.1   Cardiotonic glycosides and drugs of similar action
       Digitalis glycosides
       Digoxin
       Strophanthins

    972.2   Antilipemic and antiarteriosclerotic drugs
       Clofibrate
       Nicotinic acid derivatives

    972.3   Ganglion-blocking agents
       Pentamethonium bromide

    972.4   Coronary vasodilators
       Dipyridamole
       Nitrates [nitroglycerin]
       Nitrites

    972.5   Other vasodilators
       Cyclandelate
       Diazoxide
       Papaverine
       Excludes   *nicotinic acid (972.2)*

    972.6   Other antihypertensive agents
       Clonidine
       Guanethidine
       Rauwolfia alkaloids
       Reserpine

    972.7   Antivaricose drugs, including sclerosing agents
       Sodium morrhuate
       Zinc salts

    972.8   Capillary-active drugs
       Adrenochrome derivatives
       Metaraminol

    972.9   Other and unspecified agents primarily affecting the cardiovascular system

● **973   Poisoning by agents primarily affecting the gastrointestinal system**

    973.0   Antacids and antigastric secretion drugs
       Aluminum hydroxide
       Magnesium trisilicate
       Coding Clinic: 2003, Q1, P19

    973.1   Irritant cathartics
       Bisacodyl
       Castor oil
       Phenolphthalein

    973.2   Emollient cathartics
       Dioctyl sulfosuccinates

    973.3   Other cathartics, including intestinal atonia drugs
       Magnesium sulfate

    973.4   Digestants
       Pancreatin   Pepsin
       Papain

    973.5   Antidiarrheal drugs
       Kaolin
       Pectin
       Excludes   *anti-infectives (960.0–961.9)*

    973.6   Emetics

    973.8   Other specified agents primarily affecting the gastrointestinal system

    973.9   Unspecified agent primarily affecting the gastrointestinal system

● **974   Poisoning by water, mineral, and uric acid metabolism drugs**

    974.0   Mercurial diuretics
       Chlormerodrin
       Mercaptomerin
       Mersalyl

    974.1   Purine derivative diuretics
       Theobromine
       Theophylline
       Excludes   *aminophylline [theophylline ethylenediamine] (975.7)*
           caffeine (969.71) ◄

    974.2   Carbonic acid anhydrase inhibitors
       Acetazolamide

    974.3   Saluretics
       Benzothiadiazides
       Chlorothiazide group

    974.4   Other diuretics
       Ethacrynic acid
       Furosemide

    974.5   Electrolytic, caloric, and water-balance agents

    974.6   Other mineral salts, not elsewhere classified

    974.7   Uric acid metabolism drugs
       Allopurinol
       Colchicine
       Probenecid

INJURY AND POISONING (800–999)

N Newborn Age: 0   **P** Pediatric Age: 0–17   **M** Maternity Age: 12–55   **A** Adult Age: 15–124   ♀ Females Only   ♂ Males Only

Ⓔⓧ CC Exclusions   Complication\Comorbidity   Major C\C   Present on Admission Requirement   Hospital-Acquired Condition   **1113**

●975 **Poisoning by agents primarily acting on the smooth and skeletal muscles and respiratory system**

975.0 **Oxytocic agents**
Ergot alkaloids
Oxytocin
Prostaglandins

975.1 **Smooth muscle relaxants**
Adiphenine
Metaproterenol [orciprenaline]
Excludes *papaverine (972.5)*

975.2 **Skeletal muscle relaxants**

975.3 **Other and unspecified drugs acting on muscles**

975.4 **Antitussives**
Dextromethorphan
Pipazethate

975.5 **Expectorants**
Acetylcysteine
Guaifenesin
Terpin hydrate

975.6 **Anti-common cold drugs**

975.7 **Antiasthmatics**
Aminophylline [theophylline ethylenediamine]

975.8 **Other and unspecified respiratory drugs**

●976 **Poisoning by agents primarily affecting skin and mucous membrane, ophthalmological, otorhinolaryngological, and dental drugs**

976.0 **Local anti-infectives and anti-inflammatory drugs**

976.1 **Antipruritics**

976.2 **Local astringents and local detergents**

976.3 **Emollients, demulcents, and protectants**

976.4 **Keratolytics, keratoplastics, other hair treatment drugs and preparations**

976.5 **Eye anti-infectives and other eye drugs**
Idoxuridine

976.6 **Anti-infectives and other drugs and preparations for ear, nose, and throat**

976.7 **Dental drugs topically applied**
Excludes *anti-infectives (976.0)*
local anesthetics (968.5)

976.8 **Other agents primarily affecting skin and mucous membrane**
Spermicides [vaginal contraceptives]

976.9 **Unspecified agent primarily affecting skin and mucous membrane**

●977 **Poisoning by other and unspecified drugs and medicinal substances**

977.0 **Dietetics**
Central appetite depressants

977.1 **Lipotropic drugs**

977.2 **Antidotes and chelating agents, not elsewhere classified**

977.3 **Alcohol deterrents**

977.4 **Pharmaceutical excipients**
Pharmaceutical adjuncts

977.8 **Other specified drugs and medicinal substances**
Contrast media used for diagnostic x-ray procedures
Diagnostic agents and kits

977.9 **Unspecified drug or medicinal substance**
Coding Clinic: 1986, Mar-April, P12

●978 **Poisoning by bacterial vaccines**

978.0 **BCG**

978.1 **Typhoid and paratyphoid**

978.2 **Cholera**

978.3 **Plague**

978.4 **Tetanus**

978.5 **Diphtheria**

978.6 **Pertussis vaccine, including combinations with a pertussis component**

978.8 **Other and unspecified bacterial vaccines**

978.9 **Mixed bacterial vaccines, except combinations with a pertussis component**

●979 **Poisoning by other vaccines and biological substances**
Excludes *gamma globulin (964.6)*

979.0 **Smallpox vaccine**

979.1 **Rabies vaccine**

979.2 **Typhus vaccine**

979.3 **Yellow fever vaccine**

979.4 **Measles vaccine**

979.5 **Poliomyelitis vaccine**

979.6 **Other and unspecified viral and rickettsial vaccines**
Mumps vaccine

979.7 **Mixed viral-rickettsial and bacterial vaccines, except combinations with a pertussis component**
Excludes *combinations with a pertussis component (978.6)*

979.9 **Other and unspecified vaccines and biological substances**
OGCR Section I.C.17.e.3
When a harmful substance is ingested or comes in contact with a person, this is classified as a toxic effect. The toxic effect codes are in categories 980-989. A toxic effect code should be sequenced first, followed by the code(s) that identify the result of the toxic effect. An external cause code from categories E860-E869 for accidental exposure, codes E950.6 or E950.7 for intentional self-harm, category E962 for assault, or categories E980-E982, for undetermined, should also be assigned to indicate intent.

TOXIC EFFECTS OF SUBSTANCES CHIEFLY NONMEDICINAL AS TO SOURCE (980–989)

Excludes *burns from chemical agents (ingested) (947.0–947.9)*
localized toxic effects indexed elsewhere (001.0–799.9)
respiratory conditions due to external agents (506.0–508.9)

Use additional code to specify the nature of the toxic effect

●980 **Toxic effect of alcohol**

980.0 **Ethyl alcohol**
Denatured alcohol
Ethanol
Grain alcohol

Use additional code to identify any associated:
acute alcohol intoxication (305.0)
in alcoholism (303.0)
drunkenness (simple) (305.0)
pathological (291.4)
Coding Clinic: 1996, Q3, P16; 1991, Q3, P14

980.1 **Methyl alcohol**
Methanol
Wood alcohol

◀ New ◀▥ Revised ~~deleted~~ Deleted ● Unacceptable Principal Diagnosis ● Use Additional Digit(s)
▶ Manifestation Code OGCR Official Guidelines **Coding Clinic** Excludes Includes Use additional Code first Omit code

980.2 Isopropyl alcohol
　Dimethyl carbinol
　Isopropanol
　Rubbing alcohol

980.3 Fusel oil
　Alcohol:
　　amyl
　　butyl
　　propyl

980.8 Other specified alcohols

980.9 Unspecified alcohol

981 Toxic effect of petroleum products
　Benzine
　Gasoline
　Kerosene
　Paraffin wax
　Petroleum:
　　ether
　　naphtha
　　spirit

● **982 Toxic effect of solvents other than petroleum based**

982.0 Benzene and homologues

982.1 Carbon tetrachloride

982.2 Carbon disulfide
　Carbon bisulfide

982.3 Other chlorinated hydrocarbon solvents
　Tetrachloroethylene
　Trichloroethylene

　| **Excludes** | *chlorinated hydrocarbon preparations other than solvents (989.2)* |

　Coding Clinic: 2008, Q3, P6, 7x2

982.4 Nitroglycol

982.8 Other nonpetroleum-based solvents
　Acetone

● **983 Toxic effect of corrosive aromatics, acids, and caustic alkalis**

983.0 Corrosive aromatics
　Carbolic acid or phenol
　Cresol

983.1 Acids
　Acid:
　　hydrochloric
　　nitric
　　sulfuric

983.2 Caustic alkalis
　Lye
　Potassium hydroxide
　Sodium hydroxide

983.9 Caustic, unspecified

● **984 Toxic effect of lead and its compounds (including fumes)**

　| **Includes** | that from all sources except medicinal substances |

984.0 Inorganic lead compounds
　Lead dioxide
　Lead salts

984.1 Organic lead compounds
　Lead acetate
　Tetraethyl lead

984.8 Other lead compounds

984.9 Unspecified lead compound

● **985 Toxic effect of other metals**

　| **Includes** | that from all sources except medicinal substances |

985.0 Mercury and its compounds
　Minamata disease

985.1 Arsenic and its compounds

985.2 Manganese and its compounds

985.3 Beryllium and its compounds

985.4 Antimony and its compounds

985.5 Cadmium and its compounds

985.6 Chromium

985.8 Other specified metals
　Brass fumes
　Copper salts
　Iron compounds
　Nickel compounds

985.9 Unspecified metal

986 Toxic effect of carbon monoxide

● **987 Toxic effect of other gases, fumes, or vapors**

987.0 Liquefied petroleum gases
　Butane
　Propane

987.1 Other hydrocarbon gas

987.2 Nitrogen oxides
　Nitrogen dioxide
　Nitrous fumes

987.3 Sulfur dioxide

987.4 Freon
　Dichloromonofluoromethane

987.5 Lacrimogenic gas
　Bromobenzyl cyanide
　Chloroacetophenone
　Ethyliodoacetate

987.6 Chlorine gas

987.7 Hydrocyanic acid gas

987.8 Other specified gases, fumes, or vapors
　Phosgene
　Polyester fumes

987.9 Unspecified gas, fume, or vapor
　Coding Clinic: 2005, Q3, P10-11

● **988 Toxic effect of noxious substances eaten as food**

Excludes	*allergic reaction to food, such as:*
	*　gastroenteritis (558.3)*
	*　rash (692.5, 693.1)*
	food poisoning (bacterial) (005.0–005.9)
	toxic effects of food contaminants, such as:
	*　aflatoxin and other mycotoxin (989.7)*
	*　mercury (985.0)*

988.0 Fish and shellfish

988.1 Mushrooms

988.2 Berries and other plants

988.8 Other specified noxious substances eaten as food

988.9 Unspecified noxious substance eaten as food

N Newborn Age: 0   **P** Pediatric Age: 0–17   **M** Maternity Age: 12–55   **A** Adult Age: 15–124   ♀ Females Only   ♂ Males Only

(Ex) CC Exclusions   ● Complication\Comorbidity   Major C\C   Present on Admission Requirement   Hospital-Acquired Condition   **1115**

INJURY AND POISONING (800–999)

● 989   **Toxic effect of other substances, chiefly nonmedicinal as to source**

989.0   **Hydrocyanic acid and cyanides**
Potassium cyanide
Sodium cyanide
    Excludes | *gas and fumes (987.7)*

989.1   **Strychnine and salts**

989.2   **Chlorinated hydrocarbons**
Aldrin
Chlordane
DDT
Dieldrin
    Excludes | *chlorinated hydrocarbon solvents (982.0–982.3)*

989.3   **Organophosphate and carbamate**
Carbaryl   Parathion
Dichlorvos   Phorate
Malathion   Phosdrin

989.4   **Other pesticides, not elsewhere classified**
Mixtures of insecticides

989.5   **Venom**
Bites of venomous snakes, lizards, and spiders
Tick paralysis

989.6   **Soaps and detergents**

989.7   **Aflatoxin and other mycotoxin [food contaminants]**

● 989.8   **Other substances, chiefly nonmedicinal as to source**

989.81   **Asbestos**
    Excludes | *asbestosis (501)*
              exposure to asbestos (V15.84)

989.82   **Latex**

989.83   **Silicone**
    Excludes | *silicone used in medical devices, implants and grafts (996.00–996.79)*

989.84   **Tobacco**

989.89   **Other**

989.9   **Unspecified substance, chiefly nonmedicinal as to source**

OTHER AND UNSPECIFIED EFFECTS OF EXTERNAL CAUSES (990–995)

990   **Effects of radiation, unspecified**
Complication of:
photochemotherapy
radiation therapy
Radiation sickness
    Excludes | *specified adverse effects of radiation. Such conditions are to be classified according to the nature of the adverse effect, as:*
              burns (940.0–949.5)
              dermatitis (692.7–692.8)
              leukemia (204.0–208.9)
              pneumonia (508.0)
              sunburn (692.71, 692.76–692.77)
              [The type of radiation giving rise to the adverse effect may be identified by use of the E codes.]

● 991   **Effects of reduced temperature**

991.0   **Frostbite of face** 🅒 🅝
    Ex: 991.6, 991.3

991.1   **Frostbite of hand** 🅒 🅝
    Ex: 991.1, 991.3

991.2   **Frostbite of foot** 🅒 🅝
    Ex: 991.2–991.3

991.3   **Frostbite of other and unspecified sites** 🅒 🅝
    Ex: 991.0–991.4

991.4   **Immersion foot** 🅒 🅝
Trench foot
    Ex: 991.3–991.4

991.5   **Chilblains** 🅝
Erythema pernio
Perniosis

991.6   **Hypothermia** 🅝
Hypothermia (accidental)
    Excludes | *hypothermia following anesthesia (995.89)*
              hypothermia not associated with low environmental temperature (780.65)

991.8   **Other specified effects of reduced temperature** 🅝

991.9   **Unspecified effect of reduced temperature** 🅝
Effects of freezing or excessive cold NOS

● 992   **Effects of heat and light**
    Excludes | *burns (940.0–949.5)*
              diseases of sweat glands due to heat (705.0–705.9)
              malignant hyperpyrexia following anesthesia (995.86)
              sunburn (692.71, 692.76–692.77)

992.0   **Heat stroke and sunstroke** 🅒 🅝
Heat apoplexy
Heat pyrexia
Ictus solaris
Siriasis
Thermoplegia
    Ex: 992.0–992.9

992.1   **Heat syncope** 🅝
Heat collapse

992.2   **Heat cramps** 🅝

992.3   **Heat exhaustion, anhydrotic** 🅝
Heat prostration due to water depletion
    Excludes | *that associated with salt depletion (992.4)*

992.4   **Heat exhaustion due to salt depletion** 🅝
Heat prostration due to salt (and water) depletion

992.5   **Heat exhaustion, unspecified** 🅝
Heat prostration NOS

992.6   **Heat fatigue, transient** 🅝

992.7   **Heat edema** 🅝

992.8   **Other specified heat effects** 🅝

992.9   **Unspecified** 🅝

● 993   **Effects of air pressure**

993.0   **Barotrauma, otitic** 🅝
Aero-otitis media
Effects of high altitude on ears

993.1   **Barotrauma, sinus** 🅝
Aerosinusitis
Effects of high altitude on sinuses

993.2   **Other and unspecified effects of high altitude** 🅝
Alpine sickness
Andes disease
Anoxia due to high altitude
Hypobaropathy
Mountain sickness

◀ New   ◀═ Revised   ~~deleted~~ Deleted   ● Unacceptable Principal Diagnosis   ● Use Additional Digit(s)
▶ Manifestation Code   OGCR Official Guidelines   Coding Clinic   Excludes   Includes   Use additional   Code first   Omit code

993.3 Caisson disease 🦴 🦴
    Bends
    Compressed-air disease
    Decompression sickness
    Divers' palsy or paralysis
    (Ex) 993.3-993.9

993.4 Effects of air pressure caused by explosion 🦴

993.8 Other specified effects of air pressure 🦴

993.9 Unspecified effect of air pressure 🦴

● **994 Effects of other external causes**
    Excludes *certain adverse effects not elsewhere classified*
         (995.0–995.8)

994.0 Effects of lightning 🦴
    Shock from lightning
    Struck by lightning NOS
    Excludes *burns (940.0–949.5)*

994.1 Drowning and nonfatal submersion 🦴 🦴
    Bathing cramp
    Immersion
    (Ex) 994.1

994.2 Effects of hunger 🦴
    Deprivation of food
    Starvation

994.3 Effects of thirst 🦴
    Deprivation of water

994.4 Exhaustion due to exposure 🦴

994.5 Exhaustion due to excessive exertion 🦴
    Exhaustion due to overexertion

994.6 Motion sickness 🦴
    Air sickness
    Seasickness
    Travel sickness

994.7 Asphyxiation and strangulation 🦴 🦴
    Suffocation (by):
        bedclothes
        cave-in
        constriction
        mechanical
        plastic bag
        pressure
        strangulation
    Excludes *asphyxia from:*
        carbon monoxide (986)
        inhalation of food or foreign body
          (932–934.9)
        other gases, fumes, and vapors
          (987.0–987.9)
    (Ex) 994.7

994.8 Electrocution and nonfatal effects of electric current 🦴
    Shock from electric current
    Shock from electroshock gun (taser)
    Excludes *electric burns (940.0–949.5)*

994.9 Other effects of external causes 🦴
    Effects of:
        abnormal gravitational [G] forces or states
        weightlessness

● **995 Certain adverse effects not elsewhere classified**
    Excludes *complications of surgical and medical care*
        (996.0–999.9)
    Coding Clinic: 2008, Q1, P12-13

995.0 Other anaphylactic shock 🦴
    Allergic shock NOS or due to adverse effect
        of correct medicinal substance properly
        administered
    Anaphylactic reaction NOS or due to adverse
        effect of correct medicinal substance properly
        administered
    Anaphylaxis NOS or due to adverse effect of
        correct medicinal substance properly
        administered
    Excludes *anaphylactic reaction to serum (999.4)*
        anaphylactic shock due to adverse food
          reaction (995.60–995.69)
    Use additional E code to identify external cause,
        such as:
        adverse effects of correct medicinal substance
          properly administered [E930–E949]
    (Ex) 995.60-995.69

995.1 Angioneurotic edema
    Giant urticaria
    Excludes *urticaria:*
        due to serum (999.5)
        other specified (698.2, 708.0–708.9,
          757.33)

● **995.2 Other and unspecified adverse effect of drug, medicinal and biological substance (due) to correct medicinal substance properly administered**
    Adverse effect to correct medicinal substance
        properly administered
    Allergic reaction to correct medicinal substance
        properly administered
    Hypersensitivity to correct medicinal substance
        properly administered
    Idiosyncrasy due to correct medicinal substance
        properly administered
    Drug:
        hypersensitivity NOS
        reaction NOS
    Excludes *pathological drug intoxication (292.2)*
    Coding Clinic: 2006, Q4, P112-113; 1997, Q2, P12; 1995, Q3, P13;
        1992, Q3, P16-17

995.20 Unspecified adverse effect of unspecified drug, medicinal and biological substance

995.21 Arthus phenomenon
    Arthus reaction
    Hypersensitivity reaction resulting from
        immune complex reactions

995.22 Unspecified adverse effect of anesthesia

995.23 Unspecified adverse effect of insulin

995.24 Failed moderate sedation during procedure ◄
    Failed conscious sedation during
        procedure ◄

995.27 Other drug allergy
    Drug allergy NOS
    Drug hypersensitivity NOS

995.29 Unspecified adverse effect of other drug, medicinal and biological substance

N Newborn Age: 0   **P** Pediatric Age: 0–17   **M** Maternity Age: 12–55   **A** Adult Age: 15–124   ♀ Females Only   ♂ Males Only

(Ex) CC Exclusions   🦴 Complication\Comorbidity   🦴 Major C\C   🦴 Present on Admission Requirement   🦴 Hospital-Acquired Condition   **1117**

INJURY AND POISONING (800–999)

995.3 Allergy, unspecified
Allergic reaction NOS
Hypersensitivity NOS
Idiosyncrasy NOS

> **Excludes** | *allergic reaction NOS to correct medicinal substance properly administered (995.27)*
> *allergy to existing dental restorative materials (525.66)*
> *specific types of allergic reaction, such as:*
> *allergic diarrhea (558.3)*
> *dermatitis (691.0–693.9)*
> *hayfever (477.0–477.9)*

995.4 Shock due to anesthesia🦻
Shock due to anesthesia in which the correct substance was properly administered

> **Excludes** | *complications of anesthesia in labor or delivery (668.0–668.9)*
> *overdose or wrong substance given (968.0–969.9)*
> *postoperative shock NOS (998.0)*
> *specified adverse effects of anesthesia classified elsewhere, such as:*
> *anoxic brain damage (348.1)*
> *hepatitis (070.0–070.9), etc.*
> *unspecified adverse effect of anesthesia (995.22)*

(Ex:) 958.4, 995.4, 997.91-998.13, 998.81, 998.83-998.9

● **995.5 Child maltreatment syndrome**
Use additional code(s), if applicable, to identify any associated injuries

Use additional E code to identify:
nature of abuse (E960–E968)
perpetrator (E967.0–E967.9)
Coding Clinic: 1998, Q1, P11; 1984, Sept-Oct, P16; 1984, Nov-Dec, P9

995.50 Child abuse, unspecified🦻   P
(Ex:) 995.50-995.59, 995.80-995.85

995.51 Child emotional/psychological abuse🦻   P
(Ex:) 995.50-995.59, 995.80-995.85

995.52 Child neglect (nutritional)🦻   P
Use additional code to identify intent of neglect (E904.0,E968.4)
(Ex:) 995.50-995.59, 995.80-995.85

995.53 Child sexual abuse🦻   P
(Ex:) 995.50-995.59, 995.80-995.85

995.54 Child physical abuse🦻   P
Battered baby or child syndrome

> **Excludes** | *Shaken infant syndrome (995.55)*

(Ex:) 995.50-995.59, 995.80-995.85
Coding Clinic: 1999, Q3, P14-15

995.55 Shaken infant syndrome🦻   P
Use additional code(s) to identify any associated injuries
(Ex:) 995.50-995.59, 995.80-995.85
Coding Clinic: 1996, Q4, P43-44

995.59 Other child abuse and neglect🦻   P
Multiple forms of abuse
Use additional code to identify intent of neglect (E904.0,E968.4)
(Ex:) 995.50-995.59, 995.80-995.85

● **995.6 Anaphylactic shock due to adverse food reaction**
Anaphylactic reaction due to food
Anaphylactic shock due to nonpoisonous foods

995.60 Due to unspecified food🦻
(Ex:) 995.60-995.69

995.61 Due to peanuts🦻
(Ex:) 995.60-995.69

995.62 Due to crustaceans🦻
(Ex:) 995.60-995.69

995.63 Due to fruits and vegetables🦻
(Ex:) 995.60-995.69

995.64 Due to tree nuts and seeds🦻
(Ex:) 995.60-995.69
Coding Clinic: 2008, Q1, P12-13

995.65 Due to fish🦻
(Ex:) 995.60-995.69

995.66 Due to food additives🦻
(Ex:) 995.60-995.69

995.67 Due to milk products🦻
(Ex:) 995.60-995.69

995.68 Due to eggs🦻
(Ex:) 995.60-995.69

995.69 Due to other specified food🦻
(Ex:) 995.60-995.69

995.7 Other adverse food reactions, not elsewhere classified
Use additional code to identify the type of reaction, such as:
hives (708.0)
wheezing (786.07)

> **Excludes** | *anaphylactic shock due to adverse food reaction (995.6)*
> *asthma (493.0, 493.9)*
> *dermatitis due to food (693.1)*
> *in contact with the skin (692.5)*
> *gastroenteritis and colitis due to food (558.3)*
> *rhinitis due to food (477.1)*

● **995.8 Other specified adverse effects, not elsewhere classified**

995.80 Adult maltreatment, unspecified🦻   A
Abused person NOS

Use additional code to identify:
any associated injury
nature of abuse (E960–E968)
perpetrator (E967.0–E967.9)
(Ex:) 995.80

995.81 Adult physical abuse🦻   A
Battered:
person syndrome NEC
man
spouse
woman

Use additional code to identify:
any associated injury
nature of abuse (E960–E968)
perpetrator (E967.0–E967.9)
(Ex:) 995.50-995.59, 995.80-995.85
Coding Clinic: 1996, Q4, P43-44; 1984, Sept-Oct, P16

995.82 Adult emotional/psychological abuse   A
Use additional E code to identify perpetrator (E967.0–E967.9)

995.83 Adult sexual abuse🦻   A
Use additional code to identify:
any associated injury
perpetrator (E967.0–E967.9)
(Ex:) 995.50-995.59, 995.80 -995.85

995.84 Adult neglect (nutritional)🦻   A
Use additional code to identify:
intent of neglect (E904.0–E968.4)
perpetrator (E967.0–E967.9)
(Ex:) 995.50-995.59, 995.80-995.85

◀ New   ◀▦ Revised   ~~deleted~~ Deleted   ● Unacceptable Principal Diagnosis   ● Use Additional Digit(s)
▶ Manifestation Code   OGCR Official Guidelines   Coding Clinic   Excludes   Includes   Use additional   Code first   Omit code

995.85 Other adult abuse and neglect 🔖   A
Multiple forms of abuse and neglect

Use additional code to identify:
any associated injury
intent of neglect (E904.0, E968.4)
nature of abuse (E960–E968)
perpetrator (E967.0–E967.9)
(Ex:) 995.50-995.59, 995.80-995.85

995.86 Malignant hyperthermia 🔖
Malignant hyperpyrexia due to anesthesia
*Extremely high body temperature—greater
than 106° F or 41.1° C*
(Ex:) 958.4, 995.4, 995.86, 997.91-998.13, 998.81, 998.83-998.9

995.89 Other
Hypothermia due to anesthesia
Coding Clinic: 2004, Q2, P18; 2003, Q3, P12

● **995.9 Systemic inflammatory response syndrome (SIRS)**
Coding Clinic: 2006, Q4, P113-116; 2005, Q3, P23; 2004, Q2, P16;
2002, Q4, P71-73

**995.90 Systemic inflammatory response syndrome,
unspecified SIRS NOS** 🔖
(Ex:) 003.1, 020.2, 036.2, 038.0-038.9, 040.82-041.9, 054.5, 139.8,
995.90-995.94, V09.0-V09.91

● **995.91 Sepsis** 🔖
Systemic inflammatory response syndrome
due to infectious process without
acute organ dysfunction

Code first underlying infection

| **Excludes** | *sepsis with acute organ dysfunction (995.92)
sepsis with multiple organ dysfunction (995.92)
severe sepsis (995.92)* |

(Ex:) 003.1, 020.2, 036.2, 038.0-038.9, 040.82-041.9, 054.5, 139.8,
995.90-995.94, V09.0-V09.91
Coding Clinic: 2008, Q4, P69-73; 2007, Q4, P84-86; 2004,
Q2, P16

OGCR Section I.C.1.b.2.12

Only one code from subcategory 995.9
should be assigned. Therefore, when
a non-infectious condition leads to an
infection resulting in sepsis or severe
sepsis, assign either code 995.91 or 995.92.
Do not additionally assign code 995.93,
Systemic inflammatory response syndrome
due to non-infectious process without
acute organ dysfunctiion, or 995.94,
Systemic inflammatory response syndrome
with acute organ dysfunction.

995.92 Severe sepsis 🔖
Sepsis with acute organ dysfunction
Sepsis with multiple organ dysfunction
(MOD)
Systemic inflammatory response syndrome
due to infectious process with acute
organ dysfunction

Code first underlying infection

Use additional code to specify acute organ
dysfunction, such as:
acute ~~renal~~ kidney failure (584.5–584.9) ◀▥
acute respiratory failure (518.81)
critical illness myopathy (359.81)
critical illness polyneuropathy (357.82)
disseminated intravascular coagulopathy
(DIC) syndrome (286.6)
encephalopathy (348.31)
hepatic failure (570)
septic shock (785.52)
(Ex:) 003.1, 020.2, 036.2, 038.0-038.9, 040.82-041.9, 054.5, 139.8,
995.90-995.94, V09.0-V09.91
Coding Clinic: 2007, Q4, P96-97; 2005, Q2, P18-20x2;
2004, Q2, P16; 2003, Q4, P73, 79-81

**995.93 Systemic inflammatory response syndrome
due to noninfectious process without acute
organ dysfunction** 🔖

Code first underlying conditions, such as:
acute pancreatitis (577.0)
trauma

| **Excludes** | *systemic inflammatory
response syndrome due to
noninfectious process with
acute organ dysfunction
(995.94)* |

(Ex:) 003.1, 020.2, 036.2, 038.0-038.9, 040.82-041.9, 054.5, 139.8,
995.90-995.94, V09.0-V09.91

OGCR Section I.C.19.a.7

An external cause code(s) may be used
with codes 995.93 if trauma was the
initiating insult that precipitated the
SIRS. The external cause(s) code should
correspond to the most serious injury
resulting from the trauma. The external
cause code(s) should only be assigned if the
trauma necessitated the admission in which
the patient also developed SIRS. If a patient
is admitted with SIRS but the trauma has
been treated previously, the external cause
codes should not be used.

**995.94 Systemic inflammatory response syndrome
due to non-infectious process with acute
organ dysfunction** 🔖

Code first underlying conditions, such as:
acute pancreatitis (577.0)
trauma

Use additional code to specify acute organ
dysfunction, such as:
acute ~~renal~~ kidney failure
(584.5–584.9)   ◀▥
acute respiratory failure (518.81)
critical illness myopathy (359.81)
critical illness polyneuropathy (357.82)
disseminated intravascular coagulopathy
(DIC) syndrome (286.6)
encephalopathy (348.31)
hepatic failure (570)

| **Excludes** | *severe sepsis (995.92)* |

(Ex:) 003.1, 020.2, 036.2, 038.0-038.9, 040.82-041.9, 054.5, 139.8,
995.90-995.94, V09.0-V09.91
Coding Clinic: 2005, Q2, P19-20

OGCR Section I.C.19.a.7

An external cause code(s) may be used with
codes 995.94 if trauma was the initiating
insult that precipitated the SIRS. The
external cause(s) code should correspond to
the most serious injury resulting from the
trauma. The external cause code(s) should
only be assigned if the trauma necessitated
the admission in which the patient also
developed SIRS. If a patient is admitted
with SIRS but the trauma has been treated
previously, the external cause codes should
not be used.

INJURY AND POISONING (800–999)

COMPLICATIONS OF SURGICAL AND MEDICAL CARE, NOT ELSEWHERE CLASSIFIED (996–999)

Excludes	adverse effects of medicinal agents (001.0–799.9, 995.0–995.8)

burns from local applications and irradiation (940.0–949.5)
complications of:
conditions for which the procedure was performed
surgical procedures during abortion, labor, and delivery (630–676.9)
poisoning and toxic effects of drugs and chemicals (960.0–989.9)
postoperative conditions in which no complications are present, such as:
artificial opening status (V44.0–V44.9)
closure of external stoma (V55.0–V55.9)
fitting of prosthetic device (V52.0–V52.9)
specified complications classified elsewhere:
anesthetic shock (995.4)
electrolyte imbalance (276.0–276.9)
postlaminectomy syndrome (722.80–722.83)
postmastectomy lymphedema syndrome (457.0)
postoperative psychosis (293.0–293.9)
any other condition classified elsewhere in the Alphabetic Index when described as due to a procedure

● **996 Complications peculiar to certain specified procedures**

Includes	complications, not elsewhere classified, in the use of artificial substitutes [e.g., Dacron, metal, Silastic, Teflon] or natural sources [e.g., bone] involving:

anastomosis (internal)
graft (bypass) (patch)
implant
internal device:
  catheter
  electronic
  fixation
  prosthetic
reimplant
transplant

Excludes	accidental puncture or laceration during procedure (998.2)

capsular contracture of breast implant (611.83)
complications of internal anastomosis of:
gastrointestinal tract (997.4)
urinary tract (997.5)
endosseous dental implant failures (525.71–525.79)
intraoperative floppy iris syndrome (IFIS) (364.81)
mechanical complication of respirator (V46.14)
other specified complications classified elsewhere, such as:
hemolytic anemia (283.1)
functional cardiac disturbances (429.4)
serum hepatitis (070.2–070.3)

● **996.0 Mechanical complication of cardiac device, implant, and graft**

Breakdown (mechanical)   Obstruction, mechanical
Displacement   Perforation
Leakage   Protrusion
Coding Clinic: 2007, Q3, P7-8

996.00 Unspecified device, implant, and graft
(Ex:) 996.00, 996.04, 996.61-996.62, 996.70-996.74, 997.91-997.99, 998.81, 998.83-998.9

996.01 Due to cardiac pacemaker (electrode)
(Ex:) 996.01, 997.91-997.99, 998.81, 998.83-998.9
Coding Clinic: 2006, Q2, P15-16; 1999, Q2, P11-12

996.02 Due to heart valve prosthesis
(Ex:) 996.02, 997.91-997.99, 998.81, 998.83-998.9
Coding Clinic: 1999, Q2, P4

996.03 Due to coronary bypass graft

Excludes	atherosclerosis of graft (414.02, 414.03)

embolism [occlusion NOS] [thrombus] of graft (996.72)
(Ex:) 996.03, 997.91-997.99, 998.81, 998.83-998.9
Coding Clinic: 1993, Q4, P40-41

996.04 Due to automatic implantable cardiac defibrillator
(Ex:) 996.04, 997.91-997.99, 998.81, 998.83-998.9
Coding Clinic: 2005, Q2, P3

996.09 Other
(Ex:) 996.09, 997.91-997.99, 998.81, 998.83-998.9
Coding Clinic: 1993, Q2, P9

996.1 Mechanical complication of other vascular device, implant, and graft
Mechanical complications involving:
aortic (bifurcation) graft (replacement)
arteriovenous:
  dialysis catheter
  fistula surgically created
  shunt surgically created
balloon (counterpulsation) device, intra-aortic
carotid artery bypass graft
femoral-popliteal bypass graft
umbrella device, vena cava

Excludes	atherosclerosis of biological graft (440.30–440.32)

embolism [occlusion NOS] [thrombus] of (biological) (synthetic) graft (996.74)
peritoneal dialysis catheter (996.56)
(Ex:) 996.1, 997.91-997.99, 998.81, 998.83-998.9
Coding Clinic: 2006, Q1, P10-11; 2005, Q2, P8; 2002, Q1, P13; 1995, Q1, P3

996.2 Mechanical complication of nervous system device, implant, and graft
Mechanical complications involving:
dorsal column stimulator
electrodes implanted in brain [brain "pacemaker"]
peripheral nerve graft
ventricular (communicating) shunt
(Ex:) 996.2, 996.63, 996.75, 997.91-997.99, 998.81, 998.83-998.9
Coding Clinic: 1987, Sept-Oct, P10

● **996.3 Mechanical complication of genitourinary device, implant, and graft**

996.30 Unspecified device, implant, and graft
(Ex:) 996.30, 996.64-996.65, 996.76, 997.91-997.99, 998.81, 998.83-998.9

996.31 Due to urethral [indwelling] catheter

996.32 Due to intrauterine contraceptive device ♀

996.39 Other
Cystostomy catheter
Prosthetic reconstruction of vas deferens
Repair (graft) of ureter without mention of resection

Excludes	complications due to:

external stoma of urinary tract (997.5)
internal anastomosis of urinary tract (997.5)
(Ex:) 996.39, 996.64-996.65, 996.76, 997.91-997.99, 998.81, 998.83-998.9

◀ New   ◀ Revised   deleted Deleted   ● Unacceptable Principal Diagnosis   Use Additional Digit(s)
▶ Manifestation Code   OGCR Official Guidelines   Coding Clinic   Excludes   Includes   Use additional   Code first   Omit code

INJURY AND POISONING (800–999)

● **996.4 Mechanical complication of internal orthopedic device, implant, and graft**

Mechanical complications involving:

external (fixation) device utilizing internal screw(s), pin(s) or other methods of fixation

grafts of bone, cartilage, muscle, or tendon

internal (fixation) device such as nail, plate, rod, etc.

Use additional code to identify prosthetic joint with mechanical complication (V43.60–V43.69)

Excludes | complications of external orthopedic device, such as:

pressure ulcer due to cast (707.00–707.09)

Coding Clinic: 2005, Q4, P91-93, 110-112; 1999, Q2, P10-11; 1998, Q2, P19; 1996, Q2, P11; 1985, Nov-Dec, P11; 1984, Nov-Dec, P18

996.40 Unspecified mechanical complication of internal orthopedic device, implant, and graft

(Ex:) 996.40-996.49, 996.66-996.67, 996.77-996.78, 997.91-997.99, 998.81, 998.83-998.9

996.41 Mechanical loosening of prosthetic joint

Aseptic loosening

(Ex:) 996.40-996.49, 996.66-996.67, 996.77-996.78, 997.91-997.99, 998.81, 998.83-998.9

Coding Clinic: 2005, Q4, P91-93

996.42 Dislocation of prosthetic joint

Instability of prosthetic joint

Subluxation of prosthetic joint

(Ex:) 996.40-996.49, 996.66-996.67, 996.77-996.78, 997.91-997.99, 998.81, 998.83-998.9

996.43 ~~Prosthetic joint implant failure~~ Broken prosthetic joint implant ◀┉

Breakage (fracture) of prosthetic joint

(Ex:) 996.40-996.49, 996.66-996.67, 996.77-996.78, 997.91-997.99, 998.81, 998.83-998.9

996.44 Peri-prosthetic fracture around prosthetic joint

(Ex:) 996.40-996.49, 996.66-996.67, 996.77-996.78, 997.91-997.99, 998.81, 998.83-998.9

Coding Clinic: 2005, Q4, P91-93

996.45 Peri-prosthetic osteolysis

Use additional code to identify major osseous defect, if applicable (731.3)

(Ex:) 996.40-996.49, 996.66 -996.67, 996.77-996.78, 997.91-997.99, 998.81, 998.83-998.9

Coding Clinic: 2006, Q4, P103-104

996.46 Articular bearing surface wear of prosthetic joint

(Ex:) 996.40-996.49, 996.66-996.67, 996.77-996.78, 997.91-997.99, 998.81, 998.83-998.9

996.47 Other mechanical complication of prosthetic joint implant

Mechanical complication of prosthetic joint NOS

Prosthetic joint implant failure NOS ◀

(Ex:) 996.40-996.49, 996.66-996.67, 996.77-996.78, 997.91-997.99, 998.81, 998.83-998.9

996.49 Other mechanical complication of other internal orthopedic device, implant, and graft

Breakage of internal fixation device in bone

Dislocation of internal fixation device in bone

Excludes | mechanical complication of prosthetic joint implant (996.41–996.46)

(Ex:) 996.40-996.49, 996.66-996.67, 996.77-996.78, 997.91-997.99, 998.81, 998.83-998.9

● **996.5 Mechanical complication of other specified prosthetic device, implant, and graft**

Mechanical complications involving:

prosthetic implant in:

bile duct

breast

chin

orbit of eye

nonabsorbable surgical material NOS

other graft, implant, and internal device, not elsewhere classified

996.51 Due to corneal graft

(Ex:) 996.51, 997.91-997.99

996.52 Due to graft of other tissue, not elsewhere classified

Skin graft failure or rejection

Excludes | failure of artificial skin graft (996.55)

failure of decellularized allodermis (996.55)

sloughing of temporary skin allografts or xenografts (pigskin)- omit code

(Ex:) 996.52, 996.55, 997.91-99.799

Coding Clinic: 1996, Q1, P10; 1990, Q3, P15

996.53 Due to ocular lens prosthesis

Excludes | contact lenses—code to condition

(Ex:) 996.53, 997.91-997.99

Coding Clinic: 2000, Q1, P9-10

996.54 Due to breast prosthesis

Breast capsule (prosthesis)

Mammary implant

(Ex:) 996.54, 997.91-997.99

Coding Clinic: 1998, Q2, P14; 1992, Q3, P4-5

996.55 Due to artificial skin graft and decellularized allodermis

Dislodgement

Displacement

Failure

Non-adherence

Poor incorporation

Shearing

(Ex:) 996.52, 996.55-996.60, 996.68-996.70, 996.79, 997.91-997.99

Coding Clinic: 1998, Q4, P52-53

996.56 Due to peritoneal dialysis catheter

Excludes | mechanical complication of arteriovenous dialysis catheter (996.1)

(Ex:) 996.56-996.60, 996.68-996.70, 996.79, 997.91-997.99

Coding Clinic: 1998, Q4, P54

INJURY AND POISONING (800–999)

996.57　Due to insulin pump 🗘
(Ex:) 996.00-996.30, 996.39-996.79, 997.91-997.99, 998.81, 998.83-998.9
Coding Clinic: 2003, Q4, P81-82

OGCR Section I.C.3.a.6.a

An underdose of insulin due to an insulin pump failure should be assigned 996.57, Mechanical complication due to insulin pump, as the principal or first listed code, followed by the appropriate diabetes mellitus code based on documentation.

OGCR Section I.C.3.a.6.b

The principal or first listed code for an encounter due to an insulin pump malfunction resulting in an overdose of insulin, should also be 996.57, Mechanical complication due to insulin pump, followed by 962.3, Poisoning by insulins and antidiabetic agents, and the appropriate diabetes mellitus code based on documentation.

996.59　Due to other implant and internal device, not elsewhere classified 🗘
Nonabsorbable surgical material NOS
Prosthetic implant in:
　bile duct
　chin
　orbit of eye
(Ex:) 996.56-996.60, 996.68-996.70, 996.79, 997.91-997.99
Coding Clinic: 1999, Q2, P13-14; 1997, Q3, P7; 1994, Q3, P7x2

● **996.6　Infection and inflammatory reaction due to internal prosthetic device, implant, and graft**
Infection (causing obstruction) due to (presence of) any device, implant, and graft classifiable to 996.0–996.5
Inflammation due to (presence of) any device, implant, and graft classifiable to 996.0–996.5

Use additional code to identify specified infections
Coding Clinic: 2008, Q2, P9-10; 1987, Jan-Feb, P14-15

996.60　Due to unspecified device, implant and graft 🗘
(Ex:) 996.00-996.30, 996.39-996.79, 997.91-997.99, 998.81, 998.83-998.9

996.61　Due to cardiac device, implant and graft 🗘
Cardiac pacemaker or defibrillator:
　electrode(s), lead(s)
　pulse generator
　subcutaneous pocket
Coronary artery bypass graft
Heart valve prosthesis
(Ex:) 996.00-996.1, 996.52, 996.55-996.62, 996.68-996.74, 996.79, 997.91-997.99, 998.81, 998.83-998.9

996.62　Due to vascular device, implant and graft 🗘
Arterial graft
Arteriovenous fistula or shunt
Infusion pump
Vascular catheter (arterial) (dialysis) (peripheral venous)

Excludes　*infection due to:*
　　central venous catheter (999.31)
　　Hickman catheter (999.31)
　　peripherally inserted central catheter (PICC) (999.31)
　　portacath (port-a-cath) (999.31)
　　triple lumen catheter (999.31)
　　umbilical venous catheter (999.31)
(Ex:) 996.00-996.1, 996.52, 996.55-996.62, 996.68-996.74, 996.79, 997.91-997.99, 998.81, 998.83-998.9
Coding Clinic: 2007, Q4, P84-86; 2004, Q2, P16; Q1, P5; 2003, Q4, P111-112; Q2, P7-8; 1994, Q2, P13

996.63　Due to nervous system device, implant and graft 🗘
Electrodes implanted in brain
Peripheral nerve graft
Spinal canal catheter
Ventricular (communicating) shunt (catheter)
(Ex:) 996.2, 996.52, 996.55-996.60, 996.63, 996.68-996.70, 996.75, 996.79, 997.91-997.99, 998.81, 998.83-998.9

996.64　Due to indwelling urinary catheter 🗘 🗘
Use additional code to identify specified infections, such as:
cystitis (595.0–595.9)
sepsis (038.0–038.9)
HAC: Also excludes the following from acting as a CC/MCC:112.2 (CC), 590.10 (CC), 590.11 (MCC), 590.2 (MCC), 590.3 (CC), 590.80 (CC), 590.81 (CC), 595.0 (CC), 597.0 (CC), 599.0 (CC)
(Ex:) 599.0, 996.30, 996.39, 996.56-996.60, 996.64-996.65, 996.68-996.70, 996.76, 996.79, 997.91-997.99, 998.81, 998.83-998.9
Coding Clinic: 1993, Q3, P6

996.65　Due to other genitourinary device, implant and graft 🗘
Intrauterine contraceptive device
(Ex:) 996.30, 996.39, 996.52, 996.55-996.60, 996.64-996.65, 996.68-996.70, 996.76, 996.79, 997.91 -997.99, 998.81, 998.83-998.9
Coding Clinic: 2000, Q1, P15-16

996.66　Due to internal joint prosthesis 🗘
Use additional code to identify infected prosthetic joint (V43.60–V43.69)
(Ex:) 996.40-996.49, 996.52, 996.55-996.60, 996.66-996.70, 996.77-996.79, 997.91-997.99, 998.81, 998.83-998.9
Coding Clinic: 2008, Q2, P3-5x3; 2007, Q2, P8-9; 2005, Q4, P110-112; 1991, Q2, P18

◀ New　　◀▥ Revised　　d̶e̶l̶e̶t̶e̶d̶ Deleted　　● Unacceptable Principal Diagnosis　　● Use Additional Digit(s)
▶ Manifestation Code　　OGCR Official Guidelines　　Coding Clinic　　Excludes　　Includes　　Use additional　　Code first　　Omit code

996.67 Due to other internal orthopedic device, implant and graft 🅒 🅜
Bone growth stimulator (electrode)
Internal fixation device (pin) (rod) (screw)
HAC: And one of the following procedure
codes: 81.01-81.08, 81.23, 81.24,
81.31-81.38, 81.83, 81.85
Ⓔ 996.40-996.49, 996.52, 996.55-996.60, 996.66-996.70,
996.77-996.79, 997.91-997.99, 998.81, 998.83-998.9

996.68 Due to peritoneal dialysis catheter 🅒
Exit-site infection or inflammation
Ⓔ 996.56-996.60, 996.68-996.70, 996.79, 997.91-997.99
Coding Clinic: 2001, Q2, P11; 1998, Q4, P55

996.69 Due to other internal prosthetic device, implant, and graft 🅒
Breast prosthesis
Ocular lens prosthesis
Prosthetic orbital implant
Ⓔ 996.00-996.30, 996.39-996.79, 997.91-997.99, 998.81,
998.83-998.9
Coding Clinic: 2008, Q2, P9-11; 2003, Q4, P108; 1998, Q4,
P52-53

● **996.7 Other complications of internal (biological) (synthetic) prosthetic device, implant, and graft**
Complication NOS due to (presence of) any device,
implant, and graft classifiable to 996.0–996.5
occlusion NOS
Embolism due to (presence of) any device, implant,
and graft classifiable to 996.0–996.5
Fibrosis due to (presence of) any device, implant,
and graft classifiable to 996.0–996.5
Hemorrhage due to (presence of) any device,
implant, and graft classifiable to 996.0–996.5
Pain due to (presence of) any device, implant, and
graft classifiable to 996.0–996.5
Stenosis due to (presence of) any device, implant,
and graft classifiable to 996.0–996.5
Thrombus due to (presence of) any device, implant,
and graft classifiable to 996.0–996.5
Use additional code to identify complication,
such as:
pain due to presence of device, implant or graft
(338.18–338.19, 338.28–338.29)
venous embolism and thrombosis
(453.2-453.9) ◀

Excludes   *disruption (dehiscence) of internal suture
material (998.31)
transplant rejection (996.8)*
Coding Clinic: 2007, Q2, P13-15; 2004, Q2, P7-8; 1989, Q1, P9&10;
1984, Nov-Dec, P18

996.70 Due to unspecified device, implant, and graft

996.71 Due to heart valve prosthesis 🅒
Ⓔ 996.00, 996.02, 996.09-996.1, 996.52, 996.55-996.62,
996.68-996.74, 996.79, 997.91-997.99, 998.81,
998.83-998.9
Coding Clinic: 2008, Q2, P9-10

996.72 Due to other cardiac device, implant, and graft 🅒
Cardiac pacemaker or defibrillator:
electrode(s), lead(s)
subcutaneous pocket
Coronary artery bypass (graft)
Excludes   *occlusion due to atherosclerosis
(414.00–414.07)*
Ⓔ 996.00-996.02, 996.04-996.1, 996.52, 996.55-996.62,
996.68-996.74, 996.79, 997.91-997.99, 998.81,
998.83-998.9
Coding Clinic: 2008, Q3, P10-11; 2006, Q3, P8-9, 25; 2001,
Q3, P20

996.73 Due to renal dialysis device, implant, and graft 🅒
Ⓔ 996.1, 996.52, 996.55-996.60, 996.68-996.70, 996.73, 996.79,
997.91-997.99, 998.81, 998.83-998.9
Coding Clinic: 1991, Q2, P18

996.74 Due to vascular device, implant, and graft 🅒
Excludes   *occlusion of biological graft
due to atherosclerosis
(440.30–440.32)*
Ⓔ 996.00-996.1, 996.52, 996.55-996.62, 996.68-996.74, 996.79,
997.91-997.99, 998.81, 998.83-998.9
Coding Clinic: 2003, Q1, P16-18x2; 2000, Q1, P10

996.75 Due to nervous system device, implant, and graft 🅒
Ⓔ 996.2, 996.52, 996.55-996.60, 996.63, 996.68-996.70, 996.75,
996.79, 997.91-997.99, 998.81, 998.83-998.9

996.76 Due to genitourinary device, implant, and graft 🅒
Ⓔ 996.30, 996.39, 996.52, 996.55-996.60, 996.64-996.65,
996.68-996.70, 996.76, 996.79, 997.91-997.99, 998.81,
998.83-998.9
Coding Clinic: 2009, Q1, P13; 2000, Q1, P15-16

996.77 Due to internal joint prosthesis 🅒
Use additional code to identify prosthetic
joint (V43.60–V43.69)
Ⓔ 996.40-996.49, 996.52, 996.55-996.60, 996.66-996.70,
996.77-996.79, 997.91-997.99, 998.81, 998.83-998.9

996.78 Due to other internal orthopedic device, implant, and graft 🅒
Ⓔ 996.40-996.49, 996.52, 996.55-996.60, 996.66-996.70,
996.77-996.79, 997.91-997.99, 998.81, 998.83-998.9
Coding Clinic: 2003, Q2, P14

996.79 Due to other internal prosthetic device, implant, and graft 🅒
Ⓔ 996.00-996.30, 996.39-996.79, 997.91-997.99, 998.81,
998.83-998.9
Coding Clinic: 2004, Q2, P7; 2001, Q1, P8-9; 1995, Q3, P14;
1992, Q3, P4-5

● **996.8 Complications of transplanted organ**
Transplant failure or rejection

Use additional code to identify nature of complication, such as:
cytomegalovirus [CMV] infection (078.5)
graft-versus-host disease (279.50-279.53)
malignancy associated with organ transplant (199.2)
post-transplant lymphoproliferative disorder (PTLD) (238.77)

Coding Clinic: 2003, Q1, P11; 2002, Q4, P53-54; 2001, Q3, P12-13; 1993, Q2, P11; Q1, P24

OGCR Section I.C.17.f.1.a

Transplant complications other than kidney: Codes under subcategory 996.8, Complications of transplanted organ, are for use for both complications and rejection of transplanted organs. A transplant complication code is only assigned if the complication affects the function of the transplanted organ. Two codes are required to fully describe a transplant complication, the appropriate code from subcategory 996.8 and a secondary code that identifies the complication. Pre-existing conditions or conditions that develop after the transplant are not coded as complications unless they affect the function of the transplanted organs.
See I.C.18.d.3) for transplant organ removal status
See I.C.2.i for malignant neoplasm associated with transplanted organ.

996.80 Transplanted organ, unspecified 🔓
(Ex:) 238.77, 996.80, 996.87, 997.91-997.99

996.81 Kidney 🔓
(Ex:) 996.81, 997.91-997.99
Coding Clinic: 2008, Q4, P82-83; 2003, Q3, P16-17; 1998, Q3, P6x2&7; 1994, Q3, P8; Q2, P9; 1993, Q4, P32-33; Q1, P24-25

996.82 Liver 🔓
(Ex:) 996.82, 997.91-997.99
Coding Clinic: 2008, Q4, P82-83, 97-100; 2003, Q3, P16x2&17; 1998, Q3, P4

996.83 Heart 🔓
(Ex:) 996.83, 997.91-997.99
Coding Clinic: 2003, Q3, P16; 2002, Q4, P53-54; 2001, Q3, P13-14x2; 1998, Q3, P5; 1993, Q3, P13

996.84 Lung 🔓
(Ex:) 996.84, 997.91-997.99
Coding Clinic: 2003, Q2, P12; 1998, Q3, P5

996.85 Bone marrow 🔓
(Ex:) 279.50-279.53, 996.85, 997.91-997.99
Coding Clinic: 2008, Q4, P90-91

996.86 Pancreas 🔓
(Ex:) 996.86, 997.91-997.99

996.87 Intestine 🔓
(Ex:) 238.77, 996.80, 996.87, 997.91-997.99
Coding Clinic: 2000, Q4, P47-48

996.89 Other specified transplanted organ 🔓
(Ex:) 996.89, 997.91-997.99
Coding Clinic: 1994, Q3, P5

● **996.9 Complications of reattached extremity or body part**

996.90 Unspecified extremity 🔓
(Ex:) 996.90, 997.91-997.99, 998.81, 998.83-998.9

996.91 Forearm 🔓
(Ex:) 996.91, 997.91-997.99, 998.81, 998.83-998.9

996.92 Hand 🔓
(Ex:) 996.92, 997.91-997.99, 998.81, 998.83-998.9

996.93 Finger(s) 🔓
(Ex:) 996.93, 997.91-997.99, 998.81, 998.83-998.9

996.94 Upper extremity, other and unspecified 🔓
(Ex:) 996.94, 997.91-997.99, 998.81, 998.83-998.9

996.95 Foot and toe(s) 🔓
(Ex:) 996.95, 997.91-997.99, 998.81, 998.83-998.9

996.96 Lower extremity, other and unspecified 🔓
(Ex:) 996.96, 997.91-997.99, 998.81, 998.83-998.9

996.99 Other specified body part 🔓
(Ex:) 996.99, 997.91-997.99, 998.81, 998.83-998.9

● **997 Complications affecting specified body systems, not elsewhere classified**

Use additional code to identify complication

Excludes the listed conditions when specified as:
causing shock (998.0)
complications of:
anesthesia:
adverse effect (001.0–799.9, 995.0–995.8)
in labor or delivery (668.0–668.9)
poisoning (968.0–969.9)
implanted device or graft (996.0–996.9)
obstetrical procedures (669.0–669.4)
reattached extremity (996.90–996.96)
transplanted organ (996.80–996.89)

Coding Clinic: 1995, Q2, P7; 1993, Q2, P9-10; 1992, Q1, P13

● **997.0 Nervous system complications**

997.00 Nervous system complication, unspecified

997.01 Central nervous system complication 🔓
Anoxic brain damage
Cerebral hypoxia

Excludes Cerebrovascular hemorrhage or infarction (997.02)
(Ex:) 997.00-997.09, 997.91-997.99, 998.81, 998.83-998.9
Coding Clinic: 2007, Q1, P22-23; 2006, Q1, P15-16

997.02 Iatrogenic cerebrovascular infarction or hemorrhage 🔓
Postoperative stroke
(Ex:) 997.00-997.09, 997.91-997.99, 998.81, 998.83-998.9
Coding Clinic: 2006, Q3, P6; 2004, Q2, P8-9

OGCR Section I.C.7.c

A cerebrovascular hemorrhage or infarction that occurs as a result of medical intervention is coded to 997.02. Documentation should clearly specify cause-and-effect relationship between the medical intervention and the cerebrovascular accident in order to assign this code. A secondary code from the code range 430-432 or from a code from subcategories 433 or 434 with a fifth digit of "1" should also be used to identify the type of hemorrhage or infarct.

997.09 Other nervous system complications 🔓
(Ex:) 997.00-997.09, 997.91-997.99, 998.81, 998.83-998.9

◀ New   ◀▥ Revised   ~~deleted~~ Deleted   ● Unacceptable Principal Diagnosis   ● Use Additional Digit(s)
▶ Manifestation Code   **OGCR** Official Guidelines   **Coding Clinic**   Excludes   Includes   Use additional   Code first   Omit code

INJURY AND POISONING (800–999)

997.1 Cardiac complications🔵

Cardiac:
   arrest during or resulting from a procedure
   insufficiency during or resulting from a
      procedure
Cardiorespiratory failure during or resulting from
   a procedure
Heart failure during or resulting from a procedure

| **Excludes** | the listed conditions as long-term effects of
cardiac surgery or due to the presence
of cardiac prosthetic device (429.4) |

(Ex) 997.1, 997.91-997.99, 998.81, 998.83-998.9
Coding Clinic: 2008, Q4, P177-180; 2000, Q2, P12; 1994, Q3, P9; Q1,
   P20; 1993, Q4, P37, 39-43; 5th Issue, P6-7

997.2 Peripheral vascular complications🔵

Phlebitis or thrombophlebitis during or resulting
   from a procedure

| **Excludes** | the listed conditions due to:
implant or catheter device (996.62)
infusion, perfusion, or transfusion
(999.2)
complications affecting blood vessels
(997.71–997.79) |

(Ex) 997.2, 997.79-997.99, 998.81, 998.83-998.9
Coding Clinic: 2003, Q1, P6-7; 2002, Q3, P24-27; 1993, Q1, P26

●**997.3 Respiratory complications**

| **Excludes** | iatrogenic [postoperative] pneumothorax
(512.1)
iatrogenic pulmonary embolism (415.11)
Mendelson's syndrome in labor and delivery
(668.0)
   Aspiration into the lungs of gastric
      contents following vomiting or
      regurgitation
specified complications classified elsewhere,
   such as:
adult respiratory distress syndrome
   (518.5)
pulmonary edema, postoperative (518.4)
respiratory insufficiency, acute,
   postoperative (518.5)
shock lung (518.5)
tracheostomy complications
   (519.00–519.09)
transfusion related acute lung injury
   (TRALI) (518.7) |

Coding Clinic: 1997, Q1, P10; 1993, Q4, P 43; Q2, P9-10; Q2, P3-4;
   1990, Q4, P25x2; 1989, Q1, P10

997.31 Ventilator associated pneumonia🔵

Ventilator associated pneumonitis   ◄

Use additional code to identify organism
(Ex) 518.7, 997.31 -997.39, 997.91-997.99, 998.81, 998.83-998.9
Coding Clinic: 2008, Q4, P148-149; 2006, Q2, P25

997.39 Other respiratory complications🔵

Mendelson's syndrome resulting from a
   procedure

Pneumonia (aspiration) resulting from a
   procedure
(Ex) 518.7, 997.31-997.39, 997.91-997.99, 998.81, 998.83-998.9

997.4 Digestive system complications🔵

Complications of:
   intestinal (internal) anastomosis and bypass, not
      elsewhere classified, except that involving
      urinary tract
Hepatic failure specified as due to a procedure
Hepatorenal syndrome specified as due to a
   procedure
   *Acute renal failure occurring along with cirrhosis or
      fulminant liver failure associated with portal
      hypertension*
Intestinal obstruction NOS specified as due to a
   procedure

| **Excludes** | specified gastrointestinal complications
classified elsewhere, such as:
blind loop syndrome (579.2)
colostomy or enterostomy complications
   (569.60–569.69)
complications of intestinal pouch
   (569.71-569.79)   ◄
gastrojejunal ulcer (534.0–534.9)
gastrostomy complications
   (536.40–536.49)
infection of esophagostomy (530.86)
infection of external stoma (569.61)
mechanical complication of
   esophagostomy (530.87)
pelvic peritoneal adhesions, female
   (614.6)
peritoneal adhesions (568.0)
peritoneal adhesions with obstruction
   (560.81)
postcholecystectomy syndrome (576.0)
postgastric surgery syndromes (564.2)
pouchitis (569.71)   ◄
vomiting following gastrointestinal
   surgery (564.3) |

(Ex) 530.86-530.87, 536.40-536.49, 997.4, 997.71, 997.91-997.99, 998.81,
   998.83-998.9
Coding Clinic: 2003, Q1, P18; 2001, Q2, P4-6x2; 1999, Q3, P4-5; Q2,
   P14; 1997, Q3, P7; Q1, P11; 1995, Q3, P7, 16; Q2, P7; 1993,
   Q1, P26; 1992, Q3, P15; 1989, Q2, P15; 1988, Q1, P14;
   1987, Nov-Dec, P9; 1985, Sept-Oct, P11; Mar-April, P11

997.5 Urinary complications

Complications of:
   external stoma of urinary tract
   internal anastomosis and bypass of urinary tract,
      including that involving intestinal tract
Oliguria or anuria specified as due to procedure   ◄▬▬
Renal (kidney):
   failure (acute) specified as due to procedure
   insufficiency (acute) specified as due to
      procedure
Tubular necrosis (acute) specified as due to
   procedure

| **Excludes** | specified complications classified elsewhere,
such as:
postoperative stricture of:
   ureter (593.3)
   urethra (598.2) |

Coding Clinic: 2003, Q3, P13; 1996, Q3, P10-11,15; 1995, Q4,
   P72-73; 1994, Q1, P20; 1992, Q1, P13; 1989, Q2, P16

INJURY AND POISONING (800–999)

● **997.6 Amputation stump complication**

> Excludes | *admission for treatment for a current traumatic amputation - code to complicated traumatic amputation phantom limb (syndrome) (353.6)*
> Coding Clinic: 1996, Q4, P45-46

997.60 Unspecified complication

997.61 Neuroma of amputation stump

997.62 Infection (chronic) 🔾

> Use additional code to identify the organism
> Ex: 997.60, 997.62-997.69, 997.91-997.99, 998.81, 998.83-998.9
> Coding Clinic: 2005, Q1, P14-15; 2003, Q3, P14; 1996, Q4, P45-46

997.69 Other
> Coding Clinic: 2005, Q1, P15

● **997.7 Vascular complications of other vessels**

> Excludes | *peripheral vascular complications (997.2)*

997.71 Vascular complications of mesenteric artery 🔾
> Ex: 997.2, 997.71-997.99, 998.81, 998.83-998.9
> Coding Clinic: 2001, Q4, P53

997.72 Vascular complications of renal artery 🔾
> Ex: 997.2, 997.71-997.99, 998.81, 998.83-998.9

997.79 Vascular complications of other vessels 🔾
> Ex: 997.2, 997.71-997.99, 998.81, 998.83-998.9

● **997.9 Complications affecting other specified body systems, not elsewhere classified**

> Excludes | *specified complications classified elsewhere, such as:*
> *broad ligament laceration syndrome (620.6)*
> *postartificial menopause syndrome (627.4)*
> *postoperative stricture of vagina (623.2)*
> Coding Clinic: 1994, Q1, P16; 1993, Q4, P41-42

997.91 Hypertension

> Excludes | *Essential hypertension (401.0–401.9)*

997.99 Other 🔾
> Vitreous touch syndrome
> Ex: 997.91-997.99, 998.81, 998.83-998.9
> Coding Clinic: 1994, Q2, P12; Q1, P17; Q1, P16-17

● **998 Other complications of procedures, NEC**

998.0 Postoperative shock 🔾
> Collapse NOS during or resulting from a surgical procedure
> Shock (endotoxic) (hypovolemic) (septic) during or resulting from a surgical procedure

> Excludes | *shock:*
> *anaphylactic due to serum (999.4)*
> *anesthetic (995.4)*
> *electric (994.8)*
> *following abortion (639.5)*
> *obstetric (669.1)*
> *traumatic (958.4)*
> Ex: 958.4, 995.4, 997.91-998.13, 998.81, 998.83-998.9

● **998.1 Hemorrhage or hematoma or seroma complicating a procedure**

> Excludes | *hemorrhage, hematoma or seroma:*
> *complicating cesarean section or puerperal perineal wound (674.3)*
> *due to implanted device or graft (996.70–996.79)*
> Coding Clinic: 2003, Q3, P13; 1993, Q1, P26; 1992, Q2, P15-16; 1987, Sept-Oct, P8

998.11 Hemorrhage complicating a procedure 🔾
> Ex: 456.0, 456.20, 530.81-530.83, 530.89, 531.00-531.01, 531.20-531.21, 531.40-531.41, 531.60-531.61, 532.00-532.01, 532.20-532.21, 532.40-532.41, 532.60-532.61, 533.00-533.01, 533.20-533.21, 533.40-533.41, 533.60-533.61, 534.00-534.01, 534.20-534.21, 534.40-534.41, 534.60-534.61, 535.01, 535.11, 535.21, 535.31, 535.41, 535.51, 535.61, 535.71, 537.83, 562.02-562.03, 562.12-562.13, 569.3, 569.85, 578.0-578.9, 772.4, 997.91 -998.13, 998.81, 998.89-998.9
> Coding Clinic: 2003, Q3, P13; Q1, P4; 1997, Q4, P52; Q1, P10; 1994, Q1, P19-20

998.12 Hematoma complicating a procedure 🔾
> Ex: 456.0, 456.20, 530.81-530.83, 530.89, 531.00-531.01, 531.20-531.21, 531.40-531.41, 531.60-531.61, 532.00-532.01, 532.20-532.21, 532.40-532.41, 532.60-532.61, 533.00-533.01, 533.20-533.21, 533.40-533.41, 533.60-533.61, 534.00-534.01, 534.20-534.21, 534.40-534.41, 534.60-534.61, 535.01, 535.11, 535.21, 535.31, 535.41, 535.51, 535.61, 535.71, 537.83, 562.02-562.03, 562.12-562.13, 569.3, 569.85, 578.0-578.9, 772.4, 997.91 -998.13, 998.81, 998.89-998.9
> Coding Clinic: 2006, Q3, P12; 2003, Q1, P6-7; 2002, Q3, P24-25; 1994, Q1, P20

998.13 Seroma complicating a procedure 🔾
> *Pocket of clear serous fluid that sometimes develops in the body after surgery*
> Ex: 456.0, 456.20, 530.81-530.83, 530.89, 531.00-531.01, 531.20-531.21, 531.40-531 .41, 531.60-531.61, 532.00-532.01, 532.20 -532.21, 532.40-532.41, 532.60-532.61, 533.00-533.01, 533.20-533.21, 533.40-533.41, 533.60-533.61, 534.00-534.01, 534.20-534.21, 534.40-534.41, 534.60-534.61, 535.01, 535.11, 535.21, 535.31, 535.41, 535.51, 535.61, 535.71, 537.83, 562.02-562.03, 562.12-562.13, 569.3, 569.85, 578.0-578.9, 772.4, 997.91-998.13, 998.81, 998.89-998.9
> Coding Clinic: 1996, Q4, P46

998.2 Accidental puncture or laceration during a procedure 🔾
> Accidental perforation by catheter or other instrument during a procedure on:
> blood vessel
> nerve
> organ

> Excludes | *iatrogenic [postoperative] pneumothorax (512.1)*
> *puncture or laceration caused by implanted device intentionally left in operation wound (996.0–996.5)*
> *specified complications classified elsewhere, such as:*
> *broad ligament laceration syndrome (620.6)*
> *dural tear (349.31)*
> *incidental durotomy (349.31)*
> *trauma from instruments during delivery (664.0–665.9)*
> Ex: 349.31-349.39, 997.91-997.99, 998.2, 998.81, 998.83-998.9
> Coding Clinic: 2007, Q2, P11-12; 2006, Q1, P15; 2002, Q3, P24-27; 1994, Q3, P6; 1994, Q1, P17; 1990, Q3, P17-18; 1984, Nov-Dec, P12

INJURY AND POISONING (800–999)

◀ New ◀≡ Revised ~~deleted~~ Deleted ● Unacceptable Principal Diagnosis ● Use Additional Digit(s)
▶ Manifestation Code OGCR Official Guidelines Coding Clinic | Excludes | Includes | Use additional | Code first | Omit code

● **998.3   Disruption of wound**
     Dehiscence of operation wound
        Splitting open
     Disruption of any suture materials or other closure
        method
     Rupture of operation wound

     | **Excludes** | *disruption of:*
                  amputation of stump (997.69)
                  cesarean wound (674.1)
                  perineal wound, puerperal (674.2)

     Coding Clinic: 2008, Q4, P149-152; 2002, Q4, P73; 1993, Q1, P19

    998.30   Disruption of wound, unspecified
        Disruption of wound NOS
        (Ex:) 997.91-997.99, 998.30-998.33, 998.81, 998.83-998.9

    998.31   Disruption of internal operation surgical wound
        Disruption or dehiscence of closure of:
           fascia, superficial or muscular
           internal organ
           muscle or muscle flap
           ribs or rib cage
           skull or craniotomy
           sternum or sternotomy
           tendon or ligament
        Deep disruption or dehiscence of
           operation wound NOS
        (Ex:) 997.91-997.99, 998.30-998.33, 998.81, 998.83-998.9

        | **Excludes** | *complications of internal*
                  anastomosis of:
                  gastrointestinal tract (997.4)
                  urinary tract (997.5)

    998.32   Disruption of external operation (surgical) wound
        Disruption of operation wound NOS
        Disruption or dehiscence of closure of:
           cornea
           mucosa
           skin
           subcutaneous tissue
        Full-thickness skin disruption or
           dehiscence
        Superficial disruption or dehiscence
           of operation wound
        (Ex:) 997.91-997.99, 998.30-998.33, 998.81, 998.83-998.9
        Coding Clinic: 2006, Q1, P8; 2005, Q1, P11; 2003, Q4, P104-107

    998.33   Disruption of traumatic injury wound repair
        Disruption or dehiscence of closure of
           traumatic laceration (external)
           (internal)
        (Ex:) 997.91-997.99, 998.30-998.33, 998.81, 998.83-998.9

998.4   Foreign body accidentally left during a procedure
     Adhesions due to foreign body accidentally left
        in operative wound or body cavity during a
        procedure
     Obstruction due to foreign body accidentally left
        in operative wound or body cavity during a
        procedure
     Perforation due to foreign body accidentally left
        in operative wound or body cavity during a
        procedure

     | **Excludes** | *obstruction or perforation caused by*
                  implanted device intentionally left in
                  body (996.0–996.5)

     (Ex:) 997.91-997.99, 998.4, 998.81, 998.83-998.9
     Coding Clinic: 2009, Q1, P13; 1989, Q1, P9

● **998.5   Postoperative infection**

     | **Excludes** | *bleb associated endophthalmitis (379.63)*
                  infection due to:
                  implanted device (996.60–996.69)
                  infusion, perfusion, or transfusion
                  (999.31–999.39)
                  postoperative obstetrical wound infection
                  (674.3)

     Coding Clinic: 1996, Q4, P45-46; 1995, Q2, P7; 1994, Q3, P6; 1987, Jan-Feb, P13-14

    998.51   Infected postoperative seroma
        Use additional code to identify organism
        (Ex:) 997.91-997.99, 998.51-998.59, 998.81, 998.89-998.9
        Coding Clinic: 1996, Q4, P46

    998.59   Other postoperative infection
        Abscess: postoperative
           intra-abdominal postoperative
           stitch postoperative
           subphrenic postoperative
           wound postoperative
        Septicemia postoperative

        Use additional code to identify infection
        HAC: And one of the following procedure
           codes: 81.01-81.08, 81.23, 81.24,
           81.31-81.38, 81.83, 81.85
        HAC: Principal Diagnosis 278.01, 998.59
           (CC), and one of the following
           procedure codes: 44.38, 44.39, or
           44.95
        (Ex:) 997.91-997.99, 998.51-998.59, 998.81, 998.89-998.9
        Coding Clinic: 2006, Q2, P23-24; 2004, Q4, P75-76; 2003, Q4, P104-107; 1995, Q3, P5; Q2, P7, 11; 1993, Q1, P19

       OGCR Section I.C.1.b.10.b
        Sepsis due to postprocedural infection:
        In cases of postprocedural sepsis, the
        complication code, such as code 998.59,
        Other postoperative infection, or 674.3x,
        Other complications of obstetrical surgical
        wounds should be coded first followed
        by the appropriate sepsis codes (systemic
        infection code and either code 995.91 or
        995.92). An additional code(s) for any acute
        organ dysfunction should also be assigned
        for cases of severe sepsis.

998.6   Persistent postoperative fistula
     (Ex:) 997.91-997.99, 998.6, 998.81, 998.83-998.9
     Coding Clinic: 1987, Jan-Feb, P14

998.7   Acute reaction to foreign substance accidentally left during a procedure
     Peritonitis:
       aseptic
       chemical
     (Ex:) 997.91-997.99, 998.7-998.81, 998.83-998.9

● **998.8   Other specified complications of procedures, not elsewhere classified**
     Coding Clinic: 1993, 5th Issue, P8, 15; 1989, Q1, P9; 1987, Jan-Feb, P13

    998.81   Emphysema (subcutaneous) (surgical) resulting from a procedure

    998.82   Cataract fragments in eye following cataract surgery

    998.83   Non-healing surgical wound
        (Ex:) 997.91-997.99, 998.81, 998.83-998.9
        Coding Clinic: 1996, Q4, P47

    998.89   Other specified complications
        Coding Clinic: 2009, Q2, P13x2, 15; 2006, Q3, P9-10; 2005, Q3, P16-17; 1999, Q3, P13; 1998, Q2, P16

INJURY AND POISONING (800–999)

998.9 Unspecified complication of procedure, not elsewhere classified
Postoperative complication NOS

| Excludes | *complication NOS of obstetrical surgery or procedure (669.4)*
Coding Clinic: 1993, Q4, P41-42

● **999 Complications of medical care, not elsewhere classified**

| Includes | complications, not elsewhere classified, of:
dialysis (hemodialysis) (peritoneal) (renal)
extracorporeal circulation
hyperalimentation therapy
immunization
infusion
inhalation therapy
injection
inoculation
perfusion
transfusion
vaccination
ventilation therapy

Use additional code, where applicable, to identify specific complication

| Excludes | *specified complications classified elsewhere such as:*
complications of implanted device (996.0–996.9)
contact dermatitis due to drugs (692.3)
dementia dialysis (294.8)
transient (293.9)
dialysis disequilibrium syndrome (276.0–276.9)
poisoning and toxic effects of drugs and chemicals (960.0–989.9)
postvaccinal encephalitis (323.51)
water and electrolyte imbalance (276.0–276.9)

999.0 Generalized vaccinia 🦠

| Excludes | *vaccinia not from vaccine (051.02)*
(Ex:) 999.0

999.1 Air embolism 🦠 🦠
Air embolism to any site following infusion, perfusion, or transfusion

| Excludes | *embolism specified as:*
complicating:
abortion (634–638 with .6, 639.6)
ectopic or molar pregnancy (639.6)
pregnancy, childbirth, or the puerperium (673.0)
due to implanted device (996.7)
traumatic (958.0)
(Ex:) 958.0, 999.1

999.2 Other vascular complications 🦠
Phlebitis following infusion, perfusion, or transfusion
Thromboembolism following infusion, perfusion, or transfusion
Thrombophlebitis following infusion, perfusion, or transfusion

| Excludes | *extravasation of vesicant drugs (999.81, 999.82)*
the listed conditions when specified as:
due to implanted device (996.61–996.62, 996.72–996.74)
postoperative NOS (997.2, 997.71–997.79)
(Ex:) 999.2, 999.81-999.88
Coding Clinic: 1997, Q2, P5

● **999.3 Other infection**
Infection following infusion, injection, transfusion, or vaccination
Sepsis following infusion, injection, transfusion, or vaccination
Septicemia following infusion, injection, transfusion, or vaccination

Use additional code to identify the specified infection, such as:
septicemia (038.0–038.9)

| Excludes | *the listed conditions when specified as:*
due to implanted device (996.60–996.69)
postoperative NOS (998.51–998.59)
Coding Clinic: 2001, Q2, P11-12; 1987, Jan-Feb, P14-15

999.31 Infection due to central venous catheter 🦠 🦠
Catheter-related bloodstream infection (CRBSI) NOS
Infection due to:
Hickman catheter
peripherally inserted central catheter (PICC)
portacath (port-a-cath)
triple lumen catheter
umbilical venous catheter

| Excludes | *infection due to:*
arterial catheter (996.62)
catheter NOS (996.69)
peripheral venous catheter (996.62)
urinary catheter (996.64)
(Ex:) 996.62, 999.31-999.39
Coding Clinic: 2008, Q4, P69-73, 192-193; 2007, Q4, P96-97

999.39 Infection following other infusion, injection, transfusion, or vaccination 🦠
(Ex:) 996.62, 999.31-999.39

999.4 Anaphylactic shock due to serum 🦠
Anaphylactic reaction due to serum

| Excludes | *shock:*
allergic NOS (995.0)
anaphylactic:
NOS (995.0)
due to drugs and chemicals (995.0)
(Ex:) 999.4

999.5 Other serum reaction 🦠
Intoxication by serum
Protein sickness
Serum rash
Serum sickness
Urticaria due to serum

| Excludes | *serum hepatitis (070.2–070.3)*
(Ex:) 999.5

999.6 ABO incompatibility reaction 🦠 🦠
Incompatible blood transfusion
Reaction to blood group incompatibility in infusion or transfusion

| Excludes | *minor blood group antigens reactions (Duffy) (E) (K(ell)) (Kidd) (Lewis) (M) (N) (P) (S) (999.89)* ◀
(Ex:) 999.6

999.7 Rh incompatibility reaction 🦠
Reactions due to Rh factor in infusion or transfusion
(Ex:) 999.7

◀ New   ◀▥ Revised   ~~deleted~~ Deleted   ● Unacceptable Principal Diagnosis   ● Use Additional Digit(s)
▶ Manifestation Code   **OGCR** Official Guidelines   **Coding Clinic**   Excludes   Includes   Use additional   Code first   Omit code

● **999.8 Other infusion and transfusion reaction**

> | **Excludes** | *postoperative shock (998.0)*
> *transfusion related acute lung injury*
> *(TRALI) (518.7)*

Coding Clinic: 2008, Q4, P152-155; 2000, Q3, P9

999.81 Extravasation of vesicant chemotherapy 🔖
Infiltration of vesicant chemotherapy
(Ex) 999.2, 999.81-999.88
Coding Clinic: 2008, Q4, P152-155

999.82 Extravasation of other vesicant agent 🔖
Infiltration of other vesicant agent
(Ex) 999.2, 999.81-999.88

999.88 Other infusion reaction

999.89 Other transfusion reaction
Transfusion reaction NOS

Use additional code to identify
graft-versus-host reaction (279.5)

999.9 Other and unspecified complications of medical care, not elsewhere classified
Complications, not elsewhere classified, of:
electroshock therapy   ultrasound therapy
inhalation therapy   ventilation therapy
Unspecified misadventure of medical care

> | **Excludes** | *unspecified complication of:*
> *phototherapy (990)*
> *radiation therapy (990)*
> *ventilator associated pneumonia (997.31)*

MCE: Questionable admission, principal diagnosis
only
Coding Clinic: 2006, Q2, P25; 2003, Q1, P19; 1997, Q2, P5; 1994,
Q3, P9

INJURY AND POISONING (800–999)

SUPPLEMENTARY CLASSIFICATION OF FACTORS INFLUENCING HEALTH STATUS AND CONTACT WITH HEALTH SERVICES (V01–V89)

This classification is provided to deal with occasions when circumstances other than a disease or injury classifiable to categories 001–999 (the main part of ICD) are recorded as "diagnoses" or "problems." This can arise mainly in three ways:

a) When a person who is not currently sick encounters the health services for some specific purpose, such as to act as a donor of an organ or tissue, to receive prophylactic vaccination, or to discuss a problem which is in itself not a disease or injury. This will be a fairly rare occurrence among hospital inpatients, but will be relatively more common among hospital outpatients and patients of family practitioners, health clinics, etc.

b) When a person with a known disease or injury, whether it is current or resolving, encounters the health care system for a specific treatment of that disease or injury (e.g., dialysis for renal disease; chemotherapy for malignancy; cast change).

c) When some circumstance or problem is present which influences the person's health status but is not in itself a current illness or injury. Such factors may be elicited during population surveys, when the person may or may not be currently sick, or be recorded as an additional factor to be borne in mind when the person is receiving care for some current illness or injury classifiable to categories 001–999.

In the latter circumstances the V code should be used only as a supplementary code and should not be the one selected for use in primary, single cause tabulations. Examples of these circumstances are a personal history of certain diseases, or a person with an artificial heart valve in situ.

OGCR Section I.C.18.b

> V codes are for use in any healthcare setting as either a first listed (principal diagnosis code in the inpatient setting) or secondary code, depending on the circumstances of the encounter. Certain V codes may only be used as first listed, others only as secondary codes.

PERSONS WITH POTENTIAL HEALTH HAZARDS RELATED TO COMMUNICABLE DISEASES (V01–V06)

Excludes   *family history of infectious and parasitic diseases (V18.8)*
personal history of infectious and parasitic diseases (V12.0)

OGCR Section I.C.18.d.1

> Category V01 indicates contact with or exposure to communicable diseases. These codes are for patients who do not show any sign or symptom of a disease but have been exposed to it by close personal contact with an infected individual or are in an area where a disease is epidemic. These codes may be used as a first listed code to explain an encounter for testing, or, more commonly, as a secondary code to identify a potential risk.

● **V01   Contact with or exposure to communicable diseases**
Coding Clinic: 2001, Q1, P10

● ⑩ **V01.0   Cholera**
Conditions classifiable to 001

● ⑩ **V01.1   Tuberculosis**
Conditions classifiable to 010–018

● ⑩ **V01.2   Poliomyelitis**
Conditions classifiable to 045

● ⑩ **V01.3   Smallpox**
Conditions classifiable to 050

● ⑩ **V01.4   Rubella**
Conditions classifiable to 056

● ⑩ **V01.5   Rabies**
Conditions classifiable to 071

● ⑩ **V01.6   Venereal diseases**
Conditions classifiable to 090–099
Coding Clinic: 2007, Q4, P124-125x2

● **V01.7   Other viral diseases**
Conditions classifiable to 042–078, and V08, except as above

    ⑩ **V01.71   Varicella**

    ⑩ **V01.79   Other viral diseases**
Coding Clinic: 1992, Q2, P11

● **V01.8   Other communicable diseases**
Conditions classifiable to 001–136, except as above

● ⑩ **V01.81   Anthrax**

    ⑩ **V01.82   Exposure to SARS-associated coronavirus**
Coding Clinic: 2003, Q4, P46-48

    ⑩ **V01.83   Escherichia coli (E. coli)**

    ⑩ **V01.84   Meningococcus**

● ⑩ **V01.89   Other communicable diseases**

● ⑩ **V01.9   Unspecified communicable disease**

● **V02   Carrier or suspected carrier of infectious diseases**
Includes   Colonization status

● ⑩ **V02.0   Cholera** ⑩

● ⑩ **V02.1   Typhoid** ⑩

● ⑩ **V02.2   Amebiasis** ⑩

● ⑩ **V02.3   Other gastrointestinal pathogens** ⑩

● ⑩ **V02.4   Diphtheria** ⑩

● **V02.5   Other specified bacterial diseases**

● ⑩ **V02.51   Group B streptococcus** ⑩
Coding Clinic: 2006, Q3, P14; 2002, Q1, P14-15; 1998, Q4, P56; 1994, Q3, P4

● ⑩ **V02.52   Other streptococcus** ⑩

● ⑩ **V02.53   Methicillin susceptible Staphylococcus aureus** ⑩
MSSA colonization
Coding Clinic: 2008, Q4, P69-73

● ⑩ **V02.54   Methicillin resistant Staphylococcus aureus** ⑩
MRSA colonization
Coding Clinic: 2008, Q4, P69-73

● ⑩ **V02.59   Other specified bacterial diseases** ⑩
Meningococcal
Staphylococcal

● **V02.6   Viral hepatitis**

● ⑩ **V02.60   Viral hepatitis carrier, unspecified** ⑩

● ⑩ **V02.61   Hepatitis B carrier** ⑩

● ⑩ **V02.62   Hepatitis C carrier** ⑩

● ⑩ **V02.69   Other viral hepatitis carrier** ⑩

● ⑩ **V02.7   Gonorrhea** ⑩

● ⑩ **V02.8   Other venereal diseases** ⑩

● ⑩ **V02.9   Other specified infectious organism** ⑩
Coding Clinic: 1994, Q4, P36; 1993, Q1, P22

Ⓔⓧ CC Exclusions   ◀ New   ◀▥ Revised   ~~deleted~~ Deleted   ● Use Additional Digit(s)   ❶ First Listed   ⑩ First Listed or Additional
❷ Additional Only   ▶ Manifestation Code   **OGCR** Official Guidelines   Coding Clinic   Excludes   Includes   Use additional   Code first

OGCR Section I.C.18.d.2

> Categories V03-V06 are for encounters for inoculations and vaccinations. They indicate that a patient is being seen to receive a prophylactic inoculation against a disease. The injection itself must be represented by the appropriate procedure code. A code from V03-V06 may be used as a secondary code if the inoculation is given as a routine part of preventive health care, such as a well-baby visit.

● **V03**   Need for prophylactic vaccination and inoculation against bacterial diseases

> | Excludes | *vaccination not carried out (V64.00–V64.09)*
> *vaccines against combinations of diseases (V06.0–V06.9)*

- ● V03.0   Cholera alone
- ● V03.1   Typhoid-paratyphoid alone [TAB]
- ● V03.2   Tuberculosis [BCG]
- ● V03.3   Plague
- ● V03.4   Tularemia
- ● V03.5   Diphtheria alone
- ● V03.6   Pertussis alone
- ● V03.7   Tetanus toxoid alone
- ● V03.8   Other specified vaccinations against single bacterial diseases
  - ● V03.81   Hemophilus influenza, type B [Hib]
  - ● V03.82   Streptococcus pneumoniae [pneumococcus]
  - ● V03.89   Other specified vaccination
    Coding Clinic: 2000, Q2, P9
- ● V03.9   Unspecified single bacterial disease

● **V04**   Need for prophylactic vaccination and inoculation against certain diseases

> | Excludes | *vaccines against combinations of diseases (V06.0–V06.9)*

- ● V04.0   Poliomyelitis
- ● V04.1   Smallpox
- ● V04.2   Measles alone
- ● V04.3   Rubella alone
- ● V04.4   Yellow fever
- ● V04.5   Rabies
- ● V04.6   Mumps alone
- ● V04.7   Common cold
- ● V04.8   Other viral diseases
  - ● V04.81   Influenza
  - ● V04.82   Respiratory syncytial virus (RSV)
    Coding Clinic: 2009, Q1, P5; 2001, Q1, P4
  - ● V04.89   Other viral diseases
    Coding Clinic: 2007, Q2, P11

● **V05**   Need for prophylactic vaccination and inoculation against single diseases

> | Excludes | *vaccines against combinations of diseases (V06.0–V06.9)*

- ● V05.0   Arthropod-borne viral encephalitis
- ● V05.1   Other arthropod-borne viral diseases
- ● V05.2   Leishmaniasis
- ● V05.3   Viral hepatitis
- ● V05.4   Varicella
  Chicken pox
- ● V05.8   Other specified disease
  Coding Clinic: 2001, Q1, P4; 1991, Q3, P20-21
- ● V05.9   Unspecified single disease

● **V06**   Need for prophylactic vaccination and inoculation against combinations of diseases

> **Note:** Use additional single vaccination codes from categories V03–V05 to identify any vaccinations not included in a combination code.

- ● V06.0   Cholera with typhoid-paratyphoid [cholera TAB]
- ● V06.1   Diphtheria-tetanus-pertussis, combined [DTP] [DTaP]
  Coding Clinic: 1998, Q3, P13-14
- ● V06.2   Diphtheria-tetanus-pertussis with typhoid-paratyphoid [DTP TAB]
- ● V06.3   Diphtheria-tetanus-pertussis with poliomyelitis [DTP+polio]
- ● V06.4   Measles-mumps-rubella [MMR]
- ● V06.5   Tetanus-diphtheria [Td] [DT]
- ● V06.6   Streptococcus pneumoniae [pneumococcus] and influenza
- ● V06.8   Other combinations
  > | Excludes | *multiple single vaccination codes (V03.0–V05.9)*
  Coding Clinic: 1994, Q1, P19
- ● V06.9   Unspecified combined vaccine

PERSONS WITH NEED FOR ISOLATION, OTHER POTENTIAL HEALTH HAZARDS AND PROPHYLACTIC MEASURES (V07–V09)

● **V07**   Need for isolation and other prophylactic measures

> | Excludes | *prophylactic organ removal (V50.41–V50.49)*

- V07.0   Isolation
  Admission to protect the individual from his surroundings or for isolation of individual after contact with infectious diseases
- ● V07.1   Desensitization to allergens
- ● V07.2   Prophylactic immunotherapy
  Administration of:
      antivenin
      immune sera [gamma globulin]
      RhoGAM
      tetanus antitoxin

N Newborn Age: 0   **P** Pediatric Age: 0–17   **M** Maternity Age: 12–55   **A** Adult Age: 15–124   ♀ Females Only   ♂ Males Only   1131
● Unacceptable Principal Diagnosis   Complication\Comorbidity   Major C\C   Present on Admission Requirement   Hospital-Acquired Condition

V01-V89

● V07.3   Other prophylactic chemotherapy
   ● ℞ V07.31   Prophylactic fluoride administration ℞
   ℞ V07.39   Other prophylactic chemotherapy ℞
      Excludes   *maintenance chemotherapy*
                     following disease
                     (V58.11)

● ❷ V07.4   Hormone replacement therapy
             (postmenopausal) ♀ ℞

● V07.5   Prophylactic use of agents affecting estrogen
          receptors and estrogen levels
      Code first, if applicable:
         malignant neoplasm of breast (174.0-174.9,
            175.0-175.9)
         malignant neoplasm of prostate (185)

      Use additional code, if applicable, to
         identify:
         estrogen receptor positive status (V86.0)
         family history of breast cancer (V16.3)
         genetic susceptibility to cancer
            (V84.01-V84.09)
         personal history of breast cancer (V10.3)
         personal history of prostate cancer
            (V10.46)
         postmenopausal status (V49.81)
      Excludes   *hormone replacement therapy*
                     (postmenopausal) (V07.4)

   ● ❷ V07.51   Prophylactic use of selective estrogen
                receptor modulators (SERMs) ℞
                   Prophylactic use of:
                      raloxifene (Evista)
                      tamoxifen (Nolvadex)
                      toremifene (Fareston)

   ● ❷ V07.52   Prophylactic use of aromatase
                inhibitors ℞
                   Prophylactic use of:
                      anastrozole (Arimidex)
                      exemestane ~~exemestar~~
                         (Aromasin)   ◀▥
                      letrozole (Femara)

   ● ❷ V07.59   Prophylactic use of other agents
                affecting estrogen receptors and
                estrogen levels ℞
                   Prophylactic use of:
                      estrogen receptor downregulators
                      fulvestrant (Faslodex)
                      gonadotropin-releasing hormone
                         (GnRH) agonist
                      goserelin acetate (Zoladex)
                      leuprolide acetate (leuprorelin)
                         (Lupron)
                      megestrol acetate (Megace)

   ℞ V07.8   Other specified prophylactic measure ℞
             Coding Clinic: 1992, Q1, P11

● ℞ V07.9   Unspecified prophylactic measure ℞

OGCR   Section I.C.2.d
      V08, Asymptomatic human immunodeficiency virus
      [HIV] infection, is to be applied when the patient
      without any documentation of symptoms is listed
      as being "HIV positive," "known HIV," "HIV test
      positive," or similar terminology. Do not use this code
      if the term "AIDS" is used or if the patient is treated
      for any HIV-related illness or is described as having
      any condition(s) resulting from HIV positive status;
      use 042 in these cases.

℞ V08   Asymptomatic human immunodeficiency virus [HIV]
         infection status
         HIV positive NOS

      Note: This code is ONLY to be used when NO HIV
                  infection symptoms or conditions are present. If
                  any HIV infection symptoms or conditions are
                  present, see code 042.

      Excludes   *AIDS (042)*
                     human immunodeficiency virus [HIV] disease
                        (042)
                     exposure to HIV (V01.79)
                     nonspecific serologic evidence of HIV (795.71)
                     symptomatic human immunodeficiency virus
                        [HIV] infection (042)
      MCE: Questionable admission, principal diagnosis only
      Coding Clinic: 2004, Q2, P11; 1999, Q2, P8

● V09   Infection with drug-resistant microorganisms

      Note: This category is intended for use as an
                  additional code for infectious conditions
                  classified elsewhere to indicate the presence of
                  drug-resistance of the infectious organism.
      Coding Clinic: 2008, Q4, P69-73

   ● ❷ V09.0   Infection with microorganisms resistant to
               penicillins
                  Coding Clinic: 2006, Q2, P16-17; 2003, Q4, P104-107;
                                     1994, Q3, P4

   ● ❷ V09.1   Infection with microorganisms resistant to
               cephalosporins and other B-lactam antibiotics

   ● ❷ V09.2   Infection with microorganisms resistant to
               macrolides

   ● ❷ V09.3   Infection with microorganisms resistant to
               tetracyclines

   ● ❷ V09.4   Infection with microorganisms resistant to
               aminoglycosides

   ● V09.5   Infection with microorganisms resistant to
             quinolones and fluoroquinolones

      ● ❷ V09.50   Without mention of resistance to
                   multiple quinolones and fluoroquinoles

      ● ❷ V09.51   With resistance to multiple quinolones
                   and fluoroquinoles

   ● ❷ V09.6   Infection with microorganisms resistant to
               sulfonamides

   ● V09.7   Infection with microorganisms resistant to other
             specified antimycobacterial agents
      Excludes   *Amikacin (V09.4)*
                     Kanamycin (V09.4)
                     Streptomycin [SM] (V09.4)

      ● ❷ V09.70   Without mention of resistance to
                   multiple antimycobacterial agents

      ● ❷ V09.71   With resistance to multiple
                   antimycobacterial agents

(Ex) CC Exclusions   ◀ New   ◀▥ Revised   ~~deleted~~ Deleted   ● Use Additional Digit(s)   ❶ First Listed   ℞ First Listed or Additional
❷ Additional Only   ▶ Manifestation Code   OGCR Official Guidelines   Coding Clinic   Excludes   Includes   Use additional   Code first

● **V09.8 Infection with microorganisms resistant to other specified drugs**
Vancomycin (glycopeptide) intermediate staphylococcus aureus (VISA/GISA)
Vancomycin (glycopeptide) resistant enterococcus (VRE)
Vancomycin (glycopeptide) resistant staphylococcus aureus (VRSA/GRSA)

● ❷ **V09.80 Without mention of resistance to multiple drugs**

● ❷ **V09.81 With resistance to multiple drugs**

● **V09.9 Infection with drug-resistant microorganisms, unspecified**
Drug resistance NOS

● ❷ **V09.90 Without mention of multiple drug resistance**

● ❷ **V09.91 With multiple drug resistance**
Multiple drug resistance NOS

PERSONS WITH POTENTIAL HEALTH HAZARDS RELATED TO PERSONAL AND FAMILY HISTORY (V10–V19)

Excludes *obstetric patients where the possibility that the fetus might be affected is the reason for observation or management during pregnancy (655.0–655.9)*

OGCR Section I.C.2.d
When a primary malignancy has been previously excised or eradicated from its site and there is no further treatment directed to that site and there is no evidence of any existing primary malignancy, a code from category V10 should be used to indicate the former site of the malignancy. Any mention of extension, invasion, or metastasis to another site is coded as a secondary malignant neoplasm to that site. The secondary site may be the principal or first-listed with the V10 code used as a secondary code.

● **V10 Personal history of malignant neoplasm**
~~Code first any continuing functional activity, such as:~~
~~carcinoid syndrome (259.2)~~
Coding Clinic: 1994, Q2, P8

OGCR Section I.C.18.d.3
Personal history codes explain a patient's past medical condition that no longer exists and is not receiving any treatment, but that has the potential for recurrence, and therefore may require continued monitoring.

● **V10.0 Gastrointestinal tract**
History of conditions classifiable to 140–159
Excludes *personal history of malignant carcinoid tumor (V10.91)* ◄
personal history of malignant neuroendocrine tumor (V10.91) ◄

● ⓥ **V10.00 Gastrointestinal tract, unspecified** ⓒ

● ⓥ **V10.01 Tongue** ⓒ

● ⓥ **V10.02 Other and unspecified oral cavity and pharynx** ⓒ

● ⓥ **V10.03 Esophagus** ⓒ

● ⓥ **V10.04 Stomach** ⓒ

● ⓥ **V10.05 Large intestine** ⓒ
Coding Clinic: 1999, Q3, P7-8; 1995, Q1, P3-4

● ⓥ **V10.06 Rectum, rectosigmoid junction, and anus** ⓒ

● ⓥ **V10.07 Liver** ⓒ

● ⓥ **V10.09 Other** ⓒ
Coding Clinic: 2003, Q4, P111

● **V10.1 Trachea, bronchus, and lung**
History of conditions classifiable to 162
Excludes *personal history of malignant carcinoid tumor (V10.91)* ◄
personal history of malignant neuroendocrine tumor (V10.91) ◄

● ⓥ **V10.11 Bronchus and lung** ⓒ

● ⓥ **V10.12 Trachea** ⓒ

● **V10.2 Other respiratory and intrathoracic organs**
History of conditions classifiable to 160, 161, 163–165

● ⓥ **V10.20 Respiratory organ, unspecified** ⓒ

● ⓥ **V10.21 Larynx** ⓒ
Coding Clinic: 2003, Q4, P108,110

● ⓥ **V10.22 Nasal cavities, middle ear, and accessory sinuses** ⓒ

● ⓥ **V10.29 Other** ⓒ

● ⓥ **V10.3 Breast** ⓒ
History of conditions classifiable to 174 and 175
Coding Clinic: 2007, Q3, P4; Q1, P3-8; 2003, Q2, P3-5; 2001, Q4, P66; 1997, Q4, P50; 1995, Q4, P53; 1990, Q1, P21

● **V10.4 Genital organs**
History of conditions classifiable to 179–187

● ⓥ **V10.40 Female genital organ, unspecified ♀** ⓒ

● ⓥ **V10.41 Cervix uteri ♀** ⓒ
Coding Clinic: 2007, Q4, P99-101

● ⓥ **V10.42 Other parts of uterus ♀** ⓒ

● ⓥ **V10.43 Ovary ♀** ⓒ

● ⓥ **V10.44 Other female genital organs ♀** ⓒ

● ⓥ **V10.45 Male genital organ, unspecified ♂** ⓒ

● ⓥ **V10.46 Prostate ♂** ⓒ
Coding Clinic: 2009, Q1, P5; 1994, Q2, P12; 1984, May-June, P10

● ⓥ **V10.47 Testis ♂** ⓒ

● ⓥ **V10.48 Epididymis ♂** ⓒ

● ⓥ **V10.49 Other male genital organs ♂** ⓒ

● **V10.5 Urinary organs**
History of conditions classifiable to 188 and 189
Coding Clinic: 1995, Q2, P8

● ⓥ **V10.50 Urinary organ, unspecified** ⓒ

● ⓥ **V10.51 Bladder** ⓒ
Coding Clinic: 1995, Q2, P8;1985, July-Aug, P16

● ⓥ **V10.52 Kidney** ⓒ
Excludes *renal pelvis (V10.53)*
Coding Clinic: 2004, Q2, P4

● ⓥ **V10.53 Renal pelvis** ⓒ

● ⓥ **V10.59 Other** ⓒ

● **V10.6 Leukemia**
Conditions classifiable to 204–208
Excludes *leukemia in remission (204–208)*
Coding Clinic: 1992, Q2, P13; 1985, May-June, P8-9

● ⓥ **V10.60 Leukemia, unspecified** ⓒ

● ⓥ **V10.61 Lymphoid leukemia** ⓒ

● ⓥ **V10.62 Myeloid leukemia** ⓒ

● ⓥ **V10.63 Monocytic leukemia** ⓒ

● ⓥ **V10.69 Other** ⓒ

N Newborn Age: 0   P Pediatric Age: 0–17   M Maternity Age: 12–55   A Adult Age: 15–124   ♀ Females Only   ♂ Males Only   1133

● Unacceptable Principal Diagnosis   ⓒ Complication\Comorbidity   ⓥ Major C\C   Present on Admission Requirement   Hospital-Acquired Condition

V01-V89

● **V10.7　Other lymphatic and hematopoietic neoplasms**
　　　Conditions classifiable to 200–203
　　　　Excludes *listed conditions in 200–203 in remission*
　　　Coding Clinic: 1985, May-June, P8-9

●◐ **V10.71　Lymphosarcoma and reticulosarcoma** ◌

●◐ **V10.72　Hodgkin's disease** ◌

●◐ **V10.79　Other** ◌

● **V10.8　Personal history of malignant neoplasm of other sites**
　　　History of conditions classifiable to 170–173, 190–195
　　　　Excludes *personal history of malignant carcinoid tumor (V10.91)* ◀
　　　　　　personal history of malignant neuroendocrine tumor (V10.91) ◀

●◐ **V10.81　Bone** ◌
　　　Coding Clinic: 2003, Q2, P13

●◐ **V10.82　Malignant melanoma of skin** ◌

●◐ **V10.83　Other malignant neoplasm of skin** ◌

●◐ **V10.84　Eye** ◌

●◐ **V10.85　Brain** ◌
　　　Coding Clinic: 2001, Q1, P6-7

●◐ **V10.86　Other parts of nervous system** ◌
　　　　Excludes *peripheral, sympathetic, and parasympathetic nerves (V10.89)*

●◐ **V10.87　Thyroid** ◌

●◐ **V10.88　Other endocrine glands and related structures** ◌

●◐ **V10.89　Other** ◌

● **V10.9　Other and ~~U~~unspecified personal history of malignant neoplasm** ◀▥

●◐ **V10.90　Personal history of unspecified malignant neoplasm** ◌ ◀
　　　Personal history of malignant neoplasm NOS ◀
　　　　Excludes *personal history of malignant carcinoid tumor (V10.91)* ◀
　　　　　　personal history of malignant neuroendocrine tumor (V10.91) ◀
　　　　　　personal history of Merkel cell carcinoma (V10.91) ◀

●◐ **V10.91　Personal history of malignant neuroendocrine tumor** ◌ ◀
　　　Personal history of malignant carcinoid tumor NOS ◀
　　　Personal history of malignant neuroendocrine tumor NOS ◀
　　　Personal history of Merkel cell carcinoma NOS ◀
　　　Code first any continuing functional activity, such as: ◀
　　　　carcinoid syndrome (259.2) ◀

● **V11　Personal history of mental disorder**

● **V11.0　Schizophrenia** ◌
　　　　Excludes *that in remission (295.0–295.9 with fifth-digit 5)*
　　　Coding Clinic: 1995, Q3, P6

● **V11.1　Affective disorders** ◌
　　　Personal history of manic-depressive psychosis
　　　　Excludes *that in remission (296.0–296.6 with fifth-digit 5, 6)*

● **V11.2　Neurosis** ◌

● **V11.3　Alcoholism** ◌

● **V11.8　Other mental disorders** ◌

● **V11.9　Unspecified mental disorder** ◌

● **V12　Personal history of certain other diseases**
　　　Coding Clinic: 2005, Q4, P94-100; 1992, Q3, P11

● **V12.0　Infectious and parasitic diseases**
　　　　Excludes *personal history of infectious diseases specific to a body system*

●◐ **V12.00　Unspecified infectious and parasitic disease** ◌

●◐ **V12.01　Tuberculosis** ◌

●◐ **V12.02　Poliomyelitis** ◌

●◐ **V12.03　Malaria** ◌

●◐ **V12.04　Methicillin resistant Staphylococcus aureus** ◌
　　　MRSA
　　　Coding Clinic: 2008, Q4, P69-73

●◐ **V12.09　Other** ◌

●◐ **V12.1　Nutritional deficiency** ◌

●◐ **V12.2　Endocrine, metabolic, and immunity disorders** ◌
　　　　Excludes *history of allergy (V14.0–V14.9, V15.01–V15.09)*
　　　Coding Clinic: 2007, Q3, P5-6

●◐ **V12.3　Diseases of blood and blood-forming organs** ◌

● **V12.4　Disorders of nervous system and sense organs**

●◐ **V12.40　Unspecified disorder of nervous system and sense organs** ◌

●◐ **V12.41　Benign neoplasm of the brain** ◌

●◐ **V12.42　Infections of the central nervous system** ◌
　　　Encephalitis
　　　Meningitis

●◐ **V12.49　Other disorders of nervous system and sense organs** ◌
　　　Coding Clinic: 1998, Q4, P59-60

● **V12.5　Diseases of circulatory system**
　　　　Excludes *old myocardial infarction (412)*
　　　　　postmyocardial infarction syndrome (411.0)

●◐ **V12.50　Unspecified circulatory disease** ◌

●◐ **V12.51　Venous thrombosis and embolism** ◌
　　　Pulmonary embolism
　　　Coding Clinic: 2006, Q3, P12; 2003, Q4, P108; 2002, Q1, P15-16

●◐ **V12.52　Thrombophlebitis** ◌

●◐ **V12.53　Sudden cardiac arrest** ◌
　　　Sudden cardiac death successfully resuscitated
　　　Coding Clinic: 2007, Q4, P99-101

(Ex) CC Exclusions　　◀ New　　◀▥ Revised　　~~deleted~~ Deleted　　● Use Additional Digit(s)　　❶ First Listed　　◐ First Listed or Additional
❷ Additional Only　　▶ Manifestation Code　　OGCR Official Guidelines　　Coding Clinic　　Excludes　　Includes　　Use additional　　Code first

● ⬚V12.54　**Transient ischemic attack (TIA), and cerebral infarction without residual deficits** ⬚
　　　　Prolonged reversible ischemic neurological deficit (PRIND)
　　　　Reversible ischemic neurologic deficit (RIND)
　　　　Stroke NOS without residual deficits
　　　　| Excludes | *history of traumatic brain injury (V15.52)* ◄
　　　　　　　　　late effects of cerebrovascular disease (438.0–438.9)
　　　　Coding Clinic: 2007, Q4, P99-101; 2007, Q2, P3

　　　OGCR Section I.C.7.d.3
　　　Assign code V12.54, Transient ischemic attack (TIA), and cerebral infarction without residual deficits (and not a code from category 438) as an additional code for history of cerebrovascular disease when no neurologic deficits are present.

● ⬚V12.59　**Other** ⬚
　　　Coding Clinic: 2007, Q2, P3; 1997, Q4, P35-37

● V12.6　**Diseases of respiratory system**
　　　| Excludes | *tuberculosis (V12.01)*
　　● ⬚V12.60　**Unspecified disease of respiratory system** ⬚
　　● ⬚V12.61　**Pneumonia (recurrent)** ⬚
　　● ⬚V12.69　**Other diseases of respiratory system** ⬚

● V12.7　**Diseases of digestive system**
　　　Coding Clinic: 1995, Q1, P3; 1992, Q3, P11; 1989, Q2, P16
　　● ⬚V12.70　**Unspecified digestive disease** ⬚
　　● ⬚V12.71　**Peptic ulcer disease** ⬚
　　● ⬚V12.72　**Colonic polyps** ⬚
　　　　Coding Clinic: 2002, Q3, P14-15
　　● ⬚V12.79　**Other** ⬚

● V13　**Personal history of other diseases**
　● V13.0　**Disorders of urinary system**
　　● ⬚V13.00　**Unspecified urinary disorder** ⬚
　　● ⬚V13.01　**Urinary calculi** ⬚
　　● ⬚V13.02　**Urinary (tract) infection** ⬚
　　● ⬚V13.03　**Nephrotic syndrome** ⬚
　　● ⬚V13.09　**Other** ⬚
　　　　Coding Clinic: 1996, Q2, P7x2
　● ⬚V13.1　**Trophoblastic disease** ♀ ⬚
　　　| Excludes | *supervision during a current pregnancy (V23.1)*

　● V13.2　**Other genital system and obstetric disorders**
　　　| Excludes | *supervision during a current pregnancy of a woman with poor obstetric history (V23.0–V23.9)*
　　　　　habitual aborter (646.3)
　　　　　without current pregnancy (629.81)
　　● ⬚V13.21　**Personal history of pre-term labor** ♀ ⬚
　　　　| Excludes | *current pregnancy with history of pre-term labor (V23.41)*
　　● ⬚V13.22　**Personal history of cervical dysplasia** ♀ ⬚
　　　　Personal history of conditions classifiable to 622.10–622.12
　　　　| Excludes | *personal history of malignant neoplasm of cervix uteri (V10.41)*
　　　　Coding Clinic: 2007, Q4, P99-101
　　● ⬚V13.29　**Other genital system and obstetric disorders** ♀ ⬚

● ⬚V13.3　**Diseases of skin and subcutaneous tissue** ⬚
● V13.4　**Arthritis** ⬚
● V13.5　**Other musculoskeletal disorders**
　● ⬚V13.51　**Pathologic fracture** ⬚
　　　Healed pathologic fracture
　　　| Excludes | *personal history of traumatic fracture (V15.51)*
　● ⬚V13.52　**Stress fracture** ⬚
　　　Healed stress fracture
　　　| Excludes | *personal history of traumatic fracture (V15.51)*
　● ⬚V13.59　**Other musculoskeletal disorders** ⬚
● V13.6　**Congenital malformations**
　● ❷V13.61　**Hypospadias** ♂ ⬚
　● V13.69　**Other congenital malformations** ⬚
　　　Coding Clinic: 2004, Q1, P16-17
● ⬚V13.7　**Perinatal problems** ⬚
　　　| Excludes | *low birth weight status (V21.30–V21.35)*
● ⬚V13.8　**Other specified diseases** ⬚
● V13.9　**Unspecified disease** ⬚

● V14　**Personal history of allergy to medicinal agents**
　● ❷V14.0　**Penicillin** ⬚
　● ❷V14.1　**Other antibiotic agent** ⬚
　● ❷V14.2　**Sulfonamides** ⬚
　● ❷V14.3　**Other anti-infective agent** ⬚
　● ❷V14.4　**Anesthetic agent** ⬚
　● ❷V14.5　**Narcotic agent** ⬚
　● ❷V14.6　**Analgesic agent** ⬚
　● ❷V14.7　**Serum or vaccine** ⬚
　● ❷V14.8　**Other specified medicinal agents** ⬚
　● ❷V14.9　**Unspecified medicinal agent** ⬚

● V15　**Other personal history presenting hazards to health**
　　　| Excludes | *personal history of drug therapy (V87.41–V87.49)*
　● V15.0　**Allergy, other than to medicinal agents**
　　　| Excludes | *allergy to food substance used as base for medicinal agent (V14.0–V14.9)*
　　● ❷V15.01　**Allergy to peanuts** ⬚
　　● ❷V15.02　**Allergy to milk products** ⬚
　　　　| Excludes | *lactose intolerance (271.3)*
　　　　Coding Clinic: 2003, Q1, P12
　　● ❷V15.03　**Allergy to eggs** ⬚
　　● ❷V15.04　**Allergy to seafood** ⬚
　　　　Seafood (octopus) (squid) ink
　　　　Shellfish
　　● ❷V15.05　**Allergy to other foods** ⬚
　　　　Food additives
　　　　Nuts other than peanuts
　　● ❷V15.06　**Allergy to insects and arachnids** ⬚ ◄
　　　　Bugs
　　　　Insect bites and stings
　　　　Spiders
　　● ❷V15.07　**Allergy to latex** ⬚
　　　　Latex sensitivity
　　● ❷V15.08　**Allergy to radiographic dye** ⬚
　　　　Contrast media used for diagnostic x-ray procedures
　　● ❷V15.09　**Other allergy, other than to medicinal agents** ⬚

N Newborn Age: 0　　**P** Pediatric Age: 0–17　　**M** Maternity Age: 12–55　　**A** Adult Age: 15–124　　♀ Females Only　　♂ Males Only　　　**1135**
● Unacceptable Principal Diagnosis　　⬚ Complication\Comorbidity　　⬚ Major C\C　　⬚ Present on Admission Requirement　　⬚ Hospital-Acquired Condition

V01-V89

● ❷ **V15.1 Surgery to heart and great vessels** 🖿
> **Excludes** *replacement by transplant or other means (V42.1–V42.2, V43.2–V43.4)*

> Coding Clinic: 2004, Q1, P16-17

● **V15.2 Surgery to other organs**
> **Excludes** *replacement by transplant or other means (V42.0–V43.8)*

● ❷ **V15.21 Personal history of undergoing in utero procedure during pregnancy** ♀ 🖿

● ❷ **V15.22 Personal history of undergoing in utero procedure while a fetus** 🖿

● ❷ **V15.29 Surgery to other organs** 🖿

● ❷ **V15.3 Irradiation** 🖿
> Previous exposure to therapeutic or other ionizing radiation

● **V15.4 Psychological trauma**
> **Excludes** *history of condition classifiable to 290–316 (V11.0–V11.9)*

● ❷ **V15.41 History of physical abuse** 🖿
> Rape
> Coding Clinic: 1999, Q3, P15

● ❷ **V15.42 History of emotional abuse** 🖿
> Neglect
> Coding Clinic: 1999, Q3, P15

● ❷ **V15.49 Other** 🖿
> Coding Clinic: 1999, Q3, P15

● **V15.5 Injury**

● ❷ **V15.51 Traumatic fracture** 🖿
> Healed traumatic fracture
> **Excludes** *personal history of pathologic and stress fracture (V13.51, V13.52)*

● ❷ **V15.52 History of traumatic brain injury** 🖿 ◀
> **Excludes** *personal history of cerebrovascular accident (cerebral infarction) without residual deficits (V12.54)* ◀

● ❷ **V15.59 Other injury** 🖿

● ❷ **V15.6 Poisoning** 🖿

● **V15.7 Contraception** 🖿
> **Excludes** *current contraceptive management (V25.0–V25.4)*
> *presence of intrauterine contraceptive device as incidental finding (V45.5)*

● **V15.8 Other specified personal history presenting hazards to health**
> **Excludes** *contact with and (suspected) exposure to:*
> *aromatic compounds and dyes (V87.11-V87.19)*
> *arsenic and other metals (V87.01-V87.09)*
> *molds (V87.31)*

● ❷ **V15.80 History of failed moderate sedation** ◀
> History of failed conscious sedation ◀

● ❷ **V15.81 Noncompliance with medical treatment** 🖿
> **Excludes** *noncompliance with renal dialysis (V45.12)*
> Coding Clinic: 2007, Q3, P11; 2006, Q4, P136; 2003, Q2, P7-8; 2001, Q2, P13; 1999, Q2, P17; Q1, P13-14; 1997, Q2, P11; 1996, Q3, P9

● ❷ **V15.82 History of tobacco use** 🖿
> **Excludes** *tobacco dependence (305.1)*
> Coding Clinic: 2009, Q1, P15

● ❷ **V15.83 Underimmunization status** ◀
> Delinquent immunization status ◀
> Lapsed immunization schedule status ◀

● ❷ **V15.84 Contact with and (suspected) exposure to ~~Exposure to~~ asbestos** ◀┅

● ❷ **V15.85 Contact with and (suspected) exposure to ~~Exposure to~~ potentially hazardous body fluids** ◀┅

● ❷ **V15.86 Contact with and (suspected) exposure to ~~Exposure to~~ lead** ◀┅

● ❷ **V15.87 History of extracorporeal membrane oxygenation [ECMO]**

● 🅥ₐ **V15.88 History of fall** 🖿
> At risk for falling
> Coding Clinic: 2005, Q4, P94-100

● ❷ **V15.89 Other** 🖿
> **Excludes** *contact with and (suspected) exposure to other potentially hazardous chemicals (V87.2)*
> *contact with and (suspected) exposure to other potentially hazardous substances (V87.39)*
> Coding Clinic: 2008, Q3, P6-7; 2007, Q3, P6; 1990, Q1, P21

● ❷ **V15.9 Unspecified personal history presenting hazards to health** 🖿

> **OGCR** Section I.C.18.d.3
> Family history codes are for use when a patient has a family member(s) who has had a particular disease that causes the patient to be at higher risk of also contracting the disease.

● **V16 Family history of malignant neoplasm**
> Coding Clinic: 1985, Nov-Dec, P13

● 🅥ₐ **V16.0 Gastrointestinal tract** 🖿
> Family history of condition classifiable to 140–159
> Coding Clinic: 1999, Q1, P4

● 🅥ₐ **V16.1 Trachea, bronchus, and lung** 🖿
> Family history of condition classifiable to 162

● 🅥ₐ **V16.2 Other respiratory and intrathoracic organs** 🖿
> Family history of condition classifiable to 160–161, 163–165

● 🅥ₐ **V16.3 Breast** 🖿
> Family history of condition classifiable to 174
> Coding Clinic: 2004, Q4, P106-107; 2003, Q2, P3-5; 2000, Q2, P8-9; 1995, Q4, P61; 1992, Q1, P11; 1990, Q1, P21

● **V16.4 Genital organs**
> Family history of condition classifiable to 179–187

● 🅥ₐ **V16.40 Genital organ, unspecified** 🖿

● 🅥ₐ **V16.41 Ovary** 🖿

● 🅥ₐ **V16.42 Prostate** 🖿

● 🅥ₐ **V16.43 Testis** 🖿

● 🅥ₐ **V16.49 Other** 🖿
> Coding Clinic: 2006, Q2, P3,4

● **V16.5 Urinary organs**
> Family history of condition classifiable to 188–189

● 🅥ₐ **V16.51 Kidney** 🖿

● 🅥ₐ **V16.52 Bladder** 🖿

● 🅥ₐ **V16.59 Other** 🖿

| (Ex) CC Exclusions | ◀ New | ◀┅ Revised | ~~deleted~~ Deleted | ● Use Additional Digit(s) | ❶ First Listed | 🅥ₐ First Listed or Additional |
| ❷ Additional Only | ▶ Manifestation Code | **OGCR** Official Guidelines | Coding Clinic | Excludes | Includes | Use additional | Code first |

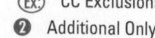

● V16.6 **Leukemia**
         Family history of condition classifiable to 204–208

● V16.7 **Other lymphatic and hematopoietic neoplasms**
         Family history of condition classifiable to 200–203

● V16.8 **Other specified malignant neoplasm**
         Family history of other condition classifiable to 140–199

● V16.9 **Unspecified malignant neoplasm**

● V17 **Family history of certain chronic disabling diseases**
     Coding Clinic: 1985, Nov-Dec, P13

● V17.0 **Psychiatric condition**

       Excludes   *family history of mental retardation (V18.4)*

● V17.1 **Stroke (cerebrovascular)**

● V17.2 **Other neurological diseases**
         Epilepsy
         Huntington's chorea

● V17.3 **Ischemic heart disease**

● V17.4 **Other cardiovascular diseases**
     Coding Clinic: 2004, Q1, P6-7

     ● V17.41 **Family history of sudden cardiac death (SCD)**

         Excludes   *family history of ischemic heart disease (V17.3)*
                       family history of myocardial infarction (V17.3)

     ● V17.49 **Family history of other cardiovascular diseases**
         Family history of cardiovascular disease NOS

● V17.5 **Asthma**

● V17.6 **Other chronic respiratory conditions**

● V17.7 **Arthritis**

● V17.8 **Other musculoskeletal diseases**

     ● V17.81 **Osteoporosis**

     ● V17.89 **Other musculoskeletal diseases**

● V18 **Family history of certain other specific conditions**
     Coding Clinic: 1985, Nov-Dec, P13

● V18.0 **Diabetes mellitus**
     Coding Clinic: 2005, Q2, P21; 2004, Q1, P8

● V18.1 **Other endocrine and metabolic diseases**

     ● V18.11 **Multiple endocrine neoplasia [MEN] syndrome**

     ● V18.19 **Other endocrine and metabolic diseases**

● V18.2 **Anemia**

● V18.3 **Other blood disorders**

● V18.4 **Mental retardation**

● V18.5 **Digestive disorders**

     ● V18.51 **Colonic polyps**

         Excludes   *family history of malignant neoplasm of gastrointestinal tract (V16.0)*

     ● V18.59 **Other digestive disorders**

● V18.6 **Kidney diseases**

     ● V18.61 **Polycystic kidney**

     ● V18.69 **Other kidney diseases**

● V18.7 **Other genitourinary diseases**

● V18.8 **Infectious and parasitic diseases**

● V18.9 **Genetic disease carrier**

● V19 **Family history of other conditions**
     Coding Clinic: 1985, Nov-Dec, P13

● V19.0 **Blindness or visual loss**

● V19.1 **Other eye disorders**

● V19.2 **Deafness or hearing loss**

● V19.3 **Other ear disorders**

● V19.4 **Skin conditions**

● V19.5 **Congenital anomalies**

● V19.6 **Allergic disorders**

● V19.7 **Consanguinity**

● V19.8 **Other condition**

PERSONS ENCOUNTERING HEALTH SERVICES IN CIRCUMSTANCES RELATED TO REPRODUCTION AND DEVELOPMENT (V20–V29)

● V20 **Health supervision of infant or child**

❶ V20.0 **Foundling**   P

● ❶ V20.1 **Other healthy infant or child receiving care**   P
         Medical or nursing care supervision of healthy infant in cases of:
            maternal illness, physical or psychiatric
            socioeconomic adverse condition at home
            too many children at home preventing or interfering with normal care
     Coding Clinic: 2000, Q1, P25; 1993, Q4, P36; 1989, Q3, P14

● ❶ V20.2 **Routine infant or child health check**   P
         Developmental testing of infant or child
         Health check for child over 28 days old ◄
         Immunizations appropriate for age
         ~~Initial and subsequent routine newborn check~~
         Routine vision and hearing testing

       Excludes   *health check for child under 29 days old (V20.31-V20.32)* ◄
                 newborn health supervision (V20.31-V20.32) ◄
                 special screening for developmental handicaps (V79.3)

       Use additional code(s) to identify:
         Special screening examination(s) performed (V73.0–V82.9)
     Coding Clinic: 2009, Q1, P15; 2004, Q1, P15-16x2

● V20.3 **Newborn health supervision**   ◄
         Health check for child under 29 days old ◄

       Excludes   *health check for child over 28 days old (V20.2)* ◄

     ● ❷ V20.31 **Health supervision for newborn under 8 days old**   N◄
         Health check for newborn under 8 days old   N◄

     ● ❷ V20.32 **Health supervision for newborn 8 to 28 days old**   N◄
         Health check for newborn 8 to 28 days old ◄
         Newborn weight check ◄

● V21 **Constitutional states in development**

● ❷ V21.0 **Period of rapid growth in childhood**

● ❷ V21.1 **Puberty**

● ❷ V21.2 **Other adolescence**

● V21.3 **Low birth weight status**

       Excludes   *history of perinatal problems (V13.7)*

     ● ❷ V21.30 **Low birth weight status, unspecified**

     ● ❷ V21.31 **Low birth weight status, less than 500 grams**

     ● ❷ V21.32 **Low birth weight status, 500–999 grams**

N Newborn Age: 0   **P** Pediatric Age: 0–17   **M** Maternity Age: 12–55   **A** Adult Age: 15–124   ♀ Females Only   ♂ Males Only

● Unacceptable Principal Diagnosis   Complication\Comorbidity   Major C\C   Present on Admission Requirement   Hospital-Acquired Condition

1137

V01-V89

● ❷ **V21.33**   **Low birth weight status, 1000–1499 grams** 🖎

● ❷ **V21.34**   **Low birth weight status, 1500–1999 grams** 🖎

● ❷ **V21.35**   **Low birth weight status, 2000–2500 grams** 🖎

● ❷ **V21.8**   **Other specified constitutional states in development** 🖎

● ❷ **V21.9**   **Unspecified constitutional state in development** 🖎

● **V22**   **Normal pregnancy**

> | Excludes | *pregnancy examination or test, pregnancy unconfirmed (V72.40)* |

> Coding Clinic: 2007, Q4, P124-125

> **OGCR**   Section I.C.11.b.1
>
> For routine outpatient prenatal visits when no complications are present codes V22.0, Supervision of normal first pregnancy, and V22.1, Supervision of other normal pregnancy, should be used as the first-listed diagnoses. These codes should not be used in conjunction with chapter 11 codes.

● ❶ **V22.0**   **Supervision of normal first pregnancy** ♀ 🖎

> Coding Clinic: 1999, Q3, P16; 1990, Q1, P10; 1984, Nov-Dec, P18

● ❶ **V22.1**   **Supervision of other normal pregnancy** ♀ 🖎

> Coding Clinic: 1999, Q3, P16; 1990, Q1, P10

● ❷ **V22.2**   **Pregnant state, incidental** ♀ 🖎

> Pregnant state NOS
>
> Coding Clinic: 1998, Q2, P13-14; 1994, Q2, P14

> **OGCR**   Section I.C.11.b.2
>
> For prenatal outpatient visits for patients with high-risk pregnancies, a code from category V23, Supervision of high-risk pregnancy, should be used as the principal or first-listed diagnosis. Secondary chapter 11 codes may be used in conjunction with these codes if appropriate.

● **V23**   **Supervision of high-risk pregnancy**

> Coding Clinic: 1990, Q1, P10

● 🅥 **V23.0**   **Pregnancy with history of infertility** ♀ 🖎   M

● 🅥 **V23.1**   **Pregnancy with history of trophoblastic disease** ♀ 🖎   M

> Pregnancy with history of:
>   hydatidiform mole
>   vesicular mole

> | Excludes | *that without current pregnancy (V13.1)* |

● 🅥 **V23.2**   **Pregnancy with history of abortion** ♀ 🖎   M

> Pregnancy with history of conditions classifiable to 634–638

> | Excludes | *habitual aborter:* |
> | | *care during pregnancy (646.3)* |
> | | *that without current pregnancy (629.81)* |

● 🅥 **V23.3**   **Grand multiparity** ♀ 🖎   M

> | Excludes | *care in relation to labor and delivery (659.4)* |
> | | *that without current pregnancy (V61.5)* |

● **V23.4**   **Pregnancy with other poor obstetric history**

> Pregnancy with history of other conditions classifiable to 630–676

● 🅥 **V23.41**   **Pregnancy with history of pre-term labor** ♀ 🖎   M

● 🅥 **V23.49**   **Pregnancy with other poor obstetric history** ♀ 🖎   M

● 🅥 **V23.5**   **Pregnancy with other poor reproductive history** ♀ 🖎   M

> Pregnancy with history of stillbirth or neonatal death

● 🅥 **V23.7**   **Insufficient prenatal care** ♀ 🖎   M

> History of little or no prenatal care

● **V23.8**   **Other high-risk pregnancy**

> Coding Clinic: 1998, Q4, P50-51

● 🅥 **V23.81**   **Elderly primigravida** ♀ 🖎   M

> First pregnancy in a woman who will be 35 years of age or older at expected date of delivery

> | Excludes | *elderly primigravida complicating pregnancy (659.5)* |

> Coding Clinic: 1998, Q4, P58

● 🅥 **V23.82**   **Elderly multigravida** ♀ 🖎   M

> Second or more pregnancy in a woman who will be 35 years of age or older at expected date of delivery

> | Excludes | *elderly multigravida complicating pregnancy (659.6)* |

● 🅥 **V23.83**   **Young primigravida** ♀ 🖎   M

> First pregnancy in a female less than 16 years old at expected date of delivery

> | Excludes | *young primigravida complicating pregnancy (659.8)* |

● 🅥 **V23.84**   **Young multigravida** ♀ 🖎   M

> Second or more pregnancy in a female less than 16 years old at expected date of delivery

> | Excludes | *young multigravida complicating pregnancy (659.8)* |

● 🅥 **V23.85**   **Pregnancy resulting from assisted reproductive technology** ♀ 🖎   M A

> Pregnancy resulting from in vitro fertilization

● 🅥 **V23.86**   **Pregnancy with history of in utero procedure during previous pregnancy** ♀ 🖎   M

> | Excludes | *management of pregnancy affected by in utero procedure during current pregnancy (679.0–679.1)* | ◀▥

● 🅥 **V23.89**   **Other high-risk pregnancy** ♀ 🖎   M

> Coding Clinic: 2006, Q3, P14

● 🅥 **V23.9**   **Unspecified high-risk pregnancy** ♀ 🖎   M

Ⓔⓧ CC Exclusions   ◀ New   ◀▥ Revised   ~~deleted~~ Deleted   ● Use Additional Digit(s)   ❶ First Listed   🅥 First Listed or Additional
❷ Additional Only   ▶ Manifestation Code   **OGCR** Official Guidelines   **Coding Clinic**   Excludes   Includes   Use additional   Code first

OGCR Section I.C.18.d.8

The follow-up codes (V24, V67 and V89), are used to explain continuing surveillance following completed treatment of a disease, condition, or injury. They imply that the condition has been fully treated and no longer exists. They should not be confused with aftercare codes that explain current treatment for a healing condition or its sequelae. Follow-up codes may be used in conjunction with history codes to provide the full picture of the healed condition and its treatment. The follow-up code is sequenced first, followed by the history code. A follow-up code may be used to explain repeated visits. Should a condition be found to have recurred on the follow-up visit, then the diagnosis code should be used in place of the follow-up code.

● **V24   Postpartum care and examination**

   ❶ **V24.0   Immediately after delivery** ♀ 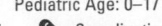   **M**
   Care and observation in uncomplicated cases
   Coding Clinic: 2006, Q3, P11

   OGCR Section I.C.10.i.5

   When the mother delivers outside the hospital prior to admission and is admitted for routine postpartum care and no complications are noted, code V24.0, Postpartum care and examination immediately after delivery, should be assigned as the principal diagnosis.

   ● ❶ **V24.1   Lactating mother** ♀
   Supervision of lactation

   ● ❶ **V24.2   Routine postpartum follow-up** ♀

● **V25   Encounter for contraceptive management**

   ● **V25.0   General counseling and advice**

      ● **V25.01   Prescription of oral contraceptives** ♀

      ● **V25.02   Initiation of other contraceptive measures**
      Fitting of diaphragm
      Prescription of foams, creams, or other agents
      Coding Clinic: 1997, Q3, P7

      ● **V25.03   Encounter for emergency contraceptive counseling and prescription**
      Encounter for postcoital contraceptive counseling and prescription

      ● **V25.04   Counseling and instruction in natural family planning to avoid pregnancy**
      Coding Clinic: 2007, Q4, P99-101

      ● **V25.09   Other**
      Family planning advice

   ● **V25.1   Insertion of intrauterine contraceptive device** ♀

   V25.2   Sterilization
   Admission for interruption of fallopian tubes or vas deferens

   V25.3   Menstrual extraction ♀
   Menstrual regulation

● **V25.4   Surveillance of previously prescribed contraceptive methods**
   Checking, reinsertion, or removal of contraceptive device
   Repeat prescription for contraceptive method
   Routine examination in connection with contraceptive maintenance

   > **Excludes** *presence of intrauterine contraceptive device as incidental finding (V45.5)*

   ● **V25.40   Contraceptive surveillance, unspecified**

   ● **V25.41   Contraceptive pill** ♀

   ● **V25.42   Intrauterine contraceptive device** ♀
   Checking, reinsertion, or removal of intrauterine device

   ● **V25.43   Implantable subdermal contraceptive** ♀

   ● **V25.49   Other contraceptive method**
   Coding Clinic: 1997, Q3, P7

● **V25.5   Insertion of implantable subdermal contraceptive** ♀

● **V25.8   Other specified contraceptive management**
   Postvasectomy sperm count

   > **Excludes** *sperm count following sterilization reversal (V26.22)*
   > *sperm count for fertility testing (V26.21)*

   Coding Clinic: 1996, Q3, P9

● **V25.9   Unspecified contraceptive management**

● **V26   Procreative management**

   V26.0   Tuboplasty or vasoplasty after previous sterilization
   Coding Clinic: 1995, Q2, P10

● **V26.1   Artificial insemination** ♀

● **V26.2   Investigation and testing**

   > **Excludes** *postvasectomy sperm count (V25.8)*

   Coding Clinic: 1996, Q2, P9; 1985, Nov-Dec, P15

   ● **V26.21   Fertility testing**
   Fallopian insufflation
   Sperm count for fertility testing

   > **Excludes** *genetic counseling and testing (V26.31–V26.39)*

   ● **V26.22   Aftercare following sterilization reversal**
   Fallopian insufflation following sterilization reversal
   Sperm count following sterilization reversal

   ● **V26.29   Other investigation and testing**

N Newborn Age: 0   **P** Pediatric Age: 0–17   **M** Maternity Age: 12–55   **A** Adult Age: 15–124   ♀ Females Only   ♂ Males Only

● Unacceptable Principal Diagnosis   Complication\Comorbidity   Major C\C   Present on Admission Requirement   Hospital-Acquired Condition

V01-V89

1139

● V26.3   Genetic counseling and testing

   Excludes   *fertility testing (V26.21)*
      nonprocreative genetic screening
        (V82.71, V82.79)

   Coding Clinic: 2006, Q4, P117; 2005, Q4, P94-100

   OGCR   Section I.C.18.d.3

     If the purpose of the encounter is genetic counseling associated with procreative management, a code from subcategory V26.3 should be assigned as the first-listed code, followed by a code from category V84, Genetic susceptibility to disease. Additional codes should be assigned for any applicable family or personal history.

   ● V26.31   Testing of female genetic disease carrier status ♀

   ● V26.32   Other genetic testing of female ♀

      Use additional code to identify habitual aborter (629.81, 646.3)

   ● V26.33   Genetic counseling

   ● V26.34   Testing of male genetic disease carrier status ♂

   ● V26.35   Encounter for testing of male partner of habitual aborter ♂

   ● V26.39   Other genetic testing of male ♂

● V26.4   General counseling and advice

   ● V26.41   Procreative counseling and advice using natural family planning

      Coding Clinic: 2007, Q4, P99-101

   ● V26.42   Encounter for fertility preservation counseling ◄

      Encounter for fertility preservation counseling prior to cancer therapy ◄

      Encounter for fertility preservation counseling prior to surgical removal of gonads ◄

   ● V26.49   Other procreative management counseling and advice

● V26.5   Sterilization status

   ● ❷ V26.51   Tubal ligation status ♀

      Excludes   *infertility not due to previous tubal ligation (628.0–628.9)*

   ● ❷ V26.52   Vasectomy status ♂

● V26.8   Other specified procreative management

   ● ❶ V26.81   Encounter for assisted reproductive fertility procedure cycle ♀

      Patient undergoing in vitro fertilization cycle

      Use additional code to identify the type of infertility

      Excludes   *pre-cycle diagnosis and testing - code to reason for encounter*

      Coding Clinic: 2007, Q4, P99-101

   ● V26.82   Encounter for fertility preservation procedure ◄

      Encounter for fertility preservation counseling prior to cancer therapy ◄

      Encounter for fertility preservation procedure prior to surgical removal of gonads ◄

   ● V26.89   Other specified procreative management

● V26.9   Unspecified procreative management

   OGCR   Section I.C.10.h.3

     V27.0, Single liveborn, is the only outcome of delivery code appropriate for use with 650.

   OGCR   Section I.C.10.k.4

     When an attempted termination of pregnancy results in a liveborn fetus assign code 644.21 with an appropriate code from category V27, Outcome of Delivery. The procedure code for the attempted termination of pregnancy should also be assigned.

   OGCR   Section I.C.11.b.5

     An outcome of delivery code, V27.0-V27.9, should be included on every maternal record when a delivery has occurred. These codes are not to be used on subsequent records or on the newborn record.

● V27   Outcome of delivery

   Note: This category is intended for the coding of the outcome of delivery on the mother's record.

   Coding Clinic: 1991, Q2, P16

   ● ❷ V27.0   Single liveborn ♀   M

      Coding Clinic: 2008, Q4, P192; 2005, Q4, P81; 2003, Q2, P9; 2002, Q2, P10; 2000, Q3, P5; 1998, Q4, P76-77

   ● ❷ V27.1   Single stillborn ♀   M

      Coding Clinic: 2001, Q1, P11-12

   ● ❷ V27.2   Twins, both liveborn ♀   M

      Coding Clinic: 1992, Q3, P10

   ● ❷ V27.3   Twins, one liveborn and one stillborn ♀   M

   ● ❷ V27.4   Twins, both stillborn ♀   M

   ● ❷ V27.5   Other multiple birth, all liveborn ♀   M

   ● ❷ V27.6   Other multiple birth, some liveborn ♀   M

   ● ❷ V27.7   Other multiple birth, all stillborn ♀   M

   ● ❷ V27.9   Unspecified outcome of delivery ♀   M

      routine prenatal care (V22.0–V23.9)

● V28   Encounter for antenatal screening of mother

   Excludes   *abnormal findings on screening - code to findings*
      suspected fetal conditions affecting management of pregnancy (655.00–655.93, 656.00–656.93, 657.00–657.03, 658.00–658.93)
      suspected fetal conditions not found (V89.01-V89.09)

   OGCR   Section I.C.18.d.5

     See V73-V82 to report special screening examinations.

   ● V28.0   Screening for chromosomal anomalies by amniocentesis ♀   M

   ● V28.1   Screening for raised alpha-fetoprotein levels in amniotic fluid ♀   M

   ● V28.2   Other screening based on amniocentesis ♀   M

   ● V28.3   Encounter for routine screening for malformation using ultrasonics ♀

      Encounter for routine fetal ultrasound NOS

      Excludes   *encounter for fetal anatomic survey (V28.81)*
        genetic counseling and testing (V26.31–V26.39)

   ● V28.4   Screening for fetal growth retardation using ultrasonics ♀

   ● V28.5   Screening for isoimmunization ♀

   ● V28.6   Screening for Streptococcus B ♀   M

(Ex.)   CC Exclusions   ◄   New   ◀▬   Revised   ~~deleted~~   Deleted   ●   Use Additional Digit(s)   ❶   First Listed   First Listed or Additional

❷   Additional Only   ▶   Manifestation Code   **OGCR**   Official Guidelines   **Coding Clinic**   Excludes   Includes   Use additional   Code first

● V28.8   **Other specified antenatal screening**
Coding Clinic: 1999, Q3, P16

    ● V28.81   **Encounter for fetal anatomic survey** ♀   **M**

    ● V28.82   **Encounter for screening for risk of pre-term labor** ♀   **M**

    ● V28.89   **Other specified antenatal screening** ♀   **M**
       Chorionic villus sampling
       Genomic screening
       Nuchal translucency testing
       Proteomic screening

● V28.9   **Unspecified antenatal screening** ♀

OGCR Section I.C.15.d.1
Assign a code from category V29 to identify those instances when a healthy newborn is evaluated for a suspected condition that is determined after study not to be present. Do not use a code from category V29 when the patient has identified signs or symptoms of a suspected problem; in such cases, code the sign or symptom. A code from category V29 may also be assigned as a principal code for readmissions or encounters when the V30 code no longer applies. Codes from category V29 are for use only for healthy newborns and infants for which no condition after study is found to be present.

OGCR Section I.C.15.d.2
A V29 code is to be used as a secondary code after the V30.

OGCR Section I.C.18.d.6
Observation codes V29, V71 and V89 are for use in very limited circumstances when a person is being observed for a suspected condition that is ruled out. The observation codes are not for use if an injury or illness or any signs or symptoms related to the suspected condition are present. In such cases the diagnosis/symptom code is used with the corresponding E code to identify any external cause. The observation codes are to be used as principal diagnosis only. The only exception to this is when the principal diagnosis is required to be a code from the V30, Live born infant, category. Then the V29 observation code is sequenced after the V30 code. Additional codes may be used in addition to the observation code but only if they are unrelated to the suspected condition being observed.

● V29   **Observation and evaluation of newborns for suspected condition not found**

    Note: This category is to be used for newborns, within the neonatal period (the first 28 days of life), who are suspected of having an abnormal condition resulting from exposure from the mother or the birth process, but without signs or symptoms, and which, after examination and observation, is found not to exist.

    Excludes   suspected fetal conditions not found (V89.01–V89.09)
    Coding Clinic: 2000, Q1, P25-26

V29.0   **Observation for suspected infectious condition**   **N**
    Coding Clinic: 2001, Q1, P10

V29.1   **Observation for suspected neurological condition**   **N**

V29.2   **Observation for suspected respiratory condition**   **N**

● V29.3   **Observation for suspected genetic or metabolic condition**   **N**
    Coding Clinic: 2005, Q2, P21; 2004, Q1, P8; 1998, Q4, P59

V29.8   **Observation for other specified suspected condition**   **N**
    Coding Clinic: 2003, Q2, P15-16

● V29.9   **Observation for unspecified suspected condition**   **N**
    Coding Clinic: 2002, Q1, P6-7

LIVEBORN INFANTS ACCORDING TO TYPE OF BIRTH (V30–V39)

OGCR Section I.C.15.b
When coding the birth of an infant, assign a code from categories V30-V39, according to the type of birth. A code from this series is assigned as a principal diagnosis, and assigned only once to a newborn at the time of birth.

OGCR Section I.C.15.c
If the newborn is transferred to another institution, the V30 series is not used at the receiving hospital.

Note: These categories are intended for the coding of liveborn infants who are consuming health care [e.g., crib or bassinet occupancy].

The following fourth-digit subdivisions are for use with categories V30–V39:

> 0   Born in hospital
> 1   Born before admission to hospital
> ● 2   Born outside hospital and not hospitalized

The following two fifths-digits are for use with the fourth-digit .0, Born in hospital:

> 0   delivered without mention of cesarean delivery
> 1   delivered by cesarean delivery

❶ ● V30   **Single liveborn**   **N**
    ● V30.2
      Coding Clinic: 2006, Q3, P10-11; 2005, Q4, P83-89; Q2, P21; 2004, Q1, P8, 16; 2003, Q4, P67-68; Q2, P9; 2001, Q4, P50-51; 2000, Q1, P25-26; 1998, Q4, P46-47, 59; 1994, Q3, P4; 1993, Q4, P36

❶ ● V31   **Twin, mate liveborn**   **N**
    ● V30.2
      Coding Clinic: 1992, Q3, P10

❶ ● V32   **Twin, mate stillborn**   **N**
    ● V32.2

❶ ● V33   **Twin, unspecified**   **N**
    ● V33.2

❶ ● V34   **Other multiple, mates all liveborn**   **N**
    ● V34.2

❶ ● V35   **Other multiple, mates all stillborn**   **N**
    ● V35.2

❶ ● V36   **Other multiple, mates live- and stillborn**   **N**
    ● V36.2

❶ ● V37   **Other multiple, unspecified**   **N**
    ● V37.2

❶ ● V39   **Unspecified**
    ● V39.1 and V39.2

N Newborn Age: 0   **P** Pediatric Age: 0–17   **M** Maternity Age: 12–55   **A** Adult Age: 15–124   ♀ Females Only   ♂ Males Only
● Unacceptable Principal Diagnosis   Complication\Comorbidity   Major C\C   Present on Admission Requirement   Hospital-Acquired Condition

1141

V01-V89

PERSONS WITH A CONDITION INFLUENCING THEIR HEALTH STATUS (V40–V49)

Note: These categories are intended for use when these conditions are recorded as "diagnoses" or "problems."

● **V40　Mental and behavioral problems**
- ● **V40.0　Problems with learning**
- ● **V40.1　Problems with communication [including speech]**
- ● **V40.2　Other mental problems**
- ● **V40.3　Other behavioral problems**
- ● **V40.9　Unspecified mental or behavioral problem**

● **V41　Problems with special senses and other special functions**
- ● **V41.0　Problems with sight**
- ● **V41.1　Other eye problems**
- ● **V41.2　Problems with hearing**
- ● **V41.3　Other ear problems**
- ● **V41.4　Problems with voice production**
- ● **V41.5　Problems with smell and taste**
- ● **V41.6　Problems with swallowing and mastication**
- ● **V41.7　Problems with sexual function**
    - Excludes　*marital problems (V61.10)*
    - 　　　　　*psychosexual disorders (302.0–302.9)*
- ● **V41.8　Other problems with special functions**
- ● **V41.9　Unspecified problem with special functions**

● **V42　Organ or tissue replaced by transplant**
- Includes　homologous or heterologous (animal) (human) transplant organ status
- Coding Clinic: 1998, Q3, P5
- **OGCR** Section I.C.17.f.2.a

    Transplant complications other than kidney: Codes under subcategory 996.8, Complications of transplanted organ, are for use for both complications and rejection of transplanted organs. A transplant complication code is only assigned if the complication affects the function of the transplanted organ. Two codes are required to fully describe a transplant complication, the appropriate code from subcategory 996.8 and a secondary code that identifies the complication.

    Pre-existing conditions or conditions that develop after the transplant are not coded as complications unless they affect the function of the transplanted organs.

    See I.C.18.d.3) for transplant organ removal status.

    See I.C.2.i for malignant neoplasm associated with transplanted organ.

● ❷ **V42.0　Kidney** 🖎 🕻
- Ex: 238.77, 996.80-996.81, 996.87, V42.0, V42.89-V42.9
- Coding Clinic: 2008, Q1, P10-13; 2003, Q1, P10-11; 2001, Q3, P12-13; 1994, Q2, P9x2
- **OGCR** Section I.C.17.f.2.b

    Patients who have undergone kidney transplant may still have some form of chronic kidney disease (CKD) because the kidney transplant may not fully restore kidney function. Code 996.81 should be assigned for documented complications of a kidney transplant, such as transplant failure or rejection or other transplant complication. Code 996.81 should not be assigned for post kidney transplant patients who have chronic kidney (CKD) unless a transplant complication such as transplant failure or rejection is documented. If the documentation is unclear as to whether the patient has a complication of the transplant, query the provider. For patients with CKD following a kidney transplant, but who do not have a complication such as failure or rejection, see section I.C.10.a.2, Chronic kidney disease and kidney transplant status.

● ❷ **V42.1　Heart** 🖎 🕻
- Ex: 238.77, 996.80, 996.83, 996.87, V42.1, V42.89-V42.9
- Coding Clinic: 2003, Q3, P16; 2001, Q3, P13-14x2; 1994, Q2, P13

● ❷ **V42.2　Heart valve** 🖎

● ❷ **V42.3　Skin** 🖎

● ❷ **V42.4　Bone** 🖎

● ❷ **V42.5　Cornea** 🖎

● ❷ **V42.6　Lung** 🖎 🕻
- Ex: 238.77, 999.80, 996.84, 996.87, V42.6, V42.89-V42.9

● ❷ **V42.7　Liver** 🖎 🕻
- Ex: 238.77, 996.80, 996.82, 996.87, V42.7, V42.89-V42.9

● **V42.8　Other specified organ or tissue**
- ● ❷ **V42.81　Bone marrow** 🖎 🕻
    - Ex: 238.77, 279.50-279.53, 996.80, 996.85, 996.87, V42.9
- ● ❷ **V42.82　Peripheral stem cells** 🖎 🕻
    - Ex: 238.77, 996.80, 996.87, V42.9
- ● ❷ **V42.83　Pancreas** 🖎 🕻
    - Ex: 238.77, 996.80, 996.86-996.87, V42.83, V42.9
    - Coding Clinic: 2003, Q1, P10-11; 2001, Q2, P16
- ● ❷ **V42.84　Intestines** 🖎 🕻
    - Ex: 238.77, 996.80, 996.89, V42.84-V42.9
    - Coding Clinic: 2000, Q4, P47-48
- ● ❷ **V42.89　Other** 🖎

● ❷ **V42.9　Unspecified organ or tissue** 🖎

● V43   **Organ or tissue replaced by other means**

    Includes   organ or tissue assisted by other means

          replacement of organ by:

            artificial device

            mechanical device

            prosthesis

    Excludes   *cardiac pacemaker in situ (V45.01)*

          fitting and adjustment of prosthetic device

            (V52.0–V52.9)

          renal dialysis status (V45.11)

●❷ V43.0   **Eye globe** ⬡

●❷ V43.1   **Lens** ⬡

        Pseudophakos

● V43.2   **Heart**

   ●❷ V43.21   **Heart assist device** ⬡ ⬡

         (Ex) 238.77, 996.80, 996.83, 996.87, V42.1, V43.21-V43.22

   ●⬡ V43.22   **Fully implantable artificial heart** ⬡ ⬡

         (Ex) 238.77, 996.80, 996.83, 996.87, V42.1, V43.21-V43.22

●❷ V43.3   **Heart valve** ⬡

      Coding Clinic: 2006, Q3, P7; 2002, Q3, P13-15

●❷ V43.4   **Blood vessel** ⬡

●❷ V43.5   **Bladder** ⬡

● V43.6   **Joint**

      Coding Clinic: 1991, Q1, P15

   ●❷ V43.60   **Unspecified joint** ⬡

   ●❷ V43.61   **Shoulder** ⬡

   ●❷ V43.62   **Elbow** ⬡

   ●❷ V43.63   **Wrist** ⬡

   ●❷ V43.64   **Hip** ⬡

        Coding Clinic: 2009, Q1, P15; 2008, Q2, P3-5; 2006,

           Q3, P4-5; 2005, Q4, P83-89, 110-112; 2004,

           Q2, P15

   ●❷ V43.65   **Knee** ⬡

        Coding Clinic: 2006, Q3, P5

   ●❷ V43.66   **Ankle** ⬡

   ●❷ V43.69   **Other** ⬡

●❷ V43.7   **Limb** ⬡

● V43.8   **Other organ or tissue**

   ●❷ V43.81   **Larynx** ⬡

   ●❷ V43.82   **Breast** ⬡

   ●❷ V43.83   **Artificial skin** ⬡

   ●❷ V43.89   **Other** ⬡

● V44   **Artificial opening status**

    Excludes   *artificial openings requiring attention or*

          management (V55.0–V55.9)

●❷ V44.0   **Tracheostomy** ⬡

      Coding Clinic: 2003, Q4, P103-104, 107, 111; 2001, Q1, P6-7

●❷ V44.1   **Gastrostomy** ⬡

      Coding Clinic: 2003, Q4, P103-104, 107-108, 110; 2001, Q1,

        P12; 1998, Q4, P42-44; 1997, Q3, P12-13; 1993, Q1,

        P26

●❷ V44.2   **Ileostomy** ⬡

      Coding Clinic: 1988, Q2, P9-10

●❷ V44.3   **Colostomy** ⬡

      Coding Clinic: 2003, Q4, P110

●❷ V44.4   **Other artificial opening of gastrointestinal tract** ⬡

●❷ V44.5   **Cystostomy**

   ●❷ V44.50   **Cystostomy, unspecified** ⬡

   ●❷ V44.51   **Cutaneous-vesicostomy** ⬡

   ●❷ V44.52   **Appendico-vesicostomy** ⬡

   ●❷ V44.59   **Other cystostomy** ⬡

●❷ V44.6   **Other artificial opening of urinary tract** ⬡

        Nephrostomy

        Ureterostomy

        Urethrostomy

●❷ V44.7   **Artificial vagina** ⬡

●❷ V44.8   **Other artificial opening status** ⬡

●❷ V44.9   **Unspecified artificial opening status** ⬡

● V45   **Other postprocedural states**

    Excludes   *aftercare management (V51–V58.9)*

          malfunction or other complication-code to

            condition

● V45.0   **Cardiac device in situ**

    Excludes   *artificial heart (V43.22)*

          heart assist device (V43.21)

      Coding Clinic: 1994, Q2, P10x2; 1993, 5th Issue, P12

   ●❷ V45.00   **Unspecified cardiac device** ⬡

   ●❷ V45.01   **Cardiac pacemaker** ⬡

   ●❷ V45.02   **Automatic implantable cardiac defibrillator** ⬡

   ●❷ V45.09   **Other specified cardiac device** ⬡

        Carotid sinus pacemaker in situ

● V45.1   **Renal dialysis status**

    Excludes   *admission for dialysis treatment or*

          session (V56.0)

      Coding Clinic: 2008, Q1, P7-8; 2007, Q4, P84-86; Q3, P11; 2006,

        Q4, P136; 2004, Q1, P22,23; 2001, Q2, P12-13; 1987,

        Sept-Oct, P8; Jan-Feb, P15

   ●❷ V45.11   **Renal dialysis status** ⬡

        Hemodialysis status

        Patient requiring intermittent renal

          dialysis

        Peritoneal dialysis status

        Presence of arterial-venous shunt

          (for dialysis)

        Coding Clinic: 2008, Q4, P193; 2004, Q1, P23

   ●❷ V45.12   **Noncompliance with renal dialysis** ⬡

        Coding Clinic: 2006, Q4, P136

●❷ V45.2   **Presence of cerebrospinal fluid drainage device** ⬡

        Cerebral ventricle (communicating) shunt,

        valve, or device in situ

    Excludes   *malfunction (996.2)*

      Coding Clinic: 2003, Q4, P106-107

●❷ V45.3   **Intestinal bypass or anastomosis status** ⬡

    Excludes   *bariatric surgery status (V45.86)*

          gastric bypass status (V45.86)

          obesity surgery status (V45.86)

●❷ V45.4   **Arthrodesis status** ⬡

      Coding Clinic: 1984, Nov-Dec, P18

● V45.5   **Presence of contraceptive device**

    Excludes   *checking, reinsertion, or removal of*

          device (V25.42)

          complication from device (996.32)

          insertion of device (V25.1)

   ●❷ V45.51   **Intrauterine contraceptive device** ♀ ⬡

   ●❷ V45.52   **Subdermal contraceptive implant** ⬡

        Coding Clinic: 1995, Q3, P14

   ●❷ V45.59   **Other** ⬡

N Newborn Age: 0   **P** Pediatric Age: 0–17   **M** Maternity Age: 12–55   **A** Adult Age: 15–124   ♀ Females Only   ♂ Males Only   **1143**

● Unacceptable Principal Diagnosis   ⬡ Complication\Comorbidity   ⬡ Major C\C   ⬡ Present on Admission Requirement   ⬡ Hospital-Acquired Condition

V01-V89

● V45.6 States following surgery of eye and adnexa

> Excludes aphakia (379.31)
> artificial:
> eye globe (V43.0)

● ❷ V45.61 Cataract extraction status ◎

> Use additional code for associated
> artificial lens status (V43.1)

● ❷ V45.69 Other states following surgery of eye and adnexa ◎
> Coding Clinic: 2001, Q2, P16-17

● V45.7 Acquired absence of organ

◐ V45.71 Acquired absence of breast and nipple ◎

> Excludes congenital absence of breast
> and nipple (757.6) ◀
> Coding Clinic: 2001, Q4, P66; 1997, Q4, P50

● ◐ V45.72 Acquired absence of intestine (large) (small) ◎

● ◐ V45.73 Acquired absence of kidney ◎

● ◐ V45.74 Other parts of urinary tract ◎
> Bladder

● ◐ V45.75 Stomach ◎

● ◐ V45.76 Lung ◎

● ◐ V45.77 Genital organs ◎

> Excludes acquired absence of cervix
> and uterus
> (V88.01–V88.03)
> female genital mutilation
> status
> (629.20–629.29)
> Coding Clinic: 2003, Q1, P13-14x2

● ◐ V45.78 Eye ◎

● ◐ V45.79 Other acquired absence of organ ◎

● V45.8 Other postprocedural status

● ❷ V45.81 Aortocoronary bypass status ◎
> Coding Clinic: 2003, Q4, P105-106; 2001, Q3, P15; 1997, Q3, P16

● ❷ V45.82 Percutaneous transluminal coronary angioplasty status ◎
> Coding Clinic: 1995, Q2, P18

● ❷ V45.83 Breast implant removal status ◎

● ❷ V45.84 Dental restoration status ◎
> Dental crowns status
> Dental fillings status

● ❷ V45.85 Insulin pump status ◎

● ❷ V45.86 Bariatric surgery status ◎
> Gastric banding status
> Gastric bypass status for obesity
> Obesity surgery status

> Excludes bariatric surgery status
> complicating pregnancy,
> childbirth or the
> puerperium (649.2)
> intestinal bypass or
> anastomosis status
> (V45.3)

> Coding Clinic: 2009, Q2, P13

● ❷ V45.87 Transplanted organ removal status ◎
> Transplanted organ previously
> removed due to complication,
> failure, rejection or infection

> Excludes encounter for removal of
> transplanted organ –
> code to complication
> of transplanted organ
> (996.80–996.89)

● ❷ V45.88 Status post administration of tPA (rtPA) in a different facility within the last 24 hours prior to admission to the current facility ◎

> Code first condition requiring tPA
> administration, such as:
> acute cerebral infarction (433.0–433.9
> with fifth-digit 1, 434.0–434.9
> with fifth digit 1)
> acute myocardial infarction
> (410.00–410.92)

● ❷ V45.89 Other ◎
> Presence of neuropacemaker or other
> electronic device

> Excludes artificial heart valve in situ
> (V43.3)
> vascular prosthesis in situ
> (V43.4)
> Coding Clinic: 1995, Q1, P11

● V46 Other dependence on machines and devices

● ❷ V46.0 Aspirator ◎

● V46.1 Respirator [Ventilator]
> Iron lung
> Coding Clinic: 2005, Q4, P94-100; 2004, Q4, P100-101

❷ V46.11 Dependence on respirator, status ◎ ◔
> (Ex) V46.0-V46.2, V46.8-V46.9
> Coding Clinic: 2003, Q4, P104-105; 2001, Q1, P12

❶ V46.12 Encounter for respirator dependence during power failure ◎ ◔
> (Ex) V46.0-V46.2, V46.8-V46.9

❶ V46.13 Encounter for weaning from respirator [ventilator] ◎ ◔
> (Ex) V46.0-V46.2, V46.8-V46.9

◐ V46.14 Mechanical complication of respirator [ventilator] ◎ ◔
> Mechanical failure of respirator
> [ventilator]
> (Ex) V46.0-V46.2, V46.8-V46.9

● ❷ V46.2 Supplemental oxygen ◎
> Long-term oxygen therapy

● ❷ V46.3 Wheelchair dependence ◎
> Wheelchair confinement status

> Code first cause of dependence, such as:
> muscular dystrophy (359.1)
> obesity (278.00, 278.01)

● ❷ V46.8 Other enabling machines ◎
> Hyperbaric chamber
> Possum [Patient-Operated-Selector-Mechanism]

> Excludes cardiac pacemaker (V45.0)
> kidney dialysis machine (V45.11)

● V46.9 Unspecified machine dependence ◎

● V47 Other problems with internal organs

● V47.0 Deficiencies of internal organs

● V47.1 Mechanical and motor problems with internal organs

● V47.2 Other cardiorespiratory problems
> Cardiovascular exercise intolerance with pain
> (with):
> at rest
> less than ordinary activity
> ordinary activity

● V47.3 Other digestive problems

● V47.4 Other urinary problems

● V47.5 Other genital problems

● V47.9 Unspecified

(Ex) CC Exclusions   ◀ New   ◀━ Revised   deleted Deleted   ● Use Additional Digit(s)   ❶ First Listed   ◐ First Listed or Additional
❷ Additional Only   ▶ Manifestation Code   OGCR Official Guidelines   Coding Clinic   Excludes   Includes   Use additional   Code first

● **V48   Problems with head, neck, and trunk**
  ● **V48.0   Deficiencies of head**
    Excludes *deficiencies of ears, eyelids, and nose (V48.8)*
  ● **V48.1   Deficiencies of neck and trunk**
  ● **V48.2   Mechanical and motor problems with head**
  ● **V48.3   Mechanical and motor problems with neck and trunk**
  ● **V48.4   Sensory problem with head**
  ● **V48.5   Sensory problem with neck and trunk**
  ● **V48.6   Disfigurements of head**
  ● **V48.7   Disfigurements of neck and trunk**
  ● **V48.8   Other problems with head, neck, and trunk**
  ● **V48.9   Unspecified problem with head, neck, or trunk**

● **V49   Other conditions influencing health status**
  ● **V49.0   Deficiencies of limbs**
  ● **V49.1   Mechanical problems with limbs**
  ● **V49.2   Motor problems with limbs**
  ● **V49.3   Sensory problems with limbs**
  ● **V49.4   Disfigurements of limbs**
  ● **V49.5   Other problems of limbs**
  ● **V49.6   Upper limb amputation status**
       Coding Clinic: 1998, Q4, P42-44
    ● **V49.60   Unspecified level**
    ● **V49.61   Thumb**
    ● **V49.62   Other finger(s)**
         Coding Clinic: 2005, Q2, P7
    ● **V49.63   Hand**
    ● **V49.64   Wrist**
         Disarticulation of wrist
    ● **V49.65   Below elbow**
    ● **V49.66   Above elbow**
         Disarticulation of elbow
    ● **V49.67   Shoulder**
         Disarticulation of shoulder
  ● **V49.7   Lower limb amputation status**
       Coding Clinic: 2006, Q3, P5; 1998, Q4, P42-44
    ● **V49.70   Unspecified level**
    ● **V49.71   Great toe**
    ● **V49.72   Other toe(s)**
    ● **V49.73   Foot**
    ● **V49.74   Ankle**
         Disarticulation of ankle
    ● **V49.75   Below knee**
    ● **V49.76   Above knee**
         Disarticulation of knee
         Coding Clinic: 2005, Q2, P14
    ● **V49.77   Hip**
         Disarticulation of hip

● **V49.8   Other specified conditions influencing health status**
    ● **V49.81   Asymptomatic postmenopausal status (age-related) (natural) ♀**   A
      Excludes *menopausal and premenopausal disorders (627.0–627.9)*
                postsurgical menopause (256.2)
                premature menopause (256.31)
                symptomatic menopause (627.0–627.9)
         Coding Clinic: 2000, Q4, P53-54
    ● ❷ **V49.82   Dental sealant status**
    ● ❷ **V49.83   Awaiting organ transplant status**
         Coding Clinic: 2004, Q4, P101
    ● **V49.84   Bed confinement status**
         Coding Clinic: 2005, Q4, P94-100
    ● ❷ **V49.85   Dual sensory impairment**
         Blindness with deafness
         Combined visual hearing impairment
      Code first:
         hearing impairment (389.00–389.9)

         visual impairment (369.00–369.9)
         Coding Clinic: 2007, Q4, P99-101
    ● **V49.89   Other specified conditions influencing health status**
  ● **V49.9   Unspecified**

PERSONS ENCOUNTERING HEALTH SERVICES FOR SPECIFIC PROCEDURES AND AFTERCARE (V50–V59)

  Note: Categories V51–V58 are intended for use to indicate a reason for care in patients who may have already been treated for some disease or injury not now present, or who are receiving care to consolidate the treatment, to deal with residual states, or to prevent recurrence.
  Excludes *follow-up examination for medical surveillance following treatment (V67.0–V67.9)*

● **V50   Elective surgery for purposes other than remedying health states**
  V50.0   Hair transplant
  V50.1   Other plastic surgery for unacceptable cosmetic appearance
         Breast augmentation or reduction
         Face-lift
      Excludes *encounter for breast reduction (611.1)*
                plastic surgery following healed injury or operation (V51.0–V51.8)
  V50.2   Routine or ritual circumcision ♂
         Circumcision in the absence of significant medical indication
  ● **V50.3   Ear piercing**

N Newborn Age: 0   **P** Pediatric Age: 0–17   **M** Maternity Age: 12–55   **A** Adult Age: 15–124   ♀ Females Only   ♂ Males Only
● Unacceptable Principal Diagnosis   Complication\Comorbidity   Major C\C   Present on Admission Requirement   Hospital-Acquired Condition

V01-V89   1145

● **V50.4 Prophylactic organ removal**

> **Excludes** *organ donations (V59.0–V59.9)*
> *therapeutic organ removal-code to*
> *condition*

    V50.41 Breast
       Coding Clinic: 2004, Q4, P106-107

    V50.42 Ovary ♀

    V50.49 Other

    OGCR Section I.C.18.d.14

> For encounters specifically for prophylactic removal of breasts, ovaries, or another organ due to a genetic susceptibility to cancer or a family history of cancer, the principal or first listed code should be a code from subcategory V50.4, Prophylactic organ removal, followed by the appropriate genetic susceptibility code and the appropriate family history code.

● **V50.8 Other**

● **V50.9 Unspecified**

● **V51 Aftercare involving the use of plastic surgery**
    Plastic surgery following healed injury or operation

> **Includes** plastic surgery following healed injury or
> operation

> **Excludes** *cosmetic plastic surgery (V50.1)*
> *plastic surgery as treatment for current*
> *condition or injury - code to condition or*
> *injury*
> *repair of scar tissue - code to scar*

❶ **V51.0 Encounter for breast reconstruction following**
       mastectomy   A

> **Excludes** *deformity and disproportion*
> *of reconstructed breast*
> *(612.0–612.1)*

V51.8 Other aftercare involving the use of plastic
       surgery

● **V52 Fitting and adjustment of prosthetic device and implant**

> **Includes** removal of device

> **Excludes** *malfunction or complication of prosthetic device*
> *(996.0–996.7)*
> *status only, without need for care*
> *(V43.0–V43.8)*

    V52.0 Artificial arm (complete) (partial)

    V52.1 Artificial leg (complete) (partial)

    V52.2 Artificial eye

    V52.3 Dental prosthetic device

    V52.4 Breast prosthesis and implant ♀
       Elective implant exchange (different material)
       (different size)
       Removal of tissue expander without
       synchronous insertion of permanent
       implant

> **Excludes** *admission for initial breast implant*
> *insertion for breast augmentation*
> *(V50.1)*
> *complications of breast implant (996.54,*
> *996.69, 996.79)*
> *encounter for breast reconstruction*
> *following mastectomy (V51.0)*
> Coding Clinic: 1995, Q4, P80.81

    V52.8 Other specified prosthetic device
       Coding Clinic: 2002, Q3, P12; Q2, P16-17

● **V52.9 Unspecified prosthetic device**

● **V53 Fitting and adjustment of other device**

> **Includes** removal of device
> replacement of device

> **Excludes** *status only, without need for care*
> *(V45.0–V45.8)*

● **V53.0 Devices related to nervous system and special**
    senses

    V53.01 Fitting and adjustment of cerebral
       ventricle (communicating) shunt
       Coding Clinic: 1997, Q4, P51

    V53.02 Neuropacemaker (brain) (peripheral
       nerve) (spinal cord)

    V53.09 Fitting and adjustment of other devices
       related to nervous system and special
       senses
       Auditory substitution device
       Visual substitution device
       Coding Clinic: 1999, Q2, P3-4

● **V53.1 Spectacles and contact lenses**

● **V53.2 Hearing aid**

● **V53.3 Cardiac device**
    Reprogramming
    Coding Clinic: 1992, Q3, P3

    V53.31 Cardiac pacemaker

> **Excludes** *mechanical complication*
> *of cardiac pacemaker*
> *(996.01)*
> MCE: Questionable admission, principal
> diagnosis only
> Coding Clinic: 2002, Q1, P3; 1984, Nov-Dec, P18

    V53.32 Automatic implantable cardiac
       defibrillator
       MCE: Questionable admission, principal
       diagnosis only
       Coding Clinic: 2005, Q3, P3-9

    V53.39 Other cardiac device
       MCE: Questionable admission, principal
       diagnosis only
       Coding Clinic: 2008, Q2, P9-10; 2007, Q1, P20

● **V53.4 Orthodontic devices**

● **V53.5 Other gastrointestinal appliance**
    and device ◀▥

> **Excludes** *colostomy (V55.3)*
> *ileostomy (V55.2)*
> *other artifical opening of digestive tract*
> *(V55.4)*

    ● **V53.50 Fitting and adjustment of intestinal**
       appliance and device ◀

    ● **V53.51 Fitting and adjustment of gastric**
       lap band ◀

    ● **V53.59 Fitting and adjustment of other**
       gastrointestinal appliance and
       device ◀

● **V53.6 Urinary devices**
    Urinary catheter

> **Excludes** *cystostomy (V55.5)*
> *nephrostomy (V55.6)*
> *ureterostomy (V55.6)*
> *urethrostomy (V55.6)*

● **V53.7 Orthopedic devices**
    Orthopedic:
       brace
       cast
       corset
       shoes

> **Excludes** *other orthopedic aftercare (V54)*

(Ex:) CC Exclusions   ◀ New   ◀▥ Revised   ~~deleted~~ Deleted   ● Use Additional Digit(s)   ❶ First Listed   First Listed or Additional
❷ Additional Only   ▶ Manifestation Code   **OGCR** Official Guidelines   **Coding Clinic**   Excludes   Includes   Use additional   Code first

 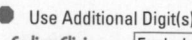

V01-V89

● **V53.8 Wheelchair**

● **V53.9 Other and unspecified device**
Coding Clinic: 2003, Q2, P6-7

● **V53.90 Unspecified device**

● **V53.91 Fitting and adjustment of insulin pump**
Insulin pump titration

● **V53.99 Other device**
Coding Clinic: 2009, Q2, P17

● **V54 Other orthopedic aftercare**
| **Excludes** | fitting and adjustment of orthopedic devices (V53.7)
malfunction of internal orthopedic device (996.40–996.49)
other complication of nonmechanical nature (996.60–996.79)

● **V54.0 Aftercare involving internal fixation device**
| **Excludes** | malfunction of internal orthopedic device (996.40–996.49)
other complication of nonmechanical nature (996.60–996.79)
removal of external fixation device (V54.89)

V54.01 Encounter for removal of internal fixation device

V54.02 Encounter for lengthening/adjustment of growth rod

V54.09 Other aftercare involving internal fixation device
Coding Clinic: 2009, Q1, P15

● **V54.1 Aftercare for healing traumatic fracture**
| **Excludes** | aftercare following joint replacement (V54.81)
aftercare for amputation stump (V54.89)

V54.10 Aftercare for healing traumatic fracture of arm, unspecified

V54.11 Aftercare for healing traumatic fracture of upper arm

V54.12 Aftercare for healing traumatic fracture of lower arm
Coding Clinic: 2007, Q1, P3-8

V54.13 Aftercare for healing traumatic fracture of hip
Coding Clinic: 2009, Q1, P15; 2007, Q1, P3-8; 2003, Q4, P103-105

V54.14 Aftercare for healing traumatic fracture of leg, unspecified

V54.15 Aftercare for healing traumatic fracture of upper leg
| **Excludes** | aftercare for healing traumatic fracture of hip (V54.13)
Coding Clinic: 2006, Q3, P6

V54.16 Aftercare for healing traumatic fracture of lower leg
Coding Clinic: 2009, Q1, P14

V54.17 Aftercare for healing traumatic fracture of vertebrae

V54.19 Aftercare for healing traumatic fracture of other bone
Coding Clinic: 2005, Q1, P13

● **V54.2 Aftercare for healing pathologic fracture**
| **Excludes** | aftercare following joint replacement (V54.81) ◄

V54.20 Aftercare for healing pathologic fracture of arm, unspecified

V54.21 Aftercare for healing pathologic fracture of upper arm

V54.22 Aftercare for healing pathologic fracture of lower arm

V54.23 Aftercare for healing pathologic fracture of hip

V54.24 Aftercare for healing pathologic fracture of leg, unspecified

V54.25 Aftercare for healing pathologic fracture of upper leg
| **Excludes** | aftercare for healing pathologic fracture of hip (V54.23)

V54.26 Aftercare for healing pathologic fracture of lower leg

V54.27 Aftercare for healing pathologic fracture of vertebrae
Coding Clinic: 2008, Q3, P4; 2003, Q4, P108-109

V54.29 Aftercare for healing pathologic fracture of other bone

● **V54.8 Other orthopedic aftercare**
Coding Clinic: 2001, Q3, P19; 1999, Q4, P5x2; 1990, Q1, P10, 20

V54.81 Aftercare following joint replacement
Use additional code to identify joint replacement site (V43.60–V43.69)
Coding Clinic: 2009, Q1, P14; 2006, Q3, P4; 2004, Q3, P12; Q2, P15

V54.89 Other orthopedic aftercare
Aftercare for healing fracture NOS
Coding Clinic: 2007, Q2, P8-9

● **V54.9 Unspecified orthopedic aftercare**

● **V55 Attention to artificial openings**
| **Includes** | adjustment or repositioning of catheter
closure
passage of sounds or bougies
reforming
removal or replacement of catheter
toilet or cleansing
| **Excludes** | complications of external stoma (519.00–519.09, 569.60–569.69, 997.4, 997.5)
status only, without need for care (V44.0–V44.9)
Coding Clinic: 1995, Q3, P13

V55.0 Tracheostomy

V55.1 Gastrostomy
(Ex:) V55.1
Coding Clinic: 1999, Q4, P9; 1997, Q3, P7-8; 1996, Q1, P14; 1995, Q3, P13

V55.2 Ileostomy

V55.3 Colostomy
Coding Clinic: 2009, Q1, P14; 2005, Q2, P4-5; 1997, Q3, P9-10

V55.4 Other artificial opening of digestive tract
Coding Clinic: 2005, Q2, P14; 2003, Q1, P10

V55.5 Cystostomy

V55.6 Other artificial opening of urinary tract
Nephrostomy
Ureterostomy
Urethrostomy

V55.7 Artificial vagina

V55.8 Other specified artificial opening

● **V55.9 Unspecified artificial opening**

N Newborn Age: 0   **P** Pediatric Age: 0–17   **M** Maternity Age: 12–55   **A** Adult Age: 15–124   ♀ Females Only   ♂ Males Only
● Unacceptable Principal Diagnosis   Complication\Comorbidity   Major C\C   Present on Admission Requirement   Hospital-Acquired Condition

1147

V01-V89

● **V56 Encounter for dialysis and dialysis catheter care**

> Use additional code to identify the associated condition
>
> **Excludes** *dialysis preparation-code to condition*
>
> Coding Clinic: 1993, Q1, P29

❶ **V56.0 Extracorporeal dialysis** 🔖

Dialysis (renal) NOS

> **Excludes** *dialysis status (V45.11)*
>
> Coding Clinic: 2005, Q4, P77-79; 2004, Q1, P23; 2000, Q4, P39-40; 1998, Q3, P6; Q2, P20-21; 1993, Q4, P34

🔖 **V56.1 Fitting and adjustment of extracorporeal dialysis catheter** 🔖

Removal or replacement of catheter
Toilet or cleansing

> Use additional code for any concurrent extracorporeal dialysis (V56.0)
>
> Coding Clinic: 1998, Q2, P20-21

● 🔖 **V56.2 Fitting and adjustment of peritoneal dialysis catheter** 🔖

> Use additional code for any concurrent peritoneal dialysis (V56.8)
>
> Coding Clinic: 1998, Q4, P55

● **V56.3 Encounter for adequacy testing for dialysis**

  ● 🔖 **V56.31 Encounter for adequacy testing for hemodialysis** 🔖

  ● 🔖 **V56.32 Encounter for adequacy testing for peritoneal dialysis** 🔖

Peritoneal equilibration test

🔖 **V56.8 Other dialysis** 🔖

Peritoneal dialysis

> Coding Clinic: 1998, Q4, P55

● **V57 Care involving use of rehabilitation procedures**

> Use additional code to identify underlying condition
>
> Coding Clinic: 2002, Q1, P18-19; 1997, Q3, P12

● ❶ **V57.0 Breathing exercises** 🔖

● ❶ **V57.1 Other physical therapy** 🔖

Therapeutic and remedial exercises, except breathing

> Coding Clinic: 2006, Q3, P4; 2004, Q2, P15; 2002, Q4, P56; 1999, Q4, P5

● **V57.2 Occupational therapy and vocational rehabilitation**

  ● ❶ **V57.21 Encounter for occupational therapy** 🔖

> Coding Clinic: 1999, Q4, P7

  ● ❶ **V57.22 Encounter for vocational therapy** 🔖

● ❶ **V57.3 Speech-language therapy** 🔖 ◀▥

> Coding Clinic: 1997, Q4, P35-37

● ❶ **V57.4 Orthoptic training** 🔖

● **V57.8 Other specified rehabilitation procedure**

  ● ❶ **V57.81 Orthotic training** 🔖

Gait training in the use of artificial limbs

  ● ❶ **V57.89 Other** 🔖

Multiple training or therapy

> Coding Clinic: 2007, Q4, P92-95; 2006, Q3, P6; 2003, Q4, P105-106, 108-109; Q2, P16; 2002, Q1, P16; 2001, Q3, P21; 1997, Q3, P11-13

● ❶ **V57.9 Unspecified rehabilitation procedure** 🔖

OGCR Section I.C.2.e.2

> If a patient admission/encounter is solely for the administration of chemotherapy, immunotherapy or radiation therapy assign code V58.0, Encounter for radiation therapy, or V58.11, Encounter for antineoplastic chemotherapy, or V58.12, Encounter for antineoplastic immunotherapy as the first-listed or principal diagnosis. If a patient receives more than one of these therapies during the same admission more than one of these codes may be assigned, in any sequence.

● **V58 Encounter for other and unspecified procedures and aftercare**

> **Excludes** *convalescence and palliative care (V66.0–V66.9)*

❶ **V58.0 Radiotherapy** 🔖

Encounter or admission for radiotherapy

> **Excludes** *encounter for radioactive implant-code to condition*
> *radioactive iodine therapy-code to condition*
>
> Coding Clinic: 1994, Q2, P10x2; 1993, Q4, P 36; 1987, Jan-Feb, P13

● **V58.1 Encounter for chemotherapy and immunotherapy for neoplastic conditions**

Encounter or admission for chemotherapy

> **Excludes** *chemotherapy and immunotherapy for nonneoplastic conditions-code to condition*
>
> Coding Clinic: 2005, Q4, P94-100; 2004, Q1, P13-14; 2003, Q2, P16-17; 2000, Q1, P23; 1993, Q4, P34, 36; Q3, P4x5; 1992, Q2, P16-17; 1991, Q2, P17; 1987, Sept-Oct, P8

  ❶ **V58.11 Encounter for antineoplastic chemotherapy** 🔖

> Coding Clinic: 2008, Q4, P82-83, 152-155; 2007, Q4, P103-104; 2006, Q2, P20-22; 2004, Q1, P13-14

  ❶ **V58.12 Encounter for antineoplastic immunotherapy** 🔖

> Coding Clinic: 2004, Q1, P13-14

● **V58.2 Blood transfusion, without reported diagnosis** 🔖

> Coding Clinic: 1994, Q1, P22

● **V58.3 Attention to dressings and sutures**

Change or removal of wound packing

> **Excludes** *attention to drains (V58.49)*
> *planned postoperative wound closure (V58.41)*
>
> Coding Clinic: 2006, Q4, P117-118; 2005, Q2, P14

  ● 🔖 **V58.30 Encounter for change or removal of nonsurgical wound dressing** 🔖

Encounter for change or removal of wound dressing NOS

  ● 🔖 **V58.31 Encounter for change or removal of surgical wound dressing** 🔖

  ● 🔖 **V58.32 Encounter for removal of sutures** 🔖

Encounter for removal of staples

V01-V89

(Ex:) CC Exclusions   ◀ New   ◀▥ Revised   ~~deleted~~ Deleted   ● Use Additional Digit(s)   ❶ First Listed   🔖 First Listed or Additional
❷ Additional Only   ▶ Manifestation Code   **OGCR** Official Guidelines   **Coding Clinic**   Excludes   Includes   Use additional   Code first

● **V58.4 Other aftercare following surgery**

> **Note:** Codes from this subcategory should be used in conjunction with other aftercare codes to fully identify the reason for the aftercare encounter.
>
> **Excludes** *aftercare following sterilization reversal surgery (V26.22)*
> *attention to artificial openings (V55.0–V55.9)*
> *orthopedic aftercare (V54.0–V54.9)*
>
> Coding Clinic: 1999, Q4, P8-9

V58.41 Encounter for planned post-operative wound closure

> **Excludes** *disruption of operative wound (998.31–998.32)*
> *encounter for dressings and suture aftercare (V58.30–V58.32)*
>
> Coding Clinic: 1999, Q4, P15

V58.42 Aftercare following surgery for neoplasm

> Conditions classifiable to 140–239

V58.43 Aftercare following surgery for injury and trauma

> Conditions classifiable to 800–999
>
> **Excludes** *aftercare for healing traumatic fracture (V54.10–V54.19)*
>
> Coding Clinic: 2007, Q2, P8-9; 1987, Nov-Dec, P9

V58.44 Aftercare following organ transplant

> Use additional code to identify the organ transplanted (V42.0–V42.9)
>
> Coding Clinic: 2004, Q4, P101

V58.49 Other specified aftercare following surgery

> Change or removal of drains
> Coding Clinic: 1996, Q1, P8-9x2

V58.5 Orthodontics

> **Excludes** *fitting and adjustment of orthodontic device (V53.4)*

OGCR Section I.C.18.d.3

> This subcategory (V58.6) indicates a patient's continuous use of a prescribed drug (including such things as aspirin therapy) for the long-term treatment of a condition or for prophylactic use. It is not for use for patients who have addictions to drugs. This subcategory is not for use of medications for detoxification or maintenance programs to prevent withdrawal symptoms in patients with drug dependence (e.g., methadone maintenance for opiate dependence). Assign the appropriate code for the drug dependence instead.
>
> Assign a code from subcategory V58.6 if the patient is receiving a medication for an extended period as a prophylactic measure (such as for the prevention of deep vein thrombosis) or as treatment of a chronic condition (such as arthritis) or a disease requiring a lengthy course of treatment (such as cancer). Do not assign a code from subcategory V58.6 for medication being administered for a brief period of time to treat an acute illness or injury (such as a course of antibiotics to treat acute bronchitis).

● **V58.6 Long-term (current) drug use**

> **Excludes** *drug abuse (305.00–305.93)*
> *drug abuse and dependence complicating pregnancy (648.3–648.4)*
> *drug dependence (304.00–304.93)*
> *hormone replacement therapy (postmenopausal) (V07.4)*
> *prophylactic use of agents affecting estrogen receptors and estrogen levels (V07.51–V07.59)*

❷ **V58.61 Long-term (current) use of anticoagulants**

> **Excludes** *long-term (current) use of aspirin (V58.66)*
>
> Coding Clinic: 2008, Q4, P134-136; 2006, Q3, P13; 2004, Q3, P7; 2003, Q4, P108; 2003, Q1, P11-12; 2002, Q3, P13-16; Q1, P16

● ❷ **V58.62 Long-term (current) use of antibiotics**
> Coding Clinic: 1998, Q4, P59-60

● ❷ **V58.63 Long-term (current) use of antiplatelets/antithrombotics**

> **Excludes** *long-term (current) use of aspirin (V58.66)*

● ❷ **V58.64 Long-term (current) use of non-steroidal anti-inflammatories (NSAID)**

> **Excludes** *long-term (current) use of aspirin (V58.66)*

● ❷ **V58.65 Long-term (current) use of steroids**

❷ **V58.66 Long-term (current) use of aspirin**
> Coding Clinic: 2004, Q4, P102-103; 2003, Q1, P11-12

❷ **V58.67 Long-term (current) use of insulin**
> Coding Clinic: 2004, Q4, P53-56

❷ **V58.69 Long-term (current) use of other medications**

> Long term current use of methadone
> Long term current use of opiate analgesic
> Other high-risk medications
> Coding Clinic: 2004, Q2, P10; Q1, P13-14; 2003, Q1, P11-12; 2000, Q2, P8-9; 1999, Q3, 13-14; 1996, Q3, P20; Q2, P7x2; 1995, Q4, P51,61

N Newborn Age: 0　　**P** Pediatric Age: 0–17　　**M** Maternity Age: 12–55　　**A** Adult Age: 15–124　　♀ Females Only　　♂ Males Only

● Unacceptable Principal Diagnosis　　 Complication\Comorbidity　　 Major C\C　　 Present on Admission Requirement　　 Hospital-Acquired Condition

1149

V01-V89

● **V58.7** **Aftercare following surgery to specified body systems, not elsewhere classified**

> **Note:** Codes from this subcategory should be used in conjunction with other aftercare codes to fully identify the reason for the aftercare encounter.
>
> **Excludes** *aftercare following organ transplant (V58.44)*
> *aftercare following surgery for neoplasm (V58.42)*
>
> Coding Clinic: 2003, Q4, P104-105

V58.71 **Aftercare following surgery of the sense organs, NEC** 🔊
> Conditions classifiable to 360–379, 380–389

V58.72 **Aftercare following surgery of the nervous system, NEC** 🔊
> Conditions classifiable to 320–359
>
> **Excludes** *aftercare following surgery of the sense organs, NEC (V58.71)*

V58.73 **Aftercare following surgery of the circulatory system, NEC** 🔊
> Conditions classifiable to 390–459
> Coding Clinic: 2009, Q2, P17

V58.74 **Aftercare following surgery of the respiratory system, NEC** 🔊
> Conditions classifiable to 460–519

V58.75 **Aftercare following surgery of the teeth, oral cavity and digestive system, NEC** 🔊
> Conditions classifiable to 520–579
> Coding Clinic: 2005, Q2, P14

V58.76 **Aftercare following surgery of the genitourinary system, NEC** 🔊
> Conditions classifiable to 580–629
>
> **Excludes** *aftercare following sterilization reversal (V26.22)*
>
> Coding Clinic: 2005, Q1, P11,12

V58.77 **Aftercare following surgery of the skin and subcutaneous tissue, NEC** 🔊
> Conditions classifiable to 680–709

V58.78 **Aftercare following surgery of the musculoskeletal system, NEC** 🔊
> Conditions classifiable to 710–739
>
> **Excludes** *orthopedic aftercare (V54.01–V54.9)*

● **V58.8** **Other specified procedures and aftercare**
> Coding Clinic: 1994, Q2, P8x2

V58.81 **Fitting and adjustment of vascular catheter** 🔊
> Removal or replacement of catheter
> Toilet or cleansing
>
> **Excludes** *complications of renal dialysis (996.73)*
> *complications of vascular catheter (996.74)*
> *dialysis preparation—code to condition*
> *encounter for dialysis (V56.0–V56.8)*
> *fitting and adjustment of dialysis catheter (V56.1)*

V58.82 **Fitting and adjustment of non-vascular catheter NEC** 🔊
> Removal or replacement of catheter
> Toilet or cleansing
>
> **Excludes** *fitting and adjustment of peritoneal dialysis catheter (V56.2)*
> *fitting and adjustment of urinary catheter (V53.6)*

V58.83 **Encounter for therapeutic drug monitoring** 🔊
> Use additional code for any associated long-term (current) drug use (V58.61–V58.69)
>
> **Excludes** *blood-drug testing for medicolegal reasons (V70.4)*
>
> Coding Clinic: 2004, Q2, P10-11; Q1, P13-14; 2002, Q3, P13-16

V58.89 **Other specified aftercare** 🔊
> Coding Clinic: 2003, Q4, P106-107; 1998, Q4, P59-60

● **V58.9** **Unspecified aftercare** 🔊

> **OGCR** Section I.C.18.d.9
>
> Category V59 is the donor codes. They are used for living individuals who are donating blood or other body tissue. These codes are only for individuals donating for others, not for self donations. They are not for use to identify cadaveric donations.

● **V59** **Donors**

> **Excludes** *examination of potential donor (V70.8)*
> *self-donation of organ or tissue--code to condition*
>
> Coding Clinic: 2008, Q2, P8-9; 1995, Q4, P50x2

● **V59.0** **Blood**
> Coding Clinic: 1990, Q1, P9-10

● ❶ **V59.01** **Whole blood** 🔊

● ❶ **V59.02** **Stem cells** 🔊
> Coding Clinic: 1995, Q4, P51

● ❶ **V59.09** **Other** 🔊

❶ **V59.1** **Skin** 🔊

❶ **V59.2** **Bone** 🔊

❶ **V59.3** **Bone marrow** 🔊
> Coding Clinic: 1985, Jan-Feb, P15

❶ **V59.4** **Kidney** 🔊

❶ **V59.5** **Cornea** 🔊

❶ **V59.6** **Liver** 🔊

● **V59.7** **Egg (oocyte) (ovum)**

● ❶ **V59.70** **Egg (oocyte) (ovum) donor, unspecified** ♀ 🔊

● ❶ **V59.71** **Egg (oocyte) (ovum) donor, under age 35, anonymous recipient** ♀ 🔊
> Egg donor, under age 35 NOS

● ❶ **V59.72** **Egg (oocyte) (ovum) donor, under age 35, designated recipient** ♀ 🔊

● ❶ **V59.73** **Egg (oocyte) (ovum) donor, age 35 and over, anonymous recipient** ♀ 🔊
> Egg donor, age 35 and over NOS

● ❶ **V59.74** **Egg (oocyte) (ovum) donor, age 35 and over, designated recipient** ♀ 🔊

❶ **V59.8** **Other specified organ or tissue** 🔊
> Coding Clinic: 2002, Q3, P20-21

❶ **V59.9** **Unspecified organ or tissue** 🔊

Ⓔ CC Exclusions   ◀ New   ◀ Revised   ~~deleted~~ Deleted   ● Use Additional Digit(s)   ❶ First Listed   First Listed or Additional

❷ Additional Only   ▶ Manifestation Code   **OGCR** Official Guidelines   **Coding Clinic**   Excludes   Includes   Use additional   Code first

V01-V89

PERSONS ENCOUNTERING HEALTH SERVICES IN OTHER CIRCUMSTANCES (V60–V69)

● **V60 Housing, household, and economic circumstances**

  ● ❷ **V60.0 Lack of housing**
      Hobos
      Social migrants
      Tramps
      Transients
      Vagabonds

  ● ❷ **V60.1 Inadequate housing**
      Lack of heating
      Restriction of space
      Technical defects in home preventing adequate
         care

  ● ❷ **V60.2 Inadequate material resources**
      Economic problem
      Poverty NOS

  ● ❷ **V60.3 Person living alone**

  ● ❷ **V60.4 No other household member able to render care**
      Person requiring care (has) (is):
         family member too handicapped, ill, or
            otherwise unsuited to render care
         partner temporarily away from home
         temporarily away from usual place of abode
      Excludes *holiday relief care (V60.5)*

  ● ❷ **V60.5 Holiday relief care**
      Provision of health care facilities to a person
         normally cared for at home, to enable
         relatives to take a vacation

  ● ❷ **V60.6 Person living in residential institution**
      Boarding school resident

  ● **V60.8 Other specified housing or economic circumstances** ◀|||
    ● ❷ **V60.81 Foster care (status)** ◀
    ● ❷ **V60.89 Other specified housing or economic circumstances** ◀

  ● ❷ **V60.9 Unspecified housing or economic circumstance**

● **V61 Other family circumstances**
    Includes when these circumstances or fear of them,
         affecting the person directly involved
         or others, are mentioned as the
         reason, justified or not, for seeking or
         receiving medical advice or care

  ● **V61.0 Family disruption**
    ● 🔶 **V61.01 Family disruption due to family member on military deployment**
        Individual or family affected by
           other family member being on
           deployment
      Excludes *family disruption due to family*
            member on non-military
            extended absence from
            home (V61.08) ◀

    ● 🔶 **V61.02 Family disruption due to return of family member from military deployment**
        Individual or family affected by other
           family member having returned
           from deployment (current or past
           conflict)

    ● 🔶 **V61.03 Family disruption due to divorce or legal separation**

    ● 🔶 **V61.04 Family disruption due to parent-child estrangement**
      Excludes *other family estrangement*
            (V61.09)

    ● 🔶 **V61.05 Family disruption due to child in welfare custody**

    ● 🔶 **V61.06 Family disruption due to child in foster care or in care of non-parental family member**

    ● 🔶 **V61.07 Family disruption due to death of family member** ◀
      Excludes *bereavement (V62.82)* ◀

    ● 🔶 **V61.08 Family disruption due to other extended absence of family member** ◀
      Excludes *family disruption due to family*
            member on military
            deployment (V61.01) ◀

    ● 🔶 **V61.09 Other family disruption**
      Family estrangement NOS

  ● **V61.1 Counseling for marital and partner problems**
    Excludes *problems related to:*
        psychosexual disorders
          (302.0–302.9)
        sexual function (V41.7)

    ● 🔶 **V61.10 Counseling for marital and partner problems, unspecified**
      Marital conflict
      Marital relationship problem
      Partner conflict
      Partner relationship problem

    ● 🔶 **V61.11 Counseling for victim of spousal and partner abuse**
      Excludes *encounter for treatment of*
            current injuries due to
            abuse (995.80–995.85)

    ● 🔶 **V61.12 Counseling for perpetrator of spousal and partner abuse**

  ● **V61.2 Parent-child problems**
    ● 🔶 **V61.20 Counseling for parent-child problem, unspecified**
      Concern about behavior of child
      Parent-child conflict
      Parent-child relationship problem

    🔶 **V61.21 Counseling for victim of child abuse**
      Child battering
      Child neglect
      Excludes *current injuries due to abuse*
            (995.50–995.59)

    ● 🔶 **V61.22 Counseling for perpetrator of parental child abuse**
      Excludes *counseling for non-parental*
            abuser (V62.83)

    ● 🔶 **V61.23 Counseling for parent-biological child problem** ◀
      Concern about behavior of biological
         child ◀
      Parent-biological child conflict ◀
      Parent-biological child relationship
         problem ◀

    ● 🔶 **V61.24 Counseling for parent-adopted child problem** ◀
      Concern about behavior of adopted
         child ◀
      Parent-adopted child conflict ◀
      Parent-adopted child relationship
         problem ◀

N Newborn Age: 0   **P** Pediatric Age: 0–17   **M** Maternity Age: 12–55   **A** Adult Age: 15–124   ♀ Females Only   ♂ Males Only

● Unacceptable Principal Diagnosis   🔶 Complication\Comorbidity   🔶 Major C\C   Present on Admission Requirement   Hospital-Acquired Condition

1151

V01-V89

● **V61.25 Counseling for parent (guardian)-foster child problem** ◄

    Concern about behavior of foster child ◄

    Parent (guardian)-foster child conflict ◄

    Parent (guardian)-foster child relationship problem ◄

● **V61.29 Other parent-child problems** ◄▥

    ~~Problem concerning adopted or foster child~~

    Coding Clinic: 1999, Q3, P16

● **V61.3 Problems with aged parents or in-laws**

● **V61.4 Health problems within family**

● **V61.41 Alcoholism in family**

● **V61.42 Substance abuse in family** ◄

● **V61.49 Other**

    Care of sick or handicapped person in family or household

    Presence of sick or handicapped person in family or household

● **V61.5 Multiparity**

● **V61.6 Illegitimacy or illegitimate pregnancy** ♀   M

● **V61.7 Other unwanted pregnancy** ♀   M

● **V61.8 Other specified family circumstances**

    Problems with family members NEC

    Sibling relationship problem

    Coding Clinic: 1994, Q1, P21

● **V61.9 Unspecified family circumstance**

● **V62 Other psychosocial circumstances**

    Includes   those circumstances or fear of them, affecting the person directly involved or others, mentioned as the reason, justified or not, for seeking or receiving medical advice or care

    Excludes   *previous psychological trauma (V15.41–V15.49)*

● **V62.0 Unemployment**

    Excludes   *circumstances when main problem is economic inadequacy or poverty (V60.2)*

● **V62.1 Adverse effects of work environment**

● **V62.2 Other occupational circumstances or maladjustment**

● **V62.21 Personal current military deployment status**   A

    Individual (civilian or military) currently deployed in theater or in support of military war, peacekeeping and humanitarian operations

● **V62.22 Personal history of return from military deployment**   A

    Individual (civilian or military) with past history of military war, peacekeeping and humanitarian deployment (current or past conflict)

● **V62.29 Other occupational circumstances or maladjustment**   A

    Career choice problem

    Dissatisfaction with employment

    Occupational problem

● **V62.3 Educational circumstances**

    Academic problem

    Dissatisfaction with school environment

    Educational handicap

● **V62.4 Social maladjustment**

    Acculturation problem

    Cultural deprivation

    Political, religious, or sex discrimination

    Social:

        isolation

        persecution

● **V62.5 Legal circumstances**

    Imprisonment

    Legal investigation

    Litigation

    Prosecution

● **V62.6 Refusal of treatment for reasons of religion or conscience**

● **V62.8 Other psychological or physical stress, not elsewhere classified**

● **V62.81 Interpersonal problems, not elsewhere classified**

    Relational problem NOS

● **V62.82 Bereavement, uncomplicated**

    Excludes   *bereavement as adjustment reaction (309.0)*

    family disruption due to death of family member (V61.07) ◄

● **V62.83 Counseling for perpetrator of physical/sexual abuse**

    Excludes   *counseling for perpetrator of parental child abuse (V61.22)*

    counseling for perpetrator of spousal and partner abuse (V61.12)

● **V62.84 Suicidal ideation**

    Excludes   *suicidal tendencies (300.9)*

    (Ex:) 290.11, 290.3, 293.0

    Coding Clinic: 2005, Q4, P94-100

● **V62.89 Other**

    Borderline intellectual functioning

    Life circumstance problems

    Phase of life problems

    Religious or spiritual problem

● **V62.9 Unspecified psychosocial circumstance**

● **V63 Unavailability of other medical facilities for care**

● **V63.0 Residence remote from hospital or other health care facility**

● **V63.1 Medical services in home not available**

    Excludes   *no other household member able to render care (V60.4)*

    Coding Clinic: 2001, Q4, P67; Q1, P12

● **V63.2 Person awaiting admission to adequate facility elsewhere**

    Coding Clinic: 1994, Q1, P22-23

● **V63.8 Other specified reasons for unavailability of medical facilities**

    Person on waiting list undergoing social agency investigation

● **V63.9 Unspecified reason for unavailability of medical facilities**

● **V64 Persons encountering health services for specific procedures, not carried out**

● **V64.0 Vaccination not carried out**

● **V64.00 Vaccination not carried out, unspecified reason**

● **V64.01 Vaccination not carried out because of acute illness**

    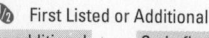

(Ex:) CC Exclusions   ◄ New   ◄▥ Revised   ~~deleted~~ Deleted   ● Use Additional Digit(s)   ❶ First Listed   First Listed or Additional

❷ Additional Only   ▶ Manifestation Code   **OGCR** Official Guidelines   Coding Clinic   Excludes   Includes   Use additional   Code first

V01-V89

● ❷ **V64.02** Vaccination not carried out because of chronic illness or condition 🔖

● ❷ **V64.03** Vaccination not carried out because of immune compromised state 🔖

● ❷ **V64.04** Vaccination not carried out because of allergy to vaccine or component 🔖

● ❷ **V64.05** Vaccination not carried out because of caregiver refusal 🔖
　　Guardian refusal
　　Parent refusal

> **Excludes** | *vaccination not carried out because of caregiver refusal for religious reasons (V64.07)*

> Coding Clinic: 2007, Q1, P12

● ❷ **V64.06** Vaccination not carried out because of patient refusal 🔖

● ❷ **V64.07** Vaccination not carried out for religious reasons 🔖

● ❷ **V64.08** Vaccination not carried out because patient had disease being vaccinated against 🔖

● ❷ **V64.09** Vaccination not carried out for other reason 🔖

● ❷ **V64.1** Surgical or other procedure not carried out because of contraindication 🔖
> Coding Clinic: 1993, 5th Issue, P9-10; 1985, Mar-April, P13; 1984, May-June, P11

● ❷ **V64.2** Surgical or other procedure not carried out because of patient's decision 🔖
> Coding Clinic: 2001, Q2, P8-9; 1999, Q1, P13-14; 1987, Jan-Feb, P13; 1985, July-Aug, P14

● ❷ **V64.3** Procedure not carried out for other reasons 🔖

● **V64.4** Closed surgical procedure converted to open procedure

● ❷ **V64.41** Laparoscopic surgical procedure converted to open procedure 🔖
> Coding Clinic: 1997, Q4, P52

● ❷ **V64.42** Thoracoscopic surgical procedure converted to open procedure 🔖

● ❷ **V64.43** Arthroscopic surgical procedure converted to open procedure 🔖

● **V65** Other persons seeking consultation

🔖**V65.0** Healthy person accompanying sick person 🔖
　　Boarder
> Coding Clinic: 1993, Q4, P36

● **V65.1** Person consulting on behalf of another person
　　Advice or treatment for nonattending third party

> **Excludes** | *concern (normal) about sick person in family (V61.41–V61.49)*

● 🔖**V65.11** Pediatric pre-birth visit for expectant ~~mother~~ parent(s) ♀ 🔖　　　　M ◀▥
　　Pre-adoption visit for adoptive parent(s)　　　◀

● 🔖**V65.19** Other person consulting on behalf of another person 🔖

🔖**V65.2** Person feigning illness 🔖
　　Malingerer
　　Peregrinating patient
> Coding Clinic: 1999, Q3, P20

● 🔖**V65.3** Dietary surveillance and counseling 🔖
　　Dietary surveillance and counseling (in):
　　　NOS
　　　colitis
　　　diabetes mellitus
　　　food allergies or intolerance
　　　gastritis
　　　hypercholesterolemia
　　　hypoglycemia
　　　obesity

> Use additional code to identify Body Mass Index (BMI), if known (V85.0–V85.54)

● **V65.4** Other counseling, not elsewhere classified
　　Health:
　　　advice
　　　education
　　　instruction

> **Excludes** | *counseling (for):*
> *contraception (V25.40–V25.49)*
> *genetic (V26.31–V26.39)*
> *on behalf of third party (V65.11–V65.19)*
> *procreative management (V26.41–V26.49)*

● 🔖**V65.40** Counseling NOS 🔖

● 🔖**V65.41** Exercise counseling 🔖

● 🔖**V65.42** Counseling on substance use and abuse 🔖

● 🔖**V65.43** Counseling on injury prevention 🔖

● 🔖**V65.44** Human immunodeficiency virus [HIV] counseling 🔖
> Coding Clinic: 1994, Q4, P35x3

> **OGCR** Section I.C.1.h
> When a patient returns to be informed of HIV test results use V65.44 if the results of the test are negative.

● 🔖**V65.45** Counseling on other sexually transmitted diseases 🔖

● 🔖**V65.46** Encounter for insulin pump training 🔖

● 🔖**V65.49** Other specified counseling 🔖
> Coding Clinic: 2000, Q2, P8-9

● 🔖**V65.5** Person with feared complaint in whom no diagnosis was made 🔖
　　Feared condition not demonstrated
　　Problem was normal state
　　"Worried well"
> Coding Clinic: 1984, July-Aug, P20

● 🔖**V65.8** Other reasons for seeking consultation 🔖
> **Excludes** | *specified symptoms*
> Coding Clinic: 1992, Q3, P4

● 🔖**V65.9** Unspecified reason for consultation 🔖

● **V66** Convalescence and palliative care

❶ **V66.0** Following surgery 🔖

❶ **V66.1** Following radiotherapy 🔖

❶ **V66.2** Following chemotherapy 🔖

❶ **V66.3** Following psychotherapy and other treatment for mental disorder 🔖

❶ **V66.4** Following treatment of fracture 🔖

● ❶ **V66.5** Following other treatment 🔖

❶ **V66.6** Following combined treatment 🔖

N Newborn Age: 0　　**P** Pediatric Age: 0–17　　**M** Maternity Age: 12–55　　**A** Adult Age: 15–124　　♀ Females Only　　♂ Males Only
● Unacceptable Principal Diagnosis　🔖 Complication\Comorbidity　🔖 Major C\C　🔖 Present on Admission Requirement　🔖 Hospital-Acquired Condition

1153

V01-V89

● ❷ **V66.7 Encounter for palliative care** 🔖
    End-of-life care
    Hospice care
    Terminal care
    Code first underlying disease
    Coding Clinic: 2008, Q3, P13-14; 2005, Q2, P9-10; 2003, Q4,
    P107; 1996, Q4, P47-48

● ❶ **V66.9 Unspecified convalescence** 🔖
    Coding Clinic: 1999, Q4, P8

OGCR Section I.C.18.d.8

> The follow-up codes, V24 and V67, are used to explain continuing surveillance following completed treatment of a disease, condition, or injury. They imply that the condition has been fully treated and no longer exists. They should not be confused with aftercare codes that explain current treatment for a healing condition or its sequelae. Follow-up codes may be used in conjunction with history codes to provide the full picture of the healed condition and its treatment. The follow-up code is sequenced first, followed by the history code. A follow-up code may be used to explain repeated visits. Should a condition be found to have recurred on the follow-up visit, then the diagnosis code should be used in place of the follow-up code.

● **V67 Follow-up examination**
    Includes surveillance only following completed treatment
    Excludes surveillance of contraception (V25.40–V25.49)
    Coding Clinic: 2009, Q1, P14; 2003, Q2, P5

  ● **V67.0 Following surgery**
    Coding Clinic: 1997, Q4, P50; 1995, Q1, P4; 1992, Q3, P11; 1985, July-Aug, P16

    🔖 **V67.00 Following surgery, unspecified** 🔖

    🔖 **V67.01 Follow-up vaginal pap smear** ♀ 🔖
        Vaginal pap smear, status-post hysterectomy for malignant condition
        Use additional code to identify: acquired absence of uterus (V88.01–V88.03)
        personal history of malignant neoplasm (V10.40–V10.44)
        Excludes vaginal pap smear status-post hysterectomy for non-malignant condition (V76.47)

    🔖 **V67.09 Following other surgery** 🔖
        Excludes sperm count following sterilization reversal (V26.22)
        sperm count for fertility testing (V26.21)
        Coding Clinic: 2008, Q3, P6; 2003, Q3, P16; 2002, Q3, P14-15; 1995, Q4, P53; Q2, P8; 1993, Q4, P32; 1992, Q3, P11; 1984, May-June, P10

  🔖 **V67.1 Following radiotherapy** 🔖
    Coding Clinic: 1985, July-Aug, P16

  🔖 **V67.2 Following chemotherapy** 🔖
    Cancer chemotherapy follow-up
    Coding Clinic: 1985, July-Aug, P16

  🔖 **V67.3 Following psychotherapy and other treatment for mental disorder** 🔖

🔖 **V67.4 Following treatment of healed fracture** 🔖
    Excludes current (healing) fracture aftercare (V54.0–V54.9)
    Coding Clinic: 2009, Q1, P14

● **V67.5 Following other treatment**
  🔖 **V67.51 Following completed treatment with high-risk medication, not elsewhere classified** 🔖
    Excludes long-term (current) drug use (V58.61–V58.69)
    Coding Clinic: 1999, Q1, P5-6x2; 1990, Q1, P18

  🔖 **V67.59 Other** 🔖

🔖 **V67.6 Following combined treatment** 🔖

● 🔖 **V67.9 Unspecified follow-up examination** 🔖

● **V68 Encounters for administrative purposes**
  ● **V68.0 Issue of medical certificates**
    Excludes encounter for general medical examination (V70.0–V70.9)

    ● ❶ **V68.01 Disability examination** 🔖
        Use additional code(s) to identify: specific examination(s), screening and testing performed (V72.0–V82.9)
        Coding Clinic: 2007, Q4, P99-101

    ● ❶ **V68.09 Other issue of medical certificates** 🔖

  ● ❶ **V68.1 Issue of repeat prescriptions** 🔖
    Issue of repeat prescription for:
      appliance
      glasses
      medications
    Excludes repeat prescription for contraceptives (V25.41–V25.49)

  ● ❶ **V68.2 Request for expert evidence** 🔖

  ● **V68.8 Other specified administrative purpose**
    ● ❶ **V68.81 Referral of patient without examination or treatment** 🔖
    ● ❶ **V68.89 Other** 🔖

  ● ❶ **V68.9 Unspecified administrative purpose** 🔖

● **V69 Problems related to lifestyle**
  ● 🔖 **V69.0 Lack of physical exercise** 🔖
  ● 🔖 **V69.1 Inappropriate diet and eating habits** 🔖
    Excludes anorexia nervosa (307.1)
    bulimia (783.6)
    malnutrition and other nutritional deficiencies (260–269.9)
    other and unspecified eating disorders (307.50–307.59)

  ● 🔖 **V69.2 High-risk sexual behavior** 🔖
  ● 🔖 **V69.3 Gambling and betting** 🔖
    Excludes pathological gambling (312.31)

  🔖 **V69.4 Lack of adequate sleep** 🔖
    Sleep deprivation
    Excludes insomnia (780.52)
    Coding Clinic: 2004, Q4, P104

  ● 🔖 **V69.5 Behavioral insomnia of childhood** 🔖   P
  ● 🔖 **V69.8 Other problems related to lifestyle** 🔖
    Self-damaging behavior
  ● 🔖 **V69.9 Problem related to lifestyle, unspecified** 🔖

V01-V89

(Ex) CC Exclusions   ◀ New   ◀▥ Revised   ~~deleted~~ Deleted   ● Use Additional Digit(s)   ❶ First Listed   🔖 First Listed or Additional
❷ Additional Only   ▶ Manifestation Code   **OGCR** Official Guidelines   **Coding Clinic**   Excludes   Includes   Use additional   Code first

PERSONS WITHOUT REPORTED DIAGNOSIS ENCOUNTERED DURING EXAMINATION AND INVESTIGATION OF INDIVIDUALS AND POPULATIONS (V70–V82)

Note: Nonspecific abnormal findings disclosed at the time of these examinations are classifiable to categories 790–796.

● **V70 General medical examination**

Use additional code(s) to identify any special screening examination(s) performed (V73.0–V82.9)
Coding Clinic: 1993, Q1, P28; 1985, Nov-Dec, P13

●❶ **V70.0 Routine general medical examination at a health care facility** 🔖
Health checkup

Excludes | *health checkup of infant or child over 28 days old (V20.2)* ◀▥
health supervision of newborn 8 to 28 days old (V20.32) ◀
health supervision of newborn under 8 days old (V20.31) ◀
pre-procedural general physical examination (V72.83)

❶ **V70.1 General psychiatric examination, requested by the authority** 🔖

●❶ **V70.2 General psychiatric examination, other and unspecified** 🔖

●❶ **V70.3 Other medical examination for administrative purposes** 🔖
General medical examination for:
admission to old age home
adoption
camp
driving license
immigration and naturalization
insurance certification
marriage
prison
school admission
sports competition

Excludes | *attendance for issue of medical certificates (V68.0)*
pre-employment screening (V70.5)
Coding Clinic: 2008, Q3, P6

❶ **V70.4 Examination for medicolegal reasons** 🔖
Blood-alcohol tests
Blood-drug tests
Paternity testing

Excludes | *examination and observation following:*
accidents (V71.3, V71.4)
assault (V71.6)
rape (V71.5)

❶ **V70.5 Health examination of defined subpopulations** 🔖
Armed forces personnel
Inhabitants of institutions
Occupational health examinations
Pre-employment screening
Preschool children
Prisoners
Prostitutes
Refugees
School children
Students

●❶ **V70.6 Health examination in population surveys** 🔖

Excludes | *special screening (V73.0–V82.9)*

🔖 **V70.7 Examination of participant in clinical trial** 🔖
Examination of participant or control in clinical research
Coding Clinic: 2006, Q2, P5-6

●❶ **V70.8 Other specified general medical examinations** 🔖
Examination of potential donor of organ or tissue

●❶ **V70.9 Unspecified general medical examination** 🔖

OGCR Section I.C.18.d.6

Observation codes V29, V71 and V89 are for use in very limited circumstances when a person is being observed for a suspected condition that is ruled out. The observation codes are not for use if an injury or illness or any signs or symptoms related to the suspected condition are present. In such cases the diagnosis/symptom code is used with the corresponding E code to identify any external cause. The observation codes are to be used as principal diagnosis only. The only exception to this is when the principal diagnosis is required to be a code from the V30, Live born infant, category. Then the V29 observation code is sequenced after the V30 code. Additional codes may be used in addition to the observation code but only if they are unrelated to the suspected condition being observed.

● **V71 Observation and evaluation for suspected conditions not found**

Note: This category is to be used when persons without a diagnosis are suspected of having an abnormal condition, without signs or symptoms, which requires study, but after examination and observation, is found not to exist. This category is also for use for administrative and legal observation status.

Excludes | *suspected maternal and fetal conditions not found (V89.01–V89.09)*
Coding Clinic: 1990, Q1, P19; 1985, Nov-Dec, P10, 13

● **V71.0 Observation for suspected mental condition**

❶ **V71.01 Adult antisocial behavior** 🔖   A
Dyssocial behavior or gang activity in adult without manifest psychiatric disorder

❶ **V71.02 Childhood or adolescent antisocial behavior** 🔖
Dyssocial behavior or gang activity in child or adolescent without manifest psychiatric disorder

❶ **V71.09 Other suspected mental condition** 🔖

❶ **V71.1 Observation for suspected malignant neoplasm** 🔖
Coding Clinic: 1990, Q1, P21

❶ **V71.2 Observation for suspected tuberculosis** 🔖

❶ **V71.3 Observation following accident at work** 🔖

❶ **V71.4 Observation following other accident** 🔖
Examination of individual involved in motor vehicle traffic accident
Coding Clinic: 2006, Q1, P9; 2004, Q1, P6-7

❶ **V71.5 Observation following alleged rape or seduction** 🔖
Examination of victim or culprit

❶ **V71.6 Observation following other inflicted injury** 🔖
Examination of victim or culprit

❶ **V71.7 Observation for suspected cardiovascular disease** 🔖
Coding Clinic: 2004, Q1, P6-7; 1993, 5th Issue, P17-24; 1990, Q1, P19; 1987, Sept-Oct, P10

N Newborn Age: 0   **P** Pediatric Age: 0–17   **M** Maternity Age: 12–55   **A** Adult Age: 15–124   ♀ Females Only   ♂ Males Only   **1155**

● Unacceptable Principal Diagnosis   🔖 Complication\Comorbidity   🔖 Major C\C   🔖 Present on Admission Requirement   🔖 Hospital-Acquired Condition

V01-V89

● **V71.8 Observation and evaluation for other specified suspected conditions**

> **Excludes** *contact with and (suspected) exposure to (potentially) hazardous substances (V15.84–V15.86, V87.0–V87.31)*
>
> Coding Clinic: 1990, Q1, P19

❶ **V71.81 Abuse and neglect** 🔖

> **Excludes** *adult abuse and neglect (995.80–995.85)*
> *child abuse and neglect (995.50–995.59)*
>
> Coding Clinic: 2000, Q4, P54-55

❶ **V71.82 Observation and evaluation for suspected exposure to anthrax** 🔖

❶ **V71.83 Observation and evaluation for suspected exposure to other biological agent** 🔖

> Coding Clinic: 2003, Q4, P46-48

❶ **V71.89 Other specified suspected conditions** 🔖

> Coding Clinic: 2008, Q3, P6-7; 2003, Q2, P15-16

●●❶ **V71.9 Observation for unspecified suspected condition** 🔖

> Coding Clinic: 2002, Q1, P6-7

● **V72 Special investigations and examinations**

> **Includes** routine examination of specific system
>
> **Excludes** *general medical examination (V70.0–70.4)*
> *general screening examination of defined population groups (V70.5, V70.6, V70.7)*
> *health supervision of newborn 8 to 28 days old (V20.32)* ◀▥
> *health supervision of newborn under 8 days old (V20.31)* ◀▥
> *routine examination of infant or child over 28 days old (V20.2)* ◀▥
>
> Use additional code(s) to identify any special screening examination(s) performed (V73.0–V82.9)
>
> Coding Clinic: 2004, Q1, P15-16; 1985, Nov-Dec, P13

▥ **V72.0 Examination of eyes and vision** 🔖

● **V72.1 Examination of ears and hearing**

> Coding Clinic: 2004, Q1, P15-16

● ▥ **V72.11 Encounter for hearing examination following failed hearing screening** 🔖

> Coding Clinic: 2006, Q4, P118

● ▥ **V72.12 Encounter for hearing conservation and treatment** 🔖

> Coding Clinic: 2007, Q4, P99-101

● ▥ **V72.19 Other examination of ears and hearing** 🔖

● ▥ **V72.2 Dental examination** 🔖

● **V72.3 Gynecological examination**

> **Excludes** *cervical Papanicolaou smear without general gynecological examination (V76.2)*
> *routine examination in contraceptive management (V25.40–V25.49)*
>
> Coding Clinic: 2004, Q4, P104-105

▥ **V72.31 Routine gynecological examination ♀** 🔖

> General gynecological examination with or without Papanicolaou cervical smear
> Pelvic examination (annual) (periodic)
>
> Use additional code to identify:
> human papillomavirus (HPV) screening (V73.81)
> routine vaginal Papanicolaou smear (V76.47)
>
> Coding Clinic: 2006, Q2, P3,4

▥ **V72.32 Encounter for Papanicolaou cervical smear to confirm findings of recent normal smear following initial abnormal smear ♀** 🔖

> Coding Clinic: 2006, Q2, P3-4

● **V72.4 Pregnancy examination or test**

> Coding Clinic: 2005, Q4, P94-100; 2004, Q4, P105

▥ **V72.40 Pregnancy examination or test, pregnancy unconfirmed ♀** 🔖

> Possible pregnancy, not (yet) confirmed

▥ **V72.41 Pregnancy examination or test, negative result ♀** 🔖

▥ **V72.42 Pregnancy examination or test, positive result ♀** 🔖   **M**

● ▥ **V72.5 Radiological examination, not elsewhere classified** 🔖

> Routine chest x-ray
>
> **Excludes** ~~*examination for suspected tuberculosis (V71.2)*~~
> *radiologic examinations as part of pre-procedural testing (V72.81-V72.84)* ◀
>
> Coding Clinic: 1990, Q1, P8, 10, 19-21; 1985, Nov-Dec, P13

> **OGCR** Section I.C.18.d.15 (outpatient)
> V72.5 is not to be used if any sign or symptoms, or reason for a test is documented.

● **V72.6 Laboratory examination** ◀▥

> Encounters for blood and urine testing ◀
>
> **Excludes** ~~*that for suspected disorder (V71.0–V71.9)*~~
>
> Coding Clinic: 2006, Q2, P4; 1994, Q4, P35; 1990, Q1, P22; 1985, Nov-Dec, P13

> **OGCR** Section I.C.18.d.15 (outpatient)
> V72.6 is not to be used if any sign or symptoms, or reason for a test is documented.

● ▥ **V72.60 Laboratory examination, unspecified** 🔖   ◀

● ▥ **V72.61 Antibody response examination** 🔖   ◀

> Immunity status testing ◀
>
> **Excludes** *encounter for allergy testing (V72.7)* ◀

● ▥ **V72.62 Laboratory examination ordered as part of a routine general medical examination** 🔖   ◀

> Blood tests for routine general physical examination ◀

● ▥ **V72.63 Pre-procedural laboratory examination** 🔖   ◀

> Blood tests prior to treatment or procedure ◀
> Pre-operative laboratory examination ◀

● ▥ **V72.69 Other laboratory examination** 🔖   ◀

● ▥ **V72.7 Diagnostic skin and sensitization tests** 🔖

> Allergy tests
> Skin tests for hypersensitivity
>
> **Excludes** *diagnostic skin tests for bacterial diseases (V74.0–V74.9)*
>
> Coding Clinic: 1985, Nov-Dec, P13

● **V72.8 Other specified examinations**

> **Excludes** *pre-procedural laboratory examinations (V72.63)* ◀
>
> Coding Clinic: 1995, Q4, P51-52; 1990, Q1, P10; 1985, Nov-Dec, P13

▥ **V72.81 Preoperative cardiovascular examination** 🔖

> Pre-procedural cardiovascular examination
>
> Coding Clinic: 1995, Q4, P51-52

V01-V89

(Ex) CC Exclusions   ◀ New   ◀▥ Revised   ~~deleted~~ Deleted   ● Use Additional Digit(s)   ❶ First Listed   ▥ First Listed or Additional
❷ Additional Only   ▶ Manifestation Code   **OGCR** Official Guidelines   **Coding Clinic**   Excludes   Includes   Use additional   Code first

V72.82　Preoperative respiratory examination
Pre-procedural respiratory examination
Coding Clinic: 1996, Q3, P14

V72.83　Other specified preoperative examination ◄
Examination prior to chemotherapy
Other pre-procedural examination
Pre-procedural general physical examination
Excludes *routine general medical examination (V70.0)*
Coding Clinic: 1996, Q3, P14; 1995, Q4, P52

V72.84　Preoperative examination, unspecified
Pre-procedural examination, unspecified
Coding Clinic: 1995, Q4, P52

V72.85　Other specified examination
Coding Clinic: 2004, Q1, P12-13

V72.86　Encounter for blood typing

V72.9　Unspecified examination

V73　Special screening examination for viral and chlamydial diseases

V73.0　Poliomyelitis

V73.1　Smallpox

V73.2　Measles

V73.3　Rubella

V73.4　Yellow fever

V73.5　Other arthropod-borne viral diseases
Dengue fever
Hemorrhagic fever
Viral encephalitis:
mosquito-borne
tick-borne

V73.6　Trachoma

V73.8　Other specified viral and chlamydial diseases

V73.81　Human papillomavirus (HPV)
Coding Clinic: 2007, Q4, P99-101

V73.88　Other specified chlamydial diseases
Coding Clinic: 2007, Q4, P124-125

V73.89　Other specified viral diseases
OGCR Section I.C.1.h.

If a patient is being seen to determine HIV status, use V73.89, Screening for other specified viral disease. Use V69.8, Other problems related to lifestyle, as a secondary code if an asymptomatic patient is in a known high risk group for HIV. Should a patient with signs or symptoms or illness, or a confirmed HIV related diagnosis be tested for HIV, code the signs and symptoms or the diagnosis. An additional counseling code V65.44 may be used if counseling is provided during the encounter for the test.

V73.9　Unspecified viral and chlamydial disease

V73.98　Unspecified chlamydial disease

V73.99　Unspecified viral disease

V74　Special screening examination for bacterial and spirochetal diseases
Includes diagnostic skin tests for these diseases

V74.0　Cholera

V74.1　Pulmonary tuberculosis

V74.2　Leprosy [Hansen's disease]

V74.3　Diphtheria

V74.4　Bacterial conjunctivitis

V74.5　Venereal disease
Screening for bacterial and spirochetal sexually transmitted diseases
Screening for sexually transmitted diseases NOS
Excludes *special screening for nonbacterial sexually transmitted diseases (V73.81–V73.89, V75.4, V75.8)*
Coding Clinic: 2007, Q4, P124-125

V74.6　Yaws

V74.8　Other specified bacterial and spirochetal diseases
Brucellosis
Leptospirosis
Plague
Tetanus
Whooping cough

V74.9　Unspecified bacterial and spirochetal disease

V75　Special screening examination for other infectious diseases

V75.0　Rickettsial diseases

V75.1　Malaria

V75.2　Leishmaniasis

V75.3　Trypanosomiasis
Chagas' disease
Sleeping sickness

V75.4　Mycotic infections

V75.5　Schistosomiasis

V75.6　Filariasis

V75.7　Intestinal helminthiasis

V75.8　Other specified parasitic infections

V75.9　Unspecified infectious disease

V76　Special screening for malignant neoplasms

V76.0　Respiratory organs

V76.1　Breast

V76.10　Breast screening, unspecified

V76.11　Screening mammogram for high-risk patient ♀
Coding Clinic: 2003, Q2, P3-5

V76.12　Other screening mammogram
Coding Clinic: 2006, Q2, P10; Q2, P3-5

V76.19　Other screening breast examination

V76.2　Cervix ♀
Routine cervical Papanicolaou smear
Excludes *special screening for human papillomavirus (V73.81)*
that as part of a general gynecological examination (V72.31)

V76.3　Bladder

V76.4　Other sites

V76.41　Rectum

V76.42　Oral cavity

V76.43　Skin

V76.44　Prostate ♂

V76.45　Testis ♂

V76.46　Ovary ♀

● ⓥ V76.47 **Vagina** ♀
     Vaginal pap smear status-post hysterectomy for non-malignant condition
     Use additional code to identify acquired absence of uterus (V88.01–V88.03)
     Excludes *vaginal pap smear status-post hysterectomy for malignant condition (V67.01)*

● ⓥ V76.49 **Other sites**
     Coding Clinic: 1999, Q1, P4

● V76.5 **Intestine**

   ● ⓥ V76.50 **Intestine, unspecified**

   ● ⓥ V76.51 **Colon**
     Excludes *rectum (V76.41)*
     Coding Clinic: 2004, Q1, P11-12; 2001, Q4, P55-56x2

   ● ⓥ V76.52 **Small intestine**

● V76.8 **Other neoplasm**

   ● ⓥ V76.81 **Nervous system**

   ● ⓥ V76.89 **Other neoplasm**

● ⓥ V76.9 **Unspecified**

● V77 **Special screening for endocrine, nutritional, metabolic, and immunity disorders**

   ● ⓥ V77.0 **Thyroid disorders**

   ● ⓥ V77.1 **Diabetes mellitus**

   ● ⓥ V77.2 **Malnutrition**

   ● ⓥ V77.3 **Phenylketonuria [PKU]**

   ● ⓥ V77.4 **Galactosemia**

   ● ⓥ V77.5 **Gout**

   ● ⓥ V77.6 **Cystic fibrosis**
     Screening for mucoviscidosis

   ● ⓥ V77.7 **Other inborn errors of metabolism**

   ● ⓥ V77.8 **Obesity**

   ● V77.9 **Other and unspecified endocrine, nutritional, metabolic, and immunity disorders**

     ● ⓥ V77.91 **Screening for lipoid disorders**
       Screening cholesterol level
       Screening for hypercholesterolemia
       Screening for hyperlipidemia

     ● ⓥ V77.99 **Other and unspecified endocrine, nutritional, metabolic, and immunity disorders**

● V78 **Special screening for disorders of blood and blood-forming organs**

   ● ⓥ V78.0 **Iron deficiency anemia**

   ● ⓥ V78.1 **Other and unspecified deficiency anemia**

   ● ⓥ V78.2 **Sickle-cell disease or trait**

   ● ⓥ V78.3 **Other hemoglobinopathies**

   ● ⓥ V78.8 **Other disorders of blood and blood-forming organs**

   ● ⓥ V78.9 **Unspecified disorder of blood and blood-forming organs**

● V79 **Special screening for mental disorders and developmental handicaps**

   ● ⓥ V79.0 **Depression**

   ● ⓥ V79.1 **Alcoholism**

   ● ⓥ V79.2 **Mental retardation**

   ● ⓥ V79.3 **Developmental handicaps in early childhood**

   ● ⓥ V79.8 **Other specified mental disorders and developmental handicaps**

   ● ⓥ V79.9 **Unspecified mental disorder and developmental handicap**

● V80 **Special screening for neurological, eye, and ear diseases**

   ● V80.0 **Neurological conditions** ◀▥

     ● ⓥ V80.01 **Traumatic brain injury** ◀

     ● ⓥ V80.09 **Other neurological conditions** ◀

   ● ⓥ V80.1 **Glaucoma**

   ● ⓥ V80.2 **Other eye conditions**
     Screening for:
       cataract
       congenital anomaly of eye
       senile macular lesions
     Excludes *general vision examination (V72.0)*

   ● ⓥ V80.3 **Ear diseases**
     Excludes *general hearing examination (V72.11–V72.19)*

● V81 **Special screening for cardiovascular, respiratory, and genitourinary diseases**

   ● ⓥ V81.0 **Ischemic heart disease**

   ● ⓥ V81.1 **Hypertension**

   ● ⓥ V81.2 **Other and unspecified cardiovascular conditions**

   ● ⓥ V81.3 **Chronic bronchitis and emphysema**

   ● ⓥ V81.4 **Other and unspecified respiratory conditions**
     Excludes *screening for:*
       lung neoplasm (V76.0)
       pulmonary tuberculosis (V74.1)

   ● ⓥ V81.5 **Nephropathy**
     Screening for asymptomatic bacteriuria

   ● ⓥ V81.6 **Other and unspecified genitourinary conditions**

● V82 **Special screening for other conditions**

   ● ⓥ V82.0 **Skin conditions**

   ● ⓥ V82.1 **Rheumatoid arthritis**

   ● ⓥ V82.2 **Other rheumatic disorders**

   ● ⓥ V82.3 **Congenital dislocation of hip**

   ● ⓥ V82.4 **Maternal postnatal screening for chromosomal anomalies** ♀
     Excludes *antenatal screening by amniocentesis (V28.0)*

   ● ⓥ V82.5 **Chemical poisoning and other contamination**
     Screening for:
       heavy metal poisoning
       ingestion of radioactive substance
       poisoning from contaminated water supply
       radiation exposure

   ● ⓥ V82.6 **Multiphasic screening**

   ● V82.7 **Genetic screening**
     Excludes *genetic testing for procreative management (V26.31–V26.39)*
     Coding Clinic: 2006, Q4, P118

     ● ⓥ V82.71 **Screening for genetic disease carrier status**

     ● ⓥ V82.79 **Other genetic screening**

Ⓔ CC Exclusions   ◀ New   ◀▥ Revised   ~~deleted~~ Deleted   ● Use Additional Digit(s)   ❶ First Listed   ⓥ First Listed or Additional
❷ Additional Only   ▶ Manifestation Code   **OGCR** Official Guidelines   **Coding Clinic**   Excludes   Includes   Use additional   Code first
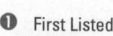

● V82.8　Other specified conditions

　● ◐V82.81　Osteoporosis ◌

　　　　Use additional code to identify:
　　　　hormone replacement therapy
　　　　　(postmenopausal) status
　　　　　(V07.4)
　　　　postmenopausal (natural) status
　　　　　(V49.81)
　　　　Coding Clinic: 2000, Q4, P53-54

　● ◐V82.89　Other specified conditions ◌

● ◐V82.9　Unspecified condition ◌

GENETICS (V83–V84)

OGCR Section I.C.18.d.3

Genetic carrier status indicates that a person carries a
gene, associated with a particular disease, which may
be passed to offspring who may develop that disease.
The person does not have the disease and is not at
risk of developing the disease.

● V83　Genetic carrier status

　● V83.0　Hemophilia A carrier

　　● ◐V83.01　Asymptomatic hemophilia A carrier ◌

　　● ◐V83.02　Symptomatic hemophilia A carrier ◌

　● V83.8　Other genetic carrier status

　　● ◐V83.81　Cystic fibrosis gene carrier ◌

　　● ◐V83.89　Other genetic carrier status ◌

OGCR Section I.C.18.d.3

Genetic susceptibility indicates that a person has a
gene that increases the risk of that person developing
the disease. Codes from category V84, Genetic
susceptibility to disease, should not be used as
principal or first-listed codes.

● V84　Genetic susceptibility to disease

　Includes　Confirmed abnormal gene

　Use additional code, if applicable, for any associated
　family history of the disease (V16–V19)

　● V84.0　Genetic susceptibility to malignant neoplasm

　　　Code first, if applicable, any current malignant
　　　　neoplasms (140.0–195.8, 200.0–208.9,
　　　　230.0–234.9)

　　　Use additional code, if applicable, for any
　　　　personal history of malignant neoplasm
　　　　(V10.0–V10.9)

　　● ❷V84.01　Genetic susceptibility to malignant
　　　　neoplasm of breast ◌
　　　　Coding Clinic: 2004, Q4, P106-107

　　● ❷V84.02　Genetic susceptibility to malignant
　　　　neoplasm of ovary ♀ ◌

　　● ❷V84.03　Genetic susceptibility to malignant
　　　　neoplasm of prostate ♂ ◌

　　● ❷V84.04　Genetic susceptibility to malignant
　　　　neoplasm of endometrium ♀ ◌

　　● ❷V84.09　Genetic susceptibility to other malignant
　　　　neoplasm ◌

　● V84.8　Genetic susceptibility to other disease

　　● ❷V84.81　Genetic susceptibility to multiple
　　　　endocrine neoplasia [MEN] ◌
　　　　Coding Clinic: 2007, Q4, P99-101

　　● ❷V84.89　Genetic susceptibility to other disease ◌

BODY MASS INDEX (V85)

● V85　Body mass index (BMI)
　　Kilograms per meters squared
　　Note: BMI adult codes are for use for persons over
　　　20 years old
　　Coding Clinic: 2008, Q4, P191; 2005, Q4, P94-100

　● ❷V85.0　Body Mass Index less than 19, adult ◌ ◌　　　A
　　　Ex: 278.00-278.01, V77.8, V85.0-V85.54

　● ❷V85.1　Body Mass Index between 19–24, adult ◌　　　A

　● V85.2　Body Mass Index between 25–29, adult

　　● ❷V85.21　Body Mass Index 25.0–25.9, adult ◌　　A

　　● ❷V85.22　Body Mass Index 26.0–26.9, adult ◌　　A

　　● ❷V85.23　Body Mass Index 27.0–27.9, adult ◌　　A

　　● ❷V85.24　Body Mass Index 28.0–28.9, adult ◌　　A

　　● ❷V85.25　Body Mass Index 29.0–29.9, adult ◌　　A

　● V85.3　Body Mass Index between 30–39, adult

　　● ❷V85.30　Body Mass Index 30.0–30.9, adult ◌　　A

　　● ❷V85.31　Body Mass Index 31.0–31.9, adult ◌　　A

　　● ❷V85.32　Body Mass Index 32.0–32.9, adult ◌　　A

　　● ❷V85.33　Body Mass Index 33.0–33.9, adult ◌　　A

　　● ❷V85.34　Body Mass Index 34.0–34.9, adult ◌　　A

　　● ❷V85.35　Body Mass Index 35.0–35.9, adult ◌　　A

　　● ❷V85.36　Body Mass Index 36.0–36.9, adult ◌　　A

　　● ❷V85.37　Body Mass Index 37.0–37.9, adult ◌　　A

　　● ❷V85.38　Body Mass Index 38.0–38.9, adult ◌　　A

　　● ❷V85.39　Body Mass Index 39.0–39.9, adult ◌　　A

　● ❷V85.4　Body Mass Index 40 and over, adult ◌ ◌　　　A
　　　Ex: 278.00-278.01, 278.1, V85.0-V85.39, V85.51-V85.54

　● V85.5　Body Mass Index, pediatric

　　　Note: BMI pediatric codes are for use for
　　　　persons age 2–20 years old. These
　　　　percentiles are based on the growth charts
　　　　published by the Centers for Disease
　　　　Control and Prevention (CDC)

　　● ❷V85.51　Body Mass Index, pediatric, less than
　　　　5th percentile for age ◌　　　　　　　　　P

　　● ❷V85.52　Body Mass Index, pediatric, 5th
　　　　percentile to less than 85th percentile
　　　　for age ◌　　　　　　　　　　　　　　P

　　● ❷V85.53　Body Mass Index, pediatric, 85th
　　　　percentile to less than 95th percentile
　　　　for age ◌　　　　　　　　　　　　　　P

　　● ❷V85.54　Body Mass Index, pediatric, greater
　　　　than or equal to 95th percentile for
　　　　age ◌　　　　　　　　　　　　　　　P

ESTROGEN RECEPTOR STATUS (V86)

● V86　Estrogen receptor status

　　Code first malignant neoplasm of breast (174.0–174.9,
　　　175.0–175.9)

　● ❷V86.0　Estrogen receptor positive status [ER+] ◌

　● ❷V86.1　Estrogen receptor negative status [ER-] ◌

OTHER SPECIFIED PERSONAL EXPOSURES AND HISTORY PRESENTING HAZARDS TO HEALTH (V87)

● **V87**   Other specified personal exposures and history presenting hazards to health

  ● **V87.0**   Contact with and (suspected) exposure to hazardous metals

     Excludes   *exposure to lead (V15.86)*
              toxic effect of metals (984.0-985.9)

    ● **V87.01**   Arsenic

    ● **V87.09**   Other hazardous metals
           Chromium compounds
           Nickel dust

  ● **V87.1**   Contact with and (suspected) exposure to hazardous aromatic compounds

     Excludes   *toxic effects of aromatic compounds (982.0, 983.0)*

    ● **V87.11**   Aromatic amines

    ● **V87.12**   Benzene

    ● **V87.19**   Other hazardous aromatic compounds
           Aromatic dyes NOS
           Polycyclic aromatic hydrocarbons

  ● **V87.2**   Contact with and (suspected) exposure to other potentially hazardous chemicals
       Dyes NOS

     Excludes   *exposure to asbestos (V15.84)*
              toxic effect of chemicals (980–989)

  ● **V87.3**   Contact with and (suspected) exposure to other potentially hazardous substances

     Excludes   *contact with and (suspected) exposure to potentially hazardous body fluids (V15.85)*
              toxic effect of substances (980–989)

    ● **V87.31**   Exposure to mold

    ● **V87.32**   Contact with and (suspected) exposure to algae bloom ◀

    ● **V87.39**   Contact with and (suspected) exposure to other potentially hazardous substances

  ● **V87.4**   Personal history of drug therapy

     Excludes   *long-term (current) drug use (V58.61-V58.69)*

    ●❷ **V87.41**   Personal history of antineoplastic chemotherapy

    ●❷ **V87.42**   Personal history of monoclonal drug therapy

    ●❷ **V87.43**   Personal history of estrogen therapy ◀

    ●❷ **V87.44**   Personal history of inhaled steroid therapy ◀

    ●❷ **V87.45**   Personal history of systemic steroid therapy ◀
           Personal history of steroid therapy NOS ◀

    ●❷ **V87.46**   Personal history of immunosuppression therapy ◀

         Excludes   *personal history of steroid therapy (V87.44, V87.45)* ◀

    ●❷ **V87.49**   Personal history of other drug therapy

ACQUIRED ABSENCE OF OTHER ORGANS AND TISSUE (V88)

● **V88**   Acquired absence of other organs and tissue

  ● **V88.0**   Acquired absence of cervix and uterus

    ●❷ **V88.01**   Acquired absence of both cervix and uterus ♀
           Acquired absence of uterus NOS
           Status post total hysterectomy

    ●❷ **V88.02**   Acquired absence of uterus with remaining cervical stump ♀
           Status post partial hysterectomy with remaining cervical stump

    ●❷ **V88.03**   Acquired absence of cervix with remaining uterus ♀

OTHER SUSPECTED CONDITIONS NOT FOUND (V89)

● **V89**   Other suspected conditions not found

  ● **V89.0**   Suspected maternal and fetal conditions not found

     Excludes   *known or suspected fetal anomalies affecting management of mother, not ruled out (655.00 655.93, 656.00–656.93, 657.00–657.03, 658.00–658.93)*
              newborn and perinatal conditions – code to condition

    ● **V89.01**   Suspected problem with amniotic cavity and membrane not found ♀   **M**
           Suspected oligohydramnios not found
           Suspected polyhydramnios not found

    ● **V89.02**   Suspected placental problem not found ♀   **M**

    ● **V89.03**   Suspected fetal anomaly not found ♀   **M**

    ● **V89.04**   Suspected problem with fetal growth not found ♀   **M**

    ● **V89.05**   Suspected cervical shortening not found ♀   **M**

    ● **V89.09**   Other suspected maternal and fetal condition not found ♀   **M**

Ⓔⓧ CC Exclusions   ◀ New   ◀▥ Revised   ~~deleted~~ Deleted   ● Use Additional Digit(s)   ❶ First Listed   ⓥ First Listed or Additional
❷ Additional Only   ▶ Manifestation Code   **OGCR** Official Guidelines   **Coding Clinic**   Excludes   Includes   Use additional   Code first

SUPPLEMENTARY CLASSIFICATION OF EXTERNAL CAUSES OF INJURY AND POISONING (E000-E999)

This section is provided to permit the classification of environmental events, circumstances, and conditions as the cause of injury, poisoning, and other adverse effects. Where a code from this section is applicable, it is intended that it shall be used in addition to a code from one of the main chapters of ICD-9-CM, indicating the nature of the condition. Certain other conditions which may be stated to be due to external causes are classified in Chapters 1 to 16 of ICD-9-CM. For these, the "E" code classification should be used as an additional code for more detailed analysis.

Machinery accidents [other than those connected with transport] are classifiable to category E919, in which the fourth digit allows a broad classification of the type of machinery involved. If a more detailed classification of type of machinery is required, it is suggested that the "Classification of Industrial Accidents according to Agency," prepared by the International Labor Office, be used in addition; it is included in this publication.

Categories for "late effects" of accidents and other external causes are to be found at E929, E959, E969, E977, E989, and E999.

Definitions and examples related to transport accidents

(a) A transport accident (E800–E848) is any accident involving a device designed primarily for, or being used at the time primarily for, conveying persons or goods from one place to another.

> **Includes** accidents involving:
> aircraft and spacecraft (E840–E845)
> watercraft (E830–E838)
> motor vehicle (E810–E825)
> railway (E800–E807)
> other road vehicles (E826–E829)

In classifying accidents which involve more than one kind of transport, the above order of precedence of transport accidents should be used.

Accidents involving agricultural and construction machines, such as tractors, cranes, and bulldozers, are regarded as transport accidents only when these vehicles are under their own power on a highway [otherwise the vehicles are regarded as machinery]. Vehicles which can travel on land or water, such as hovercraft and other amphibious vehicles, are regarded as watercraft when on the water, as motor vehicles when on the highway, and as off-road motor vehicles when on land, but off the highway.

> **Excludes** accidents:
> *in sports which involve the use of transport but where the transport vehicle itself was not involved in the accident*
> *involving vehicles which are part of industrial equipment used entirely on industrial premises*
> *occurring during transportation but unrelated to the hazards associated with the means of transportation [e.g., injuries received in a fight on board ship; transport vehicle involved in a cataclysm such as an earthquake]*
> *to persons engaged in the maintenance or repair of transport equipment or vehicle not in motion, unless injured by another vehicle in motion*

(b) A railway accident is a transport accident involving a railway train or other railway vehicle operated on rails, whether in motion or not.

> **Excludes** accidents:
> *in repair shops*
> *in roundhouse or on turntable*
> *on railway premises but not involving a train or other railway vehicle*

(c) A railway train or railway vehicle is any device with or without cars coupled to it, designed for traffic on a railway.

> **Includes** interurban:
> electric car (operated chiefly on its own right-of-way, not open to other traffic)
> streetcar (operated chiefly on its own right-of-way, not open to other traffic)
> railway train, any power [diesel] [electric] [steam]
> funicular
> monorail or two-rail
> subterranean or elevated
> other vehicle designed to run on a railway track

> **Excludes** *interurban electric cars [streetcars] specified to be operating on a right-of-way that forms part of the public street or highway [definition (n)]*

(d) A railway or railroad is a right-of-way designed for traffic on rails, which is used by carriages or wagons transporting passengers or freight, and by other rolling stock, and which is not open to other public vehicular traffic

(e) A motor vehicle accident is a transport accident involving a motor vehicle. It is defined as a motor vehicle traffic accident or as a motor vehicle nontraffic accident according to whether the accident occurs on a public highway or elsewhere.

> **Excludes** *injury or damage due to cataclysm*
> *injury or damage while a motor vehicle, not under its own power, is being loaded on, or unloaded from, another conveyance*

(f) A motor vehicle traffic accident is any motor vehicle accident occurring on a public highway [i.e., originating, terminating, or involving a vehicle partially on the highway]. A motor vehicle accident is assumed to have occurred on the highway unless another place is specified, except in the case of accidents involving only off-road motor vehicles which are classified as nontraffic accidents unless the contrary is stated.

(g) A motor vehicle nontraffic accident is any motor vehicle accident which occurs entirely in any place other than a public highway.

(h) A public highway [trafficway] or street is the entire width between property lines [or other boundary lines] of every way or place, of which any part is open to the use of the public for purposes of vehicular traffic as a matter of right or custom. A roadway is that part of the public highway designed, improved, and ordinarily used, for vehicular travel.

> **Includes** approaches (public) to:
> docks
> public building
> station

> **Excludes** *driveway (private)*
> *parking lot*
> *ramp*
> *roads in:*
> *airfield*
> *farm*
> *industrial premises*
> *mine*
> *private grounds*
> *quarry*

N Newborn Age: 0　　**P** Pediatric Age: 0–17　　**M** Maternity Age: 12–55　　**A** Adult Age: 15–124　　♀ Females Only　　♂ Males Only　　**1161**

(Ex) CC Exclusions　　Complication\Comorbidity　　Major C\C　　Present on Admission Requirement　　Hospital-Acquired Condition

E000-E999

(i) A motor vehicle is any mechanically or electrically powered device, not operated on rails, upon which any person or property may be transported or drawn upon a highway. Any object such as a trailer, coaster, sled, or wagon being towed by a motor vehicle is considered a part of the motor vehicle.

Includes	automobile [any type]
	bus
	construction machinery, farm and industrial machinery, steam roller, tractor, army tank, highway grader, or similar vehicle on wheels or treads, while in transport under own power
	fire engine (motorized)
	motorcycle
	motorized bicycle [moped] or scooter
	trolley bus not operating on rails
	truck
	van

Excludes	*devices used solely to move persons or materials within the confines of a building and its premises, such as:*
	building elevator
	coal car in mine
	electric baggage or mail truck used solely within a railroad station
	electric truck used solely within an industrial plant
	moving overhead crane

(j) A motorcycle is a two-wheeled motor vehicle having one or two riding saddles and sometimes having a third wheel for the support of a sidecar. The sidecar is considered part of the motorcycle.

Includes	motorized:
	bicycle [moped]
	scooter
	tricycle

(k) An off-road motor vehicle is a motor vehicle of special design, to enable it to negotiate rough or soft terrain or snow. Examples of special design are high construction, special wheels and tires, driven by treads, or support on a cushion of air.

Includes	all terrain vehicle [ATV]
	army tank
	hovercraft, on land or swamp
	snowmobile

(l) A driver of a motor vehicle is the occupant of the motor vehicle operating it or intending to operate it. A motorcyclist is the driver of a motorcycle. Other authorized occupants of a motor vehicle are passengers.

(m) An other road vehicle is any device, except a motor vehicle, in, on, or by which any person or property may be transported on a highway.

Includes	animal carrying a person or goods
	animal-drawn vehicle
	animal harnessed to conveyance
	bicycle [pedal cycle]
	streetcar
	tricycle (pedal)

Excludes	*pedestrian conveyance [definition (q)]*

(n) A streetcar is a device designed and used primarily for transporting persons within a municipality, running on rails, usually subject to normal traffic control signals, and operated principally on a right-of-way that forms part of the traffic way. A trailer being towed by a streetcar is considered a part of the streetcar.

Includes	interurban or intraurban electric or streetcar, when specified to be operating on a street or public highway
	tram (car)
	trolley (car)

(o) A pedal cycle is any road transport vehicle operated solely by pedals.

Includes	bicycle
	pedal cycle
	tricycle

Excludes	*motorized bicycle [definition (i)]*

(p) A pedal cyclist is any person riding on a pedal cycle or in a sidecar attached to such a vehicle.

(q) A pedestrian conveyance is any human powered device by which a pedestrian may move other than by walking or by which a walking person may move another pedestrian.

Includes	baby carriage
	coaster wagon
	heelies
	ice skates
	perambulator
	pushcart
	pushchair
	roller skates
	scooter
	skateboard
	skis
	sled
	wheelchair
	wheelies

(r) A pedestrian is any person involved in an accident who was not at the time of the accident riding in or on a motor vehicle, railroad train, streetcar, animal-drawn or other vehicle, or on a bicycle or animal.

Includes	person:
	changing tire of vehicle
	in or operating a pedestrian conveyance
	making adjustment to motor of vehicle
	on foot

(s) A watercraft is any device for transporting passengers or goods on the water.

(t) A small boat is any watercraft propelled by paddle, oars, or small motor, with a passenger capacity of less than ten.

Includes	boat NOS
	canoe
	coble
	dinghy
	punt
	raft
	rowboat
	rowing shell
	scull
	skiff
	small motorboat

Excludes	*barge*
	lifeboat (used after abandoning ship)
	raft (anchored) being used as a diving platform
	yacht

E000-E999

◀ New   ◀▥ Revised   ~~deleted~~ Deleted   ● Unacceptable Principal Diagnosis   ● Use Additional Digit(s)

▶ Manifestation Code   **OGCR** Official Guidelines   **Coding Clinic**   Excludes   Includes   Use additional   Code first   Omit code

(u) An aircraft is any device for transporting passengers or goods in the air.

> **Includes**   airplane [any type]
>   balloon
>   bomber
>   dirigible
>   glider (hang)
>   military aircraft
>   parachute

(v) A commercial transport aircraft is any device for collective passenger or freight transportation by air, whether run on commercial lines for profit or by government authorities, with the exception of military craft.

EXTERNAL CAUSE STATUS (E000) ◄

Note: A code from category E000 should be used in conjunction with the external cause code(s) assigned to a record to indicate the status of the person at the time the event occurred. A single code from category E000 should be assigned for an encounter. ◄

● **E000   External cause status** ◄

E000.0   Civilian activity done for income or pay ◄
Civilian activity done for financial or other compensation ◄
> **Excludes**   *military activity (E000.1)* ◄

E000.1   Military activity ◄
> **Excludes**   *activity of off duty military personnel (E000.8)* ◄

E000.8   Other external cause status ◄
Activity NEC ◄
Hobby not done for income ◄
Leisure activity ◄
Off-duty activity of military personnel ◄
Recreation or sport not for income or while a student ◄
Student activity ◄
Volunteer activity ◄
> **Excludes**   *civilian activity done for income or compensation (E000.0)* ◄
> *military activity (E000.1)* ◄

E000.9   Unspecified external cause status ◄

ACTIVITY (E001-E030) ◄

Note: Categories E001 to E030 are provided for use to indicate the activity of the person seeking healthcare for an injury or health condition, such as a heart attack while shoveling snow, which resulted from, or was contributed to, by the activity. These codes are appropriate for use for both acute injuries, such as those from chapter 17, and conditions that are due to the long-term, cumulative effects of an activity, such as those from chapter 13. They are also appropriate for use with external cause codes for cause and intent if identifying the activity provides additional information on the event. ◄

These codes should be used in conjunction with other external cause codes for external cause status (E000) and place of occurrence (E849). ◄

This section contains the following broad activity categories: ◄

E001 Activities involving walking and running ◄
E002 Activities involving water and water craft ◄

E003 Activities involving ice and snow ◄
E004 Activities involving climbing, rappelling, and jumping off ◄
E005 Activities involving dancing and other rhythmic movement ◄
E006 Activities involving other sports and athletics played individually ◄
E007 Activities involving other sports and athletics played as a team or group ◄
E008 Activities involving other specified sports and athletics ◄
E009 Activity involving other cardiorespiratory exercise ◄
E010 Activity involving other muscle strengthening exercises ◄
E011 Activities involving computer technology and electronic devices ◄
E012 Activities involving arts and handcrafts ◄
E013 Activities involving personal hygiene and household maintenance ◄
E014 Activities involving person providing caregiving ◄
E015 Activities involving food preparation, cooking and grilling ◄
E016 Activities involving property and land maintenance, building and construction ◄
E017 Activities involving roller coasters and other types of external motion ◄
E018 Activities involving playing musical instrument ◄
E019 Activities involving animal care ◄
E029 Other activity ◄
E030 Unspecified activity ◄

● **E001   Activities involving walking and running** ◄
> **Excludes**   *walking an animal (E019.0)* ◄
> *walking or running on a treadmill (E009.0)* ◄

E001.0   Walking, marching and hiking ◄
Walking, marching and hiking on level or elevated terrain ◄
> **Excludes**   *mountain climbing (E004.0)* ◄

E001.1   Running ◄

● **E002   Activities involving water and water craft** ◄
> **Excludes**   *activities involving ice (E003.0-E003.9)* ◄
> *boating and other watercraft transport accidents (E830-E838)* ◄

E002.0   Swimming ◄
E002.1   Springboard and platform diving ◄
E002.2   Water polo ◄
E002.3   Water aerobics and water exercise ◄
E002.4   Underwater diving and snorkeling ◄
SCUBA diving ◄
E002.5   Rowing, canoeing, kayaking, rafting and tubing ◄
Canoeing, kayaking, rafting and tubing in calm and turbulent water ◄

N Newborn Age: 0   **P** Pediatric Age: 0–17   **M** Maternity Age: 12–55   **A** Adult Age: 15–124   ♀ Females Only   ♂ Males Only
(Ex) CC Exclusions   🅒 Complication\Comorbidity   🅜 Major C\C   🅟 Present on Admission Requirement   🅗 Hospital-Acquired Condition   **1163**

E000-E999

E002.6 Water skiing and wake boarding ◄

E002.7 Surfing, windsurfing and boogie boarding ◄

E002.8 Water sliding ◄

E002.9 Other activity involving water and watercraft ◄
Activity involving water NOS
Parasailing
Water survival training and testing ◄

● **E003** Activities involving ice and snow ◄
Excludes shoveling ice and snow (E016.0) ◄

E003.0 Ice skating
Figure skating (singles) (pairs) ◄
Ice dancing ◄
Excludes ice hockey (E003.1) ◄

E003.1 Ice hockey ◄

E003.2 Snow (alpine) (downhill) skiing, snow boarding, sledding, tobogganing and snow tubing ◄
Excludes cross country skiing (E003.3) ◄

E003.3 Cross country skiing ◄
Nordic skiing ◄

E003.9 Other activity involving ice and snow ◄
Activity involving ice and snow NOS ◄

● **E004** Activities involving climbing, rappelling and jumping off ◄
Excludes hiking on level or elevated terrain (E001.0) ◄
jumping rope (E006.5) ◄
sky diving (E840-E844) ◄
trampoline jumping (E005.3) ◄

E004.0 Mountain climbing, rock climbing and wall climbing ◄

E004.1 Rappelling ◄

E004.2 BASE jumping ◄
Building, Antenna, Span, Earth jumping ◄

E004.3 Bungee jumping ◄

E004.4 Hang gliding ◄

E004.9 Other activity involving climbing, rappelling and jumping off ◄

● **E005** Activities involving dancing and other rhythmic movement ◄
Excludes martial arts (E008.4) ◄

E005.0 Dancing ◄

E005.1 Yoga ◄

E005.2 Gymnastics ◄
Rhythmic gymnastics ◄
Excludes trampoline (E005.3) ◄

E005.3 Trampoline ◄

E005.4 Cheerleading ◄

E005.9 Other activity involving dancing and other rhythmic movements ◄

● **E006** Activities involving other sports and athletics played individually ◄
Excludes dancing (E005.0) ◄
gymnastics (E005.2) ◄
trampoline (E005.3) ◄
yoga (E005.1) ◄

E006.0 Roller skating (inline) and skateboarding ◄

E006.1 Horseback riding ◄

E006.2 Golf ◄

E006.3 Bowling ◄

E006.4 Bike riding ◄
Excludes transport accident involving bike riding (E800-E829) ◄

E006.5 Jumping rope ◄

E006.6 Non-running track and field events ◄
Excludes running (any form) (E001.1) ◄

E006.9 Other activity involving other sports and athletics played individually ◄
Excludes activities involving climbing, rappelling, and jumping (E004.0-E004.9) ◄
activities involving ice and snow (E003.0-E003.9) ◄
activities involving walking and running (E001.0-E001.9) ◄
activities involving water and watercraft (E002.0-E002.9) ◄

● **E007** Activities involving other sports and athletics played as a team or group ◄
Excludes ice hockey (E003.1) ◄
water polo (E002.2) ◄

E007.0 American tackle football ◄
Football NOS ◄

E007.1 American flag or touch football ◄

E007.2 Rugby ◄

E007.3 Baseball ◄
Softball ◄

E007.4 Lacrosse and field hockey ◄

E007.5 Soccer ◄

E007.6 Basketball ◄

E007.7 Volleyball (beach) (court) ◄

E007.8 Physical games generally associated with school recess, summer camp and children ◄
Capture the flag
Dodge ball
Four square
Kickball

E007.9 Other activity involving other sports and athletics played as a team or group ◄
Cricket

● **E008** Activities involving other specified sports and athletics ◄

E008.0 Boxing ◄

E008.1 Wrestling ◄

E008.2 Racquet and hand sports ◄
Handball ◄
Racquetball ◄
Squash ◄
Tennis ◄

E008.3 Frisbee ◄
Ultimate frisbee ◄

E008.4 Martial arts ◄
Combatives ◄

E008.9 Other specified sports and athletics activity ◄
Excludes sports and athletics activities specified in categories E001-E007 ◄

◄ New   ◄▥ Revised   ~~deleted~~ Deleted   ● Unacceptable Principal Diagnosis   ● Use Additional Digit(s)
▶ Manifestation Code   **OGCR** Official Guidelines   **Coding Clinic**   Excludes   Includes   Use additional   Code first   Omit code

● **E009 Activity involving other cardiorespiratory exercise** ◄
　　Activity involving physical training ◄

　　E009.0 Exercise machines primarily for cardiorespiratory conditioning ◄
　　　　Elliptical and stepper machines ◄
　　　　Stationary bike ◄
　　　　Treadmill ◄

　　E009.1 Calisthenics ◄
　　　　Jumping jacks ◄
　　　　Warm up and cool down ◄

　　E009.2 Aerobic and step exercise ◄

　　E009.3 Circuit training ◄

　　E009.4 Obstacle course ◄
　　　　Challenge course ◄
　　　　Confidence course ◄

　　E009.5 Grass drills ◄
　　　　Guerilla drills ◄

　　E009.9 Other activity involving other cardiorespiratory exercise ◄
　　　　　Excludes *activities involving cardiorespiratory exercise specified in categories E001-E008* ◄

● **E010 Activity involving other muscle strengthening exercises** ◄

　　E010.0 Exercise machines primarily for muscle strengthening ◄

　　E010.1 Push-ups, pull-ups, sit-ups ◄

　　E010.2 Free weights ◄
　　　　Barbells ◄
　　　　Dumbbells ◄

　　E010.3 Pilates ◄

　　E010.9 Other activity involving other muscle strengthening exercises ◄
　　　　　Excludes *activities involving muscle strengthening specified in categories E001-E009* ◄

● **E011 Activities involving computer technology and electronic devices** ◄
　　　Excludes *electronic musical keyboard or instruments (E018.0)* ◄

　　E011.0 Computer keyboarding ◄
　　　　Electronic game playing using keyboard or other stationary device ◄

　　E011.1 Hand held interactive electronic device ◄
　　　　Cellular telephone and communication device ◄
　　　　Electronic game playing using interactive device ◄
　　　　　Excludes *electronic game playing using keyboard or other stationary device (E011.0)* ◄

　　E011.9 Other activity involving computer technology and electronic devices ◄

● **E012 Activities involving arts and handcrafts** ◄
　　　Excludes *activities involving playing musical instrument (E018.0-E018.3)* ◄

　　E012.0 Knitting and crocheting ◄

　　E012.1 Sewing ◄

　　E012.2 Furniture building and finishing ◄
　　　　Furniture repair ◄

　　E012.9 Activity involving other arts and handcrafts ◄

● **E013 Activities involving personal hygiene and household maintenance** ◄
　　　Excludes *activities involving cooking and grilling (E015.0-E015.9)* ◄
　　　　activities involving property and land maintenance, building and construction (E016.0-E016.9) ◄
　　　　activity involving persons providing caregiving (E014.0-E014.9) ◄
　　　　dishwashing (E015.0) ◄
　　　　food preparation (E015.0) ◄
　　　　gardening (E016.1) ◄

　　E013.0 Personal bathing and showering ◄

　　E013.1 Laundry ◄

　　E013.2 Vacuuming ◄

　　E013.3 Ironing ◄

　　E013.4 Floor mopping and cleaning ◄

　　E013.5 Residential relocation ◄
　　　　Packing up and unpacking involved in moving to a new residence ◄

　　E013.8 Other personal hygiene activity ◄

　　E013.9 Other household maintenance ◄

● **E014 Activities involving person providing caregiving** ◄

　　E014.0 Caregiving involving bathing ◄

　　E014.1 Caregiving involving lifting ◄

　　E014.9 Other activity involving person providing caregiving ◄

● **E015 Activities involving food preparation, cooking and grilling** ◄

　　E015.0 Food preparation and clean up ◄
　　　　Dishwashing ◄

　　E015.1 Grilling and smoking food ◄

　　E015.2 Cooking and baking ◄
　　　　Use of stove, oven and microwave oven ◄

　　E015.9 Other activity involving cooking and grilling ◄

● **E016 Activities involving property and land maintenance, building and construction** ◄

　　E016.0 Digging, shoveling and raking ◄
　　　　Dirt digging ◄
　　　　Raking leaves ◄
　　　　Snow shoveling ◄

　　E016.1 Gardening and landscaping ◄
　　　　Pruning, trimming shrubs, weeding ◄

　　E016.2 Building and construction ◄

　　E016.9 Other activity involving property and land maintenance, building and construction ◄

● **E017 Activities involving roller coasters and other types of external motion** ◄

　　E017.0 Rollercoaster riding ◄

　　E017.9 Other activity involving external motion ◄

● **E018 Activities involving playing musical instrument** ◄
　　Activity involving playing electric musical instrument ◄

　　E018.0 Piano playing ◄
　　　　Musical keyboard (electronic) playing ◄

　　E018.1 Drum and other percussion instrument playing ◄

　　E018.2 String instrument playing ◄

　　E018.3 Wind and brass instrument playing ◄

E000-E999

● **E019　Activities involving animal care** ◄

　　| **Excludes** | *horseback riding (E006.1)* ◄

　　E019.0　**Walking an animal** ◄

　　E019.1　**Milking an animal** ◄

　　E019.2　**Grooming and shearing an animal** ◄

　　E019.9　**Other activity involving animal care** ◄

● **E029　Other activity** ◄

　　E029.0　**Refereeing a sports activity** ◄

　　E029.1　**Spectator at an event** ◄

　　E029.2　**Rough housing and horseplay** ◄

　　E029.9　**Other activity** ◄

　　E030　**Unspecified activity** ◄

TRANSPORT ACCIDENTS (E800-E848) ◄

Definitions and examples related to transport accidents ◄

(a) A transport accident (E800-E848) is any accident involving a device designed primarily for, or being used at the time primarily for, conveying persons or goods from one place to another. ◄

RAILWAY ACCIDENTS (E800-E807)

Note:　For definitions of railway accident and related terms see definitions (a) to (d).

| **Excludes** | *accidents involving railway train and:*
aircraft (E840.0-E845.9)
motor vehicle (E810.0-E825.9)
watercraft (E830.0-E838.9)

The following fourth-digit subdivisions are for use with categories E800-E807 to identify the injured person:

0　Railway employee
　Any person who by virtue of his employment in connection with a railway, whether by the railway company or not, is at increased risk of involvement in a railway accident, such as:
　　catering staff of train
　　driver
　　guard
　　porter
　　postal staff on train
　　railway fireman
　　shunter
　　sleeping car attendant

1　Passenger on railway
　Any authorized person traveling on a train, except a railway employee.

　　| **Excludes** | *intending passenger waiting at station (8)*
　　　unauthorized rider on railway vehicle (8)

2　Pedestrian
　See definition (r)

3　Pedal cyclist
　See definition (p)

8　Other specified person
　Intending passenger or bystander waiting at station
　Unauthorized rider on railway vehicle

9　Unspecified person

● **E800　Railway accident involving collision with rolling stock** 🔊

　　Requires fourth digit. See beginning of section E800-E845 for codes and definitions.

　　| **Includes** | collision between railway trains or railway vehicles, any kind
collision NOS on railway
derailment with antecedent collision with rolling stock or NOS

● **E801　Railway accident involving collision with other object** 🔊

　　Requires fourth digit. See beginning of section E800-E845 for codes and definitions.

　　| **Includes** | collision of railway train with:
　　　buffers
　　　fallen tree on railway
　　　gates
　　　platform
　　　rock on railway
　　　streetcar
　　　other nonmotor vehicle
　　　other object

　　| **Excludes** | *collision with:*
　　　aircraft (E840.0-E842.9)
　　　motor vehicle (E810.0-E810.9,
　　　　E820.0-E822.9)

● **E802　Railway accident involving derailment without antecedent collision** 🔊

　　Requires fourth digit. See beginning of section E800-E845 for codes and definitions.

● **E803　Railway accident involving explosion, fire, or burning** 🔊

　　Requires fourth digit. See beginning of section E800-E845 for codes and definitions.

　　| **Excludes** | *explosion or fire, with antecedent derailment (E802.0-E802.9)*
　　　explosion or fire, with mention of antecedent collision (E800.0-E801.9)

● **E804　Fall in, on, or from railway train** 🔊

　　Requires fourth digit. See beginning of section E800-E845 for codes and definitions.

　　| **Includes** | fall while alighting from or boarding railway train

　　| **Excludes** | *fall related to collision, derailment, or explosion of railway train (E800.0-E803.9)*

● **E805　Hit by rolling stock** 🔊

　　Requires fourth digit. See beginning of section E800-E845 for codes and definitions.

　　| **Includes** | crushed by railway train or part
injured by railway train or part
killed by railway train or part
knocked down by railway train or part
run over by railway train or part

　　| **Excludes** | *pedestrian hit by object set in motion by railway train (E806.0-E806.9)*

◄ New　　◄⫽ Revised　　~~deleted~~ Deleted　　● Unacceptable Principal Diagnosis　　● Use Additional Digit(s)
▶ Manifestation Code　　OGCR Official Guidelines　　Coding Clinic　　| Excludes |　　| Includes |　　Use additional　　Code first　　Omit code

● **E806 Other specified railway accident** 🔖

> Requires fourth digit. See beginning of section
> E800-E845 for codes and definitions.
>
> > **Includes** hit by object falling in railway train
> > injured by door or window on railway
> > train
> > nonmotor road vehicle or pedestrian hit by
> > object set in motion by railway train
> > railway train hit by falling:
> > earth NOS
> > rock
> > tree
> > other object
>
> > **Excludes** *railway accident due to cataclysm (E908-E909)*

● **E807 Railway accident of unspecified nature** 🔖

> Requires fourth digit. See beginning of section
> E800-E845 for codes and definitions.
>
> > **Includes** found dead on railway right-of-way NOS
> > injured on railway right-of-way NOS
> > railway accident NOS

MOTOR VEHICLE TRAFFIC ACCIDENTS (E810-E819)

> **Note:** For definitions of motor vehicle traffic accident,
> and related terms, see definitions (e) to (k).
>
> > **Excludes** *accidents involving motor vehicle and aircraft*
> > *(E840.0-E845.9)*

The following fourth-digit subdivisions are for use
with categories E810-E819 to identify the injured
person:

> 0 **Driver of motor vehicle other than motorcycle**
>   See definition (l)
> 1 **Passenger in motor vehicle other than motorcycle**
>   See definition (l)
> 2 **Motorcyclist**
>   See definition (l)
> 3 **Passenger on motorcycle**
>   See definition (l)
> 4 **Occupant of streetcar**
> 5 **Rider of animal; occupant of animal-drawn vehicle**
> 6 **Pedal cyclist**
>   See definition (p)
> 7 **Pedestrian**
>   See definition (r)
> 8 **Other specified person**
>   Occupant of vehicle other than above
>   Person in railway train involved in accident
>   Unauthorized rider of motor vehicle
> 9 **Unspecified person**

● **E810 Motor vehicle traffic accident involving collision with
train** 🔖

> Requires fourth digit. See beginning of section
> E800-E845 for codes and definitions.
>
> > **Excludes** *motor vehicle collision with object set in*
> > *motion by railway train (E815.0-E815.9)*
> > *railway train hit by object set in motion by*
> > *motor vehicle (E818.0-E818.9)*

● **E811 Motor vehicle traffic accident involving re-entrant
collision with another motor vehicle** 🔖

> Requires fourth digit. See beginning of section
> E800-E845 for codes and definitions.
>
> > **Includes** collision between motor vehicle which
> > accidentally leaves the roadway
> > then re-enters the same roadway, or
> > the opposite roadway on a divided
> > highway, and another motor vehicle
>
> > **Excludes** *collision on the same roadway when none of the*
> > *motor vehicles involved have left and*
> > *re-entered the roadway (E812.0-E812.9)*

● **E812 Other motor vehicle traffic accident involving collision
with motor vehicle** 🔖

> Requires fourth digit. See beginning of section
> E800-E845 for codes and definitions.
>
> > **Includes** collision with another motor vehicle
> > parked, stopped, stalled, disabled, or
> > abandoned on the highway
> > motor vehicle collision NOS
>
> > **Excludes** *collision with object set in motion by another*
> > *motor vehicle (E815.0-E815.9)*
> > *re-entrant collision with another motor vehicle*
> > *(E811.0-E811.9)*
>
> **Coding Clinic: 2007, Q4, P105-107; 1996, Q4, P36.37**

● **E813 Motor vehicle traffic accident involving collision with
other vehicle** 🔖

> Requires fourth digit. See beginning of section
> E800-E845 for codes and definitions.
>
> > **Includes** collision between motor vehicle, any kind,
> > and:
> > other road (nonmotor transport)
> > vehicle, such as:
> > animal carrying a person
> > animal-drawn vehicle
> > pedal cycle
> > streetcar
>
> > **Excludes** *collision with:*
> > *object set in motion by nonmotor road*
> > *vehicle (E815.0-E815.9)*
> > *pedestrian (E814.0-E814.9)*
> > *nonmotor road vehicle hit by object set in*
> > *motion by motor vehicle (E818.0-E818.9)*

● **E814 Motor vehicle traffic accident involving collision with
pedestrian** 🔖

> Requires fourth digit. See beginning of section
> E800-E845 for codes and definitions.
>
> > **Includes** collision between motor vehicle, any kind,
> > and pedestrian
> > pedestrian dragged, hit, or run over by
> > motor vehicle, any kind
>
> > **Excludes** *pedestrian hit by object set in motion by motor*
> > *vehicle (E818.0-E818.9)*
>
> **Coding Clinic: 1996, Q4, P36.37**

N Newborn Age: 0   **P** Pediatric Age: 0–17   **M** Maternity Age: 12–55   **A** Adult Age: 15–124   ♀ Females Only   ♂ Males Only

(Ex) CC Exclusions   🔖 Complication\Comorbidity   🔖 Major C\C   🔖 Present on Admission Requirement   🔖 Hospital-Acquired Condition

1167

E000-E999

● **E815 Other motor vehicle traffic accident involving collision on the highway** 🖉

    Requires fourth digit. See beginning of section E800-E845 for codes and definitions.

    Includes   collision (due to loss of control) (on highway) between motor vehicle, any kind, and:
         abutment (bridge) (overpass)
         animal (herded) (unattended)
         fallen stone, traffic sign, tree, utility pole
         guard rail or boundary fence
         interhighway divider
         landslide (not moving)
         object set in motion by railway train or road vehicle (motor) (nonmotor)
         object thrown in front of motor vehicle
         safety island
         temporary traffic sign or marker
         wall of cut made for road
         other object, fixed, movable, or moving

    Excludes   *collision with:*
         any object off the highway (resulting from loss of control) (E816.0-E816.9)
         any object which normally would have been off the highway and is not stated to have been on it (E816.0-E816.9)
         motor vehicle parked, stopped, stalled, disabled, or abandoned on highway (E812.0-E812.9)
         moving landslide (E909.2)

        motor vehicle hit by object:
         set in motion by railway train or road vehicle (motor) (nonmotor) (E818.0-E818.9)
         thrown into or on vehicle (E818.0-E818.9)

● **E816 Motor vehicle traffic accident due to loss of control, without collision on the highway** 🖉

    Requires fourth digit. See beginning of section E800-E845 for codes and definitions.

    Includes   motor vehicle:
        failing to make curve and:
         colliding with object off the highway
         overturning
         stopping abruptly off the highway
        going out of control (due to)
         blowout and:
           colliding with object off the highway
           overturning
           stopping abruptly off the highway
         burst tire and:
           colliding with object off the highway
           overturning
           stopping abruptly off the highway
        driver falling asleep and:
           colliding with object off the highway
           overturning
           stopping abruptly off the highway
        driver inattention and:
           colliding with object off the highway
           overturning
           stopping abruptly off the highway
        excessive speed and:
           colliding with object off the highway
           overturning
           stopping abruptly off the highway
        failure of mechanical part and:
           colliding with object off the highway
           overturning
           stopping abruptly off the highway

    Excludes   *collision on highway following loss of control (E810.0-E815.9)*

        loss of control of motor vehicle following collision on the highway (E810.0-E815.9)

● **E817 Noncollision motor vehicle traffic accident while boarding or alighting** 🖉

    Requires fourth digit. See beginning of section E800-E845 for codes and definitions.

    Includes   fall down stairs of motor bus while boarding or alighting
        fall from car in street while boarding or alighting
        injured by moving part of the vehicle while boarding or alighting
        trapped by door of motor bus boarding or alighting while boarding or alighting

◀ New   ◀▥ Revised   ~~deleted~~ Deleted   ● Unacceptable Principal Diagnosis   ● Use Additional Digit(s)
▶ Manifestation Code   **OGCR** Official Guidelines   **Coding Clinic**   Excludes   Includes   Use additional   Code first   Omit code

● **E818   Other noncollision motor vehicle traffic accident** 🔲

> Requires fourth digit. See beginning of section E800-E845 for codes and definitions.

> | Includes | accidental poisoning from exhaust gas generated by motor vehicle while in motion |
> |---|---|

> breakage of any part of motor vehicle while in motion
> explosion of any part of motor vehicle while in motion
> fall, jump, or being accidentally pushed from motor vehicle while in motion
> fire starting in motor vehicle while in motion
> hit by object thrown into or on motor vehicle while in motion
> injured by being thrown against some part of, or object in motor vehicle while in motion
> injury from moving part of motor vehicle while in motion
> object falling in or on motor vehicle while in motion
> object thrown on motor vehicle while in motion
> collision of railway train or road vehicle except motor vehicle, with object set in motion by motor vehicle
> motor vehicle hit by object set in motion by railway train or road vehicle (motor) (nonmotor)
> pedestrian, railway train, or road vehicle (motor) (nonmotor) hit by object set in motion by motor vehicle

> | Excludes | *collision between motor vehicle and:* |
> |---|---|

> *object set in motion by railway train or road vehicle (motor) (nonmotor) (E815.0-E815.9)*
> *object thrown towards the motor vehicle (E815.0-E815.9)*
> *person overcome by carbon monoxide generated by stationary motor vehicle off the roadway with motor running (E868.2)*

● **E819   Motor vehicle traffic accident of unspecified nature** 🔲

> Requires fourth digit. See beginning of section E800-E845 for codes and definitions.

> | Includes | motor vehicle traffic accident NOS |
> |---|---|

> traffic accident NOS

> Coding Clinic: 2008, Q4, P96-97; 2006, Q4, P100-102; 2003, Q1, P7; 1999, Q4, P11-12; Q1, P10; 1993, Q2, P4-5

MOTOR VEHICLE NONTRAFFIC ACCIDENTS (E820-E825)

Note: For definitions of motor vehicle nontraffic accident and related terms see definition (a) to (k).

> | Includes | accidents involving motor vehicles being used in recreational or sporting activities off the highway |
> |---|---|

> collision and noncollision motor vehicle accidents occurring entirely off the highway

> | Excludes | *accidents involving motor vehicle and:* |
> |---|---|

> *aircraft (E840.0-E845.9)*
> *watercraft (E830.0-E838.9)*
> *accidents, not on the public highway, involving agricultural and construction machinery but not involving another motor vehicle (E919.0, E919.2, E919.7)*

The following fourth-digit subdivisions are for use with categories E820-E825 to identify the injured person:

> **0   Driver of motor vehicle other than motorcycle**
>   See definition (l)
> **1   Passenger in motor vehicle other than motorcycle**
>   See definition (l)
> **2   Motorcyclist**
>   See definition (l)
> **3   Passenger on motorcycle**
>   See definition (l)
> **4   Occupant of streetcar**
> **5   Rider of animal; occupant of animal-drawn vehicle**
> **6   Pedal cyclist**
>   See definition (p)
> **7   Pedestrian**
>   See definition (r)
> **8   Other specified person**
>   Occupant of vehicle other than above
>   Person on railway train involved in accident
>   Unauthorized rider of motor vehicle
> **9   Unspecified person**

● **E820   Nontraffic accident involving motor-driven snow vehicle** 🔲

> Requires fourth digit. See beginning of section E800-E845 for codes and definitions.

> | Includes | breakage of part of motor-driven snow vehicle (not on public highway) |
> |---|---|

> fall from motor-driven snow vehicle (not on public highway)
> hit by motor-driven snow vehicle (not on public highway)
> overturning of motor-driven snow vehicle (not on public highway)
> run over or dragged by motor-driven snow vehicle (not on public highway)
> collision of motor-driven snow vehicle with:
>   animal (being ridden) (-drawn vehicle)
>   another off-road motor vehicle
>   other motor vehicle, not on public highway
>   railway train
>   other object, fixed or movable
> injury caused by rough landing of motor-driven snow vehicle (after leaving ground on rough terrain)

> | Excludes | *accident on the public highway involving motor driven snow vehicle (E810.0-E819.9)* |
> |---|---|

N Newborn Age: 0   **P** Pediatric Age: 0–17   **M** Maternity Age: 12–55   **A** Adult Age: 15–124   ♀ Females Only   ♂ Males Only

(Ex) CC Exclusions   🔲 Complication\Comorbidity   🔲 Major C\C   🔲 Present on Admission Requirement   🔲 Hospital-Acquired Condition

1169

E000-E999

● **E821 Nontraffic accident involving other off-road motor vehicle** 🔖

> Requires fourth digit. See beginning of section E800-E845 for codes and definitions.

> **Includes** breakage of part of off-road motor vehicle, except snow vehicle (not on public highway)
> fall from off-road motor vehicle, except snow vehicle (not on public highway)
> hit by off-road motor vehicle, except snow vehicle (not on public highway)
> overturning of off-road motor vehicle, except snow vehicle (not on public highway)
> run over or dragged by off-road motor vehicle, except snow vehicle (not on public highway)
> thrown against some part of or object in off-road motor vehicle, except snow vehicle (not on public highway)
> collision with:
>   animal (being ridden) (-drawn vehicle)
>   another off-road motor vehicle, except snow vehicle
>   other motor vehicle, not on public highway
>   other object, fixed or movable

> **Excludes** *accident on public highway involving off-road motor vehicle (E810.0-E819.9)*
> *collision between motor driven snow vehicle and other off-road motor vehicle (E820.0-E820.9)*
> *hovercraft accident on water (E830.0-E838.9)*

● **E822 Other motor vehicle nontraffic accident involving collision with moving object** 🔖

> Requires fourth digit. See beginning of section E800-E845 for codes and definitions.

> **Includes** collision, not on public highway, between motor vehicle, except off-road motor vehicle and:
>   animal
>   nonmotor vehicle
>   other motor vehicle, except off-road motor vehicle
>   pedestrian
>   railway train
>   other moving object

> **Excludes** *collision with:*
> *motor-driven snow vehicle (E820.0-E820.9)*
> *other off-road motor vehicle (E821.0-E821.9)*

● **E823 Other motor vehicle nontraffic accident involving collision with stationary object** 🔖

> Requires fourth digit. See beginning of section E800-E845 for codes and definitions.

> **Includes** collision, not on public highway, between motor vehicle, except off-road motor vehicle, and any object, fixed or movable, but not in motion

● **E824 Other motor vehicle nontraffic accident while boarding and alighting** 🔖

> Requires fourth digit. See beginning of section E800-E845 for codes and definitions.

> **Includes** fall while boarding or alighting from motor vehicle except off-road motor vehicle, not on public highway
> injury from moving part of motor vehicle while boarding or alighting from motor vehicle except off-road motor vehicle, not on public highway
> trapped by door of motor vehicle while boarding or alighting from motor vehicle except off-road motor vehicle, not on public highway

● **E825 Other motor vehicle nontraffic accident of other and unspecified nature** 🔖

> Requires fourth digit. See beginning of section E800-E845 for codes and definitions.

> **Includes** accidental poisoning from carbon monoxide generated by motor vehicle while in motion, not on public highway
> breakage of any part of motor vehicle while in motion, not on public highway
> explosion of any part of motor vehicle while in motion, not on public highway
> fall, jump, or being accidentally pushed from motor vehicle while in motion, not on public highway
> fire starting in motor vehicle while in motion, not on public highway
> hit by object thrown into, towards, or on motor vehicle while in motion, not on public highway
> injured by being thrown against some part of, or object in motor vehicle while in motion, not on public highway
> injury from moving part of motor vehicle while in motion, not on public highway
> object falling in or on motor vehicle while in motion, not on public highway
> motor vehicle nontraffic accident NOS

> **Excludes** *fall from or in stationary motor vehicle (E884.9, E885.9)*
> *overcome by carbon monoxide or exhaust gas generated by stationary motor vehicle off the roadway with motor running (E868.2)*
> *struck by falling object from or in stationary motor vehicle (E916)*

◀ New   ◀▥ Revised   ~~deleted~~ Deleted   ● Unacceptable Principal Diagnosis   ● Use Additional Digit(s)
▶ Manifestation Code   **OGCR** Official Guidelines   **Coding Clinic**   Excludes   Includes   Use additional   Code first   Omit code

E000-E999

OTHER ROAD VEHICLE ACCIDENTS (E826-E829)

Note: Other road vehicle accidents are transport accidents involving road vehicles other than motor vehicles. For definitions of other road vehicle and related terms see definitions (m) to (o).

Includes   accidents involving other road vehicles being used in recreational or sporting activities

Excludes   *collision of other road vehicle [any] with:*
aircraft (E840.0-E845.9)
motor vehicle (E813.0-E813.9, E820.0-E822.9)
railway train (E801.0-E801.9)

The following fourth-digit subdivisions are for use with categories E826-E829 to identify the injured person:

> 0 **Pedestrian**
>   See definition (r)
> 1 **Pedal cyclist**
>   See definition (p)
> 2 **Rider of animal**
> 3 **Occupant of animal-drawn vehicle**
> 4 **Occupant of streetcar**
> 8 **Other specified person**
> 9 **Unspecified person**

● **E826** **Pedal cycle accident** 🔎
[0-9]

   Requires fourth digit. See beginning of section E800-E845 for codes and definitions.

Includes   breakage of any part of pedal cycle
collision between pedal cycle and:
   animal (being ridden) (herded) (unattended)
   another pedal cycle
   nonmotor road vehicle, any
   pedestrian
   other object, fixed, movable, or moving, not set in motion by motor vehicle, railway train, or aircraft
entanglement in wheel of pedal cycle
fall from pedal cycle
hit by object falling or thrown on the pedal cycle
pedal cycle accident NOS
pedal cycle overturned

● **E827** **Animal-drawn vehicle accident** 🔎
[0,2-4,8,9]

   Requires fourth digit. See beginning of section E800-E845 for codes and definitions.

Includes   breakage of any part of vehicle
collision between animal-drawn vehicle and:
   animal (being ridden) (herded) (unattended)
   nonmotor road vehicle, except pedal cycle
   pedestrian, pedestrian conveyance, or pedestrian vehicle
   other object, fixed, movable, or moving, not set in motion by motor vehicle, railway train, or aircraft
fall from animal-drawn vehicle
knocked down by animal-drawn vehicle
overturning of animal-drawn vehicle
run over by animal-drawn vehicle
thrown from animal-drawn vehicle

Excludes   *collision of animal-drawn vehicle with pedal cycle (E826.0-E826.9)*

● **E828** **Accident involving animal being ridden** 🔎
[0,2,4,8,9]

   Requires fourth digit. See beginning of section E800-E845 for codes and definitions.

Includes   collision between animal being ridden and:
   another animal
   nonmotor road vehicle, except pedal cycle, and animal-drawn vehicle
   pedestrian, pedestrian conveyance, or pedestrian vehicle
   other object, fixed, movable, or moving, not set in motion by motor vehicle, railway train, or aircraft
fall from animal being ridden
knocked down by animal being ridden
thrown from animal being ridden
trampled by animal being ridden
ridden animal stumbled and fell

Excludes   *collision of animal being ridden with:*
animal-drawn vehicle (E827.0-E827.9)
pedal cycle (E826.0-E826.9)

● **E829** **Other road vehicle accidents** 🔎
[0,4,8,9]

   Requires fourth digit. See beginning of section E800-E845 for codes and definitions.

Includes   accident while boarding or alighting from
   streetcar
   nonmotor road vehicle not classifiable to E826-E828
blow from object in
   streetcar
   nonmotor road vehicle not classifiable to E826-E828
breakage of any part of
   streetcar
   nonmotor road vehicle not classifiable to E826-E828
caught in door of
   streetcar
   nonmotor road vehicle not classifiable to E826-E828
derailment of
   streetcar
   nonmotor road vehicle not classifiable to E826-E828
fall in, on, or from
   streetcar
   nonmotor road vehicle not classifiable to E826-E828
fire in
   streetcar
   nonmotor road vehicle not classifiable to E826-E828
collision between streetcar or nonmotor road vehicle, except as in E826-E828, and:
   animal (not being ridden)
   another nonmotor road vehicle not classifiable to E826-E828
   pedestrian
   other object, fixed, movable, or moving, not set in motion by motor vehicle, railway train, or aircraft
nonmotor road vehicle accident NOS
streetcar accident NOS

Excludes   *collision with:*
animal being ridden (E828.0-E828.9)
animal-drawn vehicle (E827.0-E827.9)
pedal cycle (E826.0-E826.9)

N Newborn Age: 0   **P** Pediatric Age: 0–17   **M** Maternity Age: 12–55   **A** Adult Age: 15–124   ♀ Females Only   ♂ Males Only

(Ex) CC Exclusions   🔎 Complication\Comorbidity   🔎 Major C\C   🔎 Present on Admission Requirement   🔎 Hospital-Acquired Condition   **1171**

E000-E999

WATER TRANSPORT ACCIDENTS (E830-E838)

Note: For definitions of water transport accident and related terms see definitions (a), (s), and (t).

Includes   watercraft accidents in the course of recreational activities

Excludes   *accidents involving both aircraft, including objects set in motion by aircraft, and watercraft (E840.0-E845.9)*

The following fourth-digit subdivisions are for use with categories E830-E838 to identify the injured person:

> 0 **Occupant of small boat, unpowered**
> 1 **Occupant of small boat, powered**
>   See definition (t)
>
> **Excludes**   *water skier (4)*
>
> 2 **Occupant of other watercraft-crew**
>   Persons:
>   engaged in operation of watercraft
>   providing passenger services [cabin attendants, ship's physician, catering personnel]
>   working on ship during voyage in other capacity [musician in band, operators of shops and beauty parlors]
> 3 **Occupant of other watercraft -- other than crew**
>   Passenger
>   Occupant of lifeboat, other than crew, after abandoning ship
> 4 **Water skier**
> 5 **Swimmer**
> 6 **Dockers, stevedores**
>   Longshoreman employed on the dock in loading and unloading ships
> 7 **Occupant of military watercraft, any type** ◀
> 8 **Other specified person**
>   Immigration and custom officials on board ship
>   Person:
>   accompanying passenger or member of crew visiting boat
>   Pilot (guiding ship into port)
> 9 **Unspecified person**

● **E830   Accident to watercraft causing submersion** 🔖

Requires fourth digit. See beginning of section E800-E845 for codes and definitions.

Includes   submersion and drowning due to:
    boat overturning
    boat submerging
    falling or jumping from burning ship
    falling or jumping from crushed watercraft
    ship sinking
    other accident to watercraft

● **E831   Accident to watercraft causing other injury** 🔖

Requires fourth digit. See beginning of section E800-E845 for codes and definitions.

Includes   any injury, except submersion and drowning, as a result of an accident to watercraft
    burned while ship on fire
    crushed between ships in collision
    crushed by lifeboat after abandoning ship
    fall due to collision or other accident to watercraft
    hit by falling object due to accident to watercraft
    injured in watercraft accident involving collision
    struck by boat or part thereof after fall or jump from damaged boat

Excludes   *burns from localized fire or explosion on board ship (E837.0-E837.9)*

● **E832   Other accidental submersion or drowning in water transport accident** 🔖

Requires fourth digit. See beginning of section E800-E845 for codes and definitions.

Includes   submersion or drowning as a result of an accident other than accident to the watercraft, such as:
    fall:
        from gangplank
        from ship
        overboard
    thrown overboard by motion of ship
    washed overboard

Excludes   *submersion or drowning of swimmer or diver who voluntarily jumps from boat not involved in an accident (E910.0-E910.9)*

● **E833   Fall on stairs or ladders in water transport** 🔖

Requires fourth digit. See beginning of section E800-E845 for codes and definitions.

Excludes   *fall due to accident to watercraft (E831.0-E831.9)*

● **E834   Other fall from one level to another in water transport** 🔖

Requires fourth digit. See beginning of section E800-E845 for codes and definitions.

Excludes   *fall due to accident to watercraft (E831.0-E831.9)*

● **E835   Other and unspecified fall in water transport** 🔖

Requires fourth digit. See beginning of section E800-E845 for codes and definitions.

Excludes   *fall due to accident to watercraft (E831.0-E831.9)*

● **E836   Machinery accident in water transport** 🔖

Requires fourth digit. See beginning of section E800-E845 for codes and definitions.

Includes   injuries in water transport caused by:
    deck machinery
    engine room machinery
    galley machinery
    laundry machinery
    loading machinery

● **E837　Explosion, fire, or burning in watercraft** 🔍

> Requires fourth digit. See beginning of section E800-E845 for codes and definitions.

> **Includes**　explosion of boiler on steamship
> localized fire on ship

> **Excludes**　*burning ship (due to collision or explosion) resulting in:*
> *submersion or drowning (E830.0-E830.9)*
> *other injury (E831.0-E831.9)*

● **E838　Other and unspecified water transport accident** 🔍

> Requires fourth digit. See beginning of section E800-E845 for codes and definitions.

> **Includes**　accidental poisoning by gases or fumes on ship
> atomic power plant malfunction in watercraft
> crushed between ship and stationary object [wharf]
> crushed between ships without accident to watercraft
> crushed by falling object on ship or while loading or unloading
> hit by boat while water skiing
> struck by boat or part thereof (after fall from boat)
> watercraft accident NOS

AIR AND SPACE TRANSPORT ACCIDENTS (E840-E845)

Note:　For definition of aircraft and related terms see definitions (u) and (v).

The following fourth-digit subdivisions are for use with categories E840-E845 to identify the injured person:

> **0　Occupant of spacecraft**
> **1　Occupant of military aircraft, any**
> Crew in military aircraft [air force] [army] [national guard] [navy]
> Passenger (civilian) (military) in military aircraft [air force] [army] [national guard] [navy]
> Troops in military aircraft [air force] [army] [national guard] [navy]
>
> > **Excludes**　*occupants of aircraft operated under jurisdiction of police departments (5)*
> > *parachutist (7)*
>
> **2　Crew of commercial aircraft (powered) in surface-to-surface transport**
> **3　Other occupant of commercial aircraft (powered) in surface-to-surface transport**
> Flight personnel:
> not part of crew
> on familiarization flight
> Passenger on aircraft (powered) NOS
> **4　Occupant of commercial aircraft (powered) in surface-to-air transport**
> Occupant [crew] [passenger] of aircraft (powered) engaged in activities, such as:
> aerial spraying (crops) (fire retardants)
> air drops of emergency supplies
> air drops of parachutists, except from military craft
> crop dusting
> lowering of construction material [bridge or telephone pole]
> sky writing

> **5　Occupant of other powered aircraft**
> Occupant [crew] [passenger] of aircraft [powered] engaged in activities, such as:
> aerobatic flying
> aircraft racing
> rescue operation
> storm surveillance
> traffic surveillance
> Occupant of private plane NOS
> **6　Occupant of unpowered aircraft, except parachutist**
> Occupant of aircraft classifiable to E842
> **7　Parachutist (military) (other)**
> Person making voluntary descent
>
> > **Excludes**　*person making descent after accident to aircraft (.1–.6)*
>
> **8　Ground crew, airline employee**
> Persons employed at airfields (civil) (military) or launching pads, not occupants of aircraft
> **9　Other person**

● **E840　Accident to powered aircraft at takeoff or landing** 🔍

> Requires fourth digit. See beginning of section E800-E845 for codes and definitions.

> **Includes**　collision of aircraft with any object, fixed, movable, or moving while taking off or landing
> crash while taking off or landing
> explosion on aircraft while taking off or landing
> fire on aircraft while taking off or landing
> forced landing

● **E841　Accident to powered aircraft, other and unspecified** 🔍

> Requires fourth digit. See beginning of section E800-E845 for codes and definitions.

> **Includes**　aircraft accident NOS
> aircraft crash or wreck NOS
> any accident to powered aircraft while in transit or when not specified whether in transit, taking off, or landing
> collision of aircraft with another aircraft, bird, or any object, while in transit
> explosion on aircraft while in transit
> fire on aircraft while in transit

● **E842　Accident to unpowered aircraft** 🔍
[6-9]

> Requires fourth digit. See beginning of section E800-E845 for codes and definitions.

> **Includes**　any accident, except collision with powered aircraft, to:
> balloon
> glider
> hang glider
> kite carrying a person
> hit by object falling from unpowered aircraft

● **E843　Fall in, on, or from aircraft** 🔍
[0-9]

> Requires fourth digit. See beginning of section E800-E845 for codes and definitions.

> **Includes**　accident in boarding or alighting from aircraft, any kind
> fall in, on, or from aircraft [any kind], while in transit, taking off, or landing, except when as a result of an accident to aircraft

E000-E999

● **E844 Other specified air transport accidents** 🔍

[0-9]   Requires fourth digit. See beginning of section E800-E845 for codes and definitions.

> **Includes**   hit by aircraft without accident to aircraft
> hit by object falling from aircraft without accident to aircraft
> injury by or from machinery on aircraft without accident to aircraft
> injury by or from rotating propeller without accident to aircraft
> injury by or from voluntary parachute descent without accident to aircraft
> poisoning by carbon monoxide from aircraft while in transit without accident to aircraft
> sucked into jet without accident to aircraft
> any accident involving other transport vehicle (motor) (nonmotor) due to being hit by object set in motion by aircraft (powered)

> **Excludes**   *air sickness (E903)*
> *effects of:*
>   *high altitude (E902.0-E902.1)*
>   *pressure change (E902.0-E902.1)*
> *injury in parachute descent due to accident to aircraft (E840.0-E842.9)*

● **E845 Accident involving spacecraft** 🔍

[0,8,9]   Requires fourth digit. See beginning of section E800-E845 for codes and definitions.

> **Includes**   launching pad accident

> **Excludes**   *effects of weightlessness in spacecraft (E928.0)*

VEHICLE ACCIDENTS NOT ELSEWHERE CLASSIFIABLE (E846-E848)

E846 Accidents involving powered vehicles used solely within the buildings and premises of industrial or commercial establishment 🔍

Accident to, on, or involving:
   battery-powered airport passenger vehicle
   battery-powered trucks (baggage) (mail)
   coal car in mine
   logging car
   self-propelled truck, industrial
   station baggage truck (powered)
   tram, truck, or tub (powered) in mine or quarry
Breakage of any part of vehicle
Collision with:
   pedestrian
   other vehicle or object within premises
Explosion of powered vehicle, industrial or commercial
Fall from powered vehicle, industrial or commercial
Overturning of powered vehicle, industrial or commercial
Struck by powered vehicle, industrial or commercial

> **Excludes**   *accidental poisoning by exhaust gas from vehicle not elsewhere classifiable (E868.2)*
> *injury by crane, lift (fork), or elevator (E919.2)*

E847 Accidents involving cable cars not running on rails 🔍

Accident to, on, or involving:
   cable car, not on rails
   ski chair-lift
   ski-lift with gondola
   teleferique
Breakage of cable
   caught or dragged by cable car, not on rails
   fall or jump from cable car, not on rails
   object thrown from or in cable car not on rails

E848 Accidents involving other vehicles, not elsewhere classifiable 🔍

Accident to, on, or involving:
   ice yacht
   land yacht
   nonmotor, nonroad vehicle NOS

> **OGCR**   Section I.C.19.b
> Use an additional code from category E849 to indicate the Place of Occurrence for injuries and poisonings. The Place of Occurrence describes the place where the event occurred and not the patient's activity at the time of the event. Do not use E849.9 if the place of occurrence is not stated.

PLACE OF OCCURRENCE (E849)

● **E849 Place of Occurrence**

Note: The following category is for use to denote the place where the injury or poisoning occurred.

E849.0 Home 🔍

Apartment
Boarding house
Farm house
Home premises
House (residential)
Noninstitutional place of residence
Private:
   driveway
   garage
   garden
   home
   walk
Swimming pool in private house or garden
Yard of home

> **Excludes**   *home under construction but not yet occupied (E849.3)*
> *institutional place of residence (E849.7)*

E849.1 Farm 🔍

Buildings
Land under cultivation

> **Excludes**   *farm house and home premises of farm (E849.0)*

E849.2 Mine and quarry 🔍

Gravel pit
Sand pit
Tunnel under construction

◀ New   ◀◀◀ Revised   ~~deleted~~ Deleted   ● Unacceptable Principal Diagnosis   ● Use Additional Digit(s)
▶ Manifestation Code   **OGCR** Official Guidelines   **Coding Clinic**   Excludes   Includes   Use additional   Code first   Omit code

E000-E999

E849.3   Industrial place and premises 🔊
  Building under construction
  Dockyard
  Dry dock
  Factory
    building
    premises
  Garage (place of work)
  Industrial yard
  Loading platform (factory) (store)
  Plant, industrial
  Railway yard
  Shop (place of work)
  Warehouse
  Workhouse
  Coding Clinic: 2003, Q4, P76-78

E849.4   Place for recreation and sport 🔊

Amusement park	Playground, including
Baseball field	school playground
Basketball court	Public park
Beach resort	Racecourse
Cricket ground	Resort NOS
Fives court	Riding school
Football field	Rifle range
Golf course	Seashore resort
Gymnasium	Skating rink
Hockey field	Sports palace
Holiday camp	Stadium
Ice palace	Swimming pool, public
Lake resort	Tennis court
Mountain resort	Vacation resort

> **Excludes**   *that in private house or garden*
> *(E849.0)*

E849.5   Street and highway 🔊
  Coding Clinic: 1995, Q1, P10

E849.6   Public building 🔊
  Building (including adjacent grounds) used
    by the general public or by a particular
    group of the public, such as:
    airport
    bank
    cafe
    casino
    church
    cinema
    clubhouse
    courthouse
    dance hall
    garage building (for car storage)
    hotel
    market (grocery or other commodity)
    movie house
    music hall
    nightclub
    office
    office building
    opera house
    post office
    public hall
    radio broadcasting station
    restaurant
    school (state) (public) (private)
    shop, commercial
    station (bus) (railway)
    store
    theater

> **Excludes**   *home garage (E849.0)*
> *industrial building or workplace*
> *(E849.3)*

E849.7   Residential institution
  Children's home
  Dormitory
  Hospital
  Jail
  Old people's home
  Orphanage
  Prison
  Reform School

E849.8   Other specified places 🔊
  Beach NOS
  Canal
  Caravan site NOS
  Derelict house
  Desert
  Dock
  Forest
  Harbor
  Hill
  Lake NOS
  Mountain
  Parking lot
  Parking place
  Pond or pool (natural)
  Prairie
  Public place NOS
  Railway line
  Reservoir
  River
  Sea
  Seashore NOS
  Stream
  Swamp
  Trailer court
  Woods

E849.9   Unspecified place 🔊

ACCIDENTAL POISONING BY DRUGS, MEDICINAL SUBSTANCES, AND BIOLOGICALS (E850-E858)

> **Includes**   accidental overdose of drug, wrong drug
> given or taken in error, and drug
> taken inadvertently
> accidents in the use of drugs and
> biologicals in medical and surgical
> procedures

> **Excludes**   *administration with suicidal or homicidal*
> *intent or intent to harm, or in*
> *circumstances classifiable to E980-E989*
> *(E950.0-E950.5, E962.0, E980.0-E980.5)*
> *correct drug properly administered in*
> *therapeutic or prophylactic dosage, as the*
> *cause of adverse effect (E930.0-E949.9)*

Note: See Alphabetic Index for more complete
  list of specific drugs to be classified under
  the fourth-digit subdivisions. The American
  Hospital Formulary numbers can be used to
  classify new drugs listed by the American
  Hospital Formulary Service (AHFS). See
  Appendix C.

● **E850   Accidental poisoning by analgesics, antipyretics, and antirheumatics**
  Coding Clinic: 2008, Q3, P21

E850.0   Heroin
  Diacetylmorphine

E850.1   Methadone

E850.2 **Other opiates and related narcotics**
Codeine [methylmorphine]
Meperidine [pethidine]
Morphine
Opium (alkaloids)

E850.3 **Salicylates**
Acetylsalicylic acid [aspirin]
Amino derivatives of salicylic acid
Salicylic acid salts

E850.4 **Aromatic analgesics, not elsewhere classified**
Acetanilid
Paracetamol [acetaminophen]
Phenacetin [acetophenetidin]

E850.5 **Pyrazole derivatives**
Aminophenazone [amidopyrine]
Phenylbutazone

E850.6 **Antirheumatics [antiphlogistics]**
Gold salts
Indomethacin
> **Excludes** *salicylates (E850.3)*
> *steroids (E858.0)*

E850.7 **Other non-narcotic analgesics**
Pyrabital

E850.8 **Other specified analgesics and antipyretics**
Pentazocine

E850.9 **Unspecified analgesic or antipyretic**

E851 **Accidental poisoning by barbiturates**
Amobarbital [amylobarbitone]
Barbital [barbitone]
Butabarbital [butabarbitone]
Pentobarbital [pentobarbitone]
Phenobarbital [phenobarbitone]
Secobarbital [quinalbarbitone]
> **Excludes** *thiobarbiturates (E855.1)*

● **E852** **Accidental poisoning by other sedatives and hypnotics**

E852.0 **Chloral hydrate group**

E852.1 **Paraldehyde**

E852.2 **Bromine compounds**
Bromides
Carbromal (derivatives)

E852.3 **Methaqualone compounds**

E852.4 **Glutethimide group**

E852.5 **Mixed sedatives, not elsewhere classified**

E852.8 **Other specified sedatives and hypnotics**

E852.9 **Unspecified sedative or hypnotic**
Sleeping:
drug NOS
pill NOS
tablet NOS

● **E853** **Accidental poisoning by tranquilizers**

E853.0 **Phenothiazine-based tranquilizers**
Chlorpromazine
Fluphenazine
Prochlorperazine
Promazine

E853.1 **Butyrophenone-based tranquilizers**
Haloperidol
Spiperone
Trifluperidol

E853.2 **Benzodiazepine-based tranquilizers**
Chlordiazepoxide   Lorazepam
Diazepam   Medazepam
Flurazepam   Nitrazepam
Coding Clinic: 1991, Q3, P14

E853.8 **Other specified tranquilizers**
Hydroxyzine
Meprobamate

E853.9 **Unspecified tranquilizer**

● **E854** **Accidental poisoning by other psychotropic agents**

E854.0 **Antidepressants**
Amitriptyline
Imipramine
Monoamine oxidase [MAO] inhibitors
Coding Clinic: 1991, Q3, P14

E854.1 **Psychodysleptics [hallucinogens]**
Cannabis derivatives
Lysergide [LSD]
Marihuana (derivatives)
Mescaline
Psilocin
Psilocybin

E854.2 **Psychostimulants**
Amphetamine
Caffeine
> **Excludes** *central appetite depressants (E858.8)*
Coding Clinic: 2003, Q2, P11

E854.3 **Central nervous system stimulants**
Analeptics
Opiate antagonists

E854.8 **Other psychotropic agents**

● **E855** **Accidental poisoning by other drugs acting on central and autonomic nervous system**

E855.0 **Anticonvulsant and anti-Parkinsonism drugs**
Amantadine
Hydantoin derivatives
Levodopa [L-dopa]
Oxazolidine derivatives [paramethadione]
[trimethadione]
Succinimides

E855.1 **Other central nervous system depressants**
Ether
Gaseous anesthetics
Halogenated hydrocarbon derivatives
Intravenous anesthetics
Thiobarbiturates, such as thiopental sodium

E855.2 **Local anesthetics**
Cocaine
Lidocaine [lignocaine]
Procaine
Tetracaine

E855.3 **Parasympathomimetics [cholinergics]**
Acetylcholine
Anticholinesterase:
organophosphorus
reversible
Pilocarpine

E855.4 **Parasympatholytics [anticholinergics and antimuscarinics] and spasmolytics**
Atropine
Homatropine
Hyoscine [scopolamine]
Quaternary ammonium derivatives

◀ New   ◀▥ Revised   ~~deleted~~ Deleted   ● Unacceptable Principal Diagnosis   ● Use Additional Digit(s)

▶ Manifestation Code   **OGCR** Official Guidelines   **Coding Clinic**   Excludes   Includes   Use additional   Code first   Omit code

E855.5 Sympathomimetics [adrenergics]
Epinephrine [adrenalin]
Levarterenol [noradrenalin]

E855.6 Sympatholytics [antiadrenergics]
Phenoxybenzamine
Tolazoline hydrochloride

E855.8 Other specified drugs acting on central and autonomic nervous systems

E855.9 Unspecified drug acting on central and autonomic nervous systems

E856 Accidental poisoning by antibiotics

E857 Accidental poisoning by other anti-infectives

● **E858 Accidental poisoning by other drugs**
Coding Clinic: 2008, Q3, P21

E858.0 Hormones and synthetic substitutes

E858.1 Primarily systemic agents

E858.2 Agents primarily affecting blood constituents

E858.3 Agents primarily affecting cardiovascular system

E858.4 Agents primarily affecting gastrointestinal system

E858.5 Water, mineral, and uric acid metabolism drugs

E858.6 Agents primarily acting on the smooth and skeletal muscles and respiratory system

E858.7 Agents primarily affecting skin and mucous membrane, ophthalmological, otorhinolaryngological, and dental drugs

E858.8 Other specified drugs
Central appetite depressants

E858.9 Unspecified drug

ACCIDENTAL POISONING BY OTHER SOLID AND LIQUID SUBSTANCES, GASES, AND VAPORS (E860-E869)

Note: Categories in this section are intended primarily to indicate the external cause of poisoning states classifiable to 980–989. They may also be used to indicate external causes of localized effects classifiable to 001–799.

● **E860 Accidental poisoning by alcohol, not elsewhere classified**

E860.0 Alcoholic beverages
Alcohol in preparations intended for consumption
Coding Clinic: 1996, Q3, P161; 1991, Q3, P14

E860.1 Other and unspecified ethyl alcohol and its products
Denatured alcohol
Ethanol NOS
Grain alcohol NOS
Methylated spirit

E860.2 Methyl alcohol
Methanol
Wood alcohol

E860.3 Isopropyl alcohol
Dimethyl carbinol
Isopropanol
Rubbing alcohol substitute
Secondary propyl alcohol

E860.4 Fusel oil
Alcohol:
amyl
butyl
propyl

E860.8 Other specified alcohols

E860.9 Unspecified alcohol

● **E861 Accidental poisoning by cleansing and polishing agents, disinfectants, paints, and varnishes**

E861.0 Synthetic detergents and shampoos

E861.1 Soap products

E861.2 Polishes

E861.3 Other cleansing and polishing agents
Scouring powders

E861.4 Disinfectants
Household and other disinfectants not ordinarily used on the person
| Excludes | *carbolic acid or phenol (E864.0)*

E861.5 Lead paints

E861.6 Other paints and varnishes
Lacquers
Oil colors
Paints, other than lead
Whitewashes

E861.9 Unspecified

● **E862 Accidental poisoning by petroleum products, other solvents and their vapors, not elsewhere classified**

E862.0 Petroleum solvents
Petroleum:
ether
benzine
naphtha

E862.1 Petroleum fuels and cleaners
Antiknock additives to petroleum fuels
Gas oils
Gasoline or petrol
Kerosene
| Excludes | *kerosene insecticides (E863.4)*

E862.2 Lubricating oils

E862.3 Petroleum solids
Paraffin wax

E862.4 Other specified solvents
Benzene
Coding Clinic: 2008, Q3, P6-7

E862.9 Unspecified solvent

● **E863 Accidental poisoning by agricultural and horticultural chemical and pharmaceutical preparations other than plant foods and fertilizers**
| Excludes | *plant foods and fertilizers (E866.5)*

E863.0 Insecticides of organochlorine compounds
Benzene hexachloride   Dieldrin
Chlordane   Endrine
DDT Toxaphene

E863.1 Insecticides of organophosphorus compounds
Demeton   Parathion
Diazinon   Phenylsulphthion
Dichlorvos   Phorate
Malathion   Phosdrin
Methyl parathion

N Newborn Age: 0   **P** Pediatric Age: 0–17   **M** Maternity Age: 12–55   **A** Adult Age: 15–124   ♀ Females Only   ♂ Males Only

(Ex) CC Exclusions   Complication\Comorbidity   Major C\C   Present on Admission Requirement   Hospital-Acquired Condition   **1177**

E000-E999

E863.2 **Carbamates**
    Aldicarb
    Carbaryl
    Propoxur

E863.3 **Mixtures of insecticides**

E863.4 **Other and unspecified insecticides**
    Kerosene insecticides

E863.5 **Herbicides**
    2,4-Dichlorophenoxyacetic acid [2, 4-D]
    2,4,5-Trichlorophenoxyacetic acid [2, 4, 5-T]
    Chlorates
    Diquat
    Mixtures of plant foods and fertilizers with
        herbicides
    Paraquat

E863.6 **Fungicides**
    Organic mercurials (used in seed dressing)
    Pentachlorophenols

E863.7 **Rodenticides**
    Fluoroacetates   Warfarin
    Squill and derivatives   Zinc phosphide
    Thallium

E863.8 **Fumigants**
    Cyanides   Phosphine
    Methyl bromide

E863.9 **Other and unspecified**

● E864 **Accidental poisoning by corrosives and caustics, not elsewhere classified**

> **Excludes** *those as components of disinfectants (E861.4)*

E864.0 **Corrosive aromatics**
    Carbolic acid or phenol

E864.1 **Acids**
    Acid:
      hydrochloric
      nitric
      sulfuric

E864.2 **Caustic alkalis**
    Lye

E864.3 **Other specified corrosives and caustics**

E864.4 **Unspecified corrosives and caustics**

● E865 **Accidental poisoning from poisonous foodstuffs and poisonous plants**

> **Includes** any meat, fish, or shellfish
>   plants, berries, and fungi eaten as, or in
>   mistake for food, or by a child

> **Excludes** *anaphlyactic shock due to adverse food reaction
>   (995.60–995.69)
>   food poisoning (bacterial) (005.0–005.9)
>   poisoning and toxic reactions to venomous
>   plants (E905.6–E905.7)*

E865.0 **Meat**

E865.1 **Shellfish**

E865.2 **Other fish**

E865.3 **Berries and seeds**

E865.4 **Other specified plants**

E865.5 **Mushrooms and other fungi**

E865.8 **Other specified foods**

E865.9 **Unspecified foodstuff or poisonous plant**

● E866 **Accidental poisoning by other and unspecified solid and liquid substances**

> **Excludes** *these substances as a component of:*
>   *medicines (E850.0-E858.9)*
>   *paints (E861.5-E861.6)*
>   *pesticides (E863.0-E863.9)*
>   *petroleum fuels (E862.1)*

E866.0 **Lead and its compounds and fumes**

E866.1 **Mercury and its compounds and fumes**

E866.2 **Antimony and its compounds and fumes**

E866.3 **Arsenic and its compounds and fumes**

E866.4 **Other metals and their compounds and fumes**
    Beryllium (compounds)
    Brass fumes
    Cadmium (compounds)
    Copper salts
    Iron (compounds)
    Manganese (compounds)
    Nickel (compounds)
    Thallium (compounds)

E866.5 **Plant foods and fertilizers**

> **Excludes** *mixtures with herbicides (E863.5)*

E866.6 **Glues and adhesives**

E866.7 **Cosmetics**

E866.8 **Other specified solid or liquid substances**
    Coding Clinic: 1990, Q4, P25

E866.9 **Unspecified solid or liquid substance**

E867 **Accidental poisoning by gas distributed by pipeline**
    Carbon monoxide from incomplete combustion of
      piped gas
    Coal gas NOS
    Liquefied petroleum gas distributed through pipes
      (pure or mixed with air)
    Piped gas (natural) (manufactured)

● E868 **Accidental poisoning by other utility gas and other carbon monoxide**

E868.0 **Liquefied petroleum gas distributed in mobile containers**
    Butane or carbon monoxide from incomplete
      combustion of these gases
    Liquefied hydrocarbon gas NOS or carbon
      monoxide from incomplete combustion
      of these gases
    Propane or carbon monoxide from incomplete
      combustion of these gases

E868.1 **Other and unspecified utility gas**
    Acetylene or carbon monoxide from
      incomplete combustion of these gases
    Gas NOS used for lighting, heating, or
      cooking or carbon monoxide from
      incomplete combustion of these gases
    Water gas or carbon monoxide from
      incomplete combustion of these gases

E000-E999

◀ New   ◀▥ Revised   ~~deleted~~ Deleted   ● Unacceptable Principal Diagnosis   ● Use Additional Digit(s)
▶ Manifestation Code   **OGCR** Official Guidelines   **Coding Clinic**   Excludes   Includes   Use additional   Code first   Omit code

E868.2 **Motor vehicle exhaust gas**
Exhaust gas from:
   farm tractor, not in transit
   gas engine
   motor pump
   motor vehicle, not in transit
   any type of combustion engine not in
     watercraft

| Excludes | *poisoning by carbon monoxide from:*
aircraft while in transit
  (E844.0-E844.9)
motor vehicle while in transit
  (E818.0-E818.9)
watercraft whether or not in transit
  (E838.0-E838.9)

E868.3 **Carbon monoxide from incomplete combustion of other domestic fuels**
Carbon monoxide from incomplete
  combustion of:
   coal in domestic stove or fireplace
   coke in domestic stove or fireplace
   kerosene in domestic stove or fireplace
   wood in domestic stove or fireplace

| Excludes | *carbon monoxide from smoke and fumes due to conflagration (E890.0-E893.9)*

E868.8 **Carbon monoxide from other sources**
Carbon monoxide from:
   blast furnace gas
   incomplete combustion of fuels in
     industrial use
   kiln vapor

E868.9 **Unspecified carbon monoxide**

● E869 **Accidental poisoning by other gases and vapors**

| Excludes | *effects of gases used as anesthetics (E855.1, E938.2)*
fumes from heavy metals (E866.0-E866.4)
smoke and fumes due to conflagration or explosion (E890.0-E899)

E869.0 **Nitrogen oxides**

E869.1 **Sulfur dioxide**

E869.2 **Freon**

E869.3 **Lacrimogenic gas [tear gas]**
   Bromobenzyl cyanide
   Chloroacetophenone
   Ethyliodoacetate

E869.4 **Second-hand tobacco smoke**
   Coding Clinic: 1996, Q2, P10

E869.8 **Other specified gases and vapors**
   Chlorine
   Hydrocyanic acid gas

E869.9 **Unspecified gases and vapors**

MISADVENTURES TO PATIENTS DURING SURGICAL AND MEDICAL CARE (E870-E876)

| Excludes | *accidental overdose of drug and wrong drug given in error (E850.0-E858.9)*
surgical and medical procedures as the cause of abnormal reaction by the patient, without mention of misadventure at the time of procedure (E878.0-E879.9)

OGCR Section I.C.19.i.1
Assign a code in the range of E870-E876 if misadventures are stated by the provider.

● E870 **Accidental cut, puncture, perforation, or hemorrhage during medical care**

E870.0 **Surgical operation**

E870.1 **Infusion or transfusion**

E870.2 **Kidney dialysis or other perfusion**

E870.3 **Injection or vaccination**

E870.4 **Endoscopic examination**

E870.5 **Aspiration of fluid or tissue, puncture, and catheterization**
   Abdominal paracentesis
   Aspirating needle biopsy
   Blood sampling
   Lumbar puncture
   Thoracentesis

| Excludes | *heart catheterization (E870.6)*

E870.6 **Heart catheterization**

E870.7 **Administration of enema**

E870.8 **Other specified medical care**

E870.9 **Unspecified medical care**

● E871 **Foreign object left in body during procedure**

E871.0 **Surgical operation**

E871.1 **Infusion or transfusion**

E871.2 **Kidney dialysis or other perfusion**

E871.3 **Injection or vaccination**

E871.4 **Endoscopic examination**

E871.5 **Aspiration of fluid or tissue, puncture, and catheterization**
   Abdominal paracentesis
   Aspiration needle biopsy
   Blood sampling
   Lumbar puncture
   Thoracentesis

| Excludes | *heart catheterization (E871.6)*

E871.6 **Heart catheterization**

E871.7 **Removal of catheter or packing**

E871.8 **Other specified procedures**

E871.9 **Unspecified procedure**

N Newborn Age: 0   **P** Pediatric Age: 0–17   **M** Maternity Age: 12–55   **A** Adult Age: 15–124   ♀ Females Only   ♂ Males Only

(Ex) CC Exclusions   Complication\Comorbidity   Major C\C   Present on Admission Requirement   Hospital-Acquired Condition   1179

● **E872 Failure of sterile precautions during procedure**

     E872.0   Surgical operation

     E872.1   Infusion or transfusion

     E872.2   Kidney dialysis and other perfusion

     E872.3   Injection or vaccination

     E872.4   Endoscopic examination

     E872.5   Aspiration of fluid or tissue, puncture, and catheterization
         Abdominal paracentesis
         Aspirating needle biopsy
         Blood sampling
         Lumbar puncture
         Thoracentesis
         Excludes *heart catheterization (E872.6)*

     E872.6   Heart catheterization

     E872.8   Other specified procedures

     E872.9   Unspecified procedure

● **E873 Failure in dosage**

     Excludes *accidental overdose of drug, medicinal or biological substance (E850.0-E858.9)*

     E873.0   Excessive amount of blood or other fluid during transfusion or infusion

     E873.1   Incorrect dilution of fluid during infusion

     E873.2   Overdose of radiation in therapy

     E873.3   Inadvertent exposure of patient to radiation during medical care

     E873.4   Failure in dosage in electroshock or insulin-shock therapy

     E873.5   Inappropriate [too hot or too cold] temperature in local application and packing

     E873.6   Nonadministration of necessary drug or medicinal substance

     E873.8   Other specified failure in dosage

     E873.9   Unspecified failure in dosage

● **E874 Mechanical failure of instrument or apparatus during procedure**

     E874.0   Surgical operation

     E874.1   Infusion and transfusion
         Air in system

     E874.2   Kidney dialysis and other perfusion

     E874.3   Endoscopic examination

     E874.4   Aspiration of fluid or tissue, puncture, and catheterization
         Abdominal paracentesis
         Aspirating needle biopsy
         Blood sampling
         Lumbar puncture
         Thoracentesis
         Excludes *heart catheterization (E874.5)*

     E874.5   Heart catheterization

     E874.8   Other specified procedures

     E874.9   Unspecified procedure

● **E875 Contaminated or infected blood, other fluid, drug, or biological substance**

     Includes presence of:
         bacterial pyrogens
         endotoxin-producing bacteria
         serum hepatitis-producing agent

     E875.0   Contaminated substance transfused or infused

     E875.1   Contaminated substance injected or used for vaccination

     E875.2   Contaminated drug or biological substance administered by other means

     E875.8   Other

     E875.9   Unspecified

● **E876 Other and unspecified misadventures during medical care**

     E876.0   Mismatched blood in transfusion

     E876.1   Wrong fluid in infusion

     E876.2   Failure in suture and ligature during surgical operation

     E876.3   Endotracheal tube wrongly placed during anesthetic procedure

     E876.4   Failure to introduce or to remove other tube or instrument
         Excludes *foreign object left in body during procedure (E871.0-E871.9)*

     E876.5   Performance of ~~inappropriate~~ wrong operation (procedure) on correct patient ◀▥
         Wrong device implanted into correct surgical site   ◀
         Excludes *correct operation (procedure) performed on wrong body part (E876.7)* ◀
         Coding Clinic: 2006, Q3, P9-10

     E876.6   Performance of operation (procedure) on patient not scheduled for surgery   ◀
         Performance of operation (procedure) intended for another patient   ◀
         Performance of operation (procedure) on wrong patient   ◀

     E876.7   Performance of correct operation (procedure) on wrong side/body part   ◀
         Performance of correct operation (procedure) on wrong side   ◀
         Performance of correct operation (procedure) on wrong site   ◀

     E876.8   Other specified misadventures during medical care
         Performance of inappropriate treatment, NEC
         Coding Clinic: 2009, Q2, P13x12, 15; 2008, Q4, P152-155

     E876.9   Unspecified misadventure during medical care

SURGICAL AND MEDICAL PROCEDURES AS THE CAUSE OF ABNORMAL REACTION OF PATIENT OR LATER COMPLICATION, WITHOUT MENTION OF MISADVENTURE AT THE TIME OF PROCEDURE (E878-E879)

     Includes procedures as the cause of abnormal reaction, such as:
         displacement or malfunction of prosthetic device
         hepatorenal failure, postoperative
         malfunction of external stoma
         postoperative intestinal obstruction
         rejection of transplanted organ

     Excludes *anesthetic management properly carried out as the cause of adverse effect (E937.0-E938.9)*
         infusion and transfusion, without mention of misadventure in the technique of procedure (E930.0-E949.9)

     OGCR Section I.C.19.i.2
     Assign a code in the range of E878-E879 if the provider attributes an abnormal reaction or later complication to a surgical or medical procedure, but does not mention misadventure at the time of the procedure as the cause of the reaction.

E000-E999

● **E878** **Surgical operation and other surgical procedures as the cause of abnormal reaction of patient, or of later complication, without mention of misadventure at the time of operation**

　　E878.0 **Surgical operation with transplant of whole organ**
　　　　　Transplantation of:
　　　　　　heart
　　　　　　kidney
　　　　　　liver

　　E878.1 **Surgical operation with implant of artificial internal device**
　　　　　Cardiac pacemaker
　　　　　Electrodes implanted in brain
　　　　　Heart valve prosthesis
　　　　　Internal orthopedic device

　　E878.2 **Surgical operation with anastomosis, bypass, or graft, with natural or artificial tissues used as implant**
　　　　　Anastomosis:
　　　　　　arteriovenous
　　　　　　gastrojejunal
　　　　　Graft of blood vessel, tendon, or skin
　　　　　Excludes *external stoma (E878.3)*

　　E878.3 **Surgical operation with formation of external stoma**
　　　　　Colostomy
　　　　　Cystostomy
　　　　　Duodenostomy
　　　　　Gastrostomy
　　　　　Ureterostomy

　　E878.4 **Other restorative surgery**

　　E878.5 **Amputation of limb(s)**

　　E878.6 **Removal of other organ (partial) (total)**

　　E878.8 **Other specified surgical operations and procedures**

　　E878.9 **Unspecified surgical operations and procedures**

　　OGCR Section I.C.19.i.2
　　　　Assign a code in the range of E878-E879 if the provider attributes an abnormal reaction or later complication to a surgical or medical procedure, but does not mention misadventure at the time of the procedure as the cause of the reaction.

● **E879** **Other procedures, without mention of misadventure at the time of procedure, as the cause of abnormal reaction of patient, or of later complication**

　　E879.0 **Cardiac catheterization**

　　E879.1 **Kidney dialysis**
　　　　　Coding Clinic: 2003, Q4, P60-61; 1994, Q3, P9

　　E879.2 **Radiological procedure and radiotherapy**
　　　　　Excludes *radio-opaque dyes for diagnostic x-ray procedures (E947.8)*
　　　　　Coding Clinic: 2006, Q4, P88-91

　　E879.3 **Shock therapy**
　　　　　Electroshock therapy
　　　　　Insulin-shock therapy

　　E879.4 **Aspiration of fluid**
　　　　　Lumbar puncture
　　　　　Thoracentesis

　　E879.5 **Insertion of gastric or duodenal sound**

　　E879.6 **Urinary catheterization**

　　E879.7 **Blood sampling**

　　E879.8 **Other specified procedures**
　　　　　Blood transfusion
　　　　　Coding Clinic: 1993, Q2, P3-4

　　E879.9 **Unspecified procedure**

ACCIDENTAL FALLS (E880-E888)

　　Excludes *falls (in or from):*
　　　　burning building (E890.8, E891.8)
　　　　into fire (E890.0-E899)
　　　　into water (with submersion or drowning) (E910.0-E910.9)
　　　　machinery (in operation) (E919.0-E919.9)
　　　　on edged, pointed, or sharp object (E920.0-E920.9)
　　　　transport vehicle (E800.0-E845.9)
　　　　vehicle not elsewhere classifiable (E846-E848)

● **E880** **Fall on or from stairs or steps**

　　E880.0 **Escalator**

　　E880.1 **Fall on or from sidewalk curb**
　　　　　Excludes *fall from moving sidewalk (E885.9)*

　　E880.9 **Other stairs or steps**

● **E881** **Fall on or from ladders or scaffolding**

　　E881.0 **Fall from ladder**
　　　　　Coding Clinic: 2007, Q1, P3-8

　　E881.1 **Fall from scaffolding**
　　　　　Coding Clinic: 1999, Q4, P13

　　E882 **Fall from or out of building or other structure**
　　　　　Fall from:
　　　　　　balcony
　　　　　　bridge
　　　　　　building
　　　　　　flagpole
　　　　　　tower
　　　　　　turret
　　　　　　viaduct
　　　　　　wall
　　　　　　window
　　　　　Fall through roof
　　　　　Excludes *collapse of a building or structure (E916)*
　　　　　　fall or jump from burning building (E890.8, E891.8)

● **E883** **Fall into hole or other opening in surface**

　　Includes fall into:
　　　　　cavity
　　　　　dock
　　　　　hole
　　　　　pit
　　　　　quarry
　　　　　shaft
　　　　　swimming pool
　　　　　tank
　　　　　well

　　Excludes *fall into water NOS (E910.9)*
　　　　that resulting in drowning or submersion without mention of injury (E910.0-E910.9)

　　E883.0 **Accident from diving or jumping into water [swimming pool]**
　　　　　Strike or hit:
　　　　　　against bottom when jumping or diving into water
　　　　　　wall or board of swimming pool
　　　　　　water surface
　　　　　Excludes *diving with insufficient air supply (E913.2)*
　　　　　　effects of air pressure from diving (E902.2)

N Newborn Age: 0　　**P** Pediatric Age: 0–17　　**M** Maternity Age: 12–55　　**A** Adult Age: 15–124　　♀ Females Only　　♂ Males Only
(Ex) CC Exclusions　　Complication\Comorbidity　　Major C\C　　Present on Admission Requirement　　Hospital-Acquired Condition

E000-E999

1181

E883.1   Accidental fall into well 🔍

E883.2   Accidental fall into storm drain or manhole 🔍

E883.9   Fall into other hole or other opening in surface

● **E884**   **Other fall from one level to another**

E884.0   **Fall from playground equipment** 🔍

> Excludes   *recreational machinery (E919.8)*
>
> **Coding Clinic: 2007, Q1, P3-8**

E884.1   **Fall from cliff** 🔍

E884.2   **Fall from chair**

E884.3   **Fall from wheelchair**

E884.4   **Fall from bed**

E884.5   **Fall from other furniture**

E884.6   **Fall from commode**
> Toilet

E884.9   **Other fall from one level to another**
> Fall from:
>   embankment
>   haystack
>   stationary vehicle
>   tree

● **E885**   **Fall on same level from slipping, tripping, or stumbling**

E885.0   **Fall from (nonmotorized) scooter** 🔍
> **Coding Clinic: 2002, Q4, P73**

E885.1   **Fall from roller skates** 🔍
> Heelies
> In-line skates
> Wheelies

E885.2   **Fall from skateboard** 🔍
> **Coding Clinic: 2000, Q4, P61**

E885.3   **Fall from skis** 🔍
> **Coding Clinic: 2007, Q2, P3-4**

E885.4   **Fall from snowboard** 🔍

E885.9   **Fall from other slipping, tripping, or stumbling**
> Fall on moving sidewalk

● **E886**   **Fall on same level from collision, pushing, or shoving, by or with other person**

> Excludes   *crushed or pushed by a crowd or human stampede (E917.1, E917.6)*

E886.0   **In sports** 🔍
> Tackles in sports
>
> > Excludes   *kicked, stepped on, struck by object, in sports (E917.0, E917.5)*
> >
> > **Coding Clinic: 2007, Q2, P3-4**

E886.9   **Other and unspecified**
> Fall from collision of pedestrian (conveyance) with another pedestrian (conveyance)

E887   **Fracture, cause unspecified**

● **E888**   **Other and unspecified fall**
> Accidental fall NOS
> Fall on same level NOS
> **Coding Clinic: 1993, Q4, P25-26**

E888.0   **Fall resulting in striking against sharp object**
> Use additional   external cause code to identify object (E920)

E888.1   **Fall resulting in striking against other object**

E888.8   **Other fall**

E888.9   **Unspecified fall**
> Fall NOS

ACCIDENTS CAUSED BY FIRE AND FLAMES (E890-E899)

> Includes   asphyxia or poisoning due to conflagration or ignition
>   burning by fire
>   secondary fires resulting from explosion

> Excludes   *arson (E968.0)*
>   *fire in or on:*
>   *machinery (in operation) (E919.0-E919.9)*
>   *transport vehicle other than stationary vehicle (E800.0-E845.9)*
>   *vehicle not elsewhere classifiable (E846-E848)*

● **E890**   **Conflagration in private dwelling**

> Includes   conflagration in: conflagration in:
>   apartment   lodging house
>   boarding house   mobile home
>   camping place   private garage
>   caravan   rooming house
>   farmhouse   tenement
>   house
>   conflagration originating from sources classifiable to E893-E898 in the above buildings

E890.0   **Explosion caused by conflagration** 🔍

E890.1   **Fumes from combustion of polyvinylchloride [PVC] and similar material in conflagration** 🔍

E890.2   **Other smoke and fumes from conflagration** 🔍
> Carbon monoxide from conflagration in private building
> Fumes NOS from conflagration in private building
> Smoke NOS from conflagration in private building
> **Coding Clinic: 2005, Q3, P10-11**

E890.3   **Burning caused by conflagration** 🔍

E890.8   **Other accident resulting from conflagration** 🔍
> Collapse of burning private building
> Fall from burning private building
> Hit by object falling from burning private building
> Jump from burning private building

E890.9   **Unspecified accident resulting from conflagration in private dwelling** 🔍

● **E891**   **Conflagration in other and unspecified building or structure**
> Conflagration in:
>   barn
>   church
>   convalescent and other residential home
>   dormitory of educational institution
>   factory
>   farm outbuildings
>   hospital
>   hotel
>   school
>   store
>   theater
> Conflagration originating from sources classifiable to E893-E898, in the above buildings

E891.0   **Explosion caused by conflagration**

E891.1   **Fumes from combustion of polyvinylchloride [PVC] and similar material in conflagration**

E000-E999

◀ New   ◀▥ Revised   ~~deleted~~ Deleted   ● Unacceptable Principal Diagnosis   ● Use Additional Digit(s)
▶ Manifestation Code   **OGCR** Official Guidelines   **Coding Clinic**   Excludes   Includes   Use additional   Code first   Omit code

E891.2 Other smoke and fumes from conflagration
Carbon monoxide from conflagration in building or structure
Fumes NOS from conflagration in building or structure
Smoke NOS from conflagration in building or structure

E891.3 Burning caused by conflagration

E891.8 Other accident resulting from conflagration
Collapse of burning building or structure
Fall from burning building or structure
Hit by object falling from burning building or structure
Jump from burning building or structure

E891.9 Unspecified accident resulting from conflagration of other and unspecified building or structure

E892 Conflagration not in building or structure
Fire (uncontrolled) (in) (of):
forest
grass
hay
lumber
mine
prairie
transport vehicle [any], except while in transit
tunnel

● **E893 Accident caused by ignition of clothing**
> **Excludes** ignition of clothing:
> from highly inflammable material (E894)
> with conflagration (E890.0-E892)

E893.0 From controlled fire in private dwelling 🔖
Ignition of clothing from:
normal fire (charcoal) (coal) (electric) (gas) (wood) in:
brazier in private dwelling (as listed in E890)
fireplace in private dwelling (as listed in E890)
furnace in private dwelling (as listed in E890)
stove in private dwelling (as listed in E890)

E893.1 From controlled fire in other building or structure
Ignition of clothing from:
normal fire (charcoal) (coal) (electric) (gas) (wood) in:
brazier in other building or structure (as listed in E891)
fireplace in other building or structure (as listed in E891)
furnace in other building or structure (as listed in E891)
stove in other building or structure (as listed in E891)

E893.2 From controlled fire not in building or structure 🔖
Ignition of clothing from:
bonfire (controlled)
brazier fire (controlled), not in building or structure
trash fire (controlled)
> **Excludes** conflagration not in building (E892)
> trash fire out of control (E892)

E893.8 From other specified sources
Ignition of clothing from:
blowlamp
blowtorch
burning bedspread
candle
cigar
cigarette
lighter
matches
pipe
welding torch

E893.9 Unspecified source
Ignition of clothing (from controlled fire NOS) (in building NOS) NOS

E894 Ignition of highly inflammable material 🔖
Ignition of:
benzine (with ignition of clothing)
gasoline (with ignition of clothing)
fat (with ignition of clothing)
kerosene (with ignition of clothing)
paraffin (with ignition of clothing)
petrol (with ignition of clothing)
> **Excludes** ignition of highly inflammable material with:
> conflagration (E890.0-E892)
> explosion (E923.0-E923.9)

E895 Accident caused by controlled fire in private dwelling 🔖
Burning by (flame of) normal fire (charcoal) (coal) (electric) (gas) (wood) in:
brazier in private dwelling (as listed in E890)
fireplace in private dwelling (as listed in E890)
furnace in private dwelling (as listed in E890)
stove in private dwelling (as listed in E890)
> **Excludes** burning by hot objects not producing fire or flames (E924.0-E924.9)
> ignition of clothing from these sources (E893.0)
> poisoning by carbon monoxide from incomplete combustion of fuel (E867-E868.9)
> that with conflagration (E890.0-E890.9)

E896 Accident caused by controlled fire in other and unspecified building or structure
Burning by (flame of) normal fire (charcoal) (coal) (electric) (gas) (wood) in:
brazier in other building or structure (as listed in E891)
fireplace in other building or structure (as listed in E891)
furnace in other building or structure (as listed in E891)
stove in other building or structure (as listed in E891)
> **Excludes** burning by hot objects not producing fire or flames (E924.0-E924.9)
> ignition of clothing from these sources (E893.1)
> poisoning by carbon monoxide from incomplete combustion of fuel (E867-E868.9)
> that with conflagration (E891.0-E891.9)

E897 Accident caused by controlled fire not in building or structure 🔖
Burns from flame of:
bonfire (controlled)
brazier fire (controlled), not in building or structure
trash fire (controlled)
> **Excludes** ignition of clothing from these sources (E893.2)
> trash fire out of control (E892)
> that with conflagration (E892)

N Newborn Age: 0   P Pediatric Age: 0–17   M Maternity Age: 12–55   A Adult Age: 15–124   ♀ Females Only   ♂ Males Only
(Ex) CC Exclusions   🔖 Complication\Comorbidity   🔖 Major C\C   🔖 Present on Admission Requirement   🔖 Hospital-Acquired Condition

1183

E000-E999

● **E898 Accident caused by other specified fire and flames**

> **Excludes** *conflagration (E890.0-E892)*
> *that with ignition of:*
> *clothing (E893.0-E893.9)*
> *highly inflammable material (E894)*

    E898.0 Burning bedclothes 🔲
        Bed set on fire NOS

    E898.1 Other 🔲

Burning by:	Burning by:
blowlamp	lamp
blowtorch	lighter
candle	matches
cigar	pipe
cigarette	welding torch
fire in room NOS	

E899 Accident caused by unspecified fire
    Burning NOS

ACCIDENTS DUE TO NATURAL AND ENVIRONMENTAL FACTORS (E900-E909)

● **E900 Excessive heat**

    E900.0 Due to weather conditions
        Excessive heat as the external cause of:
            ictus solaris
            siriasis
            sunstroke

    E900.1 Of man-made origin
        Heat (in):
            boiler room
            drying room
            factory
            furnace room
            generated in transport vehicle
            kitchen

    E900.9 Of unspecified origin

● **E901 Excessive cold**

    E901.0 Due to weather conditions
        Excessive cold as the cause of:
            chilblains NOS
            immersion foot

    E901.1 Of man-made origin
        Contact with or inhalation of:
            dry ice
            liquid air
            liquid hydrogen
            liquid nitrogen
        Prolonged exposure in:
            deep freeze unit
            refrigerator

    E901.8 Other specified origin

    E901.9 Of unspecified origin

● **E902 High and low air pressure and changes in air pressure**

    E902.0 Residence or prolonged visit at high altitude
        Residence or prolonged visit at high altitude
            as the cause of:
            Acosta syndrome
            Alpine sickness
            altitude sickness
            Andes disease
            anoxia, hypoxia
            barotitis, barodontalgia, barosinusitis, otitic
              barotrauma
            hypobarism, hypobaropathy
            mountain sickness
            range disease

    E902.1 In aircraft
        Sudden change in air pressure in aircraft
            during ascent or descent as the cause of:
            aeroneurosis
            aviators' disease

    E902.2 Due to diving
        High air pressure from rapid descent in water
            as the cause of:
            caisson disease
            divers' disease
            divers' palsy or paralysis
        Reduction in atmospheric pressure while
            surfacing from deep water diving as the
            cause of:
            caisson disease
            divers' disease
            divers' palsy or paralysis

    E902.8 Due to other specified causes
        Reduction in atmospheric pressure while
            surfacing from under ground

    E902.9 Unspecified cause

    E903 Travel and motion

● **E904 Hunger, thirst, exposure, and neglect**

> **Excludes** *any condition resulting from homicidal intent*
> *(E968.0-E968.9)*
> *hunger, thirst, and exposure resulting from*
> *accidents connected with transport*
> *(E800.0-E848)*

    E904.0 Abandonment or neglect of infants and helpless persons
        Desertion of newborn
        Exposure to weather conditions resulting from
            abandonment or neglect
        Hunger or thirst resulting from abandonment
            or neglect
        Inattention at or after birth
        Lack of care (helpless person) (infant)

> **Excludes** *criminal [purposeful] neglect (E968.4)*

    OGCR Section I.C.19.e.2
    In cases of neglect when the intent is
    determined to be accidental E code E904.0
    should be the first listed E code.

    E904.1 Lack of food
        Lack of food as the cause of:
            inanition
            insufficient nourishment
            starvation

> **Excludes** *hunger resulting from abandonment*
> *or neglect (E904.0)*

    E904.2 Lack of water
        Lack of water as the cause of:
            dehydration
            inanition

> **Excludes** *dehydration due to acute fluid loss*
> *(276.51)*

    E904.3 Exposure (to weather conditions), not elsewhere classifiable
        Exposure NOS
        Humidity
        Struck by hailstones

> **Excludes** *struck by lightning (E907)*

    E904.9 Privation, unqualified
        Destitution

◀ New   ◀▥ Revised   ~~deleted~~ Deleted   ● Unacceptable Principal Diagnosis   ● Use Additional Digit(s)

▷ Manifestation Code   **OGCR** Official Guidelines   **Coding Clinic**   Excludes   Includes   Use additional   Code first   Omit code

● **E905 Venomous animals and plants as the cause of poisoning and toxic reactions**

> **Includes**   chemical released by animal
> insects
> release of venom through fangs, hairs, spines, tentacles, and other venom apparatus

> **Excludes**   *eating of poisonous animals or plants (E865.0-E865.9)*

E905.0 Venomous snakes and lizards
     Cobra
     Copperhead snake
     Coral snake
     Fer de lance
     Gila monster
     Krait
     Mamba
     Rattlesnake
     Sea snake
     Snake (venomous)
     Viper
     Water moccasin

> **Excludes**   *bites of snakes and lizards known to be nonvenomous (E906.2)*

E905.1 Venomous spiders
     Black widow spider
     Brown spider
     Tarantula (venomous)

E905.2 Scorpion

E905.3 Hornets, wasps, and bees
     Yellow jacket

E905.4 Centipede and venomous millipede (tropical)

E905.5 Other venomous arthropods
     Sting of:
         ant
         caterpillar

E905.6 Venomous marine animals and plants
     Puncture by sea urchin spine
     Sting of:
         coral
         jelly fish
         nematocysts
         sea anemone
         sea cucumber
         other marine animal or plant

> **Excludes**   *bites and other injuries caused by nonvenomous marine animal (E906.2-E906.8)*
> *bite of sea snake (venomous) (E905.0)*

E905.7 Poisoning and toxic reactions caused by other plants
     Injection of poisons or toxins into or through skin by plant thorns, spines, or other mechanisms

> **Excludes**   *puncture wound NOS by plant thorns or spines (E920.8)*

E905.8 Other specified

E905.9 Unspecified
     Sting NOS
     Venomous bite NOS

● **E906 Other injury caused by animals**

> **Excludes**   *poisoning and toxic reactions caused by venomous animals and insects (E905.0-E905.9)*
> *road vehicle accident involving animals (E827.0-E828.9)*
> *tripping or falling over an animal (E885.9)*

E906.0 Dog bite

E906.1 Rat bite

E906.2 Bite of nonvenomous snakes and lizards

E906.3 Bite of other animal except arthropod
     Cats
     Moray eel
     Rodents, except rats
     Shark

E906.4 Bite of nonvenomous arthropod
     Insect bite NOS

E906.5 Bite by unspecified animal
     Animal bite NOS

E906.8 Other specified injury caused by animal
     Butted by animal
     Fallen on by horse or other animal, not being ridden
     Gored by animal
     Implantation of quills of porcupine
     Pecked by bird
     Run over by animal, not being ridden
     Stepped on by animal, not being ridden

> **Excludes**   *injury by animal being ridden (E828.0-E828.9)*

E906.9 Unspecified injury caused by animal

E907 Lightning

> **Excludes**   *injury from:*
> *fall of tree or other object caused by lightning (E916)*
> *fire caused by lightning (E890.0-E892)*

● **E908 Cataclysmic storms, and floods resulting from storms**

> **Excludes**   *collapse of dam or man-made structure causing flood (E909.3)*

E908.0 Hurricane
     Storm surge
     "Tidal wave" caused by storm action
     Typhoon

E908.1 Tornado
     Cyclone   Twisters

E908.2 Floods
     Torrential rainfall   Flash flood

> **Excludes**   *collapse of dam or man-made structure causing flood (E909.3)*

E908.3 Blizzard (snow) (ice)

E908.4 Dust storm

E908.8 Other cataclysmic storms

E908.9 Unspecified cataclysmic storms, and floods resulting from storms
     Storm NOS

N Newborn Age: 0   **P** Pediatric Age: 0–17   **M** Maternity Age: 12–55   **A** Adult Age: 15–124   ♀ Females Only   ♂ Males Only

(Ex) CC Exclusions   �», Complication\Comorbidity   🌮 Major C\C   🌮 Present on Admission Requirement   🌮 Hospital-Acquired Condition   **1185**

E000-E999

● **E909 Cataclysmic earth surface movements and eruptions**

E909.0 Earthquakes

E909.1 Volcanic eruptions
    Burns from lava   Ash inhalation

E909.2 Avalanche, landslide, or mudslide

E909.3 Collapse of dam or man-made structure

E909.4 Tidal wave caused by earthquake
    Tidal wave NOS   Tsunami

    | Excludes | *tidal wave caused by tropical storm (E908.0)*

E909.8 Other cataclysmic earth surface movements and eruptions

E909.9 Unspecified cataclysmic earth surface movements and eruptions

---

ACCIDENTS CAUSED BY SUBMERSION, SUFFOCATION, AND FOREIGN BODIES (E910-E915)

● **E910 Accidental drowning and submersion**

    | Includes | immersion
                  swimmers' cramp

    | Excludes | *diving accident (NOS) (resulting in injury except drowning) (E883.0)*
               diving with insufficient air supply (E913.2)
               drowning and submersion due to:
                  cataclysm (E908-E909)
                  machinery accident (E919.0-E919.9)
                  transport accident (E800.0-E845.9)
               effect of high and low air pressure (E902.2)
               injury from striking against objects while in running water (E917.2)

E910.0 While water-skiing
    Fall from water skis with submersion or drowning

    | Excludes | *accident to water-skier involving a watercraft and resulting in submersion or other injury (E830.4, E831.4)*

E910.1 While engaged in other sport or recreational activity with diving equipment
    Scuba diving NOS
    Skin diving NOS
    Underwater spear fishing NOS

E910.2 While engaged in other sport or recreational activity without diving equipment
    Fishing or hunting, except from boat or with diving equipment
    Ice skating
    Playing in water
    Surfboarding
    Swimming NOS
    Voluntarily jumping from boat, not involved in accident, for swim NOS
    Wading in water

    | Excludes | *jumping into water to rescue another person (E910.3)*

E910.3 While swimming or diving for purposes other than recreation or sport
    Marine salvage (with diving equipment)
    Pearl diving (with diving equipment)
    Placement of fishing nets (with diving equipment)
    Rescue (attempt) of another person (with diving equipment)
    Underwater construction or repairs (with diving equipment)

E910.4 In bathtub

E910.8 Other accidental drowning or submersion
    Drowning in:
        quenching tank
        swimming pool

E910.9 Unspecified accidental drowning or submersion
    Accidental fall into water NOS
    Drowning NOS

E911 Inhalation and ingestion of food causing obstruction of respiratory tract or suffocation
    Aspiration and inhalation of food [any] (into respiratory tract) NOS
    Asphyxia by food [including bone, seed in food, regurgitated food]
    Choked on food [including bone, seed in food, regurgitated food]
    Suffocation by food [including bone, seed in food, regurgitated food]
    Compression of trachea by food lodged in esophagus
    Interruption of respiration by food lodged in esophagus
    Obstruction of respiration by food lodged in esophagus
    Obstruction of pharynx by food (bolus)

    | Excludes | *injury, except asphyxia and obstruction of respiratory passage, caused by food (E915)*
             obstruction of esophagus by food without mention of asphyxia or obstruction of respiratory passage (E915)

E912 Inhalation and ingestion of other object causing obstruction of respiratory tract or suffocation
    Aspiration and inhalation of foreign body except food (into respiratory tract) NOS
    Compression by foreign body in esophagus
    Foreign object [bean] [marble] in nose
    Interruption of respiration by foreign body in esophagus
    Obstruction of pharynx by foreign body
    Obstruction of respiration by foreign body in esophagus

    | Excludes | *injury, except asphyxia and obstruction of respiratory passage, caused by foreign body (E915)*
             obstruction of esophagus by foreign body without mention of asphyxia or obstruction in respiratory passage (E915)

◀ New   ◀ Revised   ~~deleted~~ Deleted   ● Unacceptable Principal Diagnosis   ● Use Additional Digit(s)
▶ Manifestation Code   **OGCR** Official Guidelines   **Coding Clinic** | Excludes | | Includes | | Use additional | | Code first | | Omit code |

● **E913 Accidental mechanical suffocation**

     Excludes *mechanical suffocation from or by:*
           accidental inhalation or ingestion of:
              food (E911)
              foreign object (E912)
           cataclysm (E908-E909)
           explosion (E921.0-E921.9, E923.0-E923.9)
           machinery accident (E919.0-E919.9)

E913.0 In bed or cradle

     Excludes *suffocation by plastic bag (E913.1)*

E913.1 By plastic bag

E913.2 Due to lack of air (in closed place)
     Accidentally closed up in refrigerator or other
         airtight enclosed space
     Diving with insufficient air supply

     Excludes *suffocation by plastic bag (E913.1)*

E913.3 By falling earth or other substance
     Cave-in NOS

     Excludes *cave-in caused by cataclysmic*
             earth surface movements and
             eruptions (E909.8)
            struck by cave-in without
             asphyxiation or suffocation
             (E916)

E913.8 Other specified means
     Accidental hanging, except in bed or cradle

E913.9 Unspecified means
     Asphyxia, mechanical NOS
     Strangulation NOS
     Suffocation NOS

E914 Foreign body accidentally entering eye and adnexa

     Excludes *corrosive liquid (E924.1)*

E915 Foreign body accidentally entering other orifice

     Excludes *aspiration and inhalation of foreign body,*
            any, (into respiratory tract) NOS
            (E911-E912)

OTHER ACCIDENTS (E916-E928)

E916 Struck accidentally by falling object
     Collapse of building, except on fire
     Falling:
         rock
         snowslide NOS
         stone
         tree
     Object falling from:
         machine, not in operation
         stationary vehicle

     Code first collapse of building on fire (E890.0-E891.9)
         falling object in:
             cataclysm (E908-E909)
             machinery accidents (E919.0-E919.9)
             transport accidents (E800.0-E845.9)
             vehicle accidents not elsewhere classifiable
                (E846-E848)
         object set in motion by:
             explosion (E921.0-E921.9, E923.0-E923.9)
             firearm (E922.0-E922.9)
             projected object (E917.0-E917.9)

● **E917 Striking against or struck accidentally by objects or persons**

     Includes bumping into or against
           object (moving) (projected) (stationary)
           pedestrian conveyance
           person
         colliding with
           object (moving) (projected) (stationary)
           pedestrian conveyance
           person
         kicking against
           object (moving) (projected) (stationary)
           pedestrian conveyance
           person
         stepping on
           object (moving) (projected) (stationary)
           pedestrian conveyance
           person
         struck by
           object (moving) (projected) (stationary)
           pedestrian conveyance
           person

     Excludes *fall from:*
           collision with another person, except when
             caused by a crowd (E886.0-E886.9)
           stumbling over object (E885.9)
           fall resulting in striking against object
             (E888.0-E888.1)
           injury caused by:
             assault (E960.0-E960.1, E967.0-E967.9)
             cutting or piercing instrument
                (E920.0-E920.9)
             explosion (E921.0-E921.9,
                E923.0-E923.9)
             firearm (E922.0-E922.9)
             machinery (E919.0-E919.9)
             transport vehicle (E800.0-E845.9)
             vehicle not elsewhere classifiable
                (E846-E848)

E917.0 In sports without subsequent fall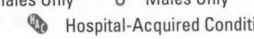
     Kicked or stepped on during game (football)
         (rugby)
     Struck by hit or thrown ball
     Struck by hockey stick or puck
     Coding Clinic: 2007, Q2, P3-4; 2006, Q1, P8; 2004, Q1, P9

E917.1 Caused by a crowd, by collective fear or panic without subsequent fall
     Crushed by crowd or human stampede
     Pushed by crowd or human stampede
     Stepped on by crowd or human stampede

E917.2 In running water without subsequent fall

     Excludes *drowning or submersion*
            (E910.0-E910.9) that in sports
            (E917.0, E917.5)

E917.3 Furniture without subsequent fall

     Excludes *fall from furniture (E884.2,*
            E884.4–E884.5)

E917.4 Other stationary object without subsequent fall
     Bath tub
     Fence
     Lamp-post

E917.5 Object in sports with subsequent fall
     Knocked down while boxing
     Coding Clinic: 2007, Q2, P3-4

E917.6 Caused by a crowd, by collective fear or panic with subsequent fall

E917.7 Furniture with subsequent fall

     Excludes *fall from furniture (E884.2,*
            E884.4–E884.5)

E000-E999

N Newborn Age: 0   **P** Pediatric Age: 0–17   **M** Maternity Age: 12–55   **A** Adult Age: 15–124   ♀ Females Only   ♂ Males Only
ⒺⓍ CC Exclusions   Complication\Comorbidity   Major C\C   Present on Admission Requirement   Hospital-Acquired Condition   **1187**

E917.8 Other stationary object with subsequent fall
> Bath tub
> Fence
> Lamp-post

E917.9 Other striking against with or without subsequent fall

E918 Caught accidentally in or between objects
> Caught, crushed, jammed, or pinched in or between moving or stationary objects, such as:
> escalator
> folding object
> hand tools, appliances, or implements
> sliding door and door frame
> under packing crate
> washing machine wringer

Excludes *injury caused by:*
> *cutting or piercing instrument (E920.0-E920.9)*
> *machinery (E919.0-E919.9)*
> *mechanism or component of firearm and air gun (E928.7)* ◄
> *transport vehicle (E800.0-E845.9)*
> *vehicle not elsewhere classifiable (E846-E848)*
> *struck accidentally by:*
> *falling object (E916)*
> *object (moving) (projected) (E917.0-E917.9)*

● **E919 Accidents caused by machinery**

Includes burned by machinery (accident)
> caught between machinery and other object
> caught in (moving parts of) machinery (accident)
> collapse of machinery (accident)
> crushed by machinery (accident)
> cut or pierced by machinery (accident)
> drowning or submersion caused by machinery (accident)
> explosion of, on, in machinery (accident)
> fall from or into moving part of machinery (accident)
> fire starting in or on machinery (accident)
> mechanical suffocation caused by machinery (accident)
> object falling from, on, in motion by machinery (accident)
> overturning of machinery (accident)
> pinned under machinery (accident)
> run over by machinery (accident)
> struck by machinery (accident)
> thrown from machinery (accident)
> machinery accident NOS

Excludes *accidents involving machinery, not in operation (E884.9, E916-E918)*
> *injury caused by:*
> *electric current in connection with machinery (E925.0-E925.9)*
> *escalator (E880.0, E918)*
> *explosion of pressure vessel in connection with machinery (E921.0-E921.9)*
> *mechanism or component of firearm and air gun (E928.7)* ◄
> *moving sidewalk (E885.9)*
> *powered hand tools, appliances, and implements (E916-E918, E920.0-E921.9, E923.0-E926.9)*
> *transport vehicle accidents involving machinery (E800.0-E848.9)*
> *poisoning by carbon monoxide generated by machine (E868.8)*

E919.0 Agricultural machines ⊚
> Animal-powered agricultural machine
> Combine
> Derrick, hay
> Farm machinery NOS
> Farm tractor
> Harvester
> Hay mower or rake
> Reaper
> Thresher

Excludes *that being towed by another vehicle on the highway (E810.0-E819.9, E827.0-E827.9, E829.0-E829.9)*
> *that in transport under own power on the highway (E810.0-E819.9)*
> *that involved in accident classifiable to E820-E829 (E820.0-E829.9)*

E919.1 Mining and earth-drilling machinery ⊚
> Bore or drill (land) (seabed)
> Shaft hoist
> Shaft lift
> Under-cutter

Excludes *coal car, tram, truck, and tub in mine (E846)*

E919.2 Lifting machines and appliances
> Chain hoist except in agricultural or mining operations
> Crane except in agricultural or mining operations
> Derrick except in agricultural or mining operations
> Elevator (building) (grain) except in agricultural or mining operations
> Forklift truck except in agricultural or mining operations
> Lift except in agricultural or mining operations
> Pulley block except in agricultural or mining operations
> Winch except in agricultural or mining operations

Excludes *that being towed by another vehicle on the highway (E810.0-E819.9, E827.0-E827.9, E829.0-E829.9)*
> *that in transport under own power on the highway (E810.0-E819.9)*
> *that involved in accident classifiable to E820-E829 (E820.0-E829.9)*

E919.3 Metalworking machines ⊚

Abrasive wheel	Metal:
Forging machine	milling machine
Lathe	power press
Mechanical shears	rolling-mill
Metal:	sawing machine
drilling machine	

Coding Clinic: 2003, Q4, P76-78

E919.4 Woodworking and forming machines ⊚

Band saw	Overhead plane
Bench saw	Powered saw
Circular saw	Radial saw
Molding machine	Sander

Excludes *hand saw (E920.1)*

◄ New   ◄‖‖‖ Revised   ~~deleted~~ Deleted   ● Unacceptable Principal Diagnosis   ● Use Additional Digit(s)
▶ Manifestation Code   **OGCR** Official Guidelines   **Coding Clinic**   Excludes   Includes   Use additional   Code first   Omit code

E000-E999

E919.5 Prime movers, except electrical motors 🔹
    Gas turbine
    Internal combustion engine
    Steam engine
    Water driven turbine

> **Excludes** *that being towed by other vehicle on the highway (E810.0–E819.9, E827.0–E827.9, E829.0–E829.9)*
> *that in transport under own power on the highway (E810.0–E819.9)*

E919.6 Transmission machinery 🔹
    Transmission: Transmission:
      belt   pinion
      cable   pulley
      chain   shaft
      gear

E919.7 Earth moving, scraping, and other excavating machines 🔹
    Bulldozer   Steam shovel
    Road scraper

> **Excludes** *that being towed by other vehicle on the highway (E810.0–E819.9)*
> *that in transport under own power on the highway (E810.0–E819.9)*

E919.8 Other specified machinery 🔹
    Machines for manufacture of:
      clothing
      foodstuffs and beverages
      paper
    Printing machine
    Recreational machinery
    Spinning, weaving, and textile machines

E919.9 Unspecified machinery 🔹

● **E920 Accidents caused by cutting and piercing instruments or objects**

> **Includes** accidental injury (by) object:
>   edged
>   pointed
>   sharp

> **Excludes** *injury caused by mechanism or component of firearm and air gun (E928.7)* ◄

E920.0 Powered lawn mower

E920.1 Other powered hand tools
    Any powered hand tool [compressed air] [electric] [explosive cartridge] [hydraulic power], such as:
      drill
      hand saw
      hedge clipper
      rivet gun
      snow blower
      staple gun

> **Excludes** *band saw (E919.4)*
> *bench saw (E919.4)*

E920.2 Powered household appliances and implements
    Blender
    Electric:
      beater or mixer
      can opener
      fan
      knife
      sewing machine
    Garbage disposal appliance

E920.3 Knives, swords, and daggers

E920.4 Other hand tools and implements
    Axe
    Can opener NOS
    Chisel
    Fork
    Hand saw
    Hoe
    Ice pick
    Needle (sewing)
    Paper cutter
    Pitchfork
    Rake
    Scissors
    Screwdriver
    Sewing machine, not powered
    Shovel

E920.5 Hypodermic needle
    Contaminated needle
    Needle stick

E920.8 Other specified cutting and piercing instruments or objects
    Arrow   Nail
    Broken glass   Plant thorn
    Dart   Splinter
    Edge of stiff paper   Tin can lid
    Lathe turnings

> **Excludes** *animal spines or quills (E906.8)*
> *flying glass due to explosion (E921.0–E923.9)*

Coding Clinic: 2001, Q3, P10

E920.9 Unspecified cutting and piercing instrument or object

● **E921 Accident caused by explosion of pressure vessel**

> **Includes** accidental explosion of pressure vessels, whether or not part of machinery

> **Excludes** *explosion of pressure vessel on transport vehicle (E800.0–E845.9)*

E921.0 Boilers 🔹
Coding Clinic: 2005, Q3, P10-11

E921.1 Gas cylinders 🔹
    Air tank
    Pressure gas tank

E921.8 Other specified pressure vessels 🔹
    Aerosol can
    Automobile tire
    Pressure cooker

E921.9 Unspecified pressure vessel 🔹

● **E922 Accident caused by firearm and air gun missile**

> **Excludes** *injury caused by mechanism or component of firearm and air gun (E928.7)* ◄

E922.0 Handgun 🔹
    Pistol
    Revolver

> **Excludes** *Verey pistol (E922.8)*

E922.1 Shotgun (automatic) 🔹

E922.2 Hunting rifle 🔹

E922.3 Military firearms 🔹
    Army rifle
    Machine gun

E922.4 Air gun 🔹
    BB gun
    Pellet gun

N Newborn Age: 0   **P** Pediatric Age: 0–17   **M** Maternity Age: 12–55   **A** Adult Age: 15–124   ♀ Females Only   ♂ Males Only

 CC Exclusions   🔹 Complication\Comorbidity   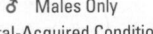 Major C\C   🔹 Present on Admission Requirement   🔹 Hospital-Acquired Condition   **1189**

E000–E999

E922.5 Paintball gun 🔍
Coding Clinic: 2002, Q4, P74

E922.8 Other specified firearm missile 🔍
Verey pistol [flare]

E922.9 Unspecified firearm missile 🔍
Gunshot wound NOS
Shot NOS

● **E923 Accident caused by explosive material**

Includes flash burns and other injuries resulting
from explosion of explosive material
ignition of highly explosive material with
explosion

Excludes *explosion:*
in or on machinery (E919.0-E919.9)
on any transport vehicle, except stationary
motor vehicle (E800.0-E848)
with conflagration (E890.0, E891.0, E892)
injury caused by mechanism or component
of firearm and air gun (E928.7) ◄
secondary fires resulting from explosion
(E890.0-E899)

E923.0 Fireworks

E923.1 Blasting materials
Blasting cap   Explosive [any]
Detonator   used in blasting
Dynamite   operations

E923.2 Explosive gases
Acetylene
Butane
Coal gas
Explosion in mine NOS
Fire damp
Gasoline fumes
Methane
Propane

E923.8 Other explosive materials
Bomb   Torpedo
Explosive missile   Explosion in munitions:
Grenade   dump
Mine   factory
Shell

E923.9 Unspecified explosive material
Explosion NOS

● **E924 Accident caused by hot substance or object, caustic or corrosive material, and steam**

Excludes *burning NOS (E899)*
chemical burn resulting from swallowing a
corrosive substance (E860.0-E864.4)
fire caused by these substances and objects
(E890.0-E894)
radiation burns (E926.0-E926.9)
therapeutic misadventures (E870.0-E876.9)

E924.0 Hot liquids and vapors, including steam
Burning or scalding by:
boiling water
hot or boiling liquids not primarily caustic
or corrosive
liquid metal
other hot vapor
steam

Excludes *hot (boiling) tap water (E924.2)*

E924.1 Caustic and corrosive substances 🔍
Burning by:
acid [any kind]
ammonia
caustic oven cleaner or other substance
corrosive substance
lye
vitriol

E924.2 Hot (boiling) tap water

E924.8 Other
Burning by:
heat from electric heating appliance
hot object NOS
light bulb
steam pipe

E924.9 Unspecified

● **E925 Accident caused by electric current**

Includes electric current from exposed wire, faulty
appliance, high voltage cable, live
rail, or open electric socket as the
cause of:
burn
cardiac fibrillation
convulsion
electric shock
electrocution
puncture wound
respiratory paralysis

Excludes *burn by heat from electrical appliance (E924.8)*
lightning (E907)

E925.0 Domestic wiring and appliances

E925.1 Electric power generating plants, distribution stations, transmission lines
Broken power line

E925.2 Industrial wiring, appliances, and electrical machinery
Conductors
Control apparatus
Electrical equipment and machinery
Transformers

E925.8 Other electric current
Wiring and appliances in or on:
farm [not farmhouse]
outdoors
public building
residential institutions
schools

E925.9 Unspecified electric current
Burns or other injury from electric current
NOS
Electric shock NOS
Electrocution NOS

◄ New   ◄▥ Revised   ~~deleted~~ Deleted   ● Unacceptable Principal Diagnosis   ● Use Additional Digit(s)
▶ Manifestation Code   OGCR Official Guidelines   **Coding Clinic**   Excludes   Includes   Use additional   Code first   Omit code

● **E926 Exposure to radiation**

> | Excludes | abnormal reaction to or complication
> of treatment without mention of
> misadventure (E879.2)
> atomic power plant malfunction in water
> transport (E838.0-E838.9)
> misadventure to patient in surgical and
> medical procedures (E873.2-E873.3)
> use of radiation in war operations
> (E996-E997.9)

E926.0 Radiofrequency radiation
> Overexposure to:
> microwave radiation from:
>> high-powered radio and television
>> transmitters
>> industrial radiofrequency induction
>> heaters
>> radar installations
> radar radiation from:
>> high-powered radio and television
>> transmitters
>> industrial radiofrequency induction
>> heaters
>> radar installations
> radiofrequency from:
>> high-powered radio and television
>> transmitters
>> industrial radiofrequency induction
>> heaters
>> radar installations
> radiofrequency radiation [any] from:
>> high-powered radio and television
>> transmitters
>> industrial radiofrequency induction
>> heaters
>> radar installations

E926.1 Infra-red heaters and lamps
> Exposure to infra-red radiation from heaters
> and lamps as the cause of:
> blistering   charring
> burning   inflammatory change
>
> | Excludes | physical contact with heater or lamp
> (E924.8)

E926.2 Visible and ultraviolet light sources 🌕
> Arc lamps
> Black light sources
> Electrical welding arc
> Oxygas welding torch
> Sun rays
> Tanning bed
>
> | Excludes | excessive heat from these sources
> (E900.1-E900.9)
>
> Coding Clinic: 1996, Q3, P6

**E926.3 X-rays and other electromagnetic ionizing
radiation**
> Gamma rays
> X-rays (hard) (soft)

E926.4 Lasers

E926.5 Radioactive isotopes
> Radiobiologicals
> Radiopharmaceuticals

E926.8 Other specified radiation
> Artificially accelerated beams of ionized
> particles generated by:
> betatrons
> synchrotrons

E926.9 Unspecified radiation
> Radiation NOS

● **E927 Overexertion and strenuous and repetitive
movements or loads**

> Use additional code to identify activity (E001-E030) ◄
> Coding Clinic: 2008, Q3, P21

**E927.0 Overexertion from sudden strenuous
movement**
> Sudden trauma from strenuous movement

E927.1 Overexertion from prolonged static position
> Overexertion from maintaining prolonged
> positions, such as:
> holding
> sitting
> standing

**E927.2 Excessive physical exertion from prolonged
activity**

E927.3 Cumulative trauma from repetitive motion
> Cumulative trauma from repetitive
> movements

E927.4 Cumulative trauma from repetitive impact

**E927.8 Other overexertion and strenuous and
repetitive movements or loads**

**E927.9 Unspecified overexertion and strenuous and
repetitive movements or loads**

● **E928 Other and unspecified environmental and accidental
causes**

E928.0 Prolonged stay in weightless environment 🌕
> Weightlessness in spacecraft (simulator)

E928.1 Exposure to noise 🌕
> Noise (pollution)
> Sound waves
> Supersonic waves

E928.2 Vibration 🌕

E928.3 Human bite 🌕

E928.4 External constriction caused by hair 🌕

E928.5 External constriction caused by other object 🌕

E928.6 Environmental exposure to harmful algae 🌕
and toxins
> Algae bloom NOS
> Blue-green algae bloom
> Brown tide
> Cyanobacteria bloom
> Florida red tide
> Harmful algae bloom
> Pfiesteria piscicida
> Red tide
> Coding Clinic: 2007, Q4, P101-102

E928.7 Mechanism or component of firearm and 🌕 ◄
air gun 🌕 ◄
> Injury due to: ◄
> explosion of gun parts ◄
> recoil ◄
> Pierced, cut, crushed, or pinched by slide
> trigger mechanism, scope or other gun
> part ◄
> Powder burn from firearm or air gun ◄
>
> | Excludes | accident caused by firearm and air
> gun missile (E922.0-E922.9) ◄

N Newborn Age: 0   **P** Pediatric Age: 0–17   **M** Maternity Age: 12–55   **A** Adult Age: 15–124   ♀ Females Only   ♂ Males Only   **1191**

(Ex) CC Exclusions   🌕 Complication\Comorbidity   🌕 Major C\C   🌕 Present on Admission Requirement   🌕 Hospital-Acquired Condition

E000-E999

E928.8 Other 🔍

E928.9 Unspecified accident

Accident NOS stated as accidentally inflicted
Blow NOS stated as accidentally inflicted
Casualty (not due to war) stated as
  accidentally inflicted
Decapitation stated as accidentally inflicted
Injury [any part of body, or unspecified]
  stated as accidentally inflicted, but not
  otherwise specified
Killed stated as accidentally inflicted, but not
  otherwise specified
Knocked down stated as accidentally inflicted,
  but not otherwise specified
Mangled stated as accidentally inflicted, but
  not otherwise specified
Wound stated as accidentally inflicted, but not
  otherwise specified

Excludes *fracture, cause unspecified (E887)*
          injuries undetermined whether
          accidentally or purposely
          inflicted (E980.0-E989)

Coding Clinic: 1996, Q3, P7; 1985, Nov-Dec, P15; 1984,
Nov-Dec, P15

LATE EFFECTS OF ACCIDENTAL INJURY (E929)

Note: This category is to be used to indicate accidental
injury as the cause of death or disability from late
effects, which are themselves classifiable elsewhere.
The "late effects" include conditions reported as
such or as sequelae, which may occur at any time
after the acute accidental injury.

● E929 Late effects of accidental injury

Excludes *late effects of:*
          surgical and medical procedures
          (E870.0-E879.9)
          therapeutic use of drugs and medicines
          (E930.0-E949.9)

E929.0 Late effects of motor vehicle accident 🔍
Late effects of accidents classifiable to
  E810-E825
Coding Clinic: 2008, Q4, P102-109; 1997, Q3, P12-13; 1995,
Q1, P10; 1994, Q3, P4

E929.1 Late effects of other transport accident 🔍
Late effects of accidents classifiable to
  E800-E807, E826-E838, E840-E848

E929.2 Late effects of accidental poisoning 🔍
Late effects of accidents classifiable to
  E850-E858, E860-E869

E929.3 Late effects of accidental fall 🔍
Late effects of accidents classifiable to
  E880-E888

E929.4 Late effects of accident caused by fire 🔍
Late effects of accidents classifiable to
  E890-E899

E929.5 Late effects of accident due to natural and
environmental factors 🔍
Late effects of accidents classifiable to
  E900-E909

E929.8 Late effects of other accidents 🔍
Late effects of accidents classifiable to
  E910-E928.8

E929.9 Late effects of unspecified accident 🔍
Late effects of accidents classifiable to E928.9

OGCR Section I.C.17.e.1

Adverse Effect: When the drug was correctly
prescribed and properly administered, code
the reaction plus the appropriate code from the
E930-E949 series. Codes from the E930-E949 series
must be used to identify the causative substance for
an adverse effect of drug, medicinal and biological
substances, correctly prescribed and properly
administered. The effect, such as tachycardia,
delirium, gastrointestinal hemorrhaging, vomiting,
hypokalemia, hepatitis, renal failure, or respiratory
failure, is coded and followed by the appropriate
code from the E930-E949 series.

DRUGS, MEDICINAL AND BIOLOGICAL SUBSTANCES CAUSING ADVERSE EFFECTS IN THERAPEUTIC USE (E930-E949)

Includes   correct drug properly administered in
           therapeutic or prophylactic dosage,
           as the cause of any adverse effect
           including allergic or hypersensitivity
           reactions

Excludes   *accidental overdose of drug and wrong drug*
           given or taken in error (E850.0-E858.9)
           accidents in the technique of administration
           of drug or biological substance such as
           accidental puncture during injection, or
           contamination of drug (E870.0-E876.9)
           administration with suicidal or homicidal
           intent or intent to harm, or in
           circumstances classifiable to
           E980-E989 (E950.0-E950.5,
           E962.0, E980.0-E980.5) ◀▥

*See Alphabetic Index for more complete list of specific drugs
to be classified under the fourth-digit subdivisions.
The American Hospital Formulary numbers can be
used to classify new drugs listed by the American
Hospital Formulary Service (AHFS). See appendix C.*

● E930 Antibiotics

Excludes   *that used as eye, ear, nose, and throat [ENT],*
           and local anti-infectives (E946.0-E946.9)

Coding Clinic: 2008, Q3, P21

E930.0 Penicillins
Natural
Synthetic
Semisynthetic, such as:
  ampicillin
  cloxacillin
  nafcillin
  oxacillin
Coding Clinic: 2008, Q4, P128-131

E930.1 Antifungal antibiotics
Amphotericin B
Griseofulvin
Hachimycin [trichomycin]
Nystatin

E930.2 Chloramphenicol group
Chloramphenicol
Thiamphenicol

E930.3 Erythromycin and other macrolides
Oleandomycin
Spiramycin

◀ New   ◀▥ Revised   ~~deleted~~ Deleted   ● Unacceptable Principal Diagnosis   ● Use Additional Digit(s)
▶ Manifestation Code   OGCR Official Guidelines   Coding Clinic   Excludes   Includes   Use additional   Code first   Omit code

E930.4 Tetracycline group
Doxycycline
Minocycline
Oxytetracycline
Coding Clinic: 1988, Q2, P9-10

E930.5 Cephalosporin group
Cephalexin
Cephaloglycin
Cephaloridine
Cephalothin

E930.6 Antimycobacterial antibiotics
Cycloserine
Kanamycin
Rifampin
Streptomycin

E930.7 Antineoplastic antibiotics
Actinomycins, such as:
bleomycin
cactinomycin
dactinomycin
daunorubicin
mitomycin

Excludes *other antineoplastic drugs (E933.1)*

Coding Clinic: 2007, Q2, P9-10

E930.8 Other specified antibiotics
Coding Clinic: 1993, Q1, P29

E930.9 Unspecified antibiotic

● **E931 Other anti-infectives**

Excludes *ENT, and local anti-infectives (E946.0-E946.9)*

E931.0 Sulfonamides
Sulfadiazine
Sulfafurazole
Sulfamethoxazole

E931.1 Arsenical anti-infectives

E931.2 Heavy metal anti-infectives
Compounds of:
antimony
bismuth
lead
mercury

Excludes *mercurial diuretics (E944.0)*

E931.3 Quinoline and hydroxyquinoline derivatives
Chiniofon
Diiodohydroxyquin

Excludes *antimalarial drugs (E931.4)*

E931.4 Antimalarials and drugs acting on other blood protozoa
Chloroquine phosphate
Cycloguanil
Primaquine
Proguanil [chloroguanide]
Pyrimethamine
Quinine (sulphate)

E931.5 Other antiprotozoal drugs
Emetine

E931.6 Anthelmintics
Hexylresorcinol
Male fern oleoresin
Piperazine
Thiabendazole

E931.7 Antiviral drugs
Methisazone

Excludes *amantadine (E936.4)*
cytarabine (E933.1)
idoxuridine (E946.5)

E931.8 Other antimycobacterial drugs
Ethambutol
Ethionamide
Isoniazid
Para-aminosalicylic acid derivatives
Sulfones

E931.9 Other and unspecified anti-infectives
Flucytosine
Nitrofuran derivatives

● **E932 Hormones and synthetic substitutes**

E932.0 Adrenal cortical steroids
Cortisone derivatives
Desoxycorticosterone derivatives
Fluorinated corticosteroids
Coding Clinic: 2008, Q4, P91-95; 2003, Q4, P108-109; 2000, Q3, P4-5

E932.1 Androgens and anabolic congeners
Nandrolone phenpropionate
Oxymetholone
Testosterone and preparations
Coding Clinic: 1985, July-Aug, P8

E932.2 Ovarian hormones and synthetic substitutes
Contraceptives, oral
Estrogens
Estrogens and progestogens combined
Progestogens

E932.3 Insulins and antidiabetic agents
Acetohexamide
Biguanide derivatives, oral
Chlorpropamide
Glucagon
Insulin
Phenformin
Sulfonylurea derivatives, oral
Tolbutamide

Excludes *adverse effect of insulin administered for shock therapy (E879.3)*

E932.4 Anterior pituitary hormones
Corticotropin
Gonadotropin
Somatotropin [growth hormone]
Coding Clinic: 1995, Q3, P15

E932.5 Posterior pituitary hormones
Vasopressin

Excludes *oxytocic agents (E945.0)*

E932.6 Parathyroid and parathyroid derivatives

E932.7 Thyroid and thyroid derivatives
Dextrothyroxine
Levothyroxine sodium
Liothyronine
Thyroglobulin

N Newborn Age: 0   **P** Pediatric Age: 0–17   **M** Maternity Age: 12–55   **A** Adult Age: 15–124   ♀ Females Only   ♂ Males Only .
(Ex) CC Exclusions   🅒 Complication\Comorbidity   🅜 Major C\C   Present on Admission Requirement   Hospital-Acquired Condition   1193

E000-E999

E932.8 Antithyroid agents
Iodides
Thiouracil
Thiourea

E932.9 Other and unspecified hormones and synthetic substitutes

● **E933 Primarily systemic agents**

E933.0 Antiallergic and antiemetic drugs
Antihistamines
Chlorpheniramine
Diphenhydramine
Diphenylpyraline
Thonzylamine
Tripelennamine

> **Excludes** phenothiazine-based tranquilizers (E939.1)
> **Coding Clinic:** 1997, Q2, P9-10

E933.1 Antineoplastic and immunosuppressive drugs
Azathioprine
Busulfan
Chlorambucil
Cyclophosphamide
Cytarabine
Fluorouracil
Mechlorethamine hydrochloride
Mercaptopurine
Triethylenethiophosphoramide [thio-TEPA]

> **Excludes** antineoplastic antibiotics (E930.7)
> **Coding Clinic:** 2008, Q2, P6, 10-11; 2006, Q4, P69-73; Q2, P20; 2005, Q3, P11-12; 1999, Q3, P6-7; Q2, P9; 1996, Q2, P12; 1985, Mar-April, P14

E933.2 Acidifying agents

E933.3 Alkalizing agents

E933.4 Enzymes, not elsewhere classified
Penicillinase

E933.5 Vitamins, not elsewhere classified
Vitamin A
Vitamin D

> **Excludes** nicotinic acid (E942.2)
>   vitamin K (E934.3)

E933.6 Oral bisphosphonates
Coding Clinic: 2007, Q4, P91-92, 102

E933.7 Intravenous bisphosphonates
Coding Clinic: 2007, Q4, P102

E933.8 Other systemic agents, not elsewhere classified
Heavy metal antagonists

E933.9 Unspecified systemic agent

● **E934 Agents primarily affecting blood constituents**
Coding Clinic: 1993, 5th Issue, P16

E934.0 Iron and its compounds
Ferric salts
Ferrous sulphate and other ferrous salts

E934.1 Liver preparations and other antianemic agents
Folic acid

E934.2 Anticoagulants
Coumarin
Heparin
Phenindione
Prothrombin synthesis inhibitor
Warfarin sodium
Coding Clinic: 2008, Q4, P134-136; 2006, Q3, P12-13; Q2, P17; 2004, Q3, P7; 1994, Q1, P22; 1990, Q3, P14

E934.3 Vitamin K [phytonadione]

E934.4 Fibrinolysis-affecting drugs
Aminocaproic acid
Streptodornase
Streptokinase
Urokinase

E934.5 Anticoagulant antagonists and other coagulants
Hexadimethrine bromide
Protamine sulfate

E934.6 Gamma globulin

E934.7 Natural blood and blood products
Blood plasma
Human fibrinogen
Packed red cells
Whole blood
Coding Clinic: 2006, Q4, P91-92; 2000, Q3, P9; 1997, Q2, P11

E934.8 Other agents affecting blood constituents
Macromolecular blood substitutes

E934.9 Unspecified agent affecting blood constituents

● **E935 Analgesics, antipyretics, and antirheumatics**

E935.0 Heroin
Diacetylmorphine

E935.1 Methadone

E935.2 Other opiates and related narcotics
Codeine [methylmorphine]
Morphine
Opium (alkaloids)
Meperidine [pethidine]

E935.3 Salicylates
Acetylsalicylic acid [aspirin]
Amino derivatives of salicylic acid
Salicylic acid salts
Coding Clinic: 1984, Nov-Dec, P15

E935.4 Aromatic analgesics, not elsewhere classified
Acetanilid
Paracetamol [acetaminophen]
Phenacetin [acetophenetidin]

E935.5 Pyrazole derivatives
Aminophenazone [aminopyrine]
Phenylbutazone
Coding Clinic: 1990, Q4, P26

E935.6 Antirheumatics [antiphlogistics]
Gold salts
Indomethacin

> **Excludes** salicylates (E935.3)
>   steroids (E932.0)

E935.7 Other non-narcotic analgesics
Pyrabital

E935.8 Other specified analgesics and antipyretics
Pentazocine
Coding Clinic: 1992, Q3, P16-17

E935.9 Unspecified analgesic and antipyretic

● **E936 Anticonvulsants and anti-Parkinsonism drugs**

E936.0 Oxazolidine derivatives
Paramethadione
Trimethadione

E936.1 Hydantoin derivatives
Phenytoin

E936.2 Succinimides
Ethosuximide
Phensuximide

E936.3 Other and unspecified anticonvulsants
Beclamide
Primidone

E936.4 Anti-Parkinsonism drugs
Amantadine
Ethopropazine [profenamine]
Levodopa [L-dopa]

● **E937 Sedatives and hypnotics**

E937.0 Barbiturates
Amobarbital [amylobarbitone]
Barbital [barbitone]
Butabarbital [butabarbitone]
Pentobarbital [pentobarbitone]
Phenobarbital [phenobarbitone]
Secobarbital [quinalbarbitone]
Excludes *thiobarbiturates (E938.3)*

E937.1 Chloral hydrate group

E937.2 Paraldehyde

E937.3 Bromine compounds
Bromide
Carbromal (derivatives)

E937.4 Methaqualone compounds

E937.5 Glutethimide group

E937.6 Mixed sedatives, not elsewhere classified

E937.8 Other sedatives and hypnotics

E937.9 Unspecified
Sleeping:
    drug NOS
    pill NOS
    tablet NOS

● **E938 Other central nervous system depressants and anesthetics**

E938.0 Central nervous system muscle-tone depressants
Chlorphenesin (carbamate)
Mephenesin
Methocarbamol

E938.1 Halothane

E938.2 Other gaseous anesthetics
Ether
Halogenated hydrocarbon derivatives, except halothane
Nitrous oxide

E938.3 Intravenous anesthetics
Ketamine
Methohexital [methohexitone]
Thiobarbiturates, such as thiopental sodium

E938.4 Other and unspecified general anesthetics

E938.5 Surface and infiltration anesthetics
Cocaine
Lidocaine [lignocaine]
Procaine
Tetracaine

E938.6 Peripheral nerve- and plexus-blocking anesthetics

E938.7 Spinal anesthetics
Coding Clinic: 2004, Q2, P18; 2003, Q3, P12; 1987, Jan-Feb, P13-14

E938.9 Other and unspecified local anesthetics

● **E939 Psychotropic agents**

E939.0 Antidepressants
Amitriptyline
Imipramine
Monoamine oxidase [MAO] inhibitors
Coding Clinic: 2003, Q4, P75-76; 1992, Q3, P16

E939.1 Phenothiazine-based tranquilizers
Chlorpromazine   Prochlorperazine
Fluphenazine   Promazine
Phenothiazine

E939.2 Butyrophenone-based tranquilizers
Haloperidol
Spiperone
Trifluperidol

E939.3 Other antipsychotics, neuroleptics, and major tranquilizers
Coding Clinic: 2006, Q4, P76-78

E939.4 Benzodiazepine-based tranquilizers
Chlordiazepoxide   Lorazepam
Diazepam   Medazepam
Flurazepam   Nitrazepam

E939.5 Other tranquilizers
Hydroxyzine
Meprobamate

E939.6 Psychodysleptics [hallucinogens]
Cannabis (derivatives)
Lysergide [LSD]
Marihuana (derivatives)
Mescaline
Psilocin
Psilocybin

E939.7 Psychostimulants
Amphetamine
Caffeine
Excludes *central appetite depressants (E947.0)*

E939.8 Other psychotropic agents

E939.9 Unspecified psychotropic agent

● **E940 Central nervous system stimulants**

E940.0 Analeptics
Lobeline
Nikethamide

E940.1 Opiate antagonists
Levallorphan
Nalorphine
Naloxone

E940.8 Other specified central nervous system stimulants

E940.9 Unspecified central nervous system stimulant

● **E941 Drugs primarily affecting the autonomic nervous system**

E941.0 Parasympathomimetics [cholinergics]
Acetylcholine
Anticholinesterase:
    organophosphorus
    reversible
Pilocarpine

E941.1 Parasympatholytics [anticholinergics and antimuscarinics] and spasmolytics
Atropine
Homatropine
Hyoscine [scopolamine]
Quaternary ammonium derivatives
Excludes *papaverine (E942.5)*

N Newborn Age: 0   P Pediatric Age: 0–17   M Maternity Age: 12–55   A Adult Age: 15–124   ♀ Females Only   ♂ Males Only
Ⓔⓧ CC Exclusions   Complication\Comorbidity   Major C\C   Present on Admission Requirement   Hospital-Acquired Condition   1195

E000-E999

E941.2　Sympathomimetics [adrenergics]
　　Epinephrine [adrenalin]
　　Levarterenol [noradrenalin]
　　Coding Clinic: 2002, Q3, P12

E941.3　Sympatholytics [antiadrenergics]
　　Phenoxybenzamine
　　Tolazoline hydrochloride
　　Coding Clinic: 2007, Q4, P77-79

E941.9　Unspecified drug primarily affecting the autonomic nervous system

● **E942　Agents primarily affecting the cardiovascular system**

E942.0　Cardiac rhythm regulators
　　Practolol
　　Procainamide
　　Propranolol
　　Quinidine
　　Coding Clinic: 1986, Mar-April, P11-12

E942.1　Cardiotonic glycosides and drugs of similar action
　　Digitalis glycosides
　　Digoxin
　　Strophanthins

E942.2　Antilipemic and antiarteriosclerotic drugs
　　Cholestyramine
　　Clofibrate
　　Nicotinic acid derivatives
　　Sitosterols
　　　Excludes　*dextrothyroxine (E932.7)*

E942.3　Ganglion-blocking agents
　　Pentamethonium bromide

E942.4　Coronary vasodilators
　　Dipyridamole
　　Nitrates [nitroglycerin]
　　Nitrites
　　Prenylamine

E942.5　Other vasodilators
　　Cyclandelate
　　Diazoxide
　　Hydralazine
　　Papaverine

E942.6　Other antihypertensive agents
　　Clonidine
　　Guanethidine
　　Rauwolfia alkaloids
　　Reserpine

E942.7　Antivaricose drugs, including sclerosing agents
　　Monoethanolamine
　　Zinc salts

E942.8　Capillary-active drugs
　　Adrenochrome derivatives
　　Bioflavonoids
　　Metaraminol

E942.9　Other and unspecified agents primarily affecting the cardiovascular system

● **E943　Agents primarily affecting gastrointestinal system**

E943.0　Antacids and antigastric secretion drugs
　　Aluminum hydroxide
　　Magnesium trisilicate

E943.1　Irritant cathartics
　　Bisacodyl
　　Castor oil
　　Phenolphthalein

E943.2　Emollient cathartics
　　Sodium dioctyl sulfosuccinate

E943.3　Other cathartics, including intestinal atonia drugs
　　Magnesium sulfate

E943.4　Digestants
　　Pancreatin
　　Papain
　　Pepsin

E943.5　Antidiarrheal drugs
　　Bismuth subcarbonate
　　Kaolin
　　Pectin
　　　Excludes　*anti-infectives (E930.0-E931.9)*

E943.6　Emetics

E943.8　Other specified agents primarily affecting the gastrointestinal system

E943.9　Unspecified agent primarily affecting the gastrointestinal system

● **E944　Water, mineral, and uric acid metabolism drugs**

E944.0　Mercurial diuretics
　　Chlormerodrin
　　Mercaptomerin
　　Mercurophylline
　　Mersalyl

E944.1　Purine derivative diuretics
　　Theobromine
　　Theophylline
　　　Excludes　*aminophylline [theophylline ethylenediamine] (E945.7)*

E944.2　Carbonic acid anhydrase inhibitors
　　Acetazolamide

E944.3　Saluretics
　　Benzothiadiazides
　　Chlorothiazide group

E944.4　Other diuretics
　　Ethacrynic acid
　　Furosemide

E944.5　Electrolytic, caloric, and water-balance agents

E944.6　Other mineral salts, not elsewhere classified

E944.7　Uric acid metabolism drugs
　　Cinchophen and congeners
　　Colchicine
　　Phenoquin
　　Probenecid

● **E945　Agents primarily acting on the smooth and skeletal muscles and respiratory system**

E945.0　Oxytocic agents
　　Ergot alkaloids
　　Prostaglandins

E945.1　Smooth muscle relaxants
　　Adiphenine
　　Metaproterenol [orciprenaline]
　　　Excludes　*papaverine (E942.5)*

◀ New　　⬅ Revised　　~~deleted~~ Deleted　　● Unacceptable Principal Diagnosis　　● Use Additional Digit(s)
▶ Manifestation Code　　**OGCR** Official Guidelines　　**Coding Clinic**　　Excludes　　Includes　　Use additional　　Code first　　Omit code

E000-E999

E945.2 Skeletal muscle relaxants
Alcuronium chloride
Suxamethonium chloride

E945.3 Other and unspecified drugs acting on muscles

E945.4 Antitussives
Dextromethorphan
Pipazethate hydrochloride

E945.5 Expectorants
Acetylcysteine
Cocillana
Guaifenesin [glyceryl guaiacolate]
Ipecacuanha
Terpin hydrate

E945.6 Anti-common cold drugs

E945.7 Antiasthmatics
Aminophylline [theophylline ethylenediamine]

E945.8 Other and unspecified respiratory drugs

● **E946 Agents primarily affecting skin and mucous membrane, ophthalmological, otorhinolaryngological, and dental drugs**

E946.0 Local anti-infectives and anti-inflammatory drugs

E946.1 Antipruritics

E946.2 Local astringents and local detergents

E946.3 Emollients, demulcents, and protectants

E946.4 Keratolytics, keratoplastics, other hair treatment drugs and preparations

E946.5 Eye anti-infectives and other eye drugs
Idoxuridine

E946.6 Anti-infectives and other drugs and preparations for ear, nose, and throat

E946.7 Dental drugs topically applied

E946.8 Other agents primarily affecting skin and mucous membrane
Spermicides

E946.9 Unspecified agent primarily affecting skin and mucous membrane

● **E947 Other and unspecified drugs and medicinal substances**

E947.0 Dietetics

E947.1 Lipotropic drugs

E947.2 Antidotes and chelating agents, not elsewhere classified

E947.3 Alcohol deterrents

E947.4 Pharmaceutical excipients

E947.8 Other drugs and medicinal substances
Contrast media used for diagnostic x-ray procedures
Diagnostic agents and kits

E947.9 Unspecified drug or medicinal substance

● **E948 Bacterial vaccines**

E948.0 BCG vaccine

E948.1 Typhoid and paratyphoid

E948.2 Cholera

E948.3 Plague

E948.4 Tetanus

E948.5 Diphtheria

E948.6 Pertussis vaccine, including combinations with a pertussis component

E948.8 Other and unspecified bacterial vaccines

E948.9 Mixed bacterial vaccines, except combinations with a pertussis component

● **E949 Other vaccines and biological substances**

Excludes	*gamma globulin (E934.6)*

Coding Clinic: 2008, Q3, P21

E949.0 Smallpox vaccine

E949.1 Rabies vaccine

E949.2 Typhus vaccine

E949.3 Yellow fever vaccine

E949.4 Measles vaccine

E949.5 Poliomyelitis vaccine

E949.6 Other and unspecified viral and rickettsial vaccines
Mumps vaccine

E949.7 Mixed viral-rickettsial and bacterial vaccines, except combinations with a pertussis component

Excludes	*combinations with a pertussis component (E948.6)*

E949.9 Other and unspecified vaccines and biological substances

---

SUICIDE AND SELF-INFLICTED INJURY (E950-E959)

Includes	injuries in suicide and attempted suicide self-inflicted injuries specified as intentional

● **E950 Suicide and self-inflicted poisoning by solid or liquid substances**

E950.0 Analgesics, antipyretics, and antirheumatics
Coding Clinic: 1998, Q4, P50-51

E950.1 Barbiturates

E950.2 Other sedatives and hypnotics

E950.3 Tranquilizers and other psychotropic agents

E950.4 Other specified drugs and medicinal substances

E950.5 Unspecified drug or medicinal substance

E950.6 Agricultural and horticultural chemical and pharmaceutical preparations other than plant foods and fertilizers

E950.7 Corrosive and caustic substances
Suicide and self-inflicted poisoning by substances classifiable to E864

E950.8 Arsenic and its compounds

E950.9 Other and unspecified solid and liquid substances

● **E951 Suicide and self-inflicted poisoning by gases in domestic use**

E951.0 Gas distributed by pipeline

E951.1 Liquefied petroleum gas distributed in mobile containers

E951.8 Other utility gas

● **E952 Suicide and self-inflicted poisoning by other gases and vapors**

E952.0 Motor vehicle exhaust gas

E952.1 Other carbon monoxide

E952.8 Other specified gases and vapors

E952.9 Unspecified gases and vapors

N Newborn Age: 0   **P** Pediatric Age: 0–17   **M** Maternity Age: 12–55   **A** Adult Age: 15–124   ♀ Females Only   ♂ Males Only

(Ex) CC Exclusions   ● Complication\Comorbidity   ● Major C\C   ● Present on Admission Requirement   ● Hospital-Acquired Condition   **1197**

E000-E999

● **E953**   **Suicide and self-inflicted injury by hanging, strangulation, and suffocation**

    E953.0   **Hanging**

    E953.1   **Suffocation by plastic bag**

    E953.8   **Other specified means**

    E953.9   **Unspecified means**

E954   **Suicide and self-inflicted injury by submersion [drowning]**

● **E955**   **Suicide and self-inflicted injury by firearms, air guns and explosives**

    E955.0   **Handgun**

    E955.1   **Shotgun**

    E955.2   **Hunting rifle**

    E955.3   **Military firearms**

    E955.4   **Other and unspecified firearm**
         Gunshot NOS
         Shot NOS

    E955.5   **Explosives**

    E955.6   **Air gun**
         BB gun
         Pellet gun

    E955.7   **Paintball gun**

    E955.9   **Unspecified**

E956   **Suicide and self-inflicted injury by cutting and piercing instrument**

● **E957**   **Suicide and self-inflicted injuries by jumping from high place**

    E957.0   **Residential premises**

    E957.1   **Other man-made structures**

    E957.2   **Natural sites**

    E957.9   **Unspecified**

● **E958**   **Suicide and self-inflicted injury by other and unspecified means**

    E958.0   **Jumping or lying before moving object**

    E958.1   **Burns, fire**

    E958.2   **Scald**

    E958.3   **Extremes of cold**

    E958.4   **Electrocution**

    E958.5   **Crashing of motor vehicle**

    E958.6   **Crashing of aircraft**

    E958.7   **Caustic substances, except poisoning**

       | **Excludes** | *poisoning by caustic substance (E950.7)*

    E958.8   **Other specified means**

    E958.9   **Unspecified means**

E959   **Late effects of self-inflicted injury** ✎

    Note: This category is to be used to indicate circumstances classifiable to E950-E958 as the cause of death or disability from late effects, which are themselves classifiable elsewhere. The "late effects" include conditions reported as such or as sequelae which may occur at any time after the attempted suicide or self-inflicted injury.

OGCR   Section I.C.19.e

When the cause of an injury or neglect is intentional child or adult abuse, the first listed E code should be assigned from categories E960-E968, Homicide and injury purposely inflicted by other persons, (except category E967). An E code from category E967, Child and adult battering and other maltreatment, should be added as an additional code to identify the perpetrator, if known.

HOMICIDE AND INJURY PURPOSELY INFLICTED BY OTHER PERSONS (E960-E969)

| Includes | injuries inflicted by another person with intent to injure or kill, by any means

| Excludes | *injuries due to:*
       legal intervention (E970-E978)
       operations of war (E990-E999)
       terrorism (E979)

● **E960**   **Fight, brawl, rape**

    E960.0   **Unarmed fight or brawl**
         Beatings NOS
         Brawl or fight with hands, fists, feet
         Injured or killed in fight NOS

       | **Excludes** | *homicidal:*
         injury by weapons (E965.0-E966, E969)
         strangulation (E963)
         submersion (E964)

    E960.1   **Rape**
       Coding Clinic: 1999, Q3, P15

E961   **Assault by corrosive or caustic substance, except poisoning**
    Injury or death purposely caused by corrosive or caustic substance, such as:
    acid [any]
    corrosive substance
    vitriol

    | **Excludes** | *burns from hot liquid (E968.3)*
       chemical burns from swallowing a corrosive substance (E962.0-E962.9)

● **E962**   **Assault by poisoning**

    E962.0   **Drugs and medicinal substances**
         Homicidal poisoning by any drug or medicinal substance

    E962.1   **Other solid and liquid substances**

    E962.2   **Other gases and vapors**

    E962.9   **Unspecified poisoning**

E963   **Assault by hanging and strangulation**
    Homicidal (attempt):
       garrotting or ligature
       hanging
       strangulation
       suffocation

E964   **Assault by submersion [drowning]**

● **E965**   **Assault by firearms and explosives**

    E965.0   **Handgun**
         Pistol
         Revolver

    E965.1   **Shotgun**

    E965.2   **Hunting rifle**

E965.3   Military firearms

E965.4   Other and unspecified firearm

E965.5   Antipersonnel bomb

E965.6   Gasoline bomb

E965.7   Letter bomb

E965.8   Other specified explosive
     Bomb NOS (placed in):
         car
         house
     Dynamite

E965.9   Unspecified explosive

E966   Assault by cutting and piercing instrument
     Assassination (attempt), homicide (attempt) by any
         instrument classifiable under E920
     Homicidal:
         cut any part of body
         puncture any part of body
         stab any part of body
     Stabbed any part of body
     Coding Clinic: 1993, Q2, P4-5

● **E967   Perpetrator of child and adult abuse**
     Note: selection of the correct perpetrator code
         is based on the relationship between the
         perpetrator and the victim.

E967.0   By father, stepfather, or boyfriend
     Male partner of child's parent or guardian

E967.1   By other specified person
     Coding Clinic: 1999, Q3, P14-15

E967.2   By mother, stepmother, or girlfriend
     Female partner of child's parent or guardian
     Coding Clinic: 1996, Q4, P43-44

E967.3   By spouse or partner
     Abuse of spouse or partner by ex-spouse or
         ex-partner
     Coding Clinic: 1996, Q4, P43-44

E967.4   By child

E967.5   By sibling

E967.6   By grandparent

E967.7   By other relative

E967.8   By non-related caregiver

E967.9   By unspecified person

● **E968   Assault by other and unspecified means**

E968.0   Fire
     Arson
     Homicidal burns NOS
     | **Excludes** | *burns from hot liquid (E968.3)* |

E968.1   Pushing from a high place

E968.2   Striking by blunt or thrown object
     Coding Clinic: 1996, Q4, P43-44

E968.3   Hot liquid
     Homicidal burns by scalding

E968.4   Criminal neglect
     Abandonment of child, infant, or other
         helpless person with intent to injure or
         kill

E968.5   Transport vehicle
     Being struck by other vehicle or run down
         with intent to injure
     Pushed in front of, thrown from, or dragged
         by moving vehicle with intent to injure

E968.6   Air gun
     BB gun
     Pellet gun

E968.7   Human bite

E968.8   Other specified means
     Coding Clinic: 1999, Q3, P14-15x2

E968.9   Unspecified means
     Assassination (attempt) NOS
     Homicidal (attempt):
         injury NOS
         wound NOS
     Manslaughter (nonaccidental)
     Murder (attempt) NOS
     Violence, non-accidental

E969   Late effects of injury purposely inflicted by other person
     Note: This category is to be used to indicate
         circumstances classifiable to E960-E968 as the
         cause of death or disability from late effects,
         which are themselves classifiable elsewhere.
         The "late effects" include conditions reported
         as such, or as sequelae which may occur at
         any time after the injury purposely inflicted by
         another person.

LEGAL INTERVENTION (E970-E978)

| **Includes** | injuries inflicted by the police or other law-enforcing agents, including military on duty, in the course of arresting or attempting to arrest lawbreakers, suppressing disturbances, maintaining order, and other legal action |
| | legal execution |

| **Excludes** | *injuries caused by civil insurrections (E990.0-E999)* |

E970   Injury due to legal intervention by firearms 🔾
     Gunshot wound
     Injury by:
         machine gun
         revolver
         rifle pellet or rubber bullet
         shot NOS

E971   Injury due to legal intervention by explosives 🔾
     Injury by:
         dynamite
         explosive shell
         grenade
         motor bomb

E972   Injury due to legal intervention by gas 🔾
     Asphyxiation by gas
     Injury by tear gas
     Poisoning by gas

E973   Injury due to legal intervention by blunt object 🔾
     Hit, struck by:
         baton (nightstick)
         blunt object
         stave

E000-E999

N Newborn Age: 0   **P** Pediatric Age: 0–17   **M** Maternity Age: 12–55   **A** Adult Age: 15–124   ♀ Females Only   ♂ Males Only   **1199**

(Ex) CC Exclusions   🔾 Complication\Comorbidity   🔾 Major C\C   🔾 Present on Admission Requirement   🔾 Hospital-Acquired Condition

E974 Injury due to legal intervention by cutting and piercing instrument 🔖
>Cut
>Incised wound
>Injured by bayonet
>Stab wound

E975 Injury due to legal intervention by other specified means 🔖
>Blow
>Manhandling

E976 Injury due to legal intervention by unspecified means 🔖

E977 Late effects of injuries due to legal intervention 🔖

>**Note:** This category is to be used to indicate circumstances classifiable to E970-E976 as the cause of death or disability from late effects, which are themselves classifiable elsewhere. The "late effects" include conditions reported as such, or as sequelae which may occur at any time after the injury due to legal intervention.

E978 Legal execution 🔖
>All executions performed at the behest of the judiciary or ruling authority [whether permanent or temporary] as:
>asphyxiation by gas
>beheading, decapitation (by guillotine)
>capital punishment
>electrocution
>hanging
>poisoning
>shooting
>other specified means

>**OGCR** Section I.C.19.j.1-3
>>When the cause of an injury is identified by the Federal Government (FBI) as terrorism, the first-listed E-code should be a code from category E979, Terrorism. The definition of terrorism employed by the FBI is found at the inclusion note at E979. The terrorism E-code is the only E-code that should be assigned. Additional E codes from the assault categories should not be assigned.
>>
>>When the cause of an injury is suspected to be the result of terrorism a code from category E979 should not be assigned. Assign a code in the range of E codes based circumstances on the documentation of intent and mechanism.
>>
>>Assign code E979.9, Terrorism, secondary effects, for conditions occurring subsequent to the terrorist event. This code should not be assigned for conditions that are due to the initial terrorist act.

TERRORISM (E979)

● **E979 Terrorism**
>Injuries resulting from the unlawful use of force or violence against persons or property to intimidate or coerce a Government, the civilian population, or any segment thereof, in furtherance of political or social objective
>Coding Clinic: 2002, Q4, P74-77

E979.0 Terrorism involving explosion of marine weapons 🔖
>Depth-charge
>Marine mine
>>Mine NOS, at sea or in harbour
>Sea-based artillery shell
>Torpedo
>Underwater blast

E979.1 Terrorism involving destruction of aircraft 🔖
>Aircraft:
>>burned
>>exploded
>>shot down
>Aircraft used as a weapon
>Crushed by falling aircraft

E979.2 Terrorism involving other explosions and fragments 🔖
>Antipersonnel bomb (fragments)
>Blast NOS
>Explosion (of):
>>artillery shell
>>breech-block
>>cannon block
>>mortar bomb
>>munitions being used in terrorism
>>NOS
>Fragments from:
>>artillery shell
>>bomb
>>grenade
>>guided missile
>>land-mine
>>rocket
>>shell
>>shrapnel
>Mine NOS

E979.3 Terrorism involving fires, conflagration and hot substances 🔖
>Burning building or structure:
>>collapse of
>>fall from
>>hit by falling object in
>>jump from
>Conflagration NOS
>Fire (causing):
>>asphyxia
>>burns
>>NOS
>>other injury
>Melting of fittings and furniture in burning
>Petrol bomb
>Smouldering building or structure

E979.4 Terrorism involving firearms 🔖
>Bullet:
>>carbine
>>machine gun
>>pistol
>>rifle
>>rubber (rifle)
>Pellets (shotgun)

E979.5 Terrorism involving nuclear weapons 🔖
>Blast effects
>Exposure to ionizing radiation from nuclear weapon
>Fireball effects
>Heat from nuclear weapon
>Other direct and secondary effects of nuclear weapons

E979.6 Terrorism involving biological weapons 🔖
>Anthrax
>Cholera
>Smallpox

E979.7 Terrorism involving chemical weapons 🔖
>Gases, fumes, chemicals
>Hydrogen cyanide
>Phosgene
>Sarin

◀ New   ◀▥ Revised   ~~deleted~~ Deleted   ● Unacceptable Principal Diagnosis   ● Use Additional Digit(s)

▶ Manifestation Code   **OGCR** Official Guidelines   **Coding Clinic**   Excludes   Includes   Use additional   Code first   Omit code

E979.8 Terrorism involving other means 🔍
Drowning and submersion
Lasers
Piercing or stabbing instruments
Terrorism NOS

E979.9 Terrorism secondary effects 🔍

> **Note:** This code is for use to identify conditions occurring subsequent to a terrorist attack not those that are due to the initial terrorist attack

> **Excludes** *late effect of terrorist attack (E999.1)*

INJURY UNDETERMINED WHETHER ACCIDENTALLY OR PURPOSELY INFLICTED (E980-E989)

> **Note:** Categories E980-E989 are for use when it is unspecified or it cannot be determined whether the injuries are accidental (unintentional), suicide (attempted), or assault.

● **E980 Poisoning by solid or liquid substances, undetermined whether accidentally or purposely inflicted**

     E980.0 Analgesics, antipyretics, and antirheumatics

     E980.1 Barbiturates

     E980.2 Other sedatives and hypnotics

     E980.3 Tranquilizers and other psychotropic agents

     E980.4 Other specified drugs and medicinal substances

     E980.5 Unspecified drug or medicinal substance

     E980.6 Corrosive and caustic substances
         Poisoning, undetermined whether accidental or purposeful, by substances classifiable to E864

     E980.7 Agricultural and horticultural chemical and pharmaceutical preparations other than plant foods and fertilizers

     E980.8 Arsenic and its compounds

     E980.9 Other and unspecified solid and liquid substances

● **E981 Poisoning by gases in domestic use, undetermined whether accidentally or purposely inflicted**

     E981.0 Gas distributed by pipeline 🔍

     E981.1 Liquefied petroleum gas distributed in mobile containers 🔍

     E981.8 Other utility gas 🔍

● **E982 Poisoning by other gases, undetermined whether accidentally or purposely inflicted**

     E982.0 Motor vehicle exhaust gas 🔍

     E982.1 Other carbon monoxide 🔍

     E982.8 Other specified gases and vapors 🔍

     E982.9 Unspecified gases and vapors 🔍

● **E983 Hanging, strangulation, or suffocation, undetermined whether accidentally or purposely inflicted**

     E983.0 Hanging

     E983.1 Suffocation by plastic bag

     E983.8 Other specified means

     E983.9 Unspecified means

E984 Submersion [drowning], undetermined whether accidentally or purposely inflicted

● **E985 Injury by firearms, air guns and explosives, undetermined whether accidentally or purposely inflicted**

     E985.0 Handgun 🔍

     E985.1 Shotgun 🔍

     E985.2 Hunting rifle 🔍

     E985.3 Military firearms 🔍

     E985.4 Other and unspecified firearm 🔍

     E985.5 Explosives 🔍

     E985.6 Air gun 🔍
         BB gun
         Pellet gun

     E985.7 Paintball gun 🔍

E986 Injury by cutting and piercing instruments, undetermined whether accidentally or purposely inflicted

● **E987 Falling from high place, undetermined whether accidentally or purposely inflicted**

     E987.0 Residential premises 🔍

     E987.1 Other man-made structures

     E987.2 Natural sites 🔍

     E987.9 Unspecified site

● **E988 Injury by other and unspecified means, undetermined whether accidentally or purposely inflicted**

     E988.0 Jumping or lying before moving object

     E988.1 Burns, fire

     E988.2 Scald

     E988.3 Extremes of cold

     E988.4 Electrocution

     E988.5 Crashing of motor vehicle

     E988.6 Crashing of aircraft

     E988.7 Caustic substances, except poisoning

     E988.8 Other specified means

     E988.9 Unspecified means

E989 Late effects of injury, undetermined whether accidentally or purposely inflicted 🔍

> **Note:** This category is to be used to indicate circumstances classifiable to E980-E988 as the cause of death or disability from late effects, which are themselves classifiable elsewhere. The "late effects" include conditions reported as such or as sequelae which may occur at any time after injury, undetermined whether accidentally or purposely inflicted.

N Newborn Age: 0   **P** Pediatric Age: 0–17   **M** Maternity Age: 12–55   **A** Adult Age: 15–124   ♀ Females Only   ♂ Males Only

(Ex) CC Exclusions   🔍 Complication\Comorbidity   🔍 Major C\C   🔍 Present on Admission Requirement   🔍 Hospital-Acquired Condition

1201

E000-E999

INJURY RESULTING FROM OPERATIONS OF WAR (E990-E999)

Includes   injuries to military personnel and civilians caused by war and civil insurrections and occurring during the time of war and insurrection, and peacekeeping missions

Excludes   *accidents during training of military personnel, manufacture of war material and transport, unless attributable to enemy action*

● **E990   Injury due to war operations by fires and conflagrations**

Includes   asphyxia, burns, or other injury originating from fire caused by a fire-producing device or indirectly by any conventional weapon

E990.0   From gasoline bomb 🖐
     Incendiary bomb ◄

E990.1   From flamethrower 🖐 ◄

E990.2   From incendiary bullet 🖐 ◄

E990.3   From fire caused indirectly from conventional weapon 🖐 ◄

     Excludes   *fire aboard military aircraft (E994.3)* ◄

E990.9   From other and unspecified source 🖐

● **E991   Injury due to war operations by bullets and fragments**

Excludes   *injury due to bullets and fragments due to war operations, but occurring after cessation of hostilities (E998.0)* ◄
     injury due to explosion of artillery shells and mortars (E993.2) ◄
     injury due to explosion of improvised explosive device [IED] (E993.3-E993.5) ◄
     injury due to sea-based artillery shell (E992.3) ◄

E991.0   Rubber bullets (rifle) 🖐

E991.1   Pellets (rifle) 🖐

E991.2   Other bullets 🖐
     Bullet [any, except rubber bullets and pellets]
        carbine
        machine gun
        pistol
        rifle
        shotgun

E991.3   Antipersonnel bomb (fragments) 🖐

E991.4   Fragments from munitions 🖐 ◄
     Fragments from:
        artillery shell ◄
        bombs, except antipersonnel ◄
        detonation of unexploded ordnance [UXO] ◄
        grenade ◄
        guided missile ◄
        land mine ◄
        rockets ◄
        shell ◄

E991.5   Fragments from person-borne improvised explosive device [IED] 🖐 ◄

E991.6   Fragments from vehicle-borne improvised explosive device [IED] 🖐 ◄
     IED borne by land, air, or water transport vehicle ◄

E991.7   Fragments from other improvised explosive device [IED] ◄
     Roadside IED ◄

E991.8   Fragments from weapons 🖐 ◄
     Fragments from:
        artillery ◄
        autocannons ◄
        automatic grenade launchers ◄
        missile launchers ◄
        mortars ◄
        small arms ◄

E991.9   Other and unspecified fragments 🖐
     ~~Fragments from:~~
        ~~artillery shell~~
        ~~bombs, except antipersonnel~~
        ~~grenade~~
        ~~guided missile~~
        ~~land mine~~
        ~~rockets~~
        ~~shell~~
     Shrapnel NOS ◄

● **E992   Injury due to war operations by explosion of marine weapons** ◄
     ~~Depth charge~~
     ~~Marine mines~~
     ~~Mine NOS, at sea or in harbor~~
     ~~Sea-based artillery shell~~
     ~~Torpedo~~
     ~~Underwater blast~~

E992.0   Torpedo 🖐 ◄

E992.1   Depth charge 🖐 ◄

E992.2   Marine mines 🖐 ◄
     Marine mines at sea or in harbor ◄

E992.3   Sea-based artillery shell 🖐 ◄

E992.8   Other by other marine weapons 🖐 ◄

E992.9   Unspecified marine weapon 🖐 ◄
     Underwater blast NOS ◄

● **E993   Injury due to war operations by other explosion** ◄
     ~~Accidental explosion of munitions being used in war~~
     ~~Accidental explosion of own weapons~~
     ~~Air blast NOS~~
     ~~Blast NOS~~
     ~~Explosion NOS~~
     ~~Explosion of:~~
        ~~artillery shell~~
        ~~breech block~~
        ~~cannon block~~
        ~~mortar bomb~~
     ~~Injury by weapon burst~~
     Injuries due to direct or indirect pressure or air blast of an explosion occurring during war operations ◄

     Excludes   *injury due to fragments resulting from an explosion (E991.0-E991.9)* ◄
     injury due to detonation of unexploded ordnance but occurring after cessation of hostilities (E998.0-E998.9) ◄
     injury due to nuclear weapons (E996.0-E996.9) ◄

E993.0   Aerial bomb 🖐 ◄

E993.1   Guided missile 🖐 ◄

E993.2   Mortar 🖐 ◄
     Artillery shell ◄

◄ New   ◄▥ Revised   ~~deleted~~ Deleted   ● Unacceptable Principal Diagnosis   ● Use Additional Digit(s)

▶ Manifestation Code   **OGCR** Official Guidelines   **Coding Clinic**   Excludes   Includes   Use additional   Code first   Omit code

E000-E999

E993.3 Person-borne improvised explosive device [IED] ◀

E993.4 Vehicle-borne improvised explosive device [IED] ◀
    IED borne by land, air, or water transport vehicle ◀

E993.5 Other improvised explosive device [IED] ◀
    Roadside IED ◀

E993.6 Unintentional detonation of own munitions ◀
    Unintentional detonation of own ammunition (artillery) (mortars) ◀

E993.7 Unintentional discharge of own munitions launch device ◀
    Unintentional explosion of own: ◀
      autocannons ◀
      automatic grenade launchers ◀
      missile launchers ◀
      small arms ◀

E993.8 Other specified explosion ◀
    Bomb ◀
    Grenade ◀
    Land mine ◀

E993.9 Unspecified explosion ◀
    Air blast NOS ◀
    Blast NOS ◀
    Blast wave NOS ◀
    Blast wind NOS ◀
    Explosion NOS ◀

● **E994 Injury due to war operations by destruction of aircraft** ◀▥
    ~~Airplane:~~
      ~~burned~~
      ~~exploded~~
      ~~shot down~~
    ~~Crushed by falling airplane~~

E994.0 Destruction of aircraft due to enemy fire or explosives ◀
    Air to air missile ◀
    Explosive device placed on aircraft ◀
    Rocket propelled grenade [RPG] ◀
    Small arms fire ◀
    Surface to air missile ◀

E994.1 Unintentional destruction of aircraft due to own onboard explosives ◀

E994.2 Destruction of aircraft due to collision with other aircraft ◀

E994.3 Destruction of aircraft due to onboard fire ◀

E994.8 Other destruction of aircraft ◀

E994.9 Unspecified destruction of aircraft ◀

● **E995 Injury due to war operations by other and unspecified forms of conventional warfare** ◀▥
    ~~Battle wounds~~
    ~~Bayonet injury~~
    ~~Drowned in war operations~~

E995.0 Unarmed hand-to-hand combat ◀
    | **Excludes** | intentional restriction of airway (E995.3) ◀

E995.1 Struck by blunt object ◀
    Baton (nightstick) ◀
    Stave ◀

E995.2 Piercing object ◀
    Bayonet ◀
    Knife ◀
    Sword ◀

E995.3 Intentional restriction of air and airway ◀
    Intentional submersion ◀
    Strangulation ◀
    Suffocation ◀

E995.4 Unintentional drowning due to inability to surface or obtain air ◀
    Submersion ◀

E995.8 Other forms of conventional warfare ◀

E995.9 Unspecified form of conventional warfare ◀

● **E996 Injury due to war operations by nuclear weapons** ◀▥
    ~~Blast effects~~
    ~~Exposure to ionizing radiation from nuclear weapons~~
    ~~Fireball effects~~
    ~~Heat~~
    ~~Other direct and secondary effects of nuclear weapons~~
    Dirty bomb NOS ◀
    | **Excludes** | *late effects of injury due to nuclear weapons (E999.1, E999.0)* ◀

E996.0 Direct blast effect of nuclear weapon ◀
    Injury to bodily organs due to blast pressure ◀

E996.1 Indirect blast effect of nuclear weapon ◀
    Injury due to being thrown by blast ◀
    Injury due to being struck or crushed by blast debris ◀

E996.2 Thermal radiation effect of nuclear weapon ◀
    Burns due to thermal radiation ◀
    Fireball effects ◀
    Flash burns ◀
    Heat effects ◀

E996.3 Nuclear radiation effects ◀
    Acute radiation exposure ◀
    Beta burns ◀
    Fallout exposure ◀
    Radiation sickness ◀
    Secondary effects of nuclear weapons ◀

E996.8 Other effects of nuclear weapons ◀

E996.9 Unspecified effect of nuclear weapon ◀

● **E997 Injury due to war operations by other forms of unconventional warfare**

E997.0 Lasers

E997.1 Biological warfare

E997.2 Gases, fumes, and chemicals

E997.3 Weapon of mass destruction [WMD], unspecified ◀

E997.8 Other specified forms of unconventional warfare

E997.9 Unspecified form of unconventional warfare

N Newborn Age: 0   **P** Pediatric Age: 0–17   **M** Maternity Age: 12–55   **A** Adult Age: 15–124   ♀ Females Only   ♂ Males Only

Ⓔⓧ CC Exclusions   ✎ Complication\Comorbidity   ✎ Major C\C   ✎ Present on Admission Requirement   ✎ Hospital-Acquired Condition   **1203**

E000–E999

● **E998 Injury due to war operations but occurring after cessation of hostilities** ◀▥

   Injuries due to operations of war but occurring after cessation of hostilities by any means classifiable under E990-E997

   Injuries by explosion of bombs or mines placed in the course of operations of war, if the explosion occurred after cessation of hostilities

E998.0 Explosion of mines 🔗 ◀

E998.1 Explosion of bombs 🔗 ◀

E998.8 Injury due to other war operations but occurring after cessation of hostilities 🔗 ◀

E998.9 Injury due to unspecified war operations but occurring after cessation of hostilities 🔗 ◀

● **E999 Late effect of injury due to war operations and terrorism**

   Note: This category is to be used to indicate circumstances classifiable to E979, E990-E998 as the cause of death or disability from late effects, which are themselves classifiable elsewhere. The "late effects" include conditions reported as such or as sequelae which may occur at any time after injury resulting from operations of war or terrorism.

E999.0 Late effect of injury due to war operations 🔗
     Coding Clinic: 1998, Q1, P4; 1996, Q2, P12

E999.1 Late effect of injury due to terrorism 🔗

◀ New   ◀▥ Revised   ~~deleted~~ Deleted   ● Unacceptable Principal Diagnosis   ● Use Additional Digit(s)
▶ Manifestation Code   **OGCR** Official Guidelines   **Coding Clinic**   Excludes   Includes   Use additional   Code first   Omit code

MORPHOLOGY OF NEOPLASMS

The World Health Organization has published an adaptation of the International Classification of Diseases for Oncology (ICD-O). It contains a coded nomenclature for the morphology of neoplasms, which is reproduced here for those who wish to use it in conjunction with Chapter 2 of the International Classification of Diseases, 9th Revision, Clinical Modification.

The morphology code numbers consist of five digits; the first four identify the histological type of the neoplasm and the fifth indicates its behavior. The one-digit behavior code is as follows:

/0   Benign
/1   Uncertain whether benign or malignant
        Borderline malignancy
/2   Carcinoma in situ
        Intraepithelial
        Noninfiltrating
        Noninvasive
/3   Malignant, primary site
/6   Malignant, metastatic site
        Secondary site
/9   Malignant, uncertain whether primary or metastatic site

In the nomenclature below, the morphology code numbers include the behavior code appropriate to the histological type of neoplasm, but this behavior code should be changed if other reported information makes this necessary. For example, "chordoma (M9370/3)" is assumed to be malignant; the term "benign chordoma" should be coded M9370/0. Similarly, "superficial spreading adenocarcinoma (M8143/3)" described as "noninvasive" should be coded M8143/2 and "melanoma (M8720/3)" described as "secondary" should be coded M8720/6.

The following table shows the correspondence between the morphology code and the different sections of Chapter 2:

Morphology Code Histology/Behavior		ICD-9-CM Chapter 2	
Any	0	210-229	Benign neoplasms
M8000-M8004	1	239	Neoplasms of unspecified nature
M8010+	1	235-238	Neoplasms of uncertain behavior
Any	2	230-234	Carcinoma in situ
Any	3	140-195 200-208	Malignant neoplasms, stated or presumed to be primary
Any	6	196-198	Malignant neoplasms, stated or presumed to be secondary

The ICD-O behavior digit /9 is inapplicable in an ICD context, since all malignant neoplasms are presumed to be primary (/3) or secondary (/6) according to other information on the medical record.

Only the first-listed term of the full ICD-O morphology nomenclature appears against each code number in the list below. The ICD-9-CM Alphabetical Index (Volume 2), however, includes all the ICD-O synonyms as well as a number of other morphological names still likely to be encountered on medical records but omitted from ICD-O as outdated or otherwise undesirable.

A coding difficulty sometimes arises where a morphological diagnosis contains two qualifying adjectives that have different code numbers. An example is "transitional cell epidermoid carcinomas." "Transitional cell carcinoma NOS" is M8120/3 and "epidermoid carcinoma NOS" is M8070/3. In such circumstances, the higher number (M8120/3 in this example) should be used, as it is usually more specific.

CODED NOMENCLATURE FOR MORPHOLOGY OF NEOPLASMS

M800	**Neoplasms NOS**
M8000/0	*Neoplasm, benign*
M8000/1	*Neoplasm, uncertain whether benign or malignant*
M8000/3	*Neoplasm, malignant*
M8000/6	*Neoplasm, metastatic*
M8000/9	*Neoplasm, malignant, uncertain whether primary or metastatic*
M8001/0	*Tumor cells, benign*
M8001/1	*Tumor cells, uncertain whether benign or malignant*
M8001/3	*Tumor cells, malignant*
M8002/3	*Malignant tumor, small cell type*
M8003/3	*Malignant tumor, giant cell type*
M8004/3	*Malignant tumor, fusiform cell type*

M801-M804	**Epithelial neoplasms NOS**
M8010/0	*Epithelial tumor, benign*
M8010/2	*Carcinoma in situ NOS*
M8010/3	*Carcinoma NOS*
M8010/6	*Carcinoma, metastatic NOS*
M8010/9	*Carcinomatosis*
M8011/0	*Epithelioma, benign*
M8011/3	*Epithelioma, malignant*
M8012/3	*Large cell carcinoma NOS*
M8020/3	*Carcinoma, undifferentiated type NOS*
M8021/3	*Carcinoma, anaplastic type NOS*
M8022/3	*Pleomorphic carcinoma*
M8030/3	*Giant cell and spindle cell carcinoma*
M8031/3	*Giant cell carcinoma*
M8032/3	*Spindle cell carcinoma*
M8033/3	*Pseudosarcomatous carcinoma*
M8034/3	*Polygonal cell carcinoma*
M8035/3	*Spheroidal cell carcinoma*
M8040/1	*Tumorlet*
M8041/3	*Small cell carcinoma NOS*
M8042/3	*Oat cell carcinoma*
M8043/3	*Small cell carcinoma, fusiform cell type*

M805-M808	**Papillary and squamous cell neoplasms**
M8050/0	*Papilloma NOS (except Papilloma of urinary bladder M8120/1)*
M8050/2	*Papillary carcinoma in situ*
M8050/3	*Papillary carcinoma NOS*
M8051/0	*Verrucous papilloma*
M8051/3	*Verrucous carcinoma NOS*
M8052/0	*Squamous cell papilloma*
M8052/3	*Papillary squamous cell carcinoma*
M8053/0	*Inverted papilloma*
M8060/0	*Papillomatosis NOS*
M8070/2	*Squamous cell carcinoma in situ NOS*
M8070/3	*Squamous cell carcinoma NOS*
M8070/6	*Squamous cell carcinoma, metastatic NOS*
M8071/3	*Squamous cell carcinoma, keratinizing type NOS*
M8072/3	*Squamous cell carcinoma, large cell, nonkeratinizing type*
M8073/3	*Squamous cell carcinoma, small cell, nonkeratinizing type*
M8074/3	*Squamous cell carcinoma, spindle cell type*
M8075/3	*Adenoid squamous cell carcinoma*
M8076/2	*Squamous cell carcinoma in situ with questionable stromal invasion*
M8076/3	*Squamous cell carcinoma, microinvasive*
M8080/2	*Queyrat's erythroplasia*
M8081/2	*Bowen's disease*
M8082/3	*Lymphoepithelial carcinoma*

M809-M811	**Basal cell neoplasms**
M8090/1	*Basal cell tumor*
M8090/3	*Basal cell carcinoma NOS*
M8091/3	*Multicentric basal cell carcinoma*
M8092/3	*Basal cell carcinoma, morphea type*
M8093/3	*Basal cell carcinoma, fibroepithelial type*
M8094/3	*Basosquamous carcinoma*
M8095/3	*Metatypical carcinoma*
M8096/0	*Intraepidermal epithelioma of Jadassohn*
M8100/0	*Trichoepithelioma*
M8101/0	*Trichofolliculoma*
M8102/0	*Tricholemmoma*
M8110/0	*Pilomatrixoma*

M812-M813	**Transitional cell papillomas and carcinomas**
M8120/0	*Transitional cell papilloma NOS*
M8120/1	*Urothelial papilloma*
M8120/2	*Transitional cell carcinoma in situ*
M8120/3	*Transitional cell carcinoma NOS*
M8121/0	*Schneiderian papilloma*
M8121/1	*Transitional cell papilloma, inverted type*
M8121/3	*Schneiderian carcinoma*
M8122/3	*Transitional cell carcinoma, spindle cell type*
M8123/3	*Basaloid carcinoma*
M8124/3	*Cloacogenic carcinoma*
M8130/3	*Papillary transitional cell carcinoma*
M814-M838	**Adenomas and adenocarcinomas**
M8140/0	*Adenoma NOS*
M8140/1	*Bronchial adenoma NOS*
M8140/2	*Adenocarcinoma in situ*
M8140/3	*Adenocarcinoma NOS*
M8140/6	*Adenocarcinoma, metastatic NOS*
M8141/3	*Scirrhous adenocarcinoma*
M8142/3	*Linitis plastica*
M8143/3	*Superficial spreading adenocarcinoma*
M8144/3	*Adenocarcinoma, intestinal type*
M8145/3	*Carcinoma, diffuse type*
M8146/0	*Monomorphic adenoma*
M8147/0	*Basal cell adenoma*
M8150/0	*Islet cell adenoma*
M8150/3	*Islet cell carcinoma*
M8151/0	*Insulinoma NOS*
M8151/3	*Insulinoma, malignant*
M8152/0	*Glucagonoma NOS*
M8152/3	*Glucagonoma, malignant*
M8153/1	*Gastrinoma NOS*
M8153/3	*Gastrinoma, malignant*
M8154/3	*Mixed islet cell and exocrine adenocarcinoma*
M8160/0	*Bile duct adenoma*
M8160/3	*Cholangiocarcinoma*
M8161/0	*Bile duct cystadenoma*
M8161/3	*Bile duct cystadenocarcinoma*
M8170/0	*Liver cell adenoma*
M8170/3	*Hepatocellular carcinoma NOS*
M8180/0	*Hepatocholangioma, benign*
M8180/3	*Combined hepatocellular carcinoma and cholangio-carcinoma*
M8190/0	*Trabecular adenoma*
M8190/3	*Trabecular adenocarcinoma*
M8191/0	*Embryonal adenoma*
M8200/0	*Eccrine dermal cylindroma*
M8200/3	*Adenoid cystic carcinoma*
M8201/3	*Cribriform carcinoma*
M8210/0	*Adenomatous polyp NOS*
M8210/3	*Adenocarcinoma in adenomatous polyp*
M8211/0	*Tubular adenoma NOS*
M8211/3	*Tubular adenocarcinoma*
M8220/0	*Adenomatous polyposis coli*
M8220/3	*Adenocarcinoma in adenomatous polyposis coli*
M8221/0	*Multiple adenomatous polyps*
M8230/3	*Solid carcinoma NOS*
M8231/3	*Carcinoma simplex*
M8240/1	*Carcinoid tumor NOS*
M8240/3	*Carcinoid tumor, malignant*
M8241/1	*Carcinoid tumor, argentaffin NOS*
M8241/3	*Carcinoid tumor, argentaffin, malignant*
M8242/1	*Carcinoid tumor, nonargentaffin NOS*
M8242/3	*Carcinoid tumor, nonargentaffin, malignant*
M8243/3	*Mucocarcinoid tumor, malignant*
M8244/3	*Composite carcinoid*
M8250/1	*Pulmonary adenomatosis*
M8250/3	*Bronchiolo-alveolar adenocarcinoma*
M8251/0	*Alveolar adenoma*
M8251/3	*Alveolar adenocarcinoma*
M8260/0	*Papillary adenoma NOS*
M8260/3	*Papillary adenocarcinoma NOS*
M8261/1	*Villous adenoma NOS*
M8261/3	*Adenocarcinoma in villous adenoma*

M8262/3	*Villous adenocarcinoma*
M8263/0	*Tubulovillous adenoma*
M8270/0	*Chromophobe adenoma*
M8270/3	*Chromophobe carcinoma*
M8280/0	*Acidophil adenoma*
M8280/3	*Acidophil carcinoma*
M8281/0	*Mixed acidophil-basophil adenoma*
M8281/3	*Mixed acidophil-basophil carcinoma*
M8290/0	*Oxyphilic adenoma*
M8290/3	*Oxyphilic adenocarcinoma*
M8300/0	*Basophil adenoma*
M8300/3	*Basophil carcinoma*
M8310/0	*Clear cell adenoma*
M8310/3	*Clear cell adenocarcinoma NOS*
M8311/1	*Hypernephroid tumor*
M8312/3	*Renal cell carcinoma*
M8313/0	*Clear cell adenofibroma*
M8320/3	*Granular cell carcinoma*
M8321/0	*Chief cell adenoma*
M8322/0	*Water-clear cell adenoma*
M8322/3	*Water-clear cell adenocarcinoma*
M8323/0	*Mixed cell adenoma*
M8323/3	*Mixed cell adenocarcinoma*
M8324/0	*Lipoadenoma*
M8330/0	*Follicular adenoma*
M8330/3	*Follicular adenocarcinoma NOS*
M8331/3	*Follicular adenocarcinoma, well differentiated type*
M8332/3	*Follicular adenocarcinoma, trabecular type*
M8333/0	*Microfollicular adenoma*
M8334/0	*Macrofollicular adenoma*
M8340/3	*Papillary and follicular adenocarcinoma*
M8350/3	*Nonencapsulated sclerosing carcinoma*
M8360/1	*Multiple endocrine adenomas*
M8361/1	*Juxtaglomerular tumor*
M8370/0	*Adrenal cortical adenoma NOS*
M8370/3	*Adrenal cortical carcinoma*
M8371/0	*Adrenal cortical adenoma, compact cell type*
M8372/0	*Adrenal cortical adenoma, heavily pigmented variant*
M8373/0	*Adrenal cortical adenoma, clear cell type*
M8374/0	*Adrenal cortical adenoma, glomerulosa cell type*
M8375/0	*Adrenal cortical adenoma, mixed cell type*
M8380/0	*Endometrioid adenoma NOS*
M8380/1	*Endometrioid adenoma, borderline malignancy*
M8380/3	*Endometrioid carcinoma*
M8381/0	*Endometrioid adenofibroma NOS*
M8381/1	*Endometrioid adenofibroma, borderline malignancy*
M8381/3	*Endometrioid adenofibroma, malignant*
M839-M842	**Adnexal and skin appendage neoplasms**
M8390/0	*Skin appendage adenoma*
M8390/3	*Skin appendage carcinoma*
M8400/0	*Sweat gland adenoma*
M8400/1	*Sweat gland tumor NOS*
M8400/3	*Sweat gland adenocarcinoma*
M8401/0	*Apocrine adenoma*
M8401/3	*Apocrine adenocarcinoma*
M8402/0	*Eccrine acrospiroma*
M8403/0	*Eccrine spiradenoma*
M8404/0	*Hidrocystoma*
M8405/0	*Papillary hydradenoma*
M8406/0	*Papillary syringadenoma*
M8407/0	*Syringoma NOS*
M8410/0	*Sebaceous adenoma*
M8410/3	*Sebaceous adenocarcinoma*
M8420/0	*Ceruminous adenoma*
M8420/3	*Ceruminous adenocarcinoma*
M843	**Mucoepidermoid neoplasms**
M8430/1	*Mucoepidermoid tumor*
M8430/3	*Mucoepidermoid carcinoma*
M844-M849	**Cystic, mucinous, and serous neoplasms**
M8440/0	*Cystadenoma NOS*
M8440/3	*Cystadenocarcinoma NOS*
M8441/0	*Serous cystadenoma NOS*
M8441/1	*Serous cystadenoma, borderline malignancy*
M8441/3	*Serous cystadenocarcinoma NOS*

APPX A

M8450/0	Papillary cystadenoma NOS
M8450/1	Papillary cystadenoma, borderline malignancy
M8450/3	Papillary cystadenocarcinoma NOS
M8460/0	Papillary serous cystadenoma NOS
M8460/1	Papillary serous cystadenoma, borderline malignancy
M8460/3	Papillary serous cystadenocarcinoma
M8461/0	Serous surface papilloma NOS
M8461/1	Serous surface papilloma, borderline malignancy
M8461/3	Serous surface papillary carcinoma
M8470/0	Mucinous cystadenoma NOS
M8470/1	Mucinous cystadenoma, borderline malignancy
M8470/3	Mucinous cystadenocarcinoma NOS
M8471/0	Papillary mucinous cystadenoma NOS
M8471/1	Papillary mucinous cystadenoma, borderline malignancy
M8471/3	Papillary mucinous cystadenocarcinoma
M8480/0	Mucinous adenoma
M8480/3	Mucinous adenocarcinoma
M8480/6	Pseudomyxoma peritonei
M8481/3	Mucin-producing adenocarcinoma
M8490/3	Signet ring cell carcinoma
M8490/6	Metastatic signet ring cell carcinoma

M850-M854 Ductal, lobular, and medullary neoplasms

M8500/2	Intraductal carcinoma, noninfiltrating NOS
M8500/3	Infiltrating duct carcinoma
M8501/2	Comedocarcinoma, noninfiltrating
M8501/3	Comedocarcinoma NOS
M8502/3	Juvenile carcinoma of the breast
M8503/0	Intraductal papilloma
M8503/3	Noninfiltrating intraductal papillary adenocarcinoma
M8504/0	Intracystic papillary adenoma
M8504/2	Noninfiltrating intracystic carcinoma
M8505/0	Intraductal papillomatosis NOS
M8506/0	Subareolar duct papillomatosis
M8510/3	Medullary carcinoma NOS
M8511/3	Medullary carcinoma with amyloid stroma
M8512/3	Medullary carcinoma with lymphoid stroma
M8520/2	Lobular carcinoma in situ
M8520/3	Lobular carcinoma NOS
M8521/3	Infiltrating ductular carcinoma
M8530/3	Inflammatory carcinoma
M8540/3	Paget's disease, mammary
M8541/3	Paget's disease and infiltrating duct carcinoma of breast
M8542/3	Paget's disease, extramammary (except Paget's disease of bone)

M855 Acinar cell neoplasms

M8550/0	Acinar cell adenoma
M8550/1	Acinar cell tumor
M8550/3	Acinar cell carcinoma

M856-M858 Complex epithelial neoplasms

M8560/3	Adenosquamous carcinoma
M8561/0	Adenolymphoma
M8570/3	Adenocarcinoma with squamous metaplasia
M8571/3	Adenocarcinoma with cartilaginous and osseous metaplasia
M8572/3	Adenocarcinoma with spindle cell metaplasia
M8573/3	Adenocarcinoma with apocrine metaplasia
M8580/0	Thymoma, benign
M8580/3	Thymoma, malignant

M859-M867 Specialized gonadal neoplasms

M8590/1	Sex cord-stromal tumor
M8600/0	Thecoma NOS
M8600/3	Theca cell carcinoma
M8610/0	Luteoma NOS
M8620/1	Granulosa cell tumor NOS
M8620/3	Granulosa cell tumor, malignant
M8621/1	Granulosa cell-theca cell tumor
M8630/0	Androblastoma, benign
M8630/1	Androblastoma NOS
M8630/3	Androblastoma, malignant
M8631/0	Sertoli-Leydig cell tumor
M8632/1	Gynandroblastoma
M8640/0	Tubular androblastoma NOS
M8640/3	Sertoli cell carcinoma

M8641/0	Tubular androblastoma with lipid storage
M8650/0	Leydig cell tumor, benign
M8650/1	Leydig cell tumor NOS
M8650/3	Leydig cell tumor, malignant
M8660/0	Hilar cell tumor
M8670/0	Lipid cell tumor of ovary
M8671/0	Adrenal rest tumor

M868-M871 Paragangliomas and glomus tumors

M8680/1	Paraganglioma NOS
M8680/3	Paraganglioma, malignant
M8681/1	Sympathetic paraganglioma
M8682/1	Parasympathetic paraganglioma
M8690/1	Glomus jugulare tumor
M8691/1	Aortic body tumor
M8692/1	Carotid body tumor
M8693/1	Extra-adrenal paraganglioma NOS
M8693/3	Extra-adrenal paraganglioma, malignant
M8700/0	Pheochromocytoma NOS
M8700/3	Pheochromocytoma, malignant
M8710/3	Glomangiosarcoma
M8711/0	Glomus tumor
M8712/0	Glomangioma

M872-M879 Nevi and melanomas

M8720/0	Pigmented nevus NOS
M8720/3	Malignant melanoma NOS
M8721/3	Nodular melanoma
M8722/0	Balloon cell nevus
M8722/3	Balloon cell melanoma
M8723/0	Halo nevus
M8724/0	Fibrous papule of the nose
M8725/0	Neuronevus
M8726/0	Magnocellular nevus
M8730/0	Nonpigmented nevus
M8730/3	Amelanotic melanoma
M8740/0	Junctional nevus
M8740/3	Malignant melanoma in junctional nevus
M8741/2	Precancerous melanosis NOS
M8741/3	Malignant melanoma in precancerous melanosis
M8742/2	Hutchinson's melanotic freckle
M8742/3	Malignant melanoma in Hutchinson's melanotic freckle
M8743/3	Superficial spreading melanoma
M8750/0	Intradermal nevus
M8760/0	Compound nevus
M8761/1	Giant pigmented nevus
M8761/3	Malignant melanoma in giant pigmented nevus
M8770/0	Epithelioid and spindle cell nevus
M8771/3	Epithelioid cell melanoma
M8772/3	Spindle cell melanoma NOS
M8773/3	Spindle cell melanoma, type A
M8774/3	Spindle cell melanoma, type B
M8775/3	Mixed epithelioid and spindle cell melanoma
M8780/0	Blue nevus NOS
M8780/3	Blue nevus, malignant
M8790/0	Cellular blue nevus

M880 Soft tissue tumors and sarcomas NOS

M8800/0	Soft tissue tumor, benign
M8800/3	Sarcoma NOS
M8800/9	Sarcomatosis NOS
M8801/3	Spindle cell sarcoma
M8802/3	Giant cell sarcoma (except of bone M9250/3)
M8803/3	Small cell sarcoma
M8804/3	Epithelioid cell sarcoma

M881-M883 Fibromatous neoplasms

M8810/0	Fibroma NOS
M8810/3	Fibrosarcoma NOS
M8811/0	Fibromyxoma
M8811/3	Fibromyxosarcoma
M8812/0	Periosteal fibroma
M8812/3	Periosteal fibrosarcoma
M8813/0	Fascial fibroma
M8813/3	Fascial fibrosarcoma
M8814/3	Infantile fibrosarcoma
M8820/0	Elastofibroma

M8821/1	Aggressive fibromatosis
M8822/1	Abdominal fibromatosis
M8823/1	Desmoplastic fibroma
M8830/0	Fibrous histiocytoma NOS
M8830/1	Atypical fibrous histiocytoma
M8830/3	Fibrous histiocytoma, malignant
M8831/0	Fibroxanthoma NOS
M8831/1	Atypical fibroxanthoma
M8831/3	Fibroxanthoma, malignant
M8832/0	Dermatofibroma NOS
M8832/1	Dermatofibroma protuberans
M8832/3	Dermatofibrosarcoma NOS

M884   **Myxomatous neoplasms**

M8840/0	Myxoma NOS
M8840/3	Myxosarcoma

M885-M888   **Lipomatous neoplasms**

M8850/0	Lipoma NOS
M8850/3	Liposarcoma NOS
M8851/0	Fibrolipoma
M8851/3	Liposarcoma, well differentiated type
M8852/0	Fibromyxolipoma
M8852/3	Myxoid liposarcoma
M8853/3	Round cell liposarcoma
M8854/3	Pleomorphic liposarcoma
M8855/3	Mixed type liposarcoma
M8856/0	Intramuscular lipoma
M8857/0	Spindle cell lipoma
M8860/0	Angiomyolipoma
M8860/3	Angiomyoliposarcoma
M8861/0	Angiolipoma NOS
M8861/1	Angiolipoma, infiltrating
M8870/0	Myelolipoma
M8880/0	Hibernoma
M8881/0	Lipoblastomatosis

M889-M892   **Myomatous neoplasms**

M8890/0	Leiomyoma NOS
M8890/1	Intravascular leiomyomatosis
M8890/3	Leiomyosarcoma NOS
M8891/1	Epithelioid leiomyoma
M8891/3	Epithelioid leiomyosarcoma
M8892/1	Cellular leiomyoma
M8893/0	Bizarre leiomyoma
M8894/0	Angiomyoma
M8894/3	Angiomyosarcoma
M8895/0	Myoma
M8895/3	Myosarcoma
M8900/0	Rhabdomyoma NOS
M8900/3	Rhabdomyosarcoma NOS
M8901/3	Pleomorphic rhabdomyosarcoma
M8902/3	Mixed type rhabdomyosarcoma
M8903/0	Fetal rhabdomyoma
M8904/0	Adult rhabdomyoma
M8910/3	Embryonal rhabdomyosarcoma
M8920/3	Alveolar rhabdomyosarcoma

M893-M899   **Complex mixed and stromal neoplasms**

M8930/3	Endometrial stromal sarcoma
M8931/1	Endolymphatic stromal myosis
M8932/0	Adenomyoma
M8940/0	Pleomorphic adenoma
M8940/3	Mixed tumor, malignant NOS
M8950/3	Mullerian mixed tumor
M8951/3	Mesodermal mixed tumor
M8960/1	Mesoblastic nephroma
M8960/3	Nephroblastoma NOS
M8961/3	Epithelial nephroblastoma
M8962/3	Mesenchymal nephroblastoma
M8970/3	Hepatoblastoma
M8980/3	Carcinosarcoma NOS
M8981/3	Carcinosarcoma, embryonal type
M8982/0	Myoepithelioma
M8990/0	Mesenchymoma, benign
M8990/1	Mesenchymoma NOS

M8990/3	Mesenchymoma, malignant
M8991/3	Embryonal sarcoma

M900-M903   **Fibroepithelial neoplasms**

M9000/0	Brenner tumor NOS
M9000/1	Brenner tumor, borderline malignancy
M9000/3	Brenner tumor, malignant
M9010/0	Fibroadenoma NOS
M9011/0	Intracanalicular fibroadenoma NOS
M9012/0	Pericanalicular fibroadenoma
M9013/0	Adenofibroma NOS
M9014/0	Serous adenofibroma
M9015/0	Mucinous adenofibroma
M9020/0	Cellular intracanalicular fibroadenoma
M9020/1	Cystosarcoma phyllodes NOS
M9020/3	Cystosarcoma phyllodes, malignant
M9030/0	Juvenile fibroadenoma

M904   **Synovial neoplasms**

M9040/0	Synovioma, benign
M9040/3	Synovial sarcoma NOS
M9041/3	Synovial sarcoma, spindle cell type
M9042/3	Synovial sarcoma, epithelioid cell type
M9043/3	Synovial sarcoma, biphasic type
M9044/3	Clear cell sarcoma of tendons and aponeuroses

M905   **Mesothelial neoplasms**

M9050/0	Mesothelioma, benign
M9050/3	Mesothelioma, malignant
M9051/0	Fibrous mesothelioma, benign
M9051/3	Fibrous mesothelioma, malignant
M9052/0	Epithelioid mesothelioma, benign
M9052/3	Epithelioid mesothelioma, malignant
M9053/0	Mesothelioma, biphasic type, benign
M9053/3	Mesothelioma, biphasic type, malignant
M9054/0	Adenomatoid tumor NOS

M906-M909   **Germ cell neoplasms**

M9060/3	Dysgerminoma
M9061/3	Seminoma NOS
M9062/3	Seminoma, anaplastic type
M9063/3	Spermatocytic seminoma
M9064/3	Germinoma
M9070/3	Embryonal carcinoma NOS
M9071/3	Endodermal sinus tumor
M9072/3	Polyembryoma
M9073/1	Gonadoblastoma
M9080/0	Teratoma, benign
M9080/1	Teratoma NOS
M9080/3	Teratoma, malignant NOS
M9081/3	Teratocarcinoma
M9082/3	Malignant teratoma, undifferentiated type
M9083/3	Malignant teratoma, intermediate type
M9084/0	Dermoid cyst
M9084/3	Dermoid cyst with malignant transformation
M9090/0	Struma ovarii NOS
M9090/3	Struma ovarii, malignant
M9091/1	Strumal carcinoid

M910   **Trophoblastic neoplasms**

M9100/0	Hydatidiform mole NOS
M9100/1	Invasive hydatidiform mole
M9100/3	Choriocarcinoma
M9101/3	Choriocarcinoma combined with teratoma
M9102/3	Malignant teratoma, trophoblastic

M911   **Mesonephromas**

M9110/0	Mesonephroma, benign
M9110/1	Mesonephric tumor
M9110/3	Mesonephroma, malignant
M9111/1	Endosalpingioma

M912-M916   **Blood vessel tumors**

M9120/0	Hemangioma NOS
M9120/3	Hemangiosarcoma
M9121/0	Cavernous hemangioma
M9122/0	Venous hemangioma
M9123/0	Racemose hemangioma
M9124/3	Kupffer cell sarcoma

APPX A

M9130/0   Hemangioendothelioma, benign
M9130/1   Hemangioendothelioma NOS
M9130/3   Hemangioendothelioma, malignant
M9131/0   Capillary hemangioma
M9132/0   Intramuscular hemangioma
M9140/3   Kaposi's sarcoma
M9141/0   Angiokeratoma
M9142/0   Verrucous keratotic hemangioma
M9150/0   Hemangiopericytoma, benign
M9150/1   Hemangiopericytoma NOS
M9150/3   Hemangiopericytoma, malignant
M9160/0   Angiofibroma NOS
M9161/1   Hemangioblastoma

M917   **Lymphatic vessel tumors**
M9170/0   Lymphangioma NOS
M9170/3   Lymphangiosarcoma
M9171/0   Capillary lymphangioma
M9172/0   Cavernous lymphangioma
M9173/0   Cystic lymphangioma
M9174/0   Lymphangiomyoma
M9174/1   Lymphangiomyomatosis
M9175/0   Hemolymphangioma

M918-M920   **Osteomas and osteosarcomas**
M9180/0   Osteoma NOS
M9180/3   Osteosarcoma NOS
M9181/3   Chondroblastic osteosarcoma
M9182/3   Fibroblastic osteosarcoma
M9183/3   Telangiectatic osteosarcoma
M9184/3   Osteosarcoma in Paget's disease of bone
M9190/3   Juxtacortical osteosarcoma
M9191/0   Osteoid osteoma NOS
M9200/0   Osteoblastoma

M921-M924   **Chondromatous neoplasms**
M9210/0   Osteochondroma
M9210/1   Osteochondromatosis NOS
M9220/0   Chondroma NOS
M9220/1   Chondromatosis NOS
M9220/3   Chondrosarcoma NOS
M9221/0   Juxtacortical chondroma
M9221/3   Juxtacortical chondrosarcoma
M9230/0   Chondroblastoma NOS
M9230/3   Chondroblastoma, malignant
M9240/3   Mesenchymal chondrosarcoma
M9241/0   Chondromyxoid fibroma

M925   **Giant cell tumors**
M9250/1   Giant cell tumor of bone NOS
M9250/3   Giant cell tumor of bone, malignant
M9251/1   Giant cell tumor of soft parts NOS
M9251/3   Malignant giant cell tumor of soft parts

M926   **Miscellaneous bone tumors**
M9260/3   Ewing's sarcoma
M9261/3   Adamantinoma of long bones
M9262/0   Ossifying fibroma

M927-M934   **Odontogenic tumors**
M9270/0   Odontogenic tumor, benign
M9270/1   Odontogenic tumor NOS
M9270/3   Odontogenic tumor, malignant
M9271/0   Dentinoma
M9272/0   Cementoma NOS
M9273/0   Cementoblastoma, benign
M9274/0   Cementifying fibroma
M9275/0   Gigantiform cementoma
M9280/0   Odontoma NOS
M9281/0   Compound odontoma
M9282/0   Complex odontoma
M9290/0   Ameloblastic fibro-odontoma
M9290/3   Ameloblastic odontosarcoma
M9300/0   Adenomatoid odontogenic tumor
M9301/0   Calcifying odontogenic cyst
M9310/0   Ameloblastoma NOS
M9310/3   Ameloblastoma, malignant
M9311/0   Odontoameloblastoma
M9312/0   Squamous odontogenic tumor

M9320/0   Odontogenic myxoma
M9321/0   Odontogenic fibroma NOS
M9330/0   Ameloblastic fibroma
M9330/3   Ameloblastic fibrosarcoma
M9340/0   Calcifying epithelial odontogenic tumor

M935-M937   **Miscellaneous tumors**
M9350/1   Craniopharyngioma
M9360/1   Pinealoma
M9361/1   Pineocytoma
M9362/3   Pineoblastoma
M9363/0   Melanotic neuroectodermal tumor
M9370/3   Chordoma

M938-M948   **Gliomas**
M9380/3   Glioma, malignant
M9381/3   Gliomatosis cerebri
M9382/3   Mixed glioma
M9383/1   Subependymal glioma
M9384/1   Subependymal giant cell astrocytoma
M9390/0   Choroid plexus papilloma NOS
M9390/3   Choroid plexus papilloma, malignant
M9391/3   Ependymoma NOS
M9392/3   Ependymoma, anaplastic type
M9393/1   Papillary ependymoma
M9394/1   Myxopapillary ependymoma
M9400/3   Astrocytoma NOS
M9401/3   Astrocytoma, anaplastic type
M9410/3   Protoplasmic astrocytoma
M9411/3   Gemistocytic astrocytoma
M9420/3   Fibrillary astrocytoma
M9421/3   Pilocytic astrocytoma
M9422/3   Spongioblastoma NOS
M9423/3   Spongioblastoma polare
M9430/3   Astroblastoma
M9440/3   Glioblastoma NOS
M9441/3   Giant cell glioblastoma
M9442/3   Glioblastoma with sarcomatous component
M9443/3   Primitive polar spongioblastoma
M9450/3   Oligodendroglioma NOS
M9451/3   Oligodendroglioma, anaplastic type
M9460/3   Oligodendroblastoma
M9470/3   Medulloblastoma NOS
M9471/3   Desmoplastic medulloblastoma
M9472/3   Medullomyoblastoma
M9480/3   Cerebellar sarcoma NOS
M9481/3   Monstrocellular sarcoma

M949-M952   **Neuroepitheliomatous neoplasms**
M9490/0   Ganglioneuroma
M9490/3   Ganglioneuroblastoma
M9491/0   Ganglioneuromatosis
M9500/3   Neuroblastoma NOS
M9501/3   Medulloepithelioma NOS
M9502/3   Teratoid medulloepithelioma
M9503/3   Neuroepithelioma NOS
M9504/3   Spongioneuroblastoma
M9505/1   Ganglioglioma
M9506/0   Neurocytoma
M9507/0   Pacinian tumor
M9510/3   Retinoblastoma NOS
M9511/3   Retinoblastoma, differentiated type
M9512/3   Retinoblastoma, undifferentiated type
M9520/3   Olfactory neurogenic tumor
M9521/3   Esthesioneurocytoma
M9522/3   Esthesioneuroblastoma
M9523/3   Esthesioneuroepithelioma

M953   **Meningiomas**
M9530/0   Meningioma NOS
M9530/1   Meningiomatosis NOS
M9530/3   Meningioma, malignant
M9531/0   Meningotheliomatous meningioma
M9532/0   Fibrous meningioma
M9533/0   Psammomatous meningioma
M9534/0   Angiomatous meningioma

APPX A

M9535/0	*Hemangioblastic meningioma*
M9536/0	*Hemangiopericytic meningioma*
M9537/0	*Transitional meningioma*
M9538/1	*Papillary meningioma*
M9539/3	*Meningeal sarcomatosis*

M954-M957 Nerve sheath tumor

M9540/0	*Neurofibroma NOS*
M9540/1	*Neurofibromatosis NOS*
M9540/3	*Neurofibrosarcoma*
M9541/0	*Melanotic neurofibroma*
M9550/0	*Plexiform neurofibroma*
M9560/0	*Neurilemmoma NOS*
M9560/1	*Neurinomatosis*
M9560/3	*Neurilemmoma, malignant*
M9570/0	*Neuroma NOS*

M958 Granular cell tumors and alveolar soft part sarcoma

M9580/0	*Granular cell tumor NOS*
M9580/3	*Granular cell tumor, malignant*
M9581/3	*Alveolar soft part sarcoma*

M959-M963 Lymphomas, NOS or diffuse

M9590/0	*Lymphomatous tumor, benign*
M9590/3	*Malignant lymphoma NOS*
M9591/3	*Malignant lymphoma, non Hodgkin's type*
M9600/3	*Malignant lymphoma, undifferentiated cell type NOS*
M9601/3	*Malignant lymphoma, stem cell type*
M9602/3	*Malignant lymphoma, convoluted cell type NOS*
M9610/3	*Lymphosarcoma NOS*
M9611/3	*Malignant lymphoma, lymphoplasmacytoid type*
M9612/3	*Malignant lymphoma, immunoblastic type*
M9613/3	*Malignant lymphoma, mixed lymphocytic-histiocytic NOS*
M9614/3	*Malignant lymphoma, centroblastic-centrocytic, diffuse*
M9615/3	*Malignant lymphoma, follicular center cell NOS*
M9620/3	*Malignant lymphoma, lymphocytic, well differentiated NOS*
M9621/3	*Malignant lymphoma, lymphocytic, intermediate differentiation NOS*
M9622/3	*Malignant lymphoma, centrocytic*
M9623/3	*Malignant lymphoma, follicular center cell, cleaved NOS*
M9630/3	*Malignant lymphoma, lymphocytic, poorly differentiated NOS*
M9631/3	*Prolymphocytic lymphosarcoma*
M9632/3	*Malignant lymphoma, centroblastic type NOS*
M9633/3	*Malignant lymphoma, follicular center cell, noncleaved NOS*

M964 Reticulosarcomas

M9640/3	*Reticulosarcoma NOS*
M9641/3	*Reticulosarcoma, pleomorphic cell type*
M9642/3	*Reticulosarcoma, nodular*

M965-M966 Hodgkin's disease

M9650/3	*Hodgkin's disease NOS*
M9651/3	*Hodgkin's disease, lymphocytic predominance*
M9652/3	*Hodgkin's disease, mixed cellularity*
M9653/3	*Hodgkin's disease, lymphocytic depletion NOS*
M9654/3	*Hodgkin's disease, lymphocytic depletion, diffuse fibrosis*
M9655/3	*Hodgkin's disease, lymphocytic depletion, reticular type*
M9656/3	*Hodgkin's disease, nodular sclerosis NOS*
M9657/3	*Hodgkin's disease, nodular sclerosis, cellular phase*
M9660/3	*Hodgkin's paragranuloma*
M9661/3	*Hodgkin's granuloma*
M9662/3	*Hodgkin's sarcoma*

M969 Lymphomas, nodular or follicular

M9690/3	*Malignant lymphoma, nodular NOS*
M9691/3	*Malignant lymphoma, mixed lymphocytic-histiocytic, nodular*
M9692/3	*Malignant lymphoma, centroblastic-centrocytic, follicular*
M9693/3	*Malignant lymphoma, lymphocytic, well differentiated, nodular*
M9694/3	*Malignant lymphoma, lymphocytic, intermediate differentiation, nodular*
M9695/3	*Malignant lymphoma, follicular center cell, cleaved, follicular*
M9696/3	*Malignant lymphoma, lymphocytic, poorly differentiated, nodular*
M9697/3	*Malignant lymphoma, centroblastic type, follicular*
M9698/3	*Malignant lymphoma, follicular center cell, noncleaved, follicular*

M970 Mycosis fungoides

M9700/3	*Mycosis fungoides*
M9701/3	*Sezary's disease*

M971-M972 Miscellaneous reticuloendothelial neoplasms

M9710/3	*Microglioma*
M9720/3	*Malignant histiocytosis*
M9721/3	*Histiocytic medullary reticulosis*
M9722/3	*Letterer-Siwe's disease*

M973 Plasma cell tumors

M9730/3	*Plasma cell myeloma*
M9731/0	*Plasma cell tumor, benign*
M9731/1	*Plasmacytoma NOS*
M9731/3	*Plasma cell tumor, malignant*

M974 Mast cell tumors

M9740/1	*Mastocytoma NOS*
M9740/3	*Mast cell sarcoma*
M9741/3	*Malignant mastocytosis*

M975 Burkitt's tumor

M9750/3	*Burkitt's tumor*

M980-M994 Leukemias

M980 Leukemias NOS

M9800/3	*Leukemia NOS*
M9801/3	*Acute leukemia NOS*
M9802/3	*Subacute leukemia NOS*
M9803/3	*Chronic leukemia NOS*
M9804/3	*Aleukemic leukemia NOS*

M981 Compound leukemias

M9810/3	*Compound leukemia*

M982 Lymphoid leukemias

M9820/3	*Lymphoid leukemia NOS*
M9821/3	*Acute lymphoid leukemia*
M9822/3	*Subacute lymphoid leukemia*
M9823/3	*Chronic lymphoid leukemia*
M9824/3	*Aleukemic lymphoid leukemia*
M9825/3	*Prolymphocytic leukemia*

M983 Plasma cell leukemias

M9830/3	*Plasma cell leukemia*

M984 Erythroleukemias

M9840/3	*Erythroleukemia*
M9841/3	*Acute erythremia*
M9842/3	*Chronic erythremia*

M985 Lymphosarcoma cell leukemias

M9850/3	*Lymphosarcoma cell leukemia*

M986 Myeloid leukemias

M9860/3	*Myeloid leukemia NOS*
M9861/3	*Acute myeloid leukemia*
M9862/3	*Subacute myeloid leukemia*
M9863/3	*Chronic myeloid leukemia*
M9864/3	*Aleukemic myeloid leukemia*
M9865/3	*Neutrophilic leukemia*
M9866/3	*Acute promyelocytic leukemia*

M987 Basophilic leukemias

M9870/3	*Basophilic leukemia*

M988 Eosinophilic leukemias

M9880/3	*Eosinophilic leukemia*

M989 Monocytic leukemias

M9890/3	*Monocytic leukemia NOS*
M9891/3	*Acute monocytic leukemia*
M9892/3	*Subacute monocytic leukemia*

APPX A

M9893/3	*Chronic monocytic leukemia*
M9894/3	*Aleukemic monocytic leukemia*
M990-M994	**Miscellaneous leukemias**
M9900/3	*Mast cell leukemia*
M9910/3	*Megakaryocytic leukemia*
M9920/3	*Megakaryocytic myelosis*
M9930/3	*Myeloid sarcoma*
M9940/3	*Hairy cell leukemia*

M995-M997	**Miscellaneous myeloproliferative and lymphoproliferative disorders**
M9950/1	*Polycythemia vera*
M9951/1	*Acute panmyelosis*
M9960/1	*Chronic myeloproliferative disease*
M9961/1	*Myelosclerosis with myeloid metaplasia*
M9962/1	*Idiopathic thrombocythemia*
M9970/1	*Chronic lymphoproliferative disease*

GLOSSARY OF MENTAL DISORDERS

Deleted as of October 1, 2004

APPENDIX C

CLASSIFICATION OF DRUGS BY AMERICAN HOSPITAL FORMULARY SERVICES LIST NUMBER AND THEIR ICD-9-CM EQUIVALENTS

The coding of adverse effects of drugs is keyed to the continually revised Hospital Formulary of the American Hospital Formulary Service (AHFS) published under the direction of the American Society of Hospital Pharmacists.

The following section gives the ICD-9-CM diagnosis code for each AHFS list.

AHFS List		ICD-9-CM Diagnosis Code
4:00	**ANTIHISTAMINE DRUGS**	**963.0**
8:00	**ANTI-INFECTIVE AGENTS**	
8:04	Amebicides	961.5
	hydroxyquinoline derivatives	961.3
	arsenical anti-infectives	961.1
8:08	Anthelmintics	961.6
	quinoline derivatives	961.3
8:12.04	Antifungal Antibiotics	960.1
	nonantibiotics	961.9
8:12.06	Cephalosporins	960.5
8:12.08	Chloramphenicol	960.2
8:12.12	The Erythromycins	960.3
8:12.16	The Penicillins	960.0
8:12.20	The Streptomycins	960.6
8:12.24	The Tetracyclines	960.4
8:12.28	Other Antibiotics	960.8
	antimycobacterial antibiotics	960.6
	macrolides	960.3
8:16	Antituberculars	961.8
	antibiotics	960.6
8:18	Antivirals	961.7
8:20	Plasmodicides (antimalarials)	961.4
8:24	Sulfonamides	961.0
8:26	The Sulfones	961.8
8:28	Treponemicides	961.2
8:32	Trichomonacides	961.5
	hydroxyquinoline derivatives	961.3
	nitrofuran derivatives	961.9
8:36	Urinary Germicides	961.9
	quinoline derivatives	961.3
8:40	Other Anti-Infectives	961.9
10:00	**ANTINEOPLASTIC AGENTS**	**963.1**
	antibiotics	960.7
	progestogens	962.2
12:00	**AUTONOMIC DRUGS**	
12:04	Parasympathomimetic (Cholinergic) Agents	971.0
12:08	Parasympatholytic (Cholinergic Blocking) Agents	971.1
12:12	Sympathomimetic (Adrenergic) Agents	971.2
12:16	Sympatholytic (Adrenergic Blocking) Agents	971.3
12:20	Skeletal Muscle Relaxants	975.2
	central nervous system muscle-tone depressants	968.0
16:00	**BLOOD DERIVATIVES**	**964.7**
20:00	**BLOOD FORMATION AND COAGULATION**	
20:04	Antianemia Drugs	964.1
20:04.04	Iron Preparations	964.0
20:04.08	Liver and Stomach Preparations	964.1
20:12.04	Anticoagulants	964.2
20:12.08	Antiheparin agents	964.5
20:12.12	Coagulants	964.5
20:12.16	Hemostatics	964.5
	capillary-active drugs	972.8
	fibrinolysis-affecting agents	964.4
	natural products	964.7

AHFS List		ICD-9-CM Diagnosis Code
24:00	**CARDIOVASCULAR DRUGS**	
24:04	Cardiac Drugs	972.9
	cardiotonic agents	972.1
	rhythm regulators	972.0
24:06	Antilipemic Agents	972.2
	thyroid derivatives	962.7
24:08	Hypotensive Agents	972.6
	adrenergic blocking agents	971.3
	ganglion-blocking agents	972.3
	vasodilators	972.5
24:12	Vasodilating Agents	972.5
	coronary	972.4
	nicotinic acid derivatives	972.2
24:16	Sclerosing Agents	972.7
28:00	**CENTRAL NERVOUS SYSTEM DRUGS**	
28:04	General Anesthetics	968.4
	gaseous anesthetics	968.2
	halothane	968.1
	intravenous anesthetics	968.3
28:08	Analgesics and Antipyretics	965.9
	antirheumatics	965.6
	aromatic analgesics	965.4
	non-narcotics NEC	965.7
	opium alkaloids	965.00
	heroin	965.01
	methadone	965.02
	specified type NEC	965.09
	pyrazole derivatives	965.5
	salicylates	965.1
	specified type NEC	965.8
28:10	Narcotic Antagonists	970.1
28:12	Anticonvulsants	966.3
	barbiturates	967.0
	benzodiazepine-based tranquilizers	969.4
	bromides	967.3
	hydantoin derivatives	966.1
	oxazolidine derivative	966.0
	succinimides	966.2
28:16.04	Antidepressants	969.0
28:16.08	Tranquilizers	969.5
	benzodiazepine-based	969.4
	butyrophenone-based	969.2
	major NEC	969.3
	phenothiazine-based	969.1
28:16.12	Other Psychotherapeutic Agents	969.8
28:20	Respiratory and Cerebral Stimulants	970.9
	analeptics	970.0
	anorexigenic agents	977.0
	psychostimulants	969.7
	specified type NEC	970.8
28:24	Sedatives and Hypnotics	967.9
	barbiturates	967.0
	benzodiazepine-based tranquilizers	969.4
	chloral hydrate group	967.1
	glutethimide group	967.5
	intravenous anesthetics	968.3
	methaqualone	967.4
	paraldehyde	967.2
	phenothiazine-based tranquilizers	969.1
	specified type NEC	967.8
	thiobarbiturates	968.3
	tranquilizer NEC	969.5
36:00	**DIAGNOSTIC AGENTS**	**977.8**
40:00	**ELECTROLYTE, CALORIC, AND WATER BALANCE AGENTS NEC**	**974.5**
40:04	Acidifying Agents	963.2

1213

40:08	Alkalinizing Agents	963.3
40:10	Ammonia Detoxicants	974.5
40:12	Replacement Solutions NEC	974.5
	plasma volume expanders	964.8
40:16	Sodium-Removing Resins	974.5
40:18	Potassium-Removing Resins	974.5
40:20	Caloric Agents	974.5
40:24	Salt and Sugar Substitutes	974.5
40:28	Diuretics NEC	974.4
	carbonic acid anhydrase inhibitors	974.2
	mercurials	974.0
	purine derivatives	974.1
	saluretics	974.3
40:36	Irrigating Solutions	974.5
40:40	Uricosuric Agents	974.7
44:00	**ENZYMES NEC**	**963.4**
	fibrinolysis-affecting agents	964.4
	gastric agents	973.4
48:00	**EXPECTORANTS AND COUGH PREPARATIONS**	
	antihistamine agents	963.0
	antitussives	975.4
	codeine derivatives	965.09
	expectorants	975.5
	narcotic agents NEC	965.09
52:00	**EYE, EAR, NOSE, AND THROAT PREPARATIONS**	
52:04	Anti-Infectives	
	ENT	976.6
	ophthalmic	976.5
52:04.04	Antibiotics	
	ENT	976.6
	ophthalmic	976.5
52:04.06	Antivirals	
	ENT	976.6
	ophthalmic	976.5
52:04.08	Sulfonamides	
	ENT	976.6
	ophthalmic	976.5
52:04.12	Miscellaneous Anti-Infectives	
	ENT	976.6
	ophthalmic	976.5
52:08	Anti-Inflammatory Agents	
	ENT	976.6
	ophthalmic	976.5
52:10	Carbonic Anhydrase Inhibitors	974.2
52:12	Contact Lens Solutions	976.5
52:16	Local Anesthetics	968.5
52:20	Miotics	971.0
52:24	Mydriatics	
	adrenergics	971.2
	anticholinergics	971.1
	antimuscarinics	971.1
	parasympatholytics	971.1
	spasmolytics	971.1
	sympathomimetics	971.2
52:28	Mouth Washes and Gargles	976.6
52:32	Vasoconstrictors	971.2
52:36	Unclassified Agents	
	ENT	976.6
	ophthalmic	976.5
56:00	**GASTROINTESTINAL DRUGS**	
56:04	Antacids and Absorbents	973.0
56:08	Anti-Diarrhea Agents	973.5
56:10	Antiflatulents	973.8
56:12	Cathartics NEC	973.3
	emollients	973.2
	irritants	973.1
56:16	Digestants	973.4
56:20	Emetics and Antiemetics	
	antiemetics	963.0
	emetics	973.6
56:24	Lipotropic Agents	977.1

60:00	**GOLD COMPOUNDS**	**965.6**
64:00	**HEAVY METAL ANTAGONISTS**	**963.8**
68:00	**HORMONES AND SYNTHETIC SUBSTITUTES**	
68:04	Adrenals	962.0
68:08	Androgens	962.1
68:12	Contraceptives	962.2
68:16	Estrogens	962.2
68:18	Gonadotropins	962.4
68:20	Insulins and Antidiabetic Agents	962.3
68:20.08	Insulins	962.3
68:24	Parathyroid	962.6
68:28	Pituitary	
	anterior	962.4
	posterior	962.5
68:32	Progestogens	962.2
68:34	Other Corpus Luteum Hormones	962.2
68:36	Thyroid and Antithyroid	
	antithyroid	962.8
	thyroid	962.7
72:00	**LOCAL ANESTHETICS NEC**	**968.9**
	topical (surface) agents	968.5
	infiltrating agents (intradermal) (subcutaneous) (submucosal)	968.5
	nerve blocking agents (peripheral) (plexus) (regional)	968.6
	spinal	968.7
76:00	**OXYTOCICS**	**975.0**
78:00	**RADIOACTIVE AGENTS**	**990**
80:00	**SERUMS, TOXOIDS, AND VACCINES**	
80:04	Serums	979.9
	immune globulin (gamma) (human)	964.6
80:08	Toxoids NEC	978.8
	diphtheria	978.5
	and tetanus	978.9
	with pertussis component	978.6
	tetanus	978.4
	and diphtheria	978.9
	with pertussis component	978.6
80:12	Vaccines NEC	979.9
	bacterial NEC	978.8
	with	
	other bacterial component	978.9
	pertussis component	978.6
	viral and rickettsial component	979.7
	rickettsial NEC	979.6
	with	
	bacterial component	979.7
	pertussis component	978.6
	viral component	979.7
	viral NEC	979.6
	with	
	bacterial component	979.7
	pertussis component	978.6
	rickettsial component	979.7
84:00	**SKIN AND MUCOUS MEMBRANE PREPARATIONS**	
84:04	Anti-Infectives	976.0
84:04.04	Antibiotics	976.0
84:04.08	Fungicides	976.0
84:04.12	Scabicides and Pediculicides	976.0
84:04.16	Miscellaneous Local Anti-Infectives	976.0
84:06	Anti-Inflammatory Agents	976.0
84:08	Antipruritics and Local Anesthetics	
	antipruritics	976.1
	local anesthetics	968.5
84:12	Astringents	976.2
84:16	Cell Stimulants and Proliferants	976.8
84:20	Detergents	976.2
84:24	Emollients, Demulcents, and Protectants	976.3
84:28	Keratolytic Agents	976.4

APPENDIX D

CLASSIFICATION OF INDUSTRIAL ACCIDENTS ACCORDING TO AGENCY

Annex B to the Resolution concerning Statistics of Employment Injuries adopted by the Tenth International Conference of Labor Statisticians on 12 October 1962

1 MACHINES

11   Prime-Movers, except Electrical Motors
111 *Steam engines*
112 *Internal combustion engines*
119 *Others*

12   Transmission Machinery
121 *Transmission shafts*
122 *Transmission belts, cables, pulleys, pinions, chains, gears*
129 *Others*

13   Metalworking Machines
131 *Power presses*
132 *Lathes*
133 *Milling machines*
134 *Abrasive wheels*
135 *Mechanical shears*
136 *Forging machines*
137 *Rolling-mills*
139 *Others*

14   Wood and Assimilated Machines
141 *Circular saws*
142 *Other saws*
143 *Molding machines*
144 *Overhand planes*
149 *Others*

15   Agricultural Machines
151 *Reapers (including combine reapers)*
152 *Threshers*
159 *Others*

16   Mining Machinery
161 *Under-cutters*
169 *Others*

19   Other Machines Not Elsewhere Classified
191 *Earth-moving machines, excavating and scraping machines, except means of transport*
192 *Spinning, weaving and other textile machines*
193 *Machines for the manufacture of foodstuffs and beverages*
194 *Machines for the manufacture of paper*
195 *Printing machines*
199 *Others*

2 MEANS OF TRANSPORT AND LIFTING EQUIPMENT

21   Lifting Machines and Appliances
211 *Cranes*
212 *Lifts and elevators*
213 *Winches*
214 *Pulley blocks*
219 *Others*

22   Means of Rail Transport
221 *Inter-urban railways*
222 *Rail transport in mines, tunnels, quarries, industrial establishments, docks, etc.*
229 *Others*

23   Other Wheeled Means of Transport, Excluding Rail Transport
231 *Tractors*
232 *Lorries*
233 *Trucks*
234 *Motor vehicles, not elsewhere classified*
235 *Animal-drawn vehicles*
236 *Hand-drawn vehicles*
239 *Others*

24   Means of Air Transport

25   Means of Water Transport
251 *Motorized means of water transport*
252 *Non-motorized means of water transport*

26   Other Means of Transport
261 *Cable-cars*
262 *Mechanical conveyors, except cable-cars*
269 *Others*

3 OTHER EQUIPMENT

31   Pressure Vessels
311 *Boilers*
312 *Pressurized containers*
313 *Pressurized piping and accessories*
314 *Gas cylinders*
315 *Caissons, diving equipment*
319 *Others*

32   Furnaces, Ovens, Kilns
321 *Blast furnaces*
322 *Refining furnaces*
323 *Other furnaces*
324 *Kilns*
325 *Ovens*

33   Refrigerating Plants

34   Electrical Installations, Including Electric Motors, but Excluding Electric Hand Tools
341 *Rotating machines*
342 *Conductors*
343 *Transformers*
344 *Control apparatus*
349 *Others*

35   Electric Hand Tools

36   Tools, Implements, and Appliances, Except Electric Hand Tools
361 *Power-driven hand tools, except electric hand tools*
362 *Hand tools, not power-driven*
369 *Others*

37   Ladders, Mobile Ramps

38   Scaffolding

39   Other Equipment, Not Elsewhere Classified

4 MATERIALS, SUBSTANCES, AND RADIATIONS

41   Explosives

42   Dusts, Gases, Liquids and Chemicals, Excluding Explosives
421 *Dusts*
422 *Gases, vapors, fumes*
423 *Liquids, not elsewhere classified*
424 *Chemicals, not elsewhere classified*

43   Flying Fragments

44   Radiations
441 *Ionizing radiations*
449 *Others*

49   Other Materials and Substances Not Elsewhere
        Classified

5 WORKING ENVIRONMENT

51   **Outdoor**
        511 *Weather*
        512 *Traffic and working surfaces*
        513 *Water*
        519 *Others*

52   **Indoor**
        521 *Floors*
        522 *Confined quarters*
        523 *Stairs*
        524 *Other traffic and working surfaces*
        525 *Floor openings and wall openings*
        526 *Environmental factors (lighting, ventilation, temperature,
             noise, etc.)*
        529 *Others*

53   **Underground**
        531 *Roofs and faces of mine roads and tunnels, etc.*
        532 *Floors of mine roads and tunnels, etc.*
        533 *Working-faces of mines, tunnels, etc.*
        534 *Mine shafts*
        535 *Fire*
        536 *Water*
        539 *Others*

6 OTHER AGENCIES, NOT ELSEWHERE CLASSIFIED

61   **Animals**
        611 *Live animals*
        612 *Animals products*

69   **Other Agencies, Not Elsewhere Classified**

7 AGENCIES NOT CLASSIFIED FOR LACK OF SUFFICIENT DATA

LIST OF THREE-DIGIT CATEGORIES

1. INFECTIOUS AND PARASITIC DISEASES

Intestinal infectious diseases (001–009)
001 Cholera
002 Typhoid and paratyphoid fevers
003 Other salmonella infections
004 Shigellosis
005 Other food poisoning (bacterial)
006 Amebiasis
007 Other protozoal intestinal diseases
008 Intestinal infections due to other organisms
009 Ill-defined intestinal infections

Tuberculosis (010–018)
010 Primary tuberculous infection
011 Pulmonary tuberculosis
012 Other respiratory tuberculosis
013 Tuberculosis of meninges and central nervous system
014 Tuberculosis of intestines, peritoneum, and mesenteric glands
015 Tuberculosis of bones and joints
016 Tuberculosis of genitourinary system
017 Tuberculosis of other organs
018 Miliary tuberculosis

Zoonotic bacterial diseases (020–027)
020 Plague
021 Tularemia
022 Anthrax
023 Brucellosis
024 Glanders
025 Melioidosis
026 Rat-bite fever
027 Other zoonotic bacterial diseases

Other bacterial diseases (030–041)
030 Leprosy
031 Diseases due to other mycobacteria
032 Diphtheria
033 Whooping cough
034 Streptococcal sore throat and scarlet fever
035 Erysipelas
036 Meningococcal infection
037 Tetanus
038 Septicemia
039 Actinomycotic infections
040 Other bacterial diseases
041 Bacterial infection in conditions classified elsewhere and of unspecified site

Human immunodeficiency virus (042)
042 Human immunodeficiency virus [HIV] disease

Poliomyelitis and other non-arthropod-borne viral diseases of central nervous system (045–049)
045 Acute poliomyelitis
046 Slow virus infection of central nervous system
047 Meningitis due to enterovirus
048 Other enterovirus diseases of central nervous system
049 Other non-arthropod-borne viral diseases of central nervous system

Viral diseases accompanied by exanthem (050–059)
050 Smallpox
051 Cowpox and paravaccinia
052 Chickenpox
053 Herpes zoster
054 Herpes simplex
055 Measles
056 Rubella
057 Other viral exanthemata
058 Other human herpesvirus
059 Other poxvirus infections

Arthropod-borne viral diseases (060–066)
060 Yellow fever
061 Dengue
062 Mosquito-borne viral encephalitis
063 Tick-borne viral encephalitis
064 Viral encephalitis transmitted by other and unspecified arthropods
065 Arthropod-borne hemorrhagic fever
066 Other arthropod-borne viral diseases

Other diseases due to viruses and Chlamydiae (070–079)
070 Viral hepatitis
071 Rabies
072 Mumps
073 Ornithosis
074 Specific diseases due to Coxsackie virus
075 Infectious mononucleosis
076 Trachoma
077 Other diseases of conjunctiva due to viruses and Chlamydiae
078 Other diseases due to viruses and Chlamydiae
079 Viral infection in conditions classified elsewhere and of unspecified site

Rickettsioses and other arthropod-borne diseases (080–088)
080 Louse-borne [epidemic] typhus
081 Other typhus
082 Tick-borne rickettsioses
083 Other rickettsioses
084 Malaria
085 Leishmaniasis
086 Trypanosomiasis
087 Relapsing fever
088 Other arthropod-borne diseases

Syphilis and other venereal diseases (090–099)
090 Congenital syphilis
091 Early syphilis, symptomatic
092 Early syphilis, latent
093 Cardiovascular syphilis
094 Neurosyphilis
095 Other forms of late syphilis, with symptoms
096 Late syphilis, latent
097 Other and unspecified syphilis
098 Gonococcal infections
099 Other venereal diseases

Other spirochetal diseases (100–104)
100 Leptospirosis
101 Vincent's angina
102 Yaws
103 Pinta
104 Other spirochetal infection

Mycoses (110–118)
110 Dermatophytosis
111 Dermatomycosis, other and unspecified
112 Candidiasis
114 Coccidioidomycosis
115 Histoplasmosis
116 Blastomycotic infection
117 Other mycoses
118 Opportunistic mycoses

Helminthiases (120–129)
120 Schistosomiasis [bilharziasis]
121 Other trematode infections
122 Echinococcosis
123 Other cestode infection
124 Trichinosis
125 Filarial infection and dracontiasis
126 Ancylostomiasis and necatoriasis
127 Other intestinal helminthiases

128 Other and unspecified helminthiases ·
129 Intestinal parasitism, unspecified

Other infectious and parasitic diseases (130–136)
130 Toxoplasmosis
131 Trichomoniasis
132 Pediculosis and phthirus infestation
133 Acariasis
134 Other infestation
135 Sarcoidosis
136 Other and unspecified infectious and parasitic diseases

Late effects of infectious and parasitic diseases (137–139)
137 Late effects of tuberculosis
138 Late effects of acute poliomyelitis
139 Late effects of other infectious and parasitic diseases

2. NEOPLASMS

Malignant neoplasm of lip, oral cavity, and pharynx (140–149)
140 Malignant neoplasm of lip
141 Malignant neoplasm of tongue
142 Malignant neoplasm of major salivary glands
143 Malignant neoplasm of gum
144 Malignant neoplasm of floor of mouth
145 Malignant neoplasm of other and unspecified parts of mouth
146 Malignant neoplasm of oropharynx
147 Malignant neoplasm of nasopharynx
148 Malignant neoplasm of hypopharynx
149 Malignant neoplasm of other and ill-defined sites within the lip, oral cavity, and pharynx

Malignant neoplasm of digestive organs and peritoneum (150–159)
150 Malignant neoplasm of esophagus
151 Malignant neoplasm of stomach
152 Malignant neoplasm of small intestine, including duodenum
153 Malignant neoplasm of colon
154 Malignant neoplasm of rectum, rectosigmoid junction, and anus
155 Malignant neoplasm of liver and intrahepatic bile ducts
156 Malignant neoplasm of gallbladder and extrahepatic bile ducts
157 Malignant neoplasm of pancreas
158 Malignant neoplasm of retroperitoneum and peritoneum
159 Malignant neoplasm of other and ill-defined sites within the digestive organs and peritoneum

Malignant neoplasm of respiratory and intrathoracic organs (160–165)
160 Malignant neoplasm of nasal cavities, middle ear, and accessory sinuses
161 Malignant neoplasm of larynx
162 Malignant neoplasm of trachea, bronchus, and lung
163 Malignant neoplasm of pleura
164 Malignant neoplasm of thymus, heart, and mediastinum
165 Malignant neoplasm of other and ill-defined sites within the respiratory system and intrathoracic organs

Malignant neoplasm of bone, connective tissue, skin, and breast (170–176)
170 Malignant neoplasm of bone and articular cartilage
171 Malignant neoplasm of connective and other soft tissue
172 Malignant melanoma of skin
173 Other malignant neoplasm of skin
174 Malignant neoplasm of female breast
175 Malignant neoplasm of male breast

Kaposi's sarcoma (176)
176 Kaposi's sarcoma

Malignant neoplasm of genitourinary organs (179–189)
179 Malignant neoplasm of uterus, part unspecified
180 Malignant neoplasm of cervix uteri
181 Malignant neoplasm of placenta

182 Malignant neoplasm of body of uterus
183 Malignant neoplasm of ovary and other uterine adnexa
184 Malignant neoplasm of other and unspecified female genital organs
185 Malignant neoplasm of prostate
186 Malignant neoplasm of testis
187 Malignant neoplasm of penis and other male genital organs
188 Malignant neoplasm of bladder
189 Malignant neoplasm of kidney and other and unspecified urinary organs

Malignant neoplasm of other and unspecified sites (190–199)
190 Malignant neoplasm of eye
191 Malignant neoplasm of brain
192 Malignant neoplasm of other and unspecified parts of nervous system
193 Malignant neoplasm of thyroid gland
194 Malignant neoplasm of other endocrine glands and related structures
195 Malignant neoplasm of other and ill-defined sites
196 Secondary and unspecified malignant neoplasm of lymph nodes
197 Secondary malignant neoplasm of respiratory and digestive systems
198 Secondary malignant neoplasm of other specified sites
199 Malignant neoplasm without specification of site

Malignant neoplasm of lymphatic and hematopoietic tissue (200–208)
200 Lymphosarcoma and reticulosarcoma
201 Hodgkin's disease
202 Other malignant neoplasm of lymphoid and histiocytic tissue
203 Multiple myeloma and immunoproliferative neoplasms
204 Lymphoid leukemia
205 Myeloid leukemia
206 Monocytic leukemia
207 Other specified leukemia
208 Leukemia of unspecified cell type

Neuroendocrine tumors (209)
209 Neuroendocrine tumors

Benign neoplasms (210–229)
210 Benign neoplasm of lip, oral cavity, and pharynx
211 Benign neoplasm of other parts of digestive system
212 Benign neoplasm of respiratory and intrathoracic organs
213 Benign neoplasm of bone and articular cartilage
214 Lipoma
215 Other benign neoplasm of connective and other soft tissue
216 Benign neoplasm of skin
217 Benign neoplasm of breast
218 Uterine leiomyoma
219 Other benign neoplasm of uterus
220 Benign neoplasm of ovary
221 Benign neoplasm of other female genital organs
222 Benign neoplasm of male genital organs
223 Benign neoplasm of kidney and other urinary organs
224 Benign neoplasm of eye
225 Benign neoplasm of brain and other parts of nervous system
226 Benign neoplasm of thyroid gland
227 Benign neoplasm of other endocrine glands and related structures
228 Hemangioma and lymphangioma, any site
229 Benign neoplasm of other and unspecified sites

Carcinoma in situ (230–234)
230 Carcinoma in situ of digestive organs
231 Carcinoma in situ of respiratory system
232 Carcinoma in situ of skin
233 Carcinoma in situ of breast and genitourinary system
234 Carcinoma in situ of other and unspecified sites

Neoplasms of uncertain behavior (235–238)

235 Neoplasm of uncertain behavior of digestive and respiratory systems
236 Neoplasm of uncertain behavior of genitourinary organs
237 Neoplasm of uncertain behavior of endocrine glands and nervous system
238 Neoplasm of uncertain behavior of other and unspecified sites and tissues

Neoplasms of unspecified nature (239)

239 Neoplasm of unspecified nature

3. ENDOCRINE, NUTRITIONAL AND METABOLIC DISEASES, AND IMMUNITY DISORDERS

Disorders of thyroid gland (240–246)

240 Simple and unspecified goiter
241 Nontoxic nodular goiter
242 Thyrotoxicosis with or without goiter
243 Congenital hypothyroidism
244 Acquired hypothyroidism
245 Thyroiditis
246 Other disorders of thyroid

Diseases of other endocrine glands (249–259)

249 Secondary diabetes mellitus
250 Diabetes mellitus
251 Other disorders of pancreatic internal secretion
252 Disorders of parathyroid gland
253 Disorders of the pituitary gland and its hypothalamic control
254 Diseases of thymus gland
255 Disorders of adrenal glands
256 Ovarian dysfunction
257 Testicular dysfunction
258 Polyglandular dysfunction and related disorders
259 Other endocrine disorders

Nutritional deficiencies (260–269)

260 Kwashiorkor
261 Nutritional marasmus
262 Other severe protein-calorie malnutrition
263 Other and unspecified protein-calorie malnutrition
264 Vitamin A deficiency
265 Thiamine and niacin deficiency states
266 Deficiency of B-complex components
267 Ascorbic acid deficiency
268 Vitamin D deficiency
269 Other nutritional deficiencies

Other metabolic disorders and immunity disorders (270–279)

270 Disorders of amino-acid transport and metabolism
271 Disorders of carbohydrate transport and metabolism
272 Disorders of lipoid metabolism
273 Disorders of plasma protein metabolism
274 Gout
275 Disorders of mineral metabolism
276 Disorders of fluid, electrolyte, and acid-base balance
277 Other and unspecified disorders of metabolism
278 Obesity and other hyperalimentation
279 Disorders involving the immune mechanism

4. DISEASES OF BLOOD AND BLOOD-FORMING ORGANS

Diseases of the blood and blood-forming organs (280–289)

280 Iron deficiency anemias
281 Other deficiency anemias
282 Hereditary hemolytic anemias
283 Acquired hemolytic anemias
284 Aplastic anemia
285 Other and unspecified anemias
286 Coagulation defects
287 Purpura and other hemorrhagic conditions
288 Diseases of white blood cells
289 Other diseases of blood and blood-forming organs

5. MENTAL DISORDERS

Organic psychotic conditions (290–294)

290 Senile and presenile organic psychotic conditions
291 Alcoholic psychoses
292 Drug psychoses
293 Transient organic psychotic conditions
294 Other organic psychotic conditions (chronic)

Other psychoses (295–299)

295 Schizophrenic psychoses
296 Affective psychoses
297 Paranoid states
298 Other nonorganic psychoses
299 Psychoses with origin specific to childhood

Neurotic disorders, personality disorders, and other nonpsychotic mental disorders (300–316)

300 Neurotic disorders
301 Personality disorders
302 Sexual deviations and disorders
303 Alcohol dependence syndrome
304 Drug dependence
305 Nondependent abuse of drugs
306 Physiological malfunction arising from mental factors
307 Special symptoms or syndromes, not elsewhere classified
308 Acute reaction to stress
309 Adjustment reaction
310 Specific nonpsychotic mental disorders following organic brain damage
311 Depressive disorder, not elsewhere classified
312 Disturbance of conduct, not elsewhere classified
313 Disturbance of emotions specific to childhood and adolescence
314 Hyperkinetic syndrome of childhood
315 Specific delays in development
316 Psychic factors associated with diseases classified elsewhere

Mental retardation (317–319)

317 Mild mental retardation
318 Other specified mental retardation
319 Unspecified mental retardation

6. DISEASES OF THE NERVOUS SYSTEM AND SENSE ORGANS

Inflammatory diseases of the central nervous system (320–326)

320 Bacterial meningitis
321 Meningitis due to other organisms
322 Meningitis of unspecified cause
323 Encephalitis, myelitis, and encephalomyelitis
324 Intracranial and intraspinal abscess
325 Phlebitis and thrombophlebitis of intracranial venous sinuses
326 Late effects of intracranial abscess or pyogenic infection
327 Organic sleep disorders

Hereditary and degenerative diseases of the central nervous system (330–337)

330 Cerebral degenerations usually manifest in childhood
331 Other cerebral degenerations
332 Parkinson's disease
333 Other extrapyramidal disease and abnormal movement disorders
334 Spinocerebellar disease
335 Anterior horn cell disease
336 Other diseases of spinal cord
337 Disorders of the autonomic nervous system

Pain (338)

338 Pain, not elsewhere classified

Other headache syndromes (339)

339 Other headache syndromes

Other disorders of the central nervous system (340–349)

340 Multiple sclerosis
341 Other demyelinating diseases of central nervous system
342 Hemiplegia and hemiparesis
343 Infantile cerebral palsy
344 Other paralytic syndromes
345 Epilepsy
346 Migraine
347 Cataplexy and narcolepsy
348 Other conditions of brain
349 Other and unspecified disorders of the nervous system

Disorders of the peripheral nervous system (350–359)

350 Trigeminal nerve disorders
351 Facial nerve disorders
352 Disorders of other cranial nerves
353 Nerve root and plexus disorders
354 Mononeuritis of upper limb and mononeuritis multiplex
355 Mononeuritis of lower limb
356 Hereditary and idiopathic peripheral neuropathy
357 Inflammatory and toxic neuropathy
358 Myoneural disorders
359 Muscular dystrophies and other myopathies

Disorders of the eye and adnexa (360–379)

360 Disorders of the globe
361 Retinal detachments and defects
362 Other retinal disorders
363 Chorioretinal inflammations and scars and other disorders of choroid
364 Disorders of iris and ciliary body
365 Glaucoma
366 Cataract
367 Disorders of refraction and accommodation
368 Visual disturbances
369 Blindness and low vision
370 Keratitis
371 Corneal opacity and other disorders of cornea
372 Disorders of conjunctiva
373 Inflammation of eyelids
374 Other disorders of eyelids
375 Disorders of lacrimal system
376 Disorders of the orbit
377 Disorders of optic nerve and visual pathways
378 Strabismus and other disorders of binocular eye movements
379 Other disorders of eye

Diseases of the ear and mastoid process (380–389)

380 Disorders of external ear
381 Nonsuppurative otitis media and Eustachian tube disorders
382 Suppurative and unspecified otitis media
383 Mastoiditis and related conditions
384 Other disorders of tympanic membrane
385 Other disorders of middle ear and mastoid
386 Vertiginous syndromes and other disorders of vestibular system
387 Otosclerosis
388 Other disorders of ear
389 Hearing loss

7. DISEASES OF THE CIRCULATORY SYSTEM

Acute rheumatic fever (390–392)

390 Rheumatic fever without mention of heart involvement
391 Rheumatic fever with heart involvement
392 Rheumatic chorea

Chronic rheumatic heart disease (393–398)

393 Chronic rheumatic pericarditis
394 Diseases of mitral valve
395 Diseases of aortic valve
396 Diseases of mitral and aortic valves
397 Diseases of other endocardial structures
398 Other rheumatic heart disease

Hypertensive disease (401–405)

401 Essential hypertension
402 Hypertensive heart disease
403 Hypertensive renal disease
404 Hypertensive heart and renal disease
405 Secondary hypertension

Ischemic heart disease (410–414)

410 Acute myocardial infarction
411 Other acute and subacute form of ischemic heart disease
412 Old myocardial infarction
413 Angina pectoris
414 Other forms of chronic ischemic heart disease

Diseases of pulmonary circulation (415–417)

415 Acute pulmonary heart disease
416 Chronic pulmonary heart disease
417 Other diseases of pulmonary circulation

Other forms of heart disease (420–429)

420 Acute pericarditis
421 Acute and subacute endocarditis
422 Acute myocarditis
423 Other diseases of pericardium
424 Other diseases of endocardium
425 Cardiomyopathy
426 Conduction disorders
427 Cardiac dysrhythmias
428 Heart failure
429 Ill-defined descriptions and complications of heart disease

Cerebrovascular disease (430–438)

430 Subarachnoid hemorrhage
431 Intracerebral hemorrhage
432 Other and unspecified intracranial hemorrhage
433 Occlusion and stenosis of precerebral arteries
434 Occlusion of cerebral arteries
435 Transient cerebral ischemia
436 Acute but ill-defined cerebrovascular disease
437 Other and ill-defined cerebrovascular disease
438 Late effects of cerebrovascular disease

Diseases of arteries, arterioles, and capillaries (440–448)

440 Atherosclerosis
441 Aortic aneurysm and dissection
442 Other aneurysm
443 Other peripheral vascular disease
444 Arterial embolism and thrombosis
445 Atheroembolism
446 Polyarteritis nodosa and allied conditions
447 Other disorders of arteries and arterioles
448 Diseases of capillaries

Diseases of veins and lymphatics, and other diseases of circulatory system (451–459)

451 Phlebitis and thrombophlebitis
452 Portal vein thrombosis
453 Other venous embolism and thrombosis
454 Varicose veins of lower extremities
455 Hemorrhoids
456 Varicose veins of other sites
457 Noninfective disorders of lymphatic channels
458 Hypotension
459 Other disorders of circulatory system

8. DISEASES OF THE RESPIRATORY SYSTEM

Acute respiratory infections (460–466)

460 Acute nasopharyngitis [common cold]
461 Acute sinusitis
462 Acute pharyngitis
463 Acute tonsillitis
464 Acute laryngitis and tracheitis
465 Acute upper respiratory infections of multiple or unspecified sites
466 Acute bronchitis and bronchiolitis

Other diseases of upper respiratory tract (470–478)
470 Deviated nasal septum
471 Nasal polyps
472 Chronic pharyngitis and nasopharyngitis
473 Chronic sinusitis
474 Chronic disease of tonsils and adenoids
475 Peritonsillar abscess
476 Chronic laryngitis and laryngotracheitis
477 Allergic rhinitis
478 Other diseases of upper respiratory tract

Pneumonia and influenza (480–488)
480 Viral pneumonia
481 Pneumococcal pneumonia [*Streptococcus pneumoniae* pneumonia]
482 Other bacterial pneumonia
483 Pneumonia due to other specified organism
484 Pneumonia in infectious diseases classified elsewhere
485 Bronchopneumonia, organism unspecified
486 Pneumonia, organism unspecified
487 Influenza
488 Influenza due to identified avian influenza virus

Chronic obstructive pulmonary disease and allied conditions (490–496)
490 Bronchitis, not specified as acute or chronic
491 Chronic bronchitis
492 Emphysema
493 Asthma
494 Bronchiectasis
495 Extrinsic allergic alveolitis
496 Chronic airways obstruction, not elsewhere classified

Pneumoconioses and other lung diseases due to external agents (500–508)
500 Coalworkers' pneumoconiosis
501 Asbestosis
502 Pneumoconiosis due to other silica or silicates
503 Pneumoconiosis due to other inorganic dust
504 Pneumopathy due to inhalation of other dust
505 Pneumoconiosis, unspecified
506 Respiratory conditions due to chemical fumes and vapors
507 Pneumonitis due to solids and liquids
508 Respiratory conditions due to other and unspecified external agents

Other diseases of respiratory system (510–519)
510 Empyema
511 Pleurisy
512 Pneumothorax
513 Abscess of lung and mediastinum
514 Pulmonary congestion and hypostasis
515 Postinflammatory pulmonary fibrosis
516 Other alveolar and parietoalveolar pneumopathy
517 Lung involvement in conditions classified elsewhere
518 Other diseases of lung
519 Other diseases of respiratory system

9. DISEASES OF THE DIGESTIVE SYSTEM

Diseases of oral cavity, salivary glands, and jaws (520–529)
520 Disorders of tooth development and eruption
521 Diseases of hard tissues of teeth
522 Diseases of pulp and periapical tissues
523 Gingival and periodontal diseases
524 Dentofacial anomalies, including malocclusion
525 Other diseases and conditions of the teeth and supporting structures
526 Diseases of the jaws
527 Diseases of the salivary glands
528 Diseases of the oral soft tissues, excluding lesions specific for gingiva and tongue
529 Diseases and other conditions of the tongue

Diseases of esophagus, stomach, and duodenum (530–538)
530 Diseases of esophagus
531 Gastric ulcer
532 Duodenal ulcer
533 Peptic ulcer, site unspecified
534 Gastrojejunal ulcer
535 Gastritis and duodenitis
536 Disorders of function of stomach
537 Other disorders of stomach and duodenum
538 Gastrointestinal mucositis (ulcerative)

Appendicitis (540–543)
540 Acute appendicitis
541 Appendicitis, unqualified
542 Other appendicitis
543 Other diseases of appendix

Hernia of abdominal cavity (550–553)
550 Inguinal hernia
551 Other hernia of abdominal cavity, with gangrene
552 Other hernia of abdominal cavity, with obstruction, but without mention of gangrene
553 Other hernia of abdominal cavity without mention of obstruction or gangrene

Noninfective enteritis and colitis (555–558)
555 Regional enteritis
556 Ulcerative colitis
557 Vascular insufficiency of intestine
558 Other noninfective gastroenteritis and colitis

Other diseases of intestines and peritoneum (560–569)
560 Intestinal obstruction without mention of hernia
562 Diverticula of intestine
564 Functional digestive disorders, not elsewhere classified
565 Anal fissure and fistula
566 Abscess of anal and rectal regions
567 Peritonitis
568 Other disorders of peritoneum
569 Other disorders of intestine

Other diseases of digestive system (570–579)
570 Acute and subacute necrosis of liver
571 Chronic liver disease and cirrhosis
572 Liver abscess and sequelae of chronic liver disease
573 Other disorders of liver
574 Cholelithiasis
575 Other disorders of gallbladder
576 Other disorders of biliary tract
577 Diseases of pancreas
578 Gastrointestinal hemorrhage
579 Intestinal malabsorption

10. DISEASES OF THE GENITOURINARY SYSTEM

Nephritis, nephrotic syndrome, and nephrosis (580–589)
580 Acute glomerulonephritis
581 Nephrotic syndrome
582 Chronic glomerulonephritis
583 Nephritis and nephropathy, not specified as acute or chronic
584 Acute renal failure
585 Chronic renal failure
586 Renal failure, unspecified
587 Renal sclerosis, unspecified
588 Disorders resulting from impaired renal function
589 Small kidney of unknown cause

Other diseases of urinary system (590–599)
590 Infections of kidney
591 Hydronephrosis
592 Calculus of kidney and ureter
593 Other disorders of kidney and ureter
594 Calculus of lower urinary tract
595 Cystitis

596 Other disorders of bladder
597 Urethritis, not sexually transmitted, and urethral syndrome
598 Urethral stricture
599 Other disorders of urethra and urinary tract

Diseases of male genital organs (600–608)
600 Hyperplasia of prostate
601 Inflammatory diseases of prostate
602 Other disorders of prostate
603 Hydrocele
604 Orchitis and epididymitis
605 Redundant prepuce and phimosis
606 Infertility, male
607 Disorders of penis
608 Other disorders of male genital organs

Disorders of breast (610–611)
610 Benign mammary dysplasias
611 Other disorders of breast
612 Deformity and disproportion of reconstructed breast

Inflammatory disease of female pelvic organs (614–616)
614 Inflammatory disease of ovary, fallopian tube, pelvic cellular tissue, and peritoneum
615 Inflammatory diseases of uterus, except cervix
616 Inflammatory disease of cervix, vagina, and vulva

Other disorders of female genital tract (617–629)
617 Endometriosis
618 Genital prolapse
619 Fistula involving female genital tract
620 Noninflammatory disorders of ovary, fallopian tube, and broad ligament
621 Disorders of uterus, not elsewhere classified
622 Noninflammatory disorders of cervix
623 Noninflammatory disorders of vagina
624 Noninflammatory disorders of vulva and perineum
625 Pain and other symptoms associated with female genital organs
626 Disorders of menstruation and other abnormal bleeding from female genital tract
627 Menopausal and postmenopausal disorders
628 Infertility, female
629 Other disorders of female genital organs

11. COMPLICATIONS OF PREGNANCY, CHILDBIRTH, AND THE PUERPERIUM

Ectopic and molar pregnancy and other pregnancy with abortive outcome (630–639)
630 Hydatidiform mole
631 Other abnormal product of conception
632 Missed abortion
633 Ectopic pregnancy
634 Spontaneous abortion
635 Legally induced abortion
636 Illegally induced abortion
637 Unspecified abortion
638 Failed attempted abortion
639 Complications following abortion and ectopic and molar pregnancies

Complications mainly related to pregnancy (640–649)
640 Hemorrhage in early pregnancy
641 Antepartum hemorrhage, abruptio placentae, and placenta previa
642 Hypertension complicating pregnancy, childbirth, and the puerperium
643 Excessive vomiting in pregnancy
644 Early or threatened labor
645 Prolonged pregnancy
646 Other complications of pregnancy, not elsewhere classified
647 Infective and parasitic conditions in the mother classifiable elsewhere but complicating pregnancy, childbirth, and the puerperium

648 Other current conditions in the mother classifiable elsewhere but complicating pregnancy, childbirth, and the puerperium
649 Other conditions or status of the mother complicating pregnancy, childbirth, or the puerperium

Normal delivery, and other indications for care in pregnancy, labor, and delivery (650–659)
650 Normal delivery
651 Multiple gestation
652 Malposition and malpresentation of fetus
653 Disproportion
654 Abnormality of organs and soft tissues of pelvis
655 Known or suspected fetal abnormality affecting management of mother
656 Other fetal and placental problems affecting management of mother
657 Polyhydramnios
658 Other problems associated with amniotic cavity and membranes
659 Other indications for care or intervention related to labor and delivery and not elsewhere classified

Complications occurring mainly in the course of labor and delivery (660–669)
660 Obstructed labor
661 Abnormality of forces of labor
662 Long labor
663 Umbilical cord complications
664 Trauma to perineum and vulva during delivery
665 Other obstetrical trauma
666 Postpartum hemorrhage
667 Retained placenta or membranes, without hemorrhage
668 Complications of the administration of anesthetic or other sedation in labor and delivery
669 Other complications of labor and delivery, not elsewhere classified

Complications of the puerperium (670–677)
670 Major puerperal infection
671 Venous complications in pregnancy and the puerperium
672 Pyrexia of unknown origin during the puerperium
673 Obstetrical pulmonary embolism
674 Other and unspecified complications of the puerperium, not elsewhere classified
675 Infections of the breast and nipple associated with childbirth
676 Other disorders of the breast associated with childbirth, and disorders of lactation
677 Late effect of complication of pregnancy, childbirth, and the puerperium

Other Maternal and Fetal Complications (678-679)
678 Other fetal conditions
679 Complications of in utero procedures

12. DISEASES OF THE SKIN AND SUBCUTANEOUS TISSUE

Infections of skin and subcutaneous tissue (680–686)
680 Carbuncle and furuncle
681 Cellulitis and abscess of finger and toe
682 Other cellulitis and abscess
683 Acute lymphadenitis
684 Impetigo
685 Pilonidal cyst
686 Other local infections of skin and subcutaneous tissue

Other inflammatory conditions of skin and subcutaneous tissue (690–698)
690 Erythematosquamous dermatosis
691 Atopic dermatitis and related conditions
692 Contact dermatitis and other eczema
693 Dermatitis due to substances taken internally
694 Bullous dermatoses

695 Erythematous conditions
696 Psoriasis and similar disorders
697 Lichen
698 Pruritus and related conditions

Other diseases of skin and subcutaneous tissue (700–709)
700 Corns and callosities
701 Other hypertrophic and atrophic conditions of skin
702 Other dermatoses
703 Diseases of nail
704 Diseases of hair and hair follicles
705 Disorders of sweat glands
706 Diseases of sebaceous glands
707 Chronic ulcer of skin
708 Urticaria
709 Other disorders of skin and subcutaneous tissue

13. DISEASES OF THE MUSCULOSKELETAL SYSTEM AND CONNECTIVE TISSUE

Arthropathies and related disorders (710–719)
710 Diffuse diseases of connective tissue
711 Arthropathy associated with infections
712 Crystal arthropathies
713 Arthropathy associated with other disorders classified elsewhere
714 Rheumatoid arthritis and other inflammatory polyarthropathies
715 Osteoarthrosis and allied disorders
716 Other and unspecified arthropathies
717 Internal derangement of knee
718 Other derangement of joint
719 Other and unspecified disorder of joint

Dorsopathies (720–724)
720 Ankylosing spondylitis and other inflammatory spondylopathies
721 Spondylosis and allied disorders
722 Intervertebral disc disorders
723 Other disorders of cervical region
724 Other and unspecified disorders of back

Rheumatism, excluding the back (725–729)
725 Polymyalgia rheumatica
726 Peripheral enthesopathies and allied syndromes
727 Other disorders of synovium, tendon, and bursa
728 Disorders of muscle, ligament, and fascia
729 Other disorders of soft tissues

Osteopathies, chondropathies, and acquired musculoskeletal deformities (730–739)
730 Osteomyelitis, periostitis, and other infections involving bone
731 Osteitis deformans and osteopathies associated with other disorders classified elsewhere
732 Osteochondropathies
733 Other disorders of bone and cartilage
734 Flat foot
735 Acquired deformities of toe
736 Other acquired deformities of limbs
737 Curvature of spine
738 Other acquired deformity
739 Nonallopathic lesions, not elsewhere classified

14. CONGENITAL ANOMALIES

Congenital anomalies (740–759)
740 Anencephalus and similar anomalies
741 Spina bifida
742 Other congenital anomalies of nervous system
743 Congenital anomalies of eye
744 Congenital anomalies of ear, face, and neck
745 Bulbus cordis anomalies and anomalies of cardiac septal closure
746 Other congenital anomalies of heart
747 Other congenital anomalies of circulatory system
748 Congenital anomalies of respiratory system
749 Cleft palate and cleft lip
750 Other congenital anomalies of upper alimentary tract
751 Other congenital anomalies of digestive system
752 Congenital anomalies of genital organs
753 Congenital anomalies of urinary system
754 Certain congenital musculoskeletal deformities
755 Other congenital anomalies of limbs
756 Other congenital musculoskeletal anomalies
757 Congenital anomalies of the integument
758 Chromosomal anomalies
759 Other and unspecified congenital anomalies

15. CERTAIN CONDITIONS ORIGINATING IN THE PERINATAL PERIOD

Maternal causes of perinatal morbidity and mortality (760–763)
760 Fetus or newborn affected by maternal conditions which may be unrelated to present pregnancy
761 Fetus or newborn affected by maternal complications of pregnancy
762 Fetus or newborn affected by complications of placenta, cord, and membranes
763 Fetus or newborn affected by other complications of labor and delivery

Other conditions originating in the perinatal period (764–779)
764 Slow fetal growth and fetal malnutrition
765 Disorders relating to short gestation and unspecified low birthweight
766 Disorders relating to long gestation and high birthweight
767 Birth trauma
768 Intrauterine hypoxia and birth asphyxia
769 Respiratory distress syndrome
770 Other respiratory conditions of fetus and newborn
771 Infections specific to the perinatal period
772 Fetal and neonatal hemorrhage
773 Hemolytic disease of fetus or newborn, due to isoimmunization
774 Other perinatal jaundice
775 Endocrine and metabolic disturbances specific to the fetus and newborn
776 Hematological disorders of fetus and newborn
777 Perinatal disorders of digestive system
778 Conditions involving the integument and temperature regulation of fetus and newborn
779 Other and ill-defined conditions originating in the perinatal period

16. SYMPTOMS, SIGNS, AND ILL-DEFINED CONDITIONS

Symptoms (780–789)
780 General symptoms
781 Symptoms involving nervous and musculoskeletal systems
782 Symptoms involving skin and other integumentary tissue
783 Symptoms concerning nutrition, metabolism, and development
784 Symptoms involving head and neck
785 Symptoms involving cardiovascular system
786 Symptoms involving respiratory system and other chest symptoms
787 Symptoms involving digestive system
788 Symptoms involving urinary system
789 Other symptoms involving abdomen and pelvis

Nonspecific abnormal findings (790–796)
790 Nonspecific findings on examination of blood
791 Nonspecific findings on examination of urine
792 Nonspecific abnormal findings in other body substances
793 Nonspecific abnormal findings on radiological and other examination of body structure
794 Nonspecific abnormal results of function studies

795 Nonspecific abnormal histological and immunological findings
796 Other nonspecific abnormal findings

Ill-defined and unknown causes of morbidity and mortality (797–799)
797 Senility without mention of psychosis
798 Sudden death, cause unknown
799 Other ill-defined and unknown causes of morbidity and mortality

17. INJURY AND POISONING

Fracture of skull (800–804)
800 Fracture of vault of skull
801 Fracture of base of skull
802 Fracture of face bones
803 Other and unqualified skull fractures
804 Multiple fractures involving skull or face with other bones

Fracture of spine and trunk (805–809)
805 Fracture of vertebral column without mention of spinal cord lesion
806 Fracture of vertebral column with spinal cord lesion
807 Fracture of rib(s), sternum, larynx, and trachea
808 Fracture of pelvis
809 Ill-defined fractures of bones of trunk

Fracture of upper limb (810–819)
810 Fracture of clavicle
811 Fracture of scapula
812 Fracture of humerus
813 Fracture of radius and ulna
814 Fracture of carpal bone(s)
815 Fracture of metacarpal bone(s)
816 Fracture of one or more phalanges of hand
817 Multiple fractures of hand bones
818 Ill-defined fractures of upper limb
819 Multiple fractures involving both upper limbs, and upper limb with rib(s) and sternum

Fracture of lower limb (820–829)
820 Fracture of neck of femur
821 Fracture of other and unspecified parts of femur
822 Fracture of patella
823 Fracture of tibia and fibula
824 Fracture of ankle
825 Fracture of one or more tarsal and metatarsal bones
826 Fracture of one or more phalanges of foot
827 Other, multiple, and ill-defined fractures of lower limb
828 Multiple fractures involving both lower limbs, lower with upper limb, and lower limb(s) with rib(s) and sternum
829 Fracture of unspecified bones

Dislocation (830–839)
830 Dislocation of jaw
831 Dislocation of shoulder
832 Dislocation of elbow
833 Dislocation of wrist
834 Dislocation of finger
835 Dislocation of hip
836 Dislocation of knee
837 Dislocation of ankle
838 Dislocation of foot
839 Other, multiple, and ill-defined dislocations

Sprains and strains of joints and adjacent muscles (840–848)
840 Sprains and strains of shoulder and upper arm
841 Sprains and strains of elbow and forearm
842 Sprains and strains of wrist and hand
843 Sprains and strains of hip and thigh
844 Sprains and strains of knee and leg
845 Sprains and strains of ankle and foot
846 Sprains and strains of sacroiliac region
847 Sprains and strains of other and unspecified parts of back
848 Other and ill-defined sprains and strains

Intracranial injury, excluding those with skull fracture (850–854)
850 Concussion
851 Cerebral laceration and contusion
852 Subarachnoid, subdural, and extradural hemorrhage, following injury
853 Other and unspecified intracranial hemorrhage following injury
854 Intracranial injury of other and unspecified nature

Internal injury of chest, abdomen, and pelvis (860–869)
860 Traumatic pneumothorax and hemothorax
861 Injury to heart and lung
862 Injury to other and unspecified intrathoracic organs
863 Injury to gastrointestinal tract
864 Injury to liver
865 Injury to spleen
866 Injury to kidney
867 Injury to pelvic organs
868 Injury to other intra-abdominal organs
869 Internal injury to unspecified or ill-defined organs

Open wound of head, neck, and trunk (870–879)
870 Open wound of ocular adnexa
871 Open wound of eyeball
872 Open wound of ear
873 Other open wound of head
874 Open wound of neck
875 Open wound of chest (wall)
876 Open wound of back
877 Open wound of buttock
878 Open wound of genital organs (external), including traumatic amputation
879 Open wound of other and unspecified sites, except limbs

Open wound of upper limb (880–887)
880 Open wound of shoulder and upper arm
881 Open wound of elbow, forearm, and wrist
882 Open wound of hand except finger(s) alone
883 Open wound of finger(s)
884 Multiple and unspecified open wound of upper limb
885 Traumatic amputation of thumb (complete) (partial)
886 Traumatic amputation of other finger(s) (complete) (partial)
887 Traumatic amputation of arm and hand (complete) (partial)

Open wound of lower limb (890–897)
890 Open wound of hip and thigh
891 Open wound of knee, leg [except thigh], and ankle
892 Open wound of foot except toe(s) alone
893 Open wound of toe(s)
894 Multiple and unspecified open wound of lower limb
895 Traumatic amputation of toe(s) (complete) (partial)
896 Traumatic amputation of foot (complete) (partial)
897 Traumatic amputation of leg(s) (complete) (partial)

Injury to blood vessels (900–904)
900 Injury to blood vessels of head and neck
901 Injury to blood vessels of thorax
902 Injury to blood vessels of abdomen and pelvis
903 Injury to blood vessels of upper extremity
904 Injury to blood vessels of lower extremity and unspecified sites

Late effects of injuries, poisonings, toxic effects, and other external causes (905–909)
905 Late effects of musculoskeletal and connective tissue injuries
906 Late effects of injuries to skin and subcutaneous tissues
907 Late effects of injuries to the nervous system
908 Late effects of other and unspecified injuries
909 Late effects of other and unspecified external causes

Superficial injury (910–919)
910 Superficial injury of face, neck, and scalp except eye
911 Superficial injury of trunk
912 Superficial injury of shoulder and upper arm

APPX E

913 Superficial injury of elbow, forearm, and wrist
914 Superficial injury of hand(s) except finger(s) alone
915 Superficial injury of finger(s)
916 Superficial injury of hip, thigh, leg, and ankle
917 Superficial injury of foot and toe(s)
918 Superficial injury of eye and adnexa
919 Superficial injury of other, multiple, and unspecified sites

Contusion with intact skin surface (920–924)
920 Contusion of face, scalp, and neck except eye(s)
921 Contusion of eye and adnexa
922 Contusion of trunk
923 Contusion of upper limb
924 Contusion of lower limb and of other and unspecified sites

Crushing injury (925–929)
925 Crushing injury of face, scalp, and neck
926 Crushing injury of trunk
927 Crushing injury of upper limb
928 Crushing injury of lower limb
929 Crushing injury of multiple and unspecified sites

Effects of foreign body entering through orifice (930–939)
930 Foreign body on external eye
931 Foreign body in ear
932 Foreign body in nose
933 Foreign body in pharynx and larynx
934 Foreign body in trachea, bronchus, and lung
935 Foreign body in mouth, esophagus, and stomach
936 Foreign body in intestine and colon
937 Foreign body in anus and rectum
938 Foreign body in digestive system, unspecified
939 Foreign body in genitourinary tract

Burns (940–949)
940 Burn confined to eye and adnexa
941 Burn of face, head, and neck
942 Burn of trunk
943 Burn of upper limb, except wrist and hand
944 Burn of wrist(s) and hand(s)
945 Burn of lower limb(s)
946 Burns of multiple specified sites
947 Burn of internal organs
948 Burns classified according to extent of body surface involved
949 Burn, unspecified

Injury to nerves and spinal cord (950–957)
950 Injury to optic nerve and pathways
951 Injury to other cranial nerve(s)
952 Spinal cord injury without evidence of spinal bone injury
953 Injury to nerve roots and spinal plexus
954 Injury to other nerve(s) of trunk excluding shoulder and pelvic girdles
955 Injury to peripheral nerve(s) of shoulder girdle and upper limb
956 Injury to peripheral nerve(s) of pelvic girdle and lower limb
957 Injury to other and unspecified nerves

Certain traumatic complications and unspecified injuries (958–959)
958 Certain early complications of trauma
959 Injury, other and unspecified

Poisoning by drugs, medicinals and biological substances (960–979)
960 Poisoning by antibiotics
961 Poisoning by other anti-infectives
962 Poisoning by hormones and synthetic substitutes
963 Poisoning by primarily systemic agents
964 Poisoning by agents primarily affecting blood constituents
965 Poisoning by analgesics, antipyretics, and antirheumatics
966 Poisoning by anticonvulsants and anti-Parkinsonism drugs
967 Poisoning by sedatives and hypnotics
968 Poisoning by other central nervous system depressants and anesthetics

969 Poisoning by psychotropic agents
970 Poisoning by central nervous system stimulants
971 Poisoning by drugs primarily affecting the autonomic nervous system
972 Poisoning by agents primarily affecting the cardiovascular system
973 Poisoning by agents primarily affecting the gastrointestinal system
974 Poisoning by water, mineral, and uric acid metabolism drugs
975 Poisoning by agents primarily acting on the smooth and skeletal muscles and respiratory system
976 Poisoning by agents primarily affecting skin and mucous membrane, ophthalmological, otorhinolaryngological, and dental drugs
977 Poisoning by other and unspecified drugs and medicinals
978 Poisoning by bacterial vaccines
979 Poisoning by other vaccines and biological substances

Toxic effects of substances chiefly nonmedicinal as to source (980–989)
980 Toxic effect of alcohol
981 Toxic effect of petroleum products
982 Toxic effect of solvents other than petroleum-based
983 Toxic effect of corrosive aromatics, acids, and caustic alkalis
984 Toxic effect of lead and its compounds (including fumes)
985 Toxic effect of other metals
986 Toxic effect of carbon monoxide
987 Toxic effect of other gases, fumes, or vapors
988 Toxic effect of noxious substances eaten as food
989 Toxic effect of other substances, chiefly nonmedicinal as to source

Other and unspecified effects of external causes (990–995)
990 Effects of radiation, unspecified
991 Effects of reduced temperature
992 Effects of heat and light
993 Effects of air pressure
994 Effects of other external causes
995 Certain adverse effects, not elsewhere classified

Complications of surgical and medical care, not elsewhere classified (996–999)
996 Complications peculiar to certain specified procedures
997 Complications affecting specified body systems, not elsewhere classified
998 Other complications of procedures, not elsewhere classified
999 Complications of medical care, not elsewhere classified

SUPPLEMENTARY CLASSIFICATION OF FACTORS INFLUENCING HEALTH STATUS AND CONTACT WITH HEALTH SERVICES (V01–V86)

Persons with potential health hazards related to communicable diseases (V01–V09)
V01 Contact with or exposure to communicable diseases
V02 Carrier or suspected carrier of infectious diseases
V03 Need for prophylactic vaccination and inoculation against bacterial diseases
V04 Need for prophylactic vaccination and inoculation against certain viral diseases
V05 Need for other prophylactic vaccination and inoculation against single diseases
V06 Need for prophylactic vaccination and inoculation against combinations of diseases
V07 Need for isolation and other prophylactic measures
V08 Asymptomatic human immunodeficiency virus [HIV] infection status
V09 Infection with drug-resistant microorganisms

Persons with potential health hazards related to personal and family history (V10–V19)
V10 Personal history of malignant neoplasm
V11 Personal history of mental disorder
V12 Personal history of certain other diseases
V13 Personal history of other diseases

APPX E

V14   Personal history of allergy to medicinal agents
V15   Other personal history presenting hazards to health
V16   Family history of malignant neoplasm
V17   Family history of certain chronic disabling diseases
V18   Family history of certain other specific conditions
V19   Family history of other conditions

Persons encountering health services in circumstances related to reproduction and development (V20–V29)
V20   Health supervision of infant or child
V21   Constitutional states in development
V22   Normal pregnancy
V23   Supervision of high-risk pregnancy
V24   Postpartum care and examination
V25   Encounter for contraceptive management
V26   Procreative management
V27   Outcome of delivery
V28   Antenatal screening
V29   Observation and evaluation of newborns and infants for suspected condition not found

Liveborn infants according to type of birth (V30–V39)
V30   Single liveborn
V31   Twin, mate liveborn
V32   Twin, mate stillborn
V33   Twin, unspecified
V34   Other multiple, mates all liveborn
V35   Other multiple, mates all stillborn
V36   Other multiple, mates live- and stillborn
V37   Other multiple, unspecified
V39   Unspecified

Persons with a condition influencing their health status (V40–V49)
V40   Mental and behavioral problems
V41   Problems with special senses and other special functions
V42   Organ or tissue replaced by transplant
V43   Organ or tissue replaced by other means
V44   Artificial opening status
V45   Other postsurgical states
V46   Other dependence on machines
V47   Other problems with internal organs
V48   Problems with head, neck, and trunk
V49   Problems with limbs and other problems

Persons encountering health services for specific procedures and aftercare (V50–V59)
V50   Elective surgery for purposes other than remedying health states
V51   Aftercare involving the use of plastic surgery
V52   Fitting and adjustment of prosthetic device
V53   Fitting and adjustment of other device
V54   Other orthopedic aftercare
V55   Attention to artificial openings
V56   Encounter for dialysis and dialysis catheter care
V57   Care involving use of rehabilitation procedures
V58   Other and unspecified aftercare
V59   Donors

Persons encountering health services in other circumstances (V60–V69)
V60   Housing, household, and economic circumstances
V61   Other family circumstances
V62   Other psychosocial circumstances
V63   Unavailability of other medical facilities for care
V64   Persons encountering health services for specific procedures, not carried out
V65   Other persons seeking consultation without complaint or sickness
V66   Convalescence and palliative care
V67   Follow-up examination
V68   Encounters for administrative purposes
V69   Problems related to lifestyle

Persons without reported diagnosis encountered during examination and investigation of individuals and populations (V70–V82)
V70   General medical examination
V71   Observation and evaluation for suspected conditions
V72   Special investigations and examinations
V73   Special screening examination for viral and chlamydial diseases
V74   Special screening examination for bacterial and spirochetal diseases
V75   Special screening examination for other infectious diseases
V76   Special screening for malignant neoplasms
V77   Special screening for endocrine, nutritional, metabolic, and immunity disorders
V78   Special screening for disorders of blood and blood-forming organs
V79   Special screening for mental disorders and developmental handicaps
V80   Special screening for neurological, eye, and ear diseases
V81   Special screening for cardiovascular, respiratory, and genitourinary diseases
V82   Special screening for other conditions

Genetics (V83–V84)
V83   Genetic carrier status
V84   Genetic susceptibility to malignant neoplasm

Body Mass Index (V85)
V85   Body mass index

Estrogen Receptor Status (V86)
V86   Estrogen receptor status

Other specified personal exposures and history presenting hazards to health (V87)
V87   Other specified personal exposures and history presenting hazards to health

Acquired absence of other organs and tissue (V88)
V88   Acquired absence of other organs and tissue

Other suspected conditions not found (V89)
V89   Other suspected conditions not found

SUPPLEMENTARY CLASSIFICATION OF EXTERNAL CAUSES OF INJURY AND POISONING (E800–E899)

Railway accidents (E800–E807)
E800   Railway accident involving collision with rolling stock
E801   Railway accident involving collision with other object
E802   Railway accident involving derailment without antecedent collision
E803   Railway accident involving explosion, fire, or burning
E804   Fall in, on, or from railway train
E805   Hit by rolling stock
E806   Other specified railway accident
E807   Railway accident of unspecified nature

Motor vehicle traffic accidents (E810–E819)
E810   Motor vehicle traffic accident involving collision with train
E811   Motor vehicle traffic accident involving re-entrant collision with another motor vehicle
E812   Other motor vehicle traffic accident involving collision with another motor vehicle
E813   Motor vehicle traffic accident involving collision with other vehicle
E814   Motor vehicle traffic accident involving collision with pedestrian
E815   Other motor vehicle traffic accident involving collision on the highway
E816   Motor vehicle traffic accident due to loss of control, without collision on the highway
E817   Noncollision motor vehicle traffic accident while boarding or alighting
E818   Other noncollision motor vehicle traffic accident
E819   Motor vehicle traffic accident of unspecified nature

Motor vehicle nontraffic accidents (E820–E825)

E820   Nontraffic accident involving motor-driven snow vehicle
E821   Nontraffic accident involving other off-road motor vehicle
E822   Other motor vehicle nontraffic accident involving collision with moving object
E823   Other motor vehicle nontraffic accident involving collision with stationary object
E824   Other motor vehicle nontraffic accident while boarding and alighting
E825   Other motor vehicle nontraffic accident of other and unspecified nature

Other road vehicle accidents (E826–E829)

E826   Pedal cycle accident
E827   Animal-drawn vehicle accident
E828   Accident involving animal being ridden
E829   Other road vehicle accidents

Water transport accidents (E830–E838)

E830   Accident to watercraft causing submersion
E831   Accident to watercraft causing other injury
E832   Other accidental submersion or drowning in water transport accident
E833   Fall on stairs or ladders in water transport
E834   Other fall from one level to another in water transport
E835   Other and unspecified fall in water transport
E836   Machinery accident in water transport
E837   Explosion, fire, or burning in watercraft
E838   Other and unspecified water transport accident

Air and space transport accidents (E840–E845)

E840   Accident to powered aircraft at takeoff or landing
E841   Accident to powered aircraft, other and unspecified
E842   Accident to unpowered aircraft
E843   Fall in, on, or from aircraft
E844   Other specified air transport accidents
E845   Accident involving spacecraft

Vehicle accidents, not elsewhere classifiable (E846–E849)

E846   Accidents involving powered vehicles used solely within the buildings and premises of an industrial or commercial establishment
E847   Accidents involving cable cars not running on rails
E848   Accidents involving other vehicles, not elsewhere classifiable
E849   Place of occurrence

Accidental poisoning by drugs, medicinal substances, and biologicals (E850–E858)

E850   Accidental poisoning by analgesics, antipyretics, and antirheumatics
E851   Accidental poisoning by barbiturates
E852   Accidental poisoning by other sedatives and hypnotics
E853   Accidental poisoning by tranquilizers
E854   Accidental poisoning by other psychotropic agents
E855   Accidental poisoning by other drugs acting on central and autonomic nervous systems
E856   Accidental poisoning by antibiotics
E857   Accidental poisoning by anti-infectives
E858   Accidental poisoning by other drugs

Accidental poisoning by other solid and liquid substances, gases, and vapors (E860–E869)

E860   Accidental poisoning by alcohol, not elsewhere classified
E861   Accidental poisoning by cleansing and polishing agents, disinfectants, paints, and varnishes
E862   Accidental poisoning by petroleum products, other solvents and their vapors, not elsewhere classified
E863   Accidental poisoning by agricultural and horticultural chemical and pharmaceutical preparations other than plant foods and fertilizers
E864   Accidental poisoning by corrosives and caustics, not elsewhere classified
E865   Accidental poisoning from poisonous foodstuffs and poisonous plants

E866   Accidental poisoning by other and unspecified solid and liquid substances
E867   Accidental poisoning by gas distributed by pipeline
E868   Accidental poisoning by other utility gas and other carbon monoxide
E869   Accidental poisoning by other gases and vapors

Misadventures to patients during surgical and medical care (E870–E876)

E870   Accidental cut, puncture, perforation, or hemorrhage during medical care
E871   Foreign object left in body during procedure
E872   Failure of sterile precautions during procedure
E873   Failure in dosage
E874   Mechanical failure of instrument or apparatus during procedure
E875   Contaminated or infected blood, other fluid, drug, or biological substance
E876   Other and unspecified misadventures during medical care

Surgical and medical procedures as the cause of abnormal reaction of patient or later complication, without mention of misadventure at the time of procedure (E878–E879)

E878   Surgical operation and other surgical procedures as the cause of abnormal reaction of patient, or of later complication, without mention of misadventure at the time of operation
E879   Other procedures, without mention of misadventure at the time of procedure, as the cause of abnormal reaction of patient, or of later complication

Accidental falls (E880–E888)

E880   Fall on or from stairs or steps
E881   Fall on or from ladders or scaffolding
E882   Fall from or out of building or other structure
E883   Fall into hole or other opening in surface
E884   Other fall from one level to another
E885   Fall on same level from slipping, tripping, or stumbling
E886   Fall on same level from collision, pushing, or shoving, by or with other person
E887   Fracture, cause unspecified
E888   Other and unspecified fall

Accidents caused by fire and flames (E890–E899)

E890   Conflagration in private dwelling
E891   Conflagration in other and unspecified building or structure
E892   Conflagration not in building or structure
E893   Accident caused by ignition of clothing
E894   Ignition of highly inflammable material
E895   Accident caused by controlled fire in private dwelling
E896   Accident caused by controlled fire in other and unspecified building or structure
E897   Accident caused by controlled fire not in building or structure
E898   Accident caused by other specified fire and flames
E899   Accident caused by unspecified fire

Accidents due to natural and environmental factors (E900–E909)

E900   Excessive heat
E901   Excessive cold
E902   High and low air pressure and changes in air pressure
E903   Travel and motion
E904   Hunger, thirst, exposure, and neglect
E905   Venomous animals and plants as the cause of poisoning and toxic reactions
E906   Other injury caused by animals
E907   Lightning
E908   Cataclysmic storms, and floods resulting from storms
E909   Cataclysmic earth surface movements and eruptions

Accidents caused by submersion, suffocation, and foreign bodies (E910–E915)

E910 Accidental drowning and submersion
E911 Inhalation and ingestion of food causing obstruction of respiratory tract or suffocation
E912 Inhalation and ingestion of other object causing obstruction of respiratory tract or suffocation
E913 Accidental mechanical suffocation
E914 Foreign body accidentally entering eye and adnexa
E915 Foreign body accidentally entering other orifice

Other accidents (E916–E928)

E916 Struck accidentally by falling object
E917 Striking against or struck accidentally by objects or persons
E918 Caught accidentally in or between objects
E919 Accidents caused by machinery
E920 Accidents caused by cutting and piercing instruments or objects
E921 Accident caused by explosion of pressure vessel
E922 Accident caused by firearm missile
E923 Accident caused by explosive material
E924 Accident caused by hot substance or object, caustic or corrosive material, and steam
E925 Accident caused by electric current
E926 Exposure to radiation
E927 Overexertion and strenuous movements
E928 Other and unspecified environmental and accidental causes

Late effects of accidental injury (E929)

E929 Late effects of accidental injury

Drugs, medicinal and biological substances causing adverse effects in therapeutic use (E930–E949)

E930 Antibiotics
E931 Other anti-infectives
E932 Hormones and synthetic substitutes
E933 Primarily systemic agents
E934 Agents primarily affecting blood constituents
E935 Analgesics, antipyretics, and antirheumatics
E936 Anticonvulsants and anti-Parkinsonism drugs
E937 Sedatives and hypnotics
E938 Other central nervous system depressants and anesthetics
E939 Psychotropic agents
E940 Central nervous system stimulants
E941 Drugs primarily affecting the autonomic nervous system
E942 Agents primarily affecting the cardiovascular system
E943 Agents primarily affecting gastrointestinal system
E944 Water, mineral, and uric acid metabolism drugs
E945 Agents primarily acting on the smooth and skeletal muscles and respiratory system
E946 Agents primarily affecting skin and mucous membrane, ophthalmological, otorhinolaryngological, and dental drugs
E947 Other and unspecified drugs and medicinal substances
E948 Bacterial vaccines
E949 Other vaccines and biological substances

Suicide and self-inflicted injury (E950–E959)

E950 Suicide and self-inflicted poisoning by solid or liquid substances
E951 Suicide and self-inflicted poisoning by gases in domestic use
E952 Suicide and self-inflicted poisoning by other gases and vapors
E953 Suicide and self-inflicted injury by hanging, strangulation, and suffocation
E954 Suicide and self-inflicted injury by submersion [drowning]
E955 Suicide and self-inflicted injury by firearms and explosives
E956 Suicide and self-inflicted injury by cutting and piercing instruments
E957 Suicide and self-inflicted injuries by jumping from high place

E958 Suicide and self-inflicted injury by other and unspecified means
E959 Late effects of self-inflicted injury

Homicide and injury purposely inflicted by other persons (E960–E969)

E960 Fight, brawl, and rape
E961 Assault by corrosive or caustic substance, except poisoning
E962 Assault by poisoning
E963 Assault by hanging and strangulation
E964 Assault by submersion [drowning]
E965 Assault by firearms and explosives
E966 Assault by cutting and piercing instrument
E967 Child and adult battering and other maltreatment
E968 Assault by other and unspecified means
E969 Late effects of injury purposely inflicted by other person

Legal intervention (E970–E978)

E970 Injury due to legal intervention by firearms
E971 Injury due to legal intervention by explosives
E972 Injury due to legal intervention by gas
E973 Injury due to legal intervention by blunt object
E974 Injury due to legal intervention by cutting and piercing instruments
E975 Injury due to legal intervention by other specified means
E976 Injury due to legal intervention by unspecified means
E977 Late effects of injuries due to legal intervention
E978 Legal execution
E979 Terrorism

Injury undetermined whether accidentally or purposely inflicted (E980–E989)

E980 Poisoning by solid or liquid substances, undetermined whether accidentally or purposely inflicted
E981 Poisoning by gases in domestic use, undetermined whether accidentally or purposely inflicted
E982 Poisoning by other gases, undetermined whether accidentally or purposely inflicted
E983 Hanging, strangulation, or suffocation, undetermined whether accidentally or purposely inflicted
E984 Submersion [drowning], undetermined whether accidentally or purposely inflicted
E985 Injury by firearms and explosives, undetermined whether accidentally or purposely inflicted
E986 Injury by cutting and piercing instruments, undetermined whether accidentally or purposely inflicted
E987 Falling from high place, undetermined whether accidentally or purposely inflicted
E988 Injury by other and unspecified means, undetermined whether accidentally or purposely inflicted
E989 Late effects of injury, undetermined whether accidentally or purposely inflicted

Injury resulting from operations of war (E990–E999)

E990 Injury due to war operations by fires and conflagrations
E991 Injury due to war operations by bullets and fragments
E992 Injury due to war operations by explosion of marine weapons
E993 Injury due to war operations by other explosion
E994 Injury due to war operations by destruction of aircraft
E995 Injury due to war operations by other and unspecified forms of conventional warfare
E996 Injury due to war operations by nuclear weapons
E997 Injury due to war operations by other forms of unconventional warfare
E998 Injury due to war operations but occurring after cessation of hostilities
E999 Late effects of injury due to war operations

TABLE A

TABLE OF BACTERIAL FOOD POISONING

Bacteria Responsible	Description	Habitat	Types of Foods	Symptoms	Cause	Temperature Sensitivity
Staphylococcus aureus	Produces a heat-stable toxin.	Nose and throat of 30 to 50 percent of healthy population; also skin and superficial wounds.	Meat and seafood salads, sandwich spreads, and high salt foods.	Nausea, vomiting, and diarrhea within 4 to 6 hours. No fever.	Poor personal hygiene and subsequent temperature abuse.	No growth below 40° F. Bacteria are destroyed by normal cooking, but toxin is heat-stable.
Clostridium perfringens	Produces a spore and prefers low oxygen atmosphere. Live cells must be ingested.	Dust, soil, and gastrointestinal tracts of animals and man.	Meat and poultry dishes, sauces and gravies.	Cramps and diarrhea within 12 to 24 hours. No vomiting or fever.	Improper temperature control of hot foods and recontamination.	No growth below 40° F. Bacteria are killed by normal cooking, but a heat-stable spore can survive.
Clostridium botulinum	Produces a spore and requires a low oxygen atmosphere. Produces a heat-sensitive toxin.	Soils, plants, marine sediments, and fish.	Home-canned foods.	Blurred vision, respiratory distress, and possible DEATH.	Improper methods of home-processing foods.	Type E and Type B can grow at 38° F. Bacteria destroyed by cooking and the toxin is destroyed by boiling for 5 to 10 minutes. Heat-resistant spore can survive.
Vibrio parahaemolyticus	Requires salt for growth.	Fish and shellfish.	Raw and cooked seafood.	Diarrhea, cramps, vomiting, headache, and fever within 12 to 24 hours.	Recontamination of cooked foods or eating raw seafood.	No growth below 40° F. Bacteria killed by normal cooking.

PART IV

Procedures
Volume 3

A

Abbe operation
  construction of vagina 70.61
    with graft or prosthesis 70.63
  intestinal anastomosis - *see*
    Anastomosis, intestine
Abciximab, infusion 99.20
Abdominocentesis 54.91
Abdominohysterectomy 68.49
  laparoscopic 68.41
Abdominoplasty 86.83
Abdominoscopy 54.21
Abdominouterotomy 68.0
  obstetrical 74.99
Abduction, arytenoid 31.69
AbioCor® total replacement heart
  37.52
Ablation
  biliary tract (lesion) by ERCP 51.64
  endometrial (hysteroscopic) 68.23
  inner ear (cryosurgery) (ultrasound)
    20.79
    by injection 20.72
  lesion
    esophagus 42.39
      endoscopic 42.33
    heart
      by peripherally inserted catheter
        37.34
      endovascular approach 37.34
      maze procedure (Cox-maze)
        endovascular approach
          37.34
        open (trans-thoracic) approach
          37.33
        trans-thoracic approach
          37.33
    intestine
      large 45.49
        endoscopic 45.43
    large intestine 45.49
      endoscopic 45.43
    liver 50.26
      laparoscopic 50.25
      open 50.23
      percutaneous 50.24
    lung 32.26
      open 32.23
      percutaneous 32.24
      thoracoscopic 32.25
    renal 55.35
      laparoscopic 55.34
      open 55.32
      percutaneous 55.33
  pituitary 07.69
    by
      Cobalt-60 92.32
      implantation (strontium-yttrium)
        (Y) NEC 07.68
        transfrontal approach 07.64
        transphenoidal approach 07.65
      proton beam (Bragg peak) 92.33
  prostate
    by
      cryoablation 60.62
      laser, transurethral 60.21
      radical cryosurgical ablation
        (RCSA) 60.62
      radiofrequency thermotherapy
        60.97
      transurethral needle ablation
        (TUNA) 60.97

Ablation (*Continued*)
  tissue
    heart - *see* Ablation, lesion, heart
    liver – *see* Ablation, lesion, liver
    lung – *see* Ablation, lesion, lung
    renal – *see* Ablation, lesion, renal
Abortion, therapeutic 69.51
  by
    aspiration curettage 69.51
    dilation and curettage 69.01
    hysterectomy - *see* Hysterectomy
    hysterotomy 74.91
    insertion
      laminaria 69.93
      prostaglandin suppository
        96.49
    intra-amniotic injection (saline)
      75.0
Abrasion
  corneal epithelium 11.41
    for smear or culture 11.21
  epicardial surface 36.39
  pleural 34.6
  skin 86.25
Abscission, cornea 11.49
Absorptiometry
  photon (dual) (single) 88.98
Aburel operation (intra-amniotic injection
  for abortion) 75.0
Accouchement forcé 73.99
Acetabulectomy 77.85
Acetabuloplasty NEC 81.40
  with prosthetic implant 81.52
Achillorrhaphy 83.64
  delayed 83.62
Achillotenotomy 83.11
  plastic 83.85
Achillotomy 83.11
  plastic 83.85
Acid peel, skin 86.24
Acromionectomy 77.81
Acromioplasty 81.83
  for recurrent dislocation of shoulder
    81.82
  partial replacement 81.81
  total replacement 81.80
Actinotherapy 99.82
Activities of daily living (ADL)
  therapy 93.83
  training for the blind 93.78
Acupuncture 99.92
  with smouldering moxa 93.35
  for anesthesia 99.91
Adams operation
  advancement of round ligament
    69.22
  crushing of nasal septum 21.88
  excision of palmar fascia 82.35
Adenectomy - *see also* Excision, by site
  prostate NEC 60.69
  retropubic 60.4
Adenoidectomy (without tonsillectomy)
  28.6
  with tonsillectomy 28.3
Adhesiolysis - *see also* Lysis, adhesions
  for collapse of lung 33.39
  middle ear 20.23
Adipectomy 86.83
Adjustment
  cardiac pacemaker program
    (reprogramming) - <mark>*omit code*</mark>
  cochlear prosthetic device (external
    components) 95.49

Adjustment (*Continued*)
  dental 99.97
  gastric restrictive device (laparoscopic)
    44.98
  occlusal 24.8
  orthopedic device (noninvasive) ◀
    external fixator - <mark>*omit code*</mark> ◀
  spectacles 95.31
Administration (of) - *see also* Injection
  Activase® 99.10
  adhesion barrier substance 99.77
  Alteplase (tPA, generic) 99.10
  Anistreplase (tPA, generic) 99.10
  antitoxins NEC 99.58
    botulism 99.57
    diphtheria 99.58
    gas gangrene 99.58
    scarlet fever 99.58
    tetanus 99.56
  Bender Visual-Motor Gestalt test 94.02
  Benton Visual Retention test 94.02
  DrotAA 00.11
  Eminase® 99.10
  inhaled nitric oxide 00.12
  intelligence test or scale (Stanford-
    Binet) (Wechsler) (adult)
    (children) 94.01
    Minnesota Multiphasic Personality
      Inventory (MMPI) 94.02
    MMPI (Minnesota Multiphasic
      Personality Inventory) 94.02
  neuroprotective agent 99.75
  Proleukin® (low-dose) 99.28
    high-dose 00.15
  psychologic test 94.02
  Retavase® 99.10
  Reteplase (tPA, generic) 99.10
  Stanford-Binet test 94.01
  Streptase® 99.10
  Streptokinase (tPA, generic) 99.10
  Tenecteplase (tPA, generic) 99.10
  TNKase™ 99.10
  toxoid
    diphtheria 99.36
      with tetanus and pertussis,
        combined (DTP) 99.39
    tetanus 99.38
      with diphtheria and pertussis,
        combined (DTP) 99.39
  vaccine - *see also* Vaccination
    BCG 99.33
    measles-mumps-rubella (MMR)
      99.48
    poliomyelitis 99.41
    TAB 99.32
  Wechsler
    Intelligence Scale (adult) (children)
      94.01
    Memory Scale 94.02
  Xigris® 00.11
Adrenalectomy (unilateral) 07.22
  with partial removal of remaining
    gland 07.29
  bilateral 07.3
    partial 07.29
    subtotal 07.29
  complete 07.3
  partial NEC 07.29
  remaining gland 07.3
  subtotal NEC 07.29
  total 07.3
Adrenalorrhaphy 07.44
Adrenalotomy (with drainage) 07.41

◀ New   ⫷ Revised   ~~deleted~~ Deleted   ● Use Additional Digit(s)   <mark></mark> Omit code

Anastomosis (*Continued*)
  bronchotracheal 33.48
  bronchus 33.48
  carotid-subclavian artery 39.22
  caval-mesenteric vein 39.1
  caval-pulmonary artery 39.21
  cervicoesophageal 42.59
  colohypopharyngeal (intrathoracic)
      42.55
    antesternal or antethoracic 42.65
  common bile duct 51.39
  common pulmonary trunk and left
      atrium (posterior wall) 35.82
  cystic bile duct 51.39
  cystocolic 57.88
  epididymis to vas deferens 63.83
  esophagocolic (intrathoracic) NEC
      42.56
    with interposition 42.55
    antesternal or antethoracic NEC
        42.66
      with interposition 42.65
  esophagocologastric (intrathoracic)
      42.55
    antesternal or antethoracic 42.65
  esophagoduodenal (intrathoracic) NEC
      42.54
    with interposition 42.53
  esophagoenteric (intrathoracic) NEC -
      see also Anastomosis, esophagus,
      to intestinal segment 42.54
    antesternal or antethoracic NEC - see
        also Anastomosis, esophagus,
        antesternal, to intestinal
        segment 42.64
  esophagoesophageal (intrathoracic)
      42.51
    antesternal or antethoracic 42.61
  esophagogastric (intrathoracic) 42.52
    antesternal or antethoracic 42.62
  esophagus (intrapleural) (intrathoracic)
      (retrosternal) NEC 42.59
    with
      gastrectomy (partial) 43.5
        complete or total 43.99
      interposition (of) NEC 42.58
        colon 42.55
        jejunum 42.53
        small bowel 42.53
    antesternal or antethoracic NEC
        42.69
      with
        interposition (of) NEC 42.68
          colon 42.65
          jejunal loop 42.63
          small bowel 42.63
        rubber tube 42.68
      to intestinal segment NEC 42.64
        with interposition 42.68
        colon NEC 42.66
          with interposition 42.65
        small bowel NEC 42.64
          with interposition 42.63
    to intestinal segment (intrathoracic)
        NEC 42.54
      with interposition 42.58
      antesternal or antethoracic NEC
          42.64
        with interposition 42.68
      colon (intrathoracic) NEC 42.56
        with interposition 42.55
        antesternal or antethoracic
            42.66
          with interposition 42.65

Anastomosis (*Continued*)
  esophagus NEC (*Continued*)
    to intestinal segment NEC
        (*Continued*)
      small bowel NEC 42.54
        with interposition 42.53
        antesternal or antethoracic
            42.64
          with interposition 42.63
  facial-accessory nerve 04.72
  facial-hypoglossal nerve 04.71
  fallopian tube 66.73
    by reanastomosis 66.79
  gallbladder 51.35
    to
      hepatic ducts 51.31
      intestine 51.32
      pancreas 51.33
      stomach 51.34
  gastroepiploic artery to coronary artery
      36.17
  hepatic duct 51.39
  hypoglossal-accessory nerve 04.73
  hypoglossal-facial nerve 04.71
  ileal loop to bladder 57.87 [45.51]
  ileoanal 45.95
  ileorectal 45.93
  inferior vena cava and portal vein
      39.1
  internal mammary artery (to)
    coronary artery (single vessel)
        36.15
      double vessel 36.16
    myocardium 36.2
  intestine 45.90
    large-to-anus 45.95
    large-to-large 45.94
    large-to-rectum 45.94
    large-to-small 45.93
    small-to-anus 45.95
    small-to-large 45.93
    small-to-rectal stump 45.92
    small-to-small 45.91
  intrahepatic 51.79
  intrathoracic vessel NEC 39.23
  kidney (pelvis) 55.86
  lacrimal sac to conjunctiva 09.82
  left-to-right (systemic-pulmonary
      artery) 39.0
  lymphatic (channel) (peripheral) 40.9
  mesenteric-caval 39.1
  mesocaval 39.1
  nasolacrimal 09.81
  nerve (cranial) (peripheral) NEC
      04.74
    accessory-facial 04.72
    accessory-hypoglossal 04.73
    hypoglossal-facial 04.71
  pancreas (duct) (to) 52.96
    bile duct 51.39
    gall bladder 51.33
    intestine 52.96
    jejunum 52.96
    stomach 52.96
  pleurothecal (with valve) 03.79
  portacaval 39.1
  portal vein to inferior vena cava 39.1
  pulmonary-aortic (Pott's) 39.0
  pulmonary artery and superior vena
      cava 39.21
  pulmonary-innominate artery (Blalock)
      39.0
  pulmonary-subclavian artery (Blalock-
      Taussig) 39.0

Anastomosis (*Continued*)
  pulmonary vein and azygos vein
      39.23
  pyeloileocutaneous 56.51
  pyeloureterovesical 55.86
  radial artery 36.19
  rectum, rectal NEC 48.74
    stump to small intestine 45.92
  renal (pelvis) 55.86
    vein and splenic vein 39.1
  renoportal 39.1
  salpingothecal (with valve) 03.79
  splenic to renal veins 39.1
  splenorenal (venous) 39.1
    arterial 39.26
  subarachnoid-peritoneal (with valve)
      03.71
  subarachnoid-ureteral (with valve)
      03.72
  subclavian-aortic 39.22
  superior vena cava to pulmonary
      artery 39.21
  systemic-pulmonary artery 39.0
  thoracic artery (to)
    coronary artery (single) 36.15
      double 36.16
    myocardium 36.2
  ureter (to) NEC 56.79
    bladder 56.74
    colon 56.71
    ileal pouch (bladder) 56.51
    ileum 56.71
    intestine 56.71
    skin 56.61
  ureterocalyceal 55.86
  ureterocolic 56.71
  ureterovesical 56.74
  urethra (end-to-end) 58.44
  vas deferens 63.82
  veins (suture of proximal to distal end)
      (with bypass graft) 39.29
    with excision or resection of vessel -
        see Phlebectomy, with
        anastomosis, by site
    mesenteric to vena cava 39.1
    portal to inferior vena cava 39.1
    revision 39.49
    splenic and renal 39.1
  ventricle, ventricular (intracerebral)
      (with valve) - see also Shunt,
      ventricular 02.2
  ventriculoatrial (with valve) 02.32
  ventriculocaval (with valve) 02.32
  ventriculomastoid (with valve) 02.31
  ventriculopleural (with valve) 02.33
  vesicle - see Anastomosis, bladder
Anderson operation (tibial lengthening)
    78.37
Anel operation (dilation of lacrimal duct)
    09.42
Anesthesia
  acupuncture for 99.91
  cryoanalgesia nerve (cranial)
      (peripheral) 04.2
  spinal - omit code
Aneurysmectomy 38.60
  with
    anastomosis 38.30
      abdominal
        artery 38.36
        vein 38.37
      aorta (arch) (ascending)
          (descending) 38.34
      head and neck NEC 38.32

◀ New   ◀▥ Revised   ~~deleted~~ Deleted   ● Use Additional Digit(s)   ▨ Omit code

Aneurysmectomy (Continued)
with (Continued)
anastomosis (Continued)
intracranial NEC 38.31
lower limb
artery 38.38
vein 38.39
thoracic NEC 38.35
upper limb (artery) (vein) 38.33
graft replacement (interposition)
38.40
abdominal
aorta
endovascular approach
39.71
open approach 38.44
Zenith® Renu™ AAA graft
39.71
artery 38.46
vein 38.47
aorta (arch) (ascending)
(descending thoracic)
abdominal 38.44
thoracic 38.45
thoracoabdominal 38.45
[38.44]
head and neck NEC 38.42
intracranial NEC 38.41
lower limb
artery 38.48
vein 38.49
thoracic NEC 38.45
upper limb (artery) (vein)
38.43
abdominal
artery 38.66
vein 38.67
aorta (arch) (ascending) (descending)
38.64
atrial, auricular 37.32
head and neck NEC 38.62
heart 37.32
intracranial NEC 38.61
lower limb
artery 38.68
vein 38.69
sinus of Valsalva 35.39
thoracic NEC 38.65
upper limb (artery) (vein) 38.63
ventricle (myocardium) 37.32
Aneurysmoplasty - see
Aneurysmorrhaphy
Aneurysmorrhaphy NEC 39.52
by or with
anastomosis - see Aneurysmectomy,
with anastomosis, by site
clipping 39.51
coagulation 39.52
electrocoagulation 39.52
endovascular graft
abdominal aorta 39.71
lower extremity artery(s) 39.79
thoracic aorta 39.73
upper extremity artery(s) 39.79
excision or resection - see also
Aneurysmectomy, by site
with
anastomosis - see
Aneurysmectomy, with
anastomosis, by site
graft replacement - see
Aneurysmectomy, with
graft replacement, by
site

Aneurysmorrhaphy NEC (Continued)
by or with (Continued)
filipuncture 39.52
graft replacement - see
Aneurysmectomy, with graft
replacement, by site
methyl methacrylate 39.52
suture 39.52
wiring 39.52
wrapping 39.52
Matas' 39.52
Aneurysmotomy - see Aneurysmectomy
Angiectomy
with
anastomosis 38.30
abdominal
artery 38.36
vein 38.37
aorta (arch) (ascending)
(descending) 38.34
head and neck NEC 38.32
intracranial NEC 38.31
lower limb
artery 38.38
vein 38.39
thoracic vessel NEC 38.35
upper limb (artery) (vein) 38.33
graft replacement (interposition)
38.40
abdominal
aorta 38.44
artery 38.46
vein 38.47
aorta (arch) (ascending)
(descending thoracic)
abdominal 38.44
thoracic 38.45
thoracoabdominal 38.45 [38.44]
head and neck NEC 38.42
intracranial NEC 38.41
lower limb
artery 38.48
vein 38.49
thoracic vessel NEC 38.45
upper limb (artery) (vein) 38.43
Angiocardiography (selective) 88.50
carbon dioxide (negative contrast)
88.58
combined right and left heart 88.54
intra-operative fluorescence vascular
88.59
left heart (aortic valve) (atrium)
(ventricle) (ventricular outflow
tract) 88.53
combined with right heart 88.54
right heart (atrium) (pulmonary valve)
(ventricle) (ventricular outflow
tract) 88.52
combined with left heart 88.54
SPY 88.59
vena cava (inferior) (superior) 88.51
Angiography (arterial) - see also
Arteriography 88.40
by C.A.T. – see Scan, C.A.T., by site
by computed tomography – see Scan,
C.A.T., by site
by radioisotope - see Scan, radioisotope,
by site
by ultrasound - see Ultrasonography,
by site
basilar 88.41
brachial 88.49
carotid (internal) 88.41
celiac 88.47

Angiography (Continued)
cerebral (posterior circulation) 88.41
coronary NEC 88.57
intra-operative fluorescence
vascular 88.59
eye (fluorescein) 95.12
femoral 88.48
heart 88.50
intra-abdominal NEC 88.47
intracranial 88.41
intrathoracic vessels NEC 88.44
lower extremity NEC 88.48
neck 88.41
placenta 88.46
pulmonary 88.43
renal 88.45
specified artery NEC 88.49
transfemoral 88.48
upper extremity NEC 88.49
veins - see Phlebography
vertebral 88.41
Angioplasty (laser) - see also Repair, blood
vessel

Note: Also use 00.40, 00.41, 00.42, or
00.43 to show the total number of
vessels treated. Use code 00.44 once to
show procedure on a bifurcated vessel.
In addition, use 00.45, 00.46, 00.47, or
00.48 to show the number of vascular
stents inserted.

balloon (percutaneous transluminal)
NEC 39.50
coronary artery 00.66
coronary 36.09
open chest approach 36.03
percutaneous transluminal (balloon)
00.66
percutaneous transluminal (balloon)
(single vessel)
basilar 00.61
carotid 00.61
cerebral (intracranial) 00.62
cerebrovascular
cerebral (intracranial) 00.62
precerebral (extracranial) 00.61
carotid 00.61
coronary (balloon) 00.66
femoropopliteal 39.50
iliac 39.50
lower extremity NOS 39.50
mesenteric 39.50
peripheral NEC 39.50
precerebral (extracranial) 00.61
carotid 00.61
renal 39.50
subclavian 39.50
upper extremity NOS 39.50
vertebral 00.61
specified site NEC 39.50
cerebrovascular
cerebral (intracranial) 00.62
precerebral (extracranial) 00.61
peripheral 39.50
Angiorrhaphy 39.30
artery 39.31
vein 39.32
Angioscopy, percutaneous 38.22
eye (fluorescein) 95.12
Angiotomy 38.00
abdominal
artery 38.06
vein 38.07

◀ New   ◀|||| Revised   ~~deleted~~ Deleted   ● Use Additional Digit(s)   ▢ Omit code

Application (Continued)
  substance, adhesion barrier 99.77
  Thomas collar 93.52
    with reduction of fracture or
      dislocation - see Reduction,
      fracture and Reduction,
      dislocation
  traction
    with reduction of fracture or
      dislocation - see Reduction,
      fracture and Reduction,
      dislocation
    adhesive tape (skin) 93.46
    boot 93.46
    Bryant's 93.44
    Buck's 93.46
    Cotrel's 93.42
    Dunlop's 93.44
    gallows 93.46
    Lyman Smith 93.44
    Russell's 93.44
    skeletal NEC 93.44
      intermittent 93.43
    skin, limbs NEC 93.46
    spinal NEC 93.42
      with skull device (caliper)
        (Crutchfield) (Gardner-
        Wells) (halo) (Vinke)
        (tongs) 93.41
        with synchronous insertion
          02.94
    Thomas' splint 93.45
  Unna's paste boot 93.53
  vasopneumatic device 93.58
  Velpeau dressing 93.59
  Vinke tongs (skull) (with synchronous
    skeletal traction) 02.94
  wound dressing NEC 93.57
Aquapheresis 99.78
Arc lamp - see Photocoagulation
Arcuplasty 81.66
Arrest
  bone growth (epiphyseal) 78.20
    by stapling - see Stapling,
      epiphyseal plate
    femur 78.25
    fibula 78.27
    humerus 78.22
    radius 78.23
    tibia 78.27
    ulna 78.23
  cardiac, induced (anoxic)
    (circulatory) 39.63
  circulatory, induced (anoxic)
    39.63
  hemorrhage - see Control,
    hemorrhage
Arslan operation (fenestration of inner
  ear) 20.61
Arteriectomy 38.60
  with
    anastomosis 38.30
      abdominal 38.36
      aorta (arch) (ascending)
        (descending) 38.34
      head and neck NEC 38.32
      intracranial NEC 38.31
      lower limb 38.38
      thoracic NEC 38.35
      upper limb 38.33
    graft replacement (interposition)
      38.40
      abdominal
        aorta 38.44

Arteriectomy (Continued)
  with (Continued)
    graft replacement (Continued)
      aorta (arch) (ascending)
        (descending thoracic)
        (thoracic)
        abdominal 38.44
        thoracic 38.45
        thoracoabdominal 38.45 [38.44]
      head and neck NEC 38.42
      intracranial NEC 38.41
      lower limb 38.48
      thoracic NEC 38.45
      upper limb 38.43
    abdominal 38.66
    aorta (arch) (ascending) (descending)
      38.64
    head and neck NEC 38.62
    intracranial NEC 38.61
    lower-limb 38.68
    thoracic NEC 38.65
    upper limb 38.63
Arteriography (contrast) (fluoroscopic)
  (retrograde) 88.40
  by
    radioisotope - see Scan, radioisotope
    ultrasound (Doppler) - see
      Ultrasonography, by site
  aorta (arch) (ascending) (descending)
    88.42
  basilar 88.41
  brachial 88.49
  carotid (internal) 88.41
  cerebral (posterior circulation) 88.41
  coronary (direct) (selective) NEC
    88.57
    double catheter technique
      (Judkins) (Ricketts and
      Abrams) 88.56
    intra-operative fluorescence
      vascular 88.59
    single catheter technique (Sones)
      88.55
  Doppler (ultrasonic) - see
    Ultrasonography, by site
  femoral 88.48
  head and neck 88.41
  intra-abdominal NEC 88.47
  intrathoracic NEC 88.44
  lower extremity 88.48
  placenta 88.46
  pulmonary 88.43
  radioisotope - see Scan, radioisotope
  renal 88.45
  specified site NEC 88.49
  SPY 88.59
  superior mesenteric artery 88.47
  transfemoral 88.48
  ultrasound - see Ultrasonography, by
    site
  upper extremity 88.49
Arterioplasty - see Repair, artery
Arteriorrhaphy 39.31
Arteriotomy 38.00
  abdominal 38.06
  aorta (arch) (ascending) (descending)
    38.04
  head and neck NEC 38.02
  intracranial NEC 38.01
  lower limb 38.08
  thoracic NEC 38.05
  upper limb 38.03
Arteriovenostomy 39.29
  for renal dialysis 39.27

Arthrectomy 80.90
  ankle 80.97
  elbow 80.92
  foot and toe 80.98
  hand and finger 80.94
  hip 80.95
  intervertebral disc - see category 80.5●
  knee 80.96
  semilunar cartilage 80.6
  shoulder 80.91
  specified site NEC 80.99
  spine NEC 80.99
  wrist 80.93
Arthrocentesis 81.91
  for arthrography - see Arthrogram
Arthrodesis (compression) (extra-
  articular) (intra-articular) (with bone
  graft) (with fixation device) 81.20
  ankle 81.11
  carporadial 81.25
  cricoarytenoid 31.69
  elbow 81.24
  finger 81.28
  foot NEC 81.17
  hip 81.21
  interphalangeal
    finger 81.28
    toe NEC 77.58
      claw toe repair 77.57
      hammer toe repair 77.56
  ischiofemoral 81.21
  knee 81.22
  lumbosacral, lumbar NEC 81.08
    ALIF (anterior lumbar interbody
      fusion) 81.06
    anterior (interbody), anterolateral
      technique 81.06
    lateral transverse process technique
      81.07
    PLIF (posterior lumbar interbody
      fusion) 81.08
    posterior (interbody), posterolateral
      technique 81.08
    TLIF (transforaminal lumbar
      interbody fusion) 81.08
  McKeever (metatarsophalangeal)
    81.16
  metacarpocarpal 81.26
  metacarpophalangeal 81.27
  metatarsophalangeal 81.16
  midtarsal 81.14
  pantalar 81.11
  sacroiliac 81.08
  shoulder 81.23
  specified joint NEC 81.29
  spinal - see also Fusion, spinal 81.00
  subtalar 81.13
  tarsometatarsal 81.15
  tibiotalar 81.11
  toe NEC 77.58
    claw toe repair 77.57
    hammer toe repair 77.56
  triple 81.12
  wrist 81.26
Arthroendoscopy - see Arthroscopy
Arthroereisis, subtalar joint 81.18
Arthrogram, arthrography 88.32
  temporomandibular 87.13
Arthrolysis 93.26
Arthroplasty (with fixation device) (with
  traction) 81.96
  ankle 81.49
  carpals 81.75
    with prosthetic implant 81.74

Arthroplasty (Continued)
carpocarpal, carpometacarpal 81.75
  with prosthetic implant 81.74
Carroll and Taber (proximal
    interphalangeal joint) 81.72
cup (partial hip) 81.52
Curtis (interphalangeal joint) 81.72
elbow 81.85
  with prosthetic replacement (partial)
    (total) 81.84 ◀
femoral head NEC 81.40
  with prosthetic implant 81.52
finger(s) 81.72
  with prosthetic implant 81.71
foot (metatarsal) with joint replacement
  81.57
Fowler (metacarpophalangeal joint)
  81.72
hand (metacarpophalangeal)
  (interphalangeal) 81.72
  with prosthetic implant 81.71
hip (with bone graft) 81.40
  cup (partial hip) 81.52
  femoral head NEC 81.40
    with prosthetic implant 81.52
      with total replacement 81.51
  partial replacement 81.52
  total replacement 81.51
interphalangeal joint 81.72
  with prosthetic implant 81.71
Kessler (carpometacarpal joint) 81.74
knee - see also Repair, knee 81.47
  prosthetic replacement
    (bicompartmental) (hemijoint)
    (partial) (total)
    (tricompartmental)
    (unicompartmental) 81.54
  revision 81.55
metacarpophalangeal joint 81.72
  with prosthetic implant 81.71
shoulder 81.83
  prosthetic replacement (partial) 81.81
    total 81.80
  for recurrent dislocation 81.82
temporomandibular 76.5
toe NEC 77.58
  with prosthetic replacement 81.57
  for hallux valgus repair 77.59
wrist 81.75
  with prosthetic implant 81.74
    total replacement 81.73
Arthroscopy 80.20
ankle 80.27
elbow 80.22
finger 80.24
foot 80.28
hand 80.24
hip 80.25
knee 80.26
shoulder 80.21
specified site NEC 80.29
toe 80.28
wrist 80.23
Arthrostomy - see also Arthrotomy 80.10
Arthrotomy 80.10
as operative approach - omit code
with
  arthrography - see Arthrogram
  arthroscopy - see Arthroscopy
  injection of drug 81.92
  removal of prosthesis without
    replacement - see also Removal,
    prosthesis, joint structures
    80.00 ◀

Arthrotomy (Continued)
ankle 80.17
elbow 80.12
foot and toe 80.18
hand and finger 80.14
hip 80.15
knee 80.16
shoulder 80.11
specified site NEC 80.19
spine 80.19
wrist 80.13
Artificial
heart 37.52
  AbioCor® 37.52
  CardioWest™ (TAH-t) 37.52
insemination 69.92
kidney 39.95
rupture of membranes 73.09
Arytenoidectomy 30.29
Arytenoidopexy 31.69
Asai operation (larynx) 31.75
Aspiration
abscess - see Aspiration, by site
anterior chamber, eye (therapeutic) 12.91
  diagnostic 12.21
aqueous (eye) (humor) (therapeutic)
  12.91
  diagnostic 12.21
ascites 54.91
Bartholin's gland (cyst)
  (percutaneous) 71.21
biopsy - see Biopsy, by site
bladder (catheter) 57.0
  percutaneous (needle) 57.11
bone marrow (for biopsy) 41.31
  from donor for transplant 41.91
  stem cell 99.79
branchial cleft cyst 29.0
breast 85.91
bronchus 96.05
  with lavage 96.56
bursa (percutaneous) 83.94
  hand 82.92
calculus, bladder 57.0
cataract 13.3
  with
    phacoemulsification 13.41
    phacofragmentation 13.43
      posterior route 13.42
chest 34.91
cisternal 01.01
cranial (puncture) 01.09
craniobuccal pouch 07.72
craniopharyngioma 07.72
cul-de-sac (abscess) 70.0
curettage, uterus 69.59
  after abortion or delivery 69.52
  diagnostic 69.59
  to terminate pregnancy 69.51
cyst - see Aspiration, by site
diverticulum, pharynx 29.0
endotracheal 96.04
  with lavage 96.56
extradural 01.09
eye (anterior chamber) (therapeutic)
  12.91
  diagnostic 12.21
fallopian tube 66.91
fascia 83.95
  hand 82.93
gallbladder (percutaneous) 51.01
hematoma - see also Aspiration, by site
  obstetrical 75.92
    incisional 75.91

Aspiration (Continued)
hydrocele, tunica vaginalis 61.91
hygroma - see Aspiration, by site
hyphema 12.91
hypophysis 07.72
intracranial space (epidural)
  (extradural) (subarachnoid)
  (subdural) (ventricular) 01.09
through previously implanted catheter
  or reservoir (Ommaya) (Rickham)
  01.02
joint 81.91
  for arthrography - see Arthrogram
kidney (cyst) (pelvis) (percutaneous)
  (therapeutic) 55.92
  diagnostic 55.23
liver (percutaneous) 50.91
lung (percutaneous) (puncture)
  (needle) (trocar) 33.93
  thoracoscopic 33.20
middle ear 20.09
  with intubation 20.01
muscle 83.95
  hand 82.93
nail 86.01
nasal sinus 22.00
  by puncture 22.01
  through natural ostium 22.02
nasotracheal 96.04
  with lavage 96.56
orbit, diagnostic 16.22
ovary 65.91
percutaneous - see Aspiration, by
  site
pericardium (wound) 37.0
pituitary gland 07.72
pleural cavity 34.91
prostate (percutaneous) 60.91
Rathke's pouch 07.72
seminal vesicles 60.71
seroma - see Aspiration, by site
skin 86.01
soft tissue NEC 83.95
  hand 82.93
spermatocele 63.91
spinal (puncture) 03.31
spleen (cyst) 41.1
stem cell 99.79
subarachnoid space (cerebral)
  01.09
subcutaneous tissue 86.01
subdural space (cerebral) 01.09
tendon 83.95
  hand 82.93
testis 62.91
thymus 07.92
  thoracoscopic 07.95
thyroid (field) (gland) 06.01
  postoperative 06.02
trachea 96.04
  with lavage 96.56
  percutaneous 31.99
tunica vaginalis (hydrocele)
  (percutaneous) 61.91
vitreous (and replacement)
  14.72
  diagnostic 14.11
Assessment
fitness to testify 94.11
mental status 94.11
nutritional status 89.39
personality 94.03
temperament 94.02
vocational 93.85

◀ New   ◀ Revised   deleted Deleted   ● Use Additional Digit(s)   Omit code

Assistance
    cardiac - *see also* Resuscitation,
        cardiac extracorporeal circulation
        39.61
    endotracheal respiratory - *see* category
        96.7
    hepatic, extracorporeal 50.92
    respiratory (endotracheal)
        (mechanical) - *see* Ventilation,
        mechanical
Astragalectomy 77.98
Asymmetrogammagram - *see* Scan,
    radioisotope
Atherectomy
    cerebrovascular - *see* Angioplasty
    coronary - *see* Angioplasty
    peripheral 39.50
Atriocommissuropexy (mitral valve)
    35.12
Atrioplasty NEC 37.99
    combined with repair of valvular and
        ventricular septal defects - *see*
        Repair, endocardial cushion
        defect
    septum (heart) NEC 35.71
Atrioseptopexy - *see also* Repair, atrial
    septal defect 35.71
Atrioseptoplasty - *see also* Repair, atrial
    septal defect 35.71
Atrioseptostomy (balloon) 35.41
Atriotomy 37.11
Atrioventriculostomy (cerebral-heart)
    02.32

Attachment
    abutment (screw) for prosthetic ear
        device
        percutaneous 20.99
    eye muscle
        orbicularis oculi to eyebrow
            08.36
        rectus to frontalis 15.9
    pedicle (flap) graft 86.74
        hand 86.73
        lip 27.57
        mouth 27.57
    pharyngeal flap (for cleft palate repair)
        27.62
        secondary or subsequent 27.63
    prosthetic ear device, abutment
        20.99
    retina - *see* Reattachment, retina
Atticoantrostomy (ear) 20.49
Atticoantrotomy (ear) 20.49
Atticotomy (ear) 20.23
Audiometry (Bekesy 5-tone) (impedance)
    (stapedial reflex response)
    (subjective) 95.41
Augmentation
    bladder 57.87
    breast - *see* Mammoplasty,
        augmentation
    buttock ("fanny-lift") 86.89
    chin 76.68
    genioplasty 76.68
    mammoplasty - *see* Mammoplasty,
        augmentation

Augmentation *(Continued)*
    outflow tract (pulmonary valve)
        (gusset type) 35.26
        in total repair of tetralogy of Fallot
        35.81
    vocal cord(s) 31.0
Auriculectomy 18.39
Autograft - *see* Graft
Autologous - *see* Blood, transfusion
Autopsy 89.8
Autotransfusion (whole blood) 99.02 - *see*
    Blood, transfusion
Autotransplant, autotransplantation - *see*
    also Reimplantation
    adrenal tissue (heterotopic)
        (orthotopic) 07.45
    kidney 55.61
    lung - *see* Transplant, transplantation,
        lung 33.5●
    ovary 65.72
        laparoscopic 65.75
    pancreatic tissue 52.81
    parathyroid tissue (heterotopic)
        (orthotopic) 06.95
    thyroid tissue (heterotopic) (orthotopic)
        06.94
    tooth 23.5
Avulsion, nerve (cranial) (peripheral)
    NEC 04.07
    acoustic 04.01
    phrenic 33.31
    sympathetic 05.29
Azygography 88.63

B

Bacterial smear - *see* Examination, microscopic
Baffes operation (interatrial transposition of venous return) 35.91
Baffle, atrial or interatrial 35.91
Balanoplasty 64.69
Baldy-Webster operation (uterine suspension) 69.22
Ballistocardiography 89.59
Balloon
    angioplasty - *see* Angioplasty, balloon
    pump, intra-aortic 37.61
    systostomy (atrial) 35.41
Ball operation
    herniorrhaphy - *see* Repair, hernia, inguinal
    undercutting 40.92
Bandage 93.37
    elastic 93.56
Banding
    gastric 44.68
        vertical 44.68
    pulmonary artery 38.85
Bankhart operation (capsular repair into glenoid, for shoulder dislocation) 81.82
Bardenheurer operation (ligation of innominate artery) 38.85
Barium swallow 87.61
Barkan operation (goniotomy) 12.52
    with goniopuncture 12.53
Barr operation (transfer of tibialis posterior tendon) 83.75
Barsky operation (closure of cleft hand) 82.82
Basal metabolic rate 89.39
Basiotripsy 73.8
Bassett operation (vulvectomy with inguinal lymph node dissection) 71.5 [40.3]
Bassini operation - *see* Repair, hernia, inguinal
Batch-Spittler-McFaddin operation (knee disarticulation) 84.16
Batista operation (partial ventriculectomy) (ventricular reduction) (ventricular remodeling) 37.35
Bearing surface, hip
    ceramic-on-ceramic 00.76
    ceramic-on-polyethylene 00.77
    metal-on-metal 00.75
    metal-on-polyethylene 00.74
Beck operation
    aorta-coronary sinus shunt 36.39
    epicardial poudrage 36.39
Beck-Jianu operation (permanent gastrostomy) 43.19
Behavior modification 94.33
Bell-Beuttner operation (subtotal abdominal hysterectomy) 68.39
    laparoscopic 68.31
Belsey operation (esophagogastric sphincter) 44.65
Benenenti operation (rotation of bulbous urethra) 58.49
Berke operation (levator resection of eyelid) 08.33
Bicuspidization of heart valve 35.10
    aortic 35.11
    mitral 35.12
Bicycle dynamometer 93.01
Biesenberger operation (size reduction of breast, bilateral) 85.32
    unilateral 85.31

Bifurcation, bone - *see also* Osteotomy 77.30
Bigelow operation (litholapaxy) 57.0
Bililite therapy (ultraviolet) 99.82
Billroth I operation (partial gastrectomy with gastroduodenostomy) 43.6
Billroth II operation (partial gastrectomy with gastrojejunostomy) 43.7
Binnie operation (hepatopexy) 50.69
Biofeedback, psychotherapy 94.39
Biopsy
    abdominal wall 54.22
    adenoid 28.11
    adrenal gland NEC 07.11
        closed 07.11
        open 07.12
        percutaneous (aspiration) (needle) 07.11
    alveolus 24.12
    anus 49.23
    appendix 45.26
    artery (any site) 38.21
    aspiration - *see* Biopsy, by site
    bile ducts 51.14
        closed (endoscopic) 51.14
        open 51.13
        percutaneous (needle) 51.12
    bladder 57.33
        closed 57.33
        open 57.34
        transurethral 57.33
    blood vessel (any site) 38.21
    bone 77.40
        carpal, metacarpal 77.44
        clavicle 77.41
        facial 76.11
        femur 77.45
        fibula 77.47
        humerus 77.42
        marrow 41.31
        patella 77.46
        pelvic 77.49
        phalanges (foot) (hand) 77.49
        radius 77.43
        scapula 77.41
        specified site NEC 77.49
        tarsal, metatarsal 77.48
        thorax (ribs) (sternum) 77.41
        tibia 77.47
        ulna 77.43
        vertebrae 77.49
    bowel - *see* Biopsy, intestine
    brain NEC 01.13
        closed 01.13
        open 01.14
        percutaneous (needle) 01.13
    breast 85.11
        blind 85.11
        closed 85.11
        open 85.12
        percutaneous (needle) (Vimm-Silverman) 85.11
    bronchus NEC 33.24
        brush 33.24
        closed (endoscopic) 33.24
        open 33.25
        transbronchoscopic needle aspiration (TBNA) 33.24 ◄
        Wang needle (transbronchoscopic) 33.24 ◄
        washings 33.24
    bursa 83.21
    cardioesophageal (junction) 44.14
        closed (endoscopic) 44.14
        open 44.15

Biopsy *(Continued)*
    cecum 45.25
        brush 45.25
        closed (endoscopic) 45.25
        open 45.26
    cerebral meninges NEC 01.11
        closed 01.11
        open 01.12
        percutaneous (needle) 01.11
    cervix (punch) 67.12
        conization (sharp) 67.2
    chest wall 34.23
    clitoris 71.11
    colon 45.25
        brush 45.25
        closed (endoscopic) 45.25
        open 45.26
    conjunctiva 10.21
    cornea 11.22
    cul-de-sac 70.23
    diaphragm 34.27
    duodenum 45.14
        brush 45.14
        closed (endoscopic) 45.14
        open 45.15
    ear (external) 18.12
        middle or inner 20.32
    endocervix 67.11
    endometrium NEC 68.16
        by
            aspiration curettage 69.59
            dilation and curettage 69.09
        closed (endoscopic) 68.16
        open 68.13
    epididymis 63.01
    esophagus 42.24
        closed (endoscopic) 42.24
        open 42.25
    extraocular muscle or tendon 15.01
    eye 16.23
        muscle (oblique) (rectus) 15.01
    eyelid 08.11
    fallopian tube 66.11
    fascia 83.21
    fetus 75.33
    gallbladder 51.12
        closed (endoscopic) 51.14
        open 51.13
        percutaneous (needle) 51.12
    ganglion (cranial) (peripheral) NEC 04.11
        closed 04.11
        open 04.12
        percutaneous (needle) 04.11
        sympathetic nerve 05.11
    gum 24.11
    heart 37.25
    hypophysis - *see also* Biopsy, pituitary gland 07.15
    ileum 45.14
        brush 45.14
        closed (endoscopic) 45.14
        open 45.15
    intestine NEC 45.27
        large 45.25
            brush 45.25
            closed (endoscopic) 45.25
            open 45.26
        small 45.14
            brush 45.14
            closed (endoscopic) 45.14
            open 45.15

◄ New   ◄▌ Revised   ~~deleted~~ Deleted   ● Use Additional Digit(s)   ▨ Omit code

Biopsy (Continued)
  intra-abdominal mass 54.24
    closed 54.24
    percutaneous (needle) 54.24
  iris 12.22
  jejunum 45.14
    brush 45.14
    closed (endoscopic) 45.14
    open 45.15
  joint structure (aspiration) 80.30
    ankle 80.37
    elbow 80.32
    foot and toe 80.38
    hand and finger 80.34
    hip 80.35
    knee 80.36
    shoulder 80.31
    specified site NEC 80.39
    spine 80.39
    wrist 80.33
  kidney 55.23
    closed 55.23
    open 55.24
    percutaneous (aspiration) (needle)
      55.23
  labia 71.11
  lacrimal
    gland 09.11
    sac 09.12
  larynx 31.43
    brush 31.43
    closed (endoscopic) 31.43
    open 31.45
  lip 27.23
  liver 50.11
    closed 50.11
    laparoscopic 50.14
    open 50.12
    percutaneous (aspiration) (needle)
      50.11
    transjugular 50.13
    transvenous 50.13
  lung NEC 33.27
    brush 33.24
    closed (percutaneous) (needle) 33.26
      brush 33.24
      endoscopic 33.27
        brush 33.24
    endoscopic 33.27
      brush 33.24
    open 33.28
    thoracoscopic 33.20
    transbronchial 33.27
    transthoracic 33.26
  lymphatic structure (channel) (node)
    (vessel) 40.11
  mediastinum NEC 34.25
    closed 34.25
    open 34.26
    percutaneous (needle) 34.25
  meninges (cerebral) NEC 01.11
    closed 01.11
    open 01.12
    percutaneous (needle) 01.11
    spinal 03.32
  mesentery 54.23
  mouth NEC 27.24
  muscle 83.21
    extraocular 15.01
    ocular 15.01
  nasopharynx 29.12
  nerve (cranial) (peripheral) NEC 04.11
    closed 04.11
    open 04.12

Biopsy (Continued)
  nerve NEC (Continued)
    percutaneous (needle) 04.11
    sympathetic 05.11
  nose, nasal 21.22
    sinus 22.11
      closed (endoscopic) (needle)
        22.11
      open 22.12
  ocular muscle or tendon 15.01
  omentum
    closed 54.24
    open 54.23
    percutaneous (needle) 54.24
  orbit 16.23
    by aspiration 16.22
  ovary 65.12
    by aspiration 65.11
    laparoscopic 65.13
  palate (bony) 27.21
    soft 27.22
  pancreas 52.11
    closed (endoscopic) 52.11
    open 52.12
    percutaneous (aspiration) (needle)
      52.11
  pancreatic duct 52.14
    closed (endoscopic) 52.14
  parathyroid gland 06.13
  penis 64.11
  perianal tissue 49.22
  pericardium 37.24
  periprostatic 60.15
  perirectal tissue 48.26
  perirenal tissue 59.21
  peritoneal implant
    closed 54.24
    open 54.23
    percutaneous (needle) 54.24
  peritoneum
    closed 54.24
    open 54.23
    percutaneous (needle) 54.24
  periurethral tissue 58.24
  perivesical tissue 59.21
  pharynx, pharyngeal 29.12
  pineal gland 07.17
  pituitary gland 07.15
    transfrontal approach 07.13
    transsphenoidal approach 07.14
  pleura, pleural 34.24
    thoracoscopic 34.20
  prostate NEC 60.11
    closed (transurethral) 60.11
    open 60.12
    percutaneous (needle) 60.11
    transrectal 60.11
  rectum 48.24
    brush 48.24
    closed (endoscopic) 48.24
    open 48.25
  retroperitoneal tissue 54.24
  salivary gland or duct 26.11
    closed (needle) 26.11
    open 26.12
  scrotum 61.11
  seminal vesicle NEC 60.13
    closed 60.13
    open 60.14
    percutaneous (needle) 60.13
  sigmoid colon 45.25
    brush 45.25
    closed (endoscopic) 45.25
    open 45.26

Biopsy (Continued)
  sinus, nasal 22.11
    closed (endoscopic) (needle) 22.11
    open 22.12
  skin (punch) 86.11
  skull 01.15
  soft palate 27.22
  soft tissue NEC 83.21
  spermatic cord 63.01
  sphincter of Oddi 51.14
    closed (endoscopic) 51.14
    open 51.13
  spinal cord (meninges) 03.32
  spleen 41.32
    closed 41.32
    open 41.33
    percutaneous (aspiration) (needle)
      41.32
  stomach 44.14
    brush 44.14
    closed (endoscopic) 44.14
    open 44.15
  subcutaneous tissue (punch) 86.11
  supraglottic mass 29.12
  sympathetic nerve 05.11
  tendon 83.21
    extraocular 15.01
    ocular 15.01
  testis NEC 62.11
    closed 62.11
    open 62.12
    percutaneous (needle) 62.11
  thymus 07.16
  thyroid gland NEC 06.11
    closed 06.11
    open 06.12
    percutaneous (aspiration) (needle)
      06.11
      tongue 25.01
    closed (needle) 25.01
    open 25.02
  tonsil 28.11
  trachea 31.44
    brush 31.44
    closed (endoscopic) 31.44
    open 31.45
  tunica vaginalis 61.11
  umbilicus 54.22
  ureter 56.33
    closed (percutaneous) 56.32
      endoscopic 56.33
    open 56.34
    transurethral 56.33
  urethra 58.23
  uterus, uterine (endometrial) 68.16
    by
      aspiration curettage 69.59
      dilation and curettage 69.09
    closed (endoscopic) 68.16
    ligaments 68.15
      closed (endoscopic) 68.15
      open 68.14
    open 68.13
  uvula 27.22
  vagina 70.24
  vas deferens 63.01
  vein (any site) 38.21
  vulva 71.11
BiPAP 93.90
  delivered by
    endotracheal tube - see category 96.7●
    tracheostomy - see category 96.7●
BIS (bispectral index) monitoring 00.94 ◄
  [89.14]

Bischoff operation
    (ureteroneocystostomy) 56.74
Bisection - *see also* Excision
    hysterectomy 68.39
        laparoscopic 68.31
    ovary 65.29
        laparoscopic 65.25
    stapes foot plate 19.79
        with incus replacement 19.11
Bischoff operation (spinal myelotomy)
    03.29
Blalock operation (systemic-pulmonary
    anastomosis) 39.0
Blalock-Hanlon operation (creation of
    atrial septal defect) 35.42
Blalock-Taussig operation (subclavian-
    pulmonary anastomosis) 39.0
Blascovic operation (resection and
    advancement of levator palpebrae
    superioris) 08.33
Blepharectomy 08.20
Blepharoplasty - *see also* Reconstruction,
    eyelid 08.70
    extensive 08.44
Blepharorrhaphy 08.52
    division or severing 08.02
Blepharotomy 08.09
Blind rehabilitation therapy NEC 93.78
Block
    caudal - *see* Injection, spinal celiac
        ganglion or plexus 05.31
    dissection
        breast
            bilateral 85.46
            unilateral 85.45
        bronchus 32.6
        larynx 30.3
        lymph nodes 40.50
        neck 40.40
        vulva 71.5
    epidural, spinal - *see* Injection, spinal
    gasserian ganglion 04.81
    intercostal nerves 04.81
    intrathecal - *see* Injection, spinal
    nerve (cranial) (peripheral) NEC
        04.81
    paravertebral stellate ganglion 05.31
    peripheral nerve 04.81
    spinal nerve root (intrathecal) - *see*
        Injection, spinal
    stellate (ganglion) 05.31
    subarachnoid, spinal - *see* Injection,
        spinal
    sympathetic nerve 05.31
    trigeminal nerve 04.81
Blood
    flow study, Doppler-type (ultrasound) -
        see Ultrasonography
    patch, spine (epidural) 03.95
    transfusion
        antihemophilic factor 99.06
        autologous
            collected prior to surgery
                99.02
            intraoperative 99.00
            perioperative 99.00
            postoperative 99.00
            previously collected 99.02
            salvage 99.00
        blood expander 99.08
        blood surrogate 99.09
        coagulation factors 99.06
        exchange 99.01
        granulocytes 99.09

Blood (*Continued*)
    transfusion (*Continued*)
        hemodilution 99.03
        other substance 99.09
        packed cells 99.04
        plasma 99.07
        platelets 99.05
        serum, other 99.07
        thrombocytes 99.05
Blount operation
    femoral shortening (with blade plate)
        78.25
        by epiphyseal stapling 78.25
Boari operation (bladder flap) 56.74
Bobb operation (cholelithotomy) 51.04
Bone
    age studies 88.33
    mineral density study 88.98
Bonney operation (abdominal
    hysterectomy) 68.49
    laparoscopic 68.41
Borthen operation (iridotasis) 12.63
Bost operation
    plantar dissection 80.48
    radiocarpal fusion 81.26
Bosworth operation
    arthroplasty for acromioclavicular
        separation 81.83
    fusion of posterior lumbar and
        lumbosacral spine 81.08
        for pseudarthrosis 81.38
    resection of radial head ligaments (for
        tennis elbow) 80.92
    shelf procedure, hip 81.40
Bottle repair of hydrocele, tunica-
    vaginalis 61.2
Boyd operation (hip disarticulation)
    84.18
Brachytherapy
    intravascular 92.27
Brauer operation (cardiolysis) 37.10
Breech extraction - *see* Extraction, breech
Bricker operation (ileoureterostomy)
    56.51
Brisement (forcé) 93.26
Bristow operation (repair of shoulder
    dislocation) 81.82
Brock operation (pulmonary valvotomy)
    35.03
Brockman operation (soft tissue release
    for clubfoot) 83.84
Bronchogram, bronchography 87.32
    endotracheal 87.31
    transcricoid 87.32
Bronchoplasty 33.48
Bronchorrhaphy 33.41
Bronchoscopy NEC 33.23
    with biopsy 33.24
        lung 33.27
            brush 33.24
    fiberoptic 33.22
        with biopsy 33.24
            lung 33.27
                brush 33.24
    through tracheostomy 33.21
        with biopsy 33.24
            lung 33.27
                brush 33.24
Bronchospirometry 89.38
Bronchostomy 33.0
    closure 33.42
Bronchotomy 33.0
Browne (-Denis) operation (hypospadias
    repair) 58.45

Brunschwig operation (temporary
    gastrostomy) 43.19
Buckling, scleral 14.49
    with
        air tamponade 14.49
        implant (silicone) (vitreous) 14.41
        resection of sclera 14.49
        vitrectomy 14.49
        vitreous implant (silicone) 14.41
Bunionectomy (radical) 77.59
    with
        arthrodesis 77.52
        osteotomy of first metatarsal 77.51
        resection of joint with prosthetic
            implant 77.59
        soft tissue correction NEC 77.53
Bunnell operation (tendon transfer)
    82.56
Burch procedure (retropubic urethral
    suspension for urinary stress
    incontinence) 59.5
Burgess operation (amputation of ankle)
    84.14
Burn dressing 93.57
Burr holes 01.24
Bursectomy 83.5
    hand 82.31
Bursocentesis 83.94
    hand 82.92
Bursotomy 83.03
    hand 82.03
Burying of fimbriae in uterine wall
    66.97
Bypass
    abdominal - coronary artery 36.17
    aortocoronary (catheter stent) (with
        prosthesis) (with saphenous vein
        graft) (with vein graft) 36.10
        one coronary vessel 36.11
        two coronary vessels 36.12
        three coronary vessels 36.13
        four coronary vessels 36.14
    arterial (graft) (mandril grown graft)
        (vein graft) NEC 39.29
        carotid-cerebral 39.28
        carotid-vertebral 39.28
        extracranial-intracranial [EC-IC]
            39.28
        intra-abdominal NEC 39.26
        intrathoracic NEC 39.23
        peripheral NEC 39.29
    cardiopulmonary 39.61
        open 39.61
        percutaneous (closed) 39.66
    carotid-cerebral 39.28
    carotid-vertebral 39.28
    coronary - *see also* Bypass,
        aortocoronary 36.10
    extracranial-intracranial [EC-IC]
        39.28
    gastric 44.39
        high 44.31
        laparoscopic 44.38
        Printen and Mason 44.31
    gastroduodenostomy (Jaboulay's)
        44.39
        laparoscopic 44.38
        percutaneous [endoscopic] 44.32
    gastroenterostomy 44.39
        laparoscopic 44.38
    gastroepiploic - coronary artery 36.17
    gastrogastrostomy 44.39
        laparoscopic 44.38
    graft, pressurized treatment 00.16

Bypass *(Continued)*
  heart-lung (complete) (partial) 39.61
    open 39.61
    percutaneous (closed) 39.66
  high gastric 44.31
  ileo-jejunal 45.91
  internal mammary-coronary artery
      (single) 36.13
    double vessel 36.16
  jejunal-ileum 45.91
  pulmonary 39.61
    open 39.61
    percutaneous (closed) 39.66
  shunt
    intestine
      large-to-large 45.94
      small-to-large 45.93
      small-to-small 45.91
    stomach 44.39
      high gastric 44.31
      laparoscopic 44.38
  terminal ileum 45.93
  vascular (arterial) (graft) (mandril
      grown graft) (vein graft) NEC
      39.29
    aorta-carotid-brachial 39.22
    aorta-iliac-femoral 39.25
    aorta-renal 39.24
    aorta-subclavian-carotid 39.22

Bypass *(Continued)*
  vascular NEC *(Continued)*
    aortic-superior mesenteric 39.26
    aortocarotid 39.22
    aortoceliac 39.26
    aortocoronary - *see also* Bypass,
        aortocoronary 36.10
    aortofemoral 39.25
    aortofemoral-popliteal 39.25
    aortoiliac 39.25
      to popliteal 39.25
    aortoiliofemoral 39.25
    aortomesenteric 39.26
    aortopopliteal 39.25
    aortorenal 39.24
    aortosubclavian 39.22
    axillary-brachial 39.29
    axillary-femoral (superficial)
        39.29
    axillofemoral (superficial) 39.29
    carotid-cerebral 39.28
    carotid-vertebral 39.28
    carotid to subclavian artery
        39.22
    common hepatic-common iliac-
        renal 39.26
    coronary - *see also* Bypass,
        aortocoronary 36.10

Bypass *(Continued)*
  vascular NEC *(Continued)*
    extracranial-intracranial [EC-IC]
        39.28
    femoral-femoral 39.29
    femoroperoneal 39.29
    femoropopliteal (reversed
        saphenous vein) (saphenous)
        39.29
    femorotibial (anterior) (posterior)
        39.29
    iliofemoral 39.25
    ilioiliac 39.26
    internal mammary-coronary
        artery (single) 36.15
      double vessel 36.16
    intra-abdominal (arterial) NEC 39.26
      venous NEC 39.1
    intrathoracic NEC 39.23
    peripheral artery NEC 39.29
    popliteal-tibial 39.29
    renal artery 39.24
    splenorenal (venous) 39.1
      arterial 39.26
    subclavian-axillary 39.29
    subclavian-carotid 39.22
    subclavian-subclavian 39.22
    Y graft to renal arteries 39.24

C

Caldwell operation (sulcus extension) 24.91
Caldwell-Luc operation (maxillary sinusotomy) 22.39
 with removal of membrane lining 22.31
Calibration, urethra 89.29
Calicectomy (renal) 55.4
Callander operation (knee disarticulation) 84.16
Caloric test, vestibular function 95.44
Calycectomy (renal) 55.4
Calyco-ileoneocystostomy 55.86
Calycotomy (renal) 55.11
Campbell operation
 bone block, ankle 81.11
 fasciotomy (iliac crest) 83.14
 reconstruction of anterior cruciate ligament 81.45
Campimetry 95.05
Canaliculodacryocystorhinostomy 09.81
Canaliculoplasty 09.73
Canaliculorhinostomy 09.81
Canaloplasty, external auditory meatus 18.6
Cannulation - see also Insertion, catheter
 ampulla of Vater 51.99
 antrum 22.01
 arteriovenous 39.93
 artery 38.91
 caval-mesenteric vein 39.1
 cisterna chyli 40.61
 Eustachian tube 20.8
 lacrimal apparatus 09.42
 lymphatic duct, left (thoracic) 40.61
 nasal sinus (by puncture) 22.01
  through natural ostium 22.02
 pancreatic duct 52.92
  by retrograde endoscopy (ERP) 52.93
 renoportal 39.1
 sinus (nasal) (by puncture) 22.01
  through natural ostium 22.02
 splenorenal (venous) 39.1
  arterial 39.26
 thoracic duct (cervical approach) (thoracic approach) 40.61
Cannulization - see Cannulation
Canthocystostomy 09.82
Canthoplasty 08.59
Canthorrhaphy 08.52
 division or severing 08.02
Canthotomy 08.51
Capsulectomy
 joint - see also Arthrectomy 80.90
 kidney 55.91
 lens 13.65
  with extraction of lens 13.51
 ovary 65.29
  laparoscopic 65.25
Capsulo-iridectomy 13.65
Capsuloplasty - see Arthroplasty
Capsulorrhaphy 81.96
 with arthroplasty - see Arthroplasty
 ankle 81.94
 foot 81.94
 lower extremity NEC 81.95
 upper extremity 81.93
Capsulotomy
 joint - see also Division, joint capsule 80.40
 for claw toe repair 77.57

Capsulotomy (Continued)
 lens 13.64
 with
  discission of lens 13.2
  removal of foreign body 13.02
   by magnet extraction 13.01
Cardiac
 mapping 37.27
 massage (external) (closed chest) 99.63
  open chest 37.91
 retraining 93.36
Cardiac support device (CSD) 37.41
Cardiectomy (stomach) 43.5
Cardiocentesis 37.0
Cardiography - see also Angiocardiography 88.50
Cardiolysis 37.10
Cardiomyopexy 36.39
Cardiomyotomy 42.7
Cardio-omentopexy 36.39
Cardiopericardiopexy 36.39
Cardioplasty (stomach and esophagus) 44.65
 stomach alone 44.66
  laparoscopic 44.67
Cardioplegia 39.63
Cardiopneumopexy 36.39
Cardiorrhaphy 37.49
Cardioschisis 37.12
Cardiosplenopexy 36.39
Cardiotomy (exploratory) 37.11
Cardiovalvulotomy - see Valvulotomy, heart
Cardioversion (external) 99.62
 atrial 99.61
CardioWest™ Total Temporary Artificial Heart (TAH-t) 37.52
Carotid pulse tracing with ECG lead 89.56
Carpectomy (partial) 77.84
 total 77.94
Carroll and Taber arthroplasty (proximal interphalangeal joint) 81.72
Casting (for immobilization) NEC 93.53
 with fracture-reduction - see Reduction, fracture
Castration
 female (oophorectomy, bilateral) 65.51
  laparoscopic 65.53
 male 62.41
C.A.T. (computerized axial tomography) - see also Scan, C.A.T. 88.38
Catheterization - see also Insertion, catheter
 arteriovenous 39.93
 artery 38.91
 bladder, indwelling 57.94
  percutaneous (cystostomy) 57.17
  suprapubic NEC 57.18
 bronchus 96.05
  with lavage 96.56
 cardiac (right) 37.21
  combined left and right 37.23
  left 37.22
   combined with right heart 37.23
  right 37.21
   combined with left heart 37.23
 central venous NEC 38.93
  peripherally inserted central catheter (PICC) 38.93

Catheterization (Continued)
 chest 34.04
  revision (with lysis of adhesions) 34.04
  thoracoscopic 34.06
  thoracoscopic 34.06
 Eustachian tube 20.8
 heart (right) 37.21
  combined left and right 37.23
  left 37.22
   combined with right heart 37.23
  right 37.21
   combined with left heart 37.23
 hepatic vein 38.93
 inferior vena cava 38.93
 intercostal space (with water seal), for drainage 34.04
  revision (with lysis of adhesions) 34.04
  thoracoscopic 34.06
  thoracoscopic 34.06
 lacrimonasal duct 09.44
 laryngeal 96.05
 nasolacrimal duct 09.44
 pancreatic cyst 52.01
 renal vein 38.93
 Swan-Ganz (pulmonary) 89.64
 transtracheal for oxygenation 31.99
 umbilical vein 38.92
 ureter (to kidney) 59.8
  for retrograde pyelogram 87.74
 urethra, indwelling 57.94
 vein NEC 38.93
  for renal dialysis 38.95
Cattell operation (herniorrhaphy) 53.51
Cauterization - see also Destruction, lesion, by site
 anus NEC 49.39
  endoscopic 49.31
 Bartholin's gland 71.24
 broad ligament 69.19
 bronchus 32.09
  endoscopic 32.01
 canaliculi 09.73
 cervix 67.32
 chalazion 08.25
 choroid plexus 02.14
 conjunctiva 10.33
  lesion 10.32
 cornea (fistula) (ulcer) 11.42
 ear, external 18.29
 endometrial implant - see Excision, lesion, by site
 entropion 08.41
 esophagus 42.39
  endoscopic 42.33
 eyelid 08.25
  for entropion or ectropion 08.41
 fallopian tube 66.61
  by endoscopy (hysteroscopy) (laparoscopy) 66.29
 hemorrhoids 49.43
 iris 12.41
 lacrimal
  gland 09.21
  punctum 09.72
   for eversion 09.71
  sac 09.6
 larynx 30.09
 liver 50.29
 lung 32.29
  endoscopic 32.28
  thoracoscopic 32.20
 meibomian gland 08.25
 nose, for epistaxis (with packing) 21.03

◀ New   ◀·· Revised   ~~deleted~~ Deleted   ● Use Additional Digit(s)   ▨ Omit code

Cauterization *(Continued)*
  ovary 65.29
    laparoscopic 65.25
  palate (bony) 27.31
  pannus (superficial) 11.42
  pharynx 29.39
  punctum, lacrimal 09.72
    for eversion 09.71
  rectum 48.32
    radical 48.31
  round ligament 69.19
  sclera 12.84
    with iridectomy 12.62
  skin 86.3
  subcutaneous tissue 86.3
  tonsillar fossa 28.7
  urethra 58.39
    endoscopic 58.31
  uterosacral ligament 69.19
  uterotubal ostia 66.61
  uterus 68.29
  vagina 70.33
  vocal cords 30.09
  vulva 71.3
Cavernoscopy 34.21
Cavernostomy 33.1
Cavernotomy, kidney 55.39
Cavography (inferior vena cava) 88.51
CCM (implantation of cardiac
  contractility modulation) ◀
  rechargeable pulse generator only
    17.52 ◀
  total system 17.51 ◀
Cecectomy (with resection of terminal
  ileum)
  laparoscopic 17.32
  open and other 45.72
Cecil operation (urethral reconstruction)
  58.46
Cecocolopicopexy 46.63
Cecocolostomy 45.94
Cecofixation 46.64
Ceco-ileostomy 45.93
Cecopexy 46.64
Cecoplication 46.62
Cecorrhaphy 46.75
Cecosigmoidostomy 45.94
Cecostomy (tube) - *see also* Colostomy 46.10
Cecotomy 45.03
Celiocentesis 54.91
Celioscopy 54.21
Celiotomy, exploratory 54.11
Cell block and Papanicolaou smear - *see*
  Examination, microscopic
CentriMag® acute circulatory support
  device 37.62
Cephalogram 87.17
  dental 87.12
  orthodontic 87.12
Cephalometry, cephalometrics 87.17
  echo 88.78
  orthodontic 87.12
  ultrasound (sonar) 88.78
  x-ray 87.81
Cephalotomy, fetus 73.8
Cerclage
  anus 49.72
  cervix 67.51
    transabdominal 67.51
    transvaginal 67.59
  isthmus uteri (cervix) 67.59
  retinal reattachment - *see also* Buckling,
    scleral 14.49
  sclera - *see also* Buckling, scleral 14.49

Cervicectomy (with synchronous
  colporrhaphy) 67.4
Cervicoplasty 67.69
Cesarean section 74.99
  classical 74.0
  corporeal 74.0
  extraperitoneal 74.2
  fundal 74.0
  laparotrachelotomy 74.1
  Latzko 74.2
  low cervical 74.1
  lower uterine segment 74.1
  peritoneal exclusion 74.4
  specified type NEC 74.4
  supravesical 74.2
  transperitoneal 74.4
    classical 74.0
    low cervical 74.1
  upper uterine segment 74.0
  vaginal 74.4
  Waters 74.2
Chamberlain procedure - *see*
  Mediastinotomy ◀
Chandler operation (hip fusion) 81.21
Change - *see also* Replacement
  cast NEC 97.13
    lower limb 97.12
    upper limb 97.11
  cystostomy catheter or tube 59.94
  gastrostomy tube 97.02
  length
    bone - *see either category* 78.2
      Shortening, bone *or category*
      78.3 ● Lengthening, bone
    muscle 83.85
      hand 82.55
    tendon 83.85
      hand 82.55
  nephrostomy catheter or tube 55.93
  pyelostomy catheter or tube 55.94
  splint 97.14
  tracheostomy tube 97.23
  ureterostomy catheter or tube 59.93
  urethral catheter, indwelling 57.95
Character analysis, psychologic 94.03
Charles operation (correction of
  lymphedema) 40.9
Charnley operation (compression
  arthrodesis)
  ankle 81.11
  hip 81.21
  knee 81.22
Cheatle-Henry operation - *see* Repair,
  hernia, femoral
Check
  automatic implantable cardioverter/
    defibrillator (AICD)
    (interrogation only) 89.49
  CRT-D (cardiac resynchronization
    defibrillator) (interrogation only)
    89.49
  CRT-P (cardiac resynchronization
    pacemaker) (interrogation only)
    89.45
  pacemaker, artificial (cardiac)
    (function) (interrogation only)
    (rate) 89.45
    amperage threshold 89.48
    artifact wave form 89.46
    electrode impedance 89.47
    voltage threshold 89.48
  vision NEC 95.09
Cheiloplasty 27.59
Cheilorrhaphy 27.51

Cheilostomatoplasty 27.59
Cheilotomy 27.0
Chemical peel, skin 86.24
Chemocauterization - *see also* Destruction,
  lesion, by site
  corneal epithelium 11.41
  palate 27.31
Chemodectomy 39.8
Chemoembolization 99.25
Chemolysis
  nerve (peripheral) 04.2
  spinal canal structure 03.8
Chemoneurolysis 04.2
Chemonucleolysis (nucleus pulposus)
  80.52
Chemopallidectomy 01.42
Chemopeel (skin) 86.24
Chemosurgery
  esophagus 42.39
    endoscopic 42.33
  Mohs' 86.24
  skin (superficial) 86.24
  stomach 43.49
    endoscopic 43.41
Chemothalamectomy 01.41
Chemotherapy - *see also* Immunotherapy
  Antabuse 94.25
  for cancer NEC 99.25
    brain wafer implantation 00.10
    CLO 17.70 ◀
    clofarabine 17.70 ◀
    CLOLAR® 17.70 ◀
    implantation of chemotherapeutic
      agent 00.10
    interstitial implantation 00.10
    intracavitary implantation 00.10
    wafer chemotherapy 00.10
  ithium 94.22
  methadone 94.25
  palate (bony) 27.31
Chevalier-Jackson operation (partial
  laryngectomy) 30.29
Child operation (radical subtotal
  pancreatectomy) 52.53
Cholangiocholangiostomy 51.39
Cholangiocholecystocholedochectomy
  51.22
Cholangio-enterostomy 51.39
Cholangiogastrostomy 51.39
Cholangiogram 87.54
  endoscopic retrograde (ERC) 51.11
  intraoperative 87.53
  intravenous 87.52
  percutaneous hepatic 87.51
  transhepatic 87.53
Cholangiography - *see also*
  Cholangiogram 87.54
Cholangiojejunostomy (intrahepatic) 51.39
Cholangiopancreatography, endoscopic
  retrograde (ERCP) 51.10
Cholangiostomy 51.59
Cholangiotomy 51.59
Cholecystectomy (total) 51.22
  partial 51.21
    laparoscopic 51.24
  total 51.22
    laparoscopic 51.23
Cholecystenterorrhaphy 51.91
Cholecystocecostomy 51.32
Cholecystocholangiogram 87.59
Cholecystocolostomy 51.32
Cholecystoduodenostomy 51.32
Cholecystoenterostomy (Winiwater) 51.32
Cholecystogastrostomy 51.34

Cholecystogram 87.59
Cholecystoileostomy 51.32
Cholecystojejunostomy (Roux-en-Y)
    (with jejunojejunostomy) 51.32
Cholecystopancreatostomy 51.33
Cholecystopexy 51.99
Cholecystorrhaphy 51.91
Cholecystostomy NEC 51.03
    by trocar 51.02
Cholecystotomy 51.04
    percutaneous 51.01
Choledochectomy 51.63
Choledochoduodenostomy 51.36
Choledochoenterostomy 51.36
Choledochojejunostomy 51.36
Choledocholithotomy 51.41
    endoscopic 51.88
Choledocholithotripsy 51.41
    endoscopic 51.88
Choledochopancreatostomy 51.39
Choledochoplasty 51.72
Choledochorrhaphy 51.71
Choledochoscopy 51.11
Choledochostomy 51.51
Choledochotomy 51.51
Cholelithotomy 51.04
Chondrectomy 80.90
    ankle 80.97
    elbow 80.92
    foot and toe 80.98
    hand and finger 80.94
    hip 80.95
    intervertebral cartilage - see category
        80.5●
    knee (semilunar cartilage) 80.6
    nasal (submucous) 21.5
    semilunar cartilage (knee) 80.6
    shoulder 80.91
    specified site NEC 80.99
    spine - see category 80.5●
    wrist 80.93
Chondroplasty - see Arthroplasty
Chondrosternoplasty (for pectus
    excavatum repair) 34.74
Chondrotomy - see also Division, cartilage
    nasal 21.1
Chopart operation (midtarsal
    amputation) 84.12
Chordectomy, vocal 30.22
Chordotomy (spinothalamic) (anterior)
    (posterior) NEC 03.29
    percutaneous 03.21
    stereotactic 03.21
Ciliarotomy 12.55
Ciliectomy (ciliary body) 12.44
    eyelid margin 08.20
Cinch, cinching
    for scleral buckling - see also Buckling,
        scleral 14.49
    ocular muscle (oblique) (rectus) 15.22
        multiple (two or more muscles) 15.4
Cineangiocardiography - see also
    Angiocardiography 88.50
Cineplasty, cineplastic prosthesis
    amputation - see Amputation
    arm 84.44
    biceps 84.44
    extremity 84.40
        lower 84.48
        upper 84.44
    leg 84.48
Cineradiograph - see Radiography
Cingulumotomy (brain) (percutaneous
    radiofrequency) 01.32

Circumcision (male) 64.0
    female 71.4
CISH [classic infrafascial SEMM
    hysterectomy] 68.31
Clagett operation (closure of chest wall
    following open flap drainage)
    34.72
Clamp and cautery, hemorrhoids 49.43
Clamping
    aneurysm (cerebral) 39.51
    blood vessel - see Ligation, blood vessel
    ventricular shunt 02.43
Clavicotomy 77.31
    fetal 73.8
Claviculectomy (partial) 77.81
    total 77.91
Clayton operation (resection of
    metatarsal heads and bases of
    phalanges) 77.88
Cleaning, wound 96.59
Clearance
    bladder (transurethral) 57.0
    pelvic
        female 68.8
        male 57.71
    prescalene fat pad 40.21
    renal pelvis (transurethral) 56.0
    ureter (transurethral) 56.0
Cleidotomy 77.31
    fetal 73.8
Clipping
    aneurysm (basilar) (carotid)
        (cerebellar) (cerebellopontine)
        (communicating artery)
        (vertebral) 39.51
    arteriovenous fistula 39.53
    frenulum, frenum
        labia (lips) 27.91
        lingual (tongue) 25.91
    left atrial appendage 37.36
    tip of uvula 27.72
Clitoridectomy 71.4
Clitoridotomy 71.4
Clivogram 87.02
Closure - see also Repair
    abdominal wall 54.63
        delayed (granulating wound) 54.62
        secondary 54.61
        tertiary 54.62
    amputation stump, secondary 84.3
    anular disc 80.54
        with graft or prosthesis 80.53
    anulus fibrosus 80.54
        with graft or prosthesis 80.53
    aorticopulmonary fenestration
        (fistula) 39.59
    appendicostomy 47.92
    artificial opening
        bile duct 51.79
        bladder 57.82
        bronchus 33.42
        common duct 51.72
        esophagus 42.83
        gallbladder 51.92
        hepatic duct 51.79
        intestine 46.50
            large 46.52
            small 46.51
        kidney 55.82
        larynx 31.62
        rectum 48.72
        stomach 44.62
        thorax 34.72
        trachea 31.72

Closure (Continued)
    artificial opening (Continued)
        ureter 56.83
        urethra 58.42
    atrial septal defect - see also Repair,
        atrial septal defect 35.71
        with umbrella device (King-Mills
            type) 35.52
        combined with repair of valvular
            and ventricular septal
            defects - see Repair,
            endocardial cushion
            defect
    bronchostomy 33.42
    cecostomy 46.52
    cholecystostomy 51.92
    cleft hand 82.82
    colostomy 46.52
    cystostomy 57.82
    diastema (alveolar) (dental) 24.8
    disrupted abdominal wall
        (postoperative) 54.61
    duodenostomy 46.51
    encephalocele 02.12
    endocardial cushion defect - see also
        Repair, endocardial cushion
        defect 35.73
    enterostomy 46.50
    esophagostomy 42.83
    fenestration
        aorticopulmonary 39.59
        septal, heart - see also Repair, heart,
            septum 35.70
    filtering bleb, corneoscleral
        (postglaucoma) 12.66
    fistula
        abdominothoracic 34.83
        anorectal 48.73
        anovaginal 70.73
        antrobuccal 22.71
        anus 49.73
        aorticopulmonary (fenestration) 39.59
        aortoduodenal 39.59
        appendix 47.92
        biliary tract 51.79
        bladder NEC 57.84
        branchial cleft 29.52
        bronchocutaneous 33.42
        bronchoesophageal 33.42
        bronchomediastinal 34.73
        bronchopleural 34.73
        bronchopleurocutaneous 34.73
        bronchopleuromediastinal 34.73
        bronchovisceral 33.42
        bronchus 33.42
        cecosigmoidal 46.76
        cerebrospinal fluid 02.12
        cervicoaural 18.79
        cervicosigmoidal 67.62
        cervicovesical 57.84
        cervix 67.62
        cholecystocolic 51.93
        cholecystoduodenal 51.93
        cholecystoenteric 51.93
        cholecystogastric 51.93
        cholecystojejunal 51.93
        cisterna chyli 40.63
        colon 46.76
        colovaginal 70.72
        common duct 51.72
        cornea 11.49
            with lamellar graft (homograft)
                11.62
            autograft 11.61

◀ New   ◀▥ Revised   ~~deleted~~ Deleted   ● Use Additional Digit(s)   ▨ Omit code

Closure *(Continued)*
  fistula *(Continued)*
    diaphragm 34.83
    duodenum 46.72
    ear, middle 19.9
    ear drum 19.4
    enterocolic 46.74
    enterocutaneous 46.74
    enterouterine 69.42
    enterovaginal 70.74
    enterovesical 57.83
    esophagobronchial 33.42
    esophagocutaneous 42.84
    esophagopleurocutaneous 34.73
    esophagotracheal 31.73
    esophagus NEC 42.84
    fecal 46.79
    gallbladder 51.93
    gastric NEC 44.63
    gastrocolic 44.63
    gastroenterocolic 44.63
    gastroesophageal 42.84
    gastrojejunal 44.63
    gastrojejunocolic 44.63
    heart valve - *see* Repair, heart, valve
    hepatic duct 51.79
    hepatopleural 34.73
    hepatopulmonary 34.73
    ileorectal 46.74
    ileosigmoidal 46.74
    ileovesical 57.83
    ileum 46.74
    in ano 49.73
    intestine 46.79
      large 46.76
      small NEC 46.74
    intestinocolonic 46.74
    intestinoureteral 56.84
    intestinouterine 69.42
    intestinovaginal 70.74
    intestinovesical 57.83
    jejunum 46.74
    kidney 55.83
    lacrimal 09.99
    laryngotracheal 31.62
    larynx 31.62
    lymphatic duct, left (thoracic) 40.63
    mastoid (antrum) 19.9
    mediastinobronchial 34.73
    mediastinocutaneous 34.73
    mouth (external) 27.53
    nasal 21.82
      sinus 22.71
    nasolabial 21.82
    nasopharyngeal 21.82
    oroantral 22.71
    oronasal 21.82
    oval window (ear) 20.93
    pancreaticoduodenal 52.95
    perilymph 20.93
    perineorectal 48.73
    perineosigmoidal 46.76
    perineourethroscrotal 58.43
    perineum 71.72
    perirectal 48.93
    pharyngoesophageal 29.53
    pharynx NEC 29.53
    pleura, pleural NEC 34.93
    pleurocutaneous 34.73
    pleuropericardial 37.49
    pleuroperitoneal 34.83
    pulmonoperitoneal 34.83
    rectolabial 48.73
    rectoureteral 56.84

Closure *(Continued)*
  fistula *(Continued)*
    rectourethral 58.43
    rectovaginal 70.73
    rectovesical 57.83
    rectovesicovaginal 57.83
    rectovulvar 48.73
    rectum NEC 48.73
    renal 55.83
    reno-intestinal 55.83
    round window 20.93
    salivary (gland) (duct) 26.42
    scrotum 61.42
    sigmoidovaginal 70.74
    sigmoidovesical 57.83
    splenocolic 41.95
    stomach NEC 44.63
    thoracic duct 40.63
    thoracoabdominal 34.83
    thoracogastric 34.83
    thoracointestinal 34.83
    thorax NEC 34.73
    trachea NEC 31.73
    tracheoesophageal 31.73
    tympanic membrane - *see also*
      Tympanoplasty 19.4
    umbilicourinary 57.51
    ureter 56.84
    ureterocervical 56.84
    ureterorectal 56.84
    ureterosigmoidal 56.84
    ureterovaginal 56.84
    ureterovesical 56.84
    urethra 58.43
    urethroperineal 58.43
    urethroperineovesical 57.84
    urethrorectal 58.43
    urethroscrotal 58.43
    urethrovaginal 58.43
    uteroenteric 69.42
    uterointestinal 69.42
    uterorectal 69.42
    uteroureteric 56.84
    uterovaginal 69.42
    uterovesical 57.84
    vagina 70.75
    vaginocutaneous 70.75
    vaginoenteric 70.74
    vaginoperineal 70.75
    vaginovesical 57.84
    vesicocervicovaginal 57.84
    vesicocolic 57.83
    vesicocutaneous 57.84
    vesicoenteric 57.83
    vesicometrorectal 57.83
    vesicoperineal 57.84
    vesicorectal 57.83
    vesicosigmoidal 57.83
    vesicosigmoidovaginal 57.83
    vesicoureteral 56.84
    vesicoureterovaginal 56.84
    vesicourethral 57.84
    vesicourethrorectal 57.83
    vesicouterine 57.84
    vesicovaginal 57.84
    vulva 71.72
    vulvorectal 48.73
  foramen ovale (patent) 35.71
    with
      prosthesis (open heart
        technique) 35.51
        closed heart technique
        35.52
      tissue graft 35.61

Closure *(Continued)*
  gastroduodenostomy 44.5
  gastrojejunostomy 44.5
  gastrostomy 44.62
  ileostomy 46.51
  jejunostomy 46.51
  laceration - *see also* Suture, by site
    liver 50.61
  laparotomy, delayed 54.62
  meningocele (spinal) 03.51
    cerebral 02.12
  myelomeningocele 03.52
  nephrostomy 55.82
  palmar cleft 82.82
  patent ductus arteriosus 38.85
  pelviostomy 55.82
  peptic ulcer (bleeding) (perforated)
    44.40
  perforation
    ear drum - *see also* Tympanoplasty
      19.4
    esophagus 42.82
    nasal septum 21.88
    tympanic membrane - *see also*
      Tympanoplasty 19.4
  proctostomy 48.72
  punctum, lacrimal (papilla) 09.91
  pyelostomy 55.82
  rectostomy 48.72
  septum defect (heart) - *see also* Repair,
    heart, septum 35.70
  sigmoidostomy 46.52
  skin (V-Y type) 86.59
  stoma
    bile duct 51.79
    bladder 57.82
    bronchus 33.42
    common duct 51.72
    esophagus 42.83
    gallbladder 51.92
    hepatic duct 51.79
    intestine 46.50
      large 46.52
      small 46.51
    kidney 55.82
    larynx 31.62
    rectum 48.72
    stomach 44.62
    thorax 34.72
    trachea 31.72
    ureter 56.83
    urethra 58.42
  thoracostomy 34.72
  tracheostomy 31.72
  ulcer (bleeding) (peptic) (perforated)
    44.40
    duodenum 44.42
    gastric 44.41
    intestine (perforated) 46.79
    skin 86.59
    stomach 44.41
  ureterostomy 56.83
  urethrostomy 58.42
  vagina 70.8
  vascular
    percutaneous puncture - *omit code*
  vesicostomy 57.22
  wound - *see also* Suture, by site
    with graft - *see* Graft
    with tissue adhesive 86.59
Coagulation, electrocoagulation - *see also*
  Destruction, lesion, by site
  aneurysm (cerebral) (peripheral vessel)
    39.52

Coagulation, electrocoagulation
(Continued)
arteriovenous fistula 39.53
brain tissue (incremental)
(radiofrequency) 01.59
broad ligament 69.19
cervix 67.32
ear
external 18.29
inner 20.79
middle 20.51
fallopian tube 66.61
gasserian ganglion 04.05
nose, for epistaxis (with packing)
21.03
ovary 65.29
laparoscopic 65.25
pharynx (by diathermy) 29.39
prostatic bed 60.94
rectum (polyp) 48.32
radical 48.31
retina (for)
destruction of lesion 14.21
reattachment 14.51
repair for tear 14.31
round ligament 69.19
semicircular canals 20.79
spinal cord (lesion) 03.4
urethrovesical junction, transurethral
57.49
uterosacral ligament 69.19
uterus 68.29
vagina 70.33
vulva 71.3
Coating, aneurysm of brain 39.52
Cobalt-60 therapy (treatment)
92.23
Coccygectomy (partial) 77.89
total 77.99
Coccygotomy 77.39
"Cocked hat" procedure (metacarpal
lengthening and transfer of local
flap) 82.69
Cockett operation (varicose vein)
lower limb 38.59
upper limb 38.53
Cody tack (perforation of footplate)
19.0
Coffey operation (uterine suspension)
(Meig's modification) 69.22
Cole operation (anterior tarsal wedge
osteotomy) 77.28
Colectomy (partial) (segmental)
(subtotal)
cecum (with terminal ileum)
laparoscopic 17.32
open and other 45.72
laparoscopic 17.39
left (Hartmann) (lower) (radical)
laparoscopic 17.35
open and other 45.75
multiple segmental
laparoscopic 17.31
open and other 45.71
open and other 45.79
right (radical)
laparoscopic 17.33
open and other 45.73
sigmoid
laparoscopic 17.36
open and other 45.76
terminal ileum with cecum
laparoscopic 17.32
open and other 45.72

Colectomy (Continued)
total
laparoscopic 45.81
open 45.82
other 45.83
unspecified 45.83
transverse
laparoscopic 17.34
open and other 45.74
Collapse, lung, surgical 33.39
by
destruction of phrenic nerve
33.31
pneumoperitoneum 33.33
pneumothorax, artificially-induced
33.32
thoracoplasty 33.34
Collection, sperm for artificial
insemination 99.96
Collis-Nissen operation (hiatal hernia
repair with esophagogastroplasty
53.80
Colocentesis 45.03
Colocolostomy 45.94
proximal to distal segment 45.79
Colocystoplasty 57.87 [45.52]
Colofixation 46.64
Coloileotomy 45.00
Colonna operation
adductor tenotomy (first stage) 83.1
hip arthroplasty (second stage) 81.4
reconstruction of hip (second stage)
81.40
Colonoscopy 45.23
with biopsy 45.25
biopsy 45.25   ◄
rectum 48.24   ◄▥
stent - see Insertion, stent, color ◄
fiberoptic (flexible) 45.23
intraoperative 45.21
through stoma (artificial) 45.22
transabdominal 45.21
Colopexy 46.63
Coloplication 46.64
Coloproctostomy 45.94
Colorectosigmoidostomy 45.94
Colorectostomy 45.94
Colorrhaphy 46.75
Coloscopy - see Colonoscopy
Colosigmoidostomy 45.94
Colostomy (ileo-ascending)
(ileotransverse) (perineal)
(transverse) 46.10
with anterior rectal resection 48.6
delayed opening 46.14
loop 46.03
permanent (magnetic) 46.13
temporary 46.11
Colotomy 45.03
Colpectomy 70.4
Colpoceliocentesis 70.0
Colpocentesis 70.0
Colpocleisis (complete) (partial) 70.8
Colpohysterectomy 68.59
laparoscopically assisted (LAVH)
68.51
Colpoperineoplasty 70.79
with repair of urethrocele 70.51
with graft or prosthesis 70.53
Colpoperineorrhaphy 70.71
following delivery 75.69
Colpopexy 70.77
with graft or prosthesis 70.78
Colpoplasty 70.79

Colpopoiesis 70.61
vaginal construction 70.61
with graft or prosthesis 70.63
Colporrhaphy 70.71
anterior (cystocele repair) 70.51
with graft or prosthesis 70.54
for repair of
cystocele 70.51
with rectocele 70.50
with graft or prosthesis 70.53
enterocele 70.92
with graft or prosthesis 70.93
rectocele 70.52
with cystocele 70.50
with graft or prosthesis 70.53
urethrocele 70.51
with graft or prosthesis 70.54
posterior (rectocele repair) 70.52
with graft or prosthesis 70.55
Colposcopy 70.21
Colpotomy 70.14
for pelvic peritoneal drainage 70.12
Commando operation (radical
glossectomy) 25.4
Commissurotomy
closed heart technique - see
Valvulotomy, heart
open heart technique - see
Valvuloplasty, heart
Compression, trigeminal nerve 04.02
Conchectomy 21.69
Conchotomy 21.1
Conduction study, nerve 89.15
Conduitogram, ileum 87.78
Condylectomy - see category 77.8●
mandible 76.5
Condylotomy NEC - see also Division,
joint capsule 80.40
mandible (open) 76.62
closed 76.61
Conization
cervix (knife) (sharp) (biopsy) 67.2
by
cryosurgery 67.33
electroconization 67.32
Conjunctivocystorhinostomy 09.82
with insertion of tube or stent 09.83
Conjunctivodacryocystorhinostomy
09.82
with insertion of tube or stent 09.83
Conjunctivodacryocystostomy 09.82
with insertion of tube or stent 09.83
Conjunctivoplasty 10.49
Conjunctivorhinostomy 09.82
with insertion of tube or stent 09.83
Constriction of globe, for scleral
buckling see also Buckling, scleral
70
Construction
auricle, ear (with graft) (with implant)
18.71
ear, auricle (with graft) (with implant)
18.71
endorectal (osseous) (skin-lined) 18.6
ileal bladder ileal pouch (H-pouch)
(J-pouch) (S-pouch) (with
anastomosis to anus) 45.95
esophagus, artificial - see Anastomosis,
esophagus
ileal bladder (open) 56.51
closed 57.87 [45.51]
ileal conduit 56.51
larynx, artificial 31.75

Construction *(Continued)*
    patent meatus (ear) 18.6
    penis (rib graft) (skin graft)
        (myocutaneous flap) 64.43
    pharyngeal valve, artificial 31.75
    urethra 58.46
    vagina, artificial 70.61
        with graft or prosthesis 70.63
    venous valves (peripheral) 39.59
Consultation 89.09
    comprehensive 89.07
    limited (single organ system) 89.06
    specified type NEC 89.08
Continuous positive airway pressure
    [CPAP] (non-invasive) 93.90
    delivered by
        endotracheal tube - *see* category
            96.7●
        tracheostomy – *see* category 96.7●
Control
    atmospheric pressure and composition
        NEC 93.98
        antigen-free air conditioning 93.98
        decompression chamber 93.97
        mountain sanatorium 93.98
    epistaxis 21.00
        by
            cauterization (and packing) 21.03
            coagulation (with packing) 21.03
            electrocoagulation (with packing)
                21.03
            excision of nasal mucosa with
                grafting 21.07
            ligation of artery 21.09
                ethmoidal 21.04
                external carotid 21.06
                maxillary (transantral) 21.05
            packing (nasal) (anterior) 21.01
                posterior (and anterior) 21.02
            specified means NEC 21.09
    hemorrhage 39.98
        abdominal cavity 54.19
        adenoids (postoperative) 28.7
        anus (postoperative) 49.95
        bladder (postoperative) 57.93
        chest 34.09
        colon 45.49
            endoscopic 45.43
        duodenum (ulcer) 44.49
            by
                embolization (transcatheter)
                    44.44
                suture (ligation) 44.42
            endoscopic 44.43
        esophagus 42.39
            endoscopic 42.33
        gastric (ulcer) 44.49
            by
                embolization (transcatheter)
                    44.44
                suture (ligation) 44.41
            endoscopic 44.43
        intrapleural 34.09
            postoperative (recurrent) 34.03
        laparotomy site 54.12
        nose - *see also* Control, epistaxis 21.00
        peptic (ulcer) 44.49
            by
                embolization (transcatheter)
                    44.44
                suture (ligation) 44.40
            endoscopic 44.43
        pleura, pleural cavity 34.09
            postoperative (recurrent) 34.03

Control *(Continued)*
    hemorrhage *(Continued)*
        postoperative NEC 39.98
        postvascular surgery 39.41
        prostate 60.94
        specified site NEC 39.98
        stomach - *see* Control, hemorrhage,
            gastric
        thorax NEC 34.09
            postoperative (recurrent)
                34.03
        thyroid (postoperative) 06.02
        tonsils (postoperative) 28.7
Conversion
    anastomosis - *see* Revision, anastomosis
    atrial rhythm (to sinus rhythm)
        99.61 ◄
    cardiac rhythm NEC 99.69
        to sinus rhythm 99.62
    gastrostomy to jejunostomy
        (endoscopic)
        for feeding tube placement
            46.32
    obstetrical position - *see* Version
Cooling, gastric 96.31
CorCap™ 37.41
Cordectomy, vocal 30.22
Cordopexy, vocal 31.69
Cordotomy
    spinal (bilateral) NEC 03.29
        percutaneous 03.21
    vocal 31.3
Corectomy 12.12
Corelysis 12.35
Coreoplasty 12.35
Corneoconjunctivoplasty 11.53
Corpectomy, (vertebral) 80.99
    with diskectomy 80.99
Correction - *see also* Repair
    atresia
        esophageal 42.85
            by magnetic forces 42.99
        external meatus (ear) 18.6
        nasopharynx, nasopharyngeal 29.4
        rectum 48.0
        tricuspid 35.94
    atrial septal defect - *see also* Repair,
        atrial septal defect 35.71
        combined with repair of valvular and
            ventricular septal defects - *see*
            Repair, endocardial cushion
            defect
    blepharoptosis - *see also* Repair,
        blepharoptosis 08.36
    bunionette (with osteotomy) 77.54
    chordee 64.42
    claw toe 77.57
    cleft
        lip 27.54
        palate 27.62
    clubfoot NEC 83.84
    coarctation of aorta
        with
            anastomosis 38.34
            graft replacement 38.44
    cornea NEC 11.59
        refractive NEC 11.79
            epikeratophakia 11.76
            keratomileusis 11.71
            keratophakia 11.72
            radial keratotomy 11.75
    esophageal atresia 42.85
        by magnetic forces 42.99
    everted lacrimal punctum 09.71

Correction *(Continued)*
    eyelid
        ptosis - *see also* Repair,
            blepharoptosis 08.36
        retraction 08.38
    fetal defect 75.36
    forcible, of musculoskeletal deformity
        NEC 93.29
    hammer toe 77.56
    hydraulic pressure, open surgery
        for penile inflatable prosthesis
        64.99
        urinary artificial sphincter 58.99
    intestinal malrotation 46.80
        large 46.82
        small 46.81
    inverted uterus - *see* Repair, inverted
        uterus
    lymphedema (of limb) 40.9
        excision with graft 40.9
        obliteration of lymphatics 40.9
        transplantation of autogenous
            lymphatics 40.9
    nasopharyngeal atresia 29.4
    overlapping toes 77.58
    palate (cleft) 27.62
    prognathism NEC 76.64
    prominent ear 18.5
    punctum (everted) 09.71
    spinal pseudarthrosis - *see* Refusion,
        spinal
    syndactyly 86.85
    tetralogy of Fallot
        one-stage 35.81
        partial - *see* specific procedure
        total 35.81
    total anomalous pulmonary venous
        connection
        one-stage 35.82
        partial - *see* specific procedure
        total 35.82
    transposition, great arteries, total
        35.84
    tricuspid atresia 35.94
    truncus arteriosus
        one-stage 35.83
        partial - *see* specific procedure
        total 35.83
    ureteropelvic junction 55.87
    ventricular septal defect - *see also*
        Repair, ventricular septal defect
        35.72
        combined with repair of valvular
            and atrial septal defects - *see*
            Repair, endocardial cushion
            defect
Costectomy 77.91
    with lung excision - *see* Excision, lung
    associated with thoracic
        operation - *omit code*
Costochondrectomy 77.91
    associated with thoracic
        operation - *omit code*
Costosternoplasty (pectus excavatum
    repair) 34.74
Costotomy 77.31
Costotransversectomy 77.91
    associated with thoracic
        operation - *omit code*
Counseling (for) NEC 94.49
    alcoholism 94.46
    drug addiction 94.45
    employers 94.49
    family (medical) (social) 94.49

Counseling NEC (*Continued*)
 marriage 94.49
 ophthalmologic (with instruction)
  95.36
 pastoral 94.49
Countershock, cardiac NEC 99.62
Coventry operation (tibial wedge
  osteotomy) 77.27
CPAP (continuous positive airway
  pressure) 93.90
 delivered by
  endotracheal tube - *see* category
   96.7●
  tracheostomy – *see* category 96.7●
Craniectomy 01.25
 linear (opening of cranial suture) 02.01
 reopening of site 01.23
 strip (opening of cranial suture) 02.01
Cranioclasis, fetal 73.8
Cranioplasty 02.06
 with synchronous repair of
  encephalocele 02.12
Craniotomy 01.24
 as operative approach - *omit code*
 fetal 73.8
 for decompression of fracture 02.02
 reopening of site 01.23
Craterization, bone - *see also* Excision,
  lesion, bone 77.60
Crawford operation (tarso-frontalis sling
  of eyelid) 08.32
Creation - *see also* Formation
 cardiac device (defibrillator)
   (pacemaker) pocket
  with initial insertion of cardiac
   device - *omit code*
  new site (skin) (subcutaneous) 37.79
 conduit
  ileal (urinary) 56.51
  left ventricle and aorta 35.93
  right atrium and pulmonary artery
   35.94
  right ventricle and pulmonary
   (distal) artery 35.92
   in repair of
    pulmonary artery atresia 35.92
    transposition of great vessels
     35.92
    truncus arteriosus 35.83
 endorectal ileal pouch (H-pouch) (J-
   pouch) (S-pouch) (with
   anastomosis to anus) 45.95
 esophagogastric sphincteric
   competence NEC 44.66
  laparoscopic 44.67
 Hartmann pouch - *see* Colectomy, by
   site
 interatrial fistula 35.42
 pericardial window 37.12
 pleural window, for drainage 34.09
 pocket
  cardiac device (defibrillator)
   (pacemaker)
   with initial insertion of cardiac
    device - *omit code*
   new site (skin) (subcutaneous)
    37.79
  loop recorder 37.79
  thalamic stimulator pulse
   generator
   with initial insertion of battery
    package - *omit code*
   new site (skin) (subcutaneous)
    86.09

Creation (*Continued*)
 shunt - *see also* Shunt
  arteriovenous fistula, for dialysis
   39.93
  left-to-right (systemic to pulmonary
   circulation) 39.0
 subcutaneous tunnel for esophageal
   anastomosis 42.86
  with anastomosis - *see* Anastomosis,
   esophagus, antesternal
 syndactyly (finger) (toe) 86.89
 thalamic stimulator pulse generator
  with initial insertion of battery
   package - *omit code*
  new site (skin) (subcutaneous) 86.09
 tracheoesophageal fistula 31.95
 window
  pericardial 37.12
  pleura, for drainage 34.09
Credé maneuver 73.59
Cricoidectomy 30.29
Cricothyreotomy (for assistance in
  breathing) 31.1
Cricothyroidectomy 30.29
Cricothyrostomy 31.1
Cricothyrotomy (for assistance in
  breathing) 31.1
Cricotomy (for assistance in breathing)
  31.1
Cricotracheotomy (for assistance in
  breathing) 31.1
Crisis intervention 94.35
Croupette, croup tent 93.94
Crown, dental (ceramic) (gold) 23.41
Crushing
 bone - *see* category 78.4●
 calculus
  bile (hepatic) passage 51.49
   endoscopic 51.88
  bladder (urinary) 57.0
  pancreatic duct 52.09
   endoscopic 52.94
 fallopian tube - *see also* Ligation,
   fallopian tube 66.39
 ganglion - *see* Crushing, nerve
 hemorrhoids 49.45
 nasal septum 21.88
 nerve (cranial) (peripheral) NEC
   04.03
  acoustic 04.01
  auditory 04.01
  phrenic 04.03
   for collapse of lung 33.31
  sympathetic 05.0
  trigeminal 04.02
  vestibular 04.01
 vas deferens 63.71
Cryoablation - *see* Ablation
Cryoanalgesia nerve (cranial) (peripheral)
  04.2
Cryoconization, cervix 67.33
Cryodestruction - *see* Destruction, lesion,
  by site
Cryoextraction, lens - *see also* Extraction,
  cataract, intracapsular 13.19
Cryohypophysectomy (complete) (total) -
  see also Hypophysectomy 07.69
Cryoleucotomy 01.32
Cryopexy, retinal - *see* Cryotherapy, retina
Cryoprostatectomy 60.62
Cryoretinopexy (for)
 reattachment 14.52
 repair of tear or defect 14.32
Cryosurgery - *see* Cryotherapy

Cryothalamectomy 01.41
Cryotherapy - *see also* Destruction, lesion,
  by site
 bladder 57.59
 brain 01.59
 cataract 13.19
 cervix 67.33
 choroid - *see* Cryotherapy, retina
 ciliary body 12.72
 corneal lesion (ulcer) 11.43
  to reshape cornea 11.79
 ear
  external 18.29
  inner 20.79
 esophagus 42.39
  endoscopic 42.33
 eyelid 08.25
 hemorrhoids 49.44
 iris 12.41
 nasal turbinates 21.61
 palate (bony) 27.31
 prostate 60.62
 retina (for)
  destruction of lesion 14.22
  reattachment 14.52
  repair of tear 14.32
 skin 86.3
 stomach 43.49
  endoscopic 43.41
 subcutaneous tissue 86.3
 turbinates (nasal) 21.61
 warts 86.3
  genital 71.3
Cryptectomy (anus) 49.39
 endoscopic 49.31
Cryptorchidectomy (unilateral) 62.3
 bilateral 62.41
Cryptotomy (anus) 49.39
 endoscopic 49.31
Cuirass 93.99
Culdocentesis 70.0
Culdoplasty 70.92
 with graft or prosthesis 70.93
Culdoscopy (exploration) (removal of
  foreign body or lesion) 70.22
Culdotomy 70.12
Culp-Deweerd operation (spiral flap
  pyeloplasty) 55.87
Culp-Scardino operation (ureteral flap
  pyeloplasty) 55.87
Culture (and sensitivity) - *see*
  Examination, microscopic
Curettage (with packing) (with secondary
  closure) - *see also* Dilation and
  curettage
 adenoids 28.6
 anus 49.39
  endoscopic 49.31
 bladder 57.59
  transurethral 57.49
 bone - *see also* Excision, lesion, bone
   77.60
 brain 01.59
 bursa 83.39
  hand 82.29
 cartilage - *see also* Excision, lesion, joint
   80.80
 cerebral meninges 01.51
 chalazion 08.25
 conjunctiva (trachoma follicles) 10.33
 corneal epithelium 11.41
  for smear or culture 11.21
 ear, external 18.29
 eyelid 08.25

◄ New   ◄▥ Revised   ~~deleted~~ Deleted   ● Use Additional Digit(s)   ▨ Omit code

Curettage *(Continued)*
  joint - *see also* Excision, lesion, joint
    80.80
  meninges (cerebral) 01.51
    spinal 03.4
  muscle 83.32
    hand 82.22
  nerve (peripheral) 04.07
    sympathetic 05.29
  sclera 12.84
  skin 86.3
  spinal cord (meninges) 03.4
  subgingival 24.31
  tendon 83.39
    sheath 83.31
      hand 82.21
  uterus (with dilation) 69.09
    aspiration (diagnostic) NEC 69.59
      after abortion or delivery 69.52
      to terminate pregnancy 69.51
    following delivery or abortion
      69.02
Curette evacuation, lens 13.2
Curtis operation (interphalangeal joint
  arthroplasty) 81.72
Cutaneolipectomy 86.83
Cutdown, venous 38.94
Cutting
  nerve (cranial) (peripheral) NEC 04.03
    acoustic 04.01
    auditory 04.01
    root, spinal 03.1
    sympathetic 05.0
    trigeminal 04.02
    vestibular 04.01
  pedicle (flap) graft 86.71
  pylorus (with wedge resection) 43.3

Cutting *(Continued)*
  spinal nerve root 03.1
  ureterovesical orifice 56.1
  urethral sphincter 58.5
CVP (central venous pressure
  monitoring) 89.62
Cyclectomy (ciliary body) 12.44
  eyelid margin 08.20
Cyclicotomy 12.55
Cycloanemization 12.74
Cyclocryotherapy 12.72
Cyclodialysis (initial) (subsequent)
  12.55
Cyclodiathermy (penetrating) (surface)
  12.71
Cycloelectrolysis 12.71
Cyclophotocoagulation 12.73
Cyclotomy 12.55
Cystectomy - *see also* Excision, lesion, by
  site
  gallbladder - *see* Cholecystectomy
  urinary (partial) (subtotal) 57.6
    complete (with urethrectomy)
      57.79
    radical 57.71
      with pelvic exenteration
        (female) 68.8
    total (with urethrectomy)
      57.79
Cystocolostomy 57.88
Cystogram, cystography NEC
  87.77
Cystolitholapaxy 57.0
Cystolithotomy 57.19
Cystometrogram 89.22
Cystopexy NEC 57.89
Cystoplasty NEC 57.89

Cystoproctostomy 57.88
Cystoprostatectomy, radical 57.71
Cystopyelography 87.74
Cystorrhaphy 57.81
Cystoscopy (transurethral) 57.32
  with biopsy 57.33
  for
    control of hemorrhage
      bladder 57.93
      prostate 60.94
    retrograde pyelography 87.74
  ileal conduit 56.35
  through stoma (artificial) 57.31
Cystostomy
  closed (suprapubic) (percutaneous)
    57.17
  open (suprapubic) 57.18
  percutaneous (closed) (suprapubic)
    57.17
  suprapubic
    closed 57.17
    open 57.18
Cystotomy (open) (for removal of calculi)
  57.19
Cystourethrogram (retrograde) (voiding)
  87.76
Cystourethropexy (by) 59.79
  levator muscle sling 59.71
  retropubic suspension 59.5
  suprapubic suspension 59.4
Cystourethroplasty 57.85
Cystourethroscopy 57.32
  with biopsy
    bladder 57.33
    ureter 56.33
Cytology - *see* Examination, microscopic

D

Dacryoadenectomy 09.20
  partial 09.22
  total 09.23
Dacryoadenotomy 09.0
Dacryocystectomy (complete) (partial) 09.6
Dacryocystogram 87.05
Dacryocystorhinostomy (DCR) (by intubation) (external) (intranasal) 09.81
Dacryocystostomy 09.53
Dacryocystosyringotomy 09.53
Dacryocystotomy 09.53
Dahlman operation (excision of esophageal diverticulum) 42.31
Dana operation (posterior rhizotomy) 03.1
Danforth operation (fetal) 73.8
Darrach operation (ulnar resection) 77.83
da Vinci® (S HD) Surgical System – see category 17.4
Davis operation (intubated ureterotomy) 56.2
Deaf training 95.49
Debridement
  abdominal wall 54.3
  bone - see also Excision, lesion, bone 77.60
    fracture - see Debridement, open fracture
  brain 01.59
  burn (skin) 86.28
    excisional 86.22
    nonexcisional 86.28
  bursa 83.5
  cerebral meninges 01.51
  dental 96.54
  fascia 83.39
  flap graft 86.75
  graft (flap) (pedicle) 86.75
  heart valve (calcified) - see Valvuloplasty, heart
  infection (skin) 86.28
    excisional 86.22
    nail (bed) (fold) 86.27
    nonexcisional 86.28
  joint - see Excision, lesion, joint
  meninges (cerebral) 01.51
    spinal 03.4
  muscle 83.45
    hand 82.36
  nail (bed) (fold) 86.27
  nerve (peripheral) 04.07
  open fracture (compound) 79.60
    arm NEC 79.62
    carpal, metacarpal 79.63
    facial bone 76.2
    femur 79.65
    fibula 79.66
    foot NEC 79.67
    hand NEC 79.63
    humerus 79.61
    leg NEC 79.66
    phalanges
      foot 79.68
      hand 79.64
    radius 79.62
    specified site NEC 79.69
    tarsal, metatarsal 79.67
    tibia 79.66
    ulna 79.62

Debridement (Continued)
  patella 77.66
  pedicle graft 86.75
  skin or subcutaneous tissue (burn) (infection) (wound) 86.28
    cardioverter/defibrillator (automatic) pocket 37.79
    excisional 86.22
    graft 86.75
    nail, nail bed, or nail fold 86.27
    nonexcisional 86.28
    pacemaker pocket 37.79
    pocket
      cardiac device NEC 37.79
      cardiac pacemaker 37.79
      cardioverter/defibrillator (automatic) 37.79
  skull 01.25
    compound fracture 02.02
  spinal cord (meninges) 03.4
  tendon 83.39
  VersaJet™ 86.28
  wound (skin) 86.28
    excisional 86.22
    nonexcisional 86.28
Decapitation, fetal 73.8
Decapsulation, kidney 55.91
Declotting - see also Removal, thrombus
  arteriovenous cannula or shunt 39.49
Decompression
  anus (imperforate) 48.0
  biliary tract 51.49
    by intubation 51.43
      endoscopic 51.87
      percutaneous 51.98
  brain 01.24
  carpal tunnel 04.43
  cauda equina 03.09
  chamber 93.97
  colon 96.08
    by incision 45.03
    endoscopic (balloon) 46.85
  common bile duct 51.42
    by intubation 51.43
      endoscopic 51.87
      percutaneous 51.98
  cranial 01.24
    for skull fracture 02.02
  endolymphatic sac 20.79
  ganglion (peripheral) NEC 04.49
    cranial NEC 04.42
  gastric 96.07
  heart 37.0
  intestine 96.08
    by incision 45.00
    endoscopic (balloon) 46.85
  intracranial 01.24
  labyrinth 20.79
  laminectomy 03.09
  laminotomy 03.09
  median nerve 04.43
  muscle 83.02
    hand 82.02
  nerve (peripheral) NEC 04.49
    auditory 04.42
    cranial NEC 04.42
    median 04.43
    trigeminal (root) 04.41
  orbit - see also Orbitotomy 16.09
  pancreatic duct 52.92
    endoscopic 52.93
  pericardium 37.0
  rectum 48.0

Decompression (Continued)
  skull fracture 02.02
  spinal cord (canal) 03.09
  tarsal tunnel 04.44
  tendon (sheath) 83.01
    hand 82.01
  thoracic outlet
    by
      myotomy (division of scalenus anticus muscle) 83.19
      tenotomy 83.13
  trigeminal (nerve root) 04.41
Decortication
  arterial 05.25
  brain 01.51
  cerebral meninges 01.51
  heart 37.31
  kidney 55.91
  lung (partial) (total) 34.51
    thoracoscopic 34.52
  nasal turbinates - see Turbinectomy
  nose 21.89
  ovary 65.29
    laparoscopic 65.25
  periarterial 05.25
  pericardium 37.31
  ventricle, heart (complete) 37.31
Decoy, E2F 00.16
Deepening
  alveolar ridge 24.5
  buccolabial sulcus 24.91
  lingual sulcus 24.91
Defatting, flap or pedicle graft 86.75
Defibrillation, electric (external) (internal) 99.62
  automatic cardioverter/defibrillator - see category 37.9●
de Grandmont operation (tarsectomy) 08.35
Delaying of pedicle graft 86.71
Delivery (with)
  assisted spontaneous 73.59
  breech extraction (assisted) 72.52
    partial 72.52
      with forceps to aftercoming head 72.51
    total 72.54
      with forceps to aftercoming head 72.53
    unassisted (spontaneous delivery) - omit code
  cesarean section - see Cesarean section
  Credé maneuver 73.59
  De Lee maneuver 72.4
  forceps 72.9
    application to aftercoming head (Piper) 72.6
      with breech extraction
        partial 72.51
        total 72.53
    Barton's 72.4
    failed 73.3
    high 72.39
      with episiotomy 72.31
    low (outlet) 72.0
      with episiotomy 72.1
    mid 72.29
      with episiotomy 72.21
    outlet (low) 72.0
      with episiotomy 72.1
    rotation of fetal head 72.4
    trial 73.3
  instrumental NEC 72.9
    specified NEC 72.8

◀ New   ◀▥ Revised   deleted Deleted   ● Use Additional Digit(s)   Omit code

Delivery *(Continued)*
 key-in-lock rotation 72.4
 Kielland rotation 72.4
 Malstrom's extraction 72.79
  with episiotomy 72.71
 manually assisted (spontaneous) 73.59
 spontaneous (unassisted) 73.59
  assisted 73.59
 vacuum extraction 72.79
  with episiotomy 72.71
Delorme operation
 pericardiectomy 37.31
 proctopexy 48.76
 repair of prolapsed rectum 48.76
 thoracoplasty 33.34
Denervation
 aortic body 39.8
 carotid body 39.8
 facet, percutaneous (radiofrequency)
  03.96
 ovarian 65.94
 paracervical uterine 69.3
 uterosacral 69.3
Denker operation (radical maxillary
 antrotomy) 22.31
Dennis-Barco operation - *see* Repair,
 hernia, femoral
Denonvillier operation (limited
 rhinoplasty) 21.86
Densitometry, bone (serial)
 (radiographic) 88.98
Depilation, skin 86.92
Derlacki operation (tympanoplasty)
 19.4
Dermabond 86.59
Dermabrasion (laser) 86.25
 for wound debridement 86.28
Derotation - *see* Reduction, torsion
Desensitization
 allergy 99.12
 psychologic 94.33
Desmotomy - *see also* Division, ligament
 80.40
Destruction
 breast 85.20
 chorioretinopathy - *see also* Destruction,
  lesion, choroid 14.29
 ciliary body 12.74
 epithelial downgrowth, anterior
  chamber 12.93
 fallopian tube 66.39
  with
   crushing (and ligation) 66.31
    by endoscopy (laparoscopy)
     66.21
   division (and ligation) 66.32
    by endoscopy (culdoscopy)
     (hysteroscopy)
     (laparoscopy)
     (peritoneoscopy)
     66.22
   ligation 66.39
    with
     crushing 66.31
      by endoscopy
       (laparoscopy)
       66.21
     division 66.32
      by endoscopy
       (culdoscopy)
       (hysteroscopy)
       (laparoscopy)
       (peritoneoscopy)
       66.22

Destruction *(Continued)*
 fetus 73.8
 hemorrhoids 49.49
  by
   cryotherapy 49.44
   sclerotherapy 49.42
 inner ear NEC 20.79
  by injection 20.72
 intervertebral disc (NOS) 80.50
  by injection 80.52
  by other specified method 80.59
  herniated (nucleus pulposus)
   80.51
 LAA 37.36
 lacrimal sac 09.6
 left atrial appendage 37.36
 lesion (local)
  anus 49.39
   endoscopic 49.31
  Bartholin's gland 71.24
   by
    aspiration 71.21
    excision 71.24
    incision 71.22
    marsupialization 71.23
  biliary ducts 51.69
   endoscopic 51.64
  bladder 57.59
   transurethral 57.49
  bone - *see* Excision, lesion, bone
  bowel - *see* Destruction, lesion,
   intestine
  brain (transtemporal approach)
   NEC 01.59
   by stereotactic radiosurgery 92.30
    cobalt 60 92.32
    linear accelerator (LINAC)
     92.31
    multi-source 92.32
    particle beam 92.33
    particulate 92.33
    radiosurgery NEC 92.39
    single source photon 92.31
  breast NEC 85.20
  bronchus NEC 32.09
   endoscopic 32.01
  cerebral NEC 01.59
   meninges 01.51
  cervix 67.39
   by
    cauterization 67.32
    cryosurgery, cryoconization
     67.33
    electroconization 67.32
  choroid 14.29
   by
    cryotherapy 14.22
    diathermy 14.21
    implantation of radiation
     source 14.27
    photocoagulation 14.25
     laser 14.24
     xenon arc 14.23
    radiation therapy 14.26
  ciliary body (nonexcisional) 12.43
   by excision 12.44
  conjunctiva 10.32
   by excision 10.31
  cornea NEC 11.49
   by
    cryotherapy 11.43
    electrocauterization 11.42
    thermocauterization 11.42
  cul-de-sac 70.32

Destruction *(Continued)*
 lesion *(Continued)*
  duodenum NEC 45.32
   by excision 45.31
    endoscopic 45.30
   endoscopic 45.30
  esophagus (chemosurgery)
   (cryosurgery) (electroresection)
   (fulguration) NEC 42.39
   by excision 42.32
    endoscopic 42.33
   endoscopic 42.33
  eye NEC 16.93
  eyebrow 08.25
  eyelid 08.25
   excisional - *see* Excision, lesion,
    eyelid
  heart
   by catheter ablation 37.34
   by endovascular approach
    37.34
   by open approach 37.33
   left atrial appendage 37.36
  intestine (large) 45.49
   by excision 45.41
    endoscopic 45.43
     polypectomy 45.42
   endoscopic 45.43
    polypectomy 45.42
   small 45.34
    by excision 45.33
  intranasal 21.31
  iris (nonexcisional) NEC 12.41
   by excision 12.42
  kidney 55.39
   by marsupialization 55.31
  lacrimal sac 09.6
  larynx 30.09
  liver 50.29
  lung 32.29
   endoscopic 32.28
   thoracoscopic 32.20
  meninges (cerebral) 01.51
   spinal 03.4
  nerve (peripheral) 04.07
   sympathetic 05.29
  nose 21.30
   intranasal 21.31
   specified NEC 21.32
  ovary
   by
    aspiration 65.91
    excision 65.29
     laparoscopic 65.25
   cyst by rupture (manual) 65.93
  palate (bony) (local) 27.31
   wide 27.32
  pancreas 52.22
   by marsupialization 52.3
   endoscopic 52.21
  pancreatic duct 52.22
   endoscopic 52.21
  penis 64.2
  pharynx (excisional) 29.39
  pituitary gland
   by stereotactic radiosurgery 92.30
    cobalt 60 92.32
    linear accelerator (LINAC)
     92.31
    multi-source 92.32
    particle beam 92.33
    particulate 92.33
    radiosurgery NEC 92.39
    single source photon 92.31

Destruction *(Continued)*
  lesion *(Continued)*
    rectum (local) 48.32
      by
        cryosurgery 48.34
        electrocoagulation 48.32
        excision 48.35
        fulguration 48.32
        laser (Argon) 48.33
      polyp 48.36
      radical 48.31
    retina 14.29
      by
        cryotherapy 14.22
        diathermy 14.21
        implantation of radiation
          source 14.27
        photocoagulation 14.25
          laser 14.24
          xenon arc 14.23
        radiation therapy 14.26
    salivary gland NEC 26.29
      by marsupialization 26.21
    sclera 12.84
    scrotum 61.3
    skin NEC 86.3
    sphincter of Oddi 51.69
      endoscopic 51.64
    spinal cord (meninges) 03.4
    spleen 41.42
      by marsupialization 41.41
    stomach NEC 43.49
      by excision 43.42
        endoscopic 43.41
      endoscopic 43.41
    subcutaneous tissue NEC 86.3
    testis 62.2
    tongue 25.1
    urethra (excisional) 58.39
      endoscopic 58.31
    uterus 68.29
  nerve (cranial) (peripheral) (by
    cryoanalgesia) (by
    radiofrequency) 04.2
  sympathetic, by injection of
    neurolytic agent 05.32
  neuroma
    acoustic 04.01
      by craniotomy 04.01
      by stereotactic radiosurgery 92.30
        cobalt 60 92.32
        linear accelerator (LINAC)
          92.31
        multi-source 92.32
        particle beam 92.33
        particulate 92.33
        radiosurgery NEC 92.39
        single source photon 92.31
    cranial 04.07
    Morton's 04.07
    peripheral
      Morton's 04.07
  prostate (prostatic tissue)
    by
      cryotherapy 60.62
      microwave 60.96
      radiofrequency 60.97
    transurethral microwave
      thermotherapy (TUMT) 60.96
    transurethral needle ablation
      (TUNA) 60.97
    TULIP (transurethral (ultrasound)
      guided laser induced
      prostatectomy) 60.21

Destruction *(Continued)*
  prostate *(Continued)*
    TUMT (transurethral microwave
      thermotherapy) 60.96
    TUNA (transurethral needle
      ablation) 60.97
  semicircular canals, by injection
    20.72
  vestibule, by injection 20.72
Detachment, uterosacral ligaments
  69.3
Determination
  mental status (clinical) (medicolegal)
    (psychiatric) NEC 94.11
    psychologic NEC 94.09
  vital capacity (pulmonary) 89.37
Detorsion
  intestine (twisted) (volvulus) 46.80
    large 46.82
      endoscopic (balloon) 46.85
    small 46.81
  kidney 55.84
  ovary 65.95
  spermatic cord 63.52
    with orchiopexy 62.5
  testis 63.52
    with orchiopexy 62.5
  volvulus 46.80
    endoscopic (balloon) 46.85
Detoxification therapy 94.25
  alcohol 94.62
    with rehabilitation 94.63
    combined alcohol and drug 94.68
      with rehabilitation 94.69
  drug 94.65
    with rehabilitation 94.66
    combined alcohol and drug 94.68
      with rehabilitation 94.69
Devascularization, stomach 44.99
Device
  CorCap™ 37.41
  external fixator - *see* Fixator, external
Dewebbing
  esophagus 42.01
  syndactyly (fingers) (toes) 86.85
Dextrorotation - *see* Reduction, torsion
Dialysis
  hemodiafiltration, hemofiltration
    (extracorporeal) 39.95
  kidney (extracorporeal) 39.95
  liver 50.92
  peritoneal 54.98
  renal (extracorporeal) 39.95
Diaphanoscopy
  nasal sinuses 89.35
  skull (newborn) 89.16
Diaphysectomy - *see* category 77.8●
Diathermy 93.34
  choroid - *see* Diathermy, retina
  nasal turbinates 21.61
  retina
    for
      destruction of lesion 14.21
      reattachment 14.51
      repair of tear 14.31
  surgical - *see* Destruction, lesion, by site
  turbinates (nasal) 21.61
Dickson operation (fascial transplant)
  83.82
Dickson-Diveley operation (tendon
  transfer and arthrodesis to correct
  claw toe) 77.57
Dieffenbach operation (hip
  disarticulation) 84.18

Dilation
  achalasia 42.92
  ampulla of Vater 51.81
    endoscopic 51.84
  anus, anal (sphincter) 96.23
  biliary duct
    endoscopic 51.84
    pancreatic duct 52.99
      endoscopic 52.98
    percutaneous (endoscopy) 51.98
    sphincter
      of Oddi 51.81
        endoscopic 51.84
      pancreatic 51.82
        endoscopic 51.85
  bladder 96.25
    neck 57.92
  bronchus 33.91
  cervix (canal) 67.0
    obstetrical 73.1
    to assist delivery 73.1
  choanae (nasopharynx) 29.91
  colon (endoscopic) (balloon) 46.85
    with insertion of colonic stent   ◀
      endoscopic 46.86   ◀
      other 46.87   ◀
  colostomy stoma 96.24
  duodenum (endoscopic) (balloon) 46.85
    with insertion of colonic stent   ◀
      endoscopic 46.86   ◀
      other 46.87   ◀
  endoscopic - *see* Dilation, by site
  enterostomy stoma 96.24
  esophagus (by bougie) (by sound) 42.92
  fallopian tube 66.96
  foreskin (newborn) 99.95
  frontonasal duct 96.21
  gastrojejunostomy site, endoscopic 44.22
  heart valve - *see* Valvulotomy, heart
  ileostomy stoma 96.24
  ileum (endoscopic) (balloon) 46.85
    with insertion of colonic stent   ◀
      endoscopic 46.86   ◀
      other 46.87   ◀
  intestinal stoma (artificial) 96.24
  intestine (endoscopic) (balloon) 46.85
    with insertion of colonic stent   ◀
      endoscopic 46.86   ◀
      other 46.87   ◀
  jejunum (endoscopic) (balloon) 46.85
    with insertion of colonic stent   ◀
      endoscopic 46.86   ◀
      other 46.87   ◀
  lacrimal
    duct 09.42
    punctum 09.41
  larynx 31.98
  lymphatic structure(s) (peripheral) 40.9
  nares 21.99
  nasolacrimal duct (retrograde) 09.43
    with insertion of tube or stent 09.44
  nasopharynx 29.91
  pancreatic duct 52.99
    endoscopic 52.98
  pharynx 29.91
  prostatic urethra (transurethral)
    (balloon) 60.95
  punctum, lacrimal papilla 09.41
  pylorus
    by incision 44.21
    endoscopic 44.22
  rectum 96.22
  salivary duct 26.91
  sphenoid ostia 22.52

◀ New   ⦉ Revised   deleted Deleted   ● Use Additional Digit(s)   ▮ Omit code

Dilation *(Continued)*
  sphincter
    anal 96.23
    cardiac 42.92
    of Oddi 51.81
      endoscopic 51.84
    pancreatic 51.82
      endoscopic 51.85
    pylorus, endoscopic 44.22
      by incision 44.21
  Stenson's duct 26.91
  trachea 31.99
  ureter 59.8
    meatus 56.91
  ureterovesical orifice 59.8
  urethra 58.6
    prostatic (transurethral) (balloon)
      60.95
  urethrovesical junction 58.6
  vagina (instrumental) (manual) NEC
    96.16
  vesical neck 57.92
  Wharton's duct 26.91
  Wirsung's duct 52.99
    endoscopic 52.98
Dilation and curettage, uterus
  (diagnostic) 69.09
  after
    abortion 69.02
    delivery 69.02
  to terminate pregnancy 69.01
Diminution, ciliary body 12.74
Disarticulation 84.91
  ankle 84.13
  elbow 84.06
  finger, except thumb 84.01
    thumb 84.02
  hip 84.18
  knee 84.16
  shoulder 84.08
  thumb 84.02
  toe 84.11
  wrist 84.04
Discectomy - *see* Diskectomy
Discission
  capsular membrane 13.64
  cataract (Wheeler knife) (Ziegler knife)
    13.2
    congenital 13.69
    secondary membrane 13.64
  iris 12.12
  lens (capsule) (Wheeler knife) (Ziegler
    knife) (with capsulotomy) 13.2
  orbitomaxillary, radical 16.51
  pupillary 13.2
  secondary membrane (after cataract)
    13.64
  vitreous strands (posterior approach)
    14.74
    anterior approach 14.73
Discogram, diskogram 87.21
Discolysis (by injection) 80.52
Diskectomy (discectomy), intervertebral
  80.51
  with corpectomy 80.99
  herniated (nucleus pulposus) 80.51
  percutaneous 80.59
Dispensing (with fitting)
  contact lens 95.32
  low vision aids NEC 95.33
  spectacles 95.31
Disruption
  blood brain barrier via infusion [BBBD]
    00.19

Dissection - *see also* Excision
  aneurysm 38.60
  artery-vein-nerve bundle 39.91
  branchial cleft fistula or sinus 29.52
  bronchus 32.1
  femoral hernia 53.29
  groin, radical 40.54
  larynx block (en bloc) 30.3
  mediastinum with pneumonectomy
    32.59
    thoracoscopic 32.50
  neck, radical 40.40
    with laryngectomy 30.4
    bilateral 40.42
    unilateral 40.41
  orbital fibrous bands 16.92
  pterygium (with reposition) 11.31
  radical neck - *see* Dissection, neck,
    radical
  retroperitoneal NEC 59.00
  thoracic structures (block) (en bloc)
    (radical) (brachial plexus,
    bronchus, lobe of lung, ribs, and
    sympathetic nerves) 32.6
  vascular bundle 39.91
Distention, bladder (therapeutic)
  (intermittent) 96.25
Diversion
  biliopancreatic (BPD) 43.7 *[45.51]*
    [45.91]
    with duodenal switch 43.89 *[45.51]*
      [45.91]
  urinary
    cutaneous 56.61
    ileal conduit 56.51
    internal NEC 56.71
    ureter to
      intestine 56.71
      skin 56.61
    uretero-ileostomy 56.51
Diversional therapy 93.81
Diverticulectomy
  bladder (suprapubic) 57.59
    transurethral approach 57.49
  duodenum 45.31
    endoscopic 45.30
  esophagus 42.31
    endoscopic 42.33
  esophagomyotomy 42.7
  hypopharyngeal (by cricopharyngeal
    myotomy) 29.32
  intestine
    large 45.41
      endoscopic 45.43
    small 45.33
  kidney 55.39
  Meckel's 45.33
  pharyngeal (by cricopharyngeal
    myotomy) 29.32
  pharyngoesophageal (by
    cricopharyngeal myotomy) 29.32
  stomach 43.42
    endoscopic 43.41
  urethra 58.39
    endoscopic 58.31
Division
  Achilles tendon 83.11
  adductor tendon (hip) 83.12
  adhesions - *see* Lysis, adhesions
  angle of mandible (open) 76.62
    closed 76.61
  anterior synechiae 12.32
  aponeurosis 83.13
  arcuate ligament (spine) - *omit code*

Division *(Continued)*
  arteriovenous fistula (with ligation)
    39.53
  artery (with ligation) 38.80
    abdominal 38.86
    aorta (arch) (ascending)
      (descending) 38.84
    head and neck NEC 38.82
    intracranial NEC 38.81
    lower limb 38.88
    thoracic NEC 38.85
    upper limb 38.83
  bladder neck 57.91
  blepharorrhaphy 08.02
  blood vessels, cornea 10.1
  bone - *see also* Osteotomy 77.30
  brain tissue 01.32
    cortical adhesions 02.91
  canaliculus 09.52
  canthorrhaphy 08.02
  cartilage 80.40
    ankle 80.47
    elbow 80.42
    foot and toe 80.48
    hand and finger 80.44
    hip 80.45
    knee 80.46
    shoulder 80.41
    specified site NEC 80.49
    spine 80.49
    wrist 80.43
  cerebral tracts 01.32
  chordae tendineae 35.32
  common wall between posterior left
    atrium and coronary sinus (with
    roofing of resultant defect with
    patch graft) 35.82
  congenital web
    larynx 31.98
    pharynx 29.54
  endometrial synechiae 68.21
  fallopian tube - *see* Ligation, fallopian
    tube
  fascia 83.14
    hand 82.12
  frenulum, frenum
    labial 27.91
    lingual 25.91
    tongue 25.91
  ganglion, sympathetic 05.0
  glossopharyngeal nerve 29.92
  goniosynechiae 12.31
  hypophyseal stalk - *see also*
    Hypophysectomy, partial 07.63
  iliotibial band 83.14
  isthmus
    horseshoe kidney 55.85
    thyroid 06.91
  joint capsule 80.40
    ankle 80.47
    elbow 80.42
    foot and toe 80.48
    hand and finger 80.44
    hip 80.45
    knee 80.46
    shoulder 80.41
    specified site NEC 80.49
    wrist 80.43
  labial frenum 27.91
  lacrimal ductules 09.0
  laryngeal nerve (external) (recurrent)
    (superior) 31.91
  ligament 80.40
    ankle 80.47

Division *(Continued)*
 ligament *(Continued)*
  arcuate (spine) - *omit code*
  canthal 08.36
  elbow 80.42
  foot and toe 80.48
  hand and finger 80.44
  hip 80.45
  knee 80.46
  palpebrae 08.36
  shoulder 80.41
  specified site NEC 80.49
  spine 80.49
   arcuate - *omit code*
   flavum - *omit code*
  uterosacral 69.3
  wrist 80.43
 ligamentum flavum (spine) - *omit code*
 meninges (cerebral) 01.31
 muscle 83.19
  hand 82.19
 nasolacrimal duct stricture (with
   drainage) 09.59
 nerve (cranial) (peripheral) NEC 04.03
  acoustic 04.01
  adrenal gland 07.42
  auditory 04.01
  glossopharyngeal 29.92
  lacrimal branch 05.0
  laryngeal (external) (recurrent)
    (superior) 31.91
  phrenic 04.03
   for collapse of lung 33.31
  root, spinal or intraspinal 03.1
  sympathetic 05.0
  tracts
   cerebral 01.32
   spinal cord 03.29
    percutaneous 03.21
  trigeminal 04.02
  vagus - *see also* Vagotomy 44.00
  vestibular 04.01
 otosclerotic process or material, middle
   ear 19.0
 papillary muscle (heart) 35.31
 patent ductus arteriosus 38.85
 penile adhesions 64.93
 posterior synechiae 12.33
 pylorus (with wedge resection) 43.3
 rectum (stricture) 48.91
 scalenus anticus muscle 83.19
 Skene's gland 71.3
 soft tissue NEC 83.19
  hand 82.19
 sphincter
  anal (external) (internal) 49.59
   left lateral 49.51
   posterior 49.52
  cardiac 42.7
  of Oddi 51.82
   endoscopic 51.85
  pancreatic 51.82
   endoscopic 51.85
 spinal
  cord tracts 03.29
   percutaneous 03.21
  nerve root 03.1
 symblepharon (with insertion of
   conformer) 10.5
 synechiae
  endometrial 68.21
  iris (posterior) 12.33
   anterior 12.32
 tarsorrhaphy 08.02

Division *(Continued)*
 tendon 83.13
  Achilles 83.11
  adductor (hip) 83.12
  hand 82.11
 trabeculae carneae cordis (heart) 35.35
 tympanum 20.23
 uterosacral ligaments 69.3
 vaginal septum 70.14
 vas deferens 63.71
 vein (with ligation) 38.80
  abdominal 38.87
  head and neck NEC 38.82
  intracranial NEC 38.81
  lower limb 38.89
   varicose 38.59
  thoracic NEC 38.85
  upper limb 38.83
  varicose 38.50
   abdominal 38.57
   head and neck NEC 38.52
   intracranial NEC 38.51
   lower limb 38.59
   thoracic NEC 38.55
   upper limb 38.53
 vitreous, cicatricial bands (posterior
   approach) 14.74
  anterior approach 14.73
Doleris operation (shortening of round
   ligaments) 69.22
D'Ombrain operation (excision of
   pterygium with corneal graft) 11.32
Domestic tasks therapy 93.83
Dopplergram, Doppler flow mapping -
   see also Ultrasonography
  aortic arch 88.73
  head and neck 88.71
  heart 88.72
  thorax NEC 88.73
Dorrance operation (push-back
   operation for cleft palate) 27.62
Dotter operation (transluminal
   angioplasty) 39.59
Douche, vagina 96.44
Douglas' operation (suture of tongue to
   lip for micrognathia) 25.59
Downstream® System (AO therapy)
   (aqueous oxygen) 00.49
Doyle operation (paracervical uterine
   denervation) 69.3
Drainage
 by
  anastomosis - *see* Anastomosis
  aspiration - *see* Aspiration
  incision - *see* Incision
 abdomen 54.19
  percutaneous 54.91
 abscess - *see also* Drainage, by site and
   Incision, by site
  appendix 47.2
   with appendectomy 47.09
    laparoscopic 47.01
  parapharyngeal (oral) (transcervical)
    28.0
  peritonsillar (oral) (transcervical)
    28.0
  retropharyngeal (oral)
    (transcervical) 28.0
  thyroid (field) (gland) 06.09
   percutaneous (needle) 06.01
   postoperative 06.02
  tonsil, tonsillar (oral) (transcervical)
    28.0
 antecubital fossa 86.04

Drainage *(Continued)*
 appendix 47.91
  with appendectomy 47.09
   laparoscopic 47.01
  abscess 47.2
   with appendectomy 47.09
    laparoscopic 47.01
 axilla 86.04
 bladder (without incision) 57.0
  by indwelling catheter 57.94
   percutaneous suprapubic (closed)
     57.17
   suprapubic NEC 57.18
 buccal space 27.0
 bursa 83.03
  by aspiration 83.94
   hand 82.92
  hand 82.03
   by aspiration 82.92
  radial 82.03
  ulnar 82.03
 cerebrum, cerebral (meninges)
   (ventricle) (incision)
   (trephination) 01.39
  by
   anastomosis - *see* Shunt,
     ventricular
   aspiration 01.09
    through previously implanted
      catheter 01.02
 chest (closed) 34.04
  open (by incision) 34.09
  thoracoscopic 34.06
 cranial sinus (incision) (trephination)
   01.21
  by aspiration 01.09
 cul-de-sac 70.12
  by aspiration 70.0
 cyst - *see also* Drainage, by site and
   Incision, by site
  pancreas (by catheter) 52.01
   by marsupialization 52.3
   internal (anastomosis) 52.4
  pilonidal 86.03
  spleen, splenic (by marsupialization)
    41.41
 duodenum (tube) 46.39
  by incision 45.01
 ear
  external 18.09
  inner 20.79
  middle (by myringotomy) 20.09
   with intubation 20.01
 epidural space, cerebral (incision)
   (trephination) 01.24
  by aspiration 01.09
 extradural space, cerebral (incision)
   (trephination) 01.24
  by aspiration 01.09
 extraperitoneal 54.0
 facial region 27.0
 fascial compartments, head and neck
   27.0
 fetal hydrocephalic head (needling)
   (trocar) 73.8
 gallbladder 51.04
  by
   anastomosis 51.35
   aspiration 51.01
   incision 51.04
 groin region (abdominal wall)
   (inguinal) 54.0
  skin 86.04
  subcutaneous tissue 86.04

◀ New   ◀▥ Revised   ~~deleted~~ Deleted   ● Use Additional Digit(s)   ▨ Omit code

Drainage (Continued)

hematoma - see Drainage, by site and Incision, by site

hydrocephalic head (needling) (trocar) 73.8

hypochondrium 54.0
  intra-abdominal 54.19

iliac fossa 54.0

infratemporal fossa 27.0

intracranial space (epidural) (extradural) (incision) (trephination) 01.24
  by aspiration 01.09
  subarachnoid or subdural (incision) (trephination) 01.31
    by aspiration 01.09

intraperitoneal 54.19
  percutaneous 54.91

kidney (by incision) 55.01
  by
    anastomosis 55.86
    catheter 59.8
  pelvis (by incision) 55.11

liver 50.0
  by aspiration 50.91

Ludwig's angina 27.0

lung (by incision) 33.1
  by punch (needle) (trocar) 33.93

midpalmar space 82.04

mouth floor 27.0

mucocele, nasal sinus 22.00
  by puncture 22.01
  through natural ostium 22.02

omentum 54.19
  percutaneous 54.91

ovary (aspiration) 65.91
  by incision 65.09
  laparoscopic 65.01

palmar space (middle) 82.04

pancreas (by catheter) 52.01
  by anastomosis 52.96

parapharyngeal 28.0

paronychia 86.04

parotid space 27.0

pelvic peritoneum (female) 70.12
  male 54.19

pericardium 37.0

perigastric 54.19
  percutaneous 54.91

perineum
  female 71.09
  male 86.04

perisplenic tissue 54.19
  percutaneous 54.91

peritoneum 54.19
  pelvic (female) 70.12
  percutaneous 54.91

peritonsillar 28.0

pharyngeal space, lateral 27.0

Drainage (Continued)

pilonidal cyst or sinus 86.03

pleura (closed) 34.04
  open (by incision) 34.09
  thoracoscopic 34.06

popliteal space 86.04

postural 93.99

postzygomatic space 27.0

pseudocyst, pancreas 52.3
  by anastomosis 52.4

pterygopalatine fossa 27.0

retropharyngeal 28.0

scrotum 61.0

skin 86.04

spinal (canal) (cord) 03.09
  by anastomosis - see Shunt, spinal
  diagnostic 03.31

spleen 41.2
  cyst (by marsupialization) 41.41

subarachnoid space, cerebral (incision) (trephination) 01.31
  by aspiration 01.09

subcutaneous tissue 86.04

subdiaphragmatic 54.19
  percutaneous 54.91

subdural space, cerebral (incision) (trephination) 01.31
  by aspiration 01.09

subhepatic space 54.19
  percutaneous 54.91

sublingual space 27.0

submental space 27.0

subphrenic space 54.19
  percutaneous 54.91

supraclavicular fossa 86.04

temporal pouches 27.0

tendon (sheath) 83.01
  hand 82.01

thenar space 82.04

thorax (closed) 34.04
  open (by incision) 34.09
  thoracoscopic 34.06

thyroglossal tract (by incision) 06.09
  by aspiration 06.01

thyroid (field) (gland) (by incision) 06.09
  by aspiration 06.01
  postoperative 06.02

tonsil 28.0

tunica vaginalis 61.0

ureter (by catheter) 59.8
  by
    anastomosis NEC - see also Anastomosis, ureter 56.79
    incision 56.2

ventricle (cerebral) (incision) NEC 02.39
  by
    anastomosis - see Shunt, ventricular

Drainage (Continued)

ventricle NEC (Continued)
  by (Continued)
    aspiration 01.09
      through previously implanted catheter 01.02

vertebral column 03.09

Drawing test 94.08

Dressing
  burn 93.57
  ulcer 93.56
  wound 93.57

Drilling
  bone - see also Incision, bone 77.10
  ovary 65.99

Drotrecogin alfa (activated), infusion 00.11

Ductogram, mammary 87.35

Duhamel operation (abdominoperineal pull-through) 48.65

Duhrssen's
  incisions (cervix, to assist delivery) 73.93
  operation (vaginofixation of uterus) 69.22

Dunn operation (triple arthrodesis) 81.12

Duodenectomy 45.62
  with
    gastrectomy - see Gastrectomy
    pancreatectomy - see Pancreatectomy

Duodenocholedochotomy 51.51

Duodenoduodenostomy 45.91
  proximal to distal segment 45.62

Duodenoileostomy 45.91

Duodenojejunostomy 45.91

Duodenoplasty 46.79

Duodenorrhaphy 46.71

Duodenoscopy 45.13
  through stoma (artificial) 45.12
  transabdominal (operative) 45.11

Duodenostomy 46.39

Duodenotomy 45.01

Dupuytren operation
  fasciectomy 82.35
  fasciotomy 82.12
    with excision 82.35
  shoulder disarticulation 84.08

Durabond 86.59

Duraplasty 02.12

Durham (-Caldwell) operation (transfer of biceps femoris tendon) 83.75

DuToit and Roux operation (staple capsulorrhaphy of shoulder) 81.82

DuVries operation (tenoplasty) 83.88

Dwyer operation
  fasciotomy 83.14
  soft tissue release NEC 83.84
  wedge osteotomy, calcaneus 77.28

E

E2F decoy 00.16
Eagleton operation (extrapetrosal
    drainage) 20.22
ECG - *see* Electrocardiogram
Echocardiography 88.72
    intracardiac (heart chambers) (ICE)
        37.28
    intravascular (coronary vessels) 00.24
    transesophageal 88.72
        monitoring (Doppler) (ultrasound)
            89.68
Echoencephalography 88.71
Echography - *see* Ultrasonography
Echogynography 88.79
Echoplacentogram 88.78
ECMO (extracorporeal membrane
    oxygenation) 39.65
Eden-Hybinette operation (glenoid bone
    block) 78.01
Educational therapy (bed-bound
    children) (handicapped) 93.82
EEG (electroencephalogram) 89.14
    monitoring (radiographic) (video)
        89.19
Effler operation (heart) 36.2
Effleurage 93.39
EGD (esophagogastroduodenoscopy)
    45.13
    with closed biopsy 45.16
Eggers operation
    tendon release (patellar retinacula)
        83.13
    tendon transfer (biceps femoris tendon)
        (hamstring tendon) 83.75
EKG - *see also* Electrocardiogram 89.52
Elastic hosiery 93.59
Electrocardiogram (with 12 or more
    leads) 89.52
    with vectorcardiogram 89.53
    fetal (scalp), intrauterine 75.32
    rhythm (with one to three leads) 89.51
Electrocautery - *see also* Cauterization
    cervix 67.32
    corneal lesion (ulcer) 11.42
    esophagus 42.39
        endoscopic 42.33
Electrocoagulation - *see also* Destruction,
    lesion, by site
    aneurysm (cerebral) (peripheral
        vessels) 39.52
    cervix 67.32
    cystoscopic 57.49
    ear
        external 18.29
        inner 20.79
        middle 20.51
    fallopian tube (lesion) 66.61
        for tubal ligation - *see* Ligation,
            fallopian tube
    gasserian ganglion 04.02
    nasal turbinates 21.61
    nose, for epistaxis (with packing)
        21.03
    ovary 65.29
        laparoscopic 65.25
    prostatic bed 60.94
    rectum (polyp) 48.32
        radical 48.31
    retina (for)
        destruction of lesion 14.21
        reattachment 14.51
        repair of tear 14.31

Electrocoagulation (*Continued*)
    round ligament 69.19
    semicircular canals 20.79
    urethrovesical junction, transurethral
        57.49
    uterine ligament 69.19
    uterosacral ligament 69.19
    uterus 68.29
    vagina 70.33
    vulva 71.3
Electrocochleography 20.31
Electroconization, cervix 67.32
Electroconvulsive therapy (ECT)
    94.27
Electroencephalogram (EEG) 89.14
    monitoring (radiographic) (video)
        89.19
Electrogastrogram 44.19
Electrokeratotomy 11.49
Electrolysis
    ciliary body 12.71
    hair follicle 86.92
    retina (for)
        destruction of lesion 14.21
        reattachment 14.51
        repair of tear 14.31
    skin 86.92
    subcutaneous tissue 86.92
Electromyogram, electromyography
    (EMG) (muscle) 93.08
    eye 95.25
    urethral sphincter 89.23
Electronarcosis 94.29
Electronic gaiter 93.59
Electronystagmogram (ENG) 95.24
Electro-oculogram (EOG) 95.22
Electroresection - *see also* Destruction,
    lesion, by site
    bladder neck (transurethral) 57.49
    esophagus 42.39
        endoscopic 42.33
    prostate (transurethral) 60.29
    stomach 43.49
        endoscopic 43.41
Electroretinogram (ERG) 95.21
Electroshock therapy (EST) 94.27
    subconvulsive 94.26
Elevation
    bone fragments (fractured)
    orbit 76.79
        sinus (nasal)
            frontal 22.79
            maxillary 22.79
        skull (with debridement) 02.02
        spinal 03.53
    pedicle graft 86.71
Elliot operation (scleral trephination
    with iridectomy) 12.61
Ellis Jones operation (repair of peroneal
    tendon) 83.88
Ellison operation (reinforcement of
    collateral ligament) 81.44
Elmslie-Cholmeley operation (tarsal
    wedge osteotomy) 77.28
Eloesser operation
    thoracoplasty 33.34
    thoracostomy 34.09
Elongation - *see* Lengthening
Embolectomy 38.00
    with endarterectomy - *see*
        Endarterectomy
    abdominal
        artery 38.06
        vein 38.07

Embolectomy (*Continued*)
    aorta (arch) (ascending) (descending)
        38.04
    arteriovenous shunt or cannula 39.49
    bovine graft 39.49
    head and neck NEC 38.02
    intracranial NEC 38.01
    lower limb
        artery 38.08
        vein 38.09
    mechanical
        endovascular
            head and neck 39.74
    pulmonary (artery) (vein) 38.05
    thoracic NEC 38.05
    upper limb (artery) (vein) 38.03
Embolization (transcatheter)
    adhesive (glue) 39.79
        head and neck 39.72
    arteriovenous fistula 39.53
        endovascular 39.72
    artery (selective) 38.80
        by
            endovascular approach 39.79
                head and neck vessels 39.72 ⬅
                    bare coils 39.75 ◀
                    bioactive coils 39.76 ◀
            percutaneous transcatheter
                infusion 99.29
        abdominal NEC 38.86
            duodenal (transcatheter) 44.44
            gastric (transcatheter) 44.44
            renal (transcatheter) 38.86
        aorta (arch) (ascending)
            (descending) 38.84
        duodenal (transcatheter) 44.44
        gastric (transcatheter) 44.44
        head and neck NEC 38.82
        intracranial NEC 38.81
        lower limb 38.88
        renal (transcatheter) 38.86
        thoracic NEC 38.85
        upper limb 38.83
        uterine (transcatheter) 99.29
    AVM, intracranial, endovascular
        approach 39.72
    carotid cavernous fistula 39.53
    chemoembolization 99.25
    coil, endovascular 39.79
        head and neck 39.72 ⬅
            bare coils 39.75 ◀
            bioactive coils 39.76 ◀
    vein (selective) 38.80
        by
            endovascular approach 39.79
                head and neck 39.72
        abdominal NEC 38.87
            duodenal (transcatheter) 44.44
            gastric (transcatheter) 44.44
        duodenal (transcatheter) 44.44
        gastric (transcatheter) 44.44
Embryotomy 73.8
EMG - *see* Electromyogram
Emmet operation (cervix) 67.61
Encephalocentesis - *see also* Puncture
    01.09
    fetal head, transabdominal 73.8
Encephalography (cisternal puncture)
    (fractional) (lumbar)
    (pneumoencephalogram) 87.01
Encephalopuncture 01.09
Encircling procedure - *see also* Cerclage
    sclera, for buckling 14.49
        with implant 14.41

◀ New   ⬅ Revised   ~~deleted~~ Deleted   ● Use Additional Digit(s)   ▨ Omit code

Endarterectomy (gas) (with patch graft) 38.10
    abdominal 38.16
    aorta (arch) (ascending) (descending) 38.14
    coronary artery - *see* category 36.0 ●
        open chest approach 36.03
    head and neck (open) NEC 38.12

> Note: Also use 00.40, 00.41, 00.42, or 00.43 to show the total number of vessels treated. Use code 00.44 once to show procedure on a bifurcated vessel. In addition, use 00.45, 00.46, 00.47, or 00.48 to show the number of vascular stents inserted.

        percutaneous approach, intracranial vessel(s) 00.62
        percutaneous approach, precerebral (extracranial) vessel(s) 00.61
    intracranial (open) NEC 38.11

> Note: Also use 00.40, 00.41, 00.42, or 00.43 to show the total number of vessels treated. Use code 00.44 once to show procedure on a bifurcated vessel. In addition, use 00.45, 00.46, 00.47, or 00.48 to show the number of vascular stents inserted.

        percutaneous approach, intracranial vessel(s) 00.62
    lower limb 38.18
    thoracic NEC 38.15
    upper limb 38.13
Endoaneurysmorrhaphy - *see also* Aneurysmorrhaphy 39.52
    by or with
        endovascular graft
            abdominal aorta 39.71
            lower extremity artery(s) 39.79
            thoracic aorta 39.73
            upper extremity artery(s) 39.79
Endolymphatic (-subarachnoid) shunt 20.71
Endometrectomy (uterine) (internal) 68.29
    bladder 57.59
    cul-de-sac 70.32
Endoprosthesis
    bile duct 51.87
    femoral head (bipolar) 81.52
Endoscopy
    with biopsy - *see* Biopsy, by site, closed
    anus 49.21
    biliary tract (operative) 51.11
        by retrograde cholangiography (ERC) 51.11
        by retrograde cholangiopancreatography (ERCP) 51.10
        intraoperative 51.11
        percutaneous (via T-tube or other tract) 51.98
            with removal of common duct stones 51.96
    bladder 57.32
        through stoma (artificial) 57.31
    bronchus NEC 33.23
        with biopsy 33.24
        fiberoptic 33.22
        through stoma (artificial) 33.21
    colon 45.23
        through stoma (artificial) 45.22
        transabdominal (operative) 45.21
    cul-de-sac 70.22

Endoscopy *(Continued)*
    ear 18.11
    esophagus NEC 42.23
        through stoma (artificial) 42.22
        transabdominal (operative) 42.21
    ileum 45.13
        through stoma (artificial) 45.12
        transabdominal (operative) 45.11
    intestine NEC 45.24
        large 45.24
            fiberoptic (flexible) 45.23
            through stoma (artificial) 45.22
            transabdominal (intraoperative) 45.21
        small 45.13
            esophagogastroduodenoscopy (EGD) 45.13
                with closed biopsy 45.16
            through stoma (artificial) 45.12
            transabdominal (operative) 45.11
    jejunum 45.13
        through stoma (artificial) 45.12
        transabdominal (operative) 45.11
    kidney 55.21
    larynx 31.42
        through stoma (artificial) 31.41
    lung - *see* Bronchoscopy
    mediastinum (transpleural) 34.22
    nasal sinus 22.19
    nose 21.21
    pancreatic duct 52.13
    pelvis 55.22
    peritoneum 54.21
    pharynx 29.11
    rectum 48.23
        through stoma (artificial) 48.22
        transabdominal (operative) 48.21
    sinus, nasal 22.19
    stomach NEC 44.13
        through stoma (artificial) 44.12
        transabdominal (operative) 44.11
    thorax (transpleural) 34.21
    trachea NEC 31.42
        through stoma (artificial) 31.41
    transpleural
        mediastinum 34.22
        thorax 34.21
    ureter 56.31
    urethra 58.22
    uterus 68.12
    vagina 70.21
Enema (transanal) NEC 96.39
    for removal of impacted feces 96.38
ENG (electronystagmogram) 95.24
Enlargement
    aortic lumen, thoracic 38.14
    atrial septal defect (pre-existing) 35.41
        in repair of total anomalous pulmonary venous connection 35.82
    eye socket 16.64
    foramen ovale (pre-existing) 35.41
        in repair of total anomalous pulmonary venous connection 35.82
    intestinal stoma 46.40
        large intestine 46.43
        small intestine 46.41
    introitus 96.16
    orbit (eye) 16.64
    palpebral fissure 08.51
    punctum 09.41
    sinus tract (skin) 86.89

Enterectomy NEC 45.63
Enteroanastomosis
    large-to-large intestine 45.94
    small-to-large intestine 45.93
    small-to-small intestine 45.91
Enterocelectomy 53.9
    female 70.92
        with graft or prosthesis 70.93
    vaginal 70.92
        with graft or prosthesis 70.93
Enterocentesis 45.00
    duodenum 45.01
    large intestine 45.03
    small intestine NEC 45.02
Enterocholecystostomy 51.32
Enteroclysis (small bowel) 96.43
Enterocolectomy NEC 45.79
Enterocolostomy 45.93
Enteroentectropy 46.99
Enteroenterostomy 45.90
    small-to-large intestine 45.93
    small-to-small intestine 45.91
Enterogastrostomy 44.39
    laparoscopic 44.38
Enterolithotomy 45.00
Enterolysis 54.59
    laparoscopic 54.51
Enteropancreatostomy 52.96
Enterorrhaphy 46.79
    large intestine 46.75
    small intestine 46.73
Enterostomy NEC 46.39
    cecum - *see also* Colostomy 46.10
    colon (transverse) - *see also* Colostomy 46.10
        loop 46.03
    delayed opening 46.31
    duodenum 46.39
        loop 46.01
    feeding NEC 46.39
        percutaneous (endoscopic) 46.32
    ileum (Brooke) (Dragstedt) 46.20
        loop 46.01
    jejunum (feeding) 46.39
        loop 46.01
        percutaneous (endoscopic) 46.32
    sigmoid colon - *see also* Colostomy 46.10
        loop 46.03
    transverse colon - *see also* Colostomy 46.10
        loop 46.03
Enterotomy 45.00
    large intestine 45.03
    small intestine 45.02
Enucleation - *see also* Excision, lesion, by site
    cyst
        broad ligament 69.19
        dental 24.4
        liver 50.29
        ovarian 65.29
            laparoscopic 65.25
        parotid gland 26.29
        salivary gland 26.29
        skin 86.3
        subcutaneous tissue 86.3
    eyeball 16.49
        with implant (into Tenon's capsule) 16.42
        with attachment of muscles 16.41
EOG (electro-oculogram) 95.22
Epicardiectomy 36.39

Epididymectomy 63.4
  with orchidectomy (unilateral) 62.3
    bilateral 62.41
Epididymogram 87.93
Epididymoplasty 63.59
Epididymorrhaphy 63.81
Epididymotomy 63.92
Epididymovasostomy 63.83
Epiglottidectomy 30.21
Epikeratophakia 11.76
Epilation
  eyebrow (forceps) 08.93
    cryosurgical 08.92
    electrosurgical 08.91
  eyelid (forceps) NEC 08.93
    cryosurgical 08.92
    electrosurgical 08.91
  skin 86.92
Epiphysiodesis - see also Arrest, bone
  growth - see category 78.2●
Epiphysiolysis - see also Arrest, bone
  growth - see category 78.2●
Epiploectomy 54.4
Epiplopexy 54.74
Epiplorrhaphy 54.74
Episioperineoplasty 71.79
Episioperineorrhaphy 71.71
  obstetrical 75.69
Episioplasty 71.79
Episioproctotomy 73.6
Episiorrhaphy 71.71
  following episiotomy - see
    Episiotomy
  for obstetrical laceration 75.69
Episiotomy (with subsequent
    episiorrhaphy) 73.6
  high forceps 72.31
  low forceps 72.1
  mid forceps 72.21
  nonobstetrical 71.09
  outlet forceps 72.1
EPS (electrophysiologic stimulation)
  as part of intraoperative testing - omit
    code
  catheter based invasive
    electrophysiologic testing
    37.26
  device interrogation only without
    arrhythmia induction (bedside
    check) 89.45-89.49
  noninvasive programmed electrical
    stimulation (NIPS) 37.20
Eptifibatide, infusion 99.20
Equalization, leg
  lengthening - see category 78.3●
  shortening - see category 78.2●
Equilibration (occlusal) 24.8
Equiloudness balance 95.43
ERC (endoscopic retrograde
    cholangiography) 51.11
ERCP (endoscopic retrograde
    cholangiopancreatography)
    51.10
  cannulation of pancreatic duct
    52.93
ERG (electroretinogram) 95.21
ERP (endoscopic retrograde
    pancreatography) 52.13
Eruption, tooth, surgical 24.6
Erythrocytapheresis, therapeutic 99.73
Escharectomy 86.22
Escharotomy 86.09
Esophageal voice training
    (postlaryngectomy) 93.73

Esophagectomy 42.40
  abdominothoracocervical (combined)
    (synchronous) 42.42
  partial or subtotal 42.41
  total 42.42
Esophagocologastrostomy (intrathoracic)
    42.55
  antesternal or antethoracic 42.65
Esophagocolostomy (intrathoracic) NEC
    42.56
  with interposition of colon 42.55
  antesternal or antethoracic NEC 42.66
    with interposition of colon 42.65
Esophagoduodenostomy (intrathoracic)
    NEC 42.54
  with
    complete gastrectomy 43.99
    interposition of small bowel 42.53
Esophagoenterostomy (intrathoracic)
    NEC - see also Anastomosis,
    esophagus, to intestinal segment
    42.54
  antesternal or antethoracic - see also
    Anastomosis, esophagus,
    antesternal, to intestinal segment
    42.64
Esophagoesophagostomy (intrathoracic)
    42.51
  antesternal or antethoracic 42.61
Esophagogastrectomy 43.99
Esophagogastroduodenoscopy (EGD)
    45.13
  with closed biopsy 45.16
  through stoma (artificial) 45.12
  transabdominal (operative) 45.11
Esophagogastromyotomy 42.7
Esophagogastropexy 44.65
Esophagogastroplasty 44.65
Esophagogastroscopy NEC 44.13
  through stoma (artificial) 44.12
  transabdominal (operative) 44.11
Esophagogastrostomy (intrathoracic) 42.52
  with partial gastrectomy 43.5
  antesternal or antethoracic 42.62
Esophagoileostomy (intrathoracic) NEC
    42.54
  with interposition of small bowel 42.53
  antesternal or antethoracic NEC 42.64
    with interposition of small bowel
    42.63
Esophagojejunostomy (intrathoracic)
    NEC 42.54
  with
    complete gastrectomy 43.99
    interposition of small bowel 42.53
  antesternal or antethoracic NEC 42.64
    with interposition of small bowel
    42.63
Esophagomyotomy 42.7
Esophagoplasty NEC 42.89
Esophagorrhaphy 42.82
Esophagoscopy NEC 42.23
  by incision (operative) 42.21
  with closed biopsy 42.24
  through stoma (artificial) 42.22
  transabdominal (operative) 42.21
Esophagostomy 42.10
  cervical 42.11
  thoracic 42.19
Esophagotomy NEC 42.09
Estes operation (ovary) 65.72
  laparoscopic 65.75
Estlander operation (thoracoplasty)
    33.34

ESWL (extracorporeal shockwave
    lithotripsy) NEC 98.59
  bile duct 98.52
  bladder 98.51
  gallbladder 98.52
  kidney 98.51
  Kock pouch (urinary diversion) 98.51
  renal pelvis 98.51
  specified site NEC 98.59
  ureter 98.51
Ethmoidectomy 22.63
Ethmoidotomy 22.51
Evacuation
  abscess - see Drainage, by site
  anterior chamber (eye) (aqueous)
    (hyphema) 12.91
  cyst - see also Excision, lesion, by site
    breast 85.91
    kidney 55.01
    liver 50.29
  hematoma - see also Incision, hematoma
    obstetrical 75.92
    incisional 75.91
  hemorrhoids (thrombosed) 49.47
  pelvic blood clot (by incision) 54.19
    by
      culdocentesis 70.0
      culdoscopy 70.22
  retained placenta
    with curettage 69.02
    manual 75.4
  streptothrix from lacrimal duct 09.42
Evaluation (of)
  audiological 95.43
  cardiac rhythm device (CRT-D)
    (CRT-P) (AICD) (pacemaker) -
    see Interrogation
  criminal responsibility, psychiatric
    94.11
  functional (physical therapy) 93.01
  hearing NEC 95.49
  orthotic (for brace fitting) 93.02
  prosthetic (for artificial limb fitting)
    93.03
  psychiatric NEC 94.19
    commitment 94.13
  psychologic NEC 94.08
  testimentary capacity, psychiatric
    94.11
Evans operation (release of clubfoot)
    83.84
Evisceration
  eyeball 16.39
    with implant (into scleral shell)
    16.31
  ocular contents 16.39
    with implant (into scleral shell)
    16.31
  orbit - see also Exenteration, orbit
    16.59
  pelvic (anterior) (posterior) (partial)
    (total) (female) 68.8
    male 57.71
Evulsion
  nail (bed) (fold) 86.23
  skin 86.3
  subcutaneous tissue 86.3
Examination (for)
  breast
    manual 89.36
    radiographic NEC 87.37
    thermographic 88.85
    ultrasonic 88.73
  cervical rib (by x-ray) 87.43

◀ New   ◀▥ Revised   deleted Deleted   ● Use Additional Digit(s)   ▨ Omit code

Examination *(Continued)*
　colostomy stoma (digital) 89.33
　dental (oral mucosa) (peridontal) 89.31
　　radiographic NEC 87.12
　enterostomy stoma (digital) 89.33
　eye 95.09
　　color vision 95.06
　　comprehensive 95.02
　　dark adaptation 95.07
　　limited (with prescription of
　　　spectacles) 95.01
　　under anesthesia 95.04
　fetus, intrauterine 75.35
　general physical 89.7
　glaucoma 95.03
　gynecological 89.26
　hearing 95.47
　microscopic (specimen) (of) 91.9●

Note: Use the following fourth-digit subclassification with categories 90-91 to identify type of examination:

1　bacterial smear
2　culture
3　culture and sensitivity
4　parasitology
5　toxicology
6　cell block and Papanicolaou
　　smear
9　other microscopic examination

　　adenoid 90.3●
　　adrenal gland 90.1●
　　amnion 91.4●
　　anus 90.9●
　　appendix 90.9●
　　bile ducts 91.0●
　　bladder 91.3●
　　blood 90.5●
　　bone 91.5●
　　　marrow 90.6●
　　brain 90.0●
　　breast 91.6●
　　bronchus 90.4●
　　bursa 91.5●
　　cartilage 91.5●
　　cervix 91.4●
　　chest wall 90.4●
　　chorion 91.4●
　　colon 90.9●
　　cul-de-sac 91.1●
　　dental 90.8●
　　diaphragm 90.4●
　　duodenum 90.8●
　　ear 90.3●
　　endocrine gland NEC 90.1●
　　esophagus 90.8●
　　eye 90.2●
　　fallopian tube 91.4●
　　fascia 91.5●
　　female genital tract 91.4●
　　fetus 91.4●
　　gallbladder 91.0●
　　hair 91.6●
　　ileum 90.9●
　　jejunum 90.9●
　　joint fluid 91.5●
　　kidney 91.2●
　　large intestine 90.9●
　　larynx 90.3●
　　ligament 91.5●
　　liver 91.0●
　　lung 90.4●
　　lymph (node) 90.7●

Examination *(Continued)*
　microscopic *(Continued)*
　　meninges 90.0●
　　mesentery 91.1●
　　mouth 90.8●
　　muscle 91.5●
　　musculoskeletal system 91.5●
　　nails 91.6●
　　nerve 90.0●
　　nervous system 90.0●
　　nose 90.3●
　　omentum 91.1●
　　operative wound 91.7●
　　ovary 91.4●
　　pancreas 91.0●
　　parathyroid gland 90.1●
　　penis 91.3●
　　perirenal tissue 91.2●
　　peritoneum (fluid) 91.1●
　　periureteral tissue 91.2●
　　perivesical (tissue) 91.3●
　　pharynx 90.3●
　　pineal gland 90.1●
　　pituitary gland 90.1●
　　placenta 91.4●
　　pleura (fluid) 90.4●
　　prostate 91.3●
　　rectum 90.9●
　　retroperitoneum 91.1●
　　semen 91.3●
　　seminal vesicle 91.3●
　　sigmoid 90.9●
　　skin 91.6●
　　small intestine 90.9●
　　specified site NEC 91.8●
　　spinal fluid 90.0●
　　spleen 90.6●
　　sputum 90.4●
　　stomach 90.8●
　　stool 90.9●
　　synovial membrane 91.5●
　　tendon 91.5●
　　thorax NEC 90.4●
　　throat 90.3●
　　thymus 90.1●
　　thyroid gland 90.1●
　　tonsil 90.3●
　　trachea 90.4●
　　ureter 91.2●
　　urethra 91.3●
　　urine 91.3●
　　uterus 91.4●
　　vagina 91.4●
　　vas deferens 91.3●
　　vomitus 90.8●
　　vulva 91.4●
　neurologic 89.13
　neuro-ophthalmology 95.03
　ophthalmoscopic 16.21
　panorex, mandible 87.12
　pelvic (manual) 89.26
　　instrumental (by pelvimeter) 88.25
　　pelvimetric 88.25
　physical, general 89.7
　postmortem 89.8
　rectum (digital) 89.34
　　endoscopic 48.23
　　　through stoma (artificial) 48.22
　　　transabdominal 48.21
　retinal disease 95.03
　specified type (manual) NEC 89.39
　thyroid field, postoperative 06.02
　uterus (digital) 68.11
　　endoscopic 68.12

Examination *(Continued)*
　vagina 89.26
　　endoscopic 70.21
　visual field 95.05
Exchange transfusion 99.01
　intrauterine 75.2
Excision
　aberrant tissue - *see* Excision, lesion, by
　　site of tissue origin
　abscess - *see* Excision, lesion, by site
　accessory tissue - *see also* Excision,
　　lesion, by site of tissue origin
　　lung 32.29
　　　endoscopic 32.28
　　　thoracoscopic 32.20
　　spleen 41.93
　adenoids (tag) 28.6
　　with tonsillectomy 28.3
　adenoma - *see* Excision, lesion, by site
　adrenal gland - *see also* Adrenalectomy
　　07.22
　ampulla of Vater (with reimplantation
　　of common duct) 51.62
　anal papilla 49.39
　　endoscopic 49.31
　aneurysm (arteriovenous) - *see also*
　　Aneurysmectomy 38.60
　　coronary artery 36.91
　　heart 37.32
　　myocardium 37.32
　　sinus of Valsalva 35.39
　　ventricle (heart) 37.32
　anus (complete) (partial) 49.6
　aortic subvalvular ring 35.35
　apocrine gland 86.3
　aponeurosis 83.42
　　hand 82.33
　appendage, left atrial 37.36
　appendiceal stump 47.09
　　laparoscopic 47.01
　appendices epiploicae 54.4
　appendix - *see also* Appendectomy
　　epididymis 63.3
　　testis 62.2
　arcuate ligament (spine) - *omit code*
　arteriovenous fistula - *see also*
　　Aneurysmectomy 38.60
　artery - *see also* Arteriectomy
　　38.60
　Baker's cyst, knee 83.39
　Bartholin's gland 71.24
　basal ganglion 01.59
　bile duct 51.69
　　endoscopic 51.64
　bladder - *see also* Cystectomy
　bleb (emphysematous), lung 32.29
　　endoscopic 32.28
　　thoracoscopic 32.20
　blood vessel - *see also* Angiectomy
　　38.60
　bone (ends) (partial), except facial - *see*
　　category 77.8●
　　facial NEC 76.39
　　　total 76.45
　　　　with reconstruction 76.44
　　for graft (autograft) (homograft) -
　　　see category 77.7●
　　fragments (chips) - *see also* Incision,
　　　bone 77.10
　　joint - *see also* Arthrotomy
　　　80.10
　　necrotic - *see also*
　　　Sequestrectomy, bone
　　　77.00

Excision (Continued)

bone, except facial (Continued)
  heterotopic, from
    muscle 83.32
      hand 82.22
    skin 86.3
    tendon 83.31
      hand 82.21
  mandible 76.31
    with arthrodesis - see Arthrodesis
    total 76.42
      with reconstruction 76.41
  spur - see Excision, lesion, bone
  total, except facial - see category
    77.9●
    facial NEC 76.45
      with reconstruction 76.44
    mandible 76.42
      with reconstruction 76.41
brain 01.59
  hemisphere 01.52
  lobe 01.53
branchial cleft cyst or vestige 29.2
breast - see also Mastectomy 85.41
  aberrant tissue 85.24
  accessory 85.24
  ectopic 85.24
  nipple 85.25
    accessory 85.24
  segmental 85.23
  supernumerary 85.24
  wedge 85.21
broad ligament 69.19
bronchogenic cyst 32.09
  endoscopic 32.01
bronchus (wide sleeve) NEC 32.1
buccal mucosa 27.49
bulbourethral gland 58.92
bulbous tuberosities (mandible)
    (maxilla) (fibrous) (osseous)
    24.31
bunion - see also Bunionectomy 77.59
bunionette (with osteotomy) 77.54
bursa 83.5
  hand 82.31
canal of Nuck 69.19
cardioma 37.33
carotid body (lesion) (partial) (total) 39.8
cartilage - see also Chondrectomy 80.90
  intervertebral - see category 80.5●
  knee (semilunar) 80.6
  larynx 30.29
  nasal (submucous) 21.5
caruncle, urethra 58.39
  endoscopic 58.31
cataract - see also Extraction, cataract
    13.19
  secondary membrane (after cataract)
    13.65
cervical
  rib 77.91
  stump 67.4
cervix (stump) NEC 67.4
  cold (knife) 67.2
  conization 67.2
  cryoconization 67.33
  electroconization 67.32
chalazion (multiple) (single) 08.21
cholesteatoma - see Excision, lesion, by
    site
choroid plexus 02.14
cicatrix (skin) 86.3
cilia base 08.20
ciliary body, prolapsed 12.98

Excision (Continued)

clavicle (head) (partial) 77.81
  total (complete) 77.91
clitoris 71.4
coarctation of aorta (end-to-end
    anastomosis) 38.64
  with
    graft replacement (interposition)
      abdominal 38.44
      thoracic 38.45
      thoracoabdominal 38.45 [38.44]
common
  duct 51.63
  wall between posterior and coronary
    sinus (with roofing or resultant
    defect with patch graft) 35.82
condyle - see category 77.8●
  mandible 76.5
conjunctival ring 10.31
cornea 11.49
  epithelium (with
    chemocauterization) 11.41
    for smear or culture 11.21
costal cartilage 80.99
cul-de-sac (Douglas') 70.92
  with graft or prosthesis 70.93
cusp, heart valve 35.10
  aortic 35.11
  mitral 35.12
  tricuspid 35.14
cyst - see also Excision, lesion, by site
  apical (tooth) 23.73
    with root canal therapy 23.72
  Baker's (popliteal) 83.39
  breast 85.21
  broad ligament 69.19
  bronchogenic 32.09
    endoscopic 32.01
  cervix 67.39
  dental 24.4
  dentigerous 24.4
  epididymis 63.2
  fallopian tube 66.61
  Gartner's duct 70.33
  hand 82.29
  labia 71.3
  lung 32.29
    endoscopic 32.28
    thoracoscopic 32.20
  mesonephric duct 69.19
  Morgagni
    female 66.61
    male 62.2
  mullerian duct 60.73
  nasolabial 27.49
  nasopalatine 27.31
    by wide excision 27.32
  ovary 65.29
    laparoscopic 65.25
  parovarian 69.19
  pericardium 37.31
  periodontal (apical) (lateral) 24.4
  popliteal (Baker's), knee 83.39
  radicular 24.4
  spleen 41.42
  synovial (membrane) 83.39
  thyroglossal (with resection of hyoid
    bone) 06.7
  urachal (bladder) 57.51
    abdominal wall 54.3
  vagina (Gartner's duct) 70.33
cystic
  duct remnant 51.61
  hygroma 40.29

Excision (Continued)

dentinoma 24.4
diaphragm 34.81
disc, intervertebral NOS 80.50
  herniated (nucleus pulposus) 80.51
  other specified (diskectomy) 80.51
diverticulum
  ampulla of Vater 51.62
  anus 49.39
    endoscopic 49.31
  bladder 57.59
    transurethral 57.49
  duodenum 45.31
    endoscopic 45.30
  esophagus (local) 42.31
    endoscopic 42.33
  hypopharyngeal (by
    cricopharyngeal myotomy)
    29.32
  intestine
    large 45.41
      endoscopic 45.43
    small NEC 45.33
  Meckel's 45.33
  pharyngeal (by cricopharyngeal
    myotomy) 29.32
  pharyngoesophageal (by
    cricopharyngeal myotomy)
    29.32
  stomach 43.42
    endoscopic 43.41
  urethra 58.39
    endoscopic 58.31
  ventricle, heart 37.33
duct
  mullerian 69.19
  paramesonephric 69.19
  thyroglossal (with resection of hyoid
    bone) 06.7
ear, external (complete) NEC 18.39
  partial 18.29
  radical 18.31
ectopic
  abdominal fetus 74.3
  tissue - see also Excision, lesion, by
    site of tissue origin
    bone, from muscle 83.32
    breast 85.24
    lung 32.29
      endoscopic 32.28
      thoracoscopic 32.20
    spleen 41.93
empyema pocket, lung 34.09
epididymis 63.4
epiglottis 30.21
epithelial downgrowth, anterior
    chamber (eye) 12.93
epulis (gingiva) 24.31
esophagus - see also Esophagectomy
    42.40
exostosis - see also Excision, lesion, bone
    77.60
  auditory canal, external 18.29
  facial bone 76.2
  first metatarsal (hallux valgus
    repair) - see Bunionectomy
eye 16.49
  with implant (into Tenon's capsule)
    16.42
  with attachment of muscles
    16.41
eyelid 08.20
  redundant skin 08.86
falciform ligament 54.4

◄ New   ◄▥ Revised   deleted Deleted   ● Use Additional Digit(s)   ▨ Omit code

Excision *(Continued)*
  fallopian tube - *see* Salpingectomy
  fascia 83.44
    for graft 83.43
      hand 82.34
    hand 82.35
      for graft 82.34
  fat pad NEC 86.3
    knee (infrapatellar) (prepatellar)
      86.3
    scalene 40.21
  fibroadenoma, breast 85.21
  fissure, anus 49.39
    endoscopic 49.31
  fistula - *see also* Fistulectomy
    anal 49.12
    arteriovenous - *see also*
      Aneurysmectomy 38.60
    ileorectal 46.74
    lacrimal
      gland 09.21
      sac 09.6
    rectal 48.73
    vesicovaginal 57.84
  frenulum, frenum
    labial (lip) 27.41
    lingual (tongue) 25.92
  ganglion (hand) (tendon sheath) (wrist)
    82.21
    gasserian 04.05
    site other than hand or nerve
      83.31
    sympathetic nerve 05.29
    trigeminal nerve 04.05
  gastrocolic ligament 54.4
  gingiva 24.31
  glomus jugulare tumor 20.51
  goiter - *see* Thyroidectomy
  gum 24.31
  hallux valgus - *see also* Bunionectomy
    with prosthetic implant 77.59
  hamartoma, mammary 85.21
  heart assist system - *see* Removal
  hematocele, tunica vaginalis 61.92
  hematoma - *see* Drainage, by site
  hemorrhoids (external) (internal) (tag)
    49.46
  heterotopic bone, from
    muscle 83.32
      hand 82.22
    skin 86.3
    tendon 83.31
      hand 82.21
  hydatid of Morgagni
    female 66.61
    male 62.2
  hydatid cyst, liver 50.29
  hydrocele
    canal of Nuck (female) 69.19
    male 63.1
    round ligament 69.19
    spermatic cord 63.1
    tunica vaginalis 61.2
  hygroma, cystic 40.29
  hymen (tag) 70.31
  hymeno-urethral fusion 70.31
  intervertebral disc - *see* Excision,
    disc, intervertebral (NOS)
    80.50
  intestine - *see also* Resection,
    intestine
    for interposition 45.50
      large 45.52
      small 45.51

Excision *(Continued)*
  intestine *(Continued)*
    large (total)
      for interposition 45.52
      laparoscopic 45.81
      local 45.41
        endoscopic 45.43
      open 45.82
      other 45.83
      segmental
        laparoscopic 17.39
        multiple
          laparoscopic 17.31
          open and other 45.71
        open and other 45.79
      unspecified 45.83
    small (total) 45.63
      for interposition 45.51
      local 45.33
      partial 45.62
      segmental 45.62
        multiple 45.61
  intraductal papilloma 85.21
  iris prolapse 12.13
  joint - *see also* Arthrectomy 80.90
  keloid (scar), skin 86.3
  LAA 37.36
  labia - *see* Vulvectomy
  lacrimal
    gland 09.20
      partial 09.22
      total 09.23
    passage 09.6
    sac 09.6
  left atrial appendage 37.36
  lesion (local)
    abdominal wall 54.3
    accessory sinus - *see* Excision, lesion,
      nasal sinus
    adenoids 28.92
    adrenal gland(s) 07.21
    alveolus 24.4
    ampulla of Vater 51.62
    anterior chamber (eye) NEC 12.40
    anus 49.39
      endoscopic 49.31
    apocrine gland 86.3
    artery 38.60
      abdominal 38.66
      aorta (arch) (ascending)
        (descending thoracic) 38.64
        with end-to-end anastomosis
          38.45
          abdominal 38.44
          thoracic 38.45
          thoracoabdominal 38.45
          [38.44]
        with graft interposition graft
          replacement 38.45
          abdominal 38.44
          thoracic 38.45
          thoracoabdominal 38.45
          [38.44]
      head and neck NEC 38.62
      intracranial NEC 38.61
      lower limb 38.68
      thoracic NEC 38.65
      upper limb 38.63
    atrium 37.33
    auditory canal or meatus, external
      18.29
      radical 18.31
    auricle, ear 18.29
      radical 18.31

Excision *(Continued)*
  lesion *(Continued)*
    biliary ducts 51.69
      endoscopic 51.64
    bladder (transurethral) 57.49
      open 57.59
      suprapubic 57.59
    blood vessel 38.60
      abdominal
        artery 38.66
        vein 38.67
      aorta (arch) (ascending)
        (descending) 38.64
      head and neck NEC 38.62
      intracranial NEC 38.61
      lower limb
        artery 38.68
        vein 38.69
      thoracic NEC 38.65
      upper limb (artery) (vein) 38.63
    bone 77.60
      carpal, metacarpal 77.64
      clavicle 77.61
      facial 76.2
      femur 77.65
      fibula 77.67
      humerus 77.62
      jaw 76.2
        dental 24.4
      patella 77.66
      pelvic 77.69
      phalanges (foot) (hand) 77.69
      radius 77.63
      scapula 77.61
      skull 01.6
      specified site NEC 77.69
      tarsal, metatarsal 77.68
      thorax (ribs) (sternum) 77.61
      tibia 77.67
      ulna 77.63
      vertebrae 77.69
    brain (transtemporal approach)
      NEC 01.59
      by stereotactic radiosurgery
        92.30
        cobalt 60 92.32
        linear accelerator (LINAC)
          92.31
        multi-source 92.32
        particle beam 92.33
        particulate 92.33
        radiosurgery NEC 92.39
        single source photon 92.31
    breast (segmental) (wedge) 85.21
    broad ligament 69.19
    bronchus NEC 32.09
      endoscopic 32.01
    cerebral (cortex) NEC 01.59
      meninges 01.51
    cervix (myoma) 67.39
    chest wall 34.4
    choroid plexus 02.14
    ciliary body 12.44
    colon 45.41
      endoscopic NEC 45.43
        polypectomy 45.42
    conjunctiva 10.31
    cornea 11.49
    cranium 01.6
    cul-de-sac (Douglas') 70.32
    dental (jaw) 24.4
    diaphragm 34.81
    duodenum (local) 45.31
      endoscopic 45.30

Excision *(Continued)*
 lesion *(Continued)*
  ear, external 18.29
   radical 18.31
  endometrium 68.29
  epicardium 37.31
  epididymis 63.3
  epiglottis 30.09
  esophagus NEC 42.32
   endoscopic 42.33
  eye, eyeball 16.93
   anterior segment NEC 12.40
  eyebrow (skin) 08.20
  eyelid 08.20
   by
     halving procedure 08.24
     wedge resection 08.24
    major
     full-thickness 08.24
     partial-thickness 08.23
    minor 08.22
  fallopian tube 66.61
  fascia 83.39
   hand 82.29
  groin region (abdominal wall)
     (inguinal) 54.3
   skin 86.3
   subcutaneous tissue 86.3
  gum 24.31
  heart 37.33
  hepatic duct 51.69
  inguinal canal 54.3
  intestine
   large 45.41
     endoscopic NEC 45.43
      polypectomy 45.42
    small NEC 45.33
  intracranial NEC 01.59
  intranasal 21.31
  intraspinal 03.4
  iris 12.42
  jaw 76.2
   dental 24.4
  joint 80.80
   ankle 80.87
   elbow 80.82
   foot and toe 80.88
   hand and finger 80.84
   hip 80.85
   knee 80.86
   shoulder 80.81
   specified site NEC 80.89
   spine 80.89
   wrist 80.83
  kidney 55.39
   with partial nephrectomy
     55.4
  labia 71.3
  lacrimal
   gland (frontal approach) 09.21
   passage 09.6
   sac 09.6
  larynx 30.09
  ligament (joint) - *see also* Excision,
     lesion, joint 80.80
   broad 69.19
   round 69.19
   uterosacral 69.19
  lip 27.43
   by wide excision 27.42
  liver 50.29
  lung NEC 32.29
   by lung volume reduction
     surgery 32.22

Excision *(Continued)*
 lesion *(Continued)*
  lung NEC *(Continued)*
   by wide excision 32.39
     thoracoscopic 32.30
    endoscopic 32.28
    thoracoscopic 32.20
  lymph structure(s) (channel) (vessel)
     NEC 40.29
   node - *see* Excision, lymph, node
  mammary duct 85.21
  mastoid (bone) 20.49
  mediastinum 34.3
  meninges (cerebral) 01.51
   spinal 03.4
  mesentery 54.4
  middle ear 20.51
  mouth NEC 27.49
  muscle 83.32
   hand 82.22
   ocular 15.13
  myocardium 37.33
  nail 86.23
  nasal sinus 22.60
   antrum 22.62
     with Caldwell-Luc approach
      22.61
     specified approach NEC 22.62
    ethmoid 22.63
    frontal 22.42
    maxillary 22.62
     with Caldwell-Luc approach
      22.61
     specified approach NEC 22.62
    sphenoid 22.64
  nasopharynx 29.3●
  nerve (cranial) (peripheral) 04.07
   sympathetic 05.29
  nonodontogenic 24.31
  nose 21.30
   intranasal 21.31
   polyp 21.31
   skin 21.32
   specified site NEC 21.32
  odontogenic 24.4
  omentum 54.4
  orbit 16.92
  ovary 65.29
   by wedge resection 65.22
     laparoscopic 65.24
    that by laparoscope 65.25
  palate (bony) 27.31
   by wide excision 27.32
   soft 27.49
  pancreas (local) 52.22
   endoscopic 52.21
  parathyroid 06.89
  parotid gland or duct NEC 26.29
  pelvic wall 54.3
  pelvirectal tissue 48.82
  penis 64.2
  pericardium 37.31
  perineum (female) 71.3
   male 86.3
  periprostatic tissue 60.82
  perirectal tissue 48.82
  perirenal tissue 59.91
  peritoneum 54.4
  perivesical tissue 59.91
  pharynx 29.39
   diverticulum 29.32
  pineal gland 07.53
  pinna 18.29
   radical 18.31

Excision *(Continued)*
 lesion *(Continued)*
  pituitary (gland) - *see also*
     Hypophysectomy, partial
     07.63
   by stereotactic radiosurgery
     92.30
    cobalt 60 92.32
    linear accelerator (LINAC)
     92.31
    multi-source 92.32
    particle beam 92.33
    particulate 92.33
    radiosurgery NEC 92.39
    single source photon 92.31
  pleura 34.59
  pouch of Douglas 70.32
  preauricular (ear) 18.21
  presacral 54.4
  prostate (transurethral) 60.61
  pulmonary (fibrosis) 32.29
   endoscopic 32.28
   thoracoscopic 32.20
  rectovaginal septum 48.82
  rectum 48.35
   polyp (endoscopic) 48.36
  retroperitoneum 54.4
  salivary gland or duct NEC 26.29
   en bloc 26.32
  sclera 12.84
  scrotum 61.3
  sinus (nasal) - *see* Excision, lesion,
     nasal sinus
  Skene's gland 71.3
  skin 86.3
   breast 85.21
   nose 21.32
   radical (wide) (involving
      underlying or adjacent
      structure) (with flap
      closure) 86.4
   scrotum 61.3
  skull 01.6
  soft tissue NEC 83.39
   hand 82.29
  spermatic cord 63.3
  sphincter of Oddi 51.62
   endoscopic 51.64
  spinal cord (meninges) 03.4
  spleen (cyst) 41.42
  stomach NEC 43.42
   endoscopic 43.41
     polyp 43.41
   polyp (endoscopic) 43.41
  subcutaneous tissue 86.3
   breast 85.21
  subgingival 24.31
  sweat gland 86.3
  tendon 83.39
   hand 82.29
   ocular 15.13
   sheath 83.31
     hand 82.21
  testis 62.2
  thorax 34.4
  thymus
   partial (open) (other) 07.81
     thoracoscopic 07.83
   total (open) (other) 07.82
     thoracoscopic 07.84
  thyroid 06.31
   substernal or transsternal route
     06.51
  tongue 25.1

◀ New   ◀▥ Revised   ~~deleted~~ Deleted   ● Use Additional Digit(s)   ▥ Omit code

◀ New   ◀▦ Revised   ~~deleted~~ Deleted   ● Use Additional Digit(s)   ▦ Omit code

Excision (Continued)
  polyp (Continued)
    nose 21.31
    rectum (endoscopic) 48.36
    stomach (endoscopic) 43.41
  preauricular
    appendage (remnant) 18.29
    cyst, fistula, or sinus (congenital) 18.21
    remnant 18.29
  prolapsed iris (in wound) 12.13
  prostate - see Prostatectomy
  pterygium (simple) 11.39
    with corneal graft 11.32
  radius (head) (partial) 77.83
    total 77.93
  ranula, salivary gland NEC 26.29
  rectal mucosa 48.35
  rectum - see Resection, rectum
  redundant mucosa
    colostomy 45.41
      endoscopic 45.43
    duodenostomy 45.31
      endoscopic 45.30
    ileostomy 45.33
    jejunostomy 45.33
    perineum 71.3
    rectum 48.35
    vulva 71.3
  renal vessel, aberrant 38.66
  rib (cervical) 77.91
  ring of conjunctiva around cornea 10.31
  round ligament 69.19
  salivary gland 26.30
    complete 26.32
    partial 26.31
    radical 26.32
  scalene fat pad 40.21
  scar - see also Excision, lesion, by site
    epicardium 37.31
    mastoid 20.92
    pericardium 37.31
    pleura 34.59
    skin 86.3
    thorax 34.4
  secondary membrane, lens 13.65
  seminal vesicle 60.73
    with radical prostatectomy 60.5
  septum - see also Excision, by site
    uterus (congenital) 68.22
    vagina 70.33
  sinus - see also Excision, lesion, by site
    nasal - see Sinusectomy
    pilonidal 86.21
    preauricular (ear) (radical) 18.21
    tarsi 80.88
    thyroglossal (with resection of hyoid bone) 06.7
    urachal (bladder) 57.51
      abdominal wall 54.3
  Skene's gland 71.3
  skin (local) 86.3
    for graft (with closure of donor site) 86.91
    radical (wide) (involving underlying or adjacent structure) (with flap closure) 86.4
    tags
      perianal 49.03
      periauricular 18.29
  soft tissue NEC 83.49
    hand 82.39
  spermatocele 63.2

Excision (Continued)
  spinous process 77.89
  spleen (total) 41.5
    accessory 41.93
    partial 41.43
  stomach - see Gastrectomy
  sublingual gland (salivary) - see also Excision, salivary gland 26.30
  submaxillary gland - see also Excision, salivary gland 26.30
  supernumerary
    breast 85.24
    digits 86.26
  sweat gland 86.3
  synechiae - see also Lysis, synechiae
    endometrial 68.21
  tarsal plate (eyelid) 08.20
    by wedge resection 08.24
  tattoo 86.3
    by dermabrasion 86.25
  tendon (sheath) 83.42
    for graft 83.41
      hand 82.32
    hand 82.33
      for graft 82.32
  thymus - see also Thymectomy 07.80
  thyroglossal duct or tract (with resection of hyoid bone) 06.7
  thyroid NEC - see also Thyroidectomy 06.39
  tongue (complete) (total) 25.3
    partial or subtotal 25.2
    radical 25.4
  tonsil 28.2
    with adenoidectomy 28.3
    lingual 28.5
    tag 28.4
  tooth NEC - see also Removal, tooth, surgical 23.19
    from nasal sinus 22.60
  torus
    lingual 76.2
    mandible, mandibularis 76.2
    palate, palatinus 27.31
      by wide excision 27.32
  trabeculae carneae cordis (heart) 35.35
  trochanteric lipomatosis 86.83
  tumor - see Excision, lesion, by site
  ulcer - see also Excision, lesion, by site
    duodenum 45.31
      endoscopic 45.30
    stomach 43.42
      endoscopic 43.41
  umbilicus 54.3
  urachus, urachal (cyst) (bladder) 57.51
    abdominal wall 54.3
  ureter, ureteral 56.40
    with nephrectomy - see Nephrectomy
    partial 56.41
    stricture 56.41
    total 56.42
  ureterocele 56.41
  urethra, urethral 58.39
    with complete cystectomy 57.79
    endoscopic 58.31
    septum 58.0
    stricture 58.39
      endoscopic 58.31
    valve (congenital) 58.39
      endoscopic (transurethral) (transvesical) 58.31

Excision (Continued)
  urethrovaginal septum 70.33
  uterus (corpus) - see also Hysterectomy 68.9
    cervix 67.4
      lesion 67.39
    lesion 68.29
    septum 68.22
  uvula 27.72
  vagina (total) 70.4
  varicocele, spermatic cord 63.1
  vein - see also Phlebectomy 38.60
    varicose 38.50
      abdominal 38.57
      head and neck NEC 38.52
      intracranial NEC 38.51
      lower limb 38.59
      ovarian 38.67
      thoracic NEC 38.55
      upper limb 38.53
  verucca - see also Excision, lesion, by site
    eyelid 08.22
  vesicovaginal septum 70.33
  vitreous opacity 14.74
    anterior approach 14.73
  vocal cord(s) (submucous) 30.22
  vulva (bilateral) (simple) - see also Vulvectomy 71.62
  wart - see also Excision, lesion, by site
    eyelid 08.22
  wolffian duct 69.19
  xanthoma (tendon sheath, hand) 82.21
    site other than hand 83.31
Excisional biopsy - see Biopsy
Exclusion
  left atrial appendage 37.36
  pyloric
    laparoscopic 44.38
    open 44.39
Exenteration
  ethmoid air cells 22.63
  orbit 16.59
    with
      removal of adjacent structures 16.51
      temporalis muscle transplant 16.59
      therapeutic removal of bone 16.52
  pelvic (organs) (female) 68.8
    male 57.71
  petrous pyramid air cells 20.59
Exercise (physical therapy) NEC 93.19
  active musculoskeletal NEC 93.12
  assisting 93.11
    in pool 93.31
  breathing 93.18
  musculoskeletal
    active NEC 93.12
    passive NEC 93.17
  neurologic 89.13
  passive musculoskeletal NEC 93.17
  resistive 93.13
Exfoliation, skin, by chemical 86.24
Exostectomy - see also Excision, lesion, bone 77.60
  first metatarsal (hallux valgus repair) - see Bunionectomy
  hallux valgus repair (with wedge osteotomy) - see Bunionectomy
Expiratory flow rate 89.38
Explant, explanation - see Removal

◀ New   ◀‖‖ Revised   deleted Deleted   ● Use Additional Digit(s)   ▨ Omit code

Exploration - *see also* Incision
abdomen 54.11
abdominal wall 54.0
adrenal (gland) 07.41
  field 07.00
    bilateral 07.02
    unilateral 07.01
artery 38.00
  abdominal 38.06
  aorta (arch) (ascending)
    (descending) 38.04
  head and neck NEC 38.02
  intracranial NEC 38.01
  lower limb 38.08
  thoracic NEC 38.05
  upper limb 38.03
auditory canal, external 18.02
axilla 86.09
bile duct(s) 51.59
  common duct 51.51
    endoscopic 51.11
    for
      relief of obstruction 51.42
        endoscopic 51.84
      removal of calculus 51.41
        endoscopic 51.88
    laparoscopic 51.11
  for relief of obstruction 51.49
    endoscopic 51.84
bladder (by incision) 57.19
  endoscopic 57.32
    through stoma (artificial)
      57.31
bone - *see also* Incision, bone 77.10
brain (tissue) 01.39
breast 85.0
bronchus 33.0
  endoscopic - *see* Bronchoscopy
bursa 83.03
  hand 82.03
carotid body 39.8
carpal tunnel 04.43
choroid 14.9
ciliary body 12.44
colon 45.03
common bile duct 51.51
  endoscopic 51.11
  for
    relief of obstruction 51.42
      endoscopic 51.84
    removal of calculus 51.41
      endoscopic 51.88
coronary artery 36.99
cranium 01.24
cul-de-sac 70.12
  endoscopic 70.22
disc space 03.09
duodenum 45.01
  endoscopic - *see* Endoscopy, by
    site
epididymis 63.92
esophagus (by incision) NEC 42.09
  endoscopic - *see* Esophagoscopy
ethmoid sinus 22.51
eyelid 08.09
fallopian tube 66.01
fascia 83.09
  hand 82.09
flank 54.0
fossa (superficial) NEC 86.09
  pituitary 07.71
frontal sinus 22.41
frontonasal duct 96.21
gallbladder 51.04

Exploration (*Continued*)
groin (region) (abdominal wall)
  (inguinal) 54.0
  skin and subcutaneous tissue 86.09
heart 37.11
hepatic duct 51.59
hypophysis 07.72
ileum 45.02
inguinal canal (groin) 54.0
intestine (by incision) NEC 45.00
  large 45.03
  small 45.02
intrathoracic 34.02
jejunum 45.02
joint structures - *see also* Arthrotomy
  80.10
kidney 55.01
  pelvis 55.11
labia 71.09
lacrimal
  gland 09.0
  sac 09.53
laparotomy site 54.12
larynx (by incision) 31.3
  endoscopic 31.42
liver 50.0
lung (by incision) 33.1
lymphatic structure(s) (channel) (node)
  (vessel) 40.0
mastoid 20.21
maxillary antrum or sinus (Caldwell-
  Luc approach) 22.39
mediastinum 34.1
  endoscopic 34.22
middle ear (transtympanic) 20.23
muscle 83.02
  hand 82.02
neck - *see also* Exploration, thyroid
  06.09
nerve (cranial) (peripheral) NEC
  04.04
  auditory 04.01
  root (spinal) 03.09
nose 21.1
orbit - *see also* Orbitotomy 16.09
pancreas 52.09
  endoscopic 52.13
pancreatic duct 52.09
  endoscopic 52.13
pelvis (by laparotomy) 54.11
  by colpotomy 70.12
penis 64.92
perinephric area 59.09
perineum (female) 71.09
  male 86.09
peripheral vessels
  lower limb
    artery 38.08
    vein 38.09
  upper limb (artery) (vein) 38.03
periprostatic tissue 60.81
perirenal tissue 59.09
perivesical tissue 59.19
petrous pyramid air cells 20.22
pilonidal sinus 86.03
pineal (gland) 07.52
  field 07.51
pituitary (gland) 07.72
  fossa 07.71
pleura 34.09
popliteal space 86.09
prostate 60.0
rectum - *see also* Proctoscopy 48.23
  by incision 48.0

Exploration (*Continued*)
retroperitoneum 54.0
retropubic 59.19
salivary gland 26.0
sclera (by incision) 12.89
scrotum 61.0
shunt
  ventriculoperitoneal at
    peritoneal site 54.95
    ventricular site 02.41
sinus
  ethmoid 22.51
  frontal 22.41
  maxillary (Caldwell-Luc approach)
    22.39
  sphenoid 22.52
  tract, skin and subcutaneous tissue
    86.09
skin 86.09
soft tissue NEC 83.09
  hand 82.09
spermatic cord 63.93
sphenoidal sinus 22.52
spinal (canal) (nerve root) 03.09
spleen 41.2
stomach (by incision) 43.0
  endoscopic - *see* Gastroscopy
subcutaneous tissue 86.09
subdiaphragmatic space 54.11
superficial fossa 86.09
tarsal tunnel 04.44
tendon (sheath) 83.01
  hand 82.01
testes 62.0
thymus (gland) 07.92
  field 07.91
  thoracoscopic 07.95
thyroid (field) (gland) (by incision)
  06.09
  postoperative 06.02
trachea (by incision) 31.3
  endoscopic - *see* Tracheoscopy
tunica vaginalis 61.0
tympanum 20.09
  transtympanic route 20.23
ureter (by incision) 56.2
  endoscopic 56.31
urethra (by incision) 58.0
  endoscopic 58.22
uterus (corpus) 68.0
  cervix 69.95
  digital 68.11
  postpartal, manual 75.7
vagina (by incision) 70.14
  endoscopic 70.21
vas deferens 63.6
vein 38.00
  abdominal 38.07
  head and neck NEC 38.02
  intracranial NEC 38.01
  lower limb 38.09
  thoracic NEC 38.05
  upper limb 38.03
vulva (by incision) 71.09
Exposure - *see also* Incision, by site
tooth (for orthodontic treatment)
  24.6
Expression, trachoma follicles 10.33
Exsanguination transfusion 99.01
Extension
buccolabial sulcus 24.91
limb, forced 93.25
lingual sulcus 24.91
mandibular ridge 76.43

Exteriorization
esophageal pouch 42.12
intestine 46.03
large 46.03
small 46.01
maxillary sinus 22.9
pilonidal cyst or sinus (open
excision) (with partial closure)
86.21
Extirpation - *see also* Excision, by site
aneurysm - *see* Aneurysmectomy
arteriovenous fistula - *see*
Aneurysmectomy
lacrimal sac 09.6
larynx 30.3
with radical neck dissection (with
synchronous thyroidectomy)
(with synchronous
tracheostomy) 30.4
nerve, tooth - *see also* Therapy, root canal
23.70
varicose vein (peripheral) (lower limb)
38.59
upper limb 38.53
Extracorporeal
circulation (regional), except hepatic
39.61
hepatic 50.92
percutaneous 39.66
hemodialysis 39.95
membrane oxygenation (ECMO) 39.65
photopheresis, therapeutic 99.88
shockwave lithotripsy (ESWL) NEC
98.59
bile duct 98.52
bladder 98.51
gallbladder 98.52
kidney 98.51
renal pelvis 98.51
specified site NEC 98.59
ureter 98.51
Extracranial-intracranial bypass [EC-IC]
39.28
Extraction
breech (partial) 72.52
with forceps to aftercoming head
72.51
total 72.54
with forceps to aftercoming head
72.53
cataract 13.19
after cataract (by)
capsulectomy 13.65
capsulotomy 13.64
discission 13.64
excision 13.65
iridocapsulectomy 13.65

Extraction (*Continued*)
cataract (*Continued*)
after cataract (*Continued*)
mechanical fragmentation 13.66
needling 13.64
phacofragmentation (mechanical)
13.66
aspiration (simple) (with irrigation)
13.3
cryoextraction (intracapsular
approach) 13.19
temporal inferior route (in
presence of fistulization
bleb) 13.11
curette evacuation (extracapsular
approach) 13.2
emulsification (and aspiration) 13.41
erysiphake (intracapsular approach)
13.19
temporal inferior route (in
presence of fistulization
bleb) 13.11
extracapsular approach (with
iridectomy) NEC 13.59
by temporal inferior route (in
presence of fistulization
bleb) 13.51
aspiration (simple) (with
irrigation) 13.3
curette evacuation 13.2
emulsification (and aspiration)
13.41
linear extraction 13.2
mechanical fragmentation with
aspiration by
posterior route 13.42
specified route NEC 13.43
phacoemulsification (ultrasonic)
(with aspiration) 13.41
phacofragmentation (mechanical)
with aspiration by
posterior route 13.42
specified route NEC 13.43
ultrasonic (with aspiration)
13.41
rotoextraction (mechanical)
with aspiration by
posterior route 13.42
specified route NEC 13.43
intracapsular (combined) (simple)
(with iridectomy) (with suction)
(with zonulolysis) 13.19
by temporal inferior route (in
presence of fistulization
bleb) 13.11
linear extraction (extracapsular
approach) 13.2

Extraction (*Continued*)
cataract (*Continued*)
phacoemulsification (and aspiration)
13.41
phacofragmentation (mechanical)
with aspiration by
posterior route 13.42
specified route NEC
13.43
ultrasonic 13.41
rotoextraction (mechanical)
with aspiration by
posterior route 13.42
specified route NEC 13.43
secondary membranous (after
cataract) (by)
capsulectomy 13.65
capsulotomy 13.64
discission 13.64
excision 13.65
iridocapsulectomy 13.65
mechanical fragmentation
13.66
needling 13.64
phacofragmentation
(mechanical) 13.66
common duct stones (percutaneous)
(through sinus tract) (with
basket) 51.96
foreign body - *see* Removal, foreign
body
kidney stone(s), percutaneous
55.03
with fragmentation procedure
55.04
lens (eye) - *see also* Extraction,
cataract 13.19
Malstrom's 72.79
with episiotomy 72.71
menstrual, menses 69.6
milk from lactating breast (manual)
(pump) 99.98
tooth (by forceps) (multiple) (single)
NEC 23.09
with mucoperiosteal flap elevation
23.19
deciduous 23.01
surgical NEC - *see also* Removal,
tooth, surgical 23.19
vacuum, fetus 72.79
with episiotomy 72.71
vitreous - *see also* Removal, vitreous
14.72

◀ New   ◀▥ Revised   ~~deleted~~ Deleted   ● Use Additional Digit(s)   ▭ Omit code

F

Face lift 86.82
Facetectomy 77.89
Facilitation, intraocular circulation NEC 12.59
Failed (trial) forceps 73.3
Family
  counselling (medical) (social) 94.49
  therapy 94.42
Farabeuf operation (ischiopubiotomy) 77.39
Fasanella-Servatt operation (blepharoptosis repair) 08.35
Fasciaplasty - see Fascioplasty
Fascia sling operation - see Operation, sling
Fasciectomy 83.44
  for graft 83.43
    hand 82.34
  hand 82.35
    for graft 82.34
  palmar (release of Dupuytren's contracture) 82.35
Fasciodesis 83.89
  hand 82.89
Fascioplasty - see also Repair, fascia 83.89
  hand - see also Repair, fascia, hand 82.89
Fasciorrhaphy - see Suture, fascia
Fasciotomy 83.14
  Dupuytren's 82.12
    with excision 82.35
  Dwyer 83.14
  hand 82.12
  Ober-Yount 83.14
  orbital - see also Orbitotomy 16.09
  palmar (release of Dupuytren's contracture) 82.12
    with excision 82.35
Fenestration
  aneurysm (dissecting), thoracic aorta 39.54
  aortic aneurysm 39.54
  cardiac valve 35.10
  chest wall 34.01
  ear
    inner (with graft) 20.61
      revision 20.62
    tympanic 19.55
  labyrinth (with graft) 20.61
  Lempert's (endaural) 19.9
  operation (aorta) 39.54
  oval window, ear canal 19.55
  palate 27.1
  pericardium 37.12
  semicircular canals (with graft) 20.61
  stapes foot plate (with vein graft) 19.19
    with incus replacement 19.11
  tympanic membrane 19.55
  vestibule (with graft) 20.61
Ferguson operation (hernia repair) 53.00
Fetography 87.81
Fetoscopy 75.31
Fiberoscopy - see Endoscopy, by site
Fibroidectomy, uterine 68.29
Fick operation (perforation of foot plate) 19.0
Filipuncture (aneurysm) (cerebral) 39.52
Filleting
  hammer toe 77.56
  pancreas 52.3

Filling, tooth (amalgam) (plastic) (silicate) 23.2
  root canal - see also Therapy, root canal 23.70
Fimbriectomy - see also Salpingectomy, partial 66.69
  Uchida (with tubal ligation) 66.32
Finney operation (pyloroplasty) 44.29
Fissurectomy, anal 49.39
  endoscopic 49.31
  skin (subcutaneous tissue) 49.04
Fistulectomy - see also Closure, fistula, by site
  abdominothoracic 34.83
  abdominouterine 69.42
  anus 49.12
  appendix 47.92
  bile duct 51.79
  biliary tract NEC 51.79
  bladder (transurethral approach) 57.84
  bone - see also Excision, lesion, bone 77.60
  branchial cleft 29.52
  bronchocutaneous 33.42
  bronchoesophageal 33.42
  bronchomediastinal 34.73
  bronchopleural 34.73
  bronchopleurocutaneous 34.73
  bronchopleuromediastinal 34.73
  bronchovisceral 33.42
  cervicosigmoidal 67.62
  cholecystogastroenteric 51.93
  cornea 11.49
  diaphragm 34.83
  enterouterine 69.42
  esophagopleurocutaneous 34.73
  esophagus NEC 42.84
  fallopian tube 66.73
  gallbladder 51.93
  gastric NEC 44.63
  hepatic duct 51.79
  hepatopleural 34.73
  hepatopulmonary 34.73
  intestine
    large 46.76
    small 46.74
  intestinouterine 69.42
  joint - see also Excision, lesion, joint 80.80
  lacrimal
    gland 09.21
    sac 09.6
  laryngotracheal 31.62
  larynx 31.62
  mediastinocutaneous 34.73
  mouth NEC 27.53
  nasal 21.82
    sinus 22.71
  nasolabial 21.82
  nasopharyngeal 21.82
  oroantral 22.71
  oronasal 21.82
  pancreas 52.95
  perineorectal 71.72
  perineosigmoidal 71.72
  perirectal, not opening into rectum 48.93
  pharyngoesophageal 29.53
  pharynx NEC 29.53
  pleura 34.73
  rectolabial 71.72
  rectourethral 58.43
  rectouterine 69.42

Fistulectomy (Continued)
  rectovaginal 70.73
  rectovesical 57.83
  rectovulvar 71.72
  rectum 48.73
  salivary (duct) (gland) 26.42
  scrotum 61.42
  skin 86.3
  stomach NEC 44.63
  subcutaneous tissue 86.3
  thoracoabdominal 34.83
  thoracogastric 34.83
  thoracointestinal 34.83
  thorax NEC 34.73
  trachea NEC 31.73
  tracheoesophageal 31.73
  ureter 56.84
  urethra 58.43
  uteroenteric 69.42
  uterointestinal 69.42
  uterorectal 69.42
  uterovaginal 69.42
  vagina 70.75
  vesicosigmoidovaginal 57.83
  vocal cords 31.62
  vulvorectal 71.72
Fistulization
  appendix 47.91
  arteriovenous 39.27
  cisterna chyli 40.62
  endolymphatic sac (for decompression) 20.79
  esophagus, external 42.10
    cervical 42.11
      specified technique NEC 42.19
  interatrial 35.41
  labyrinth (for decompression) 20.79
  lacrimal sac into nasal cavity 09.81
  larynx 31.29
  lymphatic duct, left (thoracic) 40.62
  orbit 16.09
  peritoneal 54.93
  salivary gland 26.49
  sclera 12.69
    by trephination 12.61
    with iridectomy 12.65
  sinus, nasal NEC 22.9
  subarachnoid space 02.2
  thoracic duct 40.62
  trachea 31.29
  tracheoesophageal 31.95
  urethrovaginal 58.0
  ventricle, cerebral - see also Shunt, ventricular 02.2
Fistulogram
  abdominal wall 88.03
  chest wall 87.38
  retroperitoneum 88.14
  specified site NEC 88.49
Fistulotomy, anal 49.11
Fitting
  arch bars (orthodontic) 24.7
    for immobilization (fracture) 93.55
  artificial limb 84.40
  contact lens 95.32
  denture (total) 99.97
    bridge (fixed) 23.42
      removable 23.43
    partial (fixed) 23.42
      removable 23.43
  hearing aid 95.48
  obturator (orthodontic) 24.7
  ocular prosthetics 95.34

Fitting *(Continued)*
    orthodontic
        appliance 24.7
        obturator 24.7
        wiring 24.7
    orthotic device 93.23
    periodontal splint (orthodontic)
        24.7
    prosthesis, prosthetic device
        above knee 84.45
        arm 84.43
            lower (and hand) 84.42
            upper (and shoulder) 84.41
        below knee 84.46
        hand (and lower arm) 84.42
        leg 84.47
            above knee 84.45
            below knee 84.46
        limb NEC 84.40
        ocular 95.34
        penis (external) 64.94
        shoulder (and upper arm) 84.41
    spectacles 95.31
Five-in-one repair, knee 81.42
Fixation
    bone
        external, without reduction 93.59
            with fracture reduction - *see*
                Reduction, fracture
            cast immobilization NEC
                93.53
            external fixator - *see* Fixator,
                external
            splint 93.54
            traction (skeletal) NEC 93.44
                intermittent 93.43
        internal (without fracture
            reduction) 78.50
            with fracture reduction - *see*
                Reduction, fracture
            carpal, metacarpal 78.54
            clavicle 78.51
            femur 78.55
            fibula 78.57
            humerus 78.52
            patella 78.56
            pelvic 78.59
            phalanges (foot) (hand) 78.59
            radius 78.53
            scapula 78.51
            specified site NEC 78.59
            tarsal, metatarsal 78.58
            thorax (ribs) (sternum) 78.51
            tibia 78.57
            ulna 78.53
            vertebrae 78.59
    breast (pendulous) 85.6
    cardinal ligaments 69.22
    cervical collar 93.52
    duodenum 46.62
        to abdominal wall 46.61
    external (without manipulation for
        reduction) 93.59
        with fracture reduction - *see*
            Reduction, fracture
        cast immobilization NEC 93.53
        pressure dressing 93.56
        splint 93.54
        strapping (non-traction) 93.59
        traction (skeletal) NEC 93.44
            intermittent 93.43
    hip 81.40
    ileum 46.62
        to abdominal wall 46.61

Fixation *(Continued)*
    internal
        with fracture reduction - *see*
            Reduction, fracture
        without fracture reduction - *see*
            Fixation, bone, internal
    intestine 46.60
        large 46.64
            to abdominal wall 46.63
        small 46.62
            to abdominal wall 46.61
        to abdominal wall 46.60
    iris (bombé) 12.11
    jejunum 46.62
        to abdominal wall 46.61
    joint - *see* Arthroplasty
    kidney 55.7
    ligament
        cardinal 69.22
        palpebrae 08.36
    omentum 54.74
    parametrial 69.22
    plaster jacket 93.51
        other cast 93.53
    rectum (sling) 48.76
    spine, with fusion - *see also* Fusion,
        spinal 81.00
    spleen 41.95
    splint 93.54
    tendon 83.88
        hand 82.85
    testis in scrotum 62.5
    tongue 25.59
    urethrovaginal (to Cooper's ligament)
        70.77
        with graft or prosthesis 70.78
    uterus (abdominal) (vaginal)
        (ventrofixation) 69.22
    vagina 70.77
        with graft or prosthesis 70.78
Fixator, external
    computer assisted (dependent) 84.73
    hybrid device or system 84.73
    Ilizarov type 84.72
    monoplanar system 84.71
    ring device or system 84.72
    Sheffield type 84.72
Flooding (psychologic desensitization) 94.33
Flowmetry, Doppler (ultrasonic) - *see also*
    Ultrasonography
    aortic arch 88.73
    head and neck 88.71
    heart 88.72
    thorax NEC 88.73
Fluoroscopy - *see* Radiography
Fog therapy (respiratory) 93.94
Folding, eye muscle 15.22
    multiple (two or more muscles) 15.4
Foley operation (pyeloplasty) 55.87
Fontan operation (creation of conduit
    between right atrium and
    pulmonary artery) 35.94
Foraminotomy 03.09
Forced extension, limb 93.25
Forceps delivery - *see* Delivery, forceps
Formation
    adhesions
        pericardium 36.39
        pleura 34.6
    anus, artificial - *see also* Colostomy
        46.13 ◀▭
        duodenostomy 46.39
        ileostomy - *see also* Ileostomy
            46.23 ◀▭

Formation *(Continued)*
    anus, artificial *(Continued)*
        jejunostomy 46.39
            percutaneous (endoscopic) (PEJ)
                46.32
        arteriovenous fistula (for kidney
            dialysis) (peripheral) (shunt)
            39.27
        external cannula 39.93
    bone flap, cranial 02.03
    cardiac device (defibrillator)
        (pacemaker) pocket
        with initial insertion of cardiac
            device - *omit code*
        new site (skin) (subcutaneous) 37.79
    colostomy - *see also* Colostomy 46.13 ◀▭
    conduit
        ileal (urinary) 56.51
        left ventricle and aorta 35.93
        right atrium and pulmonary artery
            35.94
        right ventricle and pulmonary
            (distal) artery 35.92
            in repair of
                pulmonary artery atresia 35.92
                transposition of great vessels
                    35.92
                truncus arteriosus 35.83
    endorectal ileal pouch (H-pouch) (J-
        pouch) (S-pouch) (with
        anastomosis to anus) 45.95
    fistula
        arteriovenous (for kidney dialysis)
            (peripheral shunt) 39.27
            external cannula 39.93
        bladder to skin NEC 57.18
            with bladder flap 57.21
            percutaneous 57.17
        cutaneoperitoneal 54.93
        gastric 43.19
            percutaneous (endoscopic)
                (transabdominal) 43.11
        mucous - *see also* Colostomy 46.13 ◀▭
        rectovaginal 48.99
        tracheoesophageal 31.95
        tubulovalvular (Beck-Jianu)
            (Frank's) (Janeway) (Spivack's)
            (Ssabanejew-Frank) 43.19
        urethrovaginal 58.0
    ileal
        bladder
            closed 57.87 [45.51]
            open 56.51
        conduit 56.51
    interatrial fistula 35.42
    mucous fistula - *see also* Colostomy
        46.13 ◀▭
    pericardial
        baffle, interatrial 35.91
        window 37.12
    pleural window (for drainage) 34.09
    pocket
        cardiac device (defibrillator)
            (pacemaker)
            with initial insertion of cardiac
                device - *omit code*
            new site (skin) (subcutaneous)
                37.79
        loop recorder 37.79
        thalamic stimulator pulse generator
            with initial insertion of battery
                package - *omit code*
            new site (skin) (subcutaneous)
                86.09

◀ New   ◀▭ Revised   deleted Deleted   ● Use Additional Digit(s)   Omit code

Formation *(Continued)*
  pupil 12.39
    by iridectomy 12.14
  rectovaginal fistula 48.99
  reversed gastric tube (intrathoracic)
      (retrosternal) 42.58
    antesternal or antethoracic 42.68
  septal defect, interatrial 35.42
  shunt
    abdominovenous 54.94
    arteriovenous 39.93
    peritoneojugular 54.94
    peritoneo-vascular 54.94
    pleuroperitoneal 34.05
    transjugular intrahepatic
        portosystemic (TIPS) 39.1
  subcutaneous tunnel
    esophageal 42.86
      with anastomosis - *see*
          Anastomosis, esophagus,
          antesternal
    pulse generator lead wire 86.99
      with initial procedure - omit code
    thalamic stimulator pulse generator
        pocket
      with initial insertion of battery
          package - omit code
    new site (skin) (subcutaneous)
        86.09
  syndactyly (finger) (toe) 86.89
  tracheoesophageal 31.95
  tubulovalvular fistula (Beck-Jianu)
      (Frank's) (Janeway) (Spivak's)
      (Ssabanejew-Frank) 43.19
  uretero-ileostomy, cutaneous 56.51
  ureterostomy, cutaneous 56.61
    ileal 56.51
  urethrovaginal fistula 58.0
  window
    pericardial 37.12
    pleural (for drainage) 34.09
      thoracoscopic 34.06
Fothergill (-Donald) operation (uterine
    suspension) 69.22
Fowler operation
  arthroplasty of metacarpophalangeal
      joint 81.72
  release (mallet finger repair) 82.84
  tenodesis (hand) 82.85
  thoracoplasty 33.34
Fox operation (entropion repair with
    wedge resection) 08.43
Fracture, surgical - *see also* Osteoclasis
    78.70
  turbinates (nasal) 21.62
Fragmentation
  lithotriptor - *see* Lithotripsy
  mechanical
    cataract (with aspiration) 13.43
      posterior route 13.42
      secondary membrane 13.66
      secondary membrane (after cataract)
          13.66
  ultrasonic
    cataract (with aspiration) 13.41
    stones, urinary (Kock pouch) 59.95
    urinary stones 59.95
      percutaneous nephrostomy 55.04
Franco operation (suprapubic cystotomy)
    57.18
Frank operation (permanent gastrostomy)
    43.19
Frazier (-Spiller) operation (subtemporal
    trigeminal rhizotomy) 04.02

Fredet-Ramstedt operation
    (pyloromyotomy) (with wedge
    resection) 43.3
Freeing
  adhesions - *see* Lysis, adhesions
  anterior synechiae (with injection of air
      or liquid) 12.32
  artery-vein-nerve bundle 39.91
  extraocular muscle, entrapped 15.7
  goniosynechiae (with injection of air or
      liquid) 12.31
  intestinal segment for interposition
      45.50
    large 45.52
    small 45.51
  posterior synechiae 12.33
  synechiae (posterior) 12.33
    anterior (with injection of air or
        liquid) 12.32
  vascular bundle 39.91
  vessel 39.91
Freezing
  gastric 96.32
  prostate 60.62
Frenckner operation (intrapetrosal
    drainage) 20.22
Frenectomy
  labial 27.41
  lingual 25.92
  lip 27.41
  maxillary 27.41
  tongue 25.92
Frenotomy
  labial 27.91
  lingual 25.91
Frenulumectomy - *see* Frenectomy
Frickman operation (abdominal
    proctopexy) 48.75
Frommel operation (shortening of
    uterosacral ligaments) 69.22
Fulguration - *see also* Electrocoagulation
    and Destruction, lesion, by site
  adenoid fossa 28.7
  anus 49.39
    endoscopic 49.31
  bladder (transurethral) 57.49
    suprapubic 57.59
  choroid 14.21
  duodenum 45.32
    endoscopic 45.30
  esophagus 42.39
    endoscopic 42.33
  large intestine 45.49
    endoscopic 45.43
      polypectomy 45.42
  penis 64.2
  perineum, female 71.3
  prostate, transurethral 60.29
  rectum 48.32
    radical 48.31
  retina 14.21
  scrotum 61.3
  Skene's gland 71.3
  skin 86.3
  small intestine NEC 45.34
    duodenum 45.32
      endoscopic 45.30
  stomach 43.49
    endoscopic 43.41
  subcutaneous tissue 86.3
  tonsillar fossa 28.7
  urethra 58.39
    endoscopic 58.31
  vulva 71.3

Function
  study - *see also* Scan, radioisotope
    gastric 89.39
    muscle 93.08
      ocular 95.25
    nasal 89.12
    pulmonary - *see* categories
        89.37-89.38
    renal 92.03
    thyroid 92.01
    urethral sphincter 89.23
Fundectomy, uterine 68.39
Fundoplication (esophageal) (Nissen's)
    44.66
  laparoscopic 44.67
Fundusectomy, gastric 43.89
Fusion
  atlas-axis (spine) - *see* Fusion, spinal,
      atlas-axis
  bone - *see also* Osteoplasty 78.40
  cervical (spine) (C2 level or below) - *see*
      Fusion, spinal, cervical
  claw toe 77.57
  craniocervical - *see* Fusion, spinal,
      craniocervical
  dorsal, dorsolumbar - *see* Fusion,
      spinal, dorsal, dorsolumbar
  epiphyseal-diaphyseal - *see also* Arrest,
      bone growth 78.20
  epiphysiodesis - *see also* Arrest, bone
      growth 78.20
  hammer toe 77.56
  joint (with bone graft) - *see also*
      Arthrodesis 81.20
    ankle 81.11
    claw toe 77.57
    foot NEC 81.17
    hammer toe 77.56
    hip 81.21
    interphalangeal, finger 81.28
    ischiofemoral 81.21
    metatarsophalangeal 81.16
    midtarsal 81.14
    overlapping toe(s) 77.58
    pantalar 81.11
    spinal - *see also* Fusion, spinal
        81.00
    subtalar 81.13
    tarsal joints NEC 81.17
    tarsometatarsal 81.15
    tibiotalar 81.11
    toe NEC 77.58
      claw toe 77.57
      hammer toe 77.56
      overlapping toe(s) 77.58
  lip to tongue 25.59
  lumbar, lumbosacral - *see* Fusion,
      spinal, lumbar, lumbosacral
  occiput-C2 (spinal) - *see* Fusion, spinal,
      occiput
  spinal (with graft) (with internal
      fixation) (with instrumentation)
      81.00
    anterior lumbar interbody fusion
        (ALIF) 81.06
    atlas-axis (anterior transoral)
        (posterior) 81.01
      for pseudarthrosis 81.31
    cervical (C2 level or below) NEC
        81.02
      anterior (interbody),
          anterolateral technique
          81.02
        for pseudarthrosis 81.32

Fusion *(Continued)*
    spinal *(Continued)*
        cervical NEC *(Continued)*
            C1-C2 level (anterior) (posterior)
                81.01
                for pseudarthrosis 81.31
            for pseudarthrosis 81.32
            posterior (interbody),
                posterolateral technique
                81.03
                for pseudarthrosis 81.33
        craniocervical (anterior transoral)
            (posterior) 81.01
            for pseudarthrosis
                81.31
        dorsal, dorsolumbar NEC 81.05
            anterior (interbody),
                anterolateral technique
                81.04
                for pseudarthrosis 81.34

Fusion *(Continued)*
    spinal *(Continued)*
        dorsal, dorsolumbar NEC *(Continued)*
            for pseudarthrosis 81.35
            posterior (interbody),
                posterolateral technique
                81.05
                for pseudarthrosis 81.35
        lumbar, lumbosacral NEC 81.08
            anterior (interbody), anterolarteral
                technique 81.06
                for pseudarthrosis 81.36
            for pseudarthrosis 81.38
            lateral transverse process
                technique 81.07
                for pseudarthrosis 81.37
            posterior (interbody),
                posterolateral technique
                81.08
                for pseudarthrosis 81.38

Fusion *(Continued)*
    spinal *(Continued)*
        number of vertebrae - *see* codes
            81.62-81.64
        occiput-C2 (anterior transoral)
            (posterior) 81.01
            for pseudarthrosis 81.31
        posterior lumbar interbody fusion
            (PLIF) 81.08
        transforaminal lumbar interbody
            fusion (TLIF) 81.08

> Note: Also use either 81.62, 81.63, or 81.64 as an additional code to show the total number of vertebrae fused.

    tongue (to lip) 25.59

◀ New   ◀ा Revised   ~~deleted~~ Deleted   ● Use Additional Digit(s)   ▨ Omit code

G

Graft, grafting *(Continued)*
   bone (autogenous) (bone bank) (dual
      onlay) (heterogeneous) (inlay)
      (massive onlay) (multiple)
      (osteoperiosteal) (peg)
      (subperiosteal) (with metallic
      fixation) 78.00
     with
       arthrodesis - *see* Arthrodesis
       arthroplasty - *see* Arthroplasty
       gingivoplasty 24.2
       lengthening - *see* Lengthening,
        bone
     carpals, metacarpals 78.04
     clavicle 78.01
     facial NEC 76.91
      with total ostectomy 76.44
     femur 78.05
     fibula 78.07
     humerus 78.02
     joint - *see* Arthroplasty
     mandible 76.91
      with total mandibulectomy 76.41
     marrow - *see* Transplant, bone,
      marrow
     nose - *see* Graft, nose
     patella 78.06
     pelvic 78.09
     pericranial 02.04
     phalanges (foot) (hand) 78.09
     radius 78.03
     scapula 78.01
     skull 02.04
     specified site NEC 78.09
     spine 78.09
      with fusion - *see* Fusion, spinal
     tarsal, metatarsal 78.08
     thorax (ribs) (sternum) 78.01
     thumb (with transfer of skin flap)
      82.69
     tibia 78.07
     ulna 78.03
     vertebrae 78.09
      with fusion - *see* Fusion, spinal
   breast - *see also* Mammoplasty 85.89
   buccal sulcus 27.99
   cartilage (joint) - *see also* Arthroplasty
     nose - *see* Graft, nose
   chest wall (mesh) (silastic) 34.79
   conjunctiva (free) (mucosa) 10.44
     for symblepharon repair 10.41
   cornea - *see also* Keratoplasty 11.60
   dermal-fat 86.69
   dermal regenerative 86.67
   dura 02.12
   ear
     auricle 18.79
     external auditory meatus 18.6
     inner 20.61
     pedicle preparation 86.71
   esophagus NEC 42.87
     with interposition (intrathoracic)
      NEC 42.58
      antesternal or antethoracic NEC
       42.68
      colon (intrathoracic) 42.55
       antesternal or antethoracic
        42.65
      small bowel (intrathoracic)
       42.53
       antesternal or antethoracic
        42.63
   eyebrow - *see also* Reconstruction,
     eyelid, with graft 08.69

Graft, grafting *(Continued)*
   eyelid - *see also* Reconstruction, eyelid,
     with graft 08.69
     free mucous membrane 08.62
   eye socket (skin) (cartilage) (bone)
     16.63
   fallopian tube 66.79
   fascia 83.82
     with hernia repair - *see* Repair,
      hernia
     eyelid 08.32
     hand 82.72
     tarsal cartilage 08.69
   fat pad NEC 86.89
     with skin graft - *see* Graft, skin, full-
      thickness
   flap (advanced) (rotating) (sliding) - *see*
     also Graft, skin, pedicle
     tarsoconjunctival 08.64
   hair-bearing skin 86.64
   hand
     fascia 82.72
     free skin 86.62
     muscle 82.72
     pedicle (flap) 86.73
     tendon 82.79
   heart, for revascularization - *see*
     category 36.3●
   joint - *see* Arthroplasty
   larynx 31.69
   lip 27.56
     full-thickness 27.55
   lymphatic structure(s) (channel) (node)
     (vessel) 40.9
   mediastinal fat to myocardium 36.39
   meninges (cerebral) 02.12
   mouth, except palate 27.56
     full-thickness 27.55
   muscle 83.82
     hand 82.72
   myocardium, for revascularization 36.39
   nasolabial flaps 21.86
   nerve (cranial) (peripheral) 04.5
   nipple 85.86
   nose 21.89
     with
      augmentation 21.85
      rhinoplasty - *see* Rhinoplasty
      total reconstruction 21.83
     septum 21.88
     tip 21.86
   omentum 54.74
     to myocardium 36.39
   orbit (bone) (cartilage) (skin) 16.63
   outflow tract (patch) (pulmonary
     valve) 35.26
     in total repair of tetralogy of Fallot
      35.81
   ovary 65.92
   palate 27.69
     for cleft palate repair 27.62
   pedicle - *see* Graft, skin, pedicle
   penis (rib) (skin) 64.49
   pigskin 86.65
   pinch - *see* Graft, skin, free
   pocket - *see* Graft, skin, pedicle
   porcine 86.65
   postauricular (Wolff) 18.79
   razor - *see* Graft, skin, free
   rope - *see* Graft, skin, pedicle
   saphenous vein in aortocoronary
     bypass - *see* Bypass, aorto-
     coronary
   scrotum 61.49

Graft, grafting *(Continued)*
   skin (partial-thickness) (split-thickness)
     86.69
     amnionic membrane 86.66
     auditory meatus (ear) 18.6
     dermal-fat 86.69
      for breast augmentation 85.50
     dermal regenerative 86.67
     ear
      auditory meatus 18.6
      postauricular 18.79
     eyelid 08.61
     flap - *see* Graft, skin, pedicle
     free (autogenous) NEC 86.60 ◀
      breast
       deep inferior epigastric artery
        perforator (DIEP) flap,
        free 85.74 ◀
       gluteal artery perforator
        [GAP] flap, free 85.76 ◀
       superficial inferior epigastric
        artery (SIEA) flap, free
        85.75 ◀
       transverse rectus abdominis
        musculocutaneous
        (TRAM) flap, free 85.73 ◀
      lip 27.56
      thumb 86.62
       for
       pollicization 82.61
       reconstruction 82.69
     full-thickness 86.63
      breast 85.83
      hand 86.61
     hair-bearing 86.64
      eyelid or eyebrow 08.63
     hand 86.62
      full-thickness 86.61
     heterograft 86.65
     homograft 86.66
     island flap 86.70
     mucous membrane 86.69
      eyelid 08.62
     nose - *see* Graft, nose
     pedicle (flap) (tube) 86.70
      advancement 86.72
      attachment to site (advanced)
       (double) (rotating) (sliding)
       86.74
       hand (cross finger) (pocket)
        86.73
       lip 27.57
       mouth 27.57
       thumb 86.73
        for
        pollicization 82.61
        reconstruction NEC 82.69
      breast 85.84
       deep inferior epigastric artery
        perforator (DIEP) flap,
        free 85.74
       gluteal artery perforator (GAP)
        flap, free 85.76
       latissimus dorsi myocutaneous
        flap 85.71
       superficial inferior epigastric
        artery (SIEA) flap, free
        85.75
      transverse rectus abdominis
       musculocutaneous (TRAM)
       flap, free 85.73
      transverse rectus abdominis
       myocutaneous (TRAM)
       flap, pedicled 85.72

Graft, grafting *(Continued)*
  skin *(Continued)*
    pedicle *(Continued)*
      defatting 86.75
      delayed 86.71
      design and raising 86.71
      elevation 86.71
      preparation of (cutting) 86.71
      revision 86.75
      sculpturing 86.71
      transection 86.71
      transfer 86.74
      trimming 86.71
    postauricular 18.79
    rotation flap 86.70
    specified site NEC 86.69
      full-thickness 86.63
  tarsal cartilage 08.69
  temporalis muscle to orbit 16.63
    with exenteration of orbit 16.59
  tendon 83.81
    for joint repair - *see* Arthroplasty
    hand 82.79

Graft, grafting *(Continued)*
  testicle 62.69
  thumb (for reconstruction) NEC 82.69
  tongue (mucosal) (skin) 25.59
  trachea 31.79
  tubular (tube) - *see* Graft, skin, pedicle
  tunnel - *see* Graft, skin, pedicle
  tympanum - *see* also Tympanoplasty 19.4
  ureter 56.89
  vagina
    biological 70.94
    synthetic 70.95
  vein (patch) 39.58
    with
      excision or resection of vessel - *see*
        Phlebectomy, with graft
        replacement
      synthetic patch (Dacron) (Teflon)
        39.57
        tissue patch (vein)
          (autogenous)
          (homograft) 39.56
  vermilion border (lip) 27.56

Grattage, conjunctiva 10.31
Green operation (scapulopexy) 78.41
Grice operation (subtalar arthrodesis)
  81.13
Grip, strength 93.04
Gritti-Stokes operation (knee
  disarticulation) 84.16
Gross operation (herniorrhaphy)
  laparoscopic 53.43
    with graft or prosthesis 53.42
  other and open with graft or prosthesis
    53.41
  other open 53.49
Group therapy 94.44
Guttering, bone - *see* also Excision, lesion,
  bone 77.60
Guyon operation (amputation of ankle)
  84.13

H

Hagner operation (epididymotomy) 63.92

Halsted operation - *see* Repair, hernia, inguinal

Hampton operation (anastomosis small intestine to rectal stump) 45.92

Hanging hip operation (muscle release) 83.19

Harelip operation 27.54

Harrison-Richardson operation (vaginal suspension) 70.77
  with graft or prosthesis 70.78

Hartmann resection (of intestine) (with pouch) - *see* Colectomy, by site

Harvesting
  bone marrow 41.91
  stem cells 99.79

Hauser operation
  achillotenotomy 83.11
  bunionectomy with adductor tendon transfer 77.53
  stabilization of patella 81.44

Heaney operation (vaginal hysterectomy) 68.59
  laparoscopically assisted (LAVH) 68.51

Hearing aid (with battery replacement) 95.49

Hearing test 95.47

HeartMate® implantable heart assist system 37.66

HeartMate® II left ventricular assist system [LVAS] 37.66

Hegar operation (perineorrhaphy) 71.79

Heine operation (cyclodialysis) 12.55

Heineke-Mikulicz operation (pyloroplasty) 44.29

Heller operation (esophagomyotomy) 42.7

Hellström operation (transplantation of aberrant renal vessel) 39.55

Hemicolectomy
  left
    laparoscopic 17.35
    open and other 45.75
  right (extended)
    laparoscopic 17.33
    open and other 45.73

Hemicystectomy 57.6

Hemigastrectomy - *see* Gastrectomy

Hemiglossectomy 25.2

Hemilaminectomy (decompression) (exploration) 03.09

Hemilaryngectomy (anterior) (lateral) (vertical) 30.1

Hemimandibulectomy 76.31

Hemimastectomy (radical) 85.23

Hemimaxillectomy (with bone graft) (with prosthesis) 76.39

Heminephrectomy 55.4

Hemipelvectomy 84.19

Hemispherectomy (cerebral) 01.52

Hemithyroidectomy (with removal of isthmus) (with removal of portion of remaining lobe) 06.2

Hemodiafiltration (extracorporeal) 39.95

Hemodialysis (extracorporeal) 39.95

Hemodilution 99.03

Hemofiltration (extracorporeal) 39.95

Hemorrhage control - *see* Control, hemorrhage

Hemorrhoidectomy 49.46
  by
    cautery, cauterization 49.43
    crushing 49.45
    cryotherapy, cryosurgery 49.44
    excision 49.46
    injection 49.42
    ligation 49.45

Hemostasis - *see* Control, hemorrhage

Henley operation (jejunal transposition) 43.81

Hepatectomy (complete) (total) 50.4
  partial or subtotal 50.22

Hepatic assistance, extracorporeal 50.92

Hepaticocholangiojejunostomy 51.37

Hepaticocystoduodenostomy 51.37

Hepaticodochotomy 51.59

Hepaticoduodenostomy 51.37

Hepaticojejunostomy 51.37

Hepaticolithectomy 51.49
  endoscopic 51.88

Hepaticolithotomy 51.49
  endoscopic 51.88

Hepaticostomy 51.59

Hepaticotomy 51.59

Hepatocholangiocystoduodenostomy 51.37

Hepatocholedochostomy 51.43
  endoscopic 51.87

Hepatoduodenostomy 50.69

Hepatogastrostomy 50.69

Hepatojejunostomy 50.69

Hepatolithotomy
  hepatic duct 51.49
  liver 50.0

Hepatopexy 50.69

Hepatorrhaphy 50.61

Hepatostomy (external) (internal) 50.69

Hepatotomy (with packing) 50.0

Hernioplasty - *see* Repair, hernia

Herniorrhaphy - *see* Repair, hernia

Herniotomy - *see* Repair, hernia

Heterograft - *see* Graft

Heterotransplant, heterotransplantation - *see* Transplant

Hey operation (amputation of foot) 84.12

Hey-Groves operation (reconstruction of anterior cruciate ligament) 81.45

Heyman operation (soft tissue release for clubfoot) 83.84

Heyman-Herndon (-Strong) operation (correction of metatarsus varus) 80.48

Hibbs operation (lumbar spinal fusion) - *see* Fusion, lumbar

Higgins operation - *see* Repair, hernia, femoral

High forceps delivery 72.39
  with episiotomy 72.31

Hill-Allison operation (hiatal hernia repair, transpleural approach) 53.80

Hinging, mitral valve 35.12

His bundle recording 37.29

Hitchcock operation (anchoring tendon of biceps) 83.88

Hofmeister operation (gastrectomy) 43.7

Hoke operation
  midtarsal fusion 81.14
  triple arthrodesis 81.12

Holth operation
  iridencleisis 12.63
  sclerectomy 12.65

Homans operation (correction of lymphedema) 40.9

Homograft - *see* Graft

Homotransplant, homotransplantation - *see* Transplant

Hosiery, elastic 93.59

Hutch operation (ureteroneocystostomy) 56.74

Hybinette-Eden operation (glenoid bone block) 78.01

Hydrocelectomy
  canal of Nuck (female) 69.19
    male 63.1
  round ligament 69.19
  spermatic cord 63.1
  tunica vaginalis 61.2

Hydrotherapy 93.33
  assisted exercise in pool 93.31
  whirlpool 93.32

Hymenectomy 70.31

Hymenoplasty 70.76

Hymenorrhaphy 70.76

Hymenotomy 70.11

Hyperalimentation (parenteral) 99.15

Hyperbaric oxygenation 93.95
  wound 93.59

Hyperextension, joint 93.25

Hyperthermia NEC 93.35
  for cancer treatment (interstitial) (local) (radiofrequency) (regional) (ultrasound) (whole-body) 99.85

Hypnodrama, psychiatric 94.32

Hypnosis (psychotherapeutic) 94.32
  for anesthesia - *omit code*

Hypnotherapy 94.32

Hypophysectomy (complete) (total) 07.69
  partial or subtotal 07.63
    transfrontal approach 07.61
    transsphenoidal approach 07.62
  specified approach NEC 07.68
  transfrontal approach (complete) (total) 07.64
    partial 07.61
  transsphenoidal approach (complete) (total) 07.65
    partial 07.62

Hypothermia (central) (local) 99.81
  gastric (cooling) 96.31
    freezing 96.32
  systemic (in open heart surgery) 39.62

Hypotympanotomy 20.23

Hysterectomy 68.9
  abdominal 68.49
    laparoscopic (total) [TLH] 68.41
    partial or subtotal (supracervical) (supravaginal) 68.39
    radical (modified) (Wertheim's) 68.69
      laparoscopic (total) [TLRH] 68.61
    supracervical 68.39
      classic infrafasical SEMM hysterectomy [CISH] 68.31
      laparoscopically assisted [LASH] 68.31

◀ New ◀▥ Revised ~~deleted~~ Deleted ● Use Additional Digit(s) ▨ Omit code

Hysterectomy (*Continued*)
  vaginal (complete) (partial) (subtotal)
    (total) 68.59
    laparoscopically assisted (LAVH)
      68.51
    radical (Schauta) 68.79
      laparoscopic [LRVH] 68.71
Hysterocolpectomy (radical) (vaginal)
  68.79
  abdominal 68.69
    laparoscopic 68.61
  laparoscopic 68.71
Hysterogram NEC 87.85
  percutaneous 87.84

Hysterolysis 54.59
  laparoscopic 54.51
Hysteromyomectomy 68.29
Hysteropexy 69.22
Hysteroplasty 69.49
Hysterorrhaphy 69.41
Hysterosalpingography gas (contrast)
  87.82
  opaque dye (contrast) 87.83
Hysterosalpingostomy 66.74
Hysteroscopy 68.12
  with
    ablation
      endometrial 68.23
    biopsy 68.16

Hysterotomy (with removal of foreign
  body) (with removal of
  hydatidiform mole) 68.0
  for intrauterine transfusion
    75.2
  obstetrical 74.99
    for termination of pregnancy
      74.91
Hysterotrachelectomy 67.4
Hysterotracheloplasty 69.49
Hysterotrachelorrhaphy 69.41
Hysterotrachelotomy 69.95

I

IAEMT (intraoperative anesthetic effect monitoring and titration) 00.94 [89.14] ◄

ICCE (intracapsular cataract extraction) 13.19

Ileal
  bladder
    closed 57.87 [45.51]
    open (ileoureterostomy) 56.51
  conduit (ileoureterostomy) 56.51

Ileocecostomy 45.93

Ileocolectomy
  laparoscopic 17.33
  open and other 45.73

Ileocolostomy 45.93

Ileocolotomy 45.00

Ileocystoplasty (isolated segment anastomosis) (open loop) 57.87 [45.51]

Ileoduodenotomy 45.01

Ileoectomy (partial) 45.62
  with cecectomy
    laparoscopic 17.32
    open and other 45.72

Ileoentectropy 46.99

Ileoesophagostomy 42.54

Ileoileostomy 45.91
  proximal to distal segment 45.62

Ileoloopogram 87.78

Ileopancreatostomy 52.96

Ileopexy 46.61

Ileoproctostomy 45.95

Ileorectostomy 45.93

Ileorrhaphy 46.73

Ileoscopy 45.13
  through stoma (artificial) 45.12
  transabdominal (operative) 45.11

Ileosigmoidostomy 45.93

Ileostomy 46.20
  continent (permanent) 46.22
    for urinary diversion 56.51
  delayed opening 46.24
  Hendon (temporary) 46.21
  loop 46.01
  Paul (temporary) 46.21
  permanent 46.23
    continent 46.22
  repair 46.41
  revision 46.41
  tangential (temporary) 46.21
  temporary 46.21
  transplantation to new site 46.23
  tube (temporary) 46.21
  ureteral
    external 56.51
    internal 56.71

Ileotomy 45.02

Ileotransversostomy 45.93

Ileoureterostomy (Bricker's) (ileal bladder) 56.51

Imaging (diagnostic) ◄
  by
    optical coherence tomography (OCT) - see OCT and Tomography, optical coherence ◄
  diagnostic, not elsewhere classified 88.90
  endovascular ultrasound - see Imaging, intravascular ultrasound
  intraoperative
    iMRI - see Imaging, magnetic resonance
    intravascular - see Imaging, intravascular ultrasound

Imaging (Continued)
  intravascular ultrasound (IVUS) 00.29
    aorta 00.22
    aortic arch 00.22
    carotid vessel 00.21
    cerebral vessel, extracranial 00.21
    coronary vessel 00.24
    intrathoracic vessel 00.22
    other specified vessel 00.28
    peripheral vessel 00.23
    renal vessel 00.25
    vena cava (inferior) (superior) 00.22
  magnetic resonance (nuclear) (proton) NEC 88.97
    abdomen 88.97
    bladder (urinary) 88.95
    bone marrow blood supply 88.94
    brain (brain stem) 88.91
      intraoperative (iMRI) 88.96
      real-time 88.96
    chest (hilar) (mediastinal) 88.92
    computer assisted surgery (CAS) with MR/MRA 00.32
    extremity (lower) (upper) 88.94
    eye orbit 88.97
    face 88.97
    head NEC 88.97
    musculoskeletal 88.94
    myocardium 88.92
    neck 88.97
    orbit of eye 88.97
    prostate 88.95
    specified site NEC 88.97
    spinal canal (cord) (spine) 88.93
  VH™ - IVUS - see Imaging (diagnostic), intravascular ultrasound (IVUS), by site ◄
  virtual histology intravascular ultrasound - see Imaging (diagnostic), intravascular ultrasound (IVUS), by site ◄

Immobilization (by)
  with fracture-reduction - see Reduction, fracture
  bandage 93.59
  bone 93.53
  cast NEC 93.53
    with reduction of fracture or dislocation - see Reduction, fracture, and Reduction, dislocation
  device NEC 93.59
  pressure dressing 93.56
  splint (plaster) (tray) 93.54
    with reduction of fracture or dislocation - see Reduction, fracture, and Reduction, dislocation
  stereotactic head frame 93.59
  strapping (non-traction) 93.59

Immunoadsorption
  extracorporeal (ECI) 99.76

Immunization - see also Vaccination
  allergy 99.12
  autoimmune disease 99.13
  BCG 99.33
  brucellosis 99.55
  cholera 99.31
  diphtheria 99.36
  DPT 99.39
  epidemic parotitis 99.46
  German measles 99.47
  Hemophilus influenzae 99.52

Immunization (Continued)
  influenza 99.52
  measles 99.45
  meningococcus 99.55
  mumps 99.46
  pertussis 99.37
  plague 99.34
  poliomyelitis 99.41
  rabies 99.44
  rubella 99.47
  salmonella 99.55
  smallpox 99.42
  staphylococcus 99.55
  TAB 99.32
  tetanus 99.38
  triple vaccine 99.48
  tuberculosis 99.33
  tularemia 99.35
  typhoid-paratyphoid 99.32
  typhus 99.55
  viral NEC 99.55
  whooping cough 99.37
  yellow fever 99.43

Immunotherapy, antineoplastic 99.28
  C-Parvum 99.28
  Interferon 99.28
  Interleukin-2 (low-dose) 99.28
    high-dose 00.15
  Levamisole 99.28
  Proleukin (low-dose) 99.28
    high-dose 00.15
  Thymosin 99.28

Impella® percutaneous external heart assist device 37.68 ◄

Implant, implantation
  abdominal artery to coronary artery 36.17
  artery
    aortic branches to heart muscle 36.2
    mammary to ventricular wall (Vineberg) 36.2
  baffle, atrial or interatrial 35.91
  biliary fistulous tract into stomach or intestine 51.39
  bipolar endoprosthesis (femoral head) 81.52
  bladder sphincter, artificial (inflatable) 58.93
  blood vessels to myocardium 36.2
  bone growth stimulator (invasive) (percutaneous) (semi-invasive) - see category 78.9●
  bone morphogenetic protein (Infuse™ (OP-1™) (recombinant) (rhBMP) 84.52
  bone void filler 84.55
    that with percutaneous vertebral augmentation 81.66
    that with percutaneous vertebroplasty 81.65
  breast (for augmentation) (bilateral) 85.54
    unilateral 85.53
  cardiac contractility modulation (CCM) ◄
    rechargeable pulse generator only 17.52 ◄
    total system 17.51 ◄
  cardiac resynchronization device defibrillator (biventricular) (BiV ICD) (BiV pacemaker with defibrillator) (BiV pacing with defibrillator) (CRT-D) (device and one or more leads) (total system) 00.51

◄ New   ◄▥ Revised   ~~deleted~~ Deleted   ● Use Additional Digit(s)   ▨ Omit code

Implant, implantation (Continued)
  cardiac resynchronization device
      (Continued)
    defibrillator (Continued)
      left ventricular coronary venous
          lead only 00.52
      pulse generator only 00.54
    pacemaker (BiV) (biventricular)
        (CRT-P) (device and one or
        more leads) (total system)
        00.50
      left ventricular coronary venous
          lead only 00.52
      pulse generator only 00.53
  cardiac support device (CSD) 37.41
  cardiomyostimulation system 37.67
  cardioverter/defibrillator (automatic)
      37.94
    leads only (patch electrode) (pacing)
        (sensing) 37.95
    pulse generator only 37.96
    total system 37.94
  CCM (cardiac contractility
      modulation)   ◄
    rechargeable pulse generator
        only 17.52   ◄
    total system 17.51   ◄
  chest wall (mesh) (silastic) 34.79
  chin (polyethylene) (silastic) 76.68
  cochlear (electrode) 20.96
    prosthetic device (electrode and
        receiver) 20.96
      channel (single) 20.97
        multiple 20.98
      electrode only 20.99
      internal coil only 20.99
  coil(s), endovascular 39.79   ◄
    head or neck vessels   ◄
      bare metal 39.75   ◄
      bioactive 39.76   ◄
  CorCap™ 37.41
  cornea 11.73
  CRT-D (biventricular defibrillator)
      (BiV ICD) (BiV pacemaker with
      defibrillator) (BiV pacing with
      defibrillator) (cardiac
      resynchronization defibrillator)
      (device and one or more leads)
      00.51
    left ventricular coronary venous
        lead only 00.52
    pulse generator only 00.54
  CRT-P (biventricular pacemaker)
      (BiV pacemaker) (cardiac
      resynchronization pacemaker)
      (device and one or more leads)
      00.50
    left ventricular coronary venous
        lead only 00.52
    pulse generator only 00.53
  custodis eye 14.41
  dental (endosseous) (prosthetic) 23.6
  device
    adjustable gastric band and port
        44.95
    bronchial device NOS 33.79
    bronchial substance NOS 33.79
    bronchial valve 33.71   ◄▥
      multiple lobes 33.73   ◄
      single lobe 33.71   ◄
    cardiac support device (CSD) 37.41
    CorCap™ 37.41
    epicardial support device 37.41
    Lap-Band™ 44.95

Implant, implantation (Continued)
  electrode(s) (Continued)
    left atrial appendage 37.36
    left atrial filter 37.36
    left atrial occluder 37.36
    prosthetic cardiac support device
        37.41
    subcutaneous for intracardiac or
        great vessel hemodynamic
        monitoring 00.57   ◄▥
    vascular access 86.07
    ventricular support device 37.41
  diaphragmatic pacemaker 34.85
  Dynesys® 84.82
  electrode(s)
    brain 02.93
      depth 02.93
      foramen ovale 02.93
      sphenoidal 02.96
    cardiac (initial) (transvenous) 37.70
      atrium (initial) 37.73
        replacement 37.76
      atrium and ventricle (initial)
          37.72
        replacement 37.76
      epicardium (sternotomy or
          thoracotomy approach)
          37.74
      left ventricular coronary venous
          system 00.52
      temporary transvenous
          pacemaker system
          37.78
        during and immediately
            following cardiac
            surgery 39.64
      ventricle (initial) 37.71
        replacement 37.76
    carotid sinus 39.8
    depth 02.93
    foramen ovale 02.93
    gastric 04.92
    heart - see also Implant, electrode(s),
        cardiac 37.70
    intracranial 02.93
    osteogenic (invasive) for bone
        growth stimulation - see
        category 78.9 ●
    peripheral nerve 04.92
    sacral nerve 04.92
    sphenoidal 02.96
    spine 03.93
  electroencephalographic receiver
    brain 02.93
    intracranial 02.93
  electronic stimulator
    anus (subcutaneous) 49.92
    bladder 57.96
    bone growth (invasive)
        (percutaneous) (semi-invasive)
        78.9 ●
    brain - see Implant, neurostimulator,
        brain
    carotid sinus 39.8
    cochlear 20.96
      channel (single) 20.97
        multiple 20.98
    gastric 04.92
    intracranial - see Implant,
        neurostimulator,
        intracranial
    peripheral nerve - see Implant,
        neurostimulator, peripheral
        nerve

Implant, implantation (Continued)
  electronic stimulator (Continued)
    phrenic nerve 34.85
    skeletal muscle 83.92
    spine - see Implant, neurostimulator,
        spine
    ureter 56.92
  electrostimulator - see Implant,
      electronic stimulator, by site
  endoprosthesis
    bile duct 51.87
    femoral head (bipolar)
        81.52
    pancreatic duct 52.93
  endosseous (dental) 23.6
  epidural pegs 02.93
  epikeratoprosthesis 11.73
  estradiol (pellet) 99.23
  eye (Iowa type) 16.61
    integrated 16.41
  facial bone, synthetic (alloplastic)
      76.92
  fallopian tube (Mulligan hood)
      (silastic tube) (stent) 66.93
    into uterus 66.74
  gastroepiploic artery to coronary
      artery 36.17
  hearing device, electromagnetic 20.95
  heart
    artificial 37.52
      total internal biventricular
          replacement system 37.52
        AbioCor® 37.52
        CardioWest™ (TAH-t) 37.52
    assist system
      CentriMag® – see Insertion,
          circulatory support device
      external heart assist device,
          percutaneous – see
          Insertion, circulatory
          support device
      external heart assist system, open
          approach 37.65
      extrinsic 37.68
      HeartMate® implantable heart
          assist system 37.66
      HeartMate® II left ventricular
          assist system [LVAS] 37.66
      Impella® percutaneous external
          circulatory assist device -
          see Insertion, circulatory
          support device   ◄
      implantable 37.66
      non-implantable – see Insertion,
          circulatory support device
      percutaneous external
          circulatory assist device –
          see Insertion, circulatory
          support device
      pulsation balloon 37.61
      pVAD (percutaneous VAD) – see
          Insertion, circulatory
          support device
      TandemHeart® - see Insertion,
          circulatory support
          device
      temporary non-implantable
          circulatory assist device -
          see Insertion, circulatory
          support device
      that for destination therapy (DT)
          37.66
    auxiliary ventricle 37.62
    cardiac support device (CSD) 37.41

Implant, implantation (*Continued*)
  heart (*Continued*)
    circulatory assist system - *see*
      Implant, heart, assist system
    CorCap™ 37.41
    epicardial support device 37.41
    pacemaker - *see also* Implant,
      pacemaker, cardiac 37.80
    prosthetic cardiac support device
      37.41
    total internal biventricular
      replacement system 37.52
    valve(s)
      prosthesis or synthetic device
        (partial) (synthetic) (total)
        35.20
        aortic 35.22
        mitral 35.24
        pulmonary 35.26
        tricuspid 35.28
      tissue graft 35.20
        aortic 35.21
        mitral 35.23
        pulmonary 35.25
        tricuspid 35.27
    ventricular support device 37.41
  inert material
    breast (for augmentation) (bilateral)
      85.54
      unilateral 85.53
    larynx 31.0
    nose 21.85
    orbit (eye socket) 16.69
      reinsertion 16.62
    scleral shell (cup) (with evisceration
      of eyeball) 16.31
      reinsertion 16.62
    Tenon's capsule (with enucleation of
      eyeball) 16.42
      with attachment of muscles 16.41
      reinsertion 16.62
    urethra 59.79
    vocal cord(s) 31.0
  infusion pump 86.06
  interbody spinal fusion device 84.51
  intracardiac or great vessel
    hemodynamic monitor,
      subcutaneous 00.57 ◀▥
  joint (prosthesis) (silastic) (Swanson
    type) NEC 81.96
    ankle (total) 81.56
      revision 81.59
    carpocarpal, carpometacarpal 81.74
    elbow (total) 81.84
      revision 81.97
    extremity (bioelectric) (cineplastic)
      (kineplastic) 84.40
      lower 84.48
        revision 81.59
      upper 84.44
        revision 81.97
    femoral (bipolar endoprosthesis) 81.52
      revision NOS 81.53
        acetabular and femoral
          components (total) 00.70
        acetabular component only
          00.71
        acetabular liner and/or
          femoral head only 00.73
        femoral component only 00.72
        femoral head only and/or
          acetabular liner 00.73
        total (acetabular and femoral
          components) 00.70

Implant, implantation (*Continued*)
  joint (*Continued*)
    finger 81.71
    hand (metacarpophalangeal)
      (interphalangeal) 81.71
      revision 81.97
    hip (partial) 81.52
      revision NOS 81.53
        acetabular and femoral
          components (total) 00.70
        acetabular component only
          00.71
        acetabular liner and/or
          femoral head only 00.73
        femoral component only 00.72
        femoral head only and/or
          acetabular liner 00.73
        partial
          acetabular component only
            00.71
          acetabular liner and/or
            femoral head only
            00.73
          femoral component only
            00.72
          femoral head only and/or
            acetabular liner 00.73
          total (acetabular and
            femoral components)
            00.70
      total 81.51
        revision (acetabular and
          femoral components)
    interphalangeal 81.71
      revision 81.97
    knee (partial) (total) 81.54
      revision NOS 81.55
        femoral component 00.82
        partial
          femoral component 00.82
          patellar component 00.83
          tibial component 00.81
          tibial insert 00.84
        patellar component 00.83
        tibial component 00.81
        tibial insert 00.84
        total (all components) 00.80
    metacarpophalangeal 81.71
      revision 81.97
    shoulder (partial) 81.81
      revision 81.97
      total replacement 81.80
    toe 81.57
      for hallux valgus repair 77.59
      revision 81.59
    wrist (partial) 81.74
      revision 81.97
      total replacement 81.73
  kidney, mechanical 55.97
  Lap-Band™ 44.95
  larynx 31.0
  leads (cardiac) - *see* Implant,
    electrode(s), cardiac
  limb lengthening device, internal
    (NOS) 84.54
    with kinetic distraction 84.53
  mammary artery
    in ventricle (Vineberg) 36.2
    to coronary artery (single vessel)
      36.15
      double vessel 36.16
  M-Brace™ 84.82
  Mulligan hood, fallopian tube 66.93
  nerve (peripheral) 04.79

Implant, implantation (*Continued*)
  neuropacemaker - *see* Implant,
    neurostimulator, by site
  neurostimulator
    electrodes
      brain 02.93
      carotid sinus 39.8
      gastric 04.92
      intracranial 02.93
      peripheral nerve 04.92
      sacral nerve 04.92
      spine 03.93
    pulse generator 86.96
      dual array 86.95
        rechargeable 86.98
      single array 86.94
        rechargeable 86.97
  nose 21.85
  Ommaya reservoir 02.2
  orbit 16.69
    reinsertion 16.62
  outflow tract prosthesis (heart) (gusset
    type)
    in
      pulmonary valvuloplasty
        35.26
      total repair of tetralogy of
        Fallot 35.81
  ovary into uterine cavity 65.72
    laparoscopic 65.75
  pacemaker
    brain - *see* Implant,
      neurostimulator, brain
    cardiac (device) (initial)
      (permanent) (replacement)
      37.80
      dual-chamber device (initial)
        37.83
        replacement 37.87
      resynchronization device
        (biventricular pacemaker)
        (BiV pacemaker) (CRT-P)
        device only (initial)
          (replacement) 00.53
        total system (device and one
          or more leads) 00.50
        transvenous lead into left
          ventricular coronary
          venous system 00.52
      single-chamber device (initial)
        37.81
        rate responsive 37.82
        replacement 37.85
          rate responsive 37.86
      temporary transvenous
        pacemaker system
        37.78
        during and immediately
          following cardiac
          surgery 39.64
    carotid sinus 39.8
    diaphragm 34.85
    gastric 04.92
    intracranial - *see* Implant,
      neurostimulator, intracranial
    neural - *see* Implant,
      neurostimulator, by site
    peripheral nerve - *see* Implant,
      neurostimulator, peripheral
      nerve
    spine - *see* Implant,
      neurostimulator,
      spine
  pancreas (duct) 52.96

◀ New   ◀▥ Revised   ~~deleted~~ Deleted   ● Use Additional Digit(s)   ▨ Omit code

Implant, implantation *(Continued)*
  penis, prosthesis (internal)
    inflatable 64.97
    non-inflatable 64.95
  port, vascular access device 86.07
  premaxilla 76.68
  progesterone (subdermal) 99.23
  prosthesis, prosthetic device
    acetabulum (Aufranc-Turner)
      81.52
    ankle (total) 81.56
    arm (bioelectric) (cineplastic)
      (kineplastic) 84.44
    breast (bilateral) (Cronin) (Dow-
      Corning) (Perras-Pappillon)
      85.54
      unilateral 85.53
    cardiac support device (CSD)
      (CorCap™) 37.41
    cochlear 20.96
      channel (single) 20.97
        multiple 20.98
    extremity (bioelectric) (cineplastic)
      (kineplastic) 84.40
      lower 84.48
      upper 84.44
    fallopian tube (Mulligan hood)
      (stent) 66.93
    femoral head (Austin-Moore)
      (bipolar) (Eicher) (Thompson)
      81.52
      revision NOS 81.53
        acetabular and femoral
          components (total)
          00.70
        acetabular component only
          00.71
        acetabular liner and/or
          femoral head only
          00.73
        femoral component only
          00.72
        femoral head only and/or
          acetabular liner 00.73
        partial
          acetabular component only
            00.71
          acetabular liner and/or
            femoral head only
            00.73
          femoral component only
            00.72
          femoral head only and/or
            acetabular liner
            00.73
        total (acetabular and
          femoral components
          00.70
    joint (Swanson type) NEC 81.96
      ankle (total) 81.56
      carpocarpal, carpometacarpal
        81.74
      elbow (total) 81.84
      finger 81.71
      hand (metacarpophalangeal)
        (interphalangeal) 81.71
      hip (partial) 81.52
        revision NOS 81.53
          acetabular and femoral
            components (total)
            00.70
          acetabular component only
            00.71

Implant, implantation *(Continued)*
  prosthesis, prosthetic device
    (Continued)
    joint NEC *(Continued)*
      hip *(Continued)*
        acetabular liner and/or
          femoral head only 00.73
        femoral component only
          00.72
        femoral head only and/or
          acetabular liner
          00.73
        partial
          acetabular component
            only 00.71
          acetabular liner and/or
            femoral head only
            00.73
          femoral component only
            00.72
          femoral head only and/
            or acetabular liner
            00.73
        total (acetabular and
          femoral components)
          00.70
      total 81.51
        revision (acetabular and
          femoral components)
          00.70
    interphalangeal 81.71
    knee (partial) (total) 81.54
      revision NOS 81.55
        femoral component 00.82
        partial
          femoral component 00.82
          patellar component 00.83
          tibial component 00.81
          tibial insert 00.84
        patellar component 00.83
        tibial component 00.81
        tibial insert 00.84
        total (all components) 00.80
    metacarpophalangeal 81.71
    shoulder (partial) 81.81
      total 81.80
    toe 81.57
      for hallux valgus repair 77.59
    wrist (partial) 81.74
      total 81.73
  leg (bioelectric) (cineplastic)
    (kineplastic) 84.48
  lens 13.91
  outflow tract (heart) (gusset type)
    in
      pulmonary valvuloplasty 35.26
      total repair of tetralogy of
        Fallot 35.81
  penis (internal) (non-inflatable)
    64.95
    inflatable (internal) 64.97
  skin (dermal regenerative) (matrix)
    86.67
  testicular (bilateral) (unilateral) 62.7
  pulsation balloon (phase-shift) 37.61
  pump, infusion 86.06
  radial artery 36.19
  radioactive isotope 92.27
  radium (radon) 92.27
  retinal attachment 14.41
    with buckling 14.41
  Rheos™ carotid sinus baroreflex
    activation device 39.8
  Rickham reservoir 02.2

Implant, implantation *(Continued)*
  silicone
    breast (bilateral) 85.54
      unilateral 85.53
    skin (for filling of defect) 86.02
      for augmentation NEC 86.89
  spine NEC 84.59
    facet replacement device(s) 84.84
    interspinous process decompression
      device 84.80
    pedicle-based dynamic stabilization
      device(s) 84.82
    posterior motion preservation
      device(s) - *see* category 84.8●
  stimoceiver - *see* Implant,
    neurostimulator, by site
  stimulator
    carotid sinus 39.8
  sudural
    grids 02.93
    strips 02.93
  Swanson prosthesis (joint) (silastic)
    NEC 81.96
    carpocarpal, carpometacarpal 81.74
    finger 81.71
    hand (interphalangeal)
      (metacarpophalangeal) 81.71
    interphalangeal 81.71
    knee (partial) (total) 81.54
      revision 81.55
    metacarpophalangeal 81.71
    toe 81.57
      for hallux valgus repair 77.59
    wrist (partial) 81.74
      total 81.73
  systemic arteries into myocardium
    (Vineberg type operation) 36.2
  Tandem™ heart 37.68
  telescope (IMT) (miniature) 13.91
  testicular prosthesis (bilateral)
    (unilateral) 62.7
  tissue expander (skin) NEC 86.93
    breast 85.95
  tissue mandril (for vascular graft)
    39.99
    with
      blood vessel repair 39.56
      vascular bypass or shunt - *see*
        Bypass, vascular
  tooth (bud) (germ) 23.5
    prosthetic 23.6
  umbrella, vena cava 38.7
  ureters into
    bladder 56.74
    intestine 56.71
      external diversion 56.51
    skin 56.61
  urethra
    for repair of urinary stress
      incontinence
      collagen 59.72
      fat 59.72
      polytef 59.72
  urethral sphincter, artificial (inflatable)
    58.93
  urinary sphincter, artificial (inflatable)
    58.93
  vascular access device 86.07
  vitreous (silicone) 14.75
    for retinal reattachment 14.41
      with buckling 14.41
  vocal cord(s) (paraglottic) 31.98
  X Stop™ 84.80

Implosion (psychologic desensitization) 94.33
Incision (and drainage)
  with
    exploration - *see* Exploration
    removal of foreign body - *see* Removal, foreign body
  abdominal wall 54.0
    as operative approach - *omit code*
  abscess - *see also* Incision, by site
    antecubital fossa 86.04
    appendix 47.2
      with appendectomy 47.09
        laparoscopic 47.01
    axilla 86.04
    cheek 86.04
    extraperitoneal 54.0
    face 86.04
    gluteal 86.04
    groin region (abdominal wall) (inguinal) 54.0
      skin 86.04
      subcutaneous tissue 86.04
    hair follicle 86.04
    ischiorectal 49.01
    lip 27.0
    nailbed or nailfold 86.04
    neck 86.04
    omental 54.19
    paronychia 86.04
    perianal 49.01
    perigastric 54.19
    perineum (female) 71.09
      male 86.04
    perisplenic 54.19
    peritoneal NEC 54.19
      pelvic (female) 70.12
    popliteal space 86.04
    retroperitoneal 54.0
    sclera 12.89
    skin 86.04
    subcutaneous tissue 86.04
    subdiaphragmatic 54.19
    subhepatic 54.19
    submaxillary 86.04
    subphrenic 54.19
    supraclavicular fossa 86.04
    vas deferens 63.6
  adrenal gland 07.41
  alveolus, alveolar bone 24.0
  antecubital fossa 86.09
  anus NEC 49.93
    fistula 49.11
    septum 49.91
  appendix 47.2
  artery 38.00
    abdominal 38.06
      aorta (arch) (ascending) (descending) 38.04
    head and neck NEC 38.02
    intracranial NEC 38.01
    lower limb 38.08
    thoracic NEC 38.05
    upper limb 38.03
  atrium (heart) 37.11
  auditory canal or meatus, external 18.02
  auricle 18.09
  axilla 86.09
  Bartholin's gland or cyst 71.22
  bile duct (with T or Y tube insertion) NEC 51.59
    common (exploratory) 51.51
      for

Incision *(Continued)*
  bile duct NEC *(Continued)*
    common *(Continued)*
      for *(Continued)*
        relief of obstruction NEC 51.42
        removal of calculus 51.41
      for
        exploration 51.59
        relief of obstruction 51.49
  bladder 57.19
    neck (transurethral) 57.91
    percutaneous suprapubic (closed) 57.17
    suprapubic NEC 57.18
  blood vessel - *see also* Angiotomy 38.00
  bone 77.10
    alveolus, alveolar 24.0
    carpals, metacarpals 77.14
    clavicle 77.11
    facial 76.09
    femur 77.15
    fibula 77.17
    humerus 77.12
    patella 77.16
    pelvic 77.19
    phalanges (foot) (hand) 77.19
    radius 77.13
    scapula 77.11
    skull 01.24
    specified site NEC 77.19
    tarsals, metatarsals 77.18
    thorax (ribs) (sternum) 77.11
    tibia 77.17
    ulna 77.13
    vertebrae 77.19
  brain 01.39
    cortical adhesions 02.91
  breast (skin) 85.0
    with removal of tissue expander 85.96
  bronchus 33.0
  buccal space 27.0
  bulbourethral gland 58.91
  bursa 83.03
    hand 82.03
    pharynx 29.0
  carotid body 39.8
  cerebral (meninges) 01.39
    epidural or extradural space 01.24
    subarachnoid or subdural space 01.31
  cerebrum 01.39
  cervix 69.95
    to
      assist delivery 73.93
      replace inverted uterus 75.93
  chalazion 08.09
    with removal of capsule 08.21
  cheek 86.09
  chest wall (for extrapleural drainage) (for removal of foreign body) 34.01
    as operative approach - *omit code*
  common bile duct (for exploration) 51.51
    for
      relief of obstruction 51.42
      removal of calculus 51.41
  common wall between posterior left atrium and coronary sinus (with roofing of resultant defect with patch graft) 35.82
  conjunctiva 10.1

Incision *(Continued)*
  cornea 11.1
    radial (refractive) 11.75
  cranial sinus 01.21
  craniobuccal pouch 07.72
  cul-de-sac 70.12
  cyst
    dentigerous 24.0
    radicular (apical) (periapical) 24.0
  Duhrssen's (cervix, to assist delivery) 73.93
  duodenum 45.01
  ear
    external 18.09
    inner 20.79
    middle 20.23
  endocardium 37.11
  endolymphatic sac 20.79
  epididymis 63.92
  epidural space, cerebral 01.24
  epigastric region 54.0
    intra-abdominal 54.19
  esophagus, esophageal NEC 42.09
    web 42.01
  exploratory - *see* Exploration
  extradural space (cerebral) 01.24
  extrapleural 34.01
  eyebrow 08.09
  eyelid 08.09
    margin (trichiasis) 08.01
  face 86.09
  fallopian tube 66.01
  fascia 83.09
    with division 83.14
      hand 82.12
    hand 82.09
      with division 82.12
  fascial compartments, head and neck 27.0
  fistula, anal 49.11
  flank 54.0
  furuncle - *see* Incision, by site
  gallbladder 51.04
  gingiva 24.0
  gluteal 86.09
  groin region (abdominal wall) (inguinal) 54.0
    skin 86.09
    subcutaneous tissue 86.09
  gum 24.0
  hair follicles 86.09
  heart 37.10
    valve - *see* Valvulotomy
  hematoma - *see also* Incision, by site
    axilla 86.04
    broad ligament 69.98
    ear 18.09
    episiotomy site 75.91
    fossa (superficial) NEC 86.04
    groin region (abdominal wall) (inguinal) 54.0
      skin 86.04
      subcutaneous tissue 86.04
    laparotomy site 54.12
    mediastinum 34.1
    perineum (female) 71.09
      male 86.04
    popliteal space 86.04
    scrotum 61.0
    skin 86.04
    space of Retzius 59.19
    subcutaneous tissue 86.04
    vagina (cuff) 70.14
      episiotomy site 75.91
      obstetrical NEC 75.92

◀ New ◀▦ Revised ~~deleted~~ Deleted ● Use Additional Digit(s) ▨ Omit code

Incision *(Continued)*
  hepatic ducts 51.59
  hordeolum 08.09
  hygroma - *see also* Incision, by site
    cystic 40.0
  hymen 70.11
  hypochondrium 54.0
    intra-abdominal 54.19
  hypophysis 07.72
  iliac fossa 54.0
  infratemporal fossa 27.0
  ingrown nail 86.09
  intestine 45.00
    large 45.03
    small 45.02
  intracerebral 01.39
  intracranial (epidural space)
      (extradural space) 01.24
    subarachnoid or subdural space
        01.31
  intraperitoneal 54.19
  ischiorectal tissue 49.02
    abscess 49.01
  joint structures - *see also* Arthrotomy
      80.10
  kidney 55.01
    pelvis 55.11
  labia 71.09
  lacrimal
    canaliculus 09.52
    gland 09.0
    passage NEC 09.59
    punctum 09.51
    sac 09.53
  larynx NEC 31.3
  ligamentum flavum (spine) - omit code
  liver 50.0
  lung 33.1
  lymphangioma 40.0
  lymphatic structure (channel) (node)
      (vessel) 40.0
  mastoid 20.21
  mediastinum 34.1
  meibomian gland 08.09
  meninges (cerebral) 01.31
    spinal 03.09
  midpalmar space 82.04
  mouth NEC 27.92
    floor 27.0
  muscle 83.02
    with division 83.19
      hand 82.19
    hand 82.02
      with division 82.19
  myocardium 37.11
  nailbed or nailfold 86.09
  nasolacrimal duct (stricture) 09.59
  neck 86.09
  nerve (cranial) (peripheral) NEC
      04.04
    root (spinal) 03.1
  nose 21.1
  omentum 54.19
  orbit - *see also* Orbitotomy 16.09
  ovary 65.09
    laparoscopic 65.01
  palate 27.1
  palmar space (middle) 82.04
  pancreas 52.09
  pancreatic sphincter 51.82
    endoscopic 51.85
  parapharyngeal (oral) (transcervical)
      28.0
  paronychia 86.09

Incision *(Continued)*
  parotid
    gland or duct 26.0
    space 27.0
  pelvirectal tissue 48.81
  penis 64.92
  perianal (skin) (tissue) 49.02
    abscess 49.01
  perigastric 54.19
  perineum (female) 71.09
    male 86.09
  peripheral vessels
    lower limb
      artery 38.08
      vein 38.09
    upper limb (artery) (vein) 38.03
  periprostatic tissue 60.81
  perirectal tissue 48.81
  perirenal tissue 59.09
  perisplenic 54.19
  peritoneum 54.95
    by laparotomy 54.19
    pelvic (female) 70.12
      male 54.19
  periureteral tissue 59.09
  periurethral tissue 58.91
  perivesical tissue 59.19
  petrous pyramid (air cells) (apex)
      (mastoid) 20.22
  pharynx, pharyngeal (bursa) 29.0
    space, lateral 27.0
  pilonidal sinus (cyst) 86.03
  pineal gland 07.52
  pituitary (gland) 07.72
  pleura NEC 34.09
  popliteal space 86.09
  postzygomatic space 27.0
  pouch of Douglas 70.12
  prostate (perineal approach)
      (transurethral approach) 60.0
  pterygopalatine fossa 27.0
  pulp canal (tooth) 24.0
  Rathke's pouch 07.72
  rectovaginal septum 48.81
  rectum 48.0
    stricture 48.91
  renal pelvis 55.11
  retroperitoneum 54.0
  retropharyngeal (oral) (transcervical)
      28.0
  salivary gland or duct 26.0
  sclera 12.89
  scrotum 61.0
  sebaceous cyst 86.04
  seminal vesicle 60.72
  sinus - *see* Sinusotomy
  Skene's duct or gland 71.09
  skin 86.09
    with drainage 86.04
    breast 85.0
    cardiac pacemaker pocket, new site
        37.79
    ear 18.09
    nose 21.1
    subcutaneous tunnel for pulse
        generator lead wire 86.99
      with initial procedure - omit code
    thalamic stimulator pulse generator
        pocket, new site 86.09
      with initial insertion of battery
          package - omit code
    tunnel, subcutaneous for pulse
        generator lead wire 86.99
      with initial procedure - omit code

Incision *(Continued)*
  skull (bone) 01.24
  soft tissue NEC 83.09
    with division 83.19
      hand 82.19
    hand 82.09
      with division 82.19
  space of Retzius 59.19
  spermatic cord 63.93
  sphincter of Oddi 51.82
    endoscopic 51.85
  spinal
    cord 03.09
    nerve root 03.1
  spleen 41.2
  stomach 43.0
  stye 08.09
  subarachnoid space, cerebral 01.31
  subcutaneous tissue 86.09
    with drainage 86.04
    tunnel
      esophageal   42.86
        with anastomosis - *see*
            Anastomosis, esophagus,
            antesternal
      pulse generator lead wire 86.99
        with initial procedure - omit
            code
  subdiaphragmatic space 54.19
  subdural space, cerebral 01.31
  sublingual space 27.0
  submandibular space 27.0
  submaxillary 86.09
    with drainage 86.04
  submental space 27.0
  subphrenic space 54.19
  supraclavicular fossa 86.09
    with drainage 86.04
  sweat glands, skin 86.04
  temporal pouches 27.0
  tendon (sheath) 83.01
    with division 83.13
      hand 82.11
    hand 82.01
      with division 82.11
  testis 62.0
  thenar space 82.04
  thymus (open) (other) 07.92
    thoracoscopic 07.95
  thyroid (field) (gland) NEC 06.09
    postoperative 06.02
  tongue NEC 25.94
    for tongue tie 25.91
  tonsil 28.0
  trachea NEC 31.3
  tunica vaginalis 61.0
  umbilicus 54.0
  urachal cyst 54.0
  ureter 56.2
  urethra 58.0
  uterus (corpus) 68.0
    cervix 69.96
    for termination of pregnancy
        74.91
    septum (congenital) 68.22
  uvula 27.71
  vagina (cuff) (septum) (stenosis)
      70.14
    for
      incisional hematoma
          (episiotomy) 75.91
      obstetrical hematoma NEC
          75.92
      pelvic abscess 70.12

◄ New   ◄▬ Revised   ~~deleted~~ Deleted   ● Use Additional Digit(s)   Omit code

Injection *(Continued)*
immune sera 99.14
inert material - *see* Implant, inert
material
inner ear, for destruction 20.72
insulin 99.17
intervertebral space for herniated disc
80.52
intra-amniotic
for induction of
abortion 75.0
labor 73.1
intrathecal - *see* Injection, spinal
joint (therapeutic agent) 81.92
temporomandibular 76.96
kidney (cyst) (therapeutic substance)
NEC 55.96
larynx 31.0
ligament (joint) (therapeutic substance)
81.92
liver 50.94
lung, for surgical collapse 33.32
Methotrexate, for cancer chemotherapy
99.25
nerve (cranial) (peripheral) 04.80
agent NEC 04.89
alcohol 04.2
anesthetic for analgesia 04.81
for operative anesthesia - *omit
code*
neurolytic 04.2
phenol 04.2
laryngeal (external) (recurrent)
(superior) 31.91
optic 16.91
sympathetic 05.39
alcohol 05.32
anesthetic for analgesia 05.31
neurolytic agent 05.32
phenol 05.32
nesiritide 00.13
neuroprotective agent 99.75
nimodipine 99.75
orbit 16.91
pericardium 37.93
peritoneal cavity
air 54.96
locally-acting therapeutic substance
54.97
platelet inhibitor
direct coronary artery 36.04
intravenous 99.20
prophylactic substance NEC 99.29
prostate 60.92
radioimmunoconjugate 92.28
radioimmunotherapy 92.28
radioisotopes (intracavitary)
(intravenous) 92.28
renal pelvis (cyst) 55.96
retrobulbar (therapeutic substance)
16.91
for anesthesia - *omit code*
Rh immune globulin 99.11
RhoGAM 99.11
sclerosing agent NEC 99.29
esophageal varices (endoscopic)
42.33
hemorrhoids 49.42
pleura 34.92
treatment of malignancy (cytotoxic
agent) 34.92 [99.25]
with tetracycline 34.92 [99.21]
varicose vein 39.92
vein NEC 39.92

Injection *(Continued)*
semicircular canals, for destruction
20.72
silicone - *see* Implant, inert material
skin (sclerosing agent) (filling material)
86.02
soft tissue 83.98
hand 82.96
spinal (canal) NEC 03.92
alcohol 03.8
anesthetic agent for analgesia 03.91
for operative anesthesia - *omit code*
contrast material (for myelogram)
87.21
destructive agent NEC 03.8
neurolytic agent NEC 03.8
phenol 03.8
proteolytic enzyme (chymodiactin)
(chymopapain) 80.52
saline (hypothermic) 03.92
steroid NEC 03.92
spinal nerve root (intrathecal) - *see*
Injection, spinal
steroid NEC 99.23
subarachnoid, spinal - *see* Injection,
spinal
subconjunctival 10.91
tendon 83.97
hand 82.95
testis 62.92
therapeutic agent NEC 99.29
thoracic cavity 34.92
thrombolytic agent (enzyme)
(streptokinase) 99.10
with percutaneous transluminal
angioplasty

> Note: Also use 00.40, 00.41, 00.42, or
> 00.43 to show the total number of
> vessels treated.

coronary 00.66
noncoronary vessels 39.50
specified site NEC 39.50
direct intracoronary artery 36.04
trachea 31.94
tranquilizer 99.26
tunica vaginalis (with aspiration) 61.91
tympanum 20.94
urethra (inert material)
for repair of urinary stress
incontinence
collagen implant 59.72
endoscopic injection of implant
59.72
fat implant 59.72
polytef implant 59.72
vaccine
tumor 99.28
varices, esophagus (endoscopic)
(sclerosing agent) 42.33
varicose vein (sclerosing agent) 39.92
esophagus (endoscopic) 42.33
vestibule, for destruction 20.72
vitreous substitute (silicone) 14.75
for reattachment of retina 14.59
vocal cords 31.0
Inlay, tooth 23.3
Inoculation
antitoxins - *see* Administration,
antitoxins
toxoids - *see* Administration, toxoids
vaccine - *see* Administration, vaccine
Insemination, artificial 69.92

Insertion
airway
esophageal obturator 96.03
nasopharynx 96.01
oropharynx 96.02
Allen-Brown cannula 39.93
arch bars (orthodontic) 24.7
for immobilization (fracture) 93.55
atrial septal umbrella 35.52
Austin-Moore prosthesis 81.52
baffle, heart (atrial) (interatrial) (intra-
atrial) 35.91
bag, cervix (nonobstetrical) 67.0
after delivery or abortion 75.8
to assist delivery or induce labor
73.1
Baker's (tube) (for stenting) 46.85
balloon
gastric 44.93
heart (pulsation-type) (Kantrowitz)
37.61
intestine (for decompression) (for
dilation) 46.85
with insertion of colonic stent ◄
endoscopic 46.86 ◄
other 46.87 ◄
band (adjustable)
gastric, laparoscopic 44.95
Lap-Band™ 44.95
Barton's tongs (skull) (with
synchronous skeletal traction)
02.94
bipolar endoprosthesis (femoral head)
81.52
Blakemore-Sengstaken tube 96.06
bone growth stimulator (invasive)
(percutaneous) (semi-invasive) -
see category 78.9 ●
bone morphogenetic protein (Infuse™)
(OP-1™) (recombinant) (rhBMP)
84.52
bone void filler 84.55
that with percutaneous vertebral
augmentation 81.66
that with percutaneous
vertebroplasty 81.65
bougie, cervix, nonobstetrical 67.0
to assist delivery or induce labor 73.1
breast implant (for augmentation)
(bilateral) 85.54
unilateral 85.53
bridge (dental) (fixed) 23.42
removable 23.43
bubble (balloon), stomach 44.93
caliper tongs (skull) (with synchronous
skeletal traction) 02.94
cannula
Allen-Brown 39.93
for extracorporeal membrane
oxygenation (ECMO) - *omit
code*
nasal sinus (by puncture) 22.01
through natural ostium 22.02
pancreatic duct 52.92
endoscopic 52.93
vessel to vessel 39.93
cardiac resynchronization device
defibrillator (biventricular
defibrillator) (BiV ICD) (BiV
pacemaker with defibrillator)
(BiV pacing with defibrillator)
(CRT- D) (device and one or
more leads) (total system)
00.51

Insertion (Continued)
cardiac resynchronization device
(Continued)
defibrillator (Continued)
left ventricular coronary venous
lead only 00.52
pulse generator only 00.54
pacemaker (biventricular
pacemaker) (BiV pacemaker)
(CRT-P) (device and one or
more leads) (total system)
00.50
left ventricular coronary venous
lead only 00.52
pulse generator only 00.53
cardiac support device (CSD)
(CorCap™) 37.41
carotid artery stent(s) (stent graft)
00.63

Note: Also use 00.40, 00.41, 00.42, or
00.43 to show the total number of
vessels treated. Use code 00.44 once to
show procedure on a bifurcated vessel.
In addition, use 00.45, 00.46, 00.47, or
00.48 to show the number of vascular
stents inserted.

catheter
abdomen of fetus, for intrauterine
transfusion 75.2
anterior chamber (eye), for
permanent drainage
(glaucoma) 12.79
artery 38.91
bile duct(s) 51.59
common 51.51
endoscopic 51.87
endoscopic 51.87
bladder, indwelling 57.94
suprapubic 57.18
percutaneous (closed)
57.17
bronchus 96.05
with lavage 96.56
central venous NEC 38.93
for
hemodialysis 38.95
pressure monitoring 89.62
peripherally inserted central
catheter (PICC) 38.93
chest 34.04
revision (with lysis of adhesions)
34.04
thoracoscopic 34.06
thoracoscopic 34.06
cranial cavity 01.26
placement via burr hole(s)
01.28
esophagus (nonoperative) 96.06
permanent tube 42.81
intercostal (with water seal), for
drainage 34.04
revision (with lysis of adhesions)
34.04
thoracoscopic 34.06
thoracoscopic 34.06
intracerebral 01.26
placement via burr hole(s)
01.28
spinal canal space (epidural)
(subarachnoid) (subdural) for
infusion of therapeutic or
palliative substances 03.90

Insertion (Continued)
catheter (Continued)
Swan-Ganz (pulmonary) 89.64
transtracheal for oxygenation 31.99
vein NEC 38.93
for renal dialysis 38.95
chest tube 34.04
thoracoscopic 34.06
choledochohepatic tube (for
decompression) 51.43
endoscopic 51.87
circulatory support device
CentriMag® 37.62
external heart assist device
biventricular 37.60
Impella® 37.68   ◀
percutaneous 37.68
temporary 37.62
non-implantable 37.62
pVAD (percutaneous VAD) 37.68
TandemHeart® 37.68
temporary non-implantable
circulatory assist device 37.62
cochlear prosthetic device - see Implant,
cochlear prosthetic device
contraceptive device (intrauterine) 69.7
CorCap™ 37.41
cordis cannula 54.98
coronary (artery)

Note: Also use 00.40, 00.41, 00.42, or
00.43 to show the total number of
vessels treated. Use code 00.44 once to
show procedure on a bifurcated vessel.
In addition, use 00.45, 00.46, 00.47, or
00.48 to show the number of vascular
stents inserted.

stent, drug-eluting 36.07
stent, non-drug-eluting 36.06
Crosby-Cooney button 54.98
CRT-D (biventricular defibrillator) (BiV
ICD) (BiV pacemaker with
defibrillator) (BiV pacing with
defibrillator) (cardiac
resynchronization defibrillator)
(device and one or more leads)
00.51
left ventricular coronary venous
lead only 00.52
pulse generator only 00.54
CRT-P (biventricular pacemaker) (BiV
pacemaker) (cardiac
resynchronization pacemaker)
(device and one or more leads)
00.50
left ventricular coronary venous
lead only 00.52
pulse generator only 00.53
Crutchfield tongs (skull) (with
synchronous skeletal traction)
02.94
Davidson button 54.98
denture (total) 99.97
device
adjustable gastric band and port 44.95
bronchial device NOS 33.79
bronchial substance NOS 33.79
bronchial valve(s) 33.71   ◀▥
multiple lobes 33.73   ◀
single lobe 33.71   ◀
cardiac resynchronization - see
Insertion, cardiac
resynchronization device

Insertion (Continued)
device (Continued)
cardiac support device (CSD) 37.41
CorCap™ 37.41
epicardial support device 37.41
Lap-Band™ 44.95
left atrial appendage 37.90
left atrial filter 37.90
left atrial occluder 37.90
prosthetic cardiac support device
37.41
vascular access 86.07
ventricular support device 37.41
diaphragm, vagina 96.17
drainage tube
kidney 55.02
pelvis 55.12
renal pelvis 55.12
Dynesys® 84.82
elbow prosthesis (total) 81.84
revision 81.97
electrode(s)
bone growth stimulator (invasive)
(percutaneous) (semi-
invasive) - see category 78.9●
brain 02.93
depth 02.93
foramen ovale 02.93
sphenoidal 02.96
depth 02.93
foramen ovale 02.93
gastric 04.92
heart (initial) (transvenous) 37.70
atrium (initial) 37.73
replacement 37.76
atrium and ventricle (initial)
37.72
replacement 37.76
epicardium (sternotomy or
thoracotomy approach)
37.74
left ventricular coronary venous
system 00.52
temporary transvenous
pacemaker system 37.78
during and immediately
following cardiac
surgery 39.64
ventricle (initial) 37.71
replacement 37.76
intracranial 02.93
osteogenic (for bone growth
stimulation) - see category
78.9●
peripheral nerve 04.92
sacral nerve 04.92
sphenoidal 02.96
spine 03.93
electroencephalographic receiver - see
Implant, electroencephalographic
receiver, by site
electronic stimulator - see Implant,
electronic stimulator, by site
electrostimulator - see Implant,
electronic stimulator, by site
endograft(s), endovascular graft(s)
endovascular, abdominal aorta
39.71
endovascular, head and neck vessels
39.72
endovascular, other vessels (for
aneurysm) 39.79
endovascular, thoracic aorta
39.73

◀ New   ◀▥ Revised   ~~deleted~~ Deleted   ● Use Additional Digit(s)   ▥ Omit code

Insertion *(Continued)*

   endoprosthesis
     bile duct 51.87
     femoral head (bipolar) 81.52
     pancreatic duct 52.93
   epidural pegs 02.93
   external fixation device (bone) - *see*
     category 78.1 ●
   facial bone implant (alloplastic)
     (synthetic) 76.92
   filling material, skin (filling of defect)
     86.02
   filter
     vena cava (inferior) (superior)
      (transvenous) 38.7
   fixator, mini device (bone) - *see*
     category 78.1 ●
   frame (stereotactic)
     for radiosurgery 93.59
   Gardner Wells tongs (skull) (with
     synchronous skeletal traction)
     02.94
   gastric bubble (balloon) 44.93
   globe, into eye socket 16.69
   Greenfield filter 38.7
   halo device (skull) (with synchronous
     skeletal traction) 02.94
   Harrington rod - *see also* Fusion, spinal,
     by level
     with dorsal, dorsolumbar fusion
      81.05
   Harris pin 79.15
   heart
     assist system - *see* Implant, heart
      assist system
     cardiac support device (CSD) 37.41
     circulatory assist system - *see*
      Implant, heart assist system
     CorCap™ 37.41
     epicardial support device 37.41
     Impella® 37.68   ◄
     pacemaker - *see* Insertion,
      pacemaker, cardiac
     prosthetic cardiac support device
      37.41
     pump (Kantrowitz) 37.62
     valve - *see* Replacement, heart valve
     ventricular support device 37.41
   hip prosthesis (partial) 81.52
     revision NOS 81.53
      acetabular and femoral
       components (total) 00.70
      acetabular component only 00.71
      acetabular liner and/or femoral
       head only 00.73
      femoral component only 00.72
      femoral head only and/or
       acetabular liner 00.73
      partial
       acetabular component only
        00.71
       acetabular liner and/or
        femoral head only 00.73
       femoral component only 00.72
       femoral head only and/or
        acetabular liner 00.73
      total (acetabular and femoral
       components) 00.70
     total 81.51
      revision
       acetabular and femoral
        components (total) 00.70
       total (acetabular and femoral
        components) 00.70

Insertion *(Continued)*

   Holter valve 02.2
   Hufnagel valve - *see* Replacement,
     heart valve
   implant - *see* Insertion, prosthesis
   infusion pump 86.06
   interbody spinal fusion device 84.51
   intercostal catheter (with water seal)
     for drainage 34.04
     revision (with lysis of adhesions)
      34.04
      thoracoscopic 34.06
   intra-arterial blood gas monitoring
     system 89.60
   intrauterine
     contraceptive device 69.7
     radium (intracavitary) 69.91
     tamponade (nonobstetric) 69.91
   Kantrowitz
     heart pump 37.62
     pulsation balloon (phase-shift)
      37.61
   keratoprosthesis 11.73
   King-Mills umbrella device (heart)
     35.52
   Kirschner wire 93.44
     with reduction of fracture or
      dislocation - *see* Reduction,
      fracture *and* Reduction,
      dislocation
   knee prosthesis (partial) (total) 81.54
     revision NOS 81.55
      femoral component 00.82
      partial
       femoral component 00.82
       patellar component 00.83
       tibial component 00.81
       tibial insert 00.84
      patellar component 00.83
      tibial component 00.81
      tibial insert 00.84
      total (all components) 00.80
   laminaria, cervix 69.93
   Lap-Band™ 44.95
   larynx, valved tube 31.75
   leads - *see* Insertion, electrode(s)
   lens, prosthetic (intraocular) 13.70
     with cataract extraction, one-stage
      13.71
     secondary (subsequent to cataract
      extraction) 13.72
   limb lengthening device, internal, NOS
     84.54
     with kinetic distraction 84.53
   loop recorder 37.79
   metal staples into epiphyseal plate - *see*
     also Stapling, epiphyseal plate
     78.20
   minifixator device (bone) - *see* category
     78.1 ●
   M-Brace™ 84.82
   Mobitz-Uddin umbrella, vena cava 38.7
   mold, vagina 96.15
   Moore (cup) 81.52
   myringotomy device (button) (tube)
     20.01
     with intubation 20.01
   nasobiliary drainage tube (endoscopic)
     51.86
   nasogastric tube
     for
      decompression, intestinal 96.07
      feeding 96.6
   naso-intestinal tube 96.08

Insertion *(Continued)*

   nasolacrimal tube or stent 09.44
   nasopancreatic drainage tube
     (endoscopic) 52.97
   neuropacemaker - *see* Implant,
     neurostimulator, by site
   neurostimulator - *see* Implant,
     neurostimulator, by site
   non-coronary vessel
     stent(s) (stent graft)

> Note: Also use 00.40, 00.41, 00.42, or
> 00.43 to show the total number of
> vessels treated. Use code 00.44 once to
> show procedure on a bifurcated vessel.
> In addition, use 00.45, 00.46, 00.47, or
> 00.48 to show the number of vascular
> stents inserted.

     with angioplasty or atherectomy
      39.50
     with bypass - *omit code*
     basilar 00.64
     carotid 00.63
     extracranial 00.64
     intracranial 00.65
     peripheral 39.90
      bare, drug-coated 39.90
      drug-eluting 00.55
     vertebral 00.64
   non-invasive (surface)
     (transcutaneous)
     stimulator 99.86
   obturator (orthodontic) 24.7
   ocular implant
     with synchronous
      enucleation 16.42
       with muscle attachment to
        implant 16.41
      evisceration 16.31
     following or secondary to
      enucleation 16.61
      evisceration 16.61
   Ommaya reservoir 02.2
   orbital implant (stent) (outside muscle
     cone) 16.69
     with orbitotomy 16.02
   orthodontic appliance (obturator)
     (wiring) 24.7
   outflow tract prosthesis (gusset type)
     (heart)
     in
      pulmonary valvuloplasty 35.26
      total repair of tetralogy of
       Fallot 35.81
   pacemaker
     brain - *see* Implant, neurostimulator,
      brain
     cardiac (device) (initial) (permanent)
      (replacement) 37.80
      dual-chamber device (initial)
       37.83
       replacement 37.87
      during and immediately
       following cardiac surgery
       39.64
      resynchronization (biventricular
       pacemaker) (BiV
       pacemaker) (CRT-P)
       (device)
       device only (initial)
        (replacement) 00.53
       total system (device and one
        or more leads) 00.50

Insertion *(Continued)*
  pacemaker *(Continued)*
    cardiac *(Continued)*
      resynchronization *(Continued)*
        transvenous lead into left
          ventricular coronary
          venous system 00.52
        single-chamber device (initial)
          37.81
          rate responsive 37.82
          replacement 37.85
            rate responsive 37.86
        temporary transvenous
          pacemaker system 37.78
          during and immediately
            following cardiac
            surgery 39.64
    carotid 39.8
    gastric 04.92
    heart - *see* Insertion, pacemaker,
      cardiac
    intracranial - *see* Implant,
      neurostimulator, intracranial
    neural - *see* Implant,
      neurostimulator, by site
    peripheral nerve - *see* Implant,
      neurostimulator, peripheral
      nerve
    spine - *see* Implant, neurostimulator,
      spine
  pacing catheter - *see* Insertion,
    pacemaker, cardiac
  pack
    auditory canal, external 96.11
    cervix (nonobstetrical) 67.0
      after delivery or abortion 75.8
      to assist delivery or induce labor
        73.1
    rectum 96.19
    sella turcica 07.79
    vagina (nonobstetrical) 96.14
      after delivery or abortion 75.8
  palatal implant 27.64
  penile prosthesis (internal) (non-
    inflatable) 64.95
    inflatable (internal) 64.97
  periodontal splint (orthodontic) 24.7
  peripheral blood vessel - *see* non-
    coronary
  pessary
    cervix 96.18
      to assist delivery or induce labor
        73.1
    vagina 96.18
  pharyngeal valve, artificial 31.75
  port, vascular access 86.07
  prostaglandin suppository (for
    abortion) 96.49
  prosthesis, prosthetic device
    acetabulum (partial) 81.52
      hip 81.52
        revision NOS 81.53
          acetabular and femoral
            components (total)
            00.70
          acetabular component only
            00.71
          acetabular liner and/or
            femoral head only
            00.73
          femoral component only
            00.72
          femoral head only and/or
            acetabular liner 00.73

Insertion *(Continued)*
  prosthesis, prosthetic device *(Continued)*
    acetabulum *(Continued)*
      hip *(Continued)*
        revision NOS *(Continued)*
          partial
            acetabular component
              only 00.71
            acetabular liner and/or
              femoral head only
              00.73
            femoral component only
              00.72
            femoral head only and/
              or acetabular liner
              00.73
          total (acetabular and
            femoral components)
            00.70
        revision 81.53
    ankle (total) 81.56
    arm (bioelectric) (cineplastic)
      (kineplastic) 84.44
    biliary tract 51.99
    breast (bilateral) 85.54
      unilateral 85.53
    cardiac support device (CSD)
      (CorCap™) 37.41
    chin (polyethylene) (silastic) 76.68
    elbow (total) 81.84
      revision 81.97
    extremity (bioelectric) (cineplastic)
      (kineplastic) 84.40
      lower 84.48
      upper 84.44
    fallopian tube 66.93
    femoral head (Austin-Moore)
      (bipolar) (Eicher) (Thompson)
      81.52
    hip (partial) 81.52
      revision NOS 81.53
        acetabular and femoral
          components (total) 00.70
        acetabular component only
          00.71
        acetabular liner and/or
          femoral head only 00.73
        femoral component only 00.72
        femoral head only and/or
          acetabular liner 00.73
        partial
          acetabular component only
           00.71
          acetabular liner and/or
           femoral head only
           00.73
          femoral component only
           00.72
          femoral head only and/or
           acetabular liner 00.73
        total (acetabular and femoral
          components) 00.70
      total 81.51
        revision
          acetabular and femoral
           components (total)
           00.70
          total (acetabular and
           femoral components)
           00.70
    joint - *see* Arthroplasty
    knee (partial) (total) 81.54
      revision NOS 81.55
        femoral component 00.82

Insertion *(Continued)*
  prosthesis, prosthetic device *(Continued)*
    knee *(Continued)*
      revision NOS *(Continued)*
        partial
          femoral component 00.82
          patellar component 00.83
          tibial component 00.81
          tibial insert 00.84
        patellar component 00.83
        tibial component 00.81
        tibial insert 00.84
        total (all components) 00.80
    leg (bioelectric) (cineplastic)
      (kineplastic) 84.48
    lens 13.91
    ocular (secondary) 16.61
      with orbital exenteration 16.42
    outflow tract (gusset type) (heart)
      in
        pulmonary valvuloplasty 35.26
        total repair of tetralogy of
          Fallot 35.81
    penis (internal) (noninflatable) 64.95
      with
        construction 64.43
        reconstruction 64.44
      inflatable (internal) 64.97
    Rosen (for urinary incontinence)
      59.79
    shoulder
      partial 81.81
      revision 81.97
      total 81.80
    spine
      artificial disc, NOS 84.60
        cervical 84.62
          nucleus 84.61
          partial 84.61
          total 84.62
        lumbar, lumbosacral 84.65
          nucleus 84.64
          partial 84.64
          total 84.65
        thoracic (partial) (total) 84.63
      other device 84.59
    testicular (bilateral) (unilateral) 62.7
    toe 81.57
      hallux valgus repair 77.59
    vagina
      synthetic 70.95
  pseudophakos - *see also* Insertion, lens
    13.70
  pump, infusion 86.06
  radioactive isotope 92.27
  radium 92.27
  radon seeds 92.27,
  Reuter bobbin (with intubation) 20.01
  Rickham reservoir 02.2
  Rosen prosthesis (for urinary
    incontinence) 59.79
  Scribner shunt 39.93
  Sengstaken-Blakemore tube 96.06
  sensor (lead)
    intra-aneurysm sac pressure
      monitoring device 00.58
    intra-arterial, for continuous blood
      gas monitoring 89.60
    intracardiac or great vessel
      hemodynamic monitoring
      00.56 ◀▥
  shunt - *see* Shunt ◀
  sieve, vena cava 38.7
  skeletal muscle stimulator 83.92

Insertion (Continued)
skull
plate 02.05
stereotactic frame 93.59
tongs (Barton) (caliper) (Garder Wells) (Vinke) (with synchronous skeletal traction) 02.94
spacer (cement) (joint) (methylmethacrylate) 84.56
spine 84.51
sphenoidal electrodes 02.96
spine
bone void filler 84.55 ◄▥
that with percutaneous vertebral augmentation 81.66
that with percutaneous vertebroplasty 81.65
cage (BAK) 84.51
facet replacement device(s) 84.84
interbody spinal fusion device 84.51
interspinous process decompression device 84.80
non-fusion stabilization device - see category 84.8 ●
pedicle-based dynamic stabilization device(s) 84.82
posterior motion preservation device(s) - see category 84.8 ●
spacer 84.51
Spitz-Holter valve 02.2
Steinmann pin 93.44
with reduction of fracture or dislocation - see Reduction, fracture and Reduction, dislocation
stent(s) (stent graft)
artery (bare) (bonded) (drug coated) (non-drug-eluting)

Note: Also use 00.40, 00.41, 00.42, or 00.43 to show the total number of vessels treated. Use code 00.44 once to show procedure on a bifurcated vessel. In addition, use 00.45, 00.46, 00.47, or 00.48 to show the number of vascular stents inserted.

basilar 00.64
carotid 00.63
cerebrovascular
cerebral (intracranial) 00.65
precerebral (extracranial) 00.64
carotid 00.63
coronary (bare) (bonded) (drug coated) (non-drug-eluting) 36.06
drug-eluting 36.07
extracranial 00.64
carotid 00.63
intracranial 00.65
non-coronary vessel
basilar 00.64
carotid 00.63
extracranial 00.64
intracranial 00.65
peripheral 39.90
bare, drug-coated 39.90
drug-eluting 00.55
vertebral 00.64
bile duct 51.43
endoscopic 51.87
percutaneous transhepatic 51.98

Insertion (Continued)
stent(s) (Continued)
colon ◄
endoscopic (fluoroscopic guidance) 46.86 ◄
other 46.87 ◄
coronary (artery) (bare) (bonded) (drug coated) (non-drug-eluting) 36.06

Note: Also use 00.40, 00.41, 00.42, or 00.43 to show the total number of vessels treated. Use code 00.44 once to show procedure on a bifurcated vessel. In addition, use 00.45, 00.46, 00.47, or 00.48 to show the number of vascular stents inserted.

drug-eluting 36.07
esophagus (endoscopic) (fluoroscopic) 42.81
mesenteric 39.90
bare, drug-coated 39.90
drug-eluting 00.55
non-coronary vessel

Note: Also use 00.40, 00.41, 00.42, or 00.43 to show the total number of vessels treated. Use code 00.44 once to show procedure on a bifurcated vessel. In addition, use 00.45, 00.46, 00.47, or 00.48 to show the number of vascular stents inserted.

with angioplasty or atherectomy 39.50
with bypass - omit code
basilar 00.64
carotid 00.63
extracranial 00.64
intracranial 00.65
mesenteric 39.90
bare, drug-coated 39.90
drug-eluting 00.55
peripheral 39.90
bare, drug-coated 39.90
drug-eluting 00.55
renal 39.90
bare, drug-coated 39.90
drug-eluting 00.55
vertebral 00.64
pancreatic duct 52.92
endoscopic 52.93
peripheral 39.90

Note: Also use 00.40, 00.41, 00.42, or 00.43 to show the total number of vessels treated. Use code 00.44 once to show procedure on a bifurcated vessel. In addition, use 00.45, 00.46, 00.47, or 00.48 to show the number of vascular stents inserted.

bare, drug-coated 39.90
drug-eluting 00.55
precerebral 00.64

Note: Also use 00.40, 00.41, 00.42 or 00.43 to show the total number of vessels treated. Use code 00.44 once to show procedure on a bifurcated vessel. In addition, use 00.45, 00.46, 00.47, or 00.48 to show the number of vascular stents inserted.

Insertion (Continued)
stent(s) (Continued)
renal 39.90
bare, drug-coated 39.90
drug-eluting 00.55
subclavian 39.90

Note: Also use 00.40, 00.41, 00.42, or 00.43 to show the total number of vessels treated. Use code 00.44 once to show procedure on a bifurcated vessel. In addition, use 00.45, 00.46, 00.47, or 00.48 to show the number of vascular stents inserted.

bare, drug-coated 39.90
drug-eluting 00.55
tracheobronchial 96.05
vertebral 00.64

Note: Also use 00.40, 00.41, 00.42, or 00.43 to show the total number of vessels treated. Use code 00.44 once to show procedure on a bifurcated vessel. In addition, use 00.45, 00.46, 00.47, or 00.48 to show the number of vascular stents inserted.

stimoceiver - see Implant, neurostimulator, by site
stimulator for bone growth - see category 78.9 ●
subdural
grids 02.93
strips 02.93
suppository
prostaglandin (for abortion) 96.49
vagina 96.49
Swan-Ganz catheter (pulmonary) 89.64
tampon
esophagus 96.06
uterus 69.91
vagina 96.14
after delivery or abortion 75.8
Tandem™ heart 37.68
telescope (IMT) (miniature) 13.91
testicular prosthesis (bilateral) (unilateral) 62.7
tissue expander (skin) NEC 86.93
breast 85.95
tissue mandril (peripheral vessel) (Dacron) (Spark's type) 39.99
with
blood vessel repair 39.56
vascular bypass or shunt - see Bypass, vascular
tongs, skull (with synchronous skeletal traction) 02.94
totally implanted device for bone growth (invasive) - see category 78.9 ●
tube - see also Catheterization and Intubation
bile duct 51.43
endoscopic 51.87
chest 34.04
revision (with lysis of adhesions) 34.04
thoracoscopic 34.06
thoracoscopic 34.06
endotracheal 96.04
esophagus (nonoperative) (Sengstaken) 96.06
permanent (silicone) (Souttar) 42.81

IOM (intra-operative neurophysiologic
    monitoring) 00.94
Ionization, medical 99.27
Iontherapy 99.27
Iontophoresis 99.27
Iridectomy (basal) (buttonhole) (optical)
    (peripheral) (total) 12.14
   with
      capsulectomy 13.65
      cataract extraction - *see* Extraction,
        cataract
      filtering operation (for glaucoma)
        NEC 12.65
      scleral
        fistulization 12.65
        thermocauterization 12.62
        trephination 12.61
Iridencleisis 12.63
Iridesis 12.63
Irido-capsulectomy 13.65
Iridocyclectomy 12.44
Iridocystectomy 12.42
Iridodesis 12.63
Iridoplasty NEC 12.39
Iridosclerectomy 12.65
Iridosclerotomy 12.69
Iridotasis 12.63
Iridotomy 12.12
   by photocoagulation 12.12
   with transfixion 12.11
   for iris bombé 12.11
   specified type NEC 12.12
Iron lung 93.99

Irradiation
   gamma, stereotactic 92.32
Irrigation
   anterior chamber (eye) 12.91
   bronchus NEC 96.56
   canaliculus 09.42
   catheter
      ureter 96.46
      urinary, indwelling NEC 96.48
      vascular 96.57
      ventricular 02.41
      wound 96.58
   cholecystostomy 96.41
   cornea 96.51
      with removal of foreign body 98.21
   corpus cavernosum 64.98
   cystostomy 96.47
   ear (removal of cerumen) 96.52
   enterostomy 96.36
   eye 96.51
      with removal of foreign body
        98.21
   gastrostomy 96.36
   lacrimal
      canaliculi 09.42
      punctum 09.41
   muscle 83.02
      hand 82.02
   nasal
      passages 96.53
      sinus 22.00
   nasolacrimal duct 09.43
      with insertion of tube or stent 09.44

Irrigation *(Continued)*
   nephrostomy 96.45
   peritoneal 54.25
   pyelostomy 96.45
   rectal 96.39
   stomach 96.33
   tendon (sheath) 83.01
      hand 82.01
   trachea NEC 96.56
   traumatic cataract 13.3
   tube
      biliary NEC 96.41
      nasogastric NEC 96.34
      pancreatic 96.42
   ureterostomy 96.46
   ventricular shunt 02.41
   wound (cleaning) NEC 96.59
Irving operation (tubal ligation) 66.32
Irwin operation - *see also* Osteotomy 77.30
Ischiectomy (partial) 77.89
   total 77.99
Ischiopubiotomy 77.39
Isolation
   after contact with infectious disease
      99.84
   ileal loop 45.51
   intestinal segment or pedicle flap
      large 45.52
      small 45.51
Isthmectomy, thyroid - *see also*
      Thyroidectomy, partial 06.39
IVUS - *see* Ultrasound, intravascular, by
   site ◀

J

Jaboulay operation
    (gastroduodenostomy) 44.39
  laparoscopic 44.38
Janeway operation (permanent
    gastrostomy) 43.19
Jatene operation (arterial switch)
    35.84
Jejunectomy 45.62
Jejunocecostomy 45.93
Jejunocholecystostomy 51.32
Jejunocolostomy 45.93

Jejunoileostomy 45.91
Jejunojejunostomy 45.91
Jejunopexy 46.61
Jejunorrhaphy 46.73
Jejunostomy (feeding) 46.39
  delayed opening 46.31
  loop 46.01
  percutaneous (endoscopic) (PEJ)
    46.32
  revision 46.41
Jejunotomy 45.02
Johanson operation (urethral
    reconstruction) 58.46

Jones operation
  claw toe (transfer of extensor hallucis
    longus tendon) 77.57
    modified (with arthrodesis) 77.57
  dacryocystorhinostomy 09.81
  hammer toe (interphalangeal fusion)
    77.56
  modified (tendon transfer with
    arthrodesis) 77.57
  repair of peroneal tendon 83.88
Joplin operation (exostectomy with
    tendon transfer) 77.53

◀ New   ◀▥ Revised   ~~deleted~~ Deleted   ● Use Additional Digit(s)   ▨ Omit code

K

Kader operation (temporary gastrostomy) 43.19

Kasai portoenterostomy 51.37

Kaufman operation (for urinary stress incontinence) 59.79

Kazanjiian operation (buccal vestibular sulcus extension) 24.91

Kehr operation (hepatopexy) 50.69

Keller operation (bunionectomy) 77.59

Kelly (-Kennedy) operation (urethrovesical plication) 59.3

Kelly-Stoeckel operation (urethrovesical plication) 59.3

Kelotomy 53.9

Keratectomy (complete) (partial) (superficial) 11.49
  for pterygium 11.39
    with corneal graft 11.32

Keratocentesis (for hyphema) 12.91

Keratomileusis 11.71

Keratophakia 11.72

Keratoplasty (tectonic) (with autograft) (with homograft) 11.60
  lamellar (nonpenetrating) (with homograft) 11.62
    with autograft 11.61

Keratoplasty (Continued)
  penetrating (full-thickness) (with homograft) 11.64
    with autograft 11.63
  perforating - see Keratoplasty, penetrating
  refractive 11.71
  specified type NEC 11.69

Keratoprosthesis 11.73

Keratotomy (delimiting) (posterior) 11.1
  radial (refractive) 11.75

Kerr operation (low cervical cesarean section) 74.1

Kessler operation (arthroplasty, carpometacarpal joint) 81.74

Kidner operation (excision of accessory navicular bone) (with tendon transfer) 77.98

Killian operation (frontal sinusotomy) 22.41

Kineplasty - see Cineplasty

King-Steelquist operation (hind-quarter amputation) 84.19

Kirk operation (amputation through thigh) 84.17

Kock pouch
  bowel anastomosis - *omit code*
  continent ileostomy 46.22

Kock pouch (Continued)
  cutaneous uretero-ileostomy 56.51
  ESWL (electrocorporeal shockwave lithotripsy) 98.51
  removal, calculus 57.19
  revision, cutaneous uretero-ileostomy 56.52
  urinary diversion procedure 56.51

Kockogram (ileal conduitogram) 87.78

Kockoscopy 45.12

Kondoleon operation (correction of lymph-edema) 40.9

Krause operation (sympathetic denervation) 05.29

Kroener operation (partial salpingectomy) 66.69

Kroenlein operation (lateral orbitotomy) 16.01

Kronig operation (low cervical cesarean section) 74.1

Krunkenberg operation (reconstruction of below-elbow amputation) 82.89

Kuhnt-Szymanowski operation (ectropion repair with lid reconstruction) 08.44

Kyphoplasty 81.66

L

Labbe operation (gastrotomy) 43.0
Labiectomy (bilateral) 71.62
  unilateral 71.61
Labyrinthectomy (transtympanic) 20.79
Labyrinthotomy (transtympanic) 20.79
Ladd operation (mobilization of intestine) 54.95
Lagrange operation (iridosclerectomy) 12.65
Lambrinudi operation (triple arthrodesis) 81.12
Laminectomy (decompression) (for exploration) 03.09
  as operative approach - omit code
  with
    excision of herniated intervertebral disc (nucleus pulposus) 80.51
    excision of other intraspinal lesion (tumor) 03.4
  reopening of site 03.02
Laminography - see Radiography
Laminoplasty, expansile 03.09
Laminotomy (decompression) (for exploration) 03.09
  as operative approach - omit code
  reopening of site 03.02
Langenbeck operation (cleft palate repair) 27.62
Laparoamnioscopy 75.31
Laparorrhaphy 54.63
Laparoscopy 54.21
  with
    biopsy (intra-abdominal) 54.24
      uterine ligaments 68.15
      uterus 68.16
    destruction of fallopian tubes - see Destruction, fallopian tube
Laparotomy NEC 54.19
  as operative approach - omit code
  exploratory (pelvic) 54.11
  reopening of recent operative site (for control of hemorrhage) (for exploration) (for incision of hematoma) 54.12
Laparotrachelotomy 74.1
Lapidus operation (bunionectomy with metatarsal osteotomy) 77.51
Larry operation (shoulder disarticulation) 84.08
Laryngectomy
  with radical neck dissection (with synchronous thyroidectomy) (with synchronous tracheostomy) 30.4
  complete (with partial laryngectomy) (with synchronous tracheostomy) 30.3
    with radical neck dissection (with synchronous thyroidectomy) (with synchronous tracheostomy) 30.4
  frontolateral partial (extended) 30.29
  glottosupraglottic partial 30.29
  lateral partial 30.29
  partial (frontolateral) (glottosupraglottic) (lateral) (submucous) (supraglottic) (vertical) 30.29
  radical (with synchronous thyroidectomy) (with synchronous tracheostomy) 30.4

Laryngectomy (Continued)
  submucous (partial) 30.29
  supraglottic partial 30.29
  total (with partial pharyngectomy) (with synchronous tracheostomy) 30.3
    with radical neck dissection (with synchronous thyroidectomy) (with synchronous tracheostomy) 30.4
  vertical partial 30.29
  wide field 30.3
Laryngocentesis 31.3
Laryngoesophagectomy 30.4
Laryngofissure 30.29
Laryngogram 87.09
  contrast 87.07
Laryngopharyngectomy (with synchronous tracheostomy) 30.3
  radical (with synchronous thyroidectomy) 30.4
Laryngopharyngoesophagectomy (with synchronous tracheostomy) 30.3
  with radical neck dissection (with synchronous thyroidectomy) 30.4
Laryngoplasty 31.69
Laryngorrhaphy 31.61
Laryngoscopy (suspension) (through artificial stoma) 31.42
Laryngostomy (permanent) 31.29
  revision 31.63
  temporary (emergency) 31.1
Laryngotomy 31.3
Laryngotracheobronchoscopy 33.23
  with biopsy 33.24
Laryngotracheoscopy 31.42
Laryngotracheostomy (permanent) 31.29
  temporary (emergency) 31.1
Laryngotracheotomy (temporary) 31.1
  permanent 31.29
Laser - see also Coagulation, Destruction, and Photocoagulation by site
  angioplasty, percutaneous transluminal 39.59
    coronary - see Angioplasty, coronary
Laser interstitial thermal therapy (LITT)
  under guidance ◀
  lesion ◀
    brain 17.61 ◀
    breast 17.69 ◀
    head and neck 17.62 ◀
    liver 17.63 ◀
    lung 17.69 ◀
    prostate 17.69 ◀
    thyroid 17.62 ◀
Lash operation
  internal cervical os repair 67.59
  laparoscopic supracervical hysterectomy 68.31
LASIK (Laser-assisted in situ keratomileusis) 11.71
Latzko operation
  cesarean section 74.2
  colpocleisis 70.8
Lavage
  antral 22.00
  bronchus NEC 96.56
    diagnostic (endoscopic) bronchoalveolar lavage (BAL) 33.24
  endotracheal 96.56

Lavage (Continued)
  gastric 96.33
  lung (total) (whole) 33.99
    diagnostic (endoscopic) bronchoalveolar lavage (BAL) 33.24
  nasal sinus(es) 22.00
    by puncture 22.01
    through natural ostium 22.02
  peritoneal (diagnostic) 54.25
  trachea NEC 96.56
Leadbetter operation (urethral reconstruction) 58.46
Leadbetter-Politano operation (ureteroneocystostomy) 56.74
LEEP (loop electrosurgical excision procedure) of cervix 67.32
Le Fort operation (colpocleisis) 70.8
LeMesurier operation (cleft lip repair) 27.54
Lengthening
  bone (with bone graft) 78.30
    femur 78.35
    for reconstruction of thumb 82.69
    specified site NEC 78.39 - see also category 78.3●
    tibia 78.37
    ulna 78.33
  extraocular muscle NEC 15.21
    multiple (two or more muscles) 15.4
  fascia 83.89
    hand 82.89
  hamstring NEC 83.85
  heel cord 83.85
  leg
    femur 78.35
    tibia 78.37
  levator palpebrae muscle 08.38
  muscle 83.85
    extraocular 15.21
      multiple (two or more muscles) 15.4
    hand 82.55
  palate 27.62
    secondary or subsequent 27.63
  tendon 83.85
    for claw toe repair 77.57
    hand 82.55
Leriche operation (periarterial sympathectomy) 05.25
Leucotomy, leukotomy 01.32
Leukopheresis, therapeutic 99.72
Lid suture operation (blepharoptosis) 08.31
Ligation
  adrenal vessel (artery) (vein) 07.43
  aneurysm 39.52
  appendages, dermal 86.26
  arteriovenous fistula 39.53
    coronary artery 36.99
  artery 38.80
    abdominal 38.86
    adrenal 07.43
    aorta (arch) (ascending) (descending) 38.84
    coronary (anomalous) 36.99
    ethmoidal 21.04
    external carotid 21.06
    for control of epistaxis - see Control, epistaxis
    head and neck NEC 38.82
    intracranial NEC 38.81
    lower limb 38.88

◀ New   ◀▥ Revised   deleted Deleted   ● Use Additional Digit(s)   ▨ Omit code

Ligation (Continued)
  artery (Continued)
    maxillary (transantral) 21.05
    middle meningeal 02.13
    thoracic NEC 38.85
    thyroid 06.92
    upper limb 38.83
  atrium, heart 37.99
  auricle, heart 37.99
  bleeding vessel - see Control,
    hemorrhage
  blood vessel 38.80
    abdominal
      artery 38.86
      vein 38.87
    adrenal 07.43
    aorta (arch) (ascending)
      (descending) 38.84
    esophagus 42.91
      endoscopic 42.33
    head and neck 38.82
    intracranial NEC 38.81
    lower limb
      artery 38.88
      vein 38.89
    meningeal (artery) (longitudinal
      sinus) 02.13
    thoracic NEC 38.85
    thyroid 06.92
    upper limb (artery) (vein) 38.83
  bronchus 33.92
  cisterna chyli 40.64
  coronary
    artery (anomalous) 36.99
    sinus 36.39
  dermal appendage 86.26
  ductus arteriosus, patent 38.85
  esophageal vessel 42.91
    endoscopic 42.33
  ethmoidal artery 21.04
  external carotid artery 21.06
  fallopian tube (bilateral) (remaining)
    (solitary) 66.39
    by endoscopy (culdoscopy)
      (hysteroscopy) (laparoscopy)
      (peritoneoscopy) 66.29
    with
      crushing 66.31
        by endoscopy (laparoscopy)
          66.21
      division 66.32
        by endoscopy (culdoscopy)
          (laparoscopy)
          (peritoneoscopy) 66.22
      Falope ring 66.39
        by endoscopy (laparoscopy)
          66.29
    unilateral 66.92
  fistula, arteriovenous 39.53
    coronary artery 36.99
  gastric
    artery 38.86
    varices 44.91
      endoscopic 43.41
  hemorrhoids 49.45
  longitudinal sinus (superior) 02.13
  lymphatic (channel) (peripheral) 40.9
    thoracic duct 40.64
  maxillary artery 21.05
  meningeal vessel 02.13
  spermatic
    cord 63.72
      varicocele 63.1
    vein (high) 63.1

Ligation (Continued)
  splenic vessels 38.86
  subclavian artery 38.85
  superior longitudinal sinus 02.13
  supernumerary digit 86.26
  thoracic duct 40.64
  thyroid vessel (artery) (vein) 06.92
  toes (supernumerary) 86.26
  tooth 93.55
    impacted 24.6
  ulcer (peptic) (base) (bed) (bleeding
    vessel) 44.40
    duodenal 44.42
    gastric 44.41
  ureter 56.95
  varices
    esophageal 42.91
      endoscopic 42.33
    gastric 44.91
      endoscopic 43.41
    peripheral vein (lower limb) 38.59
      upper limb 38.53
  varicocele 63.1
  vas deferens 63.71
  vein 38.80
    abdominal 38.87
    adrenal 07.43
    head and neck NEC 38.82
    intracranial NEC 38.81
    lower limb 38.89
    spermatic, high 63.1
    thoracic NEC 38.85
    thyroid 06.92
    upper limb 38.83
    varicose 38.50
      abdominal 38.57
      esophagus 42.91
        endoscopic 42.33
      gastric 44.91
        endoscopic 43.41
      head and neck 38.52
      intracranial NEC 38.51
      lower limb 38.59
      stomach 44.91
      thoracic NEC 38.55
      upper limb 38.53
  vena cava, inferior 38.7
  venous connection between anomalous
    vein to
    left innominate vein 35.82
    superior vena cava 35.82
  wart 86.26
Light coagulation - see Photocoagulation
Lindholm operation (repair of ruptured
  tendon) 83.88
Lingulectomy, lung 32.39
Linton operation (varicose vein) 38.59
Lipectomy (subcutaneous tissue)
  (abdominal) (submental) 86.83
Liposuction 86.83
Lip reading training 95.49
Lip shave 27.43
Lisfranc operation
  foot amputation 84.12
  shoulder disarticulation 84.08
Litholapaxy, bladder 57.0
  by incision 57.19
Lithotomy
  bile passage 51.49
  bladder (urinary) 57.19
  common duct 51.41
    percutaneous 51.96
  gallbladder 51.04
  hepatic duct 51.49

Lithotomy (Continued)
  kidney 55.01
    percutaneous 55.03
  ureter 56.2
Lithotripsy
  bile duct NEC 51.49
    extracorporeal shockwave (ESWL)
      98.52
  bladder 57.0
    with ultrasonic fragmentation 57.0
      [59.95]
    extracorporeal shockwave (ESWL)
      98.51
  extracorporeal shockwave (ESWL)
    NEC 98.59
    bile duct 98.52
    bladder (urinary) 98.51
    gallbladder 98.52
    kidney 98.51
    Kock pouch 98.51
    renal pelvis 98.51
    specified site NEC 98.59
    ureter 98.51
  gallbladder NEC 51.04
    endoscopic 51.88
    extracorporeal shockwave (ESWL)
      98.52
  kidney 56.0
    extracorporeal shockwave (ESWL)
      98.51
    percutaneous nephrostomy with
      fragmentation (laser)
      (ultrasound) 55.04
  renal pelvis 56.0
    extracorporeal shockwave (ESWL)
      98.51
    percutaneous nephrostomy with
      fragmentation (laser)
      (ultrasound) 55.04
  ureter 56.0
    extracorporeal shock wave (ESWL)
      98.51
LITT (laser interstitial thermal therapy) ◀
  under guidance ◀
  lesion ◀
    brain 17.61 ◀
    breast 17.69 ◀
    head and neck 17.62 ◀
    liver 17.63 ◀
    lung 17.69 ◀
    prostate 17.69 ◀
    thyroid 17.62 ◀
Littlewood operation (forequarter
  amputation) 84.09
LLETZ (large loop excision of the
  transformation zone) of cervix 67.32
Lloyd-Davies operation
  (abdominoperineal resection), NOS
  48.50
  laparoscopic 48.51
  open 48.52
  other 48.59
Lobectomy
  brain 01.53
    partial 01.59
  liver (with partial excision of adjacent
    lobes) 50.3
  lung (complete) 32.49
    partial 32.39
      thoracoscopic 32.30
    segmental (with resection of
      adjacent lobes) 32.49
      thoracoscopic 32.41
    thoracoscopic 32.41

Lobectomy (Continued)
 thyroid (total) (unilateral) (with
  removal of isthmus) (with
  removal of portion of remaining
  lobe) 06.2
  partial - see also Thyroidectomy,
   partial 06.39
  substernal 06.51
  subtotal - see also Thyroidectomy,
   partial 06.39
Lobotomy, brain 01.32
Localization, placenta 88.78
 by RISA injection 92.17
Longmire operation (bile duct
  anastomosis) 51.39
Loop ileal stoma (see also Ileostomy)
  46.01
Loopogram 87.78
Looposcopy (ileal conduit) 56.35
Lord operation
 dilation of anal canal for hemorrhoids
  49.49
 hemorrhoidectomy 49.49
 orchidopexy 62.5
Lower GI series (x-ray) 87.64
Lucas and Murray operation (knee
  arthrodesis with plate) 81.22
Lumpectomy
 breast 85.21
 specified site - see Excision, lesion, by
  site
Lymphadenectomy (simple) - see also
  Excision, lymph, node 40.29
Lymphadenotomy 40.0
Lymphangiectomy (radical) - see also
  Excision, lymph, node, by site,
  radical 40.50
Lymphangiogram
 abdominal 88.04
 cervical 87.08
 intrathoracic 87.34
 lower limb 88.36
 pelvic 88.04
 upper limb 88.34
Lymphangioplasty 40.9
Lymphangiorrhaphy 40.9
Lymphangiotomy 40.0
Lymphaticostomy 40.9
 thoracic duct 40.62
Lysis
 adhesions

> Note: blunt - *omit code*
> digital - *omit code*
> manual - *omit code*
> mechanical - *omit code*
> without instrumentation - *omit*
> *code*

  abdominal 54.59
   laparoscopic 54.51
  appendiceal 54.59
   laparoscopic 54.51
  artery-vein-nerve bundle 39.91
  biliary tract 54.59
   laparoscopic 54.51

Lysis (Continued)
 adhesions (Continued)
  bladder (neck) (intraluminal) 57.12
   external 59.11
    laparoscopic 59.12
   transurethral 57.41
  blood vessels 39.91
  bone - see category 78.4●
  bursa 83.91
   by stretching or manipulation
    93.28
   hand 82.91
  cartilage of joint 93.26
  chest wall 33.99
  choanae (nasopharynx) 29.54
  conjunctiva 10.5
  corneovitreal 12.34
  cortical (brain) 02.91
  ear, middle 20.23
  Eustachian tube 20.8
  extraocular muscle 15.7
  extrauterine 54.59
   laparoscopic 54.51
  eyelid 08.09
   and conjunctiva 10.5
  eye muscle 15.7
  fallopian tube 65.89
   laparoscopic 65.81
  fascia 83.91
   hand 82.91
    by stretching or manipulation
     93.26
  gallbladder 54.59
   laparoscopic 54.51
  ganglion (peripheral) NEC 04.49
   cranial NEC 04.42
  hand 82.91
   by stretching or manipulation
    93.26
  heart 37.10
  intestines 54.59
   laparoscopic 54.51
  iris (posterior) 12.33
   anterior 12.32
  joint (capsule) (structure) - see also
    Division, joint capsule 80.40
  kidney 59.02
   laparoscopic 59.03
  labia (vulva) 71.01
  larynx 31.92
  liver 54.59
   laparoscopic 54.51
  lung (for collapse of lung) 33.39
  mediastinum 34.99
  meninges (spinal) 03.6
   cortical 02.91
  middle ear 20.23
  muscle 83.91
   by stretching or manipulation
    93.27
   extraocular 15.7
   hand 82.91
    by stretching or manipulation
     93.26
  nasopharynx 29.54

Lysis (Continued)
 adhesions (Continued)
  nerve (peripheral) NEC 04.49
   cranial NEC 04.42
   roots, spinal 03.6
   trigeminal 04.41
  nose, nasal 21.91
  ocular muscle 15.7
  ovary 65.89
   laparoscopic 65.81
  pelvic 54.59
   laparoscopic 54.51
  penile 64.93
  pericardium 37.12
  perineal (female) 71.01
  peripheral vessels 39.91
  perirectal 48.81
  perirenal 59.02
   laparoscopic 59.03
  peritoneum (pelvic) 54.59
   laparoscopic 54.51
  periureteral 59.02
   laparoscopic 59.03
  perivesical 59.11
   laparoscopic 59.12
  pharynx 29.54
  pleura (for collapse of lung) 33.39
  spermatic cord 63.94
  spinal (cord) (meninges) (nerve
    roots) 03.6
  spleen 54.59
   laparoscopic 54.51
  tendon 83.91
   by stretching or manipulation
    93.27
   hand 82.91
    by stretching or manipulation
     93.26
  thorax 34.99
  tongue 25.93
  trachea 31.92
  tubo-ovarian 65.89
   laparoscopic 65.81
  ureter 59.02
   with freeing or repositioning of
    ureter 59.02
   intraluminal 56.81
   laparoscopic 59.03
  urethra (intraluminal) 58.5
  uterus 54.59
   intraluminal 68.21
   laparoscopic 54.51
   peritoneal 54.59
    laparoscopic 54.51
  vagina (intraluminal) 70.13
  vitreous (posterior approach) 14.74
   anterior approach 14.73
  vulva 71.01
 goniosynechiae (with injection of air or
   liquid) 12.31
 synechiae (posterior) 12.33
  anterior (with injection of air or
    liquid) 12.32

◀ New   ◀▥ Revised   deleted Deleted   ● Use Additional Digit(s)   ▨ Omit code

M

Madlener operation (tubal ligation) 66.31
Magnet extraction
    foreign body
        anterior chamber, eye 12.01
        choroid 14.01
        ciliary body 12.01
        conjunctiva 98.22
        cornea 11.0
        eye, eyeball NEC 98.21
            anterior segment 12.01
            posterior segment 14.01
        intraocular (anterior segment) 12.01
        iris 12.01
        lens 13.01
        orbit 98.21
        retina 14.01
        sclera 12.01
        vitreous 14.01
Magnetic resonance imaging (nuclear) -
    see Imaging, magnetic resonance
Magnuson (-Stack) operation
    (arthroplasty for recurrent shoulder
    dislocation) 81.82
Mako Tactile Guidance System™ [TGS] -
    see category 17.4●
Malleostapediopexy 19.19
    with incus replacement 19.11
Malström's vacuum extraction 72.79
    with episiotomy 72.71
Mammaplasty - see Mammoplasty
Mammectomy - see also Mastectomy
    subcutaneous (unilateral) 85.34
        with synchronous implant 85.33
        bilateral 85.36
            with synchronous implant 85.35
Mammilliplasty 85.87
Mammography NEC 87.37
Mammoplasty 85.89
    with
        full-thickness graft 85.83
        muscle flap 85.85
        pedicle graft 85.84
        split-thickness graft 85.82
    amputative (reduction) (bilateral) 85.32
        unilateral 85.31
    augmentation 85.50
        with
            breast implant (bilateral) 85.54
                unilateral 85.53
            injection into breast (bilateral)
                85.52
                unilateral 85.51
    reduction (bilateral) 85.32
        unilateral 85.31
    revision 85.89
    size reduction (gynecomastia)
        (bilateral) 85.32
        unilateral 85.31
Mammotomy 85.0
Manchester (-Donald) (-Fothergill)
    operation (uterine suspension)
    69.22
Mandibulectomy (partial) 76.31
    total 76.42
        with reconstruction 76.41
Maneuver (method)
    Bracht 72.52
    Credé 73.59
    De Lee (key-in-lock) 72.4
    Kristeller 72.54
    Loveset's (extraction of arms in breech
        birth) 72.52

Maneuver (Continued)
    Mauriceau (-Smellie-Veit) 72.52
    Pinard (total breech extraction) 72.54
    Prague 72.52
    Ritgen 73.59
    Scanzoni (rotation) 72.4
    Van Hoorn 72.52
    Wigand-Martin 72.52
Manipulation
    with reduction of fracture or
        dislocation - see Reduction,
        fracture and Reduction,
        dislocation
    enterostomy stoma (with dilation)
        96.24
    intestine (intra-abdominal) 46.80
        large 46.82
        small 46.81
    joint
        adhesions 93.26
            temporomandibular 76.95
        dislocation - see Reduction,
            dislocation
    lacrimal passage (tract) NEC 09.49
    muscle structures 93.27
    musculoskeletal (physical therapy)
        NEC 93.29
    nasal septum, displaced 21.88
    osteopathic NEC 93.67
        for general mobilization (general
            articulation) 93.61
        high-velocity, low-amplitude forces
            (thrusting) 93.62
        indirect forces 93.65
        isotonic, isometric forces 93.64
        low-velocity, high-amplitude forces
            (springing) 93.63
        to move tissue fluids 93.66
    rectum 96.22
    salivary duct 26.91
    stomach, intraoperative 44.92
    temporomandibular joint NEC 76.95
    ureteral calculus by catheter
        with removal 56.0
        without removal 59.8
    uterus NEC 69.98
        gravid 75.99
        inverted
            manual replacement (following
                delivery) 75.94
            surgical - see Repair, inverted
                uterus
Manometry
    esophageal 89.32
    spinal fluid 89.15
    urinary 89.21
Manual arts therapy 93.81
Mapping
    cardiac (electrophysiologic) 37.27
    doppler (flow) 88.72
    electrocardiogram only 89.52
Marckwald operation (cervical os repair)
    67.59
Marshall-Marchetti (-Krantz) operation
    (retropubic urethral suspension)
    59.5
Marsupialization - see also Destruction,
    lesion, by site
    cyst
        Bartholin's 71.23
        brain 01.59
        cervical (nabothian) 67.31
        dental 24.4
        dentigerous 24.4

Marsupialization (Continued)
    cyst (Continued)
        kidney 55.31
        larynx 30.01
        liver 50.21
        ovary 65.21
            laparoscopic 65.23
        pancreas 52.3
        pilonidal (open excision) (with
            partial closure) 86.21
        salivary gland 26.21
        spinal (intraspinal) (meninges)
            03.4
        spleen, splenic 41.41
    lesion
        brain 01.59
        cerebral 01.59
        liver 50.21
    pilonidal cyst or sinus (open excision)
        (with partial closure) 86.21
    pseudocyst, pancreas 52.3
    ranula, salivary gland 26.21
Massage
    cardiac (external) (manual) (closed)
        99.63
        open 37.91
    prostatic 99.94
    rectal (for levator spasm) 99.93
MAST (military anti-shock trousers)
    93.58
Mastectomy (complete) (prophylactic)
    (simple) (unilateral) 85.41
    with
        excision of regional lymph nodes
            85.43
            bilateral 85.44
        preservation of skin and nipple
            85.34
            with synchronous implant 85.33
            bilateral 85.36
                with synchronous implant
                    85.35
    bilateral 85.42
    extended
        radical (Urban) (unilateral) 85.47
            bilateral 85.48
        simple (with regional
            lymphadenectomy)
            (unilateral) 85.43
            bilateral 85.44
    modified radical (unilateral) 85.43
        bilateral 85.44
    partial 85.23
    radical (Halsted) (Meyer) (unilateral)
        85.45
        bilateral 85.46
        extended (Urban) (unilateral) 85.47
            bilateral 85.48
        modified (unilateral) 85.43
            bilateral 85.44
    subcutaneous 85.34
        with synchronous implant 85.33
        bilateral 85.36
            with synchronous implant
                85.35
    subtotal 85.23
Masters' stress test (two-step) 89.42
Mastoidectomy (cortical) (conservative)
    20.49
    complete (simple) 20.41
    modified radical 20.49
    radical 20.42
        modified 20.49
    simple (complete) 20.41

◀ New   ◀▥ Revised   ~~deleted~~ Deleted   ● Use Additional Digit(s)   ▨ Omit code

Monitoring *(Continued)*
   fetus *(Continued)*
      intrapartum *(Continued)*
         pulsed ultrasound (Doppler)
            88.78
         transcervical fetal oxygen
            saturation monitoring 75.38
         transcervical fetal SpO$_2$
            monitoring 75.38
   Holter-type device (cardiac) 89.50
   IAEMT (intraoperative anesthetic effect
      monitoring and titration) 00.94
      [89.14] ◄
   intra-aneursym sac pressure 00.58
   intracranial oxygen 01.16
   intracranial pressure 01.10
   intraoperative anesthetic effect
      monitoring and titration
      (IAEMT) 00.94 *[89.14]* ◄
   intravascular pressure 00.69
      coronary 00.59
      iliac 00.69
      intra-abdominal 00.69
      intrathoracic 00.67
         aorta 00.67
         aortic arch 00.67
         carotid 00.67
      mesenteric 00.69
      peripheral 00.68
      renal 00.69
   neurophysiologic
      intra-operative 00.94
   partial pressure of brain oxygen
      (PbtO$_2$) 01.16
   pulmonary artery
      pressure 89.63
      wedge 89.64
   sleep (recording) - *see* categories 89.17–
      89.18
   systemic arterial pressure 89.61
      intra-aneursym sac pressure 00.58
   telemetry (cardiac) 89.54
   transesophageal cardiac output
      (Doppler) 89.68
   ventricular pressure (cardiac) 89.62
Moore operation (arthroplasty) 81.52

Moschowitz
   enterocele repair 70.92
      with graft or prosthesis 70.93
   herniorrhaphy - *see* Repair, hernia,
      femoral
   sigmoidopexy 46.63
Mountain resort sanitarium 93.98
Mouth-to-mouth resuscitation 93.93
Moxibustion 93.35
MRI - *see* Imaging, magnetic resonance
Muller operation (banding of pulmonary
   artery) 38.85
Multiple sleep latency test (MSLT)
   89.18
Mumford operation (partial
   claviculectomy) 77.81
Musculoplasty - *see also* Repair, muscle
   83.87
   hand - *see also* Repair, muscle, hand
      82.89
Music therapy 93.84
Mustard operation (interatrial
   transposition of venous return) 35.91
Myectomy 83.45
   anorectal 48.92
   eye muscle 15.13
      multiple 15.3
   for graft 83.43
      hand 82.34
   hand 82.36
      for graft 82.34
   levator palpebrae 08.33
   rectal 48.92
Myelogram, myelography (air) (gas)
   87.21
   posterior fossa 87.02
Myelotomy
   spine, spinal (cord) (tract) (one-stage)
      (two-stage) 03.29
      percutaneous 03.21
Myocardiectomy (infarcted area) 37.33
Myocardiotomy 37.11
Myoclasis 83.99
   hand 82.99
Myomectomy (uterine) 68.29
   broad ligament 69.19

Myoplasty - *see also* Repair, muscle 83.87
   hand - *see also* Repair, muscle, hand
      82.89
   mastoid 19.9
Myorrhaphy 83.65
   hand 82.46
Myosuture 83.65
   hand 82.46
Myotasis 93.27
Myotenontoplasty - *see also* Repair,
   tendon 83.88
   hand 82.86
Myotenoplasty - *see also* Repair, tendon
   83.88
   hand 82.86
Myotenotomy 83.13
   hand 82.11
Myotomy 83.02
   with division 83.19
      hand 82.19
   colon NEC 46.92
      sigmoid 46.91
   cricopharyngeal 29.31
      that for pharyngeal
         (pharyngoesophageal)
         diverticulectomy 29.32
   esophagus 42.7
   eye (oblique) (rectus) 15.21
      multiple (two or more muscles) 15.4
   hand 82.02
      with division 82.19
   levator palpebrae 08.38
   sigmoid (colon) 46.91
Myringectomy 20.59
Myringodectomy 20.59
Myringomalleolabyrinthopexy
   19.52
Myringoplasty (epitympanic, type I)
   (by cauterization) (by graft) 19.4
   revision 19.6
Myringostapediopexy 19.53
Myringostomy 20.01
Myringotomy (with aspiration) (with
   drainage) 20.09
   with insertion of tube or drainage
      device (button) (grommet) 20.01

M

N

Nailing, intramedullary
  with fracture reduction - *see*
    Reduction, fracture with
    internal fixation
  internal (without fracture
    reduction) 78.50
Narcoanalysis 94.21
Narcosynthesis 94.21
Narrowing, palpebral fissure 08.51
Nasopharyngogram 87.09
  contrast 87.06
Necropsy 89.8
Needleoscopy (fetus) 75.31
Needling
  Bartholin's gland (cyst) 71.21
  cataract (secondary) 13.64
  fallopian tube 66.91
  hydrocephalic head 73.8
  lens (capsule) 13.2
  pupillary membrane (iris) 12.35
Nephrectomy (complete) (total)
    (unilateral) 55.51
  bilateral 55.54
  partial (wedge) 55.4
  remaining or solitary kidney 55.52
  removal transplanted kidney 55.53
Nephrocolopexy 55.7
Nephrocystanastomosis NEC 56.73
Nephrolithotomy 55.01
Nephrolysis 59.02
  laparoscopic 59.03
Nephropexy 55.7
Nephroplasty 55.89
Nephropyeloplasty 55.87
Nephropyeloureterostomy 55.86
Nephrorrhaphy 55.81
Nephroscopy 55.21
Nephrostolithotomy, percutaneous 55.03

Nephrostomy (with drainage tube) 55.02
  closure 55.82
  percutaneous 55.03
    with fragmentation (ultrasound)
      55.04
Nephrotomogram, nephrotomography
  NEC 87.72
Nephrotomy 55.01
Nephroureterectomy (with bladder cuff)
  55.51
Nephroureterocystectomy 55.51 [57.79]
Nerve block (cranial) (peripheral) NEC -
  see also Block, by site 04.81
Neurectasis (cranial) (peripheral) 04.91
Neurectomy (cranial) (infraorbital)
    (occipital) (peripheral) (spinal) NEC
    04.07
  gastric (vagus) - *see also* Vagotomy
    44.00
  opticociliary 12.79
  paracervical 05.22
  presacral 05.24
  retrogasserian 04.07
  sympathetic - *see* Sympathectomy
  trigeminal 04.07
  tympanic 20.91
Neurexeresis NEC 04.07
Neuroablation
  radiofrequency 04.2
Neuroanastomosis (cranial) (peripheral)
    NEC 04.74
  accessory-facial 04.72
  accessory-hypoglossal 04.73
  hypoglossal-facial 04.71
Neurolysis (peripheral nerve) NEC 04.49
  carpal tunnel 04.43
  cranial nerve NEC 04.42
  spinal (cord) (nerve roots) 03.6
  tarsal tunnel 04.44
  trigeminal nerve 04.41

Neuromonitoring
  intra-operative 00.94
Neuroplasty (cranial) (peripheral) NEC
    04.79
  of old injury (delayed repair) 04.76
  revision 04.75
Neurorrhaphy (cranial) (peripheral)
    04.3
Neurotomy (cranial) (peripheral) (spinal)
    NEC 04.04
  acoustic 04.01
  glossopharyngeal 29.92
  lacrimal branch 05.0
  retrogasserian 04.02
  sympathetic 05.0
  vestibular 04.01
Neurotripsy (peripheral) NEC 04.03
  trigeminal 04.02
Nicola operation (tenodesis for
    recurrent dislocation of shoulder)
    81.82
Nimodipine, infusion 99.75
NIPS (non-invasive programmed
    electrical stimulation) 37.20
Nissen operation (fundoplication of
    stomach) 44.66
  laparoscopic 44.67
Noble operation (plication of small
    intestine) 46.62
Norman Miller operation (vaginopexy)
    70.77
  with graft or prosthesis 70.78
Norton operation (extraperitoneal
    cesarean section) 74.2
Nuclear magnetic resonance imaging -
  see Imaging, magnetic resonance
Nutrition, concentrated substances
  enteral infusion (of) 96.6
    parenteral, (total) 99.15
    peripheral parenteral 99.15

O

Ober (-Yount) operation (gluteal-iliotibial fasciotomy) 83.14
Obliteration
  bone cavity - *see also* Osteoplasty 78.40
  calyceal diverticulum 55.39
  canaliculi 09.6
  cerebrospinal fistula 02.12
  cul-de-sac 70.92
    with graft or prosthesis 70.93
  frontal sinus (with fat) 22.42
  lacrimal punctum 09.91
  lumbar pseudomeningocele 03.51
  lymphatic structure(s) (peripheral) 40.9
  maxillary sinus 22.31
  meningocele (sacral) 03.51
  pelvic 68.8
  pleural cavity 34.6
  sacral meningocele 03.51
  Skene's gland 71.3
  tympanomastoid cavity 19.9
  vagina, vaginal (partial) (total) 70.4
  vault 70.8
Occlusal molds (dental) 89.31
Occlusion
  artery
    by embolization - *see* Embolization, artery
    by endovascular approach - *see* Embolization, artery
    by ligation - *see* Ligation, artery
  fallopian tube - *see* Ligation, fallopian tube
  patent ductus arteriosus (PDA) 38.85
  vein
    by embolization - *see* Embolization, vein
    by endovascular approach - *see* Embolization, vein
    by ligation - *see* Ligation, vein
  vena cava (surgical) 38.7
Occupational therapy 93.83
OCT (optical coherence tomography) (intavascular imaging) ◀
  coronary vessel(s) 38.24 ◀
  non-coronary vessel(s) 38.25 ◀
O'Donoghue operation (triad knee repair) 81.43
Odontectomy NEC - *see also* Removal, tooth, surgical 23.19
Oleothorax 33.39
Olshausen operation (uterine suspension) 69.22
Omentectomy 54.4
Omentofixation 54.74
Omentopexy 54.74
Omentoplasty 54.74
Omentorrhaphy 54.74
Omentotomy 54.19
Omphalectomy 54.3
Onychectomy 86.23
Onychoplasty 86.86
Onychotomy 86.09
  with drainage 86.04
Oophorectomy (unilateral) 65.39
  with salpingectomy 65.49
    laparoscopic 65.41
  bilateral (same operative episode) 65.51
    laparoscopic 65.53
    with salpingectomy 65.61
      laparoscopic 65.63
  laparoscopic 65.31

Oophorectomy (Continued)
  partial 65.29
    laparoscopic 65.25
    wedge 65.22
      that by laparoscope 65.24
  remaining ovary 65.52
    laparoscopic 65.54
    with tube 65.62
      laparoscopic 65.64
Oophorocystectomy 65.29
  laparoscopic 65.25
Oophoropexy 65.79
Oophoroplasty 65.79
Oophororrhaphy 65.71
  laparoscopic 65.74
Oophorostomy 65.09
  laparoscopic 65.01
Oophorotomy 65.09
  laparoscopic 65.01
Opening
  bony labyrinth (ear) 20.79
  cranial suture 02.01
  heart valve
    closed heart technique - *see* Valvulotomy, by site
    open heart technique - *see* Valvuloplasty, by site
  spinal dura 03.09
Operation
  Abbe
    construction of vagina 70.61
      with graft or prosthesis 70.63
    intestinal anastomosis - *see* Anastomosis, intestine
  abdominal (region) NEC 54.99
  abdominoperineal, NOS 48.50
    laparoscopic 48.51
    open 48.52
    other 48.59
  Aburel (intra-amniotic injection for abortion) 75.0
  Adams
    advancement of round ligament 69.22
    crushing of nasal septum 21.88
    excision of palmar fascia 82.35
  adenoids NEC 28.99
  adrenal (gland) (nerve) (vessel) NEC 07.49
  Albee
    bone peg, femoral neck 78.05
    graft for slipping patella 78.06
    sliding inlay graft, tibia 78.07
  Albert (arthrodesis, knee) 81.22
  Aldridge (-Studdiford) (urethral sling) 59.5
  Alexander
    prostatectomy
      perineal 60.62
      suprapubic 60.3
    shortening of round ligaments of uterus 69.22
  Alexander-Adams (shortening of round ligaments of uterus) 69.22
  Almoor (extrapetrosal drainage) 20.22
  Altemeier (perineal rectal pull-through) 48.49
  Ammon (dacryocystotomy) 09.53
  Anderson (tibial lengthening) 78.37
  Anel (dilation of lacrimal duct) 09.42
  anterior chamber (eye) NEC 12.99
  anti-incontinence NEC 59.79
  antrum window (nasal sinus) 22.2
    with Caldwell-Luc approach 22.39

Operation (Continued)
  anus NEC 49.99
  aortic body NEC 39.8
  aorticopulmonary window 39.59
  appendix NEC 47.99
  Arslan (fenestration of inner ear) 20.61
  artery NEC 39.99
  Asai (larynx) 31.75
  Baffes (interatrial transposition of venous return) 35.91
  Baldy-Webster (uterine suspension) 69.22
  Ball
    herniorrhaphy - *see* Repair, hernia, inguinal
    undercutting 49.02
  Bankhart (capsular repair into glenoid, for shoulder dislocation) 81.82
  Bardenheurer (ligation of innominate artery) 38.85
  Barkan (goniotomy) 12.52
    with goniopuncture 12.53
  Barr (transfer of tibialis posterior tendon) 83.75
  Barsky (closure of cleft hand) 82.82
  Bassett (vulvectomy with inguinal lymph node dissection) 71.5 [40.3]
  Bassini (herniorrhaphy) - *see* Repair, hernia, inguinal
  Batch-Spittler-McFaddin (knee disarticulation) 84.16
  Batista (partial ventriculectomy) (ventricular reduction) (ventricular remodeling) 37.35
  Beck I (epicardial poudrage) 36.39
  Beck II (aorta-coronary sinus shunt) 36.39
  Beck-Jianu (permanent gastrostomy) 43.19
  Bell-Beuttner (subtotal abdominal hysterectomy) 68.39
  Belsey (esophagogastric sphincter) 44.65
  Benenenti (rotation of bulbous urethra) 58.49
  Berke (levator resection eyelid) 08.33
  Biesenberger (size reduction of breast, bilateral) 85.32
    unilateral 85.31
  Bigelow (litholapaxy) 57.0
  biliary (duct) (tract) NEC 51.99
  Billroth I (partial gastrectomy with gastroduodenostomy) 43.6
  Billroth II (partial gastrectomy with gastrojejunostomy) 43.7
  Binnie (hepatopexy) 50.69
  Bischoff (ureteroneocystostomy) 56.74
  bisection hysterectomy 68.39
    laparoscopic 68.31
  Bishoff (spinal myelotomy) 03.29
  bladder NEC 57.99
    flap 56.74
  Blalock (systemic-pulmonary anastomosis) 39.0
  Blalock-Hanlon (creation of atrial septal defect) 35.42
  Blalock-Taussig (subclavian-pulmonary anastomosis) 39.0
  Blascovic (resection and advancement of levator palpebrae superioris) 08.33
  blood vessel NEC 39.99

Operation *(Continued)*

Blount
femoral shortening (with blade plate) 78.25
by epiphyseal stapling 78.25
Boari (bladder flap) 56.74
Bobb (cholelithotomy) 51.04
bone NEC - *see* category 78.4●
facial 76.99
injury NEC - *see* category 79.9●
marrow NEC 41.98
skull NEC 02.99
Bonney (abdominal hysterectomy) 68.49
laparoscopic 68.41
Borthen (iridotasis) 12.63
Bost
plantar dissection 80.48
radiocarpal fusion 81.26
Bosworth
arthroplasty for acromioclavicular separation 81.83
fusion of posterior lumbar spine 81.08
for pseudarthrosis 81.38
resection of radial head ligaments (for tennis elbow) 80.92
shelf procedure, hip 81.40
Bottle (repair of hydrocele of tunica vaginalis) 61.2
Boyd (hip disarticulation) 84.18
brain NEC 02.99
Brauer (cardiolysis) 37.10
breast NEC 85.99
Bricker (ileoureterostomy) 56.51
Bristow (repair of shoulder dislocation) 81.82
Brock (pulmonary valvulotomy) 35.03
Brockman (soft tissue release for clubfoot) 83.84
bronchus NEC 33.98
Browne (-Denis) (hypospadias repair) 58.45
Brunschwig (temporary gastrostomy) 43.19
buccal cavity NEC 27.99
Bunnell (tendon transfer) 82.56
Burch procedure (retropubic urethral suspension for urinary stress incontinence) 59.5
Burgess (amputation of ankle) 84.14
bursa NEC 83.99
hand 82.99
bypass - *see* Bypass
Caldwell (sulcus extension) 24.91
Caldwell-Luc (maxillary sinusotomy) 22.39
with removal of membrane lining 22.31
Callander (knee disarticulation) 84.16
Campbell
bone block, ankle 81.11
fasciotomy (iliac crest) 83.14
reconstruction of anterior cruciate ligaments 81.45
canthus NEC 08.99
cardiac NEC 37.99
septum NEC 35.98
valve NEC 35.99
carotid body or gland NEC 39.8
Carroll and Taber (arthroplasty proximal interphalangeal joint) 81.72

Operation *(Continued)*

Cattell (herniorrhaphy) 53.51
Cecil (urethral reconstruction) 58.46
cecum NEC 46.99
cerebral (meninges) NEC 02.99
cervix NEC 69.99
Chandler (hip fusion) 81.21
Charles (correction of lymphedema) 40.9
Charnley (compression arthrodesis)
ankle 81.11
hip 81.21
knee 81.22
Cheatle-Henry - *see* Repair, hernia, femoral
chest cavity NEC 34.99
Chevalier-Jackson (partial laryngectomy) 30.29
Child (radical subtotal pancreatectomy) 52.53
Chopart (midtarsal amputation) 84.12
chordae tendineae NEC 35.32
choroid NEC 14.9
ciliary body NEC 12.98
cisterna chyli NEC 40.69
Clagett (closure of chest wall following open flap drainage) 34.72
Clayton (resection of metatarsal heads and bases of phalanges) 77.88
clitoris NEC 71.4
cocked hat (metacarpal lengthening and transfer of local flap) 82.69
Cockett (varicose vein)
lower limb 38.59
upper limb 38.53
Cody tack (perforation of footplate) 19.0
Coffey (uterine suspension) (Meigs' modification) 69.22
Cole (anterior tarsal wedge osteotomy) 77.28
Collis-Nissen (hiatal hernia repair) 53.80
colon NEC 46.99
Colonna
adductor tenotomy (first stage) 83.12
hip arthroplasty (second stage) 81.40
reconstruction of hip (second stage) 81.40
commando (radical glossectomy) 25.4
conjunctiva NEC 10.99
destructive NEC 10.33
cornea NEC 11.99
Coventry (tibial wedge osteotomy) 77.27
Cox-maze procedure (ablation or destruction of heart tissue) - *see* maze procedure
Crawford (tarso-frontalis sling of eyelid) 08.32
cul-de-sac NEC 70.92
Culp-Deweerd (spiral flap pyeloplasty) 55.87
Culp-Scardino (ureteral flap pyeloplasty) 55.87
Curtis (interphalangeal joint arthroplasty) 81.72
cystocele NEC 70.51
Dahlman (excision of esophageal diverticulum) 42.31
Dana (posterior rhizotomy) 03.1
Danforth (fetal) 73.8

Operation *(Continued)*

Darrach (ulnar resection) 77.83
Davis (intubated ureterotomy) 56.2
de Grandmont (tarsectomy) 08.35
Delorme
pericardiectomy 37.31
proctopexy 48.76
repair of prolapsed rectum 48.76
thoracoplasty 33.34
Denker (radical maxillary antrotomy) 22.31
Dennis-Varco (herniorrhaphy) - *see* Repair, hernia, femoral
Denonvillier (limited rhinoplasty) 21.86
dental NEC 24.99
orthodontic NEC 24.8
Derlacki (tympanoplasty) 19.4
diaphragm NEC 34.89
Dickson (fascial transplant) 83.82
Dickson-Diveley (tendon transfer and arthrodesis to correct claw toe) 77.57
Dieffenbach (hip disarticulation) 84.18
digestive tract NEC 46.99
Doleris (shortening of round ligaments) 69.22
D'Ombrain (excision of pterygium with corneal graft) 11.32
Dorrance (push-back operation for cleft palate) 27.62
Dotter (transluminal angioplasty) 39.59
Douglas (suture of tongue to lip for micrognathia) 25.59
Doyle (paracervical uterine denervation) 69.3
Dühamel (abdominoperineal pull-through) 48.65
Duhrssen (vaginofixation of uterus) 69.22
Dunn (triple arthrodesis) 81.12
duodenum NEC 46.99
Dupuytren
fasciectomy 82.35
fasciotomy 82.12
with excision 82.35
shoulder disarticulation 84.08
Durham (-Caldwell) (transfer of biceps femoris tendon) 83.75
DuToit and Roux (staple capsulorrhaphy of shoulder) 81.82
DuVries (tenoplasty) 83.88
Dwyer
fasciotomy 83.14
soft tissue release NEC 83.84
wedge osteotomy, calcaneus 77.28
Eagleton (extrapetrosal drainage) 20.22
ear (external) NEC 18.9
middle or inner NEC 20.99
Eden-Hybinette (glenoid bone block) 78.01
Effler (heart) 36.2
Eggers
tendon release (patellar retinacula) 83.13
tendon transfer (biceps femoris tendon) (hamstring tendon) 83.75
Elliot (scleral trephination with iridectomy) 12.61

Operation (Continued)

Ellis Jones (repair of peroneal tendon) 83.88

Ellison (reinforcement of collateral ligament) 81.44

Elmslie-Cholmeley (tarsal wedge osteotomy) 77.28

Eloesser
    thoracoplasty 33.34
    thoracostomy 34.09

Emmet (cervix) 67.61

endorectal pull-through 48.41

epididymis NEC 63.99

esophagus NEC 42.99

Estes (ovary) 65.72
    laparoscopic 65.75

Estlander (thoracoplasty) 33.34

Evans (release of clubfoot) 83.84

extraocular muscle NEC 15.9
    multiple (two or more muscles) 15.4
        with temporary detachment from globe 15.3
        revision 15.6
    single 15.29
        with temporary detachment from globe 15.19

eyeball NEC 16.99

eyelid(s) NEC 08.99

face NEC 27.99

facial bone or joint NEC 76.99

fallopian tube NEC 66.99

Farabeuf (ischiopubiotomy) 77.39

Fasanella-Servatt (blepharoptosis repair) 08.35

fascia NEC 83.99
    hand 82.99

female (genital organs) NEC 71.9
    hysterectomy NEC 68.9

fenestration (aorta) 39.54

Ferguson (hernia repair) 53.00

Fick (perforation of footplate) 19.0

filtering (for glaucoma) 12.79
    with iridectomy 12.65

Finney (pyloroplasty) 44.29

fistulizing, sclera NEC 12.69

Foley (pyeloplasty) 55.87

Fontan (creation of conduit between right atrium and pulmonary artery) 35.94

Fothergill (-Donald) (uterine suspension) 69.22

Fowler
    arthroplasty of metacarpophalangeal joint 81.72
    release (mallet finger repair) 82.84
    tenodesis (hand) 82.85
    thoracoplasty 33.34

Fox (entropion repair with wedge resection) 08.43

Franco (suprapubic cystotomy) 57.19

Frank (permanent gastrostomy) 43.19

Frazier (-Spiller) (subtemporal trigeminal rhizotomy) 04.02

Fredet-Ramstedt (pyloromyotomy) (with wedge resection) 43.3

Frenckner (intrapetrosal drainage) 20.22

Frickman (abdominal proctopexy) 48.75

Frommel (shortening of uterosacral ligaments) 69.22

Operation (Continued)

Gabriel (abdominoperineal resection of rectum), NOS 48.50
    laparoscopic 48.51
    open 48.52
    other 48.59

gallbladder NEC 51.99

ganglia NEC 04.99
    sympathetic 05.89

Gant (wedge osteotomy of trochanter) 77.25

Garceau (tibial tendon transfer) 83.75

Gardner (spinal meningocele repair) 03.51

gastric NEC 44.99

Gelman (release of clubfoot) 83.84

genital organ NEC
    female 71.9
    male 64.99

Ghormley (hip fusion) 81.21

Giffod
    destruction of lacrimal sac 09.6
    keratotomy (delimiting) 11.1

Gill
    arthrodesis of shoulder 81.23
    laminectomy 03.09

Gill-Stein (carporadial arthrodesis) 81.25

Gilliam (uterine suspension) 69.22

Girdlestone
    laminectomy with spinal fusion 81.00
    muscle transfer for claw toe 77.57
    resection of femoral head and neck (without insertion of joint prosthesis) 77.85
        with replacement prosthesis - see Implant, joint, hip
    resection of hip prosthesis 80.05
        with replacement prosthesis - see Implant, joint, hip

Girdlestone-Taylor (muscle transfer for claw toe repair) 77.57

glaucoma NEC 12.79

Glenn (anastomosis of superior vena cava to right pulmonary artery) 39.21

globus pallidus NEC 01.42

Goebel-Frangenheim-Stoeckel (urethrovesical suspension) 59.4

Goldner (clubfoot release) 80.48

Goldthwaite
    ankle stabilization 81.11
    patella stabilization 81.44
    tendon transfer for patella dislocation 81.44

Goodall-Power (vagina) 70.4

Gordon-Taylor (hindquarter amputation) 84.19

Graber-Duvernay (drilling femoral head) 77.15

Green (scapulopexy) 78.41

Grice (subtalar arthrodesis) 81.13

Gritti-Stokes (knee disarticulation) 84.16

Gross (herniorrhaphy)
    laparoscopic 53.43
        with graft or prosthesis 53.42
    other and open with graft or prosthesis 53.41
    other open 53.49

gum NEC 24.39

Guyon (amputation of ankle) 84.13

Operation (Continued)

Hagner (epididymotomy) 63.92

Halsted - see Repair, hernia, inguinal

Halsted mastectomy 85.45

Hampton (anastomosis small intestine to rectal stump) 45.92

hanging hip (muscle release) 83.19

harelip 27.54

Harrison-Richardson (vaginal suspension) 70.77
    with graft or prosthesis 70.78

Hartmann - see Colectomy, by site

Hauser
    achillotenotomy 83.11
    bunionectomy with adductor tendon transfer 77.53
    stabilization of patella 81.44

Heaney (vaginal hysterectomy) 68.59
    laparoscopically assisted (LAVH) 68.51

heart NEC 37.99
    valve NEC 35.99
        adjacent structure NEC 35.39

Hegar (perineorrhaphy) 71.79

Heine (cyclodialysis) 12.55

Heineke-Mikulicz (pyloroplasty) - see category 44.2●

Heller (esophagomyotomy) 42.7

Hellström (transplantation of aberrant renal vessel) 39.55

hemorrhoids NEC 49.49

Henley (jejunal transposition) 43.81

hepatic NEC 50.99

hernia - see Repair, hernia

Hey (amputation of foot) 84.12

Hey-Groves (reconstruction of anterior cruciate ligament) 81.45

Heyman (soft tissue release for clubfoot) 83.84

Heyman-Herndon (-Strong) (correction of metatarsus varus) 80.48

Hibbs (lumbar spinal fusion) - see Fusion, lumbar

Higgins - see Repair, hernia, femoral

Hill-Allison (hiatal hernia repair, transpleural approach) 53.80

Hitchcock (anchoring tendon of biceps) 83.88

Hofmeister (gastrectomy) 43.7

Hoke
    midtarsal fusion 81.14
    triple arthrodesis 81.12

Holth
    iridencleisis 12.63
    sclerectomy 12.65

Homan (correction of lymphedema) 40.9

Hutch (ureteroneocystostomy) 56.74

Hybinette-Eden (glenoid bone block) 78.01

hymen NEC 70.91

hypopharynx NEC 29.99

hypophysis NEC 07.79

ileal loop 56.51

ileum NEC 46.99

intestine NEC 46.99

iris NEC 12.97
    inclusion 12.63

Irving (tubal ligation) 66.32

Irwin - see also Osteotomy 77.30

Jaboulay (gastroduodenostomy) 44.39
    laparoscopic 44.38

Operation (Continued)
  Janeway (permanent gastrostomy) 43.19
  Jatene (arterial switch) 35.84
  jejunum NEC 46.99
  Johanson (urethral reconstruction) 58.46
  joint (capsule) (ligament) (structure) NEC 81.99
    facial NEC 76.99
  Jones
    claw toe (transfer of extensor hallucis longus tendon) 77.57
      modified (with arthrodesis) 77.57
    dacryocystorhinostomy 09.81
    hammer toe (interphalangeal fusion) 77.56
      modified (tendon transfer with arthrodesis) 77.57
    repair of peroneal tendon 83.88
  Joplin (exostectomy with tendon transfer) 77.53
  Kader (temporary gastrostomy) 43.19
  Kaufman (for urinary stress incontinence) 59.79
  Kazanjiian (buccal vestibular sulcus extension) 24.91
  Kehr (hepatopexy) 50.69
  Keller (bunionectomy) 77.59
  Kelly (-Kennedy) (urethrovesical plication) 59.3
  Kelly-Stoeckel (urethrovesical plication) 59.3
  Kerr (cesarean section) 74.1
  Kessler (arthroplasty, carpometacarpal joint) 81.74
  Kidner (excision of accessory navicular bone) (with tendon transfer) 77.98
  kidney NEC 55.99
  Killian (frontal sinusotomy) 22.41
  King-Steelquist (hindquarter amputation) 84.19
  Kirk (amputation through thigh) 84.17
  Kock pouch
    bowel anastomosis - omit code
    continent ileostomy 46.22
    cutaneous uretero-ileostomy 56.51
    ESWL (electrocorporeal shock wave lithotripsy) 98.51
    removal, calculus 57.19
    revision, cutaneous uretero-ileostomy 56.52
    urinary diversion procedure 56.51
  Kondoleon (correction of lymphedema) 40.9
  Krause (sympathetic denervation) 05.29
  Kroener (partial salpingectomy) 66.69
  Kroenlein (lateral orbitotomy) 16.01
  Kronig (low cervical cesarean section) 74.1
  Krukenberg (reconstruction of below-elbow amputation) 82.89
  Kuhnt-Szymanowski (ectropion repair with lid reconstruction) 08.44
  Labbe (gastrotomy) 43.0
  labia NEC 71.8
  lacrimal
    gland 09.3
    system NEC 09.99
  Ladd (mobilization of intestine) 54.95

Operation (Continued)
  Lagrange (iridosclerectomy) 12.65
  Lambrinudi (triple arthrodesis) 81.12
  Langenbeck (cleft palate repair) 27.62
  Lapidus (bunionectomy with metatarsal osteotomy) 77.51
  Larry (shoulder disarticulation) 84.08
  larynx NEC 31.98
  Lash
    internal cervical os repair 67.59
    laparoscopic supracervical hysterectomy 68.31
  Latzko
    cesarean section, extraperitoneal 74.2
    colpocleisis 70.8
  Le Fort (colpocleisis) 70.8
  Leadbetter (urethral reconstruction) 58.46
  Leadbetter-Politano (ureteroneocystostomy) 56.74
  Le Fort (colpocleisis) 70.8
  LeMesurier (cleft lip repair) 27.54
  lens NEC 13.90
  Leriche (periarterial sympathectomy) 05.25
  levator muscle sling
    eyelid ptosis repair 08.33
    urethrovesical suspension 59.71
    urinary stress incontinence 59.71
  lid suture (blepharoptosis) 08.31
  ligament NEC 81.99
    broad NEC 69.98
    round NEC 69.98
    uterine NEC 69.98
  Lindholm (repair of ruptured tendon) 83.88
  Linton (varicose vein) 38.59
  lip NEC 27.99
  Lisfranc
    foot amputation 84.12
    shoulder disarticulation 84.08
  Littlewood (forequarter amputation) 84.09
  liver NEC 50.99
  Lloyd-Davies (abdominoperineal resection), NOS 48.50
    laparoscopic 48.51
    open 48.52
    other 48.59
  Longmire (bile duct anastomosis) 51.39
  Lord
    dilation of anal canal for hemorrhoids 49.49
    hemorrhoidectomy 49.49
    orchidopexy 62.5
  Lucas and Murray (knee arthrodesis with plate) 81.22
  lung NEC 33.99
  lung volume reduction 32.22
    biologic lung volume reduction (BLVR) - see category 33.7●
  lymphatic structure(s) NEC 40.9
    duct, left (thoracic) NEC 40.69
  Madlener (tubal ligation) 66.31
  Magnuson (-Stack) (arthroplasty for recurrent shoulder dislocation) 81.82
  male genital organs NEC 64.99
  Manchester (-Donald) (-Fothergill) (uterine suspension) 69.22
  mandible NEC 76.99
    orthognathic 76.64

Operation (Continued)
  Marckwald (cervical os repair) 67.59
  Marshall-Marchetti (-Krantz) (retropubic urethral suspension) 59.5
  Matas (aneurysmorrhaphy) 39.52
  Mayo
    bunionectomy 77.59
    herniorrhaphy
      laparoscopic 53.43
        with graft or prosthesis 53.42
      other and open with graft or prosthesis 53.41
      other open 53.49
    vaginal hysterectomy 68.59
      laparoscopically assisted (LAVH) 68.51
  maze procedure (ablation or destruction of heart tissue)
    by incision (open) 37.33
    by peripherally inserted catheter 37.34
    endovascular approach 37.34
    trans-thoracic approach 37.33
  Mazet (knee disarticulation) 84.16
  McBride (bunionectomy with soft tissue correction) 77.53
  McBurney - see Repair, hernia, inguinal
  McCall (enterocele repair) 70.92
    with graft or prosthesis 70.93
  McCauley (release of clubfoot) 83.84
  McDonald (encirclement suture, cervix) 67.59
  McIndoe (vaginal construction) 70.61
    with graft or prosthesis 70.63
  McKeever (fusion of first metatarsophalangeal joint for hallux valgus repair) 77.52
  McKissock (breast reduction) 85.33
  McReynolds (transposition of pterygium) 11.31
  McVay
    femoral hernia - see Repair, hernia, femoral
    inguinal hernia - see Repair, hernia, inguinal
  meninges (spinal) NEC 03.99
    cerebral NEC 02.99
  mesentery NEC 54.99
  Mikulicz (exteriorization of intestine) (first stage) 46.03
    second stage 46.04
  Miles (complete proctectomy), NOS 48.50
    laparoscopic 48.51
    open 48.52
    other 48.59
  Millard (cheiloplasty) 27.54
  Miller
    midtarsal arthrodesis 81.14
    urethrovesical suspension 59.4
  Millin-Read (urethrovesical suspension) 59.4
  Mitchell (hallux valgus repair) 77.51
  Mohs (chemosurgical excision of skin) 86.24
  Moore (arthroplasty) 81.52
  Moschowitz
    enterocele repair 70.92
      with graft or prosthesis 70.93
    herniorrhaphy - see Repair, hernia, femoral
    sigmoidopexy 46.63

◀ New　◀▥ Revised　deleted Deleted　● Use Additional Digit(s)　▥ Omit code

Operation (Continued)
  mouth NEC 27.99
  Muller (banding of pulmonary artery)
    38.85
  Mumford (partial claviculectomy)
    77.81
  muscle NEC 83.99
    extraocular - see Operation,
      extraocular
    hand NEC 82.99
    papillary heart NEC 35.31
  musculoskeletal system NEC 84.99
  Mustard (interatrial transposition of
    venous return) 35.91
  nail (finger) (toe) NEC 86.99
  nasal sinus NEC 22.9
  nasopharynx NEC 29.99
  nerve (cranial) (peripheral) NEC
    04.99
    adrenal NEC 07.49
    sympathetic NEC 05.89
  nervous system NEC 05.9
  Nicola (tenodesis for recurrent
    dislocation of shoulder) 81.82
  nipple NEC 85.99
  Nissen (fundoplication of stomach)
    44.66
    laparoscopic 44.67
  Noble (plication of small intestine)
    46.62
  node (lymph) NEC 40.9
  Norman Miller (vaginopexy) 70.77
    with graft or prosthesis 70.78
  Norton (extraperitoneal cesarean
    operation) 74.2
  nose, nasal NEC 21.99
    sinus NEC 22.9
  Ober (-Yount) (gluteal-iliotibial
    fasciotomy) 83.14
  obstetric NEC 75.99
  ocular NEC 16.99
    muscle - see Operation, extraocular
      muscle
  O'Donoghue (triad knee repair) 81.43
  Olshausen (uterine suspension) 69.22
  omentum NEC 54.99
  ophthalmologic NEC 16.99
  oral cavity NEC 27.99
  orbicularis muscle sling 08.36
  orbit NEC 16.98
  oropharynx NEC 29.99
  orthodontic NEC 24.8
  orthognathic NEC 76.69
  Oscar Miller (midtarsal arthrodesis)
    81.14
  Osmond-Clark (soft tissue release with
    peroneus brevis tendon transfer)
    83.75
  ovary NEC 65.99
  Oxford (for urinary incontinence)
    59.4
  palate NEC 27.99
  palpebral ligament sling 08.36
  Panas (linear proctotomy) 48.0
  Pancoast (division of trigeminal nerve
    at foramen ovale) 04.02
  pancreas NEC 52.99
  pantaloon (revision of gastric
    anastomosis) 44.5
  papillary muscle (heart) NEC 35.31
  Paquin (ureteroneocystostomy)
    56.74
  parathyroid gland(s) NEC 06.99
  parotid gland or duct NEC 26.99

Operation (Continued)
  Partsch (marsupialization of dental
    cyst) 24.4
  Pattee (auditory canal) 18.6
  Peet (splanchnic resection) 05.29
  Pemberton
    osteotomy of ilium 77.39
    rectum (mobilization and fixation
      for prolapse repair) 48.76
  penis NEC 64.98
  Pereyra (paraurethral suspension)
    59.6
  pericardium NEC 37.99
  perineum (female) NEC 71.8
    male NEC 86.99
  perirectal tissue NEC 48.99
  perirenal tissue NEC 59.92
  peritoneum NEC 54.99
  periurethral tissue NEC 58.99
  perivesical tissue NEC 59.92
  pharyngeal flap (cleft palate repair)
    27.62
    secondary or subsequent 27.63
  pharynx, pharyngeal (pouch) NEC
    29.99
  pineal gland NEC 07.59
  Pinsker (obliteration of nasoseptal
    telangiectasia) 21.07
  Piper (forceps) 72.6
  Pirogoff (ankle amputation through
    malleoli of tibia and fibula)
    84.14
  pituitary gland NEC 07.79
  plastic - see Repair, by site
  pleural cavity NEC 34.99
  Politano-Leadbetter
    (ureteroneocystostomy) 56.74
  pollicization (with nerves and blood
    supply) 82.61
  Polya (gastrectomy) 43.7
  Pomeroy (ligation and division of
    fallopian tubes) 66.32
  Poncet
    lengthening of Achilles tendon 83.85
    urethrostomy, perineal 58.0
  Porro (cesarean section) 74.99
  posterior chamber (eye) NEC 14.9
  Potts-Smith (descending aorta-left
    pulmonary artery anastomosis)
    39.0
  Printen and Mason (high gastric
    bypass) 44.31
  prostate NEC - see also Prostatectomy
    60.69
    specified type 60.99
  pterygium 11.39
    with corneal graft 11.32
  Puestow (pancreaticojejunostomy)
    52.96
  pull-through NEC 48.49
  pulmonary NEC 33.99
  push-back (cleft palate repair) 27.62
  Putti-Platt (capsulorrhaphy of
    shoulder for recurrent
    dislocation) 81.82
  pyloric exclusion 44.39
    laparoscopic 44.38
  pyriform sinus NEC 29.99
  "rabbit ear" (anterior urethropexy)
    (Tudor) 59.79
  Ramadier (intrapetrosal drainage)
    20.22
  Ramstedt (pyloromyotomy) (with
    wedge resection) 43.3

Operation (Continued)
  Rankin
    exteriorization of intestine 46.03
    proctectomy (complete), NOS
      48.50
      laparoscopic 48.51
      open 48.52
      other 48.59
  Rashkind (balloon septostomy) 35.41
  Rastelli (creation of conduit between
    right ventricle and pulmonary
    artery) 35.92
    in repair of
      pulmonary artery atresia 35.92
      transposition of great vessels
        35.92
      truncus arteriosus 35.83
  Raz-Pereyra procedure (bladder neck
    suspension) 59.79
  rectal NEC 48.99
  rectocele NEC 70.52
  re-entry (aorta) 39.54
  renal NEC 55.99
  respiratory (tract) NEC 33.99
  retina NEC 14.9
  Ripstein (repair of rectal prolapse)
    48.75
  Rodney Smith (radical subtotal
    pancreatectomy) 52.53
  Roux-en-Y
    bile duct 51.36
    cholecystojejunostomy 51.32
    esophagus (intrathoracic) 42.54
    gastroenterostomy 44.39
      laparoscopic 44.38
    gastrojejunostomy 44.39
      laparoscopic 44.38
    pancreaticojejunostomy 52.96
  Roux-Goldthwait (repair of patellar
    dislocation) 81.44
  Roux-Herzen-Judine (jejunal loop
    interposition) 42.63
  Ruiz-Mora (proximal phalangectomy
    for hammer toe) 77.99
  Russe (bone graft of scaphoid) 78.04
  Saemisch (corneal section) 11.1
  salivary gland or duct NEC 26.99
  Salter (innominate osteotomy) 77.39
  Sauer-Bacon (abdominoperineal
    resection), NOS 48.50
    laparoscopic 48.51
    open 48.52
    other 48.59
  Schanz (femoral osteotomy) 77.35
  Schauta (-Amreich) (radical vaginal
    hysterectomy) 68.79
    laparoscopic 68.71
  Schede (thoracoplasty) 33.34
  Scheie
    cautery of sclera 12.62
    sclerostomy 12.62
  Schlatter (total gastrectomy) 43.99
  Schroeder (endocervical excision)
    67.39
  Schuchardt (nonobstetrical episiotomy)
    71.09
  Schwartze (simple mastoidectomy)
    20.41
  sclera NEC 12.89
  Scott
    intestinal bypass for obesity
      45.93
    jejunocolostomy (bypass) 45.93
  scrotum NEC 61.99

Operation (*Continued*)

Seddon-Brooks (transfer of pectoralis major tendon) 83.75
Semb (apicolysis of lung) 33.39
seminal vesicle NEC 60.79
Senning (correction of transposition of great vessels) 35.91
Sever (division of soft tissue of arm) 83.19
Sewell (heart) 36.2
sex transformation NEC 64.5
Sharrard (iliopsoas muscle transfer) 83.77
shelf (hip arthroplasty) 81.40
Shirodkar (encirclement suture, cervix) 67.59
sigmoid NEC 46.99
Silver (bunionectomy) 77.59
Sistrunk (excision of thyroglossal cyst) 06.7
Skene's gland NEC 71.8
skin NEC 86.99
skull NEC 02.99
sling
   eyelid
      fascia lata, palpebral 08.36
      frontalis fascial 08.32
      levator muscle 08.33
      orbicularis muscle 08.36
      palpebrae ligament, fascia lata 08.36
      tarsus muscle 08.35
   fascial (fascia lata)
      eye 08.32
      for facial weakness (trigeminal nerve paralysis) 86.81
      palpebral ligament 08.36
      tongue 25.59
   tongue (fascial) 25.59
   urethra (suprapubic) 59.4
      retropubic 59.5
   urethrovesical 59.5
Slocum (pes anserinus transfer) 81.47
Sluder (tonsillectomy) 28.2
Smith (open osteotomy of mandible) 76.62
Smith-Peterson (radiocarpal arthrodesis) 81.25
Smithwick (sympathectomy) 05.29
Soave (endorectal pull-through) 48.41
soft tissue NEC 83.99
   hand 82.99
Sonneberg (inferior maxillary neurectomy) 04.07
Sorondo-Ferré (hindquarter amputation) 84.19
Soutter (iliac crest fasciotomy) 83.14
Spalding-Richardson (uterine suspension) 69.22
spermatic cord NEC 63.99
sphincter of Oddi NEC 51.89
spinal (canal) (cord) (structures) NEC 03.99
Spinelli (correction of inverted uterus) 75.93
Spivack (permanent gastrostomy) 43.19
spleen NEC 41.99
S.P. Rogers (knee disarticulation) 84.16
Ssabanejew-Frank (permanent gastrostomy) 43.19
Stacke (simple mastoidectomy) 20.41

Operation (*Continued*)

Stallard (conjunctivocystorhinostomy) 09.82
   with insertion of tube or stent 09.83
Stamm (-Kader) (temporary gastrostomy) 43.19
Steinberg 44.5
Steindler
   fascia stripping (for cavus deformity) 83.14
   flexorplasty (elbow) 83.77
   muscle transfer 83.77
sterilization NEC
   female - *see also* specific operation 66.39
   male - *see also* Ligation, vas deferens 63.70
Stewart (renal plication with pyeloplasty) 55.87
stomach NEC 44.99
Stone (anoplasty) 49.79
Strassman (metroplasty) 69.49
   metroplasty (Jones modification) 69.49
   uterus 68.22
Strayer (gastrocnemius recession) 83.72
stress incontinence - *see* Repair, stress incontinence
Stromeyer-Little (hepatotomy) 50.0
Strong (unbridling of celiac artery axis) 39.91
Sturmdorf (conization of cervix) 67.2
subcutaneous tissue NEC 86.99
sublingual gland or duct NEC 26.99
submaxillary gland or duct NEC 26.99
Summerskill (dacryocystorhinostomy by intubation) 09.81
Surmay (jejunostomy) 46.39
Swenson
   bladder reconstruction 57.87
   proctectomy 48.49
Swinney (urethral reconstruction) 58.46
Syme
   ankle amputation through malleoli of tibia and fibula 84.14
   urethrotomy, external 58.0
sympathetic nerve NEC 05.89
Taarnhoj (trigeminal nerve root decompression) 04.41
Tack (sacculotomy) 20.79
Talma-Morison (omentopexy) 54.74
Tanner (devascularization of stomach) 44.99
TAPVC NEC 35.82
tarsus NEC 08.99
   muscle sling 08.35
tendon NEC 83.99
   extraocular NEC 15.9
   hand NEC 82.99
testis NEC 62.99
tetralogy of Fallot
   partial repair - *see* specific procedure
   total (one-stage) 35.81
Thal (repair of esophageal stricture) 42.85
thalamus 01.41
   by stereotactic radiosurgery 92.32
      cobalt 60 92.32
      linear accelerator (LINAC) 92.31
      multi-source 92.32
      particle beam 92.33
      particulate 92.33
      radiosurgery NEC 92.39
      single source photon 92.31

Operation (*Continued*)

Thiersch
   anus 49.79
      skin graft 86.69
      hand 86.62
Thompson
   cleft lip repair 27.54
   correction of lymphedema 40.9
   quadricepsplasty 83.86
   thumb apposition with bone graft 82.69
thoracic duct NEC 40.69
thorax NEC 34.99
Thorek (partial cholecystectomy) 51.21
three-snip, punctum 09.51
thymus NEC 07.99
   thoracoscopic, NEC 07.98
thyroid gland NEC 06.98
TKP (thermokeratoplasty) 11.74
Tomkins (metroplasty) 69.49
tongue NEC 25.99
   flap, palate 27.62
   tie 25.91
tonsil NEC 28.99
Torek (-Bevan) (orchidopexy) (first stage) (second stage) 62.5
Torkildsen (ventriculocisternal shunt) 02.2
Torpin (cul-de-sac resection) 70.92
Toti (dacryocystorhinostomy) 09.81
Touchas 86.83
Touroff (ligation of subclavian artery) 38.85
trabeculae corneae cordis (heart) NEC 35.35
trachea NEC 31.99
Trauner (lingual sulcus extension) 24.91
truncus arteriosus NEC 35.83
Tsuge (macrodactyly repair) 82.83
Tudor "rabbit ear" (anterior urethropexy) 59.79
Tuffier
   apicolysis of lung 33.39
   vaginal hysterectomy 68.59
      laparoscopically assisted (LAVH) 68.51
tunica vaginalis NEC 61.99
Turco (release of joint capsules in clubfoot) 80.48
Uchida (tubal ligation with or without fimbriectomy) 66.32
umbilicus NEC 54.99
urachus NEC 57.51
Urban (mastectomy) (unilateral) 85.47
   bilateral 85.48
ureter NEC 56.99
urethra NEC 58.99
urinary system NEC 59.99
uterus NEC 69.99
   supporting structures NEC 69.98
uvula NEC 27.79
vagina NEC 70.91
vascular NEC 39.99
vas deferens NEC 63.99
   ligation NEC 63.71
vein NEC 39.99
vena cava sieve 38.7
vertebra NEC 78.49
vesical (bladder) NEC 57.99
vessel NEC 39.99
   cardiac NEC 36.99

◀ New   ◀▥ Revised   ~~deleted~~ Deleted   ● Use Additional Digit(s)   ▥ Omit code

Osteoplasty NEC (*Continued*)
  specified site NEC 78.49
  tarsal, metatarsal 78.48
  thorax (ribs) (sternum) 78.41
  tibia 78.47
  ulna 78.43
  vertebrae 78.49
Osteorrhaphy - *see also* Osteoplasty
  78.40
Osteosynthesis (fracture) - *see* Reduction,
  fracture
Osteotomy (adduction) (angulation)
  (block) (derotational) (displacement)
  (partial) (rotational) 77.30
  carpals, metacarpals 77.34
    wedge 77.24
  clavicle 77.31
    wedge 77.21
  facial bone NEC 76.69
  femur 77.35
    wedge 77.25
  fibula 77.37
    wedge 77.27
  humerus 77.32
    wedge 77.22
  mandible (segmental) (subapical) 76.64
    angle (open) 76.62
      closed 76.61
    body 76.63
    Gigli saw 76.61
    ramus (open) 76.62
      closed 76.61
  maxilla (segmental) 76.65
    total 76.66
  metatarsal 77.38
    wedge 77.28
      for hallux valgus repair 77.51
  patella 77.36
    wedge 77.26

Osteotomy (*Continued*)
  pelvic 77.39
    wedge 77.29
  phalanges (foot) (hand) 77.39
    for repair of
      bunion - *see* Bunionectomy
      bunionette 77.54
      hallux valgus - *see*
        Bunionectomy
    wedge 77.29
      for repair of
        bunion - *see* Bunionectomy
        bunionette 77.54
        hallux valgus - *see*
          Bunionectomy
  radius 77.33
    wedge 77.23
  scapula 77.31
    wedge 77.21
  specified site NEC 77.39
    wedge 77.29
  tarsal 77.38
    wedge 77.28
  thorax (ribs) (sternum) 77.31
    wedge 77.21
  tibia 77.37
    wedge 77.27
  toe 77.39
    for repair of
      bunion - *see* Bunionectomy
      bunionette 77.54
      hallux valgus - *see*
        Bunionectomy
    wedge 77.29
      for repair of
        bunion - *see* Bunionectomy
        bunionette 77.54
        hallux valgus - *see*
          Bunionectomy

Osteotomy (*Continued*)
  ulna 77.33
    wedge 77.23
  vertebrae 77.39
    wedge 77.29
Otonecrectomy (inner ear) 20.79
Otoplasty (external) 18.79
  auditory canal or meatus 18.6
  auricle 18.79
  cartilage 18.79
    reconstruction 18.71
  prominent or protruding 18.5
Otoscopy 18.11
Outfolding, sclera, for buckling - *see also*
  Buckling, scleral 14.49
Outfracture, turbinates (nasal) 21.62
Output and clearance, circulatory 92.05
Overdistension, bladder (therapeutic)
  96.25
Overlapping, sclera, for buckling - *see*
  also Buckling, scleral 14.49
Oversewing
  left atrial appendage (LAA) 37.36
  pleural bleb 32.21
  ulcer crater (peptic) 44.40
    duodenum 44.42
    stomach 44.41
Oxford operation (for urinary
  incontinence) 59.4
Oximetry
  fetal pulse 75.38
Oxygenation 93.96
  extracorporeal membrane (ECMO) 39.65
  hyperbaric 93.95
    wound 93.59
  infusion therapy, Super 00.49
Oxygen therapy (catalytic) (pump) 93.96
  hyperbaric 93.95
  SuperSaturated 00.49

◄ New   ◄▦ Revised   ~~deleted~~ Deleted   ● Use Additional Digit(s)   ▦ Omit code

P

Pacemaker
cardiac - *see also* Insertion, pacemaker, cardiac
intraoperative (temporary) 39.64
temporary (during and immediately following cardiac surgery) 39.64
Packing - *see also* Insertion, pack
auditory canal 96.11
nose, for epistaxis (anterior) 21.01
posterior (and anterior) 21.02
rectal 96.19
sella turcica 07.79
vaginal 96.14
Palatoplasty 27.69
for cleft palate 27.62
secondary or subsequent 27.63
Palatorrhaphy 27.61
for cleft palate 27.62
Pallidectomy 01.42
Pallidoansotomy 01.42
Pallidotomy 01.42
by stereotactic radiosurgery 92.32
cobalt 60 92.32
linear accelerator (LINAC) 92.31
multi-source 92.32
particle beam 92.33
particulate 92.33
radiosurgery NEC 92.39
single source photon 92.31
Panas operation (linear proctotomy) 48.0
Pancoast operation (division of trigeminal nerve at foramen ovale) 04.02
Pancreatectomy (total) (with synchronous duodenectomy) 52.6
partial NEC 52.59
distal (tail) (with part of body) 52.52
proximal (head) (with part of body) (with synchronous duodenectomy) 52.51
radical 52.53
subtotal 52.53
radical 52.7
subtotal 52.53
Pancreaticocystoduodenostomy 52.4
Pancreaticocystoenterostomy 52.4
Pancreaticocystogastrostomy 52.4
Pancreaticocystojejunostomy 52.4
Pancreaticoduodenectomy (total) 52.6
partial NEC 52.59
proximal 52.51
radical subtotal 52.53
radical (one-stage) (two-stage) 52.7
subtotal 52.53
Pancreaticoduodenostomy 52.96
Pancreaticoenterostomy 52.96
Pancreaticogastrostomy 52.96
Pancreaticoileostomy 52.96
Pancreaticojejunostomy 52.96
Pancreatoduodenectomy (total) 52.6
partial NEC 52.59
radical (one-stage) (two-stage) 52.7
subtotal 52.53
Pancreatogram 87.66
endoscopic retrograde (ERP) 52.13
Pancreatolithotomy 52.09
endoscopic 52.94
Pancreatotomy 52.09
Pancreolithotomy 52.09
endoscopic 52.94

Panendoscopy 57.32
specified site, other than bladder - *see* Endoscopy, by site
through artificial stoma 57.31
Panhysterectomy (abdominal) 68.49
laparoscopic 68.41
vaginal 68.59
laparoscopically assisted (LAVH) 68.51
Panniculectomy 86.83
Panniculotomy 86.83
Pantaloon operation (revision of gastric anastomosis) 44.5
Papillectomy, anal 49.39
endoscopic 49.31
Papillotomy (pancreas) 51.82
endoscopic 51.85
Paquin operation (ureteroneocystostomy) 56.74
Paracentesis
abdominal (percutaneous) 54.91
anterior chamber, eye 12.91
bladder 57.11
cornea 12.91
eye (anterior chamber) 12.91
thoracic, thoracis 34.91
tympanum 20.09
with intubation 20.01
Parasitology - *see* Examination, microscopic
Parathyroidectomy (partial) (subtotal) NEC 06.89
complete 06.81
ectopic 06.89
global removal 06.81
mediastinal 06.89
total 06.81
Parenteral nutrition, total 99.15
peripheral 99.15
Parotidectomy 26.30
complete 26.32
partial 26.31
radical 26.32
Partsch operation (marsupialization of dental cyst) 24.4
Passage - *see* Insertion and Intubation
Passage of sounds, urethra 58.6
Patch
blood, spinal (epidural) 03.95
graft - *see* Graft
spinal, blood (epidural) 03.95
subdural, brain 02.12
Patellapexy 78.46
Patellaplasty NEC 78.46
Patellectomy 77.96
partial 77.86
Pattee operation (auditory canal) 18.6
Pectenotomy - *see also* Sphincterotomy, anal 49.59
PDT (percutaneous dilatational tracheostomy) – *see* Tracheostomy
Pedicle flap - *see* Graft, skin, pedicle
Peet operation (splanchnic resection) 05.29
PEG (percutaneous endoscopic gastrostomy) 43.11
PEGJJ (percutaneous [endoscopic] gastrojejunostomy) 44.32
PEJ (percutaneous endoscopic jejunostomy) 46.32
Pelvectomy, kidney (partial) 55.4
Pelvimetry 88.25
gynecological 89.26
Pelviolithotomy 55.11

Pelvioplasty, kidney 55.87
Pelviostomy 55.12
closure 55.82
Pelviotomy 77.39
to assist delivery 73.94
Pelvi-ureteroplasty 55.87
Pemberton operation
osteotomy of ilium 77.39
rectum (mobilization and fixation for prolapse repair) 48.76
Penectomy 64.3
Pereyra operation (paraurethral suspension) 59.6
Perforation
stapes footplate 19.0
Perfusion NEC 39.97
carotid artery 39.97
coronary artery 39.97
for
chemotherapy NEC 99.25
hormone therapy NEC 99.24
head 39.97
hyperthermic (lymphatic), localized region or site 93.35
intestine (large) (local) 46.96
small 46.95
kidney, local 55.95
limb (lower) (upper) 39.97
liver, localized 50.93
neck 39.97
subarachnoid (spinal cord) (refrigerated saline) 03.92
total body 39.96
Pericardiectomy 37.31
Pericardiocentesis 37.0
Pericardiolysis 37.12
Pericardioplasty 37.49
Pericardiorrhaphy 37.49
Pericardiostomy (tube) 37.12
Pericardiotomy 37.12
Peridectomy 10.31
Perilimbal suction 89.11
Perimetry 95.05
Perineoplasty 71.79
Perineorrhaphy 71.71
obstetrical laceration (current) 75.69
Perineotomy (nonobstetrical) 71.09
to assist delivery - *see* Episiotomy
Periosteotomy - *see also* Incision, bone 77.10
facial bone 76.09
Perirectofistulectomy 48.93
Peritectomy 10.31
Peritomy 10.1
Peritoneocentesis 54.91
Peritoneoscopy 54.21
Peritoneotomy 54.19
Peritoneumectomy 54.4
Phacoemulsification (ultrasonic) (with aspiration) 13.41
Phacofragmentation (mechanical) (with aspiration) 13.43
posterior route 13.42
ultrasonic 13.41
Phalangectomy (partial) 77.89
claw toe 77.57
cockup toe 77.58
hammer toe 77.56
overlapping toe 77.58
total 77.99
Phalangization (fifth metacarpal) 82.81
Pharyngeal flap operation (cleft palate repair) 27.62
secondary or subsequent 27.63

◀ New ◀▥ Revised ~~deleted~~ Deleted ● Use Additional Digit(s) ▥ Omit code

Plication (Continued)
superior vena cava 38.7
tendon 83.85
hand 82.55
tricuspid valve (with repositioning)
35.14
ureter 56.89
urethra 58.49
urethrovesical junction 59.3
vein (peripheral) 39.59
vena cava (inferior) (superior) 38.7
ventricle (heart)
aneurysm 37.32
Plicotomy, tympanum 20.23
Plombage, lung 33.39
Pneumocentesis 33.93
Pneumocisternogram 87.02
Pneumoencephalogram 87.01
Pneumogram, pneumography
extraperitoneal 88.15
mediastinal 87.33
orbit 87.14
pelvic 88.13
peritoneum NEC 88.13
presacral 88.15
retroperitoneum 88.15
Pneumogynecography 87.82
Pneumomediastinography 87.33
Pneumonectomy (extended) (radical)
(standard) (total) (with mediastinal
dissection) 32.59
partial
complete excision, one lobe
32.49
resection (wedge), one lobe
32.39
thoracoscopic 32.50
Pneumonolysis (for collapse of lung)
33.39
Pneumonotomy (with exploration) 33.1
Pneumoperitoneum (surgically-induced)
54.96
for collapse of lung 33.33
pelvic 88.12
Pneumothorax (artificial) (surgical) 33.32
intrapleural 33.32
Pneumoventriculogram 87.02
Politano-Leadbetter operation
(ureteroneocystostomy) 56.74
Politzerization, Eustachian tube 20.8
Pollicization (with carry over of nerves
and blood supply) 82.61
Polya operation (gastrectomy) 43.7
Polypectomy - see also Excision, lesion, by
site
esophageal 42.32
endoscopic 42.33
gastric (endoscopic) 43.41
large intestine (colon) 45.42
nasal 21.31
rectum (endoscopic) 48.36
Polysomnogram 89.17
Pomeroy operation (ligation and division
of fallopian tubes) 66.32
Poncet operation
lengthening of Achilles tendon 83.85
urethrostomy, perineal 58.0
Porro operation (cesarean section)
74.99
Portoenterostomy (Kasai) 51.37
Positrocephalogram 92.11
Positron emission tomography (PET) - see
Scan, radioisotope
Postmortem examination 89.8

Potts-Smith operation (descending aorta-
left pulmonary artery anastomosis)
39.0
Poudrage
intrapericardial 36.39
pleural 34.6
PPN (peripheral parenteral nutrition)
99.15
Preparation (cutting), pedicle (flap) graft
86.71
Preputiotomy 64.91
Prescription for glasses 95.31
Pressurized
graft treatment 00.16
Printen and Mason operation (high
gastric bypass) 44.31
Probing
canaliculus, lacrimal (with irrigation)
09.42
lacrimal
canaliculi 09.42
punctum (with irrigation) 09.41
nasolacrimal duct (with irrigation)
09.43
with insertion of tube or stent
09.44
salivary duct (for dilation of duct) (for
removal of calculus) 26.91
with incision 26.0
Procedure - see also specific procedure
diagnostic NEC
abdomen (region) 54.29
adenoid 28.19
adrenal gland 07.19
alveolus 24.19
amnion 75.35
anterior chamber, eye 12.29
anus 49.29
appendix 45.28
biliary tract 51.19
bladder 57.39
blood vessel (any site) 38.29
bone 78.80
carpal, metacarpal 78.84
clavicle 78.81
facial 76.19
femur 78.85
fibula 78.87
humerus 78.82
marrow 41.38
patella 78.86
pelvic 78.89
phalanges (foot) (hand) 78.89
radius 78.83
scapula 78.81
specified site NEC 78.89
tarsal, metatarsal 78.88
thorax (ribs) (sternum) 78.81
tibia 78.87
ulna 78.83
vertebrae 78.89
brain 01.18
breast 85.19
bronchus 33.29
buccal 27.24
bursa 83.29
canthus 08.19
cecum 45.28
cerebral meninges 01.18
cervix 67.19
chest wall 34.28
choroid 14.19
ciliary body 12.29
clitoris 71.19

Procedure (Continued)
diagnostic NEC (Continued)
colon 45.28
conjunctiva 10.29
cornea 11.29
cul-de-sac 70.29
dental 24.19
diaphragm 34.28
duodenum 45.19
ear
external 18.19
inner and middle 20.39
epididymis 63.09
esophagus 42.29
Eustachian tube 20.39
extraocular muscle or tendon
15.09
eye 16.29
anterior chamber 12.29
posterior chamber 14.19
eyeball 16.29
eyelid 08.19
fallopian tube 66.19
fascia (any site) 83.29
fetus 75.35
gallbladder 51.19
ganglion (cranial) (peripheral)
04.19
sympathetic 05.19
gastric 44.19
globus pallidus 01.18
gum 24.19
heart 37.29
hepatic 50.19
hypophysis 07.19
ileum 45.19
intestine 45.29
large 45.28
small 45.19
iris 12.29
jejunum 45.19
joint (capsule) (ligament) (structure)
NEC 81.98
facial 76.19
kidney 55.29
labia 71.19
lacrimal (system) 09.19
large intestine 45.28
larynx 31.48
ligament 81.98
uterine 68.19
liver 50.19
lung 33.29
lymphatic structure (channel)
(gland) (node) (vessel) 40.19
mediastinum 34.29
meninges (cerebral) 01.18
spinal 03.39
mouth 27.29
muscle 83.29
extraocular (oblique) (rectus)
15.09
papillary (heart) 37.29
nail 86.19
nasopharynx 29.19
nerve (cranial) (peripheral) NEC
04.19
sympathetic 05.19
nipple 85.19
nose, nasal 21.29
sinus 22.19
ocular 16.29
muscle 15.09
omentum 54.29

Procedure *(Continued)*
  diagnostic NEC *(Continued)*
    ophthalmologic 16.29
    oral (cavity) 27.29
    orbit 16.29
    orthodontic 24.19
    ovary 65.19
      laparoscopic 65.14
    palate 27.29
    pancreas 52.19
    papillary muscle (heart) 37.29
    parathyroid gland 06.19
    penis 64.19
    perianal tissue 49.29
    pericardium 37.29
    periprostatic tissue 60.18
    perirectal tissue 48.29
    perirenal tissue 59.29
    peritoneum 54.29
    periurethral tissue 58.29
    perivesical tissue 59.29
    pharynx 29.19
    pineal gland 07.19
    pituitary gland 07.19
    pleura 34.28
    posterior chamber, eye 14.19
    prostate 60.18
    pulmonary 33.29
    rectosigmoid 48.29
    rectum 48.29
    renal 55.29
    respiratory 33.29
    retina 14.19
    retroperitoneum 59.29
    salivary gland or duct 26.19
    sclera 12.29
    scrotum 61.19
    seminal vesicle 60.19
    sigmoid 45.28
    sinus, nasal 22.19
    skin 86.19
    skull 01.19
    soft tissue 83.29
    spermatic cord 63.09
    sphincter of Oddi 51.19
    spine, spinal (canal) (cord)
        (meninges) (structure)
        03.39
    spleen 41.39
    stomach 44.19
    subcutaneous tissue 86.19
    sympathetic nerve 05.19
    tarsus 09.19
    tendon NEC 83.29
      extraocular 15.09
    testicle 62.19
    thalamus 01.18
    thoracic duct 40.19
    thorax 34.28
    thymus 07.19
    thyroid gland 06.19
    tongue 25.09
    tonsils 28.19
    tooth 24.19
    trachea 31.49
    tunica vaginalis 61.19
    ureter 56.39
    urethra 58.29
    uterus and supporting structures
        68.19
    uvula 27.29
    vagina 70.29
    vas deferens 63.09
    vesical 57.39

Procedure *(Continued)*
  diagnostic NEC *(Continued)*
    vessel (blood) (any site) 38.29
    vitreous 14.19
    vulva 71.19
  fistulizing, sclera NEC 12.69
  miscellaneous (nonoperative) NEC
      99.99
  respiratory (nonoperative) NEC 93.99
  surgical - *see* Operation
Proctectasis 96.22
Proctectomy (partial) - *see also* Resection,
    rectum 48.69
  abdominoperineal, NOS 48.50
    laparoscopic 48.51
    open 48.52
    other 48.59
  complete (Miles) (Rankin), NOS
      48.50
    laparoscopic 48.51
    open 48.52
    other 48.59
  pull-through
    laparoscopic 48.42
    not otherwise specified 48.40
    open 48.43
    other 48.49
Proctoclysis 96.37
Proctolysis 48.99
Proctopexy (Delorme) 48.76
  abdominal (Ripstein) 48.75
Proctoplasty 48.79
Proctorrhaphy 48.71
Proctoscopy 48.23
  with biopsy 48.24
  through stoma (artificial) 48.22
  transabdominal approach 48.21
Proctosigmoidectomy - *see also* Resection,
    rectum 48.69
Proctosigmoidopexy 48.76
Proctosigmoidoscopy (rigid) 48.23
  with biopsy 48.24
  flexible 45.24
  through stoma (artificial) 48.22
  transabdominal approach 48.21
Proctostomy 48.1
Proctotomy (decompression) (linear)
    48.0
Production - *see also* Formation *and*
    Creation
  atrial septal defect 35.42
  subcutaneous tunnel for esophageal
      anastomosis 42.86
    with anastomosis - *see* Anastomosis,
        esophagus, antesternal
Prognathic recession 76.64
Prophylaxis, dental (scaling) (polishing)
    96.54
Prostatectomy (complete) (partial) NEC
    60.69
  loop 60.29
  perineal 60.62
  radical (any approach) 60.5
  retropubic (punch) (transcapsular)
      60.4
  suprapubic (punch) (transvesical)
      60.3
  transcapsular NEC 60.69
    retropubic 60.4
  transperineal 60.62
  transurethral 60.29
    ablation (contact) (noncontact) by
        laser 60.21
    electrovaporization 60.29

Prostatectomy *(Continued)*
  transurethral *(Continued)*
    enucleative 60.29
    resection of prostate (TURP) 60.29
    ultrasound guided laser induced
        (TULIP) 60.21
  transvesical punch (suprapubic) 60.3
Prostatocystotomy 60.0
Prostatolithotomy 60.0
Prostatotomy (perineal) 60.0
Prostatovesiculectomy 60.5
Protection (of)
  individual from his surroundings
      99.84
  surroundings from individual 99.84
Psychoanalysis 94.31
Psychodrama 94.43
Psychotherapy NEC 94.39
  biofeedback 94.39
  exploratory verbal 94.37
  group 94.44
    for psychosexual dysfunctions
        94.41
  play 94.36
  psychosexual dysfunctions 94.34
  supportive verbal 94.38
PTCA (percutaneous transluminal
    coronary angioplasty) - *see*
    Angioplasty, balloon, coronary
Ptyalectasis 26.91
Ptyalithotomy 26.0
Ptyalolithotomy 26.0
Pubiotomy 77.39
  assisting delivery 73.94
Pubococcygeoplasty 59.71
Puestow operation
    (pancreaticojejunostomy) 52.96
Pull-through
  abdomino-anal 48.49
  abdominoperineal 48.49
    Duhamel type 48.65
  endorectal 48.41
Pulmowrap 93.99
Pulpectomy - *see also* Therapy, root canal
    23.70
Pulpotomy - *see also* Therapy, root canal
    23.70
Pump-oxygenator, for extracorporeal
    circulation 39.61
  percutaneous 39.66
Punch
  operation
    bladder neck, transurethral 57.49
    prostate - *see* Prostatectomy
  resection, vocal cords 30.22
Puncture
  antrum (nasal) (bilateral) (unilateral)
      22.01
  artery NEC 38.98
    for
      arteriography - *see also*
          Arteriography 88.40
    for
      coronary arteriography - *see also*
          Arteriography, coronary
          88.57
      percutaneous vascular closure - *omit*
          code
  bladder, suprapubic (for drainage)
      NEC 57.18
    needle 57.11
    percutaneous (suprapubic) 57.17
  bursa 83.94
    hand 82.92

◀ New   ◀▥ Revised   ~~deleted~~ Deleted   ● Use Additional Digit(s)   ▬ Omit code

Puncture (*Continued*)
cisternal 01.01
with contrast media 87.02
cranial 01.09
with contrast media 87.02
craniobuccal pouch 07.72
craniopharyngioma 07.72
fallopian tube 66.91
fontanel, anterior 01.09
heart 37.0
for intracardiac injection 37.92
hypophysis 07.72
iris 12.12
joint 81.91
kidney (percutaneous) 55.92
larynx 31.98
lumbar (diagnostic) (removal of dye)
03.31
lung (for aspiration) 33.93
nasal sinus 22.01
pericardium 37.0
pituitary gland 07.72
pleural cavity 34.91
Rathke's pouch 07.72
spinal 03.31
spleen 41.1
for biopsy 41.32

Puncture (*Continued*)
sternal (for bone marrow biopsy)
41.31
donor for bone marrow transplant
41.91
vein NEC 38.99
for
phlebography - *see also*
Phlebography 88.60
transfusion - *see* Transfusion
ventricular shunt tubing 01.02
Pupillotomy 12.35
Push-back operation (cleft palate repair)
27.62
Putti-Platt operation (capsulorrhaphy of
shoulder for recurrent dislocation)
81.82
pVAD (percutaneous ventricular assist
device) 37.68
Pyelogram (intravenous) 87.73
infusion (continuous) (diuretic)
87.73
percutaneous 87.75
retrograde 87.74
Pyeloileostomy 56.71
Pyelolithotomy 55.11
Pyeloplasty 55.87

Pyelorrhaphy 55.81
Pyeloscopy 55.22
Pyelostolithotomy, percutaneous
55.03
Pyelostomy 55.12
closure 55.82
Pyelotomy 55.11
Pyeloureteroplasty 55.87
Pylorectomy 43.6
Pyloroduodenotomy - *see* category 44.2●
Pyloromyotomy (Ramstedt) (with wedge
resection) 43.3
Pyloroplasty (Finney) (Heineke-Mikulicz)
44.29
dilation, endoscopic 44.22
by incision 44.21
not elsewhere classified 44.29
revision 44.29
Pylorostomy - *see* Gastrostomy

Q

Quadrant resection of breast 85.22
Quadricepsplasty (Thompson) 83.86
Quarantine 99.84
Quenuthoracoplasty 77.31
Quotient, respiratory 89.38

R

Rachicentesis 03.31
Rachitomy 03.09
Radiation therapy - *see also* Therapy, radiation
  teleradiotherapy - *see* Teleradiotherapy
Radical neck dissection - *see* Dissection, neck
Radicotomy 03.1
Radiculectomy 03.1
Radiculotomy 03.1
Radiography (diagnostic) NEC 88.39
  abdomen, abdominal (flat plate) NEC 88.19
    wall (soft tissue) NEC 88.09
  adenoid 87.09
  ankle (skeletal) 88.28
    soft tissue 88.37
  bone survey 88.31
  bronchus 87.49
  chest (routine) 87.44
    wall NEC 87.39
  clavicle 87.43
  computer assisted surgery (CAS) with fluoroscopy 00.33
  contrast (air) (gas) (radio-opaque substance) NEC
    abdominal wall 88.03
    arteries (by fluoroscopy) - *see* Arteriography
    bile ducts NEC 87.54
    bladder NEC 87.77
    brain 87.02
    breast 87.35
    bronchus NEC (transcricoid) 87.32
      endotracheal 87.31
    epididymis 87.93
    esophagus 87.61
    fallopian tubes
      gas 87.82
      opaque dye 87.83
    fistula (sinus tract) - *see also* Radiography, contrast, by site
      abdominal wall 88.03
      chest wall 87.38
    gallbladder NEC 87.59
    intervertebral disc(s) 87.21
    joints 88.32
    larynx 87.07
    lymph - *see* Lymphangiogram
    mammary ducts 87.35
    mediastinum 87.33
    nasal sinuses 87.15
    nasolacrimal ducts 87.05
    nasopharynx 87.06
    orbit 87.14
    pancreas 87.66
    pelvis
      gas 88.12
      opaque dye 88.11
    peritoneum NEC 88.13
    retroperitoneum NEC 88.15
    seminal vesicles 87.91
    sinus tract - *see also* Radiography, contrast, by site
      abdominal wall 88.03
      chest wall 87.38
      nose 87.15
    skull 87.02
    spinal disc(s) 87.21
    trachea 87.32

Radiography NEC (*Continued*)
  contrast (*Continued*)
    uterus
      gas 87.82
      opaque dye 87.83
    vas deferens 87.94
    veins (by fluoroscopy) - *see* Phlebography
    vena cava (inferior) (superior) 88.51
  dental NEC 87.12
  diaphragm 87.49
  digestive tract NEC 87.69
    barium swallow 87.61
    lower GI series 87.64
    small bowel series 87.63
    upper GI series 87.62
  elbow (skeletal) 88.22
    soft tissue 88.35
  epididymis NEC 87.95
  esophagus 87.69
    barium-swallow 87.61
  eye 95.14
  face, head, and neck 87.09
  facial bones 87.16
  fallopian tubes 87.85
  foot 88.28
  forearm (skeletal) 88.22
    soft tissue 88.35
  frontal area, facial 87.16
  genital organs
    female NEC 87.89
    male NEC 87.99
  hand (skeletal) 88.23
    soft tissue 88.35
  head NEC 87.09
  heart 87.49
  hip (skeletal) 88.26
    soft tissue 88.37
  intestine NEC 87.65
  kidney-ureter-bladder (KUB) 87.79
  knee (skeletal) 88.27
    soft tissue 88.37
  KUB (kidney-ureter-bladder) 87.79
  larynx 87.09
  lower leg (skeletal) 88.27
    soft tissue 88.37
  lower limb (skeletal) NEC 88.29
    soft tissue NEC 88.37
  lung 87.49
  mandible 87.16
  maxilla 87.16
  mediastinum 87.49
  nasal sinuses 87.16
  nasolacrimal duct 87.09
  nasopharynx 87.09
  neck NEC 87.09
  nose 87.16
  orbit 87.16
  pelvis (skeletal) 88.26
    pelvimetry 88.25
    soft tissue 88.19
  prostate NEC 87.92
  retroperitoneum NEC 88.16
  ribs 87.43
  root canal 87.12
  salivary gland 87.09
  seminal vesicles NEC 87.92
  shoulder (skeletal) 88.21
    soft tissue 88.35
  skeletal NEC 88.33
    series (whole or complete) 88.31
  skull (lateral, sagittal or tangential projection) NEC 87.17

Radiography NEC (*Continued*)
  spine NEC 87.29
    cervical 87.22
    lumbosacral 87.24
    sacrococcygeal 87.24
    thoracic 87.23
  sternum 87.43
  supraorbital area 87.16
  symphysis menti 87.16
  teeth NEC 87.12
    full-mouth 87.11
  thigh (skeletal) 88.27
    soft tissue 88.37
  thyroid region 87.09
  tonsils and adenoids 87.09
  trachea 87.49
  ultrasonic - *see* Ultrasonography
  upper arm (skeletal) 88.21
    soft tissue 88.35
  upper limb (skeletal) NEC 88.24
    soft tissue NEC 88.35
  urinary system NEC 87.79
  uterus NEC 87.85
    gravid 87.81
  uvula 87.09
  vas deferens NEC 87.95
  wrist 88.23
  zygomaticomaxillary complex 87.16
Radioimmunotherapy 92.28
Radioisotope
  scanning - *see* Scan, radioisotope
  therapy - *see* Therapy, radioisotope
Radiology
  diagnostic - *see* Radiography
  therapeutic - *see* Therapy, radiation
Radiosurgery, stereotactic 92.30
  cobalt 60 92.32
  linear accelerator (LINAC) 92.31
  multi-source 92.32
  particle beam 92.33
  particulate 92.33
  radiosurgery NEC 92.39
  single source photon 92.31
Raising, pedicle graft 86.71
Ramadier operation (intrapetrosal drainage) 20.22
Ramisection (sympathetic) 05.0
Ramstedt operation (pyloromyotomy) (with wedge resection) 43.3
Range of motion testing 93.05
Rankin operation
  exteriorization of intestine 46.03
  proctectomy (complete), NOS 48.50
    laparoscopic 48.51
    open 48.52
    other 48.59
Rashkind operation (balloon septostomy) 35.41
Rastelli operation (creation of conduit between right ventricle and pulmonary artery) 35.92
  in repair of
    pulmonary artery atresia 35.92
    transposition of great vessels 35.92
    truncus arteriosus 35.83
Raz-Pereyra procedure (bladder neck suspension) 59.79
RCSA (radical cryosurgical ablation) of prostate 60.62
Readjustment - *see* Adjustment
Reamputation, stump 84.3
Reanastomosis - *see* Anastomosis

◄ New   ◄▥ Revised   ~~deleted~~ Deleted   ● Use Additional Digit(s)   ▬ Omit code

Reattachment
  amputated ear 18.72
  ankle 84.27
  arm (upper) NEC 84.24
  choroid and retina NEC 14.59
    by
        cryotherapy 14.52
        diathermy 14.51
        electrocoagulation 14.51
        photocoagulation 14.55
            laser 14.54
            xenon arc 14.53
  ear (amputated) 18.72
  extremity 84.29
    ankle 84.27
    arm (upper) NEC 84.24
    fingers, except thumb 84.22
        thumb 84.21
    foot 84.26
    forearm 84.23
    hand 84.23
    leg (lower) NEC 84.27
    thigh 84.28
    thumb 84.21
    toe 84.25
    wrist 84.23
  finger 84.22
    thumb 84.21
  foot 84.26
  forearm 84.23
  hand 84.23
  joint capsule - see also Arthroplasty
    81.96
  leg (lower) NEC 84.27
  ligament - see also Arthroplasty
    uterosacral 69.22
  muscle 83.74
    hand 82.54
    papillary (heart) 35.31
  nerve (peripheral) 04.79
  nose (amputated) 21.89
  papillary muscle (heart) 35.31
  penis (amputated) 64.45
  retina (and choroid) NEC 14.59
    by
        cryotherapy 14.52
        diathermy 14.51
        electrocoagulation 14.51
        photocoagulation 14.55
            laser 14.54
            xenon arc 14.53
  tendon (to tendon) 83.73
    hand 82.53
    to skeletal attachment 83.88
        hand 82.85
  thigh 84.28
  thumb 84.21
  toe 84.25
  tooth 23.5
  uterosacral ligament(s) 69.22
  vessels (peripheral) 39.59
    renal, aberrant 39.55
  wrist 84.23
Recession
  extraocular muscle 15.11
    multiple (two or more muscles)
        (with advancement or
        resection) 15.3
  gastrocnemius tendon (Strayer
    operation) 83.72
  levator palpebrae (superioris) muscle
    08.38
  prognathic jaw 76.64
  tendon 83.72
    hand 82.52

Reclosure - see also Closure
  disrupted abdominal wall
    (postoperative) 54.61
Reconstruction (plastic) - see also
    Construction and Repair, by site
  alveolus, alveolar (process) (ridge)
    (with graft or implant) 24.5
  artery (graft) - see Graft, artery
  artificial stoma, intestine 46.40
  auditory canal (external) 18.6
  auricle (ear) 18.71
  bladder 57.87
    with
        ileum 57.87 [45.51]
        sigmoid 57.87 [45.52]
  bone, except facial - see also Osteoplasty
    78.40
    facial NEC 76.46
        with total ostectomy 76.44
    mandible 76.43
        with total mandibulectomy
        76.41
  breast, total, NOS 85.70
    deep inferior epigastric artery
        perforator (DIEP) flap, free
        85.74
    gluteal artery perforator (GAP) flap,
        free 85.76
    latissimus dorsi myocutaneous flap
        85.71
    other 85.79   ◄
    superficial inferior epigastric artery
        (SIEA) flap, free 85.75
    transverse rectus abdominis
        musculocutaneous (TRAM)
        flap, free 85.73
    transverse rectus abdominis
        myocutaneous (TRAM) flap,
        pedicled 85.72
  bronchus 33.48
  canthus (lateral) 08.59
  cardiac annulus 35.33
  chest wall (mesh) (silastic) 34.79
  cleft lip 27.54
  conjunctival cul-de-sac 10.43
    with graft (buccal mucous
        membrane) (free) 10.42
  cornea NEC 11.79
  diaphragm 34.84
  ear (external) (auricle) 18.71
    external auditory canal 18.6
    meatus (new) (osseous skin-lined)
        18.6
    ossicles 19.3
    prominent or protruding 18.5
  eyebrow 08.70
  eyelid 08.70
    with graft or flap 08.69
        hair follicle 08.63
        mucous membrane 08.62
        skin 08.61
        tarsoconjunctival (one-stage)
            (two-stage) 08.64
    full-thickness 08.74
        involving lid margin 08.73
    partial-thickness 08.72
        involving lid margin 08.71
  eye socket 16.64
    with graft 16.63
  fallopian tube 66.79
  foot and toes (with fixation device)
    81.57
    with prosthetic implant 81.57
  frontonasal duct 22.79
  hip (total) (with prosthesis) 81.51

Reconstruction (Continued)
  intraoral 27.59
  joint - see Arthroplasty
  lymphatic (by transplantation) 40.9
  mandible 76.43
    with total mandibulectomy 76.41
  mastoid cavity 19.9
  mouth 27.59
  nipple NEC 85.87
  nose (total) (with arm flap) (with
    forehead flap) 21.83
  ossicles (graft) (prosthesis) NEC 19.3
    with
        stapedectomy 19.19
        tympanoplasty 19.53
  pelvic floor 71.79
  penis (rib graft) (skin graft)
    (myocutaneous flap) 64.44
  pharynx 29.4
  scrotum (with pedicle flap) (with
    rotational flap) 61.49
  skin (plastic) (without graft) NEC
    86.89
    with graft - see Graft, skin
  subcutaneous tissue (plastic) (without
    skin graft) NEC 86.89
    with graft - see Graft, skin
  tendon pulley (with graft) (with local
    tissue) 83.83
    for opponensplasty 82.71
        hand 82.71
  thumb (osteoplastic) (with bone graft)
    (with skin graft) 82.69
  trachea (with graft) 31.75
  umbilicus
    laparoscopic 53.43
        with graft or prosthesis 53.42
    other and open with graft or
        prosthesis 53.41
    other open 53.49
  ureteropelvic junction 55.87
  urethra 58.46
  vagina 70.62
    with graft or prosthesis 70.64
  vas deferens, surgically divided
    63.82
Recontour, gingiva 24.2
Recreational therapy 93.81
Rectectomy - see also Resection, rectum
  48.69
Rectopexy (Delorme) 48.76
  abdominal (Ripstein) 48.75
Rectoplasty 48.79
Rectorectostomy 48.74
Rectorrhaphy 48.71
Rectosigmoidectomy - see also Resection,
  rectum 48.69
  transsacral 48.61
Rectosigmoidostomy 45.94
Rectostomy 48.1
  closure 48.72
Red cell survival studies 92.05
Reduction - see also Excision, by site
  adipose tissue 86.83
  batwing arms 86.83
  breast (bilateral) 85.32
    unilateral 85.31
  bulbous tuberosities (mandible)
    (maxilla) (fibrous) (osseous)
    24.31
  buttocks 86.83
  diastasis, ankle mortise (closed)
    79.77
    open 79.87

Reduction *(Continued)*
  dislocation (of joint) (manipulation) (with cast) (with splint) (with traction device) (closed) 79.70
    with fracture - *see* Reduction, fracture, by site
    ankle (closed) 79.77
      open 79.87
    elbow (closed) 79.72
      open 79.82
    finger (closed) 79.74
      open 79.84
    foot (closed) 79.78
      open 79.88
    hand (closed) 79.74
      open 79.84
    hip (closed) 79.75
      open 79.85
    knee (closed) 79.76
      open 79.86
    open (with external fixation) (with internal fixation) 79.80
      specified site NEC 79.89
    shoulder (closed) 79.71
      open 79.81
    specified site (closed) NEC 79.79
      open 79.89
    temporomandibular (closed) 76.93
      open 76.94
    toe (closed) 79.78
      open 79.88
    wrist (closed) 79.73
      open 79.83
  elephantiasis, scrotum 61.3
  epistaxis - *see also* Control, epistaxis 21.00
  fracture (bone) (with cast) (with splint) (with traction device) (closed) 79.00
    with internal fixation 79.10
    alveolar process (with stabilization of teeth)
      mandible (closed) 76.75
        open 76.77
      maxilla (closed) 76.73
        open 76.77
      open 76.77
    ankle - *see* Reduction, fracture, leg
    arm (closed) NEC 79.02
      with internal fixation 79.12
      open 79.22
        with internal fixation 79.32
    blow-out - *see* Reduction, fracture, orbit
    carpal, metacarpal (closed) 79.03
      with internal fixation 79.13
      open 79.23
        with internal fixation 79.33
    epiphysis - *see* Reduction, separation
    facial (bone) NEC 76.70
      closed 76.78
      open 76.79
    femur (closed) 79.05
      with internal fixation 79.15
      open 79.25
        with internal fixation 79.35
    fibula (closed) 79.06
      with internal fixation 79.16
      open 79.26
        with internal fixation 79.36
    foot (closed) NEC 79.07
      with internal fixation 79.17
      open 79.27
        with internal fixation 79.37

Reduction *(Continued)*
  fracture *(Continued)*
    hand (closed) NEC 79.03
      with internal fixation 79.13
      open 79.23
        with internal fixation 79.33
    humerus (closed) 79.01
      with internal fixation 79.11
      open 79.21
        with internal fixation 79.31
    jaw (lower) - *see also* Reduction, fracture, mandible
      upper - *see* Reduction, fracture, maxilla
    larynx 31.64
    leg (closed) NEC 79.06
      with internal fixation 79.16
      open 79.26
        with internal fixation 79.36
    malar (closed) 76.71
      open 76.72
    mandible (with dental wiring) (closed) 76.75
      open 76.76
    maxilla (with dental wiring) (closed) 76.73
      open 76.74
    nasal (closed) 21.71
      open 21.72
    open 79.20
      with internal fixation 79.30
      specified site NEC 79.29
        with internal fixation 79.39
    orbit (rim) (wall) (closed) 76.78
      open 76.79
    patella (open) (with internal fixation) 79.36
    phalanges
      foot (closed) 79.08
        with internal fixation 79.18
        open 79.28
          with internal fixation 79.38
      hand (closed) 79.04
        with internal fixation 79.14
        open 79.24
          with internal fixation 79.34
    radius (closed) 79.02
      with internal fixation 79.12
      open 79.22
        with internal fixation 79.32
    skull 02.02
    specified site (closed) NEC 79.09
      with internal fixation 79.19
      open 79.29
        with internal fixation 79.39
    spine 03.53
    tarsal, metatarsal (closed) 79.07
      with internal fixation 79.17
      open 79.27
        with internal fixation 79.37
    tibia (closed) 79.06
      with internal fixation 79.16
      open 79.26
        with internal fixation 79.36
    ulna (closed) 79.02
      with internal fixation 79.12
      open 79.22
        with internal fixation 79.32
    vertebra 03.53
    zygoma, zygomatic arch (closed) 76.71
      open 76.72

Reduction *(Continued)*
  fracture dislocation - *see* Reduction, fracture
  heart volume 37.35
  hemorrhoids (manual) 49.41
  hernia - *see also* Repair, hernia
    manual 96.27
  intussusception (open) 46.80
    with
      fluoroscopy 96.29
      ionizing radiation enema 96.29
      ultrasonography guidance 96.29
    hydrostatic 96.29
    large intestine 46.82
      endoscopic (balloon) 46.85
    pneumatic 96.29
    small intestine 46.81
  lung volume 32.22
    biologic lung volume reduction (BLVR) - *see* category 33.7 ●
  malrotation, intestine (manual) (surgical) 46.80
    large 46.82
      endoscopic (balloon) 46.85
    small 46.81
  mammoplasty (bilateral) 85.32
    unilateral 85.31
  prolapse
    anus (operative) 49.94
    colostomy (manual) 96.28
    enterostomy (manual) 96.28
    ileostomy (manual) 96.28
    rectum (manual) 96.26
    uterus
      by pessary 96.18
      surgical 69.22
  ptosis overcorrection 08.37
  retroversion, uterus by pessary 96.18
  separation, epiphysis (with internal fixation) (closed) 79.40
    femur (closed) 79.45
      open 79.55
    fibula (closed) 79.46
      open 79.56
    humerus (closed) 79.41
      open 79.51
    open 79.50
    specified site (closed) NEC - *see also* category 79.4 ●
      open - *see* category 79.5 ●
    tibia (closed) 79.46
      open 79.56
  size
    abdominal wall (adipose) (pendulous) 86.83
    arms (adipose) (batwing) 86.83
    breast (bilateral) 85.32
      unilateral 85.31
    buttocks (adipose) 86.83
    finger (macrodactyly repair) 82.83
    skin 86.83
    subcutaneous tissue 86.83
    thighs (adipose) 86.83
  torsion
    intestine (manual) (surgical) 46.80
      large 46.82
        endoscopic (balloon) 46.85
      small 46.81
    kidney pedicle 55.84
    omentum 54.74
    spermatic cord 63.52
      with orchiopexy 62.5

◀ New   ◀▦ Revised   ~~deleted~~ Deleted   ● Use Additional Digit(s)   ▦ Omit code

Reduction (Continued)
  torsion (Continued)
    testis 63.52
      with orchiopexy 62.5
    uterus NEC 69.98
      gravid 75.99
    ventricular 37.35
  volvulus
    intestine 46.80
      large 46.82
        endoscopic (balloon) 46.85
      small 46.81
    stomach 44.92
Reefing, joint capsule - see also
    Arthroplasty 81.96
Re-entry operation (aorta) 39.54
Re-establishment, continuity - see also
    Anastomosis
  bowel 46.50
  fallopian tube 66.79
  vas deferens 63.82
Referral (for)
  psychiatric aftercare (halfway house)
      (outpatient clinic) 94.52
  psychotherapy 94.51
  rehabilitation
    alcoholism 94.53
    drug addiction 94.54
    psychologic NEC 94.59
    vocational 94.55
Reformation
  cardiac pacemaker pocket, new site
      (skin) (subcutaneous) 37.79
  cardioverter/defibrillator (automatic)
      pocket, new site (skin)
      (subcutaneous) 37.79
  chamber of eye 12.99
Refracture
  bone (for faulty union) - see also
      Osteoclasis 78.70
  nasal bones 21.88
Refusion
  spinal, NOS 81.30
    atlas-axis (anterior) (transoral)
        (posterior) 81.31
    cervical (C2 level or below) NEC
        81.32
      anterior (interbody), anterolateral
          technique 81.32
      C1-C2 level (anterior) (posterior)
          81.31
      posterior (interbody),
          posterolateral technique
          81.33
    craniocervical (anterior) (transoral)
        (posterior) 81.31
    dorsal, dorsolumbar NEC 81.35
      anterior (interbody),
          anterolateral technique
          81.34
      posterior (interbody),
          posterolateral technique
          81.35
    lumbar, lumbosacral NEC 81.38
      anterior (interbody),
          anterolateral technique
          81.36
      anterior lumbar interbody fusion
          (ALIF) 81.36
      lateral transverse process
          technique 81.37
      posterior (interbody),
          posterolateral technique
          81.38

Refusion (Continued)
  spinal, NOS (Continued)
    lumbar, lumbosacral NEC
        (Continued)
      posterior lumbar interbody
          fusion (PLIF) 81.38
      transforaminal lumbar interbody
          fusion (TLIF) 81.38
    number of vertebrae - see codes
        81.62–81.64
    occiput–C2 (anterior) (transoral)
        (posterior) 81.31
    refusion NEC 81.39

> Note: Also use either 81.62, 81.63, or
> 81.64 as an additional code to show the
> total number of vertebrae fused

Regional blood flow study 92.05
Regulation, menstrual 69.6
Rehabilitation programs NEC 93.89
  alcohol 94.61
    with detoxification 94.63
    combined alcohol and drug 94.67
      with detoxification 94.69
  drug 94.64
    with detoxification 94.66
    combined drug and alcohol 94.67
      with detoxification 94.69
  sheltered employment 93.85
  vocational 93.85
Reimplantation
  adrenal tissue (heterotopic)
      (orthotopic) 07.45
  artery 39.59
    renal, aberrant 39.55
  bile ducts following excision of
      ampulla of Vater 51.62
  extremity - see Reattachment,
      extremity
  fallopian tube into uterus 66.74
  kidney 55.61
  lung 33.5 ●
  ovary 65.72
    laparoscopic 65.75
  pancreatic tissue 52.81
  parathyroid tissue (heterotopic)
      (orthotopic) 06.95
  pulmonary artery for hemitruncus
      repair 35.83
  renal vessel, aberrant 39.55
  testis in scrotum 62.5
  thyroid tissue (heterotopic) (orthotopic)
      06.94
  tooth 23.5
  ureter into bladder 56.74
Reinforcement - see also Repair, by site
  sclera NEC 12.88
    with graft 12.87
Reinsertion - see also Insertion or
    Revision
  cystostomy tube 59.94
  fixation device (internal) - see also
      Fixation, bone, internal 78.50
  heart valve (prosthetic) 35.95
  Holter (-Spitz) valve 02.42
  implant (expelled) (extruded)
    eyeball (with conjunctival graft)
        16.62
    orbital 16.62
  nephrostomy tube 55.93
  pyelostomy tube 55.94
  ureteral stent (transurethral) 59.8
    with ureterotomy 59.8 [56.2]

Reinsertion (Continued)
  ureterostomy tube 59.93
  valve
    heart (prosthetic) 35.95
    ventricular (cerebral) 02.42
Relaxation - see also Release training
    94.33
Release
  carpal tunnel (for nerve
      decompression) 04.43
  celiac artery axis 39.91
  central slip, extensor tendon hand
      (mallet finger repair) 82.84
  chordee 64.42
  clubfoot NEC 83.84
  de Quervain's tenosynovitis 82.01
  Dupuytren's contracture (by palmar
      fasciectomy) 82.35
    by fasciotomy (subcutaneous)
        82.12
    with excision 82.35
  Fowler (mallet finger repair) 82.84
  joint (capsule) (adherent)
      (constrictive) - see also Division,
      joint capsule 80.40
  laryngeal 31.92
  ligament - see also Division, ligament
      80.40
    median arcuate 39.91
  median arcuate ligament 39.91
  muscle (division) 83.19
    hand 82.19
  nerve (peripheral) NEC 04.49
    cranial NEC 04.42
    trigeminal 04.41
  pressure, intraocular 12.79
  scar tissue
    skin 86.84
    stoma - see Revision, stoma
  tarsal tunnel 04.44
  tendon 83.13
    hand 82.11
      extensor, central slip (repair
          mallet finger) 82.84
    sheath 83.01
      hand 82.01
  tenosynovitis 83.01
    abductor pollicis longus 82.01
    de Quervain's 82.01
    external pollicis brevis 82.01
    hand 82.01
  torsion
    intestine 46.80
      large 46.82
        endoscopic (balloon) 46.85
      small 46.81
    kidney pedicle 55.84
    ovary 65.95
    testes 63.52
  transverse carpal ligament (for nerve
      decompression) 04.43
  trigger finger or thumb 82.01
  urethral stricture 58.5
  Volkmann's contracture
    excision of scar, muscle 83.32
    fasciotomy 83.14
    muscle transplantation 83.77
  web contracture (skin) 86.84
Relief - see Release
Relocation - see also Revision
  cardiac device (CRT-D) (CRT-P)
      (defibrillator) (pacemaker)
      pocket, new site (skin)
      (subcutaneous) 37.79

Relocation *(Continued)*
  CRT-D pocket 37.79
  CRT-P pocket 37.79
  subcutaneous device pocket NEC 86.09
Remobilization
  joint 93.16
  stapes 19.0
Remodel
  ventricle 37.35
Removal - *see also* Excision
  Abrams bar (chest wall) 34.01
  abscess - *see* Incision, by site
  adenoid tag(s) 28.6
  anal sphincter
    with revision 49.75
    without revision 49.76
  arch bars (orthodontic) 24.8
    immobilization device 97.33
  arterial graft or prosthesis 39.49
  arteriovenous shunt (device) 39.43
    with creation of new shunt 39.42
  artificial heart
    internal biventricular replacement
      system 37.55
  Barton's tongs (skull) 02.95
    with synchronous replacement
      02.94
  bladder sphincter, artificial 58.99
    with replacement 58.93
  blood clot - *see also* Incision, by site
    bladder (by incision) 57.19
      without incision 57.0
    kidney (without incision) 56.0
      by incision 55.01
    ureter
      by incision 56.2
  bone fragment (chip) - *see also* Incision,
    bone 77.10
    joint - *see also* Arthrotomy 80.10
    necrotic - *see also* Sequestrectomy,
      bone 77.00
      joint - *see also* Arthrotomy 80.10
    skull 01.25
      with debridement of compound
        fracture 02.02
  bone growth stimulator - *see* category
    78.6●
  bony spicules, spinal canal 03.53
  brace 97.88
  breast implant 85.94
    tissue expander 85.96
  bronchial device or substance
    endoscopic 33.78
  calcareous deposit
    bursa 83.03
      hand 82.03
    tendon, intratendinous 83.39
      hand 82.29
  calcification, heart valve leaflets - *see*
    Valvuloplasty, heart
  calculus
    bile duct (by incision) 51.49
      endoscopic 51.88
      laparoscopic 51.88
      percutaneous 51.98
    bladder (by incision) 57.19
      without incision 57.0
    common duct (by incision) 51.41
      endoscopic 51.88
      laparoscopic 51.88
      percutaneous 51.96
    gallbladder 51.04
      endoscopic 51.88
      laparoscopic 51.88

Removal *(Continued)*
  calculus *(Continued)*
    kidney (by incision) 55.01
      without incision (transurethral)
        56.0
      percutaneous 55.03
        with fragmentation
          (ultrasound) 55.04
      renal pelvis (by incision) 55.11
        percutaneous nephostomy
          55.03
          with fragmentation
            55.04
      transurethral 56.0
    lacrimal
      canaliculi 09.42
        by incision 09.52
      gland 09.3
        by incision 09.0
      passage(s) 09.49
        by incision 09.59
      punctum 09.41
        by incision 09.51
      sac 09.49
        by incision 09.53
    pancreatic duct (by incision)
      52.09
      endoscopic 52.94
    perirenal tissue 59.09
    pharynx 29.39
    prostate 60.0
    salivary gland (by incision) 26.0
      by probe 26.91
    ureter (by incision) 56.2
      without incision 56.0
    urethra (by incision) 58.0
      without incision 58.6
  caliper tongs (skull) 02.95
  cannula
    for extracorporeal membrane
      oxygenation (ECMO) - *omit*
      code
  cardiac pacemaker (device) (initial)
    (permanent) (cardiac
    resynchronization device,
    CRT-P) 37.89
    with replacement (by)
      cardiac resynchronization
        pacemaker (CRT-P)
      device only 00.53
      total system 00.50
      dual chamber device 37.87
      single-chamber device 37.85
      rate responsive 37.86
  cardioverter/defibrillator pulse
    generator
    without replacement (cardiac
      resynchronization
      defibrillator device
      (CRT-D)) 37.79
  cast 97.88
    with reapplication 97.13
      lower limb 97.12
      upper limb 97.11
  catheter (indwelling) - *see also*
    Removal, tube
    bladder 97.64
    cranial cavity 01.27
    middle ear (tympanum) 20.1
    ureter 97.62
    urinary 97.64
    ventricular (cerebral) 02.43
      with synchronous replacement
        02.42

Removal *(Continued)*
  CCM (cardiac contractility
    modulatioin) without
    replacement (rechargeable pulse
    generator) (total system) 37.79 ◄
  cerclage material, cervix 69.96
  cerumen, ear 96.52
  corneal epithelium 11.41
    for smear or culture 11.21
  coronary artery obstruction (thrombus)
    36.09
    direct intracoronary artery infusion
      36.04
    open chest approach 36.03
    percutaneous transluminal (balloon)

> **Note:** Also use 00.40, 00.41, 00.42, or 00.43 to show the total number of vessels treated. Use code 00.44 once to show procedure on a bifurcated vessel. In addition, use 00.45, 00.46, 00.47, or 00.48 to show the number of vascular stents inserted.

  Crutchfield tongs (skull) 02.95
    with synchronous replacement
      02.94
  cyst - *see also* Excision, lesion, by site
    dental 24.4
    lung 32.29
      endoscopic 32.28
      thoracoscopic 32.20
  cystic duct remnant 51.61
  decidua (by)
    aspiration curettage 69.52
    curettage (D and C) 69.02
    manual 75.4
  dental wiring (immobilization device)
    97.33
    orthodontic 24.8
  device (therapeutic) NEC 97.89
    abdomen NEC 97.86
    bronchus 33.78
      valve 33.78
    digestive system NEC 97.59
    drainage - *see* Removal, tube
    external fixation device 97.88
      mandibular NEC 97.36
      minifixator (bone) - *see* category
        78.6●
    for musculoskeletal immobilization
      NEC 97.88
    genital tract NEC 97.79
    head and neck NEC 97.39
    intrauterine contraceptive 97.71
    spine 80.09
    thorax NEC 97.49
    trunk NEC 97.87
    urinary system NEC 97.69
  diaphragm, vagina 97.73
  drainage device - *see* Removal, tube
  dye, spinal canal 03.31
  ectopic fetus (from) 66.02
    abdominal cavity 74.3
    extraperitoneal (intraligamentous)
      74.3
    fallopian tube (by salpingostomy)
      66.02
      by salpingotomy 66.01
      with salpingectomy 66.62
    intraligamentous 74.3
    ovarian 74.3
    peritoneal (following uterine or
      tubal rupture) 74.3

Removal *(Continued)*
　ectopic fetus *(Continued)*
　　site NEC 74.3
　　tubal (by salpingostomy) 66.02
　　　by salpingotomy 66.01
　　　with salpingectomy 66.62
　electrodes
　　bone growth stimulator - *see*
　　　category 78.6●
　　brain 01.22
　　　depth 01.22
　　　　with synchronous replacement
　　　　　02.93
　　　foramen ovale 01.22
　　　　with synchronous replacement
　　　　　02.93
　　　sphenoidal - *omit code*
　　　　with synchronous replacement
　　　　　02.96
　　cardiac pacemaker (atrial)
　　　(transvenous) (ventricular)
　　　37.77
　　　with replacement 37.76
　　carotid sinus 04.93
　　　with synchronous replacement
　　　　04.92
　　depth 01.22
　　　with synchronous replacement
　　　　02.93
　　epicardial (myocardial) 37.77
　　　with replacement (by)
　　　　atrial and/or ventricular
　　　　　lead(s) (electrode)
　　　　　37.76
　　　　epicardial lead 37.74
　　epidural pegs 01.22
　　　with synchronous replacement
　　　　02.93●
　　foramen ovale 01.22
　　　with synchronous replacement
　　　　02.93
　　gastric 04.93
　　　with synchronous replacement
　　　　04.92
　　intracranial 01.22
　　　with synchronous replacement
　　　　02.93
　　peripheral nerve 04.93
　　　with synchronous replacement
　　　　04.92
　　sacral nerve 04.93
　　sphenoidal - *omit code*
　　　with synchronous replacement
　　　　02.96
　　spinal 03.94
　　　with synchronous replacement
　　　　03.93
　　temporary transvenous pacemaker
　　　system - *omit code*
　electroencephalographic receiver
　　(brain) (intracranial) 01.22
　　with synchronous replacement
　　　02.93
　electronic
　　stimulator - *see* Removal,
　　　neurostimulator, by site
　　　bladder 57.98
　　　bone 78.6●
　　　skeletal muscle 83.93
　　　　with synchronous replacement
　　　　　83.92
　　　ureter 56.94
　electrostimulator - *see* Removal,
　　electronic, stimulator, by site

Removal *(Continued)*
　embolus 38.00
　　with endarterectomy - *see*
　　　Endarterectomy
　　abdominal
　　　artery 38.06
　　　vein 38.07
　　aorta (arch) (ascending)
　　　(descending) 38.04
　　arteriovenous shunt or cannula
　　　39.49
　　bovine graft 39.49
　　head and neck vessel
　　　endovascular approach 39.74
　　　open approach, intracranial
　　　　vessels 38.01
　　　open approach, other vessels of
　　　　head and neck 38.02
　　intracranial vessel
　　　endovascular approach 39.74
　　　open approach, intracranial
　　　　vessels 38.01
　　　open approach, other vessels of
　　　　head and neck 38.02
　　lower limb
　　　artery 38.08
　　　vein 38.09
　　pulmonary (artery) (vein) 38.05
　　thoracic vessel NEC 38.05
　　upper limb (artery) (vein) 38.03
　embryo - *see* Removal, ectopic fetus
　encircling tube, eye (episcleral) 14.6
　epithelial downgrowth, anterior
　　chamber 12.93
　external fixation device 97.88
　　mandibular NEC 97.36
　　minifixator (bone) - *see* category
　　　78.6●
　extrauterine embryo - *see* Removal,
　　ectopic fetus
　eyeball 16.49
　　with implant 16.42
　　　with attachment of muscles
　　　　16.41
　fallopian tube - *see* Salpingectomy
　feces (impacted) (by flushing) (manual)
　　96.38
　fetus, ectopic - *see* Removal, ectopic
　　fetus
　fingers, supernumerary 86.26
　fixation device
　　external 97.88
　　　mandibular NEC 97.36
　　　minifixator (bone) - *see* category
　　　　78.6●
　　internal 78.60
　　　carpal, metacarpal 78.64
　　　clavicle 78.61
　　　facial (bone) 76.97
　　　femur 78.65
　　　fibula 78.67
　　　humerus 78.62
　　　patella 78.66
　　　pelvic 78.69
　　　phalanges (foot) (hand) 78.69
　　　radius 78.63
　　　scapula 78.61
　　　specified site NEC 78.69
　　　tarsal, metatarsal 78.68
　　　thorax (ribs) (sternum) 78.61
　　　tibia 78.67
　　　ulna 78.63
　　　vertebrae 78.69

Removal *(Continued)*
　foreign body NEC - *see also* Incision, by
　　site 98.20
　　abdominal (cavity) 54.92
　　　wall 54.0
　　adenoid 98.13
　　　by incision 28.91
　　alveolus, alveolar bone 98.22
　　　by incision 24.0
　　antecubital fossa 98.27
　　　by incision 86.05
　　anterior chamber 12.00
　　　by incision 12.02
　　　with use of magnet 12.01
　　anus (intraluminal) 98.05
　　　by incision 49.93
　　artificial stoma (intraluminal)
　　　98.18
　　auditory canal, external 18.02
　　axilla 98.27
　　　by incision 86.05
　　bladder (without incision) 57.0
　　　by incision 57.19
　　bone, except fixation device - *see also*
　　　Incision, bone 77.10
　　　alveolus, alveolar 98.22
　　　　by incision 24.0
　　brain 01.39
　　　without incision into brain 01.24
　　breast 85.0
　　bronchus (intraluminal) 98.15
　　　by incision 33.0
　　bursa 83.03
　　　hand 82.03
　　canthus 98.22
　　　by incision 08.51
　　cerebral meninges 01.31
　　cervix (intraluminal) NEC 98.16
　　　penetrating 69.97
　　choroid (by incision) 14.00
　　　with use of magnet 14.01
　　　without use of magnet 14.02
　　ciliary body (by incision) 12.00
　　　with use of magnet 12.01
　　　without use of magnet 12.02
　　conjunctiva (by magnet) 98.22
　　　by incision 10.0
　　cornea 98.21
　　　by
　　　　incision 11.1
　　　　magnet 11.0
　　duodenum 98.03
　　　by incision 45.01
　　ear (intraluminal) 98.11
　　　with incision 18.09
　　epididymis 63.92
　　esophagus (intraluminal) 98.02
　　　by incision 42.09
　　extrapleural (by incision) 34.01
　　eye, eyeball (by magnet) 98.21
　　　anterior segment (by incision)
　　　　12.00
　　　　with use of magnet 12.01
　　　　without use of magnet 12.02
　　　posterior segment (by incision)
　　　　14.00
　　　　with use of magnet 14.01
　　　　without use of magnet 14.02
　　　superficial 98.21
　　eyelid 98.22
　　　by incision 08.09
　　fallopian tube
　　　by salpingostomy 66.02
　　　by salpingotomy 66.01

Removal *(Continued)*
  foreign body NEC *(Continued)*
    fascia 83.09
      hand 82.09
    foot 98.28
    gallbladder 51.04
    groin region (abdominal wall)
      (inguinal) 54.0
    gum 98.22
      by incision 24.0
    hand 98.26
    head and neck NEC 98.22
    heart 37.11
    internal fixation device - *see* Removal,
      fixation device, internal
    intestine
      by incision 45.00
      large (intraluminal) 98.04
        by incision 45.03
      small (intraluminal) 98.03
        by incision 45.02
    intraocular (by incision) 12.00
      with use of magnet 12.01
      without use of magnet 12.02
    iris (by incision) 12.00
      with use of magnet 12.01
      without use of magnet 12.02
    joint structures - *see also*
      Arthrotomy 80.10
    kidney (transurethral) (by
      endoscopy) 56.0
      by incision 55.01
      pelvis (transurethral) 56.0
        by incision 55.11
    labia 98.23
      by incision 71.09
    lacrimal
      canaliculi 09.42
        by incision 09.52
      gland 09.3
        by incision 09.0
      passage(s) 09.49
        by incision 09.59
      punctum 09.41
        by incision 09.51
      sac 09.49
        by incision 09.53
    large intestine (intraluminal) 98.04
      by incision 45.03
    larynx (intraluminal) 98.14
      by incision 31.3
    lens 13.00
      by incision 13.02
        with use of magnet 13.01
    liver 50.0
    lower limb, except foot 98.29
      foot 98.28
    lung 33.1
    mediastinum 34.1
    meninges (cerebral) 01.31
      spinal 03.01
    mouth (intraluminal) 98.01
      by incision 27.92
    muscle 83.02
      hand 82.02
    nasal sinus 22.50
      antrum 22.2
        with Caldwell-Luc approach
          22.39
      ethmoid 22.51
      frontal 22.41
      maxillary 22.2
        with Caldwell-Luc approach
          22.39
      sphenoid 22.52

Removal *(Continued)*
  foreign body NEC *(Continued)*
    nerve (cranial) (peripheral) NEC
      04.04
      root 03.01
    nose (intraluminal) 98.12
      by incision 21.1
    oral cavity (intraluminal) 98.01
      by incision 27.92
    orbit (by magnet) 98.21
      by incision 16.1
    palate (penetrating) 98.22
      by incision 27.1
    pancreas 52.09
    penis 98.24
      by incision 64.92
    pericardium 37.12
    perineum (female) 98.23
      by incision 71.09
      male 98.25
        by incision 86.05
    perirenal tissue 59.09
    peritoneal cavity 54.92
    perivesical tissue 59.19
    pharynx (intraluminal) 98.13
      by pharyngotomy 29.0
    pleura (by incision) 34.09
    popliteal space 98.29
      by incision 86.05
    rectum (intraluminal) 98.05
      by incision 48.0
    renal pelvis (transurethral) 56.0
      by incision 56.1
    retina (by incision) 14.00
      with use of magnet 14.01
      without use of magnet 14.02
    retroperitoneum 54.92
    sclera (by incision) 12.00
      with use of magnet 12.01
      without use of magnet 12.02
    scrotum 98.24
      by incision 61.0
    sinus (nasal) 22.50
      antrum 22.2
        with Caldwell-Luc approach
          22.39
      ethmoid 22.51
      frontal 22.41
      maxillary 22.2
        with Caldwell-Luc approach
          22.39
      sphenoid 22.52
    skin NEC 98.20
      by incision 86.05
    skull 01.24
      with incision into brain 01.39
    small intestine (intraluminal)
      98.03
      by incision 45.02
    soft tissue NEC 83.09
      hand 82.09
    spermatic cord 63.93
    spinal (canal) (cord) (meninges)
      03.01
    stomach (intraluminal) 98.03
      bubble (balloon) 44.94
      by incision 43.0
    subconjunctival (by magnet)
      98.22
      by incision 10.0
    subcutaneous tissue NEC 98.20
      by incision 86.05
    supraclavicular fossa 98.27
      by incision 86.05

Removal *(Continued)*
  foreign body NEC *(Continued)*
    tendon (sheath) 83.01
      hand 82.01
    testis 62.0
    thorax (by incision) 34.09
    thyroid (field) (gland) (by incision)
      06.09
    tonsil 98.13
      by incision 28.91
    trachea (intraluminal) 98.15
      by incision 31.3
    trunk NEC 98.25
    tunica vaginalis 98.24
    upper limb, except hand 98.27
      hand 98.26
    ureter (transurethral) 56.0
      by incision 56.2
    urethra (intraluminal) 98.19
      by incision 58.0
    uterus (intraluminal) 98.16
    vagina (intraluminal) 98.17
      by incision 70.14
    vas deferens 63.6
    vitreous (by incision) 14.00
      with use of magnet 14.01
      without use of magnet
        14.02
    vulva 98.23
      by incision 71.09
  gallstones
    bile duct (by incision) NEC 51.49
      endoscopic 51.88
    common duct (by incision) 51.41
      endoscopic 51.88
      percutaneous 51.96
    duodenum 45.01
    gallbladder 51.04
      endoscopic 51.88
      laparoscopic 51.88
    hepatic ducts 51.49
      endoscopic 51.88
    intestine 45.00
      large 45.03
      small NEC 45.02
    liver 50.0
  Gardner Wells tongs (skull) 02.95
    with synchronous replacement
      02.94
  gastric band (adjustable), laparoscopic
    44.97
  gastric bubble (balloon) 44.94
  granulation tissue - *see also* Excision,
    lesion, by site
    with repair - *see* Repair, by site
    cranial 01.6
    skull 01.6
  halo traction device (skull) 02.95
    with synchronous replacement
      02.94
  heart assist system
    with replacement 37.63
    intra-aortic balloon pump (IABP)
      97.44
    nonoperative 97.44
    open removal 37.64
    percutaneous external device
      97.44
  heart replacement system
    internal biventricular 37.55
  hematoma - *see* Drainage, by site
  Hoffman minifixator device (bone) - *see*
    category 78.6●
  hydatidiform mole 68.0

◀ New   ◀||| Revised   deleted Deleted   ● Use Additional Digit(s)   �757 Omit code

Removal *(Continued)*

impacted
    feces (rectum) (by flushing)
      (manual) 96.38
    tooth 23.19
    from nasal sinus (maxillary) 22.61
implant
    breast 85.94
    cochlear prosthetic device 20.99
    cornea 11.92
    lens (prosthetic) 13.8
    middle ear NEC 20.99
    ocular 16.71
      posterior segment 14.6
    orbit 16.72
    retina 14.6
    tympanum 20.1
implantable hemodynamic sensor
    (lead) and monitor device
    37.79
internal biventricular heart
    replacement system 37.55
internal fixation device - *see* Removal,
    fixation device, internal
intra-aortic balloon pump (IABP)
    97.44
intrauterine contraceptive device (IUD)
    97.71
joint (structure) NOS 80.90
    ankle 80.97
    elbow 80.92
    foot and toe 80.98
    hand and finger 80.94
    hip 80.95
    knee 80.96
    other specified sites 80.99
    shoulder 80.91
    spine 80.99
    toe 80.98
    wrist 80.93
Kantrowitz heart pump 37.64
    nonoperative 97.44
keel (tantalum plate), larynx 31.98
kidney - *see also* Nephrectomy
    mechanical 55.98
    transplanted or rejected 55.53
laminaria (tent), uterus 97.79
leads (cardiac) - *see* Removal,
    electrodes, cardiac pacemaker
lesion - *see* Excision, lesion, by site
ligamentum flavum (spine) - `omit code`
ligature
    fallopian tube 66.79
    ureter 56.86
    vas deferens 63.84
limb lengthening device, internal - *see*
    category 78.6 ●
loop recorder 86.05
loose body
    bone - *see* Sequestrectomy, bone
    joint 80.10
mesh (surgical) - *see* Removal,
    foreign body, by site
lymph node - *see* Excision, lymph,
    node
minifixator device (bone) - *see* category
    78.6 ●
    external fixation device 97.88
Mulligan hood, fallopian tube 66.94
    with synchronous replacement
    66.93
muscle stimulator (skeletal) 83.93
    with replacement 83.92
myringotomy device or tube 20.1

Removal *(Continued)*

nail (bed) (fold) 86.23
    internal fixation device - *see*
      Removal, fixation device,
      internal
necrosis
    skin 86.28
      excisional 86.22
neuropacemaker - *see* Removal,
    neurostimulator, by site
neurostimulator
    electrodes
      brain 01.22
        with synchronous replacement
        02.93
      carotid sinus 04.93
        with synchronous replacement
        04.92
      gastric 04.93
      intracranial 01.22
        with synchronous replacement
        02.93
      peripheral nerve 04.93
        with synchronous replacement
        04.92
      sacral nerve 04.93
        with synchronous replacement
        04.92
      spinal 03.94
        with synchronous replacement
        03.93
    pulse generator (single array, dual
      array) 86.05
    with synchronous replacement
      86.96
      dual array 86.95
        rechargeable 86.98
      single array 86.94
        rechargeable 86.97
nonabsorbable surgical material
    NEC - *see* Removal, foreign
    body, by site
odontoma (tooth) 24.4
orbital implant 16.72
osteocartilagenous loose body, joint
    structures - *see also* Arthrotomy
    80.10
outer attic wall (middle ear) 20.59
ovo-testis (unilateral) 62.3
    bilateral 62.41
pacemaker
    brain (intracranial) - *see* Removal,
      neurostimulator
    cardiac (device) (initial) (permanent)
      37.89
      with replacement
        dual-chamber device 37.87
        single-chamber device 37.85
          rate responsive 37.86
      electrodes (atrial) (transvenous)
        (ventricular) 37.77
        with replacement 37.76
      epicardium (myocardium)
        37.77
        with replacement (by)
          atrial and/or ventricular
            lead(s) (electrode)
            37.76
          epicardial lead 37.74
      temporary transvenous
        pacemaker system - *omit
        code*
    intracranial - *see* Removal,
      neurostimulator

Removal *(Continued)*

pacemaker *(Continued)*
    neural - *see* Removal,
      neurostimulator
    peripheral nerve - *see* Removal,
      neurostimulator
    spinal - *see* Removal,
      neurostimulator
pack, packing
    dental 97.34
    intrauterine 97.72
    nasal 97.32
    rectum 97.59
    trunk NEC 97.85
    vagina 97.75
    vulva 97.75
pantopaque dye, spinal canal 03.31
patella (complete) 77.96
    partial 77.86
pectus deformity implant device
    34.01
pelvic viscera, en masse (female) 68.8
    male 57.71
pessary, vagina NEC 97.74
pharynx (partial) 29.33
phlebolith - *see* Removal, embolus
placenta (by)
    aspiration curettage 69.52
    D and C 69.02
    manual 75.4
plaque, dental 96.54
plate, skull 02.07
    with synchronous replacement 02.05
polyp - *see also* Excision, lesion, by site
    esophageal 42.32
      endoscopic 42.33
    gastric (endoscopic) 43.41
    intestine 45.41
      endoscopic 45.42
    nasal 21.31
prosthesis
    bile duct 51.95
      nonoperative 97.55
    cochlear prosthetic device 20.99
    dental 97.35
    eye 97.31
    facial bone 76.99
    fallopian tube 66.94
      with synchronous replacement
      66.93
    joint structures 80.00 ◀▥
      with replacement – *see* Revision,
        joint replacement by site
      without replacement ◀
        ankle 80.07 ◀▥
        elbow 80.02 ◀▥
        foot and toe 80.08 ◀▥
        hand and finger 80.04 ◀▥
        hip 80.05 ◀▥
        knee 80.06 ◀▥
        shoulder 80.01 ◀▥
        specified site NEC 80.09 ◀▥
        spine 80.09 ◀▥
        unspecified site 80.00 ◀
        wrist 80.03 ◀▥
    lens 13.8
    penis (internal) without replacement
      64.96
    Rheos™ carotid sinus baroreflex
      activation device 86.05
    Rosen (urethra) 59.99
    testicular, by incision 62.0
    urinary sphincter, artificial 58.99
      with replacement 58.93

◀ New   ◀▥ Revised   ~~deleted~~ Deleted   ● Use Additional Digit(s)   ▥ Omit code

Removal *(Continued)*
pseudophakos 13.8
pterygium 11.39
  with corneal graft 11.32
pulse generator
  cardiac pacemaker 37.86
  cardioverter/defibrillator 37.79
  neurostimulator - *see* Removal,
    neurostimulator, pulse
    generator
pump assist device, heart 37.64
  with replacement 37.63
  nonoperative 97.44
radioactive material - *see* Removal,
  foreign body, by site
redundant skin, eyelid 08.86
rejected organ
  kidney 55.53
  testis 62.42
reservoir, ventricular (Ommaya)
  (Rickham) 02.43
  with synchronous replacement
    02.42
retained placenta (by)
  aspiration curettage 69.52
  D and C 69.02
  manual 75.4
retinal implant 14.6
Rheos™ carotid sinus baroreflex
  activation device 86.05
rhinolith 21.31
rice bodies, tendon sheaths 83.01
  hand 82.01
Roger-Anderson minifixator device
  (bone) - *see* category 78.6●
root, residual (tooth) (buried) (retained)
  23.11
Rosen prosthesis (urethra) 59.99
scleral buckle or implant 14.6
Scribner shunt 39.43
secondary membranous cataract (with
  iridectomy) 13.65
secundines (by)
  aspiration curettage 69.52
  D and C 69.02
  manual 75.4
sequestrum - *see* Sequestrectomy
seton, anus 49.93
Shepard's tube (ear) 20.1
Shirodkar suture, cervix 69.96
shunt
  arteriovenous 39.43
    with creation of new shunt
      39.42
  lumbar-subarachnoid NEC 03.98
  pleurothecal 03.98
  salpingothecal 03.98
  spinal (thecal) NEC 03.98
  subarachnoid-peritoneal 03.98
  subarachnoid-ureteral 03.98
silastic tubes
  ear 20.1
  fallopian tubes 66.94
    with synchronous replacement
      66.93
skin
  necrosis or slough 86.28
    excisional 86.22
    superficial layer (by
      dermabrasion) 86.25
skull tongs 02.95
  with synchronous replacement 02.94
spacer (cement) (joint)
  (methylmethacrylate) 84.57

Removal *(Continued)*
splint 97.88
stent
  bile duct 97.55
  larynx 31.98
  ureteral 97.62
  urethral 97.65
stimoceiver - *see* Removal,
  neurostimulator
subdural
  grids 01.22
  strips 01.22
supernumerary digit(s) 86.26
suture(s) NEC 97.89
  abdominal wall 97.83
  by incision - *see* Incision, by site
  genital tract 97.79
  head and neck 97.38
  thorax 97.43
  trunk NEC 97.84
symblepharon - *see* Repair,
  symblepharon
temporary transvenous pacemaker
  system - *omit code*
testis (unilateral) 62.3
  bilateral 62.41
  remaining or solitary 62.42
thrombus 38.00
  with endarterectomy - *see*
    Endarterectomy
  abdominal
    artery 38.06
    vein 38.07
  aorta (arch) (ascending)
    (descending) 38.04
  arteriovenous shunt or cannula
    39.49
  bovine graft 39.49
  coronary artery 36.09
  head and neck vessel NEC 38.02
  intracranial vessel NEC 38.01
  lower limb
    artery 38.08
    vein 38.09
  pulmonary (artery) (vein) 38.05
  thoracic vessel NEC 38.05
  upper limb (artery) (vein) 38.03
tissue expander (skin) NEC 86.05
  breast 85.96
toes, supernumerary 86.26
tongs, skull 02.95
  with synchronous replacement
    02.94
tonsil tag 28.4
tooth (by forceps) (multiple) (single)
  NEC 23.09
  deciduous 23.01
  surgical NEC 23.19
    impacted 23.19
    residual root 23.11
    root apex 23.73
      with root canal therapy
        23.72
trachoma follicles 10.33
T-tube (bile duct) 97.55
tube
  appendix 97.53
  bile duct (T-tube) NEC 97.55
  cholecystostomy 97.54
  cranial cavity 01.27
  cystostomy 97.63
  ear (button) 20.1
  gastrostomy 97.51
  large intestine 97.53

Removal *(Continued)*
tube *(Continued)*
  liver 97.55
  mediastinum 97.42
  nephrostomy 97.61
  pancreas 97.56
  peritoneum 97.82
  pleural cavity 97.41
  pyelostomy 97.61
  retroperitoneum 97.81
  small intestine 97.52
  thoracotomy 97.41
  tracheostomy 97.37
  tympanostomy 20.1
  tympanum 20.1
  ureterostomy 97.62
ureteral splint (stent) 97.62
urethral sphincter, artificial 58.99
  with replacement 58.93
urinary sphincter, artificial 58.99
  with replacement 58.93
utricle 20.79
valve
  vas deferens 63.85
  ventricular (cerebral) 02.43
vascular graft or prosthesis 39.49
ventricular shunt or reservoir 02.43
  with synchronous replacement
    02.42
Vinke tongs (skull) 02.95
  with synchronous replacement
    02.94
vitreous (with replacement) 14.72
  anterior approach (partial) 14.71
  open sky technique 14.71
Wagner-Brooker minifixator device
  (bone) - *see* category 78.6●
wiring, dental (immobilization device)
  97.33
  orthodontic 24.8
Renipuncture (percutaneous) 55.92
Renogram 92.03
Renotransplantation NEC 55.69

Note: To report donor source:
      cadaver 00.93
      live non-related donor 00.92
      live related donor 00.91
      live unrelated donor 00.92

Reopening - *see also* Incision, by site
blepharorrhaphy 08.02
canthorrhaphy 08.02
cilia base 08.71
craniotomy or craniectomy site
  01.23
fallopian tube (divided) 66.79
iris in anterior chambers 12.97
laminectomy or laminotomy site
  03.02
laparotomy site 54.12
osteotomy site - *see also* Incision, bone
  77.10
  facial bone 76.09
tarsorrhaphy 08.02
thoracotomy site (for control of
  hemorrhage) (for examination)
  (for exploration) 34.03
thyroid field wound (for control of
  hemorrhage) (for examination)
  (for exploration) (for removal of
  hematoma) 06.02
Repacking - *see* Replacement, pack, by
  site

Repair
- abdominal wall 54.72
- adrenal gland 07.44
- alveolus, alveolar (process) (ridge)
  (with graft) (with implant)
  24.5
- anal sphincter 49.79
  - artificial sphincter
    - implantation 49.75
    - revision 49.75
  - laceration (by suture) 49.71
    - obstetric (current) 75.62
    - old 49.79
- aneurysm (false) (true) 39.52
  - by or with
    - clipping 39.51
    - coagulation 39.52
    - coil, NEC (endovascular
      approach) 39.79 ◀⟸
    - head and neck 39.72 ◀⟸
      - bare coils 39.75 ◀
      - bioactive coils 39.76 ◀
    - electrocoagulation 39.52
    - excision or resection of vessel -
      see also Aneurysmectomy,
      by site
    - with
      - anastomosis - see
        Aneurysmectomy,
        with anastomosis, by
        site
      - graft replacement - see
        Aneurysmectomy,
        with graft
        replacement, by site
    - endovascular graft 39.79
      - abdominal aorta 39.71
      - head and neck 39.72
      - lower extremity artery(s)
        39.79
      - thoracic aorta 39.73
      - upper extremity artery(s)
        39.79
    - filipuncture 39.52
    - graft replacement - see
      Aneurysmectomy, with
      graft
      replacement, by site
    - ligation 39.52
    - liquid tissue adhesive (glue)
      39.79
      - endovascular approach
        39.79
        - head and neck 39.72
    - methyl methacrylate 39.52
      - endovascular approach 39.79
        - head and neck 39.72
    - occlusion 39.52
      - endovascular approach 39.79
        - head and neck 39.72
    - suture 39.52
    - trapping 39.52
    - wiring 39.52
    - wrapping (gauze) (methyl
      methacrylate) (plastic)
      39.52
  - coronary artery 36.91
  - heart 37.32
  - sinus of Valsalva 35.39
  - thoracic aorta (dissecting), by
    fenestration 39.54
- anomalous pulmonary venous
  connection (total)
  one-stage 35.82

Repair (Continued)
- anomalous pulmonary venous
  connection (Continued)
  - partial - see specific procedure
  - total 35.82
- anular disc 80.54
  - with graft or prosthesis 80.53
- anulus fibrosus 80.54
  - with graft or prosthesis 80.53
- anus 49.79
  - laceration (by suture) 49.71
    - obstetric (current) 75.62
    - old 49.79
- aorta 39.31
- aorticopulmonary window 39.59
- arteriovenous fistula 39.53
  - by or with
    - clipping 39.53
    - coagulation 39.53
    - coil, NEC (endovascular
      approach) 39.79 ◀⟸
    - head and neck vessels 39.72 ◀⟸
      - bare coils 39.75 ◀
      - bioactive coils 39.76 ◀
    - division 39.53
    - excision or resection - see also
      Aneurysmectomy, by site
    - with
      - anastomosis - see
        Aneurysmectomy,
        with anastomosis, by
        site
      - graft replacement - see
        Aneurysmectomy,
        with graft
        replacement, by site
    - ligation 39.53
      - coronary artery 36.99
    - occlusion 39.53
      - endovascular approach 39.79
        - head and neck 39.72
    - suture 39.53
- artery NEC 39.59
  - by
    - endovascular approach
      - abdominal aorta 39.71
      - head and neck (embolization
        or occlusion) 39.72
      - other repair (of aneurysm) 39.79
      - percutaneous repair of
        intracranial vessel(s)
        (for stent insertion) 00.62

> Note: Also use 00.40, 00.41, 00.42, or
> 00.43 to show the total number of
> vessels treated. Use code 00.44 once to
> show procedure on a bifurcated vessel.
> In addition, use 00.45, 00.46, 00.47, or
> 00.48 to show the number of vascular
> stents inserted.

- percutaneous repair of
  precerebral (extracranial)
  vessel(s) (for stent
  insertion) 00.61

> Note: Also use 00.40, 00.41, 00.42, or
> 00.43 to show the total number of
> vessels treated. Use code 00.44 once to
> show procedure on a bifurcated vessel.
> In addition, use 00.45, 00.46, 00.47, or
> 00.48 to show the number of vascular
> stents inserted.

Repair (Continued)
- artery NEC (Continued)
  - by (Continued)
    - non-coronary percutaneous
      transluminal angioplasty or
      atherectomy

> Note: Also use 00.40, 00.41, 00.42, or
> 00.43 to show the total number of
> vessels treated. Use code 00.44 once to
> show procedure on a bifurcated vessel.
> In addition, use 00.45, 00.46, 00.47, or
> 00.48 to show the number of vascular
> stents inserted.

      - basilar 00.61
      - carotid 00.61
      - femoropopliteal 39.50
      - iliac 39.50
      - lower extremity NOS
        39.50
      - mesenteric 39.50
      - renal 39.50
      - upper extremity NOS
        39.50
      - vertebral 00.61
  - with
    - patch graft 39.58
      - with excision or resection of
        vessel - see Arteriectomy,
        with graft replacement,
        by site
      - synthetic (Dacron) (Teflon)
        39.57
      - tissue (vein) (autogenous)
        (homograft) 39.56
    - suture 39.31
  - coronary NEC 36.99
    - by angioplasty - see Angioplasty,
      coronary
    - by atherectomy - see Angioplasty,
      coronary
- artificial opening - see Repair, stoma
- atrial septal defect 35.71
  - with
    - prosthesis (open heart technique)
      35.51
      - closed heart technique 35.52
    - tissue graft 35.61
  - combined with repair of valvular
    and ventricular septal defects -
    see Repair, endocardial cushion
    defect
  - in total repair of total anomalous
    pulmonary venous connection
    35.82
- atrioventricular canal defect (any type)
  35.73
  - with
    - prosthesis 35.54
    - tissue graft 35.63
- bifid digit (finger) 82.89
- bile duct NEC 51.79
  - laceration (by suture) NEC 51.79
    - common bile duct 51.71
- bladder NEC 57.89
  - exstrophy 57.86
  - for stress incontinence - see Repair,
    stress incontinence
  - laceration (by suture) 57.81
    - obstetric (current) 75.61
    - old 57.89
  - neck 57.85
- blepharophimosis 08.59

◀ New   ◀⟸ Revised   ~~deleted~~ Deleted   ● Use Additional Digit(s)   Omit code

Repair *(Continued)*
blepharoptosis 08.36
  by
      frontalis muscle technique (with)
          fascial sling 08.32
          suture 08.31
      levator muscle technique 08.34
          with resection or advancement 08.33
      orbicularis oculi muscle sling 08.36
      tarsal technique 08.35
blood vessel NEC 39.59
    with
        patch graft 39.58
            with excision or resection - *see* Angiectomy, with graft replacement
            synthetic (Dacron) (Teflon) 39.57
            tissue (vein) (autogenous) (homograft) 39.56
        resection - *see* Angiectomy
        suture 39.30
    coronary artery NEC 36.99
        by angioplasty - *see* Angioplasty, coronary
        by atherectomy - *see* Angioplasty, coronary
    peripheral vessel NEC 39.59
        by angioplasty 39.50

> Note: Also use 00.40, 00.41, 00.42, or 00.43 to show the total number of vessels treated. Use code 00.44 once to show procedure on a bifurcated vessel. In addition, use 00.45, 00.46, 00.47, or 00.48 to show the number of vascular stents inserted.

        by atherectomy 39.50

> Note: Also use 00.40, 00.41, 00.42, or 00.43 to show the total number of vessels treated. Use code 00.44 once to show procedure on a bifurcated vessel. In addition, use 00.45, 00.46, 00.47, or 00.48 to show the number of vascular stents inserted.

        by endovascular approach 39.79
bone NEC - *see also* Osteoplasty - *see* category 78.4●
    by synostosis technique - *see* Arthrodesis
    accessory sinus 22.79
    cranium NEC 02.06
        with
            flap (bone) 02.03
            graft (bone) 02.04
    for malunion, nonunion, or delayed union of fracture - *see* Repair, fracture, malunion or nonunion
    nasal 21.89
    skull NEC 02.06
        with
            flap (bone) 02.03
            graft (bone) 02.04
bottle, hydrocele of tunica vaginalis 61.2
brain (trauma) NEC 02.92
breast (plastic) - *see also* Mammoplasty 85.89

Repair *(Continued)*
broad ligament 69.29
bronchus NEC 33.48
    laceration (by suture) 33.41
bunionette (with osteotomy) 77.54
canaliculus, lacrimal 09.73
canthus (lateral) 08.59
cardiac pacemaker NEC 37.89
    electrode(s) (lead) NEC 37.75
cardioverter/defibrillator (automatic) pocket, (skin) (subcutaneous) 37.99
cerebral meninges 02.12
cervix 67.69
    internal os 67.59
        transabdominal 67.51
        transvaginal 67.59
    aceration (by suture) 67.61
        obstetric (current) 75.51
        old 67.69
chest wall (mesh) (silastic) NEC 34.79
chordae tendineae 35.32
choroid NEC 14.9
    with retinal repair - *see* Repair, retina
cisterna chyli 40.69
claw toe 77.57
cleft
    hand 82.82
    laryngotracheal 31.69
    lip 27.54
    palate 27.62
        secondary or subsequent 27.63
coarctation of aorta - *see* Excision, coarctation of aorta
cochlear prosthetic device 20.99
    external components only 95.49
cockup toe 77.58
colostomy 46.43
conjunctiva NEC 10.49
    with scleral repair 12.81
    laceration 10.6
        with repair of sclera 12.81
    late effect of trachoma 10.49
cornea NEC 11.59
    with
        conjunctival flap 11.53
        transplant - *see* Keratoplasty
    postoperative dehiscence 11.52
coronary artery NEC 36.99
    by angioplasty - *see* Angioplasty, coronary
    by atherectomy - *see* Angioplasty, coronary
cranium NEC 02.06
    with
        flap (bone) 02.03
        graft (bone) 02.04
cusp, valve - *see* Repair, heart, valve
cystocele 70.51
    with graft or prosthesis 70.54
    and rectocele 70.50
        with graft or prosthesis 70.53
dental arch 24.8
diaphragm NEC 34.84
diastasis recti 83.65
diastematomyelia 03.59
ear (external) 18.79
    auditory canal or meatus 18.6
    auricle NEC 18.79
    cartilage NEC 18.79
    laceration (by suture) 18.4
    lop ear 18.79
    middle NEC 19.9
    prominent or protruding 18.5

Repair *(Continued)*
ectropion 08.49
    by or with
        lid reconstruction 08.44
        suture (technique) 08.42
        thermocauterization 08.41
        wedge resection 08.43
encephalocele (cerebral) 02.12
endocardial cushion defect 35.73
    with
        prosthesis (grafted to septa) 35.54
        tissue graft 35.63
enterocele (female) 70.92
    with graft or prosthesis 70.93
    male 53.9
enterostomy 46.40
entropion 08.49
    by or with
        lid reconstruction 08.44
        suture (technique) 08.42
        thermocauterization 08.41
        wedge resection 08.43
epicanthus (fold) 08.59
epididymis (and spermatic cord) NEC 63.59
    with vas deferens 63.89
epiglottis 31.69
episiotomy
    routine following delivery - *see* Episiotomy
    secondary 75.69
epispadias 58.45
esophagus, esophageal NEC 42.89
    fistula NEC 42.84
    stricture 42.85
exstrophy of bladder 57.86
eye, eyeball 16.89
    multiple structures 16.82
    rupture 16.82
    socket 16.64
        with graft 16.63
eyebrow 08.89
    linear 08.81
eyelid 08.89
    full-thickness 08.85
        involving lid margin 08.84
    laceration 08.81
        full-thickness 08.85
            involving lid margin 08.84
        partial-thickness 08.83
            involving lid margin 08.82
    linear 08.81
    partial-thickness 08.83
        involving lid margin 08.82
    retraction 08.38
fallopian tube (with prosthesis) 66.79
    by
        reanastomosis 66.79
        reimplantation into
            ovary 66.72
            uterus 66.74
        suture 66.71
false aneurysm - *see* Repair, aneurysm
fascia 83.89
    by or with
        arthroplasty - *see* Arthroplasty
        graft (fascial) (muscle) 83.82
            hand 82.72
        tendon 83.81
            hand 82.79
        suture (direct) 83.65
            hand 82.46

Repair *(Continued)*
   fascia *(Continued)*
      hand 82.89
         by
            graft NEC 82.79
               fascial 82.72
               muscle 82.72
            suture (direct) 82.46
   joint - *see* Arthroplasty
   filtering bleb (corneal) (scleral) (by
      excision) 12.82
      by
         corneal graft - *see also*
            Keratoplasty 11.60
         scleroplasty 12.82
         suture 11.51
         with conjunctival flap 11.53
   fistula - *see also* Closure, fistula
      anovaginal 70.73
      arteriovenous 39.53
         clipping 39.53
         coagulation 39.53
            endovascular approach
               39.79
               head and neck 39.72
         division 39.53
         excision or resection - *see also*
            Aneurysmectomy, by site
            with
               anastomosis - *see*
                  Aneurysmectomy,
                  with anastomosis, by
                  site
               graft replacement - *see*
                  Aneurysmectomy,
                  with graft
                  replacement, by site
         ligation 39.53
            coronary artery 36.99
         occlusion 39.53
            endovascular approach
               39.79
               head and neck 39.72
         suture 39.53
      cervicovesical 57.84
      cervix 67.62
      choledochoduodenal 51.72
      colovaginal 70.72
      enterovaginal 70.74
      enterovesical 57.83
      esophagocutaneous 42.84
      ileovesical 57.83
      intestinovaginal 70.74
      intestinovesical 57.83
      oroantral 22.71
      perirectal 48.93
      pleuropericardial 37.49
      rectovaginal 70.73
      rectovesical 57.83
      rectovesicovaginal 57.83
      scrotum 61.42
      sigmoidovaginal 70.74
      sinus
         nasal 22.71
         of Valsalva 35.39
      splenocolic 41.95
      urethroperineovesical 57.84
      urethrovesical 57.84
      urethrovesicovaginal 57.84
      uterovesical 57.84
      vagina NEC 70.75
      vaginocutaneous 70.75
      vaginoenteric NEC 70.74
      vaginoileal 70.74

Repair *(Continued)*
   fistula *(Continued)*
      vaginoperineal 70.75
      vaginovesical 57.84
      vesicocervicovaginal 57.84
      vesicocolic 57.83
      vesicocutaneous 57.84
      vesicoenteric 57.83
      vesicointestinal 57.83
      vesicometrorectal 57.83
      vesicoperineal 57.84
      vesicorectal 57.83
      vesicosigmoidal 57.83
      vesicosigmoidovaginal 57.83
      vesicourethral 57.84
      vesicourethrorectal 57.83
      vesicouterine 57.84
      vesicovaginal 57.84
      vulva 71.72
      vulvorectal 48.73
   foramen ovale (patent) 35.71
      with
         prosthesis (open heart
            technique) 35.51
            closed heart technique
               35.52
         tissue graft 35.61
   fracture - *see also* Reduction, fracture
      larynx 31.64
      malunion or nonunion
         (delayed) NEC - *see*
            category 78.4●
      with
         graft - *see* Graft, bone
         insertion (of)
            bone growth stimulator
               (invasive) - *see*
               category 78.9●
            internal fixation device
               78.5●
         manipulation for realignment -
            see Reduction, fracture,
            by site, closed
         osteotomy
            with
               correction of alignment -
                 see category 77.3●
               with internal fixation
                 device - *see*
                 categories 77.3●
                 [78.5]●
               with intramedullary
                 rod - *see* categories
                 77.3● [78.5]●
         replacement arthroplasty - *see*
            Arthroplasty
         sequestrectomy - *see* category
            77.0●
         Sofield type procedure - *see*
            categories 77.3● [78.5]●
         synostosis technique - *see*
            Arthrodesis
      vertebra 03.53
   funnel chest (with implant) 34.74
   gallbladder 51.91
   gastroschisis 54.71
   great vessels NEC 39.59
      laceration (by suture) 39.30
         artery 39.31
         vein 39.32
   hallux valgus NEC 77.59
      resection of joint with prosthetic
         implant 77.59
   hammer toe 77.56

Repair *(Continued)*
   hand 82.89
      with graft or implant 82.79
         fascia 82.72
         muscle 82.72
         tendon 82.79
   heart 37.49
      assist system 37.63
      septum 35.70
         with
            prosthesis 35.50
            tissue graft 35.60
         atrial 35.71
            with
               prosthesis (open heart
                 technique) 35.51
                 closed heart technique
                   35.52
               tissue graft 35.61
            combined with repair of
               valvular and ventricular
               septal defects - *see*
               Repair, endocardial
               cushion defect
            in total repair of
               tetralogy of Fallot 35.81
               total anomalous pulmonary
                 venous connection
                 35.82
               truncus arteriosus 35.83
         combined with repair of
            valvular defect - *see*
            Repair,
            endocardial cushion
            defect
         ventricular 35.72
            with
               prosthesis (open heart
                 technique) 35.53
                 closed heart technique
                   35.55
               tissue graft 35.62
            combined with repair of
               valvular and atrial septal
               defects - *see* Repair,
               endocardial cushion
               defect
            in total repair of
               tetralogy of Fallot 35.81
               total anomalous pulmonary
                 venous connection
                 35.82
               truncus arteriosus 35.83
      total internal biventricular
         replacement system 37.52
      implantable battery 37.54
      implantable controller 37.54
      thoracic unit 37.53
      transcutaneous energy transfer
         [TET] device 37.54
      valve (cusps) (open heart technique)
         35.10
         with prosthesis or tissue graft
            35.20
         aortic (without replacement)
            35.11
            with
               prosthesis 35.22
               tissue graft 35.21
            combined with repair of atrial
               and ventricular septal
               defects - *see* Repair,
               endocardial cushion
               defect

Repair *(Continued)*
  heart *(Continued)*
    valve *(Continued)*
      mitral (without replacement) 35.12
        with
          prosthesis 35.24
          tissue graft 35.23
      pulmonary (without replacement) 35.13
        with
          prosthesis 35.26
            in total repair of tetralogy of Fallot 35.81
          tissue graft 35.25
      tricuspid (without replacement) 35.14
        with
          prosthesis 35.28
          tissue graft 35.27
  hepatic duct 51.79
  hernia NEC 53.9
    anterior abdominal wall NEC 53.59
      with prosthesis or graft
        laparoscopic 53.63
        other and open 53.69
    colostomy 46.42
    crural 53.29
    cul-de-sac (Douglas') 70.92
    diaphragmatic
      abdominal approach
        laparoscopic 53.71
        other and open 53.72
        unspecified 53.75
      thoracic, thoracoabdominal approach 53.80
        laparoscopic 53.83
        other and open 53.84
    epigastric 53.59
      with prosthesis or graft 53.69
    esophageal hiatus
      abdominal approach
        laparoscopic 53.71
        other and open 53.72
        unspecified 53.75
      thoracic, thoracoabdominal approach 53.80
    fascia 83.89
      hand 82.89
    femoral (unilateral) 53.29
      with prosthesis or graft 53.21
      bilateral 53.39
        with prosthesis or graft 53.31
    Ferguson 53.00
    Halsted 53.00
    Hill-Allison (hiatal hernia repair, transpleural approach) 53.80
    hypogastric 53.59
      with prosthesis or graft 53.69
    incisional 53.51
      laparoscopic with prosthesis or graft 53.62
      other open with prosthesis or graft 53.61
    inguinal (unilateral) 53.00
      with prosthesis or graft 53.05
      bilateral 53.10
        with prosthesis or graft 53.17
          laparoscopic 17.24

Repair *(Continued)*
  hernia NEC *(Continued)*
    inguinal *(Continued)*
      bilateral *(Continued)*
        direct
          laparoscopic with graft or prosthesis 17.21
          other and open 53.11
            with prosthesis or graft 53.14
        direct and indirect
          laparoscopic with graft or prosthesis 17.23
          other and open 53.13
            with prosthesis or graft 53.16
        indirect
          laparoscopic with graft or prosthesis 17.22
          other and open 53.12
            with prosthesis or graft 53.15
      direct (unilateral)
        with prosthesis or graft 53.03
        and indirect (unilateral)
          laparoscopic with graft or prosthesis 17.11
          other and open 53.01
            with prosthesis or graft 53.03
        laparoscopic with graft or prosthesis 17.11
        other and open 53.01
          with prosthesis or graft 53.03
      indirect (unilateral)
        laparoscopic with graft or prosthesis 17.12
        other and open 53.02
          with prosthesis or graft 53.04
    internal 53.9
    ischiatic 53.9
    ischiorectal 53.9
    laparoscopic with graft or prosthesis, NOS 17.13
    lumbar 53.9
    manual 96.27
    obturator 53.9
    omental 53.9
    paraesophageal
      laparoscopic 53.71
      other and open 53.72
      unspecified 53.75
    parahiatal
      laparoscopic 53.71
      other and open 53.72
      unspecified 53.75
    paraileostomy 46.41
    parasternal 53.82
    paraumbilical
      laparoscopic 53.43
        with graft or prosthesis 53.42
      other and open with graft or prosthesis 53.41
      other open 53.49
    pericolostomy 46.42
    perineal (enterocele) 53.9
    preperitoneal 53.29
    pudendal 53.9
    retroperitoneal 53.9
    sciatic 53.9

Repair *(Continued)*
  hernia NEC *(Continued)*
    scrotal - *see* Repair, hernia, inguinal
    spigelian 53.59
      with prosthesis or graft 53.69
    umbilical
      laparoscopic 53.43
        with graft or prosthesis 53.42
      other and open with graft or prosthesis 53.41
      other open 53.49
    uveal 12.39
    ventral 53.59
      with prosthesis or graft
        laparoscopic 53.63
        other and open 53.69
      incisional 53.51
        other open with prosthesis or graft 53.61
  hydrocele
    round ligament 69.19
    spermatic cord 63.1
    tunica vaginalis 61.2
  hymen 70.76
  hypospadias 58.45
  ileostomy 46.41
  ingrown toenail 86.23
  intestine, intestinal NEC 46.79
    fistula - *see* Closure, fistula, intestine
    laceration
      large intestine 46.75
      small intestine NEC 46.73
    stoma - *see* Repair, stoma
  inverted uterus NEC 69.29
    manual
      nonobstetric 69.94
      obstetric 75.94
    obstetrical
      manual 75.94
      surgical 75.93
    vaginal approach 69.23
  iris (rupture) NEC 12.39
  jejunostomy 46.41
  joint (capsule) (cartilage) NEC - *see also* Arthroplasty 81.96
  kidney NEC 55.89
  knee (joint) NEC 81.47
    collateral ligaments 81.46
    cruciate ligaments 81.45
    five-in-one 81.42
    triad 81.43
  labia - *see* Repair, vulva
  laceration - *see* Suture, by site
  lacrimal system NEC 09.99
    canaliculus 09.73
    punctum 09.72
      for eversion 09.71
  laryngostomy 31.62
  laryngotracheal cleft 31.69
  larynx 31.69
    fracture 31.64
    laceration 31.61
  leads (cardiac) NEC 37.75
  ligament - *see also* Arthroplasty 81.96
    broad 69.29
    collateral, knee NEC 81.46
    cruciate, knee NEC 81.45
    round 69.29
    uterine 69.29
  lip NEC 27.59
    cleft 27.54
    laceration (by suture) 27.51

◀ New   ◀▥ Revised   ~~deleted~~ Deleted   ● Use Additional Digit(s)   ▧ Omit code

Repair *(Continued)*
liver NEC 50.69
   laceration 50.61
lop ear 18.79
lung NEC 33.49
lymphatic (channel) (peripheral) NEC
   40.9
   duct, left (thoracic) NEC 40.69
macrodactyly 82.83
mallet finger 82.84
mandibular ridge 76.64
mastoid (antrum) (cavity) 19.9
meninges (cerebral) NEC 02.12
   spinal NEC 03.59
      meningocele 03.51
      myelomeningocele 03.52
meningocele (spinal) 03.51
   cranial 02.12
mesentery 54.75
mouth NEC 27.59
   laceration NEC 27.52
muscle NEC 83.87
   by
      graft or implant (fascia) (muscle)
        83.82
        hand 82.72
        tendon 83.81
          hand 82.79
      suture (direct) 83.65
        hand 82.46
      transfer or transplantation
        (muscle) 83.77
        hand 82.58
   hand 82.89
      by
        graft or implant NEC 82.79
          fascia 82.72
        suture (direct) 82.46
        transfer or transplantation
          (muscle) 82.58
musculotendinous cuff, shoulder
   83.63
myelomeningocele 03.52
nasal
   septum (perforation) NEC 21.88
   sinus NEC 22.79
      fistula 22.71
nasolabial flaps (plastic) 21.86
nasopharyngeal atresia 29.4
nerve (cranial) (peripheral) NEC
   04.79
   old injury 04.76
   revision 04.75
   sympathetic 05.81
nipple NEC 85.87
nose (external) (internal) (plastic)
   NEC - *see also* Rhinoplasty
   21.89
   laceration (by suture) 21.81
notched lip 27.59
omentum 54.74
omphalocele
   laparoscopic 53.43
      with graft or prosthesis 53.42
   other and open with graft or
      prosthesis 53.41
   other open 53.49
orbit 16.89
   wound 16.81
ostium
   primum defect 35.73
      with
        prosthesis 35.54
        tissue graft 35.63

Repair *(Continued)*
ostium *(Continued)*
   secundum defect 35.71
      with
        prosthesis (open heart
          technique) 35.51
        closed heart technique
          35.52
        tissue graft 35.61
ovary 65.79
   with tube 65.73
      laparoscopic 65.76
overlapping toe 77.58
pacemaker
   cardiac
      device (permanent) 37.89
      electrodes (leads) NEC 37.75
      pocket (skin) (subcutaneous)
        37.79
palate NEC 27.69
   cleft 27.62
      secondary or subsequent 27.63
   laceration (by suture) 27.61
pancreas NEC 52.95
   Wirsung's duct 52.99
papillary muscle (heart) 35.31
patent ductus arteriosus 38.85
pectus deformity (chest) (carinatum)
   (excavatum) 34.74
pelvic floor NEC 70.79
   obstetric laceration (current)
      75.69
   old 70.79
penis NEC 64.49
   for epispadias or hypospadias
      58.45
   inflatable prosthesis 64.99
   laceration 64.41
pericardium 37.49
perineum (female) 71.79
   laceration (by suture) 71.71
      obstetric (current) 75.69
      old 71.79
   male NEC 86.89
      laceration (by suture) 86.59
peritoneum NEC 54.73
   by suture 54.64
pharynx NEC 29.59
   laceration (by suture) 29.51
   plastic 29.4
pleura NEC 34.93
postcataract wound dehiscence
   11.52
   with conjunctival flap 11.53
pouch of Douglas 70.52
primum ostium defect 35.73
   with
      prosthesis 35.54
      tissue graft 35.63
prostate 60.93
ptosis, eyelid - *see* Repair, blepharoptosis
punctum, lacrimal NEC 09.72
   for correction of eversion 09.71
quadriceps (mechanism) 83.86
rectocele (posterior colporrhaphy)
   70.52
   with graft or prosthesis 70.55
   and cystocele 70.50
      with graft or prosthesis 70.53
rectum NEC 48.79
   laceration (by suture) 48.71
   prolapse NEC 48.76
      abdominal approach 48.75
   STARR procedure 48.74

Repair *(Continued)*
retina, retinal
   detachment 14.59
      by
        cryotherapy 14.52
        diathermy 14.51
        photocoagulation 14.55
          laser 14.54
          xenon arc 14.53
        scleral buckling - *see also*
          Buckling, scleral
          14.49
   tear or defect 14.39
      by
        cryotherapy 14.32
        diathermy 14.31
        photocoagulation 14.35
          laser 14.34
          xenon arc 14.33
retroperitoneal tissue 54.73
rotator cuff (graft) (suture) 83.63
round ligament 69.29
ruptured tendon NEC 83.88
   hand 82.86
salivary gland or duct NEC 26.49
sclera, scleral 12.89
   fistula 12.82
   staphyloma NEC 12.86
      with graft 12.85
scrotum 61.49
sinus
   nasal NEC 22.79
   of Valsalva (aneurysm) 35.39
skin (plastic) (without graft) 86.89
   laceration (by suture) 86.59
skull NEC 02.06
   with
      flap (bone) 02.03
      graft (bone) 02.04
spermatic cord NEC 63.59
   laceration (by suture) 63.51
sphincter ani 49.79
   laceration (by suture) 49.71
      obstetric (current) 75.62
      old 49.79
spina bifida NEC 03.59
   meningocele 03.51
   myelomeningocele 03.52
spinal (cord) (meninges) (structures)
   NEC 03.59
   meningocele 03.51
   myelomeningocele 03.52
spleen 41.95
sternal defect 78.41
stoma
   bile duct 51.79
   bladder 57.22
   bronchus 33.42
   common duct 51.72
   esophagus 42.89
   gallbladder 51.99
   hepatic duct 51.79
   intestine 46.40
      large 46.43
      small 46.41
   kidney 55.89
   larynx 31.63
   rectum 48.79
   stomach 44.69
      laparoscopic 44.68
   thorax 34.79
   trachea 31.74
   ureter 56.62
   urethra 58.49

Repair *(Continued)*
  stomach NEC 44.69
    laceration (by suture) 44.61
      laparoscopic 44.68
  stress incontinence (urinary) NEC 59.79
    by
      anterior urethropexy 59.79
      Burch 59.5
      cystourethropexy (with levator
        muscle sling) 59.71
      injection of implant (fat)
        (collagen) (polytef) 59.72
      paraurethral suspension
        (Pereyra) 59.6
      periurethral suspension 59.6
      plication of urethrovesical
        junction 59.3
      pubococcygeal sling 59.71
      retropubic urethral suspension
        59.5
      suprapubic sling 59.4
      tension free vaginal tape 59.79
      urethrovesical suspension 59.4
        gracilis muscle transplant
          59.71
        levator muscle sling 59.71
  subcutaneous tissue (plastic)
    (without skin graft) 86.89
    laceration (by suture) 86.59
  supracristal defect (heart) 35.72
    with
      prosthesis (open heart technique)
        35.53
        closed heart technique 35.55
      tissue graft 35.62
  symblepharon NEC 10.49
    by division (with insertion of
      conformer) 10.5
    with free graft 10.41
  syndactyly 86.85
  synovial membrane, joint - *see*
    Arthroplasty
  telecanthus 08.59
  tendon 83.88
    by or with
      arthroplasty - *see* Arthroplasty
      graft or implant (tendon) 83.81
        fascia 83.82
          hand 82.72
        hand 82.79
        muscle 83.82
          hand 82.72
      suture (direct) (immediate)
        (primary) - *see also* Suture,
        tendon 83.64
        hand 82.45
      transfer for transplantation
        (tendon) 83.75
        hand 82.56
    hand 82.86
      by
        graft or implant (tendon)
          82.79
        suture (direct) (immediate)
          (primary) - *see also*
          Suture, tendon, hand)
          82.45
        transfer or transplantation
          (tendon) 82.56
    rotator cuff (direct suture) 83.63
    ruptured NEC 83.88
      hand 82.86
    sheath (direct suture) 83.61
      hand 82.41

Repair *(Continued)*
  testis NEC 62.69
  tetralogy of Fallot
    partial - *see* specific procedure
    total (one-stage) 35.81
  thoracic duct NEC 40.69
  thoracostomy 34.72
  thymus (gland) 07.93
  tongue NEC 25.59
  tooth NEC 23.2
    by
      crown (artificial) 23.41
      filling (amalgam) (plastic)
        (silicate) 23.2
      inlay 23.3
  total anomalous pulmonary venous
    connection
    partial - *see* specific procedure
    total (one-stage) 35.82
  trachea NEC 31.79
    laceration (by suture) 31.71
  tricuspid atresia 35.94
  truncus arteriosus
    partial - *see* specific procedure
    total (one-stage) 35.83
  tunica vaginalis 61.49
    laceration (by suture) 61.41
  tympanum - *see* Tympanoplasty
  ureter NEC 56.89
    laceration (by suture) 56.82
  ureterocele 56.89
  urethra NEC 58.49
    laceration (by suture) 58.41
      obstetric (current) 75.61
      old 58.49
    meatus 58.47
  urethrocele (anterior colporrhaphy)
    (female) 70.51
    with graft or prosthesis 70.54
    and rectocele 70.50
      with graft or prosthesis 70.53
  urinary sphincter, artificial
    (component) 58.99
  urinary stress incontinence - *see* Repair,
    stress incontinence
  uterus, uterine 69.49
    inversion - *see* Repair, inverted
      uterus
    laceration (by suture) 69.41
      obstetric (current) 75.50
      old 69.49
    ligaments 69.29
      by
        interposition 69.21
        plication 69.22
  uvula 27.73
    with synchronous cleft palate repair
      27.62
  vagina, vaginal (cuff) (wall) NEC 70.79
    anterior 70.51
      with graft or prosthesis 70.54
      with posterior repair 70.50
        with graft or prosthesis
          70.53
    cystocele 70.51
      with graft or prosthesis 70.54
      and rectocele 70.50
        with graft or prosthesis
          70.53
    enterocele 70.92
      with graft or prosthesis 70.93
    laceration (by suture) 70.71
      obstetric (current) 75.69
      old 70.79

Repair *(Continued)*
  vagina, vaginal NEC *(Continued)*
    posterior 70.52
      with anterior repair 70.50
        with graft or prosthesis
          70.53
    rectocele 70.52
      with graft or prosthesis 70.55
      and cystocele 70.50
        with graft or prosthesis 70.53
    urethrocele 70.51
      with graft or prosthesis 70.54
      and rectocele 70.50
        with graft or prosthesis
          70.53
  varicocele 63.1
  vas deferens 63.89
    by
      anastomosis 63.82
        to epididymis 63.83
      reconstruction 63.82
    laceration (by suture) 63.81
  vein NEC 39.59
    by
      endovascular approach
        head and neck (embolization
          or occlusion) 39.72
    with
      patch graft 39.58
        with excision or resection of
          vessel - *see* Phlebectomy,
          with graft replacement,
          by site
          synthetic (Dacron) (Teflon)
            39.57
          tissue (vein) (autogenous)
            (homograft) 39.56
      suture 39.32
  ventricular septal defect 35.72
    with
      prosthesis (open heart technique)
        35.53
        closed heart technique 35.55
        in total repair of tetralogy of
          Fallot 35.81
      tissue graft 35.62
    combined with repair of valvular
      and atrial septal defects - *see*
      Repair, endocardial cushion
      defect
    in total repair of
      tetralogy of Fallot 35.81
      truncus arteriosus 35.83
  vertebral arch defect (spina bifida)
    03.59
  vulva NEC 71.79
    laceration (by suture) 71.71
      obstetric (current) 75.69
      old 71.79
  Wirsung's duct 52.99
  wound (skin) (without graft) 86.59
    abdominal wall 54.63
      dehiscence 54.61
    postcataract dehiscence (corneal)
      11.52

Replacement
  acetabulum (with prosthesis) 81.52
  ankle, total 81.56
    revision 81.59
  aortic valve (with prosthesis) 35.22
    with tissue graft 35.21
  artery - *see* Graft, artery
  bag - *see* Replacement, pack or bag
  Barton's tongs (skull) 02.94

◀ New   ◀▥ Revised   ~~deleted~~ Deleted   ● Use Additional Digit(s)   ▥ Omit code

Replacement (*Continued*)
bladder
  with
    ileal loop 57.87 [45.51]
    sigmoid 57.87 [45.52]
    sphincter, artificial 58.93
bronchial device NOS 33.79
bronchial substance NOS 33.79
bronchial valve(s) 33.71 ◄▥
  multiple lobes 33.73 ◄
  single lobe 33.71 ◄
caliper tongs (skull) 02.94
cannula
  arteriovenous shunt 39.94
  pancreatic duct 97.05
  vessel-to-vessel (arteriovenous) 39.94
cardiac contractility modulation
  (CCM) ◄
  rechargeable pulse generator
    only 17.52 ◄
  total system 17.51 ◄
cardiac resynchronization device
  defibrillator (biventricular
    defibrillator) (BiV ICD) (BiV
    pacemaker with defibrillator)
    (BiV pacing with defibrillator)
    (CRT-D) (device and one or
    more leads) (total system)
    00.51
    left ventricular coronary venous
      lead only 00.52
    pulse generator only 00.54
  pacemaker (biventricular
    pacemaker) (BiV pacemaker)
    (CRT-P) (device and one or
    more leads) (total system)
    00.50
    left ventricular coronary venous
      lead only 00.52
    pulse generator only 00.53
cardioverter/defibrillator (total
  system) 37.94
  leads only (electrodes) (sensing)
    (pacing) 37.97
  pulse generator only 37.98
cast NEC 97.13
  lower limb 97.12
  upper limb 97.11
catheter
  bladder (indwelling) 57.95
  cystostomy 59.94
  ventricular shunt (cerebral) 02.42
  wound 97.15
CCM (cardiac contractility
  modulation) ◄
  rechargeable pulse generator
    only 17.52 ◄
  total system 17.51 ◄
CRT-D (biventricular defibrillator)
  (BiV ICD) (BiV pacemaker with
  defibrillator) (BiV pacing with
  defibrillator) (cardiac
  resynchronization defibrillator)
  (device and one or more leads)
  00.51
  left ventricular coronary venous
    lead only 00.52
  pulse generator only 00.54
CRT-P (biventricular pacemaker)
  (BiV pacemaker) (cardiac
  resynchronization pacemaker)
  (device and one or more leads)
  00.50
  left ventricular coronary venous
    lead only 00.52
  pulse generator only 00.53

Replacement (*Continued*)
Crutchfield tongs (skull) 02.94
cystostomy tube (catheter) 59.94
device
  subcutaneous for intracardiac or
    great vessel hemodynamic
    monitoring 00.57 ◄▥
diaphragm, vagina 97.24
disc - *see* Replacement, intervertebral
  disc
drain - *see also* Replacement, tube
  vagina 97.26
  vulva 97.26
  wound, musculoskeletal or skin
    97.16
ear (prosthetic) 18.71
elbow (joint), total 81.84
electrode(s) - *see* Implant, electrode or
  lead by site or name of device
  brain
    depth 02.93
    foramen ovale 02.93
    sphenoidal 02.96
  carotid sinus 04.92
  depth 02.93
  foramen ovale 02.93
  gastric 04.92
  intracranial 02.93
  pacemaker - *see* Replacement,
    pacemaker, electrode(s)
  peripheral nerve 04.92
  sacral nerve 04.92
  sphenoidal 02.96
  spine 03.93
electroencephalographic receiver
  (brain) (intracranial) 02.93
electronic
  cardioverter/defibrillator - *see*
    Replacement, cardioverter/
    defibrillator
  leads (electrode)(s) - *see*
    Replacement, electrode(s)
  stimulator - *see also* Implant,
    electronic stimulator, by site
    bladder 57.97
    muscle (skeletal) 83.92
    ureter 56.93
electrostimulator - *see* Implant,
  electronic stimulator, by site
enterostomy device (tube)
  large intestine 97.04
  small intestine 97.03
epidural pegs 02.93
femoral head, by prosthesis 81.52
  revision 81.53
Gardner Wells tongs (skull) 02.94
gastric band, laparoscopic 44.96
gastric port device (subcutaneous)
  44.96
graft - *see* Graft
halo traction device (skull) 02.94
Harrington rod (with refusion of
  spine) - *see* Refusion, spinal
heart
  artificial
    total internal biventricular
      replacement system
      37.52
      implantable battery 37.54
      implantable controller 37.54
      thoracic unit 37.53
      transcutaneous energy
        transfer [TET] device
        37.54

Replacement (*Continued*)
heart (*Continued*)
  total internal biventricular
    replacement system 37.52
    implantable battery 37.54
    implantable controller 37.54
    thoracic unit 37.53
    transcutaneous energy transfer
      [TET] device 37.54
  valve (with prosthesis) (with tissue
    graft) 35.20
    aortic (with prosthesis) 35.22
      with tissue graft 35.21
    mitral (with prosthesis) 35.24
      with tissue graft 35.23
    poppet (prosthetic) 35.95
    pulmonary (with prosthesis) 35.26
      with tissue graft 35.25
      in total repair of tetralogy of
        Fallot 35.81
    tricuspid (with prosthesis) 35.28
      with tissue graft 35.27
hip (partial) (with fixation device)
  (with prosthesis) (with traction)
  81.52
  acetabulum 81.52
    revision 81.53
  femoral head 81.52
    revision 81.53
  total 81.51
    revision 81.53
intervertebral disc
  artificial, NOS 84.60
    cervical 84.62
      nucleus 84.61
      partial 84.61
      total 84.62
    lumbar, lumbosacral 84.65
      nucleus 84.64
      partial 84.64
      total 84.65
    thoracic (partial) (total) 84.63
inverted uterus - *see* Repair, inverted
  uterus
iris NEC 12.39
kidney, mechanical 55.97
knee (bicompartmental) (hemijoint)
  (partial) (total)
  (tricompartmental)
  (unicompartmental) 81.54
  revision 81.55
laryngeal stent 31.93
leads (electrode)(s) - *see* Replacement,
  electrode(s)
mechanical kidney 55.97
mitral valve (with prosthesis) 35.24
  with tissue graft 35.23
Mulligan hood, fallopian tube 66.93
muscle stimulator (skeletal) 83.92
nephrostomy tube 55.93
neuropacemaker - *see* Implant,
  neurostimulator, by site
neurostimulator - *see also* Implant,
  neurostimulator, by site
  skeletal muscle 83.92
pacemaker
  brain - *see* Implant, neurostimulator,
    brain
  cardiac device (initial) (permanent)
    dual-chamber device 37.87
    resynchronization - *see*
      Replacement, CRT-P
    single-chamber device 37.85
      rate responsive 37.86

◀ New   ◀‖‖ Revised   ~~deleted~~ Deleted   ● Use Additional Digit(s)   ▨ Omit code

Resection *(Continued)*
  breast - *see also* Mastectomy
    quadrant 85.22
    segmental 85.23
  broad ligament 69.19
  bronchus (sleeve) (wide sleeve) 32.1
    block (en bloc) (with radical
        dissection of brachial plexus,
        bronchus, lobe of lung, ribs,
        and sympathetic nerves) 32.6
  bursa 83.5
    hand 82.31
  cecum (and terminal ileum)
    laparoscopic 17.32
    open and other 45.72
  cerebral meninges 01.51
  chest wall 34.4
  clavicle 77.81
  clitoris 71.4
  colon (partial) (segmental)
    ascending (cecum and terminal
        ileum)
      laparoscopic 17.32
      open and other 45.72
    cecum (and terminal ileum)
      laparoscopic 17.32
      open and other 45.72
    complete
      laparoscopic 45.81
      open 45.82
      other 45.83
      unspecified 45.83
    descending (sigmoid)
      laparoscopic 17.36
      open and other 45.76
    for interposition 45.52
    Hartmann
      laparoscopic 17.35
      open and other 45.75
    hepatic flexure
      laparoscopic 17.33
      open and other 45.73
    laparoscopic 17.39
    left radical (hemicolon)
      laparoscopic 17.35
      open and other 45.75
    multiple segmental
      laparoscopic 17.31
      open and other 45.71
    open and other 45.79
    right radical (hemicolon)
        (ileocolectomy)
      laparoscopic 17.33
      open and other 45.73
    segmental NEC
      laparoscopic 17.39
      multiple
        laparoscopic 17.31
        open and other 45.71
      open and other 45.79
    sigmoid
      laparoscopic 17.36
      open and other 45.76
    splenic flexure
      laparoscopic 17.35
      open and other 45.75
    total
      laparoscopic 45.81
      open 45.82
      other 45.83
      unspecified 45.83
    transverse
      laparoscopic 17.34
      open and other 45.74

Resection *(Continued)*
  conjunctiva, for pterygium 11.39
    corneal graft 11.32
  cornual (fallopian tube) (unilateral) 66.69
    bilateral 66.63
  diaphragm 34.81
  endaural 20.79
  endorectal (pull-through) (Soave) 48.41
    combined abdominal, NOS 48.50
      laparoscopic 48.51
      open 48.52
      other 48.59
  esophagus (partial) (subtotal) - *see also*
      Esophagectomy 42.41
    total 42.42
  exteriorized intestine - *see* Resection,
      intestine, exteriorized
  fascia 83.44
    for graft 83.43
      hand 82.34
    hand 82.35
      for graft 82.34
  gallbladder (total) 51.22
  gastric (partial) (sleeve) (subtotal)
      NEC - *see also* Gastrectomy 43.89
    with anastomosis NEC 43.89
      esophagogastric 43.5
      gastroduodenal 43.6
      gastrogastric 43.89
      gastrojejunal 43.7
    complete or total NEC 43.99
      with intestinal interposition 43.91
    radical NEC 43.99
      with intestinal interposition 43.91
    wedge 43.42
      endoscopic 43.41
  hallux valgus (joint) - *see also*
      Bunionectomy with prosthetic
      implant 77.59
  hepatic
    duct 51.69
    flexure (colon)
      laparoscopic 17.33
      open and other 45.73
  infundibula, heart (right) 35.34
  intestine (partial) NEC
    cecum (with terminal ileum)
      laparoscopic 17.32
      open and other 45.72
    exteriorized (large intestine) 46.04
      small intestine 46.02
    for interposition 45.50
      large intestine 45.52
      small intestine 45.51
    hepatic flexure
      laparoscopic 17.33
      open and other 45.73
    ileum 45.62
      with cecum
        laparoscopic 17.32
        open and other 45.72
    laparoscopic 17.39
    large (partial) (segmental) NEC
      for interposition 45.52
      laparoscopic 17.39
      multiple segmental
        laparoscopic 17.31
        open and other 45.71
      other 45.79
      total
        laparoscopic 45.81
        open 45.82
        other 45.83
        unspecified 45.83
      unspecified 45.79

Resection *(Continued)*
  intestine NEC *(Continued)*
    left hemicolon
      laparoscopic 17.35
      open and other 45.75
    multiple segmental (large
        intestine)
      laparoscopic 17.31
      open and other 45.71
      small intestine 45.61
    open and other 45.79
    right hemicolon
      laparoscopic 17.33
      open and other 45.73
    segmental (large intestine)
      laparoscopic 17.39
      multiple
        laparoscopic 17.31
        open and other 45.71
      open and other 45.79
      small intestine 45.62
        multiple 45.61
    sigmoid
      laparoscopic 17.36
      open and other 45.76
    small (partial) (segmental) NEC
        45.62
      for interposition 45.51
      multiple segmental 45.61
      total 45.63
    total
      large intestine
        laparoscopic 45.81
        open 45.82
        other 45.83
        unspecified 45.83
      small intestine 45.63
  joint structure NEC - *see also*
      Arthrectomy 80.90
  kidney (segmental) (wedge) 55.4
  larynx - *see also* Laryngectomy
    submucous 30.29
  lesion - *see* Excision, lesion, by site
  levator palpebrae muscle 08.33
  ligament - *see also* Arthrectomy 80.90
    broad 69.19
    round 69.19
    uterine 69.19
  lip (wedge) 27.43
  liver (partial) (wedge) 50.22
    lobe (total) 50.3
    total 50.4
  lung (wedge) NEC 32.29
    endoscopic 32.28
    segmental (any part) 32.39
      thoracoscopic 32.30
    thoracoscopic 32.20
    volume reduction 32.22
      biologic lung volume reduction
          (BLVR) - *see* category 33.7●
  meninges (cerebral) 01.51
    spinal 03.4
  mesentery 54.4
  muscle 83.45
    extraocular 15.13
      with
        advancement or recession of
            other eye muscle 15.3
        suture of original insertion
            15.13
      levator palpebrae 08.33
      Muller's, for blepharoptosis 08.35
      orbicularis oculi 08.20
      tarsal, for blepharoptosis 08.35

Resection *(Continued)*
    muscle *(Continued)*
        for graft 83.43
            hand 82.34
        hand 82.36
            for graft 82.34
        ocular - *see* Resection, muscle,
            extraocular
    myocardium 37.33
    nasal septum (submucous) 21.5
    nerve (cranial) (peripheral) NEC 04.07
        phrenic 04.03
            for collapse of lung 33.31
        sympathetic 05.29
        vagus - *see* Vagotomy
    nose (complete) (extended) (partial)
        (radical) 21.4
    omentum 54.4
    orbitomaxillary, radical 16.51
    ovary - *see also* Oophorectomy
        wedge 65.22
            laparoscopic 65.24
    palate (bony) (local) 27.31
        by wide excision 27.32
        soft 27.49
    pancreas (total) (with synchronous
        duodenectomy) 52.6
        partial NEC 52.59
            distal (tail) (with part of body)
                52.52
            proximal (head) (with part of
                body) (with synchronous
                duodenectomy) 52.51
            radical subtotal 52.53
        radical (one-stage) (two-stage) 52.7
        subtotal 52.53
    pancreaticoduodenal - *see also*
        Pancreatectomy 52.6
    pelvic viscera (en masse) (female) 68.8
        male 57.71
    penis 64.3
    pericardium (partial) (for)
        chronic constrictive pericarditis
            37.31
        drainage 37.12
        removal of adhesions 37.31
    peritoneum 54.4
    pharynx (partial) 29.33
    phrenic nerve 04.03
        for collapse of lung 33.31
    prostate - *see also* Prostatectomy
        transurethral (punch) 60.29
    pterygium 11.39
    radial head 77.83
    rectosigmoid - *see also* Resection,
        rectum 48.69
    rectum (partial) NEC 48.69
        with
            pelvic exenteration 68.8
            transsacral sigmoidectomy 48.61
        abdominoendorectal (combined),
            NOS 48.50
            laparoscopic 48.51
            open 48.52
            other 48.59
        abdominoperineal, NOS 48.50
            laparoscopic 48.51
            open 48.52
            other 48.59
            pull-through NEC 48.49
                Duhamel type 48.65
                laparoscopic 48.42
                not otherwise specified 48.40
                open 48.43

Resection *(Continued)*
    rectum NEC *(Continued)*
        anterior 48.63
            with colostomy (synchronous)
                48.62
        Duhamel 48.65
        endorectal 48.41
            combined abdominal, NOS
                48.50
            laparoscopic 48.51
            open 48.52
            other 48.59
        posterior 48.64
        pull-through NEC 48.49
            endorectal 48.41
            laparoscopic 48.42
            not otherwise specified 48.40
            open 48.43
        STARR procedure 48.74
        submucosal (Soave) 48.41
            combined abdominal, NOS
                48.50
            laparoscopic 48.51
            open 48.52
            other 48.59
    rib (transaxillary) 77.91
        as operative approach - *omit code*
        incidental to thoracic
            operation - *omit code*
    right ventricle (heart), for infundibular
        stenosis 35.34
    root (tooth) (apex) 23.73
        with root canal therapy 23.72
        residual or retained 23.11
    round ligament 69.19
    sclera 12.65
        with scleral buckling - *see also*
            Buckling, scleral 14.49
        lamellar (for retinal reattachment)
            14.49
            with implant 14.41
    scrotum 61.3
    soft tissue NEC 83.49
        hand 82.39
    sphincter of Oddi 51.89
    spinal cord (meninges) 03.4
    splanchnic 05.29
    splenic flexure (colon) 45.75
    sternum 77.81
    stomach (partial) (sleeve) (subtotal)
        NEC - *see also* Gastrectomy
        43.89
        with anastomosis NEC 43.89
            esophagogastric 43.5
            gastroduodenal 43.6
            gastrogastric 43.89
            gastrojejunal 43.7
        complete or total NEC 43.99
            with intestinal interposition
                43.91
        fundus 43.89
        radical NEC 43.99
            with intestinal interposition
                43.91
        wedge 43.42
            endoscopic 43.41
    submucous
        larynx 30.29
        nasal septum 21.5
        vocal cords 30.22
    synovial membrane (complete)
        (partial) - *see also* Synovectomy
        80.70
    tarsolevator 08.33

Resection *(Continued)*
    tendon 83.42
        hand 82.33
    thoracic structures (block) (en bloc)
        (radical) (brachial plexus,
        bronchus, lobes of lung, ribs, and
        sympathetic nerves) 32.6
    thorax 34.4
    tongue 25.2
        wedge 25.1
    tooth root 23.73
        with root canal therapy 23.72
        apex (abscess) 23.73
            with root canal therapy 23.72
        residual or retained 23.11
    trachea 31.5
    transurethral
        bladder NEC 57.49
        prostate 60.29
    transverse colon
        laparoscopic 17.34
        open and other 45.74
    turbinates - *see* Turbinectomy
    ureter (partial) 56.41
        total 56.42
    uterus - *see* Hysterectomy
    vein - *see* Phlebectomy
    ventricle (heart) 37.35
        infundibula 35.34
    vesical neck 57.59
        transurethral 57.49
    vocal cords (punch) 30.22
Respirator, volume-controlled (Bennett)
    (Byrd) - *see* Ventilation
Restoration
    cardioesophageal angle 44.66
        laparoscopic 44.67
    dental NEC 23.49
        by
            application of crown (artificial)
                23.41
            insertion of bridge (fixed)
                23.42
                removable 23.43
    extremity - *see* Reattachment,
        extremity
    eyebrow 08.70
        with graft 08.63
    eye socket 16.64
        with graft 16.63
    tooth NEC 23.2
        by
            crown (artificial) 23.41
            filling (amalgam) (plastic)
                (silicate) 23.2
            inlay 23.3
Restrictive
    gastric band, laparoscopic 44.95
Resurfacing, hip 00.86
    acetabulum 00.87
        with femoral head 00.85
    femoral head 00.86
        with acetabulum 00.85
    partial NOS 00.85
        acetabulum 00.87
        femoral head 00.86
    total (acetabulum and femoral head)
        00.85
Resuscitation
    artificial respiration 93.93
    cardiac 99.60
        cardioversion 99.62
            atrial 99.61
        defibrillation 99.62

◀ New ◀▥ Revised ~~deleted~~ Deleted ● Use Additional Digit(s) ▥ Omit code

Resuscitation *(Continued)*
 cardiac *(Continued)*
  external massage 99.63
   open chest 37.91
  intracardiac injection 37.92
 cardiopulmonary 99.60
 endotracheal intubation 96.04
 manual 93.93
 mouth-to-mouth 93.93
 pulmonary 93.93
Resuture
 abdominal wall 54.61
 cardiac septum prosthesis 35.95
 chest wall 34.71
 heart valve prosthesis (poppet) 35.95
 wound (skin and subcutaneous tissue)
  (without graft) NEC 86.59
Retavase, infusion 99.10
Reteplase, infusion 99.10
Retightening (noninvasive) ◄
 external fixator device - *omit code* ◄
Retinaculotomy NEC - *see also* Division,
  ligament 80.40
 carpal tunnel (flexor) 04.43
Retraining
 cardiac 93.36
 vocational 93.85
Retrogasserian neurotomy 04.02
Revascularization
 cardiac (heart muscle) (myocardium)
  (direct) 36.10
  with
   bypass anastomosis
    abdominal artery to coronary
     artery 36.17
    aortocoronary (catheter stent)
     (homograft) (prosthesis)
     (saphenous vein graft)
     36.10
     one coronary vessel 36.11
     two coronary vessels 36.12
     three coronary vessels 36.13
     four coronary vessels 36.14
    gastroepiploic artery to
     coronary artery 36.17
    internal mammary-coronary
     artery (single vessel)
     36.15
     double vessel 36.16
    specified type NEC 36.19
    thoracic artery-coronary artery
     (single vessel) 36.15
     double vessel 36.16
   implantation of artery into heart
    (muscle) (myocardium)
    (ventricle) 36.2
  indirect 36.2
  specified type NEC 36.39
  transmyocardial
   endoscopic 36.33
   endovascular 36.34
   open chest 36.31
   percutaneous 36.34
   specified type NEC 36.32
   thoracoscopic 36.33
Reversal, intestinal segment 45.50
 large 45.52
 small 45.51
Revision
 amputation stump 84.3
  current traumatic - *see* Amputation
 anastomosis
  biliary tract 51.94
  blood vessel 39.49

Revision *(Continued)*
 anastomosis *(Continued)*
  gastric, gastrointestinal (with jejunal
   interposition) 44.5
  intestine (large) 46.94
   small 46.93
  pleurothecal 03.97
  pyelointestinal 56.72
  salpingothecal 03.97
  subarachnoid-peritoneal 03.97
  subarachnoid-ureteral 03.97
  ureterointestinal 56.72
 ankle replacement (prosthesis) 81.59
 anterior segment (eye) wound
  (operative) NEC 12.83
 arteriovenous shunt (cannula) (for
  dialysis) 39.42
 arthroplasty - *see* Arthroplasty
 bone flap, skull 02.06
 breast implant 85.93
 bronchostomy 33.42
 bypass graft (vascular) 39.49
  abdominal - coronary artery
   36.17
  aortocoronary (catheter stent)
   (with prosthesis) (with
   saphenous vein graft) (with
   vein graft) 36.10
   one coronary vessel 36.11
   two coronary vessels 36.12
   three coronary vessels 36.13
   four coronary vessels 36.14
  CABG - *see* Revision, aortocoronary
   bypass graft
  chest tube - *see* intercostal catheter
  coronary artery bypass graft (CABG)
   - *see* Revision, aortocoronary
   bypass graft, abdominal -
   coronary artery bypass, and
   internal mammary - coronary
   artery bypass
  intercostal catheter (with lysis of
   adhesions) 34.04
   thoracoscopic 34.06
  internal mammary - coronary artery
   (single) 36.15
   double vessel 36.16
 cannula, vessel-to-vessel
  (arteriovenous) 39.94
 canthus, lateral 08.59
 cardiac pacemaker
  device (permanent) 37.89
  electrode(s) (atrial) (transvenous)
   (ventricular) 37.75
  pocket 37.79
 cardiac resynchronization defibrillator
  (CRT-D)
  device 37.79
  electrode(s) 37.75
  pocket 37.79
 cardiac resynchronization pacemaker
  (CRT-P)
  device (permanent) 37.89
  electrode(s) (atrial) (transvenous)
   (ventricular) 37.75
  pocket 37.79
 cardioverter/defibrillator (automatic)
  pocket 37.79
 cholecystostomy 51.99
 cleft palate repair 27.63
 colostomy 46.43
 conduit, urinary 56.52
 cystostomy (stoma) 57.22
 disc - *see* Revision, intervertebral disc

Revision *(Continued)*
 elbow replacement (prosthesis) 81.97
 enterostomy (stoma) 46.40
  large intestine 46.43
  small intestine 46.41
 enucleation socket 16.64
  with graft 16.63
 esophagostomy 42.83
 exenteration cavity 16.66
  with secondary graft 16.65
 extraocular muscle surgery 15.6
 fenestration, inner ear 20.62
 filtering bleb 12.66
 fixation device (broken) (displaced) -
  see also Fixation, bone, internal
  78.50
 flap or pedicle graft (skin) 86.75
 foot replacement (prosthesis) 81.59
 gastric anastomosis (with jejunal
  interposition) 44.5
 gastric band, laparoscopic 44.96
 gastric port device
  laparoscopic 44.96
 gastroduodenostomy (with jejunal
  interposition) 44.5
 gastrointestinal anastomosis (with
  jejunal interposition) 44.5
 gastrojejunostomy 44.5
 gastrostomy 44.69
  laparoscopic 44.68
 hand replacement (prosthesis) 81.97
 heart procedure NEC 35.95
 hip replacement NOS 81.53
  acetabular and femoral components
   (total) 00.70
  acetabular component only 00.71
  acetabular liner and/or femoral
   head only 00.73
  femoral component only 00.72
  femoral head only and/or
   acetabular liner 00.73
  partial
   acetabular component only
    00.71
   acetabular liner and/or femoral
    head only 00.73
   femoral component only 00.72
   femoral head only and/or
    acetabular liner 00.73
   total (acetabular and femoral
    components) 00.70
 Holter (-Spitz) valve 02.42
 ileal conduit 56.52
 ileostomy 46.41
 intervertebral disc, artificial (partial)
  (total) NOS 84.69
  cervical 84.66
  lumbar, lumbosacral 84.68
  thoracic 84.67
 Jejunoileal bypass 46.93
 jejunostomy 46.41
 joint replacement
  acetabular and femoral components
   (total) 00.70
  acetabular component only 00.71
  acetabular liner and/or femoral
   head only 00.73
  ankle 81.59
  elbow 81.97
  femoral component only 00.72
  femoral head only and/or
   acetabular liner 00.73
  foot 81.59
  hand 81.97

Revision (Continued)
  joint replacement (Continued)
    hip 81.53
      acetabular and femoral
        components (total) 00.70
      acetabular component only
        00.71
      acetabular liner and/or femoral
        head only 00.73
      femoral component only 00.72
      femoral head only and/or
        acetabular liner 00.73
      partial
        acetabular component only
          00.71
        acetabular liner and/or
          femoral head only 00.73
        femoral component only
          00.72
        femoral head only and/or
          acetabular liner 00.73
        total (acetabular and femoral
          components) 00.70
    knee 81.55
    knee replacement NOS 81.55
      femoral component 00.82
      partial
        femoral component 00.82
        patellar component 00.83
        tibial component 00.81
        tibial insert 00.84
      patellar component 00.83
      tibial component 00.81
      tibial insert 00.84
      total (all components) 00.80
    lower extremity NEC 81.59
    toe 81.59
    upper extremity 81.97
    wrist 81.97
  knee replacement (prosthesis) NOS
    81.55
    femoral component 00.82
    partial
      femoral component 00.82
      patellar component 00.83
      tibial component 00.81
      tibial insert 00.84
    patellar component 00.83
    tibial component 00.81
    tibial insert 00.84
    total (all components) 00.80
  laryngostomy 31.63
  lateral canthus 08.59
  mallet finger 82.84
  mastoid antrum 19.9
  mastoidectomy 20.92
  nephrostomy 55.89
  neuroplasty 04.75
  ocular implant 16.62
  orbital implant 16.62
  pocket
    cardiac device (defibrillator)
      (pacemaker)
      with initial insertion of cardiac
        device - omit code
      new site (cardiac device pocket)
        (skin) (subcutaneous)
        37.79
    intracardiac hemodynamic
      monitoring 37.79
    subcutaneous device pocket NEC
      with initial insertion of generator
        or device - omit code
      new site 86.09

Revision (Continued)
  pocket (Continued)
    thalamic stimulator pulse generator
      with initial insertion of battery
      package - omit code
    new site (skin) (subcutaneous)
      86.09
  previous mastectomy site - see
    categories 85.0–85.99
  proctostomy 48.79
  prosthesis
    acetabular and femoral components
      (total) 00.70
    acetabular component only 00.71
    acetabular liner and/or femoral
      head only 00.73
    ankle 81.59
    breast 85.93
    elbow 81.97
    femoral component only 00.72
    femoral head only and/or
      acetabular liner 00.73
    foot 81.59
    hand 81.97
    heart valve (poppet) 35.95
    hip 81.53
      acetabular component only
        00.71
      acetabular liner and/or femoral
        head only 00.73
      femoral component only 00.72
      femoral head only and/or
        acetabular liner 00.73
      partial
        acetabular component only
          00.71
        acetabular liner and/or
          femoral head only
          00.73
        femoral component only
          00.72
        femoral head only and/or
          acetabular liner 00.73
      acetabular and femoral
        components (total) 00.70
      total (acetabular and femoral
        components) 00.70
    knee NOS 81.55
      femoral component 00.82
      partial
        femoral component 00.82
        patellar component 00.83
        tibial component 00.81
        tibial insert 00.84
      patellar component 00.83
      tibial component 00.81
      tibial insert 00.84
      total (all components) 00.80
    lower extremity NEC 81.59
    shoulder 81.97
    spine
      facet replacement device(s)
        84.85
      interspinous process device(s)
        84.81
      pedicle-based dynamic
        stabilization device(s)
        84.83
    toe 81.59
    upper extremity 81.97
    wrist 81.97
  ptosis overcorrection 08.37
  pyelostomy 55.12
  pyloroplasty 44.29

Revision (Continued)
  rhinoplasty 21.84
  scar
    skin 86.84
      with excision 86.3
  scleral fistulization 12.66
  shoulder replacement (prosthesis) 81.97
  shunt
    arteriovenous (cannula) (for
      dialysis) 39.42
    lumbar-subarachnoid NEC 03.97
    peritoneojugular 54.99
    peritoneovascular 54.99
    pleurothecal 03.97
    salpingothecal 03.97
    spinal (thecal) NEC 03.97
    subarachnoid-peritoneal 03.97
    subarachnoid-ureteral 03.97
    ventricular (cerebral) 02.42
    ventriculoperitoneal
      at peritoneal site 54.95
      at ventricular site 02.42
  stapedectomy NEC 19.29
    with incus replacement (homograft)
      (prosthesis) 19.21
  stoma
    bile duct 51.79
    bladder (vesicostomy) 57.22
    bronchus 33.42
    common duct 51.72
    esophagus 42.89
    gallbladder 51.99
    hepatic duct 51.79
    intestine 46.40
      large 46.43
      small 46.41
    kidney 55.89
    larynx 31.63
    rectum 48.79
    stomach 44.69
      laparoscopic 44.68
    thorax 34.79
    trachea 31.74
    ureter 56.62
    urethra 58.49
  tack operation 20.79
  toe replacement (prosthesis) 81.59
  tracheostomy 31.74
  tunnel
    pulse generator lead wire 86.99
      with initial procedure - omit code
  tympanoplasty 19.6
  uretero-ileostomy, cutaneous 56.52
  ureterostomy (cutaneous) (stoma) NEC
    56.62
    ileal 56.52
  urethrostomy 58.49
  urinary conduit 56.52
  vascular procedure (previous) NEC
    39.49
  ventricular shunt (cerebral) 02.42
  vesicostomy stoma 57.22
  wrist replacement (prosthesis) 81.97
Rhinectomy 21.4
Rhinocheiloplasty 27.59
  cleft lip 27.54
Rhinomanometry 89.12
Rhinoplasty (external) (internal) NEC 21.87
  augmentation (with graft) (with
    synthetic implant) 21.85
  limited 21.86
  revision 21.84
  tip 21.86
  twisted nose 21.84

◀ New   ◀▦ Revised   ~~deleted~~ Deleted   ● Use Additional Digit(s)   ▨ Omit code

Rhinorrhaphy (external) (internal)
21.81
for epistaxis 21.09
Rhinoscopy 21.21
Rhinoseptoplasty 21.84
Rhinotomy 21.1
Rhizotomy (radiofrequency) (spinal)
03.1
acoustic 04.01
trigeminal 04.02
Rhytidectomy (facial) 86.82
eyelid
lower 08.86
upper 08.87
Rhytidoplasty (facial) 86.82
Ripstein operation (repair of prolapsed
rectum) 48.75
Robotic assisted surgery
endoscopic 17.44
laparoscopic 17.42
open 17.41
other and unspecified 17.49
percutaneous 17.43
thoracoscopic 17.45

Rodney Smith operation (radical subtotal
pancreatectomy) 52.53
Roentgenography - *see also* Radiography
cardiac, negative contrast 88.58
Rolling of conjunctiva 10.33
Root
canal (tooth) (therapy) 23.70
with
apicoectomy 23.72
irrigation 23.71
resection (tooth) (apex) 23.73
with root canal therapy 23.72
residual or retained 23.11
Rotation of fetal head
forceps (instrumental) (Kielland)
(Scanzoni) (key-in-lock) 72.4
manual 73.51
Routine
chest x-ray 87.44
psychiatric visit 94.12
Roux-en-Y operation
bile duct 51.36
cholecystojejunostomy 51.32
esophagus (intrathoracic) 42.54

Roux-en-Y operation (*Continued*)
gastroenterostomy 44.39
laparoscopic 44.38
gastrojejunostomy 44.39
laparoscopic 44.38
pancreaticojejunostomy 52.96
Roux-Goldthwait operation (repair of
recurrent patellar dislocation)
81.44
Roux-Herzen-Judine operation (jejunal
loop interposition) 42.63
Rubin test (insufflation of fallopian tube)
66.8
Ruiz-Mora operation (proximal
phalangectomy for hammer toe)
77.99
Rupture
esophageal web 42.01
joint adhesions, manual 93.26
membranes, artificial 73.09
for surgical induction of labor 73.01
ovarian cyst, manual 65.93
Russe operation (bone graft of scaphoid)
78.04

S

Sacculotomy (tack) 20.79
Sacrectomy (partial) 77.89
　total 77.99
Saemisch operation (corneal section)
　11.1
Salpingectomy (bilateral) (total)
　(transvaginal) 66.51
　with oophorectomy 65.61
　　laparoscopic 65.63
　partial (unilateral) 66.69
　　with removal of tubal pregnancy
　　　66.62
　bilateral 66.63
　　for sterilization 66.39
　　　by endoscopy 66.29
　remaining or solitary tube 66.52
　　with ovary 65.62
　　　laparoscopic 65.64
　unilateral (total) 66.4
　　with
　　　oophorectomy 65.49
　　　　laparoscopic 65.41
　　　removal of tubal pregnancy
　　　　66.62
　　partial 66.69
Salpingography 87.85
Salpingohysterostomy 66.74
Salpingo-oophorectomy (unilateral)
　65.49
　that by laparoscope 65.41
　bilateral (same operative episode)
　　65.61
　　laparoscopic 65.63
　remaining or solitary tube and ovary
　　65.62
　　laparoscopic 65.64
Salpingo-oophoroplasty 65.73
　laparoscopic 65.76
Salpingo-oophororrhaphy 65.79
Salpingo-oophorostomy 66.72
Salpingo-oophorotomy 65.09
　laparoscopic 65.01
Salpingoplasty 66.79
Salpingorrhaphy 66.71
Salpingosalpingostomy 66.73
Salpingostomy (for removal of non-
　ruptured ectopic pregnancy)
　66.02
Salpingotomy 66.01
Salpingo-uterostomy 66.74
Salter operation (innominate osteotomy)
　77.39
Salvage (autologous blood)
　(intraoperative) (perioperative)
　(postoperative) 99.00
Sampling, blood for genetic
　determination of fetus 75.33
Sandpapering (skin) 86.25
Saucerization
　bone - see also Excision, lesion, bone
　　77.60
　rectum 48.99
Sauer-Bacon operation
　(abdominoperineal resection), NOS
　48.50
　laparoscopic 48.51
　open 48.52
　other 48.59
Scalenectomy 83.45
Scalenotomy 83.19
Scaling and polishing, dental
　96.54

Scan, scanning
　C.A.T. (computerized axial
　　tomography) 88.38
　　with computer assisted surgery
　　　(CAS) 00.31
　　abdomen 88.01
　　bone 88.38
　　　mineral density 88.98
　　brain 87.03
　　cardiac 87.41
　　coronary 87.41
　　head 87.03
　　kidney 87.71
　　skeletal 88.38
　　　mineral density 88.98
　　thorax 87.41
　computerized axial tomography
　　(C.A.T.) - see also Scan, C.A.T.
　　88.38
　C.T. - see Scan, C.A.T.
　gallium - see Scan, radioisotope
　liver 92.02
　MUGA (multiple gated acquisition) -
　　see Scan, radioiostope
　positron emission tomography (PET) -
　　see Scan, radioisotope
　radioisotope
　　adrenal 92.09
　　bone 92.14
　　　marrow 92.05
　　bowel 92.04
　　cardiac output 92.05
　　cardiovascular 92.05
　　cerebral 92.11
　　circulation time 92.05
　　eye 95.16
　　gastrointestinal 92.04
　　head NEC 92.12
　　hematopoietic 92.05
　　intestine 92.04
　　iodine-131 92.01
　　kidney 92.03
　　liver 92.02
　　lung 92.15
　　lymphatic system 92.16
　　myocardial infarction 92.05
　　pancreatic 92.04
　　parathyroid 92.13
　　pituitary 92.11
　　placenta 92.17
　　protein-bound iodine 92.01
　　pulmonary 92.15
　　radio-iodine uptake 92.01
　　renal 92.03
　　specified site NEC 92.19
　　spleen 92.05
　　thyroid 92.01
　　total body 92.18
　　uterus 92.19
　renal 92.03
　thermal - see Thermography
Scapulectomy (partial) 77.81
　total 77.91
Scapulopexy 78.41
Scarification
　conjunctiva 10.33
　nasal veins (with packing) 21.03
　pericardium 36.39
　pleura 34.6
　　chemical 34.92
　　　with cancer chemotherapy
　　　　substance 34.92
　　　　[99.25]
　　　　tetracycline 34.92 [99.21]

Schanz operation (femoral osteotomy)
　77.35
Schauta (-Amreich) operation (radical
　vaginal hysterectomy) 68.79
　laparoscopic 68.71
Schede operation (thoracoplasty) 33.34
Scheie operation
　cautery of sclera 12.62
　sclerostomy 12.62
Schlatter operation (total gastrectomy)
　43.99
Schroeder operation (endocervical
　excision) 67.39
Schuchardt operation (nonobstetrical
　episiotomy) 71.09
Schwartze operation (simple
　mastoidectomy) 20.41
Scintiphotography - see Scan,
　radioisotope
Scintiscan - see Scan, radioisotope
Sclerectomy (punch) (scissors) 12.65
　for retinal reattachment 14.49
　Holth's 12.65
　trephine 12.61
　　with implant 14.41
Scleroplasty 12.89
Sclerosis - see Sclerotherapy
Sclerostomy (Scheie's) 12.62
Sclerotherapy
　esophageal varices (endoscopic) 42.33
　hemorrhoids 49.42
　pleura 34.92
　　treatment of malignancy (cytotoxic
　　　agent) 34.92 [99.25]
　　　with tetracycline 34.92 [99.21]
　varicose vein 39.92
　vein NEC 39.92
Sclerotomy (exploratory) 12.89
　anterior 12.89
　　with
　　　iridectomy 12.65
　　　removal of vitreous 14.71
　posterior 12.89
　　with
　　　iridectomy 12.65
　　　removal of vitreous 14.72
Scott operation
　intestinal bypass for obesity 45.93
　jejunocolostomy (bypass) 45.93
Scraping
　corneal epithelium 11.41
　　for smear or culture 11.21
　trachoma follicles 10.33
Scrotectomy (partial) 61.3
Scrotoplasty 61.49
Scrotorrhaphy 61.41
Scrototomy 61.0
Scrub, posterior nasal (adhesions)
　21.91
Sculpturing, heart valve - see
　Valvuloplasty, heart
Section - see also Division and Incision
　cesarean - see Cesarean section
　ganglion, sympathetic 05.0
　hypophyseal stalk - see also
　　Hypophysectomy, partial 07.63
　ligamentum flavum (spine) - *omit code*
　nerve (cranial) (peripheral) NEC
　　04.03
　　acoustic 04.01
　　spinal root (posterior) 03.1
　　sympathetic 05.0
　　trigeminal tract 04.02
　Saemisch (corneal) 11.1

◄ New　◄═ Revised　deleted Deleted　● Use Additional Digit(s)　▨ Omit code

Section *(Continued)*
    spinal ligament 80.49
        arcuate - *omit code*
        flavum - *omit code*
    tooth (impacted) 23.19
Seddon-Brooks operation (transfer of
    pectoralis major tendon) 83.75
Semb operation (apicolysis of lung)
    33.39
Senning operation (correction of
    transposition of great vessels) 35.91
Separation
    twins (attached) (conjoined) (Siamese)
        84.93
        asymmetrical (unequal) 84.93
        symmetrical (equal) 84.92
Septectomy
    atrial (closed) 35.41
        open 35.42
        transvenous method (balloon)
            35.41
    submucous (nasal) 21.5
Septoplasty NEC 21.88
    with submucous resection of septum
        21.5
Septorhinoplasty 21.84
Septostomy (atrial) (balloon) 35.41
Septotomy, nasal 21.1
Sequestrectomy
    bone 77.00
        carpals, metacarpals 77.04
        clavicle 77.01
        facial 76.01
        femur 77.05
        fibula 77.07
        humerus 77.02
        nose 21.32
        patella 77.06
        pelvic 77.09
        phalanges (foot) (hand) 77.09
        radius 77.03
        scapula 77.01
        skull 01.25
        specified site NEC 77.09
        tarsals, metatarsals 77.08
        thorax (ribs) (sternum) 77.01
        tibia 77.07
        ulna 77.03
        vertebrae 77.09
    nose 21.32
    skull 01.25
Sesamoidectomy 77.98
Setback, ear 18.5
Sever operation (division of soft tissue of
    arm) 83.19
Severing of blepharorrhaphy 08.02
Sewell operation (heart) 36.2
Sharrard operation (iliopsoas muscle
    transfer) 83.77
Shaving
    bone - *see also* Excision, lesion, bone
        77.60
    cornea (epithelium) 11.41
        for smear or culture 11.21
    patella 77.66
Shelf operation (hip arthroplasty) 81.40
Shirodkar operation (encirclement
    suture, cervix) 67.59
Shock therapy
    chemical 94.24
    electroconvulsive 94.27
    electrotonic 94.27
    insulin 94.24
    subconvulsive 94.26

Shortening
    bone (fusion) 78.20
        femur 78.25
        specified site NEC - *see* category
            78.2●
        tibia 78.27
        ulna 78.23
    endopelvic fascia 69.22
    extraocular muscle NEC 15.22
        multiple (two or more muscles) 15.4
    eyelid margin 08.71
    eye muscle NEC 15.22
        multiple (two or more muscles)
            (with lengthening) 15.4
    finger (macrodactyly repair) 82.83
    heel cord 83.85
    levator palpebrae muscle 08.33
    ligament - *see also* Arthroplasty
        round 69.22
        uterosacral 69.22
    muscle 83.85
        extraocular 15.22
            multiple (two or more muscles)
                15.4
        hand 82.55
    sclera (for repair of retinal detachment)
        14.59
        by scleral buckling - *see also*
            Buckling, scleral 14.49
    tendon 83.85
        hand 82.55
    ureter (with reimplantation) 56.41
Shunt - *see also* Anastomosis and Bypass,
    vascular
    abdominovenous 54.94
    aorta-coronary sinus 36.39
    aorta (descending)-pulmonary (artery)
        39.0
    aortocarotid 39.22
    aortoceliac 39.26
    aortofemoral 39.25
    aortoiliac 39.25
    aortoiliofemoral 39.25
    aortomesenteric 39.26
    aorto-myocardial (graft) 36.2
    aortorenal 39.24
    aortosubclavian 39.22
    apicoaortic 35.93
    arteriovenous NEC 39.29
        for renal dialysis (by)
            anastomosis 39.27
            external cannula 39.93
    ascending aorta to pulmonary artery
        (Waterston) 39.0
    axillary-femoral 39.29
    carotid-carotid 39.22
    carotid-subclavian 39.22
    caval-mesenteric 39.1
    corpora cavernosa-corpus spongiosum
        64.98
    corpora-saphenous 64.98
    descending aorta to pulmonary artery
        (Potts-Smith) 39.0
    endolymphatic (-subarachnoid) 20.71
    endolymph-perilymph 20.71
    extracranial-intracranial (EC-IC) 39.28
    femoroperoneal 39.29
    femoropopliteal 39.29
    iliofemoral 39.25
    ilioiliac 39.25
    intestinal
        large-to-large 45.94
        small-to-large 45.93
        small-to-small 45.91

Shunt *(Continued)*
    left subclavian to descending aorta
        (Blalock-Park) 39.0
    left-to-right (systemic-pulmonary
        artery) 39.0
    left ventricle (heart) (apex) and aorta
        35.93
    lienorenal 39.1
    lumbar-subarachnoid (with valve)
        NEC 03.79
    mesocaval 39.1
    peritoneal-jugular 54.94
    peritoneo-vascular 54.94
    peritoneovenous 54.94
    pleuroperitoneal 34.05
    pleurothecal (with valve) 03.79
    portacaval (double) 39.1
    portal-systemic 39.1
    portal vein to vena cava 39.1
    pulmonary-innominate 39.0
    pulmonary vein to atrium 35.82
    renoportal 39.1
    right atrium and pulmonary artery
        35.94
    right ventricle and pulmonary artery
        (distal) 35.92
        in repair of
            pulmonary artery atresia 35.92
            transposition of great vessels
                35.92
            truncus arteriosus 35.83
    salpingothecal (with valve) 03.79
    semicircular subarachnoid 20.71
    spinal (thecal) (with valve) NEC 03.79
        subarachnoid-peritoneal 03.71
        subarachnoid-ureteral 03.72
    splenorenal (venous) 39.1
        arterial 39.26
    subarachnoid-peritoneal (with valve)
        03.71
    subarachnoid-ureteral (with valve)
        03.72
    subclavian-pulmonary 39.0
    subdural-peritoneal (with valve) 02.34
    superior mesenteric-caval 39.1
    systemic-pulmonary artery 39.0
    transjugular intrahepatic portosystemic
        [TIPS] 39.1
    vena cava to pulmonary artery (Green)
        39.21
    ventricular (cerebral) (with valve)
        02.2
        to
            abdominal cavity or organ 02.34
            bone marrow 02.39
            cervical subarachnoid space
                02.2
            circulatory system 02.32
            cisterna magna 02.2
            extracranial site NEC 02.39
            gallbladder 02.34
            head or neck structure 02.31
            intracerebral site NEC 02.2
            lumbar site 02.39
            mastoid 02.31
            nasopharynx 02.31
            peritoneal 02.34
            thoracic cavity 02.33
            ureter 02.35
            urinary system 02.35
            venous system 02.32
    ventriculoatrial (with valve) 02.32
    ventriculocaval (with valve) 02.32
    ventriculocisternal (with valve) 02.2

◄

S

Shunt (*Continued*)
  ventriculolumbar (with valve) 02.39
  ventriculomastoid (with valve) 02.31
  ventriculonasopharyngeal 02.31
  ventriculopleural (with valve) 02.33
Sialoadenectomy (parotid) (sublingual) (submaxillary) 26.30
  complete 26.32
  partial 26.31
  radical 26.32
Sialoadenolithotomy 26.0
Sialoadenotomy 26.0
Sialodochoplasty NEC 26.49
Sialogram 87.09
Sialolithotomy 26.0
Sieve, vena cava 38.7
Sigmoid bladder 57.87 [45.52]
Sigmoidectomy
  laparoscopic 17.36
  open and other 45.76
Sigmoidomyotomy 46.91
Sigmoidopexy (Moschowitz) 46.63
Sigmoidoproctectomy - *see also* Resection, rectum 48.69
Sigmoidoproctostomy 45.94
Sigmoidorectostomy 45.94
Sigmoidorrhaphy 46.75
Sigmoidoscopy (rigid) 48.23
  with biopsy 45.25
  flexible 45.24
  through stoma (artificial) 45.22
  transabdominal 45.21
Sigmoidosigmoidostomy 45.94
  proximal to distal segment
    laparoscopic 17.36
    open and other 45.76
Sigmoidostomy - *see also* Colostomy 46.10
Sigmoidotomy 45.03
Sign language 93.75
Silver operation (bunionectomy) 77.59
Sinogram
  abdominal wall 88.03
  chest wall 87.38
  retroperitoneum 88.14
Sinusectomy (nasal) (complete) (partial) (with turbinectomy) 22.60
  antrum 22.62
    with Caldwell-Luc approach 22.61
  ethmoid 22.63
  frontal 22.42
  maxillary 22.62
    with Caldwell-Luc approach 22.61
  sphenoid 22.64
Sinusotomy (nasal) 22.50
  antrum (intranasal) 22.2
    with external approach (Caldwell-Luc) 22.39
      radical (with removal of membrane lining) 22.31
  ethmoid 22.51
  frontal 22.41
  maxillary (intranasal) 22.2
    external approach (Caldwell-Luc) 22.39
      radical (with removal of membrane lining) 22.31
  multiple 22.53
  perinasal 22.50
  sphenoid 22.52
Sistrunk operation (excision of thyroglossal cyst) 06.7

Size reduction
  abdominal wall (adipose) (pendulous) 86.83
  arms (adipose) (batwing) 86.83
  breast (bilateral) 85.32
    unilateral 85.31
  buttocks (adipose) 86.83
  skin 86.83
  subcutaneous tissue 86.83
  thighs (adipose) 86.83
Skeletal series (x-ray) 88.31
SKyphoplasty 81.66
Sling - *see also* Operation, sling
  fascial (fascia lata)
    for facial weakness (trigeminal nerve paralysis) 86.81
    mouth 86.81
    orbicularis (mouth) 86.81
    tongue 25.59
  levator muscle (urethrocystopexy) 59.71
  pubococcygeal 59.71
  rectum (puborectalis) 48.76
  tongue (fascial) 25.59
Slitting
  canaliculus for
    passage of tube 09.42
    removal of streptothrix 09.42
  lens 13.2
  prepuce (dorsal) (lateral) 64.91
Slocum operation (pes anserinus transfer) 81.47
Sluder operation (tonsillectomy) 28.2
Small bowel series (x-ray) 87.63
Smith operation (open osteotomy of mandible) 76.62
Smith-Peterson operation (radiocarpal arthrodesis) 81.25
Smithwick operation (sympathectomy) 05.29
Snaring, polyp, colon (endoscopic) 45.42
Snip, punctum (with dilation) 09.51
Soave operation (endorectal pull-through) 48.41
Somatotherapy, psychiatric NEC 94.29
Sonneberg operation (inferior maxillary neurectomy) 04.07
Sorondo-Ferré operation (hindquarter amputation) 84.19
Soutter operation (iliac crest fasciotomy) 83.14
Spaulding-Richardson operation (uterine suspension) 69.22
Spectrophotometry NEC 89.39
  blood 89.39
  placenta 89.29
  urine 89.29
Spectroscopy
  intravascular 38.23
  near infrared (NIR) 38.23
Speech therapy NEC 93.75
Spermatocelectomy 63.2
Spermatocystectomy 60.73
Spermatocystotomy 60.72
Sphenoidectomy 22.64
Sphenoidotomy 22.52
Sphincterectomy, anal 49.6
Sphincteroplasty
  anal 49.79
    obstetrical laceration (current) 75.62
    old 49.79
  bladder neck 57.85
  pancreas 51.83
  sphincter of Oddi 51.83

Sphincterorrhaphy, anal 49.71
  obstetrical laceration (current) 75.62
  old 49.79
Sphincterotomy
  anal (external) (internal) 49.59
    left lateral 49.51
    posterior 49.52
  bladder (neck) (transurethral) 57.91
  choledochal 51.82
    endoscopic 51.85
  iris 12.12
  pancreatic 51.82
    endoscopic 51.85
  sphincter of Oddi 51.82
    endoscopic 51.85
  transduodenal ampullary 51.82
    endoscopic 51.85
Spinal anesthesia - *omit code*
Spinelli operation (correction of inverted uterus) 75.93
Spineoplasty 81.66
Spirometry (incentive) (respiratory) 89.37
Spivack operation (permanent gastrostomy) 43.19
Splanchnicectomy 05.29
Splanchnicotomy 05.0
Splenectomy (complete) (total) 41.5
  partial 41.43
Splenogram 88.64
  radioisotope 92.05
Splenolysis 54.59
  laparoscopic 54.51
Splenopexy 41.95
Splenoplasty 41.95
Splenoportogram (by splenic arteriography) 88.64
Splenorrhaphy 41.95
Splenotomy 41.2
Splinting
  dental (for immobilization) 93.55
    orthodontic 24.7
  musculoskeletal 93.54
  ureteral 56.2
Splitting - *see also* Division
  canaliculus 09.52
  lacrimal papilla 09.51
  spinal cord tracts 03.29
    percutaneous 03.21
  tendon sheath 83.01
    hand 82.01
Spondylosyndesis - *see also* Fusion, spinal 81.00
S.P. Rogers operation (knee disarticulation) 84.16
Ssabanejew-Frank operation (permanent gastrostomy) 43.19
Stab, intercostal 34.09
Stabilization, joint - *see also* Arthrodesis
  patella (for recurrent dislocation) 81.44
Stacke operation (simple mastoidectomy) 20.41
Stallard operation (conjunctivocystorhinostomy) 09.82
  with insertion of tube or stent 09.83
Stamm (-Kader) operation (temporary gastrostomy) 43.19
Stapedectomy 19.19
  with incus replacement (homograft) (prosthesis) 19.11
  revision 19.29
    with incus replacement 19.21

◀ New   ◀▥ Revised   ~~deleted~~ Deleted   ● Use Additional Digit(s)   ▩ Omit code

Stapediolysis 19.0
Stapling
    artery 39.31
    blebs, lung (emphysematous) 32.21
    diaphysis - *see also* Stapling, epiphyseal
        plate 78.20
    epiphyseal plate 78.20
        femur 78.25
        fibula 78.27
        humerus 78.22
        radius 78.23
        specified site NEC 78.29
        tibia 78.27
        ulna 78.23
    gastric varices 44.91
    graft - *see* Graft
    left atrial appendage 37.36
    vein 39.32
STARR (stapled transanal rectal resection)
    48.74
StaXx® FX Structural Kyphoplasty
    System 81.66
Steinberg operation 44.5
Steindler operation
    fascia stripping (for cavus deformity)
        83.14
    flexorplasty (elbow) 83.77
    muscle transfer 83.77
Stereotactic radiosurgery 92.30
    cobalt 60 92.32
    linear accelerator (LINAC) 92.31
    multi-source 92.32
    particle beam 92.33
    particulate 92.33
    radiosurgery NEC 92.39
    single source photon 92.31
Stereotactic head frame application
    93.59
Sterilization
    female - *see also* specific operation
        66.39
    male NEC - *see also* Ligation, vas
        deferens 63.70
Sternotomy 77.31
    as operative approach - *omit code*
    for bone marrow biopsy 41.31
Stewart operation (renal plication with
    pyeloplasty) 55.87
Stimulation (electronic) - *see also* Implant,
    electronic stimulator
    bone growth (percutaneous) - *see*
        category 78.9●
        transcutaneous (surface) 99.86
    cardiac (external) 99.62
        internal 37.91
    carotid sinus 99.64
    CaverMap™ 89.58
    defibrillator
        as part of intraoperative testing
            - *omit code*
        catheter based invasive
            electrophysiologic testing
            37.26
        device interrogation only without
            arrhythmia induction (bedside
            check) 89.45–89.49
        non-invasive programmed electrical
            stimulation (NIPS) 37.20
    electrophysiologic, cardiac
        as part of intraoperative testing
            - *omit code*
        catheter based invasive
            electrophysiologic testing
            37.26

Stimulation *(Continued)*
    electrophysiologic, cardiac *(Continued)*
        device interrogation only without
            arrhythmia induction (bedside
            check) 89.45–89.49
        noninvasive programmed electrical
            stimulation (NIPS) 37.20
    nerve
        CaverMap™ 89.58
        penile 89.58
        peripheral or spinal cord,
            transcutaneous 93.39
Stitch, Kelly-Stoeckel (urethra) 59.3
Stomatoplasty 27.59
Stomatorrhaphy 27.52
Stone operation (anoplasty) 49.79
Strapping (non-traction) 93.59
Strassman operation (metroplasty)
    69.49
Strayer operation (gastrocnemius
    recession) 83.72
Stretching
    eyelid (with elongation) 08.71
    fascia 93.28
    foreskin 99.95
    iris 12.63
    muscle 93.27
    nerve (cranial) (peripheral) 04.91
    tendon 93.27
Stripping
    bone - *see also* Incision, bone 77.10
    carotid sinus 39.8
    cranial suture 02.01
    fascia 83.14
        hand 82.12
    membranes for surgical induction of
        labor 73.1
    meninges (cerebral) 01.51
        spinal 03.4
    saphenous vein, varicose 38.59
    subdural membrane (cerebral)
        01.51
        spinal 03.4
    varicose veins (lower limb) 38.59
        upper limb 38.53
    vocal cords 30.09
Stromeyer-Little operation (hepatotomy)
    50.0
Strong operation (unbridling of celiac
    artery axis) 39.91
Stryker frame 93.59
Study
    bone mineral density 88.98
    bundle of His 37.29
    color vision 95.06
    conduction, nerve (median) 89.15
    dark adaptation, eye 95.07
    electrophysiologic stimulation and
        recording, cardiac
        as part of intraoperative testing
            - *omit code*
        catheter based invasive
            electrophysiologic testing
            37.26
        device interrogation only without
            arrhythmia induction (bedside
            check) 89.45–89.49
        noninvasive programmed electrical
            stimulation (NIPS) 37.20
    function - *see also* Function, study
    radioisotope - *see* Scan,
        radioisotope
    lacrimal flow (radiographic) 87.05
    ocular motility 95.15

Study *(Continued)*
    pulmonary
        airway flow measurement,
            endoscopic 33.72
        function - *see* categories 89.37-89.38
    radiographic - *see* Radiography
    radio-iodinated triolein 92.04
    renal clearance 92.03
    spirometer 89.37
    tracer - *see also* Scan, radioisotope eye
        (P32) 95.16
    ultrasonic - *see* Ultrasonography
    visual field 95.05
    xenon flow NEC 92.19
        cardiovascular 92.05
        pulmonary 92.15
Sturmdorf operation (conization of
    cervix) 67.2
Submucous resection
    larynx 30.29
    nasal septum 21.5
Summerskill operation
    (dacryocystorhinostomy by
    intubation) 09.81
Surgery
    computer assisted (CAS) 00.39
        with robotics – *see* category 17.4●
        CAS with CT/CTA 00.31
        CAS with fluoroscopy 00.33
        CAS with MR/MRA 00.32
        CAS with multiple datasets 00.35
            imageless 00.34
            other CAS 00.39
        IGS - *see* Surgery, computer assisted
        image guided - *see* Surgery,
            computer assisted
        navigation (CT-free, IGN image
            guided, imageless) - *see*
            Surgery, computer assisted
    robotic assisted – *see* category 17.4●
Surmay operation (jejunostomy) 46.39
Suspension
    balanced, for traction 93.45
    bladder NEC 57.89
    diverticulum, pharynx 29.59
    kidney 55.7
    Olshausen (uterus) 69.22
    ovary 65.79
    paraurethral (Pereyra) 59.6
    periurethral 59.6
    urethra (retropubic) (sling) 59.5
    urethrovesical
        Goebel-Frangenheim-Stoeckel 59.4
        gracilis muscle transplant 59.71
        levator muscle sling 59.71
        Marshall-Marchetti (-Krantz) 59.5
        Millin-Read 59.4
        suprapubic 59.4
    uterus (abdominal or vaginal
        approach) 69.22
    vagina 70.77
        with graft or prosthesis 70.78
Suture (laceration)
    abdominal wall 54.63
        secondary 54.61
    adenoid fossa 28.7
    adrenal (gland) 07.44
    aneurysm (cerebral) (peripheral) 39.52
    anus 49.71
        obstetric laceration (current) 75.62
        old 49.79
    aorta 39.31
    aponeurosis - *see also* Suture, tendon
        83.64

Suture (Continued)
  arteriovenous fistula 39.53
  artery 39.31
    percutaneous puncture
      closure - omit code
  bile duct 51.79
  bladder 57.81
    obstetric laceration (current) 75.61
  blood vessel NEC 39.30
    artery 39.31
      percutaneous puncture
        closure - omit code
    vein 39.32
  breast (skin) 85.81
  bronchus 33.41
  bursa 83.99
    hand 82.99
  canaliculus 09.73
  cecum 46.75
  cerebral meninges 02.11
  cervix (traumatic laceration) 67.61
    internal os, encirclement 67.59
    obstetric laceration (current) 75.51
      old 67.69
  chest wall 34.71
  cleft palate 27.62
  clitoris 71.4
  colon 46.75
  common duct 51.71
  conjunctiva 10.6
  cornea 11.51
    with conjunctival flap 11.53
  corneoscleral 11.51
    with conjunctival flap 11.53
  diaphragm 34.82
  duodenum 46.71
    ulcer (bleeding) (perforated) 44.42
      endoscopic 44.43
  dura mater (cerebral) 02.11
    spinal 03.59
  ear, external 18.4
  enterocele 70.92
    with graft or prosthesis 70.93
  entropion 08.42
  epididymis (and)
    spermatic cord 63.51
    vas deferens 63.81
  episiotomy - see Episiotomy
  esophagus 42.82
  eyeball 16.89
  eyebrow 08.81
  eyelid 08.81
    with entropion or ectropion repair
      08.42
  fallopian tube 66.71
  fascia 83.65
    hand 82.46
    to skeletal attachment 83.89
      hand 82.89
  gallbladder 51.91
  ganglion, sympathetic 05.81
  gingiva 24.32
  great vessel 39.30
    artery 39.31
    vein 39.32
  gum 24.32
  heart 37.49
  hepatic duct 51.79
  hymen 70.76
  ileum 46.73
  intestine 46.79
    large 46.75
    small 46.73
  jejunum 46.73

Suture (Continued)
  joint capsule 81.96
    with arthroplasty - see Arthroplasty
    ankle 81.94
    foot 81.94
    lower extremity NEC 81.95
    upper extremity 81.93
  kidney 55.81
  labia 71.71
  laceration - see Suture, by site
  larynx 31.61
  ligament 81.96
    with arthroplasty - see Arthroplasty
    ankle 81.94
    broad 69.29
    Cooper's 54.64
    foot and toes 81.94
    gastrocolic 54.73
    knee 81.95
    lower extremity NEC 81.95
    sacrouterine 69.29
    upper extremity 81.93
    uterine 69.29
  ligation - see Ligation
  lip 27.51
  liver 50.61
  lung 33.43
  meninges (cerebral) 02.11
    spinal 03.59
  mesentery 54.75
  mouth 27.52
  muscle 83.65
    hand 82.46
    ocular (oblique) (rectus) 15.7
  nerve (cranial) (peripheral) 04.3
    sympathetic 05.81
  nose (external) (internal) 21.81
    for epistaxis 21.09
  obstetric laceration NEC 75.69
    bladder 75.61
    cervix 75.51
    corpus uteri 75.52
    pelvic floor 75.69
    perineum 75.69
    periurethral 75.69
    rectum 75.62
    sphincter ani 75.62
    urethra 75.61
    uterus 75.50
    vagina 75.69
    vulva 75.69
  omentum 54.64
  ovary 65.71
    laparoscopic 65.74
  palate 27.61
    cleft 27.62
  palpebral fissure 08.59
  pancreas 52.95
  pelvic floor 71.71
    obstetric laceration (current) 75.69
  penis 64.41
  peptic ulcer (bleeding) (perforated)
    44.40
  pericardium 37.49
  perineum (female) 71.71
    after delivery 75.69
      episiotomy repair - see
        Episiotomy
    male 86.59
  periosteum 78.20
    carpal, metacarpal 78.24
    femur 78.25
    fibula 78.27
    humerus 78.22

◄

Suture (Continued)
  periosteum (Continued)
    pelvic 78.29
    phalanges (foot) (hand) 78.29
    radius 78.23
    specified site NEC 78.29
    tarsal, metatarsal 78.28
    tibia 78.27
    ulna 78.23
    vertebrae 78.29
  peritoneum 54.64
  periurethral tissue to symphysis pubis
    59.5
  pharynx 29.51
  pleura 34.93
  rectum 48.71
    obstetric laceration (current) 75.62
  retina (for reattachment) 14.59
  sacrouterine ligament 69.29
  salivary gland 26.41
  scalp 86.59
    replantation 86.51
  sclera (with repair of conjunctiva)
    12.81
  scrotum (skin) 61.41
  secondary
    abdominal wall 54.61
    episiotomy 75.69
    peritoneum 54.64
  sigmoid 46.75
  skin (mucous membrane) (without
      graft) 86.59
    with graft - see Graft, skin
    breast 85.81
    ear 18.4
    eyebrow 08.81
    eyelid 08.81
    nose 21.81
    penis 64.41
    scalp 86.59
      replantation 86.51
    scrotum 61.41
    vulva 71.71
  specified site NEC - see Repair, by site
  spermatic cord 63.51
  sphincter ani 49.71
    obstetric laceration (current) 75.62
    old 49.79
  spinal meninges 03.59
  spleen 41.95
  stomach 44.61
    ulcer (bleeding) (perforated)
      44.41
      endoscopic 44.43
  subcutaneous tissue (without skin
      graft) 86.59
    with graft - see Graft, skin
  tendon (direct) (immediate) (primary)
      83.64
    delayed (secondary) 83.62
      hand NEC 82.43
        flexors 82.42
    hand NEC 82.45
      delayed (secondary) 82.43
      flexors 82.44
        delayed (secondary) 82.42
    ocular 15.7
    rotator cuff 83.63
    sheath 83.61
      hand 82.41
    supraspinatus (rotator cuff repair)
      83.63
    to skeletal attachment 83.88
      hand 82.85

Suture (*Continued*)
  Tenon's capsule 15.7
  testis 62.61
  thymus 07.93
  thyroid gland 06.93
  tongue 25.51
  tonsillar fossa 28.7
  trachea 31.71
  tunica vaginalis 61.41
  ulcer (bleeding) (perforated) (peptic)
      44.40
    duodenum 44.42
      endoscopic 44.43
    gastric 44.41
      endoscopic 44.43
    intestine 46.79
    skin 86.59
    stomach 44.41
      endoscopic 44.43
  ureter 56.82
  urethra 58.41
    obstetric laceration (current) 75.61
  uterosacral ligament 69.29
  uterus 69.41
    obstetric laceration (current) 75.50
    old 69.49
  uvula 27.73
  vagina 70.71
    obstetric laceration (current) 75.69
    old 70.79
  vas deferens 63.81
  vein 39.32

Suture (*Continued*)
  vulva 71.71
    obstetric laceration (current) 75.69
    old 71.79
Suture-ligation - *see also* Ligation
  blood vessel - *see* Ligation, blood vessel
Sweep, anterior iris 12.97
Swenson operation
  bladder reconstruction 57.87
  proctectomy 48.49
Swinney operation (urethral
    reconstruction) 58.46
Switch, switching
  coronary arteries 35.84
  great arteries, total 35.84
Syme operation
  ankle amputation through malleoli of
      tibia and fibula 84.14
  urethrotomy, external 58.0
Sympathectomy NEC 05.29
  cervical 05.22
  cervicothoracic 05.22
  lumbar 05.23
  periarterial 05.25
  presacral 05.24
  renal 05.29
  thoracolumbar 05.23
  tympanum 20.91
Sympatheticotripsy 05.0
Symphysiotomy 77.39
  assisting delivery (obstetrical) 73.94
  kidney (horseshoe) 55.85

Symphysis, pleural 34.6
Synchondrotomy - *see also* Division,
    cartilage 80.40
Syndactylization 86.89
Syndesmotomy - *see also* Division,
    ligament 80.40
Synechiotomy
  endometrium 68.21
  iris (posterior) 12.33
    anterior 12.32
Synovectomy (joint) (complete) (partial)
    80.70
  ankle 80.77
  elbow 80.72
  foot and toe 80.78
  hand and finger 80.74
  hip 80.75
  knee 80.76
  shoulder 80.71
  specified site NEC 80.79
  spine 80.79
  tendon sheath 83.42
    hand 82.33
  wrist 80.73
Syringing
  lacrimal duct or sac 09.43
  nasolacrimal duct 09.43
    with
      dilation 09.43
      insertion of tube or stent 09.44

◄ New　◄||| Revised　~~deleted~~ Deleted　● Use Additional Digit(s)　▓ Omit code

T

Taarnhoj operation (trigeminal nerve root decompression) 04.41
Tack operation (sacculotomy) 20.79
Tactile Guidance System™ [TGS] – *see* category 17.4●
Take-down
  anastomosis
    arterial 39.49
    blood vessel 39.49
    gastric, gastrointestinal 44.5
    intestine 46.93
    stomach 44.5
    vascular 39.49
    ventricular 02.43
  arterial bypass 39.49
  arteriovenous shunt 39.43
    with creation of new shunt 39.42
  cecostomy 46.52
  colostomy 46.52
  duodenostomy 46.51
  enterostomy 46.50
  esophagostomy 42.83
  gastroduodenostomy 44.5
  gastrojejunostomy 44.5
  ileostomy 46.51
  intestinal stoma 46.50
    large 46.52
    small 46.51
  jejunoileal bypass 46.93
  jejunostomy 46.51
  laryngostomy 31.62
  sigmoidostomy 46.52
  stoma
    bile duct 51.79
    bladder 57.82
    bronchus 33.42
    common duct 51.72
    esophagus 42.83
    gallbladder 51.92
    hepatic duct 51.79
    intestine 46.50
      large 46.52
      small 46.51
    kidney 55.82
    larynx 31.62
    rectum 48.72
    stomach 44.62
    thorax 34.72
    trachea 31.72
    ureter 56.83
    urethra 58.42
  systemic-pulmonary artery anastomosis 39.49
    in total repair of tetralogy of Fallot 35.81
  tracheostomy 31.72
  vascular anastomosis or bypass 39.49
  ventricular shunt (cerebral) 02.43
Talectomy 77.98
Talma-Morison operation (omentopexy) 54.74
Tamponade
  esophageal 96.06
  intrauterine (nonobstetric) 69.91
    after delivery or abortion 75.8
    antepartum 73.1
  vagina 96.14
    after delivery or abortion 75.8
    antepartum 73.1
Tanner operation (devascularization of stomach) 44.99

Tap
  abdomen 54.91
  chest 34.91
  cisternal 01.01
  cranial 01.09
  joint 81.91
  lumbar (diagnostic) (removal of dye) 03.31
  perilymphatic 20.79
  spinal (diagnostic) 03.31
  subdural (through fontanel) 01.09
  thorax 34.91
Tarsectomy 08.20
  de Grandmont 08.35
Tarsoplasty - *see also* Reconstruction, eyelid 08.70
Tarsorrhaphy (lateral) 08.52
  division or severing 08.02
Tattooing
  cornea 11.91
  skin 86.02
Tautening, eyelid for entropion 08.42
Telemetry (cardiac) 89.54
Teleradiotherapy
  beta particles 92.25
    intra-operative 92.41
  Betatron 92.24
  cobalt-60 92.23
  electrons 92.25
    intra-operative 92.41
  iodine-125 92.23
  linear accelerator 92.24
  neutrons 92.26
  particulate radiation NEC 92.26
  photons 92.24
  protons 92.26
  radioactive cesium 92.23
  radioisotopes NEC 92.23
Temperament assessment 94.02
Temperature gradient study - *see also* Thermography 88.89
Tendinoplasty - *see* Repair, tendon
Tendinosuture (immediate) (primary) - *see also* Suture, tendon 83.64
  hand - *see also* Suture, tendon, hand 82.45
Tendolysis 83.91
  hand 82.91
Tendoplasty - *see* Repair, tendon
Tenectomy 83.39
  eye 15.13
    levator palpebrae 08.33
    multiple (two or more tendons) 15.3
  hand 82.29
  levator palpebrae 08.33
  tendon sheath 83.31
    hand 82.21
Tenodesis (tendon fixation to skeletal attachment) 83.88
  Fowler 82.85
  hand 82.85
Tenolysis 83.91
  hand 82.91
Tenomyoplasty - *see also* Repair, tendon 83.88
  hand - *see also* Repair, tendon, hand 82.86
Tenomyotomy - *see* Tenonectomy
Tenonectomy 83.42
  for graft 83.41
    hand 82.32
  hand 82.33
    for graft 82.32

Tenontomyoplasty - *see* Repair, tendon
Tenontoplasty - *see* Repair, tendon
Tenoplasty - *see also* Repair, tendon 83.88
  hand - *see also* Repair, tendon, hand 82.86
Tenorrhaphy - *see also* Suture, tendon 83.64
  hand - *see also* Suture, tendon, hand 82.45
  to skeletal attachment 83.88
    hand 82.85
Tenosuspension 83.88
  hand 82.86
Tenosuture - *see also* Suture, tendon 83.64
  hand - *see also* Suture, tendon, hand 82.45
  to skeletal attachment 83.88
    hand 82.85
Tenosynovectomy 83.42
  hand 82.33
Tenotomy 83.13
  Achilles tendon 83.11
  adductor (hip) (subcutaneous) 83.12
  eye 15.12
    levator palpebrae 08.38
    multiple (two or more tendons) 15.4
  hand 82.11
  levator palpebrae 08.38
  pectoralis minor tendon (decompression thoracic outlet) 83.13
  stapedius 19.0
  tensor tympani 19.0
Tenovaginotomy - *see* Tenotomy
Tensing, orbicularis oculi 08.59
Termination of pregnancy
  by
    aspiration curettage 69.51
    dilation and curettage 69.01
    hysterectomy - *see* Hysterectomy
    hysterotomy 74.91
    intra-amniotic injection (saline) 75.0
Test, testing (for)
  14 C-Urea breath 89.39
  auditory function NEC 95.46
  Bender Visual-Motor Gestalt 94.02
  Benton Visual Retention 94.02
  cardiac (vascular)
    function NEC 89.59
    stress 89.44
      bicycle ergometer 89.43
      Masters' two-step 89.42
      treadmill 89.41
  Denver developmental (screening) 94.02
  fetus, fetal
    nonstress (fetal activity acceleration determinations) 75.34
    oxytocin challenge (contraction stress) 75.35
    sensitivity (to oxytocin) - omit code
  function
    cardiac NEC 89.59
    hearing NEC 95.46
    muscle (by)
      electromyography 93.08
      manual 93.04
    neurologic NEC 89.15
    vestibular 95.46
      clinical 95.44

◀ New   ◀▥ Revised   ~~deleted~~ Deleted   ● Use Additional Digit(s)   ▨ Omit code

Test, testing *(Continued)*
    glaucoma NEC 95.26
    hearing 95.47
      clinical NEC 95.42
    intelligence 94.01
    internal jugular-subclavian venous
      reflux 89.62
    intracarotid amobarbital (Wada) 89.10
    Masters' two-step stress (cardiac) 89.42
    muscle function (by)
      electromyography 93.08
      manual 93.04
    neurologic function NEC 89.15
    neurophysiologic monitoring
      intra-operative 00.94
    nocturnal penile tumescence 89.29
    provocative, for glaucoma 95.26
    psychologic NEC 94.08
    psychometric 94.01
    radio-cobalt B12 Schilling 92.04
    range of motion 93.05
    rotation (Bárány chair) (hearing) 95.45
    sleep disorder function - *see* categories
      89.17–89.18
    Stanford-Binet 94.01
    Thallium stress (transesophageal
      pacing) 89.44
    tuning fork (hearing) 95.42
    Urea breath, (14 C) 89.39
    vestibular function NEC 95.46
      thermal 95.44
    Wada (hemispheric function) 89.10
    whispered speech (hearing) 95.42
TEVAP (transurethral electrovaporization
    of prostate) 60.29
Thalamectomy 01.41
Thalamotomy 01.41
    by stereotactic radiosurgery 92.32
      cobalt 60 92.32
      linear accelerator (LINAC) 92.31
      multi-source 92.32
      particle beam 92.33
      particulate 92.33
      radiosurgery NEC 92.39
      single source photon 92.31
Thal operation (repair of esophageal
    stricture) 42.85
Theleplasty 85.87
Therapy
    Antabuse 94.25
    aqueous oxygen (AO) 00.49
    art 93.89
    aversion 94.33
    behavior 94.33
    Bennett respirator - *see* category 96.7●
    blind rehabilitation NEC 93.78
    Byrd respirator - *see* category 96.7●
    carbon dioxide 94.25
    cobalt-60 92.23
    conditioning, psychiatric 94.33
    continuous positive airway pressure
      (CPAP) 93.90
      delivered by
        endotracheal tube - *see* category
          96.7●
        tracheostomy – *see* category
          96.7●
    croupette, croup tent 93.94
    daily living activities 93.83
      for the blind 93.78
    dance 93.89
    desensitization 94.33
    detoxification 94.25
    diversional 93.81

Therapy *(Continued)*
    domestic tasks 93.83
      for the blind 93.78
    Downstream® system 00.49
    educational (bed-bound children)
      (handicapped) 93.82
    electroconvulsive (ECT) 94.27
    electroshock (EST) 94.27
      subconvulsive 94.26
    electrotonic (ETT) 94.27
    encounter group 94.44
    extinction 94.33
    family 94.42
    fog (inhalation) 93.94
    gamma ray 92.23
    group NEC 94.44
      for psychosexual dysfunctions 94.41
    hearing NEC 95.49
    heat NEC 93.35
      for cancer treatment 99.85
    helium 93.98
    hot pack(s) 93.35
    hyperbaric oxygen 93.95
      wound 93.59
    hyperthermia NEC 93.35
      for cancer treatment 99.85
    individual, psychiatric NEC 94.39
      for psychosexual dysfunction
        94.34
    industrial 93.89
    infrared irradiation 93.35
    inhalation NEC 93.96
      nitric oxide 00.12
    insulin shock 94.24
    intermittent positive pressure
      breathing (IPPB) 93.91
    IPPB (intermittent positive pressure
      breathing) 93.91
    leech 99.99
    lithium 94.22
    LITT (laser interstitial thermal therapy)
      under guidance ◀
      lesion ◀
        brain 17.61 ◀
        breast 17.69 ◀
        head and neck 17.62 ◀
        liver 17.63 ◀
        lung 17.69 ◀
        prostate 17.69 ◀
        thyroid 17.62 ◀
    maggot 86.28
    manipulative, osteopathic - *see also*
      Manipulation, osteopathic
      93.67
    manual arts 93.81
    methadone 94.25
    mist (inhalation) 93.94
    music 93.84
    nebulizer 93.94
    neuroleptic 94.23
    nitric oxide 00.12
    occupational 93.83
    oxygen 93.96
      aqueous 00.49
      catalytic 93.96
      hyperbaric 93.95
        wound 93.59
      SuperSaturated 00.49
      wound (hyperbaric) 93.59
    paraffin bath 93.35
    physical NEC 93.39
      combined (without mention of
        components) 93.38
      diagnostic NEC 93.09

Therapy *(Continued)*
    play 93.81
      psychotherapeutic 94.36
    positive and expiratory pressure - *see*
      category 96.7●
    psychiatric NEC 94.39
      drug NEC 94.25
        lithium 94.22
    radiation 92.29
      contact (150 KVP or less) 92.21
      deep (200-300 KVP) 92.22
      electron, intra-operative 92.41
      high voltage (200-300 KVP) 92.22
      low voltage (150 KVP or less) 92.21
      megavoltage 92.24
      orthovoltage 92.22
      particle source NEC 92.26
      photon 92.24
      radioisotope (teleradiotherapy)
        92.23
      retinal lesion 14.26
      superficial (150 KVP or less) 92.21
      supervoltage 92.24
    radioisotope, radioisotopic NEC 92.29
      implantation or insertion 92.27
      injection or instillation 92.28
      teleradiotherapy 92.23
    radium (radon) 92.23
    recreational 93.81
    rehabilitation NEC 93.89
    respiratory NEC 93.99
      bi-level positive airway pressure
        [BiPAP] 93.90
        delivered by
          endotracheal tube - *see*
            category 96.7●
          tracheostomy – *see* category
            96.7●
      continuous positive airway pressure
        [CPAP] 93.90
        delivered by
          endotracheal tube - *see*
            category 96.7●
          tracheostomy – *see* category
            96.7●
      endotracheal respiratory assistance -
        see category 96.7●
      intermittent positive pressure
        breathing [IPPB] 93.91
      negative pressure (continuous)
        [CNP] 93.99
      nitric oxide 00.12
      non-invasive positive pressure
        (NIPPV) 93.90
      other continuous invasive
        (unspecified duration)
        96.70
        for less than 96 consecutive hours
          96.71
        for 96 consecutive hours or more
          96.72
      positive end expiratory pressure
        [PEEP]
        invasive - *see* category 96.7●
        non-invasive 93.90
    root canal 23.70
      with
        apicoectomy 23.72
        irrigation 23.71
    shock
      chemical 94.24
      electric 94.27
        subconvulsive 94.26
      insulin 94.24

Therapy (Continued)
   speech 93.75
      for correction of defect 93.74
   SuperOxygenation (SSO$_2$) 00.49
   SuperSaturated oxygen 00.49
   ultrasound
      heat therapy 93.35
      hyperthermia for cancer treatment
         99.85
      physical therapy 93.35
      therapeutic - see Ultrasound
   ultraviolet light 99.82
Thermocautery - see Cauterization
Thermography 88.89
   blood vessel 88.86
   bone 88.83
   breast 88.85
   cerebral 88.81
   eye 88.82
   lymph gland 88.89
   muscle 88.84
   ocular 88.82
   osteoarticular 88.83
   specified site NEC 88.89
   vein, deep 88.86
Thermokeratoplasty 11.74
Thermosclerectomy 12.62
Thermotherapy (hot packs) (paraffin
      bath) NEC 93.35
   prostate
      by
         microwave 60.96
         radiofrequency 60.97
      transurethral microwave
         thermotherapy (TUMT) 60.96
      transurethral needle ablation
         (TUNA) 60.97
      TUMT (transurethral microwave
         thermotherapy) 60.96
      TUNA (transurethral needle
         ablation) 60.97
Thiersch operation
   anus 49.79
   skin graft 86.69
      hand 86.62
Thompson operation
   cleft lip repair 27.54
   correction of lymphedema 40.9
   quadricepsplasty 83.86
   thumb apposition with bone graft 82.69
Thoracectomy 34.09
   for lung collapse 33.34
Thoracentesis 34.91
Thoracocentesis 34.91
Thoracolysis (for collapse of lung) 33.39
Thoracoplasty (anterior) (extrapleural)
      (paravertebral) (posterolateral)
      (complete) partial) 33.34
Thoracoscopy, transpleural (for
      exploration) 34.21
Thoracostomy 34.09
   for lung collapse 33.32
Thoracotomy (with drainage) 34.09
   as operative approach - omit code
   exploratory 34.02
Thoratec® implantable ventricular assist
      device (IVAD™) 37.66
Thoratec® ventricular assist device
      (VAD) system 37.66
Three-snip operation, punctum 09.51
Thrombectomy 38.00
   with endarterectomy - see
      Endarterectomy
   abdominal
      artery 38.06
      vein 38.07

Thrombectomy (Continued)
   aorta (arch) (ascending) (descending)
      38.04
   arteriovenous shunt or cannula 39.49
   bovine graft 39.49
   coronary artery 36.09
   head and neck vessel NEC 38.02
   intracranial vessel NEC 38.01
   lower limb
      artery 38.08
      vein 38.09
   mechanical
      endovascular
         head and neck 39.74
   pulmonary vessel 38.05
   thoracic vessel NEC 38.05
   upper limb (artery) (vein) 38.03
Thromboendarterectomy 38.10
   abdominal 38.16
   aorta (arch) (ascending) (descending)
      38.14
   coronary artery 36.09
      open chest approach 36.03
   head and neck NEC 38.12
   intracranial NEC 38.11
   lower limb 38.18
   thoracic NEC 38.15
   upper limb 38.13
Thymectomy 07.80
   partial (open) (other) 07.81
      thoracoscopic 07.83
   total (open) (other) 07.82
      thoracoscopic 07.84
   transcervical 07.99
Thyrochondrotomy 31.3
Thyrocricoidectomy 30.29
Thyrocricotomy (for assistance in
      breathing) 31.1
Thyroidectomy NEC 06.39
   by mediastinotomy - see also
      Thyroidectomy, substernal
      06.50
   with laryngectomy - see Laryngectomy
   complete or total 06.4
      substernal (by mediastinotomy)
         (transsternal route) 06.52
      transoral route (lingual) 06.6
   lingual (complete) (partial) (subtotal)
      (total) 06.6
   partial or subtotal NEC 06.39
      with complete removal of remaining
         lobe 06.2
      submental route (lingual) 06.6
      substernal (by mediastinotomy)
         (transsternal route) 06.51
   remaining tissue 06.4
   submental route (lingual) 06.6
   substernal (by mediastinotomy)
      (transsternal route) 06.50
      complete or total 06.52
      partial or subtotal 06.51
   transoral route (lingual) 06.6
   transsternal route - see also
      Thyroidectomy, substernal
      06.50
   unilateral (with removal of isthmus)
      (with removal of portion of other
      lobe) 06.2
Thyroidorrhaphy 06.93
Thyroidotomy (field) (gland) NEC 06.09
   postoperative 06.02
Thyrotomy 31.3
   with tantalum plate 31.69
Tirofiban (HCL), infusion 99.20

Toilette
   skin - see Debridement, skin or
      subcutaneous tissue
   tracheostomy 96.55
Token economy (behavior therapy) 94.33
Tomkins operation (metroplasty) 69.49
Tomography - see also Radiography
   abdomen NEC 88.02
   cardiac 87.42
   computerized axial NEC 88.38
      abdomen 88.01
      bone 88.38
         quantitative 88.98
      brain 87.03
      cardiac 87.41
      coronary 87.41
      head 87.03
      kidney 87.71
      skeletal 88.38
         quantitative 88.98
      thorax 87.41
   head NEC 87.04
   kidney NEC 87.72
   lung 87.42
   optical coherence (intravascular
      imaging)   ◀
      coronary vessel(s) 38.24   ◀
      non-coronary vessel(s) 38.25   ◀
   thorax NEC 87.42
Tongue tie operation 25.91
Tonography 95.26
Tonometry 89.11
Tonsillectomy 28.2
   with adenoidectomy 28.3
Tonsillotomy 28.0
Topectomy 01.32
Torek (-Bevan) operation (orchidopexy)
      (first stage) (second stage) 62.5
Torkildsen operation (ventriculocisternal
      shunt) 02.2
Torpin operation (cul-de-sac resection)
      70.92
Toti operation (dacryocystorhinostomy)
      09.81
Touchas operation 86.83
Touroff operation (ligation of subclavian
      artery) 38.85
Toxicology - see Examination, microscopic
TPN (total parenteral nutrition) 99.15
Trabeculectomy ab externo 12.64
Trabeculodialysis 12.59
Trabeculotomy ab externo 12.54
Trachelectomy 67.4
Trachelopexy 69.22
Tracheloplasty 67.69
Trachelorrhaphy (Emmet) (suture) 67.61
   obstetrical 75.51
Trachelotomy 69.95
   obstetrical 73.93
Tracheocricotomy (for assistance in
      breathing) 31.1
Tracheofissure 31.1
Tracheography 87.32
Tracheolaryngotomy (emergency) 31.1
   permanent opening 31.29
Tracheoplasty 31.79
   with artificial larynx 31.75
Tracheorrhaphy 31.71
Tracheoscopy NEC 31.42
   through tracheotomy (stoma) 31.41
Tracheostomy (emergency) (temporary)
      (for assistance in breathing) 31.1
   mediastinal 31.21
   percutaneous dilatational
      other permanent 31.29
      temporary 31.1

◀ New   ◀▥ Revised   ~~deleted~~ Deleted   ● Use Additional Digit(s)   ▨ Omit code

Tracheostomy (*Continued*)
  permanent NEC 31.29
  revision 31.74
Tracheotomy (emergency) (temporary)
      (for assistance in breathing) 31.1
  percutaneous dilatational
      other permanent 31.29
      temporary 31.1
  permanent 31.29
Tracing, carotid pulse with ECG lead
    89.56
Traction
  with reduction of fracture or
      dislocation - *see* Reduction,
      fracture *and* Reduction,
      dislocation
  adhesive tape (skin) 93.46
  boot 93.46
  Bryant's (skeletal) 93.44
  Buck's 93.46
  caliper tongs 93.41
      with synchronous insertion of
          device 02.94
  Cortel's (spinal) 93.42
  Crutchfield tongs 93.41
      with synchronous insertion of
          device 02.94
  Dunlop's (skeletal) 93.44
  gallows 93.46
  Gardner Wells 93.41
      with synchronous insertion of
          device 02.94
  halo device, skull 93.41
      with synchronous insertion of
          device 02.94
  Lyman Smith (skeletal) 93.44
  manual, intermittent 93.21
  mechanical, intermittent 93.21
  Russell's (skeletal) 93.44
  skeletal NEC 93.44
      intermittent 93.43
  skin, limbs NEC 93.46
  spinal NEC 93.42
      with skull device (halo) (caliper)
          (Crutchfield) (Gardner Wells)
          (Vinke) (tongs) 93.41
      with synchronous insertion of
          device 02.94
  Thomas' splint 93.45
  Vinke tongs 93.41
      with synchronous insertion of
          device 02.94
Tractotomy
  brain 01.32
  medulla oblongata 01.32
  mesencephalon 01.32
  percutaneous 03.21
  spinal cord (one-stage) (two-stage)
      03.29
  trigeminal (percutaneous)
      (radiofrequency) 04.02
Training (for) (in)
  ADL (activities of daily living) 93.83
      for the blind 93.78
  ambulation 93.22
  braille 93.77
  crutch walking 93.24
  dyslexia 93.71
  dysphasia 93.72
  esophageal speech (postlaryngectomy)
      93.73
  gait 93.22
  joint movements 93.14
  lip reading 93.75

Training (*Continued*)
  Moon (blind reading) 93.77
  orthoptic 95.35
  prenatal (natural childbirth) 93.37
  prosthetic or orthotic device usage
      93.24
  relaxation 94.33
  speech NEC 93.75
      esophageal type 93.73
      for correction of defect 93.74
  use of lead dog for the blind 93.76
  vocational 93.85
TRAM (transverse rectus abdominis
      musculocutaneous) flap of breast
  free 85.73
  pedicled 85.72
Transactional analysis
  group 94.44
  individual 94.39
Transection - *see also* Division
  artery (with ligation) - *see also* Division,
      artery 38.80
      renal, aberrant (with reimplantation)
          39.55
  bone - *see also* Osteotomy 77.30
  fallopian tube (bilateral) (remaining)
      (solitary) 66.39
      by endoscopy 66.22
      unilateral 66.92
  isthmus, thyroid 06.91
  muscle 83.19
      eye 15.13
          multiple (two or more muscles)
              15.3
      hand 82.19
  nerve (cranial) (peripheral) NEC 04.03
      acoustic 04.01
      root (spinal) 03.1
      sympathetic 05.0
      tracts in spinal cord 03.29
      trigeminal 04.02
      vagus (transabdominal) - *see also*
          Vagotomy 44.00
  pylorus (with wedge resection) 43.3
  renal vessel, aberrant (with
      reimplantation) 39.55
  spinal
      cord tracts 03.29
      nerve root 03.1
  tendon 83.13
      hand 82.11
  uvula 27.71
  vas deferens 63.71
  vein (with ligation) - *see also* Division,
      vein 38.80
      renal, aberrant (with reimplantation)
          39.55
      varicose (lower limb) 38.59
Transfer, transference
  bone shaft, fibula into tibia 78.47
  digital (to replace absent thumb)
      82.69
      finger (to thumb) (same hand)
          82.61
      to
          finger, except thumb 82.81
          opposite hand (with
              amputation) 82.69
              [84.01]
          toe (to thumb) (with amputation)
              82.69 [84.11]
          to finger, except thumb 82.81
              [84.11]
  fat pad NEC 86.89
      with skin graft - *see* Graft, skin, full-
          thickness

Transfer, transference (*Continued*)
  finger (to replace absent thumb) (same
      hand) 82.61
  to
      finger, except thumb 82.81
      opposite hand (with amputation)
          82.69 [84.01]
  muscle origin 83.77
      hand 82.58
  nerve (cranial) (peripheral) (radial
      anterior) (ulnar) 04.6
  pedicle graft 86.74
  pes anserinus (tendon) (repair of knee)
      81.47
  tarsoconjunctival flap, from opposing
      lid 08.64
  tendon 83.75
      hand 82.56
      pes anserinus (repair of knee) 81.47
  toe to thumb (free) (pedicle) (with
      amputation) 82.69 [84.11]
Transfixion - *see also* Fixation
  iris (bombé) 12.11
Transfusion (of) 99.03
  antihemophilic factor 99.06
  antivenin 99.16
  autologous blood
      collected prior to surgery 99.02
      intraoperative 99.00
      perioperative 99.00
      postoperative 99.00
      previously collected 99.02
      salvage 99.00
  blood (whole) NOS 99.03
      expander 99.08
      surrogate 99.09
  bone marrow 41.00
      allogeneic 41.03
          with purging 41.02
      allograft 41.03
          with purging 41.02
      autograft 41.01
          with purging 41.09
      autologous 41.01
          with purging 41.09
  coagulation factors 99.06
  Dextran 99.08
  exchange 99.01
      intraperitoneal 75.2
      in utero (with hysterotomy) 75.2
  exsanguination 99.01
  gamma globulin 99.14
  granulocytes 99.09
  hemodilution 99.03
  intrauterine 75.2
  packed cells 99.04
  plasma 99.07
  platelets 99.05
  replacement, total 99.01
  serum NEC 99.07
  substitution 99.01
  thrombocytes 99.05
Transillumination
  nasal sinuses 89.35
  skull (newborn) 89.16
Translumbar aortogram 88.42
Transplant, transplantation

Note:	To report donor source:
	cadaver 00.93
	live non-related donor 00.92
	live related donor 00.91
	live unrelated donor 00.92

Transplant, transplantation (Continued)
artery 39.59
   renal, aberrant 39.55
autotransplant - see Reimplantation
blood vessel 39.59
   renal, aberrant 39.55
bone - see also Graft, bone 78.00
   marrow 41.00
      allogeneic 41.03
         with purging 41.02
      allograft 41.03
         with purging 41.02
      autograft 41.01
         with purging 41.09
      autologous 41.01
         with purging 41.09
      stem cell
         allogeneic (hematopoietic)
           41.05
           with purging 41.08
         autologous (hematopoietic)
           41.04
           with purging 41.07
      cord blood 41.06
   stem cell
      allogeneic (hematopoietic) 41.05
         with purging 41.08
      autologous (hematopoietic)
         41.04
         with purging 41.07
      cord blood 41.06
combined heart-lung 33.6
conjunctiva, for pterygium 11.39
corneal - see also Keratoplasty 11.60
dura 02.12
fascia 83.82
   hand 82.72
finger (replacing absent thumb) (same
   hand) 82.61
   to
      finger, except thumb 82.81
      opposite hand (with amputation)
         82.69 [84.01]
gracilis muscle (for) 83.77
   anal incontinence 49.74
   urethrovesical suspension 59.71
hair follicles
   eyebrow 08.63
   eyelid 08.63
   scalp 86.64
heart (orthotopic) 37.51
   combined with lung 33.6
ileal stoma to new site 46.23
intestine 46.97
Islets of Langerhans (cells) 52.86
   allotransplantation of cells 52.85
   autotransplantation of cells 52.84
   heterotransplantation 52.85
   homotransplantation 52.84
kidney NEC 55.69
liver 50.59
   auxiliary (permanent) (temporary)
      (recipient's liver in situ) 50.51
   cells into spleen via percutaneous
      catheterization 38.91
lung 33.50
   bilateral 33.50
   combined with heart 33.6
   double 33.52
   single 33.51
   unilateral 33.51
lymphatic structure(s) (peripheral) 40.9
mammary artery to myocardium or
   ventricular wall 36.2

Transplant, transplantation (Continued)
muscle 83.77
   gracilis (for) 83.77
      anal incontinence 49.74
      urethrovesical suspension
         59.71
   hand 82.58
   temporalis 83.77
      with orbital exenteration 16.59
nerve (cranial) (peripheral) 04.6
ovary 65.92
pancreas 52.80
   heterotransplant 52.83
   homotransplant 52.82
   Islets of Langerhans (cells) 52.86
      allotransplantation of cells
         52.85
      autotransplantation of cells
         52.84
      heterotransplantation 52.85
      homotransplantation 52.84
      reimplantation 52.81
pes anserinus (tendon) (repair of knee)
   81.47
renal NEC 55.69
   vessel, aberrant 39.55
salivary duct opening 26.49
skin - see Graft, skin
spermatic cord 63.53
spleen 41.94
stem cells
   allogeneic (hematopoietic) 41.05
      with purging 41.08
   autologous (hematopoietic) 41.04
      with purging 41.07
   cord blood 41.06
tendon 83.75
   hand 82.56
   pes anserinus (repair of knee)
      81.47
   superior rectus (blepharoptosis)
      08.36
testis to scrotum 62.5
thymus 07.94
thyroid tissue 06.94
toe (replacing absent thumb) (with
   amputation) 82.69 [84.11]
   to finger, except thumb 82.81
      [84.11]
tooth 23.5
ureter to
   bladder 56.74
   ileum (external diversion) 56.51
      internal diversion only 56.71
   intestine 56.71
   skin 56.61
vein (peripheral) 39.59
   renal, aberrant 39.55
vitreous 14.72
   anterior approach 14.71
Transposition
extraocular muscles 15.5
eyelash flaps 08.63
eye muscle (oblique) (rectus) 15.5
finger (replacing absent thumb) (same
   hand) 82.61
   to
      finger, except thumb 82.81
      opposite hand (with amputation)
         82.69 [84.01]
interatrial venous return 35.91
jejunal (Henley) 43.81
joint capsule - see also Arthroplasty
   81.96

Transposition (Continued)
muscle NEC 83.79
   extraocular 15.5
   hand 82.59
nerve (cranial) (peripheral) (radial
   anterior) (ulnar) 04.6
nipple 85.86
pterygium 11.31
tendon NEC 83.76
   hand 82.57
vocal cords 31.69
Transureteroureterostomy 56.75
Transversostomy - see also Colostomy
   46.10
Trapping, aneurysm (cerebral)
   39.52
Trauner operation (lingual sulcus
   extension) 24.91
Trephination, trephining
   accessory sinus - see Sinusotomy
   corneoscleral 12.89
   cranium 01.24
   nasal sinus - see Sinusotomy
   sclera (with iridectomy) 12.61
Trial (failed) forceps 73.3
Trigonectomy 57.6
Trimming, amputation stump 84.3
Triple arthrodesis 81.12
Trochanterplasty 81.40
Tsuge operation (macrodactyly repair)
   82.83
Tuck, tucking - see also Plication
   eye muscle 15.22
      multiple (two or more muscles)
         15.4
   levator palpebrae, for blepharoptosis
      08.34
Tudor "rabbit ear" operation (anterior
   urethropexy) 59.79
Tuffier operation
   apicolysis of lung 33.39
   vaginal hysterectomy 68.59
      laparoscopically assisted (LAVH)
         68.51
TULIP (transurethral ultrasound guided
   laser induced prostectomy) 60.21
TUMT (transurethral microwave
   thermotherapy) of prostate 60.96
TUNA (transurethral needle ablation) of
   prostate 60.97
Tunnel, subcutaneous (antethoracic)
   42.86
   esophageal 42.68
      with anastomosis - see
         Anastomosis, esophagus,
         antesternal 42.68
   pulse generator lead wire 86.99
      with initial procedure - omit code
Turbinectomy (complete) (partial) NEC
   21.69
   by
      cryosurgery 21.61
      diathermy 21.61
   with sinusectomy - see Sinusectomy
Turco operation (release of joint capsules
   in clubfoot) 80.48
TURP (transurethral resection of prostate)
   60.29
Tylectomy (breast) (partial) 85.21
Tympanectomy 20.59
   with tympanoplasty - see
      Tympanoplasty
Tympanogram 95.41
Tympanomastoidectomy 20.42

◀ New   ◀▦ Revised   deleted Deleted   ● Use Additional Digit(s)   ▨ Omit code

U

Uchida operation (tubal ligation with or without fimbriectomy) 66.32
UFR (uroflowmetry) 89.24
Ultrafiltration 99.78
    hemodiafiltration 39.95
    hemodialysis (kidney) 39.95
    removal, plasma water 99.78
    therapeutic plasmapheresis 99.71
Ultrasonography
    abdomen 88.76
    aortic arch 88.73
    biliary tract 88.74
    breast 88.73
    deep vein thrombosis 88.77
    digestive system 88.74
    eye 95.13
    head and neck 88.71
    heart 88.72
    intestine 88.74
    intravascular - see Ultrasound, intravascular (IVUS)
    lung 88.73
    midline shift, brain 88.71
    multiple sites 88.79
    peripheral vascular system 88.77
    retroperitoneum 88.76
    therapeutic - see Ultrasound
    thorax NEC 88.73
    total body 88.79
    urinary system 88.75
    uterus 88.79
        gravid 88.78
Ultrasound
    diagnostic - see Ultrasonography
    fragmentation (of)
        cataract (with aspiration) 13.41
        urinary calculus, stones (Kock pouch) 59.95
    heart
        intracardiac (heart chambers) (ICE) 37.28
        intravascular (coronary vessels) (IVUS) 00.24
        non-invasive 88.72
    inner ear 20.79
    intravascular (IVUS) (VH™-IVUS) 00.29
        aorta 00.22
        aortic arch 00.22
        cerebral vessel, extracranial 00.21
        coronary vessel 00.24
        intrathoracic vessel 00.22
        other specified vessel 00.28
        peripheral vessel 00.23
        renal vessel 00.25
        vena cava (inferior) (superior) 00.22
    VH™-IVUS - see Ultrasound, intravascular, by site ◄
    virtual histology intravascular ultrasound - see Ultrasound, intravascular, by site ◄

Ultrasound (Continued)
    therapeutic
        head 00.01
        heart 00.02
        neck 00.01
        other therapeutic ultrasound 00.09
        peripheral vascular vessels 00.03
        vessels of head and neck 00.01
    therapy 93.35
Umbilectomy 54.3
Unbridling
    blood vessel, peripheral 39.91
    celiac artery axis 39.91
Uncovering - see Incision, by site
Undercutting
    hair follicle 86.09
    perianal tissue 49.02
Unroofing - see also Incision, by site
    external
        auditory canal 18.02
        ear NEC 18.09
    kidney cyst 55.39
UPP (urethral pressure profile) 89.25
Upper GI series (x-ray) 87.62
UPPP (uvulopalatopharyngoplasty) 27.69 [29.4]
Uranoplasty (for cleft palate repair) 27.62
Uranorrhaphy (for cleft palate repair) 27.62
Uranostaphylorrhaphy 27.62
Urban operation (mastectomy) (unilateral) 85.47
    bilateral 85.48
Ureterectomy 56.40
    with nephrectomy 55.51
    partial 56.41
    total 56.42
Ureterocecostomy 56.71
Ureterocelectomy 56.41
Ureterocolostomy 56.71
Ureterocystostomy 56.74
Ureteroenterostomy 56.71
Ureteroileostomy (internal diversion) 56.71
    external diversion 56.51
Ureterolithotomy 56.2
Ureterolysis 59.02
    with freeing or repositioning of ureter 59.02
    laparoscopic 59.03
Ureteroneocystostomy 56.74
Ureteropexy 56.85
Ureteroplasty 56.89
Ureteroplication 56.89
Ureteroproctostomy 56.71
Ureteropyelography (intravenous) (diuretic infusion) 87.73
    percutaneous 87.75
    retrograde 87.74
Ureteropyeloplasty 55.87
Ureteropyelostomy 55.86

Ureterorrhaphy 56.82
Ureteroscopy 56.31
    with biopsy 56.33
Ureterosigmoidostomy 56.71
Ureterostomy (cutaneous) (external) (tube) 56.61
    closure 56.83
    ileal 56.51
Ureterotomy 56.2
Ureteroureterostomy (crossed) 56.75
    lumbar 56.41
    resection with end-to-end anastomosis 56.41
    spatulated 56.41
Urethral catheterization, indwelling 57.94
Urethral pressure profile (UPP) 89.25
Urethrectomy (complete) (partial) (radical) 58.39
    with
        complete cystectomy 57.79
        pelvic exenteration 68.8
        radical cystectomy 57.71
Urethrocystography (retrograde) (voiding) 87.76
Urethrocystopexy (by) 59.79
    levator muscle sling 59.71
    retropubic suspension 59.5
    suprapubic suspension 59.4
Urethrolithotomy 58.0
Urethrolysis 58.5
Urethropexy 58.49
    anterior 59.79
Urethroplasty 58.49
    augmentation 59.79
        collagen implant 59.72
        fat implant 59.72
        injection (endoscopic) of implant into urethra 59.72
        polytef implant 59.72
Urethrorrhaphy 58.41
Urethroscopy 58.22
    for control of hemorrhage of prostate 60.94
    perineal 58.21
Urethrostomy (perineal) 58.0
Urethrotomy (external) 58.0
    internal (endoscopic) 58.5
Uroflowmetry (UFR) 89.24
Urography (antegrade) (excretory) (intravenous) 87.73
    retrograde 87.74
Uteropexy (abdominal approach) (vaginal approach) 69.22
UVP (uvulopalatopharyngoplasty) 27.69 [29.4]
Uvulectomy 27.72
Uvulopalatopharyngoplasty (UPPP) 27.69 [29.4]
Uvulotomy 27.71

◄ New   ◄▥ Revised   ~~deleted~~ Deleted   ● Use Additional Digit(s)   ▨ Omit code

V

Vaccination (prophylactic) (against)
99.59
anthrax 99.55
brucellosis 99.55
cholera 99.31
common cold 99.51
disease NEC 99.55
arthropod-borne viral NEC 99.54
encephalitis, arthropod-borne viral
99.53
German measles 99.47
hydrophobia 99.44
infectious parotitis 99.46
influenza 99.52
measles 99.45
mumps 99.46
paratyphoid fever 99.32
pertussis 99.37
plague 99.34
poliomyelitis 99.41
rabies 99.44
Rocky Mountain spotted fever 99.55
rubella 99.47
rubeola 99.45
smallpox 99.42
Staphylococcus 99.55
Streptococcus 99.55
tuberculosis 99.33
tularemia 99.35
tumor 99.28
typhoid 99.32
typhus 99.55
undulant fever 99.55
yellow fever 99.43
Vacuum extraction, fetal head 72.79
with episiotomy 72.71
VAD
vascular access device - see Vascular
access device, totally implantable
ventricular assist device – see Implant,
heart assist system
Vagectomy (subdiaphragmatic) - see also
Vagotomy 44.00
Vaginal douche 96.44
Vaginectomy 70.4
Vaginofixation 70.77
with graft or prosthesis 70.78
Vaginoperineotomy 70.14
Vaginoplasty 70.79
Vaginorrhaphy 70.71
obstetrical 75.69
Vaginoscopy 70.21
Vaginotomy 70.14
for
culdocentesis 70.0
pelvic abscess 70.12
Vagotomy (gastric) 44.00
parietal cell 44.02
selective NEC 44.03
highly 44.02
Holle's 44.02
proximal 44.02
truncal 44.01
Valvotomy - see Valvulotomy
Valvulectomy, heart - see Valvuloplasty,
heart
Valvuloplasty
heart (open heart technique) (without
valve replacement) 35.10
with prosthesis or tissue graft - see
Replacement, heart, valve, by
site

Valvuloplasty (Continued)
heart (Continued)
aortic valve 35.11
percutaneous (balloon) 35.96
combined with repair of atrial and
ventricular septal defects - see
Repair, endocardial cushion
defect
mitral valve 35.12
percutaneous (balloon) 35.96
pulmonary valve 35.13
in total repair of tetralogy of
Fallot 35.81
percutaneous (balloon)
35.96
tricuspid valve 35.14
Valvulotomy
heart (closed heart technique)
(transatrial) (transventricular)
35.00
aortic valve 35.01
mitral valve 35.02
open heart technique - see
Valvuloplasty, heart
pulmonary valve 35.03
in total repair of tetralogy of
Fallot 35.81
tricuspid valve 35.04
Varicocelectomy, spermatic cord
63.1
Varicotomy, peripheral vessels (lower
limb) 38.59
upper limb 38.53
Vascular access device, totally
implantable 86.07
Vascular closure, percutaneous
puncture - omit code
Vascularization - see Revascularization
Vasectomy (complete) (partial)
63.73
Vasogram 87.94
Vasoligation 63.71
gastric 38.86
Vasorrhaphy 63.81
Vasostomy 63.6
Vasotomy 63.6
Vasotripsy 63.71
Vasovasostomy 63.82
Vectorcardiogram (VCG) (with ECG)
89.53
Vectra® vascular access graft 86.07
Venectomy - see Phlebectomy
Venipuncture NEC 38.99
for injection of contrast material - see
Phlebography
Venography - see Phlebography
Venorrhaphy 39.32
Venotomy 38.00
abdominal 38.07
head and neck NEC 38.02
intracranial NEC 38.01
lower limb 38.09
thoracic NEC 38.05
upper limb 38.03
Venotripsy 39.98
Venovenostomy 39.29
Ventilation
bi-level positive airway pressure
[BiPAP] 93.90
delivered by
endotracheal tube - see category
96.7●
tracheostomy – see category
96.7●

Ventilation (Continued)
continuous positive airway pressure
[CPAP] 93.90
delivered by
endotracheal tube - see category
96.7●
tracheostomy – see category 96.7●
endotracheal respiratory assistance - see
category 96.7●
intermittent positive pressure
breathing [IPPB] 93.91
mechanical, NOS 93.90
by endotracheal tube - see category
96.7●
by tracheostomy - see category
96.7●
endotracheal respiratory assistance -
see category 96.7●
invasive - see category 96.7●
non-invasive [NIPPV] 93.90
other continuous invasive
(unspecified duration) 96.70
for less than 96 consecutive hours
96.71
for 96 consecutive hours or more
96.72
negative pressure (continuous) [CNP]
93.99
non-invasive positive pressure
(NIPPV) 93.90
positive end expiratory pressure
[PEEP]
invasive - see category 96.7●
non-invasive 93.90
Ventriculectomy, heart
partial 37.35
Ventriculocholecystostomy 02.34
Ventriculocisternostomy 02.2
Ventriculocordectomy 30.29
Ventriculogram, ventriculography
(cerebral) 87.02
cardiac
left ventricle (outflow tract) 88.53
combined with right heart 88.54
right ventricle (outflow tract) 88.52
combined with left heart 88.54
radionuclide cardiac 92.05
Ventriculomyocardiotomy 37.11
Ventriculoperitoneostomy 02.34
Ventriculopuncture 01.09
through previously implanted catheter
or reservoir (Ommaya) (Rickham)
01.02
Ventriculoseptopexy - see also Repair,
ventricular septal defect 35.72
Ventriculoseptoplasty - see also Repair,
ventricular septal defect 35.72
Ventriculostomy 02.2
Ventriculotomy
cerebral 02.2
heart 37.11
Ventriculoureterostomy 02.35
Ventriculovenostomy 02.32
Ventrofixation, uterus 69.22
Ventrohysteropexy 69.22
Ventrosuspension, uterus 69.22
VEP (visual evoked potential) 95.23
Version, obstetrical (bimanual) (cephalic)
(combined) (internal) (podalic)
73.21
with extraction 73.22
Braxton Hicks 73.21
with extraction 73.22
external (bipolar) 73.91

◄ New   ◄▥ Revised   deleted Deleted   ● Use Additional Digit(s)   ▨ Omit code   1349

Version, obstetrical (*Continued*)
    Potter's (podalic) 73.21
      with extraction 73.22
    Wigand's (external) 73.91
    Wright's (cephalic) 73.21
      with extraction 73.22
Vertebroplasty, percutaneous 81.65
Vesicolithotomy (suprapubic) 57.19
Vesicostomy 57.21
Vesicourethroplasty 57.85
Vesiculectomy 60.73
    with radical prostatectomy 60.5
Vesiculogram, seminal 87.92
    contrast 87.91
Vesiculotomy 60.72
Vestibuloplasty (buccolabial) (lingual) 24.91
Vestibulotomy 20.79
VH™-IVUS - *see* Ultrasound, intravascular, by site ◀

Vicq D'azyr operation (larynx) 31.1
Vidal operation (varicocele ligation) 63.1
Vidianectomy 05.21
Villusectomy - *see also* Synovectomy 80.70
Vision check 95.09
Visual evoked potential (VEP) 95.23
Vitrectomy (mechanical) (posterior approach) 14.74
    with scleral buckling 14.49
    anterior approach 14.73
Vocational
    assessment 93.85
    retraining 93.85
    schooling 93.82
Voice training (postlaryngectomy) 93.73
von Kraske operation (proctectomy) 48.64
Voss operation (hanging hip operation) 83.19

Vulpius (-Compere) operation (lengthening of gastrocnemius muscle) 83.85
Vulvectomy (bilateral) (simple) 71.62
    partial (unilateral) 71.61
    radical (complete) 71.5
    unilateral 71.61
V-Y operation (repair)
    bladder 57.89
      neck 57.85
    ectropion 08.44
    lip 27.59
    skin (without graft) 86.89
    subcutaneous tissue (without skin graft) 86.89
    tongue 25.59

◀ New   ◀▥ Revised   ~~deleted~~ Deleted   ● Use Additional Digit(s)   ▨ Omit code

W

Wada test (hemispheric function) 89.10
Wang needle aspiration biopsy
   bronchus 33.24 ◀
Ward-Mayo operation (vaginal
   hysterectomy) 68.59
   laparoscopically assisted (LAVH)
     68.51
Washing - see Lavage and Irrigation
Waterston operation (aorta-right
   pulmonary artery anastomosis) 39.0
Watkins (-Wertheim) operation (uterus
   interposition) 69.21
Watson-Jones operation
   hip arthrodesis 81.21
   reconstruction of lateral ligaments,
     ankle 81.49
   shoulder arthrodesis (extra-articular)
     81.23
   tenoplasty 83.88
Webbing (syndactylization) 86.89
Weir operation
   appendicostomy 47.91
   correction of nostrils 21.86
Wertheim operation (radical
   hysterectomy) 68.69
   laparoscopic 68.61
West operation (dacryocystorhinostomy)
   09.81
Wheeler operation
   entropion repair 08.44
   halving procedure (eyelid) 08.24
Whipple operation (radical
   pancreaticoduodenectomy) 52.7
   Child modification (radical subtotal
     pancreatectomy) 52.53
   Rodney Smith modification (radical
     subtotal pancreatectomy) 52.53
White operation (lengthening of tendo
   calcaneus by incomplete tenotomy)
   83.11
Whitehead operation
   glossectomy, radical 25.4
   hemorrhoidectomy 49.46

Whitman operation
   foot stabilization (talectomy) 77.98
   hip reconstruction 81.40
   repair of serratus anterior muscle 83.87
   talectomy 77.98
   trochanter wedge osteotomy 77.25
Wier operation (entropion repair) 08.44
Williams-Richardson operation (vaginal
   construction) 70.61
   with graft or prosthesis 70.63
Wilms operation (thoracoplasty) 33.34
Wilson operation (angulation osteotomy
   for hallux valgus) 77.51
Window operation
   antrum (nasal sinus) - see Antrotomy,
     maxillary
   aorticopulmonary 39.59
   bone cortex - see also Incision, bone
     77.10
     facial 76.09
   nasoantral - see Antrotomy, maxillary
   pericardium 37.12
   pleura 34.09
Winiwarter operation
   (cholecystoenterostomy) 51.32
Wiring
   aneurysm 39.52
   dental (for immobilization) 93.55
     with fracture-reduction - see
       Reduction, fracture
     orthodontic 24.7
Wirsungojejunostomy 52.96
Witzel operation (temporary
   gastrostomy) 43.19
Woodward operation (release of high
   riding scapula) 81.83
Wrapping, aneurysm (gauze) (methyl
   methacrylate) (plastic) 39.52

X

Xenograft 86.65
Xerography, breast 87.36

Xeromammography 87.36
Xiphoidectomy 77.81
X-ray
   chest (routine) 87.44
     wall NEC 87.39
   contrast - see Radiography, contrast
   diagnostic - see Radiography
   injection of radio-opaque substance -
     see Radiography, contrast
   skeletal series, whole or complete
     88.31
   therapeutic - see Therapy, radiation

Y

Young operation
   epispadias repair 58.45
   tendon transfer (anterior tibialis)
     (repair of flat foot) 83.75
Yount operation (division of iliotibial
   band) 83.14

Z

Zancolli operation
   capsuloplasty 81.72
   tendon transfer (biceps) 82.56
Zeus® Robotic Surgical System – see
   category 17.4 ●
Ziegler operation (iridectomy) 12.14
Zonulolysis (with lens extraction) - see
   also Extraction, cataract,
   intracapsular 13.19
Z-plasty
   epicanthus 08.59
   eyelid - see also Reconstruction, eyelid
     08.70
   hypopharynx 29.4
   skin (scar) (web contracture)
     86.84
   with excision of lesion 86.3

Code also note: This instruction is used in the Tabular List for two purposes:

1) To code components of a procedure that are performed at the same time, and

2) To code the use of special adjunctive procedures or equipment.

Includes note: This note appears immediately under a two- or three-digit code title. The information further defines, or gives examples of, the contents of the category.

Excludes note: Terms following the word "Excludes" are to be coded elsewhere as indicated in each case.

CLASSIFICATION OF PROCEDURES

0. PROCEDURES AND INTERVENTIONS, NOT ELSEWHERE CLASSIFIED (00)

00 Procedures and interventions, Not Elsewhere Classified

● **00.0 Therapeutic ultrasound**

> Excludes | diagnostic ultrasound (non-invasive)
> (88.71–88.79)
> intracardiac echocardiography [ICE]
> (heart chamber(s)) (37.28)
> intravascular imaging (adjunctive)
> (00.21–00.29)
> Coding Clinic: 2002, Q4, P90-92

00.01 Therapeutic ultrasound of vessels of head and neck
Anti-restenotic ultrasound
Intravascular non-ablative ultrasound

> Excludes | diagnostic ultrasound of:
> eye (95.13)
> head and neck (88.71)
> that of inner ear (20.79)
> ultrasonic:
> angioplasty of non-coronary vessel
> (39.50)
> embolectomy (38.01, 38.02)
> endarterectomy (38.11, 38.12)
> thrombectomy (38.01, 38.02)

00.02 Therapeutic ultrasound of heart
Anti-restenotic ultrasound
Intravascular non-ablative ultrasound

> Excludes | diagnostic ultrasound of heart (88.72)
> ultrasonic ablation of heart lesion
> (37.34)
> ultrasonic angioplasty of coronary
> vessels (00.66, 36.09)

00.03 Therapeutic ultrasound of peripheral vascular vessels
Anti-restenotic ultrasound
Intravascular non-ablative ultrasound

> Excludes | diagnostic ultrasound of peripheral
> vascular system (88.77)
> ultrasonic angioplasty of:
> non-coronary vessel (39.50)

00.09 Other therapeutic ultrasound

> Excludes | ultrasonic:
> fragmentation of urinary stones
> (59.95)
> percutaneous nephrostomy with
> fragmentation (55.04)
> physical therapy (93.35)
> transurethral guided laser induced
> prostatectomy (TULIP)
> (60.21)

● **00.1 Pharmaceuticals**

00.10 Implantation of chemotherapeutic agent
Brain wafer chemotherapy
Interstitial/intracavitary

> Excludes | injection or infusion of cancer
> chemotherapeutic substance
> (99.25)
> Coding Clinic: 2002, Q4, P93
> ◆Non-OR Procedure that affects MS-DRG
> assignment to MDC 01, MS-DRG 023

00.11 Infusion of drotrecogin alfa (activated)
Infusion of recombinant protein
Coding Clinic: 2002, Q4, P93-94

00.12 Administration of inhaled nitric oxide
Nitric oxide therapy
Coding Clinic: 2002, Q4, P94

00.13 Injection or infusion of nesiritide
Human B-type natriuretic peptide (hBNP)
Coding Clinic: 2002, Q4, P94

00.14 Injection or infusion of oxazolidinone class of antibiotics
Linezolid injection
Coding Clinic: 2002, Q4, P95

00.15 High-dose infusion interleukin-2 [IL-2]
Infusion (IV bolus, CIV) interleukin
Injection of aldesleukin

> Excludes | low-dose infusion interleukin-2 (99.28)
> Coding Clinic: 2003, Q4, P92
> ◆Non-OR Procedure that affects MS-DRG
> assignment to MDC 17, MS-DRG 837-838

00.16 Pressurized treatment of venous bypass graft [conduit] with pharmaceutical substance
Ex-vivo treatment of vessel
Hyperbaric pressurized graft [conduit]
Coding Clinic: 2004, Q4, P108

00.17 Infusion of vasopressor agent
Coding Clinic: 2004, Q4, P108-109

00.18 Infusion of immunosuppressive antibody therapy

> Includes | during induction phase of solid
> organ transplantation
> monoclonal antibody therapy
> polyclonal antibody therapy
> Coding Clinic: 2005, Q4, P101

00.19 Disruption of blood brain barrier via infusion [BBBD]
Infusion of substance to disrupt blood
brain barrier

> Code also chemotherapy (99.25)

> Excludes | other perfusion (39.97)
> Coding Clinic: 2007, Q4, P103-104

● **00.2 Intravascular imaging of blood vessels**
Endovascular ultrasonography
Intravascular [ultrasound] imaging of blood vessels
Intravascular ultrasound (IVUS)
Virtual histology intravascular ultrasound
(VH-IVUS) ◀
Note: Real-time imaging of lumen of blood vessel(s)
using sound waves

> Code also any synchronous diagnostic or therapeutic
> procedures

> Excludes | adjunct vascular system procedures, number
> of vessels treated (00.40–00.43)
> diagnostic procedures on blood vessels
> (38.21–38.29)
> diagnostic ultrasound of peripheral vascular
> system (88.77)
> intravascular imaging of vessel(s) by OCT
> (38.24-38.25) ◀
> magnetic resonance imaging (MRI)
> (88.91–88.97)
> therapeutic ultrasound (00.01–00.09)
> Coding Clinic: 2004, Q4, P109-111

00.21 Intravascular imaging of extracranial cerebral vessels
Common carotid vessels and branches
Intravascular ultrasound (IVUS), extracranial
cerebral vessels

> Excludes | diagnostic ultrasound (non-invasive) of
> head and neck (88.71)

◀ New   ◀▥ Revised   ~~deleted~~ Deleted   ● Use Additional Digit(s)   ✱ Valid O.R. Procedure
◆ Non-O.R. Procedure   ♀ Females Only   ♂ Males Only

PROCEDURES AND INTERVENTIONS, NEC (00)

00.22   Intravascular imaging of intrathoracic vessels
     Aorta and aortic arch
     Intravascular ultrasound (IVUS), intrathoracic
       vessels
     Vena cava (superior) (inferior)

> **Excludes** | *diagnostic ultrasound (non-invasive) of*
> *other sites of thorax (88.73)*

00.23   Intravascular imaging of peripheral vessels
     Imaging of:
       vessels of arm(s)
       vessels of leg(s)
     Intravascular ultrasound (IVUS), peripheral
       vessels

> **Excludes** | *diagnostic ultrasound (non-invasive)*
> *of peripheral vascular system*
> *(88.77)*

00.24   Intravascular imaging of coronary vessels
     Intravascular ultrasound (IVUS), coronary
       vessels

> **Excludes** | *diagnostic ultrasound (non-invasive) of*
> *heart (88.72)*
> *intracardiac echocardiography [ICE]*
> *(ultrasound of heart chamber(s))*
> *(37.28)*

     Coding Clinic: 2006, Q3, P8-9

00.25   Intravascular imaging of renal vessels
     Intravascular ultrasound (IVUS), renal vessels
     Renal artery

> **Excludes** | *diagnostic ultrasound (non-invasive) of*
> *urinary system (88.75)*

00.28   Intravascular imaging, other specified vessel(s)

00.29   Intravascular imaging, unspecified vessel(s)

● **00.3   Computer assisted surgery [CAS]**
     CT-free navigation
     Image guided navigation (IGN)
     Image guided surgery (IGS)
     Imageless navigation
     That without the use of robotic(s) technology

> Code also   diagnostic or therapeutic procedure

> **Excludes** | *robotic assisted procedures (17.41–17.49)*
> *stereotactic frame application only (93.59)*

00.31   Computer assisted surgery with CT/CTA

00.32   Computer assisted surgery with MR/MRA
     Coding Clinic: 2004, Q4, P111-113

00.33   Computer assisted surgery with fluoroscopy

00.34   Imageless computer assisted surgery

00.35   Computer assisted surgery with multiple datasets

00.39   Other computer assisted surgery
     Computer assisted surgery NOS

● **00.4   Adjunct vascular system procedures**
     Note: These codes can apply to both coronary and
       peripheral vessels. These codes are to be used
       in conjunction with other therapeutic procedure
       codes to provide additional information on the
       number of vessels upon which a procedure
       was performed and/or the number of stents
       inserted. As appropriate, code both the number
       of vessels operated on (00.40–00.43), and the
       number of stents inserted (00.45–00.48).

> Code also   any:
>   angioplasty or atherectomy (00.61–00.62, 00.66,
>   39.50)
>   endarterectomy (38.10–38.18)
>   insertion of vascular stent(s) (00.55, 00.63–00.65,
>   36.06–36.07, 39.90)
>   other removal of coronary artery obstruction (36.09)

00.40   Procedure on single vessel
     Number of vessels, unspecified

> **Excludes** | *(aorto)coronary bypass (36.10–36.19)*
> *intravascular imaging of blood vessels*
> *(00.21–00.29)*

     Coding Clinic: 2009, Q2, P12; 2007, Q1, P17; 2006, Q3, P8-9;
     2005, Q4, P69-72, 103-106

00.41   Procedure on two vessels

> **Excludes** | *(aorto)coronary bypass (36.10–36.19)*
> *intravascular imaging of blood vessels*
> *(00.21–00.29)*

     Coding Clinic: 2006, Q4, P119; 2005, Q4, P101-106

00.42   Procedure on three vessels

> **Excludes** | *(aorto)coronary bypass (36.10–36.19)*
> *intravascular imaging of blood vessels*
> *(00.21–00.29)*

00.43   Procedure on four or more vessels

> **Excludes** | *(aorto)coronary bypass (36.10–36.19)*
> *intravascular imaging of blood vessels*
> *(00.21–00.29)*

     ◆ Non-OR Procedure that affects MS-DRG
       assignment to MDC 05, MS-DRG 246, 248

00.44   Procedure on vessel bifurcation
     Note: This code is to be used to identify the
       presence of a vessel bifurcation; it does
       not describe a specific bifurcation stent.
       Use this code only once per operative
       episode, irrespective of the number of
       bifurcations in vessels.

     Coding Clinic: 2006, Q4, P119

00.45   Insertion of one vascular stent
     Number of stents, unspecified
     Coding Clinic: 2005, Q4, P69-72

00.46   Insertion of two vascular stents
     Coding Clinic: 2009, Q2, P12; 2005, Q4, P103-106

00.47   Insertion of three vascular stents
     Coding Clinic: 2006, Q4, P119

00.48   Insertion of four or more vascular stents
     ◆ Non-OR Procedure that affects MS-DRG
       assignment to MDC 05, MS-DRG 246, 248

00.49   SuperSaturated oxygen therapy
     Aqueous oxygen (AO) therapy
     SSO_2
     SuperOxygenation infusion therapy

> Code also   any:
>   injection or infusion of thrombolytic agent
>   (99.10)
>   insertion of coronary artery stent(s)
>   (36.06-36.07)
>   intracoronary artery thrombolytic infusion
>   (36.04)
>   number of vascular stents inserted
>   (00.45-00.48)
>   number of vessels treated (00.40-00.43)
>   open chest coronary artery angioplasty
>   (36.03)
>   other removal of coronary obstruction
>   (36.09)
>   percutaneous transluminal coronary
>   angioplasty [PTCA] (00.66)
>   procedure on vessel bifurcation (00.44)

> **Excludes** | *other oxygen enrichment (93.96)*
> *other perfusion (39.97)*

     Coding Clinic: 2008, Q4, P162-163

PROCEDURES AND INTERVENTIONS, NEC (00)

Excludes	Includes	Use additional	Code also	Omit code

● **00.5 Other cardiovascular procedures**
Coding Clinic: 2008, Q3, P18; 2002, Q4, P95-101

✖ **00.50 Implantation of cardiac resynchronization pacemaker without mention of defibrillation, total system [CRT-P]**

BiV pacemaker
Biventricular pacemaker
Biventricular pacing without internal cardiac defibrillator
Implantation of cardiac resynchronization (biventricular) pulse generator pacing device, formation of pocket, transvenous leads including placement of lead into left ventricular coronary venous system, and intraoperative procedures for evaluation of lead signals.
That with CRT-P generator and one or more leads
Note: Device testing during procedure – *omit code*

Excludes *implantation of cardiac resynchronization defibrillator, total system [CRT-D] (00.51)*
insertion or replacement of any type pacemaker device (37.80–37.87)
replacement of cardiac resynchronization defibrillator pulse generator only [CRT-D] (00.54)
replacement of cardiac resynchronization pacemaker pulse generator only [CRT-P] (00.53)
Coding Clinic: 2008, Q3, P18; 2005, Q3, P3-9

✖ **00.51 Implantation of cardiac resynchronization defibrillator, total system [CRT-D]**

BiV defibrillator
BiV ICD
BiV pacemaker with defibrillator
BiV pacing with defibrillator
Biventricular defibrillator
Biventricular pacing with internal cardiac defibrillator
Implantation of a cardiac resynchronization (biventricular) pulse generator with defibrillator [AICD], formation of pocket, transvenous leads, including placement of lead into left ventricular coronary venous system, intraoperative procedures for evaluation of lead signals, and obtaining defibrillator threshold measurements.
That with CRT-D generator and one or more leads
Note: Device testing during procedure – *omit code*

Excludes *implantation of cardiac resynchronization pacemaker, total system [CRT-P] (00.50)*
implantation or replacement of automatic cardioverter/defibrillator, total system [AICD] (37.94)
replacement of cardiac resynchronization defibrillator pulse generator, only [CRT-D] (00.54)
Coding Clinic: 2008, Q3, P18; 2007, Q1, P16-17x2; 2005, Q3, P3-9; 2002, Q4, P99-100

✖ **00.52 Implantation or replacement of transvenous lead [electrode] into left ventricular coronary venous system**

Excludes *implantation of cardiac resynchronization defibrillator, total system [CRT-D] (00.51)*
implantation of cardiac resynchronization pacemaker, total system [CRT-P] (00.50)
initial insertion of transvenous lead [electrode] (37.70–37.72)
replacement of transvenous atrial and/or ventricular lead(s) [electrodes] (37.76)
Coding Clinic: 2008, Q3, P18; 2005, Q3, P3-9
MS-DRG: Refer to Part VI, Appendix E, Table 6, Lead/Device Reference Table

✖ **00.53 Implantation or replacement of cardiac resynchronization pacemaker pulse generator only [CRT-P]**

Implantation of CRT-P device with removal of any existing CRT-P or other pacemaker device
Note: Device testing during procedure – *omit code*

Excludes *implantation of cardiac resynchronization pacemaker, total system [CRT-P] (00.50)*
implantation or replacement of cardiac resynchronization defibrillator pulse generator only [CRT-D] (00.54)
insertion or replacement of any type pacemaker device (37.80–37.87)
Coding Clinic: 2005, Q3, P3-9
MS-DRG: Refer to Part VI, Appendix E, Table 6, Lead/Device Reference Table

✖ **00.54 Implantation or replacement of cardiac resynchronization defibrillator pulse generator device only [CRT-D]**

Implantation of CRT-D device with removal of any existing CRT-D, CRT-P, pacemaker, or defibrillator device
Note: Device testing during procedure – *omit code*

Excludes *implantation of automatic cardioverter/defibrillator pulse generator only (37.96)*
implantation of cardiac resynchronization defibrillator, total system [CRT-D] (00.51)
implantation or replacement of cardiac resynchronization pacemaker pulse generator only [CRT-P] (00.53)
Coding Clinic: 2005, Q3, P3-9; 2002, Q4, P100
MS-DRG: Refer to Part VI, Appendix E, Table 6, Lead/Device Reference Table

◀ New ◀◀ Revised ~~deleted~~ Deleted ● Use Additional Digit(s) ✖ Valid O.R. Procedure
◆ Non-O.R. Procedure ♀ Females Only ♂ Males Only

00.55 **Insertion of drug-eluting peripheral vessel stent(s)**
Endograft(s)
Endovascular graft(s)
Stent grafts

Code also any:
angioplasty or atherectomy of other non-coronary vessel(s) (39.50)
number of vascular stents inserted (00.45–00.48)
number of vessels treated (00.40–00.43)
procedure on vessel bifurcation (00.44)

Excludes   *drug-coated peripheral stents, e.g., heparin coated (39.90)*
insertion of cerebrovascular stent(s) (00.63–00.65)
insertion of drug-eluting coronary artery stent (36.07)
insertion of non-drug-eluting stent(s): coronary artery (36.06)
peripheral vessel (39.90)
that for aneurysm repair (39.71–39.79)
Coding Clinic: 2002, Q4, P101-103

✖ 00.56 **Insertion or replacement of implantable pressure sensor (lead) for intracardiac or great vessel hemodynamic monitoring** ⬅

Code also any associated implantation or replacement of monitor (00.57)

Excludes   *circulatory monitoring (blood gas, arterial or venous pressure, cardiac output and coronary blood flow) (89.60–89.69)*
Coding Clinic: 2006, Q4, P119-120
MS-DRG: Refer to Part VI, Appendix E, Table 6, Lead/Device Reference Table

✖ 00.57 **Implantation or replacement of subcutaneous device for intracardiac hemodynamic or great vessel monitoring** ⬅
Implantation of monitoring device with formation of subcutaneous pocket and connection to intracardiac pressure sensor (lead)

Code also any associated insertion or replacement of implanted pressure sensor (lead) (00.56)
Coding Clinic: 2006, Q4, P119-120
MS-DRG: Refer to Part VI, Appendix E, Table 6, Lead/Device Reference Table

00.58 **Insertion of intra-aneurysm sac pressure monitoring device (intraoperative)**
Insertion of pressure sensor during endovascular repair of abdominal or thoracic aortic aneurysm(s)
Coding Clinic: 2008, Q4, P163-165

00.59 **Intravascular pressure measurement of coronary arteries**

Includes   fractional flow reserve (FFR)

Code also any synchronous diagnostic or therapeutic procedures

Excludes   *intravascular pressure measurement of intrathoracic arteries (00.67)*
Coding Clinic: 2008, Q4, P163-165

● 00.6 **Procedures on blood vessels**
Coding Clinic: 2004, Q4, P114-116

✖ 00.61 **Percutaneous angioplasty or atherectomy of precerebral (extracranial) vessel(s)**
Basilar
Carotid
Vertebral

Code also any:
injection or infusion of thrombolytic agent (99.10)
number of vascular stents inserted (00.45–00.48)
number of vessels treated (00.40–00.43)
percutaneous insertion of carotid artery stent(s) (00.63)
percutaneous insertion of other precerebral artery stent(s) (00.64)
procedure on vessel bifurcation (00.44)

Excludes   *angioplasty or atherectomy of other non-coronary vessel(s) (39.50)*
removal of cerebrovascular obstruction of vessel(s) by open approach (38.01–38.02, 38.11–38.12, 38.31–38.32, 38.41–38.42)

✖ 00.62 **Percutaneous angioplasty or atherectomy of intracranial vessel(s)**

Code also any:
injection or infusion of thrombolytic agent (99.10)
number of vascular stents inserted (00.45–00.48)
number of vessels treated (00.40–00.43)
percutaneous insertion of intracranial stent(s) (00.65)
procedure on vessel bifurcation (00.44)

Excludes   *angioplasty or atherectomy of other non-coronary vessel(s) (39.50)*
removal of cerebrovascular obstruction of vessel(s) by open approach (38.01–38.02, 38.11–38.12, 38.31–38.32, 38.41–38.42)
MCE: Non-covered procedure except when combined with 00.65

00.63 **Percutaneous insertion of carotid artery stent(s)**
Includes the use of any embolic protection device, distal protection device, filter device, or stent delivery system
Non-drug-eluting stent

Code also any:
number of vascular stents inserted (00.45–00.48)
number of vessels treated (00.40–00.43)
percutaneous angioplasty or atherectomy of precerebral vessel(s) (00.61)
procedure on vessel bifurcation (00.44)

Excludes   *angioplasty or atherectomy of other non-coronary vessel(s) (39.50)*
insertion of drug-eluting peripheral vessel stent(s) (00.55)
◆ Non-OR Procedure that affects MS-DRG assignment to MDC 01, MS-DRG 034-036

PROCEDURES AND INTERVENTIONS, NEC (00)

00.64 **Percutaneous insertion of other precerebral (extracranial) artery stent(s)**
Includes the use of any embolic protection device, distal protection device, filter device, or stent delivery system
Basilar stent
Vertebral stent

Code also any:
number of vascular stents inserted (00.45–00.48)
number of vessels treated (00.40–00.43)
percutaneous angioplasty or atherectomy of precerebral vessel(s) (00.61)
procedure on vessel bifurcation (00.44)

Excludes   *angioplasty or atherectomy of other non-coronary vessel(s) (39.50)*
insertion of drug-eluting peripheral vessel stent(s) (00.55)

00.65 **Percutaneous insertion of intracranial vascular stent(s)**
Includes the use of any embolic protection device, distal protection device, filter device, or stent delivery system

Code also any:
number of vascular stents inserted (00.45–00.48)
number of vessels treated (00.40–00.43)
percutaneous angioplasty or atherectomy of intracranial vessel(s) (00.62)
procedure on vessel bifurcation (00.44)

Excludes   *angioplasty or atherectomy of other non-coronary vessel(s) (39.50)*
insertion of drug-eluting peripheral vessel stent(s) (00.55)

✖ 00.66 **Percutaneous transluminal coronary angioplasty [PTCA] or coronary atherectomy**
Balloon angioplasty of coronary artery
Coronary atherectomy
Percutaneous coronary angioplasty NOS
PTCA NOS

Code also any:
injection or infusion of thrombolytic agent (99.10)
insertion of coronary artery stent(s) (36.06–36.07)
intracoronary artery thrombolytic infusion (36.04)
number of vascular stents inserted (00.45–00.48)
number of vessels treated (00.40–00.43)
procedure on vessel bifurcation (00.44)
SuperSaturated oxygen therapy (00.49)
Coding Clinic: 2009, Q2, P12; 2007, Q1, P17; 2006, Q3, P8-9; 2005, Q4, 69-72, P101-103; 2004, Q1, P10; Q2, P3

00.67 **Intravascular pressure measurement of intrathoracic arteries**
Assessment of:
aorta and aortic arch
carotid

Code also any synchronous diagnostic or therapeutic procedures
Coding Clinic: 2008, Q4, P163-165

00.68 **Intravascular pressure measurement of peripheral arteries**
Other peripheral vessels
Vessels of arm(s)
Vessels of leg(s)

Code also any synchronous diagnostic or therapeutic procedures
Coding Clinic: 2008, Q4, P163-165

00.69 **Intravascular pressure measurement, other specified and unspecified vessels**
Iliac vessels
Intra-abdominal vessels
Mesenteric vessels
Renal vessels

Code also any synchronous diagnostic or therapeutic procedures

Excludes   *intravascular pressure measurement of:*
coronary arteries (00.59)
intrathoracic arteries (00.67)
peripheral arteries (00.68)
Coding Clinic: 2008, Q4, P163-165

● 00.7 **Other hip procedures**
Coding Clinic: 2005, Q4, P106-113

✖ 00.70 **Revision of hip replacement, both acetabular and femoral components**
Total hip revision

Code also any:
removal of (cement) (joint) spacer (84.57)
type of bearing surface, if known (00.74–00.77)

Excludes   *revision of hip replacement, acetabular component only (00.71)*
revision of hip replacement, femoral component only (00.72)
revision of hip replacement, Not Otherwise Specified (81.53)
revision with replacement of acetabular liner and/or femoral head only (00.73)
Coding Clinic: 2008, Q2, P3-4; 2008, Q1, P6; 2005, Q4, P110-112

MCE: Bilateral procedure when 2+ different joint procedures are reported with principal diagnosis causes assigned to MDC 8

✖ 00.71 **Revision of hip replacement, acetabular component**
Partial, acetabular component only
That with:
exchange of acetabular cup and liner
exchange of femoral head

Code also any type of bearing surface, if known (00.74–00.77)

Excludes   *revision of hip replacement, both acetabular and femoral components (00.70)*
revision of hip replacement, femoral component (00.72)
revision of hip replacement, Not Otherwise Specified (81.53)
revision with replacement of acetabular liner and/or femoral head only (00.73)
Coding Clinic: 2005, Q4, P110-112

◄ New   ◄ Revised   ~~deleted~~ Deleted   ● Use Additional Digit(s)   ✖ Valid O.R. Procedure
◆ Non-O.R. Procedure   ♀ Females Only   ♂ Males Only

✖ **00.72** **Revision of hip replacement, femoral component**
Partial, femoral component only
That with:
    exchange of acetabular liner
    exchange of femoral stem and head

Code also any type of bearing surface, if known (00.74–00.77)

Excludes | *revision of hip replacement, acetabular component (00.71)*
revision of hip replacement, both acetabular and femoral components (00.70)
revision of hip replacement, not otherwise specified (81.53)
revision with replacement of acetabular liner and/or femoral head only (00.73)

✖ **00.73** **Revision of hip replacement, acetabular liner and/or femoral head only**

Code also any type of bearing surface, if known (00.74–00.77)

00.74 **Hip bearing surface, metal on polyethylene**

00.75 **Hip bearing surface, metal-on-metal**
Coding Clinic: 2006, Q4, P120-121

00.76 **Hip bearing surface, ceramic-on-ceramic**
Coding Clinic: 2005, Q4, P110-112

00.77 **Hip bearing surface, ceramic-on-polyethylene**

● **00.8** **Other knee and hip procedures**
Note: Report up to two components using 00.81–00.83 to describe revision of knee replacements. If all three components are revised, report 00.80.
Coding Clinic: 2005, Q4, P113-117

✖ **00.80** **Revision of knee replacement, total (all components)**
Replacement of femoral, tibial, and patellar components (all components)

Code also any removal of (cement) (joint) spacer (84.57)

Excludes | *revision of only one or two components (tibial, femoral or patellar component) (00.81–00.84)*
Coding Clinic: 2008, Q1, P6
MCE: Bilateral procedure when 2+ different joint procedures are reported with principal diagnosis causes assigned to MDC 9

✖ **00.81** **Revision of knee replacement, tibial component**
Replacement of tibial baseplate and tibial insert (liner)

Excludes | *revision of knee replacement, total (all components) (00.80)*
Coding Clinic: 2006, Q4, P103-104; 2005, Q4, P113-117

✖ **00.82** **Revision of knee replacement, femoral component**
That with replacement of tibial insert (liner)

Excludes | *revision of knee replacement, total (all components) (00.80)*
Coding Clinic: 2006, Q3, P9-10; 2005, Q4, P113-117

✖ **00.83** **Revision of knee replacement, patellar component**

Excludes | *revision of knee replacement, total (all components) (00.80)*

✖ **00.84** **Revision of total knee replacement, tibial insert (liner)**
Replacement of tibial insert (liner)

Excludes | *that with replacement of tibial component (tibial baseplate and liner) (00.81)*

✖ **00.85** **Resurfacing hip, total, acetabulum and femoral head**
Hip resurfacing arthroplasty, total
Coding Clinic: 2006, Q4, P121-122
MCE: Bilateral procedure when 2+ different joint procedures are reported with principal diagnosis causes assigned to MDC 9

✖ **00.86** **Resurfacing hip, partial, femoral head**
Hip resurfacing arthroplasty, NOS
Hip resurfacing arthroplasty, partial, femoral head

Excludes | *that with resurfacing of acetabulum (00.85)*

MCE: Bilateral procedure when 2+ different joint procedures are reported with principal diagnosis causes assigned to MDC 9

✖ **00.87** **Resurfacing hip, partial, acetabulum**
Hip resurfacing arthroplasty, partial, acetabulum

Excludes | *that with resurfacing of femoral head (00.85)*

MCE: Bilateral procedure when 2+ different joint procedures are reported with principal diagnosis causes assigned to MDC 9

● **00.9** **Other procedures and interventions**

00.91 **Transplant from live related donor**

Code also organ transplant procedure

00.92 **Transplant from live non-related donor**

Code also organ transplant procedure
Coding Clinic: 2008, Q2, P8-9; 2004, Q4, P116-117

00.93 **Transplant from cadaver**

Code also organ transplant procedure

00.94 **Intra-operative neurophysiologic monitoring**
Intra-operative neurophysiologic testing
IOM
Nerve monitoring
Neuromonitoring

Includes | Cranial nerve, peripheral nerve and spinal cord testing performed intra-operatively

Excludes | *brain temperature monitoring (01.17)*
intracranial oxygen monitoring (01.16)
intracranial pressure monitoring (01.10)
plethysmogram (89.58)
Coding Clinic: 2009, Q2, P4; 2007, Q4, P104-105

Excludes   Includes   Use additional   Code also   Omit code

PROCEDURES AND INTERVENTIONS, NEC (00)

(See Plates 86, 118, 472, 473, 500, 501, 502, 544, and 545 on pages NAP-6–NAP-14.)

1. OPERATIONS ON THE NERVOUS SYSTEM (01–05)

● **01 Incision and excision of skull, brain, and cerebral meninges**

  ● **01.0 Cranial puncture**

    01.01 Cisternal puncture
Cisternal tap

      Excludes   *pneumocisternogram (87.02)*

    01.02 Ventriculopuncture through previously implanted catheter
Puncture of ventricular shunt tubing

    01.09 Other cranial puncture
Aspiration of:
   subarachnoid space
   subdural space
Cranial aspiration NOS
Puncture of anterior fontanel
Subdural tap (through fontanel)
Coding Clinic: 2007, Q4, P105-107

  ● **01.1 Diagnostic procedures on skull, brain, and cerebral meninges**

    01.10 Intracranial pressure monitoring

      Includes   insertion of catheter or probe for monitoring
Coding Clinic: 2007, Q4, P105-107

    01.11 Closed [percutaneous] [needle] biopsy of cerebral meninges
Burr hole approach
MCE: Closed biopsy procedure

    ✖ **01.12 Open biopsy of cerebral meninges**
MCE: Open biopsy procedure

    01.13 Closed [percutaneous] [needle] biopsy of brain
Burr hole approach
Stereotactic method
Coding Clinic: 1987, Mar-April, P9
MCE: Closed biopsy procedure

    ✖ **01.14 Open biopsy of brain**
MCE: Open biopsy procedure

    ✖ **01.15 Biopsy of skull**

    01.16 Intracranial oxygen monitoring
Partial pressure of brain oxygen (PbtO$_2$)

      Includes   insertion of catheter or probe for monitoring
Coding Clinic: 2007, Q4, P105-107

    01.17 Brain temperature monitoring

      Includes   insertion of catheter or probe for monitoring
Coding Clinic: 2007, Q4, P105-107

    ✖ **01.18 Other diagnostic procedures on brain and cerebral meninges**

      Excludes   *brain temperature monitoring (01.17)*
cerebral:
  arteriography (88.41)
  thermography (88.81)
contrast radiogram of brain (87.01–87.02)
echoencephalogram (88.71)
electroencephalogram (89.14)
intracranial oxygen monitoring (01.16)
intracranial pressure monitoring (01.10)
microscopic examination of specimen from nervous system and of spinal fluid (90.01–90.09)
neurologic examination (89.13)
phlebography of head and neck (88.61)
pneumoencephalogram (87.01)
radioisotope scan:
  cerebral (92.11)
  head NEC (92.12)
tomography of head:
  C.A.T. scan (87.03)
  other (87.04)
Coding Clinic: 1998, Q3, P12-13

    ✖ **01.19 Other diagnostic procedures on skull**

      Excludes   *transillumination of skull (89.16)*
x-ray of skull (87.17)

  ● **01.2 Craniotomy and craniectomy**

      Excludes   *decompression of skull fracture (02.02)*
exploration of orbit (16.01–16.09)
that as operative approach – omit code

    ✖ **01.21 Incision and drainage of cranial sinus**

    ✖ **01.22 Removal of intracranial neurostimulator lead(s)**

      Code also any removal of neurostimulator pulse generator (86.05)

      Excludes   *removal with synchronous replacement (02.93)*

    ✖ **01.23 Reopening of craniotomy site**

    ✖ **01.24 Other craniotomy**
Cranial:
  decompression
  exploration
  trephination
Craniotomy NOS
Craniotomy with removal of:
  epidural abscess
  extradural hematoma
  foreign body of skull

      Excludes   *removal of foreign body with incision into brain (01.39)*
Coding Clinic: 1991, Q1, P14; 1984, July-Aug, P20

    ✖ **01.25 Other craniectomy**
Debridement of skull NOS
Sequestrectomy of skull

      Excludes   *debridement of compound fracture of skull (02.02)*
strip craniectomy (02.01)
Coding Clinic: 2006, Q1, P6

OPERATIONS ON THE NERVOUS SYSTEM (01–05)

◀ New   ◀▓ Revised   ~~deleted~~ Deleted   ● Use Additional Digit(s)   ✖ Valid O.R. Procedure
◆ Non-O.R. Procedure   ♀ Females Only   ♂ Males Only

01.26   Insertion of catheter(s) into cranial cavity or tissue

> Code also any concomitant procedure (e.g. resection (01.59))

> | Excludes | placement of intracerebral catheter(s) via burr hole(s) (01.28)

> Coding Clinic: 2005, Q4, P117-119

01.27   Removal of catheter(s) from cranial cavity or tissue

> Coding Clinic: 2005, Q4, P117-119

✖ 01.28   Placement of intracerebral catheter(s) via burr hole(s)

> Convection enhanced delivery
> Stereotactic placement of intracerebral catheter(s)

> Code also infusion of medication

> | Excludes | insertion of catheter(s) into cranial cavity or tissue(s) (01.26)

> Coding Clinic: 2006, Q4, P122-123

● **01.3   Incision of brain and cerebral meninges**

  ✖ 01.31   Incision of cerebral meninges

> Drainage of:
>   intracranial hygroma
>   subarachnoid abscess (cerebral)
>   subdural empyema

  ✖ 01.32   Lobotomy and tractotomy

> Division of:
>   brain tissue
>   cerebral tracts
> Percutaneous (radiofrequency) cingulotomy

  ✖ 01.39   Other incision of brain

> Amygdalohippocampotomy
> Drainage of intracerebral hematoma
> Incision of brain NOS

> | Excludes | division of cortical adhesions (02.91)

● **01.4   Operations on thalamus and globus pallidus**

  ✖ 01.41   Operations on thalamus

> Chemothalamectomy
> Thalamotomy

> | Excludes | that by stereotactic radiosurgery (92.30–92.39)

  ✖ 01.42   Operations on globus pallidus

> Pallidoansectomy
> Pallidotomy

> | Excludes | that by stereotactic radiosurgery (92.30–92.39)

● **01.5   Other excision or destruction of brain and meninges**

  ✖ 01.51   Excision of lesion or tissue of cerebral meninges

> Decortication of (cerebral) meninges
> Resection of (cerebral) meninges
> Stripping of subdural membrane of (cerebral) meninges

> | Excludes | biopsy of cerebral meninges (01.11–01.12)

  ✖ 01.52   Hemispherectomy

  ✖ 01.53   Lobectomy of brain

✖ 01.59   Other excision or destruction of lesion or tissue of brain

> Curettage of brain
> Debridement of brain
> Marsupialization of brain cyst
> Transtemporal (mastoid) excision of brain tumor

> | Excludes | biopsy of brain (01.13–01.14)
> laser interstitial therapy [LITT] of lesion or tissue of brain under guidance 17.61 ◀
> that by stereotactic radiosurgery (92.30–92.39)

> Coding Clinic: 2005, Q4, P117-119; 1999, Q3, P7-8; Q1, P9-10; 1998, Q3, P12-13; Q1, P6-7; 1993, Q4, P33

✖ 01.6   Excision of lesion of skull

> Removal of granulation tissue of cranium

> | Excludes | biopsy of skull (01.15)
> sequestrectomy (01.25)

● **02   Other operations on skull, brain, and cerebral meninges**

● **02.0   Cranioplasty**

> | Excludes | that with synchronous repair of encephalocele (02.12)

  ✖ 02.01   Opening of cranial suture

> Linear craniectomy
> Strip craniectomy

  ✖ 02.02   Elevation of skull fracture fragments

> Debridement of compound fracture of skull
> Decompression of skull fracture
> Reduction of skull fracture

> Code also any synchronous debridement of brain (01.59)

> | Excludes | debridement of skull NOS (01.25)
> removal of granulation tissue of cranium (01.6)

  ✖ 02.03   Formation of cranial bone flap

> Repair of skull with flap

  ✖ 02.04   Bone graft to skull

> Pericranial graft (autogenous) (heterogenous)

  ✖ 02.05   Insertion of skull plate

> Replacement of skull plate

  ✖ 02.06   Other cranial osteoplasty

> Repair of skull NOS
> Revision of bone flap of skull
> Coding Clinic: 2006, Q1, P6-7; 2005, Q1, P11; 1998, Q3, P9-10

  ✖ 02.07   Removal of skull plate

> | Excludes | removal with synchronous replacement (02.05)

● **02.1   Repair of cerebral meninges**

> | Excludes | marsupialization of cerebral lesion (01.59)

  ✖ 02.11   Simple suture of dura mater of brain

  ✖ 02.12   Other repair of cerebral meninges

> Closure of fistula of cerebrospinal fluid
> Dural graft
> Repair of encephalocele including synchronous cranioplasty
> Repair of meninges NOS
> Subdural patch

  ✖ 02.13   Ligation of meningeal vessel

> Ligation of:
>   longitudinal sinus
>   middle meningeal artery

  ✖ 02.14   Choroid plexectomy

> Cauterization of choroid plexus

OPERATIONS ON THE NERVOUS SYSTEM (01–05)

✖ 02.2 Ventriculostomy
Anastomosis of ventricle to:
   cervical subarachnoid space
   cisterna magna
Insertion of Holter valve
Ventriculocisternal intubation

● 02.3 Extracranial ventricular shunt
> **Includes**   that with insertion of valve
> Coding Clinic: 1985, Sept-Oct, P12

✖ 02.31 Ventricular shunt to structure in head and neck
Ventricle to nasopharynx shunt
Ventriculomastoid anastomosis
Coding Clinic: 2004, Q4, P111-113

✖ 02.32 Ventricular shunt to circulatory system
Ventriculoatrial anastomosis
Ventriculocaval shunt

✖ 02.33 Ventricular shunt to thoracic cavity
Ventriculopleural anastomosis

✖ 02.34 Ventricular shunt to abdominal cavity and organs
Ventriculocholecystostomy
Ventriculoperitoneostomy

✖ 02.35 Ventricular shunt to urinary system
Ventricle to ureter shunt

✖ 02.39 Other operations to establish drainage of ventricle
Ventricle to bone marrow shunt
Ventricular shunt to extracranial site NEC

● 02.4 Revision, removal, and irrigation of ventricular shunt
> **Excludes** revision of distal catheter of ventricular shunt (54.95)

02.41 Irrigation and exploration of ventricular shunt
Exploration of ventriculoperitoneal shunt at ventricular site
Re-programming of ventriculoperitoneal shunt

✖ 02.42 Replacement of ventricular shunt
Reinsertion of Holter valve
Replacement of ventricular catheter
Revision of ventriculoperitoneal shunt at ventricular site

✖ 02.43 Removal of ventricular shunt

● 02.9 Other operations on skull, brain, and cerebral meninges
> **Excludes** operations on:
>   pineal gland (07.17, 07.51–07.59)
>   pituitary gland [hypophysis] (07.13–07.15, 07.61–07.79)

✖ 02.91 Lysis of cortical adhesions

✖ 02.92 Repair of brain

✖ 02.93 Implantation or replacement of intracranial neurostimulator lead(s)
Implantation, insertion, placement, or replacement of intracranial:
  brain pacemaker [neuropacemaker]
  depth electrodes
  epidural pegs
  electroencephalographic receiver
  foramen ovale electrodes
  intracranial electrostimulator
  subdural grids
  subdural strips
> Code also any insertion of neurostimulator pulse generator (86.94–86.98)

✖ 02.94 Insertion or replacement of skull tongs or halo traction device
Coding Clinic: 2001, Q3, P8; 1996, Q3, P14

02.95 Removal of skull tongs or halo traction device

02.96 Insertion of sphenoidal electrodes

✖ 02.99 Other
> **Excludes** chemical shock therapy (94.24)
>   electroshock therapy:
>   subconvulsive (94.26)
>   other (94.27)

● 03 Operations on spinal cord and spinal canal structures
> Code also any application or administration of an adhesion barrier substance (99.77)

● 03.0 Exploration and decompression of spinal canal structures

✖ 03.01 Removal of foreign body from spinal canal

✖ 03.02 Reopening of laminectomy site

✖ 03.09 Other exploration and decompression of spinal canal
Decompression:
  laminectomy
  laminotomy
Expansile laminoplasty
Exploration of spinal nerve root
Foraminotomy
> Code also any synchronous insertion, replacement and revision of posterior spinal motion preservation device(s), if performed (84.80–84.85)
> **Excludes** drainage of spinal fluid by anastomosis (03.71–03.79)
>   laminectomy with excision of intervertebral disc (80.51)
>   spinal tap (03.31)
>   that as operative approach – omit code

Coding Clinic: 2008, Q4, P109-110; Q2, P12; 2007, Q4, P116-120; Q1, P10; 2004, Q3, P6-7; 2002, Q4, P109-110; 2002, Q2, P15; 1999, Q4, P13-14; 1995, Q2, P9-10; 1990, 1997, Q2, P6; Q2, P23

✖ 03.1 Division of intraspinal nerve root
Rhizotomy

● 03.2 Chordotomy

✖ 03.21 Percutaneous chordotomy
Stereotactic chordotomy

✖ 03.29 Other chordotomy
Chordotomy NOS
Tractotomy (one-stage) (two-stage) of spinal cord
Transection of spinal cord tracts

● 03.3 Diagnostic procedures on spinal cord and spinal canal structures

03.31 Spinal tap
Lumbar puncture for removal of dye
> **Excludes** lumbar puncture for injection of dye [myelogram] (87.21)
> Coding Clinic: 1990, Q2, P23

✖ 03.32 Biopsy of spinal cord or spinal meninges

✖ 03.39 Other diagnostic procedures on spinal cord and spinal canal structures
> **Excludes** microscopic examination of specimen from nervous system or of spinal fluid (90.01–90.09)
>   x-ray of spine (87.21–87.29)

OPERATIONS ON THE NERVOUS SYSTEM (01–05)

◀ New   ◀▮▮ Revised   ~~deleted~~ Deleted   ● Use Additional Digit(s)   ✖ Valid O.R. Procedure
◆ Non-O.R. Procedure   ♀ Females Only   ♂ Males Only

✖ **03.4 Excision or destruction of lesion of spinal cord or spinal meninges**
Curettage of spinal cord or spinal meninges
Debridement of spinal cord or spinal meninges
Marsupialization of cyst of spinal cord or spinal meninges
Resection of spinal cord or spinal meninges

Excludes | *biopsy of spinal cord or meninges (03.32)*

Coding Clinic: 2008, Q2, P10; 1995, Q3, P5-6

● **03.5 Plastic operations on spinal cord structures**

✖ **03.51 Repair of spinal meningocele**
Repair of meningocele NOS

✖ **03.52 Repair of spinal myelomeningocele**

✖ **03.53 Repair of vertebral fracture**
Elevation of spinal bone fragments
Reduction of fracture of vertebrae
Removal of bony spicules from spinal canal

Excludes | *percutaneous vertebral augmentation (81.66)*
percutaneous vertebroplasty (81.65)

Coding Clinic: 2007, Q1, P20-21; 2004, Q4, P125-126; 2003, Q2, P22; 2002, Q2, P14; 1999, Q4, P12-13; 1996, Q3, P14

✖ **03.59 Other repair and plastic operations on spinal cord structures**
Repair of:
diastematomyelia
spina bifida NOS
spinal cord NOS
spinal meninges NOS
vertebral arch defect
Coding Clinic: 2008, Q4, P109-110

✖ **03.6 Lysis of adhesions of spinal cord and nerve roots**
Coding Clinic: 1998, Q2, P18

● **03.7 Shunt of spinal theca**

Includes | that with valve

✖ **03.71 Spinal subarachnoid-peritoneal shunt**

✖ **03.72 Spinal subarachnoid-ureteral shunt**

✖ **03.79 Other shunt of spinal theca**
Lumbar-subarachnoid shunt NOS
Pleurothecal anastomosis
Salpingothecal anastomosis
Coding Clinic: 1997, Q1, P7

03.8 Injection of destructive agent into spinal canal
Coding Clinic: 2003, Q2, P6

● **03.9 Other operations on spinal cord and spinal canal structures**

03.90 Insertion of catheter into spinal canal for infusion of therapeutic or palliative substances
Insertion of catheter into epidural, subarachnoid, or subdural space of spine with intermittent or continuous infusion of drug (with creation of any reservoir)

Code also any implantation of infusion pump (86.06)

03.91 Injection of anesthetic into spinal canal for analgesia

Excludes | *that for operative anesthesia — omit code*

Coding Clinic: 2000, Q3, P15; 1999, Q1, P7-8; 1998, Q2, P18; 1985, Mar-April, P15; 1984, May-June, P14; 1984, July-Aug, P20

03.92 Injection of other agent into spinal canal
Intrathecal injection of steroid
Subarachnoid perfusion of refrigerated saline

Excludes | *injection of:*
contrast material for myelogram (87.21)
destructive agent into spinal canal (03.8)

Coding Clinic: 2003, Q2, P6; 2000, Q3, P15; 1998, Q2, P18

✖ **03.93 Implantation or replacement of spinal neurostimulator lead(s)**

Code also any insertion of neurostimulator pulse generator (86.94–86.98)
Coding Clinic: 2000, Q1, P19-20

✖ **03.94 Removal of spinal neurostimulator lead(s)**

Code also any removal of neurostimulator pulse generator (86.05)

03.95 Spinal blood patch

03.96 Percutaneous denervation of facet

✖ **03.97 Revision of spinal thecal shunt**
Coding Clinic: 1999, Q2, P4

✖ **03.98 Removal of spinal thecal shunt**

✖ **03.99 Other**
Coding Clinic: 1985, Mar-April, P15; 1984, May-June, P14; 1984, July-Aug, P20

● **04 Operations on cranial and peripheral nerves**

● **04.0 Incision, division, and excision of cranial and peripheral nerves**

Excludes | *opticociliary neurectomy (12.79)*
sympathetic ganglionectomy (05.21–05.29)

✖ **04.01 Excision of acoustic neuroma**
That by craniotomy

Excludes | *that by stereotactic radiosurgery (92.30–92.39)*

Coding Clinic: 1998, Q2, P20; 1995, Q2, P8

✖ **04.02 Division of trigeminal nerve**
Retrogasserian neurotomy

✖ **04.03 Division or crushing of other cranial and peripheral nerves**

Excludes | *that of:*
glossopharyngeal nerve (29.92)
laryngeal nerve (31.91)
nerves to adrenal glands (07.42)
phrenic nerve for collapse of lung (33.31)
vagus nerve (44.00–44.03)

Coding Clinic: 1998, Q2, P20

✖ **04.04 Other incision of cranial and peripheral nerves**

✖ **04.05 Gasserian ganglionectomy**

✖ **04.06 Other cranial or peripheral ganglionectomy**

Excludes | *sympathetic ganglionectomy (05.21–05.29)*

✖ **04.07 Other excision or avulsion of cranial and peripheral nerves**
Curettage of peripheral nerve
Debridement of peripheral nerve
Resection of peripheral nerve
Excision of peripheral neuroma [Morton's]

Excludes | *biopsy of cranial or peripheral nerve (04.11–04.12)*

Coding Clinic: 1995, Q2, P8

OPERATIONS ON THE NERVOUS SYSTEM (01–05)

Excludes   Includes   Use additional   Code also   Omit code

OPERATIONS ON THE NERVOUS SYSTEM (01–05)

● 04.1 Diagnostic procedures on peripheral nervous system

04.11 Closed [percutaneous] [needle] biopsy of cranial or peripheral nerve or ganglion
MCE: Closed biopsy procedure

✖ 04.12 Open biopsy of cranial or peripheral nerve or ganglion
MCE: Open biopsy procedure

✖ 04.19 Other diagnostic procedures on cranial and peripheral nerves and ganglia

Excludes microscopic examination of specimen from nervous system (90.01–90.09)
neurologic examination (89.13)

04.2 Destruction of cranial and peripheral nerves
Destruction of cranial or peripheral nerves by:
cryoanalgesia
injection of neurolytic agent
radiofrequency
Radiofrequency ablation
Coding Clinic: 2002, Q3, P10-11

✖ 04.3 Suture of cranial and peripheral nerves

● 04.4 Lysis of adhesions and decompression of cranial and peripheral nerves

✖ 04.41 Decompression of trigeminal nerve root

✖ 04.42 Other cranial nerve decompression
Coding Clinic: 2002, Q3, P11-13; 1987, Mar-April, P8

✖ 04.43 Release of carpal tunnel
Coding Clinic: 1985, Nov-Dec, P11

✖ 04.44 Release of tarsal tunnel

✖ 04.49 Other peripheral nerve or ganglion decompression or lysis of adhesions
Peripheral nerve neurolysis NOS
Coding Clinic: 1993, Q2, P8

✖ 04.5 Cranial or peripheral nerve graft

✖ 04.6 Transposition of cranial and peripheral nerves
Nerve transplantation

● 04.7 Other cranial or peripheral neuroplasty

✖ 04.71 Hypoglossal-facial anastomosis

✖ 04.72 Accessory-facial anastomosis

✖ 04.73 Accessory-hypoglossal anastomosis

✖ 04.74 Other anastomosis of cranial or peripheral nerve

✖ 04.75 Revision of previous repair of cranial and peripheral nerves

✖ 04.76 Repair of old traumatic injury of cranial and peripheral nerves

✖ 04.79 Other neuroplasty
Coding Clinic: 2006, Q1, P11

● 04.8 Injection into peripheral nerve

Excludes destruction of nerve (by injection of neurolytic agent) (04.2)

04.80 Peripheral nerve injection, not otherwise specified

04.81 Injection of anesthetic into peripheral nerve for analgesia

Excludes that for operative anesthesia – omit code
Coding Clinic: 2000, Q1, P7-8

04.89 Injection of other agent, except neurolytic

Excludes injection of neurolytic agent (04.2)

● 04.9 Other operations on cranial and peripheral nerves

✖ 04.91 Neurectasis

✖ 04.92 Implantation or replacement of peripheral neurostimulator lead(s)

Code also any insertion of neurostimulator pulse generator (86.94–86.98)
Coding Clinic: 2007, Q2, P10-11; 2006, Q2, P5-6; 2004, Q2, P7; 2001, Q3, P16-17; 1996, Q3, P12

✖ 04.93 Removal of peripheral neurostimulator lead(s)

Code also any removal of neurostimulator pulse generator (86.05)
Coding Clinic: 2001, Q3, P16-17

✖ 04.99 Other

● 05 Operations on sympathetic nerves or ganglia

Excludes paracervical uterine denervation (69.3)

✖ 05.0 Division of sympathetic nerve or ganglion

Excludes that of nerves to adrenal glands (07.42)

● 05.1 Diagnostic procedures on sympathetic nerves or ganglia
Coding Clinic: 2006, Q2, P7

✖ 05.11 Biopsy of sympathetic nerve or ganglion

✖ 05.19 Other diagnostic procedures on sympathetic nerves or ganglia

● 05.2 Sympathectomy

✖ 05.21 Sphenopalatine ganglionectomy

✖ 05.22 Cervical sympathectomy

✖ 05.23 Lumbar sympathectomy

✖ 05.24 Presacral sympathectomy

✖ 05.25 Periarterial sympathectomy

✖ 05.29 Other sympathectomy and ganglionectomy
Excision or avulsion of sympathetic nerve NOS
Sympathetic ganglionectomy NOS

Excludes biopsy of sympathetic nerve or ganglion (05.11)
opticociliary neurectomy (12.79)
periarterial sympathectomy (05.25)
tympanosympathectomy (20.91)

● 05.3 Injection into sympathetic nerve or ganglion

Excludes injection of ciliary sympathetic ganglion (12.79)

05.31 Injection of anesthetic into sympathetic nerve for analgesia

05.32 Injection of neurolytic agent into sympathetic nerve

05.39 Other injection into sympathetic nerve or ganglion

● 05.8 Other operations on sympathetic nerves or ganglia

✖ 05.81 Repair of sympathetic nerve or ganglion

✖ 05.89 Other

✖ 05.9 Other operations on nervous system

◀ New   ◀⁞⁞ Revised   deleted Deleted   ● Use Additional Digit(s)   ✖ Valid O.R. Procedure
◆ Non-O.R. Procedure   ♀ Females Only   ♂ Males Only

2.   OPERATIONS ON THE ENDOCRINE SYSTEM (06–07)

● 06   **Operations on thyroid and parathyroid glands**

> **Includes**   incidental resection of hyoid bone

● 06.0   **Incision of thyroid field**

> **Excludes**   *division of isthmus (06.91)*

06.01   **Aspiration of thyroid field**
Percutaneous or needle drainage of thyroid field

> **Excludes**   *aspiration biopsy of thyroid (06.11)*
> *drainage by incision (06.09)*
> *postoperative aspiration of field (06.02)*

✖ 06.02   **Reopening of wound of thyroid field**
Reopening of wound of thyroid field for:
control of (postoperative) hemorrhage
examination
exploration
removal of hematoma

✖ 06.09   **Other incision of thyroid field**
Drainage of hematoma by incision
Drainage of thyroglossal tract by incision
Exploration:
neck by incision
thyroid (field) by incision
Removal of foreign body by incision
Thyroidotomy NOS by incision

> **Excludes**   *postoperative exploration (06.02)*
> *removal of hematoma by aspiration (06.01)*

● 06.1   **Diagnostic procedures on thyroid and parathyroid glands**

06.11   **Closed [percutaneous] [needle] biopsy of thyroid gland**
Aspiration biopsy of thyroid
MCE: Closed biopsy procedure

✖ 06.12   **Open biopsy of thyroid gland**
MCE: Open biopsy procedure

✖ 06.13   **Biopsy of parathyroid gland**

✖ 06.19   **Other diagnostic procedures on thyroid and parathyroid glands**

> **Excludes**   *radioisotope scan of:*
> *parathyroid (92.13)*
> *thyroid (92.01)*
> *soft tissue x-ray of thyroid field (87.09)*

✖ 06.2   **Unilateral thyroid lobectomy**
Complete removal of one lobe of thyroid (with removal of isthmus or portion of other lobe)
Hemithyroidectomy

> **Excludes**   *partial substernal thyroidectomy (06.51)*

● 06.3   **Other partial thyroidectomy**

✖ 06.31   **Excision of lesion of thyroid**

> **Excludes**   *biopsy of thyroid (06.11–06.12)*
> *laser interstitial thermal therapy [LITT] of lesion or tissue at neck under guidance (17.62)* ◀

✖ 06.39   **Other**
Isthmectomy
Partial thyroidectomy NOS

> **Excludes**   *partial substernal thyroidectomy (06.51)*

✖ 06.4   **Complete thyroidectomy**

> **Excludes**   *complete substernal thyroidectomy (06.52)*
> *that with laryngectomy (30.3–30.4)*

● 06.5   **Substernal thyroidectomy**

✖ 06.50   **Substernal thyroidectomy, not otherwise specified**

✖ 06.51   **Partial substernal thyroidectomy**

✖ 06.52   **Complete substernal thyroidectomy**

✖ 06.6   **Excision of lingual thyroid**
Excision of thyroid by:
submental route
transoral route

✖ 06.7   **Excision of thyroglossal duct or tract**

● 06.8   **Parathyroidectomy**

✖ 06.81   **Complete parathyroidectomy**

✖ 06.89   **Other parathyroidectomy**
Parathyroidectomy NOS
Partial parathyroidectomy

> **Excludes**   *biopsy of parathyroid (06.13)*

● 06.9   **Other operations on thyroid (region) and parathyroid**

✖ 06.91   **Division of thyroid isthmus**
Transection of thyroid isthmus

✖ 06.92   **Ligation of thyroid vessels**

✖ 06.93   **Suture of thyroid gland**

✖ 06.94   **Thyroid tissue reimplantation**
Autotransplantation of thyroid tissue

✖ 06.95   **Parathyroid tissue reimplantation**
Autotransplantation of parathyroid tissue
Coding Clinic: 1995, Q1, P9

✖ 06.98   **Other operations on thyroid glands**

✖ 06.99   **Other operations on parathyroid glands**

● 07   **Operations on other endocrine glands**

> **Includes**   operations on:
> adrenal glands
> pineal gland
> pituitary gland
> thymus

> **Excludes**   *operations on:*
> *aortic and carotid bodies (39.8)*
> *ovaries (65.0–65.99)*
> *pancreas (52.01–52.99)*
> *testes (62.0–62.99)*

● 07.0   **Exploration of adrenal field**

> **Excludes**   *incision of adrenal (gland) (07.41)*

✖ 07.00   **Exploration of adrenal field, not otherwise specified**

✖ 07.01   **Unilateral exploration of adrenal field**

✖ 07.02   **Bilateral exploration of adrenal field**

● 07.1   **Diagnostic procedures on adrenal glands, pituitary gland, pineal gland, and thymus**

07.11   **Closed [percutaneous] [needle] biopsy of adrenal gland**
MCE: Closed biopsy procedure

✖ 07.12   **Open biopsy of adrenal gland**
MCE: Open biopsy procedure

✖ 07.13   **Biopsy of pituitary gland, transfrontal approach**

✖ 07.14   **Biopsy of pituitary gland, transsphenoidal approach**

✖ 07.15   **Biopsy of pituitary gland, unspecified approach**

✖ 07.16   **Biopsy of thymus**

✖ 07.17   **Biopsy of pineal gland**

✖ 07.19   **Other diagnostic procedures on adrenal glands, pituitary gland, pineal gland, and thymus**

> **Excludes**   *microscopic examination of specimen from endocrine gland (90.11–90.19)*
> *radioisotope scan of pituitary gland (92.11)*

● **07.2 Partial adrenalectomy**
  ✖ **07.21 Excision of lesion of adrenal gland**
       Excludes *biopsy of adrenal gland (07.11–07.12)*
  ✖ **07.22 Unilateral adrenalectomy**
       Adrenalectomy NOS
       Excludes *excision of remaining adrenal gland (07.3)*
  ✖ **07.29 Other partial adrenalectomy**
       Partial adrenalectomy NOS
       Coding Clinic: 2005, Q2, P4-5
✖ **07.3 Bilateral adrenalectomy**
     Excision of remaining adrenal gland
     Excludes *bilateral partial adrenalectomy (07.29)*
● **07.4 Other operations on adrenal glands, nerves, and vessels**
  ✖ **07.41 Incision of adrenal gland**
       Adrenalotomy (with drainage)
  ✖ **07.42 Division of nerves to adrenal glands**
  ✖ **07.43 Ligation of adrenal vessels**
  ✖ **07.44 Repair of adrenal gland**
  ✖ **07.45 Reimplantation of adrenal tissue**
       Autotransplantation of adrenal tissue
  ✖ **07.49 Other**
● **07.5 Operations on pineal gland**
  ✖ **07.51 Exploration of pineal field**
       Excludes *that with incision of pineal gland (07.52)*
  ✖ **07.52 Incision of pineal gland**
  ✖ **07.53 Partial excision of pineal gland**
       Excludes *biopsy of pineal gland (07.17)*
  ✖ **07.54 Total excision of pineal gland**
       Pinealectomy (complete) (total)
  ✖ **07.59 Other operations on pineal gland**
● **07.6 Hypophysectomy**
  ✖ **07.61 Partial excision of pituitary gland, transfrontal approach**
       Cryohypophysectomy, partial transfrontal approach
       Division of hypophyseal stalk transfrontal approach
       Excision of lesion of pituitary [hypophysis] transfrontal approach
       Hypophysectomy, subtotal transfrontal approach
       Infundibulectomy, hypophyseal transfrontal approach
       Excludes *biopsy of pituitary gland, transfrontal approach (07.13)*
  ✖ **07.62 Partial excision of pituitary gland, transsphenoidal approach**
       Excludes *biopsy of pituitary gland, transsphenoidal approach (07.14)*
       Coding Clinic: 1992, Q3, P13
  ✖ **07.63 Partial excision of pituitary gland, unspecified approach**
       Excludes *biopsy of pituitary gland NOS (07.15)*
  ✖ **07.64 Total excision of pituitary gland, transfrontal approach**
       Ablation of pituitary by implantation (strontium-yttrium) (Y) transfrontal approach
       Cryohypophysectomy, complete transfrontal approach

  ✖ **07.65 Total excision of pituitary gland, transsphenoidal approach**
  ✖ **07.68 Total excision of pituitary gland, other specified approach**
  ✖ **07.69 Total excision of pituitary gland, unspecified approach**
       Hypophysectomy NOS
       Pituitectomy NOS
● **07.7 Other operations on hypophysis**
  ✖ **07.71 Exploration of pituitary fossa**
       Excludes *exploration with incision of pituitary gland (07.72)*
  ✖ **07.72 Incision of pituitary gland**
       Aspiration of:
         craniobuccal pouch
         craniopharyngioma
         hypophysis
         pituitary gland
         Rathke's pouch
  ✖ **07.79 Other**
       Insertion of pack into sella turcica
● **07.8 Thymectomy**
  ✖ **07.80 Thymectomy, not otherwise specified**
  ✖ **07.81 Other partial excision of thymus**
       Open partial excision of thymus
       Excludes *biopsy of thymus (07.16)*
       thoracoscopic partial excision of thymus (07.83)
  ✖ **07.82 Other total excision of thymus**
       Open total excision of thymus
       Excludes *thoracoscopic total excision of thymus (07.84)*
  ✖ **07.83 Thoracoscopic partial excision of thymus**
       Excludes *other partial excision of thymus (07.81)*
       Coding Clinic: 2007, Q4, P108-109
  ✖ **07.84 Thoracoscopic total excision of thymus**
       Excludes *other total excision of thymus (07.82)*
       Coding Clinic: 2007, Q4, P108-109
● **07.9 Other operations on thymus**
  ✖ **07.91 Exploration of thymus field**
       Excludes *exploration with incision of thymus (07.92)*
  ✖ **07.92 Other incision of thymus**
       Open incision of thymus
       Excludes *thoracoscopic incision of thymus (07.95)*
  ✖ **07.93 Repair of thymus**
  ✖ **07.94 Transplantation of thymus**
  ✖ **07.95 Thoracoscopic incision of thymus**
       Excludes *other incision of thymus (07.92)*
       Coding Clinic: 2007, Q4, P108-109
  ✖ **07.98 Other and unspecified thoracoscopic operations on thymus**
  ✖ **07.99 Other and unspecified operations on thymus**
       Transcervical thymectomy
       Excludes *other thoracoscopic operations on thymus (07.98)*

OPERATIONS ON THE ENDOCRINE SYSTEM (06–07)

◀ New   ◀▥ Revised   ~~deleted~~ Deleted   ● Use Additional Digit(s)   ✖ Valid O.R. Procedure
◆ Non-O.R. Procedure   ♀ Females Only   ♂ Males Only

(See Plates 81, 82, 87, and 90 on pages NAP-15–NAP-19.)

03. OPERATIONS ON THE EYE (08–16)

● 08 **Operations on eyelids**

    Includes   operations on the eyebrow

● 08.0 **Incision of eyelid**

    08.01 **Incision of lid margin**

    08.02 **Severing of blepharorrhaphy**

    08.09 **Other incision of eyelid**

● 08.1 **Diagnostic procedures on eyelid**

    ✖ 08.11 **Biopsy of eyelid**

    08.19 **Other diagnostic procedures on eyelid**

● 08.2 **Excision or destruction of lesion or tissue of eyelid**

    Code also any synchronous reconstruction (08.61–08.74)

    Excludes *biopsy of eyelid (08.11)*

    ✖ 08.20 **Removal of lesion of eyelid, not otherwise specified**
        Removal of meibomian gland NOS

    ✖ 08.21 **Excision of chalazion**

    ✖ 08.22 **Excision of other minor lesion of eyelid**
        Excision of:
          verucca
          wart

    ✖ 08.23 **Excision of major lesion of eyelid, partial-thickness**
        Excision involving one-fourth or more of lid margin, partial-thickness

    ✖ 08.24 **Excision of major lesion of eyelid, full-thickness**
        Excision involving one-fourth or more of lid margin, full-thickness
        Wedge resection of eyelid

    ✖ 08.25 **Destruction of lesion of eyelid**

● 08.3 **Repair of blepharoptosis and lid retraction**

    ✖ 08.31 **Repair of blepharoptosis by frontalis muscle technique with suture**

    ✖ 08.32 **Repair of blepharoptosis by frontalis muscle technique with fascial sling**

    ✖ 08.33 **Repair of blepharoptosis by resection or advancement of levator muscle or aponeurosis**

    ✖ 08.34 **Repair of blepharoptosis by other levator muscle techniques**

    ✖ 08.35 **Repair of blepharoptosis by tarsal technique**

    ✖ 08.36 **Repair of blepharoptosis by other techniques**
        Correction of eyelid ptosis NOS
        Orbicularis oculi muscle sling for correction of blepharoptosis

    ✖ 08.37 **Reduction of overcorrection of ptosis**

    ✖ 08.38 **Correction of lid retraction**

● 08.4 **Repair of entropion or ectropion**

    ✖ 08.41 **Repair of entropion or ectropion by thermocauterization**

    ✖ 08.42 **Repair of entropion or ectropion by suture technique**

    ✖ 08.43 **Repair of entropion or ectropion with wedge resection**

    ✖ 08.44 **Repair of entropion or ectropion with lid reconstruction**

    ✖ 08.49 **Other repair of entropion or ectropion**

● 08.5 **Other adjustment of lid position**

    ✖ 08.51 **Canthotomy**
        Enlargement of palpebral fissure

    ✖ 08.52 **Blepharorrhaphy**
        Canthorrhaphy
        Tarsorrhaphy

    ✖ 08.59 **Other**
        Canthoplasty NOS
        Repair of epicanthal fold

● 08.6 **Reconstruction of eyelid with flaps or grafts**

    Excludes *that associated with repair of entropion and ectropion (08.44)*

    ✖ 08.61 **Reconstruction of eyelid with skin flap or graft**

    ✖ 08.62 **Reconstruction of eyelid with mucous membrane flap or graft**

    ✖ 08.63 **Reconstruction of eyelid with hair follicle graft**

    ✖ 08.64 **Reconstruction of eyelid with tarsoconjunctival flap**
        Transfer of tarsoconjunctival flap from opposing lid

    ✖ 08.69 **Other reconstruction of eyelid with flaps or grafts**

● 08.7 **Other reconstruction of eyelid**

    Excludes *that associated with repair of entropion and ectropion (08.44)*
    Coding Clinic: 1996, Q2, P11

    ✖ 08.70 **Reconstruction of eyelid, not otherwise specified**

    ✖ 08.71 **Reconstruction of eyelid involving lid margin, partial-thickness**

    ✖ 08.72 **Other reconstruction of eyelid, partial-thickness**

    ✖ 08.73 **Reconstruction of eyelid involving lid margin, full-thickness**

    ✖ 08.74 **Other reconstruction of eyelid, full-thickness**

● 08.8 **Other repair of eyelid**

    08.81 **Linear repair of laceration of eyelid or eyebrow**

    08.82 **Repair of laceration involving lid margin, partial-thickness**

    08.83 **Other repair of laceration of eyelid, partial-thickness**

    08.84 **Repair of laceration involving lid margin, full-thickness**

    08.85 **Other repair of laceration of eyelid, full-thickness**

    08.86 **Lower eyelid rhytidectomy**

    08.87 **Upper eyelid rhytidectomy**
        Coding Clinic: 1996, Q2, P11

    08.89 **Other eyelid repair**
        Coding Clinic: 2000, Q1, P22-23

● 08.9 **Other operations on eyelids**

    ✖ 08.91 **Electrosurgical epilation of eyelid**

    ✖ 08.92 **Cryosurgical epilation of eyelid**

    ✖ 08.93 **Other epilation of eyelid**

    ✖ 08.99 **Other**

OPERATIONS ON THE EYE (08–16)

● 09 Operations on lacrimal system

✱ 09.0 Incision of lacrimal gland
Incision of lacrimal cyst (with drainage)

● 09.1 Diagnostic procedures on lacrimal system

✱ 09.11 Biopsy of lacrimal gland

✱ 09.12 Biopsy of lacrimal sac

✱ 09.19 Other diagnostic procedures on lacrimal system
Excludes *contrast dacryocystogram (87.05)*
*soft tissue x-ray of nasolacrimal duct
(87.09)*

● 09.2 Excision of lesion or tissue of lacrimal gland

✱ 09.20 Excision of lacrimal gland, not otherwise
specified

✱ 09.21 Excision of lesion of lacrimal gland
Excludes *biopsy of lacrimal gland (09.11)*

✱ 09.22 Other partial dacryoadenectomy
Excludes *biopsy of lacrimal gland (09.11)*

✱ 09.23 Total dacryoadenectomy

✱ 09.3 Other operations on lacrimal gland

● 09.4 Manipulation of lacrimal passage
Includes removal of calculus
that with dilation
Excludes *contrast dacryocystogram (87.05)*

✱ 09.41 Probing of lacrimal punctum

✱ 09.42 Probing of lacrimal canaliculi

✱ 09.43 Probing of nasolacrimal duct
Excludes *that with insertion of tube or stent
(09.44)*

✱ 09.44 Intubation of nasolacrimal duct
Insertion of stent into nasolacrimal duct
Coding Clinic: 1994, Q2, P11

✱ 09.49 Other manipulation of lacrimal passage

● 09.5 Incision of lacrimal sac and passages

✱ 09.51 Incision of lacrimal punctum

✱ 09.52 Incision of lacrimal canaliculi

✱ 09.53 Incision of lacrimal sac

✱ 09.59 Other incision of lacrimal passages
Incision (and drainage) of nasolacrimal duct
NOS

✱ 09.6 Excision of lacrimal sac and passage
Excludes *biopsy of lacrimal sac (09.12)*

● 09.7 Repair of canaliculus and punctum
Excludes *repair of eyelid (08.81–08.89)*

✱ 09.71 Correction of everted punctum

✱ 09.72 Other repair of punctum

✱ 09.73 Repair of canaliculus

● 09.8 Fistulization of lacrimal tract to nasal cavity

✱ 09.81 Dacryocystorhinostomy [DCR]

✱ 09.82 Conjunctivocystorhinostomy
Conjunctivodacryocystorhinostomy [CDCR]
Excludes *that with insertion of tube or stent
(09.83)*

✱ 09.83 Conjunctivorhinostomy with insertion of tube
or stent

● 09.9 Other operations on lacrimal system

✱ 09.91 Obliteration of lacrimal punctum

✱ 09.99 Other
Coding Clinic: 1994, Q2, P11

● 10 Operations on conjunctiva

✱ 10.0 Removal of embedded foreign body from conjunctiva
by incision
Excludes *removal of:*
*embedded foreign body without incision
(98.22)*
superficial foreign body (98.21)

✱ 10.1 Other incision of conjunctiva

● 10.2 Diagnostic procedures on conjunctiva

✱ 10.21 Biopsy of conjunctiva

✱ 10.29 Other diagnostic procedures on conjunctiva

● 10.3 Excision or destruction of lesion or tissue of conjunctiva

✱ 10.31 Excision of lesion or tissue of conjunctiva
Excision of ring of conjunctiva around cornea
Excludes *biopsy of conjunctiva (10.21)*
Coding Clinic: 2000, Q4, P41; 1996, Q3, P7

✱ 10.32 Destruction of lesion of conjunctiva
Excludes *excision of lesion (10.31)*
*thermocauterization for entropion
(08.41)*

✱ 10.33 Other destructive procedures on conjunctiva
Removal of trachoma follicles

● 10.4 Conjunctivoplasty

✱ 10.41 Repair of symblepharon with free graft
Coding Clinic: 1996, Q3, P7

✱ 10.42 Reconstruction of conjunctival cul-de-sac with
free graft
Excludes *revision of enucleation socket with graft
(16.63)*

✱ 10.43 Other reconstruction of conjunctival cul-de-sac
Excludes *revision of enucleation socket (16.64)*

✱ 10.44 Other free graft to conjunctiva

✱ 10.49 Other conjunctivoplasty
Excludes *repair of cornea with conjunctival flap
(11.53)*

✱ 10.5 Lysis of adhesions of conjunctiva and eyelid
Division of symblepharon (with insertion of
conformer)

✱ 10.6 Repair of laceration of conjunctiva
Excludes *that with repair of sclera (12.81)*

● 10.9 Other operations on conjunctiva

✱ 10.91 Subconjunctival injection
Coding Clinic: 1996, Q3, P7

✱ 10.99 Other

● 11 Operations on cornea

✱ 11.0 Magnetic removal of embedded foreign body from
cornea
Excludes *that with incision (11.1)*

✱ 11.1 Incision of cornea
Incision of cornea for removal of foreign body

● 11.2 Diagnostic procedures on cornea

✱ 11.21 Scraping of cornea for smear or culture

✱ 11.22 Biopsy of cornea

✱ 11.29 Other diagnostic procedures on cornea

● 11.3 Excision of pterygium

✱ 11.31 Transposition of pterygium

✱ 11.32 Excision of pterygium with corneal graft

✱ 11.39 Other excision of pterygium

◀ New   ◀═ Revised   ~~deleted~~ Deleted   ● Use Additional Digit(s)   ✱ Valid O.R. Procedure
◆ Non-O.R. Procedure   ♀ Females Only   ♂ Males Only

● **11.4 Excision or destruction of tissue or other lesion of cornea**

✷ **11.41 Mechanical removal of corneal epithelium**
That by chemocauterization

> **Excludes** *that for smear or culture (11.21)*

Coding Clinic: 2002, Q3, P20-21

✷ **11.42 Thermocauterization of corneal lesion**

✷ **11.43 Cryotherapy of corneal lesion**

✷ **11.49 Other removal or destruction of corneal lesion**
Excision of cornea NOS

> **Excludes** *biopsy of cornea (11.22)*

● **11.5 Repair of cornea**

✷ **11.51 Suture of corneal laceration**
Coding Clinic: 1996, Q3, P7

✷ **11.52 Repair of postoperative wound dehiscence of cornea**

✷ **11.53 Repair of corneal laceration or wound with conjunctival flap**

✷ **11.59 Other repair of cornea**

● **11.6 Corneal transplant**

> **Excludes** *excision of pterygium with corneal graft (11.32)*

✷ **11.60 Corneal transplant, not otherwise specified**
Keratoplasty NOS
Note: To report donor source - *see* codes 00.91–00.93

✷ **11.61 Lamellar keratoplasty with autograft**

✷ **11.62 Other lamellar keratoplasty**

✷ **11.63 Penetrating keratoplasty with autograft**
Perforating keratoplasty with autograft

✷ **11.64 Other penetrating keratoplasty**
Perforating keratoplasty (with homograft)

✷ **11.69 Other corneal transplant**

● **11.7 Other reconstructive and refractive surgery on cornea**

✷ **11.71 Keratomileusis**
MCE: Non-covered procedure

✷ **11.72 Keratophakia**
MCE: Non-covered procedure

✷ **11.73 Keratoprosthesis**

✷ **11.74 Thermokeratoplasty**

✷ **11.75 Radial keratotomy**
MCE: Non-covered procedure

✷ **11.76 Epikeratophakia**
MCE: Non-covered procedure

✷ **11.79 Other**

● **11.9 Other operations on cornea**

✷ **11.91 Tattooing of cornea**

✷ **11.92 Removal of artificial implant from cornea**

✷ **11.99 Other**
Coding Clinic: 2002, Q3, P20-21

● **12 Operations on iris, ciliary body, sclera, and anterior chamber**

> **Excludes** *operations on cornea (11.0–11.99)*

● **12.0 Removal of intraocular foreign body from anterior segment of eye**

✷ **12.00 Removal of intraocular foreign body from anterior segment of eye, not otherwise specified**

✷ **12.01 Removal of intraocular foreign body from anterior segment of eye with use of magnet**

✷ **12.02 Removal of intraocular foreign body from anterior segment of eye without use of magnet**

● **12.1 Iridotomy and simple iridectomy**

> **Excludes** *iridectomy associated with:*
> *cataract extraction (13.11–13.69)*
> *removal of lesion (12.41–12.42)*
> *scleral fistulization (12.61–12.69)*

✷ **12.11 Iridotomy with transfixion**

✷ **12.12 Other iridotomy**
Corectomy
Discission of iris
Iridotomy NOS

✷ **12.13 Excision of prolapsed iris**

✷ **12.14 Other iridectomy**
Iridectomy (basal) (peripheral) (total)

● **12.2 Diagnostic procedures on iris, ciliary body, sclera, and anterior chamber**

✷ **12.21 Diagnostic aspiration of anterior chamber of eye**

✷ **12.22 Biopsy of iris**

✷ **12.29 Other diagnostic procedures on iris, ciliary body, sclera, and anterior chamber**

● **12.3 Iridoplasty and coreoplasty**

✷ **12.31 Lysis of goniosynechiae**
Lysis of goniosynechiae by injection of air or liquid

✷ **12.32 Lysis of other anterior synechiae**
Lysis of anterior synechiae:
NOS
by injection of air or liquid

✷ **12.33 Lysis of posterior synechiae**
Lysis of iris adhesions NOS

✷ **12.34 Lysis of corneovitreal adhesions**

✷ **12.35 Coreoplasty**
Needling of pupillary membrane

✷ **12.39 Other iridoplasty**

● **12.4 Excision or destruction of lesion of iris and ciliary body**

✷ **12.40 Removal of lesion of anterior segment of eye, not otherwise specified**

✷ **12.41 Destruction of lesion of iris, nonexcisional**
Destruction of lesion of iris by:
cauterization
cryotherapy
photocoagulation

✷ **12.42 Excision of lesion of iris**

> **Excludes** *biopsy of iris (12.22)*

✷ **12.43 Destruction of lesion of ciliary body, nonexcisional**

✷ **12.44 Excision of lesion of ciliary body**

● **12.5 Facilitation of intraocular circulation**

✷ **12.51 Goniopuncture without goniotomy**

✷ **12.52 Goniotomy without goniopuncture**

✷ **12.53 Goniotomy with goniopuncture**

✷ **12.54 Trabeculotomy ab externo**

✷ **12.55 Cyclodialysis**

✷ **12.59 Other facilitation of intraocular circulation**
Coding Clinic: 1999, Q4, P13-14

OPERATIONS ON THE EYE (08–16)

| Excludes | Includes | Use additional | Code also | Omit code |

● **12.6 Scleral fistulization**

> **Excludes** *exploratory sclerotomy (12.89)*

✖ **12.61 Trephination of sclera with iridectomy**

✖ **12.62 Thermocauterization of sclera with iridectomy**

✖ **12.63 Iridencleisis and iridotasis**

✖ **12.64 Trabeculectomy ab externo**

✖ **12.65 Other scleral fistulization with iridectomy**

✖ **12.66 Postoperative revision of scleral fistulization procedure**
Revision of filtering bleb

> **Excludes** *repair of fistula (12.82)*

Coding Clinic: 2001, Q2, P16-17

✖ **12.69 Other fistulizing procedure**
Coding Clinic: 1996, Q3, P4

● **12.7 Other procedures for relief of elevated intraocular pressure**

✖ **12.71 Cyclodiathermy**

✖ **12.72 Cyclocryotherapy**

✖ **12.73 Cyclophotocoagulation**

✖ **12.74 Diminution of ciliary body, not otherwise specified**

✖ **12.79 Other glaucoma procedures**
Coding Clinic: 1998, Q2, P16

● **12.8 Operations on sclera**

> **Excludes** *those associated with:*
> *retinal reattachment (14.41–14.59)*
> *scleral fistulization (12.61–12.69)*

✖ **12.81 Suture of laceration of sclera**
Suture of sclera with synchronous repair of conjunctiva

✖ **12.82 Repair of scleral fistula**

> **Excludes** *postoperative revision of scleral fistulization procedure (12.66)*

✖ **12.83 Revision of operative wound of anterior segment, not elsewhere classified**

> **Excludes** *postoperative revision of scleral fistulization procedure (12.66)*

✖ **12.84 Excision or destruction of lesion of sclera**

✖ **12.85 Repair of scleral staphyloma with graft**

✖ **12.86 Other repair of scleral staphyloma**

✖ **12.87 Scleral reinforcement with graft**

✖ **12.88 Other scleral reinforcement**

✖ **12.89 Other operations on sclera**
Exploratory sclerotomy

● **12.9 Other operations on iris, ciliary body, and anterior chamber**

✖ **12.91 Therapeutic evacuation of anterior chamber**
Paracentesis of anterior chamber

> **Excludes** *diagnostic aspiration (12.21)*

✖ **12.92 Injection into anterior chamber**
Injection of:
air into anterior chamber
liquid into anterior chamber
medication into anterior chamber

✖ **12.93 Removal or destruction of epithelial downgrowth from anterior chamber**

> **Excludes** *that with iridectomy (12.41–12.42)*

✖ **12.97 Other operations on iris**

✖ **12.98 Other operations on ciliary body**

✖ **12.99 Other operations on anterior chamber**

● **13 Operations on lens**

● **13.0 Removal of foreign body from lens**

> **Excludes** *removal of pseudophakos (13.8)*

✖ **13.00 Removal of foreign body from lens, not otherwise specified**

✖ **13.01 Removal of foreign body from lens with use of magnet**

✖ **13.02 Removal of foreign body from lens without use of magnet**

● **13.1 Intracapsular extraction of lens**

Code also any synchronous insertion of pseudophakos (13.71)

✖ **13.11 Intracapsular extraction of lens by temporal inferior route**

✖ **13.19 Other intracapsular extraction of lens**
Cataract extraction NOS
Cryoextraction of lens
Erysiphake extraction of cataract
Extraction of lens NOS

✖ **13.2 Extracapsular extraction of lens by linear extraction technique**

Code also any synchronous insertion of pseudophakos (13.71) ◄

✖ **13.3 Extracapsular extraction of lens by simple aspiration (and irrigation) technique**
Irrigation of traumatic cataract

Code also any synchronous insertion of pseudophakos (13.71) ◄

● **13.4 Extracapsular extraction of lens by fragmentation and aspiration technique**

Code also any synchronous insertion of pseudophakos (13.71) ◄

✖ **13.41 Phacoemulsification and aspiration of cataract**
Coding Clinic: 1996, Q3, P4; 1994, Q1, P16

✖ **13.42 Mechanical phacofragmentation and aspiration of cataract by posterior route**

Code also any synchronous vitrectomy (14.74)

✖ **13.43 Mechanical phacofragmentation and other aspiration of cataract**

● **13.5 Other extracapsular extraction of lens**

Code also any synchronous insertion of pseudophakos (13.71)

✖ **13.51 Extracapsular extraction of lens by temporal inferior route**

✖ **13.59 Other extracapsular extraction of lens**

● **13.6 Other cataract extraction**

Code also any synchronous insertion of pseudophakos (13.71)

✖ **13.64 Discission of secondary membrane [after cataract]**

✖ **13.65 Excision of secondary membrane [after cataract]**
Capsulectomy

✖ **13.66 Mechanical fragmentation of secondary membrane [after cataract]**

✖ **13.69 Other cataract extraction**

● **13.7 Insertion of prosthetic lens [pseudophakos]**

> **Excludes** *implantation of intraocular telescope prosthesis (13.91)*

✖ **13.70 Insertion of pseudophakos, not otherwise specified**

✖ **13.71 Insertion of intraocular lens prosthesis at time of cataract extraction, one-stage**

Code also synchronous extraction of cataract (13.11–13.69)
Coding Clinic: 1996, Q3, P4

✖ **13.72 Secondary insertion of intraocular lens prosthesis**

◄ New   ◄▥ Revised   ~~deleted~~ Deleted   ● Use Additional Digit(s)   ✖ Valid O.R. Procedure
◆ Non-O.R. Procedure   ♀ Females Only   ♂ Males Only

✖ **13.8   Removal of implanted lens**
Removal of pseudophakos

● **13.9   Other operations on lens**
Coding Clinic: 2000, Q1, P9-10

✖ **13.90   Operation on lens, Not Elsewhere Classified**

✖ **13.91   Implantation of intraocular telescope prosthesis**
Implantable miniature telescope
> **Includes**   removal of lens, any method
> **Excludes**   *secondary insertion of ocular implant (16.61)*
Coding Clinic: 2006, Q4, P123-124

● **14   Operations on retina, choroid, vitreous, and posterior chamber**

● **14.0   Removal of foreign body from posterior segment of eye**
> **Excludes**   *removal of surgically implanted material (14.6)*

✖ **14.00   Removal of foreign body from posterior segment of eye, not otherwise specified**

✖ **14.01   Removal of foreign body from posterior segment of eye with use of magnet**

✖ **14.02   Removal of foreign body from posterior segment of eye without use of magnet**

● **14.1   Diagnostic procedures on retina, choroid, vitreous, and posterior chamber**

✖ **14.11   Diagnostic aspiration of vitreous**

✖ **14.19   Other diagnostic procedures on retina, choroid, vitreous, and posterior chamber**

● **14.2   Destruction of lesion of retina and choroid**
> **Includes**   destruction of chorioretinopathy or isolated chorioretinal lesion
> **Excludes**   *that for repair of retina (14.31–14.59)*

✖ **14.21   Destruction of chorioretinal lesion by diathermy**

✖ **14.22   Destruction of chorioretinal lesion by cryotherapy**

14.23   Destruction of chorioretinal lesion by xenon arc photocoagulation

14.24   Destruction of chorioretinal lesion by laser photocoagulation

14.25   Destruction of chorioretinal lesion by photocoagulation of unspecified type

✖ **14.26   Destruction of chorioretinal lesion by radiation therapy**

✖ **14.27   Destruction of chorioretinal lesion by implantation of radiation source**

✖ **14.29   Other destruction of chorioretinal lesion**
Destruction of lesion of retina and choroid NOS

● **14.3   Repair of retinal tear**
> **Includes**   repair of retinal defect
> **Excludes**   *repair of retinal detachment (14.41–14.59)*

✖ **14.31   Repair of retinal tear by diathermy**

✖ **14.32   Repair of retinal tear by cryotherapy**

14.33   Repair of retinal tear by xenon arc photocoagulation

14.34   Repair of retinal tear by laser photocoagulation
Coding Clinic: 1994, Q1, P17

14.35   Repair of retinal tear by photocoagulation of unspecified type

✖ **14.39   Other repair of retinal tear**

● **14.4   Repair of retinal detachment with scleral buckling and implant**

✖ **14.41   Scleral buckling with implant**
Coding Clinic: 1996, Q3, P6

✖ **14.49   Other scleral buckling**
Scleral buckling with:
air tamponade
resection of sclera
vitrectomy
Coding Clinic: 1994, Q1, P16-17

● **14.5   Other repair of retinal detachment**
> **Includes**   that with drainage

✖ **14.51   Repair of retinal detachment with diathermy**

✖ **14.52   Repair of retinal detachment with cryotherapy**

✖ **14.53   Repair of retinal detachment with xenon arc photocoagulation**

✖ **14.54   Repair of retinal detachment with laser photocoagulation**
Coding Clinic: 1987, Nov-Dec, P10

✖ **14.55   Repair of retinal detachment with photocoagulation of unspecified type**

✖ **14.59   Other**

✖ **14.6   Removal of surgically implanted material from posterior segment of eye**

● **14.7   Operations on vitreous**

✖ **14.71   Removal of vitreous, anterior approach**
Open sky technique
Removal of vitreous, anterior approach (with replacement)

✖ **14.72   Other removal of vitreous**
Aspiration of vitreous by posterior sclerotomy

✖ **14.73   Mechanical vitrectomy by anterior approach**
Coding Clinic: 1996, Q3, P4-5

✖ **14.74   Other mechanical vitrectomy**
Posterior approach
Coding Clinic: 1996, Q3, P5

✖ **14.75   Injection of vitreous substitute**
> **Excludes**   *that associated with removal (14.71–14.72)*
Coding Clinic: 1998, Q1, P6; 1996, Q3, P5; 1994, Q1, P17

✖ **14.79   Other operations on vitreous**
Coding Clinic: 1999, Q3, P12; 1999, Q1, P11; 1998, Q1, P6

✖ **14.9   Other operations on retina, choroid, and posterior chamber**
Coding Clinic: 1996, Q3, P5; 1993, 5th Issue, P13-14

● **15   Operations on extraocular muscles**

● **15.0   Diagnostic procedures on extraocular muscles or tendons**

✖ **15.01   Biopsy of extraocular muscle or tendon**

✖ **15.09   Other diagnostic procedures on extraocular muscles and tendons**

● **15.1   Operations on one extraocular muscle involving temporary detachment from globe**

✖ **15.11   Recession of one extraocular muscle**
Coding Clinic: 1996, Q3, P3-4

✖ **15.12   Advancement of one extraocular muscle**

✖ **15.13   Resection of one extraocular muscle**
Coding Clinic: 1996, Q3, P4

✖ **15.19   Other operations on one extraocular muscle involving temporary detachment from globe**
> **Excludes**   *transposition of muscle (15.5)*

OPERATIONS ON THE EYE (08–16)

● **15.2 Other operations on one extraocular muscle**

✖ **15.21 Lengthening procedure on one extraocular muscle**

✖ **15.22 Shortening procedure on one extraocular muscle**

✖ **15.29 Other**

✖ **15.3 Operations on two or more extraocular muscles involving temporary detachment from globe, one or both eyes**
Coding Clinic: 1996, Q3, P3-4x2

✖ **15.4 Other operations on two or more extraocular muscles, one or both eyes**

✖ **15.5 Transposition of extraocular muscles**
| Excludes | *that for correction of ptosis (08.31–08.36)*

✖ **15.6 Revision of extraocular muscle surgery**

✖ **15.7 Repair of injury of extraocular muscle**
Freeing of entrapped extraocular muscle
Lysis of adhesions of extraocular muscle
Repair of laceration of extraocular muscle, tendon, or Tenon's capsule

✖ **15.9 Other operations on extraocular muscles and tendons**

● **16 Operations on orbit and eyeball**
| Excludes | *reduction of fracture of orbit (76.78–76.79)*

● **16.0 Orbitotomy**

✖ **16.01 Orbitotomy with bone flap**
Orbitotomy with lateral approach

✖ **16.02 Orbitotomy with insertion of orbital implant**
| Excludes | *that with bone flap (16.01)*

✖ **16.09 Other orbitotomy**

✖ **16.1 Removal of penetrating foreign body from eye, not otherwise specified**
| Excludes | *removal of nonpenetrating foreign body (98.21)*

● **16.2 Diagnostic procedures on orbit and eyeball**

16.21 Ophthalmoscopy

✖ **16.22 Diagnostic aspiration of orbit**

✖ **16.23 Biopsy of eyeball and orbit**

✖ **16.29 Other diagnostic procedures on orbit and eyeball**
| Excludes | *examination of form and structure of eye (95.11–95.16)*
general and subjective eye examination (95.01–95.09)
microscopic examination of specimen from eye (90.21–90.29)
objective functional tests of eye (95.21–95.26)
ocular thermography (88.82)
tonometry (89.11)
x-ray of orbit (87.14, 87.16)

● **16.3 Evisceration of eyeball**

✖ **16.31 Removal of ocular contents with synchronous implant into scleral shell**

✖ **16.39 Other evisceration of eyeball**

● **16.4 Enucleation of eyeball**

✖ **16.41 Enucleation of eyeball with synchronous implant into Tenon's capsule with attachment of muscles**
Integrated implant of eyeball

✖ **16.42 Enucleation of eyeball with other synchronous implant**

✖ **16.49 Other enucleation of eyeball**
Removal of eyeball NOS

● **16.5 Exenteration of orbital contents**

✖ **16.51 Exenteration of orbit with removal of adjacent structures**
Radical orbitomaxillectomy

✖ **16.52 Exenteration of orbit with therapeutic removal of orbital bone**

✖ **16.59 Other exenteration of orbit**
Evisceration of orbit NOS
Exenteration of orbit with temporalis muscle transplant

● **16.6 Secondary procedures after removal of eyeball**
| Excludes | *that with synchronous:*
enucleation of eyeball (16.41–16.42)
evisceration of eyeball (16.31)

✖ **16.61 Secondary insertion of ocular implant**

✖ **16.62 Revision and reinsertion of ocular implant**

✖ **16.63 Revision of enucleation socket with graft**

✖ **16.64 Other revision of enucleation socket**

✖ **16.65 Secondary graft to exenteration cavity**

✖ **16.66 Other revision of exenteration cavity**

✖ **16.69 Other secondary procedures after removal of eyeball**

● **16.7 Removal of ocular or orbital implant**

✖ **16.71 Removal of ocular implant**

✖ **16.72 Removal of orbital implant**

● **16.8 Repair of injury of eyeball and orbit**

✖ **16.81 Repair of wound of orbit**
| Excludes | *reduction of orbital fracture (76.78–76.79)*
repair of extraocular muscles (15.7)

✖ **16.82 Repair of rupture of eyeball**
Repair of multiple structures of eye
| Excludes | *repair of laceration of:*
cornea (11.51–11.59)
sclera (12.81)

✖ **16.89 Other repair of injury of eyeball or orbit**

● **16.9 Other operations on orbit and eyeball**
| Excludes | *irrigation of eye (96.51)*
prescription and fitting of low vision aids (95.31–95.33)
removal of:
eye prosthesis NEC (97.31)
nonpenetrating foreign body from eye without incision (98.21)

16.91 Retrobulbar injection of therapeutic agent
| Excludes | *injection of radiographic contrast material (87.14)*
opticociliary injection (12.79)

✖ **16.92 Excision of lesion of orbit**
| Excludes | *biopsy of orbit (16.23)*

✖ **16.93 Excision of lesion of eye, unspecified structure**
| Excludes | *biopsy of eye NOS (16.23)*

✖ **16.98 Other operations on orbit**

✖ **16.99 Other operations on eyeball**

◀ New   ◀▦ Revised   ~~deleted~~ Deleted   ● Use Additional Digit(s)   ✖ Valid O.R. Procedure
◆ Non-O.R. Procedure   ♀ Females Only   ♂ Males Only

3A. OTHER MISCELLANEOUS DIAGNOSTIC AND THERAPEUTIC PROCEDURES

● **17   Other miscellaneous procedures**

● **17.1   Laparoscopic unilateral repair of inguinal hernia**

> **Excludes** *other and open unilateral repair of hernia (53.00 – 53.05)*
>
> Coding Clinic: 2008, Q4, P165-169

✖ **17.11   Laparoscopic repair of direct inguinal hernia with graft or prosthesis**
Laparoscopic repair of direct and indirect inguinal hernia with graft or prosthesis

✖ **17.12   Laparoscopic repair of indirect inguinal hernia with graft or prosthesis**

✖ **17.13   Laparoscopic repair of inguinal hernia with graft or prosthesis, not otherwise specified**

● **17.2   Laparoscopic bilateral repair of inguinal hernia**

> **Excludes** *other and open bilateral repair of hernia (53.10 – 53.17)*
>
> Coding Clinic: 2008, Q4, P165-169

✖ **17.21   Laparoscopic bilateral repair of direct inguinal hernia with graft or prosthesis**

✖ **17.22   Laparoscopic bilateral repair of indirect inguinal hernia with graft or prosthesis**

✖ **17.23   Laparoscopic bilateral repair of inguinal hernia, one direct and one indirect, with graft or prosthesis**

✖ **17.24   Laparoscopic bilateral repair of inguinal hernia with graft or prosthesis, not otherwise specified**

● **17.3   Laparoscopic partial excision of large intestine**

> **Excludes** *other and open partial excision of large intestine (45.71- 45.79)*
>
> Coding Clinic: 2008, Q4, P169-172

✖ **17.31   Laparoscopic multiple segmental resection of large intestine**

✖ **17.32   Laparoscopic cecectomy**

✖ **17.33   Laparoscopic right hemicolectomy**

✖ **17.34   Laparoscopic resection of transverse colon**

✖ **17.35   Laparoscopic left hemicolectomy**

✖ **17.36   Laparoscopic sigmoidectomy**

✖ **17.39   Other laparoscopic partial excision of large intestine**

● **17.4   Robotic assisted procedures**
Computer assisted robotic surgery
Computer-enhanced robotic surgery
Robotic procedure with computer assistance
Surgeon-controlled robotic surgery

Code first primary procedure

> **Excludes** *computer assisted surgery (00.31-00.35, 00.39)*

Note: This category includes use of a computer console with (3-D) imaging, software, camera(s), visualization and instrumentation *combined* with the use of robotic arms, device(s), or system(s) at the time of the procedure.
Coding Clinic: 2008, Q4, P172-174

17.41   Open robotic assisted procedure
Robotic assistance in open procedure

17.42   Laparoscopic robotic assisted procedure
Robotic assistance in laparoscopic procedure

17.43   Percutaneous robotic assisted procedure
Robotic assistance in percutaneous procedure

17.44   Endoscopic robotic assisted procedure
Robotic assistance in endoscopic procedure

17.45   Thoracoscopic robotic assisted procedure
Robotic assistance in thoracoscopic procedure

17.49   Other and unspecified robotic assisted procedure
Robotic assistance in other and unspecified procedure

> **Excludes** *endoscopic robotic assisted procedure (17.44)*
> *laparoscopic robotic assisted procedure (17.42)*
> *open robotic assisted procedure (17.41)*
> *percutaneous robotic assisted procedure (17.43)*
> *thoracoscopic robotic assisted procedure (17.45)*

● **17.5   Additional cardiovascular procedures** ◄

✖ **17.51   Implantation of rechargeable cardiac contractility modulation [CCM], total system** ◄
Note: Device testing during procedure – *omit code* ◄
Implantation of CCM system includes formation of pocket, transvenous leads, including placement of leads, placement of catheter into left ventricle, intraoperative procedures for evaluation of lead signals, obtaining sensing threshold measurements, obtaining defibrillator threshold measurements. ◄

> **Includes** implantation of device with removal of existing device ◄

Code also any concomitant: ◄
coronary bypass (36.10 – 36.19) ◄
extracorporeal circulation (39.61)
insertion or replacement of automatic cardioverter/defibrillator, total system [AICD] (37.94) ◄

> **Excludes** *implantation of CCM pulse generator only (17.52)* ◄

MS-DRG: Refer to Part VI, Appendix E, Table 3, Cardioverter-Defibrillator Lead/Generator Reference Table

✖ **17.52   Implantation or replacement of cardiac contractility modulation [CCM] rechargeable pulse generator only** ◄
Implantation of CCM device with removal of any existing CCM device ◄
Note: Device testing during procedure – *omit code* ◄

Code also any concomitant: ◄
revision of device pocket (37.79) ◄
revision of lead [electrode] (37.75) ◄
MS-DRG: Refer to Part VI, Appendix E, Table 3, Cardioverter-Defibrillator Lead/Generator Reference Table

OTHER MISCELLANEOUS DIAGNOSTIC AND THERAPEUTIC PROCEDURES

Excludes   Includes   Use additional   Code also   Omit code

● **17.6** **Laser interstitial thermal therapy [LITT] under guidance** ◀

Focused laser interstitial thermal therapy [f-LITT] under MRI guidance ◀

MRI-guided LITT ◀

✖ **17.61** **Laser interstitial thermal therapy [LITT] of lesion or tissue of brain under guidance** ◀

Focused laser interstitial thermal therapy [f-LITT] under MRI guidance ◀

MRI-guided LITT of lesion or tissue of brain ◀

> **Excludes**   *laser interstitial thermal therapy [LITT] of lesion or tissue of head under guidance (17.62)* ◀

✖ **17.62** **Laser interstitial thermal therapy [LITT] of lesion or tissue of head and neck under guidance** ◀

Focused laser interstitial thermal therapy [f-LITT] under MRI guidance ◀

MRI-guided LITT of lesion or tissue of head and neck ◀

> **Excludes**   *laser interstitial thermal therapy [LITT] of lesion or tissue of brain under guidance (17.61)* ◀

✖ **17.63** **Laser interstitial thermal therapy [LITT] of lesion or tissue of liver under guidance** ◀

Focused laser interstitial thermal therapy [f-LITT] under MRI guidance ◀

MRI-guided LITT of lesion or tissue of liver ◀

✖ **17.69** **Laser interstitial thermal therapy [LITT] of lesion or tissue of other and unspecified site under guidance** ◀

Focused laser interstitial thermal therapy [f-LITT] under MRI guidance ◀

MRI-guided LITT of lesion or tissue of breast ◀

MRI-guided LITT of lesion or tissue of lung ◀

MRI-guided LITT of lesion or tissue of prostate ◀

> **Excludes**   *laser interstitial thermal therapy [LITT] of lesion or tissue of brain under guidance (17.61)* ◀
>
> *laser interstitial thermal therapy [LITT] of lesion or tissue of head and neck under guidance (17.62)* ◀
>
> *laser interstitial thermal therapy [LITT] of lesion or tissue of liver under guidance (17.63)* ◀

● **17.7** **Other diagnostic and therapeutic procedures** ◀

17.70 **Intravenous infusion of clofarabine** ◀

> **Excludes**   *injection or infusion of cancer chemotherapeutic substance (99.25)* ◀

◀ New   ◀▥ Revised   ~~deleted~~ Deleted   ● Use Additional Digit(s)   ✖ Valid O.R. Procedure

◆ Non-O.R. Procedure   ♀ Females Only   ♂ Males Only

OTHER MISCELLANEOUS DIAGNOSTIC AND THERAPEUTIC PROCEDURES

(See Plates 92 and 93 on pages NAP-20–NAP-21.)

4.   OPERATIONS ON THE EAR (18–20)

● **18   Operations on external ear**

Includes   operations on:
external auditory canal
skin and cartilage of:
auricle
meatus

● **18.0   Incision of external ear**

Excludes   *removal of intraluminal foreign body (98.11)*

18.01   Piercing of ear lobe
Piercing of pinna

18.02   Incision of external auditory canal

18.09   Other incision of external ear

● **18.1   Diagnostic procedures on external ear**

18.11   Otoscopy

18.12   Biopsy of external ear

18.19   Other diagnostic procedures on external ear

Excludes   *microscopic examination of specimen from ear (90.31–90.39)*

● **18.2   Excision or destruction of lesion of external ear**

✖ **18.21   Excision of preauricular sinus**
Radical excision of preauricular sinus or cyst

Excludes   *excision of preauricular remnant [appendage] (18.29)*

18.29   Excision or destruction of other lesion of external ear
Cauterization of external ear
Coagulation of external ear
Cryosurgery of external ear
Curettage of external ear
Electrocoagulation of external ear
Enucleation of external ear
Excision of:
exostosis of external auditory canal
preauricular remnant [appendage]
Partial excision of ear

Excludes   *biopsy of external ear (18.12)*
radical excision of lesion (18.31)
removal of cerumen (96.52)

● **18.3   Other excision of external ear**

Excludes   *biopsy of external ear (18.12)*

✖ **18.31   Radical excision of lesion of external ear**

Excludes   *radical excision of preauricular sinus (18.21)*

✖ **18.39   Other**
Amputation of external ear

Excludes   *excision of lesion (18.21–18.29, 18.31)*

18.4   Suture of laceration of external ear

✖ **18.5   Surgical correction of prominent ear**
Ear:
pinning
setback

✖ **18.6   Reconstruction of external auditory canal**
Canaloplasty of external auditory meatus
Construction [reconstruction] of external meatus of ear:
osseous portion
skin-lined portion (with skin graft)

● **18.7   Other plastic repair of external ear**

✖ **18.71   Construction of auricle of ear**
Prosthetic appliance for absent ear
Reconstruction:
auricle
ear

✖ **18.72   Reattachment of amputated ear**

✖ **18.79   Other plastic repair of external ear**
Otoplasty NOS
Postauricular skin graft
Repair of lop ear
Coding Clinic: 2003, Q3, P12-13

✖ **18.9   Other operations on external ear**

Excludes   *irrigation of ear (96.52)*
packing of external auditory canal (96.11)
removal of:
cerumen (96.52)
foreign body (without incision) (98.11)

● **19   Reconstructive operations on middle ear**

✖ **19.0   Stapes mobilization**
Division, otosclerotic:
material
process
Remobilization of stapes
Stapediolysis
Transcrural stapes mobilization

Excludes   *that with synchronous stapedectomy (19.11–19.19)*

● **19.1   Stapedectomy**

Excludes   *revision of previous stapedectomy (19.21–19.29)*
stapes mobilization only (19.0)

✖ **19.11   Stapedectomy with incus replacement**
Stapedectomy with incus:
homograft
prosthesis

✖ **19.19   Other stapedectomy**

● **19.2   Revision of stapedectomy**

✖ **19.21   Revision of stapedectomy with incus replacement**

✖ **19.29   Other revision of stapedectomy**

✖ **19.3   Other operations on ossicular chain**
Incudectomy NOS
Ossiculectomy NOS
Reconstruction of ossicles, second stage

✖ **19.4   Myringoplasty**
Epitympanic, type I
Myringoplasty by:
cauterization
graft
Tympanoplasty (type I)

● **19.5   Other tympanoplasty**

✖ **19.52   Type II tympanoplasty**
Closure of perforation with graft against incus or malleus

✖ **19.53   Type III tympanoplasty**
Graft placed in contact with mobile and intact stapes
Coding Clinic: 1985, Mar-April, P15

✖ **19.54   Type IV tympanoplasty**
Mobile footplate left exposed with air pocket between round window and graft

✖ **19.55   Type V tympanoplasty**
Fenestra in horizontal semicircular canal covered by graft

Excludes   Includes   Use additional   Code also   Omit code

✖ **19.6 Revision of tympanoplasty**

✖ **19.9 Other repair of middle ear**
     Closure of mastoid fistula
     Mastoid myoplasty
     Obliteration of tympanomastoid cavity

● **20 Other operations on middle and inner ear**

  ● **20.0 Myringotomy**

    ✖ **20.01 Myringotomy with insertion of tube**
         Myringostomy

     20.09 Other myringotomy
         Aspiration of middle ear NOS

     20.1 Removal of tympanostomy tube
         Coding Clinic: 1994, Q3, P7; 1987, Nov-Dec, P9

  ● **20.2 Incision of mastoid and middle ear**

    ✖ **20.21 Incision of mastoid**

    ✖ **20.22 Incision of petrous pyramid air cells**

    ✖ **20.23 Incision of middle ear**
         Atticotomy
         Division of tympanum
         Lysis of adhesions of middle ear
         | Excludes | *division of otosclerotic process (19.0)*
                   stapediolysis (19.0)
                   that with stapedectomy (19.11–19.19)

  ● **20.3 Diagnostic procedures on middle and inner ear**

     20.31 Electrocochleography

    ✖ **20.32 Biopsy of middle and inner ear**

    ✖ **20.39 Other diagnostic procedures on middle and inner ear**
         | Excludes | *auditory and vestibular function tests (89.13, 95.41–95.49)*
                   microscopic examination of specimen from ear (90.31–90.39)

  ● **20.4 Mastoidectomy**
       Code also any:
         skin graft (18.79)
         tympanoplasty (19.4–19.55)
       | Excludes | *that with implantation of cochlear prosthetic device (20.96–20.98)*

    ✖ **20.41 Simple mastoidectomy**

    ✖ **20.42 Radical mastoidectomy**

    ✖ **20.49 Other mastoidectomy**
         Atticoantrostomy
         Mastoidectomy:
           NOS
           modified radical

  ● **20.5 Other excision of middle ear**
       | Excludes | *that with synchronous mastoidectomy (20.41–20.49)*

    ✖ **20.51 Excision of lesion of middle ear**
         | Excludes | *biopsy of middle ear (20.32)*

    ✖ **20.59 Other**
         Apicectomy of petrous pyramid
         Tympanectomy

  ● **20.6 Fenestration of inner ear**

    ✖ **20.61 Fenestration of inner ear (initial)**
         Fenestration of:
           labyrinth with graft (skin) (vein)
           semicircular canals with graft (skin) (vein)
           vestibule with graft (skin) (vein)
         | Excludes | *that with tympanoplasty, type V (19.55)*

    ✖ **20.62 Revision of fenestration of inner ear**

● **20.7 Incision, excision, and destruction of inner ear**

    ✖ **20.71 Endolymphatic shunt**

    ✖ **20.72 Injection into inner ear**
         Destruction by injection (alcohol):
           inner ear
           semicircular canals
           vestibule

    ✖ **20.79 Other incision, excision, and destruction of inner ear**
         Decompression of labyrinth
         Drainage of inner ear
         Fistulization:
           endolymphatic sac
           labyrinth
         Incision of endolymphatic sac
         Labyrinthectomy (transtympanic)
         Opening of bony labyrinth
         Perilymphatic tap
         | Excludes | *biopsy of inner ear (20.32)*

     20.8 Operations on Eustachian tube
         Catheterization of Eustachian tube
         Inflation of Eustachian tube
         Injection (Teflon paste) of Eustachian tube
         Insufflation (boric acid-salicylic acid)
         Intubation of Eustachian tube
         Politzerization of Eustachian tube

● **20.9 Other operations on inner and middle ear**

    ✖ **20.91 Tympanosympathectomy**

    ✖ **20.92 Revision of mastoidectomy**
         Coding Clinic: 1998, Q2, P20

    ✖ **20.93 Repair of oval and round windows**
         Closure of fistula:
           oval window
           perilymph
           round window

     20.94 Injection of tympanum

    ✖ **20.95 Implantation of electromagnetic hearing device**
         Bone conduction hearing device
         | Excludes | *cochlear prosthetic device (20.96–20.98)*
         Coding Clinic: 2007, Q3, P5

    ✖ **20.96 Implantation or replacement of cochlear prosthetic device, not otherwise specified**
         Implantation of receiver (within skull) and insertion of electrode(s) in the cochlea
         | Includes | mastoidectomy
         | Excludes | *electromagnetic hearing device (20.95)*

    ✖ **20.97 Implantation or replacement of cochlear prosthetic device, single channel**
         Implantation of receiver (within skull) and insertion of electrode in the cochlea
         | Includes | mastoidectomy
         | Excludes | *electromagnetic hearing device (20.95)*

    ✖ **20.98 Implantation or replacement of cochlear prosthetic device, multiple channel**
         Implantation of receiver (within skull) and insertion of electrodes in the cochlea
         | Includes | mastoidectomy
         | Excludes | *electromagnetic hearing device (20.95)*

    ✖ **20.99 Other operations on middle and inner ear**
         Attachment of percutaneous abutment (screw) for prosthetic device
         Repair or removal of cochlear prosthetic device (receiver) (electrode)
         | Excludes | *adjustment (external components) of cochlear prosthetic device (95.49)*
                   fitting of hearing aid (95.48)
         Coding Clinic: 2007, Q3, P5

◀ New   ◀▦ Revised   ~~deleted~~ Deleted   ● Use Additional Digit(s)   ✖ Valid O.R. Procedure
         ◆ Non-O.R. Procedure   ♀ Females Only   ♂ Males Only

OPERATIONS ON THE EAR (18–20)

(See Plates 49, 57, 58, and 61 on pages NAP-22–NAP-25.)

5. OPERATIONS ON THE NOSE, MOUTH, AND PHARYNX (21–29)

● 21 Operations on nose

> **Includes** operations on:
> bone of nose
> skin of nose

● 21.0 Control of epistaxis

21.00 Control of epistaxis, not otherwise specified

21.01 Control of epistaxis by anterior nasal packing

21.02 Control of epistaxis by posterior (and anterior) packing
Coding Clinic: 1995, Q1, P5

21.03 Control of epistaxis by cauterization (and packing)

✖ 21.04 Control of epistaxis by ligation of ethmoidal arteries

✖ 21.05 Control of epistaxis by (transantral) ligation of the maxillary artery

✖ 21.06 Control of epistaxis by ligation of the external carotid artery

✖ 21.07 Control of epistaxis by excision of nasal mucosa and skin grafting of septum and lateral nasal wall

✖ 21.09 Control of epistaxis by other means
Coding Clinic: 1995, Q1, P5

21.1 Incision of nose
Chondrotomy
Incision of skin of nose
Nasal septotomy

● 21.2 Diagnostic procedures on nose

21.21 Rhinoscopy

21.22 Biopsy of nose

21.29 Other diagnostic procedures on nose

> **Excludes** microscopic examination of specimen from nose (90.31–90.39)
> nasal:
> function study (89.12)
> x-ray (87.16)
> rhinomanometry (89.12)

● 21.3 Local excision or destruction of lesion of nose

> **Excludes** biopsy of nose (21.22)
> nasal fistulectomy (21.82)

21.30 Excision or destruction of lesion of nose, not otherwise specified

21.31 Local excision or destruction of intranasal lesion
Nasal polypectomy

21.32 Local excision or destruction of other lesion of nose
Coding Clinic: 1989, Q2, P16

✖ 21.4 Resection of nose
Amputation of nose

✖ 21.5 Submucous resection of nasal septum

● 21.6 Turbinectomy

✖ 21.61 Turbinectomy by diathermy or cryosurgery

✖ 21.62 Fracture of the turbinates

✖ 21.69 Other turbinectomy

> **Excludes** turbinectomy associated with sinusectomy (22.31–22.39, 22.42, 22.60–22.64)

● 21.7 Reduction of nasal fracture

21.71 Closed reduction of nasal fracture

✖ 21.72 Open reduction of nasal fracture

● 21.8 Repair and plastic operations on the nose

21.81 Suture of laceration of nose

✖ 21.82 Closure of nasal fistula
Nasolabial fistulectomy
Nasopharyngeal fistulectomy
Oronasal fistulectomy

✖ 21.83 Total nasal reconstruction
Reconstruction of nose with:
arm flap
forehead flap

✖ 21.84 Revision rhinoplasty
Rhinoseptoplasty
Twisted nose rhinoplasty

✖ 21.85 Augmentation rhinoplasty
Augmentation rhinoplasty with:
graft
synthetic implant

✖ 21.86 Limited rhinoplasty
Plastic repair of nasolabial flaps
Tip rhinoplasty

✖ 21.87 Other rhinoplasty
Rhinoplasty NOS

✖ 21.88 Other septoplasty
Crushing of nasal septum
Repair of septal perforation

> **Excludes** septoplasty associated with submucous resection of septum (21.5)

✖ 21.89 Other repair and plastic operations on nose
Reattachment of amputated nose

● 21.9 Other operations on nose

21.91 Lysis of adhesions of nose
Posterior nasal scrub

✖ 21.99 Other

> **Excludes** dilation of frontonasal duct (96.21)
> irrigation of nasal passages (96.53)
> removal of:
> intraluminal foreign body without incision (98.12)
> nasal packing (97.32)
> replacement of nasal packing (97.21)

● 22 Operations on nasal sinuses

● 22.0 Aspiration and lavage of nasal sinus

22.00 Aspiration and lavage of nasal sinus, not otherwise specified

22.01 Puncture of nasal sinus for aspiration or lavage

22.02 Aspiration or lavage of nasal sinus through natural ostium

● 22.1 Diagnostic procedures on nasal sinus

22.11 Closed [endoscopic] [needle] biopsy of nasal sinus
MCE: Closed biopsy procedure

✖ 22.12 Open biopsy of nasal sinus
MCE: Open biopsy procedure

22.19 Other diagnostic procedures on nasal sinuses
Endoscopy without biopsy

> **Excludes** transillumination of sinus (89.35)
> x-ray of sinus (87.15–87.16)

22.2 Intranasal antrotomy

> **Excludes** antrotomy with external approach (22.31–22.39)

● 22.3   **External maxillary antrotomy**

   ✖ **22.31   Radical maxillary antrotomy**
       Removal of lining membrane of maxillary
         sinus using Caldwell-Luc approach

   ✖ **22.39   Other external maxillary antrotomy**
       Exploration of maxillary antrum with
         Caldwell-Luc approach

● 22.4   **Frontal sinusotomy and sinusectomy**

   ✖ **22.41   Frontal sinusotomy**

   ✖ **22.42   Frontal sinusectomy**
       Excision of lesion of frontal sinus
       Obliteration of frontal sinus (with fat)

       | **Excludes** | *biopsy of nasal sinus (22.11–22.12)*

● 22.5   **Other nasal sinusotomy**

   ✖ **22.50   Sinusotomy, not otherwise specified**

   ✖ **22.51   Ethmoidotomy**

   ✖ **22.52   Sphenoidotomy**

   ✖ **22.53   Incision of multiple nasal sinuses**

● 22.6   **Other nasal sinusectomy**

       | **Includes** | that with incidental turbinectomy
       | **Excludes** | *biopsy of nasal sinus (22.11–22.12)*

   ✖ **22.60   Sinusectomy, not otherwise specified**

   ✖ **22.61   Excision of lesion of maxillary sinus with**
        Caldwell-Luc approach

   ✖ **22.62   Excision of lesion of maxillary sinus with other**
        approach

   ✖ **22.63   Ethmoidectomy**

   ✖ **22.64   Sphenoidectomy**

● 22.7   **Repair of nasal sinus**

   ✖ **22.71   Closure of nasal sinus fistula**
       Repair of oro-antral fistula

   ✖ **22.79   Other repair of nasal sinus**
       Reconstruction of frontonasal duct
       Repair of bone of accessory sinus

   ✖ **22.9   Other operations on nasal sinuses**
       Exteriorization of maxillary sinus
       Fistulization of sinus

       | **Excludes** | *dilation of frontonasal duct (96.21)*

● 23   **Removal and restoration of teeth**

● 23.0   **Forceps extraction of tooth**

   23.01   Extraction of deciduous tooth

   23.09   Extraction of other tooth
       Extraction of tooth NOS

● 23.1   **Surgical removal of tooth**

   23.11   Removal of residual root

   23.19   Other surgical extraction of tooth
       Odontectomy NOS
       Removal of impacted tooth
       Tooth extraction with elevation of
         mucoperiosteal flap

   23.2   Restoration of tooth by filling

   23.3   Restoration of tooth by inlay

● 23.4   **Other dental restoration**

   23.41   Application of crown

   23.42   Insertion of fixed bridge

   23.43   Insertion of removable bridge

   23.49   Other

   23.5   Implantation of tooth

   23.6   Prosthetic dental implant
       Endosseous dental implant

● 23.7   **Apicoectomy and root canal therapy**

   23.70   Root canal, not otherwise specified

   23.71   Root canal therapy with irrigation

   23.72   Root canal therapy with apicoectomy

   23.73   Apicoectomy

● 24   **Other operations on teeth, gums, and alveoli**

   24.0   Incision of gum or alveolar bone
       Apical alveolotomy

● 24.1   **Diagnostic procedures on teeth, gums, and alveoli**

   24.11   Biopsy of gum

   24.12   Biopsy of alveolus

   24.19   Other diagnostic procedures on teeth, gums, and
        alveoli

       | **Excludes** | *dental:*
          examination (89.31)
          x-ray:
            full-mouth (87.11)
            other (87.12)
          microscopic examination of dental
            specimen (90.81–90.89)

   ✖ **24.2   Gingivoplasty**
       Gingivoplasty with bone or soft tissue graft

● 24.3   **Other operations on gum**

   24.31   Excision of lesion or tissue of gum

       | **Excludes** | *biopsy of gum (24.11)*
          excision of odontogenic lesion (24.4)

   24.32   Suture of laceration of gum

   24.39   Other

   ✖ **24.4   Excision of dental lesion of jaw**
       Excision of odontogenic lesion

   ✖ **24.5   Alveoloplasty**
       Alveolectomy (interradicular) (intraseptal) (radical)
         (simple) (with graft or implant)

       | **Excludes** | *biopsy of alveolus (24.12)*
          en bloc resection of alveolar process and palate
            (27.32)

   24.6   Exposure of tooth

   24.7   Application of orthodontic appliance
       Application, insertion, or fitting of:
         arch bars
         orthodontic obturator
         orthodontic wiring
         periodontal splint

       | **Excludes** | *nonorthodontic dental wiring (93.55)*

   24.8   Other orthodontic operation
       Closure of diastema (alveolar) (dental)
       Occlusal adjustment
       Removal of arch bars
       Repair of dental arch

       | **Excludes** | *removal of nonorthodontic wiring (97.33)*

OPERATIONS ON THE NOSE, MOUTH, AND PHARYNX (21–29)

◀ New   ◀▥ Revised   ~~deleted~~ Deleted   ● Use Additional Digit(s)   ✖ Valid O.R. Procedure

◆ Non-O.R. Procedure   ♀ Females Only   ♂ Males Only

● **24.9 Other dental operations**

     24.91 Extension or deepening of buccolabial or lingual sulcus

     24.99 Other

> **Excludes**   *dental:*
> *debridement (96.54)*
> *examination (89.31)*
> *prophylaxis (96.54)*
> *scaling and polishing (96.54)*
> *wiring (93.55)*
> *fitting of dental appliance [denture]*
>   *(99.97)*
> *microscopic examination of dental*
>   *specimen (90.81–90.89)*
> *removal of dental:*
>   *packing (97.34)*
>   *prosthesis (97.35)*
>   *wiring (97.33)*
> *replacement of dental packing (97.22)*

● **25 Operations on tongue**

● **25.0 Diagnostic procedures on tongue**

     25.01 Closed [needle] biopsy of tongue
         MCE: Closed biopsy procedure

     ✖ **25.02 Open biopsy of tongue**
         Wedge biopsy
         MCE: Open biopsy procedure

     25.09 Other diagnostic procedures on tongue

✖ **25.1 Excision or destruction of lesion or tissue of tongue**

> **Excludes**   *biopsy of tongue (25.01–25.02)*
> *frenumectomy:*
>   *labial (27.41)*
>   *lingual (25.92)*

     Coding Clinic: 2002, Q2, P5-6

✖ **25.2 Partial glossectomy**

✖ **25.3 Complete glossectomy**
     Glossectomy NOS

> Code also any neck dissection (40.40–40.42)

✖ **25.4 Radical glossectomy**

> Code also any:
> neck dissection (40.40–40.42)
> tracheostomy (31.1–31.29)

● **25.5 Repair of tongue and glossoplasty**

     25.51 Suture of laceration of tongue

     ✖ **25.59 Other repair and plastic operations on tongue**
         Fascial sling of tongue
         Fusion of tongue (to lip)
         Graft of mucosa or skin to tongue

> **Excludes**   *lysis of adhesions of tongue (25.93)*

         Coding Clinic: 1997, Q1, P5

● **25.9 Other operations on tongue**

     25.91 Lingual frenotomy

> **Excludes**   *labial frenotomy (27.91)*

     25.92 Lingual frenectomy

> **Excludes**   *labial frenectomy (27.41)*

     25.93 Lysis of adhesions of tongue

     ✖ **25.94 Other glossotomy**

     ✖ **25.99 Other**

● **26 Operations on salivary glands and ducts**

> **Includes**   operations on:
> lesser salivary gland and duct
> parotid gland and duct
> sublingual gland and duct
> submaxillary gland and duct

> Code also any neck dissection (40.40–40.42)

     26.0 Incision of salivary gland or duct

● **26.1 Diagnostic procedures on salivary glands and ducts**

     26.11 Closed [needle] biopsy of salivary gland or duct
         MCE: Closed biopsy procedure

     ✖ **26.12 Open biopsy of salivary gland or duct**
         MCE: Open biopsy procedure

     26.19 Other diagnostic procedures on salivary glands and ducts

> **Excludes**   *x-ray of salivary gland (87.09)*

● **26.2 Excision of lesion of salivary gland**

     ✖ **26.21 Marsupialization of salivary gland cyst**

     ✖ **26.29 Other excision of salivary gland lesion**

> **Excludes**   *biopsy of salivary gland (26.11–26.12)*
> *salivary fistulectomy (26.42)*

● **26.3 Sialoadenectomy**

     ✖ **26.30 Sialoadenectomy, not otherwise specified**

     ✖ **26.31 Partial sialoadenectomy**

     ✖ **26.32 Complete sialoadenectomy**
         En bloc excision of salivary gland lesion
         Radical sialoadenectomy

● **26.4 Repair of salivary gland or duct**

     ✖ **26.41 Suture of laceration of salivary gland**

     ✖ **26.42 Closure of salivary fistula**

     ✖ **26.49 Other repair and plastic operations on salivary gland or duct**
         Fistulization of salivary gland
         Plastic repair of salivary gland or duct NOS
         Transplantation of salivary duct opening

● **26.9 Other operations on salivary gland or duct**

     26.91 Probing of salivary duct

     ✖ **26.99 Other**

● **27 Other operations on mouth and face**

> **Includes**   operations on:
> lips
> palate
> soft tissue of face and mouth, except tongue
>   and gingiva

> **Excludes**   *operations on:*
> *gingiva (24.0–24.99)*
> *tongue (25.01–25.99)*

     ✖ **27.0 Drainage of face and floor of mouth**
         Drainage of:
         facial region (abscess)
         fascial compartment of face
         Ludwig's angina

> **Excludes**   *drainage of thyroglossal tract (06.09)*

     ✖ **27.1 Incision of palate**

OPERATIONS ON THE NOSE, MOUTH, AND PHARYNX (21–29)

- **27.2　Diagnostic procedures on oral cavity**
  - ✖ **27.21　Biopsy of bony palate**
  - ✖ **27.22　Biopsy of uvula and soft palate**
  - **27.23　Biopsy of lip**
  - **27.24　Biopsy of mouth, unspecified structure**
  - **27.29　Other diagnostic procedures on oral cavity**
    - **Excludes** *soft tissue x-ray (87.09)*
- **27.3　Excision of lesion or tissue of bony palate**
  - ✖ **27.31　Local excision or destruction of lesion or tissue of bony palate**
    - Local excision or destruction of palate by:
      - cautery
      - chemotherapy
      - cryotherapy
    - **Excludes** *biopsy of bony palate (27.21)*
  - ✖ **27.32　Wide excision or destruction of lesion or tissue of bony palate**
    - En bloc resection of alveolar process and palate
- **27.4　Excision of other parts of mouth**
  - **27.41　Labial frenectomy**
    - **Excludes** *division of labial frenum (27.91)*
  - ✖ **27.42　Wide excision of lesion of lip**
  - ✖ **27.43　Other excision of lesion or tissue of lip**
  - ✖ **27.49　Other excision of mouth**
    - **Excludes** *biopsy of mouth NOS (27.24)*
      excision of lesion of:
      palate (27.31–27.32)
      tongue (25.1)
      uvula (27.72)
      fistulectomy of mouth (27.53)
      frenectomy of:
      lip (27.41)
      tongue (25.92)
    - Coding Clinic: 2005, Q2, P8-9
- **27.5　Plastic repair of lip and mouth** ⬅||||
  - **Excludes** *palatoplasty (27.61–27.69)*
  - **27.51　Suture of laceration of lip**
  - **27.52　Suture of laceration of other part of mouth**
  - ✖ **27.53　Closure of fistula of mouth**
    - **Excludes** *fistulectomy:*
      nasolabial (21.82)
      oro-antral (22.71)
      oronasal (21.82)
  - ✖ **27.54　Repair of cleft lip**
  - ✖ **27.55　Full-thickness skin graft to lip and mouth**
  - ✖ **27.56　Other skin graft to lip and mouth**
  - ✖ **27.57　Attachment of pedicle or flap graft to lip and mouth**
  - ✖ **27.59　Other plastic repair of mouth**
- **27.6　Palatoplasty**
  - ✖ **27.61　Suture of laceration of palate**
  - ✖ **27.62　Correction of cleft palate**
    - Correction of cleft palate by push-back operation
    - **Excludes** *revision of cleft palate repair (27.63)*
  - ✖ **27.63　Revision of cleft palate repair**
    - Secondary:
      - attachment of pharyngeal flap
      - lengthening of palate
    - Coding Clinic: 1996, Q1, P14

- ✖ **27.64　Insertion of palatal implant**
  - Coding Clinic: 2004, Q4, P117-118
- ✖ **27.69　Other plastic repair of palate**
  - Code also any insertion of palatal implant (27.64)
  - **Excludes** *fistulectomy of mouth (27.53)*
  - Coding Clinic: 1999, Q3, P22; 1997, Q1, P5; 1985, Mar-April, P12
- **27.7　Operations on uvula**
  - ✖ **27.71　Incision of uvula**
  - ✖ **27.72　Excision of uvula**
    - **Excludes** *biopsy of uvula (27.22)*
  - ✖ **27.73　Repair of uvula**
    - **Excludes** *that with synchronous cleft palate repair (27.62)*
      uranostaphylorrhaphy (27.62)
  - ✖ **27.79　Other operations on uvula**
    - Coding Clinic: 1992, Q3, P18; 1985, Mar-April, P12
- **27.9　Other operations on mouth and face**
  - **27.91　Labial frenotomy**
    - Division of labial frenum
    - **Excludes** *lingual frenotomy (25.91)*
  - ✖ **27.92　Incision of mouth, unspecified structure**
    - **Excludes** *incision of:*
      gum (24.0)
      palate (27.1)
      salivary gland or duct (26.0)
      tongue (25.94)
      uvula (27.71)
  - ✖ **27.99　Other operations on oral cavity**
    - Graft of buccal sulcus
    - **Excludes** *removal of:*
      intraluminal foreign body (98.01)
      penetrating foreign body from mouth without incision (98.22)
- **28　Operations on tonsils and adenoids**
  - ✖ **28.0　Incision and drainage of tonsil and peritonsillar structures**
    - Drainage (oral) (transcervical) of:
      - parapharyngeal abscess
      - peritonsillar abscess
      - retropharyngeal abscess
      - tonsillar abscess
  - **28.1　Diagnostic procedures on tonsils and adenoids**
    - ✖ **28.11　Biopsy of tonsils and adenoids**
    - ✖ **28.19　Other diagnostic procedures on tonsils and adenoids**
      - **Excludes** *soft tissue x-ray (87.09)*
  - ✖ **28.2　Tonsillectomy without adenoidectomy**
    - Coding Clinic: 1997, Q1, P5; 1990, Q2, P23
  - ✖ **28.3　Tonsillectomy with adenoidectomy**
    - Coding Clinic: 2005, Q2, P16
  - ✖ **28.4　Excision of tonsil tag**
  - ✖ **28.5　Excision of lingual tonsil**
  - ✖ **28.6　Adenoidectomy without tonsillectomy**
    - Excision of adenoid tag
  - ✖ **28.7　Control of hemorrhage after tonsillectomy and adenoidectomy**
    - Coding Clinic: 2005, Q2, P16

◀ New　　⬅|||| Revised　　deleted Deleted　　● Use Additional Digit(s)　　✖ Valid O.R. Procedure
◆ Non-O.R. Procedure　　♀ Females Only　　♂ Males Only

OPERATIONS ON THE NOSE, MOUTH, AND PHARYNX (21–29)

● **28.9 Other operations on tonsils and adenoids**

✖ **28.91 Removal of foreign body from tonsil and adenoid by incision**

> Excludes │ *that without incision (98.13)*

✖ **28.92 Excision of lesion of tonsil and adenoid**

> Excludes │ *biopsy of tonsil and adenoid (28.11)*

✖ **28.99 Other**

Coding Clinic: 1990, Q2, P23

● **29 Operations on pharynx**

> Includes │ operations on:
> hypopharynx
> nasopharynx
> oropharynx
> pharyngeal pouch
> pyriform sinus

✖ **29.0 Pharyngotomy**

Drainage of pharyngeal bursa

> Excludes │ *incision and drainage of retropharyngeal*
> *abscess (28.0)*
> *removal of foreign body (without incision)*
> *(98.13)*

● **29.1 Diagnostic procedures on pharynx**

29.11 Pharyngoscopy

29.12 Pharyngeal biopsy

Biopsy of supraglottic mass

29.19 Other diagnostic procedures on pharynx

> Excludes │ *x-ray of nasopharynx:*
> *contrast (87.06)*
> *other (87.09)*

✖ **29.2 Excision of branchial cleft cyst or vestige**

> Excludes │ *branchial cleft fistulectomy (29.52)*

● **29.3 Excision or destruction of lesion or tissue of pharynx**

✖ **29.31 Cricopharyngeal myotomy**

> Excludes │ *that with pharyngeal diverticulectomy*
> *(29.32)*

✖ **29.32 Pharyngeal diverticulectomy**

✖ **29.33 Pharyngectomy (partial)**

> Excludes │ *laryngopharyngectomy (30.3)*

✖ **29.39 Other excision or destruction of lesion or tissue of pharynx**

✖ **29.4 Plastic operation on pharynx**

Correction of nasopharyngeal atresia

> Excludes │ *pharyngoplasty associated with cleft palate*
> *repair (27.62–27.63)*

Coding Clinic: 1999, Q3, P22; 1997, Q1, P5; 1992, Q3, P18; 1985, Mar-April, P12

● **29.5 Other repair of pharynx**

✖ **29.51 Suture of laceration of pharynx**

✖ **29.52 Closure of branchial cleft fistula**

✖ **29.53 Closure of other fistula of pharynx**

Pharyngoesophageal fistulectomy

✖ **29.54 Lysis of pharyngeal adhesions**

✖ **29.59 Other**

● **29.9 Other operations on pharynx**

29.91 Dilation of pharynx

Dilation of nasopharynx

✖ **29.92 Division of glossopharyngeal nerve**

✖ **29.99 Other**

> Excludes │ *insertion of radium into pharynx and*
> *nasopharynx (92.27)*
> *removal of intraluminal foreign body*
> *(98.13)*

OPERATIONS ON THE NOSE, MOUTH, AND PHARYNX (21–29)

6. OPERATIONS ON THE RESPIRATORY SYSTEM (30–34)

● **30 Excision of larynx**

  ● **30.0 Excision or destruction of lesion or tissue of larynx**

    ✖ **30.01 Marsupialization of laryngeal cyst**

    ✖ **30.09 Other excision or destruction of lesion or tissue of larynx**
      Stripping of vocal cords

      Excludes *biopsy of larynx (31.43)*
        laryngeal fistulectomy (31.62)
        laryngotracheal fistulectomy (31.62)

  ✖ **30.1 Hemilaryngectomy**

  ● **30.2 Other partial laryngectomy**

    ✖ **30.21 Epiglottidectomy**

    ✖ **30.22 Vocal cordectomy**
      Excision of vocal cords

    ✖ **30.29 Other partial laryngectomy**
      Excision of laryngeal cartilage

  ✖ **30.3 Complete laryngectomy**
    Block dissection of larynx (with thyroidectomy) (with synchronous tracheostomy)
    Laryngopharyngectomy

    Excludes *that with radical neck dissection (30.4)*

  ✖ **30.4 Radical laryngectomy**
    Complete [total] laryngectomy with radical neck dissection (with thyroidectomy) (with synchronous tracheostomy)

● **31 Other operations on larynx and trachea**

  31.0 Injection of larynx
    Injection of inert material into larynx or vocal cords

  31.1 Temporary tracheostomy
    Temporary percutaneous dilatational tracheostomy [PDT]
    Tracheotomy for assistance in breathing

    Code also any synchronous bronchoscopy, if performed (33.21–33.24, 33.27)
    Coding Clinic: 1997, Q1, P6

    ◆ Non-OR Procedure that affects MS-DRG assignment to MS-DRG 003-004, 011-013

  ● **31.2 Permanent tracheostomy**

    ✖ **31.21 Mediastinal tracheostomy**

    ✖ **31.29 Other permanent tracheostomy**
      Permanent percutaneous dilatational tracheostomy [PDT]

      Excludes *that with laryngectomy (30.3–30.4)*

      Code also any synchronous bronchoscopy, if performed (33.21–33.24, 33.27)
      Coding Clinic: 2005, Q2, P8-9; 2002, Q2, P6

  ✖ **31.3 Other incision of larynx or trachea**

    Excludes *that for assistance in breathing (31.1–31.29)*

  ● **31.4 Diagnostic procedures on larynx and trachea**

    31.41 Tracheoscopy through artificial stoma

      Excludes *that with biopsy (31.43–31.44)*

    31.42 Laryngoscopy and other tracheoscopy

      Excludes *that with biopsy (31.43–31.44)*

    31.43 Closed [endoscopic] biopsy of larynx
      MCE: Closed biopsy procedure

    31.44 Closed [endoscopic] biopsy of trachea
      MCE: Closed biopsy procedure

    ✖ **31.45 Open biopsy of larynx or trachea**
      MCE: Open biopsy procedure

    31.48 Other diagnostic procedures on larynx

      Excludes *contrast laryngogram (87.07)*
        microscopic examination of specimen from larynx (90.31–90.39)
        soft tissue x-ray of larynx NEC (87.09)

    31.49 Other diagnostic procedures on trachea

      Excludes *microscopic examination of specimen from trachea (90.41–90.49)*
        x-ray of trachea (87.49)

  ✖ **31.5 Local excision or destruction of lesion or tissue of trachea**

    Excludes *biopsy of trachea (31.44–31.45)*
      laryngotracheal fistulectomy (31.62)
      tracheoesophageal fistulectomy (31.73)

  ● **31.6 Repair of larynx**

    ✖ **31.61 Suture of laceration of larynx**

    ✖ **31.62 Closure of fistula of larynx**
      Laryngotracheal fistulectomy
      Take-down of laryngostomy

    ✖ **31.63 Revision of laryngostomy**

    ✖ **31.64 Repair of laryngeal fracture**

    ✖ **31.69 Other repair of larynx**
      Arytenoidopexy
      Graft of larynx
      Transposition of vocal cords

      Excludes *construction of artificial larynx (31.75)*

  ● **31.7 Repair and plastic operations on trachea**

    ✖ **31.71 Suture of laceration of trachea**

    ✖ **31.72 Closure of external fistula of trachea**
      Closure of tracheotomy

    ✖ **31.73 Closure of other fistula of trachea**
      Tracheoesophageal fistulectomy

      Excludes *laryngotracheal fistulectomy (31.62)*

    ✖ **31.74 Revision of tracheostomy**

    ✖ **31.75 Reconstruction of trachea and construction of artificial larynx**
      Tracheoplasty with artificial larynx

    ✖ **31.79 Other repair and plastic operations on trachea**

  ● **31.9 Other operations on larynx and trachea**

    ✖ **31.91 Division of laryngeal nerve**

    ✖ **31.92 Lysis of adhesions of trachea or larynx**

    31.93 Replacement of laryngeal or tracheal stent

    31.94 Injection of locally-acting therapeutic substance into trachea

    31.95 Tracheoesophageal fistulization

    ✖ **31.98 Other operations on larynx**
      Dilation of larynx
      Division of congenital web of larynx
      Removal of keel or stent of larynx

      Excludes *removal of intraluminal foreign body from larynx without incision (98.14)*

    ✖ **31.99 Other operations on trachea**

      Excludes *removal of:*
        intraluminal foreign body from trachea without incision (98.15)
        tracheostomy tube (97.37)
        replacement of tracheostomy tube (97.23)
        tracheostomy toilette (96.55)

◄ New   ◄▬ Revised   ~~deleted~~ Deleted   ● Use Additional Digit(s)   ✖ Valid O.R. Procedure
◆ Non-O.R. Procedure   ♀ Females Only   ♂ Males Only

OPERATIONS ON THE RESPIRATORY SYSTEM (30–34)

● **32 Excision of lung and bronchus**

> **Includes**   rib resection as operative approach
> sternotomy as operative approach
> sternum-splitting incision as operative
>   approach
> thoracotomy as operative approach

> Code also   any synchronous bronchoplasty (33.48)
> Coding Clinic: 1988, Q4, P11

● **32.0 Local excision or destruction of lesion or tissue of bronchus**

> **Excludes**   *biopsy of bronchus (33.24–33.25)*
> *bronchial fistulectomy (33.42)*

  32.01 Endoscopic excision or destruction of lesion or tissue of bronchus

✖ **32.09 Other local excision or destruction of lesion or tissue of bronchus**

> **Excludes**   *that by endoscopic approach (32.01)*

✖ **32.1 Other excision of bronchus**
> Resection (wide sleeve) of bronchus

> **Excludes**   *radical dissection [excision] of bronchus (32.6)*

● **32.2 Local excision or destruction of lesion or tissue of lung**
> Coding Clinic: 2006, Q4, P124-126

✖ **32.20 Thoracoscopic excision of lesion or tissue of lung**
> Thoracoscopic wedge resection
> Coding Clinic: 2007, Q4, P109-113

✖ **32.21 Plication of emphysematous bleb**

✖ **32.22 Lung volume reduction surgery**
> Coding Clinic: 1997, Q1, P6; 1995, Q4, P64
> MCE: Limited coverage

✖ **32.23 Open ablation of lung lesion or tissue**

✖ **32.24 Percutaneous ablation of lung lesion or tissue**

✖ **32.25 Thoracoscopic ablation of lung lesion or tissue**

> **Excludes**   *thoracoscopic excision of lesion or*
> *tissue of lung (32.20)*

✖ **32.26 Other and unspecified ablation of lung lesion or tissue**

  32.28 Endoscopic excision or destruction of lesion or tissue of lung

> **Excludes**   *ablation of lung lesion or tissue:*
> *open (32.23)*
> *other (32.26)*
> *percutaneous (32.24)*
> *thoracoscopic (32.25)*
> *biopsy of lung (33.26–33.27)*

✖ **32.29 Other local excision or destruction of lesion or tissue of lung**
> Resection of lung:
>   NOS
>   wedge

> **Excludes**   *ablation of lung lesion or tissue:*
> *open (32.23)*
> *other (32.26)*
> *percutaneous (32.24)*
> *thoracoscopic (32.25)*
> *biopsy of lung (33.26–33.27)*
> *laser interstitial thermal therapy*
>   *[LITT] of lesion or tissue of*
>   *lung under guidance (17.69)* ◄
> *that by endoscopic approach (32.28)*
> *thoracoscopic excision of lesion or*
>   *tissue of lung (32.20)*
> *wide excision of lesion of lung (32.3)*
> Coding Clinic: 1999, Q3, P3-4

● **32.3 Segmental resection of lung**
> Partial lobectomy

✖ **32.30 Thoracoscopic segmental resection of lung**
> Coding Clinic: 2007, Q4, P109-113

✖ **32.39 Other and unspecified segmental resection of lung**

> **Excludes**   *thoracoscopic segmental resection of*
> *lung (32.30)*

● **32.4 Lobectomy of lung**
> Lobectomy with segmental resection of adjacent lobes
>   of lung

> **Excludes**   *that with radical dissection [excision] of*
> *thoracic structures (32.6)*

✖ **32.41 Thoracoscopic lobectomy of lung**
> Coding Clinic: 2007, Q4, P109-113

✖ **32.49 Other lobectomy of lung**

> **Excludes**   *thoracoscopic lobectomy of lung (32.41)*

● **32.5 Pneumonectomy**
> Excision of lung NOS
> Pneumonectomy (with mediastinal dissection)
> Coding Clinic: 1999, Q1, P6

✖ **32.50 Thoracoscopic pneumonectomy**
> Coding Clinic: 2007, Q4, P109-113

✖ **32.59 Other and unspecified pneumonectomy**

> **Excludes**   *thoracoscopic pneumonectomy (32.50)*

✖ **32.6 Radical dissection of thoracic structures**
> Block [en bloc] dissection of bronchus, lobe of lung,
>   brachial plexus, intercostal structure, ribs
>   (transverse process), and sympathetic nerves

✖ **32.9 Other excision of lung**

> **Excludes**   *biopsy of lung and bronchus (33.24–33.27)*
> *pulmonary decortication (34.51)*

● **33 Other operations on lung and bronchus**

> **Includes**   rib resection as operative approach
> sternotomy as operative approach
> sternum-splitting incision as operative
>   approach
> thoracotomy as operative approach

✖ **33.0 Incision of bronchus**

✖ **33.1 Incision of lung**

> **Excludes**   *puncture of lung (33.93)*

● **33.2 Diagnostic procedures on lung and bronchus**

✖ **33.20 Thoracoscopic lung biopsy**

> **Excludes**   *closed endoscopic biopsy of lung*
>   *(33.27)*
> *closed [percutaneous] [needle] biopsy of*
>   *lung (33.26)*
> *open biopsy of lung (33.28)*
> Coding Clinic: 2007, Q4, P109-113

  33.21 Bronchoscopy through artificial stoma

> **Excludes**   *that with biopsy (33.24, 33.27)*

  33.22 Fiber-optic bronchoscopy

> **Excludes**   *that with biopsy (33.24, 33.27)*
> Coding Clinic: 2004, Q1, P4-5; 1986, Sept-Oct, P11

  33.23 Other bronchoscopy

> **Excludes**   *that for:*
> *aspiration (96.05)*
> *biopsy (33.24, 33.27)*
> Coding Clinic: 2002, Q3, P18; 1999, Q1, P6

OPERATIONS ON THE RESPIRATORY SYSTEM (30–34)

33.24   Closed [endoscopic] biopsy of bronchus
Bronchoscopy (fiberoptic) (rigid) with:
    brush biopsy of "lung"
    brushing or washing for specimen collection
    excision (bite) biopsy
Diagnostic bronchoalveolar lavage (BAL)
Transbronchoscopic needle aspiration [TBNA] ◄

> **Excludes**   *closed biopsy of lung, other than brush*
> *biopsy of "lung" (33.26, 33.27)*
> *whole lung lavage (33.99)*

Coding Clinic: 2009, Q2, P10; 2006, Q2, P20; 2004, Q3, P9;
2002, Q3, P16-17; 1991, Q3, P15; Q2, P15
MCE: Closed biopsy procedure

✖ **33.25   Open biopsy of bronchus**

> **Excludes**   *open biopsy of lung (33.28)*

MCE: Open biopsy procedure

33.26   Closed [percutaneous] [needle] biopsy of lung
Fine needle aspiration (FNA) of lung
Transthoracic needle biopsy of lung (TTNB)

> **Excludes**   *endoscopic biopsy of lung (33.27)*
> *thoracoscopic lung biopsy (33.20)*

Coding Clinic: 1992, Q3, P12-13
MCE: Closed biopsy procedure

✖ **33.27   Closed endoscopic biopsy of lung**
Fiber-optic (flexible) bronchoscopy with
    fluoroscopic guidance with biopsy
Transbronchial lung biopsy

> **Excludes**   *brush biopsy of "lung" (33.24)*
> *percutaneous biopsy of lung (33.26)*
> *thoracoscopic lung biopsy (33.20)*

Coding Clinic: 2009, Q2, P10; 2004, Q3, P9; 2002, Q3, P16-17;
1991, Q3, P15; 1986, Sept-Oct, P11

✖ **33.28   Open biopsy of lung**
Coding Clinic: 1999, Q3, P3-4; 1992, Q3, P12-13
MCE: Open biopsy procedure

✖ **33.29   Other diagnostic procedures on lung and
bronchus**

> **Excludes**   *contrast bronchogram:*
> *endotracheal (87.31)*
> *other (87.32)*
> *endoscopic pulmonary airway flow*
> *measurement (33.72)*
> *lung scan (92.15)*
> *magnetic resonance imaging (88.92)*
> *microscopic examination of specimen*
> *from bronchus or lung*
> *(90.41–90.49)*
> *routine chest x-ray (87.44)*
> *ultrasonography of lung (88.73)*
> *vital capacity determination (89.37)*
> *x-ray of bronchus or lung NOS (87.49)*

● **33.3   Surgical collapse of lung**

33.31   Destruction of phrenic nerve for collapse of lung

33.32   Artificial pneumothorax for collapse of lung
Thoracotomy for collapse of lung

33.33   Pneumoperitoneum for collapse of lung

✖ **33.34   Thoracoplasty**

✖ **33.39   Other surgical collapse of lung**
Collapse of lung NOS

● **33.4   Repair and plastic operation on lung and bronchus**

✖ **33.41   Suture of laceration of bronchus**

✖ **33.42   Closure of bronchial fistula**
Closure of bronchostomy
Fistulectomy:
    bronchocutaneous
    bronchoesophageal
    bronchovisceral

> **Excludes**   *closure of fistula:*
> *bronchomediastinal (34.73)*
> *bronchopleural (34.73)*
> *bronchopleuromediastinal (34.73)*

✖ **33.43   Closure of laceration of lung**

✖ **33.48   Other repair and plastic operations on bronchus**

✖ **33.49   Other repair and plastic operations on lung**

> **Excludes**   *closure of pleural fistula (34.73)*

● **33.5   Lung transplant**
Note: To report donor source - *see* codes 00.91–00.93

> **Excludes**   *combined heart-lung transplantation (33.6)*

Code also cardiopulmonary bypass [extracorporeal
circulation] [heart-lung machine] (39.61)

✖ **33.50   Lung transplantation, not otherwise specified**
MCE: Limited coverage

✖ **33.51   Unilateral lung transplantation**
MCE: Limited coverage

✖ **33.52   Bilateral lung transplantation**
Double-lung transplantation
En bloc transplantation

> Code also cardiopulmonary bypass
> [extracorporeal circulation] [heart-lung
> machine] (39.61)

MCE: Limited coverage

✖ **33.6   Combined heart-lung transplantation**
Note: To report donor source - *see* codes 00.91–00.93

Code also cardiopulmonary bypass [extracorporeal
circulation] [heart-lung machine] (39.61)
MCE: Limited coverage

● **33.7   Other endoscopic procedures in bronchus or lung**

> **Excludes**   *insertion of tracheobronchial stent (96.05)*

Coding Clinic: 2006, Q4, P126-127

**33.71   Endoscopic insertion or replacement of
bronchial valve(s), single lobe** ◄▥
Endobronchial airflow redirection valve
Intrabronchial airflow redirection valve

> **Excludes**   *endoscopic insertion or replacement of*
> *bronchial valve(s), single*
> *lobe (33.73)* ◄

Coding Clinic: 2008, Q4, P174-175

**33.72   Endoscopic pulmonary airway flow
measurement**
Assessment of pulmonary airway flow

> Code also any diagnostic or therapeutic
> procedure if performed

Coding Clinic: 2008, Q4, P174-175

**33.73   Endoscopic insertion or replacement of
bronchial valve(s), multiple lobes** ◄

> **Excludes**   *endoscopic insertion or replacement of*
> *bronchial valve(s), single*
> *lobe (33.71)* ◄

**33.78   Endoscopic removal of bronchial device(s) or
substances**

**33.79   Endoscopic insertion of other bronchial device
or substances**
Biologic Lung Volume Reduction NOS (BLVR)

◄ New   ◄▥ Revised   ~~deleted~~ Deleted   ● Use Additional Digit(s)   ✖ Valid O.R. Procedure
◆ Non-O.R. Procedure   ♀ Females Only   ♂ Males Only

OPERATIONS ON THE RESPIRATORY SYSTEM (30–34)

● **33.9 Other operations on lung and bronchus**

    33.91 Bronchial dilation
       Coding Clinic: 1997, Q1, P14

✖ **33.92 Ligation of bronchus**

✖ **33.93 Puncture of lung**
       Excludes   *needle biopsy (33.26)*

✖ **33.98 Other operations on bronchus**
       Excludes   *bronchial lavage (96.56)*
           removal of intraluminal foreign body
             from bronchus without incision
             (98.15)

✖ **33.99 Other operations on lung**
       Whole lung lavage
       Excludes   *other continuous mechanical*
             ventilation (96.70–96.72)
             respiratory therapy (93.90–93.99)
       Coding Clinic: 2002, Q3, P17

● **34 Operations on chest wall, pleura, mediastinum, and diaphragm**
       Excludes   *operations on breast (85.0–85.99)*

● **34.0 Incision of chest wall and pleura**
       Excludes   *that as operative approach — omit code*

    34.01 Incision of chest wall
       Extrapleural drainage
       Excludes   *incision of pleura (34.09)*
       Coding Clinic: 2000, Q3, P12; 1992, Q1, P13

✖ **34.02 Exploratory thoracotomy**

✖ **34.03 Reopening of recent thoracotomy site**

    34.04 Insertion of intercostal catheter for drainage
       Chest tube
       Closed chest drainage
       Revision of intercostal catheter (chest tube)
           (with lysis of adhesions)
       Excludes   *thoracoscopic drainage of pleural cavity*
             (34.06)
       Coding Clinic: 2007, Q1, P14; 2003, Q2, P7-8; 1999, Q2,
             P12-13; Q1, P10; 1995, Q1, P5-6; 1992, Q1, P12

    34.05 Creation of pleuroperitoneal shunt

✖ **34.06 Thoracoscopic drainage of pleural cavity**
       Evacuation of empyema
       Coding Clinic: 2007, Q4, P109-113

    34.09 Other incision of pleura
       Creation of pleural window for drainage
       Intercostal stab
       Open chest drainage
       Excludes   *thoracoscopy (34.21)*
             thoracotomy for collapse of lung
             (33.32)
       Coding Clinic: 2002, Q3, P22-23x2; 1994, Q1, P8

✖ **34.1 Incision of mediastinum**
       Excludes   *mediastinoscopy (34.22)*
             mediastinotomy associated with
             pneumonectomy (32.5)
       Code also any biopsy, if performed   ◄

● **34.2 Diagnostic procedures on chest wall, pleura, mediastinum, and diaphragm**

✖ **34.20 Thoracoscopic pleural biopsy**
       Coding Clinic: 2007, Q4, P109-113

✖ **34.21 Transpleural thoracoscopy**
       Coding Clinic: 2002, Q3, P27

✖ **34.22 Mediastinoscopy**
       Code also any ~~lymph node~~ biopsy, if
           performed (40.11)   ◄═

    34.23 Biopsy of chest wall

    34.24 Other pleural biopsy
       Excludes   *thoracoscopic pleural biopsy (34.20)*
       Coding Clinic: 2002, Q3, P22-23, 27

    34.25 Closed [percutaneous] [needle] biopsy of mediastinum
       MCE: Closed biopsy procedure

✖ **34.26 Open mediastinal biopsy**
       MCE: Open biopsy procedure

✖ **34.27 Biopsy of diaphragm**

✖ **34.28 Other diagnostic procedures on chest wall, pleura, and diaphragm**
       Excludes   *angiocardiography (88.50–88.58)*
             aortography (88.42)
             arteriography of:
                intrathoracic vessels NEC (88.44)
                pulmonary arteries (88.43)
             microscopic examination of specimen
                from chest wall, pleura, and
                diaphragm (90.41–90.49)
             phlebography of:
                intrathoracic vessels NEC (88.63)
                pulmonary veins (88.62)
             radiological examinations of thorax:
             C.A.T. scan (87.41)
             diaphragmatic x-ray (87.49)
             intrathoracic lymphangiogram
                (87.34)
             routine chest x-ray (87.44)
             sinogram of chest wall (87.38)
             soft tissue x-ray of chest wall NEC
                (87.39)
             tomogram of thorax NEC (87.42)
             ultrasonography of thorax 88.73)

✖ **34.29 Other diagnostic procedures on mediastinum**
       Excludes   *mediastinal:*
             pneumogram (87.33)
             x-ray NEC (87.49)

✖ **34.3 Excision or destruction of lesion or tissue of mediastinum**
       Excludes   *biopsy of mediastinum (34.25–34.26)*
             mediastinal fistulectomy (34.73)

✖ **34.4 Excision or destruction of lesion of chest wall**
       Excision of lesion of chest wall NOS (with excision
          of ribs)
       Excludes   *biopsy of chest wall (34.23)*
             costectomy not incidental to thoracic
                procedure (77.91)
             excision of lesion of:
                breast (85.20–85.25)
                cartilage (80.89)
                skin (86.2–86.3)
             fistulectomy (34.73)

OPERATIONS ON THE RESPIRATORY SYSTEM (30-34)

● **34.5**   **Pleurectomy**

  ✖ **34.51**   **Decortication of lung**

     Excludes   *thoracoscopic decortication of lung (34.52)*

  ✖ **34.52**   **Thoracoscopic decortication of lung**
     Coding Clinic: 2007, Q4, P109-113

  ✖ **34.59**   **Other excision of pleura**
     Excision of pleural lesion

     Excludes   *biopsy of pleura (34.24)*
                  pleural fistulectomy (34.73)

✖ **34.6**   **Scarification of pleura**
   Pleurosclerosis

     Excludes   *injection of sclerosing agent (34.92)*

     Coding Clinic: 1992, Q1, P12

● **34.7**   **Repair of chest wall**

   34.71   **Suture of laceration of chest wall**

     Excludes   *suture of skin and subcutaneous tissue alone (86.59)*

   34.72   **Closure of thoracostomy**

  ✖ **34.73**   **Closure of other fistula of thorax**
     Closure of:
       bronchopleural fistula
       bronchopleurocutaneous fistula
       bronchopleuromediastinal fistula

  ✖ **34.74**   **Repair of pectus deformity**
     Repair of:
       pectus carinatum (with implant)
       pectus excavatum (with implant)
     Coding Clinic: 2004, Q2, P6-7

  ✖ **34.79**   **Other repair of chest wall**
     Repair of chest wall NOS
     Coding Clinic: 2004, Q2, P6; 1987, Jan-Feb, P13

● **34.8**   **Operations on diaphragm**

  ✖ **34.81**   **Excision of lesion or tissue of diaphragm**

     Excludes   *biopsy of diaphragm (34.27)*

  ✖ **34.82**   **Suture of laceration of diaphragm**

  ✖ **34.83**   **Closure of fistula of diaphragm**
     Thoracicoabdominal fistulectomy
     Thoracicogastric fistulectomy
     Thoracicointestinal fistulectomy

  ✖ **34.84**   **Other repair of diaphragm**

     Excludes   *repair of diaphragmatic hernia (53.7–53.82)*

  ✖ **34.85**   **Implantation of diaphragmatic pacemaker**

  ✖ **34.89**   **Other operations on diaphragm**

● **34.9**   **Other operations on thorax**

   34.91   **Thoracentesis**

   34.92   **Injection into thoracic cavity**
     Chemical pleurodesis
     Injection of cytotoxic agent or tetracycline
     Coding Clinic: 2007, Q4, P109-113; 2007, Q1, P14; 1992, Q1, P12; 1989, Q2, P17
     Instillation into thoracic cavity
     Requires additional code for any cancer chemotherapeutic substance (99.25)

     Excludes   *that for collapse of lung (33.32)*

     Coding Clinic: 2007, Q4, P109-113; Q1, P14; 1992, Q1, P12; 1989, Q2, P17

  ✖ **34.93**   **Repair of pleura**

  ✖ **34.99**   **Other**

     Excludes   *removal of:*
           mediastinal drain (97.42)
           sutures (97.43)
           thoracotomy tube (97.41)
     Coding Clinic: 2000, Q1, P17; 1988, Q1, P9

OPERATIONS ON THE RESPIRATORY SYSTEM (30–34)

◄ New   ◄▥▥ Revised   ~~deleted~~ Deleted   ● Use Additional Digit(s)   ✖ Valid O.R. Procedure   ◆ Non-O.R. Procedure   ♀ Females Only   ♂ Males Only

(See Plates 141, 218, 219, 473, 500, 501, 502, 544, and
545 on pages NAP-9–NAP-14 and NAP-26–NAP-28.)

7.   **OPERATIONS ON THE
       CARDIOVASCULAR SYSTEM (35–39)**

● 35 **Operations on valves and septa of heart**

Includes   sternotomy (median) (transverse) as operative
               approach
               thoracotomy as operative approach

Code also cardiopulmonary bypass [extracorporeal
              circulation] [heart-lung machine] (39.61)

● 35.0 **Closed heart valvotomy**

    Excludes   *percutaneous (balloon) valvuloplasty (35.96)*

✖ 35.00 **Closed heart valvotomy, unspecified valve**

✖ 35.01 **Closed heart valvotomy, aortic valve**

✖ 35.02 **Closed heart valvotomy, mitral valve**

✖ 35.03 **Closed heart valvotomy, pulmonary valve**

✖ 35.04 **Closed heart valvotomy, tricuspid valve**

● 35.1 **Open heart valvuloplasty without replacement**

    Includes   open heart valvotomy

    Excludes   *that associated with repair of:*
               endocardial cushion defect (35.54, 35.63,
               35.73)
               percutaneous (balloon) valvuloplasty
               (35.96)
               valvular defect associated with atrial and
               ventricular septal defects (35.54,
               35.63, 35.73)

    Code also cardiopulmonary bypass if performed
              [extracorporeal circulation] [heart-lung
              machine] (39.61)
              Coding Clinic: 2008, Q2, P13

✖ 35.10 **Open heart valvuloplasty without replacement,
          unspecified valve**

✖ 35.11 **Open heart valvuloplasty of aortic valve without
          replacement**

✖ 35.12 **Open heart valvuloplasty of mitral valve
          without replacement**
          Coding Clinic: 1997, Q1, P13; 1988, Q1, P10

✖ 35.13 **Open heart valvuloplasty of pulmonary valve
          without replacement**

✖ 35.14 **Open heart valvuloplasty of tricuspid valve
          without replacement**

● 35.2 **Replacement of heart valve**

    Includes   excision of heart valve with replacement

    Code also cardiopulmonary bypass [extracorporeal
              circulation] [heart-lung machine] (39.61)

    Excludes   *that associated with repair of:*
               endocardial cushion defect (35.54, 35.63,
               35.73)
               valvular defect associated with atrial and
               ventricular septal defects (35.54,
               35.63, 35.73)

✖ 35.20 **Replacement of unspecified heart valve**
          Repair of unspecified heart valve with tissue
          graft or prosthetic implant

✖ 35.21 **Replacement of aortic valve with tissue graft**
          Repair of aortic valve with tissue graft
          (autograft) (heterograft) (homograft)
          Coding Clinic: 1997, Q2, P8

✖ 35.22 **Other replacement of aortic valve**
          Repair of aortic valve with replacement:
          NOS
          prosthetic (partial) (synthetic) (total)
          Coding Clinic: 2008, Q4, P177-180; 1996, Q1, P11

✖ 35.23 **Replacement of mitral valve with tissue graft**
          Repair of mitral valve with tissue graft
          (autograft) (heterograft) (homograft)

✖ 35.24 **Other replacement of mitral valve**
          Repair of mitral valve with replacement:
          NOS
          prosthetic (partial) (synthetic) (total)
          Coding Clinic: 1997, Q4, P54-55

✖ 35.25 **Replacement of pulmonary valve with tissue
          graft**
          Repair of pulmonary valve with tissue graft
          (autograft) (heterograft) (homograft)
          Coding Clinic: 2007, Q1, P14-15; 2004, Q1, P16-17; 1997,
          Q2, P8

✖ 35.26 **Other replacement of pulmonary valve**
          Repair of pulmonary valve with replacement:
          NOS
          prosthetic (partial) (synthetic) (total)

✖ 35.27 **Replacement of tricuspid valve with tissue graft**
          Repair of tricuspid valve with tissue graft
          (autograft) (heterograft) (homograft)

✖ 35.28 **Other replacement of tricuspid valve**
          Repair of tricuspid valve with replacement:
          NOS
          prosthetic (partial) (synthetic) (total)

● 35.3 **Operations on structures adjacent to heart valves**

    Code also cardiopulmonary bypass [extracorporeal
              circulation] [heart-lung machine] (39.61)

✖ 35.31 **Operations on papillary muscle**
          Division of papillary muscle
          Reattachment of papillary muscle
          Repair of papillary muscle

✖ 35.32 **Operations on chordae tendineae**
          Division of chordae tendineae
          Repair of chordae tendineae

✖ 35.33 **Annuloplasty**
          Plication of annulus
          Coding Clinic: 1997, Q1, P13; 1988, Q1, P10

✖ 35.34 **Infundibulectomy**
          Right ventricular infundibulectomy

✖ 35.35 **Operations on trabeculae carneae cordis**
          Division of trabeculae carneae cordis
          Excision of trabeculae carneae cordis
          Excision of aortic subvalvular ring

✖ 35.39 **Operations on other structures adjacent to
          valves of heart**
          Repair of sinus of Valsalva (aneurysm)

● 35.4 **Production of septal defect in heart**

35.41 **Enlargement of existing atrial septal defect**
        Rashkind procedure
        Septostomy (atrial) (balloon)

✖ 35.42 **Creation of septal defect in heart**
          Blalock-Hanlon operation

● 35.5 **Repair of atrial and ventricular septa with prosthesis**

    Includes   repair of septa with synthetic implant or
               patch

    Code also cardiopulmonary bypass [extracorporeal
              circulation] [heart-lung machine] (39.61)

✖ 35.50 **Repair of unspecified septal defect of heart with
          prosthesis**

    Excludes   *that associated with repair of:*
               endocardial cushion defect (35.54)
               septal defect associated with
               valvular defect (35.54)

Excludes   Includes   Use additional   Code also   Omit code

✖ 35.51 Repair of atrial septal defect with prosthesis, open technique
Atrioseptoplasty with prosthesis
Correction of atrial septal defect with
    prosthesis
Repair:
    foramen ovale (patent)
    with prosthesis ostium secundum defect
        with prosthesis

> **Excludes** *that associated with repair of:*
> *atrial septal defect associated with*
> *valvular and ventricular*
> *septal defects (35.54)*
> *endocardial cushion defect (35.54)*

✖ 35.52 Repair of atrial septal defect with prosthesis, closed technique
Insertion of atrial septal umbrella [King-Mills]
Coding Clinic: 2005, Q2, 17-18; 1998, Q3, P11

✖ 35.53 Repair of ventricular septal defect with prosthesis, open technique
Correction of ventricular septal defect with
    prosthesis
Repair of supracristal defect with prosthesis

> **Excludes** *that associated with repair of:*
> *endocardial cushion defect (35.54)*
> *ventricular defect associated with*
> *valvular and atrial septal*
> *defects (35.54)*

Coding Clinic: 2007, Q1, P14-15

✖ 35.54 Repair of endocardial cushion defect with prosthesis
Repair:
    atrioventricular canal with prosthesis
        (grafted to septa)
    ostium primum defect with prosthesis
        (grafted to septa)
    valvular defect associated with atrial
        and ventricular septal defects with
        prosthesis (grafted to septa)

> **Excludes** *repair of isolated:*
> *atrial septal defect (35.51–35.52)*
> *valvular defect (35.20, 35.22, 35.24,*
> *35.26, 35.28)*
> *ventricular septal defect (35.53)*

✖ 35.55 Repair of ventricular septal defect with prosthesis, closed technique

● 35.6 Repair of atrial and ventricular septa with tissue graft

Code also cardiopulmonary bypass [extracorporeal
    circulation] [heart-lung machine] (39.61)

✖ 35.60 Repair of unspecified septal defect of heart with tissue graft

> **Excludes** *that associated with repair of:*
> *endocardial cushion defect (35.63)*
> *septal defect associated with*
> *valvular defect (35.63)*

✖ 35.61 Repair of atrial septal defect with tissue graft
Atrioseptoplasty with tissue graft
Correction of atrial septal defect with tissue
    graft
Repair:
    foramen ovale (patent) with tissue graft
    ostium secundum defect with tissue graft

> **Excludes** *that associated with repair of:*
> *atrial septal defect associated with*
> *valvular and ventricular*
> *septal defects (35.63)*
> *endocardial cushion defect (35.63)*

✖ 35.62 Repair of ventricular septal defect with tissue graft
Correction of ventricular septal defect with
    tissue graft
Repair of supracristal defect with tissue graft

> **Excludes** *that associated with repair of:*
> *endocardial cushion defect (35.63)*
> *ventricular defect associate with*
> *valvular and atrial septal*
> *defects (35.63)*

✖ 35.63 Repair of endocardial cushion defect with tissue graft
Repair of:
    atrioventricular canal with tissue graft
    ostium primum defect with tissue graft
    valvular defect associated with atrial and
        ventricular septal defects with tissue
        graft

> **Excludes** *repair of isolated:*
> *atrial septal defect (35.61)*
> *valvular defect (35.20–35.21, 35.23,*
> *35.25, 35.27)*
> *ventricular septal defect (35.62)*

● 35.7 Other and unspecified repair of atrial and ventricular septa

Code also cardiopulmonary bypass [extracorporeal
    circulation] [heart-lung machine] (39.61)

✖ 35.70 Other and unspecified repair of unspecified septal defect of heart
Repair of septal defect NOS

> **Excludes** *that associated with repair of:*
> *endocardial cushion defect (35.73)*
> *septal defect associated with*
> *valvular defect (35.73)*

✖ 35.71 Other and unspecified repair of atrial septal defect
Repair NOS:
    atrial septum
    foramen ovale (patent)
    ostium secundum defect

> **Excludes** *that associated with repair of:*
> *atrial septal defect associated with*
> *valvular ventricular septal*
> *defects (35.73)*
> *endocardial cushion defect (35.73)*

✖ 35.72 Other and unspecified repair of ventricular septal defect
Repair NOS:
    supracristal defect
    ventricular septum

> **Excludes** *that associated with repair of:*
> *endocardial cushion defect (35.73)*
> *ventricular septal defect associated*
> *with valvular and atrial septal*
> *defects (35.73)*

✖ 35.73 Other and unspecified repair of endocardial cushion defect
Repair NOS:
    atrioventricular canal
    ostium primum defect
    valvular defect associated with atrial and
        ventricular septal defects

> **Excludes** *repair of isolated:*
> *atrial septal defect (35.71)*
> *valvular defect (35.20, 35.22, 35.24,*
> *35.26, 35.28)*
> *ventricular septal defect (35.72)*

◀ New   ◀▥ Revised   ~~deleted~~ Deleted   ● Use Additional Digit(s)   ✖ Valid O.R. Procedure
◆ Non-O.R. Procedure   ♀ Females Only   ♂ Males Only

OPERATIONS ON THE CARDIOVASCULAR SYSTEM (35–39)

● **35.8 Total repair of certain congenital cardiac anomalies**
  Note: For partial repair of defect [e.g. repair of atrial septal defect in tetralogy of Fallot] — *code to specific procedure*

✖ **35.81 Total repair of tetralogy of Fallot**
  One-stage total correction of tetralogy of Fallot with or without:
    commissurotomy of pulmonary valve
    infundibulectomy
    outflow tract prosthesis
    patch graft of outflow tract
    prosthetic tube for pulmonary artery
    repair of ventricular septal defect (with prosthesis)
    take-down of previous systemic-pulmonary artery anastomosis

✖ **35.82 Total repair of total anomalous venous connection**
  One-stage total correction of total anomalous pulmonary venous connection with or without:
    anastomosis between (horizontal) common pulmonary trunk and posterior wall of left atrium (side-to-side)
    enlargement of foramen ovale
    incision [excision] of common wall between posterior left atrium and coronary sinus and roofing of resultant defect with patch graft (synthetic)
    ligation of venous connection (descending anomalous vein) (to left innominate vein) (to superior vena cava)
    repair of atrial septal defect (with prosthesis)

✖ **35.83 Total repair of truncus arteriosus**
  One-stage total correction of truncus arteriosus with or without:
    construction (with aortic homograft) (with prosthesis) of a pulmonary artery placed from right ventricle to arteries supplying the lung
    ligation of connections between aorta and pulmonary artery
    repair of ventricular septal defect (with prosthesis)

✖ **35.84 Total correction of transposition of great vessels, not elsewhere classified**
  Arterial switch operation [Jatene]
  Total correction of transposition of great arteries at the arterial level by switching the great arteries, including the left or both coronary arteries, implanted in the wall of the pulmonary artery

  | Excludes | *baffle operation [Mustard] [Senning] (35.91)* |
  | | *creation of shunt between right ventricle and pulmonary artery [Rastelli] (35.92)* |

● **35.9 Other operations on valves and septa of heart**

  Code also cardiopulmonary bypass, if performed [extracorporeal circulation] [heart-lung machine] (39.61)

✖ **35.91 Interatrial transposition of venous return**
  Baffle:
    atrial
    interatrial
  Mustard's operation
  Resection of atrial septum and insertion of patch to direct systemic venous return to tricuspid valve and pulmonary venous return to mitral valve

✖ **35.92 Creation of conduit between right ventricle and pulmonary artery**
  Creation of shunt between right ventricle and (distal) pulmonary artery

  | Excludes | *that associated with total repair of truncus arteriosus (35.83)* |
  Coding Clinic: 2007, Q1, P14-15

✖ **35.93 Creation of conduit between left ventricle and aorta**
  Creation of apicoaortic shunt
  Shunt between apex of left ventricle and aorta
  Coding Clinic: 2009, Q2, P9

✖ **35.94 Creation of conduit between atrium and pulmonary artery**
  Fontan procedure

✖ **35.95 Revision of corrective procedure on heart**
  Replacement of prosthetic heart valve poppet
  Resuture of prosthesis of:
    septum
    valve

Excludes	*complete revision — code to specific procedure*
	replacement of prosthesis or graft of:
	septum (35.50–35.63)
	valve (35.20–35.28)

✖ **35.96 Percutaneous valvuloplasty**
  Percutaneous balloon valvuloplasty
  Coding Clinic: 2004, Q3, P10

✖ **35.98 Other operations on septa of heart**
  Coding Clinic: 2007, Q1, P11-12

✖ **35.99 Other operations on valves of heart**

● **36 Operations on vessels of heart**

  | Includes | sternotomy (median) (transverse) as operative approach |
  | | thoracotomy as operative approach |

  Code also any:
    cardiopulmonary bypass, if performed [extracorporeal circulation] [heart-lung machine] (39.61)
    injection or infusion of platelet inhibitor (99.20)
    injection or infusion of thrombolytic agent (99.10)
  Coding Clinic: 1990, Q2, P23-24; 1985, July-Aug, P8-9

● **36.0 Removal of coronary artery obstruction and insertion of stent(s)**
  Coding Clinic: 1994, Q2, P14; 1993, 5th Issue, P3

✖ **36.03 Open chest coronary artery angioplasty**
  Coronary (artery):
    endarterectomy (with patch graft)
    thromboendarterectomy (with patch graft)
  Open surgery for direct relief of coronary artery obstruction

  | Excludes | *that with coronary artery bypass graft (36.10–36.19)* |

  Code also any:
    insertion of drug-eluting coronary stent(s) (36.07)
    insertion of non-drug-eluting coronary stent(s) (36.06)
    number of vascular stents inserted (00.45–00.48)
    number of vessels treated (00.40–00.43)
    procedure on vessel bifurcation (00.44)
  Coding Clinic: 1994, Q1, P6; 1993, Q3, P7-8

OPERATIONS ON THE CARDIOVASCULAR SYSTEM (35–39)

36.04   Intracoronary artery thrombolytic infusion

That by direct coronary artery injection, infusion, or catheterization

Enzyme infusion

Platelet inhibitor

> **Excludes** *infusion of platelet inhibitor (99.20)*
> *infusion of thrombolytic agent (99.10)*
> *that associated with any procedure in 36.03*

Coding Clinic: 2002, Q3, P20

36.06   Insertion of non-drug-eluting coronary artery stent(s)

Bare stent(s)

Bonded stent(s)

Drug-coated stent(s), i.e. heparin coated

Endograft(s)

Endovascular graft(s)

Stent grafts

> Code also any:
> number of vascular stents inserted (00.45–00.48)
> number of vessels treated (00.40–00.43)
> open chest coronary artery angioplasty (36.03)
> percutaneous transluminal coronary angioplasty [PTCA] or coronary atherectomy (00.66)
> procedure on vessel bifurcation (00.44)

> **Excludes** *insertion of drug-eluting coronary artery stent(s) (36.07)*

Coding Clinic: 2009, Q2, P12; 2005, Q4, P69-72; 2001, Q2, P24; 2001, Q1, P9-10; 2000, Q1, P11-12; 1999, Q1, P17-18

◆Non-OR Procedure that affects MS-DRG assignment to MDC 05, MS-DRG 248-249

36.07   Insertion of drug-eluting coronary artery stent(s)

Endograft(s)

Endovascular graft(s)

Stent graft(s)

> Code also any:
> number of vascular stents inserted (00.45–00.48)
> number of vessels treated (00.40–00.43)
> open chest coronary artery angioplasty (36.03)
> percutaneous transluminal coronary angioplasty [PTCA] or coronary atherectomy (00.66)
> procedure on vessel bifurcation (00.44)

> **Excludes** *drug-coated stents, e.g., heparin coated (36.06)*
> *insertion of non-drug-eluting coronary artery stent(s) (36.06)*

Coding Clinic: 2005, Q4, P103-106; 2002, Q4, P101-103

◆Non-OR Procedure that affects MS-DRG assignment to MDC 05, MS-DRG 246-247

✖ 36.09   Other removal of coronary artery obstruction

Coronary angioplasty NOS

> Code also any:
> number of vascular stents inserted (00.45–00.48)
> number of vessels treated (00.40–00.43)
> procedure on vessel bifurcation (00.44)

> **Excludes** *that by open angioplasty (36.03)*
> *that by percutaneous transluminal coronary angioplasty [PTCA] or coronary atherectomy (00.66)*

Coding Clinic: 1990, Q2, P23

● 36.1   Bypass anastomosis for heart revascularization

Note: Do not assign codes from series 00.40–00.43 with codes from series 36.10–36.19

> Code also
> cardiopulmonary bypass [extracorporeal circulation] [heart-lung machine] (39.61)
> pressurized treatment of venous bypass graft [conduit] with pharmaceutical substance, if performed (00.16)

Coding Clinic: 2002, Q3, P3-91; 1993, Q3, P7-8; 1990, Q2, P24

✖ 36.10   Aortocoronary bypass for heart revascularization, not otherwise specified

Direct revascularization:
cardiac with catheter stent, prosthesis, or vein graft
coronary with catheter stent, prosthesis, or vein graft
heart muscle with catheter stent, prosthesis, or vein graft
myocardial with catheter stent, prosthesis, or vein graft

Heart revascularization NOS

✖ 36.11   (Aorto)coronary bypass of one coronary artery

Coding Clinic: 2002, Q3, P4-5,9; 1996, Q2, P7-8

✖ 36.12   (Aorto)coronary bypass of two coronary arteries

Coding Clinic: 2007, Q4, P121-122; 2002, Q3, P8; 1999, Q4, P15-16; 1996, Q2, P7-8; 1993, 5th Issue, P17-24

✖ 36.13   (Aorto)coronary bypass of three coronary arteries

Coding Clinic: 2002, Q3, P6-9; 1996, Q2, P7-8; 1993, 5th Issue, P17-24

✖ 36.14   (Aorto)coronary bypass of four or more coronary arteries

Coding Clinic: 2002, Q3, P5; 1996, Q2, P7-8

✖ 36.15   Single internal mammary-coronary artery bypass

Anastomosis (single):
mammary artery to coronary artery
thoracic artery to coronary artery

Coding Clinic: 2002, Q3, P4-9; 1999, Q4, P15-16; 1996, Q2, P7-8

✖ 36.16   Double internal mammary-coronary artery bypass

Anastomosis, double:
mammary artery to coronary artery
thoracic artery to coronary artery

Coding Clinic: 2002, Q3, P6,8-9; 1996, Q2, P7-8

✖ 36.17   Abdominal - coronary artery bypass

Anastomosis:
gastroepiploic - coronary artery

✖ 36.19   Other bypass anastomosis for heart revascularization

Coding Clinic: 1996, Q2, P7-8

✖ 36.2   Heart revascularization by arterial implant

Implantation of:
aortic branches [ascending aortic branches] into heart muscle
blood vessels into myocardium
internal mammary artery [internal thoracic artery] into:
heart muscle
myocardium
ventricle
ventricular wall

Indirect heart revascularization NOS

◄ New   ◄▥ Revised   ~~deleted~~ Deleted   ● Use Additional Digit(s)   ✖ Valid O.R. Procedure
◆ Non-O.R. Procedure   ♀ Females Only   ♂ Males Only

●36.3 **Other heart revascularization**

✖36.31 **Open chest transmyocardial revascularization**

✖36.32 **Other transmyocardial revascularization**
Coding Clinic: 1998, Q4, P73-75

✖36.33 **Endoscopic transmyocardial revascularization**
Thoracoscopic transmyocardial revascularization
Coding Clinic: 2006, Q4, P127-128

✖36.34 **Percutaneous transmyocardial revascularization**
Endovascular transmyocardial revascularization
Coding Clinic: 2006, Q4, P127-128

✖36.39 **Other heart revascularization**
Abrasion of epicardium
Cardio-omentopexy
Intrapericardial poudrage
Myocardial graft:
mediastinal fat
omentum
pectoral muscles

●36.9 **Other operations on vessels of heart**

Code also cardiopulmonary bypass [extracorporeal circulation] [heart-lung machine] (39.61)

✖36.91 **Repair of aneurysm of coronary vessel**
Coding Clinic: 2008, Q2, P13

✖36.99 **Other operations on vessels of heart**
Exploration of coronary artery
Incision of coronary artery
Ligation of coronary artery
Repair of arteriovenous fistula
Coding Clinic: 2003, Q3, P18; 1999, Q4, P15-16

●37 **Other operations on heart and pericardium**

Code also any injection or infusion of platelet inhibitor (99.20)
Coding Clinic: 2007, Q1, P11-12

37.0 **Pericardiocentesis**

●37.1 **Cardiotomy and pericardiotomy**

Code also cardiopulmonary bypass [extracorporeal circulation] [heart-lung machine] (39.61)

✖37.10 **Incision of heart, not otherwise specified**
Cardiolysis NOS

✖37.11 **Cardiotomy**
Incision of:
atrium
endocardium
myocardium
ventricle

✖37.12 **Pericardiotomy**
Pericardial window operation
Pericardiolysis
Pericardiotomy
Coding Clinic: 1995, Q3, P7

●37.2 **Diagnostic procedures on heart and pericardium**

37.20 **Noninvasive programmed electrical stimulation (NIPS)**

Excludes *that as part of intraoperative testing – omit code*
catheter based invasive electrophysiologic testing (37.26)
device interrogation only without arrhythmia induction (bedside check) (89.45–89.49)
Coding Clinic: 2006, Q4, P128-129

37.21 **Right heart cardiac catheterization**
Cardiac catheterization NOS

Excludes *that with catheterization of left heart (37.23)*
Coding Clinic: 2004, Q3, P10; 2003, Q3, P9-10; 1984, Nov-Dec, P12, 19; 1984, July-Aug, P19x2
◆Non-OR Procedure that affects MS-DRG assignment to MDC 05, MS-DRG 216-218, 222-225, 233-234, 286-287

37.22 **Left heart cardiac catheterization**

Excludes *that with catheterization of right heart (37.23)*
Coding Clinic: 2006, Q1, P69-72; 2005, Q4, P69-72; Q2, P10-11, 17-18; Q3, P14; 2004, Q3, P10; Q2, P3; 2000, Q1, P21; 1993, 5th Issue, P17-24
◆Non-OR Procedure that affects MS-DRG assignment to MDC 05, MS-DRG 216-218, 222-225, 233-234, 286-287

37.23 **Combined right and left heart cardiac catheterization**
Coding Clinic: 2007, Q1, P11-12; 2005, Q2, P17-18; 2004, Q3, P10; 2001, Q2, P8-9; 2000, Q1, P20-21; 1998, Q3, P11; 1996, Q1, P8; 1993, 5th Issue, P17-24; 1984, Nov-Dec, P19; 1984, July-Aug, P19
◆Non-OR Procedure that affects MS-DRG assignment to MDC 05, MS-DRG 216-218, 222-225, 233-234, 286-287

✖37.24 **Biopsy of pericardium**

37.25 **Biopsy of heart**
Coding Clinic: 2003, Q3, P16; 1994, Q3, P7-8

37.26 **Catheter based invasive electrophysiologic testing**
Electrophysiologic studies [EPS]

Code also any concomitant procedure

Excludes *that as part of intraoperative testing – omit code*
device interrogation only without arrhythmia induction (bedside check) (89.45–89.49)
His bundle recording (37.29)
noninvasive programmed electrical stimulation (NIPS) (37.20)
Coding Clinic: 2003, Q3, P23; Q2, P19; 2002, Q1, P8-9; 1999, Q1, P3x21; 997, Q2, P10
◆Non-OR Procedure that affects MS-DRG assignment to MDC 05, MS-DRG 216-218, 246-251

37.27 **Cardiac mapping**

Code also any concomitant procedure

Excludes *electrocardiogram (89.52)*
His bundle recording (37.29)
◆Non-OR Procedure that affects MS-DRG assignment to MDC 05, MS-DRG 246-251

37.28 **Intracardiac echocardiography**
Echocardiography of heart chambers
ICE

Code also any synchronous Doppler flow mapping (88.72)

Excludes *intravascular imaging of coronary vessels (intravascular ultrasound) (IVUS) (00.24)*

OPERATIONS ON THE CARDIOVASCULAR SYSTEM (35–39)

OPERATIONS ON THE CARDIOVASCULAR SYSTEM (35–39)

37.29 Other diagnostic procedures on heart and pericardium

Excludes | *angiocardiography (88.50–88.58)*
cardiac function tests (89.41–89.69)
cardiovascular radioisotopic scan and
function study (92.05)
coronary arteriography (88.55–88.57)
diagnostic pericardiocentesis (37.0)
diagnostic ultrasound of heart (88.72)
x-ray of heart (87.49)

● **37.3 Pericardiectomy and excision of lesion of heart**

Code also cardiopulmonary bypass [extracorporeal circulation] [heart-lung machine] (39.61)

✖ **37.31 Pericardiectomy**
Excision of:
adhesions of pericardium
constricting scar of:
epicardium
pericardium

✖ **37.32 Excision of aneurysm of heart**
Repair of aneurysm of heart

✖ **37.33 Excision or destruction of other lesion or tissue of heart, open approach**
Ablation of heart tissue (cryoablation)
(electrocurrent) (laser) (microwave)
(radiofrequency) (resection), open chest
approach
Cox-maze procedure
Maze procedure
Modified maze procedure, trans-thoracic
approach

Excludes | *ablation, excision, or destruction*
of lesion or tissue of heart,
endovascular approach (37.34)
excision or destruction of left atrial
appendate (LAA) (37.36)
Coding Clinic: 2006, Q3, P13-14; 2003, Q4, P93-95; 1994, Q2,
P12

✖ **37.34 Excision or destruction of other lesion or tissue of heart, other approach**
Ablation of heart tissue (cryoablation)
(electrocurrent) (laser) (microwave)
(radiofrequency) (resection), via
peripherally inserted catheter
Modified maze procedure, endovascular
approach
Coding Clinic: 2003, Q4, P93-95; 2000, Q1, P20-21

✖ **37.35 Partial ventriculectomy**
Ventricular reduction surgery
Ventricular remodeling

Code also any synchronous:
mitral valve repair (35.02, 35.12)
mitral valve replacement (35.23–35.24)
Coding Clinic: 2008, Q3, P9-10; 1997, Q4, P54-55
MCE: Non-covered procedure

37.36 Excision or destruction of left atrial appendage (LAA)

Includes | Thoracoscopic approach,
minithoracotomy approach
Clipping of left atrial appendage
Exclusion of left atrial appendage
Oversewing of left atrial
appendage
Stapling of left atrial appendage

Code also any concomitant procedure
performed

Excludes | *ablation, excision or destruction*
of lesion or tissue of heart,
endovascular approach (37.34)
Coding Clinic: 2008, Q4, P176; 2006, Q3, P13-14

● **37.4 Repair of heart and pericardium**
Coding Clinic: 1990, Q2, P24

✖ **37.41 Implantation of prosthetic cardiac support device around the heart**
Cardiac support device (CSD)
Epicardial support device
Fabric (textile) (mesh) device
Ventricular support device on surface of heart

Code also any:
cardiopulmonary bypass [extracorporeal
circulation] [heart-lung machine] if
performed (39.61)
mitral valve repair (35.02, 35.12)
mitral valve replacement (35.23–35.24)
transesophageal echocardiography (88.72)

Excludes | *circulatory assist systems*
(37.61–37.68)
Coding Clinic: 2005, Q4, P119-120

✖ **37.49 Other repair of heart and pericardium**
Coding Clinic: 2008, Q3, P9-10

● **37.5 Heart replacement procedures**
Coding Clinic: 2003, Q4, P96-98

✖ **37.51 Heart transplantation**

Excludes | *combined heart-lung transplantation*
(33.6)
Coding Clinic: 2008, Q4, P180-182; 2005, Q2, P14-15
MCE: Limited coverage

✖ **37.52 Implantation of total internal biventricular heart replacement system**
Artificial heart

Excludes | *implantation of heart assist system*
[VAD] (37.62, 37.65, 37.66,
37.68)

Note: This procedure includes substantial
removal of part or all of the biological
heart. Both ventricles are resected, and
the native heart is no longer intact.
Ventriculectomy is included in this
procedure; do not code separately.
MCE: Non-covered procedure except when
combined with V70.7. Limited coverage
when combined with diagnosis V70.7

✖ **37.53 Replacement or repair of thoracic unit of (total) replacement heart system**

Excludes | *replacement and repair of heart assist*
system [VAD] (37.63)
MCE: Non-covered procedure

✖ **37.54 Replacement or repair of other implantable component of (total) replacement heart system**
Implantable battery
Implantable controller
Transcutaneous energy transfer [TET] device

Excludes | *replacement and repair of heart assist*
system [VAD] (37.63)
replacement or repair of thoracic unit of
(total) replacement heart system
(37.53)
MCE: Non-covered procedure

◀ New   ◀◀◀ Revised   deleted Deleted   ● Use Additional Digit(s)   ✖ Valid O.R. Procedure
◆ Non-O.R. Procedure   ♀ Females Only   ♂ Males Only

�острий **37.55 Removal of internal biventricular heart replacement system**
    Explanation of artificial heart

> Code also any concomitant procedure, such as:
>> combined heart-lung transplantation (33.6)
>> heart transplantation (37.51)
>> implantation of internal biventricular heart replacement system (37.52)

> **Excludes**   *explantation [removal] of external heart assist system (37.64)*
>> *explantation [removal] of percutaneous external heart assist device (97.44)*
>> *nonoperative removal of heart assist system (97.44)*
>> *that with replacement or repair of heart replacement system (37.53, 37.54)*

> Coding Clinic: 2008, Q4, P180-182

● **37.6 Implantation of heart and circulatory assist system(s)**

> **Excludes**   *implantation of prosthetic cardiac support system (37.41)*

> Coding Clinic: 2008, Q4, P177-180; 2004, Q4, P118-120

✱ **37.60 Implantation or insertion of biventricular external heart assist system**
    Temporary cardiac support for both left and right ventricles, inserted in the same operative episode

> **Includes**   open chest (sternotomy) procedure for cannulae attachments

> **Note:** Device (outside the body but connected to heart) with external circulation pump. Ventriculotomy is included; do not code separately.

> **Excludes**   *implantation of internal biventricular heart replacement system (artificial heart) (37.52)*
>> *implant of pulsation balloon (37.61)*
>> *insertion of percutaneous external heart assist device (37.68)*
>> *insertion of temporary non-implantable extracorporeal circulatory assist device (37.62)*

✱ **37.61 Implant of pulsation balloon**
> Coding Clinic: 2005, Q3, P14

✱ **37.62 Insertion of temporary non-implantable extracorporeal circulatory assist device**
    Acute circulatory support device
    Insertion of heart assist system, NOS
    Insertion of heart pump
    Short-term circulatory support (up to six hours)

> **Excludes**   *implantation of total internal biventricular heart replacement system [artificial heart] (37.52)*
>> *implant of external heart assist system (37.65)*
>> *insertion of implantable extracorporeal heart assist system (37.66)*
>> *insertion of percutaneous external heart assist device (37.68)*
>> *removal of heart assist system (37.64)*

> **Note:** Includes explanation of this device; do not code separately.
> Coding Clinic: 2003, Q4, P116-117; 1990, Q2, P23

✱ **37.63 Repair of heart assist system**
    Replacement of parts of an existing ventricular assist device (VAD)

> **Excludes**   *replacement or repair of other implantable component of (total) replacement heart system [artificial heart] (37.54)*
>> *replacement or repair of thoracic unit of (total) replacement heart system [artificial heart] (37.53)*

✱ **37.64 Removal of external heart assist system(s) or device(s)**
    Explanation of external device(s) providing left and right ventricular support
    Explanation of single external device and cannulae

> **Excludes**   *explantation [removal] of percutaneous external heart assist device (97.44)*
>> *nonoperative removal of heart assist system (97.44)*
>> *temporary non-implantable extracorporeal circulatory assist device (37.62)*
>> *that with replacement of implant (37.63)*

> Coding Clinic: 2008, Q4, P177-180

✱ **37.65 Implant of single ventricular (extracorporeal) external heart assist system**
    Insertion of one device into one ventricle

> **Includes**   open chest (sternotomy) procedure for cannulae attachments

> **Excludes**   *implant of pulsation balloon (37.61)*
>> *implantation of total internal biventricular heart replacement system (37.52)*
>> *insertion of implantable heart assist system (37.66)*
>> *insertion of implantation of two external VADs for simultaneous right and left heart support (37.60)*
>> *insertion of percutaneous external heart assist device (37.68)*
>> *that without sternotomy (37.62)*

> **Note:** Insertion or implantation of one external VAD for left or right heart support.
> **Note:** Device (outside the body but connected to heart) with external circulation and pump.

OPERATIONS ON THE CARDIOVASCULAR SYSTEM (35–39)

✖ **37.66 Insertion of implantable heart assist system**
Axial flow heart assist system
Diagonal pump heart assist system
Left ventricular assist device (LVAD)
Pulsatile heart assist system
Right ventricular assist device (RVAD)
Rotary pump heart assist system
Transportable, implantable heart assist system.
Ventricular assist device (VAD) not otherwise
    specified
Note: Device directly connected to the
    heart and implanted in the upper left
    quadrant of peritoneal cavity.
Note: This device can be used for
    either destination therapy (DT) or
    bridge-to-transplant (BTT)

> **Excludes** | *implant of pulsation balloon (37.61)*
> *implantation of total internal*
>   *biventricular heart replacement*
>   *system [artificial heart] (37.52)*
> *insertion of percutaneous external heart*
>   *assist device (37.68)*

Coding Clinic: 2003, Q4, P116-117; 1998, Q1, P8
MCE: Limited coverage

✖ **37.67 Implantation of cardiomyostimulation system**
Note: Two-step open procedure consisting
    of transfer of one end of the latissimus
    dorsi muscle; wrapping it around the
    heart; rib resection; implantation of
    epicardial cardiac pacing leads into the
    right ventricle; tunneling and pocket
    creation for the cardiomyostimulator.
Coding Clinic: 1998, Q43, P75-76

✖ **37.68 Insertion of percutaneous external heart assist
device**
Includes percutaneous [femoral] insertion of
    cannulae attachments
Circulatory assist device
Extrinsic heart assist device
pVAD
Percutaneous heart assist device
Coding Clinic: 2008, Q2, P12

● **37.7 Insertion, revision, replacement, and removal of leads;
insertion of temporary pacemaker system; or revision
of cardiac device pocket**

Code also any insertion and replacement of
    pacemaker device (37.80–37.87)

> **Excludes** | *implantation or replacement of transvenous*
> *lead [electrode] into left ventricular*
> *cardiac venous system (00.52)*

**37.70 Initial insertion of lead [electrode], not
otherwise specified**

> **Excludes** | *insertion of temporary transvenous*
> *pacemaker system (37.78)*
> *replacement of atrial and/or ventricular*
>   *lead(s) (37.76)*

◆ Non-OR Procedure that affects MS-DRG
    assignment to MDC 01, 05, 21; refer to
    Part VI, Appendix E, Table 1, Pacemaker/
    Lead Device Reference Table and Table
    3, Cardio-Defibrillator Lead/Generator
    Reference Table

**37.71 Initial insertion of transvenous lead [electrode]
into ventricle**

> **Excludes** | *insertion of temporary transvenous*
> *pacemaker system (37.78)*
> *replacement of atrial and/or ventricular*
>   *lead(s) (37.76)*

◆ Non-OR Procedure that affects MS-DRG
    assignment to MDC 01, 05, 21; refer to Part
    VI, Appendix E, Table 1, Pacemaker/Lead
    Device Reference Table and Table 3, Cardio-
    Defibrillator Lead/Generator Reference Table

**37.72 Initial insertion of transvenous leads
[electrodes] into atrium and ventricle**

> **Excludes** | *insertion of temporary transvenous*
> *pacemaker system (37.78)*
> *replacement of atrial and/or ventricular*
>   *lead(s) (37.76)*

Coding Clinic: 2008, Q4, P101-102; 1997, Q2, P4
◆ Non-OR Procedure that affects MS-DRG
    assignment to MDC 01, 05, 21; refer to Part
    VI, Appendix E, Table 1, Pacemaker/Lead
    Device Reference Table and Table 3, Cardio-
    Defibrillator Lead/Generator Reference Table

**37.73 Initial insertion of transvenous lead [electrode]
into atrium**

> **Excludes** | *insertion of temporary transvenous*
> *pacemaker system (37.78)*
> *replacement of atrial and/or ventricular*
>   *lead(s) (37.76)*

◆ Non-OR Procedure that affects MS-DRG
    assignment to MDC 01, 05, 21; refer to Part
    VI, Appendix E, Table 1, Pacemaker/Lead
    Device Reference Table and Table 3, Cardio-
    Defibrillator Lead/Generator Reference Table

✖ **37.74 Insertion or replacement of epicardial lead
[electrode] into epicardium**
Insertion or replacement of epicardial by:
    sternotomy
    thoracotomy

> **Excludes** | *replacement of atrial and/or ventricular*
> *lead(s) (37.76)*

Coding Clinic: 2007, Q1, P20; 2005, Q3, P3-9
MS-DRG: Refer to Part VI, Appendix E, Table 1,
    Pacemaker/Lead Device Reference Table
    and Table 3, Cardioverter-Defibrillator
    Lead/Generator Reference Table

✖ **37.75 Revision of lead [electrode]**
Repair of electrode [removal with re-insertion]
Repositioning of lead(s) (AICD) (cardiac
    device) (CRT-D) (CRT-P) (defibrillator)
    (pacemaker) (pacing) (sensing)
    [electrode]
Revision of lead NOS

> **Excludes** | *repositioning of temporary transvenous*
> *pacemaker system — omit code*

Coding Clinic: 2005, Q3, P3-9; 1999, Q2, P11-12

✖ **37.76 Replacement of transvenous atrial and/or
ventricular lead(s) [electrode]**
Removal or abandonment of existing
    transvenous or epicardial lead(s) with
    transvenous lead(s) replacement

> **Excludes** | *replacement of epicardial lead*
> *[electrode] (37.74)*

Coding Clinic: 2005, Q3, P3-9
MS-DRG: Refer to Part VI, Appendix E, Table 1,
    Pacemaker/Lead Device Reference Table
    and Table 3, Cardioverter-Defibrillator
    Lead/Generator Reference Table

OPERATIONS ON THE CARDIOVASCULAR SYSTEM (35–39)

◀ New   ◀▥ Revised   deleted Deleted   ● Use Additional Digit(s)   ✖ Valid O.R. Procedure
◆ Non-O.R. Procedure   ♀ Females Only   ♂ Males Only

✖ **37.77   Removal of lead(s) [electrode] without replacement**
Removal:
epicardial lead (transthoracic approach)
transvenous lead(s)

> **Excludes**   *removal of temporary transvenous pacemaker system —* omit code
> *that with replacement of:*
> *atrial and/or ventricular lead(s)*
> *[electrode] (37.76)*
> *epicardial lead [electrode] (37.74)*

37.78   Insertion of temporary transvenous pacemaker system

> **Excludes**   *intraoperative cardiac pacemaker (39.64)*

Coding Clinic: 2005, Q3, P3-9; 1993, Q3, P12

✖ **37.79   Revision or relocation of cardiac device pocket**
Debridement and reforming pocket (skin and subcutaneous tissue)
Insertion of loop recorder
Relocation of pocket [creation of new pocket] pacemaker or CRT-P
Removal of cardiac device/pulse generator without replacement
Removal of implantable hemodynamic pressure sensor (lead) and monitor device
Removal without replacement of cardiac resynchronization defibrillator device
Repositioning of implantable hemodynamic pressure sensor (lead) and monitor device
Repositioning of pulse generator
Revision of cardioverter/defibrillator (automatic) pocket
Revision of pocket for intracardiac hemodynamic monitoring
Revision or relocation of CRT-D pocket
Revision or relocation of pacemaker, defibrillator, or other implanted cardiac device pocket

> **Excludes**   *removal of loop recorder (86.05)*

Coding Clinic: 2005, Q3, P3-9; 1994, Q2, P10x2

● **37.8   Insertion, replacement, removal, and revision of pacemaker device**
Note: Device testing during procedure – omit code
Code also any lead insertion, lead replacement, lead removal and/or lead revision (37.70–37.77)

> **Excludes**   *implantation of cardiac resynchronization pacemaker [CRT-P] (00.50)*
> *implantation or replacement of cardiac resynchronization pacemaker pulse generator only [CRT-P] (00.53)*

✖ **37.80   Insertion of permanent pacemaker, initial or replacement, type of device not specified**
MS-DRG: Refer to Part VI, Appendix E, Table 1, Pacemaker/Lead Reference Table

37.81   Initial insertion of single-chamber device, not specified as rate responsive

> **Excludes**   *replacement of existing pacemaker device (37.85–37.87)*

◆Non-OR Procedure that affects MS-DRG assignment to MDC 01, 05, 21; refer to Part VI, Appendix E, Table 1, Pacemaker/Lead Device Reference Table

37.82   Initial insertion of single-chamber device, rate responsive
Rate responsive to physiologic stimuli other than atrial rate

> **Excludes**   *replacement of existing pacemaker device (37.85–37.87)*

◆Non-OR Procedure that affects MS-DRG assignment to MDC 01, 05, 21; refer to Part VI, Appendix E, Table 1, Pacemaker/Lead Device Reference Table

37.83   Initial insertion of dual-chamber device
Atrial ventricular sequential device

> **Excludes**   *replacement of existing pacemaker device (37.85–37.87)*

Coding Clinic: 2008, Q4, P101-102; 1997, Q2, P4; 1997, Q2, P4

◆Non-OR Procedure that affects MS-DRG assignment to MDC 01, 05, 21; refer to Part VI, Appendix E, Table 1, Pacemaker/Lead Device Reference Table

✖ **37.85   Replacement of any type pacemaker device with single-chamber device, not specified as rate responsive**
MS-DRG: Refer to Part VI, Appendix E, Table 1, Pacemaker/Lead Reference Table

✖ **37.86   Replacement of any type of pacemaker device with single-chamber device, rate responsive**
Rate responsive to physiologic stimuli other than atrial rate
MS-DRG: Refer to Part VI, Appendix E, Table 1, Pacemaker/Lead Reference Table

✖ **37.87   Replacement of any type pacemaker device with dual-chamber device**
Atrial ventricular sequential device
MS-DRG: Refer to Part VI, Appendix E, Table 1, Pacemaker/Lead Reference Table

✖ **37.89   Revision or removal of pacemaker device**
Removal without replacement of cardiac resynchronization pacemaker device [CRT-P]
Repair of pacemaker device

> **Excludes**   *removal of temporary transvenous pacemaker system —* omit code
> *replacement of existing pacemaker device (37.85–37.87)*
> *replacement of existing pacemaker device with CRT-P pacemaker device (00.53)*

● **37.9   Other operations on heart and pericardium**

37.90   Insertion of left atrial appendage device
Left atrial filter
Left atrial occluder
Transseptal catheter technique
Coding Clinic: 2004, Q4, P121-122

◆Non-OR Procedure that affects MS-DRG assignment to MDC 05, MS-DRG 250-251

✖ **37.91   Open chest cardiac massage**

> **Excludes**   *closed chest cardiac massage (99.63)*

Coding Clinic: 1988, Q4, P12

37.92   Injection of therapeutic substance into heart

37.93   Injection of therapeutic substance into pericardium

OPERATIONS ON THE CARDIOVASCULAR SYSTEM (35–39)

| Excludes | Includes | Use additional | Code also | Omit code |

✖ **37.94 Implantation or replacement of automatic cardioverter/defibrillator, total system [AICD]**

Implantation of defibrillator with leads (epicardial patches), formation of pocket (abdominal fascia) (subcutaneous), any transvenous leads, intraoperative procedures for evaluation of lead signals, and obtaining defibrillator threshold measurements

Techniques:
    lateral thoracotomy
    medial sternotomy
    subxiphoid procedure

Note: Device testing during procedure – *omit code*

Code also
    extracorporeal circulation, if performed (39.61)
    any concomitant procedure [e.g., coronary bypass] (36.01–36.19) or CCM, total system (17.51)] ◀▥

Excludes   *implantation of cardiac resynchronization defibrillator, total system [CRT-D] (00.51)*

Coding Clinic: 2003, Q2, P19; 2001, Q3, P5-7; 1999, Q3, P12-13; Q1, P3; 1994, Q2, P12

✖ **37.95 Implantation of automatic cardioverter/defibrillator lead(s) only**

MS-DRG: Refer to Part VI, Appendix E, Table 3, Cardioverter-Defibrillator Lead/Generator Reference Table

✖ **37.96 Implantation of automatic cardioverter/defibrillator pulse generator only**

Note: Device testing during procedure – *omit code*

Excludes   *implantation or replacement of cardiac resynchronization defibrillator, pulse generator device only [CRT-D] (00.54)*

MS-DRG: Refer to Part VI, Appendix E, Table 3, Cardioverter-Defibrillator Lead/Generator Reference Table

✖ **37.97 Replacement of automatic cardioverter/defibrillator lead(s) only**

Excludes   *replacement of epicardial lead [electrode] into epicardium (37.74)*
replacement of transvenous lead [electrode] into left ventricular coronary venous system (00.52

Coding Clinic: 2005, Q3, P3-9

MS-DRG: Refer to Part VI, Appendix E, Table 3, Cardioverter-Defibrillator Lead/Generator Reference Table

✖ **37.98 Replacement of automatic cardioverter/defibrillator pulse generator only**

Note: Device testing during procedure – *omit code*

Excludes   *replacement of cardiac resynchronization defibrillator, pulse generator device only [CRT-D] (00.54)*

Coding Clinic: 1999, Q1, P3

MS-DRG: Refer to Part VI, Appendix E, Table 3, Cardioverter-Defibrillator Lead/Generator Reference Table

✖ **37.99 Other**

Excludes   *cardiac retraining (93.36)*
conversion of cardiac rhythm (99.60–99.69)
implantation of prosthetic cardiac support device (37.41)
insertion of left atrial appendage device (37.90)
maze procedure (Cox-maze), open (37.33)
maze procedure, endovascular approach (37.34)
repositioning of pulse generator (37.79)
revision of lead(s) (37.75)
revision or relocation of pacemaker, defibrillator, or other implanted cardiac device pocket (37.79)

Coding Clinic: 2005, Q3, P3-9; Q2, P14-15; 1997, Q1, P12; 1994, Q1, P19; 1993, Q3, P12; 1989, Q1, P11

● **38   Incision, excision, and occlusion of vessels**

Code also
    any application or administration of an adhesion barrier substance (99.77)
    cardiopulmonary bypass [extracorporeal circulation] [heart-lung machine] (39.61)

Excludes   *that of coronary vessels (00.66, 36.03, 36.04, 36.09, 36.10–36.99)*

Coding Clinic: 1988, Q1, P11

The following fourth-digit subclassification is for use with appropriate categories in section 38.0, 38.1, 38.3, 38.5, 38.6, 38.8, and 38.9 according to site. Valid fourth-digits are in [brackets] at the end of each code/description.

0   unspecified site

1   intracranial vessels
    Cerebral (anterior) (middle)
    Circle of Willis
    Posterior communicating artery

2   other vessels of head and neck
    Carotid artery (common) (external) (internal)
    Jugular vein (external) (internal)

3   upper limb vessels
    Axillary
    Brachial
    Radial
    Ulnar

4   aorta

5   other thoracic vessels
    Innominate
    Pulmonary (artery) (vein)
    Subclavian
    Vena cava, superior

6   abdominal arteries
    Celiac
    Gastric
    Hepatic
    Iliac
    Mesenteric
    Renal
    Splenic
    Umbilical

    Excludes   *abdominal aorta (4)*

7   abdominal veins
    Iliac
    Portal
    Renal
    Splenic
    Vena cava (inferior)

◀ New   ◀▥ Revised   ~~deleted~~ Deleted   ● Use Additional Digit(s)   ✖ Valid O.R. Procedure

◆ Non-O.R. Procedure   ♀ Females Only   ♂ Males Only

---

8 lower limb arteries
    Femoral (common) (superficial)
    Popliteal
    Tibial
9 lower limb veins
    Femoral
    Popliteal
    Saphenous
    Tibial

✖ ● **38.0 Incision of vessel**
[0-9]   Embolectomy
    Thrombectomy

      Excludes *endovascular removal of obstruction from head and neck vessel(s) (39.74)*
        puncture or catheterization of any:
          artery (38.91, 38.98)
          vein (38.92–38.95, 38.99)
      Coding Clinic: 2003, Q1, P17-18; 1998, Q2, P23

✖ ● **38.1 Endarterectomy**
[0-6, 8]   Endarterectomy with:
    embolectomy
    patch graft
    temporary bypass during procedure
    thrombectomy

    Code also any:
      number of vascular stents inserted (00.45–00.48)
      number of vessels treated (00.40–00.43)
      procedure on vessel bifurcation (00.44)
    Coding Clinic: 2006, Q3, P20; 2002, Q1, P10-11; 2000, Q1, P16; 1999, Q2, P5; 1995, Q2, P16; 1985, Mar-April, P15

● **38.2 Diagnostic procedures on blood vessels**

      Excludes *adjunct vascular system procedures (00.40–00.43)*

✖ **38.21 Biopsy of blood vessel**

38.22 Percutaneous angioscopy

      Excludes *angioscopy of eye (95.12)*

38.23 Intravascular spectroscopy
    Intravascular chemography
    Near infrared (NIR) spectroscopy

      Includes imaging spectroscopy of both coronary and peripheral vessels ◄▦

      Excludes *intravascular imaging of:*
        coronary vessels (00.24, 38.24) ◄▦
        peripheral vessels (00.23, 38.25) ◄▦
      Coding Clinic: 2008, Q4, P182-183

38.24 Intravascular imaging of coronary vessel(s) by optical coherence tomography [OCT] ◄

38.25 Intravascular imaging of non-coronary vessel(s) by optical coherence tomograpy [OCT] ◄

      Excludes *intravascular imaging of coronary vessel(s) by OCT (38.24)* ◄

✖ **38.29 Other diagnostic procedures on blood vessels**

      Excludes *blood vessel thermography (88.86)*
        circulatory monitoring (89.61–89.69)
        contrast:
          angiocardiography (88.50–88.58)
          arteriography (88.40–88.49)
          phlebography (88.60–88.67)
        impedance phlebography (88.68)
        peripheral vascular ultrasonography (88.77)
        plethysmogram (89.58)
      Coding Clinic: 2000, Q3, P16; 1999, Q1, P7

✖ ● **38.3 Resection of vessel with anastomosis**
[0-9]   Angiectomy
    Excision of:
      aneurysm (arteriovenous) with anastomosis
      blood vessel (lesion) with anastomosis
    Coding Clinic: 1985, Mar-April, P15; 1984, Nov-Dec, P10

✖ ● **38.4 Resection of vessel with replacement**
[0-9]   Angiectomy
    Excision of:
      aneurysm (arteriovenous) or blood vessel (lesion) with replacement
    Partial resection with replacement

      Excludes *endovascular repair of aneurysm (39.71–39.79)*

    Coding Clinic: 2008, Q2, P13; 2006, Q3, P15-16; 1999, Q2, P5-6; Q1, P15; 1992, Q3, P10-11; 1985, Mar-April, P15; 1984, Nov-Dec, P10

    MS-DRG: Refer to Part VI, Appendix E, Table 2, Abdominal Aorta/Thoracic Vessel Resection Reference Table for 38.44 and 38.45

    Requires the use of one of the following fourth-digit subclassifications to identify site:

---

0 unspecified site
1 intracranial vessels
    Cerebral (anterior) (middle)
    Circle of Willis
    Posterior communicating artery
2 other vessels of head and neck
    Carotid artery (common) (external) (internal)
    Jugular vein (external) (internal)
3 upper limb vessels
    Axillary
    Brachial
    Radial
    Ulnar
4 aorta, abdominal
    Code also any thoracic vessel involvement (thoracoabdominal procedure) (38.45)
5 thoracic vessels
    Aorta (thoracic)
    Innominate
    Pulmonary (artery) (vein)
    Subclavian
    Vena cava, superior
    Code also any abdominal aorta involvement (thoracoabdominal procedure) (38.44)
6 abdominal arteries
    Celiac
    Gastric
    Hepatic
    Iliac
    Mesenteric
    Renal
    Splenic
    Umbilical
      Excludes *abdominal aorta (4)*
7 abdominal veins
    Iliac
    Portal
    Renal
    Splenic
    Vena cava (inferior)
8 lower limb arteries
    Femoral (common) (superficial)
    Popliteal
    Tibial
9 lower limb veins
    Femoral
    Popliteal
    Saphenous
    Tibial

OPERATIONS ON THE CARDIOVASCULAR SYSTEM (35–39)

Excludes   Includes   Use additional   Code also   Omit code

OPERATIONS ON THE CARDIOVASCULAR SYSTEM (35–39)

✖ ● **38.5 Ligation and stripping of varicose veins**
[0-3, 5, 7, 9]

Excludes *ligation of varices:*
esophageal (42.91)
gastric (44.91)

Coding Clinic: 1997, Q2, P7

✖ ● **38.6 Other excision of vessel**
[0-9] Excision of blood vessel (lesion) NOS

Excludes *excision of vessel for aortocoronary bypass*
(36.10–36.14)
excision with:
anastomosis (38.30–38.39)
graft replacement (38.40–38.49)
implant (38.40–38.49)

Coding Clinic: 1995, Q3, P5-6; 1990, Q3, P17

✖ **38.7 Interruption of the vena cava**
Insertion of implant or sieve in vena cava
Ligation of vena cava (inferior) (superior)
Plication of vena cava

Coding Clinic: 2007, Q2, P5; 1994, Q2, P9

✖ ● **38.8 Other surgical occlusion of vessels**
[0-9] Clamping of blood vessel
Division of blood vessel
Ligation of blood vessel
Occlusion of blood vessel

Excludes *adrenal vessels (07.43)*
esophageal varices (42.91)
gastric or duodenal vessel for ulcer
(44.40–44.49)
gastric varices (44.91)
meningeal vessel (02.13)
percutaneous transcatheter infusion
embolization (99.29)
spermatic vein for varicocele (63.1)
surgical occlusion of vena cava (38.7)
that for chemoembolization (99.25)
that for control of (postoperative) hemorrhage:
anus (49.95)
bladder (57.93)
following vascular procedure (39.41)
nose (21.00–21.09)
prostate (60.94)
tonsil (28.7)
thyroid vessel (06.92)
transcatheter (infusion) (99.29)

Coding Clinic: 2005, Q1, P14; 2003, Q1, P15-16; 2000, Q3, P16; 2005,
Q1, P14; 1999, Q1, P17-18; 1996, Q2, P7-8; 1996, Q1, P8;
1987, Mar-April, P9

● **38.9 Puncture of vessel**

Excludes *that for circulatory monitoring (89.60–89.69)*

38.91 Arterial catheterization
Coding Clinic: 2005, Q1, P14; 1998, Q2, P24; 1995, Q1, P3;
1990, Q2, P23; 1988, Q1, P8; 1984, May-June, P11

38.92 Umbilical vein catheterization

38.93 Venous catheterization, not elsewhere classified

Excludes *that for cardiac catheterization*
(37.21–37.23)
that for renal dialysis (38.95)
Coding Clinic: 2000, Q3, P9; 1998, Q2, P24; 1996, Q1, P5-6;
1992, Q2, P15-16; 1990, Q2, P24; 1985, July-Aug, P11

38.94 Venous cutdown

38.95 Venous catheterization for renal dialysis

Excludes *insertion of totally implantable*
vascular access device [VAD]
(86.07)
Coding Clinic: 2008, Q4, P193; 1998, Q3, P13; 1994, Q2, P11

38.98 Other puncture of artery

Excludes *that for:*
arteriography (88.40–88.49)
coronary arteriography
(88.55–88.57)

38.99 Other puncture of vein
Phlebotomy

Excludes *that for:*
angiography of veins (88.60–88.68)
extracorporeal circulation (39.61,
50.92)
injection or infusion of:
sclerosing solution (39.92)
therapeutic or prophylactic
substance (99.11–99.29)
perfusion (39.96–39.97)
phlebography (88.60–88.68)
transfusion (99.01–99.09)

Coding Clinic: 1988, Q1, P11

● **39 Other operations on vessels**

Excludes *those on coronary vessels (36.03–36.99)*

✖ **39.0 Systemic to pulmonary artery shunt**
Descending aorta-pulmonary artery anastomosis
(graft)
Left to right anastomosis (graft)
Subclavian-pulmonary anastomosis (graft)

Code also cardiopulmonary bypass [extracorporeal
circulation] [heart-lung machine] (39.61)

✖ **39.1 Intra-abdominal venous shunt**
Anastomosis:
mesocaval
portacaval
portal vein to inferior vena cava
splenic and renal veins
transjugular intrahepatic portosystemic shunt
(TIPS)

Excludes *peritoneovenous shunt (54.94)*

Coding Clinic: 2002, Q2, P4; 1993, Q4, P31; Q2, P8

● **39.2 Other shunt or vascular bypass**

Code also pressurized treatment of venous bypass
graft [conduit] with pharmaceutical substance,
if performed (00.16)

✖ **39.21 Caval-pulmonary artery anastomosis**

Code also cardiopulmonary bypass (39.61)

✖ **39.22 Aorta-subclavian-carotid bypass**
Bypass (arterial):
aorta to carotid and brachial
aorta to subclavian and carotid
carotid to subclavian

✖ **39.23 Other intrathoracic vascular shunt or bypass**
Intrathoracic (arterial) bypass graft NOS

Excludes *coronary artery bypass (36.10–36.19)*

✖ **39.24 Aorta-renal bypass**

✖ **39.25 Aorta-iliac-femoral bypass**
Bypass:
aortofemoral
aortoiliac
aortoiliac to popliteal
aortopopliteal
iliofemoral [iliac-femoral]
Coding Clinic: 2003, Q1, P16-17; 1988, Q1, P10

✖ **39.26 Other intra-abdominal vascular shunt or bypass**
Bypass:
aortoceliac
aortic-superior mesenteric
common hepatic-common iliac-renal
Intra-abdominal arterial bypass graft NOS

Excludes *peritoneovenous shunt (54.94)*

◄ New ◄⃫ Revised ~~deleted~~ Deleted ● Use Additional Digit(s) ✖ Valid O.R. Procedure
◆ Non-O.R. Procedure ♀ Females Only ♂ Males Only

✖ **39.27   Arteriovenostomy for renal dialysis**
Anastomosis for renal dialysis
Formation of (peripheral) arteriovenous
fistula for renal [kidney] dialysis

> Code also any renal dialysis (39.95)
> **Coding Clinic: 2007, Q1, P18; 2006, Q1, P10-11; 1985,
> Sept-Oct, P12**

✖ **39.28   Extracranial-intracranial (EC-IC) vascular bypass**
Coding Clinic: 1992, Q2, P7
MCE: Non-covered procedure

✖ **39.29   Other (peripheral) vascular shunt or bypass**
Bypass (graft):
    axillary-brachial
    axillary-femoral [axillofemoral] (superficial)
    brachial
    femoral-femoral
    femoroperoneal
    femoropopliteal (arteries)
    femorotibial (anterior) (posterior)
    popliteal
    vascular NOS

> **Excludes**   *peritoneovenous shunt (54.94)*
>
> **Coding Clinic: 2003, Q1, P17-18; 2002, Q2, P8; Q1, P13; 1985,
> Sept-Oct, P13; 1984, July-Aug, P20**

● **39.3   Suture of vessel**
Repair of laceration of blood vessel

> **Excludes**   *any other vascular puncture closure device —
> omit code*
>   *suture of aneurysm (39.52)*
>   *that for control of hemorrhage (postoperative):*
>   *anus (49.95)*
>   *bladder (57.93)*
>   *following vascular procedure (39.41)*
>   *nose (21.00–21.09)*
>   *prostate (60.94)*
>   *tonsil (28.7)*

✖ **39.30   Suture of unspecified blood vessel**

✖ **39.31   Suture of artery**
Coding Clinic: 2006, Q3, P9; 1998, Q2, P22

✖ **39.32   Suture of vein**

● **39.4   Revision of vascular procedure**

✖ **39.41   Control of hemorrhage following vascular
surgery**

> **Excludes**   *that for control of hemorrhage (post
> operative):*
>   *anus (49.95)*
>   *bladder (57.93)*
>   *nose (21.00–21.09)*
>   *prostate (60.94)*
>   *tonsil (28.7)*

✖ **39.42   Revision of arteriovenous shunt for renal dialysis**
Conversion of renal dialysis:
    end-to-end anastomosis to end-to-side
    end-to-side anastomosis to end-to-end
    vessel-to-vessel cannula to arteriovenous
        shunt
Removal of old arteriovenous shunt and
    creation of new shunt

> **Excludes**   *replacement of vessel-to-vessel cannula
> (39.94)*
>
> **Coding Clinic: 1994, Q2, P15; 1993, Q4, P33**

✖ **39.43   Removal of arteriovenous shunt for renal dialysis**

> **Excludes**   *that with replacement [revision] of
> shunt (39.42)*

✖ **39.49   Other revision of vascular procedure**
Declotting (graft)
Revision of:
    anastomosis of blood vessel
    vascular procedure (previous)

● **39.5   Other repair of vessels**
**Coding Clinic: 2002, Q1, P13; 2000, Q4, P63-64; 1998, Q2, P17; 1996,
Q4, P63**

✖ **39.50   Angioplasty or atherectomy of other
non-coronary vessel(s)**
Percutaneous transluminal angioplasty (PTA)
    of non-coronary vessels:
    Lower extremity vessels
    Mesenteric artery
    Renal artery
    Upper extremity vessels

> Code also any:
>   injection or infusion of thrombolytic agent
>   (99.10)
>   insertion of drug-eluting peripheral vessel
>   stent (00.55)   ◄
>   insertion of non-~~coronary~~ drug-eluting
>   peripheral vessel stent(s) or stent
>   grafts(s) (39.90)
>   number of vascular stents inserted
>   (00.45–00.48)
>   number of vessels treated (00.40–00.43)
>   procedure on vessel bifurcation (00.44)

> **Excludes**   *percutaneous angioplasty or
> atherectomy of precerebral or
> cerebral vessel(s) (00.61–00.62)*
>
> **Coding Clinic: 2006, Q4, P119; 2003, Q3, P10; 2001, Q2,
> P23x2, 24; 2000, Q2, P10-11; Q1, P12; 1993, 5th
> Issue, P11**

✖ **39.51   Clipping of aneurysm**

> **Excludes**   *clipping of arteriovenous fistula (39.53)*

✖ **39.52   Other repair of aneurysm**
Repair of aneurysm by:
    coagulation
    electrocoagulation
    filipuncture
    methyl methacrylate
    suture
    wiring
    wrapping

> **Excludes**   *endovascular repair of aneurysm
> (39.71–39.79)*
>   *re-entry operation (aorta) (39.54)*
>   *that with:*
>   *graft replacement (38.40–38.49)*
>   *resection (38.30–38.49,*
>   *38.60–38.69)*
>
> **Coding Clinic: 2002, Q3, P25-27x2; 1999, Q1, P15-17 x2; 1988,
> Q1, P10**

OPERATIONS ON THE CARDIOVASCULAR SYSTEM (35–39)

✖ 39.53   Repair of arteriovenous fistula
Embolization of carotid cavernous fistula
Repair of arteriovenous fistula by:
    clipping
    coagulation
    ligation and division

> **Excludes** *repair of:*
>   *arteriovenous shunt for renal*
>   *dialysis (39.42)*
>   *head and neck vessels, endovascular*
>   *approach (39.72)*
>   *that with:*
>   *graft replacement (38.40–38.49)*
>   *resection (38.30–38.49,*
>   *38.60–38.69)*

Coding Clinic: 2006, Q3, P15-16; 2000, Q1, P8-9

✖ 39.54   Re-entry operation (aorta)
Fenestration of dissecting aneurysm of thoracic
    aorta

Code also cardiopulmonary bypass
    [extracorporeal circulation] [heart-lung
    machine] (39.61)

✖ 39.55   Reimplantation of aberrant renal vessel

✖ 39.56   Repair of blood vessel with tissue patch graft

> **Excludes** *that with resection (38.40–38.49)*

Coding Clinic: 2004, Q1, P16-17

✖ 39.57   Repair of blood vessel with synthetic patch graft

> **Excludes** *that with resection (38.40–38.49)*

**✖ 39.58   Repair of blood vessel with unspecified type of
patch graft**

> **Excludes** *that with resection (38.40–38.49)*

✖ 39.59   Other repair of vessel
Aorticopulmonary window operation
Arterioplasty NOS
Construction of venous valves (peripheral)
Plication of vein (peripheral)
Reimplantation of artery

Code also cardiopulmonary bypass
    [extracorporeal circulation] [heart-lung
    machine] (39.61)

> **Excludes** *interruption of the vena cava (38.7)*
>   *reimplantation of renal artery (39.55)*
>   *that with:*
>   *graft (39.56–39.58)*
>   *resection (38.30–38.49,*
>   *38.60–38.69)*

Coding Clinic: 1993, Q4, P31-32; 5th Issue, P5; 1989, Q2, P17;
    1985, July-Aug, P8-9; Mar-April, P15

**● 39.6   Extracorporeal circulation and procedures auxiliary to
heart surgery**

**39.61   Extracorporeal circulation auxiliary to open
heart surgery**
Artificial heart and lung
Cardiopulmonary bypass
Pump oxygenator

> **Excludes** *extracorporeal hepatic assistance*
>   *(50.92)*
>   *extracorporeal membrane oxygenation*
>   *[ECMO] (39.65)*
>   *hemodialysis (39.95)*
>   *percutaneous cardiopulmonary bypass*
>   *(39.66)*

Coding Clinic: 2009, Q2, P9; 2008, Q3, P9-10; 2006, Q2, P13;
    2004, Q1, P16-17; 2002, Q3, P5; 1997, Q4, P54-55;
    1997, Q2, P8; 1995, Q1, P5-6; 1993, 5th Issue, P17-24;
    1990, Q2, P24; 1985, July-Aug, P8-9

**39.62   Hypothermia (systemic) incidental to open heart
surgery**
Coding Clinic: 1995, Q1, P5-6

39.63   Cardioplegia
Arrest:
    anoxic
    circulatory
Coding Clinic: 1995, Q1, P5-6

39.64   Intraoperative cardiac pacemaker
Temporary pacemaker used during and
    immediately following cardiac surgery
Coding Clinic: 1995, Q1, P5-6

✖ 39.65   Extracorporeal membrane oxygenation [ECMO]

> **Excludes** *extracorporeal circulation auxiliary to*
>   *open heart surgery (39.61)*
>   *percutaneous cardiopulmonary bypass*
>   *(39.66)*

Coding Clinic: 1990, Q2, P23; 1989, Q2, P17

39.66   Percutaneous cardiopulmonary bypass
Closed chest

> **Excludes** *extracorporeal circulation auxiliary to*
>   *open heart surgery (39.61)*
>   *extracorporeal hepatic assistance*
>   *(50.92)*
>   *extracorporeal membrane oxygenation*
>   *[ECMO] (39.65)*
>   *hemodialysis (39.95)*

Coding Clinic: 1996, Q3, P11-12

● 39.7   Endovascular repair procedures on of vessel(s)   ◄═
Embolization   ◄
Endoluminal repair
Implantation   ◄
Occlusion   ◄
Removal   ◄
Repair   ◄

> **Excludes** *angioplasty or atherectomy of other*
>   *non-coronary vessel(s) (39.50)*
>   *insertion of non-drug-eluting peripheral vessel*
>   *stent(s) (39.90)*
>   *other repair of aneurysm (39.52)*
>   *percutaneous insertion of carotid artery*
>   *stent(s) (00.63)*
>   *percutaneous insertion of intracranial stent(s)*
>   *(00.65)*
>   *percutaneous insertion of other precerebral*
>   *artery stent(s) (00.64)*
>   *resection of abdominal aorta with replacement*
>   *(38.44)*
>   *resection of lower limb arteries with*
>   *replacement (38.48)*
>   *resection of thoracic aorta with replacement*
>   *(38.45)*
>   *resection of upper limb vessels with*
>   *replacement (38.43)*

Coding Clinic: 2000, Q4, P63-64

**✖ 39.71   Endovascular implantation of graft in
abdominal aorta**
Endovascular repair of abdominal aortic
    aneurysm with graft
Stent graft(s)

Code also intra-aneurysm sac pressure
    monitoring (intraoperative) (00.58)
Coding Clinic: 2002, Q1, P13; 2000, Q4, P63-64

◄ New   ◄═ Revised   ~~deleted~~ Deleted   ● Use Additional Digit(s)   ✖ Valid O.R. Procedure
◆ Non-O.R. Procedure   ♀ Females Only   ♂ Males Only

OPERATIONS ON THE CARDIOVASCULAR SYSTEM (35–39)

✖ **39.72** Endovascular ~~repair~~ embolization or occlusion of head and neck vessels ◀
~~Coil embolization or occlusion~~ ◀
Endograft(s)
Endovascular graft(s)
Liquid tissue adhesive (glue) embolization or occlusion
Other implant or substance for repair, embolization or occlusion
That for repair of aneurysm, arteriovenous malformation [AVM], or fistula

> **Excludes** *embolization of head or neck vessels using bare coils (39.75)* ◀
> *embolization of head or neck vessels using bioactive coils (39.76)* ◀
> *mechanical thrombectomy of pre-cerebral and cerebral vessels (39.74)*

Coding Clinic: 2002, Q4, P103-105

✖ **39.73** Endovascular implantation of graft in thoracic aorta
Endograft(s)
Endovascular graft(s)
Endovascular repair of defect of thoracic aorta with graft(s) or device(s)
Stent graft(s) or device(s)
That for repair of aneurysm, dissection, or injury

> **Excludes** *fenestration of dissecting aneurysm of thoracic aorta (39.54)*

> **Code also** intra-aneurysm sac pressure monitoring (intraoperative) (00.58)

Coding Clinic: 2005, Q4, P120-121

✖ **39.74** Endovascular removal of obstruction from head and neck vessel(s)
Endovascular embolectomy
Endovascular thrombectomy of pre-cerebral and cerebral vessels
Mechanical embolectomy or thrombectomy

> **Code also**:
> any injection or infusion of thrombolytic agent (99.10)
> number of vessels treated (00.40–00.43)
> procedure on vessel bifurcation (00.44)

> **Excludes** *endarterectomy of intracranial vessels and other vessels of head and neck (38.11–38.12)*
> *occlusive endovascular ~~repair~~ embolization of head or neck vessel(s) ~~(39.72)~~ (39.75)* ◀
> *occlusive endovascular embolization of head or neck vessel(s) using bioactive coils (39.76)* ◀
> *open embolectomy or thrombectomy (38.01– 38.02)*

Coding Clinic: 2006, Q4, P129-130

✖ **39.75** Endovascular embolization or occlusion of vessel(s) of head or neck using bare coils ◀
Bare metal coils ◀
Bare platinum coils [BPC] ◀
That for treatment of aneurysm, arteriovenous malformation [AVM] or fistula ◀

✖ **39.76** Endovascular embolization or occlusion of vessel(s) of head or neck using bioactive coils ◀
Biodegradable inner luminal polymer coils ◀
Coil embolization or occlusion utilizing bioactive coils ◀
Coils containing polyglycolic acid [PGA] ◀
That for treatment of aneurysm, arteriovenous malformation [AVM] or fistula ◀

✖ **39.79** Other endovascular ~~repair~~ procedures ~~(of aneurysm)~~ of on other vessels ◀
Endograft(s)
Endovascular graft(s)
Liquid tissue adhesive (glue) embolization or occlusion
Other ~~C~~coil embolization or occlusion ◀
Other implant or substance for repair, embolization or occlusion
Repair of aneurysm ◀

> **Excludes** *abdominal aortic aneurysm resection [AAA] (38.44)* ◀
> *endovascular implantation of graft in abdominal aorta (39.71)* ◀
> *endovascular implantation of graft in thoracic aorta (39.73)*
> *endovascular ~~repair~~ embolism or occlusion of head and neck vessels, bare metal coils ~~(39.72)~~ 39.75* ◀
> *endovascular embolization or occlusion of head and neck vessels, bioactive coils (39.76)* ◀
> *insertion of drug-eluting peripheral vessel stent(s) (00.55)*
> *insertion of non-drug-eluting peripheral vessel(s) (for other than aneurysm repair) (39.90)*
> *non-endovascular repair of arteriovenous fistula (39.53)*
> *other surgical occlusion of vessels - see category 38.8*
> *percutaneous transcatheter infusion (99.29)*
> *thoracic aortic aneurysm resection (38.45)* ◀
> *transcatheter embolization for gastric or duodenal bleeding (44.44)*

Coding Clinic: 2009, Q2, P7-8; 2006, Q2, P22, 23x2; 2002, Q4, P103-105; 2001, Q3, P17-18

✖ **39.8** Operations on carotid body, carotid sinus and other vascular bodies
Chemodectomy
Denervation of:
aortic body
carotid body
Electronic stimulator
Glomectomy, carotid
Implantation or replacement of carotid sinus baroreflex activation device

> **Excludes** *excision of glomus jugulare (20.51)*
> *replacement of carotid sinus lead(s) only (04.92)*

Coding Clinic: 2007, Q2, P10-11

● **39.9   Other operations on vessels**
Coding Clinic: 1996, Q4, P63

     39.90   Insertion of non-drug-eluting, peripheral (non-coronary) vessel stent(s) ⇐
         Bare stent(s)
         Bonded stent(s)
         Drug-coated stent(s), i.e., heparin coated
         Endograft(s)
         Endovascular graft(s)
         Endovascular recanalization techniques
         Stent graft(s)

         Code also any:
            non-coronary angioplasty or atherectomy (39.50)
            number of vascular stents inserted (00.45–00.48)
            number of vessels treated (00.40–00.43)
            procedure on vessel bifurcation (00.44)

         Excludes   *insertion of drug-eluting peripheral vessel stent(s) (00.55)*
            percutaneous insertion of carotid artery stent(s) (00.63)
            percutaneous insertion of intracranial stent(s) (00.65)
            percutaneous insertion of other precerebral artery stent(s) (00.64)
            that for aneurysm repair (39.71–39.79)
         Coding Clinic: 2006, Q4, P119; 2001, Q2, P23-24; 2000, Q1, P12

     ✖ **39.91   Freeing of vessel**
         Dissection and freeing of adherent tissue:
            artery-vein-nerve bundle
            vascular bundle
         Coding Clinic: 2002, Q3, P12-13

     ✖ **39.92   Injection of sclerosing agent into vein**
         Excludes   *injection:*
            esophageal varices (42.33)
            hemorrhoids (49.42)
         Coding Clinic: 1992, Q2, P17-18

     ✖ **39.93   Insertion of vessel-to-vessel cannula**
         Formation of:
            arteriovenous:
                fistula by external cannula
                shunt by external cannula
         Code also any renal dialysis (39.95)
         Coding Clinic: 1985, Sept-Oct, P12

     ✖ **39.94   Replacement of vessel-to-vessel cannula**
         Revision of vessel-to-vessel cannula

     39.95   Hemodialysis
         Artificial kidney
         Hemodiafiltration
         Hemofiltration
         Renal dialysis
         Excludes   *peritoneal dialysis (54.98)*
         Coding Clinic: 2008, Q4, P193; 2007, Q3, P11; 2004, Q1, P22; 2003, Q4, P111-112; 2001, Q2, P4-6, 13; 2000, Q4, P39-40; 1998, Q2, P20-21; 1986, Sept-Oct, P10-11

     39.96   Total body perfusion
         Code also substance perfused (99.21–99.29)

     39.97   Other perfusion
         Perfusion NOS
         Perfusion, local [regional] of:
            carotid artery
            coronary artery
            head
            lower limb
            neck
            upper limb
         Code also substance perfused (99.21–99.29)
         Excludes   *perfusion of:*
            kidney (55.95)
            large intestine (46.96)
            Coding Clinic: 2007, Q4, P103-104; 1996, Q3, P11-12
            liver (50.93)
            small intestine (46.95)
            SuperSaturated oxygen therapy (00.49)
         Coding Clinic: 2007, Q4, P103-104; 1996, Q3, P11-12

     ✖ **39.98   Control of hemorrhage, not otherwise specified**
         Angiotripsy
         Control of postoperative hemorrhage NOS
         Venotripsy
         Excludes   *control of hemorrhage (postoperative):*
            anus (49.95)
            bladder (57.93)
            following vascular procedure (39.41)
            nose (21.00–21.09)
            prostate (60.94)
            tonsil (28.7)
            that by:
            ligation (38.80–38.89)
            suture (39.30–39.32)

     ✖ **39.99   Other operations on vessels**
         Excludes   *injection or infusion of therapeutic or prophylactic substance (99.11–99.29)*
            transfusion of blood and blood components (99.01–99.09)
         Coding Clinic: 1989, Q1, P11

OPERATIONS ON THE CARDIOVASCULAR SYSTEM (35–39)

◀ New   ⇐ Revised   ~~deleted~~ Deleted   ● Use Additional Digit(s)   ✖ Valid O.R. Procedure
◆ Non-O.R. Procedure   ♀ Females Only   ♂ Males Only

8. OPERATIONS ON THE HEMIC AND LYMPHATIC SYSTEM (40–41)

● **40   Operations on lymphatic system**
    Coding Clinic: 1993, Q3, P12

✖ **40.0   Incision of lymphatic structures**

● **40.1   Diagnostic procedures on lymphatic structures**

    ✖ **40.11   Biopsy of lymphatic structure**
       Coding Clinic: 2008, Q4, P90-91; 1984, Nov-Dec, P12

    ✖ **40.19   Other diagnostic procedures on lymphatic structures**

       | Excludes | *lymphangiogram:*
                    abdominal (88.04)
                    cervical (87.08)
                    intrathoracic (87.34)
                    lower limb (88.36)
                    upper limb (88.34)
                    microscopic examination of specimen (90.71–90.79)
                    radioisotope scan (92.16)
                    thermography (88.89)

● **40.2   Simple excision of lymphatic structure**

      | Excludes | *biopsy of lymphatic structure (40.11)*

    ✖ **40.21   Excision of deep cervical lymph node**

    ✖ **40.22   Excision of internal mammary lymph node**

    ✖ **40.23   Excision of axillary lymph node**
       Coding Clinic: 2002, Q2, P7

    ✖ **40.24   Excision of inguinal lymph node**

    ✖ **40.29   Simple excision of other lymphatic structure**
       Excision of:
         cystic hygroma
         lymphangioma
       Simple lymphadenectomy
       Coding Clinic: 1999, Q1, P6

✖ **40.3   Regional lymph node excision**
    Extended regional lymph node excision
    Regional lymph node excision with excision of lymphatic drainage area including skin, subcutaneous tissue, and fat
    Coding Clinic: 1992, Q2, P7

● **40.4   Radical excision of cervical lymph nodes**
    Resection of cervical lymph nodes down to muscle and deep fascia

      | Excludes | *that associated with radical laryngectomy (30.4)*

    ✖ **40.40   Radical neck dissection, not otherwise specified**

    ✖ **40.41   Radical neck dissection, unilateral**
       Coding Clinic: 2005, Q2, P8-9; 1999, Q2, P6-7

    ✖ **40.42   Radical neck dissection, bilateral**

● **40.5   Radical excision of other lymph nodes**

      | Excludes | *that associated with radical mastectomy (85.45–85.48)*

    ✖ **40.50   Radical excision of lymph nodes, not otherwise specified**
       Radical (lymph) node dissection NOS

    ✖ **40.51   Radical excision of axillary lymph nodes**

    ✖ **40.52   Radical excision of periaortic lymph nodes**

    ✖ **40.53   Radical excision of iliac lymph nodes**

    ✖ **40.54   Radical groin dissection**

    ✖ **40.59   Radical excision of other lymph nodes**

       | Excludes | *radical neck dissection (40.40–40.42)*

● **40.6   Operations on thoracic duct**

    ✖ **40.61   Cannulation of thoracic duct**

    ✖ **40.62   Fistulization of thoracic duct**

    ✖ **40.63   Closure of fistula of thoracic duct**

    ✖ **40.64   Ligation of thoracic duct**

    ✖ **40.69   Other operations on thoracic duct**

✖ **40.9   Other operations on lymphatic structures**
    Anastomosis of peripheral lymphatics
    Dilation of peripheral lymphatics
    Ligation of peripheral lymphatics
    Obliteration of peripheral lymphatics
    Reconstruction of peripheral lymphatics
    Repair of peripheral lymphatics
    Transplantation of peripheral lymphatics
    Correction of lymphedema of limb, NOS

      | Excludes | *reduction of elephantiasis of scrotum (61.3)*

● **41   Operations on bone marrow and spleen**
    Coding Clinic: 1985, May-June, P18-19

● **41.0   Bone marrow or hematopoietic stem cell transplant**
    Note: To report donor source - *see* codes 00.91–00.93

      | Excludes | *aspiration of bone marrow from donor (41.91)*

    ✖ **41.00   Bone marrow transplant, not otherwise specified**

    ✖ **41.01   Autologous bone marrow transplant without purging**

       | Excludes | *that with purging (41.09)*

       MCE: Non-covered procedure only when principal or secondary diagnosis of 204.00, 205.00, 205.10, 205.11, 206.00, 207.00, 208.00

    ✖ **41.02   Allogeneic bone marrow transplant with purging**
       Allograft of bone marrow with in vitro removal (purging) of T-cells
       MCE: Non-covered procedure only when principal or secondary diagnosis of 203.00, 203.01

    ✖ **41.03   Allogeneic bone marrow transplant without purging**
       Allograft of bone marrow NOS
       MCE: Non-covered procedure only when principal or secondary diagnosis of 203.00, 203.01

    ✖ **41.04   Autologous hematopoietic stem cell transplant without purging**

       | Excludes | *that with purging (41.07)*

       MCE: Non-covered procedure only when principal or secondary diagnosis of 204.00, 205.00, 205.10, 205.11, 206.00, 207.00, 208.00

    ✖ **41.05   Allogeneic hematopoietic stem cell transplant without purging**

       | Excludes | *that with purging (41.08)*

       Coding Clinic: 2009, Q1, P9

       MCE: Non-covered procedure only when principal or secondary diagnosis of 203.00, 203.01

    ✖ **41.06   Cord blood stem cell transplant**

| Excludes | Includes   Use additional   Code also   Omit code

✖ **41.07 Autologous hematopoietic stem cell transplant with purging**
Cell depletion
Coding Clinic: 2006, Q2, P20-22
MCE: Non-covered procedure only when principal or secondary diagnosis of 204.00, 205.00, 205.10, 205.11, 206.00, 207.00, 208.00

✖ **41.08 Allogeneic hematopoietic stem cell transplant**
Cell depletion
MCE: Non-covered procedure only when principal or secondary diagnosis of 203.00, 203.01

✖ **41.09 Autologous bone marrow transplant with purging**
With extracorporeal purging of malignant cells from marrow
Cell depletion
MCE: Non-covered procedure only when principal or secondary diagnosis of 204.00, 205.00, 205.10, 205.11, 206.00, 207.00, 208.00

41.1 Puncture of spleen
> **Excludes** *aspiration biopsy of spleen (41.32)*

✖ **41.2 Splenotomy**

● **41.3 Diagnostic procedures on bone marrow and spleen**

41.31 Biopsy of bone marrow
Coding Clinic: 1985, Jan-Feb, P15

41.32 Closed [aspiration] [percutaneous] biopsy of spleen
MCE: Closed biopsy procedure

✖ **41.33 Open biopsy of spleen**
MCE: Open biopsy procedure

41.38 Other diagnostic procedures on bone marrow
> **Excludes** *microscopic examination of specimen from bone marrow (90.61–90.69)*
> *radioisotope scan (92.05)*

41.39 Other diagnostic procedures on spleen
> **Excludes** *microscopic examination of specimen from spleen (90.61–90.69)*
> *radioisotope scan (92.05)*

● **41.4 Excision or destruction of lesion or tissue of spleen**
Code also any application or administration of an adhesion barrier substance (99.77)
> **Excludes** *excision of accessory spleen (41.93)*

✖ **41.41 Marsupialization of splenic cyst**

✖ **41.42 Excision of lesion or tissue of spleen**
> **Excludes** *biopsy of spleen (41.32–41.33)*

✖ **41.43 Partial splenectomy**

✖ **41.5 Total splenectomy**
Splenectomy NOS
Code also any application or administration of an adhesion barrier substance (99.77)

● **41.9 Other operations on spleen and bone marrow**
Code also any application or administration of an adhesion barrier substance (99.77)

41.91 Aspiration of bone marrow from donor for transplant
> **Excludes** *biopsy of bone marrow (41.31)*
> Coding Clinic: 1985, Jan-Feb, P15

41.92 Injection into bone marrow
> **Excludes** *bone marrow transplant (41.00–41.03)*
> Coding Clinic: 1996, Q3, P17

✖ **41.93 Excision of accessory spleen**

✖ **41.94 Transplantation of spleen**

✖ **41.95 Repair and plastic operations on spleen**

41.98 Other operations on bone marrow
Coding Clinic: 2008, Q3, P19; 1994, Q3, P10

✖ **41.99 Other operations on spleen**

◀ New   ◀▥ Revised   ~~deleted~~ Deleted   ● Use Additional Digit(s)   ✖ Valid O.R. Procedure
◆ Non-O.R. Procedure   ♀ Females Only   ♂ Males Only

(See Plate 284 on page NAP-29.)

9. OPERATIONS ON THE DIGESTIVE SYSTEM (42–54)

● **42 Operations on esophagus**

● **42.0 Esophagotomy**

✖ **42.01 Incision of esophageal web**

✖ **42.09 Other incision of esophagus**
Esophagotomy NOS

Excludes *esophagomyotomy (42.7)*
esophagostomy (42.10–42.19)

● **42.1 Esophagostomy**

✖ **42.10 Esophagostomy, not otherwise specified**

✖ **42.11 Cervical esophagostomy**

✖ **42.12 Exteriorization of esophageal pouch**

✖ **42.19 Other external fistulization of esophagus**
Thoracic esophagostomy
Code also any resection (42.40–42.42)

● **42.2 Diagnostic procedures on esophagus**

✖ **42.21 Operative esophagoscopy by incision**

✖ **42.22 Esophagoscopy through artificial stoma**

Excludes *that with biopsy (42.24)*

42.23 Other esophagoscopy

Excludes *that with biopsy (42.24)*

Coding Clinic: 2000, Q1, P20-21; 1998, Q3, P11

42.24 Closed [endoscopic] biopsy of esophagus
Brushing or washing for specimen collection
Esophagoscopy with biopsy
Suction biopsy of the esophagus

Excludes *esophagogastroduodenoscopy [EGD]*
with closed biopsy (45.16)

MCE: Closed biopsy procedure

✖ **42.25 Open biopsy of esophagus**
MCE: Open biopsy procedure

42.29 Other diagnostic procedures on esophagus

Excludes *barium swallow (87.61)*
esophageal manometry (89.32)
microscopic examination of specimen
from esophagus (90.81–90.89)

Coding Clinic: 1996, Q3, P12-13

● **42.3 Local excision or destruction of lesion or tissue of esophagus**

✖ **42.31 Local excision of esophageal diverticulum**

✖ **42.32 Local excision of other lesion or tissue of esophagus**

Excludes *biopsy of esophagus (42.24–42.25)*
esophageal fistulectomy (42.84)

42.33 Endoscopic excision or destruction of lesion or tissue of esophagus
Ablation of esophageal neoplasm by
endoscopic approach
Control of esophageal bleeding by endoscopic
approach
Esophageal polypectomy by endoscopic
approach
Esophageal varices by endoscopic approach
Injection of esophageal varices by endoscopic
approach

Excludes *biopsy of esophagus (42.24–42.25)*
fistulectomy (42.84)
open ligation of esophageal varices
(42.91)

✖ **42.39 Other destruction of lesion or tissue of esophagus**

Excludes *that by endoscopic approach (42.33)*

● **42.4 Excision of esophagus**

Excludes *esophagogastrectomy NOS (43.99)*

✖ **42.40 Esophagectomy, not otherwise specified**

✖ **42.41 Partial esophagectomy**

Code also any synchronous:
anastomosis other than end-to-end
(42.51–42.69)
esophagostomy (42.10–42.19)
gastrostomy (43.11–43.19)

✖ **42.42 Total esophagectomy**

Code also any synchronous:
gastrostomy (43.11–43.19)
interposition or anastomosis other than
end-to-end (42.51–42.69)

Excludes *esophagogastrectomy (43.99)*

Coding Clinic: 1988, Q4, P11

● **42.5 Intrathoracic anastomosis of esophagus**

Code also any synchronous:
esophagectomy (42.40–42.42)
gastrostomy (43.1)

✖ **42.51 Intrathoracic esophagoesophagostomy**

✖ **42.52 Intrathoracic esophagogastrostomy**

✖ **42.53 Intrathoracic esophageal anastomosis with interposition of small bowel**

✖ **42.54 Other intrathoracic esophagoenterostomy**
Anastomosis of esophagus to intestinal
segment NOS

✖ **42.55 Intrathoracic esophageal anastomosis with interposition of colon**

✖ **42.56 Other intrathoracic esophagocolostomy**
Esophagocolostomy NOS

✖ **42.58 Intrathoracic esophageal anastomosis with other interposition**
Construction of artificial esophagus
Retrosternal formation of reversed gastric tube

✖ **42.59 Other intrathoracic anastomosis of esophagus**
Coding Clinic: 1988, Q4, P11

● **42.6 Antesternal anastomosis of esophagus**

Code also any synchronous:
esophagectomy (42.40–42.42)
gastrostomy (43.1)

✖ **42.61 Antesternal esophagoesophagostomy**

✖ **42.62 Antesternal esophagogastrostomy**

✖ **42.63 Antesternal esophageal anastomosis with interposition of small bowel**

✖ **42.64 Other antesternal esophagoenterostomy**
Antethoracic:
esophagoenterostomy
esophagoileostomy
esophagojejunostomy

✖ **42.65 Antesternal esophageal anastomosis with interposition of colon**

✖ **42.66 Other antesternal esophagocolostomy**
Antethoracic esophagocolostomy

✖ **42.68 Other antesternal esophageal anastomosis with interposition**

✖ **42.69 Other antesternal anastomosis of esophagus**

✖ **42.7 Esophagomyotomy**

● **42.8 Other repair of esophagus**

42.81 Insertion of permanent tube into esophagus
Coding Clinic: 1997, Q1, P15

✖ **42.82 Suture of laceration of esophagus**

✖ **42.83 Closure of esophagostomy**

OPERATIONS ON THE DIGESTIVE SYSTEM (42–54)

�825 42.84   **Repair of esophageal fistula, not elsewhere classified**

> **Excludes**   *repair of fistula:*
> *bronchoesophageal (33.42)*
> *esophagopleurocutaneous (34.73)*
> *pharyngoesophageal (29.53)*
> *tracheoesophageal (31.73)*

�825 42.85   **Repair of esophageal stricture**

�825 42.86   **Production of subcutaneous tunnel without esophageal anastomosis**

�825 42.87   **Other graft of esophagus**

> **Excludes**   *antesternal esophageal anastomosis*
> *with interposition of:*
> *colon (42.65)*
> *small bowel (42.63)*
> *antesternal esophageal anastomosis*
> *with other interposition (42.68)*
> *intrathoracic esophageal anastomosis*
> *with interposition of:*
> *colon (42.55)*
> *small bowel (42.53)*
> *intrathoracic esophageal anastomosis*
> *with other interposition (42.58)*

�825 42.89   **Other repair of esophagus**

● 42.9   **Other operations on esophagus**

�825 42.91   **Ligation of esophageal varices**

> **Excludes**   *that by endoscopic approach (42.33)*

42.92   **Dilation of esophagus**
Dilation of cardiac sphincter

> **Excludes**   *intubation of esophagus (96.03,*
> *96.06–96.08)*

42.99   **Other**

> **Excludes**   *insertion of Sengstaken tube (96.06)*
> *intubation of esophagus (96.03,*
> *96.06–96.08)*
> *removal of intraluminal foreign body*
> *from esophagus without incision*
> *(98.02)*
> *tamponade of esophagus (96.06)*

● 43   **Incision and excision of stomach**

> Code also any application or administration of an
> adhesion barrier substance (99.77)
> Coding Clinic: 1989, Q3, P14

�825 43.0   **Gastrotomy**

> **Excludes**   *gastrostomy (43.11–43.19)*
> *that for control of hemorrhage (44.49)*

● 43.1   **Gastrostomy**

43.11   **Percutaneous [endoscopic] gastrostomy [PEG]**
Percutaneous transabdominal gastrostomy
Coding Clinic: 1994, Q2, P10-11

43.19   **Other gastrostomy**

> **Excludes**   *percutaneous [endoscopic] gastrostomy*
> *[PEG] (43.11)*
> Coding Clinic: 1992, Q1, P13-14; 1989, Q3, P14

�825 43.3   **Pyloromyotomy**

● 43.4   **Local excision or destruction of lesion or tissue of stomach**

43.41   **Endoscopic excision or destruction of lesion or tissue of stomach**
Gastric polypectomy by endoscopic approach
Gastric varices by endoscopic approach

> **Excludes**   *biopsy of stomach (44.14–44.15)*
> *control of hemorrhage (44.43)*
> *open ligation of gastric varices (44.91)*
> Coding Clinic: 1996, Q3, P10

�825 43.42   **Local excision of other lesion or tissue of stomach**

> **Excludes**   *biopsy of stomach (44.14–44.15)*
> *gastric fistulectomy (44.62–44.63)*
> *partial gastrectomy (43.5–43.89)*

�825 43.49   **Other destruction of lesion or tissue of stomach**

> **Excludes**   *that by endoscopic approach (43.41)*

�825 43.5   **Partial gastrectomy with anastomosis to esophagus**
Proximal gastrectomy

�825 43.6   **Partial gastrectomy with anastomosis to duodenum**
Billroth I operation
Distal gastrectomy
Gastropylorectomy

�825 43.7   **Partial gastrectomy with anastomosis to jejunum**
Billroth II operation
Coding Clinic: 2003, Q3, P3-8

● 43.8   **Other partial gastrectomy**

�825 43.81   **Partial gastrectomy with jejunal transposition**
Henley jejunal transposition operation

> Code also any synchronous intestinal
> resection (45.51)

�825 43.89   **Other**
Partial gastrectomy with bypass
gastrogastrostomy
Sleeve resection of stomach
Coding Clinic: 2003, Q3, P3-8

● 43.9   **Total gastrectomy**

�825 43.91   **Total gastrectomy with intestinal interposition**

�825 43.99   **Other total gastrectomy**
Complete gastroduodenectomy
Esophagoduodenostomy with complete
gastrectomy
Esophagogastrectomy NOS
Esophagojejunostomy with complete
gastrectomy
Radical gastrectomy

● 44   **Other operations on stomach**

> Code also any application or administration of an
> adhesion barrier substance (99.77)

● 44.0   **Vagotomy**

�825 44.00   **Vagotomy, not otherwise specified**
Division of vagus nerve NOS

�825 44.01   **Truncal vagotomy**

�825 44.02   **Highly selective vagotomy**
Parietal cell vagotomy
Selective proximal vagotomy

�825 44.03   **Other selective vagotomy**

● 44.1   **Diagnostic procedures on stomach**

�825 44.11   **Transabdominal gastroscopy**
Intraoperative gastroscopy

> **Excludes**   *that with biopsy (44.14)*

44.12   **Gastroscopy through artificial stoma**

> **Excludes**   *that with biopsy (44.14)*

44.13   **Other gastroscopy**

> **Excludes**   *that with biopsy (44.14)*

44.14   **Closed [endoscopic] biopsy of stomach**
Brushing or washing for specimen collection

> **Excludes**   *esophagogastroduodenoscopy [EGD]*
> *with closed biopsy (45.16)*
> MCE: Closed biopsy procedure

�825 44.15   **Open biopsy of stomach**
MCE: Open biopsy procedure

◀ New   ◀|||| Revised   ~~deleted~~ Deleted   ● Use Additional Digit(s)   ✗ Valid O.R. Procedure
◆ Non-O.R. Procedure   ♀ Females Only   ♂ Males Only

44.19   Other diagnostic procedures on stomach

> **Excludes**   *gastric lavage (96.33)*
> *microscopic examination of specimen*
> *from stomach (90.81–90.89)*
> *upper GI series (87.62)*

● **44.2   Pyloroplasty**

✱ **44.21   Dilation of pylorus by incision**

44.22   Endoscopic dilation of pylorus
Dilation with balloon endoscope
Endoscopic dilation of gastrojejunostomy site
Coding Clinic: 2001, Q2, P17-18

✱ **44.29   Other pyloroplasty**
Pyloroplasty NOS
Revision of pylorus
Coding Clinic: 1999, Q3, P3

● **44.3   Gastroenterostomy without gastrectomy**

✱ **44.31   High gastric bypass**
Printen and Mason gastric bypass

✱ **44.32   Percutaneous [endoscopic] gastrojejunostomy**
Bypass:
     gastroduodenostomy
PEGJJ

> **Excludes**   *percutaneous (endoscopic) feeding*
> *jejunostomy (46.32)*

✱ **44.38   Laparoscopic gastroenterostomy**
Bypass:
     gastroduodenostomy
     gastroenterostomy
     gastrogastrostomy
Laparoscopic gastrojejunostomy without
     gastrectomy NEC

> **Excludes**   *gastroenterostomy, open approach*
> *(44.39)*

Coding Clinic: 2004, Q4, P122

✱ **44.39   Other gastroenterostomy**
Bypass:
     gastroduodenostomy
     gastroenterostomy
     gastrogastrostomy
Gastrojejunostomy without gastrectomy NOS
Coding Clinic: 2003, Q3, P3-8; 2001, Q1, P16-17x2

● **44.4   Control of hemorrhage and suture of ulcer of stomach
or duodenum**

✱ **44.40   Suture of peptic ulcer, not otherwise specified**

✱ **44.41   Suture of gastric ulcer site**

> **Excludes**   *ligation of gastric varices (44.91)*

✱ **44.42   Suture of duodenal ulcer site**
Coding Clinic: 1987, Jan-Feb, P11

**44.43   Endoscopic control of gastric or duodenal
bleeding**
Coding Clinic: 2004, Q2, P12-13; 1992, Q2, P17-18

**44.44   Transcatheter embolization for gastric or
duodenal bleeding**

> **Excludes**   *surgical occlusion of abdominal vessels*
> *(38.86–38.87)*

**44.49   Other control of hemorrhage of stomach or
duodenum**
That with gastrotomy

✱ **44.5   Revision of gastric anastomosis**
Closure of:
     gastric anastomosis
     gastroduodenostomy
     gastrojejunostomy
Pantaloon operation

● **44.6   Other repair of stomach**

✱ **44.61   Suture of laceration of stomach**

> **Excludes**   *that of ulcer site (44.41)*

44.62   Closure of gastrostomy

✱ **44.63   Closure of other gastric fistula**
Closure of:
     gastrocolic fistula
     gastrojejunocolic fistula

✱ **44.64   Gastropexy**

✱ **44.65   Esophagogastroplasty**
Belsey operation
Esophagus and stomach cardioplasty

✱ **44.66   Other procedures for creation of esophagogastric
sphincteric competence**
Fundoplication
Gastric cardioplasty
Nissen's fundoplication
Restoration of cardio-esophageal angle

> **Excludes**   *that by laparoscopy (44.67)*

**Coding Clinic: 2003, Q2, P12; 2001, Q2, P4, 5x2, 6x3; 1998,
Q3, P10**

✱ **44.67   Laparoscopic procedures for creation of
esophagogastric sphincteric competence**
Fundoplication
Gastric cardioplasty
Nissen's fundoplication
Restoration of cardio-esophageal angle
Coding Clinic: 2004, Q4, P122

✱ **44.68   Laparoscopic gastroplasty**
Banding
Silastic vertical banding
Vertical banded gastroplasty (VBG)

> Code also   any synchronous laparoscopic
> gastroenterostomy (44.38)

> **Excludes**   *insertion, laparoscopic adjustable*
> *gastric band (restrictive*
> *procedure) (44.95)*
> *other repair of stomach, open approach*
> *(44.61–44.65, 44.69)*

Coding Clinic: 2004, Q4, P123-124

✱ **44.69   Other**
Inversion of gastric diverticulum
Repair of stomach NOS
**Coding Clinic: 2003, Q3, P3-8; 1999, Q3, P3;
1984, Nov-Dec, P13**

● **44.9   Other operations on stomach**

✱ **44.91   Ligation of gastric varices**

> **Excludes**   *that by endoscopic approach (43.41)*

✱ **44.92   Intraoperative manipulation of stomach**
Reduction of gastric volvulus

44.93   Insertion of gastric bubble (balloon)
MCE: Non-covered procedure

44.94   Removal of gastric bubble (balloon)

✱ **44.95   Laparoscopic gastric restrictive procedure**
Adjustable gastric band and port insertion

> **Excludes**   *laparoscopic gastroplasty (44.68)*
> *other repair of stomach (44.69)*

Coding Clinic: 2004, Q4, P123-124

✱ **44.96   Laparoscopic revision of gastric restrictive
procedure**
Revision or replacement of:
     adjustable gastric band
     subcutaneous gastric port device
Coding Clinic: 2004, Q4, P123-124

OPERATIONS ON THE DIGESTIVE SYSTEM (42–54)

✖ 44.97   Laparoscopic removal of gastric restrictive device(s)

Removal of either or both:
    adjustable gastric band
    subcutaneous port device

> **Excludes**   *nonoperative removal of gastric restrictive device(s) (97.86)*
> *open removal of gastric restrictive device(s) (44.99)*

Coding Clinic: 2004, Q4, P123-124

✖ 44.98   (Laparoscopic) adjustment of size of adjustable gastric restrictive device

Infusion of saline for device tightening
Withdrawal of saline for device loosening

Code also any:
    abdominal ultrasound (88.76)
    abdominal wall fluoroscopy (88.09)
    barium swallow (87.61)

Coding Clinic: 2004, Q4, P123-124

✖ 44.99   Other

> **Excludes**   *change of gastrostomy tube (97.02)*
> *dilation of cardiac sphincter (42.92)*
> *gastric:*
>   *cooling (96.31)*
>   *freezing (96.32)*
>   *gavage (96.35)*
>   *hypothermia (96.31)*
>   *lavage (96.33)*
> *insertion of nasogastric tube (96.07)*
> *irrigation of gastrostomy (96.36)*
> *irrigation of nasogastric tube (96.34)*
> *removal of:*
>   *gastrostomy tube (97.51)*
>   *intraluminal foreign body from stomach without incision (98.03)*
> *replacement of:*
>   *gastrostomy tube (97.02)*
>   *(naso-)gastric tube (97.01)*

Coding Clinic: 2004, Q3, P5; 1985, Jan-Feb, P14-15

● 45   Incision, excision, and anastomosis of intestine

Code also any application or administration of an adhesion barrier substance (99.77)

● 45.0   Enterotomy

> **Excludes**   *duodenocholedochotomy (51.41–51.42, 51.51)*
> *that for destruction of lesion (45.30–45.34)*
> *that of exteriorized intestine (46.14, 46.24, 46.31)*

✖ 45.00   Incision of intestine, not otherwise specified

✖ 45.01   Incision of duodenum

✖ 45.02   Other incision of small intestine

✖ 45.03   Incision of large intestine

> **Excludes**   *proctotomy (48.0)*

● 45.1   Diagnostic procedures on small intestine

Code also any laparotomy (54.11–54.19)

✖ 45.11   Transabdominal endoscopy of small intestine

Intraoperative endoscopy of small intestine

> **Excludes**   *that with biopsy (45.14)*

45.12   Endoscopy of small intestine through artificial stoma

> **Excludes**   *that with biopsy (45.14)*

45.13   Other endoscopy of small intestine

Esophagogastroduodenoscopy [EGD]

> **Excludes**   *that with biopsy (45.14, 45.16)*

Coding Clinic: 2004, Q3, P5

45.14   Closed [endoscopic] biopsy of small intestine

Brushing or washing for specimen collection

> **Excludes**   *esophagogastroduodenoscopy [EGD] with closed biopsy (45.16)*

MCE: Closed biopsy procedure

✖ 45.15   Open biopsy of small intestine

Coding Clinic: 2005, Q2, P12; 2001, Q2, P9-11

MCE: Open biopsy procedure

45.16   Esophagogastroduodenoscopy [EGD] with closed biopsy

Biopsy of one or more sites involving esophagus, stomach, and/or duodenum

Coding Clinic: 2005, Q3, P17-18

45.19   Other diagnostic procedures on small intestine

> **Excludes**   *microscopic examination of specimen from small intestine (90.91–90.99)*
> *radioisotope scan (92.04)*
> *ultrasonography (88.74)*
> *x-ray (87.61–87.69)*

● 45.2   Diagnostic procedures on large intestine

Code also any laparotomy (54.11–54.19)

✖ 45.21   Transabdominal endoscopy of large intestine

Intraoperative endoscopy of large intestine

> **Excludes**   *that with biopsy (45.25)*

45.22   Endoscopy of large intestine through artificial stoma

> **Excludes**   *that with biopsy (45.25)*

45.23   Colonoscopy

Flexible fiberoptic colonoscopy

> **Excludes**   *endoscopy of large intestine through artificial stoma (45.22)*
> *flexible sigmoidoscopy (45.24)*
> *rigid proctosigmoidoscopy (48.23)*
> *transabdominal endoscopy of large intestine (45.21)*

Coding Clinic: 2005, Q3, P17-18; 1995, Q1, P3-4

45.24   Flexible sigmoidoscopy

Endoscopy of descending colon

> **Excludes**   *rigid proctosigmoidoscopy (48.23)*

45.25   Closed [endoscopic] biopsy of large intestine

Biopsy, closed, of unspecified intestinal site
Brushing or washing for specimen collection
Colonoscopy with biopsy

> **Excludes**   *proctosigmoidoscopy with biopsy (48.24)*

Coding Clinic: 2003, Q1, P10-11

MCE: Closed biopsy procedure

✖ 45.26   Open biopsy of large intestine

MCE: Open biopsy procedure

45.27   Intestinal biopsy, site unspecified

45.28   Other diagnostic procedures on large intestine

45.29   Other diagnostic procedures on intestine, site unspecified

> **Excludes**   *microscopic examination of specimen (90.91–90.99)*
> *scan and radioisotope function study (92.04)*
> *ultrasonography (88.74)*
> *x-ray (87.61–87.69)*

OPERATIONS ON THE DIGESTIVE SYSTEM (42–54)

◀ New   ◀|||| Revised   ~~deleted~~ Deleted   ● Use Additional Digit(s)   ✖ Valid O.R. Procedure
◆ Non-O.R. Procedure   ♀ Females Only   ♂ Males Only

●**45.3** **Local excision or destruction of lesion or tissue of small intestine**

  45.30 **Endoscopic excision or destruction of lesion of duodenum**

  Excludes *biopsy of duodenum (45.14–45.15)*
  control of hemorrhage (44.43)
  fistulectomy (46.72)

✖**45.31** **Other local excision of lesion of duodenum**

  Excludes *biopsy of duodenum (45.14–45.15)*
  fistulectomy (46.72)
  multiple segmental resection (45.61)
  that by endoscopic approach (45.30)

✖**45.32** **Other destruction of lesion of duodenum**

  Excludes *that by endoscopic approach (45.30)*

✖**45.33** **Local excision of lesion or tissue of small intestine, except duodenum**
  Excision of redundant mucosa of ileostomy

  Excludes *biopsy of small intestine (45.14–45.15)*
  fistulectomy (46.74)
  multiple segmental resection (45.61)

✖**45.34** **Other destruction of lesion of small intestine, except duodenum**

●**45.4** **Local excision or destruction of lesion or tissue of large intestine**

✖**45.41** **Excision of lesion or tissue of large intestine**
  Excision of redundant mucosa of colostomy

  Excludes *biopsy of large intestine (45.25–45.27)*
  endoscopic polypectomy of large intestine (45.42)
  fistulectomy (46.76)
  multiple segmental resection (17.31, 45.71)
  that by endoscopic approach (45.42–45.43)

  Coding Clinic: 1987, Nov-Dec, P11

  45.42 **Endoscopic polypectomy of large intestine**

  Excludes *that by open approach (45.41)*

  Coding Clinic: 2005, Q2, P16-17; 1990, Q2, P25

  45.43 **Endoscopic destruction of other lesion or tissue of large intestine**
  Endoscopic ablation of tumor of large intestine
  Endoscopic control of colonic bleeding

  Excludes *endoscopic polypectomy of large intestine (45.42)*

  Coding Clinic: 2002, Q4, P61

✖**45.49** **Other destruction of lesion of large intestine**

  Excludes *that by endoscopic approach (45.43)*

  Coding Clinic: 1987, Nov-Dec, P11

●**45.5** **Isolation of intestinal segment**

  Code also any synchronous:
  anastomosis other than end-to-end (45.90–45.94)
  enterostomy (46.10–46.39)

✖**45.50** **Isolation of intestinal segment, not otherwise specified**
  Isolation of intestinal pedicle flap
  Reversal of intestinal segment

✖**45.51** **Isolation of segment of small intestine**
  Isolation of ileal loop
  Resection of small intestine for interposition
  Coding Clinic: 2005, Q2, P12-13x2; 2003, Q3, P3-8; Q2, P11-12; 2000, Q3, P7-8

✖**45.52** **Isolation of segment of large intestine**
  Resection of colon for interposition

●**45.6** **Other excision of small intestine**

  Code also any synchronous:
  anastomosis other than end-to-end (45.90–45.93, 45.95)
  colostomy (46.10–46.13)
  enterostomy (46.10–46.39)

  Excludes *cecectomy (17.32, 45.72)*
  enterocolectomy (17.39, 45.79)
  gastroduodenectomy (43.6–43.99)
  ileocolectomy (17.33, 45.73)
  pancreatoduodenectomy (52.51–52.7)

✖**45.61** **Multiple segmental resection of small intestine**
  Segmental resection for multiple traumatic lesions of small intestine

✖**45.62** **Other partial resection of small intestine**
  Duodenectomy
  Ileectomy
  Jejunectomy

  Excludes *duodenectomy with synchronous pancreatectomy (52.51–52.7)*
  resection of cecum and terminal ileum (17.32, 45.72)

  Coding Clinic: 2004, Q1, P10-11; 2003, Q1, P18

✖**45.63** **Total removal of small intestine**

●**45.7** **Open and other partial excision of large intestine**

  Code also any synchronous:
  anastomosis other than end-to-end (45.92–45.94)
  enterostomy (46.10–46.39)

  Excludes *laparoscopic partial excision of large intestine (17.31–17.39)*

  Coding Clinic: 2009, Q1, P10x2

✖**45.71** **Open and other multiple segmental resection of large intestine**
  Segmental resection for multiple traumatic lesions of large intestine

✖**45.72** **Open and other cecectomy**
  Resection of cecum and terminal ileum

✖**45.73** **Open and other right hemicolectomy**
  Ileocolectomy
  Right radical colectomy
  Coding Clinic: 1999, Q3, P10-11

✖**45.74** **Open and other resection of transverse colon**

✖**45.75** **Open and other left hemicolectomy**

  Excludes *proctosigmoidectomy (48.41–48.69)*
  second stage Mikulicz operation (46.04)

  Coding Clinic: 2002, Q4, P105-106

✖**45.76** **Open and other sigmoidectomy**
  Coding Clinic: 1996, Q1, P9; 1989, Q3, P15; 2002, Q4, P105-106

✖**45.79** **Other and unspecified partial excision of large intestine**
  Enterocolectomy NEC
  Coding Clinic: 2009, Q1, P11; 2003, Q1, P18; 1997, Q3, P9-10; 1991, Q1, P11

●**45.8** **Total intra-abdominal colectomy**
  Excision of cecum, colon, and sigmoid

  Excludes *coloproctectomy (48.41–48.69)*

  Coding Clinic: 2008, Q4, P169-172

✖**45.81** **Laparoscopic total intra-abdominal colectomy**

✖**45.82** **Open total intra-abdominal colectomy**

✖**45.83** **Other and unspecified total intra-abdominal colectomy**

| Excludes | Includes | Use additional | Code also | Omit code |

OPERATIONS ON THE DIGESTIVE SYSTEM (42–54)

● **45.9   Intestinal anastomosis**

Code also any synchronous resection (45.31–45.8, 48.41–48.69)

Excludes   *end-to-end anastomosis — omit code*

Coding Clinic: 1999, Q3, P10-11

✖ **45.90   Intestinal anastomosis, not otherwise specified**

✖ **45.91   Small-to-small intestinal anastomosis**
Coding Clinic: 2003, Q3, P3-8

✖ **45.92   Anastomosis of small intestine to rectal stump**
Hampton procedure
Coding Clinic: 2009, Q1, P5

✖ **45.93   Other small-to-large intestinal anastomosis**
Coding Clinic: 2009, Q1, P5; 2003, Q1, P18; 1986, Nov-Dec, P11

✖ **45.94   Large-to-large intestinal anastomosis**

Excludes   *rectorectostomy (48.74)*

Coding Clinic: 2009, Q1, P5; 1989, Q3, P15

✖ **45.95   Anastomosis to anus**
Formation of endorectal ileal pouch (H-pouch) (J-pouch) (S-pouch) with anastomosis of small intestine to anus
Coding Clinic: 2005, Q2, P13-14

● **46   Other operations on intestine**

Code also any application or administration of an adhesion barrier substance (99.77)

● **46.0   Exteriorization of intestine**

Includes   loop enterostomy
multiple stage resection of intestine

✖ **46.01   Exteriorization of small intestine**
Loop ileostomy

✖ **46.02   Resection of exteriorized segment of small intestine**

✖ **46.03   Exteriorization of large intestine**
Exteriorization of intestine NOS
First stage Mikulicz exteriorization of intestine
Loop colostomy

✖ **46.04   Resection of exteriorized segment of large intestine**
Resection of exteriorized segment of intestine NOS
Second stage Mikulicz operation

● **46.1   Colostomy**

Code also any synchronous resection (45.49, 45.71–45.79, 45.8)

Excludes   *loop colostomy (46.03)*
that with abdominoperineal resection of rectum (48.5)
that with synchronous anterior rectal resection (48.62)

✖ **46.10   Colostomy, not otherwise specified**

✖ **46.11   Temporary colostomy**

✖ **46.13   Permanent colostomy**

46.14   Delayed opening of colostomy

● **46.2   Ileostomy**

Code also any synchronous resection (45.34, 45.61–45.63)

Excludes   *loop ileostomy (46.01)*

✖ **46.20   Ileostomy, not otherwise specified**

✖ **46.21   Temporary ileostomy**

✖ **46.22   Continent ileostomy**

✖ **46.23   Other permanent ileostomy**

46.24   Delayed opening of ileostomy

● **46.3   Other enterostomy**

Code also any synchronous resection (45.61–45.8)

46.31   Delayed opening of other enterostomy

46.32   Percutaneous (endoscopic) jejunostomy [PEJ]
Endoscopic conversion of gastrostomy to jejunostomy
Percutaneous (endoscopic) feeding enterostomy

Excludes   *percutaneous [endoscopic] gastrojejunostomy (bypass) (44.32)*

46.39   Other
Duodenostomy
Feeding enterostomy
Coding Clinic: 1989, Q3, P15

● **46.4   Revision of intestinal stoma**

✖ **46.40   Revision of intestinal stoma, not otherwise specified**
Plastic enlargement of intestinal stoma
Reconstruction of stoma of intestine
Release of scar tissue of intestinal stoma

Excludes   *excision of redundant mucosa (45.41)*

✖ **46.41   Revision of stoma of small intestine**

Excludes   *excision of redundant mucosa (45.33)*

Coding Clinic: 2005, Q2, P11-12

✖ **46.42   Repair of pericolostomy hernia**

✖ **46.43   Other revision of stoma of large intestine**

Excludes   *excision of redundant mucosa (45.41)*

Coding Clinic: 2002, Q2, P9-10

● **46.5   Closure of intestinal stoma**

Code also any synchronous resection (45.34, 45.49, 45.61–45.8)

✖ **46.50   Closure of intestinal stoma, not otherwise specified**

✖ **46.51   Closure of stoma of small intestine**

✖ **46.52   Closure of stoma of large intestine**
Closure or take-down of:
    cecostomy
    colostomy
    sigmoidostomy
Coding Clinic: 2009, Q1, P5; 2005, Q2, P4-5; 1997, Q3, P9-10; 1987, Nov-Dec, P8

● **46.6   Fixation of intestine**

✖ **46.60   Fixation of intestine, not otherwise specified**
Fixation of intestine to abdominal wall

✖ **46.61   Fixation of small intestine to abdominal wall**
Ileopexy

✖ **46.62   Other fixation of small intestine**
Noble plication of small intestine
Plication of jejunum

✖ **46.63   Fixation of large intestine to abdominal wall**
Cecocoloplicopexy
Sigmoidopexy (Moschowitz)

✖ **46.64   Other fixation of large intestine**
Cecofixation
Colofixation

● **46.7   Other repair of intestine**

Excludes   *closure of:*
ulcer of duodenum (44.42)
vesicoenteric fistula (57.83)

✖ **46.71   Suture of laceration of duodenum**

✖ **46.72   Closure of fistula of duodenum**

✖ **46.73   Suture of laceration of small intestine, except duodenum**

◀ New   ◀▥ Revised   ~~deleted~~ Deleted   ● Use Additional Digit(s)   ✖ Valid O.R. Procedure
◆ Non-O.R. Procedure   ♀ Females Only   ♂ Males Only

OPERATIONS ON THE DIGESTIVE SYSTEM (42–54)

✖ **46.74 Closure of fistula of small intestine, except duodenum**

> | Excludes | *closure of:*
> *artificial stoma (46.51)*
> *vaginal fistula (70.74)*
> *repair of gastrojejunocolic fistula (44.63)*

✖ **46.75 Suture of laceration of large intestine**

✖ **46.76 Closure of fistula of large intestine**

> | Excludes | *closure of:*
> *gastrocolic fistula (44.63)*
> *rectal fistula (48.73)*
> *sigmoidovesical fistula (57.83)*
> *stoma (46.52)*
> *vaginal fistula (70.72–70.73)*
> *vesicocolic fistula (57.83)*
> *vesicosigmoidovaginal fistula (57.83)*

Coding Clinic: 1999, Q3, P8

✖ **46.79 Other repair of intestine**
Duodenoplasty

● **46.8 Dilation and manipulation of intestine**
Coding Clinic: 2003, Q1, P14-15; 1998, Q43, P82-83

✖ **46.80 Intra-abdominal manipulation of intestine, not otherwise specified**
Correction of intestinal malrotation
Reduction of:
intestinal torsion
intestinal volvulus
intussusception

> | Excludes | *reduction of intussusception with:*
> *fluoroscopy (96.29)*
> *ionizing radiation enema (96.29)*
> *ultrasonography guidance (96.29)*

✖ **46.81 Intra-abdominal manipulation of small intestine**

✖ **46.82 Intra-abdominal manipulation of large intestine**

46.85 Dilation of intestine
Dilation (balloon) of duodenum
Dilation (balloon) of jejunum
Endoscopic dilation (balloon) of large intestine
That through rectum or colostomy

> | Excludes | *with insertion of colonic stent (46.86–46.87)* ◄

Coding Clinic: 2007, Q3, P6-7; 1989, Q3, P15

46.86 Endoscopic insertion of colonic stent(s) ◄
Colonoscopy (flexible) (through stoma) with transendoscopic stent placement ◄
Combined with fluoroscopic-guided insertion ◄
Stent endoprosthesis of colon ◄
Through the scope [TTS] technique ◄

> | Excludes | *other non-endoscopic insertion of colonic stent (46.87)* ◄

46.87 Other insertion of colonic stent(s) ◄

> | Includes | *that by:* ◄
> *fluoroscopic guidance only* ◄
> *rectal guiding tube* ◄
> Non-endoscopic insertion ◄

> Code also any synchronous diagnostic procedure(s) ◄

> | Excludes | *endoscopic insertion of colonic stent (46.86)* ◄

● **46.9 Other operations on intestines**

✖ **46.91 Myotomy of sigmoid colon**

✖ **46.92 Myotomy of other parts of colon**

✖ **46.93 Revision of anastomosis of small intestine**

✖ **46.94 Revision of anastomosis of large intestine**

46.95 Local perfusion of small intestine
> Code also substance perfused (99.21–99.29)

46.96 Local perfusion of large intestine
> Code also substance perfused (99.21–99.29)

✖ **46.97 Transplant of intestine**
Note: To report donor source - *see* codes 00.91–00.93
MCE: Limited coverage

✖ **46.99 Other**
Ileoentectropy

> | Excludes | *diagnostic procedures on intestine (45.11–45.29)*
> *dilation of enterostomy stoma (96.24)*
> *intestinal intubation (96.08)*
> *removal of:*
> *intraluminal foreign body from large intestine without incision (98.04)*
> *intraluminal foreign body from small intestine without incision (98.03)*
> *tube from large intestine (97.53)*
> *tube from small intestine (97.52)*
> *replacement of:*
> *large intestine tube or enterostomy device (97.04)*
> *small intestine tube or enterostomy device (97.03)*

Coding Clinic: 1999, Q3, P11; 1989, Q1, P11

● **47 Operations on appendix**

> | Includes | appendiceal stump

> Code also any application or administration of an adhesion barrier substance (99.77)

● **47.0 Appendectomy**

> | Excludes | *incidental appendectomy, so described*
> *laparoscopic (47.11)*
> *other (47.19)*

Coding Clinic: 1992, Q3, P12

✖ **47.01 Laparoscopic appendectomy**
Coding Clinic: 2001, Q1, P15-16; 1996, Q4, P64-65

✖ **47.09 Other appendectomy**
Coding Clinic: 1997, Q4, P52

● **47.1 Incidental appendectomy**
Coding Clinic: 1987, Jan-Feb, P11-12

✖ **47.11 Laparoscopic incidental appendectomy**

✖ **47.19 Other incidental appendectomy**
Coding Clinic: 1996, Q4, P64-65; 1984, Nov-Dec, P12

✖ **47.2 Drainage of appendiceal abscess**

> | Excludes | *that with appendectomy (47.0)*

● **47.9 Other operations on appendix**

✖ **47.91 Appendicostomy**

✖ **47.92 Closure of appendiceal fistula**

✖ **47.99 Other**
Anastomosis of appendix

> | Excludes | *diagnostic procedures on appendix (45.21–45.29)*

Coding Clinic: 2001, Q3, P16

| Excludes | Includes | Use additional | Code also | Omit code |

OPERATIONS ON THE DIGESTIVE SYSTEM (42–54)

● **48   Operations on rectum, rectosigmoid and perirectal tissue**

     Code also any application or administration of an adhesion barrier substance (99.77)

     Coding Clinic: 1999, Q3, P8-9

✖ **48.0   Proctotomy**

     Decompression of imperforate anus

     Panas' operation [linear proctotomy]

     Excludes   incision of perirectal tissue (48.81)

✖ **48.1   Proctostomy**

● **48.2   Diagnostic procedures on rectum, rectosigmoid and perirectal tissue**

     ✖ **48.21   Transabdominal proctosigmoidoscopy**

         Intraoperative proctosigmoidoscopy

         Excludes   that with biopsy (48.24)

     48.22   Proctosigmoidoscopy through artificial stoma

         Excludes   that with biopsy (48.24)

     48.23   Rigid proctosigmoidoscopy

         Excludes   flexible sigmoidoscopy (45.24)

         Coding Clinic: 2001, Q1, P8

     48.24   Closed [endoscopic] biopsy of rectum

         Brushing or washing for specimen collection

         Proctosigmoidoscopy with biopsy

         Coding Clinic: 2003, Q1, P12

         MCE: Closed biopsy procedure

     ✖ **48.25   Open biopsy of rectum**

         MCE: Open biopsy procedure

     48.26   Biopsy of perirectal tissue

     48.29   Other diagnostic procedures on rectum, rectosigmoid and perirectal tissue

         Excludes   digital examination of rectum (89.34)

             lower GI series (87.64)

             microscopic examination of specimen from rectum (90.91–90.99)

● **48.3   Local excision or destruction of lesion or tissue of rectum**

     48.31   Radical electrocoagulation of rectal lesion or tissue

     48.32   Other electrocoagulation of rectal lesion or tissue

         Coding Clinic: 1998, Q2, P18; 1987, Nov-Dec, P11

     48.33   Destruction of rectal lesion or tissue by laser

     48.34   Destruction of rectal lesion or tissue by cryosurgery

     ✖ **48.35   Local excision of rectal lesion or tissue**

         Excludes   biopsy of rectum (48.24–48.25)

             excision of perirectal tissue (48.82)

             hemorrhoidectomy (49.46)

             [endoscopic] polypectomy of rectum (48.36)

             rectal fistulectomy (48.73)

     48.36   [Endoscopic] polypectomy of rectum

● **48.4   Pull-through resection of rectum**

     Code also any synchronous anastomosis other than end-to-end (45.90, 45.92–45.95)

     Coding Clinic: 2008, Q4, P169-172

     ✖ **48.40   Pull-through resection of rectum, not otherwise specified**

         Pull-through resection NOS

         Excludes   abdominoperineal pull-through NOS (48.50)

     ✖ **48.41   Soave submucosal resection of rectum**

         Endorectal pull-through operation

     ✖ **48.42   Laparoscopic pull-through resection of rectum**

✖ **48.43   Open pull-through resection of rectum**

✖ **48.49   Other pull-through resection of rectum**

     Abdominoperineal pull-through

     Altemeier operation

     Swenson proctectomy

     Excludes   Duhamel abdominoperineal pull-through (48.65)

         laparoscopic pull-through resection of rectum (48.42)

         open pull-through resection of rectum (48.43)

         pull-through resection of rectum, not otherwise specified (48.40)

     Coding Clinic: 2001, Q3, P8-9; 1999, Q2, P13

● **48.5   Abdominoperineal resection of rectum**

     Combined abdominoendorectal resection

     Complete proctectomy

     Includes   with synchronous colostomy

     Code also any synchronous anastomosis other than end-to-end (45.90, 45.92–45.95)

     Excludes   Duhamel abdominoperineal pull-through (48.65)

         that as part of pelvic exenteration (68.8)

     Coding Clinic: 1997, Q2, P5

     ✖ **48.50   Abdominoperineal resection of the rectum, not otherwise specified**

     ✖ **48.51   Laparoscopic abdominoperineal resection of the rectum**

     ✖ **48.52   Open abdominoperineal resection of the rectum**

     ✖ **48.59   Other abdominoperineal resection of the rectum**

         Excludes   abdominoperineal resection of the rectum, NOS (48.50)

             laparoscopic abdominoperineal resection of the rectum (48.51)

             open abdominoperineal resection of the rectum (48.52)

● **48.6   Other resection of rectum**

     Code also any synchronous anastomosis other than end-to-end (45.90, 45.92–45.95)

     ✖ **48.61   Transsacral rectosigmoidectomy**

     ✖ **48.62   Anterior resection of rectum with synchronous colostomy**

         Coding Clinic: 1997, Q2, P5

     ✖ **48.63   Other anterior resection of rectum**

         Excludes   that with synchronous colostomy (48.62)

         Coding Clinic: 1996, Q1, P9

     ✖ **48.64   Posterior resection of rectum**

     ✖ **48.65   Duhamel resection of rectum**

         Duhamel abdominoperineal pull-through

     ✖ **48.69   Other**

         Partial proctectomy

         Rectal resection NOS

         Coding Clinic: 2005, Q2, P13-14; 1987, Jan-Feb, P11; 1986, Nov-Dec, P11

● **48.7   Repair of rectum**

     Excludes   repair of:

         current obstetric laceration (75.62)

         vaginal rectocele (70.50, 70.52, 70.53, 70.55)

     ✖ **48.71   Suture of laceration of rectum**

     ✖ **48.72   Closure of proctostomy**

◀ New   ◀═ Revised   ~~deleted~~ Deleted   ● Use Additional Digit(s)   ✖ Valid O.R. Procedure

◆ Non-O.R. Procedure   ♀ Females Only   ♂ Males Only

✖ **48.73 Closure of other rectal fistula**

> **Excludes** *fistulectomy:*
> *perirectal (48.93)*
> *rectourethral (58.43)*
> *rectovaginal (70.73)*
> *rectovesical (57.83)*
> *rectovesicovaginal (57.83)*

✖ **48.74 Rectorectostomy**
Rectal anastomosis NOS
Stapled transanal rectal resection (STARR)

✖ **48.75 Abdominal proctopexy**
Frickman procedure
Ripstein repair of rectal prolapse

✖ **48.76 Other proctopexy**
Delorme repair of prolapsed rectum
Proctosigmoidopexy
Puborectalis sling operation

> **Excludes** *manual reduction of rectal prolapse*
> *(96.26)*

✖ **48.79 Other repair of rectum**
Repair of old obstetric laceration of rectum

> **Excludes** *anastomosis to:*
> *large intestine (45.94)*
> *small intestine (45.92–45.93)*
> *repair of:*
> *current obstetrica laceration (75.62)*
> *vaginal rectocele (70.50, 70.52)*

● **48.8 Incision or excision of perirectal tissue or lesion**

> **Includes** pelvirectal tissue
> rectovaginal septum

✖ **48.81 Incision of perirectal tissue**
Incision of rectovaginal septum

✖ **48.82 Excision of perirectal tissue**

> **Excludes** *perirectal biopsy (48.26)*
> *perirectofistulectomy (48.93)*
> *rectal fistulectomy (48.73)*

● **48.9 Other operations on rectum and perirectal tissue**

✖ **48.91 Incision of rectal stricture**

✖ **48.92 Anorectal myectomy**

✖ **48.93 Repair of perirectal fistula**

> **Excludes** *that opening into rectum (48.73)*

> Coding Clinic: 2007, Q1, P13

✖ **48.99 Other**

> **Excludes** *digital examination of rectum (89.34)*
> *dilation of rectum (96.22)*
> *insertion of rectal tube (96.09)*
> *irrigation of rectum (96.38–96.39)*
> *manual reduction of rectal prolapse*
> *(96.26)*
> *proctoclysis (96.37)*
> *rectal massage (99.93)*
> *rectal packing (96.19)*
> *removal of:*
> *impacted feces (96.38)*
> *intraluminal foreign body from*
> *rectum without incision*
> *(98.05)*
> *rectal packing (97.59)*
> *transanal enema (96.39)*

● **49 Operations on anus**

> Code also any application or administration of an
> adhesion barrier substance (99.77)

● **49.0 Incision or excision of perianal tissue**

✖ **49.01 Incision of perianal abscess**
> Coding Clinic: 2005, Q2, P10

✖ **49.02 Other incision of perianal tissue**
Undercutting of perianal tissue

> **Excludes** *anal fistulotomy (49.11)*

49.03 Excision of perianal skin tags

✖ **49.04 Other excision of perianal tissue**

> **Excludes** *anal fistulectomy (49.12)*
> *biopsy of perianal tissue (49.22)*

> Coding Clinic: 2001, Q1, P8

● **49.1 Incision or excision of anal fistula**

> **Excludes** *closure of anal fistula (49.73)*

✖ **49.11 Anal fistulotomy**

✖ **49.12 Anal fistulectomy**

● **49.2 Diagnostic procedures on anus and perianal tissue**

49.21 Anoscopy

49.22 Biopsy of perianal tissue

49.23 Biopsy of anus

**49.29 Other diagnostic procedures on anus and
perianal tissue**

> **Excludes** *microscopic examination of specimen*
> *from anus (90.91–90.99)*

● **49.3 Local excision or destruction of other lesion or tissue
of anus**
Anal cryptotomy
Cauterization of lesion of anus

> **Excludes** *biopsy of anus (49.23)*
> *control of (postoperative) hemorrhage of anus*
> *(49.95)*
> *hemorrhoidectomy (49.46)*

**49.31 Endoscopic excision or destruction of lesion or
tissue of anus**

✖ **49.39 Other local excision or destruction of lesion or
tissue of anus**

> **Excludes** *that by endoscopic approach (49.31)*

> Coding Clinic: 2001, Q1, P8

● **49.4 Procedures on hemorrhoids**

49.41 Reduction of hemorrhoids

49.42 Injection of hemorrhoids

49.43 Cauterization of hemorrhoids
Clamp and cautery of hemorrhoids

✖ **49.44 Destruction of hemorrhoids by cryotherapy**

✖ **49.45 Ligation of hemorrhoids**

✖ **49.46 Excision of hemorrhoids**
Hemorrhoidectomy NOS
> Coding Clinic: 2007, Q1, P13

49.47 Evacuation of thrombosed hemorrhoids

✖ **49.49 Other procedures on hemorrhoids**
Lord procedure

● **49.5 Division of anal sphincter**

✖ **49.51 Left lateral anal sphincterotomy**

✖ **49.52 Posterior anal sphincterotomy**

✖ **49.59 Other anal sphincterotomy**
Division of sphincter NOS

✖ **49.6 Excision of anus**

OPERATIONS ON THE DIGESTIVE SYSTEM (42–54)

● **49.7   Repair of anus**

> **Excludes**   *repair of current obstetric laceration (75.62)*

✖ **49.71   Suture of laceration of anus**

✖ **49.72   Anal cerclage**

✖ **49.73   Closure of anal fistula**

> **Excludes**   *excision of anal fistula (49.12)*

✖ **49.74   Gracilis muscle transplant for anal incontinence**

✖ **49.75   Implantation or revision of artificial anal sphincter**
> Removal with subsequent replacement
> Replacement during same or subsequent
>   operative episode

✖ **49.76   Removal of artificial anal sphincter**
> Explantation or removal without replacement

> **Excludes**   *revision with implantation during*
>   *same operative episode (49.75)*

✖ **49.79   Other repair of anal sphincter**
> Repair of old obstetric laceration of anus

> **Excludes**   *anoplasty with synchronous*
>   *hemorrhoidectomy (49.46)*
>   *repair of current obstetric laceration*
>   *(75.62)*

> Coding Clinic: 1998, Q2, P16-17; 1997, Q1, P9-10

● **49.9   Other operations on anus**

> **Excludes**   *dilation of anus (sphincter) (96.23)*

✖ **49.91   Incision of anal septum**

✖ **49.92   Insertion of subcutaneous electrical anal stimulator**

✖ **49.93   Other incision of anus**
> Removal of:
>   foreign body from anus with incision
>   seton from anus

> **Excludes**   *anal fistulotomy (49.11)*
>   *removal of intraluminal foreign body*
>   *without incision (98.05)*

✖ **49.94   Reduction of anal prolapse**

> **Excludes**   *manual reduction of rectal prolapse*
>   *(96.26)*

✖ **49.95   Control of (postoperative) hemorrhage of anus**

✖ **49.99   Other**

● **50   Operations on liver**

> Code also   any application or administration of an
>   adhesion barrier substance (99.77)

✖ **50.0   Hepatotomy**
> Incision of abscess of liver
> Removal of gallstones from liver
> Stromeyer-Little operation

● **50.1   Diagnostic procedures on liver**

50.11   Closed (percutaneous) [needle] biopsy of liver
> Diagnostic aspiration of liver
> Coding Clinic: 2005, Q3, P24; 1994, Q3, P11; 1988, Q4, P12
> MCE: Closed biopsy procedure

✖ **50.12   Open biopsy of liver**
> Wedge biopsy
> Coding Clinic: 2005, Q2, P13-14; 1984, Nov-Dec, P12
> MCE: Open biopsy procedure

50.13   Transjugular liver biopsy
> Transvenous liver biopsy

> **Excludes**   *closed (percutaneous) [needle] biopsy of*
>   *liver (50.11)*
>   *laparoscopic liver biopsy (50.14)*
> Coding Clinic: 2007, Q4, P113-114

✖ **50.14   Laparoscopic liver biopsy**

> **Excludes**   *closed (percutaneous) [needle] biopsy of*
>   *liver (50.11)*
>   *open biopsy of liver (50.12)*
>   *transjugular liver biopsy (50.13)*
> Coding Clinic: 2007, Q4, P113-114

✖ **50.19   Other diagnostic procedures on liver**

> **Excludes**   *laparoscopic liver biopsy (50.14)*
>   *liver scan and radioisotope function*
>   *study (92.02)*
>   *microscopic examination of specimen*
>   *from liver (91.01–91.09)*
>   *transjugular liver biopsy (50.13)*

● **50.2   Local excision or destruction of liver tissue or lesion**
> Coding Clinic: 2006, Q4, P124-126

✖ **50.21   Marsupialization of lesion of liver**

✖ **50.22   Partial hepatectomy**
> Wedge resection of liver

> **Excludes**   *biopsy of liver (50.11–50.12)*
>   *hepatic lobectomy (50.3)*

✖ **50.23   Open ablation of liver lesion or tissue**

✖ **50.24   Percutaneous ablation of liver lesion or tissue**

✖ **50.25   Laparoscopic ablation of liver lesion or tissue**

✖ **50.26   Other and unspecified ablation of liver lesion or tissue**

✖ **50.29   Other destruction of lesion of liver**
> Cauterization of hepatic lesion
> Enucleation of hepatic lesion
> Evacuation of hepatic lesion

> **Excludes**   *ablation of liver lesion or tissue:*
>   *laparoscopic (50.25)*
>   *open (50.23)*
>   *other (50.26)*
>   *percutaneous (50.24)*
>   *laser interstitial thermal therapy*
>   *[LITT] of lesion or tissue of liver*
>   *under guidance (17.63)* ◄
>   *percutaneous aspiration of lesion*
>   *(50.91)*
> Coding Clinic: 2003, Q2, P9

✖ **50.3   Lobectomy of liver**
> Total hepatic lobectomy with partial excision of other
> lobe

✖ **50.4   Total hepatectomy**
> Coding Clinic: 2008, Q2, P8-9

● **50.5   Liver transplant**
> Note: To report donor source - *see* codes 00.91–00.93

✖ **50.51   Auxiliary liver transplant**
> Auxiliary hepatic transplantation leaving
>   patient's own liver in situ
> MCE: Non-Covered procedure

✖ **50.59   Other transplant of liver**
> Coding Clinic: 2008, Q4, P120; Q2, P8-9
> MCE: Limited coverage

● **50.6   Repair of liver**

✖ **50.61   Closure of laceration of liver**

✖ **50.69   Other repair of liver**
> Hepatopexy

◄ New   ◄▥ Revised   ~~deleted~~ Deleted   ● Use Additional Digit(s)   ✖ Valid O.R. Procedure
     ◆ Non-O.R. Procedure   ♀ Females Only   ♂ Males Only

OPERATIONS ON THE DIGESTIVE SYSTEM (42–54)

● **50.9 Other operations on liver**

> Excludes   *lysis of adhesions (54.5)*

    50.91 Percutaneous aspiration of liver

> > Excludes   *percutaneous biopsy (50.11)*

    50.92 Extracorporeal hepatic assistance
       Liver dialysis
       Coding Clinic: 2001, Q2, P21-22

    50.93 Localized perfusion of liver

    50.94 Other injection of therapeutic substance into liver

    50.99 Other

● **51 Operations on gallbladder and biliary tract**

> Includes   operations on:
> > ampulla of Vater
> > common bile duct
> > cystic duct
> > hepatic duct
> > intrahepatic bile duct
> > sphincter of Oddi

> Code also any application or administration of an adhesion barrier substance (99.77)

● **51.0 Cholecystotomy and cholecystostomy**

    51.01 Percutaneous aspiration of gallbladder
       Percutaneous cholecystotomy for drainage
       That by: needle or catheter

> > Excludes   *needle biopsy (51.12)*

    ✶ **51.02 Trocar cholecystostomy**

    ✶ **51.03 Other cholecystostomy**

    ✶ **51.04 Other cholecystotomy**
       Cholelithotomy NOS

● **51.1 Diagnostic procedures on biliary tract**

> Excludes   *that for endoscopic procedures classifiable to 51.64, 51.84–51.88, 52.14, 52.21, 52.93–52.94, 52.97–52.98*

    Coding Clinic: 1997, Q2, P7

    51.10 Endoscopic retrograde cholangiopancreatography [ERCP]

> > Excludes   *endoscopic retrograde:*
> > *cholangiography [ERC] (51.11)*
> > *pancreatography [ERP] (52.13)*

       Coding Clinic: 2003, Q3, P17-18; 2001, Q1, P8-9; 1999, Q2, P13-14; 1993, 5th Issue, P12

    51.11 Endoscopic retrograde cholangiography [ERC]
       Laparoscopic exploration of common bile duct

> > Excludes   *endoscopic retrograde:*
> > *cholangiopancreatography [ERCP] (51.10)*
> > *pancreatography [ERP] (52.13)*

       Coding Clinic: 1996, Q1, P12-13; 1993, 5th Issue, P12; 1988, Q4, P7

    51.12 Percutaneous biopsy of gallbladder or bile ducts
       Needle biopsy of gallbladder
       MCE: Closed biopsy procedure

    ✶ **51.13 Open biopsy of gallbladder or bile ducts**
       MCE: Open biopsy procedure

    51.14 Other closed [endoscopic] biopsy of biliary duct or sphincter of Oddi
       Brushing or washing for specimen collection
       Closed biopsy of biliary duct or sphincter of Oddi by procedures classifiable to 51.10–51.11, 52.13

51.15 Pressure measurement of sphincter of Oddi
       Pressure measurement of sphincter by procedures classifiable to 51.10–51.11, 52.13

    ✶ **51.19 Other diagnostic procedures on biliary tract**

> > Excludes   *biliary tract x-ray (87.51–87.59)*
> > *microscopic examination of specimen from biliary tract (91.01–91.09)*

● **51.2 Cholecystectomy**

    ✶ **51.21 Other partial cholecystectomy**
       Revision of prior cholecystectomy

> > Excludes   *that by laparoscope (51.24)*

    ✶ **51.22 Cholecystectomy**

> > Excludes   *laparoscopic cholecystectomy (51.23)*

       Coding Clinic: 1997, Q4, P52; 1995, Q2, P11; 1993, 5th Issue, P11; 1992, Q2, P16; 1988, Q4, P7

    ✶ **51.23 Laparoscopic cholecystectomy**
       That by laser
       Coding Clinic: 2008, Q4, P172-174; 1998, Q3, P10; 1997, Q4, P52; 1996, Q1, P12-13; 1995, Q2, P11; 1994, Q3, P11

    ✶ **51.24 Laparoscopic partial cholecystectomy**
       Coding Clinic: 1996, Q4, P69

● **51.3 Anastomosis of gallbladder or bile duct**

> Excludes   *resection with end-to-end anastomosis (51.61–51.69)*

    ✶ **51.31 Anastomosis of gallbladder to hepatic ducts**

    ✶ **51.32 Anastomosis of gallbladder to intestine**

    ✶ **51.33 Anastomosis of gallbladder to pancreas**

    ✶ **51.34 Anastomosis of gallbladder to stomach**

    ✶ **51.35 Other gallbladder anastomosis**
       Gallbladder anastomosis NOS

    ✶ **51.36 Choledochoenterostomy**

    ✶ **51.37 Anastomosis of hepatic duct to gastrointestinal tract**
       Kasai portoenterostomy
       Coding Clinic: 2002, Q2, P12

    ✶ **51.39 Other bile duct anastomosis**
       Anastomosis of bile duct NOS
       Anastomosis of unspecified bile duct to:
         intestine
         liver
         pancreas
         stomach

● **51.4 Incision of bile duct for relief of obstruction**

    ✶ **51.41 Common duct exploration for removal of calculus**

> > Excludes   *percutaneous extraction (51.96)*

       Coding Clinic: 1996, Q1, P12-13; 1988, Q4, P7

    ✶ **51.42 Common duct exploration for relief of other obstruction**

    ✶ **51.43 Insertion of choledochohepatic tube for decompression**
       Hepatocholedochostomy
       Coding Clinic: 1988, Q4, P7

    ✶ **51.49 Incision of other bile ducts for relief of obstruction**

● **51.5 Other incision of bile duct**

> Excludes   *that for relief of obstruction (51.41–51.49)*

    ✶ **51.51 Exploration of common duct**
       Incision of common bile duct
       Coding Clinic: 1996, Q1, P12
       MCE: Non-covered procedure

    ✶ **51.59 Incision of other bile duct**

OPERATIONS ON THE DIGESTIVE SYSTEM (42–54)

● **51.6   Local excision or destruction of lesion or tissue of biliary ducts and sphincter of Oddi**

> **Code also** anastomosis other than end-to-end (51.31, 51.36–51.39)
>
> **Excludes**   *biopsy of bile duct (51.12–51.13)*

✖ **51.61   Excision of cystic duct remnant**

✖ **51.62   Excision of ampulla of Vater (with reimplantation of common duct)**

✖ **51.63   Other excision of common duct**
Choledochectomy

> **Excludes**   *fistulectomy (51.72)*

51.64   Endoscopic excision or destruction of lesion of biliary ducts or sphincter of Oddi
Excision or destruction of lesion of biliary duct by procedures classifiable to 51.10–51.11, 52.13
Coding Clinic: 1993, 5th Issue, P14

✖ **51.69   Excision of other bile duct**
Excision of lesion of bile duct NOS

> **Excludes**   *fistulectomy (51.79)*

● **51.7   Repair of bile ducts**

✖ **51.71   Simple suture of common bile duct**

✖ **51.72   Choledochoplasty**
Repair of fistula of common bile duct

✖ **51.79   Repair of other bile ducts**
Closure of artificial opening of bile duct NOS
Suture of bile duct NOS

> **Excludes**   *operative removal of prosthetic device (51.95)*

● **51.8   Other operations on biliary ducts and sphincter of Oddi**

✖ **51.81   Dilation of sphincter of Oddi**
Dilation of ampulla of Vater

> **Excludes**   *that by endoscopic approach (51.84)*

✖ **51.82   Pancreatic sphincterotomy**
Incision of pancreatic sphincter
Transduodenal ampullary sphincterotomy

> **Excludes**   *that by endoscopic approach (51.85)*

✖ **51.83   Pancreatic sphincteroplasty**

51.84   Endoscopic dilation of ampulla and biliary duct
Dilation of ampulla and biliary duct by procedures classifiable to 51.10–51.11, 52.13

51.85   Endoscopic sphincterotomy and papillotomy
Sphincterotomy and papillotomy by procedures classifiable to 51.10–51.11, 52.13
Coding Clinic: 2003, Q3, P17.18; 1993, 5th Issue, P14

51.86   Endoscopic insertion of nasobiliary drainage tube
Insertion of nasobiliary tube by procedures classifiable to 51.10–51.11, 52.13

51.87   Endoscopic insertion of stent (tube) into bile duct
Endoprosthesis of bile duct
Insertion of stent into bile duct by procedures classifiable to 51.10–51.11, 52.13

> **Excludes**   *nasobiliary drainage tube (51.86)*
> *replacement of stent (tube) (97.05)*
> Coding Clinic: 2003, Q3, P17

51.88   Endoscopic removal of stone(s) from biliary tract
Laparoscopic removal of stone(s) from biliary tract
Removal of biliary tract stone(s) by procedures classifiable to 51.10–51.11, 52.13

> **Excludes**   *percutaneous extraction of common duct stones (51.96)*
> Coding Clinic: 2000, Q2, P11; 1997, Q2, P7; 1993, 5th Issue, P12

✖ **51.89   Other operations on sphincter of Oddi**

● **51.9   Other operations on biliary tract**

✖ **51.91   Repair of laceration of gallbladder**

✖ **51.92   Closure of cholecystostomy**

✖ **51.93   Closure of other biliary fistula**
Cholecystogastroenteric fistulectomy

✖ **51.94   Revision of anastomosis of biliary tract**

✖ **51.95   Removal of prosthetic device from bile duct**

> **Excludes**   *nonoperative removal (97.55)*

51.96   Percutaneous extraction of common duct stones
Coding Clinic: 1988, Q4, P7

51.98   Other percutaneous procedures on biliary tract
Percutaneous biliary endoscopy via existing T-tube or other tract for:
dilation of biliary duct stricture
removal of stone(s) except common duct stone
exploration (postoperative)
Percutaneous transhepatic biliary drainage

> **Excludes**   *percutaneous aspiration of gallbladder (51.01)*
> *percutaneous biopsy and/or collection of specimen by brushing or washing (51.12)*
> *percutaneous removal of common duct stone(s) (51.96)*
> Coding Clinic: 1997, Q1, P14

✖ **51.99   Other**
Insertion or replacement of biliary tract prosthesis

> **Excludes**   *biopsy of gallbladder (51.12–51.13)*
> *irrigation of cholecystostomy and other biliary tube (96.41)*
> *lysis of peritoneal adhesions (54.5)*
> *nonoperative removal of:*
> *cholecystostomy tube (97.54)*
> *tube from biliary tract or liver (97.55)*

● **52   Operations on pancreas**

> **Includes**   operations on pancreatic duct
>
> **Code also** any application or administration of an adhesion barrier substance (99.77)

● **52.0   Pancreatotomy**

✖ **52.01   Drainage of pancreatic cyst by catheter**

✖ **52.09   Other pancreatotomy**
Pancreatolithotomy

> **Excludes**   *drainage by anastomosis (52.4, 52.96)*
> *incision of pancreatic sphincter (51.82)*
> *marsupialization of cyst (52.3)*

● **52.1   Diagnostic procedures on pancreas**

52.11   Closed [aspiration] [needle] [percutaneous] biopsy of pancreas
MCE: Closed biopsy procedure

✖ **52.12   Open biopsy of pancreas**
MCE: Open biopsy procedure

52.13   Endoscopic retrograde pancreatography [ERP]

> **Excludes**   *endoscopic retrograde:*
> *cholangiography [ERC] (51.11)*
> *cholangiopancreatography [ERCP] (51.10)*
> *that for procedures classifiable to 51.14–51.15, 51.64, 51.84–51.88, 52.14, 52.21, 52.92–52.94, 52.97–52.98*
> Coding Clinic: 1993, 5th Issue, P12

◀ New   ◀▦ Revised   ~~deleted~~ Deleted   ● Use Additional Digit(s)   ✖ Valid O.R. Procedure

◆ Non-O.R. Procedure   ♀ Females Only   ♂ Males Only

52.14 Closed [endoscopic] biopsy of pancreatic duct
Closed biopsy of pancreatic duct by procedures classifiable to 51.10–51.11, 52.13

✖**52.19 Other diagnostic procedures on pancreas**

| Excludes | contrast pancreatogram (87.66)
endoscopic retrograde pancreatography [ERP] (52.13)
microscopic examination of specimen from pancreas (91.01–91.09) |

●**52.2 Local excision or destruction of pancreas and pancreatic duct**

| Excludes | biopsy of pancreas (52.11–52.12, 52.14)
pancreatic fistulectomy (52.95) |

52.21 Endoscopic excision or destruction of lesion or tissue of pancreatic duct
Excision or destruction of lesion or tissue of pancreatic duct by procedures classifiable to 51.10–51.11, 52.13

✖**52.22 Other excision or destruction of lesion or tissue of pancreas or pancreatic duct**

✖**52.3 Marsupialization of pancreatic cyst**

| Excludes | drainage of cyst by catheter (52.01) |

✖**52.4 Internal drainage of pancreatic cyst**
Pancreaticocystoduodenostomy
Pancreaticocystogastrostomy
Pancreaticocystojejunostomy

●**52.5 Partial pancreatectomy**

| Excludes | pancreatic fistulectomy (52.95) |

✖**52.51 Proximal pancreatectomy**
Excision of head of pancreas (with part of body)
Proximal pancreatectomy with synchronous duodenectomy

✖**52.52 Distal pancreatectomy**
Excision of tail of pancreas (with part of body)

✖**52.53 Radical subtotal pancreatectomy**
Coding Clinic: 2001, Q1, P13

✖**52.59 Other partial pancreatectomy**

✖**52.6 Total pancreatectomy**
Pancreatectomy with synchronous duodenectomy
Coding Clinic: 1996, Q4, P70-71

✖**52.7 Radical pancreaticoduodenectomy**
One-stage pancreaticoduodenal resection with choledochojejunal anastomosis, pancreaticojejunal anastomosis, and gastrojejunostomy
Two-stage pancreaticoduodenal resection (first stage) (second stage)
Radical resection of the pancreas
Whipple procedure

| Excludes | radical subtotal pancreatectomy (52.53) |

Coding Clinic: 2001, Q1, P13

●**52.8 Transplant of pancreas**
Note: To report donor source - *see* codes 00.91–00.93

✖**52.80 Pancreatic transplant, not otherwise specified**
MS-DRG: Refer to Part VI, Appendix E, Table 5, Kidney/Pancreas Transplant Reference Table.
MCE: Non-covered procedure when reported alone (without 55.69); Limited coverage when combined with at least one principal or secondary diagnosis of 250.01, 250.03, 250.11, 250.13, 250.21, 250.23, 250.31, 250.33, 250.41, 250.43, 250.51, 250.53, 250.61, 250.63, 250.71, 250.73, 250.81, 250.83, 250.91, 250.93
MCE: Limited coverage

✖**52.81 Reimplantation of pancreatic tissue**

✖**52.82 Homotransplant of pancreas**
MS-DRG: Refer to Part VI, Appendix E, Table 5, Kidney/Pancreas Transplant Reference Table.
MCE: Non-covered procedure when reported alone (without 55.69); Limited coverage when combined with at least one principal or secondary diagnosis of 250.01, 250.03, 250.11, 250.13, 250.21, 250.23, 250.31, 250.33, 250.41, 250.43, 250.51, 250.53, 250.61, 250.63, 250.71, 250.73, 250.81, 250.83, 250.91, 250.93
MCE: Limited coverage

✖**52.83 Heterotransplant of pancreas**
MCE: Non-covered procedure

52.84 Autotransplantation of cells of Islets of Langerhans
Homotransplantation of islet cells of pancreas
Coding Clinic: 1996, Q4, P70-71
◆ Non-OR Procedure that affects MS-DRG assignment to MDC 11, MS-DRG 673-675

52.85 Allotransplantation of cells of Islets of Langerhans
Heterotransplantation of islet cells of pancreas
Coding Clinic: 1996, Q4, P70-71
◆ Non-OR Procedure that affects MS-DRG assignment to MDC 11, MS-DRG 673-675

52.86 Transplantation of cells of Islets of Langerhans, not otherwise specified

●**52.9 Other operations on pancreas**

✖**52.92 Cannulation of pancreatic duct**

| Excludes | that by endoscopic approach (52.93) |

52.93 Endoscopic insertion of stent (tube) into pancreatic duct
Insertion of cannula or stent into pancreatic duct by procedures classifiable to 51.10–51.11, 52.13

| Excludes | endoscopic insertion of nasopancreatic drainage tube (52.97)
replacement of stent (tube) (97.05) |

Coding Clinic: 1997, Q2, P7

52.94 Endoscopic removal of stone(s) from pancreatic duct
Removal of stone(s) from pancreatic duct by procedures classifiable to 51.10–51.11, 52.13

✖**52.95 Other repair of pancreas**
Fistulectomy of pancreas
Simple suture of pancreas

✖**52.96 Anastomosis of pancreas**
Anastomosis of pancreas (duct) to:
intestine
jejunum
stomach

| Excludes | anastomosis to:
bile duct (51.39)
gallbladder (51.33) |

52.97 Endoscopic insertion of nasopancreatic drainage tube
Insertion of nasopancreatic drainage tube by procedures classifiable to 51.10–51.11, 52.13

| Excludes | drainage of pancreatic cyst by catheter (52.01)
replacement of stent (tube) (97.05) |

OPERATIONS ON THE DIGESTIVE SYSTEM (42–54)

| Excludes | Includes | Use additional | Code also | Omit code |

52.98 Endoscopic dilation of pancreatic duct
Dilation of Wirsung's duct by procedures classifiable to 51.10–51.11, 52.13

✖ **52.99 Other**
Dilation of pancreatic [Wirsung's] duct by open approach
Repair of pancreatic [Wirsung's] duct by open approach

Excludes	*irrigation of pancreatic tube (96.42)*
	removal of pancreatic tube (97.56)

● **53 Repair of hernia**

Includes	hernioplasty
	herniorrhaphy

Code also any application or administration of an adhesion barrier substance (99.77)

Excludes	*manual reduction of hernia (96.27)*

● **53.0 Other unilateral repair of inguinal hernia**

Excludes	*laparoscopic unilateral repair of inguinal hernia (17.11–17.13)*

Coding Clinic: 1994, Q3, P8

✖ **53.00 Unilateral repair of inguinal hernia, not otherwise specified**
Inguinal herniorrhaphy NOS
Coding Clinic: 2008, Q4, P165-169; 2003, Q3, P10-11

✖ **53.01 Other and open repair of direct inguinal hernia**
Direct and indirect inguinal hernia
Coding Clinic: 1996, Q4, P65-66

✖ **53.02 Other and open repair of indirect inguinal hernia**

✖ **53.03 Other and open repair of direct inguinal hernia with graft or prosthesis**

✖ **53.04 Other and open repair of indirect inguinal hernia with graft or prosthesis**

✖ **53.05 Repair of inguinal hernia with graft or prosthesis, not otherwise specified**

● **53.1 Other bilateral repair of inguinal hernia**

Excludes	*laparoscopic bilateral repair of inguinal hernia (17.21–17.24)*

✖ **53.10 Bilateral repair of inguinal hernia, not otherwise specified**

✖ **53.11 Other and open bilateral repair of direct inguinal hernia**
Coding Clinic: 1988, Q1, P9

✖ **53.12 Other and open bilateral repair of indirect inguinal hernia**

✖ **53.13 Other and open bilateral repair of inguinal hernia, one direct and one indirect**

✖ **53.14 Other and open bilateral repair of direct inguinal hernia with graft or prosthesis**

✖ **53.15 Other and open bilateral repair of indirect inguinal hernia with graft or prosthesis**

✖ **53.16 Other and open bilateral repair of inguinal hernia, one direct and one indirect, with graft or prosthesis**

✖ **53.17 Bilateral inguinal hernia repair with graft or prosthesis, not otherwise specified**

● **53.2 Unilateral repair of femoral hernia**

✖ **53.21 Unilateral repair of femoral hernia with graft or prosthesis**

✖ **53.29 Other unilateral femoral herniorrhaphy**

● **53.3 Bilateral repair of femoral hernia**

✖ **53.31 Bilateral repair of femoral hernia with graft or prosthesis**

✖ **53.39 Other bilateral femoral herniorrhaphy**

● **53.4 Repair of umbilical hernia**

Excludes	*repair of gastroschisis (54.71)*

✖ **53.41 Other and open repair of umbilical hernia with graft or prosthesis**

✖ **53.42 Laparoscopic repair of umbilical hernia with graft or prosthesis**

✖ **53.43 Other laparoscopic umbilical herniorrhaphy**

✖ **53.49 Other open umbilical herniorrhaphy**

Excludes	*other laparoscopic umbilical herniorrhaphy (53.43)*
	repair of umbilical hernia with graft or prosthesis (53.41, 53.42)

● **53.5 Repair of other hernia of anterior abdominal wall (without graft or prosthesis)**

✖ **53.51 Incisional hernia repair**
Coding Clinic: 2003, Q3, P6

✖ **53.59 Repair of other hernia of anterior abdominal wall**
Repair of hernia:
epigastric
hypogastric
spigelian
ventral
Coding Clinic: 1996, Q3, P15

● **53.6 Repair of other hernia of anterior abdominal wall with graft or prosthesis**

✖ **53.61 Other open incisional hernia repair with graft or prosthesis**

Excludes	*laparoscopic incisional hernia repair with graft or prosthesis (53.62)*

Coding Clinic: 2006, Q2, P10-11

✖ **53.62 Laparoscopic incisional hernia repair with graft or prosthesis**
Coding Clinic: 2003, Q3, P11

✖ **53.63 Other laparoscopic repair of other hernia of anterior abdominal wall with graft or prosthesis**

✖ **53.69 Other and open repair of other hernia of anterior abdominal wall with graft or prosthesis**

Excludes	*other laparoscopic repair of other hernia of anterior abdominal wall with graft or prothesis (53.63)*

● **53.7 Repair of diaphragmatic hernia, abdominal approach**

✖ **53.71 Laparoscopic repair of diaphragmatic hernia, abdominal approach**

✖ **53.72 Other and open repair of diaphragmatic hernia, abdominal approach**

✖ **53.75 Repair of diaphragmatic hernia, abdominal approach, not otherwise specified**

Excludes	*laparoscopic repair of diaphragmatic hernia (53.71)*
	other and open repair of diaphragmatic hernia (53.72)

◀ New   ◀▥ Revised   ~~deleted~~ Deleted   ● Use Additional Digit(s)   ✖ Valid O.R. Procedure
◆ Non-O.R. Procedure   ♀ Females Only   ♂ Males Only

OPERATIONS ON THE DIGESTIVE SYSTEM (42–54)

● **53.8 Repair of diaphragmatic hernia, thoracic approach**

✖ **53.80 Repair of diaphragmatic hernia with thoracic approach, not otherwise specified**
Thoracoabdominal repair of diaphragmatic hernia

✖ **53.81 Plication of the diaphragm**

✖ **53.82 Repair of parasternal hernia**

✖ **53.83 Laparoscopic repair of diaphragmatic hernia, with thoracic approach**

✖ **53.84 Other and open repair of diaphragmatic hernia, with thoracic approach**

| Excludes | *repair of diaphragmatic hernia with thoracic approach, NOS (53.80)* |

✖ **53.9 Other hernia repair**

Repair of hernia:
  ischiatic
  ischiorectal
  lumbar
  obturator

Repair of hernia:
  omental
  retroperitoneal
  sciatic

Excludes	*relief of strangulated hernia with exteriorization of intestine (46.01, 46.03)*
	repair of pericolostomy hernia (46.42)
	repair of vaginal enterocele (70.92)

● **54 Other operations on abdominal region**

| Includes | operations on: |

epigastric region
flank
groin region
hypochondrium
inguinal region
loin region
pelvic cavity
mesentery
omentum
peritoneum
retroperitoneal tissue space

Code also any application or administration of an adhesion barrier substance (99.77)

Excludes	*hernia repair (53.00–53.9)*
	obliteration of cul-de-sac (70.92)
	retroperitoneal tissue dissection (59.00–59.09)
	skin and subcutaneous tissue of abdominal wall (86.01–86.99)

Coding Clinic: 1997, Q1, P11; 1987, Nov-Dec, P12

✖ **54.0 Incision of abdominal wall**

Drainage of:
  abdominal wall
  extraperitoneal abscess
  retroperitoneal abscess

| Excludes | *incision of peritoneum (54.95)* |
| | *laparotomy (54.11–54.19)* |

Coding Clinic: 2006, Q2, P23-24; 2005, Q4, P74-77; 1993, 5th Issue, P9-10

● **54.1 Laparotomy**

✖ **54.11 Exploratory laparotomy**

| Excludes | *exploration incidental to intra-abdominal surgery —* omit code |

Coding Clinic: 1989, Q3, P14; 1988, Q4, P12; 1987, Jan-Feb, P11-12; 1984, Nov-Dec, P12

✖ **54.12 Reopening of recent laparotomy site**

Reopening of recent laparotomy site for:
  control of hemorrhage
  exploration
  incision of hematoma

✖ **54.19 Other laparotomy**

Drainage of intraperitoneal abscess or hematoma

Excludes	*culdocentesis (70.0)*
	drainage of appendiceal abscess (47.2)
	exploration incidental to intra abdominal surgery — omit code
	Ladd operation (54.95)
	percutaneous drainage of abdomen (54.91)
	removal of foreign body (54.92)

Coding Clinic: 2003, Q3, P16-17; 1992, Q1, P14

● **54.2 Diagnostic procedures of abdominal region**

✖ **54.21 Laparoscopy**

Peritoneoscopy

| Excludes | *laparoscopic cholecystectomy (51.23)* |
| | *that incidental to destruction of fallopian tubes (66.21–66.29)* |

Coding Clinic: 1996, Q4, P64-66

✖ **54.22 Biopsy of abdominal wall or umbilicus**

✖ **54.23 Biopsy of peritoneum**

Biopsy of:
  mesentery
  omentum
  peritoneal implant

Excludes	*closed biopsy of:*
	omentum (54.24)
	peritoneum (54.24)

MCE: Open biopsy procedure

54.24 Closed [percutaneous] [needle] biopsy of intra-abdominal mass

Closed biopsy of:
  omentum
  peritoneal implant
  peritoneum

Excludes	*that of:*
	fallopian tube (66.11)
	ovary (65.11)
	uterine ligaments (68.15)
	uterus (68.16)

Coding Clinic: 1997, Q4, P57

MCE: Closed biopsy procedure

54.25 Peritoneal lavage

Diagnostic peritoneal lavage

| Excludes | *peritoneal dialysis (54.98)* |

Coding Clinic: 1998, Q2, P19-20; 1993, Q4, P31

✖ **54.29 Other diagnostic procedures on abdominal region**

Excludes	*abdominal lymphangiogram (88.04)*
	abdominal x-ray NEC (88.19)
	angiocardiography of venae cava (88.51)
	C.A.T. scan of abdomen (88.01)
	contrast x-ray of abdominal cavity (88.11–88.15)
	intra-abdominal arteriography NEC (88.47)
	microscopic examination of peritoneal and retroperitoneal specimen (91.11–91.19)
	phlebography of:
	intra-abdominal vessels NEC (88.65)
	portal venous system (88.64)
	sinogram of abdominal wall (88.03)
	soft tissue x-ray of abdominal wall NEC (88.09)
	tomography of abdomen NEC (88.02)
	ultrasonography of abdomen and retroperitoneum (88.76)

| Excludes | Includes | Use additional | Code also | Omit code |

OPERATIONS ON THE DIGESTIVE SYSTEM (42–54)

✖ **54.3 Excision or destruction of lesion or tissue of abdominal wall or umbilicus**
Debridement of abdominal wall
Omphalectomy

> **Excludes**   *biopsy of abdominal wall or umbilicus (54.22)*
> *size reduction operation (86.83)*
> *that of skin of abdominal wall (86.22, 86.26, 86.3)*

Coding Clinic: 1989, Q1, P11

✖ **54.4 Excision or destruction of peritoneal tissue**
Excision of:
     appendices epiploicae
     falciform ligament
     gastrocolic ligament
     lesion of:
         mesentery
         omentum
         peritoneum
     presacral lesion NOS
     retroperitoneal lesion NOS

> **Excludes**   *biopsy of peritoneum (54.23)*
> *endometrectomy of cul-de-sac (70.32)*

● **54.5 Lysis of peritoneal adhesions**
Freeing of adhesions of:
     biliary tract
     intestines
     liver
     pelvic peritoneum
     peritoneum
     spleen
     uterus

> **Excludes**   *lysis of adhesions of:*
> *bladder (59.11)*
> *fallopian tube and ovary*
> *laparoscopic (65.81)*
> *other (65.89)*
> *kidney (59.02)*
> *ureter (59.02)*

✖ **54.51 Laparoscopic lysis of peritoneal adhesions**
Coding Clinic: 2006, Q4, P130-134; 2003, Q3, P6-7; 1996, Q4, P65-66

✖ **54.59 Other lysis of peritoneal adhesions**
Coding Clinic: 2006, Q3, P15-16; 2003, Q3, P11; Q1, P14-15; 1996, Q4, P65-66; 1994, Q3, P8

● **54.6 Suture of abdominal wall and peritoneum**

✖ **54.61 Reclosure of postoperative disruption of abdominal wall**

✖ **54.62 Delayed closure of granulating abdominal wound**
Tertiary subcutaneous wound closure

✖ **54.63 Other suture of abdominal wall**
Suture of laceration of abdominal wall

> **Excludes**   *closure of operative wound —*
> *omit code*

✖ **54.64 Suture of peritoneum**
Secondary suture of peritoneum

> **Excludes**   *closure of operative wound —*
> *omit code*

● **54.7 Other repair of abdominal wall and peritoneum**

✖ **54.71 Repair of gastroschisis**
Coding Clinic: 2002, Q2, P9

✖ **54.72 Other repair of abdominal wall**

✖ **54.73 Other repair of peritoneum**
Suture of gastrocolic ligament

✖ **54.74 Other repair of omentum**
Epiplorrhaphy
Graft of omentum
Omentopexy
Reduction of torsion of omentum

> **Excludes**   *cardio-omentopexy (36.39)*

Coding Clinic: 1987, Jan-Feb, P11

✖ **54.75 Other repair of mesentery**
Mesenteric plication
Mesenteropexy

● **54.9 Other operations of abdominal region**

> **Excludes**   *removal of ectopic pregnancy (74.3)*

54.91 Percutaneous abdominal drainage
Paracentesis

> **Excludes**   *creation of cutaneoperitoneal fistula (54.93)*

Coding Clinic: 2007, Q4, P95-96; 1999, Q3, P9; 1999, Q2, P14; 1998, Q3, P12; 1990, Q2, P25

✖ **54.92 Removal of foreign body from peritoneal cavity**
Coding Clinic: 1989, Q1, P11

✖ **54.93 Creation of cutaneoperitoneal fistula**
Coding Clinic: 1995, Q2, P10

✖ **54.94 Creation of peritoneovascular shunt**
Peritoneovenous shunt
Coding Clinic: 1988, Q1, P9

✖ **54.95 Incision of peritoneum**
Exploration of ventriculoperitoneal shunt at peritoneal site
Ladd operation
Revision of distal catheter of ventricular shunt
Revision of ventriculoperitoneal shunt at peritoneal site

> **Excludes**   *that incidental to laparotomy (54.11–54.19)*

54.96 Injection of air into peritoneal cavity
Pneumoperitoneum

> **Excludes**   *that for:*
> *collapse of lung (33.33)*
> *radiography (88.12–88.13, 88.15)*

54.97 Injection of locally-acting therapeutic substance into peritoneal cavity

> **Excludes**   *peritoneal dialysis (54.98)*

54.98 Peritoneal dialysis

> **Excludes**   *peritoneal lavage (diagnostic) (54.25)*

Coding Clinic: 1993, Q4, P31

54.99 Other

> **Excludes**   *removal of:*
> *abdominal wall suture (97.83)*
> *peritoneal drainage device (97.82)*
> *retroperitoneal drainage device (97.81)*

Coding Clinic: 1999, Q1, P4

◄ New   ◄▥ Revised   ~~deleted~~ Deleted   ● Use Additional Digit(s)   ✖ Valid O.R. Procedure
◆ Non-O.R. Procedure   ♀ Females Only   ♂ Males Only

10. OPERATIONS ON THE URINARY SYSTEM (55–59)

● **55 Operations on kidney**

> **Includes** operations on renal pelvis
>
> **Code also** any application or administration of an adhesion barrier substance (99.77)
>
> **Excludes** *perirenal tissue (59.00–59.09, 59.21–59.29, 59.91–59.92)*

● **55.0 Nephrotomy and nephrostomy**

> **Excludes** *drainage by:*
> *anastomosis (55.86)*
> *aspiration (55.92)*
> *incision of kidney pelvis (55.11–55.12)*

✖ **55.01 Nephrotomy**
Evacuation of renal cyst
Exploration of kidney
Nephrolithotomy

✖ **55.02 Nephrostomy**
Coding Clinic: 1997, Q2, P4; 1986, Sept-Oct, P11-12

✖ **55.03 Percutaneous nephrostomy without fragmentation**
Nephrostolithotomy, percutaneous (nephroscopic)
Percutaneous removal of kidney stone(s) by:
basket extraction
forceps extraction (nephroscopic)
Pyelostolithotomy, percutaneous (nephroscopic)
With placement of catheter down ureter

> **Excludes** *percutaneous removal by fragmentation (55.04)*
> *repeat nephroscopic removal during current episode (55.92)*

Coding Clinic: 1996, Q2, P5

✖ **55.04 Percutaneous nephrostomy with fragmentation**
Percutaneous nephrostomy with disruption of kidney stone by ultrasonic energy and extraction (suction) through endoscope
With placement of catheter down ureter
With fluoroscopic guidance

> **Excludes** *repeat fragmentation during current episode (59.95)*

Coding Clinic: 1986, Sept-Oct, P11-12

● **55.1 Pyelotomy and pyelostomy**

> **Excludes** *drainage by anastomosis (55.86)*
> *percutaneous pyelostolithotomy (55.03)*
> *removal of calculus without incision (56.0)*

✖ **55.11 Pyelotomy**
Exploration of renal pelvis
Pyelolithotomy

✖ **55.12 Pyelostomy**
Insertion of drainage tube into renal pelvis

● **55.2 Diagnostic procedures on kidney**

55.21 Nephroscopy

55.22 Pyeloscopy

55.23 Closed [percutaneous] [needle] biopsy of kidney
Endoscopic biopsy via existing nephrostomy, nephrotomy, pyelostomy, or pyelotomy
MCE: Closed biopsy procedure

✖ **55.24 Open biopsy of kidney**
MCE: Open biopsy procedure

✖ **55.29 Other diagnostic procedures on kidney**

> **Excludes** *microscopic examination of specimen from kidney (91.21–91.29)*
> *pyelogram:*
> *intravenous (87.73)*
> *percutaneous (87.75)*
> *retrograde (87.74)*
> *radioisotope scan (92.03)*
> *renal arteriography (88.45)*
> *tomography:*
> *C.A.T. scan (87.71)*
> *other (87.72)*

● **55.3 Local excision or destruction of lesion or tissue of kidney**
Coding Clinic: 2006, Q4, P124-126

✖ **55.31 Marsupialization of kidney lesion**

✖ **55.32 Open ablation of renal lesion or tissue**

✖ **55.33 Percutaneous ablation of renal lesion or tissue**

✖ **55.34 Laparoscopic ablation of renal lesion or tissue**

✖ **55.35 Other and unspecified ablation of renal lesion or tissue**

✖ **55.39 Other local destruction or excision of renal lesion or tissue**
Obliteration of calyceal diverticulum

> **Excludes** *ablation of renal lesion or tissue:*
> *laparoscopic (55.34)*
> *open (55.32)*
> *other (55.35)*
> *percutaneous (55.33)*
> *biopsy of kidney (55.23–55.24)*
> *partial nephrectomy (55.4)*
> *percutaneous aspiration of kidney (55.92)*
> *wedge resection of kidney (55.4)*

Coding Clinic: 1996, Q1, P10-11

✖ **55.4 Partial nephrectomy**
Calycectomy
Wedge resection of kidney

> **Code also** any synchronous resection of ureter (56.40–56.42)

● **55.5 Complete nephrectomy**

> **Code also** any synchronous excision of:
> adrenal gland (07.21–07.3)
> bladder segment (57.6)
> lymph nodes (40.3, 40.52–40.59)

✖ **55.51 Nephroureterectomy**
Nephroureterectomy with bladder cuff
Total nephrectomy (unilateral)

> **Excludes** *removal of transplanted kidney (55.53)*

Coding Clinic: 2005, Q2, P4-5

✖ **55.52 Nephrectomy of remaining kidney**
Removal of solitary kidney

> **Excludes** *removal of transplanted kidney (55.53)*

✖ **55.53 Removal of transplanted or rejected kidney**
Coding Clinic: 2008, Q4, P82-83

✖ **55.54 Bilateral nephrectomy**

> **Excludes** *complete nephrectomy NOS (55.51)*

● **55.6 Transplant of kidney**
Note: To report donor source - *see* codes 00.91–00.93

✖ **55.61 Renal autotransplantation**

✖ **55.69 Other kidney transplantation**
Coding Clinic: 2004, Q4, P116-117; 1996, Q4, P70-71
MS-DRG: Refer to Part VI, Appendix E, Table 5, Kidney/Pancreas Transplant Reference Table.
MCE: Limited coverage

OPERATIONS ON THE URINARY SYSTEM (55–59)

✖ **55.7   Nephropexy**
Fixation or suspension of movable [floating] kidney

● **55.8   Other repair of kidney**

✖ **55.81   Suture of laceration of kidney**

✖ **55.82   Closure of nephrostomy and pyelostomy**

✖ **55.83   Closure of other fistula of kidney**

✖ **55.84   Reduction of torsion of renal pedicle**

✖ **55.85   Symphysiotomy for horseshoe kidney**

✖ **55.86   Anastomosis of kidney**
Nephropyeloureterostomy
Pyeloureterovesical anastomosis
Ureterocalyceal anastomosis

     | Excludes | *nephrocystanastomosis NOS (56.73)*

✖ **55.87   Correction of ureteropelvic junction**

✖ **55.89   Other**

● **55.9   Other operations on kidney**

     | Excludes | *lysis of perirenal adhesions (59.02)*

✖ **55.91   Decapsulation of kidney**
Capsulectomy of kidney
Decortication of kidney

55.92   Percutaneous aspiration of kidney (pelvis)
Aspiration of renal cyst
Renipuncture

     | Excludes | *percutaneous biopsy of kidney (55.23)*

     Coding Clinic: 1984, Nov-Dec, P20

55.93   Replacement of nephrostomy tube

55.94   Replacement of pyelostomy tube

55.95   Local perfusion of kidney

55.96   Other injection of therapeutic substance into kidney
Injection into renal cyst

✖ **55.97   Implantation or replacement of mechanical kidney**

✖ **55.98   Removal of mechanical kidney**

✖ **55.99   Other**

     | Excludes | *removal of pyelostomy or nephrostomy tube (97.61)*

● **56   Operations on ureter**

Code also any application or administration of an adhesion barrier substance (99.77)
Coding Clinic: 1986, Sept-Oct, P11-12

✖ **56.0   Transurethral removal of obstruction from ureter and renal pelvis**
Removal of:
     blood clot from ureter or renal pelvis without incision
     calculus from ureter or renal pelvis without incision
     foreign body from ureter or renal pelvis without incision

     | Excludes | *manipulation without removal of obstruction (59.8)*
     that by incision (55.11, 56.2)
     transurethral insertion of ureteral stent for passage of calculus (59.8)

✖ **56.1   Ureteral meatotomy**

✖ **56.2   Ureterotomy**
Incision of ureter for:
     drainage
     exploration
     removal of calculus

     | Excludes | *cutting of ureterovesical orifice (56.1)*
     removal of calculus without incision (56.0)
     transurethral insertion of ureteral stent for passage of calculus (59.8)
     urinary diversion (56.51–56.79)

     Coding Clinic: 1986, Sept-Oct, P10

● **56.3   Diagnostic procedures on ureter**

56.31   Ureteroscopy

56.32   Closed percutaneous biopsy of ureter

     | Excludes | *endoscopic biopsy of ureter (56.33)*

     MCE: Closed biopsy procedure

56.33   Closed endoscopic biopsy of ureter
Cystourethroscopy with ureteral biopsy
Transurethral biopsy of ureter
Ureteral endoscopy with biopsy through ureterotomy
Ureteroscopy with biopsy

     | Excludes | *percutaneous biopsy of ureter (56.32)*

✖ **56.34   Open biopsy of ureter**
MCE: Open biopsy procedure

56.35   Endoscopy (cystoscopy) (looposcopy) of ileal conduit

✖ **56.39   Other diagnostic procedures on ureter**

     | Excludes | *microscopic examination of specimen from ureter (91.21–91.29)*

● **56.4   Ureterectomy**

Code also anastomosis other than end-to-end (56.51–56.79)

     | Excludes | *fistulectomy (56.84)*
     nephroureterectomy (55.51–55.54)

✖ **56.40   Ureterectomy, not otherwise specified**

✖ **56.41   Partial ureterectomy**
Excision of lesion of ureter
Shortening of ureter with reimplantation

     | Excludes | *biopsy of ureter (56.32–56.34)*

✖ **56.42   Total ureterectomy**

● **56.5   Cutaneous uretero-ileostomy**

✖ **56.51   Formation of cutaneous uretero-ileostomy**
Construction of ileal conduit
External ureteral ileostomy
Formation of open ileal bladder
Ileal loop operation
Ileoureterostomy (Bricker's) (ileal bladder)
Transplantation of ureter into ileum with external diversion

     | Excludes | *closed ileal bladder (57.87)*
     replacement of ureteral defect by ileal segment (56.89)

✖ **56.52   Revision of cutaneous uretero-ileostomy**
     Coding Clinic: 1996, Q3, P15; 1988, Q4, P7

● **56.6   Other external urinary diversion**

✖ **56.61   Formation of other cutaneous ureterostomy**
Anastomosis of ureter to skin
Ureterostomy NOS

✖ **56.62   Revision of other cutaneous ureterostomy**
Revision of ureterostomy stoma

     | Excludes | *nonoperative removal of ureterostomy tube (97.62)*

◀ New   ◀▥ Revised   ~~deleted~~ Deleted   ● Use Additional Digit(s)   ✖ Valid O.R. Procedure
◆ Non-O.R. Procedure   ♀ Females Only   ♂ Males Only

● **56.7   Other anastomosis or bypass of ureter**

> | Excludes | *ureteropyelostomy (55.86)*

✖ **56.71   Urinary diversion to intestine**
Anastomosis of ureter to intestine
Internal urinary diversion NOS

> Code also   any synchronous colostomy
> (46.10–46.13)

> | Excludes | *external ureteral ileostomy (56.51)*

✖ **56.72   Revision of ureterointestinal anastomosis**

> | Excludes | *revision of external ureteral ileostomy
> (56.52)*

✖ **56.73   Nephrocystanastomosis, not otherwise specified**

✖ **56.74   Ureteroneocystostomy**
Replacement of ureter with bladder flap
Ureterovesical anastomosis

✖ **56.75   Transureteroureterostomy**

> | Excludes | *ureteroureterostomy associated with
> partial resection (56.41)*

✖ **56.79   Other**

● **56.8   Repair of ureter**

✖ **56.81   Lysis of intraluminal adhesions of ureter**

> | Excludes | *lysis of periureteral adhesions
> (59.02–59.03)
> ureterolysis (59.02–59.03)*

✖ **56.82   Suture of laceration of ureter**

✖ **56.83   Closure of ureterostomy**

✖ **56.84   Closure of other fistula of ureter**

✖ **56.85   Ureteropexy**

✖ **56.86   Removal of ligature from ureter**

✖ **56.89   Other repair of ureter**
Graft of ureter
Replacement of ureter with ileal segment
implanted into bladder
Ureteroplication

● **56.9   Other operations on ureter**

56.91   Dilation of ureteral meatus

✖ **56.92   Implantation of electronic ureteral stimulator**

✖ **56.93   Replacement of electronic ureteral stimulator**

✖ **56.94   Removal of electronic ureteral stimulator**

> | Excludes | *that with synchronous replacement
> (56.93)*

✖ **56.95   Ligation of ureter**

✖ **56.99   Other**

> | Excludes | *removal of ureterostomy tube and
> ureteral catheter (97.62)
> ureteral catheterization (59.8)*

● **57   Operations on urinary bladder**

> Code also   any application or administration of an
> adhesion barrier substance (99.77)

> | Excludes | *perivesical tissue (59.11–59.29, 59.91–59.92)
> ureterovesical orifice (56.0–56.99)*

Coding Clinic: 1986, Sept-Oct, P11-12

57.0   Transurethral clearance of bladder
Drainage of bladder without incision
Removal of:
   blood clots from bladder without incision
   calculus from bladder without incision
   foreign body from bladder without incision

> | Excludes | *that by incision (57.19)*

● **57.1   Cystotomy and cystostomy**

> | Excludes | *cystotomy and cystostomy as operative
> approach —* omit code

57.11   Percutaneous aspiration of bladder

✖ **57.12   Lysis of intraluminal adhesions with incision
into bladder**

> | Excludes | *transurethral lysis of intraluminal
> adhesions (57.41)*

57.17   Percutaneous cystostomy
Closed cystostomy
Percutaneous suprapubic cystostomy

> | Excludes | *removal of cystostomy tube (97.63)
> replacement of cystostomy tube (59.94)*

✖ **57.18   Other suprapubic cystostomy**

> | Excludes | *percutaneous cystostomy (57.17)
> removal of cystostomy tube (97.63)
> replacement of cystostomy tube (59.94)*

✖ **57.19   Other cystotomy**
Cystolithotomy

> | Excludes | *percutaneous cystostomy (57.17)
> suprapubic cystostomy (57.18)*

Coding Clinic: 1986, Sept-Oct, P11-12

● **57.2   Vesicostomy**

> | Excludes | *percutaneous cystostomy (57.17)
> suprapubic cystostomy (57.18)*

✖ **57.21   Vesicostomy**
Creation of permanent opening from bladder
to skin using a bladder flap

✖ **57.22   Revision or closure of vesicostomy**

> | Excludes | *closure of cystostomy (57.82)*

● **57.3   Diagnostic procedures on bladder**

57.31   Cystoscopy through artificial stoma

57.32   Other cystoscopy
Transurethral cystoscopy

> | Excludes | *cystourethroscopy with ureteral biopsy
> (56.33)
> retrograde pyelogram (87.74)
> that for control of hemorrhage
> (postoperative):
> bladder (57.93)
> prostate (60.94)*

Coding Clinic: 2001, Q1, P14; 1984, May-June, P10

✖ **57.33   Closed [transurethral] biopsy of bladder**
MCE: Closed biopsy procedure

✖ **57.34   Open biopsy of bladder**
Coding Clinic: 2005, Q2, P12
MCE: Open biopsy procedure

✖ **57.39   Other diagnostic procedures on bladder**

> | Excludes | *cystogram NEC (87.77)
> microscopic examination of specimen
> from bladder (91.31–91.39)
> retrograde cystourethrogram (87.76)
> therapeutic distention of bladder
> (96.25)*

● **57.4   Transurethral excision or destruction of bladder tissue**

✖ **57.41   Transurethral lysis of intraluminal adhesions**

✖ **57.49   Other transurethral excision or destruction of
lesion or tissue of bladder**
Endoscopic resection of bladder lesion

> | Excludes | *transurethral biopsy of bladder (57.33)
> transurethral fistulectomy
> (57.83–57.84)*

Coding Clinic: 1996, Q1, P10-11

| Excludes   Includes   Use additional   Code also   Omit code

OPERATIONS ON THE URINARY SYSTEM (55–59)

● **57.5   Other excision or destruction of bladder tissue**

> **Excludes** | *that with transurethral approach (57.41–57.49)*

✸ **57.51   Excision of urachus**
Excision of urachal sinus of bladder

> **Excludes** | *excision of urachal cyst of abdominal wall (54.3)*

✸ **57.59   Open excision or destruction of other lesion or tissue of bladder**
Endometrectomy of bladder
Suprapubic excision of bladder lesion

> **Excludes** | *biopsy of bladder (57.33–57.34)*
> *fistulectomy of bladder (57.83–57.84)*

✸ **57.6   Partial cystectomy**
Excision of bladder dome
Trigonectomy
Wedge resection of bladder

● **57.7   Total cystectomy**

> **Includes**   total cystectomy with urethrectomy

✸ **57.71   Radical cystectomy**
Pelvic exenteration in male
Removal of bladder, prostate, seminal vesicles, and fat
Removal of bladder, urethra, and fat in a female

> Code also any:
> lymph node dissection (40.3, 40.5)
> urinary diversion (56.51–56.79)

> **Excludes** | *that as part of pelvic exenteration in female (68.8)*

✸ **57.79   Other total cystectomy**

● **57.8   Other repair of urinary bladder**

> **Excludes** | *repair of:*
> *current obstetric laceration (75.61)*
> *cystocele (70.50–70.51)*
> *that for stress incontinence (59.3–59.79)*

✸ **57.81   Suture of laceration of bladder**

✸ **57.82   Closure of cystostomy**

✸ **57.83   Repair of fistula involving bladder and intestine**
Rectovesicovaginal fistulectomy
Vesicosigmoidovaginal fistulectomy

✸ **57.84   Repair of other fistula of bladder**
Cervicovesical fistulectomy
Urethroperineovesical fistulectomy
Uterovesical fistulectomy
Vaginovesical fistulectomy

> **Excludes** | *vesicoureterovaginal fistulectomy (56.84)*

✸ **57.85   Cystourethroplasty and plastic repair of bladder neck**
Plication of sphincter of urinary bladder
V-Y plasty of bladder neck

✸ **57.86   Repair of bladder exstrophy**

✸ **57.87   Reconstruction of urinary bladder**
Anastomosis of bladder with isolated segment of ileum
Augmentation of bladder
Replacement of bladder with ileum or sigmoid [closed ileal bladder]

> Code also resection of intestine (45.50–45.52)

> **Coding Clinic: 2005, Q2, P12-13x2; 2003, Q2, P11-12; 2000, Q3, P7-8**

✸ **57.88   Other anastomosis of bladder**
Anastomosis of bladder to intestine NOS
Cystocolic anastomosis

> **Excludes** | *formation of closed ileal bladder (57.87)*

✸ **57.89   Other repair of bladder**
Bladder suspension, not elsewhere classified
Cystopexy NOS
Repair of old obstetric laceration of bladder

> **Excludes** | *repair of current obstetric laceration (75.61)*

● **57.9   Other operations on bladder**

✸ **57.91   Sphincterotomy of bladder**
Division of bladder neck
Coding Clinic: 1994, Q3, P12; 1990, Q2, P23

57.92   Dilation of bladder neck

✸ **57.93   Control of (postoperative) hemorrhage of bladder**

57.94   Insertion of indwelling urinary catheter

57.95   Replacement of indwelling urinary catheter

✸ **57.96   Implantation of electronic bladder stimulator**
MCE: Non-covered procedure

✸ **57.97   Replacement of electronic bladder stimulator**
MCE: Non-covered procedure

✸ **57.98   Removal of electronic bladder stimulator**

> **Excludes** | *that with synchronou replacement (57.97)*

✸ **57.99   Other**

> **Excludes** | *irrigation of:*
> *cystostomy (96.47)*
> *other indwelling urinary catheter (96.48)*
> *lysis of external adhesions (59.11)*
> *removal of:*
> *cystostomy tube (97.63)*
> *other urinary drainage device (97.64)*
> *therapeutic distention of bladder (96.25)*

● **58   Operations on urethra**

> **Includes**   operations on:
> bulbourethral gland [Cowper's gland]
> periurethral tissue

> Code also any application or administration of an adhesion barrier substance (99.77)

✸ **58.0   Urethrotomy**
Excision of urethral septum
Formation of urethrovaginal fistula
Perineal urethrostomy
Removal of calculus from urethra by incision

> **Excludes** | *drainage of bulbourethral gland or periurethral tissue (58.91)*
> *internal urethral meatotomy (58.5)*
> *removal of urethral calculus without incision (58.6)*

✸ **58.1   Urethral meatotomy**

> **Excludes** | *internal urethral meatotomy (58.5)*

● **58.2   Diagnostic procedures on urethra**

58.21   Perineal urethroscopy

58.22   Other urethroscopy

58.23   Biopsy of urethra

58.24   Biopsy of periurethral tissue

58.29   Other diagnostic procedures on urethra and periurethral tissue

> **Excludes** | *microscopic examination of specimen from urethra (91.31–91.39)*
> *retrograde cystourethrogram (87.76)*
> *urethral pressure profile (89.25)*
> *urethral sphincter electromyogram (89.23)*

OPERATIONS ON THE URINARY SYSTEM (55–59)

◀ New   ◀▥ Revised   ~~deleted~~ Deleted   ● Use Additional Digit(s)   ✸ Valid O.R. Procedure
◆ Non-O.R. Procedure   ♀ Females Only   ♂ Males Only

● **58.3 Excision or destruction of lesion or tissue of urethra**

> Excludes | *biopsy of urethra (58.23)*
> *excision of bulbourethral gland (58.92)*
> *fistulectomy (58.43)*
> *urethrectomy as part of:*
> *complete cystectomy (57.79)*
> *pelvic evisceration (68.8)*
> *radical cystectomy (57.71)*

    58.31 Endoscopic excision or destruction of lesion or tissue of urethra
        Fulguration of urethral lesion

    58.39 Other local excision or destruction of lesion or tissue of urethra
        Excision of:
          congenital valve of urethra
          lesion of urethra
          stricture of urethra
        Urethrectomy

> Excludes | *that by endoscopic approach (58.31)*

● **58.4 Repair of urethra**

> Excludes | *repair of current obstetric laceration (75.61)*

   ✖ **58.41 Suture of laceration of urethra**

   ✖ **58.42 Closure of urethrostomy**

   ✖ **58.43 Closure of other fistula of urethra**

> Excludes | *repair of urethroperineovesical fistula (57.84)*

   ✖ **58.44 Reanastomosis of urethra**
        Anastomosis of urethra

   ✖ **58.45 Repair of hypospadias or epispadias**
        Coding Clinic: 1997, Q3, P6; 1996, Q4, P34-35

   ✖ **58.46 Other reconstruction of urethra**
        Urethral construction

   ✖ **58.47 Urethral meatoplasty**

   ✖ **58.49 Other repair of urethra**
        Benenenti rotation of bulbous urethra
        Repair of old obstetric laceration of urethra
        Urethral plication

> Excludes | *repair of:*
> *current obstetric laceration (75.61)*
> *urethrocele (70.50–70.51)*

        Coding Clinic: 2009, Q1, P5

✖ **58.5 Release of urethral stricture**
    Cutting of urethral sphincter
    Internal urethral meatotomy
    Urethrolysis
    Coding Clinic: 1997, Q1, P13-14

58.6 Dilation of urethra
    Dilation of urethrovesical junction
    Passage of sounds through urethra
    Removal of calculus from urethra without incision

> Excludes | *urethral calibration (89.29)*

    Coding Clinic: 2001, Q1, P14; 1997, Q1, P13-14

● **58.9 Other operations on urethra and periurethral tissue**

   ✖ **58.91 Incision of periurethral tissue**
        Drainage of bulbourethral gland

   ✖ **58.92 Excision of periurethral tissue**

> Excludes | *biopsy of periurethral tissue (58.24)*
> *lysis of periurethral adhesions*
> *laparoscopic (59.12)*
> *other (59.11)*

   ✖ **58.93 Implantation of artificial urinary sphincter [AUS]**
        Placement of inflatable:
          bladder sphincter
          urethral sphincter
        Removal with replacement of sphincter device [AUS]
        With pump and/or reservoir

✖ **58.99 Other**
    Removal of inflatable urinary sphincter without replacement
    Repair of inflatable sphincter pump and/or reservoir
    Surgical correction of hydraulic pressure of inflatable sphincter device

> Excludes | *removal of:*
> *intraluminal foreign body from urethra without incision (98.19)*
> *urethral stent (97.65)*

    Coding Clinic: 2009, Q1, P5; 1995, Q4, P72-73

● **59 Other operations on urinary tract**

> Code also any application or administration of an adhesion barrier substance (99.77)

● **59.0 Dissection of retroperitoneal tissue**

   ✖ **59.00 Retroperitoneal dissection, not otherwise specified**

   ✖ **59.02 Other lysis of perirenal or periureteral adhesions**

> Excludes | *that by laparoscope (59.03)*

   ✖ **59.03 Laparoscopic lysis of perirenal or periureteral adhesions**
        Coding Clinic: 2006, Q4, P130-134

   ✖ **59.09 Other incision of perirenal or periureteral tissue**
        Exploration of perinephric area
        Incision of perirenal abscess

● **59.1 Incision of perivesical tissue**

   ✖ **59.11 Other lysis of perivesical adhesions**

   ✖ **59.12 Laparoscopic lysis of perivesical adhesions**

   ✖ **59.19 Other incision of perivesical tissue**
        Exploration of perivesical tissue
        Incision of hematoma of space of Retzius
        Retropubic exploration

● **59.2 Diagnostic procedures on perirenal and perivesical tissue**

   ✖ **59.21 Biopsy of perirenal or perivesical tissue**

   ✖ **59.29 Other diagnostic procedures on perirenal tissue, perivesical tissue, and retroperitoneum**

> Excludes | *microscopic examination of specimen from:*
> *perirenal tissue (91.21–91.29)*
> *perivesical tissue (91.31–91.39)*
> *retroperitoneum NEC (91.11–91.19)*
> *retroperitoneal x-ray (88.14–88.16)*

✖ **59.3 Plication of urethrovesical junction**
    Kelly-Kennedy operation on urethra
    Kelly-Stoeckel urethral plication

✖ **59.4 Suprapubic sling operation**
    Goebel-Frangenheim-Stoeckel urethrovesical suspension
    Millin-Read urethrovesical suspension
    Oxford operation for urinary incontinence
    Urethrocystopexy by suprapubic suspension

✖ **59.5 Retropubic urethral suspension**
    Burch procedure
    Marshall-Marchetti-Krantz operation
    Suture of periurethral tissue to symphysis pubis
    Urethral suspension NOS
    Coding Clinic: 1997, Q1, P11-12

✖ **59.6 Paraurethral suspension**
    Pereyra paraurethral suspension
    Periurethral suspension

OPERATIONS ON THE URINARY SYSTEM (55–59)

Excludes	Includes	Use additional	Code also	Omit code

● **59.7   Other repair of urinary stress incontinence**

✖ **59.71   Levator muscle operation for urethrovesical suspension**
        Cystourethropexy with levator muscle sling
        Gracilis muscle transplant for urethrovesical suspension
        Pubococcygeal sling

59.72   Injection of implant into urethra and/or bladder neck
        Collagen implant
        Endoscopic injection of implant
        Fat implant
        Polytef implant
        Coding Clinic: 1995, Q4, P72-73

✖ **59.79   Other**
        Anterior urethropexy
        Repair of stress incontinence NOS
        Tudor "rabbit ear" urethropexy
        Coding Clinic: 2001, Q2, P20; 2000, Q1, P14-15, 19-20; 1995, Q4, P72-73

59.8   Ureteral catheterization
        Drainage of kidney by catheter
        Insertion of ureteral stent
        Ureterovesical orifice dilation

        Code also any ureterotomy (56.2)

        Excludes *that for:*
                retrograde pyelogram (87.74)
                transurethral removal of calculus or clot from ureter and renal pelvis (56.0)
        Coding Clinic: 2005, Q2, P12-13; 2003, Q2, P11-12; 2000, Q3, P7-8; 1994, Q3, P8

● **59.9   Other operations on urinary system**

        Excludes *nonoperative removal of therapeutic device (97.61–97.69)*

✖ **59.91   Excision of perirenal or perivesical tissue**
        Excludes *biopsy of perirenal or perivesical tissue (59.21)*

✖ **59.92   Other operations on perirenal or perivesical tissue**

59.93   Replacement of ureterostomy tube
        Change of ureterostomy tube
        Reinsertion of ureterostomy tube
        Excludes *nonoperative removal of ureterostomy tube (97.62)*

59.94   Replacement of cystostomy tube
        Excludes *nonoperative removal of cystostomy tube (97.63)*

59.95   Ultrasonic fragmentation of urinary stones
        Shattered urinary stones
        Excludes *percutaneous nephrostomy with fragmentation (55.04)*
                shock-wave disintegration (98.51)
        Coding Clinic: 1986, Sept-Oct, P11-12; 1984, Nov-Dec, P20

59.99   Other
        Excludes *instillation of medication into urinary tract (96.49)*
                irrigation of urinary tract (96.45–96.48)
        Coding Clinic: 2008, Q2, P14

OPERATIONS ON THE URINARY SYSTEM (55–59)

◀ New   ◀▥ Revised   deleted Deleted   ● Use Additional Digit(s)   ✖ Valid O.R. Procedure
◆ Non-O.R. Procedure   ♀ Females Only   ♂ Males Only

11. OPERATIONS ON THE MALE GENITAL ORGANS (60–64)

● **60 Operations on prostate and seminal vesicles**

     Includes operations on periprostatic tissue

     Code also any application or administration of an adhesion barrier substance (99.77)

     Excludes *that associated with radical cystectomy (57.71)*

✖ **60.0 Incision of prostate** ♂
     Drainage of prostatic abscess
     Prostatolithotomy

     Excludes *drainage of periprostatic tissue only (60.81)*

● **60.1 Diagnostic procedures on prostate and seminal vesicles**

     60.11 Closed [percutaneous] [needle] biopsy of prostate ♂
         Approach:
           transrectal
           transurethral
         Punch biopsy
         MCE: Closed biopsy procedure

     ✖ **60.12 Open biopsy of prostate** ♂
         MCE: Open biopsy procedure

     60.13 Closed [percutaneous] biopsy of seminal vesicles ♂
         Needle biopsy of seminal vesicles
         MCE: Closed biopsy procedure

     ✖ **60.14 Open biopsy of seminal vesicles** ♂
         MCE: Open biopsy procedure

     ✖ **60.15 Biopsy of periprostatic tissue** ♂

     ✖ **60.18 Other diagnostic procedures on prostate and periprostatic tissue** ♂

         Excludes *microscopic examination of specimen from prostate (91.31–91.39)*
           x-ray of prostate (87.92)

     ✖ **60.19 Other diagnostic procedures on seminal vesicles** ♂

         Excludes *microscopic examination of specimen from seminal vesicles (91.31–91.39)*
           x-ray:
             contrast seminal vesiculogram (87.91)
             other (87.92)

● **60.2 Transurethral prostatectomy**

     Excludes *local excision of lesion of prostate (60.61)*

     Coding Clinic: 1993, 5th Issue, P9; 1985, Sept-Oct, P10

     ✖ **60.21 Transurethral (ultrasound) guided laser induced prostatectomy (TULIP)** ♂
         Ablation (contact) (noncontact) by laser
         Coding Clinic: 1995, Q4, P71; 1994, Q2, P9; 1992, Q3, P13

     ✖ **60.29 Other transurethral prostatectomy** ♂
         Excision of median bar by transurethral approach
         Transurethral electrovaporization of prostrate (TEVAP)
         Transurethral enucleative procedure
         Transurethral prostatectomy NOS
         Transurethral resection of prostate (TURP)
         Coding Clinic: 1997, Q3, P3; 1994, Q3, P12

✖ **60.3 Suprapubic prostatectomy** ♂
     Transvesical prostatectomy

     Excludes *local excision of lesion of prostate (60.61)*
         radical prostatectomy (60.5)

✖ **60.4 Retropubic prostatectomy** ♂

     Excludes *local excision of lesion of prostate (60.61)*
         radical prostatectomy (60.5)

✖ **60.5 Radical prostatectomy** ♂
     Prostatovesiculectomy
     Radical prostatectomy by any approach

     Excludes *cystoprostatectomy (57.71)*

     Coding Clinic: 1993, Q3, P12

● **60.6 Other prostatectomy**

     ✖ **60.61 Local excision of lesion of prostate** ♂
         ~~Excision of prostatic lesion by any approach~~ ◀▥

         Excludes *biopsy of prostate (60.11–60.12)*
           laser interstitial thermal therapy [LITT] of lesion or tissue of prostate under guidance (17.69) ◀

     ✖ **60.62 Perineal prostatectomy** ♂
         Cryoablation of prostate
         Cryoprostatectomy
         Cryosurgery of prostate
         Radical cryosurgical ablation of prostate (RCSA)

         Excludes *local excision of lesion of prostate (60.61)*

     ✖ **60.69 Other** ♂

● **60.7 Operations on seminal vesicles**

     60.71 Percutaneous aspiration of seminal vesicle ♂

         Excludes *needle biopsy of seminal vesicle (60.13)*

     ✖ **60.72 Incision of seminal vesicle** ♂

     ✖ **60.73 Excision of seminal vesicle** ♂
         Excision of Müllerian duct cyst
         Spermatocystectomy

         Excludes *biopsy of seminal vesicle (60.13–60.14)*
           prostatovesiculectomy (60.5)

     ✖ **60.79 Other operations on seminal vesicles** ♂

● **60.8 Incision or excision of periprostatic tissue**

     ✖ **60.81 Incision of periprostatic tissue** ♂
         Drainage of periprostatic abscess

     ✖ **60.82 Excision of periprostatic tissue** ♂
         Excision of lesion of periprostatic tissue

         Excludes *biopsy of periprostatic tissue (60.15)*

● **60.9 Other operations on prostate**

     60.91 Percutaneous aspiration of prostate ♂

         Excludes *needle biopsy of prostate (60.11)*

     60.92 Injection into prostate test link ♂

     ✖ **60.93 Repair of prostate** ♂

     ✖ **60.94 Control of (postoperative) hemorrhage of prostate** ♂
         Coagulation of prostatic bed
         Cystoscopy for control of prostatic hemorrhage

     ✖ **60.95 Transurethral balloon dilation of the prostatic urethra** ♂

     ✖ **60.96 Transurethral destruction of prostate tissue by microwave thermotherapy** ♂
         Transurethral microwave thermotherapy (TUMT) of prostate

         Excludes *prostatectomy:*
           other (60.61–60.69)
           radical (60.5)
           retropubic (60.4)
           suprapubic (60.3)
           transurethral (60.21–60.29)

     Excludes   Includes   Use additional   Code also   Omit code

✖ **60.97 Other transuretheral destruction of prostate tissue by other thermotherapy** ♂
Radiofrequency thermotherapy
Transurethral needle ablation (TUNA) of prostate

> **Excludes** | *prostatectomy:*
> *other (60.61–60.69)*
> *radical (60.5)*
> *retropubic (60.4)*
> *suprapubic (60.3)*
> *transurethral (60.21–60.29)*

✖ **60.99 Other** ♂

> **Excludes** | *prostatic massage (99.94)*
> **Coding Clinic: 1990, Q3, P13**

● **61 Operations on scrotum and tunica vaginalis**

61.0 Incision and drainage of scrotum and tunica vaginalis ♂

> **Excludes** | *percutaneous aspiration of hydrocele (61.91)*

● **61.1 Diagnostic procedures on scrotum and tunica vaginalis**

61.11 Biopsy of scrotum or tunica vaginalis ♂

61.19 Other diagnostic procedures on scrotum and tunica vaginalis ♂

✖ **61.2 Excision of hydrocele (of tunica vaginalis)** ♂
Bottle repair of hydrocele of tunica vaginalis

> **Excludes** | *percutaneous aspiration of hydrocele (61.91)*

61.3 Excision or destruction of lesion or tissue of scrotum ♂
Fulguration of lesion of scrotum
Reduction of elephantiasis of scrotum
Partial scrotectomy of scrotum

> **Excludes** | *biopsy of scrotum (61.11)*
> *scrotal fistulectomy (61.42)*

● **61.4 Repair of scrotum and tunica vaginalis**

61.41 Suture of laceration of scrotum and tunica vaginalis ♂

✖ **61.42 Repair of scrotal fistula** ♂

✖ **61.49 Other repair of scrotum and tunica vaginalis** ♂
Reconstruction with rotational or pedicle flaps

● **61.9 Other operations on scrotum and tunica vaginalis**

61.91 Percutaneous aspiration of tunica vaginalis ♂
Aspiration of hydrocele of tunica vaginalis

✖ **61.92 Excision of lesion of tunica vaginalis other than hydrocele** ♂
Excision of hematocele of tunica vaginalis

✖ **61.99 Other** ♂

> **Excludes** | *removal of foreign body from scrotum without incision (98.24)*

● **62 Operations on testes**

✖ **62.0 Incision of testis** ♂

● **62.1 Diagnostic procedures on testes**

62.11 Closed [percutaneous] [needle] biopsy of testis ♂
MCE: Closed biopsy procedure

✖ **62.12 Open biopsy of testis** ♂
MCE: Open biopsy procedure

✖ **62.19 Other diagnostic procedures on testes** ♂

✖ **62.2 Excision or destruction of testicular lesion** ♂
Excision of appendix testis
Excision of cyst of Morgagni in the male

> **Excludes** | *biopsy of testis (62.11–62.12)*

✖ **62.3 Unilateral orchiectomy** ♂
Orchidectomy (with epididymectomy) NOS

● **62.4 Bilateral orchiectomy**
Male castration
Radical bilateral orchiectomy (with epididymectomy)

> **Code also** any synchronous lymph node dissection (40.3, 40.5)

✖ **62.41 Removal of both testes at same operative episode** ♂
Bilateral orchidectomy NOS

✖ **62.42 Removal of remaining testis** ♂
Removal of solitary testis

✖ **62.5 Orchiopexy** ♂
Mobilization and replacement of testis in scrotum
Orchiopexy with detorsion of testis
Torek (-Bevan) operation (orchidopexy) (first stage) (second stage)
Transplantation to and fixation of testis in scrotum

● **62.6 Repair of testes**

> **Excludes** | *reduction of torsion (63.52)*

✖ **62.61 Suture of laceration of testis** ♂

✖ **62.69 Other repair of testis** ♂
Testicular graft

✖ **62.7 Insertion of testicular prosthesis** ♂

● **62.9 Other operations on testes**

62.91 Aspiration of testis ♂

> **Excludes** | *percutaneous biopsy of testis (62.11)*

62.92 Injection of therapeutic substance into testis ♂

✖ **62.99 Other** ♂

● **63 Operations on spermatic cord, epididymis, and vas deferens**

● **63.0 Diagnostic procedures on spermatic cord, epididymis, and vas deferens**

63.01 Biopsy of spermatic cord, epididymis, or vas deferens ♂

✖ **63.09 Other diagnostic procedures on spermatic cord, epididymis, and vas deferens** ♂

> **Excludes** | *contrast epididymogram (87.93)*
> *contrast vasogram (87.94)*
> *other x-ray of epididymis and vas deferens (87.95)*

✖ **63.1 Excision of varicocele and hydrocele of spermatic cord** ♂
High ligation of spermatic vein
Hydrocelectomy of canal of Nuck

✖ **63.2 Excision of cyst of epididymis** ♂
Spermatocelectomy

✖ **63.3 Excision of other lesion or tissue of spermatic cord and epididymis** ♂
Excision of appendix epididymis

> **Excludes** | *biopsy of spermatic cord or epididymis (63.01)*

✖ **63.4 Epididymectomy** ♂

> **Excludes** | *that synchronous with orchiectomy (62.3–62.42)*

● **63.5 Repair of spermatic cord and epididymis**

✖ **63.51 Suture of laceration of spermatic cord and epididymis** ♂

63.52 Reduction of torsion of testis or spermatic cord ♂

> **Excludes** | *that associated with orchiopexy (62.5)*

✖ **63.53 Transplantation of spermatic cord** ♂

✖ **63.59 Other repair of spermatic cord and epididymis** ♂

63.6 Vasotomy ♂
Vasostomy

◄ New   ⇐ Revised   ~~deleted~~ Deleted   ● Use Additional Digit(s)   ✖ Valid O.R. Procedure
◆ Non-O.R. Procedure   ♀ Females Only   ♂ Males Only

OPERATIONS ON THE MALE GENITAL ORGANS (60–64)

● **63.7   Vasectomy and ligation of vas deferens**

    63.70   Male sterilization procedure, not otherwise specified ♂
       MCE: Non-covered procedure

    63.71   Ligation of vas deferens ♂
       Crushing of vas deferens
       Division of vas deferens
       MCE: Non-covered procedure

    63.72   Ligation of spermatic cord ♂
       MCE: Non-covered procedure

    63.73   Vasectomy ♂
       Coding Clinic: 1998, Q2, P13
       MCE: Non-covered procedure

● **63.8   Repair of vas deferens and epididymis**

    ✖ **63.81   Suture of laceration of vas deferens and epididymis** ♂

    ✖ **63.82   Reconstruction of surgically divided vas deferens** ♂

    ✖ **63.83   Epididymovasostomy** ♂

    63.84   Removal of ligature from vas deferens ♂

    ✖ **63.85   Removal of valve from vas deferens** ♂

    ✖ **63.89   Other repair of vas deferens and epididymis** ♂

● **63.9   Other operations on spermatic cord, epididymis, and vas deferens**

    63.91   Aspiration of spermatocele ♂

    ✖ **63.92   Epididymotomy** ♂

    ✖ **63.93   Incision of spermatic cord** ♂

    ✖ **63.94   Lysis of adhesions of spermatic cord** ♂

    ✖ **63.95   Insertion of valve in vas deferens** ♂

    ✖ **63.99   Other** ♂

● **64   Operations on penis**

    | Includes | operations on:
          corpora cavernosa
          glans penis
          prepuce

    64.0   Circumcision ♂

● **64.1   Diagnostic procedures on the penis**

    ✖ **64.11   Biopsy of penis** ♂

    64.19   Other diagnostic procedures on penis ♂

✖ **64.2   Local excision or destruction of lesion of penis** ♂

    | Excludes | *biopsy of penis (64.11)*

✖ **64.3   Amputation of penis** ♂

● **64.4   Repair and plastic operation on penis**

    ✖ **64.41   Suture of laceration of penis** ♂

    ✖ **64.42   Release of chordee** ♂
       Coding Clinic: 1996, Q4, P34-35

✖ **64.43   Construction of penis** ♂

✖ **64.44   Reconstruction of penis** ♂

✖ **64.45   Replantation of penis** ♂
       Reattachment of amputated penis

✖ **64.49   Other repair of penis** ♂

    | Excludes | *repair of epispadias and hypospadias (58.45)*

✖ **64.5   Operations for sex transformation, not elsewhere classified** ♂
    MCE: Non-covered procedure

● **64.9   Other operations on male genital organs**

    64.91   Dorsal or lateral slit of prepuce ♂

    ✖ **64.92   Incision of penis** ♂

    64.93   Division of penile adhesions ♂

    64.94   Fitting of external prosthesis of penis ♂
       Penile prosthesis NOS

    ✖ **64.95   Insertion or replacement of non-inflatable penile prosthesis** ♂
       Insertion of semi-rigid rod prosthesis into shaft of penis

       | Excludes | *external penile prosthesis (64.94)*
          inflatable penile prosthesis (64.97)
          plastic repair, penis (64.43–64.49)
          that associated with:
             construction (64.43)
             reconstruction (64.44)

    ✖ **64.96   Removal of internal prosthesis of penis** ♂
       Removal without replacement of non-inflatable or inflatable penile prosthesis

    ✖ **64.97   Insertion or replacement of inflatable penile prosthesis** ♂
       Insertion of cylinders into shaft of penis and placement of pump and reservoir

       | Excludes | *external penile prosthesis (64.94)*
          non-inflatable penile prosthesis (64.95)
          plastic repair, penis (64.43–64.49)
       Coding Clinic: 1990, Q2, P26

    ✖ **64.98   Other operations on penis** ♂
       Corpora cavernosa-corpus spongiosum shunt
       Corpora-saphenous shunt
       Irrigation of corpus cavernosum

       | Excludes | *removal of foreign body:*
          intraluminal (98.19)
          without incision (98.24)
          stretching of foreskin (99.95)
       Coding Clinic: 1992, Q3, P9-10

    ✖ **64.99   Other** ♂

       | Excludes | *collection of sperm for artificial insemination (99.96)*

12. OPERATIONS ON THE FEMALE GENITAL ORGANS (65–71)

● 65   Operations on ovary

     Code also any application or administration of an adhesion barrier substance (99.77)

● 65.0   Oophorotomy
     Salpingo-oophorotomy

✖ 65.01   Laparoscopic oophorotomy ♀

✖ 65.09   Other oophorotomy ♀

● 65.1   Diagnostic procedures on ovaries

✖ 65.11   Aspiration biopsy of ovary ♀

✖ 65.12   Other biopsy of ovary ♀

✖ 65.13   Laparoscopic biopsy of ovary ♀
     Coding Clinic: 1996, Q4, P66-67

✖ 65.14   Other laparoscopic diagnostic procedures on ovaries ♀

✖ 65.19   Other diagnostic procedures on ovaries ♀
     Excludes   microscopic examination of specimen from ovary (91.41–91.49)

● 65.2   Local excision or destruction of ovarian lesion or tissue

✖ 65.21   Marsupialization of ovarian cyst ♀
     Excludes   that by laparoscope (65.23)

✖ 65.22   Wedge resection of ovary ♀
     Excludes   that by laparoscope (65.24)

✖ 65.23   Laparoscopic marsupialization of ovarian cyst ♀

✖ 65.24   Laparoscopic wedge resection of ovary ♀

✖ 65.25   Other laparoscopic local excision or destruction of ovary ♀

✖ 65.29   Other local excision or destruction of ovary ♀
     Bisection of ovary
     Cauterization of ovary
     Partial excision of ovary
     Excludes   biopsy of ovary (65.11–65.13)
     that by laparoscope (65.25)

● 65.3   Unilateral oophorectomy
     Coding Clinic: 1995, Q3, P15

✖ 65.31   Laparoscopic unilateral oophorectomy ♀

✖ 65.39   Other unilateral oophorectomy ♀
     Excludes   that by laparoscope (65.31)

● 65.4   Unilateral salpingo-oophorectomy

✖ 65.41   Laparoscopic unilateral salpingo-oophorectomy ♀
     Coding Clinic: 1996, Q4, P66-67

✖ 65.49   Other unilateral salpingo-oophorectomy ♀

● 65.5   Bilateral oophorectomy

✖ 65.51   Other removal of both ovaries at same operative episode ♀
     Female castration
     Excludes   that by laparoscope (65.53)

✖ 65.52   Other removal of remaining ovary ♀
     Removal of solitary ovary
     Excludes   that by laparoscope (65.54)

✖ 65.53   Laparoscopic removal of both ovaries at same operative episode ♀

✖ 65.54   Laparoscopic removal of remaining ovary ♀

● 65.6   Bilateral salpingo-oophorectomy

✖ 65.61   Other removal of both ovaries and tubes at same operative episode ♀
     Excludes   that by laparoscope (65.63)
     Coding Clinic: 1996, Q4, P64-65

✖ 65.62   Other removal of remaining ovary and tube ♀
     Removal of solitary ovary and tube
     Excludes   that by laparoscope (65.64)

✖ 65.63   Laparoscopic removal of both ovaries and tubes at same operative episode ♀
     Coding Clinic: 2006, Q4, P130-134; 1996, Q4, P68

✖ 65.64   Laparoscopic removal of remaining ovary and tube ♀

● 65.7   Repair of ovary
     Excludes   salpingo-oophorostomy (66.72)

✖ 65.71   Other simple suture of ovary ♀
     Excludes   that by laparoscope (65.74)

✖ 65.72   Other reimplantation of ovary ♀
     Excludes   that by laparoscope (65.75)

✖ 65.73   Other salpingo-oophoroplasty ♀
     Excludes   that by laparoscope (65.76)

✖ 65.74   Laparoscopic simple suture of ovary ♀

✖ 65.75   Laparoscopic reimplantation of ovary ♀

✖ 65.76   Laparoscopic salpingo-oophoroplasty ♀

✖ 65.79   Other repair of ovary ♀
     Oophoropexy

● 65.8   Lysis of adhesions of ovary and fallopian tube

✖ 65.81   Laparoscopic lysis of adhesions of ovary and fallopian tube ♀
     Coding Clinic: 1996, Q4, P66-67

✖ 65.89   Other lysis of adhesions of ovary and fallopian tube ♀
     Excludes   that by laparoscope (65.81)

● 65.9   Other operations on ovary

✖ 65.91   Aspiration of ovary ♀
     Excludes   aspiration biopsy of ovary (65.11)

✖ 65.92   Transplantation of ovary ♀
     Excludes   reimplantation of ovary
     laparoscopic (65.75)
     other (65.72)

✖ 65.93   Manual rupture of ovarian cyst ♀

✖ 65.94   Ovarian denervation ♀

✖ 65.95   Release of torsion of ovary ♀

✖ 65.99   Other ♀
     Ovarian drilling
     Coding Clinic: 1986, Nov-Dec, P9

● 66   Operations on fallopian tubes

     Code also any application or administration of an adhesion barrier substance (99.77)

● 66.0   Salpingotomy and salpingostomy

✖ 66.01   Salpingotomy ♀

✖ 66.02   Salpingostomy ♀

◄ New   ⬅ Revised   ~~deleted~~ Deleted   ● Use Additional Digit(s)   ✖ Valid O.R. Procedure
◆ Non-O.R. Procedure   ♀ Females Only   ♂ Males Only

OPERATIONS ON THE FEMALE GENITAL ORGANS (65–71)

● **66.1 Diagnostic procedures on fallopian tubes**

✖ **66.11 Biopsy of fallopian tube** ♀

✖ **66.19 Other diagnostic procedures on fallopian tubes** ♀

> **Excludes** *microscopic examination of specimen from fallopian tubes (91.41–91.49)*
> *radiography of fallopian tubes (87.82–87.83, 87.85)*
> *Rubin's test (66.8)*

● **66.2 Bilateral endoscopic destruction or occlusion of fallopian tubes**

> **Includes** bilateral endoscopic destruction or occlusion of fallopian tubes by:
> culdoscopy
> endoscopy
> hysteroscopy
> laparoscopy
> peritoneoscopy
> endoscopic destruction of solitary fallopian tube

✖ **66.21 Bilateral endoscopic ligation and crushing of fallopian tubes** ♀
> MCE: Non-covered procedure

✖ **66.22 Bilateral endoscopic ligation and division of fallopian tubes** ♀
> MCE: Non-covered procedure

✖ **66.29 Other bilateral endoscopic destruction or occlusion of fallopian tubes** ♀
> MCE: Non-covered procedure

● **66.3 Other bilateral destruction or occlusion of fallopian tubes**

> **Includes** destruction of solitary fallopian tube
> **Excludes** *endoscopic destruction or occlusion of fallopian tubes (66.21–66.29)*

✖ **66.31 Other bilateral ligation and crushing of fallopian tubes** ♀
> MCE: Non-covered procedure

✖ **66.32 Other bilateral ligation and division of fallopian tubes** ♀
> Pomeroy operation
> MCE: Non-covered procedure

✖ **66.39 Other bilateral destruction or occlusion of fallopian tubes** ♀
> Female sterilization operation NOS
> MCE: Non-covered procedure

✖ **66.4 Total unilateral salpingectomy** ♀

● **66.5 Total bilateral salpingectomy**

> **Excludes** *bilateral partial salpingectomy for sterilization (66.39)*
> *that with oophorectomy (65.61–65.64)*

✖ **66.51 Removal of both fallopian tubes at same operative episode** ♀

✖ **66.52 Removal of remaining fallopian tube** ♀
> Removal of solitary fallopian tube

● **66.6 Other salpingectomy**

> **Includes** salpingectomy by:
> cauterization
> coagulation
> electrocoagulation
> excision
> **Excludes** *fistulectomy (66.73)*

✖ **66.61 Excision or destruction of lesion of fallopian tube** ♀

> **Excludes** *biopsy of fallopian tube (66.11)*

✖ **66.62 Salpingectomy with removal of tubal pregnancy** ♀

> **Code also** any synchronous oophorectomy (65.31, 65.39)
> Coding Clinic: 1995, Q3, P15; 1985, Sept-Oct, P14

✖ **66.63 Bilateral partial salpingectomy, not otherwise specified** ♀

✖ **66.69 Other partial salpingectomy** ♀

● **66.7 Repair of fallopian tube**

✖ **66.71 Simple suture of fallopian tube** ♀

✖ **66.72 Salpingo-oophorostomy** ♀

✖ **66.73 Salpingo-salpingostomy** ♀

✖ **66.74 Salpingo-uterostomy** ♀

✖ **66.79 Other repair of fallopian tube** ♀
> Graft of fallopian tube
> Reopening of divided fallopian tube
> Salpingoplasty
> Coding Clinic: 1995, Q2, P10

66.8 Insufflation of fallopian tube ♀
> Insufflation of fallopian tube with:
> air
> dye
> gas
> saline
> Rubin's test

> **Excludes** *insufflation of therapeutic agent (66.95)*
> *that for hysterosalpingography (87.82–87.83)*
> Coding Clinic: 1990, Q2, P26

● **66.9 Other operations on fallopian tubes**

66.91 Aspiration of fallopian tube ♀

✖ **66.92 Unilateral destruction or occlusion of fallopian tube** ♀

> **Excludes** *that of solitary tube (66.21–66.39)*

✖ **66.93 Implantation or replacement of prosthesis of fallopian tube** ♀

✖ **66.94 Removal of prosthesis of fallopian tube** ♀

✖ **66.95 Insufflation of therapeutic agent into fallopian tubes** ♀

✖ **66.96 Dilation of fallopian tube** ♀

✖ **66.97 Burying of fimbriae in uterine wall** ♀

✖ **66.99 Other** ♀

> **Excludes** *lysis of adhesions of ovary and tube laparoscopic (65.81)*
> *other (65.89)*
> Coding Clinic: 1994, Q2, P11

● **67 Operations on cervix**

> **Code also** any application or administration of an adhesion barrier substance (99.77)

67.0 Dilation of cervical canal ♀

> **Excludes** *dilation and curettage (69.01–69.09)*
> *that for induction of labor (73.1)*

● **67.1 Diagnostic procedures on cervix**

✖ **67.11 Endocervical biopsy** ♀

> **Excludes** *conization of cervix (67.2)*

✖ **67.12 Other cervical biopsy** ♀
> Punch biopsy of cervix NOS

> **Excludes** *conization of cervix (67.2)*

✖ **67.19 Other diagnostic procedures on cervix** ♀

> **Excludes** *microscopic examination of specimen from cervix (91.41–91.49)*

Excludes	Includes	Use additional	Code also	Omit code

✖ 67.2   Conization of cervix ♀

> **Excludes**   *that by:*
>> *cryosurgery (67.33)*
>> *electrosurgery (67.32)*

● 67.3   Other excision or destruction of lesion or tissue of cervix

> **✖ 67.31   Marsupialization of cervical cyst ♀**

> **✖ 67.32   Destruction of lesion of cervix by cauterization ♀**
>> Electroconization of cervix
>> LEEP (loop electrosurgical excision procedure)
>> LLETZ (large loop excision of the transformation zone)
>> Coding Clinic: 1998, Q1, P3

> **✖ 67.33   Destruction of lesion of cervix by cryosurgery ♀**
>> Cryoconization of cervix

> **✖ 67.39   Other excision or destruction of lesion or tissue of cervix ♀**
>> **Excludes**   *biopsy of cervix (67.11–67.12)*
>>> *cervical fistulectomy (67.62)*
>>> *conization of cervix (67.2)*

✖ 67.4   Amputation of cervix ♀
> Cervicectomy with synchronous colporrhaphy

● 67.5   Repair of internal cervical os
> Coding Clinic: 2000, Q3, P11-12

> **✖ 67.51   Transabdominal cerclage of cervix ♀**

> **✖ 67.59   Other repair of internal cervical os ♀**
>> Cerclage of isthmus uteri
>> McDonald operation
>> Shirodkar operation
>> Transvaginal cerclage
>>> **Excludes**   *laparoscopically assisted supracervical hysterectomy [LASH] (68.31)*
>>>> *transabdominal cerclage of cervix (67.51)*
>>> Coding Clinic: 2008, Q4, P124-125

● 67.6   Other repair of cervix
> **Excludes**   *repair of current obstetric laceration (75.51)*

> **✖ 67.61   Suture of laceration of cervix ♀**

> **✖ 67.62   Repair of fistula of cervix ♀**
>> Cervicosigmoidal fistulectomy
>>> **Excludes**   *fistulectomy:*
>>>> *cervicovesical (57.84)*
>>>> *ureterocervical (56.84)*
>>>> *vesicocervicovaginal (57.84)*

> **✖ 67.69   Other repair of cervix ♀**
>> Repair of old obstetric laceration of cervix

● 68   Other incision and excision of uterus
> Code also any application or administration of an adhesion barrier substance (99.77)

✖ 68.0   Hysterotomy ♀
> Hysterotomy with removal of hydatidiform mole
>> **Excludes**   *hysterotomy for termination of pregnancy (74.91)*

● 68.1   Diagnostic procedures on uterus and supporting structures

> **68.11   Digital examination of uterus ♀**
>> **Excludes**   *pelvic examination, so described (89.26)*
>>> *postpartal manual exploration of uterine cavity (75.7)*

68.12   Hysteroscopy ♀
> **Excludes**   *that with biopsy (68.16)*
> Coding Clinic: 1990, Q2, P26

✖ 68.13   Open biopsy of uterus ♀
> **Excludes**   *closed biopsy of uterus (68.16)*
> MCE: Open biopsy procedure

✖ 68.14   Open biopsy of uterine ligaments ♀
> **Excludes**   *closed biopsy of uterine ligaments (68.15)*
> MCE: Open biopsy procedure

✖ 68.15   Closed biopsy of uterine ligaments ♀
> Endoscopic (laparoscopy) biopsy of uterine adnexa, except ovary and fallopian tube
> MCE: Closed biopsy procedure

✖ 68.16   Closed biopsy of uterus ♀
> Endoscopic (laparoscopy) (hysteroscopy) biopsy of uterus
>> **Excludes**   *open biopsy of uterus (68.13)*
> MCE: Closed biopsy procedure

✖ 68.19   Other diagnostic procedures on uterus and supporting structures ♀
> **Excludes**   *diagnostic:*
>> *aspiration curettage (69.59)*
>> *dilation and curettage (69.09)*
>> *microscopic examination of specimen from uterus (91.41–91.49)*
>> *pelvic examination (89.26)*
>> *radioisotope scan of:*
>>> *placenta (92.17)*
>>> *uterus (92.19)*
>> *ultrasonography of uterus (88.78–88.79)*
>> *x-ray of uterus (87.81–87.89)*

● 68.2   Excision or destruction of lesion or tissue of uterus

> **✖ 68.21   Division of endometrial synechiae ♀**
>> Lysis of intraluminal uterine adhesions

> **✖ 68.22   Incision or excision of congenital septum of uterus ♀**

> **✖ 68.23   Endometrial ablation ♀**
>> Dilation and curettage
>> Hysteroscopic endometrial ablation

> **✖ 68.29   Other excision or destruction of lesion of uterus ♀**
>> Uterine myomectomy
>>> **Excludes**   *biopsy of uterus (68.13, 68.16)*
>>>> *uterine fistulectomy (69.42)*
>>> Coding Clinic: 2006, Q3, P18-19; 1996, Q1, P15

● 68.3   Subtotal abdominal hysterectomy

> **✖ 68.31   Laparoscopic supracervical hysterectomy [LSH] ♀**
>> Classic infrafascial SEMM hysterectomy [CISH]
>> Laparoscopically assisted supracervical hysterectomy [LASH]
>> Coding Clinic: 2003, Q4, P98-99

> **✖ 68.39   Other and unspecified subtotal abdominal hysterectomy ♀**
>> Supracervical hysterectomy
>>> **Excludes**   *classic infrafascial SEMM hysterectomy [CISH] (68.31)*
>>>> *laparoscopic supracervical hysterectomy [LSH] (68.31)*

◀ New   ◀▥ Revised   ~~deleted~~ Deleted   ● Use Additional Digit(s)   ✖ Valid O.R. Procedure
◆ Non-O.R. Procedure   ♀ Females Only   ♂ Males Only

OPERATIONS ON THE FEMALE GENITAL ORGANS (65–71)

● **68.4　Total abdominal hysterectomy**

　Code also any synchronous removal of tubes and ovaries (65.31–65.64)

　　Excludes　*laparoscopic total abdominal hysterectomy (68.41)*
　　　　radical abdominal hysterectomy, any approach (68.61–68.69)

　　Coding Clinic: 1996, Q4, P64-65

✖ **68.41　Laparoscopic total abdominal hysterectomy ♀**
　Total laparoscopic hysterectomy [TLH]
　Coding Clinic: 2006, Q4, P130-134

✖ **68.49　Other and unspecified total abdominal hysterectomy ♀**
　Hysterectomy:
　　extended

● **68.5　Vaginal hysterectomy**

　Code also any synchronous:
　　removal of tubes and ovaries (65.31–65.64)
　　repair of cystocele or rectocele (70.50–70.52)
　　repair of pelvic floor (70.79)

✖ **68.51　Laparoscopically assisted vaginal hysterectomy (LAVH) ♀**
　Coding Clinic: 1996, Q4, P68

✖ **68.59　Other and unspecified vaginal hysterectomy ♀**
　　Excludes　*laparoscopically assisted vaginal hysterectomy (LAVH) (68.51)*
　　　　radical vaginal hysterectomy (68.7)

● **68.6　Radical abdominal hysterectomy**

　Code also any synchronous:
　　lymph gland dissection (40.3, 40.5)
　　removal of tubes and ovaries (65.31–65.64)

　　Excludes　*pelvic evisceration (68.8)*

✖ **68.61　Laparoscopic radical abdominal hysterectomy ♀**
　Laparoscopic modified radical hysterectomy
　Total laparoscopic radical hysterectomy [TLRH]
　Coding Clinic: 2006, Q4, P130-134

✖ **68.69　Other and unspecified radical abdominal hysterectomy ♀**
　Modified radical hysterectomy
　Wertheim's operation
　　Excludes　*laparoscopic total abdominal hysterectomy (68.41)*
　　　　laparoscopic radical abdominal hysterectomy (68.61)

● **68.7　Radical vaginal hysterectomy**

　Code also any synchronous:
　　lymph gland dissection (40.3, 40.5)
　　removal of tubes and ovaries (65.31–65.64)

　　Excludes　*abdominal hysterectomy, any approach (68.31–68.39, 68.41–68.49, 68.61–68.69, 68.9)*

✖ **68.71　Laparoscopic radical vaginal hysterectomy [LRVH] ♀**
　Coding Clinic: 2006, Q4, P130-134

✖ **68.79　Other and unspecified radical vaginal hysterectomy ♀**
　Hysterocolpectomy
　Schauta operation

✖ **68.8　Pelvic evisceration ♀**
　Removal of ovaries, tubes, uterus, vagina, bladder, and urethra (with removal of sigmoid colon and rectum)
　Code also any synchronous:
　　colostomy (46.12–46.13)
　　lymph gland dissection (40.3, 40.5)
　　urinary diversion (56.51–56.79)

✖ **68.9　Other and unspecified hysterectomy ♀**
　Hysterectomy, NOS
　　Excludes　*abdominal hysterectomy, any approach (68.31–68.39, 68.41–68.49, 68.61–68.69)*
　　　　vaginal hysterectomy, any approach (68.51–68.59, 68.71–68.79)

● **69　Other operations on uterus and supporting structures**

　Code also any application or administration of an adhesion barrier substance (99.77)

● **69.0　Dilation and curettage of uterus**

　　Excludes　*aspiration curettage of uterus (69.51–69.59)*

✖ **69.01　Dilation and curettage for termination of pregnancy ♀**
　Coding Clinic: 1993, Q3, P6

✖ **69.02　Dilation and curettage following delivery or abortion ♀**
　Coding Clinic: 1993, Q3, P6

✖ **69.09　Other dilation and curettage ♀**
　Diagnostic D and C
　Coding Clinic: 1998, Q1, P4

● **69.1　Excision or destruction of lesion or tissue of uterus and supporting structures**

✖ **69.19　Other excision or destruction of uterus and supporting structures ♀**
　　Excludes　*biopsy of uterine ligament (68.14)*

● **69.2　Repair of uterine supporting structures**

✖ **69.21　Interposition operation ♀**
　Watkins procedure

✖ **69.22　Other uterine suspension ♀**
　Hysteropexy
　Manchester operation
　Plication of uterine ligament

✖ **69.23　Vaginal repair of chronic inversion of uterus ♀**

✖ **69.29　Other repair of uterus and supporting structures ♀**

✖ **69.3　Paracervical uterine denervation ♀**

● **69.4　Uterine repair**

　　Excludes　*repair of current obstetric laceration (75.50–75.52)*

✖ **69.41　Suture of laceration of uterus ♀**

✖ **69.42　Closure of fistula of uterus ♀**
　　Excludes　*uterovesical fistulectomy (57.84)*

✖ **69.49　Other repair of uterus ♀**
　Repair of old obstetric laceration of uterus

● **69.5　Aspiration curettage of uterus**

　　Excludes　*menstrual extraction (69.6)*

✖ **69.51　Aspiration curettage of uterus for termination of pregnancy ♀**
　Therapeutic abortion NOS

✖ **69.52　Aspiration curettage following delivery or abortion ♀**

　69.59　Other aspiration curettage of uterus ♀
　Coding Clinic: 1998, Q1, P7

　69.6　Menstrual extraction or regulation ♀

　69.7　Insertion of intrauterine contraceptive device ♀

OPERATIONS ON THE FEMALE GENITAL ORGANS (65–71)

Excludes　Includes　Use additional　Code also　Omit code

● **69.9   Other operations on uterus, cervix, and supporting structures**

> **Excludes**   *obstetric dilation or incision of cervix (73.1, 73.93)*

> **69.91   Insertion of therapeutic device into uterus ♀**

>> **Excludes**   *insertion of:*
>> *intrauterine contraceptive device (69.7)*
>> *laminaria (69.93)*
>> *obstetric insertion of bag, bougie, or pack (73.1)*

> **69.92   Artificial insemination ♀**

> **69.93   Insertion of laminaria ♀**

> **69.94   Manual replacement of inverted uterus ♀**

>> **Excludes**   *that in immediate postpartal period (75.94)*

> ✖ **69.95   Incision of cervix ♀**

>> **Excludes**   *that to assist delivery (73.93)*

> **69.96   Removal of cerclage material from cervix ♀**

> ✖ **69.97   Removal of other penetrating foreign body from cervix ♀**

>> **Excludes**   *removal of intraluminal foreign body from cervix (98.16)*

> ✖ **69.98   Other operations on supporting structures of uterus ♀**

>> **Excludes**   *biopsy of uterine ligament (68.14)*

> ✖ **69.99   Other operations on cervix and uterus ♀**

>> **Excludes**   *removal of:*
>> *foreign body (98.16)*
>> *intrauterine contraceptive device (97.71)*
>> *obstetric bag, bougie, or pack (97.72)*
>> *packing (97.72)*

● **70   Operations on vagina and cul-de-sac**

> Code also any application or administration of an adhesion barrier substance (99.77)
> **Coding Clinic: 1990, Q2, P26**

> **70.0   Culdocentesis ♀**

● **70.1   Incision of vagina and cul-de-sac**

> **70.11   Hymenotomy ♀**

> ✖ **70.12   Culdotomy ♀**

> ✖ **70.13   Lysis of intraluminal adhesions of vagina ♀**

> ✖ **70.14   Other vaginotomy ♀**
> Division of vaginal septum
> Drainage of hematoma of vaginal cuff

● **70.2   Diagnostic procedures on vagina and cul-de-sac**

> **70.21   Vaginoscopy ♀**

> **70.22   Culdoscopy ♀**

> ✖ **70.23   Biopsy of cul-de-sac ♀**

> ✖ **70.24   Vaginal biopsy ♀**

> ✖ **70.29   Other diagnostic procedures on vagina and cul-de-sac ♀**

● **70.3   Local excision or destruction of vagina and cul-de-sac**

> ✖ **70.31   Hymenectomy ♀**

> ✖ **70.32   Excision or destruction of lesion of cul-de-sac ♀**
> Endometrectomy of cul-de-sac

>> **Excludes**   *biopsy of cul-de-sac (70.23)*

> ✖ **70.33   Excision or destruction of lesion of vagina ♀**

>> **Excludes**   *biopsy of vagina (70.24)*
>> *vaginal fistulectomy (70.72–70.75)*

> ✖ **70.4   Obliteration and total excision of vagina ♀**
> Vaginectomy

>> **Excludes**   *obliteration of vaginal vault (70.8)*

● **70.5   Repair of cystocele and rectocele**

> ✖ **70.50   Repair of cystocele and rectocele ♀**

>> **Excludes**   *repair of cystocele and rectocele with graft or prosthesis (70.53)*

> ✖ **70.51   Repair of cystocele ♀**
> Anterior colporrhaphy (with urethrocele repair)

>> **Excludes**   *repair of cystocele and rectocele with graft or prosthesis (70.53)*
>> *repair of cystocele with graft or prosthesis (70.54)*
>> **Coding Clinic: 1984, Nov-Dec, P20**

> ✖ **70.52   Repair of rectocele ♀**
> Posterior colporrhaphy

>> **Excludes**   *repair of cystocele and rectocele with graft or prosthesis (70.53)*
>> *repair of rectocele with graft or prosthesis (70.55)*
>> *STARR procedure (48.74)*
>> **Coding Clinic: 2006, Q1, P12**

> ✖ **70.53   Repair of cystocele and rectocele with graft or prosthesis ♀**

>> Use additional code for biological substance (70.94) or synthetic substance (70.95), if known

> ✖ **70.54   Repair of cystocele with graft or prosthesis ♀**
> Anterior colporrhaphy (with urethrocele repair)

>> Use additional code for biological substance (70.94) or synthetic substance (70.95), if known

> ✖ **70.55   Repair of rectocele with graft or prosthesis ♀**
> Posterior colporrhaphy

>> Use additional code for biological substance (70.94) or synthetic substance (70.95), if known

● **70.6   Vaginal construction and reconstruction**

> Code also episiotomy, if performed (73.6)

> ✖ **70.61   Vaginal construction ♀**
> **Coding Clinic: 2006, Q3, P18-19**

> ✖ **70.62   Vaginal reconstruction ♀**
> **Coding Clinic: 1984, Nov-Dec, P20**

> ✖ **70.63   Vaginal construction with graft or prosthesis**

>> Use additional code for biological substance (70.94) or synthetic substance (70.95), if known

>> **Excludes**   *vaginal construction (70.61)*

> ✖ **70.64   Vaginal reconstruction with graft or prosthesis**

>> Use additional code for biological substance (70.94) or synthetic substance (70.95), if known

>> **Excludes**   *vaginal reconstruction (70.62)*

● **70.7   Other repair of vagina**

> **Excludes**   *lysis of intraluminal adhesions (70.13)*
> *repair of current obstetric laceration (75.69)*
> *that associated with cervical amputation (67.4)*

✖ **70.71   Suture of laceration of vagina ♀**
     Coding Clinic: 1984, Nov-Dec, P20

✖ **70.72   Repair of colovaginal fistula ♀**

✖ **70.73   Repair of rectovaginal fistula ♀**

✖ **70.74   Repair of other vaginoenteric fistula ♀**

✖ **70.75   Repair of other fistula of vagina ♀**

> **Excludes**   *repair of fistula:*
> *rectovesicovaginal (57.83)*
> *ureterovaginal (56.84)*
> *urethrovaginal (58.43)*
> *uterovaginal (69.42)*
> *vesicocervicovaginal (57.84)*
> *vesicosigmoidovaginal (57.83)*
> *vesicoureterovaginal (56.84)*
> *vesicovaginal (57.84)*

✖ **70.76   Hymenorrhaphy ♀**

✖ **70.77   Vaginal suspension and fixation ♀**

✖ **70.78   Vaginal suspension and fixation with graft or prosthesis ♀**

> Use additional code for biological substance (70.94) or synthetic substance (70.95), if known

✖ **70.79   Other repair of vagina ♀**
Colpoperineoplasty
Repair of old obstetric laceration of vagina

✖ **70.8   Obliteration of vaginal vault ♀**
LeFort operation

● **70.9   Other operations on vagina and cul-de-sac**

✖ **70.91   Other operations on vagina ♀**

> **Excludes**   *insertion of:*
> *diaphragm (96.17)*
> *mold (96.15)*
> *pack (96.14)*
> *pessary (96.18)*
> *suppository (96.49)*
> *removal of:*
> *diaphragm (97.73)*
> *foreign body (98.17)*
> *pack (97.75)*
> *pessary (97.74)*
> *replacement of:*
> *diaphragm (97.24)*
> *pack (97.26)*
> *pessary (97.25)*
> *vaginal dilation (96.16)*
> *vaginal douche (96.44)*

✖ **70.92   Other operations on cul-de-sac ♀**
Obliteration of cul-de-sac
Repair of vaginal enterocele

✖ **70.93   Other operations on cul-de-sac with graft or prosthesis ♀**
Repair of vaginal enterocele with graft or prosthesis

> Use additional code for biological substance (70.94) or synthetic substance (70.95), if known

70.94   Insertion of biological graft ♀
Allogenic material or substance
Allograft
Autograft
Autologous material or substance
Heterograft
Xenogenic material or substance

> Code first these procedures when done with graft or prosthesis:
> Other operations on cul-de-sac (70.93)
> Repair of cystocele (70.54)
> Repair of cystocele and rectocele (70.53)
> Repair of rectocele (70.55)
> Vaginal construction (70.63)
> Vaginal reconstruction (70.64)
> Vaginal suspension and fixation (70.78)

70.95   Insertion of synthetic graft or prosthesis ♀
Artificial tissue

> Code first these procedures when done with graft or prosthesis:
> Other operations on cul-de-sac (70.93)
> Repair of cystocele (70.54)
> Repair of cystocele and rectocele (70.53)
> Repair of rectocele (70.55)
> Vaginal construction (70.63)
> Vaginal reconstruction (70.64)
> Vaginal suspension and fixation (70.78)

● **71   Operations on vulva and perineum**

> Code also any application or administration of an adhesion barrier substance (99.77)

● **71.0   Incision of vulva and perineum**

✖ **71.01   Lysis of vulvar adhesions ♀**

✖ **71.09   Other incision of vulva and perineum ♀**
Enlargement of introitus NOS

> **Excludes**   *removal of foreign body without incision (98.23)*

● **71.1   Diagnostic procedures on vulva**

✖ **71.11   Biopsy of vulva ♀**

✖ **71.19   Other diagnostic procedures on vulva ♀**

● **71.2   Operations on Bartholin's gland**

71.21   Percutaneous aspiration of Bartholin's gland (cyst) ♀

✖ **71.22   Incision of Bartholin's gland (cyst) ♀**

✖ **71.23   Marsupialization of Bartholin's gland (cyst) ♀**

✖ **71.24   Excision or other destruction of Bartholin's gland (cyst) ♀**

✖ **71.29   Other operations on Bartholin's gland ♀**

✖ **71.3   Other local excision or destruction of vulva and perineum ♀**
Division of Skene's gland

> **Excludes**   *biopsy of vulva (71.11)*
> *vulvar fistulectomy (71.72)*

     Coding Clinic: 2007, Q4, P90-91

✖ **71.4   Operations on clitoris ♀**
Amputation of clitoris
Clitoridotomy
Female circumcision

✖ **71.5   Radical vulvectomy ♀**

> Code also any synchronous lymph gland dissection (40.3, 40.5)

● **71.6   Other vulvectomy**

✖ **71.61   Unilateral vulvectomy** ♀
Coding Clinic: 2006, Q2, P19

✖ **71.62   Bilateral vulvectomy** ♀
Vulvectomy NOS

● **71.7   Repair of vulva and perineum**

⬚ Excludes *repair of current obstetric laceration (75.69)*

✖ **71.71   Suture of laceration of vulva or perineum** ♀

✖ **71.72   Repair of fistula of vulva or perineum** ♀

⬚ Excludes *repair of fistula:*
urethroperineal (58.43)
urethroperineovesical (57.84)
vaginoperineal (70.75)

✖ **71.79   Other repair of vulva and perineum** ♀
Repair of old obstetric laceration of vulva or
perineum
Coding Clinic: 1997, Q1, P9-10

✖ **71.8   Other operations on vulva** ♀

⬚ Excludes *removal of:*
foreign body without incision (98.23)
packing (97.75)
replacement of packing (97.26)

✖ **71.9   Other operations on female genital organs** ♀
Coding Clinic: 2004, Q4, P88-90; 2003, Q1, P13-14

◀ New   ◀▥ Revised   ~~deleted~~ Deleted   ● Use Additional Digit(s)   ✖ Valid O.R. Procedure
◆ Non-O.R. Procedure   ♀ Females Only   ♂ Males Only

13. OBSTETRICAL PROCEDURES (72–75)

● **72 Forceps, vacuum, and breech delivery**

72.0 Low forceps operation ♀
Outlet forceps operation

72.1 Low forceps operation with episiotomy ♀
Outlet forceps operation with episiotomy

● **72.2 Mid forceps operation**

72.21 Mid forceps operation with episiotomy ♀

72.29 Other mid forceps operation ♀

● **72.3 High forceps operation**

72.31 High forceps operation with episiotomy ♀

72.39 Other high forceps operation ♀

72.4 Forceps rotation of fetal head ♀
DeLee maneuver
Key-in-lock rotation
Kielland rotation
Scanzoni's maneuver

Code also any associated forceps extraction
(72.0–72.39)

● **72.5 Breech extraction**

72.51 Partial breech extraction with forceps to aftercoming head ♀

72.52 Other partial breech extraction ♀

72.53 Total breech extraction with forceps to aftercoming head ♀

72.54 Other total breech extraction ♀

72.6 Forceps application to aftercoming head ♀
Piper forceps operation

Excludes *partial breech extraction with forceps to aftercoming head (72.51)*
total breech extraction with forceps to aftercoming head (72.53)

● **72.7 Vacuum extraction**

Includes Malström's extraction

72.71 Vacuum extraction with episiotomy ♀

72.79 Other vacuum extraction ♀
Coding Clinic: 2006, Q2, P5

72.8 Other specified instrumental delivery ♀

72.9 Unspecified instrumental delivery ♀

● **73 Other procedures inducing or assisting delivery**

● **73.0 Artificial rupture of membranes**

73.01 Induction of labor by artificial rupture of membranes ♀
Surgical induction NOS

Excludes *artificial rupture of membranes after onset of labor (73.09)*
Coding Clinic: 2000, Q3, P5

73.09 Other artificial rupture of membranes ♀
Artificial rupture of membranes at time of delivery

73.1 Other surgical induction of labor ♀
Induction by cervical dilation

Excludes *injection for abortion (75.0)*
insertion of suppository for abortion (96.49)

● **73.2 Internal and combined version and extraction**

73.21 Internal and combined version without extraction ♀
Version NOS

73.22 Internal and combined version with extraction ♀

73.3 Failed forceps ♀
Application of forceps without delivery
Trial forceps

73.4 Medical induction of labor ♀

Excludes *medication to augment active labor — omit code*

● **73.5 Manually assisted delivery**

73.51 Manual rotation of fetal head ♀

73.59 Other manually assisted delivery ♀
Assisted spontaneous delivery
Crede maneuver
Coding Clinic: 1998, Q4, P76-77

73.6 Episiotomy ♀
Episioproctotomy
Episiotomy with subsequent episiorrhaphy

Excludes *that with:*
high forceps (72.31)
low forceps (72.1)
mid forceps (72.21)
outlet forceps (72.1)
vacuum extraction (72.71)
Coding Clinic: 2008, Q4, P192; 2006, Q2, P5; 1992, Q1, P10-11

73.8 Operations on fetus to facilitate delivery ♀
Clavicotomy on fetus
Destruction of fetus
Needling of hydrocephalic head

● **73.9 Other operations assisting delivery**

73.91 External version ♀

73.92 Replacement of prolapsed umbilical cord ♀

73.93 Incision of cervix to assist delivery ♀
Dührssen's incisions

✖ **73.94 Pubiotomy to assist delivery** ♀
Obstetrical symphysiotomy

✖ **73.99 Other** ♀

Excludes *dilation of cervix, obstetrical to induce labor (73.1)*
insertion of bag or bougie to induce labor (73.1)
removal of cerclage material (69.96)

● **74 Cesarean section and removal of fetus**

Code also any synchronous:
hysterectomy (68.3–68.4, 68.6, 68.8)
myomectomy (68.29)
sterilization (66.31–66.39, 66.63)

✖ **74.0 Classical cesarean section** ♀
Transperitoneal classical cesarean section

✖ **74.1 Low cervical cesarean section** ♀
Lower uterine segment cesarean section
Coding Clinic: 2001, Q1, P11-12

✖ **74.2 Extraperitoneal cesarean section** ♀
Supravesical cesarean section

✖ **74.3 Removal of extratubal ectopic pregnancy** ♀
Removal of:
ectopic abdominal pregnancy
fetus from peritoneal or extraperitoneal cavity following uterine or tubal rupture

Excludes *that by salpingostomy (66.02)*
that by salpingotomy (66.01)
that with synchronous salpingectomy (66.62)
Coding Clinic: 1990, Q2, P25, 27; 1989, Q1, P11; 1985, Sept-Oct, P14

✖ **74.4 Cesarean section of other specified type** ♀
Peritoneal exclusion cesarean section
Transperitoneal cesarean section NOS
Vaginal cesarean section

Excludes Includes Use additional Code also Omit code

● 74.9   Cesarean section of unspecified type

  ✖ 74.91   Hysterotomy to terminate pregnancy ♀
      Therapeutic abortion by hysterotomy

  ✖ 74.99   Other cesarean section of unspecified type ♀
      Cesarean section NOS
      Obstetrical abdominouterotomy
      Obstetrical hysterotomy

● 75   Other obstetric operations

   75.0   Intra-amniotic injection for abortion ♀
      Injection of:
        prostaglandin for induction of abortion
        saline for induction of abortion
      Termination of pregnancy by intrauterine injection

     Excludes   *insertion of prostaglandin suppository for abortion (96.49)*

   75.1   Diagnostic amniocentesis ♀

   75.2   Intrauterine transfusion ♀
      Exchange transfusion in utero
      Insertion of catheter into abdomen of fetus for transfusion

     Code also   any hysterotomy approach (68.0)

● 75.3   Other intrauterine operations on fetus and amnion

     Code also   any hysterotomy approach (68.0)

     75.31   Amnioscopy ♀
        Fetoscopy
        Laparoamnioscopy
        Coding Clinic: 2006, Q3, P16-18

     75.32   Fetal EKG (scalp) ♀

     75.33   Fetal blood sampling and biopsy ♀

     75.34   Other fetal monitoring ♀
        Antepartum fetal nonstress test
        Fetal monitoring, not otherwise specified

       Excludes   *fetal pulse oximetry (75.38)*

     75.35   Other diagnostic procedures on fetus and amnion ♀
        Intrauterine pressure determination

       Excludes   *amniocentesis (75.1)*
            diagnostic procedures on gravid uterus and placenta (87.81, 88.46, 88.78, 92.17)

       Coding Clinic: 2006, Q3, P16-18

  ✖ 75.36   Correction of fetal defect ♀

     OGCR   Section I.C.10.a.2

     In cases when in utero surgery is performed on the fetus, a code from category 655 should be assigned identifying the fetal condition. Procedure code 75.36, Correction of fetal defect, should be assigned on the hospital inpatient record. No code from Chapter 15, the perinatal codes, should be used on the mother's record to identify fetal conditions. Surgery performed in utero on a fetus is still to be coded as an obstetric encounter.

     75.37   Amnioinfusion

       Code also   injection of antibiotic (99.21)
       Coding Clinic: 1998, Q4, P76-77

     75.38   Fetal pulse oximetry
        Transcervical fetal oxygen saturation monitoring
        Transcervical fetal SpO_2 monitoring

   75.4   Manual removal of retained placenta ♀

     Excludes   *aspiration curettage (69.52)*
            dilation and curettage (69.02)
     Coding Clinic: 2006, Q3, P11

● 75.5   Repair of current obstetric laceration of uterus

  ✖ 75.50   Repair of current obstetric laceration of uterus, not otherwise specified ♀

  ✖ 75.51   Repair of current obstetric laceration of cervix ♀

  ✖ 75.52   Repair of current obstetric laceration of corpus uteri ♀
       Coding Clinic: 2008, Q2, P7-8

● 75.6   Repair of other current obstetric laceration

     Code also   episiotomy, if performed (73.6)
     Coding Clinic: 2008, Q4, P192; 1992, Q1, P10-11

  ✖ 75.61   Repair of current obstetric laceration of bladder and urethra ♀

     75.62   Repair of current obstetric laceration of rectum and sphincter ani ♀

     75.69   Repair of other current obstetric laceration ♀
        Episioperineorrhaphy
        Repair of:
          pelvic floor
          perineum
          vagina
          vulva
        Secondary repair of episiotomy
        Coding Clinic: 2008, Q4, P192; 2007, Q4, P125

   75.7   Manual exploration of uterine cavity, postpartum ♀

   75.8   Obstetric tamponade of uterus or vagina ♀
     Excludes   *antepartum tamponade (73.1)*

● 75.9   Other obstetric operations

     75.91   Evacuation of obstetrical incisional hematoma of perineum ♀
        Evacuation of hematoma of:
          episiotomy
          perineorrhaphy

     75.92   Evacuation of other hematoma of vulva or vagina ♀

  ✖ 75.93   Surgical correction of inverted uterus ♀
        Spintelli operation

       Excludes   *vaginal repair of chronic inversion of uterus (69.23)*

     75.94   Manual replacement of inverted uterus ♀

  ✖ 75.99   Other ♀
       Coding Clinic: 2006, Q3, P16-18

◀ New   ◀▥ Revised   ~~deleted~~ Deleted   ● Use Additional Digit(s)   ✖ Valid O.R. Procedure
     ◆ Non-O.R. Procedure   ♀ Females Only   ♂ Males Only

(See Plates 244 and 509 on pages NAP-30–NAP-31.)

14. OPERATIONS ON THE MUSCULOSKELETAL SYSTEM (76–84)

● **76   Operations on facial bones and joints**

> **Excludes** *accessory sinuses (22.00–22.9)*
> *nasal bones (21.00–21.99)*
> *skull (01.01–02.99)*

● **76.0   Incision of facial bone without division**

✖ **76.01   Sequestrectomy of facial bone**
Removal of necrotic bone chip from facial bone

✖ **76.09   Other incision of facial bone**
Reopening of osteotomy site of facial bone

> **Excludes** *osteotomy associated with orthognathic surgery (76.61–76.69)*
> *removal of internal fixation device (76.97)*

● **76.1   Diagnostic procedures on facial bones and joints**

✖ **76.11   Biopsy of facial bone**

✖ **76.19   Other diagnostic procedures on facial bones and joints**

> **Excludes** *contrast arthrogram of temporomandibular joint (87.13)*
> *other x-ray (87.11–87.12, 87.14–87.16)*
> **Coding Clinic: 1987, Nov-Dec, P12**

✖ **76.2   Local excision or destruction of lesion of facial bone**

> **Excludes** *biopsy of facial bone (76.11)*
> *excision of odontogenic lesion (24.4)*

● **76.3   Partial ostectomy of facial bone**

✖ **76.31   Partial mandibulectomy**
Hemimandibulectomy

> **Excludes** *that associated with temporomandibular arthroplasty (76.5)*
> **Coding Clinic: 2005, Q2, P8-9**

✖ **76.39   Partial ostectomy of other facial bone**
Hemimaxillectomy (with bone graft or prosthesis)
Coding Clinic: 1987, Jan-Feb, P14

● **76.4   Excision and reconstruction of facial bones**

✖ **76.41   Total mandibulectomy with synchronous reconstruction**

✖ **76.42   Other total mandibulectomy**

✖ **76.43   Other reconstruction of mandible**

> **Excludes** *genioplasty (76.67–76.68)*
> *that with synchronous total mandibulectomy (76.41)*
> **Coding Clinic: 2003, Q2, P13**

✖ **76.44   Total ostectomy of other facial bone with synchronous reconstruction**
Coding Clinic: 1993, Q3, P6

✖ **76.45   Other total ostectomy of other facial bone**

✖ **76.46   Other reconstruction of other facial bone**

> **Excludes** *that with synchronous total ostectomy (76.44)*

✖ **76.5   Temporomandibular arthroplasty**

● **76.6   Other facial bone repair and orthognathic surgery**

> **Code also** any synchronous:
> bone graft (76.91)
> synthetic implant (76.92)

> **Excludes** *reconstruction of facial bones (76.41–76.46)*

✖ **76.61   Closed osteoplasty [osteotomy] of mandibular ramus**
Gigli saw osteotomy

✖ **76.62   Open osteoplasty [osteotomy] of mandibular ramus**

✖ **76.63   Osteoplasty [osteotomy] of body of mandible**

✖ **76.64   Other orthognathic surgery on mandible**
Mandibular osteoplasty NOS
Segmental or subapical osteotomy
Coding Clinic: 2004, Q2, P9,10

✖ **76.65   Segmental osteoplasty [osteotomy] of maxilla**
Maxillary osteoplasty NOS

✖ **76.66   Total osteoplasty [osteotomy] of maxilla**

✖ **76.67   Reduction genioplasty**
Reduction mentoplasty

✖ **76.68   Augmentation genioplasty**
Mentoplasty:
NOS
with graft or implant

✖ **76.69   Other facial bone repair**
Osteoplasty of facial bone NOS

● **76.7   Reduction of facial fracture**

> **Includes** internal fixation

> **Code also** any synchronous:
> bone graft (76.91)
> synthetic implant (76.92)

> **Excludes** *that of nasal bones (21.71–21.72)*

✖ **76.70   Reduction of facial fracture, not otherwise specified**

76.71   Closed reduction of malar and zygomatic fracture

✖ **76.72   Open reduction of malar and zygomatic fracture**

76.73   Closed reduction of maxillary fracture

✖ **76.74   Open reduction of maxillary fracture**

76.75   Closed reduction of mandibular fracture

✖ **76.76   Open reduction of mandibular fracture**

✖ **76.77   Open reduction of alveolar fracture**
Reduction of alveolar fracture with stabilization of teeth

76.78   Other closed reduction of facial fracture
Closed reduction of orbital fracture

> **Excludes** *nasal bone (21.71)*

✖ **76.79   Other open reduction of facial fracture**
Open reduction of orbit rim or wall

> **Excludes** *nasal bone (21.72)*

● **76.9   Other operations on facial bones and joints**

✖ **76.91   Bone graft to facial bone**
Autogenous graft to facial bone
Bone bank graft to facial bone
Heterogenous graft to facial bone

✖ **76.92   Insertion of synthetic implant in facial bone**
Alloplastic implant to facial bone

76.93   Closed reduction of temporomandibular dislocation

✖ **76.94   Open reduction of temporomandibular dislocation**

76.95   Other manipulation of temporomandibular joint

76.96   Injection of therapeutic substance into temporomandibular joint

| Excludes | Includes | Use additional | Code also | Omit code |

OPERATIONS ON THE MUSCULOSKELETAL SYSTEM (76–84)

✖ **76.97** **Removal of internal fixation device from facial bone**

> **Excludes** *removal of:*
> *dental wiring (97.33)*
> *external mandibular fixation device NEC (97.36)*

✖ **76.99** **Other**

● **77** **Incision, excision, and division of other bones**

> **Excludes** *laminectomy for decompression (03.09)*
> *operations on:*
> *accessory sinuses (22.00–22.9)*
> *ear ossicles (19.0–19.55)*
> *facial bones (76.01–76.99)*
> *joint structures (80.00–81.99)*
> *mastoid (19.9–20.99)*
> *nasal bones (21.00–21.99)*
> *skull (01.01–02.99)*

The following fourth-digit subclassification is for use with appropriate categories in section 77 to identify the site. Valid fourth-digit categories are in brackets under each code.

> 0   unspecified site
> 1   scapula, clavicle, and thorax [ribs and sternum]
> 2   humerus
> 3   radius and ulna
> 4   carpals and metacarpals
> 5   femur
> 6   patella
> 7   tibia and fibula
> 8   tarsals and metatarsals
> 9   other
>   Pelvic bones
>   Phalanges (of foot) (of hand)
>   Vertebrae

✖● **77.0** **Sequestrectomy**
[0-9]

✖● **77.1** **Other incision of bone without division**
[0-9]   Reopening of osteotomy site

> **Excludes** *aspiration of bone marrow (41.31, 41.91)*
> *removal of internal fixation device (78.60–78.69)*

Coding Clinic: 2002, Q1, P3-4

✖● **77.2** **Wedge osteotomy**
[0-9]
> **Excludes** *that for hallux valgus (77.51)*

✖● **77.3** **Other division of bone**
[0-9]   Osteoarthrotomy

> **Excludes** *clavicotomy of fetus (73.8)*
> *laminotomy or incision of vertebra (03.01–03.09)*
> *pubiotomy to assist delivery (73.94)*
> *sternotomy incidental to thoracic operation — omit code*

✖● **77.4** **Biopsy of bone**
[0-9]   Coding Clinic: 2006, Q3, P13; 1998, Q2, P12

● **77.5** **Excision and repair of bunion and other toe deformities**

✖ **77.51** **Bunionectomy with soft tissue correction and osteotomy of the first metatarsal**

✖ **77.52** **Bunionectomy with soft tissue correction and arthrodesis**

✖ **77.53** **Other bunionectomy with soft tissue correction**

✖ **77.54** **Excision or correction of bunionette**
> That with osteotomy

✖ **77.56** **Repair of hammer toe**
> Filleting of hammer toe
> Fusion of hammer toe
> Phalangectomy (partial) of hammer toe

✖ **77.57** **Repair of claw toe**
> Capsulotomy of claw toe
> Fusion of claw toe
> Phalangectomy (partial) of claw toe
> Tendon lengthening of claw toe

✖ **77.58** **Other excision, fusion, and repair of toes**
> Cockup toe repair
> Overlapping toe repair
> That with use of prosthetic materials

✖ **77.59** **Other bunionectomy**
> Resection of hallux valgus joint with insertion of prosthesis

✖● **77.6** **Local excision of lesion or tissue of bone**
[0-9]
> **Excludes** *biopsy of bone (77.40–77.49)*
> *debridement of compound fracture (79.60–79.69)*

Coding Clinic: 2008, Q1, P3-4; 2004, Q4, P128-129; 2002, Q1, P3-49; 2001, Q3, P9; 2000, Q2, P18-19; 1999, Q1, P8-9

✖● **77.7** **Excision of bone for graft**
[0-9]   Coding Clinic: 2008, Q1, P5-6; 2007, Q2, P6; 2003, Q3, P19; 2003, Q2, P13; 2002, Q4, P107-110; 2002, Q2, P16; 2000, Q2, P12-13; 1999, Q4, P12-13; 1995, Q2, P9;1994, Q2; P7

✖● **77.8** **Other partial ostectomy**
[0-9]   Condylectomy

> **Excludes** *amputation (84.00–84.19, 84.91)*
> *arthrectomy (80.90–80.99)*
> *excision of bone ends associated with:*
> *arthrodesis (81.00–81.39, 81.62–81.66)*
> *arthroplasty (81.40–81.59, 81.71–81.85)*
> *excision of cartilage (80.5–80.6, 80.80–80.99)*
> *excision of head of femur with synchronous replacement (00.70–00.73, 81.51–81.53)*
> *hemilaminectomy (03.01–03.09)*
> *laminectomy (03.01–03.09)*
> *ostectomy for hallux valgus (77.51–77.59)*
> *partial amputation:*
> *finger (84.01)*
> *thumb (84.02)*
> *toe (84.11)*
> *resection of ribs incidental to thoracic operation — omit code*
> *that incidental to other operation — omit code*

Coding Clinic: 2002, Q2, P8

✖● **77.9** **Total ostectomy**
[0-9]
> **Excludes** *amputation of limb (84.00–84.19, 84.91)*
> *that incidental to other operation — omit code*

◀ New   ⫷ Revised   ~~deleted~~ Deleted   ● Use Additional Digit(s)   ✖ Valid O.R. Procedure
◆ Non-O.R. Procedure   ♀ Females Only   ♂ Males Only

● **78 Other operations on bones, except facial bones**

> **Excludes** *operations on:*
> *accessory sinuses (22.00–22.9)*
> *facial bones (76.01–76.99)*
> *joint structures (80.00–81.99)*
> *nasal bones (21.00–21.99)*
> *skull (01.01–02.99)*

Coding Clinic: 2002, Q2, P11

The following fourth-digit subclassification is for use with categories in section 78 to identify the site. Valid fourth-digit categories are in [brackets] under each code.

> 0   unspecified site
> 1   scapula, clavicle, and thorax [ribs and sternum]
> 2   humerus
> 3   radius and ulna
> 4   carpals and metacarpals
> 5   femur
> 6   patella
> 7   tibia and fibula
> 8   tarsals and metatarsals
> 9   other
>   Pelvic bones
>   Phalanges (of foot) (of hand)
>   Vertebrae

✘● **78.0 Bone graft**
[0-9]   Bone:
      bank graft
      graft (autogenous) (heterogenous)
     That with debridement of bone graft site (removal of sclerosed, fibrous, or necrotic bone or tissue)
     Transplantation of bone

> Code also any excision of bone for graft (77.70–77.79)

> **Excludes** *that for bone lengthening (78.30–78.39)*

Coding Clinic: 2006, Q4, P103-104; 1998, Q2, P12; 1994, Q3, P10; 1994, Q2, P7

✘● **78.1 Application of external fixator device**
[0-9]   Fixator with insertion of pins/wires/screws into bone

> Code also any type of fixator device, if known (84.71–84.73)

> **Excludes** *other immobilization, pressure, and attention to wound (93.51–93.59)*

Coding Clinic: 2005, Q4, P127-129; 1994, Q2, P5

✘● **78.2 Limb shortening procedures**
[0, 2-5, 7-9]   Epiphyseal stapling
     Open epiphysiodesis
     Percutaneous epiphysiodesis
     Resection/osteotomy

✘● **78.3 Limb lengthening procedures**
[0, 2-5, 7-9]   Bone graft with or without internal fixation devices or osteotomy
     Distraction technique with or without corticotomy/osteotomy

> Code also any application of an external fixation device (78.10–78.19)

✘● **78.4 Other repair or plastic operations on bone**
[0-9]   Other operation on bone NEC
     Repair of malunion or nonunion fracture NEC

> **Excludes** *application of external fixation device (78.10–78.19)*
> *limb lengthening procedures (78.30–78.39)*
> *limb shortening procedures (78.20–78.29)*
> *osteotomy (77.3)*
> *reconstruction of thumb (82.61–82.69)*
> *repair of pectus deformity (34.74)*
> *repair with bone graft (78.00–78.09)*

Coding Clinic: 2004, Q3, P9-10; 2002, Q3, P12; Q2, P14-16; 1999, Q4, P22; 1997, Q1, P5; 1991, Q3, P20; Q2, P20

✘● **78.5 Internal fixation of bone without fracture reduction**
[0-9]   Internal fixation of bone (prophylactic)
     Reinsertion of internal fixation device
     Revision of displaced or broken fixation device

> **Excludes** *arthroplasty and arthrodesis (81.00–81.85)*
> *bone graft (78.00–78.09)*
> *limb shortening procedures (78.20–78.29)*
> *that for fracture reduction (79.10–79.19, 79.30–79.59)*

Coding Clinic: 2004, Q3, P6-7; 2003, Q2, P15; 1999, Q4, P13-14; 1995, Q3, P12

✘● **78.6 Removal of implanted devices from bone**
[0-9]   External fixator device (invasive)
     Internal fixation device
     Removal of bone growth stimulator (invasive)
     Removal of internal limb lengthening device
     Removal of pedicle screw(s) used in spinal fusion

> **Excludes** *removal of cast, splint, and traction device (Kirschner wire) (Steinmann pin) (97.88)*
> *removal of posterior spinal motion preservation (facet replacement, pedicle-based dynamic stabilization, interspinous process) device(s) (80.09)*
> *removal of skull tongs or halo traction device (02.95)*

Coding Clinic: 2003, Q2, P14; 2002, Q4, P110; 2000, Q2, P18-19; Q1, P15-16; 1995, Q1, P10

✘● **78.7 Osteoclasis**
[0-9]

✘● **78.8 Diagnostic procedures on bone, not elsewhere**
[0-9] **classified**

> **Excludes** *biopsy of bone (77.40–77.49)*
> *magnetic resonance imaging (88.94)*
> *microscopic examination of specimen from bone (91.51–91.59)*
> *radioisotope scan (92.14)*
> *skeletal x-ray (87.21–87.29, 87.43, 88.21–88.33)*
> *thermography (88.83)*

✘● **78.9 Insertion of bone growth stimulator**
[0-9]   Insertion of:
     bone stimulator (electrical) to aid bone healing
     osteogenic electrodes for bone growth stimulation
     totally implanted device (invasive)

> **Excludes** *non-invasive (transcutaneous) (surface) stimulator (99.86)*

OPERATIONS ON THE MUSCULOSKELETAL SYSTEM (76–84)

● **79   Reduction of fracture and dislocation**

> **Includes**   application of cast or splint reduction with insertion of traction device (Kirschner wire) (Steinmann pin)

> **Code also** any:
> application of external fixator device (78.10–78.19)
> type of fixator device, if known (84.71–84.73)

> **Excludes**   *external fixation alone for immobilization of fracture (93.51–93.56, 93.59)*
>
> *internal fixation without reduction of fracture (78.50–78.59)*
>
> *operations on:*
> *facial bones (76.70–76.79)*
> *nasal bones (21.71–21.72)*
> *orbit (76.78–76.79)*
> *skull (02.02)*
> *vertebrae (03.53)*
>
> *removal of cast or splint (97.88)*
>
> *replacement of cast or splint (97.11–97.14)*
>
> *traction alone for reduction of fracture (93.41–93.46)*

The following fourth-digit subclassification is for use with appropriate categories in section 79 to identify the site. Valid fourth-digit categories are in [brackets] under each code.

> 0   unspecified site
> 1   humerus
> 2   radius and ulna
>   Arm NOS
> 3   carpals and metacarpals
>   Hand NOS
> 4   phalanges of hand
> 5   femur
> 6   tibia and fibula
>   Leg NOS
> 7   tarsals and metatarsals
>   Foot NOS
> 8   phalanges of foot
> 9   other specified bone

● **79.0   Closed reduction of fracture without internal fixation**
[0-9]
> **Excludes**   *that for separation of epiphysis (79.40–79.49)*
> Coding Clinic: 2005, Q4, P127-129; 1989, Q3, P16; 1988, Q4, P11

✖ ● **79.1   Closed reduction of fracture with internal fixation**
[0-9]
> **Excludes**   *that for separation of epiphysis (79.40–79.49)*
> Coding Clinic: 1994, Q2, P6-7; 1993, Q4, P35; 1993, Q1, P27; 1984, May-June, P11

✖ ● **79.2   Open reduction of fracture without internal fixation**
[0-9]
> **Excludes**   *that for separation of epiphysis (79.50–79.59)*

✖ ● **79.3   Open reduction of fracture with internal fixation**
[0-9]
> **Excludes**   *that for separation of epiphysis (79.50–79.59)*
> Coding Clinic: 2007, Q1, P3-8; 2004, Q1, P9; 1998, Q2, P12; 1994, Q3, P10; Q2, P5, 7

✖ ● **79.4   Closed reduction of separated epiphysis**
[0-2, 5, 6, 9]   Reduction with or without internal fixation

✖ ● **79.5   Open reduction of separated epiphysis**
[0-2, 5, 6, 9]   Reduction with or without internal fixation

✖ ● **79.6   Debridement of open fracture site**
[0-9]   Debridement of compound fracture
> Coding Clinic: 1995, Q3, P12

● **79.7   Closed reduction of dislocation**

> **Includes**   closed reduction (with external traction device)

> **Excludes**   *closed reduction of dislocation of temporomandibular joint (76.93)*

   79.70   Closed reduction of dislocation of unspecified site

   79.71   Closed reduction of dislocation of shoulder

   79.72   Closed reduction of dislocation of elbow

   79.73   Closed reduction of dislocation of wrist

   79.74   Closed reduction of dislocation of hand and finger

   79.75   Closed reduction of dislocation of hip

   79.76   Closed reduction of dislocation of knee

   79.77   Closed reduction of dislocation of ankle

   79.78   Closed reduction of dislocation of foot and toe

   79.79   Closed reduction of dislocation of other specified sites

● **79.8   Open reduction of dislocation**

> **Includes**   open reduction (with internal and external fixation devices)

> **Excludes**   *open reduction of dislocation of temporomandibular joint (76.94)*

✖ **79.80   Open reduction of dislocation of unspecified site**

✖ **79.81   Open reduction of dislocation of shoulder**

✖ **79.82   Open reduction of dislocation of elbow**

✖ **79.83   Open reduction of dislocation of wrist**

✖ **79.84   Open reduction of dislocation of hand and finger**

✖ **79.85   Open reduction of dislocation of hip**

✖ **79.86   Open reduction of dislocation of knee**

✖ **79.87   Open reduction of dislocation of ankle**
> Coding Clinic: 2004, Q1, P9

✖ **79.88   Open reduction of dislocation of foot and toe**

✖ **79.89   Open reduction of dislocation of other specified sites**

✖ ● **79.9   Unspecified operation on bone injury**
[0-9]

● **80   Incision and excision of joint structures**

> **Includes**   operations on:
> capsule of joint
> cartilage
> condyle
> ligament
> meniscus
> synovial membrane

> **Excludes**   *cartilage of:*
> *ear (18.01–18.9)*
> *nose (21.00–21.99)*
> *temporomandibular joint (76.01–76.99)*

◄ New   ◄▥ Revised   ~~deleted~~ Deleted   ● Use Additional Digit(s)   ✖ Valid O.R. Procedure
◆ Non-O.R. Procedure   ♀ Females Only   ♂ Males Only

The following fourth-digit subclassification is for use with appropriate categories in section 80 to identify the site:

> 0   **unspecified site**
> 1   **shoulder**
> 2   **elbow**
> 3   **wrist**
> 4   **hand and finger**
> 5   **hip**
> 6   **knee**
> 7   **ankle**
> 8   **foot and toe**
> 9   **other specified sites**
>   **Spine**

✖ ● **80.0**   **Arthrotomy for removal of prosthesis without**
[0-9]   **replacement**

> Includes   removal of posterior spinal motion preservation (dynamic stabilization, facet replacement, interspinous process) device(s)

> Code also any:
>   insertion of (cement) (joint) (methylmethacrylate) spacer (84.56)
>   removal of (cement) (joint) (methylmethacrylate) spacer (84.57)

> Excludes   *removal of pedicle screws used in spinal fusion (78.69)*

> Coding Clinic: 2008, Q2, P3-5; 1997, Q2, P10; 1992, Q2, P18; 1990, Q2, P27

✖ ● **80.1**   **Other arthrotomy**
[0-9]   Arthrostomy

> Excludes   *that for:*
>   *arthrography (88.32)*
>   *arthroscopy (80.20–80.29)*
>   *injection of drug (81.92)*
>   *operative approach —* omit code

> Coding Clinic: 2006, Q3, P22-23

✖ ● **80.2**   **Arthroscopy**
[0-9]

● **80.3**   **Biopsy of joint structure**
[0-9]   Aspiration biopsy

> Coding Clinic: 2005, Q3, P13-14x2

✖ ● **80.4**   **Division of joint capsule, ligament, or cartilage**
[0-9]   Goldner clubfoot release
     Heyman-Herndon(-Strong) correction of metatarsus varus
     Release of:
         adherent or constrictive joint capsule
         joint
         ligament

> Excludes   *symphysiotomy to assist delivery (73.94)*
>   *that for:*
>   *carpal tunnel syndrome (04.43)*
>   *tarsal tunnel syndrome (04.44)*

> Coding Clinic: 2002, Q2, P16

● **80.5**   **Excision, destruction and other repair of intervertebral disc**

> Coding Clinic: 1986, Sept-Oct, P11-12

✖ **80.50**   **Excision or destruction of intervertebral disc, unspecified**
     Unspecified as to excision or destruction

✖ **80.51**   **Excision of intervertebral disc**
     Diskectomy
     Removal of herniated nucleus pulposus
     Level:
         cervical
         thoracic
         lumbar (lumbosacral)
     That by laminotomy or hemilaminectomy
     That with decompression of spinal nerve root at same level
     Requires additional code for any concomitant decompression of spinal nerve root at different level from excision site

> Code also any
>   concurrent spinal fusion (81.00–81.09)
>   repair of the anulus fibrosus (80.53–80.54)

> Excludes   *intervertebral chemonucleolysis (80.52)*
>   *laminectomy for exploration of intraspinal canal (03.09)*
>   *laminotomy for decompression of spinal nerve root only (03.09)*
>   *that for insertion of (non-fusion) spinal disc replacement device (84.60–84.69)*
>   *that with corpectomy, (vertebral) (80.99)*

> Coding Clinic: 2009, Q2, P4x2; 2008, Q4, P183-184; Q4, P14-15; 2008, Q1, P5-6; 2008, Q1, P3-5; 2007, Q1, P9; 2006, Q1, P12-13; 2004, Q4, P129-133; 2003, Q3, P12; 1996, Q1, P7 x2; 1995, Q2, P9

80.52   **Intervertebral chemonucleolysis**
     With aspiration of disc fragments
     With diskography
     Injection of proteolytic enzyme into intervertebral space (chymopapain)

> Excludes   *injection of anestheti substance (03.91)*
>   *injection of other substances (03.92)*

✖ **80.53**   **Repair of the anulus fibrosus with graft or prosthesis**
     Anular disc repair
     Closure (sealing) of the anulus fibrosus defect

> Includes   microsurgical suture repair with fascial autograft
>   soft tissue re-approximation repair with tension bands
>   surgical mesh repair

> Code also any:
>   application or administration of adhesion barrier substance, if performed (99.77)
>   intervertebral discectomy, if performed (80.51)
>   locally harvested fascia for graft (83.43)

> Coding Clinic: 2008, Q4, P183-184

✖ **80.54**   **Other and unspecified repair of the anulus fibrosus**
     Anular disc repair
     Closure (sealing) of the anulus fibrosus defect
     Microsurgical suture repair without fascial autograft
     Percutaneous repair of the anulus fibrosus

> Code also any:
>   application or administration of adhesion barrier substance, if performed (99.77)
>   intervertebral discectomy, if performed (80.51)

> Coding Clinic: 2008, Q4, P183-184

✖ **80.59 Other destruction of intervertebral disc**
Destruction NEC
That by laser
Coding Clinic: 2002, Q3, P10; 1989, Q1, P11; 1988, Q4, P11

✖ **80.6 Excision of semilunar cartilage of knee**
Excision of meniscus of knee
Coding Clinic: 2003, Q2, P18; 2000, Q3, P4; 1996, Q2, P4; 1993, Q1, P23

✖● **80.7 Synovectomy**
[0-9] Complete or partial resection of synovial membrane
Excludes excision of Baker's cyst (83.39)
Coding Clinic: 1984, Nov-Dec, P9

✖● **80.8 Other local excision or destruction of lesion of joint**
[0-9] Coding Clinic: 2008, Q1, P7

✖● **80.9 Other excision of joint**
[0-9] **Excludes** cheilectomy of joint (77.80–77.89)
excision of bone ends (77.80–77.89)
Coding Clinic: 2007, Q1, P20-21

●**81 Repair and plastic operations on joint structures**

●**81.0 Spinal fusion**
Includes arthrodesis of spine with:
bone graft
internal fixation
Code also:
any insertion of interbody spinal fusion device (84.51)
any insertion of recombinant bone morphogenetic protein (84.52)
any synchronous excision of (locally) harvested bone for graft (77.70–77.79)
the total number of vertebrae fused (81.62–81.64)
Excludes correction of pseudarthrosis of spine (81.30–81.39)
refusion of spine (81.30–81.39)
Coding Clinic: 2009, Q2, P4

✖ **81.00 Spinal fusion, not otherwise specified**
MS-DRG: Refer to Part VI, Appendix E, Table 4, Spinal Fusion Reference Table

✖ **81.01 Atlas-axis spinal fusion**
Craniocervical fusion by anterior, transoral, or posterior technique
C1-C2 fusion by anterior, transoral, or posterior technique
Occiput C2 fusion by anterior, transoral, or posterior technique
MS-DRG: Refer to Part VI, Appendix E, Table 4, Spinal Fusion Reference Table

✖ **81.02 Other cervical fusion, anterior technique**
Arthrodesis of C2 level or below:
anterior (interbody) technique
anterolateral technique
Coding Clinic: 2003, Q4, P99-101; 2001, Q1, P6; 1996, Q1, P7x2
MS-DRG: Refer to Part VI, Appendix E, Table 4, Spinal Fusion Reference Table

✖ **81.03 Other cervical fusion, posterior technique**
Arthrodesis of C2 level or below:
posterior (interbody) technique
posterolateral technique
MS-DRG: Refer to Part VI, Appendix E, Table 4, Spinal Fusion Reference Table

✖ **81.04 Dorsal and dorsolumbar fusion, anterior technique**
Arthrodesis of thoracic or thoracolumbar region:
anterior (interbody) technique
anterolateral technique
Coding Clinic: 2003, Q3, P19
MS-DRG: Refer to Part VI, Appendix E, Table 4, Spinal Fusion Reference Table

✖ **81.05 Dorsal and dorsolumbar fusion, posterior technique**
Arthrodesis of thoracic or thoracolumbar region:
posterior (interbody) technique
posterolateral technique
MS-DRG: Refer to Part VI, Appendix E, Table 4, Spinal Fusion Reference Table

✖ **81.06 Lumbar and lumbosacral fusion, anterior technique**
Anterior lumbar interbody fusion (ALIF)
Arthrodesis of lumbar or lumbosacral region:
anterior (interbody) technique
anterolateral technique
Coding Clinic: 2008, Q2, P14-15; 2007, Q1, P9-10,20-21; 2002, Q4, P107-108
MS-DRG: Refer to Part VI, Appendix E, Table 4, Spinal Fusion Reference Table

✖ **81.07 Lumbar and lumbosacral fusion, lateral transverse process technique**
Coding Clinic: 2009, Q2, P4; 2002, Q4, P108
MS-DRG: Refer to Part VI, Appendix E, Table 4, Spinal Fusion Reference Table

✖ **81.08 Lumbar and lumbosacral fusion, posterior technique**
Arthrodesis of lumbar or lumbosacral region:
posterior (interbody) technique
posterolateral technique
Posterior lumbar interbody fusion (PLIF)
Transforaminal lumbar interbody fusion (TLIF)
Coding Clinic: 2009, Q2, P4x2, 5; 2008, Q1, P5-6; 2006, Q1, P12-14x2; 2005, Q4, P122-123; 2002, Q4, P107-110; 2000, Q2, P12-13; 1999, Q4, P12-13; 1995, Q2, P9
MS-DRG: Refer to Part VI, Appendix E, Table 4, Spinal Fusion Reference Table

●**81.1 Arthrodesis and arthroereisis of foot and ankle**
Includes arthrodesis of foot and ankle with:
bone graft
external fixation device

✖ **81.11 Ankle fusion**
Tibiotalar fusion

✖ **81.12 Triple arthrodesis**
Talus to calcaneus and calcaneus to cuboid and navicular

✖ **81.13 Subtalar fusion**
Excludes arthroereisis (81.18)

✖ **81.14 Midtarsal fusion**

✖ **81.15 Tarsometatarsal fusion**

✖ **81.16 Metatarsophalangeal fusion**

✖ **81.17 Other fusion of foot**

✖ **81.18 Subtalar joint arthroereisis**
Coding Clinic: 2005, Q4, P124

◀ New   ◀▥ Revised   ~~deleted~~ Deleted   ● Use Additional Digit(s)   ✖ Valid O.R. Procedure
◆ Non-O.R. Procedure   ♀ Females Only   ♂ Males Only

● **81.2 Arthrodesis of other joint**

Includes arthrodesis with:
>> bone graft
>> external fixation device
>> excision of bone ends and compression

✖ **81.20 Arthrodesis of unspecified joint**

✖ **81.21 Arthrodesis of hip**

✖ **81.22 Arthrodesis of knee**

✖ **81.23 Arthrodesis of shoulder**

✖ **81.24 Arthrodesis of elbow**

✖ **81.25 Carporadial fusion**

✖ **81.26 Metacarpocarpal fusion**

✖ **81.27 Metacarpophalangeal fusion**

✖ **81.28 Interphalangeal fusion**

✖ **81.29 Arthrodesis of other specified joints**

● **81.3 Refusion of spine**

Includes arthrodesis of spine with:
>> bone graft
>> internal fixation
>> correction of pseudarthrosis of spine

Code also:
>> any insertion of interbody spinal fusion device
>> (84.51)
>> any insertion of recombinant bone morphogenetic
>> protein (84.52)
>> any synchronous excision of (locally) harvested
>> bone for graft (77.70–77.79)
>> the total number of vertebrae fused (81.62–81.64)
Coding Clinic: 2005, Q4, P122-123

✖ **81.30 Refusion of spine, not otherwise specified**
MS-DRG: Refer to Part VI, Appendix E, Table 4,
Spinal Fusion Reference Table

✖ **81.31 Refusion of atlas-axis spine**
Craniocervical fusion by anterior, transoral, or
posterior technique
C1-C2 fusion by anterior, transoral, or posterior
technique
Occiput C2 fusion by anterior, transoral, or
posterior technique
MS-DRG: Refer to Part VI, Appendix E, Table 4,
Spinal Fusion Reference Table

✖ **81.32 Refusion of other cervical spine, anterior
technique**
Arthrodesis of C2 level or below:
anterior (interbody) technique
anterolateral technique
MS-DRG: Refer to Part VI, Appendix E, Table 4,
Spinal Fusion Reference Table

✖ **81.33 Refusion of other cervical spine, posterior
technique**
Arthrodesis of C2 level or below:
posterior (interbody) technique
posterolateral technique
MS-DRG: Refer to Part VI, Appendix E, Table 4,
Spinal Fusion Reference Table

✖ **81.34 Refusion of dorsal and dorsolumbar spine,
anterior technique**
Arthrodesis of thoracic or thoracolumbar
region:
anterior (interbody) technique
anterolateral technique
MS-DRG: Refer to Part VI, Appendix E, Table 4,
Spinal Fusion Reference Table

✖ **81.35 Refusion of dorsal and dorsolumbar spine,
posterior technique**
Arthrodesis of thoracic or thoracolumbar
region:
posterior (interbody) technique
posterolateral technique
MS-DRG: Refer to Part VI, Appendix E, Table 4,
Spinal Fusion Reference Table

✖ **81.36 Refusion of lumbar and lumbosacral spine,
anterior technique**
Anterior lumbar interbody fusion (ALIF)
Arthrodesis of lumbar or lumbosacral region:
anterior (interbody) technique
anterolateral technique
MS-DRG: Refer to Part VI, Appendix E, Table 4,
Spinal Fusion Reference Table

✖ **81.37 Refusion of lumbar and lumbosacral spine,
lateral transverse process technique**
MS-DRG: Refer to Part VI, Appendix E, Table 4,
Spinal Fusion Reference Table

✖ **81.38 Refusion of lumbar and lumbosacral spine,
posterior technique**
Arthrodesis of lumbar or lumbosacral region:
posterior (interbody) technique
posterolateral technique
Posterior lumbar interbody fusion (PLIF)
Transforaminal lumbar interbody fusion (TLIF)
MS-DRG: Refer to Part VI, Appendix E, Table 4,
Spinal Fusion Reference Table

✖ **81.39 Refusion of spine, not elsewhere classified**
MS-DRG: Refer to Part VI, Appendix E, Table 4,
Spinal Fusion Reference Table

● **81.4 Other repair of joint of lower extremity**

Includes arthroplasty of lower extremity with:
>> external traction or fixation
>> graft of bone (chips) or cartilage
>> internal fixation device

✖ **81.40 Repair of hip, not elsewhere classified**

✖ **81.42 Five-in-one repair of knee**
Medial meniscectomy, medial collateral
ligament repair, vastus medialis
advancement, semitendinosus
advancement, and pes anserinus transfer

✖ **81.43 Triad knee repair**
Medial meniscectomy with repair of the
anterior cruciate ligament and the medial
collateral ligament
O'Donoghue procedure

✖ **81.44 Patellar stabilization**
Roux-Goldthwait operation for recurrent
dislocation of patella

✖ **81.45 Other repair of the cruciate ligaments**

✖ **81.46 Other repair of the collateral ligaments**
Coding Clinic: 1995, Q1, P8

✖ **81.47 Other repair of knee**
Coding Clinic: 2006, Q2, P13-14; 2003, Q2, P18; 2000, Q1,
P12-13; 1996, Q2, P4; 1995, Q1, P8; 1993, Q3, P5

✖ **81.49 Other repair of ankle**
Coding Clinic: 2001, Q2, P14-15; 2000, Q3, P4

● **81.5 Joint replacement of lower extremity**
Note: Removal of prior prosthesis - *omit code* ◄

Includes arthroplasty of lower extremity with:
>> external traction or fixation
>> graft of bone (chips) or cartilage
>> internal fixation device or prosthesis

OPERATIONS ON THE MUSCULOSKELETAL SYSTEM (76–84)

✖ **81.51 Total hip replacement**
Replacement of both femoral head and
acetabulum by prosthesis
Total reconstruction of hip
> Code also any type of bearing surface, if
> known (00.74–00.77)
> Coding Clinic: 2009, Q2, P11; 2004, Q4, P111-113; 1992, Q2, P18
> MCE: Bilateral procedure when 2+ different joint
> procedures are reported with principal
> diagnosis causes assigned to MDC 10

✖ **81.52 Partial hip replacement**
Bipolar endoprosthesis
> Code also any type of bearing surface, if
> known (00.74–00.77)
> Coding Clinic: 1992, Q2, P18
> MCE: Bilateral procedure when 2+ different joint
> procedures are reported with principal
> diagnosis causes assigned to MDC 10

✖ **81.53 Revision of hip replacement, not otherwise
specified**
Revision of hip replacement, not specified as
to components(s) replaced (acetabular,
femoral, or both)
> Code also any:
> removal of (cement) (joint) spacer (84.57)
> type of bearing surface, if known
> (00.74–00.77)
> > Excludes *revision of hip replacement,
> > components specified
> > (00.70–00.73)*
> Coding Clinic: 2005, Q4, P106-113; 1997, Q3, P13

✖ **81.54 Total knee replacement**
Bicompartmental
Partial knee replacement ◀
Tricompartmental
Unicompartmental (hemijoint)
> Coding Clinic: 1985, Nov-Dec, P11
> MCE: Bilateral procedure when 2+ different joint
> procedures are reported with principal
> diagnosis causes assigned to MDC 10

✖ **81.55 Revision of knee replacement, not otherwise
specified**
> Code also any removal of (cement) spacer
> (84.57)
> > Excludes *arthrodesis of knee (81.22)
> > revision of knee replacement,
> > components specified
> > (00.80–00.84)*
> Coding Clinic: 2005, Q4, P113-117; 1997, Q2, P10

✖ **81.56 Total ankle replacement**
> MCE: Bilateral procedure when 2+ different joint
> procedures are reported with principal
> diagnosis causes assigned to MDC 11

✖ **81.57 Replacement of joint of foot and toe**

✖ **81.59 Revision of joint replacement of lower
extremity, not elsewhere classified**
> Coding Clinic: 1988, Q1, P9

● **81.6 Other procedures on spine**
Note: Number of vertebrae
The vertebral spine consists of 25 vertebrae in the
following order and number:
Cervical: C1 (atlas), C2 (axis), C3, C4, C5, C6, C7
Thoracic or Dorsal: T1, T2, T3, T4, T5, T6, T7, T8,
T9, T10, T11, T12
Lumbar and Sacral: L1, L2, L3, L4, L5, S1
Coders should report only one code from the series
81.62 or 81.63 or 81.64 to show the total number
of vertebrae fused on the patient.
> Code also the level and approach of the fusion or
> refusion (81.00–81.08, 81.30–81.39)
> Coding Clinic: 2009, Q2, P4

81.62 Fusion or refusion of 2–3 vertebrae
> Coding Clinic: 2009, Q2, P4; 2008, Q2, P14-15; 2008, Q1, P5-6;
> 2006, Q1, P12-14x2; 2005, Q4, P122-123

81.63 Fusion or refusion of 4–8 vertebrae
> Coding Clinic: 2007, Q1, P20-21; 2003, Q4, P99-101

81.64 Fusion or refusion of 9 or more vertebrae
◆ Non-OR Procedure that affects MS-DRG
assignment to MDC 08, MS-DRG 456-458

✖ **81.65 Percutaneous vertebroplasty**
Injection of bone void filler (cement)
(polymethylmethacrylate) (PMMA) into
the diseased or fractured vertebral body
> > Excludes *kyphoplasty (81.66)
> > percutaneous vertebral augmentation
> > (81.66)*
> Coding Clinic: 2008, Q2, P14-15; 2004, Q4, P125-126; 2002,
> Q2, P14-15

✖ **81.66 Percutaneous vertebral augmentation**
Insertion of inflatable balloon, bone tamp, or
other device displacing (removing)
(compacting) bone to create a space
(cavity) (void) prior to the injection of
bone void filler (cement)
(polymethylmethacrylate) (PMMA) or
other substance
Arcuplasty
Kyphoplasty
SKyphoplasty
Spineoplasty
> > Excludes *percutaneous vertebroplasty (81.65)*
> Coding Clinic: 2008, Q2, P15; 2007, Q1, P3-8x2; 2006, Q3, P13;
> 2004, Q4, P125-126; 2002, Q2, P14

● **81.7 Arthroplasty and repair of hand, fingers and wrist**
> Includes arthroplasty of hand and finger with:
> external traction or fixation
> graft of bone (chips) or cartilage
> internal fixation device or prosthesis
> > Excludes *operations on muscle, tendon and fascia of
> > hand (82.01–82.99)*

✖ **81.71 Arthroplasty of metacarpophalangeal and
interphalangeal joint with implant**

✖ **81.72 Arthroplasty of metacarpophalangeal and
interphalangeal joint without implant**
> Coding Clinic: 1993, Q1, P28

✖ **81.73 Total wrist replacement**

✖ **81.74 Arthroplasty of carpocarpal or carpometacarpal
joint with implant**

✖ **81.75 Arthroplasty of carpocarpal or carpometacarpal
joint without implant**
> Coding Clinic: 1993, Q3, P8

✖ **81.79 Other repair of hand, fingers and wrist**

● **81.8 Arthroplasty and repair of shoulder and elbow**
> Includes arthroplasty of upper limb NEC with:
> external traction or fixation
> graft of bone (chips) or cartilage
> internal fixation device or prosthesis

✖ **81.80 Total shoulder replacement**
> Coding Clinic: 2008, Q2, P5-6

✖ **81.81 Partial shoulder replacement**

✖ **81.82 Repair of recurrent dislocation of shoulder**
> Coding Clinic: 1995, Q3, P15

✖ **81.83 Other repair of shoulder**
Revision of arthroplasty of shoulder
> Coding Clinic: 2004, Q1, P12; 2002, Q4, P110; Q1, P9-10;
> 2001, Q4, P52; 2000, Q2, P14-15; 1993, Q3, P5

OPERATIONS ON THE MUSCULOSKELETAL SYSTEM (76–84)

◀ New   ◀▥ Revised   ~~deleted~~ Deleted   ● Use Additional Digit(s)   ✖ Valid O.R. Procedure
◆ Non-O.R. Procedure   ♀ Females Only   ♂ Males Only

✱ **81.84 Total elbow replacement**
Partial elbow replacement ◄

✱ **81.85 Other repair of elbow**

● **81.9 Other operations on joint structures**

81.91 Arthrocentesis
Joint aspiration
| Excludes | that for:
         arthrography (88.32)
         biopsy of joint structure
            (80.30–80.39)
         injection of drug (81.92)

81.92 Injection of therapeutic substance into joint or ligament
Coding Clinic: 2000, Q2, P14-15; 1989, Q3, P16

✱ **81.93 Suture of capsule or ligament of upper extremity**
| Excludes | that associated with arthroplasty
         (81.71–81.75, 81.80–81.81,
         81.84)

✱ **81.94 Suture of capsule or ligament of ankle and foot**
| Excludes | that associated with arthroplasty
         (81.56–81.59)

✱ **81.95 Suture of capsule or ligament of other lower extremity**
| Excludes | that associated with arthroplasty
         (81.51–81.55, 81.59)

✱ **81.96 Other repair of joint**

✱ **81.97 Revision of joint replacement of upper extremity**
Partial
Removal of cement spacer
Total
Coding Clinic: 2004, Q1, P12

✱ **81.98 Other diagnostic procedures on joint structures**
| Excludes | arthroscopy (80.20–80.29)
         biopsy of joint structure (80.30–80.39)
         microscopic examination of specimen
            from joint (91.51–91.59)
         thermography (88.83)
         x-ray (87.21–87.29, 88.21–88.33)

✱ **81.99 Other**

● **82 Operations on muscle, tendon, and fascia of hand**
| Includes | operations on:
         aponeurosis
         synovial membrane (tendon sheath)
         tendon sheath

● **82.0 Incision of muscle, tendon, fascia, and bursa of hand**

✱ **82.01 Exploration of tendon sheath of hand**
Incision of tendon sheath of hand
Removal of rice bodies in tendon sheath of hand
| Excludes | division of tendon (82.11)

✱ **82.02 Myotomy of hand**
| Excludes | myotomy for division (82.19)

✱ **82.03 Bursotomy of hand**

82.04 Incision and drainage of palmar or thenar space

✱ **82.09 Other incision of soft tissue of hand**
| Excludes | incision of skin and subcutaneous
         tissue alone (86.01–86.09)
Coding Clinic: 1987, Nov-Dec, P10

● **82.1 Division of muscle, tendon, and fascia of hand**

✱ **82.11 Tenotomy of hand**
Division of tendon of hand

✱ **82.12 Fasciotomy of hand**
Division of fascia of hand

✱ **82.19 Other division of soft tissue of hand**
Division of muscle of hand

● **82.2 Excision of lesion of muscle, tendon, and fascia of hand**

✱ **82.21 Excision of lesion of tendon sheath of hand**
Ganglionectomy of tendon sheath (wrist)

✱ **82.22 Excision of lesion of muscle of hand**

✱ **82.29 Excision of other lesion of soft tissue of hand**
| Excludes | excision of lesion of skin and
         subcutaneous tissue (86.21–86.3)

● **82.3 Other excision of soft tissue of hand**
| Code also | any skin graft (86.61–86.62, 86.73)
| Excludes | excision of skin and subcutaneous tissue
         (86.21–86.3)

✱ **82.31 Bursectomy of hand**

✱ **82.32 Excision of tendon of hand for graft**

✱ **82.33 Other tenonectomy of hand**
Tenosynovectomy of hand
| Excludes | excision of lesion of:
         tendon (82.29)
         sheath (82.21)

✱ **82.34 Excision of muscle or fascia of hand for graft**

✱ **82.35 Other fasciectomy of hand**
Release of Dupuytren's contracture
| Excludes | excision of lesion of fascia (82.29)

✱ **82.36 Other myectomy of hand**
| Excludes | excision of lesion of muscle (82.22)

✱ **82.39 Other excision of soft tissue of hand**
| Excludes | excision of skin (86.21–86.3)
         excision of soft tissue lesion (82.29)

● **82.4 Suture of muscle, tendon, and fascia of hand**

✱ **82.41 Suture of tendon sheath of hand**

✱ **82.42 Delayed suture of flexor tendon of hand**

✱ **82.43 Delayed suture of other tendon of hand**

✱ **82.44 Other suture of flexor tendon of hand**
| Excludes | delayed suture of flexor tendon of hand
         (82.42)

✱ **82.45 Other suture of other tendon of hand**
| Excludes | delayed suture of other tendon of hand
         (82.43)

✱ **82.46 Suture of muscle or fascia of hand**

● **82.5 Transplantation of muscle and tendon of hand**

✱ **82.51 Advancement of tendon of hand**

✱ **82.52 Recession of tendon of hand**

✱ **82.53 Reattachment of tendon of hand**

✱ **82.54 Reattachment of muscle of hand**

✱ **82.55 Other change in hand muscle or tendon length**

✱ **82.56 Other hand tendon transfer or transplantation**
| Excludes | pollicization of thumb (82.61)
         transfer of finger, except thumb (82.81)
Coding Clinic: 1999, Q2, P10; 1998, Q43, P39-40

✱ **82.57 Other hand tendon transposition**
Coding Clinic: 1993, Q3, P8; Q1, P28

✱ **82.58 Other hand muscle transfer or transplantation**

✱ **82.59 Other hand muscle transposition**

● **82.6 Reconstruction of thumb**
| Includes | digital transfer to act as thumb
| Code also | any amputation for digital transfer (84.01, 84.11)

OPERATIONS ON THE MUSCULOSKELETAL SYSTEM (76–84)

OPERATIONS ON THE MUSCULOSKELETAL SYSTEM (76–84)

�ö **82.61 Pollicization operation carrying over nerves and blood supply**

✖ **82.69 Other reconstruction of thumb**
"Cocked-hat" procedure [skin flap and bone]
Grafts:
bone to thumb skin (pedicle) to thumb

● **82.7 Plastic operation on hand with graft or implant**

✖ **82.71 Tendon pulley reconstruction**
Reconstruction for opponensplasty

✖ **82.72 Plastic operation on hand with graft of muscle or fascia**

✖ **82.79 Plastic operation on hand with other graft or implant**
Tendon graft to hand

● **82.8 Other plastic operations on hand**

✖ **82.81 Transfer of finger, except thumb**
| **Excludes** | *pollicization of thumb (82.61)* |
Coding Clinic: 2005, Q2, P7

✖ **82.82 Repair of cleft hand**

✖ **82.83 Repair of macrodactyly**

✖ **82.84 Repair of mallet finger**

✖ **82.85 Other tenodesis of hand**
Tendon fixation of hand NOS

✖ **82.86 Other tenoplasty of hand**
Myotenoplasty of hand

✖ **82.89 Other plastic operations on hand**
Plication of fascia
Repair of fascial hernia
| **Excludes** | *that with graft or implant (82.71–82.79)* |

● **82.9 Other operations on muscle, tendon, and fascia of hand**
| **Excludes** | *diagnostic procedures on soft tissue of hand (83.21–83.29)* |

✖ **82.91 Lysis of adhesions of hand**
Freeing of adhesions of fascia, muscle, and tendon of hand
| **Excludes** | *decompression of carpal tunnel (04.43)* |
| | *that by stretching or manipulation only (93.26)* |

82.92 Aspiration of bursa of hand

82.93 Aspiration of other soft tissue of hand
| **Excludes** | *skin and subcutaneous tissue (86.01)* |

82.94 Injection of therapeutic substance into bursa of hand

82.95 Injection of therapeutic substance into tendon of hand

82.96 Other injection of locally-acting therapeutic substance into soft tissue of hand
| **Excludes** | *subcutaneous or intramuscular injection (99.11–99.29)* |

✖ **82.99 Other operations on muscle, tendon, and fascia of hand**

● **83 Operations on muscle, tendon, fascia, and bursa, except hand**
| **Includes** | operations on: |
aponeurosis
synovial membrane of bursa and tendon sheaths
tendon sheaths
Excludes	*diaphragm (34.81–34.89)*
	hand (82.01–82.99)
	muscles of eye (15.01–15.9)

● **83.0 Incision of muscle, tendon, fascia, and bursa**

✖ **83.01 Exploration of tendon sheath**
Incision of tendon sheath
Removal of rice bodies from tendon sheath

✖ **83.02 Myotomy**
| **Excludes** | *cricopharyngeal myotomy (29.31)* |
Coding Clinic: 2008, Q4, P134-136

✖ **83.03 Bursotomy**
Removal of calcareous deposit of bursa
| **Excludes** | *aspiration of bursa (percutaneous) (83.94)* |

✖ **83.09 Other incision of soft tissue**
Incision of fascia
| **Excludes** | *incision of skin and subcutaneous tissue alone (86.01–86.09)* |
Coding Clinic: 2009, Q1, P15

● **83.1 Division of muscle, tendon, and fascia**

✖ **83.11 Achillotenotomy**

✖ **83.12 Adductor tenotomy of hip**

✖ **83.13 Other tenotomy**
Aponeurotomy
Division of tendon
Tendon release
Tendon transection
Tenotomy for thoracic outlet decompression

✖ **83.14 Fasciotomy**
Division of fascia
Division of iliotibial band
Fascia stripping
Release of Volkmann's contracture by fasciotomy
Coding Clinic: 2006, Q4, P100-102

✖ **83.19 Other division of soft tissue**
Division of muscle
Muscle release
Myotomy for thoracic outlet decompression
Myotomy with division
Scalenotomy
Transection of muscle

● **83.2 Diagnostic procedures on muscle, tendon, fascia, and bursa, including that of hand**

✖ **83.21 Biopsy of soft tissue**
| **Excludes** | *biopsy of chest wall (34.23)* |
| | *biopsy of skin and subcutaneous tissue (86.11)* |

✖ **83.29 Other diagnostic procedures on muscle, tendon, fascia, and bursa, including that of hand**
Excludes	*microscopic examination of specimen (91.51–91.59)*
	soft tissue x-ray (87.09, 87.38–87.39, 88.09, 88.35, 88.37)
	thermography of muscle (88.84)

● **83.3 Excision of lesion of muscle, tendon, fascia, and bursa**
| **Excludes** | *biopsy of soft tissue (83.21)* |

✖ **83.31 Excision of lesion of tendon sheath**
Excision of ganglion of tendon sheath, except of hand

✖ **83.32 Excision of lesion of muscle**
Excision of:
heterotopic bone
muscle scar for release of Volkmann's contracture
myositis ossificans

◀ New   ◀ⅢⅢ Revised   ~~deleted~~ Deleted   ● Use Additional Digit(s)   ✖ Valid O.R. Procedure
◆ Non-O.R. Procedure   ♀ Females Only   ♂ Males Only

✖ **83.39 Excision of lesion of other soft tissue**
Excision of Baker's cyst

> **Excludes** *bursectomy (83.5)*
> *excision of lesion of skin and*
> *subcutaneous tissue (86.3)*
> *synovectomy (80.70–80.79)*
> Coding Clinic: 2005, Q2, P3-4; 1997, Q2, P6

● **83.4 Other excision of muscle, tendon, and fascia**

✖ **83.41 Excision of tendon for graft**

✖ **83.42 Other tenonectomy**
Excision of:
    aponeurosis
    tendon sheath
Tenosynovectomy

✖ **83.43 Excision of muscle or fascia for graft**

✖ **83.44 Other fasciectomy**

✖ **83.45 Other myectomy**
Debridement of muscle NOS
Scalenectomy
Coding Clinic: 1999, Q1, P8-9

✖ **83.49 Other excision of soft tissue**

✖ **83.5 Bursectomy**
Coding Clinic: 2006, Q2, P15x2; 1999, Q2, P10-11

● **83.6 Suture of muscle, tendon, and fascia**

✖ **83.61 Suture of tendon sheath**

✖ **83.62 Delayed suture of tendon**

✖ **83.63 Rotator cuff repair**
Coding Clinic: 2006, Q1, P6; 1993, Q2, P8

✖ **83.64 Other suture of tendon**
Achillorrhaphy
Aponeurorrhaphy

> **Excludes** *delayed suture of tendon (83.62)*

✖ **83.65 Other suture of muscle or fascia**
Repair of diastasis recti

● **83.7 Reconstruction of muscle and tendon**

> **Excludes** *reconstruction of muscle and tendon associated*
> *with arthroplasty*

✖ **83.71 Advancement of tendon**

✖ **83.72 Recession of tendon**

✖ **83.73 Reattachment of tendon**

✖ **83.74 Reattachment of muscle**

✖ **83.75 Tendon transfer or transplantation**

✖ **83.76 Other tendon transposition**

✖ **83.77 Muscle transfer or transplantation**
Release of Volkmann's contracture by muscle
    transplantation

✖ **83.79 Other muscle transposition**

● **83.8 Other plastic operations on muscle, tendon, and fascia**

> **Excludes** *plastic operations on muscle, tendon, and*
> *fascia associated with arthroplasty*

✖ **83.81 Tendon graft**

✖ **83.82 Graft of muscle or fascia**
Coding Clinic: 2001, Q3, P9

✖ **83.83 Tendon pulley reconstruction**

✖ **83.84 Release of clubfoot, not elsewhere classified**
Evans operation on clubfoot

✖ **83.85 Other change in muscle or tendon length**
Hamstring lengthening
Heel cord shortening
Plastic achillotenotomy
Tendon plication

✖ **83.86 Quadricepsplasty**

✖ **83.87 Other plastic operations on muscle**
Musculoplasty
Myoplasty
Coding Clinic: 1997, Q1, P9-10

✖ **83.88 Other plastic operations on tendon**
Myotenoplasty
Tendon fixation
Tenodesis
Tenoplasty

✖ **83.89 Other plastic operations on fascia**
Fascia lengthening
Fascioplasty
Plication of fascia

● **83.9 Other operations on muscle, tendon, fascia, and bursa**

> **Excludes** *nonoperative:*
> *manipulation (93.25–93.29)*
> *stretching (93.27–93.29)*

✖ **83.91 Lysis of adhesions of muscle, tendon, fascia, and
bursa**

> **Excludes** *that for tarsal tunnel syndrome (04.44)*

✖ **83.92 Insertion or replacement of skeletal muscle
stimulator**
Implantation, insertion, placement, or
    replacement of skeletal muscle:
    electrodes
    stimulator
Coding Clinic: 1999, Q2, P10

✖ **83.93 Removal of skeletal muscle stimulator**

83.94 Aspiration of bursa

83.95 Aspiration of other soft tissue

> **Excludes** *that of skin and subcutaneous tissue*
> *(86.01)*

83.96 Injection of therapeutic substance into bursa

83.97 Injection of therapeutic substance into tendon

**83.98 Injection of locally-acting therapeutic substance
into other soft tissue**

> **Excludes** *subcutaneous or intramuscular*
> *injection (99.11–99.29)*
> Coding Clinic: 2006, Q2, P11

✖ **83.99 Other operations on muscle, tendon, fascia, and
bursa**
Suture of bursa

● **84 Other procedures on musculoskeletal system**

● **84.0 Amputation of upper limb**

> **Excludes** *revision of amputation stump (84.3)*

✖ **84.00 Upper limb amputation, not otherwise specified**
Closed flap amputation of upper limb NOS
Kineplastic amputation of upper limb NOS
Open or guillotine amputation of upper limb
    NOS
Revision of current traumatic amputation of
    upper limb NOS

✖ **84.01 Amputation and disarticulation of finger**

> **Excludes** *ligation of supernumerary finger*
> *(86.26)*

✖ **84.02 Amputation and disarticulation of thumb**

✖ **84.03 Amputation through hand**
Amputation through carpals

✖ **84.04 Disarticulation of wrist**

✖ **84.05 Amputation through forearm**
Forearm amputation

✖ **84.06 Disarticulation of elbow**

✖ **84.07 Amputation through humerus**
Upper arm amputation

✖ **84.08 Disarticulation of shoulder**

✖ **84.09 Interthoracoscapular amputation**
Forequarter amputation

● **84.1 Amputation of lower limb**

> Excludes revision of amputation stump (84.3)

✖ **84.10 Lower limb amputation, not otherwise specified**
Closed flap amputation of lower limb NOS
Kineplastic amputation of lower limb NOS
Open or guillotine amputation of lower limb NOS
Revision of current traumatic amputation of lower limb NOS

✖ **84.11 Amputation of toe**
Amputation through metatarsophalangeal joint
Disarticulation of toe
Metatarsal head amputation
Ray amputation of foot (disarticulation of the metatarsal head of the toe extending across the forefoot just proximal to the metatarsophalangeal crease)

> Excludes ligation of supernumerary toe (86.26)

Coding Clinic: 2005, Q2, P7

✖ **84.12 Amputation through foot**
Amputation of forefoot
Amputation through middle of foot
Chopart's amputation
Midtarsal amputation
Transmetatarsal amputation (amputation of the forefoot, including all the toes)

> Excludes ray amputation of foot (84.11)

✖ **84.13 Disarticulation of ankle**

✖ **84.14 Amputation of ankle through malleoli of tibia and fibula**

✖ **84.15 Other amputation below knee**
Amputation of leg through tibia and fibula NOS

✖ **84.16 Disarticulation of knee**
Batch, Spitler, and McFaddin amputation
Mazet amputation
S.P. Roger's amputation

✖ **84.17 Amputation above knee**
Amputation of leg through femur
Amputation of thigh
Conversion of below-knee amputation into above-knee amputation
Supracondylar above-knee amputation
Coding Clinic: 2005, Q1, P16; 2003, Q3, P14-15; 1995, Q1, P10; 1988, Q4, P12

✖ **84.18 Disarticulation of hip**

✖ **84.19 Abdominopelvic amputation**
Hemipelvectomy
Hindquarter amputation

● **84.2 Reattachment of extremity**

✖ **84.21 Thumb reattachment**

✖ **84.22 Finger reattachment**

✖ **84.23 Forearm, wrist, or hand reattachment**

✖ **84.24 Upper arm reattachment**
Reattachment of arm NOS

✖ **84.25 Toe reattachment**

✖ **84.26 Foot reattachment**

✖ **84.27 Lower leg or ankle reattachment**
Reattachment of leg NOS
Coding Clinic: 1995, Q1, P8

✖ **84.28 Thigh reattachment**

✖ **84.29 Other reattachment**

✖ **84.3 Revision of amputation stump**
Reamputation of stump
Secondary closure of stump
Trimming of stump

> Excludes revision of current traumatic amputation [revision by further amputation of current injury] (84.00–84.19, 84.91)

Coding Clinic: 2005, Q1, P14,16; 1999, Q4, P15; 1998, Q4, P12; Q2, P15

● **84.4 Implantation or fitting of prosthetic limb device**

✖ **84.40 Implantation or fitting of prosthetic limb device, not otherwise specified**

84.41 Fitting of prosthesis of upper arm and shoulder

84.42 Fitting of prosthesis of lower arm and hand

84.43 Fitting of prosthesis of arm, not otherwise specified

✖ **84.44 Implantation of prosthetic device of arm**

84.45 Fitting of prosthesis above knee

84.46 Fitting of prosthesis below knee

84.47 Fitting of prosthesis of leg, not otherwise specified

✖ **84.48 Implantation of prosthetic device of leg**

● **84.5 Implantation of other musculoskeletal devices and substances**

> Excludes insertion of (non-fusion) spinal disc replacement device (84.60–84.69)

84.51 Insertion of interbody spinal fusion device
Insertion of: cages (carbon, ceramic, metal, plastic or titanium)
interbody fusion cage
synthetic cages or spacers
threaded bone dowels

> Code also refusion of spine (81.30–81.39)

> Code also spinal fusion (81.00–81.08)

Coding Clinic: 2009, Q2, P4; 2008, Q2, P14-15; 2007, Q1, P20-21; 2005, Q4, P122-123; 2004, Q1, P21-22; 2003, Q2, P20; 2002, Q4, P108-110

84.52 Insertion of recombinant bone morphogenetic protein rhBMP
That via collagen sponge, coral, ceramic and other carriers

> Code also primary procedure performed:
fracture repair (79.00–79.99)
spinal fusion (81.00–81.08)
spinal refusion (81.30–81.39)

Coding Clinic: 2009, Q2, P4x2; 2006, Q1, P13-14; 2002, Q4, P110-111

84.53 Implantation of internal limb lengthening device with kinetic distraction

> Code also limb lengthening procedure (78.30–78.39)

Coding Clinic: 2004, Q4, P127

84.54 Implantation of other internal limb lengthening device
Implantation of internal limb lengthening device, Not Otherwise Specified (NOS)

> Code also limb lengthening procedure (78.30–78.39)

Coding Clinic: 2004, Q4, P127

◄ New   ◄ Revised   ~~deleted~~ Deleted   ● Use Additional Digit(s)   ✖ Valid O.R. Procedure
◆ Non-O.R. Procedure   ♀ Females Only   ♂ Males Only

OPERATIONS ON THE MUSCULOSKELETAL SYSTEM (76–84)

84.55   Insertion of bone void filler
Insertion of:
    acrylic cement (PMMA)
    bone void cement
    calcium based bone void filler
    polymethylmethacrylate (PMMA)

> **Excludes** | *that with percutaneous vertebral*
> *augmentation (81.66)*
> *that with percutaneous vertebroplasty*
> *(81.65)*

Coding Clinic: 2004, Q4, P128-129

84.56   Insertion or replacement of (cement) spacer
Insertion or replacement of joint
    (methylmethacrylate) spacer
Coding Clinic: 2008, Q2, P3-4; 2005, Q4, P124-125

84.57   Removal of (cement) spacer
Removal of joint (methylmethacrylate)
    spacer
Coding Clinic: 2008, Q2, P3-6; 2005, Q4, P124-125

✖84.59   Insertion of other spinal devices

> **Excludes** | *initial insertion of pedicle screws with*
> *spinal fusion— omit code*
> *insertion of facet replacement device(s)*
> *(84.84)*
> *insertion of interspinous process*
> *device(s) (84.80)*
> *insertion of pedicle-based dynamic*
> *stabilization device(s) (84.82)*

Coding Clinic: 2007, Q1, P9-10

●84.6   Replacement of spinal disc

> **Includes**   non-fusion arthroplasty of the spine with
> insertion of artificial disc prosthesis

✖84.60   Insertion of spinal disc prosthesis, not otherwise specified
Replacement of spinal disc, NOS

> **Includes**   diskectomy (discectomy)

✖84.61   Insertion of partial spinal disc prosthesis, cervical
Nuclear replacement device, cervical
Partial artificial disc prosthesis (flexible),
    cervical
Replacement of nuclear disc (nucleus
    pulposus), cervical

> **Includes**   diskectomy (discectomy)

✖84.62   Insertion of total spinal disc prosthesis, cervical
Replacement of cervical spinal disc, NOS
Replacement of total spinal disc, cervical
Total artificial disc prosthesis (flexible),
    cervical

> **Includes**   diskectomy (discectomy)

✖84.63   Insertion of spinal disc prosthesis, thoracic
Artificial disc prosthesis (flexible), thoracic
Replacement of thoracic spinal disc, partial or
    total

> **Includes**   diskectomy (discectomy)

✖84.64   Insertion of partial spinal disc prosthesis, lumbosacral
Nuclear replacement device, lumbar
Partial artificial disc prosthesis (flexible),
    lumbar
Replacement of nuclear disc (nucleus
    pulposus), lumbar

> **Includes**   diskectomy (discectomy)

✖84.65   Insertion of total spinal disc prosthesis, lumbosacral
Replacement of lumbar spinal disc, NOS
Replacement of total spinal disc, lumbar
Total artificial disc prosthesis (flexible), lumbar

> **Includes**   diskectomy (discectomy)

Coding Clinic: 2004, Q4, P129-133
MCE: Non-covered procedure when beneficiary
    age >60

✖84.66   Revision or replacement of artificial spinal disc prosthesis, cervical
Removal of (partial) (total) spinal disc
    prosthesis with synchronous insertion
    of new (partial) (total) spinal disc
    prosthesis, cervical
Repair of previously inserted spinal disc
    prosthesis, cervical

✖84.67   Revision or replacement of artificial spinal disc prosthesis, thoracic
Removal of (partial) (total) spinal disc
    prosthesis with synchronous insertion
    of new (partial) (total) spinal disc
    prosthesis, thoracic
Repair of previously inserted spinal disc
    prosthesis, thoracic

✖84.68   Revision or replacement of artificial spinal disc prosthesis, lumbosacral
Removal of (partial) (total) spinal disc
    prosthesis with synchronous insertion
    of new (partial) (total) spinal disc
    prosthesis, lumbosacral
Repair of previously inserted spinal disc
    prosthesis, lumbosacral

✖84.69   Revision or replacement of artificial spinal disc prosthesis, not otherwise specified
Removal of (partial) (total) spinal disc
    prosthesis with synchronous insertion of
    new (partial) (total) spinal disc prosthesis
Repair of previously inserted spinal disc
    prosthesis

●84.7   Adjunct codes for external fixator devices

> Code also   any primary procedure performed:
> application of external fixator device (78.10,
>   78.12–78.13, 78.15, 78.17–78.19)
> reduction of fracture and dislocation (79.00–79.89)

84.71   Application of external fixator device, monoplanar system

> **Excludes** | *other hybrid device or system (84.73)*
> *ring device or system (84.72)*

Coding Clinic: 2005, Q4, P127-129

84.72   Application of external fixator device, ring system
Ilizarov type
Sheffield type

> **Excludes** | *monoplanar device or system (84.71)*
> *other hybrid device or system (84.73)*

84.73   Application of hybrid external fixator device
Computer (assisted) (dependent) external
    fixator device
Hybrid system using both ring and
    monoplanar devices

> **Excludes** | *monoplanar device or system, when*
> *used alone (84.71)*
> *ring device or system, when used alone*
> *(84.72)*

OPERATIONS ON THE MUSCULOSKELETAL SYSTEM (76–84)

● **84.8 Insertion, replacement and revision of posterior spinal motion preservation device(s)**

Dynamic spinal stabilization device(s)

Includes any synchronous facetectomy (partial, total) performed at the same level

Code also any synchronous surgical decompression (foraminotomy, laminectomy, laminotomy), if performed (03.09)

Excludes *fusion of spine (81.00–81.08, 81.30–81.39)*
insertion of artificial disc prosthesis (84.60–84.69)
insertion of interbody spinal fusion device (84.51)

Coding Clinic: 2007, Q1, P9

✖ **84.80 Insertion or replacement of interspinous process device(s)**

Interspinous process decompression device(s)
Interspinous process distraction device(s)

Excludes *insertion or replacement of facet replacement device (84.84)*
insertion or replacement of pedicle-based dynamic stabilization device (84.82)

Coding Clinic: 2007, Q4, P116-120

✖ **84.81 Revision of interspinous process device(s)**

Repair of previously inserted interspinous process device(s)

Excludes *revision of facet replacement device(s) (84.85)*
revision of pedicle-based dynamic stabilization device (84.83)

✖ **84.82 Insertion or replacement of pedicle-based dynamic stabilization device(s)**

Excludes *initial insertion of pedicle screws with spinal fusion — omit code*
insertion or replacement of facet replacement device(s) (84.84)
insertion or replacement of interspinous process device(s) (84.80)
replacement of pedicle screws used in spinal fusion (78.59)

Coding Clinic: 2007, Q4, P116-120

✖ **84.83 Revision of pedicle-based dynamic stabilization device(s)**

Repair of previously inserted pedicle-based dynamic stabilization device(s)

Excludes *removal of pedicle screws used in spinal fusion (78.69)*
replacement of pedicle screws used in spinal fusion (78.59)
revision of facet replacement device(s) (84.85)
revision of interspinous process device(s) (84.81)

✖ **84.84 Insertion or replacement of facet replacement device(s)**

Facet arthroplasty

Excludes *initial insertion of pedicle screws with spinal fusion — omit code*
insertion or replacement of interspinous process device(s) (84.80)
insertion or replacement of pedicle-based dynamic stabilization device(s) (84.82)
replacement of pedicle screws used in spinal fusion (78.59)

Coding Clinic: 2007, Q4, P116-120

✖ **84.85 Revision of facet replacement device(s)**

Repair of previously inserted facet replacement device(s)

Excludes *removal of pedicle screws used in spinal fusion (78.69)*
replacement of pedicle screws used in spinal fusion (78.59)
revision of interspinous process device(s) (84.81)
revision of pedicle-based dynamic stabilization device(s) (84.83)

● **84.9 Other operations on musculoskeletal system**

Excludes *nonoperative manipulation (93.25–93.29)*

✖ **84.91 Amputation, not otherwise specified**

✖ **84.92 Separation of equal conjoined twins**

✖ **84.93 Separation of unequal conjoined twins**

Separation of conjoined twins NOS

✖ **84.99 Other**

◀ New ◀▥ Revised ~~deleted~~ Deleted ● Use Additional Digit(s) ✖ Valid O.R. Procedure
◆ Non-O.R. Procedure ♀ Females Only ♂ Males Only

15. OPERATIONS ON THE INTEGUMENTARY SYSTEM (85–86)

● **85 Operations on the breast**

> **Includes**   operations on the skin and subcutaneous tissue of:
> breast female or male
> previous mastectomy site female or male
> revision of previous mastectomy site

85.0 Mastotomy
Incision of breast (skin)
Mammotomy

> **Excludes** *aspiration of breast (85.91)*
> *removal of implant (85.94)*

Coding Clinic: 2004, Q1, P3-4; 1990, Q2, P27

● **85.1 Diagnostic procedures on breast**

85.11 Closed [percutaneous] [needle] biopsy of breast
Coding Clinic: 2000, Q2, P10; 1989, Q3, P17
MCE: Closed biopsy procedure

✖ **85.12 Open biopsy of breast**
Coding Clinic: 1989, Q3, P17; 1986, Mar-April, P11
MCE: Open biopsy procedure

85.19 Other diagnostic procedures on breast

> **Excludes** *mammary ductogram (87.35)*
> *mammography NEC (87.37)*
> *manual examination (89.36)*
> *microscopic examination of specimen (91.61–91.69)*
> *thermography (88.85)*
> *ultrasonography (88.73)*
> *xerography (87.36)*

● **85.2 Excision or destruction of breast tissue**

> **Excludes** *mastectomy (85.41–85.48)*
> *reduction mammoplasty (85.31–85.32)*

✖ **85.20 Excision or destruction of breast tissue, not otherwise specified**

> **Excludes** *laser interstitial thermal therapy [LITT] of lesion or tissue of breast under guidance (17.69)* ◀

✖ **85.21 Local excision of lesion of breast**
Lumpectomy
Removal of area of fibrosis from breast

> **Excludes** *biopsy of breast (85.11–85.12)*

Coding Clinic: 1990, Q2, P27; 1989, Q3, P17; 1985, Sept-Oct, P12

✖ **85.22 Resection of quadrant of breast**
Coding Clinic: 1985, Sept-Oct, P12

✖ **85.23 Subtotal mastectomy**

> **Excludes** *quadrant resection (85.22)*

Coding Clinic: 1992, Q2, P7; 1985, Sept-Oct, P12

✖ **85.24 Excision of ectopic breast tissue**
Excision of accessory nipple

✖ **85.25 Excision of nipple**

> **Excludes** *excision of accessory nipple (85.24)*

● **85.3 Reduction mammoplasty and subcutaneous mammectomy**
Coding Clinic: 1995, Q4, P79-80

✖ **85.31 Unilateral reduction mammoplasty**
Unilateral:
amputative mammoplasty
size reduction mammoplasty

✖ **85.32 Bilateral reduction mammoplasty**
Amputative mammoplasty
Reduction mammoplasty (for gynecomastia)

✖ **85.33 Unilateral subcutaneous mammectomy with synchronous implant**

> **Excludes** *that without synchronous implant (85.34)*

✖ **85.34 Other unilateral subcutaneous mammectomy**
Removal of breast tissue with preservation of skin and nipple
Subcutaneous mammectomy NOS

✖ **85.35 Bilateral subcutaneous mammectomy with synchronous implant**

> **Excludes** *that without synchronous implant (85.36)*

✖ **85.36 Other bilateral subcutaneous mammectomy**

● **85.4 Mastectomy**

✖ **85.41 Unilateral simple mastectomy**
Mastectomy:
NOS
complete

✖ **85.42 Bilateral simple mastectomy**
Bilateral complete mastectomy

✖ **85.43 Unilateral extended simple mastectomy**
Extended simple mastectomy NOS
Modified radical mastectomy
Simple mastectomy with excision of regional lymph nodes
Coding Clinic: 1984, May-June, P11

✖ **85.44 Bilateral extended simple mastectomy**

✖ **85.45 Unilateral radical mastectomy**
Excision of breast, pectoral muscles, and regional lymph nodes [axillary, clavicular, supraclavicular]
Radical mastectomy NOS

✖ **85.46 Bilateral radical mastectomy**

✖ **85.47 Unilateral extended radical mastectomy**
Excision of breast, muscles, and lymph nodes [axillary, clavicular, supraclavicular, internal mammary, and mediastinal]
Extended radical mastectomy NOS

✖ **85.48 Bilateral extended radical mastectomy**

● **85.5 Augmentation mammoplasty**

> **Excludes** *that associated with subcutaneous mammectomy (85.33, 85.35)*

Coding Clinic: 1995, Q4, P80

✖ **85.50 Augmentation mammoplasty, not otherwise specified**

85.51 Unilateral injection into breast for augmentation
Coding Clinic: 1997, Q3, P13

85.52 Bilateral injection into breast for augmentation
Injection into breast for augmentation NOS

✖ **85.53 Unilateral breast implant**
Coding Clinic: 2000, Q2, P18; 1998, Q2, P14

✖ **85.54 Bilateral breast implant**
Breast implant NOS

✖ **85.6 Mastopexy**

● **85.7 Total reconstruction of breast**
Coding Clinic: 2008, Q4, P185-187; 1993, Q1, P27-28

✖ **85.70 Total reconstruction of breast, not otherwise specified**
Perforator flap, free

✖ **85.71 Latissimus dorsi myocutaneous flap**

✖ **85.72 Transverse rectus abdominis myocutaneous (TRAM) flap, pedicled**

> **Excludes** *transverse rectus abdominis myocutaneous (TRAM) flap, free (85.73)*

Excludes   Includes   Use additional   Code also   Omit code

✖ **85.73 Transverse rectus abdominis myocutaneous (TRAM) flap, free**

> **Excludes** *transverse rectus abdominis myocutaneous (TRAM) flap, pedicled (85.72)*

✖ **85.74 Deep inferior epigastric artery perforator (DIEP) flap, free**

✖ **85.75 Superficial inferior epigastric artery (SIEA) flap, free**

✖ **85.76 Gluteal artery perforator (GAP) flap, free**

✖ **85.79 Other total reconstruction of breast**

> **Excludes** *deep inferior epigastric artery perforator (DIEP) flap, free (85.74)*
> *gluteal artery perforator (GAP) flap, free (85.76)*
> *latissimus dorsi myocutaneous flap (85.71)*
> *perforator flap, free (85.70)*
> *superficial inferior epigastric artery (SIEA) flap, free (85.75)*
> *total reconstruction of breast, not otherwise specified (85.70)*
> *transverse rectus abdominis myocutaneous (TRAM) flap, free (85.73)*
> *transverse rectus abdominis myocutaneous (TRAM) flap, pedicled (85.72)*

● **85.8 Other repair and plastic operations on breast**

> **Excludes** *that for:*
> *augmentation (85.50–85.54)*
> *reconstruction (85.70–85.76, 85.79)*
> *reduction (85.31–85.32)*

85.81 Suture of laceration of breast

✖ **85.82 Split-thickness graft to breast**

✖ **85.83 Full-thickness graft to breast**

✖ **85.84 Pedicle graft to breast**

✖ **85.85 Muscle flap graft to breast**

✖ **85.86 Transposition of nipple**
Coding Clinic: 1995, Q4, P79-80

✖ **85.87 Other repair or reconstruction of nipple**

✖ **85.89 Other mammoplasty**

● **85.9 Other operations on the breast**

85.91 Aspiration of breast

> **Excludes** *percutaneous biopsy of breast (85.11)*

85.92 Injection of therapeutic agent into breast

> **Excludes** *that for augmentation of breast (85.51–85.52)*

✖ **85.93 Revision of implant of breast**
Coding Clinic: 1998, Q2, P14

✖ **85.94 Removal of implant of breast**
Coding Clinic: 1998, Q2, P14; 1992, Q3, P4-5

✖ **85.95 Insertion of breast tissue expander**
Insertion (soft tissue) of tissue expander (one or more) under muscle or platysma to develop skin flaps for donor use

✖ **85.96 Removal of breast tissue expander**
Coding Clinic: 2000, Q2, P18

✖ **85.99 Other**
Coding Clinic: 1986, Nov-Dec, P9

● **86 Operations on skin and subcutaneous tissue**

Includes operations on:
> hair follicles
> male perineum
> nails
> sebaceous glands
> subcutaneous fat pads
> sudoriferous glands
> superficial fossae

> **Excludes** *those on skin of:*
> *anus (49.01–49.99)*
> *breast (mastectomy site) (85.0–85.99)*
> *ear (18.01–18.9)*
> *eyebrow (08.01–08.99)*
> *eyelid (08.01–08.99)*
> *female perineum (71.01–71.9)*
> *lips (27.0–27.99)*
> *nose (21.00–21.99)*
> *penis (64.0–64.99)*
> *scrotum (61.0–61.99)*
> *vulva (71.01–71.9)*

● **86.0 Incision of skin and subcutaneous tissue**

86.01 Aspiration of skin and subcutaneous tissue
Aspiration of:
> abscess of nail, skin, or subcutaneous tissue
> hematoma of nail, skin, or subcutaneous tissue
> seroma of nail, skin, or subcutaneous tissue
Coding Clinic: 1989, Q3, P16

86.02 Injection or tattooing of skin lesion or defect
Injection of filling material
Insertion of filling material
Pigmenting of skin of filling material

86.03 Incision of pilonidal sinus or cyst

> **Excludes** *marsupialization (86.21)*

86.04 Other incision with drainage of skin and subcutaneous tissue

> **Excludes** *drainage of:*
> *fascial compartments of face and mouth (27.0)*
> *palmar or thenar space (82.04)*
> *pilonidal sinus or cyst (86.03)*
Coding Clinic: 2009, Q1, P15; 2008, Q3, P8-9; 2004, Q4, P75-76

86.05 Incision with removal of foreign body or device from skin and subcutaneous tissue
Removal of carotid sinus baroreflex activation device
Removal of loop recorder
Removal of neurostimulator pulse generator (single array, dual array)
Removal of tissue expander(s) from skin or soft tissue other than breast tissue

> **Excludes** *removal of foreign body without incision (98.20–98.29)*
Coding Clinic: 1992, Q3, P9; 1986, Nov-Dec, P9

✖ **86.06 Insertion of totally implantable infusion pump**

Code also any associated catheterization

> **Excludes** *insertion of totally implantable vascular access device (86.07)*
Coding Clinic: 1999, Q2, P4; 1993, 5th Issue, P11; 1988, Q1, P8

86.07 Insertion of totally implantable vascular access device [VAD]
Totally implanted port

> **Excludes** *insertion of totally implantable infusion pump (86.06)*
Coding Clinic: 2001, Q1, P13-14; 1996, Q1, P5-6x2; 1994, Q2, P11; 1993, 5th Issue, P11

> ◆ Non-OR Procedure that affects MS-DRG assignment to MDC 09, MS-DRG 579-581; MDC 11, MS-DRG 673-675

◀ New   ◀■ Revised   ~~deleted~~ Deleted   ● Use Additional Digit(s)   ✖ Valid O.R. Procedure
◆ Non-O.R. Procedure   ♀ Females Only   ♂ Males Only

86.09 Other incision of skin and subcutaneous tissue
Creation of thalamic stimulator pulse generator
pocket, new site
Escharotomy
Exploration:
sinus tract, skin
superficial fossa
Relocation of subcutaneous device pocket
NEC
Reopening subcutaneous pocket for device
revision without replacement
Undercutting of hair follicle

> **Excludes** *creation of loop recorder pocket, new*
> *site, and insertion/relocation of*
> *device (37.79)*
> *creation of pocket for implantable,*
> *patient-activated cardiac event*
> *recorder and insertion/relocation*
> *of device (37.79)*
> *removal of catheter from cranial cavity*
> *(01.27)*
> *that for drainage (86.04)*
> *that of:*
> *cardiac pacemaker pocket, new site*
> *(37.79)*
> *fascial compartments of face and*
> *mouth (27.0)*

Coding Clinic: 2005, Q1, P17; 2004, Q2, P3, 7-8x2; 1999, Q4,
P21; 1995, Q3, P14; 1993, 5th Issue, P11; 1989, Q3,
P17; 1985, July-Aug, P11; 1985, Mar-April, P15; 1984,
May-June, P11, 14

◆Non-OR Procedure that affects MS-DRG
assignment to MDC 09, MS-DRG 579-581

● **86.1 Diagnostic procedures on skin and subcutaneous tissue**

86.11 Biopsy of skin and subcutaneous tissue
Coding Clinic: 2008, Q4, P97-100

86.19 Other diagnostic procedures on skin and subcutaneous tissue

> **Excludes** *microscopic examination of specimen*
> *from skin and subcutaneous*
> *tissue (91.61–91.79)*

● **86.2 Excision or destruction of lesion or tissue of skin and subcutaneous tissue**

✖ **86.21 Excision of pilonidal cyst or sinus**
Marsupialization of cyst

> **Excludes** *incision of pilonidal cyst or sinus*
> *(86.03)*

✖ **86.22 Excisional debridement of wound, infection, or burn**
Removal by excision of:
devitalized tissue
necrosis
slough

> **Excludes** *debridement of:*
> *abdominal wall (wound) (54.3)*
> *bone (77.60–77.69)*
> *muscle (83.45)*
> *of hand (82.36)*
> *nail (bed) (fold) (86.27)*
> *nonexcisional debridement of*
> *wound, infection, or burn*
> *(86.28)*
> *open fracture site (79.60–79.69)*
> *pedicle or flap graft (86.75)*

Coding Clinic: 2008, Q3, P8-9; Q1, P3-4; 2006, Q3, P19-20; Q2,
P11; 2005, Q2, P3-4; 2004, Q4, P138-139; Q2, P5;
2002, Q3, P23; Q1, P14-15; 2000, Q2, P9; 1999, Q1,
P8-9; 1998, Q2, P15; 1995, Q3, P12; 1992, Q2, P17;
1991, Q3, P18-19; Q2, P18-19; 1989, Q3, P16

OGCR Section I.C.17.d
> Excisional debridement involves surgical
> removal or cutting away, as opposed to a
> mechanical (brushing, scrubbing, washing)
> debridement. For coding purposes, excisional
> debridement is assigned to code 86.22.
> Nonexcisional debridement is assigned to
> code 86.28.

86.23 Removal of nail, nail bed, or nail fold

86.24 Chemosurgery of skin
Chemical peel of skin

✖ **86.25 Dermabrasion**
That with laser

> **Excludes** *dermabrasion of wound to remove*
> *embedded debris (86.28)*

86.26 Ligation of dermal appendage

> **Excludes** *excision of preauricular appendage*
> *(18.29)*

86.27 Debridement of nail, nail bed, or nail fold
Removal of:
necrosis
slough

> **Excludes** *removal of nail, nail bed, or nail fold*
> *(86.23)*

86.28 Nonexcisional debridement of wound, infection or burn
Debridement NOS
Maggot therapy
Removal of devitalized tissue, necrosis, and
slough by such methods as:
brushing
irrigation (under pressure)
scrubbing
washing
Water scalpel (jet)

Coding Clinic: 2007, Q1, P10-11; 2005, Q1, P14-15; 2004, Q2,
P5,6; 2003, Q2, P15; 2002, Q3, P23; 2001, Q2, P18;
1991, Q3, P18-19; Q2, P18-19

OGCR Section I.C.17.d
> Excisional debridement involves surgical
> removal or cutting away, as opposed to a
> mechanical (brushing, scrubbing, washing)
> debridement. For coding purposes, excisional
> debridement is assigned to code 86.22.
> Nonexcisional debridement is assigned to
> code 86.28.

86.3 Other local excision or destruction of lesion or tissue of skin and subcutaneous tissue
Destruction of skin by:
cauterization cryosurgery
fulguration
laser beam
That with Z-plasty

> **Excludes** *adipectomy (86.83)*
> *biopsy of skin (86.11)*
> *wide or radical excision of skin (86.4)*
> *Z-plasty without excision (86.84)*

Coding Clinic: 1996, Q1, P9; 1995, Q3, P14; 1990, Q2, P27; 1989, Q1,
P12

◆Non-OR Procedure that affects MS-DRG assignment to
MDC 09, MS-DRG 579-581

Excludes   Includes   Use additional   Code also   Omit code

✖ **86.4   Radical excision of skin lesion**
Wide excision of skin lesion involving underlying or adjacent structure
Code also any lymph node dissection (40.3–40.5)

● **86.5   Suture or other closure of skin and subcutaneous tissue**

     86.51   Replantation of scalp

     86.59   Closure of skin and subcutaneous tissue of other sites
Adhesives (surgical) (tissue)
Staples
Sutures
Excludes | *application of adhesive strips (butterfly)* — omit code

● **86.6   Free skin graft**

Includes   excision of skin for autogenous graft

Excludes | *construction or reconstruction of:*
     penis (64.43–64.44)
     trachea (31.75)
     vagina (70.61–70.64)

✖ **86.60   Free skin graft, not otherwise specified**

✖ **86.61   Full-thickness skin graft to hand**
Excludes | *heterograft (86.65)*
     homograft (86.66)

✖ **86.62   Other skin graft to hand**
Excludes | *heterograft (86.65)*
     homograft (86.66)

✖ **86.63   Full-thickness skin graft to other sites**
Excludes | *heterograft (86.65)*
     homograft (86.66)

     86.64   Hair transplant
Excludes | *hair follicle transplant to eyebrow or eyelash (08.63)*

✖ **86.65   Heterograft to skin**
Pigskin graft
Porcine graft
Excludes | *application of dressing only (93.57)*
Coding Clinic: 2002, Q3, P23

✖ **86.66   Homograft to skin**
Graft to skin of:
     amnionic membrane from donor skin from donor

✖ **86.67   Dermal regenerative graft**
Artificial skin, NOS
Creation of "neodermis"
Decellularized allodermis
Integumentary matrix implants
Prosthetic implant of dermal layer of skin
Regenerate dermal layer of skin
Excludes | *heterograft to skin (86.65)*
     homograft to skin (86.66)
Coding Clinic: 2006, Q3, P19-20; 1998, Q43, P77-79

✖ **86.69   Other skin graft to other sites**
Excludes | *heterograft (86.65)*
     homograft (86.66)
Coding Clinic: 1999, Q4, P15; 1998, Q43, P77-79

● **86.7   Pedicle grafts or flaps**

Excludes | *construction or reconstruction of:*
     penis (64.43–64.44)
     trachea (31.75)
     vagina (70.61–70.64)

✖ **86.70   Pedicle or flap graft, not otherwise specified**

✖ **86.71   Cutting and preparation of pedicle grafts or flaps**
Elevation of pedicle from its bed
Flap design and raising
Partial cutting of pedicle or tube
Pedicle delay
Excludes | *pollicization or digital transfer (82.61, 82.81)*
     revision of pedicle (86.75)
Coding Clinic: 2001, Q4, P66

✖ **86.72   Advancement of pedicle graft**
Coding Clinic: 1999, Q3, P9-10

✖ **86.73   Attachment of pedicle or flap graft to hand**
Excludes | *pollicization or digital transfer (82.61, 82.81)*

✖ **86.74   Attachment of pedicle or flap graft to other sites**
Attachment by:
     advanced flap
     double pedicled flap
     pedicle graft
     rotating flap
     sliding flap
     tube graft
Coding Clinic: 1999, Q3, P10; 1996, Q1, P15; 1993, Q2, P11

✖ **86.75   Revision of pedicle or flap graft**
Debridement of pedicle or flap graft
Defatting of pedicle or flap graft

● **86.8   Other repair and reconstruction of skin and subcutaneous tissue**

✖ **86.81   Repair for facial weakness**

✖ **86.82   Facial rhytidectomy**
Face lift
Excludes | *rhytidectomy of eyelid (08.86–08.87)*

✖ **86.83   Size reduction plastic operation**
Liposuction
Reduction of adipose tissue of:
     abdominal wall (pendulous)
     arms (batwing)
     buttock
     thighs (trochanteric lipomatosis)
Excludes | *breast (85.31–85.32)*
Coding Clinic: 2006, Q2, P10-11

✖ **86.84   Relaxation of scar or web contracture of skin**
Z-plasty of skin
Excludes | *Z-plasty with excision of lesion (86.3)*

✖ **86.85   Correction of syndactyly**

✖ **86.86   Onychoplasty**

✖ **86.89   Other repair and reconstruction of skin and subcutaneous tissue**
Excludes | *mentoplasty (76.67–76.68)*
Coding Clinic: 2002, Q4, P107-108; 2000, Q1, P26; 1998, Q2, P20; 1993, Q2, P11; 1992, Q2, P17

OPERATIONS ON THE INTEGUMENTARY SYSTEM (85–86)

◀ New   ◀‖‖ Revised   ~~deleted~~ Deleted   ● Use Additional Digit(s)   ✖ Valid O.R. Procedure
◆ Non-O.R. Procedure   ♀ Females Only   ♂ Males Only

● **86.9   Other operations on skin and subcutaneous tissue**

✖ **86.91   Excision of skin for graft**

Excision of skin with closure of donor site

> **Excludes**   *that with graft at same operative episode (86.60- 86.69)*

86.92   Electrolysis and other epilation of skin

> **Excludes**   *epilation of eyelid (08.91–08.93)*

✖ **86.93   Insertion of tissue expander**

Insertion (subcutaneous) (soft tissue) of expander (one or more) in scalp (subgaleal space), face, neck, trunk except breast, and upper and lower extremities for development of skin flaps for donor use

> **Excludes**   *flap graft preparation (86.71)*
> *tissue expander, breast (85.95)*

✖ **86.94   Insertion or replacement of single array neurostimulator pulse generator, not specified as rechargeable**

Pulse generator (single array, single channel) for intracranial, spinal, and peripheral neurostimulator

> Code also   any associated lead implantation (02.93, 03.93, 04.92)

> **Excludes**   *insertion or replacement of single array rechargeable neurostimulator pulse generator (86.97)*

Coding Clinic: 2004, Q4, P133-135

✖ **86.95   Insertion or replacement of dual array neurostimulator pulse generator, not specified as rechargeable**

Pulse generator (dual array, dual channel) for intracranial, spinal, and peripheral neurostimulator

> Code also   any associated lead implantation (02.93, 03.93, 04.92)

> **Excludes**   *insertion or replacement of dual array rechargeable neurostimulator pulse generator (86.98)*

Coding Clinic: 2004, Q4, P133-135

✖ **86.96   Insertion or replacement of other neurostimulator pulse generator**

> Code also   any associated lead implantation (02.93, 03.93, 04.92)

> **Excludes**   *insertion of dual array neurostimulator pulse generator (86.95, 86.98)*
> *insertion of single array neurostimulator pulse generator (86.94, 86.97)*

Coding Clinic: 2007, Q2, P10-11; 2006, Q2, P5-6; 2004, Q4, P133-135

✖ **86.97   Insertion or replacement of single array rechargeable neurostimulator pulse generator**

Rechargeable pulse generator (single array, single channel) for intracranial, spinal, and peripheral neurostimulator

> Code also   any associated lead implantation (02.93, 03.93, 04.92)

Coding Clinic: 2005, Q4, P130-131

✖ **86.98   Insertion or replacement of dual array rechargeable neurostimulator pulse generator**

Rechargeable pulse generator (dual array, dual channel) for intracranial, spinal, and peripheral neurostimulator

> Code also   any associated lead implantation (02.93, 03.93, 04.92)

Coding Clinic: 2005, Q4, P130-131

86.99   Other

> **Excludes**   *removal of sutures from:*
> *abdomen (97.83)*
> *head and neck (97.38)*
> *thorax (97.43)*
> *trunk NEC (97.84)*
> *wound catheter:*
> *irrigation (96.58)*
> *replacement (97.15)*

OPERATIONS ON THE INTEGUMENTARY SYSTEM (85–86)

16. MISCELLANEOUS DIAGNOSTIC AND THERAPEUTIC PROCEDURES (87–99)

● **87 Diagnostic Radiology**

● **87.0 Soft tissue x-ray of face, head, and neck**

Excludes *angiography (88.40–88.68)*

87.01 Pneumoencephalogram

87.02 Other contrast radiogram of brain and skull
Pneumocisternogram
Pneumoventriculogram
Posterior fossa myelogram

87.03 Computerized axial tomography of head
C.A.T. scan of head
Coding Clinic: 2005, Q3, P12-13; 1999, Q3, P7-8

87.04 Other tomography of head

87.05 Contrast dacryocystogram

87.06 Contrast radiogram of nasopharynx

87.07 Contrast laryngogram

87.08 Cervical lymphangiogram

87.09 Other soft tissue x-ray of face, head, and neck
Noncontrast x-ray of:
adenoid
larynx
nasolacrimal duct
nasopharynx
salivary gland
thyroid region
uvula
Excludes *x-ray study of eye (95.14)*

● **87.1 Other x-ray of face, head, and neck**

Excludes *angiography (88.40–88.68)*

87.11 Full-mouth x-ray of teeth

87.12 Other dental x-ray
Orthodontic cephalogram or cephalometrics
Panorex examination of mandible
Root canal x-ray

87.13 Temporomandibular contrast arthrogram

87.14 Contrast radiogram of orbit

87.15 Contrast radiogram of sinus

87.16 Other x-ray of facial bones
X-ray of:
frontal area
mandible
maxilla
nasal sinuses
nose
orbit
supraorbital area
symphysis menti
zygomaticomaxillary complex

87.17 Other x-ray of skull
Lateral projection of skull
Sagittal projection
Tangential projection

● **87.2 X-ray of spine**

87.21 Contrast myelogram

87.22 Other x-ray of cervical spine

87.23 Other x-ray of thoracic spine

87.24 Other x-ray of lumbosacral spine
Sacrococcygeal x-ray

87.29 Other x-ray of spine
Spinal x-ray NOS

● **87.3 Soft tissue x-ray of thorax**

Excludes *angiocardiography (88.50–88.58)*
angiography (88.40–88.68)

87.31 Endotracheal bronchogram

87.32 Other contrast bronchogram
Transcricoid bronchogram

87.33 Mediastinal pneumogram

87.34 Intrathoracic lymphangiogram

87.35 Contrast radiogram of mammary ducts

87.36 Xerography of breast

87.37 Other mammography
Coding Clinic: 1989, Q3, P17

87.38 Sinogram of chest wall
Fistulogram of chest wall

87.39 Other soft tissue x-ray of chest wall

● **87.4 Other x-ray of thorax**

Excludes *angiocardiography (88.50–88.58)*
angiography (88.40–88.68)

87.41 Computerized axial tomography of thorax
C.A.T. scan of
heart
thorax
Crystal linear scan of x-ray beam of thorax
Electronic subtraction of thorax
Photoelectric response of thorax
Tomography with use of computer, x-rays, and
camera of thorax

87.42 Other tomography of thorax
Cardiac tomogram
Excludes *C.A.T. scan of heart (87.41)*

87.43 X-ray of ribs, sternum, and clavicle
Examination for:
cervical rib
fracture

87.44 Routine chest x-ray, so described
X-ray of chest NOS

87.49 Other chest x-ray
X-ray of:
bronchus NOS
diaphragm NOS
heart NOS
lung NOS
mediastinum NOS
trachea NOS

● **87.5 Biliary tract x-ray**

87.51 Percutaneous hepatic cholangiogram
Coding Clinic: 1990, Q2, P28

87.52 Intravenous cholangiogram

✖ **87.53 Intraoperative cholangiogram**
Coding Clinic: 1996, Q1, P12-13; Q1, P12-13; 1990, Q2, P28

87.54 Other cholangiogram
Coding Clinic: 1988, Q4, P7

87.59 Other biliary tract x-ray
Cholecystogram

● **87.6 Other x-ray of digestive system**

87.61 Barium swallow

87.62 Upper GI series

87.63 Small bowel series

87.64 Lower GI series

87.65 Other x-ray of intestine

87.66 Contrast pancreatogram

87.69 Other digestive tract x-ray

◀ New   ◀▥ Revised   ~~deleted~~ Deleted   ● Use Additional Digit(s)   ✖ Valid O.R. Procedure
◆ Non-O.R. Procedure   ♀ Females Only   ♂ Males Only

● **87.7　X-ray of urinary system**

> **Excludes** *angiography of renal vessels (88.45, 88.65)*

87.71　Computerized axial tomography of kidney
C.A.T. scan of kidney

87.72　Other nephrotomogram

87.73　Intravenous pyelogram
Diuretic infusion pyelogram

87.74　Retrograde pyelogram

87.75　Percutaneous pyelogram

87.76　Retrograde cystourethrogram

87.77　Other cystogram

87.78　Ileal conduitogram

87.79　Other x-ray of the urinary system
KUB x-ray

● **87.8　X-ray of female genital organs**

87.81　X-ray of gravid uterus ♀
Intrauterine cephalometry by x-ray

87.82　Gas contrast hysterosalpingogram ♀

87.83　Opaque dye contrast hysterosalpingogram ♀

87.84　Percutaneous hysterogram ♀

87.85　Other x-ray of fallopian tubes and uterus ♀

87.89　Other x-ray of female genital organs ♀

● **87.9　X-ray of male genital organs**

87.91　Contrast seminal vesiculogram ♂

87.92　Other x-ray of prostate and seminal vesicles ♂

87.93　Contrast epididymogram ♂

87.94　Contrast vasogram ♂

87.95　Other x-ray of epididymis and vas deferens ♂

87.99　Other x-ray of male genital organs ♂

● **88　Other diagnostic radiology and related techniques**

● **88.0　Soft tissue x-ray of abdomen**

> **Excludes** *angiography (88.40–88.68)*

88.01　Computerized axial tomography of abdomen
C.A.T. scan of abdomen

> **Excludes** *C.A.T. scan of kidney (87.71)*

Coding Clinic: 1998, Q2, P13

88.02　Other abdomen tomography

> **Excludes** *nephrotomogram (87.72)*

88.03　Sinogram of abdominal wall
Fistulogram of abdominal wall

88.04　Abdominal lymphangiogram

88.09　Other soft tissue x-ray of abdominal wall

● **88.1　Other x-ray of abdomen**

88.11　Pelvic opaque dye contrast radiography

88.12　Pelvic gas contrast radiography
Pelvic pneumoperitoneum

88.13　Other peritoneal pneumogram

88.14　Retroperitoneal fistulogram
Coding Clinic: 1998, Q3, P8-9

88.15　Retroperitoneal pneumogram

88.16　Other retroperitoneal x-ray

88.19　Other x-ray of abdomen
Flat plate of abdomen
Coding Clinic: 1999, Q3, P9

● **88.2　Skeletal x-ray of extremities and pelvis**

> **Excludes** *contrast radiogram of joint (88.32)*

88.21　Skeletal x-ray of shoulder and upper arm

88.22　Skeletal x-ray of elbow and forearm

88.23　Skeletal x-ray of wrist and hand

88.24　Skeletal x-ray of upper limb, not otherwise specified

88.25　Pelvimetry

88.26　Other skeletal x-ray of pelvis and hip

88.27　Skeletal x-ray of thigh, knee, and lower leg

88.28　Skeletal x-ray of ankle and foot
Coding Clinic: 2003, Q4, P110

88.29　Skeletal x-ray of lower limb, not otherwise specified

● **88.3　Other x-ray**

88.31　Skeletal series
X-ray of whole skeleton

88.32　Contrast arthrogram

> **Excludes** *that of temporomandibular joint (87.13)*

88.33　Other skeletal x-ray

> **Excludes** *skeletal x-ray of:*
> *extremities and pelvis (88.21–88.29)*
> *face, head, and neck (87.11–87.17)*
> *spine (87.21–87.29)*
> *thorax (87.43)*

88.34　Lymphangiogram of upper limb

88.35　Other soft tissue x-ray of upper limb

88.36　Lymphangiogram of lower limb

88.37　Other soft tissue x-ray of lower limb

> **Excludes** *femoral angiography (88.48, 88.66)*

88.38　Other computerized axial tomography
C.A.T. scan NOS

> **Excludes** *C.A.T. scan of:*
> *abdomen (88.01)*
> *head (87.03)*
> *heart (87.41)*
> *kidney (87.71)*
> *thorax (87.41)*

Coding Clinic: 2005, Q3, P13-14

88.39　X-ray, other and unspecified

● **88.4　Arteriography using contrast material**

> **Includes** angiography of arteries
> arterial puncture for injection of
> contrast material
> radiography of arteries (by
> fluoroscopy)
> retrograde arteriography

Note: The fourth-digit subclassification identifies the site to be viewed, not the site of injection.

> **Excludes** *arteriography using:*
> *radioisotopes or radionuclides (92.01–92.19)*
> *ultrasound (88.71–88.79)*
> *fluorescein angiography of eye (95.12)*

Coding Clinic: 1985, Nov-Dec, P14

88.40　Arteriography using contrast material, unspecified site

88.41　Arteriography of cerebral arteries
Angiography of:
basilar artery
carotid (internal)
posterior cerebral circulation
vertebral artery
Coding Clinic: 2000, Q1, P16; 1999, Q1, P7; 1995, Q2, P12

88.42　Aortography
Arteriography of aorta and aortic arch
Coding Clinic: 1999, Q1, P17

88.43　Arteriography of pulmonary arteries

Excludes　　Includes　　Use additional　　Code also　　Omit code

MISCELLANEOUS DIAGNOSTIC AND THERAPEUTIC PROCEDURES (87–99)

88.44 Arteriography of other intrathoracic vessels

> **Excludes** *angiocardiography (88.50–88.58)*
> *arteriography of coronary arteries*
> *(88.55–88.57)*

88.45 Arteriography of renal arteries

88.46 Arteriography of placenta ♀
Placentogram using contrast material

88.47 Arteriography of other intra-abdominal arteries
Coding Clinic: 2009, Q2, P7; 2000, Q1, P18-19

88.48 Arteriography of femoral and other lower extremity arteries
Coding Clinic: 2006, Q2, P22-23; 2003, Q3, P10x2; Q1, P17-18; 1996, Q2, P7-8; 1989, Q2, P17

88.49 Arteriography of other specified sites

● **88.5 Angiocardiography using contrast material**

> **Includes** arterial puncture and insertion of arterial catheter for injection of contrast material
> cineangiocardiography
> selective angiocardiography

> Code also synchronous cardiac catheterization (37.21–37.23)

> **Excludes** *angiography of pulmonary vessels (88.43, 88.62)*

Coding Clinic: 2008, Q3, P18; 2002, Q3, P20

88.50 Angiocardiography, not otherwise specified

88.51 Angiocardiography of venae cavae
Inferior vena cavography
Phlebography of vena cava (inferior) (superior)

88.52 Angiocardiography of right heart structures
Angiocardiography of:
pulmonary valve
right atrium
right ventricle (outflow tract)

> **Excludes** *intra-operative fluorescence vascular angiography (88.59)*
> *that combined with left heart angiocardiography (88.54)*

Coding Clinic: 2008, Q3, P18; 2007, Q1, P16-17

◆ Non-OR Procedure that affects MS-DRG assignment to MDC 05, MS-DRG 216-218, 222-225, 233-234, 286-287

88.53 Angiocardiography of left heart structures
Angiocardiography of:
aortic valve
left atrium
left ventricle (outflow tract)

> **Excludes** *intra-operative fluorescence vascular angiography (88.59)*
> *that combined with right heart angiocardiography (88.54)*

Coding Clinic: 2007, Q1, P11-12, 17; 2005, Q4, P69-72; Q3, P14; 2000, Q1, P20-21

◆ Non-OR Procedure that affects MS-DRG assignment to MDC 05, MS-DRG 216-218, 222-225, 233-234, 286-287

88.54 Combined right and left heart angiocardiography

> **Excludes** *intra-operative fluorescence vascular angiography (88.59)*

◆ Non-OR Procedure that affects MS-DRG assignment to MDC 05, MS-DRG 216-218, 222-225, 233-234, 286-287

88.55 Coronary arteriography using a single catheter
Coronary arteriography by Sones technique
Direct selective coronary arteriography using a single catheter

> **Excludes** *intra-operative fluorescence vascular angiography (88.59)*

Coding Clinic: 2006, Q2, P25-26; 2002, Q3, P20; 1992, Q3, P10, 17-18

◆ Non-OR Procedure that affects MS-DRG assignment to MDC 05, MS-DRG 216-218, 222-225, 233-234, 286-287

88.56 Coronary arteriography using two catheters
Coronary arteriography by:
Judkins technique
Ricketts and Abrams technique
Direct selective coronary arteriography using two catheters

> **Excludes** *intra-operative fluorescence vascular angiography (88.59)*

Coding Clinic: 2006, Q3, P8-9; 2000, Q1, P20-21; 1992, Q3, P17-18; Q3, P10

◆ Non-OR Procedure that affects MS-DRG assignment to MDC 05, MS-DRG 216-218, 222-225, 233-234, 286-287

88.57 Other and unspecified coronary arteriography
Coronary arteriography NOS

> **Excludes** *intra-operative fluorescence vascular angiography (88.59)*

Coding Clinic: 2007, Q1, P15-16; 2006, Q2, P25-26; 2005, Q4, P69-72; Q2, P10; Q3, P14; 2000, Q1, P21; 1992, Q3, P10, 17-18

◆ Non-OR Procedure that affects MS-DRG assignment to MDC 05, MS-DRG 216-218, 222-225, 233-234, 286-287

88.58 Negative-contrast cardiac roentgenography
Cardiac roentgenography with injection of carbon dioxide

◆ Non-OR Procedure that affects MS-DRG assignment to MDC 05, MS-DRG 216-218, 222-225, 233-234, 286-287

88.59 Intra-operative fluorescence vascular angiography
Intraoperative laser arteriogram (SPY)
SPY arteriogram
SPY arteriography
Coding Clinic: 2007, Q4, P121-122; 2006, Q2, P25-26

● **88.6 Phlebography**

> **Includes** angiography of veins
> radiography of veins (by fluoroscopy)
> retrograde phlebography
> venipuncture for injection of contrast material
> venography using contrast material

Note: The fourth-digit subclassification (88.60–88.67) identifies the site to be viewed, not the site of injection.

> **Excludes** *angiography using:*
> *radioisotopes or radionuclides (92.01–92.19)*
> *ultrasound (88.71–88.79)*
> *fluorescein angiography of eye (95.12)*

88.60 Phlebography using contrast material, unspecified site

88.61 Phlebography of veins of head and neck using contrast material

88.62 Phlebography of pulmonary veins using contrast material

88.63 Phlebography of other intrathoracic veins using contrast material
Coding Clinic: 2008, Q3, P18

◀ New   ◀▥ Revised   deleted Deleted   ● Use Additional Digit(s)   ✖ Valid O.R. Procedure
◆ Non-O.R. Procedure   ♀ Females Only   ♂ Males Only

88.64 **Phlebography of the portal venous system using contrast material**
Splenoportogram (by splenic arteriography)

88.65 **Phlebography of other intra-abdominal veins using contrast material**
Coding Clinic: 2000, Q3, P9

88.66 **Phlebography of femoral and other lower extremity veins using contrast material**
Coding Clinic: 2006, Q2, P22-23

88.67 **Phlebography of other specified sites using contrast material**

88.68 **Impedance phlebography**

● **88.7** **Diagnostic ultrasound**

> **Includes** Echography
> Non-invasive ultrasound
> Ultrasonic angiography
> Ultrasonography

> **Excludes** *intravascular imaging (adjunctive) (IVUS)*
> *(00.21–00.29)*
> *therapeutic ultrasound (00.01–00.09)*

88.71 **Diagnostic ultrasound of head and neck**
Determination of midline shift of brain
Echoencephalography

> **Excludes** *eye (95.13)*

Coding Clinic: 2002, Q1, P10-11; 1992, Q1, P11x2

88.72 **Diagnostic ultrasound of heart**
Echocardiography
Transesophageal echocardiography

> **Excludes** *echocardiography of heart chambers*
> *(37.28)*
> *intracardiac echocardiography (ICE)*
> *(37.28)*
> *intravascular (IVUS) imaging of*
> *coronary vessels (00.24)*

Coding Clinic: 2007, Q1, P11-12; 2005, Q2, P17-18; Q3, P14; 2004, Q4, P121-122; Q1, P16-17; 2000, Q1, P20-21; 1999, Q1, P6; 1998, Q3, P11

88.73 **Diagnostic ultrasound of other sites of thorax**
Aortic arch ultrasonography
Breast ultrasonography
Lung ultrasonography

88.74 **Diagnostic ultrasound of digestive system**

88.75 **Diagnostic ultrasound of urinary system**

88.76 **Diagnostic ultrasound of abdomen and retroperitoneum**
Coding Clinic: 1999, Q2, P14

88.77 **Diagnostic ultrasound of peripheral vascular system**
Deep vein thrombosis ultrasonic scanning

> **Excludes** *adjunct vascular system procedures*
> *(00.40–00.43)*

Coding Clinic: 1999, Q4, P17-18; Q1, P13; Q1, P12-13; 1993, 5th Issue, P5; 1992, Q1, P11

88.78 **Diagnostic ultrasound of gravid uterus ♀**
Intrauterine cephalometry:
echo
ultrasonic
Placental localization by ultrasound
Coding Clinic: 2008, Q4, P124-125

88.79 **Other diagnostic ultrasound**
Ultrasonography of:
multiple sites
nongravid uterus
total body

● **88.8** **Thermography**

88.81 **Cerebral thermography**

88.82 **Ocular thermography**

88.83 **Bone thermography**
Osteoarticular thermography

88.84 **Muscle thermography**

88.85 **Breast thermography**

88.86 **Blood vessel thermography**
Deep vein thermography

88.89 **Thermography of other sites**
Lymph gland thermography
Thermography NOS

● **88.9** **Other diagnostic imaging**
Coding Clinic: 2006, Q2, P25-26

88.90 **Diagnostic imaging, not elsewhere classified**

88.91 **Magnetic resonance imaging of brain and brain stem**

> **Excludes** *intraoperative magnetic resonance*
> *imaging (88.96)*
> *laser interstitial thermal therapy*
> *[LITT] of lesion or tissue of*
> *brain under guidance (17.61)* ◄
> *real-time magnetic resonance imaging*
> *(88.96)*

88.92 **Magnetic resonance imaging of chest and myocardium**
For evaluation of hilar and mediastinal
lymphadenopathy

> **Excludes** *laser interstitial thermal therapy*
> *[LITT] of lesion or tissue of*
> *breast under guidance (17.69)* ◄
> *laser interstitial thermal therapy*
> *[LITT] of lesion or tissue of*
> *lung under guidance (17.69)* ◄

88.93 **Magnetic resonance imaging of spinal canal**
Spinal cord levels:
cervical
thoracic
lumbar (lumbosacral)
Spinal cord
Spine

88.94 **Magnetic resonance imaging of musculoskeletal**
Bone marrow blood supply
Extremities (upper) (lower)

88.95 **Magnetic resonance imaging of pelvis, prostate, and bladder**

> **Excludes** *laser interstitial thermal therapy*
> *[LITT] of lesion or tissue of*
> *prostate under guidance*
> *(17.69)* ◄

88.96 **Other intraoperative magnetic resonance imaging**
iMRI
Real-time magnetic resonance imaging
Coding Clinic: 2002, Q4, P111

88.97 **Magnetic resonance imaging of other and unspecified sites**
Abdomen
Eye orbit
Face
Neck

> **Excludes** *laser interstitial thermal therapy*
> *[LITT] of lesion* ◄
> *or tissue of other and unspecified* ◄
> *site under guidance (17.69)* ◄

88.98 **Bone mineral density studies**
Dual photon absorptiometry
Quantitative computed tomography (CT)
studies
Radiographic densitometry
Single photon absorptiometry

MISCELLANEOUS DIAGNOSTIC AND THERAPEUTIC PROCEDURES (87–99)

● 89 **Interview, evaluation, consultation, and examination**

  ● 89.0 **Diagnostic interview, consultation, and evaluation**

    Excludes *psychiatric diagnostic interview (94.11–94.19)*

    89.01 **Interview and evaluation, described as brief**
      Abbreviated history and evaluation

    89.02 **Interview and evaluation, described as limited**
      Interval history and evaluation

    89.03 **Interview and evaluation, described as comprehensive**
      History and evaluation of new problem

    89.04 **Other interview and evaluation**

    89.05 **Diagnostic interview and evaluation, not otherwise specified**

    89.06 **Consultation, described as limited**
      Consultation on a single organ system

    89.07 **Consultation, described as comprehensive**

    89.08 **Other consultation**

    89.09 **Consultation, not otherwise specified**

  ● 89.1 **Anatomic and physiologic measurements and manual examinations — nervous system and sense organs**

    Excludes *ear examination (95.41–95.49)*
      eye examination (95.01–95.26)
      the listed procedures when done as part of a general physical examination (89.7)

    89.10 **Intracarotid amobarbital test**
      Wada test

    89.11 **Tonometry**

    89.12 **Nasal function study**
      Rhinomanometry

    89.13 **Neurologic examination**

    89.14 **Electroencephalogram**
      Excludes *that with polysomnogram (89.17)*
      Coding Clinic: 2005, Q3, P12-13

    89.15 **Other nonoperative neurologic function tests**
      Coding Clinic: 1995, Q3, P5-6; 1991, Q1, P14; 1987, Jan-Feb, P15-16

    89.16 **Transillumination of newborn skull**

    89.17 **Polysomnogram**
      Sleep recording

    89.18 **Other sleep disorder function tests**
      Multiple sleep latency test [MSLT]

    89.19 **Video and radio-telemetered electroencephalographic monitoring**
      Radiographic EEG monitoring
      Video EEG monitoring
      Coding Clinic: 1992, Q1, P17; 1991, Q1, P14

  ● 89.2 **Anatomic and physiologic measurements and manual examinations — genitourinary system**

    Excludes *the listed procedures when done as part of a general physical examination (89.7)*

    89.21 **Urinary manometry**
      Manometry through:
        indwelling ureteral catheter
        nephrostomy
        pyelostomy
        ureterostomy

    89.22 **Cystometrogram**
      Coding Clinic: 1990, Q2, P27

    89.23 **Urethral sphincter electromyogram**
      Coding Clinic: 1990, Q2, P27

    89.24 **Uroflowmetry [UFR]**
      Coding Clinic: 1990, Q2, P27

    89.25 **Urethral pressure profile [UPP]**
      Coding Clinic: 1990, Q2, P27

    89.26 **Gynecological examination ♀**
      Pelvic examination

    89.29 **Other nonoperative genitourinary system measurements**
      Bioassay of urine
      Renal clearance
      Urine chemistry

  ● 89.3 **Other anatomic and physiologic measurements and manual examinations**

    Excludes *the listed procedures when done as part of a general physical examination (89.7)*

    89.31 **Dental examination**
      Oral mucosal survey
      Periodontal survey

    89.32 **Esophageal manometry**
      Coding Clinic: 1996, Q3, P13

    89.33 **Digital examination of enterostomy stoma**
      Digital examination of colostomy stoma

    89.34 **Digital examination of rectum**

    89.35 **Transillumination of nasal sinuses**

    89.36 **Manual examination of breast**

    89.37 **Vital capacity determination**
      Excludes *endoscopic pulmonary airway flow measurement (33.72)*

    89.38 **Other nonoperative respiratory measurements**
      Plethysmography for measurement of respiratory function
      Thoracic impedance plethysmography
      Excludes *endoscopic pulmonary airway flow measurement (33.72)*

    89.39 **Other nonoperative measurements and examinations**
      14 C-Urea breath test
      Basal metabolic rate [BMR]
      Gastric:
        analysis
        function NEC
      Excludes *body measurement (93.07)*
      cardiac tests (89.41–89.69)
      fundus photography (95.11)
      limb length measurement (93.06)
      Coding Clinic: 2001, Q2, P9-11; 2000, Q3, P9; 1996, Q3, P12-13; 1994, Q1, P18

  ● 89.4 **Cardiac stress tests, pacemaker and defibrillator checks**

    89.41 **Cardiovascular stress test using treadmill**
      Coding Clinic: 1988, Q1, P11

    89.42 **Masters' two-step stress test**
      Coding Clinic: 1988, Q1, P11

    89.43 **Cardiovascular stress test using bicycle ergometer**
      Coding Clinic: 1988, Q1, P11

    89.44 **Other cardiovascular stress test**
      Thallium stress test with or without transesophageal pacing

    89.45 **Artificial pacemaker rate check**
      Artificial pacemaker function check NOS
      Bedside device check of pacemaker or cardiac resynchronization pacemaker [CRT-P]
      Interrogation only without arrhythmia induction
      Excludes *catheter based invasive electrophysiologic testing (37.26)*
      noninvasive programmed electrical stimulation [NIPS] (arrhythmia induction) (37.20)
      Coding Clinic: 2002, Q1, P3

MISCELLANEOUS DIAGNOSTIC AND THERAPEUTIC PROCEDURES (87–99)

◄ New   ◄▦ Revised   ~~deleted~~ Deleted   ● Use Additional Digit(s)   ✖ Valid O.R. Procedure
◆ Non-O.R. Procedure   ♀ Females Only   ♂ Males Only

89.46   **Artificial pacemaker artifact wave form check**

89.47   **Artificial pacemaker electrode impedance check**

89.48   **Artificial pacemaker voltage or amperage threshold check**

89.49   **Automatic implantable cardioverter/defibrillator (AICD) check**
Bedside check of an AICD or cardiac resynchronization defibrillator [CRT-D]
Checking pacing thresholds of device
Interrogation only without arrhythmia induction

> **Excludes**   *catheter based invasive electrophysiologic testing (37.26)*
> *noninvasive programmed electrical stimulation [NIPS] (arrhythmia induction) (37.20)*

Coding Clinic: 2004, Q4, P135-136; 2002, Q1, P9

● 89.5   **Other nonoperative cardiac and vascular diagnostic procedures**

> **Excludes**   *fetal EKG (75.32)*

Coding Clinic: 1984, July-Aug, P19

89.50   **Ambulatory cardiac monitoring**
Analog devices [Holter-type]
Coding Clinic: 1999, Q4, P21

89.51   **Rhythm electrocardiogram**
Rhythm EKG (with one to three leads)

89.52   **Electrocardiogram**
ECG NOS
EKG (with 12 or more leads)
Coding Clinic: 1988, Q1, P11

89.53   **Vectorcardiogram (with ECG)**

89.54   **Electrographic monitoring**
Telemetry

> **Excludes**   *ambulatory cardiac monitoring (89.50)*
> *electrographic monitoring during surgery — omit code*

Coding Clinic: 1988, Q1, P11; 1984, Nov-Dec, P12

89.55   **Phonocardiogram with ECG lead**

89.56   **Carotid pulse tracing with ECG lead**

> **Excludes**   *oculoplethysmography (89.58)*

89.57   **Apexcardiogram (with ECG lead)**
Coding Clinic: 1987, Jan-Feb, P15-16

89.58   **Plethysmogram**
Penile plethysmography with nerve stimulation

> **Excludes**   *plethysmography (for):*
> *measurement of respiratory function (89.38)*
> *thoracic impedance (89.38)*

89.59   **Other nonoperative cardiac and vascular measurements**
Coding Clinic: 2005, Q3, P21; 2004, Q4, P135-136; 2003, Q3, P23; 1992, Q2, P12

● 89.6   **Circulatory monitoring**

> **Excludes**   *electrocardiographic monitoring during surgery — omit code*
> *implantation or replacement of subcutaneous device for intracardiac hemodynamic monitoring (00.57)*
> *insertion or replacement of implantable pressure sensor (lead) for intracardiac hemodynamic monitoring (00.56)*

Coding Clinic: 1984, July-Aug, P19

89.60   **Continuous intra-arterial blood gas monitoring**
Insertion of blood gas monitoring system and continuous monitoring of blood gases through an intra-arterial sensor
Coding Clinic: 2002, Q4, P111-112

89.61   **Systemic arterial pressure monitoring**

> **Excludes**   *intra-aneurysm sac pressure monitoring (intraoperative) (00.58)*
> *intravascular pressure measurement of intrathoracic arteries (00.67)*
> *intravascular pressure measurement of peripheral arteries (00.68)*

89.62   **Central venous pressure monitoring**

> **Excludes**   *intravascular pressure measurement, other specified and unspecified vessels (00.69)*

89.63   **Pulmonary artery pressure monitoring**

> **Excludes**   *pulmonary artery wedge monitoring (89.64)*

Coding Clinic: 1984, Nov-Dec, P19

89.64   **Pulmonary artery wedge monitoring**
Pulmonary capillary wedge [PCW] monitoring
Swan-Ganz catheterization
Coding Clinic: 1984, Nov-Dec, P19; July-Aug, P19

89.65   **Measurement of systemic arterial blood gases**

> **Excludes**   *continuous intra-arterial blood gas monitoring (89.60)*

89.66   **Measurement of mixed venous blood gases**

89.67   **Monitoring of cardiac output by oxygen consumption technique**
Fick method

89.68   **Monitoring of cardiac output by other technique**
Cardiac output monitor by thermodilution indicator

89.69   **Monitoring of coronary blood flow**
Coronary blood flow monitoring by coincidence counting technique

> **Excludes**   *intravascular pressure measurement of coronary arteries (00.59)*

89.7   **General physical examination**

89.8   **Autopsy**

● 90   **Microscopic examination-I**
The following fourth-digit subclassification is for use with categories in section 90 to identify type of examination:

> 1   **bacterial smear**
> 2   **culture**
> 3   **culture and sensitivity**
> 4   **parasitology**
> 5   **toxicology**
> 6   **cell block and Papanicolaou smear**
> 9   **other microscopic examination**

● 90.0   **Microscopic examination of specimen from nervous system and of spinal fluid**

● 90.1   **Microscopic examination of specimen from endocrine gland, not elsewhere classified**

● 90.2   **Microscopic examination of specimen from eye**

● 90.3   **Microscopic examination of specimen from ear, nose, throat, and larynx**

● 90.4   **Microscopic examination of specimen from trachea, bronchus, pleura, lung, and other thoracic specimen, and of sputum**

● 90.5   **Microscopic examination of blood**

● 90.6   **Microscopic examination of specimen from spleen and of bone marrow**

● 90.7   **Microscopic examination of specimen from lymph node and of lymph**

● 90.8   **Microscopic examination of specimen from upper gastrointestinal tract and of vomitus**

● 90.9   **Microscopic examination of specimen from lower gastrointestinal tract and of stool**

Excludes	Includes	Use additional	Code also	Omit code

MISCELLANEOUS DIAGNOSTIC AND THERAPEUTIC PROCEDURES (87–99)

● **91 Microscopic examination-II**
The following fourth-digit subclassification is for use with categories in section 91 to identify type of examination

> 1 bacterial smear
> 2 culture
> 3 culture and sensitivity
> 4 parasitology
> 5 toxicology
> 6 cell block and Papanicolaou smear
> 9 other microscopic examination

● **91.0 Microscopic examination of specimen from liver, biliary tract, and pancreas**

● **91.1 Microscopic examination of peritoneal and retroperitoneal specimen**

● **91.2 Microscopic examination of specimen from kidney, ureter, perirenal, and periureteral tissue**

● **91.3 Microscopic examination of specimen from bladder, urethra, prostate, seminal vesicle, perivesical tissue, and of urine and semen**

● **91.4 Microscopic examination of specimen from female genital tract ♀**
Amnionic sac
Fetus

● **91.5 Microscopic examination of specimen from musculoskeletal system and of joint fluid**
Microscopic examination of:
bone   ligament
bursa   muscle
cartilage   synovial membrane
fascia   tendon

● **91.6 Microscopic examination of specimen from skin and other integument**
Microscopic examination of:
hair   skin
nails

> **Excludes** *mucous membrane — code to organ site that of operative wound (91.71–91.79)*

● **91.7 Microscopic examination of specimen from operative wound**

● **91.8 Microscopic examination of specimen from other site**

● **91.9 Microscopic examination of specimen from unspecified site**

● **92 Nuclear medicine**

● **92.0 Radioisotope scan and function study**

92.01 Thyroid scan and radioisotope function studies
Iodine-131 uptake
Protein-bound iodine
Radio-iodine uptake

92.02 Liver scan and radioisotope function study

92.03 Renal scan and radioisotope function study
Renal clearance study

92.04 Gastrointestinal scan and radioisotope function study
Radio-cobalt B12 Schilling test
Radio-iodinated triolein study

92.05 Cardiovascular and hematopoietic scan and radioisotope function study
Bone marrow scan or function study
Cardiac output scan or function study
Circulation time scan or function study
Radionuclide cardiac ventriculogram scan or function study
Spleen scan or function study
Coding Clinic: 1992, Q2, P7-8; 1988, Q1, P11

92.09 Other radioisotope function studies

● **92.1 Other radioisotope scan**

92.11 Cerebral scan
Pituitary

92.12 Scan of other sites of head
> **Excludes** *eye (95.16)*

92.13 Parathyroid scan

92.14 Bone scan

92.15 Pulmonary scan

92.16 Scan of lymphatic system

92.17 Placental scan ♀

92.18 Total body scan

92.19 Scan of other sites

● **92.2 Therapeutic radiology and nuclear medicine**
> **Excludes** *that for:*
> *ablation of pituitary gland (07.64–07.69)*
> *destruction of chorioretinal lesion (14.26–14.27)*

92.20 Infusion of liquid brachytherapy radioisotope
I-125 radioisotope
Intracavitary brachytherapy
> **Includes** removal of radioisotope
> Coding Clinic: 2005, Q4, P117-119; 2004, Q1, P3-5x2; 2000, Q1, P11-12; 1994, Q3, P11; 1994, Q2, P10

92.21 Superficial radiation
Contact radiation [up to 150 KVP]

92.22 Orthovoltage radiation
Deep radiation [200–300 KVP]

92.23 Radioisotopic teleradiotherapy
Teleradiotherapy using:
cobalt-60
iodine-125
radioactive cesium

92.24 Teleradiotherapy using photons
Megavoltage NOS
Supervoltage NOS
Use of:
Betatron
linear accelerator

92.25 Teleradiotherapy using electrons
Beta particles
> **Excludes** *intra-operative electron radiation therapy (92.41)*

92.26 Teleradiotherapy of other particulate radiation
Neutrons
Protons NOS

✖ **92.27 Implantation or insertion of radioactive elements**
Intravascular brachytherapy
> **Code also** incision of site
> **Excludes** *infusion of liquid brachytherapy radioisotope (92.20)*
> Coding Clinic: 2004, Q1, P3-5

92.28 Injection or instillation of radioisotopes
Injection or infusion of radioimmunoconjugate
Intracavitary injection or instillation
Intravenous injection or instillation
Iodine-131 [I-131] tositumomab
Radioimmunotherapy
Ytrium-90 [Y-90] ibritumomab tiuxetan
> **Excludes** *infusion of liquid brachytherapy radioisotope (92.20)*

92.29 Other radiotherapeutic procedure
Coding Clinic: 2006, Q3, P14-15

◀ New   ◀▥ Revised   ~~deleted~~ Deleted   ● Use Additional Digit(s)   ✖ Valid O.R. Procedure
◆ Non-O.R. Procedure   ♀ Females Only   ♂ Males Only

● **92.3   Stereotactic radiosurgery**

> Code also stereotactic head frame application (93.59)
>
> **Excludes** *stereotactic biopsy*

92.30   Stereotactic radiosurgery, not otherwise specified

◆ Non-OR Procedure that affects MS-DRG assignment to MDC 01, MS-DRG 040-042; MDC 10, MS-DRG 628-630; MDC 17, MS-DRG 823-825, 829-830

92.31   Single source photon radiosurgery

High energy x-rays
Linear accelerator (LINAC)

◆ Non-OR Procedure that affects MS-DRG assignment to MDC 01, MS-DRG 040-042; MDC 10, MS-DRG 628-630; MDC 17, MS-DRG 823-825, 829-830

92.32   Multi-source photon radiosurgery

Cobalt 60 radiation
Gamma irradiation

◆ Non-OR Procedure that affects MS-DRG assignment to MDC 01, MS-DRG 040-042; MDC 10, MS-DRG 628-630; MDC 17, MS-DRG 823-825, 829-830

92.33   Particulate radiosurgery

Particle beam radiation (cyclotron)
Proton accelerator

◆ Non-OR Procedure that affects MS-DRG assignment to MDC 01, MS-DRG 040-042; MDC 10, MS-DRG 628-630; MDC 17, MS-DRG 823-825, 829-830

92.39   Stereotactic radiosurgery, not elsewhere classified

◆ Non-OR Procedure that affects MS-DRG assignment to MDC 01, MS-DRG 040-042; MDC 10, MS-DRG 628-630; MDC 17, MS-DRG 823-825, 829-830

● **92.4   Intra-operative radiation procedures**

92.41   Intra-operative electron radiation therapy

IOERT
That using a mobile linear accelerator
Coding Clinic: 2007, Q4, P122

● **93   Physical therapy, respiratory therapy, rehabilitation, and related procedures**

● **93.0   Diagnostic physical therapy**

93.01   Functional evaluation

93.02   Orthotic evaluation

93.03   Prosthetic evaluation

93.04   Manual testing of muscle function
Coding Clinic: 1987, Jan-Feb, P15-16

93.05   Range of motion testing
Coding Clinic: 1987, Jan-Feb, P15-16

93.06   Measurement of limb length

93.07   Body measurement
Girth measurement
Measurement of skull circumference

93.08   Electromyography

> **Excludes** *eye EMG (95.25)*
> *that with polysomnogram (89.17)*
> *urethral sphincter EMG (89.23)*

Coding Clinic: 1987, Jan-Feb, P15-16

93.09   Other diagnostic physical therapy procedure

● **93.1   Physical therapy exercises**
Coding Clinic: 1987, Jan-Feb, P15-16

93.11   Assisting exercise

> **Excludes** *assisted exercise in pool (93.31)*

93.12   Other active musculoskeletal exercise

93.13   Resistive exercise

93.14   Training in joint movements

93.15   Mobilization of spine

93.16   Mobilization of other joints

> **Excludes** *manipulation of temporomandibular joint (76.95)*

93.17   Other passive musculoskeletal exercise

93.18   Breathing exercise

93.19   Exercise, not elsewhere classified

● **93.2   Other physical therapy musculoskeletal manipulation**

93.21   Manual and mechanical traction

> **Excludes** *skeletal traction (93.43–93.44)*
> *skin traction (93.45–93.46)*
> *spinal traction (93.41–93.42)*

93.22   Ambulation and gait training

93.23   Fitting of orthotic device

93.24   Training in use of prosthetic or orthotic device
Training in crutch walking

93.25   Forced extension of limb

93.26   Manual rupture of joint adhesions

93.27   Stretching of muscle or tendon

93.28   Stretching of fascia

93.29   Other forcible correction of deformity
Coding Clinic: 1985, Nov-Dec, P11

● **93.3   Other physical therapy therapeutic procedures**

93.31   Assisted exercise in pool

93.32   Whirlpool treatment

93.33   Other hydrotherapy

93.34   Diathermy

93.35   Other heat therapy
Acupuncture with smouldering moxa
Hot packs
Hyperthermia NEC
Infrared irradiation
Moxibustion
Paraffin bath

> **Excludes** *hyperthermia for treatment of cancer (99.85)*

93.36   Cardiac retraining

93.37   Prenatal training
Training for natural childbirth

93.38   Combined physical therapy without mention of the components

93.39   Other physical therapy
Coding Clinic: 2005, Q2, P6-7; 2003, Q4, P105-106, 108-110; 1997, Q3, P12-13; 1991, Q3, P15; Q2, P15

● **93.4   Skeletal traction and other traction**

93.41   Spinal traction using skull device
Traction using:
caliper tongs
Crutchfield tongs
halo device
Vinke tongs

> **Excludes** *insertion of tongs or halo traction device (02.94)*

Coding Clinic: 2001, Q3, P8; 1996, Q3, P14

MISCELLANEOUS DIAGNOSTIC AND THERAPEUTIC PROCEDURES (87–99)

93.42   Other spinal traction
Cotrel's traction

> **Excludes** cervical collar (93.52)

93.43   Intermittent skeletal traction

93.44   Other skeletal traction
Bryant's traction
Dunlop's traction
Lyman Smith traction
Russell's traction
Coding Clinic: 1989, Q3, P16

93.45   Thomas' splint traction

93.46   Other skin traction of limbs
Adhesive tape traction
Boot traction
Buck's traction
Gallows traction

● **93.5   Other immobilization, pressure, and attention to wound**

> **Excludes** external fixator device (84.71–84.73)
> wound cleansing (96.58–96.59)

93.51   Application of plaster jacket

> **Excludes** Minerva jacket (93.52)

93.52   Application of neck support
Application of:
cervical collar
Minerva jacket
molded neck support

93.53   Application of other cast

93.54   Application of splint
Plaster splint
Tray splint

> **Excludes** periodontal splint (24.7)

93.55   Dental wiring

> **Excludes** that for orthodontia (24.7)

93.56   Application of pressure dressing
Application of:
Gibney bandage
Robert Jones' bandage
Shanz dressing

93.57   Application of other wound dressing
Porcine wound dressing
Coding Clinic: 2002, Q3, P23

93.58   Application of pressure trousers
Application of:
anti-shock trousers
MAST trousers
vasopneumatic device
Coding Clinic: 1996, Q3, P13-14

93.59   Other immobilization, pressure, and attention to wound
Elastic stockings
Electronic gaiter
Intermittent pressure device
Oxygenation of wound (hyperbaric)
Stereotactic head frame application
Strapping (non-traction)
Velpeau dressing
Coding Clinic: 1999, Q3, P7-8; Q1, P12-13; 1991, Q1, P3-4; 1989, Q1, P12; 1988, Q4, P11

● **93.6   Osteopathic manipulative treatment**

93.61   Osteopathic manipulative treatment for general mobilization
General articulatory treatment

93.62   Osteopathic manipulative treatment using high- velocity, low-amplitude forces
Thrusting forces

93.63   Osteopathic manipulative treatment using low- velocity, high-amplitude forces
Springing forces

93.64   Osteopathic manipulative treatment using isotonic, isometric forces

93.65   Osteopathic manipulative treatment using indirect forces

93.66   Osteopathic manipulative treatment to move tissue fluids
Lymphatic pump

93.67   Other specified osteopathic manipulative treatment

● **93.7   Speech and reading rehabilitation and rehabilitation of the blind**

93.71   Dyslexia training

93.72   Dysphasia training

93.73   Esophageal speech training

93.74   Speech defect training

93.75   Other speech training and therapy
Coding Clinic: 2003, Q4, P105-106, 109-110; 1997, Q4, P35-37; Q3, P12-13

93.76   Training in use of lead dog for the blind

93.77   Training in braille or Moon

93.78   Other rehabilitation for the blind

● **93.8   Other rehabilitation therapy**

93.81   Recreation therapy
Diversional therapy
Play therapy

> **Excludes** play psychotherapy (94.36)

93.82   Educational therapy
Education of bed-bound children
Special schooling for the handicapped

93.83   Occupational therapy
Daily living activities therapy

> **Excludes** training in activities of daily living for the blind (93.78)

Coding Clinic: 2005, Q2, P6-7; 2003, Q4, P105-106, 108; 1997, Q3, P12-13

93.84   Music therapy

93.85   Vocational rehabilitation
Sheltered employment
Vocational:
assessment
retraining
training

93.89   Rehabilitation, not elsewhere classified
Coding Clinic: 2005, Q2, P6-7

◀ New   ◀▥ Revised   ~~deleted~~ Deleted   ● Use Additional Digit(s)   ✖ Valid O.R. Procedure
◆ Non-O.R. Procedure   ♀ Females Only   ♂ Males Only

● **93.9 Respiratory therapy**

> **Excludes** *insertion of airway (96.01–96.05)*
> *other continuous invasive (through*
> *endotracheal tube or tracheostomy)*
> *mechanical ventilation (96.70–96.72)*
>
> Coding Clinic: 2004, Q3, P3; 2002, Q1, P12.-13; 1998, Q3, P14

93.90   Non-invasive mechanical ventilation
    Bi-level airway pressure
    BiPAP without (delivery through) endotracheal
      tube or tracheostomy
    CPAP without (delivery through) endotracheal
      tube or tracheostomy
    Mechanical ventilation NOS
    Non-invasive positive pressure (NIPPV)
    Non-invasive PPV
    NPPV
    That delivered by non-invasive interface:
      face mask
      nasal mask
      nasal pillow
      oral mouthpiece
      oronasal mask

> **Excludes** *invasive (through endotracheal tube*
> *or tracheostomy) continuous*
> *mechanical ventilation*
> *(96.70–96.72)*

> **Note:** Patients admitted on *non-invasive*
> mechanical ventilation that subsequently
> require *invasive* mechanical ventilation;
> code both types of mechanical
> ventilation.
> Coding Clinic: 2008, Q4, P187-190; Q1, P8-9; 2004, Q3, P3

93.91   Intermittent positive pressure breathing [IPPB]

93.93   Nonmechanical methods of resuscitation
    Artificial respiration
    Manual resuscitation
    Mouth-to-mouth resuscitation
    Coding Clinic: 2003, Q2, P17

**93.94   Respiratory medication administered by
nebulizer**
    Mist therapy

93.95   Hyperbaric oxygenation

> **Excludes** *oxygenation of wound (93.59)*

93.96   Other oxygen enrichment
    Catalytic oxygen therapy
    Cytoreductive effect
    Oxygenators
    Oxygen therapy

> **Excludes** *oxygenation of wound (93.59)*
> *SuperSaturated oxygen therapy*
> *(00.49)*

93.97   Decompression chamber

**93.98   Other control of atmospheric pressure and
composition**
    Antigen-free air conditioning
    Helium therapy

> **Excludes** *inhaled nitric oxide therapy (INO)*
> *(00.12)*
> Coding Clinic: 2002, Q1, P14

93.99   Other respiratory procedures
    Continuous negative pressure ventilation [CNP]
    Postural drainage
    Coding Clinic: 2003, Q4, P108-109; 1999, Q3, P11-12

● **94 Procedures related to the psyche**

● **94.0 Psychologic evaluation and testing**

94.01   Administration of intelligence test
    Administration of:
      Stanford-Binet
      Wechsler Adult Intelligence Scale
      Wechsler Intelligence Scale for Children

94.02   Administration of psychologic test
    Administration of:
      Bender Visual-Motor Gestalt Test
      Benton Visual Retention Test
      Minnesota Multiphasic Personality Inventory
      Wechsler Memory Scale

94.03   Character analysis

94.08   Other psychologic evaluation and testing

**94.09   Psychologic mental status determination, not
otherwise specified**

● **94.1 Psychiatric interviews, consultations, and evaluations**

94.11   Psychiatric mental status determination
    Clinical psychiatric mental status
      determination
    Evaluation for criminal responsibility
    Evaluation for testimentary capacity
    Medicolegal mental status determination
    Mental status determination NOS

94.12   Routine psychiatric visit, not otherwise specified

94.13   Psychiatric commitment evaluation
    Pre-commitment interview

94.19   Other psychiatric interview and evaluation
    Follow-up psychiatric interview NOS

● **94.2 Psychiatric somatotherapy**

94.21   Narcoanalysis
    Narcosynthesis

94.22   Lithium therapy

94.23   Neuroleptic therapy

94.24   Chemical shock therapy

94.25   Other psychiatric drug therapy

94.26   Subconvulsive electroshock therapy

94.27   Other electroshock therapy
    Electroconvulsive therapy (ECT)
    EST

94.29   Other psychiatric somatotherapy

● **94.3 Individual psychotherapy**

94.31   Psychoanalysis

94.32   Hypnotherapy
    Hypnodrome
    Hypnosis

94.33   Behavior therapy
    Aversion therapy
    Behavior modification
    Desensitization therapy
    Extinction therapy
    Relaxation training
    Token economy

**94.34   Individual therapy for psychosexual
dysfunction**

> **Excludes** *that performed in group setting (94.41)*

94.35   Crisis intervention

94.36   Play psychotherapy

94.37   Exploratory verbal psychotherapy

94.38   Supportive verbal psychotherapy

94.39   Other individual psychotherapy
    Biofeedback

MISCELLANEOUS DIAGNOSTIC AND THERAPEUTIC PROCEDURES (87–99)

Excludes	Includes	Use additional	Code also	Omit code

● 94.4   Other psychotherapy and counseling

    94.41   Group therapy for psychosexual dysfunction

    94.42   Family therapy

    94.43   Psychodrama

    94.44   Other group therapy

    94.45   Drug addiction counseling

    94.46   Alcoholism counseling

    94.49   Other counseling

● 94.5   Referral for psychologic rehabilitation

    94.51   Referral for psychotherapy

    94.52   Referral for psychiatric aftercare:
         That in:
            halfway house
            outpatient (clinic) facility

    94.53   Referral for alcoholism rehabilitation

    94.54   Referral for drug addiction rehabilitation

    94.55   Referral for vocational rehabilitation

    94.59   Referral for other psychologic rehabilitation

● 94.6   Alcohol and drug rehabilitation and detoxification

    94.61   Alcohol rehabilitation
       ◆ Non-OR Procedure that affects MS-DRG
           assignment to MDC 20, MS-DRG 895

    94.62   Alcohol detoxification

    94.63   Alcohol rehabilitation and detoxification
       ◆ Non-OR Procedure that affects MS-DRG
           assignment to MDC 20, MS-DRG 895

    94.64   Drug rehabilitation
       ◆ Non-OR Procedure that affects MS-DRG
           assignment to MDC 20, MS-DRG 895

    94.65   Drug detoxification

    94.66   Drug rehabilitation and detoxification
       ◆ Non-OR Procedure that affects MS-DRG
           assignment to MDC 20, MS-DRG 895

    94.67   Combined alcohol and drug rehabilitation
       ◆ Non-OR Procedure that affects MS-DRG
           assignment to MDC 20, MS-DRG 895

    94.68   Combined alcohol and drug detoxification

    94.69   Combined alcohol and drug rehabilitation and detoxification
       ◆ Non-OR Procedure that affects MS-DRG
           assignment to MDC 20, MS-DRG 895

● 95   Ophthalmologic and otologic diagnosis and treatment

● 95.0   General and subjective eye examination

    95.01   Limited eye examination
         Eye examination with prescription of
            spectacles

    95.02   Comprehensive eye examination
         Eye examination covering all aspects of the
            visual system

    95.03   Extended ophthalmologic work-up
         Examination (for):
            glaucoma
            neuro-ophthalmology
            retinal disease

✖ 95.04   Eye examination under anesthesia
         Code also type of examination

    95.05   Visual field study

    95.06   Color vision study

    95.07   Dark adaptation study

    95.09   Eye examination, not otherwise specified
         Vision check NOS

● 95.1   Examinations of form and structure of eye

    95.11   Fundus photography

    95.12   Fluorescein angiography or angioscopy of eye

    95.13   Ultrasound study of eye

    95.14   X-ray study of eye

    95.15   Ocular motility study

    95.16   P32 and other tracer studies of eye

● 95.2   Objective functional tests of eye
       Excludes   *that with polysomnogram (89.17)*

    95.21   Electroretinogram [ERG]

    95.22   Electro-oculogram [EOG]

    95.23   Visual evoked potential [VEP]

    95.24   Electronystagmogram [ENG]

    95.25   Electromyogram of eye [EMG]

    95.26   Tonography, provocative tests, and other
         glaucoma testing

● 95.3   Special vision services

    95.31   Fitting and dispensing of spectacles

    95.32   Prescription, fitting, and dispensing of contact
         lens

    95.33   Dispensing of other low vision aids

    95.34   Ocular prosthetics

    95.35   Orthoptic training

    95.36   Ophthalmologic counseling and instruction
         Counseling in:
            adaptation to visual loss
            use of low vision aids

● 95.4   Nonoperative procedures related to hearing

    95.41   Audiometry
         Békésy 5-tone audiometry
         Impedance audiometry
         Stapedial reflex response
         Subjective audiometry
         Tympanogram

    95.42   Clinical test of hearing
         Tuning fork test
         Whispered speech test

    95.43   Audiological evaluation
         Audiological evaluation by:
            Bárány noise machine
            blindfold test
            delayed feedback
            masking
            Weber lateralization

    95.44   Clinical vestibular function tests
         Thermal test of vestibular function

    95.45   Rotation tests
         Bárány chair

    95.46   Other auditory and vestibular function tests

    95.47   Hearing examination, not otherwise specified

    95.48   Fitting of hearing aid
       Excludes   *implantation of electromagnetic*
            hearing device (20.95)

    95.49   Other nonoperative procedures related to
         hearing
         Adjustment (external components) of cochlear
            prosthetic device

● 96   Nonoperative intubation and irrigation

● 96.0   Nonoperative intubation of gastrointestinal and
      respiratory tracts

    96.01   Insertion of nasopharyngeal airway

    96.02   Insertion of oropharyngeal airway

MISCELLANEOUS DIAGNOSTIC AND THERAPEUTIC PROCEDURES (87–99)

◀ New   ◀▥ Revised   ~~deleted~~ Deleted   ● Use Additional Digit(s)   ✖ Valid O.R. Procedure
          ◆ Non-O.R. Procedure   ♀ Females Only   ♂ Males Only

96.03 **Insertion of esophageal obturator airway**

96.04 **Insertion of endotracheal tube**
Coding Clinic: 2007, Q1, P11; 2006, Q2, P8-9; 2005, Q4,
  P83-89; Q3, P10-11; Q2, P19-20; 2003, Q2, P17;
  1993, 5th Issue, P11

96.05 **Other intubation of respiratory tract**
> **Excludes** *endoscopic insertion or replacement
> of bronchial device or substance
> (33.71, 33.79)*
Coding Clinic: 1997, Q1, P14

96.06 **Insertion of Sengstaken tube**
Esophageal tamponade

96.07 **Insertion of other (naso-)gastric tube**
Intubation for decompression
> **Excludes** *that for enteral infusion of nutritional
> substance (96.6)*
Coding Clinic: 2008, Q4, P138-140

96.08 **Insertion of (naso-)intestinal tube**
Miller-Abbott tube (for decompression)

96.09 **Insertion of rectal tube**
Replacement of rectal tube

● 96.1 **Other nonoperative insertion**
> **Excludes** *nasolacrimal intubation (09.44)*

96.11 **Packing of external auditory canal**

96.14 **Vaginal packing** ♀

96.15 **Insertion of vaginal mold** ♀

96.16 **Other vaginal dilation** ♀

96.17 **Insertion of vaginal diaphragm** ♀

96.18 **Insertion of other vaginal pessary** ♀

96.19 **Rectal packing**

● 96.2 **Nonoperative dilation and manipulation**

96.21 **Dilation of frontonasal duct**

96.22 **Dilation of rectum**

96.23 **Dilation of anal sphincter**

96.24 **Dilation and manipulation of enterostomy stoma**

96.25 **Therapeutic distention of bladder**
Intermittent distention of bladder

96.26 **Manual reduction of rectal prolapse**

96.27 **Manual reduction of hernia**

96.28 **Manual reduction of enterostomy prolapse**
Coding Clinic: 1987, Nov-Dec, P11

96.29 **Reduction of intussusception of alimentary tract**
With:
   fluoroscopy
   ionizing radiation enema
   ultrasonography guidance
Hydrostatic reduction
Pneumatic reduction
> **Excludes** *intra-abdominal manipulation of
> intestine, not otherwise specified
> (46.80)*
Coding Clinic: 1998, Q43, P82-83

● 96.3 **Nonoperative alimentary tract irrigation, cleaning, and local instillation**

96.31 **Gastric cooling**
Gastric hypothermia

96.32 **Gastric freezing**

96.33 **Gastric lavage**

96.34 **Other irrigation of (naso-)gastric tube**

96.35 **Gastric gavage**

96.36 **Irrigation of gastrostomy or enterostomy**

96.37 **Proctoclysis**

96.38 **Removal of impacted feces**
Removal of impaction:
   by flushing
   manually

96.39 **Other transanal enema**
Rectal irrigation
> **Excludes** *reduction of intussusception of
> alimentary tract by ionizing
> radiation enema (96.29)*

● 96.4 **Nonoperative irrigation, cleaning, and local instillation of other digestive and genitourinary organs**

96.41 **Irrigation of cholecystostomy and other biliary tube**

96.42 **Irrigation of pancreatic tube**

96.43 **Digestive tract instillation, except gastric gavage**

96.44 **Vaginal douche** ♀

96.45 **Irrigation of nephrostomy and pyelostomy**

96.46 **Irrigation of ureterostomy and ureteral catheter**
Coding Clinic: 1985, July-Aug, P15

96.47 **Irrigation of cystostomy**

96.48 **Irrigation of other indwelling urinary catheter**

96.49 **Other genitourinary instillation**
Insertion of prostaglandin suppository
Coding Clinic: 2001, Q1, P5

● 96.5 **Other nonoperative irrigation and cleaning**

96.51 **Irrigation of eye**
Irrigation of cornea
> **Excludes** *irrigation with removal of foreign body
> (98.21)*

96.52 **Irrigation of ear**
Irrigation with removal of cerumen

96.53 **Irrigation of nasal passages**

96.54 **Dental scaling, polishing, and debridement**
Dental prophylaxis
Plaque removal

96.55 **Tracheostomy toilette**

96.56 **Other lavage of bronchus and trachea**
> **Excludes** *diagnostic bronchoalveolar lavage
> (BAL) (33.24)
> whole lung lavage (33.99)*
Coding Clinic: 2002, Q3, P18

96.57 **Irrigation of vascular catheter**
Coding Clinic: 1993, Q3, P5

96.58 **Irrigation of wound catheter**

96.59 **Other irrigation of wound**
Wound cleaning NOS
> **Excludes** *debridement (86.22, 86.27–86.28)*

96.6 **Enteral infusion of concentrated nutritional substances**

MISCELLANEOUS DIAGNOSTIC AND THERAPEUTIC PROCEDURES (87–99)

● **96.7 Other continuous invasive mechanical ventilation**

Includes BiPAP delivered through endotracheal tube or tracheostomy (invasive interface)

CPAP delivered through endotracheal tube or tracheostomy (invasive interface)

Endotracheal respiratory assistance

Invasive positive pressure ventilation [IPPV]

Mechanical ventilation through invasive interface

That by tracheostomy

Weaning of an intubated (endotracheal tube) patient

Excludes *continuous negative pressure ventilation [CNP] (iron lung) (cuirass) (93.99)*

intermittent positive pressure breathing [IPPB] (93.91)

non-invasive bi-level positive airway pressure [BiPAP] (93.90)

non-invasive continuous positive airway pressure [CPAP] (93.90)

non-invasive positive pressure (NIPPV) (93.90)

that by face mask (93.90–93.99)

that by nasal cannula (93.90–93.99)

that by nasal catheter (93.90–93.99)

Code also any associated:
endotracheal tube insertion (96.04)
tracheostomy (31.1–31.29)

Note: Endotracheal Intubation

To calculate the number of hours (duration) of continuous mechanical ventilation during a hospitalization, begin the count from the start of the (endotracheal) intubation. The duration ends with (endotracheal) extubation.

If a patient is intubated prior to admission, begin counting the duration from the time of the admission. If a patient is transferred (discharged) while intubated, the duration would end at the time of transfer (discharge).

For patients who begin on (endotracheal) intubation and subsequently have a tracheostomy performed for mechanical ventilation, the duration begins with the (endotracheal) intubation and ends when the mechanical ventilation is turned off (after the weaning period).

Tracheostomy

To calculate the number of hours of continuous mechanical ventilation during a hospitalization, begin counting the duration when mechanical ventilation is started. The duration ends when the mechanical ventilator is turned off (after the weaning period).

If a patient has received a tracheostomy prior to admission and is on mechanical ventilation at the time of admission, begin counting the duration from the time of admission. If a patient is transferred (discharged) while still on mechanical ventilation via tracheostomy, the duration would end at the time of the transfer (discharge).

Coding Clinic: 2008, Q4, P187-190; 2004, Q3, P3, 11; 2003, Q2, P17; 2002, Q2, P19; 1998, Q3, P14

96.70 Continuous invasive mechanical ventilation of unspecified duration

Invasive mechanical ventilation NOS
Coding Clinic: 1992, Q2, P13-14x3

◆ Non-OR Procedure that affects MS-DRG assignment to MDC 04, MS-DRG 208

96.71 Continuous invasive mechanical ventilation for less than 96 consecutive hours
Coding Clinic: 2009, Q2, P12; 2007, Q3, P7-8; 2006, Q2, P8-9x2; 2005, Q3, P10-11; 2004, Q3, P3, 11; 2003, Q2, P17; 2002, Q1, P12-13; 2001, Q1, P6-7; 1993, 5th Issue, P11; 1992, Q2, P13-14x3

◆ Non-OR Procedure that affects MS-DRG assignment to MDC 04, MS-DRG 208

96.72 Continuous invasive mechanical ventilation for 96 consecutive hours or more
Coding Clinic: 2005, Q2, P19-20; 1992, Q2, P13-14x3

◆ Non-OR Procedure that affects MS-DRG assignment to MS-DRG 003-004, MDC 04, MS-DRG 207, MDC 18, MS-DRG 870, MDC 22, MS-DRG 927, 933

● **97 Replacement and removal of therapeutic appliances**

● **97.0 Nonoperative replacement of gastrointestinal appliance**

97.01 Replacement of (naso-)gastric or esophagostomy tube

97.02 Replacement of gastrostomy tube
Coding Clinic: 1997, Q1, P11

97.03 Replacement of tube or enterostomy device of small intestine
Coding Clinic: 2003, Q1, P10

97.04 Replacement of tube or enterostomy device of large intestine

97.05 Replacement of stent (tube) in biliary or pancreatic duct
Coding Clinic: 1999, Q2, P13-14

● **97.1 Nonoperative replacement of musculoskeletal and integumentary system appliance**

97.11 Replacement of cast on upper limb

97.12 Replacement of cast on lower limb

97.13 Replacement of other cast

97.14 Replacement of other device for musculoskeletal immobilization
Splinting
Strapping

97.15 Replacement of wound catheter

97.16 Replacement of wound packing or drain
Excludes *repacking of:*
dental wound (97.22)
vulvar wound (97.26)

● **97.2 Other nonoperative replacement**

97.21 Replacement of nasal packing

97.22 Replacement of dental packing

97.23 Replacement of tracheostomy tube
Coding Clinic: 1987, Nov-Dec, P11

97.24 Replacement and refitting of vaginal diaphragm ♀

97.25 Replacement of other vaginal pessary ♀

97.26 Replacement of vaginal or vulvar packing or drain ♀

97.29 Other nonoperative replacements
Coding Clinic: 1999, Q3, P9; 1998, Q3, P12; 1985, Mar-April, P11

● **97.3 Nonoperative removal of therapeutic device from head and neck**

97.31 Removal of eye prosthesis
Excludes *removal of ocular implant (16.71)*
removal of orbital implant (16.72)

97.32 Removal of nasal packing

97.33 Removal of dental wiring

◀ New   ◀▦ Revised   ~~deleted~~ Deleted   ● Use Additional Digit(s)   ✖ Valid O.R. Procedure
◆ Non-O.R. Procedure   ♀ Females Only   ♂ Males Only

97.34   **Removal of dental packing**

97.35   **Removal of dental prosthesis**

97.36   **Removal of other external mandibular fixation device**

97.37   **Removal of tracheostomy tube**

97.38   **Removal of sutures from head and neck**

97.39   **Removal of other therapeutic device from head and neck**

> **Excludes**   *removal of skull tongs (02.94)*

● **97.4**   **Nonoperative removal of therapeutic device from thorax**

97.41   **Removal of thoracotomy tube or pleural cavity drain**
> Coding Clinic: 1999, Q1, P10

97.42   **Removal of mediastinal drain**

97.43   **Removal of sutures from thorax**

97.44   **Nonoperative removal of heart assist system**
> Explantation [removal] of circulatory assist device
> Explantation [removal] of percutaneous external heart assist device
> Intra-aortic balloon pump [IABP]
> Removal of extrinsic heart assist device
> Removal of pVAD
> Removal of percutaneous heart assist device
> Coding Clinic: 2001, Q4, P65

97.49   **Removal of other device from thorax**

> **Excludes**   *endoscopic removal of bronchial device(s) or substances (33.78)*
> Coding Clinic: 1986, Nov-Dec, P9

● **97.5**   **Nonoperative removal of therapeutic device from digestive system**

97.51   **Removal of gastrostomy tube**

97.52   **Removal of tube from small intestine**

97.53   **Removal of tube from large intestine or appendix**

97.54   **Removal of cholecystostomy tube**

97.55   **Removal of T-tube, other bile duct tube, or liver tube**
> Removal of bile duct stent
> Coding Clinic: 2001, Q1, P8-9

97.56   **Removal of pancreatic tube or drain**

97.59   **Removal of other device from digestive system**
> Removal of rectal packing

● **97.6**   **Nonoperative removal of therapeutic device from urinary system**

97.61   **Removal of pyelostomy and nephrostomy tube**

97.62   **Removal of ureterostomy tube and ureteral catheter**

97.63   **Removal of cystostomy tube**

97.64   **Removal of other urinary drainage device**
> Removal of indwelling urinary catheter

97.65   **Removal of urethral stent**

97.69   **Removal of other device from urinary system**

● **97.7**   **Nonoperative removal of therapeutic device from genital system**

97.71   **Removal of intrauterine contraceptive device ♀**

97.72   **Removal of intrauterine pack ♀**

97.73   **Removal of vaginal diaphragm ♀**

97.74   **Removal of other vaginal pessary ♀**

97.75   **Removal of vaginal or vulvar packing ♀**

97.79   **Removal of other device from genital tract**
> Removal of sutures

● **97.8**   **Other nonoperative removal of therapeutic device**

97.81   **Removal of retroperitoneal drainage device**

97.82   **Removal of peritoneal drainage device**
> Coding Clinic: 1993, 5th Issue, P8-9; 1990, Q2, P28; 1986, Sept-Oct, P12

97.83   **Removal of abdominal wall sutures**

97.84   **Removal of sutures from trunk, not elsewhere classified**

97.85   **Removal of packing from trunk, not elsewhere classified**

97.86   **Removal of other device from abdomen**

97.87   **Removal of other device from trunk**

97.88   **Removal of external immobilization device**
> Removal of:
> brace
> cast
> splint

97.89   **Removal of other therapeutic device**

● **98**   **Nonoperative removal of foreign body or calculus**

● **98.0**   **Removal of intraluminal foreign body from digestive system without incision**

> **Excludes**   *removal of therapeutic device (97.51–97.59)*

98.01   **Removal of intraluminal foreign body from mouth without incision**

98.02   **Removal of intraluminal foreign body from esophagus without incision**

98.03   **Removal of intraluminal foreign body from stomach and small intestine without incision**
> Coding Clinic: 1985, Jan-Feb, P14-15

98.04   **Removal of intraluminal foreign body from large intestine without incision**

98.05   **Removal of intraluminal foreign body from rectum and anus without incision**

● **98.1**   **Removal of intraluminal foreign body from other sites without incision**

> **Excludes**   *removal of therapeutic device (97.31–97.49, 97.61–97.89)*

98.11   **Removal of intraluminal foreign body from ear without incision**

98.12   **Removal of intraluminal foreign body from nose without incision**

98.13   **Removal of intraluminal foreign body from pharynx without incision**

98.14   **Removal of intraluminal foreign body from larynx without incision**

98.15   **Removal of intraluminal foreign body from trachea and bronchus without incision**

> **Excludes**   *endoscopic removal of bronchial device(s) or substances (33.78)*

98.16   **Removal of intraluminal foreign body from uterus without incision ♀**

> **Excludes**   *removal of intrauterine contraceptive device (97.71)*

98.17   **Removal of intraluminal foreign body from vagina without incision ♀**

98.18   **Removal of intraluminal foreign body from artificial stoma without incision**

98.19   **Removal of intraluminal foreign body from urethra without incision**

Excludes   Includes   Use additional   Code also   Omit code

● **98.2 Removal of other foreign body without incision**

> | Excludes | *removal of intraluminal foreign body (98.01–98.19)*

98.20 Removal of foreign body, not otherwise specified

98.21 Removal of superficial foreign body from eye without incision

98.22 Removal of other foreign body without incision from head and neck
Removal of embedded foreign body from eyelid or conjunctiva without incision

98.23 Removal of foreign body from vulva without incision ♀

98.24 Removal of foreign body from scrotum or penis without incision ♂

98.25 Removal of other foreign body without incision from trunk except scrotum, penis, or vulva

98.26 Removal of foreign body from hand without incision
Coding Clinic: 1987, Nov-Dec, P10

98.27 Removal of foreign body without incision from upper limb, except hand

98.28 Removal of foreign body from foot without incision

98.29 Removal of foreign body without incision from lower limb, except foot

● **98.5 Extracorporeal shockwave lithotripsy [ESWL]**
Lithotriptor tank procedure
Disintegration of stones by extracorporeal induced shockwaves
That with insertion of stent

98.51 Extracorporeal shockwave lithotripsy [ESWL] of the kidney, ureter, and/or bladder
◆Non-OR Procedure that affects MS-DRG assignment to MDC 11, MS-DRG 691-692

98.52 Extracorporeal shockwave lithotripsy [ESWL] of the gallbladder and/or bile duct
MCE: Non-covered procedure

98.59 Extracorporeal shockwave lithotripsy of other sites
MCE: Non-covered procedure

● **99 Other nonoperative procedures**

● **99.0 Transfusion of blood and blood components**

> | Use additional | code for that done via catheter or cutdown (38.92–38.94)

99.00 Perioperative autologous transfusion of whole blood or blood components
Intraoperative blood collection
Postoperative blood collection
Salvage

99.01 Exchange transfusion
Transfusion:
exsanguination
replacement
Coding Clinic: 1989, Q2, P15

99.02 Transfusion of previously collected autologous blood
Blood component
Coding Clinic: 1990, Q1, P10; 1985, July-Aug, P16

99.03 Other transfusion of whole blood
Transfusion:
blood NOS
hemodilution
NOS

99.04 Transfusion of packed cells
Coding Clinic: 2006, Q4, P91-92

99.05 Transfusion of platelets
Transfusion of thrombocytes

99.06 Transfusion of coagulation factors
Transfusion of antihemophilic factor

99.07 Transfusion of other serum
Transfusion of plasma

> | Excludes | *injection [transfusion] of:*
> *antivenin (99.16)*
> *gamma globulin (99.14)*
Coding Clinic: 1985, Nov-Dec, P14

99.08 Transfusion of blood expander
Transfusion of Dextran

99.09 Transfusion of other substance
Transfusion of:
blood surrogate
granulocytes

> | Excludes | *transplantation [transfusion] of bone marrow (41.0)*

● **99.1 Injection or infusion of therapeutic or prophylactic substance**

> | Includes | injection or infusion given:
> hypodermically acting locally or systemically
> intramuscularly acting locally or systemically
> intravenously acting locally or systemically
Coding Clinic: 2005, Q4, P101-103

99.10 Injection or infusion of thrombolytic agent
Alteplase
Anistreplase
Reteplase
Streptokinase
Tenecteplase
Tissue plasminogen activator (TPA)
Urokinase

> | Excludes | *aspirin — omit code*
> *GP IIB/IIIa platelet inhibitors (99.20)*
> *heparin (99.19)*
> *SuperSaturated oxygen therapy (00.49)*
> *warfarin — omit code*
Coding Clinic: 2006, Q2, P22; 2001, Q2, P8-9; Q2, P7-8, 23
◆Non-OR Procedure that affects MS-DRG assignment to MDC 01, MS-DRG 061-063

99.11 Injection of Rh immune globulin
Injection of:
Anti-D (Rhesus) globulin
RhoGAM

99.12 Immunization for allergy
Desensitization

99.13 Immunization for autoimmune disease

99.14 Injection or infusion of gamma globulin
Injection of immune sera

99.15 Parenteral infusion of concentrated nutritional substances
Hyperalimentation
Total parenteral nutrition [TPN]
Peripheral parenteral nutrition [PPN]
Coding Clinic: 2003, Q4, P104-105

99.16 Injection of antidote
Injection of:
antivenin
heavy metal antagonist

99.17 Injection of insulin

99.18 Injection or infusion of electrolytes

99.19 Injection of anticoagulant

> | Excludes | *infusion of drotrecogin alfa (activated) (00.11)*

◀ New   ◀▥ Revised   ~~deleted~~ Deleted   ● Use Additional Digit(s)   ✖ Valid O.R. Procedure
◆ Non-O.R. Procedure   ♀ Females Only   ♂ Males Only

● **99.2 Injection or infusion of other therapeutic or prophylactic substance**

> **Includes** injection or infusion given:
> > hypodermically acting locally or systemically
> > intramuscularly acting locally or systemically
> > intravenously acting locally or systemically
>
> **Excludes** *SuperSaturated oxygen therapy (00.49)*

Use additional code for:
> injection (into):
> > breast (85.92)
> > bursa (82.94, 83.96)
> > intraperitoneal (cavity) (54.97)
> > intrathecal (03.92)
> > joint (76.96, 81.92)
> > kidney (55.96)
> > liver (50.94)
> > orbit (16.91)
> > other sites — see Alphabetic Index
> perfusion:
> > NOS (39.97)
> > intestine (46.95, 46.96)
> > kidney (55.95)
> > liver (50.93)
> > total body (39.96)

Coding Clinic: 2004, Q4, P138; 2002, Q3, P20; 1998, Q43, P85-86

99.20 Injection or infusion of platelet inhibitor
> Glycoprotein IIB/IIIa inhibitor
> GP IIB/IIIa inhibitor
> GP IIB-IIIa inhibitor
>
> **Excludes** *infusion of heparin (99.19)*
> > *injection or infusion of thrombolytic agent (99.10)*

Coding Clinic: 2006, Q3, P8-9; 2004, Q2, P3

99.21 Injection of antibiotic
> **Excludes** *injection or infusion of oxazolidinone class of antibiotics (00.14)*

Coding Clinic: 1998, Q43, P76-77; 1990, Q2, P24; 1989, Q3, P16; 1987, Mar-April, P9

99.22 Injection of other anti-infective
> **Excludes** *injection or infusion of oxazolidinone class of antibiotics (00.14)*

99.23 Injection of steroid
> Injection of cortisone
> Subdermal implantation of progesterone

Coding Clinic: 2000, Q3, P15; 1999, Q1, P7-8; 1996, Q3, P7; 1992, Q3, P9

99.24 Injection of other hormone
Coding Clinic: 2006, Q1, P9-10

99.25 Injection or infusion of cancer chemotherapeutic substance
> Chemoembolization
> Injection or infusion of antineoplastic agent
>
> **Use additional** code for disruption of blood brain barrier, if performed [BBBD] (00.19)
>
> **Excludes** *immunotherapy, antineoplastic (00.15, 99.28)*
> > *implantation of chemotherapeutic agent (00.10)*
> > *injection of radioisotope (92.28)*
> > *injection or infusion of biological response modifier [BRM] as an antineoplastic agent (99.28)*
> > *intravenous infusion of clofarabine (17.70)* ◄

Coding Clinic: 2008, Q4, P82-83; 2007, Q4, P103-104; 2003, Q2, P6, 16-17; 2000, Q1, P23-24; 1999, Q1, P4; 1998, Q1, P6-7; 1996, Q3, P11-12; 1992, Q2, P6-7; Q1, P12; 1988, Q1, P8; 1986, Nov-Dec, P11; 1985, July-Aug, P11; 1984, May-June, P11

99.26 Injection of tranquilizer

99.27 Iontophoresis

99.28 Injection or infusion of biological response modifier [BRM] as an antineoplastic agent
> Immunotherapy, antineoplastic
> Infusion of cintredekin besudotox
> Interleukin therapy
> Low-dose interleukin-2 (IL-2) therapy
> Tumor vaccine
>
> **Excludes** *high-dose infusion interleukin-2 [IL-2] (00.15)*

Coding Clinic: 2006, Q4, P122-123; 1999, Q2, P8; 1998, Q2, P10-11

99.29 Injection or infusion of other therapeutic or prophylactic substance
> **Excludes** *administration of neuroprotective agent (99.75)*
> > *immunization (99.31–99.59)*
> > *infusion of blood brain barrier disruption substance (00.19)*
> > *injection of sclerosing agent into:*
> > > *esophageal varices (42.33)*
> > > *hemorrhoids (49.42)*
> > > *veins (39.92)*
> > *injection or infusion of human B-type natriuretic peptide (hBNP) (00.13)*
> > *injection or infusion of nesiritide (00.13)*
> > *injection or infusion of platelet inhibitor (99.20)*
> > *injection or infusion of thrombolytic agent (99.10)*

Coding Clinic: 2007, Q1, P11; 2004, Q4, P138; 2003, Q2, P10; 2002, Q3, P24-25; 2001, Q1, P15, 19-20; 2000, Q2, P14-15; Q1, P8-9, 18-19, 23-24; 1999, Q4, P17-18; 1998, Q2, P17-18, 23-24; Q1, P6; 1997, Q2, P11; 1996, Q3, P21; 1995, Q2, P12; 1990, Q2, P23-24; 1989, Q2, P17; 1988, Q1, P9; 1987, Sept-Oct, P11; 1984, Nov-Dec, P12

● **99.3 Prophylactic vaccination and inoculation against certain bacterial diseases**

99.31 Vaccination against cholera

99.32 Vaccination against typhoid and paratyphoid fever
> Administration of TAB vaccine

99.33 Vaccination against tuberculosis
> Administration of BCG vaccine

Coding Clinic: 1988, Q1, P8

MISCELLANEOUS DIAGNOSTIC AND THERAPEUTIC PROCEDURES (87–99)

99.34   **Vaccination against plague**

99.35   **Vaccination against tularemia**

99.36   **Administration of diphtheria toxoid**

> **Excludes**   *administration of:*
> *diphtheria antitoxin (99.58)*
> *diphtheria-tetanus-pertussis,*
> *combined (99.39)*

99.37   **Vaccination against pertussis**

> **Excludes**   *administration of*
> *diphtheria-tetanus-pertussis,*
> *combined (99.39)*

99.38   **Administration of tetanus toxoid**

> **Excludes**   *administration of:*
> *diphtheria-tetanus-pertussis,*
> *combined (99.39)*
> *tetanus antitoxin (99.56)*

99.39   **Administration of diphtheria-tetanus-pertussis, combined**

● **99.4 Prophylactic vaccination and inoculation against certain viral diseases**

99.41   **Administration of poliomyelitis vaccine**

99.42   **Vaccination against smallpox**

99.43   **Vaccination against yellow fever**

99.44   **Vaccination against rabies**

99.45   **Vaccination against measles**

> **Excludes**   *administration of measles-mumps rubella vaccine (99.48)*

99.46   **Vaccination against mumps**

> **Excludes**   *administration of measles-mumps rubella vaccine (99.48)*

99.47   **Vaccination against rubella**

> **Excludes**   *administration of measles-mumps rubella vaccine (99.48)*

99.48   **Administration of measles-mumps-rubella vaccine**

● **99.5 Other vaccination and inoculation**

99.51   **Prophylactic vaccination against the common cold**

99.52   **Prophylactic vaccination against influenza**

99.53   **Prophylactic vaccination against arthropod-borne viral encephalitis**

99.54   **Prophylactic vaccination against other arthropod-borne viral diseases**

99.55   **Prophylactic administration of vaccine against other diseases**

Vaccination against:
  anthrax
  brucellosis
  Rocky Mountain spotted fever
  Staphylococcus
  Streptococcus
  typhus
Coding Clinic: 1994, Q1, P19

99.56   **Administration of tetanus antitoxin**

99.57   **Administration of botulism antitoxin**

99.58   **Administration of other antitoxins**

Administration of:
  diphtheria antitoxin
  gas gangrene antitoxin
  scarlet fever antitoxin

99.59   **Other vaccination and inoculation**

Vaccination NOS

> **Excludes**   *injection of:*
> *gamma globulin (99.14)*
> *Rh immune globulin (99.11)*
> *immunization for:*
> *allergy (99.12)*
> *autoimmune disease (99.13)*

● **99.6 Conversion of cardiac rhythm**

> **Excludes**   *open chest cardiac:*
> *electric stimulation (37.91)*
> *massage (37.91)*

99.60   **Cardiopulmonary resuscitation, not otherwise specified**
Coding Clinic: 1994, Q1, P16

99.61   **Atrial cardioversion**
Coding Clinic: 1993, Q3, P12

99.62   **Other electric countershock of heart**
Cardioversion:
  NOS
  external
Conversion to sinus rhythm
Defibrillation
External electrode stimulation
Coding Clinic: 2007, Q1, P17-18

99.63   **Closed chest cardiac massage**
Cardiac massage NOS
Manual external cardiac massage

99.64   **Carotid sinus stimulation**

99.69   **Other conversion of cardiac rhythm**
Coding Clinic: 1988, Q4, P11

● **99.7 Therapeutic apheresis or other injection, administration, or infusion of other therapeutic or prophylactic substance**

99.71   **Therapeutic plasmapheresis**

> **Excludes**   *extracorporeal immunoadsorption [ECI] (99.76)*

99.72   **Therapeutic leukopheresis**
Therapeutic leukocytapheresis

99.73   **Therapeutic erythrocytapheresis**
Therapeutic erythropheresis
Coding Clinic: 1994, Q1, P20-21

99.74   **Therapeutic plateletpheresis**

99.75   **Administration of neuroprotective agent**

99.76   **Extracorporeal immunoadsorption**
Removal of antibodies from plasma with protein A columns
Coding Clinic: 2002, Q4, P112-113

99.77   **Application or administration of adhesion barrier substance**
Coding Clinic: 2002, Q4, P113

99.78   **Aquapheresis**
Plasma water removal
Ultrafiltration [for water removal]

> **Excludes**   *hemodiafiltration (39.95)*
> *hemodialysis (39.95)*
> *therapeutic plasmapheresis (99.71)*

99.79   **Other**
Apheresis (harvest) of stem cells
Coding Clinic: 2008, Q3, P19; 2006, Q1, P12-14x2; 2005, Q1, P16-17; 1997, Q4, P55

MISCELLANEOUS DIAGNOSTIC AND THERAPEUTIC PROCEDURES (87–99)

◄ New   ◄▥ Revised   deleted Deleted   ● Use Additional Digit(s)   ✖ Valid O.R. Procedure
◆ Non-O.R. Procedure   ♀ Females Only   ♂ Males Only

● **99.8 Miscellaneous physical procedures**

    99.81 Hypothermia (central) (local)

        | Excludes | *gastric cooling (96.31)*
                     gastric freezing (96.32)
                     that incidental to open heart surgery (39.62)

    99.82 Ultraviolet light therapy
         Actinotherapy

    99.83 Other phototherapy
         Phototherapy of the newborn

        | Excludes | *extracorporeal photochemotherapy (99.88)*
                     photocoagulation of retinal lesion (14.23–14.25, 14.33–14.35, 14.53–14.55)

        Coding Clinic: 1989, Q2, P15

    99.84 Isolation
         Isolation after contact with infectious disease
         Protection of individual from his surroundings
         Protection of surroundings from individual

    99.85 Hyperthermia for treatment of cancer
         Hyperthermia (adjunct therapy) induced by microwave, ultrasound, low energy radio frequency, probes (interstitial), or other means in the treatment of cancer

        Code also any concurrent chemotherapy or radiation therapy
        Coding Clinic: 1996, Q3, P11-12; 1989, Q3, P17

    99.86 Non-invasive placement of bone growth stimulator
         Transcutaneous (surface) placement of pads or patches for stimulation to aid bone healing

        | Excludes | *insertion of invasive or semi-invasive bone growth stimulators (device) (percutaneous electrodes) (78.90–78.99)*

    99.88 Therapeutic photopheresis
         Extracorporeal photochemotherapy
         Extracorporeal photopheresis

        | Excludes | *other phototherapy (99.83)*
                     ultraviolet light therapy (99.82)
        Coding Clinic: 1999, Q2, P7-8

● **99.9 Other miscellaneous procedures**

    99.91 Acupuncture for anesthesia

    99.92 Other acupuncture

        | Excludes | *that with smouldering mox (93.35)*

    99.93 Rectal massage (for levator spasm)

    99.94 Prostatic massage ♂

    99.95 Stretching of foreskin ♂

    99.96 Collection of sperm for artificial insemination ♂

    99.97 Fitting of denture

    99.98 Extraction of milk from lactating breast ♀

    99.99 Other
         Leech therapy

MISCELLANEOUS DIAGNOSTIC AND THERAPEUTIC PROCEDURES (87–99)

PART V

2009 Inpatient Procedures

2009 FINAL INPATIENT PROCEDURES

The following list is part of the changes to the Hospital Outpatient Prospective Payment System for Calendar Year 2009. Specifically, the file is Addendum E that lists the codes that are only payable as inpatient procedures as displayed at http://www.cms.hhs.gov/HospitalOutpatientPPS/HORD/list.asp#TopOfPage

For the 2010 updates, see the companion website in December 2009 at: http://codingupdates.com

00176	01634	21154	22212	22865	27156	27488	31760	32661
00192	01636	21155	22214	23200	27158	27495	31766	32662
00211	01638	21159	22216	23210	27161	27506	31770	32663
00214	01652	21160	22220	23220	27165	27507	31775	32664
00215	01654	21179	22224	23221	27170	27511	31780	32665
00452	01656	21180	22226	23222	27175	27513	31781	32800
00474	01756	21182	22318	23332	27176	27514	31786	32810
00524	01990	21183	22319	23472	27177	27519	31800	32815
00540	11004	21184	22325	23900	27178	27535	31805	32820
00542	11005	21188	22326	23920	27179	27536	32035	32850
00546	11006	21193	22327	24900	27181	27540	32036	32851
00560	11008	21194	22328	24920	27185	27556	32095	32852
00561	15756	21196	22532	24930	27187	27557	32100	32853
00562	15757	21247	22533	24931	27222	27558	32110	32854
00567	15758	21255	22534	24940	27226	27580	32120	32855
00580	16036	21256	22548	25900	27227	27590	32124	32856
00604	19271	21268	22554	25905	27228	27591	32140	32900
00622	19272	21343	22556	25909	27232	27592	32141	32905
00632	19305	21344	22558	25915	27236	27596	32150	32906
00670	19306	21346	22585	25920	27240	27598	32151	32940
00792	19361	21347	22590	25924	27244	27645	32160	32997
00794	19364	21348	22595	25927	27245	27646	32200	33015
00796	19367	21366	22600	26551	27248	27702	32215	33020
00802	19368	21395	22610	26553	27253	27703	32220	33025
00844	19369	21422	22630	26554	27254	27712	32225	33030
00846	20661	21423	22632	26556	27258	27715	32310	33031
00848	20664	21431	22800	26992	27259	27724	32320	33050
00864	20802	21432	22802	27005	27268	27725	32402	33120
00865	20805	21433	22804	27025	27269	27727	32440	33130
00866	20808	21435	22808	27030	27280	27880	32442	33140
00868	20816	21436	22810	27036	27282	27881	32445	33141
00882	20824	21510	22812	27054	27284	27882	32480	33202
00904	20827	21615	22818	27070	27286	27886	32482	33203
00908	20838	21616	22819	27071	27290	27888	32484	33236
00932	20930	21620	22830	27075	27295	28800	32486	33237
00934	20931	21627	22840	27076	27303	28805	32488	33238
00936	20936	21630	22841	27077	27365	31225	32491	33243
00944	20937	21632	22842	27078	27445	31230	32500	33250
01140	20938	21705	22843	27079	27447	31290	32501	33251
01150	20955	21740	22844	27090	27448	31291	32503	33254
01212	20956	21750	22845	27091	27450	31360	32504	33255
01214	20957	21810	22846	27120	27454	31365	32540	33256
01232	20962	21825	22847	27122	27455	31367	32650	33257
01234	20969	22010	22848	27125	27457	31368	32651	33258
01272	20970	22015	22849	27130	27465	31370	32652	33259
01274	21045	22110	22850	27132	27466	31375	32653	33261
01402	21141	22112	22852	27134	27468	31380	32654	33265
01404	21142	22114	22855	27137	27470	31382	32655	33266
01442	21143	22116	22856	27138	27472	31390	32656	33300
01444	21145	22206	22857	27140	27477	31395	32657	33305
01486	21146	22207	22861	27146	27485	31584	32658	33310
01502	21147	22208	22862	27147	27486	31587	32659	33315
01632	21151	22210	22864	27151	27487	31725	32660	33320

33321	33535	33788	34451	35331	35623	38381	43314	43880
33322	33536	33800	34502	35341	35626	38382	43320	43881
33330	33542	33802	34800	35351	35631	38562	43324	43882
33332	33545	33803	34802	35355	35632	38564	43325	44005
33335	33548	33813	34803	35361	35633	38724	43326	44010
33400	33572	33814	34804	35363	35634	38746	43330	44015
33401	33600	33820	34805	35371	35636	38747	43331	44020
33403	33602	33822	34806	35372	35637	38765	43340	44021
33404	33606	33824	34808	35390	35638	38770	43341	44025
33405	33608	33840	34812	35400	35642	38780	43350	44050
33406	33610	33845	34813	35450	35645	39000	43351	44055
33410	33611	33851	34820	35452	35646	39010	43352	44110
33411	33612	33852	34825	35454	35647	39200	43360	44111
33412	33615	33853	34826	35456	35650	39220	43361	44120
33413	33617	33860	34830	35480	35651	39499	43400	44121
33414	33619	33861	34831	35481	35654	39501	43401	44125
33415	33641	33863	34832	35482	35656	39502	43405	44126
33416	33645	33864	34833	35483	35661	39503	43410	44127
33417	33647	33870	34834	35501	35663	39520	43415	44128
33420	33660	33875	34900	35506	35665	39530	43425	44130
33422	33665	33877	35001	35508	35666	39531	43460	44132
33425	33670	33880	35002	35509	35671	39540	43496	44133
33426	33675	33881	35005	35510	35681	39541	43500	44135
33427	33676	33883	35013	35511	35682	39545	43501	44136
33430	33677	33884	35021	35512	35683	39560	43502	44137
33460	33681	33886	35022	35515	35691	39561	43520	44139
33463	33684	33889	35045	35516	35693	39599	43605	44140
33464	33688	33891	35081	35518	35694	41130	43610	44141
33465	33690	33910	35082	35521	35695	41135	43611	44143
33468	33692	33915	35091	35522	35697	41140	43620	44144
33470	33694	33916	35092	35523	35700	41145	43621	44145
33471	33697	33917	35102	35525	35701	41150	43622	44146
33472	33702	33920	35103	35526	35721	41153	43631	44147
33474	33710	33922	35111	35531	35741	41155	43632	44150
33475	33720	33924	35112	35533	35800	42426	43633	44151
33476	33722	33925	35121	35535	35820	42845	43634	44155
33478	33724	33926	35122	35536	35840	42894	43635	44156
33496	33726	33930	35131	35537	35870	42953	43640	44157
33500	33730	33933	35132	35538	35901	42961	43641	44158
33501	33732	33935	35141	35539	35905	42971	43644	44160
33502	33735	33940	35142	35540	35907	43045	43645	44187
33503	33736	33944	35151	35548	36660	43100	43770	44188
33504	33737	33945	35152	35549	36822	43101	43771	44202
33505	33750	33960	35182	35551	36823	43107	43772	44203
33506	33755	33961	35189	35556	37140	43108	43773	44204
33507	33762	33967	35211	35558	37145	43112	43774	44205
33510	33764	33968	35216	35560	37160	43113	43800	44210
33511	33766	33970	35221	35563	37180	43116	43810	44211
33512	33767	33971	35241	35565	37181	43117	43820	44212
33513	33768	33973	35246	35566	37182	43118	43825	44227
33514	33770	33974	35251	35570	37215	43121	43832	44300
33516	33771	33975	35271	35571	37616	43122	43840	44310
33517	33774	33976	35276	35583	37617	43123	43843	44314
33518	33775	33977	35281	35585	37618	43124	43845	44316
33519	33776	33978	35301	35587	37660	43135	43846	44320
33521	33777	33979	35302	35600	37788	43279	43847	44322
33522	33778	33980	35303	35601	38100	43300	43848	44345
33523	33779	34001	35304	35606	38101	43305	43850	44346
33530	33780	34051	35305	35612	38102	43310	43855	44602
33533	33781	34151	35306	35616	38115	43312	43860	44603
33534	33786	34401	35311	35621	38380	43313	43865	44604

44605	47010	48145	50240	51525	57305	59855	61526	61624
44615	47015	48146	50250	51530	57307	59856	61530	61630
44620	47100	48148	50280	51550	57308	59857	61531	61635
44625	47120	48150	50290	51555	57311	60254	61533	61680
44626	47122	48152	50300	51565	57531	60270	61534	61682
44640	47125	48153	50320	51570	57540	60505	61535	61684
44650	47130	48154	50323	51575	57545	60521	61536	61686
44660	47133	48155	50325	51580	58140	60522	61537	61690
44661	47135	48400	50327	51585	58146	60540	61538	61692
44680	47136	48500	50328	51590	58150	60545	61539	61697
44700	47140	48510	50329	51595	58152	60600	61540	61698
44715	47141	48520	50340	51596	58180	60605	61541	61700
44720	47142	48540	50360	51597	58200	60650	61542	61702
44721	47143	48545	50365	51800	58210	61105	61543	61703
44800	47144	48547	50370	51820	58240	61107	61544	61705
44820	47145	48548	50380	51840	58267	61108	61545	61708
44850	47146	48551	50400	51841	58275	61120	61546	61710
44899	47147	48552	50405	51865	58280	61140	61548	61711
44900	47300	48554	50500	51900	58285	61150	61550	61735
44950	47350	48556	50520	51920	58293	61151	61552	61750
44955	47360	49000	50525	51925	58400	61154	61556	61751
44960	47361	49002	50526	51940	58410	61156	61557	61760
45110	47362	49010	50540	51960	58520	61210	61558	61850
45111	47380	49020	50545	51980	58540	61250	61559	61860
45112	47381	49040	50546	53415	58548	61253	61563	61863
45113	47400	49060	50547	53448	58605	61304	61564	61864
45114	47420	49062	50548	54125	58611	61305	61566	61867
45116	47425	49203	50600	54130	58700	61312	61567	61868
45119	47460	49204	50605	54135	58720	61313	61570	61870
45120	47480	49205	50610	54390	58740	61314	61571	61875
45121	47550	49215	50620	54411	58750	61315	61575	62005
45123	47570	49220	50630	54417	58752	61316	61576	62010
45126	47600	49255	50650	54430	58760	61320	61580	62100
45130	47605	49425	50660	54650	58822	61321	61581	62115
45135	47610	49428	50700	55605	58825	61322	61582	62116
45136	47612	49605	50715	55650	58940	61323	61583	62117
45395	47620	49606	50722	55801	58943	61332	61584	62120
45397	47700	49610	50725	55810	58950	61333	61585	62121
45400	47701	49611	50728	55812	58951	61340	61586	62140
45402	47711	49900	50740	55815	58952	61343	61590	62141
45540	47712	49904	50750	55821	58953	61345	61591	62142
45550	47715	49905	50760	55831	58954	61440	61592	62143
45562	47720	49906	50770	55840	58956	61450	61595	62145
45563	47721	50010	50780	55842	58957	61458	61596	62146
45800	47740	50040	50782	55845	58958	61460	61597	62147
45805	47741	50045	50783	55862	58960	61470	61598	62148
45820	47760	50060	50785	55865	59120	61480	61600	62161
45825	47765	50065	50800	55866	59121	61490	61601	62162
46705	47780	50070	50810	56630	59130	61500	61605	62163
46710	47785	50075	50815	56631	59135	61501	61606	62164
46712	47800	50100	50820	56632	59136	61510	61607	62165
46715	47801	50120	50825	56633	59140	61512	61608	62180
46716	47802	50125	50830	56634	59325	61514	61609	62190
46730	47900	50130	50840	56637	59350	61516	61610	62192
46735	48000	50135	50845	56640	59514	61517	61611	62200
46740	48001	50205	50860	57110	59525	61518	61612	62201
46742	48020	50220	50900	57111	59620	61519	61613	62220
46744	48100	50225	50920	57112	59830	61520	61615	62223
46746	48105	50230	50930	57270	59850	61521	61616	62256
46748	48120	50234	50940	57280	59851	61522	61618	62258
46751	48140	50236	51060	57296	59852	61524	61619	63043

63044	63172	63266	63290	63740	75957	99462	0077T	0196T
63050	63173	63267	63295	64752	75958	99468	0078T	G0341
63051	63180	63268	63300	64755	75959	99469	0079T	G0342
63076	63182	63270	63301	64760	92970	99471	0080T	G0343
63077	63185	63271	63302	64809	92971	99472	0081T	G0406
63078	63190	63272	63303	64818	92975	99475	0092T	G0407
63081	63191	63273	63304	64866	92992	99476	0095T	G0408
63082	63194	63275	63305	64868	92993	99477	0098T	G0412
63085	63195	63276	63306	65273	99190	99478	0157T	G0414
63086	63196	63277	63307	69155	99191	99479	0158T	G0415
63087	63197	63278	63308	69535	99192	99480	0163T	
63088	63198	63280	63700	69554	99251	0048T	0164T	
63090	63199	63281	63702	69950	99252	0050T	0165T	
63091	63200	63282	63704	75900	99253	0051T	0166T	
63101	63250	63283	63706	75952	99254	0052T	0167T	
63102	63251	63285	63707	75953	99255	0053T	0169T	
63103	63252	63286	63709	75954	99356	0075T	0184T	
63170	63265	63287	63710	75956	99357	0076T	0195T	

2010 MS-DRG, Version 27 (Proposed)

MS-DRG, APPENDIX A

List of Medicare Severity Diagnosis Related Groups, Version 27 (Proposed)

Appendix A contains a list of each MS-DRG with a specification of the MDC and whether the MS-DRG is medical or surgical. Some MS-DRGs which contain patients from multiple MDCs (e.g., 009 Bone Marrow Transplant) do not have an MDC specified. The letter "M" is used to designate a medical MS-DRG and the letter "P" is used to designate a surgical MS-DRG.

001	PRE	P	HEART TRANSPLANT OR IMPLANT OF HEART ASSIST SYSTEM W MCC
002	PRE	P	HEART TRANSPLANT OR IMPLANT OF HEART ASSIST SYSTEM W/O MCC
003	PRE	P	ECMO OR TRACH W MV 96+ HRS OR PDX EXC FACE, MOUTH & NECK W MAJ O.R.
004	PRE	P	TRACH W MV 96+ HRS OR PDX EXC FACE, MOUTH & NECK W/O MAJ O.R.
005	PRE	P	LIVER TRANSPLANT W MCC OR INTESTINAL TRANSPLANT
006	PRE	P	LIVER TRANSPLANT W/O MCC
007	PRE	P	LUNG TRANSPLANT
008	PRE	P	SIMULTANEOUS PANCREAS/KIDNEY TRANSPLANT
009	PRE	P	BONE MARROW TRANSPLANT
010	PRE	P	PANCREAS TRANSPLANT
011	PRE	P	TRACHEOSTOMY FOR FACE, MOUTH & NECK DIAGNOSES W MCC
012	PRE	P	TRACHEOSTOMY FOR FACE, MOUTH & NECK DIAGNOSES W CC
013	PRE	P	TRACHEOSTOMY FOR FACE, MOUTH & NECK DIAGNOSES W/O CC/MCC
020	MDC 01	P	INTRACRANIAL VASCULAR PROCEDURES W PDX HEMORRHAGE W MCC
021	MDC 01	P	INTRACRANIAL VASCULAR PROCEDURES W PDX HEMORRHAGE W CC
022	MDC 01	P	INTRACRANIAL VASCULAR PROCEDURES W PDX HEMORRHAGE W/O CC/MCC
023	MDC 01	P	CRANIO W MAJOR DEV IMPL/ACUTE COMPLEX CNS PDX W MCC OR CHEMO IMPLANT
024	MDC 01	P	CRANIO W MAJOR DEV IMPL/ACUTE COMPLEX CNS PDX W/O MCC
025	MDC 01	P	CRANIOTOMY & ENDOVASCULAR INTRACRANIAL PROCEDURES W MCC
026	MDC 01	P	CRANIOTOMY & ENDOVASCULAR INTRACRANIAL PROCEDURES W CC
027	MDC 01	P	CRANIOTOMY & ENDOVASCULAR INTRACRANIAL PROCEDURES W/O CC/MCC
028	MDC 01	P	SPINAL PROCEDURES W MCC
029	MDC 01	P	SPINAL PROCEDURES W CC OR SPINAL NEUROSTIMULATORS
030	MDC 01	P	SPINAL PROCEDURES W/O CC/MCC
031	MDC 01	P	VENTRICULAR SHUNT PROCEDURES W MCC
032	MDC 01	P	VENTRICULAR SHUNT PROCEDURES W CC
033	MDC 01	P	VENTRICULAR SHUNT PROCEDURES W/O CC/MCC
034	MDC 01	P	CAROTID ARTERY STENT PROCEDURE W MCC
035	MDC 01	P	CAROTID ARTERY STENT PROCEDURE W CC
036	MDC 01	P	CAROTID ARTERY STENT PROCEDURE W/O CC/MCC
037	MDC 01	P	EXTRACRANIAL PROCEDURES W MCC
038	MDC 01	P	EXTRACRANIAL PROCEDURES W CC
039	MDC 01	P	EXTRACRANIAL PROCEDURES W/O CC/MCC
040	MDC 01	P	PERIPH/CRANIAL NERVE & OTHER NERV SYST PROC W MCC
041	MDC 01	P	PERIPH/CRANIAL NERVE & OTHER NERV SYST PROC W CC OR PERIPH NEUROSTIM
042	MDC 01	P	PERIPH/CRANIAL NERVE & OTHER NERV SYST PROC W/O CC/MCC
052	MDC 01	M	SPINAL DISORDERS & INJURIES W CC/MCC
053	MDC 01	M	SPINAL DISORDERS & INJURIES W/O CC/MCC
054	MDC 01	M	NERVOUS SYSTEM NEOPLASMS W MCC
055	MDC 01	M	NERVOUS SYSTEM NEOPLASMS W/O MCC
056	MDC 01	M	DEGENERATIVE NERVOUS SYSTEM DISORDERS W MCC
057	MDC 01	M	DEGENERATIVE NERVOUS SYSTEM DISORDERS W/O MCC
058	MDC 01	M	MULTIPLE SCLEROSIS & CEREBELLAR ATAXIA W MCC
059	MDC 01	M	MULTIPLE SCLEROSIS & CEREBELLAR ATAXIA W CC
060	MDC 01	M	MULTIPLE SCLEROSIS & CEREBELLAR ATAXIA W/O CC/MCC
061	MDC 01	M	ACUTE ISCHEMIC STROKE W USE OF THROMBOLYTIC AGENT W MCC
062	MDC 01	M	ACUTE ISCHEMIC STROKE W USE OF THROMBOLYTIC AGENT W CC
063	MDC 01	M	ACUTE ISCHEMIC STROKE W USE OF THROMBOLYTIC AGENT W/O CC/MCC
064	MDC 01	M	INTRACRANIAL HEMORRHAGE OR CEREBRAL INFARCTION W MCC
065	MDC 01	M	INTRACRANIAL HEMORRHAGE OR CEREBRAL INFARCTION W CC
066	MDC 01	M	INTRACRANIAL HEMORRHAGE OR CEREBRAL INFARCTION W/O CC/MCC
067	MDC 01	M	NONSPECIFIC CVA & PRECEREBRAL OCCLUSION W/O INFARCT W MCC
068	MDC 01	M	NONSPECIFIC CVA & PRECEREBRAL OCCLUSION W/O INFARCT W/O MCC
069	MDC 01	M	TRANSIENT ISCHEMIA
070	MDC 01	M	NONSPECIFIC CEREBROVASCULAR DISORDERS W MCC
071	MDC 01	M	NONSPECIFIC CEREBROVASCULAR DISORDERS W CC
072	MDC 01	M	NONSPECIFIC CEREBROVASCULAR DISORDERS W/O CC/MCC
073	MDC 01	M	CRANIAL & PERIPHERAL NERVE DISORDERS W MCC
074	MDC 01	M	CRANIAL & PERIPHERAL NERVE DISORDERS W/O MCC
075	MDC 01	M	VIRAL MENINGITIS W CC/MCC
076	MDC 01	M	VIRAL MENINGITIS W/O CC/MCC
077	MDC 01	M	HYPERTENSIVE ENCEPHALOPATHY W MCC
078	MDC 01	M	HYPERTENSIVE ENCEPHALOPATHY W CC
079	MDC 01	M	HYPERTENSIVE ENCEPHALOPATHY W/O CC/MCC
080	MDC 01	M	NONTRAUMATIC STUPOR & COMA W MCC
081	MDC 01	M	NONTRAUMATIC STUPOR & COMA W/O MCC
082	MDC 01	M	TRAUMATIC STUPOR & COMA, COMA >1 HR W MCC
083	MDC 01	M	TRAUMATIC STUPOR & COMA, COMA >1 HR W CC
084	MDC 01	M	TRAUMATIC STUPOR & COMA, COMA >1 HR W/O CC/MCC
085	MDC 01	M	TRAUMATIC STUPOR & COMA, COMA <1 HR W MCC

086	MDC 01	M	TRAUMATIC STUPOR & COMA, COMA <1 HR W CC
087	MDC 01	M	TRAUMATIC STUPOR & COMA, COMA <1 HR W/O CC/MCC
088	MDC 01	M	CONCUSSION W MCC
089	MDC 01	M	CONCUSSION W CC
090	MDC 01	M	CONCUSSION W/O CC/MCC
091	MDC 01	M	OTHER DISORDERS OF NERVOUS SYSTEM W MCC
092	MDC 01	M	OTHER DISORDERS OF NERVOUS SYSTEM W CC
093	MDC 01	M	OTHER DISORDERS OF NERVOUS SYSTEM W/O CC/MCC
094	MDC 01	M	BACTERIAL & TUBERCULOUS INFECTIONS OF NERVOUS SYSTEM W MCC
095	MDC 01	M	BACTERIAL & TUBERCULOUS INFECTIONS OF NERVOUS SYSTEM W CC
096	MDC 01	M	BACTERIAL & TUBERCULOUS INFECTIONS OF NERVOUS SYSTEM W/O CC/MCC
097	MDC 01	M	NON-BACTERIAL INFECT OF NERVOUS SYS EXC VIRAL MENINGITIS W MCC
098	MDC 01	M	NON-BACTERIAL INFECT OF NERVOUS SYS EXC VIRAL MENINGITIS W CC
099	MDC 01	M	NON-BACTERIAL INFECT OF NERVOUS SYS EXC VIRAL MENINGITIS W/O CC/MCC
100	MDC 01	M	SEIZURES W MCC
101	MDC 01	M	SEIZURES W/O MCC
102	MDC 01	M	HEADACHES W MCC
103	MDC 01	M	HEADACHES W/O MCC
113	MDC 02	P	ORBITAL PROCEDURES W CC/MCC
114	MDC 02	P	ORBITAL PROCEDURES W/O CC/MCC
115	MDC 02	P	EXTRAOCULAR PROCEDURES EXCEPT ORBIT
116	MDC 02	P	INTRAOCULAR PROCEDURES W CC/MCC
117	MDC 02	P	INTRAOCULAR PROCEDURES W/O CC/MCC
121	MDC 02	M	ACUTE MAJOR EYE INFECTIONS W CC/MCC
122	MDC 02	M	ACUTE MAJOR EYE INFECTIONS W/O CC/MCC
123	MDC 02	M	NEUROLOGICAL EYE DISORDERS
124	MDC 02	M	OTHER DISORDERS OF THE EYE W MCC
125	MDC 02	M	OTHER DISORDERS OF THE EYE W/O MCC
129	MDC 03	P	MAJOR HEAD & NECK PROCEDURES W CC/MCC OR MAJOR DEVICE
130	MDC 03	P	MAJOR HEAD & NECK PROCEDURES W/O CC/MCC
131	MDC 03	P	CRANIAL/FACIAL PROCEDURES W CC/MCC
132	MDC 03	P	CRANIAL/FACIAL PROCEDURES W/O CC/MCC
133	MDC 03	P	OTHER EAR, NOSE, MOUTH & THROAT O.R. PROCEDURES W CC/MCC
134	MDC 03	P	OTHER EAR, NOSE, MOUTH & THROAT O.R. PROCEDURES W/O CC/MCC
135	MDC 03	P	SINUS & MASTOID PROCEDURES W CC/MCC
136	MDC 03	P	SINUS & MASTOID PROCEDURES W/O CC/MCC
137	MDC 03	P	MOUTH PROCEDURES W CC/MCC
138	MDC 03	P	MOUTH PROCEDURES W/O CC/MCC
139	MDC 03	P	SALIVARY GLAND PROCEDURES
146	MDC 03	M	EAR, NOSE, MOUTH & THROAT MALIGNANCY W MCC
147	MDC 03	M	EAR, NOSE, MOUTH & THROAT MALIGNANCY W CC
148	MDC 03	M	EAR, NOSE, MOUTH & THROAT MALIGNANCY W/O CC/MCC
149	MDC 03	M	DYSEQUILIBRIUM
150	MDC 03	M	EPISTAXIS W MCC
151	MDC 03	M	EPISTAXIS W/O MCC
152	MDC 03	M	OTITIS MEDIA & URI W MCC
153	MDC 03	M	OTITIS MEDIA & URI W/O MCC
154	MDC 03	M	OTHER EAR, NOSE, MOUTH & THROAT DIAGNOSES W MCC
155	MDC 03	M	OTHER EAR, NOSE, MOUTH & THROAT DIAGNOSES W CC
156	MDC 03	M	OTHER EAR, NOSE, MOUTH & THROAT DIAGNOSES W/O CC/MCC
157	MDC 03	M	DENTAL & ORAL DISEASES W MCC
158	MDC 03	M	DENTAL & ORAL DISEASES W CC
159	MDC 03	M	DENTAL & ORAL DISEASES W/O CC/MCC
163	MDC 04	P	MAJOR CHEST PROCEDURES W MCC
164	MDC 04	P	MAJOR CHEST PROCEDURES W CC
165	MDC 04	P	MAJOR CHEST PROCEDURES W/O CC/MCC
166	MDC 04	P	OTHER RESP SYSTEM O.R. PROCEDURES W MCC
167	MDC 04	P	OTHER RESP SYSTEM O.R. PROCEDURES W CC
168	MDC 04	P	OTHER RESP SYSTEM O.R. PROCEDURES W/O CC/MCC
175	MDC 04	M	PULMONARY EMBOLISM W MCC
176	MDC 04	M	PULMONARY EMBOLISM W/O MCC
177	MDC 04	M	RESPIRATORY INFECTIONS & INFLAMMATIONS W MCC
178	MDC 04	M	RESPIRATORY INFECTIONS & INFLAMMATIONS W CC
179	MDC 04	M	RESPIRATORY INFECTIONS & INFLAMMATIONS W/O CC/MCC
180	MDC 04	M	RESPIRATORY NEOPLASMS W MCC
181	MDC 04	M	RESPIRATORY NEOPLASMS W CC
182	MDC 04	M	RESPIRATORY NEOPLASMS W/O CC/MCC
183	MDC 04	M	MAJOR CHEST TRAUMA W MCC
184	MDC 04	M	MAJOR CHEST TRAUMA W CC
185	MDC 04	M	MAJOR CHEST TRAUMA W/O CC/MCC
186	MDC 04	M	PLEURAL EFFUSION W MCC
187	MDC 04	M	PLEURAL EFFUSION W CC
188	MDC 04	M	PLEURAL EFFUSION W/O CC/MCC

189	MDC 04	M	PULMONARY EDEMA & RESPIRATORY FAILURE
190	MDC 04	M	CHRONIC OBSTRUCTIVE PULMONARY DISEASE W MCC
191	MDC 04	M	CHRONIC OBSTRUCTIVE PULMONARY DISEASE W CC
192	MDC 04	M	CHRONIC OBSTRUCTIVE PULMONARY DISEASE W/O CC/MCC
193	MDC 04	M	SIMPLE PNEUMONIA & PLEURISY W MCC
194	MDC 04	M	SIMPLE PNEUMONIA & PLEURISY W CC
195	MDC 04	M	SIMPLE PNEUMONIA & PLEURISY W/O CC/MCC
196	MDC 04	M	INTERSTITIAL LUNG DISEASE W MCC
197	MDC 04	M	INTERSTITIAL LUNG DISEASE W CC
198	MDC 04	M	INTERSTITIAL LUNG DISEASE W/O CC/MCC
199	MDC 04	M	PNEUMOTHORAX W MCC
200	MDC 04	M	PNEUMOTHORAX W CC
201	MDC 04	M	PNEUMOTHORAX W/O CC/MCC
202	MDC 04	M	BRONCHITIS & ASTHMA W CC/MCC
203	MDC 04	M	BRONCHITIS & ASTHMA W/O CC/MCC
204	MDC 04	M	RESPIRATORY SIGNS & SYMPTOMS
205	MDC 04	M	OTHER RESPIRATORY SYSTEM DIAGNOSES W MCC
206	MDC 04	M	OTHER RESPIRATORY SYSTEM DIAGNOSES W/O MCC
207	MDC 04	M	RESPIRATORY SYSTEM DIAGNOSIS W VENTILATOR SUPPORT 96+ HOURS
208	MDC 04	M	RESPIRATORY SYSTEM DIAGNOSIS W VENTILATOR SUPPORT <96 HOURS
215	MDC 05	P	OTHER HEART ASSIST SYSTEM IMPLANT
216	MDC 05	P	CARDIAC VALVE & OTH MAJ CARDIOTHORACIC PROC W CARD CATH W MCC
217	MDC 05	P	CARDIAC VALVE & OTH MAJ CARDIOTHORACIC PROC W CARD CATH W CC
218	MDC 05	P	CARDIAC VALVE & OTH MAJ CARDIOTHORACIC PROC W CARD CATH W/O CC/MCC
219	MDC 05	P	CARDIAC VALVE & OTH MAJ CARDIOTHORACIC PROC W/O CARD CATH W MCC
220	MDC 05	P	CARDIAC VALVE & OTH MAJ CARDIOTHORACIC PROC W/O CARD CATH W CC
221	MDC 05	P	CARDIAC VALVE & OTH MAJ CARDIOTHORACIC PROC W/O CARD CATH W/O CC/MCC
222	MDC 05	P	CARDIAC DEFIB IMPLANT W CARDIAC CATH W AMI/HF/SHOCK W MCC
223	MDC 05	P	CARDIAC DEFIB IMPLANT W CARDIAC CATH W AMI/HF/SHOCK W/O MCC
224	MDC 05	P	CARDIAC DEFIB IMPLANT W CARDIAC CATH W/O AMI/HF/SHOCK W MCC
225	MDC 05	P	CARDIAC DEFIB IMPLANT W CARDIAC CATH W/O AMI/HF/SHOCK W/O MCC
226	MDC 05	P	CARDIAC DEFIBRILLATOR IMPLANT W/O CARDIAC CATH W MCC
227	MDC 05	P	CARDIAC DEFIBRILLATOR IMPLANT W/O CARDIAC CATH W/O MCC
228	MDC 05	P	OTHER CARDIOTHORACIC PROCEDURES W MCC
229	MDC 05	P	OTHER CARDIOTHORACIC PROCEDURES W CC
230	MDC 05	P	OTHER CARDIOTHORACIC PROCEDURES W/O CC/MCC
231	MDC 05	P	CORONARY BYPASS W PTCA W MCC
232	MDC 05	P	CORONARY BYPASS W PTCA W/O MCC
233	MDC 05	P	CORONARY BYPASS W CARDIAC CATH W MCC
234	MDC 05	P	CORONARY BYPASS W CARDIAC CATH W/O MCC
235	MDC 05	P	CORONARY BYPASS W/O CARDIAC CATH W MCC
236	MDC 05	P	CORONARY BYPASS W/O CARDIAC CATH W/O MCC
237	MDC 05	P	MAJOR CARDIOVASC PROCEDURES W MCC OR THORACIC AORTIC ANEURYSM REPAIR
238	MDC 05	P	MAJOR CARDIOVASC PROCEDURES W/O MCC
239	MDC 05	P	AMPUTATION FOR CIRC SYS DISORDERS EXC UPPER LIMB & TOE W MCC
240	MDC 05	P	AMPUTATION FOR CIRC SYS DISORDERS EXC UPPER LIMB & TOE W CC
241	MDC 05	P	AMPUTATION FOR CIRC SYS DISORDERS EXC UPPER LIMB & TOE W/O CC/MCC
242	MDC 05	P	PERMANENT CARDIAC PACEMAKER IMPLANT W MCC
243	MDC 05	P	PERMANENT CARDIAC PACEMAKER IMPLANT W CC
244	MDC 05	P	PERMANENT CARDIAC PACEMAKER IMPLANT W/O CC/MCC
245	MDC 05	P	AICD GENERATOR PROCEDURES
246	MDC 05	P	PERC CARDIOVASC PROC W DRUG-ELUTING STENT W MCC OR 4+ VESSELS/STENTS
247	MDC 05	P	PERC CARDIOVASC PROC W DRUG-ELUTING STENT W/O MCC
248	MDC 05	P	PERC CARDIOVASC PROC W NON-DRUG-ELUTING STENT W MCC OR 4+ VES/STENTS
249	MDC 05	P	PERC CARDIOVASC PROC W NON-DRUG-ELUTING STENT W/O MCC
250	MDC 05	P	PERC CARDIOVASC PROC W/O CORONARY ARTERY STENT W MCC
251	MDC 05	P	PERC CARDIOVASC PROC W/O CORONARY ARTERY STENT W/O MCC
252	MDC 05	P	OTHER VASCULAR PROCEDURES W MCC
253	MDC 05	P	OTHER VASCULAR PROCEDURES W CC
254	MDC 05	P	OTHER VASCULAR PROCEDURES W/O CC/MCC
255	MDC 05	P	UPPER LIMB & TOE AMPUTATION FOR CIRC SYSTEM DISORDERS W MCC
256	MDC 05	P	UPPER LIMB & TOE AMPUTATION FOR CIRC SYSTEM DISORDERS W CC
257	MDC 05	P	UPPER LIMB & TOE AMPUTATION FOR CIRC SYSTEM DISORDERS W/O CC/MCC
258	MDC 05	P	CARDIAC PACEMAKER DEVICE REPLACEMENT W MCC
259	MDC 05	P	CARDIAC PACEMAKER DEVICE REPLACEMENT W/O MCC
260	MDC 05	P	CARDIAC PACEMAKER REVISION EXCEPT DEVICE REPLACEMENT W MCC
261	MDC 05	P	CARDIAC PACEMAKER REVISION EXCEPT DEVICE REPLACEMENT W CC

262	MDC 05	P	CARDIAC PACEMAKER REVISION EXCEPT DEVICE REPLACEMENT W/O CC/MCC
263	MDC 05	P	VEIN LIGATION & STRIPPING
264	MDC 05	P	OTHER CIRCULATORY SYSTEM O.R. PROCEDURES
265	MDC 05	P	AICD LEAD PROCEDURES
280	MDC 05	M	ACUTE MYOCARDIAL INFARCTION, DISCHARGED ALIVE W MCC
281	MDC 05	M	ACUTE MYOCARDIAL INFARCTION, DISCHARGED ALIVE W CC
282	MDC 05	M	ACUTE MYOCARDIAL INFARCTION, DISCHARGED ALIVE W/O CC/MCC
283	MDC 05	M	ACUTE MYOCARDIAL INFARCTION, EXPIRED W MCC
284	MDC 05	M	ACUTE MYOCARDIAL INFARCTION, EXPIRED W CC
285	MDC 05	M	ACUTE MYOCARDIAL INFARCTION, EXPIRED W/O CC/MCC
286	MDC 05	M	CIRCULATORY DISORDERS EXCEPT AMI, W CARD CATH W MCC
287	MDC 05	M	CIRCULATORY DISORDERS EXCEPT AMI, W CARD CATH W/O MCC
288	MDC 05	M	ACUTE & SUBACUTE ENDOCARDITIS W MCC
289	MDC 05	M	ACUTE & SUBACUTE ENDOCARDITIS W CC
290	MDC 05	M	ACUTE & SUBACUTE ENDOCARDITIS W/O CC/MCC
291	MDC 05	M	HEART FAILURE & SHOCK W MCC
292	MDC 05	M	HEART FAILURE & SHOCK W CC
293	MDC 05	M	HEART FAILURE & SHOCK W/O CC/MCC
294	MDC 05	M	DEEP VEIN THROMBOPHLEBITIS W CC/MCC
295	MDC 05	M	DEEP VEIN THROMBOPHLEBITIS W/O CC/MCC
296	MDC 05	M	CARDIAC ARREST, UNEXPLAINED W MCC
297	MDC 05	M	CARDIAC ARREST, UNEXPLAINED W CC
298	MDC 05	M	CARDIAC ARREST, UNEXPLAINED W/O CC/MCC
299	MDC 05	M	PERIPHERAL VASCULAR DISORDERS W MCC
300	MDC 05	M	PERIPHERAL VASCULAR DISORDERS W CC
301	MDC 05	M	PERIPHERAL VASCULAR DISORDERS W/O CC/MCC
302	MDC 05	M	ATHEROSCLEROSIS W MCC
303	MDC 05	M	ATHEROSCLEROSIS W/O MCC
304	MDC 05	M	HYPERTENSION W MCC
305	MDC 05	M	HYPERTENSION W/O MCC
306	MDC 05	M	CARDIAC CONGENITAL & VALVULAR DISORDERS W MCC
307	MDC 05	M	CARDIAC CONGENITAL & VALVULAR DISORDERS W/O MCC
308	MDC 05	M	CARDIAC ARRHYTHMIA & CONDUCTION DISORDERS W MCC
309	MDC 05	M	CARDIAC ARRHYTHMIA & CONDUCTION DISORDERS W CC
310	MDC 05	M	CARDIAC ARRHYTHMIA & CONDUCTION DISORDERS W/O CC/MCC
311	MDC 05	M	ANGINA PECTORIS
312	MDC 05	M	SYNCOPE & COLLAPSE
313	MDC 05	M	CHEST PAIN
314	MDC 05	M	OTHER CIRCULATORY SYSTEM DIAGNOSES W MCC
315	MDC 05	M	OTHER CIRCULATORY SYSTEM DIAGNOSES W CC
316	MDC 05	M	OTHER CIRCULATORY SYSTEM DIAGNOSES W/O CC/MCC
326	MDC 06	P	STOMACH, ESOPHAGEAL & DUODENAL PROC W MCC
327	MDC 06	P	STOMACH, ESOPHAGEAL & DUODENAL PROC W CC
328	MDC 06	P	STOMACH, ESOPHAGEAL & DUODENAL PROC W/O CC/MCC
329	MDC 06	P	MAJOR SMALL & LARGE BOWEL PROCEDURES W MCC
330	MDC 06	P	MAJOR SMALL & LARGE BOWEL PROCEDURES W CC
331	MDC 06	P	MAJOR SMALL & LARGE BOWEL PROCEDURES W/O CC/MCC
332	MDC 06	P	RECTAL RESECTION W MCC
333	MDC 06	P	RECTAL RESECTION W CC
334	MDC 06	P	RECTAL RESECTION W/O CC/MCC
335	MDC 06	P	PERITONEAL ADHESIOLYSIS W MCC
336	MDC 06	P	PERITONEAL ADHESIOLYSIS W CC
337	MDC 06	P	PERITONEAL ADHESIOLYSIS W/O CC/MCC
338	MDC 06	P	APPENDECTOMY W COMPLICATED PRINCIPAL DIAG W MCC
339	MDC 06	P	APPENDECTOMY W COMPLICATED PRINCIPAL DIAG W CC
340	MDC 06	P	APPENDECTOMY W COMPLICATED PRINCIPAL DIAG W/O CC/MCC
341	MDC 06	P	APPENDECTOMY W/O COMPLICATED PRINCIPAL DIAG W MCC
342	MDC 06	P	APPENDECTOMY W/O COMPLICATED PRINCIPAL DIAG W CC
343	MDC 06	P	APPENDECTOMY W/O COMPLICATED PRINCIPAL DIAG W/O CC/MCC
344	MDC 06	P	MINOR SMALL & LARGE BOWEL PROCEDURES W MCC
345	MDC 06	P	MINOR SMALL & LARGE BOWEL PROCEDURES W CC
346	MDC 06	P	MINOR SMALL & LARGE BOWEL PROCEDURES W/O CC/MCC
347	MDC 06	P	ANAL & STOMAL PROCEDURES W MCC
348	MDC 06	P	ANAL & STOMAL PROCEDURES W CC
349	MDC 06	P	ANAL & STOMAL PROCEDURES W/O CC/MCC
350	MDC 06	P	INGUINAL & FEMORAL HERNIA PROCEDURES W MCC
351	MDC 06	P	INGUINAL & FEMORAL HERNIA PROCEDURES W CC
352	MDC 06	P	INGUINAL & FEMORAL HERNIA PROCEDURES W/O CC/MCC
353	MDC 06	P	HERNIA PROCEDURES EXCEPT INGUINAL & FEMORAL W MCC
354	MDC 06	P	HERNIA PROCEDURES EXCEPT INGUINAL & FEMORAL W CC
355	MDC 06	P	HERNIA PROCEDURES EXCEPT INGUINAL & FEMORAL W/O CC/MCC
356	MDC 06	P	OTHER DIGESTIVE SYSTEM O.R. PROCEDURES W MCC
357	MDC 06	P	OTHER DIGESTIVE SYSTEM O.R. PROCEDURES W CC
358	MDC 06	P	OTHER DIGESTIVE SYSTEM O.R. PROCEDURES W/O CC/MCC

368	MDC 06	M	MAJOR ESOPHAGEAL DISORDERS W MCC
369	MDC 06	M	MAJOR ESOPHAGEAL DISORDERS W CC
370	MDC 06	M	MAJOR ESOPHAGEAL DISORDERS W/O CC/MCC
371	MDC 06	M	MAJOR GASTROINTESTINAL DISORDERS & PERITONEAL INFECTIONS W MCC
372	MDC 06	M	MAJOR GASTROINTESTINAL DISORDERS & PERITONEAL INFECTIONS W CC
373	MDC 06	M	MAJOR GASTROINTESTINAL DISORDERS & PERITONEAL INFECTIONS W/O CC/MCC
374	MDC 06	M	DIGESTIVE MALIGNANCY W MCC
375	MDC 06	M	DIGESTIVE MALIGNANCY W CC
376	MDC 06	M	DIGESTIVE MALIGNANCY W/O CC/MCC
377	MDC 06	M	G.I. HEMORRHAGE W MCC
378	MDC 06	M	G.I. HEMORRHAGE W CC
379	MDC 06	M	G.I. HEMORRHAGE W/O CC/MCC
380	MDC 06	M	COMPLICATED PEPTIC ULCER W MCC
381	MDC 06	M	COMPLICATED PEPTIC ULCER W CC
382	MDC 06	M	COMPLICATED PEPTIC ULCER W/O CC/MCC
383	MDC 06	M	UNCOMPLICATED PEPTIC ULCER W MCC
384	MDC 06	M	UNCOMPLICATED PEPTIC ULCER W/O MCC
385	MDC 06	M	INFLAMMATORY BOWEL DISEASE W MCC
386	MDC 06	M	INFLAMMATORY BOWEL DISEASE W CC
387	MDC 06	M	INFLAMMATORY BOWEL DISEASE W/O CC/MCC
388	MDC 06	M	G.I. OBSTRUCTION W MCC
389	MDC 06	M	G.I. OBSTRUCTION W CC
390	MDC 06	M	G.I. OBSTRUCTION W/O CC/MCC
391	MDC 06	M	ESOPHAGITIS, GASTROENT & MISC DIGEST DISORDERS W MCC
392	MDC 06	M	ESOPHAGITIS, GASTROENT & MISC DIGEST DISORDERS W/O MCC
393	MDC 06	M	OTHER DIGESTIVE SYSTEM DIAGNOSES W MCC
394	MDC 06	M	OTHER DIGESTIVE SYSTEM DIAGNOSES W CC
395	MDC 06	M	OTHER DIGESTIVE SYSTEM DIAGNOSES W/O CC/MCC
405	MDC 07	P	PANCREAS, LIVER& SHUNT PROCEDURES W MCC
406	MDC 07	P	PANCREAS, LIVER & SHUNT PROCEDURES W CC
407	MDC 07	P	PANCREAS, LIVER& SHUNT PROCEDURES W/O CC/MCC
408	MDC 07	P	BILIARY TRACT PROC EXCEPT ONLY CHOLECYST W OR W/O C.D.E. W MCC
409	MDC 07	P	BILIARY TRACT PROC EXCEPT ONLY CHOLECYST W OR W/O C.D.E. W CC
410	MDC 07	P	BILIARY TRACT PROC EXCEPT ONLY CHOLECYST W OR W/O C.D.E. W/O CC/MCC
411	MDC 07	P	CHOLECYSTECTOMY W C.D.E. W MCC
412	MDC 07	P	CHOLECYSTECTOMY W C.D.E. W CC
413	MDC 07	P	CHOLECYSTECTOMY W C.D.E. W/O CC/MCC
414	MDC 07	P	CHOLECYSTECTOMY EXCEPT BY LAPAROSCOPE W/O C.D.E. W MCC
415	MDC 07	P	CHOLECYSTECTOMY EXCEPT BY LAPAROSCOPE W/O C.D.E. W CC
416	MDC 07	P	CHOLECYSTECTOMY EXCEPT BY LAPAROSCOPE W/O C.D.E. W/O CC/MCC
417	MDC 07	P	LAPAROSCOPIC CHOLECYSTECTOMY W/O C.D.E. W MCC
418	MDC 07	P	LAPAROSCOPIC CHOLECYSTECTOMY W/O C.D.E. W CC
419	MDC 07	P	LAPAROSCOPIC CHOLECYSTECTOMY W/O C.D.E. W/O CC/MCC
420	MDC 07	P	HEPATOBILIARY DIAGNOSTIC PROCEDURES W MCC
421	MDC 07	P	HEPATOBILIARY DIAGNOSTIC PROCEDURES W CC
422	MDC 07	P	HEPATOBILIARY DIAGNOSTIC PROCEDURES W/O CC/MCC
423	MDC 07	P	OTHER HEPATOBILIARY OR PANCREAS O.R. PROCEDURES W MCC
424	MDC 07	P	OTHER HEPATOBILIARY OR PANCREAS O.R. PROCEDURES W CC
425	MDC 07	P	OTHER HEPATOBILIARY OR PANCREAS O.R. PROCEDURES W/O CC/MCC
432	MDC 07	M	CIRRHOSIS & ALCOHOLIC HEPATITIS W MCC
433	MDC 07	M	CIRRHOSIS & ALCOHOLIC HEPATITIS W CC
434	MDC 07	M	CIRRHOSIS & ALCOHOLIC HEPATITIS W/O CC/MCC
435	MDC 07	M	MALIGNANCY OF HEPATOBILIARY SYSTEM OR PANCREAS W MCC
436	MDC 07	M	MALIGNANCY OF HEPATOBILIARY SYSTEM OR PANCREAS W CC
437	MDC 07	M	MALIGNANCY OF HEPATOBILIARY SYSTEM OR PANCREAS W/O CC/MCC
438	MDC 07	M	DISORDERS OF PANCREAS EXCEPT MALIGNANCY W MCC
439	MDC 07	M	DISORDERS OF PANCREAS EXCEPT MALIGNANCY W CC
440	MDC 07	M	DISORDERS OF PANCREAS EXCEPT MALIGNANCY W/O CC/MCC
441	MDC 07	M	DISORDERS OF LIVER EXCEPT MALIG, CIRR, ALC HEPA W MCC
442	MDC 07	M	DISORDERS OF LIVER EXCEPT MALIG, CIRR, ALC HEPA W CC
443	MDC 07	M	DISORDERS OF LIVER EXCEPT MALIG, CIRR, ALC HEPA W/O CC/MCC
444	MDC 07	M	DISORDERS OF THE BILIARY TRACT W MCC
445	MDC 07	M	DISORDERS OF THE BILIARY TRACT W CC
446	MDC 07	M	DISORDERS OF THE BILIARY TRACT W/O CC/MCC
453	MDC 08	P	COMBINED ANTERIOR/POSTERIOR SPINAL FUSION W MCC
454	MDC 08	P	COMBINED ANTERIOR/POSTERIOR SPINAL FUSION W CC
455	MDC 08	P	COMBINED ANTERIOR/POSTERIOR SPINAL FUSION W/O CC/MCC
456	MDC 08	P	SPINAL FUS EXC CERV W SPINAL CURV/MALIG/INFEC OR 9+ FUS W MCC
457	MDC 08	P	SPINAL FUS EXC CERV W SPINAL CURV/MALIG/INFEC OR 9+ FUS W CC
458	MDC 08	P	SPINAL FUS EXC CERV W SPINAL CURV/MALIG/INFEC OR 9+ FUS W/O CC/MCC
459	MDC 08	P	SPINAL FUSION EXCEPT CERVICAL W MCC
460	MDC 08	P	SPINAL FUSION EXCEPT CERVICAL W/O MCC

PART VI, MS-DRG, APPENDIX A

461	MDC 08	P	BILATERAL OR MULTIPLE MAJOR JOINT PROCS OF LOWER EXTREMITY W MCC
462	MDC 08	P	BILATERAL OR MULTIPLE MAJOR JOINT PROCS OF LOWER EXTREMITY W/O MCC
463	MDC 08	P	WND DEBRID & SKN GRFT EXC HAND, FOR MUSCULO-CONN TISS DIS W MCC
464	MDC 08	P	WND DEBRID & SKN GRFT EXC HAND, FOR MUSCULO-CONN TISS DIS W CC
465	MDC 08	P	WND DEBRID & SKN GRFT EXC HAND, FOR MUSCULO-CONN TISS DIS W/O CC/MCC
466	MDC 08	P	REVISION OF HIP OR KNEE REPLACEMENT W MCC
467	MDC 08	P	REVISION OF HIP OR KNEE REPLACEMENT W CC
468	MDC 08	P	REVISION OF HIP OR KNEE REPLACEMENT W/O CC/MCC
469	MDC 08	P	MAJOR JOINT REPLACEMENT OR REATTACHMENT OF LOWER EXTREMITY W MCC
470	MDC 08	P	MAJOR JOINT REPLACEMENT OR REATTACHMENT OF LOWER EXTREMITY W/O MCC
471	MDC 08	P	CERVICAL SPINAL FUSION W MCC
472	MDC 08	P	CERVICAL SPINAL FUSION W CC
473	MDC 08	P	CERVICAL SPINAL FUSION W/O CC/MCC
474	MDC 08	P	AMPUTATION FOR MUSCULOSKELETAL SYS & CONN TISSUE DIS W MCC
475	MDC 08	P	AMPUTATION FOR MUSCULOSKELETAL SYS & CONN TISSUE DIS W CC
476	MDC 08	P	AMPUTATION FOR MUSCULOSKELETAL SYS & CONN TISSUE DIS W/O CC/MCC
477	MDC 08	P	BIOPSIES OF MUSCULOSKELETAL SYSTEM & CONNECTIVE TISSUE W MCC
478	MDC 08	P	BIOPSIES OF MUSCULOSKELETAL SYSTEM & CONNECTIVE TISSUE W CC
479	MDC 08	P	BIOPSIES OF MUSCULOSKELETAL SYSTEM & CONNECTIVE TISSUE W/O CC/MCC
480	MDC 08	P	HIP & FEMUR PROCEDURES EXCEPT MAJOR JOINT W MCC
481	MDC 08	P	HIP & FEMUR PROCEDURES EXCEPT MAJOR JOINT W CC
482	MDC 08	P	HIP & FEMUR PROCEDURES EXCEPT MAJOR JOINT W/O CC/MCC
483	MDC 08	P	MAJOR JOINT & LIMB REATTACHMENT PROC OF UPPER EXTREMITY W CC/MCC
484	MDC 08	P	MAJOR JOINT & LIMB REATTACHMENT PROC OF UPPER EXTREMITY W/O CC/MCC
485	MDC 08	P	KNEE PROCEDURES W PDX OF INFECTION W MCC
486	MDC 08	P	KNEE PROCEDURES W PDX OF INFECTION W CC
487	MDC 08	P	KNEE PROCEDURES W PDX OF INFECTION W/O CC/MCC
488	MDC 08	P	KNEE PROCEDURES W/O PDX OF INFECTION W CC/MCC
489	MDC 08	P	KNEE PROCEDURES W/O PDX OF INFECTION W/O CC/MCC
490	MDC 08	P	BACK & NECK PROC EXC SPINAL FUSION W CC/MCC OR DISC DEVICE/NEUROSTIM
491	MDC 08	P	BACK & NECK PROC EXC SPINAL FUSION W/O CC/MCC
492	MDC 08	P	LOWER EXTREM & HUMER PROC EXCEPT HIP, FOOT, FEMUR W MCC
493	MDC 08	P	LOWER EXTREM & HUMER PROC EXCEPT HIP, FOOT, FEMUR W CC
494	MDC 08	P	LOWER EXTREM & HUMER PROC EXCEPT HIP, FOOT, FEMUR W/O CC/MCC
495	MDC 08	P	LOCAL EXCISION & REMOVAL INT FIX DEVICES EXC HIP & FEMUR W MCC
496	MDC 08	P	LOCAL EXCISION & REMOVAL INT FIX DEVICES EXC HIP & FEMUR W CC
497	MDC 08	P	LOCAL EXCISION & REMOVAL INT FIX DEVICES EXC HIP & FEMUR W/O CC/MCC
498	MDC 08	P	LOCAL EXCISION & REMOVAL INT FIX DEVICES OF HIP & FEMUR W CC/MCC
499	MDC 08	P	LOCAL EXCISION & REMOVAL INT FIX DEVICES OF HIP & FEMUR W/O CC/MCC
500	MDC 08	P	SOFT TISSUE PROCEDURES W MCC
501	MDC 08	P	SOFT TISSUE PROCEDURES W CC
502	MDC 08	P	SOFT TISSUE PROCEDURES W/O CC/MCC
503	MDC 08	P	FOOT PROCEDURES W MCC
504	MDC 08	P	FOOT PROCEDURES W CC
505	MDC 08	P	FOOT PROCEDURES W/O CC/MCC
506	MDC 08	P	MAJOR THUMB OR JOINT PROCEDURES
507	MDC 08	P	MAJOR SHOULDER OR ELBOW JOINT PROCEDURES W CC/MCC
508	MDC 08	P	MAJOR SHOULDER OR ELBOW JOINT PROCEDURES W/O CC/MCC
509	MDC 08	P	ARTHROSCOPY
510	MDC 08	P	SHOULDER, ELBOW OR FOREARM PROC, EXC MAJOR JOINT PROC W MCC
511	MDC 08	P	SHOULDER, ELBOW OR FOREARM PROC, EXC MAJOR JOINT PROC W CC
512	MDC 08	P	SHOULDER, ELBOW OR FOREARM PROC, EXC MAJOR JOINT PROC W/O CC/MCC
513	MDC 08	P	HAND OR WRIST PROC, EXCEPT MAJOR THUMB OR JOINT PROC W CC/MCC
514	MDC 08	P	HAND OR WRIST PROC, EXCEPT MAJOR THUMB OR JOINT PROC W/O CC/MCC
515	MDC 08	P	OTHER MUSCULOSKELET SYS & CONN TISS O.R. PROC W MCC
516	MDC 08	P	OTHER MUSCULOSKELET SYS & CONN TISS O.R. PROC W CC
517	MDC 08	P	OTHER MUSCULOSKELET SYS & CONN TISS O.R. PROC W/O CC/MCC
533	MDC 08	M	FRACTURES OF FEMUR W MCC
534	MDC 08	M	FRACTURES OF FEMUR W/O MCC
535	MDC 08	M	FRACTURES OF HIP & PELVIS W MCC
536	MDC 08	M	FRACTURES OF HIP & PELVIS W/O MCC
537	MDC 08	M	SPRAINS, STRAINS, & DISLOCATIONS OF HIP, PELVIS & THIGH W CC/MCC

538	MDC 08	M	SPRAINS, STRAINS, & DISLOCATIONS OF HIP, PELVIS & THIGH W/O CC/MCC
539	MDC 08	M	OSTEOMYELITIS W MCC
540	MDC 08	M	OSTEOMYELITIS W CC
541	MDC 08	M	OSTEOMYELITIS W/O CC/MCC
542	MDC 08	M	PATHOLOGICAL FRACTURES & MUSCULOSKELET & CONN TISS MALIG W MCC
543	MDC 08	M	PATHOLOGICAL FRACTURES & MUSCULOSKELET & CONN TISS MALIG W CC
544	MDC 08	M	PATHOLOGICAL FRACTURES & MUSCULOSKELET & CONN TISS MALIG W/O CC/MCC
545	MDC 08	M	CONNECTIVE TISSUE DISORDERS W MCC
546	MDC 08	M	CONNECTIVE TISSUE DISORDERS W CC
547	MDC 08	M	CONNECTIVE TISSUE DISORDERS W/O CC/MCC
548	MDC 08	M	SEPTIC ARTHRITIS W MCC
549	MDC 08	M	SEPTIC ARTHRITIS W CC
550	MDC 08	M	SEPTIC ARTHRITIS W/O CC/MCC
551	MDC 08	M	MEDICAL BACK PROBLEMS W MCC
552	MDC 08	M	MEDICAL BACK PROBLEMS W/O MCC
553	MDC 08	M	BONE DISEASES & ARTHROPATHIES W MCC
554	MDC 08	M	BONE DISEASES & ARTHROPATHIES W/O MCC
555	MDC 08	M	SIGNS & SYMPTOMS OF MUSCULOSKELETAL SYSTEM & CONN TISSUE W MCC
556	MDC 08	M	SIGNS & SYMPTOMS OF MUSCULOSKELETAL SYSTEM & CONN TISSUE W/O MCC
557	MDC 08	M	TENDONITIS, MYOSITIS & BURSITIS W MCC
558	MDC 08	M	TENDONITIS, MYOSITIS & BURSITIS W/O MCC
559	MDC 08	M	AFTERCARE, MUSCULOSKELETAL SYSTEM & CONNECTIVE TISSUE W MCC
560	MDC 08	M	AFTERCARE, MUSCULOSKELETAL SYSTEM & CONNECTIVE TISSUE W CC
561	MDC 08	M	AFTERCARE, MUSCULOSKELETAL SYSTEM & CONNECTIVE TISSUE W/O CC/MCC
562	MDC 08	M	FX, SPRN, STRN & DISL EXCEPT FEMUR, HIP, PELVIS & THIGH W MCC
563	MDC 08	M	FX, SPRN, STRN & DISL EXCEPT FEMUR, HIP, PELVIS & THIGH W/O MCC
564	MDC 08	M	OTHER MUSCULOSKELETAL SYS & CONNECTIVE TISSUE DIAGNOSES W MCC
565	MDC 08	M	OTHER MUSCULOSKELETAL SYS & CONNECTIVE TISSUE DIAGNOSES W CC
566	MDC 08	M	OTHER MUSCULOSKELETAL SYS & CONNECTIVE TISSUE DIAGNOSES W/O CC/MCC
573	MDC 09	P	SKIN GRAFT &/OR DEBRID FOR SKN ULCER OR CELLULITIS W MCC
574	MDC 09	P	SKIN GRAFT &/OR DEBRID FOR SKN ULCER OR CELLULITIS W CC
575	MDC 09	P	SKIN GRAFT &/OR DEBRID FOR SKN ULCER OR CELLULITIS W/O CC/MCC
576	MDC 09	P	SKIN GRAFT &/OR DEBRID EXC FOR SKIN ULCER OR CELLULITIS W MCC
577	MDC 09	P	SKIN GRAFT &/OR DEBRID EXC FOR SKIN ULCER OR CELLULITIS W CC
578	MDC 09	P	SKIN GRAFT &/OR DEBRID EXC FOR SKIN ULCER OR CELLULITIS W/O CC/MCC
579	MDC 09	P	OTHER SKIN, SUBCUT TISS & BREAST PROC W MCC
580	MDC 09	P	OTHER SKIN, SUBCUT TISS & BREAST PROC W CC
581	MDC 09	P	OTHER SKIN, SUBCUT TISS & BREAST PROC W/O CC/MCC
582	MDC 09	P	MASTECTOMY FOR MALIGNANCY W CC/MCC
583	MDC 09	P	MASTECTOMY FOR MALIGNANCY W/O CC/MCC
584	MDC 09	P	BREAST BIOPSY, LOCAL EXCISION & OTHER BREAST PROCEDURES W CC/MCC
585	MDC 09	P	BREAST BIOPSY, LOCAL EXCISION & OTHER BREAST PROCEDURES W/O CC/MCC
592	MDC 09	M	SKIN ULCERS W MCC
593	MDC 09	M	SKIN ULCERS W CC
594	MDC 09	M	SKIN ULCERS W/O CC/MCC
595	MDC 09	M	MAJOR SKIN DISORDERS W MCC
596	MDC 09	M	MAJOR SKIN DISORDERS W/O MCC
597	MDC 09	M	MALIGNANT BREAST DISORDERS W MCC
598	MDC 09	M	MALIGNANT BREAST DISORDERS W CC
599	MDC 09	M	MALIGNANT BREAST DISORDERS W/O CC/MCC
600	MDC 09	M	NON-MALIGNANT BREAST DISORDERS W CC/MCC
601	MDC 09	M	NON-MALIGNANT BREAST DISORDERS W/O CC/MCC
602	MDC 09	M	CELLULITIS W MCC
603	MDC 09	M	CELLULITIS W/O MCC
604	MDC 09	M	TRAUMA TO THE SKIN, SUBCUT TISS & BREAST W MCC
605	MDC 09	M	TRAUMA TO THE SKIN, SUBCUT TISS & BREAST W/O MCC
606	MDC 09	M	MINOR SKIN DISORDERS W MCC
607	MDC 09	M	MINOR SKIN DISORDERS W/O MCC
614	MDC 10	P	ADRENAL & PITUITARY PROCEDURES W CC/MCC
615	MDC 10	P	ADRENAL & PITUITARY PROCEDURES W/O CC/MCC
616	MDC 10	P	AMPUTAT OF LOWER LIMB FOR ENDOCRINE, NUTRIT, & METABOL DIS W MCC
617	MDC 10	P	AMPUTAT OF LOWER LIMB FOR ENDOCRINE, NUTRIT, & METABOL DIS W CC
618	MDC 10	P	AMPUTAT OF LOWER LIMB FOR ENDOCRINE, NUTRIT, & METABOL DIS W/O CC/MCC
619	MDC 10	P	O.R. PROCEDURES FOR OBESITY W MCC
620	MDC 10	P	O.R. PROCEDURES FOR OBESITY W CC

621	MDC 10	P	O.R. PROCEDURES FOR OBESITY W/O CC/MCC
622	MDC 10	P	SKIN GRAFTS & WOUND DEBRID FOR ENDOC, NUTRIT & METAB DIS W MCC
623	MDC 10	P	SKIN GRAFTS & WOUND DEBRID FOR ENDOC, NUTRIT & METAB DIS W CC
624	MDC 10	P	SKIN GRAFTS & WOUND DEBRID FOR ENDOC, NUTRIT & METAB DIS W/O CC/MCC
625	MDC 10	P	THYROID, PARATHYROID & THYROGLOSSAL PROCEDURES W MCC
626	MDC 10	P	THYROID, PARATHYROID & THYROGLOSSAL PROCEDURES W CC
627	MDC 10	P	THYROID, PARATHYROID & THYROGLOSSAL PROCEDURES W/O CC/MCC
628	MDC 10	P	OTHER ENDOCRINE, NUTRIT & METAB O.R. PROC W MCC
629	MDC 10	P	OTHER ENDOCRINE, NUTRIT & METAB O.R. PROC W CC
630	MDC 10	P	OTHER ENDOCRINE, NUTRIT & METAB O.R. PROC W/O CC/MCC
637	MDC 10	M	DIABETES W MCC
638	MDC 10	M	DIABETES W CC
639	MDC 10	M	DIABETES W/O CC/MCC
640	MDC 10	M	NUTRITIONAL & MISC METABOLIC DISORDERS W MCC
641	MDC 10	M	NUTRITIONAL & MISC METABOLIC DISORDERS W/O MCC
642	MDC 10	M	INBORN ERRORS OF METABOLISM
643	MDC 10	M	ENDOCRINE DISORDERS W MCC
644	MDC 10	M	ENDOCRINE DISORDERS W CC
645	MDC 10	M	ENDOCRINE DISORDERS W/O CC/MCC
652	MDC 11	P	KIDNEY TRANSPLANT
653	MDC 11	P	MAJOR BLADDER PROCEDURES W MCC
654	MDC 11	P	MAJOR BLADDER PROCEDURES W CC
655	MDC 11	P	MAJOR BLADDER PROCEDURES W/O CC/MCC
656	MDC 11	P	KIDNEY & URETER PROCEDURES FOR NEOPLASM W MCC
657	MDC 11	P	KIDNEY & URETER PROCEDURES FOR NEOPLASM W CC
658	MDC 11	P	KIDNEY & URETER PROCEDURES FOR NEOPLASM W/O CC/MCC
659	MDC 11	P	KIDNEY & URETER PROCEDURES FOR NON-NEOPLASM W MCC
660	MDC 11	P	KIDNEY & URETER PROCEDURES FOR NON-NEOPLASM W CC
661	MDC 11	P	KIDNEY & URETER PROCEDURES FOR NON-NEOPLASM W/O CC/MCC
662	MDC 11	P	MINOR BLADDER PROCEDURES W MCC
663	MDC 11	P	MINOR BLADDER PROCEDURES W CC
664	MDC 11	P	MINOR BLADDER PROCEDURES W/O CC/MCC
665	MDC 11	P	PROSTATECTOMY W MCC
666	MDC 11	P	PROSTATECTOMY W CC
667	MDC 11	P	PROSTATECTOMY W/O CC/MCC
668	MDC 11	P	TRANSURETHRAL PROCEDURES W MCC
669	MDC 11	P	TRANSURETHRAL PROCEDURES W CC
670	MDC 11	P	TRANSURETHRAL PROCEDURES W/O CC/MCC
671	MDC 11	P	URETHRAL PROCEDURES W CC/MCC
672	MDC 11	P	URETHRAL PROCEDURES W/O CC/MCC
673	MDC 11	P	OTHER KIDNEY & URINARY TRACT PROCEDURES W MCC
674	MDC 11	P	OTHER KIDNEY & URINARY TRACT PROCEDURES W CC
675	MDC 11	P	OTHER KIDNEY & URINARY TRACT PROCEDURES W/O CC/MCC
682	MDC 11	M	RENAL FAILURE W MCC
683	MDC 11	M	RENAL FAILURE W CC
684	MDC 11	M	RENAL FAILURE W/O CC/MCC
685	MDC 11	M	ADMIT FOR RENAL DIALYSIS
686	MDC 11	M	KIDNEY & URINARY TRACT NEOPLASMS W MCC
687	MDC 11	M	KIDNEY & URINARY TRACT NEOPLASMS W CC
688	MDC 11	M	KIDNEY & URINARY TRACT NEOPLASMS W/O CC/MCC
689	MDC 11	M	KIDNEY & URINARY TRACT INFECTIONS W MCC
690	MDC 11	M	KIDNEY & URINARY TRACT INFECTIONS W/O MCC
691	MDC 11	M	URINARY STONES W ESW LITHOTRIPSY W CC/MCC
692	MDC 11	M	URINARY STONES W ESW LITHOTRIPSY W/O CC/MCC
693	MDC 11	M	URINARY STONES W/O ESW LITHOTRIPSY W MCC
694	MDC 11	M	URINARY STONES W/O ESW LITHOTRIPSY W/O MCC
695	MDC 11	M	KIDNEY & URINARY TRACT SIGNS & SYMPTOMS W MCC
696	MDC 11	M	KIDNEY & URINARY TRACT SIGNS & SYMPTOMS W/O MCC
697	MDC 11	M	URETHRAL STRICTURE
698	MDC 11	M	OTHER KIDNEY & URINARY TRACT DIAGNOSES W MCC
699	MDC 11	M	OTHER KIDNEY & URINARY TRACT DIAGNOSES W CC
700	MDC 11	M	OTHER KIDNEY & URINARY TRACT DIAGNOSES W/O CC/MCC
707	MDC 12	P	MAJOR MALE PELVIC PROCEDURES W CC/MCC
708	MDC 12	P	MAJOR MALE PELVIC PROCEDURES W/O CC/MCC
709	MDC 12	P	PENIS PROCEDURES W CC/MCC
710	MDC 12	P	PENIS PROCEDURES W/O CC/MCC
711	MDC 12	P	TESTES PROCEDURES W CC/MCC
712	MDC 12	P	TESTES PROCEDURES W/O CC/MCC
713	MDC 12	P	TRANSURETHRAL PROSTATECTOMY W CC/MCC
714	MDC 12	P	TRANSURETHRAL PROSTATECTOMY W/O CC/MCC
715	MDC 12	P	OTHER MALE REPRODUCTIVE SYSTEM O.R. PROC FOR MALIGNANCY W CC/MCC
716	MDC 12	P	OTHER MALE REPRODUCTIVE SYSTEM O.R. PROC FOR MALIGNANCY W/O CC/MCC

717	MDC 12	P	OTHER MALE REPRODUCTIVE SYSTEM O.R. PROC EXC MALIGNANCY W CC/MCC
718	MDC 12	P	OTHER MALE REPRODUCTIVE SYSTEM O.R. PROC EXC MALIGNANCY W/O CC/MCC
722	MDC 12	M	MALIGNANCY, MALE REPRODUCTIVE SYSTEM W MCC
723	MDC 12	M	MALIGNANCY, MALE REPRODUCTIVE SYSTEM W CC
724	MDC 12	M	MALIGNANCY, MALE REPRODUCTIVE SYSTEM W/O CC/MCC
725	MDC 12	M	BENIGN PROSTATIC HYPERTROPHY W MCC
726	MDC 12	M	BENIGN PROSTATIC HYPERTROPHY W/O MCC
727	MDC 12	M	INFLAMMATION OF THE MALE REPRODUCTIVE SYSTEM W MCC
728	MDC 12	M	INFLAMMATION OF THE MALE REPRODUCTIVE SYSTEM W/O MCC
729	MDC 12	M	OTHER MALE REPRODUCTIVE SYSTEM DIAGNOSES W CC/MCC
730	MDC 12	M	OTHER MALE REPRODUCTIVE SYSTEM DIAGNOSES W/O CC/MCC
734	MDC 13	P	PELVIC EVISCERATION, RAD HYSTERECTOMY & RAD VULVECTOMY W CC/MCC
735	MDC 13	P	PELVIC EVISCERATION, RAD HYSTERECTOMY & RAD VULVECTOMY W/O CC/MCC
736	MDC 13	P	UTERINE & ADNEXA PROC FOR OVARIAN OR ADNEXAL MALIGNANCY W MCC
737	MDC 13	P	UTERINE & ADNEXA PROC FOR OVARIAN OR ADNEXAL MALIGNANCY W CC
738	MDC 13	P	UTERINE & ADNEXA PROC FOR OVARIAN OR ADNEXAL MALIGNANCY W/O CC/MCC
739	MDC 13	P	UTERINE, ADNEXA PROC FOR NON-OVARIAN/ADNEXAL MALIG W MCC
740	MDC 13	P	UTERINE, ADNEXA PROC FOR NON-OVARIAN/ADNEXAL MALIG W CC
741	MDC 13	P	UTERINE, ADNEXA PROC FOR NON-OVARIAN/ADNEXAL MALIG W/O CC/MCC
742	MDC 13	P	UTERINE & ADNEXA PROC FOR NON-MALIGNANCY W CC/MCC
743	MDC 13	P	UTERINE & ADNEXA PROC FOR NON-MALIGNANCY W/O CC/MCC
744	MDC 13	P	D&C, CONIZATION, LAPAROSCOPY & TUBAL INTERRUPTION W CC/MCC
745	MDC 13	P	D&C, CONIZATION, LAPAROSCOPY & TUBAL INTERRUPTION W/O CC/MCC
746	MDC 13	P	VAGINA, CERVIX & VULVA PROCEDURES W CC/MCC
747	MDC 13	P	VAGINA, CERVIX & VULVA PROCEDURES W/O CC/MCC
748	MDC 13	P	FEMALE REPRODUCTIVE SYSTEM RECONSTRUCTIVE PROCEDURES
749	MDC 13	P	OTHER FEMALE REPRODUCTIVE SYSTEM O.R. PROCEDURES W CC/MCC
750	MDC 13	P	OTHER FEMALE REPRODUCTIVE SYSTEM O.R. PROCEDURES W/O CC/MCC
754	MDC 13	M	MALIGNANCY, FEMALE REPRODUCTIVE SYSTEM W MCC
755	MDC 13	M	MALIGNANCY, FEMALE REPRODUCTIVE SYSTEM W CC
756	MDC 13	M	MALIGNANCY, FEMALE REPRODUCTIVE SYSTEM W/O CC/MCC
757	MDC 13	M	INFECTIONS, FEMALE REPRODUCTIVE SYSTEM W MCC
758	MDC 13	M	INFECTIONS, FEMALE REPRODUCTIVE SYSTEM W CC
759	MDC 13	M	INFECTIONS, FEMALE REPRODUCTIVE SYSTEM W/O CC/MCC
760	MDC 13	M	MENSTRUAL & OTHER FEMALE REPRODUCTIVE SYSTEM DISORDERS W CC/MCC
761	MDC 13	M	MENSTRUAL & OTHER FEMALE REPRODUCTIVE SYSTEM DISORDERS W/O CC/MCC
765	MDC 14	P	CESAREAN SECTION W CC/MCC
766	MDC 14	P	CESAREAN SECTION W/O CC/MCC
767	MDC 14	P	VAGINAL DELIVERY W STERILIZATION &/OR D&C
768	MDC 14	P	VAGINAL DELIVERY W O.R. PROC EXCEPT STERIL &/OR D&C
769	MDC 14	P	POSTPARTUM & POST ABORTION DIAGNOSES W O.R. PROCEDURE
770	MDC 14	P	ABORTION W D&C, ASPIRATION CURETTAGE OR HYSTEROTOMY
774	MDC 14	M	VAGINAL DELIVERY W COMPLICATING DIAGNOSES
775	MDC 14	M	VAGINAL DELIVERY W/O COMPLICATING DIAGNOSES
776	MDC 14	M	POSTPARTUM & POST ABORTION DIAGNOSES W/O O.R. PROCEDURE
777	MDC 14	M	ECTOPIC PREGNANCY
778	MDC 14	M	THREATENED ABORTION
779	MDC 14	M	ABORTION W/O D&C
780	MDC 14	M	FALSE LABOR
781	MDC 14	M	OTHER ANTEPARTUM DIAGNOSES W MEDICAL COMPLICATIONS
782	MDC 14	M	OTHER ANTEPARTUM DIAGNOSES W/O MEDICAL COMPLICATIONS
789	MDC 15	M	NEONATES, DIED OR TRANSFERRED TO ANOTHER ACUTE CARE FACILITY
790	MDC 15	M	EXTREME IMMATURITY OR RESPIRATORY DISTRESS SYNDROME NEONATE
791	MDC 15	M	PREMATURITY W MAJOR PROBLEMS
792	MDC 15	M	PREMATURITY W/O MAJOR PROBLEMS
793	MDC 15	M	FULL TERM NEONATE W MAJOR PROBLEMS
794	MDC 15	M	NEONATE W OTHER SIGNIFICANT PROBLEMS
795	MDC 15	M	NORMAL NEWBORN
799	MDC 16	P	SPLENECTOMY W MCC
800	MDC 16	P	SPLENECTOMY W CC
801	MDC 16	P	SPLENECTOMY W/O CC/MCC
802	MDC 16	P	OTHER O.R. PROC OF THE BLOOD & BLOOD FORMING ORGANS W MCC
803	MDC 16	P	OTHER O.R. PROC OF THE BLOOD & BLOOD FORMING ORGANS W CC
804	MDC 16	P	OTHER O.R. PROC OF THE BLOOD & BLOOD FORMING ORGANS W/O CC/MCC
808	MDC 16	M	MAJOR HEMATOL/IMMUN DIAG EXC SICKLE CELL CRISIS & COAGUL W MCC
809	MDC 16	M	MAJOR HEMATOL/IMMUN DIAG EXC SICKLE CELL CRISIS & COAGUL W CC

810	MDC 16	M	MAJOR HEMATOL/IMMUN DIAG EXC SICKLE CELL CRISIS & COAGUL W/O CC/MCC
811	MDC 16	M	RED BLOOD CELL DISORDERS W MCC
812	MDC 16	M	RED BLOOD CELL DISORDERS W/O MCC
813	MDC 16	M	COAGULATION DISORDERS
814	MDC 16	M	RETICULOENDOTHELIAL & IMMUNITY DISORDERS W MCC
815	MDC 16	M	RETICULOENDOTHELIAL & IMMUNITY DISORDERS W CC
816	MDC 16	M	RETICULOENDOTHELIAL & IMMUNITY DISORDERS W/O CC/MCC
820	MDC 17	P	LYMPHOMA & LEUKEMIA W MAJOR O.R. PROCEDURE W MCC
821	MDC 17	P	LYMPHOMA & LEUKEMIA W MAJOR O.R. PROCEDURE W CC
822	MDC 17	P	LYMPHOMA & LEUKEMIA W MAJOR O.R. PROCEDURE W/O CC/MCC
823	MDC 17	P	LYMPHOMA & NON-ACUTE LEUKEMIA W OTHER O.R. PROC W MCC
824	MDC 17	P	LYMPHOMA & NON-ACUTE LEUKEMIA W OTHER O.R. PROC W CC
825	MDC 17	P	LYMPHOMA & NON-ACUTE LEUKEMIA W OTHER O.R. PROC W/O CC/MCC
826	MDC 17	P	MYELOPROLIF DISORD OR POORLY DIFF NEOPL W MAJ O.R. PROC W MCC
827	MDC 17	P	MYELOPROLIF DISORD OR POORLY DIFF NEOPL W MAJ O.R. PROC W CC
828	MDC 17	P	MYELOPROLIF DISORD OR POORLY DIFF NEOPL W MAJ O.R. PROC W/O CC/MCC
829	MDC 17	P	MYELOPROLIF DISORD OR POORLY DIFF NEOPL W OTHER O.R. PROC W CC/MCC
830	MDC 17	P	MYELOPROLIF DISORD OR POORLY DIFF NEOPL W OTHER O.R. PROC W/O CC/MCC
834	MDC 17	M	ACUTE LEUKEMIA W/O MAJOR O.R. PROCEDURE W MCC
835	MDC 17	M	ACUTE LEUKEMIA W/O MAJOR O.R. PROCEDURE W CC
836	MDC 17	M	ACUTE LEUKEMIA W/O MAJOR O.R. PROCEDURE W/O CC/MCC
837	MDC 17	M	CHEMO W ACUTE LEUKEMIA AS SDX OR W HIGH DOSE CHEMO AGENT W MCC
838	MDC 17	M	CHEMO W ACUTE LEUKEMIA AS SDX W CC OR HIGH DOSE CHEMO AGENT
839	MDC 17	M	CHEMO W ACUTE LEUKEMIA AS SDX W/O CC/MCC
840	MDC 17	M	LYMPHOMA & NON-ACUTE LEUKEMIA W MCC
841	MDC 17	M	LYMPHOMA & NON-ACUTE LEUKEMIA W CC
842	MDC 17	M	LYMPHOMA & NON-ACUTE LEUKEMIA W/O CC/MCC
843	MDC 17	M	OTHER MYELOPROLIF DIS OR POORLY DIFF NEOPL DIAG W MCC
844	MDC 17	M	OTHER MYELOPROLIF DIS OR POORLY DIFF NEOPL DIAG W CC
845	MDC 17	M	OTHER MYELOPROLIF DIS OR POORLY DIFF NEOPL DIAG W/O CC/MCC
846	MDC 17	M	CHEMOTHERAPY W/O ACUTE LEUKEMIA AS SECONDARY DIAGNOSIS W MCC
847	MDC 17	M	CHEMOTHERAPY W/O ACUTE LEUKEMIA AS SECONDARY DIAGNOSIS W CC
848	MDC 17	M	CHEMOTHERAPY W/O ACUTE LEUKEMIA AS SECONDARY DIAGNOSIS W/O CC/MCC
849	MDC 17	M	RADIOTHERAPY
853	MDC 18	P	INFECTIOUS & PARASITIC DISEASES W O.R. PROCEDURE W MCC
854	MDC 18	P	INFECTIOUS & PARASITIC DISEASES W O.R. PROCEDURE W CC
855	MDC 18	P	INFECTIOUS & PARASITIC DISEASES W O.R. PROCEDURE W/O CC/MCC
856	MDC 18	P	POSTOPERATIVE OR POST-TRAUMATIC INFECTIONS W O.R. PROC W MCC
857	MDC 18	P	POSTOPERATIVE OR POST-TRAUMATIC INFECTIONS W O.R. PROC W CC
858	MDC 18	P	POSTOPERATIVE OR POST-TRAUMATIC INFECTIONS W O.R. PROC W/O CC/MCC
862	MDC 18	M	POSTOPERATIVE & POST-TRAUMATIC INFECTIONS W MCC
863	MDC 18	M	POSTOPERATIVE & POST-TRAUMATIC INFECTIONS W/O MCC
864	MDC 18	M	FEVER
865	MDC 18	M	VIRAL ILLNESS W MCC
866	MDC 18	M	VIRAL ILLNESS W/O MCC
867	MDC 18	M	OTHER INFECTIOUS & PARASITIC DISEASES DIAGNOSES W MCC
868	MDC 18	M	OTHER INFECTIOUS & PARASITIC DISEASES DIAGNOSES W CC
869	MDC 18	M	OTHER INFECTIOUS & PARASITIC DISEASES DIAGNOSES W/O CC/MCC
870	MDC 18	M	SEPTICEMIA OR SEVERE SEPSIS W MV 96+ HOURS
871	MDC 18	M	SEPTICEMIA OR SEVERE SEPSIS W/O MV 96+ HOURS W MCC
872	MDC 18	M	SEPTICEMIA OR SEVERE SEPSIS W/O MV 96+ HOURS W/O MCC
876	MDC 19	P	O.R. PROCEDURE W PRINCIPAL DIAGNOSES OF MENTAL ILLNESS
880	MDC 19	M	ACUTE ADJUSTMENT REACTION & PSYCHOSOCIAL DYSFUNCTION
881	MDC 19	M	DEPRESSIVE NEUROSES
882	MDC 19	M	NEUROSES EXCEPT DEPRESSIVE
883	MDC 19	M	DISORDERS OF PERSONALITY & IMPULSE CONTROL
884	MDC 19	M	ORGANIC DISTURBANCES & MENTAL RETARDATION
885	MDC 19	M	PSYCHOSES
886	MDC 19	M	BEHAVIORAL & DEVELOPMENTAL DISORDERS
887	MDC 19	M	OTHER MENTAL DISORDER DIAGNOSES
894	MDC 20	M	ALCOHOL/DRUG ABUSE OR DEPENDENCE LEFT AMA
895	MDC 20	M	ALCOHOL/DRUG ABUSE OR DEPENDENCE W REHABILITATION THERAPY
896	MDC 20	M	ALCOHOL/DRUG ABUSE OR DEPENDENCE W/O REHABILITATION THERAPY W MCC
897	MDC 20	M	ALCOHOL/DRUG ABUSE OR DEPENDENCE W/O REHABILITATION THERAPY W/O MCC
901	MDC 21	P	WOUND DEBRIDEMENTS FOR INJURIES W MCC
902	MDC 21	P	WOUND DEBRIDEMENTS FOR INJURIES W CC

903	MDC 21	P	WOUND DEBRIDEMENTS FOR INJURIES W/O CC/MCC
904	MDC 21	P	SKIN GRAFTS FOR INJURIES W CC/MCC
905	MDC 21	P	SKIN GRAFTS FOR INJURIES W/O CC/MCC
906	MDC 21	P	HAND PROCEDURES FOR INJURIES
907	MDC 21	P	OTHER O.R. PROCEDURES FOR INJURIES W MCC
908	MDC 21	P	OTHER O.R. PROCEDURES FOR INJURIES W CC
909	MDC 21	P	OTHER O.R. PROCEDURES FOR INJURIES W/O CC/MCC
913	MDC 21	M	TRAUMATIC INJURY W MCC
914	MDC 21	M	TRAUMATIC INJURY W/O MCC
915	MDC 21	M	ALLERGIC REACTIONS W MCC
916	MDC 21	M	ALLERGIC REACTIONS W/O MCC
917	MDC 21	M	POISONING & TOXIC EFFECTS OF DRUGS W MCC
918	MDC 21	M	POISONING & TOXIC EFFECTS OF DRUGS W/O MCC
919	MDC 21	M	COMPLICATIONS OF TREATMENT W MCC
920	MDC 21	M	COMPLICATIONS OF TREATMENT W CC
921	MDC 21	M	COMPLICATIONS OF TREATMENT W/O CC/MCC
922	MDC 21	M	OTHER INJURY, POISONING & TOXIC EFFECT DIAG W MCC
923	MDC 21	M	OTHER INJURY, POISONING & TOXIC EFFECT DIAG W/O MCC
927	MDC 22	P	EXTENSIVE BURNS OR FULL THICKNESS BURNS W MV 96+ HRS W SKIN GRAFT
928	MDC 22	P	FULL THICKNESS BURN W SKIN GRAFT OR INHAL INJ W CC/MCC
929	MDC 22	P	FULL THICKNESS BURN W SKIN GRAFT OR INHAL INJ W/O CC/MCC
933	MDC 22	M	EXTENSIVE BURNS OR FULL THICKNESS BURNS W MV 96+ HRS W/O SKIN GRAFT
934	MDC 22	M	FULL THICKNESS BURN W/O SKIN GRFT OR INHAL INJ
935	MDC 22	M	NON-EXTENSIVE BURNS
939	MDC 23	P	O.R. PROC W DIAGNOSES OF OTHER CONTACT W HEALTH SERVICES W MCC
940	MDC 23	P	O.R. PROC W DIAGNOSES OF OTHER CONTACT W HEALTH SERVICES W CC
941	MDC 23	P	O.R. PROC W DIAGNOSES OF OTHER CONTACT W HEALTH SERVICES W/O CC/MCC
945	MDC 23	M	REHABILITATION W CC/MCC
946	MDC 23	M	REHABILITATION W/O CC/MCC
947	MDC 23	M	SIGNS & SYMPTOMS W MCC
948	MDC 23	M	SIGNS & SYMPTOMS W/O MCC
949	MDC 23	M	AFTERCARE W CC/MCC
950	MDC 23	M	AFTERCARE W/O CC/MCC
951	MDC 23	M	OTHER FACTORS INFLUENCING HEALTH STATUS
955	MDC 24	P	CRANIOTOMY FOR MULTIPLE SIGNIFICANT TRAUMA
956	MDC 24	P	LIMB REATTACHMENT, HIP & FEMUR PROC FOR MULTIPLE SIGNIFICANT TRAUMA
957	MDC 24	P	OTHER O.R. PROCEDURES FOR MULTIPLE SIGNIFICANT TRAUMA W MCC
958	MDC 24	P	OTHER O.R. PROCEDURES FOR MULTIPLE SIGNIFICANT TRAUMA W CC
959	MDC 24	P	OTHER O.R. PROCEDURES FOR MULTIPLE SIGNIFICANT TRAUMA W/O CC/MCC
963	MDC 24	M	OTHER MULTIPLE SIGNIFICANT TRAUMA W MCC
964	MDC 24	M	OTHER MULTIPLE SIGNIFICANT TRAUMA W CC
965	MDC 24	M	OTHER MULTIPLE SIGNIFICANT TRAUMA W/O CC/MCC
969	MDC 25	P	HIV W EXTENSIVE O.R. PROCEDURE W MCC
970	MDC 25	P	HIV W EXTENSIVE O.R. PROCEDURE W/O MCC
974	MDC 25	M	HIV W MAJOR RELATED CONDITION W MCC
975	MDC 25	M	HIV W MAJOR RELATED CONDITION W CC
976	MDC 25	M	HIV W MAJOR RELATED CONDITION W/O CC/MCC
977	MDC 25	M	HIV W OR W/O OTHER RELATED CONDITION
981		P	EXTENSIVE O.R. PROCEDURE UNRELATED TO PRINCIPAL DIAGNOSIS W MCC
982		P	EXTENSIVE O.R. PROCEDURE UNRELATED TO PRINCIPAL DIAGNOSIS W CC
983		P	EXTENSIVE O.R. PROCEDURE UNRELATED TO PRINCIPAL DIAGNOSIS W/O CC/MCC
984		P	PROSTATIC O.R. PROCEDURE UNRELATED TO PRINCIPAL DIAGNOSIS W MCC
985		P	PROSTATIC O.R. PROCEDURE UNRELATED TO PRINCIPAL DIAGNOSIS W CC
986		P	PROSTATIC O.R. PROCEDURE UNRELATED TO PRINCIPAL DIAGNOSIS W/O CC/MCC
987		P	NON-EXTENSIVE O.R. PROC UNRELATED TO PRINCIPAL DIAGNOSIS W MCC
988		P	NON-EXTENSIVE O.R. PROC UNRELATED TO PRINCIPAL DIAGNOSIS W CC
989		P	NON-EXTENSIVE O.R. PROC UNRELATED TO PRINCIPAL DIAGNOSIS W/O CC/MCC
998			PRINCIPAL DIAGNOSIS INVALID AS DISCHARGE DIAGNOSIS
999			UNGROUPABLE

Diagnosis Code/MDC/
MS-DRG Index

The Diagnosis Code/MDC/MS-DRG Index lists each diagnosis code, as well as the MDC, and the MS-DRGs to which the diagnosis is assigned when used as the principal diagnosis. The Diagnosis Code/MDC/MS-DRG Index assumes that the secondary diagnoses do not cause assignment to MDCs 24 or 25, and that the procedures do not cause assignment to the Heart Transplant/Heart Assist System Implant, Liver or Intestinal Transplant, Lung Transplant, Bone Marrow Transplant, ECMO, Tracheostomy, Simultaneous Pancreas/Kidney Transplant or Pancreas Transplant DRGs.

DX	MDC	MS-DRG	DX	MDC	MS-DRG	DX	MDC	MS-DRG
0010	06	371-373	00847	06	371-373	01131	04	177-179
0011	06	371-373	00849	06	371-373	01132	04	177-179
0019	06	371-373	0085	06	371-373	01133	04	177-179
0020	18	867-869	00861	06	391-392	01134	04	177-179
0021	18	867-869	00862	06	391-392	01135	04	177-179
0022	18	867-869	00863	06	391-392	01136	04	177-179
0023	18	867-869	00864	06	391-392	01140	04	177-179
0029	18	867-869	00865	06	391-392	01141	04	177-179
0030	06	371-373	00866	06	391-392	01142	04	177-179
0031	18	870-872	00867	06	391-392	01143	04	177-179
00320	18	867-869	00869	06	391-392	01144	04	177-179
00321	01	023-024, 094-096	0088	06	391-392	01145	04	177-179
00322	04	177-179	0090	06	391-392	01146	04	177-179
00323	08	548-550	0091	06	391-392	01150	04	177-179
00324	08	539-541	0092	06	391-392	01151	04	177-179
00329	18	867-869	0093	06	391-392	01152	04	177-179
0038	18	867-869	01000	04	177-179	01153	04	177-179
0039	18	867-869	01001	04	177-179	01154	04	177-179
0040	06	371-373	01002	04	177-179	01155	04	177-179
0041	06	371-373	01003	04	177-179	01156	04	177-179
0042	06	371-373	01004	04	177-179	01160	04	177-179
0043	06	371-373	01005	04	177-179	01161	04	177-179
0048	06	371-373	01006	04	177-179	01162	04	177-179
0049	06	371-373	01010	04	177-179	01163	04	177-179
0050	06	371-373	01011	04	177-179	01164	04	177-179
0051	18	867-869	01012	04	177-179	01165	04	177-179
0052	06	371-373	01013	04	177-179	01166	04	177-179
0053	06	371-373	01014	04	177-179	01170	04	177-179
0054	06	371-373	01015	04	177-179	01171	04	177-179
00581	06	371-373	01016	04	177-179	01172	04	177-179
00589	06	371-373	01080	04	177-179	01173	04	177-179
0059	06	391-392	01081	04	177-179	01174	04	177-179
0060	06	371-373	01082	04	177-179	01175	04	177-179
0061	06	371-373	01083	04	177-179	01176	04	177-179
0062	06	371-373	01084	04	177-179	01180	04	177-179
0063	07	441-443	01085	04	177-179	01181	04	177-179
0064	04	177-179	01086	04	177-179	01182	04	177-179
0065	01	023-024, 097-099	01090	04	177-179	01183	04	177-179
			01091	04	177-179	01184	04	177-179
			01092	04	177-179	01185	04	177-179
0066	09	606-607	01093	04	177-179	01186	04	177-179
0068	18	867-869	01094	04	177-179	01190	04	177-179
0069	18	867-869	01095	04	177-179	01191	04	177-179
0070	06	371-373	01096	04	177-179	01192	04	177-179
0071	06	371-373	01100	04	177-179	01193	04	177-179
0072	06	371-373	01101	04	177-179	01194	04	177-179
0073	06	371-373	01102	04	177-179	01195	04	177-179
0074	06	371-373	01103	04	177-179	01196	04	177-179
0075	06	371-373	01104	04	177-179	01200	04	177-179
0078	06	371-373	01105	04	177-179	01201	04	177-179
0079	06	371-373	01106	04	177-179	01202	04	177-179
00800	06	371-373	01110	04	177-179	01203	04	177-179
00801	06	371-373	01111	04	177-179	01204	04	177-179
00802	06	371-373	01112	04	177-179	01205	04	177-179
00803	06	371-373	01113	04	177-179	01206	04	177-179
00804	06	371-373	01114	04	177-179	01210	04	177-179
00809	06	371-373	01115	04	177-179	01211	04	177-179
0081	06	371-373	01116	04	177-179	01212	04	177-179
0082	06	371-373	01120	04	177-179	01213	04	177-179
0083	06	371-373	01121	04	177-179	01214	04	177-179
00841	06	371-373	01122	04	177-179	01215	04	177-179
00842	06	371-373	01123	04	177-179	01216	04	177-179
00843	06	371-373	01124	04	177-179	01220	04	177-179
00844	06	371-373	01125	04	177-179	01221	04	177-179
00845	06	371-373	01126	04	177-179	01222	04	177-179
00846	06	371-373	01130	04	177-179	01223	04	177-179

DX	MDC	MS-DRG
01224	04	177-179
01225	04	177-179
01226	04	177-179
01230	03	154-156
01231	03	154-156
01232	03	154-156
01233	03	154-156
01234	03	154-156
01235	03	154-156
01236	03	154-156
01280	04	177-179
01281	04	177-179
01282	04	177-179
01283	04	177-179
01284	04	177-179
01285	04	177-179
01286	04	177-179
01300	01	023-024, 094-096
01301	01	023-024, 094-096
01302	01	023-024, 094-096
01303	01	023-024, 094-096
01304	01	023-024, 094-096
01305	01	023-024, 094-096
01306	01	023-024, 094-096
01310	01	023-024, 094-096
01311	01	023-024, 094-096
01312	01	023-024, 094-096
01313	01	023-024, 094-096
01314	01	023-024, 094-096
01315	01	023-024, 094-096
01316	01	023-024, 094-096
01320	01	023-024, 094-096
01321	01	023-024, 094-096
01322	01	023-024, 094-096
01323	01	023-024, 094-096
01324	01	023-024, 094-096
01325	01	023-024, 094-096
01326	01	023-024, 094-096
01330	01	023-024, 094-096
01331	01	023-024, 094-096
01332	01	023-024, 094-096

DX	MDC	MS-DRG
01333	01	023-024, 094-096
01334	01	023-024, 094-096
01335	01	023-024, 094-096
01336	01	023-024, 094-096
01340	01	023-024, 094-096
01341	01	023-024, 094-096
01342	01	023-024, 094-096
01343	01	023-024, 094-096
01344	01	023-024, 094-096
01345	01	023-024, 094-096
01346	01	023-024, 094-096
01350	01	023-024, 094-096
01351	01	023-024, 094-096
01352	01	023-024, 094-096
01353	01	023-024, 094-096
01354	01	023-024, 094-096
01355	01	023-024, 094-096
01356	01	023-024, 094-096
01360	01	023-024, 094-096
01361	01	023-024, 094-096
01362	01	023-024, 094-096
01363	01	023-024, 094-096
01364	01	023-024, 094-096
01365	01	023-024, 094-096
01366	01	023-024, 094-096
01380	01	023-024, 094-096
01381	01	023-024, 094-096
01382	01	023-024, 094-096
01383	01	023-024, 094-096
01384	01	023-024, 094-096
01385	01	023-024, 094-096
01386	01	023-024, 094-096
01390	01	023-024, 094-096

DX	MDC	MS-DRG
01391	01	023-024, 094-096
01392	01	023-024, 094-096
01393	01	023-024, 094-096
01394	01	023-024, 094-096
01395	01	023-024, 094-096
01396	01	023-024, 094-096
01400	06	371-373
01401	06	371-373
01402	06	371-373
01403	06	371-373
01404	06	371-373
01405	06	371-373
01406	06	371-373
01480	06	371-373
01481	06	371-373
01482	06	371-373
01483	06	371-373
01484	06	371-373
01485	06	371-373
01486	06	371-373
01500	08	539-541
01501	08	539-541
01502	08	456-458, 539-541
01503	08	539-541
01504	08	456-458, 539-541
01505	08	456-458, 539-541
01506	08	539-541
01510	08	548-550
01511	08	548-550
01512	08	548-550
01513	08	548-550
01514	08	548-550
01515	08	548-550
01516	08	548-550
01520	08	548-550
01521	08	548-550
01522	08	548-550
01523	08	548-550
01524	08	548-550
01525	08	548-550
01526	08	548-550
01550	08	539-541
01551	08	539-541
01552	08	539-541
01553	08	539-541
01554	08	539-541
01555	08	539-541
01556	08	539-541
01560	03	154-156
01561	03	154-156
01562	03	154-156
01563	03	154-156
01564	03	154-156
01565	03	154-156
01566	03	154-156
01570	08	539-541
01571	08	539-541

DX	MDC	MS-DRG	DX	MDC	MS-DRG	DX	MDC	MS-DRG
01572	08	539-541	01662	13	742-743, 757-759	01750	10	643-645
01573	08	539-541				01751	10	643-645
01574	08	539-541	01663	13	742-743, 757-759	01752	10	643-645
01575	08	539-541				01753	10	643-645
01576	08	539-541	01664	13	742-743, 757-759	01754	10	643-645
01580	08	548-550				01755	10	643-645
01581	08	548-550	01665	13	742-743, 757-759	01756	10	643-645
01582	08	548-550				01760	10	643-645
01583	08	548-550	01666	13	742-743, 757-759	01761	10	643-645
01584	08	548-550				01762	10	643-645
01585	08	548-550	01670	13	742-743, 757-759	01763	10	643-645
01586	08	548-550				01764	10	643-645
01590	08	548-550	01671	13	742-743, 757-759	01765	10	643-645
01591	08	548-550				01766	10	643-645
01592	08	548-550	01672	13	742-743, 757-759	01770	16	814-816
01593	08	548-550				01771	16	814-816
01594	08	548-550	01673	13	742-743, 757-759	01772	16	814-816
01595	08	548-550				01773	16	814-816
01596	08	548-550	01674	13	742-743, 757-759	01774	16	814-816
01600	11	689-690				01775	16	814-816
01601	11	689-690	01675	13	742-743, 757-759	01776	16	814-816
01602	11	689-690				01780	06	368-370
01603	11	689-690	01676	13	742-743, 757-759	01781	06	368-370
01604	11	689-690				01782	06	368-370
01605	11	689-690	01690	11	689-690	01783	06	368-370
01606	11	689-690	01691	11	689-690	01784	06	368-370
01610	11	689-690	01692	11	689-690	01785	06	368-370
01611	11	689-690	01693	11	689-690	01786	06	368-370
01612	11	689-690	01694	11	689-690	01790	18	867-869
01613	11	689-690	01695	11	689-690	01791	18	867-869
01614	11	689-690	01696	11	689-690	01792	18	867-869
01615	11	689-690	01700	09	606-607	01793	18	867-869
01616	11	689-690	01701	09	606-607	01794	18	867-869
01620	11	689-690	01702	09	606-607	01795	18	867-869
01621	11	689-690	01703	09	606-607	01796	18	867-869
01622	11	689-690	01704	09	606-607	01800	18	867-869
01623	11	689-690	01705	09	606-607	01801	18	867-869
01624	11	689-690	01706	09	606-607	01802	18	867-869
01625	11	689-690	01710	09	595-596	01803	18	867-869
01626	11	689-690	01711	09	595-596	01804	18	867-869
01630	11	689-690	01712	09	595-596	01805	18	867-869
01631	11	689-690	01713	09	595-596	01806	18	867-869
01632	11	689-690	01714	09	595-596	01880	18	867-869
01633	11	689-690	01715	09	595-596	01881	18	867-869
01634	11	689-690	01716	09	595-596	01882	18	867-869
01635	11	689-690	01720	16	814-816	01883	18	867-869
01636	11	689-690	01721	16	814-816	01884	18	867-869
01640	12	727-728	01722	16	814-816	01885	18	867-869
01641	12	727-728	01723	16	814-816	01886	18	867-869
01642	12	727-728	01724	16	814-816	01890	18	867-869
01643	12	727-728	01725	16	814-816	01891	18	867-869
01644	12	727-728	01726	16	814-816	01892	18	867-869
01645	12	727-728	01730	02	124-125	01893	18	867-869
01646	12	727-728	01731	02	124-125	01894	18	867-869
01650	12	727-728	01732	02	124-125	01895	18	867-869
01651	12	727-728	01733	02	124-125	01896	18	867-869
01652	12	727-728	01734	02	124-125	0200	18	867-869
01653	12	727-728	01735	02	124-125	0201	18	867-869
01654	12	727-728	01736	02	124-125	0202	18	870-872
01655	12	727-728	01740	03	154-156	0203	04	177-179
01656	12	727-728	01741	03	154-156	0204	04	177-179
01660	13	742-743, 757-759	01742	03	154-156	0205	04	177-179
			01743	03	154-156	0208	18	867-869
01661	13	742-743, 757-759	01744	03	154-156	0209	18	867-869
			01745	03	154-156	0210	18	867-869
			01746	03	154-156	0211	06	371-373

DX	MDC	MS-DRG
0212	04	177-179
0213	18	867-869
0218	18	867-869
0219	18	867-869
0220	09	606-607
0221	04	177-179
0222	06	371-373
0223	18	870-872
0228	18	867-869
0229	18	867-869
0230	18	867-869
0231	18	867-869
0232	18	867-869
0233	18	867-869
0238	18	867-869
0239	18	867-869
024	18	867-869
025	18	867-869
0260	18	867-869
0261	18	867-869
0269	18	867-869
0270	18	867-869
0271	18	867-869
0272	18	867-869
0278	18	867-869
0279	18	867-869
0300	18	867-869
0301	18	867-869
0302	18	867-869
0303	18	867-869
0308	18	867-869
0309	18	867-869
0310	04	177-179
0311	09	606-607
0312	18	867-869
0318	18	867-869
0319	18	867-869
0320	03	154-156
0321	03	154-156
0322	03	154-156
0323	03	154-156
03281	02	124-125
03282	05	314-316
03283	06	371-373
03284	11	689-690
03285	09	606-607
03289	18	867-869
0329	18	867-869
0330	04	202-203
0331	04	202-203
0338	04	202-203
0339	04	202-203
0340	03	152-153
0341	18	867-869
035	09	602-603
0360	01	023-024, 094-096
0361	01	023-024, 094-096
0362	18	870-872
0363	18	870-872
03640	05	314-316
03641	05	314-316
03642	05	288-290
03643	05	314-316
03681	02	123

DX	MDC	MS-DRG
03682	08	548-550
03689	18	870-872
0369	18	870-872
037	18	867-869
0380	18	870-872
03810	18	870-872
03811	18	870-872
03812	18	870-872
03819	18	870-872
0382	18	870-872
0383	18	870-872
03840	18	870-872
03841	18	870-872
03842	18	870-872
03843	18	870-872
03844	18	870-872
03849	18	870-872
0388	18	870-872
0389	18	870-872
0390	09	606-607
0391	04	177-179
0392	06	371-373
0393	09	606-607
0394	09	606-607
0398	18	867-869
0399	18	867-869
0400	18	867-869
0401	18	867-869
0402	06	393-395
0403	18	867-869
04041	18	867-869
04042	18	867-869
04081	08	557-558
04082	18	867-869
04089	18	867-869
04100	18	867-869
04101	18	867-869
04102	18	867-869
04103	18	867-869
04104	18	867-869
04105	18	867-869
04109	18	867-869
04110	18	867-869
04111	18	867-869
04112	18	867-869
04119	18	867-869
0412	18	867-869
0413	18	867-869
0414	18	867-869
0415	18	867-869
0416	18	867-869
0417	18	867-869
04181	18	867-869
04182	18	867-869
04183	18	867-869
04184	18	867-869
04185	18	867-869
04186	18	867-869
04189	18	867-869
0419	18	867-869
042	25	974-977
04500	01	023-024, 097-099
04501	01	023-024, 097-099

DX	MDC	MS-DRG
04502	01	023-024, 097-099
04503	01	023-024, 097-099
04510	01	023-024, 097-099
04511	01	023-024, 097-099
04512	01	023-024, 097-099
04513	01	023-024, 097-099
04520	18	865-866
04521	18	865-866
04522	18	865-866
04523	18	865-866
04590	01	023-024, 097-099
04591	01	023-024, 097-099
04592	01	023-024, 097-099
04593	01	023-024, 097-099
0460	01	056-057
04611	01	056-057
04619	01	056-057
0462	01	056-057
0463	01	056-057
04671	01	056-057
04672	01	056-057
04679	01	056-057
0468	01	056-057
0469	01	056-057
0470	01	075-076
0471	01	075-076
0478	01	075-076
0479	01	075-076
048	01	075-076
0490	01	075-076
0491	01	075-076
0498	01	097-099
0499	01	097-099
0500	18	865-866
0501	18	865-866
0502	18	865-866
0509	18	865-866
05101	18	865-866
05102	18	865-866
0511	09	606-607
0512	09	606-607
0519	18	865-866
0520	01	097-099
0521	04	177-179
0522	01	023-024, 097-099
0527	18	865-866
0528	18	865-866
0529	18	865-866
0530	01	075-076
05310	01	073-074
05311	01	073-074
05312	01	073-074
05313	01	073-074
05314	01	023-024, 097-099

DX	MDC	MS-DRG	DX	MDC	MS-DRG	DX	MDC	MS-DRG
05319	01	073-074	05881	09	606-607	0701	07	441-443
05320	02	124-125	05882	09	606-607	07020	07	441-443
05321	02	124-125	05889	09	606-607	07021	07	441-443
05322	02	124-125	05900	18	865-866	07022	07	441-443
05329	02	124-125	05901	18	865-866	07023	07	441-443
05371	03	154-156	05909	18	865-866	07030	07	441-443
05379	18	865-866	05910	18	865-866	07031	07	441-443
0538	18	865-866	05911	18	865-866	07032	07	441-443
0539	09	595-596	05912	18	865-866	07033	07	441-443
0540	09	606-607	05919	18	865-866	07041	07	441-443
05410	12	727-728	05920	18	865-866	07042	07	441-443
05410	13	742-743, 757-759	05921	18	865-866	07043	07	441-443
05411	13	742-743, 757-759	05922	18	865-866	07044	07	441-443
05412	13	742-743, 757-759	0598	18	865-866	07049	07	441-443
			0599	18	865-866	07051	07	441-443
05413	12	727-728	0600	18	865-866	07052	07	441-443
05419	12	727-728	0601	18	865-866	07053	07	441-443
05419	13	742-743, 757-759	0609	18	865-866	07054	07	441-443
			061	18	865-866	07059	07	441-443
0542	03	157-159	0620	01	023-024, 097-099	0706	07	441-443
0543	01	023-024, 097-099	0621	01	023-024, 097-099	07070	07	441-443
05440	02	124-125	0622	01	023-024, 097-099	07071	07	441-443
05441	02	124-125				0709	07	441-443
05442	02	124-125	0623	01	023-024, 097-099	071	01	023-024, 097-099
05443	02	124-125	0624	01	023-024, 097-099			
05444	02	124-125				0720	12	727-728
05449	02	124-125	0625	01	023-024, 097-099	0721	01	023-024, 075-076
0545	18	870-872	0628	01	023-024, 097-099	0722	01	023-024, 097-099
0546	09	606-607						
05471	06	393-395	0629	01	023-024, 097-099	0723	07	438-440
05472	01	023-024, 075-076	0630	01	023-024, 097-099	07271	07	441-443
						07272	01	073-074
05473	03	154-156	0631	01	023-024, 097-099	07279	18	865-866
05474	01	023-024, 097-099	0632	01	023-024, 097-099	0728	18	865-866
						0729	18	865-866
05479	18	865-866	0638	01	023-024, 097-099	0730	04	177-179
0548	18	865-866				0737	18	865-866
0549	09	606-607	0639	01	023-024, 097-099	0738	18	865-866
0550	01	023-024, 097-099	064	01	023-024, 097-099	0739	18	865-866
						0740	03	152-153
0551	04	177-179	0650	18	865-866	0741	04	193-195
0552	03	152-153	0651	18	865-866	07420	05	314-316
05571	02	124-125	0652	18	865-866	07421	05	314-316
05579	18	865-866	0653	18	865-866	07422	05	306-307
0558	18	865-866	0654	18	865-866	07423	05	314-316
0559	18	865-866	0658	18	865-866	0743	18	865-866
05600	01	073-074	0659	18	865-866	0748	18	865-866
05601	01	097-099	0660	18	865-866	075	18	865-866
05609	01	097-099	0661	18	865-866	0760	02	124-125
05671	08	553-554	0662	01	023-024, 097-099	0761	02	124-125
05679	18	865-866				0769	02	124-125
0568	18	865-866	0663	18	865-866	0770	02	124-125
0569	18	865-866	06640	18	865-866	0771	02	124-125
0570	18	865-866	06641	18	865-866	0772	02	124-125
0578	18	865-866	06642	18	865-866	0773	02	124-125
0579	18	865-866	06649	18	865-866	0774	02	124-125
05810	18	865-866	0668	18	865-866	0778	02	124-125
05811	18	865-866	0669	18	865-866	07798	02	124-125
05812	18	865-866	0700	07	441-443	07799	02	124-125
05821	01	023-024, 097-099				0780	09	606-607
						07810	09	606-607
05829	01	023-024, 097-099				07811	09	606-607
						07812	09	606-607
						07819	09	606-607
						0782	18	865-866

DX	MDC	MS-DRG
0783	16	814-816
0784	18	865-866
0785	18	865-866
0786	11	689-690
0787	18	865-866
07881	01	091-093
07882	06	391-392
07888	18	865-866
07889	18	865-866
0790	18	865-866
0791	18	865-866
0792	18	865-866
0793	18	865-866
0794	18	865-866
07950	18	865-866
07951	18	865-866
07952	18	865-866
07953	18	865-866
07959	18	865-866
0796	18	865-866
07981	18	865-866
07982	18	865-866
07983	18	865-866
07988	18	865-866
07989	18	865-866
07998	18	865-866
07999	18	865-866
080	18	867-869
0810	18	867-869
0811	18	867-869
0812	18	867-869
0819	18	867-869
0820	18	867-869
0821	18	867-869
0822	18	867-869
0823	18	867-869
08240	18	867-869
08241	18	867-869
08249	18	867-869
0828	18	867-869
0829	18	867-869
0830	18	867-869
0831	18	867-869
0832	18	867-869
0838	18	867-869
0839	18	867-869
0840	18	867-869
0841	18	867-869
0842	18	867-869
0843	18	867-869
0844	18	867-869
0845	18	867-869
0846	18	867-869
0847	18	867-869
0848	18	867-869
0849	18	867-869
0850	18	867-869
0851	09	606-607
0852	09	606-607
0853	09	606-607
0854	09	606-607
0855	09	606-607
0859	18	867-869
0860	05	314-316
0861	18	867-869
0862	18	867-869

DX	MDC	MS-DRG
0863	18	867-869
0864	18	867-869
0865	18	867-869
0869	18	867-869
0870	18	867-869
0871	18	867-869
0879	18	867-869
0880	18	867-869
08881	18	867-869
08882	18	867-869
08889	18	867-869
0889	18	867-869
0900	18	867-869
0901	18	867-869
0902	18	867-869
0903	02	124-125
09040	01	097-099
09041	01	097-099
09042	01	097-099
09049	01	097-099
0905	18	867-869
0906	18	867-869
0907	18	867-869
0909	18	867-869
0910	12	727-728
0910	13	742-743, 757-759
0911	06	393-395
0912	18	867-869
0913	09	606-607
0914	16	814-816
09150	02	124-125
09151	02	124-125
09152	02	124-125
09161	08	539-541
09162	07	441-443
09169	06	393-395
0917	18	867-869
09181	01	023-024, 097-099
09182	09	606-607
09189	18	867-869
0919	18	867-869
0920	18	867-869
0929	18	867-869
0930	05	306-307
0931	05	306-307
09320	05	288-290
09321	05	306-307
09322	05	306-307
09323	05	306-307
09324	05	306-307
09381	05	314-316
09382	05	314-316
09389	05	314-316
0939	05	314-316
0940	01	056-057
0941	01	056-057
0942	01	023-024, 097-099
0943	01	097-099
09481	01	023-024, 097-099
09482	01	056-057
09483	02	124-125
09484	02	124-125

DX	MDC	MS-DRG
09485	01	056-057
09486	03	154-156
09487	01	020-022, 091-093
09489	01	056-057
0949	01	056-057
0950	02	124-125
0951	04	177-179
0952	06	371-373
0953	07	441-443
0954	11	689-690
0955	08	539-541
0956	08	557-558
0957	08	557-558
0958	18	867-869
0959	18	867-869
096	18	867-869
0970	18	867-869
0971	18	867-869
0979	18	867-869
0980	12	727-728
0980	13	742-743, 757-759
09810	12	727-728
09810	13	742-743, 757-759
09811	11	689-690
09812	12	727-728
09813	12	727-728
09814	12	727-728
09815	13	742-743, 757-759
09816	13	742-743, 757-759
09817	13	742-743, 757-759
09819	12	727-728
09819	13	742-743, 757-759
0982	12	727-728
0982	13	742-743, 757-759
09830	11	689-690
09831	11	689-690
09832	12	727-728
09833	12	727-728
09834	12	727-728
09835	13	742-743, 757-759
09836	13	742-743, 757-759
09837	13	742-743, 757-759
09839	12	727-728
09839	13	742-743, 757-759
09840	02	124-125
09841	02	124-125
09842	02	124-125
09843	02	124-125
09849	02	124-125
09850	08	548-550
09851	08	548-550
09852	08	548-550
09853	08	539-541
09859	08	548-550

DX	MDC	MS-DRG	DX	MDC	MS-DRG	DX	MDC	MS-DRG
0986	03	152-153	1028	18	867-869	11590	18	867-869
0987	06	393-395	1029	18	867-869	11591	01	023-024,
09881	02	124-125	1030	09	606-607			097-099
09882	01	023-024,	1031	09	606-607	11592	02	124-125
		094-096	1032	18	867-869	11593	05	314-316
09883	05	314-316	1033	09	606-607	11594	05	288-290
09884	05	288-290	1039	18	867-869	11595	04	177-179
09885	05	314-316	1040	18	867-869	11599	18	867-869
09886	06	371-373	1048	18	867-869	1160	18	867-869
09889	18	867-869	1049	18	867-869	1161	18	867-869
0990	12	727-728	1100	09	606-607	1162	18	867-869
0990	13	742-743,	1101	09	606-607	1170	18	867-869
		757-759	1102	09	606-607	1171	18	867-869
0991	12	727-728	1103	09	606-607	1172	18	867-869
0991	13	742-743,	1104	09	606-607	1173	18	867-869
		757-759	1105	09	606-607	1174	18	867-869
0992	12	727-728	1106	09	606-607	1175	18	867-869
0992	13	742-743,	1108	09	606-607	1176	18	867-869
		757-759	1109	09	606-607	1177	18	867-869
0993	08	545-547	1110	09	606-607	1178	18	867-869
09940	12	727-728	1111	09	606-607	1179	18	867-869
09940	13	742-743,	1112	09	606-607	118	18	867-869
		757-759	1113	09	606-607	1200	11	689-690
09941	12	727-728	1118	09	606-607	1201	07	441-443
09941	13	742-743,	1119	09	606-607	1202	18	867-869
		757-759	1120	03	157-159	1203	09	606-607
09949	12	727-728	1121	13	742-743,	1208	18	867-869
09949	13	742-743,			757-759	1209	18	867-869
		757-759	1122	12	727-728	1210	07	441-443
09950	12	727-728	1122	13	742-743,	1211	07	441-443
09950	13	742-743,			757-759	1212	04	177-179
		757-759	1123	09	606-607	1213	07	441-443
09951	03	152-153	1124	04	177-179	1214	07	441-443
09952	06	393-395	1125	18	867-869	1215	18	867-869
09953	12	727-728	11281	05	288-290	1216	18	867-869
09953	13	742-743,	11282	03	154-156	1218	18	867-869
		757-759	11283	01	023-024,	1219	18	867-869
09954	11	689-690			097-099	1220	07	441-443
09955	12	727-728	11284	06	368-370	1221	04	177-179
09955	13	742-743,	11285	06	391-392	1222	10	643-645
		757-759	11289	18	867-869	1223	18	867-869
09956	06	393-395	1129	18	867-869	1224	18	867-869
09959	12	727-728	1140	04	177-179	1225	07	441-443
09959	13	742-743,	1141	09	606-607	1226	18	867-869
		757-759	1142	01	023-024,	1227	18	867-869
0998	12	727-728			097-099	1228	07	441-443
0998	13	742-743,	1143	18	867-869	1229	18	867-869
		757-759	1144	04	177-179	1230	06	391-392
0999	12	727-728	1145	04	177-179	1231	06	371-373
0999	13	742-743,	1149	18	867-869	1232	06	391-392
		757-759	11500	18	867-869	1233	06	391-392
1000	18	867-869	11501	01	023-024,	1234	06	391-392
10081	01	023-024,			097-099	1235	06	371-373
		097-099	11502	02	124-125	1236	06	371-373
10089	01	023-024,	11503	05	314-316	1238	06	371-373
		097-099	11504	05	288-290	1239	06	371-373
1009	18	867-869	11505	04	177-179	124	18	867-869
101	03	152-153	11509	18	867-869	1250	18	867-869
1020	09	606-607	11510	18	867-869	1251	18	867-869
1021	09	606-607	11511	01	023-024,	1252	18	867-869
1022	09	606-607			097-099	1253	18	867-869
1023	09	606-607	11512	02	124-125	1254	18	867-869
1024	09	606-607	11513	05	314-316	1255	18	867-869
1025	03	154-156	11514	05	288-290	1256	18	867-869
1026	08	548-550	11515	04	177-179	1257	18	867-869
1027	18	867-869	11519	18	867-869	1259	18	867-869

PART VI, MS-DRG, APPENDIX B

DX	MDC	MS-DRG	DX	MDC	MS-DRG	DX	MDC	MS-DRG
1260	06	371-373	1368	18	867-869	1480	03	146-148
1261	06	371-373	1369	18	867-869	1481	03	146-148
1262	06	371-373	1370	04	196-198	1482	03	146-148
1263	06	371-373	1371	01	091-093	1483	03	146-148
1268	06	371-373	1372	11	689-690	1488	03	146-148
1269	06	371-373	1373	08	564-566	1489	03	146-148
1270	06	391-392	1374	18	867-869	1490	03	146-148
1271	06	391-392	138	01	091-093	1491	03	146-148
1272	06	391-392	1390	01	091-093	1498	03	146-148
1273	06	391-392	1391	02	124-125	1499	03	146-148
1274	06	391-392	1398	18	867-869	1500	06	374-376
1275	06	391-392	1400	03	146-148	1501	06	374-376
1276	06	391-392	1401	03	146-148	1502	06	374-376
1277	06	391-392	1403	03	146-148	1503	06	374-376
1278	18	867-869	1404	03	146-148	1504	06	374-376
1279	06	391-392	1405	03	146-148	1505	06	374-376
1280	18	867-869	1406	03	146-148	1508	06	374-376
1281	18	867-869	1408	03	146-148	1509	06	374-376
1288	18	867-869	1409	03	146-148	1510	06	374-376
1289	18	867-869	1410	03	146-148	1511	06	374-376
129	06	391-392	1411	03	146-148	1512	06	374-376
1300	01	023-024,	1412	03	146-148	1513	06	374-376
		097-099	1413	03	146-148	1514	06	374-376
1301	02	124-125	1414	03	146-148	1515	06	374-376
1302	02	124-125	1415	03	146-148	1516	06	374-376
1303	05	314-316	1416	03	146-148	1518	06	374-376
1304	04	177-179	1418	03	146-148	1519	06	374-376
1305	07	441-443	1419	03	146-148	1520	06	374-376
1307	18	867-869	1420	03	146-148	1521	06	374-376
1308	18	867-869	1421	03	146-148	1522	06	374-376
1309	18	867-869	1422	03	146-148	1523	06	374-376
13100	12	727-728	1428	03	146-148	1528	06	374-376
13100	13	742-743,	1429	03	146-148	1529	06	374-376
		757-759	1430	03	146-148	1530	06	374-376
13101	13	742-743,	1431	03	146-148	1531	06	374-376
		757-759	1438	03	146-148	1532	06	374-376
13102	12	727-728	1439	03	146-148	1533	06	374-376
13102	13	742-743,	1440	03	146-148	1534	06	374-376
		757-759	1441	03	146-148	1535	06	338-340,
13103	12	727-728	1448	03	146-148			374-376
13109	12	727-728	1449	03	146-148	1536	06	374-376
13109	13	742-743,	1450	03	146-148	1537	06	374-376
		757-759	1451	03	146-148	1538	06	374-376
1318	18	867-869	1452	03	146-148	1539	06	374-376
1319	18	867-869	1453	03	146-148	1540	06	374-376
1320	09	606-607	1454	03	146-148	1541	06	374-376
1321	09	606-607	1455	03	146-148	1542	06	374-376
1322	09	606-607	1456	03	146-148	1543	06	374-376
1323	09	606-607	1458	03	146-148	1548	06	374-376
1329	09	606-607	1459	03	146-148	1550	07	435-437
1330	09	606-607	1460	03	146-148	1551	07	435-437
1338	09	606-607	1461	03	146-148	1552	07	435-437
1339	09	606-607	1462	03	146-148	1560	07	435-437
1340	09	606-607	1463	03	146-148	1561	07	435-437
1341	09	606-607	1464	03	146-148	1562	07	435-437
1342	09	606-607	1465	03	146-148	1568	07	435-437
1348	09	606-607	1466	03	146-148	1569	07	435-437
1349	09	606-607	1467	03	146-148	1570	07	435-437
135	04	196-198	1468	03	146-148	1571	07	435-437
1360	18	867-869	1469	03	146-148	1572	07	435-437
1361	08	545-547	1470	03	146-148	1573	07	435-437
13621	18	867-869	1471	03	146-148	1574	07	435-437
13629	18	867-869	1472	03	146-148	1578	07	435-437
1363	04	177-179	1473	03	146-148	1579	07	435-437
1364	18	867-869	1478	03	146-148	1580	17	843-845
1365	18	867-869	1479	03	146-148	1588	06	374-376

DX	MDC	MS-DRG	DX	MDC	MS-DRG	DX	MDC	MS-DRG
1589	06	374-376	1726	09	595-596	1832	13	736-738, 754-756
1590	06	374-376	1727	09	595-596	1833	13	736-738, 754-756
1591	17	820-825, 840-842	1728	09	595-596	1834	13	736-738, 754-756
			1729	09	595-596			
1598	06	374-376	1730	09	606-607	1835	13	736-738, 754-756
1599	06	374-376	1731	02	124-125			
1600	03	146-148	1732	09	606-607	1838	13	736-738, 754-756
1601	03	146-148	1733	09	606-607			
1602	03	146-148	1734	09	606-607	1839	13	736-738, 754-756
1603	03	146-148	1735	09	606-607			
1604	03	146-148	1736	09	606-607	1840	13	739-741, 754-756
1605	03	146-148	1737	09	606-607			
1608	03	146-148	1738	09	606-607	1841	13	739-741, 754-756
1609	03	146-148	1739	09	606-607			
1610	03	146-148	1740	09	582-583, 597-599	1842	13	739-741, 754-756
1611	03	146-148						
1612	03	146-148	1741	09	582-583, 597-599	1843	13	739-741, 754-756
1613	03	146-148						
1618	03	146-148	1742	09	582-583, 597-599	1844	13	739-741, 754-756
1619	03	146-148						
1620	04	180-182	1743	09	582-583, 597-599	1848	13	739-741, 754-756
1622	04	180-182						
1623	04	180-182	1744	09	582-583, 597-599	1849	13	739-741, 754-756
1624	04	180-182						
1625	04	180-182	1745	09	582-583, 597-599	185	12	715-716, 722-724
1628	04	180-182						
1629	04	180-182	1746	09	582-583, 597-599	1860	12	715-716, 722-724
1630	04	180-182						
1631	04	180-182	1748	09	582-583, 597-599	1869	12	715-716, 722-724
1638	04	180-182						
1639	04	180-182	1749	09	582-583, 597-599	1871	12	715-716, 722-724
1640	17	843-845						
1641	05	314-316	1750	09	582-583, 597-599	1872	12	715-716, 722-724
1642	04	180-182						
1643	04	180-182	1759	09	582-583, 597-599	1873	12	715-716, 722-724
1648	04	180-182						
1649	04	180-182	1760	09	606-607	1874	12	715-716, 722-724
1650	03	146-148	1761	09	606-607			
1658	04	180-182	1762	03	146-148	1875	12	715-716, 722-724
1659	04	180-182	1763	06	374-376			
1700	08	542-544	1764	04	180-182	1876	12	715-716, 722-724
1701	08	542-544	1765	17	820-825, 840-842			
1702	08	456-458, 542-544				1877	12	715-716, 722-724
			1768	09	606-607			
1703	08	542-544	1769	09	606-607	1878	12	715-716, 722-724
1704	08	542-544	179	13	739-741, 754-756			
1705	08	542-544				1879	12	715-716, 722-724
1706	08	542-544	1800	13	739-741, 754-756			
1707	08	542-544				1880	11	656-658, 686-688
1708	08	542-544	1801	13	739-741, 754-756			
1709	08	542-544				1881	11	656-658, 686-688
1710	08	542-544	1808	13	739-741, 754-756			
1712	08	542-544				1882	11	656-658, 686-688
1713	08	542-544	1809	13	739-741, 754-756			
1714	08	542-544				1883	11	656-658, 686-688
1715	08	542-544	181	13	739-741, 754-756			
1716	08	542-544				1884	11	656-658, 686-688
1717	08	542-544	1820	13	739-741, 754-756			
1718	08	542-544				1885	11	656-658, 686-688
1719	08	542-544	1821	13	739-741, 754-756			
1720	09	595-596				1886	11	656-658, 686-688
1721	02	124-125	1828	13	739-741, 754-756			
1722	09	595-596				1887	11	656-658, 686-688
1723	09	595-596	1830	13	736-738, 754-756			
1724	09	595-596						
1725	09	595-596						

DX	MDC	MS-DRG	DX	MDC	MS-DRG	DX	MDC	MS-DRG
1888	11	656-658, 686-688	1961	17	820-825, 840-842	20011	17	820-825, 840-842
1889	11	656-658, 686-688	1962	17	820-825, 840-842	20012	17	820-825, 840-842
1890	11	656-658, 686-688	1963	17	820-825, 840-842	20013	17	820-825, 840-842
1891	11	656-658, 686-688	1965	17	820-825, 840-842	20014	17	820-825, 840-842
1892	11	656-658, 686-688	1966	17	820-825, 840-842	20015	17	820-825, 840-842
1893	11	656-658, 686-688	1968	17	820-825, 840-842	20016	17	820-825, 840-842
1894	11	656-658, 686-688	1969	17	820-825, 840-842	20017	17	820-825, 840-842
1898	11	656-658, 686-688	1970	04	180-182	20018	17	820-825, 840-842
1899	11	656-658, 686-688	1971	04	180-182	20020	17	820-825, 840-842
1900	02	124-125	1972	04	180-182	20021	17	820-825, 840-842
1901	02	124-125	1973	04	180-182	20022	17	820-825, 840-842
1902	02	124-125	1974	06	374-376	20023	17	820-825, 840-842
1903	02	124-125	1975	06	374-376	20024	17	820-825, 840-842
1904	02	124-125	1976	06	374-376	20025	17	820-825, 840-842
1905	02	124-125	1977	07	435-437	20026	17	820-825, 840-842
1906	02	124-125	1978	06	374-376	20027	17	820-825, 840-842
1907	02	124-125	1980	11	656-658, 686-688	20028	17	820-825, 840-842
1908	02	124-125	1981	11	656-658, 686-688	20030	17	820-825, 840-842
1909	02	124-125	1982	09	582-583, 597-599	20031	17	820-825, 840-842
1910	01	054-055	1983	01	054-055	20032	17	820-825, 840-842
1911	01	054-055	1984	01	054-055	20033	17	820-825, 840-842
1912	01	054-055	1985	08	456-458, 542-544	20034	17	820-825, 840-842
1913	01	054-055	1986	13	736-738, 754-756	20035	17	820-825, 840-842
1914	01	054-055	1987	10	643-645	20036	17	820-825, 840-842
1915	01	054-055	19881	09	582-583, 597-599	20037	17	820-825, 840-842
1916	01	054-055	19882	12	715-716, 722-724	20038	17	820-825, 840-842
1917	01	054-055	19882	13	739-741, 754-756	20040	17	820-825, 840-842
1918	01	054-055	19889	17	843-845	20041	17	820-825, 840-842
1919	01	054-055	1990	17	843-845	20042	17	820-825, 840-842
1920	01	054-055	1991	17	843-845	20043	17	820-825, 840-842
1921	01	054-055	1992	17	843-845	20044	17	820-825, 840-842
1922	01	054-055	20000	17	820-825, 840-842	20045	17	820-825, 840-842
1923	01	054-055	20001	17	820-825, 840-842	20046	17	820-825, 840-842
1928	01	054-055	20002	17	820-825, 840-842			
1929	01	054-055	20003	17	820-825, 840-842			
193	10	643-645	20004	17	820-825, 840-842			
1940	10	643-645	20005	17	820-825, 840-842			
1941	10	643-645	20006	17	820-825, 840-842			
1943	10	643-645	20007	17	820-825, 840-842			
1944	01	054-055	20008	17	820-825, 840-842			
1945	01	054-055	20010	17	820-825, 840-842			
1946	01	054-055						
1948	10	643-645						
1949	10	643-645						
1950	03	146-148						
1951	04	180-182						
1952	06	374-376						
1953	12	715-716, 722-724						
1953	13	739-741, 754-756						
1954	17	843-845						
1955	17	843-845						
1958	17	843-845						
1960	17	820-825, 840-842						

DX	MDC	MS-DRG	DX	MDC	MS-DRG	DX	MDC	MS-DRG
20047	17	820-825, 840-842	20084	17	820-825, 840-842	20141	17	820-825, 840-842
20048	17	820-825, 840-842	20085	17	820-825, 840-842	20142	17	820-825, 840-842
20050	17	820-825, 840-842	20086	17	820-825, 840-842	20143	17	820-825, 840-842
20051	17	820-825, 840-842	20087	17	820-825, 840-842	20144	17	820-825, 840-842
20052	17	820-825, 840-842	20088	17	820-825, 840-842	20145	17	820-825, 840-842
20053	17	820-825, 840-842	20100	17	820-825, 840-842	20146	17	820-825, 840-842
20054	17	820-825, 840-842	20101	17	820-825, 840-842	20147	17	820-825, 840-842
20055	17	820-825, 840-842	20102	17	820-825, 840-842	20148	17	820-825, 840-842
20056	17	820-825, 840-842	20103	17	820-825, 840-842	20150	17	820-825, 840-842
20057	17	820-825, 840-842	20104	17	820-825, 840-842	20151	17	820-825, 840-842
20058	17	820-825, 840-842	20105	17	820-825, 840-842	20152	17	820-825, 840-842
20060	17	820-825, 840-842	20106	17	820-825, 840-842	20153	17	820-825, 840-842
20061	17	820-825, 840-842	20107	17	820-825, 840-842	20154	17	820-825, 840-842
20062	17	820-825, 840-842	20108	17	820-825, 840-842	20155	17	820-825, 840-842
20063	17	820-825, 840-842	20110	17	820-825, 840-842	20156	17	820-825, 840-842
20064	17	820-825, 840-842	20111	17	820-825, 840-842	20157	17	820-825, 840-842
20065	17	820-825, 840-842	20112	17	820-825, 840-842	20158	17	820-825, 840-842
20066	17	820-825, 840-842	20113	17	820-825, 840-842	20160	17	820-825, 840-842
20067	17	820-825, 840-842	20114	17	820-825, 840-842	20161	17	820-825, 840-842
20068	17	820-825, 840-842	20115	17	820-825, 840-842	20162	17	820-825, 840-842
20070	17	820-825, 840-842	20116	17	820-825, 840-842	20163	17	820-825, 840-842
20071	17	820-825, 840-842	20117	17	820-825, 840-842	20164	17	820-825, 840-842
20072	17	820-825, 840-842	20118	17	820-825, 840-842	20165	17	820-825, 840-842
20073	17	820-825, 840-842	20120	17	820-825, 840-842	20166	17	820-825, 840-842
20074	17	820-825, 840-842	20121	17	820-825, 840-842	20167	17	820-825, 840-842
20075	17	820-825, 840-842	20122	17	820-825, 840-842	20168	17	820-825, 840-842
20076	17	820-825, 840-842	20123	17	820-825, 840-842	20170	17	820-825, 840-842
20077	17	820-825, 840-842	20124	17	820-825, 840-842	20171	17	820-825, 840-842
20078	17	820-825, 840-842	20125	17	820-825, 840-842	20172	17	820-825, 840-842
20080	17	820-825, 840-842	20126	17	820-825, 840-842	20173	17	820-825, 840-842
20081	17	820-825, 840-842	20127	17	820-825, 840-842	20174	17	820-825, 840-842
20082	17	820-825, 840-842	20128	17	820-825, 840-842	20175	17	820-825, 840-842
20083	17	820-825, 840-842	20140	17	820-825, 840-842	20176	17	820-825, 840-842

DX	MDC	MS-DRG	DX	MDC	MS-DRG	DX	MDC	MS-DRG
20177	17	820-825, 840-842	20224	17	820-825, 840-842	20265	17	820-825, 840-842
20178	17	820-825, 840-842	20225	17	820-825, 840-842	20266	17	820-825, 840-842
20190	17	820-825, 840-842	20226	17	820-825, 840-842	20267	17	820-825, 840-842
20191	17	820-825, 840-842	20227	17	820-825, 840-842	20268	17	820-825, 840-842
20192	17	820-825, 840-842	20228	17	820-825, 840-842	20270	17	820-825, 840-842
20193	17	820-825, 840-842	20230	17	820-825, 840-842	20271	17	820-825, 840-842
20194	17	820-825, 840-842	20231	17	820-825, 840-842	20272	17	820-825, 840-842
20195	17	820-825, 840-842	20232	17	820-825, 840-842	20273	17	820-825, 840-842
20196	17	820-825, 840-842	20233	17	820-825, 840-842	20274	17	820-825, 840-842
20197	17	820-825, 840-842	20234	17	820-825, 840-842	20275	17	820-825, 840-842
20198	17	820-825, 840-842	20235	17	820-825, 840-842	20276	17	820-825, 840-842
20200	17	820-825, 840-842	20236	17	820-825, 840-842	20277	17	820-825, 840-842
20201	17	820-825, 840-842	20237	17	820-825, 840-842	20278	17	820-825, 840-842
20202	17	820-825, 840-842	20238	17	820-825, 840-842	20280	17	820-825, 840-842
20203	17	820-825, 840-842	20240	17	820-825, 840-842	20281	17	820-825, 840-842
20204	17	820-825, 840-842	20241	17	820-825, 840-842	20282	17	820-825, 840-842
20205	17	820-825, 840-842	20242	17	820-825, 840-842	20283	17	820-825, 840-842
20206	17	820-825, 840-842	20243	17	820-825, 840-842	20284	17	820-825, 840-842
20207	17	820-825, 840-842	20244	17	820-825, 840-842	20285	17	820-825, 840-842
20208	17	820-825, 840-842	20245	17	820-825, 840-842	20286	17	820-825, 840-842
20210	17	820-825, 840-842	20246	17	820-825, 840-842	20287	17	820-825, 840-842
20211	17	820-825, 840-842	20247	17	820-825, 840-842	20288	17	820-825, 840-842
20212	17	820-825, 840-842	20248	17	820-825, 840-842	20290	17	820-825, 840-842
20213	17	820-825, 840-842	20250	17	843-845	20291	17	820-825, 840-842
20214	17	820-825, 840-842	20251	17	843-845	20292	17	820-825, 840-842
20215	17	820-825, 840-842	20252	17	843-845	20293	17	820-825, 840-842
20216	17	820-825, 840-842	20253	17	843-845	20294	17	820-825, 840-842
			20254	17	843-845			
			20255	17	843-845			
20217	17	820-825, 840-842	20256	17	843-845	20295	17	820-825, 840-842
			20257	17	843-845			
20218	17	820-825, 840-842	20258	17	843-845	20296	17	820-825, 840-842
			20260	17	820-825, 840-842			
20220	17	820-825, 840-842	20261	17	820-825, 840-842	20297	17	820-825, 840-842
20221	17	820-825, 840-842	20262	17	820-825, 840-842	20298	17	820-825, 840-842
20222	17	820-825, 840-842	20263	17	820-825, 840-842	20300	17	820-825, 840-842
20223	17	820-825, 840-842	20264	17	820-825, 840-842	20301	17	820-825, 840-842

DX	MDC	MS-DRG	DX	MDC	MS-DRG	DX	MDC	MS-DRG
20302	17	820-825, 840-842	20532	17	820-825, 840-842	20782	17	820-825, 840-842
20310	17	820-825, 840-842	20580	17	820-825, 840-842	20800	17	820-822, 834-836
20311	17	820-825, 840-842	20581	17	820-825, 840-842	20801	17	820-822, 834-836
20312	17	820-825, 840-842	20582	17	820-825, 840-842	20802	17	820-822, 834-836
20380	17	820-825, 840-842	20590	17	820-825, 840-842	20810	17	820-825, 840-842
20381	17	820-825, 840-842	20591	17	820-825, 840-842	20811	17	820-825, 840-842
20382	17	820-825, 840-842	20592	17	820-825, 840-842	20812	17	820-825, 840-842
20400	17	820-822, 834-836	20600	17	820-822, 834-836	20820	17	820-825, 840-842
20401	17	820-822, 834-836	20601	17	820-822, 834-836	20821	17	820-825, 840-842
20402	17	820-822, 834-836	20602	17	820-822, 834-836	20822	17	820-825, 840-842
20410	17	820-825, 840-842	20610	17	820-825, 840-842	20880	17	820-825, 840-842
20411	17	820-825, 840-842	20611	17	820-825, 840-842	20881	17	820-825, 840-842
20412	17	820-825, 840-842	20612	17	820-825, 840-842	20882	17	820-825, 840-842
20420	17	820-825, 840-842	20620	17	820-825, 840-842	20890	17	820-825, 840-842
20421	17	820-825, 840-842	20621	17	820-825, 840-842	20891	17	820-825, 840-842
20422	17	820-825, 840-842	20622	17	820-825, 840-842	20892	17	820-825, 840-842
20480	17	820-825, 840-842	20680	17	820-825, 840-842	20900	06	374-376
						20901	06	374-376
20481	17	820-825, 840-842	20681	17	820-825, 840-842	20902	06	374-376
						20903	06	374-376
20482	17	820-825, 840-842	20682	17	820-825, 840-842	20910	06	374-376
20490	17	820-825, 840-842	20690	17	820-825, 840-842	20911	06	338-340, 374-376
20491	17	820-825, 840-842	20691	17	820-825, 840-842	20912	06	374-376
						20913	06	374-376
20492	17	820-825, 840-842	20692	17	820-825, 840-842	20914	06	374-376
						20915	06	374-376
20500	17	820-822, 834-836	20700	17	820-822, 834-836	20916	06	374-376
						20917	06	374-376
20501	17	820-822, 834-836	20701	17	820-822, 834-836	20920	17	843-845
						20921	04	180-182
20502	17	820-822, 834-836	20702	17	820-822, 834-836	20922	17	843-845
						20923	06	374-376
20510	17	820-825, 840-842	20710	17	820-825, 840-842	20924	11	656-658, 686-688
20511	17	820-825, 840-842	20711	17	820-825, 840-842	20925	06	374-376
						20926	06	374-376
20512	17	820-825, 840-842	20712	17	820-825, 840-842	20927	06	374-376
						20929	17	843-845
20520	17	820-825, 840-842	20720	17	820-825, 840-842	20930	17	843-845
						20931	09	595-596 ◄
20521	17	820-825, 840-842	20721	17	820-825, 840-842	20932	09	595-596 ◄
						20933	09	595-596 ◄
20522	17	820-825, 840-842	20722	17	820-825, 840-842	20934	09	595-596 ◄
						20935	09	595-596 ◄
20530	17	820-825, 840-842	20780	17	820-825, 840-842	20936	09	595-596 ◄
						20940	06	393-395
20531	17	820-825, 840-842	20781	17	820-825, 840-842	20941	06	393-395
						20942	06	393-395
						20943	06	393-395

DX	MDC	MS-DRG		DX	MDC	MS-DRG		DX	MDC	MS-DRG
20950	06	393-395		2136	08	564-566		2230	11	656-658,
20951	06	393-395		2137	08	564-566				686-688
20952	06	393-395		2138	08	564-566		2231	11	656-658,
20953	06	393-395		2139	08	564-566				686-688
20954	06	393-395		2140	09	606-607		2232	11	656-658,
20955	06	393-395		2141	09	606-607				686-688
20956	06	393-395		2142	04	180-182		2233	11	656-658,
20957	06	393-395		2143	06	393-395				686-688
20960	17	843-845		2144	12	729-730		22381	11	656-658,
20961	04	180-182		2148	09	606-607				686-688
20962	16	814-816		2149	09	606-607		22389	11	656-658,
20963	06	393-395		2150	08	564-566				686-688
20964	11	656-658,		2152	08	564-566		2239	11	656-658,
		686-688		2153	08	564-566				686-688
20965	06	393-395		2154	08	564-566		2240	02	124-125
20966	06	393-395		2155	08	564-566		2241	02	124-125
20967	06	393-395		2156	08	564-566		2242	02	124-125
20969	17	843-845		2157	08	564-566		2243	02	124-125
20970	17	826-830, ◄		2158	08	564-566		2244	02	124-125
		843-845		2159	08	564-566		2245	02	124-125
20771	17	826-830, ◄		2160	09	606-607		2246	02	124-125
		843-845		2161	02	124-125		2247	02	124-125
20772	07	435-437 ◄		2162	09	606-607		2248	02	124-125
20973	08	456-458,		2163	09	606-607		2249	02	124-125
		542-544		2164	09	606-607		2250	01	054-055
20974	06	374-376 ◄		2165	09	606-607		2251	01	054-055
20975	09	595-596 ◄		2166	09	606-607		2252	01	054-055
20979	17	826-830, ◄		2167	09	606-607		2253	01	054-055
		843-845		2168	09	606-607		2254	01	054-055
2100	03	157-159		2169	09	606-607		2258	01	054-055
2101	03	157-159		217	09	606-607		2259	01	054-055
2102	03	154-156		2180	13	742-743,		226	10	643-645
2103	03	157-159				760-761		2270	10	643-645
2104	03	157-159		2181	13	742-743,		2271	10	643-645
2105	03	154-156				760-761		2273	10	643-645
2106	03	154-156		2182	13	742-743,		2274	01	054-055
2107	03	154-156				760-761		2275	01	054-055
2108	03	154-156		2189	13	742-743,		2276	01	054-055
2109	03	154-156				760-761		2278	10	643-645
2110	06	393-395		2190	13	742-743,		2279	10	643-645
2111	06	393-395				760-761		22800	05	314-316
2112	06	393-395		2191	13	742-743,		22801	09	666-607
2113	06	393-395				760-761		22802	01	091-093
2114	06	393-395		2198	13	742-743,		22803	02	124-125
2115	07	441-443				760-761		22804	06	391-392
2116	07	438-440		2199	13	742-743,		22809	05	314-316
2117	10	643-645				760-761		2281	16	814-816
2118	06	393-395		220	13	742-743,		2290	16	814-816
2119	06	393-395				760-761		2298	17	843-845
2120	03	154-156		2210	13	742-743,		2299	17	843-845
2121	03	154-156				760-761		2300	03	146-148
2122	04	180-182		2211	13	742-743,		2301	06	374-376
2123	04	180-182				760-761		2302	06	374-376
2124	04	180-182		2212	13	742-743,		2303	06	374-376
2125	04	180-182				760-761		2304	06	374-376
2126	16	814-816		2218	13	742-743,		2305	06	374-376
2127	05	314-316				760-761		2306	06	374-376
2128	04	180-182		2219	13	742-743,		2307	06	374-376
2129	04	180-182				760-761		2308	07	435-437
2130	08	564-566		2220	12	729-730		2309	06	374-376
2131	03	157-159		2221	12	729-730		2310	03	146-148
2132	08	456-458,		2222	12	729-730		2311	04	180-182
		564-566		2223	12	729-730		2312	04	180-182
2133	04	180-182		2224	12	729-730		2318	04	180-182
2134	08	564-566		2228	12	729-730		2319	04	180-182
2135	08	564-566		2229	12	729-730		2320	09	606-607

DX	MDC	MS-DRG	DX	MDC	MS-DRG	DX	MDC	MS-DRG
2321	02	124-125	23699	11	656-658, 686-688	24240	10	643-645
2322	09	606-607				24241	10	643-645
2323	09	606-607	2370	10	643-645	24280	10	643-645
2324	09	606-607	2371	01	054-055	24281	10	643-645
2325	09	606-607	2372	10	643-645	24290	10	643-645
2326	09	606-607	2373	01	054-055	24291	10	643-645
2327	09	606-607	2374	10	643-645	243	10	643-645
2328	09	606-607	2375	01	054-055	2440	10	643-645
2329	09	606-607	2376	01	054-055	2441	10	643-645
2330	09	582-583, 597-599	23770	01	091-093	2442	10	643-645
			23771	01	091-093	2443	10	643-645
2331	13	739-741, 754-756	23772	01	091-093	2448	10	643-645
			2379	01	054-055	2449	10	643-645
2332	13	739-741, 754-756	2380	08	456-458, 542-544	2450	10	643-645
						2451	10	643-645
23330	13	739-741, 754-756	2381	08	564-566	2452	10	643-645
			2382	09	606-607	2453	10	643-645
23331	13	739-741, 754-756	2383	09	582-583, 597-599	2454	10	643-645
						2458	10	643-645
23332	13	739-741, 754-756	2384	17	820-825, 840-842	2459	10	643-645
						2460	10	643-645
23339	13	739-741, 754-756	2385	17	820-825, 840-842	2461	10	643-645
						2462	10	643-645
2334	12	715-716, 722-724	2386	17	820-825, 840-842	2463	10	643-645
						2468	10	643-645
2335	12	715-716, 722-724	23871	16	814-816	2469	10	643-645
			23872	16	811-812	24900	10	637-639
2336	12	715-716, 722-724	23873	16	811-812	24901	10	637-639
			23874	16	811-812	24910	10	637-639
2337	11	656-658, 686-688	23875	16	811-812	24911	10	637-639
			23876	17	820-825, 840-842	24920	10	637-639
2339	11	656-658, 686-688				24921	10	637-639
			23877	21	919-921	24930	10	637-639
2340	02	124-125	23879	17	820-825, 840-842	24931	10	637-639
2348	17	843-845				24940	11	698-700
2349	17	843-845	2388	17	843-845	24941	11	698-700
2350	03	146-148	2389	17	843-845	24950	02	124-125
2351	03	146-148	2390	06	374-376	24951	02	124-125
2352	06	374-376	2391	04	180-182	24960	01	073-074
2353	07	435-437	2392	08	456-458, 564-566	24961	01	073-074
2354	06	374-376				24970	05	299-301
2355	06	374-376	2393	09	600-601	24971	05	299-301
2356	03	146-148	2394	11	656-658, 686-688	24980	10	637-639
2357	04	180-182				24981	10	637-639
2358	04	180-182	2395	11	656-658, 686-688	24990	10	637-639
2359	04	180-182				24991	10	637-639
2360	13	739-741, 754-756	2396	01	054-055	25000	10	637-639
			2397	10	643-645	25001	10	637-639
2361	13	739-741, 754-756	23981	17	826-830, 843-845 ◄	25002	10	637-639
						25003	10	637-639
2362	13	736-738, 754-756	23989	17	826-830, 843-845 ◄	25010	10	637-639
			2399	17	843-845	25011	10	637-639
2363	13	739-741, 754-756	2400	10	643-645	25012	10	637-639
			2409	10	643-645	25013	10	637-639
2364	12	715-716, 722-724	2410	10	643-645	25020	10	637-639
			2411	10	643-645	25021	10	637-639
2365	12	715-716, 722-724	2419	10	643-645	25022	10	637-639
			24200	10	643-645	25023	10	637-639
2366	12	715-716, 722-724	24201	10	643-645	25030	10	637-639
			24210	10	643-645	25031	10	637-639
2367	11	656-658, 686-688	24211	10	643-645	25032	10	637-639
			24220	10	643-645	25033	10	637-639
23690	11	656-658, 686-688	24221	10	643-645	25040	11	698-700
			24230	10	643-645	25041	11	673-675, 698-700
23691	11	656-658, 686-688	24231	10	643-645	25042	11	698-700

DX	MDC	MS-DRG	DX	MDC	MS-DRG	DX	MDC	MS-DRG
25043	11	673-675, 698-700	2560	13	742-743, 760-761	2689	10	640-641
25050	02	124-125	2561	13	742-743, 760-761	2690	10	640-641
25051	02	124-125	2562	13	742-743, 760-761	2691	10	640-641
25052	02	124-125				2692	10	640-641
25053	02	124-125	25631	13	742-743, 760-761	2693	10	640-641
25060	01	073-074				2698	10	640-641
25061	01	073-074	25639	13	742-743, 760-761	2699	10	640-641
25062	01	073-074				2700	10	642
25063	01	073-074	2564	13	742-743, 760-761	2701	10	642
25070	05	299-301				2702	10	642
25071	05	299-301	2568	13	742-743, 760-761	2703	10	642
25072	05	299-301				2704	10	642
25073	05	299-301	2569	13	742-743, 760-761	2705	10	642
25080	10	637-639				2706	10	642
25081	10	637-639	2570	10	643-645	2707	10	642
25082	10	637-639	2571	10	643-645	2708	10	642
25083	10	637-639	2572	10	643-645	2709	10	642
25090	10	637-639	2578	10	643-645	2710	10	642
25091	10	637-639	2579	10	643-645	2711	10	642
25092	10	637-639	25801	10	643-645	2712	06	391-392
25093	10	637-639	25802	10	643-645	2713	06	391-392
2510	10	640-641	25803	10	643-645	2714	10	642
2511	10	643-645	2581	10	643-645	2718	10	642
2512	10	640-641	2588	10	643-645	2719	10	642
2513	10	640-641	2589	10	643-645	2720	10	642
2514	10	643-645	2590	10	643-645	2721	10	642
2515	06	380-382	2591	10	643-645	2722	10	642
2518	10	643-645	2592	10	643-645	2723	10	642
2519	10	643-645	2593	10	643-645	2724	10	642
25200	10	643-645	2594	10	643-645	2725	10	642
25201	10	643-645	25950	10	643-645	2726	10	642
25202	10	643-645	25951	10	643-645	2727	10	642
25208	10	643-645	25952	10	643-645	2728	10	642
2521	10	643-645	2598	10	643-645	2729	10	642
2528	10	643-645	2599	10	643-645	2730	16	814-816
2529	10	643-645	260	10	640-641	2731	16	814-816
2530	10	643-645	261	10	640-641	2732	17	820-825, 840-842
2531	10	643-645	262	10	640-641			
2532	10	643-645	2630	10	640-641	2733	17	820-825, 840-842
2533	10	643-645	2631	10	640-641			
2534	10	643-645	2632	10	640-641	2734	10	642
2535	10	643-645	2638	10	640-641	2738	17	843-845
2536	10	643-645	2639	10	640-641	2739	17	843-845
2537	10	643-645	2640	02	124-125	27400	08	553-554
2538	10	643-645	2641	02	124-125	27401	08	553-554 ◄
2539	10	643-645	2642	02	124-125	27402	08	553-554 ◄
2540	16	814-816	2643	02	124-125	27403	08	553-554 ◄
2541	16	814-816	2644	02	124-125	27410	11	698-700
2548	16	814-816	2645	02	124-125	27411	11	691-694
2549	16	814-816	2646	02	124-125	27419	11	698-700
2550	10	643-645	2647	02	124-125	27481	08	553-554
25510	10	643-645	2648	10	640-641	27482	08	553-554
25511	10	643-645	2649	10	640-641	27489	08	553-554
25512	10	643-645	2650	10	640-641	2749	08	553-554
25513	10	643-645	2651	10	640-641	2750	10	642
25514	10	643-645	2652	10	640-641	2751	10	642
2552	10	643-645	2660	10	640-641	2752	10	640-641
2553	10	643-645	2661	10	640-641	2753	10	642
25541	10	643-645	2662	10	640-641	27540	10	640-641
25542	10	643-645	2669	10	640-641	27541	10	640-641
2555	10	643-645	267	10	640-641	27542	10	640-641
2556	10	643-645	2680	08	553-554	27549	10	640-641
2558	10	643-645	2681	08	553-554	2755	10	640-641
2559	10	643-645	2682	08	553-554	2758	10	642
						2759	10	642
						2760	10	640-641

DX	MDC	MS-DRG
2761	10	640-641
2762	10	640-641
2763	10	640-641
2764	10	640-641
27650	10	640-641
27651	10	640-641
27652	10	640-641
2766	10	640-641
2767	10	640-641
2768	10	640-641
2769	10	640-641
27700	10	640-641
27701	15	791,793
27702	04	177-179
27703	06	393-395
27709	10	640-641
2771	10	642
2772	10	642
27730	08	545-547
27731	08	545-547
27739	08	545-547
2774	07	441-443
2775	10	642
2776	10	642
2777	10	642
27781	10	642
27782	10	642
27783	10	642
27784	10	642
27785	10	642
27786	10	642
27787	10	642
27789	10	642
2779	10	642
27800	10	640-641
27801	10	640-641
27802	10	640-641
2781	10	640-641
2782	10	640-641
2783	10	640-641
2784	10	640-641
2788	10	640-641
27900	16	814-816
27901	16	814-816
27902	16	814-816
27903	16	814-816
27904	16	814-816
27905	16	814-816
27906	16	814-816
27909	16	814-816
27910	16	814-816
27911	16	808-810
27912	16	808-810
27913	16	808-810
27919	16	808-810
2792	16	808-810
2793	16	814-816
27941	08	545-547,
	25	977
27949	08	545-547, ◄
	25	977
27950	16	808-810
27951	16	808-810
27952	16	808-810
27953	16	808-810
2798	16	814-816

DX	MDC	MS-DRG
2799	16	814-816
2800	16	811-812
2801	16	811-812
2808	16	811-812
2809	16	811-812
2810	16	811-812
2811	16	811-812
2812	16	811-812
2813	16	811-812
2814	16	811-812
2818	16	811-812
2819	16	811-812
2820	16	811-812
2821	16	811-812
2822	16	811-812
2823	16	811-812
28241	16	811-812
28242	16	811-812
28249	16	811-812
2825	16	811-812
28260	16	811-812
28261	16	811-812
28262	16	811-812
28263	16	811-812
28264	16	811-812
28268	16	811-812
28269	16	811-812
2827	16	811-812
2828	16	811-812
2829	16	811-812
2830	16	808-810
28310	16	808-810
28311	16	811-812
28319	16	808-810
2832	16	808-810
2839	16	808-810
28401	16	808-810
28409	16	808-810
2841	16	811-812
2842	17	820-825,
		840-842
28481	16	808-810
28489	16	808-810
2849	16	808-810
2850	16	811-812
2851	16	811-812
28521	16	811-812
28522	16	811-812
28529	16	811-812
2853	16	811-812 ◄
2858	16	811-812
2859	16	811-812
2860	16	813
2861	16	813
2862	16	813
2863	16	813
2864	16	813
2865	16	813
2866	16	813
2867	16	813
2869	16	813
2870	16	813
2871	16	813
2872	16	813
28730	16	813
28731	16	813

DX	MDC	MS-DRG
28732	16	813
28733	16	813
28739	16	813
2874	16	813
2875	16	813
2878	16	813
2879	16	813
28800	16	808-810
28801	16	808-810
28802	16	808-810
28803	16	808-810
28804	16	808-810
28809	16	808-810
2881	16	808-810
2882	16	808-810
2883	16	814-816
2884	16	814-816
28850	16	814-816
28851	16	814-816
28859	16	814-816
28860	16	814-816
28861	16	814-816
28862	16	814-816
28863	16	814-816
28864	16	814-816
28865	16	814-816
28866	16	814-816
28869	16	814-816
2888	16	814-816
2889	16	814-816
2890	16	814-816
2891	16	814-816
2892	06	393-395
2893	16	814-816
2894	16	814-816
28950	16	814-816
28951	16	814-816
28952	16	814-816
28953	16	814-816
28959	16	814-816
2896	16	814-816
2897	16	811-812
28981	16	814-816
28982	16	814-816
28983	17	820-825,
		840-842
28984	16	813
28989	16	814-816
2899	16	814-816
2900	19	884
29010	19	884
29011	19	884
29012	19	884
29013	19	884
29020	19	884
29021	19	884
2903	19	884
29040	19	884
29041	19	884
29042	19	884
29043	19	884
2908	19	884
2909	19	884
2910	20	894-897
2911	20	894-897
2912	20	894-897

DX	MDC	MS-DRG
2913	20	894-897
2914	20	894-897
2915	20	894-897
29181	20	894-897
29182	20	894-897
29189	20	894-897
2919	20	894-897
2920	20	894-897
29211	20	894-897
29212	20	894-897
2922	20	894-897
29281	20	894-897
29282	20	894-897
29283	20	894-897
29284	20	894-897
29285	20	894-897
29289	20	894-897
2929	20	894-897
2930	19	880
2931	19	880
29381	19	884
29382	19	884
29383	19	884
29384	19	884
29389	19	884
2939	19	880
2940	19	884
29410	19	884
29411	19	884
2948	19	884
2949	19	884
29500	19	885
29501	19	885
29502	19	885
29503	19	885
29504	19	885
29505	19	885
29510	19	885
29511	19	885
29512	19	885
29513	19	885
29514	19	885
29515	19	885
29520	19	885
29521	19	885
29522	19	885
29523	19	885
29524	19	885
29525	19	885
29530	19	885
29531	19	885
29532	19	885
29533	19	885
29534	19	885
29535	19	885
29540	19	885
29541	19	885
29542	19	885
29543	19	885
29544	19	885
29545	19	885
29550	19	885
29551	19	885
29552	19	885
29553	19	885
29554	19	885
29555	19	885
29560	19	885
29561	19	885
29562	19	885
29563	19	885
29564	19	885
29565	19	885
29570	19	885
29571	19	885
29572	19	885
29573	19	885
29574	19	885
29575	19	885
29580	19	885
29581	19	885
29582	19	885
29583	19	885
29584	19	885
29585	19	885
29590	19	885
29591	19	885
29592	19	885
29593	19	885
29594	19	885
29595	19	885
29600	19	885
29601	19	885
29602	19	885
29603	19	885
29604	19	885
29605	19	885
29606	19	885
29610	19	885
29611	19	885
29612	19	885
29613	19	885
29614	19	885
29615	19	885
29616	19	885
29620	19	885
29621	19	885
29622	19	885
29623	19	885
29624	19	885
29625	19	885
29626	19	885
29630	19	885
29631	19	885
29632	19	885
29633	19	885
29634	19	885
29635	19	885
29636	19	885
29640	19	885
29641	19	885
29642	19	885
29643	19	885
29644	19	885
29645	19	885
29646	19	885
29650	19	885
29651	19	885
29652	19	885
29653	19	885
29654	19	885
29655	19	885
29656	19	885
29660	19	885
29661	19	885
29662	19	885
29663	19	885
29664	19	885
29665	19	885
29666	19	885
2967	19	885
29680	19	885
29681	19	885
29682	19	885
29689	19	885
29690	19	885
29699	19	885
2970	19	885
2971	19	885
2972	19	885
2973	19	885
2978	19	885
2979	19	885
2980	19	885
2981	19	885
2982	19	887
2983	19	885
2984	19	885
2988	19	885
2989	19	885
29900	19	884
29901	19	884
29910	19	884
29911	19	884
29980	19	885
29981	19	885
29990	19	885
29991	19	885
30000	19	880
30001	19	880
30002	19	880
30009	19	880
30010	19	880
30011	19	880
30012	19	880
30013	19	880
30014	19	883
30015	19	880
30016	19	880
30019	19	880
30020	19	882
30021	19	882
30022	19	882
30023	19	882
30029	19	882
3003	19	882
3004	19	881
3005	19	882
3006	19	882
3007	19	882
30081	19	882
30082	19	882
30089	19	882
3009	19	880
3010	19	883
30110	19	883
30111	19	883
30112	19	881

DX	MDC	MS-DRG	DX	MDC	MS-DRG	DX	MDC	MS-DRG
30113	19	883	30440	20	894-897	30650	11	698-700
30120	19	883	30441	20	894-897	30651	13	742-743, 760-761
30121	19	883	30442	20	894-897			
30122	19	883	30443	20	894-897	30652	13	742-743, 760-761
3013	19	883	30450	20	894-897			
3014	19	883	30451	20	894-897	30653	11	698-700
30150	19	883	30452	20	894-897	30659	11	698-700
30151	19	883	30453	20	894-897	3066	10	643-645
30159	19	883	30460	20	894-897	3067	19	882
3016	19	883	30461	20	894-897	3068	19	887
3017	19	883	30462	20	894-897	3069	19	882
30181	19	883	30463	20	894-897	3070	19	887
30182	19	883	30470	20	894-897	3071	19	883
30183	19	883	30471	20	894-897	30720	01	091-093
30184	19	883	30472	20	894-897	30721	01	091-093
30189	19	883	30473	20	894-897	30722	01	091-093
3019	19	883	30480	20	894-897	30723	01	091-093
3020	19	887	30481	20	894-897	3073	19	887
3021	19	887	30482	20	894-897	30740	19	887
3022	19	887	30483	20	894-897	30741	19	887
3023	19	887	30490	20	894-897	30742	19	887
3024	19	887	30491	20	894-897	30743	19	887
30250	19	887	30492	20	894-897	30744	19	887
30251	19	887	30493	20	894-897	30745	19	887
30252	19	887	30500	20	894-897	30746	19	887
30253	19	887	30501	20	894-897	30747	19	887
3026	19	887	30502	20	894-897	30748	19	887
30270	19	887	30503	20	894-897	30749	19	887
30271	19	887	3051	23	951	30750	19	887
30272	19	887	30520	20	894-897	30751	19	887
30273	19	887	30521	20	894-897	30752	19	886
30274	19	887	30522	20	894-897	30753	19	882
30275	19	887	30523	20	894-897	30754	19	882
30276	19	887	30530	20	894-897	30759	19	887
30279	19	887	30531	20	894-897	3076	19	886
30281	19	887	30532	20	894-897	3077	19	886
30282	19	887	30533	20	894-897	30780	19	882
30283	19	887	30540	20	894-897	30781	01	102-103
30284	19	887	30541	20	894-897	30789	19	882
30285	19	887	30542	20	894-897	3079	19	884
30289	19	887	30543	20	894-897	3080	19	880
3029	19	887	30550	20	894-897	3081	19	880
30300	20	894-897	30551	20	894-897	3082	19	880
30301	20	894-897	30552	20	894-897	3083	19	880
30302	20	894-897	30553	20	894-897	3084	19	880
30303	20	894-897	30560	20	894-897	3089	19	880
30390	20	894-897	30561	20	894-897	3090	19	881
30391	20	894-897	30562	20	894-897	3091	19	881
30392	20	894-897	30563	20	894-897	30921	19	882
30393	20	894-897	30570	20	894-897	30922	19	882
30400	20	894-897	30571	20	894-897	30923	19	882
30401	20	894-897	30572	20	894-897	30924	19	882
30402	20	894-897	30573	20	894-897	30928	19	882
30403	20	894-897	30580	20	894-897	30929	19	882
30410	20	894-897	30581	20	894-897	3093	19	882
30411	20	894-897	30582	20	894-897	3094	19	882
30412	20	894-897	30583	20	894-897	30981	19	882
30413	20	894-897	30590	20	894-897	30982	19	882
30420	20	894-897	30591	20	894-897	30983	19	882
30421	20	894-897	30592	20	894-897	30989	19	882
30422	20	894-897	30593	20	894-897	3099	19	882
30423	20	894-897	3060	08	557-558	3100	19	884
30430	20	894-897	3061	04	205-206	3101	19	884
30431	20	894-897	3062	05	314-316	3102	01	102-103
30432	20	894-897	3063	09	606-607	3108	19	884
30433	20	894-897	3064	06	391-392	3109	19	884

DX	MDC	MS-DRG	DX	MDC	MS-DRG	DX	MDC	MS-DRG
311	19	881	3202	01	023-024, 094-096	325	01	023-024, 091-093
31200	19	886				326	01	091-093
31201	19	886	3203	01	023-024, 094-096	32700	19	887
31202	19	886	3207	01	023-024, 094-096	32701	19	887
31203	19	886				32702	19	887
31210	19	886	32081	01	023-024, 094-096	32709	19	887
31211	19	886				32710	19	887
31212	19	886	32082	01	023-024, 094-096	32711	19	887
31213	19	886				32712	19	887
31220	19	886	32089	01	023-024, 094-096	32713	19	887
31221	19	886				32714	19	887
31222	19	886	3209	01	023-024, 094-096	32715	19	887
31223	19	886				32719	19	887
31230	19	886	3210	01	023-024, 097-099	32720	03	154-156
31231	19	883				32721	01	091-093
31232	19	883	3211	01	023-024, 097-099	32722	04	204
31233	19	886	3212	01	023-024, 097-099	32723	03	154-156
31234	19	883				32724	03	154-156
31235	19	883	3213	01	023-024, 097-099	32725	01	091-093
31239	19	883				32726	03	154-156
3124	19	886	3214	01	097-099	32727	01	091-093
31281	19	886	3218	01	097-099	32729	03	154-156
31282	19	886	3220	01	097-099	32730	01	091-093
31289	19	886	3221	01	097-099	32731	01	091-093
3129	19	886	3222	01	097-099	32732	01	091-093
3130	19	882	3229	01	097-099	32733	01	091-093
3131	19	882	32301	01	023-024, 097-099	32734	01	091-093
31321	19	886				32735	01	091-093
31322	19	886	32302	01	023-024, 097-099	32736	01	091-093
31323	19	886				32737	01	091-093
3133	19	886	3231	01	023-024, 097-099	32739	01	091-093
31381	19	886				32740	03	154-156
31382	19	886	3232	01	023-024, 097-099	32741	01	091-093
31383	19	886				32742	03	154-156
31389	19	886	32341	01	023-024, 097-099	32743	01	091-093
3139	19	886				32744	03	154-156
31400	19	886	32342	01	023-024, 097-099	32749	03	154-156
31401	19	886				32751	01	091-093
3141	19	886	32351	01	023-024, 097-099	32752	01	091-093
3142	19	886				32753	03	154-156
3148	19	886	32352	01	023-024, 097-099	32759	03	154-156
3149	19	886				3278	03	154-156
31500	19	886	32361	01	023-024, 097-099	3300	01	056-057
31501	19	886				3301	01	056-057
31502	19	886	32362	01	023-024, 097-099	3302	01	056-057
31509	19	886				3303	01	056-057
3151	19	886	32363	01	023-024, 097-099	3308	01	056-057
3152	19	886				3309	01	056-057
31531	19	886	32371	01	023-024, 091-093	3310	01	056-057
31532	19	886				33111	01	056-057
31534	19	886	32372	01	023-024, 091-093	33119	01	056-057
31539	19	886				3312	01	056-057
3154	19	886	32381	01	023-024, 097-099	3313	01	056-057
3155	19	886				3314	01	056-057
3158	19	886	32382	01	023-024, 097-099	3315	01	056-057
3159	19	886				3317	01	056-057
316	19	884	3239	01	023-024, 097-099	33181	01	091-093
317	19	884				33182	01	056-057
3180	19	884	3240	01	023-024, 094-096	33183	01	056-057
3181	19	884				33189	01	056-057
3182	19	884	3241	01	023-024, 094-096	3319	01	056-057
319	19	884				3320	01	056-057
3200	01	023-024, 094-096	3249	01	023-024, 094-096	3321	01	056-057
						3330	01	056-057
3201	01	023-024, 094-096				3331	01	091-093

DX	MDC	MS-DRG	DX	MDC	MS-DRG	DX	MDC	MS-DRG
3332	01	091-093	33900	01	102-103	34441	01	091-093
3333	01	091-093	33901	01	102-103	34442	01	091-093
3334	01	056-057	33902	01	102-103	3445	01	091-093
3335	01	056-057	33903	01	102-103	34460	01	073-074
3336	01	056-057	33904	01	102-103	34461	11	698-700
33371	01	056-057	33905	01	102-103	34481	01	091^093
33372	01	091-093	33909	01	102-103	34489	01	091-093
33379	01	091-093	33910	01	102-103	3449	01	091-093
33381	02	124-125	33911	01	102-103	34500	01	100-101
33382	01	091-093	33912	01	102-103	34501	01	100-101
33383	01	091-093	33920	01	102-103	34510	01	100-101
33384	01	091-093	33921	01	102-103	34511	01	100-101
33385	01	091-093	33922	01	102-103	3452	01	100-101
33389	01	091-093	3393	01	102-103	3453	01	100-101
33390	01	056-057	33941	01	102-103	34540	01	100-101
33391	01	091-093	33942	01	102-103	34541	01	100-101
33392	01	091-093	33943	01	102-103	34550	01	100-101
33393	01	091-093	33944	01	102-103	34551	01	100-101
33394	01	056-057	33981	01	102-103	34560	01	100-101
33399	01	056-057	33982	01	102-103	34561	01	100-101
3340	01	058-060	33983	01	102-103	34570	01	100-101
3341	01	058-060	33984	01	102-103	34571	01	100-101
3342	01	058-060	33985	01	102-103	34580	01	100-101
3343	01	058-060	33989	01	102-103	34581	01	100-101
3344	01	058-060	340	01	058-060	34590	01	100-101
3348	01	058-060	3410	01	058-060	34591	01	100-101
3349	01	058-060	3411	01	058-060	34600	01	102-103
3350	01	056-057	34120	01	023-024, 097-099	34601	01	102-103
33510	01	056-057				34602	01	102-103
33511	01	056-057	34121	01	023-024, 097-099	34603	01	102-103
33519	01	056-057				34610	01	102-103
33520	01	056-057	34122	01	023-024, 097-099	34611	01	102-103
33521	01	056-057				34612	01	102-103
33522	01	056-057	3418	01	058-060	34613	01	102-103
33523	01	056-057	3419	01	058-060	34620	01	102-103
33524	01	056-057	34200	01	056-057	34621	01	102-103
33529	01	056-057	34201	01	056-057	34622	01	102-103
3358	01	056-057	34202	01	056-057	34623	01	102-103
3359	01	056-057	34210	01	056-057	34630	01	102-103
3360	01	056-057	34211	01	056-057	34631	01	102-103
3361	01	091-093	34212	01	056-057	34632	01	102-103
3362	01	091-093	34280	01	056-057	34633	01	102-103
3363	01	091-093	34281	01	056-057	34640	01	102-103
3368	01	091-093	34282	01	056-057	34641	01	102-103
3369	01	091-093	34290	01	056-057	34642	01	102-103
33700	01	073-074	34291	01	056-057	34643	01	102-103
33701	01	073-074	34292	01	056-057	34650	01	102-103
33709	01	073-074	3430	01	052-053	34651	01	102-103
3371	01	073-074	3431	01	052-053	34652	01	102-103
33720	01	073-074	3432	01	052-053	34653	01	102-103
33721	01	073-074	3433	01	091-093	34660	01	102-103
33722	01	073-074	3434	01	052-053	34661	01	102-103
33729	01	073-074	3438	01	091-093	34662	01	102-103
3373	01	073-074	3439	01	091-093	34663	01	102-103
3379	01	073-074	34400	01	052-053	34670	01	102-103
3380	01	091-093	34401	01	052-053	34671	01	102-103
33811	23	947-948	34402	01	052-053	34672	01	102-103
33812	23	947-948	34403	01	052-053	34673	01	102-103
33818	23	947-948	34404	01	052-053	34680	01	102-103
33819	23	947-948	34409	01	052-053	34681	01	102-103
33821	01	091-093	3441	01	052-053	34682	01	102-103
33822	01	091-093	3442	01	052-053	34683	01	102-103
33828	01	091-093	34430	01	091-093	34690	01	102-103
33829	01	091-093	34431	01	091-093	34691	01	102-103
3383	23	947-948	34432	01	091-093	34692	01	102-103
3384	01	091-093	34440	01	091-093	34693	01	102-103

DX	MDC	MS-DRG	DX	MDC	MS-DRG	DX	MDC	MS-DRG
34700	01	091-093	3558	01	073-074	36043	02	124-125
34701	01	091-093	3559	01	073-074	36044	02	124-125
34710	01	091-093	3560	01	073-074	36050	02	124-125
34711	01	091-093	3561	01	073-074	36051	02	124-125
3480	01	091-093	3562	01	073-074	36052	02	124-125
3481	01	091-093	3563	01	091-093	36053	02	124-125
3482	01	102-103	3564	01	073-074	36054	02	124-125
34830	01	070-072	3568	01	073-074	36055	02	124-125
34831	01	070-072	3569	01	073-074	36059	02	124-125
34839	01	070-072	3570	01	094-096	36060	02	124-125
3484	01	080-081	3571	01	073-074	36061	02	124-125
3485	01	080-081	3572	01	073-074	36062	02	124-125
34881	01	070-072	3573	01	073-074	36063	02	124-125
34889	01	070-072 ◀	3574	01	073-074	36064	02	124-125
3489	01	070-072	3575	01	073-074	36065	02	124-125
3490	01	102-103	3576	01	073-074	36069	02	124-125
3491	01	091-093	3577	01	073-074	36081	02	124-125
3492	01	091-093	35781	01	073-074	36089	02	124-125
34931	21	919-921	35782	01	073-074	3609	02	124-125
34939	21	919-921	35789	01	073-074	36100	02	124-125
34981	01	091-093	3579	01	073-074	36101	02	124-125
34982	01	091-093	35800	01	056-057	36102	02	124-125
34989	01	070-072	35801	01	056-057	36103	02	124-125
3499	01	070-072	3581	01	056-057	36104	02	124-125
3501	01	073-074	3582	01	073-074	36105	02	124-125
3502	01	073-074	3588	01	073-074	36106	02	124-125
3508	01	073-074	3589	01	073-074	36107	02	124-125
3509	01	073-074	3590	01	091-093	36110	02	124-125
3510	01	073-074	3591	01	091-093	36111	02	124-125
3511	01	073-074	35921	01	091-093	36112	02	124-125
3518	01	073-074	35922	01	091-093	36113	02	124-125
3519	01	073-074	35923	01	091-093	36114	02	124-125
3520	01	073-074	35924	01	091-093	36119	02	124-125
3521	01	073-074	35929	01	091-093	3612	02	124-125
3522	01	073-074	3593	01	091-093	36130	02	124-125
3523	01	073-074	3594	01	091-093	36131	02	124-125
3524	01	073-074	3595	01	091-093	36132	02	124-125
3525	01	073-074	3596	01	091-093	36133	02	124-125
3526	01	073-074	35971	08	545-547 ◀	36181	02	124-125
3529	01	073-074	35979	08	545-547 ◀	36189	02	124-125
3530	01	073-074	35981	01	091-093	3619	02	124-125
3531	01	073-074	35989	01	091-093	36201	02	124-125
3532	01	073-074	3599	01	091-093	36202	02	124-125
3533	01	073-074	36000	02	121-122	36203	02	124-125
3534	01	073-074	36001	02	121-122	36204	02	124-125
3535	01	073-074	36002	02	121-122	36205	02	124-125
3536	01	073-074	36003	02	124-125	36206	02	124-125
3538	01	073-074	36004	02	121-122	36207	02	124-125
3539	01	073-074	36011	02	124-125	36210	02	124-125
3540	01	073-074	36012	02	124-125	36211	02	124-125
3541	01	073-074	36013	02	121-122	36212	02	124-125
3542	01	073-074	36014	02	124-125	36213	02	124-125
3543	01	073-074	36019	02	121-122	36214	02	124-125
3544	01	073-074	36020	02	124-125	36215	02	124-125
3545	01	073-074	36021	02	124-125	36216	02	124-125
3548	01	073-074	36023	02	124-125	36217	02	124-125
3549	01	073-074	36024	02	124-125	36218	02	124-125
3550	01	073-074	36029	02	124-125	36220	02	124-125
3551	01	073-074	36030	02	124-125	36221	02	124-125
3552	01	073-074	36031	02	124-125	36222	02	124-125
3553	01	073-074	36032	02	124-125	36223	02	124-125
3554	01	073-074	36033	02	124-125	36224	02	124-125
3555	01	073-074	36034	02	124-125	36225	02	124-125
3556	01	073-074	36040	02	124-125	36226	02	124-125
35571	01	073-074	36041	02	124-125	36227	02	124-125
35579	01	073-074	36042	02	124-125	36229	02	124-125

DX	MDC	MS-DRG	DX	MDC	MS-DRG	DX	MDC	MS-DRG
36230	02	123	36341	02	124-125	36512	02	123
36231	02	123	36342	02	124-125	36513	02	124-125
36232	02	123	36343	02	124-125	36514	02	124-125
36233	02	123	36350	02	124-125	36515	02	124-125
36234	02	123	36351	02	124-125	36520	02	124-125
36235	02	123	36352	02	124-125	36521	02	124-125
36236	02	123	36353	02	124-125	36522	02	124-125
36237	02	123	36354	02	124-125	36523	02	124-125
36240	02	124-125	36355	02	124-125	36524	02	124-125
36241	02	124-125	36356	02	124-125	36531	02	124-125
36242	02	124-125	36357	02	124-125	36532	02	124-125
36243	02	124-125	36361	02	124-125	36541	02	124-125
36250	02	124-125	36362	02	124-125	36542	02	124-125
36251	02	124-125	36363	02	124-125	36543	02	124-125
36252	02	124-125	36370	02	124-125	36544	02	124-125
36253	02	124-125	36371	02	124-125	36551	02	124-125
36254	02	124-125	36372	02	124-125	36552	02	124-125
36255	02	124-125	3638	02	124-125	36559	02	124-125
36256	02	124-125	3639	02	124-125	36560	02	124-125
36257	02	124-125	36400	02	124-125	36561	02	124-125
36260	02	124-125	36401	02	124-125	36562	02	124-125
36261	02	124-125	36402	02	124-125	36563	02	124-125
36262	02	124-125	36403	02	124-125	36564	02	124-125
36263	02	124-125	36404	02	124-125	36565	02	124-125
36264	02	124-125	36405	02	124-125	36581	02	124-125
36265	02	124-125	36410	02	124-125	36582	02	124-125
36266	02	124-125	36411	02	124-125	36583	02	124-125
36270	02	124-125	36421	02	124-125	36589	02	124-125
36271	02	124-125	36422	02	124-125	3659	02	124-125
36272	02	124-125	36423	02	124-125	36600	02	124-125
36273	02	124-125	36424	02	124-125	36601	02	124-125
36274	02	124-125	3643	02	124-125	36602	02	124-125
36275	02	124-125	36441	02	124-125	36603	02	124-125
36276	02	124-125	36442	02	124-125	36604	02	124-125
36277	02	124-125	36451	02	124-125	36609	02	124-125
36281	02	124-125	36452	02	124-125	36610	02	124-125
36282	02	124-125	36453	02	124-125	36611	02	124-125
36283	02	124-125	36454	02	124-125	36612	02	124-125
36284	02	124-125	36455	02	124-125	36613	02	124-125
36285	02	124-125	36456	02	124-125	36614	02	124-125
36289	02	124-125	36457	02	124-125	36615	02	124-125
3629	02	124-125	36459	02	124-125	36616	02	124-125
36300	02	124-125	36460	02	124-125	36617	02	124-125
36301	02	124-125	36461	02	124-125	36618	02	124-125
36303	02	124-125	36462	02	124-125	36619	02	124-125
36304	02	124-125	36463	02	124-125	36620	02	124-125
36305	02	124-125	36464	02	124-125	36621	02	124-125
36306	02	124-125	36470	02	124-125	36622	02	124-125
36307	02	124-125	36471	02	124-125	36623	02	124-125
36308	02	124-125	36472	02	124-125	36630	02	124-125
36310	02	124-125	36473	02	124-125	36631	02	124-125
36311	02	124-125	36474	02	124-125	36632	02	124-125
36312	02	124-125	36475	02	124-125	36633	02	124-125
36313	02	124-125	36476	02	124-125	36634	02	124-125
36314	02	124-125	36477	02	124-125	36641	02	124-125
36315	02	124-125	36481	02	124-125	36642	02	124-125
36320	02	124-125	36482	02	124-125	36643	02	124-125
36321	02	124-125	36489	02	124-125	36644	02	124-125
36322	02	124-125	3649	02	124-125	36645	02	124-125
36330	02	124-125	36500	02	124-125	36646	02	124-125
36331	02	124-125	36501	02	124-125	36650	02	124-125
36332	02	124-125	36502	02	124-125	36651	02	124-125
36333	02	124-125	36503	02	124-125	36652	02	124-125
36334	02	124-125	36504	02	124-125	36653	02	124-125
36335	02	124-125	36510	02	124-125	3668	02	124-125
36340	02	124-125	36511	02	124-125	3669	02	124-125

DX	MDC	MS-DRG	DX	MDC	MS-DRG	DX	MDC	MS-DRG
3670	02	124-125	36915	02	124-125	37102	02	124-125
3671	02	124-125	36916	02	124-125	37103	02	124-125
36720	02	124-125	36917	02	124-125	37104	02	124-125
36721	02	124-125	36918	02	124-125	37105	02	124-125
36722	02	124-125	36920	02	124-125	37110	02	124-125
36731	02	124-125	36921	02	124-125	37111	02	124-125
36732	02	124-125	36922	02	124-125	37112	02	124-125
3674	02	124-125	36923	02	124-125	37113	02	124-125
36751	02	124-125	36924	02	124-125	37114	02	124-125
36752	02	123	36925	02	124-125	37115	02	124-125
36753	02	124-125	3693	02	124-125	37116	02	124-125
36781	02	124-125	3694	02	124-125	37120	02	124-125
36789	02	124-125	36960	02	124-125	37121	02	124-125
3679	02	124-125	36961	02	124-125	37122	02	124-125
36800	02	124-125	36962	02	124-125	37123	02	124-125
36801	02	124-125	36963	02	124-125	37124	02	124-125
36802	02	124-125	36964	02	124-125	37130	02	124-125
36803	02	124-125	36965	02	124-125	37131	02	124-125
36810	02	124-125	36966	02	124-125	37132	02	124-125
36811	02	123	36967	02	124-125	37133	02	124-125
36812	02	123	36968	02	124-125	37140	02	124-125
36813	02	124-125	36969	02	124-125	37141	02	124-125
36814	02	124-125	36970	02	124-125	37142	02	124-125
36815	02	124-125	36971	02	124-125	37143	02	124-125
36816	02	124-125	36972	02	124-125	37144	02	124-125
3682	02	123	36973	02	124-125	37145	02	124-125
36830	02	124-125	36974	02	124-125	37146	02	124-125
36831	02	124-125	36975	02	124-125	37148	02	124-125
36832	02	124-125	36976	02	124-125	37149	02	124-125
36833	02	124-125	3698	02	124-125	37150	02	124-125
36834	02	124-125	3699	02	124-125	37151	02	124-125
36840	02	123	37000	02	121-122	37152	02	124-125
36841	02	123	37001	02	124-125	37153	02	124-125
36842	02	124-125	37002	02	124-125	37154	02	124-125
36843	02	123	37003	02	121-122	37155	02	124-125
36844	02	123	37004	02	121-122	37156	02	124-125
36845	02	123	37005	02	121-122	37157	02	124-125
36846	02	123	37006	02	121-122	37158	02	124-125
36847	02	123	37007	02	124-125	37160	02	124-125
36851	02	124-125	37020	02	124-125	37161	02	124-125
36852	02	124-125	37021	02	124-125	37162	02	124-125
36853	02	124-125	37022	02	124-125	37170	02	124-125
36854	02	124-125	37023	02	124-125	37171	02	124-125
36855	02	123	37024	02	124-125	37172	02	124-125
36859	02	124-125	37031	02	124-125	37173	02	124-125
36860	02	124-125	37032	02	124-125	37181	02	124-125
36861	02	124-125	37033	02	124-125	37182	02	124-125
36862	02	124-125	37034	02	124-125	37189	02	124-125
36863	02	124-125	37035	02	124-125	3719	02	124-125
36869	02	124-125	37040	02	124-125	37200	02	124-125
3688	02	124-125	37044	02	124-125	37201	02	124-125
3689	02	124-125	37049	02	124-125	37202	02	124-125
36900	02	124-125	37050	02	124-125	37203	02	124-125
36901	02	124-125	37052	02	124-125	37204	02	124-125
36902	02	124-125	37054	02	124-125	37205	02	124-125
36903	02	124-125	37055	02	121-122	37206	02	124-125 ◀
36904	02	124-125	37059	02	124-125	37210	02	124-125
36905	02	124-125	37060	02	124-125	37211	02	124-125
36906	02	124-125	37061	02	124-125	37212	02	124-125
36907	02	124-125	37062	02	124-125	37213	02	124-125
36908	02	124-125	37063	02	124-125	37214	02	124-125
36910	02	124-125	37064	02	124-125	37215	02	124-125
36911	02	124-125	3708	02	124-125	37220	02	124-125
36912	02	124-125	3709	02	124-125	37221	02	124-125
36913	02	124-125	37100	02	124-125	37222	02	124-125
36914	02	124-125	37101	02	124-125	37230	02	124-125

DX	MDC	MS-DRG	DX	MDC	MS-DRG	DX	MDC	MS-DRG
37231	02	124-125	37443	02	124-125	37633	02	124-125
37233	02	124-125	37444	02	124-125	37634	02	123
37234	02	124-125	37445	02	123	37635	02	123
37239	02	124-125	37446	02	124-125	37636	02	123
37240	02	124-125	37450	02	124-125	37640	02	124-125
37241	02	124-125	37451	09	606-607	37641	02	124-125
37242	02	124-125	37452	02	124-125	37642	02	124-125
37243	02	124-125	37453	02	124-125	37643	02	124-125
37244	02	124-125	37454	02	124-125	37644	02	124-125
37245	02	124-125	37455	02	124-125	37645	02	124-125
37250	02	124-125	37456	02	124-125	37646	02	124-125
37251	02	124-125	37481	02	124-125	37647	02	124-125
37252	02	124-125	37482	02	124-125	37650	02	124-125
37253	02	124-125	37483	02	124-125	37651	02	124-125
37254	02	124-125	37484	02	124-125	37652	02	124-125
37255	02	124-125	37485	02	124-125	3766	02	124-125
37256	02	124-125	37486	02	124-125	37681	02	124-125
37261	02	124-125	37487	02	124-125	37682	02	123
37262	02	124-125	37489	02	124-125	37689	02	124-125
37263	02	124-125	3749	02	124-125	3769	02	124-125
37264	02	124-125	37500	02	124-125	37700	01	091-093
37271	02	124-125	37501	02	121-122	37701	01	091-093
37272	02	124-125	37502	02	124-125	37702	02	124-125
37273	02	124-125	37503	02	124-125	37703	02	124-125
37274	02	124-125	37511	02	124-125	37704	01	091-093
37275	02	124-125	37512	02	124-125	37710	02	123
37281	02	124-125	37513	02	124-125	37711	02	123
37289	02	124-125	37514	02	124-125	37712	02	123
3729	02	124-125	37515	02	124-125	37713	02	124-125
37300	02	124-125	37516	02	124-125	37714	02	124-125
37301	02	124-125	37520	02	124-125	37715	02	123
37302	02	124-125	37521	02	124-125	37716	02	123
37311	02	124-125	37522	02	124-125	37721	02	123
37312	02	124-125	37530	02	124-125	37722	02	124-125
37313	02	124-125	37531	02	121-122	37723	02	124-125
3732	02	124-125	37532	02	121-122	37724	02	123
37331	02	124-125	37533	02	124-125	37730	02	123
37332	02	124-125	37541	02	124-125	37731	02	123
37333	02	124-125	37542	02	124-125	37732	02	123
37334	02	124-125	37543	02	124-125	37733	02	123
3734	02	124-125	37551	02	124-125	37734	02	123
3735	02	124-125	37552	02	124-125	37739	02	123
3736	02	124-125	37553	02	124-125	37741	02	123
3738	02	124-125	37554	02	124-125	37742	02	123
3739	02	124-125	37555	02	124-125	37743	02	123
37400	02	124-125	37556	02	124-125	37749	02	123
37401	02	124-125	37557	02	124-125	37751	01	091-093
37402	02	124-125	37561	02	124-125	37752	01	091-093
37403	02	124-125	37569	02	124-125	37753	01	091-093
37404	02	124-125	37581	02	124-125	37754	01	091-093
37405	02	124-125	37589	02	124-125	37761	01	091-093
37410	02	124-125	3759	02	124-125	37762	01	091-093
37411	02	124-125	37600	02	124-125	37763	01	091-093
37412	02	124-125	37601	02	121-122	37771	01	091-093
37413	02	124-125	37602	02	121-122	37772	01	091-093
37414	02	124-125	37603	02	121-122	37773	01	091-093
37420	02	124-125	37604	02	121-122	37775	01	091-093
37421	02	124-125	37610	02	124-125	3779	01	091-093
37422	02	124-125	37611	02	124-125	37800	02	124-125
37423	02	124-125	37612	02	124-125	37801	02	124-125
37430	02	123	37613	02	124-125	37802	02	124-125
37431	02	123	37621	02	124-125	37803	02	124-125
37432	02	123	37622	02	124-125	37804	02	124-125
37433	02	124-125	37630	02	124-125	37805	02	124-125
37434	02	124-125	37631	02	124-125	37806	02	124-125
37441	02	124-125	37632	02	124-125	37807	02	124-125

1520

DX	MDC	MS-DRG
37808	02	124-125
37810	02	124-125
37811	02	124-125
37812	02	124-125
37813	02	124-125
37814	02	124-125
37815	02	124-125
37816	02	124-125
37817	02	124-125
37818	02	124-125
37820	02	124-125
37821	02	124-125
37822	02	124-125
37823	02	124-125
37824	02	124-125
37830	02	124-125
37831	02	124-125
37832	02	124-125
37833	02	124-125
37834	02	124-125
37835	02	124-125
37840	02	124-125
37841	02	124-125
37842	02	124-125
37843	02	124-125
37844	02	124-125
37845	02	124-125
37850	02	123
37851	02	123
37852	02	123
37853	02	123
37854	02	123
37855	02	123
37856	02	123
37860	02	124-125
37861	02	124-125
37862	02	124-125
37863	02	124-125
37871	02	124-125
37872	02	123
37873	02	123
37881	02	124-125
37882	02	124-125
37883	02	124-125
37884	02	124-125
37885	02	124-125
37886	01	091-093
37887	02	123
3789	02	124-125
37900	02	124-125
37901	02	124-125
37902	02	124-125
37903	02	124-125
37904	02	124-125
37905	02	124-125
37906	02	124-125
37907	02	124-125
37909	02	124-125
37911	02	124-125
37912	02	124-125
37913	02	124-125
37914	02	124-125
37915	02	124-125
37916	02	124-125
37919	02	124-125
37921	02	124-125

DX	MDC	MS-DRG
37922	02	124-125
37923	02	124-125
37924	02	124-125
37925	02	124-125
37926	02	124-125
37929	02	124-125
37931	02	124-125
37932	02	124-125
37933	02	124-125
37934	02	124-125
37939	02	124-125
37940	02	123
37941	02	123
37942	02	123
37943	02	123
37945	01	056-057
37946	02	123
37949	02	123
37950	02	123
37951	02	124-125
37952	02	123
37953	02	124-125
37954	02	123
37955	02	123
37956	02	124-125
37957	02	123
37958	02	123
37959	02	124-125
37960	02	124-125
37961	02	124-125
37962	02	124-125
37963	02	124-125
3798	02	124-125
37990	02	124-125
37991	02	124-125
37992	02	124-125
37993	02	124-125
37999	02	124-125
38000	03	152-153
38001	08	564-566
38002	08	564-566
38003	08	564-566
38010	03	154-156
38011	03	154-156
38012	03	154-156
38013	03	154-156
38014	03	154-156
38015	03	154-156
38016	03	154-156
38021	03	154-156
38022	03	154-156
38023	03	154-156
38030	03	154-156
38031	03	154-156
38032	03	154-156
38039	03	154-156
3804	03	154-156
38050	03	154-156
38051	03	154-156
38052	03	154-156
38053	03	154-156
38081	03	154-156
38089	03	154-156
3809	03	154-156
38100	03	152-153
38101	03	152-153

DX	MDC	MS-DRG
38102	03	152-153
38103	03	152-153
38104	03	152-153
38105	03	152-153
38106	03	152-153
38110	03	152-153
38119	03	152-153
38120	03	152-153
38129	03	152-153
3813	03	152-153
3814	03	152-153
38150	03	152-153
38151	03	152-153
38152	03	152-153
38160	03	154-156
38161	03	154-156
38162	03	154-156
38163	03	154-156
3817	03	154-156
38181	03	154-156
38189	03	154-156
3819	03	154-156
38200	03	152-153
38201	03	152-153
38202	03	152-153
3821	03	152-153
3822	03	152-153
3823	03	152-153
3824	03	152-153
3829	03	152-153
38300	03	152-153
38301	03	152-153
38302	03	152-153
3831	03	152-153
38320	03	152-153
38321	03	152-153
38322	03	152-153
38330	03	154-156
38331	03	154-156
38332	03	154-156
38333	03	154-156
38381	03	154-156
38389	03	154-156
3839	03	152-153
38400	03	152-153
38401	03	152-153
38409	03	152-153
3841	03	152-153
38420	03	154-156
38421	03	154-156
38422	03	154-156
38423	03	154-156
38424	03	154-156
38425	03	154-156
38481	03	154-156
38482	03	154-156
3849	03	154-156
38500	03	154-156
38501	03	154-156
38502	03	154-156
38503	03	154-156
38509	03	154-156
38510	03	154-156
38511	03	154-156
38512	03	154-156
38513	03	154-156

PART VI, MS-DRG, APPENDIX B

DX	MDC	MS-DRG	DX	MDC	MS-DRG	DX	MDC	MS-DRG
38519	03	154-156	3885	03	154-156	40200	05	304-305
38521	03	154-156	38860	03	154-156	40201	05	222-223, 291-293
38522	03	154-156	38861	01	091-093	40210	05	304-305
38523	03	154-156	38869	03	154-156	40211	05	222-223, 291-293
38524	03	154-156	38870	03	154-156	40290	05	304-305
38530	03	154-156	38871	03	154-156	40291	05	222-223, 291-293
38531	03	154-156	38872	03	154-156	40300	11	673-675, 682-684
38532	03	154-156	3888	03	154-156	40301	11	673-675, 682-684
38533	03	154-156	3889	03	154-156	40310	11	673-675, 682-684
38535	03	154-156	38900	03	154-156	40311	11	673-675, 682-684
38582	03	154-156	38901	03	154-156	40390	11	673-675, 682-684
38583	03	154-156	38902	03	154-156	40391	11	673-675, 682-684
38589	03	154-156	38903	03	154-156	40400	05	304-305
3859	03	154-156	38904	03	154-156	40401	05	222-223, 291-293
38600	03	149	38905	03	154-156	40402	11	673-675, 682-684
38601	03	149	38906	03	154-156	40403	05	222-223, 291-293
38602	03	149	38908	03	154-156	40410	05	304-305
38603	03	149	38910	03	154-156	40411	05	222-223, 291-293
38604	03	149	38911	03	154-156	40412	11	673-675, 682-684
38610	03	149	38912	03	154-156	40413	05	222-223, 291-293
38611	03	149	38913	03	154-156	40490	05	304-305
38612	03	149	38914	03	154-156	40491	05	222-223, 291-293
38619	03	149	38915	03	154-156	40492	11	673-675, 682-684
3862	03	149	38916	03	154-156	40493	05	222-223, 291-293
38630	03	149	38917	03	154-156	40501	05	304-305
38631	03	149	38918	03	154-156	40509	05	304-305
38632	03	149	38920	03	154-156	40511	05	304-305
38633	03	149	38921	03	154-156	40519	05	304-305
38634	03	149	38922	03	154-156	40591	05	304-305
38635	03	149	3897	03	154-156	40599	05	304-305
38640	03	154-156	3898	03	154-156	41000	05	314-316
38641	03	154-156	3899	03	154-156	41001	05	222-223, 280-285
38642	03	154-156	390	08	545-547	41002	05	314-316
38643	03	154-156	3910	05	314-316	41010	05	314-316
38648	03	154-156	3911	05	306-307	41011	05	222-223, 280-285
38650	03	149	3912	05	314-316	41012	05	314-316
38651	03	149	3918	05	314-316	41020	05	314-316
38652	03	149	3919	05	314-316	41021	05	222-223, 280-285
38653	03	149	3920	05	314-316	41022	05	314-316
38654	03	149	3929	05	314-316	41030	05	314-316
38655	03	149	393	05	314-316	41031	05	222-223, 280-285
38656	03	149	3940	05	306-307	41032	05	314-316
38658	03	149	3941	05	306-307	41040	05	314-316
3868	03	149	3942	05	306-307			
3869	03	149	3949	05	306-307			
3870	03	154-156	3950	05	306-307			
3871	03	154-156	3951	05	306-307			
3872	03	154-156	3952	05	306-307			
3878	03	154-156	3959	05	306-307			
3879	03	154-156	3960	05	306-307			
38800	03	154-156	3961	05	306-307			
38801	03	154-156	3962	05	306-307			
38802	03	154-156	3963	05	306-307			
38810	03	154-156	3968	05	306-307			
38811	03	154-156	3969	05	306-307			
38812	03	154-156	3970	05	306-307			
3882	03	154-156	3971	05	306-307			
38830	03	154-156	3979	05	306-307			
38831	03	154-156	3980	05	314-316			
38832	03	154-156	39890	05	314-316			
38840	03	154-156	39891	05	222-223, 291-293			
38841	03	154-156	39899	05	314-316			
38842	03	154-156	4010	05	304-305			
38843	03	154-156	4011	05	304-305			
38844	03	154-156	4019	05	304-305			
38845	19	886						

DX	MDC	MS-DRG	DX	MDC	MS-DRG	DX	MDC	MS-DRG
41041	05	222-223, 280-285	4211	05	288-290	4281	05	222-223, 291-293
41042	05	314-316	4219	05	288-290	42820	05	222-223, 291-293
41050	05	314-316	4220	05	314-316			
41051	05	222-223, 280-285	42290	05	314-316	42821	05	222-223, 291-293
41052	05	314-316	42291	05	314-316	42822	05	222-223, 291-293
41060	05	314-316	42292	05	314-316			
41061	05	222-223, 280-285	42293	05	314-316	42823	05	222-223, 291-293
41062	05	314-316	42299	05	314-316	42830	05	222-223, 291-293
41070	05	314-316	4230	05	314-316			
41071	05	222-223, 280-285	4231	05	314-316	42831	05	222-223, 291-293
41072	05	314-316	4232	05	314-316	42832	05	222-223, 291-293
41080	05	314-316	4233	05	314-316			
41081	05	222-223, 280-285	4238	05	314-316	42833	05	222-223, 291-293
41082	05	314-316	4239	05	314-316	42840	05	222-223, 291-293
41090	05	314-316	4240	05	306-307			
41091	05	222-223, 280-285	4241	05	306-307	42841	05	222-223, 291-293
41092	05	314-316	4242	05	306-307	42842	05	222-223, 291-293
4110	05	314-316	4243	05	306-307			
4111	05	311	42490	05	306-307	42843	05	222-223, 291-293
41181	05	311	42491	05	306-307	4289	05	222-223, 291-293
41189	05	311	42499	05	306-307			
412	05	302-303	4250	05	314-316	4290	05	314-316
4130	05	311	4251	05	314-316	4291	05	314-316
4131	05	311	4252	05	314-316	4292	05	302-303
4139	05	311	4253	05	314-316	4293	05	302-303
41400	05	302-303	4254	05	314-316	4294	05	314-316
41401	05	302-303	4255	05	314-316	4295	05	306-307
41402	05	302-303	4257	05	314-316	4296	05	306-307
41403	05	302-303	4258	05	314-316	42971	05	314-316
41404	05	302-303	4259	05	314-316	42979	05	314-316
41405	05	302-303	4260	05	308-310	42981	05	306-307
41406	05	302-303	42610	05	308-310	42982	05	314-316
41407	05	302-303	42611	05	308-310	42983	05	314-316
41410	05	314-316	42612	05	308-310	42989	05	302-303
41411	05	314-316	42613	05	308-310	4299	05	302-303
41412	05	314-316	4262	05	308-310	430	01	020-024, 064-066
41419	05	314-316	4263	05	308-310			
4142	05	302-303	4264	05	308-310	431	01	020-024, 064-066
4143	05	302-303	42650	05	308-310			
4148	05	302-303	42651	05	308-310	4320	01	020-022, 064-066
4149	05	302-303	42652	05	308-310			
4150	05	314-316	42653	05	308-310	4321	01	020-022, 064-066
41511	04	175-176	42654	05	308-310			
41512	04	175-176	4266	05	308-310	4329	01	020-024, 064-066
41519	04	175-176	4267	05	308-310			
4160	05	314-316	42681	05	308-310	43300	01	067-068
4161	05	314-316	42682	05	308-310	43301	01	023-024, 061-066
4162	04	175-176,	42689	05	308-310			
	15	791, 793	4269	05	308-310	43310	01	067-068
4168	05	314-316	4270	05	308-310	43311	01	023-024, 061-066
4169	05	314-316	4271	05	308-310			
4170	05	314-316	4272	05	308-310	43320	01	067-068
4171	05	314-316	42731	05	308-310	43321	01	023-024, 061-066
4178	05	314-316	42732	05	308-310			
4179	05	314-316	42741	05	308-310	43330	01	067-068
4200	05	314-316	42742	05	308-310	43331	01	023-024, 061-066
42090	05	314-316	4275	05	296-298			
42091	05	314-316	42760	05	308-310	43380	01	067-068
42099	05	314-316	42761	05	308-310			
4210	05	288-290	42769	05	308-310			
			42781	05	308-310			
			42789	05	308-310			
			4279	05	308-310			
			4280	05	222-223, 291-293			

◀

DX	MDC	MS-DRG	DX	MDC	MS-DRG	DX	MDC	MS-DRG
43381	01	023-024, 061-066	44024	05	299-301	4474	06	391-392
43390	01	067-068	44029	05	299-301	4475	05	299-301
43391	01	023-024, 061-066	44030	05	299-301	4476	08	545-547
			44031	05	299-301	4478	05	299-301
43400	01	067-068	44032	05	299-301	4479	05	299-301
43401	01	023-024, 061-066	4404	05	299-301	4480	05	299-301
			4408	05	299-301	4481	09	606-607
43410	01	067-068	4409	05	299-301	4489	05	299-301
43411	01	023-024, 061-066	44100	05	299-301	449	05	299-301
			44101	05	299-301	4510	05	299-301
43490	01	067-068	44102	05	299-301	45111	05	294-295
43491	01	023-024, 061-066	44103	05	299-301	45119	05	294-295
			4411	05	299-301	4512	05	294-295
4350	01	069	4412	05	299-301	45181	05	294-295
4351	01	069	4413	05	299-301	45182	05	299-301
4352	01	069	4414	05	299-301	45183	05	299-301
4353	01	069	4415	05	299-301	45184	05	299-301
4358	01	069	4416	05	299-301	45189	05	299-301
4359	01	069	4417	05	299-301	4519	05	299-301
436	01	067-068	4419	05	299-301	452	07	441-443
4370	01	070-072	4420	05	299-301	4530	07	441-443
4371	01	069	4421	11	698-700	4531	05	299-301
4372	01	077-079	4422	05	299-301	4532	05	294-295
4373	01	091-093	4423	05	299-301	4533	11	698-700
4374	01	102-103	44281	05	299-301	45340	05	299-301
4375	01	091-093	44282	05	299-301	45341	05	299-301
4376	01	091-093	44283	05	299-301	45342	05	299-301
4377	01	070-072	44284	05	299-301	45350	05	299-301 ◄
4378	01	070-072	44289	05	299-301	45351	05	299-301 ◄
4379	01	070-072	4429	05	299-301	45252	05	299-301 ◄
4380	01	056-057	4430	08	545-547	45371	05	299-301 ◄
43810	01	056-057	4431	05	299-301	45372	05	299-301 ◄
43811	01	056-057	44321	05	299-301	45373	05	299-301 ◄
43812	01	056-057	44322	05	299-301	45374	05	299-301 ◄
43813	01	056-057 ◄	44323	11	698-700	45375	05	299-301 ◄
43814	01	056-057 ◄	44324	05	299-301	45376	05	299-301 ◄
43819	01	056-057	44329	05	299-301	45377	05	299-301 ◄
43820	01	056-057	44381	05	299-301	45379	05	299-301 ◄
43821	01	056-057	44382	05	299-301	45381	05	299-301
43822	01	056-057	44389	05	299-301	45382	05	299-301 ◄
43830	01	056-057	4439	05	299-301	45383	05	299-301 ◄
43831	01	056-057	4440	05	299-301	45384	05	299-301 ◄
43832	01	056-057	4441	05	299-301	45385	05	299-301 ◄
43840	01	056-057	44421	05	299-301	45386	05	299-301 ◄
43841	01	056-057	44422	05	299-301	45387	05	299-301 ◄
43842	01	056-057	44481	05	299-301	45389	05	299-301 ◄
43850	01	056-057	44489	05	299-301	4539	05	299-301
43851	01	056-057	4449	05	299-301	4540	05	299-301
43852	01	056-057	44501	05	299-301	4541	05	299-301
43853	01	056-057	44502	05	299-301	4542	05	299-301
4386	01	056-057	44581	11	698-700	4548	05	299-301
4387	01	056-057	44589	05	299-301	4549	05	299-301
43881	01	056-057	4460	08	545-547	4550	06	393-395
43882	01	056-057	4461	08	545-547	4551	06	393-395
43883	01	056-057	44620	08	545-547	4552	06	393-395
43884	01	056-057	44621	08	545-547	4553	06	393-395
43885	01	056-057	44629	08	545-547	4554	06	393-395
43889	01	056-057	4463	08	542-544	4555	06	393-395
4389	01	056-057	4464	08	542-544	4556	06	393-395
4400	05	299-301	4465	08	545-547	4557	06	393-395
4401	11	698-700	4466	08	545-547	4558	06	393-395
44020	05	299-301	4467	08	545-547	4559	06	393-395
44021	05	299-301	4470	05	299-301	4560	06	368-370
44022	05	299-301	4471	05	299-301	4561	06	368-370
44023	05	299-301	4472	05	299-301	45620	06	368-370
			4473	11	698-700	45621	06	393-395

DX	MDC	MS-DRG	DX	MDC	MS-DRG	DX	MDC	MS-DRG
4563	05	299-301	4721	03	152-153	48242	04	177-179
4564	12	729-730	4722	03	152-153	48249	04	177-179
4565	12	729-730	4730	03	152-153	48281	04	177-179
4565	13	742-743, 760-761	4731	03	152-153	48282	04	177-179
			4732	03	152-153	48283	04	177-179
4566	13	742-743, 760-761	4733	03	152-153	48284	04	177-179
			4738	03	152-153	48289	04	177-179
4568	05	299-301	4739	03	152-153	4829	04	193-195
4570	09	600-601	47400	03	152-153	4830	04	193-195
4571	09	606-607	47401	03	152-153	4831	04	193-195
4572	09	602-603	47402	03	152-153	4838	04	193-195
4578	16	814-816	47410	03	154-156	4841	04	177-179
4579	16	814-816	47411	03	154-156	4843	04	177-179
4580	05	312	47412	03	154-156	4845	04	177-179
4581	05	314-316	4742	03	154-156	4846	04	177-179
45821	05	312	4748	03	154-156	4847	04	177-179
45829	05	312	4749	03	154-156	4848	04	177-179
4588	05	314-316	475	03	152-153	485	04	193-195
4589	05	314-316	4760	03	152-153	486	04	193-195
4590	05	314-316	4761	03	152-153	4870	04	193-195
45910	05	299-301	4770	03	152-153	4871	03	152-153
45911	05	299-301	4771	03	152-153	4878	18	865-866
45912	05	299-301	4772	03	152-153	488	03	152-153
45913	05	299-301	4778	03	152-153	490	04	202-203
45919	05	299-301	4779	03	152-153	4910	04	202-203
4592	05	299-301	4780	03	154-156	4911	04	190-192
45930	05	299-301	47811	03	154-156	49120	04	190-192
45931	05	299-301	47819	03	154-156	49121	04	190-192
45932	05	299-301	47820	03	154-156	49122	04	190-192
45933	05	299-301	47821	03	152-153	4918	04	190-192
45939	05	299-301	47822	03	152-153	4919	04	190-192
45981	05	299-301	47824	03	152-153	4920	04	190-192
45989	05	302-303	47825	03	154-156	4928	04	190-192
4599	05	302-303	47826	03	154-156	49300	04	202-203
460	03	152-153	47829	03	154-156	49301	04	202-203
4610	03	152-153	47830	03	154-156	49302	04	202-203
4611	03	152-153	47831	03	154-156	49310	04	202-203
4612	03	152-153	47832	03	154-156	49311	04	202-203
4613	03	152-153	47833	03	154-156	49312	04	202-203
4618	03	152-153	47834	03	154-156	49320	04	190-192
4619	03	152-153	4784	03	154-156	49321	04	190-192
462	03	152-153	4785	03	154-156	49322	04	190-192
463	03	152-153	4786	03	154-156	49381	04	202-203
46400	03	152-153	47870	03	154-156	49382	04	202-203
46401	03	152-153	47871	03	152-153	49390	04	202-203
46410	04	202-203	47874	03	154-156	49391	04	202-203
46411	04	202-203	47875	03	154-156	49392	04	202-203
46420	03	152-153	47879	03	154-156	4940	04	190-192
46421	03	152-153	4788	03	152-153	4941	04	190-192
46430	03	152-153	4789	03	152-153	4950	04	196-198
46431	03	152-153	4800	04	193-195	4951	04	196-198
4644	03	152-153	4801	04	193-195	4952	04	196-198
46450	03	152-153	4802	04	193-195	4953	04	196-198
46451	03	152-153	4803	04	193-195	4954	04	196-198
4650	03	152-153	4808	04	193-195	4955	04	196-198
4658	03	152-153	4809	04	193-195	4956	04	196-198
4659	03	152-153	481	04	193-195	4957	04	196-198
4660	04	202-203	4820	04	177-179	4958	04	196-198
46611	04	202-203	4821	04	177-179	4959	04	196-198
46619	04	202-203	4822	04	193-195	496	04	190-192
470	03	154-156	48230	04	193-195	500	04	196-198
4710	03	154-156	48231	04	193-195	501	04	196-198
4711	03	154-156	48232	04	193-195	502	04	196-198
4718	03	154-156	48239	04	193-195	503	04	196-198
4719	03	154-156	48240	04	177-179	504	04	196-198
4720	03	152-153	48241	04	177-179	505	04	196-198

DX	MDC	MS-DRG	DX	MDC	MS-DRG	DX	MDC	MS-DRG
5060	04	205-206	5205	03	157-159	52333	03	157-159
5061	04	189	5206	03	157-159	52340	03	157-159
5062	04	205-206	5207	03	157-159	52341	03	157-159
5063	04	205-206	5208	03	157-159	52342	03	157-159
5064	04	190-192	5209	03	157-159	5235	03	157-159
5069	04	190-192	52100	03	157-159	5236	03	157-159
5070	04	177-179	52101	03	157-159	5238	03	157-159
5071	04	177-179	52102	03	157-159	5239	03	157-159
5078	04	177-179	52103	03	157-159	52400	03	157-159
5080	04	205-206	52104	03	157-159	52401	03	157-159
5081	04	196-198	52105	03	157-159	52402	03	157-159
5088	04	205-206	52106	03	157-159	52403	03	157-159
5089	04	205-206	52107	03	157-159	52404	03	157-159
5100	04	177-179	52108	03	157-159	52405	03	157-159
5109	04	177-179	52109	03	157-159	52406	03	157-159
5110	04	193-195	52110	03	157-159	52407	03	157-159
5111	04	177-179	52111	03	157-159	52409	03	157-159
51181	04	180-182	52112	03	157-159	52410	03	157-159
51189	04	186-188	52113	03	157-159	52411	03	157-159
5119	04	186-188	52114	03	157-159	52412	03	157-159
5120	04	199-201	52115	03	157-159	52419	03	157-159
5121	04	199-201	52120	03	157-159	52420	03	157-159
5128	04	199-201	52121	03	157-159	52421	03	157-159
5130	04	177-179	52122	03	157-159	52422	03	157-159
5131	04	177-179	52123	03	157-159	52423	03	157-159
514	04	189	52124	03	157-159	52424	03	157-159
515	04	196-198	52125	03	157-159	52425	03	157-159
5160	04	196-198	52130	03	157-159	52426	03	157-159
5161	04	196-198	52131	03	157-159	52427	03	157-159
5162	04	196-198	52132	03	157-159	52428	03	157-159
5163	04	196-198	52133	03	157-159	52429	03	157-159
5168	04	196-198	52134	03	157-159	52430	03	157-159
5169	04	196-198	52135	03	157-159	52431	03	157-159
5171	04	196-198	52140	03	157-159	52432	03	157-159
5172	04	196-198	52141	03	157-159	52433	03	157-159
5173	04	196-198	52142	03	157-159	52434	03	157-159
5178	04	196-198	52149	03	157-159	52435	03	157-159
5180	04	205-206	5215	03	157-159	52436	03	157-159
5181	04	199-201	5216	03	157-159	52437	03	157-159
5182	04	205-206	5217	03	157-159	52439	03	157-159
5183	04	196-198	52181	03	157-159	5244	03	157-159
5184	04	189	52189	03	157-159	52450	03	157-159
5185	04	189	5219	03	157-159	52451	03	157-159
5186	04	196-198	5220	03	157-159	52452	03	157-159
5187	04	205-206	5221	03	157-159	52453	03	157-159
51881	04	189	5222	03	157-159	52454	03	157-159
51882	04	204	5223	03	157-159	52455	03	157-159
51883	04	189	5224	03	157-159	52456	03	157-159
51884	04	189	5225	03	157-159	52457	03	157-159
51889	04	205-206	5226	03	157-159	52459	03	157-159
51900	04	205-206	5227	03	157-159	52460	03	157-159
51901	04	205-206	5228	03	157-159	52461	03	157-159
51902	04	205-206	5229	03	157-159	52462	03	157-159
51909	04	205-206	52300	03	157-159	52463	03	157-159
51911	04	202-203	52301	03	157-159	52464	03	157-159
51919	04	202-203	52310	03	157-159	52469	03	157-159
5192	04	177-179	52311	03	157-159	52470	03	157-159
5193	04	205-206	52320	03	157-159	52471	03	157-159
5194	04	205-206	52321	03	157-159	52472	03	157-159
5198	04	205-206	52322	03	157-159	52473	03	157-159
5199	04	205-206	52323	03	157-159	52474	03	157-159
5200	03	157-159	52324	03	157-159	52475	03	157-159
5201	03	157-159	52325	03	157-159	52476	03	157-159
5202	03	157-159	52330	03	157-159	52479	03	157-159
5203	03	157-159	52331	03	157-159	52481	03	157-159
5204	03	157-159	52332	03	157-159	52482	03	157-159

DX	MDC	MS-DRG	DX	MDC	MS-DRG	DX	MDC	MS-DRG
52489	03	157-159	52802	03	157-159	53220	06	377-379
5249	03	157-159	52809	03	157-159	53221	06	377-379
5250	03	157-159	5281	03	157-159	53230	06	383-384
52510	03	157-159	5282	03	157-159	53231	06	380-382
52511	03	157-159	5283	03	157-159	53240	06	377-379
52512	03	157-159	5284	03	157-159	53241	06	377-379
52513	03	157-159	5285	03	157-159	53250	06	380-382
52519	03	157-159	5286	03	157-159	53251	06	380-382
52520	03	157-159	52871	03	157-159	53260	06	377-379
52521	03	157-159	52872	03	157-159	53261	06	377-379
52522	03	157-159	52879	03	157-159	53270	06	383-384
52523	03	157-159	5288	03	157-159	53271	06	380-382
52524	03	157-159	5289	03	157-159	53290	06	383-384
52525	03	157-159	5290	03	157-159	53291	06	380-382
52526	03	157-159	5291	03	157-159	53300	06	377-379
5253	03	157-159	5292	03	157-159	53301	06	377-379
52540	03	157-159	5293	03	157-159	53310	06	380-382
52541	03	157-159	5294	03	157-159	53311	06	380-382
52542	03	157-159	5295	03	157-159	53320	06	377-379
52543	03	157-159	5296	03	157-159	53321	06	377-379
52544	03	157-159	5298	03	157-159	53330	06	383-384
52550	03	157-159	5299	03	157-159	53331	06	380-382
52551	03	157-159	5300	06	391-392	53340	06	377-379
52552	03	157-159	53010	06	391-392	53341	06	377-379
52553	03	157-159	53011	06	391-392	53350	06	380-382
52554	03	157-159	53012	06	391-392	53351	06	380-382
52560	03	157-159	53013	06	391-392	53360	06	377-379
52561	03	157-159	53019	06	391-392	53361	06	377-379
52562	03	157-159	53020	06	380-382	53370	06	383-384
52563	03	157-159	53021	06	380-382	53371	06	380-382
52564	03	157-159	5303	06	391-392	53390	06	383-384
52565	03	157-159	5304	06	368-370	53391	06	380-382
52566	03	157-159	5305	06	391-392	53400	06	377-379
52567	03	157-159	5306	06	391-392	53401	06	377-379
52569	03	157-159	5307	06	368-370	53410	06	380-382
52571	03	157-159	53081	06	391-392	53411	06	380-382
52572	03	157-159	53082	06	368-370	53420	06	377-379
52573	03	157-159	53083	06	391-392	53421	06	377-379
52579	03	157-159	53084	06	368-370	53430	06	380-382
5258	03	157-159	53085	06	380-382	53431	06	380-382
5259	03	157-159	53086	06	393-395	53440	06	377-379
5260	03	157-159	53087	06	393-395	53441	06	377-379
5261	03	157-159	53089	06	391-392	53450	06	380-382
5262	03	157-159	5309	06	391-392	53451	06	380-382
5263	03	157-159	53100	06	377-379	53460	06	377-379
5264	03	157-159	53101	06	377-379	53461	06	377-379
5265	03	157-159	53110	06	380-382	53470	06	380-382
52661	03	157-159	53111	06	380-382	53471	06	380-382
52662	03	157-159	53120	06	377-379	53490	06	380-382
52663	03	157-159	53121	06	377-379	53491	06	380-382
52669	03	157-159	53130	06	383-384	53500	06	391-392
52681	03	157-159	53131	06	380-382	53501	06	377-379
52689	03	157-159	53140	06	377-379	53510	06	391-392
5269	03	157-159	53141	06	377-379	53511	06	377-379
5270	03	154-156	53150	06	380-382	53520	06	391-392
5271	03	154-156	53151	06	380-382	53521	06	377-379
5272	03	154-156	53160	06	377-379	53530	06	391-392
5273	03	154-156	53161	06	377-379	53531	06	377-379
5274	03	154-156	53170	06	383-384	53540	06	391-392
5275	03	154-156	53171	06	380-382	53541	06	377-379
5276	03	154-156	53190	06	383-384	53550	06	391-392
5277	03	154-156	53191	06	380-382	53551	06	377-379
5278	03	154-156	53200	06	377-379	53560	06	391-392
5279	03	154-156	53201	06	377-379	53561	06	377-379
52800	03	157-159	53210	06	380-382	53570	06	391-392
52801	03	157-159	53211	06	380-382	53571	06	377-379

DX	MDC	MS-DRG	DX	MDC	MS-DRG	DX	MDC	MS-DRG
5360	06	391-392	5529	06	393-395	5651	06	393-395
5361	06	391-392	55300	06	393-395	566	06	393-395
5362	06	391-392	55301	06	393-395	5670	06	371-373
5363	06	391-392	55302	06	393-395	5671	06	371-373
53640	06	393-395	55303	06	393-395	56721	06	371-373
53641	06	393-395	5531	06	393-395	56722	06	371-373
53642	06	393-395	55320	06	393-395	56723	06	371-373
53649	06	393-395	55321	06	393-395	56729	06	371-373
5368	06	391-392	55329	06	393-395	56731	06	371-373
5369	06	391-392	5533	06	391-392	56738	06	371-373
5370	06	380-382	5538	06	393-395	56739	06	371-373
5371	06	391-392	5539	06	393-395	56781	06	393-395
5372	06	391-392	5550	06	385-387	56782	06	393-395
5373	06	380-382	5551	06	385-387	56789	06	371-373
5374	06	391-392	5552	06	385-387	5679	06	371-373
5375	06	391-392	5559	06	385-387	5680	06	393-395
5376	06	391-392	5560	06	385-387	56881	06	393-395
53781	06	391-392	5561	06	385-387	56882	06	393-395
53782	06	391-392	5562	06	385-387	56889	06	393-395
53783	06	377-379	5563	06	385-387	5689	06	393-395
53784	06	377-379	5564	06	385-387	5690	06	393-395
53789	06	391-392	5565	06	385-387	5691	06	393-395
5379	06	391-392	5566	06	385-387	5692	06	393-395
538	06	391-392	5568	06	385-387	5693	06	377-379
5400	06	338-340, 371-373	5569	06	385-387	56941	06	393-395
5401	06	338-340, 371-373	5570	06	393-395	56942	06	393-395
			5571	06	393-395	56943	06	393-395
5409	06	393-395	5579	06	393-395	56944	06	393-395
541	06	393-395	5581	06	393-395	56949	06	393-395
542	06	393-395	5582	06	393-395	5695	06	371-373
5430	06	393-395	5583	06	391-392	56960	06	393-395
5439	06	393-395	55841	06	391-392	56961	06	393-395
55000	06	393-395	55842	06	391-392	56962	06	393-395
55001	06	393-395	5589	06	391-392	56969	06	393-395
55002	06	393-395	5600	06	388-390	56971	06	393-395, ◄
55003	06	393-395	5601	06	388-390		15	791,793 ◄
55010	06	393-395	5602	06	388-390	56979	06	393-395, ◄
55011	06	393-395	56030	06	388-390		15	791,793 ◄
55012	06	393-395	56031	06	388-390	56981	06	393-395
55013	06	393-395	56039	06	388-390	56982	06	393-395
55090	06	393-395	56081	06	388-390	56983	06	393-395
55091	06	393-395	56089	06	388-390	56984	06	393-395
55092	06	393-395	5609	06	388-390	56985	06	377-379
55093	06	393-395	56200	06	391-392	56986	06	393-395
55100	06	393-395	56201	06	391-392	56987	06	393-395 ◄
55101	06	393-395	56202	06	377-379	56989	06	393-395
55102	06	393-395	56203	06	377-379	5699	06	393-395
55103	06	393-395	56210	06	391-392	570	07	441-443
5511	06	393-395	56211	06	391-392	5710	07	441-443
55120	06	393-395	56212	06	377-379	5711	07	432-434
55121	06	393-395	56213	06	377-379	5712	07	432-434
55129	06	393-395	56400	06	391-392	5713	07	432-434
5513	06	393-395	56401	06	391-392	57140	07	441-443
5518	06	393-395	56402	06	391-392	57141	07	441-443
5519	06	393-395	56409	06	391-392	57142	07	441-443
55200	06	393-395	5641	06	391-392	57149	07	441-443
55201	06	393-395	5642	06	391-392	5715	07	432-434
55202	06	393-395	5643	06	391-392	5716	07	432-434
55203	06	393-395	5644	06	391-392	5718	07	441-443
5521	06	393-395	5645	06	391-392	5719	07	441-443
55220	06	393-395	5646	06	391-392	5720	07	441-443
55221	06	393-395	5647	06	393-395	5721	07	441-443
55229	06	393-395	56481	06	391-392	5722	07	441-443
5523	06	391-392	56489	06	391-392	5723	07	441-443
			5649	06	391-392		15	791,793 ◄
5528	06	393-395	5650	06	393-395	5724	07	441-443

DX	MDC	MS-DRG
5728	07	441-443
5730	07	441-443
5731	07	441-443
5732	07	441-443
5733	07	441-443
5734	07	441-443
5738	07	441-443
5739	07	441-443
57400	07	444-446
57401	07	444-446
57410	07	444-446
57411	07	444-446
57420	07	444-446
57421	07	444-446
57430	07	444-446
57431	07	444-446
57440	07	444-446
57441	07	444-446
57450	07	444-446
57451	07	444-446
57460	07	444-446
57461	07	444-446
57470	07	444-446
57471	07	444-446
57480	07	444-446
57481	07	444-446
57490	07	444-446
57491	07	444-446
5750	07	444-446
57510	07	444-446
57511	07	444-446
57512	07	444-446
5752	07	444-446
5753	07	444-446
5754	07	444-446
5755	07	444-446
5756	07	444-446
5758	07	444-446
5759	07	444-446
5760	07	444-446
5761	07	444-446
5762	07	444-446
5763	07	444-446
5764	07	444-446
5765	07	444-446
5768	07	444-446
5769	07	444-446
5770	07	438-440
5771	07	438-440
5772	07	438-440
5778	07	438-440
5779	07	438-440
5780	06	377-379
5781	06	377-379
5789	06	377-379
5790	06	391-392
5791	06	391-392
5792	06	391-392
5793	06	391-392
5794	06	391-392
5798	06	391-392
5799	06	391-392
5800	11	698-700
5804	11	698-700
58081	11	698-700
58089	11	698-700

DX	MDC	MS-DRG
5809	11	698-700
5810	11	698-700
5811	11	698-700
5812	11	698-700
5813	11	698-700
58181	11	698-700
58189	11	698-700
5819	11	698-700
5820	11	698-700
5821	11	698-700
5822	11	698-700
5824	11	698-700
58281	11	698-700
58289	11	698-700
5829	11	698-700
5830	11	698-700
5831	11	698-700
5832	11	698-700
5834	11	698-700
5836	11	698-700
5837	11	698-700
58381	11	698-700
58389	11	698-700
5839	11	698-700
5845	11	673-675, 682-684
	15	791,793 ◄▪▪▪
5846	11	673-675, 682-684
	15	791,793 ◄▪▪▪
5847	11	673-675, 682-684
	15	791,793 ◄▪▪▪
5848	11	673-675, 682-684
	15	791,793 ◄▪▪▪
5849	11	673-675, 682-684
5851	11	673-675, 682-684
5852	11	673-675, 682-684
5853	11	673-675, 682-684
5854	11	673-675, 682-684
5855	11	673-675, 682-684
5856	11	673-675, 682-684
5859	11	673-675, 682-684
586	11	673-675, 682-684
587	11	698-700
5880	11	698-700
5881	11	698-700
58881	11	698-700
58889	11	698-700
5889	11	698-700
5890	11	698-700
5891	11	698-700
5899	11	698-700
59000	11	689-690
59001	11	689-690
59010	11	689-690

DX	MDC	MS-DRG
59011	11	689-690
5902	11	689-690
5903	11	689-690
59080	11	689-690
59081	11	689-690
5909	11	689-690
591	11	691-694
5920	11	691-694
5921	11	691-694
5929	11	691-694
5930	11	698-700
5931	11	698-700
5932	11	698-700
5933	11	689-690
5934	11	691-694
5935	11	691-694
5936	11	698-700
59370	11	698-700
59371	11	698-700
59372	11	698-700
59373	11	698-700
59381	11	698-700
59382	11	698-700
59389	11	698-700
5939	11	698-700
5940	11	698-700
5941	11	691-694
5942	11	691-694
5948	11	691-694
5949	11	691-694
5950	11	689-690
5951	11	689-690
5952	11	689-690
5953	11	689-690
5954	11	689-690
59581	11	689-690
59582	11	698-700
59589	11	689-690
5959	11	689-690
5960	11	698-700
5961	11	698-700
5962	11	698-700
5963	11	698-700
5964	11	698-700
59651	11	698-700
59652	11	698-700
59653	11	698-700
59654	11	698-700
59655	11	698-700
59659	11	698-700
5966	11	698-700
5967	11	698-700
5968	11	698-700
5969	11	698-700
5970	11	689-690
59780	11	689-690
59781	11	689-690
59789	11	689-690
59800	11	697
59801	11	697
5981	11	697
5982	11	697
5988	11	697
5989	11	697
5990	11	689-690
5991	11	698-700

DX	MDC	MS-DRG	DX	MDC	MS-DRG	DX	MDC	MS-DRG
5992	11	698-700	60823	12	729-730	61610	13	742-743, 757-759
5993	11	698-700	60824	12	729-730	61611	13	742-743, 757-759
5994	11	698-700	6083	12	729-730	6162	13	742-743, 760-761
5995	11	698-700	6084	12	727-728	6163	13	742-743, 757-759
59960	11	698-700	60881	12	729-730	6164	13	742-743, 757-759
59969	11	698-700	60882	12	729-730	61650	13	742-743, 760-761
59970	11	695-696	60883	12	729-730	61651	13	742-743, 760-761
59971	11	695-696	60884	12	729-730	61681	13	742-743, 757-759
59972	11	695-696	60885	12	729-730	61689	13	742-743, 757-759
59981	11	698-700	60886	12	729-730	6169	13	742-743, 757-759
59982	11	698-700	60887	12	729-730	6170	13	742-743, 760-761
59983	11	698-700	60889	12	729-730	6171	13	742-743, 760-761
59984	11	698-700	6089	12	729-730	6172	13	742-743, 760-761
59989	11	698-700	6100	09	600-601	6173	13	742-743, 760-761
5999	11	698-700	6101	09	600-601	6174	13	742-743, 760-761
60000	12	725-726	6102	09	600-601	6175	06	391-392
60001	12	725-726	6103	09	600-601	6176	09	606-607
60010	12	725-726	6104	09	600-601	6178	13	742-743, 760-761
60011	12	725-726	6108	09	600-601	6179	13	742-743, 760-761
60020	12	725-726	6109	09	600-601	61800	13	742-743, 760-761
60021	12	725-726	6110	09	600-601	61801	13	742-743, 760-761
6003	12	725-726	6111	09	600-601	61802	13	742-743, 760-761
60090	12	725-726	6112	09	600-601	61803	13	742-743, 760-761
60091	12	725-726	6113	09	600-601	61804	13	742-743, 760-761
6010	12	727-728	6114	09	600-601	61805	13	742-743, 760-761
6011	12	727-728	6115	09	600-601	61809	13	742-743, 760-761
6012	12	727-728	6116	09	600-601	6181	13	742-743, 760-761
6013	12	727-728	61171	09	600-601	6182	13	742-743, 760-761
6014	12	727-728	61172	09	600-601	6183	13	742-743, 760-761
6018	12	727-728	61179	09	600-601	6184	13	742-743, 760-761
6019	12	727-728	61181	09	600-601	6185	13	742-743, 760-761
6020	12	729-730	61182	09	600-601	6186	13	742-743, 760-761
6021	12	729-730	61183	09	600-601	6187	13	742-743, 760-761
6022	12	729-730	61189	09	600-601	61881	13	742-743, 760-761
6023	12	729-730	6119	09	600-601			
6028	12	729-730	6120	09	600-601			
6029	12	729-730	6121	09	600-601			
6030	12	729-730	6140	13	742-743, 757-759			
6031	12	727-728	6141	13	742-743, 757-759			
6038	12	729-730	6142	13	742-743, 757-759			
6039	12	729-730	6143	13	742-743, 757-759			
6040	12	727-728	6144	13	742-743, 757-759			
60490	12	727-728	6145	13	742-743, 757-759			
60491	12	727-728	6146	13	742-743, 760-761			
60499	12	727-728	6147	13	742-743, 757-759			
605	12	727-728	6148	13	742-743, 757-759			
6060	12	729-730	6149	13	742-743, 757-759			
6061	12	729-730	6150	13	742-743, 757-759			
6068	12	729-730	6151	13	742-743, 757-759			
6069	12	729-730	6159	13	742-743, 757-759			
6070	12	729-730	6160	13	742-743, 757-759			
6071	12	727-728						
6072	12	727-728						
6073	12	729-730						
60781	12	727-728						
60782	12	729-730						
60783	12	729-730						
60784	12	729-730						
60785	12	729-730						
60789	12	729-730						
6079	12	729-730						
6080	12	727-728						
6081	12	729-730						
60820	12	729-730						
60821	12	729-730						
60822	12	729-730						

DX	MDC	MS-DRG		DX	MDC	MS-DRG		DX	MDC	MS-DRG
61882	13	742-743, 760-761		6218	13	742-743, 760-761		6248	13	742-743, 760-761
61883	13	742-743, 760-761		6219	13	742-743, 760-761		6249	13	742-743, 760-761
61884	13	742-743, 760-761		6220	13	742-743, 760-761		6250	13	742-743, 760-761
61889	13	742-743, 760-761		62210	13	742-743, 760-761		6251	13	742-743, 760-761
6189	13	742-743, 760-761		62211	13	742-743, 760-761		6252	13	742-743, 760-761
6190	13	742-743, 760-761		62212	13	742-743, 760-761		6253	13	742-743, 760-761
6191	06	393-395		6222	13	742-743, 760-761		6254	13	742-743, 760-761
6192	13	742-743, 760-761		6223	13	742-743, 760-761		6255	13	742-743, 760-761
6198	13	742-743, 760-761		6224	13	742-743, 760-761		6256	13	742-743, 760-761
6199	13	742-743, 760-761		6225	13	742-743, 760-761		62570	13	742-743, 760-761
6200	13	742-743, 760-761		6226	13	742-743, 760-761		62571	13	742-743, 757-759
6201	13	742-743, 760-761		6227	13	742-743, 760-761		62579	13	742-743, 760-761
6202	13	742-743, 760-761		6228	13	742-743, 760-761		6258	13	742-743, 760-761
6203	13	742-743, 760-761		6229	13	742-743, 760-761		6259	13	742-743, 760-761
6204	13	742-743, 760-761		6230	13	742-743, 760-761		6260	13	742-743, 760-761
6205	13	742-743, 760-761		6231	13	742-743, 760-761		6261	13	742-743, 760-761
6206	13	742-743, 760-761		6232	13	742-743, 760-761		6262	13	742-743, 760-761
6207	13	742-743, 760-761		6233	13	742-743, 760-761		6263	13	742-743, 760-761
6208	13	742-743, 760-761		6234	13	742-743, 760-761		6264	13	742-743, 760-761
6209	13	742-743, 760-761		6235	13	742-743, 760-761		6265	13	742-743, 760-761
6210	13	742-743, 760-761		6236	13	742-743, 760-761		6266	13	742-743, 760-761
6211	13	742-743, 760-761		6237	13	742-743, 760-761		6267	13	742-743, 760-761
6212	13	742-743, 760-761		6238	13	742-743, 760-761		6268	13	742-743, 760-761
62130	13	742-743, 760-761		6239	13	742-743, 760-761		6269	13	742-743, 760-761
62131	13	742-743, 760-761		62401	13	742-743, 760-761		6270	13	742-743, 760-761
62132	13	742-743, 760-761		62402	13	742-743, 760-761		6271	13	742-743, 760-761
62133	13	742-743, 760-761		62409	13	742-743, 760-761		6272	13	742-743, 760-761
62134 ◄	13	742-743, 760-761		6241	13	742-743, 760-761		6273	13	742-743, 760-761
62135 ◄	13	742-743, 760-761		6242	13	742-743, 760-761		6274	13	742-743, 760-761
6214	13	742-743, 760-761		6243	13	742-743, 760-761		6278	13	742-743, 760-761
6215	13	742-743, 760-761		6244	13	742-743, 760-761		6279	13	742-743, 760-761
6216	13	742-743, 760-761		6245	13	742-743, 760-761		6280	13	742-743, 760-761
6217	13	742-743, 760-761		6246	13	742-743, 760-761		6281	13	742-743, 760-761

DX	MDC	MS-DRG	DX	MDC	MS-DRG	DX	MDC	MS-DRG
6282	13	742-743, 760-761	63472	14	770,779	63692	14	770,779
6283	13	742-743, 760-761	63480	14	770,779	63700	14	770,779
6284	13	742-743, 760-761	63481	14	770,779	63701	14	770,779
6288	13	742-743, 760-761	63482	14	770,779	63702	14	770,779
6289	13	742-743, 760-761	63490	14	770,779	63710	14	770,779
6290	13	742-743, 760-761	63491	14	770,779	63711	14	770,779
6291	13	742-743, 760-761	63492	14	770,779	63712	14	770,779
62920	13	742-743, 760-761	63500	14	770,779	63720	14	770,779
62921	13	742-743, 760-761	63501	14	770,779	63721	14	770,779
62922	13	742-743, 760-761	63502	14	770,779	63722	14	770,779
62923	13	742-743, 760-761	63510	14	770,779	63730	14	770,779
62929	13	742-743, 760-761	63511	14	770,779	63731	14	770,779
62981	13	742-743, 760-761	63512	14	770,779	63732	14	770,779
62989	13	742-743, 760-761	63520	14	770,779	63740	14	770,779
6299	13	742-743, 760-761	63521	14	770,779	63741	14	770,779
630	14	781-782	63522	14	770,779	63742	14	770,779
631	14	781-782	63530	14	770,779	63750	14	770,779
632	14	770,779	63531	14	770,779	63751	14	770,779
63300	14	777	63532	14	770,779	63752	14	770,779
63301	14	777	63540	14	770,779	63760	14	770,779
63310	14	777	63541	14	770,779	63761	14	770,779
63311	14	777	63542	14	770,779	63762	14	770,779
63320	14	777	63550	14	770,779	63770	14	770,779
63321	14	777	63551	14	770,779	63771	14	770,779
63380	14	777	63552	14	770,779	63772	14	770,779
63381	14	777	63560	14	770,779	63780	14	770,779
63390	14	777	63561	14	770,779	63781	14	770,779
63391	14	777	63562	14	770,779	63782	14	770,779
63400	14	770,779	63570	14	770,779	63790	14	770,779
63401	14	770,779	63571	14	770,779	63791	14	770,779
63402	14	770,779	63572	14	770,779	63792	14	770,779
63410	14	770,779	63580	14	770,779	6380	14	770,779
63411	14	770,779	63581	14	770,779	6381	14	770,779
63412	14	770,779	63582	14	770,779	6382	14	770,779
63420	14	770,779	63590	14	770,779	6383	14	770,779
63421	14	770,779	63591	14	770,779	6384	14	770,779
63422	14	770,779	63592	14	770,779	6385	14	770,779
63430	14	770,779	63600	14	770,779	6386	14	770,779
63431	14	770,779	63601	14	770,779	6387	14	770,779
63432	14	770,779	63602	14	770,779	6388	14	770,779
63440	14	770,779	63610	14	770,779	6389	14	770,779
63441	14	770,779	63611	14	770,779	6390	14	769,776
63442	14	770,779	63612	14	770,779	6391	14	769,776
63450	14	770,779	63620	14	770,779	6392	14	769,776
63451	14	770,779	63621	14	770,779	6393	14	769,776
63452	14	770,779	63622	14	770,779	6394	14	769,776
63460	14	770,779	63630	14	770,779	6395	14	769,776
63461	14	770,779	63631	14	770,779	6396	14	769,776
63462	14	770,779	63632	14	770,779	6398	14	769,776
63470	14	770,779	63640	14	770,779	6399	14	769,776
63471	14	770,779	63641	14	770,779	64000	14	778
			63642	14	770,779	64001	14	765-768, 774-775
			63650	14	770,779			
			63651	14	770,779	64003	14	778
			63652	14	770,779	64080	14	778
			63660	14	770,779	64081	14	765-768, 774-775
			63661	14	770,779			
			63662	14	770,779	64083	14	778
			63670	14	770,779	64090	14	778
			63671	14	770,779	64091	14	765-768, 774-775
			63672	14	770,779			
			63680	14	770,779	64093	14	778
			63681	14	770,779	64100	14	998
			63682	14	770,779	64101	14	765-768,774
			63690	14	770,779	64103	14	781-782
			63691	14	770,779	64110	14	998

DX	MDC	MS-DRG
64111	14	765-768,774
64113	14	781-782
64120	14	998
64121	14	765-768,774
64123	14	781-782
64130	14	998
64131	14	765-768,774
64133	14	781
64180	14	998
64181	14	765-768,774
64183	14	781-782
64190	14	998
64191	14	765-768,774
64193	14	781-782
64200	14	998
64201	14	765-768,774
64202	14	765-768,774
64203	14	781
64204	14	769,776
64210	14	998
64211	14	765-768,774
64212	14	765-768,774
64213	14	781
64214	14	769,776
64220	14	998
64221	14	765-768,774
64222	14	765-768,774
64223	14	781
64224	14	769,776
64230	14	998
64231	14	765-768, 774-775
64232	14	765-768, 774-775
64233	14	781-782
64234	14	769,776
64240	14	998
64241	14	765-768,774
64242	14	765-768,774
64243	14	781
64244	14	769,776
64250	14	998
64251	14	765-768,774
64252	14	765-768,774
64253	14	781
64254	14	769,776
64260	14	998
64261	14	765-768,774
64262	14	765-768,774
64263	14	781
64264	14	769,776
64270	14	998
64271	14	765-768,774
64272	14	765-768,774
64273	14	781
64274	14	769,776
64290	14	998
64291	14	765-768,774
64292	14	765-768,774
64293	14	781
64294	14	769,776
64300	14	998
64301	14	765-768, 774-775
64303	14	781
64310	14	998

DX	MDC	MS-DRG
64311	14	765-768, 774-775
64313	14	781
64320	14	998
64321	14	765-768, 774-775
64323	14	781
64380	14	998
64381	14	765-768, 774-775
64383	14	781
64390	14	998
64391	14	765-768, 774-775
64393	14	781
64400	14	778
64403	14	778
64410	14	780
64413	14	780
64420	14	781-782
64421	14	765-768, 774-775
64510	14	998
64511	14	765-768, 774-775
64513	14	781-782
64520	14	998
64521	14	765-768, 774-775
64523	14	781-782
64600	14	765-768, 774-775
64601	14	765-768, 774-775
64603	14	781-782
64610	14	998
64611	14	765-768, 774-775
64612	14	765-768, 774-775
64613	14	781
64614	14	769,776
64620	14	998
64621	14	765-768, 774-775
64622	14	765-768, 774-775
64623	14	781
64624	14	769,776
64630	14	998
64631	14	765-768, 774-775
64633	14	781-782
64640	14	998
64641	14	765-768, 774-775
64642	14	765-768, 774-775
64643	14	781
64644	14	769,776
64650	14	998
64651	14	765-768, 774-775
64652	14	765-768, 774-775
64653	14	781-782

DX	MDC	MS-DRG
64654	14	769,776
64660	14	998
64661	14	765-768, 774-775
64662	14	765-768, 774-775
64663	14	781
64664	14	769,776
64670	14	998
64671	14	765-768, 774-775
64673	14	781
64680	14	998
64681	14	765-768, 774-775
64682	14	765-768, 774-775
64683	14	781
64684	14	769,776
64690	14	998
64691	14	765-768, 774-775
64693	14	781-782
64700	14	998
64701	14	765-768,774
64702	14	765-768,774
64703	14	781
64704	14	769,776
64710	14	998
64711	14	765-768,774
64712	14	765-768,774
64713	14	781
64714	14	769,776
64720	14	998
64721	14	765-768,774
64722	14	765-768,774
64723	14	781
64724	14	769,776
64730	14	998
64731	14	765-768,774
64732	14	765-768,774
64733	14	781
64734	14	769,776
64740	14	998
64741	14	765-768,774
64742	14	765-768,774
64743	14	781
64744	14	769,776
64750	14	998
64751	14	765-768,774
64752	14	765-768,774
64753	14	781
64754	14	769,776
64760	14	998
64761	14	765-768,774
64762	14	765-768,774
64763	14	781
64764	14	769,776
64780	14	998
64781	14	765-768,774
64782	14	765-768,774
64783	14	781
64784	14	769,776
64790	14	998
64791	14	765-768,774
64792	14	765-768,774

DX	MDC	MS-DRG	DX	MDC	MS-DRG	DX	MDC	MS-DRG
64793	14	781	64900	14	998	65131	14	765-768, 774-775
64794	14	769,776	64901	14	765-768, 774-775	65133	14	781-782
64800	14	998				65140	14	998
64801	14	765-768,774	64902	14	765-768, 774-775	65141	14	765-768, 774-775
64802	14	765-768,774	64903	14	781-782			
64803	14	781	64904	14	769,776	65143	14	781-782
64804	14	769,776	64910	14	998	65150	14	998
64810	14	998	64911	14	765-768, 774-775	65151	14	765-768, 774-775
64811	14	765-768, 774-775	64912	14	765-768, 774-775	65153	14	781-782
64812	14	765-768, 774-775				65160	14	998
64813	14	781	64913	14	781-782	65161	14	765-768, 774-775
64814	14	769,776	64914	14	769,776			
64820	14	998	64920	14	998	65163	14	781-782
64821	14	765-768, 774-775	64921	14	765-768, 774-775	65170	14	998
64822	14	765-768, 774-775	64922	14	765-768, 774-775	65171	14	765-768, 774-775
64823	14	781	64923	14	781-782	65173	14	781-782
64824	14	769,776	64924	14	769,776	65180	14	998
64830	14	998	64930	14	998	65181	14	765-768, 774-775
64831	14	765-768, 774-775	64931	14	765-768, 774-775	65183	14	781-782
64832	14	765-768, 774-775	64932	14	765-768, 774-775	65190	14	998
64833	14	781	64933	14	781-782	65191	14	765-768, 774-775
64834	14	769,776	64934	14	769,776			
64840	14	998	64940	14	998	65193	14	781-782
64841	14	765-768, 774-775	64941	14	765-768, 774-775	65200	14	998
64842	14	765-768, 774-775	64942	14	765-768, 774-775	65201	14	765-768, 774-775
64843	14	781	64943	14	781-782	65203	14	781-782
64844	14	769,776	64944	14	769,776	65210	14	998
64850	14	998	64950	14	998	65211	14	765-768, 774-775
64851	14	765-768,774	64951	14	765-768, 774-775			
64852	14	765-768,774				65213	14	781-782
64853	14	781	64953	14	781-782	65220	14	998
64854	14	769,776	64960	14	998	65221	14	765-768, 774-775
64860	14	998	64961	14	765-768, 774-775	65223	14	781-782
64861	14	765-768,774	64962	14	765-768, 774-775	65230	14	998
64862	14	765-768,774				65231	14	765-768, 774-775
64863	14	781	64963	14	781-782	65233	14	781-782
64864	14	769,776	64964	14	769,776	65240	14	998
64870	14	998	64970	14	998	65241	14	765-768, 774-775
64871	14	765-768, 774-775	64971	14	765-768, 774-775	65243	14	781-782
64872	14	765-768, 774-775	64973	14	781-782	65250	14	998
64873	14	781	650	14	765-768, 774-775	65251	14	765-768, 774-775
64874	14	769,776				65253	14	781-782
64880	14	998	65100	14	998	65260	14	998
64881	14	765-768, 774-775	65101	14	765-768, 774-775	65261	14	765-768, 774-775
64882	14	765-768, 774-775	65103	14	781-782	65263	14	781-782
64883	14	781	65110	14	998	65270	14	998
64884	14	769,776	65111	14	765-768, 774-775	65271	14	765-768, 774-775
64890	14	998	65113	14	781-782	65273	14	781-782
64891	14	765-768, 774-775	65120	14	998	65280	14	998
64892	14	765-768, 774-775	65121	14	765-768, 774-775	65281	14	765-768, 774-775
64893	14	781	65123	14	781-782	65283	14	781-782
64894	14	769,776	65130	14	998	65290	14	998
						65291	14	765-768, 774-775

DX	MDC	MS-DRG	DX	MDC	MS-DRG	DX	MDC	MS-DRG
65293	14	781-782	65440	14	998	65560	14	998
65300	14	998	65441	14	765-768,	65561	14	765-768,
65301	14	765-768,			774-775			774-775
		774-775	65442	14	765-768,	65563	14	781-782
65303	14	781-782			774-775	65570	14	998
65310	14	998	65443	14	781-782	65571	14	765-768,
65311	14	765-768,	65444	14	769,776			774-775
		774-775	65450	14	998	65573	14	781-782
65313	14	781-782	65451	14	765-768,	65580	14	998
65320	14	998			774-775	65581	14	765-768,
65321	14	765-768,	65452	14	765-768,			774-775
		774-775			774-775	65583	14	781-782
65323	14	781-782	65453	14	781-782	65590	14	998
65330	14	998	65454	14	769,776	65591	14	765-768,
65331	14	765-768,	65460	14	998			774-775
		774-775	65461	14	765-768,	65593	14	781-782
65333	14	781-782			774-775	65600	14	998
65340	14	998	65462	14	765-768,	65601	14	765-768,
65341	14	765-768,			774-775			774-775
		774-775	65463	14	781-782	65603	14	781-782
65343	14	781-782	65464	14	769,776	65610	14	998
65350	14	998	65470	14	998	65611	14	765-768,
65351	14	765-768,	65471	14	765-768,			774-775
		774-775			774-775	65613	14	781-782
65353	14	781-782	65472	14	765-768,	65620	14	998
65360	14	998			774-775	65621	14	765-768,
65361	14	765-768,	65473	14	781-782			774-775
		774-775	65474	14	769,776	65623	14	781-782
65363	14	781-782	65480	14	998	65630	14	765-768,
65370	14	998	65481	14	765-768,			774-775
65371	14	765-768,			774-775	65631	14	765-768,
		774-775	65482	14	765-768,			774-775
65373	14	781-782			774-775	65633	14	781-782
65380	14	998	65483	14	781-782	65640	14	765-768,
65381	14	765-768,	65484	14	769,776			774-775
		774-775	65490	14	998	65641	14	765-768,
65383	14	781-782	65491	14	765-768,			774-775
65390	14	998			774-775	65643	14	781-782
65391	14	765-768,	65492	14	765-768,	65650	14	998
		774-775			774-775	65651	14	765-768,
65393	14	781-782	65493	14	781-782			774-775
65400	14	998	65494	14	769,776	65653	14	781-782
65401	14	765-768,	65500	14	998	65660	14	998
		774-775	65501	14	765-768,	65661	14	765-768,
65402	14	765-768,			774-775			774-775
		774-775	65503	14	781-782	65663	14	781-782
65403	14	781-782	65510	14	998	65670	14	998
65404	14	769,776	65511	14	765-768,	65671	14	765-768,
65410	14	998			774-775			774-775
65411	14	765-768,	65513	14	781-782	65673	14	781-782
		774-775	65520	14	998	65680	14	998
65412	14	765-768,	65521	14	765-768,	65681	14	765-768,
		774-775			774-775			774-775
65413	14	781-782	65523	14	781-782	65683	14	781-782
65414	14	769,776	65530	14	998	65690	14	998
65420	14	998	65531	14	765-768,	65691	14	765-768,
65421	14	765-768,			774-775			774-775
		774-775	65533	14	781-782	65693	14	781-782
65423	14	781-782	65540	14	998	65700	14	998
65430	14	998	65541	14	765-768,	65701	14	765-768,
65431	14	765-768,			774-775			774-775
		774-775	65543	14	781-782	65703	14	781-782
65432	14	765-768,	65550	14	998	65800	14	998
		774-775	65551	14	765-768,	65801	14	765-768,
65433	14	781-782			774-775			774-775
65434	14	769,776	65553	14	781-782	65803	14	781-782

DX	MDC	MS-DRG	DX	MDC	MS-DRG	DX	MDC	MS-DRG
65810	14	765-768, 774-775	65980	14	765-768, 774-775	66110	14	765-768, 774-775
65811	14	765-768, 774-775	65981	14	765-768, 774-775	66111	14	765-768, 774-775
65813	14	781-782	65983	14	781-782	66113	14	781-782
65820	14	765-768, 774-775	65990	14	765-768, 774-775	66120	14	765-768, 774-775
65821	14	765-768, 774-775	65991	14	765-768, 774-775	66121	14	765-768, 774-775
65823	14	781-782	65993	14	781-782	66123	14	781-782
65830	14	765-768, 774-775	66000	14	765-768, 774-775	66130	14	765-768, 774-775
65831	14	765-768, 774-775	66001	14	765-768, 774-775	66131	14	765-768, 774-775
65833	14	781-782	66003	14	781-782	66133	14	781-782
65840	14	765-768, 774-775	66010	14	765-768, 774-775	66140	14	765-768, 774-775
65841	14	765-768, 774-775	66011	14	765-768, 774-775	66141	14	765-768, 774-775
65843	14	781-782	66013	14	781-782	66143	14	781-782
65880	14	998	66020	14	765-768, 774-775	66190	14	765-768, 774-775
65881	14	765-768, 774-775	66021	14	765-768, 774-775	66191	14	765-768, 774-775
65883	14	781-782	66023	14	781-782	66193	14	781-782
65890	14	998	66030	14	765-768, 774-775	66200	14	765-768, 774-775
65891	14	765-768, 774-775	66031	14	765-768, 774-775	66201	14	765-768, 774-775
65893	14	781-782	66033	14	781-782	66203	14	781-782
65900	14	765-768, 774-775	66040	14	765-768, 774-775	66210	14	765-768, 774-775
65901	14	765-768, 774-775	66041	14	765-768, 774-775	66211	14	765-768, 774-775
65903	14	781-782	66043	14	781-782	66213	14	781-782
65910	14	765-768, 774-775	66050	14	765-768, 774-775	66220	14	765-768, 774-775
65911	14	765-768, 774-775	66051	14	765-768, 774-775	66221	14	765-768, 774-775
65913	14	781-782	66053	14	781-782	66223	14	781-782
65920	14	765-768, 774-775	66060	14	765-768, 774-775	66230	14	765-768, 774-775
65921	14	765-768,774	66061	14	765-768, 774-775	66231	14	765-768, 774-775
65923	14	781-782	66063	14	781-782	66233	14	781-782
65930	14	765-768, 774-775	66070	14	765-768, 774-775	66300	14	765-768, 774-775
65931	14	765-768,774	66071	14	765-768, 774-775	66301	14	765-768, 774-775
65933	14	781-782	66073	14	781-782	66303	14	781-782
65940	14	998	66080	14	765-768, 774-775	66310	14	765-768, 774-775
65941	14	765-768, 774-775	66081	14	765-768, 774-775	66311	14	765-768, 774-775
65943	14	781-782	66083	14	781-782	66313	14	781-782
65950	14	765-768, 774-775	66090	14	765-768, 774-775	66320	14	765-768, 774-775
65951	14	765-768, 774-775	66091	14	765-768, 774-775	66321	14	765-768, 774-775
65953	14	781-782	66093	14	781-782	66323	14	781-782
65960	14	765-768, 774-775	66100	14	765-768, 774-775	66330	14	765-768, 774-775
65961	14	765-768, 774-775	66101	14	765-768, 774-775	66331	14	765-768, 774-775
65963	14	781-782	66103	14	781-782	66333	14	781-782
65970	14	765-768, 774-775						
65971	14	765-768, 774-775						
65973	14	781-782						

PART VI, MS-DRG, APPENDIX B

DX	MDC	MS-DRG
66340	14	765-768, 774-775
66341	14	765-768, 774-775
66343	14	781-782
66350	14	765-768, 774-775
66351	14	765-768, 774-775
66353	14	781-782
66360	14	765-768, 774-775
66361	14	765-768, 774-775
66363	14	781-782
66380	14	765-768, 774-775
66381	14	765-768, 774-775
66383	14	781-782
66390	14	765-768, 774-775
66391	14	765-768, 774-775
66393	14	781-782
66400	14	765-768, 774-775
66401	14	765-768, 774-775
66404	14	769,776
66410	14	765-768, 774-775
66411	14	765-768, 774-775
66414	14	769,776
66420	14	765-768, 774-775
66421	14	765-768, 774-775
66424	14	769,776
66430	14	765-768, 774-775
66431	14	765-768, 774-775
66434	14	769,776
66440	14	765-768, 774-775
66441	14	765-768, 774-775
66444	14	769,776
66450	14	765-768, 774-775
66451	14	765-768, 774-775
66454	14	769,776
66460	14	765-768, 774-775
66461	14	765-768, 774-775
66464	14	769,776
66480	14	765-768, 774-775
66481	14	765-768, 774-775
66484	14	769,776

DX	MDC	MS-DRG
66490	14	765-768, 774-775
66491	14	765-768, 774-775
66494	14	769,776
66500	14	765-768, 774-775
66501	14	765-768, 774-775
66503	14	781-782
66510	14	765-768, 774-775
66511	14	765-768, 774-775
66520	14	765-768, 774-775
66522	14	765-768, 774-775
66524	14	769,776
66530	14	765-768, 774-775
66531	14	765-768, 774-775
66534	14	769,776
66540	14	765-768, 774-775
66541	14	765-768, 774-775
66544	14	769,776
66550	14	765-768, 774-775
66551	14	765-768, 774-775
66554	14	769,776
66560	14	765-768, 774-775
66561	14	765-768, 774-775
66564	14	769,776
66570	14	765-768, 774-775
66571	14	765-768, 774-775
66572	14	765-768, 774-775
66574	14	769,776
66580	14	765-768, 774-775
66581	14	765-768, 774-775
66582	14	765-768, 774-775
66583	14	781-782
66584	14	769,776
66590	14	765-768, 774-775
66591	14	765-768, 774-775
66592	14	765-768, 774-775
66593	14	781-782
66594	14	769,776
66600	14	998
66602	14	765-768,774
66604	14	769,776
66610	14	998

DX	MDC	MS-DRG
66612	14	765-768,774
66614	14	769,776
66620	14	998
66622	14	765-768,774
66624	14	769,776
66630	14	998
66632	14	765-768,774
66634	14	769,776
66700	14	998
66702	14	765-768,774
66704	14	769,776
66710	14	998
66712	14	765-768,774
66714	14	769,776
66800	14	765-768, 774-775
66801	14	765-768,774
66802	14	765-768,774
66803	14	781-782
66804	14	769,776
66810	14	765-768, 774-775
66811	14	765-768,774
66812	14	765-768,774
66813	14	781-782
66814	14	769,776
66820	14	765-768, 774-775
66821	14	765-768,774
66822	14	765-768,774
66823	14	781-782
66824	14	769,776
66880	14	765-768, 774-775
66881	14	765-768,774
66882	14	765-768,774
66883	14	781-782
66884	14	769,776
66890	14	765-768, 774-775
66891	14	765-768,774
66892	14	765-768,774
66893	14	781-782
66894	14	769,776
66900	14	765-768, 774-775
66901	14	765-768, 774-775
66902	14	765-768, 774-775
66903	14	781-782
66904	14	769,776
66910	14	765-768, 774-775
66911	14	765-768,774
66912	14	765-768,774
66913	14	781-782
66914	14	769,776
66920	14	765-768, 774-775
66921	14	765-768, 774-775
66922	14	765-768, 774-775
66923	14	781-782
66924	14	769,776

DX	MDC	MS-DRG	DX	MDC	MS-DRG	DX	MDC	MS-DRG
66930	14	765-768, 774-775	67111	14	765-768, 774-775	67400	14	998
66932	14	765-768,774	67112	14	765-768, 774-775	67401	14	765-768,774
66934	14	769,776				67402	14	765-768,774
66940	14	765-768, 774-775	67113	14	781-782	67403	14	781-782
			67114	14	769,776	67404	14	769,776
66941	14	765-768,774	67120	14	998	67410	14	998
66942	14	765-768,774	67121	14	765-768, 774-775	67412	14	765-768,774
66943	14	781-782				67414	14	769,776
66944	14	769,776	67122	14	765-768, 774-775	67420	14	998
66950	14	765-768, 774-775				67422	14	765-768,774
			67123	14	781-782	67424	14	769,776
66951	14	765-768, 774-775	67124	14	769,776	67430	14	998
			67130	14	998	67432	14	765-768,774
66960	14	765-768, 774-775	67131	14	765-768,774	67434	14	769,776
			67133	14	781-782	67440	14	998
66961	14	765-768, 774-775	67140	14	998	67442	14	765-768, 774-775
			67142	14	765-768,774			
66970	14	765-768, 774-775	67144	14	769,776	67444	14	769,776
			67150	14	998	67450	14	998
66971	14	765-768, 774-775	67151	14	765-768,774	67451	14	765-768,774
			67152	14	765-768,774	67452	14	765-768,774
66980	14	765-768, 774-775	67153	14	781-782	67453	14	781-782
			67154	14	769,776	67454	14	769,776
66981	14	765-768, 774-775	67180	14	998	67480	14	998
			67181	14	765-768, 774-775	67482	14	765-768,774
66982	14	765-768, 774-775				67484	14	769,776
			67182	14	765-768, 774-775	67490	14	998
66983	14	781-782				67492	14	765-768, 774-775
66984	14	769,776	67183	14	781-782			
66990	14	765-768, 774-775	67184	14	769,776	67494	14	769,776
			67190	14	998	67500	14	998
66991	14	765-768, 774-775	67191	14	765-768, 774-775	67501	14	765-768,774
						67502	14	765-768,774
66992	14	765-768, 774-775	67192	14	765-768, 774-775	67503	14	781-782
						67504	14	769,776
66993	14	781-782	67193	14	781-782	67510	14	998
66994	14	769,776	67194	14	769,776	67511	14	765-768,774
67000	14	998	67200	14	998	67512	14	765-768,774
67002	14	765-768,774	67202	14	765-768,774	67513	14	781-782
67004	14	769,776	67204	14	769,776	67514	14	769,776
67010	14	998 ◄	67300	14	998	67520	14	998
67012	14	765-768, 774 ◄	67301	14	765-768,774	67521	14	765-768,774
			67302	14	765-768,774	67522	14	765-768,774
67014	14	769,776 ◄	67303	14	781-782	67523	14	781-782
67020	14	998 ◄	67304	14	769,776	67524	14	769,776
67022	14	765-768, 774 ◄	67310	14	998	67580	14	998
			67311	14	765-768,774	67581	14	765-768, 774-775
67024	14	769,776 ◄	67312	14	765-768,774			
67030	14	998 ◄	67313	14	781-782	67582	14	765-768, 774-775
67032	14	765-768, 774 ◄	67314	14	769,776			
			67320	14	998	67583	14	781-782
67034	14	769,776 ◄	67321	14	765-768,774	67584	14	769,776
67080	14	998 ◄	67322	14	765-768,774	67590	14	998
67082	14	765-768, 774 ◄	67323	14	781-782	67591	14	765-768, 774-775
			67324	14	769,776			
67084	14	769,776 ◄	67330	14	998	67592	14	765-768, 774-775
67100	14	998	67331	14	765-768,774			
67101	14	765-768, 774-775	67332	14	765-768,774	67593	14	781-782
			67333	14	781-782	67594	14	769,776
67102	14	765-768, 774-775	67334	14	769,776	67600	14	998
			67380	14	998	67601	14	765-768, 774-775
67103	14	781-782	67381	14	765-768,774			
67104	14	769,776	67382	14	765-768,774	67602	14	765-768, 774-775
67110	14	998	67383	14	781-782	67603	14	781-782
			67384	14	769,776	67604	14	769,776

DX	MDC	MS-DRG
67610	14	998
67611	14	765-768, 774-775
67612	14	765-768, 774-775
67613	14	781-782
67614	14	769,776
67620	14	998
67621	14	765-768, 774-775
67622	14	765-768, 774-775
67623	14	781-782
67624	14	769,776
67630	14	998
67631	14	765-768, 774-775
67632	14	765-768, 774-775
67633	14	781-782
67634	14	769,776
67640	14	998
67641	14	765-768, 774-775
67642	14	765-768, 774-775
67643	14	781-782
67644	14	769,776
67650	14	998
67651	14	765-768, 774-775
67652	14	765-768, 774-775
67653	14	781-782
67654	14	769,776
67660	14	998
67661	14	765-768, 774-775
67662	14	765-768, 774-775
67663	14	781-782
67664	14	769,776
67680	14	998
67681	14	765-768, 774-775
67682	14	765-768, 774-775
67683	14	781-782
67684	14	769,776
67690	14	998
67691	14	765-768, 774-775
67692	14	765-768, 774-775
67693	14	781-782
67694	14	769,776
677	14	998
67800	14	998
67801	14	765-768, 774-775
67803	14	781-782
67810	14	998
67811	14	765-768, 774-775
67813	14	781-782

DX	MDC	MS-DRG
67900	14	765-768, 774-775
67901	14	765-768,774
67902	14	765-768,774
67903	14	781-782
67904	14	769,776
67910	14	998
67911	14	765-768, 774-775
67912	14	765-768, 774-775
67913	14	781-782
67914	14	769,776
6800	09	602-603
6801	09	602-603
6802	09	602-603
6803	09	602-603
6804	09	602-603
6805	09	602-603
6806	09	602-603
6807	09	602-603
6808	09	602-603
6809	09	602-603
68100	09	573-575, 602-603
68101	09	573-575, 602-603
68102	09	573-575, 602-603
68110	09	573-575, 602-603
68111	09	573-575, 602-603
6819	09	573-575, 757-759
6820	09	573-575, 602-603
6821	09	573-575, 602-603
6822	09	573-575, 602-603
6823	09	573-575, 602-603
6824	09	573-575, 602-603
6825	09	573-575, 602-603
6826	09	573-575, 602-603
6827	09	573-575, 602-603
6828	09	573-575, 602-603
6829	09	573-575, 602-603
683	16	814-816
684	09	602-603
6850	09	602-603
6851	09	602-603
68600	09	602-603
68601	09	602-603
68609	09	602-603
6861	09	602-603
6868	09	602-603
6869	09	602-603
69010	09	606-607

DX	MDC	MS-DRG
69011	09	606-607
69012	09	606-607
69018	09	606-607
6908	09	606-607
6910	09	606-607
6918	09	606-607
6920	09	606-607
6921	09	606-607
6922	09	606-607
6923	09	606-607
6924	09	606-607
6925	09	606-607
6926	09	606-607
69270	09	606-607
69271	09	606-607
69272	09	606-607
69273	09	606-607
69274	09	606-607
69275	09	606-607
69276	09	606-607
69277	09	606-607
69279	09	606-607
69281	09	606-607
69282	09	606-607
69283	09	606-607
69284	MDC	606-607
69289	09	606-607
6929	09	606-607
6930	09	606-607
6931	09	606-607
6938	09	606-607
6939	09	606-607
6940	09	606-607
6941	09	606-607
6942	09	606-607
6943	09	606-607
6944	09	595-596
6945	09	595-596
69460	09	595-596
69461	02	124-125
6948	09	595-596
6949	09	595-596
6950	09	595-596
69510	09	595-596
69511	09	595-596
69512	09	595-596
69513	09	595-596
69514	09	595-596
69515	09	595-596
69519	09	595-596
6952	09	595-596
6953	09	606-607
6954	09	595-596
69550	09	606-607
69551	09	606-607
69552	09	606-607
69553	09	606-607
69554	09	606-607
69555	09	606-607
69556	09	606-607
69557	09	606-607
69558	09	606-607
69559	09	606-607
69581	09	595-596
69589	09	606-607
6959	09	606-607

DX	MDC	MS-DRG	DX	MDC	MS-DRG	DX	MDC	MS-DRG
6960	08	545-547	70703	09	573-575, 592-594	7109	08	545-547
6961	09	595-596				71100	08	548-550
6962	09	595-596	70704	09	573-575, 592-594	71101	08	548-550
6963	09	606-607				71102	08	548-550
6964	09	606-607	70705	09	573-575, 592-594	71103	08	548-550
6965	09	606-607				71104	08	548-550
6968	09	606-607	70706	09	573-575, 592-594	71105	08	548-550
6970	09	606-607				71106	08	485-487, 548-550
6971	09	606-607	70707	09	573-575, 592-594			
6978	09	606-607				71107	08	548-550
6979	09	606-607	70709	09	573-575, 592-594	71108	08	548-550
6980	09	606-607				71109	08	548-550
6981	12	729-730	70710	09	573-575, 592-594	71110	08	545-547
6981	13	742-743, 602-603				71111	08	545-547
			70711	09	573-575, 592-594	71112	08	545-547
6982	09	606-607				71113	08	545-547
6983	09	606-607	70712	09	573-575, 592-594	71114	08	545-547
6984	09	606-607				71115	08	545-547
6988	09	606-607	70713	09	573-575, 592-594	71116	08	545-547
6989	09	606-607				71117	08	545-547
700	09	606-607	70714	09	573-575, 592-594	71118	08	545-547
7010	09	606-607				71119	08	545-547
7011	09	606-607	70715	09	573-575, 592-594	71120	08	545-547
7012	09	606-607				71121	08	545-547
7013	09	606-607	70719	09	573-575, 592-594	71122	08	545-547
7014	09	606-607				71123	08	545-547
7015	09	606-607	70720	09	573-575, 592-594	71124	08	545-547
7018	09	606-607				71125	08	545-547
7019	09	606-607	70721	09	573-575, 592-594	71126	08	545-547
7020	09	606-607				71127	08	545-547
70211	09	606-607	70722	09	573-575, 592-594	71128	08	545-547
70219	09	606-607				71129	08	545-547
7028	09	606-607	70723	09	573-575, 592-594	71130	08	553-554
7030	09	606-607				71131	08	553-554
7038	09	606-607	70724	09	573-575, 592-594	71132	08	553-554
7039	09	606-607				71133	08	553-554
70400	09	606-607	70725	09	573-575, 592-594	71134	08	553-554
70401	09	606-607				71135	08	553-554
70402	09	606-607	7078	09	573-575, 592-594	71136	08	553-554
70409	09	606-607				71137	08	553-554
7041	09	606-607	7079	09	573-575, 592-594	71138	08	553-554
7042	09	606-607				71139	08	553-554
7043	09	606-607	7080	09	606-607	71140	08	548-550
7048	09	606-607	7081	09	606-607	71141	08	548-550
7049	09	606-607	7082	09	606-607	71142	08	548-550
7050	09	606-607	7083	09	606-607	71143	08	548-550
7051	09	606-607	7084	09	606-607	71144	08	548-550
70521	09	606-607	7085	09	606-607	71145	08	548-550
70522	09	606-607	7088	09	606-607	71146	08	548-550
70581	09	606-607	7089	09	606-607	71147	08	548-550
70582	09	606-607	70900	09	606-607	71148	08	548-550
70583	09	606-607	70901	09	606-607	71149	08	548-550
70589	09	606-607	70909	09	606-607	71150	08	553-554
7059	09	606-607	7091	09	606-607	71151	08	553-554
7060	09	606-607	7092	09	606-607	71152	08	553-554
7061	09	606-607	7093	09	606-607	71153	08	553-554
7062	09	606-607	7094	09	606-607	71154	08	553-554
7063	09	606-607	7098	09	606-607	71155	08	553-554
7068	09	606-607	7099	09	606-607	71156	08	553-554
7069	09	606-607	7100	08	545-547	71157	08	553-554
70700	09	573-575, 592-594	7101	08	545-547	71158	08	553-554
			7102	08	545-547	71159	08	553-554
70701	09	573-575, 592-594	7103	08	545-547	71160	08	548-550
			7104	08	545-547	71161	08	548-550
70702	09	573-575, 592-594	7105	08	545-547	71162	08	548-550
			7108	08	545-547	71163	08	548-550

DX	MDC	MS-DRG	DX	MDC	MS-DRG	DX	MDC	MS-DRG
71164	08	548-550	71280	08	553-554	71535	08	553-554
71165	08	548-550	71281	08	553-554	71536	08	553-554
71166	08	548-550	71282	08	553-554	71537	08	553-554
71167	08	548-550	71283	08	553-554	71538	08	553-554
71168	08	548-550	71284	08	553-554	71580	08	553-554
71169	08	548-550	71285	08	553-554	71589	08	553-554
71170	08	548-550	71286	08	553-554	71590	08	553-554
71171	08	548-550	71287	08	553-554	71591	08	553-554
71172	08	548-550	71288	08	553-554	71592	08	553-554
71173	08	548-550	71289	08	553-554	71593	08	553-554
71174	08	548-550	71290	08	553-554	71594	08	553-554
71175	08	548-550	71291	08	553-554	71595	08	553-554
71176	08	548-550	71292	08	553-554	71596	08	553-554
71177	08	548-550	71293	08	553-554	71597	08	553-554
71178	08	548-550	71294	08	553-554	71598	08	553-554
71179	08	548-550	71295	08	553-554	71600	08	553-554
71180	08	548-550	71296	08	553-554	71601	08	553-554
71181	08	548-550	71297	08	553-554	71602	08	553-554
71182	08	548-550	71298	08	553-554	71603	08	553-554
71183	08	548-550	71299	08	553-554	71604	08	553-554
71184	08	548-550	7130	08	553-554	71605	08	553-554
71185	08	548-550	7131	08	553-554	71606	08	553-554
71186	08	548-550	7132	08	553-554	71607	08	553-554
71187	08	548-550	7133	08	553-554	71608	08	553-554
71188	08	548-550	7134	08	553-554	71609	08	553-554
71189	08	548-550	7135	08	553-554	71610	08	553-554
71190	08	548-550	7136	08	553-554	71611	08	553-554
71191	08	548-550	7137	08	553-554	71612	08	553-554
71192	08	548-550	7138	08	553-554	71613	08	553-554
71193	08	548-550	7140	08	545-547	71614	08	553-554
71194	08	548-550	7141	08	545-547	71615	08	553-554
71195	08	548-550	7142	08	545-547	71616	08	553-554
71196	08	548-550	71430	08	545-547	71617	08	553-554
71197	08	548-550	71431	08	545-547	71618	08	553-554
71198	08	548-550	71432	08	545-547	71619	08	553-554
71199	08	548-550	71433	08	545-547	71620	08	553-554
71210	08	553-554	7144	08	553-554	71621	08	553-554
71211	08	553-554	71481	04	196-198	71622	08	553-554
71212	08	553-554	71489	08	545-547	71623	08	553-554
71213	08	553-554	7149	08	553-554	71624	08	553-554
71214	08	553-554	71500	08	553-554	71625	08	553-554
71215	08	553-554	71504	08	553-554	71626	08	553-554
71216	08	553-554	71509	08	553-554	71627	08	553-554
71217	08	553-554	71510	08	553-554	71628	08	553-554
71218	08	553-554	71511	08	553-554	71629	08	553-554
71219	08	553-554	71512	08	553-554	71630	08	553-554
71220	08	553-554	71513	08	553-554	71631	08	553-554
71221	08	553-554	71514	08	553-554	71632	08	553-554
71222	08	553-554	71515	08	553-554	71633	08	553-554
71223	08	553-554	71516	08	553-554	71634	08	553-554
71224	08	553-554	71517	08	553-554	71635	08	553-554
71225	08	553-554	71518	08	553-554	71636	08	553-554
71226	08	553-554	71520	08	553-554	71637	08	553-554
71227	08	553-554	71521	08	553-554	71638	08	553-554
71228	08	553-554	71522	08	553-554	71639	08	553-554
71229	08	553-554	71523	08	553-554	71640	08	553-554
71230	08	553-554	71524	08	553-554	71641	08	553-554
71231	08	553-554	71525	08	553-554	71642	08	553-554
71232	08	553-554	71526	08	553-554	71643	08	553-554
71233	08	553-554	71527	08	553-554	71644	08	553-554
71234	08	553-554	71528	08	553-554	71645	08	553-554
71235	08	553-554	71530	08	553-554	71646	08	553-554
71236	08	553-554	71531	08	553-554	71647	08	553-554
71237	08	553-554	71532	08	553-554	71648	08	553-554
71238	08	553-554	71533	08	553-554	71649	08	553-554
71239	08	553-554	71534	08	553-554	71650	08	553-554

DX	MDC	MS-DRG	DX	MDC	MS-DRG	DX	MDC	MS-DRG
71651	08	553-554	71810	08	564-566	71885	08	564-566
71652	08	553-554	71811	08	564-566	71886	08	564-566
71653	08	553-554	71812	08	564-566	71887	08	564-566
71654	08	553-554	71813	08	564-566	71888	08	564-566
71655	08	553-554	71814	08	564-566	71889	08	564-566
71656	08	553-554	71815	08	564-566	71890	08	564-566
71657	08	553-554	71817	08	564-566	71891	08	564-566
71658	08	553-554	71818	08	564-566	71892	08	564-566
71659	08	553-554	71819	08	564-566	71893	08	564-566
71660	08	553-554	71820	08	562-563	71894	08	564-566
71661	08	553-554	71821	08	562-563	71895	08	564-566
71662	08	553-554	71822	08	562-563	71897	08	564-566
71663	08	553-554	71823	08	562-563	71898	08	564-566
71664	08	553-554	71824	08	562-563	71899	08	564-566
71665	08	553-554	71825	08	564-566	71900	08	564-566
71666	08	553-554	71826	08	562-563	71901	08	564-566
71667	08	553-554	71827	08	562-563	71902	08	564-566
71668	08	553-554	71828	08	564-566	71903	08	564-566
71680	08	553-554	71829	08	564-566	71904	08	564-566
71681	08	553-554	71830	08	564-566	71905	08	564-566
71682	08	553-554	71831	08	562-563	71906	08	564-566
71683	08	553-554	71832	08	562-563	71907	08	564-566
71684	08	553-554	71833	08	562-563	71908	08	564-566
71685	08	553-554	71834	08	562-563	71909	08	564-566
71686	08	553-554	71835	08	564-566	71910	08	553-554
71687	08	553-554	71836	08	562-563	71911	08	553-554
71688	08	553-554	71837	08	562-563	71912	08	553-554
71689	08	553-554	71838	08	564-566	71913	08	553-554
71690	08	553-554	71839	08	564-566	71914	08	553-554
71691	08	553-554	71840	08	564-566	71915	08	553-554
71692	08	553-554	71841	08	564-566	71916	08	553-554
71693	08	553-554	71842	08	564-566	71917	08	553-554
71694	08	553-554	71843	08	564-566	71918	08	553-554
71695	08	553-554	71844	08	564-566	71919	08	553-554
71696	08	553-554	71845	08	564-566	71920	08	553-554
71697	08	553-554	71846	08	564-566	71921	08	553-554
71698	08	553-554	71847	08	564-566	71922	08	553-554
71699	08	553-554	71848	08	564-566	71923	08	553-554
7170	08	562-563	71849	08	564-566	71924	08	553-554
7171	08	562-563	71850	08	553-554	71925	08	553-554
7172	08	562-563	71851	08	553-554	71926	08	553-554
7173	08	562-563	71852	08	553-554	71927	08	553-554
71740	08	562-563	71853	08	553-554	71928	08	553-554
71741	08	562-563	71854	08	553-554	71929	08	553-554
71742	08	562-563	71855	08	553-554	71930	08	553-554
71743	08	562-563	71856	08	553-554	71931	08	553-554
71749	08	562-563	71857	08	553-554	71932	08	553-554
7175	08	562-563	71858	08	553-554	71933	08	553-554
7176	08	564-566	71859	08	553-554	71934	08	553-554
7177	08	562-563	71860	08	564-566	71935	08	553-554
71781	08	562-563	71865	08	564-566	71936	08	553-554
71782	08	562-563	71870	08	564-566	71937	08	553-554
71783	08	562-563	71871	08	564-566	71938	08	553-554
71784	08	562-563	71872	08	564-566	71939	08	553-554
71785	08	562-563	71873	08	564-566	71940	08	555-556
71789	08	562-563	71874	08	564-566	71941	08	555-556
7179	08	562-563	71875	08	564-566	71942	08	555-556
71800	08	564-566	71876	08	564-566	71943	08	555-556
71801	08	562-563	71877	08	564-566	71944	08	555-556
71802	08	562-563	71878	08	564-566	71945	08	555-556
71803	08	562-563	71879	08	564-566	71946	08	555-556
71804	08	562-563	71880	08	564-566	71947	08	555-556
71805	08	564-566	71881	08	564-566	71948	08	555-556
71807	08	562-563	71882	08	564-566	71949	08	555-556
71808	08	564-566	71883	08	564-566	71950	08	555-556
71809	08	564-566	71884	08	564-566	71951	08	555-556

DX	MDC	MS-DRG
71952	08	555-556
71953	08	555-556
71954	08	555-556
71955	08	555-556
71956	08	555-556
71957	08	555-556
71958	08	555-556
71959	08	555-556
71960	08	555-556
71961	08	555-556
71962	08	555-556
71963	08	555-556
71964	08	555-556
71965	08	555-556
71966	08	555-556
71967	08	555-556
71968	08	555-556
71969	08	555-556
7197	08	555-556
71980	08	555-556
71981	08	555-556
71982	08	555-556
71983	08	555-556
71984	08	555-556
71985	08	555-556
71986	08	555-556
71987	08	555-556
71988	08	555-556
71989	08	555-556
71990	08	555-556
71991	08	555-556
71992	08	555-556
71993	08	555-556
71994	08	555-556
71995	08	555-556
71996	08	555-556
71997	08	555-556
71998	08	555-556
71999	08	555-556
7200	08	545-547
7201	08	551-552
7202	08	551-552
72081	08	551-552
72089	08	551-552
7209	08	551-552
7210	08	551-552
7211	08	551-552
7212	08	551-552
7213	08	551-552
72141	08	551-552
72142	08	551-552
7215	08	551-552
7216	08	551-552
7217	08	551-552
7218	08	551-552
72190	08	551-552
72191	08	551-552
7220	08	551-552
72210	08	551-552
72211	08	551-552
7222	08	551-552
72230	08	551-552
72231	08	551-552
72232	08	551-552
72239	08	551-552
7224	08	551-552

DX	MDC	MS-DRG
72251	08	551-552
72252	08	551-552
7226	08	551-552
72270	08	551-552
72271	08	551-552
72272	08	551-552
72273	08	551-552
72280	08	551-552
72281	08	551-552
72282	08	551-552
72283	08	551-552
72290	08	551-552
72291	08	551-552
72292	08	551-552
72293	08	551-552
7230	08	551-552
7231	08	551-552
7232	01	073-074
7233	01	073-074
7234	01	073-074
7235	08	551-552
7236	09	606-607
7237	08	551-552
7238	08	551-552
7239	08	551-552
72400	08	551-552
72401	08	551-552
72402	08	551-552
72409	08	551-552
7241	08	551-552
7242	08	551-552
7243	08	551-552
7244	08	551-552
7245	08	551-552
7246	08	551-552
72470	08	551-552
72471	08	551-552
72479	08	551-552
7248	08	551-552
7249	08	551-552
725	08	545-547
7260	08	557-558
72610	08	557-558
72611	08	557-558
72612	08	557-558
72619	08	557-558
7262	08	557-558
72630	08	557-558
72631	08	557-558
72632	08	557-558
72633	08	557-558
72639	08	557-558
7264	08	557-558
7265	08	557-558
72660	08	557-558
72661	08	557-558
72662	08	557-558
72663	08	557-558
72664	08	557-558
72665	08	557-558
72669	08	557-558
72670	08	557-558
72671	08	557-558
72672	08	557-558
72673	08	564-566
72679	08	557-558

DX	MDC	MS-DRG
7268	08	557-558
72690	08	557-558
72691	08	557-558
72700	08	557-558
72701	08	557-558
72702	08	564-566
72703	08	557-558
72704	08	557-558
72705	08	557-558
72706	08	557-558
72709	08	557-558
7271	08	564-566
7272	08	557-558
7273	08	557-558
72740	08	557-558
72741	08	557-558
72742	08	557-558
72743	08	557-558
72749	08	557-558
72750	08	557-558
72751	08	557-558
72759	08	557-558
72760	08	557-558
72761	08	557-558
72762	08	557-558
72763	08	557-558
72764	08	557-558
72765	08	557-558
72766	08	557-558
72767	08	557-558
72768	08	557-558
72769	08	557-558
72781	08	557-558
72782	08	557-558
72783	08	557-558
72789	08	557-558
7279	08	557-558
7280	08	557-558
72810	08	557-558
72811	08	557-558
72812	08	557-558
72813	08	557-558
72819	08	557-558
7282	08	557-558
7283	08	557-558
7284	08	557-558
7285	08	557-558
7286	08	557-558
72871	08	557-558
72879	08	557-558
72881	08	557-558
72882	08	557-558
72883	08	557-558
72884	08	557-558
72885	08	555-556
72886	08	557-558
72887	08	555-556
72888	08	557-558
72889	08	557-558
7289	08	557-558
7290	08	555-556
7291	08	555-556
7292	01	073-074
72930	09	606-607
72931	09	606-607
72939	09	606-607

DX	MDC	MS-DRG	DX	MDC	MS-DRG	DX	MDC	MS-DRG
7294	08	557-558	73076	08	564-566	7335	08	553-554
7295	08	555-556	73077	08	564-566	7336	04	205-206
7296	08	564-566	73078	08	564-566	7337	08	564-566
72971	08	557-558	73079	08	564-566	73381	08	564-566
72972	08	557-558	73080	08	539-541	73382	08	564-566
72973	08	557-558	73081	08	539-541	73390	08	564-566
72979	08	557-558	73082	08	539-541	73391	08	564-566
72981	08	555-556	73083	08	539-541	73392	08	553-554
72982	08	555-556	73084	08	539-541	73393	08	542-544
72989	08	555-556	73085	08	539-541	73394	08	542-544
72990	08	555-556	73086	08	539-541	73395	08	542-544
72991	08	555-556	73087	08	539-541	73396	08	542-544
72992	08	555-556	73088	08	539-541	73397	08	542-544
72999	08	555-556	73089	08	539-541	73398	08	542-544
73000	08	539-541	73090	08	539-541	73399	08	564-566
73001	08	539-541	73091	08	539-541	734	08	564-566
73002	08	539-541	73092	08	539-541	7350	08	564-566
73003	08	539-541	73093	08	539-541	7351	08	564-566
73004	08	539-541	73094	08	539-541	7352	08	564-566
73005	08	539-541	73095	08	539-541	7353	08	564-566
73006	08	485-487, 539-541	73096	08	539-541	7354	08	564-566
			73097	08	539-541	7355	08	564-566
73007	08	539-541	73098	08	539-541	7358	08	564-566
73008	08	456-458, 539-541	73099	08	539-541	7359	08	564-566
			7310	08	553-554	73600	08	564-566
73009	08	539-541	7311	08	553-554	73601	08	564-566
73010	08	539-541	7312	08	553-554	73602	08	564-566
73011	08	539-541	7313	08	553-554	73603	08	564-566
73012	08	539-541	7318	08	553-554	73604	08	564-566
73013	08	539-541	7320	08	456-458, 553-554	73605	01	073-074
73014	08	539-541				73606	01	073-074
73015	08	539-541	7321	08	553-554	73607	01	073-074
73016	08	485-487, 539-541	7322	08	553-554	73609	08	564-566
			7323	08	553-554	7361	08	564-566
73017	08	539-541	7324	08	553-554	73620	08	564-566
73018	08	456-458, 539-541	7325	08	553-554	73621	08	564-566
			7326	08	553-554	73622	08	564-566
73019	08	539-541	7327	08	553-554	73629	08	564-566
73020	08	539-541	7328	08	553-554	73630	08	564-566
73021	08	539-541	7329	08	553-554	73631	08	564-566
73022	08	539-541	73300	08	553-554	73632	08	564-566
73023	08	539-541	73301	08	553-554	73639	08	564-566
73024	08	539-541	73302	08	553-554	73641	08	564-566
73025	08	539-541	73303	08	553-554	73642	08	564-566
73026	08	485-487, 539-541	73309	08	553-554	7365	08	564-566
			73310	08	542-544	7366	08	564-566
73027	08	539-541	73311	08	542-544	73670	08	564-566
73028	08	456-458, 539-541	73312	08	542-544	73671	08	564-566
			73313	08	456-458, 542-544	73672	08	564-566
73029	08	539-541				73673	08	564-566
73030	08	553-554	73314	08	542-544	73674	01	073-074
73031	08	553-554	73315	08	542-544	73675	08	564-566
73032	08	553-554	73316	08	542-544	73676	08	564-566
73033	08	553-554	73319	08	542-544	73679	08	564-566
73034	08	553-554	73320	08	553-554	73681	08	564-566
73035	08	553-554	73321	08	553-554	73689	08	564-566
73036	08	553-554	73322	08	553-554	7369	08	564-566
73037	08	564-566	73329	08	553-554	7370	08	456-458, 551-552
73038	08	564-566	7333	08	564-566			
73039	08	564-566	73340	08	553-554	73710	08	456-458, 551-552
73070	08	564-566	73341	08	553-554			
73071	08	564-566	73342	08	553-554	73711	08	456-458, 551-552
73072	08	564-566	73343	08	553-554			
73073	08	564-566	73344	08	553-554	73712	08	456-458, 551-552
73074	08	564-566	73345	08	553-554			
73075	08	564-566	73349	08	553-554			

DX	MDC	MS-DRG	DX	MDC	MS-DRG	DX	MDC	MS-DRG
73719	08	456-458, 551-552	7422	01	091-093	7443	03	154-156
73720	08	456-458, 551-552	7423	01	091-093	74441	03	154-156
			7424	01	091-093	74442	03	154-156
73721	08	456-458, 551-552	74251	01	091-093	74443	03	154-156
73722	08	456-458, 551-552	74253	01	091-093	74446	03	154-156
			74259	01	091-093	74447	03	154-156
73729	08	456-458, 551-552	7428	01	091-093	74449	03	154-156
			7429	01	091-093	7445	09	606-607
73730	08	456-458, 551-552	74300	02	124-125	74481	03	157-159
			74303	02	124-125	74482	03	157-159
73731	08	456-458, 551-552	74306	02	124-125	74483	03	157-159
			74310	02	124-125	74484	03	157-159
73732	08	456-458, 551-552	74311	02	124-125	74489	03	154-156
			74312	02	124-125	7449	09	606-607
73733	08	456-458, 551-552	74320	02	124-125	7450	05	306-307
			74321	02	124-125	74510	05	306-307
73734	08	456-458, 551-552	74322	02	124-125	74511	05	306-307
			74330	02	124-125	74512	05	306-307
73739	08	456-458, 551-552	74331	02	124-125	74519	05	306-307
			74332	02	124-125	7452	05	306-307
73740	08	551-552	74333	02	124-125	7453	05	306-307
73741	08	551-552	74334	02	124-125	7454	05	306-307
73742	08	551-552	74335	02	124-125	7455	05	306-307
73743	08	551-552	74336	02	124-125	74560	05	306-307
7378	08	456-458, 551-552	74337	02	124-125	74561	05	306-307
			74339	02	124-125	74569	05	306-307
7379	08	456-458, 551-552	74341	02	124-125	7457	05	306-307
			74342	02	124-125	7458	05	306-307
7380	03	154-156	74343	02	124-125	7459	05	306-307
73810	08	564-566	74344	02	124-125	74600	05	306-307
73811	08	564-566	74345	02	124-125	74601	05	306-307
73812	08	564-566	74346	02	124-125	74602	05	306-307
73819	08	564-566	74347	02	124-125	74609	05	306-307
7382	08	564-566	74348	02	124-125	7461	05	306-307
7383	08	564-566	74349	02	124-125	7462	05	306-307
7384	08	551-552	74351	02	124-125	7463	05	306-307
7385	08	551-552	74352	02	124-125	7464	05	306-307
7386	08	564-566	74353	02	124-125	7465	05	306-307
7387	03	154-156	74354	02	124-125	7466	05	306-307
7388	08	564-566	74355	02	124-125	7467	05	306-307
7389	08	564-566	74356	02	124-125	74681	05	306-307
7390	08	555-556	74357	02	124-125	74682	05	306-307
7391	08	551-552	74358	02	124-125	74683	05	306-307
7392	08	551-552	74359	02	124-125	74684	05	306-307
7393	08	551-552	74361	02	124-125	74685	05	306-307
7394	08	551-552	74362	02	124-125	74686	05	308-310
7395	08	555-556	74363	02	124-125	74687	05	306-307
7396	08	555-556	74364	02	124-125	74689	05	306-307
7397	08	555-556	74365	02	124-125	7469	05	306-307
7398	08	555-556	74366	02	124-125	7470	05	306-307
7399	08	555-556	74369	02	124-125	74710	05	306-307
7400	01	091-093	7438	02	124-125	74711	05	306-307
7401	01	091-093	7439	02	124-125	74720	05	306-307
7402	01	091-093	74400	03	154-156	74721	05	306-307
74100	01	091-093	74401	03	154-156	74722	05	306-307
74101	01	091-093	74402	03	154-156	74729	05	306-307
74102	01	091-093	74403	03	154-156	7473	05	306-307
74103	01	091-093	74404	03	154-156	74740	05	306-307
74190	01	091-093	74405	03	154-156	74741	05	306-307
74191	01	091-093	74409	03	154-156	74742	05	306-307
74192	01	091-093	7441	03	154-156	74749	05	306-307
74193	01	091-093	74421	03	154-156	7475	05	299-301
7420	01	091-093	74422	03	154-156	74760	05	299-301
7421	01	091-093	74423	03	154-156	74761	05	299-301
			74424	03	154-156	74762	05	299-301
			74429	03	154-156	74763	05	299-301

DX	MDC	MS-DRG	DX	MDC	MS-DRG	DX	MDC	MS-DRG
74764	05	299-301	75169	07	441-443	7542	08	456-458, 564-566
74769	05	299-301	7517	07	438-440			
74781	01	091-093	7518	06	393-395	75430	08	564-566
74782	01	091-093	7519	06	393-395	75431	08	564-566
74783	15	791,793	7520	13	742-743, 760-761	75432	08	564-566
74789	05	299-301				75433	08	564-566
7479	05	299-301	75210	13	742-743, 760-761	75435	08	564-566
7480	03	154-156				75440	08	564-566
7481	03	154-156	75211	13	742-743, 760-761	75441	08	562-563
7482	03	154-156				75442	08	564-566
7483	03	154-156	75219	13	742-743, 760-761	75443	08	564-566
7484	04	205-206				75444	08	564-566
7485	04	205-206	7522	13	742-743, 760-761	75450	08	564-566
74860	04	205-206				75451	08	564-566
74861	04	190-192	7523	13	742-743, 760-761	75452	08	564-566
74869	04	205-206				75453	08	564-566
7488	04	205-206	75240	13	742-743, 760-761	75459	08	564-566
7489	04	205-206				75460	08	564-566
74900	03	157-159	75241	13	742-743, 760-761	75461	08	564-566
74901	03	157-159				75462	08	564-566
74902	03	157-159	75242	13	742-743, 760-761	75469	08	564-566
74903	03	157-159				75470	08	564-566
74904	03	157-159	75249	13	742-743, 760-761	75471	08	564-566
74910	03	157-159				75479	08	564-566
74911	03	157-159	75251	12	729-730	75481	04	205-206
74912	03	157-159	75252	12	729-730	75482	04	205-206
74913	03	157-159	75261	12	729-730	75489	08	564-566
74914	03	157-159	75262	12	729-730	75500	08	564-566
74920	03	157-159	75263	12	729-730	75501	08	564-566
74921	03	157-159	75264	12	729-730	75502	08	564-566
74922	03	157-159	75265	12	729-730	75510	08	564-566
74923	03	157-159	75269	12	729-730	75511	08	564-566
74924	03	157-159	7527	12	729-730	75512	08	564-566
74925	03	157-159	7527	13	742-743, 760-761	75513	08	564-566
7500	03	157-159				75514	08	564-566
75010	03	157-159	75281	12	729-730	75520	08	564-566
75011	03	157-159	75289	12	729-730	75521	08	564-566
75012	03	157-159	75289	13	742-743, 760-761	75522	08	564-566
75013	03	157-159				75523	08	564-566
75015	03	157-159	7529	12	729-730	75524	08	564-566
75016	03	157-159	7529	13	742-743, 760-761	75525	08	564-566
75019	03	157-159				75526	08	564-566
75021	03	154-156	7530	11	698-700	75527	08	564-566
75022	03	154-156	75310	11	698-700	75528	08	564-566
75023	03	154-156	75311	11	698-700	75529	08	564-566
75024	03	154-156	75312	11	698-700	75530	08	564-566
75025	03	157-159	75313	11	698-700	75531	08	564-566
75026	03	157-159	75314	11	698-700	75532	08	564-566
75027	03	154-156	75315	11	698-700	75533	08	564-566
75029	03	154-156	75316	11	698-700	75534	08	564-566
7503	06	368-370	75317	11	698-700	75535	08	564-566
7504	06	368-370	75319	11	698-700	75536	08	564-566
7505	06	393-395	75320	11	698-700	75537	08	564-566
7506	06	393-395	75321	11	698-700	75538	08	564-566
7507	06	393-395	75322	11	698-700	75539	08	564-566
7508	06	393-395	75323	11	698-700	7554	08	564-566
7509	06	393-395	75329	11	698-700	75550	08	564-566
7510	06	380-382	7533	11	698-700	75551	08	564-566
7511	06	393-395	7534	11	698-700	75552	08	564-566
7512	06	393-395	7535	11	698-700	75553	08	564-566
7513	06	393-395	7536	11	698-700	75554	08	564-566
7514	06	393-395	7537	11	698-700	75555	08	564-566
7515	06	393-395	7538	11	698-700	75556	08	564-566
75160	07	444-446	7539	11	698-700	75557	08	564-566
75161	07	444-446	7540	08	564-566	75558	08	564-566
75162	07	441-443	7541	08	564-566	75559	08	564-566

DX	MDC	MS-DRG	DX	MDC	MS-DRG	DX	MDC	MS-DRG
75560	08	564-566	7585	23	951	7629	15	794
75561	08	564-566	7586	12	729-730	7630	15	795
75562	08	564-566	7586	13	742-743,	7631	15	795
75563	08	564-566			760-761	7632	15	795
75564	08	564-566	7587	12	729-730	7633	15	795
75565	08	564-566	75881	12	729-730	7634	15	791,793
75566	08	564-566	75881	13	742-743,	7635	15	794
75567	08	564-566			760-761	7636	15	795
75569	08	564-566	75889	12	729-730	7637	15	794
7558	08	564-566	75889	13	742-743,	76381	15	794
7559	08	564-566			760-761	76382	15	794
7560	08	564-566	7589	23	951	76383	15	794
75610	08	551-552	7590	16	814-816	76384	15	794
75611	08	551-552	7591	10	643-645	76389	15	794
75612	08	551-552	7592	10	643-645	7639	15	795
75613	08	551-552	7593	06	393-395	76400	15	794
75614	08	551-552	7594	06	393-395	76401	15	794
75615	08	551-552	7595	01	091-093	76402	15	794
75616	08	564-566	7596	17	843-845	76403	15	794
75617	01	091-093	7597	08	564-566	76404	15	794
75619	08	551-552	75981	08	564-566	76405	15	794
7562	08	564-566	75982	05	306-307	76406	15	794
7563	04	205-206	75983	19	884	76407	15	794
7564	08	564-566	75989	08	564-566	76408	15	795
75650	08	564-566	7599	23	951	76409	15	795
75651	08	456-458,	7600	15	794	76410	15	794
		564-566	7601	15	794	76411	15	791,793
75652	08	564-566	7602	15	794	76412	15	791,793
75653	08	564-566	7603	15	794	76413	15	791,793
75654	08	564-566	7604	15	794	76414	15	791,793
75655	08	564-566	7605	15	794	76415	15	791,793
75656	08	564-566	76061	15	794	76416	15	791,793
75659	08	564-566	76062	15	794	76417	15	791,793
7566	04	205-206	76063	15	794	76418	15	791,793
75670	06	393-395	76064	15	794	76419	15	794
75671	06	393-395	76070	15	794	76420	15	794
75672	06	393-395 ◄	76071	15	794	76421	15	791,793
	15	791,793 ◄	76072	15	794	76422	15	791,793
75673	06	393-395 ◄	76073	15	794	76423	15	791,793
	15	791,793 ◄	76074	15	794	76424	15	791,793
75679	06	393-395	76075	15	794	76425	15	791,793
75681	08	564-566	76076	15	794	76426	15	791,793
75682	08	564-566	76077	15	794	76427	15	791,793
75683	08	564-566	76078	15	794	76428	15	791,793
75689	08	564-566	76079	15	794	76429	15	794
7569	08	564-566	7608	15	794	76490	15	794
7570	09	606-607	7609	15	794	76491	15	794
7571	09	606-607	7610	15	794	76492	15	794
7572	09	606-607	7611	15	794	76493	15	794
75731	09	606-607	7612	15	794	76494	15	794
75732	09	606-607	7613	15	794	76495	15	794
75733	09	606-607	7614	15	794	76496	15	794
75739	09	606-607	7615	15	794	76497	15	794
7574	09	606-607	7616	15	794	76498	15	795
7575	09	606-607	7617	15	794	76499	15	795
7576	09	600-601	7618	15	794	76500	15	791-792
7578	09	606-607	7619	15	794	76501	15	790
7579	09	606-607	7620	15	794	76502	15	790
7580	19	884	7621	15	794	76503	15	790
7581	19	884	7622	15	794	76504	15	790
7582	19	884	7623	15	794	76505	15	790
75831	19	884	7624	15	795	76506	15	791-792
75832	19	884	7625	15	795	76507	15	791-792
75833	19	884	7626	15	795	76508	15	791-792
75839	19	884	7627	15	794	76509	15	999
7584	23	951	7628	15	794	76510	15	791-792

DX	MDC	MS-DRG	DX	MDC	MS-DRG	DX	MDC	MS-DRG
76511	15	791-792	77084	15	791,793	7767	15	794
76512	15	791-792	77085	15	791,793	7768	15	794
76513	15	791-792	77086	15	791,793	7769	15	794
76514	15	791-792	77087	15	794	7771	15	791,793
76515	15	791-792	77088	15	794	7772	15	791,793
76516	15	791-792	77089	15	794	7773	15	794
76517	15	791-792	7709	15	794	7774	15	794
76518	15	791-792	7710	15	791,793	77750	15	791,793
76519	15	791-792	7711	15	791,793	77751	15	791,793
76520	15	795	7712	15	791,793	77752	15	791,793
76521	15	790	7713	15	794	77753	15	791,793
76522	15	790	7714	15	791,793	7776	15	791,793
76523	15	790	7715	15	791,793	7778	15	794
76524	15	791-792	7716	15	794	7779	15	794
76525	15	791-792	7717	15	794	7780	15	791,793
76526	15	791-792	77181	15	791,793	7781	15	794
76527	15	791-792	77182	15	791,793	7782	15	794
76528	15	791-792	77183	15	791,793	7783	15	794
76529	15	795	77189	15	791,793	7784	15	794
7660	15	795	7720	15	791,793	7785	15	794
7661	15	795	77210	15	791,793	7786	15	794
76621	15	795	77211	15	791,793	7787	15	794
76622	15	795	77212	15	791,793	7788	15	795
7670	15	791,793	77213	15	791,793	7789	15	794
76711	15	791,793	77214	15	791,793	7790	15	791,793
76719	15	795	7722	15	791,793	7791	15	791,793
7672	15	794	7723	15	794	7792	15	791,793
7673	15	794	7724	15	791,793	77931	15	795
7674	15	791,793	7725	15	791,793	77932	15	791,793 ◄
7675	15	794	7726	15	795	77933	15	795 ◄
7676	15	794	7728	15	794	77934	10	640-641 ◄
7677	15	791,793	7729	15	794		25	977 ◄
7678	15	794	7730	15	794	7794	15	791,793
7679	15	794	7731	15	794	7795	15	791,793
7680	15	794	7732	15	791,793	7796	15	794
7681	15	794	7733	15	791,793	7797	01	091-093
7682	15	794	7734	15	791,793	77981	15	794
7683	15	794	7735	15	791,793	77982	15	794
7684	15	794	7740	15	794	77983	15	795
7685	15	791,793	7741	15	794	77984	15	794
7686	15	795	7742	15	794	77985	15	791,793
76870	15	794	77430	15	795	77989	15	794
76871	15	794 ◄	77431	15	795	7799	15	794
76872	15	791,793 ◄	77439	15	795	78001	01	080-081
76873	15	791,793 ◄	7744	15	791,793	78002	19	884
7689	15	794	7745	15	795	78003	01	080-081
769	15	790	7746	15	795	78009	01	080-081
7700	15	791,793	7747	15	791,793	7801	19	880
77010	15	791,793	7750	15	794	7802	05	312
77011	15	791,793	7751	15	791,793	78031	01	100-101
77012	15	791,793	7752	15	791,793	78032	01	100-101
77013	15	791,793	7753	15	791,793	78039	01	100-101
77014	15	791,793	7754	15	791,793	7804	03	149
77015	15	791,793	7755	15	791,793	78050	19	887
77016	15	791,793	7756	15	791,793	78051	03	154-156
77017	15	791,793	7757	15	791,793	78052	19	887
77018	15	791,793	77581	15	794	78053	03	154-156
7702	15	791,793	77589	15	794	78054	19	887
7703	15	791,793	7759	15	794	78055	19	887
7704	15	791,793	7760	15	791,793	78056	19	887
7705	15	794	7761	15	791,793	78057	03	154-156
7706	15	794	7762	15	791,793	78058	19	887
7707	04	196-198	7763	15	791,793	78059	19	887
77081	15	794	7764	15	794	78060	18	864
77082	15	794	7765	15	794	78061	18	864
77083	15	794	7766	15	791,793	78062	18	864

DX	MDC	MS-DRG	DX	MDC	MS-DRG	DX	MDC	MS-DRG
78063	18	864	78461	19	886	78833	11	695-696
78064	23	947-948	78469	19	886	78834	11	695-696
78065	23	947-948	7847	03	150-151	78835	11	695-696
78071	23	947-948	7848	03	154-156	78836	11	695-696
78072	01	052-053	78491	03	154-156	78837	11	695-696
78079	23	947-948	78499	03	154-156	78838	11	695-696
7808	09	606-607	7850	05	308-310	78839	11	695-696
78091	23	947-948	7851	05	308-310	78841	11	695-696
78092	23	947-948	7852	05	306-307	78842	11	695-696
78093	23	947-948	7853	05	314-316	78843	11	695-696
78094	23	947-948	7854	05	299-301	7885	11	673-675,
78095	23	947-948	78550	05	222-223,			682-684
78096	23	947-948			291-293	78861	11	695-696
78097	23	947-948	78551	05	222-223,	78862	11	695-696
78099	23	947-948			291-293	78863	11	695-696
7810	01	091-093	78552	18	870-872	78864	11	695-696
7811	01	091-093	78559	18	870-872	78865	11	695-696
7812	01	091-093	7856	16	814-816	78869	11	695-696
7813	01	091-093	7859	05	314-316	7887	11	695-696
7814	01	091-093	78600	04	204	7888	11	695-696
7815	04	205-206	78601	04	204	78891	11	695-696
7816	01	091-093	78602	04	204	78899	11	695-696
7817	10	640-641	78603	04	204	78900	06	391-392
7818	01	091-093	78604	04	204	78901	06	391-392
78191	01	091-093	78605	04	204	78902	06	391-392
78192	01	091-093	78606	04	204	78903	06	391-392
78193	08	551-552	78607	04	204	78904	06	391-392
78194	01	091-093	78609	04	204	78905	06	391-392
78199	01	091-093	7861	04	204	78906	06	391-392
7820	01	091-093	7862	04	204	78907	06	391-392
7821	09	606-607	7863	04	204	78909	06	391-392
7822	09	606-607	7864	04	204	7891	07	441-443
7823	23	947-948	78650	05	313	7892	16	814-816
7824	07	441-443	78651	05	313	78930	06	391-392
7825	23	947-948	78652	04	204	78931	06	391-392
78261	23	947-948	78659	05	313	78932	06	391-392
78262	23	947-948	7866	04	204	78933	06	391-392
7827	16	813	7867	04	204	78934	06	391-392
7828	09	606-607	7868	04	204	78935	06	391-392
7829	09	606-607	7869	04	204	78936	06	391-392
7830	10	640-641	78701	06	391-392	78937	06	391-392
7831	10	640-641	78702	06	391-392	78939	06	391-392
78321	10	640-641	78703	06	391-392	78940	06	393-395
78322	10	640-641	78704	06	391-392 ◀	78941	06	393-395
7833	10	640-641	7871	06	391-392	78942	06	393-395
78340	10	640-641	78720	06	391-392	78943	06	393-395
78341	10	640-641	78721	06	391-392	78944	06	393-395
78342	10	640-641	78722	06	391-392	78945	06	393-395
78343	10	640-641	78723	06	391-392	78946	06	393-395
7835	10	640-641	78724	06	391-392	78947	06	393-395
7836	10	640-641	78729	06	391-392	78949	06	393-395
7837	10	640-641	7873	06	391-392	78951	23	947-948
7839	10	640-641	7874	06	391-392	78959	23	947-948
7840	01	102-103	7875	06	391-392	78960	06	391-392
7841	03	154-156	7876	06	391-392	78961	06	391-392
7842	09	606-607	7877	06	391-392	78962	06	391-392
7843	01	091-093	78791	06	391-392	78963	06	391-392
78440	03	154-156	78799	06	391-392	78964	06	391-392
78441	03	154-156	7880	11	691-694	78965	06	391-392
78442	03	154-156 ◀	7881	11	695-696	78966	06	391-392
78443	03	154-156 ◀	78820	11	695-696	78967	06	391-392
78444	03	154-156 ◀	78821	11	695-696	78969	06	391-392
78449	03	154-156	78829	11	695-696	7897	06	391-392 ◀
78451	01	091-093	78830	11	695-696	7899	06	391-392
78459	01	091-093 ◀	78831	11	695-696	79001	16	811-812
78460	19	887	78832	11	695-696	79009	16	811-812

DX	MDC	MS-DRG	DX	MDC	MS-DRG	DX	MDC	MS-DRG
7901	23	947-948	7948	07	441-443	79678	06	393-395
79021	10	640-641	7949	11	695-696	79679	06	393-395
79022	10	640-641	79500	13	742-743, 760-761	7969	23	947-948
79029	10	640-641				797	19	884
7903	20	894-897	79501	13	742-743, 760-761	7980	01	091-093
7904	23	947-948	79502	13	742-743, 760-761	7981	05	296-298
7905	23	947-948				7982	05	296-298
7906	23	947-948	79503	13	742-743, 760-761	7989	23	951
7907	18	870-872				79901	04	205-206
7908	18	865-866	79504	13	742-743, 760-761	79902	04	205-206
79091	23	947-948				7991	04	205-206
79092	23	947-948	79505	13	742-743, 760-761	79921	19	880
79093	23	947-948	79506	13	742-743, 760-761	79922	19	880 ◄
79094	23	947-948				79923	19	882 ◄
79095	23	947-948	79507	13	742-743, 760-761	79924	19	883 ◄
79099	23	947-948				79925	19	880 ◄
7910	11	695-696	79508	13	742-743, 760-761	79929	19	880 ◄
7911	11	695-696				7993	23	947-948
7912	11	695-696	79509	13	742-743, 760-761	7994	23	947-948
7913	23	947-948				79981	23	951
7914	07	441-443	79510	13	742-743, 760-761	79982	23	951 ◄
7915	10	637-639				79989	23	951
7916	10	640-641	79511	13	742-743, 760-761	7999	23	951
7917	11	695-696				80000	01	082-087
7919	11	695-696	79512	13	742-743, 760-761	80001	01	082-087
7920	01	091-093				80002	01	082-087
7921	06	391-392	79513	13	742-743, 760-761	80003	01	082-084
7922	12	729-730				80004	01	082-084
7923	14	781-782	79514	13	742-743, 760-761	80005	01	082-084
7924	03	154-156				80006	01	082-084
7925	23	947-948	79515	13	742-743, 760-761	80009	01	082-087
7929	23	947-948				80010	01	082-087
7930	01	091-093	79516	13	742-743, 760-761	80011	01	082-087
7931	04	204				80012	01	082-087
7932	05	302-303	79518	13	742-743, 760-761	80013	01	082-084
7933	07	444-446				80014	01	082-084
7934	06	391-392	79519	13	742-743, 760-761	80015	01	082-084
7935	11	695-696				80016	01	082-084
7936	06	391-392	7952	23	951	80019	01	082-087
7937	08	564-566	79531	18	867-869	80020	01	082-087
79380	09	600-601	79539	18	867-869	80021	01	082-087
79381	09	600-601	7954	23	947-948	80022	01	082-087
79389	09	600-601	7955	04	177-179	80023	01	082-084
79391	23	947-948	7956	08	545-547	80024	01	082-084
79399	23	947-948	79571	16	814-816	80025	01	082-084
79400	01	091-093	79579	16	814-816	80026	01	082-084
79401	01	091-093	79581	23	947-948	80029	01	082-087
79402	01	091-093	79582	23	947-948	80030	01	082-087
79409	01	091-093	79589	23	947-948	80031	01	082-087
79410	01	091-093	7960	21	922-923	80032	01	082-087
79411	02	124-125	7961	01	091-093	80033	01	082-084
79412	02	124-125	7962	05	314-316	80034	01	082-084
79413	02	124-125	7963	05	314-316	80035	01	082-084
79414	02	124-125	7964	23	947-948	80036	01	082-084
79415	03	154-156	7965	14	781-782	80039	01	082-087
79416	03	154-156	7966	23	947-948	80040	01	082-087
79417	08	564-566	79670	06	393-395	80041	01	082-087
79419	01	091-093	79671	06	393-395	80042	01	082-087
7942	04	205-206	79672	06	393-395	80043	01	082-084
79430	05	314-316	79673	06	393-395	80044	01	082-084
79431	05	314-316	79674	06	393-395	80045	01	082-084
79439	05	314-316	79675	06	393-395	80046	01	082-084
7944	11	695-696	79676	06	393-395	80049	01	082-087
7945	10	643-645	79677	06	393-395	80050	01	082-087
7946	10	643-645				80051	01	082-087
7947	10	643-645				80052	01	082-087

DX	MDC	MS-DRG	DX	MDC	MS-DRG	DX	MDC	MS-DRG
80053	01	082-084	80135	01	082-084	80233	03	157-159
80054	01	082-084	80136	01	082-084	80234	03	157-159
80055	01	082-084	80139	01	082-087	80235	03	157-159
80056	01	082-084	80140	01	082-087	80236	03	157-159
80059	01	082-087	80141	01	082-087	80237	03	157-159
80060	01	082-087	80142	01	082-087	80238	03	157-159
80061	01	082-087	80143	01	082-084	80239	03	157-159
80062	01	082-087	80144	01	082-084	8024	03	157-159
80063	01	082-084	80145	01	082-084	8025	03	157-159
80064	01	082-084	80146	01	082-084	8026	02	124-125
80065	01	082-084	80149	01	082-087	8027	02	124-125
80066	01	082-084	80150	01	082-087	8028	08	564-566
80069	01	082-087	80151	01	082-087	8029	08	564-566
80070	01	082-087	80152	01	082-087	80300	01	082-087
80071	01	082-087	80153	01	082-084	80301	01	082-087
80072	01	082-087	80154	01	082-084	80302	01	082-087
80073	01	082-084	80155	01	082-084	80303	01	082-084
80074	01	082-084	80156	01	082-084	80304	01	082-084
80075	01	082-084	80159	01	082-087	80305	01	082-084
80076	01	082-084	80160	01	082-087	80306	01	082-084
80079	01	082-087	80161	01	082-087	80309	01	082-087
80080	01	082-087	80162	01	082-087	80310	01	082-087
80081	01	082-087	80163	01	082-084	80311	01	082-087
80082	01	082-087	80164	01	082-084	80312	01	082-087
80083	01	082-084	80165	01	082-084	80313	01	082-084
80084	01	082-084	80166	01	082-084	80314	01	082-084
80085	01	082-084	80169	01	082-087	80315	01	082-084
80086	01	082-084	80170	01	082-087	80316	01	082-084
80089	01	082-087	80171	01	082-087	80319	01	082-087
80090	01	082-087	80172	01	082-087	80320	01	082-087
80091	01	082-087	80173	01	082-084	80321	01	082-087
80092	01	082-087	80174	01	082-084	80322	01	082-087
80093	01	082-084	80175	01	082-084	80323	01	082-084
80094	01	082-084	80176	01	082-084	80324	01	082-084
80095	01	082-084	80179	01	082-087	80325	01	082-084
80096	01	082-084	80180	01	082-087	80326	01	082-084
80099	01	082-087	80181	01	082-087	80329	01	082-087
80100	01	082-087	80182	01	082-087	80330	01	082-087
80101	01	082-087	80183	01	082-084	80331	01	082-087
80102	01	082-087	80184	01	082-084	80332	01	082-087
80103	01	082-084	80185	01	082-084	80333	01	082-084
80104	01	082-084	80186	01	082-084	80334	01	082-084
80105	01	082-084	80189	01	082-087	80335	01	082-084
80106	01	082-084	80190	01	082-087	80336	01	082-084
80109	01	082-087	80191	01	082-087	80339	01	082-087
80110	01	082-087	80192	01	082-087	80340	01	082-087
80111	01	082-087	80193	01	082-084	80341	01	082-087
80112	01	082-087	80194	01	082-084	80342	01	082-087
80113	01	082-084	80195	01	082-084	80343	01	082-084
80114	01	082-084	80196	01	082-084	80344	01	082-084
80115	01	082-084	80199	01	082-087	80345	01	082-084
80116	01	082-084	8020	03	154-156	80346	01	082-084
80119	01	082-087	8021	03	154-156	80349	01	082-087
80120	01	082-087	80220	03	157-159	80350	01	082-087
80121	01	082-087	80221	03	157-159	80351	01	082-087
80122	01	082-087	80222	03	157-159	80352	01	082-087
80123	01	082-084	80223	03	157-159	80353	01	082-084
80124	01	082-084	80224	03	157-159	80354	01	082-084
80125	01	082-084	80225	03	157-159	80355	01	082-084
80126	01	082-084	80226	03	157-159	80356	01	082-084
80129	01	082-087	80227	03	157-159	80359	01	082-087
80130	01	082-087	80228	03	157-159	80360	01	082-087
80131	01	082-087	80229	03	157-159	80361	01	082-087
80132	01	082-087	80230	03	157-159	80362	01	082-087
80133	01	082-084	80231	03	157-159	80363	01	082-084
80134	01	082-084	80232	03	157-159	80364	01	082-084

DX	MDC	MS-DRG	DX	MDC	MS-DRG	DX	MDC	MS-DRG
80365	01	082-084	80449	01	082-087	8059	08	551-552
80366	01	082-084	80450	01	082-087	80600	01	052-053
80369	01	082-087	80451	01	082-087	80601	01	052-053
80370	01	082-087	80452	01	082-087	80602	01	052-053
80371	01	082-087	80453	01	082-084	80603	01	052-053
80372	01	082-087	80454	01	082-084	80604	01	052-053
80373	01	082-084	80455	01	082-084	80605	01	052-053
80374	01	082-084	80456	01	082-084	80606	01	052-053
80375	01	082-084	80459	01	082-087	80607	01	052-053
80376	01	082-084	80460	01	082-087	80608	01	052-053
80379	01	082-087	80461	01	082-087	80609	01	052-053
80380	01	082-087	80462	01	082-087	80610	01	052-053
80381	01	082-087	80463	01	082-084	80611	01	052-053
80382	01	082-087	80464	01	082-084	80612	01	052-053
80383	01	082-084	80465	01	082-084	80613	01	052-053
80384	01	082-084	80466	01	082-084	80614	01	052-053
80385	01	082-084	80469	01	082-087	80615	01	052-053
80386	01	082-084	80470	01	082-087	80616	01	052-053
80389	01	082-087	80471	01	082-087	80617	01	052-053
80390	01	082-087	80472	01	082-087	80618	01	052-053
80391	01	082-087	80473	01	082-084	80619	01	052-053
80392	01	082-087	80474	01	082-084	80620	01	052-053
80393	01	082-084	80475	01	082-084	80621	01	052-053
80394	01	082-084	80476	01	082-084	80622	01	052-053
80395	01	082-084	80479	01	082-087	80623	01	052-053
80396	01	082-084	80480	01	082-087	80624	01	052-053
80399	01	082-087	80481	01	082-087	80625	01	052-053
80400	01	082-087	80482	01	082-087	80626	01	052-053
80401	01	082-087	80483	01	082-084	80627	01	052-053
80402	01	082-087	80484	01	082-084	80628	01	052-053
80403	01	082-084	80485	01	082-084	80629	01	052-053
80404	01	082-084	80486	01	082-084	80630	01	052-053
80405	01	082-084	80489	01	082-087	80631	01	052-053
80406	01	082-084	80490	01	082-087	80632	01	052-053
80409	01	082-087	80491	01	082-087	80633	01	052-053
80410	01	082-087	80492	01	082-087	80634	01	052-053
80411	01	082-087	80493	01	082-084	80635	01	052-053
80412	01	082-087	80494	01	082-084	80636	01	052-053
80413	01	082-084	80495	01	082-084	80637	01	052-053
80414	01	082-084	80496	01	082-084	80638	01	052-053
80415	01	082-084	80499	01	082-087	80639	01	052-053
80416	01	082-084	80500	08	551-552	8064	01	052-053
80419	01	082-087	80501	08	551-552	8065	01	052-053
80420	01	082-087	80502	08	551-552	80660	01	052-053
80421	01	082-087	80503	08	551-552	80661	01	052-053
80422	01	082-087	80504	08	551-552	80662	01	052-053
80423	01	082-084	80505	08	551-552	80669	01	052-053
80424	01	082-084	80506	08	551-552	80670	01	052-053
80425	01	082-084	80507	08	551-552	80671	01	052-053
80426	01	082-084	80508	08	551-552	80672	01	052-053
80429	01	082-087	80510	08	551-552	80679	01	052-053
80430	01	082-087	80511	08	551-552	8068	01	052-053
80431	01	082-087	80512	08	551-552	8069	01	052-053
80432	01	082-087	80513	08	551-552	80700	04	205-206
80433	01	082-084	80514	08	551-552	80701	04	205-206
80434	01	082-084	80515	08	551-552	80702	04	205-206
80435	01	082-084	80516	08	551-552	80703	04	183-185
80436	01	082-084	80517	08	551-552	80704	04	183-185
80439	01	082-087	80518	08	551-552	80705	04	183-185
80440	01	082-087	8052	08	551-552	80706	04	183-185
80441	01	082-087	8053	08	551-552	80707	04	183-185
80442	01	082-087	8054	08	551-552	80708	04	183-185
80443	01	082-084	8055	08	551-552	80709	04	183-185
80444	01	082-084	8056	08	551-552	80710	04	183-185
80445	01	082-084	8057	08	551-552	80711	04	183-185
80446	01	082-084	8058	08	551-552	80712	04	183-185

DX	MDC	MS-DRG	DX	MDC	MS-DRG	DX	MDC	MS-DRG
80713	04	183-185	81250	08	562-563	81410	08	562-563
80714	04	183-185	81251	08	562-563	81411	08	562-563
80715	04	183-185	81252	08	562-563	81412	08	562-563
80716	04	183-185	81253	08	562-563	81413	08	562-563
80717	04	183-185	81254	08	562-563	81414	08	562-563
80718	04	183-185	81259	08	562-563	81415	08	562-563
80719	04	183-185	81300	08	562-563	81416	08	562-563
8072	04	183-185	81301	08	562-563	81417	08	562-563
8073	04	183-185	81302	08	562-563	81418	08	562-563
8074	04	183-185	81303	08	562-563	81419	08	562-563
8075	03	154-156	81304	08	562-563	81500	08	562-563
8076	03	154-156	81305	08	562-563	81501	08	562-563
8080	08	535-536	81306	08	562-563	81502	08	562-563
8081	08	535-536	81307	08	562-563	81503	08	562-563
8082	08	535-536	81308	08	562-563	81504	08	562-563
8083	08	535-536	81310	08	562-563	81509	08	562-563
80841	08	535-536	81311	08	562-563	81510	08	562-563
80842	08	535-536	81312	08	562-563	81511	08	562-563
80843	08	535-536	81313	08	562-563	81512	08	562-563
80849	08	535-536	81314	08	562-563	81513	08	562-563
80851	08	535-536	81315	08	562-563	81514	08	562-563
80852	08	535-536	81316	08	562-563	81519	08	562-563
80853	08	535-536	81317	08	562-563	81600	08	562-563
80859	08	535-536	81318	08	562-563	81601	08	562-563
8088	08	535-536	81320	08	562-563	81602	08	562-563
8089	08	535-536	81321	08	562-563	81603	08	562-563
8090	08	564-566	81322	08	562-563	81610	08	562-563
8091	08	564-566	81323	08	562-563	81611	08	562-563
81000	08	562-563	81330	08	562-563	81612	08	562-563
81001	08	562-563	81331	08	562-563	81613	08	562-563
81002	08	562-563	81332	08	562-563	8170	08	562-563
81003	08	562-563	81333	08	562-563	8171	08	562-563
81010	08	562-563	81340	08	562-563	8180	08	562-563
81011	08	562-563	81341	08	562-563	8181	08	562-563
81012	08	562-563	81342	08	562-563	8190	21	913-914
81013	08	562-563	81343	08	562-563	8191	21	913-914
81100	08	562-563	81344	08	562-563	82000	08	535-536
81101	08	562-563	81345	08	562-563	82001	08	535-536
81102	08	562-563		24	963-965 ◄▥	82002	08	535-536
81103	08	562-563	81346	08	562-563, ◄	82003	08	535-536
81109	08	564-566		24	963-965	82009	08	535-536
81110	08	562-563	81347	08	562-563, ◄	82010	08	535-536
81111	08	562-563		24	963-965	82011	08	535-536
81112	08	562-563	81350	08	562-563	82012	08	535-536
81113	08	562-563	81351	08	562-563	82013	08	535-536
81119	08	564-566	81352	08	562-563	82019	08	535-536
81200	08	562-563	81353	08	562-563	82020	08	535-536
81201	08	562-563	81354	08	562-563	82021	08	535-536
81202	08	562-563	81380	08	562-563	82022	08	535-536
81203	08	562-563	81381	08	562-563	82030	08	535-536
81209	08	562-563	81382	08	562-563	82031	08	535-536
81210	08	562-563	81383	08	562-563	82032	08	535-536
81211	08	562-563	81390	08	562-563	8208	08	535-536
81212	08	562-563	81391	08	562-563	8209	08	535-536
81213	08	562-563	81392	08	562-563	82100	08	533-534
81219	08	562-563	81393	08	562-563	82101	08	533-534
81220	08	562-563	81400	08	562-563	82110	08	533-534
81221	08	562-563	81401	08	562-563	82111	08	533-534
81230	08	562-563	81402	08	562-563	82120	08	533-534
81231	08	562-563	81403	08	562-563	82121	08	533-534
81240	08	562-563	81404	08	562-563	82122	08	533-534
81241	08	562-563	81405	08	562-563	82123	08	533-534
81242	08	562-563	81406	08	562-563	82129	08	533-534
81243	08	562-563	81407	08	562-563	82130	08	533-534
81244	08	562-563	81408	08	562-563	82131	08	533-534
81249	08	562-563	81409	08	562-563	82132	08	533-534

DX	MDC	MS-DRG	DX	MDC	MS-DRG	DX	MDC	MS-DRG
82133	08	533-534	83109	08	562-563	8370	08	562-563
82139	08	533-534	83110	08	562-563	8371	08	562-563
8220	08	562-563	83111	08	562-563	83800	08	562-563
8221	08	562-563	83112	08	562-563	83801	08	562-563
82300	08	562-563	83113	08	562-563	83802	08	562-563
82301	08	562-563	83114	08	562-563	83803	08	562-563
82302	08	562-563	83119	08	562-563	83804	08	562-563
82310	08	562-563	83200	08	562-563	83805	08	562-563
82311	08	562-563	83201	08	562-563	83806	08	562-563
82312	08	562-563	83202	08	562-563	83809	08	562-563
82320	08	562-563	83203	08	562-563	83810	08	562-563
82321	08	562-563	83204	08	562-563	83811	08	562-563
82322	08	562-563	83209	08	562-563	83812	08	562-563
82330	08	562-563	83210	08	562-563	83813	08	562-563
82331	08	562-563	83211	08	562-563	83814	08	562-563
82332	08	562-563	83212	08	562-563	83815	08	562-563
82340	08	562-563	83213	08	562-563	83816	08	562-563
82341	08	562-563	83214	08	562-563	83819	08	562-563
82342	08	562-563	83219	08	562-563	83900	08	551-552
82380	08	562-563	8322	08	562-563 ◄	83901	08	551-552
82381	08	562-563		24	963-965	83902	08	551-552
82382	08	562-563	83300	08	562-563	83903	08	551-552
82390	08	562-563	83301	08	562-563	83904	08	551-552
82391	08	562-563	83302	08	562-563	83905	08	551-552
82392	08	562-563	83303	08	562-563	83906	08	551-552
8240	08	562-563	83304	08	562-563	83907	08	551-552
8241	08	562-563	83305	08	562-563	83908	08	551-552
8242	08	562-563	83309	08	562-563	83910	08	551-552
8243	08	562-563	83310	08	562-563	83911	08	551-552
8244	08	562-563	83311	08	562-563	83912	08	551-552
8245	08	562-563	83312	08	562-563	83913	08	551-552
8246	08	562-563	83313	08	562-563	83914	08	551-552
8247	08	562-563	83314	08	562-563	83915	08	551-552
8248	08	562-563	83315	08	562-563	83916	08	551-552
8249	08	562-563	83319	08	562-563	83917	08	551-552
8250	08	562-563	83400	08	562-563	83918	08	551-552
8251	08	562-563	83401	08	562-563	83920	08	551-552
82520	08	562-563	83402	08	562-563	83921	08	551-552
82521	08	562-563	83410	08	562-563	83930	08	551-552
82522	08	562-563	83411	08	562-563	83931	08	551-552
82523	08	562-563	83412	08	562-563	83940	08	551-552
82524	08	562-563	83500	08	537-538	83941	08	551-552
82525	08	562-563	83501	08	537-538	83942	08	551-552
82529	08	562-563	83502	08	537-538	83949	08	551-552
82530	08	562-563	83503	08	537-538	83950	08	551-552
82531	08	562-563	83510	08	537-538	83951	08	551-552
82532	08	562-563	83511	08	537-538	83952	08	551-552
82533	08	562-563	83512	08	537-538	83959	08	551-552
82534	08	562-563	83513	08	537-538	83961	04	183-185
82535	08	562-563	8360	08	562-563	83969	08	562-563
82539	08	562-563	8361	08	562-563	83971	04	183-185
8260	08	562-563	8362	08	562-563	83979	08	562-563
8261	08	562-563	8363	08	562-563	8398	08	562-563
8270	08	562-563	8364	08	562-563	8399	08	562-563
8271	08	562-563	83650	08	562-563	8400	08	562-563
8280	21	913-914	83651	08	562-563	8401	08	562-563
8281	21	913-914	83652	08	562-563	8402	08	562-563
8290	08	562-563	83653	08	562-563	8403	08	562-563
8291	08	562-563	83654	08	562-563	8404	08	562-563
8300	03	157-159	83659	08	562-563	8405	08	562-563
8301	03	157-159	83660	08	562-563	8406	08	562-563
83100	08	562-563	83661	08	562-563	8407	08	562-563
83101	08	562-563	83662	08	562-563	8408	08	562-563
83102	08	562-563	83663	08	562-563	8409	08	562-563
83103	08	562-563	83664	08	562-563	8410	08	562-563
83104	08	562-563	83669	08	562-563	8411	08	562-563

PART VI, MS-DRG, APPENDIX B

DX	MDC	MS-DRG	DX	MDC	MS-DRG	DX	MDC	MS-DRG
8412	08	562-563	85102	01	082-087	85152	01	023-024, 082-087
8413	08	562-563	85103	01	082-084	85153	01	023-024, 082-084
8418	08	562-563	85104	01	082-084			
8419	08	562-563	85105	01	082-084	85154	01	023-024, 082-084
84200	08	562-563	85106	01	082-084			
84201	08	562-563	85109	01	082-087	85155	01	023-024, 082-084
84202	08	562-563	85110	01	023-024, 082-087			
84209	08	562-563				85156	01	023-024, 082-084
84210	08	562-563	85111	01	023-024, 082-087			
84211	08	562-563				85159	01	023-024, 082-087
84212	08	562-563	85112	01	023-024, 082-087			
84213	08	562-563				85160	01	023-024, 082-087
84219	08	562-563	85113	01	023-024, 082-084			
8430	08	537-538				85161	01	023-024, 082-087
8431	08	537-538	85114	01	023-024, 082-084			
8438	08	537-538				85162	01	023-024, 082-087
8439	08	537-538	85115	01	023-024, 082-084			
8440	08	562-563				85163	01	023-024, 082-084
8441	08	562-563	85116	01	023-024, 082-084			
8442	08	562-563				85164	01	023-024, 082-084
8443	08	562-563	85119	01	023-024, 082-087			
8448	08	562-563				85165	01	023-024, 082-084
8449	08	562-563	85120	01	023-024, 082-087			
84500	08	562-563				85166	01	023-024, 082-084
84501	08	562-563	85121	01	023-024, 082-087			
84502	08	562-563				85169	01	023-024, 082-087
84503	08	562-563	85122	01	023-024, 082-087			
84509	08	562-563				85170	01	023-024, 082-087
84510	08	562-563	85123	01	023-024, 082-084			
84511	08	562-563				85171	01	023-024, 082-087
84512	08	562-563	85124	01	023-024, 082-084			
84513	08	562-563				85172	01	023-024, 082-087
84519	08	562-563	85125	01	023-024, 082-084			
8460	08	551-552				85173	01	023-024, 082-084
8461	08	551-552	85126	01	023-024, 082-084			
8462	08	551-552				85174	01	023-024, 082-084
8463	08	551-552	85129	01	023-024, 082-087			
8468	08	551-552				85175	01	023-024, 082-084
8469	08	551-552	85130	01	023-024, 082-087			
8470	08	551-552				85176	01	023-024, 082-084
8471	08	551-552	85131	01	023-024, 082-087			
8472	08	551-552				85179	01	023-024, 082-087
8473	08	551-552	85132	01	023-024, 082-087			
8474	08	551-552				85180	01	023-024, 082-087
8479	08	551-552	85133	01	023-024, 082-084			
8480	08	564-566				85181	01	023-024, 082-087
8481	03	157-159	85134	01	023-024, 082-084			
8482	08	564-566				85182	01	023-024, 082-087
8483	04	205-206	85135	01	023-024, 082-084			
84840	04	205-206				85183	01	023-024, 082-084
84841	04	205-206	85136	01	023 024, 082-084			
84842	04	205-206				85184	01	023-024, 082-084
84849	04	205-206	85139	01	023-024, 082-087			
8485	08	537-538				85185	01	023-024, 082-084
8488	08	562-563	85140	01	082-087			
8489	08	562-563	85141	01	082-087	85186	01	023-024, 082-084
8500	01	088-090	85142	01	082-087			
85011	01	088-090	85143	01	082-084	85189	01	023-024, 082-087
85012	01	088-090	85144	01	082-084			
8502	01	088-090	85145	01	082-084	85190	01	023-024, 082-087
8503	01	088-090	85146	01	082-084			
8504	01	088-090	85149	01	082-087	85191	01	023-024, 082-087
8505	01	088-090	85150	01	023-024, 082-087			
8509	01	088-090				85192	01	023-024, 082-087
85100	01	082-087	85151	01	023-024, 082-087			
85101	01	082-087						

DX	MDC	MS-DRG	DX	MDC	MS-DRG	DX	MDC	MS-DRG
85193	01	023-024, 082-084	85240	01	082-087	85415	01	023-024, 082-084
85194	01	023-024, 082-084	85241	01	082-087	85416	01	023-024, 082-084
			85242	01	082-087			
85195	01	023-024, 082-084	85243	01	082-084	85419	01	023-024, 082-087
85196	01	023-024, 082-084	85244	01	082-084	8600	04	199-201
			85245	01	082-084	8601	04	199-201
85199	01	023-024, 082-087	85246	01	082-084	8602	04	199-201
			85249	01	082-087	8603	04	199-201
85200	01	023-024, 082-087	85250	01	082-087	8604	04	199-201
			85251	01	082-087	8605	04	199-201
85201	01	023-024, 082-087	85252	01	082-087	86100	05	314-316
			85253	01	082-084	86101	05	314-316
85202	01	023-024, 082-087	85254	01	082-084	86102	05	314-316
			85255	01	082-084	86103	05	314-316
85203	01	023-024, 082-084	85256	01	082-084	86110	05	314-316
			85259	01	082-087	86111	05	314-316
85204	01	023-024, 082-084	85300	01	023-024, 082-087	86112	05	314-316
						86113	05	314-316
85205	01	023-024, 082-084	85301	01	023-024, 082-087	86120	04	205-206
						86121	04	205-206
85206	01	023-024, 082-084	85302	01	023-024, 082-087	86122	04	183-185
						86130	04	205-206
85209	01	023-024, 082-087	85303	01	023-024, 082-084	86131	04	205-206
						86132	04	183-185
85210	01	023-024, 082-087	85304	01	023-024, 082-084	8620	04	183-185
						8621	04	183-185
85211	01	023-024, 082-087	85305	01	023-024, 082-084	86221	04	183-185
						86222	06	368-370
85212	01	023-024, 082-087	85306	01	023-024, 082-084	86229	04	205-206
						86231	04	183-185
85213	01	023-024, 082-084	85309	01	023-024, 082-087	86232	06	393-395
						86239	04	205-206
85214	01	023-024, 082-084	85310	01	023-024, 082-087	8628	21	913-914
						8629	21	913-914
85215	01	023-024, 082-084	85311	01	023-024, 082-087	8630	06	393-395
						8631	06	393-395
85216	01	023-024, 082-084	85312	01	023-024, 082-087	86320	06	393-395
						86321	06	393-395
85219	01	023-024, 082-087	85313	01	023-024, 082-084	86329	06	393-395
						86330	06	393-395
85220	01	082-087	85314	01	023-024, 082-084	86331	06	393-395
85221	01	082-087				86339	06	393-395
85222	01	082-087	85315	01	023-024, 082-084	86340	06	393-395
85223	01	082-084				86341	06	393-395
85224	01	082-084	85316	01	023-024, 082-084	86342	06	393-395
85225	01	082-084				86343	06	393-395
85226	01	082-084	85319	01	023-024, 082-087	86344	06	393-395
85229	01	082-087	85400	01	082-087	86345	06	393-395
85230	01	023-024, 082-087	85401	01	082-087	86346	06	393-395
			85402	01	082-087	86349	06	393-395
85231	01	023-024, 082-087	85403	01	082-084	86350	06	393-395
			85404	01	082-084	86351	06	393-395
85232	01	023-024, 082-087	85405	01	082-084	86352	06	393-395
			85406	01	082-084	86353	06	393-395
85233	01	023-024, 082-084	85409	01	082-087	86354	06	393-395
			85410	01	023-024, 082-087	86355	06	393-395
85234	01	023-024, 082-084				86356	06	393-395
			85411	01	023-024, 082-087	86359	06	393-395
85235	01	023-024, 082-084	85412	01	023-024, 082-087	86380	06	393-395
						86381	07	438-440
85236	01	023-024, 082-084	85413	01	023-024, 082-084	86382	07	438-440
						86383	07	438-440
85239	01	023-024, 082-087	85414	01	023-024, 082-084	86384	07	438-440
						86385	06	393-395

PART VI, MS-DRG, APPENDIX B

DX	MDC	MS-DRG
86389	06	393-395
86390	06	393-395
86391	07	438-440
86392	07	438-440
86393	07	438-440
86394	07	438-440
86395	06	393-395
86399	06	393-395
86400	07	441-443
86401	07	441-443
86402	07	441-443
86403	07	441-443
86404	07	441-443
86405	07	441-443
86409	07	441-443
86410	07	441-443
86411	07	441-443
86412	07	441-443
86413	07	441-443
86414	07	441-443
86415	07	441-443
86419	07	441-443
86500	16	814-816
86501	16	814-816
86502	16	814-816
86503	16	814-816
86504	16	814-816
86509	16	814-816
86510	16	814-816
86511	16	814-816
86512	16	814-816
86513	16	814-816
86514	16	814-816
86519	16	814-816
86600	11	698-700
86601	11	698-700
86602	11	698-700
86603	11	698-700
86610	11	698-700
86611	11	698-700
86612	11	698-700
86613	11	698-700
8670	11	698-700
8671	11	698-700
8672	11	698-700
8673	11	698-700
8674	13	742-743, 760-761
8675	13	742-743, 760-761
8676	12	729-730
8676	13	742-743, 760-761
8677	12	729-730
8677	13	742-743, 760-761
8678	12	729-730
8678	13	742-743, 760-761
8679	12	729-730
8679	13	742-743, 760-761
86800	06	393-395
86801	10	643-645
86802	07	444-446
86803	06	393-395

DX	MDC	MS-DRG
86804,	11	698-700
86809	21	913-914
86810	06	393-395
86811	10	643-645
86812	07	444-446
86813	06	393-395
86814	11	698-700
86819	21	913-914
8690	21	913-914
8691	21	913-914
8700	02	124-125
8701	02	124-125
8702	02	124-125
8703	02	124-125
8704	02	124-125
8708	02	124-125
8709	02	124-125
8710	02	124-125
8711	02	124-125
8712	02	124-125
8713	02	124-125
8714	02	124-125
8715	02	124-125
8716	02	124-125
8717	02	124-125
8719	02	124-125
87200	03	154-156
87201	03	154-156
87202	03	154-156
87210	03	154-156
87211	03	154-156
87212	03	154-156
87261	03	154-156
87262	03	154-156
87263	03	154-156
87264	03	154-156
87269	03	154-156
87271	03	154-156
87272	03	154-156
87273	03	154-156
87274	03	154-156
87279	03	154-156
8728	03	154-156
8729	03	154-156
8730	09	604-605
8731	09	604-605
87320	03	154-156
87321	03	154-156
87322	03	154-156
87323	03	154-156
87329	03	154-156
87330	03	154-156
87331	03	154-156
87332	03	154-156
87333	03	154-156
87339	03	154-156
87340	09	604-605
87341	09	604-605
87342	09	604-605
87343	03	157-159
87344	03	157-159
87349	09	604-605
87350	09	604-605
87351	09	604-605
87352	09	604-605
87353	03	157-159

DX	MDC	MS-DRG
87354	03	157-159
87359	09	604-605
87360	03	157-159
87361	03	157-159
87362	03	157-159
87363	03	157-159
87364	03	157-159
87365	03	157-159
87369	03	157-159
87370	03	157-159
87371	03	157-159
87372	03	157-159
87373	03	157-159
87374	03	157-159
87375	03	157-159
87379	03	157-159
8738	09	604-605
8739	09	604-605
87400	03	154-156
87401	03	154-156
87402	04	183-185
87410	03	154-156
87411	03	154-156
87412	04	183-185
8742	10	643-645
8743	10	643-645
8744	03	154-156
8745	03	154-156
8748	09	604-605
8749	09	604-605
8750	09	604-605
8751	21	913-914
8760	09	604-605
8761	09	604-605
8770	09	604-605
8771	09	604-605
8780	12	729-730
8781	12	729-730
8782	12	729-730
8783	12	729-730
8784	13	742-743, 760-761
8785	13	742-743, 760-761
8786	13	742-743, 760-761
8787	13	742-743, 760-761
8788	12	729-730
8788	13	742-743, 760-761
8789	12	729-730
8789	13	742-743, 760-761
8790	09	604-605
8791	09	604-605
8792	09	604-605
8793	21	913-914
8794	09	604-605
8795	21	913-914
8796	09	604-605
8797	21	913-914
8798	09	604-605
8799	21	913-914
88000	09	604-605
88001	09	604-605

DX	MDC	MS-DRG	DX	MDC	MS-DRG	DX	MDC	MS-DRG
88002	09	604-605	8972	21	913-914	9032	21	913-914
88003	09	604-605	8973	21	913-914	9033	21	913-914
88009	09	604-605	8974	21	913-914	9034	21	913-914
88010	21	913-914	8975	21	913-914	9035	21	913-914
88011	21	913-914	8976	21	913-914	9038	21	913-914
88012	21	913-914	8977	21	913-914	9039	21	913-914
88013	21	913-914	90000	21	913-914	9040	21	913-914
88019	21	913-914	90001	21	913-914	9041	21	913-914
88020	08	564-566	90002	21	913-914	9042	21	913-914
88021	08	564-566	90003	21	913-914	9043	21	913-914
88022	08	564-566	9001	21	913-914	90440	21	913-914
88023	08	564-566	90081	21	913-914	90441	21	913-914
88029	08	564-566	90082	21	913-914	90442	21	913-914
88100	09	604-605	90089	21	913-914	90450	21	913-914
88101	09	604-605	9009	21	913-914	90451	21	913-914
88102	09	604-605	9010	21	913-914	90452	21	913-914
88110	21	913-914	9011	21	913-914	90453	21	913-914
88111	21	913-914	9012	21	913-914	90454	21	913-914
88112	21	913-914	9013	21	913-914	9046	21	913-914
88120	08	564-566	90140	21	913-914	9047	21	913-914
88121	08	564-566	90141	21	913-914	9048	21	913-914
88122	08	564-566	90142	21	913-914	9049	21	913-914
8820	09	604-605	90181	21	913-914	9050	01	091-093
8821	21	913-914	90182	21	913-914	9051	08	551-552
8822	08	564-566	90183	21	913-914	9052	08	559-561
8830	09	604-605	90189	21	913-914	9053	08	559-561
8831	21	913-914	9019	21	913-914	9054	08	559-561
8832	08	564-566	9020	21	913-914	9055	08	559-561
8840	09	604-605	90210	21	913-914	9056	08	562-563
8841	21	913-914	90211	21	913-914	9057	08	562-563
8842	08	564-566	90219	21	913-914	9058	08	559-561
8850	21	913-914	90220	21	913-914	9059	08	559-561
8851	21	913-914	90221	21	913-914	9060	09	604-605
8860	21	913-914	90222	21	913-914	9061	09	604-605
8861	21	913-914	90223	21	913-914	9062	09	604-605
8870	21	913-914	90224	21	913-914	9063	09	604-605
8871	21	913-914	90225	21	913-914	9064	09	604-605
8872	21	913-914	90226	21	913-914	9065	09	604-605
8873	21	913-914	90227	21	913-914	9066	09	604-605
8874	21	913-914	90229	21	913-914	9067	09	604-605
8875	21	913-914	90231	21	913-914	9068	09	604-605
8876	21	913-914	90232	21	913-914	9069	09	604-605
8877	21	913-914	90233	21	913-914	9070	01	091-093
8900	09	604-605	90234	21	913-914	9071	01	091-093
8901	21	913-914	90239	21	913-914	9072	01	052-053
8902	08	564-566	90240	21	913-914	9073	01	091-093
8910	09	604-605	90241	21	913-914	9074	01	091-093
8911	21	913-914	90242	21	913-914	9075	01	091-093
8912	08	564-566	90249	21	913-914	9079	01	091-093
8920	09	604-605	90250	21	913-914	9080	04	205-206
8921	21	913-914	90251	21	913-914	9081	06	393-395
8922	08	564-566	90252	21	913-914	9082	12	729-730
8930	09	604-605	90253	21	913-914	9082	13	742-743, 760-761
8931	21	913-914	90254	21	913-914			
8932	08	564-566	90255	21	913-914	9083	05	299-301
8940	09	604-605	90256	21	913-914	9084	05	299-301
8941	21	913-914	90259	21	913-914	9085	21	913-914
8942	08	564-566	90281	21	913-914	9086	21	913-914
8950	21	913-914	90282	21	913-914	9089	21	913-914
8951	21	913-914	90287	21	913-914	9090	21	922-923
8960	21	913-914	90289	21	913-914	9091	21	922-923
8961	21	913-914	9029	21	913-914	9092	21	922-923
8962	21	913-914	90300	21	913-914	9093	21	922-923
8963	21	913-914	90301	21	913-914	9094	21	922-923
8970	21	913-914	90302	21	913-914	9095	21	922-923
8971	21	913-914	9031	21	913-914	9099	21	922-923

1558

DX	MDC	MS-DRG	DX	MDC	MS-DRG	DX	MDC	MS-DRG
9100	09	604-605	9166	09	604-605	9248	09	604-605
9101	09	602-603	9167	09	602-603	9249	09	604-605
9102	09	606-607	9168	09	604-605	9251	21	913-914
9103	09	606-607	9169	09	602-603	9252	21	913-914
9104	09	606-607	9170	09	604-605	9260	12	729-730
9105	09	602-603	9171	09	602-603	9260	13	742-743,
9106	09	604-605	9172	09	606-607			760-761
9107	09	602-603	9173	09	602-603	92611	21	913-914
9108	09	604-605	9174	09	606-607	92612	21	913-914
9109	09	602-603	9175	09	602-603	92619	21	913-914
9110	09	604-605	9176	09	604-605	9268	21	913-914
9111	09	602-603	9177	09	602-603	9269	21	913-914
9112	09	606-607	9178	09	604-605	92700	21	913-914
9113	09	602-603	9179	09	602-603	92701	21	913-914
9114	09	606-607	9180	02	124-125	92702	21	913-914
9115	09	602-603	9181	02	124-125	92703	21	913-914
9116	09	604-605	9182	02	124-125	92709	21	913-914
9117	09	602-603	9189	02	124-125	92710	21	913-914
9118	09	604-605	9190	09	604-605	92711	21	913-914
9119	09	602-603	9191	09	602-603	92720	21	913-914
9120	09	604-605	9192	09	606-607	92721	21	913-914
9121	09	602-603	9193	09	602-603	9273	21	913-914
9122	09	604-605	9194	09	606-607	9278	21	913-914
9123	09	602-603	9195	09	602-603	9279	21	913-914
9124	09	606-607	9196	09	604-605	92800	21	913-914
9125	09	602-603	9197	09	602-603	92801	21	913-914
9126	09	604-605	9198	09	604-605	92810	21	913-914
9127	09	602-603	9199	09	602-603	92811	21	913-914
9128	09	604-605	920	09	604-605	92820	21	913-914
9129	09	602-603	9210	02	124-125	92821	21	913-914
9130	09	604-605	9211	02	124-125	9283	21	913-914
9131	09	602-603	9212	02	124-125	9288	21	913-914
9132	09	606-607	9213	02	124-125	9289	21	913-914
9133	09	602-603	9219	02	124-125	9290	21	913-914
9134	09	606-607	9220	09	604-605	9299	21	913-914
9135	09	602-603	9221	09	604-605	9300	02	124-125
9136	09	604-605	9222	09	604-605	9301	02	124-125
9137	09	602-603	92231	09	604-605	9302	02	124-125
9138	09	604-605	92232	09	604-605	9308	02	124-125
9139	09	602-603	92233	09	604-605	9309	02	124-125
9140	09	604-605	9224	12	729-730	931	03	154-156
9141	09	602-603	9224	13	742-743,	932	03	154-156
9142	09	606-607			760-761	9330	03	154-156
9143	09	602-603	9228	09	604-605	9331	03	154-156
9144	09	606-607	9229	09	604-605	9340	04	205-206
9145	09	602-603	92300	09	604-605	9341	04	205-206
9146	09	604-605	92301	09	604-605	9348	04	205-206
9147	09	602-603	92302	09	604-605	9349	04	205-206
9148	09	604-605	92303	09	604-605	9350	03	157-159
9149	09	602-603	92309	09	604-605	9351	06	393-395
9150	09	604-605	92310	09	604-605	9352	06	393-395
9151	09	602-603	92311	09	604-605	936	06	393-395
9152	09	606-607	92320	09	604-605	937	06	393-395
9153	09	602-603	92321	09	604-605	938	06	393-395
9154	09	606-607	9233	09	604-605	9390	11	698-700
9155	09	602-603	9238	09	604-605	9391	13	742-743,
9156	09	604-605	9239	09	604-605			760-761
9157	09	602-603	92400	09	604-605	9392	13	742-743,
9158	09	604-605	92401	09	604-605			760-761
9159	09	602-603	92410	09	604-605	9393	12	729-730
9160	09	604-605	92411	09	604-605	9399	11	698-700
9161	09	602-603	92420	09	604-605	9400	02	124-125
9162	09	606-607	92421	09	604-605	9401	02	124-125
9163	09	602-603	9243	09	604-605	9402	02	124-125
9164	09	606-607	9244	09	604-605	9403	02	124-125
9165	09	602-603	9245	09	604-605	9404	02	124-125

DX	MDC	MS-DRG	DX	MDC	MS-DRG	DX	MDC	MS-DRG
9405	02	124-125	94148	22	927-929, 933-934	94244	22	927-929, 933-934
9409	02	124-125	94149	22	927-929, 933-934	94245	22	927-929, 933-934
94100	22	935						
94101	22	935	94150	22	927-929, 933-934	94249	22	927-929, 933-934
94102	02	124-125	94151	22	927-929, 933-934	94250	22	927-929, 933-934
94103	22	935						
94104	22	935	94152	02	124-125	94251	22	927-929, 933-934
94105	22	935	94153	22	927-929, 933-934			
94106	22	935				94252	22	927-929, 933-934
94107	22	935	94154	22	927-929, 933-934			
94108	22	935				94253	22	927-929, 933-934
94109	22	935	94155	22	927-929, 933-934			
94110	22	935				94254	22	927-929, 933-934
94111	22	935	94156	22	927-929, 933-934			
94112	02	124-125				94255	22	927-929, 933-934
94113	22	935	94157	22	927-929, 933-934			
94114	22	935				94259	22	927-929, 933-934
94115	22	935	94158	22	927-929, 933-934			
94116	22	935				94300	22	935
94117	22	935	94159	22	927-929, 933-934	94301	22	935
94118	22	935				94302	22	935
94119	22	935	94200	22	935	94303	22	935
94120	22	935	94201	22	935	94304	22	935
94121	22	935	94202	22	935	94305	22	935
94122	02	124-125	94203	22	935	94306	22	935
94123	22	935	94204	22	935	94309	22	935
94124	22	935	94205	22	935	94310	22	935
94125	22	935	94209	22	935	94311	22	935
94126	22	935	94210	22	935	94312	22	935
94127	22	935	94211	22	935	94313	22	935
94128	22	935	94212	22	935	94314	22	935
94129	22	935	94213	22	935	94315	22	935
94130	22	927-929, 933-934	94214	22	935	94316	22	935
			94215	22	935	94319	22	935
94131	22	927-929, 933-934	94219	22	935	94320	22	935
			94220	22	935	94321	22	935
94132	02	124-125	94221	22	935	94322	22	935
94133	22	927-929, 933-934	94222	22	935	94323	22	935
			94223	22	935	94324	22	935
94134	22	927-929, 933-934	94224	22	935	94325	22	935
			94225	22	935	94326	22	935
94135	22	927-929, 933-934	94229	22	935	94329	22	935
94136	22	927-929, 933-934	94230	22	927-929, 933-934	94330	22	927-929, 933-934
94137	22	927-929, 933-934	94231	22	927-929, 933-934	94331	22	927-929, 933-934
94138	22	927-929, 933-934	94232	22	927-929, 933-934	94332	22	927-929, 933-934
94139	22	927-929, 933-934	94233	22	927-929, 933-934	94333	22	927-929, 933-934
94140	22	927-929, 933-934	94234	22	927-929, 933-934	94334	22	927-929, 933-934
94141	22	927-929, 933-934	94235	22	927-929, 933-934	94335	22	927-929, 933-934
94142	02	124-125	94239	22	927-929, 933-934	94336	22	927-929, 933-934
94143	22	927-929, 933-934	94240	22	927-929, 933-934	94339	22	927-929, 933-934
94144	22	927-929, 933-934	94241	22	927-929, 933-934	94340	22	927-929, 933-934
94145	22	927-929, 933-934	94242	22	927-929, 933-934	94341	22	927-929, 933-934
94146	22	927-929, 933-934	94243	22	927-929, 933-934	94342	22	927-929, 933-934
94147	22	927-929, 933-934						

DX	MDC	MS-DRG		DX	MDC	MS-DRG		DX	MDC	MS-DRG
94343	22	927-929, 933-934		94436	22	927-929, 933-934		94530	22	927-929, 933-934
94344	22	927-929, 933-934		94437	22	927-929, 933-934		94531	22	927-929, 933-934
94345	22	927-929, 933-934		94438	22	927-929, 933-934		94532	22	927-929, 933-934
94346	22	927-929, 933-934		94440	22	927-929, 933-934		94533	22	927-929, 933-934
94349	22	927-929, 933-934		94441	22	927-929, 933-934		94534	22	927-929, 933-934
94350	22	927-929, 933-934		94442	22	927-929, 933-934		94535	22	927-929, 933-934
94351	22	927-929, 933-934		94443	22	927-929, 933-934		94536	22	927-929, 933-934
94352	22	927-929, 933-934		94444	22	927-929, 933-934		94539	22	927-929, 933-934
94353	22	927-929, 933-934		94445	22	927-929, 933-934		94540	22	927-929, 933-934
94354	22	927-929, 933-934		94446	22	927-929, 933-934		94541	22	927-929, 933-934
94355	22	927-929, 933-934		94447	22	927-929, 933-934		94542	22	927-929, 933-934
94356	22	927-929, 933-934		94448	22	927-929, 933-934		94543	22	927-929, 933-934
94359	22	927-929, 933-934		94450	22	927-929, 933-934		94544	22	927-929, 933-934
94400	22	935		94451	22	927-929, 933-934		94545	22	927-929, 933-934
94401	22	935		94452	22	927-929, 933-934		94546	22	927-929, 933-934
94402	22	935		94453	22	927-929, 933-934		94549	22	927-929, 933-934
94403	22	935		94454	22	927-929, 933-934		94550	22	927-929, 933-934
94404	22	935		94455	22	927-929, 933-934		94551	22	927-929, 933-934
94405	22	935		94456	22	927-929, 933-934		94552	22	927-929, 933-934
94406	22	935		94457	22	927-929, 933-934		94553	22	927-929, 933-934
94407	22	935		94458	22	927-929, 933-934		94554	22	927-929, 933-934
94408	22	935		94500	22	935		94555	22	927-929, 933-934
94410	22	935		94501	22	935		94556	22	927-929, 933-934
94411	22	935		94502	22	935		94559	22	927-929, 933-934
94412	22	935		94503	22	935		9460	22	935
94413	22	935		94504	22	935		9461	22	935
94414	22	935		94505	22	935		9462	22	935
94415	22	935		94506	22	935		9463	22	927-929, 933-934
94416	22	935		94509	22	935		9464	22	927-929, 933-934
94417	22	935		94510	22	935		9465	22	927-929, 933-934
94418	22	935		94511	22	935				
94420	22	935		94512	22	935		9470	03	154-156
94421	22	935		94513	22	935		9471	04	205-206
94422	22	935		94514	22	935		9472	06	368-370
94423	22	935		94515	22	935		9473	06	393-395
94424	22	935		94516	22	935		9474	13	742-743, 760-761
94425	22	935		94519	22	935				
94426	22	935		94520	22	935		9478	22	935
94427	22	935		94521	22	935		9479	22	935
94428	22	935		94522	22	935		94800	22	935
94430	22	927-929, 933-934		94523	22	935				
94431	22	927-929, 933-934		94524	22	935				
94432	22	927-929, 933-934		94525	22	935				
94433	22	927-929, 933-934		94526	22	935				
94434	22	927-929, 933-934		94529	22	935				
94435	22	927-929, 933-934								

DX	MDC	MS-DRG	DX	MDC	MS-DRG	DX	MDC	MS-DRG
94810	22	935	9502	01	091-093	9568	01	073-074
94811	22	927-929, 933-934	9503	01	091-093	9569	01	073-074
			9509	01	091-093	9570	01	073-074
94820	22	935	9510	01	073-074	9571	01	073-074
94821	22	927,933	9511	01	073-074	9578	01	073-074
94822	22	927,933	9512	01	073-074	9579	01	073-074
94830	22	935	9513	01	073-074	9580	04	175-176
94831	22	927,933	9514	01	073-074	9581	04	175-176
94832	22	927,933	9515	03	154-156	9582	21	922-923
94833	22	927,933	9516	01	073-074	9583	18	856-858, 862-863
94840	22	935	9517	01	073-074			
94841	22	927,933	9518	01	073-074	9584	21	922-923
94842	22	927,933	9519	01	073-074	9585	11	673-675, 682-684
94843	22	927,933	95200	01	052-053			
94844	22	927,933	95201	01	052-053	9586	08	564-566
94850	22	935	95202	01	052-053	9587	04	199-201
94851	22	927,933	95203	01	052-053	9588	21	922-923
94852	22	927,933	95204	01	052-053	95890	21	922-923
94853	22	927,933	95205	01	052-053	95891	21	922-923
94854	22	927,933	95206	01	052-053	95892	21	922-923
94855	22	927,933	95207	01	052-053	95893	21	922-923
94860	22	935	95208	01	052-053	95899	21	922-923
94861	22	927,933	95209	01	052-053	95901	21	913-914
94862	22	927,933	95210	01	052-053	95909	21	913-914
94863	22	927,933	95211	01	052-053	95911	21	913-914
94864	22	927,933	95212	01	052-053	95912	21	913-914
94865	22	927,933	95213	01	052-053	95913	21	913-914
94866	22	927,933	95214	01	052-053	95914	21	913-914
94870	22	935	95215	01	052-053	95919	21	913-914
94871	22	927,933	95216	01	052-053	9592	21	913-914
94872	22	927,933	95217	01	052-053	9593	21	913-914
94873	22	927,933	95218	01	052-053	9594	21	913-914
94874	22	927,933	95219	01	052-053	9595	21	913-914
94875	22	927,933	9522	01	052-053	9596	21	913-914
94876	22	927,933	9523	01	052-053	9597	21	913-914
94877	22	927,933	9524	01	052-053	9598	21	913-914
94880	22	935	9528	01	052-053	9599	21	913-914
94881	22	927,933	9529	01	052-053	9600	21	917-918
94882	22	927,933	9530	01	073-074	9601	21	917-918
94883	22	927,933	9531	01	073-074	9602	21	917-918
94884	22	927,933	9532	01	073-074	9603	21	917-918
94885	22	927,933	9533	01	073-074	9604	21	917-918
94886	22	927,933	9534	01	073-074	9605	21	917-918
94887	22	927,933	9535	01	073-074	9606	21	917-918
94888	22	927,933	9538	01	073-074	9607	21	917-918
94890	22	935	9539	01	073-074	9608	21	917-918
94891	22	927,933	9540	01	073-074	9609	21	917-918
94892	22	927,933	9541	01	073-074	9610	21	917-918
94893	22	927,933	9548	01	073-074	9611	21	917-918
94894	22	927,933	9549	01	073-074	9612	21	917-918
94895	22	927,933	9550	01	073-074	9613	21	917-918
94896	22	927,933	9551	01	073-074	9614	21	917-918
94897	22	927,933	9552	01	073-074	9615	21	917-918
94898	22	927,933	9553	01	073-074	9616	21	917-918
94899	22	927,933	9554	01	073-074	9617	21	917-918
9490	22	935	9555	01	073-074	9618	21	917-918
9491	22	935	9556	01	073-074	9619	21	917-918
9492	22	935	9557	01	073-074	9620	21	917-918
9493	22	927-929, 933-934	9558	01	073-074	9621	21	917-918
			9559	01	073-074	9622	21	917-918
9494	22	927-929, 933-934	9560	01	073-074	9623	21	917-918
			9561	01	073-074	9624	21	917-918
9495	22	927-929, 933-934	9562	01	073-074	9625	21	917-918
			9563	01	073-074	9626	21	917-918
9500	02	124-125	9564	01	073-074	9627	21	917-918
9501	01	091-093	9565	01	073-074	9628	21	917-918

DX	MDC	MS-DRG		DX	MDC	MS-DRG		DX	MDC	MS-DRG
9629	21	917-918		9696	21	917-918		9773	21	917-918
9630	21	917-918		96970	21	917-918		9774	21	917-918
9631	21	917-918		96971	21	917-918 ◄		9778	21	917-918
9632	21	917-918		96972	21	917-918 ◄		9779	21	917-918
9633	21	917-918		96973	21	917-918 ◄		9780	21	917-918
9634	21	917-918		96979	21	917-918 ◄		9781	21	917-918
9635	21	917-918		9698	21	917-918		9782	21	917-918
9638	21	917-918		9699	21	917-918		9783	21	917-918
9639	21	917-918		9700	21	917-918		9784	21	917-918
9640	21	917-918		9701	21	917-918		9785	21	917-918
9641	21	917-918		9708	21	917-918		9786	21	917-918
9642	21	917-918		9709	21	917-918		9788	21	917-918
9643	21	917-918		9710	21	917-918		9789	21	917-918
9644	21	917-918		9711	21	917-918		9790	21	917-918
9645	21	917-918		9712	21	917-918		9791	21	917-918
9646	21	917-918		9713	21	917-918		9792	21	917-918
9647	21	917-918		9719	21	917-918		9793	21	917-918
9648	21	917-918		9720	21	917-918		9794	21	917-918
9649	21	917-918		9721	21	917-918		9795	21	917-918
96500	21	917-918		9722	21	917-918		9796	21	917-918
96501	21	917-918		9723	21	917-918		9797	21	917-918
96502	21	917-918		9724	21	917-918		9799	21	917-918
96509	21	917-918		9725	21	917-918		9800	21	917-918
9651	21	917-918		9726	21	917-918		9801	21	917-918
9654	21	917-918		9727	21	917-918		9802	21	917-918
9655	21	917-918		9728	21	917-918		9803	21	917-918
96561	21	917-918		9729	21	917-918		9808	21	917-918
96569	21	917-918		9730	21	917-918		9809	21	917-918
9657	21	917-918		9731	21	917-918		981	21	917-918
9658	21	917-918		9732	21	917-918		9820	21	917-918
9659	21	917-918		9733	21	917-918		9821	21	917-918
9660	21	917-918		9734	21	917-918		9822	21	917-918
9661	21	917-918		9735	21	917-918		9823	21	917-918
9662	21	917-918		9736	21	917-918		9824	21	917-918
9663	21	917-918		9738	21	917-918		9828	21	917-918
9664	21	917-918		9739	21	917-918		9830	21	917-918
9670	21	917-918		9740	21	917-918		9831	21	917-918
9671	21	917-918		9741	21	917-918		9832	21	917-918
9672	21	917-918		9742	21	917-918		9839	21	917-918
9673	21	917-918		9743	21	917-918		9840	21	917-918
9674	21	917-918		9744	21	917-918		9841	21	917-918
9675	21	917-918		9745	21	917-918		9848	21	917-918
9676	21	917-918		9746	21	917-918		9849	21	917-918
9678	21	917-918		9747	21	917-918		9850	21	917-918
9679	21	917-918		9750	21	917-918		9851	21	917-918
9680	21	917-918		9751	21	917-918		9852	21	917-918
9681	21	917-918		9752	21	917-918		9853	21	917-918
9682	21	917-918		9753	21	917-918		9854	21	917-918
9683	21	917-918		9754	21	917-918		9855	21	917-918
9684	21	917-918		9755	21	917-918		9856	21	917-918
9685	21	917-918		9756	21	917-918		9858	21	917-918
9686	21	917-918		9757	21	917-918		9859	21	917-918
9687	21	917-918		9758	21	917-918		986	21	917-918
9689	21	917-918		9760	21	917-918		9870	21	917-918
96900	21	917-918		9761	21	917-918		9871	21	917-918
96901	21	917-918 ◄		9762	21	917-918		9872	21	917-918
96902	21	917-918 ◄		9763	21	917-918		9873	21	917-918
96903	21	917-918 ◄		9764	21	917-918		9874	21	917-918
96904	21	917-918 ◄		9765	02	124-125		9875	21	917-918
96905	21	917-918 ◄		9766	21	917-918		9876	21	917-918
96909	21	917-918 ◄		9767	21	917-918		9877	21	917-918
9691	21	917-918		9768	21	917-918		9878	21	917-918
9692	21	917-918		9769	21	917-918		9879	21	917-918
9693	21	917-918		9770	21	917-918		9880	21	917-918
9694	21	917-918		9771	21	917-918		9881	21	917-918
9695	21	917-918		9772	21	917-918		9882	21	917-918

DX	MDC	MS-DRG	DX	MDC	MS-DRG	DX	MDC	MS-DRG
9888	21	917-918	99553	21	922-923	99667	08	485-487, 559-561
9889	21	917-918	99554	21	922-923			
9890	21	917-918	99555	21	922-923	99668	21	919-921
9891	21	917-918	99559	21	922-923	99669	21	919-921
9892	21	917-918	99560	21	915-916	99670	21	919-921
9893	21	917-918	99561	21	915-916	99671	05	314-316
9894	21	917-918	99562	21	915-916	99672	05	314-316
9895	21	917-918	99563	21	915-916	99673	05	314-316
9896	21	917-918	99564	21	915-916	99674	05	314-316
9897	21	917-918	99565	21	915-916	99675	01	091-093
98981	21	917-918	99566	21	915-916	99676	11	698-700
98982	21	917-918	99567	21	915-916	99677	08	559-561
98983	21	917-918	99568	21	915-916	99678	08	559-561
98984	21	917-918	99569	21	915-916	99679	21	919-921
98989	21	917-918	9957	21	922-923	99680	21	919-921
9899	21	917-918	99580	21	922-923	99681	11	698-700
990	21	922-923	99581	21	922-923	99682	07	441-443
9910	21	922-923	99582	21	922-923	99683	05	314-316
9911	21	922-923	99583	21	922-923	99684	04	205-206
9912	21	922-923	99584	21	922-923	99685	16	808-810
9913	21	922-923	99585	21	922-923	99686	07	438-440
9914	21	922-923	99586	21	922-923	99687	21	919-921
9915	21	922-923	99589	21	922-923	99689	21	919-921
9916	21	922-923	99590	18	870-872	99690	08	559-561
9918	21	922-923	99591	18	870-872	99691	08	559-561
9919	21	922-923	99592	18	870-872	99692	08	559-561
9920	21	922-923	99593	18	870-872	99693	08	559-561
9921	21	922-923	99594	18	870-872	99694	08	559-561
9922	21	922-923	99600	05	314-316	99695	08	559-561
9923	21	922-923	99601	05	308-310	99696	08	559-561
9924	21	922-923	99602	05	306-307	99699	08	559-561
9925	21	922-923	99603	05	314-316	99700	01	091-093
9926	21	922-923	99604	05	308-310	99701	01	091-093
9927	21	922-923	99609	05	314-316	99702	01	091-093
9928	21	922-923	9961	05	314-316	99709	01	091-093
9929	21	922-923	9962	01	091-093	9971	05	314-316
9930	03	152-153	99630	11	698-700	9972	05	299-301
9931	03	152-153	99631	11	698-700	99731	04	205-206
9932	21	922-923	99632	13	742-743, 760-761	99739	04	205-206
9933	21	922-923				9974	06	393-395
9934	21	922-923	99639	11	698-700	9975	11	698-700
9938	21	922-923	99640	08	559-561	99760	08	564-566
9939	21	922-923	99641	08	559-561	99761	08	564-566
9940	21	922-923	99642	08	559-561	99762	08	564-566
9941	21	922-923	99643	08	559-561	99769	08	564-566
9942	21	922-923	99644	08	559-561	99771	06	393-395
9943	21	922-923	99645	08	559-561	99772	11	698-700
9944	21	922-923	99646	08	559-561	99779	05	299-301
9945	21	922-923	99647	08	559-561	99791	21	919-921
9946	03	149	99649	08	559-561	99799	21	919-921
9947	21	922-923	99651	02	124-125	9980	21	919-921
9948	21	922-923	99652	21	919-921	99811	21	919-921
9949	21	922-923	99653	02	124-125	99812	21	919-921
9950	21	915-916	99654	09	600-601	99813	21	919-921
9951	21	915-916	99655	21	919-921	9982	21	919-921
99520	21	917-918	99656	21	919-921	99830	21	919-921
99521	21	917-918	99657	21	919-921	99831	21	919-921
99522	21	917-918	99659	21	919-921	99832	21	919-921
99523	21	917-918	99660	21	919-921	99833	21	919-921
99527	21	917-918	99661	05	314-316	9984	21	919-921
99529	21	917-918	99662	05	314-316	99851	18	856-858, 862-863
9953	21	915-916	99663	01	091-093			
9954	21	922-923	99664	11	698-700	99859	18	856-858, 862-863
99550	21	922-923	99665	11	698-700			
99551	21	922-923	99666	08	485-487, 559-561	9986	21	919-921
99552	21	922-923				9987	21	919-921

DX	MDC	MS-DRG
99881	21	919-921
99882	02	124-125
99883	21	919-921
99889	21	919-921
9989	21	919-921
9990	18	865-866
9991	04	175-176
9992	05	314-316
99931	05	314-316
99939	18	856-858, 867-869
9994	21	915-916
9995	21	915-916
9996	16	811-812
9997	16	811-812
99981	05	314-316
99982	05	314-316
99988	05	314-316
99989	16	811-812
9999	21	919-921
V010	23	951
V0-11	23	951
V012	23	951
V013	23	951
V014	23	951
V015	23	951
V016	23	951
V0171	23	951
V0179	23	951
V0181	23	951
V0182	23	951
V0183	23	951
V0184	23	951
V0189	23	951
V019	23	951
V020	23	951
V021	23	951
V022	23	951
V023	23	951
V024	23	951
V0251	23	951
V0252	23	951
V0253	23	951
V0254	23	951
V0259	23	951
V0260	07	441-443
V0261	07	441-443
V0262	07	441-443
V0269	07	441-443
V027	23	951
V028	23	951
V029	23	951
V030	23	951
V031	23	951
V032	23	951
V033	23	951
V034	23	951
V035	23	951
V036	23	951
V037	23	951
V0381	23	951
V0382	23	951
V0389	23	951
V039	23	951
V040	23	951
V041	23	951
V042	23	951
V043	23	951
V044	23	951
V045	23	951
V046	23	951
V047	23	951
V0481	23	951
V0482	23	951
V0489	23	951
V050	23	951
V051	23	951
V052	23	951
V053	23	951
V054	23	951
V058	23	951
V059	23	951
V060	23	951
V061	23	951
V062	23	951
V063	23	951
V064	23	951
V065	23	951
V066	23	951
V068	23	951
V069	23	951
V070	23	951
V071	23	951
V072	23	951
V0731	23	951
V0739	23	951
V074	23	951
V0751	23	951
V0752	23	951
V0759	23	951
V078	23	951
V079	23	951
V08	18	865-866
V090	18	867-869
V091	18	867-869
V092	18	867-869
V093	18	867-869
V094	18	867-869
V0950	18	867-869
V0951	18	867-869
V096	18	867-869
V0970	18	867-869
V0971	18	867-869
V0980	18	867-869
V0981	18	867-869
V0990	18	867-869
V0991	18	867-869
V1000	17	843-845
V1001	17	843-845
V1002	17	843-845
V1003	17	843-845
V1004	17	843-845
V1005	17	843-845
V1006	17	843-845
V1007	17	843-845
V1009	17	843-845
V1011	17	843-845
V1012	17	843-845
V1020	17	843-845
V1021	17	843-845
V1022	17	843-845
V1029	17	843-845
V103	17	843-845
V1040	17	843-845
V1041	17	843-845
V1042	17	843-845
V1043	17	843-845
V1044	17	843-845
V1045	17	843-845
V1046	17	843-845
V1047	17	843-845
V1048	17	843-845
V1049	17	843-845
V1050	17	843-845
V1051	17	843-845
V1052	17	843-845
V1053	17	843-845
V1059	17	843-845
V1060	17	843-845
V1061	17	843-845
V1062	17	843-845
V1063	17	843-845
V1069	17	843-845
V1071	17	843-845
V1072	17	843-845
V1079	17	843-845
V1081	17	843-845
V1082	17	843-845
V1083	17	843-845
V1084	17	843-845
V1085	17	843-845
V1086	17	843-845
V1087	17	843-845
V1088	17	843-845
V1089	17	843-845
V1090	17	826-830, 843-845
V1091	17	826-830, 843-845
V110	23	951
V111	23	951
V112	23	951
V113	23	951
V118	23	951
V119	23	951
V1200	23	951
V1201	23	951
V1202	23	951
V1203	23	951
V1204	23	951
V1209	23	951
V121	23	951
V122	23	951
V123	23	951
V1240	23	951
V1241	23	951
V1242	23	951
V1249	23	951
V1250	23	951
V1251	23	951
V1252	23	951
V1253	23	951
V1254	23	951
V1259	23	951
V1260	23	951
V1261	23	951
V1269	23	951
V1270	23	951

DX	MDC	MS-DRG	DX	MDC	MS-DRG	DX	MDC	MS-DRG
V1271	23	951	V161	23	951	V220	23	951
V1272	23	951	V162	23	951	V221	23	951
V1279	23	951	V163	23	951	V222	23	951
V1300	23	951	V1640	23	951	V230	14	998
V1301	23	951	V1641	23	951	V231	14	998
V1302	23	951	V1642	23	951	V232	14	998
V1303	23	951	V1643	23	951	V233	14	998
V1309	23	951	V1649	23	951	V2341	14	998
V131	23	951	V1651	23	951	V2349	14	998
V1321	23	951	V1652	23	951	V235	14	998
V1322	17	843-845	V1659	23	951	V237	14	998
V1329	23	951	V166	23	951	V2381	14	998
V133	23	951	V167	23	951	V2382	14	998
V134	23	951	V168	23	951	V2383	14	998
V1351	23	951	V169	23	951	V2384	14	998
V1352	23	951	V170	23	951	V2385	14	998
V1359	23	951	V171	23	951	V2386	14	998
V1361	23	951	V172	23	951	V2389	14	998
V1369	23	951	V173	23	951	V239	14	998
V137	23	951	V1741	23	951	V240	14	769,776
V138	23	951	V1749	23	951	V241	23	951
V139	23	951	V175	23	951	V242	23	951
V140	23	951	V176	23	951	V2501	23	951
V141	23	951	V177	23	951	V2502	23	951
V142	23	951	V1781	23	951	V2503	23	951
V143	23	951	V1789	23	951	V2504	23	951
V144	23	951	V180	23	951	V2509	23	951
V145	23	951	V1811	23	951	V251	23	951
V146	23	951	V1819	23	951	V252	12	729-730
V147	23	951	V182	23	951	V252	13	742-743, 760-761
V148	23	951	V183	23	951			
V149	23	951	V184	23	951	V253	13	742-743, 760-761
V1501	23	951	V1851	23	951			
V1502	23	951	V1859	23	951	V2540	23	951
V1503	23	951	V1861	23	951	V2541	23	951
V1504	23	951	V1869	23	951	V2542	23	951
V1505	23	951	V187	23	951	V2543	23	951
V1506	23	951	V188	23	951	V2549	23	951
V1507	23	951	V189	23	951	V255	23	951
V1508	23	951	V190	23	951	V258	23	951
V1509	23	951	V191	23	951	V259	23	951
V151	23	951	V192	23	951	V260	12	729-730
V1521	23	951	V193	23	951	V260	13	742-743, 760-761
V1522	23	951	V194	23	951			
V1529	23	951	V195	23	951	V261	23	951
V153	23	951	V196	23	951	V2621	23	951
V1541	23	951	V197	23	951	V2622	23	951
V1542	23	951	V198	23	951	V2629	23	951
V1549	23	951	V200	23	951	V2631	23	951
V1551	23	951	V201	23	951	V2632	23	951
V1552	23	951 ◄	V202	23	951	V2633	23	951
V1559	23	951	V2031	153	795 ◄	V2634	23	951
V156	23	951		23	951	V2635	23	951
V157	23	951	V2032	153	795 ◄	V2639	23	951
V1580	23	951 ◄		23	951	V2641	23	951
V1581	23	951	V210	23	951	V2642	23	951 ◄
V1582	23	951	V211	23	951	V2649	23	951
V1583	23	951 ◄	V212	23	951	V2651	23	951
V1584	23	951	V2130	23	951	V2652	23	951
V1585	23	951	V2131	23	951	V2681	23	951
V1586	23	951	V2132	23	951	V2682	23	951 ◄
V1587	23	951	V2133	23	951	V2689	23	951
V1588	23	951	V2134	23	951	V269	23	951
V1589	23	951	V2135	23	951	V270	23	951
V159	23	951	V218	23	951	V271	23	951
V160	23	951	V219	23	951	V272	23	951

DX	MDC	MS-DRG		DX	MDC	MS-DRG		DX	MDC	MS-DRG
V273	23	951		V412	23	951		V4559	23	951
V274	23	951		V413	23	951		V4561	23	951
V275	23	951		V414	23	951		V4569	23	951
V276	23	951		V415	23	951		V4571	23	951
V277	23	951		V416	23	951		V4572	23	951
V279	23	951		V417	23	951		V4573	23	951
V280	14	781-782		V418	23	951		V4574	11	698-700
V281	14	781-782		V419	23	951		V4575	23	951
V282	14	781-782		V420	11	698-700		V4576	04	205-206
V283	23	951		V421	05	314-316		V4577	12	729-730
V284	23	951		V422	05	314-316		V4577	13	742-743,
V285	23	951		V423	09	606-607				760-761
V286	23	951		V424	08	564-566		V4578	02	124-125
V2881	23	951		V425	02	124-125		V4579	23	951
V2882	23	951		V426	04	205-206		V4581	23	951
V2889	23	951		V427	07	441-443		V4582	23	951
V289	23	951		V4281	16	814-816		V4583	23	951
V290	23	951		V4282	16	814-816		V4584	23	951
V291	23	951		V4283	07	438-440		V4585	23	951
V292	23	951		V4284	23	951		V4586	23	951
V293	23	951		V4289	23	951		V4587	23	951
V298	23	951		V429	23	951		V4588	23	951
V299	23	951		V430	02	124-125		V4589	23	951
V3000	15	795		V431	02	124-125		V460	23	951
V3001	15	795		V4321	05	314-316		V4611	23	951
V301	15	795		V4322	05	314-316		V4612	23	951
V302	15	998		V433	05	314-316		V4613	23	951
V3100	15	795		V434	05	314-316		V4614	23	951
V3101	15	795		V435	11	698-700		V462	23	951
V311	15	795		V4360	08	564-566		V463	23	951
V312	15	998		V4361	08	564-566		V468	23	951
V3200	15	795		V4362	08	564-566		V469	23	951
V3201	15	795		V4363	08	564-566		V470	23	951
V321	15	795		V4364	08	564-566		V471	23	951
V322	15	998		V4365	08	564-566		V472	23	951
V3300	15	795		V4366	08	564-566		V473	23	951
V330f	15	795		V4369	08	564-566		V474	23	951
V331	15	795		V437	08	564-566		V475	23	951
V332	15	998		V4381	23	951		V479	23	951
V3400	15	795		V4382	23	951		V480	23	951
V3401	15	795		V4383	23	951		V481	23	951
V341	15	795		V4389	23	951		V482	23	951
V342	15	998		V440	23	951		V483	23	951
V3500	15	795		V441	23	951		V484	23	951
V3501	15	795		V442	23	951		V485	23	951
V351	15	795		V443	23	951		V486	23	951
V352	15	998		V444	23	951		V487	23	951
V3600	15	795		V4450	23	951		V488	23	951
V3601	15	795		V4451	23	951		V489	23	951
V361	15	795		V4452	23	951		V490	23	951
V362	15	998		V4459	23	951		V491	23	951
V3700	15	795		V446	23	951		V492	23	951
V3701	15	795		V447	23	951		V493	23	951
V371	15	795		V448	23	951		V494	23	951
V372	15	998		V449	23	951		V495	23	951
V3900	15	795		V4500	23	951		V4960	23	951
V3901	15	795		V4501	23	951		V4961	23	951
V391	15	795		V4502	23	951		V4962	23	951
V392	15	998		V4509	23	951		V4963	23	951
V400	23	951		V4511	23	951		V4964	23	951
V401	23	951		V4512	23	951		V4965	23	951
V402	23	951		V452	23	951		V4966	23	951
V403	23	951		V453	23	951		V4967	23	951
V409	23	951		V454	23	951		V4970	23	951
V410	23	951		V4551	23	951		V4971	23	951
V411	23	951		V4552	23	951		V4972	23	951

DX	MDC	MS-DRG
V4973	23	951
V4974	23	951
V4975	23	951
V4976	23	951
V4977	23	951
V4981	23	951
V4982	23	951
V4983	23	951
V4984	23	951
V4985	23	951
V4989	23	951
V499	23	951
V500	09	606-607
V501	09	606-607
V502	12	727-728
V503	23	951
V5041	09	600-601
V5042	13	742-743, 760-761
V5049	23	951
V508	23	951
V509	23	951
V510	09	606-607
V518	09	606-607
V520	08	559-561
V521	08	559-561
V522	23	951
V523	23	951
V524	23	951
V528	23	945-946
V529	23	945-946
V5301	01	091-093
V5302	01	091-093
V5309	01	091-093
V531	23	951
V532	23	951
V5331	05	314-316
V5332	05	314-316
V5339	05	314-316
V534	23	951
V5350	06	393-395
V5351	06	393-395 ◀
V5359	06	393-395 ◀
V536	11	698-700
V537	08	559-561
V538	23	951
V5390	23	951
V5391	23	951
V5399	23	951
V5401	08	559-561
V5402	08	559-561
V5409	08	559-561
V5410	08	559-561
V5411	08	559-561
V5412	08	559-561
V5413	08	559-561
V5414	08	559-561
V5415	08	559-561
V5416	08	559-561
V5417	08	559-561
V5419	08	559-561
V5420	08	559-561
V5421	08	559-561
V5422	08	559-561
V5423	08	559-561
V5424	08	559-561

DX	MDC	MS-DRG
V5425	08	559-561
V5426	08	559-561
V5427	08	559-561
V5429	08	559-561
V5481	08	559-561
V5489	08	559-561
V549	08	559-561
V550	04	205-206
V551	06	393-395
V552	06	393-395
V553	06	393-395
V554	06	393-395
V555	11	698-700
V556	11	698-700
V557	13	742-743, 760-761
V558	23	951
V559	23	951
V560	11	685
V561	11	685
V562	11	685
V5631	11	685
V5632	11	685
V568	11	685
V570	23	951
V571	23	945-946
V5721	23	945-946
V5722	23	945-946
V573	23	945-946
V574	23	951
V5781	23	951
V5789	23	945-946
V579	23	945-946
V580	17	849
V5811	17	837-839, 846-848
V5812	17	837-839, 846-848
V582	23	951
V5830	23	951
V5831	23	951
V5832	23	951
V5841	23	949-950
V5842	23	949-950
V5843	23	949-950
V5844	23	949-950
V5849	23	949-950
V585	23	949-950
V5861	23	949-950
V5862	23	949-950
V5863	23	949-950
V5864	23	949-950
V5865	23	949-950
V5866	23	949-950
V5867	23	949-950
V5869	23	949-950
V5871	23	949-950
V5872	23	949-950
V5873	23	949-950
V5874	23	949-950
V5876	23	949-950
V5877	23	949-950
V5878	23	949-950
V5881	23	949-950
V5882	23	949-950
V5883	23	949-950

DX	MDC	MS-DRG
V5889	23	949-950
V589	23	949-950
V5901	23	951
V5902	23	951
V5909	23	951
V591	09	606-607
V592	08	564-566
V593	23	951
V594	11	698-700
V595	23	951
V596	07	441-443
V5970	23	951
V5971	23	951
V5972	23	951
V5973	23	951
V5974	23	951
V598	23	951
V599	23	951
V600	23	951
V601	23	951
V602	23	951
V603	23	951
V604	23	951
V605	23	951
V606	23	951
V6081	23	951
V6089	23	951 ◀
V609	23	951
V6101	23	951
V6102	23	951
V6103	23	951
V6104	23	951
V6105	23	951
V6106	23	951
V6107	23	951 ◀
V6108	23	951 ◀
V6109	23	951
V6110	23	951
V6111	23	951
V6112	23	951
V6120	23	951
V6121	23	951
V6122	23	951
V6123	23	951 ◀
V6124	23	951 ◀
V6125	23	951 ◀
V6129	23	951
V613	23	951
V6141	23	951
V6142	23	951 ◀
V6149	23	951
V615	13	742-743, 760-761
V616	14	781-782
V617	14	770,779
V618	23	951
V619	23	951
V620	23	951
V621	23	951
V6221	23	951
V6222	23	951
V6229	23	951
V623	23	951
V624	23	951
V625	23	951
V626	23	951

PART VI, MS-DRG, APPENDIX B

DX	MDC	MS-DRG
V6281	23	951
V6282	23	951
V6283	23	951
V6284	19	880
V6289	23	951
V629	23	951
V630	23	951
V631	23	951
V632	23	951
V638	23	951
V639	23	951
V6400	23	951
V6401	23	951
V6402	23	951
V6403	23	951
V6404	23	951
V6405	23	951
V6406	23	951
V6407	23	951
V6408	23	951
V6409	23	951
V641	23	951
V642	23	951
V643	23	951
V6441	23	951
V6442	23	951
V6443	23	951
V650	23	951
V6511	23	951
V6519	23	951
V652	23	951
V653	23	951
V6540	23	951
V6541	23	951
V6542	23	951
V6543	23	951
V6544	23	951
V6545	23	951
V6546	23	951
V6549	23	951
V655	23	951
V658	23	951
V659	23	951
V660	23	951
V661	23	951
V662	23	951
V663	23	951
V664	23	951
V665	23	951
V666	23	951
V667	23	951
V669	23	951
V6700	23	949-950
V6701	23	949-950
V6709	23	949-950
V671	17	849
V672	17	837-839, 846-848
V673	23	951
V674	23	949-950
V6751	23	951
V6759	23	951
V676	23	951
V679	23	951
V6801	23	951
V6809	23	951

DX	MDC	MS-DRG
V681	23	951
V682	23	951
V6881	23	951
V6889	23	951
V689	23	951
V690	23	951
V691	23	951
V692	23	951
V693	23	951
V694	23	951
V695	23	951
V698	23	951
V699	23	951
V700	23	951
V701	23	951
V702	23	951
V703	23	951
V704	23	951
V705	23	951
V706	23	951
V707	23	951
V708	23	951
V709	23	951
V7101	19	880
V7102	19	880
V7109	19	887
V711	17	843-845
V712	04	177-179
V713	21	922-923
V714	21	922-923
V715	23	951
V716	21	922-923
V717	05	313
V7181	23	951
V7182	23	951
V7183	23	951
V7189	23	951
V719	23	951
V720	23	951
V7211	23	951
V7212	23	951
V7219	23	951
V722	23	951
V7231	23	951
V7232	23	951
V7240	23	951
V7241	23	951
V7242	23	951
V725	23	951
V7260	23	951
V7261	23	951 ◄
V7262	23	951 ◄
V7263	23	951 ◄
V7269	23	951 ◄
V727	23	951
V7281	23	951
V7282	23	951
V7283	23	951
V7284	23	951
V7285	23	951
V7286	23	951
V729	23	951
V730	23	951
V731	23	951
V732	23	951
V733	23	951

DX	MDC	MS-DRG
V734	23	951
V735	23	951
V736	23	951
V7381	23	951
V7388	23	951
V7389	23	951
V7398	23	951
V7399	23	951
V740	23	951
V741	23	951
V742	23	951
V743	23	951
V744	23	951
V745	23	951
V746	23	951
V748	23	951
V749	23	951
V750	23	951
V751	23	951
V752	23	951
V753	23	951
V754	23	951
V755	23	951
V756	23	951
V757	23	951
V758	23	951
V759	23	951
V760	23	951
V7610	23	951
V7611	23	951
V7612	23	951
V7619	23	951
V762	23	951
V763	23	951
V7641	23	951
V7642	23	951
V7643	23	951
V7644	23	951
V7645	23	951
V7646	23	951
V7647	23	951
V7649	23	951
V7650	23	951
V7651	23	951
V7652	23	951
V7681	23	951
V7689	23	951
V769	23	951
V770	23	951
V771	23	951
V772	23	951
V773	23	951
V774	23	951
V775	23	951
V776	23	951
V777	23	951
V778	23	951
V7791	23	951
V7799	23	951
V780	23	951
V781	23	951
V782	23	951
V783	23	951
V788	23	951
V789	23	951
V790	23	951

DX	MDC	MS-DRG		DX	MDC	MS-DRG		DX	MDC	MS-DRG	
V791	23	951		V8381	23	951		V860	23	951	
V792	23	951		V8389	23	951		V861	23	951	
V793	23	951		V8401	23	951		V8701	23	951	
V798	23	951		V8402	23	951		V8709	23	951	
V799	23	951		V8403	23	951		V8711	23	951	
V8001	23	951		V8404	23	951		V8712	23	951	
V8009	23	951	◄	V8409	23	951		V8719	23	951	
V801	23	951		V8481	23	951		V872	23	951	
V802	23	951		V8489	23	951		V8731	23	951	
V803	23	951		V850	23	951		V8732	23	951	◄
V810	23	951		V851	23	951		V8739	23	951	
V811	23	951		V8521	23	951		V8741	23	949-950	
V812	23	951		V8522	23	951		V8742	23	949-950	
V813	23	951		V8523	23	951		V8743	23	949-950	◄
V814	23	951		V8524	23	951		V8744	23	949-950	◄
V815	23	951		V8525	23	951		V8745	23	949-950	◄
V816	23	951		V8530	23	951		V8746	23	949-950	◄
V820	23	951		V8531	23	951		V8749	23	949-950	
V821	23	951		V8532	23	951		V8801	13	742-743, 760-761	
V822	23	951		V8533	23	951					
V823	23	951		V8534	23	951		V8802	13	742-743, 760-761	
V824	23	951		V8535	23	951					
V825	23	951		V8536	23	951		V8803	13	742-743, 760-761	
V826	23	951		V8537	23	951					
V8271	23	951		V8538	23	951		V8901	23	951	
V8279	23	951		V8539	23	951		V8902	23	951	
V8281	23	951		V854	10	640-641		V8903	23	951	
V8289	23	951		V8551	23	951		V8904	23	951	
V829	23	951		V8552	23	951		V8905	23	951	
V8301	23	951		V8553	23	951		V8909	23	951	
V8302	23	951		V8554	23	951					

MS-DRG, APPENDIX C

Complications or Comorbidities Exclusion List

Appendix C is a list of all of the codes that are defined as either a complication or comorbidity (CC) or a major complication or comorbidity (MCC) when used as a secondary diagnosis.

These codes are shown in bold print. Following each CC or MCC code is a list of diagnosis codes that, when used as the principal diagnosis, will cause the CC or MCC to be considered as only a non CC.

For any CC or MCC allowed with all principal diagnoses, the phrase "No Exclusions" follows the code.

In addition to the exclusion list, based on principal diagnosis, the following MCC exclusions also apply:

Diagnoses codes 42741 (Ventricular fibrillation), 4275 (Cardiac arrest), 78551 (Cardiogenic shock), 78559 (Other shock without mention of trauma) and 7991 (Respiratory arrest) are assigned as a major CC only for patients discharged alive, otherwise they will be assigned as a non CC.

The CC & MCC are designated within the text and not listed separately.

MS-DRG Surgical Hierarchy by MDC and MS-DRG

Since patients can have multiple procedures related to their principal diagnosis during a particular hospital stay, and a patient can be assigned to only one surgical class, the surgical classes in each MDC are defined in a hierarchical order. Patients with multiple procedures are assigned to the highest surgical class in the hierarchy to which one of the procedures is assigned. Thus, if a patient receives both a D&C and a hysterectomy, the patient is assigned to the hysterectomy surgical class because a hysterectomy is higher in the hierarchy than a D&C. Because of the surgical hierarchy, ordering of the surgical procedures on the patient abstract or claim has no influence on the assignment of the surgical class and the MS-DRG.

The surgical hierarchy for each MDC reflects the relative resource requirements of various surgical procedures. In some cases a surgical class in the hierarchy is actually an MS-DRG. For example, Arthroscopy is both a surgical class in the hierarchy and MS-DRG 509 in MDC 8, Diseases and Disorders of the Musculoskeletal System and Connective Tissue. In other cases the surgical class in the hierarchy is further partitioned based on other variables such as complications and comorbidities, or principal diagnosis to form multiple MS-DRGs. As an example, in MDC 5, Diseases and Disorders of the Circulatory System, the surgical class for permanent pacemaker implantation is divided into three MS-DRGs (242-244) based on whether or not the patient had no CCs, a CC or an MCC.

Appendix D presents the surgical hierarchy for each MDC. Appendix D is organized by MDC with a list of the surgical classes associated with that MDC listed in hierarchical order as well as the MS-DRGs that are included in each surgical class. The names given to the surgical classes in the hierarchy correspond to the names used in the MS-DRG logic tables and in the body of the Definitions Manual.

	MS-DRG
PRE MDC	
Heart Transplant or Implant of Heart Assist System	001-002
ECMO or Tracheostomy with MV 96+ Hours or PDX Except Face, Mouth and Neck	003-004
Liver or Intestinal Transplant	005-006
Lung Transplant	007
Simultaneous Pancreas/Kidney Transplant	008
Bone Marrow Transplant	009
Pancreas Transplant	010
Tracheostomy for Face, Mouth and Neck Diagnoses	011-013
MULTIPLE SIGNIFICANT TRAUMA	955-959
HIV INFECTION	969-970
MDC 01, DISEASES AND DISORDERS OF THE NERVOUS SYSTEM	
Intracranial Vascular Procedures with PDX Hemorrhage	020-022
Craniotomy	023-027
Spinal Procedures	028-030
Ventricular Shunt Procedures	031-033
Carotid Artery Stent Procedures	034-036
Extracranial Procedures	037-039
Peripheral and Cranial Nerve and Other Nervous System Procedures	040-042
MDC 02, DISEASES AND DISORDERS OF THE EYE	
Orbital Procedures	113-114
Extraocular Procedures Except Orbit	115
Intraocular Procedures	116-117
MDC 03, DISEASES AND DISORDERS OF THE EAR, NOSE, MOUTH AND THROAT	
Major Head and Neck Procedures	129-130
Cranial/facial Procedures	131-132
Other Ear, Nose, Mouth and Throat O.R. Procedures	133-134
Sinus and Mastoid Procedures	135-136
Mouth Procedures	137-138
Salivary Gland Procedures	139
MDC 04, DISEASES AND DISORDERS OF THE RESPIRATORY SYSTEM	
Major Chest Procedures	163-165
Other Respiratory System O.R. Procedures	166-168
MDC 05, DISEASES AND DISORDERS OF THE CIRCULATORY SYSTEM	
Other Heart Assist System Implant	215
Cardiac Valve and Other Major Cardiothoracic Procedures	216-221
Cardiac Defibrillator Implant	222-227
Other Cardiothoracic Procedures	228-230
Coronary Bypass	231-236
Major Cardiovascular Procedures	237-238
Amputation for Circulatory System Disorders Except Upper Limb and Toe	239-241
Permanent Cardiac Pacemaker Implant	242-244
AICD Generator Procedures	245
AICD Lead Procedures	265
Percutaneous Cardiovascular Procedures with Coronary Artery Stent	246-249
Percutaneous Cardiovasc Procedures without Coronary Artery Stent	250-251
Other Vascular Procedures	252-254
Upper Limb and Toe Amputation for Circulatory System Disorders	255-257
Cardiac Pacemaker Device Replacement	258-259
Cardiac Pacemaker Revision Except Device Replacement	260-262
Vein Ligation and Stripping	263
Other Circulatory System O.R. Procedures	264

PART VI, MS-DRG, APPENDIX D

	MS-DRG
MDC 06, DISEASES AND DISORDERS OF THE DIGESTIVE SYSTEM	
Stomach, Esophageal and Duodenal Procedures	326-328
Major Small and Large Bowel Procedures	329-331
Rectal Resection	332-334
Peritoneal Adhesiolysis	335-337
Appendectomy	338-343
Minor Small and Large Bowel Procedures	344-346
Anal and Stomal Procedures	347-349
Inguinal and Femoral Hernia Procedures	350-352
Hernia Procedures Except Inguinal and Femoral	353-355
Other Digestive System O.R. Procedures	356-358
MDC 07, DISEASES AND DISORDERS OF THE HEPATOBILIARY SYSTEM AND PANCREAS	
Pancreas, Liver and Shunt Procedures	405-407
Biliary Tract Procedures Except Only Cholecystectomy with or without C.D.E.	408-410
Cholecystectomy	411-419
Hepatobiliary Diagnostic Procedures	420-422
Other Hepatobiliary or Pancreas O.R. Procedures	423-425
MDC 08, DISEASES AND DISORDERS OF THE MUSCULOSKELETAL SYSTEM AND CONNECTIVE TISSUE	
Combined Anterior/Posterior Spinal Fusion	453-455
Spinal Fusion Except Cervical with Spinal Curvature / Malignancy / Infection or 9+ Fusions	456-458
Spinal Fusion Except Cervical	459-460
Bilateral or Multiple Major Joint Procedures of Lower Extremity	461-462
Wound Debridement and Skin Graft Except Hand, for Musculoskeletal and Connective Tissue Disorders	463-465
Revision of Hip or Knee Replacement	466-468
Major Joint Replacement or Reattachment of Lower Extremity	469-470
Cervical Spinal Fusion	471-473
Amputation for Musculoskeletal System and Connective Tissue Disorders	474-476
Biopsies of Musculoskeletal System and Connective Tissue	477-479
Hip and Femur Procedures Except Major Joint	480-482
Major Joint and Limb Reattachment Procedures of Upper Extremity	483-484
Knee Procedures	485-489
Back and Neck Procedures, Except Spinal Fusion, or Disc Devices/Neurostimulators	490-491
Lower Extremity and Humerus Procedures Except Hip,Foot,Femur	492-494
Local Excision and Removal Int Fix Devices Except Hip and Femur	495-497
Local Excision and Removal Int Fix Devices of Hip and Femur	498-499
Soft Tissue Procedures	500-502
Foot Procedures	503-505
Major Thumb or Joint Procedures	506
Major Shoulder or Elbow Joint Procedures	507-508
Arthroscopy	509
Shoulder, Elbow or Forearm Procedures, Except Major Joint Procedures	510-512
Hand or Wrist Procedures, Except Major Thumb or Joint Procedures	513-514
Other Musculoskeletal System and Connective Tissue O.R. Procedures	515-517
MDC 09, DISEASES AND DISORDERS OF THE SKIN, SUBCUTANEOUS TISSUE AND BREAST	
Skin Graft and/or Debridment	573-578
Other Skin, Subcutaneous Tissue and Breast Procedures	579-581
Mastectomy for Malignancy	582-583
Breast Biopsy, Local Excision and Other Breast Procedures	584-585

	MS-DRG
MDC 10, ENDOCRINE, NUTRITIONAL AND METABOLIC DISEASES AND DISORDERS	
Adrenal and Pituitary Procedures	614-615
Amputation of Lower Limb for Endocrine,Nutritional, and Metabolic Disorders	616-618
O.R. Procedures for Obesity	619-621
Skin Grafts and Wound Debridment for Endocrine, Nutritional and Metabolic Disorders	622-624
Thyroid, Parathyroid and Thyroglossal Procedures	625-627
Other Endocrine, Nutritional and Metabolic O.R. Procedures	628-630
MDC 11, DISEASES AND DISORDERS OF THE KIDNEY AND URINARY TRACT	
Kidney Transplant	652
Major Bladder Procedures	653-655
Kidney and Ureter Procedures	656-661
Minor Bladder Procedures	662-664
Prostatectomy	665-667
Transurethral Procedures	668-670
Urethral Procedures	671-672
Other Kidney and Urinary Tract Procedures	673-675
MDC 12, DISEASES AND DISORDERS OF THE MALE REPRODUCTIVE SYSTEM	
Major Male Pelvic Procedures	707-708
Penis Procedures	709-710
Testes Procedures	711-712
Transurethral Prostatectomy	713-714
Other Male Reproductive System O.R. Procedures	715-718
MDC 13, DISEASES AND DISORDERS OF THE FEMALE REPRODUCTIVE SYSTEM	
Pelvic Evisceration, Radical Hysterectomy and Radical Vulvectomy	734-735
Uterine and Adnexal Procedures for Malignancy	736-741
Uterine and Adnexal Procedures for Non-Malignancy	742-743
D&C, Conization, Laparascopy and Tubal Interruption	744-745
Vagina, Cervix and Vulva Procedures	746-747
Female Reproductive System Reconstructive Procedures	748
Other Female Reproductive System O.R. Procedures	749-750
MDC 14, PREGNANCY, CHILDBIRTH AND THE PUERPERIUM	
Cesarean Section	765-766
Vaginal Delivery with O.R. Procedure	767-768
Postpartum and Post Abortion Diagnoses with O.R. Procedure	769
Abortion with D&C, Aspiration Curettage or Hysterotomy	770
MDC 15, NEWBORNS AND OTHER NEONATES WITH CONDITION ORIGINATING IN PERINATAL PERIOD	
None	
MDC 16, DISEASES AND DISORDERS OF BLOOD, BLOOD FORMING ORGANS, IMMUNOLOGICAL DISORDERS	
Splenectomy	799-801
Other O.R. Procedures of the Blood and Blood Forming Organs	802-804
MDC 17, MYELOPROLIFERATIVE DISEASES AND DISORDERS, POORLY DIFFERENTIATED NEOPLASM	
Lymphoma and Leukemia with Major O.R. Procedure	820-822
Lymphoma and Non-Acute Leukemia with Other O.R. Procedure	823-825
Myeloproliferative Disorders or Poorly Differentiated Neoplasms	826-830
MDC 18, INFECTIOUS AND PARASITIC DISEASES, SYSTEMIC OR UNSPECIFIED SITES	
Postoperative or Post-Traumatic Infections with O.R. Procedure	856-858
Infectious and Parasitic Diseases with O.R. Procedure	853-855
MDC 19, MENTAL DISEASES AND DISORDERS	
O.R. Procedure with Principal Diagnoses of Mental Illness	876

	MS-DRG
MDC 20, ALCOHOL/DRUG USE AND ALCOHOL/DRUG INDUCED ORGANIC MENTAL DISORDERS	
None	
MDC 21, INJURIES, POISONINGS AND TOXIC EFFECTS OF DRUGS	
Wound Debridements for Injuries	901-903
Skin Grafts for Injuries	904-905
Hand Procedures for Injuries	906
Other O.R. Procedures for Injuries	907-909
MDC 22, BURNS	
Extensive Burns or Full Thickness Burns with MV 96+ Hours with Skin Graft	927
Full Thickness Burns with Skin Graft	928-929
MDC 23, FACTORS INFLUENCING HEALTH STATUS AND OTHER CONTACTS WITH HEALTH SERVICES	
O.R. Procedures with Diagnoses of Other Contact with Health Services	939-941
MDC 24, MULTIPLE SIGNIFICANT TRAUMA	
Craniotomy for Multiple Significant Trauma	955
Limb Reattachment, Hip and Femur Procedures for Multiple Significant Trauma	956
Other O.R. Procedures for Multiple Significant Trauma	957-959
MDC 25, HUMAN IMMUNODEFICIENCY VIRUS INFECTIONS	
HIV with Extensive O.R. Procedure	969-970

MS-DRG, APPENDIX E

MS-DRG, Procedure Code/ MS-DRG Tables

The Procedure Code/MS-DRG Index is a reference source of all ICD-9-CM procedure codes that affect MS-DRG assignment, the MDCs and MS-DRGs to which they are assigned, and a description of the surgical categories. The procedure codes are listed in code order with an asterisk indicating the non-operating room procedures. All procedures without an asterisk are considered *OPERATING ROOM PROCEDURES* by the MS-DRGs.

The first section of Appendix E contains the Pacemaker Lead/Device Reference Table, the Cardioverter-Defibrillator Lead(s) Generator Reference Table, the Abdominal Aorta/Thoracic Vessel Resection Reference Table, the Spinal Fusion Reference Table, the Pancreas Transplant Reference Table, and the Lead/Device Reference Table. The Pacemaker Lead/Device Reference Table lists codes for the initial insertion of permanent pacemaker leads and devices with their associated code descriptions. Following this list are pairs of codes, one lead and one device code, that must be used in combination in order to code the initial implantation of a permanent cardiac pacemaker.

For example, procedure codes: 3770, 3771, 3772, 3773, 3781, 3782, and 2783 are not considered operating room procedures by the MS-DRGs unless used in combination with their related codes. If used singularly, these codes will be ignored for the purpose of MS-DRG assignment:

The Abdominal Aorta/Thoracic Vessel Resection Reference Table lists codes for Abdominal Aorta and Thoracic Vessel resection with their associated code descriptions and MS-DRG assignment.

The Cardioverter-Defibrillator Lead(s)/Generator Reference Table lists codes for the implantation and replacement of automatic cardioverter-defibrillator lead(s) and generator, with their associated code descriptions and MS-DRG assignment.

The Spinal Fusion Reference Table lists codes for Spinal Fusion and Combined Anterior/ Posterior Spinal Fusion with their associated code descriptions and MS-DRG assignment.

The Pancreas Transplant Reference Table lists codes for Simultaneous Pancreas/Kidney Transplant and Pancreas Transplant with their associated code descriptions and MS-DRG assignment.

The Lead/Device Reference Table lists codes for the insertion and replacement of a intracardiac hemodynamic monitoring sensor and device, with their associated code descriptions and MS-DRG assignment.

TABLE 1 PACEMAKER LEAD/DEVICE REFERENCE TABLE

3770	Int insert pacemak lead	3781	Int insert 1-cham, non
3771	Int insert lead in vent	3782	Int insert 1-cham, rate
3772	Int inser lead atri-vent	3783	Int insert dual-cham dev
3773	Int inser lead in atrium	3785	Repl pacem w 1-cham, non
3774	Int or repl lead epicar	3786	Repl pacem 1-cham, rate
3776	Repl tv atri-vent lead	3787	Repl pacem w dual-cham
3780	Int or repl perm pacemkr		

LEAD DEVICE	MDC	MS-DRG	SURGICAL CATEGORY
3770 & 3780	01	040-042	Periph/Cranial Nerve & Other
	05	242-244	Cardiac Pacemaker Implant
	21	907-909	Other Procs for Injuries
3770 & 3781	01	040-042	Periph/Cranial Nerve & Other
	05	242-244	Cardiac Pacemaker Implant
	21	907-909	Other Procs for Injuries
3770 & 3782	01	040-042	Periph/Cranial Nerve & Other
	05	242-244	Cardiac Pacemaker Implant
	21	907-909	Other Procs for Injuries
3770 & 3785	01	040-042	Periph/Cranial Nerve & Other
	05	242-244	Cardiac Pacemaker Implant
	21	907-909	Other Procs for Injuries
3770 & 3786	01	040-042	Periph/Cranial Nerve & Other
	05	242-244	Cardiac Pacemaker Implant
	21	907-909	Other Procs for Injuries
3770 & 3787	01	040-042	Periph/Cranial Nerve & Other
	05	242-244	Cardiac Pacemaker Implant
	21	907-909	Other Procs for Injuries
3771 & 3780	01	040-042	Periph/Cranial Nerve & Other
	05	242-244	Cardiac Pacemaker Implant
	21	907-909	Other Procs for Injuries
3771 & 3781	01	040-042	Periph/Cranial Nerve & Other
	05	242-244	Cardiac Pacemaker Implant
	21	907-909	Other Procs for Injuries
3771 & 3782	01	040-042	Periph/Cranial Nerve & Other
	05	242-244	Cardiac Pacemaker Implant
	21	907-909	Other Procs for Injuries
3771 & 3785	01	040-042	Periph/Cranial Nerve & Other
	05	242-244	Cardiac Pacemaker Implant
	21	907-909	Other Procs for Injuries
3771 & 3786	01	040-042	Periph/Cranial Nerve & Other
	05	242-244	Cardiac Pacemaker Implant
	21	907-909	Other Procs for Injuries
3771 & 3787	01	040-042	Periph/Cranial Nerve & Other
	05	242-244	Cardiac Pacemaker Implant
	21	907-909	Other Procs for Injuries
3772 & 3780	01	040-042	Periph/Cranial Nerve & Other
	05	242-244	Cardiac Pacemaker Implant
	21	907-909	Other Procs for Injuries
3772 & 3783	01	040-042	Periph/Cranial Nerve & Other
	05	242-244	Cardiac Pacemaker Implant
	21	907-909	Other Procs for Injuries

LEAD DEVICE	MDC	MS-DRG	SURGICAL CATEGORY
3773 & 3780	01	040-042	Periph/Cranial Nerve & Other
	05	242-244	Cardiac Pacemaker Implant
	21	907-909	Other Procs for Injuries
3773 & 3781	01	040-042	Periph/Cranial Nerve & Other
	05	242-244	Cardiac Pacemaker Implant
	21	907-909	Other Procs for Injuries
3773 & 3782	01	040-042	Periph/Cranial Nerve & Other
	05	242-244	Cardiac Pacemaker Implant
	21	907-909	Other Procs for Injuries
3773 & 3785	01	040-042	Periph/Cranial Nerve & Other
	05	242-244	Cardiac Pacemaker Implant
	21	907-909	Other Procs for Injuries
3773 & 3786	01	040-042	Periph/Cranial Nerve & Other
	05	242-244	Cardiac Pacemaker Implant
	21	907-909	Other Procs for Injuries
3773 & 3787	01	040-042	Periph/Cranial Nerve & Other
	05	242-244	Cardiac Pacemaker Implant
	21	907-909	Other Procs for Injuries
3774 & 3780	01	040-042	Periph/Cranial Nerve & Other
	05	242-244	Cardiac Pacemaker Implant
	21	907-909	Other Procs for Injuries
3774 & 3781	01	040-042	Periph/Cranial Nerve & Other
	05	242-244	Cardiac Pacemaker Implant
	21	907-909	Other Procs for Injuries
3774 & 3782	01	040-042	Periph/Cranial Nerve & Other
	05	242-244	Cardiac Pacemaker Implant
	21	907-909	Other Procs for Injuries
3774 & 3783	01	040-042	Periph/Cranial Nerve & Other
	05	242-244	Cardiac Pacemaker Implant
	21	907-909	Other Procs for Injuries
3774 & 3785	01	040-042	Periph/Cranial Nerve & Other
	05	242-244	Cardiac Pacemaker Implant
	21	907-909	Other Procs for Injuries
3774 & 3786	01	040-042	Periph/Cranial Nerve & Other
	05	242-244	Cardiac Pacemaker Implant
	21	907-909	Other Procs for Injuries
3774 & 3787	01	040-042	Periph/Cranial Nerve & Other
	05	242-244	Cardiac Pacemaker Implant
	21	907-909	Other Procs for Injuries
3776 & 3780	01	040-042	Periph/Cranial Nerve & Other
	05	242-244	Cardiac Pacemaker Implant
	21	907-909	Other Procs for Injuries
3776 & 3785	01	040-042	Periph/Cranial Nerve & Other
	05	242-244	Cardiac Pacemaker Implant
	21	907-909	Other Procs for Injuries
3776 & 3786	01	040-042	Periph/Cranial Nerve & Other
	05	242-244	Cardiac Pacemaker Implant
	21	907-909	Other Procs for Injuries
3776 & 3787	01	040-042	Periph/Cranial Nerve & Other
	05	242-244	Cardiac Pacemaker Implant
	21	907-909	Other Procs for Injuries

TABLE 2 ABDOMINAL AORTA/THORACIC VESSEL RESECTION REFERENCE TABLE

3844	Resect abdm aorta w repl		3845	Resect thorac ves w repl

PROCEDURES	MDC	MS-DRG	SURGICAL CATEGORY
3844	05	237-238	Major Cardiovascular
3845	05	237-238	Major Cardiovascular
3844 & 3845	05	228-230	Other Cardiothoracic

TABLE 3 CARDIOVERTER-DEFIBRILLATOR LEAD/GENERATOR REFERENCE TABLE

0052	Imp/rep lead lf ven sys		3773	Int inser lead in atrium
0053	Imp/rep CRT pacemakr gen		3774	Int or repl lead epicar
0054	Imp/rep CRT defib genat		3776	Repl tv atri-vent lead
1751	Int insert cardiac implant		3795	Implt cardiodefib leads
1752	Imp generator		3796	Implt cardiodefib genatr
3770	Int insert pacemak lead		3797	Repl cardiodefib leads
3771	Int insert lead in vent		3798	Repl cardiodefib genratr
3772	Int inser lead atri-vent			

PROCEDURES	MDC	MS-DRG	SURGICAL CATEGORY
0052	05	265	AICD Lead
0053	05	258-259	Pacemaker Device Replacement
0054	05	245	AICD Generator
1751	05	222-227	Cardiac Implant
1752	05	245	Cardiac Generator
3795	05	265	AICD Lead
3796	05	245	AICD Generator
3797	05	265	AICD Lead
3798	05	245	AICD Generator
0052 & 0053	05	242-244	Cardiac Pacemaker Implant
0052 & 0054	05	222-227	Cardiac Defibrillator Implant
0053 & 3770	05	242-244	Cardiac Pacemaker Implant
0053 & 3771	05	242-244	Cardiac Pacemaker Implant
0053 & 3772	05	242-244	Cardiac Pacemaker Implant
0053 & 3773	05	242-244	Cardiac Pacemaker Implant
0053 & 3774	05	242-244	Cardiac Pacemaker Implant
0053 & 3776	05	242-244	Cardiac Pacemaker Implant
0054 & 3774	05	222-227	Cardiac Defibrillator Implant
0054 & 3795	05	222-227	Cardiac Defibrillator Implant
0054 & 3797	05	222-227	Cardiac Defibrillator Implant
3774 & 3796	05	222-227	Cardiac Defibrillator Implant
3774 & 3798	05	222-227	Cardiac Defibrillator Implant
3795 & 3796	05	222-227	Cardiac Defibrillator Implant
3797 & 3798	05	222-227	Cardiac Defibrillator Implant

TABLE 4 SPINAL FUSION REFERENCE TABLE

8100	Spinal fusion NOS	8131	Refusion of atlas-axis
8101	Atlas-axis fusion	8132	Refusion of oth cerv ant
8102	Other cervical fus ant	8133	Refus of oth cerv post
8103	Other cervical fus post	8134	Refusion of dorsal ant
8104	Dorsal/dorsolum fus ant	8135	Refusion of dorsal post
8105	Dorsal/dorsolum fus post	8136	Refusion of lumbar ant
8106	Lumbar/lumbosac fus ant	8137	Refusion of lumbar lat
8107	Lumbar/lumbosac fus lat	8138	Refusion of lumbar post
8108	Lumbar/lumbosac fus post	8139	Refusion of spine NEC
8130	Spinal refusion NOS		

PROCEDURES	MDC	MS-DRG	SURGICAL CATEGORY
8100	08	456-460	Spinal Fusion
8101	08	471-473	Cervical Spinal Fusion
8102	08	471-473	Cervical Spinal Fusion
8103	08	471-473	Cervical Spinal Fusion
8104	08	456-460	Spinal Fusion
8105	08	456-480	Spinal Fusion
8106	08	456-460	Spinal Fusion
8107	08	456-460	Spinal Fusion
8108	08	456-460	Spinal Fusion
8130	08	456-460	Spinal Fusion
8131	08	471-473	Cervical Spinal Fusion
8132	08	471-473	Cervical Spinal Fusion
8133	08	471-473	Cervical Spinal Fusion
8134	08	456-460	Spinal Fusion
8135	08	456-460	Spinal Fusion
8136	08	456-460	Spinal Fusion
8137	08	456-460	Spinal Fusion
8138	08	456-460	Spinal Fusion
8139	08	456-460	Spinal Fusion
8102 & 8103	08	453-455	Anterior/Posterior Spinal Fusion
8102 & 8105	08	453-455	Anterior/Posterior Spinal Fusion
8102 & 8107	08	453-455	Anterior/Posterior Spinal Fusion
8102 & 8108	08	453-455	Anterior/Posterior Spinal Fusion
8102 & 8133	08	453-455	Anterior/Posterior Spinal Fusion
8102 & 8135	08	453-455	Anterior/Posterior Spinal Fusion
8102 & 8137	08	453-455	Anterior/Posterior Spinal Fusion
8102 & 8138	08	453-455	Anterior/Posterior Spinal Fusion
8104 & 8103	08	453-455	Anterior/Posterior Spinal Fusion
8104 & 8105	08	453-455	Anterior/Posterior Spinal Fusion
8104 & 8107	08	453-455	Anterior/Posterior Spinal Fusion
8104 & 8108	08	453-455	Anterior/Posterior Spinal Fusion
8104 & 8133	08	453-455	Anterior/Posterior Spinal Fusion
8104 & 8135	08	453-455	Anterior/Posterior Spinal Fusion
8104 & 8137	08	453-455	Anterior/Posterior Spinal Fusion
8104 & 8138	08	453-455	Anterior/Posterior Spinal Fusion
8106 & 8103	08	453-455	Anterior/Posterior Spinal Fusion
8106 & 8105	08	453-455	Anterior/Posterior Spinal Fusion
8106 & 8107	08	453-455	Anterior/Posterior Spinal Fusion
8106 & 8108	08	453-455	Anterior/Posterior Spinal Fusion
8106 & 8133	08	453-455	Anterior/Posterior Spinal Fusion
8106 & 8135	08	453-455	Anterior/Posterior Spinal Fusion
8106 & 8137	08	453-455	Anterior/Posterior Spinal Fusion
8106 & 8138	08	453-455	Anterior/Posterior Spinal Fusion
8132 & 8103	08	453-455	Anterior/Posterior Spinal Fusion
8132 & 8105	08	453-455	Anterior/Posterior Spinal Fusion
8132 & 8107	08	453-455	Anterior/Posterior Spinal Fusion
8132 & 8108	08	453-455	Anterior/Posterior Spinal Fusion
8132 & 8133	08	453-455	Anterior/Posterior Spinal Fusion
8132 & 8135	08	453-455	Anterior/Posterior Spinal Fusion
8132 & 8137	08	453-455	Anterior/Posterior Spinal Fusion
8132 & 8138	08	453-455	Anterior/Posterior Spinal Fusion

PROCEDURES	MDC	MS-DRG	SURGICAL CATEGORY
8134 & 8103	08	453-455	Anterior/Posterior Spinal Fusion
8134 & 8105	08	453-455	Anterior/Posterior Spinal Fusion
8134 & 8107	08	453-455	Anterior/Posterior Spinal Fusion
8134 & 8108	08	453-455	Anterior/Posterior Spinal Fusion
8134 & 8133	08	453-455	Anterior/Posterior Spinal Fusion
8134 & 8135	08	453-455	Anterior/Posterior Spinal Fusion
8134 & 8137	08	453-455	Anterior/Posterior Spinal Fusion
8134 & 8138	08	453-455	Anterior/Posterior Spinal Fusion
8136 & 8103	08	453-455	Anterior/Posterior Spinal Fusion
8136 & 8105	08	453-455	Anterior/Posterior Spinal Fusion
8136 & 8107	08	453-455	Anterior/Posterior Spinal Fusion
8136 & 8108	08	453-455	Anterior/Posterior Spinal Fusion
8136 & 8133	08	453-456	Anterior/Posterior Spinal Fusion
8136 & 8135	08	453-455	Anterior/Posterior Spinal Fusion
8136 & 8137	08	453-455	Anterior/Posterior Spinal Fusion
8136 & 8138	08	453-455	Anterior/Posterior Spinal Fusion

TABLE 5 KIDNEY/PANCREAS TRANSPLANT REFERENCE TABLE

5280	Pancreat transplant NOS
5282	Pancreatic homotransplan
5569	Kidney transplant NEC

PROCEDURES	MDC	MS-DRG	SURGICAL CATEGORY
5280	Pre	010	Pancreas Transplant
	07	405-407	Pancreas, Liver and Shunt
	10	628-630	Other Endocrine/Nutrit/Metabolic
5282	Pre	010	Pancreas Transplant
	07	405-407	Pancreas, Liver and Shunt
	10	628-630	Other Endocrine/Nutrit/Metabolic
5569	11	652	Kidney Transplant
5280 & 5569	Pre	008	Simultaneous Pancreas/Kidney Transplant
5282 & 5569	Pre	008	Simultaneous Pancreas/Kidney Transplant

TABLE 6 LEAD/DEVICE REFERENCE TABLE

0056	Ins/rep impl sensor lead
0057	Imp/rep subcue card dev

PROCEDURES	MDC	MS-DRG	SURGICAL CATEGORY
0056	05	260-262	Intracard monitoring sensor insert
0057	05	258-259	Intracard monitoring device insert
0056 & 0057	05	264	Other Circulatory System

Develop a more productive and prosperous medical practice with proven coding resources from the American Medical Association (AMA)

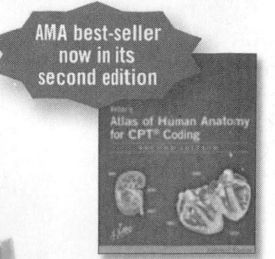

AMA best-seller now in its second edition

Netter's Atlas of Human Anatomy for CPT® Coding, second edition
Designed to provide a better understanding of anatomic structures described within CPT codes.

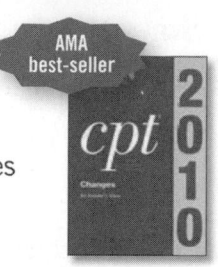

AMA best-seller

CPT® Changes 2010: An Insider's View
An indispensable guide for CPT® codebook users. Helps you understand each CPT 2010 code change in detail and helps you code CPT more accurately.

AMA best-seller now in its second edition

Stedman's CPT® Dictionary, second edition
Truly understand CPT code descriptions with this one-of-a-kind resource that now contains CPT customized Stedman's medical definitions to enhance coding efficiency.

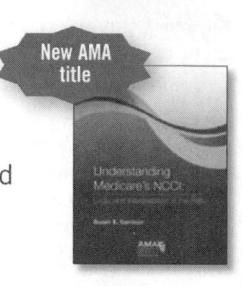

New AMA title

Understanding Medicare's NCCI
Walks users through the logic behind Medicare's National Correct Coding Initiative (NCCI) edits and teaches how to make the correct determination regarding bundling versus billing separately for edited services.

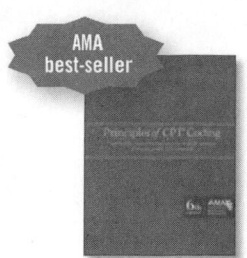

AMA best-seller

Principles of CPT® Coding, sixth edition
Provides the most in-depth review available of the entire CPT codebook. Now contains ancillary educator material, including three-levels of question-and-answer banks.

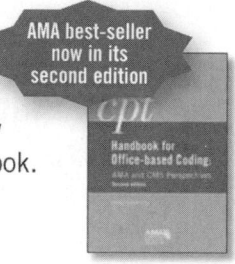

AMA best-seller now in its second edition

CPT® Handbook for Office-Based Coding, second edition
The time-saving, all-in-one reference is full of coding and Medicare policy information relevant to CPT to build understanding and help accurately report and reduce claim denials.

AMA
AMERICAN MEDICAL ASSOCIATION

For more information on these popular coding resources or to download our recent catalog, visit www.amabookstore.com. Order online or call (800) 621-8335 today!